CM07001034
1/08

CF

Contemporary Medical-Surgical Nursing

Rick Daniels, RN, PhD

Oregon Health and Science University
Ashland, Oregon

Laura John Nosek, RN, PhD

Frances Payne Bolton School of
Nursing
Case Western Reserve University
Cleveland, Ohio

Leslie H. Nicoll, PhD, MBA, RN, BC

Principal and Owner
Maine Desk, LLC
Portland, Maine

THOMSON

DELMAR LEARNING

Australia Canada Mexico Singapore Spain United Kingdom United States

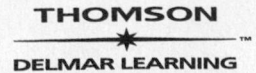

Contemporary Medical-Surgical Nursing

Rick Daniels, Laura John Nosek, and Leslie H. Nicoll

Vice President, Health Care Business Unit:
William Brottmiller

Director of Learning Solutions:
Matthew Kane

Acquisitions Editor:
Tamara Caruso

Product Manager:
Patricia Gaworecki

Editorial Assistant:
Jennifer Waters

Marketing Director:
Jennifer McAvey

Marketing Channel Manager:
Michele McTighe

Marketing Coordinator:
Danielle Pacella

Technology Director:
Laurie Davis

Technology Product Manager:
Mary Colleen Liburdi

Production Director:
Carolyn Miller

Production Manager:
Barbara Bullock

Art Director:
Robert Plante
Jack Pendleton

Content Project Manager:
Stacey Lamodi
Jessica McNavich

Library of Congress Cataloging-in-Publication Data
ISBN 1-4018-3718-2

Notice to the Reader

Publisher does not warrant or guarantee any of the products described herein or perform any independent analysis in connection with any of the product information contained herein. Publisher does not assume, and expressly disclaims, any obligation to obtain and include information other than that provided to it by the manufacturer.

The reader is expressly warned to consider and adopt all safety precautions that might be indicated by the activities described herein and to avoid all potential hazards. By following the instructions contained herein, the reader willingly assumes all risks in connection with such instructions.

The publisher makes no representations or warranties of any kind, including but not limited to, the warranties of fitness for particular purpose or merchantability, nor are any such representations implied with respect to the material set forth herein, and the publisher takes no responsibility with respect to such material. The publisher shall not be liable for any special, consequential, or exemplary damages resulting, in whole or part, from the reader's use of, or reliance upon, this material.

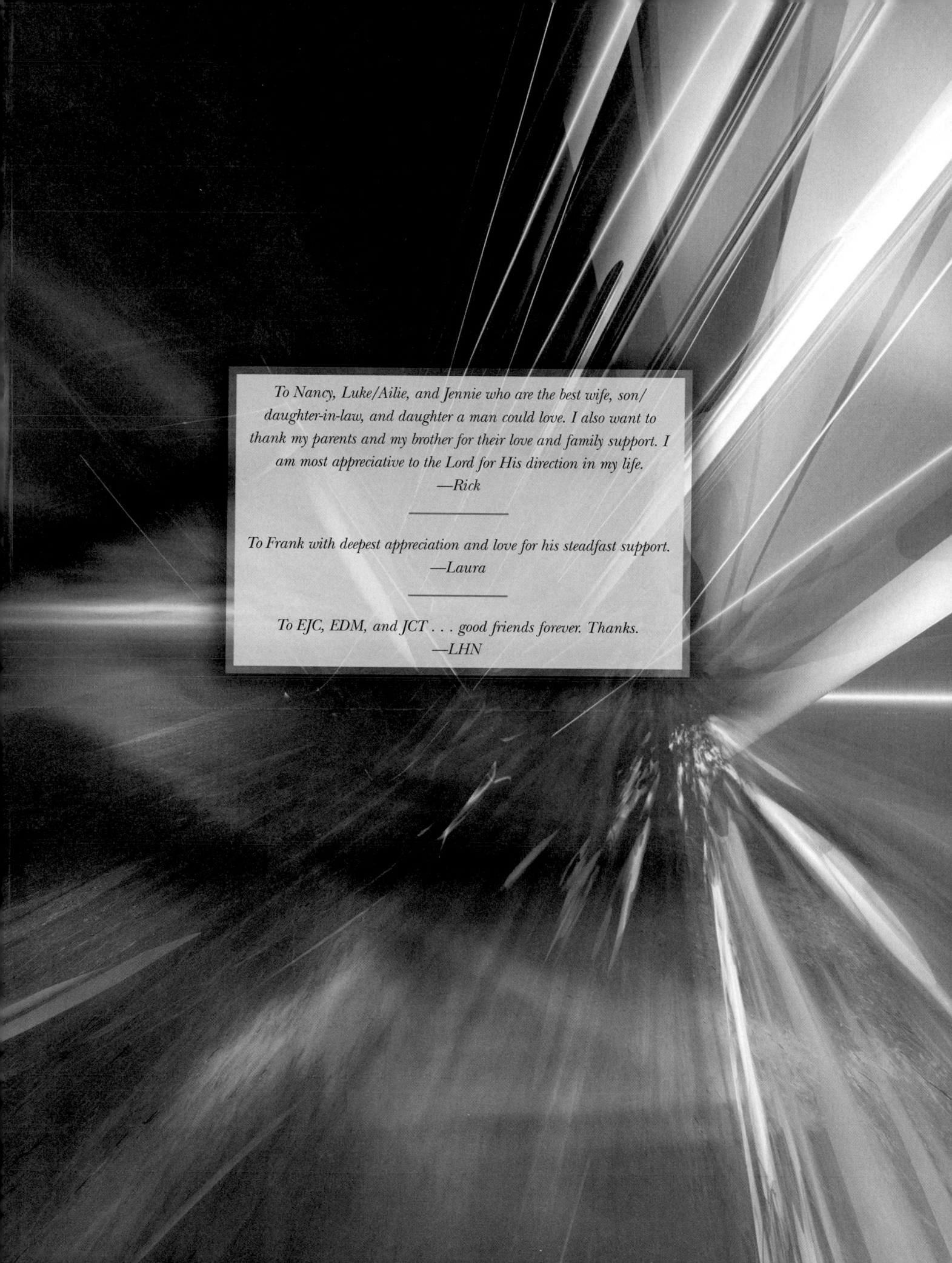

To Nancy, Luke/Ailie, and Jennie who are the best wife, son/ daughter-in-law, and daughter a man could love. I also want to thank my parents and my brother for their love and family support. I am most appreciative to the Lord for His direction in my life.
—*Rick*

———————

To Frank with deepest appreciation and love for his steadfast support.
—*Laura*

———————

To EJC, EDM, and JCT . . . good friends forever. Thanks.
—*LHN*

Contents

UNIT I: Nursing and the Health Care System   1

CHAPTER 1: The Health Care System and Contemporary Nursing   2

CHAPTER 2: Clinical Decision Making and Evidence-Based Practice   23

CHAPTER 3: Health Education and Promotion   43

CHAPTER 4: Culturally Sensitive Care   69

CHAPTER 5: Legal and Ethical Aspects of Health Care

95

CHAPTER 6: Nursing of Adults Across the Life Span   121

CHAPTER 9: Genetics and the Multiple Determinants of Health   197

CHAPTER 12: Fluid, Electrolyte, and Acid-Base Imbalances   295

CHAPTER 13: Infusion Therapy   339

CHAPTER 14: Complementary and Alternative Therapies   375

CHAPTER 15: Cancer Management   401

CHAPTER 16: Pain Management — 447

CHAPTER 17: Pharmacology: Nursing Management 483

UNIT III: Settings for Nursing Care   531

CHAPTER 18: Health Care Agencies   532

CHAPTER 19: Critical Care   559

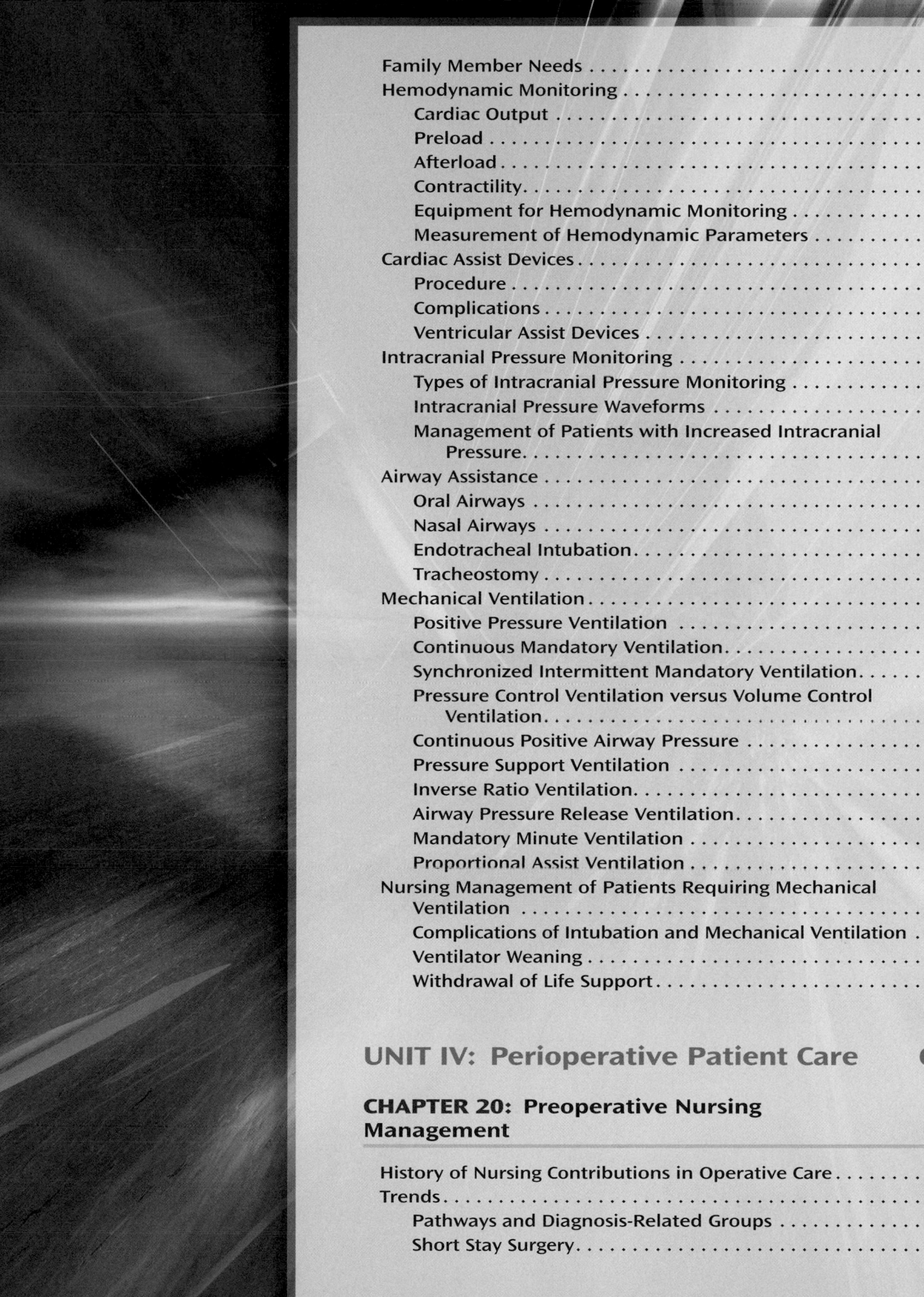

UNIT IV: Perioperative Patient Care   607

CHAPTER 20: Preoperative Nursing Management   608

CHAPTER 21: Intraoperative Nursing Management 653

CHAPTER 22: Postoperative Nursing Management 691

UNIT V: Alterations in Cardiovascular and Hematological Function 733

CHAPTER 23: Assessment of Cardiovascular and Hematological Function 734

CHAPTER 24: Coronary Artery Dysfunction: Nursing Management   769

CHAPTER 25: Heart Failure and Inflammatory Dysfunction: Nursing Management   803

CHAPTER 26: Arrhythmias: Nursing Management   835

CHAPTER 27: Vascular Dysfunction: Nursing Management   877

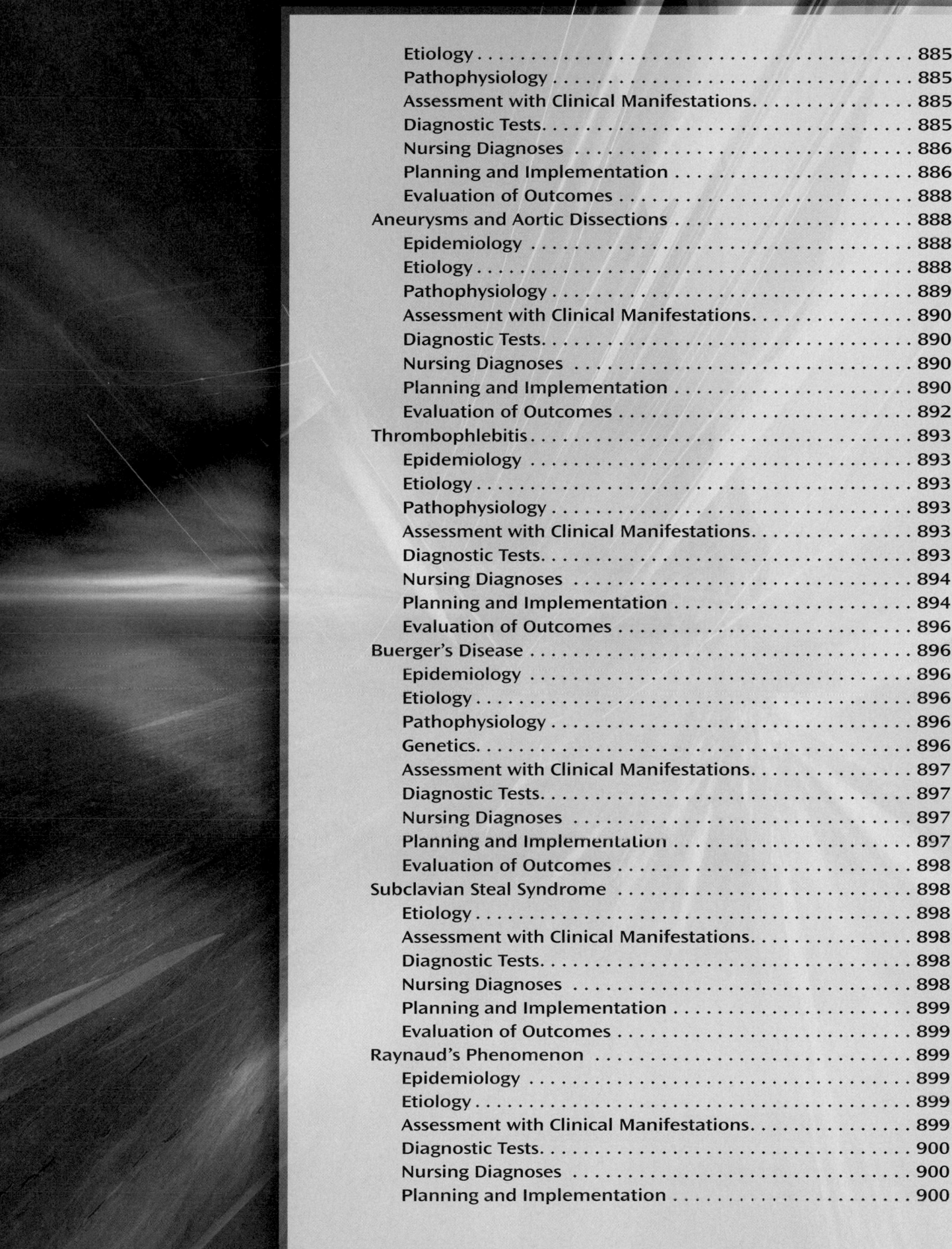

CHAPTER 28: Hypertension: Nursing Management   907

CHAPTER 29: Hematological Dysfunction: Nursing Management   929

CHAPTER 33: Obstructive Pulmonary Disease: Nursing Management   1099

UNIT VII: Alterations in Neurological Function   1135

CHAPTER 34: Assessment of Neurological Function   1136

CHAPTER 35: Dysfunction of the Brain: Nursing Management   1171

CHAPTER 36: Dysfunction of the Spinal Cord and Peripheral Nervous System: Nursing Management   1213

CHAPTER 37: Degenerative Neurological Dysfunction: Nursing Management   1261

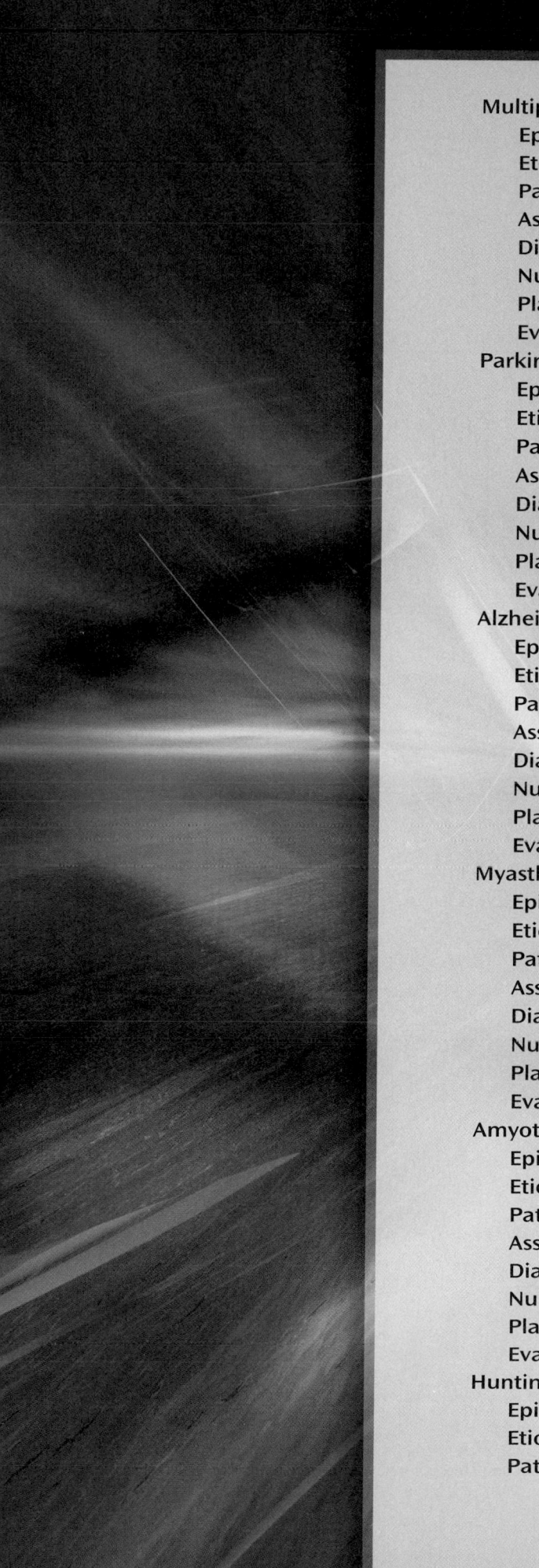

UNIT VIII: Alterations in Sensory Function   1299

CHAPTER 38: Assessment of Sensory Function   1300

CHAPTER 39: Visual Dysfunction: Nursing Management   1323

CHAPTER 40: Auditory Dysfunction: Nursing Management — 1349

UNIT X: Alterations in Integumentary Function   1475

CHAPTER 44: Assessment of Integumentary Function   1476

CHAPTER 45: Dermatological Dysfunction: Nursing Management   1495

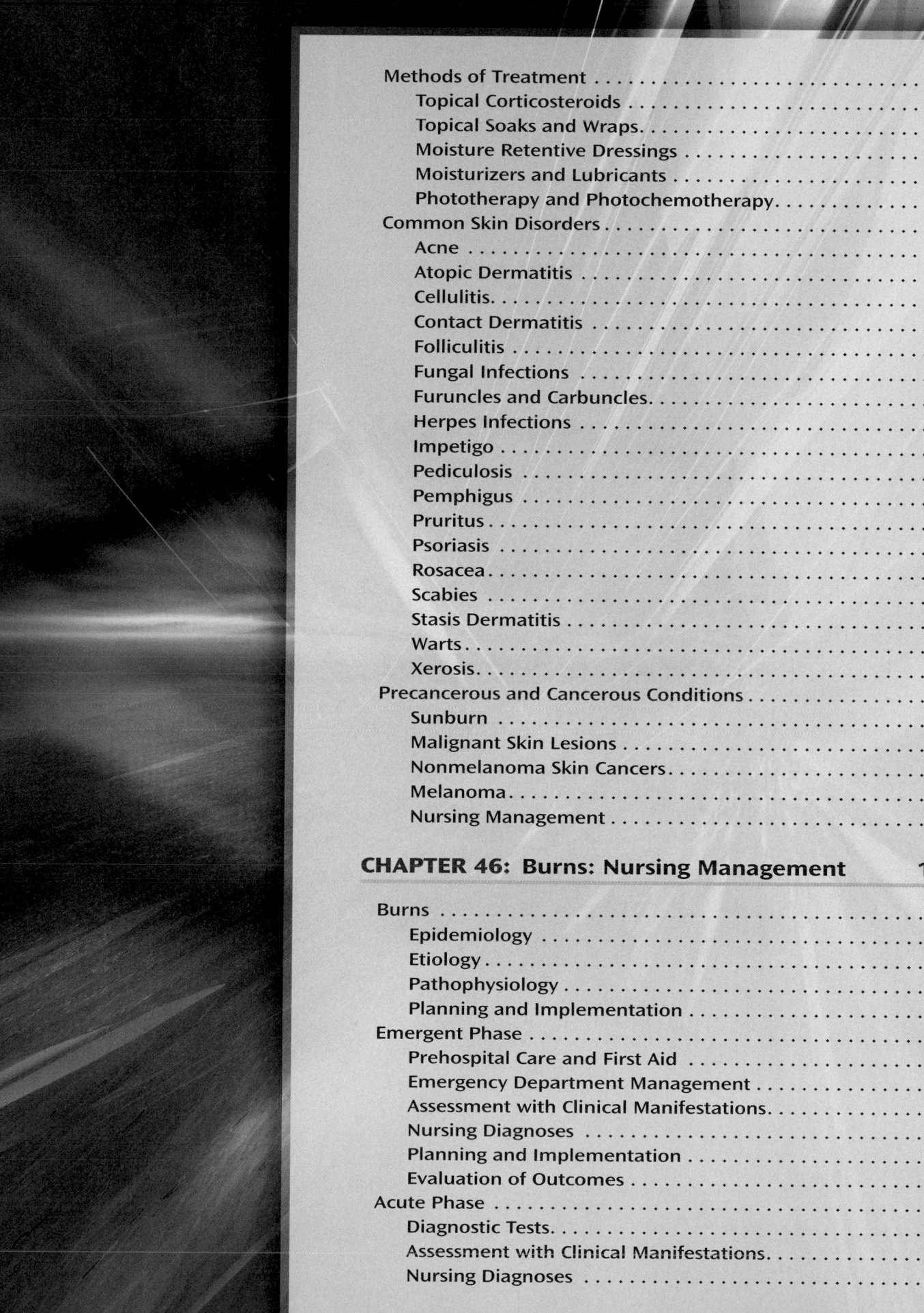

CHAPTER 46: Burns: Nursing Management   1529

UNIT XI: Alterations in Gastrointestinal Function   1567

CHAPTER 47: Assessment of Gastrointestinal Function   1568

CHAPTER 48: Nutrition, Malnutrition, and Obesity: Nursing Management   1595

CHAPTER 49: Upper Gastrointestinal Tract Dysfunction: Nursing Management   1619

UNIT XII: Alterations in Renal Function   1745

CHAPTER 52: Assessment of Renal Function   1746

CHAPTER 53: Urinary Dysfunction: Nursing Management   1765

UNIT XIII: Alterations in Endocrine Function 1847

CHAPTER 55: Assessment of Endocrine Function 1848

CHAPTER 56: Endocrine Dysfunction: Nursing Management 1863

UNIT XV: Alterations in Reproductive Function   2053

CHAPTER 64: Male Reproductive Dysfunction: Nursing Management   2163

UNIT XVI: Special Considerations in Medical and Surgical Nursing — 2201

CHAPTER 65: Multisystem Failure — 2202

CHAPTER 66: Mass Casualty Care   2235

Boxed Elements Contents

CHAPTER 54 Renal Dysfunction: Nursing Management

CHAPTER 56 Endocrine Dysfunction: Nursing Management

CHAPTER 57 Diabetes Mellitus: Nursing Management

CHAPTER 58 Assessment of Musculoskeletal Function

CHAPTER 59 Musculoskeletal Dysfunction: Nursing Management

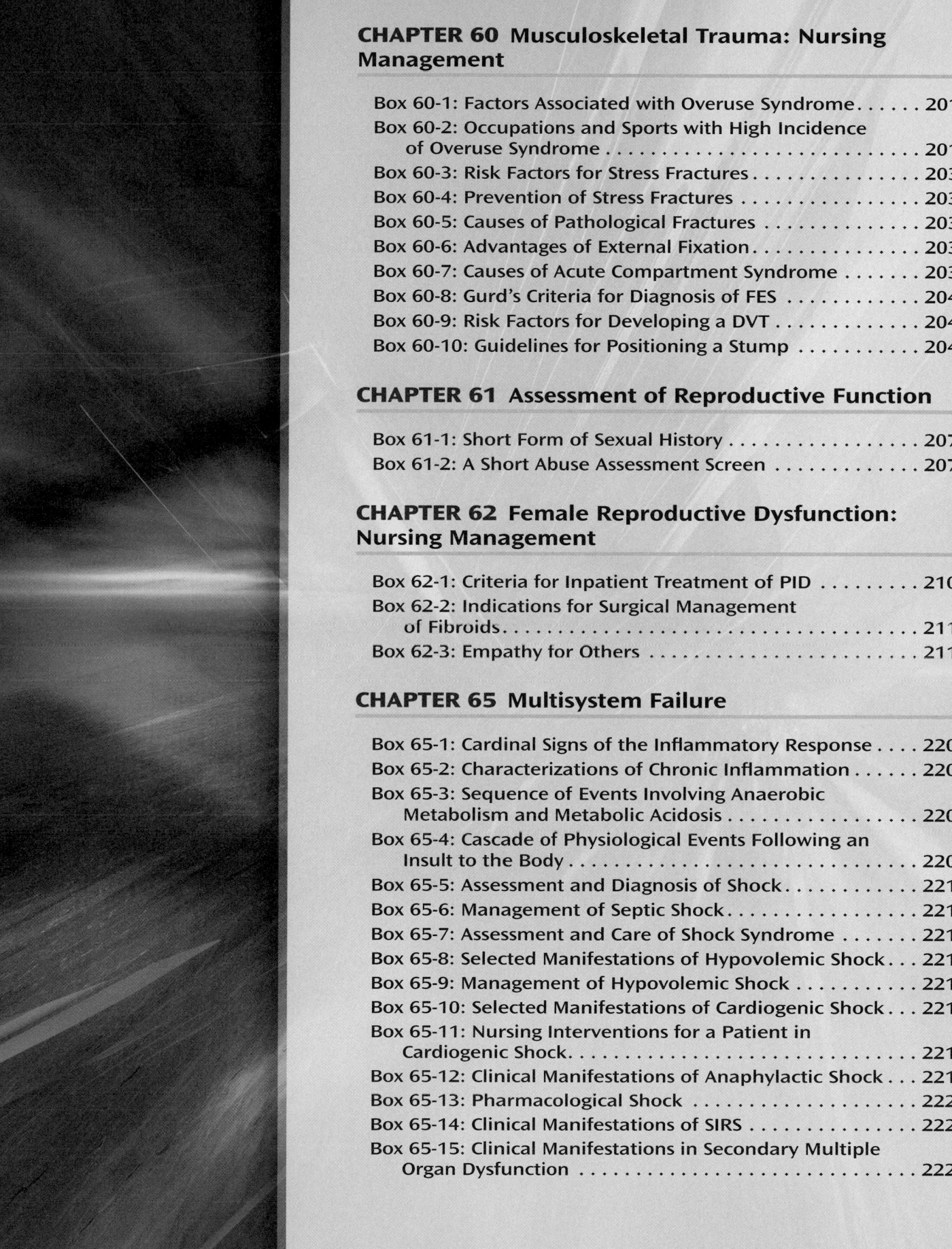

CHAPTER 66 Mass Casualty Care

Preface

Contemporary Medical-Surgical Nursing is an exciting new comprehensive text created for nursing students to address the adult health and illness topics that support the most current nursing practice. It provides a reader-oriented, logically organized source of information focused on the knowledge and skill required to become a caring and responsible practitioner.

As the century continues to unfold, the health care delivery system will increase in complexity. Staying abreast of both technological and biotechnological advancements will be challenging, but just as challenging will be ongoing changes in patient situations and in the health care system to which nurses as leaders in care management and system management must adapt. New family structures, increasing prevalence of the diseases of aging and chronic illness, and globalization will refocus the major care requirements of society. Acute care will continue to move from hospitals to community settings, including the home and alternative sites unrelated to health care. Nurses will continue to pioneer new vital roles, and critical shortages of nurse providers across all arenas will challenge the profession toward innovative practice. Nurses must embrace such challenges and prepare students to excel in providing the quality care that is required by a changing society. Our goal in creating this book was to continue Thomson Delmar Learning's commitment to help bridge the gap from nursing student to practitioner. To assist students in making this transition, we provide real-world applications, such as case studies and unique features like Dollars and Sense and Ethics or Law in Practice. In addition, we are proud to feature innovative teaching methods, such as our IV therapy animations and StudyWARE™ games, as well as PDA downloads available on our online companion. And all of this is delivered through a caring approach to the content—a central theme to fostering quality nursing care for generations to come.

CONCEPTUAL APPROACH

The concept for *Contemporary Medical-Surgical Nursing* arose from a need that the authors identified after years of instruction to nursing students, a need for a thorough, organized, and practical approach to its delivery. There is a balance created that presents pedagogical information specifically designed for the nursing student. And there are learning approaches within the text and its additional resources for the various learning styles that are unique to each student. The most current information obtained from a wide variety of sources is the underpinning for this medical-surgical textbook. In addition, there are wide varieties of important features, such as evidence from current research studies, information regarding the ethicolegal practice of nursing, and nursing education approaches that enhance the critical thinking skills of the reader.

The patient is the focus of the textbook, with an in-depth presentation of the many acute care topics that are central to the practice of nursing. There are concept maps and case study presentations throughout the book. In addition, there are review activities and review questions at the end of each chapter styled like NCLEX® questions, which provide the reader with excellent methods of mastering the content. There is a full-color visually appealing design, tables and boxes that emphasize essential points, and additional tutorial references that engage the reader in a user-friendly approach. The information and learning processes in conjunction with the active reader's critical thinking skills foster the development of a caring, ethical, and responsible practicing professional nurse.

ORGANIZATION OF THE TEXT

Contemporary Medical-Surgical Nursing consists of 66 chapters organized into 16 units. A composite of topics provides a comprehensive approach to acute care nursing within these units of study. A unique nursing perspective is threaded through each chapter of study, and the outcome of evidence-based knowledge and evidence-based practice is encouraged. As noticed in most units, the first chapter is an assessment chapter that presents the information necessary for the nurse to begin care for patients in acute care nursing. The chapters that follow in each unit have the phrase nursing management in their titles, which depicts the focus on the relationship of nursing interventions or strategies for most of the topics presented in the 16 units of study.

Unit I: Nursing and the Health Care System, Chapters 1 through 7

These seven chapters introduce the student to the foundational topics of acute care nursing. Chapter 1 is an overview of the health care delivery system. Chapter 2 emphasizes clinical decision making and the value of evidence-based nursing practice. Chapter 3 presents information on health education and promotion. Chapter 4 describes the implications of both the cultural and ethnic backgrounds of patients. Chapter 5 presents the invaluable legal and ethical issues relevant to nursing practice. Chapters 6 and 7 focus on caring for adults across the life span as well as palliative care.

Unit II: Supportive Patient Care, Chapters 8 through 17

The first chapters begin with a review of health assessment (chapter 8), genetics (chapter 9), and stress/coping (chapter 10). In addition, the next seven chapters provide information that is primarily foundational for acute patient care, with such topics as inflammation/infection (chapter 11), fluid/electrolytes (chapter 12), infusion therapy (chapter 13), complementary and alternative care (chapter 14), cancer and pain management (chapters 15 and 16), and pharmacology (chapter 17).

Unit III: Settings for Nursing Care, Chapters 18 and 19

These two chapters present information on two primary settings for acute care nursing. Chapter 18 focuses on health care agencies, and chapter 19 covers critical care nursing.

Unit IV: Perioperative Patient Care, Chapters 20 through 22

The perioperative arena of nursing is essential to acute care nursing. These three chapters present information relative to the three phases of perioperative nursing: preoperative (chapter 20), intraoperative (chapter 21), and postoperative (chapter 22).

Unit V: Alterations in Cardiovascular and Hematological Function, Chapters 23 through 29

These seven chapters present information that involves the cardiovascular and hematological systems. It begins with assessment of the systems (chapter 23) and then presents information on coronary artery dysfunction (chapter 24), heart failure (chapter 25), arrhythmias (chapter 26), vascular dysfunction (chapter 27), and hypertension (chapter 28). Chapter 29 presents information on the hematological system and its acute care topics.

Unit VI: Alterations in Respiratory Function, Chapters 30 through 33

These four chapters explain various topics pertinent to the respiratory system beginning with an assessment of respiratory function in chapter 30. Chapter 31 examines upper airway disturbances, chapter 32 covers lower airway disorders, and chapter 33 describes obstructive pulmonary diseases.

Unit VII: Alterations in Neurological Function, Chapters 34 through 37

These four chapters discuss the neurological system as related to acute care nursing. Chapter 34 describes the assessment of the neurological system. Chapter 35 presents the brain, chapter 36 discusses the spinal cord and peripheral nervous system disorders, and chapter 37 identifies the various neurological degenerative disorders.

Unit VIII: Alterations in Sensory Function, Chapters 38 through 40

These three chapters discuss the important elements organs of sensory function beginning with an assessment of these systems in chapter 38. Chapters 39 and 40 provide information on visual and auditory dysfunctions.

Unit IX: Alterations in Immunological Function, Chapters 41 through 43

These three chapters describe the acute care disorders of the immune system. The unit begins with an assessment of the immune system (chapter 41). Chapter 42 discusses immunodeficient disorders and human immunodeficiency virus (HIV), and chapter 43 presents information on allergic dysfunctions.

Unit X: Alterations in Integumentary Function, Chapters 44 through 46

These three chapters explain disorders of the integumentary system. Chapter 44 presents important information regarding the assessment of the integumentary system. Chapter 45 adds the important nursing implications of dermatological issues, and chapter 46 details an in-depth discussion of patients with burns.

Unit XI: Alterations in Gastrointestinal Function, Chapters 47 through 51

This unit presents a thorough examination of the GI system and begins with assessment strategies in chapter 47. Chapter 48 describes the essentials of nutrition and the disorders of malnutrition and obesity. Chapters 49 and 50 present the variety of upper and lower GI disorders. Chapter 51 concludes the unit with a discussion of the hepatic system, biliary tract, and pancreatic disorders.

Unit XII: Alterations in Renal Function, Chapters 52 through 54

These three chapters discuss the critical diseases of the renal system. Chapter 52 presents the assessment of the renal system. Chapter 53 explores the urinary system disorders, and chapter 54 discusses those affecting dysfunctions of the renal system.

Unit XIII: Alterations in Endocrine Function, Chapters 55 through 57

This unit describes the dysfunctions of the endocrine system; chapter 55 includes in-depth assessment information. Chapter 56 presents the variety of diseases of the endocrine system, along with the nursing strategies. Chapter 57 identifies the specific disorders under the category of diabetes mellitus and the varied implications for patients with this disorder.

Unit XIV: Alterations in Musculoskeletal Function, Chapters 58 through 60

These three chapters address the disorders of the musculoskeletal system. Chapter 58 identifies the assessment of the MS system. Chapter 59 examines MS dysfunctions, and chapter 60 presents MS trauma as it relates to patients and their conditions.

Unit XV: Alterations in Reproductive Function, Chapters 61 through 64

This unit discusses the disorders of the reproductive system, beginning with detailed assessment of the reproductive system in chapter 61. Chapter 62 presents disorders of the female. Chapter 63 presents information on breast alterations, and chapter 64 discusses disorders of the male.

Unit XVI: Special Considerations in Medical and Surgical Nursing, Chapters 65 and 66

These chapters explore complex arenas of multisystem failure (chapter 65) and mass casualty care (chapter 66).

PEDAGOGICAL FEATURES

Enlightening features in *Contemporary Medical-Surgical Nursing* stimulate critical thinking and self-reflection and assist the reader in synthesizing and applying the information provided in the text. These complements to the text information create a supportive learning environment as the student transitions to a practicing professional.

Learning Objectives

Learning objectives are located on the online companion by chapter and provide the primary specific learning goals for the reader. They offer a means of measuring the outcomes of learning the cognitive information contained in each chapter.

Chapter Topics

Chapter topics are placed at the beginning of the chapter to highlight the main points of the text. They help provide direction for study and logically organize the content.

Key Terms

Key terms are bold in the chapters to denote those terms that are of particular importance to the reader. In addition, these terms are defined in the glossary for further reference.

Key Concepts

Key concepts highlight the primary points within the chapter and direct the reader in reviewing pertinent information.

Appendices

Several appendices augment medical-surgical topics. They include the most current NANDA nursing diagnoses, abbreviations and symbols, reference laboratory values, English/Spanish words and phrases, standard precautions, concept mapping, and the detailed glossary.

References

References document a current and varied theoretical basis for the content of the text on a chapter-by-chapter basis and are organized at the back of the text.

Review Questions and Activities

Review questions and answers are located at the end of each chapter and offer readers an opportunity to evaluate their understanding of specific chapter content. There are stimulating questions that are thought provoking and challenging to help develop critical thinking skills.

The Index

The index facilitates access to material and includes special entries for tables and illustrations.

SPECIAL FEATURES

Fast Forward

These provide detailed and informative predictions of new things to come in nursing and health care.

Dollars and Sense

These explore the cost and benefits of a particular nursing intervention. They include relevant statistics, possible solutions, and recommendations.

Real World, Real Choice

These allow for a management strategy scenario discussion that involves a real-life nursing dilemma. The solution and rationale can be found on the accompanying online companion.

Uncovering the Evidence

These present a synopsis of research studies for each chapter, which emphasize evidence-based practice for the concepts fundamental to basic nursing practice. These referred journal sources support the reader in developing a knowledgeable foundation of learning.

Ethics or Law in Practice

These present real-life cases involving legal implications or ethical issues related to chapter content.

Respecting Our Differences

These highlight nursing implications of given cultural backgrounds (e.g., ethnicity, age, race, or gender) in the format of a brief narrative that informs the reader of life span issues and outcome of care.

Red Flag

These provide a concise indication of cautionary information for the nurse, including emergency management of life-threatening and serious situations.

Patient Playbook

These allow concise, relevant teaching interventions for patient, family, or support persons necessary to enhance the individual's health.

Skills 360°

These discuss professionalism, communication, and relevant nursing strategies that are pertinent to the variety of acute care disorders.

Safety First

These identify categories of potential error and outline the problem along with the strategies for nursing management.

Case Studies

These are highlighted in at least one chapter per unit at the end of the chapter and appear in one of two formats: *nursing care plans* and *concept maps*. Both formats include patient examples where pertinent history, physical assessment data, and laboratory findings emphasize the nursing role in the clinical setting. Both engage the reader by humanizing the material and helping readers continue to develop critical thinking skills. In addition, the *case study concept map* challenges the learner to create a concept map at the end of the presented case.

EXTENSIVE TEACHING AND LEARNING PACKAGE

The complete ancillary package was created to achieve two goals:
1. To assist students in learning the skills and information essential to bridging the gap to professional practice.
2. To assist instructors in planning and implementing their programs for the most efficient use of time and other resources.

Clinical Companion (ISBN 1-4018-3721-2)

The *Clinical Companion to Accompany Contemporary Medical-Surgical Nursing* is a practical and convenient manual presented in a concise and alphabetical format for quick clinical reference. Designed for portability, this resource provides nurses fast answers to the questions:
- What is the condition?
- What should I look for?
- What should I do?

Approximately 200 common diseases, disorders, acute care procedures, and treatments are covered in an easy-to-follow format.

Study Guide (ISBN 1-4018-3723-9)

Containing over 1,100 questions, the study guide is an essential tool that reinforces the content presented in *Contemporary Medical-Surgical Nursing*. The variety of questions (multiple response, multiple choice, and fill in the blank) are similar to those found on the NCLEX-RN® and will help the learner build on key concepts presented in the text on a chapter-by-chapter basis.

Electronic Classroom Manager (ISBN 1-4018-3724-7)

Instructor's Guide

Based on each chapter's learning objectives, each chapter in the *Instructor's Guide* contains a variety of instructional strategies, Internet research, discussion questions, homework assignments, and classroom activities.

Computerized Test Bank

This computerized test bank holds over 1,000 questions geared to the text content and follows the NCLEX format. Each answer is accompanied by a rationale explaining right and wrong choices.

PowerPoint Presentations

Almost 1,000 slides are available and designed to support and facilitate lecture and classroom instructions.

Image Library

The image library includes more than 500 files containing images and tables from the text.

Link to Online Companion

An online version of the *Instructor's Guide* is included, as is a wealth of additional information for instructors and students designed to complement core concepts presented in the text. Instructors will also find conversion guides available.

Online Companion

A&P Animations

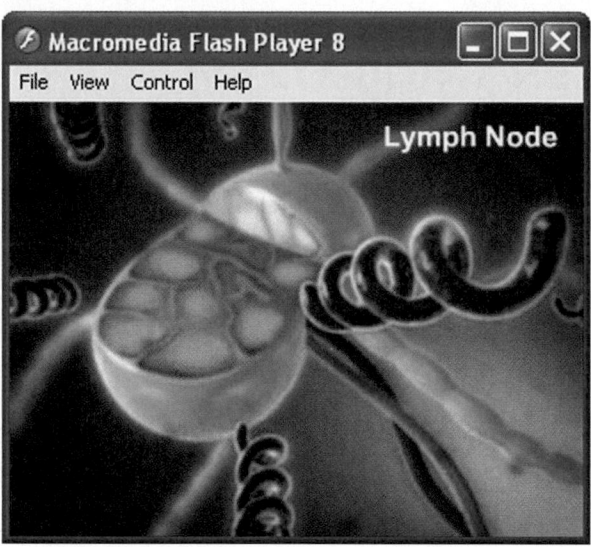

These visually demonstrate detailed anatomy and physiology concepts in an animated environment.

StudyWARE™

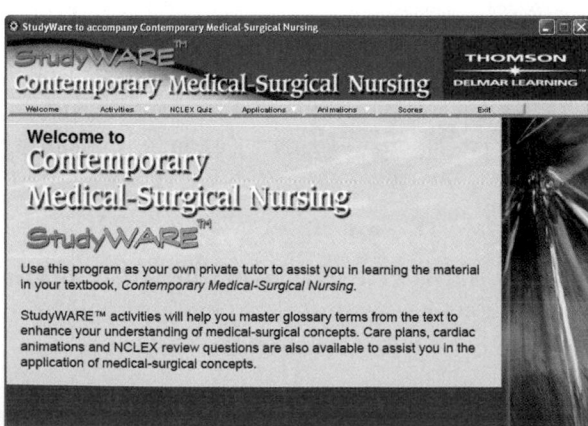

This provides activities and games to enhance the learner's understanding of medical-surgical concepts.

PDA downloads

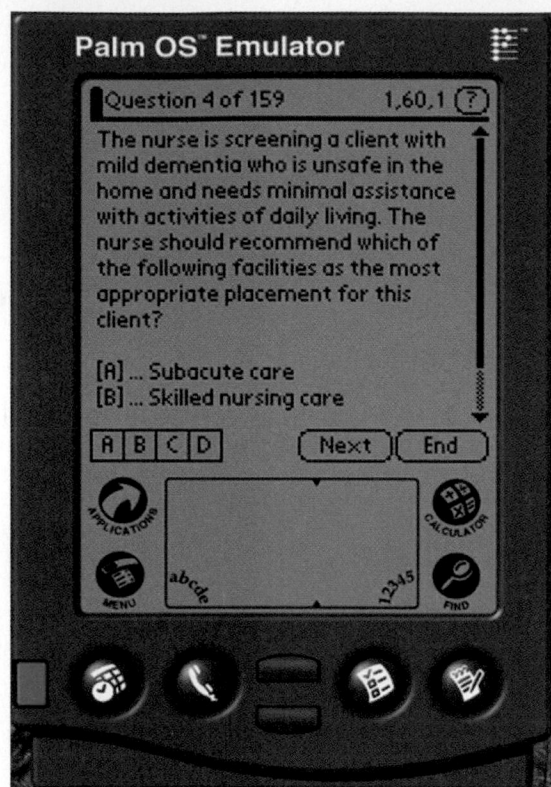

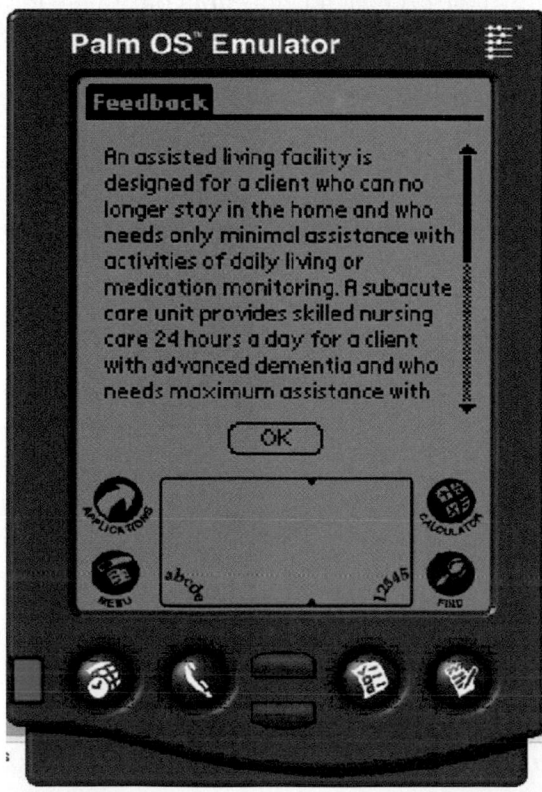

Free PDA downloads of up to 225 review questions in NCLEX style that include rationales as well as test and learning modes.

Additional Reading and Related Web Sites with Hotlinks

These provide a source of additional research on related topics organized in a chapter-by-chapter format.

Instructor's Guide

This is an online version of the *Instructor's Guide* and provides the same variety of instructional strategies, Internet research, discussion questions, homework assignments, and classroom activities.

WebTutor Advantage

Video Clips

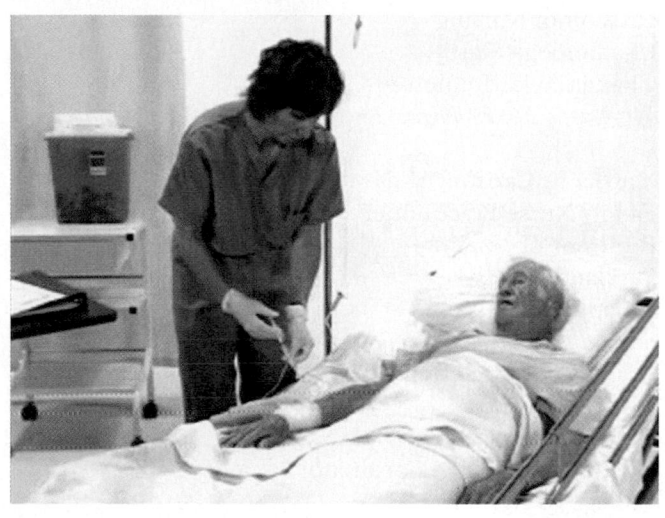

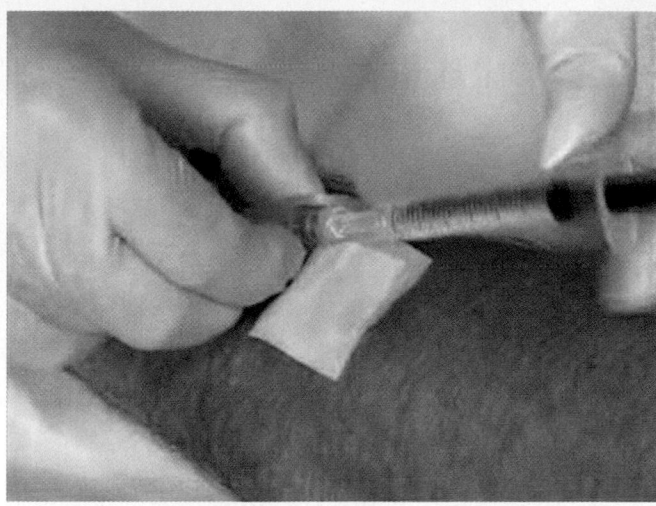

Skills-based video clips that include care of medical-surgical patients, medications administration, and IV therapy skills.

Medical-Surgical Case Studies

Using a body systems approach, this content allows additional opportunities to enhance critical thinking skills while working with medical-surgical patients and conditions.

IV Therapy Animations

Use these two- and three-dimensional animations to watch or participate in a series of specific IV therapy skills. A "Read it," "See it," and "Do it" organization offers a hands-on approach to these important skills and concepts.

Contributors and Reviewers

CONTRIBUTORS

Lisa Anderson-Shaw, DrPH, MA, MSN
Director, Clinical Ethics Consult Service
Assistant Clinical Professor
University of Illinois Medical Center
University of Illinois College of Nursing
Chicago, Illinois
Chapter 5: Legal and Ethical Aspects of Health Care

Crisamar J. Anunciado, MSN, FNP, RN
Senior Specialist
Intermediate Care Unit
Sharp HealthCare
San Diego, California
Chapter 38: Assessment of Sensory Function

Elizabeth D. Archer, MS, DSN, PhD, APRN, BC, CS, ANP, CRRN, CNRN
Clinical Nurse Specialist
Neuro/Ortho Nursing
Northwestern Memorial Hospital
Chicago, Illinois
Chapter 30: Assessment of Respiratory Function

Constance J. Ayers, PhD, RN
Associate Professor
College of Nursing
Texas Woman's University
Houston, Texas
Chapter 36: Dysfunction of the Spinal Cord and Peripheral Nervous System: Nursing Management

Kristi Bennett, RN, ANP, MS
Cardiac Specialist NP
Sharp Memorial Hospital
Escondido, California
Chapter 24: Coronary Artery Dysfunction: Nursing Management

Joyce Campbell, RN, MSN, CCRN, FNP-C
Division of Nursing
Chattanooga State
Chattanooga, Tennessee
Chapter 56: Endocrine Dysfunction: Nursing Management

Martha K. Carlson, MSN
Family Nurse Practitioner
Professor of Nursing
Parkland College
Champaign, Illinois
Chapter 55: Assessment of Endocrine Function
Chapter 57: Diabetes Mellitus: Nursing Management

Sandra K. Cesario, RNC, MS, PhD
Doctoral Program Coordinator
College of Nursing
Texas Woman's University
Houston, Texas
Chapter 9: Genetics and the Multiple Determinants of Health

Paul Chamberland, MSN, APRN, BC, CMSRN
Nurse Consultant
Scarborough, Maine
Chapter 53: Urinary Dysfunction: Nursing Management

Therese M. Clinch, RN, MSN
Academic Coordinator
St. David's Medical Center
Austin, Texas
Chapter 13: Infusion Therapy

Tammy Coffee, MSN, RN, ACNP
MetroHealth Medical Center
Comprehensive Burn Care Center
Cleveland, Ohio
Chapter 46: Burns: Nursing Management

Margaret M. Conger, RN, MSN, EdD
Professor Emeritus
School of Nursing
Northern Arizona University
Flagstaff, Arizona
Chapter 11: Inflammation and Infection Management

Debra Davis, BSN, RN
Director of Education
New Albany Surgical Hospital
New Albany, Ohio
Chapter 59: Musculoskeletal Dysfunction: Nursing Management

Doris Denison, MSN, APRN, BC, CCRN
Assistant Professor (Clinical)
Adult Health Area
College of Nursing
Wayne State University
Detroit, Michigan
Nurse Practitioner
Neurosurgery Service
William Beaumont Hospital
Royal Oak, Michigan
Chapter 28: Hypertension: Nursing Management
Chapter 34: Assessment of Neurological Function
Chapter 37: Degenerative Neurological Dysfunction: Nursing Management

Irene Eaton-Bancroft, RN, MSN, CS
Clinical Faculty
University of Southern Maine
Portland, Maine
Chapter 52: Assessment of Renal Function
Chapter 53: Urinary Dysfunction: Nursing Management
Chapter 54: Renal Dysfunction: Nursing Management

Ellen K. Fleischman, MBA, RD, RN
Manager
Diabetes Service Line
Sharp Memorial Hospital
San Diego, California
Chapter 48: Nutrition, Malnutrition, and Obesity: Nursing Management

Mary Franklin, MSN, CNM
Nurse Midwife
Paragon Health Associates
Akron, Ohio
Chapter 62: Female Reproductive Dysfunction: Nursing Management

Heather Freiheit, RN, BSN, EMT-P
Clinical Manager
Emergency Services
Rogue Valley Medical Center
Medford, Oregon
Chapter 66: Mass Casualty Care

Mary Fry, PhD, RN
Faculty
School of Nursing
University of Washington
Seattle, Washington
Chapter 61: Assessment of Reproductive Function

Amy Goodwin, RN, MSN, APRN, BC
Faculty
Department of Nursing
University of West Georgia
Carrollton, Georgia
Chapter 25: Heart Failure and Inflammatory Dysfunction: Nursing Management
Chapter 31: Upper Airway Dysfunction: Nursing Management

Ruth Grendell, MSN, RN
Professor Emerita
Point Loma Nazarene University
San Diego, California
Chapter 10: Stress, Coping, and Adaptation
Chapter 16: Pain Management
Chapter 42: Immunodeficiency and HIV Infection/AIDS: Nursing Management
Chapter 63: Breast Alterations: Nursing Management
Chapter 65: Multisystem Failure

Corinne Grimes, RN, DNSc, AOCN
Assistant Professor of Clinical Nursing
The UT Austin School of Nursing
The University of Texas at Austin
Austin, Texas
Chapter 20: Preoperative Nursing Management
Chapter 22: Postoperative Nursing Management

Darla Grimes, MS, RN
Assistant Professor
Nursing
Austin Community College
Austin, Texas
Chapter 22: Postoperative Nursing Management

Pam Hamre, RN, MS, CNM
Associate Professor
Nursing
College of St. Catherine
Minneapolis, Minnesota
Chapter 64: Male Reproductive Dysfunction: Nursing Management

Jane Harmon, PhD, MSN, CS-PMHNP
Retired
Chapter 17: Pharmacology: Nursing Management

Christine M. Henshaw, EdD, RN, CNE
Assistant Professor
Seattle Pacific University
Seattle, Washington
Staff Nurse
Highline Medical Center
Burien, Washington
  Chapter 12: Fluid, Electrolyte, and Acid-Base Imbalances

Patrick Heyman, PhD, ARNP-BC
Assistant Professor
School of Nursing
Palm Beach Atlantic University
West Palm Beach, Florida
  Chapter 41: Assessment of Immunological Function

Beth Hickey, RN, MSN, CRRN, CNA
Associate Professor
School of Nursing and Health Professions
Northern Kentucky University
Highland Heights, Kentucky
  *Chapter 35: Dysfunction of the Brain: Nursing
  Management*

Patricia Kelly, RN, MSN
Professor Emeritus
Purdue University Calumet
Hammond, Indiana
  *Chapter 33: Obstructive Pulmonary Disease: Nursing
  Management*

Adrianne J. Lane, EdD, RN, C
Professor of Nursing
University of Cincinnati College of Nursing
Cincinnati Ohio
  Chapter 15: Cancer Management

Dale Halsey Lea, RN, MPH
Southern Maine Regional Genetics Services Program
Supervisor
Foundation for Blood Research
Scarborough, Maine
  *Chapter 9: Genetics and the Multiple Determinants
  of Health*

MariJo Letizia, PhD, RN, C, APRN-BC
Associate Professor
Loyola University Chicago
Chicago, Illinois
  Chapter 7: Palliative Care

Sharon Little-Stoetzel, RN, MS
Associate Professor
Graceland Univerisity
Independence, Missouri
  Chapter 19: Critical Care
  Chapter 26: Arrhythmias: Nursing Management

Madeleine Lynch Martin, MSN, EdD, RN
Professor
Executive Director
Undergraduate and Masters Curricula
College of Nursing
University of Cincinnati
Cincinnati, Ohio
  Chapter 15: Cancer Management

Carrie A. McCoy, PhD, MSPH, RN, CEN
Professor of Nursing
Northern Kentucky University
Highland Heights, Kentucky
  Chapter 35: Dysfunction of the Brain: Nursing Management

Linda Meuleveld, BA, RN, COHN-S, CCM, DABFN,
VPS
Medical Training Coordinator
Occupational Health and Safety Consultant
Trainer
SAIF Corporation
Salem, Oregon
  Chapter 43: Allergic Dysfunction: Nursing Management

Diane Montgomery, PhD, RN
Assistant Professor
College of Nursing
Texas Woman's University
Houston, Texas
  Chapter 40: Auditory Dysfunction: Nursing Management

Marilyn Moorhouse, RN, MSN
Manager Consultative Specialty
Group Health
Redmond, Washington
University of Phoenix
Online Faculty
Adjunct Faculty
Seattle Pacific University
Seattle, Washington
  Chapter 63: Breast Alterations: Nursing Management

Linda L. Morris, PhD, APN, CCNS
Clinical Nurse Specialist, Respiratory Care
Northwestern Memorial Hospital
Assistant Professor of Clinical Anesthesiology
Feinberg School of Medicine
Northwestern University
Chicago, Illinois
  Chapter 30: Assessment of Respiratory Function

May Mui, Pharm D, BCPS
Clinical Pharmacist
St. David's Medical Center,
Austin, Texas
  *Chapter 33: Obstructive Pulmonary Disease: Nursing
  Management*

Sharon Narducci, MSN, RN, FNP-BC, CCRN
Cardiac Specialist NP
Sharp Memorial Hospital
Escondido, California
  Chapter 24: Coronary Artery Dysfunction: Nursing
  Management

Evelyn Perez, RN, MSN, ACNP
APN Critical Care
University of Chicago Hospitals
Department of Nursing Professional Development
Chicago, Illinois
  Chapter 6: Nursing of Adults Across the Life Span

Sharon Raymen, RN, MSA, CPTC, CCTC
Assistant Professor
Samaritan College of Nursing
Grand Canyon University
Phoenix, Arizona
  Chapter 8: Health Assessment

Diana Rodrigues, RN, PhD
Assistant Professor
Point Loma Nazarene University
San Diego, California
  Chapter 4: Culturally Sensitive Care

Laura M. Rogers, RNC, MSN
Clinical Nurse Manager
Swedish Covenant Hospital
Chicago, Illinois
  Chapter 18: Health Care Agencies

Kathryn Schroeter, PhD, RN, CNOR
Surgical Services Education Coordinator
Froedtert Hospital and Medical College of Wisconsin
Milwaukee, Wisconsin
Faculty
Marquette University College of Nursing
Milwaukee, Wisconsin
Editor
International Journal of Perioperative Care
Milwaukee, Wisconsin
  Chapter 21: Intraoperative Nursing Management

Carolyn M. Schwartz, RN, MSN, APRN, BC
North Austin Medical Center
Austin, Texas
  Chapter 13: Infusion Therapy

Rebecca Sears, RN
Clinical Educator
Mount Carmel St. Ann's Hospital
Westerville, Ohio
  Chapter 59: Musculoskeletal Dysfunction: Nursing
  Management
  Chapter 60: Musculoskeletal Trauma: Nursing Management

Milena Segatore, MScN, MNI-PG, CNRN
Clinical Nurse Specialist
St. Joseph's Hospital
Milwaukee, Wisconsin
  Chapter 50: Lower Gastrointestinal Tract Dysfunction:
  Nursing Management

Valerie Lindquist Stalsbroten, RN, MC
Adjunct Faculty
School of Health Sciences
Seattle Pacific University
Seattle, Washington
  Chapter 51: Hepatic, Biliary Tract, and Pancreatic
  Dysfunction: Nursing Management

Kathleen R. Stevens, RN, EdD, FAAN
Professor and Director
Academic Center for Evidence-Based Practice
The University of Texas Health Science Center
San Antonio, Texas
  Chapter 2: Clinical Decision Making and Evidence-
  Based Practice

Beth Strauss, MS, RN, APRN, BC
Clinical Assistant Professor
School of Nursing
University of Wisconsin-Madison
Madison, Wisconsin
  Chapter 32: Lower Airway Dysfunction: Nursing
  Management

Deb Topham, PhD, RN, CNS, ACRN
Assistant Professor
Oregon Health and Science University
Portland, Oregon
  Chapter 14: Complementary and Alternative Therapies
  Chapter 42: Immunodeficiency and HIV Infection/AIDS:
  Nursing Management

Elizabeth Torrence, RN, MN, EdD
Associate Professor
School of Health Sciences
Seattle Pacific University
Seattle, Washington
  Chapter 47: Assessment of Gastrointestinal Function
  Chapter 49: Upper Gastrointestinal Tract Dysfunction:
  Nursing Management

Frances Vlasses, PhD, RN
Faculty
Loyola University
Chicago, Illinois
  Chapter 18: Health Care Agencies

Barbara Voshall, RN, MN
Assistant Professor of Nursing
Graceland University
Independence, Missouri
  *Chapter 23: Assessment of Cardiovascular and
  Hematological Function*
  Chapter 26: Arrhythmias: Nursing Management

David Voshall, PhD, MD
PhD Biochemistry
Owner of Blue Springs Internal Medicine
Blue Springs, Missouri
  *Chapter 23: Assessment of Cardiovascular and
  Hematological Function*

Karen Wikoff, RN, DNS
Dameron Hospital
Stockton, California
  Chapter 39: Visual Dysfunction: Nursing Management

Tanya D. Williams, RN, BSN, MSN, CCNS, APRN-BC
Critical Care Clinical Nurse Specialist
Comprehensive Burn Center
MetroHealth Medical Center
Cleveland, Ohio
  Chapter 46: Burns: Nursing Management

Julie S. Williard, RN, MS, NP-C
Assistant Professor
University of West Georgia
Carrollton, Georgia
  *Chapter 25: Heart Failure and Inflammatory
  Dysfunction: Nursing Management*
  *Chapter 31: Upper Airway Dysfunction: Nursing
  Management*

Cynthia A. Worley, BSN, RN, WOCN
Wound, Ostomy, Continence Nurse
M.D. Anderson Cancer Center
The University of Texas
Houston, Texas
  Chapter 44: Assessment of Integumentary Function
  *Chapter 45: Dermatological Dysfunction: Nursing
  Management*

Mary J. Yoho, PhD, RN
Director of Nursing Programs
Tomball College
Tomball, Texas
  *Chapter 27: Vascular Dysfunction: Nursing
  Management*

Lynne Yurko, RN, BSN, CNA-BC
Nurse Manager
Burn Center
MetroHealth Medical Center
Cleveland, Ohio
  Chapter 46: Burns: Nursing Management

Anita M. Zehala, RN, MS, ONC, CNS
The Ohio State University
Columbus, Ohio
Excelsior College
Albany, New York
  Chapter 58: Assessment of Musculoskeletal Function
  *Chapter 59: Musculoskeletal Dysfunction: Nursing
  Management*
  *Chapter 60: Musculoskeletal Trauma: Nursing
  Management*

REVIEWERS

Patricia Allen, RN, MSN
Clinical Instructor
School of Nursing
Indiana University
Bloomington, Indiana

Lisa Anderson-Shaw, DrPH, MA, MSN
Director, Clinical Ethics Consult Service
Assistant Clinical Professor
University of Illinois Medical Center
University of Illinois College of Nursing
Chicago, Illinois

Danette Birkhimer, MS, RN, CNS, OCN
Clinical Instructor
College of Nursing
Ohio State University
Columbus, Ohio

Madeleine Buck, RN, MSc
School of Nursing
McGill University
Montreal, Quebec, Canada

Joyce Campbell, MSN, CCRN, APRN, BC
Associate Professor of Nursing
Chattanooga State Technical Community College
Chattanooga, Tennessee

Cecily Cosby PhD, FNP/PA-C
Associate Professor
FNP Program Director
Samuel Merritt College
Oakland, California

Marianne Curia, MSN, RN
Assistant Professor
Staff Nurse
University of St. Francis
University of Chicago
Chicago, Illinois

Connie Frisch, RNMA
Instructor
Department of Nursing
Central Lakes College
Brainerd, Minnesota

Karen K. Gerbasich, RN, MSN
Assistant Professor
Ivy Tech Community College
South Bend, Indiana

Stephanie Johnson, MSN, RN, BC
Assistant Professor
School of Nursing
Morehead State University
Morehead, Kentucky

Mary F. King, RN, MS
Phillips Community College
University of Arkansas
Helena, Arkansas

Anita G. Kinser, EdD, RN, BC
Associate Professor
Nursing Education Resource Specialist
Riverside Community College
Riverside, California

Pam Kohlbry, RN, PhDc
Course Coordinator
College of Nursing
San Diego State University
San Diego, California

Darlene Lacy, PhD, RN, BC
Assistant Professor
School of Nursing
Texas Tech Health Sciences Center
Lubbock, Texas

Miki Magnino-Rabig, PhD, RN
Assistant Professor
University of St. Francis
Joliet, Illinois

Patsy L. Maloney, RN, BC, EdD, MSN, MA, CNAA
Associate Professor
Director
Professional Development and Continuing Studies
Pacific Lutheran University
Tacoma, Washington

Amy Moore, RN, MSN, FNP-C
Instructor
School of Nursing
Texas Tech University
Lubbock, Texas

Jill R. Reed, MSN, APRN
Instructor
College of Nursing
Kearney Division
University of Nebraska Medical Center
Kearney, Nebraska

Amanda Reynolds, MSN, RN
Associate Professor
School of Nursing
Grambling State University
Grambling, Louisiana

Diane Reynolds, RN, MS, OCN, CNE
Assistant Professor of Nursing
Long Island University
Brooklyn, New York

Nancy Jo Ross, RN, BSN, MSN
Instructor
School of Nursing
Central Maine Medical Center
Lewiston, Maine

Bonnie Ruiz, RN, MSN, FNP-C
Instructor
School of Nursing
Health Sciences Center
Texas Tech University
Lubbock, Texas

Jacalyn M. Schaefer, MSN, RN, CNOR
Clinical Associate
College of Nursing
James Cancer Hospital and Solove Research Institute
The Ohio State University
Columbus, Ohio

Linda Schaffer, RN, MN
Chief Nursing Officer
Corporate Director
Health Science Education Programs
U.S. Education Corporation
Mission Viejo, California

Barbara Scheirer, RN, MSN
Assistant Professor
School of Nursing
Grambling State University
Grambling, Louisiana

Krista Susan Sifford, MSN, RN
Assistant Professor
College of Nursing
Arkansas State University
State University, Arkansas

Annette Smith Stacy, MSN, RN, AOCN
Associate Professor of Nursing
BSN Program Director
Arkansas State University
Jonesboro, Arkansas

Kristy Tabor, RN, MSN, AOCN
Clinical Faculty
The Ohio State University
Columbus, Ohio

Annie Thomas, RN, MSN, PhD
Assistant Professor
School of Nursing
Texas Tech University Health Sciences Center
Lubbock, Texas

Elayne Trepel, RN, MSN
Instructor
College of Nursing
University of Illinois at Chicago
Chicago, Illinois

Mary Wcisel, RN, MSN
Assistant Professor
Saint Mary's College
Notre Dame, Indiana

Paige Wimberley, MSN, RN, CS, CNE
Assistant Professor of Nursing
Arkansas State University
State University, Arkansas

Faye G. Zeigler, RN, BSN, MSN
Associate Professor
School of Nursing
Austin Peay State University
Clarksville, Tennessee

Acknowledgments

I would first like to express my appreciation to my two coauthors, Leslie Nicoll and Laura Nosek, for their tenacity and expertise in supervising contributors for this project. Each of these authors has maintained a high level of professionalism as they has pursued the completion of this first edition of this medical-surgical nursing text.

We would also like to thank all of the contributors of this comprehensive book for their time and effort in sharing their knowledge gained through the years. We also thank the reviewers for their time spent in critically reviewing the manuscripts and providing valuable comments that have been added to this text.

We would like to acknowledge and thank the members of the team at Thomson Delmar Learning who have worked with us in making this text a reality. Tamera Caruso, acquisitions editor, and Patty Gaworecki, product manager, are incredible people who have brought their knowledge and professional guidance to assist us with this project.

We particularly want to acknowledge our families for their supportive attitudes and actions as we have undertaken this project. They have encouraged us at each step of the way and enveloped us with their positive thoughts and words. For this we are thankful.

About the Authors

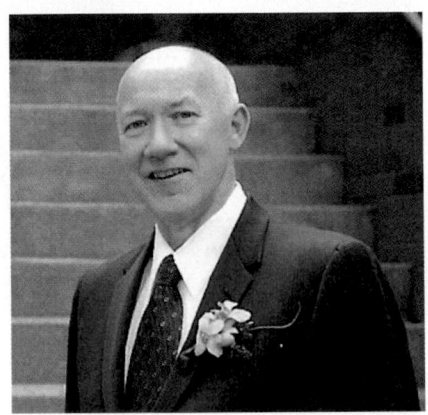

DR. RICK DANIELS

Dr. Rick Daniels obtained a Bachelor of Science in Nursing from the University of Oregon Nursing School, Portland, Oregon; a master of science in nursing from the University of San Diego, California; and a Ph.D. in nursing from the University of Texas in Austin.

He has taught nursing in associate, baccalaureate, and graduate schools of nursing, as well as RN degree completion programs. Dr. Daniels has taught fundamentals of nursing, medical-surgical nursing, pathophysiology, pharmacology, and research in a variety of programs. In addition, he has taught in several venues, including distance learning, correspondence, and traditional classroom settings. He has also taught many adult health and illness topics at seminars and has presented posters for national organizations (e.g., AORN, NLN Educators Conference). Dr. Daniels administers clinical practicum courses in critical care, emergency department, and perioperative nursing arenas.

Dr. Daniels' clinical practice is kept current by practicing nursing as a colonel in the Oregon Army National Guard. He is also serving as the deputy state commander of Oregon under the supervision of the Oregon State Surgeon.

Dr. Daniels' research is primarily associated with the concept of health promotion, and he has received three successive fundings with the Department of the Army to implement health promotion programs with national guardsmen. In addition, Dr. Daniels publishes in nursing journals and authors nursing textbooks. He has membership in a number of professional nursing organizations; such as Sigma Theta Tau and the American Nurses Association.

Dr. Daniels is currently an associate professor with tenure at Oregon Health and Science University, School of Nursing.

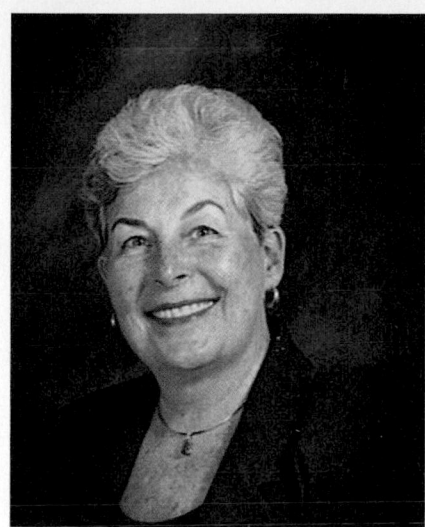

LAURA JOHN NOSEK

Laura John Nosek is a graduate of the Grace New Haven School of Nursing at Yale New Haven Medical Center, New Haven, Connecticut. She earned the bachelor of science in nursing from Frances Payne Bolton School of Nursing, Western Reserve University in Cleveland, Ohio, and the master of science in nursing and the Ph.D. in executive practice from Case Western Reserve University, Cleveland, Ohio.

Dr. Nosek's primary career has been as the chief nursing officer in academic health science centers in the private sector and as the chief nursing officer and chief operating officer in a public sector academic health science center. She currently holds academic appointments at universities in Ohio, Illinois, and New York, where she teaches various aspects of nursing administration and organizational science. She has taught in diploma, baccalaureate, masters, and doctoral nursing programs in four states, focusing on women's health, executive practice, and organizational systems, her areas of research. Dr. Nosek has made numerous presentations nationally and internationally and is published in nursing textbooks and juried nursing journals.

Dr. Nosek has served on national committees of Sigma Theta Tau and the National League for Nursing and has held multiple state and local offices in AONE, NLN, Sigma Theta Tau, and ANA. She currently sits on the national finance committee of NLN and serves as an NLN Ambassador.

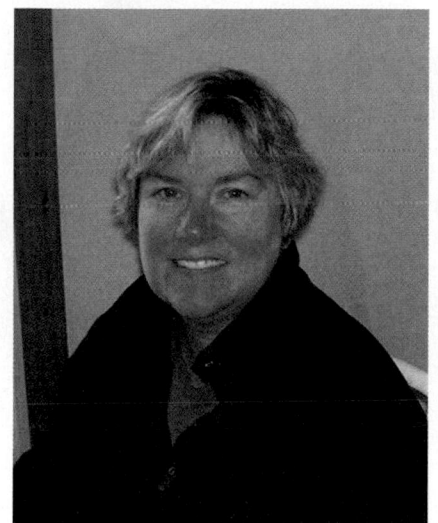

LESLIE H. NICOLL

Leslie H. Nicoll is the President and Owner of Maine Desk, LLC, a consulting and editorial services firm specializing in nursing, health, informatics, and research. Since 1995, Dr. Nicoll has been the editor-in-chief of *CIN* (formerly *Computers in Nursing*). On July 1, 2001, Dr. Nicoll was appointed editor-in-chief of the *Journal of Hospice and Palliative Nursing*, the official publication of the Hospice and Palliative Nurses Association. Prior to founding Maine Desk, Dr. Nicoll held a joint appointment as an Associate Research Professor in the College of Nursing and Health Professions and a Senior Research Associate in the Edmund S. Muskie School of Public Service, both at the University of Southern Maine, Portland, Maine. She is the author of *Nurses' Guide to the Internet* and editor of *Perspectives on Nursing Theory*. In addition, Dr. Nicoll is the author of more than 110 articles, books, editorials, and reviews. On September 8, 2003, she had a crossword puzzle published in *The New York Times*, which many consider a greater accomplishment than all her other articles combined. She is a graduate of Russell Sage College (BS, Nursing), the University of Illinois (MS, Nursing), and Case Western Reserve University (Ph.D., Nursing). As a Commonwealth Fund Executive Nurse Fellow, she pursued MBA study at the Whittemore School of Business and Economics, University of New Hampshire, graduating in 1991.

How to Use This Text

Patient Playbook

Patients benefit greatly from knowledge of self-care, and nurses presenting information in a collaborative manner promote health. These boxes present relevant teaching interventions for patient, family, or support people necessary to enhance the individual's health. Instructions on how to equip patients with knowledge of well-being or preparing for procedures or outcomes is vital.

Red Flag

As a professional nurse, you will need to be able to react immediately in selected situations to ensure the health and safety of your patients. Pay careful attention to this feature, as it will assist you to begin to identify and respond to critical situations on your own, both efficiently and effectively.

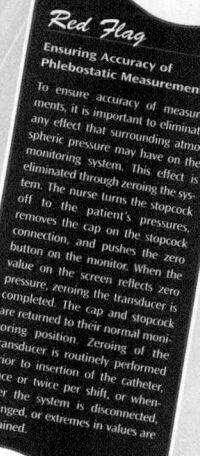

Ethics or Law in Practice

Our health care delivery system has many legal and ethical issues for the nurse to consider in the practice setting. These boxes describe patient situations that make it easier for you to see the ethicolegal implications as you provide your patient care. Incorporate these insights into your professional growth and development as an ethical practitioner.

Respecting Our Differences

It is important to recognize the specific implications for your care of patients with different cultural backgrounds. You need to review such things as the physiological and psychological implications of your different patients. This will assist you in delivering individualized nursing care.

Safety First

Error prevention is a vital consideration in contemporary practice. As you read these boxes, think about how each strategy will improve safe practice and patient care.

Uncovering the Evidence

Evidence-based practice is essential to your development of knowledge and growth as a professional nurse. As you read these boxes, focus your attention on the elements of the research that are presented and incorporate the application as appropriate to your nursing practice.

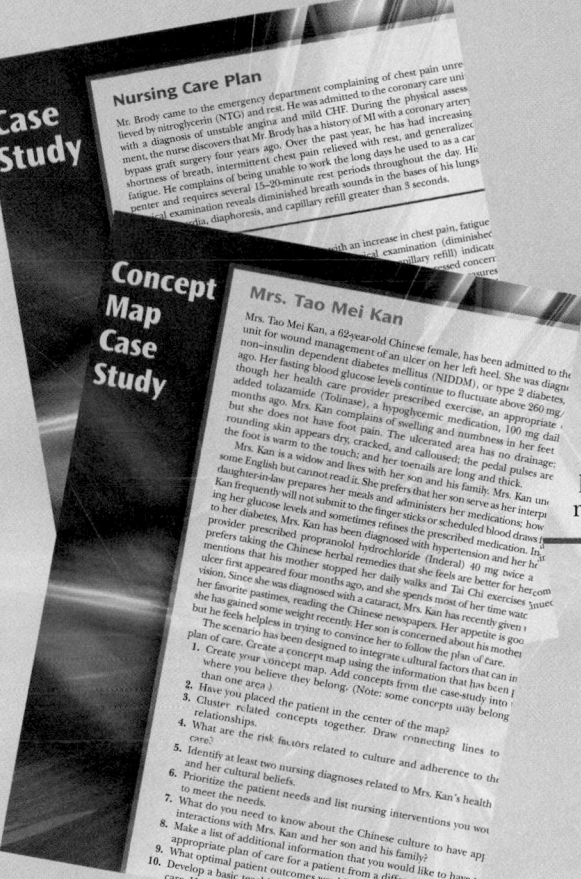

Uncovering the Evidence

Survey of Americans Living with Pain

Discussion: To determine the current awareness and understanding of pain and pain management issues among the general population of the United States, a random digit dialing system including all household telephone numbers (listed and unlisted) in the United States was used in 2002 to collect data. Data were collected through 800 telephone interviews with adults experiencing chronic pain.

The findings revealed the following:

- Seventy-two percent of respondents experiencing chronic pain had lived with it for more than 3 years; 34 percent had lived with pain for more than a decade.
- Seventy-eight percent of respondents believed that treatment with narcotic medications would cause addiction.
- Most respondents thought the typical person living with chronic pain was an adult at or above 65 years of age.
- A majority agreed that some people tend to exaggerate their pain to gain attention, avoid work, or to obtain painkillers. (More of the youngest respondents answered "strongly agree" to this statement.)
- One-third of respondents reported living with ongoing pain.
- Workplace Issues:
  1. Forty-one percent of employed persons who had chronic pain stated that it affected their ability to work a full day.
  2. Twenty-seven percent stated that the pain affected their ability to get to work.
  3. Sixteen percent stated that chronic pain affected their opportunities for career advancement.
- Pain Management:
  1. Eighty-one percent reported satisfaction with their prescribed plan of medical treatment.
  2. Eight-six percent of those taking prescription medications also reported using alternative treatments, including physical therapy (58 percent) massage (39 percent), and meditation (23 percent).
  3. Sixty-four percent of those who used over-the-counter (OTC) medications were satisfied with their relief of pain.
- Economic Fears: Three of ten persons were unable to have a prescription filled because of its cost or the lack of health insurance; they also felt it would become more difficult to obtain the needed medication in the future.

Implications for Practice: Patient education and encouraging many pain-relieving modalities available and encouraging patients and their families to become a principal part of the treatment team are very important aspects of good pain management.

Source: American Chronic Pain Association (ACPA). (2004). Nurses' pain awareness kit. Retrieved from: http://www. theacpa.org.

Case Studies

These real-life scenarios present a patient situation followed by nursing responsibilities framed in a nursing process format. Use case studies to provide a focused opportunity to refine critical thinking skills.

Skills 360°

These help to develop and enhance professionalism, communication, and skills in the workplace. Use Skills 360° to expand discussion on patient care.

Skills 360°

Professional and Caring Communication

Patients with endocrine disorders may have disfigurement related to their physical appearance (e.g., acromegaly, dwarfism, Grave's disease, or goiter). The nurse must remember to focus on maintaining an objective assessment and still provide a caring and supportive style of communication with the patient.

Review Questions and Activities

As a method of reviewing a chapter, answer the open-ended questions in this box. These activities will stimulate your learning and allow you to synthesize and evaluate the knowledge gained when you study each section.

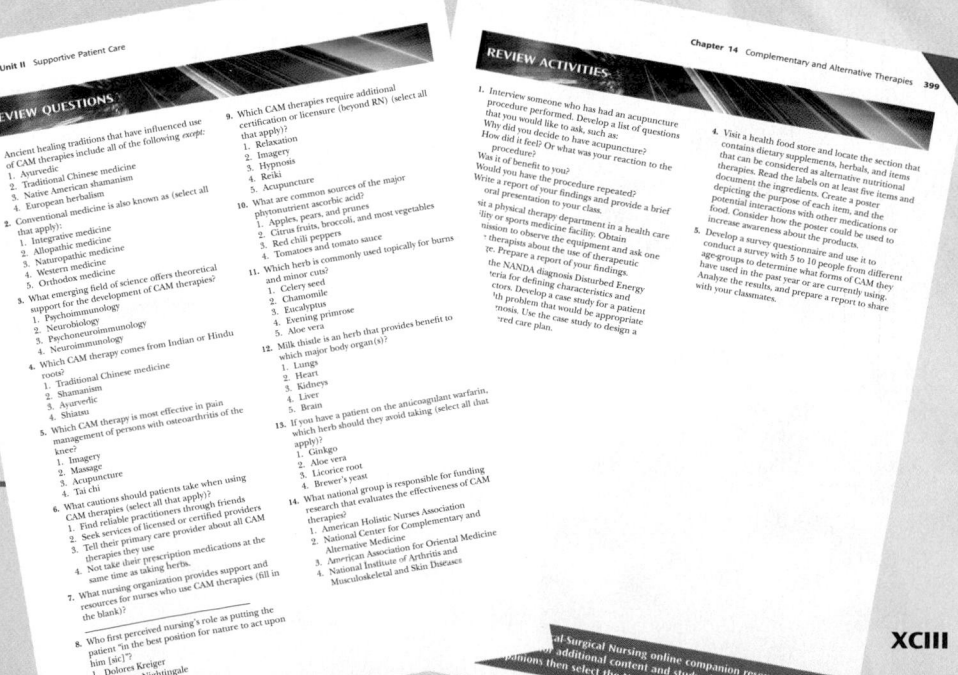

How to Use the CD-ROM

A ccess a wealth of information designed to enhance the text content

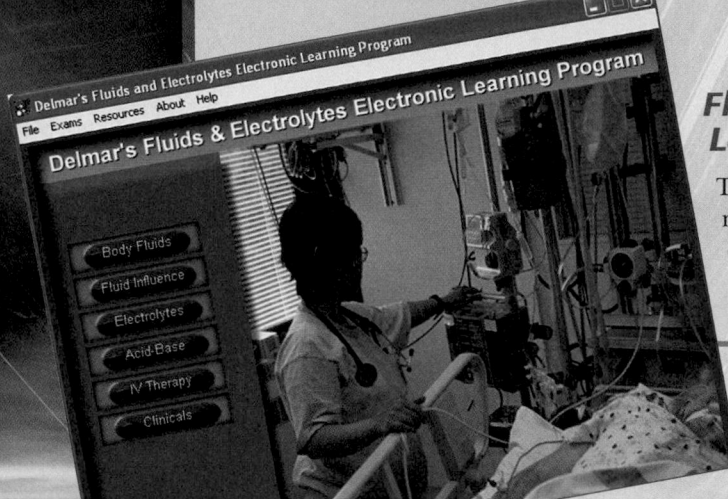

Fluids & Electrolytes Learning Program

This provides an interactive, easy-to-navigate program that simplifies difficult concepts and their application to medical-surgical nursing.

Critical Care Nursing Care Plans

These offer a unique experience to create and customize care plans in an electronic environment for the medical-surgical patient.

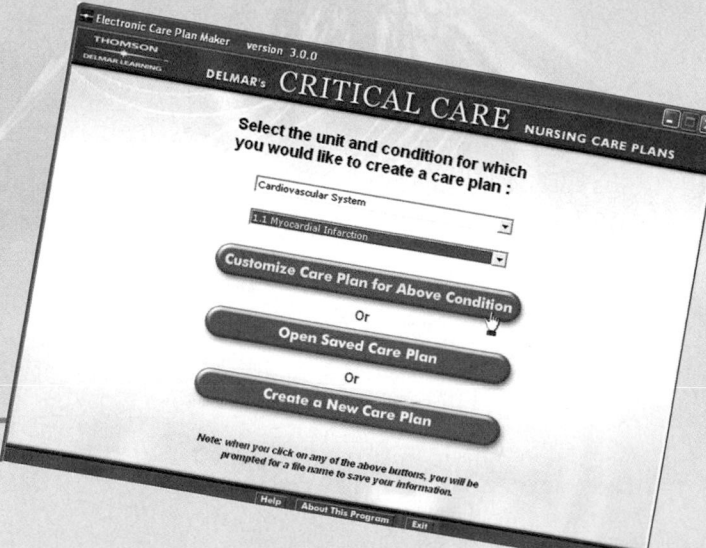

Heart & Lung Sounds Review

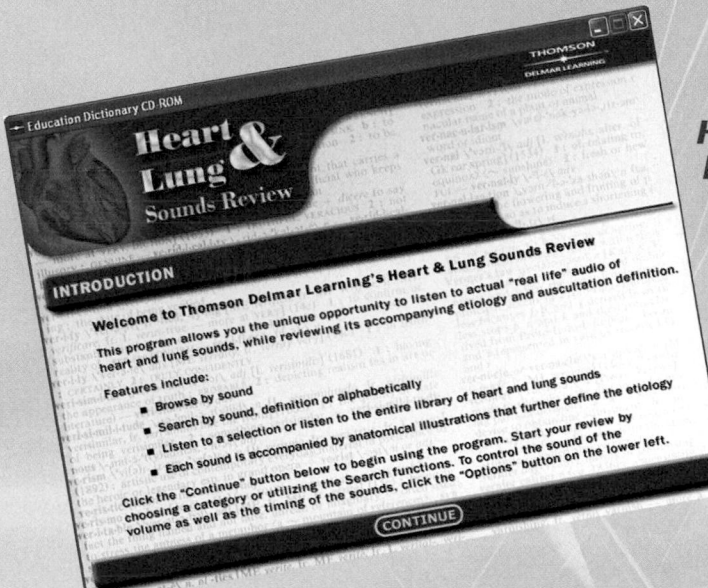

This program offers the opportunity to listen to actual real-life audio of heart and lung sounds while reviewing the accompanying etiology and auscultation definition.

NCLEX Review Tests

Two 100-question NCLEX exams are available in a test environment and focus on the areas of delegation and pharmacology. These tests have a rationale for right and wrong choices and are based on the current test plan with an emphasis on the medical-surgical patient.

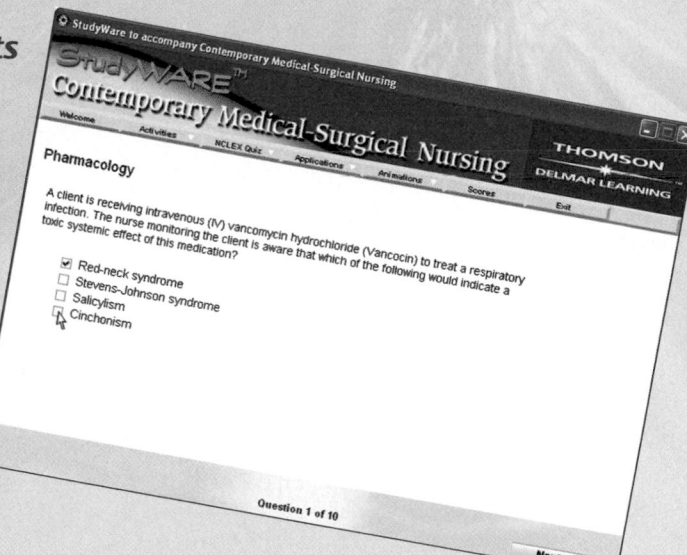

Nursing and the Health Care System

The Health Care System and Contemporary Nursing

Laura John Nosek, PhD, RN

KEY TERMS

Altruism
Autonomously
Biotechnology
Clinical decisions
Collective bargaining
Competence
Continuous quality improvement (CQI)
Culture for caring
Domains of nursing
Enterprises
Ergonomics
Globalization
Health care
Health care system
Illness care
System
Total quality management (TQM)
Wellness care
Workforce diversity

CHAPTER TOPICS

- Emergence of the Contemporary Health Care System in the United States

- Emergence of Contemporary Nursing in the United States

- Contemporary Nursing Practice in the United States

- Environment for Contemporary Nursing Practice in the United States

Caring for others who cannot or who do not care for themselves is as ancient as humankind. Over time, knowledge about causes and efficacious treatment of illness has expanded, a system for providing care has emerged, and eventually a robust and costly industry was formed. Nursing matured from the art of providing comfort to include practices rooted in science. During the late 20th century, expansion of the use of biotechnology and information technology, discovery of new medications, and focus on the need to control health care cost resulted in a paradigm shift from illness care toward strategies for maintaining and improving health and preventing illness known as **wellness care.** At the same time, nursing matured as a science and its scope of practice expanded. This chapter explores selected aspects of the evolution of the health care system in the United States, the contemporary health care system, and its impact on nurses and their practice.

EMERGENCE OF THE CONTEMPORARY HEALTH CARE SYSTEM IN THE UNITED STATES

A **system** is a set of parts linked in orderly, logical interdependence that function together as a synergistic unit. The **health care system** in the United States is the network of individuals, technologies, and processes that provide and support **health care.** Health care refers to all states of health from severe illness and injury to supreme good health and the behaviors that seek to improve an individual's health status.

Transition from Illness Care to Health Care

The term health care was adopted when expansion of **biotechnology,** the use of data and techniques of engineering to solve problems related to living organisms, and discovery of hundreds of efficacious pharmaceutical and technological therapies shifted the paradigm of care from **illness care** aimed at relieving illness to wellness care to prevent illness. This shift in terminology does not reflect a shift along a continuum toward a healthier society. Rather, it reflects paradigm shifts in society's perception about the mission of care, where care is most suitably provided, who provides the care, how care is managed and controlled, and how its cost and quality are determined.

Site for Care

The earliest site where humans cared for each other was in the home, whether that home was a cave, an igloo, a tent, or a castle. For centuries, home care predominantly sought to provide comfort for the ill or injured following the nursing care tenets of Florence Nightingale (1969 [1859]). Medieval religious orders established infirmaries to care for the aged, orphaned, poor, and disabled who could not be cared for at home or who had no home. Today such care is referred to as population-focused care.

Originally, a hospital was an inn or guest room that provided shelter and sustenance for travelers. *Hospital* was derived from the concept of hospitality provided by such inns. Gradually, simple remedies for illnesses encountered during travel were added to the services of inns, followed by surgical procedures, custodial care for mental illness, and lying-in for birthing.

For nearly 100 years hospitals have remained the site for providing care dependent on complex, costly technology and care dependent on nurses. The introduction of health insurance and subsequent shift of payment responsibility from the direct recipient of care to an insurance intermediary only willing to pay for skilled nursing services reinforced society's dependence on hospitals. Now, advanced practice nurses providing primary care are moving from hospital to community sites to provide care side-by-side with their physician colleagues.

Providers of Care

Over just the past 50 years extraordinary changes have emerged in the way health care is delivered and compensated in the United States. In the mid-20th century those who perceived themselves to be ill sought their physician, a general practitioner (GP), who usually provided care to the entire family. It was common for a single GP to provide care to an individual for several decades, often beginning at birth and lasting until the physician or patient expired.

As the biological sciences matured, knowledge about the causes, courses, and treatment of illness expanded exponentially. It became difficult, then impossible, for a single physician to manage all aspects of all illnesses. Physicians compressed the breadth of their practice to better manage the depth of that practice. Initially, the GP became the gatekeeper for accessing specialists' care, but by the 1980s it was common for patients to make a self-diagnosis about the nature of an illness and choose an appropriate specialist.

The close and trusting relationship between any individual and that individual's physician waned, replaced by fleeting acquaintances with a cadre of specialists. Allied health care providers, including therapists rooted in various disciplines and advanced practice nurses, were educated to manage selected components of care, further fragmenting that care. Together, the effect of new technologies, new therapies, and multiple care providers significantly depersonalized the care provider-patient relationship.

The medical team was traditionally perceived to be a physician and a nurse. Their mission to relieve suffering and cure disease involved three levels of care: to *sustain* the patient's life, to then assist the patient to *regain* the former level of health, and finally to *maintain* that former level of health. The shift in focus toward health care added a plethora of health promotion, disease prevention research and intervention strategies to the domains of medical and nursing knowledge and practice. Diagnosing, treating, and curing disease expanded to include a fourth level, *attaining* enhanced health and physical and mental performance. Physicians extended their ability to care for the expanded workload through implementation of a new discipline called the physician assistant (PA). This two-year university-based educational program prepares graduates to work under the direct supervision of a physician. In addition, registered nurses (RNs) with masters education practice **autonomously,** or independently, as nurse practitioners (NPs) providing primary health care within the regulations of the state in which they practice. All but 64 hospitals that employed a three-year apprentice model of nursing education rooted in learning through hands-on clinical practice are now closed and have been replaced by college-based two-year programs rooted in both liberal arts and human sciences. In addition, formal accredited educational programs, along with required examination and certification, were established for unlicensed assistive personnel (UAPs) who previously received only on-the-job (OTJ) training by their employer.

Control of Care

Health care was traditionally delivered from a paternalistic model of governance and control. Health professionals from various disciplines, led by physicians, controlled a vast body of scientific knowledge and skill rendered awesome and mystical by complex scientific language. Command of that unique body of scientific knowledge and skill required extensive and expensive education that gave its owners the privilege to be viewed and revered as professionals. Decision making about all aspects of health care was the exclusive domain of the physician, independent of the patient and, commonly independent of professional colleagues.

Virginia Henderson's (1991) reflections on the nature of nursing from 1966 through 1991 prompted her to stress that health care is a political subject. That is, health care is concerned with government, and government is concerned with it. Clearly, Florence Nightingale was immersed in political action throughout her career, prolifically corresponding and skillfully negotiating with influential members of government and business in the cause of improving illness care and the general health of society. However, few nurses providing direct clinical care recognize the influence government holds over their practice beyond their respective nurse practice acts that regulate the scope of nursing practice or beyond the more than 30-year-old Roe v. Wade decision that supports women's right to choose abortion. More and more each year, government is establishing laws that regulate what health care providers and their employers can and cannot do.

Cost regulation by government effectively put health care rationing in place. However, the effect of the regulation laws on nurses' practice has been indirect. That is, the laws did not impact the way nurses deliver care to their patients.

Over the past five years nurses have become acutely aware of the impact legislation has on the way they provide nursing care. The expansion of opportunities for RNs in the United States is contributing to the shortage of RNs to provide direct clinical care, despite the fact that approximately 2.9 million of the world's 4 million nurses are in the United States and that there are more RNs per capita in the United States than in any other country in the world (Nosek, 2004; Nosek & Androwich, 2003). Numerous states have enacted staffing ratio laws that require hospitals to hire sufficient numbers of RNs to ensure safe and high-quality care, regardless of the size of the RN pool available, and to regulate an RN's patient load. It ought to be noted that the number of patients assigned to an individual nurse (patient load) does not necessarily reflect the amount of effort required to care for those patients. The staffing laws also regulate the number of hours RNs can work each day. In addition, government has assumed the responsibility for funding more and more of the cost of education for nurses providing clinical care and for nurse educators to teach them.

The reality of practicing under the Health Insurance Portability and Accountability Act (HIPAA) of 1996 only became evident to nurses several years after its passage when the extensive requirements for maintaining patient confidentiality were interpreted and implemented. HIPAA standardizes the processing of health care data and protects the privacy of information about an individual's health status. It requires providers to adhere to an abundance of confidentiality safeguards as caregivers go about their work. HIPAA has failed to achieve its goal of reducing administrative costs through the sharing of existing data because of the lack of widespread adoption of the required eligibility, enrollment, and remittance systems by health insurance plans (American Hospital Association [AHA], 2005). In 2002 the secretary of the department of health and human services recommended 255 reforms to reduce the regulatory burden on health care providers. By the beginning of 2006 no report had been generated about the status of those reforms (AHA, 2005).

Cyclic RN shortages and abundances have plagued health care for years. However, the shortage that began to emerge around 2002 seems to be rooted in a new set of factors that cannot be readily resolved and that suggest that the shortage will worsen to a critical level by 2020. A government attempt to counter the shortage and protect society from a deadly loss of RNs is to require that enough RNs be hired to ensure that the minimum staffing ratios established by law are maintained at all times and that mandatory overtime for RNs is limited to genuine emergency situations, such as mass disasters. There is simply an inadequate number of capable RNs available to comply with such staffing mandates across all health care **enterprises,** those organizational

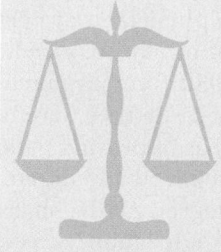

LAW IN PRACTICE

It's the Law!

In April of 2004 the New Jersey Senate passed a law requiring health care facilities to report all serious and reportable adverse events to the state and to the affected patient. Assurances have been given that the reports will not be used as a basis for litigation (AONE, 2004), but society's experience with the military's handling of admissions of same gender preference suggests that there may be strong reluctance to test such a law by both individuals and by their employers.

systems of any size in any location that provide any type of health care for compensation. Nurses are caught in a catch 22 between their professional responsibility not to abandon their patients and their personal responsibility to ensure their own self-care in order to provide safe care to patients. Nurses and their employers must find creative, safe care delivery models that are in compliance with staffing legislation.

Clinical Systems Leadership

Examination of the senior leadership of health care enterprises over the past 200 to 300 years reveals a cyclical pattern of leadership under clinical experts and business experts. Generally, the expertise required of a leader is dependent on the type of leadership that is needed to manage the current issues, clinical, or business. The earliest senior hospital administrators were nuns from the religious orders that sponsored the hospitals. The nuns' expertise was two-pronged. They were gifted with clinical expertise rooted in their religious mission to relieve physical and spiritual distress, and they also had expertise in resource management rooted in their dependence on human charity for survival.

During the pre-Nightingale era in the early 19th century hospital, leadership shifted away from the nuns and rested with physicians, the experts in medical science. Generally, physicians had neither education nor experience in business management. Physicians rose to the top administrative position because they were successful clinical practitioners who achieved above average clinical outcomes.

Florence Nightingale began her career in hospital service as Resident Lady Superintendent of the Invalid Gentlewoman's Institution, a small charity hospital in London. It was the rigorous tutoring in mathematics and statistics she had received that best prepared her to reform the management of the hospital. Nightingale's (1969 [1859]) highly successful analytic approach to administration was later emulated by other nurses who replaced physicians in hospital leadership positions.

By the early to mid-20th century physicians were again enlisted to provide leadership as the captain of the ship. As the cost of health care spiraled upward in the 1960s, however, business experts were recruited to the helm in an effort to achieve health care cost efficiencies. By the late 1980s, physicians, disenchanted with the influence of third-party insurers over clinical practice decisions and with diminishing compensation, sought business management education and began to replace the business leaders of the hospital enterprise in an effort to temper cost control initiatives. However, when the chief executive officer (CEO) of the hospital is also a physician, there is risk of conflict of interest and adversarial interactions between the physician administrator who is accountable to the hospital board and the community for achieving business goals and the clinical practitioners who expect the physician leader to be biased in favor of achieving clinicians' interests. Serving such disparate masters is truly challenging.

Nurses, as well as physicians, are clinical experts and strong advocates for making achievement of clinical excellence a priority of a health care enterprise. During the 1980s, nurses pursued masters in business administration (MBA) education, because they were highly interested in improving the work environment, as well as improving patient care processes. Nurses interested in scientific analysis of clinical and organizational issues pursued a research doctor of philosophy degree (PhD) in executive practice that included strong components of MBA education. Selected programs offered a dual MBA/PhD degree, initiating a trend toward employing nurses with advanced clinical knowledge and skill, as well as business knowledge, as the senior clinical systems leader. Interest in integrating clinical and nonclinical, or clinical support, services into a single team with the synergy to achieve high performance leads some health care enterprises to appoint nurses with clinical and business expertise as chief operating officers (COOs).

Cost of Care

By the middle of the 20th century the cost of the emerging technology, along with the burgeoning providers of that technology and the health care agencies that support their practices, significantly increased health care cost. The elderly and the indigent struggled to afford health care. The government stepped in with a series of legislative initiatives to improve access to health care through insurance coverage for the elderly and indigent and to slow the upward spiral of health care cost. Titles XVIII and XIX, amendments to the Social Security Act commonly referred to as Medicare and Medicaid, were passed by Congress in 1965, marking the beginning of health care reform. The Tax Equity and Fiscal Responsibility Act (TEFRA) of 1982 established prospective, rather than retrospective, payment for health care as an incentive to curb cost (Nosek & Androwich, 2003). When it became evident that Medicare and Medicaid program costs were continuing to rise in concert with the size of an aging population able to better survive acute illness and now vulnerable to chronic illness, health maintenance organizations (HMOs), or managed care, emerged as the answer to more efficiently manage cost while continuing to provide quality care.

The mission and vision of managed care is to provide wellness care at a minimal cost to keep people healthy and thus avoid providing illness care at a higher, even astronomical, cost. The secondary mission of managed care is to standardize diagnostic and treatment decisions across the nation. Managed care emphasizes delivery of a coordinated continuum of services across the care spectrum from wellness to death, using financial incentives to decrease length of stay and achieve cost-efficiency. Thus, over merely 40 years the transition from an illness care focus to a health care focus transpired. Yet, cost remains a major contemporary health care issue. Both the health care industry and the public reacted viscerally to the implementation of reduced lengths of hospital stays. Nearly 30 years later health care providers vehemently blame third-party insurers' regulations for diminished quality of clinical care and clinical outcomes.

Quality Measure Shift

Measures of quality have been inextricably linked with clinical care for some time. The quality health care movement began in the early 1900s with the Flexner Report urging university education be adopted as the standard for health care providers. In 1912 Codman designed and implemented the first medical audits of clinical outcomes. In 1919 the American College of Surgeons formed an accreditation body for standards development, education, and measurement of practitioner competence. That accreditation body evolved into the contemporary Joint Commission for the Accreditation of Healthcare Organizations (JCAHO) in 1952.

Strategies to control costs in the mid-1960s were quickly followed by development of strategies to measure and ensure that the quality of health care does not diminish as a result of cost cutting. By 1975 hospitals were establishing utilization review departments that use standards developed by Donabedian (1966) to measure quality against practice benchmarks. As attention shifted to controlling the cost of health care in the late 1960s, concern about ensuring the safety and quality of care began to be voiced by both patients and providers. **Total quality management (TQM)** and **continuous quality improvement (CQI)** programs were initiated to ensure society that cost management was not compromising safety or quality. Such programs, as well as JCAHO, require all stakeholders, including patients, to work together to achieve benchmarked clinical outcomes at budgeted cost. The contemporary concept of quality embraces the expectations the *patient* has for the structure, process, and outcome of care and for the goal to exceed those expectations. Through the growing access to valid

DOLLARS AND SENSE

A Patient Outcry

The headlines of a major Midwest megalopolis newspaper that October morning in 1983 sent shock waves throughout the city. Seemingly out of nowhere and effective immediately, the payment by the major nationwide health insurer for hospital stay during labor and delivery was drastically reduced. For those experiencing normal vaginal delivery, three calendar days, instead of the usual five, would be covered by health care insurance starting with the day of admission. For those experiencing Cesarean delivery, five calendar days, rather than the usual seven, would be covered. If a woman were admitted to the hospital shortly before midnight, calendar day one would soon be past. If a woman experienced prolonged labor, she risked being discharged on her first postpartum day.

As the news spread among the patients on the postpartum unit that morning, anxiety turned to panic and anger. One patient haltingly made her way toward the nurses' station clinging to the wall for support and sobbing uncontrollably. A nurse approached the patient and asked what was troubling her so much. The patient could barely stand or speak through her tears to tell the nurse that she was exhausted from a long labor, that she had two small children at home and no one to help her care for them and for her newborn, and that under the new rules she would have to go home when her baby was only two days old. That was only the first of the 36 mothers on that unit who made their way to the nurses seeking help that day.

The postpartum nurses' reactions were predominantly anger. They felt betrayed and disenfranchised by an insurance industry that had no doubt failed to consult a nurse about why hospitalization for more than three days was necessary to support safe labor and delivery followed by education and support to prepare mothers and their newborns for safe discharge. The nurses' strongest arguments centered on the impossibility for ensuring successful breastfeeding by the second postpartum day when breast milk did not even come in until the third postpartum day. However, nurses all across the country rallied and quickly reinvented the postpartum and newborn care delivery system, safely and successfully moving the preponderance of care to home and community sites.

and reliable information technology, patients are now empowered to better understand their own health, the complex technologies available to improve their health status, their options for choosing to manage the decisions about their care, and the cost implications of those decisions. Patients and members of their support system are now expected and required to perform a variety of complex procedures previously reserved by law to licensed health care providers. No longer is health care the exclusive domain of professional health care providers. The JCAHO dimensions of quality and priority focus areas are listed in Box 1-1 and Box 1-2, respectively.

As health care matures as a legitimate business the focus of quality measurement is shifting from predominantly clinical measures to predominantly business measures. The concept of a dashboard of clinical and business measures helps administrators track quality trends. Similar to the dashboard of gauges on a motor vehicle, a quality dashboard contains graphic depictions of actual performance. Alongside the depiction of each actual performance appears a depiction of the benchmark, or desired, performance for all of the quality measures of an enterprise. Turnover rates for various personnel categories, medication errors, litigation rates, morbidity and mortality rates, budget variance,

---

BOX 1-1

JCAHO DIMENSIONS OF QUALITY PERFORMANCE

- Efficacy—degree to which the intervention has been shown to accomplish the intended outcome
- Appropriateness—degree to which the intervention is relevant to patient needs
- Availability—degree to which appropriate interventions are available to meet patient needs
- Timeliness—degree to which the intervention is provided at the most beneficial time to the patient
- Effectiveness—degree to which the intervention is provided in the correct manner to achieve the intended patient outcome
- Continuity—degree to which the interventions are coordinated between organizations, among care providers, and across time
- Safety—degree to which the risk of an intervention and risk in the environment are reduced for both patient and health care provider
- Efficiency—degree to which care has the desired effect with a minimum of effort, expense, or waste
- Respect and caring—degree to which patients are involved in health care decisions and are treated with sensitivity and respect for their individual needs, expectations, and differences by health care providers

Source: Joint Commission on Accreditation of Healthcare Organizations. (2005). Accreditation manual. Retrieved July 10, 2005, from http://www.jcrinc.com/ publications.asp?durki=8142&site=4&return=77.

---

turnaround time for accounts receivable, patient falls, overtime rates, admission rates by health care provider, and length of stay for the 10 most common admitting diagnoses are just a few of the most common quality measures on the dashboard. Bar graphs, stacked bar graphs, pie graphs, exploded pie graphs, and line graphs may be included to visually depict any gap between desired and actual performance.

The Agency for Healthcare Research and Quality (AHRQ) is highly interested in the efficacy of medical treatments. By the end of 2006 AHRQ planned to provide health care enterprises with guidelines for creation of a standard patient registry to track the outcomes of medical treatments (AHA, 2005). Such registries were created as Physician Peer Review Data Committees as early as 1990 to examine clinical outcome differences related to health care provider practices in selected regions of the United States such as the combined states of New Hampshire and Vermont. A nurse executive with research expertise from each state sits on the New Hampshire/Vermont Data Committee.

EMERGENCE OF CONTEMPORARY NURSING IN THE UNITED STATES

The major concern of early civilizations was survival. Primitive health care practices were rooted in trial and error. In prehistoric times women tended to care for the sick and injured and the health care belief system was that evil spirits cause illness. Thus, illness care and religion were intertwined (Catalano, 2003). Those who provided care to the ill and infirm up until the mid-20th century generally did so out of a sense of compassion and **altruism,** unselfish concern for the welfare of others. Although nurses considered themselves to

BOX 1-2

JCAHO PRIORITY FOCUS AREAS

- Ethics, rights, and responsibilities
- Provision of care, treatment, and services
- Medication management
- Surveillance and prevention of infection
- Improving organizational performance
- Leadership
- Management of the environment for care
- Management of human resources
- Management of information

Source: Joint Commission on Accreditation of Healthcare Organizations. (2006b). Focus areas. Retrieved May 22, 2006, from http://www.soros.org/ initiatives/pdia/focusareas/grants /grantees/royal1994.

be professionals, the preponderance of nursing education was provided through three-year educational programs that combined formal classroom experience in a school of nursing with considerable clinical care and clinical management experience on a wide variety of hospital units. Nursing did, however, meet all other criteria essential for a profession. Box 1-3 shows the criteria broadly accepted by society as essential to a profession.

For the past 150 years nurses have struggled to clarify to others the work that they do so effectively, efficiently, and creatively. It is clearly difficult to articulate the complex, split-second synergy of physical, social, emotional, and spiritual assessment with critical cognitive analysis, decision making, and caring that result in selection of optimally appropriate therapeutic interventions to ease, or relieve, a patient's health care problem. Nurse theorists have struggled to capture the theoretical underpinnings of the nursing discipline.

The work of Tomey and Alligood (1998) captures the concepts of numerous nurses who were recognized as theorists at the turn of the 21st century. Nightingale's (1969 [1859]) theory of nursing focuses on the environment for care. Orem's self-care deficit theory of nursing describes and explains relationships that must be brought about and maintained for nursing to be produced. Sister Callista Roy's adaptation model is based in systems theory and an individual's ability to adapt to ever-changing adaptive responses. Influenced by Martha Rogers' principles of helicy, integrality, and resonance, Parse's theory challenges the traditional medical view of nursing and distinguishes the discipline of nursing as a unique basic science. The most recent definition of nursing promulgated by the American Nurses Association (ANA) acknowledges six essential features of professional nursing that include (a) a caring relationship, (b) attention to the full range of human health and illness experiences, (c) integration of objective and subjective data, (d) application of scientific knowledge and critical thinking, (e) advancement of nursing knowledge through scholarly inquiry, and (f) promotion of social justice (ANA, 2003a).

Perhaps Virginia Henderson's (1978) simple, yet elegant, definition of nursing is the most poignant and timeless expression of the fundamental nature of what nurses have always done, do contemporarily, and will no doubt continue to do in the future, regardless of the health care advances that evolve. That is, help people toward achievement of health, or a peaceful death, so that they can be independent from the nurse's help as quickly as possible. Henderson, world-renowned nurse scholar, author, and teacher, passionately embraced

BOX 1-3

ESSENTIAL CRITERIA FOR A PROFESSION

1. Provides practical services that are vital to human and social welfare
2. Possesses a special body of knowledge and skills
3. Educates its practitioners in institutions of higher education
4. Attracts people who emphasize service over personal gain or self-interest and recognize their occupations as long-term commitments
5. Formulates and controls its policies and activities and has practitioners who function relatively autonomously in the performance of functions and activities
6. Has a code of ethics that is usually enforced by colleagues or through licensure examinations
7. Has a professional association that promotes and ensures quality of practice

Source: Simms, L. M., Price, S. A., & Ervin, N. E. (2000). Professional practice of nursing administration (3rd ed.). Albany, NY: Thomson Delmar Learning.

nursing as a professional discipline. Importantly, Henderson defined nursing as unique and aimed both toward people who are ill and those who are well (Henderson and Nite, 1978). Regardless which of the four **domains of nursing** (clinical practice, education, administration, or research) is the focus of a nurse's effort and regardless of the site(s) where a nurse practices, Henderson's definition is relevant and applicable. Yet, extraordinary changes continue to occur in what nurses do and in the way nurses work.

CONTEMPORARY NURSING PRACTICE IN THE UNITED STATES

While physician practices have remained primarily community-based throughout history, nurses' primary practice site shifted from the home to the hospital, back to the home and, more recently, to independent practice sites in the community. The scope of nurses' practice has expanded to encompass uncomplicated aspects of illness care previously reserved to physicians by law. The insurance industry is a pivotal driver of the transition out of the hospital for care, requiring that hospitalization be restricted to the portion of illness care that can only be provided in a hospital. Hospital-based nurses refer their patients to community-based colleagues for continued recovery and rehabilitation as soon as the patient is independent of hospital nurses' care and consistent with Henderson's definition of nursing.

Leadership

Nurses' practice has expanded to a variety of nontraditional arenas in nonhospital sites. Society's growing investment in complementary and alternative medical (CAM) therapies offers nurses numerous opportunities in new health-focused fields, such as exercise, music, pet, and natural therapies. Society's recognition that nurses' knowledge and skill can contribute to improved quality of work in many fields has opened doors in such diverse areas as occupational health nurse for workers on the Alaskan pipe line, nurse astronaut, certified legal nurse consultant, retail mart walk-in clinic NP, and CEO of public and private health care enterprises (Landro, 2006). The shift toward patient education as a strategy to attain and maintain each individual's highest potential for health through an optimal lifestyle of mind and body exercise, nutrition and hydration, relaxation techniques, adequate sleep, lifelong learning, and strengthening of personal support systems is an outcome of the shift from an illness focus to a health focus.

Nursing Education

NPs' expertise in providing primary care with particular attention to patient-focused holistic care is now generally recognized. They have successfully influenced public policy for prescriptive authority and direct insurance reimbursement for their services.

In 2004 the American Association of Colleges of Nursing (AACN) issued a position paper calling for all NPs to earn a terminal clinical doctorate by 2015 (AACN, 2004). In response, Doctor of Nursing Practice (DNP) educational programs are being established by colleges and universities across the United States. The first Doctor of Nursing (ND) program, established at Case Western Reserve University (Case) in Cleveland, Ohio, more than 25 years ago, now confers the DNP through a program of intensive courses offered both on-site and at cohort sites throughout the United States taught by Case faculty.

The current nursing shortage is provoking both undergraduate and graduate nursing education to come in step with e-technology. Nontraditional sites and program formats that include online courses and intensives are moving

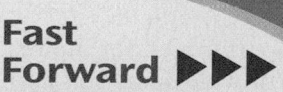

Fast Forward ▶▶▶

Innovation plus Convenience

NPs are now staffing clinics located in a variety of popular, high customer volume retail sites including drug stores and big box stores. Basic preventive care, such as flu shots, and basic primary care including treatment for simple infections, such as a sore throat, are provided. Use of a beeper accommodates shopping until the NP is available.

If taking such basic care to the patient at about 85 percent of the cost of physician care without an appointment or prolonged wait time is well received by society, NPs may soon be asked to provide a fuller scope of their practice capabilities at such convenience sites.

DOLLARS AND SENSE

Health Care Provider Gatekeeping

Patients enter home care programs and nursing homes to access nursing care. NPs with expertise in both nursing practice and primary care practice may be the most appropriate providers to admit patients to home care and nursing homes. NPs are compensated directly by insurers at 85 percent of the physician rate. Therefore, it should not be necessary for a physician to sign for admission, and cost savings, nationally, could be substantial. This concept is consistent with Nosek's (1986) suggestion that it is most appropriate for RNs to discharge patients from hospitals and refer them to the next appropriate level of nursing care.

BOX 1-4

DO YOU KNOW WHERE YOUR PLASTIC DUCKY'S BEEN?

In 1992 a cargo ship carrying 29,000 plastic toy ducks was lost at sea in a North Pacific storm. Some of those ducks have now been found on beaches in Alaska. From what is known about ocean currents and sea patterns it has been predicted that some of those ducks will also turn up on beaches along Canada, Iceland, and New England, having floated thousands of miles across the Pacific and hitching a ride on slow-moving ice around the North Pole before making it to the Atlantic.

Adapted from Rubber ducks at sea. (August 1, 2003). USA Today, 14A.

students through the educational process and into practice more rapidly. Increased sophistication, validity, and reliability of health care Web sites facilitate students' prompt access to science as it becomes available.

The shift to a therapeutic team approach to patient care is generating a fresh look at the staff nurse as a leader, not just a novice, in clinical practice and at the nurse manager as an interdisciplinary leader responsible for coordinating patient care across the team of professional and nonprofessional support staff. Such broadened scope of responsibility is bringing new recognition that the nurse manager must have knowledge and skill in business and management science (business intelligence), as well as in the clinical and behavioral sciences. Knowledge about emotional intelligence and skill in appreciative inquiry are now required in addition to finance and mediation. Ability to apply the Synergy Model described in chapter 18, Health Care Agencies, to better manage nurse staffing for improved clinical quality and financial outcomes is also required.

Globalization

Globalization is a business concept that refers to a business component that is organized or established worldwide, yet it is significantly impacting health care and nurses' practice. As world society increases its global mobility, routinely traveling around the world in a few hours, and electronic communication permeates ever more remote areas of the world via the Internet, satellite broadcasts, and cell phones, health care reaps both benefits and burdens. Extraordinary collaboration in the discovery and sharing of new knowledge about solutions to complex biological and technological health care challenges become public knowledge even as health care experts are rushing to validate their efficacy. The ability for patients to access health care expertise in distant sites through telehealth modalities that allow the manipulation of instruments to accomplish even microsurgery at distant sites nearly anywhere in the world is a reality attributable to globalization. The use of e-demonstration to teach providers vast distances away how to use contemporary technology promotes its safe and effective use without the need for an expert to be on-site.

The global marketplace offers many new opportunities for nurses to expand their clinical practice into world spheres, to provide nursing education to students in other countries, to provide health care education to members of other disciplines seeking the United States' expertise, and to serve as expert consultants about public health issues and establishment of health care enterprises. Lively competition for ownership of global marketplace segments already exists in the pharmaceutical and biotechnology industries. Brown (2004) suggests that globalization may not only offer nurses opportunities for expanded practice, it may also offer opportunities for health care cost savings.

Both new and previously remote diseases are being disseminated across the world in epidemics and pandemics, carried by infected humans, air, water, food, or fomites. Acquired immune deficiency syndrome (AIDS), river blindness, West Nile virus, tuberculosis, severe acute respiratory syndrome (SARS), and a highly resistant strain of bird flu are demonstrating the vulnerability to disease that globalization has wrought. The news story in Box 1-4 may create a strong mental image of the insidious way contamination could flow around the world. Diseases can no longer be defined in terms of a confined location. More effective strategies for halting the spread of organisms than physical isolation through quarantining must be conceptualized and operationalized. Because nurses observe patients' symptoms and their responses to treatment 24 hours a day, seven days a week, nurses have the potential to recognize patterns of symptoms and responses that could hold the key to containing the transfer of organisms.

Globalization's impact on health care generates several new challenges for nurses, not the least of which is self-protection from contamination even though the source and route of contamination may not be well understood. A number of health care workers have succumbed to SARS, despite their knowledge of infection control. Nurse leaders must prepare to manage adeptly and adroitly in the midst of a work environment highly charged with fear of death, not only among patients and their families, but also among the staff and their families. To lead in an environment charged with ambiguity and fear, all nurses must possess **competence** (that is, specialized knowledge and ability) in emotional intelligence and the ability to optimize relationships and resolve disputes under fire.

Together with their colleagues in allied health disciplines, nurse executives must ensure the readiness of their enterprise to manage an influx of contagious and deadly illness. Clinical care protocols, alternative service use designs, staff education including simulation drills, emergency staffing procedures, and access to adequate infectious disease testing, equipment, and pharmaceuticals must be in place (Nosek, 2004). Rooted in lessons learned during the 2004 hurricane disasters along the Gulf coast, in January 2005 JCAHO issued a guide for planning, establishing, and operating temporary surge hospitals to enable an existing hospital to surge in place in response to a mass casualty event, assuming that the hospital itself remains operational (AHA, 2005).

Globalization is impacting nurses' bedside practice in a number of ways. The population and mix of immigrants in the United States is enlarging, generally, and Hispanic (Americans) now comprise the second largest population in the United States. New ethnic, cultural, and religious values are challenging nurses to provide culturally responsible care for patients and to find culturally responsible ways to work collegially with a diverse workforce. Nuances of new languages and dialects bring increased risk for communication breakdown that can lead to patient morbidity and mortality or disruption to the workplace, even when interpreters are used. Immigrants may not be eligible for health insurance or may not be able to afford health insurance. As a result, they may not seek care until an illness has progressed significantly, and they experience comorbidities.

The ease and speed of worldwide travel carries increased risk for introduction of new diseases and new organisms to the United States. Never before has the risk of pandemic spread of infection to the United States been as high as it is currently. Immigrants from Europe through Ellis Island were closely screened, isolated, and treated if they were found to be ill. Such triaging of immigrants through the multiple entry portals currently used has not yet been stringently undertaken. Nurses, often the first to come in contact with the patient, must be aware of the signs and symptoms of multiple strange illnesses and take appropriate action to isolate and treat the patient.

Terrorism is a well-recognized threat of the current world unrest. A terrorism attack can emanate from multiple sources to which nurses must be alert. Nurses need to be well-versed about the bioterrorism plan of their health care enterprise to protect themselves and others.

In addition to strange new infectious diseases, nurses are encountering injuries and illnesses related to combat. Traumatic amputations, multiple organ injury, blindness, deafness, acute grief, depression, and posttraumatic stress disorders (PTSD) are examples of war-related diagnoses among soldiers and their families. Such diagnoses are not necessarily restricted to military and veterans health care agencies.

Many businesses are currently restructuring to accommodate both competition and opportunity in a global marketplace. Acquisitions, bankruptcies, and the aging workforce requiring pension payouts and more health care are prompting employers to restructure their benefit packages and to lay off employees. Many employers are shifting more responsibility for the cost of health care insurance to the covered individuals. For some, the increased personal expense forces choices about their health practices that may not serve them well in the long run. Just as in the case of immigrants, preventive care, diagnosis, and treatment may be delayed until a disease process is advanced, and there are comorbidities. Nurses are challenged to work with such patients to find creative, cost-efficient ways that patients can optimally manage their health.

Changes in Family Structure

Legislation to recognize civil partners has implications for nurses. Confidentiality about diagnoses and decisions about end-of-life care can present new ethical challenges when a civil partner is deemed next of kin or when a civil partner's decisions are contrary to those of other family members. Nurses may be torn or confused about their advocacy role in such cases and can gain direction from an ethics committee at their enterprise.

International adoptions may also cause nurses confusion about their advocacy role when there are diverse cultural considerations. An ethics committee or an ethicist can also be of assistance in these situations.

Risk-Taking Behaviors

Risk-taking behavior can take many forms and seems to be becoming more prevalent. Clearly one form is a pattern of noncompliance with a sound health care treatment plan. Others include bungee jumping, speeding and weaving in traffic, failure to wear a helmet while riding a motorcycle, use of street drugs, and practicing unprotected sexual activity. The high price of gasoline may be driving sales of Harley-Davidson motorcycles up, according to a recent news report (Wall Street Journal, 2006). Nurses may encounter more, and more serious, motorcycle injuries with more inexperienced riders on the road.

Transition from Formality to Informality

Contemporary society, particularly its younger members, embraces informality. For instance, use of professional and social titles, e.g., Dr., Mr., and Mrs., has shifted to use of first names, sometimes referred to as "palism," which seeks to blur status differences. In some instances a compromise position that combines formality with informality has been adopted. Dr. Bob, Ms. Sally, and Mr. Bill have replaced Dr. Brown, Ms. Jones, and Mr. Smith. Use of a title with a person's last name has traditionally been a sign of respect for that person's age, knowledge, or position or for a lack of familiarity with the person. The rationale given for omitting the title is that it makes the titled individual seem less formal and unreachable.

In contrast, many cultures use entirely different words to signify the closeness, or distance, of a relationship. For instance, in Spanish when *you* refers to family members and close relationships *tu* is used. When *you* refers to more distant, formal relationships, or to strangers *usted* is used. When caregivers automatically address patients or colleagues by a first name it may be interpreted as an affront or insult by that person. In both professional and social relationships asking others what they would like to be called or how they prefer to be addressed may avoid establishing an adversarial relationship detrimental to a therapeutic relationship.

Professional clothing has also become more informal and at the same time, more practical. Long-sleeved uniforms gave way to short sleeves that soiled less readily by the 1950s. Starched cotton uniform dresses were replaced by softer, more flexible, wrinkle-resistant polyester two-piece dresses in the 1960s. A few years later when women's street length skirts shifted to miniskirts that did not accommodate reaching, bending, and lifting well, professional women shifted to pant suits, and nurses gave up wearing caps that they perceived served no purpose but to tangle in bed curtains and equipment lines. Soon after, white was replaced by colors that camouflaged stains. By the 1990s roomy, flexible, wear-resistant scrub suits, long a mainstay of operating suite attire (in green to soften the harsh effect of surgical spotlights on the eyes of the staff) became de rigueur in diverse clinical settings. Worn in department-specific colors, scrubs are a badge of identification worn with pride.

Transition from Nursing as Altruism to Nursing as Business

Nurses' reaction to the increasing admonitions from their employers that they must accept responsibility for contributing to the success of the mission of their enterprise is considerably less than positive. Not only do nurses object that business is none of their business, i.e., that clinical care of patients is their business, they point out that they have no educational preparation to understand organizational science, fiscal management, or business practices. By the late 1970s health care enterprises began to allocate release time and tuition dollars to provide selected nurse employees with business education in consideration of the nurse's commitment to new management, quality assurance, continuing education, and fiscal and information system service positions that did not involve direct clinical care. Such positions were not necessarily aligned in reporting relationships to nurses, or even to managers with clinical backgrounds. The so-called silos of isolating communication and work patterns in health care enterprises were challenged. Transdisciplinary teams were charged to identify interdependent work components and design collaborative practices and processes that could enhance efficiency across the entire enterprise.

Although many nurses strongly resist the shift to business interests, others embrace the opportunity to more broadly influence the structure and function of the entire enterprise. Senior nurse executives are seeking MBA education in an attempt to level the playing field for negotiating clinical care system, as well as business system, issues with nonclinical executive colleagues. The benefit of baccalaureate- and masters-prepared nurses who can draw on a broader educational background for decision making is also recognized. These are, generally, the frontline nurses responsible for conceptualizing and negotiating improved clinical care delivery systems with colleagues whose value systems have been honed in disparate disciplines not necessary congruent with each other.

Care Delivery Models

Nurses have searched for the ideal care delivery model for decades. Work assignment by tasks, such as medication administration to a group of patients, team nursing by personnel with various levels of nursing education preparation under the supervision of an RN, modular assignments based on the physical proximity of patients, primary care that places responsibility for all aspects of a single patient's care during a specified work shift on an RN, case management that places responsibility for oversight management of a patient's care throughout that patient's interface with the health care enterprise on an RN, and various iterations that combine aspects of these models have all been lauded as the answer to multiple staffing issues.

Not only has the transition to managing nursing as a business intensified the contemporary search for the most cost-effective care delivery model, the transition in work ethic of generations X and Y has changed the way nurses are willing to work. Young, upwardly mobile professionals, including nurses, view a commitment of three years to a single employer as a long-term commitment; this is in contrast to older generations that felt successful if they worked for a single employer for their entire career and particularly proud if successive generations of their family worked for that same employer for their entire careers (PBS interview, 2006). No longer is a résumé that shows job changes every two to three years suspect; just the opposite. The younger generations are action oriented, speaking rapidly, seeking action-oriented entertainment and action-oriented work environments. They value creativity and innovation and are unwilling to tolerate the status quo. They purposely and assertively seek mentoring from an influential leader of the enterprise to rapidly propel them along a career trajectory to the top position, then early retirement to a leisurely lifestyle or to a second career (PBS interview, 2006). In addition, there has been an accelerating unwillingness among younger workers to sacrifice personal and family time to work. They unabashedly declare that they have a personal life and that they are unwilling to work additional or overtime hours (PBS interview, 2006). This value, in combination with brief interactions with patients who are facilitated to discharge; creative, flexible work schedules that often defy continuity of patient care; and a perception that providing sufficient nursing staff to manage the workload within the allotted time frame is the responsibility of the enterprise, not the responsibility of the nurse, may contribute toward a reluctance to go beyond the basic work shift.

A recent survey by the Organization for Economic Co-operation and Development revealed that Japan is no longer the world leader in the number of hours worked per year on average. In 1990 the Japanese work ethic was benchmarked to a world striving to enhance productivity. At that time Japanese workers averaged 2,031 worked hours per year, 170 hours more than U.S. workers. According to the new survey the contemporary worker in the United States works 1,825 hours per year, 36 fewer hours than in 1990, but 36 hours more than the Japanese who now average just 1,789 hours per year (Wlnlk, 2006).

Younger nurses are often unwilling to travel to multiple-day professional conferences that separate them from their family and personal activities. January, 2006 recruitment literature from a national health care traveler enterprise encourages nurses to take their spouse, their children, and their pets on assignment so as to feel right at home and take care of their family.

These changes in contemporary work ethics have significant impact on both the cost and the quality of health care. The cost to hire an RN may reach $46,000. When an enterprise experiences a vigorous turnover rate because its RNs are moving onward and upward to more dynamic, challenging, and satisfying work, the cost to recruit and replace those RNs can quickly become crippling to its budget for other operations. Not only do RNs require generic clinical knowledge and competence, they require knowledge and competence about the particular patient population for whom they will be caring, and they require knowledge and competence about how to efficiently and effectively negotiate the unique formal and informal operations of their new enterprise to deliver optimal quality nursing care.

In 1990, a cry of social outrage was heard when news media broke stories of health care waste, including syringes, being found washed up on beaches along the eastern coast of North America. Fear, not only of injury but also of disease, was at the root of the outrage. Society demanded that waste control methods immediately be improved to stop such contamination.

A registered nurse in Vermont, a landlocked but environmentally sensitive state, rose to the challenge. Hollie Shaner, AD, RN, a staff nurse who worked in critical care, dialysis, postanesthesia recovery, and the float pool on nights, laboriously collected operating room waste, organized and analyzed data, researched relevant law, and persuaded hospital management to create Hollie's unique position of clinical waste reduction coordinator assigned to the environmental services division of the hospital. In her new position Hollie initiated educational programs for all hospital employees and waste management system improvements throughout the hospital. Under her leadership the hospital met the Vermont Act 78 requirement to reduce solid waste by 40 percent. That 40 percent amounted to more than one ton per day for that hospital (Sample, 2003). Hollie seems to be the single nurse trash specialist position in the world.

The U.S. health care system is a $1.5 trillion industry which leads the world in cost but ranks 21st in life expectancy and 27th in infant mortality, has the highest drug costs in the world, and has significant distribution gaps (Brown, 2004; Cicatiello, 2004). The United States exports health care expertise and technology around the world and for various humanitarian and political reasons supports the travel and care of many foreigners who seek health care in the United States. At the same time the care of the health of the helpless, homeless, and geographically isolated in the United States is often little better than that of the helpless, poverty-stricken, and geographically isolated in Third World countries.

ENVIRONMENT FOR CONTEMPORARY NURSING PRACTICE

Although numerous new career opportunities outside of the health care industry have become available to RNs, and more nursing positions have been established in community sites for health care, more than half of all RNs continue to be employed in hospitals. Each setting where nurses work possesses a unique set of beliefs, values, assumptions, ideas, customs, verbal and nonverbal behavior norms, and skills that are shared by people in the workgroup. Known as that setting's **culture for caring,** they tend to persist over time, even when the group membership changes. Attributes and rules about the culture are usually invisible; that is, they are seldom formalized in writing.

Particularly over the past 40 years the public perception of the culture of the health care industry, in general, and of hospitals, in particular, has been growing more negative. It is common to hear nurses, themselves, refer to the way they interact with novice nurses in the work environment as eating their young. There is longstanding recognition within health care, as well as across U.S. society that, in general, nurses and physicians have an adversarial relationship. A best-selling book about the U.S. health care system calls the *system* an oxymoron, because it is perceived as fragmented and disorganized. National nursing conferences refer to navigating in treacherous waters and managing patient care in a zoo. Administrators and staff both speak in terms of we *versus* they and not in terms of we. A multitude of management theories including chaos theory have been applied to the search for strategies to improve the structure and function of health care delivery. What a bleak and negative view of a work culture that purports to promote *caring!* Yet, nurses and other health care providers speak passionately about their love for their work and for their patients and about the miracles of contemporary care.

Culture for Caring

Significant attention is being directed to improving the contemporary hospital work environment. The physical environment is receiving a facelift with more interesting colors and surfaces, purposeful artwork, live plantings in a natural light-filled atrium, known as greening, and open spaces that suggest closeness to the outdoors. Natural light is replacing florescent bulbs. Noise levels are being lowered through use of sound-absorbing materials and personal, rather than overhead, paging systems. Personal services that may include chair massages, dry cleaning and shoe repair, postal services, cosmetology and barber services, and fully prepared meals to take home for the family are available on-site. Finally, cafeterias managed by professional chefs, are serving more preferred foods that are prepared-to-order.

Employer Value System

Contemporary health care executives and other leaders recognize that they set the tone of the culture for caring through the quality and quantity of their communication, or lack of communication, and through their personal interaction, or lack of interaction, with staff. It is the leader's value system that establishes the benchmark of caring of the enterprise. If the leaders actively recognize that every employee makes a valuable contribution to the mission of the enterprise and if they actively seek and acknowledge the unique expertise each employee brings to the work at all levels, employee self-confidence, energy, creativeness, and commitment to the work and to the enterprise could be greatly enhanced.

Every day every person has the opportunity to choose an attitude for the day. The old adage that one reaps what one sows is as relevant to the hospital environment as it is to the agricultural environment. We each choose our attitude, consciously or unconsciously. A pleasant smile, respect conveyed through aligned posture, eye contact, and a tone of voice that conveys that you are "present" in the conversation and "attending" to its content may go a long way in boosting another person's self-confidence and self-esteem and "making a great day" for that person (Lundin, Paul, & Christensen, 2000).

Public recognition of an employee's expertise or special contributions to patient care and to the interests of the enterprise, specific support to facilitate the work, and giving individuals increased autonomy over how they manage their own work can establish mutually trusting relationships that contribute toward a positive culture for caring. Providing all employees with increased awareness about the nature of the overall enterprise and its work can generate work excitement among employees at all levels. Playing together actively in sporting events and celebrations, or playing together as passive spectators at some special event tends to allow everyone to relate on a level field.

Workforce Diversity

Workforce diversity simply refers to differences among members of the workforce. Those differences may be in age, gender, race, geographical background, sexual preference, education, religion, culture, language, or belief system. Diversity is a multifaceted issue that involves many aspects of people's lives. Each time two people interact they bring the wealth of their attributes, education, life experiences, culture, and belief system to the interaction. Misunderstanding can be a logical outcome unless one recognizes the differences and how they may impact the interaction, then makes adjustments for the differences to ensure effective communication and clear understanding by both individuals. The ultimate goal of diversity recognition is to enrich each individual's experience and to use each individual's unique strengths to build a stronger, more self-confident and productive work environment. When individuals feel insecure about their knowledge, skill, or appearance they may choose defensive or hostile behaviors that contribute to an uncomfortable work environment (Catalano, 2003).

Collective Bargaining

Employees' joining together to more forcefully influence their employer to improve working conditions is known as **collective bargaining.** Such unions of employees were conceptualized as an effective way to protect workers from unsavory practices of employers in the middle 1800s. Collective bargaining was not legally recognized in the United States until 1935 when the National Labor Relations Act (NLRA) was passed by Congress and the National Labor Relations Board (NLRB) was established to implement the tenets of the NLRA (Catalano, 2003). Collective bargaining reached its zenith in the mid-1950s among nonprofessional workers. The Taft-Hartley Act of 1947, an amendment to the NLRA, specifically excluded nurses employed in nonprofit hospitals from organizing collective bargaining units. In 1974 the Taft-Hartley Act was amended to allow nurses to organize.

By 1991 nurses felt strongly that they needed help to influence management of working conditions and petitioned the Supreme Court for the right to bargain collectively. The Supreme Court ruled in favor of NLRB authority to define bargaining units for health care providers in any setting, as shown in Box 1-5. Selected state nurses associations and several nonprofessional unions have been elected to represent nurses for purposes of collective bargaining. The only issues that collective bargaining agents can bargain over, by law, are working conditions, including wages. Because Congress establishes the compensation levels for nurses employed by the government, wages are not eligible for bargaining by nurses working for the government. However, government-employed nurses who are unionized have the right for representation to

BOX 1-5

EIGHT BARGAINING UNITS FOR HOSPITALS

1. Nurses
2. Physicians
3. All professionals except nurses and physicians
4. All technical employees
5. All skilled maintenance employees
6. All business office clerical employees
7. All guards
8. All other nonprofessional employees

bargain for other working conditions. There are numerous laws regulating the interactions between union members and management in the workplace and between collective bargaining agents and management representatives during contract negotiations. There are also numerous professional issues associated with collective bargaining.

Culture for Safety

Much attention is given to providing a safe environment for patients. More recently, attention has been broadened to include creating an environment of safety for employees. Not only are physical and biological threats to employees being examined, emotional threats are being examined and rectified.

Interpersonal Threats

An interpersonal threat may take the form of actual or perceived communication that involves threatening body language, touching, or verbiage. Feelings of fatigue, frustration, stress, and fear of making a clinical judgment error are commonly experienced by those working in health care. Such feelings can negatively influence the way people communicate, with or without, purposeful intent. A raised or tight voice, unpleasant words, an intent stare, a pointing finger, slamming an article down, or an embrace can all be perceived as violent and threatening. Education about strategies that can defuse, rather than escalate, harsh communication and use of mediation specialists to settle disputes are available in most health care enterprises. It is no longer acceptable to just keep quiet about negative behavior, and communication and whistle blower protection is commonly included in the value statement of the enterprise.

Ergonomic Hazards

The nurse shortage at the turn of the 21st century intensified both nurse and health care enterprise interest in providing a culture of safety in the workplace. Even one ill or injured nurse unable to work could wreak havoc in a tightly staffed enterprise. By far the most common OTJ injury to nurses is a back injury. Of the top 10 riskiest jobs for back injury 6 are in health care, according to federal studies. UAPs are at the third greatest risk for back injury, following construction workers and garbage collectors. RNs follow truck drivers as the sixth riskiest job (Gentry, 2005).

Health care facilities utilize **ergonomics,** which is the practice of designing and arranging things people use so that the people and things interact most efficiently and safely. It is common for health care enterprises to create a lift program to help decrease the risk of back injuries. Included in such programs are mechanical lift devices, belts, and boards to assist during patient transfers; staff education; and patient education. Although the cost of implementing a lift program can be substantial, most enterprises report that the expense is quickly repaid by the decreased cost of downtime and treatment of back injuries.

Another significant ergonomic hazard for RNs can be traced to a side effect of the use of computers to document patient activity. Carpal tunnel syndrome plagues nurses who must spend significant lengths of time using computers that are not ergonomically friendly. Ever since the introduction of computers the recommendation of ergonomic specialists has been that body alignment be maintained when using a computer to decrease risk of injury. However, use of a foot rest, a chair with armrests and lumbar support at the appropriate height, a wrist support bar, an elbow-high keyboard, and an eye-friendly screen is difficult to achieve for multiple users.

Toxins

Numerous toxins are present in health care workplaces. Agents of infection are continuously present. New mutations and imported organisms have become a serious threat stemming from common use of antibiotics and globalization, respectively. White-out, mercury, latex, and dioxins are the most commonly recognized chemical agents, along with chemotherapeutic agents. Toxins can be present in any body fluid, so it is essential that nurses consistently use excellent hand washing practices and don gloves automatically when providing personal care to patients.

Impaired Colleagues

Perhaps the most insidious threat to both patient and employee safety is the impaired health care provider. Chemical use across society is broadly becoming more common and more open. The national incidence of chemical dependence among nurses even 15 years ago was one in four. Increased access to street drugs has helped push that figure to a guesstimate (because of the covert nature of chemical use) of four in every seven. Ready access to narcotics and sedatives by anesthesiologists, as well as by nurses, puts them at exceptional risk for chemical abuse and dependence, also.

Chemical dependence is an illness, and the confidentiality of health care information results in naiveté about the existence and the extent of the illness among health care colleagues, how to detect chemical dependence, and how to best address it. Not only do nurses need to know how to provide clinical care to their patients who are chemically dependent, if novice or experienced nurses do not know how to recognize the signs of chemical dependence among their health care colleagues across all disciplines and how to respond to that recognition, they will remain silent and both patients' and nurses' lives will, ultimately, be at risk for loss. Health care providers who use chemical substances to ease stress, fatigue, frustration, and anger are *impaired*. They are making **clinical decisions** that critically impact others' lives while *under the influence of mind-altering chemicals.*

Use of such substances is illegal. Health care providers who use illegal substances risk the loss of their professional license and thus their career and livelihood. The need to not be discovered generates a high level of clever creativity around substance use. Colleagues who do not want to believe that an individual may be using, and even stealing money or the chemical substances to support their dependency, accept extensive subterfuges rather than accept the evidence that a colleague may be impaired. If an individual was chemically dependent when they were first met, their normal behavior when sober may never be revealed. Some of the clues that an individual may be chemically dependent are presented in Box 1-6.

The perception of a blackout is of someone losing consciousness. However, a blackout related to chemical dependence means that the person is not aware of, or cognitively engaged in, what he or she is doing, and he or she has no memory of events that occur during a blackout. For example, the individual who is unable to remember what occurred at a party after heavy alcohol consumption at that party but who was fully engaged with activities at the party, was experiencing a blackout at the party. Blackouts can last for days or even weeks. The implications for a health care worker to continue to work during a blackout are frightening.

Intervening when chemical dependence is suspected requires special training and skill. Unskilled intervention could drive the chemically dependent individual to go underground, rather than seek help, continuing to endanger self and others. Interventions must be carefully scripted and timed and are best orchestrated by a trained interventionist.

BOX 1-6

CLUES TO THE POSSIBILITY OF CHEMICAL DEPENDENCE

1. Tardiness
2. Late sick calls
3. Frequent or prolonged work breaks
4. Inability to recall recent events
5. Heavy use of fragrances
6. Clinical care omissions or errors
7. Patient complaints or requests for a change in care provider
8. Mood instability
9. Extraordinary accomplishments

KEY CONCEPTS

- Over just the past 50 years extraordinary changes have emerged in the nature of nursing care interventions, nursing education, the scope of nursing practice, the health care system, and the sites for care.
- Nurses' bedside practice is becoming more regulated by both national and state legislation.
- Nurses are contributing unique insights to improve work patterns and productivity in nonhealth care business and industry.
- In addition to knowledge of nursing and related health sciences, nurses are using business science to communicate and collaborate with transdisciplinary colleagues.
- Health care cost and quality remain major foci for health care system improvement.
- Theoretical tenets of both Nightingale and Henderson remain relevant to contemporary nursing practice.
- Society's contemporary interest in lifestyle behaviors and embrace of CAM therapies is offering nurses numerous opportunities in new health-focused fields and nontraditional arenas, such as exercise, music, pet, and natural therapy.
- The current nursing shortage is provoking nursing education to come in step with e-technology.
- Globalization is impacting nurses' bedside practice through the need to provide culturally competent care to a growing immigrant population and to families in nontraditional structures, the need to be knowledgeable about and alert to previously unfamiliar diseases and their management, the care needs of a growing number of war casualties and their families, and the care needs of a risk-taking population.
- Concern for providing a culture of safety in the workplace is growing.

REVIEW QUESTIONS

1. The care provided by nurses historically is referred to as:
   1. Wellness care
   2. Evidence-based care
   3. Comfort care
   4. Health care

2. The close trusting relationship between physicians and patients changed when:
   1. Nurse practitioners began to provide primary care.
   2. Society became aware of the high rate of medical errors.
   3. Physicians' work load expanded.
   4. Knowledge of the biological sciences grew more specialized.

3. A significant influence on the way nurses care for patients is:
   1. Legislation passed by state governments
   2. The amount of funding available for nursing research
   3. The nurse's cultural background
   4. The school the nurse attended

4. Contemporary health care reform was initiated by:
   1. The Flexner Report
   2. The Tax Equity and Fiscal Responsibility Act of 1982
   3. Titles XVIII and XIX of the Social Security Act
   4. Florence Nightingale

5. The following is not an essential feature of professional nursing, according to ANA:
   1. A caring relationship
   2. Scholarly publication
   3. Promotion of social justice
   4. Integration of objective and subjective data

6. Contemporary therapies may include:
   1. Mind and body exercise
   2. Use of poultices
   3. Grazing
   4. The North Beach Diet

7. Contemporary nurses must have knowledge and skill in:
   1. Clinical care, communication, and food preparation
   2. Biomedical engineering, faith healing, and clinical care
   3. Finance, synergy, and meditation
   4. Appreciative inquiry, clinical science, and management science

Continued

REVIEW QUESTIONS—cont'd

8. A way in which nurses' clinical practice is impacted by globalization is:
   1. Cost containment is shifting toward reusable items.
   2. Need for clinical knowledge about unfamiliar diseases is growing.
   3. Biohazardous waste disposal is no longer needed.
   4. U.S. nurses are being recruited for overseas assignment.

9. Provision of a supportive culture for caring does not include:
   1. Protection from harmful chemicals and toxins
   2. Protection from ergonomic hazards
   3. A ban on fresh flowers in health care sites
   4. Chemically dependent colleagues

10. When a chemically dependent person experiences a blackout he or she:
   1. Faints
   2. Experiences heart palpitations
   3. Experiences memory loss
   4. Experiences loss of vision

REVIEW ACTIVITIES

1. Contact the lobbyist or the executive officer for your state nurses association and explore the position the association is taking on a bill related to nursing or health care.

2. Contact your state senator or representative and explore the position that person is taking on that same legislation.

3. Read the article titled, *Will disruptive innovations kill health care?* listed in the Suggested Readings and Web Resources. What single disruptive innovation could you suggest to improve the environment for caring where you work or attend school?

4. Consider the last time you felt threatened by an individual's words or actions. Why do you think they said or did that?

5. Contact the president of your state board of nursing and discover how an accusation that a nurse may be chemically dependent is processed in your state.

Clinical Decision Making and Evidence-Based Practice

Kathleen R. Stevens, RN, EdD, FAAN

CHAPTER TOPICS

- Overview of Evidence-Based Practice (EBP)

- EBP in Nursing

- Stages of the Star Model of EBP

- Major Features of EBP

- Use of EBP for Clinical Nursing Practice

KEY TERMS

Agency for Healthcare Research and Quality (AHRQ)

Clinical practice guidelines (CPGs)

Cochrane Collaboration

Cochrane library

Evidence-based practice (EBP)

Evidence summary

Integrative review

Knowledge transformation

Meta analysis

Narrative review

National Guideline Clearinghouse

Review of literature

Science

Science of research synthesis

State-of-the-science review

Systematic review

Nurses provide care to accurately diagnose actual or potential health problems and to assist patients toward attaining desired health outcomes. The extent to which this care effectively produces accurate diagnoses and desired outcomes depends on the type of knowledge used in these clinical decisions. The past decade has witnessed a dramatic shift in professional and public expectations that health care be based on the best scientific knowledge in the form of evidence-based practice (EBP) demands. Nurses are actively engaged in reconstructing the basis for nursing care to ensure that it reflects principles of evidence-based practice.

OVERVIEW OF EVIDENCE-BASED PRACTICE

An understanding of the sources of knowledge and various external forces that contribute to the way nursing is practiced is necessary for nurses to judge whether they are practicing based on sound principles and knowledge. The concept that nursing practice is rooted in scientific evidence can be an epiphany for nurses accustomed to practicing a particular way because faculty or colleagues taught them a technical procedure.

Knowledge Bases for Clinical Decisions

Actions taken by nurses may be based on a variety of knowledge sources. This knowledge comes from one's own experience, trial and error, a nursing procedure manual, a textbook, or science produced through systematic inquiry (research). The variety of knowledge sources are often referred to as ways of knowing, each providing a level of certainty in the likelihood of producing the desired health outcome. Not all sources of knowledge are reliable or consistently produce the desired patient outcome.

Knowledge for nursing practice can be generated through either unstructured or structured approaches. Unstructured approaches include trial and error, tradition, and authority. One can easily identify clinical decisions in nursing that are based on tradition, experience, and authority. Many examples of care based on unstructured knowledge exist in nursing care manuals, unit policies, textbooks, and even care standards established by authoritative entities.

In the recent past, nursing care guidelines often reflected authority, for example nursing textbooks that provided a procedure but did not make explicit the scientific foundation for the recommended actions. In many cases, other unstructured knowledge underlies a clinical policy, such as the policy-maker's own clinical experience or tradition (it has always been done this way). While experience and trial and error are good teachers, knowledge gained through these approaches contains bias. That is, the results may be due to something other than the intervention, or the results from one situation may not be applicable to another situation or patient. Knowledge produced through unstructured approaches lacks generalizability and is fraught with systematic bias because the cause and effect of the action has been inadequately examined. The end result is that the nurse is unable to predict the extent to which a given clinical action based on this type of knowledge will produce the intended outcome.

In contrast, structured approaches, such as logical reasoning and systematic inquiry, produce knowledge of the likelihood that the nursing action will cause the intended health outcome. The scientific approach reflected in research inquiry uses logic, theory, and order in arriving at reproducible conclusions about effectiveness of nursing practices. Knowledge generated through a structured, systematic approach is more likely to be generalizable and valid than knowledge produced through unstructured approaches.

Definition of Evidence-Based Practice

Evidence-based practice (EPB) is a process through which scientific evidence is identified, appraised, and applied in health care interventions. It is the conscientious, explicit, and judicious use of current best evidence in making decisions about the care of individual patients. The objective of EBP is to apply the best available evidence in clinical care to implement interventions that will predictably move patients toward their health care goals.

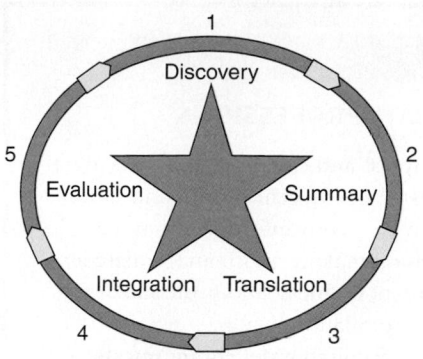

Figure 2-1 ACE Star Model of Knowledge Transformation. *Stevens, K. R. (2004). ACE star model of knowledge transformation. Retrieved May 1, 2005, from www.acestar. uthscsa.edu. Reprinted with expressed permission.*

Socio-Political Forces in Quality of Care

The current movement of evidence-based quality improvement has brought science-based care to the forefront of effective nursing care and created an unprecedented level of interest in professional duty and public accountability for the scientific basis of care. For three decades nurses addressed the importance of research in guiding nursing practice. During this early stage, the term research utilization (RU) referred to moving research findings into practice. While this approach reflected the essence of the applied science of nursing, the movement lacked essential aspects to make research into practice a widespread reality.

THE PROCESS OF EBP

EBP includes a total process. For example, the ACE Star Model of Knowledge Transformation shown in Figure 2-1 outlines a process that moves evidence through five stages: production of knowledge through original research, evidence summary, evidence translation, integration into clinical decision making, and evaluation. There are two primary features that distinguish contemporary EBP from earlier RU. First, EBP requires that practice innovations and changes be based on an evidence summary when available and that the evidential base be explicated and rated for strength (cause and effect). By contrast, the early RU approaches promoted change based on single research studies, such as Stetler and Marram (1976). EBP has demonstrated that there is greater causal strength derived from using a body of research rather than a single study; the conclusions are more stable than results from a single research study.

Also, while nurses accomplished significant work on implementation of research findings (e.g., Funk, Tournquist, & Champaign, 1989), this work represents only a portion of the total EBP process. EBP is a total, systematic process that moves newly developed knowledge through carefully planned (and evidence-based) approaches to summarize, translate, integrate, and evaluate EBP in terms of outcomes. The EBP movement has replaced RU, because it is a complete paradigm, connecting research findings to practice, health care policy, and patient outcomes. In the recent past, a number of socio-political forces emphasized that RU concepts must be evolved into the more highly developed EBP principles to address the quality of health care in the United States.

The urgency for changes in health care quality was brought into sharp focus by health care leaders with the report, *To err is human: Building a safer health system* (Institute of Medicine [IOM], 2000). This shocking analysis pointed out that as many as 98,000 hospitalized Americans die each year as a result of errors in their care. In a second report, the chasm between what we know through science to be best health care and what is actually practiced was revealed. The report drew attention to the fact that health science and technology have advanced at a rapid pace, but the health care delivery system has not maintained delivery of high-quality health care services (IOM, 2001). In this report EBP was recommended as an important solution to move the knowledge generated through science into practice.

Preparation of the future workforce was addressed in *Health professions education: A bridge to quality* (IOM, 2003). All health disciplines were urged to come together and address five core competencies essential in bridging the quality chasm. The core competencies are presented in Box 2-1 and include integrating best research with clinical expertise and patient values for optimum care (IOM, 2003, p. 4). Clearly, EBP is seen as *crucial* in nursing as the profession contributes to closing the quality chasm in health care.

Fast Forward ▶▶▶

Projected Value of EBP

In the coming decade, EBP as a component to health care quality and safety will continue to permeate health care systems, agencies, regulatory establishments, and educational programs. The resulting changes promise to be the most significant improvements in health care for the next half century.

BOX 2-1

CORE COMPETENCIES FOR HEALTH PROFESSIONS

1. *Provide patient-centered care:* Identify, respect, and care about patients' differences, values, preferences, and expressed needs; relieve pain and suffering; coordinate continuous care; listen to, clearly inform, communicate with, and educate patients; share decision making and management; and continuously advocate disease prevention, wellness, and promotion of healthy lifestyles, including a focus on population health.
2. *Work in interdisciplinary teams:* Cooperate, collaborate, communicate, and integrate care in teams to ensure that care is continuous and reliable.
3. *Employ EBP:* Integrate best research with clinical expertise and patient values for optimum care and participate in learning and research activities to the extent feasible.
4. *Apply quality improvement:* Identify errors and hazards in care; understand and implement basic safety design principles, such as standardization and simplification; continually understand and measure quality of care in terms of structure, process, and outcomes in relation to patient and community needs; and design and test interventions to change processes and systems of care with the objective of improving quality.
5. *Utilize informatics:* Communicate, manage knowledge, mitigate error, and support decision making using information technology.

Source: Institute of Medicine. (2003). Priority areas for national action: Transforming health care quality. *Washington, DC: National Academy Press.*

The evidence-based quality initiative has spread across multiple facets in health care. For example, nursing licensure rules include expectations of EBP; health care purchasers (e.g., Medicare) have begun to incorporate EBP into payment and reimbursement policy; EBP competencies have been set for undergraduate, graduate, and doctoral nursing education programs; and criteria for Magnet Recognition status of excellence in nursing service specify EBP.

While evidence and knowledge can be drawn from a variety of sources, best evidence is specifically identified as that evidence drawn from scientific investigation or research. EBPs generate more accurate diagnoses, maximally effective and efficient interventions, and the most favorable patient outcomes.

Of great importance in the definition of EBP are the three components: research evidence, clinical expertise, and patient preference. EBP is not simply applying research findings in care. It also includes factoring into the clinical guidelines clinical expertise where evidence does not yet exist. Expertise is also important as research evidence is being extrapolated to a particular patient population with which the clinician has much expertise. The third element, patient preference, is incorporated into evidence-based care as the plan of care is devised for that particular patient, individualizing the evidence-based clinical guidelines to meet the individual patient's needs and desires. Approaching EBP in this way ensures that best practice will have the highest likelihood of producing the best outcomes.

APPLYING EVIDENCE-BASED CONCEPT

The primary concept of EBP is that **science** is the most reliable source of knowledge on which to base clinical decisions. The effectiveness of care to produce desired patient outcomes improves when research results guide that care.

The benchmark, or standard, of best practice is that interventions are based on best evidence; specifically, scientific findings. EBP is a way of applying best evidence in clinical decision making to ensure the best outcome that science has been shown to produce. Individual clinician decisions about care, as well as agency systems and policies, should reflect the best evidence produced to date. The end result of applying state-of-the-science patient care is that health care status goals are effectively and efficiently met within the preferences of both the patient and the health care provider (Sackett, Straus, Richardson, Rosenberg, & Haynes, 2000).

The concept of EBP is obvious; however, multiple impediments make the *practice* of EBP difficult. Obstacles to moving research rapidly into routine patient care are as follows: (a) the *volume* and complexity of science and technology and (b) the *form* of knowledge available in the literature. Before the development of EBP methods and processes, the large volume of clinical health research was neither translated into clinical practice nor applied consistently in the delivery of health care (IOM, 2001). Not only is the volume of literature a barrier, but the form of the knowledge is a barrier as well. Research evidence is made available in forms that are not useful to clinicians in clinical decision making. For example, a research report is less useful in clinical decision making than other forms of knowledge, such as evidence-based clinical practice guidelines. The major hurdles related to the knowledge or evidence are presented in Table 2-1 along with new solutions derived from EBP processes. Support for EBP comes from newly developed EBP methods and processes.

EBP in Nursing

Evidence-based nursing can be described as a process of moving research knowledge through the full cycle of transformation and into practice (Stevens, 2004). Clearly, from past experiences with unsuccessful RU efforts, attempts to move research results from a single research report into direct clinical application underscored that new forms of knowledge were necessary to support clinical decision making more fully. Since these attempts, new processes, knowledge products, and supporting EBP entities have matured. Processes, such as methods for conducting systematic reviews, now distill volumes of evidence into a single, meaningful whole. Clinical practice guidelines are now

TABLE 2-1 Knowledge Hurdles and Solutions to Moving Research into Practice	
Hurdle — **COMPLEXITY OF LITERATURE**	**FORM OF KNOWLEDGE**
One obstacle in moving research rapidly into patient care is the growing complexity of science and technology. "No unaided human being can read, recall, and act effectively on the volume of clinically relevant scientific literature." (IOM, 2001, p. 25).	Not only is the volume of literature a hurdle, but the *form* of the knowledge is a hurdle as well. Literature contains a variety of knowledge forms, many of which are *not* suitable for direct practice application.
EBP Solution — **EVIDENCE SUMMARY**	**KNOWLEDGE TRANSFORMATION**
Evidence summaries, including systematic reviews and other forms, reduce the *complexity and volume* of evidence by integrating all research on a given topic into a single, meaningful whole.	From the point of discovery, knowledge can be transformed through a series of stages to increase meaning to the clinician and utility in clinical decision making. The stages of converting knowledge are explained by the ACE Star Model of Knowledge Transformation.

Source: Stevens, K. R. (2004). ACE star model of knowledge transformation. Retrieved May 1, 2005, from www.acestar.uthscsa.edu. Reproduced with expressed permission.

developed using systematic approaches and formats that explicate the underlying evidence. EBP changes are now understood in light of the nature of the health care system, change, and adoption of innovation. There is also a growing understanding of the nature of knowledge in the context of EBP and the transformation needed before research evidence is useful in practice.

The five star points of the ACE Star Model of Knowledge Transformation depict how knowledge transformation must occur in five sequential steps to move research from "bench to bedside." The steps of knowledge transformation are as follows: primary research, evidence summary, translation, integration, and evaluation (Stevens, 2004). Through these steps, knowledge undergoes conversion from one form of knowledge to the rest. Research findings are transformed from single studies, through a series of stages and forms, to have an impact on health outcomes by way of evidence-based care. In each stage, the nature and characteristics of knowledge are transformed into forms that are utilized in various aspects of EBP. The primary forms are as follows: research results from a single study, evidence summaries of all studies on a given topic, clinical recommendations, system practices, and quantification of the impact of EBP.

 # Uncovering the Evidence

Processes for Knowledge Transformation

Transformation of Knowledge Through Evidence Summary: If the available form of knowledge is mismatched to its use in clinical decision making, clinical implications are unclear and the evidence is difficult to manage. For example, a nurse in a community clinic wishes to establish EBPs for clinical decisions about interventions for pregnant women who smoke. The nurse searches the research literature to locate the best evidence to support such decisions and locates over 70 research studies that directly apply. Perhaps only two of these studies are available to the nurse online, and the rest of the studies are not obtained.

On review of the research findings of the first study the nurse sees that cognitive behavioral smoking cessation interventions *did not* produce differences in smoking cessation between the experimental and control groups, and the second study *did* demonstrate statistically significant differences between the experimental and control groups. Further, there were wide differences in the sample sizes, with only 86 adolescents in the first study and 231 subjects from 17 different countries in the second. The obstacle to applying the research results is because of the wrong form of knowledge (research from single studies) for the intended use of the knowledge (i.e., to guide clinical decision making). The variation in size of sample and the incongruence in the results of the two studies leave the nurse wondering what the truth is about the effectiveness of cognitive behavior intervention for smoking cessation in women. This set of research evidence is of little use to the clinician, because it has not been transformed into a package that supports clinical decision making.

With new methods in EBP this research evidence can be converted to a more useful form. Specifically, systematic reviews are conducted to produce useable evidence summaries of all relevant research on a given topic. In a specialized database of systematic reviews, the nurse locates a systematic review entitled *Interventions for Promoting Smoking Cessation during Pregnancy* (Lumley, et al., 2005). Evidence summaries transform knowledge by scientifically synthesizing all results into a single statement of what is known, with inconsistencies and sample size variations resolved through scientific methods, such as meta analytic techniques. The systematic review located indicates that a total of 64 trials, conducted between 1975 and 2003 and including over 20,000 women, were synthesized into the review conclusion:

"There was a significant reduction in smoking in the intervention groups of the 48 trials included; the authors concluded that smoking cessation programs in pregnancy reduce the proportion of women who continue to smoke, and reduce low birthweight and preterm birth; the pooled trials have inadequate power to detect reductions in perinatal mortality or very low birthweight."

Without the evidence summary, the clinician would be left to struggle with 64 research studies and without a systematic design arrive at an erroneous conclusion about whether or not cognitive behavioral interventions for smoking cessation were effective in producing the desired patient outcomes.

Lumley, J., Oliver, S. S., Chamberlain, C., & Oakley, L. (2005). Interventions for promoting smoking cessation during pregnancy. Cochrane Pregnancy and Childbirth Group, The Cochrane Database of Systematic Reviews. Cochrane Library (3). Chichester, UK: Wiley & Sons, Ltd.

Examples of Transformation of Knowledge

Because nurses are unaccustomed to distinguishing among the various forms of knowledge, examples of knowledge transformation are provided in the two accompanying Uncovering the Evidence features to clarify the process.

The ACE Star Model of Knowledge Transformation

The examples shown in the Uncovering the Evidence features call attention to the importance of the *form* of knowledge. EBP has provided nurses with new insights to the necessity of transforming knowledge in clinically useful packages. The ACE Star Model of EBP depicts various forms of knowledge in sequence as research evidence is moved through several cycles, combined with knowledge from other sources, and integrated into practice to improve patient outcomes. The ACE Star Model provides a framework for systematically putting EBP processes into operation. It is a simple, parsimonious depiction of the relationships between various stages of knowledge as newly discovered research evidence is moved through several stages and into practice. The ACE

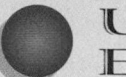 **Uncovering the Evidence**

Processes for Knowledge Transformation

Transformation of Knowledge Through Clinical Practice Guidelines:
The nurse manager of an extended care facility for elderly forms a task force to respond to the Joint Commission on Accreditation of Healthcare Organization's (JCAHO) patient safety goal: reduction in falls among patients. The task force locates a single study of the effect of group exercise. The study indicates that group exercise in a sample of frail older people living in retirement villages produced 22 percent fewer falls during the trial than in the control group (interrater reliability [IRR] = 0.78, 95 percent confidence interval [CI] = 0.62–0.99).

For most clinicians this form of knowledge holds little utility for clinical action; further transformation of this research evidence is needed before it is useful in clinical decision making. The task force locates another form of knowledge; it is an evidence-based clinical practice guideline (EB-CPG). The EB-CPG contains the following recommendation to clinicians:

> "A program of muscle strengthening and balance training, individually prescribed by a trained health professional in a New Zealand primary health care setting, reduces the frequency of falls in high risk community-dwelling older people" (Strength of Recommendation = A). (NZGG, 2003).

The task force is ensured that the CPG is, indeed, evidence-based because of the development approaches used by the developing group. It is known that the NZGG holds high credibility for their thorough approach to guideline development. The process is clearly defined, the evidence is explicated in the CPG recommendations, and the strength of the recommendation is rated. Each recommendation in the CPG is accompanied by the specific research evidence and is rated according to strength.

New Zealand Guidelines Group. (2003). Prevention of hip fracture amongst people aged 65 years and over. Retrieved June, 15, 2005, from http://www.nzgg.org.nz/.

Star Model places previous scientific work in the nursing discipline within the context of EBP, serves as an organizer for examining and applying EBP, and mainstreams nursing into the formal network of EBP.

Configured as a simple five-point star, the model illustrates five major stages of knowledge transformation: (a) knowledge discovery (primary research studies), (b) evidence summary and synthesis, (c) translation into practice recommendations, (d) integration into practice, and (e) evaluation of EBP on outcomes (see Figure 2-1). Evidence-based processes and methods vary from one point of the star model to the next (Stevens, 2004).

Definition of Knowledge Transformation

The core concept of the ACE Star Model is **knowledge transformation;** this is defined as the conversion of research findings from primary research results through a series of stages and forms to have an impact on health outcomes by way of evidence-based care.

Underlying Premises of Knowledge Transformation

The premises that form the foundation for the ACE Star Model are presented in Box 2-2.

BOX 2-2

UNDERLYING PREMISES OF KNOWLEDGE TRANSFORMATION

1. Knowledge transformation is necessary before research results are useable in clinical decision making.
2. Knowledge derives from a variety of sources. In health care, sources of knowledge include research evidence, experience, authority, trial and error, and theoretical principles.
3. The most stable and generalizable knowledge is discovered through systematic processes that control bias, namely, the research process.
4. Evidence can be classified into a hierarchy of strength of evidence. Relative strength of evidence is largely dependent on the rigor of the scientific design that produced the evidence. The value of rigor is that it strengthens cause-and-effect relationships.
5. Knowledge exists in a variety of forms. As research evidence is converted through systematic steps, knowledge from other sources (expertise or patient preference) is added, creating yet another form of knowledge.
6. The form (package) in which knowledge exists can be referenced to its use; in the case of EBP, the ultimate use is application in health care.
7. The form of knowledge determines its usability in clinical decision making. For example, research results from a primary investigation are less useful to decision making than an EB-CPG.
8. Knowledge is transformed through the following processes:
   a. Summarization into a single statement about the state of the science
   b. Translation of the state of the science into clinical recommendations, with addition of clinical expertise, application of theoretical principles, and patient preferences
   c. Implementation of recommendations through organizational and individual actions
   d. Evaluation of impact of actions on targeted outcomes

Source: Stevens, K. R. (2004). ACE star model of knowledge transformation. Retrieved May 1, 2005, from www.acestar.uthscsa.edu. Reproduced with expressed permission.

STAGES OF THE STAR MODEL

Each of the five points of the star focuses on a sequential cognitive activity. In the model the stages progress clockwise from discovery to evaluation.

Star Point 1: Discovery

In this stage, new knowledge is discovered through traditional research methodologies and scientific inquiry. Research results are generated through the conduct of a single study. This may be called a primary research study, and research designs range from descriptive to correlational to causal and from randomized control trials to qualitative. This stage builds the aggregate, or corpus, of research evidence for clinical actions.

Point 1, or primary research, is the approach with which nurses are familiar, i.e., single reports of research studies. Over the past three decades nurse scientists have produced literally thousands of research studies on a wide variety of nursing clinical topics. The cluster of primary research studies on any given topic may include both strong and weak study designs, small and large samples, and conflicting or converging results, leaving the clinician to wonder which study is the best reflection of truth.

Star Point 2: Evidence Summary

To remedy this situation EBP experts have developed the second step in EBP, **evidence summary.** In an evidence summary all primary research on a given clinical topic is gathered together and summarized into a single statement about the state of the science. This summary step is the main feature that distinguishes EBP from simple research application and RU in clinical practice. Evidence summary is the first unique step in EBP; the task is to synthesize the corpus of research evidence into a single, meaningful statement of the state of the knowledge. The most advanced EBP methods to date are those used to develop evidence summaries, i.e., evidence synthesis and systematic review from randomized control trials, such as the systematic review methods outlined in the *Cochrane Collaboration Handbook,* a highly regarded resource for EBP information. Some evidence summaries employ more rigorous methods than others, yielding more credible and reproducible results. A fuller discussion of evidence summaries follows later in this chapter.

Evidence summary produces new knowledge by combining findings from all studies to identify bias and limit chance effect in the conclusion. The systematic methodology also increases reliability and reproducibility of results and increases the power of cause and effect. Evidence summaries are also called evidence synthesis, systematic reviews, integrative reviews, and review of literature, depending on the rigor with which the summary was conducted and the group that produced it.

The rigorous evidence summary step distinguishes EBP from the old paradigm of RU and offers distinct advantages. Largely due to the work of the **Cochrane Collaboration,** an international nonprofit and independent organization founded in 1993 dedicated to making up-to-date, accurate information about the effects of health care readily available worldwide, rigorous methods for systematic reviews have been greatly advanced. The Cochrane Collaboration uses meta analytic statistical techniques and other statistical summary strategies, such as Number Needed to Treat (NNT), in its work. A systematic review accomplishes the following (Mulrow, 1994):

- Reduces large quantities of information into a manageable form
- Integrates existing information for decisions about clinical care, economic decisions, future research design, and policy formation
- Increases efficiency in time between research and clinical implementation

- Establishes generalizability across participants, settings, treatment variations, and different study designs
- Assesses consistency and explains inconsistencies of relationships across studies
- Increases power in suggesting the cause-and-effect relationship
- Reduces bias from random and systematic error, improving true reflection of reality
- Provides better continuous updates of new evidence

Star Point 3: Translation

Evidence summaries provide the base for moving evidence into actual practice. However, the summary conclusions must be translated into practice recommendations to enhance utility of the knowledge. In this third step of EBP, experts are called on to consider the evidence summary, fill in gaps, and merge research knowledge with expertise to produce **clinical practice guidelines (CPGs).** Clinical practice guidelines are commonly produced and sponsored by a clinical specialty organization.

The aim of translation is to provide a useful and relevant package of screened, summarized, and interpreted evidence to clinicians and patients in a form that suits the time, cost, and care standard. Such recommendations are generically termed CPGs and may be represented as, or embedded in, formats such as care standards, clinical pathways, protocols, and algorithms.

CPGs are tools to inform clinical decisions made by the clinician, organization, and patient. Well-developed CPGs state benefits, harms, and costs of various decision options. The strongest CPGs are developed systematically using a process that is explicit and reproducible. Summarized research evidence is interpreted and combined with other sources of knowledge (such as clinical expertise and theoretical guides) and then contextualized to the specific patient population and setting. Well-developed EB-CPGs explicitly articulate the link between the clinical recommendation and the strength of supporting evidence or strength of the recommendation.

Star Point 4: Integration

Integration is perhaps the most familiar stage of knowledge transformation in health care because of society's long-standing expectation that health care be based on the most current knowledge, thus requiring implementation of innovations. Once guidelines are produced on point 3, implementation plans are put into action to change the individual clinician practices, organizational practices, and environmental policies. This step involves changing individual and organizational practices and environmental support through formal and informal channels. Major factors addressed in this stage are those that affect the individual and organizational rate of adoption of innovation, as well as integration of the change into sustainable systems.

Star Point 5: Evaluation

The final stage in knowledge transformation is evaluation. In EBP, a broad array of endpoints and outcomes are evaluated. These include evaluation of the impact of EBP on patient health outcomes, provider and patient satisfaction, efficacy, efficiency, economic analysis, and the health status of a population.

As new knowledge is transformed through the five stages, the final outcome is evidence-based quality improvement of health care.

MAJOR FEATURES OF EBP

Several features of EBP are notable and reflect new approaches to evidence-based clinical decision making. The major features of EBP are that (a) it is heavily interdisciplinary; (b) the development of clinical practice is based on evidence summary of the topic; (c) translation of evidence into CPGs repackages the evidence for use by a clinician; (d) individual provider and organizational factors guide integration; and (e) evaluation includes determining effectiveness and efficiency in terms of patient outcomes, provider and patient satisfaction, and economy. As evidence summaries are constructed, the research reports that are assembled are gathered from across all health care disciplines that may have produced the evidence. This body of evidence yields the interdisciplinary science of care. The research evidence produced by investigators from nursing, medicine, or psychology is transparent to the discipline, because it focuses on resolving the patient's clinical problem. Therefore, all research is included in the summary.

EBP demands that CPGs be based on evidence summaries on the topic because this is the strongest level of knowledge. Even contemporary guidelines, in the form of unit policy, care procedure manuals, and such are based more on tradition and authority and less on existing research evidence. Translation of the evidence summary into practice guidelines is essential in making the evidence useful in practice. Systematic development of CPGs produces the scientifically based guidance for clinical decision making.

Evidence Summary

Because the evidence summary is central to EBP, it is discussed in further detail. Evidence summary is defined as a report of the state of scientifically produced knowledge that was developed using rigorous methods to synthesize knowledge across a number of research studies so that study variations and contradictory study results can be understood in a single conclusion statement. The evidence summary provides a state-of-the-science conclusion about what has been discovered to date. Broadly, this field of science is referred to as the **science of research synthesis.** Research synthesis is coming to be seen by scientists, clinicians, policymakers, and the public as the most reliable basis for clinical care.

As a primary feature of EBP, systematic reviews "efficiently integrate valid information and provide a basis for rational decision making [in clinical care]." (Mulrow, 1994, p. 597). Only in rare instances will a single research study offer highly reliable answers to a clinical question. For this reason it is incumbent on the clinician to (a) ensure that knowledge has been adequately transformed to include research evidence summarized to the high standard of systematic reviews and (b) explicitly translate research evidence into well-documented EB-CPGs. Because of the rigor, requisite specialized skills, and resource intensity of conducting systematic reviews, this knowledge transformation is usually beyond the capacity of clinicians. Rather, systematic reviews are conducted by specialized scientists, such as those working in the Cochrane Collaboration or **Agency for Healthcare Research and Quality (AHRQ)** Evidence-Based Practice Centers, both of which are discussed further in the following section.

Because the movement of EBP is so new, wide variations in terminology still exist. In the case of evidence summaries, this form of knowledge may be called evidence synthesis, systematic reviews, or integrative reviews, depending on which organization produces them. AHRQ uses the term evidence synthesis and the Cochrane Collaboration uses systematic review. **Meta analysis** is a statistical procedure used to summarize the results of research across multiple research reports and is typically associated with experimental research. The following terms have been used in nursing: **integrative review, narrative review,**

review of literature, and state-of-the-science review; these terms usually refer to a less rigorous and therefore less reliable summary process. The term systematic review is coming into most common usage in EBP and will be used in the remainder of this section.

Method for Producing Systematic Reviews

Those who conduct systematic reviews indicate explicitly how the literature was searched and located, how the studies were appraised, and how the study results are summarized. They use systematic and reproducible methods to identify, select, critically appraise, and analyze relevant research around a clearly formulated question. While several approaches have been outlined, there are six essential steps in conducting a systematic review: (a) formulate the question; (b) locate relevant studies; (c) select and appraise the studies; (d) summarize and synthesize results across studies; (e) interpret the findings; and (f) update the review regularly (Glasziou, Irwig, Bain, & Colditz, 2001). Such a systematic process guarantees that the knowledge is accurately and comprehensively represented. Sophisticated methods for conducting systematic reviews were developed by the Cochrane Collaboration. Alderson, Green, and Higgin's *Cochrane Handbook* (2003) is considered the gold standard for methods with which to conduct systematic reviews in EBP.

Evidence Summaries

The method of systematic review requires a review of literature that addresses a clearly formulated question. This review uses systematic and explicit methods to identify, select, and critically appraise relevant research and to collect and analyze data from the studies that are included in the review. Once data are abstracted from the primary studies, statistical analysis may or may not be used to analyze and summarize the results of the included studies. The scientific process involves: formulating a question, locating and evaluating the world's relevant research on the topic, appraising it according to specified criteria, and synthesizing the results into one harmonious statement.

This analytic approach to evidence summary sets a high standard for systematic, reproducible summaries of existing research results from all existing research. This approach renders obsolete the traditional review of literature, because those reviews were not typically conducted using rigorous scientific methods. Past reviews of literature were not adequately focused on extrapolating practice implications from existing research knowledge or sufficiently rigorous to produce comprehensive and replicable results for clinical decision making. Without scientific methods in evidence summaries, the end product is less valid, being prone to biased conclusions and open to question. The rudiments of a systematic review are:

- Review addresses an explicit clinical question including population, intervention, and outcomes of interest
- Methods for locating relevant studies are detailed in report
- Literature search is comprehensive and exhaustive, regardless of discipline of research team and regardless of language
- Selection method used to grade methodological quality and relevance of primary studies is explicit
- Primary studies included in the review are of high methodological quality
- Method of synthesizing is described and appropriate to level of evidence

Systematic reviews could be called the heart of the EBP because of the pivotal role they play in moving research evidence into practice. A systematic review increases the power and validity of the cause-and-effect relationship between interventions and outcomes, thus making it the ideal base for formulation of clinical guidelines. Evidence summaries and development of evidence-based guidelines are potent approaches to putting results of studies into action.

However, conducting a systematic review corresponds to conducting a major primary research study. Entities that conduct systematic reviews find that they often require appraisal of over 3,000 articles, a team of 6 to 12 investigators, a 12-month schedule, and $250,000 to support the work to the required level of rigor. Anything less than a high-quality, systematic review will result in less than valid conclusions for clinical decision making. Clinicians should not attempt these evidence summary studies as part of a typical EBP infrastructure. Instead, they should seek these high-quality evidence summaries and parallel EB-CPGs from credible sources that have already critically appraised and synthesized the evidence. These sources are described in the next section.

Sources of Evidence for Clinical Practice

Systematic reviews address many of the hurdles encountered by clinicians as they attempt to apply research findings in clinical decision making and practice. However, conducting evidence synthesis is a resource-intensive and rigorous process beyond the capacity of the typical clinician. For these reasons awareness of existing sources of synthesized evidence and other transformed knowledge is critical for the clinician. Two primary knowledge forms are now readily available owing to the advancements in the EBP movement and the entities that support it. These are (a) evidence summaries and (b) EB-CPGs.

Sources of Evidence Summaries

Synthesis work is conducted by several organized agencies, such as the AHRQ and the Cochrane Collaboration. Because the conduct of a systematic review requires specialized scientific methods and significant resources, it is usually a sponsored activity conducted by groups of scientists, librarians, clinicians, and statisticians. The prime sponsors are the Cochrane Collaboration (a global collaborative headquartered in the United Kingdom) and the Agency for Healthcare Research and Quality (a federally funded agency in the United States). In turn, these agencies disseminate the evidence summaries for use by clinicians, health care policymakers, and consumers of health care.

Cochrane systematic reviews follow a standard format, are regularly updated in response to newly discovered evidence, and are subject to extensive peer review. These reviews are published as part of the **Cochrane library,** in an electronic database known as the *Cochrane Database of Systematic Reviews*. This database contains both topic reports (completed systematic reviews) and protocols (systematic reviews in progress). To date there are over 1,500 topics that have been reviewed by the Cochrane Collaboration. The Cochrane library requires a subscription to access the full text report; however, abstracts of the reviews are available online free. Cochrane reviews are indexed in CINAHL bibliographic database and can be quickly located by searching with the term *systematic review*. Further information about the Cochrane Collaboration and Library is available online at http://www.cochrane.org.

The AHRQ is the second major source of systematic reviews. Presently, AHRQ has sponsored almost 70 evidence reports or evidence summaries. On the AHRQ site can be found full-text documents on evidence reports, archived CPGs, quick-reference guides, and consumer brochures. Since 1996, the Agency for Health Care Policy and Research (AHCPR) produces evidence reports only. AHRQ is the United States' premier EBP agency. In 1989 it was established by Congress as the lead federal agency charged with supporting research designed to improve the quality and safety of health care. About 15 AHRQ EBP centers contract to conduct these evidence summaries on topics nominated for review. Further information can be found online at http://www.ahrq.gov. Examples of evidence summaries from the Cochrane Database of Systematic Reviews and AHRQ evidence reports are presented in Box 2-3.

BOX 2-3

EXAMPLES OF EVIDENCE SUMMARIES FROM THE COCHRANE LIBRARY AND AHRQ

In patients with high blood pressure in ambulatory settings, simplifying dosing regimens appears to increase adherence to blood pressure–lowering medication. However, effects on subsequent blood pressure are unclear. Motivational strategies and complex interventions may improve treatment adherence, but more evidence is needed. Patient education alone does not appear to improve treatment adherence.

Source: Schroeder, K., Fahey, T., & Ebrahim, S. (2004). Interventions for improving adherence to treatment in patients with high blood pressure in ambulatory settings. The Cochrane Database of Systematic Reviews *(2), CD004804.*

There is some evidence that melatonin is effective in the management of chronic insomnia in subsets of the chronic insomnia population, and there is no evidence that melatonin poses a risk of harm. However, more research is required in this area given that the results are based on a small number of studies. Similarly, additional large-scale, randomized trials are needed to determine the efficacy of melatonin across subsets of the chronic insomnia population. There is insufficient evidence to conclude on the efficacy and safety of L-tryptophan and valerian in the management of chronic insomnia. Additional large-scale, randomized trials are needed in these areas.

Source: Buscemi, N., Vandermeer, B., Friesen, C., Bialy, L., Tubman, M., Ospina, M., et al. (2005, June). Manifestations and management of chronic insomnia in adults. Summary. *Evidence Report/Technology Assessment: Number 125. AHRQ Publication Number 05-E021-1. Retrieved June 28, 2005, from http://www.ahrq.gov/clinic/epcsums/insomnsum.htm.*

Clinical Practice Guidelines

Current EBP approaches emphasize the usefulness of CPGs in bridging the gap between primary research findings and clinical decision making. CPGs are seen as tools to help move scientific evidence to the bedside. CPGs are defined as systematically developed statements to assist clinicians and patients in making decisions about appropriate health care for specific clinical circumstances (National Health System, 2005a). It is imperative that guidelines are based on best available evidence, systematically located, appraised, and synthesized.

Locating CPGs can be challenging. Prior to the EBP movement, guidelines were developed and disseminated by clinical specialty organizations, particularly in medicine. These guidelines were not necessarily evidence-based, and many times were based on consensus opinion of clinical experts. Today AHRQ provides the **National Guideline Clearinghouse,** a searchable database of almost 1,500 CPGs entered by numerous sources. While this database can be easily used to locate a wide variety of CPGs, the user must examine the information presented with the CPG to determine that it is current, was developed systematically, and is based on best evidence.

Other guidelines can be located on the U.S. Preventive Services Task Force (USPSTF) segment of the AHRQ Web site. These recommendations focus on screening tests, counseling, immunizations, and chemoprophylaxis and are based on evidence summary work performed by AHRQ. The task force was convened by the U.S. Public Health Service in 1984 to systematically review the evidence of the effectiveness of a wide range of clinical preventive services.

Examples of EB-CPGs located through the National Guideline Clearinghouse and through the USPTF are presented in Box 2-4.

A highly credible, nursing-specific resource for CPGs is the Registered Nurses Association of Ontario (RNAO). Through the RNAO Center for Professional Nursing Excellence, this group systematically develops CPGs based on examined and explicit evidence. At this date, RNAO offers 28 guidelines, including the CPG noted in Box 2-5. Further information about RNAO can be accessed at http://rnao.org.

Crucial criteria for well-developed CPGs are that the evidence is explicitly identified and that the evidence underlying the recommendation is rated. To assist in rating evidence, several taxonomics have been developed. One such taxonomy was developed by the National Health Services of the United Kingdom. This rating system identifies systematic reviews as the uppermost strength of evidence. Also included is consensus of expert opinion. The latter is rated as having the weakest strength of evidence; however, if no other evidence exists this may serve to support clinical decision making (National Health System, 2005b). The strength of the evidence for therapy ratings uses the following coding system:

1A   Systematic review (SR) with homogeneity of randomized control trials (RCTs)

1B   Individual RCT with narrow CI

1C   All or none

2A   SR with homogeneity of cohort studies

2B   Individual cohort study

2C   "Outcomes" research

3A   SR with homogeneity of case-control studies

3B   Individual case-control study

4   Case-series, poor quality cohort and case-control

5   Expert opinion, theory, bench research

BOX 2-4

EXAMPLES OF CPGS

Assessment

Assess fall risk on admission
(Level of Evidence = Ib; Grade of Recommendation = B)
Assess fall risk after a fall
(Level of Evidence = Ib; Grade of Recommendation = B)

Intervention

Tai chi to prevent falls in the elderly is recommended for those patients whose length of stay (LOS) is greater than four months and for those patients with no history of a fall fracture. There is insufficient evidence to recommend Tai chi to prevent falls for patients with length of stay less than four months.
(Level of Evidence = Ib; Grade of Recommendation = B)
Nurses can use strength training as a component of multifactorial fall interventions; however, there is insufficient evidence to recommend it as a stand-alone intervention.
(Level of Evidence = Ib; Grade of Recommendation = I)

Source: Registered Nurses Association of Ontario. (2005). Prevention of falls and fall injuries in the older adult. *Toronto, ON: Author.*

BOX 2-5

EXAMPLES OF KNOWLEDGE FROM VARIOUS SOURCES

ACE Star Point 1: Primary Research

There were 22 percent fewer falls during the trial in the group exercise group than in the comparison group (IRR = 0.78, 95 percent CI = 0.62–0.99).

Source: Lord, S. R., Castell, S., Corcoran, J., Dayhew, J., Matters, B., Shan, A., et al. (2003). The effect of group exercise on physical functioning and falls in frail older people living in retirement villages: A randomized, controlled trial. Journal of the American Geriatrics Society, 51(12), 1685–1692.

ACE Star Point 2: Evidence Summary

This systematic review screened literature and selected 62 relevant, high-quality trials involving 21,668 people and synthesized the research evidence. Conclusions from the synthesis are as follows:

Interventions Likely to be Beneficial in Preventing Falls in the Elderly

- Multifactor health or environmental risk factor screening or intervention
- Muscle strengthening and balance retraining
- Home hazard assessment and modification
- Withdrawal of psychotropic medication
- Tai chi group exercise intervention

Source: Gillespie, L. D., Gillespie, W. J., Robertson, M. C., Lamb, S. E., Cumming, R. G., & Rowe, B. H. (2005). Interventions for preventing falls in elderly people. Oxford, UK: The Cochrane Database of Systematic Reviews.

ACE Star Point 3: CPG

Multifactorial Interventions for Preventing Falls in the Elderly

Recommendation: All older people with recurrent falls or assessed as being at increased risk of falling should be considered for an individualized multifactorial intervention.

Strength of Evidence-Level I; Strength of Recommendation-A

Recommendation: In successful multifactorial intervention programs the following specific components are common (Evidence level I):

- Strength and balance training
- Home hazard assessment and intervention
- Vision assessment and referral
- Medication review with modification or withdrawal
- Strength of Evidence-Level I; Strength of Recommendation-A

Source: National Collaborating Centre for Nursing and Supportive Care. (2004). Clinical practice guideline for the assessment and prevention of falls in older people. London, UK: National Institute for Clinical Excellence. Retrieved on June 15, 2005, from http://www.guideline.gov/.

In parallel, recommendations flowing forth from evidence are rated in terms of strength. The USPTF uses a schema rating recommendations. This schema is detailed in Box 2-6.

Fundamental to the use of EB-CPGs is the clinician's critical appraisal of those under consideration for adoption. Systematic approaches have been developed with a good example being the AGREE Instrument for Assessing Guidelines. This checklist developed by an international collaboration has been widely adopted. The instrument outlines the primary facets of the

---

BOX 2-6

STRENGTH OF RECOMMENDATIONS FROM THE U.S. PREVENTIVE SERVICES TASK FORCE

The U.S. Preventive Services Task Force (USPSTF) grades its recommendations according to one of five classifications (A, B, C, D, I) reflecting the strength of evidence and magnitude of net benefit (benefits minus harms).

A—The USPSTF strongly recommends that clinicians provide [the service] to eligible patients. *The USPSTF found good evidence that [the service] improves important health outcomes and concludes that benefits substantially outweigh harms.*

B—The USPSTF recommends that clinicians provide [this service] to eligible patients. *The USPSTF found at least fair evidence that [the service] improves important health outcomes and concludes that benefits outweigh harms.*

C—The USPSTF makes no recommendation for or against routine provision of [the service]. *The USPSTF found at least fair evidence that [the service] can improve health outcomes but concludes that the balance of benefits and harms is too close to justify a general recommendation.*

D—The USPSTF recommends against routinely providing [the service] to asymptomatic patients. *The USPSTF found at least fair evidence that [the service] is ineffective or that harms outweigh benefits.*

I—The USPSTF concludes that the evidence is insufficient to recommend for or against routinely providing [the service]. *Evidence that the [service] is effective is lacking, of poor quality, or conflicting, and the balance of benefits and harms cannot be determined.*

Source: AHRQ. (2002). What is AHRQ? *Retrieved June 15, 2005, from http://www.ahrq.gov/about/whatis.htm.*

CPG to be appraised: scope and purpose, stakeholder involvement, rigor of development, clarity and presentation, application, and editorial independence. While the instrument is not easily used by the individual clinician, it is helpful to groups and organizations charged with adoption of specific CPGs.

Priorities in Evidence-Based Changes in Health Care

Following the proposal for sweeping health care reform by the IOM (2001), the next step was to target priority health topics. A total of 20 priority areas for quality improvement were identified according to three criteria: (a) impact in terms of burden on the patient, family, health care system, and society; (b) improvability by using evidence to close gaps between best practice and usual care; and (c) inclusiveness, reflecting applicability to patients across the life span and settings and eliminating disparities (IOM, 2003). Improvability includes the existence of evidence-based standards for effective care. The 20 priority areas that were identified for national action are listed in Box 2-7.

The primary implication of these priorities for nursing is that the report emphasizes the need for evidence-based practice principles for health care practice revisions in clinical agencies. This set of priorities will likely set the agenda for change efforts for the next 5 to 10 years, and nurses must be full members of the team that sets about to improve practice.

BOX 2-7

IOM-PRIORITY AREAS FOR NATIONAL ACTION

Care coordination	Ischemic heart disease
Self-management and health literacy	Major depression
Asthma	Medication management
Evidence-based cancer screening	Nosocomial infections
Children with special health care needs	Pain control in advanced cancer
Diabetes	Pregnancy and childbirth
End-of-life organ failures	Mental illness
Frailty associated with old age	Stroke
Hypertension	Tobacco dependence
Immunizations	Obesity (emerging, does not meet improvability criterion)

Source: Institute of Medicine. (2003). Priority areas for national action: Transforming health care quality. *Washington, DC: National Academy Press.*

USE OF EBP FOR CLINICAL NURSING PRACTICE

Evidence developed through research provides the best guidelines for effective practice. As health care providers, nurses strive to apply the best available evidence in clinical decisions about the care nurses deliver. While experience is a good teacher, conclusions drawn from experience frequently contain bias arising from numerous sources. Conclusions drawn from experience will not likely represent the truth or validity of the broader reality. For example, patients in a particular geographic area or during a particular season may not represent all patients. Indeed, it is suggested that failing to use existing research evidence in clinical practice falls short of nursing's ethical mandates.

Using research evidence in nursing care increases certainty and predictability in the effect of the practice on the outcome. The reality of clinical practice is that the nurse needs evidence summaries and EB-CPGs to guide clinical decisions. In most instances, the knowledge work necessary to produce evidence summaries and guidelines is not feasible in the clinical setting, given the resources necessary. Therefore, nurses must turn to credible sources of evidence and EB-CPGs and must add to their skill set the critical appraisal of those knowledge forms. Clinical decisions that are based on science are more certain to produce the desired health outcomes. In the end, patients will be major benefactors of the evidence-based quality improvement movement.

KEY CONCEPTS

- Knowledge may come from one's own experience, trial and error, a nursing procedure manual, a textbook, or science produced through research.
- Not all sources of knowledge are reliable or consistently produce the desired patient outcome.
- Knowledge produced through unstructured approaches lacks generalizability and is fraught with systematic bias because the cause-and-effect relationship between the action and the outcome is inadequately examined.
- EBP is a process through which scientific evidence is identified, appraised, and applied in health care interventions.
- In 2000 the IOM report, *To err is human: Building a safer health system* revealed that about 98,000 hospitalized Americans die each year as a result of errors in their care. In 2001 the chasm between what we know through science to be best health care and what is actually practiced became evident.
- The objective of EBP is to apply the best available research evidence in clinical care to predictably move patients toward their health care goals.
- EBP involves applying research findings in care, factoring in clinical expertise, and individualizing practice guidelines to meet a unique patient's needs and desires.
- The primary concept of EBP is that science is the most reliable source of knowledge on which to base clinical decisions.

- Evidence-based nursing can be described as a process of moving research knowledge through the full cycle of transformation and into practice.
- The five star points of the ACE Star Model of Knowledge Transformation depict the five sequential steps of knowledge transformation.
- In an evidence summary all primary research on a given clinical topic is gathered and summarized into a single statement about the state of the science.
- Evidence summary produces new knowledge by combining findings from all studies to identify bias and limit chance effect in the conclusion.
- Once evidence summaries provide the base, experts are called on to merge the research knowledge with expertise to produce CPGs.
- Only in rare instances will a single research study offer highly reliable answers to a clinical question.
- Sophisticated methods for conducting systematic reviews were developed by the Cochrane Collaboration, an international not-for-profit organization with the goal of helping practitioners make well-informed health care decisions by preparing, maintaining, and promoting accessibility of systematic reviews of research.
- A highly credible, nursing-specific resource for CPGs is the RNAO.
- Using research evidence in nursing care increases certainty and predictability in the effect of the practice on the outcome.

REVIEW QUESTIONS

1. Examples of EBP may include:
   1. Strict adherence to written procedures
   2. Checking with a health care provider about how to carry out an order
   3. Securing the patient's preference about the care being provided
   4. Accessing an evidence summary
2. The following present obstacles to moving research rapidly into routine patient care:
   1. Time and money
   2. Volume and complexity of science and technology
   3. Lack of access to a health science library
   4. Computer-based systematic reviews of evidence

3. Knowledge transformation:
   1. Occurs when clinicians consult together about patient care
   2. Involves discovery, manipulation, and integration
   3. Is documentation about how well a nursing intervention worked for a particular patient
   4. Is necessary before research results are usable in clinical decision making
4. Major features of EBP include:
   1. Repackaging procedures for clinician use
   2. Provider and patient dissatisfaction
   3. Interdisciplinary research
   4. Budget neutrality

Continued

REVIEW QUESTIONS—cont'd

5. To obtain evidence-based practice guidance go to:
   1. http://www.ncms.gov
   2. http://www.careguidelines.gov
   3. http://www.cochrane.org
   4. http://www.hcfa.org

6. The ACE Star Model of EBP:
   1. Names various forms of knowledge in sequence
   2. Derives from a single source
   3. Suggests that knowledge emanates from five "ways of knowing"
   4. Names the steps of knowledge transformation

7. A systematic review of evidence includes:
   1. Formulating the question, surveying practitioners, and selecting relevant studies
   2. Formulating the question, locating relevant studies, selecting, and appraising the studies
   3. Formulating the question, summarizing, and synthesizing populations across studies
   4. Formulating the question, locating relevant studies, and choosing the study that best matches your clinical situation

8. Using research evidence in nursing practice:
   1. Increases certainty and predictability in the effect of the practice on the outcome
   2. Is not feasible at this time, given the resources available
   3. Is becoming more in demand by patients
   4. Is only appropriate for advanced practice nurses

9. A criterion for quality improvement through EBP identified by the Institute of Medicine is to:
   1. Cut the cost of health care
   2. Expand the care covered by Medicare and Medicaid
   3. Close gaps between best practice care and usual care
   4. Provide EBP to those who need it most, the young and the elderly

10. EBP is another name for:
    1. Science-based care
    2. Quality improvement
    3. Research utilization
    4. Expert care

REVIEW ACTIVITIES

1. Think about something that you do to help patients that seems to you to be of questionable usefulness. Go to the Cochrane Collection Web site at http://www.cochrane.org and search for an evidence report about it.

2. Go to the AHRQ Web site at http://www.ahrq.gov and search for an evidence report about the same topic.

3. What conclusion can you draw from your searches?

4. How will your conclusion impact your continued use of that nursing intervention?

5. How does your conclusion impact your thinking about what contribution you might personally make to the application of scientific knowledge for nursing practice?

Health Education and Promotion

Rick Daniels, RN, PhD

CHAPTER TOPICS

- Teaching-Learning Process
- Teaching Strategies
- Health Maintenance
- Health Promotion
- Disease Prevention

Patient education and health maintenance are integral components of nursing care. Both patient education and health maintenance are the nurse's responsibility to assist the patient to improve his or her health conditions. This chapter offers an overview of: (a) the teaching-learning process, including learning barriers and teaching responsibilities of nurses and (b) an emphasis on health promotion and disease prevention activities with an emphasis on nursing's role. Patient education is extremely important today in a health care environment that demands cost-effective measures. With shorter hospital stays, patients are being discharged to the home or other health care settings in more critical conditions than ever before. Patient education, a hallmark of quality nursing care, is a fiscally responsible intervention that encourages health care consumers to engage in self-care and to develop healthy lifestyle practices.

KEY TERMS

Affective domain
Auditory learners
Basic human needs
Cognitive domain
Disease prevention or
    health protection
Empowerment
Health maintenance
Health maintenance
    activities
Health promotion
Kinesthetic learners
Learning
Learning plateaus
Learning style
Motivation
Perception
Philosophy
Psychomotor domain
Self-efficacy
Sex roles
Sexuality
Spirituality
Teaching
Teaching-learning process
Teaching strategies
Visual learners

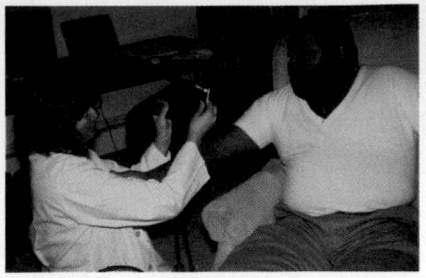

Figure 3-1 This nurse is teaching a newly admitted patient regarding hypertension and the taking of blood pressure.

THE TEACHING-LEARNING PROCESS

The **teaching-learning process** is a planned interaction promoting behavioral change that is not a result of maturation or coincidence. **Teaching** is an active process in which one individual shares information with others to provide them with the information to make behavioral changes. Teaching refers to all the activities used by a teacher to assist the learner to absorb new information; it consists of activities that promote change. Teaching is a goal-directed process that provides the opportunity for learning (Figure 3-1).

Learning is the process of assimilating information with a resultant change in behavior. Nurses and patients have shared responsibilities in the teaching-learning process. Knowledge is power. By sharing knowledge with patients, the nurse empowers patients to achieve their maximum level of wellness. The teaching-learning process will be familiar to nurses in that it mirrors the steps of the nursing process: assessment, identification of learning needs (nursing diagnosis), planning, implementation of teaching strategies, and evaluation of learner progress and teaching efficacy.

Purposes of Patient Education

According to Edelman and Mandle (2002), the goal of health education is to help individuals achieve optimum states of health through their own actions. Teaching, one of the most important nursing functions, addresses patients' need for information. Often, a knowledge deficit about the course of illness or self-care practices hinders a patient's recovering from illness or engaging in behaviors that promote health. The nurse's charge is to help bridge the gap between what a patient knows and what a patient needs to know to achieve optimum health.

Patient education is done for a variety of reasons (Table 3-1). Patient education focuses on the patient's ability to practice healthy behaviors. The patient's ability to care for self is enhanced by effective education.

To be more effective teachers, nurses need a basic understanding of learning theories. There are many schools of thought (theories) about how people learn. Table 3-2 provides an overview of major learning theories.

Each nurse needs to develop an individual **philosophy** (statement of beliefs that is the foundation for behavior) of learning. When formulating a philosophy about teaching-learning, nurses need to consider the common beliefs about learning listed in Box 3-1.

TABLE 3-1 Patient Education Topics

HEALTH PROMOTION	HEALTH RESTORATION
Parenting skills	Medication information
Nutrition	Community resources
Exercise	Information about treatment modalities
Family planning	
DISEASE OR INJURY PREVENTION	**FACILITATING COPING**
Immunizations	Safe use of medical equipment
Health screenings	Dietary modifications
Smoking cessation	Information about the disease process
Breast self-examination	Counseling related to anger, grief, or self-esteem
Safety measures (e.g., car seat and restraining devices)	Stress management

TABLE 3-2 Overview of Learning Theories

THEORIST	DESCRIPTION
John Watson	Learning is a result of conditioning and experiences, and encouraged by changing the environment.
Ivan Pavlov	The learner is passive (controlled by the environment).
B. F. Skinner	Teaching is the deliberate manipulation of the environment.
Edward L. Thorndike	Learning can be transferred from one situation to another. Assessment of learner's behavior is necessary.
John Dewey	The learner must have an understanding of the goals, and education should promote learner independence.
Jerome Bruner	Learning is affected by culture and value system, and the learner is an active participant in the learning process.
Robert Gagne	Learning occurs in an orderly fashion, from the simple to the complex, from the concrete to the abstract.
Albert Bandura	Behavior is regulated by internal mechanisms, such as self-efficacy.

Facilitators of Learning

Certain fundamental principles of education can be used by nurses to facilitate patient learning. Knowles (1984) stated four basic assumptions about adult learners, which are applicable to patient education:

- *Assumption:* An individual's personality develops in an orderly fashion from dependence to independence. *Nursing Application:* Plan teaching-learning activities that promote patient participation, thus encouraging independence; this increases patient control and self-care through empowerment.
- *Assumption:* Learning readiness is affected by developmental stage and sociocultural factors. *Nursing Application:* Conduct a thorough psychosocial assessment before planning the teaching-learning activities.
- *Assumption:* An individual's previous learning experiences can be used as a foundation for further learning. *Nursing Application:* Perform a complete assessment to determine what the patient already knows and build on that knowledge base.
- *Assumption:* Immediacy reinforces learning. *Nursing Application:* Provide opportunities for immediate application of knowledge and skills. Incorporate feedback as a continuous part of each nurse-patient interaction.

Table 3-3 describes main learning principles.

It is a good idea to keep in mind that **learning plateaus,** or peaks in effectiveness of teaching and depth of learning, will occur in relation to the patient's motivation, interest, and perception of relevance of the material. Frequent reinforcement of learning through immediate feedback and continual reassessment of effectiveness will enhance the value of the learning process for both the teacher and the learner. Making the information acquisition process as user-friendly as possible will also increase satisfaction and success. This can be done by organizing content from the simple to the complex and from the familiar to the new, making learning as creative and interesting as possible, and adopting a flexible approach to allow the learning process to be dynamic.

Barriers to Learning

Receiving information does not, in and of itself, guarantee that learning will occur. Several barriers can impede the learning process. In a nursing situation, learning barriers can be classified as either internal (psychological or physiological) or external (environmental or sociocultural). Examples of these barriers are shown in Box 3-2.

BOX 3-1

BELIEFS ABOUT LEARNING

- Each individual has the capacity to learn; learning ability varies from person to person and is situational.
- The pace of learning varies with each person.
- Learning is a continuous process, occurring throughout the life cycle.
- Learning can occur in formal and informal settings and interactions.
- Learning is an individualized process.
- Learning new information is based on previous knowledge and experiences.
- Motivation and readiness are necessary for learning to occur.
- Prompt feedback facilitates learning.

The nurse must assess for the presence of barriers to facilitate the learning process. Specific assessment information is presented later in this chapter.

Domains of Learning

Bloom, in his classic work (1977), identified three areas, or domains, in which learning occurs: the **cognitive domain** (intellectual understanding), the **affective domain** (emotions and attitudes), and the **psychomotor domain** (motor skills).

TABLE 3-3 Principles of Learning	
PRINCIPLE	**EXPLANATION**
Relevance	The material should be: • Meaningful to patient • Easily understood by patient • Related to previously learned information
Motivation	Patient should: • Want to learn • Perceive value of information
Readiness	Patient should be able and willing to learn.
Maturation	Patient should be developmentally able to learn and have requisite cognitive and psychomotor abilities.
Reinforcement	Feedback to learner should be: • Positive • Immediate
Participation	Active involvement promotes learning.
Organization	The material should: • Incorporate previously learned information • Be presented in sequence of simple to complex
Repetition	Retention of material is reinforced by practice, repetition, and presentation of same material in a variety of ways.

BOX 3-2

BARRIERS TO LEARNING

External Barriers	**Internal Barriers**
Environmental	**Psychological**
• Interruptions	• Anxiety
• Lack of privacy	• Fear
• Multiple stimuli	• Anger
• Depression	**Physiological**
• Inability to comprehend	• Pain
Sociocultural	• Fatigue
• Language	• Sensory deprivation
• Value system	
• Educational background	
• Oxygen deprivation	

TABLE 3-4	Domains of Learning	
DOMAIN	**DEFINITION**	**CLINICAL EXAMPLE**
Cognitive	Learning that involves the acquisition of facts and data. Used in problem solving and decision making.	Patient states the name and purpose of prescribed medications.
Affective	Learning that involves changing attitudes, emotions, beliefs. Used in making judgments.	Patient accepts that he or she has a chronic illness.
Psychomotor	Learning that involves gaining motor skills. Uses physical application of knowledge.	Patient gives self an injection.

Source: Casebeer, L., Strasser, S., Spettell, C., Wall, T., Weisman, N., Ray, M., et al. (2003). Designing tailored web-based instruction to improve physician's preventative practices. *Retrieved September 8, 2006, from www.jmir.org.*

Each domain responds to and processes information in different ways. Table 3-4 briefly describes the three domains of learning through clinical examples.

Teaching Strategies

Nurses need to be sensitive to all three domains of learning when developing effective teaching plans and to use **teaching strategies**, or techniques, to promote learning, which will tap into each of the domains. For instance, teaching a patient with diabetes how and why to measure the proper daily balance of insulin against glucose levels is within the cognitive domain. Helping this patient learn how to self-administer insulin falls within the psychomotor domain, and seeing that the patient learns to view diabetes as only one part of an entire individual stimulates the affective domain (Burckhardt, 2005).

Although teaching opportunities arise with any interaction with a patient, the nurse must do advanced planning for a formal teaching session. Most educators agree that a combination of teaching strategies is most beneficial for learning to take place. Proper assessment of the patient's learning needs and the way patients learn best are imperative for a teaching session to be successful. A variety of teaching strategies are presented in this section (i.e., discussion, demonstration, role-playing, visual aids, programmed instruction, and computer-assisted instruction).

Discussion

Discussion is the exchange of information both verbally and nonverbally. It involves audience participation. It requires the nurse to focus on building some sort of conversation before focusing on expanding that conversation. Discussion is effective for large groups, as it pools ideas and experiences from diverse backgrounds, allowing everyone to participate in an active process of exchanging information. It is the nurse's responsibility to act as facilitator to keep the discussion on track. Discussion also is effective for one-to-one interactions. Some patients prefer this method, especially if the topic is sensitive.

Demonstration

Demonstration and return demonstration provide a realistic learning experience. Demonstrations should be as realistic as possible. Adequate time should be allowed for this type of teaching strategy. Demonstration combined with lecture or discussion is a practical strategy when teaching a new skill—for example, insulin injection, use of equipment, wound care, or exercise. Return demonstration allows for evaluation of the patient's learning.

Role-Playing

Role-playing allows the patient to apply knowledge in a simulated environment. The nurse sets the stage, then the patient plays out the scenario with the nurse or another learner. This can be effective with adolescents. For example,

Fast Forward ▶▶▶

Simulation Manikins

Recently, simulation manikins with computer driven capabilities have created an additional learning experience for nursing students. Perhaps in the future, there will also be simulation scenarios for patients as demonstrated by these manikins. The Laerdal SimMan simulator offers the ability to provide simulation education to challenge and test students' clinical and decision-making skills during realistic patient care scenarios. Extremely realistic, yet somewhat expensive, the SimMan simulator was specifically designed to meet the scenario-based training needs of a wide variety of simulations (e.g., advanced cardiac life support [ACLS], advanced trauma life support [ATLS], difficult airway management). Future applications could use these simulator manikins to educate patients regarding their self-injections for diabetes, performing self-examinations (e.g., breast self-examinations, testicular self-examinations), and changing ostomy appliances for colorectal disorders.

The use of patient simulation is considered an educational device as many scenarios can be presented including uncommon but critical situations where a rapid response is needed. Errors can be allowed to occur and reach their conclusion without any risk to a patient. It will be interesting to see if this type of educational equipment can be applied to patient education (Platt, Parrish, & Hostler, 2004).

a teenage boy can rehearse with a partner what he will say to his parents when telling them his girlfriend is pregnant.

Role-playing is also beneficial for small children (Figure 3-2). It allows them the opportunity to deal with their fear and negative emotions about illness or hospitalization. Game playing is also useful when dealing with small children or patients with developmental delay (Antai-Otong, 2003).

Visual Aids

Visual aids come in many forms, allowing the nurse to select the one(s) most appropriate for the patient. These include flip charts, slides, television programs, pamphlets, and books, to name a few. It is important that the nurse does not rely solely on the use of visual aids. They should be used in conjunction with other teaching strategies (Yellen, 2005).

Programmed Instruction

Programmed instruction, often referred to as canned (audio) presentations, is intended for use without the nurse. This can be effective for some patients, but the nurse needs to do a thorough assessment of the patient and the instruction to make sure the two are compatible.

Computer-Assisted Instruction

Computer-assisted instruction is an aid available to nurses. The programs can be personalized to the patient. The options for this form of instruction are growing daily. They, however, come with a price. Depending on the type of computer equipment, the cost can run into the thousands. Patients also need to have some basic computer skills, and some may feel intimidated by the "modern" technology (Smith, et al., 2005; Boyington, et al., 2005).

Online Internet Support Groups

In recent years, there are an increasing number of Internet support groups for patients. These groups provide interpersonal communication for a wide variety of patients and disease-related topics. The self-motivation of the patient to participate in such a group is foundational to the success of this type of patient education. There are positive results reported from patients that interact in this type of patient program (Potts, 2005).

PROFESSIONAL RESPONSIBILITIES RELATED TO TEACHING

Through teaching, the nurse empowers patients in their self-care abilities. Teaching is the tool for providing information to patients about specific disease processes, treatment methods, and health-promoting behaviors.

Legal Aspects

The American Nurses Association, in its *Social Policy Statement* (1995), identifies health teaching as an essential function of nursing. Each state has its own definition of nursing practice; in most states, teaching is a required function of nurses.

Patient education is also mandated by several accrediting bodies, such as the Joint Commission for Accreditation of Healthcare Organizations (JCAHO, 2005). The American Hospital Association's *Patient's Bill of Rights* (1980) calls for the patient's understanding of health status and treatment approaches. Informed consent for treatment procedures can be given only by patients who are well informed. The nurse assesses the patient's level of understanding about treatment methods and corrects any knowledge deficits. The nurse is often a health care provider interpreter to the patient—explaining in easily understood terms, clarifying, and referring.

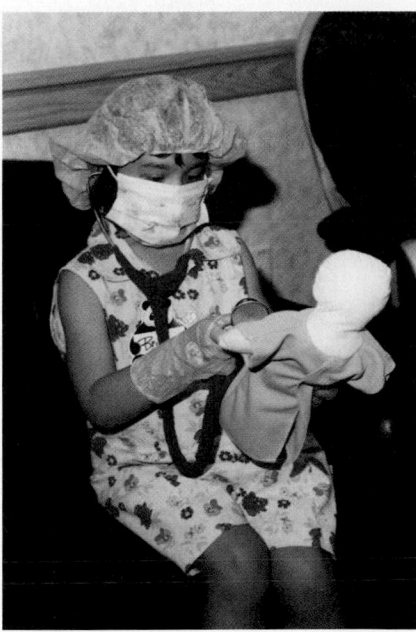

Figure 3-2 Hospitalized child using doll in her role-playing activity.

Teaching supports behavior change that leads to positive adaptation. Thus, teaching involves decreasing the fear of change. Reducing anxiety and anticipatory stress is an important component of teaching.

Patient education is an essential function of every professional nurse regardless of the practice setting. Table 3-5 outlines learning needs as they relate to the three phases of nursing care: primary, secondary, and tertiary. Patients who are hospitalized need information regarding their condition, the hospital environment, and expectations regarding treatment.

Documentation

The nurse is legally responsible to document patient education in the medical record. From a legal perspective, if the nurse teaches the patient but fails to document it, then the educational activities never occurred. Documentation of the teaching-learning event should include a summary of the learning need, the plan of action, implementation of the plan, and evaluation of the results. The evaluation phase is crucial. It must include who the nurse instructed. The nurse must document concrete evidence that the desired outcome was

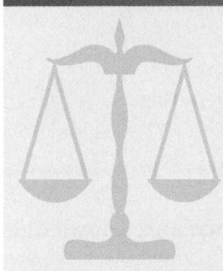

LAW IN PRACTICE

Patient Education and the Law

The nurse must remember the legal ramifications of patient education. Specific considerations are the informed consent, characteristics of the patient (e.g., age, mental condition, or anxiety), appropriate language of the information, and the timing of presenting the information. The nurse must present the information in wording that is understandable to the patient and ask the patient for clarifications regarding the information.

Source: Dempski, K. M., & Killion, S. W. (2001). Legal and ethical issues in nursing. *Thorofare, NJ: SLACK, Inc.*

TABLE 3-5 Learning Needs in Various Phases of Care		
PRIMARY: HEALTH MAINTENANCE	**SECONDARY: DIAGNOSIS AND TREATMENT**	**TERTIARY: FOLLOW-UP**
Disease prevention	Disease process	Care at home
Health care services availability	Methods of care and treatment	Medications
		Dietary modifications
Growth and development	Health care setting	Activity
		Rehabilitation plans
Safety		Prevention/recurrence of complications
First aid		
Nutrition		
Hygiene		

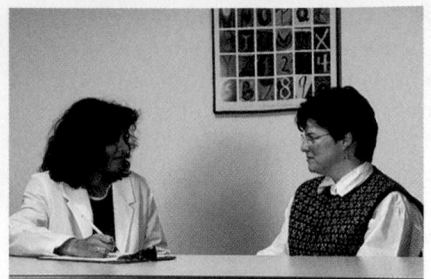

Figure 3-3 Documentation of patient education is an essential component of promoting the teaching-learning process.

achieved and what steps were taken if the outcome was not achieved. The medical record must contain evidence that the patient, caregiver, or significant other has actually learned the material taught. Documentation of teaching promotes continuity of care and facilitates accurate communication to other health care colleagues (Daniels, 2004) (Figure 3-3).

TEACHING-LEARNING AND THE NURSING PROCESS

The teaching-learning process and the nursing process are interdependent. Both are dynamic and consist of the same phases: assessment, diagnosis, planning, implementation, and evaluation.

Assessment

The nurse should assess each learning situation for every patient. Primary and secondary data sources are used by nurses for assessment of learning needs. Communicating with the patient and family or significant others is the foundation of assessment related to learning. Several factors need to be considered during assessment, including:

* Learning styles
* Learning needs
* Potential learning needs
* Ability to learn
* Readiness to learn
* Patient strengths
* Previous experience and knowledge base

Learning Styles

Each individual has a unique way of processing information. The manner in which an individual incorporates new data is called **learning style**. Some people learn by processing information visually (**visual learners**) (Figure 3-4), others by listening to words (**auditory learners**), and others by doing (**kinesthetic learners**). The nurse should use a variety of techniques, such as lecture, discussion, small group work, role-playing, modeling, return demonstration, imitation, problem solving, games, and question-and-answer sessions, to match different learning styles of patients. A good way to discover a patient's learning style is to ask the patient, "What helps you to learn?" or "What kinds of things do you enjoy doing?"

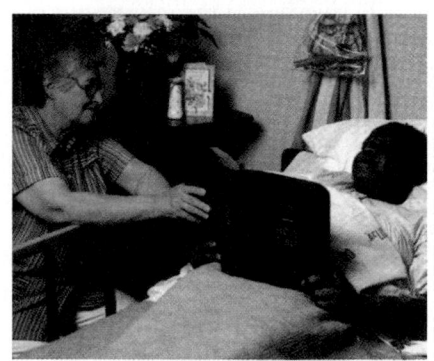

Figure 3-4 This patient is a visual learner, and the nurse is showing her written instructions for an upcoming procedure.

Learning Needs

Everyone who receives health care services has some need for learning. Patient education may be indicated when a patient:

* Expresses a need for information to make decisions
* Has a need for new skills
* Desires to make modifications in lifestyle
* Is in an unfamiliar environment

Comprehensive assessment is a mutual process between patient and nurse. A crucial step in teaching is to determine the patient's learning needs—what the patient needs to know and what the patient already knows. The nurse must evaluate the patient's knowledge about the content that is to be taught. This previous knowledge can then be used as a foundation for new concepts. If the patient is misinformed, the nurse develops a remediation plan for learning. Determination of the patient's learning needs is accomplished in a variety of ways, including:

* Questioning the patient directly
* Observing patient behaviors
* Interacting with the patient's family or significant others

It is imperative that the nurse address the patient's immediate need for knowledge first. This is facilitated by assessing the patient's perception of learning needs and prioritizing those needs on the basis of patient input and status.

Potential Learning Needs

The nurse also assesses for potential learning needs so that anticipatory planning can be done to avert a relapse in the recovery process and to maintain wellness. Some examples of anticipatory learning needs include:

- Mrs. Stone is pregnant for the first time. *Potential Learning Need:* Infant care
- Mr. Carpenter has just been diagnosed with diabetes that is currently controlled by dietary modifications. He has been told that he may have to take insulin daily in the future. *Potential Learning Need:* Self-administration of insulin

Ability to Learn

The nurse assesses the patient for characteristics that will hinder or facilitate learning. One such characteristic is the patient's developmental stage. For example, do not automatically assume that a patient who is 34 years old has mastered the developmental tasks of earlier stages. Age is not synonymous with developmental level; observation of behavior provides the clearest clue to developmental level.

The patient's maturity level greatly influences the ability to learn information. Every developmental stage is characterized by unique skills and abilities that affect the response to various teaching tools. Developmental stage greatly determines the type of data to be taught, the method(s) to be used, the language that is used, and the location for teaching. In addition to developmental stage, assessment should include evaluation of the patient's cognitive skills, problem-solving abilities, and attention span.

Readiness to Learn

Another characteristic to be assessed is the patient's learning readiness. Table 3-6 shows some factors that influence readiness.

Readiness is closely related to growth and development; for example, does the patient have the requisite cognitive and psychomotor skills for learning a particular task? Can the patient comprehend the information? Learning readiness is present when the patient asks questions. Another indicator that the patient is ready to learn is patient participation in learning activities, such as actively participating in return demonstration of a dressing change. Some behaviors that indicate lack of patient readiness are anxiety, avoidance, denial, lack of participation in discussion or demonstration, and lack of participation in self-care activities.

PATIENT PLAYBOOK

Learning Needs Assessment

Questions for the nurse to ask in determining the learning needs of the patient:
- Does the patient express uncertainty or anxiety over an upcoming procedure?
- Is the patient able to tell you about medications, purposes, and side effects?
- Can the patient describe necessary lifestyle modifications?
- Does the patient perform self-care activities correctly?
- Is the patient able to demonstrate necessary treatment procedures (e.g., colostomy irrigations, injections, or blood glucose monitoring)?

TABLE 3-6 Factors Influencing Learning Readiness

CAPABILITY	COMFORT	MOTIVATION
Maturity level	Basic physiological needs met	Care for self
Physical ability	Feelings of safety and security	Get well
Cognitive ability	Low degree (or absence of) pain	Achieve a higher level of wellness
Attitude	Pleasant surroundings with few distractions	Know and understand
	Rapport with caregiver	Return to work
		Please others
		Be a "good" patient
		Avoid complications and relapse

Closely related to readiness is patient motivation. Individuals must believe that they need to learn the information before learning occurs. Does the patient perceive relevance (meaningfulness) in the current information to be taught? If an individual sees the information as being personally valuable, the information is more likely to be learned. However, if the patient does not think that the content is relevant, learning is not likely to occur. Relevance is determined individually; the nurse must assess the personal meaning of learning content for each patient.

Albert Bandura, a psychologist, described the concept of **self-efficacy** (a belief that one will succeed in attempts to change behavior) as having a profound influence on motivation (1977). If patients feel they will not achieve the goals, they will lack motivation to try. To maximize motivation, keep the teaching-learning goals realistic. Break the content down into small steps that are achievable and provide feedback on the progress.

Patient Strengths

Identifying the patient's strengths and limitations provides a foundation for realistic expectations. An understanding of the patient's strengths and weaknesses allows the nurse to plan successful teaching-learning experiences. Determination of patient strengths assists the nurse in selecting appropriate teaching methods.

Previous Experience and Knowledge Base

The patient has a knowledge base acquired through life experiences. Previous knowledge affects the patient's attitudes about learning and perception of the importance of information to be learned and is related to the patient's type of educational experiences.

Certainly when considering a patient's previous knowledge, the nurse recognizes that culture plays an important role in knowledge acquisition. Attitudes (which are derived from a cultural context) toward what is appropriate to learn and who should teach may require alterations in the nurse's approach. The nurse's sensitivity to cultural values affects every aspect of the teaching-learning process.

Nursing Diagnoses

Several nursing diagnoses can apply to the patient when barriers to the learning process exist. When lack of knowledge is the primary barrier to learning, the diagnosis of *Deficient Knowledge* is applicable. For example:

- A patient who does not understand how to use crutches for assisted ambulation may have the diagnosis of *Deficient Knowledge: Crutchwalking*, related to inexperience as evidenced by multiple questions and hesitancy to walk.
- A patient who has had a colostomy and will be discharged soon may have a diagnosis of *Deficient Knowledge: Follow-Up Care* related to colostomy care and maintenance as evidenced by requests for information.

Deficient knowledge may also be a component of many other nursing diagnoses in which risk or impaired behavior exists. For instance, *Risk for Infection* may relate to a patient's compromised health status; this risk can be modified or reduced through certain physical and environmental changes and also through proper patient education. A patient presenting with a diagnosis of a *Self-Care Deficit: Bathing* may need assistance acquiring the physical supplies to remedy the deficit, as well as instruction in techniques related to present physical and mental abilities (Carpenito-Moyet, 2005).

Planning and Implementation

Informal teaching can occur in any setting at any time; formal teaching is planned and goal-directed. Teaching is a goal-directed, purposeful process, which means that teaching-learning activities must be planned. Learning is the process by which a person acquires or increases knowledge in a way that is measurable. It is the nurse's responsibility to adequately plan a formal teaching session. The teaching plan closely resembles a nursing care plan; both use the nursing process as a guide. Planning, an ongoing phase of the teaching process, involves consideration of the following:

- What to teach
- How to teach
- Who will teach and who will be taught
- When teaching will occur
- Where teaching will be done

Determination of *what* to teach is done through comprehensive assessment. The content to be taught depends greatly on the patient's knowledge base, readiness to learn, and current health status.

Deciding *how* to teach involves matching teaching strategies with patient's learning needs, readiness, and ability. The nurse who is an effective teacher uses methods that capture the patient's interest. A variety of teaching methods can be used to match the patient's learning styles.

Planning also means deciding *who* will teach the patient. Effective patient education is the result of a multidisciplinary effort. However, the nurse is the coordinator of the health care team's teaching activities. Responsibility for planning a comprehensive teaching approach, from admission to postdischarge, remains with the nurse. Continuity of care is greatly affected by the teaching plan.

Timing of *when* to teach should be carefully considered. The nurse recognizes that *every* interaction with the patient is an opportunity for informal teaching. Whenever a patient asks a question, there is an opportunity for teaching. These windows of teaching opportunities must be used.

In addition to capitalizing on informal teaching time, the nurse must plan time during which formal teaching can be done. Teaching must match the pace of the patient's progress. Some patients learn more quickly than others; some need more repetition. Timing of the teaching session is crucial. The more information presented, the more a patient is likely to forget. Therefore, teaching sessions must be kept brief to avoid overwhelming the patient. Throughout the teaching session, use repetition and frequently ask the patient questions to allow pacing the delivery of information.

An important part of planning in the teaching-learning process is goal setting. The patient and family or significant others must be involved in setting goals. Mutually determined learning goals promote learning. Specific learning goals should include these elements:

- Measurable behavioral change
- Time frame
- Methods and intervals for evaluation

Teaching-learning goals must be realistic, that is, based on the abilities of the learner and the teacher.

Establishing teaching-learning goals involves setting priorities. One way to prioritize goals is to teach the need-to-know information (which is necessary for survival) before moving on to the nice-to-know content. For example, Mrs. Stone, who is in her first trimester of pregnancy, *must* know guidelines for diet and exercise (need-to-know goal); learning about infant care can occur later in the pregnancy (nice-to-know goal).

Teaching Vulnerable Populations

When planning to teach individuals with special needs, it is important that the usual teaching strategies be modified according to the patient's individual needs. This section describes education of individuals who experience developmental delays, chronic illness, low literacy skills, and sensory impairments.

Developmental Delays

Individuals with limited cognitive abilities have a medical diagnosis of mental retardation if the intelligent quotient (IQ) level is 70 or less. The patient's learning depends on the degree of cognitive impairment, so teaching strategies

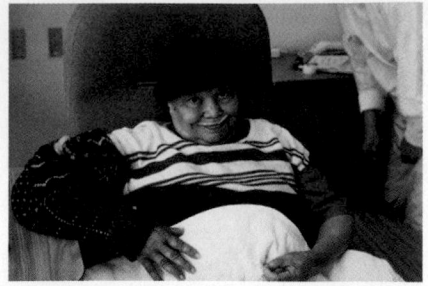

Figure 3-5 This patient is developmentally delayed and therefore requires the nurse to make specific adaptations in patient education techniques.

must be selected accordingly. For example, a patient who has mild mental retardation (IQ level of 50 to 70) may be able to learn by discussion of simple concepts that are stated in easily understood terms. Note that it is important to use concrete language and frequent repetition with patients in this category; the use of simple games is often effective. On the other hand, a patient who is profoundly mentally retarded (IQ level below 25) may be unable to learn in the traditional sense. Frequent communication and repetition are required when working with a patient with this degree of mental impairment (Figure 3-5).

Chronic Illness

Patients who experience chronic illness (e.g., arthritis, hypertension, diabetes, or asthma) have many learning needs, both actual and potential. Some chronic disorders, such as arthritis, may impair mobility and thus interfere with learning psychomotor skills as a result of decreased flexibility and dexterity of the fingers. Other chronic illnesses, such as diabetes, require ongoing assessment of the patient's level of understanding about self-care (e.g., diet, exercise, and lifestyle changes). Essential hypertension, another chronic disease process, often leads to patient's noncompliance with the prescribed treatment regimen. Ongoing education related to antihypertensive medication helps improve compliance.

Low Literacy Skills

It is imperative that nurses assess the reading and comprehension abilities of patients before using printed educational materials. The majority of health care teaching involves the use of printed materials. It is a common mistake to equate the highest educational level achieved with reading level. Typically, individuals read at three to five grade levels lower than their achieved educational level.

Sensory Impairments

Many patients have sensory impairments as a result of illness, injury, or the aging process. Effective nurses modify their teaching approaches to accommodate such impairments. A common mistake many people make when talking with someone who has a sensory impairment is to talk loudly. Screaming and yelling do not help the person who has auditory or visual impairments. See the accompanying Patient Playbook ("Guidelines for Teaching Patients with Sensory Impairments") for guidelines in working with patient's who have visual, auditory, or memory impairments.

Implementation

Implementation of the teaching plan may not go as envisioned. The nurse must constantly assess the patient's response during this phase. Fatigue, pain, fear, and ambivalence can alter the patient's ability to learn. The nurse needs to speak in terms the patient understands, be specific on what is to be covered, and keep the message short and concise. The patient may become bored or confused if too much information is given in one setting. Questions and interactive dialogue can help keep the patient engaged (Estes, 2006).

There are several characteristics of nurses that influence the outcome of the teaching-learning process. Nursing self-awareness, an all-important first step in teaching, focuses on the concepts discussed in the following sections. The Patient Playbook ("Guidelines for Effective Patient Teaching") provides some implementation guidelines for making teaching more meaningful to patients.

Knowledge Base

It is impossible for nurses to teach if they lack the knowledge or skills that are to be taught. Staying current in knowledge and proficient in skills is the first step to maintaining efficacy and credibility as a teacher. It is impossible for one individual to be an expert in every area of nursing. Therefore, knowing when to refer the patient to others for teaching can augment learning.

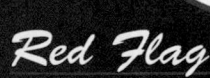

Interpersonal Skills

Effective teaching is based on the nurse's ability to establish rapport with the patient. The nurse who is empathic to the patient shows sensitivity to the patient's needs and preferences. An atmosphere in which the patient feels free to ask questions promotes learning. Activities that help establish an environment conducive to learning include:

- Showing genuine interest in the patient.
- Including the patient in *every* step of the teaching- learning process.
- Using a nonjudgmental approach.
- Communicating at the patient's level of understanding.

Evaluation of Outcomes

Evaluation of teaching-learning is a twofold process:

1. Determining what the patient has learned
2. Assessing the nurse's teaching effectiveness

Evaluation of Learning

Evaluation is the last step of the teaching process. It is a continuous and crucial step in the teaching process. Evaluation includes determining if the teaching session was successful and if the patient learned the intended information. Evaluation also provides the needed evidence that the patient received and understood the educational material. The nurse can ascertain this information by asking these questions:

- Is there a change in behavior?
- Is the behavior change related to learning activities?
- Is further change necessary?
- Will continued behavior change promote improved health?

The accompanying Patient Playbook ("Evaluation of Learning") provides guidelines for evaluating the patient's achieved learning.

Evaluation of Teaching

A major purpose of evaluation is to assess the effectiveness of the teaching activities and decide which modifications, if any, are necessary. When learning objectives are not met, reassessment is the basis for planning modification of teaching-learning activities. Several activities can evaluate teaching effectiveness, including the following:

- Feedback from the learner
- Feedback from colleagues
- Situational feedback
- Self-evaluation

Evaluation is facilitated through the use of goals that are measurable and specific. Use of the accompanying Patient Playbook ("Evaluation of Teacher Effectiveness") facilitates evaluation of teacher effectiveness.

Patient education has been proven to decrease the length of hospital days, improve the general quality of care, decrease visits needed from home care, and improve patient adherence to the plan of care (Hitchcock, Schubert, & Thomas, 2003).

HEALTH MAINTENANCE

Health maintenance is defined as behavior directed toward maintaining a current level of health. **Health maintenance activities** are the activities and behaviors an individual performs to maintain or improve a current level of health.

Characteristics of Health Maintenance

The patient can do more to maintain health than anyone else. There are no quick fixes or shortcuts to be successful in achieving health maintenance. To be successful in changing health behavior, the patient must take time to prepare and plan. Often the outcomes of health-related behaviors are the primary focus. However, it is important to also examine the role of motivation and attitudes about health status and the ability to change health status. Normal health maintenance can be conceptualized by three characteristics: (a) perception, (b) motivation, and (c) maintenance, which are examined as follows (Edelman & Mandle, 2002).

Perception

The ability of a patient to adopt and maintain healthy behaviors depends on the patient's **perception** (i.e., a person's sense and understanding of the world) of his or her current health status, and his or her level of knowledge regarding the effect of the behaviors and how to maintain these behaviors. First, the patient must identify the behavior(s) to be maintained or changed. If the patient does not perceive a problem with his or her current health maintenance activities, it would be futile for the nurse to try to intervene at this point. The nurse first must work with the patient to show how the lack of health-promotive activities is not beneficial (Daniels, 2004).

Motivation

Motivation (i.e., the internal drive or externally arising stimulus to action or thought) to maintain a current level of health or achieve an optimal level of health must come from the patient. Other factors can help or hinder the patient's success for behavior management. Environment, support or nonsupport from friends and family, and genetic makeup all affect the person's ability to manage healthy behaviors. A friend suffering a heart attack or developing a chronic illness may energize a person to reevaluate his or her current health practices. At this point, the motivation for change may be high, but the person may lack the knowledge of how to undertake this change in behavior. A motivated person will seek health information, activities, and groups or organizations that support achieving wellness. The challenge to the nurse is to identify the patient's level of motivation. Then the nurse must provide interventions that increase the patient's motivation (Edelman & Mandle, 2002).

Maintenance

The maintenance of new health behaviors is challenging for patients. Learning a new behavior is not difficult; the difficulty comes in maintaining the behavior. For the new behaviors to be beneficial, they must be practiced for the long term. Once new health behaviors have been adopted, it is crucial to have the tools needed to maintain them. Time and preparation are required to maintain healthy behaviors.

HEALTH PROMOTION AND DISEASE PREVENTION

Two basic components of health maintenance are health promotion and disease prevention or health protection. **Health promotion** is behavior motivated by the desire to increase the levels of health and well-being and actualize or maximize the health potential of individuals, families, groups, communities, and society. **Disease prevention or health protection** is behavior motivated by a desire to actively avoid illness, detect it early, or maintain functioning within the constraints of an illness (Figure 3-6). Health promotion includes activities undertaken by health professionals to promote health and includes health education and counseling.

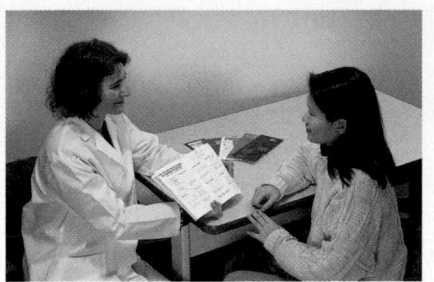

Figure 3-6 The nurse is providing disease prevention teaching strategies for this patient with juvenile diabetes.

It is often difficult to differentiate between health promotion and disease prevention because the two overlap and complement each other. The most important difference between health promotion and health protection or disease prevention is the underlying motivation for the behavior. For example, an individual who lives a sedentary lifestyle may begin an exercise program (health maintenance) and continue this behavior after attainment of his or her goals, because he or she feels better practicing these behaviors (health promotion).

Health Promotion

Health promotion begins with the mindset to shape a healthy lifestyle. Health promotion is the process of enabling people to increase control over their health and to improve their health through development of human resources and behaviors that maintain or enhance well-being. From an individual standpoint, health promotion means the practice of positive health behaviors (see Box 3-3). Health promotion also includes avoidance of unhealthy behaviors (e.g., smoking, drug use, and excessive consumption of alcohol). Health promotion efforts intervene with healthy rather than ill populations to help maximize their health status. Individuals who participate in health promotive behaviors strive toward a high level of wellness rather than just being disease free (Pender, Murdaugh, & Parsons, 2002).

HEALTH PROMOTION ON A GLOBAL LEVEL

On global, national, and local levels, health promotion is still being developed, with the World Health Organization (WHO) leading the way with international conferences and meetings and dissemination of successful health promotion strategies, programs, and policies. In 2000, the WHO, the Pan American Health Organization (PAHO), and the Ministry of Health of Mexico hosted the Fifth Global Conference on Health Promotion (5GCHP). The 5GCHP took forward the priorities for health promotion in the 21st century, which were identified at the Fourth Global Conference on Health Promotion in Jakarta in 1997 (Flynn, 1997) and confirmed by the Health Promotion Resolution adopted by the World Health Assembly in May 1998. The priorities are shown in Box 3-3.

BOX 3-3

PRIORITIES FOR HEALTH PROMOTION IN THE 21ST CENTURY

1. Promoting social responsibility for health.
2. Increasing community capacity and empowering the individual.
3. Increasing investments for health development.
4. Securing an infrastructure for health promotion.
5. Strengthening the evidence base for health promotion.
6. Reorienting health systems and health services.

Source: World Health Organization. (2002). World health report 2002: Reducing risks, promoting healthy lifestyles. *Geneva, Switzerland. Retrieved September 8, 2006, from www.who.int.*

TABLE 3-7 Healthy People 2010 Objectives

OBJECTIVE	DESCRIPTION	EXAMPLES
Promote healthy behaviors	Focuses on behaviors resulting from personal choice	Physical activity Nutrition Tobacco use
Promote healthy and safe communities	Addresses programs that have an impact on individual health through education and community-based programs	Environmental health Food safety Occupational health Injury prevention Violence prevention
Improve systems for personal health and public health	Emphasizes the need for all citizens to have access to health care services (goal: to reduce racial and ethnic disparities)	Maternal, infant, and child Family planning Medical product safety Health education Public health infrastructure
Prevent and reduce diseases and disorders	Outlines specific interventions related to chronic, prevalent health problems	Cancer Cardiovascular disease Stroke Arthritis Mental illness

Data from Chrvala, C. A., & Bulger, R. J. (1999). Leading health indicators for Healthy People 2010: Final report, Division of Health Promotion and Disease Prevention, Institute of Medicine. Washington, DC: National Academy of Press; Wilson, L. M. (1999). Healthy people—a new millennium: Progress and comparison on the Healthy People 2000 and Healthy People 2010 objectives. JONAs Healthcare Law, Ethics, and Regulation, 1(2), 29–32.

HEALTH PROMOTION IN THE UNITED STATES

The United States Public Health Service (1990), in its *Healthy People 2000* initiative, focused on the individual's responsibility in promoting health. The individual is viewed as having the ability to influence his or her own health and also that of the country.

In 1979, the U.S. Department of Health and Human Services mobilized public health agencies to work toward developing healthier Americans. This initiative, *Healthy People,* is now in its third decade and is called *Healthy People 2010.* The program, coordinated by the U.S. Public Health Service, will focus efforts on allowing equal access of all Americans to preventive health care services. Most states use the *Healthy People* framework to guide the development and implementation of local health policies and programs. *Healthy People 2010* recognizes the need to focus on improving the quality of life, as well as reducing disparities in the type of health care services received by Americans (Centers for Disease Control and Prevention, 2005a).

Healthy People 2010 has established the four objectives that are to be emphasized through the efforts of health care agencies, both public and private, for the next 20 years; see Table 3-7.

ASSESSMENT

The first functional health pattern (Gordon, 1997) is health perception–health management. The focus of this health pattern is the patient's own perception of health and well-being, and how the patient manages his or her health

(health maintenance). Applying the nursing process is instrumental in addressing the strategies for alterations in health maintenance. The nurse must begin with the assessment phase of the nursing process.

The focus of assessing health maintenance is determining the patient's health status. Examples of objective data for assessing health maintenance include such things as the potential or actual risk factors for ineffective health maintenance and laboratory and diagnostic tests. Subjective data obtained from asking questions (and listening) assists the nurse to identify functional and dysfunctional patterns of health maintenance.

Risk Factor Identification in Health Maintenance

Identifying risks that could decrease health is essential in the assessment of health maintenance. Risks to health behavior can be physical, environmental, or psychological behaviors that increase an individual's vulnerability to disease or injury. Risk factors also include the following interrelated categories: genes, physiology, age, physical environment, and lifestyle. These factors vary in intensity, and multiple risk factors may interact to develop additional risk factors. Assessing the patient's knowledge of his or her risk factors can lead to the identification of health promotion and disease prevention activities. The nurse should assess for cues during the nursing history process that warn of the presence of a risk factor. Many tools are available for risk identification, and the nurse must carefully assess for potential or actual risk factors (Edelman & Mandle, 2002).

Diagnostic Tests

Laboratory data (e.g., cholesterol levels, blood glucose, urine studies) are important pieces of information in assessing health maintenance. Health and maintenance behaviors may be measured with varieties of diagnostic tests and equipment, such as pregnancy tests, blood glucose monitors, thermometers, body fat calculators, and sphygmomanometers (Figure 3-7). It is important for nurses to make sure patients know the proper use and maintenance of the equipment. It is also necessary to educate patients on what to do with the results obtained from these tests. Patients may monitor blood pressure at home, but never contact the health care provider with elevated readings. Patients may think they are practicing health maintenance activities appropriately, while in reality, they may be putting their health in jeopardy.

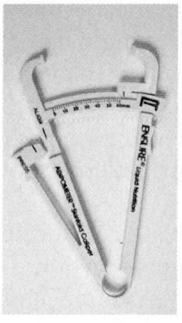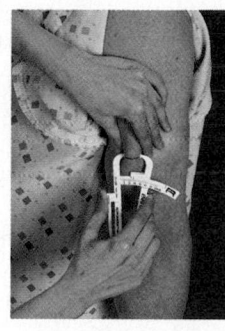

Figure 3-7 Body fat measurement device.

NURSING DIAGNOSES

Alterations in health maintenance are caused by a patient's inability to perform the daily functions needed to maintain health. The nurse's role is to first assess the patient and then to select the appropriate nursing diagnosis pertinent to the patient's condition. The selected nursing diagnoses will be identified by the defining characteristics of the patient's condition (see Box 3-4). Several nursing diagnoses are typical for the functional health pattern of health maintenance. These nursing diagnoses are *Ineffective Health Maintenance, Health-Seeking Behavior, Noncompliance, Deficient Knowledge,* and *Ineffective Therapeutic Regimen Management.* After selecting the nursing diagnoses, the nurse identifies the risk factors that contribute to the patient's dysfunctional health maintenance. Expected outcomes are developed to direct the patient in pursuit of health, and the nurse devises interventions with the patient to improve health status.

Red Flag

Health Maintenance Involving Diagnostic Tests for Diabetes

Patients with diabetes may not take appropriate measures when their blood glucose readings are high. These patients must be taught parameters for which they should contact their health care providers. For example, readings above 300 mg/dL and clinical manifestations, such as nausea and vomiting, abdominal pain, severe fatigue, and muscle cramps, should be reported to the health care provider. Out-of-control diabetic crises require immediate attention and management to prevent severe complications.

Source: Daniels, R. (2003). Delmar's manual of laboratory and diagnostic tests. Clifton Park, NY: Thomson Delmar Learning.

BOX 3-4

DEFINING CHARACTERISTICS FOR INEFFECTIVE HEALTH MAINTENANCE

The following are typical defining characteristics for the nursing diagnoses in alterations in health maintenance:

- Impairment of personal support systems
- Observed inability to take responsibility for meeting basic health practices
- Demonstrated lack of knowledge
- Failure to recognize important symptoms reflective of altered health state
- Lack of health-seeking behaviors
- Inadequate resources (e.g., equipment, finances, or care providers)

PLANNING AND IMPLEMENTATION

In identifying goals and planning nursing care for patients with alterations in health maintenance, the nurse considers patient outcomes for each nursing diagnosis and each patient. The goals that are developed will be individualized to reflect the patient's capabilities and limitations. In many ineffective health maintenance situations, the desired outcomes of care are best accomplished in small increments.

The patient outcomes for an individual patient are developed from the assessment data that led to the most appropriate nursing diagnosis (see Box 3-5). For example, if a patient with diabetes is dependent on insulin and becomes unemployed, the desired outcome for interventions could be obtaining the necessary resources to enable purchasing the insulin to not miss any doses of the medication. Achievement of the outcome resolves the problem for the patient.

Nurses play a vital role in promoting health and wellness. Through health promotion and risk reduction, the individual develops behavior patterns that promote a healthy lifestyle and reduce the risk of disease.

The challenge for nurses is to ensure policies and programs are conducive to health promotion. For example, it is not only a class on proper nutrition to enable people to change unhealthy eating patterns but also the economic and structural resources that are required for good nutrition.

Another challenge for nurses is to find a way to motivate individuals and families to develop health promoting behaviors. When behaviors that once worked for the individual are no longer effective, the individual must give up the old behaviors to be able to adopt new, healthier ones. Teaching is an intervention for promoting health along with the supportive economic and structural conditions necessary for changing a behavior. (Table 3-8) An essential component of teaching is encouraging patients to make necessary lifestyle changes to promote health.

Motivation is a vital component of achieving and maintaining health. Nurses can better help patients engage in healthy behaviors by considering the patient's beliefs and experiences when planning care. Many factors help patients feel motivated to change health behaviors:

- Perception of self as able to succeed (self-efficacy)
- Belief that health status will improve
- Response to their attempts to change in the form of feeling healthier and receiving confirmation of these changes from others

Needs and Health

To implement holistic nursing interventions in health maintenance situations, the nurse takes into account the existing human needs. Because human beings are not merely physiological creatures, basic human needs occur in

PATIENT OUTCOMES FOR INEFFECTIVE HEALTH MAINTENANCE

Examples of patient outcomes for ineffective health maintenance are:

- Follows mutually acceptable health care maintenance plan
- Meets goals for health care maintenance
- Describes positive health-maintenance behaviors
- Identifies available resources for meeting health-maintenance alterations

the emotional, sociocultural, intellectual, and spiritual realms as well as the physiological realm. The entire person (body, mind, and spirit) is influenced by satisfaction of needs. A variety of needs emerge, are met, and reemerge in each area of a person's life.

A need is anything that is absolutely *essential* for one's existence. **Basic human needs** (also known as universal needs) are those that are necessary for every person's survival. Table 3-9 provides an overview of basic needs.

Maslow (1970) classified human needs as they occur on a tier with the most basic needs at the foundation of the hierarchy (Figure 3-8). These basic needs must be met before the individual can satisfy higher level needs. For example, an individual who is starving must be fed before achieving the need for acceptance. An individual with a deficient self-esteem and who is hemorrhaging must have the biological needs met first. The satisfaction of basic needs enhances wellness. Conversely, an impairment in the satisfaction of basic needs can result in a patient's altered health status.

The following section describes implementing nursing care in addressing the basic needs related to the physiological, psychological, sociocultural, intellectual, spiritual, and sexual dimensions.

Physiological Dimension

Providing physiological care focuses on the achievement of the basic needs of a patient. The nurse must assess the patient for the alterations that are occurring and then provide interventions to meet the patient's needs. There are many physiological needs in health maintenance, and several examples of physiological interventions are provided in this section.

Physical Self-Examination Techniques

Physical self-examination is a health maintenance behavior that does not require any special equipment but requires proper instruction on the correct procedure. Breast self-examinations, testicular examinations, and skin examinations should begin at age 18 for women and age 15 for men. The examinations should be performed monthly. The nurse encourages the patient to select a day that is easy to remember (e.g., the first day of the month). Then the nurse instructs the patient

---

TABLE 3-8 Strategies for Health Promotion

HEALTH PROMOTION STRATEGIES	HEALTH PROMOTION *IS NOT*	HEALTH PROMOTION *IS*
Creating supportive environments	Recommending stress management courses for men	Creating an environment that includes men in a team approach to decision making regarding stress management
Strengthening community action and participation	Creating a women's group around an outside agenda	Responding to issues identified by women in partnership with other groups and community members
Developing healthy public policy	Imposing a policy that has been developed without consultation of the affected individuals and communities	Developing effective smoking restrictions in consultation with the affected individuals and and communities
Developing personal skills	Giving an adolescent a pamphlet or fact sheet about risky health behaviors	Offering a program that develops adolescent skills for decision making related to risky health behaviors
Reorienting health care services	A health care organization setting program priorities for families	Families defining their own health issues and creating the solutions

Adapted from Pender, J., Murdaugh, C., & Parsons, M. A. (2002). Health promotion in nursing practice (4th ed.). Upper Saddle River, NJ: Prentice-Hall.

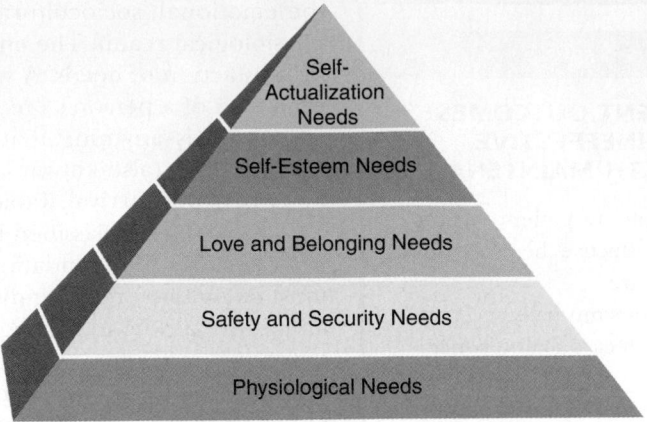

Figure 3-8 Maslow's hierarchy of needs

TABLE 3-9	**Basic Human Needs**
NEED	**EXAMPLE**
Physiological	Oxygen, water, food, temperature (shelter and clothing), elimination, sleep, activity, and sex
Psychological	Self-esteem, feelings of security, happiness, sadness
Sociocultural	Feelings of belonging, relationships
Intellectual	Thinking, learning
Spiritual	Being connected to others, having a sense of purpose

on the correct technique of the self-examination. In addition, a return demonstration by the patient is essential to ensure the patient performs the examination properly (Estes, 2006). It is important that the nurse instructs the patient in what to look for and what action to take if an abnormal finding is identified.

Health Maintenance in Nutrition Management Behaviors

Inadequate nutritional intake affects the activities of daily living. The exact number of health problems that can be directly attributed to the diet are unknown. Throughout the life cycle, nutritional needs change in relation to growth, development, and activity levels. In children, hunger compromises the ability to learn. Hungry children have a higher absentee rate, and when they do attend school, they have a difficult time concentrating. Inadequate nutrition can have a lasting effect on a child's cognitive development. Inadequate nutrition in adults impairs their ability to concentrate, which in turn can lead to poor work performance. Energy levels are also compromised. Inadequate nutrition also weakens a person's immune system, increasing susceptibility to illness and disease. Nursing interventions include such things as educating the patient with information regarding food groups and recommended nutrients, selecting a diet plan that meets the patient's nutrition needs, advising the patient to keep a food journal to monitor the dietary intake, assisting the patient and family to access resources for obtaining nutritious food, and teaching the patient the clinical manifestations associated with nutrient deficiencies or excess (Roth, 2007).

Health Maintenance and Alterations in Sleep Patterns

Another health maintenance problem that affects activities of daily living is the lack of sleep. Sleep accomplishes restoration of physical well-being, relieves anxiety and stress, and restores the ability to cope and concentrate on activities of daily living. Poor sleep patterns can affect a person's ability to concentrate at work and school, resulting in a negative effect on their performance. Exercise, smoking, alcohol consumption, illness, and stress can all affect a person's sleep patterns. The nurse can suggest that the patient monitor sleep patterns and keep a journal of hours of sleep for each 24-hour period. In addition, the patient can be encouraged to establish a routine bedtime to facilitate the transition from wakefulness to sleep.

Psychological Dimension

Individuals have psychological needs for security, a sense of belonging, and self-esteem. Nursing actions that promote a sense of emotional comfort include the following:
- Treating the patient as a unique individual
- Protecting confidentiality and privacy
- Using touch and personal space in a therapeutic manner
- Recognizing and respecting cultural differences
- Decreasing anxiety through stress management techniques

Goals for patients experiencing unmet psychological needs usually revolve around the following issues:
- Improve self-esteem
- Establish trusting relationships
- Develop social skills
- Cope with losses

Sociocultural Dimension

As social creatures, all people rely on others to some extent. Research has shown that social connection is correlated with positive health outcomes. It is difficult for some people to ask for help or to accept assistance when it is offered. It is important for nurses to assess the patient's degree of dependence. Often, the nurse becomes involved in a balancing act in an effort to maintain equilibrium between the patient's needs for dependence and independence.

Empowerment is a process of enabling others to do for themselves. It consists of encouraging the patient to be an active participant in treatment rather than a passive recipient of care. Nurses empower patients by teaching them and their families how to develop skills for self-care and for healthier living.

Intellectual Dimension

The intellectual dimension consists of cognitive functions, such as judgment, orientation, memory, and the ability to take in and process information.

Intellectual functioning can be impaired by multiple factors, including infection, exposure to toxins, substance abuse, trauma, and psychological problems. It is important for nurses to determine the patient's intellectual abilities to communicate effectively. Using words that are easily comprehended by the patient and implementing teaching strategies appropriate to developmental level promotes patient learning.

Spiritual Dimension

Spirituality is multidimensional in that it refers to one's relationship with one's self, a sense of connection with others, and a relationship with a higher power or divine source. Spirituality assists a person in determining the sense of meaning or purpose in one's life. It is an integral component, or core, of one's being. Spirituality is somewhat difficult to define, as it is determined at an individual level.

Spirituality is *not* the same as religion, which refers to a set of beliefs and practices associated with a particular church, synagogue, mosque, or other formal organized group. Spirituality is a personal, individualized set of beliefs and practices that are not church related.

Sexual Dimension

Sexuality is a complex human characteristic that refers not just to genital sex but to all the aspects of being male or female, including feelings, attitudes, beliefs, and behavior. It is an essential part of one's personality. Sexuality is a pervasive aspect of the total self from birth to death and is an important aspect of health for people of all ages. Sexuality includes a person's attitudes toward relationships with people of the same sex, relationships with those of the opposite sex, and about touching and being touched. The ways people dress, talk, and relate to others are indicators of their sexuality.

Sex roles are culturally determined patterns associated with being male and female. These patterns are developed as a result of cultural expectations, customs, norms, habits, and traditions. For example, the differences between the sexes are evident in the ways infants are treated during their first days of life. Infant boys and infant girls are talked to, handled, and, many times, dressed differently. In many cultures, the role of the man is to be strong and protective, whereas the woman is expected to be passive and nurturing. Sex roles change as societal norms change and may be accepted or rejected by individuals.

EVALUATION OF OUTCOMES

Evaluation of outcomes is essential in the health maintenance-health pattern of an individual. The patient and nurse together must measure how well the patient has achieved the goals specified in the plan of care. Factors that contribute to the patient's ability to achieve the goal are identified. This is also when goals may need to be reevaluated and adjusted accordingly.

Case Study

Nursing Care Plan

Miranda is a 23-year-old who has been an insulin-dependent diabetic since she was 15. Compliance with her diet, exercise, and insulin regimen has always been difficult for Miranda. As a teenager, Miranda did not want to be seen as different, which was a barrier to her compliance. More recently, Miranda learned she is three months pregnant. She is concerned about the health of her baby and the potential complications related to the fact that she has diabetes. Miranda comes to your outpatient diabetic education class for instruction on how to take care of herself and her developing baby. During your assessment of Miranda, you discover she could improve the technique for giving insulin injections. She also does not have a good understanding of her diabetic diet.

Assessment

Patient lacks both knowledge of proper insulin injection technique and understanding of her diabetic diet. She is expressing a desire to become proficient and educated in diabetic care for herself and the well-being of her unborn baby. Patient's blood glucose level was 192 at the clinic, and she could not verbalize the normal range of her blood glucose levels.

Nursing Diagnosis 1: *Deficient Knowledge* related to insulin injection technique and American Diabetic Association (ADA) diet as evidenced by uncontrolled blood sugars and patient's demonstration of improper injection technique.

Case Study

NOC: Knowledge of diabetes and medication therapy; health behaviors; treatment regimen

NIC: Teaching: Individual; Teaching: Diabetes Management

Expected Outcomes

The patient will:

1. Explain and return-demonstrate correct insulin injection technique (cognitive and psychomotor domains) during visit to clinic. *Learning mode of demonstration is valid for learning physical skills.*
2. Verbalize confidence in self-administration of correct insulin dosages. *Self-confidence increases level of performance.*
3. *Learn self-care of diabetes as shown through her attendance at diabetic education classes.* Reflects internal motivation and adherence to treatment regimen.
4. Explain and identify proper foods for ADA diet. *Verifies knowledge and retention of disease process information.*

Planning, Interventions, Rationales

1. Ask patient, through the interview process, what teaching strategies (discussion, visual aids, etc.) are the most effective ways for her to learn. *Matching teaching strategies to learning styles and needs increases likelihood of a successful and productive educational experience.*
2. *Explain briefly mechanics of proper insulin injection techniques and rationale for such.* Knowledge of the correct technique for insulin injection will help the patient understand the mechanics of administering insulin.
3. Demonstrate proper insulin injection techniques. *Proper injection technique is vital for insulin to work properly. Observing proper technique will help Miranda be able to perform it properly.*
4. *Encourage patient to have her husband learn proper insulin technique and ADA diet.* He will be able to give injection confidently if necessary and can help reinforce with her the proper technique. He will also be able to help with meal planning.

Evaluation

Patient verbalizes proper sequence and technique for insulin injection. Patient performs return demonstration of drawing up and administering insulin using sterile and proper technique, requiring minimal verbal cueing. Correctly identifies proper food for her prescribed ADA diet.

KEY CONCEPTS

- Patient education is done to help individuals achieve optimum states of health.
- The teaching-learning process is a planned interaction promoting behavioral change that is not a result of maturation or coincidence.
- Teaching supports behavior change that leads to positive adaptation.

- Learning is the process of assimilating information with a resultant change in behavior.
- Learning occurs in three domains: the cognitive (intellectual), the affective (emotional), and the psychomotor (motor skills).
- Elements for documenting patient education include the content taught, teaching methods used, who was taught, and response of the learners.

Continued

KEY CONCEPTS—cont'd

- The teaching-learning process and the nursing process are interdependent dynamic processes.
- Evaluation of the teaching-learning process involves two aspects: (a) determination of what the patient has learned and (b) efficacy of the teacher.
- Identify teaching strategies for patient education.
- The three approaches to health maintenance (health promotion, health protection, and disease prevention) are centered on the individual's and society's responsibility in promoting one's own health.
- Nurses play a role in helping patients to adopt healthy lifestyles and use approaches such as role modeling and formal teaching to motivate patient change.
- Nurses must focus their efforts on improving the health status of vulnerable populations.

- The satisfaction of basic human needs, such as physiological, psychological, sociocultural, intellectual, and spiritual needs, is necessary for every person's survival.
- Lifestyle, locus of control, self-efficacy, health care attitudes, and self-concept are examples of variables that influence health-promoting behaviors.
- An impairment in meeting basic needs results in an altered health status.
- Health protection, disease prevention, and health promotion are centered on individual and societal responsibilities for health.
- Nurses must focus their efforts on supporting and creating policy, structural resources, and economic resources that are conducive to health promotion.

REVIEW QUESTIONS

1. Mr. Carter reaches a learning plateau. This is a(n):
   1. Indicator that he is unwilling to learn
   2. Peak in the effectiveness of the teaching process
   3. Philosophy that adheres to the learner not being important to the teaching-learning process
   4. Time when teaching is received at its optimum level

2. Mrs. Myers learns best by understanding the material that is presented with her mind. This is which domain of learning?
   1. Affective domain
   2. Psychomotor domain
   3. Cognitive domain
   4. Emotional domain

3. The nurse allows the patient with diabetes to give an injection to a synthetic material that is similar to a real arm. This is an example of which of the following teaching strategies?
   1. Discussion
   2. Programmed instruction
   3. Role-playing
   4. Demonstration

4. Mr. Duncan learns best when he is able to physically do something. This is which type of learning style?
   1. Visual learning
   2. Auditory learning
   3. Kinesthetic learning
   4. Cognitive learning

5. Mrs. White truly believes that if she "puts her mind to it" she can quit smoking. This is an example of:
   1. Self-efficacy
   2. Self-esteem
   3. External locus of control
   4. Extrinsic motivation

6. Mr. Ladner is memory impaired. Which of the following is the best strategy in teaching him new information regarding changing his ostomy appliance?
   1. Use signals to reinforce verbal information
   2. Ask for feedback and listen actively
   3. Use repetition
   4. Use short sentences and words that are easily understood

7. Mrs. Cox does not believe that her diverticulitis is serious enough to need to change her dietary habits. This is an example of a problem with?
   1. Motivation
   2. Perception
   3. Self-esteem
   4. Disease prevention

8. Two basic components of health maintenance are:
   1. Health promotion and wellness
   2. Disease prevention and patient education
   3. Health promotion and disease prevention
   4. Disease prevention and risk factor identification

Continued

REVIEW QUESTIONS—cont'd

9. Which of the following is not a health promotion strategy?
   1. Developing an effective smoking cessation program
   2. Creating an environment that is conducive to making decisions regarding reducing stress
   3. Imposing a health policy that an individual must follow
   4. Encouraging families to define their own health solutions

10. Which of the following is accurate concerning basic human needs?
    1. The sociocultural dimension refers to being connected to others and having a sense of purpose.
    2. The intellectual dimension describes the feelings of belonging that one person has for others.
    3. The psychological dimension are those characteristics of self-esteem, feelings of security, and those feelings that create a sense of belonging.
    4. The physiological dimension is made up of the emotional and cognitive aspects of a person.

REVIEW ACTIVITIES

1. Give an example of each of the three domains of learning.

2. List four barriers to learning. What nursing interventions would you implement to overcome each barrier?

3. Why is it important for the nurse to use more than one teaching method?

4. What are some of your own learning needs right now? How are they being addressed?

5. Develop a flow sheet for patient teaching to use in one of your clinical agencies.

6. Identify two learning needs of a selected patient. What will you do to help the patient overcome the knowledge deficits?

Continued

REVIEW ACTIVITIES—cont'd

7. What are the nursing implications of Maslow's hierarchy of basic needs?

8. Select a classmate to interview. Note any relationship between attitudes and physical symptoms. Does your partner feel better physically when mentally relaxed? Vice versa?

9. Interview five people in your community. Ask them how they know when they are healthy. Compare the answers, and develop a brief list of determinants of health.

10. Think about motivation and lifestyle changes. What motivates you to engage in healthy behaviors? How can you find incentives to use in teaching patients about the need to modify habits that affect health?

Culturally Sensitive Care

Diana Rodrigues, RN, PhD

CHAPTER TOPICS

- Concepts of Culture

- Multiculturalism in the United States

- Cultural Disparities in Health and Health Care Delivery

- Transcultural Nursing

- Cultural Competence

- Cultural Competence and Nursing Process

KEY TERMS

Acculturation
Cultural assimilation
Cultural competence
Cultural context
Cultural diversity
Culture
Dominant culture
Environmental control
Ethnicity
Ethnocentrism
Extrinsic distortion
Intrinsic distortion
Minority group
Oppression
Race
Racism
Stereotyping
Subculture

As human beings we are connected with one another. There are also many differences among us; particularly differences in culture, lifestyle, ethnicity, and religion. Despite the commonalities, our differences can and do separate us from one another. In the United States nurses are predominantly Caucasian and female, and their patients are continuing to grow in cultural, religious, racial, and linguistic diversity (Spector, 2004). As the population of the United States continues to diversify, recognition of cultural and linguistic differences and their impact on health care is more critical to providing optimal nursing care. Behavior, including behavior that affects health and health promotion, is, in part, culturally determined. This chapter discusses the various concepts related to culture, the importance of diversity in American society, the influence of culture on health, transcultural nursing, and culturally competent nursing care.

CONCEPTS OF CULTURE

Each individual is culturally unique. Behavior, self-perception, and judgment of others all depend on cultural perspective. Nurses have long valued holistic care. To provide holistic care the nurse needs a thorough understanding of dominant cultural concepts.

Culture

Culture refers to knowledge, beliefs, behaviors, ideas, attitudes, values, habits, customs, languages, symbols, rituals, ceremonies, and practices that are unique to a particular group of people. A structure of knowledge, behaviors, and values provides a group with a blueprint, or general design, for living that guides them in their worldview and decision making (Figure 4-1). **Cultural context** refers to the environment or situation that is relevant to the care, beliefs, values, and practices of a culture.

Culture is not static, and it is not uniform among all members within cultural groups. Culture represents adaptive dynamic processes learned through life experiences. People have culturally predetermined values and beliefs that may change as new information is gained. Diversity from within the group results from individual perspectives and practices. For example, health seeking behaviors, such as deciding to seek medical care, use home or folk remedies, or practice health promotion activities, differ significantly across cultural groups (Spector, 2004).

People learn about cultural beliefs, values, customs, and behaviors through traditions that are transmitted from one generation to another. Grandparents, other elders, and parents teach children cultural expectations and norms through role modeling, demonstration, and discussion. Cultural messages are also transmitted through schools and churches. Various forms of communication media are also powerful transmitters and shapers of culture.

Characteristics of Culture

Differences exist among cultural groups and among individuals within a single culture. Despite these differences, all cultures exhibit the characteristics shown in Box 4-1.

Ethnicity and Race

Ethnicity is a cultural group's perception of themselves or group identity. This self-perception influences how others perceive the group's members. Ethnicity is a sense of belonging and a common social heritage that is passed from one generation to the next. Members of an ethnic group demonstrate their shared sense of identity in common customs and traits.

Race refers to a group of people based on biological similarities. Members of a racial group have similar physical characteristics, such as blood group, facial features, and color of skin, hair, and eyes. There is often overlap between racial and ethnic groups because the cultural and biological commonalities support one another (Giger & Davidhizar, 2004). The similarities of people in racial and ethnic groups reinforce a sense of commonality and cohesiveness. However, there may be differences with regard to individuals' perceptions of their racial backgrounds and their social relationships. The nurse must be careful to assess patients and their families individually when considering race and ethnicity.

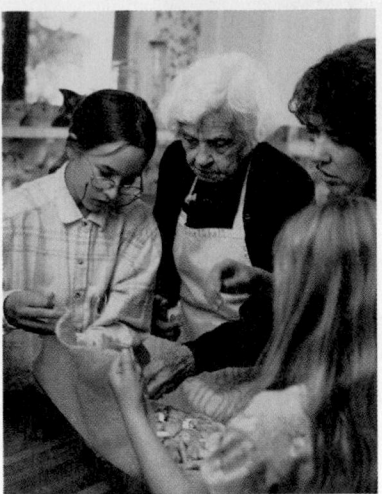

Figure 4-1 Cultural expectations and traditions are shared through formal and informal activities.

BOX 4-1

CHARACTERISTICS OF CULTURE

- Culture is learned and taught. A person is not born with cultural concepts, but instead learns such concepts through socialization as knowledge is transmitted from one generation to another.
- Culture is shared. The sharing of common practices provides a group with part of its cultural identity.
- Culture is social in nature. Culture develops in, and is communicated by, groups of people.
- Culture is dynamic, adaptive, and ever-changing. Adaptation allows cultural groups to adjust to meet environmental changes. Cultural change occurs slowly and in response to the needs of the group. This dynamic and adaptable nature allows a culture to survive.

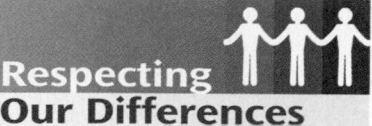

Respecting Our Differences

Life Span Considerations for the Elderly

Elderly persons may have different perspectives on the implications of their cultural heritage from the perspectives of younger people of the same culture. For example, an older African American person raised in the southern United States may have experienced a great deal of discrimination and consequently is somewhat distrustful of Caucasian health care providers. The nurse may not recognize the reasons for the elderly person's attitude of distrust and inaccurately assess its root cause. The nurse must remember to consider age and experience, as well as the patient's racial background.

BOX 4-2

WAYS IN WHICH PEOPLE DIFFER

- Age
- Gender
- Educational level
- Language
- Occupation
- Residence (rural, urban, suburban, mountains, shore, and U. S. region)
- Socioeconomic status
- Social class
- Religion
- Functional abilities
- Cognitive abilities
- Racial composition
- Nationality
- Family structure and ties
- Rituals (food, births, deaths, and holidays)

Labeling and Stereotyping

Problems arise when differences across and within cultural groups are misunderstood. Misperception, confusion, and ignorance often accompany people's expectations of each other. Some of the common ways that people are different from each other and, thus, classified by others are provided in Box 4-2.

Members of some cultural groups have historically and globally experienced bias and oppression in various forms of racism, sexism, and classism. The basic underlying premise of such biases is that one race, gender, or class is assumed to be superior and every other is perceived as inferior. **Ethnocentrism** is the belief that one's own culture is superior to all others. This belief is common to all cultural groups; all groups regard their own culture as not only the best but also the correct, moral, and only way of life. This belief is pervasive, often unconscious, and is imposed on every aspect of day-to-day interaction and health care practices. It is this attitude that can create problems between nurses and patients of diverse cultural groups.

Ethnocentrism results in oppression. **Oppression** occurs when the rules, modes, and ideals of one group are imposed on another group. Oppression is based on cultural biases that stem from values, beliefs, traditions, and cultural expectations. **Racism,** a form of oppression, is defined as discrimination directed toward individuals who are misperceived to be inferior because of biological differences.

Stereotyping is an expectation that all people within the same racial, ethnic, or cultural group act alike and share the same beliefs and attitudes. Stereotyping serves as a template that further filters out any other potential future information about a given group of individuals. Although some generalizations are positive, more often, these generalizations portray individuals within a group negatively. Nurses need to realize that stereotypes may be translated into attitudes, positive or negative, which can lead to prejudice. Stereotyping results in labeling people according to cultural preconceptions; therefore, an individual's unique identity is often ignored.

Dominant Values in the United States

Cultural differences refer to values, practices, and rituals that vary from those of the dominant culture. The dominant culture of the United States is composed of Caucasian middle-class Protestants of European ancestry. A **dominant culture** is the group whose values prevail within a society. The European value orientation has had an important influence on U.S. culture, as illustrated by the following dominant beliefs:
- Achievement and success
- Individualism, independence, and self-reliance
- Activity, work, and ownership
- Efficiency, practicality, and reliance on technology
- Material comfort
- Competition and achievement
- Youth and beauty

Frequently, these dominant values, which may be blatant or subtle, conflict with the values of minority groups. Generally, a **minority group** can be composed of an ethnic, racial, or religious group that constitutes less than a numerical majority of the population. Because of their cultural or physical characteristics, such groups are labeled and treated differently from others in the society. Minority groups are usually considered to be less powerful than the dominant group (Giger & Davidhizar, 2004).

Acculturation is the process of learning norms, beliefs, and behavioral expectations of a group. People assume the characteristics of the dominant

Fast Forward ▶▶▶

Unrecognized Cultures: The Deaf Culture

Legitimate cultures that go largely unrecognized by society exist among populations, such as people who are deaf. Literature and evidence-based practice to guide nurses providing care to the deaf population is negligible if, indeed, any can be found. Consider what policies or practice guidelines exist in your organization related to caring for a deaf woman in labor who is separated from her support system and taken to the operating room where everyone is masked, preventing her from reading their lips. Consider how terrifying that must be for that patient. The culture of deaf patients is fertile for future qualitative research by nurses.

Respecting Our Differences

Life Span Considerations: Families

The family environment and acculturation process involves how the values and communication in the families change during the intergenerational process, resulting in cultural changes in children and their families. Cultural values that are taught in the schools may conflict with values that are taught in the home. Acculturation that is encouraged in the schools may lead to acculturative conflicts and crises in the lives of children and adolescents leading to less than desired behaviors (Rodriguez, 2002). These may include, but are not limited to, problems with language, perceived discrimination, and perceived cultural incompatibilities.

culture through acculturation. Acculturation is encouraged through schools and the media. **Cultural assimilation** occurs when individuals from a minority group are absorbed by the dominant culture and take on the characteristics of the dominant culture.

MULTICULTURALISM IN THE UNITED STATES

The U.S. population is composed of many ethnic and racial subcultures. A **subculture** is a group of people within the dominant group who are functionally unified by factors, such as status, ethnic background, residence, religion, or education, resulting in experiences that differ from those of the dominant group. The U.S. population has shown an increase in ethnic and racial diversity during the last half of the 20th century, especially in the last three decades. Emigration from Latin America, Asia, and the Pacific Islands has contributed to the growing U.S. diversity, resulting in more than doubling of these groups in the last two decades of the century (Hobbs & Stoops, 2002). The population of races that are different from the Caucasian or African American populations has demonstrated significant growth, but Caucasians continue to be the most prolific race.

Data about demographic trends in the 20th century indicate the following changes in racial and ethnic demographics in the United States as shown in Box 4-3 (Hobbs & Stoops, 2002).

BOX 4-3

CHANGES IN RACIAL AND ETHNIC DEMOGRAPHICS

- Hispanic (Americans) are the fastest growing ethnic minority, having more than doubled from 1980 to 2000. In 1980 there were 14.6 million Latinos in the United States, or 6.4 percent of the total population; by 1990 there were 22.4 million Hispanic (Americans), or 9 percent of the population; and in 2000, the Hispanic (American) population was 35.3 million, or 12.5 percent of the population. Factors that contribute to the tremendous growth include high levels of immigration and high fertility levels.
- The percentage of Asian (American) and Pacific Islander populations which, in 1980, was 1.5 percent of the U.S. population, more than doubled to 3.8 percent in 2000.
- The percentage of African Americans changed slightly from 11.7 percent of the American population to 12.3 percent in 2000, as did the American Indian and Alaska Natives, only going from 0.6 to 0.9 percent in the same time frame.
- The Caucasian population, therefore, has shown a noticeable proportional decrease, going from 83.1 percent of the total U.S. population in 1980 to 75.1 percent in 2000.
- By 2000, the United States was much more racially diverse than in 1990. In 1990, approximately one out of every eight Americans was a race other than Caucasian, and by 2000, this was true of one out every four Americans.
- The population census has always included data on race and ethnicity. However, the 2000 census was the first time that individuals were allowed to identify themselves as being of more than one race. For example, prior to the 2000 census individuals who were biracial were only allowed to self-identify in one race not both. In the 2000 census biracial individuals were allowed to self-identify in more than one race.

Skills 360°

Cultural Considerations

1. Why is culturally competent care important when providing care to patients?
2. Is there a group that should not be considered for culturally competent care?
3. Why did you choose this group?
4. How do the beliefs of the dominant society compare with your personal beliefs?

Racial and ethnic groups are not evenly distributed throughout the United States (Hobbs & Stoops, 2002). All of the various groups have concentrations in various regions. The African Americans population has generally been concentrated in the South, with 9 out of 10 African Americans living there. Although during the 1970s and 1980s there was a migration toward large metropolitan areas in the Midwest and Northeast, in 2000 migration reversed and many African Americans returned to the South.

Traditionally, the Asian (American) and Pacific Islander population were highly concentrated (four out of five) in the West. Although there have been changes in migration patterns throughout the United States, in 2000 the patterns showed that Asian (Americans) and Pacific Islanders are settled in the Northeast and in the South. The American Indian and Alaska Native population has remained stable, primarily concentrated in the West. The regional distribution of the Hispanic (American) population has also remained stable through 2000 but has grown in size (Hobbs & Stoops, 2002). The majority of Hispanic (Americans) continue to live in the South and the West. The 2000 data show a slight increase in the Hispanic (American) population in the Midwest and a decline in the Hispanic (American) population in the Northeast.

Immigrants to the United States have contributed greatly to the increased diversity of the population. The U.S. Department of Homeland Security (2004) statistics show that legal emigration to the United States was lower in 2003 (705,827) than in 2002 (1,063,732). Even though total emigration was down in 2003, after three years of decline, refugee arrivals increased. Of all of the immigrants, 36 percent were born in North America (16 percent in Mexico) and 35 percent were born in Asia. Approximately one of five emigrants arrived with the intention of living in New York City or Los Angeles.

Projections indicate that the diversity in the U.S. population will only continue to increase. It is estimated that by 2045, the Hispanic (American) and the Asian (American) and Pacific Islander populations will essentially double, comprising 23.1 percent and 8.8 percent, respectively, of the total population (U.S. Census Bureau, 2003).

Value of Diversity

Cultural diversity is the difference among people that results from ethnic, racial, and cultural variables. Cultural diversity refers to the differences between people based on a shared ideology and value set of beliefs, norms, customs, and meanings evidenced in a way of life. The United States has vast human resources, whose divergent viewpoints and behaviors enrich the sociopolitical climate. New ideas, multiple viewpoints, increased problem-solving approaches, and increased tolerances are all outcomes of a diverse population. In addition to these advantages, there are also some disadvantages to living and working within such a culturally diverse environment. For example, the amount and types of differences can lead to splitting and ethnocentrism.

Cultural diversity presents special challenges for nurses who must provide care that is congruent with a patient's expectations. Nurses caring for patients who are different from themselves must remember to determine the patient's perception of the significance or meaning of an illness event. The nurse must understand that culture influences how patients are viewed and treated within health care settings and honor each individual's differences.

Organizing Phenomena of Culture

Cultural factors determine the work of behaviors, whether behaviors are acceptable, and whether behaviors are incorporated into daily living. When these behavioral concepts are applied to health, they influence the individual's expectation of health care. Diversity of expectations among cultural groups influences health care. The nurse must be sensitive to the patient's cultural context to provide care that meets individual needs. Each cultural group has the same six basic organizing factors (Box 4-4) that must be considered when delivering culturally competent care.

BOX 4-4

ORGANIZING PHENOMENA OF CULTURE

- Communication
- Space
- Orientation to time
- Social organization
- Environmental control
- Biological variations

Communication

Communication is the vehicle for transmitting and preserving culture. To share complete and accurate information nurses must be aware of the cultural variances related to communication. In 2003 almost 20 percent of the homes in the United States spoke a language other than English, with approximately the same number of homes reporting that they spoke English less than very well (U.S. Bureau of the Census, 2003).

Nurses provide information to patients by using two types of communication: verbal and nonverbal. Verbal communication consists of words, both spoken and written. When cultural variances exist, communication problems may occur. The nurse must validate the meaning of, and interpret, words to ensure that patients receive the intended message.

When the nurse and patient speak different languages there are two potential communication problems that could result in language barriers. **Intrinsic distortion** occurs when information is passed on from one person to another through an interpreter. Distortions can occur through vocal tones, eye contact, phrasing, body language, and many other things that differ from one language to another. **Extrinsic distortion** occurs when the interpreter is improperly prepared. Problems may arise because the interpreter's knowledge of medical terminology is limited, or because there are colloquial or regional dialects, even though there is a common primary language.

Even when both patient and nurse speak the same language, communication problems may occur because of varying cultural contexts in which words have different meanings to different people. Fear, compounded with illness, can affect the patient's ability to hear what is being said, greatly interfering with communication. Even though patients may have English language proficiency, during times of stress or emotional trauma they may prefer to use their primary language, when it differs from English. In 2000, the Office of Minority Health (OMH) of Health and Human Services released the "National Standards for Culturally and Linguistically Appropriate Services in Health Care" (U.S. Department of Health and Human Services Office of Minority Health, 2000) outlining 14 standards for culturally and linguistically appropriate services. The OMH developed these public policies because of the fundamental belief that cultural and linguistic minorities are entitled to equal access and the same quality of care as mainstream America. Although nursing has articulated that providing culturally and linguistically competent nursing care is a priority, it has been inconsistently achieved throughout the United States, primarily in regions where cultural and linguistic minorities concentrate. The mandate to fulfill these national standards has significant implications for nursing. Cultural and linguistic competence is defined as the ability of health care providers and health care organizations to understand and respond effectively to the cultural and linguistic needs brought by patients to the health care encounter.

Utilizing a qualified interpreter is imperative to achieving communication when the nurse and patient do not speak the same language, regardless of the practice domain or site (Figure 4-2). Simply using someone who speaks the same language is not sufficient to ensure full and accurate translation. Conversing socially with someone in a different language is different from communicating in a health care setting (Farooq & Fear, 2003).

Using family members, hospital staff not hired for interpreting, or other patients or their families, may result in less than optimal care for the patient who does not speak English. First, the ability to speak another language does not ensure that a person can accurately translate medical information. Second, using family members to translate has the potential to create a power imbalance within the family that may not be acceptable to them. Third, use of family members or others who are not interpreters may result in the interpreter not wanting

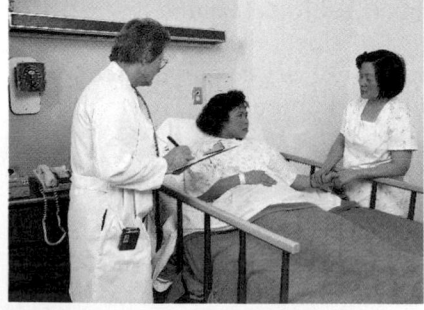

Figure 4-2 This woman is acting as an interpreter in this acute care setting.

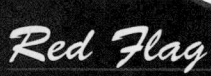

Red Flag

Miscommunication

When you assume that the patient understands the intended message and fail to confirm the patient's understanding, cultural blindness can hamper the communication and jeopardize the patient's health.

to translate sensitive information to the patient; the interpreter may even try to protect the patient by changing the information. Conversely, the information could be misinterpreted, because the family does not want the nurse to know everything, or because the family may be protective of their family member. Children should not be used as interpreters because they are not medically savvy, some information is not appropriate for them to be telling their parents, or using a child as an interpreter may violate their cultural norms.

Finally, ethical violations arise when a qualified interpreter is not utilized. Patient confidentiality is not maintained, because information about the patient is being disclosed without the consent of the patient. Furthermore, if improper translation occurs, the patient is not truly fully informed and informed consent cannot occur.

Nonverbal communication consists of body language, such as facial expressions, posture, and gestures; the use of silence; and paralinguistic cues including voice tone, pitch, and rate. Nonverbal communication can be culturally misunderstood through the presence, or absence, of eye contact. For example, in Native American and Asian (American) cultures eye contact may be considered intrusive and disrespectful. However, in the dominant U.S. cultural group eye contact between individuals indicates trustworthiness.

Another factor to consider is the assumption that patients are literate in their native language and able to accurately read written material provided in that language. Many Spanish-speaking people who cannot read English also cannot read Spanish (Dreger & Tremback, 2002). Although low levels (50 percent) of literacy occur in all minority groups, Hispanic (Americans) who are illiterate in English or Spanish, disproportionately represent adult minority groups with low literacy skills. Patients with low literacy skills may feel ashamed or embarrassed. Commonly, they do not admit their limitations in literacy to their spouse or family member, let alone to their health care provider.

Language and illiteracy barriers have potentially significant consequences. Patients who do not fully understand care instructions are at risk for poor health

Skills 360°

Nursing Strategies When Using an Interpreter

- Maintain basic knowledge of the cultural values, health beliefs, and practices for the patients you serve.
- Try to determine the level of English fluency of your patient.
- Show respect, interest, and understanding without being judgmental.
- Ask the patient how he or she prefers to be addressed.
- A smile and a nod of the head does not necessarily mean that your patient agrees or understands. Your patient may mean that what you are saying will be considered, or the nod may simply be a gesture of respect for your position. You must seriously consider that your patient may not understand or agree with what you are trying to communicate.
- Avoid potentially offensive body language.
- When addressing the patient, always speak to the patient and not to the interpreter.
- Make eye contact with the patient.
- Speak slowly and simply. Avoid the use of medical jargon.

Adapted from Tate, D. M. (2003). Cultural awareness: Bridging the gap between caregivers and Hispanic patients. Journal of Continuing Education in Nursing, 34*(5)*, 213–217.

status and poorer health outcomes, resulting in higher health care costs (Brown, et al., 2004). Patients who do not have the ability to read and understand written instructions may not be able to properly carry out the treatment plan, leading health care providers to determine that the patient is purposefully noncompliant. If a patient whose dominant language is other than English appears to be non-compliant with recommended health care followup or in taking medications, rather than assume that the patient is noncompliant, it is imperative that the nurse determine whether the patient understood the written instructions, regard-less of the language in which those instructions were written.

Space

An individual's personal space includes one's body, the surrounding environ-ment, and objects and people within that environment. Culture determines the amount of social distance tolerated by a person. Members of British, German, and American cultures usually require more personal space than do people of Hispanic or French backgrounds (Giger & Davidhizar, 2004). Nurses must be aware of the patient's degree of comfort with closeness, because diverse groups have varying norms for the use of touch. Touch may be per-ceived as invasive by patients from some cultures. Who can touch a person, when a person can be touched, and what forms of touch are appropriate are culturally determined. For example, members of the dominant U.S. culture often greet each other with handshakes, but it is commonly accepted in European cultures to greet others with a kiss on the cheek.

Orientation to Time

Time orientation (being focused on the past, the present, or the future) varies according to cultural groups. European Americans are future oriented as evi-denced by their development of plans, such as retirement savings. Many Native Americans have a different concept of time in that they tend to live in the pres-ent moment (Giger & Davidhizar, 2004). For many Native Americans, watching the clock and timeliness or tardiness have little importance. This is considered a circular, rather than a linear, process. Most health care providers value quickness and efficiency, which is interpreted by members of the Lakota tribe as insincer-ity and a lack of interest. The nurse's nonverbal behavior can be changed to build interpersonal rapport by spending time, sitting down with patients, and demonstrating presence.

Social Organization

Social organization refers to the ways in which groups determine rules of acceptable behavior and roles of individual members (Figure 4-3). Examples of social organizations include family and other kinship ties, religious groups, and ethnic groups. Just as the nurse approaches the patient with cul-turally competent care, the nurse must show the family the same cultural competence. Consideration of the family from a cultural perspective is important, because culture profoundly affects the way that families respond to threats to the health of a family member. Assumptions about how families are supposed to act when not based on knowledge of that family's cultural background can lead to erroneous conclusions. The primary factors that lead to family differences within cultural groups are related to the family life cycle, the socioeconomic and social class status of the family, and the family's degree of acculturation. The various types of family structures are described in Table 4-1. It is vital for the nurse to know who will be involved in making decisions related to health care. Including the family according to their cul-tural expectations is a hallmark of quality nursing care. Family patterns usu-ally are of one of three types: linear, collateral, or individualist. Table 4-2 provides an explanation of these types of family patterns.

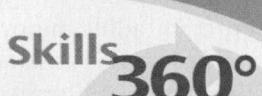

Skills 360°

Nursing Strategies When Considering Time Among Cultures

- In mainstream American culture time is a valuable commodity, and the phrase "Time is money!" is commonly used.
- Patients from diverse cultures may each view time differently.
- When a patient is late for an appointment, avoid jumping to the conclusion that the patient is lazy or inconsiderate.

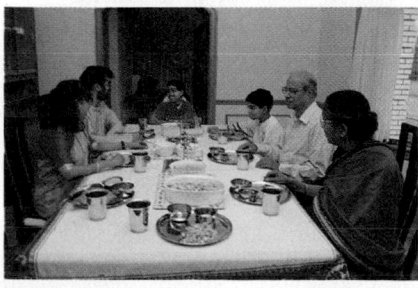

Figure 4-3 Families have their own prac-tices that are culturally driven, such as meal times together.

TABLE 4-1 Types of Family Structures

Nuclear	Parents and children
Extended	Parents, children, and other relatives, such as grandparents or cousins
Attenuated	Single parent with children
Incipient	Married couple with no children
Blended	Married couple and their children from previous unions; may indicate stepparents, step-siblings, half-siblings
Nontraditional	Same-sex partners with or without children

Adapted from DeLaune, S., & Ladner, P. (2006). Fundamentals of nursing (3rd ed.). New York: Thomson Delmar Learning.

TABLE 4-2 Family Patterns

KINSHIP PATTERN	EXPLANATION	MOST COMMON CULTURAL CONTEXT
Linear	Goals focus on needs of extended hereditary family.	Asian
	Patriarchal structure is present.	Middle Eastern
	Enculturation of children is an important function.	Upper-class Euro-American
	Elders are respected.	
Collateral	Individual member's goals are less important than those of the family.	Hispanic (American)
	Nuclear family is present.	Native American
	Men are "head of household," yet women contribute to decision making (especially about childcare).	
	Children are highly valued.	
	Socialization revolves around family groups.	
Individualist	Individual's goals take precedence over those of family.	Middle-class Euro-American
	Emphasis is on individual accountability and self-responsibility.	

In many cultures the family assumes greater importance than the individual. For example, in most Native American tribes the extended family is the basic family structure. The extended family is also extremely important in Hispanic (American) cultural groups. In some Hispanic (American) groups the family may include third and fourth cousins, as well as close friends who are not related by ties of kinship (Table 4-2). The following attributes are necessary for nurses to collaborate with families:

- Nonjudgmental attitude (i.e., do not expect all families to be alike and behave similarly to one's own)
- Self-awareness of own preconceptions about family members
- Respect for others' beliefs and values
- Recognition of families as significant providers of support
- Value the participation of families in care giving

BOX 4-5

WELLNESS AND PRAYER IN OTHER CULTURES

Various cultures emphasize the value and importance of prayer associated with their religious beliefs. The nurse must remember that patients with strong religious faiths might practice prayer regularly as part of their wellness practices. The nurse needs to create private times to facilitate a patient's religious practices. The nurse should also remember that some cultures have identified persons (e.g., herbalist, rabbi, or shaman) who are important to spiritual practices, such as prayer.

Gender roles vary according to cultural context. In families with a patriarchal structure the male husband or father is the head of the household, chief authority figure, and dominant person. Patriarchal structure is the cultural norm for Hispanic (American) and traditional Muslim families. The husband or father, therefore, may be the one who makes decisions regarding health care for all family members. In such cultures the wife is responsible for childcare and household maintenance, whereas the husband or father's role is to protect and support the family members. However, caution must be taken to individually assess families about gender roles. Changes in migration, employment patterns, and levels of acculturation have resulted in changes in the traditional role of the husband or father within the family (Rodriguez, 2002).

In addition to the heterogeneity of population groups in the United States, lifestyles are becoming more diverse. Some examples of alternative lifestyles are homosexual couples, single-parent families, and communal groups. Nurses must demonstrate respect for patients' lifestyles even when they differ radically from those of the nurse. Some specific ways in which nurses can demonstrate respect for patients with differing lifestyles are:
- Be aware of own tendency to be ethnocentric.
- Be sensitive to the patient's needs, especially those expressed nonverbally.
- Use self-awareness to determine the impact of own beliefs and values.

Often the nurse and patient are of different racial backgrounds. The nurse must be culturally sensitive to promote the development of a therapeutic nurse-patient relationship.

Religious beliefs influence a person's response to major life events, such as birth, illness, and death. Religious practices are often a source of comfort during stressful life events and provide support during the healing process (Box 4-5). Crises, such as illness and major treatment modalities, are often the catalyst for increased spiritual needs.

CULTURAL DISPARITIES IN HEALTH AND HEALTH CARE DELIVERY

Language and other cultural differences often present barriers to necessary health care including: appointment procedures, transportation, and directions written in an unfamiliar language. When such barriers are not overcome patients' health may languish. Life expectancies and overall health have improved for most Americans as a result of improvements in preventive health care and medical advances. However, among all of the minority groups there continue to be disparities in the burden of illness and death as compared with the U.S. population as a whole (U.S. Department of Health and Human Services, 2004). Efforts need to be continued in the areas of prevention, treatment, and resources toward reducing morbidity and the loss of life. Box 4-6 provides examples of health disparities identified by the U.S. Department of Health and Human Services (2004).

One of the major objectives established by the U.S. Office of Public Health in its Healthy People 2010 Objectives is the elimination of disparities in health status by providing equitable services for people of all groups. Yet, while the objectives of Healthy People 2010 call for providing equitable services for all groups of different backgrounds, the shift in health care toward a managed care model causes concern. The emphasis of the managed care model is cost-containment, which therefore has the potential for placing less priority in providing services that are culturally competent. This is concerning, because managed care organizations increasingly are serving culturally diverse, underserved populations because Medicaid recipients are enrolled into such services.

Respecting Our Differences

Life Span Considerations: Child Development

Application of child development theories to all children, regardless of their cultural or ethnic backgrounds needs to be done with caution. Normative development has been defined according to Eurocentric standards, leaving little room for any other differences in the developing child. A total of five major sources of influence impact the developmental outcome of minority children: the effects of culture, health status, socioeconomic status, family structure, and biological factors. All of these factors operate together and are difficult to isolate from each other. Children from culturally or ethnically diverse backgrounds may not meet currently established milestones for various reasons. A common child development assessment tool, the Denver Developmental II, originally developed from a Eurocentric perspective, required major revision and restandardization to determine its usefulness for ethnic groups. More recently, the Center for Disease Control and Prevention (CDC) updated the widely used growth charts using government data from the last 30 years on children from all ethnic groups (CDC, 2003c). The old chart, which was widely used prior to the updating, was developed using data from a private study of formula-fed, primarily Caucasian children in Ohio.

BOX 4-6

HEALTH DISPARITY EXAMPLES

Cancer
- African Americans have higher incidence and death rates from cancer than any other racial or ethnic group.
- Although African American women have lower cancer rates than Caucasian women, they have a higher cancer mortality rate.
- Hispanic (American) women have a higher rate of cervical cancer than other groups.
- Higher rates of stomach cancer occur among Asian (Americans), Pacific Islanders, and American Indians than among Caucasians.

Cardiovascular Disease and Stroke
- Heart disease accounts for one fourth of all deaths, making it the leading killer across most racial and ethnic minority groups.
- Approximately 40 percent of African Americans have some form of heart disease compared to 24 to 30 percent of Caucasians. Furthermore, African Americans are more likely to die from heart disease, than are Caucasians.
- More Hispanic (American) women than Caucasian women are diagnosed with heart disease. Hispanic (American) women also have a higher incidence of obesity, one of the leading causes of heart disease.
- African Americans have higher rates of strokes than Caucasians.

Diabetes
- Racial and ethnic minority groups have higher incidences of prediabetes and diabetes.
- Two million Hispanic (Americans) (8.2 percent of the population) have diabetes.
- African Americans experience higher rates of complications from diabetes than do Caucasians.

HIV/AIDS
- Racial and ethnic minorities account for almost 70 percent of new HIV and AIDS cases. Among babies born with HIV, 90 percent are from minority groups.
- In the African American community, HIV/AIDS has hit epidemic proportions with 54 percent of the new cases coming from this group.
- HIV/AIDS is the sixth leading cause of death for Asian (American) and Pacific Islander men, ages 25 to 34.

Immunizations
- Less then 50 percent of African Americans and Hispanic (Americans) receive the influenza vaccination, compared with 69 percent of Caucasians.
- The difference in pneumococcal vaccinations is even greater between the groups.

Infant Mortality
- Although the overall infant mortality rate has shown improvements, African American, American Indian, and Alaska Native populations continued to show higher rates.

Adapted from U.S. Department of Health and Human Services. (2004). HHS Fact Sheet. *Retrieved June 17, 2005, from http://raceandhealth.hhs.gov.*

Vulnerable Populations

As a result of societal changes, more people are at risk for health problems. Groups that are especially susceptible for health-related problems include the poor, the homeless, migrant workers, abused individuals, the elderly, pregnant adolescents, and people with sexually transmitted disease, such as acquired immunodeficiency syndrome (AIDS). The United States is currently facing many economic, social, and political challenges related to the delivery of health care services to vulnerable population groups (Delaune & Ladner, 2006). As a result, many vulnerable populations are underserved because of the high demand for services, lack of services, and limited availability.

Poor

Living in poverty means being unable to meet the financial demands of basic living expenses such as food, shelter, and clothing. Socioeconomic status is determined by family income, educational level, and occupation. Childhood poverty has long-lasting negative effects on one's health. Children in low-income families fare less well than children in more affluent families. Seventeen percent of American children live in poverty and a family of four with an annual income below $20,000 is below the federal poverty threshold. The poor population has more complex health problems, including a higher incidence of chronic illness. Health risk factors related to lower income are higher prevalence of cigarette smoking, greater incidence of obesity, elevated blood pressure, sedentary lifestyle, less likely to be covered by health insurance, and less likely to receive preventive health care services.

Increasing numbers of federally mandated health care initiatives are being implemented to address the historic racial and class disparities in health care. Entitlement programs imply that the government is legally mandated to provide services to the programs' eligible populations. Entitlement programs, such as Medicare, Medicaid, and Women, Infants, and Children (WIC), were developed, in part, because of social and political pressures. WIC, a special supplemental food program for women, infants, and children is a U.S. Public Health–sponsored program that targets low-income pregnant and breastfeeding mothers and their children age five years and younger. WIC links health care services, food supplements, and health education into a combined service package for eligible members. Medicaid is a program designed to provide access to health care for medically needy infants, children, and adults. Medicare is an entitlement program that finances health care services for individuals over the age of 65 or disabled at any age.

Poverty interferes with a child's ability to be housed, clothed, and fed adequately and can deprive the child of a safe (physical and psychological) environment. Children with access to health care have the possibility of getting necessary health care services. Children with health insurance (public or private) are much more likely than children without insurance to have a regular and accessible source of health care. Parents may have limited health care benefits related to employment issues or recent immigration.

Homeless

Estimates are that 350,000 to six million people in the United States are homeless (Figure 4-4). Societal factors that contribute to homelessness are lack of affordable housing, increasingly stringent criteria for public assistance, decreased availability of social services, inadequate or lack of employment, a history of psychosocial trauma, and deinstitutionalization of patients from mental health facilities without adequate community support, such as halfway houses and group homes.

Approximately 85 percent of homeless people are on the streets, because they have some form of mental illness or are addicted to alcohol or other drugs. In most instances, homeless is not a choice. It is important to understand the

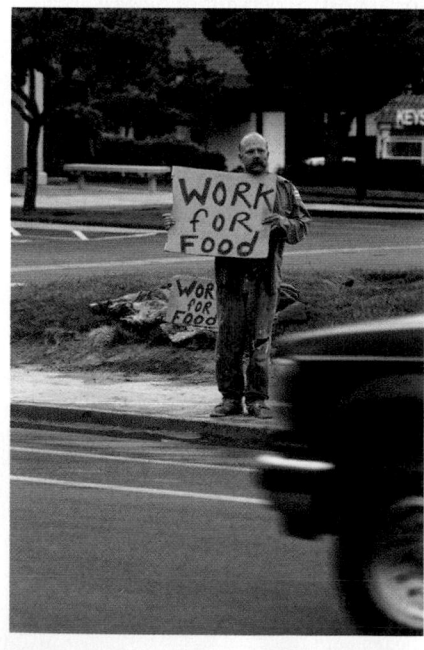

Figure 4-4 The visible homeless shape the public perception of the homeless; however, the homeless population includes diverse types of people and circumstances. Courtesy of Photodisc.

connection between homelessness and chronic mental illness, for with understanding can come the sensitivity and compassion necessary to serve this population.

Those who are homeless are at greater risk for illness and injuries (Denkins, 2005). The following major needs for health care among homeless women include mental health, sexually transmitted diseases, and substance abuse. Access to basic health care services is limited, because the homeless lack health insurance coverage. Those few facilities that do provide services to the homeless are not always accessible because of lack of transportation (Table 4-3).

Children are especially vulnerable to the perils of homelessness. Thirty six percent of U.S. households with children had housing problems, including physically inadequate housing and crowded housing. Adolescents who are homeless are at high risk for physical and mental health problems, including malnutrition, substance abuse, accidental pregnancy, and sexually transmitted disease.

The social and political reforms that are needed to create solutions to homelessness have just begun. There is great urgency to meet the immediate needs of the homeless and to provide health care that emphasizes both disease prevention and health promotion. Listed below are a few examples of nursing efforts to respond to the needs of vulnerable patients:

- Community Volunteers in Medicine is a nonprofit organization in which nurses, physicians, and dentists volunteer their time and services to treat uninsured people of all ages living in Chester County, Pennsylvania.
- Philadelphia-based Regional Nursing Centers consortium (RNCC) sees approximately 250,000 patients annually. Up to 50 percent of these patients are uninsured.

TABLE 4-3 Common Health Problems Experienced by the Homeless

PROBLEM	IMPACT OF HOMELESSNESS
Diabetes	Lack of regularly scheduled nutritious meals
	Inadequate rest
	Insufficient exercise
AIDS	Higher rate of sexual assault
	IV drug use
	Lack of treatment or inadequate follow-up
Respiratory diseases (e.g., tuberculosis, pneumonia)	Crowded living conditions
	Inadequate nutrition
	Limited or no access to treatment facilities
Cardiovascular diseases	Impaired peripheral circulation as a result of extended time of walking on the streets or sleeping in upright, seated position
	Food served in many shelters has a high sodium content
	Consumption of alcohol and tobacco products
Parasitic infestations	Shared personal items (clothing, bedding, and hair brushes)
	Close physical contact such as in a shelter
	Inability to treat all those in contact with the affected person

Adapted from Denkins, B. A. (2005). My side. Are we really helping? The problem of dual diagnoses, homelessness, & hospital-hopping. Journal of Psychosocial Nursing and Mental Health Services, 43(11), 48–50.

- The LaSalle Neighborhood Nursing Center in Philadelphia identified 300 uninsured children and enrolled them in the Children's Health Insurance Program (CHIP) or for medical assistance.
- Health Promotion Center (HPC) in the Church of the Nazarene in Mid-City, San Diego, California, a multicultural church, began in 2000. The HPC first began with student nurses and faculty from Point Loma Nazarene University (PLNU) providing screenings for diabetes, hypertension, and tuberculosis. Now it provides full service primary care for free, involving three San Diego area universities: PLNU, the University of California San Diego, and the University of San Diego.

Environmental Control

Environmental control refers to the relationships between people and nature and to a person's perceived ability to control activities of nature, such as factors causing illness. A person's belief about the causation of disease will determine the type of treatment (if any) sought. According to Andrews and Boyle (2002), there are three types of health belief systems: magicoreligious, biomedical, and holistic. The magicoreligious belief system is based on the concept that health and illness are determined by supernatural forces (such as a higher power or the gods). The biomedical belief system states that illness is a result of an impairment in physical or biochemical processes. The holistic belief system views health as a result of harmony among the elements of nature; conversely, disease is caused by disharmony.

Folk Medicine

Most cultures have preferences about health care, including: (a) the type of care that is necessary and appropriate, (b) when care or treatment should appropriately be sought, and (c) the appropriate caregiver. Because the presence of a folk medicine (also referred to as alternative medicine) can present challenges to nurses caring for patients from diverse cultures, knowledge of basic beliefs about illness, factors contributing to illness, and home remedies is necessary. Nurses must realize that patients are often using folk medicine or remedies at home but may be reluctant to disclose this information. It is important to try to obtain information about possible use of home remedies, because some home remedies may alter the function of some medical interventions. Table 4-4 presents the various healers within different cultures and describes common folk healing practices used. Nurses must be able to incorporate informal caregivers, healers, and other members of the patient's support system as allies in treatment.

Biological Variables

Biological variations that distinguish one cultural group from another include enzymatic differences and susceptibility to disease (Andrews & Boyle, 2002; Giger & Davidhizar, 2004). Enzymatic differences account for diverse responses of some groups to dietary therapy and drugs. Nutritional variations include food preferences that may contribute to health problems as shown in Table 4-5.

Immigrant Population

Exploring the health status of the immigrant population has important implications for health care. Data demonstrate that most immigrant groups have longer life expectancies when compared with U.S.-born minority groups (Singh & Miller, 2004). Hispanic (American) immigrants have several years longer life expectancy than their U.S.-born counterparts. African immigrants die 35 percent less frequently from cancer than U.S.-born Africans. However, Asian (American) immigrants have a 30 percent higher incidence of cancer

TABLE 4-4 **Folk Medicine: Healers and Practices**

CULTURAL GROUP	TRADITIONAL HEALERS	HEALING PRACTICES
African American	Elderly women healers	Herbs, roots
	"Community Mother" or "Granny"	Poultices
		Oils
	"Root doctor"	Religious healing through rituals, (e.g., laying on of hands)
	Voodoo healer ("Mambo" or "oungan")	Talismans are worn around the wrist or neck, or carried in a pouch to ward off disease
	Spiritualists	
Asian (American)	Herbalist	Use of hot and cold foods
	Health care provider	Herbs (e.g., ginseng root, which is used as a restorative potion)
		Soups
		Cupping, pinching, and rubbing
		Meditation
		Acupuncture (puncturing the skin at specified areas with metal needles)
		Acupressure (applying pressure with the fingertips to specified areas of the body)
		Application of tiger balm (a salve) to relieve muscular pains
		Energy to restore balance between yin and yang
European American	Nurse	Exercise
	Health care provider	Medication (prescribed and over-the-counter)
		Modified diets
		Amulets
		Religious healing rituals
Latino	Curandero	Hot and cold foods to treat some conditions
	Espiritualista	Herbal teas, such as Manzanilla, used to treat GI problems, insomnia, and menstrual cramps
	Yerbero (herbalist)	
	Brujo (healer who uses witchcraft)	Prayers and religious medals
		Massage
	Sobadora	Azabache, a black stone worn as a necklace or bracelet to ward off the "evil eye"
	Santiguadora	
		Some Haitian mothers practice the "three baths" ritual: they bathe for the first three postpartum days in water boiled with special leaves.
Native American	Shaman	Use of plants and herbs
	Medicine man or woman	Medicine bundle or bag filled with herbs that have been blessed by a medicine man or woman during a healing ceremony
		Sweet grass (herbs) burned to purify the ill person
		Estafiate (dried leaves) boiled to produce tea for treating stomach disorders
		The Blessingway ceremony (a healing ritual conducted by the medicine man or woman)
		In some Navajo tribes, the medicine man or woman uses sand painting as a diagnostic method

Adapted from Spector, R. E. (2004). Cultural diversity in health and illness (6th ed.). Upper Saddle River, NJ: Prentice Hall.

TABLE 4-5 Effects of Biological Variations on Selected Drugs

CULTURAL GROUP	EFFECT OF BIOLOGICAL VARIANCE ON DRUGS
African American	Isoniazid (drug used to treat tuberculosis) is rapidly metabolized, thus becoming inactive quickly; occurs in approximately 60 percent of population.
	An enzyme deficiency interferes with metabolism of primaquine (used to treat malaria); occurs in approximately 35 percent of population.
	Antihypertensive drugs (e.g., propranolol) needs to be administered in higher doses to produce same effects as in European Americans.
Asian (American)	Isoniazid (drug used to treat tuberculosis) is rapidly metabolized, thus becoming inactive quickly; occurs in approximately 85 to 90 percent of population.
	Rapid metabolism of alcohol results in excessive facial flushing and other vasomotor symptoms.
	Chinese men need only about half as much propranolol (antihypertensive drug) as European American men.
	Asian (American) people need smaller doses of alprazolam (antianxiety drug) to achieve same blood levels as their European American counterparts; the drug is also metabolized more slowly (remains in the bloodstream longer) in Asian (American) men.
European American	Because of liver enzyme differences, caffeine is metabolized and excreted faster than by people of other cultural groups.
Native American	Isoniazid (drug used to treat tuberculosis) is rapidly metabolized, thus becoming inactive quickly; occurs in approximately 60 to 90 percent of population.
	Rapid metabolism of alcohol results in excessive facial flushing and other vasomotor symptoms.

Adapted from Broyles, B. E., Reiss, B. S., & Evans, M. E. (2007). Pharmacological aspects of nursing care (7th ed.). New York: Thomson Delmar Learning; Giger, J. N., & Davidhizar, R. E. (2004). Transcultural nursing: Assessment and intervention (4th ed.). St. Louis, MO: Mosby.

deaths, along with lower life expectancies, than their U.S.-born counterparts. Low birth rates and infant mortality are lower for all immigrants. Overall, immigrants have better overall health and prenatal status, as well as lower disability and mortality than those born in the United States.

Although it is not well understood why these differences exist, there are some possible explanations. Generally, people immigrating to the United States are healthier than those who do not emigrate. Those who emigrate generally have more favorable health behaviors, such as lower rates of smoking, drinking, obesity, and dieting. Recent immigrants may have higher levels of social and familial support. Unfortunately, the protective factors that new immigrants bring are lost the longer they live in the United States. As the length of stay in United States increases, health status, mortality patterns, and health behaviors of immigrants begin to look more like that of those who were born in the United States (Singh & Miller, 2004). Acculturation into the United States seems to have undesirable effects on the health of immigrants because of lifestyle changes, including smoking, drinking, drug use, unhealthy diets, and obesity. Research needs to continue to better understand the protective factors that immigrants may bring with them (Table 4-6).

TRANSCULTURAL NURSING

Eggenberger, Grassley, and Restrepo, (2006) state that culture is a central concept of nursing. Acknowledgement and acceptance of cultural differences and understanding of culturally specific responses to illness are prerequisites for providing safe and effective care.

TABLE 4-6 Food Preferences and Related Effects on Health

CULTURAL GROUP	FOOD PREFERENCES	NUTRITIONAL EXCESS	RELATED HEALTH PROBLEM
African American	Pork	Calories	Obesity
	Greens	Cholesterol	Cardiovascular illnesses (hypertension, coronary heart disease)
	Rice	Carbohydrates	
	Fried foods	Sodium	
Asian (American)	Raw fish	Calories	Coronary heart disease
	Rice	Cholesterol	Liver disease
	Soy sauce	Carbohydrates	Stomach cancer
		Sodium	Ulcers
Hispanic (American)	Beans	Calories	Obesity
	Fried foods	Cholesterol	Coronary heart disease
	Chili	Carbohydrates	Diabetes
	Carbonated beverages	Sodium	
Native American	Blue cornmeal	Calories	Malnutrition
	Fish	Carbohydrates	Diabetes
	Game		
	Fruits and berries		

Adapted from Roth, R. (2007). Nutrition and diet therapy (9th ed.). New York: Thomson Delmar Learning.

The conceptual framework for understanding cultural diversity and providing culturally competent care is based on Madeline Leininger's (1978) transcultural nursing theory. Transcultural nursing, according to Leininger's transcultural nursing theory, focuses on the study and analysis of different cultures and subcultures with respect to cultural care, health beliefs, and health practices with the goal of providing health care within the context of the patient's culture.

A basic assumption of transcultural nursing is that when health care providers see problems from the patient's cultural viewpoint they are more open to understanding, appreciating, and working effectively with these patients. Other assumptions of Leininger's transcultural nursing theory include (a) every culture has some kind of system for health care that is based on values and behaviors and (b) cultures have certain methods for providing health care. These methods of care are often unknown to nurses from other cultures. Because of rapid globalization, every nurse must have an understanding of human conditions in diverse societies. Nurses do not need to travel to foreign countries to engage in international nursing. Nurses encounter cultural diversity everywhere—from inner-city hospitals to suburban clinics and from technologically sophisticated institutions to homes in rural, inner city, and suburban areas.

CULTURAL COMPETENCE

Community, social and kinship ties, religion, language, food, and cultural perceptions of illness are all areas that need to be considered by the nurse when working with culturally diverse patients. Cultural diversity challenges nurses to bridge cultural gaps with patients by providing culturally relevant care. An understanding of

TABLE 4-7   Elements of Cultural Competence

ELEMENT	DEFINITION
Cultural awareness	A cognitive process in which the nurse becomes aware of and sensitive to the patient's cultural values, beliefs, and practices.
Cultural knowledge	The nurse seeks a sound educational base about different cultures.
Cultural skill	The nurse's ability to perform a culturally specific assessment (i.e., physical and psychosocial).
Cultural encounters	The nurse interacts with patients from diverse cultural backgrounds.
Cultural desire	The nurse's motivation ("want") to become culturally competent.

Adapted from Furness, S. (2005). Shifting sands: Developing cultural competence.
Practice, 17(4), 247–256.

the patient's cultural context permits nurses to become familiar with the patient as a person instead of focusing only on the illness or problem.

Cultural competence is the process through which the nurse provides care that is appropriate to the patient's cultural context. Culturally competent nurses are those who demonstrate knowledge and understanding of the patient's culture, accept and respect cultural differences, and adapt care to be congruent with the patient's culture. Culturally competent nurses have knowledge about cultural values related to health and illness. Also, nurses who provide care in a culturally competent manner are flexible in their approaches and thinking. The five elements of cultural competence are presented in Table 4-7.

CULTURAL COMPETENCE AND NURSING PROCESS

Cultural competency is requisite in every phase of the nursing process. The nurse's role in providing culturally competent care includes performing a cultural assessment, formulating nursing diagnoses, identifying expected patient outcomes, planning care to assist patients in achieving the expected outcomes, intervening to address the patient's nursing diagnoses, and evaluating the plan of care. There are four elements of providing culturally sensitive care: self-reflection, facilitating patient choice, gaining cultural knowledge, and effective communication. These four elements permeate the nursing process.

Assessment

Caring for a patient from a different culture can be challenging to the nurse. Using the patient's strengths and respecting the patient's values are essential components of effective nursing care. To begin providing culturally competent care the nurse should use questions to gather information about the patient's cultural background. The factors pertinent to cultural assessment are listed in Box 4-7.

BOX 4-7

CULTURAL ASSESSMENT FACTORS

- Patient's ethnic heritage
- Family role and function
- Religious practices
- Food preferences
- Native language
- Social networks
- Educational experiences (formal and informal)
- Health care beliefs
- Family patterns of health care
- Social class status

Understanding how a patient explains and understands his or her illness is an important part of conducting a cultural assessment. When a nurse is able to understand the patient's perspective, the nurse is better able to develop culturally appropriate plans of care that are inclusive of the patient's thoughts, values, and perspectives about the illness. The Patient's Explanatory Model developed by Kleinman in 1980 is useful for assisting the nurse to explore a patient's thoughts through some or all of the questions. The model was presented in *The spirit catches you and you fall down,* a true story of a Hmong child and her family's experiences with the western health care system, by Ann Fadiman (1997). The questions in Box 4-8 can either be incorporated

---

BOX 4-8

CULTURAL ASSESSMENT INTERVIEW GUIDE

- Name/Nickname/names of special meaning attributed to your name
- Primary Language: When speaking; When writing
- Date/Place of birth
- Educational level or specialized training
- To which ethnic group do you belong?
- To what extent do you identify with your cultural group?
- Who is the spokesperson for your family?
- Describe some of the customs or beliefs that you have about the following:
    Health
    Life
    Illness
    Death
- How do you learn information best:
    Reading
    Having someone explain verbally
    Having someone demonstrate
- Describe some of your family's dietary habits and your personal food preferences.
- Are there any foods forbidden from your diet for religious or cultural reasons?
- Describe your religious affiliation.
- What role do your religious beliefs and practices play in your life during times of good health and bad health?
- Whom do you rely on for health care services or healing and what type of cultural health practices have you been exposed to?
- Are there any sanctions or restrictions in your culture that the person taking care of you should know?
- How do members of your family communicate with each other?
- Who or what is your primary source of information about your health?
- Is there anything else that is important about your cultural beliefs that you want to tell me?

Adapted from Estes, M. (2006). Health assessment and physical examination *(3rd ed.). New York: Thomson Delmar Learning.*

Skills 360°

Nursing Strategy for Determining Diagnosis

Ask the patient the following questions to explore the patient's thoughts:

- What do you call the problem?
- What do you think has caused the problem?
- Why do you think it started when it did?
- What do you think the sickness does? How does it work?
- How severe is the sickness? Will it have a short or long course?
- What kind of treatment do you think you should receive? What are the most important results you hope to gain?
- What are the chief problems the sickness has caused?
- What do you fear most about the sickness?

into a general nursing assessment tool or used separately as a cultural assessment tool.

Nursing Diagnoses

Nurses use diagnoses approved by the North American Nursing Diagnosis Association ([NANDA], 2005) extensively. However, one stated disadvantage to NANDA diagnostic statements is that sometimes the diagnoses are worded in ways that result in cultural bias. Some diagnoses that may be culturally biased are: noncompliance, impaired verbal communication, impaired social interaction, deficient knowledge, disturbed thought processes, and powerlessness. Consider the following examples of ways in which these diagnoses may be used in a culturally inappropriate manner:

- Applying the diagnosis *impaired verbal communication* to patients who speak a language different from that of the nurse
- Using the diagnosis *noncompliance* with a patient who rejects a prescribed treatment method to adhere to culturally sanctioned folk healing methods, or who may not be able to read written instructions, even those written in their primary language

It may be more appropriate to use another term instead of *noncompliant*. The term, *nonadherent* may present less of a stigma to patients than noncompliant.

Planning and Implementation

Cultural groups are not homogeneous; there are individual variations in personality, behavior, and expectations. It is important not to consider one member of a particular group to be like all the others of that same group. To develop effective plans of care, nurses need to understand the following: cultural groups' perspectives on life processes (e.g., birth and death), cultural definitions of health and illness, how cultural groups maintain wellness, culture's perspectives on the causes of illness, potential use of healers in the cure and care of illness, and the influence of the nurse's cultural background on the delivery of care.

It is also necessary to consider how the patient's beliefs may impact the plan of care. Cultural beliefs greatly influence perceptions about health and therefore, may create barriers to adhering to prescribed treatment plans. Culture influences the following: perceptions of illness versus health, responses to illness, perceptions about the significance of symptoms, and the types of treatment approaches (e.g., alternative and conventional).

Caring for culturally diverse patients requires three major nursing interventions: self-awareness, use of nonjudgmental approach, and patient education. Each of these aspects is discussed in the following section. The Respecting Our Difference features offers guidelines for providing culturally sensitive care for patients at home.

In an increasingly diverse society the nurse must be aware of the potential for bias or misunderstanding. Self-awareness can be used to help nurses recognize their own stereotypes, biases, and prejudgments about patients who are culturally different. Further experience, introspection, and study empower nurses to appreciate their own cultures and the strengths of other cultures.

A nonjudgmental attitude is essential in the provision of culturally sensitive care. When caring in a manner sensitive to the patient's cultural background, the nurse enables the patient to offer open, honest feedback, to disagree, or to discuss real or perceived problems. The patient must learn to also value the ethnicity of the health care provider (Figure 4-5). A health care partnership is the outcome of this approach.

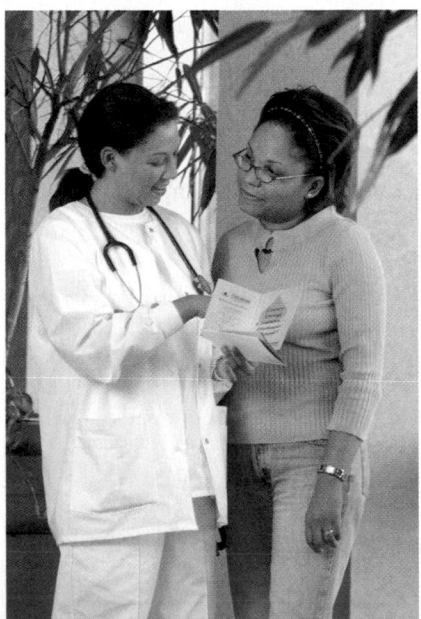

Figure 4-5 The relationship between this nurse and patient is based on mutual acceptance of each other's cultural viewpoints.

Respecting Our Differences

Community or Home Care

Remember that the setting for care is controlled by the patient and family not by the health care provider.

- The nurse is often viewed as a guest by the patient and family. Social chatter may be necessary to facilitate rapport.
- The nurse must be nonjudgmental about the condition of the home (e.g., presence of clutter and disarray).

Show respect and consideration for the patient. For example:

- Ask permission to use the sink or bathroom to wash your hands.
- Wipe your feet before entering the home.
- Ask permission before moving the patient's belongings, and replace items after you have finished the task.

Take advantage of the home environment to assess cultural values and norms. Cultural clues may include:

- Orderliness and décor of the home.
- Assignment of family roles and tasks.
- Types of interactions among family members.
- Value placed on privacy.
- Value placed on possessions.

Skills 360°

Culturally Competent Teaching

When caring for patients from diverse cultures the nurse should consider the following guidelines for patient teaching:

- Assess and incorporate family history of health care:

  Fluency in English; obtain an interpreter if necessary

  Extent of family support

  Community resources

  Level of education

  Change of social status as a result of coming to this country

- Affirm patient strengths.
- Recognize informal caregivers (family members and significant others) as an integral part of treatment.
- Evaluate the patient's current knowledge base by asking the patient to state what is known about the specific topic.
- Provide teaching in a step-by-step process, presenting the most essential information first.
- Observe the interaction between the patient and family to determine family roles and authority figures. Include the dominant family member in your teaching.
- Use language easily understood by the patient; avoid medical jargon.
- Maintain consistency in terminology used (e.g., do not use the term *bed sore* one time and then use the term *pressure ulcer* another time).
- Clarify your verbal and nonverbal messages with the patient.
- Have the patient repeat the information learned and, if possible, return any demonstration provided by the nurse.
- Inquire whether the patient has any further questions.
- Summarize at the end of the teaching segment.

Adapted from Daniels, R. (2004). Nursing fundamentals: Caring and clinical decision making. *New York: Thomson Delmar Learning; Dreger, V., & Tremback, T. (2002). Optimize patient health by treating literacy and language barriers.* Association of Operating Room Nurses Journal, 75(2), *280–293.*

Patient and Family Teaching

Educating patients is an integral part of nursing practice. Education not only must be relevant to the patient's needs, it also must be provided in a culturally sensitive manner (Figure 4-6). Culturally competent teaching guidelines are provided in the Skills 360°.

Evaluation

The final phase of the nursing process, evaluation, is extremely important in determining the patient's achievement of expected outcomes and the efficacy of nursing interventions in delivery of culturally sensitive care. Provision of culturally competent care requires that the nurse view the patient as a partner of the health care team. It is important to demonstrate caring behaviors, rather than just demonstrating toleration of cultural variations in patients' behavior. Awareness of cultural similarities and variations allow nurses to accept and appreciate the impact of culture on health care.

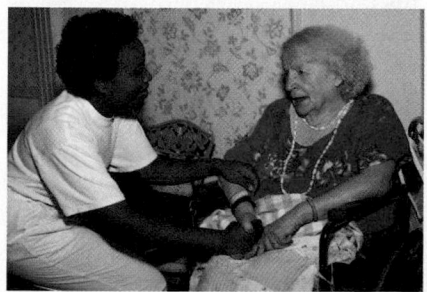

Figure 4-6 Provision of culturally sensitive care depends on establishing a therapeutic nurse-patient relationship.

Concept Map Case Study

Mrs. Tao Mei Kan

Mrs. Tao Mei Kan, a 62-year-old Chinese female, has been admitted to the medical unit for wound management of an ulcer on her left heel. She was diagnosed with non–insulin dependent diabetes mellitus (NIDDM), or type 2 diabetes, six years ago. Her fasting blood glucose levels continue to fluctuate above 260 mg/dL, even though her health care provider prescribed exercise, an appropriate diet, and added tolazamide (Tolinase), a hypoglycemic medication, 100 mg daily, several months ago. Mrs. Kan complains of swelling and numbness in her feet and legs, but she does not have foot pain. The ulcerated area has no drainage; the surrounding skin appears dry, cracked, and calloused; the pedal pulses are normal; the foot is warm to the touch; and her toenails are long and thick.

Mrs. Kan is a widow and lives with her son and his family. Mrs. Kan understands some English but cannot read it. She prefers that her son serve as her interpreter. Her daughter-in-law prepares her meals and administers her medications; however Mrs. Kan frequently will not submit to the finger sticks or scheduled blood draws for checking her glucose levels and sometimes refuses the prescribed medication. In addition to her diabetes, Mrs. Kan has been diagnosed with hypertension and her health care provider prescribed propranolol hydrochloride (Inderal) 40 mg twice a day. She prefers taking the Chinese herbal remedies that she feels are better for her. Her son mentions that his mother stopped her daily walks and Tai Chi exercises when the ulcer first appeared four months ago, and she spends most of her time watching television. Since she was diagnosed with a cataract, Mrs. Kan has recently given up one of her favorite pastimes, reading the Chinese newspapers. Her appetite is good. In fact she has gained some weight recently. Her son is concerned about his mother's health, but he feels helpless in trying to convince her to follow the plan of care.

The scenario has been designed to integrate cultural factors that can impact the plan of care. Create a concept map using the information that has been provided.

1. Create your concept map. Add concepts from the case-study into the areas where you believe they belong. (Note: some concepts may belong in more than one area.)
2. Have you placed the patient in the center of the map?
3. Cluster related concepts together. Draw connecting lines to indicate relationships.
4. What are the risk factors related to culture and adherence to the plan of care?
5. Identify at least two nursing diagnoses related to Mrs. Kan's health problem and her cultural beliefs.
6. Prioritize the patient needs and list nursing interventions you would make to meet the needs.
7. What do you need to know about the Chinese culture to have appropriate interactions with Mrs. Kan and her son and his family?
8. Make a list of additional information that you would like to have to plan an appropriate plan of care for a patient from a different culture.
9. What optimal patient outcomes would you like to see?
10. Develop a basic teaching plan related to diabetes management and wound care. How will you need to adjust the teaching plan to minimize the cultural barriers to learning and application?
11. Compare your map with other students. How do they differ?
12. Discuss how cultural sensitivity is an essential component of safe and effective nursing care.

Concept Map Case Study

Suggested References

Andrews, M., & Boyle, J. (2002). *Transcultural concepts in nursing care.* Philadelphia: Lippincott, Wilkins and Williams.

Leininger, M., & McFarland, M. (2002). *Transcultural nursing.* New York: McGraw-Hill.

Daniels, R. (2003). *Delmar's manual of laboratory and diagnostic tests.* New York: Thomson Delmar Learning.

Myers, B. (2003). *Wound management: Principles and practice.* Upper Saddle River, NJ: Prentice Hall.

KEY CONCEPTS

- Each individual is culturally unique. Behavior, self-perception, and judgment of others all depend on one's cultural perspective.
- Culture is not static, nor is it uniform among all members within cultural groups. Culture represents adaptive dynamic processes learned through life experiences.
- Communication is the vehicle for transmitting and preserving culture. To share complete and accurate information nurses must be aware of the cultural variances related to communication.
- Time orientation (being focused on the past, the present, or the future) varies according to cultural groups.
- Social organization refers to the ways in which groups determine rules of acceptable behavior and roles of individual members.
- Various cultures emphasize the value and importance of family structure, as well as the value and importance of religious beliefs.

- Health disparities exist among cultural groups, such as different incidences and deaths because of cancer, cardiovascular problems, diabetes mellitus, human immunodeficiency virus (HIV), infant mortality, and health prevention measures including immunizations.
- Vulnerable groups at higher risk for health problems include cultural groups, such as the poor and homeless, because of lifestyle, obesity, dietary habits, environmental factors, and lack of access to health care services.
- There is an urgent need to develop social and political reforms as solutions for vulnerable cultural groups.
- Folk medicine and assistance for traditional healers are practiced by various cultural groups that are specific to each group.
- Transcultural nursing focuses on the study and analysis of different cultures and subcultures with respect to cultural care, health beliefs, and health practices with the goal of providing health care within the context of the patient's culture.

REVIEW QUESTIONS

1. Cultural competency occurs when one:
   1. Has knowledge of all the cultural beliefs and practices of a patient
   2. Has memorized all of the boxes of information about Hispanic (Americans), recently immigrated Salvadorans, African Americans, Chinese immigrants, second-generation Eastern European Americans, and others
   3. Considers cultural differences exotic
   4. Has the ability to incorporate cultural preferences into nursing practice

2. Which of the following terms best describes the emotional attitude that one's own ethnic group is superior to others?
   1. Culture
   2. Ethnicity
   3. Superiority
   4. Ethnocentrism

Continued

3. What can one do to ensure culturally competent care is integrated into practice on a regular basis?
   1. Practice self-awareness attitudes, be alert to language barriers, and memorize all the specific cultural groups from the textbook
   2. Use cultural assessment tools, including assessment of family structure, traditional preferences, and medical context
   3. Be aware of assessment findings but not necessarily incorporate them into practice
   4. Treat everyone the same because that is the only fair thing to do

4. The most overwhelming adverse influence on health is which of the following?
   1. Race
   2. Customs
   3. Poverty status
   4. Genetic constitution

5. Which of the following terms best describes a group of people who share a set of values, beliefs, practices, social relationships, law, politics, economics, and norms of behavior?
   1. Race
   2. Culture
   3. Ethnicity
   4. Social group

6. The racial/ethnic diversity in the United States is projected to:
   1. Increase
   2. Decrease
   3. Not change
   4. Become a melting pot

7. Disparities in health status among minority groups have continued to persist in spite of overall improvements in health status and life expectancy in the overall population. Examples of continuing health disparities include:
   1. Caucasians are more likely to die from heart disease than African Americans.
   2. Racial and ethnic minority groups have a higher incidence of prediabetes and diabetes.
   3. Infant mortality of the African American, American Indian, and Alaska Native populations has shown improvement.
   4. The majority of babies born with HIV are born to Caucasian mothers.

8. You have a patient who requires an interpreter for discharge planning. There is no one available to interpret, so you use the patient's roommate. The roommate admits to knowing enough of your patient's language. This could result in:
   1. Intrinsic distortion
   2. Excellent communication
   3. Maintaining patient confidentiality
   4. Extrinsic distortion

9. Racism is defined as:
   1. An expectation that all people within a same culture group act alike
   2. Classifying individuals according to biological differences
   3. Extrinsic distortion of reality
   4. A form of oppression or discrimination of people perceived as inferior

10. A magicoreligious belief system is based on the concept that health and illness:
   1. Are determined by supernatural forces
   2. Are because of fate or outside of personal control
   3. Are because of disharmony of natural elements or processes
   4. Are related to appropriate personal behavior or failure to behave properly

REVIEW ACTIVITIES

1. Explain the difference between culture and ethnicity.

2. Discuss the factors that contribute to the multiculturalism environment in the United States.

3. Discuss how a nurse can provide culturally and linguistically competent nursing care.

4. Develop several questions a nurse could ask to assess patients' cultural values.

5. Develop three culturally sensitive teaching strategies to use when teaching a patient from a diverse background a self-care procedure of your choice.

6. Visit the Management Sciences and Health (subsidiary of Office of Mental Health Bureau) at: http://erc.msh.org to learn more about Kleinman's explanatory health model and be able to discuss the questions that could have been asked of the Hmong family described in *The spirit catches you and you fall down* by Ann Fadiman (1997). Review the techniques that are described for taking a patient history.

Legal and Ethical Aspects of Health Care

Lisa Anderson-Shaw, DrPH, MA, MSN

CHAPTER TOPICS

- Principles of Clinical Ethics

- Ethical Theories

- Professional Ethics

- Advance Directives

- Confidentiality and Informed Consent

- Ethical Decision Making Models

- End-of-Life Care, Euthanasia, and Assisted Suicide

- Medical Futility

- Research Ethics

KEY TERMS

Active euthanasia
Advance directives
Agency
Assisted suicide
Autonomy
Beneficence
Brain dead
Clinical ethics
Code of ethics
Coma depasse
Contextual features
Deontology
Double effect
Durable Power of Attorney for Health Care (DPAHC)
Ethics
Ethics of care
Euthanasia
Informed consent
Justice
Liberty
Living will (LW)
Medical futility
Moral distress
Morals
Nonmaleficence
Passive euthanasia
Right to die
Rights-based ethics
Surrogate decision maker
Teleology
Utilitarian

Providing care for those in need of health care has never been more complex than it is today. Innovation and technology keep pushing the limits of how, when, where, and how far to go with the health care treatment options available. Scientific research continuously provides new and improved ways of treating illness and disease, yet people continue to struggle with sickness, injury, and death. With that struggle often come legal and ethical issues that provide dilemmas of their own. The nurse's application of ethical principles to achieve the best clinical outcomes when ethical and legal dilemmas exist is the focal point of this chapter.

ETHICS IN NURSING PRACTICE OVERVIEW

Each person brings to his or her work his or her own world view, that is, how he or she looks at life and the events that happen in his or her life. This world view is cultivated throughout a lifetime and is influenced by many things, especially culture, religion, and family values and practices. How nurses view the ethical dimensions of their work is directly related to their world view. As nurses become more aware of their individual world view, they can begin to analyze the ethical and moral dimensions of who they are as individuals and who they are as nursing professionals. For example, nurses need to examine their own personal beliefs regarding specific ethical issues, such as end-of-life care, withdrawal of life-sustaining treatment, or refusal of consent to treatment, so that they can provide appropriate care to those patients who may not hold the same beliefs or world views.

ETHICS AND MORALS

To further discuss this topic, some of the common language used when speaking about the legal and ethical dimensions of nursing must be clarified. The term *ethics* is often used in the same way the word *morals* is used. Both of these terms are derived from the study of philosophy. **Ethics,** also referred to as moral philosophy, helps people examine their life and their life actions as they relate to what is right or wrong. The word ethics comes from the Greek word *ethos,* which means character, customs, and standards of conduct. The word **morals** comes from the Latin word *mores,* which means customs or habits. It is evident that these terms have similar meaning and are often used interchangeably (Green, 2005).

Clinical Ethics

Medical ethics is often used synonymously with the terms clinical ethics or bioethics. In this chapter, the term **clinical ethics** is used to denote those ethical issues that have an impact on the nurse's role in patient care and is applied to individual situations. It is, after all, in the clinical arena in which nurses work that these issues present themselves. The solutions to these issues must be applied to each individual situation so that resolution can be achieved. Thus, clinical ethics is viewed as applied ethics.

Applied solutions to ethical issues in the clinical setting are a product of increasingly advanced technology. There was little right and wrong to discuss about therapeutic interventions prior to the advancement of medical technology. However, as interventions became more invasive and the clinical outcomes less clear, ethical dilemmas began to appear, and medical professionals called on their colleagues in theology and philosophy to help analyze and find resolutions to the dilemmas. Thus, clinical ethics was born from traditional disciplines accented by legal, political, and social thought. One of the most basic questions related to clinical ethics has to do with the use of advanced technologies, and that question is: Just because we can, does that mean we should?

Ethical Issues and Ethical Dilemmas

An ethical issue in the clinical setting arises out of a dilemma between what a patient wants, or does not want, and what is actually being done for or to that person. This issue may become a dilemma and escalate into a disagreement or argument about the plan of care decision. For example, if a patient tells the nurse that a second opinion about a certain test result is desired, and the nurse facilitates this action, there is no dilemma. On the other hand, if that nurse is told by the patient's health care provider not to assist the patient to obtain a second opinion, a dilemma will result. The real ethical dilemma is related to patient autonomy and patient rights. To resolve such an ethical dilemma, some background information is needed related to the principles of clinical ethics.

PRINCIPLES OF CLINICAL ETHICS

There are four main principles of clinical ethics (Burkhardt & Nathaniel, 2002). These four principles include respect for autonomy, nonmaleficence, beneficence, and justice. The first principle deals with the concept of **autonomy,** which comes from the Greek *autos* meaning self, and *nomos* meaning rule. Personal autonomy is, at a minimum, self-rule that is free from both controlling interference by others and from limitations, such as inadequate understanding, that prevent meaningful choice. For a person to possess personal autonomy, that person must be at **liberty,** or free and independent from coercion. That person must also have **agency,** that is, he or she must have capacity for intentional action. Generally speaking, if a person is at least 18 years of age and has the ability to make reasoned choices, that person possesses autonomy and is free to make decisions regarding his or her own health care. Autonomous choices made by patients may not be the choices that their family, nurses, or other health care providers would make, but autonomous decisions must be honored.

There may be situations in which a patient may not possess personal autonomy because that person does not have the capacity to make reasoned and informed decisions about his or her health care. On the other hand, a person may be autonomous but not be at liberty because a legal guardian has been named to make health care decisions for that person. Personal autonomy is limited when a person does not have liberty or the agency to exercise his or her own autonomy.

The second principle is **nonmaleficence.** This principle mirrors the do-no-harm concept taken from the Hippocratic tradition; one uses his or her own ability, judgment, and skill to help someone else and not to cause further injury or harm. This principle is referred to in cases in which further aggressive or invasive treatments may cause injury, pain, or harm without offering any meaningful recovery. For example, providing painful dialysis treatments to a patient at the end of life may, in fact, cause more pain and harm than it provides relief and comfort. In this case, the principle of nonmaleficence may support the option of not providing dialysis but instead providing comfort care.

The third principle is the principle of **beneficence.** This principle requires that nurses be of benefit to others, not just do not harm to them as in nonmaleficence. Morality requires not only that nurses treat persons autonomously and refrain from harming them, but in addition that nurses contribute to the welfare of others. There are clinical situations in which it appears that to be of benefit to someone, nurses must first cause the other person harm. A simple example of this might be providing intravenous (IV) fluids and medications. The venipuncture itself may cause anxiety and local pain, and some medications, themselves, cause discomfort or pain, but at the same time significant benefit is provided by maintaining fluid balance or treating an illness.

The fourth and final principle of clinical ethics is the principle of **justice.** Justice in health care is a difficult concept to define. The individualized nature of health care in America contributes to this difficulty, as does the variance of skill from provider to provider. Application of the concept of justice in health care requires that like cases are treated in a like fashion, but it is impossible to secure this from institution to institution and from provider to provider. What can be used and applied from this principle is that, in general, all people who seek health care should receive the best treatment available and that all people are treated with dignity and respect.

ETHICAL THEORIES

There are several important categories of ethical theories that can assist nurses in thinking about and analyzing ethical issues that occur in the clinical setting. The ethical literature is vast. However, a brief overview can assist nurses to begin to analyze situations using ethical theory. Not all theories will fit every situation, and, more importantly, they should not. It might be the case that several theories offer a nurse insights for a particular clinical situation. As more about ethics is learned, nurses usually feel more confident about incorporating that knowledge into clinical practice decisions.

Deontology

Deontology is the first category of ethical theory for exploration. This philosophy is one of moral duty and obligation and is most concerned not with the outcomes of an action but rather with the action itself. This theory is most prominently displayed in the ideas of Immanuel Kant (1724–1804). Kantian Deontology is comparable to the Golden Rule, in that one would chose to act and behave in the way that one would want everyone to act and behave. For example, given a choice of lying or not lying to a patient about something, one would choose not to lie, because the world and society would be better off if no one ever lied. A second important point with regard to deontological thought is that one should always treat people with dignity and respect and never as a means to an end. (Mapes & Zembaty, 1986). For example, a nurse would never try to talk a patient into trying out a new piece of equipment for the sake of practicing its use and for no other reason.

Teleology and Utilitarian

Teleology is the second ethical category for discussion. **Utilitarian** is one of the more prominent teleological theories and is usually associated with the works of Jeremy Bentham (1748–1832) and John Stuart Mill (1806–1873). Utilitarianism proscribes that it is the consequences of an action that are of the utmost importance rather than the action itself. For an action to have utility, it must be of benefit to the greatest number of people affected by the action. This is what is commonly referred to as the greatest good principle (Mapes & Zembaty, 1986). A clinical example of this is immunizations. It is known that there will be a small number of people who will have negative side effects from immunizations; however, the vast majority of people will benefit. Therefore, it is argued that the end result (avoidance of future disease) justifies the action.

Rights-Based

A third category of ethical theory is **rights-based ethics.** It was previously noted that it is often difficult to provide justice and ensure that all people are treated equally. The rights-based theory of ethics proscribes that there are specific human rights to specific human goods, such as health care, that society is obligated to provide to everyone through the American system of health care (Figure 5-1). Human rights often take on moral standing, which means that "persons are entitled to be recognized and heard, and to have their views considered fairly and equally" (Bandman & Bandman, 2002, p. 91). Rights-based ethics not only applies to patients but also to nurses and other health care providers as well.

Ethics of Care

The fourth category of ethical theory is **ethics of care.** This ethical concept is one of the oldest, by far, and one at which nurses are skilled by the nature of their work. Long before there were scientifically proven cures for diseases

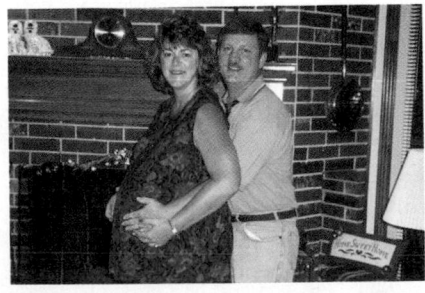

Figure 5-1 This couple is planning a home birth, because the husband recently lost his job, and they do not have health insurance. Scarce resources create the ethical dilemma exemplified in the question: Should health care benefits be a "right" for everyone in society?

nurses cared for those in need. The ethical concept of caring is so valued in the nurse-patient relationship that caring behaviors are broadly embraced by society as the core of the nurse's role (Fry & Johnstone, 2002). For the past several years nurses have been at the top of the list of people most trusted by society in nationwide surveys. It is believed that health care professionals have a moral obligation and a duty to provide care to those in need.

PROFESSIONAL ETHICS

What is professional ethics and how does it fit in with the nurse-patient relationship? Many organizations within the nursing profession have published a **code of ethics,** which guides professional practice and behavior in a specific area of nursing practice. The National Association of Neonatal Nurses, The American Association of Occupational Health Nurses, and the International Council of Nurses each have a code of ethics to guide its members. Many health care provider groups, as well as business organizations, adopt a uniquely focused code of ethics. In May of 2004 the American College of Emergency Physicians published a code of ethics for emergency physicians. This code lists the principles that express the fundamental moral responsibilities of emergency physicians (American College of Emergency Physicians, 2004). In a similar fashion, the American Nurses Association (ANA) updated and published a revision of its code of ethics for nurses in 2001. The ANA code lists nine statements that give definition and guidance to the moral sense of the nursing profession, broadly (Box 5-1).

BOX 5-1

THE ANA CODE OF ETHICS FOR NURSES

The nurse, in all professional relationships, practices with compassion and respect for the inherent dignity, worth, and uniqueness of every individual, unrestricted by considerations of social or economic status, personal attributes, or the nature of health problems.

The nurse's primary commitment is to the patient, whether an individual, family, group, or community.

The nurse promotes, advocates for, and strives to protect the health, safety, and rights of the patient.

The nurse is responsible and accountable for individual nursing practice and determines the appropriate delegation of tasks consistent with the nurse's obligation to provide optimum patient care.

The nurse owes the same duties to self as to others, including the responsibility to preserve integrity and safety, to maintain competence, and to continue personal and professional growth.

The nurse participates in establishing, maintaining, and improving health care environments and conditions of employment conducive to the provision of quality health care and consistent with the values of the profession through individual and collective action.

The nurse participates in the advancement of the profession through contributions to practice, education, administration, and knowledge development.

The nurse collaborates with other health professionals and the public in promoting community, national, and international efforts to meet health needs.

The profession of nursing, as represented by associations and their members, is responsible for articulating nursing values, for maintaining the integrity of the profession and its practice, and for shaping social policy.

Adapted from American Nurses Association. (2001). Code of ethics for nurses with interpretive statements. *Silver Springs, MD: Author.*

Professional codes of ethics focus on behavior within the work setting and often on the behavior between the nurse and the patient. For example, the second provision of the ANA code of ethics for nurses states, "The nurse's primary commitment is to the patient, whether an individual, family, group, or community" (2001). Many code statements relate to the protection of patients from both external and internal harm. Professional ethics involves the care of patients, but it also involves protecting employees and respecting colleagues at all levels of the organization (Huston & Brox, 2004).

Patient's Bill of Rights

Professional codes of ethics are statements that reflect what a particular profession believes and values and for what the profession can be held accountable. The Patient's Bill of Rights is a code of ethics that describes what the patient can expect from the health care enterprise and from that enterprise's health care providers. In addition, Patient's Bill of Rights documents articulate specific responsibilities on the part of the patient so that maximum benefit can be received from the enterprise and from the care providers (American Hospital Association [AHA], 1992). The concept of a Patient's Bill of Rights grew out of a 1969 consumer movement demanding that more attention be given to the needs and perspectives of patients by the Joint Commission on Accreditation of Hospitals (JCAHO), which is a private regulatory body. The document, adopted by the AHA in 1972 and published in 1973, was the initial step in the patient's rights movement. The document was subsequently revised in 1992.

Organizational Ethics

With corporate scandals, such as those associated with Enron and Martha Stewart, there has been increased interest in organizational ethics. Organizational ethics is broader in scope than traditional codes of ethics that focus on a specific group of professionals within an organization. Many organizations develop values statements in addition to the organization's mission and vision statements. Values statements articulate organization-wide standards for ethical behavior. Similarly, most enterprises have corporate compliance programs that guide employees regarding ethical business behavior standards and the obligations incumbent on an employee who becomes aware of infringements of the standards by fellow workers. Corporate compliance programs may be referred to as internal audits that ensure consistent adherence to the standards, policies, practices, and procedures of the enterprise through a system of checks and balances. Such programs strive to empower and support the employees to do the right thing without fear of corporate reprisal.

A NURSE'S ROLE

By the nature of their work, nurses are often caught in between the patient and other health care providers, or family members. In the acute care setting, nurses are in direct contact with the patients for longer periods of time than any other health care team members, so nurses usually have more interaction with, and receive more information from, patients and their families than other care providers. Historically, Bishop and Scudder (1985) adequately describe this in-between position as "day-to-day care through which nurses foster the patient's well-being by bringing together (1) the physician's plan of medical care, (2) the institution's policies and resources, and (3) the patient's view of the good life" (p. 30).

What happens when a patient is not able, or not willing, to carry out the health care provider's plan of medical care, and the nurse's responsibility is to advocate for the patient, yet also implement the plan of care that is believed to be in the patient's best interest medically? These can be difficult situations that are not easily resolved. There are moral obligations on the part of the nurse to both the patient and to the health care provider. When nurses feel that they cannot resolve issues that place them in this in-between position, and for which negative consequences are anticipated, moral distress can result.

Moral Distress

Moral distress in nursing occurs when the nurse is aware of the right and moral action to take in a given patient situation but is unable to carry out that action because of external constraints. External constraints may include a nurse's heavy patient workload because of a shortage of nurses or lack of synergy between the nurse's skill and knowledge and the patient's needs for nursing care, financial constraints on resources, or an institutional imbalance of power resulting in fear of conflict between the nurse and health care provider or other coworkers. This form of distress can take a heavy toll on the nurse, resulting in overall feelings of anger, guilt, and frustration. This form of distress can occur by not being able to fulfill an action the nurse believes is the right thing to do, e.g., not being able to allow a child to visit a sick parent because of organizational policies or by performing an action the nurse perceives to be morally wrong, e.g., performing cardiopulmonary resuscitation (CPR) on a person with end-stage cancer who is near death.

Overcoming moral distress in nursing practice is difficult to do, first and foremost because it is often not identified or talked about among nursing staff. Feelings of distress are often suppressed in the workplace, resulting in stress-related physical symptoms and increased job dissatisfaction. It is therefore important that when nurses feel moral distress these feelings are acknowledged and systems are in place to assist nurses to resolve such feelings. This system should include an understanding of the general principles of ethics that provide the framework for professional practice, an environment that encourages discussion among nursing staff of the ethical issues and dilemmas that are occurring and, finally, a safe environment for nurses to address organizational problems with the interdisciplinary health care team and management so that proper resolutions may be reached. There may be situations in which full resolution of the feelings of distress are not possible; however, with proper communication systems in place, moral distress may not progress to the point of despair.

Nurse as Patient Advocate

Nurses have long been associated with the patient advocate role. The word advocate itself means to act in support of something, which is what nurses do. Nurses act in many ways that support patients. Inherent to this word and its meaning is the notion that patients need an advocate, because they cannot support themselves to their fullest extent and, therefore, need another to look out for their interest, namely their health. Nurses are at the patient's bedside and consequently interact consistently with patients, their friends, and their family. Thus, nurses tend to have a holistic perspective of their patients. The ANA Code of Ethics for Nurses states the nurse promotes, advocates for, and strives to protect the health, safety, and rights of the patient (ANA, 2001). This objective can only be achieved through a holistic nursing practice.

Within the legal sense of the word, an advocate is a person who pleads another's cause. One might think of the advocacy role of nursing as that of partnering with the other health care providers in ways that promote the good of the patient, because all forms of providers are advocates in that same sense. However, the position that nurses hold by being in constant contact with their patients and families does allow the nurse to have special knowledge and a special responsibility toward the advocacy role. This unique position is intertwined in the art of nursing, which is based on ethical constructs as opposed to task-oriented behavior (DeLaune & Ladner, 2006). Advocacy in this sense has to do with a therapeutic and holistic relationship with patients and is a basis for professional nursing practice.

The nurse's position as patient advocate is not an independent role. Rather, the advocate role is uniquely and importantly integrated across all of the various roles that make up the practice of nursing. Conflict may occur within advocacy situations. For instance, the nurse does not work in isolation but rather with other nurses and health care providers, as well as being an employee of a specific institution or agency. Conflict may arise when the nurse feels a strain between what the patient needs and what the nurse is able to do within the constraints of the work environment. This is similar to the moral distress that is felt by being in between the patient and his or her health care provider or other providers.

It may be the case that the nurse feels powerless to truly advocate for patient needs because of an overall feeling of powerlessness among the nursing profession in an institutional setting. Though all team members may be advocating for a patient, they may each have different ideas on what is the best plan of action, which in turn can lead to conflict among providers and perhaps between provider and patient. However, the nurse is always obligated to protect a patient's rights and, additionally, to maintain professional practice within the nursing profession. Alternative measures, such as an interdisciplinary team meeting, can be effective in empowering nurses to advocate for patients.

CONFIDENTIALITY

Issues of confidentiality are extremely important for patients and for nurses. Personal privacy is viewed as a fundamental patient right. The nurse-patient relationship is based on trust, which includes trust that personal patient health information is only shared with people who are directly involved with the patient's care. One might think that keeping patient information confidential is not necessarily a problem; however, where and how a nurse discusses patient information may lend itself to the disclosure of confidential information. For instance, speaking about a patient in an open or public space where others may hear, such as a crowded elevator on in the cafeteria, may breach confidentiality. In addition, disclosing patient information over the phone may also be a breach of confidentiality, unless the patient has given permission to do so.

With the advancement of information technology, including electronic medical records, facsimiles, e-mail, and computer printers located in open work areas comes the added burden of keeping patient information confidential. Leaving a computer screen with patient information visible to others is a breach of confidentiality, as is leaving computer printouts containing patient information lying about a work area where it can be viewed by other staff. Awareness of patient confidentiality has never been as important as it is now. JCAHO has adopted many standards dealing with confidentiality.

In 1996, the United States Department of Health and Human Services (USDHHS) instituted oversight of legal health information confidentiality. This federal law is called the Health Insurance Portability and Accountability Act (HIPAA) of 1996 and it became effective in 2003. The law applies to health information created or maintained by health care providers who engage in certain electronic transactions, health plans, and health care clearinghouses. In essence, this law protects patients' basic rights to privacy and their control over the disclosure of their personal health information (Erlen, 2004). HIPAA protects information in the medical record, conversations providers have with other care providers, and personal insurance and billing information related to individuals' personal health information.

Personal health information can be used and shared with providers who are involved in a specific patient's care and with family and friends who the patient permits, as well as appropriate public health and police agencies as outlined in the HIPAA guidelines. Confusion over what is and what is not protected health information under the HIPAA guidelines is common. Each institution or workplace is responsible for implementing its own policies and regulations by which the nursing staff must operate with respect to the HIPAA guidelines. Every nurse must be aware of, and abide by, the operating rules and regulations at their workplace. Appropriate and ethical nursing practice should always respect the confidentiality of patient information in all settings.

INFORMED CONSENT

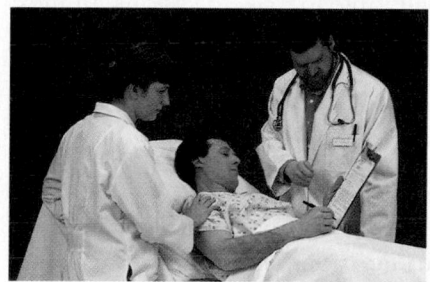

Figure 5-2 This nurse is witnessing the signing of a consent form after the health care provider has fully informed the patient about the proposed treatment.

Issues related to informed consent are often difficult to sift through, despite appearing straightforward. Simply stated, **informed consent** is the process by which a patient receives information about a specific procedure or therapy, alternative procedures and therapies, and the expected outcomes of each to deliberate the information and come to an informed, autonomous decision about which specific procedure or therapy is most appropriate for him or her (Figure 5-2). Informed consent requires respect for the informed and voluntary treatment choice of a competent patient.

The difficulty with this simple process of informed consent makes itself known in dealing with the variables that occur in real-life patient situations. First, for a patient to freely give informed consent, that patient must have the autonomy to do so. That is, the patient must be of legal age and must have the cognitive ability to understand and deliberate with reasoning skill that allows him or her to come to a conclusion. In addition, he or she must not be coerced or forced into a specific decision by family, care providers, or others. Second, the patient must be given all the pertinent information about the risks and benefits of the procedure to which they are consenting and alternative options, as well as information about what will happen if he or she chooses not to consent to the procedure or therapy in question. Third, the patient needs to have the cognitive ability to reasonably understand and deliberate among the stated choices. Finally, the patient must be able to freely consent or refuse to consent, based on the information given and his or her own personal values and wishes.

The overriding goal of informed consent is the protection of the patient and the promotion of autonomous choice. In the case of children, or adults who are not autonomous (do not have the cognitive capacity to make informed decisions), a surrogate decision maker must make health care decisions for them. For people who are not yet 18 years of age (minors), parents or legal guardians are the surrogate decision makers and are responsible for informed consent for the minor person. A rare legal exception to this rule is made when the patient is an emancipated minor, a person under 18 years of age who is self-supporting and living independently. If such a situation presents itself, the nurse should review the relevant institutional policy and contact the legal affairs officer for consultation.

Do all adults, then, retain autonomy or the right to make informed consent for themselves? Yes, in most situations, adult individuals are given the right to informed consent unless there is reason to question their cognition or the ability to make informed consent. However, a nurse might question the ability of an adult patient to fulfill the requirements of informed consent, when the health care provider does not. For example, a patient who is heavily sedated may not be able to adequately and reasonably deliberate among therapy choices while bearing in mind the risks and benefits associated with these choices. If a nurse questions the cognitive ability of an adult patient to make an informed decision about health care, the nurse needs to bring it to the attention of the health care provider and further assessment of the patient should ensue. A patient may be able to provide a reasonably legible signature on the consent form line, but the process that precedes the signing is far more important than the signature (Figure 5-3).

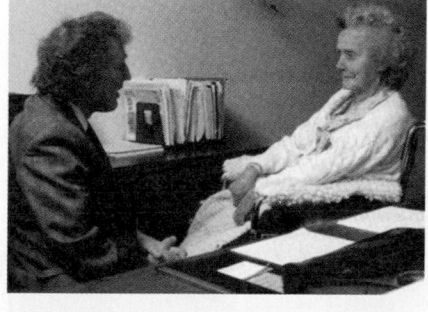

Figure 5-3 Nurse explaining a procedure to an elderly patient who is cognitively impaired.

In emergency situations where life or limb is at risk, the process of informed consent is waived in lieu of providing the needed emergency care. However, once the emergency situation is under control and if the patient has the ability, informed consent for further procedures must be obtained (see Real World, Real Choices).

If an adult patient does not have the ability to give informed consent, nurses must follow the institution's policy and the state laws regarding who must be solicited to legally give informed consent on behalf of the patient. In many states, there are surrogate decision making laws that allow next of kin to make legal decisions for a patient who is not legally able to make decisions. In most cases, there is a hierarchy of individuals who are eligible to be a patient's surrogate decision maker; therefore, nurses must be aware of policy and law related to these situations.

ADVANCE DIRECTIVES

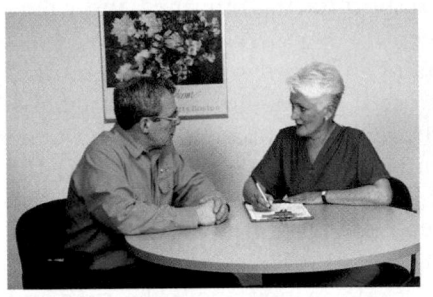

Figure 5-4 A patient and nurse discussing and completing advance directives.

Adults have the right to make autonomous decisions about their own health care, even if they become incapacitated and are unable to communicate their specific health care wishes. For this reason, over the past several decades various forms of advance directives for health care have been enacted into law. Such **advance directives** allow a person to make specific decisions about his or her future health care treatments in advance and often in advance of illness (Figure 5-4). These documents are a way of expressing one's autonomy in situations in which one may no longer be able to do so. Advance directives are typically written and take various forms such as a living will or a durable power of attorney for health care. There may also be a verbal understanding between an individual and the family or between the individual and the health care provider, which is called a verbal advance directive.

Advance directives have become so important that a federal law called the Patient Self Determination Act was enacted as part of the Omnibus Budget

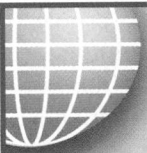

Real World, Real Choices

A 54-year-old man was admitted to the intensive care unit with acute bleeding of esophageal varices due to portal hypertension and cirrhosis of the liver. He is also suffering from chronic renal failure and has been diagnosed with mental status changes due to encephalopathy. The patient agreed to undergo endoscopy with banding procedure of his varices to stop the bleeding. Such a procedure requires that the patient be sedated and placed on mechanical ventilation. The banding procedure was successful in stopping his internal bleeding, but he lost a large amount of blood and his health care providers wish to treat his drop in hemoglobin with a blood transfusion. Because this patient is still under the influence of previous sedation, he is not able to give informed consent needed to administer the blood transfusion. The patient's wife is at his bedside. He does not have any form of written advance directive, so his wife is asked to consent for the blood transfusion. The wife is a practicing Jehovah's Witness (JW) and refuses to consent for a blood transfusion for her husband, even though she acknowledges that her husband is not of the JW faith.

1. What should the health care team do?
2. Who should make decisions for this patient?
3. How can the nurses support both this patient and his wife?
4. Which principles of clinical ethics can be applied to this case?

Reconciliation Act of 1990. The law was enacted in 1991 and requires all health care enterprises that receive federal funds to ask all patients seeking care in their facility to provide that facility with any form of advance directive for health care the patient may have. The law also requires such enterprises to provide assistance to those patients who want more information about advance directives or who want assistance to complete an advance directive.

The intent of advance directives is to allow individual autonomy in addition to assisting with difficult treatment decisions that often include end-of-life decisions. Conversations about what a person would want done in specific situations if that person were no longer able to make the decisions for themselves are difficult to initiate with family and friends. Having an advance directive, such as a durable power of attorney for health care, and knowing that health care institutions ask about such documents may ultimately open the door for people to initiate difficult, yet important, conversations with family and friends.

There are many resources available to assist people who want to execute an advance directive for health care. Most health care institutions provide various forms for patients, and the Internet has multiple resources available for research. In addition, people may consult a lawyer for assistance, but an attorney is not required in most states. The ability to express one's autonomy through an advance directive is protected under law to the extent that health care providers who ignore valid documents expressing patients' wishes regarding life-sustaining care may face civil lawsuits.

Living Will

Many states have statutes that allow an individual to write a **living will (LW).** This document is a form of advance directive for health care that allows a person to document specifically what kinds of medical treatment he or she wants or does not want in the event that he or she is assessed to be terminally ill. LWs should not be confused with any form of testamentary will or will for one's estate. An LW contains directives only about health care treatment decisions at the end of life and nothing more (Haas, 2005).

The LW document allows a person to make decisions related to life-prolonging medical treatment, including artificial ventilation, CPR, artificial food and fluid support, surgical procedures, and other such procedures. In the case of a terminal illness (which usually is defined as having six months or less to live), nurses and health care providers are directed by a valid LW. To be valid, the proper state form must be used and executed in compliance with specific state laws. Each state has its own requirements and patients, as well as care providers, need to be aware of what constitutes a valid LW in their own state.

If a patient has an LW, nursing staff need to review the document with the medical care team and secure a copy of this form in the patient's health care record. If the patient is alert and able to communicate, reviewing the form with the patient is always important to do to be sure that he or she currently supports the contents of the form and do not wish to alter or revoke it in any way. When a nurse reviews the LW with a patient, the patient and nurse both need to initial and date the review. A third person may be required to witness the patient's initials. If the patient is incapacitated, the nurse needs to review the contents with family members, particularly the surrogate decision maker, so that there is clear understanding about what the patient has expressed through the LW form.

Durable Power of Attorney for Health Care

Another form of written advance directive for health care is the **Durable Power of Attorney for Health Care (DPAHC).** This directive allows a person to appoint an agent, or proxy decision maker, to make health care decisions for that person in case decisional capacity is lost. In many states the DPAHC form includes specific medical treatment options that can be checked off, as well as

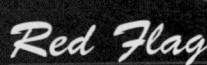

Patient Inability to Make a Decision

The nurse must remember that the lack of decisional capacity may be a temporary state for a patient. Many conditions aggravate the ability to have good cognitive decision making processes. And, sometimes, as in the case of acute illnesses, the patient's condition is alleviated with health care interventions, and the patient becomes enabled to make clear decisions again. Therefore, the nurse must assess mental status frequently and document specific findings.

space to write in specific medical treatment options that one wants to have or not have, done. The DPAHC also allows a person to name successor agents or proxy decision makers in the event that the first named agent is not available to fulfill the responsibility. In most cases the DPAHC goes into effect when a person lacks decisional capacity for any reason and is terminated when that person regains decisional capacity (Brown, Grigsby, Walsh, & Kaye, 2002).

An important difference to note between most LW documents and DPAHC documents is that an LW goes into effect when a person is assessed to have a terminal illness and lacks capacity, whereas a DPAHC is not constrained by a terminal state of health. For this reason, many people choose to hold only a DPAHC, which includes the specific treatment information that an LW contains.

What is so important to realize about initiating advance directives for health care is that people can fill these forms out and make decisions about future health care decisions while they remain able to do so and, in most cases, are not in any form of distress. The ethical quandary that is ever present has to do with all the what ifs that come to mind, specifically: What if I change my mind about my directive after I become sick? Remember that advance directives can be revoked or revised at any time that a patient has the capacity to do so. Once capacity is lost, there really is no way of knowing if a person might have changed his or her mind about a specific part of his or her advance directive. Therefore, his or her last known wishes as expressed in his or her advance directive must be honored.

Verbal Advance Directive

A person may not have any formal written advance directive for health care but may have specific wishes about his or her medical treatment. In such cases all he or she needs to do is discuss those wishes with his or her health care provider and family. The health care provider needs to clearly document what the patient has stated he or she wants or does not want done in specific situations, or the fact that the patient has named an agent to speak for him or her in the event that decisional capacity is lost.

The patient may also verbalize his or her wishes to a nurse. If this occurs, the nurse must document the patient's directive in the clinical record and review the conversation with the health care provider and care team so that everyone involved in the care of the patient is clear about the patient's wishes. A family or team meeting with the patient present is important for deciding on a clear plan of care. As with written advance directives, a verbal advance directive may be revised or rescinded by the patient as long as that patient has decisional capacity to do so. A verbal directive replaces a previously written advance directive or a written advance directive that cannot be located or produced when the patient makes the verbal wishes known. In all cases, timely, thorough documentation and communication are extremely important.

Surrogate Decision Maker

In many cases patients do not have any form of written or verbal advance directive for health care decision making at the time they lose decisional capacity. Research on advance directives consistently reports that only a small number of individuals actually have prepared any kind of advance directive (Shapiro & Bowles, 2002). There are multiple reasons that individuals do not complete formal written advance directives for health care, including lack of knowledge, lack of interest, denial, or simply not taking the time to have a conversation with family or friends or to complete the forms. There may also be cultural issues that impact advance directives. For example, not all cultures or religions value the rights of self-determination and informed consent inherent in American culture. Therefore, nurses and other health care providers need to be sensitive to the reasons that a patient may not have an advance directive.

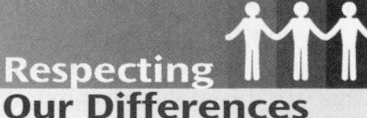

Respecting Our Differences

Same Sex Partners and Advanced Directives

Note that same sex partners are not legally recognized in most states in the next of kin surrogate decision maker hierarchy. Therefore, unless a same sex partner is specifically recognized and named as the legal surrogate in a formal written advance directive for health care, that person will not be the first in line as a choice for legal surrogate decision maker. Patients who are gay or lesbian can be given information about advance directives during routine medical visits so that they can make informed decisions regarding potential surrogate decision makers if they choose to do so.

If a patient does not have any kind of advance directive for health care and he or she does not have decisional capacity, a **surrogate decision maker** must be named on his or her behalf. The procedure for naming this surrogate, or proxy, agent for the patient may vary from state to state. Therefore, nurses must be aware of the specific state's law, as well as the specific health care enterprise's policies related to surrogate decision making. In many states, the law allows a form of next of kin hierarchy from which a surrogate decision maker may be named on behalf of the patient who lacks decisional capacity. According to this type of state statute, a surrogate decision maker can be legally named without going to the court system for approval. When a legal surrogate is named, the surrogate has the legal right to make any and all medical decisions on behalf of the patient, including the withholding or withdrawal of life-sustaining treatments. There are some restrictions noted in the law, so it is important to have knowledge of the specific state's statute and also know the institutional resources available, such as the ethics consultant or social worker.

If there is no one available to act as a patient surrogate according to law and policy, the institution would need to proceed through legal channels so that a court-appointed guardian be named for the patient without decisional capacity. If nurses identify a potential need for a surrogate decision maker early in the patient's care, a legal guardian can be appointed in a timely manner to provide the patient with an appropriate medical decision maker.

ETHICAL DECISION MAKING MODELS

There are a variety of approaches to making decisions within the health care system. There is not a single best approach to ethical decision making, and different models exist. This section will present five models for ethical decision making: medical indications, patient preferences, quality of life, contextual features, and an integrated model.

Medical Indications

Many decisions made by nurses are made because the patient is in need. For example, medications and therapy are ordered based on what it is the patient not only needs, but what will also benefit the patient. For example, a patient will receive the appropriate antibiotic therapy based on the organism that is causing the infection. In other words, the treatment is related to clinical and medical indications. Much of what nurses do is done because it is medically indicated or medically necessary to benefit the patient in need. Nurses would not provide medical treatments that were not indicated or that would be of no benefit.

One model of ethical decision making is based on medical indications and encompasses the ethical principles of beneficence and nonmaleficence. In essence, this model is rooted in the way a patient may benefit from medical and nursing care and how harm can be avoided. The ethical issues that arise for which this model is useful are issues that are often conflict based. For example, a patient requests a specific treatment or procedure that the medical team does not believe is medically indicated or of medical benefit to the patient. This type of conflict is frequently seen when discussing aggressive end-of-life treatment or resuscitative measures for a patient for whom the health care provider believes the treatment is not medically indicated or who cannot benefit from the treatment.

For instance, the surrogate decision maker for a patient with end-stage metastatic cancer may want everything possible to be done, including resuscitative measures. The health care team, however, believes that resuscitative measures would not provide any benefit and will not reverse the end-stage disease process, and therefore resuscitative measures are not indicated. The team may also believe that such measures may actually harm the patient in the process. Although these types of decisions are often difficult because of the emotions involved, ethical, as well as clinical, decisions need to be based on appropriate indications for the given situation; that is, what are the goals of treatment and the likelihood of success?

Patient Preferences

Another model used in ethical decision making is related to patient preferences and follows the ethical principle of autonomy. Care providers should allow patient autonomy unless there is reason to believe that the patient is not able to exercise autonomy, as with patients who lack decisional capacity. In cases where a patient lacks decisional capacity, the care provider must determine whether the patient has made preferences known via any form of advance directive for health care. This model strives to respect patient preferences while avoiding being overly paternalistic with regard to clinical and ethical decisions.

Quality of Life

A third model for ethical decision making relates to quality of life and is based on the principles of beneficence, nonmaleficence, and respect for autonomy. Quality of life (QOL) issues can be difficult to assess, because care providers judge a patient's QOL based on their own ideas of what is an acceptable QOL. For example, if a patient is confined to bed and cannot communicate verbally because of a stroke, care providers may judge the QOL to be poor. However, it might be that the patient is able to touch his or her loved ones and to maintain eye contact with them in a way that has meaning to him or her and that such QOL is acceptable to them. The patient may still wish for the ability to live actively as he or she once did but accepts his or her current state of health. QOL is an individualistic concept, and the range of quality that one may find acceptable in life can be quite variable. Nurses should not judge another's QOL based on their own ideals, and should try to understand their patient's QOL perspective to assist that patient to make ethical decisions.

Contextual Features

Contextual features encompass many of the social, economic, and cultural factors that make each person unique as an individual. In addition, contextual features are correlated with the principles of loyalty and fairness; however, these contextual features are also a part of the ethical principle of justice. Nurses and other medical team members cannot really assess a patient's health condition and needs without taking into account the contextual features that have had an influence on the patient's health or illness. The concept of justice takes into account various ideals that affect each person as an individual and as a member of a community, including the distribution of health care services, the ability to access health care services, how individuals are treated within the health care system, and the decisions made pertaining to health care treatment.

Health care decisions cannot be made without evaluating each patient holistically, including the contextual features that will no doubt affect treatment outcomes. If a patient does not have the ability to pay for expensive medications, treatment decisions must take this into account, and alternative treatment options must be found. All other contextual features that might affect the health and illness must be approached in the same manner. It would be unethical to disregard the individual within the context of his or her daily life.

Integrated Model

The four models discussed here are most often employed together, using the information from each model to ascertain a holistic assessment of the patient's condition so that the appropriate and ethical plan of care might be rendered. So, in essence, when the ethical nature of a specific patient issue is being assessed, the nurse needs to consider all four models: medical indications, patient preferences, QOL, and contextual features to best assist the patient toward an ethical conclusion. The approach might be started by simply listing patient information related to each model topic. Once this list is complete, the data can be analyzed according to the topic and principles involved. As in most clinical evaluations, the ethical evaluation may not give a crystal clear result, but the integrated model for ethical decision making may provide a clear picture of the individual patient who has medical decisions to make (Makoul & Clayman, 2006).

ETHICAL ISSUES OF PAIN MANAGEMENT

The alleviation of pain and suffering and the provision of comfort have long been associated with nursing as a caring profession. Comfort measures may be as simple as a therapeutic touch, applying a cool compress to a warm forehead, or supplying a warm blanket to a person who is cold. However, pain management for people who are more than just a little uncomfortable is often a complicated matter. Despite significant advances in medical technology and biology, nurses across most practice settings encounter patient pain and struggle to manage it (Hader & Guy, 2004).

Ethically, the principles of autonomy, beneficence, and nonmaleficence should all be considered in relationship to patients' pain management issues. Pain and the ability to manage pain are of great concern to the general public, as well as to nurses and health care providers. Publicity over the undertreatment of pain both in the news media and in the legal arena has gotten the attention of all who are involved in health care—patient and provider, alike. Litigation related to the undertreatment of pain is on the rise. The concerns are real; so much so that in 1999 JCAHO initiated pain treatment standards. JCAHO takes pain standards so seriously that patients and their families are provided with information for the reporting of undertreatment of pain complaints.

Why is it that patients fear that their pain will not be adequately assessed, treated, and resolved by nurses and health care providers, and why is it that nurses and health care providers are reluctant to adequately assess, treat, and follow-up with pain management issues? The reasons for both patients' and providers' concerns related to pain management are multifaceted. Patients may be reluctant to report pain symptoms because of a fear of becoming addicted to drugs, or they may have cultural reasons for not reporting or displaying pain. There is fear that if a patient complains of pain too much, they may be labeled or thought of negatively. Medical, as well as nursing, staff may not believe the patient is experiencing pain to the degree to which the patient is complaining, or staff may themselves believe that adequate pain control will lead to the patient's addiction to pain medications.

Perhaps the greatest barrier to adequate pain management is lack of understanding by both patient and provider about pain management issues, coupled with lack of skill in the assessment of pain. Since the JCAHO pain management standards have been employed, most institutions have developed standards of care and training programs to help staff better manage patients' pain. In addition, the American Pain Society has labeled pain assessment as the fifth vital sign, which emphasizes the importance of pain assessment. In his presidential

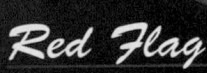
address to the American Pain Society in 1995, Dr. James Campbell asked health care professionals to consider pain as the fifth vital sign, which must be assessed each time that other vital signs (pulse, blood pressure, temperature, and respiration) are assessed. In addition, he urged providers to take their patients' complaints of pain seriously and to take the treatment of their pain seriously, as well. The ANA also acknowledges a problem with pain management and holds an ethics and human rights position statement on The Promotion of Comfort and Relief of Pain in Dying Patients.

Nurses are an important part of the pain management process for their patients. Nurses need to be educated about pain assessment techniques and the rationale for responding promptly with pain treatment when patients are in need. Nurses must follow-up and reassess patients' pain after treatment to evaluate whether pain treatment regimens are adequate or the regimen needs modification. It would be unethical for a nurse to respond to a patient's request for pain relief by stating that it is not yet time for the medication and then offer no other assistance. In such cases, the nurse must assess the patient and contact the treating health care provider so that the pain management regimen might be revised. Reassessment is vital to successful pain management. Care providers too often fall short with this ongoing activity. Pain assessment, treatment, and follow-up are essential to the basic right of patients to have their pain treated appropriately.

END-OF-LIFE CARE

Providing care for patients near the end of life is an essential part of nursing. Many issues are involved with end-of-life care, including pain control. The ethical issues that are apparent at the end of life are often complex, because nursing care not only serves the patient, but also the patient's family and loved ones. This time of transition is often emotional for all individuals involved, including the nurse. Most end-of-life decisions can be articulated by individuals through some form of advance directive for health care. It is often the case, though, that a surrogate is the one making end-of-life decisions on behalf of a loved one who lacks the capacity and who does not have an advance directive.

Hospice and Palliative Care

Hospice and palliative care are often used interchangeably in the United States to mean specific treatment at the end of one's life. The word hospice refers to a place of shelter for the sick and has been established as a program that is Medicare-sponsored to provide comfort care services for the terminally ill and their families. These programs generally provide multidisciplinary support services that may be provided in a home situation or in a health care institution. To receive hospice services, patients must qualify under specific guidelines. Therefore, the term hospice should really be reserved for those patients who will be entering the federally funded hospice service program.

Palliative care, on the other hand, should not imply a Medicare-sponsored program. Palliative care should be viewed as a process that focuses on relieving pain and other physical symptoms, enhancing psychosocial supports, and allowing patients and families to achieve meaningful resolution to their lives together. Palliative comfort care should be provided to all patients in need of such care, no matter if they are near death or simply in need of comfort. Therefore, the fear that surrounds discussing palliative care with patients because the patient might think he or she is dying needs to be dispelled by care providers.

Nurses and health care providers may generally avoid discussing the concept of hospice and palliative care, because they do not want patients to lose hope or to think that the providers have given up caring for them. However, it might be a misunderstanding of the definition of what hope is that causes reluctance to discuss palliative care. Often, when there is no further curative treatment that can be offered to a patient, the patient is well aware of that fact. The patient may continue to wish for a cure, but hope shifts from cure to an inner power that facilitates the transcendence of the present situation and movement toward new awareness and enrichment of being. Even when the patient is knowingly facing death, love of family and friends, spirituality, maintaining independence, positive relationships with care providers, humor, and uplifting memories have been shown to foster this kind of hope (Buckley & Herth, 2004).

Barriers other than general discomfort with the subject may prevent discussion of palliative care with patients and family members. Cultural and spiritual issues, social issues related to patient and family relationships, or physical and environmental issues, such as physical pain, noisy medical equipment, or a lack of privacy, may impede such discussion. It is generally acknowledged that there is an ongoing need for significant improvement in end-of-life care. Therefore nurses and health care providers must use their assessment skills and the treatment options available to them to overcome the barriers and appropriately treat patients (Fine, 2005).

Concept of Double Effect

A serious concern for people faced with a terminal condition, or for people faced with caring for someone who has a terminal illness, is the fear of pain and suffering. Recent research supports the fact that fear of pain is a reality and that unrelieved pain causes distress for both patients and families at the end of life (Jablonski & Wyatt, 2005). JCAHO standards include specific measures that address pain management, underscoring the importance of this issue for health care providers. Moreover, there is an ethical obligation for providers to assist patients by providing comfort measures that are beneficial.

There are barriers present that can hinder appropriate symptom management for patients near the end of life. Such barriers may include the environment, socio-economic status, cultural and religious issues, and the fear of causing death through the use of increased doses of pain medications. There is a general fear of pain while in the dying process, and for some, there is a fear that palliative pain therapy will, itself, hasten a person's death. This is called the principle of **double effect.** Double effect occurs when the intended use of palliation has the unintended effect of hastening a person's death. The principle of double effect acknowledges that one act can embrace two effects: an intended effect and an unintended, secondary effect. The intended effect governs the morality of the act.

An example of this principle of double effect is when a medication given to relieve pain also has the effect of depressing the patient's respiratory drive, causing loss of respiratory function and, thus, death. However, the intent of increased pain medication is to relieve pain and suffering, not to cause death, the unintended consequence of the medication. Such unintended consequence would not be viewed as euthanasia, or administering a medication to purposefully cause the death of another person.

Because pain and symptom management are such important issues for both caregivers and patients, each patient who is near death requires a well thought-out plan of care that will enable him or her to be as comfortable as possible in the final hours of life. The patient, to the fullest extent possible, should be enabled to express preferences and needs for care and be involved in developing the plan of care. In all cases, however, the differences in how patients and their families view the various aspects of pain management must be acknowledged, accepted, and respected.

Limitation of Treatment

When cure is no longer a treatment goal and the goal for patient care has turned to comfort and palliative care, patients or their surrogates may wish to limit further aggressive treatment and therapy. Generally, limitation of aggressive treatment is discussed with the patient, family, and health care team so that the plan of care may be coordinated to include the most appropriate comfort measures.

For example, a patient may have end-stage cancer for which no further cancer treatments are available. In addition, the patient may be in acute renal failure. After discussing treatment options with the family and the health care team, the decision to forego dialysis may be made. Another example of limitation of treatment is choosing not to have further blood product transfusions for a patient in fulminate hepatic failure when death is imminent but who has developed abdominal bleeding.

Ethical dilemmas can occur regarding the limitation of treatment option when either the patient or surrogate is at odds with the treatment recommendations of the medical team. It might be that the medical team recommends limiting further aggressive treatment, but the patient or the surrogate wants aggressive treatment to continue. **Medical futility** is often cited as the reason not to continue aggressive therapy, because the particular therapy offers no medical benefit. Such situations are difficult for everyone directly involved, and guidance from the institutional ethics committee or ethics consultant may be required to resolve the dilemma. Decisions to limit aggressive treatment can be emotional, because the decision usually indicates that death is near. It is therefore important to provide emotional and spiritual support to patients and their family members faced with a decision to discontinue further aggressive treatment.

Do-Not-Resuscitate Orders

It is generally accepted practice in the United States that when a patient in a health care facility experiences a cardiac or respiratory arrest providers attempt resuscitation measures unless that patient or their surrogate has expressed a desire not to have resuscitation attempted. This is one of the few directives in health care that requires consent not to do something rather than consent to do something.

Much has been written about the do-not-resuscitate (DNR) order, including the various terms used to describe such inactivity. Terms may include do-not-attempt-resuscitation (DNAR), do-not-intubate (DNI), or allow natural death (AND). Every health care enterprise has policies that describe the procedures that are not to be carried out. In addition, there are usually specific laws and policies that direct who can make these decisions. For example, some states allow a surrogate decision maker to give consent for this type of order without legal intervention or allow a health care provider to enter such an order unilaterally without specific consent from the patient or a surrogate (Anderson-Shaw, 2003). It is important to understand the laws and institutional policies that surround resuscitation orders to ensure that the appropriate steps are taken when the order is implemented.

Ethical dilemmas may occur when a conflict between provider and the patient or surrogate occurs regarding the implementation of a DNR order. It might be that the health care providers believe that resuscitative measures would be of no benefit, but the patient or family wants to have resuscitative measures provided in the event of cardiac or respiratory arrest. Again, these situations are emotional and can cause a good deal of distress to patients, surrogates, and providers. Providers need to always point out that a DNR order does not mean that care for the patient will stop or that comfort measures will not be implemented or continued.

Artificial Nutrition and Hydration

Providing food and fluid have long been associated with basic medical care. Proper nutrition and hydration are essential for healing and the homeostasis associated with general good health. However, when restoration of health is no longer a goal of care and end-of-life care is the goal, the question of providing artificial nutrition and hydration (ANH) may come up. ANH is when a person can no longer receive food and fluid orally due to illness and disease, and it must be delivered to them through artificial means, which may include a nasogastric tube, gastrostomy tube, or IV infusions.

Just as patients or their surrogates may decide to limit medical interventions at the end of life, they may also want to limit ANH. This means the patient or surrogate refuses to accept liquid nutrition, hydration, or both. Controversy surrounds the use of ANH, because some people believe that ANH should be viewed as ordinary care, while others believe that ANH is medical treatment that can be refused (Sieger, Arnold, & Ahronheim, 2002). Many states have statutes that define ANH as life-sustaining treatment, thereby allowing patients or their surrogates the right to refuse ANH.

One of the main moral dilemmas associated with ANH revolves around the notion that people suffer or have pain when ANH is withheld or removed. However, research has shown that most people in the dying process do not experience feelings of hunger and thirst or exhibit signs of pain when ANH is withheld secondary to decreased gastrointestinal activity (HPNA Board, 2004).

Because the act of taking nutrition is usually an activity shared with others i.e., surrounded by family, friends, or colleagues, or associated with the love expressed in feeding an infant, there is social and emotional significance associated with offering food and fluid to those who are ill. Providers must be mindful that continued personal contact by providers and family should be encouraged even if the act of providing food and hydration is absent. In addition, patients or surrogates may have religious preferences regarding specific aspects of ANH. The counsel of their clergy can be encouraged if patients or surrogates have specific questions.

Right to Die

Many people believe that just as there may be a right to life, there may also be a **right to die,** or at least to make decisions about how one's death might occur within the medical context. As previously explored, the use of formal advance directives for health care may assist in making end-of-life decisions even when the patient might not have the mental capacity to do so. Of course, if a person is able to make specific decisions about his or her health care, he or she is autonomous to do so and health care providers must honor autonomous decisions made by patients.

Brain Death and Organ Donation

Coma depasse, or irreversible coma, was first introduced as a clinical concept in 1959, and was used to describe patients who were unconscious, had loss of brainstem reflexes and respiration, and who had essentially flat electroencephalograms (Mollaret & Goulon, 1959). In 1968 Harvard Medical School reviewed this definition of brain death and established the classic criteria by which we now assess brain death. As a social phenomenon, the term itself is poorly understood, and the language used surrounding a person who has been declared brain dead or dead by neurological criteria, is equally confusing.

Conceptually, and by most state statutes, when a person has been assessed to be dead by neurological criteria (previously referred to as **brain dead**), the person is declared legally dead. Most institutions have their own death by neurological exam policies and protocols, but essentially, neurological death is

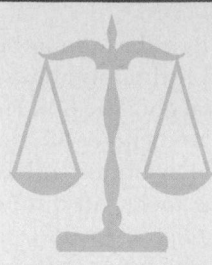

LAW IN PRACTICE

Right-to-Die Legal Cases

The landmark right-to-die legal cases in the United States span four decades. They began in 1976 with Karen Ann Quinlan, who was in a persistent vegetative state and mechanically ventilated for years. The Quinlan case was followed in 1983 by a 25-year-old woman named Nancy Beth Cruzan, who suffered irreparable brain damage in a car accident. Most recently, Terri Schiavo's husband, acting as her legal surrogate, elected to withdraw ANH following her parents' prolonged court battle to continue ANH. In all three cases, young women without formal written advance directives suffered irreparable brain damage, and family members acted as surrogates to have life-sustaining treatments withdrawn. In all three cases, clear and convincing evidence by a court of law was required before life-sustaining treatment could be withdrawn.

Most state statues have specific legal processes that must be followed so that a surrogate decision maker can withdraw life-sustaining therapy from another person. The courts have upheld the right of autonomous individuals or their legal surrogate decision maker to refuse life-sustaining medical treatment. Health care providers may not always agree with these decisions and may even feel moral distress when such decisions occur. For this reason, it is imperative that providers understand their own personal beliefs and values so that they may better understand and accept those of their patients and coproviders.

legally the same as cardiopulmonary death. This can be confusing to family members whose loved one remains mechanically ventilated after the assessment of death by neurological criteria has been made. This is because the body continues to be artificially maintained via mechanical ventilation, thereby giving the appearance of being alive. The main reason to continue mechanical ventilation is if organ donation is a consideration. Institutions have specific policies and state statutes provide guidelines about how family members should be approached about the possibility of organ donation. There may also be religious reasons that require the continuation of mechanical ventilation of a brain dead body, as seen with some orthodox Jewish groups. In all cases, care providers need to use terminology appropriate to a person who is deceased when referring to a patient who is assessed to be neurologically dead while communicating with family members about that person.

EUTHANASIA AND ASSISTED SUICIDE

The term **euthanasia** commonly defined means a good or easy death. The term itself is morally neutral. However, because of the images that the term conjures up, it is often associated with the term **active euthanasia,** which usually means that someone other than the patient performs an action that ends the patient's life. An example of active euthanasia is the act of administering a lethal injection of medication with the intent to end another person's life. The term, mercy killing, is often used to soften an act of active euthanasia.

Passive euthanasia generally means the omission of an action that could prevent death, allowing death to occur. An example of passive euthanasia is honoring a valid DNR order and not attempting to resuscitate the patient with such an order (Bandman & Bandman, 2002). **Assisted suicide** is similar to active euthanasia in that an action must be carried out by one person to help end the life of a second person. Assisted suicide is often associated with a health care provider being the person assisting another to end his or her own life. Active euthanasia and assisted suicide are illegal in most states within the United States. Several states have considered legalizing assisted suicide. Only the state of Oregon and some foreign countries, such as the Netherlands, have specific laws and guidelines which make assisted suicide legal.

Many health care providers find it offensive to think that those given the job to heal and comfort might be involved in actively taking another person's life. Morally, there is a distinction between active and passive euthanasia. However, each person must come to terms with the concepts based on his or her own individual beliefs and values. Double effect, withholding or withdrawing life-sustaining therapy, and limitation of aggressive treatments are all actions that can be viewed as forms of passive euthanasia within their specific contexts.

MEDICAL FUTILITY

The concept of futility has been recognized for centuries. The word itself is derived from the Latin *futilis* and literally means "that easily pours out." The Greek myth related to futilis depicts the daughters of the King of Argos murdering their husbands at the King's demand. The daughters were subsequently condemned by the gods to collect water in leaky containers for eternity. Thus, futile acts are those that are ineffective and that are "incapable of achieving a desired result or goal" (Civetta, 1996, p. 346).

What does futility mean within the health care arena? Technological advances in medicine continue to push the limits of what can be done, but just because something can be done, it does not mean something should be done. What does it mean when something is futile and should not be done? This is a difficult question to answer with complete certainty, because there is no generally accepted definition of medical futility. A common notion of futility is associated with the goal of medical intervention, (e.g., to improve the patient's prognosis, comfort, well-being, or general state of health). A treatment that fails to provide such a benefit, even though it produces a measurable effect, should be considered futile. The problem with the term medical futility is that it is often subjective and elusive. The reality is that making decisions about treatments that are of minimal medical benefit to a patient is difficult for patients, surrogates, and care providers.

Individual autonomy to make decisions about medical treatment is important to the western view of medical care. People have the legal and ethical right to seek appropriate medical care and to consent or refuse recommended medical care. There might be situations in which a patient or surrogate is seeking medical care that health care providers and nurses believe is not appropriate and should not be offered. In fact, the medical team may believe that a particular medical treatment will not physically benefit the patient and therefore should not be offered. Is there a right to demand medical treatment that has been assessed to be of no medical benefit? A conflict might then occur between what the patient or surrogate wishes and what the health care team believes should be done.

This dilemma related to medical futility is often difficult to resolve because of perceived values and social judgments that may be involved. The patient or surrogate may believe there is some benefit (perhaps emotional or psychological) of the treatment, but the health care providers and other health care team members may believe that the physical benefit of treatment is not worth the cost when cost is measured as pain and suffering; minimal, if any, physical

Fast Forward ▶▶▶

Perhaps at some time in the future there will be a medical futility clinical assessment that could be applied equally to all patients. However, until such an assessment tool is identified, tested, and applied with equity and fairness, we must continue to work through the issues surrounding medical futility one clinical case at a time (Svehla & Anderson-Shaw, 2006).

benefit; and the financial cost of the treatment. Because medical futility is difficult to define and because health care institutions may not have specific policies related to medical futility, medical futility dilemmas continue to challenge patients and providers alike.

To impose some kind of continuity regarding the issue of medical futility, the American Medical Association (AMA) issued a statement on medical futility and end-of-life care in 1997, urging health care enterprises to adopt a policy on medical futility. In this statement the AMA outlined a process by which patients and providers could settle disagreements related to futility issues. The AMA, though not offering a specific definition of what constitutes medical futility, stated there is no obligation by providers to offer or perform medical treatments that are without benefit (1999).

Some health care institutions have adopted versions of the AMA's guidelines, which offer steps to help resolve disputes over medical futility. Some states, such as Texas through an advance directives act, adopted legislation that also provides steps to futility conflict resolution. In most cases the process of conflict resolution involves the institutional ethics committee (Fine & Mayo, 2003).

RESEARCH ETHICS

Clinical medical research is carried out at many health care institutions throughout the world. The outcomes of research can make significant contributions to the health and welfare of society, in addition to significantly improving professional practice. Nurses, in the course of providing patient care, may be involved in research activity, such as carrying out a specific clinical protocol, providing care to a patient enrolled as a research subject, or actively enrolling potential subjects in a study that is underway in the department or institution. More and more frequently nurses are directing research projects in a quest to develop new knowledge for nursing science. Involvement with patients who are subjects of clinical research requires that nurses be aware of the ethical guidelines that are in place to protect human subjects while ensuring the integrity of the research. Nurses need to be able to assist patients who are participating in research to make informed decisions about their health and safety.

History has provided several examples of how corrupt research can be and how vulnerable people are when being used as research subjects. The 1945 Nuremberg war crimes trials exposed numerous crimes related to horrific medical research experiments carried out by health care providers who used prisoners of war as research subjects during World War II. Other unethical behavior of researchers includes the use of 23,000 American civilians in numerous experiments to study the effect of radiation on human subjects over many years without the knowledge and consent of those subjects. Researchers also used patients at an institution for mentally retarded children to test the physical outcomes of the ingesting irradiated cereal.

One of the most significant breaches in research ethics occurred in the Tuskegee Study carried out from the 1930s through the 1970s. In that research the United States Public Health Service conducted a study of the effects of untreated syphilis on African American men in Macon County, Alabama. The study continued long after penicillin was found to cure syphilis in the 1940s, yet none of the men enrolled in the study were given penicillin or were told of the available cure (Jones, 1993).

These examples emphasize the need for research ethics and for high standards within the research community so that human subjects who participate in research are protected to the utmost extent possible. Several important codes of ethics guide research. The Nuremberg Code was adopted in 1947 as an outcome of the Nuremberg trials. This code, though brief in words, is monumental in stature in setting up the foundation for human subject protection with regard to participation in research. The first statement of this code makes voluntary consent of human subjects in research essential. The code goes on to clarify that research experiments must be designed to yield results that will be of good use to society and that the researcher is, at all times, responsible for the safety and health of the human research subject.

In 1964 the World Medical Association recommended guidelines for biomedical research involving human subjects through a document titled The Declaration of Helsinki. The Declaration of Helsinki guidelines are similar to the Nuremberg Code, but specifically address physicians to safeguard the health of human subjects involved in medical research. A third significant document related to research ethics is The Belmont Report written by The National Commission for the Protection of Human Subjects of Biomedical and Behavioral Research. This report was published by the U.S. Department of Health, Education, and Welfare (now the USDHHS) in 1979 and provides ethical principles and guidelines specifically for the protection of human subjects of biomedical and behavioral research (Emanuel, Crouch, Arras, Moreno, & Grady, 2003). The Office for Human Research Protections (OHRP) of the USDHHS is responsible for providing oversight to institutions where research is conducted, or supported, by USDHHS.

All institutions provide their research staff with some form of institutional review board (IRB). An IRB is responsible for reviewing all research projects that will be sponsored by, or be carried out within, that institution. IRB membership is interdisciplinary and includes health care providers, nurses, various therapists, social workers, nutritionists, clergy, ethicists, and community members, as well as various administrative people who have responsibility for oversight of research projects.

Researchers are required to submit a research application to the IRB describing in great detail all aspects of their proposed research project, including details about human subject protection. No research activity may begin until the IRB approves the research proposal. IRB activity is paramount in the protection of human research subjects. While IRB approval cannot guarantee that a research subject will not have negative effects related to the research, it does ensure that the researcher obtains free and informed consent from that human subject prior to participation (Miller & Moreno, 2005).

The legal and ethical aspects of health care are as complex as the technology used in providing care. The intimate nature of nursing practice places the nurse in situations in which ethical issues can be at the forefront of care. A basic understanding of the ethical principles that guide nursing care is essential to ensuring professional practice. Nurses' knowledge of the federal and state laws that impact practice, as well as knowledge of specific institutional policy that regulates professional practice must be reviewed and updated often.

KEY CONCEPTS

- Nurses need to examine their own personal beliefs regarding specific ethical issues (e.g., end-of-life care or withdrawal of life support) to provide quality patient care.
- Ethics, also referred to as moral philosophy, assists relating to what is right or wrong.
- There are four main principles of clinical ethics: autonomy, nonmaleficence, beneficence, and justice.

- There are several important categories of ethical theories that can assist nurses in thinking about and analyzing ethical issues.
- Issues of confidentiality are extremely important for patients and for nurses.
- Informed consent requires respect for the informed and voluntary treatment choice of a competent patient.

Continued

KEY CONCEPTS—cont'd

- Advance directives are typically written and take various forms, such as an LW or DPAHC.
- The following are five models for ethical decision making: medical indications, patient preferences, QOL, contextual features, and an integrated model.
- Ethically, the principles of autonomy, beneficence, and nonmaleficence should all be considered in relationship to patients' pain management issues.
- The ethical issues that are apparent at the end of life are often complex because nursing care not only serves the patient but also the patient's family and loved ones.

- Euthanasia as a term is morally neutral, but when identified as either active or passive, multiple ethical issues surface for the health care provider to identify.
- There is no obligation by providers to offer or perform medical treatments that are without benefit.
- There is a need for research ethics to exist at a high standard so that human subjects who participate in research are protected to the utmost extent possible.

REVIEW QUESTIONS

1. Beneficence is the ethical principle that describes:
   1. Patient decision making capacity
   2. Patient preferences
   3. Providing care that is equal for all patients
   4. Providing care that maximizes health

2. A patient with Parkinson's disease is treated with levodopa and has severe side effects. The decision to give him the medication in the beginning of his condition was prefaced with the knowledge that most patients respond well to this medication strategy. Which ethical theory is this describing?
   1. Deontology
   2. Utilitarian
   3. Right's based
   4. Ethics of care

3. The ANA Code of Ethics for Nurses provides:
   1. General guidelines for clinical practice
   2. Definition and guidance to the moral sense of the nursing profession
   3. Definition and guidance to the social sense of the nursing profession
   4. Procedural steps for corporate compliance

4. A nurse may feel a sense of moral distress when:
   1. Not being able to fulfill an action thought to be the right thing to do
   2. Not being able to change a patient's mind about a procedure
   3. Being late for work
   4. Having a disagreement with a coworker

5. The 1996 Act known as HIPAA:
   1. Does not allow nurses to share any patient information
   2. Allows for the sharing of all electronic patient information
   3. Does not address patient information shared in public places
   4. Covers disclosure of all patient personal health information

6. A mother is emotionally positive and accepting of her child's terminal condition and the fact that the parents have agreed to not have another surgery for the genetic disorder. The ethical decision making model ascribed to by this mother is:
   1. Patient preferences
   2. Contextual features
   3. Integrated model
   4. Quality of life

7. The concept of double effect related to pain management:
   1. Is considered active euthanasia
   2. Is illegal in most states within the United States
   3. Is acceptable as a consequence of pain management in end-of-life care
   4. Should be avoided so as not to cause addiction to pain medication

Continued

REVIEW QUESTIONS—cont'd

8. Legal forms of advance directives for health care include:
   1. LW
   2. Verbal patient preferences
   3. DPAHC
   4. 1, 3
   5. 1, 2, 3

9. The first document to provide a framework for research ethics was:
   1. The Nuremberg Code
   2. JCAHO Standards
   3. The Belmont Report
   4. The Department of Health and Human Subjects report

10. Patients have the right to refuse medically necessary treatments:
    1. If they have been evaluated by a psychiatrist
    2. If they have decisional capacity
    3. For minor treatments only
    4. After the next of kin has been contacted

REVIEW ACTIVITIES

1. Contact the chairperson of an IRB and request the opportunity to attend a meeting as a student guest. Discuss your impressions in class.

2. Contact the chairperson of an ethics committee and request the opportunity to attend an ethics committee meeting as a student guest. Discuss your impressions in class.

3. Identify an ethical dilemma in the clinical setting and make a decision based on one of the ethical theories (e.g., teleology or deontology).

4. Obtain a copy of advanced directives and complete the form for yourself. Share your emotional thoughts related to filling out the form with your peer group of students.

5. Compare and contrast active euthanasia with passive euthanasia with respect to the concept of a DNR.

Nursing of Adults Across the Life Span

Evelyn Perez, RN, MSN, ACNP

CHAPTER TOPICS

- Adult Developmental Stages

- Contemporary Adult Health Behaviors and Evolving Trends of Adult Health Behaviors

- Common Adult Diseases and Treatment Linked to Contemporary Trends

- Health and Illness Trends for Young, Middle, and Older Adults

KEY TERMS

Incidence
Metabolic syndrome
Morbidity
Mortality
Prevalence
Trends

The 21st century that seemed so far in the future with its promises of a better life is here. Traditional methods of accomplishing tasks have been replaced by an abundance of electronic miracles that accomplish the work we used to do with merely a point and a click of a finger or a thumb. Nurses are now caring for adults whose lives run on battery-powered advanced technology and on jet power that speeds them around the world in a few hours. Adults of all ages rely on automation, such as remote activating devices, robots, drive-through conveniences, prepared food, and use multiple modes of transportation to accomplish both work and pleasure expediently. Time is of the essence; people desire even more conveniences to experience the ever broadening array of available activities. In America, adults are growing more diverse, living longer, becoming more sedentary, growing fatter, and threatening their health status.

ADULT DEVELOPMENTAL STAGES

Caring for adults requires understanding the stage of life each patient currently occupies and how to individualize nursing care to best facilitate achievement of the patient's health care goals. Nurses are most familiar with the developmental stages of children described by Freud's psychosexual development theory, Piaget's cognitive development theory, and the birth through adolescence stages (stages one to five) of Erickson's psychosocial life span theory. Until recently, however, less attention was devoted to understanding adult development, and it was considered to exist on a relatively stagnant plateau. An assumption made by many individuals was that between adolescence and teen years and old age there were no systematic changes occurring in adults.

Theories of Adult Development

Erik Erikson (1902–1994), a social psychologist, actually viewed the personality of the individual to develop through eight phases of conflict or confrontation between the ego and the social environment from birth to old age. This theory is a major contribution to understanding humans across the life span. Erikson designated the adult stages as: (stage 6) intimacy versus isolation during young adulthood that involves exploring personal relationships and developing a committed relationship; (stage 7) generativity versus stagnation in middle adulthood, a time of continuing to build and nurture the next generation with a focus on career and family; and (stage 8) integrity versus despair in older adulthood, a time of reflecting back on life and being proud of accomplishments, having no regrets or feeling that life goals were not met. The resolutions of the conflicts in each sequential stage, or maintaining a balance between the state of stability and the state of disorder, help to define the person's identity (Erikson, 1963).

Daniel Levinson (1978), a cultural anthropologist, developed a comprehensive theory of adult development titled Life Structure Theory based on Erikson's earlier work. Levenson also proposed that a person's life stages and structure are affected and altered by the social, cultural, and physical environment. He defined the five developmental stages of adults as: (a) young adult (18–28); (b) the thirties (29–39); (c) middle age (40–55); (d) late adulthood (56–75); and (e) old age (beyond 75) (Table 6-1).

TABLE 6-1 Levinson's Theory of Adult Developmental Stages	
Young adult (18–28)	A period of exploration. Leaving home and trying out new possibilities. It is a period marked by leaving parental control and defining oneself as an adult.
The thirties	A time to assess gains and asking if the gains were worth the price. Questions of personal satisfaction arise. The identification of the exact year is difficult, occurring as early as the 30s to 50s. Perceptions become important and how one feels about life experiences as a means of indicating life importance. This time may be marked by stress.
Middle age (40–55)	The period that begins with a midlife transition. This time can be a crisis period for many individuals.
Late adulthood (56–75)	The lower boundary of late adulthood is retirement. Considered the young old. No longer in the workforce, they may assume political or community activity. Transition into late adulthood is usually from 60–65 years of age.
Old age (beyond 75)	A period marked by declining powers, health, loss of loved ones. This can be period of waiting for death.

Adapted from Levinson, D. J., Darrow, C. N., Klein, E. B., Levinson, M. H., & McKee, B. (1978). The seasons of a man's life. New York: Knopf.

Robert Havinghurst's classic theory (1976) also proposed specific development tasks for each stage of development. He emphasized that optimal moments for mastering these tasks were dependent on the success in previous life stages. Each adult patient a nurse encounters is biologically and experientially unique. Such uniqueness influences the patient's health behavior. Scientists are continuing to develop other contemporary psychosocial adult development theories that will enhance our understanding of adult behavior in numerous circumstances including their health care needs.

Bernice Neugarten, a professor of behavioral science and a pioneer in the study of aging at the University of Chicago, focused her 1970s research on the social norms that influence a person's perception of age. Neugarten proposed that there are three times in a person's life that interact simultaneously to influence adult development (Transitions, 2006). Those three times are: life time, social time, and historic time (Table 6-2).

CONTEMPORARY TRENDS RELATED TO ADULT BEHAVIOR

There are numerous governmental and health care agencies that track, record, and disseminate information about various health and illness patterns in the population. Components of these patterns include prevalence, incidence, and trends. **Prevalence** is the number of current cases of a disease in a specific population at a given time period (Medline Plus, 2006). Prevalence is used to measure the amount of illness in the community and to determine the current or prevailing health care needs. Contributing factors to prevalence include disease incidence rate and illness duration.

Incidence is the number of new cases of a condition, symptom, death, or injury that arise during a specific period of time such as a month or a year. It is often expressed as a percentage of a population (e.g., 25 percent of American residents were diagnosed with the flu in 2002). Incidence conveys the likelihood that an individual in that population will be affected by the condition. **Trends** are the general direction or prevailing tendency in following a general course. Disease trends can be measured over a period of time and are used as statistical information for predicting national and worldwide incidences. Disease trends recently making news are the sudden acute respiratory syndrome (SARS) epidemic, West Nile virus, and Asian bird flu. Refer to the U.S. Government Web sites for the Centers for Disease Control and Prevention (CDC) at: http://www.cdc.gov and the Department of Health and Human Services (DHHS) at http://www.dhhs.gov.nchs for further information.

TABLE 6-2	Perceived Times in Adult Life
Life time	The biological clock time and chronological passage of time indicated by graying hair, menopause, and reduced levels of physical activity.
Social time	Recognized by age grading and expectations and identified as a time to go back to school, raise a family, or retire. The social time clock superimposed on the biological clock.
Historic time	A time of political, social, and economic events that influence one's life. The events affect what a person does and when.

Adapted from Transitions. (2006). Bernice Neugarten's life times theory. Retrieved July 25, 2006, from http://www.transitionalonestop.org.

Health patterns and trends have changed over the years, providing information necessary to deliver current and individualized care with appropriate nursing interventions. The 29th report on the health status of the nation, *Health, United States, 2005*, presents measures in four major areas: (a) health care status and determinants; (b) health care utilization; (c) health care resources; and (d) health care expenditures (National Center for Health Statistics [NCHS], 2006b). The report provides important information about the impact of people's health on their self-care health practices. Nurses must be equipped with multiple skills to empower individuals to learn and practice healthy lifestyles. Additional information can be gleaned from the government's Morbidity and Mortality Weekly Report at: http://www.cdc.gov/nmwr.

Dietary Habits

Dietary changes include higher consumption of fat, carbohydrates, low fiber foods, and high-caloric processed food and drinks. Moreover, people are leading sedentary lives. These practices can be linked to obesity, hypertension, risk of developing type 2 diabetes, and other chronic diseases.

Obesity Rates

Causes of obesity are multiple and complex. Environmental, genetic, and socioeconomic factors are interwoven in some causes. Obesity has increased 61 percent since 1991. The prevalence of obesity in 2000 in the United States among adults was 19.8 percent, and 38.8 million American adults who qualified for the classification of obesity. A total of 64 percent of Americans are either overweight or obese. An increasing number of Americans who are identified as obese are also diagnosed with type 2 diabetes. A recent report from the Alzheimer's Association suggests that Alzheimer's and diabetes (type 2) are closely associated. The findings of several studies were reported at the International Conference on Alzheimer's-related disorders in Spain (Grady, 2006). Refer to chapter 48 for additional information on obesity and nursing responsibilities in management of care.

A measurement of body fat used in studying obesity is the body mass index (BMI) based on the height and weight of adult men and women. The BMI uses a mathematical formula that involves a person's weight in kilograms divided by height in meters squared ($BMI=kg/m^2$). A person's waist size (male or female) is also a determining factor of obesity. The BMI is available at: http://www.consumer.gov/weightloss and includes a conversion table (to pounds and inches) for the reader to calculate his or her own BMI.

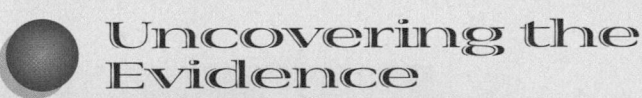

Uncovering the Evidence

Prevalence of Obesity in American Adults

Data collected in a state-based telephone survey of adults over 18 revealed the prevalence of obesity in American adults had increased from 19.8 to 20 percent between 2000 and 2001. An increase in diagnosed type 2 diabetes from 7.3 to 7.9 percent was also found with a prevalence of more than 15 percent of Americans aged 60 or older, the highest in Alabama (10.5 percent) and the lowest (5.0 percent) in Minnesota. The data were obtained by the Behavioral Risk Factor Surveillance System (BRFSS).

Source: Mokdad, A., Ford, E., Bowman, B., Dietz, W., Vinevor, F., Bales, V., et al. (2003). Prevalence of obesity, diabetes and obesity-related health risk factors, 2001. Journal of American Medical Association, 289, 76–79.

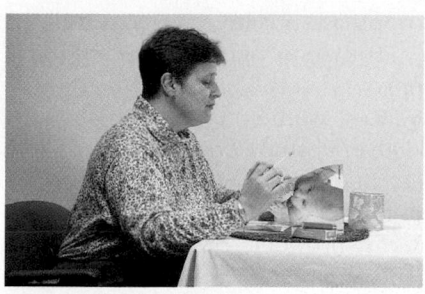

Figure 6-1 This adult patient is continuing to smoke, even though she knows that lung cancer is the leading cause of cancer death among women.

Smoking Trends

Since 1990 the percentage of adults who smoke has slightly decreased. In 2001 25 percent of men and 21 percent of women were smokers (Figure 6-1). Cigarette smoking by adults can be linked to educational levels, and adults with less than a high school education are more likely to smoke than those with a college education. Smoking during pregnancy has been linked with low birth-weight newborns and infant death. Cigarette smoking by pregnant mothers has declined to 12 percent, down from 20 percent in 1989. Recently, smoking has increased among high school age young people, particularly for Hispanic (American) and African American males (NCHS, 2006b).

Suicide Incidence Rates

Every year approximately 30,000 Americans die as a result of suicide. Over the last 100 years, suicides have outnumbered homicides by about 3:1. Many who commit suicide visit a nonmental health care provider within the last month of their lives. Recognizing those at risk for suicide and accessing appropriate health care and interventions is made difficult with the lack of data collected. Biological, genetic, psychological, and cultural factors play an important role in the risk of suicide in any individual.

Risk factors associated with an increased risk for suicide include serious mental illness, alcohol and drug abuse, childhood abuse, loss of a loved one, joblessness, loss of economic security, and posttraumatic stress disorder (PTSD). Treatment and prevention begins with the health care provider recognizing signs and symptoms of suicide ideation and providing access to appropriate treatment (NCHS, 2006b).

Morbidity and Mortality Trends

Morbidity is the proportion of ill persons in relationship to a specific population. Measures of morbidity include the incidence of specific disease processes, injury-related emergency department visits, and suicide attempts. Morbidity can be represented as the quality of life in the presence of disease. An increase in morbidity rates has paralleled the increase in the number of Americans diagnosed yearly with morbid obesity, diabetes, lung disorders, and heart disease. **Mortality** is the proportion of deaths in a given population. It is also related to life expectancy and is used to gauge the overall health of a population. In 2001, life expectancy at birth reached a record high of 77.2 years, up from 75.4 years in 1990. Americans are living longer; however, lifestyles and environmental factors contribute to a greater number of chronic illnesses, greater use of health care services and prescriptions, and higher costs (NCHS, 2006b).

EVOLVING TRENDS IN POPULATION COMPOSITION

Several changes have taken place over the last several decades. The nation has become a multicultural mixture of different age-groups, thus presenting different individual, social, and political influences on health care services.

The Aging Population

Americans are aging, and the numbers will continue to grow as the baby boomer generation reaches age 65. The oldest of the baby boomer population (born between 1946 and the 1964) reached the age of 55 in 2001. Attributable factors are the decline in births and a 20-year life span increase in the second half of the 20th century. (An aging population is determined by the proportion of older adults to the number of births and younger persons in that population.) The mean age of the world's population is increasing as well. In the United States, the proportion of the population aged 65 and older is expected to increase from 12.4 percent (approximately 35 million) in 2000 to 19.6 percent (approximately 71 million) by 2030. Women, comprising 59 percent of the population age 65 or older in 2000, are estimated to comprise only 56 percent of the population in 2030.

As the baby boomers age, public resources may become exhausted; thus placing the burden of care on families, older adult care providers, or friends. However, the traditional neighborhoods of multiple generation families and the changing marital relationships affect the degree of family support available to care for older family members. Many of the elderly population live in the community or in assisted living facilities, group homes, or senior housing. Many older women live alone, have lower incomes, and have poorer health (NCHS, 2006b).

Aging Nurse Workforce

Our aging population also includes the aging nurse workforce. In 2001, 9.1 percent of all nurses were under the age of 30; 18.3 percent were under age 35; and only 31.7 percent of all nurses were under the age of 41. The mean age of nurses in the United States in 2003 was 45.2 years. These percentages suggest that caring for a graying America may become difficult if nursing shortages are not adequately addressed.

Some of the contributing factors are older graduates from associate degree programs, decreased enrollment of younger nursing students, challenges in recruitment, financial costs in health care, and hospital restructuring and reengineering. There will continue to be a growing need for geriatric prepared nurses who will be able to work in a variety of health care settings and meet the complex needs of the elderly (Heinz, 2004; Mion, 2003).

Minority and Ethnic Population Trends

The United States is a multicultural nation. Future predictive trends include an increase in the percentage of minority groups aged 65 or older between the years 2000 and 2030 from 11.3 to 16.5 percent with Hispanic (Americans) doubling their percentage from 5.6 to 10.9 percent. Despite an overall decline in mortality rates, racial and ethnic disparities in morbidity and mortality persist because of several cultural, environmental, and social factors.

Selecting among available treatment options requires that the nurse develop culturally sensitive patient knowledge. An important diagnostic tool for nurses is knowledge of the cultural factors that affect Americans' health at different times in their adult development. Such knowledge helps nurses make an accurate diagnosis and choose appropriate treatment. See Table 6-3 depicting the ten leading causes of death in Americans.

COMMON ADULT DISEASES LINKED TO CONTEMPORARY TRENDS

The following discussion of common adult diseases is not inclusive of all disease processes. Rather, it is provided to demonstrate the interrelationship of diseases and health care practice trends. The notion of the importance of health trends and life span development is important information for nurse's practice.

Asthma

Asthma is a chronic respiratory condition of the tracheobronchial tree that causes airway inflammation and narrowing. After contact with an irritant, bronchial tubes become inflamed. People of all ages may be affected; however

TABLE 6-3 **The Ten Leading Causes of Death in Americans**

Age-Groups

RANK	15–24	25–34	35–44	45–54	55–64	65 OR OLDER
1	Unintentional injury	Unintentional injury	Malignant neoplasms	Malignant neoplasms	Malignant neoplasms	Heart disease
2	Homicide	Suicide	Unintentional injury	Heart disease	Heart disease	Malignant neoplasms
3	Suicide	Homicide	Heart disease	Unintentional injury	Chronic respiratory disease	Cerebrovascular
4	Malignant neoplasms	Malignant neoplasms	Suicide	Liver disease	Cerebrovascular	Cerebrovascular
5	Heart disease	Heart disease	HIV	Cerebrovascular	Diabetes mellitus	Chronic respiratory disease
6	Congenital anomalies	HIV	Homicide	Suicide	Unintentional injury	Diabetes mellitus
7	HIV	Diabetes mellitus	Liver disease	Diabetes mellitus	Liver disease	Alzheimer's disease
8	Cerebrovascular	Cerebrovascular	Cerebrovascular	HIV		Unintentional injury
9	Chronic respiratory disease	Congenital anomalies	Diabetes mellitus	Chronic respiratory disease	Suicide	Nephritis
10	Influenza and pneumonia	Liver disease	Influenza and pneumonia	Homicide	Septicemia	Septicemia

Source: National Center for Health Statistics. (2006b). Health, United States, 2005: 29th report on the health status of the nation. *Retrieved July 12, 2006, from http://www.cdc.gov/nchs.*

asthma occurs most frequently in childhood or early adulthood. In 1998, an estimated 17 million Americans, or 6.4 percent of the population, were diagnosed with asthma. Children accounted for 4.8 million of the Americans with asthma. Each year nearly 500,000 Americans with asthma are hospitalized and more than 4,000 die. Although asthma deaths are infrequent, they have increased significantly in the past two decades. Refer to chapter 32 for detailed information on asthma and nursing responsibilities in the management of care (NCHS, 2006b).

Metabolic Syndrome

Metabolic syndrome is diagnosed when three or more factors, such as high blood pressure, abdominal obesity, high triglyceride levels, low high-density lipoprotein (HDL) cholesterol, and high fasting blood glucose levels are present. It is also referred to as insulin resistance syndrome or syndrome X (Medline Plus, 2006). Metabolic syndrome is characterized by a combination of risk factors that also present an elevated risk of development of cardiovascular disease and type 2 diabetes mellitus.

One of every four, or 47 million U.S. adults, have a risk for the development of metabolic syndrome. Men have the highest age-adjusted prevalence of hypertension (38.2 percent), women the highest age-adjusted prevalence of

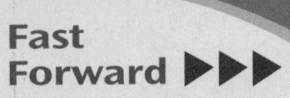

Fast Forward ▶▶▶

Vaccine for Obesity

Scientists at Scripps Research Institute in La Jolla, California, have developed a vaccine to counteract the effects of the hormone ghrelin, primarily produced in the stomach, which is thought to be involved in sensation of hunger, slowing down metabolism and increased storage of fat. It has been tested with laboratory rats, who continued to eat and drink normally, yet their weight gain was slowed dramatically in comparison with nonvaccinated rats. The vaccine uses the natural immune system to block the hormone from reaching the brain. Although the vaccine is in the early experimental stages, no serious side effects have been detected. Ghrelin has been the focus of hundreds of studies since it was discovered in 1999. Some reports suggest that the hormone is also important for memory and other brain functions; therefore its many functions remain uncertain. Still, the scientists hope that it will be a breakthrough treatment for obesity in humans (Lieberman, 2006).

abdominal obesity (46.3 percent). Prevalence increases with age. The prevalence of obesity and diabetes has increased along with the prevalence of metabolic syndrome. According to a recent World Health Organization (WHO) study metabolic syndrome is present in about 10 percent of patients with normal glucose tolerance, and it is present in about 50 percent of patients with impaired fasting glucose or impaired glucose tolerance. Metabolic syndrome is present in about 80 percent of patients with type 2 diabetes. Identifying and diagnosing metabolic syndrome early is important to prevention and treatment. Refer to chapter 57 for additional information on metabolic syndrome risk factors and nursing responsibilities in prevention and management of care.

Hypercholesterolemia

Hypercholesterolemia is one of the major modifiable risk factors for cardiovascular disease. A 10 percent reduction in cholesterol levels can decrease the risk factor by as much as 30 percent. According to the *Health, United States, 2005,* 18 percent of adults 20 years or older have high total serum cholesterol levels greater than 240 mm/dL. Many are unaware of their serum levels or the risks involved. The goal of *Healthy People 2010* is to increase screening procedures for adults age 20 and older from 63 percent in 2005 to 80 percent and provide education about treatment options. The overall outcome goal is to decrease the racial and ethnic disparities in all health outcomes. Nurses can play pivotal roles in public health campaigns in meeting these goals (NCHS, 2006b). Detailed information about hypercholesterolemia and nursing responsibilities related to prevention and management of care is in chapter 51.

Hypertension

Recently, the definition of hypertension has undergone a radical change, and new guidelines have been established for the classifications of hypertension. A persistent elevation of systolic blood pressure over 140 mm Hg or higher and a diastolic pressure of 90 mm Hg or higher are indications for careful monitoring.

It is estimated that 50 million Americans have hypertension due to multiple causes and risk factors, such as family history, age, gender, and ethnicity. Hypertension occurs at a higher rate in African Americans than in Caucasians. Hypertension is associated with elevated risks of coronary artery disease (CAD), heart attack, stroke, and renal failure, therefore accurate diagnosis is important. Modifiable risk factors include obesity, diet, and lifestyle. Assisting individuals to understand the interrelationships of diet, inactivity, and obesity is the focus of the patient-nurse relationship. Nurses need to assist patients in their navigation of obstacles to successful management of their illness (Seventh Report of Joint National Commission on Prevention, Detection and Treatment of Hypertension [JNC7], 2006). Refer to chapter 28 for detailed information on hypertension and the nurse's responsibilities in prevention and the management of care.

Diabetes Mellitus

Diabetes mellitus is a chronic disorder of metabolism in which the body cannot properly use glucose due to either a deficiency of insulin or a decreased ability of the body to use insulin that is produced. An estimated 18.2 million Americans, 6.3 percent of the population, have diabetes. Of the 18.2 million, 13 million have been diagnosed, and 5.2 million have not yet been diagnosed. People age 65 and older account for almost 40 percent of the population with diabetes, and each year about 1.3 million Americans age 20 or older are diagnosed with the disease (Figure 6-2). Obesity as well as advanced age, physical

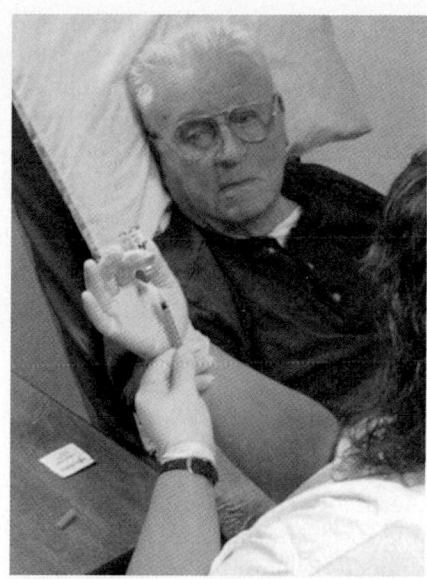

Figure 6-2 This older adult patient is learning to self-administer insulin for his newly diagnosed diabetes.

Fast Forward ▶▶▶

Child Onset of Type 2 Diabetes Poses Risk

Obesity-related type 2 diabetes in children (mean age 17) increases the risk of kidney failure and death at middle age. National Institute of Health researchers discovered that adult onset–diabetes at a younger age has been more prevalent in the last decade. Their study was conducted over a two-year period with Pima Indians, a population that has a genetic predisposition for diabetes and obesity. Weight control and exercise can help delay this phenomenon.

inactivity, unhealthy diet, and genetic predisposition have been shown as contributing factors. Diabetes increases the risk of developing hypertension, heart disease, stroke and renal failure, other comorbidities, and death (NCHS, 2005). The patient's circumstances, abilities, and desires need to be taken into consideration in developing the management plan. Refer to chapter 57 for detailed information about diabetes mellitus and the nursing responsibilities in prevention and management of care.

Coronary Artery Disease

Coronary artery disease (CAD) is the most common form of heart disease. About 13 million people in the United States have CAD. It is the number one killer of adult men and women, with more than 500,000 Americans dying from CAD each year. As Americans age, the risk for CAD increases; in men risk increases after age 45 and in women risk increases after age 55. Other risk factors that are nonmodifiable include a family history of heart disease. Modifiable risk factors include high blood cholesterol, high blood pressure, cigarette smoking, diabetes, being overweight or obese, and lack of physical activity. The more risk factors that are present, the greater are the chances of developing CAD. Management of CAD revolves around lifestyle changes, medication, and special procedures (NCHS, 2005). Refer to chapter 24 for detailed information on nursing responsibilities in prevention and management of care of patients with CAD.

Cancer

Cancer is a group of diseases that develop because of mutation of normal cells of the body. These abnormal cells can proliferate and affect many body tissues and systems. The term cancer has been traditionally linked to high morbidity and mortality rates; however, primary prevention and new technologies have resulted in considering many of the cancers as chronic diseases. Skin cancers screening is one form of preventive measures that can be used. For other cancers, preventive measures include lifestyle changes, including diet, exercise, and weight loss and avoidance of environmental exposure to mutants, such as air pollution, radiation, chemicals, pesticides, solvents, and smoke. Refer to chapter 15 for detailed information on cancer, prevention measures, and the nurse's responsibilities in prevention and management of care.

USE OF CONTEMPORARY TREATMENT MODALITIES

Many people are selecting alternative health care methods, such as complementary and alterative medicines, diets, and cosmetic surgery to improve their self-image and minimize the effects of the aging process. Bariatric surgery is available to a select group of people to correct the effects of obesity.

Complementary Alternative Medicine

In the United States 36 percent of adults use some form of complementary (integrative) or alternative medicine (CAM). Complementary medicine is used either exclusively or in combination with conventional medical modalities. Examples are the use of aromatherapy and music therapy to help lessen a patient's perception of pain. Many individuals use religious beliefs and prayer as a complementary therapy. A greater percentage of African Americans, especially women, rely on religious practices as complementary therapy than other racial groups. Alternative medicine is used in place of conventional medical modalities. An

Cosmetic Surgery and Treatments

Many people are unaware of the risks involved with cosmetic procedures. The nurse can inform them how to avoid many of these risks and suggest where additional information resources can be found.

- Any cosmetic treatment should be performed by a qualified health care provider (one who is certified by a surgical specialty organization, such as the American Society for Aesthetic Plastic Surgery [ASAPS]), and procedures should be performed in accredited facilities.
- Be leery of inexpensive prices and unrealistic claims that are made.
- Know what substances are being injected into your body. Only products approved by the Food and Drug Administration (FDA) should be used. The individual can access the quick facts on the ASAPS Web site for additional information about injectable substances.
- Provide full disclosure of your medical history, including allergies, supplements, medications, over-the-counter (OTC) drugs. These may influence the procedure outcome.
- Make sure the benefits and the risks are fully explained to you. (This is the hallmark of an informed consent.)
- Evaluate all your reasons for deciding on these therapies. Recognize that you may be requested to have a psychological consult.
- Develop realistic expectations regarding the outcomes.
- Adhere to the prescribed follow-up and self-care regimen.

Adapted from American Society for Aesthetic Plastic Surgery (ASAPS). (2006). What's new in plastic surgery? Retrieved July 26, 2006, from http://www.surgery.org.

example of alternative medicine is the use of a special diet to treat cancer instead of undergoing surgery or chemotherapy. The body of evidence supporting the efficacy of CAM is growing and much of the CAM research is being done by nurses. Refer to chapter 14 for detailed information on CAM and nursing responsibilities in management of care of patients who may use these therapies (National Center for Complementary and Alternative Medicine (NCCAM, 2005).

Cosmetic Treatments and Surgery

There is a strong trend in America to undo the physical changes that occur as the body ages by enhancing physical appearance. The way that patients perceive themselves is important and strongly influenced by the way social norms are portrayed in the media. Clearly, self-perception strongly impacts self-esteem and subsequently, emotional health.

Botox injections are currently the fastest-growing cosmetic procedure according to the American Society for Aesthetic Plastic Surgery (ASAPS, 2006). In 2001, more than 1.6 million people received injections, an increase of 46 percent over the previous year. Botox injections have become more popular than breast enhancement surgery.

Nurses need to ensure that the patient's need for self-improvement and effective self-esteem is understood and if possible, met. Cosmetic surgery and weight loss products and procedures can be expensive and difficult to access. High out-of-pocket costs can drive patients to seek practitioners who may not be particularly knowledgeable or skilled in cosmetic surgery. Complications are common and range from temporary to permanent.

Bariatric Surgery

Several types of surgery are classified as bariatric surgery. Bariatric surgery was conceptualized when health care providers noticed that patients who underwent gastric resection for cancer or peptic ulcers lost weight. The individuals must meet nationally accepted criteria before being accepted for bariatric surgery. These criteria include a comprehensive medical, psychological, nutritional, and surgical evaluation by a multidisciplinary team usually including an internist, bariatric surgeon, registered nurse educator, home care nurse, psychologist, nutritionist, physical therapist, and clinical pharmacologist. All surgeries have inherent complications. The complications of bariatric surgery can be quite serious and include severe malabsorption, uncontrollable diarrhea, electrolyte imbalance, vitamin deficiency, development of kidney stones, hepatic failure, and even death.

Bariatric surgery is considered successful if the patient loses from 50 to 75 percent of their excess weight. The amount of weight loss that can be achieved depends on the specific surgical procedure performed, the skill and technique of the surgeon, the patient's mental health, and the patient's presurgical weight. Bariatric procedures are further considered a success if the patient maintains a weight loss of at least 48 percent over the long-term (five plus years), even with a weight regain of 5 to 10 percent over that time.

Nurses must be aware of the dilemma faced by patients who are overweight and for whom every diet attempt or other program has failed. The need for bariatric surgery should be weighed against potential complications and overall cost. The individual must realize that a long-term lifestyle change is imperative. More recently insurance companies are viewing bariatric surgery as health promotion and disease prevention for the long-term. With the weight loss, diabetes and hypertension are becoming easier to manage and in some cases resolved. Joint problems also may be resolved with weight loss. Mental health can also be improved with weight loss (National Heart, Blood, and Lung Institute, 2006a).

HEALTH AND ILLNESS TRENDS FOR YOUNG AND MIDDLE-AGED ADULTS

Many of the illnesses and health care issues in this population group are related to unintentional accidents in the work, home, and recreational environments, injuries because of vehicular accidents, homicide, suicide, malignant neoplasms, and CAD. Young and middle-aged adults who are sexually active are a high-risk group for developing sexually transmitted diseases (STDs). The majority of persons with human immunodeficiency virus/acquired immune deficiency syndrome (HIV/AIDS) are in the 20 to 40 year age range. HIV has a long lag time between exposure and manifestation of symptoms that may not occur until later in life.

Stress-related health problems for this group are primarily associated with work, financial concerns, and multiple responsibilities of family, home, and social relationships. Many individuals in this age-group unexpectedly must cope with caring for their aging, ill parents while raising and caring for their children. These situations can impose heavy emotional, physical, and financial burdens on the family. A three-generation family living together in one household is a common occurrence in some cultural groups; however, geographical distances between families have limited these practices for many other U.S. families who are not prepared for this way of life. Substance and alcohol abuse, smoking, divorce, and domestic abuse are also sources of illness and are often contributing factors to chronic diseases in later life. Obesity, unhealthy diets, and insufficient exercise can also be precursors to chronic diseases in later life. Practicing health promotive behaviors can help these adults cope with the stressors of their ages (Figure 6-3).

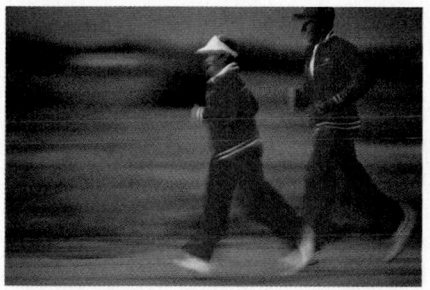

Figure 6-3 Through activities such as running, these middle-aged adults have taken responsibility for their health and are learning to cope with the physiological changes that occur during this stage.

Skills 360°

Awareness of Risk Factors Among Young Adults

The nurse should be knowledgeable of the prevalence of risk factors among young adults, be able to conduct a comprehensive history when interacting with patients in this age-group, and be prepared to provide health information. Selected examples of risk factors include:

- Exposure to infectious diseases, such as hepatitis A, during close contact with others in large gatherings, such as music concerts. (People often travel from concert to concert encountering repeated exposure to infections.)
- Smoking history. Although incidences have decreased somewhat, an increased incidence is seen in young American Indians and Alaska Natives.
- Incidence of heavy alcohol drinking and binges can be contributing factors to injuries, especially vehicular accidents and homicides.
- There has also been a significant increase for self-reported mental distress, alcohol and substance abuse, violence associated with an environment, poverty, and for some minority groups, particularly for African American and Hispanic (American) males.

Adapted from DeLaune, S., & Ladner, P. (2006). Fundamentals of nursing (3rd ed.). New York: Thomson Delmar Learning.

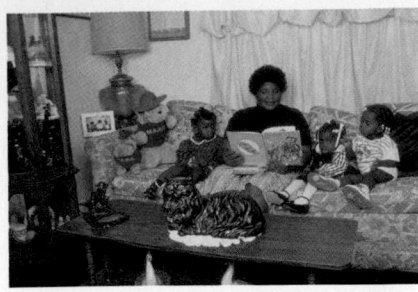

Figure 6-4 Older adults often assume new roles, such as grandparent, as they mature. They can gain immense pleasure in spending time with family and sharing wisdom and ideas with the younger generation.

HEALTH AND ILLNESS TRENDS FOR OLDER ADULTS

People are living longer and therefore experiencing more acute and chronic illness than ever before. Several social, economic, and political factors and policies must be considered. There are many definitions of *elderly*. Elderly status is frequently determined by the social values and roles within the culture, becoming a grandparent or the oldest sibling in the family (Figure 6-4). The most common definition in the United States and other modern societies is the chronological age of 65, a time of normal retirement. However, many individuals continue to be functionally active. Some of the physiological influences on functioning include sleep disturbances, sensory impairments, less mobility, and imbalance.

Health is also defined individually. One person may feel that health is the ability to live independently, to be self-reliant, and to be a functioning person in the community. Another may feel that health is defined as feeling good or having a positive outlook on life in general. Health can also mean being mentally active and not necessarily totally free from physical disease. Health, then, is a complex phenomenon comprising of physical, functional, and psychosocial factors.

Older adults also experience several stressors in their lives because of personal losses, such as social position, diminished finances, social support, independence, and inability to provide self-care because of a variety of reasons. Self-confidence can be affected by these losses and through the social prejudices and stereotyping that is often imposed by younger people in the society. Role reversal between the parent and child when the older adult is no longer able to provide self-care is a difficult transition for both individuals. Many of the older adult children can also have health problems that limit what they can do for their parents. In many instances, family members do not live close enough to provide direct care when needed. (This can be a major stress factor for both the parents and adult children.) Neglect and elder abuse can also be a major concern. The necessity to leave the home, live with family members, or live in assisted living or nursing care facilities can be difficult choices to make.

Skills 360°

Strategies to Use When Interacting with the Older Adult Patient

- Assess current knowledge and person's perception of self-participation in plan of care.
- Use all available resources to prepare for the teaching sessions. Whenever possible, contact members of the interdisciplinary team for assistance.
- Ensure that person can see and hear instructions.
- Provide a comfortable, well-lit environment.
- Choose a time for teaching when there are fewer distractions.
- Allow sufficient time for teaching, for demonstrating a skill, and for return demonstration.
- Structure teaching sessions for short periods of time to avoid tiring the person and to allow absorption of the information. Use language that patient can understand. Avoid use of medical terms. Clarify patient's understanding of the information.
- Partner with the patient and personal care provider in setting goals.
- Include a family member or personal care provider in the teaching sessions whenever possible.
- Provide written information as reinforcement.

A profile of aging in the American population provided by the U.S. Bureau of the Census at the National Center on Health Statistics (2006b) is seen in Box 6-1.

Effects of the Aging Process

The aging process involves physiological and psychological changes. The normal changes affect all body systems but do not necessarily occur at the same rate or time. The older adult has fewer reserves to draw on in time of illness or stress. The immune system is particularly vulnerable. Decreased absorption of nutrients and metabolism of drugs occurs; functioning of the renal system

---

BOX 6-1

PROFILE OF OLDER AMERICANS

- The older population (65 years of age or older) numbered 35.6 million in 2002, an increase of 3.3 million or 10.2 percent since 1992.
- The number of Americans aged 45 to 64 who will reach 65 over the next two decades increased by 38 percent from 1992 to 2002. About one in every eight, or 12.3 percent, of the total population is an older American. Over two million persons celebrated their 65th birthday in 2002.
- Persons reaching age 65 in 2002 have an average life expectancy of an additional 18.1 years (19.4 years for females and 16.4 years for males).
- Older women outnumber older men at 20.8 million older women to 14.8 million older men. Almost half (46 percent) of all older women in 2002 were widows.
- Older men were more likely to be married than older women; 73 percent of men were married compared to 41 percent of women. About 31 percent (10.5 million) of noninstitutionalized older people live alone (7.9 million women, 2.6 million men). Almost 400,000 grandparents aged 65 or older had the primary responsibility for their grandchildren who lived with them.
- By the year 2030, the growth in the older population will more than double to 71.5 million. The 85 and older population is projected to increase from 4.6 million in 2002 to 9.6 million in 2030.
- Members of minority groups are projected to represent 26.4 percent of the older population in 2030, up from 16.4 percent in 2000.
- The median income of older persons in 2002 was $19,436 for males and $11,406 for females. Median financial income of all households headed by older people (after adjusting for inflation) fell by 1.4 percent from 2001 to 2002; however, this difference was not statistically significant.
- The Social Security Administration reported that the major sources of income for older people were:
    Social Security (reported by 91 percent)
    Income from assets (reported by 58 percent)
    Public and private pensions (reported by 40 percent)
    Earnings (reported by 22 percent)
- About 3.6 million older persons lived below the poverty level in 2002. The poverty rate for older persons was 10.4 percent in 2002, which is not statistically different from the rate in 2001. Another 2.2 million, or 6.4 percent, of the elderly were classified as "near-poor" (income between the poverty level and 125 percent of this level).

Adapted from National Center for Health Statistics. (2006b). Health, United States, 2005: 29th report on the health status of the nation. *Retrieved July 12, 2006, from http://www.cdc.gov/nchs.*

BOX 6-2

MEDICATION USE BY OLDER ADULTS

Older adults frequently alter the prescribed medication regimen because they:

- Forget to take the medications as scheduled
- Use OTC medications that are less expensive.
- Use medications prescribed for someone else.
- Cut pills in half or take medications on alternate days to save money.
- Fail to understand the instructions or importance of the schedule or amount of medication to take.
- Fail to have prescriptions filled due to lack of funds.
- Refuse to take medications because of undesirable side effects.

Adapted from Broyles, B. E., Reiss, B. S., & Evans, M. E. (2007). Pharmacological aspects of nursing care (7th ed.). New York: Thomson Delmar Learning.

decreases significantly; sensory losses in vision and hearing can have a major impact on daily activities. Osteoarthritis, rheumatoid arthritis, and osteoporosis are also common for this age-group. Diminished mobility and balance place the older person at risk of falls and injuries. Middle-aged adults (over 45) are more prone to outdoor injuries; older adults have more indoor injuries (Li, Keegan, Sternfeld, Quesenberry, Jr., & Kelsey, 2006). Major surgeries for older adults include hip, knee, and shoulder joint replacement and cataract removal to improve vision. The older adult is a great risk for the common chronic diseases and health problems described previously in this chapter. Box 6-2 illustrates some of the common factors related to medication use by the older adult.

Yet, retirement and the older years can be satisfying. Many people look forward to spending time leisurely with family and at social activities. A network of social support has a major impact on physical and psychological well-being. Some enjoy small group gatherings, church groups, participating in senior center activities, and in moderate exercise activities (swimming, croquet, golf, yoga, and tai chi movements). Many people enjoy outside activities and gardening. Some people may find fulfillment in volunteer work at schools, hospitals, animal shelters, and other places; others may continue part-time employment. Many people enjoy writing or recording their life history or creating a scrapbook to reflect on their lives as legacy to the younger generation.

Legal and ethical issues are concerns for older adults. Many legal issues involve estate planning, making living wills, advance directives, and designating a power of attorney. Advance directives are now mandated when admitted to a health care facility by the Self-Determination Act of 1991 (Delaune & Ladner, 2006). Ethical issues involve the person's ability to make decisions, end-of-life care, and types of intensive care procedures. The nurse can assist the patient, family, and others in recognizing the presence of an ethical dilemma and suggest resources that are available to help resolve the issues.

Many psychological changes are related to the person's health status. Depression often occurs because of the many losses, lower self-esteem, and anxiety about their declining health. Certain types of memory diminish with aging, the attention span may be altered, and personality changes are often stress induced. Several of the mental changes are also because of the degree of social support and social interactions. Mental assessment of the older adult is a vital component in planning holistic health care. Of particular concern are the dementias that primarily appear at this stage of life.

Alzheimer's Disease

Alzheimer's disease is a major progressive neurodegenerative disorder initially affecting short-term memory and later affecting intellectual abilities. The disease seriously affects a person's ability to care for self and carry out simple, common activities of daily living. Alzheimer's disease accounts for about 50 percent of all clinical cases of dementia. The prevalence of Alzheimer's increases steadily with age and the number of newly diagnosed cases is expected to increase as the population continues to age. The disease imposes a heavy financial and care burden on the family and society. Annual costs are $100 billion annually. Scientists are searching for a drug to help the immune system fight the buildup of plaque and delay the progress of the disease. Refer to chapter 37 for detailed information on Alzheimer's disease, and nursing responsibilities in the management of care.

SUBPOPULATIONS OF OLDER ADULTS

Subpopulations of older adults include the homeless, older adult women, those who live in rural areas, the frail elderly 85 years of age, the chronically ill older adult, and the ethnic older adult. For nurses to care for patients across the life span these subpopulations provide a means of categorizing the various groups of patients.

Homeless Older Adults

Homelessness is increasing in many geographical areas because of the lack of services and housing. Approximately 14 to 15 percent of the homeless are older adults. These individuals are at great risk for multiple acute and chronic illnesses, assault, abuse, rape, malnutrition, and physical and mental illnesses. Many elderly are homeless because of an illness that depleted their funds or lack of health insurance coverage. Other problems include sleep deprivation, dental problems, upper respiratory diseases, tuberculosis, frost bite, leg ulcers, heat exhaustion, depression, and other serious mental health problems. This population is underserved. Health care workers and volunteers provide assistance; however, there is a great need for appropriate health care programs.

Older Adult Women

As mentioned earlier, many older women live alone. Many rely on Social Security as their only source of income and have less access to health insurance coverage. They also have higher incidences of one or more chronic diseases. Married older women are often the principle caregiver of ill husbands.

Older Adults Living in Rural Areas

Most of the older adults live in urban areas. Approximately 23 percent live in rural communities where weather conditions and lack of transportation limit access to a variety of resources. Lower income status is prevalent in the rural areas. Older adults in rural areas use a balance of activities to promote physical and mental health. Sometimes they are lonely, but they are comfortable with the services provided by local health care personnel who are also neighbors and friends. There is a need for innovative home health nursing care models to provide health promotion and illness prevention measures.

The Frail Elderly

The frail elderly have declining physical health and resources to draw on and are most vulnerable to complications of an existing illness or acquiring a new disease, particularly a respiratory infection. They usually respond to the additional stressful life event, such as death of a pet, and have little energy to complete the activities of daily living. They are also vulnerable to dehydration and malnutrition, skin injuries, mobility problems, falls, and cognitive decline. The older adult usually sleeps less during the night but may nap during the day; they may eat less and drink less fluid to avoid getting up during the night to urinate. In some cases older adults will become incontinent.

Chronically Ill Older Adults

It is not unusual for older adults to have two or more chronic health problems. These individuals, also, have difficulty in performing basic activities of daily living, such as dressing and hygiene practices or transferring from one position to another and walking. Impairment of instrumental activities of daily living, such as shopping, taking medications, meal preparation, managing finances, transportation, and housekeeping skills, should be carefully assessed to determine the assistance that is needed. Illnesses can be difficult to accurately diagnose as older adults often underreport their symptoms. There is a common belief that new symptoms are because of old age and are inevitable. Therefore, they must be endured.

Safety First

Climate Extremes and Older Adult Responses

Heat waves have resulted in several deaths among older adults. A chronic health problem or medications may inhibit the normal body responses to extreme heat. Measures to prevent heat exhaustion include taking a cool shower, bath, or sponge bath, wearing light loose clothing, and limiting activities. Older adults should be monitored during a heat wave, have an electric fan, or be taken to an air-conditioned location.

Severe cold weather is also a great concern for older adults who are prone to hypothermia and frostbite. Some deaths have been reported of older people who have wandered into the cold environment and were not discovered until it was too late. Careful monitoring of the confused older adult is essential.

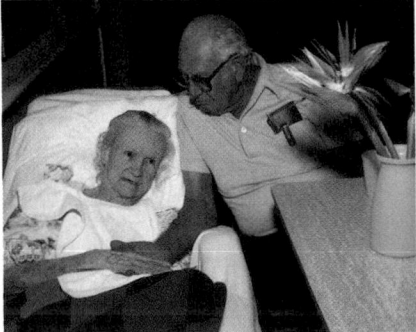

Figure 6-5 This older adult female is visited by her spouse in a long-term care facility. Long-term care can be expensive and not easily affordable by many persons.

Most of the care is provided by a family member who lives with the older adult. This can be a rewarding or burdensome and isolating experience. It is important that respite time is provided. Day care centers may be a solution if the older adult is able to attend; some people rely on part-time in-home help by other family members, friends, or paid assistants. The nurse should assess the patient for symptoms of abuse or neglect and assess the caregiver for signs of role strain. Caregivers must also receive instructions that will assist them in the care provider role.

Health problems in older adults will vary a great deal. Treatment of one disease may trigger a problem in another body system. Medication side effects can include urinary retention, dizziness, nausea, gastric upset, drowsiness, or insomnia.

Ethnic Older Adults

Attention should be given to the health care needs of the ethnic older adult who may experience many unique losses in his or her lives. The availability of ethnic foods, opportunities to worship as they choose, to visit with people from their own culture, and to use cultural remedies are sources of comfort. Unfortunately, the ethnic older adult often lives in older and poorer neighborhoods, and he or she is more socially vulnerable to unsafe living conditions and crime.

TRENDS IN USE OF HEALTH CARE SERVICES BY OLDER ADULTS

As Americans age, acute disease processes take on more chronic properties. These chronic diseases are characterized by prolonged courses and increased use of health care resources. New technologies are able to delay aging and death. Open heart surgery is being performed on people in their 80s. More elderly Americans continue to drive their cars, and the debate about the physical and cognitive capacity of older people to drive is revisited when accidents involving the elderly occur. Compromised visual, auditory, and cognitive ability, as well as slower reaction time and the increased risk of sudden onset of acute cardiac or vascular illness must be weighed against the physical agility and mental acuity enjoyed by many elderly.

It is estimated that 80 percent of Americans will live beyond the age of 65 years. These Americans may not be retiring at 62 or even at 65. The cost of health care is, in many cases, requiring that they work long past their preferred retirement age. There is a greater likelihood that more extensive and more expensive health care services will be required prior to or after retirement. These situations necessitate consideration of obtaining long-term care insurance at an earlier age. Medicare is the major health insurance coverage that elderly Americans depend on to assist them in paying for health care during retirement. Medicare health care coverage was created in 1965 with the passage of the Social Security Act to pay for acute hospital care and care in skilled nursing facilities, as well as physical rehabilitation and care in long-term mental health facilities for the elderly and disabled people (Figure 6-5). It was not designed to pay for long-term outpatient care management and the increased number of prescription drugs, particularly used by older people with chronic illnesses. There is a great concern about the availability of funds in the future.

Many people are also concerned about the costs and navigating the new Medicare prescription coverage plan that became available to 42.6 million Medicare beneficiaries in January, 2006. Meeting these extended needs requires that nurses become more involved in care planning and teaching because a preponderance of the care needs of the elderly fall within nurses' scope of practice (Baier, 2006).

Medicaid is financed jointly by state and federal governments and from general tax revenues. Medicaid is a program for the poor and disabled. It is estimated

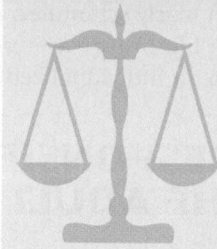

LAW IN PRACTICE

Decisions on Ability to Drive an Automobile

It is extremely stressful for anyone to relinquish a driver's license. It is a hallmark symbol of independence. Many older adults deny their physical, cognitive, and sensory limitations that pose safety issues for themselves and others and delay the process as long as possible. State regulations differ regarding this issue. Licensing exams are usually scheduled at shorter intervals; an actual driving test may be required as the examiner assesses the person's reaction time, peripheral vision acuity, judgment of distance, hearing, and other physical functions, and emotional reactions. Daytime driving limitations on surface streets may be imposed. The state driver handbook usually has information for people who are concerned for the safe driving issues of someone judged to be incapable to drive. An explanation about the specific concern, the person's name, date of birth, current address, and current driver license number can be sent to the local department of motor vehicles. The person will be contacted for a reexamination, and the license could be suspended or revoked depending on the driving record. A health care provider is also required to report people who are diagnosed with lapses of consciousness and can report a patient believed to be an unsafe driver because of a health problem.

The psychological response to these situations can be stressful for the individual and the person reporting the problem, especially if the report is made by a family member.

that about 15 percent of the population that receives Medicare benefits also receives Medicaid benefits. Nurses need to know how these benefits work and how to access them for the benefit of this particular aging population.

Many Americans do not qualify for any type of health insurance, and those that do qualify may still incur significant out-of-pocket health costs. Families may be forced to decide that they cannot afford health care. Many elderly live alone in anonymity, and the working poor, those below the poverty level, are at great risk to fall through the health care system cracks.

Health literacy is becoming a great concern. Many younger and older Americans have difficulty understanding the complicated health care forms or are unable to successfully navigate through the system. Health care literacy is the degree to which an individual can obtain, process, and understand basic health care services. When people do not understand the system, they do not use the services even when they are eligible to do so. Health care literacy is also dependent on the skill of the health care provider and how well providers can assist patients to navigate the processes.

HEALTH PROMOTION

Many of the life-threatening and chronic diseases are diseases that are the result of high-risk factors including biological (aging), genetic, and environmental factors and unhealthy lifestyles. There is a great need for geriatric nurses and geriatric nurse practitioners. Nurses must develop multiple skills to educate, motivate, and empower individuals to adopt healthy lifestyle behaviors.

PATIENT PLAYBOOK

Health Promotion Education

The nurse can ask patients the following questions in preparing a health promotion education program:

- What motivates you to learn something new?
- How do you like to learn?
- What factors do you feel will be incentives for you to learn? And what factors will be obstacles for you to learn?
- What type of environment is best for you? Do you want someone from your family to be present during the education sessions? Would you like the information provided in another language than English? Who would be a good person to translate this information for you? Would you be willing to have a professional translator present? What language would you prefer for the written materials?
- Are you able to set realistic goals? Are you willing to partner with me in developing a plan? Are you willing to be committed to reaching the goals that will be agreed upon?
- What do you believe the causes are for your current health problem? Do you feel that you can take control of your situation? What benefits do you see when you take control?

Participation in screening procedures, maintaining an appropriate immunization schedule, and regularly scheduled physical examinations with attention to obtaining a thorough life history are important elements in determining what should be included in an individualized health promotion program.

NURSING RESPONSIBILITIES IN THE CARE OF THE ADULT ACROSS THE LIFE SPAN

Providing education is one of the major roles of the nurse in health promotion, and opportunities exist in all interaction settings. Many people fear or distrust the health care system. Serving as the person's advocate is another major nursing role. Building a trusting relationship with individuals of all ages takes time and patience. The nurse must also be equipped with the knowledge about what motivates individuals to learn and the environmental influences that facilitate or inhibit learning. Knowing about the different learning styles and teaching strategies is also important. Additional factors include understanding a person's health beliefs, the perception of the causes of the health problem, and self-confidence in the ability to change behavior and take on a new lifestyle. A holistic perspective is essential in meeting the person's total needs.

The theories presented previously in this chapter provide the nurse with the tools to develop appropriate age-related education. Health promotion and self-efficacy theories are additional resources to provide a framework for planning and implementing health care education for all age-groups.

The nurse also can be a facilitator of change and must be able to evaluate the effectiveness of the educational program. As nursing continues to evolve as a scientific discipline the use of evidence-based practice (EBP) interventions must be the goal. EBP is the process by which nurses make clinical decisions using the best available research evidence, clinical expertise, and patient preferences. By carrying out the three steps shown in Box 6-3, EBP can help resolve some of the problems encountered by nurses.

Healthy People 2010 is a national health promotion and disease prevention initiative that addresses the disparities in health care. The program outlines the steps that individuals, communities, and professionals should take to ensure long and healthy lives. The major healthy activities include some sort of physical activity; a decrease in obesity, tobacco use, and substance abuse; and practicing responsible sexual behavior. Environmental quality is of great importance as is the attention to promoting mental health and access to health care.

BOX 6-3

STEPS OF EVIDENCE-BASED NURSING PRACTICE

- Clearly identify the issue or problem based on accurate analysis of current nursing knowledge and practice.
- Search the literature for relevant research.
- Evaluate the research evidence using established criteria regarding scientific merit.

Adapted from DeLaune, S., & Ladner, P. (2006). Fundamentals of nursing (3rd ed.). New York: Thomson Delmar Learning.

KEY CONCEPTS

- Each adult patient a nurse encounters is biologically and experientially unique.
- Nurses must be knowledgeable of adult developmental theories and the stage of life each patient currently occupies to tailor the plan of care to the person's unique needs.
- The health of the U.S. population has changed over the years and changing patterns and trends have evolved delivering the information necessary to deliver individualized care with appropriate nursing interventions and desired outcomes.
- Several changes have taken place over the last several decades. The nation has become a multicultural mixture of different age-groups, thus presenting different individual, social, and political influences on health care services.
- The United States is a multicultural nation. Despite an overall decline in mortality, racial and ethnic disparities in mortality persist.
- Many people are selecting alternative health care methods, such as CAM, to improve their self-image and the effects of the aging process.

- People are living longer and therefore experiencing more acute and chronic illness than ever before. Several social, economic, and political factors and policies must be considered.
- The aging process involves physiological and psychological changes.
- The normal changes affect all body systems, but they do not necessarily occur at the same rate or time. The older adult has fewer reserves to draw on in time of illness or stress.
- Many of the life-threatening and chronic diseases are diseases that are the end result of high-risk factors including biological (aging), genetic, and environmental factors and unhealthy lifestyles.
- Chronic diseases are characterized by prolonged courses and increased use of health care resources.
- As nursing continues to evolve as a scientific discipline the use of EBN interventions must be the goal.

REVIEW QUESTIONS

1. The impact on health care resources attributed to older adults is demonstrated by:
   1. Overreporting health problem symptoms and frequent hospitalizations
   2. All people over 65 have at least two chronic health problems.
   3. Older adults represent the fastest growing segment of the population.
   4. The prevalence of diabetes in older adults

2. Obesity is a major health care problem in the United States. Which of the following are the most accurate statements (select all that apply)?
   1. Obesity is primarily due to overeating.
   2. More than half of Americans are overweight or obese.
   3. The causes of obesity are multiple and complex.
   4. Current trends indicate a leveling off in obesity rates.

3. Recent trends in smoking rates indicate one of the following situations:
   1. There has been a slight decrease in the percentage of smoking by adults.
   2. Smoking is linked primarily with adults who have a higher level of education.

   3. Smoking has increased in the last decade by pregnant women.
   4. Smoking is more prevalent for people in a higher social economic status.

4. Suicide has become a serious public health concern. According to the trends data:
   1. The rates of suicide have outnumbered homicide rates in the last several decades.
   2. Many people who commit suicide have not had any recent contact with a health care provider.
   3. Symptoms of suicide intent can be easily recognizable.
   4. The primary reason for suicide ideation is the presence of a chronic disease.

5. According to the predicted trends for the future:
   1. There will be a greater increase in the percentage of older men than the increase in percentage of older women by 2030.
   2. The older adult population will comprise less than 19 percent of the population.
   3. A majority of the frail elderly population will live in skilled nursing care facilities.
   4. Older adult African Americans will be the largest racial/ethnic/group by 2030.

Continued

6. Data about metabolic syndrome, or syndrome X, indicate that:
   1. The syndrome is related to a neurological dysfunction.
   2. The syndrome is unassociated with CAD.
   3. The risk for developing the syndrome is seen primarily in adults over 65 years of age.
   4. One of four individuals in the total population is at risk for developing this health problem.

7. Certain population groups are at higher risk of developing hypertension; therefore, accurate diagnosis is important. According to statistical data, the nurse should recognize that people belonging to one of the ethnic groups below is at the greatest risk:
   1. Asian (Americans)
   2. African Americans
   3. Hispanic (Americans) from the Caribbean
   4. Americans of European descent

8. Many adults select cosmetic therapies and surgery to enhance their physical appearance and emotional health and to increase their self-esteem. The nurse can advise them how to avoid complications by:
   1. Stating that they can inquire whether the therapy providers offer special prices on specific procedures
   2. Mentioning that an informed consent is not necessary for minimally invasive procedures

3. Ensuring the individuals know what substance is being injected into their bodies
4. Stating the person can rely on the information presented by the experienced therapy provider

9. The health care team informs the patient that bariatric surgery is considered successful when (select all that apply):
   1. The patient loses approximately 25 percent of excess weight within three months.
   2. The patient maintains a weight loss of at least 48 percent over the long-term.
   3. The patient is between 24 and 40 years of age.
   4. The patient realizes the need for a lifelong change in behavior.

10. A profile of aging Americans by the U.S. Bureau of the Census indicates that:
    1. Older Americans represent approximately 12 percent of the total population today.
    2. Life expectancy has reached a plateau and will not increase for at least a decade.
    3. There are more male widowers today than in the past 20 years.
    4. The median income of older adults is approximately $27,000 and will continue to rise due to increases in Medicare benefits.

REVIEW ACTIVITIES

1. Access the Robert Havinghurst information at: http://personalwebs.oakland.edu (Search for Havinghurst) Review the following information:
   - Ten stages of adult-sibling relationships: A comparison across the late adolescence to late adult years. The topics include: Comparison of four stages of life, the impact of birth order on sibling relationships, and unraveling the typologies of adult sibling relationships.
   - Interview a middle-aged or older adult who has siblings and summarize your findings. Compare your findings with the comments mentioned on the Web site.

2. Access the body mass index (BMI) measuring instrument at: http://www.consumer.gov/weightloss.bmi.htm. This is a public access site that permits personal calculation of BMI.
   - Determine your BMI and list what risk factors you may have.
   - Determine the BMI of a family member and compare the risk factors with your own.

3. Locate the Activity Pyramid at: http://www.mypyramid.gov/pyramid Web site. There is information why exercise is important, the amount needed, tips for increasing activity, and precautions for people at risk. Design an exercise program for the inactive individual. Include how to overcome potential barriers to an exercise program, such as lack of time, no convenient access to exercise center, and such.

Continued

4. At the Activity Pyramid site, review all the topics inside the pyramid. Review information for kids, for professionals, and my pyramid tracker. Click on the pyramid areas to learn more about the new dietary pyramid guidelines. Plan a menu for one day for you that meets the guidelines.

5. Prevention of injuries and falls in the elderly is a major health promotion strategy. Locate the tool kit to prevent senior falls provided by the National Center for Injury and Prevention and Control at: http://www.cdc.gov/ncipc. Interview a friend or family member who is living independently in the community. Use the tool kit to assess vision and balance capability. Inquire what assistance is needed, if any, for accomplishing activities of daily living or impaired activities of daily living (referring to transportation and social interactions in the community, use of telephone, etc.). Explore what safety features should be addressed in the home environment as addressed in the tool kit guidelines.

6. Review the tips for care of aging parents provided by the National Safety Council at http://www.nsc.org. Create a poster using these tips and present the information to a small community group (such as a church group or PTA).

7. Review the techniques to improve patient safety (TIPS) provided by the Joint Commission Resources at: http://www.doody.com/TIPS. Click on Obese Patients. Write a summary report of the strategies that are mentioned.

8. Access one of the following resources and write a brief report on the mission or services provided:
   Aging Network at
       http://www.infaaa.org/agingnet.html.
   American Geriatric Society at:
       http://www.americangeriatrics.org.
   American Association of Retired Persons at:
       http://www.aarp.org.
   Family Caregiver Alliance at:
       http://www.caregiver.org.
   National Council of Senior Citizens at:
       http://www.ncscinc.org.

Visit the Contemporary Medical-Surgical Nursing online companion resource at www.delmarhealthcare.com for additional content and study aids. Click on Online Companions then select the Nursing discipline.

Palliative Care

MariJo Letizia, PhD, RN, C, APRN-BC

CHAPTER TOPICS

- Overview of Death and Dying

- Assessment of the Patient Receiving Hospice and Palliative Care

- Nursing Diagnoses

- Planning and Implementing Care for Patients Receiving Hospice and Palliative Care

- Special Considerations in the Home Care of the Dying

KEY TERMS

Addiction
Advance Directives
Anticipatory grieving
Assisted suicide
Bereaved
Caregiver role strain
Complementary and alternative medicine (CAM)
Do not resuscitate (DNR)
Euthanasia
Grief resolution
Hospice care
Interdisciplinary team
Living Will
Medicare Hospice Benefit
Palliative care
Physical dependence
Physician-assisted suicide
Power of Attorney for Health Care
Terminal illness
Tolerance

Death is a natural part of the cycle of life. Everyone knows that at one time or another, he or she will die. Over the past two decades, health care providers and the public have come to acknowledge the importance of improved quality care at the end of life. For example, in 1997 the International Council of Nurses mandated the unique and primary responsibility of nurses for ensuring that individuals experience a peaceful death at the end of life. The American Association of Colleges of Nursing's (AACN) Peaceful Death document outlines 15 end-of-life competencies that every undergraduate nursing student should attain before graduation (AACN, 1997). These competencies incorporate the physical, psychosocial, and spiritual dimensions of care provided to the dying patient and his or her family. The word *family* is used inclusively as those people who have a connection to the patient and who may take responsibility for some aspect of the patient's care, including a spouse, significant other, child, parent, sibling, neighbor, or close friend. From the time of diagnosis to the time of death, nurses provide person-centered care by involving patients and families at all levels of decision making. A holistic approach to end-of-life care is accomplished by enhancing the nurse's knowledge, skills, attitudes, and values. This chapter describes the philosophy and characteristics of hospice and palliative care and discusses the role of the nurse in meeting the needs of patients and their families.

OVERVIEW OF DEATH AND DYING

Dying refers to the process that ultimately ends in an event called death. Leading causes of death in the United States include heart disease, malignant neoplasm, cerebrovascular disease, and lung disease; less than 10 percent of Americans die suddenly. In contrast to accidental death, a **terminal illness** is one in which there is no possibility for a cure, resulting in the decline of the patient's physical condition and then death. Disorders causing terminal illness include altered immune disease; neoplastic conditions; neurological, cardiac, pulmonary, renal, and gastrointestinal (GI) conditions; dementia; and endocrine disorders.

Patients with terminal illnesses progress through the failure of one or more body systems until death occurs. The dying process and eventual death may be peaceful as the patient solidifies relationships and says goodbye to loved ones. Symptom management is crucial to a peaceful death; patients are much more able to devote themselves to important relationships when pain and other symptoms are well controlled. People die in a variety of settings including their homes, hospitals, emergency departments, and skilled nursing facilities. Surveys indicate that up to 90 percent of those in the United States prefer to die at home (Brown University School of Medicine, 2000).

The concept of death is often overwhelming; it is accompanied by questions and feelings of uncertainty that have wide-ranging and far-reaching effects for all involved. Nurses who care for patients who are dying and their families are impacted by their work in various ways. Helping patients and families cope and find meaning in the face of great loss often brings to mind memories from the past. An important first step is to reflect on personal experiences with death and get in touch with the feelings and reactions associated with those experiences. Nurses are encouraged to come to terms with these losses to ensure effective end-of-life care for their patients and family members.

Overview of Palliative Care

More than 15 years ago the World Health Organization (WHO) defined **palliative care** as active holistic care of patients whose disease is not responsive to curative treatment. Palliative care emphasizes control of pain and other distressing physical, psychosocial, and spiritual concerns of those with life-limiting illness (WHO, 2005a). WHO has developed principles to guide providers of care in their work with the dying that state that palliative care affirms life and regards dying as a normal process, neither hastening nor postponing death. Fundamentally, the plan of care is developed in light of the values and expressed desires of the patient and family.

The goal of palliative care is the attainment of the highest possible quality of life for patients and their families. While such care is provided to those with life-threatening or terminal illnesses, palliative care is also offered to those with chronic illness not responsive to curative treatment. Because quality of life is important during all phases of illness, patients can access palliative care at any time during their illness. In contrast to hospice care, palliative care approaches can coexist with curative interventions, such as radiation therapy, chemotherapy, and palliative surgery. Palliative treatment is designed to comfort and support the patient and family.

Palliative care is planned and delivered through the collaborative efforts of an **interdisciplinary team** (members of specific disciplines who work collaboratively) beginning at the time the illness is diagnosed and continuing through the bereavement period. The team's focus is on relieving suffering, controlling symptoms, and supporting the patient's functional capacity. Members of the team include patients, families, physicians, nurses, pharmacists, social workers, chaplains, physical, occupational, speech, and respiratory therapists, massage, music, pet, and art therapists, and volunteers. Within the personal, cultural, and religious values and practices of the patient and family, nurses providing palliative care address physical, psychosocial, and spiritual concerns.

The need for palliative care education for providers of care has been addressed in a variety of ways in the United States. Formal palliative care education is available to physicians by a program created by the American Medical Association called the Education of Physicians on End-of-Life Care (EPEC). Likewise, the AACN has supported an educational training program for nurses called the End-of-Life Nursing Education Consortium (ELNEC).

History and Overview of Hospice Care

In the United States today, hospice is a formal program that delivers end-of-life care to patients who have a limited prognosis or life expectancy. **Hospice care** is a coordinated program of services that exists within the larger umbrella of palliative care service, delivering palliative care rather than curative treatment. Hospice programs provide hospice care with sensitivity to the diverse backgrounds and needs of the people they serve and with the hope and belief that through appropriate management, patients and families can attain a degree of mental and spiritual preparation for death.

The concept of hospice is derived from medieval times, when the term hospice was used to identify particular places where travelers could find rest and comfort. The word *hospice* originates in the Latin root for *hospitality* and *hospitable*. To provide such comfort and a natural death to dying patients, Cicely Saunders established St. Christopher's Hospice in London, England in 1967. Saunders is widely recognized as a pioneer in modern-day hospice; she was first a nurse, then a social worker, and finally obtained her medical degree to promote her vision of hospice care. Saunders developed a program of care for the dying that included attention to the physical, psychosocial, and spiritual needs of the patient and family. She included physicians, nurses, counselors, chaplains, and physical therapists on her team. Her work formed the foundation for the modern day hospice movement.

In 1966 Florence Wald, who was then dean of the Yale University School of Nursing, invited Dr. Saunders to present a workshop on the care of the dying. Subsequently, in 1974, Wald opened the New Haven Hospice, the first hospice program in the United States (New Haven Hospice, 2006). About that same time a Canadian surgeon, Balfour Mount, began a hospital-based palliative care service at the Royal Victoria Hospital of McGill University in Montreal, Canada (Royal Victoria Hospital, 2006). The McGill program continues to serve as an international model in end-of-life care.

It is important to recognize that during that same period Elizabeth Kübler-Ross was working in the United States as a psychiatrist interviewing dying patients. She is well-known for her work on defining the psychological stages of dying. Her model, outlined in her book *On Death and Dying* (1969), serves as a theoretical framework and essential reading for those who care for the dying. In this work, Kübler-Ross outlines the stages that terminally ill patients may experience as they cope with impending death: denial, anger, bargaining, depression, and acceptance or resignation. Because of her testimony on the needs of the dying before Congress in 1972, the Health Care Financing Administration (HCFA) funded demonstration projects that led to subsequent legislation supporting hospice programs in the United States.

Volunteers primarily provided early hospice services in the United States, because there was no structure for reimbursement for such services. Then in 1984, the Joint Commission on Accreditation of Health Care Organizations (JCAHO) published the first standards manual for hospice programs. Since that time, hospice care has been available to patients who sign a consent form stating that they elect hospice services to provide care for their terminal illness. They may leave the hospice program to receive curative treatment at any time.

Hospice care is provided by a public agency or private organization that is primarily engaged in providing services to the terminally ill; hospice care can also be provided by homecare agencies. It is important to recognize that hospice is a concept and not a place. The patient and family may have a preference about the type of care setting, living situation, and services that can be provided. In the United States, hospice care is most often delivered in the home or extended care settings; however, more hospitals are accommodating dying patients in designated palliative care units and more freestanding facilities are being built to provide a setting for people without competent caregivers in the home.

The National Hospice Reimbursement Act of 1986 mandated that Medicare pay the cost of all health services related to the hospice patient's terminal illness. To be eligible for the **Medicare Hospice Benefit** (a reimbursement benefit for those with a prognosis of six months or less), a physician must certify that the patient has a limited life expectancy of six months or less. The hospice nurse explains the Medicare and Medicaid Hospice Benefits to the patient and the family at the time of inquiry about hospice care and also discusses options that are possible under private insurance benefit plans.

Patients who are eligible for standard Medicare are also eligible for the Medicare Hospice Benefit under Medicare Hospital Insurance Part A. This benefit entitles patients to receive noncurative medical and support services under an interdisciplinary plan of care established by the hospice team. The Medicare Hospice Benefit covers hospice services, durable medical equipment (such as a hospital bed, overbed table, commode, walker, and oxygen), and supplies (such as urinary catheters, wound care supplies, and incontinence pads and diapers), hospital admissions, and medications related to the terminal illness. Standard Medicare continues to provide coverage for medical care unrelated to the terminal illness. An example of this benefit is seen in the case of a woman diagnosed with breast cancer metastatic to the bone with concurrent diabetes. The Medicare Hospice Benefit pays 100 percent of the cost for the pain medication related to the bony metastasis and standard Medicare covers treatment for her diabetes. Patients access the Medicare Hospice Benefit by having care provided by a Medicare-certified hospice program. In addition to support provided by the entire interdisciplinary hospice team, patients who opt to die at home must have a caregiver in the home that is able, willing, and available.

Role of the Hospice and Palliative Care Nurse

Hospice and palliative care nurses focus on the management of the complex clinical problems encountered in the care of the patient. Using standardized tools, nurses assess patients' symptoms and use this information to plan care interventions and evaluate outcomes. In providing hospice and palliative care, nurses share in one of the most intimate and tumultuous times in the lives of their patients and families, assuming various roles including those of teacher, counselor, advocate, and supporter.

Nurses must examine their own attitudes about death and be cautious not to impose their own values and beliefs about the dying experience on others. Cultural background plays a major role in people's attitudes about death. Every culture has values and behaviors that influence the experience of dying for members of the group. However, such values and behaviors may vary among members of the group. Therefore, nurses must be cautious in making assumptions about the care of a dying patient solely on the basis of culture or ethnic background. Remember that culture serves as a guide for many different kinds of human interaction.

The influence and impact of culture is far more than simply the person's race and ethnicity. Culture involves the person's belief systems about sexual orientation, physical and cognitive abilities or disabilities, socioeconomic status, employment, and educational level. Such beliefs are considered in developing the plan of care. People from all cultures experience the grief that accompanies the death of a loved one. Social customs, religion, and cultural practices influence the way people mourn that loss. Rituals surrounding illness and death give structure to support the **bereaved** (a state of sadness or sorrow because of a loss or death) through this painful process when people are vulnerable and feel off balance.

Nurses should include such rituals in the plan of care. Some questions nurses can consider as they interact with each patient and family are: (a) How is family defined? (b) Who is or should be involved in the decision making? (c) Does the person have special dietary needs? (d) Are candles, music, or other special items needed to complete a ritual? (e) Is the body to be treated in any special way at the time of death? and (f) What are the patient's attitudes toward organ donation and autopsy? Table 7-1 highlights selected cultural practices that influence the dying experience, which is essential understanding for hospice and palliative care nurses.

One of the most important aspects of hospice and palliative nursing care is communication with the patient, family, and health care team members about end-of-life issues. Open, honest, and understandable communication is essential for patients to be able to make decisions about their care. Assess patients' desire for information; while patient autonomy and empowerment are a focus of care, not all patients desire full disclosure about their terminal diagnosis.

Individualize the way information is provided. For example, when sharing information consider the patient's place in the family structure and the roles of family members. Address all questions and concerns and give the patient and family accurate information. Help prepare the family for the decline in the physical, emotional, and cognitive status of the patient and assist them in coping with suffering, grief, and loss. Many hospice and palliative care programs

TABLE 7-1 Cultural Considerations Related to Dying

Native Americans

Family:	Includes immediate and extended family and friends.
Communication:	The discussion of a terminal illness varies from tribe to tribe; some do not openly discuss serious illnesses, because negative thoughts are believed to hasten death. Eye contact is avoided and respectful distance is maintained.
Sick role:	The patient tends to be quiet and stoic.
Spiritual healing:	Healers may be used.
Time of death:	The family may sing, touch, hug, and stay close to the deceased. Wailing and shrieking may also occur.
Care of the body:	Depends on the specific tribe; common practices include turning or flexing the body and purifying the body using sweet grass smoke. Family may prefer to prepare the body. The soul is believed to depart the body 36 hours after death, and the family may want the body to remain at the place of death for this period of time.
Organ donation:	Generally not desired.
Autopsy:	Generally not desired.

African Americans

Family:	Includes immediate and extended family and close friends; tends to be a matriarchal system.
Communication:	The spokesperson is usually the father or eldest family member.
Sick role:	The patient tends to desire to maintain independence and expects attention from the family.
Spiritual healing:	Faith is important; home remedies may be used for healing.
Time of death:	Expression of emotion in public varies. Some think it is bad luck to die in the home.
Care of the body:	Generally expect professionals to prepare the body; there is great respect for the deceased and afterlife; cremation is avoided.
Organ donation:	Generally taboo except for immediate family needs.
Autopsy:	Generally accepted.

Continued

TABLE 7-1   Cultural Considerations Related to Dying—cont'd

Chinese Americans

Family:	Includes extended family
Communication:	Family may prefer to tell the patient about the terminal illness themselves. It is important to include the head of the household (usually the eldest male) in the decision making. Eye contact is avoided to signify respect.
Sick role:	The patient tends to be passive; the family is expected to take care of the patient.
Spiritual healing:	Herbs, traditional Chinese medicine, and acupuncture may be used.
Time of death:	May believe that the spirit gets lost if death occurs in the hospital.
Care of the body:	Family may prefer to bathe the body.
Organ donation:	Generally uncommon.
Autopsy:	May not be allowed.

Japanese Americans

Family:	Family-oriented, person is subordinate to family unit, patriarchal system
Communication:	Spokesperson and decision maker is usually the eldest male. The patient and family may avoid discussing serious illness. DNR status typically decided by entire family.
Sick role:	Patient tends to be passive.
Spiritual healing:	Herbal medicine, prayer, and offerings may be used.
Time of death:	Prefer to die at home.
Care of the body:	Cleanliness, dignity, modesty are important; cremation possible.

Japanese Americans

Organ donation:	Highly individualized.
Autopsy:	Highly individualized.

Hispanic (Americans)

Family:	Includes extended family that is obligated to care for the sick. Caring for the dying and attending funerals are prohibited for pregnant women.
Communication:	Spokesperson is the older daughter or son; the family may want to protect patient from information about serious illness believing that knowledge and subsequent worry will hasten death. Important decisions may require consultation among entire family.
Sick role:	Illness is a social crisis; family caregiving is accepted and encouraged. Stoicism is highly regarded.
Spiritual healing:	Spiritual healers, herbalists, massage or manipulation, and spiritual ceremonies are also used, but may not be discussed with health care providers.
Time of death:	May have preference not to die in the hospital, believing that their spirit may get lost and not be able to find its way home. The hospital environment and visiting hours are considered to be restrictive.
Care of the body:	Death is an important spiritual event; extended family member may assist with the preparation of the body and may request time with the deceased person.
Organ donation:	Extreme respect for the body, which must be kept intact for burial.
Autopsy:	Decision made by the entire family.

Source: Andrews, M., & Boyle, J. (2003). Transcultural concepts in nursing care. Philadelphia: Lippincott, Williams, and Wilkins.

have developed and distribute a document that outlines the rights of the dying patient and his or her family. Box 7-1 displays one example of the dying patient's Bill of Rights. Nurses need to recognize such rights in the plan of care of every hospice and palliative care patient.

Include legal and ethical considerations in the plan of care. Encourage patients to discuss their preferences for treatment at the end of life and have them complete Advance Directives that allow those preferences to be carried out. Provide

---

BOX 7-1

DYING PATIENT'S BILL OF RIGHTS

1. I have the right to be treated as a living human being until I die.
2. I have the right to maintain a sense of hopefulness, however changing its focus may be.
3. I have the right to be cared for by those who can maintain a sense of hopefulness, however changing this may be.
4. I have the right to express my feelings and emotions about my approaching death in my own way.
5. I have the right to be in control and participate in decisions regarding my care.
6. I have the right to expect continuing medical and nursing attention even though "cure" goals have been changed to "comfort" goals.
7. I have the right not to die alone.
8. I have the right to be free of pain.
9. I have the right to have my questions answered honestly.
10. I have the right to retain my individuality and not be judged for my decisions that may be contrary to the beliefs of others.
11. I have the right to hear the truth and the right to be in denial.
12. I have the right to expect that the sanctity of my body will be respected after my death.
13. I have the right to be cared for by caring, sensitive, knowledgeable people who will attempt to understand my needs and will be able to gain some satisfaction in helping me face my death.

---

patients with the Living Will and Power of Attorney for Health Care documents. The nonprofit organization, Aging with Dignity (www.agingwithdignity.org) has developed a document that combines both the Living Will and Power of Attorney for Health care; it is the Five Wishes document now recognized by 35 states. This document is an important resource for patients and families; it promotes discussion of the patient's end-of-life wishes regarding the following: (a) the person designated by the patient to make health care decisions for the patient when the patient is unable to do so, (b) the kinds of medical treatment that the patient wants or does not want, (c) the level of comfort that the patient wants, (d) the way in which the patient wants to be treated, and (e) what the patient wants his or her loved ones to know. The Five Wishes document can be ordered from the Aging with Dignity Web site.

Nurses can foster discussion among patients and family members about Advance Directives. It is a fallacy to believe that only physicians have this role. Nurses see patients and their families throughout the illness trajectory and are in ideal positions to talk with the patient about values and issues related to end-of-life care. In addition to encouraging patients to complete Advance Directives to clarify the goals of care, nurses recognize the importance of reviewing and updating such documents on a regular basis.

While advance care planning is clearly recognized as providing great benefit to the patient, family, and health care team, such discussion and planning is unfortunately often avoided. Some of the reasons health care providers give for avoiding end-of-life discussions with patients and families include: (a) the provider believes that the patient is not sick enough for the discussion, may become upset with the discussion, will not be able to understand the discussion, or will be robbed of hope with the discussion; (b) the provider lacks confidence in being able to have the discussion; (c) the provider believes there is insufficient time for the discussion; (d) the provider believes that there are too many contingencies for patients to consider in light of what the future might hold for them. However, resources such as the Five Wishes document previously discussed can provide a format that stimulates thought and discussion about end-of-life care among patients, family members, and providers of care.

It is important that nurses recognize the American Nurses Association's (ANA) position on assisted suicide. **Assisted suicide** refers to the practice in which a person other than the patient provides medication to a patient with the intent that the patient use the medication to voluntarily commit suicide. This differs from **euthanasia,** in which a person other than the patient directly administers medication that causes the death of a patient. **Physician-assisted suicide** refers to the enabling or assisting of death by a physician in consultation with a terminally ill patient. Several states have attempted to legalize physician-assisted suicide; Oregon is the only state in the United States that has passed this legislation to date (Oregon Death with Dignity Act, 1997). Physician-assisted suicide is not synonymous with euthanasia. The significant difference between physician-assisted suicide and euthanasia is in who acts. The ANA has directed that nurses not participate in assisted suicide (ANA, 1992a).

In the 1990s the public began to be quite aware of physician-assisted suicide because of the publicity surrounding Dr. Jack Kevorkian's actions with patients having incurable diseases. Some believe that patients with incurable diseases consider assisted suicide because of inadequacies in end-of-life care. Therefore, hospice and palliative care health care providers aggressively address pain and suffering in this population.

Indeed, the ANA takes the position that nurses have an obligation to provide comprehensive and compassionate end-of-life care, which includes the promotion of comfort, the relief of pain and, at times, foregoing life-sustaining treatments (ANA, 2003b). In addition, in the early 1990s the ANA issued several position statements related to palliative care. A brief overview of each of the statements appears in the Ethics in Practice box.

Role of the Interdisciplinary Team in Hospice and Palliative Care

Patients and families benefit from the expertise of a variety of professionals who work together as a team to provide hospice and palliative care services. Staff nurses provide direct patient care, case management, and coordination of care in conjunction with the patient's attending health care provider or the medical director of the hospice or palliative care service. Medical directors and health care providers skilled in hospice and palliative care are intimately involved in treatment decisions and the development of a comprehensive plan of care. Advanced practice palliative care nurses with graduate education provide expert patient care, patient and family education, and consultation to the interdisciplinary team.

Home health aides provide hygiene and personal care to patients so they are knowledgeable about the patient's ability to perform, or assist with, activities of daily living. Social workers assess the psychosocial needs of patients and families, and coordinate the social services provided to them. Pastoral care providers assess the spiritual needs of patients and families, providing support consistent with the patient's faith needs and religious beliefs and collaborating with the personal spiritual leaders identified by patients and families. Bereavement counselors communicate with grieving families and offer support by way of counseling, support groups, and memorial services.

Volunteers are also essential members of the interdisciplinary team; they are a required component of Medicare-certified hospice programs. Volunteers provide respite care, emotional support, and companionship; they can also help with shopping, transportation, and household maintenance. Volunteers often provide administrative support by helping with filing and other work in the hospice and palliative care office. A volunteer coordinator is responsible for the training and scheduling of the volunteers.

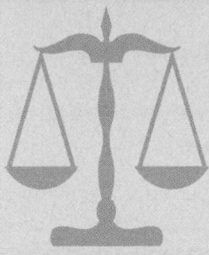

ETHICS IN PRACTICE

Legal and Ethical Considerations Related to Dying

Advance Directives

Advance care planning is a process of decision-making and communication about how and where people want to live at the end of their lives. **Advance Directives** are written documents used to plan and then communicate choices for medical treatment when people can no longer speak for themselves because of terminal illness or permanent loss of consciousness. All patients have the right to accurate information about their health status and treatment alternatives. The federal Patient Determination Act (PDA) of 1991 requires all health care agencies to provide patients with written information about their right to accept or refuse treatment. This act also requires that patients be informed of ways in which they can execute Advance Directives. The ANA's position is that nurses must play a primary role in implementation of this law (ANA, 1992b).

Living Will

A **Living Will** encodes specific instructions about what the patient does or does not want. Many Living Will forms contain a checklist of treatments, such as artificial nutrition, hydration, and mechanical ventilation.

Power of Attorney for Health Care

With the **Power of Attorney for Health Care** a person designates another person (called the health care proxy or agent) to make decisions about medical care for him or her when he or she is unable to do so. This document typically does not require that the patient be nearing death; it becomes effective whenever the patient is unable to communicate and ceases to be in effect as soon as the patient regains decision-making capacity. If there are no written directives, the care team asks the surrogate decision maker what the patient would be most likely to choose in the present situation. The patient's wishes are always the gold standard in decision making; what the patient would most likely consent to or refuse, if he or she could speak, guides treatment approaches.

Do Not Resuscitate Orders

JCAHO requires all of its members to have policies regarding **do not resuscitate (DNR)** orders. Also called a no code, a DNR order indicates that there should be no attempt to restart a failed heartbeat or apply cardiopulmonary resuscitation (CPR) to restore normal breathing. In a DNR situation comfort care is provided, and the DNR order can be changed at any time the patient wishes. The ANA has stated that nurses bear a large responsibility at the time a patient experiences cardiac arrest for either initiating resuscitation or ensuring that unwanted attempts to resuscitate do not occur (ANA, 1992c; 1992d).

DOLLARS AND SENSE

Utilization of Advanced Practice Nurses (APNs) in Hospice and Palliative Care

People in the United States are living longer in part because of increased attention to preventive care, evidence-based practice interventions, and use of technology. However, this increased life span creates a related need for sound management of chronic disease and attention to the principles of palliative care. Unfortunately, our country is experiencing a nursing shortage that impedes the delivery of that care.

One of the solutions to this situation lies in the use of advanced practice nurses in hospice and palliative care. According to well-known end-of-life expert Ira Byock (1997), advanced practice nurses who provide palliative care are a critical resource for meeting the needs of dying Americans and their families. With graduate level education, APNs provide great benefit to hospice and palliative care teams by improving patient care through their application of advanced knowledge and skill, by teaching evidence-based interventions, and by carrying out clinical research. APNs also contribute by collecting cost data and managing resources in a cost-effective manner. Under Medicare guidelines, APNs are reimbursed for their services at 85 percent of the rate for physicians (Daniels, 2004).

Members of the interdisciplinary team make regular home visits based on the needs of the patient and family. A registered nurse is available 24 hours a day, seven days a week. The team meets weekly to review the interdisciplinary plan of care and develop ongoing treatment goals. The team encourages family and friends to participate in giving care, comfort, and support to the dying patient and to each other. In the home setting, family members and supportive others are full participants in the plan of care. It is important to recognize that these individuals, themselves, may face substantial physical, emotional, and economic demands. The team assesses the capacity of the home caregiver to provide care, and offers suggestions when the primary caregiver is unreliable or additional caregiving is needed.

ASSESSMENT OF THE PATIENT RECEIVING HOSPICE AND PALLIATIVE CARE

A cornerstone and focus of hospice and palliative care is the holistic assessment and management of physical symptoms experienced by the dying patient. It is well recognized that physical symptoms that are not controlled, negatively impact quality of life. Common symptoms include pain, dyspnea, nausea, vomiting, constipation, loss of appetite, urinary urgency and incontinence, insomnia, confusion, delirium, anxiety, and depression. These symptoms can increase in intensity and frequency over the course of the illness and dying process. Patients commonly experience multiple symptoms that must be addressed concurrently.

Pain

Pain is a subjective sensation that is influenced by physical, emotional, and social circumstances. Therefore all of these aspects must be included in a complete assessment of pain in the dying patient. Chronic pain experienced by the dying is different from acute pain; it can be unrelenting and is often progressive. Because the body's autonomic nervous system adapts to chronic pain, classic signs and symptoms of discomfort, such as diaphoresis, anxiety, and increased pulse and blood pressure, may not occur. The patient experiencing chronic pain may develop adaptive coping mechanisms that mask the characteristic findings seen in people with acute pain. These include, but are not limited to, humor and distraction through conversation, music, or art.

Pain may result from a number of conditions, such as tumor progression, toxicities of chemotherapy and radiation, infection, and muscle ache. Be sure to assess all of the patient's pains, because many patients have more than one source of pain. As part of the pain assessment, obtain a pain history from the patient or caregiver. Brief and easy-to-use assessment tools, such as a visual analogue or numeric rating scale, allow patients to quantify pain; the assessment should also include the onset, location, and description of the discomfort. The well-known mnemonic ABCDE shown in Box 7-2 is a helpful guide for pain assessment.

Nurses conduct comprehensive pain assessments by teaching patients the importance of fully describing their experience of pain. Specifically, nurses teach patients to consider and respond to specific questions about the characteristics of their pain. Box 7-3 outlines the components of a comprehensive pain assessment.

Dyspnea

Dyspnea refers to an unpleasant awareness of an increased need to ventilate, such as breathlessness or difficulty breathing. Because it can cause severe suffering for the patient, it deserves serious and prompt attention. Dyspnea may result from extreme fatigue, anemia, hypoxia, respiratory muscle fatigue, heart failure, anxiety, or pain. Patients may also experience dyspnea from pulmonary effusion

---

BOX 7-2

ABCDE GUIDE TO PAIN ASSESSMENT

A: Ask about the pain regularly. Assess pain systematically.

B: Believe the patient and family in their reports of pain and what relieves it.

C: Choose pain control options appropriate for the patient, family, and setting.

D: Deliver interventions in a timely, logical, and coordinated fashion.

E: Empower patients and their families. Enable them to control their course to the greatest extent possible.

Source: Jacox, A., Carr, D., & Payne, R. (1994). Management of cancer pain. Clinical practice guidelines. No. 9, AHCPR Publication No. 94-0592. Rockville, MD: Agency for Health Care Policy and Research, U.S. Department of Health and Human Services, Public Health Service.

BOX 7-3

COMPONENTS OF A COMPREHENSIVE PAIN ASSESSMENT

Nurses ask the patient to:
1. Characterize the pain by location, quality, intensity, and duration.
   Location: Point to the area of pain and describe whether or not the pain radiates
   Quality: Describe how the pain feels (e.g., burning, aching, or throbbing).
   Intensity: Use a pain intensity scale.
   Duration: Describe the pain as constant or intermittent.
2. Describe aggravating and relieving factors.
   What makes the pain better?
   What makes the pain worse?
3. Describe how the pain interferes with activities of daily living.
4. Describe the impact of the pain on your state of mind (e.g., meaning of the pain, past experiences with pain, concerns about using opioids, or changes in mood).
5. Describe responses to previous pharmacological and nonpharmacological interventions.
6. Keep a diary that includes all of the above issues.

Source: Jacox, A., Carr, D., & Payne, R. (1994). Management of cancer pain. Clinical practice guidelines. No. 9, AHCPR Publication No. 94-0592. Rockville, MD: Agency for Health Care Policy and Research, U.S. Department of Health and Human Services, Public Health Service.

or consolidation, masses compressing bronchi, atelectasis, or central nervous system metastasis. Like pain, dyspnea is best documented by the patient's report. However, nurses can also note related signs and symptoms, including cyanosis, the use of accessory muscles, pursed lip breathing, and anxiety.

Loss of Appetite, Constipation, Nausea, and Vomiting

Loss of appetite is commonly reported as a diminished or nearly complete lack of interest in food with early satiety (the feeling of being full soon after starting to eat). It can occur from numerous underlying problems, including side effects of medications, constipation, and taste abnormalities; oral infection and disease progression are other common causes. Assessment includes noting the ability to swallow and the amount of food intake, a visual examination of the mouth and throat, and auscultation of bowel sounds.

Like loss of appetite, constipation is another common problem experienced by patients. Constipation is often the result of using opioid medications for pain relief. Decreased physical mobility and diminished fluid and fiber intake can also contribute to constipation. Intestinal obstruction can occur if there is GI or ovarian tumor extension. Symptoms of constipation include hard stools, overflow incontinence, abdominal distension and pain, and increased bowel sounds. Nursing assessment includes noting the date of the last bowel movement, stool characteristics, quality of bowel sounds, and checking the rectum for fecal impaction.

Nausea and vomiting may occur as a result of constipation, poor gastric emptying, oral and esophageal lesions, uremia, liver failure, anxiety, or as a side effect of chemotherapy. The vomiting center in the brain is stimulated by a number of nerve pathways throughout the body. Assessment involves noting abdominal tenderness or pain, auscultating bowel sounds, determining the date and consistency of the last bowel movement, and documenting the contents and color of vomitus.

Urinary Urgency and Incontinence

The etiology of urinary urgency and incontinence includes the presence of a genitourinary tumor, drug and radiation side effects, debility, urinary retention, or anxiety. Benign prostatic hypertrophy, stool impaction, and side effects of drugs can cause urinary retention. Assessment involves the subjective report of urinary urgency, nocturia, incomplete bladder emptying, dysuria, or incontinence. On physical examination, the nurse assesses for the following: localized abdominal pain, fullness or tenderness of the suprapubic area, absence of tympany on percussion, and fecal impaction.

Insomnia, Confusion, and Delirium

The etiology of insomnia in the terminally ill patient can include psychosocial distress, pain, or other symptoms that disturb sleep. Dyspnea, fear, anxiety, depression, nausea, pruritus, and urinary frequency are often contributing factors. Patients may acknowledge that they are having difficulty falling asleep at night, wake up without intention during the night, or wake up prematurely from sleep as the nurse carries out the patient assessment.

Confusion occurs frequently in the terminally ill patient. Effects of medication, metabolic abnormalities, fever or infection, pain, or withdrawal from alcohol or opiate drugs can contribute to confusion. It can result from depression, fear, anxiety, infection, metabolic factors, or pain, manifesting itself in cognitive changes, such as alteration in perception, thinking, or memory. Confusion can also manifest itself in sleep-wake cycle abnormalities and psychomotor symptoms. Assessment involves noting the patient's reality orientation, interaction with others in the environment, complaints of insomnia, and the presence of delusions or hallucinations.

Anxiety and Depression

Anxiety is a common symptom of patients receiving hospice and palliative care. Nurses must attend to both physical and psychological manifestations of anxiety. Anxiety results from various sources, including fear of pain, fear of dying, fear of being isolated, worry, and grief. Anxiety can also result from underlying diseases and treatments; for example, in the case of diminished oxygenation and uncontrolled pain and as a side effect of medications. Nursing assessment includes noting the following symptoms: insomnia, tremors, motor tension, palpitations, irritability, restlessness, appetite change, and decreased ability to concentrate. Heart and respiratory rates are also monitored for abnormalities.

While depression is commonly seen in dying patients, it is an incorrect assumption that depression is expected in this population. Nurses recognize the important distinction between sadness and sorrow that normally accompany a limited life expectancy and full-blown depression, using screening tools to demonstrate the difference. Patients may have accompanying physical indicators of depression, such as decreased appetite, fatigue, and insomnia. It is important to determine whether such symptoms stem from depression or from other aspects of the underlying disease to develop and implement an appropriate plan of care. Persistent feelings of hopelessness, worthlessness, and inadequacy and expression of thoughts of suicide need prompt evaluation and treatment.

NURSING DIAGNOSES

Hospice and palliative care nurses recognize that there are many nursing diagnoses that apply to end-of-life care. In addition to the nursing diagnoses inherent in the assessment discussion (Pain, Ineffective Airway Clearance, Constipation, Nausea, Urge Urinary Incontinence, Disturbed Sleep Pattern, Acute Confusion, Anxiety, and Ineffective Coping) other appropriate nursing diagnoses are: Fatigue, Disturbed Thought Processes (delirium), Diarrhea, Impaired Skin Integrity, Impaired Oral Mucous Membrane, Decreased Cardiac Output, Ineffective Thermoregulation, Risk for Injury, and Self-Care Deficits (NANDA, 2005).

Two important nursing diagnoses that nurses providing hospice and palliative care must also consider are related to the patient's caregiver(s); these are Caregiver Role Strain and Anticipatory Grieving. **Caregiver role strain** is the caregiver's felt difficulty in performing the family caregiver role. An expected outcome related to this diagnosis is caregiver home care readiness, defined as being prepared and ready to assume responsibility for the health care of a family member or significant other in the home (McCloskey & Bulechek, 2000). Nurses assess the level of a given caregiver's home care readiness by noting the following: a willingness to assume the care giving role, knowledge about the care giving role, demonstration of positive regard for the care recipient, knowledge of the care recipient's disease process, knowledge of the recommended treatment regimen, social support, confidence in the ability to manage care at home, evidence of plans for caregiver backup, and knowledge of equipment operation. Nursing interventions for this diagnosis center on providing caregiver support. This is accomplished by the following: determine the caregiver's level of knowledge, determine the caregiver's acceptance of the role, accept expressions of negative emotions, encourage the caregiver to assume responsibility, encourage the acceptance of interdependency among family members, provide information about the patient's condition, teach the caregiver specific components of the patient's treatment plan, monitor for indicators of stress, teach the caregiver health maintenance strategies to sustain his or her own physical and mental health, and inform the caregiver of health care and community resources (McCloskey & Bulechek, 2000).

A second important nursing diagnosis is **anticipatory grieving,** defined as the intellectual and emotional responses and behaviors by which individuals work through the process of modifying self-concept based on the perception of potential loss. An expected outcome related to this diagnosis is **grief resolution,** defined as an adjustment to actual or impending loss (NANDA, 2005). Nurses assess the level of a given caregiver's grief resolution by noting the following: an ability to express feelings about loss, express spiritual beliefs about death, verbalize the reality of the loss, verbalize acceptance of the loss, describe the meaning of the death, participate in planning the funeral, discuss unresolved conflict(s), share the loss with significant others, progress through the Kübler-Ross stages of grief, and express positive expectations about the future.

Nursing interventions for this diagnosis center on assisting the caregiver with resolution of the loss. This is accomplished by encouraging the caregiver to: express feelings about the loss, discuss previous loss experiences, verbalize memories of the previous loss, and identify the greatest fears concerning the loss. The nurse must also instruct the caregiver about the phases of the grieving process; assist in the identification of the caregiver's personal coping strategies; encourage the caregiver to implement cultural, religious, and social customs associated with the loss; discuss available bereavement groups; identify sources of community support; discuss characteristics of normal and abnormal grieving; and reinforce progress made in the grieving process.

PLANNING AND IMPLEMENTING CARE FOR PATIENTS RECEIVING HOSPICE AND PALLIATIVE CARE

While considering caregiver issues, nurses recognize that a major focus of hospice and palliative care is the control of symptoms experienced by the patient; a shift from efforts directed at curing the disease. Therefore, invasive diagnostic and therapeutic procedures are typically not performed.

Hospice and palliative nurses incorporate **complementary and alternative medicine (CAM)** in their plan of care. CAM involves those therapies that have a focus beyond specific symptom management. The National Center for Complementary and Alternative Medicine (NCCAM), founded in 1998, has worked to demonstrate the scientific basis of such therapies. NCCAM provides such information to both the lay and professional public. Specifically, acupuncture, aromatherapy, massage therapy, relaxation therapy, music therapy, and therapeutic touch have been used in end-of-life care to complement standard therapies.

Hospice and palliative care nurses use their understanding of pathophysiology and pharmacology and their communication and clinical skills to develop a sound plan of care that addresses symptom management. Interventions are evaluated for effectiveness, patient and family teaching is ongoing, and care is coordinated with the interdisciplinary team throughout.

While considering current evidence-based interventions, nurses recognize the historic roots of such care in the recommendations of Florence Nightingale. Her written work, *Notes on nursing what it is and what it is not,* first published in 1859, describes the critical need to relieve suffering and provide comfort care to the sick.

Managing Pain

Hospice and palliative nurses focus the pain management plan on preventing pain, rather than intervening in the case of a pain crisis. Principles of pain management include using the simplest dosing schedules and least invasive

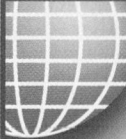

Real World, Real Choices

Complex Nursing Management of a Patient with Metastatic Bowel Obstruction

Irena is a 67-year-old woman who was admitted to a community hospital with the diagnosis of widely metastatic ovarian cancer. Irena had gone to the emergency department complaining of continuous nausea and abdominal pain and intermittent vomiting. She was found to have a partial bowel obstruction caused by her disease. Treatment for the obstruction included placing a nasogastric tube to decompress her stomach and small bowel. Because of her advanced disease, she was not a candidate for surgical removal of the obstruction. Irena was discharged from the hospital to a home hospice program with the nasogastric tube to suction and medications for symptom control.

Irena's case requires the hospice nurses to address multifaceted aspects of care.

1. Irena and her family understand that the bowel obstruction signifies advanced progression of her disease. They may want and need information about changes that are likely to occur as her death approaches. What does the hospice nurse tell them?
2. What are the primary goals of Irena's care at this point in her illness?
3. What is a crucial focus of assessment on each home visit by the hospice nurse?
4. What are crucial interventions to control Irena's symptoms?
5. How can the nurse address the psychosocial and spiritual components of Irena's care?

route; using the right drug for the specific type of pain being experienced; anticipating, preventing, and treating side effects; giving medications for persistent pain around the clock; and respecting individual differences in the treatment plan. While medications are given around the clock to provide a basal amount of medication, as needed medication should be available for pain that breaks through the basal dose.

Nurses apply the WHO approach to the management of pain as conceptualized in Figure 7-1. Using a ladder approach, nurses work with the prescribing provider and adjust the class and dose of medications to the patient's pain level. At the first rung of the ladder, treat patients who are in mild pain with around-the-clock doses of nonopioids. Remember that nonsteroidal antiinflammatory drugs (NSAIDs) have a maximal dose that cannot be exceeded. Dosing above this level causes adverse effects without increasing the amount of pain relief experienced by the patient. Many patients take acetaminophen (Tylenol) at the first rung of the ladder and in combination products. However, no patient should take more than 4 grams of acetaminophen in a given 24-hour time period because of the potential for liver toxicity.

At the second level, use opioid-acetaminophen combinations to treat mild to moderate pain. On the third rung, use strong opioids. Morphine is the gold standard at this level and along with other opioid medications, is available in both short- and long-acting preparations. The ladder also recommends the use of adjuvant agents at each step along with combining nonopioid and opioid drugs at each step. Adjuvant medications can enhance analgesic effectiveness, treat symptoms that exacerbate pain, and provide relief for specific pain. Adjuvant medications include antidepressants, anticonvulsants, and corticosteroids. These drugs are particularly effective for patients experiencing neuropathic pain in which the nerves themselves are damaged or injured.

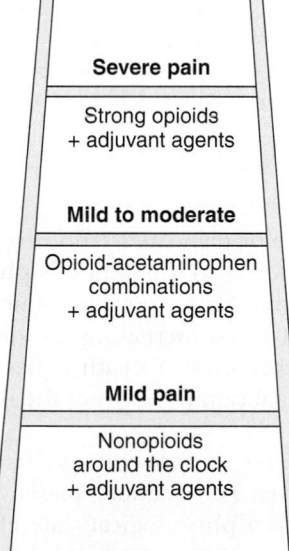

Figure 7-1 Conceptual model of ladder approach to pain management. Courtesy L. J. Nosek.

Skills 360°

Nightingale's Perspective on Nursing Related to Palliative Care

Amazingly, many of the principles of care that Nightingale described nearly 150 years ago remain pertinent for today's nurses and collaborative health care providers. Nightingale's teachings have direct application to the care of patients at the end of life; she advocated for the relief of suffering and the promotion of comfort, always. In particular, nurses can derive guidance for palliative care interventions from Nightingale's emphasis on the importance of the patient's physical environment and concern for the patient's emotional states. Relevant topics include:

1. Ventilation
   a. Provide fresh air and avoid odors in the patient's direct environment.
2. Noise Management
   a. Avoid unnecessary noise that disrupts the patient's rest and sleep.
   b. Manage the amount and volume of conversation among family, visitors, and providers who surround the patient.
   c. Do not speak in front of the patient as if he or she were not there, even if it appears that the patient is sleeping.
3. Variety in the Environment
   a. According to patient preference, provide serene, soothing or colorful, stimulating visuals in the patient's environment.
4. Food and Liquids
   a. Provide fresh, cool water in a small container that appears full even though it is a small volume.
5. Bed and Bedding
   a. Provide comfortable clothing, nightwear, and pillow support.
   b. Consider the weight and texture of bed linens and blankets.
6. Light
   a. Allow for the patient to be exposed to sunlight.
   b. Provide soothing indirect artificial light and nightlights.
7. Personal Cleanliness
   a. Provide frequent oral hygiene and warm baths.
8. Chattering hopes and advice
   a. Do not offer false promises and avoid attempting to cheer the patient; do remember how their life is to them disappointed and incomplete.

Source: Nightingale, F. (1969 [1859]). Notes on nursing what it is and what it is not. New York: Dover Publications, Inc.

Do not hesitate to use full and effective doses of pain medication to properly manage pain of the dying patient; this is crucial to the patient's physical and psychological well-being. Recognize that the ANA's position statement (2003b) on the principle of double effect means that increasing the dose of medication to achieve adequate symptom control, even if death is hastened secondarily, is ethically justified. Consider the legal ramifications of the undertreatment of pain.

It is important for the nurse to discuss myths and misconceptions surrounding use of analgesics with the patient and caregiver. For example, patients may develop tolerance to their analgesic. **Tolerance** is a physiological state characterized by a decrease in the effects of a drug that results in the patient requiring a higher dose. The dose should be adjusted to control the pain with acceptable side effects. Patients usually require higher doses because of disease progression rather than tolerance. Tolerance to the nonanalgesic effects of opioids, such as

Fast Forward ▶▶▶

Legal Ramifications of the Undertreatment of Pain

The undertreatment of pain has been a major focus of care in the United States over the past several years. In 2001, JCAHO instituted policies that mandate care providers to: (a) recognize patients' rights to pain assessment and management; (b) assess the intensity and nature of patients' pain; (c) record results of patients' pain assessment that aid in followup; (d) ensure competency in pain assessment and management; (e) appropriately prescribe pain medication; and (f) address the need for pain management in discharge planning. JCAHO has provided sound scientific evidence to guide health care providers in their management of pain.

Based on such mandates, there are predictions that increased lawsuits will occur when pain is undertreated. For example, in a landmark case in 2001, Bergman v. Chin, the children of an 85-year-old man with metastatic lung cancer sued the treating health care provider for inadequate treatment of their father's pain. The patient had been admitted to a California hospital in excruciating pain. Throughout his five-day hospitalization staff documented severe pain, yet the pain medication was never adjusted to provide him relief. The health care provider's lack of attention to the patient's pain was described as "reckless and inexcusable;" the jury awarded the family $1.5 million in what was considered a case of elder abuse. This legal precedent provides further impetus for health care providers to follow standards of care and have accountability in the pain management plan of care.

Source: Warm, E., & Weissman, D. (2002, March). The legal liability of undertreatment of pain. End-of-Life Physician Resource Center Fast Facts and Concepts #63. Retrieved June 1, 2005, from http://www.eperc.mcw.edu.

sedation, changes in breathing, and nausea, is expected after several days of use. However, tolerance to the constipating effect of opioids does not develop.

Similarly, **physical dependence** can be expected within two to three days of initiating an opioid. The body becomes dependent on the opioid and an abrupt cessation or reduction in the dose may result in withdrawal symptoms. Addiction is often confused with physical dependence and tolerance, so it is important for the nurse to clarify the term addiction with the patient and family.

Addiction is a psychological dependence on medication exhibited by a craving for the mood altering effects of the medication. The nurse should be sure to stress that addiction is rare when patients take opioids for pain relief. In the discussion with the patient, the nurse should be aware of the barriers to pain medication highlighted in Box 7-4. The nurse should recognize research findings that indicate the need for special attention to those caregivers who express concern about administering pain medications to patients receiving hospice and palliative care.

The addition of a clinical pharmacist to the health care team can facilitate improved pain management by other providers. Enhanced knowledge about drug action and efficacy across team members can ease common concerns that may lead to undertreatment of pain. All team members need to participate in frequent and thorough evaluation of the patient's comfort level.

Opioid medications are often given to the hospice and palliative care patients who experience pain. Opiate drugs are compounds derived from the poppy plant that relieve pain by blocking portions of the pain pathway in the nervous system. The most commonly used opioid is morphine; it forms the basis for equianalgesic conversions and has versatile routes of administration. There is essentially no upper limit or ceiling to the dose of an opioid medication that can be safely given

BOX 7-4

BARRIERS TO PAIN MANAGEMENT

Problems Related to Health Care Professionals

- Poor assessment and documentation of pain
- Concern about regulation of controlled substances
- Fear of patient addiction
- Concern about side effects of analgesics
- Concern about patients becoming tolerant to analgesics

Problems Related to Patients and Family Caregivers

- Reluctance to report pain
- Concern about distracting the health care provider from treatment of underlying disease
- Fear that pain means the disease is worse
- Concern about not being a good patient
- Reluctance to take pain medications
- Fear of addiction or of being thought of as an addict
- Worries about unmanageable side effects
- Inadequate knowledge of pain management
- Concern about becoming tolerant to pain medications

Problems Related to the Health Care System

- Low priority given to cancer pain treatment
- Inadequate reimbursement
- Restrictive regulation of controlled substances
- Problems of availability of treatment or access to it

Source: Jacox, A., Carr, D., & Payne, R. (1994). Management of cancer pain Clinical practice guidelines. *No. 9, AHCPR Publication No. 94-0592. Rockville, MD: Agency for Health Care Policy and Research, U.S. Department of Health and Human Services, Public Health Service.*

Safety First

Potential Liquid Oral Pain Medication Dosing Error

Causes of medication errors commonly reported to the Federal Drug Administration (FDA) include poor communication, illegible handwriting, confusion about drug names, inaccurate use of the decimal point, and lack of understanding about directions in taking the ordered medication. Another cause that is significant in hospice and palliative care is the dosing and administration of liquid oral medications. Drug manufacturers supply calibrated liquid medication cups, droppers, and calibrated spoons. Liquid oral medications may also be taken by using oral syringes or household teaspoons. It is critical that patients and caregivers fully understand how to dose accurately, use the appropriate medication administration device, and use the same device each time medication is taken or provided.

to a patient experiencing pain. However, nurses need to consider the effects on other organ systems when giving opioid medications. Such effects include sedation, cough suppression, and nausea. The nurse should recognize that these are transitory effects, because patients rapidly develop tolerance to these effects. Because patients do not develop tolerance to the constipating effect of opioid medications, institute a bowel program for patients receiving these drugs. Be aware of withdrawal symptoms that patients develop if opioids are discontinued. Withdrawal symptoms may begin within 6 to 12 hours and peak at 24 to 72 hours and include: anxiety, irritability, chills, joint pain, lacrimation, rhinorrhea, diaphoresis, nausea, vomiting, diarrhea, and abdominal cramps.

The nurse should consider alternative routes of medication administration when the patient is unable to take or tolerate oral medications. These include rectal, transdermal, nasal, intraspinal, intravenous (IV), and subcutaneous methods of administration. Dose equivalent tables should be used by the nurse when analgesics or the routes of administration are changed. The nurse should be especially careful in teaching patients and caregivers about correct dosing and medication administration when liquid oral medications are used.

Oral morphine sulfate (MS) solution is a commonly used medication in hospice and palliative care. To use this opioid medication, a dropper or spoon is provided by the manufacturer. The device is secured to the medication packaging and must be used each time the medication is taken or given to prevent inaccuracy in dosing. A different dropper or other device can alter the dose.

Uncovering the Evidence

Caregiver Concerns about Pain and Pain Medication Administration

Discussion: A study was undertaken to test a 22-item self-report instrument to measure caregiver concern about (a) reporting information about the patient's pain to the hospice nurse, (b) administering analgesics to the patient, and (c) difficulty administering analgesics to the patient.

A total of 151 caregivers in 3 Chicagoland hospice agencies completed the tool.

Only a small percent of these caregivers expressed concern about communicating information to the hospice nurse about the patient's pain. However, over 25 percent of the caregivers were concerned about administering analgesics because of their own uneasiness about addiction, tolerance, and side effects from the medication. A fourth of the caregivers expressed difficulty actually administering medications to the patient because of fear of doing something wrong and difficulty deciding which or what amount of medication to provide. Male caregivers and hired caregivers in the home had greater concerns than others about reporting information about pain and about administering analgesics. Greater levels of concern were also evident among less educated caregivers and caregivers who were homemakers or were retired. In addition, caregivers who had greater concern about addiction and tolerance and more difficulty administering medications rated the patient's pain as less completely controlled.

Implications for Practice: The findings of this study remind hospice and palliative nurses of the importance of assessing specific caregiver concerns about pain and pain medication administration. When such concerns are identified, nurses must devise appropriate strategies to reduce the concerns in order to promote appropriate and adequate pain management at the end of life.

Source: Letizia, M., Creech, S., Norton, E., Shanahan, M., & Hedges, L. (2004). Barriers to caregiver administration of pain medication in hospice care. Journal of Pain and Symptom Management, 27(2), 114–124.

Also, providers of care must recognize that this medication is available in different dosing regimens, including:

- Morphine Sulfate Immediate Release (MSIR) oral solution—each 1 mL of MSIR oral solution contains 1 mg MS

- MSIR oral solution—each 5 mL of MSIR oral solution contains 10 mg MS

- MSIR oral solution—each 5 mL of MSIR oral solution contains 20 mg MS

- MSIR oral solution concentrate—each 1 mL of MSIR oral solution concentrate contains 20 mg MS

Clearly, dosing problems and errors can occur when a patient or the caregiver have been using one of the concentrations, the order is changed by the health care provider, and the pharmacist fills the prescription using a different concentration, or a different pharmacy is used to fill the prescription and the pharmacist uses a different concentration. To address this problem, hospice and palliative care nurses insist that the health care provider write the prescription with the following two pieces of information: (a) the specific dose in milligrams with the corresponding volume in milliliters and (b) the concentration to be dispensed. An example prescription would read: Morphine Sulfate Immediate Release 20 mg/mL. Take 20 mg (1 mL) every four hours.

The nurse also considers the possibility of confusion or difficulty when patients or caregivers use a dropper to administer this medication. The nurse must carefully teach the patient or caregiver about filling the dropper to the correct calibration mark and must be sure that the person can clearly see that mark and has the psychomotor ability to fill it accurately. The nurse must ask the patient or caregiver to demonstrate the proper technique in administering this medication.

The nurse must be sure to consider nonpharmacological options in the pain management plan. Physical or massage therapy, use of heat or cold treatments, distraction, and humor can be helpful alternatives or adjuncts to pain medication. Patients with bone metastasis may achieve pain relief from palliative radiation. Others may need nerve blocks and other more aggressive interventions to control their pain. The nurse must recognize the importance of addressing psychosocial and spiritual issues related to pain.

Managing Dyspnea

Important interventions for the dyspneic patient include placing the patient in a semi-Fowler position, allaying anxiety, providing a cool mist vaporizer or bedside fan, and keeping the room temperature cool. Oxygen therapy is generally not helpful unless the patient is actually hypoxic; if oxygen is used, a nasal cannula is the preferred delivery type. Medications can also help to control dyspnea, but consideration must be given to the etiology of the breathlessness. For example, opiates, such as low-dose morphine sulfate, decrease both respiratory sensitivity and rate and may allay the anxiety associated with difficulty breathing. Anxiolytics, such as lorazepam and diazepam, can also be helpful in those cases. If the dyspnea is related to chronic obstructive pulmonary disease, bronchodilators and corticosteroids are often effective. When congestive heart failure contributes to dyspnea, diuretics and vasodilators can be provided. If dyspnea is caused by bronchial obstruction from a tumor or superior vena cava syndrome, steroids, such as dexamethasone, may be helpful. In some circumstances, blood transfusions may ease dyspnea associated with anemia.

Managing Loss of Appetite, Constipation, Nausea, and Vomiting

Nursing interventions for GI symptoms include eliminating odors, minimizing movement by the patient, supplying an emesis container within reach, providing oral hygiene, circulating room air, and administering pharmacological agents according to the underlying cause of the symptoms. The nurse must reassure the patient and family that loss of appetite is an expected symptom as the patient's energy level begins to diminish. Other recommendations include providing small frequent meals and elevating the head of the bed when the patient is eating. Note the color and consistency of foods most appealing to the patient or best tolerated by the patient. Mouth care is also an important aspect of nutritional care, including frequently applying water-based lubricants or petroleum to the lips to alleviate dryness, providing frozen tonic water, and using artificial saliva for lubrication. Iced nutritional drinks, clear cold drinks, ice chips, popsicles, fruit juices, pineapple chunks, and lemon drops are also helpful. If the mouth is ulcerated, infection may be the underlying cause and can be treated with the appropriate medication.

Yeast infection (thrush) is common in the terminally ill, with the oral mucosa appearing red, sore, and spotted with white adherent patches. If including yogurt in the diet offers insufficient control of the yeast infection, the nurse needs to obtain an order for clotrimazole troches or nystatin suspension to treat the thrush. Nurses need to also consider medications that can be given prior to meals that improve the appetite. Such medications include megestrol acetate, corticosteroids, dronabinol, and anabolic steroids. While there may be a role for nutritional support in patients receiving palliative care for chronic diseases, IV hydration and enteral tube feedings are not generally recommended in hospice care.

Constipation is so common with opioid medications that nurses should anticipate it and routinely administer stool softeners and stimulants and increase the dose as the opioid dose is increased. Be sure to institute a bowel program that includes the entire GI tract. This means providing an oral preparation for the upper GI system and enemas or suppositories, if necessary, to clear the rectum. Interventions include increasing the fluid intake and the use of bulk foods if tolerated. If the patient is receiving an opioid medication, institute a bowel protocol even if he or she is not eating.

Bulk-forming laxatives include bran products and psyllium. However, these are only used if the patient is able to ingest the recommended amount of accompanying fluid. Stool softeners include docusate calcium (Surfak) and docusate sodium (Colace). Small bowel flushers include magnesium hydroxide and lactulose. Peristaltic stimulants include bisacodyl, senna, and cascara. Enemas and suppositories are often given and it may be necessary to remove a patient's stool manually.

Nausea can be eliminated by using medications that act on the chemoreceptive trigger zone such as those from the class of butyrophenones (such as haloperidol [Haldol]) and the class of phenothiazines (such as prochlorperazine [Compazine]). Gastrokinetics, such as metoclopramide (Reglan), increase gastric motility and allow movement of secretions and foods through the lower intestine. Antihistamines, such as diphenhydramine (Benadryl), can also be helpful because of the action on the vomiting center in the medulla. If anxiety triggers nausea and vomiting, anxiolytics, such as lorazepam (Ativan) or diazepam (Valium), may also be prescribed. When a GI tumor is suspected as the cause of nausea and vomiting, a corticosteroid, such as dexamethasone can be used. In some cases, more than one antiemetic will be necessary to control distressing symptoms. If patients are unable to swallow, alternative routes of medication administration will be necessary.

Managing Urinary Urgency and Incontinence

Symptomatic treatment for urinary urgency and incontinence includes administering an antibiotic if a urinary tract infection is suspected, changing the diuretic regimen and providing medications to increase urethral sphincter tone. Medications are also available for bladder spasm and urinary retention. Hospice nurses do not hesitate to place indwelling urinary catheters if a catheter is indicated or requested by a patient or family member.

Managing Insomnia, Confusion, and Delirium

It is important to treat insomnia aggressively, because control of other symptoms in the patient is often dependent on proper rest and sleep. Nonpharmacological measures include attempting to reverse the day-night sleep patterns by allowing the patient to be as active as possible during daytime hours. Pharmacological measures include the hypnotic drugs; drugs most frequently used are those in the benzodiazepine class, such as temazepam (Restoril) and triazolam (Halcion).

Nursing interventions for the patient who is confused include providing a quiet environment and eliminating unnecessary stimuli. When interacting with the patient, speak clearly in simple short sentences, and focus on the present. During daytime hours surroundings should be well lit, with familiar objects and safety measures must be in place. Drug therapy for the patient who is confused includes haloperidol (Haldol) to decrease agitation, diphenhydramine (Benadryl) for extrapyramidal symptoms, and chlorpromazine (Thorazine) for sedation.

Managing Anxiety and Depression

Interventions for the patient who is anxious and fearful include exploring the patient's concerns and encouraging the patient to express those concerns. Nurses help patients use coping strategies that have been helpful in the past and suggest nonpharmacological interventions, such as anxiety-reducing breathing exercises. Drug therapy includes benzodiazepines, such as lorazepam (Ativan) and diazepam (Valium); beta-adrenergic blockers, such as atenolol (Tenormin) can be given if the patient has somatic symptoms, such as palpitations and tachycardia. Hospice and palliative care nurses also recognize that delirium is common among patients with advanced diseases; manifestations of delirium can be misinterpreted as anxiety. If the patient's symptoms have an acute onset and are accompanied by changes in cognitive function or level of consciousness, the diagnosis of delirium should be considered.

Treatment for depression also involves pharmacological and nonpharmacological interventions. Patients who are dying may express feelings of hopelessness. An important intervention is to encourage them to express what it is that they continue to hope for, although those hopes most certainly change over time and as the disease progresses. If the patient expresses feelings of helplessness, giving the patient more opportunities for control may help. If depression has a basis in ongoing physical symptoms, aggressive attempts at controlling those symptoms are essential. If patients express feelings of profound despair, counseling may be necessary. Classes of medication used in the treatment of depression at the end of life are the antidepressants, stimulants, nonbenzodiazepines, and steroids.

Providing Spiritual Support

In providing holistic care, nurses attending to the needs of the patients receiving hospice and palliative care must address spiritual care, as well as physical and psychosocial care. Specific religious practices are a component of spirituality. Religion provides a means for people to express common values and beliefs by way of particular systems of faith expression and worship. However, spirituality involves the broader concepts of finding meaning and purpose in life and feeling connected to a power greater than oneself. While being cured of a physical illness is not possible for patients with terminal illness, being healed is possible. Such healing involves paying special attention to those questions of meaning asked and those issues raised by the patient. In the dying process, patients and family members can indeed find solace, comfort, and hope. According to palliative care expert Byock (1997), there are five aspects of relationship completion that allow for healing; those are the statements: "I forgive you"; "Please forgive me"; "Thank you"; "I love you"; and "Goodbye."

Nurses and hospice pastoral care team members assist patients to complete a spiritual assessment. Information from such an assessment can provide the team with information about particular beliefs, values, and traditions that can bring comfort to the patient and family. Specifically, patients are asked about the importance or significance of God or a deity for them, their religious traditions and beliefs, the spiritual community or group to which they are affiliated and spiritual resources that they have found useful in the past. Asking a patient about his or her thoughts about the link between spiritual beliefs and health is also important (Highfield, 2000). Patients and family members may express a fear of suffering and of death itself and may discuss these concerns

---

BOX 7-5

SPIRITUAL CONSIDERATIONS RELATED TO DYING

Important Spiritual Work for the Dying

- Coming to terms with the meaning and purpose of one's life.
- Leaving legacies to loved ones in the form of pictures, stories, and poetry.
- Reviewing one's life; remembering the good and bad times.
- Reconciling and healing strained or broken relationships.
- Talking with family and friends to give and receive love and forgiveness.
- Reconnecting or deepening a relationship with a higher power.

Spiritual Changes That the Patient May Exhibit

- Less interest in, and eventual detachment from, material goods.
- Less tolerance for mundane and trivial conversation.
- Increased interest in reconnecting with religious beliefs.
- Preference for more time in silence.
- Detachment from concern about appearance.
- Detachment from relationships slowly over time.
- Seeing and talking with people who have died.

Nursing Interventions

- Validate the importance of the person.
- Actively listen without judgment.
- Use therapeutic communication.
- Encourage prayer and visual guided imagery as appropriate or requested.
- Refer to a religious representative, as appropriate or requested.

---

from a spiritual point of view. Box 7-5 reviews spiritual considerations related to death and dying. Identify the patient and family member's values, priorities, and cultural and spiritual perspectives in the plan of care.

One technique found useful in helping patients to find meaning and comfort at the end of life is called life review. Life review allows the patient to tell an oral or written narrative history. In this review, patients focus on what they have accomplished in the span of their lifetime. Patients are provided with an opportunity to think about and talk about the people, traditions, and circumstances that have held meaning for them. They are encouraged to discuss their hobbies and interests, and the contributions that they have made throughout their lives of which they are particularly proud.

SPECIAL CONSIDERATIONS IN THE HOME CARE OF THE DYING PATIENT

In providing personal care to terminally ill patients in the home setting, nurses need to assess the patient's ability to perform the activities of daily living. The patient's need for assistance with eating and oral hygiene, meal preparation, bathing, toileting, shopping, cleaning, and laundry should be noted by the nurse. In addition, the nurse should assess and respond to environmental and safety risks in the care of the patient and family and should advise them on adapting the home environment for safety to prevent falls, conserve energy, use equipment and medications safely, and prevent infection. The nurse should help obtain necessary medical equipment and supplies.

In the home setting, caregivers of the terminally ill are full participants in the plan of care. However, caregivers themselves face substantial physical, emotional, and economic demands. Nurses must assess the capacity of the caregiver to provide care and offer alternatives when the primary caregiver is unreliable or additional care giving is needed. The nurse should respond to the need for a change in the level of care provided or increased services by the team. Assisting the family with hiring professional caregivers when the burden of providing around the clock care becomes too great for them. The nurse should remind the caregivers that the hospice team is available 24 hours a day, seven days a week for telephone support whether that be to answer a simple question or to respond to a need for urgent assistance

Caregivers of dying patients must be given information about the expected progression of the patient's disease process. Such information can help the patient and family make decisions, plan for the future, and utilize resources. However, prediction about survival, called prognostication, is not an exact science; it is based on factors related to the patient, the disease, and the experience of the health care providers. Many believe that the patient's performance status measured by tools, such as the Karnofsky Performance Status, provides the most helpful information. Regardless of prognosis and the way in which prognosis is estimated, it is important that such information is provided to patients and families in a thoughtful and careful manner.

Providing Care in the Active Phase of Dying

If the dying patient is receiving care in the home setting, it is especially essential for the nurse to prepare the family for what to expect as death draws near. This is often referred to as the active phase of dying. Table 7-2 highlights physiological changes that occur at the end of life. Along with a general deterioration of body functions, general systems fail and cognitive changes, electrolyte imbalance, and cardiac, hepatic, renal, and pulmonary failure are common. In the last two weeks of life, the patient may experience a diminished appetite, decreased urinary output, progressive lethargy, and withdrawal from surroundings and people. The patient often becomes disoriented, picking at clothes or the bed linens, talking with the unseen, and appearing confused and agitated. At this point, the patient is generally bed bound and requires around-the-clock skilled care. Comfort continues to be the focus. Caregivers dress the patient in comfortable bedclothes, keep the skin clean and dry, provide mouth care, and reposition the patient as he or she tolerates such movement.

In the last 72 hours of life, the following symptoms occur: tachypnea and periods of apnea, increased use of accessory muscles to breathe, changes in heart rate with a weak radial pulse, hypotension, cold hands and feet, and mottling of body tissues that are in dependent positions or at the periphery. The patient may experience restlessness or may have no activity at all. Nurses prepare the family for the occasional final surprising rally by the patient in which he or she becomes temporarily more alert and responsive before retreating. Terminal congestion can occur, with a rattling sound heard in the lungs and upper throat. The nurse should not attempt to clear such congestion with nasotracheal suctioning; suctioning will not clear these deep secretions but instead cause discomfort and may induce painful coughing or vomiting. The body temperature can fluctuate and the patient is often diaphoretic.

Physical care is important as the patient approaches death. Mouth care is necessary as the patient begins mouth breathing; balm is applied to the lips. The eyes need frequent cleansing; artificial tears and lubricating ointment can be provided. Although the urine output decreases, patients are monitored for incontinence; daily baths and good skin care are provided. As death approaches, the family may take turns at the bedside of the dying patient; this is often referred to as the death vigil. Family members are encouraged to continue talking with their loved one; they are also encouraged to give their loved one permission to let go and die in a peaceful, comfortable manner.

TABLE 7-2 Physiology of Dying

Cardiovascular System

- The heart fails to pump, resulting in insufficient blood flow and ischemia.
- Insufficient peripheral blood flow results in a decrease in skin temperature and changes in skin color, such as pallor and mottling, beginning at the distal extremities, moving toward the torso.
- A decrease in circulation time between the lungs and the brain results in Cheyne-Stokes respirations.
- Signs of cardiac decompensation include decreasing blood pressure, tachycardia, irregular pulse, decreased mentation, cool extremities, reduced urinary output, pulmonary congestion, and hepatic distension. Symptoms include chest pain and dyspnea.

Pulmonary System

- Respiratory failure begins as hypoxia that leads to high carbon dioxide levels, resulting in confusion, restlessness, and eventual coma.
- Underlying causes of respiratory failure include pneumonia, pulmonary embolism, and pulmonary edema.
- Respiratory symptoms can begin with dyspnea on exertion with increased respiratory rate and depth, then progress to dyspnea at rest.
- Early signs of hypoxia include: confusion, orthopnea, irregular breathing, tachycardia, and use of accessory muscles to breathe. Symptoms of hypoxia include restlessness, irritability, and anxiety.

Central Nervous System

- Changes in level of consciousness are manifested by periods of confusion, disorientation, and lethargy progressing to stupor.
- Periods of sleep increase and periods of wakefulness decrease.
- Sluggish pupil constriction progresses to dilation in a fixed position as brain hypoxia increases.

Renal System

- Urine volume decreases and concentration increases as fluid intake decreases and kidney function and renal blood flow diminish.

Respecting Our Differences

It is critical that the nurse recognize the wide variation in customs of different groups following a patient's death. There may be specific directives for cleaning, positioning, and dressing the body. In some cultures, particular individuals have roles in the preparation of the body; be sure to be attentive to these individuals. Varying religious tenets govern timing and rituals around grieving and disposition of the body.

Signs and symptoms of death include the following: absence of heart beat and respirations, fixed and dilated pupils with eyes remaining open, lack of response to stimulation, and dropping of the body temperature. For patients who are receiving care in the home, instruct the family to notify the nursing staff at the time of death; there is no need to call emergency medical providers. After being paged, the hospice nurse assesses by phone how well those in the home are coping and then reassures the family that they do not need to do anything for the patient or to the body immediately. When the nurse arrives at the home, he or she offers support and condolence to the family and asks if they want a pastoral care person to be called. The procedures for pronouncement of death vary among states and settings. However, the pronouncement includes listening for the absence of the patient's heart and breath sounds for a full minute and checking the patient's pupil response with a flashlight. When no vital signs are noted, and the pupils are declared dilated and fixed, the official time of death is recorded.

Generally speaking, the nurse prepares the body for departure from the home by removing catheters and other devices and providing simple hygienic care in a respectful and dignified manner. Family members may want to spend time alone with the patient's body. When the funeral service provider arrives, the family often gathers in a different part of the home while the body is removed. Afterward, take the time to review the events leading up to death with the family and answer their questions. Participate in formal closure with the family by a visit, call, or card following the death of the patient.

Supporting the Bereaved

An essential element of hospice and palliative care is assessing and attending to the needs of the bereaved family. Grief is the physical and psychosocial response to a loss. While grief is experienced universally, there are wide variations in such expression, including sadness, despair, anger, guilt, or physical illness. Each person experiences loss in his or her own unique way. There is no one way to grieve, or a set timeline in the grieving process; indeed, many authors have written about the types of grief, the stages of grief, the tasks of grief work, and grief assessment to guide the provider of care.

Normal reactions include physical, cognitive, and emotional behaviors, such as palpitations, GI symptoms, fatigue, and appetite changes. Patients express feelings of anger, relief, guilt, loneliness, ambivalence, and sadness. They may say that they cannot concentrate, feel confused, perhaps cannot sleep or rest. In contrast to inward grief, the outward response to death is mourning. People mourn in many different ways according to their cultural traditions, religious beliefs, and life experiences. Lastly, the term bereavement encompasses grief, loss, and mourning as it refers to both the inward emotional and outward behavioral responses of survivors to a death.

In hospice care, the interdisciplinary team works together to develop a plan that meets bereavement needs before and after the death of the patient. Nurses use therapeutic communication as they assist family members with anticipatory grieving and recognize age-related responses that affect the grieving process. Nurses may witness anger, hostility, depression, fear, and guilt as they provide emotional support to families coping with suffering, grief, and loss.

Hospice offers bereavement services to surviving family members for up to 14 months after the patient's death. If desired, team members make visits or phone calls to provide ongoing support and supervision. Grief support groups, led by the hospice social worker or bereavement coordinator, are also available to help people cope with the loss of a loved one. Other means of bereavement support are also provided. Individual counseling, camps, and educational materials in the form of pamphlets, books, and audiovisuals may be used.

Death is seen by many as the final stage of growth. The person facing the end of life, family members, and members of the health care team all must confront their own philosophies about living and dying. Hospice and palliative care nurses are privileged to be part of this stage. Despite witnessing great loss, they are able to also experience significant personal and professional satisfaction.

KEY CONCEPTS

- Dying is a process that ultimately ends in an event called death. Death can be sudden and unexpected, or protracted and expected.
- Palliative care is the active total care of patients whose disease is not responsive to curative treatment. Palliative care is planned and delivered through the collaborative efforts of an interdisciplinary team.

- Hospice is a coordinated program of palliative care services with the goal of attaining the highest possible quality of life for patients who have a prognosis of six months to live.
- In hospice and palliative care, the patient and the family are considered a single unit of care.
- Interdisciplinary teams in hospice and palliative care are composed of individuals who work collaboratively to plan and implement care according to goals expressed by the patient and family.

Continued

KEY CONCEPTS—cont'd

- Nurses providing hospice and palliative care consider the personal, cultural, and spiritual values and practices of their patients and families in the plan of care.
- Hospice and palliative care patients experience a wide range of physiological, psychosocial, and spiritual needs that require nursing assessment and intervention.
- Common physiological problems include pain, dyspnea, loss of appetite, constipation, nausea and vomiting, insomnia, anxiety, depression, and delirium.
- Nurses use evidence-based guidelines and accepted protocols in designing interventions to minimize pain and other symptoms experienced by patients

receiving hospice and palliative care. Psychosocial and spiritual components of care are also emphasized by each member of the interdisciplinary team.
- Nurses caring for patients receiving hospice and palliative care also provide care to meet the needs of the patient's family. Nursing interventions focus on assessing the coping abilities of the family members and assisting them in preparing for the patient's death.
- Bereavement services are an integral component of hospice and palliative care. Such services are offered to those who are facing, or have experienced, the death of a significant other. Bereavement services are provided by group and individual support programs. These programs are offered to children and adults.

REVIEW QUESTIONS

1. The nurse contributes to ethical practice in end-of-life care by doing all of the following except:
   1. Working closely with other members of the interdisciplinary team to meet the holistic needs of patients and families
   2. Ensuring that patients and families are aware of treatment options and of the consequences of those options
   3. Participating in creating systems of care that specifically meet end-of-life needs of patients and families
   4. Using his or her personal values and morals to determine best courses of actions for patients and families

2. Which statement is most helpful in talking with the wife of a patient who died recently?
   1. "I know exactly how you are feeling."
   2. "It must be hard to accept that this has happened."
   3. "His suffering is over. He's in heaven now."
   4. "Most people find it takes six months before things get back to normal."

3. Which statement by the nurse indicates understanding of the best method to assess for shortness of breath experienced by a hospice patient?
   1. "I will auscultate the patient's chest."
   2. "I will count the patient's respiratory rate."
   3. "I will ask the patient about his/her breathing."
   4. "I will check the patient's oxygen saturation rate."

4. The home care nurse is caring for a patient with end-stage renal disease who has decided to forego further dialysis. The nurse provides the family with information about the physical signs and symptoms of the dying process. What is considered a universal sign of imminent death?
   1. Decrease in the swallowing reflex
   2. Change in breathing pattern
   3. Weakness and fatigue
   4. Weight loss and dehydration

5. The nurse is caring for a patient who is close to death. Of the following assessment findings, which is the most reliable sign of death?
   1. Mottling of extremities
   2. Absence of urine output
   3. Constipation
   4. Fixed, dilated pupils

6. The nurse consults with the physician to arrange a referral for hospice care for a patient with end-stage kidney disease, based on the knowledge that hospice care is indicated when:
   1. Family members can no longer care for dying patients at home.
   2. Patients and families are having difficulty coping with grief reactions.
   3. Comfort rather than cure is the goal of care.
   4. Patients have unmanageable pain and suffering as a result of their condition.

Continued

REVIEW QUESTIONS—cont'd

7. A patient is diagnosed with lung cancer that has metastasized to his brain and bone. Which information should the nurse include in the teaching plan regarding palliative care (select all that apply)?
   1. The focus of care is on symptom control and quality of life.
   2. The patient and family are seen as the unit of care.
   3. Members of a multidisciplinary team participate in the plan of care.
   4. The patient can only receive hospice and palliative care services if he or she is in the home setting.

8. Palliative care nurses care for patients whose cultural background is different from their own. In those cases, which interventions are appropriate (select all that apply)?
   1. Respect the cultural beliefs of the patient and family
   2. Include cultural practices in the plan of care
   3. Recognize that values and behaviors do not vary among members of a given group
   4. Acknowledge that people from all cultures experience grief with the death of a loved one

9. Interdisciplinary team members provide hospice and palliative services. Integral members of the team include which of the following (select all that apply)?
   1. Nurses
   2. Health care providers
   3. Social workers
   4. Nuns
   5. Volunteers

10. The palliative care nurse admits a patient to a hospice program and asks the patient if he has a document that names another person to act in his behalf about medical decisions in the event that the patient cannot act for himself. What is the name of this document?

REVIEW ACTIVITIES

1. Identify a hospice agency that serves dying patients in your community. Talk with a staff nurse at that agency. How long has the nurse worked at the agency? What does he or she find most challenging about the role and the work? What does he or she find most valuable or rewarding about the role and the work? What particular patient or family is most memorable and why? Use what you learned as a basis to discuss the career opportunities and rewards available in palliative and hospice care nursing with your classmates.

2. Access one of the end-of-life Web sites featured in the Suggested Readings and Web Resources. Select one part of the Web site that provides you with information that enhances your understanding of a particular issue faced by dying patients or their family members. How might you and your classmates apply what you learned to the nursing care all of you provide?

Continued

REVIEW ACTIVITIES—cont'd

3. Ask a fellow student who is not a member of your ethnic or religious background whether you might be able to meet with some of the student's family members or friends to learn about their beliefs and specific cultural practices related to death and dying. How does what you learn compare to your own beliefs and practices?

5. Those who ascribe to the Jehovah's Witness religion are forbidden from accepting blood from others. Access a library or web resource to discover the religious law about organ transplant for Jehovah's Witnesses.

4. Rent the movie "Life as a House." The main character in the movie, George, spends the last part of his life with his son, building a house that he has always wanted. George does not dwell on his illness; in fact, his family does not learn of his cancer until the last days of his life. What does this movie convey about communication between patients and families at the end of life? What have you learned that you can you apply to the nursing care you provide?

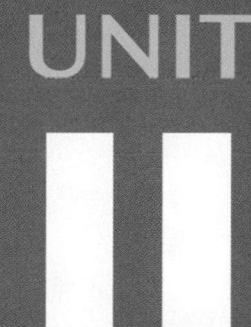

UNIT II

Supportive Patient Care

Health Assessment

Sharon Raymen, RN, MSA, CPTC, CCTC

CHAPTER TOPICS

- Health Assessment Process
- Methods of Data Collection
- Functional Health Patterns
- Health History
- Physical Examination
- Documentation

Assessment is the first step in the nursing process, which involves the systematic collection, verification, organization, interpretation, and documentation of data for use by health care professionals. A critical thinking approach to assessment is purposeful, focused, relevant, systematic, comprehensive, and accurate (Estes, 2006). Information obtained during the assessment phase contributes to a database that identifies the patient's current and past health state and provides a baseline against which future changes can be evaluated. Nursing assessments focus on human responses to health problems, perceived health needs, and health practices and values. The goal for collecting nursing assessment data is to formulate nursing diagnoses related to the patient's health status, identify outcomes, and develop nursing interventions. Assessment of the human responses is structured within the framework of functional health patterns (FHPs), which is a typology of health patterns of clients (individual patients, families, communities) that evolve from patient and environment interactions (Gordon, 1994). Effective planning and implementation of patient care depends on a complete database and accurate interpretation of information. The nurse must evaluate the ethical considerations needed to protect patient rights related to data collection. The data must be relevant to patient needs, collected from a variety of valid sources, obtained using appropriate techniques in a systematic manner, and documented in a usable format.

PURPOSE OF HEALTH ASSESSMENT

Health and physical assessment is performed on every patient. Health and physical assessment is the collection of subjective and objective data about an individual's health state. Health assessment is aimed at establishing a database against which subsequent data can be compared to evaluate physiological functioning of the body, to detect problems related to altered structure and/or function, and to identify factors that may place the patient at risk for developing health problems. Through assessment, the nurse determines patient functional abilities, the absence or presence of dysfunction, normal routine for activities of daily living, lifestyle patterns, and strengths. Data about patient strengths and functional abilities provide the nurse and other members of the treatment team information about the skills, abilities, and behaviors the patient has available to promote the treatment and recovery process.

Types of Assessment

The type and scope of information needed for assessment are usually determined by the patient's needs, health care setting, and nurse's role within that setting. Four types of assessment databases are comprehensive, focused, follow-up, and emergency (Daniels, 2004). A comprehensive assessment is desirable when initially determining a patient's need for nursing care. However, time limitations or special circumstances may dictate the need for an abbreviated data collection process. The assessment database can be expanded after the initial focused assessment. The database should be updated through out the assessment process.

Comprehensive Assessment

A comprehensive assessment, which includes a complete health history and a full physical examination, is usually completed on admission to a health care agency or first visit to a health care provider. The sources of information for the comprehensive assessment include the complete health history, the physical examination, the results of laboratory and diagnostic tests, and the information contributed by other health professionals. Collectively, this constitutes the database that provides a baseline against which changes in the patient's health status can be measured. The complete health history will include an assessment of the patient's perceived physical, emotional, social, developmental, and spiritual aspects of health, the presence of health risk factors, and the patient's coping patterns. A comprehensive assessment is most desirable to initially determine a patient's need for nursing care, but occasionally time limitations or special circumstances may dictate the need for an abbreviated data collection process.

Focused Assessment

A **focused assessment** is an assessment that is limited in scope to focus on a particular need or health care problem or potential health care risk (Figure 8-1). Focused assessments are often conducted in health care agencies in which short stays are anticipated, such as ambulatory surgery centers and emergency centers, in specialty care areas such as labor and delivery, in dialysis centers, and for purposes of screening for specific health problems (see Patient Playbook feature) or risk factors such as well child clinics or weight loss clinics.

Ongoing Assessment

An ongoing assessment is an assessment that includes systematic monitoring and observation related to specific health problems or risk factors. Systematic follow-up is required when

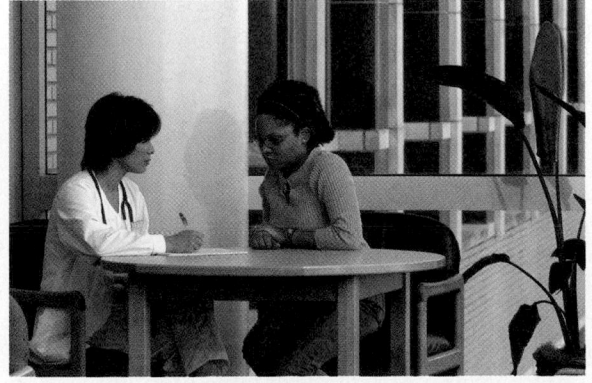

Figure 8-1 In this focused assessment, the nurse is collecting data about the patient prior to elective surgery.

Sample Focused Foot Assessment of the Patient with Type I Diabetes

To perform a focused assessment of a patient with type 1 diabetes, the nurse should:

- Assess for risk of diabetic foot problems.
  - History of previous foot ulcers
  - History of previous amputation
- Assess for abnormal skin and nail conditions.
  - Skin: cracks, ulcers
  - Toenails: thickened, ingrown nails, long nails
  - Fungal infections
- Assess for status of circulation.
  - Symptoms for claudication
  - Presence/absence of pedal or posterior tibial pulses
  - Prolonged capillary refill (>25 sec)
  - Absence/presence of hair growth on top of foot
- Assess for evidence of deformity.
  - Calluses, corns, bunions
  - Prominent metatarsal heads
  - Toe contractures: clawed toes, hammertoes, and Charcot foot
- Assess for loss of strength.
  - Ankle joint and great toe range of motion
- Assess for loss of protective sensation.
  - Numbness, burning tingling

Adapted from Estes, M. (2006). Health assessment and physical examination (3rd ed.). New York: Thomson Delmar Learning.

problems are identified during a comprehensive or focused assessment. Data from an ongoing assessment enable the nurse to broaden the database or to confirm the validity of the data obtained during the initial assessment. Ongoing assessment is especially important when problems have been identified and a plan of care has been implemented to address these problems. Systematic monitoring and observations allow the nurse to determine the response to nursing interventions and to identify any emerging problems.

Emergency Assessment

An emergency assessment is a rapid assessment of a patient who is experiencing a life-threatening problem or crisis. This problem can be of a physiological, psychological, or sociological nature. In the event of a cardiac arrest, the nurse will focus on airway patency, breathing, and cardiac status. In the event of an emotional crisis, the nurse will focus on immediate safety and coping abilities and strategies (see Red Flag feature).

Types of Data

The focus of nursing care is the diagnosis and treatment of human responses to actual or potential health problems (Estes, 2006). Health assessment data are obtained by five methods: the interview, physical examination, observation, review of records and diagnostic reports, and collaboration with colleagues. The nurse must possess cognitive, interpersonal, and technical skills to elicit appropriate information and make relevant observations during the data collection process.

The database includes information that the patient communicates concerning perceptions of personal health status and information of the observations made by the nurse. **Subjective data** are data from the patient's point of view and include feelings, perceptions, and concerns; it is the patient's story. The data are obtained through interviews with the patient. The patient may either respond to direct questioning or offer information spontaneously. The data are subjective, because the information relies on the feelings or opinions of the person experiencing them and cannot be readily observed by another. Subjective data may also be referred to as symptoms.

Objective data are observable and measurable. These types of data are obtained through standard assessment techniques including inspection, palpation, percussion, and auscultation performed during the physical examination. Objective data (also called signs) can be seen, heard, or felt by someone other than the person experiencing them. Objective data may be provided by other health care providers and diagnostic testing.

Sources of Data

A comprehensive databases should include data from every possible source. If possible, the patient should always be consulted, because he or she is always the primary source of data.

Other sources of data should also be considered. Data from sources other than the patient are considered secondary sources of information. The patient's family and significant others can provide useful information, especially if the patient is unable to verbalize or relate information. Other health care professionals who have cared for the patient may contribute valuable information. Medical records and other health care professional consults should be reviewed.

Pertinent literature should be investigated to pursue relevant information and plan appropriate nursing interventions. Written standards are valuable sources of data for comparison; for example, a standard table of infant growth to determine if an infant's weight and height are within normal growth range. Another valuable source of data is knowledge about the patient's normal parameters of functioning. The nurse's knowledge based on experience is another important source of data (Daniels, 2004).

THE INTERVIEW

A nursing health assessment interview is a patient-focused, goal-oriented, and time-limited, nonjudgmental verbal interaction between the nurse and patient. The purpose of the interview is to collect specific information about the patient and patient's health status. The nursing interview includes an assessment of physical, mental, emotional, social, cultural, and spiritual aspects of the patient. The interview enables the nurse to collect data regarding the patient's self-concept, family status and relationships, cultural background, lifestyle preferences, sexuality and reproductive processes, and developmental level. Data collected through the interview assist the nurse and the patient with identifying health problems, as well as patient strengths and resources. The nurse must function within professional, legal, ethical, and personal boundaries (Sheldon, 2004).

Creating the Climate for the Interview

Effective communication is a vital factor in interview process. The interview is more productive if the nurse has an opportunity to prepare for the interaction. Such preparation includes review of the patient's medical records, conversations with other health care team members, and research of the presenting medical diagnosis. The information can be useful in obtaining the patient's relevant history and personal information and formulating a current needs assessment.

Nurse Characteristics

The climate and tone of the initial patient interview may influence all future interactions the patient has in the health care setting. The nurse's attitude and expectations set the stage for the interview. First impressions can have a long-lasting impact on one's thoughts, feelings, and perceptions. In American culture, it is expected that nurses will present a professional appearance that is appropriate for the particular setting in which they work (Estes, 2006).

Environmental Characteristics

The patient is more likely to respond freely if the interview environment provides comfort and privacy. The environment should also enable the nurse to establish rapport with the patient. The nurse should sit or be at a level where the nurse and patient can establish eye contact (as appropriate). The environment should be free of extraneous noises and distractions so that the nurse can listen attentively.

Patient Characteristics

The nurse must include the patient as an active and equal participant in the interview process. In today's health care environment, patients are taking a more active role in both their own health care and in health care decisions. In addition the Health Insurance Portability and Accountability Act (HIPAA) of 1996, assists the health care system in aiding patient's rights (see Ethics in Practice feature). Patients expect their health care provider to be clinically and culturally competent and to provide individualized care. Patients are more apt to question health care providers, to treat themselves, and to demand a role in decision making (Walters, 2005).

A patient is able to make an informed decision about consenting or refusing a treatment regimen only if adequate information has been presented. The law requires that patients or their representatives be given sufficient infor-

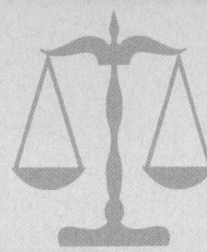

ETHICS IN PRACTICE

Health Insurance Portability and Accountability Act (HIPAA)

The Health Insurance Portability and Accountability Act (HIPAA) of 1996 protects working Americans and their families by:

- Lowering the chances of losing existing health insurance coverage because of preexisting conditions.
- Easing the ability to switch health insurance plans, because HIPAA prohibits group health plans from discriminating by denying coverage or charging extra coverage based on patient or patient family member's past or present poor health.
- Guarantying the right to purchase health insurance.

Source: Centers for Medicare and Medicaid Services. (2006). HIPAA insurance reform. *Retrieved June 15, 2006, from www.cms.hhs.gov.*

mation regarding various treatment modalities so that the consent is an informed process. Although the law does not require staff nurses to obtain a formal informed consent for nursing procedures, the nurse has the responsibility of explaining to the patient what to expect during any part of nursing care or procedures (see Ethics in Practice feature).

Phases of the Interview Process

The establishment of the nurse-patient relationship is a conscious commitment on the part of the nurse conducting the assessment interview. The nurse accepts primary responsibility for setting the structure and purpose of the assessment interview. There are three phases to the nurse-patient relationship during a health assessment interview: orientation, working, and closure. The orientation phase sets the tone for the relationship and establishes the goals for the interaction. The working phase of the interview focuses on the details of data collection. The closure phase is a time for review and evaluation of progress of interventions toward the intended goals (Sheldon, 2004).

METHODS OF DATA ORGANIZATION AND ASSESSMENT MODELS

There are many ways that nurses organize the data that they collect for assessment purposes. An assessment model is a framework that provides a systematic method for organizing data. The use of a model helps to ensure comprehensive and organized data collection. A guiding framework also provides direction for decision making about nursing diagnoses. A number of nursing and nonnursing models serve as guiding frameworks. Nursing models have been developed to focus on a wide range of human responses to alterations in health status. These models typically include psychosocial, sociocultural, behavioral, and biophysical data. Nursing models may offer the advantage of organizing information in a mode that more easily allows transition from data collection to nursing diagnoses.

There are several nursing models available, but Marjory Gordon's human functional health patterns (FHP) in *Manual of Nursing Diagnosis* (2002) serves as an example of an assessment model for clustering data. Gordon's FHP are not based on a particular theory of nursing but provides a systematic frame-

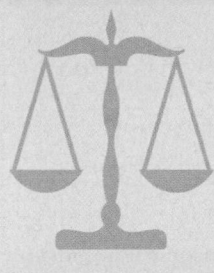

ETHICS IN PRACTICE

Should Health Care Professionals Tell the Truth?

In general, most, but not all, patients want truthfulness about their health. While nurses and physicians move toward more honest and truthful disclosure to their patients, there are arguments both for and against telling the truth. Based on a review of the literature, most patients want truthfulness about their health. Tuckett recommends that practitioners ought to ask patients and patients' families what information requirements are preferred, because there may be cultural manifestations as well as contextual conditions where telling the truth may not be preferred.

Source: Tuckett, A. G. (2004). Truth-telling in clinical practice and the arguments for and against: A review of the literature. Nursing Ethics, 11*(5), 500–513.*

work for data collection that focuses on 11 functional health patterns (Estes, 2006, review). These FHP areas allow gathering and clustering of information about a patient's usual patterns and any recent changes to determine if the patient's response is functional or dysfunctional. After data collection is completed and information is validated, the nurse organizes or clusters the information together to identify areas of strength and weakness. This process is known as data clustering.

Health History

A primary focus of the data collection interview is the health history. The health history is the collection of subjective information regarding patient health status (Box 8-1). The nursing health history focuses on the patient's functional health patterns, responses to changes in health status, and alterations in lifestyle. The medical health history concentrates on symptoms and the progression of disease. Data obtained through the health history are used to develop the plan of care and formulate nursing interventions.

The demographic information includes personal data; such as name, address, date of birth, gender, religion, race and ethnic origin, and occupation; type of health plan and insurance also should be included. This information may be useful in helping to foster understanding of the patient's perspective.

The patient's reason for seeking health care should be described in the patient's own words. The patient's perspective is important, because it explains what is significant about the event from the patient's point of view. At this point, it is also important to complete a symptom analysis, which is a means of collecting relevant data related to the symptom (Estes, 2006).

Perception of health status refers to the patient's opinion of one's own general health, well-being, and personal practices for maintaining health. This includes preventive screening activities and immunizations. It may be useful to ask patients to rate their health on a scale of 1 to 10 (with 10 being ideal and 1 being poor), together with the patients' rationale for their rating score.

The history and timing of any previous experiences with illness, surgery, or hospitalization are helpful to assess recurrent conditions and to anticipate responses to illness, because prior experiences often have an impact on current responses. The nurse needs to determine any family history of acute and chronic illnesses that tend to be passed down. Health history forms will frequently include checklists of various illnesses that the nurse can use as the basis for questions about this aspect. The patient should be instructed that family history refers to blood relatives and developing a **genogram** (a family tree related to health history) is helpful (Figure 8-2).

BOX 8-1

ELEMENTS OF HEALTH HISTORY

- Demographic information: name, age, gender, and marital status
- Reason for seeking health care; concern that initiated visit
- Perception of health status: patient's view of health
- Management of health
  - Previous illness, hospitalizations, and surgeries; any chronic illness or acute episodes that led to hospitalization or surgery
  - Family medical history: illness or cause of deaths in blood relatives (genogram)
  - Immunizations/exposure to communicable disease: childhood immunizations or relevant immunizations of adulthood; any known exposure to communicable disease
  - Allergies and side/untoward effects; prior allergic reactions to medications, food, or environmental substances
  - Current medications: prescription or over-the-counter medications, including laxatives, birth control pills, pain medications, vitamins, or herbal supplements
- Activities of daily living
  - Nutrition/metabolic patterns
  - Elimination patterns
  - Activity/exercise patterns
  - Sleep/rest patterns
  - Cognition/perception patterns
- Psychosocial history
  - Perception of self-identity and self-concept
  - Patterns of coping and stress tolerance
  - Perception of sexual identity
- Sociocultural history
- Perception of ones role to self, community, and society
- Values and beliefs systems

Adapted from Estes, M. (2006). Health assessment and physical examination (3rd ed.). New York: Thomson Delmar Learning.

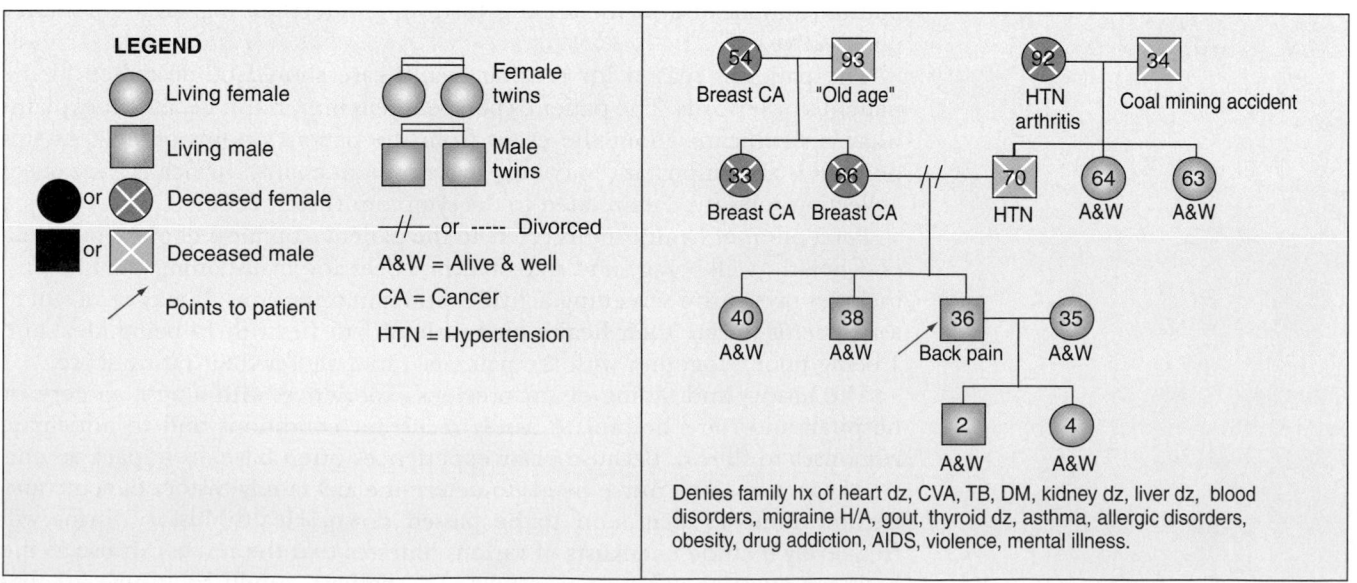

Figure 8-2 Family health history and genogram.

Any history of childhood or other communicable diseases should be noted. Additionally, a record of current immunizations should be obtained. This is particularly important with children; however, records of immunizations for tetanus, influenza, and hepatitis B can also be important for adults. If the patient has traveled out of the country, the time frame should be indicated to determine incubation periods for relevant diseases. The patient should also be asked about potential exposure to communicable diseases such as tuberculosis and human immunodeficiency virus (HIV).

Any drug, food, or environmental allergies should be noted in the health history. In addition to the name of the allergen, the type of reaction to the substance should be noted. All currently taken prescription and nonprescription medications should be recorded by name, frequency, and dosage. Remind patients that this information should include medications such as birth control pills, laxatives, hormone replacement therapy, and over-the-counter nonprescription medications such as analgesics, antihistamines, cathartics, and vitamin supplements. Ask which, if any, herbal preparations the patient uses. Patterns related to caffeine and alcohol intake and use of tobacco or recreational drugs should also be explored.

Knowledge of developmental level is essential for considering appropriate norms of behavior and for appraising the achievement of relevant developmental tasks. Any recognized theory of growth and development can be applied to determine if patients are functioning within the parameters expected for their age-group.

The activities of daily living is a description of the patient's lifestyle and capacity for self-care and is useful both as a baseline of information and as a source of insight into usual health behaviors. This database should include nutrition/metabolic patterns, elimination patterns, activity/exercise patterns, sleep/rest patterns, sexuality/reproductive patterns, and cognitive/perceptual patterns.

The goals for assessing the patient's nutrition and metabolic patterns are to determine his or her ability to attain and utilize nourishment of the body. Database information should include type of diet and foods eaten and fluids consumed regularly, food preparation, the size of portions, and the number of meals per day. Food preferences and dislikes, as well as the patient's need for assistance with food preparation or eating, should be determined. The assessment should contain data regarding and changes with skin, nail, and hair texture, wound healing, appetite, and any oral cavity problems.

The goals for assessing the patient's urinary and fecal elimination patterns are to determine one's perception and patterns of excretory function (bowel, bladder, and skin). The nurse should obtain data regarding the patient's bowel and bladder elimination patterns such as frequency, character, discomfort, the use of laxatives and enemas, and the use of any devices to control excretion, such as ostomy bags.

The nurse must assess the patient's perception of routine daily and leisure activities. These include the patient's perceived capabilities for movement, self-care (feeding, bathing, dressing, grooming, and toileting), and home management. If assistance is needed with activities such as walking, standing, or meeting hygienic needs, this information should be recorded.

Discussion of sleep habits is included as part of the regular health history. Any patient who acknowledges a sleep disturbance should be thoroughly assessed to determine sleep routines, sleep alterations, type of disturbances, and impact of sleep problems. Typically, the patient is a reliable source for this information, but a spouse or partner who shares sleeping arrangements may be able to add valuable information to the patient's report.

The nurse must assess the adequacy of sensory modes, such as vision, hearing, taste, touch, smell, pain perception, and language and cognitive func-

PATIENT PLAYBOOK

Sexual Health History Questions: Adult Patient

- Are you sexually active?
- If not, would you like to be and is something stopping you?
- If yes, with how many partners? Men? Women? Or Both?
- Is sex satisfying to you? For your partner?
- Do you have difficulty achieving erection or orgasm?
- Do you ever experience pain or bleeding with sexual activity? If yes, what kind and under what circumstances?
- Do you have any questions or concerns about your sexual functioning? About your partner's sexual functioning?

Adapted from Daniels, R. (2004). Nursing fundamentals: Caring and clinical decision making. New York: Thomson Delmar Learning.

tional abilities. Often the use of one's senses and thinking are taken for granted until deficits arise. Preventing deficits and helping patients to compensate for losses are important nursing functions.

The objective of assessment in the sexuality/reproductive arena is to describe perceived satisfaction or disturbances in sexuality or sexual relationships. Included are the female's reproductive state, premenopause or postmenopause, and any perceived problems. All patients should have a sexual health assessment. For those with more than one sexual partner, high-risk behavior, or indications of sexual dysfunction, a more detailed sexual assessment is necessary (see Patient Playbook feature).

A psychosocial history refers to assessment of dimensions such as self-concept and self-esteem, as well as usual sources of stress and the patient's ability to cope. Sources of support for patients in crisis, such as family, significant others, religion, or support groups should be explored. It is necessary to determine the patient's perception of self-concept and factors affecting it. Behavior, thoughts, and emotions are affected by self-concept. It is important to attend to the patient's verbal and nonverbal cues. Self-concept is reflected in a person's behavior and conversation.

A thorough assessment of stress and anxiety levels is assessed, which includes eliciting patient input to evaluate patterns of stressors, typical responses to stressful situations, cause-and-effect relationships between stressors and thoughts, feelings, and behaviors, and past history of successful coping mechanisms. Assessing the patient's coping abilities can be done in various ways. For example, use open-ended questions to determine previously used coping mechanisms.

When caring for an anxious patient, the nurse must first determine the patient's perception of the situation. This determination is done by directly asking for the patient's input and carefully listening to the patient's response. Because the nurse's nonverbal behavior can affect the patient's anxiety level, nurses must be aware of their own body language.

In exploring the patient's sociocultural history, it is important to inquire about the home environment, family situation, and the patient's role in the family. For example, the patient could be the parent of five children and the sole provider in a single-parent family. The responsibilities of the patient are important data through which the nurse can determine the impact of changes in health status and thus plan the most beneficial care for the patient. The concept of social support is interrelated with family theory and the roles and relationships that exist among people. Family-based social support is a naturally occurring resource for promoting individual health.

It is important to identify the patient's values and beliefs about life, death, health, illness, and spirituality. The value and belief system is the basis of a person's philosophy of life. The patient's cultural and ethnic background and spiritual dimensions influence views about health and illness. The degree to which traditional ethnic values are maintained may affect health care practices, health-related decisions, and behaviors in life-threatening situations. Spiritual assessment begins with the consideration of how spirituality develops across the life span. Spirituality is an important aspect for children who are seriously ill or dying, but their spirituality is quite different from adult spirituality. Adolescents are often spiritual seekers, and their spiritual development affects how a nurse will assess their needs. Adults, especially older adults, may have deep spiritual concerns that influence their approach to illness and dying.

PHYSICAL EXAMINATION

The purpose of the physical examination is to make direct observations of any deviations from normal and to validate subjective data gathered through the interview. Baseline measurements are obtained, and physical examination tech-

Coping with Problems

When patients are coping with a stressful situation, the nurse should ask the patient:

- Do you find yourself feeling tense? How often? What helps?
- Do you take medicines, drugs, or alcohol in response to your stress?
- Who is most helpful when you need to talk about problems?
- How available are your resources when you need to deal with problems?
- What, if any, crises or significant changes have occurred in your life in the last year or two?
- When crises or problems occur in your life, how do you handle them?

Source: Estes, M. (2006). Health assessment and physical examination (3rd ed.). New York: Thomson Delmar Learning.

Skills 360°

Parts of Hand Used for Palpation

Dorsal aspect: Best for temperature

Balls and ulnar surface of hand: Best for vibrations

Fingertips: Best for fine sensations

niques are used to gather objective data. The nurse usually takes the assessment form to the bedside to ensure accuracy of documented data. The room needs to be quiet, warm, without drafts, and adequately lit. Depending on the setting, the nurse must make the necessary adjustments to ensure privacy. Inform other personnel about the time of the examination to avoid interruptions, which are frustrating and distracting to both the patient and the nurse.

The nurse must wash hands and gather the necessary equipment. Equipment should be gathered before entering the patient's room. However, certain pieces of equipment, such as blood pressure cuff, ophthalmoscope, and otoscope, may be permanently installed in the examination and inpatient rooms. The nurse should observe what equipment is in the room during the first visit with the patient. The necessary equipment for patients who are maintained on isolation precautions should be kept inside the room, because items should not be taken in or out of isolation rooms.

Baseline data collection is the systematic organization of observations obtained during the physical examination that forms the basis for comparison and evaluation to establish the status of a patient at a given point in time. The physical assessment is initiated by performing a general survey, measuring height, weight, and vital signs (temperature, pulse, respirations, and blood pressure). These initial observations can provide data about the patient's general state of health as well as provide important information that will guide the nurse on how to proceed with the physical examination. Baseline data is important for comparison with future measurements to judge the significance of any changes (progress or regressions) over time.

The physical examination incorporates the use of visual, auditory, tactile, and olfactory senses and the use of systematic assessment techniques. The use of visual, auditory, and tactile senses will be described with each of the specific assessment techniques. Additionally, olfaction (sense of smell) is helpful in detecting characteristic odors as well as those associated with altered health states. For example, presence of infection is sometimes first detected by the change in the characteristic odor of body fluids or drainage. The four assessment techniques used in physical examination are inspection, palpation, percussion, and auscultation (Estes, 2006).

Inspection

Inspection involves careful, systematic visual observation. Inspection is more than just looking. The patient is observed first from a general point of view and then with specific attention to detail. For example, the nurse first observes for patterns of skin lesions and then focuses on the specific characteristics of individual lesions. Instruments such as a penlight and otoscope are often used to enhance visualization. Effective inspection requires adequate lighting and exposure of the body parts being observed. Beginning nurses often feel self-conscious or embarrassed using the technique of inspection; however, most become comfortable with the technique over time. Nurses must also be sensitive to the patient's feelings of embarrassment with the use of inspection and respond to this situation by discussing the technique with the patient and using measures such as draping to increase the patient's comfort level.

Palpation

Palpation involves the use of the sense of touch to assess texture, temperature, moisture, organ location and size, vibrations and pulsations, swelling, masses, and tenderness. Palpation requires a calm, gentle approach and is used systematically, with light palpation preceding deep palpation. Palpation of tender areas is performed last.

The technique of palpation uses the hands and fingers in different ways. The nurse will learn that different parts of the hand are more sensitive for spe-

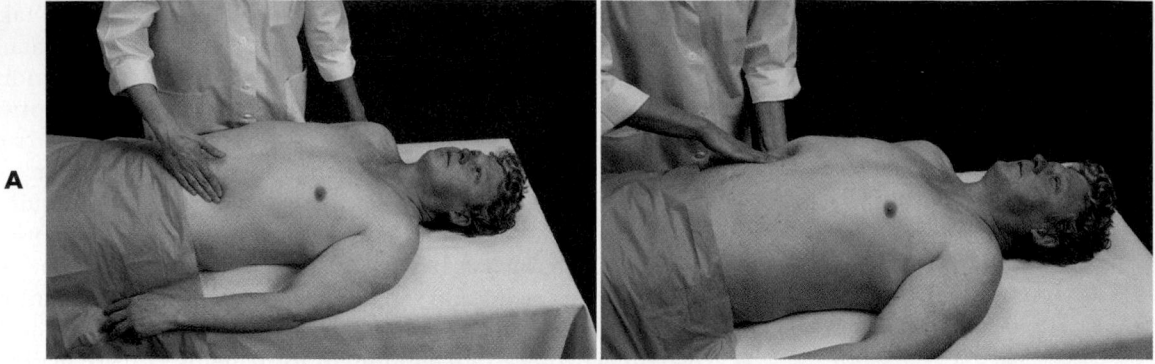

A
B

Figure 8-3 Technique of palpation: A. Light palpation, B. Deep palpation.

cific assessments. For example, the skin is thinner on the backs of the hands and more sensitive to temperature changes. The finger pads are sensitive and are used to palpate the size, position, and consistency of various body parts, such as lymph nodes and breast tissue (see Skills 360° feature). In addition, there is both light and deep palpation (Figure 8-3).

Percussion

Percussion uses short tapping strokes on the surface of the skin to create vibrations of underlying organs (Figure 8-4). It is used for assessing the density of structures or determining the location and the size of organs in the body. Structures with relatively more air (such as the lungs) produce louder, deeper, and longer sounds with percussion than denser, solid structures (such as the liver), which produce softer, higher, shorter sounds. Refer to Table 8-1 for characteristics of percussion sounds.

Auscultation

Auscultation is listening to sounds produced by the body that are created by movement of air or fluid. Areas most often auscultated include the lungs, heart, abdomen, and blood vessels. Although direct auscultation is sometimes possible, a stethoscope is usually employed to clarify the sound by blocking extrane-

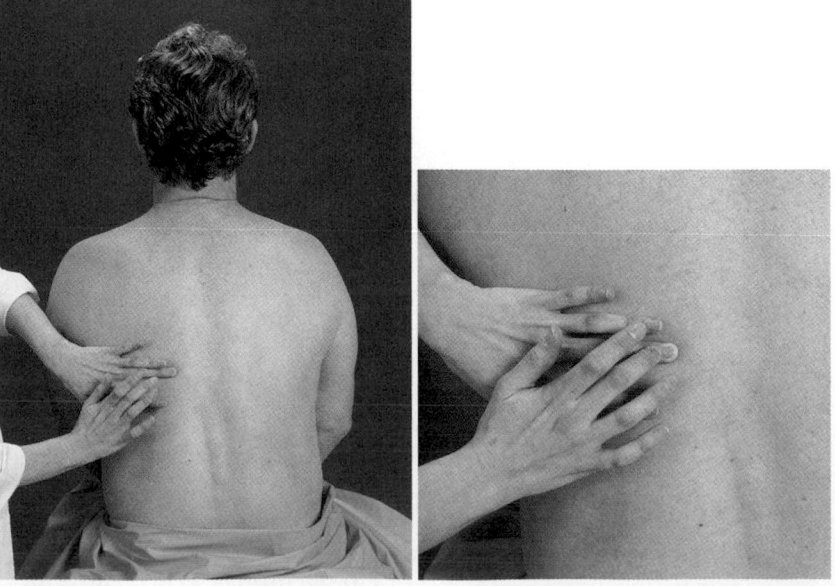

Figure 8-4 Technique of percussion.

TABLE 8-1	Characteristics of Percussion Sounds						
SOUND	**INTENSITY**	**DURATION**	**PITCH**	**QUALITY**	**NORMAL LOCATION**	**ABNORMAL LOCATION**	**DENSITY**
Flatness	Soft	Short	High	Flat	Muscle (thigh) or bone	Lungs (severe pneumonia)	Densest
Dullness	Moderate	Moderate	High	Thud	Organs (liver)	Lungs (atelectasis)	
Resonance	Loud	Moderate-long	Low	Hollow	Normal lungs	No abnormal location	
Hyperresonance	Very loud	Long	Very low	Boom	No normal location in adults; normal lungs in children	Lungs (emphysema)	
Tympany	Loud	Long	High	Drum	Gastric air bubble	Lungs (large pneumothorax)	Least dense

Source: Estes, M. (2006). Health assessment and physical examination (3rd ed.). New York: Thomson Delmar Learning.

ous sounds. The bell of the stethoscope is more sensitive to low-pitched sounds. The diaphragm of the stethoscope is more sensitive to high-pitched sounds.

Not all assessment techniques are appropriate for all body parts and systems. The physical assessment techniques are usually performed in the sequence of inspection, palpation, percussion, and auscultation except for abdominal examination. In this situation, the sequence is inspection, auscultation, percussion, and palpation. Percussion and palpation of the abdomen before auscultation can alter bowel sounds and thus produce false findings.

Head-to-Toe Assessment

The physical examination may involve a complete head-to-toe physical examination, a focused examination of a body system, or a focused examination of a body part. The procedure can vary according to the age of the patient, the severity of the illness, the preferences of the nurse, the location of the examination, and the agency's procedures. The physical examination is conducted in an aseptic, systematic, and efficient manner that requires the fewest position changes for the patient. After completion of the physical examination, give the patient a few minutes to redress in privacy. Always thank the patient for his or her time and explain what can be expected next.

Review of Systems Assessment

The **review of systems (ROS)** is a brief account from the patient of any recent signs of symptoms associated with any of the body systems. This allows the patient an opportunity to communicate any deviations from normal that have not been otherwise identified. The ROS relies on subjective information provided by the patient rather than on the nurse's own physical examination. When a symptom is encountered, either while eliciting the health history or during the physical examination of the patient, the nurse should obtain as much information as possible about the symptom.

Laboratory and Diagnostic Data

Results of laboratory and diagnostic tests can be useful objective data as these values often serve as defining characteristics for various altered health states; these can also be helpful in ruling out certain suspected problems. For example, diabetic patients who poorly control their diet, medication, or both will usually have an elevated blood glucose level. The pattern of these types of variations is useful in determining a plan of care. In addition, the effectiveness of nursing and medical interventions and progress toward health restoration are often monitored through laboratory and diagnostic test data (Daniels, 2003).

VARIATIONS RELATED TO HEALTH ASSESSMENT PRACTICES

Many factors influence health assessment practices. Age, culture, ethnicity, gender, and genetic makeup all significantly influence a person's health.

Age

It makes good sense to consider health assessment from a life cycle approach. The nurse must be familiar with the usual and expected developmental tasks for each age-group. This alerts the nurse to which physical, psychosocial, cognitive, and behavioral tasks are important for each patient. The nurse's knowledge of communication skills and health history content is enhanced as the nurse considers how they apply to individuals throughout the life cycle. The physical examination is more relevant when the nurse considers age-specific data about anatomy, method of examination, and normal and abnormal findings. Age influences normal physical characteristics. The ability to participate in some parts of the examination is also influenced by age. For each age-group, a holistic approach to health assessment arises from an orientation toward wellness and health maintenance. The nurse must be cognizant of the normal limits for the patient through out the life span.

Neonate

Immediately after delivery, a complete and thorough assessment of the neonate includes an evaluation of the neonate's reflexes and respiratory and cardiac functioning. The Apgar assessment tool is performed by the nurse at 1 minute and again at 5 minutes after birth (Estes, 2006).

Infant

Infancy (1 to 18 months) is a time of continued adaptation. During this stage, the infant experiences rapid physiological growth and psychosocial development. The parameters of weight, length or height, and head circumference are essential in serial physical growth measurements. For infants, the average birth weight is 7.5 pounds, length is 19 to 21 inches, and head circumference is 13 to 14 inches. Infants should double birth weight at 6 months and triple birth weight by 1 year of age. It is not uncommon for infants to double birth weight at 4 months. An infant's height increases about 1 inch per month for the first six months, and then slows to one-half inch per month.

The nurse's assessment must focus on safety, prevention of infection, and developmental milestones. Common health problems for infants include low birth weight, lack of prenatal care, poverty, infections, and accidents. A major factor influencing health maintenance of the infant is the provision of adequate nutrients delivered in a loving, consistent manner. Caregivers must be taught that the nutrients must be germ free and provide the recommended amounts of carbohydrates, protein, calcium, iron, and vitamins. Infants are vulnerable to infections, because their immune system is not fully matured. Nurses should confirm that infants receive all necessary immunizations. The Department of Health and Human Services, Centers of Disease Control and Prevention recommends following the schedule for infant, childhood, and adolescent immunizations (Magnusson, Sundelin, & Westerlund, 2006).

Respecting Our Differences

Acquired Lactase Deficiency

Acquired lactase deficiency, an intolerance to milk, may develop during preschool years. This condition occurs most often in African American, Asian (American), and Native-American children (Rizzo, 2006).

Toddler

Toddler (1 to 3 years) growth rate slows, the growth of subcutaneous adipose tissue decreases, and the extremities grow more rapidly compared with the trunk. The toddler's gastrointestinal (GI) tract reaches functional maturity and can handle most adult foods. Lung capacity increases, and the respiratory rate decreases to 25 breaths per minute. The anatomy of the ear and throat gradually increases in size. Tonsils are large (Rizzo, 2006).

Preschool

The preschool child (3 to 6 years) has a more mature body and is beginning to master independence. The protuberant abdomen disappears and abdominal muscles develop. Growth rate remains steady. The skin matures with minimal sebum secretion, which makes the skin fairly dry. Hair color darkens and hair becomes straighter. The GI organs continue to grow. Lung capacity continues to increase. Ears increase in size, and the incidence of otitis media decreases slightly. Tonsils and adenoids remain large, and primary teeth have erupted. Musculoskeletal and neurological system development reaches a level that allows for effortless walking, running, and climbing, with advances in fine and gross motor development skills. There are variations among cultures as the preschool child develops (see Respecting Our Differences feature).

School Age

School age (6 to 12 years) children have a slimmer shape because of the changes in the amount and distribution of fat on the body with longer legs. Growth is steady. Boys and girls are similar in size. Respirations become slower, deeper, and more regular, changing from 20 to 30 breaths per minute to 17 to 25 breaths per minute. The heart increases in size, and heart rate slows to the average adult heart rate of 70 to 100 beats per minute. Lymph tissue grows rapidly. With the rapid change in the number and type of teeth and the uneven growth in the child's jaw, malocclusion may be noted. Neurological, skeletal, and muscular changes combine to increase the child's overall motor abilities. Muscle mass increases with muscle strength. There are differences among school-aged children across cultures (see Respecting Our Differences feature).

Adolescent

The period of adolescence is difficult to define in chronological age but is often is identified by the onset of puberty and ends with the achievement of a certain level of independence. The adolescent experiences accelerated growth. Sexual characteristics develop, and sexual maturity is achieved. The heart grows in size and strength, respiratory rate decreases to 15 to 20 breaths per minute. Respiratory volume and vital capacity increase, laryngeal cartilage, larynx, and vocal cords grow, which produces the voice changes of puberty. The liver, kidneys, spleen, and digestive tract enlarge. The skin becomes tough and thick. Sweat glands become fully functional and body hair appears.

Adult

The physical attributes of height, strength, endurance, coordination, and speed of response are at their maximal levels. Physical appearance is determined by genetic endowment. Full adult stature in men is reached at approximately age 21 and in women by age 17.

Older Adult

A multitude of changes accompany the aging person (Eliopoulos, 2005; Estes, 2006). Normal aging changes are responsible for the increased risk of developing health-related problems within the geriatric population. Prevalent problems associated with older adults include health alterations in sleep/rest patterns,

Fast Forward ▶▶▶

The Aging Population and Nutrition

By the year 2030, nearly one fourth of the United States population will be older than 65. The American Dietetic Association reports that persons aged 65 and over, malnutrition is estimated at 20 to 60 percent in home care populations. Approximately 40 to 60 percent of hospitalized patients and 40 to 80 percent of nursing home populations are at risk for malnutrition. Older adults are at risk for conditions, such as excessive or inadequate caloric/nutrient intake, body weight, and inactivity that lead to chronic diseases (Figure 8-5). Eighty five percent of older adults in the United States have conditions that could be improved with nutrition intervention. Nutrition screening and intervention is imperative to the initial and long-term management of many of the chronic diseases. Evidence-based nutrition screening and interventions exist for such chronic diseases as hypertension, coronary artery disease, congestive heart failure, and diabetes. In addition, effective nutrition screening and interventions offers a cost-effective solution to rising health care costs (see Dollars and Sense feature). Healthy nutrition may help keep older adults in home- and community-based settings and may reduce the costs associated with acute care.

Source: Roth, R. (2007). Nutrition & diet therapy (9th ed.). New York: Thomson Delmar Learning.

nutrition/metabolic patterns, elimination patterns, and activity/exercise patterns. Familiarity with these commonly occurring alterations in health patterns enables the nurse to prevent unnecessary treatment-related problems and to promote optimal function of the aging patient.

Culture

Values and beliefs influence health and the patient's care. In today's multicultural environment, nurses will come in contact with patients from many different cultures (Spector, 2004). **Culture** refers to the knowledge, values, beliefs, art, morals, law, customs, and habits of the members of a society. Culture also includes the systems of technology and political practices. Cultural patterns of behavior develop over time and are shared by members of the same cultural group.

Culture is not static, and it is not uniform among all members within cultural groups. Culture represents adaptive dynamic processes learned through life experiences. Patients have culturally predetermined values and beliefs that may change as new information is gained. Culture is unconscious and has powerful influences on health and illness. Culture is first learned in the family, then in school, and then in the community and social organizations. Nurses must recognize, respect, and integrate patients' cultural beliefs and practices into their assessment and nursing care (Purnell & Paulanka, 2005).

A subculture is a group of people who have experiences different from those of the dominant culture by virtue of status, ethnic background, residence, religion, education, or other factors that functionally unify the group. To provide culturally acceptable care and to offer improved opportunities for health promotion, illness and disease prevention, and health restoration, nurses must understand their patients' cultural values, beliefs, and practices.

Cultural competence involves the complex integration of knowledge, attitudes, and skills that enable the nurse to provide culturally appropriate health care (Purnell & Paulanka, 2005).

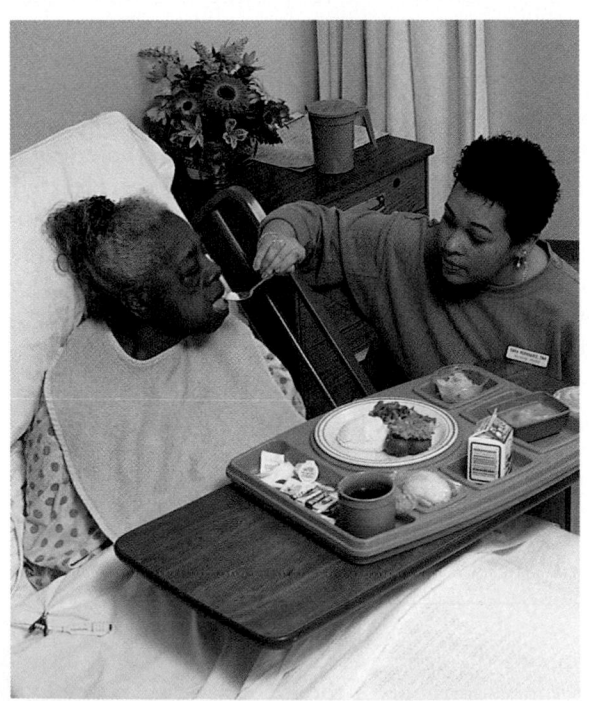

Figure 8-5 The nutritional care of this elderly patient is vital to prevent further complications during this hospitalization episode.

DOLLARS AND SENSE

The United States spends a larger share of its gross domestic product on health care than any other major industrialized country. Factors that influence increased dollars spent on health care are a larger of proportion of elderly persons, medical advances that heighten the need for nurses and other health care staff, and a greater percentage of hospitalized patients receiving care in the intensive care unit (ICU).

Nearly half of all ICU patients are over age 65. The cost of ICU care for a patient over age 65 is three to five times more per day than the cost of resources utilized for the average acute care admission.

Source: Values, Ethics and Rationing in Critical Care (VERICC) Task Force. (2005). ICU cost burdens. Retrieved June 15, 2006, from www.vericc.org.

Developing cultural competence requires cultural awareness, cultural knowledge, cultural skills, and cultural encounter.

Cultural awareness is a conscious learning process in which individuals become appreciative of and sensitive to the cultures of other people. Nurses are influenced by their own cultural background, the culture of the nursing profession, and the health care setting in which the interaction takes place. Therefore, cultural awareness involves the identification of one's own cultural background, values, and beliefs related to health and health care and the examination of ones own cultural biases toward people whose cultures differ from one's own culture.

Cultural knowledge involves the process of understanding the main aspects of a groups' culture as it relates to health and health care practices. To gain cultural knowledge, nurses must become knowledgeable about the predominant cultural groups within one's geographic area and assess for presence or absence of cultural phenomena based on the understanding of generalizations about a cultural group. The nurse may gain this knowledge through reading research literature, ethnic newspaper articles, and novels or by viewing documentaries about cultural groups.

Cultural skill is the ability to collect relevant cultural data regarding health histories and performing culturally specific assessments. Skills based on cultural knowledge can be use to create a safe environment so that patients will share information about their health-related cultural practices.

Cultural encounter is the process that encourages individuals to engage directly in cross-cultural interactions with people from culturally diverse backgrounds. Nurses who interact and work with patients from different cultures become competent in understanding how cultural beliefs and practices affect health and health care practices. For example there are some cultural sanctions against breastfeeding, and some cultures view bottle feeding as a status symbol. In addition, sexual health is influenced by culture. What may be appropriate in one culture may be considered inappropriate in other cultures. One example is the ritual of female circumcision or removal of the clitoris. This is known as female genital mutilation (FGM). In some areas of Africa, FGM is considered a cultural norm and used for the purpose of controlling women's sexual desires. This ritual is considered inappropriate in many other cultures (Daniels, 2004).

Cultural Assessment

Caring for a patient from a different culture can be challenging. Using the patient's strengths and respecting the patients values are essential components of effective nursing care. To begin providing culturally competent care, the nurse should use questions to gather information about the patient's cultural background. The questions in the cultural assessment interview guide can either be incorporated into a general nursing assessment tool or used separately as a cultural assessment instrument (see Respecting Our Differences feature).

Ethnicity

Ethnicity is a cultural group's perception of themselves (group identity). This self-perception influences how the group's members are perceived by others. Ethnicity is a sense of belongingness and a common social heritage that is passed from one generation to the next. Members of an ethnic group demonstrate their shared sense of identity in common traits.

Race

Race is a grouping of people based on biological similarities. Members of a racial group have similar physical characteristics such as blood group, facial features, and color of skin, hair, and eyes. There is often overlap between racial and ethnic groups because the cultural and biological commonalities support one another. The similarities of people in racial and ethnic groups reinforce a sense of commonality and cohesiveness. However, there may be differences with regard to individuals' perceptions of their racial backgrounds and their social relationships. The nurse must be careful to assess patients individually when considering race and ethnicity. For example, some ethnic groups are more susceptible than others to hemodynamic alterations. The incidence of hypertension is higher in African Americans than in European-Americans (African American men over the age of 35 have higher blood pressure than do European-American men of the same age). The issue of race's effect on health is complex. The nurse should examine socioeconomic factors and race and adapt health teaching to the individual patient and family's situation (Lane, Lip, & Beevers, 2005).

Gender

Assessment of appearance and behavior begins while the nurse prepares the patient for the examination. A patient's gender affects the type of examination performed and the manner in which assessments are made. Different physical features and certain illnesses are related to gender.

Gender identity refers to the biological sex of male, female, or intersexed. Intersexed people, formerly known as hermaphrodites, are people who are born with both sets of, or ambiguous, genitalia. These infants are usually surgically assigned gender by physicians who perform the most expedient surgery. Unfortunately, an increasing number of these infants grow up and find when their hormones of puberty are fully functioning, they had been assigned the wrong gender (Haas, 2004).

Gender role is the masculine or feminine role adopted by a person, which is often culturally and socially determined. While masculine and feminine roles vary among cultures around the world, the gender stereotypes of the submissive female and dominant male are most prevalent and most harmful to sexual health. Traditional gender roles may hinder communication, and often lead to violence, sexual exploitation, unplanned pregnancy, and sexually transmitted infections (STIs).

Gender research is an emerging field. Gender is a component in human nature that affects many aspects of communication between the sexes. There is sufficient data that indicates that males and females perceive life and one another differently and therefore communicate differently (Daniels, 2004). For example, there are gender differences related to expression of emotions. Men typically do not express emotions as frequently or as openly as women. Women are perceived to be more sensitive and empathic than men, because women are both biologically and socially conditioned to express emotions more easily than men. However, women are socialized to express certain emotions, such as sadness rather than anger (Scileppi, 2005).

Physical Variations Related to Gender

There are many physical variations in people, which must be considered when performing an assessment. Specifically, the vital signs, physical growth, and assessment of the breasts and axillae vary from one person to another. The nurse must be aware of these physical differences during the assessment processes.

Women usually experience greater temperature fluctuations than men because of hormonal changes. Temperature variations occur during the menstrual cycle mainly in response to the progesterone level. As the progesterone level increases during ovulation, temperature gradually rises. During menopause, the instability of the vasomotor controls may cause periods (30 seconds to 5 minutes) of intense body heat and sweating. Males in general have higher blood pressure than do females of the same age.

Studies reveal biological and behavioral differences between male and female infants. At birth, on average, boys are larger and have more muscle mass at birth. Girls are smaller, but physiologically more mature at birth and are less vulnerable to stress. Boys show more motor activity whereas girls are more responsive to tactile stimulation and pain (Bee & Boyd, 2003). By 6 months of age, girls respond to visual stimulation with longer attention spans and are more socially responsive than are boys. Girls develop language earlier and respond to speech better than do boys. Therefore, girls learn to communicate with language whereas boys use their bodies. Female infants tend to sit up, walk, and crawl earlier than do male infants.

From birth to 12 years of age, height and weight increases are similar for males and females. Rapid growth in the adolescent is called the growth spurt. Females commonly experience this between ages 10 and 14, whereas in males, it occurs somewhat later, between 12 and 16 years of age. Throughout infancy and childhood, boys are more likely to show atypical development and to be affected by some common childhood illnesses more compared with girls. Toddlers often experience otitis media (middle ear infection). Boys tend to have a ratio of 5:4 for hearing problems and a ratio of 3:2 for speech deficits. The reason for this difference is unclear. One hypothesis is that two X chromosomes protect girls not only from recessively inherited diseases, but also from commonly encountered organisms (Estes, 2006).

As adults, the breasts of men and women need to be inspected and palpated. Men have some glandular tissue beneath each nipple, a potential site for malignancy, whereas mature women have glandular tissue throughout the breast. In females, the largest portion of glandular breast tissue is located in the upper outer quadrant of each breast and extending into the axilla, called the tail of Spence.

Genetics

Genetic makeup influences biological characteristics, innate temperament, activity level, and intellectual potential. Heredity or genetic predisposition has been related to the susceptibility of specific diseases. Genetic predisposition to specific illnesses is a major physical risk factor. For example, a person with a family history of diabetes mellitus is at risk for developing the disease later in life. Other documented genetic risk factors include family history of cancer, heart disease, kidney disease, or mental illness.

ETHICAL CONSIDERATIONS RELATED TO DATA COLLECTION

As professionals, nurses are accountable for protecting the rights and interests of the patient. Consequently, sound nursing practice involves making ethical decisions. Ethics affects nurses in most health care settings, and each practice setting presents the nurse with its own set of ethical concerns (Table 8-2).

Ethics is the study of philosophical ideals of right and wrong behavior. The professional practice of nursing is guided by the American Nurses Association *Code of Ethics* (ANA, 2006). Nurses' commitment to this code guarantees the public that nurses adhere to professional practice standards. When acting as a patient advocate, the nurse's first step is to develop a meaningful relationship with the patient. The primary ethical responsibility is to protect the patients' rights to make their own decisions. Respecting the rights of others is a fundamental responsibility of the nurse. Respect for persons is the foundation of six ethical principles: justice, autonomy, beneficence, nonmaleficence, veracity, and fidelity.

Until recently, many patients did not question the information provided by their health care provider, they did not exercise their basic human rights. Now,

TABLE 8-2	**Overview of Ethical Principles**
PRINCIPLE	**EXPLANATION**
Autonomy	Respect for an individual's right to self-determination; respect for individual liberty
Nonmaleficence	Obligation to do or cause no harm to another
Beneficence	Duty to do good to others and to maintain a balance between benefits and harms
Justice	Equitable distribution of potential benefits and risks
Veracity	Obligation to tell the truth
Fidelity	Duty to do what one has promised

Source: DeLaune, S., & Ladner, P. (2006). Fundamentals of nursing (3rd ed.). New York: Thomson Delmar Learning.

patients are increasingly demanding to have a say in matters affecting their health care.

The nurse who functions as a patient advocate is adhering to the *Code of Ethics* (ANA, 2006). Examples of advocacy behaviors include empowerment of patients through education, providing support, actively listening to patient concerns, and acting as a liaison between the patient and other health care providers. Elderly patients often require nurses to fulfill the patient advocate role in a proactive manner and in ways that other groups of patients might not need.

Patient Rights

Some rights owed to patients include informed consent, the right to die, privacy, confidentiality, respectful care, and information concerning medical condition and treatment. Additionally, patients have the right to be informed if any aspect of treatment is experimental and also have the right to refuse to participate in experimental treatment (Chally & Hough, 2005).

Informed Consent

Informed consent is a patient's authorization for care based on full disclosure of risks, benefits, alternatives, and consequences of refusal (Chally & Hough, 2005). It is the nurse's responsibility to inform the patient of the purpose for collecting health assessment data and how the information will be used.

Confidentiality

Confidentiality is the protection of private information gathered about a patient during the provision of health care services. The nurse safeguards the patient's right to privacy by carefully protecting information of a confidential nature. It is the nurse's responsibility to share with the patient how the assessment data is used in the plan of care and with whom the information is shared. While the principle of confidentiality is protected by state and federal statues, there are exceptions and limitations. The nurse does have the duty to report or disclose information in the event of suspected child abuse, gunshot wounds, certain communicable diseases, and threats toward third parties. These laws may vary by state and may be the responsibility of institutions providing health care services rather than that of the individual practitioner.

The Health Insurance Portability and Accountability Act (HIPAA) of 1996, implemented in 2003, is the first federal privacy standard governing the protection of patients' medical records. HIPAA regulations offer several major patient protections including see and obtain copies of their medical records; provider's information practices and explanation of patients' rights; and limitations on length of time records can be retrieved, what information can be shared, where it can be shared, and who can be present when it is shared.

Advanced Directives

The Patient Self-Determination Act (PSDA) was enacted in 1991. The PSDA requires health care institutions to provide written information to patients concerning the patients' rights under state law to make decisions, including the right to refuse treatment and formulate advance directives. It is incumbent on the nurse to be informed of the patient's desire, if rendered incompetent, who and what health care decisions can be made on the patient's behalf (Browning, 2006).

Genetic Screening and Counseling

As our culture becomes more entrenched in the power and availability of information, individuals wish to have more. Information is perceived by many to be power and control. Health professionals who provide primary and secondary care find that they are required to understand the basics of genetics and to explain the principles to patients and to support them through genetic testing and screening. The advances of genetic testing and genetic therapy are a manifestation of these perceptions. Health care providers have gained the ability to reverse, postpone, and predict many diseases as a result of genetic testing information.

Genetic screening and testing has forced health care to address new ethical questions. **Genetic screening** refers to population screening for a genetic variation or mutation, for example PKU screening at birth. **Genetic testing** refers to testing of an individual at significant risk because of family history or because of presentation of symptoms, for example, chromosome abnormalities. The potential benefits and harms of genetic testing are debated at the same time that new technology is being developed. To avoid harm and to maximize benefits, individual and collective moral reflection is imperative. Nurses must be able to integrate genetics knowledge, skills, and attitudes into routine health care assessment and practices to provide effective care to patients and their families.

Ethical principles may serve as guidelines for the nurse or genetics team to deal with patients and family members at risk for a genetic condition. An example of the components of a genetic counseling interaction is shown in the Patient Playbook feature.

PATIENT PLAYBOOK

Components of a Genetic Counseling Interaction

The nurse can discuss issues of a genetic concern by remembering the following areas of interaction:

- Diagnosis associated with the genetic issue.
- Collect thorough information including the patient's knowledge level and the data with which the patient is familiar.
- Explain to the patient the risks involved and identify how the patient evaluates the risks.
- Present an objective list of options.
- Provide ongoing support for the patient and family members.

Source: Skirton, H., & Patch, C. (2002). Genetics for healthcare professionals: A lifestage approach. *Oxford, UK: BIOS Scientific Publishers Limited.*

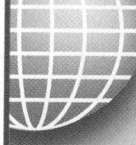

Real World, Real Choices

Genetic Counseling

Mary is 40 years old and has a 50 percent chance of inheriting Huntington's disease (HD) from her mother. Mary dreads the possibility of having HD and feels she could not cope if she knew that was awaiting her. Her son, Kevin, wants to be tested for the gene mutation that causes Huntington's disease. He is in a serious relationship and wants to know his own status before deciding to have a family.

1. What is the benefit to Mary if Kevin is tested? To Kevin?
2. What is the harm? Who may be harmed?
3. How can you support the principle of justice? Autonomy?
4. What if Mary and Kevin are not able to negotiate a solution?

Advances in molecular biology have enabled scientists to acquire extraordinary insights into genetics and human genetic development. These extraordinary developments have the potential to influence the human race in the future. Ethically, one must constantly evaluate the advances that genetic therapy can accomplish. The types of genetic therapy include eugenics (planned breeding), genetic engineering, and euthenics (euphenics). **Eugenics** involves the selection and recombination of genes already existing in the gene pool. There are two types of eugenics: positive (preferential breeding) and negative (legal prohibition of reproduction). Preferential breeding encourages the development of sperm banks for the purpose of storing frozen sperm acquired from outstanding people and cloning. Negative eugenics involves genetic counseling or the provision for abortion or sterilization on either a voluntary or an enforced basis. **Genetic engineering** entails changing a particular molecule in the structure of the gene, either to eliminate a certain bad trait or to improve the genotype. This process might be used to control genetic diseases such as sickle cell anemia. **Euthenics (euphenics)** involves the techniques for correcting defects in individuals after they have been born. For example, if a person is born with defective pancreatic cells, it might be possible to extract one or two cells, modify their DNA, and reimplant them.

Genetic therapy has great possibilities for the advancement of humankind. However, all individuals must keep two basic ethical principles in mind: the principle of human stewardship over human existence and the principle of nonmaleficence related to testing and results. Currently, the potential of genetic therapy is an exciting area of development in the health care system.

CARE OF THE PATIENT AFTER THE EXAMINATION

A health history and physical examination is taxing on the patient, especially if the complete assessment is performed in one session. The nurse should assess the patient's needs after this process and respond appropriately. The nurse should also dispose of soiled articles in the proper container, clean and store equipment appropriate for the setting, and put all furniture back in its original place. The bed should be returned to a low position, side rails up, and call light in place. Quietly check on the patient several times within the two to three hours after assessment to monitor the patient's condition. Thank the patient for cooperating during physical examination demonstrates concern and caring.

DOCUMENTATION

Health care agencies have specific forms for recording the assessment findings. Review these forms before initiating the assessment, and record the findings on the appropriate form as the data are gathered. This practice ensures accuracy in documentation of findings. Some data (e.g., vital signs) may need to be recorded on two or more forms. Reporting information is a critical part of documentation. If findings that require immediate attention—for example, bright red blood or change in the nature and character of previous symptoms—are identified, report the findings to the nursing supervisor, and document the actions taken in the medical record. Documentation should reflect the objective data obtained from the examination regarding the patient's current condition. Avoid phrases such as the patient appears lethargic, rather, record the Glasgow Coma Scale score. If the data identify areas in which the patient is at risk, such as a 36-year-old woman with a family history of breast cancer, use the appropriate resources for prevention. Likewise, abnormal findings should be addressed in planning the nursing care and patient outcomes.

KEY CONCEPTS

- Assessment is the first step in determining patient health status.
- Assessment can be comprehensive, focused, ongoing, or emergency depending on the health care setting and needs of the patient.
- Data are collected through the interview, health history, symptom analysis, physical examination, and laboratory and diagnostic tests.
- There are three phases of an assessment interview: orientation, working, and closure.
- Gordon's Functional Health Patterns is an assessment model that enables the nurse to complete a comprehensive health history, determine the patient's functional health patterns, responses to changes in health status, and alterations in lifestyle.
- The health history is a collection of subjective information regarding the patient's health status.

- The physical examination provides a complete picture of the patient's physiological functioning; when combined with a health history, the information forms a database to direct decision making.
- The four assessment techniques used in physical examination are inspection, palpation, percussion, and auscultation.
- Age, culture, ethnicity, gender, and genetic makeup may influence a patient's health and the nurses' health assessment practices.
- Nurses must be able to integrate genetics knowledge, skills, and attitudes into routine health care assessment and practices to provide effective care to patients and their families.
- Reporting information is a critical part of documentation. Findings that require instant attention should be reported immediately and documentation should reflect the action taken.

REVIEW QUESTIONS

1. The health history that is conducted on a patient who presents with suicidal tendencies would most likely be:
   1. Comprehensive assessment
   2. Focused assessment
   3. Ongoing assessment
   4. Emergency assessment

2. Which component of the physical examination is usually conducted with the patient's street clothes on?
   1. Mental status
   2. Integument
   3. Lungs
   4. Musculoskeletal

3. Your patient is describing his headache. He reports that ice packs to the neck and temporal area provide temporary relief. Which characteristic of the symptom analysis best describe the action of the ice packs?
   1. Quality
   2. Associated manifestation
   3. Alleviating factor
   4. Timing

4. The statement "I bumped my head on the floor when I fell" would be recorded in what section of the health history?
   1. Review of systems (ROS)
   2. Reason for seeking care
   3. Nutrition/metabolic pattern
   4. Values/beliefs pattern

5. A diagrammatic representation of the emotional relationships and strength of those bonds among family members is called which of the following?
   1. Family tree
   2. Ecomap
   3. Ecogram
   4. Genogram

6. A female patient needs emergency surgery and is being taken to the operating room before her significant other arrives. She asks you to pray for her. What is an appropriate response?
   1. Grab her hand and tell her that prayer is not something you are used to doing.
   2. Suddenly start wondering if you are comfortable with prayer.
   3. Hold her hand or bow your head and say a brief prayer, silently or aloud.
   4. Hold her hand and pray for her to be forgiven of her sins so she can be healed.

Continued

REVIEW QUESTIONS—cont'd

7. Which of the following ethical principles means to do no harm?
   1. Beneficence
   2. Nonmaleficence
   3. Utilitarianism
   4. Autonomy

8. Which of the following actions would make you more vulnerable to legal action?
   1. Documenting all patient interaction
   2. Knowing your state's Nurse Practice Act
   3. Respecting a patient's right to refuse an examination
   4. Discussing your patient's case in an elevator

9. Which of the following assessments are you capable of performing on a comatose patient?
   1. Corneal reflex
   2. Snellen test
   3. Cerebellar function
   4. Stepping reflex

10. Which of the following is the correct sequence for a complete physical assessment?
    1. Skin, eyes, neck, mouth, and throat
    2. Abdomen, inguinal area, lower extremities, and neurological system
    3. Neurological system, musculoskeletal system, inguinal area, anus, and rectum
    4. Anterior thorax, neck upper extremities, and breasts

11. Which variable can be altered to positively influence the health of a patient?
    1. Age
    2. Race
    3. Gender
    4. Culture

REVIEW ACTIVITIES

1. Identify the Functional Health Patterns for each piece of data in the following list:
   a. Married, no children
   b. BP: 120/80
   c. Labored respirations
   d. History of depression
   e. Requests to void every 30 minutes
   f. Refuses to eat or drink
   g. Extremities flaccid and cool to touch
   h. Husband states that he feels "helpless" and "useless"
   i. Husband demands that wife receive "the sacrament of Communion"
   j. Husband reports that wife had annual "wellness checks"

2. Identify the stage of assessment interview for each of the following statements made by the nurse. Write O for interview preparation, I for introduction, W for working, and C for closure:
   _____   "What brings you to the clinic today?"
   _____   "I spoke with your primary care physician who made the referral for your hospital admission."
   _____   "The last time we met, you told me you were on a diet. I see that your clothes fit much looser and that your face appears thinner. How much weight have you lost?"
   _____   "I have completed the physical examination and our time is about up."

3. Convert the following closed-ended questions to open-ended questions.
   Closed ended: "Do you have children?"
   Open ended:
   Closed ended: "Do you think surgery will help?"
   Open ended:
   Closed ended: "Do you have any questions about the newly prescribed medication?"
   Open ended:

4. A 60-year-old female is recently diagnosed with colon cancer and is aware of the familial risk factors related to bowel caner. She refuses to inform her siblings (who are at risk) of her situation. How could the practice nurse approach this situation?

Genetics and the Multiple Determinants of Health

CHAPTER 9

Sandra K. Cesario, RNC, MS, PhD

Dale Halsey Lea, RN, MPH

CHAPTER TOPICS

- Fundamentals of Genetics
- Patterns of Inheritance
- Screening for Genetic Disease
- Contributions of Genetics to Various Conditions across the Life Span
- Legal, Ethical, and Social Issues Associated with Genetics
- The Human Genome Project
- Gene Therapy and Genetic Engineering
- Resources for Genetic Information

KEY TERMS

Allele
Alpha-fetoprotein (AFP)
Aneuploid
Autosomes
Carrier
Chromosomes
Deletion
Deoxyribonucleic acid (DNA)
Diploid
Euploidy
Gene
Gene therapy
Genetic counseling
Genetic engineering
Genetic screening
Genomics
Genotype
Haploid
Inborn error of metabolism
Karyotype
Locus
Meiosis
Mitosis
Mosaicism
Mutation
Oncogenes
Pedigrees
Pharmacogenomics
Phenotype
Recessive trait
Teratogens
Translocation
Trisomies

The last few decades have brought an explosion in the advancement of genetics as a means to identify and treat a wide host of diseases. As the research continues in this area, new information appears in the media, health care literature, and clinical practice almost daily. With the exception of trauma, all disease has a genetic component. People at risk for certain diseases, individual responses to treatment, and human development (both physical and psychological) are all influenced by genetics. A person's genetic makeup, in combination with the environment, is a major determinant of health. It is this complex interplay of genetic and environmental factors that has led to the creation of a new discipline currently referred to as genomics. **Genomics** is the study of genome composition, structure, and function that has led to the discovery of numerous health care products by identifying new biological targets for the development of drugs and by giving scientists innovative ways to design new drugs, vaccines, and deoxyribonucleic acid (DNA) diagnostics. Information systems, databases, and computerized research tools have joined forces in the Human Genome Project (HGP), a worldwide collaborative effort to identify and record the 30,000 genes and three billion DNA segments that define the human species. The growing public interest in genetics has furthered research and clinical application of new genetic information and technologies making it an integral part of routine health care (Collins, Green, Guttmacher, & Guyer, 2003). Science is now able to map the genetic code of each human being. With this knowledge, the area of genetics provides opportunities for prevention and treatment of disease never thought possible. Advances in molecular biology and genetics have revolutionized health care and opened the door for nursing specialization in this field. These advances and opportunities, however, raise many legal, ethical, and practical questions that nurses need to understand and address if they are to provide the highest quality of care to patients based on the best available evidence.

FUNDAMENTALS OF GENETICS

Genetics is the study of the mechanisms by which genes operate. This encompasses how the DNA affects physiological reactions within the cell and the genetic transmission of various characteristics from generation to generation. This process is referred to as heredity, a complex biological process that results in offspring resembling their parents in some ways yet differing in many others. This variability creates the foundation of the science of genetics. Each person has 23 pairs of **chromosomes** (thread-like structures within the nucleus of a cell that carry the genes) with approximately 30,000 **genes** (a segment of a DNA molecule that is the heredity unit that occupies a fixed chromosomal locus). The regulation and expression of these genes is the result of a complex series of events occurring within each cell (Guttmacher & Collins, 2002; Jenkins, & Lea, 2004). When a **mutation** (a permanent change in genetic material) occurs in the genetic material of a germ cell (ova or sperm), heredity will be affected.

An individual who exhibits a disease or condition that is attributed to the hereditary process is referred to as an affected individual. A person can also be a **carrier** (an individual who is heterozygous for a normal gene and an abnormal gene) of a mutated gene and be unaware of its presence. Only when two parents contribute a similar gene will the condition appear in their offspring. When the DNA of a somatic cell undergoes mutation, only body cells reproduced from that cell will be affected. While there may be a genetic disposition to conditions, such as hypertension, diabetes, cancer, or various forms of infections, the environment often plays a role in triggering the onset of the disease. Multifactorial traits are determined by the interaction of genes and the environment.

Congenital defects are often attributed to an infant being born with too many or too few chromosomes or with one or more chromosomes that are broken or rearranged. Errors in the number or structure of chromosomes cause a wide variety of birth defects ranging from mild to severe.

Structure and Function of Chromosomes and Genes

Deoxyribonucleic acid (DNA) (the molecular basis of heredity, consisting of purine and pyrimidine nucleotides arranged in two long strands, twisted about each other to form a double helix) is the hereditary material contained in the nucleus of each somatic cell, which determines an individual's appearance and health characteristics. The DNA is comprised of tiny string-like structures present in all cells of the body known as chromosomes. Each chromosome contains an estimated 20,000 to 30,000 gene pairs that determine traits, like eye color, hair color, and blood type, as well as direct the growth and development of every part of a person's physical and biochemical systems.

Humans have 23 pairs of homologous (matched) chromosomes for a total of 46 chromosomes. One chromosome of each pair comes from the mother and the other from the father. There are 22 pairs of **autosomes** (any chromosome other than the sex chromosomes), with chromosome number one being the largest and chromosome number twenty-two being the smallest. These 22 determine the majority of traits exhibited by an individual, and one pair of sex chromosomes that determines the biological sex of the offspring. In regard to the sex chromosomes, the female partner always contributes an X chromosome, and the male partner contributes either an X or Y chromosome. Therefore, in a female, the homologous pair of sex chromosomes is XX, and for a male the homologous pair is XY.

The autosomes have the same number and arrangements of genes located on the chromosomes and are arranged neatly in a linear order. The loci of specific genes are always in the same position on the same chromosome in all individuals. **Allele** refers to one of two or more alternative forms of a gene at the same location on a chromosome that determines alternative characteristics in inheritance. When an individual has two copies of the same allele for a specified trait, that person is said to be homozygous for that trait. If the two alleles are different, the person is considered to be heterozygous for the trait.

Genotype is a term that refers to the genetic constitution, or blueprint, of an individual or the actual gene pairs that are inherited from the parents. Phenotype, on the other hand, is the physical, biochemical, and physiological nature of an individual as determined by the genotype and the environment. It is the outward expression of the individual's genes. A dominant trait is expressed whether homozygous or heterozygous. A **recessive trait** is one that is expressed only when an individual is homozygous for that specific gene.

Some characteristics are inherited through single genes; these are called simple genetic traits. There are several patterns or modes of single gene inheritance: autosomal dominant, autosomal recessive, X-linked dominant, and X-linked recessive.

Chromosomal Abnormalities

About 1 in 200 babies are born with a chromosomal abnormality. In addition, 4 to 7 percent of perinatal deaths are attributed to an abnormality in chromosome number or structure. These abnormalities may occur during **mitosis** (somatic cell division resulting in the formation of two cells, each with the same chromosome complement as the parent cell). They may also occur during **meiosis** (a series of two specialized divisions of diploid germ cells to produce four gametes containing the haploid number of chromosomes with the slightest deviation causing abnormal fetal development).

Down syndrome, a condition in which an infant is born with an extra chromosome 21, is one of the most common chromosomal abnormalities. Children with Down syndrome have varying degrees of mental retardation, characteristic facial features, and often, heart defects and other problems.

However, there are many other chromosomal abnormalities besides Down syndrome. Some abnormalities produce syndromes and conditions less severe than Down syndrome, and others are more severe or even fatal. Many individuals with chromosomal abnormalities have mental retardation, learning disabilities, and health or behavioral problems. A comprehensive understanding of chromosome structure and function is crucial in identifying the wide range of problems associated with chromosomal abnormalities.

Abnormalities of Chromosome Number

Genetic abnormalities can occur for a variety of reasons. Sometimes, an error occurs during cell division causing an error in chromosome number either before or shortly after conception. The embryo then develops from cells that have either too many or too few chromosomes. In the majority of circumstances, an embryo with the wrong number of chromosomes will not survive. Oftentimes the pregnant woman will experience a miscarriage without knowing the pregnancy had occurred. It is believed that up to 70 percent of first trimester miscarriages can be attributed to chromosomal abnormalities.

Euploidy is a term referring to the correct number of chromosomes in a cell. **Diploid** is two complete sets of chromosomes, double the number present in gametes (ova or sperm cells). In humans, the diploid number is 46, and it refers to having two complete sets of chromosomes. **Haploid** refers to having one complete set of chromosomes. The haploid number in humans is 23.

Aneuploidy is a condition in which the numerical deviation is not an exact multiple of the haploid number, resulting in an extra or missing chromosome, and is the most common chromosomal abnormality to affect humans. Pregnancy loss and genetically caused mentally retardation are frequently linked to aneuploidy. The two most commonly identified **aneuploid** conditions are monosomies and trisomies.

Monosomies

In monosomy, one member of a chromosome pair is missing. There are only 45 chromosomes in each cell. One of the more common monosomic conditions is monosomy X, or Turner syndrome. Individuals with monosomy X are phenotypically female but have gonadal dysgenesis or streak ovaries and short stature. Monosomy X is a common condition found in stillborn babies as well. Conditions of monosomy, other than monosomy X, are not compatible with extra-uterine life.

Trisomies

Trisomies (three of a given chromosome instead of the usual two) are more common than monosomies and are the result of a failure of a chromosome pair to separate properly during cell division. These individuals have 47 chromosomes in each cell. As mentioned previously, Down syndrome is the most common trisomy with an additional chromosome 21. Individuals can also be born with extra copies of chromosomes 13 or 18. The conditions produced by these trisomies are usually more severe than Down syndrome. Babies with trisomy 13 (Patau syndrome) or trisomy 18 (Edward syndrome) generally have profound mental retardation and numerous physical birth defects. Many of these infants will not survive past the first year of life.

Most trisomies are a result of maternal meiosis I errors. This is known as nondisjunction and is the product of one pair of chromosomes failing to separate during the first meiotic cell division. The result is one cell that contains both chromosomes and one cell that has none.

Mosaicism

Mosaicism (tissue composed of cells of two different genotypes or karyotypes) occurs when two different cell types are present in a single person. There are two types of mosaicism: germline and somatic. In somatic mosaicism there is an error of nondisjunction that occurs during mitosis early in embryonic development when cell lines are forming. As a result, the mosaic individual has a mixture of cells, some with a normal number of chromosomes, some with an extra chromosome, and yet others with a missing chromosome. The relative proportion of each cell line is highly variable, both between people and within different tissues and organs in the same person. The prognosis for intelligence presumably depends on the proportion of abnormal cells in the brain. In germline mosaicism the mutation is confined to a portion of the germ cells (ova or sperm). The mutation can be transmitted to offspring. Loss of a large portion of a chromosome may be lethal. However, there are cases in which a small portion of a chromosome can be lost, and the individual still survives. This **deletion** involves the loss of varying amounts of genetic material that is detectable at the DNA or chromosomal level.

In humans, a rare condition known as cri-du-chat syndrome is associated with a deletion on the short arm of chromosome 5. The name of this syndrome is French for "cry of the cat." These children have a distinctive cry caused by abnormal larynx development. Infants with cri-du-chat usually have low birth weight and respiratory difficulties during the neonatal period.

Abnormalities of Chromosome Structure

Other accidents also can occur, usually before pregnancy begins, that can alter the structure of one or more chromosomes. While such individuals may have the normal number of chromosomes, small pieces of a chromosome (or chromosomes) may be deleted, duplicated, inverted, misplaced, or exchanged with part of another chromosome. These structural rearrangements, or mutations, may result in pregnancy loss and congenital anomalies.

These uncommon abnormalities include translocations (a section of a chromosome is attached to another chromosome); deletions (small missing sections); microdeletions (a minute amount of missing material that may include only a single gene); and inversions (a section of chromosome is snipped out and reinserted upside down).

Translocation

Translocation, affecting 1 out of every 500 newborns, is the transfer of a segment of one chromosome to a nonhomologous chromosome. When no material is lost or gained, the translocation is balanced. The parts of two chromosomes are exchanged equally. Balanced translocations in which there is no net loss or gain of chromosome material are usually not associated with phenotypic abnormalities but may have an increased risk of miscarriage or chromosome abnormalities in their own children. Gene disruptions at the breakpoints of the translocation can, in some cases, cause adverse effects.

An unbalanced **translocation** occurs when a part of a chromosome is transferred to a different chromosome. There is loss of chromosomal material on one chromosome and a gain on another. This nearly always yields an abnormal phenotype. Translocations may either be inherited from a parent or arise spontaneously in a child's own chromosomes. Translocation can be caused by drugs, viruses, radiation, or for no apparent reason. A small number of parents of children with Down syndrome have a chromosomal rearrangement that does not affect their own health but can be harmful when passed on to their offspring. Following the birth of a child with a genetic condition, a counselor may recommend genetic testing to determine if the parents carry such a rearrangement so the parents can be given the most accurate picture of their risk of having another child with this type of Down syndrome.

Deletions and Microdeletions

Sometimes it is not the number of chromosomes that is the problem. Instead, one or more chromosomes are incomplete or abnormally shaped. In both deletions and microdeletions, for example, some small part of a chromosome is missing. Loss of chromosomal material at the end of a chromosome is described as terminal deletion. If the loss of chromosomal material occurs at another place along the chromosome, it is referred to as interstitial deletion.

In a microdeletion, the missing part of a chromosome is usually so small that it amounts to being just a single gene or only a few genes. These abnormalities cannot be normally be detected with standard cytogenetic techniques. A newer technology called fluorescent in situ hybridization (FISH) uses a single-stranded piece of DNA with a florescent label that will adhere to is complementary piece of DNA in the chromosome being examined and identify the missing gene or genes. Some important genetic disorders caused by deletions and microdeletions include Wolf-Hirschhorn syndrome (chromosome 4), William's syndrome (chromosome 7), Prader-Willi syndrome (chromosome 15), and DiGeorge syndrome (chromosome 22).

Inversion

Inversion is a deviation in which small parts of the DNA code seem to be snipped out and reinserted in a reverse order. Few congenital anomalies are associated with this chromosomal abnormality, but this condition may be responsible for infertility and spontaneous abortion. When it is identified, inversions are most frequently found on chromosome 9.

Chromosomal Breakage

Chromosomal breakage syndromes are a group of genetic disorders that typically are transmitted in an autosomal recessive mode of inheritance. When cultured, cells from affected individuals exhibit elevated rates of chromosomal breakage or instability, leading to chromosomal rearrangements. The disorders are characterized by a defect in DNA repair mechanisms or genomic instability, and patients with these disorders show increased predisposition to cancer.

These disorders occur infrequently. Some of the specific syndromes occur at relatively high rates in certain ethnic groups and may be lethal. Diagnosis is complicated, because the symptoms may be varied and complex. Ataxia telangiectasia (AT), or Louis-Bar syndrome, Bloom syndrome (BS), Fanconi anemia (FA), and xeroderma pigmentosum (XP) are examples of chromosomal breakage syndromes. These diagnoses are characterized by different types of cancer, including leukemia, lymphoma, and skin cancer. Other traits, such as cerebellar ataxia, immunodeficiencies, growth retardation, microcephaly, skeletal abnormalities, hypogonadism, pancytopenia, and abnormal pigmentation, are also common. Complications in these disorders make therapy difficult.

Abnormalities of Sex Chromosomes

Two of the 46 total human chromosomes are called sex chromosomes. Sex chromosomes come in two types, X and Y. Individuals with two X chromosomes are female, and those with one X and one Y chromosome are male. If a gene is located on the X chromosome, it is called X-linked. In an X-linked dominant disease, only one copy of the disease gene is necessary to cause disease in both males and females. In an X-linked recessive disease, males are affected if they carry a single copy of the disease gene on their single X chromosome, whereas females are affected only if they carry two copies of the disease gene, one on each of their two X chromosomes. Because it is more likely that someone will inherit one rather than two copies of an abnormal gene, X-linked diseases are much more common in males than in females.

Abnormalities of the sex chromosomes are caused by nondisjunction that occurs during gametogenesis in either parent. Turner syndrome (Bonnevie-Ullrich syndrome) is the most common abnormality affecting girls and occurs in about 1 in 4,000 live female births. These females have only one X chromosome and exhibit juvenile external genitalia, short stature, webbed neck, and lymphedema of the hands and feet. Turner syndrome females will also have undeveloped ovaries and learning issues. Most affected embryos are aborted spontaneously.

About 1 in 1,000 to 2,000 females has an extra X chromosome, referred to as triple X or 47,XXX. These girls, who tend to be tall, have no consistent pattern of physical abnormalities, undergo normal puberty, and appear to be fertile. Intelligence is normal, though learning disabilities are fairly common. Because these girls are healthy and have a normal appearance, parents are most likely to know their daughter has this chromosomal abnormality only if they have undergone prenatal testing.

Although rare, 48,XXXX, also known as tetra-X, and 49,XXXXX, also known as penta-X, females have been identified. There is no consistent phenotype. The risk of mental retardation and congenital abnormalities increases markedly with an increase in the number of X chromosomes.

Klinefelter syndrome is a sex chromosome alteration that affects about 1 in 600 to 800 boys. Boys with Klinefelter syndrome have two, or occasionally more, X chromosomes in addition to their Y chromosome. Affected males exhibit poorly developed secondary sex characteristics, small testes, infertility, tall stature, and learning problems. They often have more problems with judgment and impulse control than XY males. As adults, they produce lower than normal amounts of the male hormone testosterone and are infertile.

Other X-linked conditions include fragile X syndrome, hemophilia, and Duchenne muscular dystrophy. Females are usually carriers of these conditions and do not exhibit symptoms, because they also inherit a normal X chromosome. Males, on the other hand, only have one X chromosome and are almost always the ones who exhibit the disorder.

Intersex states are conditions in which the appearance of the external genitalia is either ambiguous or at variance with the chromosomal or gonadal sex of the individual. The genitalia form during the first three months of gestation. Aberrations occurring during this time period may produce genital ambiguities or inconsistencies, resulting in intersex states.

Female pseudohermaphrodites have ovaries and normal female internal genitalia but ambiguous external genitalia. They are genetically normal females with a 46,XX karyotype. The ambiguous external genitalia result from exposure to excessive amounts of androgens in utero.

Male pseudohermaphrodites have gonadal tissue that is only testicular and usually have a normal 46,XY karyotype. The external genitalia are usually ambiguous. True hermaphrodites have both ovarian and testicular tissue and mixed masculine and feminine genital structures depending on whether ovarian or testicular tissue predominates.

Assessment of affected intersex newborns is urgent, not only to establish sex because of social pressures but also to correct physiological and metabolic abnormalities. A blood sample should be drawn immediately for karyotyping, but results may require several days. Meanwhile, a pelvic ultrasound may offer parents some information regarding the biological sex of their child. Laparoscopy or surgical exploration with biopsy of gonadal tissue may be required to establish a definitive diagnosis. Sex assignment should be made as soon as possible but should not be based on what appears to be the biological sex of the infant.

PATTERNS OF INHERITANCE

Gregor Mendel first introduced the concept of heredity when he described genes in 1865. However, his findings were largely ignored, because they did not conform to the conventional beliefs of the time—that parental traits undergo blending in an offspring. Through a series of experiments involving peas, Mendel showed that there are independent units of heredity that are transmitted unchanged from generation to generation. Mendel studied traits in the pea that are characterized by single genes. These included height (tall plant versus short plant), seed shape (round versus wrinkled), and seed color (yellow versus green). When he crossed tall pea plants (homozygous TT) with short pea plants (homozygous tt), Mendel observed that the offspring were all tall (heterozygous Tt). The trait of shortness appeared to have been lost. However, in subsequent experiments, the first generation of tall pea plants (heterozygous Tt) were crossed with each other, and the short pea plant reappeared. This is the basis of the commonly used Punnett Square for illustrating homozygous and heterozygous traits.

The Punnett Square is also used to communicate the concept of genotype and phenotype (Figure 9-1). As presented previously in the chapter, genotype refers to the nature of the genes (or alleles) at a particular **locus** (the position of a gene on a chromosome) on a pair of chromosomes. **Phenotype** refers to the physical or biochemical characteristics of an organism.

The units of heredity, or genes, are DNA sequences that code for the synthesis of proteins. The DNA sequences are made of the nucleotide bases adenine, guanine, cytosine, and thymine. A gene is composed of several exons (coding sequences) and introns (intervening sequences). Like chromosomes, genes are inherited in pairs, one from each parent. The pattern in which heritable characteristics appear in subsequent generations is affected by the number of genes involved in the expression of the trait. If a phenotypic characteristic is the result of two or more genes on different chromosomes acting together, the trait is determined by multifactorial inheritance. When a single gene determines a trait, unifactorial inheritance is the mode of heredity in operation.

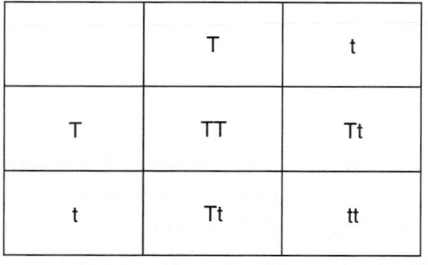

	T	t
T	TT	Tt
t	Tt	tt

Figure 9-1 The Punnett Square.

Mendelian (Single Gene) Inheritance

Some genetic problems are caused by a single gene that is present but altered in some way and may be referred to as gene mutations. The number and appearance of the larger chromosome is usually normal. Mendelian, or unifactorial, genetic disorders are disorders caused by a single gene mutation that leads to an abnormality that is generally confined to a single organ system. For example, the skeletal system is affected in achondroplasia (dwarfism), the hematological system in sickle cell disease, and the central nervous system (CNS) in Huntington disease. However, there can be widespread effects of the disorder if several tissues or organs in conditions, such as mucopolysaccharidoses, need an enzyme or protein.

The number of unifactorial gene disorders far exceeds the number of chromosomal defects. With some 30,000 genes on each of the 23 chromosomes, single gene mutations are more likely to occur than abnormalities involving the entire chromosome (Jenkins & Lea, 2004). Some of these abnormalities are so rare that they have been known to affect only a few individuals. Recently, scientists have discovered genetic links to many different diseases that historically have not been thought of as genetic, including several different types of cancer. Single gene disorders follow the patterns of inheritance as described by Mendel almost 150 years ago. These include autosomal dominant, autosomal recessive, and the X-linked modes of inheritance.

Autosomal Dominant Inheritance

Autosomal means that males or females are equally affected, because the abnormal gene that is located on one of the nonsex chromosomes. In autosomal dominant inherited disorders, only one copy of the abnormal gene is needed for phenotypic expression. If the gene is inherited it will result in an affected individual. When a parent carries an autosomal dominant gene mutation, each of his or her offspring has a 50 percent chance to inherit the mutation.

Autosomal dominant inherited conditions are often seen in multiple generations. Examples of such conditions are Huntington disease, Marfan syndrome, and neurofibromatosis. In some cases penetrance may not be complete in some individuals, resulting in a mild form of the condition. Occasionally, a condition with autosomal dominant inheritance may arise with no preceding family history because of a mutation in ova or sperm.

Autosomal Recessive Inheritance

An autosomal recessive pattern of inheritance is one in which both copies of a gene must be altered for a genetic condition or disease to become apparent or visible. Two carriers must each contribute an altered gene to the offspring. In this form of inheritance, the altered gene, located on a nonsex chromosome, is recessive, and the parents are often unaware that they are carriers of the gene. In contrast to autosomal dominant inherited conditions, autosomal recessive inherited conditions are usually seen in a single generation of a family.

A carrier is heterozygous for that characteristic. When both parents are carriers and do not express the trait, the chance for them to have an affected child will be 25 percent for each pregnancy (Figure 9-2). Except in cases of consanguineous partners, the chance of marrying a carrier of the same recessive gene is low, though the incidence of the existence of recessive genes in the population varies with condition. **Genetic counseling** (the interaction between health care provider and patient to manage the human problems associated with the occurrence, or risk of occurrence, of a genetic disorder in a family) can help to predict the occurrence for individual families.

Tay-Sachs disease, sickle cell disease, and cystic fibrosis (CF) fall in the category of autosomal recessive inherited diseases. Inborn errors of metabolism (IEM), such as phenylketonuria (PKU) and galactosemia, are inherited in this pattern as well. Defective enzyme action interrupts normal metabolism causing a series of chemical reactions in the affected individual. More than 350 IEM have been identified. While each IEM is quite rare, collectively they account for many diseases (Deodato, et al., 2004).

(A) When both parents carry the disease gene, there is a 25% chance that each child conceived will not have the disease or carry the disease. There is a 50% chance that each child conceived will carry the gene, and a 25% chance that each child conceived will have the disease.

	B	b
B	BB 25% Normal	Bb 25% Carrier
b	Bb 25% Carrier	bb 25% Disease

(B) When one parent has the disease and the other is a carrier for the disease, there is a 50% chance that each child conceived will carry the disease and a 50% chance that each child conceived will have the disease.

	b	b
B	Bb 25% Carrier	Bb 25% Carrier
b	bb 25% Disease	bb 25% Disease

Legend
b = Recessive disease gene
B = Dominant normal gene
bb = Disease state
Bb or bB = Carrier state
BB = Normal state

Figure 9-2 Autosomal recessive inheritance.

X-Linked Dominant Inheritance

X-linked dominant disorders occur in males and heterozygous females. Females are usually less severely affected, because they have a normal gene to offset the effects of the abnormal gene on the second X chromosome. An affected female will have a 50 percent chance of passing the disorder on to sons and daughters. An affected male will pass the condition on to all his daughters but not to his sons.

Examples of this type of inheritance are D-resistant Rickets, Coffin-Lowry syndrome, and fragile X syndrome (Figure 9-3). Fragile X syndrome causes a wide range of mental impairment, from mild learning disabilities to severe mental retardation. It is the most common cause of genetically inherited mental impairment. In addition to mental impairment, fragile X syndrome is associated with a number of physical and behavioral characteristics.

X-Linked Recessive Inheritance

In this situation, the abnormal gene is also located on the X chromosome. However, females may be heterozygous or homozygous for the trait, because they have two X chromosomes. Only homozygous females and hemizygous males (because they only have one X chromosome) will manifest the disease. Most often, this means that females are carriers and males are affected by the disorder. A female carrier has a 50 percent chance to pass on the gene mutation to her daughters who would be carriers, and a 50 percent chance to pass the gene mutation on to her sons, who would be affected. Affected men will not pass the condition on to their sons, but all their daughters will be carriers.

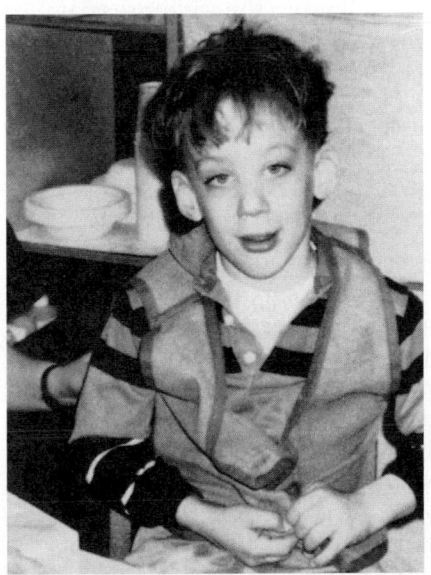

Figure 9-3 Young boy with fragile X syndrome.

Examples of X-linked recessive disorders include color blindness, Duchenne muscular dystrophy, hemophilia, and Hunter disease.

Non-Mendelian (Multifactorial, Polygenic) Inheritance

Many disorders exhibit familial clustering that does not fit into any recognized pattern of Mendelian inheritance. The list of examples is quite lengthy and includes most congenital malformations and acquired diseases that occur over the life span. Cleft lip or palate, congenital heart defects, neural tube defects, pyloric stenosis, asthma, autism, diabetes, arthritis, heart disease, and schizophrenia are some of these disorders, to name a few. It is believed that many factors, both genetic and environmental, are involved in causing these disorders to appear. Also, many genes may play a role in the development of some disorders, hence the term polygenetic. A disease state, such as insulin-dependent diabetes mellitus, probably involves many loci with some genes having more influence than others.

Multifactorial disorders are common and make a major contribution to human morbidity and mortality. Yet the genetic mechanisms underlying these disorders are not well understood. Extensive research is being done to identify clear connections between gene characteristics and the environmental triggers that cause the disorder to be manifested. This is amply demonstrated by the beneficial effect of folic acid supplementation in preventing neural tube defects.

Principles of Teratology

Teratology is a branch of the biological sciences that is concerned with the development of malformations or deviations from normal patterns of development. While this is an important field of study, many factors hinder our ability to understand **teratogens** (an agent that produces or increases the incidence of congenital malformations) and their effect on human development and disease. Among these are the limitations of animal and epidemiological studies, the lack of understanding of the mechanisms of action of most teratogens, and the variability in expression of the clinical manifestation. Dose and timing of exposure, interactions with other environmental agents, and host susceptibility influence this variable expressivity. The adverse effects on human development of exposure of an embryo or fetus to exogenous chemical agents were first recognized and studied following the widespread use of thalidomide in 1961, which resulted in numerous and profound birth defects. Wilson (1973) developed six general principles of teratology that continue to be useful today.

SCREENING FOR GENETIC DISEASE

Genetic counseling is a communication process that translates complicated medical information into understandable terms and explores the implications of this information for the individual and his or her family. The goals of genetic counseling are to help individuals and their families (a) understand the genetic condition and how it is inherited, (b) adjust to the personal and family issues related to the genetic condition, and (c) provide comprehensive information so that informed decisions about health care can be made.

The principles of **genetic screening** (a systematic search of a population for individuals with genotypes indicating they are at risk for genetic disease) were clearly defined in the report of the subcommittee on screening of the American College of Medical Genetics Clinical Practice Committee (Edgar, 2004). Screening for genetic disease or genetic predisposition to disease is an opportunity to prevent or minimize the effects of the deviation. Distinctions must be made between carrier screening, screening for predisposition to disease, screening for presymptomatic disease, and screening for those affected with disease. Newborn screening represents an example of population-based screening as opposed to selective screening where a specified subset of the population is targeted. Screening for clinical purposes should be tied to the availability of intervention, including prenatal diagnosis, counseling, reproductive decision making, lifestyle changes, and enhanced phenotype screening (Lewis, 2002).

An essential component of any screening program is a follow-up evaluation and counseling by genetic professionals. People with positive results may experience a high degree of anxiety and fear stigmatization. They require education, support, and prompt intervention. Counseling of individuals with negative results may also be necessary in some cases and should not be overlooked (Harman, 2003).

All screening results are to remain confidential. The results may only be revealed to the participant and the participant's personal health care provider. Research programs should apply for a certificate of confidentiality. Because of potential problems of insurability and employability for carriers or affected individuals, participants may not want their insurance company or employer to know they are having the screening test performed. This may place the burden of payment for the screening test on the participant. Tests should be simple, accurate, and relatively inexpensive. They should identify most of the carriers and affected people (high sensitivity) with few false positives (high specificity). Sensitivity, specificity, and predictive value should be appropriate for the screening venue. Acceptable sensitivity and specificity will depend on the a priori risk of the screened population, and may vary for individuals within the population (Ciarleglio, Bennett, Williamson, Mandell, & Marks, 2003).

Gene Testing

Gene tests, also called DNA-based tests, are the newest and most sophisticated techniques used to test for genetic disorders and involve direct examination of the DNA molecule itself (Table 9-1) (Tantravahi & Wheeler, 2003). Other genetic tests include biochemical tests for such gene products as enzymes and other proteins and for microscopic examination of stained or fluorescent chromosomes.

TABLE 9-1 Genetic Tests	
Carrier screening	Used for the identification of unaffected individuals who carry one copy of a gene for a disease that requires two copies for the disease to be expressed
Preimplantation genetic diagnosis	Genetic testing and analysis performed on early embryos (formed from in vitro fertilization) prior to implantation during pregnancy
Prenatal diagnostic testing	Testing performed during pregnancy to determine whether a congenital abnormality, genetic syndrome, or other genetic condition is present in the fetus
Newborn screening	Population-based testing designed to identify infants who are at higher risk of having or developing a metabolic or genetic disorder
Presymptomatic testing	Used for predicting adult-onset disorders, such as Huntington disease, or for estimating the risk of developing adult-onset cancers and Alzheimer's disease
Confirmational diagnosis	Used for the symptomatic individual and for confirming a practitioner's medical diagnosis
Forensic testing	Used for genetic identity testing

Adapted from Tantravahi, U., & Wheeler, P. (2003). Molecular genetic testing for prenatal diagnosis. Clinics in Laboratory Medicine, 23(2), 481–502.

DOLLARS AND SENSE

The Cost of Genetic Testing

CONDITION TESTED FOR	TESTING COST	RELATED COST ISSUES
Breast and ovarian cancer—tests for genetic changes associated with hereditary forms of these cancers	$585–$3,311	Requires testing an affected family member for most accurate result; does not include cost of genetic counseling
Thrombophilia—tests for factor V Leiden and other genetic changes associated with increased risk for thrombosis	$380	May involve additional cost of genetic counseling
Hemochromatosis—tests for genetic causes of iron overload	$199	May involve additional cost of genetic counseling
Cystic fibrosis (CF)—tests for common genetic changes associated with CF	$260	May involve testing affected relative to identify CF mutation in the family. May involved cost of genetic counseling.

Source: DNAdirect. (2006). Genetic testing. Retrieved July 10, 2006, from www.dnadirect.org.

There are advantages and disadvantages of gene testing. Gene testing has already dramatically improved many lives. Some tests are used to clarify a diagnosis and direct a health care provider toward appropriate treatments, and others allow families to avoid having children with devastating diseases or identify people at high risk for conditions that may be preventable (Braun, Roth, & McGinniss, 2003). Aggressive monitoring for, and removal of, colon growths in those inheriting a gene for familial adenomatous polyposis, for example, has saved many lives. Other genetic tests are now available that provide doctors with a simple diagnostic test for common conditions, such as thrombophilia, cancer, and hemochromatosis. Of major concern is the issue of equal access to this testing, because genetic testing may or may not be covered by insurance, Medicaid, or Medicare.

Commercialized gene tests for adult-onset disorders, such as Alzheimer's disease and some cancers, are the subject of most of the debate over gene testing. These tests are targeted to healthy (presymptomatic) people who are identified as being at high risk because of a strong family medical history for the disorder. The tests give only a probability for developing the disorder. One of the most serious limitations of these susceptibility tests is the difficulty in interpreting a positive result, because some people who carry a disease-associated mutation never develop the disease. Scientists believe that these mutations may work together with other, unknown mutations or with environmental factors to cause disease (Botstein & Risch, 2003).

A limitation of all medical testing is the possibility for laboratory errors. These might be because of sample misidentification, contamination of the chemicals used for testing, or other factors. Many in the medical establishment feel that uncertainties surrounding test interpretation, the current lack of available medical options for these diseases, the tests' potential for provoking anxiety, and risks for discrimination and social stigmatization could outweigh the benefits of testing.

Screening embryos for disease is another area of heated controversy. Preimplantation genetic diagnosis (PGD) is a test that identifies errors in genetic material in embryos used for in vitro fertilization. The embryos that were created in vitro from the egg and sperm of biological parents are analyzed for gene abnormalities that can cause genetic disorders. Fertility specialists will then select only mutation-free embryos for implantation into the mother's uterus. Before the availability of PGD, parents at high risk for conceiving a child with a genetic disorder would have to initiate the pregnancy and then undergo chorionic villus sampling (CVS) in the first trimester or amniocentesis in the second trimester to test the fetus for the presence of disease. If the fetus tested positive for the disorder, the couple would be faced with the dilemma of whether or not to terminate the pregnancy.

Family Screening

Whether a child has a rare or common chromosomal abnormality, it is important that he or she be evaluated as an individual. Even people with apparently identical chromosomal abnormalities can differ from each other substantially. New techniques of analyzing chromosomes sometimes can pinpoint exactly where missing or extra genetic material comes from. If doctors know what genes may be contained in that section and their function, they can sometimes give parents a better prediction of a child's future development.

Parents who have had a baby with a chromosomal abnormality should consult a genetic counselor. Information regarding the family history is collected for at least three generations. The historical information that is obtained from family members is then verified with medical records. Health professionals then help families understand what is known about the causes of a birth defect and the chances that it will recur in another pregnancy. The options for managing the risks associated with a genetic condition are then presented to the family in a nondirective manner. The goal of presenting these choices is to enable the family to make informed decisions appropriate for their personal situation.

In addition to the family and medical history, comprehensive clinical genetic evaluation usually involves the creation of an individual pedigree, genogram (Figure 9-4), genetic laboratory studies, such as a chromosome analysis, DNA tests, and other biochemical studies as indicated. Genetic register services can also be used to incorporate long-term care for families to improve access to care and reduce psychological stressors associated with being a carrier for some genetic diseases (Wright, et al., 2002).

Population Screening

Population genetics is a discipline studying genetic variation in defined populations, including relevant aspects of population structure and geographic variability of DNA sequences and their frequencies. Population genetics deals with

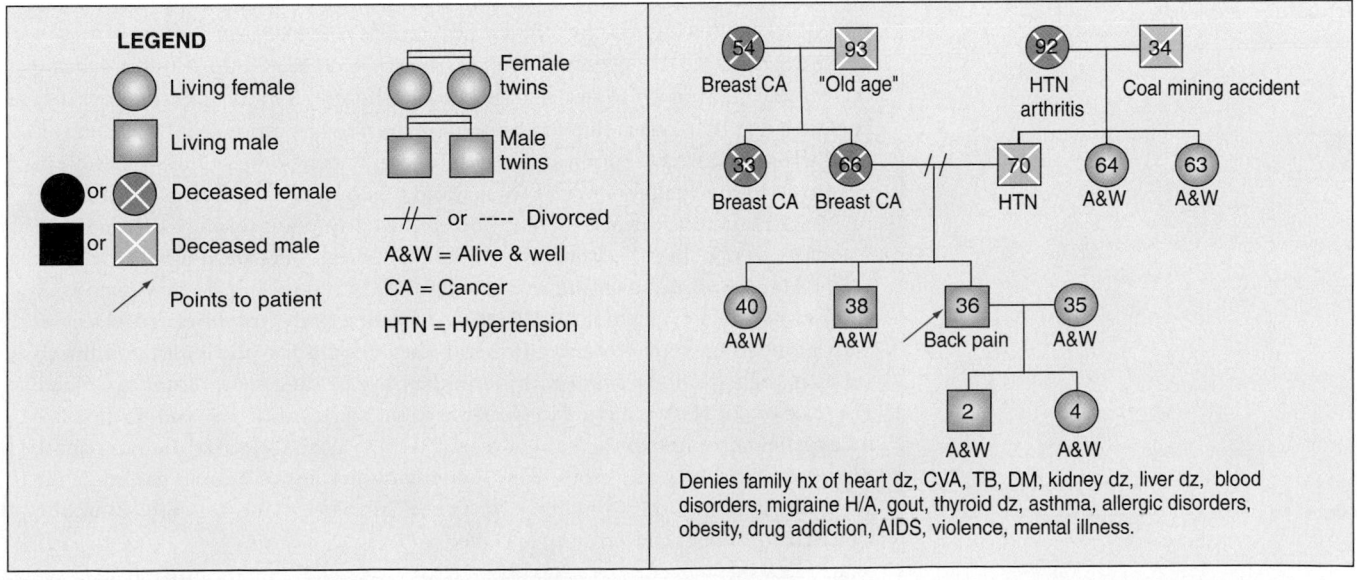

Figure 9-4 Family history and genogram.

the characteristics of genes within a population as opposed to the description of the genes in a particular individual (Khoury, McCabe, & McCabe, 2003).

Population screening programs are designed to screen large masses of people for particular disease genes. Examples of this might be screening for thalassemia in Cypress or PKU in newborns in the United States. Many of the issues in current genetic screening programs are relevant to population genetics research but differ on the notion of group consent. Therefore the ethical considerations must be carefully treated, because whole groups of asymptomatic individuals are the targets rather than single individuals who seek their own screening (Schultz, Caldwell, & Foster, 2003).

Screening in the Workplace

A special type of population screening is the screening for genetic traits in the workplace. Many countries around the world, including the United States, have considered legislation addressing the issue of genetic testing for employees. Just as companies have instituted policies on drug and alcohol screening, there have been proposals to incorporate genetic test results in making employment decisions, deny health coverage, or raise insurance premiums.

Fast Forward ▶▶▶

Genome Scanning

New genetic tests are using a laboratory method that involves a type of DNA chip called a microarray. The microarray analysis is a glass slide that has tiny dots of DNA from different genes arranged in a grid-like array. Microarray analysis allows researchers to test the activity of thousands of known genes in a cell sample. To do this, scientists isolate messenger ribonucleic acid (RNA) from the molecules to identify which of the 30,000 genes are "turned on" in a cell. The information from the messenger RNA is converted to a form of DNA called complementary DNA (cDNA). A fluorescent label is attached to the cDNA, and a robot is used to place the cDNA onto the glass slide. When the sample of cDNA matches the particular gene on the microarray, the cDNA sticks to that spot, like two pieces of Velcro coming together. Computerized detectors then measure the amount of fluorescence for each spot. The brighter the fluorescence, the more active the gene must be in that sample. Results of the microarray analysis appear as a pattern of spots showing whether the known gene is active or not.

Researchers at the National Human Genome Research Institute are using microarray technology to distinguish between hereditary and sporadic forms of breast cancer. The research team examined samples of tumors that had been surgically removed from 22 individuals with breast cancer. Some of the women were known to have hereditary breast cancer and a known mutation in either BRCA1 or BRCA2 hereditary cancer genes. The control group was women with sporadic breast cancer. Using the microarray analyses, researchers were able to quickly and accurately distinguish the women with BRCA1 mutation from women with BRCA2 hereditary changes and from the women with noninherited changes. This pioneering work is now leading to better designs for prevention and intervention strategies for women with hereditary breast cancer. Dr. Frances Collins, Director of the National Human Genome Research Institute has said this work is an excellent example of the kind of research that will characterize the next phase of the HGP, as scientists move from sequencing the entire human genetic code to understanding the functions of genes in health and disease (Tambor, Bernhardt, Rodgers, Holtzman, & Geller, 2002).

In some instances genetic screening can prevent susceptible persons from substances that are harmful. Individuals with the sickle cell trait, for example, may be at increased risk for sickle cell anemia if exposed to carbon monoxide or cyanide. Exposure to lead or benzene can be especially hazardous to the health of people with the thalassemia gene. However, as genetic testing becomes more accessible and less costly, tests able to detect a wide range of common genetic disorders, including predisposition to heart disease, cancer, and manic depression, may become commonplace.

History and Physical Examination

A person's family and medical history and physical examination can be used to screen for potential genetic conditions. A medical history indicating that a woman had a deep vein thrombosis (DVT) at an early age and who has a family history of DVT would suggest the possibility of an inherited thrombophilia, such as the factor V Leiden. Testing for the factor V Leiden gene mutation and other risk factors for thrombophilia would be indicated for this woman to prevent pregnancy complications. Such testing would also be recommended before prescribing oral contraceptives as this may increase the woman's risk for thrombosis (Jenkins & Lea, 2004).

A family history is a screening tool to identify individuals who may have a higher risk of developing a genetic condition or of having children with a genetic condition. The Centers for Disease Control (CDC) and the Surgeon General recommend that individuals record and examine their family history to look for potential health risks.

Physical examination of an infant, child, or adult may reveal variations from normal that suggest the presence of a genetic condition. As an example, the presence of low tone (hypotonia), excessive nuchal fold, and upslanting palpebral fissures in an infant suggest the possibility of Down syndrome (Figure 9-5). Identification of multiple café-au-lait spots on a child could indicate the presence of neurofibromatosis, while tall stature, mitral valve prolapse, and scoliosis may be clinical signs of Marfan syndrome. In each of these situations, further genetic evaluation and testing is indicated.

Laboratory Studies

Genetic testing laboratory studies are increasingly used for screening, diagnosis, and treatment of genetic conditions. Genetic testing is often recommended as a component of a genetic evaluation and counseling when a genetic condition is suspected. Genetic testing involves the analysis of human DNA, RNA, chromosomes, proteins, or certain metabolites to identify alterations related to a heritable disorder. Genetic testing is done by directly examining the DNA or RNA that makes up a gene (direct testing), examining markers coinherited with a disease-causing gene (linkage testing), assaying certain metabolites (biochemical testing), or examining the chromosomes (cytogenetic testing). The process of genetic testing for screening and diagnosis of a genetic condition may involve multiple testing methodologies. In some situations, other family members may need to be tested.

A **karyotype** is an organized profile of a person's chromosomes. In a karyotype, chromosomes are arranged and numbered by size, from largest to smallest. This arrangement helps scientists quickly identify chromosomal alterations that may result in a genetic disorder. To make a karyotype, scientists take a picture of someone's chromosomes, cut them out, and match them up using size, banding pattern, and centromere position as guides. Metaphase cells are required to prepare a standard karyotype, and virtually any population of dividing cells could be used. Blood is easily the most frequently sampled tissue, but at times karyotypes are prepared from cultured skin fibroblasts or bone marrow cells. None of the leukocytes in blood normally divide, but lympho-

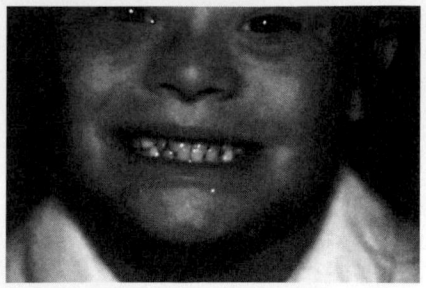

Figure 9-5 Spacing abnormality of the teeth in a patient with Down syndrome.

cytes can readily be induced to proliferate, providing an accessible source of metaphase cells (Botstein & Risch, 2003).

Once stained slides are prepared, they are scanned to identify "good" chromosome spreads (i.e., the chromosomes are not too long or too compact and are not overlapping), which are photographed. A digital image of the chromosomes is cut and pasted using a computer. If standard staining was used, the orderly arrangement is limited to grouping like-sized chromosomes together in pairs, whereas if the chromosomes were banded, they can be unambiguously paired and numbered. Karyotypes are presented in a standard form. First, the total number of chromosomes is given, followed by a comma and the sex chromosome constitution. Coding of any autosomal abnormalities follows this shorthand description.

Prenatal Procedures

There are many methods used to identify defects prenatally when a woman is at risk of delivering an infant with an abnormality (Table 9-2) (Lewis, 2002). Families at risk are those in which there is a history of anomaly, ethnic populations at high-risk for certain conditions, such as sickle-cell anemia or Tay Sachs disease, a woman of advanced age, or the parents who have previously had one child with a birth defect.

Prenatal screening for CF is a way of testing couples to find those who have a high risk of having a baby with CF. If the couple chooses to have the screening test the parents of the expected baby should send samples to the testing center as soon as possible. This test uses DNA from cheek cells not blood, so it is easy to get a sample. But sometimes not enough cells to sample are given, or too much time goes by between the day a sample is taken and the day it gets to the lab, and the test can not be performed.

Amniocentesis

Amniocentesis is a procedure by which a sample of amniotic fluid is aspirated through the uterine and abdominal wall with a sterile syringe guided by ultrasonography. The sample of fluid is then analyzed and certain biochemical, chromosomal, or neural tube defects can be identified. Results may take three to four weeks. Amniocentesis can identify single gene disorders (e.g. CF); metabolic diseases in which the affected enzyme has been previously identified; chromosome defects; and neural tube defects, such as spina bifida.

TABLE 9-2	Prenatal Diagnosis Procedures		
PROCEDURE	**TECHNIQUE (ULTRASOUND GUIDED)**	**SAMPLE**	**TIMING IN GESTATION**
Chorionic villus sampling (CVS)	Needle inserted through mother's abdomen or catheter through cervix	Chorionic villus	10–12 weeks
Early amniocentesis	Needle inserted through mother's abdomen into amniotic sac	Amniotic fluid or amniocytes	Before 15 weeks
Amniocentesis	Needle inserted through mother's abdomen into amniotic sac	Amniotic fluid or amniocytes	15–20 weeks
Placental biopsy	Needle inserted into mother's abdomen into placenta	Placental tissue	After 12 weeks
Periumbilical blood sampling (PUBS) or cordocentesis	Needle inserted through mother's abdomen into fetal umbilical vein	Fetal blood	After 18 weeks
Fetoscopy with fetal skin biopsy	Needle inserted through mother's abdomen, camera used to facilitate biopsy	Fetal skin	After 18 weeks

Adapted from Daniels, R. (2003). Delmar's manual of laboratory and diagnostic tests. *New York: Thomson Delmar Learning.*

Prenatal CF Carrier Screening: How to Use the CF Sampling Kit

If these steps are followed carefully, test results should be sufficiently attained the first time.

- Twist the opposite ends of the plastic tube to open it. Remove the swab by the handle (PINK for female, and BLUE for male).
- Place the tip of the swab between cheek and gum in the upper rear part of the patient's mouth.
- Apply gentile pressure wit the index finger of the opposite hand to the outside of the cheek so that the swab is in firm contact with the outside of the cheek.
- Timing with the 30-second sand timer, swab the inside of the cheek by twisting the handle or scrubbing up and down for a *full 30 seconds.*
- Using the same swab, sample the *other cheek* for a full 30 seconds.
- Touching only the handle, return the swab to the tube and label the tube as indicated.
- Return the tube to the plastic bag, along with a copy of the lab slip—include the pink slip with the sample from the female or the blue slip with the sample from the male.
- Do not forget: Keep swabs separately and do not touch the other person's swab, so that the cells do not mix.
- Return the tubes and lab requisition to the mailer, seal and mail the same day as the samples are taken.

Adapted from Lea, D. H., & Smith, R. S. (2003). The genetics resource guide. Scarborough, ME: Foundation for Blood Research.

Researchers have discovered that the cell-free portion of amniotic fluid that is routinely discarded after amniotic fluid analysis can also provide information about fetal gene expression. These studies also highlight that environmental exposure to cigarette smoke while in utero may serve as a trigger for the expression of some diseases later in life (de la Chica, Ribas, Giraldo, Egozcue, & Fuster, 2005; DeMarini & Preston, 2005).

Chorionic Villus Sampling

After fertilization of the ovum by the sperm, the fertilized body forms a cell mass. The inner cells of this mass form the embryo and subsequently the fetus, while the outer cells form the placenta. These outer cells become embedded in the wall of uterus forming placental material with same origin as the fetus. These chorion cells can be tested to indicate fetal abnormality. A catheter is introduced through the vagina or abdominal wall and using ultrasound scanning is guided to the chorionic villi. This test can be performed at 10 to 12 weeks gestation, and chromosome results are available within 2 weeks. Diagnosis of abnormalities or genetic conditions can be obtained earlier than by amniocentesis. CVS is able to detect metabolic defects, chromosomal defects, and some single gene defects.

Percutaneous Umbilical Blood Sampling

Percutaneous umbilical blood sampling (PUBS) is a procedure by which a spinal needle is passed through the maternal abdomen and uterine wall to withdraw blood directly from the fetal circulation via the umbilical cord. The procedure replaces fetoscopy and has revolutionized the ability to diagnose and treat the fetus in utero by direct venous access (Daniels, 2003). PUBS can be done as early as 16 to 18 weeks gestation if the cord can be visualized by ultrasound. Umbilical cord access enables the health care provider to perform a karyotype or other diagnostic blood studies. It also provides a route for the administration of gene therapies and the collection of stem cells.

Fetoscopy

Fetoscopy is a prenatal diagnostic procedure that involves the insertion of a needle (fetoscope) through a small incision that is made in the woman's abdomen. Fetal ultrasound is used to guide the placement of the fetoscope so that the fetus is not harmed. Fetoscopy is used to obtain a skin biopsy for evaluation and is used to identify birth defects and inherited diseases that cannot be detected using amniocentesis or CVS, for example hereditary skin diseases. Surgical procedures are currently being perfected using fetoscopy to correct such problems as abnormal blood flow between twins and a condition called amniotic band syndrome in which bands from the amnion can deform limbs and other fetal structures. Fetoscopy carries a significant risk to both the mother and the fetus, therefore it is performed in specialized institutions when other prenatal diagnostic techniques will not provide the diagnostic information (Lashley, 2005).

Alpha-Fetoprotein, Triple Screen, and Fluorescent In Situ Hybridization

Maternal serum **alpha-fetoprotein (AFP)** (a fetal protein produced in the yolk sac of the embryo for the first 6 weeks of gestation and then by the fetal liver) screening is done routinely at 16 to 18 weeks gestation to identify the possibility of neural tube defects, such as spina bifida and anencephaly. In addition to screening for neural tube defects, it has also been noted that elevated AFP levels are associated with multiple gestation, isoimmunization, and a wide variety of congenital defects.

When maternal AFP is done in conjunction with maternal serum human chorionic gonadotropin (hCG) estriol levels, and in some laboratories, inhibin A (DIA), the study is known as multiple marker screening, expanded AFP screening, pregnancy risk profile, or triple or quadruple screen. The use of multiple marker screening is particularly useful in the identification of trisomies. Another study referred to as fluorescent in situ hybridization (FISH) is used to detect is used to detect chromosomal abnormalities on chromosomes 12, 18, 21, and the X or Y chromosome. The results can usually be obtained within 24 to 48 hours, but it is expensive, may not be covered by insurance, and can have false negative results.

Diagnostic Imaging

Ultrasound scanning is widely used technique involving the use of ultrasonic waves (sound waves of a high frequency that cannot be heard by the human ear) to scan the fetus and measure it. The fetus can be seen on the screen enabling skeletal and other abnormalities to be identified. Fetal measurements taken at the scan can be compared with average normal fetal age measurements to identify anomalies. Scans are normally performed between 16 to 20 weeks gestation. Conditions that may be identified include spina bifida, hydrocephaly, and microcephaly. In some conditions like tuberous sclerosis, where heart tumors may contribute to the diagnosis, an additional scan may be performed at 20 to 22 weeks gestation. The technique is widely used and has no specific risks for mother or fetus.

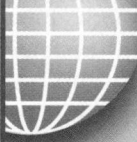

Real World, Real Choices

Supportive Care for an Unexpected Prenatal Diagnosis

Mrs. Roberts is a 25-year-old woman gravida 2, para (G2 P1). There is no family history of neural tube defects (NTD) in either Mrs. or Mr. Robert's families. During a routine 18 weeks' gestation ultrasound, performed in the doctor's office, a large lumbar neural tube defect is observed in the developing baby. Mrs. Roberts' doctor refers the couple to a perinatal center for further evaluation.

Mr. and Mrs. Roberts live in a rural part of their state and have financial and transportation concerns. They also have social concerns about this situation. To help them with all of their concerns, the physician makes a referral to public health nursing, saying that Mr. and Mrs. Roberts will need help in making both appointment and transportation arrangements and will require dependable support for whatever is learned, as well as follow-up for whatever is recommended.

The public health nurse finds Mrs. Roberts understandably upset. Mrs. Roberts asks her what will happen at the perinatal center, confiding that she is "scared to have that amniocentesis thing" because "it may tell me more bad things." She asks, "What else can I do?" and ends by asking, "What would you do?" adding, "Please tell me what to do."

1. Where is it best to start in providing the necessary support and help needed by Mr. and Mrs. Roberts?
2. How do you respond to questions about other options?
3. How do you handle her request asking you to tell her what to do?
4. What practical support can you offer this concerned and frightened couple in the face of their fears?
5. How prepared are you to provide full support and advocacy for them, regardless of whatever decisions they may reach?
6. What other questions may they have as they work their way through this crisis?

Adapted from Lea, D. H., & Smith, R. S. (2003). The genetics resource guide. Scarborough, ME: Foundation for Blood Research.

In adult populations, magnetic resonance imaging (MRI) and ultrasound are similarly used to identify structural and functional malformations. MRI is a noninvasive procedure with no known side effects that serves as an adjunct to other diagnostic methods.

GENETICS ACROSS THE LIFE SPAN

As the role of genetics becomes more clearly defined in a wide variety of clinical conditions, it is apparent that genetics has an impact on individuals across the life span. Historically, the survival rate of people with severe birth defects was low. With today's technologies, people with congenital anomalies have increased survival rates and an improved quality of life. More people with genetic conditions are now capable of parenting children to whom the condition may be passed. The genetics clinical specialty area includes physical care and diagnosis, education, and emotional support to individuals and their families when there is a genetic basis for an exhibited or potential health condition. Whether testing germ cells for mutations to prevent birth defects or predicting which healthy adults in a family will develop a life-threatening condition, genetics plays a role at all points along the life cycle (Ciarleglio, et al., 2003).

Genetic Contribution to Neonatal and Pediatric Conditions

Neonatal and pediatric conditions are often diagnosed prenatally or at the time of birth. Decision making in this population is determined by parents and often centers on genetic counseling to determine the chances of the birth of another infant with the same genetic anomaly or **inborn error of metabolism** (a condition in which the metabolism of an organism is abnormal because of the presence of one, or a pair of, abnormal alleles) (Enns & Packman, 2002). Congenital anomalies and a wide variety of syndromes are prevalent in this age-group.

Congenital Anomalies and Chromosomal Syndromes

Congenital anomalies occur frequently, but the underlying causes for most defects remains unknown. It has been estimated that around 15 to 25 percent of congenital anomalies are due to recognized genetic conditions (chromosome and single gene causes), 8 to 12 percent are due to environmental factors (maternal-related conditions, drug, or chemical exposures); 20 to 25 percent are due to multifactorial inheritance; and 40 to 60 percent of congenital anomalies have unexplained origins.

Infectious agents can be transmitted to the fetus and have an adverse effect on the genetic structure or function of the child. These are most often virus and include rubella, cytomegalovirus (CMV), varicella, and toxoplasmosis. Several drugs have demonstrated teratogenic properties when administered to pregnant women. The aforementioned thalidomide epidemic, which caused severe limb defects in the 1960s, has resulted in current monitoring for congenital anomalies due to pharmacological agents. Other known teratogenic agents include folic acid antagonists, anticonvulsants (Dilantin and Tegretol), coumarin derivatives, and retinoids (Accutane). The most commonly used teratogenic agent is alcohol. Fetal alcohol syndrome (FAS) and fetal alcohol effect (FAE) are recognized as the leading causes of preventable birth defects and developmental delay in children (Figure 9-6). An estimate of the incidence of FAS is 1:1,000 births. A wide variety of birth defects and chromosomal abnormalities have been associated with air pollution, hazardous wastes, pesticides exposure, trihalomethane by-products in public water supplies, and industrial areas heavily polluted with lead. Maternal age and health condition are risk factors for increased incidence of chromosomal abnormalities.

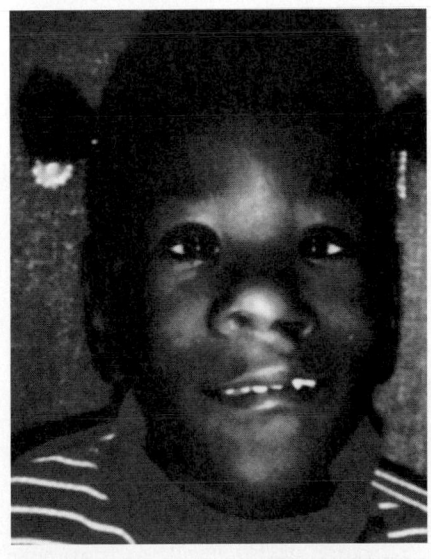

Figure 9-6 Young girl with FAS. In this case, the mother drank heavily from the onset of conception.

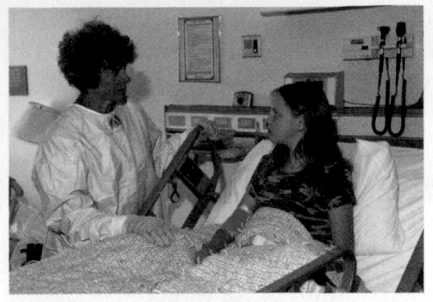

Figure 9-7 Patient education for CF should include the need for adequate nutrition, rest, and ongoing follow-up care with members of the health care team.

Women who are obese, taking anticonvulsant agents to control epilepsy, and have thyroid disease or insulin-dependent diabetes are at the highest risk of delivering an infant with genetic problems.

Strategies to minimize prenatal exposure to teratogens and promote maternal-fetal health include food fortification with folic acid, promoting multivitamin use in the periconceptional period, immunization against rubella prior to pregnancy, and programs to educate women about the adverse effects of alcohol and drug use in pregnancy. Prenatal diagnosis, fetal surgery to correct anomalies, and termination of affected pregnancies are secondary preventive strategies.

Cystic Fibrosis

Cystic fibrosis (CF) is an inherited disease of the mucous glands. It causes chronic, progressive damage to the respiratory system and digestive tract. Mutations in the *CFTR* gene alter protein, causing cells that line the passageways of the lungs, pancreas, and other organs to produce the abnormally thick mucus characteristic of CF. Accumulation of the tenacious mucus obstructs the airway, and repeated bacterial infections lead to chronic obstructive pulmonary disease. This damage is characterized the formation of scar tissue (fibrosis) and cysts in the lungs giving the condition its name. Infertility is common in adult men with CF, but infrequent in women with the condition.

CF is a common genetic disease affecting Caucasians in the United States. The disease occurs in 1 out of every 3,000 Caucasian births. It also affects other ethnic groups but is much less common; 1 in 15,000 African Americans and 1 in 31,000 Asian (Americans) have the disorder (Gill, Davies, Pringle, & Hyde, 2004). This condition is inherited in an autosomal recessive pattern. The nursing care for patients with CF involves a focus on patient education and is multidisciplinary in nature (Figure 9-7).

Mental Retardation

Numerous genetic mental retardation disorders were identified throughout the 1970s, 1980s, and 1990s. However, not all people with a specific disorder exhibit classic behaviors, and not every genetic disorder is totally distinct behaviorally from other disorders. Given recent advances in genetics, child psychiatry, and mental retardation research, etiology-based interventions are becoming increasingly possible for children with different genetic mental retardation conditions. Etiology-related cognitive-linguistic profiles and tendencies to develop distinct personalities and behavior problems are useful in planning interventions.

Autism is a severe developmental disorder marked by significant impairments in social, behavioral, and communicative functioning. Its early onset, symptom profile, and chronicity strongly argue for a biological basis, and in fact, several of lines of research implicate core biological mechanisms. About a quarter of individuals with autism exhibit a seizure disorder, and a larger number of individuals have abnormal electroencephalograms (EEGs), which typically indicate bilateral abnormalities without a consistent focus. However, the absence of consistent biological markers present across all cases and the pronounced heterogeneity of the manifestations of autism have slowed research into its pathophysiology.

Genetic Contribution to Adult Conditions

Huntington disease (HD), as mentioned previously, is an autosomal dominant inherited disorder that is only seen in adulthood (see chapter 37). When a parent has HD, each of his or her children has a 50 percent chance of inheriting the HD gene from the affected parent. This life-shortening, terminal disease will manifest itself around 40 years of age if the person carries the gene regardless of environmental influences or preventive measures (Brouwer-DudokdeWit, Savenue, Zoeteweij, Maat-Kievit, & Tibben, 2002). In 1993, HD became the first

Uncovering the Evidence

Genetic Testing

Discussion: The process of genetic testing is a family affair, affecting how people at risk understand and communicate test results and the dynamics of family relationships and communication. Evidence from studies of people at risk for hereditary breast ovarian cancer has shown that test participants may have difficulty disclosing test results because of the potential implications of these results for all of their family members.

This research was undertaken to explore and describe the experiences of disclosing test results to biological family members among individuals tested for Huntington disease (HD) or hereditary breast ovarian cancer (HBOC). Using grounded theory methodology, researchers conducted 29 open-ended, tape-recorded interviews. Twenty-four participants had received genetic test results, and five had decided not to be tested. Participants were from three countries, including the United States. The interviews were conducted two months to four years after participants had received their test results. The tapes were then transcribed and analyzed for conceptual categories describing the experience of disclosing test results.

The results revealed that participants selectively disclosed results to family members. Timing of disclosure was influenced by the specific disease and the individual's perceived need to prepare. Disclosure of genetic test results brought the risk of the disease (HD or HBOC) into the foreground for the family as well as the individual tested. The researchers conclude that this study has elucidated the perspective of the discloser and the consequences they anticipated and experienced.

Implications for Practice: This research has important significance to nurses and other health care professionals concerning genetic testing and family impact. Nurses will increasingly interact with and assist individuals and families who receive genetic information, and they must be prepared to assess and identify issues of concern and support individuals considering disclosure to family members. In this study, for example, individuals being tested expressed concern that that their positive test would shift the family perception of breast cancer from a sporadic event, related to only one family member to a family disease, creating risk for everyone. Participants expressed feelings of guilt over bringing this news into the open and being responsible for the shift in risk perception among family members. For many participants disclosure was a difficult process with careful consideration about how they would inform other family members of their potential genetic risk, and the realization that their results would bring the family disease to the foreground.

Source: Hamilton, R. J., Bowers, B. J., & Williams, J. K. (2005). Disclosing genetic test results to family members. Journal of Nursing Scholarship, 37(1), 18–24.

gene mutation to be confirmed via a blood test with a high degree of accuracy. This discovery brought with it the psychological implications of predictive, presymptomatic testing, and knowing if a person will or will not eventually develop this debilitating disease (Hicken & Tucker, 2002). The anxiety of not knowing when and how the disease will appear and the guilt that is often felt by parents who transmit this disease to their children has led to depression, anxiety, suicide, and psychological distress in many people carrying the HD gene. Anyone who has a biological parent with this disorder and is over 18 years of age may request that this test be done prior to the onset of clinical symptoms.

More recently, the discovery of susceptibly genes has moved the study of genetics in a new and challenging direction, that is, predispositional testing. Susceptibility genes are combinations of one or many genetic characteristics interacting with environmental influences that may ultimately result in disease. Cardiac disease, diabetes, mental illness, allergies, and many other conditions seen in adulthood are believed to be precipitated in this manner. Even alcoholism, sleep disorders, and back pain are now attributed, at least in part, to the presence of a susceptibility gene (Sobajima, Kim, Gilbertson, & Kang, 2004).

Cardiovascular Disease

Recent advances in genetic research have suggested that cardiovascular disease is a multifactorial genetic disease. One biological marker being investigated is Apo ε. Apo ε is a member of the apolipoprotein gene family, a group of genes that serve a variety of functions related to lipoprotein metabolism. Apo ϵ is located at chromosome 19q13.2 and is closely linked to the apo C-l/C-II gene complex. The major effect of genetic variation at this locus is its influence on cholesterol levels, one of the major risk factors for cardiovascular disease (CVD). Many studies have looked at interactions with variants of this gene as possible modifiers of other cardiovascular risks, such as high- and low-fat diets and active versus sedentary lifestyles. Interactions with lipid-lowering medications also have been investigated in relation to apo ϵ. Apo ϵ has been studied as a possible risk factor for other diseases, such as Alzheimer's disease, in some populations.

Genotyping for apo ϵ is available both for clinical purposes and for laboratory research. Several techniques have been used to determine an individual's genotype, but most involve amplification of genomic sequences containing polymorphic sites. The test is offered commercially (Eichner, et al., 2002).

Diabetes Mellitus

There are two main forms of diabetes mellitus. Type 1 diabetes mellitus (T1DM) is the less prevalent juvenile-onset insulin-dependent form (previous abbreviation IDDM) that affects 0.4 percent of the population and shows a high incidence of potentially serious renal, retinal, and vascular complications. Type 2 diabetes mellitus is more common, has a later-onset, and is the non–insulin-dependent form that affects up to 10 percent of the population. Both type 1 and type 2 show complex patterns of familial clustering, which led to diabetes being labeled as the geneticist's nightmare. The hunt for these genetic and environmental risk factors is ongoing. About 18 regions of the genome have been linked with influencing type 1 diabetes risk. These regions, each of which may contain several genes, have been labeled IDDM1 to IDDM18. The most commonly studied gene is IDDM1, which contains the histocompatibility locus antigen (HLA) genes that encode immune response proteins. Variations in HLA genes are an important genetic risk factor, but it is known that many other factors are involved in manifestation of the disease.

Initial research tended to focus on type 1 diabetes mellitus, in which there is greater evidence for familial clustering. The concordance rates in monozygotic and dizygotic twins are around 50 percent and 12 percent, respectively. These observations point to a multifactorial etiology with both environmental and genetic contributions. Known environmental factors include diet, viral exposure in early childhood, and certain drugs. The disease process involves irreversible destruction of insulin-producing islet cells in the pancreas by the body's own immune system, probably as a result of an interaction between infection and an abnormal genetically programmed immune response. The first major breakthrough came with the recognition of strong associations with the HLA region on chromosome 6p21. The original associations were with the HLA B8 and B15 that are in linkage disequilibrium with the DR3 and DR4 alleles. It is with these that the T1DM association is strongest, with 95 percent of affected individuals having DR3 or DR4 compared with 50 percent of the general population. Following the development of PCR analysis for the HLA region, it was shown that the HLA contribution to T1DM susceptibility is determined by the 57th amino acid residue at the DQ locus, where aspartic acid conveys protection, in contrast to other alleles that increase susceptibility. As this was the first susceptibility locus identified for type 1 diabetes, it was labeled IDDM1. The next locus to be identified was the insulin gene on chromosome 11p15, where it was shown that variation in the number of tandem repeats of a 14bp sequence upstream to the gene (known as the INS VNTR) influences disease susceptibility. It is hypothesized that long repeats convey protection by increasing expression of the insulin gene in the fetal thymus gland, thereby reducing the likelihood that insulin-producing cells will be viewed as foreign by the mature immune system.

The current understanding is that T1DM is indeed a multifactorial disorder with an underlying oligogenic or polygenic susceptibility consisting of one major locus (IDDM1 = HLA) and up to 20 minor loci. The products of these loci are believed to interact in a complex and poorly understood way to confer susceptibility to environmental triggers of autoimmune pancreatic cell destruction. This phenomenon of gene interaction is referred to as epistasis. The long-term research goals are to map all the IDDM loci, then to identify the relevant genes, and finally devise new strategies for prevention and possibly treatment based on a full understanding of the underlying etiology and pathogenesis.

The prevalence of type 2 diabetes mellitus (T2DM) is increasing and is predicted to reach 215 million affected worldwide by 2010. Although believed to be more benign than the earlier-onset, insulin-dependent T1DM, patients with T2DM are also prone to diabetic complications with corresponding excess morbidity and mortality. The later age of onset has made family studies difficult, but breakthroughs have been possible through genome-wide scans using hundreds of affected sibling pairs and association studies involving thousands of cases and control samples.

Gestational diabetes remains more of a mystery. Women who develop diabetes while they are pregnant are more likely to have a family history of diabetes, especially on their mothers' side. But as in other forms of diabetes, nongenetic factors play a role. Older mothers and overweight women are more likely to develop gestational diabetes.

Cancer

Researchers have identified more than 30 **oncogenes** (cancer-susceptibility genes) that greatly increase a person's odds of developing some form of malignancy. Because of this discovery, cancer is increasingly being viewed as a genetic disease. This change in views calls for new approaches to prevention, screening and diagnosis, and clinical management of many cancers (Middleton, Dimond, Calzone, Davis, & Jenkins, 2002). For example, a gene has been identified on chromosome number 9 that may be linked to a common skin cancer called basal cell carcinoma. This gene, labeled PTCH or Patched, may someday be important in screening for this type of cancer. Basal cell carcinoma is the most common malignancy in the Caucasian population, and its incidence is increasing worldwide. Risk factors include lightly pigmented skin and hair, blue or green eyes, freckling in childhood, sunburn in childhood, immunosuppressive treatment, and ingestion of arsenic (Diepgen & Mahler, 2002).

Another gene, carried by 1 out of every 300 Americans, may greatly increase an individual's chance of developing hereditary nonpolyposis colon cancer (HNPCC), the most common hereditary colon cancer syndrome. The risk of developing colorectal cancer increases with age, increased consumption of alcohol or red meat, and smoking. Mutations in the doubly dangerous gene called BRCA-1 seems to give women an 85 percent chance of developing breast cancer, as well as a 50 percent chance of ovarian tumors. BRCA-1 is a cancer susceptibility gene located on chromosome 17 and BRCA-2 is found on chromosome 13 and is often linked to breast cancer in men (Nogueira & Appling, 2000).

There are over 100 known genetic conditions involving cancer. Individuals who have a personal or family history of cancer are encouraged to review their family medical histories to identify patterns of cancer with the family, determine personal and family members' risk for cancer, learn about lifestyle changes that could be made early to avert the diagnosis of cancer, and discuss options for genetic testing, management, and surveillance. A multidisciplinary team of health care providers is essential in a comprehensive approach to cancer care. Nurses play a major role in cancer education, prevention, and screening (Middleton, et al., 2002).

Mutations that people are not born with, but that occur by chance over time in cells of the body, are acquired. Acquired mutations are not present in all cells of the body, are not inherited, and are not passed down to children. Acquired mutations are always involved in causing cancer. The formation of tumors basically results from cell growth that gets out of control. In the human genome, there are many different types of genes that control cell growth in a systematic, precise way. When these genes have an error in their DNA code, they may not work properly and are altered or mutated. An accumulation of many mutations in different genes occurring in a specific group of cells over time is required to cause malignancy.

The different types of genes, that when mutated, can lead to the development of cancer are described here. Remember, it takes mutations in several of these genes for a person to develop cancer. What specifically causes mutations to occur in these genes is largely unknown. However, mutations can be caused by a wide variety of carcinogens. The development of mutations is also a natural part of the aging process.

Oncogenes are altered forms of genes called proto-oncogenes. Proto-oncogenes, when altered or mutated, become oncogenes and promote tumor formation or growth. Oncogenes are usually acquired. Having a mutation in just one of the two copies of a particular proto-oncogene is enough to cause a change in cell growth and the formation of a tumor. For this reason, oncogenes are said to be dominant at the cellular level.

Tumor suppressor genes are normally present in human body cells. When working properly, they control the processes of cell growth and cell death (apoptosis). Both members of a gene pair of a specific tumor suppressor need to be mutated to cause a change in cell growth and the development of a tumor. For this reason, tumor suppressor genes are said to be recessive at the cellular level. Most often, mutations in tumor suppressor genes are acquired as a result of aging or environmental exposures. In a few cases, mutation of a tumor suppressor gene is inherited and may affect one or both copies of the gene.

During cell division, the DNA is constantly replicating itself. When errors are made during this fragile process, DNA repair genes correct this naturally occurring miscoding of the DNA. When the DNA repair genes themselves are altered or mutated, the errors in the DNA remain. If these mistakes occur in tumor suppressor genes or proto-oncogenes, eventually this will lead to uncontrolled cell growth and tumor formation. Mutations in DNA repair genes can be inherited or acquired and are recessive at the cellular level.

It is important to remember that it takes mutations in several of these genes for cancer to develop. In many types of cancer, all the mutations are acquired. Because of the multifactorial nature of these mutations, not all people who inherit a mutation in a tumor suppressor gene, proto-oncogene, or DNA repair gene will develop cancer.

Mental Illness

Genetic factors may be important in a general sense, but the existence of a specific genetic component to the various psychoses is not as clearly established as is sometimes reported. Most of the studies reported are evidence for a combination of genetic and environmental influences. Evidence for a genetic element to psychotic experiences comes mainly from studies that compare identical and nonidentical twins and from adoption studies that compare the biological and adoptive relatives of people who were subsequently given a diagnosis of schizophrenia or bipolar disorder (Rosenberg, Prusiner, DiMauro, Barchi, & Nestler, 2003).

The best estimate is that the risk of being given a diagnosis of schizophrenia is 46 percent for the child of two parents with the diagnosis, 13 percent for the child of one parent with the diagnosis, and 9 percent for siblings. This is compared to the overall risk of 1 percent for the general population. Similar findings have been reported for a genetic contribution to bipolar disorder.

Most scientists believe that psychiatric disorders are usually the products of multiple interacting causal factors. Studies of significant causes and processes in the development of mental illness have found physical, mental, environmental, and emotional causes for mental illness.

Researchers have been searching for specific genes, passed down through generations that may increase a person's chance of developing the illness because bipolar disorders tend to be familial. The evidence that heredity plays a role in the development of some forms of mental illness has been discovered by studying identical twins who were raised separately and studying adopted children of mothers with different forms of severe mental illness and comparing them to nonidentical twins raised separately and the general public.

Studying twins has confirmed the major role that genetics plays in the development of manic depression (Merikangans & Risch, 2003). For example, if an identical twin has manic depression, the other twin will also develop it 40 to 80 percent of the time. With nonidentical twins, when one twin is affected the chance of the other twin developing the condition is 15 to 20 percent. Close relatives, such as parents, children and siblings (first-degree relatives), have a 5 to 10 percent likelihood.

Alzheimer's Disease

Alzheimer's disease (AD) is a multifactorial hereditary disorder. More than one gene mutation can cause AD, and genes on multiple chromosomes are involved (Schutte, 2002). There are four basic classifications of AD: familial early-onset (appearing before 65 years of age), familial late-onset (appearing after 65 years of age), sporadic early-onset, and sporadic late-onset. Familial AD (FAD) is the least common form of AD, affecting less than 10 percent of AD patients (Ciarleglio, et al., 2003). It is caused by gene mutations on chromosomes 1, 14, and 21. Even if one of these mutated genes is inherited from a parent, the person will almost always develop early-onset AD. This inheritance pattern is referred to as autosomal dominant inheritance. In other words, all offspring in the same generation have a 50 percent chance of developing FAD if one of their parents had the disorder.

The majority of AD cases are late-onset, usually developing after age 65. Late-onset AD has no known cause and shows no obvious inheritance pattern. However, in some families, clusters of cases are seen. Although a specific gene has not been identified as the cause of late-onset AD, genetic factors do appear to play a role in the development of this form of AD. To date, only one risk factor gene has been identified. Apolipoprotein E gene found on chromosome 19 appears to be related to an increased risk of developing late-onset AD. This gene codes for a protein that helps carry cholesterol in the bloodstream. The APOE gene comes in several different forms, or alleles, but three occur most frequently: APOE-e2, APOE-e3, and APOE-e4. People inherit one APOE allele from each parent. Having one or two copies of the e4 allele increases a person's risk of getting AD. That is, having the e4 allele is a risk factor for AD, but it does not mean that AD is certain. Some people with two copies of the e4 allele (the highest risk group) do not develop clinical signs of AD, but others with no e4s do. The e3 allele is the most common form found in the general population and may play a neutral role in AD. The least common e2 allele appears to be associated with a lower risk of AD. The exact degree of risk of AD for any given person cannot be determined based on APOE status. Therefore, the APOE-e4 gene is called a risk factor gene for late-onset AD.

Scientists are looking for genetic risk factors for late-onset AD on other chromosomes as well. They think that additional risk factor genes may lie on regions of chromosomes 9, 10, and 12. The National Institute on Aging (NIA) has launched a major study to discover remaining genetic risk factors for late-onset AD. Geneticists from the NIA's Alzheimer's Disease Centers are working to collect genetic samples from families affected by multiple cases of late-onset AD.

In diagnosing AD, APOE testing is not a common practice. The only definite way to diagnose AD is by viewing a sample of a person's brain tissue under a microscope to determine if there are plaques and tangles present. This is usually done after the person dies. However, through a complete medical evaluation (including a medical history, laboratory tests, neuropsychological tests, and brain scans), well-trained clinicians are able to diagnose AD correctly 90 percent of the time (Roberts, et al., 2003). In some cases, APOE testing may be used in combination with these other medical tests to strengthen the diagnosis of a suspected case of AD. Currently, there is no medical test to establish if a person without the symptoms of AD is going to develop the disease.

Epilepsy

Epilepsy is a disorder in which seizures occur repeatedly without any immediate trigger. In about 25 percent of cases, a past injury to the brain (occurring more than a week before the first seizure) is likely to have caused the epilepsy, even though there is no immediate trigger of the seizures. Epilepsy caused by an identifiable injury to the brain (e.g., head trauma, stroke, or brain infection) is called symptomatic epilepsy. In the remaining 75 percent of those affected, the underlying cause is unknown, and the epilepsy is called either idiopathic epilepsy, which means of unknown cause, or cryptogenic, which means hidden cause (Bell & Sander, 2002).

Most cases of epilepsy are probably not caused by single genes, although a few rare types of epilepsy have been found to result from a single altered gene, and studying these rare types can help us to understand the causes of epilepsy and its genetic complexity. Epilepsy is highly variable, with many different types of seizures, ages at onset, responses to treatment, and other features. For this reason, as a condition it is referred to as the epilepsies to indicate that this is a group of disorders that may have many different features. The epilepsies are grouped in the following categories, according to seizure type and syndrome and include generalized seizures, partial (or focal) seizures, epilepsy syndromes, and febrile seizures. In addition, genetic predisposition plays a major role in the effectiveness of medications used to manage the disorder (Kullmann, 2003; Ramachandran & Shorvon, 2003).

Generalized seizures involve the entire brain (both sides) from the outset. Some examples are absence, myoclonic, atonic, and generalized tonic-clonic (also called primary generalized grand mal). Absence seizures are sometimes called petit mal, because they appear simply to be staring spells with no convulsive or physical movements. Partial (or focal) seizures begin in a specific part of the brain. They may then spread to involve the whole brain, in which case a secondarily generalized grand mal seizure occurs, but they may also stay in just one part of the brain. Partial seizures may also be called petit mal when they consist of staring without convulsive movements.

An epileptic syndrome is an epileptic disorder characterized by a cluster of typical signs and symptoms that usually occur together. A syndrome can include features, such as type of seizure, cause, precipitating factors, severity, age of onset, and prognosis. Generalized epilepsy syndromes are epilepsy syndromes characterized by generalized seizures, while localization-related epilepsy syndromes are syndromes characterized by partial or focal seizures.

Epilepsy is a broad term referring to a collection of many different seizure disorders with varying degrees of genetic influence. Even among genetically determined epilepsies, the genes responsible will vary. In addition, most epilepsy is not determined by simple modes of inheritance in which there is a clear, predictable relationship between having an altered gene and developing a disorder. There are many other factors that may influence whether or not the abnormal gene will cause the disorder (Kinton, et al., 2002). When inheritance of a specific gene is not sufficient to cause disease, some gene carriers will be unaffected. This is called reduced penetrance. In this case, other genes or environmental factors may be needed for the specific gene to cause disease.

Genetic and nongenetic factors (such as head injury) may work together to produce seizures. This phenomenon is known as gene-environment interaction. Alternatively, multiple genes may work together to increase the risk of developing epilepsy (Gaitatzis & Patsalos, 2002). Most of the epilepsy genes that have been discovered, which cause idiopathic or cryptogenic epilepsy, are responsible for making normal ion channels. These channels are holes in the membranes of cells that allow charged molecules to exit and enter, and are important in nerve cell function and communication between nerve cells. Mutations in these genes appear to lead to channel dysfunction and seizures.

A febrile seizure is a type of seizure that occurs in infants or young children, usually between three months and five years of age. It is associated with fever, without evidence of any brain infection or other direct cause of the seizure other than the fever itself. Febrile seizures are also, like epilepsy, probably a combination of disorders, not just one simple disease, and this makes the search for genetic or other causes difficult. The risk of febrile seizures is increased in siblings and offspring of individuals with febrile seizures. The risk of epilepsy is also increased in the relatives of people with febrile convulsions and vice versa.

In 2003 there were 11 known epilepsy genes. However, despite these findings, relatively little is known about the genetic causes of epilepsy in most people. The genes that have been identified so far either cause rare types of epilepsy or are rare causes of the more common types of epilepsy. In addition, it is believed that the common genetic epilepsies are caused by a number of genes acting together, making it much harder to identify each individual gene (Kullmann, 2003).

Allergies

People with allergies have an inherited predisposition for developing hypersensitivity to inhaled and ingested allergens that are harmless to other people. A healthy immune system is balanced between the activity of two types of white blood cells, called Th1 and Th2. Like most diseases of unknown cause, allergies and asthma were initially explained in terms of magic and mystery. In ancient times, they mere maladies popularly thought to be the result of God's wrath or possession by evil spirits. Still, health care providers recognized fairly early that exposure to environmental agents, such as dust, foods, and animals, contributed to the development of these conditions. They also realized that, unlike infections, where repeated exposure to the offending agent builds up one's immunity, repeated exposure to the agents responsible for allergies only results in an increased sensitivity and the worsening of symptoms. In addition, they noted that these diseases seemed to cluster in families.

The process by which an allergic reaction occurs is a complex chain of events. First, an individual must be exposed to an offending environmental agent. Take, for example, the house dust mite, which is a common allergen. Once in the body, the antigen presenting cells, or APCs, capture the dust mite. These APCs break the dust mite down into smaller pieces called peptides, and these peptides then combine with other proteins within the APCs called human leukocyte antigens, or HLAs. HLAs help the body distinguish self from nonself; so when a foreign substance like the dust mite appears, the body will attempt to dispose of it.

Once the connection has been made, the peptide-HLA amalgam travels to the surface of the APC, exposing itself to a neighboring immune cell called the T lymphocyte, or T cell. This sets off another chain of events in which different types of T cells are created and interact with other immune cells called B cells. The end result is the production of an antibody known as immunoglobulin E, or IgE (the gene that causes an individual to make antibodies in response to a specific allergen), which is behind every allergic reaction, from hay fever to asthma. Once produced, these IgE antibodies attach themselves to receptors located on the surfaces of particular types of white blood cells, including mast cells and basophils.

The next time the individual in question is exposed to the offending or sensitizing agent (e.g., dust mite) the IgE is primed to recognize and combine with its peptides. Once this allergen-IgE combination is made, it unlocks the mast cells and basophils, prompting them to release mediators, such as histamine, leukotrienes, and cytokines. These mediators then act on one or more of their specific target organs to produce various clinical symptoms. It is extremely difficult to identify the gene or genes that initiated this process. This is attributed to a lack of universally accepted definitions of asthma or allergy. No clinical, biochemical, or genetic criteria have been universally accepted as definitive indicators of either disease. Until the condition is clearly defined, it is impossible to pinpoint the genes involved in its transmission. However, research is moving forward in this area. There are three major approaches that researchers can use to study the genetics of complex diseases, like allergies and asthma, forward genetics, positional genetics, and the candidate gene approach.

Forward genetics is the approach geneticists use when they already have or know the protein produced by the gene causing the condition. Once the order of amino acids in that protein is determined, researchers can describe the sequence of nucleic acids that code for those amino acids. Tracing the production of the protein, the location on the chromosome can be identified, and the genetic basis of the condition under study explained. However, this process cannot be used to examine the underlying defect for asthma, because there is lack of information about the protein produced by the gene causing the condition.

Positional genetics is the opposite of the forward approach and is used when geneticists do not have a gene product to work with. This is the process being used in asthma research. The positional approach attempts to pin down the location of the gene or genes in question by studying a set of already known gene markers that are present on all chromosomes.

Certain markers always appear in people who have a particular condition or symptom. This term is synonymous with the phenotype of a given individual. Once the near location of the gene is found, its sequence, structure and, ultimately, its disease-promoting product can be identified. Because geneticists begin this process with a pool of more than 300 million strands of DNA, detailed and time-consuming research is required to identify the relatively few nucleotides that make up a particular gene.

It appears that a single gene controls neither asthma nor allergies, and so the search for their genetic basis is multifaceted. Researchers are making efforts to identify the genes behind specific IgE responses. In addition, researchers have tried to uncover the genes behind a number of other allergy and asthma phenotypes.

Attempts to find the gene behind the specific IgE immune response have been performed using the candidate gene approach. One such candidate is the gene for HLA, which is found on chromosome 6p. HLA plays a role in the development of specific immune responses to many antigens. While it appears that this genetic area is necessary, by itself it will not result in responsiveness to a particular allergen. T cell receptors, with which the allergen-HLA complex comes in contact, are additional gene candidates found on chromosome 14q. Researchers report data suggesting that the genes in this area also play a role in the development of the specific IgE immune response. Serum IgE levels have been correlated with allergy, asthma, and bronchial hyperreactivity (BHR). Twin, family, and population studies have shown that somewhere between 50 and 84 percent of the factors that determine the serum IgE levels are genetic in origin. Genes behind the variables that have already been determined to exert control over IgE responsiveness include interleukin 4 and interferon gamma. Investigations of genes on chromosomes 5q and 12q have led to suggestions that genes in both of these areas may be involved in IgE regulation. Scientists using the positional gene approach, on the other hand, have found linkages for IgE on 7q, 11q, and 16q. Research has shown that a major gene or gene family is involved in the regulation of serum IgE levels.

BHR, a condition in which the airways suddenly constrict as a sort of over-response to some environmental stimulus, seems to be a necessary condition for the development of asthma. BHR has also been noted in a large percentage of patients suffering only from allergic rhinitis, and even some people who appear not to have allergies or asthma at all. A number of different studies have demonstrated that BHR is inherited.

Scientists using the candidate gene approach say that BHR susceptibility is associated with two regions on chromosome 5q. The first is the area where a genetic variant of the beta$_2$-adrenergic receptor is found. This receptor is involved in determining the tone of the smooth muscle underlying the bronchi and bronchioles in the lungs. The second associated area is one that contains many of the genes involved in the inflammatory process, which have been linked to serum IgE levels as well. Positional genetics has shown that areas on chromosomes 4q and 7q have linkages to BHR.

Bronchial asthma is considered to be an inherited condition. Familial clusters of asthma have been observed, and family and twin studies have demonstrated its inheritability. Scientists have suggested a number of candidate gene sites, but none has been proven to have a definite relationship with the disease. A modifying gene has been associated with chromosome 5q. The gene for the beta$_2$-adrenergic receptor on chromosome 5q is linked to the development of both severe asthma and night wheezing.

Allergies and asthma are complex, multifactorial conditions involving multiple steps and pathways. These conditions are likely the result of multiple genes carrying traits that increase susceptibility as well as possible interactions with additional genes as they are influenced by the environment.

Hemoglobinopathies

The hemoglobin molecule is composed of four separate polypeptide chains of amino acids and four iron-bearing heme groups on genes of chromosomes 11 and 16. Mutations and deletions in these genes cause one of the many hemoglobinopathies. Hemoglobinopathies are divided into those in which the gene abnormality results in a qualitative change in the hemoglobin molecule, such as sickle cell disease, and those in which the change is quantitative as is found in the group of disorders known as the thalassemias. It has been estimated that one third of one million people worldwide are seriously affected by one of these genetic disorders (Nienhuis, Hanawa, Sawai, Sorrentino, & Persons, 2003).

Sickle cell anemia (SSA), an autosomal recessive disorder more common in the African American population. Approximately 1 in 400 to 1 in 600 African Americans are born with the disorder, and 1 in 10 is a carrier of one copy of the mutation. In certain parts of the African continent, the prevalence of the disease reaches 1 in 50 individuals (Stuart & Nagel, 2004). The mutation causes the hemoglobin to become a sickle-shaped cell, so that it is no longer able to pass smoothly through small capillaries (Figure 9-8). This alteration in shape obstructs blood flow and results in severe pain crises, tissue and organ damage, splenomegaly, growth retardation, and stroke. Individuals with SSA are anemic and prone to infections, particularly pneumonia, which a significant cause of death in this group.

The thalassemias are a diverse group of disorders characterized by the fact that the causative mutations result in a decrease in the amount of normal hemoglobin. Thalassemias are common in Mediterranean populations as well as in Africa, India, the Mideast, and Southeast Asia. The two main types of thalassemias are alpha-thalassemia due to mutations in the alpha polypeptide and beta-thalassemia resulting from beta chain mutations.

Because individuals possess a total of four genes for the alpha polypeptide (two genes on each of their two chromosomes 16), disease severity depends on how many of the four genes are abnormal. A defect in one or two of the genes has no clinical effect. Mild to moderately severe anemia (hemoglobin H disease) and splenomegaly are caused by abnormalities of three genes. Loss of

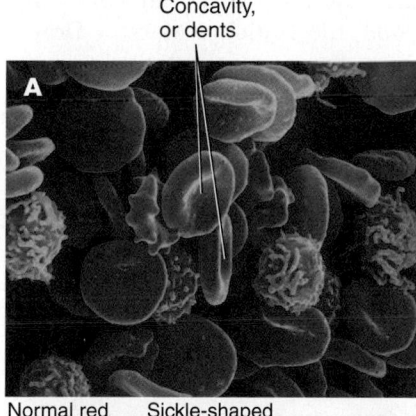

Concavity, or dents

Normal red blood cell   Sickle-shaped red blood cell

Figure 9-8 A. Side of normal red blood cells, which have a concavity (or dent) on the two slides, B. Sickle shaped (crescent-shaped) red blood cells.

function of all four genes usually causes such severe oxygen deprivation that the affected fetus does not survive. A massive accumulation of fluid in the fetus (hydrops fetalis) results in stillbirth or neonatal death.

Beta thalassemias can range from mild and clinically insignificant (beta thalassemia minor) to severe and life-threatening (beta thalassemia major, also known as Cooley's anemia), depending on the exact nature of the gene mutation and whether one or both copies of the beta gene are affected. While the milder forms may only cause slight anemia, the more severe types result in growth retardation, skeletal changes, splenomegaly, vulnerability to infections, and death as early as the first decade of life.

Treatment of sickle cell disease has improved greatly in recent years with a resulting increase in life expectancy. The use of prophylactic (preventive) antibiotic therapy has been particularly successful. Other treatments include fluid therapy to prevent dehydration, oxygen supplementation, pain relievers, blood transfusions, and several different types of medications. Recent interest has focused on bone marrow transplantation, which has been successful in selected patients.

Because the clinically important thalassemias are characterized by severe anemia, the traditional treatment has been blood transfusion, but the multiple transfusions needed to sustain life lead to an iron overload throughout the tissues of the body and eventual destruction of the heart and other organs. For this reason, transfusion therapy must also include infusions of medications, such as deferoxamine (desferrioxamine) to rid the body of excess iron. Phlebotomy is another technique that has been used with some success to lower the concentration of iron in the patient's blood. As with SSA, bone marrow therapy has been successful in some cases.

Until recently, patients being treated with bone marrow transplants had to find a sibling or other closely related donor to avoid rejection of the transplant. Advances in the preparation of the transplanted cells, however, have made the use of bone marrow from unrelated donors (URD) an option for patients with hemoglobinopathies. As of 2003, the National Marrow Donor Program reports that about 40 percent of bone marrow transplants involve a patient in the United States receiving marrow from an international donor or an international patient receiving marrow from a donor in the United States (Lea & Smith, 2003).

Emphasis is also being placed on developing drugs that treat SSA directly. The most promising of these drugs since the late 1990s is hydroxyurea, a drug that was originally designed for anticancer treatment. Hydroxyurea has been shown to reduce the frequency of painful crises and acute chest syndrome in adults and to lessen the need for blood transfusions. Hydroxyurea seems to work by inducing a higher production of fetal hemoglobin. The major side effects of the drug include decreased production of platelets, red blood cells, and certain white blood cells. The effects of long-term hydroxyurea treatment are unknown; however, a nine-year follow-up study of 299 adults with frequent painful crises reported in 2003 that taking hydroxyurea was associated with a 40 percent reduction in mortality (Davies & Gilmore, 2003).

Another promising development for the treatment of hemoglobinopathies is gene therapy, which has interested researchers since the early 1990s. In late 2001, genetic scientists reported that they had designed a gene that might lead to a future treatment of SSA. Although the gene had not been tested in humans, early results showed that the injected gene protected cells from sickling. Experiments in **gene therapy** (the process of treating or curing a genetic disorder by providing the affected individual with an intact, functional copy of the gene in question) for sickle cell disease have been carried out in mice, using lentiviral vectors to transfer the corrective gene into the mouse's stem cells.

Hemoglobinopathies are lifelong disorders. The prognosis depends on the exact nature of the mutation, the availability of effective treatment, as well as the individual's compliance with therapies. Hemoglobinopathies significantly complicate pregnancy and increase the risk of infant mortality. Because the hemoglobinopathies are inherited diseases, primary prevention involves carriers making reproductive decisions to prevent passage of the abnormal gene to their offspring. At present, most prevention is targeted toward the symptoms using treatments such as those described previously.

Hemochromatosis

Hemochromatosis is a disorder that causes the body to absorb too much iron from the diet. The excess iron is stored in the body's tissues and organs, particularly the heart, liver, pancreas, and joints. Because humans cannot increase excretion of iron, the extra iron accumulates over time and eventually can damage the tissue or organ.

The signs and symptoms of hemochromatosis result from damage to tissues and organs that experience an overload of iron. For example, iron deposits in the joints can cause joint pain. In the most common form of hemochromatosis (type 1), early symptoms are nonspecific and may include fatigue, joint pain, abdominal pain, impotence, and loss of sex drive. Later signs and symptoms include arthritis, liver disease, diabetes, heart abnormalities, and skin discoloration. The age of onset for symptoms varies with the type of hemochromatosis, from newborn (neonatal hemochromatosis) to midlife (type 1 hemochromatosis).

Type 1 hemochromatosis is one of the most common genetic disorders in the United States, affecting about one million people. It most often affects Caucasians of Northern European descent. The other types of hemochromatosis are considered rare and have been studied in only a small number of families. Mutations in the HAMP, HFE, HFE2, SLC40A1, and TFR2 genes cause hemochromatosis.

The proteins produced by hemochromatosis genes play an important role in regulating the absorption, transport, and storage of iron. Mutations in these genes disrupt their normal activities. As a result, iron accumulates in the body, which can damage tissues and organs. Mutations in additional genes, which have not yet been identified or well characterized, are suspected to cause hemochromatosis.

Hemochromatosis types 1, 2, and 3 are inherited in an autosomal recessive pattern, which means two copies of the gene must be altered for a person to be affected by the disorder. Most often, the parents of a child with an autosomal recessive disorder are not affected but are carriers of the altered gene. Type 4 hemochromatosis is distinguished by its autosomal dominant inheritance pattern. This means only one copy of the altered gene is necessary to cause the disorder. In most cases, an affected person has one affected parent, and the disorder is seen in every generation of a family.

LEGAL, ETHICAL, AND SOCIAL ISSUES

Genetics is becoming more apparent in everyday lives through applications in health care, insurance, employment, and the criminal justice system. The increased use of genetic information presents both promises and challenges for our society. The impact of genomics on current paradigms in science and medicine will depend on the response of legal, political, and social institutions.

Science has developed the capacity to test and screen for gene mutations, but there continues to be a lesser ability to cure the conditions associated with heredity and errors in genetic coding. In addition, there is a potential for misuse of genetic information by employers, insurance companies, and other agencies that has led to unfair treatment of some individuals based on their genotypes when there is no evidence of disease. This has led to some individuals declining genetic testing even when the tests might be beneficial.

The scope of genetics and the complex nature of genomics extend beyond individuals, to the family and society. It is the responsibility of scientists and health care providers to balance the patient rights of privacy and autonomy with the best interests of the family, community, and society.

The HGP has also introduced some significant new ethical and legal issues associated with predictive information about common diseases and for traits that are not diseases at all. To examine this and other issues surrounding the HGP, the Ethical, Legal, and Social Implications (ELSI) Program was established. The HGP designated 3 to 5 percent of its annual working budget to address issues of confidentiality and privacy as the science was being developed. A primary goal of ELSI is the prevention of inappropriate use of the newly discovered genetic information and ensures that the discoveries are used for the benefit of individuals and society.

Ethical Issues Surrounding Genetics

The nature of genetic information requires that the health care team must be familiar not only with its clinical significance but also the ethical implications. The caregiver and patient advocate needs to expand the application from a

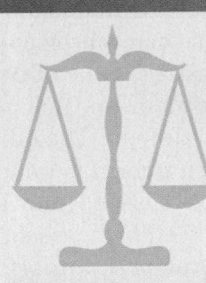

ETHICS IN PRACTICE

Genetics and Ethics

- Is the application of genetics test or procedure lawful?
- If the health care provider has a personal ethical objection to a test or procedure, should that individual advise the patient to see another provider?
- Is it safe? If it can cause harm, is the likely harm balanced by the likely benefit?
- Is it evidence-based, or still a research procedure?
- Is it cost effective?
- Who should have access to personal genetic information, and how will it be used?
- How does personal genetic information affect an individual and society's perceptions of that individual?
- Do health care personnel properly counsel parents about the risks and limitations of genetic technology?
- How reliable and useful is fetal genetic testing?
- What are the larger societal issues raised by new reproductive technologies?
- How do we prepare health care professionals for the new genetics?
- How do we prepare the public to make informed choices?
- How do we as a society balance current scientific limitations and social risk with long-term benefits?
- Should testing be performed when no treatment is available?
- Should parents have the right to have their minor children tested for adult-onset diseases?
- Do people's genes make them behave in a particular way? Can people always control their behavior? What is considered acceptable diversity?
- Are all foods and other products that have been genetically altered safe to humans and the environment?

focus on the individual to the gene analysis of parents, siblings, children, the unborn, and sometimes entire ethnic groups. This expanded responsibility to family and society may conflict with the individual's right to privacy and autonomy (Plantinga, et al., 2003). Genetics raises many questions that, right now, there may not be answers for (See Ethics in Practice).

Many of these questions arise with other tests and procedures, but occur with an unprecedented intensity in genomics. The availability of testing offers the ability to answer many questions about an individual's genetic destiny with greater certainty than revealed by family history alone. However, that information may not always be desirable, and currently, some individuals make the choice regarding tests or procedures they want done regardless of the impact the results will have on others (Chapman, 2002). The ethics of testing are different if action can be taken to prevent or treat a disease, such as hemochromatosis, as compared with conditions for which no treatments are presently available such as HD (Brouwer-DudokdeWit, et al., 2002). If prevention or early treatment is available, it is unethical not to offer testing. However, some people want and use genetic information even if there are no treatments or choices that affect reproductive options. Predictive genetic testing of children is a highly controversial issue and is generally believed to be inappropriate unless preventive or treatment interventions are available (Otlowski & Williamson, 2003).

Using information derived from genetic testing for reproductive choice adds a host of ethical dilemmas. Genetic information regarding the unborn with intent to terminate a pregnancy has been met with objection by several groups. Disability advocates, certain religions, prolife groups, and other private and political factions are concerned about approaches that treat disability as a problem, which should be eliminated using genetic information and intervention, rather than dealing with the issue of nondiscrimination of people with disease and disability. Concerns have been expressed that the range of conditions that can now be tested for will extend to sex of offspring, intelligence, attractive appearance, or athletic abilities, leading to fears of designer babies and social or ethical issues surrounding eugenics (Plomin & Spinath, 2004).

Because there is great diversity among cultures, religions, values, and belief systems, health care ethics must consider all persons during the ethical decision-making process as it relates to genetics (Table 9-3).

Legal Issues Associated with Genetics

A legal framework sets limits within which scientific development and clinical practice can operate to reasonably protect individuals from avoidable harm. The vast majority of health care providers, patients, and families want to make reasonable and safe choices. The legal framework that is used to interpret

TABLE 9-3 Four Principles Support the Ethical Decision-Making Process	
Autonomy	Educate, communicate, consult, respect, and empower the patient to make informed but independent choices regarding care. This is controversial in genetics because of the potential conflict between the rights of the individual, family, and community.
Beneficence	To do good, to provide maximal benefits
Nonmaleficence	Do no avoidable harm to individuals or groups
Justice	Promote fair distribution and accessibility of resources, respect for rights and laws; genetics is inherently not fair as individuals are genetically different and therefore needs for resources will also differ.

Adapted from Otlowski, M., & Williamson, R. (2003). Ethical and legal issues and the "new genetics." Medical Journal of Australia, 178(11), 582–585.

ethical principles, issues, and dilemmas needs to be designed to ensure that application of genomics is not unreasonably restricted as it develops. Civic and religious groups may exert political pressure to pass laws to regulate the application of genetics testing and information. However, because the science of genomics is changing so rapidly, there is a need for flexibility in the development of regulation that governs genetic research and health care applications (Otlowski & Williamson, 2003). Geneticists and health care communities, in preference to statute law, recommend guidelines and codes of practice, as the former are easier to adapt to new situations.

There are three federal laws that may, to a limited extent, restrict discrimination in employment and health insurance on the basis of genetic information. These include the Americans with Disabilities Act (ADA), The Health Insurance Portability and Accountability Act (HIPAA), and the Genetic Information Nondiscrimination Act (GINA). Genetic discrimination is defined as discrimination against an individual or against members of that individual's family solely because of real or perceived differences from the normal genome of that individual. Genetic discrimination is distinguished from discrimination based on disabilities caused by altered genes because of an inherited condition.

Patient Privacy and Confidentiality

GINA extends the same privacy protections outlined in part C of title XI of the Social Security Act and section 264 of HIPAA of 1996 to the use or disclosure of genetic information. These acts also limit the collection of genetic information prior to enrollment into health plans. The confidentiality standards only apply to insurance plans and insurers covered by the Social Security Act or HIPAA, and to individually identifiable health information as defined in those acts.

If an employer, employment agency, labor organization, or joint labor-management committee possesses genetic information, they must treat this information as part of a confidential medical record and maintain it in separate medical files. Additionally, they cannot disclose genetic information unless requested by the employee or a court order. If a group health plan, health insurer, or an issuer of a Medicare supplemental policy incidentally obtains genetic information when requesting, requiring, or purchasing of other information, they will not be considered as violating this act.

Autonomy

The availability of the new genetics has implications with regard to the health care provider's legal duty of care to patients. Providers have a responsibility to keep up to date with the new genetics so that they can provide education, recommendations, and care based on the most current research. As with any diagnostic test or procedure, the law protects the autonomy of competent individuals in making health care decisions regarding genetic testing and the lifestyle changes resulting from such tests. However, there may be conflict between the rights of individuals and the rights of the family, for whom this information may have relevance to health. In some instances, constructing a family history involves a potential breach of the privacy of other family members.

Problems can also arise with the disclosure of an individual's genetic information to other family members. At present, standard rules regarding the disclosure of health information apply, limiting disclosure to circumstances where there is a threat of serious and imminent harm to others or a serious public health risk. However, the familial nature of genetic information demands some modification of the usual principles of privacy and nondisclosure, in both directions. The information should be able to be shared with family members whose health may benefit from access to this information by alerting them to the risk of genetic disease and enabling them to institute preventive or therapeutic strategies but be protected more carefully from outsiders (Friedrich, 2002).

Fundamental questions are also being raised about the status of genetic samples collected for pathology examination, such as blood or other sources of DNA, including pathological tissue blocks and human tissue on microscope slides. At present, these are generally regarded as the property of the hospital, over which the donor may have no legally enforceable rights. Although such samples have no clear legal status as property, opinions are divided over whether it is appropriate to create legally enforceable rights, especially if the sample proves to have a commercial value. The line between research and clinical care is ethically blurred when a sample is studied by a specialist or a pathologist, and becomes even more confusing as the society moves toward an increasingly commercialized environment in which the potential for profit from genetic knowledge exists.

Prospective parents are now able to choose pregnancies that will provide an infant with a particular genetic makeup when another child develops a critical illness, such as leukemia. The new baby can then serve as a donor of cord blood stem cells to the critically ill sibling. It is important for primary health care providers to be aware of, and emphasize the difference between, the use of clinical interventions to save the lives of children with serious diseases, as compared with the use of procedures for trivial purposes, such as choosing hair or eye color.

Employment Issues

Three federal laws limit discrimination in employment and health insurance on the basis of genetic information. This legislation includes ADA, HIPAA that prohibits group health plans from denying coverage to individuals on the basis of genetic predispositions toward disease, and GINA.

In addition to disclosure of information to family members, questions about third-party access to personal genetic information have come into question. When applying for insurance, individuals are required to disclose family history and the results of any genetic tests. Insurers are then entitled to take this information into account for the purposes of underwriting for life insurance. Insurers are exempt from disability discrimination but must be able to justify the way in which they use the genetic information with regard to actuarial, statistical, or other data. In the employment arena, the challenge is to ensure that legitimate uses of genetic test information are permitted, such as offering screening for susceptibility to occupational hazards or safety issues that cannot otherwise be avoided, but to protect employees and job seekers from unfair discrimination motivated by employers' expediency and profit.

It is unlawful for employers, employment agencies, labor organizations, and training programs to hire or fire anyone because of genetic information. They cannot provide different compensation, terms, conditions, or privileges of employment to employees because of genetic information. Additionally, they cannot use genetic information to limit, segregate, or classify employees in any way that would deprive them of opportunities. Health care professionals can provide genetic information to an employer in aggregate terms that do not disclose the identity of specific employees.

Employers are able to purchase documents containing genetic information that are publicly available. Employers can request or require genetic information to comply with the Family and Medical Leave Act of 1993. An employer is allowed to use genetic information to monitor employees when required by federal or state law, if written notice of the monitoring is provided, the employee gives written authorization, and the employee is informed of the results.

Insurability

Group and individual health plans cannot restrict enrollment nor charge higher premiums because of genetic information or genetic services. Additionally, group health plans cannot request or require an individual or family member to undergo a genetic test. A group health plan, a health insurer, or an issuer of a Medicare supplemental policy shall not use or disclose genetic information for purposes of underwriting, determining enrollment eligibility, establishing premiums, or the creation, renewal or replacement of a plan, contract or coverage.

The Human Genome Project

Begun formally in 1990, the U.S. Human Genome Project (HGP) was a 13-year effort coordinated by the U.S. Department of Energy and the National Institutes of Health. The project originally was planned to last 15 years, but rapid technological advances accelerated the completion date to 2003. Several of the HGP goals were: identify all the approximately 20,000 to 25,000 genes in human DNA, determine the sequences of the three billion chemical base pairs that make up human DNA, store this information in databases, and improve tools for data analysis.

To help achieve these goals, researchers also studied the genetic makeup of several nonhuman organisms. These include the common human gut bacterium *Escherichia coli*, the fruit fly, and the laboratory mouse. A unique aspect of the U.S. HGP is that it was the first large scientific undertaking to address potential ELSI implications arising from project data. Another important feature of the project was the federal government's long-standing dedication to the transfer of technology to the private sector. By licensing technologies to private companies and awarding grants for innovative research, the project catalyzed the multibillion dollar U.S. biotechnology industry and fostered the development of new medical applications.

The HGP, sponsored in the United States by the Department of Energy and the National Institutes of Health, created the field of genomics. The health care industry is building on the knowledge, resources, and technologies emanating from the HGP to further understanding of genetic contributions to human health. As a result of this expansion of genomics into human health applications, the field of genomic medicine was born. Genetics is playing an increasingly important role in the diagnosis, monitoring, and treatment of diseases carrying with it implications for practice and policy development.

All diseases have a genetic component, whether inherited or resulting from the body's response to environmental stresses, such as viruses or toxins. The successes of the HGP have even enabled researchers to pinpoint errors in genes, the smallest units of heredity, which cause or contribute to disease. The ultimate goal is to use this information to develop new ways to treat, cure, or even prevent the thousands of diseases that afflict humankind. But the road from gene identification to effective treatments is long and fraught with challenges. In the meantime, biotechnology companies are developing diagnostic tests to identify gene mutations in people at risk for having or developing specific diseases. An increasing number of gene tests are becoming available commercially, although the scientific community continues to debate the best way to deliver them to the public and the health care professions may be unaware of their scientific and social implications. While some of these tests have greatly improved and even saved lives, scientists remain unsure of how to interpret many of them. Also, patients taking the tests may have concerns that results will jeopardize their employment or insurance status. And because genetic information is shared, these risks may extend beyond them to their family members as well.

Explorations into the function of each human gene will shed light on how faulty genes play a role in disease causation. With this knowledge, commercial efforts are shifting away from diagnostics and toward developing a new generation of therapeutics based on genes. Drug design is being revolutionized as researchers create new classes of medicines based on a reasoned approach to the use of information on gene sequence and protein structure function rather than the traditional trial-and-error method. Drugs targeted to specific sites in the body promise to have fewer side effects than many of today's medicines.

Gene Therapy

Gene therapy is the potential for using genes themselves to treat disease. The media has ignited the imaginations of the public and the biomedical community as to the benefits and challenges of this new science (Tambor, et al., 2002). This rapidly developing field holds great potential for treating or even curing genetic and acquired diseases, using normal genes to replace or supplement a defective gene or to bolster immunity to disease.

Genes are specific sequences of bases that encode instructions on how to make proteins. Although genes get a lot of attention, it is protein that performs most life functions and constitutes the majority of cellular structures. When genes are altered so that the encoded proteins are unable to carry out their normal functions, genetic disorders can result. Gene therapy is a technique for correcting defective genes responsible for disease development. Researchers may use one of several approaches for correcting faulty genes.

In most gene therapy studies, a normal gene is inserted into the genome to replace an abnormal, disease-causing gene. A carrier molecule called a vector must be used to deliver the therapeutic gene to the patient's target cells. Currently, the most common vector is a virus that has been genetically altered to carry normal human DNA. Viruses have evolved a way of encapsulating and delivering their genes to human cells in a pathogenic manner. Scientists have tried to take advantage of this capability and manipulate the virus genome to remove disease-causing genes and insert therapeutic genes.

Target cells, such as the patient's liver or lung cells, are infected with the viral vector. The vector then unloads its genetic material containing the therapeutic human gene into the target cell. The generation of a functional protein product from the therapeutic gene restores the target cell to a normal state.

Besides virus-mediated gene-delivery systems, there are several nonviral options for gene delivery. The simplest method is the direct introduction of therapeutic DNA into target cells. This approach is limited in its application, because it can be used only with certain tissues and requires large amounts of DNA. Another nonviral approach involves the creation of an artificial lipid sphere with an aqueous core. This liposome, which carries the therapeutic DNA, is capable of passing the DNA through the target cell's membrane.

Therapeutic DNA also can get inside target cells by chemically linking the DNA to a molecule that will bind to special cell receptors. Once bound to these receptors, the therapeutic DNA constructs are engulfed by the cell membrane and passed into the interior of the target cell. This delivery system tends to be less effective than other options.

Researchers also are experimenting with introducing a 47th (artificial human) chromosome into target cells. This chromosome would exist autonomously alongside the standard 46, not affecting their workings or causing any mutations. It would be a large vector capable of carrying substantial amounts of genetic code, and scientists anticipate that, because of its construction and autonomy, the body's immune systems would not attack it. A problem with this potential method is the difficulty in delivering such a large molecule to the nucleus of a target cell.

Genetic Engineering

Genetic engineering is a collective term for a group of new research techniques used to manipulate the DNA of cells. This term has come to have a broad meaning including the manipulation and alteration of the genetic constitution of an organism in such a way as to allow it to produce endogenous proteins with properties different from those of the traditional (historic and typical), or to produce entirely different (foreign) proteins altogether. The creation of synthetic forms of insulin, the development of drugs and vaccines, alterations and improvements in agricultural products, and the experimentation with bio warfare materials may have all been accomplished with some form of genetic engineering.

Other words used when referring to genetic engineering include gene splicing, gene manipulation, or recombinant DNA technology. The gene-splicing technique, which produces recombinant DNA, is a method of transporting selected genes from one species to another. For example, in this technique, the genes, which are actually portions of molecules of DNA, are removed from the donor (insect, plant, mammal, or other organism) and spliced into the genetic material of a virus; then the virus is allowed to infect recipient bacteria. In this way the bacteria become recipients of both viral and foreign genetic material. When the virus replicates within the bacteria, large quantities of the foreign as well as viral material are made. Genetic engineering is a way of directly manipulating genetic material in a cell or organism to produce desired traits or characteristics and eliminate undesirable ones.

Human cloning is a type of genetic engineering, but it is not the same as true genetic manipulation. In human cloning, the aim is to duplicate the genes of an existing person so that an identical set is inside a human egg. The result is intended to be a cloned twin. Genetic engineering in its fullest form would result in the child produced having unique genes as a result of laboratory interference, and therefore, the child would not be an identical twin.

Pharmacogenomics

Pharmacogenomics is the study of how an individual's genetic inheritance affects the body's response to drugs. The term comes from the words pharmacology and genomics and is thus the intersection of pharmaceuticals and genetics. The goal of pharmacogenomics is the individualization of drug therapy in which medications are adapted to each person's own genetic makeup. Environment, diet, age, gender, ethnicity, lifestyle, and state of health may all influence a person's response to drugs, but understanding an individual's genetic makeup is thought to be the key to creating personalized drugs with greater efficacy and safety (Weijer & Miller, 2004). This area of study combines traditional pharmaceutical sciences, such as biochemistry with annotated knowledge of genes, proteins, and single nucleotide polymorphisms.

Pharmacogenomics has many anticipated benefits. Pharmaceutical companies will be able to create drugs based on the proteins, enzymes, and RNA molecules associated with genes and diseases. This will facilitate drug discovery and allow drug makers to produce a therapy more targeted to specific diseases. This accuracy not only will maximize therapeutic effects but also decrease damage to nearby healthy cells.

Instead of the standard trial-and-error method of matching patients with the right drugs, primary care providers will be able to assess a patient's genetic profile and prescribe the best available drug therapy from the onset of symptoms or the discover of gene mutation. This approach will be more accurate, speed recovery time, and increase safety because of reduction in adverse reactions and side effects associated with inappropriate dosage. Pharmacogenomics has the potential to dramatically reduce the estimated 100,000 deaths and two million hospitalizations that occur each year in the United States as the result of adverse drug reactions (Weijer & Miller, 2004).

Current methods of basing dosages on weight and age will be replaced with dosages based on a person's genetics. Genetically individualized drugs can predetermine how the body processes specific medications and the time it takes to metabolize it. This will maximize the therapy's value and decrease the likelihood of overdose.

Knowing one's genetic code will allow a person to make adequate lifestyle and environmental changes at an early age so as to avoid or lessen the severity of a genetic disease. Likewise, advance knowledge of particular disease susceptibility will allow careful monitoring, and treatments can be introduced at the most appropriate stage to maximize their therapy.

Vaccines made of genetic material, either DNA or RNA, promise all the benefits of existing vaccines without all the risks. They will activate the immune system but will be unable to cause infections. They will be inexpensive, stable, easy to store, and capable of being engineered to carry several strains of a pathogen at once.

Pharmacogenomics also has the potential to decrease the overall cost of health care. Decreases in the number of adverse drug reactions, the number of failed drug trials, the time it takes to get a drug approved, the length of time patients are on medication, the number of medications patients must take to find an effective therapy, the effects of a disease on the body through early detection, and an increase in the range of possible drug targets will promote a net decrease in the cost of health care. However, pharmacogenomics is a developing research field that is still in its infancy and will have to be overcome many barriers before the comprehensive range of benefits can be realized.

EXPANDED ROLES FOR NURSES

Nurses around the world have entered a new era in which the reality of genetic advances and knowledge impacts the practice of every nurse (Edgar, 2004; Ehlers, 2002; Gilchrist & Hall, 2002; Terzioglu, & Dinc, 2004). No longer is it acceptable to just mention genetics in the nursing curriculum. Genetic nursing practice has been transformed from a nearly invisible specialty to critical component of clinical practice with formal recognition by the American Nurses Association (ANA), publication of scope and standards of practice, and most recently the availability of credentialing for genetic nurses (Greco & Mahon, 2003).

Genetics now plays a role in all health care settings and affects individuals across the life span. Research has indicated that human diseases, such as myocardial infarction, cancer, mental illness, diabetes, and AD are a result of complex interactions between a number of factors including the influence of one or more genes and a variety of environmental exposures. The influence of recent genetic advances on nursing practice is especially evident in oncology. Oncology nurses practicing in cancer prevention and control apply genetic principles to their clinical practice daily. For example, they assess hereditary and nonhereditary cancer risk factors, take detailed family histories, and construct **pedigrees** (diagrammatic representations of a family history, indicating the affected individuals and their relationship to proband or index case), identify individuals and families at risk for hereditary cancer syndromes, make recommendations for cancer risk reduction, surveillance, and management, and when appropriate, counsel and educate about the risks and benefits of genetic testing.

It is becoming increasingly necessary to include genetics concepts throughout the nursing curriculum at all levels of nursing education and in continuing education offerings for nursing graduates. Genetics concepts are essential components of every clinical nursing course, didactic nursing courses (research, history, and trends in nursing and human development), biology, microbiology, sociology, anthropology, ethics, and pharmacology courses with specific applications to nursing practice.

Nurses have increased responsibility for understanding the contribution of genetic factors to the development of disease to provide comprehensive nursing care. Appropriate nursing assessment techniques to identify individuals who may be predisposed to certain genetic conditions are becoming the standard of care. Early identification and up-to-date patient education ensures at-risk individuals have access to the most current diagnostic, treatment, and management therapies.

Skills 360°

The Integration of Genetics and Genomics into Nursing Practice

- Correctly identifying patients and families where there is a question of genetic condition or history.
- Taking a thorough family history.
- Carrying out a physical assessment to look for variations that suggest a genetic condition may be present (e.g., exceedingly tall stature; café-au-lait spots).
- Recommending a genetics referral.
- Explaining the genetic counseling and evaluation processes—what the patient and family can expect.
- Actively collaborating with genetics professionals.
- Coordinating genetic-related health care services.
- Giving follow-up care and support.
- Providing information on other parent and patient support resources.

Adapted from Lashley, F. (2005). Genetics in clinical nursing practice (3rd ed.). New York: Springer Publishing Company.

KEY CONCEPTS

- Chromosomes are the thread-like structures within the nucleus of each cell that carry the genes. Each person has 23 pairs of chromosomes, with one of each pair being inherited from the mother and the other from the father.
- Chromosome abnormalities are common with 1 in 200 babies born with a chromosomal abnormality.
- Genes, like chromosomes, are inherited in pairs, one from each parent. The pattern in which heritable characteristics appear in subsequent generations is affected by the number of genes involved in the expression of the trait.
- Genetic screening refers to a systematic search of a population for individuals with genotypes indicating that they are at risk for genetic disease.
- Genetics has an impact across the life span and there are clinical specialty areas when there is a genetic basis for an exhibited or potential health condition.
- Science has developed the capacity to test and screen for gene mutations, but there continues to be a lesser ability to cure conditions associated with heredity and errors in genetic coding.
- The ELSI branch of the HGP was established to address issues of confidentiality, privacy, and to prevent the inappropriate use of genetic information.
- Genetics clinical nursing practice is recognized by the ANA with publication of a scope and standards of practice and more recently the availability of credentialing for genetics nurses.

REVIEW QUESTIONS

1. Which of the following conditions of heredity are considered to be unifactorial?
   1. Sickle cell disease
   2. Cri-du-chat syndrome
   3. Down syndrome
   4. Achondroplasia (dwarfism)
   5. Neural tube defects

2. Genotype is defined as which of the following:
   1. A permanent change in genetic material
   2. The outward expression of the individual's genes
   3. The genetic constitution or blueprint of an individual
   4. Photos of chromosomes that have been arranged by group and size

3. The haploid number of chromosomes in humans is:
   1. 22
   2. 23
   3. 46
   4. 47

4. If a boy inherits a disease that is autosomal recessive, he inherited it from:
   1. His mother
   2. His father
   3. His mother and his father
   4. Neither his mother nor his father

5. An isolated neural tube defect is an example of a:
   1. Recessive condition
   2. Multifactorial condition
   3. Dominant condition
   4. X-linked condition

6. Genetic testing in children is indicated in which of the following situations?
   1. To find out if a child is a carrier for CF
   2. Predictive testing for HD
   3. Diagnosis of Down syndrome
   4. All of the above

7. Which of the following can be regarded as a screening test?
   1. Amniocentesis
   2. Prenatal AFP multiple marker testing
   3. Ultrasound examination
   4. 2 and 3

8. Nurses are involved in genetic testing in the following ways:
   1. Identifying individuals for whom genetic testing is available
   2. Refer individuals for genetic testing
   3. Assessing the impact of genetic test results on the individual and family
   4. All of the above

Continued

REVIEW QUESTIONS—cont'd

9. People with allergies have an inherited predisposition for developing hypersensitivity to allergens. A health immune system is affected by the balance of two types of white blood cells referred to as:
   1. Th1 and Th2
   2. BRCA1 and BRCA2
   3. Phagocytes and IgE
   4. Eosinophils and basophils

10. Allergies and asthma are best described as a(n):
    1. Single gene disorder
    2. Complex multifactorial disorder
    3. Autosomal recessive disease
    4. Autosomal dominant disease

REVIEW ACTIVITIES

1. Martha, a 25-year-old woman, has come for her first clinic visit at eight weeks of pregnancy. She has a 3-year-old son who is in good health at home. Her husband is 27 years old and in good health. When reviewing the family history, she tells you that her sister has a 1-year-old son with CF. What could you tell Martha about the inheritance of CF and her chance to be a CF carrier? What genetic testing would be appropriate to discuss with Martha?

2. Mrs. R. is a 35-year-old Hispanic (American) woman who is 15 weeks pregnant. This is her fourth pregnancy. All her previous children were born in Mexico. All were home births. This is her first visit to the prenatal clinic. Her mother and two sisters accompany her. What genetic testing would be appropriate to discuss with Mrs. R? What would you want to assess before talking with Mrs. R. about genetic testing and prenatal care? What resources could you use to explain genetic testing?

3. Ann is a 40-year-old woman who has a history of anxiety and depression. She has a family history of depression. Her brother, who committed suicide at age 50, her mother, and a late maternal uncle also suffered from depression. Her sister has a history of anxiety and has twin boys who have histories of depression and anxiety. Ann has taken several medications to treat her depression but has had significant side effects. She tells you that she has been looking on the Internet for better treatment and has found several sites that indicate that some people with depression do not respond to the usual dose of antidepressants, and some people have significant adverse effects with the usual dose. Genetic testing is being offered on some sites to help identify individuals who have these difficulties. She tells you that she thinks she may be one of those individuals who cannot handle the usual dose of antidepressant medication and wants to have testing to find out. What inheritance pattern for depression seems to be present in Ann's family? What type of genetic testing is Ann referring to? How would you respond to Ann's request for genetic testing?

Continued

REVIEW ACTIVITIES—cont'd

4. Susan is a 30-year-old pregnant woman who is being followed for her prenatal care by a nurse midwife in a prenatal clinic. When taking the family history, Susan informs the nurse midwife that her husband has a history of a congenital heart defect and some learning issues. His sister was born with a cleft palate, and his sister's daughter was born with a congenital heart defect and also has learning issues. Her husband's father has a history of speech difficulties, and his brother died in early infancy from complications related to a congenital heart defect. Susan tells the nurse midwife that she is concerned about the chance for her baby to be born with a heart defect or cleft palate, because "something seems to be running in my husband's family, with all of those birth defects." What could you tell Susan about the constellation of birth defects and learning issues in her husband's family? What referrals would be appropriate to discuss with Susan?

5. Jane is a 32-year-old woman who is having her annual physical evaluation with her nurse practitioner. As the nurse practitioner is reviewing the family history, Jane tells her that she is adopted but recently learned about her biological mother's family history. Her biological mother died from breast cancer at age 41. Her biological mother apparently had a sister who died in her 30s from cancer of the ovaries. Jane has also learned that she has a biological sister who was treated for breast cancer when she was 38 years old. Jane tells the nurse practitioner that she is concerned about her risk for developing breast cancer and wants to know what she can do "to know whether I will get breast cancer and what I can do." Jane's family history of breast and ovarian cancer suggest what type of inheritance pattern? How could the nurse practitioner respond to Jane's concerns?

Visit the Contemporary Medical-Surgical Nursing online companion resource at www.delmarhealthcare.com for additional content and study aids. Click on Online Companions then select the Nursing discipline.

Stress, Coping, and Adaptation

Ruth Grendell, MSN, RN

CHAPTER TOPICS

- Stress
- Coping
- Adaptation

- Stress and Illness
- Nursing and Stress

Stress (the body's reaction to any stimulus) is an inevitable part of every person's life, especially in a society that is characterized by rapid and accelerating change. Hans Selye (1956), a pioneer in stress research, referred to stress as a stimulus that arouses a reaction, and also as a nonspecific, common response of any demand on the body, whether the effect is mental or physical. According to Richard Lazarus (1990), a renowned psychologist, stress is described as a particular kind of response relationship, a process, or transaction, between the person's perceptions of harm or as a challenge imposed by the environment. Some scientists have labeled stress as the day-to-day happenings that are monotonous, positive, or undesirable, as all these events require an expenditure of energy to meet the demands. Numerous studies have been conducted to understand the complexities of the stress concept, the various sources of stressors, as well as the influence of exposure to prolonged stress and the subsequent association with psychological and physiological illnesses (Rintala, Robinson-Whelen, & Matamoros, 2005). It is estimated that 60 to 90 percent of health care visits in the United States are for stress-related illnesses. This chapter focuses on (a) the theoretical concepts related to stress, various coping strategies, and adaptation, (b) stress/illness relationships, (c) stress management strategies, (d) their significance to nursing, and (e) the impact on patient/client outcomes. The chapter begins with an overview of the several historical and theoretical perspectives believed to be causative factors of illness and disease.

KEY TERMS

Adaptation (Adjustment)
Adrenergic stress response
Anticipatory stress
Coping
Coping efficacy
Distress
Dysthymia
Empowerment
Eustress
General inhibition syndrome (GIS)
Health
Homeostasis
Hope
Posttraumatic stress disorder (PTSD)
Psychoneuroimmunoendocrinology (PNIE)
Resilience
Self-efficacy
Social support
Stress

HISTORICAL AND THEORETICAL PERSPECTIVES

The concept of stress has evolved for many years, and there have been varied factors influencing the knowledge of the stress response. From early civilization to present, there have been many ideologies on the causative nature of stress and the individual methods of adaptation and coping mechanisms to the stress response. In addition, there are a variety of theoretical developments that also add knowledge to the general concepts of stress.

Early Civilization Theories and Practices

Since ancient times, various theories have been used to explain the causative factors of disease, such as being the result of anger of the gods, evil spirits, and demons, as a matter of fate, or because human destiny was determined by the stars. Sorcerers, priests, and witch doctors used magic, exorcism, herbs, and potions to placate the evil spirits. Animal sacrifices were made to appease the gods. Trephining, the boring of holes into the skull, was often performed to allow evil spirits to leave the body. In biblical times illness was a representation of God's wrath on sinful man, and many laws were established regarding touching things that were unclean and for eliminating unclean foods from the diet. People with leprosy were quarantined away from the society (Mohr & Pelletier, 2006). Each of these theories attributed one specific causative factor for all diseases.

Oriental beliefs taught that physical and emotional health depended on the orderly flow through the body channels of Qi (Chi), a mysterious life energy source that produced a proper balance between feminine and masculine components of yin and yang. Any blockage in this energy flow resulted in disease that could be cured by acupuncture and other ancient Oriental treatments.

Aristotle, Plato, Aquinas, Hippocrates, and others considered the behavioral influence of the interaction between the human mind and body in health and illness. Hippocrates proposed that health was dependent on the harmony, or balance, between the body, the mind, and the environment; illness was the result of an imbalance or disharmony. However, in the 17th century, René Descartes, a French philosopher, considered the body a complex machine, a separate entity from the mind. Descartes' ideas became the fundamental principles for traditional Western medicine. Illness occurred when the body broke down; it was the responsibility of the doctor, or healer, to locate the faulty part and to fix it. Problems related to the mind were beyond the capabilities of man to correct, and therefore delegated to the religious priests for treatment (Daniels, 2004).

The Germ Theory

During the latter part of the 19th century, following the Renaissance period, scientists began to study the cause of infectious diseases. Ignaz Semmelweis (1818–1865), an obstetrician, claimed that puerperal, or child-birth, fever was a contagious disease and insisted on hand washing and disinfection when physicians attended women in labor. Anton Van Leeuwenhoek (1632–1723) developed the powerful microscope lens and demonstrated that minute organisms existed in a variety of substances. Louis Pasteur (1822–1895) discovered that bacteria caused disease and showed that bacteria could be controlled. Sir Joseph Lister (1827–1912) extended Pasteur's findings and introduced antiseptics into hospital surgeries for cleansing surgeons' hands and instruments. Florence Nightingale (1820–1910) declared that poor sanitation was the cause of many of the diseases experienced by the soldiers during the Crimean War. The military hospital was built over a network of cesspools, sewer lines were blocked, and privies overflowed into the hallways. Windows were closed against the cold, wind, and rain, thus trapping the stench from the sewers together with smoke from the stoves. The water supply was visibly contaminated with organic matter. Cholera, typhoid, typhus, untreated wounds, inadequate nutrition, lack of drugs, and lack of appropriate care were prominent causes of death. Nightingale worked diligently in establishing standards of care and for maintaining a clean and safe environment. The germ theory became a pivotal point in developing medical treatment, nursing interventions, and reduction of deaths (Blais, Hayes, Kozier, & Erb, 2002).

Until this time, nursing had little prestige and care for the sick in hospitals or private homes was often performed by untrained prisoners or prostitutes who had little interest in their work. In many ancient cultures, the nurturing role was provided by midwives, herbalists, wet nurses, and caregivers for children and the elderly. During the Middle Ages (A.D. 500–1500) and the time of the crusades, military, religious, and secular orders for men and women were established to care for the sick. From 1600 to 1850, hospitals and programs of nursing education were established in Europe, Canada, and the United States by various religious orders; yet, little was known about controlling contagious diseases including dysentery, smallpox, and yellow fever, which still caused deaths among patients and their caregivers (Blais et al., 2002).

The Biological Theory

In the early part of the 20th century, scientists realized that the germ theory could not explain all diseases. The biological model that evolved from the germ theory classified diseases according to cause and effect. Signs and symptoms of a disease were observable indications that something had invaded the body to cause the disease, or there was a malfunction of the body cells or organs. Because of the strong influence of Descartes' earlier philosophical beliefs on the practice of medicine, the biological model often ignored the psychosocial components of disease. Scant attention was given to the patient's subjective comments and feelings regarding the symptoms.

Multicausal Theories

Historically people did not live long enough to acquire many of the chronic diseases that are prevalent today. Scientists discovered that disease processes could be related to multiple causes, such as lifestyle, diet, genetics, and the stress response. Scientists began to link the impact of threatening environmental stimuli on the body's protective responses to the association between emotional reactions and the rapid release of epinephrine from the sympathetic nervous system (Marcus, 2004). This reaction was referred to as the body's **adrenergic stress response.**

Stress Stimulus-Response Theory

Hans Selye (1991), an endocrinologist and pioneer in stress research during the 1940s and 1950s, expanded on this biological theory through his investigations of human responses to stressful, or noxious, stimuli and primarily on the prolonged effects of **posttraumatic stress disorder (PTSD)** experienced by World War II veterans, formerly referred to as shell shock or combat fatigue. PTSD will be discussed more fully later in the chapter.

Selye (1991, p. 22) explained that stress as a stimulus could be: "a variety of dissimilar situations: emotional arousal, effort, fatigue, pain, fear, concentration, humiliation, loss of blood, and even great and unexpected success; hence, no single factor can, in itself, be pinpointed as the cause of the [person's] stress reaction." Selye stated that a certain level of stress whether positive (**eustress**) or negative (**distress**) produces changes that are needed for growth and survival. Eustress is a nonspecific stress response associated with desirable events such as marriage or a job promotion; distress is a subjective response to internal or external stimuli that are threatening or perceived as threatening to the self. Selye also found that human and animal bodies and plant life responded to any type of stress with a predictable adaptive pattern of events to maintain **homeostasis,** the "coordinated physiologic processes which maintain most of the steady states in the organism" (p. 23).

Selye (1956, 1991) postulated that the rapid biological fight or flight stress survival response to internal or external threatening stimuli was triggered by the reciprocal reaction between the autonomic nervous system (ANS) and the endocrine system. The release of epinephrine from the sympathetic branch of the ANS and activation of the hypothalamic-pituitary-adrenal (HPA) axis results in the release of cortisol from the adrenal glands, and places the person on alert (Marcus, 2004; Porth, 2003). Selye also noted that the immune system was affected by an increase in white blood cells regardless of the stressor. During the 1940s and 1950s, other researchers were investigating the effects of chemicals secreted by the ANS in regulating cardiovascular, gastrointestinal (GI), and motor responses. Like Selye, they also found that the physiological balance, or homeostasis, was often disrupted in response to stress. The researchers noted that the sympathetic nervous system of the ANS was particularly responsive to environmental stimuli and involved emotional reactions, as well.

Selye (1956, 1991) labeled the three stages of the individual's behavioral responses to stress, whether positive or negative, as the biological stress syndrome or general adaptation syndrome (GAS). The GAS associated processes are normal responses and are considered as adaptation measures to help people cope with the immediate threat. The first stage is a brief alarm reaction stage or fight or flight stage, which alerts the individual to the presence of stressful stimuli. Responses during this stage include elevation of blood pressure, tachycardia, constriction of blood vessels, and diversion of blood from nonessential organs to the heart, brain, and skeletal muscles, increased muscle tone, increased blood sugar levels, dilated pupils, increased alertness, and free-floating anxiety (Table 10-1).

The second stage, resistance, is a more prolonged stage that comprises the biological and psychological behavioral methods used to eliminate or modify the threat. During this stage, energy resources of the neuroendocrine-adrenal systems are mobilized to enhance epinephrine's vasoconstrictive effects, to help to sustain the elevated blood pressure, activate the immune system, and all unnecessary functions are temporarily shut down. The severity or persistent activity of the stress response, the frequency of threats, nonadaptive responses, or a breakdown in the body's negative feedback system that normally regulates the stress response can have health-damaging effects. The persistent elevated levels of cortisol and catecholamines, because of stimulation of the sympathetic nervous system, affect multiple organ systems of the body, including the brain, the immune system, and the cardiovascular system (Porth, 2003).

The third stage, exhaustion, is when the individual's psychological and biological resources are depleted and results in a loss of adaptability to the stressor. The person may become ill or die if resources are not replenished. However, even the stage of exhaustion need not be irreversible and can have only a limited effect when the body is able to adapt or the stressor is removed. In some cases, the individual freezes, or shuts down and is unable to respond in any manner. Neurnberger (1981) termed this reaction as the "possum response" because of overstimulation of the parasympathetic nervous system (PNS) and labeled this reaction as the **general inhibition syndrome (GIS),** which can be used as a means of survival or as a paralyzing or numbing effect when facing a life-threatening event.

More recently, technology, such as positron emission tomography (PET), has permitted observation of the living brain and the role of stress on brain function, particularly related to long-term effects of PTSD. Certain portions of the brain, particularly the frontal cortex, can be suppressed because of a cascade of events that involve many integrated levels of control between the neuroendocrine sys-

TABLE 10-1 **Fight or Flight Responses to Stress**

STAGES	BIOLOGICAL	COGNITIVE APPRAISAL	EMOTIONAL/BEHAVIORAL
Alarm Activation of sympathetic nervous system and endocrine system to mobilize resources for survival	Dilated pupils Dilated bronchioles ↑ Heart rate, pulse rate, blood pressure ↑ Vascular smooth muscle tone ↑ Blood sugar ↑ Constriction of blood vessels Diaphoresis Relaxes smooth muscle—GI system Bladder Uterus Dry mouth ↓ Hearing and pain sensations	Broad perception of multiple internal and external stimuli ↓ Alert; focused attention. Problem-solving activities ↓ Selection of response	Tense, excited Readiness for action Concerned or interested facial expression May experience shock, numbness, fear, hostility, anxiety May seek assistance and enlist all inner strengths to meet the challenge
Resistance	Above biological responses continue and increase in intensity GI symptoms—diarrhea Bladder—urgency and frequency ↓ Pain and hearing sensations	Secondary appraisal Narrowing of perception Selective focus Selective inattention to block out stress stimuli	Behavior can be extremely active or inactive Pace about, wringing hands Startles easily; feels threatened Behaviors may become disorganized Irritable, agitated Use of ego defense mechanisms (denial, repression, regression, etc.) May exhibit somatic symptoms— aches/pains Alcohol or drug abuse Withdraw/isolate self May be depressed
Exhaustion	Resources depleted Pale skin ↓ Blood pressure ↓ Muscle coordination ↓ Pain and hearing sensations Death may result unless resources are replenished or stressor is removed	Scattered thoughts Unable to respond to stimuli Dissociation may occur	Feels helplessness, terrified Crying/sobbing, scream, moan Loss of control May display anger, be combative or withdraw, run away Panic/freeze

Adapted from Daniels, R. (2004). Nursing fundamentals: Caring and clinical decision making. New York: Thomson Delmar Learning; Marcus, P. (2004). Anxiety and related disorders. In K. Fortinash & P. Holoday-Worret (Ed.), Psychiatric mental health nursing (3rd ed., pp. 112–123). St. Louis, MO: Mosby.

tem and multiple body systems. Prolonged exposure to stress causes atrophic changes in the hippocampus; decreases short-term memory storage, a potential for repeatedly reliving the event; increases risk for depression; and causes poor regulation of endocrine responses to stress. Psychological stress has been defined as all processes, whether originating in the external environment or within the person, that demand a mental appraisal of the event before the involvement or activation of any other system (Hagerty & Patusky, 2004; Marcus, 2004).

Appraisal-Transaction Theory

Psychosocial theories, such as the appraisal-transaction theory, help explain how disease or illness can occur in one person while other people remain healthy. These theories have revised many of the former concepts of disease/illness causative factors. From the 1970s to the 1990s psychosocial research was conducted on stress, stress appraisal, coping mechanisms, and adaptation. Lazarus (1990) stated that stress is mainly subjective and can change at any given time. Stress, then, is defined as "the relationship which the demands [of the stressor] tax or exceed the person's resources" (p. 4). Lazarus and Folkman (1987) viewed stress as a transaction process, rather than an event, that occurs as the person makes a cognitive appraisal of each stress encounter regarding its intensity as either harmful, a threat of harm, or as a challenge to overcome. The process is dependent on the individual's current and past experiences with stressful stimuli, or stressors, and is influenced by the person's characteristics of problem-focused or emotion-focused coping skills, and the timing of the event. Problem-focused coping skills refer to strategies used to resolve the stressful situation. Emotion-focused coping skills are the responses related to fear, anxiety, and ego defense mechanisms such as denial or repression. A secondary appraisal determines what the response will be, such as what coping method will be used to minimize the impact of the stress. The social response is actually a prerequisite to selecting a coping strategy because of the person's need for (a) understanding what is happening, (b) discovering the unique factors that may have contributed to the situation, and (c) comparing personal skills and capability with those of others with similar problems. Lazarus also stated that the degree of resistance to infectious microbes is greatly affected by the individual's methods for coping with stress and general life experiences (Stuart, 2004).

Lazarus (1990) believed that all life events are considered to evoke various degrees of stress and that many of the life's stressful events consist of the accumulation of seemingly minor daily annoyances; therefore, stress must be viewed within the total context and not in isolation. Any measurement of stress should assess the source, frequency, and degree of intensity to determine the effect that these daily hassles may have on the person over time. Hassles were defined as annoying or troublesome concerns, states of confusion or turmoil, and events that the person cannot control. The effect of an event is also influenced by the individual's perception of social support, whether it is desired or not desired or considered to be sufficient or insufficient. Hassles can also affect coping processes. Self-generated hassles and poor coping skills are more damaging to a person's health than hassles that occur by chance. Lazarus also investigated daily uplifts as buffering measures against the effect of daily hassles. Uplifts, such as meeting with friends, touching and physical contact, satisfaction in completing a task, healthy self-care, meditation, and prayer have been found to sustain or restore a balance (Figure 10-1). The findings of several studies revealed fluctuations in content and intensity of stress reactions over time. Lazarus concluded that daily hassles were more significant contributors to illness than major life events.

Life Changes and Illness Theory

Holmes and Rahe (1967) also studied the relationship of life events as stressful stimuli and the subsequent response as a transaction process. Their work focused on the universal maturational changes (childhood, adolescence,

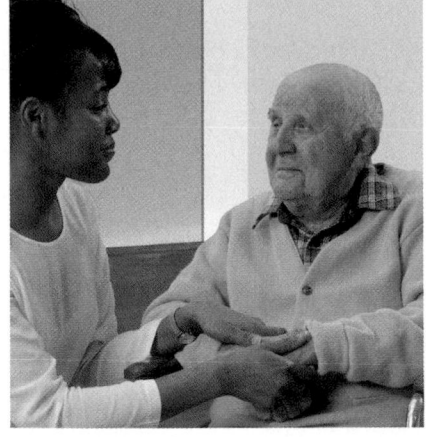

Figure 10-1 Physical contact in the form of touch is uplifting and is one means of creating a balance to the stressors of life.

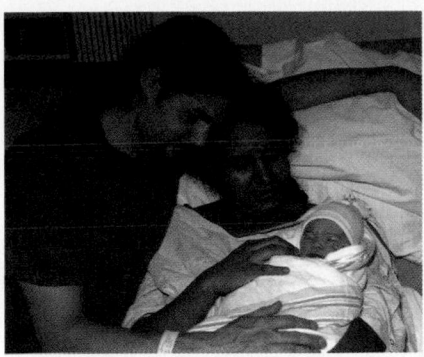

Figure 10-2 The birth experience is a normal transition change that creates varying levels of stress.

adulthood, and aging) and the transitional changes (e.g., marriage, death of spouse, changing careers) throughout life that can create varying levels of stress and the subsequent type of response (Figure 10-2). Adaptation to many significant changes over a short period of time can tax the person's energy sources. They predicted that the outcome of an individual's responses to life events was mediated by the individual's evaluation of the stimuli, previous experiences, developmental level, age, cultural background, and personal resources such as problem-solving skills. They found that effective coping was closely linked to a positive self-esteem and perceived **self-efficacy,** or internal locus of control, in mastering difficult situations and the ability to actively control one's own destiny. Ineffective coping was associated with irrational beliefs, negative outcomes of personal responses to previous stressful experiences, self-blame, and external locus of control, a feeling of no personal control over life events or one's own destiny (Fortinash & Holoday-Worret, 2004). Holmes and Rahe's social readjustment rating scale developed in 1967 has been used in numerous studies and indicated that a cluster of both positive and negative life changes within a relatively short time can be contributing factors to illness. Examples of significant life changes that require a greater level of adaptation include death of a spouse, marriage, divorce, personal injury, and retirement. Examples of events that may be perceived as a lower significance include holidays, a vacation, a change in eating habits, and a change in residence or job. However, further research is needed as the scale does not include any of the chronic life changes, monotony, anticipated stress, or unexpected events that can be significant stressors.

Stress, Organ Maladaptation, and Disease Theory

Harold Wolff (Black & Hawks, 2004) studied human responses to chronic stressors and believed that the individual's total positive and negative life experiences influence the person's susceptibility to disease. Wolff stated that the coping strategies used to maintain homeostasis, or balance, may be appropriate, but the consistent response could cause pathological changes and tissue damage in a particular body system or organ, such as the musculoskeletal or GI systems, or mucous membranes throughout the body (Black & Hawks, 2004). Wolff encouraged his psychiatry residents, including Thomas Holmes and Stewart Wolf, to practice and research the field of psychosomatic medicine. The research by Holmes and Rahe (1967) had a tremendous impact on the practice of mind-body medicine. Stewart Wolf's (1979) research demonstrated the importance of social relationships as a buffering agent against ischemic heart disease in men under the age of 55 (Black & Hawks, 2004).

Psychoneuroimmunoendocrinology

Psychoneuroimmunoendocrinology (PNIE) is a multidisciplinary paradigm involving psychosomatic, or mind-body, medicine that emerged in 1955. PNIE studies are used to define extensive links among the intricate web of neurological activity, the endocrine system, and altered immune response in stressed patients and those with depressive disorders (McCain, Gray, Walter, & Robins, 2005). Stress is the phenomenon most people encounter nearly every day and can lead to depression, feelings of helplessness, hopelessness, and loss of control and may also suppress immunity. A greater resistance to illness has been associated with lower levels of stress and anxiety. Stress has also been defined as the wear and tear on the body over time. The PNIE model provides a holistic framework for screening risk factors of health problems including consideration of stress stimuli, sociodemographic factors, lifestyle behaviors, and health history.

More recently, scientists have explored the ancient mind-body healing practices used in other societies, particularly the Oriental healing arts. Complementary

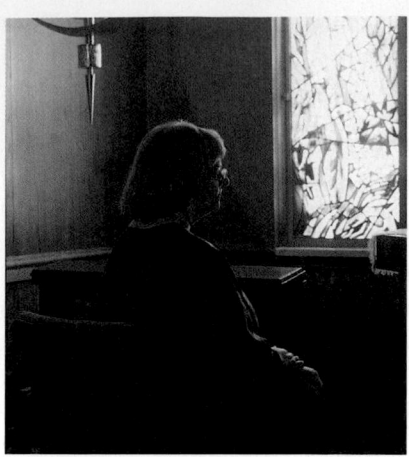

Figure 10-3 Prayer is one form of religious practice that can play an important role in maintaining health and wellness.

BOX 10-1

COMMON COMPLEMENTARY ALTERNATIVE MEDICINE AND THERAPIES

- Meditation, prayer, yoga, and exercise.
- The arts—music, dance, drama, art, literature, and humor.
- Traditional Oriental medicine—acupuncture, acupressure, moxibustion, and herbal medicine.
- Ayurvedic medicine, homeopathic medicine, naturopathy, environmental medicines, and culture-based medicines.
- Diet (food elimination, ethnic-based, and vegetarian diets) and nutrition supplements.
- Osteopathy, chiropractic medicine, massage, reflexology, and therapeutic touch.

Source: National Center for Complementary and Alternative Medicine (NCCAM). (2006). What is complementary and alternative medicine? (p. 11). Retrieved June 23, 2006, from http://nccam. nih.gov.

---

alternative medicine (CAM), such as exercise, nutrition guidelines, acupuncture, herbal remedies, and stress reduction measures, including biofeedback and meditation, is being slowly integrated into mainstream health care. The National Center for Complementary Alternative Medicine (NCCAM) was established in 1998 as a subsidiary agency of the National Institute of Health (NIH) to investigate the effectiveness of several popular CAM therapies. Kenneth Pelletier (2004), a past director of NCCAM, defined CAM as a broad range of healing philosophies, approaches, and therapies that mainstream Western (conventional) medicine does not commonly use, accept, study, understand, or make available.

However, some barriers exist including the demand by Western medicine circles for clinical studies within strictly controlled parameters and the concerns about the accuracy and dosage of herbal remedies. Additional concerns are in regard to self-diagnosis and the availability of the remedies through the Internet and over the counter. People all over the world have become disillusioned with medicine that looks at human beings as physical bodies only and are fascinated by mind-body interactions and are interested in spirituality. Consumers are not waiting for scientific studies to tell them what acceptable choices are, and the use of alternative therapies is now the fastest-growing aspect of American health care.

The focus of CAM is on the health of the total person. Illness is viewed as an imbalance. Religious and spiritual values are important aspects of health (Figure 10-3). Pelletier (2004) cautioned that Western medicine also includes some practices that have not been validated by research. To avoid a double standard, Pelletier believes all therapeutic interventions should be held to the same rigorous standards of research or evidence-based medicine. Research can also validate the benefits or identify the dangers of both types of therapy.

Resistance to incorporating CAM into mainstream medicine is still strong. Many health care providers have little knowledge about CAM interventions, and many patients do not inform their health care providers about their use of alternative medicines. In some instances this can have disastrous effects because of interactions between the herbal supplements and medications. Because of the extreme popularity of CAM therapies, it is imperative that practitioners of traditional medicine become more knowledgeable about CAM, and that there is open communication and collaboration between patient and provider (Box 10-1).

The preceding discussion is an overview of the progression in the development of stress theories, and the role that stress plays as a potential or actual contributing factor to illness and disease. The theories provide a framework for interpreting human responses to stress and for planning interventions. Primary themes include: There is now a general agreement that stress is a part of life, and no one is immune to its effects. Researchers have supported Selye's (1956) initial theory that there is a general characteristic and predictable adaptive patterned response to positive or negative stress. The response involves the biological and psychological mechanisms to maintain the person's homeostasis, or equilibrium. However, the meaning of stress is in the eye of the beholder, and each person is unique in appraising and coping with stress. The person's response is also dependent on predisposing factors such as age, developmental level, cultural background, previous stressful experiences, variations in personality style, and need for personal control. Research has shown that there is a strong association between illness and disease and exposure to the total number, frequency, and duration of positive and negative stressors. Dealing with life changes, or daily hassles, can have a greater effect on a person's attitude and health than major stressful occurrences. Self-generated hassles and poor coping skills are more damaging to a person's health than hassles that occur by chance. Illness and disease are the result of multiple factors.

The current health care model includes a greater emphasis on holistic care, which considers the person's total biopsychosocial and spiritual needs. This is especially important as a greater emphasis is placed on health promotion across the life span, promoting self-care management, providing community-based services for managing care of people with chronic illnesses, and toward cost containment. It is imperative for nurses to recognize the impact of stress and the rationale of people's responses to stress to assist them in having the optimal quality of life regardless of the circumstances.

COPING

Coping is defined as methods to deal with and attempt to overcome problems and difficulties, such as adjustment or adaptation to stressful events, violence, and illness. Conscious methods may be learned and may be adaptive or maladaptive; unconscious mechanisms are often referred to as protective ego defenses (Holloday-Worret, 2004). Adaptive conscious mechanisms include exercising, seeking social support, reading, journaling, crying, practicing relaxation techniques, and use of meditation or prayer. Maladaptive conscious mechanisms can be sleeping, withdrawing from social contacts, overeating, smoking, drug and alcohol abuse, and excessive involvement in an activity. Unconscious ego defense mechanisms include repression, denial, rationalization, regression, displacement, and a discharge of pent-up feelings, such as hostility or regression to an earlier level of adaptation. Unconscious mechanisms may prevent the individual from a realistic appraisal of self, other people, and situations. These lists of conscious and unconscious defense mechanisms are not all inclusive, because many other ego defense mechanisms can be utilized. The goal is to use strategies to minimize unnecessary sources of stress and to promote effective adaptive responses.

However, it is important to recognize that the choice of response may be the only one available or acceptable to protect the integrity to the person at the time. A response may be a temporary measure until the immediate crisis is resolved or the person can gain control of the situation. During the appraisal process, the person may use a variety of coping options, such as wondering how to alter the situation, accept it, seek more information, or resist impulsive actions. The ability to regulate emotions, behavior, and the environment are critical to successful adjustment, because heightened emotions can interfere with the thought processes necessary to effectively deal with stressors. Careful and cautious assessment of the person's behavior may be required in determining whether the coping mechanism should be supported or altered. The ultimate goal of quality nursing care is to promote a healthy outcome.

Studies have shown that after experiencing a major trauma patients reveal that the severity of the injury influenced the person's perception of the stressful event. Perceived control, satisfaction with social support, and problem-focused coping strategies play important roles in minimizing the trauma effect. Avoidance and wishful thinking coping mechanisms are predictors for PTSD (Bisson & Andrew, 2005). Studies have also found that care providers frequently underestimate the psychological effects of trauma that can contribute to costly prolonged hospital stay, decreased productivity of the person, and increased medical costs. Social support is also found to be an important factor in recovery. **Social support** is defined as the person's perception of and the degree of satisfaction with support systems. **Coping efficacy** is defined as the individual's perceived effectiveness of the coping effort to manage the stressful event. Emotion-focused coping behaviors included avoidance, wishful thinking, and self-blame. Problem-focused coping is identified as taking direct action to solve a problem, such as identifying personal strengths and accepting support when needed.

Resilience

Resilience is a dynamic process that involves protective factors against stress, such as effective problem-solving strategies and adaptability to situations that the person cannot control or change. Resilience has also been described as self-efficacy, or perseverance, of being optimistic in overcoming a stressful situation, having an internal locus of control, having a personal responsibility in managing life, and minimizing risk factors (Tusaie & Dyer, 2004). Resilience and hardiness, another concept of inner strength, are frequently used synonymously.

Kinsel (2005) studied resilience in older women. Face-to-face audiotaped interviews with 17 women between the ages of 70 and 80 were the primary data source. Paths to resilience were variously affected depending on developmental, socialstructural, historical, and individual life story influences. Among the seven factors that emerged as salient to resilience in this study were the external resource of social connectedness and internal resources, including a head-on approach to challenge and spiritual grounding. Pivotal in the women's lives were curiosity and extending self to others. Moving forward with life following adversity and nontraditional behavior facilitated preservation of the self in these resilient women. Other studies on resilience have studied the adaptation to major transitions, or turning points, in the lives of persons with traumatic incidents (e.g., battered women). Resilient strategies included seeking mentors, becoming assertive, learning to ask for help, and trying to understand the context of the traumatic events. The patients reported that the challenges of coping with crises can be lifelong. Resilience is not a static characteristic, and individuals may still require intervention to return to successful coping patterns (Kinsel, 2005).

Hope

Research with elderly adults living with chronic disease revealed that hope is a multidimensional construct that provides comfort and gives a meaning to life. **Hope** has been defined as the ability to cherish a desire with an expectation of fulfillment. Hope is future-oriented and allows the person to set goals, devise strategies for achieving the desired goals, and have a sense of being in control

 ## Uncovering the Evidence

Stress in Patients with Disabilities

Discussion: This study explores psychological, social, and physical aspects and the ability to fill social roles and deal with the stress that accompanies living with disability.

Women were recruited from various racial, marital status, socioeconomic, and impairment groups who had a physical disability that limited mobility or physical activities. A total of 18 women participated in either focus groups or were interviewed individually. A qualitative analysis of the data was used. The women were found to (a) associate perceptions of health with functional capacity, (b) acknowledge the importance of mental attitudes in promoting and maintaining health, (c) state that health was affected by the presence or absence of social support, (d) define certain health promotion behaviors in terms that fit within their level of function, and (e) express a pervasive frustration with the medical profession and how interactions with health professionals influenced their health.

Stress, for this group, had many sources including attitudes of family and health professionals, disability-related dysfunction, loss of independent living arrangements, and feeling trapped. Coping strategies to manage stress included engaging in meaningful occupations, i.e., listening to music, crafts, watching movies, and other distracting activities, social interactions, and attitude adjustment through prayer, hope, and faith. Release-escapist behaviors included crying, blowing up, smoking, anger, denial, and avoiding stressful situations.

Implications for Practice: Health care providers should be aware of the patient's expressed frustrations with health care (e.g., feelings of being shortchanged) regarding health promotion screenings and lack of information about health and health promotion in the context of disability.

Source: Nosek, M., Hughes, R., Howland, C., Young, M., Mullen, P., & Shelton, M. (2004). The meaning of health for women with physical disabilities: A qualitative analysis. Family and Community Health, 27(1), 6–21.

or having transcendence over suffering. Hope is a never-ending process when living with the unpredictable experiences of a chronic disease. Hope can be lost and regained as the distressful symptoms fluctuate. Hope is a letting go of old values, establishing new ones, learning to protect the self, having some control over pain and symptoms, and being able to enjoy what activities that can still be done (Jones, 2005). Hope is also linked to spiritual beliefs that provide an inner strength in coping with adverse circumstances. The human spirit has been referred to as the unifying inner strength and intangible motivation that nurtures hope, inner peace, and meaning and purpose to life.

All individuals deserve to have hope for their future, even if the future may include death or disability. Spiritual well-being not only predicts a better ability to cope with terminal illness, but actually has a stronger positive effect than depression has toward a negative outcome. Spiritual and physical well-being are inseparable (McClain, Rosenfeld, & Breitbart, 2003). One of the strongest themes in a study with a group of women with physical disabilities was the connection between a positive state of mind and wellness. Many of the participants mentioned the importance of salvaging hope and control out of extraordinarily depressing and oppressive circumstances (Nosek et al., 2004).

ADAPTATION

Adaptation, or **adjustment,** is defined, as an ongoing process of modifying one's behavior in changed circumstances or an altered environment to fulfill psychological, physiological, and social needs. Lazarus (1990) viewed adaptation as a process involving both cognitive and physiological neural-chemical and endocrine processes. Roy and Andrews (1991, p. 4) stated that "adaptive responses are those that promote integrity in terms of the goals of the human system; and the adaptation level is a changing point that represents the person's ability to respond positively in a situation. **Health** is referred to as a state and a process of being and becoming an integrated and whole person." Adaptation has also been referred to as homeostasis or equilibrium and stability (Carver, 2005).

STRESS AND ILLNESS

The relationship between stress and lowered immunity and potential for disease has been extensively researched. Various life events as psychological stressors (e.g., bereavement, divorce, developmental transitions, as well as work-related and caregiver stress) have been identified. Acute illnesses suddenly interrupt or limit a person's activities. Fear, anxiety, powerlessness, helplessness, hostility, and anger are common responses. A rapid recovery and a return to a sense of control over life can quickly erase these emotions.

Posttraumatic Stress Disorder

The affects of acute and chronic stress disorders have been studied extensively during the past 50 years. The results of Selye's (1956) pioneer stress research on PTSD enabled scientists to explore the associated links between stress and acute and chronic illnesses and the stress associated with life-threatening illnesses such as cancer.

Recently investigators have adapted the PTSD model of responses to traumatic events including the experiences of adult and child survivors of sexual abuse, physical abuse, disasters, and the grieving process (Bisson & Andrew, 2005). Identifying factors include: (a) the person has experienced, witnessed, or been confronted with an event or events that involve actual or threatened death or serious injury or a threat to the physical integrity of oneself or others;

Respecting Our Differences

Age-Related Responses to Catastrophic Events

Mature individuals may be inoculated against the most serious psychological consequences of trauma by previous life experiences that protect them. Adolescence is a maturational period that is characterized by stress, which can be compounded by experiencing a catastrophic event. The adolescent may not be unable to respond appropriately because of the lack of experiences to call on. Buffers to stress include cognitive understanding, self-efficacy, and social support.

Source: Daniels, R. (2004). Nursing fundamentals: Caring and clinical decision making. New York: Thomson Delmar Learning.

and (b) The person's response involved intense fear, helplessness, or horror (Stuart, 2004). The typical symptoms depicted in PTSD usually persist longer than one month and cause significant impairment in social or occupational or other significant areas of functioning.

Acute Stress Disorder

Acute stress disorder (ASD) refers to the psychological and physiological responses to a trauma or crisis event. However, the symptoms persist for a shorter duration than PTSD and do not cause prolonged impairment in social or occupational functioning. Onset of symptoms for both types of stress disorders may occur during or after the traumatic event (Stuart, 2004).

Greater attention has been given to ASD since the September 11, 2001 terrorist attacks in the United States and other recent disasters to minimize the long-lasting effects associated with PTSD (Box 10-2). Three of the following responses of ASD to traumatic, or crisis, events include symptoms of dissociation, (a) a sense of detachment or reduced awareness of surroundings, (b) depersonalization (feelings of unreality or alienation, amnesia), and (c) the inability to cope effectively. The onset of these dissociation symptoms may occur during or after the traumatic event and may continue for a few days or up to a month. Immediate psychological and spiritual counseling that allows the individual to freely express stressful feelings of fear and anxiety can assist in gaining a clearer appraisal and impact of the situation, assist with problem solving, and assist with a return to what the person considers to be a normal way of functioning. Supportive therapy includes enhancing the person's strengths and coping skills, decreasing maladaptive responses, encouraging the person to participate in decision making, and promoting the greatest independence as possible (Marcus, 2004; Stuart, 2004).

The wave of terror that has befallen the Israeli civilian population over the past two years, striking deep into the heart of towns and cities all over the country, presents a unique challenge for the health care system of Israel in general and nursing in particular. Nurses identify numerous hardships and great anxiety, particularly in areas of practice, such as emergency departments. People have experienced similar traumatic effects following losses because of recent global environmental disasters such as earthquakes, floods, fires, tornadoes, and major accidental tragedies. Such events can trigger **anticipatory stress** (a concern or worry about a potential problem or the uncertain outcome of a future event and the inability to control one's future) related to the fear of a recurring disaster and its unpredictable outcome and the inability to control one's future. The need for stress management techniques and debriefing skills is strongly recommended for nurses in these unique settings.

Stress of Chronic Illness

Quality of life within the context of chronic illness is difficult to attain for people who face a variety of needs, demands, and discomforts. Chronic illness brings a tremendous social, financial, and emotional burden worldwide. The long-term effects and unpredictability of chronic illness challenge the person's self-esteem, body image, and sexuality, as well as disrupt social relationships and usual role functions within the family, work, and community. In addition, the sense of autonomy is lost.

These chronic diseases are those that require ongoing management over a period of years or decades and include noncommunicable diseases, such as (a) cardiovascular, respiratory, and cancer diseases; (b) persistent chronic diseases (e.g., diabetes, HIV/AIDS); (c) certain long-term mental disorders such as schizophrenia and bipolar disease; and (d) ongoing impairments in structure (e.g., amputations, paralysis, blindness) that can affect persons in all age-groups (Cumbie, Conley, & Berman, 2004). These diseases leave a residual

---

BOX 10-2

POSTTRAUMATIC STRESS DISORDER (PTSD)

Diagnosis of PTSD is dependent on four general criteria: (a) cause is identifiable, (b) reliving experiences of the trauma, (c) repression of the trauma, and (d) symptoms of increased arousal.

Identifiable cause:

- Person has experienced a traumatic event prior to the appearance of symptoms. The person may have experienced or witnessed an event or has been faced by event that threatened death or serious injury or threat to physiological integrity of self or others.
- Response must have involved intense fear, feeling of helplessness, or horror. (Child may demonstrate agitated or disorganized behavior.)

Reliving experiences of the trauma:

- Reexperiencing the event via recurrent intrusive reflections of the event (flashbacks), recurrent dreams or nightmares.
- Person exhibits internal or external cues that resemble the event and physical reactivity on exposure to internal or external cues that resemble the original trauma.

Repression of the trauma:

- Person avoids stimuli that are perceived as associated with the trauma, such as avoiding thoughts, individuals, or places associated with the event or avoids entering into conversations about it.
- Person experiences a numbing of general responsiveness that was not present prior to the trauma or represses memory of an important aspect of the trauma.
- Person has a sense of detachment from life events including nonparticipation in significant activities, has a restricted range of affect, and may have no expectations of a career or normal life span.

Increased arousal (two of the following must be present):

- Sleep disturbances
- Irritability; angry outbursts
- Difficulty concentrating
- Hypervigilance
- Exaggerated startle response

Adapted from Marcus, P. (2004). Anxiety and related disorders. In K. Fortinash & P. Holoday-Worret (Eds.), Psychiatric mental health nursing *(3rd ed., pp. 112–123). St. Louis, MO: Mosby.*

---

disability and are caused by irreversible pathological alterations that require special training of the patient for rehabilitation or may be expected to require a long period of supervision, and observation or care.

Living with a chronic illness requires coping with the patterns of exacerbations of symptoms and remissions or a steady decline. Progression in the severity of symptoms or dysfunctions may be rapid or slow and may be due to side effects, complications, or failure of treatment. Adaptation is a complex and continuous demanding process in restructuring life around the chronic condition, particularly in accepting loss of independence and valued roles, and inability to participate in the anticipated normal life experiences. Uncertainty about the future and a heightened sense of mortality can lead to depression, hopelessness, and helplessness (Neville, 2003).

Some individuals take on the invalid or sick role. They may use their illness to receive attention or to avoid responsibilities. The invalid role can also be the result of self-pity. Society's attitudes have shifted during the last several years from believing that individuals were not responsible for certain illnesses to recognizing that unhealthy lifestyle and behaviors play an active role in the development of some illnesses. Beliefs today also expect individuals to maintain responsibility for personal, family, and social activities that they are capable of doing or learning. There is also the expectation that individuals will seek help in managing the health problem and be actively involved in decision making regarding the options available to them.

PATIENT PLAYBOOK

Patient Education for Managing the Stress of HF

The nurse should consider the following in managing the stress of HF:

- Inform patients that depression, worry, and anxiety are common responses when living with a serious chronic disease. They have the right to be depressed, but also have the responsibility to pull themselves out of it.
- Empower patients through education. Patients need to know enough about the disease and treatment to have a sense of control and to monitor symptoms. Inform patients about appropriate diet, exercise, and medications.
- Encourage patients to maintain a journal to record personal responses to food, activities, medications, and so on that help to identify what helped and what did not. The journal can also be a helpful tool for monitoring progress during appointments with the health care provider.
- Encourage patients to seek social support and to avoid isolation.
- Assist patients in reframing their thoughts and responses to stressful situations, which can trigger an increase in respiratory and cardiac symptoms.

Source: Mason, D. (2003). Being around for a long time: How one woman with heart failure learned to live again. American Journal of Nursing, 103(12), 35.

Many chronic conditions are accompanied by depression, anxiety, or full psychiatric disorders. A recent research study of elderly persons revealed an association of psychological distress and proneness to Alzheimer's disease (Ray, 2004). Several studies have shown that depression, anger, and anxiety and feelings of helpless can exacerbate the devastating effects of a chronic illness or disease such as heart failure (HF). People experience more mood disturbances when there is a greater uncertainty about the progress of an illness, and some individuals said they felt imprisoned in illness. These feelings are often referred to as **dysthymia,** a low-level depression that can last at least two years and can lead to more severe depression if untreated (Artinian, 2003). Not all patients with HF became angry or depressed, and many have found ways to remain engaged in pleasurable activities within their limitations. Elimination of stress was a major factor in adapting and living with HF that included learning to reframe one's thinking and responses to stressful situations.

Artinian (2003) also mentioned that younger persons with HF may experience more stress and depression because of the inability to fulfill family and career goals and facing these limitations sooner than anticipated. Patients and their families often have difficulties in accepting the disruption in their lives, wondering why the illness occurred, and coming to terms with the impact on their lives. Becoming reconciled to living with HF includes self-care management of symptoms, participating in the treatment protocols, and searching for the meaning and purpose of the illness.

Chronic Illness Across the Life Span

The stressors associated with chronic disease of early childhood and adolescence have negative impact on growth and development. Coping strategies and adaptation are often adversely affected and may interfere with maturational and transitional changes and social relationships with others. Some of the environmental and social stresses that contribute to chronic conditions are related to early disruption of attachment because of parental dysfunction; loss of a parent through divorce, death, or other reasons; living with violence and abuse; homelessness; prolonged poverty; and malnutrition. The strengths, coping skills, and available resources of the child and the family are important influences in achieving an optimal level of health.

Greater risk factors with long-term effects for adolescents are smoking, substance abuse, unsafe sexual practices, peer pressure, and stress. Children in these age ranges often practice dangerous and unsafe activities believing that no harm can come to them. Violence and access to potentially dangerous objects (e.g., guns, cars) are also important factors in injuries, which can result in chronic health problems.

Adulthood is a time of dynamic change as the person is involved in defining a new self-image, establishing a career, family, and other social roles. Several transitional stages are experienced as the person moves from entering the adult world, settling down, and entering middle and later phases of adult life. Each phase presents its unique stressors, challenges, and responsibilities. The midlife challenges of the "sandwich generation" are particularly stressful as people take on the responsibility of caring for their children and of their own aging parents. The onset of many chronic diseases occurs during these years.

Aging is also a complex process. The elderly experience many negative life events such as retirement and decreased financial resources, caring for an aging spouse, loss of significant others, and cumulative stress. Multiple health problems are common, and the person learns to adapt through various methods. Many of the former coping strategies may no longer be effective, and new adjustments are necessary. Aging also brings physiological changes that are universal and irreversible involving the body systems. The elderly are more susceptible to falls and injuries that can complicate their independent activities of daily living. Successful adaptation is the ability to let go of some of the past roles and activities, while pursuing new interests that enhance the quality of life.

However, today many elderly are well-educated, maintain better health care practices than some of the younger generation by exercising, having better dietary habits, and eliminating or minimizing the use of alcohol, tobacco, and practice stress management techniques. Many researchers predict that life expectancy will continue to increase. Nurses familiar with the problems of aging, as well as the capabilities of older adults, can help them to effectively manage the daily hassles that they encounter.

ADDITIONAL RISK FACTORS FOR STRESS-RELATED ILLNESS

Illness must always be considered as a stress-related stimulus and as a response. Stress is also referred to as the result of wear and tear over time (Selye, 1990). Additional risk populations for stress include homeless people, people with nutritional deficits, obesity with its impact on mind-body interactions, individuals in stressful occupations, critically ill patients, caregivers for chronically ill people, or people exposed to abusive situations, and age-specific stress conditions.

Cultural Factors

Social demographics within the United States have changed dramatically over the last several years. Immigrants from nations throughout the world have brought their various health care beliefs and practices with them. A person's perspective of what constitutes health and illness and what maintains a balance for the individual, family, and community can be strongly influenced by one's cultural heritage. Conflict arises when there is a mismatch between beliefs of the health care provider and the patient. The adaptive behavior chosen by the person may differ from what the health care professional believes is effective or ineffective. A particular disease may carry a stigma, or a therapeutic procedure may be forbidden. Many cultures adopt a wait-and-see attitude toward illness or use home remedies that have been passed down from generation to generation before seeking professional health care. Some cultures have elaborate systems of healing practice that use folk healers, herbal medicines, purgatives, blood-letting, leeching, and pilgrimages to sacred shrines.

Many health care providers in the United States have been socialized to believe that modern medicine is the only method for preventing and treating illnesses, and there are no alternative forms of healing. Modern technology has yielded greater scientific understanding and helped to eliminate many of the health problems of the past; therefore these advanced skills should be readily embraced by everyone. The health care provider is often unaware of the various cultural beliefs and their effects on patients' perceptions of what constitutes good health practices. The nurse's sensitivity to the various cultural beliefs and practices creates a clearer understanding of the multiple issues that influence interactions with the patient and family.

Environmental Stress

Hospitalization can be a stressful experience for anyone, especially for older individuals who cannot readily adapt to new situations. The older adult commonly experiences hospitalization for an exacerbation of a chronic health condition. Older adults now account for 47 percent of inpatient hospital days. Leaving the security of home and entering the complex and often impersonal health care system is quite stressful. The unfamiliar environment, multiple stimuli, and contacts with numerous hospital personnel can lead to exhaustion and confusion. They may also experience adverse physical or mental problems because of treatment effects, such as medication reactions, immobilization, sleep disturbances, and loss of dignity. Excessive noise, tiring procedures, and

Reducing Environmental Distress for Critically Ill Patients

The nurse can do the following to decrease environmental stimuli that increase a patient's anxiety:

- Provide private room if possible.
- Dim the lights or close window blinds.
- Maintain an environment in which the patient feels free to express emotions.
- Limit contacts with other patients to minimize contagious aspects of anxiety.
- Limit the length of stay and number of visitors at any one time.
- Limit visits with family and visitors that may contribute to patient's anxiety.
- Assist anxious family members to relax.
- Introduce supportive measures such as massage, warm baths, and relaxation techniques.
- Use soft background music if it is soothing to patient.
- Personalize the environment with patient's familiar objects.

Adapted from Hughes, F., Bryan, K., & Robbins, I. (2005). Relatives' experiences of critical care. Nursing in Critical Care, 10(1), 23–30; Aldridge, M. (2005). Decreasing parental stress in the pediatric intensive care unit: One unit's experience. Critical Care Nurse, 25(6), 40–50.

pain are additional stressful stimuli. The older patient is also more vulnerable to falls because of the unfamiliar environment, pressure ulcers because of immobility, dehydration because of the age-related decrease in thirst, or from nausea and vomiting, and inaccessible fluids, constipation because of medication side effects, reduced activity, and diet changes. Loss of functional independence can be because of stereotypical staff expectations and insufficient time for self-care. Knowledge and expertise of the holistic needs of older adults by all care providers, families, and older adults, themselves, provide the ideal model for optimum care. An excellent resource is the National Gerontological Nursing Association's *Core curriculum for gerontological nursing* (Habel, 2004).

The psychosocial needs of critically ill patients are a major concern for them and their families. There is an overwhelming need to feel safe while in the intensive care unit (ICU). Many sources of stress in the ICU have been identified including noise, lighting, sleep interruption, pain, treatments, emotional reactions to life-saving procedures, loss of dignity, and privacy. The elderly patients are particularly prone to confusion. Emotional actions can range from frustration, anger, fighting attitudes, and paranoia. Interviews took place after patients were stabilized during their ICU experience and revealed that loss of control, lack of information, hopelessness, and lack of trust were the major stressors. A model of the psychosocial needs was developed describing what measures contributed to feeling safe. Family, friends, professional staff, religious beliefs, hope, and trust were viewed as contributing factors to feelings of safety.

Caregiver Stress

In the current managed care system, patients are discharged sooner from acute care, and they are more ill. Their continuing care often requires the assistance of family care providers that sometimes results in a heavy psychological, physical, and financial burden (Figure 10-4). Family and spousal caregivers of people with chronic illness define stress as a process. An example of patient condition and caregiver stress is seen in Alzheimer patients (Gruffydd & Randle, 2006). Caregivers recognize the difficulties they encounter with patients who have Alzheimer's disease, and the caregivers learn there is a combined effect when facing stressful events. Many caregivers report that they learn how to differentiate stresses from challenges and learn to select a response to fit the situation. Appraisal of a specific stressful encounter results in a variety of coping styles, including the opposite choices of confrontational behaviors or self-control, distancing self from the situation, accepting the role as a responsibility, seeking social support, or using escape and avoidance behaviors.

Care of cancer patients most frequently takes place in the home. A qualitative study by Borneman, Stahl, Ferrell, and Smith (2002) identified several barriers to maintaining hope for family caregivers of people with cancer. Nursing interventions can include helping caregivers to realize the importance of self-care, to recognize the need for rest to keep fatigue levels at a minimum, to utilize better emotional health practices, and how to deal with anger, despair, and disappointment. Providing symptom control for the patient helps to ease the anxiety of the family caregiver. Support can be provided through listening to their concerns and by identifying measures that help the person to maintain hope.

Occupational Stress

Occupational stressors have been linked to negative physical and emotional outcomes (Hall, 2004). Police, firefighters, people in the military, business executives, nurses, and people whose work has a demanding time pressure are

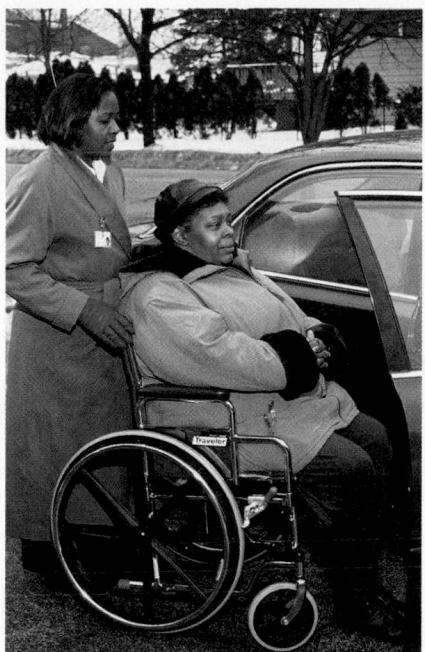

Figure 10-4 This caregiver takes care of her mother, works full time, and is a parent to her young children. The caregiver must be aware of the increased stress this produces.

Respecting Our Differences

Stress in the Home Setting

Patients who have home health care nursing needs are automatically more at risk for stress and anxiety simply because they require assistance outside themselves. Regardless of the primary needs of these patients, the home health nurse must recognize that the patient is likely to experience increased stress. This requires the nurse to carefully assess the patient for the effects of stress on the body systems and to incorporate stress management into the care plan for the patient in a home setting. The nurse must be aware of the variety of clinical manifestations of stress and design interventions accordingly.

Source: Daniels, R. (2004). Nursing fundamentals: Caring and clinical decision making. New York: Thomson Delmar Learning.

considered to be in highly stressful occupations. Additional work-related stressors include job insecurity, work overload, and repetitive tasks. Women who fulfill multiple roles are often more affected by daily stressors than men. The stressors encountered have been associated with decreased job satisfaction, burnout, high turnover rates in acute care settings, and loss of valuable workers from the profession. An increase in absences from work has been linked to work stress–related illnesses. It is imperative that nurses apply self-care principles to their own lives (Sadovich, 2005).

A study by AlRub (2004) investigated the effect of job-related stress on job performance of hospital nurses and the effect of perceived social support from coworkers on stress-performance relationship. Findings from this study supported the benefits of social support in enhancing the quality of care. It was also suggested fostering cooperation, social interaction concepts, and effective coping mechanisms among nursing students might be important for future behaviors. AlRub stated that students who learn the importance of cooperation and social integration during their education might better understand the significance of coworker support in the work place.

Stress in the job setting can lead to nurses not coming to work and taking illness-related days off of their work schedule. Nurses missing days of work can have an impact on the financial well-being of the health care system. This impact is identified in the Dollars and Sense feature, "The Financial Effects of Stress on the Health Care System."

NURSING THEORIES AND STRESS MANAGEMENT

Florence Nightingale (1859) described nursing as one of the finest arts. She proclaimed that the primary nursing skills included close observation of the patient, prevention of illness, and manipulating the patient's environment to assist in the healing, or reparative process. Virginia Henderson (1939, p. 2) defined nursing "as that service to the individual that helps him to attain or maintain a healthy state of mind and body; or, where a return to health is not possible, the relief of pain and discomfort." The work of several nurse scholars that began in the 1970s incorporated Nightingale's and Henderson's principles and are currently recognized as conceptual models for guiding the activities in stress management, nursing education, practice, and research. All nursing theoretical models have been designed as guiding frameworks for implementing nursing care. The following models are selected examples.

Adaptation Model

Sister Callista Roy (1991) viewed stress as a general term for the transaction between the environmental demands for adaptation and the person's responses. Both environmental demands and the person's responses can be of a psychological or physiological nature. Roy conceptualized coping strategies as "innate or acquired ways of responding to the changing environment". Stress can be a focal stimulus that demands the person's immediate attention to deal with it or a contextual stimulus that contributes to the effects of the focal stimulus. An example of a focal stress stimulus could be a painful procedure; contextual stressful stimuli would be a cold room, fatigue, or the illness itself. Roy cautions that stress may be an important factor that influences habits as well as current behaviors. The stress response is the process that results from any physical or psychological stimulus that disturbs the equilibrium or adaptive state. Her nursing conceptual model is based on maintaining total integrity of the individual. Physiological integrity (oxygenation, nutrition, elimination, activity, rest, and protection), and the complex processes involving the senses, fluids and electrolyte balances, and neurological and endocrine

Skills 360°

Nurses Experiencing Burnout

The following are questions to ask if you think you are experiencing burnout:

- What are behaviors and feelings that you have when you are experiencing burnout?
- What are coping mechanisms you use to protect yourself from being emotionally drained when interacting with patients?
- Who do you connect with when you are stressed?
- What are some specific actions you can do to take better care of yourself?

functions. Psychic integrity consists of the self-concept, physical and personal self, role function or social integrity, and interdependence with others in giving and receiving love, respect, and value. Each person's behavior is viewed in relation to the physiological and psychological interactive responses. Roy defines ineffective coping responses, or emotion-focused coping, as not contributing to the integrity of the person; conversely, problem-focused coping, or effective coping responses, assist in maintaining integrity of the person. Roy and Andrews (1999) expanded the original ideas to include recognizing the holistic nature of mind, body, and spirit.

An example for application of the model would identify role transition as a focal stimulus for a new first-time mother. Contextual stimuli are environmental factors that either facilitate or inhibit adaptation during the transition process. The nurse would assess the mother's patterns of expressive behavior and the methods used to gain mastery in the role. The nurse and patient would work together to facilitate the bonding process, assess the need for support in gaining confidence in the new parent role, and identify available resources when going home with the new infant.

Systems Model

The Neuman Systems Model developed in 1972 was based on Selye's (1956) definition of stress as a nonspecific response to any demand on the person's system. Adjustment to stress is dynamic and continuous (Neuman, 1982). She believed that all of life is involved in the interplay of balance and imbalance. Illness occurs when disharmony is prolonged, and the person's needs are not

Uncovering the Evidence

On the Job Stress for Registered Nurses

Discussion: The purpose of this study is to identify common work-related stressors and coping mechanisms of registered nurses within a hospital setting. Occupational stress was defined as "the harmful physical and emotional responses that occur when the requirements of the job do not match the capabilities, resources, or needs of the worker" (p. 7). The method used was a grounded theory qualitative study and was conducted with 10 nurses who worked in a trauma center. The study investigated the nurses' appraisal of events they encountered on a regular basis as stressful and identified the coping strategies were used to help resolve the stress. The study findings revealed four themes of stressful events: (a) identified barriers in meeting patient needs (i.e., time limitations, lack of medications and equipment, and sudden changes in a patient's condition); (b) the inability to meet self-expectations of the nurse; (c) the degree of quantitative workload, including a shortage of skilled labor, and pressure for immediate results in responding to the patients' condition changes; and (d) the salary was not commensurate with responsibility and lack of teamwork also contributed to their perceived stress.

The primary coping strategies for the nurses consisted of talking with and receiving help from coworkers and performing problem solving together, such as prioritizing patient needs, depending on others to help in coping, and meeting the most important need, seeking validation for actions taken. The consequences of experiencing severe occupational stress were dependent on the type of coping strategies. Perceived ineffective coping produced a feeling of being overwhelmed, exhausted, angry, difficulty sleeping, questioning their ability, and a dread of returning to work. Perceived effective coping produced a sense of accomplishment, meeting the challenges, enjoying learning new skills, feeling productive.

Implications for Nursing: Nursing administrators must recognize factors that lead to job dissatisfaction and employee turnover and nursing shortages. Findings should be incorporated into development of orientation programs for new graduates, preparation of preceptors, scheduling of an appropriate mix of skilled staff, and appropriate nurse:patient ratios. The researchers also suggested establishing programs to alleviate some stressors, to improve or provide support for coping and retain nursing staff, and enhance patient care and employee health.

Source: Hall, D. (2004). Work-related stress of registered nurses in a hospital setting. Journal for Nurses in Staff Development, 20(1), 6–14.

DOLLARS AND SENSE

The Financial Effects of Stress on the Health Care System

Nurses are susceptible to stress, particularly those working in mental health and acute care settings. Occupational stress leads to job dissatisfaction, poor morale in the workplace, decreased efficiency and performance, absenteeism, and attrition. These factors definitely contribute to increase the costs of health care. A systematic review of several studies from 1996 to 2000 was conducted in the United Kingdom to identify the sources of stress for working nurses and the effectiveness of stress management interventions. Mixed results were found related to outcomes from interventions in decreasing stress in varied groups of working nurses. Therefore, nurse employers and managers must consider the financial implications of nurses who are struggling with stressors on the job and seek appropriate intervention measures.

Source: Edwards, D., & Burnard, P. (2003). A systematic review of stress and stress management interventions for mental health nurses. Journal of Advanced Nursing, *42(2), 169–200.*

met. Neuman considered the person to be an open system interacting with the environment. Stressors were defined as tension producing stimuli. Nursing roles were described as providing primary prevention before the person encounters a stressor; secondary prevention to minimize the effect or possible effect through early diagnosis of the problem and intervention; and tertiary prevention to reduce any residual stressor effect.

An example for using this model would be an interaction between the nurse and a patient recently diagnosed with breast cancer. The nurse would assess the woman's normal lines of defense in responding to stress and maintaining stability and integrity. Identification of her lines of resistance to stress and illness would also be addressed. The nurse and patient would design a plan of action that would assist in restoring stability during and following the therapeutic treatment.

Self-Care Theory

Dorothea Orem's self-care theory developed in 1959 is one of the most popular theories used today. It is based on a person's capability of meeting own personal health care needs and the health care needs of a dependent individual (child, ill or aging family member). Orem (1995) included dependent care to facilitate application of the theory across the developmental stages of the life span. Self-care deficit is when the person does not have adequate resources to meet the self-care demands. Nursing is viewed as three types of activity systems that provide (a) wholly compensatory care when the person is unable to care for self; (b) partly compensatory care when the person is able to participate in some of the self-care activities; and (c) supportive educational activities that provide the person with additional knowledge and support. Nursing activities are designed to accommodate the patient's changing needs. The supportive educational nursing activities serve to empower the patient to manage self-care activities.

The use of the nursing process within the self-care framework permits the nurse to include the patient in (a) the assessment and identification of the self-care deficit, (b) deciding on the desired outcome, (c) identifying what internal and external resources are available, and (d) deciding on a mutual plan of

> **BOX 10-3**
>
> **OREM AND STRESS MANAGEMENT**
>
> When patients experience stress, encourage them to self-evaluate their surrounding stressors and the environment. Assist the patient in identifying the necessity for understanding their control over their circumstances. Encourage the patient to carefully follow the suggested nursing interventions that can effectively reduce the stress situation. In addition, the nurse needs to consider the patient's self-care needs when providing patient education and implementing the plan of care.
>
> Source: Orem, D. E. (1995). Nursing: Concepts of practice (5th ed.). St. Louis, MO: Mosby-Yearbook.

action. The nurse uses the implementation phase of the nursing process to facilitate the patient's participation and to promote the patient's responsibility for self-care management (Box 10-3). The evaluation phase consists of observing how well the patient is capable of performing self-care tasks, identifying if additional assistance is needed, and determining whether the patient can provide rationale for maintaining healthy self-care.

SIGNIFICANCE TO NURSING

Holistic nursing care requires understanding of a person's history and current physiological, psychological, social, cultural, and spiritual needs from both an individual and generalized view (Weiss, 2005). Each person comes to an illness with a history and knowledge of the particular situation and its impact on life. Interpretation of the event and the responses are dependent on this history, which changes with each new encounter. The person must be recognized as a whole person who is greater than the sum of the parts.

Current Practice Issues

New theory-driven health care models that give attention to acute patient-focused care are in place. However, there is a need for practice models for care of persons with chronic health problems. According to The American Holistic Nursing Association (2006) disease and distress are viewed as opportunities for increasing people's awareness of the interconnectedness of body, mind, and spirit. Nurses have a unique opportunity to provide services to facilitate wholeness.

Five million Americans have been diagnosed with HF; it is estimated that 550,000 new cases will be added each year. Related direct and indirect costs totaled more than $24 billion in 2003 (Artinian, 2003). Approximately 108 million people in the U.S. have one chronic health problem; approximately 25 percent have more than one chronic condition that can complicate management of care. This number is increasing as the large population of baby boomers become part of the older generation. It is predicted by 2020 that chronic conditions will contribute to more than 60 to 70 percent of the global burden of disease, and the social and economic burden of chronic conditions for almost 50 percent of the U.S. population is predicted by 2030 (Cumbie, et al., 2004).

In addition to new care models for treating and managing health problems, there is a need for creating care models for health promotion. The health care industry has experienced a gradual shift, from illness-focused care

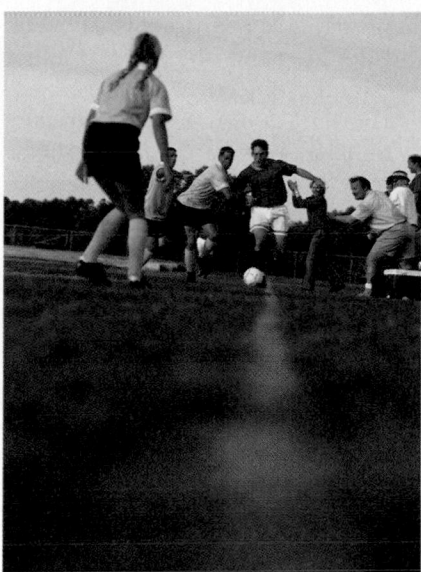

Figure 10-5 Regular physical activity is one form of maintaining and participating in a healthy lifestyle.

to health-focused care. The old paradigm that viewed sickness as just happening and being outside the person's control has been replaced by a new set of rules, which place health care in the position to assist people in adopting healthy lifestyles and participating in illness prevention (Figure 10-5). The former premise that people naturally know what behaviors contribute to health or what threatens optimal health is not true. The health-focused paradigm emphasizes educating people about participating in health-focused behaviors. The transition to the new paradigm has not been an easy one because of the strong beliefs, values, and assumptions in the old paradigm and to the reimbursement system for managing care of disease with no emphasis on reducing the incidence of illness (Thurkettle, 2003). The incentive of the new paradigm is to promote health education and adopting healthy lifestyles, as well as early diagnosis and treatment. The nurse case manager role gained prominence during the transition to the health-focused paradigm.

The nurse case manager can play a pivotal role in meeting the new paradigm goals in contributing to the quality of life for individuals whether sick or well. For instance, the case manager can suggest and assist the health care team in initiating community resources that are available to the elderly, which will aid them in remaining independent; work with at-risk populations and promote access to health screening and immunizations; and enhance self-health care management (Box 10-4).

Traditionally, nurses have had varying roles in the health status of educational institutions. Nurses have played a role in public school systems for many years. Nurses have assisted with identifying many common stressors in the students of the educational facilities and have been proponents of successfully managing stress levels (See Respecting Our Differences feature). Currently, funding problems have made nurses have to struggle to have a viable role in the many educational systems. The role of school nurse is one that continues to be affected and is a significant practice issue as related to the general topic of stress reduction.

Empowering the patient and the family caregiver is an important component of holistic nursing care. The nurse must understand the manifestations of mind-body interactions and recognize the factors that alter a person's resistance to stress. The patient and support system should be involved in decision making and development of the plan of care. The nurse also provides teaching and positive reinforcement to assist the patient and caregivers to assume self-care management. The education process must be individualized and be

---

BOX 10-4

ROLES OF THE NURSE CASE MANAGER

Nurse Managers can contribute to the well-being of the health care system by:
- Collaborating with health care providers in health promotion, health maintenance, illness care, and rehabilitation.
- Providing education related to equipping individuals to fulfill roles in all development phases of the life span including parenting, diet, exercise, stress management, safety practices, and self-care.
- Developing a monitoring program to remind people of screening practices.
- Prepare people for health care system appointments by coaching and clarifying what questions the person should ask during a health care appointment.
- Clarifying any misunderstandings the patient may have following the appointment.

Adapted from Thurkettle, M. (2003). Shifting the healthcare paradigm: The case manager's opportunity and responsibility. Case Management, 8(4), 160–165.

Respecting Our Differences

Stress on a Campus in Canada

The Campus Health Resource Center at the University of Manitoba surveyed 691 students with a health assessment instrument. The results found that many of their students showed interest specifically in stress management skills. Students were not interested in topics generally thought to be important to students such as contraception, safer sex, and STD or AIDS prevention. The implications for nurses in the health center are to address this desire for stress management in education and to further delineate the specific stressors on this population.

Source: Katz, A., Davis, P., & Findlay, S. S. (2002). Ask and ye shall plan: A health needs assessment of a university population. Canadian Journal of Public Health [Revue Canadienne de Sante Publicque], 93(1), 63–66.

appropriate to the patient's level of understanding. A self-contract is an excellent method in setting an outcome goal and defining the objectives to meet that goal. The nurse assists the patient in designing objectives that are challenging, yet within the personal capabilities (Powers, 2003). A self-contract is an agreement that an individual makes with himself or herself, individually or with the assistance of a support person. A self-contract to increase exercise level would stipulate realistic short-term and long-term goals, such as walking for 20 minutes four times a week for six weeks; then, walking/running for 30 minutes five times a week by the end of six months. The type of assistance and evaluation checkpoints would be established, and the type of expected reward would be included. Advantages of self-contracting are the reduction of the patient's passivity and dependency, increase in self-confidence, and facilitating compliance with the therapeutic regimen.

Teresa Campbell (2004) chronicled her experiences of living with multiple sclerosis for 37 years in her book, *Live as an Adventure.* In a recent journal article, she commented that a definitive diagnosis of her disease was not made for over two years after the initial symptoms began. Chronic diseases are difficult to diagnose, and many patients become overwhelmed by stress and feel they must have mental problems, as well. As a retired nursing professor and public health nurse, Campbell knew what resources were available to her. After her diagnosis was confirmed she contacted the National Multiple Sclerosis Society and located a support group, recognizing that knowledge is power, and she would have a group to share her concerns and discover how others were coping with chronic illness problems.

Campbell (2004) said that nurses are vital to those who live with a chronic disease and presented important information for nurses in her article. Nurses must be good listeners. People with chronic illnesses need to express their concerns about their illnesses. Through careful listening, nurses can encourage patients to sort out their symptoms, so they can be presented to their health care providers in a logical sequence within the context of the surrounding events. Campbell mentioned that many physically disabled people resist using assistive devices because they see them as a social stigma and a threat to their identity. Nurses should encourage patients to express these concerns about the mobility aids, assess their mobility with and without the aids, and request referrals for rehabilitation. Nurses must also question the patients about bladder and bowel function, because patients may feel embarrassed about discussing these issues. Nurses can also assist patients and their families to understand their chronic conditions and to assume responsibility for being involved in health care decisions. Family caregivers need to be included in the patient's plan of care and provided with information about caregiver support groups and respite care. Finally, Campbell commented on the financial burden of a chronic illness that can be an additional source of stress. "Nurses need to explore how patients are financially managing their disease costs and make appropriate referrals" (p. 34). Campbell concludes that "living with a chronic disease is a challenge, but it's not insurmountable. With the help of nurses, these patients can get the most out of life" (p. 34).

Future Nursing Practice Issues

Neuhauser (2003) describes three health care revolutions that have occurred during the last 30 years. The current health care system is primarily focused on providing illness care with less emphasis on health promotion. The first health care revolution refers to the replacement of fee for service reimbursement with the cost containment model of managed care. The second health care revolution is the evidence-based practice model that has become the umbrella phrase for organized care of chronic diseases, such as asthma, HF, and diabetes. This permits a primary health care provider to manage the majority of care provided to people with these diseases and the referral of patients with

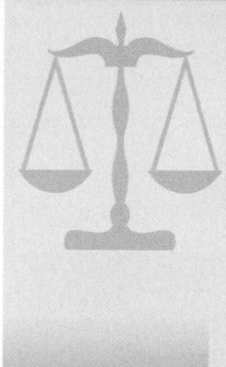

ETHICS IN PRACTICE

Confidentiality and Issues of Stress

When patients are undergoing stressful situations, the nurse must remember that there may be issues of confidentiality surrounding the patient's source of stress, particularly if the patient is actually anxious related to specific family members. The nurse must not divulge confidential information that a patient would share in regard to the family, even though the patient experiences increased anxiety. An example would be the consequences of an alternative lifestyle.

more serious conditions to specialty care. The third health care revolution is entitled as personal **empowerment** (to assist, or encourage person to be involved in decision making and development of the plan of care; the ability to assume self-care management). Self-care and hospice care are components of this model. Neuhauser believes that nurses and other health care professionals can play a leading role in this model through the use of a holistic perspective in patient education, reducing patient stress and anxiety, and being part of the patient's social support system. In this model, best practice care guidelines will be the norm in managing care of chronic diseases. This model also includes self-contracts to assist persons in successfully managing their health. A unique approach in this revolution will be the use of community coaches, individuals who have successfully managed their own health problems, and now, assist others who have similar problems. Theoretically, a nurse case manager could supervise 20 diabetic community coaches and their groups and actually manage 420 diabetics. Thurkettle (2003) suggests that case managers be proactively assigned to, or contracted with, patients in well populations to facilitate health promotion activities, as well as assisting patients with diagnosed illnesses in recovery and rehabilitation processes.

Consumers will have more access to Internet information and know more about their condition than the health care provider in the third revolution model. However, knowledge is not necessarily associated with behavioral changes, and some of the web-based information may be misleading. Health care organizations are developing their own Web sites and making them available to the public while encouraging consumers to seek information from reliable sources. An example is the web-based information provided by Sharp Health Care (2004) about the relationship of chronic stress and hypertension, self-care strategies to use, and how to seek professional help if needed. Sigma Theta Tau International (2004), the nursing honor society, commissioned a series of multinational, multidisciplinary conferences named the Arista series. The executive summary outlines a blue print for action that calls for nursing to be central in every health care system. Four suggestions for the future are: (a) nursing should be an integral partner in every health care system; (b) nursing's focus should be on delivering culturally appropriate, evidence-based, holistic and humane care; (c) nursing care involves maximizing the health of individuals, families, and communities; and (d) nursing must be involved in achievement of equitable health outcomes across the life span.

To achieve these goals, nurses will need knowledge and expertise in the sciences, i.e., anatomy, physiology, pathophysiology, the behavioral and social sciences, communication, as well as theories in nursing, human development,

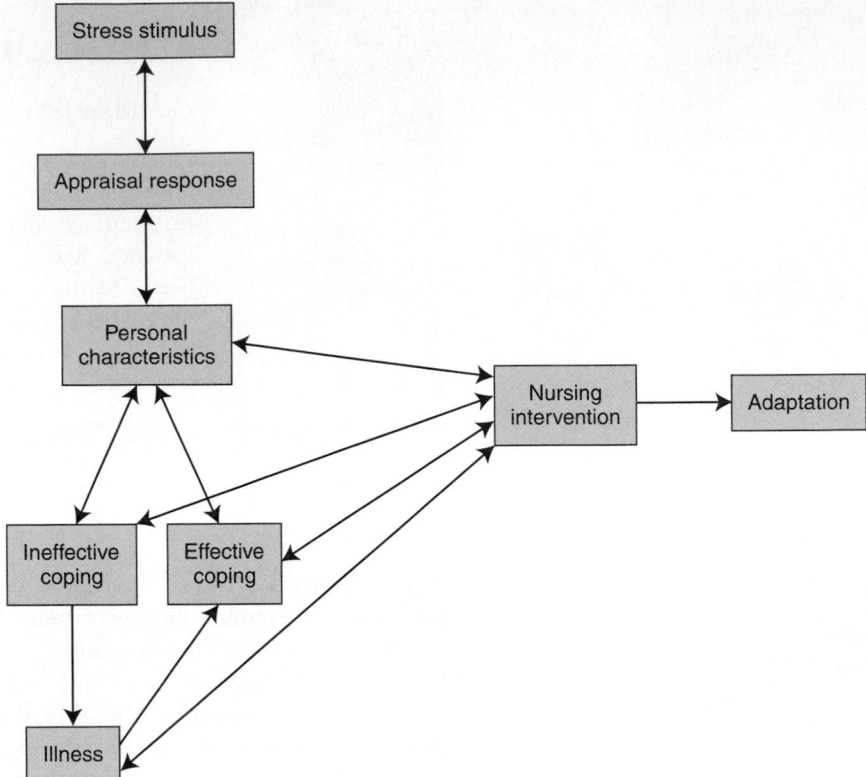

Figure 10-6 The stress adaptation model that depicts the individual's appraisal of a stressor.

learning, and stress adaptation. This knowledge will allow the nurse to address the issues related to stress that will come into his or her life.

The stress adaptation model shown in Figure 10-6 depicts the individual's perception of a stressor. The response to the stressor is influenced by the individual's characteristics, which include: internal resources i.e., (a) self-efficacy or resilience, (b) previous experience with stressful events, (c) perceived social support, and (d) knowledge of other external resources. These factors can lead to the use of effective coping skills or ineffective coping skills, which can result in physiological or psychological illness. Nursing interventions serve as a buffering process to promote use of effective coping strategies and to assist the individual to meet the individual's optimal level of adaptation to stress.

KEY CONCEPTS

- The definition of stress has changed over recent years. Selye's explanation of the concept of stress is commonly accepted.
- The general adaptation syndrome has three stages, i.e., alarm reaction, resistance, and exhaustion.
- Lazarus defined cognitive appraisal as a transactional process.
- There are both maturational and transitional changes in life that create varying levels of stress.
- Psychoneuroimmunoendocrinology is a multidisciplinary paradigm that identifies the links between the neurological, the endocrine, and the immune systems.

- Complementary alternative medicine involves healing practices that use ancient mind-body healing treatments.
- There is a wide variety of coping mechanisms with which persons adapt to stressful stimuli.
- Ineffective coping mechanisms may result in illness or maladaptation.
- Resilience is a process that assists in protecting a person in adapting to situations that the person cannot change.
- Adaptation is the ongoing process of modifying one's behavior in changed circumstances.

Continued

KEY CONCEPTS—cont'd

- Stress may cause illness as a result of lowered immunity.
- Chronic illnesses create stress, which adds to the complication of the disease processes.
- There are a variety of at-risk populations for stress, such as the elderly, adolescents, caregivers, and people from different cultures with varying health care beliefs.
- Occupations often cause stress and lead to work-related illnesses.
- The health care delivery system is changing from an illness to a health promotion model, which encourages nursing to employ stress management techniques.

- The nurse case manager continues to have the role of managing stress, which positively influences illness prevention and wellness practices.
- Several nursing theorists support the role of nursing in reducing stress, such as Orem's concept of self-care principles.
- Empowering patients is an important component of stress management.
- Future nursing practices encourage the role of nurses in holistic practices, which includes stress management.

REVIEW QUESTIONS

1. A patient is in her third postoperative day following a colostomy. As you change her dressing, you notice that she watches the procedure, but she does not make any comment. This behavior may indicate that:
   1. She is observing how others will react to her altered body image.
   2. She is using anger as a coping mechanism.
   3. She is in the exhaustion stage of the general adaptation syndrome.
   4. She is making a secondary appraisal of the situation.

2. A patient is scheduled for a breast biopsy today. She states that she feels that she has no hope for a positive outcome. Her statement indicates that:
   1. She is repressing her anxiety over this stressful situation.
   2. She has misinterpreted the physician's information to her.
   3. She is depressed regarding the outcome of the surgery.
   4. She believes she has no control over the situation.

3. As a nurse, you understand that after the discovery of a breast lump:
   1. Depression is usually not a great issue for an unmarried woman.
   2. When a marriage has a sound foundation, husbands have little difficulty adjusting to the wife's altered body image.
   3. Fantasies related to body mutilation may be initiated.
   4. A married woman's adjustment to a mastectomy may be less difficult in accepting her altered body image.

4. Hospitalization is often considered to be a stressful environment. The nurse can help the patient to be more comfortable by:
   1. Encouraging physical activity an hour prior to bedtime.
   2. Providing a mild antianxiety medication as ordered by the physician.
   3. Informing the patient about the purpose of hospital routines.
   4. Encouraging the patient to participate in decisions for the clinical plan.

5. An elderly mother was diagnosed with Alzheimer's disease three years ago. The mother's daughter was the primary caregiver during that time, because there was no one else in her family who was able to do so. Her mother died two weeks ago, and the daughter tells the nurse, "I can't believe that my mother is dead. I feel so lost." What response could the nurse use to learn more about the daughter's self-care needs?
   1. "Do you feel angry that your mother has died?"
   2. "Can you tell me more about how you feel?"
   3. "How can I help you adjust to this situation?"
   4. "I understand how you feel."

6. A 56-year-old obese gentleman has undergone a coronary artery bypass graft (CABG) procedure. He is referred to the cardiac rehabilitation program to learn about strategies he can use to promote a healthy lifestyle. The doctor informed him that he is a prime candidate for another heart attack. The patient informs the nurse that he is not really interested in a major lifestyle change, because he has been lucky all his life and is not worried about any further damage to his heart.

Continued

REVIEW QUESTIONS—cont'd

These comments refer to the use of a(n) _____ as a defense mechanism:
1. fantasy
2. undoing
3. denial
4. rationalization

7. In planning psychosocial care for the patient in question 6 the nurse realizes that he has:
   1. A realistic perception of his problem that helps him not to be troubled by it.
   2. An unrealistic pathological perception and manner of coping.
   3. Chosen to cope with the situation before making a secondary appraisal.
   4. Protected himself by using selective listening and hears only what he wishes to hear.

8. A 10-year-old boy has had frequent episodes of feeling sick at school. Noticing a pattern of these illnesses over the last several weeks, the school nurse decides to ask the child's mother to come in to visit with her. The nurse learns that the parents have been separated for two months. The mother is now considering divorce proceedings. The child and his two sisters spent a weekend with their father shortly after he moved into an apartment across town, but the father has only telephoned them twice since then. Which of the following statements may not be an indicator that the child is having difficulty adapting to the family situation?
   1. Drop in scholastic grades
   2. Increased attachment to siblings
   3. Disturbance in relations with peers
   4. Loss internal locus of control

9. A patient has been a two-pack-a-day smoker for over 30 years. He was diagnosed with chronic obstructive pulmonary disease (COPD) two years ago. He has been hospitalized several times, but refuses to quit smoking. He is currently hospitalized because of increased dyspnea on exertion during the past week, productive cough of thick yellow sputum, and fever. Nursing assessment reveals signs and symptoms including: enlarged anterior-posterior diameter of the chest (barrel chest), use of accessory breathing muscles, a temperature of 102, bilateral basilar rales, dusky nail beds, and some clubbing of fingers. He appears anxious, but says, "It is too late to give smoking up, now. It's the only pleasure I have left." Which of the following statements is *not* an explanation for his behavior?
   1. Smoking makes him feel better.
   2. Refusal to quit may be an attempt to retain control of his life.
   3. He may be denying the severity of his condition.
   4. Neurotic reactions should be expected with COPD.

10. Which of the following is true concerning the future of health care?
    1. There have been seven health care revolutions that have occurred during the last 30 years.
    2. The current health care system is primarily focused on providing wellness care with more emphasis on health promotion.
    3. The patients will know more about their condition than the health care provider in the third revolution model.
    4. The web-based information is very accurate and dependable for the patient who uses the internet as a health care information source.

REVIEW ACTIVITIES

1. You are providing care for a patient experiencing stress related to a recent diagnosis of cancer. Describe to the patient several common physiological and psychological stress responses.

2. You are acting as a consultant to a family who is providing care to their elderly grandparent. Explain to the family how the stress response is related to their difficulties in providing care.

3. A patient has been experiencing chronic stress from the financial implications of a recent surgery that has left the patient unemployed. Utilizing a nursing theorist, describe interventions for the patient adapting to the stress.

4. Evaluate your current stress levels and develop a plan of self-care to minimize your stress.

5. Interview a peer as related to coping mechanisms and write an evaluation of the effectiveness of their strategies.

Inflammation and Infection Management

Margaret M. Conger, RN, MSN, EdD

CHAPTER TOPICS

- Processes of Inflammation

- Diseases of Inflammation (Asthma, Arthritis, Myocardial Infarction [MI])

- Infectious Disease Control

- Standard Precautions

- Wound Healing

The human body is extremely complex, particularly in the processes of defense against invading organisms. There are many intricate aspects of barriers to disease and cellular processes that attempt to protect the body from illness. This chapter delineates both the general and specific qualities of the body in regard to inflammation and infection, the relationship of the science of nursing to these processes, and integrates nursing management as it relates to each topic.

KEY TERMS

Airborne transmission
Basophils
Chemotaxis
Diapedesis
Direct contact transmission
Droplet transmission
Eosinophils
Exudate
Indirect contact transmission
Leukocytes
Lymphocytes
Macrophages
Monocytes
Neutrophils
Opsonization
Phagocytosis
Primary intention
Reticuloendothethial (RE) system
Secondary intention
Standard precautions
Tertiary intention
Transmission routes
Vector-borne transmission

INFLAMMATORY PROCESS

The inflammatory process is an important protective mechanism for the body. Contact with substances that can cause injury to tissues is an experience faced by everyone daily. This tissue injury can result from contact with bacteria, trauma, chemical, heat, cold, surgery, or a multitude of other agents. When tissues damage occurs, the body's normal response is to mount an immediate reaction to repair the damage. In this way, a person is able to maintain healthy tissue despite living in an environment filled with potential threats.

Leukocytes

The **leukocytes,** the general name for all of the white blood cells (WBCs), make up a mobile defense system ready to respond to any type of foreign invasion. Normally there are about 4,500 to 11,000 WBCs per mm^3 in the blood at any given time. The WBCs consist of several types of cells; each designed to carry out different functions in combating foreign substances. Several of the leukocytes, in particular, the **neutrophils,** which are the chief phagocytic cell of the early inflammatory response, and the **monocytes,** also phagocytic cells found in the blood, are vital to initiating and sustaining the inflammatory response. These cells carry out **phagocytosis,** a process by which foreign substances are ingested and destroyed. The neutrophils have a granular appearance when studied under a microscope and thus are often referred to as granulocytes. The neutrophils make up about 56 percent of the total leukocytes circulating in the blood. The monocytes make up only 4 percent of the leukocytes in the circulation; they are primarily found in tissue sites rather than in the blood. Thus, their presence in the body is far greater than would be suggested by the laboratory values reported (McCance & Huether, 2005).

Both of these WBCs are formed in bone marrow along with other WBCs (Table 11-1). From there they are transported throughout the body via the blood and are always ready for an encounter with a foreign substance. When the body needs to destroy foreign materials, the bone marrow rapidly pours out stored neutrophils, and their blood level rises rapidly. In severe infections, it is not uncommon to see the percentage of lymphocytes rise to 75 percent of the total WBCs, with the total WBC count rising as high as 20,000/mm^3. The neutrophils are mature cells ready for action when they leave the bone mar-

TABLE 11-1	Laboratory Values: White Blood Cells	
Total Leukocyte (CBC) Count		*4,500–11,000/mm³*
Monocytes or Nongranular Leukocytes		*1,000–4,800/mm³*
Lymphocytes	34 percent	
Monocytes	4 percent	
Bands or stabs	3 percent	
(Immature neutrophils)		
Polymorphonuclears or Granulocytes		*1,800–7,000/mm³*
Neutrophils	56 percent	
Eosinophils	2.7 percent	
Basophils	0.3 percent	

Source: Daniels, R. (2003). Delmar's manual of laboratory and diagnostic tests. New York: Thomson Delmar Learning.

row unless there is a sustained inflammatory response in which the bone marrow storage of these cells is depleted. In this case, the bone marrow will put out immature cells referred to as bands. An expression often used to describe this increase in the number of immature neutrophils is a shift to the left. This expression arose from an old handwritten report of a differential WBC in which the bands were reported on the left side of the page.

The monocytes are also vital to the inflammatory response. These cells travel through the blood to various body tissues as monocytes, an immature form of the cell. They then attach to various tissues and greatly increase in size. Monocytes located in the tissue are known as **macrophages** and are the phagocytic cells found in tissues. These cells take on specific names based on the tissue in which they are deposited. For example, in the liver the macrophages are known as Kupffer cells and in the lungs as alveolar macrophages. They also are attached to cells in the spleen and many other organs lined with mucous membranes. As such, these cells are always ready to attack foreign substances that penetrate the tissue. The monocyte-macrophage cells including both those traveling in the blood from the bone marrow to specific tissue sites and those attached to cells in specific organs. These cells together are known as the **reticuloendothethial (RE) system,** a phagocytic system.

Other leukocytes include the **eosinophils,** a granulocyte that helps control the inflammatory process and is also active in destroying parasites, and **basophils,** active in allergic reactions. The fifth type of leukocyte is the **lymphocyte,** the primary cells in the immune response and for the most part, not directly involved in the inflammatory process. One type of lymphocyte, the natural killer cell, is able to directly destroy foreign invaders without the presence of other immune system components (Porth, 2005).

Chemical Response to Tissue Injury

When tissue injury occurs, from any of the sources mentioned previously, a variety of chemicals are released (Table 11-2). Mast cells that line the connective tissue alongside blood vessels contain chemicals vital to the inflammatory process. These chemicals include histamine, neutrophil chemotactic factor, and eosinophil chemotactic factor, to name a few. Also found at the site of injury are platelets from the vascular system that release serotonin. All of these chemicals cause the large blood vessels to constrict resulting in dilatation of the postcapillary venules increasing blood flow to the area. They also cause increased vascular permeability with rapid movement of fluid and cells into the injured area. These chemicals exert **chemotaxis,** a response to a chemical stimulant to attract WBCs to a specific site. It is because of chemotaxis that large numbers of neutrophils and monocytes are attracted to the area of injury. There these cells squeeze through capillary blood vessel walls by **diapedesis,** a process in which the cells adapt their shape to fit through the pores in the capillary walls and slide through one area of the cell at a time. Once through the capillary wall, they move rapidly to the injury site.

Mast cells also produce other chemicals important to the inflammatory process. These include leukotrienes, prostaglandins, and platelet-activating factor. Leukotriene action is similar to that of histamine, but it is important later in the inflammatory process causing a more prolonged action than that of histamine. Prostaglandins are involved in increasing vascular permeability and neutrophil chemotaxis, but they also cause pain. Aspirin has long been known as a chemical that inhibits prostaglandin formation and thus reduces pain. Platelet-activating factor increases the activity of platelets and is important in stemming blood loss from an injured area. Other chemicals important to the inflammatory process include protein substances found in the plasma. These are the clotting system, the kinin system, and the complement system. The clotting system is important because it forms the fibrous mass the stops bleeding at the site. It is also important in trapping foreign materials at the

TABLE 11-2   Chemicals Involved in Inflammatory Response

STAGE	CHEMICAL MEDIATOR RELEASED	ACTION
Initial Response		
Mast cell degranulation	Histamine	Increase circulation to area
	Neutrophil and eosinophil chemotactic factor	Alter arteriole vessel wall to allow for fluid and cell migration into injured tissue
Platelet breakdown	Serotonin	Attract neutrophils and monocytes to area.
Subsequent Response		
Mast cell degranulation	Leukotriene	Action similar to histamine but more prolonged
		Occurs later in inflammatory response
Mast cell degranulation	Prostaglandin	Increases vascular permeability
		Neutrophil chemotaxis
		Pain
Protein Mediators		
Clotting system-platelet break down	Platelet-activating factor	Reduces blood loss in area
		Traps foreign material at site of injury
Kinin system	Bradykinin	Dilation of blood vessels
		Pain
Complementary system	Complementary chain of proteins	Prepares bacteria for destruction by phagocytes
		Chemotaxis
Cytokines	Interleukins	Stimulate growth and function of inflammatory cells
		Stimulates hypothalamus to raise body temperature
	Interferon	Coats virus cell walls to prevent their penetration into cells
Leukocyte-activating factors	Granulocyte colony-stimulating factor (G-CSF)	Increases production and release of neutrophils
	Monocyte colony-stimulating factor (M-CSF)	Increases production and release of neutrophils
	Tumor necrosis factor	Stimulates macrophage maturation and migration
Stop the Inflammatory Response		
Eosinophils—release chemicals to inactivate vasoactive amines	Histaminase	Degrades histamine
	Arylsulfatase	Degrades leukotrienes

Adapted from McCance, K., & Huether, S. (2005). Pathophysiology: The biological basis for disease in adults and children (5th ed.). St. Louis, MO: Mosby.

site. Once trapped, these foreign materials will be subjected to phagocytic activity and destroyed. This clotting process also helps to prevent the spread of the foreign material to other areas. The kinin system produces the chemical bradykinin that causes dilation of blood vessels but also causes pain. The third protein system important in inflammation is the complement system. While the complement system is primarily activated through an immune response of antigen-antibody interaction, it can also be activated by cellular enzymes. It serves to prepare bacteria for destruction by macrophages through a process known as **opsonization,** a process that coats a foreign substance and makes it more susceptible to phagocytosis. It also has a chemotactic effect on leukocytes and causes mast cells to degranulate McCance & Huether, 2005).

Cytokines are another group of chemicals involved in the inflammatory process. These include interleukins, interferon, and several leukocyte activating factors. Interleukins are produced by macrophages or lymphocytes and stimulate the growth and function of inflammatory cells. Interleukin also raises body temperature because of its effect on the hypothalamus. Interferon protects cells from virus activity. It coats cell walls and prevents virus particles from entering a cell so protected. The leukocyte activating factors such as granulocyte colony-stimulating factor (G-CSF) and monocyte colony-stimulating factor (M-CSF) increase the production and release of neutrophils, eosinophils, and basophils. Another chemical in the inflammatory process is tumor necrosis factor (TNF), which is important in stimulating macrophage maturation and migration (Porth, 2005).

Signs of Inflammation

The inflammatory process is a protective host response to injury (see Concept Map: Inflammatory Process). It is characterized by the common phenomena known to all of redness, swelling, heat, and pain. The outcome of this process is the loss of function in the injured area. Each of these common signs of inflammation is directly related to the physiological events that occur. The redness and heat is caused by the increased blood flow to the injured area in response to the chemicals released by mast cell degranulation. The swelling seen is the result of the leaking of plasma and leukocytes into the injured area. The increase in fluid and the production of cellular chemicals causes injury to nerve endings in the area resulting in the pain that is experienced.

Phagocytosis

The first of the leukocytes to reach the injured area are the neutrophils, which carry out their phagocytic action of ingesting the foreign substances such as bacteria, the dead cells, and any other cellular debris. Also important to this process are platelets from the blood vessels, which will initiate the clotting process if injury has occurred to a blood vessel. To shut off this phagocytic process, eosinophils attracted to the area release enzymes, such as histaminase that destroys histamine and stops the inflammatory process.

The inflammatory response is enhanced by the products of the immune system discussed in chapter 42. Foreign substances such as bacteria that have been altered by specific antibody interaction are more readily phagocytized and thus brought under control more readily than if no antibody is present. This is why diseases to which a person has had prior exposure and thus has preformed antibodies are more readily controlled than ones to which the person has had no prior exposure. The type of **exudate** (accumulated fluid in a cavity) seen in the inflammation varies dependent on the stage of the inflammatory process. Early in the inflammation, the inflamed area is filled with serous fluid such as seen in a new blister. As the process progresses, the debris from phagocytosis collects, and the area becomes filled with a purulent exudate. There may also be bleeding into the area, and then the exudate is filled with erythrocytes and is known as a hemorrhagic exudate. The exudate is removed from the area either by the lymphatic system or through the epithelial tissue as when the pressure in the area becomes high, and the pus is released through the skin. At times the infected area is surgically opened and drained of the pus (McCance & Huether, 2005; Porth, 2005).

Resolution and Repair of Tissue

The end stage of the inflammatory process is resolution and repair of the involved tissue. This process may be quite short, such as in the response to a foreign object like a splinter in the finger that has been removed, or it can be quite prolonged, even up to two years. The lymphatic system is important is clearing away the materials formed by the phagocytic process. The fibrinolytic enzymes clear away fibrin from the area. The chemical mediators released by eosinophils, such as histaminase, which destroys histamine, and arylsulfatase, which destroys leukotrienes, are important in stopping the inflammatory response. They reduce vascular dilatation, chemotaxis, and vessel wall permeability. These actions prevent the inflammatory response from getting out of control.

If the tissue is one in which the normal cells can regenerate, complete function can be restored to the tissue. In tissues such as the heart muscle, which does not regenerate, the area is left with a collagen fiber filling the area. This will restore tensile strength but will not restore the function of the original cells. Specifics of wound healing will be discussed at a later point in this chapter.

Chronic Inflammation

If the inflammatory process is prolonged, usually more than two weeks, the condition is referred to as chronic inflammation. This is often caused by the persistence presence of the irritant such as a foreign object like a splinter in the skin, bacteria, such as *Mycobacterium tuberculous* that is resistant to phagocytosis, or prolonged exposure to a chemical irritant. The body will attempt to wall off the involved area with fibrous tissue and form a granuloma. Often the contents within the walled off area will die releasing enzymes that destroy the cells leaving a clear fluid. This fluid eventually diffuses out of the area leaving behind a hollow structure that may remain for the person's entire lifetime.

INFLAMMATORY DISEASE

A number of diseases commonly encountered in nursing practice produce an inflammatory effect. On the other hand, there are other diseases that are caused by an inflammatory effect. The following section separates these two categories.

Diseases That Result in an Inflammatory Process

Many diseases that initiate an inflammatory response are caused by infectious agents. These can result in serious illness and even death. In developed countries, many of these diseases have been controlled through widespread immunization programs. However, in many parts of the world these diseases still have a high mortality rate. Because many of them can be spread from person to person or by contact with an intermediate object, they are often referred to as communicable diseases. The World Health Organization (WHO) (2006) reports that 31.1 percent of deaths worldwide are caused by communicable diseases (i.e., respiratory infection, HIV/AIDS, perinatal diseases, diarrheal diseases, tuberculosis, childhood diseases, malaria, sexually transmitted infections, hepatitis, maternal diseases).

Infectious Organisms

The infectious organisms that are the cause for these communicable diseases are many. The most common organisms causing infectious diseases are viruses, bacteria, fungi, and protozoa. Others that can also cause disease are chlamydia, rickettsia, mycoplasma, and helminths. Some common diseases caused by bacteria and viruses are listed in Table 11-3.

The body's first line of defense against these microorganisms is the skin and mucous membranes lining the respiratory, digestive, and genitourinary tracts. If the organism is able to penetrate through these external barriers, the inflammatory response will be initiated, and the immune system will be activated. The introduction of antibiotics to combat infectious diseases has

TABLE 11-3 **Types of Agents Causing Disease**

COMMON AGENTS	DESCRIPTION	COMMON DISEASE(S)
Viruses	Smallest organism that can only be seen using an electron microscope. Viruses can only live inside of other cells	Hepatitis A, B, C Rubella Rubeola
Bacteria	A one-celled organism, which can reproduce independently. Needs a host to supply food	Pneumonia Urinary tract infections
Fungi	A yeast or mold. Can be either single-celled or multicelled and obtain food from other living material	Yeast infection Ringworm
Protozoa	Single cell parasitic organisms that form cysts or spores	Malaria Gastroenteritis
LESS COMMON AGENTS	**DESCRIPTION**	**COMMON DISEASE(S)**
Chlamydia	Similar to bacteria but grow only within other cells	Pneumonia Genital infections
Rickettsia	Similar to bacteria but must grow only within other cells	Typhus Rocky Mountain spotted fever
Mycoplasma	Similar to bacteria but do not have a cell wall	Pneumonia
Helminth	Worm-like animal	Tapeworm infection Pinworm infection

Adapted from Porth, C. (2005). Pathophysiology: Concepts of altered health states (7th ed.). Philadelphia: Lippincott, Williams & Wilkins; McCance, K., & Huether, S. (2005). Pathophysiology: The biological basis for disease in adults and children (5th ed.). St. Louis, MO: Mosby.

significantly reduced the mortality rate of infectious diseases. However, a number of organisms have developed resistance to multiple antibiotics and can cause significant damage to a patient. It is believed that inadequate treatment with antibiotics has allowed resistant organisms to develop selectively. This is an emerging problem and one that requires considerable research.

Antibiotic-Resistant Organisms

Antibiotic-resistant organisms are described as those organisms that are no longer destroyed by the usual antibiotics. An organism of current concern is an antibiotic-resistant strain of *M. tuberculosis*. This strain has become a particular problem in patients with HIV/AIDS. Other common organisms that have developed antibiotic resistance and have become acute problems in health care institutions include methicillin-resistant *Staphylococcus aureus* (MRSA) and vancomycin-resistant *Enterococcus* (VRE). These organisms are of particular concern because long-term care patients have become colonized with both organisms. Recent evidence suggests that genetic material from the enterococcus can join with the genetic material of the staphylococcus to form a new resistant strain of *S. aureus* known as vancomycin-resistant *S. aureus* (VRSA) (Goldrick, 2004). This newly emerging strain is resistant to penicillins, cephalosporins, and vancomycin. To prevent the emergence of new strains of antibiotic-resistant organisms, health care professionals need to be vigilant in using infection control measures at all times.

Asthma: An Allergic Disease

Asthma is an inflammatory disease that is the response to allergens or irritants found in the environment. Contact with the allergen initiates an inflammatory response similar to that seen with an infectious organism. The allergen binds to mast cells found in bronchial wall membranes and causes the mast cells to degranulate. The chemicals released, histamine, leukotrienes, prostaglandin, platelet-activating factor, and others, initiate the inflammatory response. These chemicals cause the bronchioles to spasm thus reducing airflow. They also cause increased blood flow to area as seen in other inflammatory reactions. The increased vascularity of the capillary vessels in the area brings neutrophils and monocytes to the site (see chapter 33).

The effect of the inflammatory response is to increase mucous secretions and reduce movement of air through the bronchioles. This results in increased coughing in an attempt to clear the airways. The person will complain of tightness in the chest and increased difficulty in breathing. In an acute attack, the person can become quite hypoxic with signs of restlessness and increased anxiety, pulse rate, and blood pressure. As the disease progresses, the number of allergens that can stimulate an episode seem to increase. The constant inflammatory state of the airways seems to make them hyperreactive to a number of irritants. Thus this is an inflammatory disease that becomes progressively more difficult to manage. Drug therapy is the usual management plan. Drugs that relax bronchial smooth muscle such as a beta-adrenergic agonist (Albuterol) are commonly used to manage acute episodes. Inhaled corticosteroids such as the fluticasone found in the preparation Advair and oral corticosteroids can be used to reduce response to an inflammatory reaction. A third group of drugs, cromolyn (Intal), are used to prevent mast cell degranulation when the allergen attaches. This prevents the inflammatory response from even starting.

Diseases Caused by an Inflammatory Effect

While one often thinks of inflammatory diseases as resulting from an outside of the body attack, there are a number of diseases that occur as a self-induced inflammatory reaction. The various diseases falling under the general classification of arthritis are an example of a self-induced inflammatory reaction. Other inflammatory responses that have gained considerable attention recently include the role of inflammation in myocardial infarction (MI) and obesity.

Arthritis

A number of diseases constitute the general classification of arthritis are characterized by an inflammatory condition in which the body's inflammatory system attacks its own tissue. The most common form is osteoarthritis, in which the cartilage covering the ends of bones in joints deteriorates, and the bone rubs against bone (see chapter 59). This results in an inflammatory condition, which results in pain and loss of movement in the joint. It is commonly treated with anti-inflammatory drugs such as the nonsteroidal anti-inflammatory drugs (NSAIDs) or corticoid steroids. An important nursing intervention for working with patients with arthritis is to encourage activity. Often people with this disease tend to become inactive from the joint pain, which is particularly painful after being immobile for a time. An exercise program that begins gradually often improves the quality of life for these people. The Arthritis Foundation provides guidelines for a walking program that can be used for person at a variety of stages of disease. When a person becomes too immobilized with joint pain, surgery that replaces the inflamed joint can be considered.

A more serious form is rheumatoid arthritis (RA) in which the joints become inflamed in response to an immune reaction (see chapter 42). RA occurs primarily in women. Again, medications such as NSAIDs or cortisol drugs are the major treatment. Gout is another form of arthritis in which the joints, usually in the big toe, become inflamed. The inflammatory agent in this case is an overproduction of uric acid, which is deposited in the joint as a crystal. Treatment with anti-inflammatory drugs and changes in diet that excludes purine, one of the amino acids found in protein, often relieves the symptoms.

Myocardial Infarction

Recently, research has demonstrated that a primary problem in the development of MI is related to an inflammatory reaction within the walls of arteries (see chapter 24). It has now been shown that low-density lipoproteins (LDL) collect on the intima wall of the arteriole when they are present in high levels. There they undergo oxidation and glycation. These products then attract monocytes and initiate the inflammatory response. The monocytes are changed into macrophages and ingest the fatty LDL particles until the cells are so filled with the fatty substance that they look foamy. In time, the inflammatory process remodels the arteriole wall into a large plaque area. A fibrous covering is formed over the plaque area that becomes quite thin as the plaque area expands. This cap can break open, cause bleeding, and a fibrous clot is formed. This is the most common cause of the stenosis (narrowing of opening in a blood vessel), which results in MI.

Because inflammation is now known to be a major factor in precipitating an MI, new assessment tools have become important in evaluating risk for an MI. Monitoring LDL levels is an important assessment. Recommendations for optimal LDL levels have been dropped to below 100 mg/dL. C-reactive protein is another blood test that can be used to identify the presence of an inflammatory reaction in the body. However, it is not specific for arteriole inflammatory response. However, a low level, below 1 mg/L, would be helpful in ruling out the possibility of an impending MI. Levels between 1 and 3 mg/L are considered to be at moderate risk level, while greater than 3 mg/L is high risk (American Heart Association, 2006c).

Obesity

A related problem of an inflammatory reaction detrimental to one's health is found with obesity (see chapter 48). Fat cells can produce the inflammatory chemicals and induce an inflammatory response. It is now believed that the inflammatory chemicals formed in response to excess fat cells contribute to vascular inflammation and are thus associated with heart disease.

Thus the inflammatory response, while vital to maintaining protection from a host of foreign substances, can also be a cause of disease. As research demonstrates new links with the inflammatory process, perhaps new strategies for controlling the process will be found.

NURSING RESPONSE: INFLAMMATION

Inflammation is an expected response to injury and can cause a person considerable discomfort. A number of nursing diagnoses related to alleviation of the effects of inflammation have been developed. Nursing interventions used to manage patients with an inflammatory condition and outcomes to assess the effectiveness of these interventions are also important. The goal of these nursing interventions is to support the patient while the body attempts to repair itself. Some of the nursing diagnoses used when caring for a patient with an inflammatory process include risk for infection, ineffective thermoregulation, acute pain, imbalanced nutrition, less than body requirements, fluid volume, risk for deficit, and impaired tissue integrity. Each of these nursing diagnoses will be addressed in terms of assessments needed, interventions utilized, and desired outcomes.

Risk for Infection

Strategies to prevent and assess for infection in a patient at risk is a nursing responsibility. The white blood count and the differential count are important laboratory values to monitor to detect changes in a patient's response to the inflammatory condition. Assessment of the injured site is also essential.

Frequent monitoring for localized as well as systemic signs and symptoms of infection is necessary. The consistency, color, and any odor associated with the inflamed area must be documented. The use of standard infection control precautions and any appropriate transmission-based precautions (see guidelines later in chapter) must be followed to protect the patient and others from spread of an infectious disease. Antibiotics are often ordered for a patient; however in this era of antibiotic-resistant strains of microorganisms, their use is sometimes questioned. When ordered, it is important that the patient takes the entire prescribed dose to reduce possible risk for development of an antibiotic-resistant strain. This teaching point must be emphasized with all patients.

It is particularly important to observe patients where there is reason to question their ability to initiate an inflammatory response. People who have been on prolonged steroid therapy, which inhibits the inflammatory response, can become quite septic without the usual signs of infections, such as fever. Also persons who are immunocompromised because of HIV/AIDS will not show the usual signs of inflammation. These patients should be managed with aggressive antibiotic therapy early in the disease process, because they will not initiate the normal inflammatory response. The outcome desired for managing a person at risk for infection is to prevent or reduce the severity of the infection and to maintain tissue integrity.

Thermoregulation: Ineffective

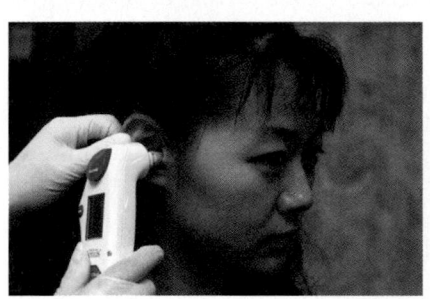

Figure 11-1 Taking a temperature with a tympanic thermometer.

Because the patient's temperature may increase in an infectious process, it is important to measure and document body temperature (Figure 11-1). However, many times the increased temperature is a positive sign of response to the injury and can be an important host defense. The administration of fever reducing drugs is generally not advocated unless the fever is greater than 39.5° C (103.1° F). However, temperatures that are higher than this should be treated to prevent possible seizure activity. The antipyretic drugs used to control fever during an inflammatory response are several. Aspirin (acetylsalicylic acid) acts by blocking prostaglandin synthesis and thus reduces the set point for elevated temperature in the hypothalamus. Acetaminophen (Tylenol) also acts on the heat regulating system in the hypothalamus. Some NSAIDs, such as ibuprofen, also can reduce fever. These drugs should be administered around the clock so that the set point in the hypothalamus remains depressed. If given intermittently, the set point can fluctuate, leading to chills, which act as a metabolic stimulant to increase body temperature and lead to patient discomfort.

Another intervention to reduce fever is the use of a cooling blanket or a cool sponge bath. These should only be used in conjunction with an antipyretic drug that reduces the temperature set point in the hypothalamus. If the set point is not reduced, the patient will attempt to compensate for the loss of heat by initiating a shivering response. This in turn will again increase metabolism and subsequently, body temperature.

Pain: Acute

There are a number of measures that can be used to reduce pain for a patient undergoing an inflammatory process. The use of both hot and cold applications is important. Understanding the timing of each is essential to achieving positive results, because their use is dependent on the stage of the inflammatory process. Initially, the use of cold is recommended to reduce swelling and thus pain. Later, the use of heat is recommended to increase circulation to the area, thus providing increased nutrients and oxygen to promote healing. Elevation of the injured area will also reduce the amount of swelling at the injured site and thus reduce pain.

Use of rest and immobilization of the area also are important to decreasing swelling and inflammation. Immobilization with a bandage, a cast, or other immobilizing device will reduce pain. Rest is important to reducing general metabolic needs and thus conserving nutrients and oxygen for the healing process.

Nutrition: Imbalanced, Less Than Body Requirements

Tissue repair places great stress on the body's metabolic needs. It is important to determine, with the help of a dietician, the number and type of calories the patient requires to promote tissue healing. The calorie needs for some type of injuries, such as a burn, are phenomenal. Protein is also needed in larger than normal amounts to provide the materials for tissue repair. Along with nutritional needs, the patient requires oxygen to utilize these nutrients. When caring for a person with a vascular disease that impairs oxygen delivery to the injured area, the use of supplemental oxygen can be helpful.

The type of feeding used to obtain optimal nutrition is dependent on the status of the patient. Whenever possible, oral feedings will be the easiest way to supply the needed nutrients. If the patient is unable to take oral or nasogastric feedings, the IV route must be considered. It is important to remember that the nutrition from a peripheral IV route is minimal and will not be adequate to supply the needed nutrients. Some type of hyperalimentation will be required.

Fluid Volume: Risk for Deficit

Another area of assessment for the person with an inflammatory response is that of fluid management. Elevated temperatures lead to increased metabolic demands and thus can lead to increased risk for fluid volume deficit. Assessments include observing for dry lips and tongue, poor skin turgor, and sunken eyes. Maintaining a careful intake and output record can also be important. However, because much of the fluid loss can be insensible through sweating, observation of the skin, the bed covers, and such can give an indication of more fluid loss than the intake and output record indicate. Careful management of fluid administration is vital. If possible the patient should be encouraged to take in up to 3 to 4 L of fluid per 24 hours. If oral fluids cannot be tolerated, this may be given the IV route. Vital signs can also be useful in determining possible dehydration. Increasing respiratory and pulse rates and a decreasing blood pressure can be indicators of impending hypovolemia (diminished blood volume).

INFECTIOUS DISEASE CONTROL

Because many infectious processes are related to bacterial or viral contamination, it is important to maintain infectious disease control practices to prevent spread of disease from the infected patient to others, both health care staff as well as other patients. There are many types of equipment (Figure 11-2), along with good hygiene practices, that can provide safe and effective care to prevent further contamination associated with infectious diseases.

Transmission Routes

Transmission routes for invading organisms are important to understand, because these are the ways by which microorganisms reach the body. Five types of transmission routes have been identified, and knowledge of these is important when planning effective strategies to prevent spread of infectious disease.

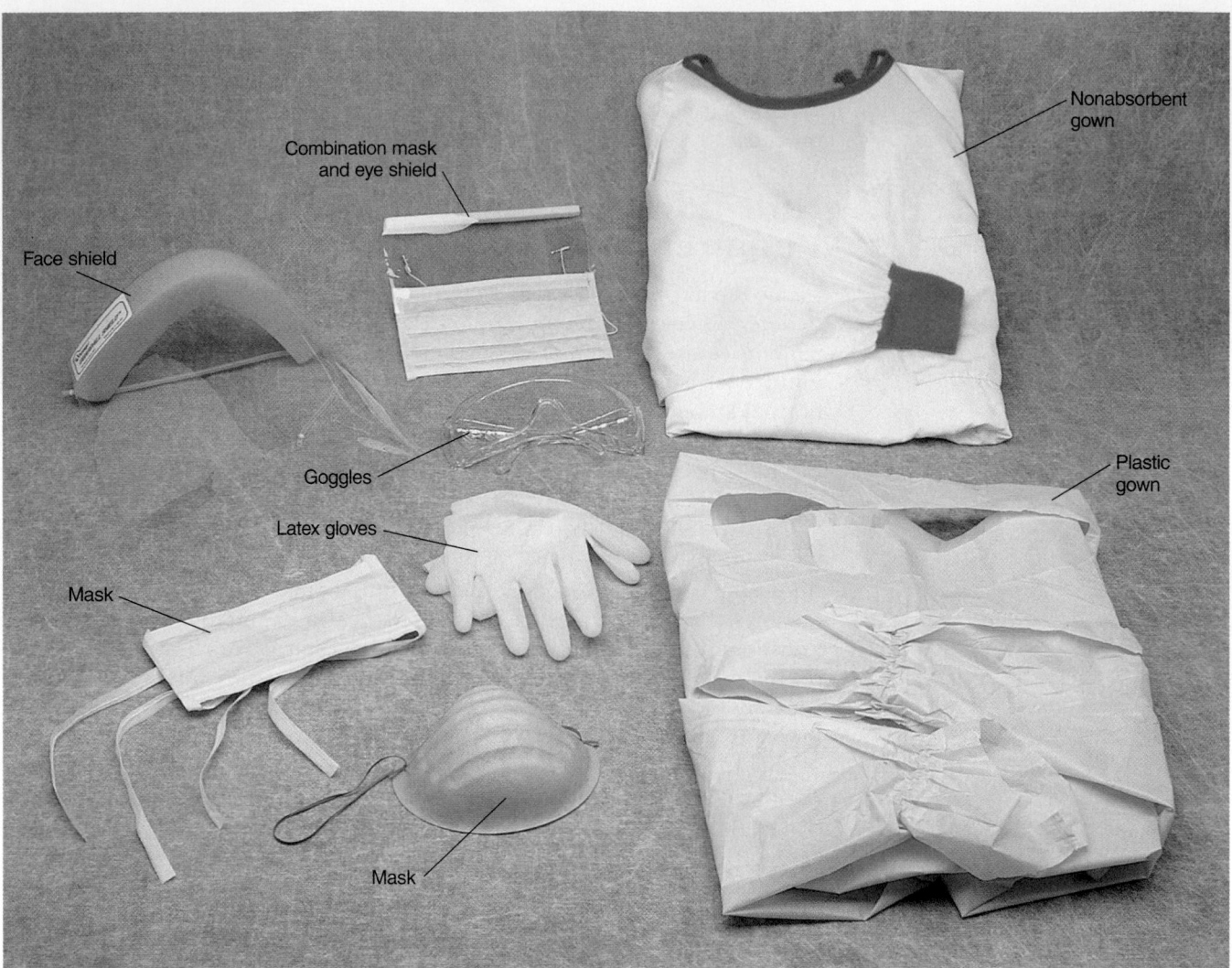

Figure 11-2 A variety of personal protective equipment available to the health care provider to prevent contamination from infectious diseases.

Contact Transmission

Contact transmission is the most common transmission route and can be either direct or indirect. With **direct contact transmission** there is body surface to body surface contact through which the infectious material is transferred such as occurs when giving direct personal care. **Indirect contact transmission** occurs when there is an inanimate object involved in the transfer. Examples of this type of transfer include contaminated instruments or even unwashed human hands (see Red Flag feature).

Droplet Transmission

Droplet transmission is also a common type of transmission in which particles are propelled through the air. These droplets are formed during coughing, sneezing, talking, or during procedures, such as suctioning. They can be propelled through the air for a short distance and then deposited on the new host. Because they rapidly fall from the air, they are not able to be transmitted over long distances.

Airborne Transmission

Airborne transmission, the third type, differs from droplet transmission in the distance the particles travel. In airborne transmission, the infectious material is trapped in dust and carried on air currents. The particles can also remain following evaporation of the liquid portion of the droplet and then travel long distances through the air. The particles in this transmission route are small, less than 5 μm and thus can be widely dispersed by air currents. Special air filtration equipment is required to prevent the spread of disease in airborne transmission.

Common Vehicle Transmission

Common vehicle transmission is similar to contact transmission in that microorganisms are disseminated on equipment, in food, water, or other commonly shared materials. Prevention of spread of disease by this route can be managed by careful housekeeping. Hand washing by all health care personnel is especially important in preventing disease transmission by this route. Careful control of hand washing procedures is essential in preventing the spread of multidrug-resistant organisms that have become prevalent in health care institutions. Organisms such as MSRA and VRE are particularly difficult organisms to treat. Patients who are infected with both organisms have recently been identified. This is particularly troublesome because of the ability of the *Enterococcus* to transfer its DNA strand that is resistant to vancomycin to the *S. aureus* bacteria, making the organism resistant to penicillin, cephalosporins, and vancomycin (Goldrick, 2004). It is imperative that health care workers are meticulous in preventing the spread of these organisms by common vectors such as hands or equipment.

Hand Washing Recommendations

Hand hygiene is an extremely important aspect in prevention of disease transmission. The Center for Disease Control and Prevention (CDC) in the United States has reviewed cleansing agents for hand hygiene and has issued recommendations for hand care. These recommendations support the use of both soap and water and alcohol-based products. When hands are contaminated with blood or other body fluids, soap and water are recommended as the preferred cleansing agent. Soap and water are also the recommended cleansing agent before eating or after using a restroom. At other times an alcohol-based hand cleanser may be used as long as it is well rubbed into the hands. A simple packet of alcohol rubbed lightly over the hands is not sufficient to remove pathogens. These cleansers can be placed directly at the bedside or carried with the health care worker so that they are always available. They should be used both before and after any contact with a patient, as well as when moving from a contaminated area on a patient to a clean area. They also must be used before putting on gloves to insert various invasive tubes, IV lines, and catheters (DeLaune & Ladner, 2006).

Vector-Borne Transmission

The last route of transmission, **vector-borne transmission,** occurs when the infectious material is carried by living organisms. It is not a common problem in health care facilities in the United States. However, when it arises, it can tax the abilities of the health care staff to the extreme. The carriers of disease in this form include mosquitoes, flies, rats, and other small animals. Recently, in the southwestern part of the United States, cases of plague carried by fleas who fed on wild rodents were reported. Another vector-borne disease that can lead to rapid death is the pneumonia caused by the Hantavirus. This virus is transmitted from the droppings of infected mice. It has become a serious disease in the American southwest. Lyme disease in the northeastern part of the United States is frequently reported; this is carried by a tick. Prevention of these vector-borne diseases is focused on interrupting the transmission route of microorganisms.

A recent report describes the dilemma faced by health care staff in New York when confronted with two cases of plague, a disease virtually unknown in this part of the country. A couple who were visiting New York from New Mexico became ill and were admitted to Beth Israel Medical Center with symptoms of a severe flu-like disease. The husband had malaise, fatigue, muscle aches, and

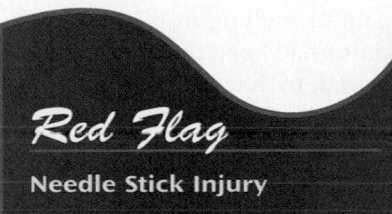

Red Flag

Needle Stick Injury

Needlestick injuries have become an area of huge concern in nursing. In this transmission route, the common vehicle between the person with a blood-borne pathogen disease, such as hepatitis B or C or HIV, is a needle that has been used for the patient. It is estimated that there are 600,000 exposures to blood by health care workers annually. Nurses make up the majority of these. Fortunately, only a small fraction of these exposures result in disease.

The federal government has legislation in place, the Needle Stick Safety and Prevention Act of 2001, and with it is attempting to diminish the exposure of health care workers to possible disease transmission episodes. This act requires the following:

1. Use of sharps injury protection devices (Figure 11-3) and greater use of needleless systems.
2. Training for employees directly at risk for injury in device evaluation and selection.
3. Maintenance of an exposure control plan available to all employees.
4. Provide hepatitis B vaccine to employees at no cost.
5. Provide testing and prophylactic treatment to all employees within two hours of an exposure.
6. Maintain a sharps injury log.

Source: Foley, M. (2004). Update on needlestick and sharps injuries. American Journal of Nursing, 104(8), 96.

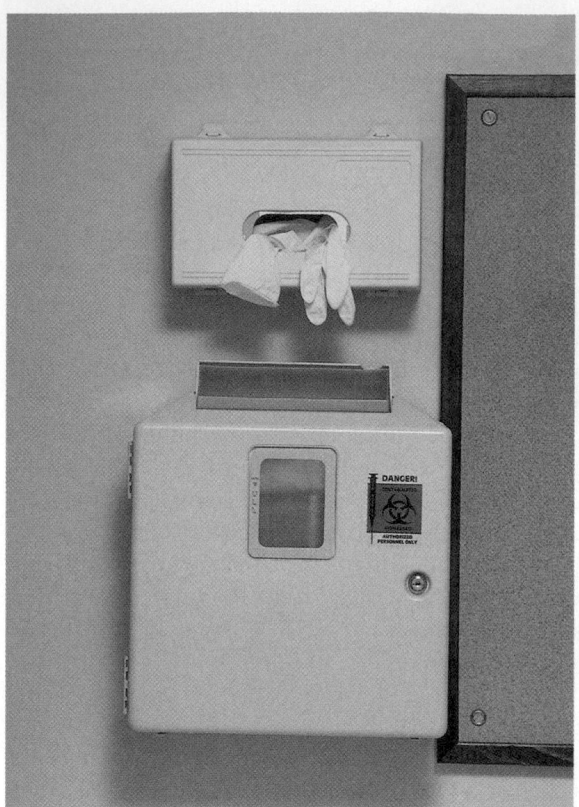

Figure 11-3 Sharps disposal and infectious waste container.

a high fever. The wife had a painful swelling in the groin. The couple did know that dead rodents had been recently found on their property and were believed to have died of bubonic plague (Drumm, Bruner, & Minutillo, 2004).

The *Yersinia pestis* bacterium is carried by fleas that have fed on infected rodents. When a person or another rodent is bitten by this infected flea, the disease is spread. In humans, plague can occur in three forms: bubonic plague characterized by infected lymph glands; pneumonic plague in which the bacterium invade the pulmonary tissue; and septicemic plague, a widespread invasion of the entire body. All forms are treated with antibiotics and life-maintaining measures to support involved body systems.

Measures to prevent transmission of the bacteria by body fluids and droplets from the respiratory track are essential. In the bubonic form of the disease, rapid administration of antibiotics can result in rapid recovery. However, in the pneumonic form, measures to maintain oxygenation are also essential. The most life-threatening form of the disease is when all body systems are invaded by the organism, and circulatory, digestive, and renal systems shut down. Nursing care for this form of disease is intensive with trying to maintain body systems and trying to protect the staff from possible cross-contamination from respiratory secretions.

To control the plague, it is essential to interrupt the cycle from the infected rodent to the flea to the next recipient. In areas of infestation of a disease like plague, the department of public health needs to monitor for infected animals and take the preventive action. Destroying fleas in areas where humans are likely to have contact with infected rodents can interrupt this cycle (Drumm, Bruner, & Minutillo, 2004).

In the spring of 1993, a previously unrecognized disease appeared in the American Southwest known as the Four Corners. Young people who had been in excellent health suddenly were appearing at emergency departments with severe respiratory disease. The mortality rate for these people was about 50 percent. The public health departments in the area quickly began investigating for possible causes of this sudden appearance of this new disease. Researchers suspected that this sudden appearance of this severe respiratory disease was related to the Hantavirus. They began trapping rodents in the areas in which the patients lived in an effort to find the source of the virus.

The deer mouse was quickly identified as the carrier of this virus. The virus was found in the urine, droppings, and saliva of these mice. People were exposed to these sources when they breathed the air contaminated with the virus. Any place in which mice were able to live was potential sources for possible exposure.

Early symptoms were flu-like, with headache, chills, dizziness, and abdominal upsets including nausea, vomiting, and diarrhea. Within a few days of these symptoms, the respiratory problems that could cause death developed. The affected people demonstrated a massive inflammatory response in the respiratory tract. They complained of coughing and shortness of breath. X-ray examination showed pulmonary infiltrates expected to be seen in severe pneumonia. The massive amount of fluid that accumulated in the respiratory tissue precluded oxygen transport into the tissues.

The disease is definitely diagnosed through laboratory means. Sputum from the person with the suspected illness can be examined for the presence of the Hantavirus. Serum samples can be tested for rising titers of Hantavirus specific immunoglobulin G.

Control of this disease is best done by educating people about how to avoid exposure to the air in which mouse droppings are present. If the mouse-to-person chain of transmission can be broken, the disease will be prevented. It has been demonstrated that other routes of transmission such as direct person-to-person does not occur (CDC National Center for Infectious Diseases, 2006).

GUIDELINES FOR INFECTION CONTROL

In the United States, the CDC has been the agency charged with developing and disseminating guidelines to reduce transmission of diseases in acute care hospitals. In 1970, guidelines for isolation practices in hospitals were developed by the CDC. Over the years, these guidelines have been refined and updated. In 1985, with the rising awareness of the HIV epidemic, a new approach to prevention of disease transmission was needed. This gave rise to isolation practices known as universal precautions (UP). The emphasis of these guidelines was to prevent transmission of disease from a patient with a diagnosed or even undiagnosed blood-borne disease to hospital staff utilizing the former guidelines of blood and body fluid precautions with all patients. In 1987, body substance isolation (BSI) was introduced to further refine infectious disease control practices. This system focused on techniques to protect health care personnel from body substances including blood, feces, urine, sputum, saliva, wound drainage, and other body fluids. The focus was on the use of gloves and did not emphasize hand washing as an important part of disease transmission prevention.

The need for new guidelines that would better protect both health care workers and patients from exposure to disease was identified, and the CDC was charged with developing new systems. This resulted in an entirely new system composed of two levels of precautions (CDC, 2006). Standard precautions were designed to be used with all patients to reduce the risk of transmission of blood-borne and other type of pathogens among health care workers and patients. In addition, another level of prevention, transmission-based precautions, are to be used with patients who have been diagnosed or are highly suspicious of having a communicable disease.

Standard Precautions

Standard precautions are actions to be used with all patients to reduce risk of transmission of disease. They are applied to all patients in acute care hospitals regardless of their diagnosis. These guidelines are summarized in Table 11-4.

TABLE 11-4 **CDC Guidelines for Infection Control: Standard Precautions for All Patients in a Health Care Setting**

SITUATION	ACTION
When touching any body fluid, secretion, or contaminated item	Nonsterile gloves Wash hands after removing gloves
Possibility of splashes or sprays from body fluids	Masks, eye protection, or face shields
Exposure to blood, body fluids, secretions, excretions	Gown: Remove prior to leaving patient room Wash hands after gown removal
Patient care equipment exposed to body fluids and secretions	Clean prior to use with another patient
Linens	Transport in closed containers Laundry facilities adequate to destroy pathogens.

Adapted from Center for Disease Control, National Center for Infectious Diseases. (2006). All about hantaviruses. Retrieved June 23, 2006, from www.cdc.gov; DeLaune, S., & Ladner, P. (2006). Fundamentals of nursing (3rd ed.). New York: Thomson Delmar Learning.

Transmission-Based Precautions

When a patient is known or suspected to have a communicable disease, transmission-based precautions are to be used. These are designed to prevent the spread of specific communicable diseases. These precautions are categorized by transmission route of airborne, droplet, or contact. A summary of these guidelines is shown in Table 11-5.

Contact Precautions

Contact precautions are to be used when caring for a patient with possible direct transmission of pathogenic microorganisms. These must be used when caring for the patient directly or when handling equipment or surfaces in the patient's environment. The patient should be placed in a private room whenever possible, and standard precautions are to be used at all times. Both a gown and gloves must be worn when caring for the patient. If there is expected to be significant contact with the infected material, such as when changing a dressing, the gloves should be changed and hands washed with a disinfectant material prior to applying the new dressing. All equipment used for the patient is ideally dedicated to just that patient. If equipment is moved among several patients, it must be cleaned and disinfected before using it with a second patient.

Droplet Precautions

Patients with a disease resulting in droplet release such as meningitis, pneumonia, diphtheria, or pertussis must be cared for using droplet precautions. The patient is to be placed in a private room if possible. If this is not possible, the patient must be kept at least 3 feet away from any other patient, preferably the other patient will have the same infectious disease. The door of the room may remain open. Health care personnel should wear a surgical mask when working within 3 feet of the patient (Figure 11-4). Again, limit transport of the patient as much as possible and place a surgical mask on the patient if transport is essential.

TABLE 11-5 CDC Guidelines for Infection Control: Transmission-Based Precautions

SITUATION	ACTION
Airborne transmission	Place patient in room in which air is filtered before entering general circulation
	Door to remain shut
	Use respiratory mask with HEPA filter
	Patient transport must be limited
	Patient must wear mask during transport
Droplet transmission	Place patient in private room if possible or keep patient at least 3 feet from another patient
	Room door can remain open
	Staff must wear mask if working within 3 feet of patient
	Limit patient transport
	Patient must wear mask during transport
Contact transmission	Place patient in private room if possible
	Wear gown and gloves when contacting patient
	Change gloves and wash hands during dressing changes—after removing old dressing and before applying new dressing
	Use of equipment should be dedicated to one patient
	Equipment must be cleaned before use with another patient

Adapted from Center for Disease Control, National Center for Infectious Diseases. (2006). All about hantaviruses. Retrieved June 23, 2006, from www.cdc.gov; DeLaune, S., & Ladner, P. (2006). Fundamentals of nursing (3rd ed.). New York: Thomson Delmar Learning.

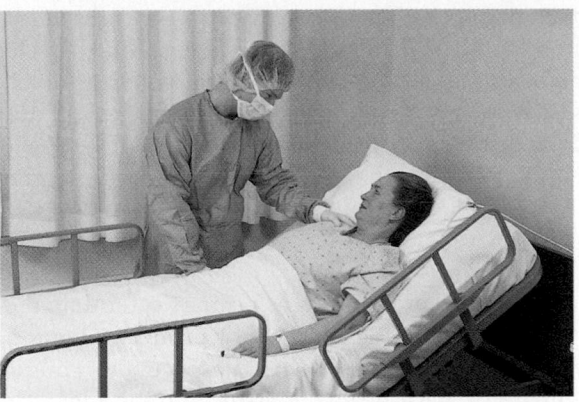

Figure 11-4 This nurse is interacting with a patient who requires isolation precautions. Although the patient and the nurse are observing isolation precautions, they are still able to communicate with one another. In planning the care of this patient, what would the expected outcomes of these interventions be?

Airborne Precautions

Airborne precautions must be utilized when caring for patients with disease such as measles, varicella, or tuberculosis in which the bacteria are contained in particles smaller than 5 μm and can become airborne over long distances. The patient must be placed in a room in which the air is filtered prior to entering the general circulation, and the door to the room must remain shut. Health care workers must wear respiratory masks that utilize a filter such as a high-efficiency particulate air (HEPA) filter. The only exception to this use of the mask is for persons who are known to be immune to the disease, such as with measles. When working with a person with active tuberculosis, the mask must always be worn. Transport of the patient out of the room should only be done when absolutely necessary, and the patient should wear a surgical mask during transport.

Nurse's Role

The nurse has a major role in preventing transmission of disease. These guidelines have been developed to provide protection to both the health care worker and all patients. Strict adherence to them is vital to preventing the spread of infectious disease. In this era of many antibiotic-resistant microorganisms, scrupulous nursing care is required to promote the health of all people. The principles outlined by Florence Nightingale (1969 [1859]) still are relevant to nurses today and are shown in Box 11-1.

WOUND HEALING

A critical function of the inflammatory system is to instigate and direct the repair process of injured tissue to maintain the integrity of the body. A wound is defined as any disruption of normal tissue structure and function. Wound healing is defined as a restoration of anatomical continuity and function. However, often in wound healing, this goal is not totally achieved. There can be delayed healing, chronic infection in the area, or formation of scar tissue. If tissue is restored to normal cell structure, the process is known as restoration. Repair occurs when destroyed cells are replaced with connective tissue that does not have the capacity to carry out the normal tissue function. A good example of this is the repair that occurs in myocardial tissue following a major

---

BOX 11-1

NIGHTINGALE AND TRANSMISSION OF DISEASE

The following are direct quotations from Florence Nightingale related to the transmission of disease:

"The very first canon of nursing, the first and the last thing upon which a nurse's attention must be fixed . . . keep the air he (the patient) breathes as pure as the external air without chilling him" (p. 12).

"It cannot be necessary to tell a nurse that she should be clean, or that she should keep her patient clean—seeing that the greater part of nursing consists in preserving cleanliness" (p. 87).

"Every nurse ought to be careful to wash her hands very frequently during the day" (p. 4).

Adapted from Nightingale, F. (1969 [1859]). Notes on nursing: What it is and what it is not. New York: Dover Publications.

disruption of blood flow and death of cells. The recovery process results in formation of connective tissue in the injured area rather than myocardial muscle; consequently there is loss of heart function. Cells in tissue which normally have rapid division such as skin, mucous membranes, or bone marrow generally heal by regeneration. Cells in tissue such as heart or nerve tend not to regenerate (McCance & Huether, 2005; Porth, 2005).

Types of Wound Healing

Wound healing occurs through either what is known as primary intention, secondary intention, or tertiary intention. Wounds that heal by **primary intention,** utilize normal wound repair processes. This type of healing occurs in wounds that are clean, i.e., not contaminated, have little loss of tissue, and the edges can be approximated using materials such as sutures, staples, or tissue adhesives. Many surgical wounds fall into this category. Wounds that do not meet these criteria are more difficult to heal, and the process is known as healing by either secondary or tertiary intention. In **secondary intention,** the wound heals by spread of granulation tissue from the base of the wound (Vermeulen, Ubbink, Goossens, de Vos, & Legemate, 2006). In **tertiary intention,** the wound must be sutured through several layers of granulation tissue to bring closure to the wound surface.

Wounds such as venous leg ulcers heal by secondary intention. In this process, the wound is allowed to remain open and granulate from the base. In wounds that are highly contaminated with microorganisms, the wound is allowed to remain open for several days and be treated with antibiotics to reduce the bacterial load. Only when the level of bacterial load is reduced, can the wound be closed surgically. Nursing management of wound care is primarily focused on wounds healing by secondary or tertiary intention. Those healing by primary intention are generally covered by a sterile dressing and allowed to heal without further intervention.

Wounds are also classified by the depth. Partial thickness wounds such as skin tears or abrasions only penetrate into the dermis and the epidermis. Full-thickness wounds penetrate much deeper and can involve the subcutaneous tissue, muscle, and even into bone. Partial thickness wounds require little more than cleansing of the site and a dressing to protect the area while it heals. Full-thickness wounds require considerable nursing intervention to promote healing in the area. The discussion of nursing interventions will focus on the management of full-thickness wounds that heal by secondary or tertiary intention.

Risk Factors for Delayed Wound Healing

Risk factors for delayed wound healing include ischemia to the area, infection, and repetitive injury (Table 11-6). Repetitive injury occurs when the damaged area is subjected to a new force while the area is still under repair. Scar tissue that is forming in the area is not as sturdy as normal tissue and is less able withstand new injury. Oxygen and nutrients are vital to the repair process; thus any ischemia to the area will prevent wound healing. The presence of bacteria in the wound stimulates the inflammatory process and also prevents the healing process (see Concept Map: Tissue Repair). Other chemical mediators such as beta-blocker drugs, smoking, or exposure to cold can also delay wound healing. All of these chemical factors reduce blood flow to the area and thus decrease both the oxygen and nutrients required for wound healing. In addition excess anti-inflammatory steroids, such as cortisol, inhibit macrophages from migrating to the injured area thus preventing their normal role in phagocytosis. They also inhibit fibroblast migration to the area and thus delay wound healing. Finally, a person's age is related to the adequacy of wound healing. Older persons tend to have a less robust inflammatory response. Their cells do not respond as well to growth factors and cytokine action thus delaying wound repair (McCance & Huether, 2005).

TABLE 11-6 **Risk Factors for Delayed Wound Healing**	
FACTOR	**ACTION**
Ischemia	Reduced flow of nutrients and oxygen to area

Chemical mediators
    Medications such as beta-blockers
    Smoking
    Exposure to cold
	All factors reduce blood flow to area

Repetitive injury	Stress of scar tissue
Altered nutrition	Lack of nutrients required for healing
Infection	Stimulates inflammatory process
Anti-inflammatory steroids	Inhibit macrophage activity
Older age	Less robust inflammatory response

Adapted from Murphy, F. (2005). Myths and realities in acute woundcare. Practice Nurse, 30(4), 52–53; Porth, C. (2005). Pathophysiology: Concepts of altered health states (7th ed.). Philadelphia: Lippincott, Williams & Wilkins; Watret, L. (2005). Teaching wound management: A collaborative model for future education. World Wide Wounds, 8(12), 13–15.

Phases of Wound Healing

Wound healing occurs along a continuum of time that follows a consistent pattern. The phases include the inflammatory, the proliferative, and the remodeling processes. Each of these will be described.

Inflammatory Phase

As previously discussed, the inflammatory phase begins with the presence of injury to a tissue caused by a multitude of possible factors. As a result of the chemical mediators, which are released in the inflammatory process, platelets are activated and the clotting cascade initiated. This results in the formation of a loose clot filled with fibrin and stems blood flow into the area. In a surgical wound, the area is usually sealed with this fibrin clot within two hours of injury and thus provides a barrier for possible bacterial contamination.

Another chemical formed in the initial inflammatory response, epidermal growth factor, stimulates mitosis of epidermal cells. Cells that border the wound area multiply and begin to move into the injured area filling the area with granulation tissue. Injured cells, microorganisms, and other foreign tissue are phagocytized by the granulocytes and the macrophages and are cleared from the area through the lymphatic system. Also, the fibrin clot must be dissolved. At this time capillary and lymphatic buds are formed to begin the process of restoring circulation to the injured tissue.

Proliferative Phase

The proliferative phase generally begins three to four days following the initial injury and is characterized by extensive fibroblast activity in which collagen is formed that will develop into connective tissue. In this way the wound is sealed off and begins to fill in with tissue. During this time wound retraction also occurs. Myofibroblasts, cells similar to fibroblasts, are composed of fibers that exert contractile strength and attach to cells on the edges of the wound. There they pull these healthy cells together and cause the wound to contract.

Remodeling Phase

The remodeling phase consists of reforming collagen fibers into a strong structure. The collagen material that is initially deposited in the wound area has a gel-like consistency. This must be remodeled into a stronger structure. The initial collagen fibers are dissolved by an enzyme, and new fibers are laid down along lines of mechanical stress. Cross-links between the collagen fibers are formed giving additional strength to the new tissue. The remodeling phase can take up to several years following injury. In this phase, the scar tissue is remodeled by removing the capillary beds and leaving the tissue avascular. The wound is healed, but usually it has only about 80 percent of the strength of the original tissue.

Dysfunctional Wound Healing

There are many factors that delay normal wound healing and thus lead to chronic wounds. The most common types of chronic wounds are pressure ulcers, diabetic foot ulcers, and venous ulcers. In addition, there are also less common factors that deter wound healing, and these will be described. An understanding of the factors that delay wound healing can explain why these ulcers are so difficult to heal.

Factors Leading to Delayed Wound Healing

If bleeding is not controlled during the initial response to the wound, several problems arise. The clot from the excessive blood in the area increases the amount of space that must be filled in with granulation tissue. The enlarged space prevents good diffusion of oxygen to the area. Also, the excess of blood cells that must be removed by phagocytosis prolongs the inflammatory phase of wound healing. These excess blood cells are also an excellent medium for bacterial growth increasing the chance for infection in the wound. Another problem in wound healing is if excess fibrin is formed. This makes it difficult for all of the fibrin to be reabsorbed and leads to formation of adhesions. These adhesions are particularly serious in the pleural, pericardial, or abdominal cavities where they can bind organs together and seriously affect their ability to function.

Hypovolemia in the affected area, the presence of steroid drugs, or decreased nutrition are additional factors that can inhibit wound healing. If adequate blood flow to the area is not present, the inflammatory cells needed for repair cannot be delivered, and the process will be hindered. This is why venous leg ulcers with inadequate perfusion to the area are so difficult to heal. Steroid drugs inhibit macrophage migration to the affected area thus hindering the inflammatory response and preventing collagen from being released to stimulate wound healing. With decreased inflammatory response, patients who have been on prolonged steroid drugs will have delayed phagocytosis and delayed wound healing.

Optimal nutrition is vital to wound healing. Both glucose and protein are necessary to the process. Tremendous amounts of adenosine triphosphate (ATP) are utilized in the inflammatory and repair processes and must be formed through the cellular oxidation process. People with diabetes mellitus often have small vessel damage and thus cannot provide adequate nutrition and oxygen to the wound, which leads to delayed healing (Anderson, 2005).

If collagen synthesis is excessive, several problems in wound healing can occur. If the excess collagen is deposited within the original boundaries of the wound, it is known as a hypertrophic scar. At times the amount of colloid formation is so excessive that it extends beyond the boundaries of the original wound. This excess scar tissue is known as a keloid. Why some people are prone to excess colloid formation is not known.

Occasionally there is a disruption of a sutured wound when the wound pulls apart opening up the area to underlying tissue. This is known as dehiscence. The most common time for this to occur is from 5 to 12 days postoperatively. The most common reason for dehiscence to occur is because of an underlying infection. Another factor known to cause suture line rupture is excessive strain placed on the wound. Obese people are more likely to have wound disruption than normal weight persons. This is because it is more difficult to suture through adipose tissue. In all cases, when dehiscence occurs, the patient must return to the surgery and have the wound attended to. Many times the wound will be dressed and allowed to heal by secondary intention.

Another problem that can occur with wound healing is when excessive contracture occurs because of excess myofibroblast activity. The resulting formation is known as an adhesion. These are particularly problematic when they bind organs together. People recovering from a burn injury often have excessive contraction of the tissue. The use of pressure dressings and body coverings helps prevent excessive formation of contracture.

Common Wounds

Several chronic wounds are commonly encountered in both community and hospital settings. As the longevity of the population increases, the number of people with chronic wound healing problems also increases. This is placing a significant financial burden on the health care industry. Any measures that can be taken to reduce wound healing problems will have a significant impact on conserving health care expenditures. The three most common wounds seen are venous ulcers, pressure ulcers, and diabetic foot ulcers.

Venous Ulcers

A common problem in older adults is the development of venous ulcers in the lower extremities. It is believed that there is disruption in normal venous return through the deep vein system in the leg because of incompetent valves in the veins. Normally, as the calf muscles contract, blood is forced upward in the venous system against gravity pressure. If the valves along the venous system cannot prevent back flow, excess blood can be pumped into the superficial venous system and increase fluid pressure in the area. The excess pressure causes fluid to leak into the tissue causing edema. Even a slight injury to this edematous area can be the cause of ulcer formation.

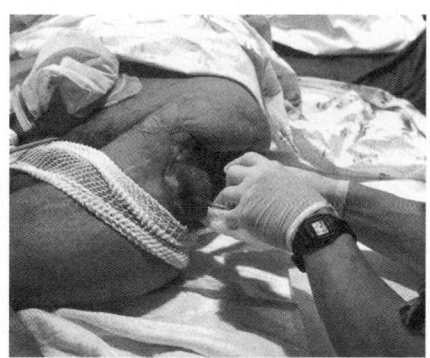

Figure 11-5 Performing a dressing change on a large pressure ulcer.

Pressure Ulcers

Pressure ulcers are an all too common occurrence in people who remain in one position for long periods of time (Figure 11-5). When caring for bedridden patients and those confined to wheel chairs for long times, the nurse must be on high alert for pressure ulcer formation. Several theories about the cause of pressure development exist. Vertical pressure over a bony prominence has long been known to be responsible for pressure ulcer development. Pressure ulcers can also develop from friction as when a person is moved across a bed surface and by shearing as when a person slides down in bed. Both of these are thought to rupture of small blood vessels as the superficial and deep tissues move in opposite directions (Moore, 2006).

Diabetic Foot Ulcers

Another common wound that nurses frequently encounter is a diabetic foot ulcer. These ulcers are most commonly found in the lower extremities involving the tibial and peroneal arteries. People with uncontrolled blood sugars for long periods experience damage to the microcirculation and nerves. The arterioles become sclerotic, and blood flow to the area is reduced leading to ischemia. The nerve damage makes the person less aware of injury to the area and thus does not take action when a minor injury occurs. With the decreased blood flow to the area, the normal inflammatory response is delayed and healing is retarded. In addition, high glucose levels inhibit leukocyte activity. All of these factors lead to a high incidence of ulcer formation in people with diabetes mellitus (Smith, 2006).

NURSING RESPONSE: WOUND HEALING

Nurses are the primary health care provider charged with the management of patients' chronic wounds. Often the nurse works alongside the physical therapist in developing and carrying out the plan of care. Much of the management of these patients occurs in community settings, such as with home health nurses or in long-term care facilities. When nurses see patients who are at risk for infection, they monitor the wound with careful skin surveillance. The nurse assesses for signs of inflammation, the type of drainage, and the size and depth of the wound. In addition, the nurses examines the laboratory results (e.g., WBC and differential counts, hemoglobin, hematocrit, wound cultures). Once a patient has a wound the nurse must then focus on care interventions, such as, debridement, wound irrigation, and the prevention of further injury. In addition, the nurse must educate and encourage the patient in the arena of maintaining good nutrition with adequate calories and protein (Carpenito, 2004).

Assessment with Clinical Manifestations

Vigilant assessment of a wound is a vital part of nursing care. The timing of the assessment is somewhat dependent on the nature and the extent of the wound. A wound healing by primary intention requires inspection of the area surrounding the wound to observe for any untoward development. Wounds healing by secondary or tertiary intention require more frequent monitoring. There is no consensus about an exact timing schedule for assessment, but a minimum is at the time of each dressing change.

There are many factors to be assessed when managing patients with a wound. The area around the wound should be assessed for signs of spreading inflammation such as redness or swelling. The drainage from the wound must be assessed for amount, color, consistency, and odor. The patient should be asked about pain in the wound area. When the dressing is changed, the wound size and depth must be assessed. Laboratory values that are important to evaluating the wound healing process include a white blood cell count, a differential count, and a hemoglobin and hematocrit. The white count will assess the ability of the person to mount the inflammatory response. The hemoglobin and hematocrit will give an indication of the ability of the person to carry oxygen to the site that is needed to promote healing.

Wound size and depth are important assessments to make; however, they are not always easy to determine. The length and width of the wound can be measured with a disposable ruler. The depth of the wound can be estimated with a disposable probe. At times it is difficult to assess the true size of the wound if the wound is undermined; that is, the area under the skin is larger than the actual skin opening. A probe can be used to estimate the size of the undermining.

Any exudates included in the wound must also be described. In the acute stage of inflammation, the exudate in the wound is usually liquid. If the wound becomes chronic, the exudate will have a more fibrous appearance. If the wound is infected, the color will vary based on the organism involved. For example, wounds infected with pseudomonas have a greenish color. A healing wound will have a reddish appearance as new capillary growth occurs. A dark black color is indicative of necrotic tissue.

If the wound appears to be infected, further assessment is needed. A nurse must differentiate between a wound that is colonized with bacteria and one that is infected. When the wound is colonized, the number of bacteria is limited, and the body immunological defenses can keep them under control and will not interfere with wound healing. If the bacterial count exceeds 100,000 organisms per gram of tissue, the wound is considered infected. Other signs of infection include redness of the skin surrounding the wound, a purulent drainage that has a foul odor, and edema. A culture of the wound must be made to determine the invading organisms and help with choosing the appropriate antibiotic. The presence of fever and leukocytosis must also be assessed. Other signs of infection such as pain, redness, heat, odor, and purulent exudate are also to be noted (Estes, 2006).

Because pressure ulcers are an enormous problem in patients who have limited mobility, every effort must be made to prevent their occurrence. Several predictive scales have been developed to assist nurses to identify patients at risk from pressure ulcer formation. The Braden scale (Bergstrom & Braden, 2002) has been extensively researched for validity of use. Brown (2004) found this scale to be highly useful in predicting patients not at risk for pressure ulcer development. The scale's ability to predict the development of a pressure ulcer increases if used between 24 and 48 hours following admission to an acute care setting rather than at the time of admission. The elements included in the Braden scale are shown in Table 11-7.

Interventions: Wound Management

The nursing management of patients who have a chronic wound either because of an infectious process or reduced blood flow to the area is always a challenge. Frantz (2004) outlines four principles to be followed in managing chronic wounds: (a) debridement, (b) provide moist environment, (c) prevent further injury, and (d) nutrition. Each of these principles will be discussed and appropriate nursing measures described.

Debridement

Debridement involves the removal of nonviable tissue from the wound. This dead tissue will serve as a source of continuous infection if not removed. Four types of debridement can be utilized: autolytic, biochemical, mechanical, and surgical.

In autolytic debridement, the body utilizes its own defenses, the inflammatory process, to remove the dead tissue. The wound is covered with an occlusive or a semiocclusive dressing and left in place for several days. During this time, the leukocytes and other body fluids collect in the wound area and begin to lyse (break down) the necrotic tissue. If the person's immune system is functional, any bacteria in the area will also be destroyed. This type of debridement is best utilized in wounds that have relatively small amounts of nonviable tissue. The type of products that can be used to provide the covering include transparent film dressings such as OpSite or Tegaderm, a hydrocolloid such as DuoDerm, or a Hydrogel such as Aquasorb. The transparent film allows for oxygen to diffuse into the wound, but yet retains inflammatory fluids within the wound. The hydrocolloid and hydrogel dressings do not allow for oxygen diffusion. All of these dressings will retain moisture within the wound allowing autolytic debridement.

Biochemical debridement employs enzymes to debride the nonviable tissue. Enzyme products that can be used include a fibrinolysin-deoxyribonuclease agent contained in Elase or a sutilain as found in Travase. After application of one of these products, the wound must be covered by gauze or a semitransparent dressing.

TABLE 11-7	**Elements in Braden Pressure Scale**
1. Sensory perception	Ability to respond meaningfully to pressure-related discomfort
2. Moisture	Degree to which skin is exposed to moisture
3. Activity	Degree of physical activity
4. Mobility	Ability to change and control body position
5. Nutrition	Usual food intake pattern
6. Friction and shear	Potential for problem during movements in bed

Source: Bergstrom, N., & Braden, B. (2002). Predictive validity of the Braden Scale among black and white subjects. Nursing Research, 51*(6), 398–403.*

Mechanical debridement is a common method used when the amount of nonviable tissue is minimal. The most common technique used is the wet-to-damp dressing in which gauze soaked in normal saline is packed into the wound and left for several hours in which time it can gradually lose some of its moisture. The entire area is then covered with a dry dressing. Several hours later, the gauze is removed and with it the wound debris. A down side of this method is that when the gauze is removed it can also remove healthy tissue. In the past, antibacterial solutions such as povidone-iodine or hydrogen peroxide have also been used to wet the gauze. This is no longer recommended because such agents can be toxic to healthy cells (Calianno & Jakubek, 2006).

Another aspect of mechanical debridement involves cleansing of the wound area (Figure 11-6). This can remove foreign materials from the wound that may have come from the dressing used. It is important to remove this foreign material to prevent a buildup of bacteria in the wound. A vigorous method of cleansing is to put the patient into a whirlpool bath and allow the agitation of the water soften the necrotic tissue. A more gentle method of cleaning is to irrigate the wound with a 35-mL syringe with a 19-gauge angiocatheter, which can deliver about 8 pounds of pressure (Frantz, 2004). This method is now recommended rather than the use of an Asepto type syringe that has been used in the past. The Asepto syringe method is unable to generate the recommended 8 pounds of pressure. The wound can also be cleansed using a gauze dressing soaked in normal saline and gently patting the wound.

The most invasive wound debridement strategy is that of surgical removal of the nonviable tissue. This method is recommended when there are large amounts of nonviable tissue, and the other methods would be too time-consuming. It requires hospitalization with its attendant issues, such as exposure to more virulent bacteria and to anesthetics. Thus it is usually used only as a last resort in a chronic wound that is not responding to less invasive treatment. Wounds caused by necrotizing fasciitis are an example in which surgical debridement must be rapidly utilized to overcome the spread of the inflammation. In this disease, a person can quickly develop overwhelming infection that leads to death within a period of days.

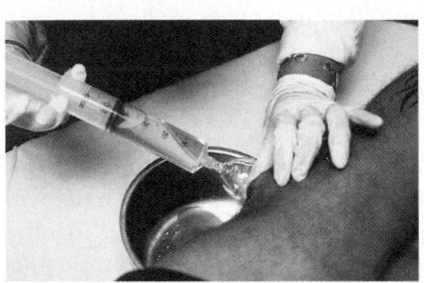

Figure 11-6 Wound irrigation.

Moist Environment

The second principle of wound management is to maintain a moist environment. This has been shown to encourage reepitheliazation and healing. If the wound is exposed to air, the surface will dry and prevent healing from occurring. Several strategies can be used to keep the wound moist. The wet-to-damp dressing previously discussed is often used. Also the semipermeable dressings that allow oxygen to diffuse into the wound but retain moisture are often used. However, a semipermeable dressing should not be used if the wound is infected.

Prevention of Further Injury

To maintain optimal conditions for wound healing, care must be taken to prevent further injury. Based on the cause of the initial wound, various nursing measures can be taken. With a pressure ulcer, pressure reducing devices such as a foam cushion, an air mattress, or an alternating-pressure mattress are often used. With wounds caused by poor venous circulation, a compression stocking that promotes venous return to the heart can be used. Another device often used to enhance venous circulation is an Unna boot that provides compression on the venous system or even a pneumatic compression stocking.

Nutrition

Appropriate nutrition is vital to promoting wound healing. Protein is needed to supply the amino acids required to build new tissue. The adequacy of protein levels is best measured by albumin levels. The albumin level needed to promote wound healing is above 3.5 g/dL. A low albumin level is a sign of chronic malnutrition, a problem often seen is the elderly who are prone to delayed wound healing. Another indicator of chronic malnutrition is a lymphocyte count of less than 800.

The patient must have an adequate caloric intake, including carbohydrates and fats so that protein is not utilized for daily metabolic needs. Another essential for wound healing is an adequate iron intake so that hemoglobin levels are maintained. Hemoglobin is the oxygen transport system, and oxygen is essential to the healing process. Other nutrients important to wound healing are vitamins, zinc, copper, and magnesium (Anderson, 2005).

Necrotizing fasciitis is a disease in which surgical debridement of the involved area is an absolute necessity. It is caused by what are commonly referred to as flesh-eating bacteria. The most common bacteria responsible for this infection are group A beta hemolytic *Streptococcus* and *Staphylococcus aureus.* These bacteria can first cause a flu-like syndrome in which the patient experiences fever, nausea, weakness, or fatigue. Within hours to days, skin lesions will appear that are bright red and indurated and can be mistaken for cellulites in the early stages of the disease. The area quickly takes on a violet color and large fluid filled blisters form. The patient also experiences severe pain in the area and appears to be much sicker than the first appearance of the wound would suggest. The infection spreads rapidly through the subcutaneous tissue and can invade the muscle and fascia.

The origin of the disease can be from an internal source, such as trauma from a kidney stone, or an external source through a wound. When the invading organism is a *Streptococcus,* the bacteria release an exotoxin, which causes high fever and toxic shock. The streptococci also block the blood vessels and the lymph glands in the area impeding the flow of leukocytes to the infected area. Fluid from the blood vessels leaks into the damaged tissue causing edema and decreased oxygen to the tissues. This hypoxic state leads to cell damage and death. Enzymes released by the bacteria cause further necrosis of the tissue. The toxins released by the streptococcal organisms cause systemic shock. The patient experiences critically low blood pressure leading to kidney failure. The shock syndrome that results can lead to massive failure of all the body organs.

Management of this disease is to rapidly identify the causative organism using a Gram's stain and a rapid strep screen. Laboratory values will indicate leukocytosis with a rapid increase in the number of band cells. Antibiotic therapy using drugs such as cleomycin or ciprofloxacin must be started immediately. Surgical debridement of the wound can reduce the mortality rate seen in this disease. This debridement may need to be done several times to remove the necrotic tissue and new areas of infection. If the infected area is a limb, amputation may be needed to save the person's life. To combat the septic shock syndrome, massive amounts of IV fluids are required to replace fluid lost in the inflamed area.

Management of chronic wounds requires a great deal of knowledge about wound healing as well as frequent assessment of the wound. This is a challenge that the nurse faces often. Nursing care will often be the difference between a wound that heals and one that goes on to be a chronic problem.

The inflammatory process is vital to maintaining the health and well-being of all people. It provides us with a means to mount an immediate response to invasion of foreign material into the body. People whose inflammatory response is diminished because of nutrition, altered immune system, drug therapy, or a multitude of other factors face risk of serious illness. However, at times the inflammatory reaction can cause disease such as arthritis. In these situations, the nursing response is focused on reducing the inflammatory response.

Because microorganisms are such an important causative factor in inducing an inflammatory response, an important focus of all nursing care is to actively reduce transmission of microorganisms between patients and health care workers. The use of standard precautions and transmission-based precautions must become a part of each nurse's daily practice. With the rise of antibiotic-resistant organisms, such practices are doubly important. Wound care is also an important nursing intervention. As the population ages, problems with wound healing will increase. Developing expertise in this area of nursing is vital to each nurse.

CONCEPT MAP

Inflammatory Process

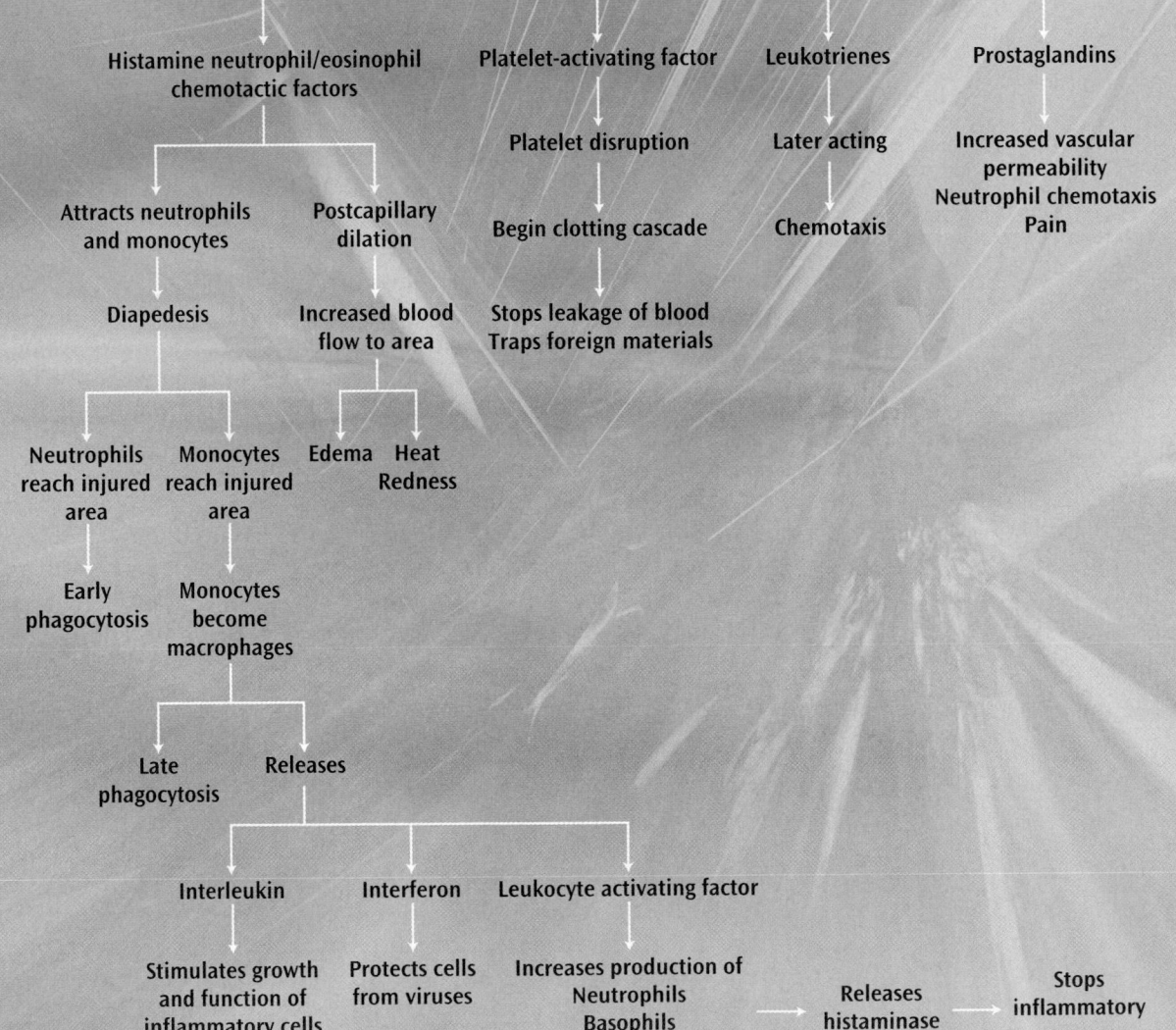

Tissue injury caused by:
Microorganisms
Trauma
Chemicals
Surgery, etc.
Heat/cold

Mast cell degranulation releases

Histamine neutrophil/eosinophil chemotactic factors

Platelet-activating factor

Leukotrienes

Prostaglandins

Attracts neutrophils and monocytes

Postcapillary dilation

Platelet disruption

Later acting

Increased vascular permeability
Neutrophil chemotaxis
Pain

Diapedesis

Increased blood flow to area

Begin clotting cascade

Chemotaxis

Neutrophils reach injured area

Monocytes reach injured area

Edema Heat Redness

Stops leakage of blood
Traps foreign materials

Early phagocytosis

Monocytes become macrophages

Late phagocytosis

Releases

Interleukin

Interferon

Leukocyte activating factor

Stimulates growth and function of inflammatory cells

Protects cells from viruses

Increases production of
Neutrophils
Basophils
Eosinophils

Releases histaminase

Stops inflammatory process

Adapted from McCance, K., & Huether, S. (2005). Pathophysiology: The biological basis for disease in adults and children (5th ed.). St. Louis, MO: Mosby; Porth, C. (2005). Pathophysiology: Concepts of altered health states (7th ed.). Philadelphia: Lippincott, Williams & Wilkins.

CONCEPT MAP

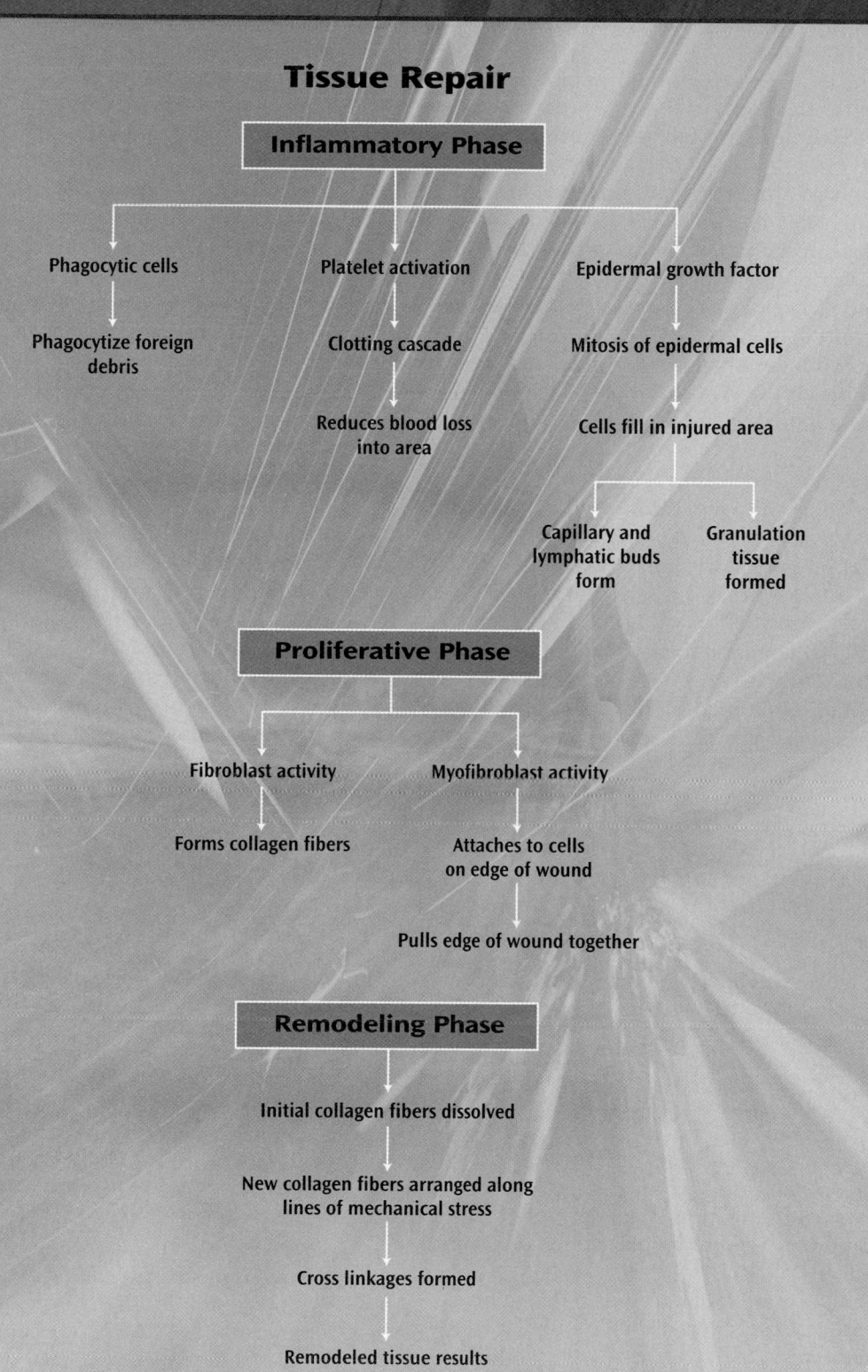

Tissue Repair

Inflammatory Phase

Phagocytic cells → Phagocytize foreign debris

Platelet activation → Clotting cascade → Reduces blood loss into area

Epidermal growth factor → Mitosis of epidermal cells → Cells fill in injured area → Capillary and lymphatic buds form / Granulation tissue formed

Proliferative Phase

Fibroblast activity → Forms collagen fibers

Myofibroblast activity → Attaches to cells on edge of wound → Pulls edge of wound together

Remodeling Phase

Initial collagen fibers dissolved

New collagen fibers arranged along lines of mechanical stress

Cross linkages formed

Remodeled tissue results

Adapted from McCance, K., & Huether, S. (2005). Pathophysiology: The biological basis for disease in adults and children (5th ed.). St. Louis, MO: Mosby; Porth, C. (2005). Pathophysiology: Concepts of altered health states (7th ed.). Philadelphia: Lippincott, Williams & Wilkins.

KEY CONCEPTS

- The inflammatory process is an important protective mechanism for the body.
- A variety of chemicals are released during inflammation.
- The inflammatory process is characterized by redness, swelling, heat, and pain.
- The end stage of the inflammatory process is resolution and repair of the involved tissue.
- If the inflammatory process is prolonged, the condition is referred to as chronic inflammation.
- The body's first line of defense against these microorganisms is the skin and mucous membranes lining the respiratory, digestive, and genitourinary tracts.
- Antibiotic-resistant organisms are described as those organisms that are no longer destroyed by the usual antibiotics.
- Asthma is an inflammatory disease that is the response to allergens or irritants found in the environment.
- One of the most common forms of an inflammatory disease is osteoarthritis, in which the cartilage covering the ends of bones in joints deteriorates and the bone rubs against bone.
- Recently research has demonstrated that a primary problem in the development of a MI is related to an inflammatory reaction within the walls of arteries.
- Transmission routes for invading organisms are important to understand because these are the ways by which microorganisms reach the body.
- Contact transmission is the most common transmission route and can be either direct or indirect.
- Hand hygiene is an extremely important aspect in prevention of disease transmission.
- The CDC has been the agency charged with developing and disseminating guidelines to reduce transmission of diseases in acute care hospitals.
- Standard precautions are actions to be used with all patients to reduce risk of transmission of disease.
- A critical function of the inflammatory system is to instigate and direct the repair process of injured tissue to maintain the integrity of the body.
- Much of the management of wound care occurs in community settings such as with home health nurses or in long-term care facilities.
- The four principles to be followed in managing chronic wounds are: debridement, providing a moist environment, preventing further injury, and ensuring healthy nutrition.

REVIEW QUESTIONS

1. The first leukocytes attracted to an injured tissue are the:
   1. Mast cells
   2. Neutrophils
   3. Lymphocytes
   4. Eosinophils

2. The correct order for these events in an inflammatory response is:
   1. Mast cell degranulation, diapedesis of leukocytes, increased vascular permeability, and capillary dilatation
   2. Mast cell degranulation, capillary dilatation, increased vascular permeability, and diapedesis of leukocytes
   3. Diapedesis of leukocytes, increased capillary dilatation, increased vascular permeability, and mast cell degranulation

   4. Increased capillary dilatation, mast cell degranulation, diapedesis of leukocytes, and increased capillary permeability

3. The classic sign of swelling seen in the inflammatory process results from:
   1. Leakage of plasma into the injured area
   2. Increased blood circulation to the area
   3. The presence of phagocytic activity in the area
   4. Response to the cytokines released

4. Fever that is seen in a patient with an infectious disease is most likely caused by:
   1. Increased release of histamine
   2. Increased release of interleukin
   3. Increased number of bacteria in the body
   4. Increased vasodilation in the area of injury

Continued

REVIEW QUESTIONS—cont'd

5. Chronic inflammation can be caused by all of these *except:*
   1. A foreign body such as a bullet lodged in the tissue
   2. A response to a normal body substance such as low-density lipoprotein lodged in excess in an arteriole wall
   3. Use of an arthritic joint
   4. A walled off tubercle

6. A nursing teaching strategy to reduce the development of an antibiotic-resistant organism is to:
   1. Wash hands before and after all patient contact
   2. Keep people with a known infection in an isolation room
   3. Stress the importance of taking all doses of an antibiotic when ordered
   4. Have a patient with a known infection wear a mask when in public areas

7. A patient with a known infection must be managed by using which identified method of precaution?
   1. Strict asepsis
   2. Standard precautions
   3. Droplet precautions
   4. Transmission-based precautions

8. All of the following are risk factors for delayed wound healing *except:*
   1. Inadequate nutrition
   2. Repetitive injury
   3. Tissue ischemia
   4. Maintaining a moist environment

9. In healing by primary intention the wound fills in from:
   1. Granulation tissue from the bottom of the wound
   2. Suturing layers of granulation tissue
   3. Cell migration from the borders of the wound
   4. All of these

10. If a person has been taking a steroid drug, wound healing will be delayed because the steroid drug:
    1. Impedes macrophage migration
    2. Reduces body temperature
    3. Reduces appetite and thus results in poor nutrition
    4. Prevents fluid from reaching the involved area

11. Rest and immobilization are important to wound healing because they:
    1. Increase circulation to involved area
    2. Increase the metabolic rate
    3. Prevent further injury to area
    4. Prevent contractures in the involved area

REVIEW ACTIVITIES

1. Evaluate the laboratory studies in a patient with an inflammatory disease.
2. Identify several nursing diagnoses for a patient who has an inflammatory disorder.
3. Select a patient with a wound and evaluate the phase of the wound healing.
4. Describe the role of the nurse in providing standard precautions for a patient with a highly contagious disease.
5. List the necessary elements for enhancing wound healing across the spectrum of patient populations.

Fluid, Electrolyte, and Acid-Base Imbalances

Christine M. Henshaw, EdD, RN, CNE

CHAPTER TOPICS

- Principles of Fluid Homeostasis

- Electrolyte Balance/Imbalance

- Fluid Imbalances

- Acid-Base Balance/Imbalance

F luid, electrolyte, and acid-base balance are critical to the maintenance of life. Minor shifts in any of these parameters can have devastating effects on the human body. Changes in fluid location or balance, changes in the relative concentrations of various electrolytes, or changes in hydrogen balance in the body can cause loss of cellular function, and if severe, cell death, and ultimately, death of the patient. The nurse is a vital member of the health care team in assessing for and identifying changes in fluid, electrolyte, and acid-base balance. Understanding the basic principles of fluid and electrolyte balance in the body is essential in assessing the patient, planning interventions, and evaluating the effects of care. The purpose of this chapter is to review these principles and to identify common and major fluid, electrolyte, and acid-base imbalances that nurses encounter.

KEY TERMS

Anion gap
Anions
Baroreceptors
Cations
Diffusion
Electrolytes
Extracellular fluid (ECF)
Hypertonic
Hypotonic
Interstitial fluid
Intracellular fluid (ICF)
Intravascular fluid
Isotonic
Oncotic pressure
Osmolality
Osmolarity
Osmosis
Osmotic pressure
Semipermeable membranes
Solutes
Transcellular fluid

TABLE 12-1	Fluid Component of Body Weight

CATEGORY	% BODY WEIGHT THAT IS FLUID
Newborn	75%
Adult	
Male	60%
Female	50%
Elderly	
Male	50%
Female	40%

Source: Kee, J. L., Paulanka, B., & Purnel, L. (2004). Fluid and electrolytes with clinical applications: A programmed approach (7th ed.). New York: Thomson Delmar Learning.

Respecting Our Differences

Body Water Percentages

Although infants have more fat cells than adults, their percentage of body water is much higher than adults. On the other hand, the percentage of body water in the elderly is considerably lower. Because of their special needs, both the young and the old are at much higher risk of fluid imbalances. Careful assessment of body fluid status and early recognition of fluid imbalances are critical at both ends of the age spectrum.

FLUID BALANCE

The average human body is comprised of 60 to 75 percent fluid (Table 12-1). Infants' bodies contain a larger percentage of body fluid; elderly have less body fluid. Adipose (fat) cells contain less fluid than other cells; therefore women, who typically have more fat cells than men, have less body fluid than men, and overweight people have less body fluid than thin people (Rizzo, 2006).

The fluid in the body is located in two major compartments: the intracellular compartment and the extracellular compartment. **Intracellular fluid (ICF)** is that fluid inside each cell in the body and accounts for approximately two thirds of the body's fluid. **Extracellular fluid (ECF)** accounts for approximately one third of the body's fluid, and includes the fluid in the bloodstream, called **intravascular fluid** (excluding the fluid within the cells inside the bloodstream), and the fluid between the cells in body tissues, called **interstitial fluid. Transcellular fluid,** that fluid outside the ICF, interstitial, and intravascular fluid, makes up a small portion of the total body water, and includes cerebrospinal fluid, joint fluid, and the fluid within the gastrointestinal (GI) tract (Guyton & Hall, 2006).

Fluid Gains and Losses

Fluid normally is added to the body through oral ingestion of fluid and through ingestion of fluids contained in solid foods. In addition, daily metabolism produces fluids. Artificially, fluids are added through administration of IV fluids and tube feedings. Fluid is removed from the body through urine output, in feces, and through perspiration and respiration. Artificial means of fluid loss include nasogastric suction, wound drainage, and loss of fluids through burns. Table 12-2 shows the typical balance of fluid gains and losses.

Principles of Concentration Regulation

Within the fluids in the body are particles, such as electrolytes and proteins, called **solutes.** Two similar measures are used to describe the concentration of solutes in fluid. **Osmolality** is the number of solutes per *kilogram* of fluid. **Osmolarity** is the number of solutes per *liter* of fluid. Although there are subtle differences between the two, the terms are often used interchangeably. Clinically, the term osmolality is used to describe the concentration of body fluids. Normal serum osmolality is 280 to 300 milliosmoles per kilogram (mOsm/kg).

Water moves between the body's fluid compartments as necessary to maintain proper concentration and balance. Separating the intracellular and extracellular compartments are cell walls, which are **semipermeable membranes.**

TABLE 12-2	Average Fluid Losses and Gains in 24 Hours		
INTAKE		**OUTPUT**	
Oral liquids	1,300 mL	Urine	1,500 mL
Water in food	1,000 mL	Stool	200 mL
Water from metabolism	300 mL	Insensible losses	
		Lungs	300 mL
		Skin	600 mL
Total	2,600 mL	Total	2,600 mL

Source: Roth, R. (2007). Nutrition and diet therapy (9th ed.). New York: Thomson Delmar Learning.

Water moves across a semipermeable membrane by the process of **osmosis.** In osmosis, to equalize the concentration in both areas, water moves from an area of low concentration of solutes (low osmolality) to an area of high concentration of solutes (high osmolality). Figure 12-1 demonstrates the principle of osmosis. Although fluids continually move back and forth between the intracellular and extracellular compartments, net shifts in fluid occur only when there is an imbalance in osmolality between the two compartments. **Diffusion** is the movement of solutes from an area of high concentration of solutes to an area of low concentration of solutes. This force works with osmosis to equalize the concentration of solutes across compartments. Figure 12-2 demonstrates the principle of diffusion.

Together, osmosis and diffusion help regulate the osmolality, or concentration, of body fluids. **Osmotic pressure** is the ability of a solution to draw water across a semipermeable membrane to affect the concentration (Figure 12-3). For example, a concentrated solution has a high osmotic pressure. If a concentrated solution, for example a **hypertonic** IV solution, is placed in the intravascular compartment, it exerts a high osmotic pressure. The high osmotic pressure will draw

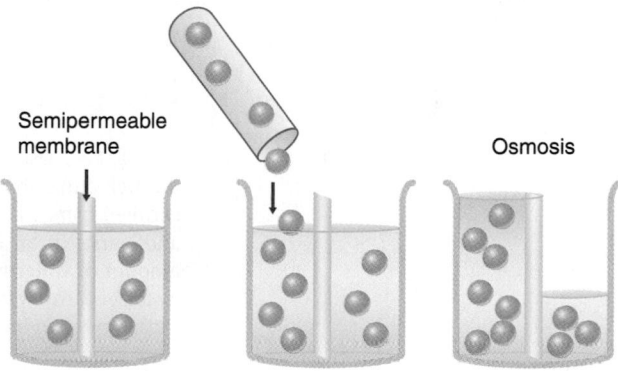

Figure 12-1 Osmosis: Water moves from an area of low concentration of solutes to an area of high concentration of solutes.

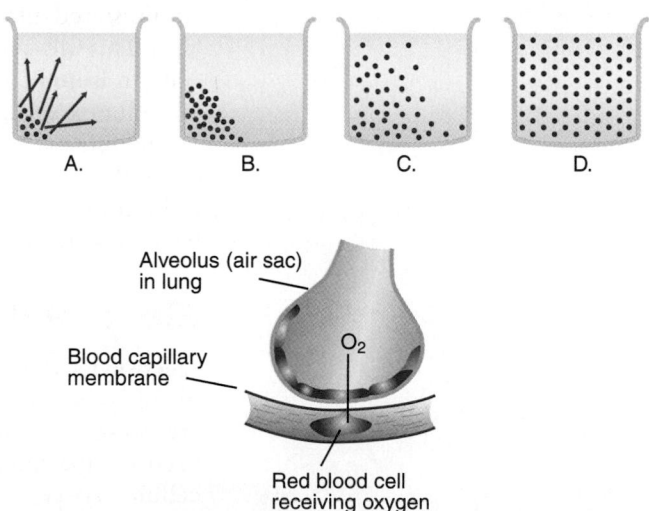

Figure 12-2 The process of diffusion. A. A small lump of sugar is placed in a beaker of water; its molecules dissolve and begin to diffuse outward. B. and C. The sugar molecules continue to diffuse through the water from an area of greater concentration to an area of lesser concentration. D. Over a long period of time, the sugar molecules are evenly distributed throughout the water, reaching a state of equilibrium. Example of diffusion in the human body: Oxygen diffuses from an alveolus in a lung, where it is in greater concentration, across the capillary membrane and into a red blood cell, where it is in lesser concentration.

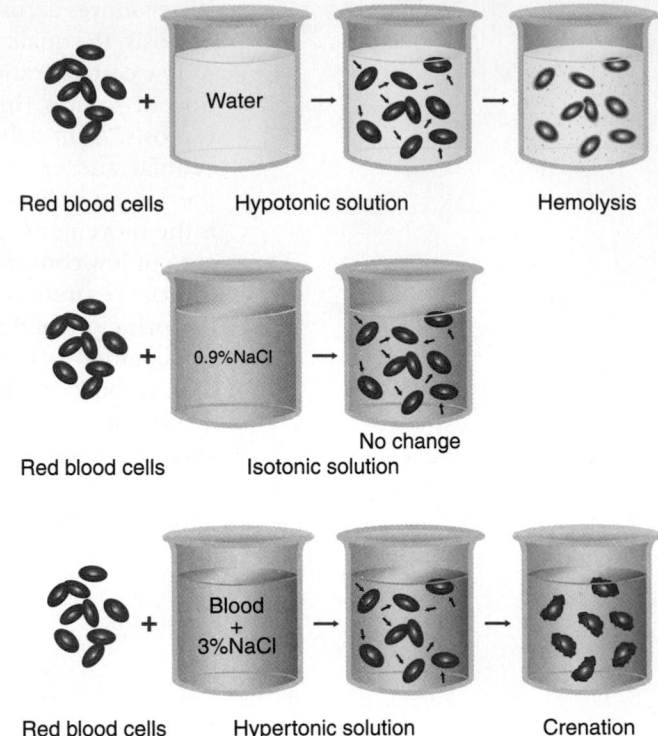

Figure 12-3 Osmosis as it relates to the osmolarity of a solution. The movement of water through a membrane from an area of a lower solute concentration to a higher concentration is called osmosis. In a hypotonic solution, water moves into the cells, causing them to swell and burst. In an isotonic solution, cells are normal in size and shape because the same amount of water is entering and leaving the cells. Cells in the hypertonic solution are losing water because water moves from a weaker concentration inside the cell to a greater concentration outside the cell membrane.

water from inside the cells, across the semipermeable cell wall into the intravascular space to dilute the high concentration of solutes. A **hypotonic** solution administered intravenously will dilute the intravascular space, lowering the osmolality. This will cause water to move across the semipermeable membrane into the cell. An **isotonic** solution is one that has the same osmotic pressure as the referent solution (e.g., plasma).

Oncotic pressure is a special type of osmotic pressure that is due to the presence of proteins. Proteins in the bloodstream exert oncotic pressure to pull fluid out of the interstitial space into the intravascular space to maintain fluid balance and osmolality.

Electrolytes

Electrolytes are charged particles found in body fluids (Table 12-3). A number of electrolytes contribute to the osmolality of body fluids. While the electrolytes are present in both the ICF and the ECF, certain electrolytes predominate in each compartment. The major positively charged ions (**cations**) in the extracellular space are sodium, calcium, and magnesium. The major negatively charged ions (**anions**) in the ECF are chloride and bicarbonate. The major ICF cations are potassium and magnesium (Kee, Paulanka, & Purnel, 2004). Phosphates, sulfates, and proteins are the major ICF anions. When assessing a patient's electrolyte levels, a sample of serum is drawn from a vein. The electrolytes are measured in the ECF of that serum sample. Clinical measures of electrolyte concentrations in ICF are not available. Normal ranges for the major electrolytes are shown in the subsequent sections on each electrolyte.

TABLE 12-3 Common Electrolytes

ELECTROLYTE ION	DISTRIBUTION IN BODY FLUID		BASIC FUNCTIONS	DIETARY SOURCES
	EXTRACELLULAR (MEQ/L)	INTRACELLULAR (MEQ/L)		
Sodium (Na⁺)	135–154	15–20	Regulates fluid volume within extracellular fluid (ECF) compartment. Regulates vascular osmotic pressure. Controls water distribution between ECF and intracellular fluid (ICF) compartments. Participates in conduction of nerve impulses. Maintains neuromuscular excitability.	Table salt (NaCl), 40% of which is sodium; cheese, milk, processed meat, poultry, shellfish, fish, eggs, and foods preserved with salt (e.g., ham and bacon)
Potassium (K⁺)	3.5–5	150–155	Regulates osmolality of ICF. Participates in transmission of nerve impulses. Promotes contraction of skeletal and smooth muscles. Promotes contraction of skeletal and smooth muscles. Promotes enzymatic action for cellular energy production by transforming carbohydrates into energy and restructuring amino acids into proteins. Regulates acid-base balance by cellular exchange of hydrogen ions.	Fruits, especially bananas, oranges, and dried fruits; vegetables, meats, and nuts
Calcium (Ca²⁺)	4.5–5.5	1–2	Provides strength and durability to bones and teeth. Establishes thickness and strength of cell membranes. Promotes transmission of nerve impulses. Maintains neuromuscular excitability. Is essential for blood coagulation. Promotes absorption and use of vitamin B₁₂. Activates enzyme reactions and hormone secretions.	Dairy products (milk, cheese, and yogurt), sardines, whole grains, and green-leafy vegetables
Magnesium (Mg²⁺)	4.5–5.5	27–29	Activates enzyme systems, mainly those associated with vitamin B metabolism and the use of potassium, calcium, and protein. Promotes regulation of serum calcium, phosphorus, and potassium levels. Promotes neuromuscular activity.	Green leafy vegetables, whole grains, fish, and nuts

Because sodium is so abundant in the ECF, it has a large impact on the overall concentration of body fluids. Because body fluids must maintain electrical neutrality, each positively charged ion is matched by a negatively charged ion. Knowing that for each positively charged sodium ion there is a matching anion, the nurse can estimate the osmolality of body fluids by doubling the serum sodium level (accounting for each sodium ion plus each matching negative ion) For example, if the serum sodium level is 140 mEq/L, the serum osmolality will be approximately 280 mOsm/kg. Large quantities of certain large molecules in the bloodstream, for example, glucose and urea nitrogen, make this estimation less accurate.

The sodium level affects and is affected by the overall amount of fluid in the body. Ingestion of increased amounts of sodium in the diet promotes water retention. On the other hand, retention of large quantities of water can dilute the serum sodium and make the value appear lower than normal, even if sodium has not been lost from the body. These processes will be discussed in more detail later in this chapter.

CONTROL OF FLUID AND ELECTROLYTE BALANCE

A number of mechanisms work together to maintain the balance of fluids and electrolytes in the body. The kidneys, the cardiovascular system, the respiratory system, and hormonal mechanisms all play a role in fluid homeostasis.

Kidneys

The kidneys are a major regulator of fluid and electrolyte balance. All the fluid in the body travels through the kidneys by way of the renal arteries many times each day, with approximately 170 L passing through the kidneys daily. Amazingly, despite the large volume that passes through the kidneys each day, only approximately 1.5 L is excreted as urine. Through the nephron functions of glomerular filtration and reabsorption, fluid is retained or excreted based on the body's needs. Impairment of normal nephron functions can rapidly lead to fluid imbalances in the body.

Besides regulating fluid balance, the kidneys also contribute to regulation of electrolyte levels. Selectively secreting or reabsorbing electrolytes achieves body balance. Two important electrolytes regulated by the kidneys are hydrogen and bicarbonate. Regulation of these two ions contributes significantly to the body's overall acid-base balance. Acid-base imbalances are discussed later in this chapter.

The kidneys also affect calcium balance by participating in the final stages of vitamin D activation. Without activation of vitamin D in the kidneys, calcium is poorly absorbed from the GI tract, and low levels of serum calcium may result.

Cardiovascular System

The pumping action of the heart propels blood through the vascular system to the kidneys. The glomerular filtration rate (GFR) is determined in part by the force of the pumping action of the heart. Anything that diminishes cardiac output, for example, heart failure, reduces GFR; if GFR is reduced, less fluid is filtered and urine output decreases. Likewise, if GFR is increased, more fluid is filtered and urine output increases.

Baroreceptors, located primarily in the arch of the aorta, sense the pressure generated in the arteries by the pumping action of the heart (that is, the blood pressure). If the blood pressure is low, the baroreceptors send fewer signals to the control centers in the brain stimulating activation of the sympathetic nervous system (SNS). Activation of the SNS causes vasoconstriction and increased heart rate. Both of these mechanisms serve to increase blood pressure and to improve circulation of the volume of blood currently in the arterioles. High pressure sensed by the baroreceptors typically result in increased firing to the brain control centers with inhibition of the SNS, resulting in vasodilation, decreased heart rate, and decreased blood pressure. However, people with chronically high blood pressure appear to experience a resetting of their baroreceptors, so the baroreceptors are not stimulated at usual blood pressure values.

Cells in the atria of the heart are sensitive to stretching of the atria. Excess fluid volume stretches these cells, causing release of a hormone called atrial natriuretic peptide (ANP). ANP prevents reabsorption of sodium by the renal tubules, resulting in excretion of sodium and water by the kidneys (Candela & Yucha, 2004).

Respiratory System

The lungs participate in the maintenance of fluid balance by excreting moisture during exhalation. Under normal conditions, this contributes about 300 mL per 24 hours to the fluid output of the body. However, in cases of increased respiratory rate, as may occur with fever or respiratory problems, such as pneumonia, the amount of fluid lost during respiration can increase significantly, potentially leading to fluid deficits. The lungs also play a role in acid-base balance by regulating excretion of carbon dioxide (CO_2).

Renin-Angiotensin-Aldosterone System

The renin-angiotensin-aldosterone system (RAAS) is a complex interaction among various substances in the body. In response to inadequate renal perfusion, the kidneys release renin, an inactive substance, into the bloodstream. Angiotensinogen, an inert substance circulating in the blood stream, is acted on by renin to produce angiotensin I. Angiotensin I is also an inactive substance, but is acted un by angiotensin converting enzyme (ACE) to produce the active substance angiotensin II. Angiotensin II is a potent vasoconstrictor that shifts blood to the central circulation to improve blood flow. As part of this system, the hormone aldosterone is released from the adrenal cortex. This mineralocorticoid causes retention of sodium by enhancing reabsorption of sodium in the renal tubules. As a result, water is also retained, resulting in an increased circulating blood volume, as well as an increase in blood pressure (Candela & Yucha, 2004). Figure 12-4 summarizes the RAAS.

Factors that reduce blood pressure stimulate both the SNS response and the RAAS response. Together, those compensatory mechanisms serve to increase blood volume and blood pressure. When excess volume is present, both the SNS and the RAAS are inhibited to reduce blood volume and blood pressure.

Posterior Pituitary Gland

Antidiuretic hormone (ADH), also known as vasopressin, is produced by the posterior pituitary gland. ADH acts on the renal tubules to promote retention of water in the kidneys. Increases in serum osmolality are sensed by osmoreceptors in the posterior pituitary that stimulate the production of more ADH, which causes water retention and dilution of the high level of osmolality. In addition, thirst is stimulated to promote oral intake of fluids to dilute the high osmolality. A 1 to 2 percent increase in osmolality stimulates thirst and release of ADH to retain water (Candela & Yucha, 2004). Likewise, a reduction in serum osmolality causes the posterior pituitary to produce less

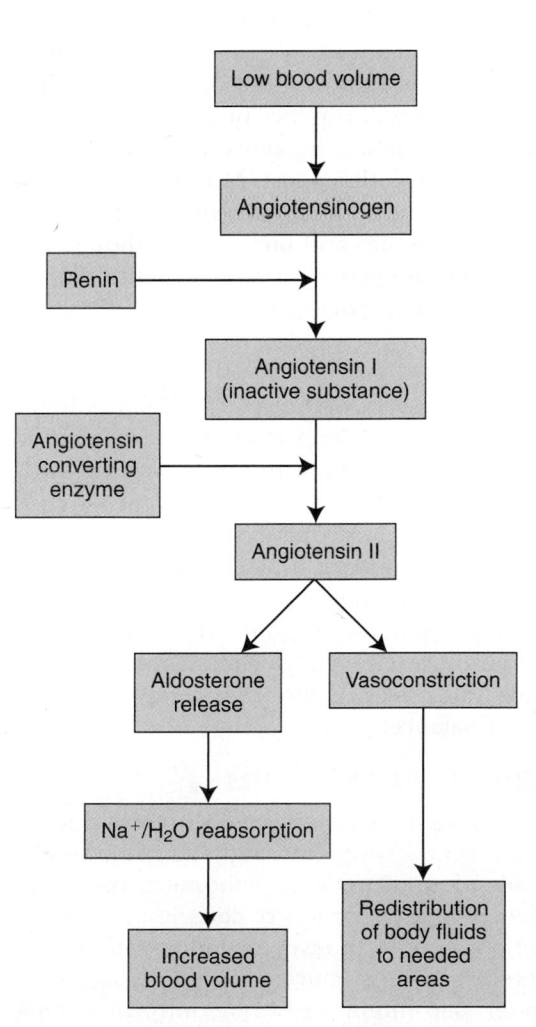

Figure 12-4 Renin-angiotensin-aldosterone system (RAAS).

ADH, which results in excretion of water and an increase in serum osmolality. Although both ADH and the RAAS work together to maintain body volume and concentration, ADH responds primarily to changes in osmolality; whereas the RAAS responds primarily to changes in overall volume of blood in the body, rather than to changes in osmolality of body fluids.

FLUID IMBALANCES

There are primarily two types of fluid imbalances (a) fluid volume deficit and (b) fluid volume excess. Both types of imbalances can be life-threatening and are often seen in acute care settings. Patients with many underlying pathologies develop one of these fluid imbalances and without careful management, serious and critical conditions may develop.

Fluid Volume Deficit (Hypovolemia)

Fluid volume deficit, or hypovolemia, occurs when there is a loss of fluid from the body. The fluids lost may be isotonic, hypotonic, or hypertonic.

Etiology

The best example of a cause of isotonic fluid volume deficit is hemorrhage. Blood (isotonic fluid) is lost from the body, leaving the body with less volume, but without changing the osmolality of the blood. Inability to ingest sufficient fluids, because of nausea or swallowing difficulties, or inability to gain access to fluids, because of physical or mental limitations as occur with immobility or dementia, may result in fluid volume deficit. Loss of fluids through vomiting, diarrhea, use of diuretic medications, diabetes insipidus, or gastric suctioning may cause fluid volume deficit. Whether or not osmolality changes with these causes depends on the concentration of the fluids lost. Movement of fluids from the vascular space to spaces such as the abdominal cavity is called third spacing. Causes of third spacing include ascites and burns. Even though the fluid still remains in the body, the patient is hypovolemic because the fluid in the third space is not available to the vascular space (Estes, 2006).

Pathophysiology

Loss of isotonic fluids results in a decrease in overall extracellular volume. Both the intravascular and the interstitial fluid compartments are reduced. If there is no change in osmolality, fluid does not shift into or out of the intracellular compartment. A change in serum osmolality results in hypernatremia or hyponatremia, discussed later in the chapter. Reduction in overall fluid volume stimulates the baroreceptors and results in activation of both the SNS and the RAAS. Sodium is reabsorbed from renal tubules, resulting in retention of both sodium and water. Vasoconstriction and increased heart rate attempt to circulate the reduced blood volume more efficiently. While these compensatory mechanisms help, significant fluid losses require replacement of fluids intravenously to restore normal fluid balance.

Assessment with Clinical Manifestations

Slow fluid loss may result in few or no signs and symptoms. More rapid losses cause earlier and more dramatic signs and symptoms. Signs of intravascular fluid loss include reduction of blood pressure and orthostatic (postural) hypotension. Patients may experience dizziness or loss of consciousness when changing from a lying to standing position. With less circulating volume, the kidneys receive less perfusion, therefore urine output may be decreased. Signs of interstitial fluid loss include poor skin turgor and dry mouth. In infants, fontanelles may be depressed. Parents may report a reduction in the number of wet diapers or lack of tears when the infant cries. Loss of fluid results in a loss of weight. One liter of fluid weighs 1 kilogram. Weight loss of more than 0.5 kg per 24 hours generally is the result of fluid loss, not loss of body mass. As a result of the compensatory mechanisms associated with fluid loss, patients also display an increase in heart rate and pale, clammy skin.

The nurse assesses each patient to evaluate the risk for fluid volume deficit (Box 12-1). Patients with nausea, vomiting, diarrhea, hemorrhage, or GI suction are all at risk for volume deficits. Infants, immobilized patients, and confused elderly are at risk for insufficient fluid intake. Identifying patients at risk allows for interventions that may prevent fluid deficits.

Assessment of the patient with actual fluid volume deficit focuses on vital signs. A low blood pressure in conjunction with an elevated heart rate may signal a fluid deficit. Repeated readings over time are most helpful in determining changes in fluid volume. Especially useful in assessing fluid status is measurement of postural vital signs. The nurse should assess postural vital signs in any patient with a history of fluid losses or in any patient who is dizzy or light-headed when sitting or standing. A decrease in systolic blood pressure of more than 20 mm Hg when going from lying to standing, along with an increase in heart rate of 10 beats per minute, or a decrease in diastolic blood pressure of more than 10 mm Hg along with a 10 beat per minute increase in heart rate is considered postural hypotension. Aside from medications that may cause postural hypotension, fluid volume deficit is the most common cause (Bradley & Davis, 2003). Assessment of skin turgor may be helpful in monitoring fluid status, however, elderly patients typically have poor skin turgor regardless of fluid status, so this sign is less helpful in that population. In infants, assessing fontanelles and questioning parents about the number of diaper changes and whether the infant produces tears when crying can help determine fluid status. In children, prolonged capillary refill time, poor skin turgor, and abnormal respiratory patterns have been found to be accurate indicators of fluid volume deficit. However, the presence or absence of any one sign or symptom of volume deficit is less useful than the presence of several signs and symptoms simultaneously (Steiner, DeWalt, & Byerley, 2004).

Potential Complications

Mild fluid losses may be reversed by the body's compensatory mechanisms. More severe losses, if not corrected, will result in significant reduction in blood pressure, lack of perfusion to vital organs, hypovolemic shock, and ultimately, death. Undetected fluid losses may be a cause of falls as patients experience dizziness, with resultant injuries such as fractures or head injuries.

Diagnostic Tests

No single laboratory test signifies fluid volume deficit. Helpful lab tests vary with the cause of the deficit. If hemorrhage is the cause, hemoglobin and hematocrit levels may be decreased. Other types of fluid losses may result in hemoconcentration, that is, an increased proportion of red blood cells because of a reduction of blood plasma. Hemoconcentration will be reflected in an increased hematocrit value. Depending on the concentration of the fluids lost, the sodium level may be increased, normal, or decreased. Sodium concentration is discussed later in the chapter.

Blood urea nitrogen (BUN) and creatinine are waste products excreted by the kidneys that exist normally in a 10:1 ratio. Loss of renal function results in a proportionate increase in both values. A BUN/creatinine ratio of greater than 10:1 generally indicates fluid volume deficit.

Nursing Diagnoses

Based on the information gathered, the primary example of nursing diagnosis in the patient with decreased fluid volume includes the following:

- Deficient fluid volume.

BOX 12-1

FLUID VOLUME DEFICIT

Intravascular Deficit
- Hypotension
- Tachycardia
- Postural hypotension
- Decreased urine output

Interstitial Deficit
- Dry mucous membranes
- Depressed fontanelles
- Decreased skin turgor

General
- Weight Loss

Source: Estes, M. (2006). Health assessment and physical examination *(3rd ed.). New York: Thomson Delmar Learning.*

Planning and Implementation

NIC interventions for deficient fluid volume include:

- Fluid management.
- Fluid monitoring.
- Hypovolemia management.
- IV therapy.
- Shock management: Volume.

Patients unable to access fluids independently warrant special attention from the nurse. Fluids should be offered regularly to those patients unable to ask for or obtain fluids on their own. This is especially true in warm environments where fluid losses are accentuated.

Sources of fluid loss are identified and stopped, if possible. Mild to moderate fluid losses may be replaced through administration of oral fluid supplements (Spandorfer, Alessandrini, Joffe, Localio, & Shaw, 2005). Replacement of significant fluid losses is accomplished by administration of IV fluids. Loss of ECF is replaced with isotonic solutions. Table 12-4 identifies characteristics of common IV solutions. Major fluid losses due to hemorrhage are replaced with blood transfusions.

Evaluation of Outcomes

NOC outcomes include fluid balance, hydration, and nutritional status: food and fluid intake. Evidence of adequate fluid volume includes return of blood pressure and heart rate to the patient's baseline levels and absence of postural hypotension. Urine output greater than 30 mL/hr signals sufficient body fluid to perfuse the kidneys. Return of skin turgor, moist mucous membranes, and absence of depressed fontanelles indicate normal volume status.

Fluid Volume Excess (Hypervolemia)

Fluid volume excess, or hypervolemia, occurs when fluids are retained or administered. An illustrative cause of fluid volume excess is administration of excessive amounts of an isotonic IV fluid, such as normal saline. This overfills the ECF compartment, both intravascular and interstitial. If no change in serum osmolality occurs, intracellular compartment is not affected.

Etiology

Additional causes of hypervolemia include renal failure, heart failure, and liver failure. Excess secretion of aldosterone, which occurs in primary aldosteronism, causes retention of sodium and water. If the fluids retained in these conditions

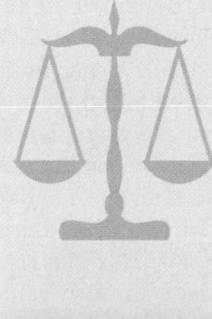

ETHICS IN PRACTICE

Fluids for Terminal Patients

When a patient refuses to take fluids, the health care provider must respect their wishes (making the assumption that the patient has an understanding of the reasons for needing the fluid intake). For example, a terminal patient with cancer may not desire to prolong their life and consequently may choose to not have forced fluids. The nurse must acknowledge the patient's right to refusal in this instance.

Source: Hospice Foundation of America. (2003). Retrieved June 24, 2006, from http://www.hospicefoundation.org.

TABLE 12-4 Common IV Solutions

TONICITY	SOLUTION	CONTENTS (MEQ/L)	CLINICAL IMPLICATIONS
Hypotonic	Sodium chloride 0.45%	77 Na$^+$, 77 Cl$^-$	Daily maintenance of body fluid and establishment of renal function
Isotonic	Dextrose 2.5% in 0.45% saline	77 Na$^+$, 77 Cl$^-$	Promotes renal function and urine output
	Dextrose 5% in 0.2% saline	38 Na$^+$, 38 Cl$^-$	Daily maintenance of body fluids when less Na$^+$ and Cl$^-$ are required
	Dextrose 5% in water (D$_5$W)		Promotes rehydration and elimination; may cause urinary Na$^+$ loss; good vehicle for K$^+$
	Ringer's lactate	130 Na$^+$, 4 K$^+$, Ca^{2+}, 109 Cl$^-$, 28 lactate	Resembles the normal composition of blood serum and plasma; K$^+$ level below body's daily requirement
	Normal saline (NS), 0.9%	154 Na$^+$, 154 Cl$^-$	Restores sodium chloride deficit and extracellular fluid volume
	Dextran 40 10% in NS (0.9%) or D$_5$W		A colloidal solution used to increase plasma volume of patients in early shock. *It should not be given* to severely dehydrated patients and patients with renal disease, thrombocytopenia, or active hemorrhaging.
	Dextran 70% in NS		A long-lived (20 hours) plasma volume expander. Used to treat shock or impending shock due to hemorrhage, surgery, or burns. *It can prolong bleeding and coats the RBCs (draw type and cross-match prior to administering).*
Hypertonic	Dextrose 5% in 0.45% saline	77 Na$^+$, 77 Cl$^-$	Daily maintenance of body fluid and nutrition; treatment of FVD
	Dextrose 5% in saline 0.9%	154 Na$^+$, 154 Cl$^-$	Fluid replacement of sodium, chloride, and calories (170)
	Dextrose 10% in saline 0.9%	154 Na$^+$, 154 Cl$^-$	Fluid replacement of sodium, chloride, and calories (340)
	Dextrose 5% in lactated Ringer's	130 Na$^+$, 4 K$^+$, 3 Ca^{2+}, 109 Cl$^-$, 28 lactate	Resembles the normal composition of blood serum and plasma; K$^+$ level below body's daily requirement; caloric value 180
	Hyperosmolar saline 3% and 5% NaCl	856 Na$^+$, 865 Cl$^-$	Treatment of hyponatremia; raises the Na$^+$ osmolarity of the blood, and reduces intracellular fluid excess
	Ionosol B with dextrose 5%	57 Na$^+$, 25 K$^+$, 49 Cl$^-$, 25 lactate, 5 Mg^{2+}, 7 PO$_4^-$	Treatment of polyionic parenteral replacement caused by vomiting-induced alkalosis, diabetic acidosis, fluid loss from burns, and postoperative FVD
	Ionosol D-CM with dextrose 5%	138 Na$^+$, 12 K$^+$, 5 Ca^{2+}, 108 Cl$^-$, 50 lactate, 3 Mg^{2+}	Treatment of electrolyte losses of duodenal fluids caused by intestinal suction or biliary or pancreatic drainage; treatment of mild acidosis.
	Aminosyn RF 5.2%	5.4 K$^+$	Restores fluid and protein and promotes wound healing.
	Aminosyn II 3.5%	18 Na$^+$	Treatment of malnourished older patients and hypoproteinemia; *it is not to be given to patients with severe liver damage.*

are in the same concentration as blood, the fluid gains are isotonic. If the fluids retained are in a concentration different from blood, changes in osmolality may occur. Syndrome of inappropriate antidiuretic hormone (SIADH) is an excess of ADH. This results in retention of water, which dilutes the bloodstream, and makes it more hypotonic (less concentrated than blood).

Pathophysiology

In fluid volume excess, the extracellular compartment is expanded. This increase in volume increases the pressure in the vasculature. Baroreceptors sense the increase in pressure and increase their firing to the central nervous system (CNS). In response, the SNS is inhibited, and RAAS functions declines. The resulting vasodilation promotes pooling of blood and lowering of blood pressure. Reabsorption of sodium in the renal tubules is reduced, and more urine is excreted.

Assessment with Clinical Manifestations

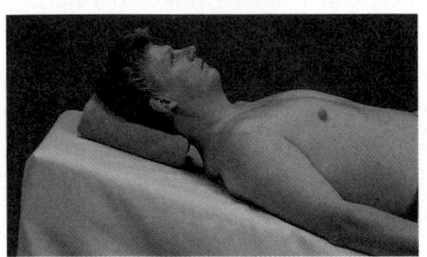

Figure 12-5 Positioning the patient to assess jugular vein distension.

Excess fluid in the intravascular space causes an elevation in blood pressure. The pulse may be bounding. Increased jugular venous pressure may be visible in distended neck veins (Figure 12-5). Increased volume circulating through the kidneys may result in increased urine output. Excess fluid in the interstitial space may produce edema, bulging fontanelles in infants, and pulmonary congestion as evidenced by dyspnea and crackles on auscultation.

Patients at risk for fluid volume excess need careful assessment for early signs of fluid accumulation. Blood pressure and pulse assessment should be done periodically with emphasis on evaluation of trends, looking for elevations in both.

Accumulation of fluid in the interstitial space will lead to edema. Edema generally accumulates in dependent tissues. Ambulatory patients will experience edema in their hands and feet. Asking patients about tightness of rings and shoes may reveal edema even if the patient is unaware of swelling. Patients in wheelchairs will accumulate fluid in the buttocks, and bedridden patients will demonstrate edema in the tissues of the back and sacrum. Pitting edema is measured by pressing the thumb or finger gently but firmly into the swollen tissues. Assessment of the depth of the indentation determines the degree of edema. This is a relatively subjective measurement. Accurate measurement of edema is accomplished by using a tape measure to assess the size of the extremity.

Accumulation of fluid in the vascular space can lead to distension of the jugular veins. When lying flat, the neck veins are normally visible. As the head of the bed is elevated, the fluid drains from the neck veins because of gravity, until, at 90° of elevation, the neck veins are flat. With fluid volume excess, the neck veins remain distended with the head of the bed at 90°.

Accumulation of fluid in the pulmonary vasculature increases hydrostatic pressure within the blood vessels, forcing fluid into the interstitial spaces in the lungs and into the alveoli. This may result in a moist cough and auscultation of the lungs may reveal crackles. Impairment of gas exchange causes hypoxia with dyspnea and rapid respiratory rate.

Potential Complications

Excess fluid volume may overload the heart leading to heart failure. With or without heart failure, fluid excess may cause pulmonary congestion leading to significant hypoxia.

Diagnostic Tests

As with fluid volume deficit, no single test identifies fluid volume excess. Excess volume in the vascular space may cause hemodilution with a lowering of hematocrit. Presence of pulmonary congestion may be seen on a chest radiograph as congestion of the pulmonary vasculature or pleural effusion. Fluid in the alveoli impairs gas exchange resulting in hypoxia as evidenced by a low PO_2 in arterial blood gases (ABGs). Chronic fluid overload that strains the heart may cause cardiomegaly that is visible on the chest radiograph.

Nursing Diagnoses

Based on the information gathered, the primary example of nursing diagnosis in the patient with decreased fluid volume includes the following:

- Excess fluid volume.

Planning and Implementation

NIC interventions for patients with excess fluid volume include:

- Fluid monitoring.
- Fluid management.

Attention to the underlying cause of the fluid excess is essential. Patients with renal failure or heart failure must be treated for those conditions. In patients with renal failure, hemodialysis or peritoneal dialysis removes excess fluid. Patients with heart failure are treated with diuretics and medications that improve heart function, which helps reduce fluid retention. Patients with excess fluid volume because of excess IV fluid administration need to have their IV fluids slowed or stopped. Daily measurement of weight and regular assessment of neck veins allows for an assessment of the amount of fluid retention.

Evaluation of Outcomes

NOC outcomes for patients with excess fluid volume include electrolyte and acid-base balance, fluid balance, and hydration. Evidence of normal fluid balance includes reduction in or absence of edema, flat neck veins with the head of the bed elevated to 45°, and clear breath sounds without crackles. Absence of cough and dyspnea and adequate oxygen saturation as measured by pulse oximetry indicate sufficient gas exchange.

ELECTROLYTE IMBALANCES

In addition to maintaining adequate fluid balance, it is essential for the body to manage electrolytes to maintain homeostasis. When any of the electrolytes are out of balance there are a wide variety of clinical manifestations that accompany those imbalances, and many of these imbalances may lead to critical conditions (Table 12-5) (Kraft, Btaiche, Sacks, & Kudsk, 2005). Balance of six major electrolytes will be discussed: sodium, potassium, calcium, magnesium, and phosphorus. Recommended dietary intake for each electrolyte is presented in Table 12-6.

Deficient Sodium Ion (Hyponatremia)

Sodium is the most abundant extracellular cation. As such, it is a major determiner of the concentration of body fluids (osmolality) (Candela & Yucha, 2004). The normal sodium level in the body ranges from 136 to 145 mEq/L. A low sodium level may be due to loss of sodium ions, or more commonly, from an excess of body water that dilutes the sodium in the bloodstream. The most common electrolyte abnormality in hospitalized patients is hyponatremia.

Etiology

Extremely low sodium diets may result in deficient sodium levels. Loss of sodium ions may occur with administration of diuretic medications that inhibit sodium reabsorption in the renal tubules. Dilutional hyponatremia occurs with retention of water as occurs with SIADH. Excessive ADH secretion causes retention of water in the renal tubules with dilution of the serum sodium level. Elective surgery is the most common cause of excess ADH that may result in

TABLE 12-5 **The Clinical Management of Patients Experiencing Common Electrolyte Disturbances**

DISTURBANCE/CAUSES	CLINICAL MANIFESTATIONS	NURSING INTERVENTIONS
Hyponatremia		
Operational definition:	Cognitive and consciousness	
• Serum NA < 135 mEq/L	• Headaches	
• Serum osmolality < 280 mOsm/kg	• Apprehension	Monitor level of consciousness.
	• Lethargy	Institute safety measures for seizures.
	• Confusion	
Nutrition and metabolism	• Depression	
• Low sodium intake	• Convulsion	
• High water intake		
• Anorexia nervosa		
• Loss of GI secretions (vomiting, diarrhea, bulimia, suctioning or drainage, tap-water enemas)	Activity/mobility • Muscular weakness	
• Loss of ECF sodium (peritonitis, burns)	Skin and mucous membranes	Administer IV isotonic solution (e.g., 0.9% NaCl) per order.
• Excessive ingestion of water or administration of IV solutions (D_5W)	• Dry, pale skin • Dry mucous membranes	Restrict free water intake (e.g., 1.2 L/24 hr).
• ECF sodium dilution (congestive heart failure [CHF], cirrhosis, nephrosis)	Oxygenation and ECG • Tachycardia	Monitor hourly vital signs and I&O (ECF excess, restrict fluids and administer diuretics).
Elimination	• Hypotension/hypertension	
• Advanced renal disorders		
• Diuretics	Nutrition and metabolism	Monitor daily intake of sodium and watch for water intoxication with SIADH (headaches and behavioral changes).
• Syndrome of inappropriate antidiuretic hormone (SIADH)	• Nausea • Vomiting • Diarrhea	
	• Abdominal cramps	Monitor serum sodium levels. Teach patient about adequate intake of sodium, side effects of diuretics, and other causes for hyponatremia.
Hypernatremia		
Operational definition	Cognitive and sensory	Monitor level of consciousness.
• Serum Na > 145 mEq/L	• Restlessness	
• Serum osmolality > 295 mOsm/kg	• Agitation	Institute safety measures for seizures.
• Urine Na < 40 mEq/L	• Delirium	
	• Twitching	
Nutrition and metabolism	• Convulsions	
• High sodium intake	• Coma	
• Low water intake		
• Severe GI loss (diarrhea and vomiting)	Activity/mobility	Maintain body alignment and assist with movement.
• Excessive insensible loss (perspiration)	• ↑ Muscle tone	
• Salt water drowning	• Hyperreflexia	

Continued

TABLE 12-5 **The Clinical Management of Patients Experiencing Common Electrolyte Disturbances—cont'd**

DISTURBANCE/CAUSES	CLINICAL MANIFESTATIONS	NURSING INTERVENTIONS
Hypernatremia—cont'd		
• Administration of IV solutions (hypertonic or isotonic saline, sodium bicarbonate) • Hypertonic saline abortions • Bladder irrigation	Skin and mucous membranes • Flushed, dry skin • Red, dry tongue • Sticky mucous membranes	Administer oral hygiene hourly.
Elimination • Renal dysfunction • Peritoneal dialysis with glucose solution • Uncompensated diabetes insipidus	Oxygenation and ECG • Tachycardia Nutrition and metabolism • Nausea • Vomiting • Anorexia	Monitor vital signs. Administer oral fluids or a parenteral hypotonic solution (e.g., 0.3% NaCl or D_5W) as ordered.
Hemostatic dysfunction • CHF ($\downarrow$ cardiac output, $\downarrow$ renal flow, $\uparrow$ sodium retention) • Nephrotic syndrome and cirrhosis ($\uparrow$ aldosterone leading to $\uparrow$ sodium retention)	Elimination • Polyuria (nephritis and uncompensated diabetes insipidus)	Monitor I&O. Monitor daily weights. Monitor laboratory findings. Teach patient about foods high in sodium and about sodium-retaining drugs (cough medicines, cortisone, and laxatives with sodium).
Hypokalemia		
Operational definition: • Serum K < 3.5 mEq/L	Nutrition and metabolism • $\downarrow$ Motility (hypoactive $\rightarrow$ absent bowel sounds)	Administer potassium replacement therapy as ordered:
Nutrition and metabolism • Malnutrition • Starvation • Crash diets • Alcoholism • Anorexia nervosa • Stress • Licorice abuse • GI loss (vomiting, diarrhea, gastric or intestinal suctioning, intestinal fistula) • NPO and potassium-free IV fluids • Diabetic ketoacidosis • Hyperaldosteronism • Adrenal tumor, cirrhosis, CHF	• Abdominal distension • Paralytic ileus • Nausea • Vomiting Cognitive and sensory • Malaise • Disorientation • Coma • Loss of tactile discrimination Activity/mobility • Muscle weakness • Hyporeflexia	• Oral potassium should be diluted in 4-8 oz of water or juice ($\downarrow$ gastric mucosa irritation). • Dilute IV potassium 20-40 mEq in 1 L of IV fluids (irritating to blood vessels and myocardium). • Never administer bolus IV potassium. Monitor IV site for phlebitis and infiltration. Protect from injury.

Continued

TABLE 12-5 The Clinical Management of Patients Experiencing Common Electrolyte Disturbances—cont'd

DISTURBANCE/CAUSES	CLINICAL MANIFESTATIONS	NURSING INTERVENTIONS
Hypokalemia—cont'd		
Elimination	Elimination	Monitor I&O hourly.
• Laxative abuse	• Constipation	
• Bulimia	• Polyuria	
• Enemas		
• Potassium-depleting diuretics (thiazide and furosemide)	Oxygenation and ECG	Monitor vital signs.
• Diuretic phase of acute renal failure	• Shallow, rapid, ineffective respirations	Monitor heart rate and rhythm.
• Dialysis	• Tachycardia	Monitor patient closely for signs of digitalis toxicity (premature atrial and ventricular beats).
• Steroids	• ↑ Sensitivity to digitalis	
• Cushing's syndrome	• ST depression	
	• T wave inverted	
Skin and cellular integrity	• U wave prominent	Teach patient about potassium-rich foods and how to prevent excessive loss (abuse of laxatives and diuretics).
• Trauma	• Heart block	
• Tissue injury	• Cardiac arrest (severe hypokalemia)	
• Surgery		
Redistribution of potassium		
• Insulin		
• Alkalotic state		
• Healing phase of burns		
Hyperkalemia		
Operational definition:	Nutrition and metabolism	Restrict oral and parenteral potassium intake as ordered.
• Serum K > 5.3 mEq/L	• Abdominal cramps (intermittent GI pain)	
	• Nausea	Administer cation-exchange resins (Kayexalate) to reduce serum potassium. Administer glucose and insulin parenteral solutions to facilitate movement of potassium into the cells as ordered.
Nutrition and metabolism	• Diarrhea	
• Oral potassium supplement	Activity/mobility	
• IV potassium supplement	• Muscular weakness	
Elimination	• Paresthesia	Assess for pain and provide comfort measures as indicated.
• Acute and chronic renal failure	• Muscle cramps and pain	
• Potassium-sparing diuretics		
• Addison's disease		
	Elimination	Monitor I&O.
Skin and cellular integrity	• Oliguria or anuria	
• Massive trauma and crushing injuries		Monitor patient closely if receiving diuretics.
• Hemolysis	Oxygenation and ECG	
• Tourniquet application	• Bradycardia → arrest	
• Phlebotomy	• T wave tented	Monitor vital signs and heart rhythm hourly for ECG changes.
• Burns	• P wave small → nonvisible	
	• QRS complex widened	

Continued

TABLE 12-5 **The Clinical Management of Patients Experiencing Common Electrolyte Disturbances—cont'd**

DISTURBANCE/CAUSES	CLINICAL MANIFESTATIONS	NURSING INTERVENTIONS
Hyperkalemia—cont'd		
	• Life-threatening dysrhythmias (supraventricular and/or ventricular tachycardia, premature ventricular beats, and ventricular fibrillation → arrest)	Institute safety measures when drawing blood: • Leave tourniquet on for 1 to 2 minutes. • Draw blood from vein away from all infusions. If the patient is to receive whole blood, indicate on the blood bank requisition the potassium level (blood 10 days or older has an elevated serum potassium due to hemolysis of aging blood). Teach patient about potassium-rich foods, potassium-containing salt substitutes, and potassium-conserving diuretics.
Hypocalcemia		
Operational definition: • Serum Ca < 4.5 mEq/L (total) • Elevated serum phosphorus • Prolonged prothrombin time	Cognitive and sensory • Anxiety, irritability • Tingling and numbness of fingers • Tetany • Convulsions	Monitor level of consciousness and breathing for laryngeal stridor.
Nutrition and metabolism • Inadequate dietary intake of calcium-rich foods (e.g., during pregnancy and lactation, when calcium requirements are high)	Activity/mobility • Abdominal and muscle cramps • Positive Trousseau's sign—carpopedal spasm	Administer 10% IV solution of calcium gluconate; observe IV solutions with calcium for infiltration.
• Poor vitamin D intake and absorption • Associated disorders: Hypoparathyroidism, pancreatitis, acute metabolic acidosis, and accidental surgical removal of parathyroid glands during a thyroidectomy	• Positive Chvostek's sign—contraction of facial muscles when facial nerve is tapped • Patholigic fractures	Teach a diet high in calcium with vitamin D supplement. Administer calcium carbonate orally.
Elimination • Diarrhea • Wound drainage • Steroid therapy	Oxygenation and ECG • ↓ Stroke volume • ECG changes: • ST segment lengthened and prolonged PR interval	Monitor ECG for changes.
Hypercalcemia		
Operational definition: • Serum Ca > 5.5 mEq/L (total)	Cognitive and sensory • Depression and lethargy	Monitor level of consciousness for safety.

Continued

TABLE 12-5 **The Clinical Management of Patients Experiencing Common Electrolyte Disturbances—cont'd**

DISTURBANCE/CAUSES	CLINICAL MANIFESTATIONS	NURSING INTERVENTIONS
Hypercalcemia—cont'd		
Activity/mobility	Activity/mobility	Encourage patient movement and exercise.
• Excessive movement of calcium out of bones: multiple fractures, bone tumors, immobility	• ↓ Muscle tone and deep tendon reflexes	Assist patient with movement to ↓ pain.
	• Osteoporosis	
	• Osteomalacia	
	• Pathologic fractures	
	• Deep bone pain	
Nutrition and metabolism	Oxygenation and ECG	Monitor for ECG changes.
• Overconsumption of milk or dietary salts	• Heart block	
• Overactivity of parathyroid glands	• Arrest (hypercalcemia crisis)	
Elimination	Nutrition and metabolism	Teach patient to ↓ calcium intake and ↑ fiber.
• Renal impairment	• Nausea, vomiting, anorexia	
• Thiazide diuretics	• Constipation	Encourage oral intake of acid-ash fluids to ↓ deposit of calcium salts.
• Steroid therapy		
	Elimination	Monitor for symptoms of digitalis toxicity; calcium enhances the action of digitalis.
	• Flank pain from calculi	
	• Polyuria	
Hypomagnesemia		
Operational definition:	Cognitive and sensory	Monitor the patient for seizure activity and laryngeal stridor.
• Serum Mg < 1.5 mEq/L	• Disorientation, confusion	
	• Vertigo	
Nutrition and metabolism	• Irritability, tremors	Administer magnesium sulphate.
• Prolonged inadequate dietary intake of magnesium (e.g., malnutrition and alcoholism)	Activity/mobility	
• Excessive losses of magnesium (e.g., vomiting, gastric suction)	• ↑ Tendon reflexes	
	• Positive Chvostek's & Trousseau's signs	
• Prolonged administration of IV solutions without magnesium additives	Oxygenation and ECG	Monitor for ECG changes and assess the patient for digitalis toxicity.
	• ↑ BP	
Elimination	• Tachycardia	
• Severe renal disease	• Dysrhythmias	Teach patient to eat magnesium-rich foods and to avoid excessive use of laxatives and diuretics.
• Thiazide diuretics	• T wave flat or inverted	
• Aldosterone excess	• ST segment depressed	
• Polyuria		
Hypermagnesemia		
Operational definition:	Cognitive and sensory	Monitor level of consciousness.
• Serum Mg > 2.5 mEq/L	• Lethargy, drowsiness	
	• Coma	

Continued

TABLE 12-5 The Clinical Management of Patients Experiencing Common Electrolyte Disturbances—cont'd

DISTURBANCE/CAUSES	CLINICAL MANIFESTATIONS	NURSING INTERVENTIONS
Hypermagnesemia—cont'd		
Nutrition and metabolism		
• Excessive treatment of magnesium deficit	Activity/mobility	Assess patellar reflexes; if absent notify practitioner.
Elimination	• Muscle weakness, paralysis	
• Renal failure	• ↓ Deep-tendon reflexes	
	Oxygenation and ECG	Monitor vital signs q15-30 minutes until stable and for ECG changes.
	• ↓ respirations, 10 to 12 per minute	
	• ↓ BP	
	• Bradycardia	Encourage fluids unless contraindicated to dilute the serum level of magnesium.
	• AV block	
	• Respiratory and cardiac arrest (severe hypermagnesemia)	Teach patient about over-the-counter drugs with magnesium content.
	• QRS complex widening	
	• QT interval prolonged	
Hypophosphatemia		
Operational definition:	Cognitive and sensory	Monitor patient's level of consciousness. Institute safety measures for seizures.
• Serum phosphate < 1.7 mEq/L	• Confusion, seizures, coma	
• Reduced WBC; platelets	• Fatigue, memory loss	
• Elevated cardiac isoenzymes	Activity/mobility	Administer pain medications and other comfort measures.
Nutrition and metabolism	• Muscle pain, weakness	
• Inadequate intake: malnutrition, chronic alcoholism	• Paresthesia	Assist the patient in maintaining proper body alignment.
• Prolonged administration of IV solutions that are phosphorus-poor or phosphorus-free	• Hyporeflexia	
	• Bone pain	
	• Joint stiffness	
• Acid-base imbalances (e.g., diabetic ketoacidosis and respiratory alkalosis)	Oxygenation and ECG	Monitor for bleeding and respiratory failure.
	• Tissue hypoxia	
• Increased secretion of parathyroid hormone	• Hyperventilation	
	• Possible bleeding	
• Overuse of aluminum-containing antacids	• Weak pulse	
	Safety	Institute precautions to prevent infection.
	• Possible infection	
	Nutrition and metabolism	Teach patient about phosphorus-rich foods and over-the-counter drugs that contain aluminum hydroxide.
	• Anorexia	
	• Dysphagia	Administer IV phosphate with caution: dilute and infuse slowly to avoid phlebitis; infiltration at the IV site may cause tissue sloughing; do not infuse with calcium.

Continued

TABLE 12-5 The Clinical Management of Patients Experiencing Common Electrolyte Disturbances—cont'd

DISTURBANCE/CAUSES	CLINICAL MANIFESTATIONS	NURSING INTERVENTIONS
Hyperphosphatemia		
Operational definition:	Activity/mobility	Monitor for tetany and other signs of hypocalcemia.
• Serum phosphate > 2.6 mEq/L	• Tetany	
• Reduced serum calcium	• Muscle weakness	
	• Flaccid paralysis	
Nutrition and metabolism	• Circumoral paraesthesia	
• Excessive administration of oral and IV solutions containing phosphate substances	• Hyperreflexia	
	Oxygenation and ECG	Monitor heart rate and assess for ECG changes.
• Hypoparathyroidism	• Tachycardia	
• Laxatives containing phosphate	• ST segment shortened	
	• QT interval shortened	
Elimination		
• Renal insufficiency	Nutrition and metabolism	Administer calcium replacement.
	• Nausea, anorexia, vomiting, diarrhea	Monitor urinary output; < 25 mL/hour will increase serum phosphorus level.
		Teach patient to avoid foods high in phosphorus (to read the labels on canned foods) and excessive use of phosphorus-containing laxatives and enemas.

TABLE 12-6 Recommended Dietary Intakes for Elements

AGE-GROUP	CALCIUM (MG/DAY)	MAGNESIUM (MG/DAY)	PHOSPHORUS (MG/DAY)	POTASSIUM (G/DAY)	SODIUM (G/DAY)	CHLORIDE (G/DAY)
0–12 months	210–270*	30–75*	100–275*	0.4–0.7*	0.12–0.37*	0.18–0.57*
1–8 years	500–800*	80–130**	460–500**	3.0–3.8*	1.0–1.2*	1.5–1.9*
9–70 years+	1,000–1,300*	240–420**	700–1,250**	4.5–4.7*	1.3–1.5*	2.0–2.3*
Older than 70 years	1,200*	320–420**	700**	4.7*	1.2*	1.8*

Adequate intake
**Recommended daily allowance*
+*Varies in males and females*
Adapted from Food and Nutrition Board, National Academy of Sciences. (2004). Dietary reference intakes table. *Retrieved June 24, 2006, from http://www.iom.edu.*

hyponatremia (Kee, et al., 2004). Pain and nausea associated with surgery increase ADH secretion, as do narcotic and anesthetic medications used during and after surgery. SIADH occurs with head injuries and in response to some medications; both physiological and psychological stress may produce SIADH; and some types of lung conditions, including tumors and tuberculosis, may produce secretion of a substance that mimics the action of ADH. An iatrogenic cause of hyponatremia is excessive administration of hypotonic IV fluids. All patients receiving hypotonic IV solutions should be monitored for developing hyponatremia, particularly elderly patients. Installation of excessive amounts of water into the body, as may occur for example through nasogastric tubes or tap water enemas, may dilute the serum and result in hyponatremia. Diuretic use may cause hyponatremia as both water and sodium are excreted. Thiazide diuretics are particularly associated with hyponatremia (Kee, et al., 2004).

Pathophysiology

Hyponatremia results in a lowering of serum osmolality. When the ECF compartment has a low osmolality compared to the intracellular space, fluid moves from the extracellular space to the intracellular space through osmosis to equalize the osmolality in the two compartments. When fluid moves into the intracellular space, the cells swell and eventually burst. Although this happens throughout the cells in the body, the most serious location for this swelling is in the brain. A change in the size of the cells in the brain causes changes in mental functioning with confusion, altered level of consciousness, and ultimately seizures and coma when the serum sodium level drops below about 115 mEq/L.

Assessment with Clinical Manifestations

The change in osmolality that occurs with hyponatremia causes fluid to shift into the intracellular space. Signs and symptoms associated with an expanded intracellular compartment include confusion, restlessness or lethargy, and seizures and coma (Estes, 2006).

Hyponatremia may occur with or without associated fluid deficit or fluid excess. If fluid imbalance is present, patients may exhibit signs of fluid imbalance as previously discussed. Typically, hyponatremia occurs because of excess fluid volume diluting the sodium. Signs of excess ECF such as edema, distended neck veins, and crackles in the lungs will be present.

In conditions that cause hyponatremia through water retention, urine will be concentrated with a high osmolality. Hyponatremia from diuretic use may produce large quantities of urine, but the urine will be concentrated as sodium ions are lost in the urine. Untreated hyponatremia will lead to death as cerebral cells swell and burst.

Assessment of the patient with hyponatremia focuses on mental status. Slight changes in serum sodium level may cause confusion and changes in level of consciousness. Confusion in elderly hospitalized patients should always trigger assessment of the serum sodium level.

Diagnostic Tests

A serum sodium level determines below 135 mEq/L indicates hyponatremia. The serum osmolality will be reduced. Urine osmolality will be increased reflecting the concentrated urine. The hematocrit and hemoglobin may be reduced from dilution of the blood.

Nursing Diagnoses

Nursing diagnoses pertinent to patients with hyponatremia include disturbed thought processes and, in patients with dilutional hyponatremia, excess fluid volume.

Planning and Implementation

NIC interventions for patients with hyponatremia include:
- Electrolyte management: Hyponatremia.
- Cerebral edema management.
- Delirium management.
- Fluid monitoring.
- Fluid management.
- Seizure precautions.

Patients receiving IV fluids should be monitored closely for signs of developing hyponatremia. Hypotonic IVs should be stopped if hyponatremia occurs. Patients may have fluids restricted (Yeates, Singer, & Morton, 2004). All fluids may be restricted, or the patient may be placed on a free water restriction.

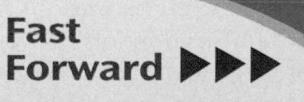

Fast Forward ▶▶▶

Medications to Treat SIADH

New drugs are being developed that counteract the effects of ADH in the body. ADH or arginine vasopressin (AVP) acts on three types of receptors. Medications that antagonize the AVP V2 receptors interfere with the action of ADH in the renal tubules, promoting excretion of free water. These new compounds are identified as promoting aquaresis, excretion of water without excretion of sodium (natriuresis) or potassium (kaliuresis) as occurs with other classes of diuretics. Clinical trials are underway to test the efficacy and safety of this new class of medication used to treat SIADH.

Source: Spratto, G. R., & Woods, A. L. (2007). 2007 PDR nurse's drug handbook. New York: Thomson Delmar Learning.

Juices are considered free water, because the glucose in the juice is rapidly metabolized, leaving only water, which has a hypotonic effect on the body. Water is also restricted. Fluids such as broth and milk might be allowed on a free water restriction. Diuretic medications may be ordered to remove excess fluid from the body. Weight is monitored to assess fluid balance. Patients must be watched closely for signs of mental status changes. Patients with low sodium levels, below about 125 mEq/L, are at high risk for seizures. Side rails should be padded to protect the patient from injury during seizures. Hypertonic saline (3% NaCl) may be given when severe neurological symptoms are present.

Treatment of hyponatremia must proceed cautiously. Too rapid correction of chronic hyponatremia may result in demyelination in the brain leading to permanent brain damage. Hyponatremia that has developed acutely may be safely corrected more quickly than chronic hyponatremia.

Evaluation of Outcomes

NOC outcomes for hyponatremia include cognitive orientation, electrolyte and acid-base balance, fluid balance, and hydration. Serum sodium level should be within normal range, and signs of fluid excess should be absent. Absence of seizure activity and normal mental status are important indicators of resolution of hyponatremia.

Excess Sodium Ion (Hypernatremia)

Hypernatremia is defined as having a serum sodium level that is above the normal range (136 to 145 mEq/L). Hypernatremia may occur when excess sodium ions are present in the body, or when water is lost from the body, leaving the sodium ions more concentrated.

Etiology

Hypernatremia may occur when patients are unable to ingest sufficient water to maintain normal serum osmolality. Excessive exercise without sufficient water replacement, extreme heat, or administration of excessive amounts of diuretic medications may result in hypernatremia. Diabetes insipidus, a condition associated with insufficient production of ADH, may result in hypernatremia.

Pathophysiology

Rarely is hypernatremia due to excess amounts of sodium in the body. More commonly, it is a signal of insufficient water in the body, leaving the body fluids too concentrated. Lack of ability to communicate thirst or to ingest water independently, as may occur in frail elderly patients or in comatose patients, may result in insufficient water intake. Inability to match water intake to need, as may occur in extreme heat or exercise, may result in hypernatremia. Diuretic use may cause excessive elimination of water, leaving body fluids more concentrated. Excessive amounts of ADH, as occurs in diabetes insipidus, causes excretion of large volumes of dilute urine, leaving the fluids in the body more concentrated than normal.

The increased osmolality that occurs because the fluids are more concentrated in the extracellular space causes fluid to shift from the intracellular compartment into the extracellular compartment to dilute the increased osmolality in the extracellular space. This leaves the cells shrunken and not able to function well. As with hyponatremia, the most devastating effects of this shrinkage of cells occur in the brain. Typically, all body compartments (vascular, interstitial, and intracellular) are low on volume in hypernatremia.

Assessment with Clinical Manifestations

Signs and symptoms of hypernatremia generally include evidence of decreased extracellular volume, such as dry mucous membranes, postural hypotension, and decreased skin turgor. In addition, signs of intracellular volume deficit are

Red Flag

Uncorrected Hypernatremia

Uncorrected hypernatremia leads to severe intracellular dehydration and will result in death if not treated. In addition, it is usually accompanied by systemic dehydration and may lead to hypovolemic shock and death. Therefore, the nurse must always assess sodium levels to quickly detect progressively lowering lab levels.

present, such as confusion, lethargy, seizures, or coma (Estes, 2006). Patients with diabetes insipidus will have high volumes of dilute urine output.

Patients at risk for hypernatremia need close monitoring. Patients unable to communicate their needs must be assessed carefully for signs of extracellular dehydration, such as dry mucous membranes, postural hypotension, and poor skin turgor, and for signs of intracellular dehydration, such as confusion and seizures. Elderly patients who develop a new onset of confusion should have their serum sodium level checked.

Diagnostic Tests

The serum sodium level will be greater than 145 mEq/L. The hematocrit may be elevated if extracellular dehydration is present.

Nursing Diagnoses

Based on the information gathered, examples of nursing diagnoses in the patient with hypernatremia may include the following:
- Disturbed thought processes.
- Deficient fluid volume.

Planning and Implementation

NIC interventions for patients with hypernatremia include:
- Electrolyte management: Hypernatremia.
- Delirium management.
- Fluid monitoring.
- Fluid management.
- Seizure precautions.

Patients with hypernatremia have elevated serum osmolality. Treatment involves administration of hypotonic fluids to dilute the high serum osmolality. If patients are able to take fluids orally, and the hypernatremia is mild, patients will be encouraged to drink hypotonic fluids. Patients with significant hypernatremia will require hypotonic IV solutions such as one-half normal saline or one-fourth normal saline. Hypotonic solutions will replenish both the extracellular and intracellular compartments. Oral care is important for comfort because of dry mucous membranes. Patients with postural hypotension should be monitored for dizziness and assisted to change positions slowly. Patients with diabetes insipidus may require supplemental ADH, administered as desmopressin (DDAVP).

Patients with high sodium levels, above 155 mEq/L, are at high risk for seizures. Side rails should be padded to protect the patient from injury during seizures.

Evaluation of Outcomes

NOC outcomes for hypernatremia include cognitive orientation, electrolyte and acid-base balance, fluid balance, and hydration. Serum sodium level should be within normal range, and signs of fluid deficit should be absent. Resolution of seizures and return of normal mental function and orientation are indicators of resolution of hypernatremia.

Deficient Potassium Ion (Hypokalemia)

Hypokalemia is defined as having a potassium level lower than the normal range of between 3.5 and 5.5 mEq/L. Hypokalemia results from anything that causes either an excessive loss of potassium from the body or from a prolonged decrease of ingestion of potassium.

Etiology

Diuretics may cause excretion of excess potassium ions. Excess aldosterone release, as occurs in heart failure, causes excretion of potassium ions. Diarrhea, vomiting or nasogastric suction, and drainage from wounds may cause hypokalemia (Verive, 2004). Patients with a limited food intake or those who are unable to ingest a sufficiently varied diet may experience hypokalemia.

Metabolic alkalosis results in loss of potassium ions in the kidneys as bicarbonate ions are excreted to reduce the amount of base in the body. In addition, in alkalosis, hydrogen ions shift into the cells from the extracellular space; in exchange intracellular potassium ions are forced out into the extracellular space.

Pathophysiology

Potassium ions are necessary for adequate neuromuscular function. A deficit of potassium ions interferes with normal smooth, skeletal, and cardiac muscle contraction and also with nerve conduction.

Assessment with Clinical Manifestations

Hypokalemia results in poor muscle contraction. Evidence of this includes fatigue, skeletal muscle weakness, poor muscle tone, hyporeflexia, and possibly paralysis. Weakening of the respiratory muscles may interfere with depth and quality of respirations. Poor smooth muscle function leads to decreased GI motility with anorexia, nausea, vomiting, and ileus with decreased bowel sounds. Neurological effects of hypokalemia include paresthesias, confusion, and lethargy. Cardiac effects include dysrhythmias. On the electrocardiogram (ECG), T wave will be flattened. Hypokalemia increases sensitivity to digitalis and the risk of digitalis toxicity.

Patients with hypokalemia should have careful assessment of neuromuscular and cardiac status. Muscle strength and tone and reflexes should be assessed at regular intervals. Assessment of GI status, including bowel sounds, is important. Auscultation of the apical pulse and assessment of peripheral pulses helps in evaluation of cardiac status.

Diagnostic Tests

Patients at risk for hypokalemia should have their serum potassium level measured regularly. Normal serum potassium falls between 3.5 and 5.5 mEq/L. Patients with potassium levels below 3.0 mEq/L should have an ECG taken and should be placed on continuous cardiac monitoring to monitor for flattened T waves.

Nursing Diagnoses

Based on the information gathered, examples of nursing diagnoses in the patient with hypokalemia may include the following:
- Decreased cardiac output related to dysrhythmias.
- Ineffective breathing pattern related to depressed respiratory muscles.
- Activity intolerance related to fatigue and muscle weakness.

Planning and Implementation

NIC interventions for patients with hypokalemia may include:
- Electrolyte management: Hypokalemia.
- Dysrhythmia management.
- Acid-base management: Metabolic alkalosis.

Raising the serum potassium level is the goal of treatment. Administration of oral potassium is effective when the serum potassium level is mildly reduced. Oral potassium supplements may cause GI upset and should be given with food when possible.

Significant potassium deficiency calls for replacement with IV potassium. Potassium is potentially fatal when given undiluted or when not diluted sufficiently. Potassium should never be pushed directly into an IV. The concentration of potassium administered through a peripheral IV site should not exceed 40 to 60 mEq/L. Potassium administered through a central IV line may be in a concentration of 60 to 80 mEq/L.

Patients with hypokalemia often have concurrent hypomagnesemia. Hypokalemia is resistant to treatment unless the hypomagnesemia is corrected. Hypokalemia associated with metabolic alkalosis also is resistant to treatment unless the alkalosis is treated.

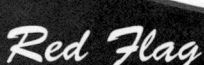

Red Flag

Hypokalemia

Significant uncorrected hypokalemia will cause serious dysrhythmias and, ultimately, cardiac arrest and death. Patients taking digoxin must be monitored closely for digitalis toxicity, which also can cause dysrhythmias.

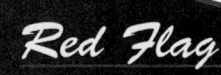

Patients with significant hypokalemia should be on continuous cardiac monitoring. Treatment of dysrhythmias may be necessary; however, correction of the hypokalemia is the definitive treatment. Patients at risk for ongoing hypokalemia should be instructed in dietary sources of potassium to supplement their potassium.

Evaluation of Outcomes

Potential patient outcomes for each of the example nursing diagnoses for the patient with hypokalemia are:

- Decreased cardiac output related to dysrhythmias. The patient maintains blood pressure within normal limits; warm dry skin; regular cardiac rhythm; clear lung sounds; strong bilateral, equal peripheral pulses.
- Ineffective breathing pattern related to depressed respiratory muscles. The patient's breathing pattern is maintained by eupnea, normal skin color, and regular respiratory rate or pattern.
- Activity intolerance related to fatigue and muscle weakness. The patient should perform physical activity independently or with assistive devices as needed. In addition, the patient should be free of complications of immobility, as evidenced by intact skin, absence of thrombophlebitis, and normal bowel patterns.

NOC outcomes pertinent to patients with hypokalemia include electrolyte and acid-base balance, mobility, and activity tolerance. Return of serum potassium level to normal range and normal ECG are major goals of treatment.

Excess Potassium Ion (Hyperkalemia)

Hyperkalemia is defined when the serum potassium is above the normal range (3.5 to 5.5 mEq/L) for serum potassium. Hyperkalemia occurs when intake of potassium exceeds normal requirements or when excretion of potassium from the body is impaired. Ingestion of excess amounts of dietary potassium or overmedication with potassium supplements may result in excessive serum potassium. Many salt substitutes contain potassium and may lead to hyperkalemia.

Etiology

The kidneys help maintain potassium balance by excreting 80% of the potassium removed from the body daily. Kidney impairment may result in hyperkalemia as the kidneys become unable to excrete sufficient potassium. Potassium-sparing diuretics such as spironolactone and triamterene encourage retention of potassium, possibly leading to hyperkalemia. Metabolic acidosis shifts potassium from the intracellular compartment into the extracellular compartment resulting in hyperkalemia.

Pathophysiology

Hyperkalemia makes cells more sensitive to electrical impulses. Initially, this results in increased muscle contractions; however, eventually it results in paralysis.

Assessment with Clinical Manifestations

Increased sensitivity to stimuli causes muscle twitching and contraction. Ultimately, weakness and paralysis result. Excessive contraction of smooth muscle in the GI tract is associated with abdominal cramping, hyperactive bowel tones, and diarrhea. Cardiac manifestations include dysrhythmias and tall, tented T waves on the ECG. Untreated hyperkalemia results in potentially fatal cardiac dysrhythmias and may lead to death.

Patients with hyperkalemia should be monitored for abnormal muscular function, either spontaneous muscle contractions or flaccid paralysis. Abdominal cramping and diarrhea may be present, and hyperactive bowel sounds may be auscultated. Assessment of apical and peripheral pulses will help determine the presence of dysrhythmias and the patient with significant hyperkalemia should be placed on continuous cardiac monitoring (Wilbanks, Wakim, Daicoff, & Monterde, 2005).

Diagnostic Tests

A serum potassium level of greater than 5.5 mEq/L indicates hyperkalemia. The ECG will demonstrate tall, peaked T waves and dysrhythmias.

Nursing Diagnoses

Based on the information gathered, examples of nursing diagnoses in the patient with hyperkalemia may include the following:
- Decreased cardiac output related to cardiac dysrhythmias.
- Ineffective breathing pattern may occur as the muscle hyperactivity progresses to respiratory muscle flaccidity and paralysis.
- Diarrhea.

Planning and Implementation

NIC interventions for patients with hyperkalemia may include:
- Electrolyte management: Hyperkalemia.
- Dysrhythmia management.
- The medication Kayexalate may be administered orally, via nasogastric tube or rectally.

Kayexalate causes exchange of sodium and potassium in the GI tract, resulting in excretion of potassium in the stool. Other medications used in the management of hyperkalemia temporarily counteract the effects of the hyperkalemia but do not remove potassium from the body.

IV calcium interrupts the action of potassium in the body. Administration of IV regular insulin causes movement of potassium into the intracellular space, lowering the potassium level in the extracellular compartment (that is, the serum potassium level). Because this lowers blood glucose level, IV glucose is administered concurrently with the IV insulin. Administration of sodium bicarbonate also promotes movement of potassium into the intracellular compartment, lowering serum potassium level. Correction of metabolic acidosis encourages movement of potassium from the extracellular space back into the cells in exchange for hydrogen ions (Spratto & Woods, 2007).

Significant levels of hyperkalemia may require dialysis to remove excess potassium ions. Patients with renal failure will require dialysis; other patients may require dialysis depending on their serum potassium level and other signs and symptoms of hyperkalemia.

Evaluation of Outcomes

Potential patient outcomes for each of the example nursing diagnoses for the patient with hyperkalemia are:
- Decreased cardiac output related to cardiac dysrhythmias. The patient maintains blood pressure within normal limits; warm dry skin; regular cardiac rhythm; clear lung sounds; strong bilateral, equal peripheral pulses.
- Ineffective breathing pattern may occur as the muscle hyperactivity progresses to respiratory muscle flaccidity and paralysis. The patient's breathing pattern is maintained by eupnea, normal skin color, and regular respiratory rate or pattern.
- Diarrhea. The patient will have normal, formed stools.

The major NOC outcome for hyperkalemia is electrolyte and acid-base balance.

Return of serum potassium level to normal and a normal ECG are the major indicators of potassium balance.

Deficient Calcium Ion (Hypocalcemia)

Hypocalcemia is defined as a serum calcium level that is below the normal range for serum calcium (8.5 to 10.5 mg/dL). Low calcium levels can have negative consequences and symptomology that depicts the condition. Hypocalcemia may result from inadequate calcium intake or excessive calcium excretion.

Etiology

Conditions that inhibit calcium absorption from the GI tract include Crohn's disease and inadequate intake of vitamin D. In addition, renal failure prevents completion of vitamin D activation, also inhibiting calcium absorption. Diarrhea and excessive wound drainage increase calcium losses from the body. Alkalosis, pancreatitis, increased phosphorous levels, and immobility decrease the proportion of calcium that is ionized, making less calcium available and resulting in signs and symptoms of hypocalcemia, even though the total amount of calcium in the body is unchanged. Removal of the parathyroid gland, which may occur during thyroidectomy, may shift calcium balance resulting in hypocalcemia.

Pathophysiology

Calcium exists in the body in ionized and unionized forms. The ionized calcium is the available portion that acts on the body. Calcium suppresses electrical activity in cells. When calcium levels are low, electrical activity occurs spontaneously and continuously.

Assessment with Clinical Manifestations

Excessive electrical activity of cells results in spontaneous and continuous contraction of muscle cells. Paresthesias, twitching, muscle cramps, and tetany may occur. Deep tendon reflexes may be hyperactive. Contraction of smooth muscle in the GI tract increases GI motility causing cramping and diarrhea. Hypocalcemia causes decreased myocardial contractility, dysrhythmias, and changes on the ECG. Ongoing excessive hypocalcemia may produce seizures and tetany of the respiratory muscles resulting in respiratory arrest or cardiac arrest.

Trousseau's sign, also called carpopedal spasm, and Chvostek's sign are evidence of hypocalcemia. Trousseau's sign is assessed by placing a blood pressure cuff on the arm. The cuff is inflated to just above the patient's systolic pressure for up to 4 minutes. If the patient is hypocalcemic, the hand will spasm. Tapping on the facial nerve assesses Chvostek's sign (Figure 12-6). A positive sign is associated with spasm of the facial muscles on the side that is tapped.

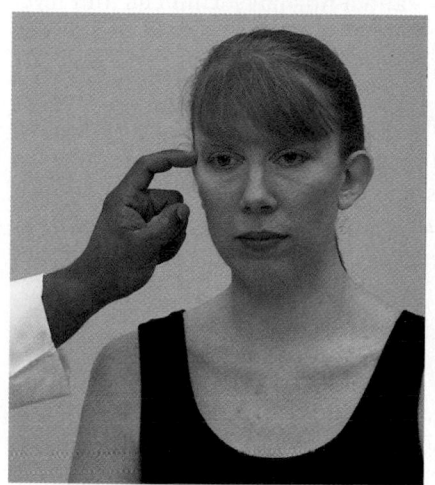

Figure 12-6 Assessing for Chvostek's sign.

Diagnostic Tests

Measurement of serum calcium allows identification of hypocalcemia. Normal serum calcium ranges from 8.5 to 10.5 mEq/L. The ECG should be examined for prolongation of the ST segment and the Q-T interval, characteristic of hypocalcemia.

Nursing Diagnoses

Based on the information gathered, examples of nursing diagnoses in the patient with hypocalcemia may include the following:
• Decreased cardiac output related to diminished contractility.
• Ineffective breathing pattern related to respiratory muscle tetany.
• Activity intolerance related to neuromuscular irritability.

Planning and Implementation

NIC interventions for patients with hypocalcemia include:
• Electrolyte management: Hypocalcemia.
• Dysrhythmia management.

Management of hypocalcemia is focused on calcium replacement. Oral replacements are given to patients with mild hypocalcemia. Medications that improve calcium absorption from the GI tract may be given, including vitamin D supplements. IV calcium is given to patients with more severe hypocalcemia. Magnesium may be administered to reduce cellular responsiveness to electrical stimuli.

Evaluation of Outcomes

Potential patient outcomes for each of the example nursing diagnoses for the patient with hypocalcemia are:

- Decreased cardiac output related to dysrhythmias. The patient maintains blood pressure within normal limits; warm dry skin; regular cardiac rhythm; clear lung sounds; strong bilateral, equal peripheral pulses.
- Ineffective breathing pattern related to depressed respiratory muscles. The patient's breathing pattern is maintained by eupnea, normal skin color, and regular respiratory rate or pattern.
- Activity intolerance related to fatigue and muscle weakness. The patient should perform physical activity independently or with assistive devices as needed. In addition, the patient should be free of complications of immobility, as evidenced by intact skin, absence of thrombophlebitis, and normal bowel patterns.

The major NOC outcome for hypocalcemia is electrolyte and acid-base balance. Absence of neuromuscular symptoms and a normal serum calcium level are the goals of treatment.

Excess Calcium Ion (Hypercalcemia)

Hypercalcemia is defined as having a calcium level above the normal range for serum calcium (8.5 to 10.5 mg/dL). There are a variety of concerns for patients with high calcium levels and significant negative consequences may occur. Hypercalcemia may result from excess calcium intake or inability to excrete calcium.

Etiology

High levels of calcium in the blood may be caused by hyperparathyroidism, which results in release of stored calcium from the bone, absorption of calcium from the GI tract, and retention of calcium by the kidneys. Malignant tumors may produce hypercalcemia by releasing a hormone similar to parathyroid hormone. Excessive ingestion of calcium supplements may cause hypercalcemia. Prolonged immobility may cause release of calcium from the bone (Shuey & Brant, 2004).

Pathophysiology

The calcium ion suppresses electrical activity in cells and is vital to the normal physiological processes of the body. Hypercalcemia suppresses cellular excitability, resulting in muscle weakness and impaired transmission of neurological signals.

Assessment with Clinical Manifestations

Suppressed cellular excitability manifests as muscular weakness, fatigue, and hyporeflexia. Suppression of smooth muscle affects the GI tract with slowed GI motility, nausea, vomiting, and constipation. Changes in neurological function may include lethargy, confusion, or coma. Suppression of cardiac muscle produces dysrhythmias. Significant hypercalcemia may result in respiratory and cardiac arrest.

Assessment of the patient centers around assessment of neuromuscular function. Assessment of muscle strength, tone, and reflexes establishes a baseline for later comparison. Assessment of the GI system includes review of symptoms and auscultation of bowel sounds. Assessment of apical and peripheral pulses provides information about cardiac function.

Diagnostic Tests

Diagnosis of hypercalcemia is made based on a serum calcium level of greater than 10.5 mEq/L. The ECG is evaluated to detect dysrhythmias.

Nursing Diagnoses

Based on the information gathered, examples of nursing diagnoses in the patient with hypercalcemia may include the following:
- Decreased cardiac output related to dysrhythmias.
- Ineffective breathing pattern related to respiratory muscle weakness.
- Activity intolerance related to neuromuscular weakness.

Planning and Implementation

NIC interventions for patients with hypercalcemia include:
- Electrolyte management: Hypercalcemia.
- Dysrhythmia management.

Management of hypercalcemia is focused on removing calcium from the body. Administration of diuretics and IV fluids promote renal elimination of calcium. In the long-term, patients with malignancies might be treated with bisphosphonates, such as etidronate, to prevent reabsorption of bone, thereby limiting the amount of calcium released into the bloodstream. In patients with significant hypercalcemia, IV sodium or potassium phosphate is administered; the phosphate binds with the calcium reducing the effects of the hypercalcemia. Continuous cardiac monitoring should be implemented in patients at risk for dysrhythmias.

Evaluation of Outcomes

Potential patient outcomes for each of the example nursing diagnoses for the patient with hypercalcemia are:
- Decreased cardiac output related to dysrhythmias. The patient maintains blood pressure within normal limits; warm dry skin; regular cardiac rhythm; clear lung sounds; strong bilateral, equal peripheral pulses.
- Ineffective breathing pattern related to depressed respiratory muscles. The patient's breathing pattern is maintained by eupnea, normal skin color, and regular respiratory rate or pattern.
- Activity intolerance related to related to neuromuscular weakness. The patient should perform physical activity independently or with assistive devices as needed. In addition, the patient should be free of complications of immobility, as evidenced by intact skin, absence of thrombophlebitis, and normal bowel patterns.

The major NOC outcome for hypocalcemia is electrolyte and acid-base balance. As with hypocalcemia, absence of neuromuscular symptoms and a normal serum calcium level are the goals of treatment.

Deficient Phosphorus Ion (Hypophosphatemia)

Hypophosphatemia is defined as having a phosphorus level below the normal range (3 to 4.5 mg/dL). Low phosphorus level is caused by decreased ingestion or absorption of phosphate or by increased renal excretion of phosphate.

Etiology

A diet deficient in phosphorous may cause hypophosphatemia and reduced absorption of phosphorous, as occurs with chronic alcoholism. Intake of magnesium or calcium containing antacids may inhibit phosphorous absorption. Administration of parenteral or enteral feedings to malnourished patients may stimulate insulin release, which promotes movement of phosphorous into cells, reducing serum phosphorous levels.

Pathophysiology

Phosphorous is important in neuromuscular and energy functions of cells. Muscle weakness and paresthesias may occur with low serum phosphorous levels. Breakdown of muscle cells, rhabdomyolysis, may occur, with release of creatinine kinase (CK). Lack of cellular energy results in cellular hypoxia (Hayes, 2004).

Assessment with Clinical Manifestations

Muscular weakness, muscle pain, paresthesias, and paralysis may occur. Decreased myocardial contractility may result in heart failure, and respiratory muscle weakness may result in respiratory failure. Neurological symptoms may include irritability, confusion, and seizures. Decreased GI motility may cause anorexia, nausea, and decreased bowel sounds. Hypophosphatemia may result in cardiac and respiratory failure and arrest. Careful assessment of neuromuscular function is important in patients with hypophosphatemia. Poor muscle tone, muscle weakness, and hyporeflexia will be seen. Decreased GI motility will be accompanied by hypoactive bowel sounds. Cardiac monitoring should be instituted to assess cardiac rhythm.

Diagnostic Tests

Hypophosphatemia is defined as a serum phosphorous level below 3 mg/dL. An ECG is helpful to assess the effects of the low phosphorous level on the heart.

Nursing Diagnoses

Based on the information gathered, examples of nursing diagnoses in the patient with hypophosphatemia may include the following:
- Decreased cardiac output related to dysrhythmias.
- Ineffective breathing pattern related to respiratory muscle weakness.
- Activity intolerance related to neuromuscular weakness.

Planning and Implementation

NIC interventions for patients with hypophosphatemia include:
- Electrolyte management: Hypophosphatemia.
- Dysrhythmia management.

Management of hypophosphatemia is focused on replacing phosphorous levels in the body. Phosphorous may be administered orally or intravenously.

Evaluation of Outcomes

Potential patient outcomes for each of the example nursing diagnoses for the patient with hypophosphatemia are:
- Decreased cardiac output related to dysrhythmias. The patient maintains blood pressure within normal limits; warm dry skin; regular cardiac rhythm; clear lung sounds; strong bilateral, equal peripheral pulses.
- Ineffective breathing pattern related to depressed respiratory muscles. The patient's breathing pattern is maintained by eupnea, normal skin color, and regular respiratory rate or pattern.
- Activity intolerance related to related to neuromuscular weakness. The patient should perform physical activity independently or with assistive devices as needed. In addition, the patient should be free of complications of immobility, as evidenced by intact skin, absence of thrombophlebitis, and normal bowel patterns.

The major NOC outcome for hypophosphatemia is electrolyte and acid-base balance. As with other electrolyte imbalances, absence of neuromuscular symptoms and a normal serum phosphorous level are the goals of treatment.

Excess Phosphorus Ion (Hyperphosphatemia)

Hyperphosphatemia is defined as having a phosphorus level above the normal range (3–4.5 mg/dL). Hyperphosphatemia may result from excess intake of phosphorous through the diet or through supplements. A major cause of hyperphosphatemia is renal failure with impaired excretion of phosphorous.

Etiology

Hyperphosphatemia can develop with exogenous or endogenous additions of phosphorus to the ECF. In addition, high levels of phosphorus are seen with cell destruction associated with treatment of metastatic tumors with chemotherapy, because it releases large amounts of phosphorus into the blood. Also, regular use of enemas and laxatives that contain phosphorus can cause hyperphosphatemia. Last, hypoparathyroidism increases renal tubular reabsorption of phosphate, which also causes hyperphosphatemia.

Pathophysiology

Effects of high phosphorous levels are actually due to the hypocalcemia that accompanies hyperphosphatemia. Because calcium suppresses cellular excitability, hypocalcemia is associated with spontaneous and sustained cellular activity.

Assessment with Clinical Manifestations

Signs and symptoms of hyperphosphatemia are those that occur with hypocalcemia, including muscle contractions and tetany, positive Trousseau's sign, and positive Chvostek's sign. Excess phosphorous levels may result in cardiac and respiratory arrest.

Diagnostic Tests

Hyperphosphatemia is indicated by a serum phosphorus level greater than 4.5 mg/dL. An ECG should be obtained to evaluate cardiac function.

Nursing Diagnoses

Based on the information gathered, examples of nursing diagnoses in the patient with hyperphosphatemia may include the following:
- Decreased cardiac output related to dysrhythmias.
- Ineffective breathing pattern related to respiratory muscle weakness.
- Activity intolerance related to neuromuscular weakness.

Planning and Implementation

NIC interventions for patients with hyperphosphatemia include:
- Electrolyte management: Hyperphosphatemia.
- Dysrhythmia management.

Management of hyperphosphatemia is focused on lowering serum phosphorous levels. Avoidance of dietary and medical sources of phosphorous is initiated. Phosphate binders, such as calcium-containing antacids, may bind phosphorous in the GI tract and promote elimination of phosphorous in the stool. Dialysis may be necessary to remove high levels of phosphorous.

Evaluation of Outcomes

Potential patient outcomes for each of the example nursing diagnoses for the patient with hyperphosphatemia are:
- Decreased cardiac output related to dysrhythmias. The patient maintains blood pressure within normal limits; warm dry skin; regular cardiac rhythm; clear lung sounds; strong bilateral, equal peripheral pulses.
- Ineffective breathing pattern related to depressed respiratory muscles. The patient's breathing pattern is maintained by eupnea, normal skin color, and regular respiratory rate or pattern.
- Activity intolerance related to related to neuromuscular weakness. The patient should perform physical activity independently or with assistive devices as needed. In addition, the patient should be free of complications of immobility, as evidenced by intact skin, absence of thrombophlebitis, and normal bowel patterns.

The major NOC outcome for hyperphosphatemia is electrolyte and acid-base balance. A normal serum phosphorous level and absence of neuromuscular signs and symptoms are indicators of normal phosphorous balance.

Deficient Magnesium Ion (Hypomagnesemia)

Hypomagnesemia is defined as having serum magnesium levels below the normal range (1.6–2.6 mg/dL). Magnesium levels may be low because of insufficient intake or absorption of and commonly occurs with chronic alcoholism.

Etiology

Loss of magnesium may occur through the GI tract with diarrhea. Loss of magnesium through the kidneys occurs with alcohol use, diuretic administration, and in diabetes (Verive, 2004).

Pathophysiology

Hypomagnesemia commonly occurs simultaneously with hypokalemia and hypocalcemia. Magnesium is important in neuromuscular function; hypomagnesemia increases cellular excitability.

Assessment with Clinical Manifestations

Because low magnesium level is associated with low potassium and calcium, signs and symptoms are similar to hypokalemia and hypocalcemia. Muscular twitching and spasms, hyperreflexia, and tetany are signs of hypomagnesemia. Cardiac dysrhythmias are common. GI signs and symptoms include anorexia, nausea, vomiting, and diarrhea. Mental status may be altered, and patients may be confused or lethargic. Seizures may occur. Major risks of hypomagnesemia are respiratory and cardiac arrest. Assessment of patients with hypomagnesemia focuses on neuromuscular function. Assessment of muscle tone and reflexes is important, as is assessment of GI function. The bowel sounds will be hyperactive. Auscultation of apical pulse and palpation of peripheral pulses provides assessment of cardiac function. Patients with cardiac dysrhythmias should be placed on continuous cardiac monitoring.

Diagnostic Tests

Hypomagnesemia is diagnosed by an elevated serum magnesium level above 2.6 mg/dL. An ECG is important to assess the effects of a low level of magnesium on the heart.

Nursing Diagnoses

Based on the information gathered, examples of nursing diagnoses in the patient with hypomagnesemia may include the following:
- Decreased cardiac output related to dysrhythmias.
- Ineffective breathing pattern related to respiratory muscle weakness.
- Activity intolerance related to neuromuscular weakness.

Planning and Implementation

NIC interventions for patients with hypomagnesemia include:
- Electrolyte management: Hypomagnesemia.
- Dysrhythmia management.

Management of hypomagnesemia is focused on replacing magnesium stores in the body. Magnesium may be administered orally or intravenously. Patients with mild magnesium deficiencies should be instructed in dietary sources of magnesium.

Evaluation of Outcomes

Potential patient outcomes for each of the example nursing diagnoses for the patient with hypomagnesemia are:

- Decreased cardiac output related to dysrhythmias. The patient maintains blood pressure within normal limits; warm dry skin; regular cardiac rhythm; clear lung sounds; strong bilateral, equal peripheral pulses.
- Ineffective breathing pattern related to depressed respiratory muscles. The patient's breathing pattern is maintained by eupnea, normal skin color, and regular respiratory rate or pattern.
- Activity intolerance related to related to neuromuscular weakness: The patient should perform physical activity independently or with assistive devices as needed. In addition, the patient should be free of complications of immobility, as evidenced by intact skin, absence of thrombophlebitis, and normal bowel patterns.

The major NOC outcome for hypomagnesemia is electrolyte and acid-base balance. As with hypocalcemia, absence of neuromuscular symptoms and a normal serum magnesium level are the goals of treatment.

Excess Magnesium Ion (Hypermagnesemia)

Hypermagnesemia is defined as having serum magnesium levels above the normal range (1.6 to 2.6 mg/dL). Elevated magnesium levels may be because of excessive ingestion of magnesium or failure to excrete magnesium.

Etiology

Elevated magnesium levels may be due to excessive ingestion of magnesium or failure to excrete magnesium. Patients receiving oral or IV magnesium supplements may develop hypermagnesemia. Excretion of magnesium is impaired in patients with renal failure. Because patients with renal failure have decreased ability to excrete magnesium, they should avoid medications that contain magnesium, such as Milk of Magnesia and magnesium-based antacids, such as Mylanta and Maalox.

Pathophysiology

Elevated magnesium levels interfere with neuromuscular function. By suppressing cellular excitability, hypermagnesemia results in muscular flaccidity and suppression of electrical impulses.

Assessment with Clinical Manifestations

Signs and symptoms of hypermagnesemia are similar to those seen with hypercalcemia. Paresthesias, muscle weakness, and hyporeflexia are seen. GI symptoms including anorexia, nausea, and constipation occur. Cardiac dysrhythmias occur. Hypermagnesemia depresses the CNS resulting in confusion, depression, lethargy, and coma. Untreated significant hypermagnesemia results in respiratory and cardiac arrest.

Patients with hypermagnesemia should be assessed for depressed neuromuscular function. Muscle strength, tone, and reflexes should all be assessed. Bowel sounds will be diminished. Mental status may be depressed. Assessment of apical and peripheral pulses and continuous cardiac monitoring are needed in patients with dysrhythmias.

Diagnostic Tests

A serum magnesium level above 2.6 mEq/L signifies hypermagnesemia. An ECG should be obtained to assess cardiac effects.

Nursing Diagnoses

Based on the information gathered, examples of nursing diagnoses in the patient with hypermagnesemia may include the following:

- Decreased cardiac output related to dysrhythmias.
- Ineffective breathing pattern related to respiratory muscle weakness.
- Activity intolerance related to neuromuscular weakness.

Planning and Implementation

NIC interventions for patients with hypermagnesemia include:

- Electrolyte management: Hypermagnesemia.
- Dysrhythmia management.

Avoidance of medications that contain magnesium is important for patients at risk for hypermagnesemia. IV calcium may be administered to counteract the effects of hypermagnesemia. Dialysis may be used to remove excess magnesium.

Evaluation of Outcomes

Potential patient outcomes for each of the example nursing diagnoses for the patient with hypermagnesemia are:

- Decreased cardiac output related to dysrhythmias. The patient maintains blood pressure within normal limits; warm dry skin; regular cardiac rhythm; clear lung sounds; strong bilateral, equal peripheral pulses.
- Ineffective breathing pattern related to depressed respiratory muscles. The patient's breathing pattern is maintained by eupnea, normal skin color, and regular respiratory rate or pattern.
- Activity intolerance related to related to neuromuscular weakness. The patient should perform physical activity independently or with assistive devices as needed. In addition, the patient should be free of complications of immobility, as evidenced by intact skin, absence of thrombophlebitis, and normal bowel patterns.

The major NOC outcome for hypermagnesemia is electrolyte and acid-base balance. As with hypomagnesemia, absence of neuromuscular symptoms and a normal serum magnesium level are the goals of treatment.

ACID-BASE BALANCE

Human cells function normally only within a narrow range of pH. Significant movement outside of the normal pH range interferes with cell function and leads to cell death. The body maintains proper pH with buffers. A number of substances act as buffers in body cells and tissues, including bicarbonates, phosphates, ammonia, and proteins (Candela & Yucha, 2004). A major buffer system in the body is the bicarbonate buffer system.

The bicarbonate buffer system uses a reversible chemical reaction to manage body pH. The equation is:

$$H^+ + HCO_3^- \leftrightarrow H_2CO_3 \leftrightarrow H_2O + CO_2$$

Hydrogen ions combine with bicarbonate ions to form carbonic acid. Carbonic acid dissociates into water and carbon dioxide. The equation goes in both directions, depending on the metabolic and pH needs of the body.

The kidneys regulate hydrogen and bicarbonate ion concentrations. If the body is too acidic, because of accumulation of hydrogen ions or loss of bicarbonate ions, the kidneys will retain or excrete hydrogen or bicarbonate to return the body's pH back to normal. These renal processes take some time to occur, but are able to compensate for wide ranges in pH. The lungs help regulate the amount of CO_2 in the body. If there is too much CO_2 in the body, the lungs exhale more CO_2; if there is too little CO_2 in the body, the lungs retain CO_2. The lungs' ability to retain or excrete CO_2 is rapid. However, there is a limit to how much CO_2 the lungs can excrete or retain; as there are limits to how much the respiratory rate can increase or decrease (Woodruff, 2006).

Many diseases and many medical interventions affect acid-base balance. The body can become either too acidotic or too alkalotic. Imbalances in acid-base occur because of respiratory causes or because of changes in the body's metabolism of acids and bases. Four imbalances are possible: respiratory acidosis, metabolic acidosis, respiratory alkalosis, and metabolic alkalosis (Table 12-7) (Figure 12-7).

Respiratory Acidosis

Respiratory acidosis occurs when the body retains too much CO_2. Anything that interferes with effective ventilation may cause respiratory acidosis. Patients who have undergone surgery may have a decreased respiratory rate because of the effects of anesthesia or because of narcotics used for pain relief. Patients undergoing thoracic or abdominal surgery are especially susceptible to inadequate ventilation because of the location of their incisions and the pain association with breathing. People with chronic obstructive pulmonary disease (COPD) may have difficulty exhaling and may retain CO_2. Patients with structural problems in the chest are at risk for shallow respirations. Rib fractures and kyphosis may impede respirations. Finally, people with neuromuscular disorders such as Guillain-Barré syndrome or amyotrophic lateral sclerosis are at risk for ineffective respirations (Daniels, 2004).

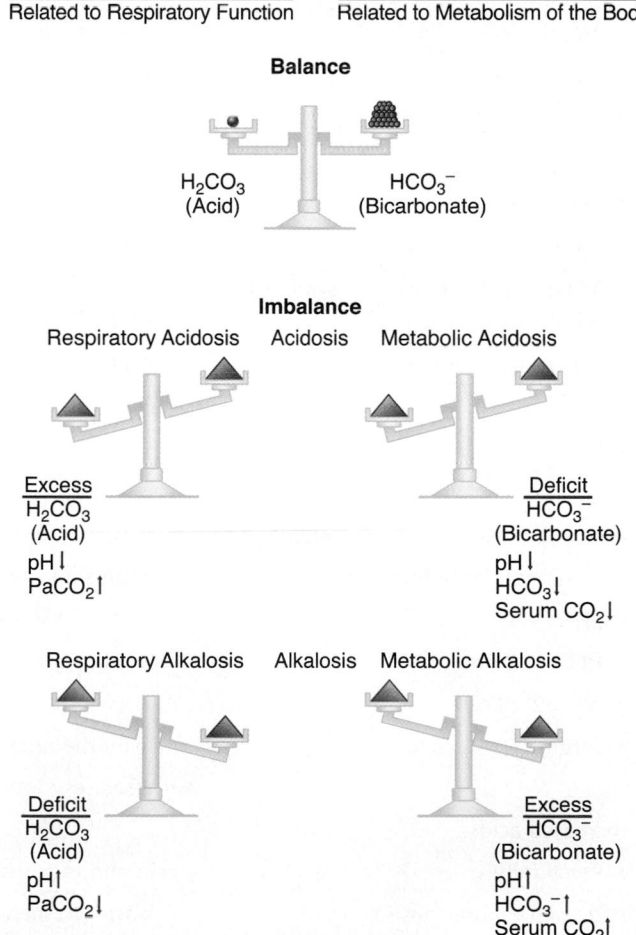

Figure 12-7 Acid-base balance and imbalance.

TABLE 12-7   Respiratory and Metabolic Acidosis and Alkalosis

IMBALANCE/CAUSES	CLINICAL MANIFESTATIONS	NURSING INTERVENTIONS
Respiratory Acidosis (Retention of Carbon Dioxide)		
Operational definition:	Cognitive and sensory	Institute safety measures.
• pH < 7.35	• Disorientation	Assist with positioning.
• $PaCO_2$ > 45 mmHg	• Depression	
• HCO_3 > 28 mEq/L (suggestive of renal compensation)	• Weakness → stupor	
	Skin and mucous membranes	Monitor I&O and administer fluids as ordered.
CNS disorders	• Flushed and warm	
Drug overdose		
Pneumonia	Oxygenation and ECG	Administer oxygen and medications per order; monitor hourly vital signs and respiratory status (may require mechanical ventilation).
Pulmonary edema	• Dyspnea	
Pneumothorax	• Tachycardia	
Restrictive lung disease	• Dysrhythmia	Monitor arterial blood gases (ABGs), pH, $PaCO_2$, HCO_3^-.
Respiratory Alkalosis (Hyperventilation)		
Operational definition:	Cognitive and sensory	Institute safety measures for the patient with vertigo or the unconscious patient. Encourage the anxious patient to verbalize fears.
• pH > 7.45	• Hyperactive reflexes	
• $PaCO_2$ < 35 mmHg	• Tetany	
	• Positive Chvostek's sign	
• Anxiety, fear	• Positive Trousseau's sign	Administer sedation as ordered to relax the patient.
• CNS disorders	• Vertigo	
• Pain	• Unconsciousness	
• Fever		
• Pneumonia, atelectasis	Skin and mucous membranes	Keep the patient warm and dry.
• Asthma	• Sweating (may occur)	
• Acute respiratory distress syndrome (ARDS)	Oxygenation and ECG	Encourage the patient to take deep, slow breaths or breathe into a brown paper bag (inspire CO_2). Monitor vital signs.
• Congestive heart failure, pulmonary edema	• Rapid, shallow breathing	
	• Palpitations	
• Pulmonary embolus		Monitor ABGs, primarily $PaCO_2$; a value ↓ 35 mm Hg indicates too little CO_2 (e.g., carbonic acid)
Metabolic Acidosis (Gain of Metabolic Acids or Loss of Base)		
Operational definition:	Cognitive and sensory	Institute safety measures.
• pH < 7.35	• Restlessness, disorientation	Monitor patient's sensorium; report alteration in level of consciousness.
• HCO_3 < 24 mEq/L	• Stupor, coma	
• BE < 2 mEq/L		
• Serum CO_2 < 22 mEq/L	Activity/mobility	Assist the patient with positioning and proper body alignment.
	• Weakness, lethargy	
Increased acids:		
• Renal failure	Skin and mucous membranes	Keep the patient comfortable.
• Diabetic ketoacidosis	• Warm, flushed skin	
• Anaerobic metabolism		

Continued

TABLE 12-7 Respiratory and Metabolic Acidosis and Alkalosis—cont'd

IMBALANCE/CAUSES	CLINICAL MANIFESTATIONS	NURSING INTERVENTIONS
Metabolic Acidosis (Gain of Metabolic Acids or Loss of Base)—cont'd		
• Drug overdose (salicylates, methanol)	Oxygenation and ECG • Kussmaul breathing (deep, rapid respirations)	Monitor vital signs and I&O. Monitor and report cardiac dysrhythmias. Administer sodium bicarbonate and fluid replacement as ordered.
Loss of base: • Diarrhea	• Bradycardia, decreased cardiac output • Dysrhythmias	
	Nutrition and metabolism • Nausea, vomiting • Abdominal pain	Provide comfort measures. Correct metabolic problem as ordered. Monitor ABGs and evaluate the metabolic indicators (HCO_3^- and BE).
Metabolic Alkalosis (Gain of Base or Loss of Metabolic Acids		
Operation definition: • pH > 7.45 • HCO_3 > 28 mEq/L • BE > 2 mEq/L • Reduced serum potassium and chloride	Cognitive and sensory • Irritability, confusion	Monitor the patient's sensorium and report increasing mental confusion.
	Activity/mobility • Tetany • Hypertonic muscles • Hypertonic reflexes	Institute safety and comfort measures. Report symptoms of tetany.
Gain of base: • Excess ingestion of antacids • Excess administration of sodium bicarbonate	Oxygenation and ECG • Depressed rate and depth of respirations	Monitor vital signs and report changes in the patient's respiratory status.
Loss of metabolic acids: • Vomiting • Nasogastric suctioning or lavage • Low potassium or chloride • Increased aldosterone • Administration of steroids or diuretics	Nutrition and metabolism • Vomiting	Monitor I&O, recording amount of fluid loss from vomiting and gastric suctioning. Administer intravenous fluid ± replacement as ordered. Monitor ABGs and evaluate the metabolic indicators (HCO_3^- and BE).

Regardless of the cause, shallow or ineffective respirations lead to retention of CO_2. CO_2 retention increases the acid load in the body, leading to respiratory acidosis. Excess acid in the body acts as a CNS depressant. Patients with acidosis may exhibit a reduced level of consciousness, confusion, lethargy, or coma. Acidosis also interferes with cell functions. Myocardial cells are particularly sensitive to acidosis, which may cause serious or fatal dysrhythmias.

Treatment for respiratory acidosis is aimed at improving ventilation. Patients with surgical pain need adequate pain medication to ensure they are able to breathe deeply. Incentive spirometers may be used to encourage patients to do deep breathing exercises. Ambulation after surgery also helps to open airways and expand alveoli, promoting effective respirations. Patients with narrowed airways may use bronchodilators to improve airflow through the lungs. Patients with poor ventilation may need mechanical ventilation to promote blowing off CO_2.

Respiratory Alkalosis

Respiratory alkalosis occurs when the lungs excrete too much CO_2. By reducing the acid load in the body, the body becomes alkalotic. Anything that increases the rate and depth of respirations has the potential to cause respiratory alkalosis. Common causes include anxiety, pain, fever, and hypoxia. Anxiety increases the rate and depth of respirations through stimulation of the SNS. Pain also increases respirations by stimulating the SNS. Fever increases the metabolic rate, which increases the need for oxygen and stimulates increased respirations. Hypoxia causes an increase in respiratory rate as the body tries to acquire more oxygen; in exchange, CO_2 is lost leaving the body alkalotic.

Alkalosis is a CNS irritant. Patients may exhibit tremors, restlessness, and irritability. When severe, seizures may occur. Alkalosis changes the amount of available calcium in the bloodstream, leading to hypocalcemia. Hypocalcemia results in muscle spasms and twitches, including carpopedal spasms (Trousseau's sign) and facial muscle spasms (Chvostek's sign).

Treatment of respiratory alkalosis involves correcting the underlying problem that caused the increased respiratory rate. Relief of anxiety through careful nursing assessment and intervention, pain management, fever reduction, and oxygen administration are all interventions for respiratory alkalosis, depending on the cause. Occasionally, anxious patients will blow off too much CO_2 and will develop tingling of lips and fingers. If the patient is unable to control his or her respirations, the nurse may have the patient breathe into a paper bag, forcing rebreathing of CO_2. This helps replenish CO_2 and diminishes the tingling sensations. This intervention is not to be taken lightly, and should be performed only under controlled circumstances where further ventilatory support is possible. Excess rebreathing of CO_2 may depress respirations or cause the patient to stop breathing.

Metabolic Acidosis

Metabolic acidosis occurs when there is addition of acid to the body or loss of base. Examples of conditions causing an excess accumulation of acid include renal failure, diabetes, and inadequate oxygenation of tissues as might occur in shock. Severe diarrhea may cause loss of significant amounts of bicarbonate (base) from the GI tract.

During normal body metabolism, the body produces large quantities of acids. One of the major functions of the kidneys is to excrete the excess acids produced every day. In renal failure, all functions of the kidneys are reduced, including the ability to manage acid-base balance. The end result is an accumulation of acids in the body leading to metabolic acidosis (Lawn, Weir, & McGuire, 2006).

In type 1 diabetes mellitus, the patient produces no insulin. This results in burning of fats for energy, producing ketones as a by-product. Ketones are acids; when excessive ketones accumulate, diabetic ketoacidosis occurs, resulting in metabolic acidosis.

Any time the body has insufficient oxygen at the tissue level, cells convert to anaerobic metabolism. A by-product of anaerobic metabolism is lactic acid. As that builds up, the body develops lactic acidosis, a form of metabolic acidosis.

Acidosis, whether respiratory or metabolic in origin, is a CNS depressant. Patients may be lethargic, confused, or comatose. Patients should be monitored for cardiac dysrhythmias. Deep, rapid respirations are noted. In diabetics, these respirations are called Kussmaul respirations.

Treatment of metabolic acidosis is focused on resolving the underlying cause. Diabetics need insulin to prevent breakdown of fats for energy and production of ketones. People with chronic renal failure need dialysis to remove the acids from their bodies. People with lactic acidosis need oxygen supplementation to prevent anaerobic metabolism. Patients with diarrhea may need antidiarrheal medications while the underlying cause is addressed.

Metabolic acidosis may also result from a loss of bases from the body. Lower GI secretions are rich in bicarbonate from the pancreas, which is used to neutralize the acidic gastric contents as they move into the duodenum. Rapid transit of GI secretions through the lower GI tract, as occurs in severe diarrhea, may cause excessive loss of bicarbonate from the body, leaving the body too acidic. Crohn's disease and intestinal bypass surgeries may also produce diarrhea and loss of bicarbonate. Treatment of the diarrhea will prevent excessive loss of the bicarbonate.

Anion gap is a measurement used to help identify the cause of metabolic acidosis. **Anion gap** is that portion of negatively charged ions not measured with routine laboratory studies. Sodium is the most abundant extracellular ion. For every positively charged sodium ion, there must be a matching negatively charged ion. The anion gap represents the negative ions that are known to be present but that are not measured. Some causes of metabolic acidosis cause the anion gap to be increased; other causes do not change the anion gap (Corey, 2003). Acidosis with a normal anion gap is usually associated with an increase in chloride ions. GI losses of bicarbonate are replaced with large volumes of normal saline (0.9% NaCl solution). Diabetic ketoacidosis, lactic acidosis, and aspirin overdose cause metabolic acidosis with a high anion gap.

Metabolic Alkalosis

Metabolic alkalosis occurs when there is a loss of acid or an accumulation of base in the body. Acid is lost primarily through the upper GI tract and may occur with vomiting or with suctioning out of GI secretions through a nasogastric tube. An accumulation of base may occur through the use of antacid medications, especially with the use of baking soda (sodium bicarbonate) as an antacid.

Metabolic alkalosis results in CNS irritability, restlessness, and tremors. Seizures may occur. Cardiac monitoring is important to detect dysrhythmias.

Treatment of metabolic alkalosis is geared primarily toward removing the underlying cause. Control of vomiting and avoidance of bicarbonate antacids are primary interventions.

Arterial Blood Gases

Assessment of the body's acid-base balance is accomplished through the evaluation of ABGs. This laboratory test involves obtaining a sample of the patient's arterial blood. ABGs assess the patient's oxygenation status and acid-base status. This discussion will focus on the acid-base information in the ABGs. The oxygenation portion of the ABGs is discussed in chapter 30.

ABGs provide information on the following blood parameters: PO_2 (the pressure exerted on the arterial wall by the oxygen gas), PCO_2 (pressure of the carbon dioxide in the bloodstream), HCO_3^- (the amount of bicarbonate ion in the blood stream), pH (the acid measurement of the blood), and O_2 saturation (the percent of hemoglobin saturated with oxygen).

Normal values are:

PO_2	80–100 mm Hg
PCO_2	35–45 mm Hg
HCO_3^-	22–26 mEq/L
pH	7.35–7.45
O_2 Sat	97–100%

Interpretation of the patient's acid-base status involves evaluation of three components of the ABGs: pH, PCO_2, and HCO_3^-. There are many methods to assess ABGs. The method described here involves four steps shown in Box 12-2 and Box 12-3.

BOX 12-2

INTERPRETATION OF ARTERIAL BLOOD GASES (ABGs)

To interpret ABG results, the nurse should use the following steps:

Step 1: Assess the pH and determine if it is acid, base, or normal. Use the midline of the pH range, 7.4, for this determination (only in this step). For example, a pH of 7.47 would be identified as base. A pH of 7.39, while within normal range, would be identified as acid for this step.

Step 2: Assess the PCO_2 and the HCO_3^- and determine if they are acid, base, or normal. CO_2 adds to the acid load in the body, so an elevation in CO_2 would be called acid, while a low CO_2 value would be called base. For example, if the PCO_2 value is 49 mm Hg, it is acid; if it is 32, it is base. Bicarbonate is a base, so elevations in HCO_3^- would be called base, and low values of HCO_3^- would be called acid. For example, a HCO_3^- of 32 mEq/L would be called base, and a HCO_3^- level of 18 would be called acid. A HCO_3^- level within normal range would be called normal.

Step 3: Determine which of the CO_2 or HCO_3^-, as labeled in step 2, match the pH, as labeled in step 1. For example, if the pH is acid, the PCO_2 is acid, and the bicarbonate is base, the PCO_2 matches the pH. If the pH is acid, and the PCO_2 is base, and the HCO_3^- is acid, the HCO_3^- and the pH match. If the $PCOo_2$ and the pH match, the underlying problem is a respiratory one, if the HCO_3^- and the pH match, the underlying problem is a metabolic one.

Step 4: Determine if compensation has occurred. If the acid-base imbalance begins with a respiratory problem, the kidneys begin retaining or excreting hydrogen ions or bicarbonate as necessary to restore balance. If the acid-base imbalance occurs because of a metabolic problem, the lungs can retain or exhale carbon dioxide as needed to restore balance. To detect compensation, assess the ABG value that does not represent the primary problem. For example, if the PCO_2 and pH are both acidic, the primary problem is respiratory, so the bicarbonate is the compensating value. The bicarbonate value reveals one of three possibilities: that compensation is complete, that compensation is partially complete, or that compensation has not begun. If the compensating value is normal, no compensation has been started, and the acid-base imbalance is uncompensated. In the example of an acidic pH and PCO_2, and normal bicarbonate, the problem is respiratory acidosis, and it is uncompensated. If the compensating value has shifted out of normal range, the body has begun compensating for the acid-base imbalance. Again, with an acidic pH and PCO_2, the kidneys would compensate for the acidic state by retaining bicarbonate. Full compensation would be achieved when the pH returns to normal range. Partial compensation exists when the compensating value has moved outside of normal range, but the pH is not yet back within normal range.

Adapted from Daniels, R. (2004). Nursing fundamentals: Caring and clinical decision making. *New York: Thomson Delmar Learning; Woodruff, D. (2006). Deciphering diagnostics. Take these 6 easy steps to ABG analysis.* Nursing Made Incredibly Easy! *4(1), 4–7.*

BOX 12-3

AN EXAMPLE OF INTERPRETING ARTERIAL BLOOD GASES (ABGs)

Sample ABGs: pH 7.31 PCO_2 50 HCO_3^- 25

Step 1: Using 7.4 as the cutoff, identify whether the pH is acid or base. (In this stage, no pH is labeled as normal, even if it falls within the normal range of 7.35–7.45.)

    pH 7.31   Acid

Step 2: Label the PCO_2 and HCO_3^- as acid, base, or normal. Remember that PCO_2 acts as an acid, and HCO_3^- acts as a base. Use the full range of normal for each value.

    PCO_2 50 HCO_3^- 25
    Acid   Normal

Step 3: Identify which label (PCO_2 or HCO_3^-) matches the pH label

Label for $PCOo_2$ matches label for pH (both Acid), therefore, the problem is primarily respiratory.

Step 4: Determine if compensation has occurred. Label the ABGs as compensated, partially compensated or uncompensated.

    HCO_3^- 25 Normal (normal range 22–26 mEq/L) = uncompensated

Name the acid base status: Uncompensated respiratory acidosis.

Concept Map Case Study

Cody Barnes

Cody Barnes has been hospitalized for treatment of dehydration and electrolyte imbalances as the result of vomiting and diarrhea and influenza-like symptoms for the past three days. Cody, who is 56, had a Koch, or continent, ileostomy eight years ago. He lives in a small townhouse in a suburb of the city, and he is employed as a manager of a small restaurant. Cody eats out frequently and does not have the best nutrients in his daily intake.

Cody's admission assessment findings included muscle weakness, dry mucous membranes and lips, tachycardia, oliguria (less than 30 mL/hour), and a temperature of 38.4° C (101.2° F). The laboratory diagnostic results reported in International System Units (SI), indicated the following electrolyte imbalances for an adult: sodium: 125 mMol/L; potassium: 2.5 mMol/L; calcium: 3 mMol/L; magnesium: 1 mMol/L; bicarbonate: 20 mMol/L; chloride: 90 mMol/L; phosphorus: 0.9 mMol/L; and proteins: 14 g/L. Intravenous replacement fluids and electrolytes have been ordered.

After reading your texts, you understand that the output from an ileostomy is a caustic enzyme rich liquid that can be yellow, green, or brown in color, and the amount of liquid output is dependent on where the stoma is located in the ileum. After a time, the stool can have a paste-like consistency. A major complication for the individual with an ileostomy is the potential for fluid and electrolyte imbalances. Dehydration, deficiencies in potassium and sodium, and acidosis due to the loss of bicarbonate can occur rapidly because of diarrhea due to antibiotics, illness, or changes in diet.

You will be Cody's nurse on his second hospital day. He tells you that he is feeling much better, although he still tires easily and prefers to remain on bed rest. The diarrhea has subsided, and his electrolytes and acid-base balance are within the normal ranges. A dietitian and discharge planning coordinator are scheduled to meet with Cody today.

Refer back to discussion of fluid and electrolytes in this chapter, review content in a current medical-surgical text related to care of the person with an ileostomy. Use a current diagnostic studies text and nursing diagnosis and intervention text as needed.

Add concepts for your map from the case study into the areas where you believe they belong (some concepts may belong in more than one area). Cluster related concepts together. Draw connecting lines to indicate relationships among the clusters and with the patient.

1. What are the normal values for the electrolytes and acid-base balance? What do the diagnostic study results indicate?
2. In your assessment, what symptoms would be related to the hypokalemia, hyponatremia, and fluid volume deficit?
3. What additional information would you like to have to help you prepare a patient-centered plan of care? How will you obtain this information?
4. What information would you expect to see included in discharge planning and home care related to:
   a. Introduction of new foods into Cody's diet?
   b. Type of foods that would help to thicken his stool?
   c. How to monitor the symptoms of dehydration and electrolyte imbalances?
   d. Prevention of fluid and electrolyte imbalances and type of fluid for rapid electrolyte replacement?
5. What other precautions should Cody take to prevent
   a. Vitamin and mineral deficiencies?
   b. Infections?
   c. Skin excoriation?
6. What instructions would you give Cody regarding side effects of antibiotics and problems encountered due to dietary changes (related to the ileostomy)?

KEY CONCEPTS

- Fluid, electrolyte, and acid-base balance is closely managed through cardiovascular, renal, respiratory, and neurohormonal mechanisms.

- Imbalances in fluids, electrolytes, or acid-base impair cellular functions and may be fatal if untreated.

- Fluid volume deficit results when fluids are lost from the body or when patients are unable to access adequate fluid intake. Postural hypotension, tachycardia, and dry mucous membranes are important features. Treatment with isotonic oral or IV fluids is needed.

- Fluid volume excess results when excessive fluids are taken in or when fluids cannot be excreted. Bounding pulse, high blood pressure, and edema are common characteristics. Fluid restriction and diuretics are common interventions.

- Hyponatremia is most often associated with an excess of free water rather than a deficit of sodium. Hyponatremia is accompanied by a decrease in serum osmolality that causes water to move from the extracellular space to the intracellular space, causing cellular edema and cell death. This is most apparent in the brain and causes confusion, lethargy, and seizures. Restriction of free water and avoidance of hypotonic IV solutions are vital.

- Hypernatremia occurs with dehydration and reflects a loss of body water. Because of the increased serum osmolality that occurs, water moves from the intracellular space to the extracellular space, shrinking cells and causing confusion, lethargy, and seizures. Administration of hypotonic fluids orally or intravenously helps replenish the intracellular dehydration.

- Disorders of potassium, calcium, and magnesium affect cellular excitability and contractility. Both high and low levels affect neuromuscular and cardiac function. Immediate treatment is focused on supporting body functions such as heart rhythm and respirations. Deficits are replaced, and excess levels of electrolytes may require dialysis for removal.

- Acid-base balance is assessed through evaluation of ABGs. A determination is made as to whether the patient is acidotic or alkalotic and whether the problem is metabolic or respiratory in nature.

- Respiratory acidosis occurs when patients are unable to exhale carbon dioxide. Increasing ventilation through deep breathing, ambulation, or use of bronchodilators may help in excreting acid and restoring normal acid-base balance.

- Respiratory alkalosis is due to hyperventilation most commonly associated with such things as pain, fever, and anxiety. Correcting the underlying cause reduces respirations and allows retention of more carbon dioxide, correctly the alkalosis.

- Metabolic acidosis is due to addition of acids to the body or loss of bases. Correcting the underlying problem is important in interfering with the acidosis. Administration of sodium bicarbonate may be used in extreme cases of acidosis.

- Metabolic alkalosis occurs with loss of acid or retention of base. Emphasis is placed on reversing the problem that led to the alkalosis.

REVIEW QUESTIONS

1. Parents report their 6-month-old daughter has had diarrhea and vomiting for 24 hours. Which assessment finding do you expect to find that suggests fluid volume deficit?
   1. Swelling of extremities
   2. Increased number of diaper changes
   3. Depressed fontanelles
   4. Weight gain

2. In prioritizing patient care, you recognize that the patient most at risk for fluid volume deficit is:
   1. A 30-year-old man with a fractured tibia
   2. An 82-year-old woman with a fractured hip
   3. A 62-year-old man with a myocardial infarction
   4. A 35-year-old woman who just delivered a baby

3. A priority assessment for patients with fluid volume excess is:
   1. Mental status
   2. Weight
   3. Postural vital signs
   4. Urine output

4. A patient presents with a serum sodium level of 115 mEq/L. A priority nursing intervention is:
   1. Seizure precautions
   2. Vital signs every two hours
   3. Frequent oral care
   4. Cardiac rhythm monitoring

5. A patient receiving D_5W at 100 mL/hr is most at risk for developing:
   1. Hypernatremia
   2. Hyponatremia
   3. Fluid volume excess
   4. Fluid volume deficit

6. A patient is exhibiting sudden onset of crackles in the lungs, moist respirations, and rapid respiratory rate. Which intervention should be performed first?
   1. Weigh the patient
   2. Assess capillary refill
   3. Measure edema
   4. Reduce IV rate

7. The assessment of a patient with hypokalemia should focus on:
   1. Blood pressure
   2. Edema
   3. Chvostek's sign
   4. Heart rhythm

8. You are caring for a patient with hyperkalemia. You prepare for administration of which medication?
   1. Kayexalate
   2. K-Lor
   3. Kaopectate
   4. Keflex

9. The most important assessment in a patient with hypocalcemia is:
   1. Heart rhythm
   2. Urine output
   3. Trousseau's sign
   4. Weight

10. A patient who has experienced cardiac arrest is most at risk for:
    1. Metabolic acidosis
    2. Respiratory alkalosis
    3. Hyponatremia
    4. Fluid volume excess

11. ABGs of a patient admitted to the emergency department shows pH 7.24, PCO_2, 65 mm Hg, and HCO_3^- 24 mEq/L. The patient is diagnosed with bacterial pneumonia and is started on antibiotics and oxygen. What is a priority nursing intervention?
    1. Encourage coughing and deep breathing
    2. Monitor vital signs frequently
    3. Monitor cardiac rhythm
    4. Encourage leg exercises

12. The patient most at risk for metabolic alkalosis is:
    1. A 30-year-old postsurgical patient with undergoing nasogastric suction
    2. A 70-year-old patient in a nursing home unable to access water freely
    3. A 2-year-old infant receiving isotonic sodium chloride IV solution
    4. A 54-year-old patient who has just experienced a stroke

13. Which set of ABGs indicate compensated respiratory alkalosis?
    1. pH 7.43, PCO_2 32, HCO_3^- 18 mEq/L
    2. pH 7.49, PCO_2 32, HCO_3^- 20 mEq/L
    3. pH 7.39, PCO_2 48, HCO_3^- 28 mEq/L
    4. pH 7.43, PCO_2 38, HCO_3^- 23 mEq/L

REVIEW ACTIVITIES

1. You are caring for a patient taking the diuretic furosemide. Yesterday, the patient's weight was 62 kg. After the dose of furosemide yesterday, the patient's urine output was 2,500 mL. What do you expect the patient's weight to be today?

2. Obtain ABG results from a patient you care for. Identify the acid-base imbalance indicated in the lab results. What is the patient's condition that led to the imbalance? What signs and symptoms did the patient exhibit? How was the patient's clinical picture similar to or different from expected?

3. What types of IV solutions would be appropriate for the patient with fluid volume deficit?

4. What type of serum osmolality will result in patients with an increased secretion of ADH?

5. What type of IV solution best benefits a patient with intracellular dehydration? Why?

Infusion Therapy

Carolyn M. Schwartz, RN, MSN, APRN, BC

Therese M. Clinch, RN, MSN

CHAPTER TOPICS

- Purpose and Administration of Infusion Therapy

- Complications of Infusion Therapy

- Central Venous Catheters

- Total Parenteral Nutrition

- Blood Components and Transfusions

- Infusion Therapy in Oncology, Pain Management, Sedation, and Hemodynamic Monitoring

- Legal and Ethical Aspects of Infusion Therapy

- Future of Infusion Therapy

KEY TERMS

Extravasation
Half-life
Hypertonic
Hypotonic
Infiltration
Isotonic
Nosocomial
Percent solution
Phlebitis
Sepsis
Total parenteral nutrition (TPN)
Vesicant

Infusion therapy is a relevantly young science, having seen rapid growth in the last 75 years. Prior to that time, infusion therapy consisted largely of experiments and crude techniques. Until the discovery of the germ theory of disease, infection and incompatibility plagued the infusion therapy world. Advances in infusion therapy continue today, resulting in changes in practice related to equipment, medications, and techniques. It remains the nurse's responsibility to maintain current knowledge related to the safe practice of infusion therapy.

ANATOMY AND PHYSIOLOGY

The skin is the largest organ of the body. The main function of the skin is to protect the body by providing a barrier between the environment and the internal structures of the body (Delaune & Ladner, 2006). Any compromise of this barrier invites infectious organisms into the body. Any break in the barrier can lead to illnesses ranging from minor local infections to major systemic life-threatening ones. Venipuncture not only violates the skin barrier but can also introduce microorganisms into the venous system. Many factors can increase the risk of developing an infection. Some, such as age, immune status, and the presence of other illnesses, cannot be controlled. There are, however, factors that the nurse can control. These include careful site preparation, vein selection, site maintenance, careful handling of equipment, tubing, fluids, and fluid containers. Reports indicate that almost all patients admitted to the hospital will receive some type of infusion therapy. Infusion therapy is one of the leading causes of **nosocomial** (or hospital acquired) infections in patients resulting in longer lengths of stay, higher cost of health care, and, sometimes, death.

Successful infusion therapy relies on a healthy and functioning peripheral vascular system. The peripheral vascular system consists of veins and arteries carrying blood, oxygenated and un-oxygenated, throughout the body providing nutrients to the tissues. Knowledge of the structure and function of the peripheral vascular system is imperative when initiating and maintaining infusion therapy.

Arteries and veins have three basic layers, ranging from the deepest layer (tunica intima), to the middle layer (tunica media) and the outer layer (tunica adventitia). Both arteries and veins contain these three layers, but variations in the structure and function of these layers occur between arteries and veins. Arteries carry oxygenated blood to the tissues. Arterial walls are under higher pressure as the heart pumps the blood though out the body. The wall of the artery contains an elastic membrane that enables the artery wall to stretch in response to the pumping of the heart. Arteries are not typically used for infusion therapy. Veins contains valves that prevent the blood from pooling, thereby moving the blood back toward the heart by utilizing the venous muscle pump. The venous pump is activated by the contraction of muscles during movement. This causes the proximal valve to open and the distal valve to close, preventing the backflow of blood. The newer, softer, more flexible IV catheters used today may be inadvertently dislodged from the vein because of this pumping action.

Veins are classified as superficial or deep. Deep veins can be found close to arteries that bear the same name. Superficial veins lie just under the surface of the skin, thereby making them the choice for infusion therapy. These veins are found in the upper extremities in the forearm and hand. The dorsal metacarpal veins are located on the back of the hand. They are typically easy to find, have less subcutaneous tissue surrounding them, and are the most distal site in the upper extremities. Venipuncture at these sites may limit the patient's use of the hand, and the patient's arm may need to be immobilized with an arm board (splint) to decrease movement of the catheter. The veins of the hand are not suitable for infusing certain medications that can cause tissue damage if they leak outside the vein. There is little subcutaneous tissue in the hands to absorb the drug, which can result in extensive damage to tendons and nerves.

There are a variety of veins that can be accessed via venipuncture. The cephalic vein runs along the thumb side of the wrist. It is a large vein that is easy to access. If the catheter is placed too close to the wrist, joint movement may cause dislodgement of the catheter, or the patient may experience numbness and tingling of the thumb and possibly permanent nerve damage, as the radial nerve lies close to the cephalic vein. It is safer to perform venipuncture higher

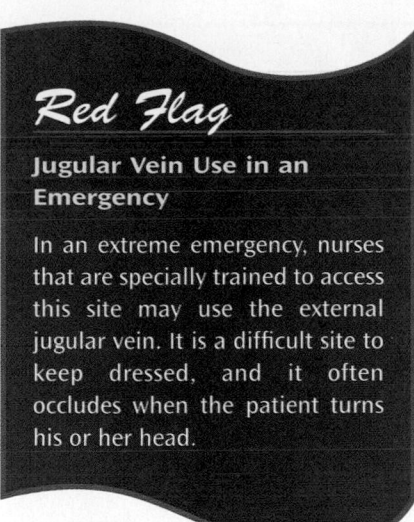

up the cephalic vein toward the antecubital fossa. The median vein is located on the anterior forearm starting at the wrist and ending just below the antecubital fossa. Although this vein maybe difficult to visualize, it is easy to stabilize and access. The lower portion of this vein closest to the wrist is a painful site for venipuncture and because of its location tends to be a short-lived site. The basilic vein runs along the little finger of the arm. It is large and often overlooked because of its location. It tends to roll when attempting to access. To utilize this site, the nurse should place the patient's forearm across his or her chest and access the vein from the opposite side of the bed. Veins in the foot and leg should not routinely be used as they may compromise circulation, potentially leading to infection or blood clots and limit the patient's ability to ambulate.

Types of Fluids

An **isotonic** solution causes no fluid shift between compartments but rather expands circulating volume in the body. These solutions have the same tonicity as plasma. **Hypertonic** solutions cause fluid to move out of the cells resulting in shrinkage of the cells. **Hypotonic** solutions cause fluid to move into the cells leading to swelling and in some instances, bursting of cells. The type of fluid prescribed for the patient will depend on the type of deficit the patient is experiencing (Table 13-1).

EQUIPMENT AND PRODUCT SELECTION

Choosing appropriate IV therapy equipment requires an understanding of the purpose of the therapy, as well as the advantages and disadvantages of the available equipment. A clear understanding of the product is imperative, as equipment should be used only for purposes specified by the manufacturer. IV therapy equipment undergoes changes according to federal safety guidelines in an effort to protect the nurse and the patient. Therefore, nurses carry the responsibility of maintaining current knowledge of equipment, products, and their uses.

There are six main types of administration sets: (a) primary sets (main tubing), which consist of a spike, a drip chamber, roller clamp, and medication ports; (b) secondary (piggyback) sets, which are used with a primary set typically for intermittent medication administration and shorter in length than primary sets; (c) vented sets, which have a small vent on the spike of the tubing that may require removing a removable cap over the vent; (d) nonvented sets, which are used with a collapsible plastic container, such as a plastic IV solution bag; (e) metered volume chamber sets that are designed to limit the amount of fluid a patient can receive and are often used for intermittent infusions (e.g., used in critical care settings, pediatric settings, and volume-restricted patients); and (f) primary Y sets which have two separate spikes for two IV solutions to be run simultaneously and are used most often in critical care, trauma, or surgery for rapid infusion of fluids. The administration set tubing is relatively standard and comes in three main types: (a) standard tubing, which is the most commonly used type, and almost all infusions can be given through standard lumen tubing; (b) macrobore tubing, which has a larger inner lumen to accommodate high flow rates as in anesthesia sets and trauma sets; and (c) microbore tubing, which has a smaller than standard inner lumen to avoid accidental bolus or rapid infusion and is commonly found in pain management, syringe pump administration, and for prolonged infusions of small amounts of medication (Altman, 2004).

The rate control devices are connected to the administration sets and are the equipment that controls the speed of infusion. The most common is the roller clamp, which is affected by the height of the fluid container, patient movement, and ambulation. There is also a slide and pinch clamp, which are not regulated by clamps but can be easily operated with one hand and provide on/off capability. In

TABLE 13-1   Common IV Therapy Solutions

COMMON IV SOLUTION	COMPONENTS	CLINICAL USE	PRECAUTIONS	NURSING ACTIONS
Volume Expanders				
D_5W (hypotonic) Also listed isotonic	Carbohydrates in water	Provides calories for essential energy	Do not administer with blood	Monitor intake and output
$D_{10}W$ (hypertonic)		Provides breakdown of protein needs	Will cause hemolysis of red cells	Monitor serum K^+
$D_{20}W$ (hypertonic)				
$D_{500}W$ (hypertonic)		Prevents dehydration	Electrolyte-free solutions may result in hypokalemia	
		Improves hepatic function		
D_5 1/3 (hypertonic)	Carbohydrates in normal saline (NS)	Hypertonic solutions useful to pull fluid from tissues into bloodstream, such as burns, increased intracranial pressure (ICP) and postoperatively to keep swelling from operative site	Do not administer to patients with cellular dehydration	Monitor intake and output
D_5 1/2 hypertonic			Use cautiously in patients with cardiac disease, congestive heart failure (CHF), hypertension, and other fluid volume excesses or deficits because additional fluid will be moved into the bloodstream	Monitor vital signs
				Monitor serum electrolytes
				Monitor for signs and symptoms of CHF
		Provides sodium chloride		
D_5NS (hypertonic)	Carbohydrates in NS	Temporary treatment for excessive fluid loss	Use with caution in patients with cardiac, renal, and hepatic disease	Monitor intake and output
		Early treatment along with plasma or albumin for fluid loss due to burns	May result in acidosis and hypokalemia	Monitor vital signs
				Monitor patient for circulatory overload and shortness of breath
		Treatment for acute adrenocortical insufficiency		Monitor serum K^+
NaCl 0.9% (isotonic; same tonicity as plasma)	Sodium chloride	Restores circulatory volume	Use with caution in patients with cardiac, renal, and hepatic disease	Monitor intake and output
		Treatment for hypovolemic hypotension	May result in acidosis and hypokalemia	Monitor vital signs
		Treatment for metabolic acidosis		Monitor patient for circulatory overload and shortness of breath
		Replaces sodium chloride deficit		Monitor serum K^+
		Initiation and termination of blood transfusions		

Continued

TABLE 13-1 Common IV Therapy Solutions—cont'd

COMMON IV SOLUTION	COMPONENTS	CLINICAL USE	PRECAUTIONS	NURSING ACTIONS
Volume Expanders—cont'd				
0.45% NS (hypotonic) 0.33% NS (hypotonic)	Sodium chloride	Replaces sodium chloride deficits Treatment for cellular dehydration	Do not administer to patients with increased ICP, burns, or edema	Monitor intake and output Monitor vital signs Monitor extremities for edema
Ringer's lactate (isotonic) Ringer's injection (isotonic)	Contains sodium chloride, potassium, calcium, and lactate Content approximates that of plasma and includes sodium, potassium, calcium, and chloride	Replaces surgical and GI losses Treats dehydration Fluid losses due to diarrhea and burns Used to replace electrolytes Provides water for hydration Often used to replace extracellular fluid losses	Use with caution in patients with renal, cardiac, and liver diseases Do not use in severe metabolic acidosis or alkalosis Does not contain calories Use with caution in patients with renal, cardiac, and liver diseases; can cause over hydration, electrolyte excess, and caloric depletion	Monitor intake and output Monitor vital signs Monitor blood gases Monitor intake and output Monitor serum electrolytes Monitor blood gases
Plasma Expanders				
Dextran 6% in NS Dextran 5% in sterile water Mannitol Hetastarch Albumin	Dextran Mannitol Hetastarch Albumin (natural plasma protein)	Increases blood volume temporarily Restores excessive fluid loss due to hypovolemic shock Promotes diuresis and excretion of toxic substances For ICP and cerebral edema Reduces intraocular pressure Increases blood volume Increase granulocyte yield during leukapheresis Used for plasma volume expansion in treating shock or impending shock related to a circulatory volume deficit 5% generally used to treat hypovolemia	Do not use as sole replacement of blood Initially administered at keep vein open rate to observe for possible reactions Can cause hypovolemia and electrolyte imbalances Extravasation can lead to skin irritation and necrosis. Preexisting conditions should be considered, such as renal or cardiac disease Can cause hypovolemia, electrolyte imbalances, tissue dehydration, anaphylactic reactions, and increased bleeding times	Observe for allergic reactions such as wheezing, mild urticaria, nausea, and vomiting Notify nurse manager and health care provider Monitor intake and output Monitor vital signs Monitor serum electrolytes Monitor IV site Monitor hydration Monitor labs for bleeding times, platelets, H & H Monitor for volume overload Monitor labs for serum protein and hematocrit

Continued

TABLE 13-1   Common IV Therapy Solutions—cont'd

COMMON IV SOLUTION	COMPONENTS	CLINICAL USE	PRECAUTIONS	NURSING ACTIONS
Plasma Expanders—cont'd				
		5% reserved for treatment when there are fluid and sodium restrictions	Preexisting conditions should be considered, such as renal or cardiac disease	
			The potential for complications should be considered if cardiac, hepatic, or renal disease is present	
			Increased circulating volume may result in fluid overload	
			Rapid influx and excretion of fluid may dilute or deplete electrolytes	
Fat emulsions intralipid 10%, 20%	Essential fatty acids	Provides a source of calories and essential fatty acids for metabolic processes	Do not administer to patients with hyperlipidemia, lipoid nephrosis, or acute pancreatitis	Observe for adverse reactions Administer only at prescribed dose and rate
			Administer with a filter and proper IV tubing. Do not add medications to fat emulsions. Do not hang for more than 16 hours	

Adapted from Broyles, B. E., Reiss, B. S., & Evans, M. E. (2007). Pharmacological aspects of nursing care (7th ed.). New York: Thomson Delmar Learning.

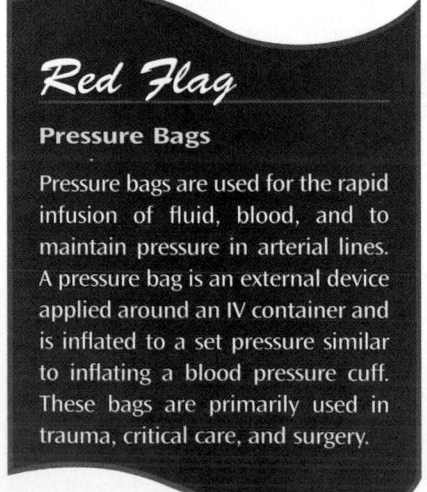

Red Flag

Pressure Bags

Pressure bags are used for the rapid infusion of fluid, blood, and to maintain pressure in arterial lines. A pressure bag is an external device applied around an IV container and is inflated to a set pressure similar to inflating a blood pressure cuff. These bags are primarily used in trauma, critical care, and surgery.

addition, there are manual flow control devices that are used to control the rate of flow of fluids instead of using the roller clamp or infusion pump. There are also resealable Y injection ports that are part of the needleless tubing system and are able to reseal after being punctured by a needle or a blunt plastic cannula. A piece of the resealable port can be removed or compromised during a single or multiple needle penetration, which allows air or bacteria to enter the infusion line. There are also back check valves, which are one-way valves that allow the fluid to flow in one direction only and are usually part of the standard IV administration tubing. There are also a variety of additional add-on devices that can be used with infusion therapy (Box 13-1).

Infusion Pumps

Infusion pumps are sensitive devices used to ensure a high likelihood of accuracy when infusing fluids into patients. There are many features to ensure patient safety. The pump will alarm when there is something wrong with the infusion, such as air in the line, occlusion, end of infusion, and low battery. The

ADD-ON DEVICES FOR INFUSION THERAPY

Stopcocks: These devices are used to direct the flow of fluid in the IV line. They are typically three- or four-way devices. They are commonly used to infuse other solutions intermittently or to inject medication into a line. There is a high risk of error using stopcocks as they may be accidentally turned, stopping the flow of fluid, may disconnect, or the portals may not be recapped and become contaminated.

Extension sets: These sets are used to add length and additional medication ports to primary tubing. These sets should not be used routinely as they may end up lying on the floor when the patient is in bed and therefore become contaminated. The set may add too much length to the primary tubing and can become entangled in the bedrails or when the patient is ambulating.

Infusion caps/Intermittent infusion loops: These caps or loops are used to convert a continuous infusion to an intermittent infusion. These devices allow the IV cannula to remain in place for use later. They can be as small as one half inch length cap, to a three- to four-inch capped loop. The set is flushed with either heparin or saline between uses to maintain patency, depending on the institution's policy.

Filters: The purpose of the filter is to eliminate air and particles of a certain size that should not be infused into the patient. Filters come in different sizes with varying capabilities of filtering particles depending on what medication is being infused. Bacteria, viruses, fungi, and particulate matter can be separated out of solutions by the use of the proper sized filter. Filters can be added as a single unit or as part of an extension set.

Needleless access devices: These are used at medication ports for safety reasons. Do not use steel needles to access the medication ports. Use needleless access devices, such as the blunt plastic cannula. Another needleless system utilizes Luer connections at the medication ports. A third type of needleless system uses the traditional injection port, but the needle used to penetrate it recessed inside a protective covering.

Adapted from Altman, G. (2004). Delmar's fundamental and advanced nursing skills *(2nd ed.). New York: Thomson Delmar Learning; Broyles, B. E., Reiss, B. S., & Evans, M. E. (2007).* Pharmacological aspects of nursing care *(7th ed.). New York: Thomson Delmar Learning.*

nurse should be comfortable with the way the pump works, so that the alarms can be resolved with no harm to the patient. The pump can be programmed to infuse at a high rate of accuracy. Many pumps can even infuse fractions of drops at a time. Other programming features include changing the rate of the infusion, infusing by volume, or infusing by time. A different rate for secondary infusions can also be programmed, and when the secondary infusion is completed, the pump resorts to the already programmed primary rate (Figure 13-1).

Patients outside of the hospital setting use ambulatory pumps. They are small enough to fit into a small backpack or fanny pack. These pumps have allowed patients who need infusions outside of the hospital to go home and to work or school. They are designed with safety features, alarms, and memory and can be programmed for different infusion rates.

Patient-controlled analgesia (PCA) pumps infuse pain medications continuously and can give intermittent doses when the patient pushes a button. This empowers patients to control their pain management, and in fact, patients use less pain medication overall because pain medication levels in the blood stay

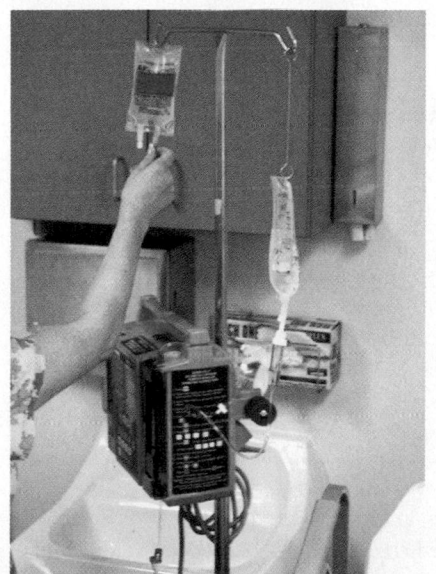

Figure 13-1 A nurse administering IV solutions using an infusion pump.

relatively constant. The pump is programmed to deliver only a set continuous dose (optional) and extra doses at prescribed intervals (also optional) with a set hourly limit to prevent accidental overdose. It is imperative that the pump is programmed according to the institution's policy to ensure accuracy and patient safety.

Multichannel and dual channel pumps allow multiple solution infusion rates to be programmed into one device and run simultaneously. This eliminates the need for multiple single channel pumps at the bedside. The advancement in technology has allowed pumps to evolve to where they can safely be used outside of the hospital setting, in the home, in the community, or in an ambulatory setting.

PROCEDURE OF INFUSION THERAPY

Prior to initiating IV therapy, the nurse must review and understand the physician's orders, assess the patient, and gather the proper equipment. Then the nurse can prepare and perform the venipuncture. Different methods of cleaning the area to make the procedure aseptic are used, and changes are made as research reveals the best practice (see Uncovering the Evidence).

Recently, there has continued to be an emphasis on the use of safe equipment and many health care workers complain about the new safety cannulas being cumbersome and difficult to use. For these reasons, there is much resistance to the federally mandated switch to safety products. Hoarding of nonsafety catheters continued until the deadline for all safety cannulas was in force. At the 2004 Annual Meeting of the American Society of Anesthesiologists, an informal meeting was held to discuss these issues. One solution proposed was to encourage the manufacturers of IV cannulas to continue to manufacture the nonsafety cannulas. Concern for patient safety was cited as the reason for this proposal. Many health care workers are concerned that in an emergency,

---

Safety First

PCA by Proxy

The nurse will frequently encounter patients who are not capable of pushing the PCA button on their own. Well-intentioned family members or nurses may push the button, believing that they are helping the patient who cannot push the button independently. When the nurse does this, it is referred to as nurse controlled analgesia (NCA), a form of PCA by proxy. The problem with PCA by proxy is that the main safeguard of the PCA system is disabled. A sedated patient would no longer push the PCA button, reducing the risk of an overdose. There have been numerous cases of patients receiving too much medication and even dying as a result of PCA by proxy. The Institute for Safe Medication Practices (ISMP) discourages PCA by proxy, but recognizes that with clear policies, NCA may be safe if additional monitoring is implemented for the patient, such as pulse oximetry and more frequent assessments of patient sedation and pain control response. Careful selection criteria should be clearly outlines to identify which patients may be appropriate for PCA by proxy.

Adapted from Broyles, B. E., Reiss, B. S., & Evans, M. E. (2007). Pharmacological aspects of nursing care (7th ed.). New York: Thomson Delmar Learning.

Uncovering the Evidence

Chlorhexidine versus Povidone-Iodine Solution

Discussion: In this study, chlorhexidine and povidone-iodine solution were compared for rates of vascular catheter-related infections. Patients were randomly placed in either the chlorhexidine group or the povidone-iodine group. Various types of catheters were studied, and all participants were in a hospital setting. The risk of central catheter-related bloodstream infections was reduced by 49 percent with the use of chlorhexidine as a skin antiseptic. This study demonstrates the advantage of using chlorhexidine as a site prep that decreases the risk of bloodstream infections. Chlorhexidine is readily available now in the United States and is recommended by the Centers for Disease Control and Prevention (CDC) as a preferred skin antiseptic prior to venipuncture.

Implications for Practice: The health care system in general will continue to have less infections related to infusion therapy. This reduces health care costs, as well as increasing the well-being of the patients. Nurses benefit by decreasing the risks of the infusion procedures and creating greater success with their nursing care.

Source: Chaiyakunapruk, N., Veenstra, D., Lipsky, B., & Saint, S. (2002). Chlorhexidine compared with povidone-iodine solution for vascular catheter-site care: A meta-analysis. Annals of Internal Medicine, 136(11), 792–801.

establishing IV access may be delayed because of the new products. A second proposal was put forth, which is to work with the manufacturers of these products to find cannulas that are easier to use, yet still provide the safety features necessary to meet the intention of the federal act. Newer, more user-friendly cannulas have continued to enter the marketplace. More reliable safety features with less change in practice are satisfying both sides of this debate (Hughes & Martin, 2005).

IV Procedure Special Considerations

When performing an IV initiation, the nurse needs to remember the effects of the fight-or-flight response. The nurse may recall that the peripheral vessels constrict to promote more blood flow to the vital organs. If the patient picks up on the nurse's nervousness or becomes anxious for any reason, the nurse is more likely to face vasoconstriction and a more difficult IV start. In addition, the nurse should use the correct size cannula for the job. Nurses should not insert a large bore cannula just because a huge vein is spotted. Besides the pain factor, it is well documented that larger catheters have a higher phlebitis rate than smaller ones. This is a mechanical response to the presence of the catheter. It can also lead to a chemical phlebitis because of less hemodilution of the medication. The smaller the catheter, the more blood flows around it, therefore diluting the medication more. If the IV is running to gravity, a larger bore will cause a larger volume of extravasate if the IV infiltrates. The nurse should also be wary of trouble spots, such as veins over joints. If the nurse has to place an IV over a joint, the nurse should think about using an arm board. Immobilizing the site will prolong the life of the IV as well as decrease mechanical phlebitis. Another consideration is for the nurse to try hanging the extremity over the side of the bed and wait a minute or so. This will promote venous distension allowing the nurse to visualize the vein. In general, the nurse might try using a warm towel or heating pad to assist with distension of elusive veins. Veins dilate in the presence of warmth, which can be an advantage for the nurse. The nurse should take time in finding the right vein. The nurse can let the patient know that he or she is looking for the right vein. This gives the nurse time to gather thoughts and find the best vein. It also puts the patient more at ease thinking that the nurse obviously knows what he or she is doing. The nurse can try rotating the arm in quarter turns, which may cause the vein to distend with the arm in a different position. The nurse can also consider an anesthetic for anxious patients. The nurse should not release the tourniquet too soon. After the flash back, the catheter can be advanced slightly. In addition, the nurse should not have the patient pump his or her fist. This has actually been shown to increase vasospasm. Instead, it is usually better to have the patient relax his or her arm. It is important to communicate effectively during the procedure as shown in the Skills 360° feature. After successfully starting the IV, secure the site well. The only way the nurse can use tape directly over the IV site and under the transparent dressing is if it is sterile tape. Secure the catheter to the skin using a chevron approach. Do not cover the connection between the IV tubing and the catheter with the transparent dressing. If the connector needs to be changed (converting a running IV to a saline lock) having to peel the dressing back can cause the catheter to dislodge and will necessitate a new dressing at a minimum.

IV COMPLICATIONS

As previously discussed in this chapter, any break in the skin barrier has the potential to cause infection. IV therapy presents many opportunities for infection to occur. Improper site preparation, contamination of equipment or fluids, and inadequate cannula stabilization are all factors within the nurse's control. Recognizing which patients are especially vulnerable to infection is another important weapon in the battle against infection. The key to reducing IV-related IV infections can be as simple as performing good hand washing prior to venipuncture. In the CDC guidelines for the prevention of catheter-related infections, proper hand hygiene is strongly recommended as the first step in reducing the risk of IV site infection. When preparing the IV equip-ment, maintain asepsis when opening packages and spiking IV fluid bags. Follow the institution's policies regarding when IV tubing and fluid containers are changed. Site preparation is the next important consideration when safe-guarding against infection. Once the site is prepped, the nurse should not touch the site unless sterile gloves are worn. The nurse should pay attention to the health of the skin on his or her hands. Nurses undergo frequent hand washing, which can lead to small breaks in the skin. These breaks can harbor bacteria, which can be transmitted to the patient. Remember to follow the institution's policy on the use of antiseptic soaps and lotions.

Monitor the IV site for signs of infection. These include pain, redness, swelling, or discharge from the site. The patient may also be febrile. If the IV is suspected of being the source of infection, remove the cannula and send it to the laboratory for culture according to the institution's policy. Occasionally, the IV tubing or IV fluid container may be the source of the infection. Add-on devices can be the source of tubing infection as each add-on device opens the system to organisms. This type of infection can be difficult to distinguish from infection from other sources; but when suspected, the nurse should send the tubing and IV bag to the laboratory for culture. Occasionally, the equipment and fluid can be contaminated in the manufacturing process. If a cluster of infections occurs, the infection control nurse should be alerted so that the products can be tracked and the manufacturer notified if indicated.

Infections that progress to the bloodstream causing systemic infections are called **sepsis.** Sepsis can lead to death, even with the best treatment. Patients with comorbid factors and then suffer from sepsis have high mortality rates (Daniels, 2004).

Phlebitis

Phlebitis refers to the inflammation of a vein. A patient with phlebitis may have redness, warmth over the IV site, pain, elevated body temperature, and a hard, palpable cord along the vein track. Phlebitis may occur in two differ-ent ways. Mechanical phlebitis occurs when the vein becomes inflamed from the cannula. The cannula may be too large for the vein, may not be well secured, allowing it to move back and forth, or may be placed over a joint, also allowing movement of the cannula within the vein. Chemical phlebitis occurs when the medication itself causes irritation of the vein wall. Some medications are acidic, and others are alkalotic. Either type of solution can irritate the vein wall. Depending on the medication being infused, a chemical buffer may be added to reduce this effect. If that is not possible or is ineffective, a larger vein should be selected. A larger vein allows more blood to flow around the can-nula, diluting the medication as it is infused, decreasing the chemical irrita-tion. It is also important to use filters when indicated, as some particles can also lead to vein wall irritation. To decrease the risk of phlebitis, the nurse should use the smallest, shortest cannula necessary to deliver the therapy. Additionally, properly secure the cannula and avoid placement over joints to minimize movement of the cannula.

Infiltration

Infiltration refers to the leakage of the IV fluid out of the vein and into the surrounding tissue. Infiltration may occur by a number of routes. A common way for an IV to infiltrate is by mechanical means. A poorly secured catheter or one placed over a joint can become easily dislodged from the vein, infusing into the tissue around the vein. Another culprit is inflammation of the vein. The factors that can lead to phlebitis can also lead to infiltration. An inflamed vein wall is weakened, making it easy to be punctured by the cannula. Additionally, the endothelial cell lining of the vein wall becomes leaky when injured because of the chemical mediators that are released when injury occurs (Hadaway, 2002).

Infiltration may cause swelling at the site, coolness to the touch, pain, and blanching of the skin. Unfortunately, not all patients show these symptoms. In patients who already have edema and circulatory compromise, swelling and coolness may not be apparent. The type of fluid may dictate the symptoms of infiltration. A hypertonic solution draws fluid out of cells and tends to cause more pain than hypotonic solutions do. Hypotonic solutions are more readily absorbed by the tissues, but as fluid is pulled back into cells, they may swell and burst, leading to additional fluid leaking into the surrounding tissue. The condition of the patient may also affect how much fluid escapes into the tissue. Elderly patients who tend to have loose skin with less subcutaneous tissue will be able to harbor more fluid in their tissues, whereas, the younger individuals have elastic skin with plenty of subcutaneous tissue, which slows the infusion down sooner. Fluids delivered by pump will tend to leak a larger volume because of the pressure of the pump infusing than will gravity delivered fluids.

The nurse should not only monitor the insertion site but also where the cannula tip is. If just the tip has come out of the vein wall, the signs of infiltration may only occur there, distal to the actual venipuncture site (Haldaway, 2002). If infiltration is suspected, the nurse should compare both arms to see if there is a significant difference in the diameter of the arms. The dominant arm should be a bit larger (approximately a half inch in diameter), but significant differences could mean infiltration. Was the patient lying on the IV site or tubing, impeding flow? If so, correct the patient's position and continue to monitor the site. The nurse should not rely solely on blood return to determine if infiltration has occurred. Blood return may still be visible with an infiltrated IV. Perhaps the cannula is still in the vein, but the wall is leaky because inflammation. Another scenario is that the cannula tip may only be partially out of the vein, still enabling blood to be aspirated from the vein. Conversely, a lack of blood return does not always mean that the cannula is no longer in the vein. Small-gauge cannulas are easily collapsed when aspirating from them and may not allow blood to flow back through them. There may be a fibrin sheath inside the cannula, blocking the flow of blood back into the cannula (Hadaway, 2002).

Extravasation

Another complication of IV therapy is **extravasation.** Although many nurses use these terms interchangeably, they are actually different processes. Infiltration, as previously described, refers to the infusion of IV fluid or medications outside of the vein into the surrounding tissue. Extravasation is similar, but it involves the infusion of a vesicant into the surrounding tissue. A **vesicant** is a solution that is capable of causing tissue injury and necrosis. Many patients have required plastic surgery to repair the damage of extravasation. The nurse follows the same precautions as outlined with infiltration but in addition knows which drugs are considered vesicants. Many chemotherapy agents, antibiotics, and vasopressor drugs are vesicants. The nurse should not infuse these drugs into the small veins of the hand, which are surrounded not by subcutaneous tissue but by tendons and nerves. Damage here can be severe. Many vesicants must be infused through a large vein in the central circulation. The nurse should be familiar with the institution's policies on infusing vesicant medications.

If extravasation occurs, the cannula should not be removed until it is determined if an antidote exists. Some medications have antidotes that limit the local damage if given in a reasonable amount of time. If an antidote exists, instill it through the cannula into the area of extravasation. After the antidote is instilled, remove the cannula and elevate the extremity. Most extravasations should have cold compresses applied to them, but a few others require warm compresses. The physician should be notified, and an incident report should be completed if the institution's policy calls for it.

Nerve Damage

Nerve damage is another type of complication that can occur with IV therapy. It occurs when nerves are injured during venipuncture. Nerves may be nicked when probing to find the vein. Nerves may also be compressed when infiltration or a hematoma occurs or when the tourniquet is left on too long. To prevent these types of injuries, which may be lifelong for the patient, the nurse chooses the venipuncture site carefully. Familiarity with normal anatomy can help the nurse avoid nerves, although anatomic differences in people do occur. Another consideration is to avoid the cephalic vein close to the wrist. If this vein must be used, the nurse chooses a site a few inches above the wrist to decrease the chance of hitting the nerve. The nurse should not spend too much time attempting to start the IV and should try another site or ask a colleague for assistance. Stabilize the vein as best as possible. If bleeding occurs, the nurse should hold pressure long enough to prevent the formation of a hematoma. Patients who experience nerve damage may complain of an electric sensation running along the nerve, numbness or tingling in the area supplied by the nerve, or pain that changes when the cannula is moved. If the patient complains of any of these symptoms, the nurse should remove the cannula, document the complaint, and notify the physician if the symptoms do not resolve with removal of the cannula.

IV THERAPY CALCULATIONS

Medication administration is often part of the patient's plan of care. The patient's physician is responsible for prescribing the appropriate medication, and it is the nurse's responsibility to ensure that the medication order is accurate and safe for the patient. The accurate and safe administration of medication depends on a variety of calculations. The nurse, health care provider, and pharmacist works closely together ensure that the medication regimen is safe and appropriate for the patient. Ultimately, the nurse will administer the medication, so the responsibility to make sure that the medication is the right drug for the right patient and administered at the correct dose, rate, route, and time lies with the nurse. Understanding the purpose of the medication, the route of administration, and the side effects of the medication is the first step in safe medication administration. The measurement system of choice by the medical profession is the metric system. It is more accurate than the household or apothecary measuring system for calculating drug dosages. Again, it is extremely important to be accurate in drug calculation especially for medication that is administered directly into the bloodstream (Broyles, et al., 2007).

The most commonly used weights range from largest to smallest: kilogram (kg), gram (g), milligram (mg), and microgram (mcg). Units of volume range from largest to smallest: liter (L) to milliliter (mL). These are the measurement of choice for calculating IV drugs. The other unit of measurement used in health care is length. Length is measured in meters, such as millimeter (mm) and centimeter (cm). However, it is seldom used in IV dose calculations (Rice, 2002).

Ratio-Proportion Method

Ratio is the comparison between two related items, and a proportion is the equality of two ratios (Rice, 2002). To set up this method, start with what you know about the drug on the label, i.e. strength of the drug on hand (H) and volume of the drug on hand (V). Take this information and set it up in a form of a ratio (H:V) on the left side of the equal sign (=):

$$\text{H:V (ratio)} = \underline{\hspace{2cm}} \text{(proportion)}$$

The ratio for the dose desired is the relationship of the dosed ordered (D) and the amount to give (G), and this is placed to the right side of the equal sign (=):

$$\text{H:V (ratio)} = \text{D:G (proportion)}$$

Thus the strength on hand (H) is related (:) to the volume (V) as the dose ordered (D) is related (:) to the amount to give (G).

The product of the means must equal the product of the extremes. In the sample above, the extremes are always the two outside number (H and G) and the means are the two inside numbers (V and D).

$$2 \text{ (H)}:4 \text{ (V)} = 4 \text{ (D)}:8 \text{ (G)}$$

Multiply the extremes together ($2 \times 8 = 16$). Multiply the means together ($4 \times 4 = 16$). The product of the extremes equals the product of the means.

When one of the numbers in the proportion is unknown, it is identified with an X. Using the sample above, the 8 is replaced with an X:

$$2 \text{ (H)}:4 \text{ (V)} = 4 \text{ (D)}:X$$

$$2X \text{ (extremes)} = 16 \text{ (means)}$$

$$X = 8$$

Formula Method

The formula method uses the same terminology as the ratio-proportion method, but the set up of the equation is different. It is as follow:

$$\text{Amount to give (G)} = \frac{\text{Dose ordered (D)}}{\text{Strength on hand (H)}} \times \text{Volume (V)}$$

Using the sample above, the formula method is express by the following:

$$X \text{ (G)} = \frac{4 \text{ (D)}}{2 \text{ (H)}} \times \frac{4}{1} \text{ (V)} = \frac{16}{2} = 16 \div 2 = 8$$

The answer is 8.

Example 1: A vial contains Keflex 500 mg/4 mL. What volume must be given to administer 250 mg?

Ratio-proportion method:

$$\text{H (mg)}:\text{V (mL)} = \text{D (mg)}:\text{G (mL)}$$

$$500{:}4 = 250{:}X$$

$$500X = 1{,}000$$

$$X = 2 \text{ mL of Keflex}$$

Formula method:

$$G = \frac{D}{H} \times V$$

$$X = \frac{250}{500} \times \frac{4}{1} = \frac{1{,}000}{500} = 1{,}000 \div 500 = 2 \text{ mL of Keflex}$$

Example 2: A vial contains ampicillin, 1.5 g/mL. What volume must be given to administer 750 mg? The dose on hand and dose ordered are not identical units of measure. Using the conversion table, convert grams to milligrams:

$$1.5g \times 1,000 = 1,500 \text{ mg}$$

Ratio-proportion method:

$$H \text{ (mg)}:V \text{ (mL)} = D \text{ (mg)}:G \text{ (mL)}$$

$$1,500:1 = 750:X$$

$$1,500X = 750$$

$$X = 0.5 \text{ mL of ampicillin}$$

Formula method:

$$X = \frac{750}{1,500} \times \frac{1}{1} = \frac{750}{1,500} = 750 \div 1,500 = 0.5 \text{ mL of Keflex}$$

Percent Solutions

A **percent solution** is a measure of parts per hundred. This means that 1 g of a drug in 100 mL of solution is 1% solution. Most solutions administered intravenously are in the form of a percent solution. The nurse can use either the ratio-proportion method or formula method when calculation percent solutions (Rice, 2002).

Ratio-proportion method:

$$g:mL = g:mL$$

$$10:100 = X:1,000$$

$$100X = 10,000$$

$$X = 100 \text{ g of drug required for a 10% solution}$$

Formula method:

$$X = \frac{10}{100} \times 1,000 = \frac{10,000}{100} = 10,000 \div 100 =$$

100 g of drug required for a 10% solution

Example: A 10 mL vial contains 10% calcium chloride. What volume must be given to administer 700 mg? (Recall that a 10% solution contains 10 g drug in 100 mL and that grams and percentages are interchangeable.)

Ratio-proportion method:

$$g:mL = g:mL$$

$$10:100 = X:10$$

$$100X = 100$$

$$X = 1 \text{ g of calcium chloride in 10 mL}$$

Formula method:

$$X = \frac{10}{100} \times 10 \text{ mL} = \frac{100}{100} = 1g \text{ of calcium chloride in 10 mL}$$

Units as Related to Infusion Therapy

A unit is defined as a measurement of a specific drug. The number of units in a specific drug is based on the strength of that drug. When administering a drug that is measured in units, accuracy is crucial so as not to give too much or too little of a drug. Example of a drug measured in units is insulin. The standard measurement of insulin is 100 units/mL. To ensure accuracy, the medication is drawn up in an insulin syringe. Although insulin can be drawn up into a tuberculosis (TB) syringe, there is too much room for error. Besides having to perform a calculation, there are two scales on the TB syringe. One scale is to measure minims and may be inadvertently used to dose insulin. This would deliver an incorrect dose to the patient. Another common drug that is measured in units is heparin.

Example: The physician orders a heparin infusion of 800 units/hour. The supply on hand is a bag containing 25,000 units in 500 mL of normal saline. At what rate do you infuse the heparin?

Ratio-proportion method:

$$units:mL = units:mL$$

$$25{,}000{:}500 = 800{:}X$$

$$800 \times 500 = 40{,}000$$

$$40{,}000/25{,}000 = 16 \; X = 16 \; mL/hour$$

Formula method:

$$X = 800/25{,}000 \times 500 = 16$$

$$X = 16 \; mL/hour$$

Body Surface Area and Body Weight

Body surface area (BSA) and body weights are both used in calculating drug dosages. BSA is one of the most accurate methods for calculating adult drug dosages, especially, chemotherapy and some antibiotics (Altman, 2004). BSA is determined by the height and weight of patient. Once the height and weight are known, the BSA can be determined by use of West nomogram are used.

Body weight is another method to determine medication dosages. It is a more accurate way to calculate dosages. A patient's body weight is measured in kg. It is important that an accurate weight is obtained, as the dosage will be based on this measurement. Too much or too little medication may be ordered if the weight is not obtained accurately. Changes in body weight may lead to changes in the medication dosages, so the patient's weight should be checked at prescribed intervals and changes should be reported to the physician.

ADMINISTRATION OF IV SOLUTIONS

The administration of IV solutions is carefully and accurately regulated by the flow rate (Figure 13-2). Flow rates are expressed in the form of infusions over a period of hours, milliliters per hour or minute, or number of drops per minute. The nurse must select the IV solution set that is appropriate for the administration of solution. When calculating the flow rate, the nurse rounds up to the next whole number, as the IV administration set cannot deliver a fraction of a drop of fluid. The drip chamber inlet of the IV administration solution set determines how many drops per minute the set can deliver. The larger the inlet, the fewer drops required to equal 1 mL. The smaller the inlet, the more drops required to equal 1 mL. The drop factor is usually determined by the set brand and can be located on the solution set package.

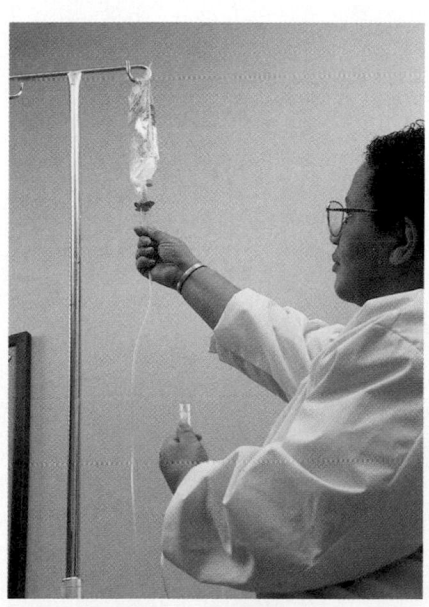

Figure 13-2 A nurse regulating an IV flow rate by adjusting the roller clamp.

Three-Step Method

The three-step method calculates the flow rate in milliliters per hour or milliliters per minute as well as the number of drops per minute for solution administration (Box 13-2).

The infusion of small volumes over a short period of time and at equal intervals within a 24-hour period is known as the intermittent infusion. An

---

BOX 13-2

EXAMPLE OF THE THREE-STEP METHOD

A physician has ordered 2,000 mL of solution to be administered over 24 hours.

Step 1: Determine the flow rate per hour.

> Total volume ÷ administration time = milliliters per hour
> 2,000 mL ÷ 24 hours = 83 mL/hr

Step 2: Determine the rate per min.

> Milliliters per hour ÷ minutes per hour (60) = milliliters per minutes
> 83 mL ÷ 60 minutes = 1.38 mL/min

Step 3: The administration set drop factor is 15 drops (gtt/mL). Determine the number of drops per minute.

> Milliliters per minutes X drop factor = drops per minute
> 1.38 mL/min × 15 gtt = 20.7 gtt/min (round up to 21 gtt/min)

Example of the ratio-proportion method: A physician has ordered 2,000 mL of a solution to be administered over 24 hours.

Step 1: Determine the flow rate per hour.

> mL:hr = mL:hr
> 2,000:24 = X:1
> 24X = 2,000
> X = 83 mL/hr

Step 2: Determine the rate per minute.

> Remember to convert hours to minutes
> mL:min = mL:min
> 83:60 = X:1
> 60X = 83
> X = 1.38 mL/min

Step 3: The administration set drop factor is 15 drops (gtt/mL). Determine thc number of drops per minute.

> gtt:mL = gtt:mL
> 15:1 = X:1.38
> 15X = 20.7 gtt/min (round up to 21 gtt/min)

Example of the formula method: A physician has ordered 2,000 mL of solution to be administered over 24 hours.

Step 1: Determine the flow rate per hour.

$$\frac{2,000 \text{ mL}}{24 \text{hr}} = X \text{ mL/hr}$$

$$2,000 \div 24 = 83 \text{ mL/hr}$$

Step 2: Determine the rate per minute. Convert 1 hour to 60 minutes

$$\frac{83 \text{ mL}}{60 \text{ min}} = 1.38 \text{ mL/min}$$

Step 3: The administration set drop factor is 15 drops (gtt/mL). Determine the number of drops per minute.

$$15 \text{ gtt} \times 1.38 \text{ mL/min} = 20.7 \text{ gtts/min (round up to 21 gtts/min)}$$

infusion of large amounts of volume over a period of hours is known as continuous infusion. The goal in administering IV solution is to calculate an accurate flow rate to infuse all of the solution in the container and IV tubing. Fluid left in the container or tubing could be a result of miscalculation of the time frame, the drip rate, problems with the IV site, or overfill of the IV container from the manufacturer. The amount of overfill present is not consistent and therefore not predictable.

The nurse should use one preferred dosage calculation method and use the same method to save time and increase accuracy of dose determination. The nurse should check and double-check his or her dosage calculation using the appropriate resources: calculator, paper and pencil, pharmacist, or another nurse to ensure safe administration of medication and IV solution to the patient.

PHARMACOLOGY

The IV route infuses medication directly into the bloodstream. This route was once reserved for emergency situations or for critically ill patients only but now has become a common route for most parenteral drug administration. With the increased use of the IV route for drug delivery, the nurse has increased responsibility to ensure safe outcomes. The nurse must administer the IV drugs, monitor the patient's responses to the IV medications, and provide patient education regarding the IV therapy (Broyles, et al., 2007).

The Nurse Practice Act, the institution's IV therapy policies, and the Infusion Nurses Standards of Practice govern and provide guidelines on who may administer IV drugs. The Nurse Practice Act defines the scope of practice for the nurses, and the institution's policies outline who may administer what drugs under what circumstances. The Infusion Nurses Standards of Practice provide information to measure the quality of IV nursing care. Institutions that provide IV drug therapy in developing IV policies use these standards.

A health care provider or approved licensed professional is responsible for prescribing IV therapy including IV drug administration. It is the nurse's responsibility to make sure the order is complete, correct, appropriate, and valid, and if there are any discrepancies, the nurse should clarify the order with the physician. A complete order should contain the name of the drug, dosage, route of administration, frequency or time of administration, date and time the order was written, and a legible signature. As the nurse is the likely person to be giving the medication, it is his or her responsibility to be aware of the actions, purpose, and side effects of the medication being administering. Additionally, the nurse should check for any contraindications, such as allergies, sensitivities, or incompatibilities. There are several ways that the physician can order IV therapy and drug therapy for the patient: written, verbal, and telephone orders. With the implementation of the patient safety goals by Joint Commission on Accreditation Health Organization (JCAHO), verbal and telephone orders are discouraged as errors can be made in transcribing these orders or in hearing the orders, especially when so many medications sound alike.

Controlled substances and investigational drugs are other areas with legal implications. The Controlled Substances Act of 1970 established five categories of controlled substances, called schedules, based on the potential for abuse and dependence and the medication indications for the drug's use. Many of the IV drugs fall under the Schedule II drugs, which require specific prescription and record keeping. Patients who undergo investigational drug therapy must sign an informed consent to participate in the clinical drug trials. Before the patient signs the informed consent, the principal investigator must inform the patient and family member of the risks, benefits, expected effects on the disease process, and alternatives to the investigational therapy.

Legal consideration must be given to medication errors. Many errors occur due to the practitioner, be it nurse, pharmacist, or physician, not adhering to the safety measures put into place to prevent errors. The institution's policies should outline the steps necessary to deliver medications to patients safely. Nurses have been taught the five rights in medication administration: right dose, right drug, right patient, right time, and right route (DeLaune & Ladner, 2006). Failure to follow one or more of these rights increases the risk of medication error. Risk management departments are implementing programs, such as the near miss card, to encourage reporting of any medication error or near error for tracking and trending purposes. This system is not intended to be punitive; rather, the data gathered should be examined for trends and sources of system error. Medications with sound-alike names, similar packaging, difficult to read dosing, and medications delivered to the unit in error are some common near miss events. Proper patient identification is another source of medication administration error. One of the patient safety goals by JCAHO is to improve the accuracy of patient identification by using at least two patient identifiers (patient's room number is not one) whenever taking blood samples or administering medications or blood products.

It is the nurse's responsibility to utilize the nursing process: assessment, planning, intervention, and evaluation. This also applies to the plan of care for medication delivery. The patient's plan of care should be reviewed and revised according to the results of the evaluation. Assessment consists of reviewing the patient's health history noting any allergies to drugs, food, and environmental factors, lifestyle, and resources available to the patient. The patient's desire to understand and follow the prescribed drug therapy can determine the patient's adherence to the plan of care. Other factors to consider include the presence of other illnesses, any genetic factors that may influence response to therapy and the patient's age. Planning is the phase in which nursing diagnoses are developed based on the patient assessment. Nursing diagnoses provide a consistent method of communicating the plan of care for that patient. Once the nursing diagnoses have been formulated, the patient's plan of care can be developed. The patient's drug therapy plan of care should consider the patient's reaction to the drug, such as single dose verses repeated doses, therapeutic drug concentration range, such as plateau (steady drug level in blood), peak time (maximum concentration of drug in the bloodstream after IV administration), and trough time (lowest concentration of drug in the bloodstream after IV administration), as well as the plasma half-life of the drug. **Half-life** refers to the amount of time required for the elimination processes to reduce the blood concentration of the drug by 50 percent. Implementation of the patient's drug therapy depends on the patient's level of understanding, drug administration, and documentation. Documentation is important in this phase as it records the actions that have been implemented. To ensure that the patient is benefiting from the prescribed therapy, the nurse must do evaluation of the patient's drug therapy. It is an ongoing process to include appropriate modification as long as the patient is receiving the therapy.

Nurses should be aware of their role in drug administration, which can vary with the health care setting. Nurses who work in an inpatient setting may be responsible for drug preparation and administration, whereas nurses in a home care setting are responsible for patient and family self-administration techniques. In the home setting, it is often the patient or family who is responsible for administering the medication, patient education, and monitoring falls to the home care nurse. Although drug preparation usually occurs in a centralized pharmacy, in emergency cases, the nurse for administration must prepare medications immediately. IV drugs and admixtures are usually prepared under a laminar flow hood in pharmacy to decrease the possibility of airborne contaminants entering the IV solution. There are considerations that need to be taken when preparing IV drugs: diluents used to reconstitute the drug, drug compatibility, and stability. Diluents are solutions used to change mediations from powder form to liquid form. Some diluents contain a preservative, which may be harmful to the patient. It is important that the nurse recognize these situations. Drug incompatibility is a reaction that occurs between the drug and the solution, the container, or another drug. There are three types of incompatibility: physical, chemical, and therapeutic. Physical incompatibility consists of a visual reaction, such as color change, or the formation of a cloudy gas within the syringe. Chemical incompatibility consists of an actual chemical change of the drug, such as reduction, oxidation, hydrolysis, or decomposition. The change is not visible, but there is still an incompatibility. Therapeutic incompatibility occurs inside the patient, because the drug being given interacts with other medications the patient is receiving. Stability refers to the pH value expressed as acidic or alkaline of the drug mixture.

After the drug is reconstituted, the nurse should verify the mode of infusion with the original order. The mode of IV drug administration depends on the drug used, the patient's condition, and the desired effects of the drug. There are four primary modes of administration: continuous infusion, intermittent infusion, direct injection, and patient-controlled analgesia. There are advantages and disadvantages to each of these modes.

Continuous infusion means that a large volume of fluid is infused over hours and days to maintain drug concentrations, or large volumes of fluids and electrolytes must be replaced. This type of infusion must be monitored to prevent fluid overload and potential incompatibilities between the infusion and IV drug administered together through the venous access devices.

Intermittent infusion means that a small volume of fluid is infused in a short amount of time (15 to 90 minutes) at intervals within a 24-hour period. These infusions are also referred to as piggyback or secondary infusions. The goal of this type of infusion is for the drug to peak at periodic intervals and to decrease the risk of fluid overload. There are four ways to provide intermittent infusions: (a) piggyback infusion; (b) simultaneous infusion; (c) volume control set; and (d) direct intermittent infusion into the venous access device. Piggyback infusion is the most common method for drug administration. The drug is infused by a shorter IV administration set into the main set. The nurse must check for compatibility between the piggyback solution and the continuous solution. Simultaneous infusion occurs when two solutions are administered together into the venous access device. This infusion must be monitored closely to prevent blood backing up into the secondary infusion set on completion of infusion from the primary infusion set resulting in the possible clotting of the venous access device. Volume control infusion is often used in patients who need to have close fluid intake monitoring. The medication is injected into a special chamber of the infusion set, mixed with a small amount of IV fluid, and administered slowly through the set into the venous access device. The fourth and last method of intermittent infusion is the direct intermittent infusion of medication into the venous access device. The medication is infused using an intermittent infusion set connected to a capped venous access device. This infusion is short in duration, occurs at intervals over 24-hours, and allows the patient freedom to continue with activities of daily living. These devices are sometimes called saline locks. They are kept patent by flushing them with saline when the intermittent infusion is completed (Altman, 2004).

Direct injection, also known as IV push or bolus, allows for the medication to enter the bloodstream directly for a quicker response. The medication is injected into the venous access device using the appropriate syringe for the volume of medication. It is extremely important that the nurse has the right drug and dose before injecting and monitors the patient's response and tolerance to the infusion. The nurse should remember that once the medication is injected, there is no way to get it back.

PCA is the fourth type of method, which gives the patient the ability to determine when pain medication will be infused. With this method, an electronic pump (PCA pump) is programmed to administer a small amount of drug when activated by the patient at certain programmed intervals. The PCA tubing is connected to the continuous infusion set. It cannot be used with intermittent infusion as the volumes are small and need a fluid carrier to get the medication into the vein. The physician determines the amount of drug—continuous or intermittent, intervals and bolus for patient, and the hourly limit the patient can receive, but the nurse must ensure that the pump is programmed according to the order and to the policies of the institution (Everett & Salamonson, 2005).

CENTRAL VENOUS CATHETERS

Central lines, once thought to be use only with critically ill people, are beginning to be used more often and in more settings than ever before. Unfortunately, too often, peripheral IVs are ordered until all sites are used up and only then are central lines considered. Some of the common reasons for this include the risks associated with central lines, the cost, and the maintenance. The misperception that peripheral IVs are completely safe also contributes to the under use of central lines. For an IV to be considered central the tip of the catheter should lie in the distal one third of the superior vena cava. Considerations for determining which central line would be best for a patient, see Box 13-3.

Tunneled Catheters

These catheters are implanted in the chest wall near the vein into which they will be inserted (typically the subclavian vein) and tunneled subcutaneously until they reach a place, typically lower on the chest, that the catheter will exit. The catheter can exit low enough on the chest to be hidden under clothing. This subcutaneous tunnel enables the catheter to dwell or remain in the vein longer. If the catheter were to become infected, it is most likely to become

---

BOX 13-3

CONSIDERATIONS FOR SELECTION OF USING A CENTRAL LINE

- Patient's diagnoses and concurrent conditions: (a) Patients with circulatory impairment; (b) immune suppression; and (c) other chronic conditions may make peripheral venipuncture difficult or may make central line therapy risky.
- Peripheral vein access options: Does the patient have anything limiting peripheral access options, such as arteriovenous fistula or graft, mastectomy with axillary's node removal, loss of sensation or an amputation?
- Length and type of therapy needed: Even with the best veins, long-term peripheral IV therapy will be limited. Some central lines are made of a material that allows them to remain in place or to dwell longer.
- Monitoring needed for therapy: Frequent laboratory studies, central pressures, core temperature, will the patient require frequent magnetic resonance imaging (MRI) or other scans?
- Long-term or short-term therapy indicated: How long is the therapy intended to last?
- Who will maintain line: Who will help if the patient is unable to care for the line? Is the line able to be easily repaired?
- Body image issues: Will an external device be difficult for the patient to accept?

Adapted from Tilton, D. (2006). Central venous access device infections in the critical care unit. Critical Care Nursing Quarterly, 29(2), 117–122.

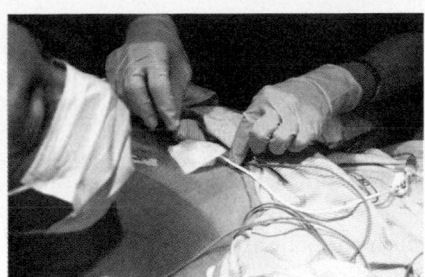

Figure 13-3 Nurse changing a central line dressing.

infected at the exit site. From there, the organisms must migrate up the tunnel prior to entering the circulatory system. If the infection is detected at the exit site, it is much easier to treat than when it is allowed to progress. Common tunneled catheters include: (a) Hickman; (b) Broviac; (c) Groshong; and (d) Hohn and may have single or multiple lumens. These types of catheters can remain in place for months at a time, as long as the catheter site remains healthy. Specific methods of applying dressings (Figure 13-3) are provided in agency procedure manuals (Bartholomay, et al., 2006).

Percutaneous Catheters

These catheters are inserted directly into the vein. These catheters are suited for short to moderate length therapy. A specially trained nurse inserts a peripherally inserted central catheter (PICC) lines at the bedside. Venipuncture is achieved much like it is for peripheral IV, but a flexible catheter is threaded through the cannula or introducer to the superior vena cava. The site of entry is typically the antecubital fossa or just above or below it. Another type of percutaneous catheter is a multilumen central line. These catheters have two to four separate lumens that can be used to infuse incompatible solutions, as the solutions never mix in the catheter. This type of catheter is typically used in the hospital setting as it is vulnerable to infection and is not suited for moderate or long-term use.

Implanted Ports

These devices are inserted in a subcutaneous pocket above the breast tissue. The catheter tubing is inserted into the subclavian vein, and the tip is advanced to the superior vena cava. These devices can be single or dual lumen. The port contains a reservoir that is accessed with a noncoring needle. This type of needle has a specially designed bevel that does not take a piece of the reservoir material into its hollow core. If the proper access is used, a port can withstand up to 2,000 punctures. This catheter is popular because of its low maintenance and low visibility. These ports can be made of plastic or titanium.

Closed-Ended Catheters

Closed-ended catheters are currently known as Groshong catheters or three-way valve catheters. As the name implies, these catheters are closed at the end. The way fluids infuse through this catheter is by a slit on the distal portion of the catheter opening in response to the change in pressure when infusing. With no pressure, the slit remains closed and with aspiration, the slit opens inward, allowing blood to be pulled back into the catheter. This functions much like the old coin purses that opened when the slit was squeezed. Because these catheters are closed when not in use, there is no need to clamp the catheter. Unless the valve is malfunctioning, the catheter should not be clamped as the pressure exerted by the clamp being applied can open the valve and allow blood to flow back into the catheter.

The nurse follows the institution's policy on changing dressings and caps of central lines. The dressing should be changed at least weekly and more frequently if it becomes loose, soiled, or wet. Complications with central lines are similar to those of peripheral IV. In addition to those, complications can occur on insertion of the central line, the most common one being pneumothorax. With percutaneous insertion in the subclavian vein, there exists the potential to pierce the apex of the lung. Additionally, air may enter the central circulation when caps on lines are changed and when lines are inserted. An additional complication with central lines is thrombus formation. As the catheter remains in the vein, it can irritate and injure the vein wall, leading to clot formation. Swelling of the upper extremity of the same side as the central line may indicate the presence of a venous thrombus.

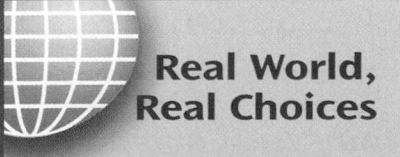

Real World, Real Choices

Selection of Central Line

John is 17 years old. He has just been diagnosed with testicular cancer and has come in for teaching regarding his chemotherapy. He has just been released from the hospital following removal of his cancerous testicle. He will need central venous access for his chemotherapy, but which line is best for him?

Troubleshooting

There are a variety of potential complications seen in the administration of central line infusions. The following are interventions for the nurse to consider when troubleshooting central lines. First, if there is difficulty flushing the line, never force any solution through the catheter, as a clot could enter the circulation or rupture and embolize a piece of the catheter. Possible causes for a nonpatent line are the clamp is on the line, clot in the injection cap, chemical obstruction (precipitate), blood clot in catheter, or kinked line. Solutions to an obstructed line are: check line from patient to IV bag for any clamps or kinks, change injection cap, be sure to flush out cap every time line is flushed, use proper amount of heparin when indicated, reposition patient, and confirm placement of catheter by X-ray before initial use and as needed. (Note: a patient who frequently experiences increases in intrathoracic pressures may have flipped the tip of the catheter leading to retrograde infusion or infusion in a different vein.)

If the patient has a fever, assume the cause is the central line until other causes are ruled out. Possible causes are contamination during insertion, dressing changes, coughing on site, food spillage, diaphoresis, and immune-compromised patient. Solutions for the febrile condition are strict technique during insertion and maintain strict technique during dressing changes, encourage patient to turn head away from site when coughing, change any loose or soiled dressing as soon as possible, and maintain good hand washing, and frequently assess catheter site.

TOTAL PARENTERAL NUTRITION

Total parenteral nutrition (TPN) or total parenteral admixture (TPA) is nutritional support supplying glucose, protein, vitamins, electrolytes, trace elements, and sometimes fats to maintain the body's growth, development, and tissue repair. Sometimes, the nurse may also hear this therapy referred to as IV hyperalimentation. Patients who cannot meet their caloric and nutritional needs by taking in nutrition because of illness or malfunction of the gastrointestinal (GI) tract can benefit from TPN. The role of nutrition in healing is well-known, but it is not always possible to meet those needs through oral intake. TPN by central line reverses starvation and adequately achieves tissue synthesis, repair, and growth. TPN solutions are always administered through a central vein because of the high concentration of dextrose and the hypertonicity and hyperosmolarity of the solution. The nursing strategies for the administration of TPN are shown in Box 13-4. By infusing this solution into the central venous system there is less incidence of

---

BOX 13-4

NURSING CONSIDERATIONS FOR PARENTERAL NUTRITION

1. Begin TPN infusion at a slow rate (40 to 60 mL per hour).
2. Gradually increase the rate until maximum infusion rate.
3. Use a rate control device to monitor the infusion (pumps are ideal).
4. Blood sugar checks should be performed every six hours, particularly during the first week of infusion.
5. Accurate intake and output recording every eight hours.
6. Check daily weight using the same scale. Ideally the weight gain for patients receiving TPN is approximately 2 lb/week.
7. Monitor vital signs at regular intervals. Look for signs of infection, such as fever.
8. Follow your institution's policy regarding laboratory studies necessary with TPN therapy.

phlebitis and the highly concentrated formula can be rapidly diluted (Roth, 2007). The advantages and disadvantages of TPN are depicted in Table 13-2.

Patient Conditions That Warrant Candidacy for TPN

Patients who would be good candidates for TPN are those who suffer from a multiplicity of problems and whose clinical course can be complicated by malnutrition and depletion of body protein. Candidates for TPN include but are not limited to postoperative complications including GI tract dysfunction; poor nutritional state at onset of medical problem; persistent ileus; GI problems (e.g., Crohn's disease, short bowel syndrome, bowel obstruction, or fistulas); trauma; severe burns; anorexia nervosa; cachexia; and hyperemesis associated with pregnancy.

Nutritional Characteristics of Parenteral Nutrition

Carbohydrates provide energy and spare the body protein. When glucose is provided parenterally, it is completely bioavailable to the body without any effects of malabsorption. During the critical phase of illness or injury, carbohydrate metabolism is radically altered. Hyperglycemia is a hallmark of stress.

Protein is included in TPN is an essential nutrient that functions to promote tissue growth and repair, wound healing, and replace body cells. Protein is also a component in antibodies, scar tissue, and clots. Enzymes, hormones, and carrier substances also require protein for development. Protein contributes to energy needs; however this is not its major purpose. Amino acids are the basic unit of protein. There are eight essential amino acids for adults.

Fats are the primary source of heat and energy. Fat provides twice as many energy calories per gram as either protein or carbohydrate. Fat is essential for structural integrity of all cell membranes. Linoleic acid is the only fatty acids essential to humans. These two acids prevent essential fatty acid deficiency (EFAD).

Electrolytes are infused either as a component already contained in the amino acid solution or as a separate additive. The electrolytes commonly found in TPN include potassium, magnesium, calcium, sodium, chloride, and phosphorus. Electrolytes must be individually compounded and can be highly

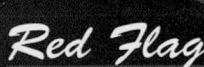

Red Flag

Fractured Line

A fractured line is a potential emergency, especially with open-ended catheters as air may get into the line and then the systemic circulation. Possible causes for this condition are the line is inadvertently cut while changing dressing (note: do not use scissors to cut old dressing off), the wrong type of clamp applied to line and caused damage, too long of a needle used to access line and punctured line, and there has been forced flushing against resistance or the syringe is too small. The solutions are to use only the clamp provided with line; use short needles or blunt tip needles to access line; use only 10 mL or larger syringes for access (note: smaller syringes exert more pounds per square inch of pressure and can rupture the catheter); teach patients going home with catheters to pinch off or clamp line when system is open or if line breaks.

TABLE 13-2 Advantages and Disadvantages of TPN	
ADVANTAGES	**DISADVANTAGES**
Dextrose solutions of 20–70% administered as calorie source	May cause metabolic complications: glucose intolerance and electrolyte imbalances
Useful for long-term therapy (usually longer than three weeks)	Fat emulsions may not be used effectively in severely stressed patients especially burn patients)
Useful for patients with large caloric and nutrient needs	
Provides calories, restores nitrogen balance, replaces essential vitamins, electrolytes, and minerals	Risk of pneumothorax or hemothorax with central line insertion.
Promotes tissue synthesis, wound healing, and normal metabolic function	
Allows bowel rest and healing	
Improves tolerance to surgery	
Is nutritionally complete	

Adapted from Roth, R. (2007). Nutrition and diet therapy (9th ed.). New York: Thomson Delmar Learning.

TABLE 13-3 Advantages and Disadvantages of PPN	
ADVANTAGES	**DISADVANTAGES**
Avoid insertion and maintenance of a central catheter	Cannot be used in nutritionally depleted patients
Delivers less hypertonic solutions than central venous TPN	Cannot be used in volume-restricted patients, as higher volumes of solution are needed to provide adequate calories
Reduces the chance of metabolic complications compared to central venous TPN	Does not generally increase a patient's weight
Increases calorie source, along with fat emulsions	May cause phlebitis owing to the osmolarity of the solution

Adapted from Roth, R. (2007). Nutrition and diet therapy (9th ed.). New York: Thomson Delmar Learning.

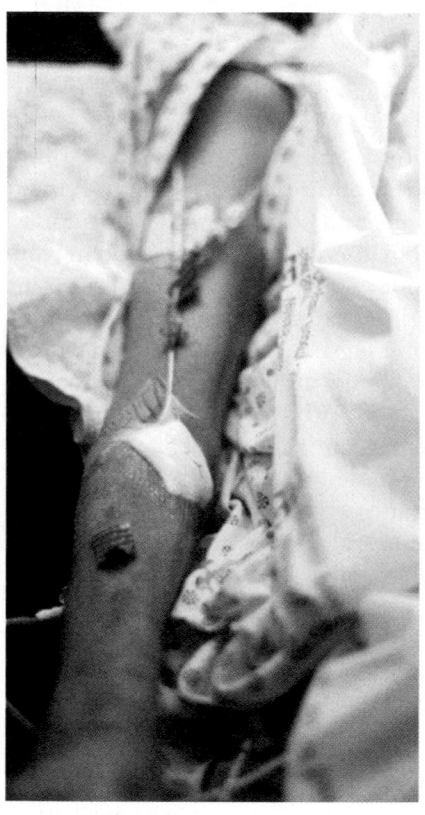

Figure 13-4 PPN may be administered through a PICC line.

variable in the patient receiving TPN. The physician in response to the patient's laboratory studies can make changes in the TPN formula.

Peripheral Parenteral Nutrition

Peripheral parenteral nutrition (PPN) is designed for mildly stressed patients who are expected to be able to resume enteral feeding within 7 to 10 days. Generally, PPN helps to maintain a patient's nutritional status, so it is not typically used for patients who are already have nutritional deficiencies (Figure 13-4). The advantages and disadvantages of PPN are shown in Table 13-3.

Metabolic Complications of TPN

Because the dextrose concentration in TPN is high, hyperglycemia and hyperosmolar syndrome are common metabolic occurrences. It is important to tell the patient that TPN will not make him a diabetic, but while on this therapy, insulin may be necessary to control his or her blood sugar. Hypoglycemia can occur if the TPN is stopped abruptly; therefore, always wean patients from TPN. Additional complications associated with metabolic imbalances when administering TPN are either avoidable or controllable. Major electrolyte imbalances occur when excessive or deficient amounts of electrolytes are supplied in the daily fluid allowance. The nurse should observe for signs and symptoms of hypophosphatemia, hypokalemia, hypomagnesemia, and hypernatremia. In addition, TPN protocols for laboratory study monitoring should be in place.

BLOOD COMPONENTS

Blood transfusions can save lives. With the discovery of the blood types (ABO system), transfusions have become a mainstay in the treatment of patients whose blood counts have reached levels low enough to compromise their lives. On any given day in the United States, approximately 32,000 units of red blood cells (RBCs) are needed for patients receiving treatment or undergoing surgery. While transfusions have become commonplace in health care today, it is important to realize that the transfusion of blood and blood products carries risks in various degrees of transfusion reactions as well as in the transmission of blood-borne pathogens and diseases.

ABO System

There are four types of blood: A, B, AB, and O. The presence of a specific antigen on the RBC determines which type of blood a person has. There are other antigens, but they represent extremely rare blood types and will not be discussed here. Some blood types can receive other types of blood without any problems; others can cause a potentially lethal reaction. The nurse should have an understanding of the compatibilities of blood and blood components to administer these therapies safely (Table 13-4).

Rh Factor

The Rh (or Rhesus) factor was discovered in 1940. The Rh factor was named for the Rhesus monkeys that were involved in experiments to uncover factors making blood transfusions incompatible. This component is a protein substance present in the RBCs of most people, capable of inducing intense antigenic reactions. A person is either Rh-negative or Rh-positive. If a person does not have the Rh factor (Rh-negative), it is important that the individual does not receive Rh-positive blood. Rh-positive blood could cause a devastating reaction to the factor. An Rh-positive person can receive Rh-negative blood safely.

Blood Components

There are several types of blood components, and which one(s) are used depend on what each patient needs. After careful screening for blood-borne pathogens and diseases, the blood is analyzed and cross-matched specifically to each patient. There are between 300 and 400 antigens in the blood system, only a few of which the function is known. Some of these antigens can trigger the immune system to react, causing minor symptoms to a major systemic reaction.

Whole Blood

Whole blood includes all the blood cells (RBCs and white blood cells [WBCs]) as well as plasma. Whole blood is rarely used anymore, as patients typically do not need all the components of blood. This component may be used for patients who lose a massive amount of blood and need replacement not only of the components of blood but volume as well. Because whole blood is not used often anymore, it can be difficult to obtain.

Packed Red Blood Cells

Packed red blood cells (PRBCs) are left after the plasma is separated out of whole blood. This component is used for routine blood replacement during surgery or for those patients who need more oxygen-carrying capability because

PATIENT PLAYBOOK

Administration of TPN/PPN

The nurse should instruct the patient in the following regarding the administration of TPN/PPN:

- Your weight will be checked every day to evaluate your fluid balance state.
- You will have frequent lab work to be sure you are getting enough nutrition.
- You will have your blood sugar checked a few times a day. TPN/PPN does not make you become diabetic, but it has high sugar content and you may need insulin while you are on it.
- A dietitian will see you periodically.
- You need to participate in good hygiene (e.g., hand washing) whenever handling the infusion site.

TABLE 13-4	**Blood Types**	
TYPE	**CAN DONATE BLOOD TO**	**CAN RECEIVE BLOOD FROM**
A+	A+, AB+	A+, A−, O+, O−
O+	O+, A+, B+, AB+	O+, O−
B+	B+, AB+	B+, B−, O+, O−
AB+	AB+	Everyone
A−	A+, A−, AB+, AB−	A−, O−
O−	Everyone	O−
B−	B+, B−, AB+, AB−	B−, O−
AB−	AB+, AB−	AB−, A−,B−, O−

Adapted from Blood type facts. *(2006). Retrieved July 11, 2006, from* http://www.bloodbook.com.

of anemia that either does not respond to medication or in those in whom waiting for pharmaceutical therapies to work is not possible. WBCs remain and are often the cause of febrile reactions to blood; therefore, the trend is now to separate or wash the blood to remove the WBCs and in some cases, the platelets. The WBCs can trigger the immune response to form antibodies, making further cross-matching a challenge as the development of new antibodies limits the number of units of blood a patient will match. This also can affect patients who may need future transplants of organs or bone marrow. If a patient has received multiple transfusions and has developed many antibodies, finding a compatible match becomes like finding a needle in a haystack.

One way to wash blood is to use a process that utilizes saline to remove platelets and cellular debris from the blood. Many, but not all, of the WBCs are removed in this process. While this decreases the components that are more likely to cause a reaction, it does not fully eliminate the WBCs. Another method used is to freeze the blood for later use. When the blood is thawed, it is washed with saline, again reducing the number of cells that may cause antibody production but does not totally eliminate them. A third method of removing these cells is to filter them through a leukocyte filter. The cells may be filtered during the initial processing of the donation or by use of an inline filter when being transfused.

Fresh frozen plasma (FFP) is made by removing plasma from the unit of donated blood and freezing it within six hours of collection. This component is thawed prior to use in a warm water bath and is rich in clotting factors. Patients who have severe liver disease who cannot produce enough of these clotting factors and patients who are on warfarin (Coumadin) therapy who need to have the effects of that drug reversed for surgery or in cases of uncontrolled bleeding are candidates for FFP transfusion.

Platelets

Platelets come as a single unit from multiple donors or multiple units from a single donor. Single donor platelets have been used mostly for patients who are at risk of developing antibodies or who may need transplantation in the future. It is now understood that the immune response that can occur with platelet transfusions is related more to the WBCs present rather than the number of donors the patient is exposed to, but single donor platelets remain popular for these types of patients. Platelets are used in patients who have bleeding disorders from illness, medications, trauma, or organ dysfunction. Platelets are not always exactly matched to the patient, although as more is learned about the role the immune system plays in response to receiving platelets, this may change. Some patients do not seem to benefit from platelet transfusions, and in these patients, the body may more readily accept a more specifically cross-matched product (Gajic, Dzik, & Toy, 2006).

Cryoprecipitate

Cryoprecipitate (cryo) is obtained when slowly thawing a unit of FFP. The cold precipitated protein recovered, cryo, is rich in certain clotting factors, such as VIII and XIII, and is used for patients with factor XIII deficiency and those with hypofibrinogenemia, which is seen during bleeding and clotting disorders, such as disseminated intravascular coagulation (DIC) syndrome.

Granulocytes

Granulocytes are prepared by separating WBCs. Some RBCs, other types of WBCs, and platelets may also be contained in this component. It is rarely used, because it must be transfused within 24 hours of collection and often testing on specimens takes longer than that. The patients who get these transfusions must have extremely low WBC counts that do not respond to other medical therapies and must have a reasonable chance of bone marrow recovery.

Albumin

Albumin is a protein manufactured by the liver that performs many functions, including maintaining the osmotic pressure that causes fluid to remain within the bloodstream instead of leaking out into the tissues. There are a number of reasons why the albumin level gets low, including liver disease in which the liver cannot manufacture enough albumin; kidney disease in which there is increased excretion of albumin; and poor diet in which the body does not get enough building blocks to make albumin. When the albumin level gets low, fluids begin to leak into the tissues and may cause peripheral edema, pulmonary edema, ascites, or other evidence of third spacing. As previously discussed, in third spacing the circulating volume is decreased, as the fluid is sequestered and not available to the body to use. Albumin is not a component that must be cross-matched, but it is considered a blood product.

TRANSFUSION RISKS

Although in a perfect world there would be no risks associated with the transfusion of blood components, this is not a perfect world. Transmission of blood-borne diseases is a known risk, including the risk of the transmission of human immunodeficiency virus (HIV), hepatitis B and C, syphilis, and the human T cell lymphotropic virus 1 and 2. Transfusion reactions can vary and may or may not trigger the immune response. Rash, fever, and back pain may not seem to be too serious but can trigger the immune response, leading to further reactions or reactions to further blood products. Acute lung injury, intravascular hemolysis, anaphylaxis, and shock can be fatal. Additionally, volume overload and hypocalcemia (from the citrate used to prevent the unit of blood from clotting) can affect the patient. Reactions can occur as rapidly as fifteen minutes into the transfusion to days later (Simmons, 2003).

The transfusion of blood components requires the informed consent of the patient receiving the blood. Some patients refuse blood because of religious beliefs, cultural beliefs, or fear of disease transmission. Regardless, patients should have the opportunity to discuss their concerns and fears related to transfusions. For those who have religious or cultural concerns, alternatives to blood components should be explored (Box 13-5) (Simmons, 2003).

Colloids, Crystalloids, Erythropoietin, Colony Factor Stimulating Products

With the rise of concern over blood-borne pathogen and disease transmission, occasional component shortages, as well as those with religious and cultural concerns over transfusions, the need for alternatives to blood component therapy (e.g., colloids and crystalloids) has also grown. Some alternatives are costly, some have undesirable side effects, and some simply take too long to become effective. Therefore, component alternatives are not ideal for all people or for all situations.

Colloids are fluids that expand the circulatory volume due to particles that cannot cross a semipermeable membrane. They pull fluid from the interstitial space into the intravascular space, increasing fluid volume. This can be a great advantage in cases of large losses of fluid, such as severe trauma and hemorrhage. The main disadvantages are cost and the risk of volume overload, including pulmonary edema. Types of colloids are dextrans and hetastarches.

Crystalloids work much like colloids but do not stay in the intravascular circulation as well as colloids do, so more of them need to be used. They are cheaper and are more convenient to use. Crystalloids provide hydration and

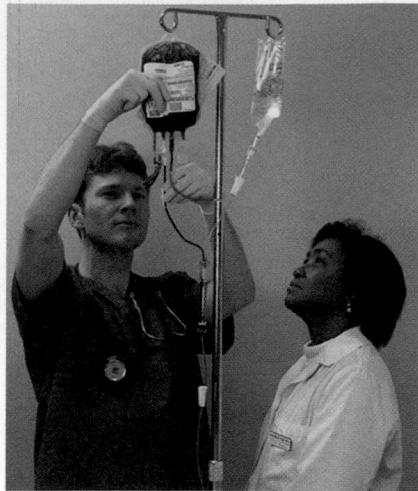

Figure 13-5 Nurses hanging a unit of PRBCs along with normal saline.

BOX 13-5

TRANSFUSION PROCESS

1. Prior to obtaining the blood component from the blood bank, the patient's vital signs should be obtained. If there is any change in the vital signs, the health care provider should be consulted regarding continuing with the transfusion.
2. Next, correctly identify the patient and ensure that consent has been obtained. Ensure a working IV of the appropriate size is available. If it is not, start one prior to obtaining the component from the blood bank. Double-check the health care provider's order.
3. Obtain the correct component from the blood bank. It should be checked at the bedside of the patient according to the institution's policy.
4. Inform the patient of the procedure, the vital sign monitoring, and the potential side effects. Be sure the patient can call you if he or she experiences any problems.
5. Obtain the proper tubing and normal saline (Figure 13-5). Apply clean gloves to protect yourself The nurse should apply clean gloves to protect himself or herself from exposure to the unit of blood or the blood product. Prime the tubing with the normal saline and then the blood. Connect the tubing to the IV and slowly begin the transfusion. Take vital signs 15 minutes after the start of the transfusion. If there is no change, increase the rate if indicated and continue to monitor the patient according to the institution's policy.
6. If a reaction is suspected, stop the blood. Obtain separate IV tubing and prime it with normal saline and begin to infuse that into the patient. Do not use the saline and tubing from the transfusion as it still contains the blood component that may have caused the reaction. Obtain the patient's vital signs, including temperature, and do a quick assessment of the patient focusing for signs of a progressing reaction. Notify the health care provider and follow the institution's policy regarding blood transfusion reaction.

Adapted from Altman, G. (2004). Delmar's fundamental and advanced nursing skills (2nd ed.). New York: Thomson Delmar Learning.

---

calories to patients and include dextrose, normal saline, and Ringer's and lactated Ringer's solutions. While colloids and crystalloids increase the circulating volume, they do not increase the RBC counts and therefore do not increase the oxygen-carrying capacity of the blood (Rudnicke, 2003).

Drugs that stimulate the bone marrow to produce more RBCs, called erythropoietin products, have been around for several years. Other products, called colony factor stimulating products, stimulate the bone marrow to produce more WBCs. These products have reduced the need for transfusions greatly but are not indicated for patients who need immediate replacement. Patients with chronic diseases or undergoing long treatments, such as chemotherapy, best utilize these products. These drugs can take up to four weeks to work and are quite costly. Genetic alterations of blood components and synthetic blood and blood products are under development. Time will tell if these types of products can limit the use of human blood and blood products (Rudnicke, 2003).

ONCOLOGY THERAPY

Cancer is a chronic disease characterized by the growth and spread of abnormal cells in the body. It is typically a long-term disease and requires that the nurse possess special knowledge to care for these patients. These therapies can cause many side effects that can be lethal. Patient monitoring is essential to the safe practice of oncology nursing. Symptom management, prevention of side effects, and management are main goals. Body image changes from hair loss to weight loss and surgical treatments, and side effects of some medications can be devastating for patients. Loved ones who want to be supportive of the patient may themselves need support and a safe environment to discuss their feelings and fears. Finally, patient education is essential in this field. Patients and their families need to know how the patient's altered immune system can lead to serious infections that can be life-threatening emergencies. They also need to understand the course of the specific type of cancer they have and in some cases, need support to make treatment decisions and to know when to stop treatment.

The medications used to treat many types of cancer are toxic and can be harmful to both the patient and the nurse who is administering medications. Nurses should have special education to administer chemotherapeutic medications, as there are many considerations in giving these drugs. The effects of the therapy as well as the actions of the drugs must be well understood by the nurse administering the medications. Some drugs are administered in some sites better than in other sites. Chemotherapy that spills must be cleaned up in a safe manner as not to expose the nurse, the patient, or the environment to any hazards. Many of these patients will have a central line. Understanding the uses of each type of access is important as well as recognizing complications associated with the central line or with the patient's disease process. For the oncology nurse, dealing with death and dying issues is a major component of the specialty.

PAIN MANAGEMENT

Pain management is another nursing specialty that requires extensive knowledge in the pathophysiology of pain and a thorough understanding of the modalities used to treat pain. Every patient has the right to have pain controlled, be it acute, chronic, or cancer pain. JCAHO requires a pain assessment and reassessment at regular intervals during the care of a patient. There are several barriers to effective pain control, including those imposed by the nurse. These barriers must be overcome for the patient to have the best pain control possible.

These barriers include inadequate knowledge of the mechanisms of pain, the modalities used to treat pain, and the cultural differences in how people experience pain. Nurses as well as other health care workers can be judgmental about a patient's report of pain, especially if the nurse does not think the patient is in pain. Many patients cope with chronic pain with distraction by watching television, doing a hobby, or talking on the phone. Others may sleep to avoid the conscious experience of the pain.

Some patients may feel they deserve the pain or that bearing the pain makes them stronger. Others see their own suffering as a means to achieve a higher level of spirituality or as the natural part of a journey. These issues are best handled by a pain management team or by a multidisciplinary approach to helping the patient work through his or her feelings and beliefs and finding a way to honor those beliefs while keeping the patient as comfortable as possible.

Pain management is another specialty area of nursing that can be rewarding. There have been tremendous breakthroughs in how pain is managed and more breakthroughs are on the horizon. Pressurized balloons that deliver precise amounts of pain medication, patches, implanted pumps, surgical interventions, and alternative therapy are a small fraction of the therapies available. Patient education can make a big difference in how autonomously the patient can control his or her pain and live life with the best quality possible (Kim, Schwartz-Barcott, Tracy, Fortin, & Sjostrom, 2005).

SEDATION

Patients undergoing medical procedures used to rely solely on anesthesia to make them comfortable and make the procedure possible. With the explosion of pharmaceuticals on the market as well as the newer, less invasive procedures available today, the need exists for faster, safer methods of sedating patients.

In many states, registered nurses (RNs) may administer certain levels of sedation. The levels of sedation are defined by the ability of the patient to maintain an airway, the patient's vital signs, and the ability of the patient to respond to verbal commands. Knowledge of the medications used in sedation as well as the reversal agents and the emergency protocols is essential to administer any level of sedation safely. Additionally, it is important to recognize when a patient is moving to a deeper level of sedation and what actions need to be taken. Sedation is always performed under the direct supervision of a physician, and the availability of emergency equipment as well as the skill in using the equipment is imperative. The patient should be monitored and recovered according to the institution's policy.

HEMODYNAMIC MONITORING

Usually reserved for critical care areas and the operating room, hemodynamic monitoring can give the health care team invaluable information regarding many aspects of a patient's current status. Core temperature, cardiac and pulmonary pressures, arterial pressures, and fluid volume status are some of the data that these monitoring systems can give to the health care team.

Special catheters and monitors enable nurses to "see" into the patient's body by providing measurements and readings and allowing other therapies, such as temporary pacemaking to take place. Arterial catheters give a constant reading of the patient's blood pressure. They also provide access to obtain blood specimens, which are obtained several times a day in a critically ill patient. These catheters can be placed at the bed side and require a pressurized solution through a special IV tubing to keep the arterial blood from backing up into the tubing. A transducer converts blood pressure into electrical impulses that can be seen on the monitor as a waveform.

A central line, whose tip lies in the distal portion of the superior vena cava, can be used to measure a patient's central venous pressure (CVP). The CVP reading is obtained with similar equipment as the arterial line described above. The CVP measurement indicates the pumping action of the right side of the heart as well as gives an indication of the circulating fluid volume. Manometers can be used to obtain a CVP reading outside of the critical care unit.

Another specialized catheter, called a pulmonary artery catheter, or a Swan-Ganz catheter, is crucial in some critical patients as it gives constant feedback by providing a number of measurements regarding heart function and fluid volume status. One port on this catheter measures pulmonary artery pressure, giving a picture of left ventricular functioning. Another lumen "wedges" the catheter tip when a balloon on the catheter is inflated; reflecting left ventricular end diastolic function. These parameters give clues to the health care team about cardiac functioning and circulatory status. Still another part of the catheter gives a continual core temperature reading. A special port on some catheters allows for temporary pacemaker wires to be inserted. Another port allows for the measurement of cardiac output. As fluid is pushed past this sensor, it reads how long it takes the fluid to reach the sensor and calculates the patient's cardiac output, telling the health care team how effectively the heart is pumping. Other ports are available for IV access and blood sampling as needed.

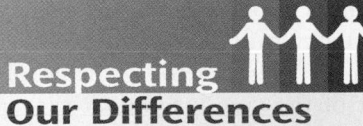

Respecting Our Differences

Respecting our Elders

Prior to initiating IV therapy in an older person, the nurse should consider the physiological changes that occur with aging. The skin becomes thinner and dryer, and subcutaneous tissue is decreased. The immune response of the skin is also decreased as a person ages. That, together with the decreased cell generation and blood supply lead to delayed wound healing and make it even more important to prep the site well. When communicating with an older adult, the nurse should approach the person from the front. Changes in vision and hearing may cause the older person to be startled if approached from the side (Estes, 2006). The nurse should also remember to use layperson terminology when interacting with an older adult. Many older adults will not question the physician or the nurse as they were raised to believe that doctors and nurses are always right and should not be bothered with questions.

SPECIAL CONSIDERATIONS

The graying of America refers to fact that people are living longer than ever before. It also means people are living with more illnesses and needing more health care. The goal of IV therapy in the older adult consists of selecting the correct venous access device, type of therapy, and medication. Nurses need to expand their understanding and knowledge to include the unique needs of the geriatric population and adjust their assessment skills. How well a person ages depends on nutritional, environmental, educational, genetic, societal, physiological, and spiritual factors. Because of the complexity of the aging process, it is more of a challenge to assess the older adult than the younger adult. The geriatric patient is classified into three major groups: (a) young-old (65 to 74 years); (b) middle-old (75 to 84 years); (c) old-old (85 years and older) (Estes, 2006).

The older adult has the right to receive the same consideration and sense of control as the younger population. The older patient should be included when developing the plan of care unless the patient is confused or does not have the ability to make decisions. However, assessment and evaluation of the older patient to make decisions regarding plan of care should be ongoing.

Considerations of IV therapy in the older adult should include vein selection, vascular access device selection, and administration equipment selection. Other special considerations for the older adult and IV therapy are skin preparation, technique, device maintenance, site monitoring, and patient education. Careful assessment and monitoring of the older adult can assist with avoiding the common pitfalls of IV therapy, including fluid volume overload and damage to the skin and vasculature. Selecting the appropriate vein for IV access in the older adult can be challenging for the nurse. The nurse must remember that the initial venipuncture should be in the most distal portion of the extremity. The nurse must also know the type and duration of IV therapy order, which can determine site choice. In addition, the nurse must provide good light when assessing for a site and then carefully palpate the veins. When selecting a site in the older adult, the top of the hand may not be the best choice because of the thinning of the skin and the decreased amount of subcutaneous tissue. The nurse should assess all parts of both extremities noting the number of potential insertion sites. The nurse palpates and assesses the condition of the veins avoiding bruised areas and previously used veins. If a tourniquet is used to distend the vein, the nurse must be careful when applying it so not to tear or pinch the fragile skin and should not leave it on for an extended length of time. Vein damage can result if the tourniquet is left on too long causing bruising or hematoma formation (Altman, 2004).

Once the extremities have been assessed and the veins have been selected, careful consideration must occur when selecting a vascular access device. The nurse must take into consideration the type and duration of the IV therapy such as hydration, antibiotic therapy, supplemental infusion, chemotherapy, and TPN. The selection of the smallest gauge size cannula applies to the older adult as well as the younger adult, because it reduces insertion-related trauma, provides greater hemodilution, and less vein irritation.

Fluid overload, electrolyte imbalance, and other problems can develop rapidly in the older patient receiving IV therapy, especially if there is compromised renal and cardiovascular function. To maintain an accurate IV infusion, the use of an IV pump, evaluation of laboratory values, and patient assessment for signs and symptoms of fluid overload is the responsibility of the nurse.

While skin prep is important in the older adult, the nurse should remember the changes in the skin discussed above. The nurse should consider the appropriate cleansing agent that is not irritating to the skin, apply enough friction so not to bruise or tear the skin, and if hair removal is necessary, clipping the hair is performed (not shaving). Stabilizing the vein is important to successful venipuncture. The older person's fragile veins and thin skin have the tendency to move or roll on insertion, resulting in possible shearing of the skin while piercing the vein. The best insertion technique is to hold the skin taut and use the direct method of inserting on top of the vein. Securing of the device is crucial to prevent the movement of the cannula, which can cause mechanical phlebitis. The IV site should be monitored often and before the start of any IV drug therapy for any indications that the IV cannula might have come out of the vein and be leaking into the tissue. Medications that are infused into the older patient's fragile skin can lead to tissue damage, irritation, and possible burns to the tissue and skin, which can result in infection.

Before venipuncture, the nurse should educate the patient on the purpose of therapy and answer any questions that the patient may have regarding the initiation of the IV. The nurse should speak slowly, clearly, and directly to the older adult as the venipuncture is performed. The patient should be taught to inform the nurse of any problems or concerns with the IV or IV site during therapy. Successful IV therapy in the older adult is dependent on good communication between the nurse and the patient. IV therapy can be administered in various health care settings outside the hospital. As the length of stay in the hospital has increased, so has the realm of the IV home care nurse. The home care IV nurse's role is to evaluate the type and duration of therapy, infusion access, and infusion delivery equipment required (Hitchcock, Schubert, & Thomas, 2003).

These factors are all crucial to determine the appropriateness of home infusion therapy. Evaluation of the patient's home environment, family support, cost of therapy, insurance coverage, and other health care providers are essential when considering home IV therapy. The IV nurse providing care in the home is a partner in the development of a safe, home-based, infusion delivery system. The home is evaluated for: (a) cleanliness; (b) place for supplies; (c) clean work area; (d) special refrigeration needs; (e) pets; (f) sufficient electrical outlets; (g) home is free of insects and parasites; (h) telephone; and (i) batteries and supplies.

LEGAL ASPECTS OF INFUSION NURSING

The professional nurse has the responsibility to deliver nursing care always according to the standards of professional practice. These standards outline what can be reasonably expected from a nurse practicing in a specialty area. These standards are measurable and can be evaluated based on what other similarly educated nurses would do. The standards may vary state to state, so it is important that nurses are familiar with the standards set in the state. Finally, the standard must be based on current nursing knowledge. As knowledge changes, so will the standards of practice, and each nurse is required to maintain a current understanding of the standards. The standards are in place to assist the nurse in delivering safe, consistent care. They also exist to protect the public by providing quality patient care. Federal, state, and local regulations may influence the standards, as well as the professional organizations to which nurses belong. For example, the infusion nurses' society plays a vital role in developing and updating the standards of practice related to IV therapy (Monarch, 2002).

Despite these standards, patients may still believe that the nursing care they received was substandard and may accuse the nurse of negligence. Negligence refers to the failure to act in a manner that a reasonable person would do. In the case of IV therapy, this can refer to the failure to recognize a complication of IV therapy or the failure to take corrective action once a complication is identified. Four things must be proved for negligence to exist. First, it must be proven that the nurse had a duty to act within a certain standard of care. Second, the existence of a breach must be shown. A breach exists when the nurse fails to act according to the standards of care. The third factor is to prove that this breach led to harm. Finally, there must be damages for which the patient may collect compensation. If all four of these conditions do not exist, then negligence cannot be proved. Emotional damages are another way that patient may recover financial compensation. This claims that a patient suffered severe emotional distress as a result of the negligence of the nurse (Monarch, 2002).

Common areas of negligence include medication administration, use of equipment, failure to act, poor communication, and the negligence of another (e.g., carrying out an incomplete order that causes harm). The nurse's best defense is to know the standards of care in the specialty area and to keep current knowledge (Monarch, 2002).

ETHICAL CONSIDERATIONS IN INFUSION NURSING

As medicine continues to evolve, so does the practice of medical ethics. Nurses are not immune to these considerations as patients are living longer and becoming sicker. Nurses are in the natural position to speak up for patients, as they are historically the advocates of the patient. Ethics refers to what is considered morally right and wrong. Terms used in the discussion of ethics include autonomy, nonmaleficence, and beneficence.

Autonomy refers to the right of each person to make decisions without coercion, bullying, or manipulation. Informed consent is based on this principle. Patients may express this right by refusing IV therapy or refusing a blood transfusion. If a patient lacks the ability to make a decision, attempts should be made to try to find out what the patient would have wanted. If the patient previously appointed someone to speak for him or her through an advance directive, that person should be consulted.

Nonmaleficence is the right of each person to be free from harm or the risk of harm being inflicted on him or her. The nurse failing to maintain competency in skills and assessments can inflict harm on a patient. The risk of harm is less defined. Being sick and needing nursing and medical care can be stressful for patients. The fear of having an incompetent or uncaring nurse or the fear of not having one's needs met can cause psychological harm. Frequent communication with patients regarding questions and concerns can help to allay many fears.

Beneficence means that a person is not only free from harm but actually is helped. Nurses are in a unique position not to only carry out physician orders but to empower patients to care for themselves. Nurses empower patients by providing them with the tools necessary to manage their illnesses and have the best quality of life possible.

These principles often come into play no matter which specialty a nurse practices. Patients with chronic illnesses or those with terminal illnesses may no longer wish to receive treatment. The patient may be in conflict with his or her family or with his or her health care provider. Nurses may be asked to participate in procedures with which they are not comfortable, such as abortions or removal of life support. Consulting the institution's ethics committee, chaplain, or social worker can be of great assistance when faced with these conflicts.

FUTURE OF INFUSION THERAPY

Medicine and nursing have seen tremendous growth and will continue to see exponential growth in the future. The key to the future of the IV nurse will lie in the amount of flexibility the profession has. The IV nurse will need to adapt to the changes in how and where therapy is delivered. With the rising costs of health care, more cost effective ways to provide therapy in alternative settings will be necessary, and the IV nurse is the best candidate for this opportunity. The growth in technology will also influence the future of the practice of the IV nurse. The IV nurse needs to keep up with the changes in product technology and become the expert in using these products. No one knows where the specialty of IV nursing will end up, but it is sure to be exciting. While there are many professional organizations that promote aspects of infusion nursing, two major organizations solely devoted to the practice of infusion nursing are the Infusion Nurses Society and The Association for Vascular Access.

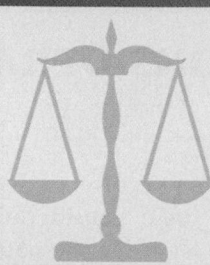

ETHICS IN PRACTICE

Patient's Right to Choice

Mrs. Jones is 72 years old, has a large, close family, and has just been diagnosed with advanced lung cancer. She expresses to you that she does not want to have chemotherapy as she would like what time she has left with her family to be good quality. Her family wants her to have chemotherapy, as they want her to be with them as long as possible. Mrs. Jones tells the physician that she will have the chemotherapy, but you suspect that she is reluctantly doing this to please her family.

The principle of autonomy tells the nurse that the patient has the right to make decisions without coercion or force. The nurse is concerned that her family is coercing Mrs. Jones. Nonmaleficence refers to the right of each person to be free from harm or to be free from the risk of harm. Mrs. Jones is aware of the side effects of the chemotherapy that is being proposed for her, and considering her advanced disease, she is at higher risk of developing these side effects. Beneficence ensures that each person will actually be helped by the nurses' actions. In this case, the nurse is aware that the patient has other wishes than what she is expressing to her physician and is concerned that this is not her true wish. The nurse can play an important role in ensuring that Mrs. Jones' rights are respected and that she makes the best decision for herself.

KEY CONCEPTS

- The skin is the largest organ of the body. It functions to protect the body.
- Arteries and veins are found next to each other in the body. Veins have valves and move blood back to the heart by means of a muscle pump.
- There is a wide variety of equipment used in infusion therapy, including but not limited to administration sets, needleless systems, and rate control devices.

- IV pumps provide an accurate means to infuse fluids or medications.
- Complications of IV therapy can be serious and include: infection, phlebitis, infiltration, extravasation, and nerve damage.
- There are two common methods for calculating drug dosages or fluid infusion rates: the rate-proportion method and the formula method.

Continued

KEY CONCEPTS—cont'd

- IV administration of medications allows for rapid absorption into the system but can also cause severe complications as these drugs work systemically more rapidly than oral medications do.
- Central venous catheters provide access to large veins and long-term access for therapy. Appropriate patient selection as well as appropriate catheter selection is essential to successful therapy.
- TPN and PPN can provide nutrition for patients unable to take nutrition orally.

- Rarely is whole blood transfused anymore, rather, components are given as needed for specific conditions.
- Oncology, pain management, sedation, and hemodynamic monitoring are examples of advance IV therapies.
- IV therapy can be found in many settings: home, acute care, long-term care, and ambulatory infusion centers.
- There are both legal and ethical considerations when involved in infusion therapy.

REVIEW QUESTIONS

1. The cephalic vein runs along the:
   1. Thumb side of the arm
   2. Little finger side of the arm
   3. Inner surface of the forearm
   4. Back of the hand

2. What is the process called that has the ability to cause fluid movement across membranes?
   1. Osmosis
   2. Hypertonic
   3. Tonicity
   4. Osmolality

3. Which type of fluid can cause cells to swell and burst?
   1. Isotonic
   2. Hypotonic
   3. Hypertonic
   4. Tonic

4. Too much of which electrolyte can lead to respiratory depression and arrest?
   1. Calcium
   2. Magnesium
   3. Potassium
   4. Chloride

5. Place the following steps of venipuncture in order: (a) Open all packages; (b) Put on gloves; (c) Verify health care provider order; (d) Prep site; and (e) Perform venipuncture:
   1. a, d, b, c, e
   2. b, c, a, d, e
   3. a, d, c, b, e
   4. c, a, b, d, e

6. Identify the two major types of phlebitis:
   1. Chemical and mechanical
   2. Infected and soft
   3. Extravasation and vesicant
   4. Infiltration and occluded

7. The tip of the central venous catheter lies in the:
   1. Right atrium
   2. Axillary vein
   3. Distal one third of the superior vena cava
   4. External jugular vein

8. Identify which of the following are components of blood (select all that apply):
   1. PRBCs
   2. Normal saline
   3. FFP
   4. Platelets

9. Which of the following is not one of the five rights of medication administration?
   1. Right medication
   2. Right patient
   3. Right room
   4. Right dose

10. Which of the following physiological change in the older adult should a nurse consider when assessing an IV site?
   1. Mental status
   2. Limited income
   3. Skin condition
   4. Mobility IV calculations

Continued

REVIEW QUESTIONS—cont'd

11. Complete the following equation. Amount and medication ordered: morphine sulfate 6 mg IV push as needed. Medication delivered by the pharmacy: morphine sulfate 10 mg/1 mL:
    1. 6 mL
    2. 0.6 mL
    3. 0.06 mL
    4. 60 mL

12. Complete the following equation. Amount and medication ordered: 1,000 mL of D_5RL to run over a 24-hour period. IV fluid available: 15 gtt/mL (drop factor):
    1. 42 mL/hr
    2. 4.2 mL/hr
    3. 0.7 mL/hr
    4. 7 mL/hr

REVIEW ACTIVITIES

1. Set up an IV infusion administration set with a macro standard infusion set.

4. Describe the types of patients that are benefited by using TPN.

2. Compare infiltration and phlebitis.

5. Select a patient that requires a blood transfusion and provide the documentation after performing the skill.

3. Calculate the drip rate of administering an IV solution and set the rate using the clamp and an infusion pump.

Visit the Contemporary Medical-Surgical Nursing online companion resource at www.delmarhealthcare.com for additional content and study aids. Click on Online Companions then select the Nursing discipline.

Complementary and Alternative Therapies

Deb Topham, PhD, RN, CNS, ACRN

CHAPTER TOPICS

- History of Complementary and Alternative Therapy

- Contemporary Trends of Complementary and Alternative Therapy

- Holism and Nursing Practice

- Comparison of Complementary and Alternative Therapy

Western society traditionally tends to look to conventional medicine for mediations, surgery, and other technological interventions. **Conventional medicine** is the common medical practice in the United States by medical doctors, doctors of osteopathy, and their adjunct practitioners: nurses, physical therapists, social workers, and such. However, in many other cultures—past and present—healing is sought through nonconventional means. In the United States, these nonconventional means are known as complementary and alternative medicine (CAM) therapies. Integrative medicine combines mainstream medical therapies and CAM therapies for which there is some high-quality scientific evidence of safety and effectiveness (National Center for Complementary and Alternative Medicine [NCCAM], 2002). This chapter discusses CAM therapies currently being used in holistic nursing practice. Nurses need to critically evaluate CAM therapies before recommending or implementing these approaches.

CURRENT HEALTH SELF-CARE PRACTICES AND COSTS

CAM therapies are diverse medical and health care systems, practices, and products that are not presently considered to be part of conventional medicine (NCCAM, 2002). Americans spend billions of dollars, mostly out-of-pocket, to pay for CAM therapies. Approximately 19 percent of Americans use a nutritional supplement, herb, or other natural product every day (Kelly, et al., 2005). Many insurance companies have increased coverage for some of these therapies, especially chiropractic, massage, and acupuncture.

CONVENTIONAL MEDICINE

Conventional (Western) medicine is relatively new in that it began about 200 years ago. It is also known as **allopathic,** mainstream, orthodox, and regular medicine. Its fundamental principle is that the mind and body are separate entities, and the human is a collection of separate body parts. This approach typically views health as the absence of disease with the goal of treatment to be curing the disease or fixing the problem, such as in the case of trauma. The Western medical model additionally focuses on ridding the body of symptoms induced by disease states or traumatic injury.

The conventional system is most effective when aggressive treatment is needed in the emergency situation. State-of-the-art technology and advanced surgical techniques have become true lifesavers for many in society. However, with its emphasis on curing disease, conventional medicine may overlook the crucial role of energy, emotions, and thoughts in manifestations of disease. Conventional medicine may be less effective in treating chronic conditions, such as hypertension and arthritis. Alternative medicine is especially perceived to be effective for people with chronic, debilitating illnesses for which conventional medicine has few, if any answers. See Table 14-1 for comparison of

TABLE 14-1 Comparison of Conventional and CAM Perspectives

CONVENTIONAL PERSPECTIVE	CAM PERSPECTIVE
Health is absence of disease	Health is a state of well-being illustrated by mind-body balance
Focus of care is on cure or prevention of disease	Focus is on optimum wellness and health
Mind and body are treated separately	Mind and body are one; what affects one affects the other
Disease has a causative agent	Disease is from within and usually a result of internal imbalances
Healing depends on outside agents or interventions; the practitioner cures the patient	The body has a natural ability to heal itself; healing is facilitated through the practitioner
Treatment is usually medications, surgery, or radiation	Treatment is a variety of noninvasive techniques
Healing is aggressive and quick	Healing is a slow and gentle process
Practitioner role is more paternalistic and authoritarian	Practitioner and patient have a more collaborative relationship

Adapted from Conboy, L., Patel, S., Koptchuk, T., Gottlieb, B., Eisenberg, D., & Acevedo-Garcia, D. (2005). Types of complementary and alternative medicines: An analysis based on nationally representative sample. Alternative and Complementary Medicine, 11(6), 977–994.

conventional medicine and CAM therapies; note that as CAM therapies become more accepted, the categorizations are less discrete.

HISTORICAL ROOTS OF CAM

For as long as history has been recorded, people have tried to cure disease and relieve pain. Early cave drawings depict healers practicing their art. Primitive healers attributed the cause of mysterious diseases and ailments to magic and superstition; as a result, religious beliefs and health practices became intertwined. Remedies and interventions from these ancient traditions are being rediscovered and implemented by contemporary holistic practitioners. This section discusses the influence of ancient healing practices on uses of CAM.

Ancient Greek Influence

The ancient Greek culture perceived health as a maintenance of balance in all dimensions of life but especially spiritual. In Greek mythology, Asclepius was the god of healing. Temples, called asclepions, were beautiful places for people to rest, restore themselves, and worship. The Greeks' elaborate healing system consisted of myths, symbols, and rites administered by rigorously trained priest-healers.

Influences from the Far East

Healing systems from the Far East integrate mind, body, and spirit into a system of balanced energy both within the individual and between the individual and the universe. The concept of life force or life energy permeates Eastern philosophies. In Chinese culture, the life force is known as *chi;* in Indian culture, it is known as *prana;* and in Japanese culture, it is known as *qi.* Chinese medicine, known as traditional Chinese medicine (TCM) and Indian medicine, known as Ayurveda, have most heavily influenced integrative therapies in conventional medicine. The concept of the human body provides a fundamental difference in perspective between Western, Eastern, and Indian cultures.

The traditional Chinese healing system is based on the **Tao.** The Tao is a spiritual belief system based upon the teachings of Lao Tzu. In essence, it is believed that everything is the Tao, and the Tao is everything. This belief leads to the understanding of oneness in all things in nature. Life energy (chi) flows through both the universe and the person, thus creating wholeness among all things and people. Chi provides warmth, protection from illness, and vitality. Chi flows along an invisible system of meridians (pathways) that link Chinese medicine's five organ systems together. Illness and injury can alter the flow of this injury by creating obstructed or blocked flow of chi. The flow of chi is enhanced by stimulating points along the meridians.

Acupuncture, acupressure, Chinese herbs, qi gong (breath work), shiatsu (massage), and tai chi (moving meditation) are all therapies within the field of TCM, which act by enhancing the flow of chi. This enhanced chi flow leads not only to healing but also to prevention of imbalances that can lead to disease. Specific TCM therapies are discussed later in this chapter.

Ayurveda is a healing system based on Hindu philosophy, which embraces the concept of an energy force in the body that seeks to maintain balance or harmony. From the Ayurvedic perspective, the body and mind are filled with a vital energy, **prana,** the life force. According to Goldberg (2002), "like all enlightened healing methods, Ayurveda emphasizes prevention above curing disease" (p. 68). The prana is transported through the body by a wind or *vata.* Vata regulates every type of movement. The various types of vata are: *prana, udana, samana, vyana,* and *apana.* Each of these regulates a part of the body's function. For example prana vata regulates the nervous system and samana vata regulates digestion.

The Hindu concept of chakras refers to seven primary energy centers in the physical body. A **chakra** is a concentrated area of energy. The chakras are vertically aligned through the center of the body from the crown of the head to the pelvis. Chakras influence the physical body, emotions, mental patterns, and spiritual awareness. Each chakra has specific functions and a corresponding relationship to body structures and organs.

Prevention of illness and restoration of health through inner search and spiritual growth are the primary goals in the Ayurvedic healing system. Union of the Divine and the Truth occurs through the physical and meditative practice of yoga. In contemporary practice, Ayurvedic interventions consist of yoga, herbs, diet, exercise, steam baths, acupuncture, cathartics, and detoxifying massage.

Shamanic Influence

Shamanism refers to the practice of entering altered states of consciousness with the intent of helping others. The **shaman,** a folk healer-priest who uses natural and supernatural forces to heal others, has an extensive knowledge of herbs, is skilled in many forms of healing, and serves as guardian of the spirits. Illness is considered to be a result of spirit loss. Shamans have the power to heal by working with the spirits to encourage their full return to the individual. The shaman functions as both healer and priest.

The shaman performs ritualized processes, which include seeking wisdom about the universe, a relationship with the creator, and avoidance of death. The shaman's practice may incorporate special objects, such as power animals, totems, and fetishes, as well as ritual songs, dances, food, and clothing. Sleep deprivation, ritual changes, isolation, imagery, drumming, and hallucinogenic drugs may be used to create a trance-like state, which is the vehicle through which the shaman contacts the spirit world. It is on behalf of the patient that the shaman requests spiritual healing. It is believed spiritual healing will lead to physical and emotional healing.

CONTEMPORARY TRENDS

The contemporary public perception of CAM therapies has changed dramatically over recent decades. In the late 1960s and early 1970s, the natural, new age, and self-help movements began to attract followers, first among consumers and later among health care practitioners. During that time, there was a growing trend toward rejection of conventional medicine because of its perceived invasiveness, painfulness, cost, and ineffectiveness, especially with chronic or unknown illnesses. A rekindled interest in Eastern religions, lifestyle, and medicine fueled use of CAM therapies in conventional medicine.

Ever-increasing numbers of consumers, seeking natural and safer approaches to health care, are using CAM therapies to cure disease, manage symptoms of disease, alleviate pain, promote health, and prevent disease. Forty percent of consumers have reported using some form of CAM therapy (Astin, 2004; Astin & Forys, 2004). The sale of natural herbs, vitamins, and other supplements is now a multimillion dollar a year industry. When combined with money spent on other nonconventional therapies, as a whole, integrative therapies are a multibillion dollar market. Based on data collected in a national survey it was estimated Americans spent more than $27 billion dollars, mostly out-of-pocket, on integrative therapies (Conboy, et. al., 2005).

Several factors contribute to the increased use of CAM therapies in the United States. Many health care consumers want to be more involved in their own healing and view CAM therapies as a way to promote this autonomy and control. People who use CAM therapies tend to be people with more education, poorer health status, a holistic view of health, and typically chronic problems, such as anxiety, pain, chronic fatigue syndrome, addictions, headaches, arthritis, back problems, and gastrointestinal (GI) issues.

Nurses need to teach patients about the best of all systems to promote positive healthy outcomes. Patients who withhold use of CAM therapies from a primary health care provider may actually be endangering their health if herbal-pharmaceutical interactions are not anticipated nor screened. The term **integrative therapy** (a clinical approach that combines conventional medicine with CAM therapies) is becoming more accepted. The integrative approach rejects neither conventional medicine or alternative and complementary medicines. Rather, it seeks to help the patient safely integrate the two approaches to health care.

As a result of the public's increased use of CAM, the unethical behavior of some CAM practitioners and a lack of scientific evidence that either supports or refutes the effectiveness of some of these therapies, the United States government established the Office of Alternative Medicine (OAM) in 1992. Today, the OAM is known as the National Center for Complementary and Alternative Medicine (NCCAM) in the National Institutes of Health (NIH). Its mission is to conduct and support research and training, and to disseminate information on these therapies to the public and health care practitioners. Since its inception, the NCCAM has greatly increased the amount of federally funded research that explores the efficacy and therapeutic benefits of various CAM therapies. Clinical trials are underway for nearly every type of CAM therapy. For a listing of clinical trials, go to the NCCAM Web site at http://nccam.nih.gov.

The NCCAM categorizes CAM therapies as: an alternative medical system, mind-body interventions, biologically based therapies, manipulative and body-based methods, and energy therapies (Pelletier, 2004). These classifications imply a discreteness and mutually exclusiveness that is not an accurate characterization of CAM therapies; for instance, the NCCAM includes qi gong as an energy therapy when it is a part of TCM. Examples of alternative medical systems include Ayurvedic medicine, homeopathy, and naturopathy. Mind-body interventions are numerous and include meditation, prayer, guided imagery, and therapies that use creative outlets such as art, music, or dance.

Biologically based therapies include nutrition, dietary supplements, and herbal products. Manipulative and body-based therapies include chiropractic, Rolfing, and massage. Energy therapies include biofield therapies, such as Reiki and therapeutic touch, and bioelectromagnetic-based therapies, such as pulsed fields and magnetic fields.

Mind-Body Research

The conventional medical model was founded on the dualistic belief that the mind and body are separate entities. However, **psychoneuroimmunology (PNI),** an emerging field of science, is studying the complex relationship between the mind and body, specifically the cognitive/affective system in the brain, neurological system, and the immune system. It is also referred to as psychoneuroimmunoendocrinology or PNIE (Anderson, 2005). Psychoneuroimmunologists are investigating how the brain transmits signals along the nerves to enhance the body's normal immune functioning. PNI research supports the idea that the human mind and psychosocial support can alter physiology.

All body cells have receptor sites for **neuropeptides** (amino acids produced in the brain and other sites in the body that act as chemical communicators) that are released when **neurotransmitters** (chemical substances produced by the body that facilitate nerve transmissions) signal emotions in the brain. Thus, it is possible for cells to be directly affected by emotions. In other words, people can affect their health by what they think and feel. The intermeshed complex system of psyche and body chemistry is now referred to as the body-mind (inseparable connection and operation of thoughts, feelings, and physiological functions).

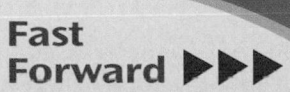

Fast Forward ▶▶▶

Increase Use of Integrative Health Services

In 2006 and beyond, there will continue to be an increase in integrative health services within acute care facilities. Facilities with current integrative therapy departments will be expanding the types of therapies and number of patient visits. Facilities without integrative therapy departments will add these services.

HOLISM AND NURSING PRACTICE

The concept of holism builds on the idea of the mind-body connection, adding a spiritual dimension. **Holism** refers to the concept that the whole is greater than the sum of its parts. Since Florence Nightingale, nursing has taken a holistic approach to patient care. Holism encompasses consideration of the physiological, psychological, sociocultural, intellectual, and spiritual aspects of each individual. Holistic nursing can be described as the art and science of caring for the whole person, knowing that each person is unique in all expressions of self. As holistic healers, nurses often employ CAM therapies to promote patients' well-being. Basic concepts of a holistic philosophy of caring are:

- Mind and body are one entity not separate entities.
- People are responsible for their own choices.
- People have the power to solve their own problems.
- Well-being is multifaceted—physical, emotional, mental, and spiritual.

The Nature of Healing

The word healing is derived from the Anglo-Saxon word *hael*, which means to make whole, to move toward, or to become whole. It is important to establish that healing is not the same as curing (ridding one of disease), but it is a process that activates the individual's healing forces from within. As a healing facilitator, the nurse enters into a relationship with the patient and can assist the patient by offering to be a guide, change agent, or instrument of healing (a means by which healing can be achieved, performed, or enhanced). From a nursing perspective, the nurse facilitates the patient's healing by assisting and supporting the patient. Nightingale (1859) said it best when she wrote, "and what nursing has to do . . . is to put the patient in the best condition for nature to act upon him" (p. 133).

CAM THERAPIES

Many CAM therapies are used in holistic nursing practice. These therapies are categorized as mind-body, body and movement, energy and body work, spiritual, nutritional, and other methodologies (Table 14-2). Although different in technique, many of the CAM therapies have common ideological threads. Conceptual threads shared among CAM therapies include: (a) therapy is geared to the whole system so that parts could be helped; (b) the person is integrated and related to his or her environment; (c) the life force or life energy is used as a part of the healing process; and (d) ritual, prescribed practice and skilled practitioners are integral parts of CAM therapies.

Mind-Body Techniques

Mind-body techniques are methods by which an individual can consciously control some functions of the sympathetic nervous system (e.g., heart rate, respiratory rate, and blood pressure). Mind-body techniques include relaxation, meditation, imagery, biofeedback, and hypnosis.

Relaxation

When confronted with a stressor, the body's flight-or-fight response is stimulated. As a result, the body releases epinephrine, speeds up metabolism, and increases heart and respiratory rates. It has been found that relaxation techniques offer a way for a person to reduce the flight-or-fight response, returning the body to a normal physiological state.

TABLE 14-2 Categories of CAM Therapies

MIND-BODY	BODY MOVEMENT	ENERGY AND BODY WORK	SPIRITUAL	NUTRITIONAL AND DIET	OTHER
Biofeedback	Chiropractic	Acupressure	Faith healing	Herbs	Aromatherapy
Hypnosis	Exercise	Acupuncture	Prayer	Nutraceuticals	Homeopathy
Imagery	Tai chi	Healing touch	Shamanism	Vitamins and supplements	Humor
Meditation	Yoga	Reflexology			Music
Relaxation		Reiki			Pet therapy
		Rolfing			
		Shiatsu			
		Therapeutic massage			
		Therapeutic touch			

Adapted from Conboy, L., Patel, S., Koptchuk, T., Gottlieb, B., Eisenberg, D., & Acevedo-Garcia, D. (2005). Types of complementary and alternative medicines: An analysis based on nationally representative sample. Alternative and Complementary Medicine, *11(6), 977–994.*

Cardiologist Herbert Benson began his studies of the effects of meditation on individuals in 1975. He then incorporated the basic elements of meditation into the therapeutic process he called the **relaxation response,** a state of increased arousal of the parasympathetic nervous system, which leads to a relaxed physiological state. Benson employed the relaxation response with individuals experiencing high blood pressure and heart disease. While initially trying to avoid a mystical flaw in his work, Benson later discovered that the techniques were more effective if individuals focused on inspirational prayer or praise (Astin, 2004; Bonadonna, 2003; Schaffer & Yucha, 2004). The basic elements that facilitate the relaxation response are: (a) a quiet environment, (b) a comfortable position, (c) focused attention, (d) passive attitude, and (e) consistent, regular practice (Schaffer & Yucha, 2004).

Relaxation techniques are skills anyone can use and can be included in the education about nutrition and exercise. One method for achieving relaxation is progressive muscle relaxation (PMR), which is the alternate tensing and relaxing of muscles. Aids to relaxation training include music or nature sounds, drumming, hypertonic saline relaxation tanks, isolation chambers, yoga, and guided imagery.

Nurses can use relaxation techniques in their work with patients to reduce anxiety, pain, and stress. Relaxation techniques are also an essential aspect of cognitive behavioral therapy when treating people with phobias, fear, and depression.

Meditation

The practice of **meditation** (quieting the mind by focusing one's attention) can bring about remarkable physiological changes (Figure 14-1). People who meditate strive for a sense of oneness within themselves and a sense of relatedness to a greater power and the universe. A person can be guided into a meditative or relaxed state by using breath coaching (assisting the patient to become aware of or focus on breathing and thus slowing respirations). Nurses can teach this therapy to patients by using verbal cues, counting the patient's inhalations and exhalations, and showing the patient how to take slow, deep breaths. Some therapeutic benefits of meditation are stress relief, relaxation,

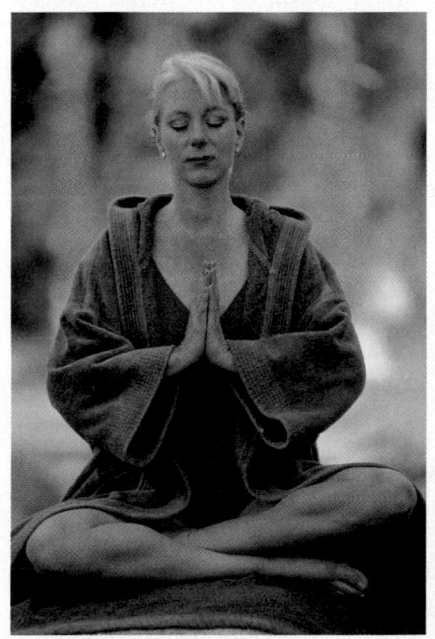

Figure 14-1 Patients may find relief from anxiety through meditation. Courtesy of Photodisc.

Safety First

Contraindications for Imagery

Imagery is not recommended for patients who are emotionally unstable or have active delusions or hallucinations. Patients with these conditions may become agitated or emotionally upset with imagery. The outcome would not be therapeutic.

reduced levels of lactic acid, slowed heart rate, decreased blood pressure, improved immune system function, and decreased oxygen consumption.

Imagery

Imagery is the use of one's sense to create an image in one's mind. The practitioner encourages the patient to use as many of the senses as possible to enhance the formation of vivid images. Table 14-3 illustrates images that can be evoked by the five senses.

Imagery is not a new concept in nursing. In the mid-1800s, Nightingale (1859) wrote about nurses helping the ill to alter their thoughts through images of nature, such as a bouquet of flowers. Imagery has been used effectively by nurses with patients of all ages in settings as varied as schools, homes, hospitals, and nursing homes.

Nurses can create guided imagery for many patients who are capable of hearing and understanding the nurse's suggestions of meaningful and physiologically correct images. For example, a nurse can show a chart of the stages of bone healing to a patient who has suffered a fracture and ask the patient to imagine this sequential activity in his or her body. Another example would be of the nurse using imagery to assist the patient in imaging the white blood cells of the immune system attacking and killing viruses in the body. Imagery has been found to reduce pain and anxiety during procedures, decrease the need for medication or restraints, and promote relaxation.

Biofeedback

Biofeedback is a mechanism of providing feedback about physiological processes to help patients learn how to manipulate those responses through mental activity. It was developed by experimental psychologists and rehabilitation clinicians in the 1960s. Biofeedback allows a person to see the effect of the mind over the body. Biofeedback can be described as a method of gaining conscious control over many bodily reactions by monitoring the emotional state with specially designed equipment. While attached to sensory devices that measure such bodily responses as skin temperature, blood pressure, galvanic skin resistance, and electrical activity in the muscles, the individual imagines stressful experiences. The person's physiological responses are then measured and recorded. Subsequent physiological responses to the relaxation response are also recorded. The individual receives an interpretation of these responses and is taught methods for practicing relaxation, while using feedback from the physiological measures to alter his or her stress response.

Biofeedback has been found to enhance relaxation in tense muscles, relieve tension headaches, reduce bruxism (teeth grinding), reduce the pain of temporomandibular joint (TMJ) syndrome, and relieve backache. Temperature

---

TABLE 14-3	Incorporating All Five Senses into Imagery			
VISUAL	**AUDITORY**	**KINESTHETIC**	**GUSTATORY**	**OLFACTORY**
See foamy water crashing against the rocks	Hear the roar of the water as it crashes onto the rocks	Feel the mist from the water spraying across your face	Taste the saltiness of the ocean wave	Smell the salty air from the ocean shore
See the plump, round orange	Hear peel being pulled from the fleshy fruit of the orange	Feel the rough texture of the orange's outer skin	Taste the orange's juicy flavor as you bite into a slice	Smell the orange with its distinctive smell

Adapted from Astin, J. (2004) Mind-body therapies for the management of pain. Clinical Journal of Pain, 20(1), 27–32.

biofeedback is useful in training people to purposefully warm their hands to treat Raynaud's disease, to lower blood pressure, and to prevent or relieve migraine headaches.

Hypnosis

Therapeutic hypnosis induces altered states of consciousness or awareness (via a trance) during which the person is more receptive to suggestion. A hypnotic state also enhances the patient's ability to form images. In 1955, the British Medical Association approved hypnotherapy as a valid medical intervention. The American Medical Association (AMA) did likewise in 1958. Approximately 15,000 American health care providers currently use hypnosis in conjunction with conventional medical interventions (Goldberg, 2002).

Once the patient is in a hypnotic state, the practitioner offers the patient therapeutic suggestions. Therapeutic use of suggestion is the heart of hypnosis. Suggestions can be phrased directly ("You will feel more comfortable") or indirectly ("You may feel different"). Once aroused from the hypnotic state, the patient's behavior may be affected according to the therapeutic suggestion introduced during the hypnotic state. For example, if the suggestion was to not smoke, a patient may decrease the amount of cigarettes smoked or stop smoking entirely.

Hypnosis is a potentially effective and powerful tool for altering pain, anxiety, and some physiological processes. Although hypnosis is useful as an adjunct to treatment, it does not magically cure such problems as nicotine addiction, alcoholism, and eating disorders, and should be used in conjunction with other therapies.

Nurses wishing to use hypnosis in their practice must be aware of the guidelines concerning this therapy in the scope of practice as defined by the respective state boards of nursing. Advanced training in hypnosis is necessary. In most states, licensure or certification is required to practice as a hypnotist.

Body-Movement Strategies

As the name implies, body-movement therapies employ techniques for moving or manipulating various body parts to achieve therapeutic outcomes. There are many body-movement strategies. The more common strategies of movement are exercise, yoga, tai chi, and chiropractic treatments.

Exercise

Movement, as a therapeutic intervention and health-promoting activity, is associated with athletic exercise and dance. Although the primary goal of exercise is fitness (muscle strength, flexibility, endurance, and cardiovascular and respiratory health), there are many other positive outcomes of exercise.

Nurses can help patients use movement as therapy in a variety of ways, such as range-of-motion exercises, water exercises, physical therapy, and stretching exercises. It is an effective method through which people of all ages can improve their level of functioning. Some of the therapeutic benefits of movement and exercise are improved circulation, enhanced respiratory function, improved elimination, enhanced immune function, and release of **endorphins** (natural brain chemicals that boost mood and help fight depression and pain).

Numerous self-help books, videotapes, magazines, and so forth, are available to assist patients with learning about exercise and movement strategies. For a sedentary patient, a complete physical examination is recommended before beginning any new exercise regimen, especially if the patient is over 40 years old. Patients should be referred to appropriate professionals to assist in learning proper movement and exercise techniques. These would include, but are not limited to, exercise physiologists, certified personal trainers, and physical therapists.

Yoga

Many cultures believe that one particular form of movement can keep the body's life forces in correct balance and flow. Yoga is one ancient ritual movement that enhances overall health, including spiritual enlightenment and well-being. Yoga involves concentration, strength, flexibility, breathing, and use of symbolic movements. Yoga began in Hindu culture around 3,000 B.C. It was formally introduced into Western cultures in the 1800s. The three main elements of yoga are breathing, movement, and posture. Yoga disciplined focus on the mind and body and involves completing a series of postures carried out in sequential order (Goldberg & Goldberg, 2002).

Yoga postures are designed to benefit the physical body. Spiritual benefits are realized when breathing techniques and meditation are incorporated into yoga practice. This enhances the flow of prana or life energy. While self-help tapes are useful, patients should be directed to an experienced yoga teacher to learn correct postures and techniques, thereby maximizing the effectiveness of yoga.

Tai Chi

As with yoga, tai chi is an ancient ritual movement that involves concentration, strength, flexibility, breathing, and use of symbolic movements. Tai chi originated in China in the13th century as a form of movement therapy practiced by Taoist monks. It is often described as a moving meditation, with the goal of gaining balance in the mind, body, and spirit. Tai chi is based on the philosophy of the quest for harmony with nature and the universe through balancing the yin and yang energies of the chi. When balance exists, everything functions with the laws of nature and chi flows. Tai chi consists of a series of sequential movements connected in a smooth flowing process (Horstman, 2006).

As with other forms of chi manipulation, tai chi improves the flow of chi through the meridians of the body. In this manner, tai chi enhances health and promotes healing. People who regularly perform tai chi find it enhances stamina, agility, and balance, as well as boosting energy and conferring a sense of well-being. Tai chi has been shown to lower blood pressure and heart rate in people in cardiac rehabilitation programs and reduces falls by improving balance in older adults (Hortsman, 2006).

Chiropractic Therapy

Chiropractic therapy was begun in 1895 by Daniel Palmer. Palmer found that deliberate and specific manipulation of the spine could improve a patient's health. The major principle underlying chiropractic therapy (the promotion of healing through manipulation of the spinal column) is that the brain sends vital energy to every organ in the body via the nerves originating from the spinal column. Disease results from interferences along these pathways; therefore, manipulation of the spinal column frees up the energy flow and thereby alleviates a variety of ills. Removing the blocks with quick thrusts and adjustments of the spine allows the body to restore its innate recuperative power.

The AMA has a long history of skepticism about chiropractic therapy, condemning it as unscientific in the 1960s. In 1987 the AMA lost a court battle to limit chiropractic therapy. Since then, chiropractic therapy has gradually been accepted by the medical community. Chiropractors are staff members of some medical centers and are commissioned to military branches as health care providers (Goldberg, 2002). As with any CAM therapy, nurses should encourage patients considering the use of chiropractic services to seek the services of board-certified chiropractors. Overwhelming research supports the use of chiropractic therapy for the treatment of acute lower back pain as well as other back injuries.

Energy Therapies

Energy and body work has greatly increased in nursing practice over the past 30 years. Energy work is a group of techniques that work with the body's energy field, using the practitioner's hands to direct or redirect the energy to enhance balance within the field. These therapies have been found to be effective for many patients and can be used to restore balance in all aspects of a person's health. Energy therapies can be used by people of all ages.

Energy therapies have their roots in TCM, ancient Eastern cultures, and Native American philosophies. The fundamental concept is that individuals are composed of a life force or energy that is not confined to the physical skin boundaries. An individual's energy field consists of layers of energy that are in constant flux. The energy layers can be diminished or otherwise adversely affected by any type of illness, trauma, or distress. The energy system can also be positively affected by the intentionally directed use of the hands of the practitioner.

A variety of energy therapies are being used by nurses today. These therapies are being effectively integrated into holistic practice. Holistic nurses were integral in helping the North American Nursing Diagnosis Association (NANDA) establish the nursing diagnosis of *Disturbed Energy Field,* defined as a disruption of the flow of energy (Williams, 2006). A slowing or blocking of the energy field can be due to pathological factors, situational factors, treatment-related factors or maturational factors. Refer to the *Nursing Diagnoses: Definitions and Classification* (2005–2006) by NANDA International for additional information.

Therapeutic Touch

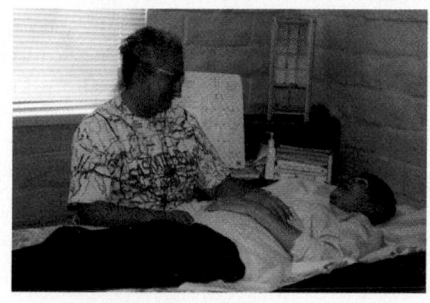

Figure 14-2 Nurse administering therapeutic touch.

Therapeutic touch (TT), which is similar to the ancient healing practice of laying on of hands, consists of assessing alterations in a person's energy field and using a hand to direct energy to achieve a balanced energy state (Figure 14-2). The practice of TT was developed in the early 1970s by Dolores Krieger, then nursing professor at New York University, and Dora Kunz, a noted healer. TT is based on four assumptions: (a) a human being is an open energy system; (b) anatomically, a human being is bilaterally symmetrical; (c) illness is an imbalance in an individual's energy field; and (d) human beings have natural abilities to transform and transcend their conditions of living (Krieger, 1993; 2002).

TT is readily learned in workshops, can be done with hands either on or off the body in the energy field, complements medical treatments, and has reasonably consistent and reliable results. Research has documented the effectiveness of TT in wound healing, relaxation, and immunological functioning. TT can decrease knee pain caused by arthritis. Those participants who received TT reported significantly less pain and more improved function than those in the control group.

Healing Touch

Healing touch (HT) is an energy-based therapeutic therapy that alters the energy field through the use of touch. HT was developed by Janet Mentgen, a nurse, in the 1980s. In 1993, HT was established as a certification program of the American Holistic Nurses Association (AHNA). The AHNA curriculum includes varied techniques for use of HT in general balancing of the body's energy field, relaxation, and for specific problems, such as headaches, spinal problems, and pain. HT recognizes the need for followup or sequential treatments, as well as discharge planning and referral to assist the patient in adequately meeting his or her care goals (Nurse Healers-Professional Associates, Inc., 2005). In both TT and HT, the practitioner uses **centering** (a process of bringing oneself to an inward focus of serenity) before initiating treatment. Centering is a useful tool to employ before performing any treatment or before any situation that may be stressful or difficult (such as a major school examination).

Reiki

Reiki is one of many forms of energy work that was founded in the 1800s when Mikao Usui, a Christian minister in Japan, sought to explain how Jesus healed through the laying on of hands. Usui studied a healing tradition of using hands by Buddhist monks. Through his study and meditation, the system of

Reiki was founded. Reiki has three levels of practitioners, with the Reiki master or master teacher being the highest level. Level I Reiki practitioners are prepared to provide healing work at the physiological/physical level and work with the patient physically present. Level II Reiki practitioners are prepared to provide healing on the emotional and spiritual levels and in absentia. Level III Reiki practitioners are the most skilled and advance to the Reiki teacher. While anyone can learn the hand positions of Reiki, Reiki attunements from a master teacher are necessary to prepare the practitioner for work with patients. Reiki attunements open the crown chakra, enhancing universal energy flow through the practitioner.

Reiki is the use of physical, emotional, and spiritual healing. The practitioner does not use his or her energy to heal the patient but rather acts as a conduit for the universal energy to flow into the person. A typical Reiki session involves the practitioner laying hands over the seven chakras of the body, both anterior and posterior. The universal energy flows through the chakras, opening the energy flow in the individual so that he or she might heal.

There is some research, mostly anecdotal, that supports the benefits of Reiki treatment. Reiki has been found to calm physiological function, increase red and white blood cell production, enhance pain relief, and reduce anxiety. Because Reiki works on physical, emotional, and spiritual levels, the patient is exhausted after a session. The Reiki practitioner should be aware of this and ensure that the patient has support to process emotional reactions after a Reiki session. The NCCAM has been conducting clinical trials on the use of Reiki since 2000. Reiki practitioners are not licensed. They do receive certificates from their Reiki master verifying completion of their training. Nurses should educate their patients to request to see the practitioner's certificate.

Acupuncture

Acupuncture is the use of needles inserted at specific points on the body that correspond to TCM meridians to promote the flow of chi, and thus healing (Figure 14-3). Treatment focuses on correcting the flow of chi when imbalances or blockages occur. TCM practitioners believe that meridians conduct chi between the body's surface and internal organs. In the case of pain, needles are inserted into meridians that affect chi in the liver. It is believed that liver stagnation results in pain. By opening the blocked liver chi, the energy is released and pain is eased. The Western corollary of this is that acupuncture points are believed to stimulate the central nervous system to release chemicals into the muscles, spinal cord, and brain. These chemicals alter the experience of pain or produce other chemicals to lessen the pain (Cherkin, Sherman, Deyo, Shekelle, 2003; NIH, 2004a).

Acupuncture is one of the oldest, most commonly used medical procedures in the world. It originated in China over 5,000 years ago and is effective in treating a variety of health problems. Acupuncture is rapidly gaining acceptance in mainstream conventional medicine. The Food and Drug Administration (FDA) has approved the use of acupuncture in the management of pain, one of the major reasons Americans use acupuncture. It has been found to be particularly useful in the treatment of chronic pain, especially lower back and arthritic pain. Several studies on acupuncture have been sponsored by the NCCAM, including a study that found over half of women with depression experienced significant improvement with acupuncture and use of acupuncture on pregnant women with breech presentations significantly increased head-first births. Several clinical trials have been completed and are available for review on the NCCAM Web site.

NCCAM (2002) reexamined the results of 49 randomized, controlled trials that evaluated massage, spinal manipulation, and acupuncture for effectiveness and costs. Results suggest that massage is an effective treatment for chronic back pain and that spinal manipulation had benefits that are similar to more traditional treatments for chronic back pain. Although acupuncture

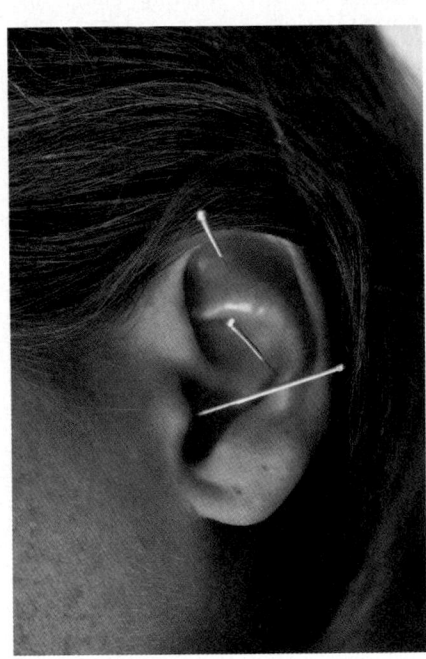

Figure 14-3 Acupuncture needles inserted for treatment of depression. Courtesy of Photodisc.

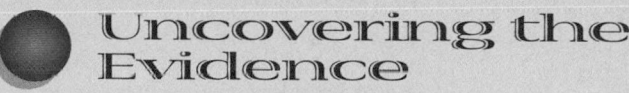

Uncovering the Evidence

Research on Effectiveness of Acupuncture

Discussion: This study is considered to be a landmark study, because it is the longest and largest randomized, controlled phase III clinical trial of acupuncture ever conducted. Rheumatologists and licensed acupuncturists enrolled 570 patients, age 50 or older, with osteoarthritis of the knee. Research subjects were randomly assigned to receive one of three treatments: acupuncture, sham acupuncture, or a control group that used self-help literature to manage their pain. Patients continued to receive conventional medical care from their health care providers, including anti-inflammatory medications and narcotics. For 24 treatment sessions over 26 weeks, 190 patients received acupuncture and 191 patients received sham acupuncture. In the education control group 189 participants attended six, two-hour group sessions over 12 weeks based on the Arthritis Foundation's Arthritis Self-Help Course. Those who received acupuncture had a 40 percent decrease in pain compared with the other two groups and a nearly 40 percent improvement in function compared to baseline assessments of the sham acupuncture and education control groups in the 26-week study period.

Implications for Practice: Acupuncture is an effective intervention in relieving pain and improving movement in people with osteoarthritis of the knee. Given recent problems with side effects from nonsteroidal anti-inflammatory drugs (NSAIDs) and COX-2 inhibitors, patients with limited choices for effective pain relief from medications may be able to get relief and benefit more from acupuncture, which has minimal and temporary side effects.

Citation: Berman, B. M., Lao, L., Langenberg, P., Lee, W. L., Gilpin, A. M. K., & Hochberg, M. C. (2004). Effectiveness of acupuncture as adjunctive therapy in osteoarthritis of the knee: A randomized, controlled trial. Annals of Internal Medicine, 141(12), 901–910.

---

is only slightly more effective than no treatment or sham treatment, the review found the quality of the studies is not high enough to draw firm conclusions. The study concludes that massage, spinal manipulation, and acupuncture are all relatively safe, but massage therapy is the most cost-effective.

Acupressure

Acupressure is similar to acupuncture in its application and effect. The difference is that rather than using fine, solid needles to stimulate acupuncture points, the practitioner uses consistent and firm pressure from fingers or other devices. Antiemetic armbands applied to specific acupuncture points on the wrist have been found to be effective in decreasing nausea both during pregnancy and chemotherapy.

Body Work Therapies

One of the most universal CAM therapies is various forms of touch. Touch, simply defined, is the means of perceiving or experiencing through tactile sensation. According to the classic work of anthropologist Montague (1986), touch is the earliest sense to develop in humans, and thus it provides a basic means of interacting with others and the environment. Tactile stimulation is necessary for survival and the healthy behavioral development of the individual. Touch carries with it taboos and prescriptions. It was used in all ancient

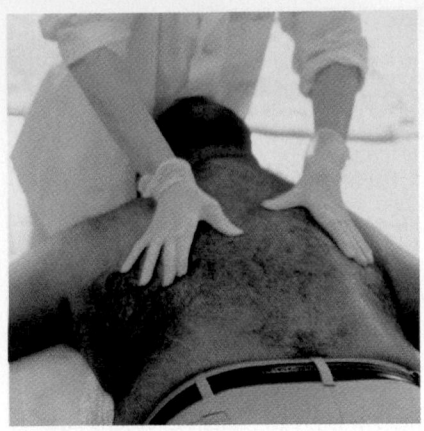

Figure 14-4 Nurse finishing a massage with effleurage—long, gliding, rhythmic strokes.

cultures and shamanistic traditions for healing. The advent of scientific medicine and Puritanism led many healers away from the purposeful use of touch. Some cultures are comfortable with physical touch; others specify that touch may be used only in certain situations within specified parameters. In addition, the use of gloves by health care providers adds to the difficulty of contact and the use of touch.

Because touch involves personal contact, the nurse must be sure to convey positive and healthy intentions. When in doubt, the nurse should withhold touch until effective communication with the patient has been established. Touch has several important uses in nursing practice: it is an integral part of assessment; it promotes bonding between nurse and patient; it is an important means of communicating caring, especially if other senses are impaired; it assists in soothing, calming, and comforting patients; and it helps keep the patient oriented.

Therapeutic Massage

Therapeutic massage is the application of pressure and motion by the hands with the intent of improving the recipient's well-being. Massage increases muscle circulation, promotes removal of toxins, and leads to muscular relaxation (Figure 14-4). It involves kneading, rubbing, and using friction (Box 14-1).

BOX 14-1

BASIC MASSAGE TECHNIQUES

Effleurage

- The whole hand is used. Gliding and long rhythmic strokes are used.
- Firm, even-pressured strokes are directed toward the heart to assist blood return.
- Lighter pressure is used when moving away from the heart.

Pétrissage

- Pressing, squeezing, kneading, and rolling movements by both hands (entire hand).
- Deep circulation is enhanced.
- C-shaped motions stimulate the muscle body.
- Promotes muscle relaxation.

Friction

- Thumb pads, heel of hand, or fingertips are used.
- Focused, deep, circular motions are used.
- Penetrates deeper muscle layers.
- Is done after effleurage and pétrissage.

Tapotement

- Palms, fingertips, and knuckles are used.
- Brisk, vigorous, rhythmic, percussive movements are used.
- Hands alternately tap, cup, slap, and pummel muscles.
- Invigorates and stimulates tired muscles.

Touch Vibrations

- Fine, rapid, shaking movements are administered by the entire hand.
- Stimulates or relaxes muscles.

Adapted from Cherkin, D. C., Sherman, K. J., Deyo, R. A., & Shekelle, P. G. (2003). A review of the evidence for the effectiveness, safety, and cost of acupuncture, massage therapy, and spinal manipulation for back pain. Annals of Internal Medicine, 138*(11), 898–906.*

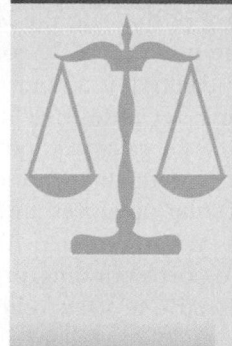

ETHICS IN PRACTICE

Professional Standards for Massage

The National Association of Nurse Massage Therapists (NANMT) was established in 1990 to promote professional ethical standards for nurse massage therapists. These standards reflect the standards of the American Nurses Associations. Boards of nursing in some states, e.g., Louisiana and Massachusetts, specifically indicate that complementary therapies including massage are within the scope of nursing practice.

For the past 30 years, many touch therapies have been assimilated into mainstream nursing practice. Massage therapy is now recognized as a highly beneficial therapy and is prescribed by a number of health care providers. In most states there are no licensing requirements for practitioners who use massage techniques. While only licensed massage therapists can perform therapeutic massage, nurses and physical therapists commonly use massage techniques to promote patient relaxation and healing.

Traditionally, back rubs are administered by nurses to provide comfort to hospitalized patients. Back rubs assist with easing back strain that accompanies prolonged time lying in bed. Massage techniques can be used with all age-groups and are especially beneficial to those who are immobilized. A back rub or massage can promote relaxation, increase circulation of the blood and lymph, and provide relief from musculoskeletal stiffness, pain, and spasm.

Shiatsu

Shiatsu is a combination of acupressure, massage, stretching, and joint manipulation. It is based on a Japanese methodology but heavily influenced and guided by TCM. Shiatsu literally means finger pressure. As with acupuncture, the focus of the shiatsu practitioner is to unblock chi flow by application of pressure, massage, and manipulation along meridians of the body. In contrast to traditional massage, shiatsu is performed with the patient fully clothed and on a low bed or floor mat.

Rolfing

Rolfing is a form of deep tissue massage and manipulation to correct body posture. The rolfer focuses on one specific body part and applies pressure to loosen connective tissue or fascia. This results in lengthening and relaxation of the fascia. These releases allow the body's correct alignment to be restored. Usually 10 sessions are required to completely restore the body's alignment. It is believed that the corrected body alignment allows the body to restore its natural healing.

Reflexology

Reflexology is also rooted in ancient healing arts. Egyptian wall paintings from approximately 2,300 B.C. show the use of reflexology. Contemporary use of reflexology is credited to the work of William H. Fitzgerald, an American physician who, in the early 1900s, discovered that applying pressure to certain parts of fingers could relieve pain in other body parts. In the 1930s, Eunice Ingham discovered that certain points on the feet were more responsive to pressure and provided better pain relief than points on the hand.

The fundamental concept of reflexology is that the body is divided into 10 equal, longitudinal zones that run the length of the body from the top of the head to the tip of the toes. These 10 zones are correlated with the 10 fingers and toes. The foot is viewed as a microcosm of the entire body. Reflexology theory posits that illness manifests itself in calcium deposits and acids in the corresponding part of the person's foot. Pressing specific points on the foot stimulates energy movement and produces relaxation, reduces stress, and promotes health by relieving pressures and accumulation of toxins in the corresponding body part. Massage of specific points on the feet and hands promotes energy flow to corresponding organs and body parts. Reflexology has been shown to be effective in stress relief. It is believed to facilitate healing in the body organs and to restore balance to the body.

Spiritual Therapies

A basic premise of spiritual therapies is that one's health is dependent on the spiritual aspects of oneself. When the body or mind is disrupted or unhealthy, it reflects a spiritual imbalance and vice versa. Thus, spiritual interventions facilitate whole-body healing. The belief that there is a relationship between spirituality and health is not new.

A core value of holistic nursing practice is adherence to preserving the wholeness and dignity of all people and their families, as well as their values, meaning, and purpose in life.

The role of the spirit in healing is witnessed in all cultures. The inseparable link between the state of one's soul (life energy or spirit) and the state of one's health is accepted by many cultures. Healers believe that biological changes are a result of therapeutic changes in a person's soul or spirit. Scientists, specifically psychoneuroimmunologists, are beginning to validate that there are inner mechanisms of healing within individuals.

Faith Healing

At the heart of spiritual or faith healing is the practitioner's belief that one has to purify one's self and reach a state of unity with God or a higher power. This process, based on religious belief, is usually done through prayer. During preparation for healing, the practitioner adopts a passive and receptive mood to be a channel for divine power. To benefit from the healer's intervention, the ill person is best healed if he or she has faith in the healer and the deity that the healer represents.

Healing Prayer

When individuals pray, they believe they are communicating directly with God or a higher power. Prayer is an integral part of a person's spiritual life and, as such, can affect well-being. Nightingale (1859) recognized that prayer helps connect individuals to nature and the environment. Many religions adhere to established rituals for organized prayer. For example, Tibetan Buddhists use prayer wheels, which are wooden and metal cylinders with prayers written on them. Islam has five periods of prayer scheduled daily. Christian Scientists rely on prayer in lieu of conventional medical therapy based on a belief that prayer alone can heal disease. Medical research is currently investigating the effects of prayer on physical health. Early research has shown that worshipping and prayer have significant health and survival implications

Shamanism

As previously described, shamanism is a form of spiritual healing. With the increased interest in CAM therapies, many patients are turning to shamans to assist in healing and well-being. Shamans, both priest and healer, work with a variety of therapies to enhance healing, but spiritual guidance underlies all

---

Respecting Our Differences

Cultural Beliefs

Recently there has been a significant increase in Hmong immigrants to the United States. A Hmong belief that interferes with the U.S. health care is that when surgery opens the body, the spirit escapes. To facilitate surgery on a Hmong patient one health care facility agreed to allow a Hmong healer to be present in the operating room. The healer carried with him a hard-boiled egg. During surgery the healer directed the man's escaping spirit into the egg. After surgery the Hmong patient ate the egg, returning his escaped spirit to his body.

shamanic practice. The shaman connects with spiritual guides and seeks healing on behalf of patients.

Nutritional and Diet Therapies

In the last 30 years nutritional interventions for prevention and treatment of disease have received increased interest from consumers and health care providers. Conventional researchers have been able to clearly demonstrate a link between diet and cardiac disease, diabetes, and some forms of cancer, specifically GI cancers. Based on this research, conventional practitioners recommend a diet high in fiber, low in fat, and high in fruits and vegetables. Nutritional therapies discussed here will focus on CAM therapies that have less but increasing scientific support.

Nutraceuticals

Currently, many foods and plants are being studied for their medicinal value. **Nutraceuticals** refer to any natural substance found in plant or animal foods that acts as a protective or healing agent. **Phytonutrients** refer to those chemicals found in plants (Table 14-4).

Foods that are being investigated by the National Cancer Institute for possible cancer preventive qualities include carrots, celery, citrus fruits, flaxseed, garlic, licorice root, parsley, and soybeans. The best source of nutrients is fresh whole foods, preferably eaten in their natural form. The standard Western diet lacks many essential nutrients because of processing and contains many harmful additives. In contrast, a TCM diet contains fresh, semiraw, and slightly cooked ingredients. The Chinese diet emphasizes natural food alchemy taking place inside the body by virtue of food enzyme activity (Chopra & Simon, 2002; Pitchford, 2002).

TABLE 14-4 Sources and Actions of Major Phytonutrients

PHYTONUTRIENT	SOURCES	ACTIONS
Ascorbic acid	Citrus fruits, broccoli, and most fruit and vegetables	Binds iron, preventing it from becoming a cancer-causing preoxidant
Capsaicin	Red chili peppers	Helps prevent carcinogens from binding with DNA at the cellular level
Catechins	Green tea and black tea	Reduce the risk of GI cancers
Fiber ligands	Soybeans, flaxseed, and nuts	Inhibit growth of tumors
Fiber pectin	Apples, pears, plums, and prunes	Improves colon health; encourages growth of beneficial intestinal flora
Lycopene	Tomatoes and tomato sauce	Protects against prostate cancer; helps block ultraviolet A (UVA) and ultraviolet B (UVB) rays
Phytoestrogens	Soy products and alfalfa sprouts	Help reduce menopausal symptoms; may block some cancers (i.e., breast)
Phytosterols	Plant oils, corn, sesame, soy, safflower, pumpkin, and wheat	Inhibit uptake of cholesterol from foods; block hormonal role in cancer production
Protease inhibitors	Soybeans and soy products, eggs, cereal, and potatoes	Protect against negative effects of radiation and free radical damage; prevent activation of certain genes that cause cancer
Sulfur compounds	Onions and garlic	Lower blood pressure; improve immune system response; fight infections; antimicrobial effect; lower cholesterol; reduce triglycerides

From Pitchford, P. (2002). Healing with whole foods: Asian traditions and Modern nutrition. Berkeley, CA: North Atlantic Books; Roth, R. (2007). Nutrition and diet therapy (9th ed.). New York: Thomson Delmar Learning.

Vitamins and Supplements: Antioxidants and Free Radicals

Vitamins and other supplements have long been believed to be effective in promoting health. While a healthy, balanced diet should provide all the vitamins and minerals the body needs, many Americans eat unbalanced diets and thus need vitamin supplementation. Vitamins and minerals for supplementation are different from vitamins used for CAM. Vitamins and minerals in CAM traditionally are used in doses higher than recommended daily doses of vitamins and minerals. Research has just begun on the health benefits of vitamins and minerals used in CAM.

Vitamin C, vitamin E, and beta-carotene, which converts to vitamin A, have been shown to possibly prevent heart disease and some forms of cancer. Antioxidants exert several beneficial effects including prevention of cancer, reduction of heart disease, and possible retardation of the aging process. Antioxidants neutralize free radicals, preventing them from damaging cells or altering deoxyribonucleic acid (DNA). Sources of dietary antioxidants include vitamin C (in fruits and vegetables), vitamin B_6 (in whole grains), vitamin A (metabolized from beta-carotene), beta-carotene (yellow-orange pigment in fruits and vegetables), and vitamin E (in polyunsaturated oils, butter, and eggs). The antioxidants devour free radicals (unstable molecules that alter genetic codes and trigger the development of cancer growth in cells).

Other vitamins, minerals, trace elements, and enzymes are being investigated for possible therapeutic value and health benefits. For instance, calcium supplements are believed to be beneficial in prevention of osteoarthritis, and calcium is also believed to have a sedative effect if taken before bedtime. Chromium is believed to play a role in blood sugar regulation via enhancement of fat metabolism. Folic acid is commonly prescribed in early pregnancy as it enhances neurodevelopment of the fetus. Iron supplements aid in treating some forms of chronic anemia. A final examination of beneficial supplements is that of omega-3 fatty acids. Omega-3 fatty acids, most commonly found in fish oils, have been found to support immune system function and help mediate allergic responses, especially in people with allergy-induced asthma (Roth, 2007).

Herbal Therapy

Herbal medicine has been a powerful tool in folk healing for centuries. Medicinal herbs have been cataloged for thousands of years. The earliest record of herbal remedies was found in ancient Egypt. More than 500 herbal remedies were recorded on papyrus during that time. Herbal remedies are prevalent throughout the world. Most herbs used are indigenous to various cultures. Only recently have herbs been transported for use by people of other cultures; an example is the increasing use of Chinese herbs by Americans. Outside of industrialized countries herbs may be the primary form of medication. Herbal medicine, also know as botanical medicine or phytotherapy, uses plant extracts for therapeutic outcomes. Many holistic practitioners incorporate the use of herbs into their practice.

Learning about herbal treatment is similar to learning pharmacology. Herbs work because of their chemical composition. Different herbs contain different compounds that can strengthen the immune system, alter the blood chemistry, or protect specific organs against disease (Duke, 2002). For instance, peppermint oil may help relieve the symptoms of irritable bowel syndrome by exerting a relaxing effect on the GI tract (Gruenwald, 2004). Echinacea is frequently used for its immune-enhancing properties (NCCAM, 2005). See Table 14-5 for a list of medicinal uses of common herbs.

Herbs should not be used indiscriminately, because their use may negatively affect the patient. In addition, some patients may experience allergic reactions to herbs. See Table 14-6 for a list of common allergic reactions to specific herbs. Patients should be taught to recognize the potential for developing

TABLE 14-5 Medicinal Value of Herbs	
HERB	**MEDICINAL USE(S)**
Aloe Vera *(Aloe vera)*	Minor cuts and abrasions
	Burns
Calendula *(Calendula officinalis)*	Cuts and abrasions
	Minor burns and sunburns
	Acne
	Athlete's foot
	Oral thrush (as mouthwash)
	Vaginal thrush (douche)
Celery seed *(Apium graveolens)*	Hypercholesterolemia
	Edema and fluid overload
Chamomile *(Matricaria chamomilla)*	Anxiety
	Nausea
	Tension headache
Dandelion *(Taraxacum officinalis)*	Edema, fluid overload
	Indigestion
Eucalyptus *(Eucalyptus globules)*	Prevent and treat bacterial infections
	Respiratory decongestant
Evening primrose *(Oenothera biennis)*	Atopic eczema
	Asthma
	Migraines
	Premenstrual syndrome (PMS)
	Arthritis
Feverfew *(Tanacetum parthenium)*	Migraines
Garlic *(Allium sativum)*	Hypercholesterolemia
	Prevent respiratory infections
	Expectorant
Ginger *(Zingiber officinale)*	Nausea related to motion sickness or pregnancy
	Poor circulation in hands and feet
	Expectorant
	Indigestion, flatulence, diarrhea
Ginkgo *(Gingko biloba)*	Dementia
	Impotence
	Peripheral vascular insufficiency
	Memory impairment
Lavender *(Lavandula angustifolia)*	Headaches
	Muscle spasms
	Tension, anxiety
Milk thistle *(Silybum marianum)*	Hepatitis, cirrhosis and other liver disorders
	Gallstones

Continued

TABLE 14-5 Medicinal Value of Herbs—cont'd	
HERB	**MEDICINAL USE(S)**
Peppermint *(Mentha X piperita)*	Headache
	Sinus congestion
	Indigestion
St. John's wort *(Hypericum pereforatum)*	Mild to moderate depression
	Sleep disorders
	Viral infections
Sage *(Salvia officinalis)*	Prevent bacterial infections
Thyme *(Thymus vulgaris, T. serpyllum)*	Prevent bacterial infections
	Common cold, bronchitis
	Cystitis
	Fungal infections, especially topically applied
	Oral thrush (as mouthwash)
Valerian *(Valeriana officinalis)*	Insomnia
White willow *(Salix alba)*	Headache
	Fever
	Muscular aches and pains

Note: The information is not intended to be a guide for self-medication. Have your patient consult an experienced herbalist before consuming herbs for medicinal purposes.
Adapted from Goldberg, B., & Goldberg, M. (2002); Alternative medicine: The definitive guide. Berkeley, CA: Celestial Arts; Gruenwald, J. (2004). PDR for herbal medicines (3rd ed.). Montvale, NJ: Medical Economics Co., Inc.

allergic reaction to herbs, identify indicators of allergic reactions, and to stop using the herbs if allergic symptoms occur. For example, apricot and arnica have contact allergy reactions; celery and motherwort have photosensitivity reactions; and garlic and tansy have systemic reactions (Mustalish, 2002).

Patients taking herbs should also understand that herbs and pharmaceutical medications may interact. Additionally, the chemical constituents of herbs may alter the effects of some medications. See Table 14-6 for a list of herb and medication interactions. The nurse should instruct patients to disclose all herbal supplements to their health care providers and pharmacists so that they may evaluate the potential for drug-herb interactions.

Aromatherapy

Aromatherapy is the therapeutic use of concentrated essences or essential oils that have been extracted from plants and flowers. When diluted in carrier oil for massage or in warm water for inhalation, essences may be stimulating, uplifting, relaxing, or soothing. Essential oils help relax the mind and the body by promoting balance between the sympathetic and parasympathetic nervous systems. They stimulate endorphins, peptides released by the brain that relieve pain, and rejuvenate the immune system. Aromatherapy is used to treat a variety of conditions and promote a sense of well-being, including: stress and anxiety related problems, muscular and rheumatic pains, digestive disorders (e.g., nausea), female sexual health conditions (e.g., premenstrual syndrome[PMS] and menopausal symptoms), upper respiratory conditions, and skin conditions.

TABLE 14-6	Interactions between Herbs and Medications	
HERB	**MEDICATION**	**EFFECT OF COMBINATION**
Aloe	Thiazide diuretics and corticosteroids	Enhanced potassium loss
	Cardiac glycosides and antiarrhythmics	Potentiated by potassium loss
Belladonna	Tricyclic antidepressants, amantadine, quinidine	Increased anticholinergic effect
Brewer's yeast	MAO inhibitors	Increased warfarin bioavailability
		Increased prothrombin time
Ginkgo	Warfarin, heparin	Increased bleeding risks
Licorice root	Acetaminophen	Accelerated excretion
	Antihypertensives	Decreased antihypertensive effect
	Estrogens	Increased estrogenic effect
	Fludrocortisone	Increased blood pressure
	Thiazide diuretics and corticosteroids	Enhanced potassium loss

Adapted from Blumenthal, M., Brinkman, J., Dinda, K., Goldberg, A., & Wolkschlaegear, B. (2004). The ABC clinical guide to herbs. *New York: Hawthorne Press, Inc.*

While aromatherapy is an essentially safe CAM therapy, certain precautions should be followed. Guidelines for using aromatherapy are: always dilute essential oils in a carrier oil; do a skin patch test for sensitivity before applying essential oils to the skin; avoid contact with the eyes or mucous membranes; inhale essential oils only for a short period of time; store oils in a dark glass bottle, tightly capped and away from heat and sunlight; and use only pure essential oils, not synthetics.

Humor

Humor is a frequently used CAM therapy and one of the therapies most often used to promote wellness (Minden, 2002). Norman Cousins (1979) was one of the first to identify the use of humor for its health benefits. Cousins attributed his recovery from an incurable connective tissue disorder by daily watching of films and movies that made him laugh. He described his experiences in his book, *Anatomy of an Illness*. Humor is found to increase an ability to cope with pain, enhance immune system function, enhance respiratory function, and reduce preprocedural anxiety (Figure 14-5).

Prior to initiating humor therapy, it is important to determine patients' perceptions of what is humorous to avoid offending them. Differentiation between humorous and offensive situations varies greatly from culture to culture and person to person. Nurses can use humor with patients in a variety of ways. A humor cart (portable cart filled with joke books and funny videos) is easy to use and allows patients to select their own humor tools. Humor should also be age appropriate.

Pet Therapy

The use of animals to enhance health status has a long history. In Britain in the 18th and 19th centuries, pets were used in institutions to give a sense of meaning and purpose to people institutionalized because of developmental delays. Nightingale (1859) stated, "a small pet is often an excellent companion for the sick, for long chronic cases especially" (p. 36). The therapeutic use of pets may

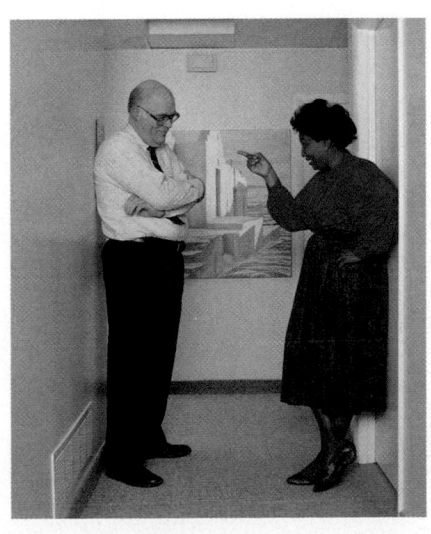

Figure 14-5 Humor and laughter are effective means of promoting wellness.

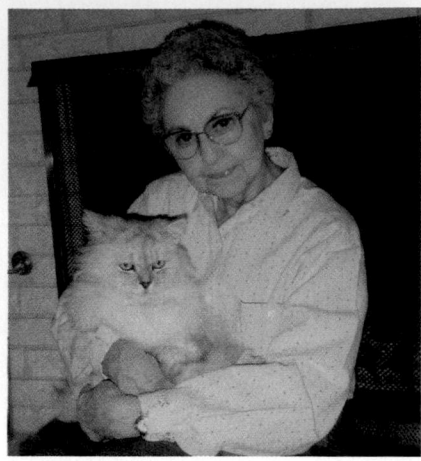

Figure 14-6 Interacting with pets can lead to therapeutic benefits.

be particularly helpful with older people (Delta Society, 2005). Playing with and petting animals can help people feel less isolated and lower blood pressure.

Pet therapy is currently used as adjunctive treatment for people in both acute and long-term care settings (Figure 14-6). Among the uses of pet therapy include helping people to overcome physical limitations, improve mood, decrease blood pressure, improve socialization skills, improve self-esteem, decrease anxiety, and provide companionship.

Music

Music enters the body-mind through the auditory sense. Therapeutic use of music is the playing of music to elicit positive changes in behavior, emotions, or physiological responses. Music complements other treatment therapies and encourages active participation of patients in their health care. Music is a good adjunct to imagery because it can enhance the relaxation response and thereby heighten images. Music can also be used to relax or stimulate—it can lull infants to sleep or it can energize a person who is lethargic and unmotivated. The therapeutic benefit derived from music will be influenced by patients' perceptions and cultural backgrounds. The basic elements of music (i.e., rhythm, pitch, and intensity) are transmitted by sensory impulses from the cochlea to the thalamus, where they are mediated, then to the cerebral cortex, affecting the autonomic nervous system (Goodal & Etters, 2005). Many therapeutic benefits can be derived from music therapy, such as reducing pain and anxiety; calming irritable infants; relaxing women during the labor process; and for relaxation and stress reduction during the rehabilitation process (Nolan, 2006). Music and imagery can be used together to reduce pain and provide greater mobility in affected rheumatoid arthritic joints. It can also be used with children with attention deficit disorder to gain longer attention spans, improved mood control, decreased impulsivity, and improved social skills.

Music delivered via headsets can be a useful tool in decreasing anxiety in patients who are immobilized, waiting for or undergoing diagnostic tests, such as magnetic resonance imaging (MRI), or awaiting surgical procedures. Some patients have benefited from having their selected music played during their surgical procedure. Pleasurable music has been shown to reduce pain, stress, anxiety, and feelings of isolation.

Although music is therapeutic for people of all stages in the life cycle, **music-thanatology** is a holistic and palliative method for use of music with dying patients. Harpists are most commonly trained to provide therapeutic music for patients in the dying process. Music-thanatology is used to help dissipate obstacles to patients' peaceful transition to death.

Homeopathy

Homeopathy, the treatment of disease with minute drug dosages, was created by a German physician, Samuel Hahnemann, in the early 1800s. The term homeopathy is derived from the Greek terms *homoios,* which means like, and *pathos,* which means pathology. The basis of homeopathy is the belief that like causes like. Thus, a substance is given to activate an illness, which then stimulates the body's normal defense system to eliminate the illness. Hanemann believed that symptoms of illness are a part of the curative process in patients. A homeopathic remedy is an extremely diluted form of a medication that serves to stimulate patients' defenses to fight disease and thus to heal.

NURSING AND CAM THERAPIES

Nurses play an important role in educating consumers about CAM therapies by providing information about the safety and efficacy of such methods. A major challenge facing nursing, today and in the future, will be the promotion of integrative care in which patients use the best of CAM and conventional medicine. An integrative approach to practice will demand that nurses promote integration rather than replacement of conventional care. Education is a major function of nurses, and it is greatly needed as consumers try to determine which CAM therapies are best matched to their own needs. Consumers should be cautioned to recognize the following signals to fraudulent CAM practices: practitioners promise immediate relief or complete cures, practitioners claim their way is the only sure therapy, practitioners refuse to work with other health care providers, practitioners place more priority on money than on the patient's well-being, practitioners who use testimonials versus research to support "amazing results," and practitioners use phrases such as "miraculous cure," "scientific breakthrough," or "secret ingredient."

Holistic nurses individualize every intervention on the basis of patients' unique needs. Nurses using CAM therapies must maintain technical expertise and critical analysis about these therapies. In addition, nurses must assist patients in differentiating between valid, science-based evidence and vague, unsupported claims.

Nurses as an Instrument of Healing

When nurses serve as an instrument of healing, the objective is to assist patients to call forth their inner resources for healing. To accomplish this goal nurses must have a solid knowledge base of CAM therapies, obtain certification or licensure for therapies requiring them, foster intentionality to consciously direct healing, respect and honor patients' culturally based health beliefs, and model health and wellness for their patients.

Nurses can use many CAM therapies without advanced preparation. Imagery, relaxation techniques, meditation, massage, touch, prayer, humor, music, and pet therapy are CAM therapies available to all nurses. Nurses who are interested in performing Reiki, TT, HT, hypnosis, biofeedback, and other such therapies need additional education and training. Nurses need to check with their individual states to determine which require additional licensure or certification. Nurses interested in pursuing use of CAM therapies should begin by contacting the American Holistic Nurses Association at http://ahna.org.

KEY CONCEPTS

- An ever-increasing number of health care consumers use CAM therapies.
- Holistic nursing practice values each patient as a unique and whole being with physiological, psychological, sociocultural, intellectual, and spiritual components.
- Healing is not the same as curing. Rather, healing is regaining balance and finding harmony and wholeness as changes take place within the individual.
- CAM practitioners do not heal the patient; they support the patient's innate healing capacity.

- CAM therapies are categorized as mind-body, body-movement, energy and body work, nutritional therapies, spiritual therapies, and other therapies.
- Nurses should only practice CAM therapies for which they are prepared.
- Every health assessment should include the assessment of the patient's use of CAM therapies, especially herbs and essential oils that might interact with medications or produce an allergic response.

REVIEW QUESTIONS

1. Ancient healing traditions that have influenced use of CAM therapies include all of the following *except:*
   1. Ayurvedic
   2. Traditional Chinese medicine
   3. Native American shamanism
   4. European herbalism

2. Conventional medicine is also known as (select all that apply):
   1. Integrative medicine
   2. Allopathic medicine
   3. Naturopathic medicine
   4. Western medicine
   5. Orthodox medicine

3. What emerging field of science offers theoretical support for the development of CAM therapies?
   1. Psychoimmunology
   2. Neurobiology
   3. Psychoneuroimmunology
   4. Neuroimmunology

4. Which CAM therapy comes from Indian or Hindu roots?
   1. Traditional Chinese medicine
   2. Shamanism
   3. Ayurvedic
   4. Shiatsu

5. Which CAM therapy is most effective in pain management of persons with osteoarthritis of the knee?
   1. Imagery
   2. Massage
   3. Acupuncture
   4. Tai chi

6. What cautions should patients take when using CAM therapies (select all that apply)?
   1. Find reliable practitioners through friends
   2. Seek services of licensed or certified providers
   3. Tell their primary care provider about all CAM therapies they use
   4. Not take their prescription medications at the same time as taking herbs.

7. What nursing organization provides support and resources for nurses who use CAM therapies (fill in the blank)?

   _____

8. Who first perceived nursing's role as putting the patient "in the best position for nature to act upon him [sic]"?
   1. Dolores Kreiger
   2. Florence Nightingale
   3. Barbara Dossey
   4. Janet Mentgen

9. Which CAM therapies require additional certification or licensure (beyond RN) (select all that apply)?
   1. Relaxation
   2. Imagery
   3. Hypnosis
   4. Reiki
   5. Acupuncture

10. What are common sources of the major phytonutrient ascorbic acid?
    1. Apples, pears, and prunes
    2. Citrus fruits, broccoli, and most vegetables
    3. Red chili peppers
    4. Tomatoes and tomato sauce

11. Which herb is commonly used topically for burns and minor cuts?
    1. Celery seed
    2. Chamomile
    3. Eucalyptus
    4. Evening primrose
    5. Aloe vera

12. Milk thistle is an herb that provides benefit to which major body organ(s)?
    1. Lungs
    2. Heart
    3. Kidneys
    4. Liver
    5. Brain

13. If you have a patient on the anticoagulant warfarin, which herb should they avoid taking (select all that apply)?
    1. Ginkgo
    2. Aloe vera
    3. Licorice root
    4. Brewer's yeast

14. What national group is responsible for funding research that evaluates the effectiveness of CAM therapies?
    1. American Holistic Nurses Association
    2. National Center for Complementary and Alternative Medicine
    3. American Association for Oriental Medicine
    4. National Institute of Arthritis and Musculoskeletal and Skin Diseases

1. Interview someone who has had an acupuncture procedure performed. Develop a list of questions that you would like to ask, such as:
   Why did you decide to have acupuncture?
   How did it feel? Or what was your reaction to the procedure?
   Was it of benefit to you?
   Would you have the procedure repeated?
   Write a report of your findings and provide a brief oral presentation to your class.

2. Visit a physical therapy department in a health care facility or sports medicine facility. Obtain permission to observe the equipment and ask one of the therapists about the use of therapeutic massage. Prepare a report of your findings.

3. Review the NANDA diagnosis Disturbed Energy Field criteria for defining characteristics and related factors. Develop a case study for a patient with a health problem that would be appropriate for this diagnosis. Use the case study to design a patient-centered care plan.

4. Visit a health food store and locate the section that contains dietary supplements, herbals, and items that can be considered as alternative nutritional therapies. Read the labels on at least five items and document the ingredients. Create a poster depicting the purpose of each item, and the potential interactions with other medications or food. Consider how the poster could be used to increase awareness about the products.

5. Develop a survey questionnaire and use it to conduct a survey with 5 to 10 people from different age-groups to determine what forms of CAM they have used in the past year or are currently using. Analyze the results, and prepare a report to share with your classmates.

Cancer Management

Madeleine Lynch Martin, MSN, EdD, RN

Adrianne J. Lane, EdD, RN, C

CHAPTER TOPICS

- Etiology of Cancer

- Physiology and Pathophysiology of Cancer

- Prevention and Diagnosis of Cancer

- Management of Cancer

- Multisymptom Management of Cancer

- Oncological Emergencies

ancer is a general term that is used for a group of diseases that affect multiple systems of the body. Cancer is a major public health problem and is second only to heart disease as a major cause of deaths in the United States. It may occur at any age; however, people over 65 are at greater risk of developing cancer. Cancer is considered to be the most feared disease, as it has been traditionally associated with pain, suffering, disfigurement, and certain death. Technological advances have helped to discover new treatments that can change the course of the disease, and in many cases, cancer can be classified as a chronic disease. Still, the etiology of cancer "is confounded by a prolonged latency period from exposure to a potential carcinogen and the development of clinically detectable disease" (Milligan, 2006, p. 15). It is essential for the nurse to be knowledgeable about prevention and detection of cancer, and the outcome goals of collaborative care. The nurse must also be competent in the nurse's role related to treatment management and in meeting the holistic and unique needs of individual patients and their families.

KEY TERMS

Adjuvant
Allogeneic
Alopecia
Angiogenesis
Antineoplastic
Autologous
Brachytherapy
Cachexia
Dehiscence
Erythropoietic
Glossitis
Grading
Harvesting
Hematopoietic
Hyperplasia
Hypertrophy
Intrathecal
Leukapheresis
Malignant
Metastasis
Mucositis
Myelosuppression
Nadir
Neoadjuvant
Neoplasm
Oncogene
Palliation
Radiotherapy
Staging
Stomatitis
Tumor markers
Tumor suppressor gene
Vesicant

OVERVIEW OF CANCER

Cancer is defined as a group of diseases characterized by the abnormal growth and spread of cells. Specifically, cell division in cancer is both abnormal and uncontrolled. Even though cancer is often thought of as a single disease, it is actually comprised of more than 100 different diseases. The ancient Egyptians have described cancer as an affliction to the human body as early as 1600 B.C. in writings. Ancient papyri describe treatments for both benign and malignant tumors. Hippocrates is known to have named cancer as karkinoma (carcinoma) because of the resemblance of a tumor to a crab: a central body with legs or extensions. Even though cancer has been continuously studied and patients have suffered its effects over the years, the most significant strides in treatment and management occurred in the twentieth century. In 1971 President Richard M. Nixon declared a war on cancer and launched a National Cancer Program. Since 1971, the U.S. Federal Government has funded biomedical research to advance the understanding of cancer. Great strides have been made identifying prevention strategies, screening activities, treatment approaches including surgery, radiation, and chemotherapy, and management of symptoms.

Incidence

Incidence is defined as the number of new cases of the disease and is reported by the American Cancer Society (ACS) on a per year basis. In the United States, breast cancer has the highest incidence of nonskin cancer among women and prostate cancer has the highest incidence for men. For men and women, lung cancer incidence is second and colon and rectal cancer incidence is third. The ACS estimated that more than 1.3 million individuals would be diagnosed with new cases of cancer in 2006 and that 564,830 people were expected to die from a diagnosis of cancer in 2006. It is estimated that one in two men and one in three women will develop cancer over a lifetime. However, since 1991 death rates for the majority of cancer types have been continuously dropping. Today, in the United States, more than 9.8 million individuals are cured of or living with a diagnosis of cancer. The majority of these survivors are older than 65 years of age. Two thirds of adults who are diagnosed today with cancer can expect to be alive in five years. Cancer is being recognized and managed more as a chronic disease.

Mortality

One in four deaths in the United States is attributed to cancer. Mortality (the number of deaths from the disease) charts published by the ACS depict that the number one cause of cancer deaths for in the United States is lung and bronchus cancer. Table 15-1 displays the leading sites of new cancer cases and cancer deaths. Even though skin cancer is not ranked in the top causes of cancer death, it is of great concern because of its increasing incidence. Each year more than one million cases of nonmelanoma skin cancer are diagnosed in the United States.

ETIOLOGY

The professional nurse needs to clearly understand the etiology of all diseases to assess which individuals are at risk for developing illness. People at risk for cancer need to be taught strategies to avoid cancer or to hinder its development. Three factors are known to contribute to the development of cancer: (a) heredity, (b) environment, and (c) lifestyle. Heredity and lifestyle are

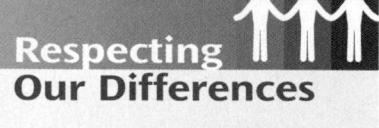

Respecting Our Differences

Mortality versus Incidence

It is important to note that mortality and incidence differ among countries of the world. For instance, the incidence of skin cancer is high in Australia, and the incidence of lung cancer is high in England. Conversely, the incidence of prostate and breast cancer is low in Asia. In the United States Hispanic (American) populations have the highest incidence of cervical cancer, and African American women have the highest death rate for breast cancer. Incidence and death rates are highest among African American men for lung, prostate, and colorectal cancer. These differences are related to a number of factors that include both environmental and lifestyle factors.

TABLE 15-1 Leading Sites of New Cancer Cases and Deaths (2006 Estimates)

ESTIMATED NEW CASES*		ESTIMATED DEATHS	
Male	*Female*	*Male*	*Female*
Prostate 234,460 (33 percent)	Breast 212,920 (31 percent)	Lung and bronchus 90,330 (31 percent)	Lung and bronchus 72,130 (26 percent)
Lung and bronchus 92,700 (13 percent)	Lung and bronchus 81,770 (12 percent)	Prostate 27,350 (9 percent)	Breast 40,970 (15 percent)
Colon and rectum 72,800 (10 percent)	Colon and rectum 75,810 (11 percent)	Colon and rectum 27,870 (10 percent)	Colon and rectum 27,300 (10 percent)
Urinary bladder 44,690 (6 percent)	Uterine corpus 41,200 (6 percent)	Pancreas 16,090 (6 percent)	Ovary 15,310 (6 percent)
Melanoma of the skin 34,260 (5 percent)	Non-Hodgkin lymphoma 28,190 (4 percent)	Leukemia 12,470 (4 percent)	Pancreas 16,210 (6 percent)
Non-Hodgkin lymphoma 30,680 (4 percent)	Melanoma of the skin 27,930 (4 percent)	Esophagus 10,730 (4 percent)	Leukemia 9,810 (4 percent)
Kidney and renal pelvis 24,650 (3 percent)	Ovary 20,180 (3 percent)	Liver and intrahepatic bile duct 10,840 (4 percent)	Non-Hodgkin lymphoma 8,840 (3 percent)
Leukemia 20,000 (3 percent)	Thyroid 22,590 (3 percent)	Non-Hodgkin lymphoma 10,000 (3 percent)	Uterine corpus 7,350 (3 percent)
Oral cavity and pharynx 20,180 (3 percent)	Urinary bladder 16,730 (2 percent)	Urinary bladder 8,990 (3 percent)	Multiple myeloma 5,630 (2 percent)
Pancreas 17,150 (2 percent)	Pancreas 16,580 (2 percent)	Kidney and renal pelvis 8,130 (3 percent)	Brain and other nervous system 5,560 (2 percent)
All sites 720,280 (100 percent)	All sites 679,510 (100 percent)	All sites 291,270 (100 percent)	All sites 273,560 (100 percent)

Excludes basal and squamous cell skin cancers and in situ carcinoma except urinary bladder.

Note: Percentages may not total 100 percent because of rounding. ©2005, American Cancer Society, Inc., Surveillance Research. Adapted from American Cancer Society. (2006b). Surveillance research. Retrieved October 4, 2006, from http://www.cancer.org.

within the host (the individual), and environment is all that is outside of the host. Because these three factors interact to initiate its development, cancer development is described as multifactorial. In addition to these three factors, aging has a direct effect on one's risk of developing cancer. The longer one lives, the greater the risk for developing cancer. This is attributed to both a decrease in the immune response over time as well as the length of exposure to carcinogens or cancer-causing agents.

Heredity

Even though all cancer has a genetic basis, all cancer is not inherited. Usually, cancer begins with a change at the deoxyribonucleic acid (DNA) level of cell. This DNA effect accounts for the genetic basis of cancer. Conversely, an inherited cancer is a cancer that passes from one generation to another generation. Only 10 to 15 percent of all cancers are inherited. Examples of cancers that can be inherited are breast cancer, colon adenocarcinoma, prostate cancer, Wilm's tumor, and retinoblastoma. An individual is at increased risk of developing breast and ovarian cancer if the individual has a mutated BRCA1 or mutated BRCA2 gene.

Environment

The environment in which an individual lives and works may contribute to the development of cancer. Environmental factors include air pollutants, bacteria, and pollutants in water, and exposures to some environmental chemicals, viruses and bacteria, radiation, asbestos, certain medical drugs, and hormones. Pollutants in the air, such as vinyl chloride, lead, and insecticides, are linked to the development of lung cancer. Certain work environments may expose individuals to chemicals that can be linked to cancers. For example, welders, chrome platers, and leather tanner workers may be exposed to chromium, which has been linked to lung cancer. Water polluted with chemicals, such as beryllium, cadmium, dioxin, or arsenic, can lead to the development of cancers, such as lung and kidney. Exposure to radiation when repeated or prolonged can cause cancer. The most common types of such radiation include ultraviolet (UV) radiation from sunlight, X-rays, and exposure to radioactive chemicals. Pesticides, such as those used by farmers and manufacturers, have been linked to blood, lymphatic, brain, lung, stomach, prostate, lip, and skin cancers (U.S. Department of Health and Human Services, 2003).

Lifestyle

Individuals make lifestyle choices that can increase risk for developing cancer. Cigarette smoking causes lung cancer; 30 percent of all cancer deaths have been linked to cigarette smoking. Cigarette smoking is also linked to pancreatic, kidney, mouth, esophagus, larynx, stomach, liver, cervix, and bladder cancer. In addition to cigarette smoking, smokeless tobacco use, and cigar and pipe smoking can also lead to cancer. Environmental tobacco smoke (ETS) has been linked to cancer. Cigarette smoke contains more than 100 cancer-causing agents. Excessive intake of alcohol, particularly two or more drinks daily, can contribute to the development of head, neck, laryngeal, esophageal, and hepatocellular cancer. Drug abuse, such as intravenous (IV) drug use, can contribute to the development of hepatocellular cancer, or marijuana smoking abuse can lead to lung cancer.

Diet may enhance the risk for cancer development. A diet high in red and preserved meats can lead to the development of colorectal and stomach cancer. A diet rich in fat can contribute to development of colorectal cancer and breast cancer. Estrogen, which is stored in body fat, is known to enhance the development of certain types of cancer, particularly breast cancer. Thus a diet high in fat or physical inactivity may promote an increase in body fat and thus enhance the risk to develop cancer. Obesity has been linked to breast, endometrial, kidney, colon, and esophageal cancers. Exposure to UV radiation from the sun, sunlamps, and tanning beds can lead to melanoma and other types of skin cancers. Thus lifeguards, construction workers, and others who work in the sun have an increased risk for skin cancer. Ionizing radiation, such as that delivered during medical procedures, particularly radiation to treat cancer is associated with increased risk of developing future cancers. Women who receive diagnostic X-rays during pregnancy have been linked to increased risk of development of childhood leukemia in their newborns.

Individuals who have increased exposure to sexually acquired viruses, such as various types of the human papillomavirus (HPV), can increase their risk to develop cervical and anal cancer. Other virus and cancer links include the Epstein-Barr virus with Burkitt's lymphoma, hepatitis B and C viruses and liver cancer, human herpes virus 8 with Kaposi sarcoma, and human T cell lymphotrophic virus to adult T cell leukemia. In addition to viruses, bacteria, such as the *Helicobacter pylori* bacterium have been linked to development of stomach cancer.

A variety of drugs have been associated with increasing the risk of cancer in adults. Drugs, such as cyclosporine, chlorambucil, and melphalan, have been linked to secondary cancers, such as leukemia. Certain immunosuppressants contribute to the development of lymphoma. Hormones, such as estrogen, have been associated with increased risk for the development of endometrial and breast cancers and a decreased risk of development of colorectal cancer. Hormone replacement therapy including progesterone and estrogen has been linked to increased incidence of endometrial cancer (National Cancer Institute, 2003a).

PHYSIOLOGY AND PATHOPHYSIOLOGY

Understanding basic cell physiology is the first step to understanding the pathophysiology of cancer. The normal cell has certain characteristics. Changes in these characteristics result in benign (not cancerous, does not spread to other parts of the body) and **malignant,** which are cells that invade and destroy nearby tissues and spread to other parts of the body. Benign and malignant cells give rise to neoplasms. A **neoplasm** or tumor is defined as an abnormal mass of cells, and it can be benign or malignant. The smallest cancer that can be detected by X-ray, examination, or scan is less than 1 cm in diameter and contains approximately one billion cells.

Normal Cell Growth

Normal cells have well-regulated cell division or mitosis. A normal cell undergoes cell division only when like cells need to be replaced because of programmed death (apoptosis) or injury. Cells of the gastrointestinal (GI) tract, skin, hair follicle, and bone marrow are cells that undergo cell division at a rapid rate. Conversely, an individual is born with a specific number of skeletal muscle cells. Skeletal muscle cells do not undergo cell division; instead, these cells grow by increasing their size **(hypertrophy)** and not their number **(hyperplasia).** Because normal cells have regulated mitosis, the ratio of the nucleus to the cytoplasm of the cell is small. The nucleus to cytoplasmic ratio changes during cell division when the nucleus enlarges to prepare and allow for division. Normal cells have a specific morphology meaning that normal cells look like and act like the cells from which they arose. An example is a beta cell from the pancreas looks and acts like other beta cells from the pancreas. Further, normal cells are highly differentiated and have a specific function. One example is that beta cells of the pancreas secrete insulin. Normal cells are cohesive and do not migrate; they secrete fibronectin and stick with like cells within the tissue. For example, normal ductal breast cells do not migrate to the pancreas. Normal cells also exhibit contact inhibition. When a normal healthy cell is surrounded on all sides by other normal healthy cells, cell division will stop.

Benign Cell Growth

Benign cells are like normal cells in many ways. Even though benign cells have regulated cell division, these cells grow at the wrong rate, time, or location. Benign cells have a small nucleus to cytoplasmic ratio, are well-differentiated, and have a specific morphology. For example, in endometriosis (a benign cell condition) the cells of the lining of the uterus are in the wrong location but look and function like normal uterine cells. Even though in endometriosis uterine cells are present outside of the uterine cavity, some researchers believe that this location was established at birth rather than by migration. Benign cells that form benign tumors tend to be surrounded by a fibrous capsule. Benign tumors are not cancerous. These tumors only grow locally; therefore, they do not spread by invasion nor metastasize. Problems that arise from benign tumors are the result of the increased size of the tumor mass causing pressure on vital organs or from changes in hormone production. A benign tumor can cause patient problems such as obstruction, pain, seizures, or overproduction of hormones.

Malignant Cells

Malignant cells differ from normal and benign cells in many ways. Malignant cells have many of the same characteristics of the early embryonic cells. Malignant cells have uncontrolled and unregulated cell division, and divide at a high rate and without regard for normal mitotic limitations. Malignant cells have a large, variably shaped nucleus because of the increased cell division activity and are anaplastic and poorly differentiated. Within the same malignant tumor, various morphological characteristics are present. As the malignancy progresses, the malignant cells appear and function less like the cells from which they arose. Malignant cells invade other tissues and metastasize. They secrete enzymes that contribute to abnormal interactions with nearby tissues allowing the malignant cell to invade those nearby tissues. Malignant cells have minimal to no fibronectin. Therefore, they break off and invade the blood and lymph vessels that carry them to distant sites. They lack contact inhibition and continue to divide even when surrounded on all sides by other malignant cells causing the malignant cells to pile on top of one another. Because malignant cells are a result of a change in the DNA structure within a cell, the chromosomes of the malignant cell are abnormal in number, shape, and function.

Carcinogenesis

The process by which a normal cell is transformed into a malignant or cancerous cell is known as carcinogenesis. Another term for this cellular transformation is oncogenesis. The process of carcinogenesis has four stages: initiation, promotion, progression, and metastasis. The first stage of carcinogenesis is initiation. Initiation is a nonreversible event that occurs when a carcinogen (chemical, radiation, viral, bacterial, or familial) invades and damages the DNA of the cell, causing a change in the DNA structure. This structural DNA change is evidenced by either a gene, such as an **oncogene** (a gene that normally directs cell growth, and if altered, can promote or allow the uncontrolled growth of cancer) being turned on, or a gene such as a **tumor suppressor gene** (gene that can block or suppress the development of cancer), being turned off.

Promotion, the second stage of carcinogenesis, must follow initiation. Promotion is a reversible event. During this stage prolonged, repeated exposure by a promoter stimulates cellular proliferation of the initiated cell. The promoter in a sense potentiates the effects of the initiator. An example is the chemicals found in tobacco smoke may be the carcinogens that initiate a cell; however, the prolonged repeated exposure to the tobacco smoke actually promotes the malignant tumor growth. In this case, cigarette smoking is termed a pure carcinogen. In other cases, a carcinogen may have initiated a cell and then years later because of prolonged, repeated exposure to smoke, the malignant tumor grows. The carcinogen then becomes a promoter. At this time the cell moves toward malignant tumor growth. Examples of promoters include but are not limited to hormones, such as estrogen, chemicals, such as chloroform, and certain drugs.

The third stage of carcinogenesis is progression. The movement between promotion and progression is not distinct. During progression the transformed cancer or malignant tumor experiences morphological change, growing in size and malignancy and becoming more anaplastic and less differentiated. During progression the primary malignant tumor is formed, and its own blood supply is established through a process of **angiogenesis** that is the establishment of blood supply through the formation of new blood vessels. By creating a blood supply the malignant tumor is able to nourish itself for sustained growth.

The fourth stage of carcinogenesis is metastasis. **Metastasis** is the spread of the malignant tumor to other locations. Metastasis can occur through the direct invading of nearby tissues or by spreading to distant sites in the body by penetration into blood and lymph vessels that circulate the cells throughout the body. Malignant tumors tend to spread either to adjacent tissues or to tissues and organs that are linked via lymph and blood channels. The presence of metastasis is not considered a second cancer. For example, a person who has been diagnosed with primary colon cancer that has metastasized to the liver through venous blood supply has colon cancer cells in both the colon and in the liver. Even though common sites of metastasis include bone, brain, lung, and liver, each specific cancer has its own specific sites of metastasis. For example, the most common site of metastasis for colon cancer is the liver, whereas pulmonary metastasis is most common for rectal cancer. Each metastasis is because of its respective venous circulation.

A crucial element in the stage of metastasis is the process of angiogenesis. Angiogenesis is a normal process that occurs in adults whenever new blood vessels are needed, such as during wound healing or tissue repair. Angiogenesis also occurs in children at specific times for normal growth and development. Tumor angiogenesis is the proliferation of blood vessels to supply nutrients and remove waste products from malignant tumors and is associated with the process of carcinogenesis. The new blood supply, stimulated by the angiogenesis-stimulating molecules of the tumor, serves to nourish the malignant tumor and enhance its growth and spread. Without this tumor angiogenesis, tumor growth would be halted because of the lack of nourishment for growth and cell division. This serves as a strategy for treatment and will be discussed later in the chapter.

Classification of Tumors

Benign tumors are classified based on their tissues of origin and usually end with the suffix *-oma*, the Greek word for *tumor*. Malignant tumors are also classified based on their tissue of origin, but often end with the suffix *sarcoma* or *carcinoma*. Tumors that are termed as sarcoma arise from connective tissue. Tumors termed carcinoma arise from epithelial tissues. An example is a benign tumor of glandular tissue termed adenoma, whereas as a malignant tumor of glandular tissue may be termed adenocarcinoma. Classification of tumors is shown in Table 15-2.

Staging and Grading

Once a tumor is classified as malignant, the tumor is staged and graded. **Staging** describes the extent or spread of the tumor within the body from the site of origin, and **grading** (the degree of malignancy or cell differentiation of the tumor cells) describes the degree of malignancy or cell differentiation of the tumor cells. Although different tumor types may have specific staging systems, the international community has provided a consistent staging system for malignant tumors to facilitate cancer management and treatment internationally. The American Joint Committee on Cancer (AJCC) recommends the use of the tumor node malignancy (TNM) system for staging solid tumors. The TNM system is used to describe the primary tumor (T), the nodal involvement (N), and the presence or absence of metastasis (M). The primary tumor is described as Tx (cannot be assessed), T0 (no evidence of tumor), Tis (tumor in situ), or T1, T2, T3, T4 (dependent on size and reflective of increasing in size). The (N) describes the regional lymph node involvement as Nx (cannot be assessed), N0 (no evidence of regional lymph node metastasis), or N1, N2, N3 (dependent on increasing extent of involvement). The presence or absence of distant metastasis is indicated by Mx (unable to assess), M0 (no presence of metastasis), or M1 (presence of metastasis). No specific size or

TABLE 15-2 Tumor Classifications	
CARCINOMA	**ARISES FROM EPITHELIAL TISSUES**
Sarcoma	Arises from bone, cartilage, fat, muscle, blood vessels, or other connective or supportive tissues
Leukemia	Caused by immature blood cells, starts in blood-forming tissues, like bone marrow
Lymphoma and multiple myeloma	Starts in the cells of the immune system

Adapted from American Joint Committee on Cancer. (2002). Staging systems. Retrieved June 16, 2005, from http://training.seer.cancer.gov.

extent guidelines are provided for T or N, because each type of cancer has its specific characteristics. The lower the stage of the tumor is, the better the chance of survival of the cancer.

The grade of the malignant tumor is indicative of its degree of malignancy or its aggressiveness. A pathologist is responsible for grading a tumor. As with staging, each cancer type will have specific characteristics. Tumor grading may be classified as I, II, III, IV or Gx, G1, G2, G3, G4. A grade of Gx indicates that the grade cannot be assessed. The key to both systems is that the primary tumor graded as I or G1 contains highly differentiated cells, which are cells that resemble the normal tissue cells from which they arose, and as the grade number increases the degree of differentiation decreases. A primary tumor graded as III or G3 contains cells that are undifferentiated, and a primary tumor graded as IV or G4 has cells that have no specific differentiation. G4 tumors are anaplastic, highly aggressive, and rapidly multiplying. Tumors that are graded as G1 have a much better prognosis than tumors graded as G4. For instance, a G1 breast cancer has greater than a 90 percent cure rate, and a G4 breast cancer has a 20 percent cure rate. The AJCC recommends the Gx to G4 system. The grading and the staging of a primary tumor is of utmost importance as the oncologist plans the treatment regimen for the patient. The nurse has the responsibility to interpret the staging and grading to the patient to assist in understanding of the disease.

PREVENTION

The professional nurse must assess each patient and determine what types of cancer preventive education and activities and screening measures are specifically recommended. Cancer prevention can be classified as primary, secondary, or tertiary. The goal of primary cancer prevention for development of cancer is by reducing one's risk for the development of cancer. Secondary cancer prevention is aimed at early detection of cancer through participation in screening activities. Tertiary cancer prevention is aimed at prevention of recurrence of cancer through use of chemo-preventive agents.

Primary Prevention

Two main strategies for primary cancer prevention include the use of vaccines and health counseling. The use of vaccines for cancer prevention is limited. Currently, a vaccine is available for the hepatitis B virus, which is associated with liver cancer. At least two thirds of cancer cases are caused by environmental factors, thus health counseling is the strategy that is commonly used. Nurses should counsel patients regarding how to reduce their risk of developing cancer. All patients should be screened for tobacco behaviors. Patients should be instructed to stop smoking and avoid secondhand smoke. Avoiding tobacco is the single best strategy for an individual to reduce the risk of developing cancer. Individuals should also be taught to protect themselves from sunlight. Death from melanoma has also risen dramatically. Individuals should be taught to wear at least SPF 15 sunscreen, to stay out of the sun between 10 am and 4 pm, and wear clothing to protect their skin from the sun.

Individuals should be taught to limit the drinking of alcohol to less than one drink per day for women and less than two drinks per day for men. Excessive alcohol intake is related to mouth, throat, and esophageal cancers. The combination of heavy drinking and smoking compounds the risk associated individually for either substance. Health counseling should include information about diet. Studies suggest that various vitamins, fiber, and other nutrients may protect against cancer. Foods containing antioxidants have been identified by a number of researchers as cancer protective or chemo-protective, a substance or agents that are used to protect healthy tissues from the effects of cancer therapies and

Fast Forward ▶▶▶

Cancer Vaccines

Cancer vaccines are considered biological therapy and are mostly available only in clinical trials. Vaccines for breast, cervical, lung, kidney, follicular B-cell non-Hodgkin's lymphoma, and melanoma are currently available only in clinical trials to patients determined to be high-risk for developing those cancers. The goal of such vaccines is to either prevent or reduce the risk of developing cancer. With the identification of the human genome, great strides in vaccine therapy are forthcoming (NCI, 2004a). A July 2006 news release by the ACS recommended that the Food and Drug Administration (FDA) approve HPV vaccine be given to all girls aged 11 to 12 in the United States. It could also be given to girls as young as 9 years if deemed necessary and to women up to 26 years of age. The vaccine, given in three injections over a period of six months is most effective against two of the most common cervical cancer-causing types of HPV when given before persons are infected with HPV through sexual intercourse. The recommendations must still be approved by the director of the Centers for Disease Control (CDC) and the secretary of the Department of Health and Human Services.

cancer (Roth, 2007). Another dietary caution concerns the consumption of large amounts of calories and foods high in fat, including red meat products, which have an increased risk for various types of cancer, such as breast and colon cancer. Individuals should be taught to exercise regularly. Regular exercise, at least 30 minutes daily, contributes to overall body reduction of fat as well as a generalized well-being. Foods that are smoked or preserved with salt have increased levels of nitrites and should be limited in the diet. Cured meats including bacon and ham and processed meats, such as deli meats, hotdogs, and lunchmeats, are some that have increased levels of nitrites.

People should also be aware that exposure to various viruses and bacteria can lead to development of cancer. A primary preventive strategy to guard against exposure to HPV, which is linked to cervical cancer, would be to practice safe sex through use of condoms and limiting exposure to multiple sex partners. Individuals should be advised to assess the home and the workplace for known carcinogens and to develop strategies to avoid those carcinogens. A potential carcinogen in the home may be the presence of radon, a radioactive gas. Simple home test kits are available for radon. Certain occupations expose workers to known carcinogens. Workers need to be counseled regarding their risks and possible options, such as protective devices or seeking alternative employment.

Secondary Prevention

Secondary cancer prevention is aimed at screening and early recognition of cancer. Early recognition of cancer can lead to early diagnosis, resulting in earlier treatment and treatment success. An example is that the treatment success rate for breast cancer diagnosed in an early stage is over 90 percent as compared to 26 percent diagnosed in a late stage. The cancer community knows that the best chance for cure or long-term management is early diagnosis (Box 15-1).

In addition, the professional nurse should inform individuals about the specific cancer screening guidelines that are appropriate for them based on their

---

BOX 15-1

WARNING SIGNS OF CANCER

The professional nurse should educate individuals about the warning signs of cancer. The seven warning signs can easily be remembered through the acronym, caution.

C: Change in bladder or bowel habits, such as absence of urination or bowel movement or a change may be excessive urination or stool.

A: A sore that does not heal within a realistic period of time.

U: Unusual bleeding or discharge from any body orifice, such as the vagina, the nipple, or the penis. The unusual discharge can be bloody, purulent, clear, or viscous. The keywords are *unusual* and *any body orifice.*

T: Thickening or the presence of a lump of the breast, testicle, or any part of the body.

I: Indigestion or difficulty swallowing for a prolonged period of time.

O: Obvious change in a wart or mole, such as color, size, texture.

N: Nagging cough or hoarseness that is prolonged.

If any of these warning signs are observed, the patient should see a health care provider.

Adapted from Daniels, R. (2004). Nursing fundamentals: Caring and clinical decision making. *New York: Thomson Delmar Learning.*

sex, age, and other identified risk factors. The ACS sets forth recommendations based on sex and age for the early detection of cancer in average-risk asymptomatic individuals. An individual who has a family history of cancer, a genetic link to cancer, or another identified high risk factor should seek the advice of the primary care provider regarding an appropriate screening timetable specific for their needs (Table 15-3).

Regular screening recommendations are outlined for breast, colorectal, prostate, cervical, and endometrial cancers (Figure 15-1). In addition to these recommendations, beginning at age 20, all men and women should be examined for cancers of the thyroid, testicles, ovaries, lymph nodes, oral cavity, and skin and receive health counseling about risk factors, sexual practices, environmental and occupational exposures, diet and nutrition, sun exposure, and tobacco during the periodic health examination. Refer to the ACS Web site regarding specific cancer screening recommendations at: http://www.cancer.org and search for cancer screening.

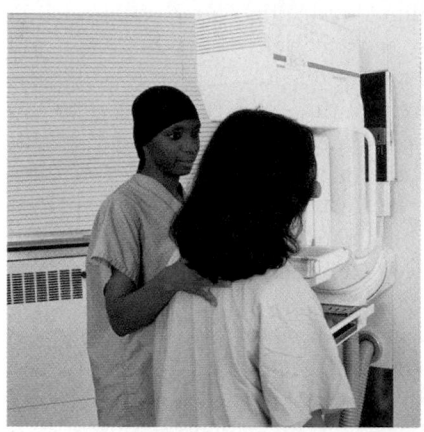

Figure 15-1 Mammograms are a vital element to wellness promotion for all women over the age of 40 years.

TABLE 15-3	High Risk Factors Associated with Different Types of Cancer
CANCER	**RISK FACTORS**
Lung	Cigarette smoking
	Passive smoking
	Occupational and environmental exposure to carcinogens, such as asbestos, arsenic, chromium, and nickel
	Exposure to radiation
Breast	Female
	Age older than 50 and increasing age
	Personal history of breast cancer
	Personal history of biopsy
	Family history of breast cancer
	Nulliparity or delayed first pregnancy
	Early menarche or late menopause
	BRCA 1 or BRCA2 mutation
	Postmenopausal obesity
	High-fat diet
	Alcohol consumption
	Prolonged exposure to exogenous estrogens
	Radiation to chest wall
Prostate	Male
	Age older than 50
	African American
	Family history
	High-fat, low-fiber diet
	Occupational exposure to chemicals or pesticides
	Occupational exposure to cadmium
	BRCA1 or BRCA 2 mutations

Continued

TABLE 15-3 High Risk Factors Associated with Different Types of Cancer—cont'd

CANCER	RISK FACTORS
Colorectal	Age older than 60
	High-fat diet
	Diet low in fruits and vegetables
	Heavy alcohol consumption
	Smoking
	Obesity
	Sedentary lifestyle
	History of polyps
	Inflammatory bowel disorders
	Family history
	Familial genetic syndromes, e.g., familial adenomatous polyposis (FAP), APC1130K mutation, or hereditary nonpolyposis colon cancer (HNPCC)
Endometrial	Prolonged estrogen stimulation
	Early menarche or late menopause
	Exogenous estrogen
	Obesity
	Increasing age
	Nulliparity or delayed pregnancy
	Family history
	Polycystic ovary syndrome (PCOS)
	History of ovarian tumors
Cervical	Multiple sex partners
	Cigarette smoking
	Early coitus
	Presence or history sexually transmitted disease
	Presence of HPV
	Immunosuppression
	Vitamin deficiencies
Skin	Exposure to ultraviolet light
	Fair skinned or red-headed
	Sun exposure
	Tanning booth use
	Family history
	Personal history
	Increasing age
	History of severe sunburns
	Chronic immunosuppression

Adapted from Milligan, L. (2006). Epidemiology and cancer. Advance for Nurses, 3(15), 15–17.

Tertiary Prevention

Tertiary cancer prevention is defined as specific activities aimed at the prevention of recurrence of cancer. Two primary strategies to teach patients to prevent recurrence of disease are health counseling and chemoprevention. Health counseling is aimed at educating patients already diagnosed with cancer or those who are survivors specifically about actions that would reduce their risk of developing the specific cancers. These activities are centered on diet, exercise, avoidance of exposure, and healthy lifestyles. Chemoprevention is the incorporation of drugs, foods, or other agents into the treatment plan to reduce the risk of cancer development or cancer recurrence. Tamoxifen is an example of a drug that is prescribed to reduce the risk of recurrence of breast cancer after breast cancer surgery (Broyles, Reiss, & Evans, 2007). Tamoxifen is a synthetic hormone. Although tamoxifen has chemo-protective actions related to recurrence of breast cancer, it has been linked to increased risk of endometrial cancer, stroke, and blood clot formation. Other drugs such as aspirin and various nonsteroidal anti-inflammatory drugs (NSAIDS) are used for chemoprevention related to decreasing the risk of colon cancer. The professional nurse must teach the patient the importance of tertiary prevention in the prevention of future disease.

DIAGNOSTIC TESTS

There are a wide variety of diagnostic tests used to identify the presence of cancer. The nurse should instruct the patients about the implications of having these diagnostic tests performed. In addition, the nurse should carefully explain the implications of each cancer screening test.

Laboratory Tests

No specific value or laboratory test is specific for cancer. Laboratory tests that might indicate the presence of cancer may include the analysis of blood, urine, and other body fluids for a variety of abnormalities that may be indicative of cancer. **Tumor markers** are substances that are expressed by the tumor or by normal tissue in response to a tumor. Tumor markers may indicate the presence of disease, although often such markers are not specific for the cancer. An example is a prostate-specific antigen (PSA) test is elevated in conditions, such as benign prostatic hypertrophy in addition to prostate cancer. Even so, the PSA is an appropriate screening test for cancer and is an excellent marker for determination of response to treatment. Tumor markers are important in the assessment of cancer, monitoring tumor response during treatment strategies, and diagnosis of recurrence of disease.

Radiographic Tests

If a tumor mass is suspected, radiographic technology may be employed. Imaging techniques assist in localizing and providing further detail about a mass or tumor (Figure 15-2). Examples of such techniques include, but are not limited to, ultrasounds, computed tomography (CT) scans, magnetic resonance imaging (MRI) with or without contrast, X-ray, bone scans, nuclear medicine imaging, and positron emission tomography (PET) scan that are useful in identifying the presence of primary tumor or metastasis. Selection procedures are specific to certain cancers, such as mammograms are useful in identifying the presence of breast cancer. The nurse should explain the purpose and the process of the procedure to the patient and instruct the patient on any specific preoperative preparation necessitated (Daniels, 2003).

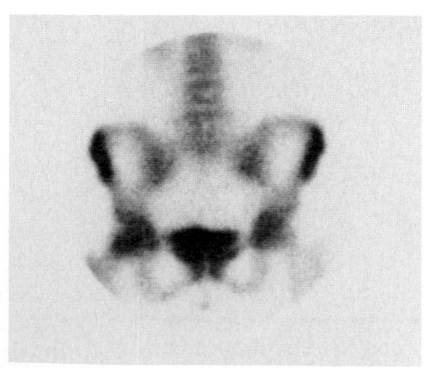

Figure 15-2 Radionuclide scan, lumbar.

Biopsy

The purpose of a biopsy, or removal of a sample of tissue, is to determine if the suspicious mass is a cancerous tumor as opposed to a cyst, an adhesion, or another structure, such as a calcification. Definitive diagnosis is accomplished only through histological or cytological proof. If the mass is determined to be a tumor, the tumor will be analyzed to determine if it is benign or malignant. The common techniques used for biopsy include needle biopsies, surgical biopsies, and bone marrow aspiration. A needle biopsy can be performed through fine needle aspiration, stereotactic needle aspiration, or core needle procedure. Such biopsies are performed when growths are easily accessible, such as those occurring in the lung, liver, breast, thyroid, or kidney. Stereotactic needle biopsy is done in conjunction with imaging to help locate the suspected mass (Daniels, 2003). A core needle procedure is undertaken when a small core of tissue needs to be obtained for accurate diagnosis. Potential postoperative complications include infection, hematoma, and pain.

Surgical biopsies are performed to secure a larger piece of tumor tissue. The types of surgical biopsy techniques include incisional, excisional, and endoscopic. These techniques can be performed using local anesthesia with possible mild sedation. The purpose of the incisional biopsy is to remove a small piece of the mass for histological examination when the mass is too large for removal, whereas with an excisional biopsy, an attempt is made to remove the entire mass and surrounding marginal tissues. Excisional biopsies are chosen when the mass is in an easily accessible area, such as a tumor of the breast, GI tract, respiratory tract, or the skin. An endoscopic biopsy is performed when the mass can be removed through the use of endoscopic entry, such as removal of a polyp through colonoscopy. Possible postoperative complications include bleeding, infection, and pain.

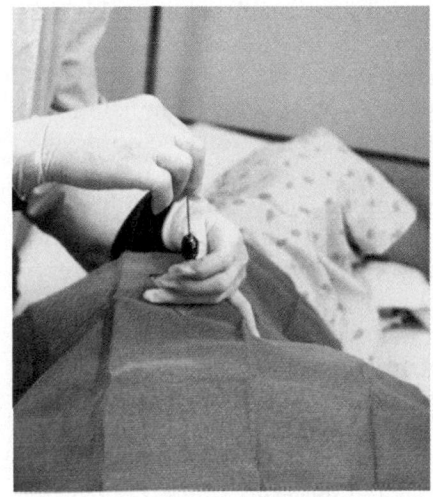

Figure 15-3 Bone marrow biopsy.

Bone Marrow Aspiration

Bone marrow aspiration is performed to procure a small amount of bone marrow for microscopic examination (Figure 15-3). Bone marrow aspiration is used for diagnosis of blood disorders, diagnosis of primary and metastatic tumors, and evaluation of treatment effectiveness. The nurse should be alert for complications that include hemorrhage and infection.

Other Diagnostic Tests

Other diagnostic tests, such as bronchoscopy, colposcopy, colonoscopy, endoscopy, and electroencephalogram (EEG) may be useful in the assessment for cancer. The responsibility of the nurse is to explain the purpose and specific procedures related to these tests to the patient. If the patient has questions, the nurse should serve as the advocate for answering any patient concerns. Refer to a laboratory and diagnostic text for further information regarding the specifics of these additional diagnostic tests.

PLANNING AND IMPLEMENTATION

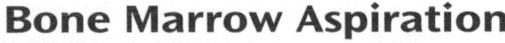

Suddenly confronted with a life-threatening diagnosis, the patient will also be faced with multiple treatment choices and the prospect of a prolonged period of single or combined therapy. It is no surprise that the patient diagnosed with cancer is often overwhelmed. The nurse may be the single most constant health provider with whom the patient and family will interact. His or her journey with the patient begins with an understanding of the most prevalent types of cancer treatment. A thorough well-documented initial assessment of the patient continues as the basis for the nurse's ongoing plan of care. In addition to a sound understanding of the patient's physical and psychological condition is the need to regularly assess the patient's level of understanding of what is happening. This understanding is one of the nurse's most important tasks for educating the patient and family and clarifying information. Throughout the course of treatment the patient will be bombarded with information, some of it in totally unfamiliar terminology. The nurse's ability to help the patient understand this information limits misunderstanding and confused expectations. Patient and family education starts before therapy and continues during and after therapy. Reinforcement helps ensure successful compliance. Appropriate written and visual teaching aids may be utilized as well as referrals to other professionals or community programs, such as cancer support groups.

Overview of Treatment

Nurses need to understand treatment alternatives so that they can assist the patient to evaluate his or her options and make informed choices. This understanding includes the goals and benefits of a treatment as well as its possible risks. Generally, the goals of cancer treatments are to: (a) cure the cancer; (b) control its spread and manage as a chronic illness; or (c) **palliation,** to ease symptoms and maximize quality of life when cure or control is not possible. The ultimate goal is cancer cure, and scientists are making progress as they continue to develop advanced technologies and treatments that extend life and prevent tumor genesis and development. The problem is that the cure for cancer is not going to show up anytime soon. In fact, there may never be a single cure, one drug that will bring every cancer patient back to glowing good health, in part because every type of cancer, from brain to breast to bowel, is different. However, it is a time of optimism. Within 10 years, predicts Robert Weinberg, a cancer biologist at the Whitehead Institute in Cambridge, Massachusetts, an analysis of the mutant genes and then treatments for that particular tumor will be found (Lee, 2005).

Chronic diseases are those that are viewed from the standpoint that they are treated, become less active, or are controlled but then may reactivate or come back. Because of advances in treatment options and successes, cancer control now includes both control of metastasis and management as a chronic disease. Examples of palliation of cancer include draining fluid collections or reopening hollow structures blocked by tumors, such as bile ducts, the kidney, or bowels. These procedures may reduce the symptoms and problems caused by the blockage. Even in cancers where cure is not possible, longer survival may be. During this time bone metastasis can occur with resulting pathological fracture, particularly of the long bones. Palliative surgical stabilization of these fractures is extremely effective in alleviating pain and allowing patients to resume an ambulatory status.

The three most common treatments for cancer are surgery, pharmacotherapy including chemotherapy, and radiation. While single treatments may be effective, most often the plan includes a combination of approaches. The selection of the treatments will vary depending on the cancer site, type, disease progression or spread, and individual patient response. The ideal is to maximize destruction or eradication of the diseased cells with a minimum of side effects that may impact quality of life. The National Comprehensive Cancer Network (NCCN) is an alliance of 19 leading cancer centers worldwide that has developed Clinical Practice Guidelines in Oncology, which are updated annually and are evidence-based. The nurse can use these guidelines as a resource for accepted treatments for specific cancers. A patient version is also available for selected cancers and may be offered as a resource to patients (NCCN, 2005).

Principles of Treatment

Surgery was the first modality to be used in the treatment of cancer. Surgery is used to diagnose; to biopsy and stage tumors; to remove, decrease size of, or destroy tumors; for hardware insertion; to help relieve the discomfort and symptoms often associated with cancer; and for reconstruction. New techniques have allowed the surgery to be minimally invasive, which has the advantage of smaller incisions with fewer traumas. Fewer traumas to the patient frequently results in shorter hospital stay and allows for the earlier start of additional therapies. The ultimate goal of surgery is complete tumor removal, but this may not be possible because of invasiveness or metastasis. Therefore, surgery today is often used in conjunction with other therapies as part of the treatment plan. Radiation or chemotherapy may be used either before or after the surgery to reduce the tumor size or to destroy metastatic cells. If there is significant tumor growth, surgery may be used as a palliative intervention to ease discomfort or support normal body function as when removing a bowel obstruction to allow normal peristalsis.

Preoperative Management

There are some special considerations for the nurse when caring for the preoperative cancer patient. The nurse needs to know if the patient has had other cancer therapies, including radiation and chemotherapy. With radiation there may be increased risk of hemorrhage or infection because of effects on the bone marrow. With some chemotherapy agents, such as doxorubicin (Adriamycin), cardiac functioning can be affected. It is important for the nurse to work with the patient and family prior to surgery to develop the best physiological and psychological status possible. A comprehensive preoperative evaluation allows the nurse to evaluate the patient and, if necessary, implement measures to prepare higher risk patients for surgery. Nutritional status can affect postoperative healing and increase the risk for **dehiscence** (the separation of a wound or scar) and evisceration (to protrude through a surgical incision or have protrusion of a part through an incision). Preoperatively the nurse should offer the patient the opportunity to talk about concerns and ask questions. There is no evidence that surgery for cancer patients leads to the disease exacerbation or an increase in aggressiveness. Often, there are cancer cells remaining in the body after the surgery even when the complete tumor has been removed. With or without surgery, these cells could grow over period of time and lead to the disease return. Such remaining cancer cells need to be managed by postoperative adjuvant therapy such as **radiotherapy** (the use of X-rays and other forms of radiation in treatment) or chemotherapy that significantly reduces the chances of disease recurrence. Preoperative education should include information about the surgical procedure and what the patient will experience before, during, and after surgery.

Postoperative Management

In management of the postoperative cancer patient, the patient and family must be fully engaged in the treatment process to increase the chance for successful recovery. Pain is assessed frequently to evaluate the effectiveness of analgesics. IV or epidural infusion of narcotic analgesics is often necessary for control of pain that can be severe. The stress of this pain can affect the patient's ability to heal and prepare for further treatment. Teaching the patient position changes and exercise can support pulmonary gas exchange. Many patients with cancer come to the surgery with weakened immune systems and in poor nutritional state. Nursing measures to promote wound healing are instituted and include good nutrition, asepsis, and frequent wound assessment

Complications

Complications of special concern for the postoperative cancer patient include alterations in bowel elimination, fear and anxiety, and infections. Alterations in bowel elimination, including both diarrhea and constipation, can occur in the postoperative period. Diarrhea is most often related to enteral feedings or chemotherapeutic agents. It may be treated with antidiarrheal agents and by addressing the causative factors. Constipation may result from narcotic analgesics, immobility, and decreased dietary intake. Consulting a dietitian can be helpful in developing an individualized nutritional plan.

Fear and anxiety are normal for any surgical patient and especially the cancer patient who is facing multiple treatments and decisions. The nurse should continue to encourage the patient and family members to express their feelings and concerns. Realistic information and reassurance and referrals to other members of the health care team, including the social worker, clinical nurse specialist, or clergy should be considered.

Infections, both wound and systemic, are potential complications in the postoperative cancer patient. The wound incision should be inspected daily. Any signs of redness, swelling, or drainage should be reported. An elevated temperature is another sign of infection.

Long-Term Implications

The nurse needs to be vigilant in observing for complications, promoting comfort, and preparing the patient for discharge. Discharge planning should begin on admission, utilizing available resources in the institution and the community to facilitate a smooth transition to the home. Desired outcomes include total removal of cancer tissue with minimal side effects. Long-term implications can be impacted by functional alterations, which may result from radical surgeries, such as amputation. Alterations in body image and disruption in activities of daily living that may be short- or long-term. As in other areas of health care, oncology surgical procedures are increasingly done on an outpatient basis. For those done as inpatient, the hospital stays have shortened. The patient may be anticipating additional surgery related to surgical reconstruction to alleviate functional or body image disruptions. This makes good preoperative teaching important, as well as effective discharge coordination and outpatient monitoring. The postoperative period is important in cancer care, because many patients will be beginning radiation or chemotherapy

Radiation Therapy

Radiation therapy is the use of high-energy ionizing rays to damage or kill cancer cells by preventing them from growing and dividing. Similar to surgery, radiation is considered a local treatment, because only cells in the area being treated are targeted. Radiation may be used in early-stage cancers to cure or control the disease as well as before surgery to shrink the tumor or after surgery to prevent the cancer recurrence. If a type of cancer is known to spread commonly to a particular area, it is sometimes assumed that even though no tumors are identified metastasis may be present and warrants irradiation (ACS, 2004f). For example, people with certain types of lung cancer may receive radiation to the brain, because this is a common site of metastasis.

External and Internal Radiation

Radiation therapy may be externally or internally delivered. External radiation delivers high-energy rays directly to the tumor site from a linear accelerator external to the body. Internal radiation, or **brachytherapy,** involves the implantation of a small amount of radioactive material in or near the cancer. Radiation used for cancer treatment is called *ionizing radiation,* because it forms ions as it passes through tissues causing cell death by genetic change.

Principles of Treatment

More than half of all cancer patients receive radiation therapy, so the nurse needs to be knowledgeable about the treatment plan as well as possible side effects. Important aspects of nursing and home care for the patient receiving external radiation therapy include early careful explanation of the treatment process. There should be opportunities offered at each visit for the patient and family to ask questions either about the treatment or side effects that may be occurring. Most often the treatment process begins with a consultation with the radiation oncologist. This consultation will include a review of all the previously collected pertinent data as well as a history and physical examination to collect additional data. Following this the patient has a simulation or a treatment planning session. Here the patient comes to the radiation department and lies down under a machine called a simulator; markings are made on the skin and various X-rays taken. Various immobilization devices, such as a headrest or a facemask, may be used to ensure the patient is positioned correctly and consistently for each treatment (NCI, 2004d). This process is integral to ensuring that the radiation is directed to areas where cancer cells are present or have the potential of being present and may require multiple visits. It is important to limit the effect of radiation on normal, healthy tissues. At the conclusion of the simulation, the treatment team then calculates a dose of radiation specific for each patient.

External Treatment

For the external radiation treatment itself, the patient lies flat on a table similar to an examining table. The table moves in multiple directions so that the patient is in the proper position for the X-rays to treat the desired area. Blocks and lead shields may be placed between the patient and the accelerator to protect normal tissues in the body and ensure that radiation is delivered principally to the tumor. External radiation is a safe and basically painless form of treatment. There is no sensation to being treated and the actual exposure to radiation is usually less than 3 minutes per visit. The patient may however be in the treatment room for 10 to 20 minutes depending on the required number of treatment angles. Radiation therapists who remain outside of the room give the treatment. This and how the patient can communicate with the therapist during treatment should be explained to the patient.

Side Effects

There are side effects of the radiation that may be anticipated and should be discussed with the patient prior to treatments. Side effects often increase as therapy progresses and can be anticipated about two weeks after treatment starts. Radiation therapy mainly affects rapidly dividing cells, such as the cells lining the GI tract, including the large and small bowel, resulting in radiation enteritis. Several factors determine the occurrence and severity of radiation enteritis. These factors include the dose of radiation, tumor size and spread, amount of normal bowel treated, concurrent chemotherapy, use of radiation implants, and individual patient factors (such as previous surgery to the abdomen or pelvis, diabetes, pelvic inflammatory disease, or poor nutrition). Patients with acute enteritis may complain of nausea, vomiting, abdominal cramping, the frequent urge to have a bowel movement, and watery diarrhea. Almost all patients undergoing radiation to the abdomen, pelvis, or rectum will show signs of acute enteritis (Leon & Pase, 2004). Acute symptoms are those that appear during the first course of radiation therapy and up to eight weeks later. Chronic radiation enteritis may appear months to years after finishing radiation therapy or it may begin as acute enteritis and continue after treatment stops. Only 5 to 15 percent of persons treated with radiation to the abdomen will develop chronic problems.

Management

A common side effect of radiation is enteritis. Management of enteritis begins with assessment. The nurse should determine usual pattern of bowel movements and ask the patient to log the pattern of diarrhea, including when it started; how long it has lasted; frequency, amount, and type of stools. Other symptoms, such as gas, cramping, bloating, urgency, bleeding, and rectal soreness, should be reported and may indicate radiation damage to the anus or rectum. With diarrhea, the GI tract does not function as efficiently and fat, lactose, bile salts, and vitamin B_{12} are not well absorbed. Nutrition assessment including height and weight, usual eating habits, any change in eating habits, amount of fiber in the diet, and signs of dehydration (such as poor skin tone, increased weakness, or fatigue) are important to determine severity of nausea and vomiting.

Treatment of acute enteritis includes treating the diarrhea, loss of fluids, poor absorption, and stomach or rectal pain. These symptoms usually get better with medications, changes in diet, and rest. If symptoms become worse even with this treatment, then cancer treatment may have to be stopped, at least temporarily. Medication may be prescribed such as antidiarrheals, narcotics to relieve pain, and steroid foams to relieve rectal inflammation and irritation. In addition to enteritis, radiation therapy may also cause nausea and vomiting. Nausea and vomiting associated with radiation therapy usually occurs half an hour to several hours after treatment. Symptoms may improve on days the patient does not receive radiation therapy (NCI, 2004e).

Fatigue and skin irritation are two additional common symptoms following radiation therapy. As with GI disturbance, fatigue can dramatically impact quality of life. It may be caused by anemia or the collection of toxic substances produced by cell death. In the case of radiation, it may be caused by the increased energy needed to repair damaged skin tissue. In addition to discussing and preparing the patient for the possibility of extreme fatigue, suggestions for dealing with it include limiting unnecessary activities, maintaining good nutrition, maintaining a regular sleep schedule, and relying on friends and family to assist with activities of daily living.

The patient should be prepared for early and late skin reactions to radiation therapy. Nutritional status and skin condition at the start of therapy have an impact on later skin reactions. The patient should be taught to use only creams or lotions approved by the radiation oncologist and to avoid sun exposure. Binding clothing at the radiation site should be avoided to limit skin irritation. Changes the nurse and patient look for include thinning, altered pigmentation, ulceration or necrosis, and other reactions. An effective skin regimen can be developed and individualized to the patient. Again, good pretreatment assessment and education are the basis for decreasing anxiety and fostering compliance with these regimens. The patient should be taught that excreta are not radioactive in patients who receive external radiation therapy.

Internal Radiation

Internal radiation, or brachytherapy, occurs when radioactive materials are delivered internally. Brachytherapy may be delivered through oral and IV routes as well as through implantation of seeds, rods, catheters, or wires via interstitial or intracavitary (within an organ or body cavity) pathway. Radiation therapy can be delivered orally such as I-131 for carcinoma of the thyroid and intravenously as with P 32 for metastasis of the bone. Examples of interstitial radiation therapy include seed implants into the prostate and wafers into the brain. Intracavity placement of cesium for gynecological cancer is another type of example of brachytherapy. Radioactive seeds can also be temporarily placed into the breast tissue following lumpectomy for breast cancer using a Mammosite RTS balloon catheter in conjunction with an after-loader.

Because the implanted radiation source emits radiation, those who come into contact with the patient need to observe the principles of time, distance, and shielding. When unsealed sources of radiation therapy are used, the excreta are considered radioactive, and radiation precautions must be taken in handling of the excreta. General guidelines include assigning the patient to a private room, postradiation precaution signage, limiting the amount of time in the room, observing a distance of at least six feet from the source when possible, and prohibiting pregnant staff, family, and visitors and children from interacting or visiting with the patient. The health care staff, patient and family should be instructed on the specific precautions to be followed, and these precautions will vary from radioisotope to radioisotope. The radiation therapy personnel should provide specific instructions to the patient and family. All health care staff should be required to wear personnel dosimeter badge to record their total personal exposure to radiation. A highlight of nursing issues related to the more significant side effects will be included in the section on multisymptom management. The nurse is also encouraged to visit NCI at www.cancernet.gov, which is an excellent source of information on side effects of radiation.

Outcomes

Desired outcomes of radiation therapy include cure, long-term remission, and improved comfort. The nurse needs to be aware of long-term negative consequences, including risk of secondary neoplasms, and work with the patient and family to seek regular annual assessments and follow-up. The 20-year cumulative risk of a second neoplasm was significantly higher (21 versus 1 percent) in radiated patients than in nonirradiated patients (Pui, et al., 2003).

Chemotherapy

The use of **antineoplastic** (a drug that prevents, kills, or blocks the growth and spread of cancer cells) agents to treat cancer is based on the physiology of normal cell division. The goal is to systemically administer specific drugs in prescribed dosages, so that the process of cell growth and replication is disrupted. Most chemotherapy is given as a combination of drugs that work together to kill cancer cells. Combining drugs that have different actions at the cellular level reduce the patient's resistance to one particular drug. Unlike radiation, which treats only the part of the body exposed to the radiation, chemotherapy treats the entire body and is considered a systemic treatment modality. This is one of chemotherapy's main advantages and disadvantages. As a result of this systemic effect, any cells that may have migrated from where the cancer originated can be treated. Conversely, noncancerous cells are also more likely to be damaged. Two terms, which are commonly heard in relation to chemotherapy, are **neoadjuvant** (adjunctive or adjuvant therapy given prior to the primary [main] therapy) and **adjuvant** (remedy that enhances the effect of another therapy). The goal of neoadjuvant therapy is to reduce the size of a tumor before surgery or radiation therapy. Adjuvant chemotherapy is administered after surgery or radiation with the goal of eliminating any cancer cells that might remain following earlier treatments. The nurse usually administers chemotherapy. The Oncology Nursing Society recommends the specially trained and certified nurses be charged with the responsibility (Varricchio, 2004). Because chemotherapy is often administered on an outpatient basis or in the patients home, all oncology nurses should be aware of their role in coordinating therapy and care and in management of side effects.

Principles of Treatment

Treatment decisions for chemotherapy include the selection of the agent, dosage, and the cycle of administration. The selection of agents is generally based on the type of cancer, age, and assessed ability to tolerate potential side effects. Antineoplastic drugs are generally classified in two ways, either by the targeted point in cell cycle (cell-cycle specific) or the effect on cellular function at any or all points within the cell cycle (non–cell-cycle specific). In other words, the medication is effective during a specific stage of the cell cycle or not (Figure 15-4). Chemotherapy doses are most commonly determined based on body surface area (BSA). The patient must be carefully weighed and the exact height known. Because of the narrow range of safe dosage for these toxic drugs, dosage is calculated precisely and administered based on a dose-response relationship where the dose administered will ideally destroy the most cancer cells while producing the least side effects. Dosages may also be adjusted for the elderly, nutritional status, other

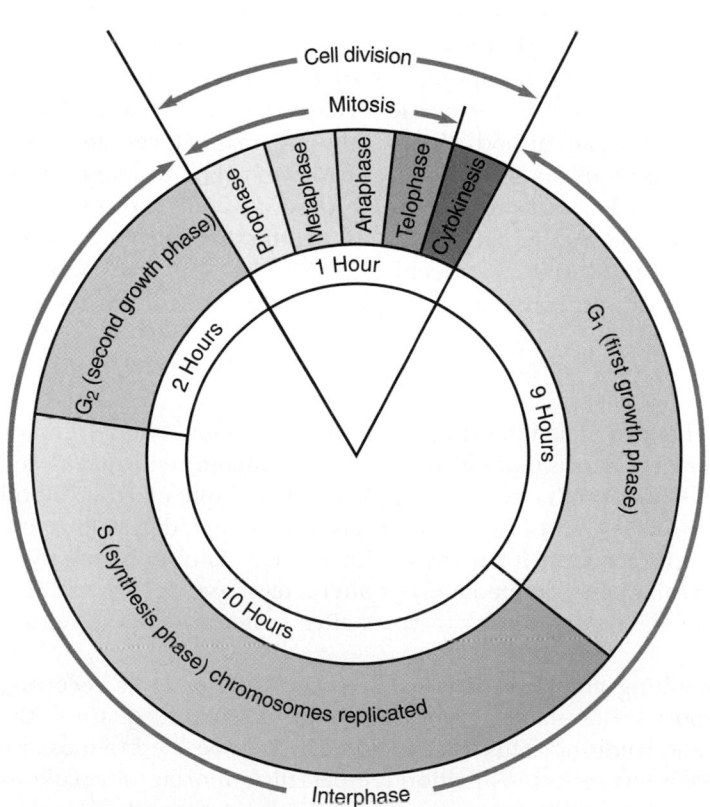

Figure 15-4 The stages of the cell cycle.

medications, concurrent therapies, such as radiation, and blood cell counts. Because the liver or kidney processes most drugs, including chemotherapeutic agents, existing organ disease should be considered.

Cycle of administration refers to the schedule of administration. Some cycles involve one dose followed by several days or weeks without treatment. This allows normal tissues time to recover from the drug's side effects. Alternatively, doses may be given several days in a row, or every other day for several days, followed by a period of rest. Some drugs work best when given continuously over several days. Administration routes are varied based on the drug and protocol but may include: (a) oral; (b) IV; (c) intramuscular; (d) intracavitary; (e) intraperitoneal; (f) **intrathecal** (within the spinal canal, the space between the double-layered covering or lining of the brain and spinal cord); (g) intrapleural; (h) intravesicular; (i) topical; and (j) intra-arterial. One complication related to administration is hypersensitivity, either local or systemic. Administration protocols are patient specific, and it would be difficult for the nurse to be aware of all possible complications. What the nurse must do is be vigilant in assessment and observation. Responses can vary from burning, erythema, ulceration, and necrosis to anaphylaxis, and immediate response should be available.

As with radiation therapy, there are specific safety considerations when handling hazardous chemicals. Chemotherapeutic agents are classified as either **vesicant** or nonvesicant. Vesicants are those agents that when they enter the subcutaneous tissue cause tissue necrosis and damage to the underlying structures, such as the tendons, veins, arteries, and nerves. This process of infiltration and tissue damage is termed extravasation. Leaking of a minute amount of a vesicant drug from the vein can immediately blister the skin. In some cases tissue breakdown may be so extreme that grafting may be needed, and even limbs may be lost (Polovich, 2004).

Because of the potential toxicities of chemotherapeutic agents, it is the nurse's responsibility to be aware of and to follow policies and procedures for handling and disposing of these materials. Drugs should be stored in a protective area. When working with the drugs the nurse should avoid spills, wash hands before and after preparation and administration, and wear protective clothing or equipment. Chemotherapy agents are recorded on material safety data (MSD) sheets and are regulated by the Occupational Safety and Health Administration (OSHA). Patient body fluids including, urine, feces, and emesis are considered hazardous for 48 hours after treatment. The primary routes for contamination exposure are inhalation, absorption, and ingestion. The patient and family should also be taught how to handle these drugs at home and to wear protective covering (Varricchio, 2004). The Oncology Nursing Society and ACS provide information and guidelines on specific drugs and safety measures.

Side Effects

Because of its mechanism of action on cell growth and division, chemotherapy has the greatest impact on cells that divide rapidly. This includes normal as well as malignant cells. Normal cells that divide rapidly include bone marrow/blood cells, cells of hair follicles, and cells in the reproductive and digestive tracts. Damage to these cells accounts for many of the side effects of chemotherapy drugs. Side effects can appear immediately or after a few days (acute), within a few weeks (intermediate), or months to years after long-term chemotherapy administration.

Nausea and vomiting are frequently experienced with patients receiving chemotherapy. Tools are available to help the nurse assess and quantify the extent of nausea and vomiting. This information can then be used to measure the effectiveness of interventions. Nutrition is especially important for patients at this time. Not only is good nutrition necessary to support physiological processes, but also the ability to tolerate foods impacts the emotional outlook

BOX 15-2

COMMON SIDE EFFECTS OF CHEMOTHERAPY

- Hair loss (alopecia)
- Dry mouth (xerostomia)
- Mouth sores (stomatitis)
- Difficulty swallowing due to esophagitis
- Nausea
- Vomiting
- Diarrhea
- Fatigue
- Bleeding
- Susceptibility to infection

Adapted from Broyles, B. E., Reiss, B. S., & Evans, M. E. (2007). Pharmacological aspects of nursing care *(7th ed.). New York: Thomson Delmar Learning.*

of the patient during this difficult process. Suggestions for the patient can include eating food at room temperature, drinking adequate fluids (three liters of fluid a day), and allowing carbonated beverages to lose their carbonation before drinking. There are some herbs and natural products that have been shown to be effective for nausea and vomiting. Nutmeg, ginger, and peppermint added to food may help decrease movement of the GI tract or improve appetite. Antiemetics, drugs that prevent or control nausea and vomiting such as ondansetron or granisetron, may be prescribed to lessen the incidence of nausea and vomiting. Antiemetics may be prescribed around the clock before, during, and after chemotherapy administration. Other common side effects are included in Box 15-2.

Until the last several years patients reported nausea and vomiting as the most distressing side effects. Recently, fatigue has emerged as the most distressing and persistent patient side effect. Cancer-related fatigue may be caused by a host of factors, including, but not limited to, an aggressive treatment regimen; insomnia; anemia; pain; medications, such as opioids, antiemetics, antidepressants; and poor nutrition. Thus, cancer-related fatigue must be thoroughly assessed, and therapy should be aimed at the causative factor(s). When fatigue is related to anemia, the patient may be managed in a variety of ways, such as being prescribed iron or folic acid replacement, receiving a blood transfusion, or being prescribed a colony-stimulating factor (CSF), such as recombinant human erythropoietin, to encourage the production of red blood cells (RBCs). If insomnia is the cause, a combination of pharmacological and nonpharmacological strategies could be used to enhance sleep. If poor nutrition is identified, a nutritional consult may be helpful as well as prescription of medications to enhance appetite, such as dronabinol (Marinol) or megestrol acetate. Effective pain management may contribute to the alleviation of fatigue. Studies have shown a decrease in stress and increased quality of life in patients who engaged in exercise during cancer therapy (NCCN, 2005). The exercise plan should take in consideration comorbidities the patient has, such as bone metastasis or cardiac involvement. Involvement of a physical or therapist or rehabilitation provider may be helpful in planning the exercise program. The main issue is that fatigue is a most distressing symptom that has a multifaceted etiology. Managing a single cause of fatigue may not be effective in overall management of the fatigue. The cancer patient must be regularly assessed for the presence of fatigue during, as well as after completion of chemotherapy.

Although fatigue, nausea, and vomiting are the symptoms that patients report cause them the most distress, the side effect related to susceptibility to infection can be deadly. Because of the effects of the chemotherapeutic agents on the bone marrow, the patient may suffer **myelosuppression** (a decrease in the production of RBCs, platelets, and some white blood cells [WBCs] by the bone marrow), resulting in pancytopenia that includes anemia, thrombocytopenia, and neutropenia. The management of anemia, thrombocytopenia, and neutropenia are addressed in the section Multisymptom Management. A number of measures should be observed to decrease the risk of infection for the patient receiving chemotherapy, including instructions for strict hand washing, screening all visitors, and ensuring adequate nutrition. Refer to chapter 11 for detailed discussion regarding infection control.

Less common problems include damage to the heart, liver, lungs, kidneys, or nerves. Changes in concentration and memory have commonly been referred to as "chemo brain" or "chemo fog" by patients following treatment. Research is only beginning to be reported on this, but patients report changes in those areas immediately following treatment to up to 10 years later. Some research implies that these brain changes are worst during or just after chemo and do get better over time (Cancer Research UK, 2004). Overall, researchers say there may well be some long-term effects on memory and concentration, but these are only likely to be slight.

When side effects occur, the nurse should assess to determine if the effects are within expected ranges or indicate a toxic reaction. This assessment can also help distinguish between side effects to the drugs and complications related to the cancer. For example, a patient with facial swelling may be experiencing minor edema or may be exhibiting signs of significant cardiac pathology (superior vena cava syndrome) or the effects of high cell death resulting in systemic toxicity (tumor lysis syndrome [TLS]). Using specific parameters and operational definitions to define the degree of a given toxicity ensures consistency in documenting observed reactions. Toxicity grading scales have been developed by the World Health Organization and various cooperative study groups to provide consistency in reporting (Cancer Source, 2003). The nurse's careful observation and documentation of side effects and individual patient responses provide data for decisions regarding the need for appropriate adjustments in the treatment plan. Data that should be documented by the nurse include side effect, severity, onset, duration, and responses to interventions. Documentation of the effectiveness of treatments helps modify nursing plans and maximize desired outcomes.

Teaching patients about their treatment helps to reduce fear, increases self-confidence, improves compliance, and can enhance their participation in self-care. The intent of teaching is more than to give information; it provides support and knowledge to empower the patient to manage self-care effectively. The Oncology Nursing Society recommends focusing educational efforts for the patient and family on the diagnosis, treatment, rehabilitation, survivorship, or recurrent phases of care. Specific teaching goals may include helping the patient adjust to the treatment; explaining how the treatment will affect the cancer; imparting the sequence of administration; and recognizing and controlling side effects. Repetition and restatement of important points may be necessary during this time of mental and physical stress. No matter how slight, side effects can be distressing to the patient. The nurse should reinforce with the patient and family that most side effects will gradually diminish over time. Opportunity for the patient to discuss side effects and other concerns should be provided at every outpatient care visit. Also, patients should be provided with information about how to contact someone on the treatment team if side effects are severe or they have concerns.

Outcomes

Consistent with the goals of therapy potential outcomes for the nursing diagnosis of a patient receiving chemotherapy are permanent destruction of the cancer cells, remission of the disease, or improved quality of life through reduction of symptoms.

It is important to discuss long-term implications of therapy with the patient throughout the treatment. Long-term effects that might occur related to nerve damage include tinnitus and hearing loss. Some patients complain of fatigue, and others may have decreased resistance to infection. There are cases in which secondary cancers appear years after the treatment, but data to date indicate that this occurs is in a small number of patients and is a lesser risk than failure to treat the current cancer effectively (Hudson, et al., 2003).

In some cases chemotherapy can cause infertility, affecting either the ovaries or the sperm. Depending on the chemotherapeutic agent, patients may be counseled regarding preservation of eggs, ovarian tissue, or sperm prior to beginning therapy. If the patient is in childbearing years, strict birth control must be observed. Chemotherapy can lead to genetic damage in the fetus. The patient should consult with the oncologist after chemotherapy to determine when pregnancy may be safe. For premenopausal women, chemotherapy may precipitate early menopause. The effects of chemotherapy on sexuality are varied, and these issues must be addressed with the patient. The nurse is a main advocate in regard to dealing with issues of sexuality.

Depression has been reported to occur in as many as 25 out every 100 patients diagnosed with cancer and may be a reaction to the diagnosis and treatment.

Ongoing assessment of depression is an important intervention. A simple depression visual analogue scale may be used during visits. The nurse needs to assess for depression, listen to the patient, provide appropriate therapy, or refer for therapy as needed.

Hormone Therapy

Hormones are chemicals produced by glands and released directly into the bloodstream. Some types of cancer are hormone responsive, meaning that hormones promote the growth of these cancers. For example, estrogen produced by the ovaries, sometimes promotes the growth of breast cancer and testosterone, produced by the testicles, has been found to promote the growth of most prostate cancers. The goal of hormone therapy is to prevent hormones from stimulating the growth of any cancer cells at the tumor site itself and those that may have migrated to other parts of the body. There are several ways to limit these hormones. One way is to remove the organs that make them: the ovaries or the testicles. More recently, however, drug therapy is being used to stop the organs from making the hormones or to prevent the hormones from affecting the cancer cells. Thus the cancer cells are kept from getting the hormones they need to grow. Patients with breast cancer or prostate cancer are the two most likely types of patients that the nurse will encounter receiving hormone therapy.

Until menopause a woman's ovaries produce the hormone estrogen, subsequently it is produced by fat tissue. Estrogen promotes the growth of about two thirds of breast cancers. Because of this several approaches to blocking the effect of estrogen or lowering estrogen levels are used to treat breast cancer. One approach is the use of selective estrogen receptor modulators (SERMs) that bind to estrogen receptors in the breast cancer cells, blocking estrogen from reaching cancer cells and thus preventing their growth. A second approach, aromatase inhibitors, blocks estrogen production by binding to the enzyme responsible for producing estrogen, the aromatase enzyme. Some aromatase inhibitors include letrozole (Femara), anastrozole (Arimidex), and exemestane (Aromasin) (Broyles, et al., 2007). Tamoxifen (Nolvadex) is the estrogen receptor–modulating drug used most often in women with both early and late stage breast cancer, for postmenopausal women at high risk of developing breast cancer and to prevent the reoccurrence of breast cancer. It is taken daily in pill form and has the advantages of maintaining bone strength and lowering cholesterol in some patients. Side effects of SERMS include those symptoms commonly encountered in menopause: hot flashes, blood clots, loss of interest in sex, and a higher risk of other cancers. Tamoxifen can increase the risk of developing endometrial cancer or uterine sarcoma. Endometrial cancer, if caught early is generally curable by surgery. Patients taking tamoxifen should be alerted to report any unusual vaginal bleeding immediately so that they can be screened quickly for these secondary cancers. Tamoxifen therapy is generally prescribed for five years. Research has shown that maximum effect is gained at five years with no noticeable effectiveness when continued; therefore tamoxifen therapy is generally stopped at five years thus reducing the continued risk of side effects. The search for other drugs with similar action, such as raloxifene, continues, with the goal being to develop drugs that have maximum effectiveness with minimal side effects.

There are several forms of hormone therapy for prostate cancer. The goal of hormone therapy, also called androgen deprivation therapy (ADT), is to lower levels of the male hormones (androgens, such as testosterone) in the body. Androgens allow prostate cancer cells to grow, thus by lowering androgen levels, prostate cancers shrink or grow more slowly. Surgery to remove the testicles (orchiectomy) acts by eliminating the main source of male hormones. Drugs, including estrogen, may also be given, which limit or prevent the testicles from producing testosterone. Hormone therapy is frequently used as a neoadjuvant therapy being given as initial treatment before surgery or radiation to shrink the cancer, making these treatments more effective. Hormone therapy given in addition to radiation therapy via permanent seed implantation has been shown to improve outcomes significantly in patients with moderate to high-risk prostate cancer.

It is important for the patient to understand that hormone therapy alone does not cure prostate cancer. For cure, hormonal therapy is used in connection with other treatments. It may be used as an initial therapy for prostate cancer if the patient is unable to have surgery or radiation, if the cancer has spread beyond the prostate gland, or after initial surgery or radiation therapy if the cancer remains or reoccurs. Antiandrogen are taken orally daily. Side effects include hot flashes, difficulty with erection, bone loss, pain, and liver damage. Nurses must address with patients issues that impact quality of life and physical functioning. Patient education, as well as emotional support to the patient and spouse for side effects should begin with screening and diagnosis and follow through treatment to cure, to palliative care, or hospice. The challenge to oncology nursing is to assist men in making appropriate decisions regarding treatment options.

Biological Therapy

Biological therapy (immunotherapy) is a relatively new weapon in the fight against cancer. Biological therapies use substances naturally produced by the immune system to fight cancer either directly or indirectly or to lessen the side effects that may be caused by some cancer treatments. The immune system is the body's natural defense mechanism that recognizes normal (self) cells from abnormal (nonself) cells. However, the abnormal, or mutated, cancer cells are derived from the natural human cells, and the immune system may not be adequate to destroy them. In some cases, the immune system responds to the antigens on the cancer cell surface and can prevent these transformed cells from developing into clinically detectable tumors.

There is debate over the exact mechanism of action, but it is thought that biological agents act by interfering with cancer cell growth, acting indirectly to help healthy immune cells control cancer, and helping to repair normal cells damaged by other forms of cancer treatment (NCI, 2004b). Biological therapies can be used alone or in conjunction with chemotherapy or radiation therapy. In general, immunotherapy is most likely to be effective when treating small cancers and will probably be less effective for more advanced disease. There are two forms of immunotherapy used to treat cancer: passive and active. Biological therapies can be used to treat cancers or used to treat side effects of other cancer treatments. Biological agents include interferon, interleukins, vaccines, CSFs, and monoclonal antibodies. These often are used in conjunction with other cancer therapies, such as chemotherapy, radiation therapy, or surgery. Interferon alpha, rituxan, herceptin, bacillus Calmette-Guérin vaccine (BCG), and IL-2 are examples of biological therapies used to treat various cancers and CSFs, such as erythropoietin for RBCs, oprelvekin for platelets, and Neupogen for WBCs are other examples of biological therapies used to manage side effects of cancer therapy.

As noted with other cancer therapies, the specific agent being administered influences nursing care. In addition to understanding the agent being given, the nurse assesses the patient's overall physical and physiological status, resources and reactions or severity of side effects. The nurse can then plan for the educational and care needs of the patient and family. The most common method of administration is parenteral. Administration may be both inpatient and outpatient requiring effective coordination plans by the nurse. Because there is the potential for environmental contamination risk, the nurse should be familiar with administration issues and follow all recommended procedures and discuss them with the family.

Side effects may vary by agent, but there are several more frequently encountered and alarming to the patient and caregiver. First is a flu-like syndrome that includes fever, headache, and general fatigue. A fever of 40° C (104° F) is not unexpected and can be accompanied by mental confusion. Fatigue affects both physical activity and mental outlook and can result from both the treatment and the disease. Mental confusion resulting from the treatment can be compounded by depression and stress. It is important for the patients and caregivers to understand that, because these agents are administered over a period of several months, the symptoms can be long-term and may vary in intensity throughput the treatment. Education includes guidelines on when to contact health care providers and how to communicate information effectively including keeping logs. Empowering knowledge includes knowing resources, how to access them, and symptom management strategies.

The need for open and comprehensive communication is crucial for all who are diagnosed with cancer and particularly those diagnosed with prostate cancer. Aggressive management of prostate cancer is coupled with significant long-term side effects for both the patient and the significant other. Such side effects may have a profound effect on quality of life. The literature reports treatment variations based on age, comorbidity pathology, and related quality of life issues. Research demonstrates that more men die with prostate cancer than of prostate cancer. For some men, an approach of watchful waiting may be offered as a treatment option for early stage prostate cancer. Watchful waiting is an alternative choice to aggressive treatment and may offer greater quality of life for some. This approach involves ongoing urological assessment, regular and periodic physical examination including PSA and digital rectal examination (DRE) testing, and annual bone scan. These patients are followed closely for changes in disease and need for aggressive management. Even so, for the period of watchful waiting, the patient is spared the side effects associated with aggressive therapy.

Blood and Bone Marrow Transplantation

Bone marrow transplantation (BMT) and peripheral blood stem cell transplantation (PBSCT) are procedures that restore cells necessary to produce blood cells. Stem cell and bone marrow transplantation are used both to counter the effects of high dose chemotherapy and radiation and to treat some forms of cancer.

Chemotherapy and radiation therapy are used to treat cancer, because cancer cells divide at a greater rate than most healthy cells. However, because bone marrow cells also divide frequently, high-dose treatments can severely damage or destroy the patient's bone marrow. Without healthy bone marrow, the patient is no longer able to make the blood cells needed to carry oxygen, fight infection, and prevent bleeding.

Bone marrow contains immature cells known as **hematopoietic** (pertaining to the formation of blood) or blood-forming stem cells. Hematopoietic stem cells either divide to form more blood-forming stem cells, or they mature into WBCs, RBCs, and platelets. Most hematopoietic stem cells are found in the bone marrow, but some cells, called peripheral blood stem cells (PBSCs), are found in the bloodstream. Blood in the umbilical cord also contains hematopoietic stem cells. Cells from any of these sources can be used in transplants.

The patient and caregivers should be aware that BMT is an intensive procedure with many risks, including death from complications of the transplant or from relapse of the original disease. There are no guarantees and cure rates are low; however transplants often result in a period of remission. The success of BMT will be influenced by a number of factors, including age, general physical condition, diagnosis, and disease stage. To minimize potential side effects transplanted stem cells that match the patient's own stem cells as closely as possible are desirable. There are three types of transplants: **autologous,** any transplant in which a person receives his or her own stem cells that he or she donated earlier; **allogeneic** (replaces a patient's blood or bone marrow with blood or bone marrow from a donor), any transplant in which hematopoietic stem cells from one person are transplanted into another the donor and recipient can be related or unrelated; and syngenic, which is a transplant in which the patient and donor are identical twins.

Information important for the nurse includes issues for both the donor and recipient. The general term for collection of the cells is **harvesting.** The procedure is the same in all three types of donation. For bone marrow transplant, the donor is given a general anesthetic for needle aspiration from the bone site (usually the hip), and the marrow is extracted. The sample is then filtered, and the cells may be frozen for later use, as needed through cryopreservation (the process of preserving by freezing). While the area may be sore for a few days or the donor may feel tired, there is limited risk to the donor other than that of other surgical procedures, primarily the effects of the general anesthetic. The stem cells used in PBSCT come from the bloodstream. A process called apheresis, which is a procedure where whole blood is removed from the body and a desired component is retained, or **leukapheresis** (the removal of blood to collect specific blood cells; the remaining blood is returned to the body) is used to obtain PBSCs for transplantation. In apheresis, blood is removed through one of the large veins or using a central line. The blood is filtered to extract the stem cells and then returned to the donor. The collected cells frozen are stored. Apheresis typically takes four to six hours.

The recipient patient receives the stem cells intravenously over one to five hours. The stem cells used for autologous transplantation must be relatively free of cancer cells, and so the harvested cells may be purged of cancer cells to minimize the chance that cancer will return. Engraftment is the process where, after entering the bloodstream, the stem cells enter the bone marrow and begin to produce new blood cells. This usually occurs within about two to four weeks after transplantation. Complete recovery of immune function can take from several months to one to two years for patients depending on the type of graft. The major risk of both treatments is an increased susceptibility to infection, bleeding, and symptoms associated with the immune system response. The patient may be given antibiotics to prevent or treat infection, and isolation procedures will be enacted. The recipients may be given transfusions of platelets to prevent bleeding and RBCs to treat anemia. Patients who undergo BMT and PBSCT may experience short-term side effects such as: (a) nausea; (b) vomiting; (c) fatigue; (d) loss of appetite; (e) mouth sores; (f) hair loss; and (g) skin reactions (NCI, 2004c).

A significant complication that should be discussed with the patient is graft-versus-host disease (GVHD). With allogeneic transplants, that is a graft from a donor other than the patient or an identical twin, GVHD sometimes develops. GVHD occurs when WBCs from the donor (the graft) identify these cells in the patient's body (the host) as foreign and cause a severe immune response. The most commonly damaged organs are the skin, liver, and intestines. This complication can develop within a few weeks of the transplant or much later. The patient may receive immunosuppressive therapy, such as cyclosporin or prednisone, to control this response. Additionally, the donated stem cells can be treated to remove the WBCs that cause GVHD in a process called T cell depletion. GVHD can be difficult to treat, but some studies suggest that patients with leukemia who develop GVHD are less likely to have the cancer come back. Clinical trials are being conducted to find ways to prevent and treat GVHD.

In some types of cancer, such as leukemia, Hodgkin disease and non-Hodgkin lymphoma, and neuroblastoma or retinoblastoma transplantation takes advantage of the graft-versus-tumor (GVT) effect that occurs after allogeneic BMT and PBSCT. Other factors to discuss with the patient include the cost of the treatment and the recovery period. The BMT procedure can require up to six months of hospitalization and extensive care that can cost $100,000 to $250,000. While health insurance usually covers most of these expenses, the family may still be responsible for a considerable amount. Recovery after BMT is slow, and for several weeks the patient may have nausea, vomiting, fever, diarrhea, and extreme weakness. Good nutrition is particularly important to recovery, and food supplements or other nutrients may be given until a healthy appetite returns. The family and patient need to be prepared after transplant for many return visits to monitor recovery and possible signs of disease return. In the posttransplant period the patient needs to be observed for late complications or those complications that can occur after 100 days. Late effects can include pneumonias, pulmonary disorders, and viral infections. Patients may also experience chronic GVT. Psychological assessments as well as support must be ongoing.

Complementary Therapies

In recent years, complementary and alternative therapies (CAM) have received increasing interest by both the public and professionals. As consumers become more informed and more involved in their health promotion and care, they have sought alternative methods by which they can impact their own health. Because of the nature of a diagnosis of cancer and the accompanying stress and fear, cancer patients may be more susceptible to such options. When properly combined with standard cancer treatments, many professionals believe that some complementary therapies can enhance wellness and quality of life, but others may be harmful during or alter treatment. (See chapter 14 for detailed information about CAM.) The nurse must act as an advocate for the patient when addressing the use of complementary therapies (Montbriand, 2005). Additional resources for the nurse and patient include the Memorial Sloan-Kettering Cancer Center at http://www.mskcc.org particularly the section called *Products,* and M.D. Anderson Cancer Center at: http://www.mdanderson.org.

Clinical Trials

Clinical trials have been an important part of the journey toward cancer cure. Because they are conducted in all areas of disease management, a nurse may be working with a patient who is part of clinical trial. Because of their impact on both the patient and treatment, the nurse should have a general understanding of the clinical trial process. A clinical trial is a research study using human volunteers to answer specific health questions. It is one of the final stages of a long and careful cancer research process. Studies are done with cancer patients to find out whether promising approaches to cancer prevention, diagnosis, and treatment are safe and effective. Carefully conducted clinical trials are the fastest and safest way to find treatments that work in people and ways to improve health.

Government agencies, such as the FDA, require companies to show that new medical products, treatments, and drugs are both safe and effective before approval. Clinical trials are the best way to demonstrate this efficacy. A patient may be included in one of several types of clinical trials. Types include treatment trials that are the most common type and test new or alternative potential treatments for specific diseases or medical conditions. Prevention trials test new ways to prevent specific diseases, evaluating new medications or lifestyle changes. Screening trials test new ways to detect specific diseases, especially diseases that may have an early stage before they produce symptoms. Diagnostic trials study tests or procedures that could be used to identify disease more accurately and at an earlier stage, and genetics studies are sometimes included as part of another clinical trial. The genetics component of the trial may focus on how genetic makeup can affect detection, diagnosis, or response to treatment (Beth Israel Deaconess Medical Center, 2004).

In addition to types of trials or therapies tested, the NCI clinical trials are conducted in phases. The trials at each phase have a different purpose and help scientists answer different questions. In phase I, researchers test an experimental drug or treatment in a small group of people (20 to 80) for the first time to evaluate its safety, determine a safe dosage range, and identify side effects. In phase II (with 100 to 300 subjects) and phase III trials (1,000 to 3,000), the drug or treatment is given to increasingly large numbers of patients to collect addition information on effectiveness and safety for broader groups. Phase IV consists of postmarketing studies which collect information on possible adverse effects over time.

Clinical trials have been proven to offer some of the most effective cancer treatments available today. Currently, there are hundreds of ongoing clinical trials in the United States, however fewer than 5 percent of cancer patients participate in them. Reasons vary but may include lack of interest or knowledge that they exist, difficulty finding an appropriate clinical trial that may be of benefit to them, or ineligibility to participate because of prior treatment interventions. The goal should be to offer all newly diagnosed patients the option to participate in a clinical trial. The choice to participate is theirs. The role of the nurse is to be the patient's advocate ensuring that the patient has the necessary information to make an informed choice that all trials are approved by appropriate review boards, that care follows clinical trial instructions, and that the patient stays informed. Other activities for the nurse caring for the patient in a clinical trial may include: collecting data; monitoring the patient's physical and emotional health; providing emotional support and comfort; administering the treatment; teaching the patient and family how to prevent complications; decreasing side effects; transition to home care; and offering referral to cancer community resources.

Patients who participate in clinical trials almost never receive a placebo, unless there is no current standard treatment for their disease. Rather, participants receive either a promising new treatment or the best available conventional treatment. An advantage may be that patients receiving the investigational therapy then may be among the first to benefit. Patients on clinical trials are monitored and may undergo more frequent testing and examinations to help evaluate their progress. There is no guarantee, however, that any new treatment will be successful. Also, there are some costs that may be part of participating and the patient should clearly understand and have the opportunity to discuss these. With intensive monitoring, there may be extra hospital visits required. All cancer treatments have side effects, but treatments being studied may have side effects that are not yet understood as well as the side effects of standard treatments.

In addition to time and physical effects, there may be financial costs. Patient care costs are those associated with providing the treatment to each patient. Costs include physician visits, hospital stays, and clinical laboratory tests. These are medical costs that occur regardless of whether a patient is participating in a clinical trial or receiving standard treatment, but additional costs brought on by the clinical trails may not be covered by a third-party health plan. Research costs of data collection and management, research health care provider and nurse time, analysis of results, and tests performed purely for research purposes are usually covered by the sponsoring organization, such as a pharmaceutical company or hospital, but this issue should be clarified prior to starting the treatment.

After agreeing to take part in a trial, the patient can still withdraw at any time. After making the decision whether or not to become part of a clinical trial, patients with cancer and their families often have mixed emotions. They may feel anger, sadness, and fear of the future or nervousness. They may always wonder if the decision affected the outcome of their treatment. Oncology nurses give the patient and family emotional support before, during, and after all treatments (refer to Law in Practice).

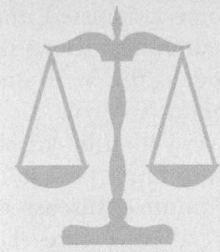

LAW IN PRACTICE

Clinical Trials

Clinical trials have played an important role in the development of many of today's successful cancer treatments. Hundreds of clinical trials are currently being conducted, but less than 5 percent of eligible patients choose to participate. One concern about participation has been the financial cost to the patient. Informed consent documents for clinical trials include statements that state the patient and the insurance company will need to pay some or all of the costs of treating the cancer in this study. The patient is informed that participating in the study may cost more than the health plan will cover. This makes the patient responsible for contacting the insurance company, and if the insurance does not pay all expenses, the patient will be financially responsible. Financial costs to patients ranged from costs for extra tests and medications to total treatment costs when health plans voided all coverage because of participation. Thus, even though the treatment may offer promise for their condition, many choose not to participate. Others have found themselves caught between the hospital and the insurance company with no coverage. To address this problem, California has passed a Clinical Trial Law (i.e., ViK Khanna NCI #CA10117 2003 ANCO MOASC and State health Policy Solutions LLC). This law requires the health plan to cover the costs of the clinical trial. Additional coverage mandated by law includes visits, hospital stays and medical testing, drugs, devices, and services related to the trial that the individuals would pay if not in the study, and any therapy needed to prevent, diagnose, or treat problems that might occur while in the trial. It does not cover experimental drugs, but the manufacturer or research institution usually covers these. In summary, the California law allows patients the opportunity to participate in a clinical trial without worrying about having to pay for the entire treatment themselves.

Adapted from Beth Israel Deaconess Medical Center. (2004). WebMD clinical trial services. Retrieved June 10, 2005, from http://my.webmd.com.

MULTISYMPTOM MANAGEMENT

Because of the aggressive nature of cancer therapies, side effects of cancer care are a significant nursing management issue. The National Institutes of Health estimates that 90 percent of patients diagnosed with cancer will experience pain; 20 to 40 percent will become depressed, and a large number will report debilitating fatigue. Professionals have begun to recognize that many of the symptoms are interrelated and in fact form symptom clusters. Such clusters are groupings of symptoms that affect the patient simultaneously and have an interactive or coreactive relationship, such as pain and fatigue. As either pain or fatigue increase during the course of the disease or treatment, the patient's energy reserves become exhausted, making him or her less able to manage both symptoms. Research also shows that in many cases cancer-related symptoms are undertreated, as the focus on care has been disease cure (DeLaune & Ladner, 2006). The nurse's role is to provide opportunities for the patient to discuss symptoms and then be knowledgeable on techniques to effectively manage them. It is also important to remember that symptom management exists across the continuum of disease stage, from diagnosis through treatment and at times during palliative care. Thus, multisymptoms dictate multimanagement strategies.

Myelosuppression

Myelosuppression is a defined as the state when one or more components of blood is decreased and is a common condition in cancer patients. Not only does it result in debilitating side effects for the patient, but also it is a common cause of treatment delays and can be life-threatening. Bone marrow is the primary producer of pluripotent (those stem cells found in developing embryos, which can give rise to all the cells found in the human body), stem cells that differentiate as they mature into WBCs, RBCs, and platelets in a process called hematopoiesis. Bone marrow suppression results in a disruption of this process and can result from the disease itself or from therapy. Bone marrow infiltration is seen in lymphomas and solid tumors as well as in leukemia cells. Many chemotherapeutic agents and radiation therapy impact rapidly dividing normal cells as well as cancer cells. Because bone marrow cells are rapidly dividing, this rapidity can cause temporary damage to the bone marrow, which prevents the differentiation of the stem cell into mature blood cells. Myelosuppression is classified according to the type of blood cell affected. Discussed here will be anemia (RBCs), neutropenia (WBCs), and thrombocytopenia (platelets).

Anemia

Anemia is defined as a hemoglobin (iron containing molecules in the RBC) value of less than 12 g/dL and a hematocrit (packed RBC volume as a percentage of total blood volume) of less than 36 percent. Anemia can occur for several reasons. The most common cause is a decrease in production of new RBCs by the bone marrow. Many of the cancer chemotherapy drugs significantly depress RBC formation. Chemotherapy agents that are likely to cause anemia via these mechanisms include alkylating agents, such as cyclophosphamide and melphalan, the antimetabolite gemcitabine, anthracyclines, such as doxorubicin, the topoisomerase I inhibitor topotecan, and taxanes, such as 24-hour infusions of paclitaxel. Not only is there systemic consequence of untreated anemia, such as fatigue, but correction of anemia by increasing oxygenation of tissues, has been shown to increase tumor response to antineoplastic agents and to radiation therapy. Local radiation therapy can cause anemia especially when directed at high functioning bone marrow (e.g., pelvis, ribs, sternum, and base of skull) by damaging early precursor cells in the bone marrow. Other causes of anemia include bleeding related to the tumor itself and insufficient intake of iron and other nutrients because of poor appetite (Wilkes, 2004).

Signs and symptoms of anemia result from lack of tissue oxygenation and the subsequent attempts by the body to compensate. Those most often seen include fatigue, shortness of breath, chest pain, tachycardia, headache, pallor, and mental status changes. Laboratory studies obtained for diagnosis include complete blood count in patients at risk for developing or suspected of having anemia. Iron studies, stool for guaiac, and liver function if jaundiced or with hepatomegaly are other laboratory tests to consider. The skin, mucous membranes, nail beds, and conjunctiva should be assessed for pallor. If anemia is chronic the lips should be assessed for color, and the tongue for atrophic **glossitis** (an inflammation of the tongue). The heart should be assessed for tachycardia (with activity as well as at rest), presence of systolic ejection murmur, and the lungs for breath sounds and tachypnea. The abdomen should be assessed for distension, hepatomegaly or splenomegaly. Lower extremity edema may be present.

Once the diagnosis and cause of the anemia have been determined, then the treatment plan is developed. The plan includes interventions directed at treating the underlying anemia if possible as well as related symptoms. Based on symptoms and blood values, the anemia is classified as mild, moderate, or severe. Hemoglobin levels between 10 and 11 g/dL are classified as mild, 8 to 10 moderate, and below 8 g/dL, severe. Treatment is directed to supporting RBC replacement. Transfusions are one option but do present risks, including transfusion reactions and infection. Epoetin alfa (Procrit) and darbepoetin alfa (Aranesp) are erythrocyte CSF agents and are used for chemotherapy-induced anemia (CIA) in patients with nonmyeloid malignancies. These drugs have reduced the need for RBC transfusions in some patients, effectively elevated hemoglobin levels, and have been associated with improvements in patient quality of life (Vadhan-Raj, et al., 2003).

Other interventions to consider are nutritional supplements that include iron, B_{12}, or folic acid and treatment of infections, inflammations, or malignancies. Nursing interventions include measures to minimize and manage fatigue. The nurse should assess severity of fatigue on a scale of 0 to 10; assess frequency of fatigue and activities associated with increased fatigue; and ability to perform activities of daily living. The nurse needs to also assist the patient with activities of daily living as necessary and encourage independence without causing exhaustion. Patient education concerning safety is important if the patient has dizziness or orthostasis. Patient education points of emphasis are (a) the process of anemia and cause; (b) importance and ways of managing anemia; (c) self-assessment and reporting of signs and symptoms; and (d) self-care strategies, including dietary modification, measures to conserve energy and manage fatigue, self-administration of medications including **erythropoietic** (relating to the formation of RBCs) agents, and safety measures.

Neutropenia

Neutropenia is a major factor in the deaths of many immunocompromised patients, including patients with cancer. Neutropenia is defined as an absolute neutrophil count (ANC) of less than 2,000/mm³. Neutrophils are responsible for phagocytosis of bacteria and cellular debris. This side effect of chemotherapy can be deadly because without sufficient neutrophils the body struggles to combat infection. Infection in the immunocompromised patient can quickly lead to septicemia and then death. As noted, in either disruptions of the hematopoiesis process, a reduction in neutrophil can be from the cancer pathology itself or a result of receiving antineoplastic agents. It may be temporary or persist for some time, with cell count continuing to fall as treatment progresses (Box 15-3). The ANC is calculated by multiplying the total WBC count times the quantity of the percentage of segs + percentage of bands (Brown, et al., 2002).

The higher the grade and the lower the ANC count, the greater the risk for developing neutropenia The ANC is usually at the **nadir,** or lowest point, 10 to 14 days after chemotherapy administration; a point when the patient is at the greatest risk for development of infection. Febrile neutropenia occurs when a patient presents with both a fever and a significant reduction in the WBC count. For the patient with neutropenia, signs of infection include a temperature greater than 38.1° C (100.5° F), chills, cough, shortness of breath, sore throat, stomatitis, redness, or swelling around any breaks in skin, changes in bowel or urination, flu-like symptoms, nausea and vomiting, or general malaise. Untreated septic shock can lead to death.

The patient who is neutropenic is severely comprised in their ability to mount an immunological response to infection, thus a temperature greater than 38.1° C (100.5° F) is of great concern. Often this low-grade temperature

---

BOX 15-3

ABSOLUTE NEUTROPHIL COUNT INFECTION RISK GRADING SYSTEM

The National Cancer Institute provides a grading system for absolute neutrophil count as follows:

- Grade 1: greater than 1,500/mm³
- Grade 2: 1,000–1,500 mm³
- Grade 3: 500–1,000 mm³
- Grade 4: less than 500/mm³

Adapted from National Cancer Institute. (2004c). Bone marrow transplantation and peripheral blood stem cell transplantation: Questions and answers. Retrieved June 10, 2005, from http://cis.nci.nih.gov.

is the only sign of infection because of the compromised immune system. The patient should call the oncologist immediately and prepare to seek medical attention. Treatment for neutropenia includes administration of antibiotics as well as administration of CSFs, such as filgrastim (Neupogen) or pegfilgrastim (Neulasta). These CSFs can be given subcutaneously or intravenously and stimulate the production of neutrophils. Often these drugs are given prophylactically in anticipation of neutropenia.

Fortunately, heightened awareness and new medications are reducing both mortality and morbidity. Assessment includes temperature and blood tests to determine the number of WBCs present. If febrile neutropenia is determined, then cultures and additional blood work will be taken to try to determine the presence and possible site of any infections. The nurse should be aware, however, that a source of infection is ultimately determined in only about one third of patients. Depending on the clinical state of the patient and the predicted length of the lowered WBC counts, a decision will be made whether the patient should be treated as an outpatient or admitted to a health care facility for observation and treatment. Whether the patient is admitted or not, treatment will usually include the use of broad-spectrum antibiotics.

The goals of nursing care focus on: (a) prevention and treatment of infection and (b) knowledge deficit. Infection control measures include strict aseptic technique during invasive measures, meticulous care of all IV devices, and avoidance of indwelling devices, such as urinary catheters, if possible. Increased monitoring of vital signs, including temperature, is part of ongoing assessment. At the first sign of infection laboratory tests, such as blood cultures, urine cultures, and chest X-ray, should be considered. Biological response modifiers (BRMs), Neupogen and Leukine can be used to manage neutropenia. In the hospital a private room is best, and the nurse should take measure to ensure a low infection risk environment (Figure 15-5). Staff, patient, and visitor education includes discouraging flowers and get well cards as they collect dust and grow mold. Bacteria may be present on fresh fruits and vegetables, so dietary staff should be alerted to the immunocompromised status. When transporting the patient the transporter should avoid crowded or confined areas, such as waiting rooms and occupied elevators. Patient education begins with teaching patients and families basic hygiene measures, such as hand washing and avoiding contact with people exposed to infectious diseases. Daily showers with mild soap and protection of skin integrity and oral hygiene are stressed, with care not to damage oral mucous membranes. Nutritional support is important to support the immune system (Byars, 2002).

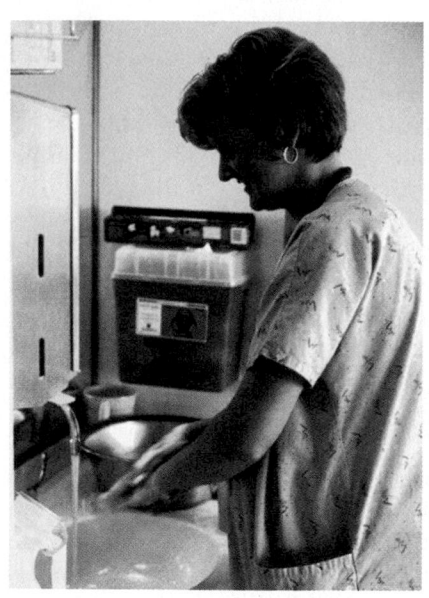

Figure 15-5 Washing hands to prevent infection for a immunosuppressed patient with cancer.

Thrombocytopenia

Thrombocytopenia is defined as a circulating platelet count of less than 100,000. Chemotherapy-related thrombocytopenia usually occurs after the nadir. Patients should be assessed for signs of thrombocytopenia, which include bruising, frank bleeding, hematoma formation, occult blood, epistaxis, petechiae, hematuria, and melena. Confusion, headache, blurred vision, changes in papillary response, and changes in cognition could be signs of an intracranial bleed associated with extremely low platelet counts. Thus, platelet counts should be closely monitored.

The patient should be taught to watch for signs of bleeding and to observe measures to reduce potential injury. The patient should be taught to use a soft-bristled toothbrush, not to floss, not to shave with a razor, to avoid falls, to avoid straining during bowel movements, and to report any signs of bleeding or hemorrhage. Nurses should be cautious in provision of care and be cognizant of bleeding precautions. All medications should be assessed to determine they contain antiaggregation properties as present with drugs containing aspirin, NSAIDs, or anticoagulants. Treatment for severe thrombocytopenia may include platelet transfusion or the administration of oprelvekin, a thrombopoietic growth factor.

Neuropathy

Peripheral neuropathy is a condition of the nervous system that usually begins in the hands or feet with symptoms of numbness, tingling, burning. The patient may also complain of mild weakness and constipation. Certain anti-cancer drugs, such as vincristine, cisplatin, and paclitaxel, which have neurological side effects can cause neuropathy. When severe, nerve damage may impair walking abilities, alter bladder dysfunction, and result in significant sensory loss. These side effects may improve or disappear after the discontinuation of chemotherapy but may take several months to do so.

Symptoms of neuropathy are temporary in most cases if caught early. Safety measures relate to risk from altered or diminished sensation. For example, if fingers become numb, the patient needs to exercise care when handling objects that are sharp, hot, or otherwise dangerous. Other safety measures include using a thermometer to test bath temperature; using skid-free shower and bathroom mats; clearing walkways of clutter; and wiping spills on the floor immediately. Protective footwear should be considered to avoid pressure points. The nurse should instruct patients that if their sense of balance is affected, they should move carefully and use handrails. Assessment of activities of daily living should include driving skills; particularly the ability to feel gas and brake pedals and changes in reaction time. For severe pain caused by peripheral neuropathy, analgesics are most effective when a fixed dose is taken at a fixed time schedule. Nonmedical therapeutic approaches include relaxation training that can reduce anxiety and stress, reduce pain, and promote sleep. Regular daily exercise, like walking and stretching exercises to keep muscles flexible, should be done as tolerated (Estes, 2006).

Cognitive Disorders

Cognitive impairment is the loss of the ability to remember certain things, learn new skills, and complete certain tasks. It is estimated that from 20 to 50 percent of cancer patients describe some cognitive changes, such as "being in a fog," inability to concentrate, and memory loss. As a health care provider one must recognize that cognitive impairment is frightening to the patient and family, but they are not clear what causes the changes. The phenomenon is often seen during and following chemotherapy and is so common that patients may refer to it as "chemo brain" or "chemo fog," which may last up to two years following treatment. Other factors that have been suggested as playing a part are stress and hormonal fluctuations, low blood counts, fatigue, depression, and medications. Specific signs and symptoms patients might report include the inability to find the right word in conversation, short-term memory lapses, prolonged learning time for new tasks, and prolonged response times. Such changes are upsetting for people in today's society who are used to performing multiple jobs quickly and simultaneously.

Interventions should be those that empower the patient and family to feel some control. Physical exercise as tolerated improves circulation, stimulates endorphins, and provides diversion. Establishing a routine also helps with memory loss. The nurse can have the patient write down when memory problems occur. By reviewing the log, patterns may emerge, which can guide intervention. For example, if forgetfulness is worst in late afternoon, perhaps it is related to fatigue, and scheduled rests may help. Cognitive changes can be embarrassing for patients. Encourage them to talk openly about the problem with staff, family, and friends who can help fill in gaps and who will reinforce that the situation is temporary. All teaching activity by the nurse should be planned when the patient is rested. Less content should be presented at one time, reinforced at later times, and the nurse should validate retention before the patient is expected to manage tasks independently (Green, Pakenham, & Gardiner, 2005).

GI System

There are several symptoms related to the GI system that significantly impact the patient with cancer. Nausea and vomiting, **mucositis** (an inflammation and ulceration of the lining of the mouth, throat, or GI tract most commonly associated with chemotherapy or radiotherapy for cancer), diarrhea, and anorexia or **cachexia** (a breakdown of muscle mass resulting from rapid weight loss or a general wasting because of illness or stress) may result from malignancies, chemotherapy, or radiation therapy, all of which may interfere with ingestion, digestion, or absorption of food.

Uncontrolled nausea and vomiting may interfere with the patient's ability to receive cancer treatment and care of himself or herself. Nausea and vomiting are controlled by the central nervous system, and the process of nausea and vomiting is a complex and physiological protective mechanism. Various triggers from along the GI tract stimulate the vomiting center located near the brainstem to indicate that there is delay in emptying the stomach contents. Smell, taste, anxiety, pain, motion, changes in the body caused by inflammation, poor blood flow, or irritation can act as triggers.

The most common causes of nausea and vomiting are certain chemotherapy drugs and radiation therapy to the GI tract, liver, or brain. Nausea and vomiting are more likely to occur if they have been severe after past chemotherapy sessions, if the patient is female, and if the patient is younger than 50 years old. When a patient has had nausea and vomiting in response to previous cancer treatments, anticipatory nausea and vomiting are likely. Other possible causes of nausea and vomiting include fluid and electrolyte imbalances, such as hypercalcemia, dehydration, edema; tumor growth in the GI tract, liver, or brain; constipation; certain drugs; infection or blood poisoning; kidney problems; and anxiety. Complications include dehydration, electrolyte imbalance, and esophageal and GI bleeding, emotional problems, torn esophagus, broken bones, and the reopening of surgical wounds (Varricchio, 2004).

Nausea and vomiting caused by cancer therapy are classified as anticipatory, acute, delayed, or chronic. Anticipatory nausea and vomiting may occur before or during chemotherapy and appear earlier than these symptoms would be expected. Anticipatory symptoms may also appear in patients who are receiving radiation therapy. Acute nausea and vomiting usually occur within 24 hours after chemotherapy has begun. Delayed nausea and vomiting occur more than 24 hours after chemotherapy. Chronic nausea and vomiting may affect people who have advanced cancer, but it is not well understood.

Interventions begin with ongoing assessment. The nurse and patient can log the severity and frequency of episodes. Taking a daily weight is used to monitor affects of antiemetic therapy. Constipation is one of the most common causes of nausea in patients with advanced cancer, so it is important to record bowel movements. The nurse should have the patient notify staff if signs and symptoms of dehydration develop. These include dry mouth, reduced urine output, concentrated urine, and weakness. Having foods prepared in a room different from where foods are consumed can ease symptoms, because odors may cause nausea. The key to controlling nausea and vomiting is to prevent it before it occurs. Many new antiemetic drugs are effective for preventing or decreasing nausea and vomiting. Antiemetics may be used alone or in combinations and are typically administered 24 hours prior to chemotherapy and then continued until 24 hours after chemotherapy. In addition, some patients may wish to consider nondrug methods to help with nausea and vomiting

Some chemotherapeutic agents have diarrhea rates as high as 50 to 80 percent. Overall rates are as high as 19 percent (NCI, 2005a). The high incidence is not surprising when considering the list of contributing factors. Chemotherapy destroys rapidly growing cells of the intestine. Surgery to the bowel or stomach, underlying cancer, responses to diet, stress and anxiety, infection, radiation, and BMT all list diarrhea as a common side effect as do many medications. Diarrhea affects quality of life, weakens the patient for therapy and healing, and can be life-threatening. Rapid recognition and assessment by the nurse are important. A common problem is that often assessments are not standardized. The NCI's Common Toxicity Criteria is a useful tool and evaluates diarrhea by number of stools and patient response (NCI, 2005a). The entire tool may be found at NCI's GI complications Web site (NCI, 2005b). For a complete assessment, it has been suggested to obtain background information from the patient that includes the type and extent of the patient's cancer, anticancer treatment, comorbid factors, coexisting symptoms, patient and provider perceptions, as well as a thorough description of the diarrhea. Stringent monitoring should be conducted at least weekly in patients at risk (Broyles, et al., 2007). Defining characteristics of diarrhea are listed as hyperactive bowel sounds; at least three loose liquid stools per day; urgency; abdominal pain; and cramping. Related factors include: (a) psychological (high stress levels and anxiety); (b) situational (alcohol abuse, toxins, laxative abuse, radiation, tube feedings, adverse effects of medications, contaminants, and travel), and (c) physiological (inflammation, malabsorption, infectious processes, irritation, and parasites).

The goals of nursing interventions for diarrhea are to decrease gastric motility. Dietary modifications, such as low-fiber diet, avoid over stimulation of the lower GI. Pharmacological interventions work to decrease motility, decrease intestinal secretions, and promote absorption. Opioids, such as loperamide, slow motility with limited cognitive effects. Diphenoxylate and atropine (Lomotil) and anticholinergics, like Levsin, diminish intestinal activity and bismuth subsalicylate (Pepto-Bismol) may help in less severe cases. Octreotide is a somatostatin analogue that has been shown effective in chemotherapy-induced diarrhea as well as that resulting from GVHD. The nurse should teach the patient to increase clear liquid intake to avoid dehydration. Parenteral nutrition and electrolyte supplementation may be necessary (Benson, et al., 2004).

Anorexia and Cachexia

Anorexia and cachexia are recognized as significant and complex problems for cancer patients. The syndrome affects an estimated 31 to 98 percent of cancer patients. Anorexia is a loss of appetite or aversion to food, which can lead to drastic weight loss. Anorexia can compromise adequate nutritional intake, forcing the body to use fat and muscle stores. Cachexia is the condition that results because of physical wasting and is defined as a rapid loss of fatty tissue and skeletal muscle.

Signs and symptoms of anorexia and cachexia include loss of appetite, rapid satiety, weight loss, muscle wasting, and metabolic abnormalities, including protein depletion. Not only can these conditions affect response to therapy and occurrence of toxicity to treatment and survival, but they are a documented cause of death. As food intake and body mass decrease, the patient develops lowered resistance to infection and slower healing. As the person becomes unable to perform simple tasks and becomes weaker and more fatigued, appetite and food intake decrease, creating a cycle that can culminate in death if untreated. The underlying physiological cause is an imbalance between caloric intake and energy output or metabolic need, but the contributing factors can be complex. Causative factors, such as treatment modalities and the cancer itself, are similar to other GI side effects and have been discussed. Other causes the nurse may consider are alterations in taste, organ enlargement with pressure causing early satiation, altered glucose metabolism, and psychological factors of grief, depression, and fear. The goal in managing the patient is to increase nutritional intake to preserve and improve the overall nutritional status of the patient. The caregiver should consider food preferences when planning dietary regimens. Mouth care, pain control, and education in relaxation techniques may help.

Mucositis

Mucositis is an inflammation of the mucous membrane of the GI tract and commonly occurs in cancer patients. Another term associated with this side affect is **stomatitis,** which is inflammation of the oral mucosa because of chemotherapy. Symptoms begin with dry mouth and chapped lips. Progression includes painful white patches and ulceration. It can be significant enough to require narcotics for pain and results in weight loss, delayed cancer treatment, and hospitalization. The cause is damage to the rapidly regenerating epithelial cells, causing epithelial thinning, inflammation, and decreased cell. High risks for developing mucositis include: (a) age younger then 20 years; (b) hematologic or head and neck cancers; (c) preexisting oral disease; and (d) chemotherapy or radiation. As with other disruptions of the GI tract discussed, objective description, and assessment are both crucial and difficult. Descriptive criteria include appearance of ulcers, redness, degree of soreness, level of pain, edema, and interference with ability to eat. Parental or enteral nutritional support may be required. Prevention of myositis other than decreasing doses of chemotherapy is not known.

There have been multiple treatment strategies offered, but it is generally agreed that effectiveness varies from case to case. There are topical agents, such as sucralfate, prostaglandin E_2, and systemic agents, including beta-carotene, propantheline that have some degree of success. Nonpharmacological actions, such as cryotherapy and soft laser therapy may also be considered. Nursing care for all patients at risk begins with good oral care. Cryotherapy is the use of ice chips in the mouth to decrease blood circulation to the area during peak time of drug concentrations. Infection prevention strategies are important for any patient with disruption of the skin and mucous membrane, but topical therapy has not proved definitively helpful in curing mucositis. It is important to instruct the patient to drink increased amounts of fluid and soft foods less likely to damage fragile tissue. The patient should avoid acidic or irritating foods. Cool or room temperature foods are less irritating.

While some interventions that are targeted to the specific GI symptom have been discussed, there are many nursing actions that can be effective for multiple GI symptoms even though their effectiveness may vary from patient to patient. Assessing and monitoring the patient for signs of malnutrition or for potential disruption in intake is an important responsibility of the nurse. The nurse should begin with determining a baseline weight, identifying appetite change, noting any specific problems, and asking about the patients nutritional concerns. Encouraging the patient to adequately complete calorie diaries and accurately report symptoms that may influence intake is helpful in planning and evaluating nutrition plans. The patient should also be evaluated via a multidisciplinary approach for potential deficits of knowledge about nutrition, nutritional support, disease symptoms, or treatment side effects. Response to treatment or dietary intervention needs to be assessed (NCI, 2005c).

Nursing interventions are directed to controlling nausea and vomiting, maintaining adequate nutrition, and stimulating appetite. The goal of nutritional support is to replenishing the body with proteins, carbohydrates, fats, vitamins, and minerals being lost through the anorexia or cachexia syndrome. Increasing the calorie or protein intake may be accomplished through oral supplementation, enteral feeding, or parenteral nutrition. Allowing others to cook and not coming to the table until after the meal is prepared are useful strategies if odors are problem triggers. Using small amounts of seasonings or flavorings may enhance taste. The patient may require more seasoning than previously noted for food to have a pleasant taste. The use of wine or beer before meals, if allowed, is also relaxing and may stimulate appetite.

A variety of appetite stimulants may help to the patient maintain adequate calorie and nutrient intake from food sources. These include dronabinol (Marinol), megestrol acetate (Megace), and dexamethasone. Marinol is part of a class of drugs called cannabinoids. Dronabinol is produced in the laboratory and is a version of a naturally occurring substance in *Cannabis sativa* L. (marijuana). Marinol is known to be an appetite stimulant. Also, Marinol is thought to block directly a receptor that is involved in chemotherapy-induced nausea and vomiting. Because of these two effects, Marinol may be beneficial to patients receiving chemotherapy treatments. Dexamethasone is a corticosteroid that is often prescribed for cancer-associated anorexia. It appears to be beneficial for some cancer patients with a poor prognosis as serious side effects are unlikely to occur in the short-term (Walsh, Nelson, & Mahmoud, 2003).

Patient education includes encouraging patient and family interaction during meals. When family members can provide the patient's favorite foods, food intake usually improves, and family bonds are strengthened. A clean, uncluttered environment can promote relaxation and result in an unhurried meal. High-protein foods should be consumed at the most tolerated time of the day. The patient should be encouraged to participate in meal planning and to choose appealing foods high in proteins. Small, frequent meals are often better tolerated than larger, infrequent ones. Pleasant food aromas and light exercise may stimulate appetite.

BOX 15-4

NURSING PLAN FOR ALTERED BODY IMAGE

Nursing Diagnosis:

Body image disturbance related to cancer diagnosis and surgery

Nursing Interventions:

- Assess ability to adjust to altered body image
- Provide opportunities for patient and family to discuss feelings of altered body image
- Emphasize that disease and surgery have no affect on patient's masculinity
- Reassure patient of ability to continue roles and relationships with family and friends
- If patient wishes, arrange for him or her to talk with someone who has had surgery for cancer
- Refer patient and family to support or self-help group if appropriate

Expected Outcome:

Patient and family will adapt to altered body image

Adapted from DeLaune, S., & Ladner, P. (2006). Fundamentals of nursing (3rd ed.). New York: Thomson Delmar Learning.

Body Image

Cancer and its treatments can affect body image in multiple ways. Surgery can cause changes in physical appearance and scarring. Radiation and chemotherapy can affect a cancer patient's body image, because they often cause hair loss, radiation burns, and unattractive changes in the patient's complexion. While hair loss caused by chemotherapy is usually a temporary condition, hair loss caused by radiation treatment may be permanent. Other treatments can cause weight loss or weight gain, fatigue, nausea, hair loss, and skin changes, which can change how the patient looks and feels. Psychological reactions, including anxiety and depression, impact the patient's sense of competence as well as his or her relationships with others. The degree of impact on body image depends on a combination of amount of change, specific change, and predisease personality of the patient.

It is the nurse's responsibility to prepare the patient in advance for potential body altering effects of treatments. Armed with knowledge the nurse and patient can plan strategies for changes prior to their onset. Both avoidance of and obsessive preoccupation with the alterations are not uncommon responses. Nurses can reassure the patient and family that fear, grief, and their physiological consequences are normal. Effective treatments can include cosmetic techniques, counseling, and guidance, and complementary therapies. Since 1989 the American Cancer Society, the Cosmetic, Toiletry, and Fragrance Association Foundation, and the National Cosmetology Association have sponsored the "Look Good . . . Feel Better" (LGFB) program, which offers classes in a number of medical centers. This program offers useful tips and teaches how to deal with changes to skin, hair, and general appearance with cosmetics, wigs, turbans, and scarves. The nurse may offer the patient the number (800-650-960) to call for more information on this program. The American Hair Loss Council offers detailed information about ways to cope with hair loss caused by cancer treatment. Plastic surgery can treat observable scars or other types of surgical disfigurement, including the loss of body parts. A prosthesis should be considered to replace a missing or damaged body part.

Patients who experience emotional problems related to changes in appearance may benefit from counseling or support groups. Individual psychotherapy, group therapy, and pastoral or spiritual counseling can help patients gain from the experiences of others and look past their physical worth. Alternative and complementary therapy may allow patients to balance the side effects of cancer treatment with relaxing and pleasant experiences (Box 15-4).

Sexuality

Sexual dysfunction is a common side effect of cancer treatment. Sexual concerns are also some of the most difficult for the patient and family to discuss. About half the women who survive breast or gynecological cancer and as many as 70 percent of men who are undergoing active treatment for localized prostate cancer report sexual problems. The most common sexual problems for people with cancer are loss of desire for sexual activity in men and women, erectile dysfunction in men, and dyspareunia (pain with intercourse) in women. It should also be recognized by the nurse and shared with the patient that sexual problems do not tend to resolve within the first year or two of disease-free survival; rather, they may remain constant and fairly severe (Ganz, Greendale, Petersen, Kahn, & Bower, 2003).

There is a variety of both physiological and psychosocial factors contributing to altered sexual functioning. Physical factors include functional damage secondary to cancer therapy, fatigue and low energy, pain, hormonal changes, altered circulation, and nerve function damage. These changes usually lower sexual interest and sexual ability. Medications used to treat pain, depression, hypertension, and metabolic conditions may all contribute to sexual dysfunction. Physical changes may also result in the patient feeling less attractive sexually. Psychological factors include false beliefs about the origin of the cancer. It is not an uncommon belief that past sexual activity, an extramarital affair, sexually transmitted disease, or abortion has caused the cancer. This belief causes guilt. Depression, worries about changes in appearance, anxiety about health, family, or finances can also impact sexuality. When the malignancy is in the pelvic or genital area another misconception is that sexual activity may promote a recurrence of the tumor.

It is difficult to find data that address the degree that sexual problems influence overall health-related quality of life, but what data exist, along with anecdotal reports do support impacting patients' lives. While it may be difficult, talking openly of sexual concerns and problems is an important part of good nursing intervention, because sexual problems can contribute to poor self-esteem and interfere with relationships. The nurse can begin by asking about a variety of quality of life issues, including relationships and sexuality as part of the regular assessment. A simple statement, such as, "Many patients dealing with cancer notice changes or problems in their sex lives. Do you have any problems or concerns related to sexuality?" may be enough to open communication. For women estrogen replacement therapy can usually reverse many sexual problems, and the nurse should discuss the risks and benefits of hormone replacement therapy with consideration of each woman's individual risk profile.

There are a variety of treatment strategies available for patients with sexual dysfunction after cancer. Education may help those who have a basic lack of understanding about normal sexual functioning. The nurse may need to provide information related to safety concerns, explaining that cancer is not transmitted through sexual contact. The patient and partner should understand that intimacy is not harmful during external beam radiation therapy or after brachytherapy is completed. Sex may not be recommended, however, during periods of extreme immunosuppression and should be discussed individually in relation to chemotherapy. Many patients fear that side effects of cancer treatment will make them less sexually attractive. Physical changes may be subtle as with a radiation tattoo, temporary as with treatment-induced **alopecia** (the loss of hair), or more radical as with head and neck surgery, mastectomy, or creation of an ostomy. In all cases the nurse should remember that it is normal for men and women to feel insecure when these changes occur. For those with ostomies, the nurse can suggest limiting food intake prior to anticipated sexual activity, watching the type of foods consumed, and planning times for intimacy when a bowel movement is less likely. Patients should be taught to empty the pouch when anticipating sexual intimacy. If the patient finds that the ostomy bag interferes with sexual intimacy, the nurse can suggest covering the bag or rolling it under a special belt. Wigs, makeup, and prosthesis are some other options to help women look and feel better. Artificial vaginal moisturizers (e.g., Replens) and water-based lubricants (e.g., Astroglide and K-Y Jelly) are options especially for women who cannot use estrogen replacement. For many of the patients' concerns, the most important role of the nurse is one of informed listener.

Sleep Disorders

It is estimated that 45 percent of people with cancer have sleep disturbance. Physical illness, pain, hospitalization, drugs, and other treatments for cancer, and the psychological impact of a malignant disease may disrupt the sleeping patterns of persons with cancer pain. The sleep disorders classification committee has defined four major categories of sleep disorders. These include: (a) disorders of initiating and maintaining sleep (insomnias); (b) disorders of the sleep-wake cycle; (c) dysfunctions associated with sleep, sleep stages, or partial arousals (parasomnias); and (d) disorders of excessive somnolence (Wagner & Cella, 2004).

The nurse should consider environmental factors that may impact sleep both at home and in the hospital. Hospitalized patients are likely to experience frequent interruptions of sleep because of treatment schedules, hospital routines, and roommates. Other factors influencing sleep-wake schedules include age, noise, temperature, comfort, pain, and anxiety. Medications commonly considered for altered sleep patterns are nonbenzodiazepine sleep aids, including antidepressants, antihistamines, and antipsychotics. Antihistamines have the anticholinergic properties that relieve nausea, vomiting, and insomnia. The nurse must remember that these agents must be used with caution because daytime sedation and delirium can occur, especially in the elderly. Barbiturates are generally not recommended for the management of sleep disturbances in cancer patients as they have a number of adverse effects, including the development of tolerance, and they also have a narrow margin of safety (Broyles, et al., 2007).

Fatigue

The fatigue coalition states the "fatigue is the most common symptom associated with cancer and cancer treatment." The nurse should realize that the level of fatigue experienced by these patients is significantly more severe than that experienced by the rest of us during normal daily routines or even at times of stress. As with pain, fatigue is a subjective experience that is what the patient says it is. Patients describe the feeling as overwhelming and that it is experienced unrelated to activity of exertion (Wagner & Cella, 2004). It affects thought process as well as activity level and is further complicated by pain and nausea that limit the ability to rest. Also, cancer-related fatigue affects activities of daily living, relationships, ability to cope, and physical and emotional responses to diagnosis and treatment. Management of fatigue begins with the nursing assessment to define the extent of fatigue. The nurse should determine the severity as well as interventions that the patient has found helpful. The best way to manage fatigue is to treat the underlying cause. Unfortunately, it is not always easy to know what the exact cause is. For the cancer patient, many factors may be involved and causes vary from patient to patient.

Nursing interventions for fatigue include the promotion of good nutrition. The patient should be encouraged to eat frequent small meals with the goal of maintaining caloric input necessary for energy expenditure. For patients with anemia, transfusions and drugs, such as epoetin, to replace hemoglobin may be considered. Both the cancer itself and the treatment lead to increased energy expenditure. Providing quiet, restful areas for treatments, such as chemotherapy,

PATIENT PLAYBOOK

Patient and Family Education on Pain Management

The nurse caring for the patient with cancer and assisting the family caregivers is to provide the following information about pain management:

- The nurse should encourage the patient to be specific when asked about the level of pain he or she is experiencing.
- The nurse should encourage the patient to provide personal information regarding the history of the pain episode (the onset, location, radiation, duration, quality, severity, and frequency).
- The nurse should encourage the patient to state how the pain impacts activities of daily living, what activities precipitate or exacerbate the pain, and what measures are used to alleviate the pain.
- Ensure the patient and family that experiencing pain does not necessarily mean that cancer is getting worse.

- Ensure the patient that using pain medicines rarely, if ever, results in addiction (provide written materials regarding pain control).
- Instruct patients and family about signs and symptoms of pain medication side effects.
- Teach patient and family safety issues of pain management routine (e.g., combinations of opioids, alcohol, and tranquilizers can be dangerous).
- Teach patients and family appropriate pain medication administration technique per the medication route. Provide opportunity for practice with equipment.
- Provide the patient and family with information on available resources (e.g., emotional support counseling, support groups, and nonpharmacological interventions).

Adapted from Daniels, R. (2004). Nursing fundamentals: Caring and clinical decision making. *New York: Thomson Delmar Learning; DeLaune, S., & Ladner, P. (2006).* Fundamentals of nursing *(3rd ed.). New York: Thomson Delmar Learning.*

is helpful. Encourage the patient to avoid physically taxing activities prior to these treatments and to allow time for rest following them. Cancer fatigue is more often a result of the treatments than the cancer itself. Explain to the patient that fatigue as a result of therapy or surgery may persist even after the cancer therapy is completed but will eventually improve (Poirier, 2006).

Pain

When asked, patients respond that pain is one of the greatest issues with which they must contend. Pain is defined as an unpleasant sensory and emotional experience arising from actual or potential tissue damage or described in terms of such damage. Onset can be sudden or slow, of any intensity, from mild to severe, constant or recurring, without an anticipated or predictable end, having duration greater than six months. Furthermore, acute pain is described as being caused by injury, surgery, illness, trauma, or painful medical procedures, and chronic pain exists beyond an expected time for healing. Research indicates that over 40 percent of patients with cancer do not get adequate relief of their pain despite that medications and other therapy currently exist to relieve almost all cancer pain. Communication between patients and health care professionals is essential. Undertreatment of pain has significant adverse effects on quality of life and has been associated with serious patient despair and depression. A report of pain should not be viewed as a sign of weakness. Refer to detailed information, especially for management of breakthrough and intractable pain in chapter 16. Additional information on cancer pain management can be obtained from NCI and ACS.

Coping

The preceding section has presented material on multiple side effects that the patient with cancer may face. Unfortunately, the list presented is only a partial one. The reality is that, in addition to dealing with the diagnosis of a chronic or life-threatening disease, the journey following diagnosis is filled with treatments and side effects that impact every aspect of the individual's life. Among the many fears at this time is loss of independence, becoming a financial burden on the family, pain, debilitating illness, the side effects of chemotherapy, radiation, or other treatments, and death. Some suggest that stress is highest immediately after the diagnosis. For others the initial treatment was the most stressful time. Some people handle the initial stress well, only to have a delayed reaction as much as six months later.

Anyone with cancer will likely experience significant amounts of stress. Each person has his or her own way of coping with cancer, and not one nursing plan of care fits all patients. The effective nurse seeks ways for cancer patients and caregivers to cope with the cancer, its side effects, grief, or end-of-life issues, and decision making. Assessment of effective coping should be ongoing throughout the care process (Mayo Clinic, 2005). The ACS is an excellent source of information for the patient and for professional and family caregivers. Interventions should be individualized, and there are many options for the nurse to consider. The patient should be encouraged to use coping skills that have worked before. Some patients find talking and being with others helpful while others find individual approaches, such as relaxation therapy and meditation, beneficial. Family and friends should be screened to select those helpful to the patient.

Family caregivers also have coping needs. Many of the same strategies apply to the caregiver. Often treatment facilities offer strategies that the patients, team, and family have found helpful. Support groups often are beneficial for sharing concerns and learning effective coping strategies. Becoming well-informed about the patient's treatment regimen and being able to consult with health care professionals is an essential component in the plan of care. The caregiver should understand that planned time away from the 24-hour task of caregiving is important. Enlisting help with household tasks and providing direct patient care may be necessary to ease daily stress. It is also important to maintain and care for one's personal physical, psychosocial, and spiritual health. Many treatment facilities have a resource center that includes information, resource lists, equipment, and supplies.

As a primary care provider the nurse should allow time for questions and treat all concerns with respect and trust. The nurse should encourage the patient to bring a friend or partner with him or her for treatment. Often, a second person will ask helpful questions to assist the patient to remember information. The patient may at times feel desperate. Information is empowering and critical in cancer treatment. Patients should have as much information about their condition and treatments as possible. ACS and NCI provide useful, mainstream, current information. The patient and designated family member should be encouraged to discuss other sources of information with health care providers as there are many sources of inaccurate information.

ONCOLOGICAL EMERGENCIES

Several emergencies may occur related to tumor obstruction or compression or edema or are associated with fluid, electrolyte, or hormone imbalances and infection. Certain emergencies are relatively rare, such as superior vena cava syndrome, which results from impairment of blood flow through the superior vena cava to the right atrium because of obstruction or compression. The role of the nurse is to understand the underlying pathology and to educate the patient and family about signs and symptoms of potential emergency conditions.

Hypercalcemia occurs in 10 to 20 percent of patients with cancer. This is most commonly associated with cancers of the lung, breast, multiple myeloma, renal, and prostate. TLS is a group of metabolic imbalances that result from acute destruction of cancer cells and release of intracellular products into the circulation. The risk of TLS depends on the type of tumors, the extent of the disease, type of treatment, and preexisting renal function. Included in this syndrome are hyperuricemia, hypocalcemia, hyperkalemia, and hyperphosphatemia. TLS is most common in hematological malignancies. Refer to chapter 12 for detailed information on etiologies and management of hypercalcemia.

The syndrome of inappropriate antidiuretical hormone (SIADH) occurs when ADH hormone secretion exceeds homeostatic control resulting in increased fluid retention and hyponatremia. This syndrome is rare, occurring in 2 percent of cancer patients. It is reversible with administering hypertonic saline solution, a diuretic, and discontinuing drugs (such as morphine) that may have contributed to the fluid retention.

Spinal cord compression is due to pressure, displacement, or compression of the spinal cord by a tumor. Fifty percent of the cases result from metastasis from the breast, lung, or prostate cancer. Pleural effusion, an abnormal accumulation of fluid in the pericardial space, can be caused by excess fluid produced by a tumor or postradiation pericarditis. The pressure of the excess fluid can result in cardiac tamponade, a mechanical compression of the heart. A rapid accumulation of fluid and sudden rise in pressure impairs diastolic filling of the heart and can create an emergency situation. A slower accumulation of fluid or blood, as in effusion related to cancer, may not produce immediate signs of trouble, because the fibrous wall of the pericardial sac can gradually stretch to accommodate a liter or more of fluid. The nurse should closely observe the patient for signs of dyspnea, restlessness, chest pain, electrocardiogram (ECG), pulse, and blood pressure changes. Refer to chapter 24 on cardiac problems for more detailed information.

Anaphylaxis, a life-threatening condition, can be due to decreased systemic vascular resistance and fluid leaking from blood vessels resulting in IV volume depletion. Some systemic therapy, such as interleukin 1, can cause severe hypotension, especially with high-dose therapy. Close monitoring of changes in respiratory status, blood pressure, and peripheral vascular status during therapy is essential (see chapter 43).

Disseminated intravascular coagulation (DIC) is widespread clotting within the arterioles or capillaries that occurs spontaneously with hemorrhage. Cancer is considered to be a triggering event that may be related to tumor necrosis factor (TNP), a cytokine with wide-range biological activity. Symptoms include petechia, ecchymosis or purpura of the skin and mucous membranes, pulse, shortness of breath, hematuria, oliguria, or renal failure. The nurse should observe for signs and symptoms of deep vein thrombosis, conduct frequent assessment of mental status and neurological checks, and monitor urinary output. For more detailed information on management of DIC refer to chapter 29.

Increased intracranial pressure (ICP) is a life-threatening situation. It can occur when a cerebral tumor reaches a mass that displaces cerebral tissue in the direction of least resistance. Sustained increases in ICP can result in compression of the brainstem, resulting in herniation of the tissue through the foramen magnum. Herniation and damage to circulation and brain function is dependent on the location of the tumor, the rate of growth, and the direction of the tissue displacement. The nurse should monitor the patient's mental status, observe for signs of respiratory distress, use measures to maintain oxygenation, and report abnormal findings immediately. The nurse should also reassure the patient and family and minimize external stimulation. Refer to chapter 35 for more detailed information.

Septic shock is a common problem for people with cancer because of the depressed immune system resulting from therapy or from cancers, such as leukemia. Health care providers must give particular attention to aseptic technique when working with central venous lines and other invasive procedures. Refer to chapter 11 for detailed information on management of patients with sepsis and septic shock.

KEY CONCEPTS

- Cancer is defined as a group of diseases characterized by abnormal growth and spread of cells.
- At least two thirds of cancer cases are caused by environmental factors, including lifestyle choices, which make health counseling an important nursing role.
- The goals of cancer treatment are to: (a) cure the cancer; (b) control its spread and manage it as a chronic illness; or (c) ease symptoms and maximize quality of life.
- There are a wide variety of diagnostic tests for cancer (e.g., laboratory tests, radiation, biopsy, and bone marrow aspiration).
- The three most common treatments for cancer are surgery, pharmacotherapy or chemotherapy, and radiation.
- Other therapy about which the nurse should be aware includes hormone therapy, biological therapy, blood and bone marrow transplantation, and complementary and alternative therapy.
- Immune system suppression is a side effect common to many cancer treatments, making risk of infection a major nursing concern.

- Fatigue has emerged as the most distressing and persistent treatment side effect, surpassing nausea and vomiting, which are also major nursing issues.
- Anemia, neutropenia, and thrombocytopenia are significant patient risk issues, which result from bone marrow suppression.
- Cognitive impairment is the loss of the ability to remember certain things, learn new skills, and complete certain tasks.
- Because of the many side effects impacting nutrition and the effect of poor nutrition on healing, outlook, and comfort, the nurse should aggressively monitor nutritional status and regular, even daily, weights are indicated.
- Throughout the diagnosis and treatment of cancer, the nurse should consider both the patient and caregiver when offering coping strategies.
- Research indicates that over 40 percent of patients with cancer do not get adequate relief from pain even though therapy exists to relive almost all cancer pain.
- While cancer is now managed as a chronic illness, there are multiple oncological emergencies.

REVIEW QUESTIONS

1. Mrs. Smith was recently diagnosed with ductal cell carcinoma of the breast. The oncologist described Mrs. Smith's cancer as T2, N1, Mx. Mrs. Smith asked the nurse to repeat to her what "all those letters and numbers mean." The nurse would reply that T2, N1, Mx, means the following:
   1. Two tumors present, one lymph node involved, and many sites of metastasis
   2. One tumor present, which is larger than 2.5 centimeters, nodal involvement in one region, and metastasis was unable to be determined
   3. One large tumor present, nodal involvement in one region, and metastasis was present
   4. Two tumors present, one lymph node involved, and metastasis was present

2. Mrs. Juarez, who also had breast cancer, called the clinic to talk with the nurse regarding her sister's diagnosis of cancer. Mrs. Juarez tells the nurse that she is extremely concerned, because she was aware that breast cancer "ran in her family," but she could not recall that any family member had been diagnosed with bone or lung cancer. The nurse's best response would be:

   1. "Well, it is apparent that your sister is not lucky. It is rare to have three such unrelated cancers at one time."
   2. "I think it is important for you to be tested for lung cancer as soon as possible, because it has a strong hereditary link."
   3. "I am sorry to hear about your sister's recent diagnosis. Most probably your sister has breast cancer that has metastasized or spread to the bone and lungs."
   4. "I am sorry to hear about your sister. I think you should meet with all of your family members and share with them their increased risk for developing both lung and bone cancer."

3. During the planning of a community-wide cancer program, the nurse shares that she wants to focus on secondary prevention. Activities, which would be included with such a focus, would include:
   1. A smoking cessation class
   2. Information on dietary guidelines that include foods rich in antioxidants
   3. Instruction on testicular self-exam
   4. Instruction on herbal supplements that are chemo-protective

Continued

4. In caring for a patient during the time of nadir, the nurse must be sure to assess for which of the following?
   1. Low potassium level
   2. High creatinine level
   3. Low absolute neutrophil count
   4. High thrombocyte count

5. In providing instruction to a patient after external beam radiation therapy for skin cancer, the nurse instructs the patient to:
   1. Wash off the all markings applied in the radiation department between treatments
   2. Apply cold to irradiated area for 15-minute intervals at least three times a day to decrease discomfort
   3. Limit creams or lotions used on irradiated areas to those that have approved by the oncology health care provider
   4. Avoid close contact with others for at least two weeks to reduce their exposure to radiation

6. As the nurse is preparing to administer doxorubicin (Adriamycin) to a patient in the outpatient cancer clinic, approximately 30 mL of the fluid leaks onto the counter. The most appropriate nursing action is:
   1. Wipe up the spill with a paper towel and then cleanse the surface with alcohol
   2. Call the pharmacy and have a technician come to the floor to clean up the spill
   3. Locate the chemotherapy spill kit on the patient unit and follow the instructions for clean up
   4. Request the patient care assistant wipe up the spill and prepare to administer the medication

7. In providing nursing care to Mrs. Brown who has a cesium implant in place for the treatment of cervical cancer, the nurse should be aware that:
   1. No special radiation precautions must be observed.
   2. Shielding oneself and visitors from the radiation is the single, most important precaution.
   3. Mrs. Brown will be up ad lib with bathroom privileges.
   4. Both the staff and visitors must limit time spent in the Mrs. Brown's room.

8. Mr. Schenley is started on the colony-stimulating factor, Neupogen, after 10 days of chemotherapy. Which of the following lab values would be most indicative of effectiveness of the Neumega (Filgrastim)?
   1. Hemoglobin: 6.5 g/dL
   2. Hemoglobin: 10 g/dL
   3. Absolute neutrophil count: $750/mm^3$
   4. Absolute neutrophil count: $1,100/mm^3$

9. Mr. Zidarisku is diagnosed with stage III colon cancer. He underwent external beam radiation prior to abdominal surgery. In considering Mr. Zidarisku's treatment approach, the nurse is aware that the patient is at increased risk for which of the following?
   1. Dehiscence
   2. Fatigue
   3. Body image disturbance
   4. Anemia

10. Cherie Link, age 54, comes to the clinic and shares that her best friend was recently diagnosed with colon cancer. Cherie says she wants to know which cancer screening tests she should have based on her age and sex. The nurse informs Cherie that ACS recommendations include the following:
    1. Flexible sigmoidoscopy every 3 to 5 years after age 50; mammogram and clinical breast exam every year after age 40; Pap smear every year after age 18; and annual physical that checks for variety of other cancers
    2. Colonoscopy every 7 years after age 45, mammogram and clinical breast exam every year after age 50; Pap smear every year after age 18; and annual physical that checks for variety of other cancers
    3. Flexible sigmoidoscopy every 10 years after age 50; mammogram and clinical breast exam every year after age 35; and Pap smear every year after age 21
    4. Colonoscopy every 3 to 5 years after age 50; mammogram and clinical breast exam every year after age 50; Pap smear every year after age 21

REVIEW ACTIVITIES

1. When someone is diagnosed with cancer, in addition to physiological effects, the diagnosis has a dramatic effect on activities of daily living and quality of life. Examine the impact of receiving one dose of chemotherapy on the life of a woman diagnosed with breast cancer that works part-time and is the mother of a 9-year-old boy and 5-year-old-girl.

2. Communication is an integral part of nursing practice. In today's fast-paced world nurses may find it hard to meet face to face on a regular basis to share innovative methods of care for the patient with cancer. As a small group project, develop a discussion board and post two cancer related topics where students at the school or college can review and respond to these topics for a two-week period. Other students can also post their own topics of interest. Tabulate the responses according to treatment ideas, assessment issues, or professional practice issues.

3. Mr. James is a 32-year-old science teacher who will be returning to work following treatment for lymphoma. As his primary nurse, develop a plan to integrate him back into his place of employment after a three-month absence.

4. Select a media item, such as a magazine of television ad, which depicts an environmental hazard for cancer (fun in the sun or smoking). Identify the type of risk factor, if it is controllable and how. Present data that contradicts common health myths related to the ad.

5. Choose a patient who has cancer and provide care for the patient in the practicum setting. Evaluate your feelings of developing a relationship with the patient and identify the thoughts that you have about the patient having cancer.

Pain Management

Ruth Grendell, MSN, RN

CHAPTER TOPICS

- Definitions, Theories, and Implications of Pain

- Factors Related to the Perception of Pain

- Human Responses to Pain

- Collaborative Management of Pain

- Medications and Nonpharmacological Methods for Providing Pain Relief

According to the American Chronic Pain Association (ACPA, 2003), pain is a major health issue, a major economic issue, and a major social issue. "Pain is the number one cause of adult disability in the United States and affects one in three people or about 50 million Americans" (ACPA, p. 14). Approximate costs related to pain total $100 billion in lost workdays, medical expenses, and other benefits. As a social issue, long-term unmanaged pain can lead to the person's withdrawal from family and social activities and can result in unsteady employment, anxiety regarding the future, and sometimes severe depression. Pain is a fundamental human experience that can affect the individual, the family, and the community.

KEY TERMS

Addiction
Breakthrough pain
Dermatome
Equianalgesia
Fast pain (rapid pain)
Homeostasis
Hyperalgesia (allodynia)
Idiopathic pain
Intractable pain
Kinesthesia
Modulation
Nociceptive pain
Nociceptor
Pain
Pain threshold
Pain tolerance
Proprioception
Referred pain
Slow pain
Somesthesia
Somatic pain
Tolerance
Transduction
Transmission
Visceral pain

DEFINITIONS AND IMPLICATIONS OF PAIN

Pain, as defined by the International Association for the Study of Pain (2004), is an unpleasant sensory and emotional experience arising from actual or potential tissue damage, or it may be described in terms related to such damage. Pain includes not only the perception of an uncomfortable stimulus but also the response to that perception. Pain is defined subjectively based on a person's own experience. Simply, pain is what the person says it is and exists when the person says it does. Pain, is currently considered as the "fifth vital sign" that should be included in the routine patient assessment (Arnstein, 2005).

We must recognize that pain is also an important component of the person's protective system. Without the sense of pain, we would not be immediately aware of injuries to tissues. Pain, through negative reinforcement, instructs us to learn about pain and the various causes of pain and to remember what it feels like and how to adapt or seek help. Examples include the automatic withdrawal reflex after touching the flame of a candle or a hot stove or feeling the cuts from a sharp knife. The person with peripheral neuropathy does not feel the tissue damage until it is too late. Simple mishaps such as an accidental cut when clipping toenails or abrasions from an ill-fitting shoe can lead to multiple complications including infections, delayed healing, and the possibility of amputation. Very few people have a genetic insensitivity to pain; those who do can experience multiple traumatic body injuries due to nonprotective or unsafe behaviors.

"Nurses play a pivotal role in assessing and implementing interventions that promote effective pain relief" (Hader & Guy, 2004, p. 23). Unfortunately, pain management continues to be a prevalent problem despite improved technology and a variety of treatment options. Effective pain management begins with a broad understanding of pain theories, anatomy and physiology, the transmission and interpretation of sensory messages, the different types of pain, the recognition of human responses to pain, and knowledge of the various pain management strategies.

PAIN THEORIES

For many years two widely accepted theories were used to explain the pain processes. More recent research findings and advances in technology have revealed new information and understanding of the pain experience. In the 1950s, the gate control theory, a scientifically based model, was introduced. This new perspective prompted additional research, which has revealed that multiple physiological and psychological factors must be considered in the assessment and management of pain.

Specificity Theory

The specificity theory was proposed in the seventeenth century by René Descartes (1596–1650), a philosopher and mathematician. He perceived the mind, or spirit, as a separate entity from a well-functioning mechanical body, with only casual communication between the two. His theory explained pain as the activity of highly specific peripheral nerve endings that receive sensory information from the environment, which is then transmitted by nerve fibers through the spinal cord to the pain center, or pineal body, in the forebrain. He believed that the "thinking" mind was not actively involved in the body's response to pain. Descartes' theory of mind-body dualism was widely accepted for hundreds of years. However, it is merely a biological explanation and does not address the multidimensional, complex pain process (Wozniak, 1992).

Pattern Theory

Pattern theory is actually a group of theories proposing that pain receptors share endings or pathways with other sensory modalities, but that different patterns of activity in the same neurons can be used to signal painful and nonpainful stimuli. The pattern theory, like that of Descartes, also does not address the motivational, cognitive, cultural, and affective components of pain and is no longer considered a major theory.

Gate Control Theory

In the mid-1900s scientists believed that the intensity of pain was related to the degree of tissue damage. However, during World War II, it was discovered that the severity of injury and intensity of pain did not correlate, since physicians observed behaviors and treated military personnel who had various severe injuries that did not prevent them from carrying out their duties during battle; they seemed, in fact, to be pain-free despite life-threatening wounds. These discoveries and later research on human anatomy and physiology were partially responsible for the development of the gate control theory (Figure 16-1). This theory was introduced by Ronald Melzack and Patrick Wall in 1965. The original theory hypothesized that a gating mechanism located in the spinal cord could be closed by the normal stimulation of fast-conducting tactile nerve fibers to prevent pain sensations from reaching the brain centers or be opened to allow certain high-volume, intense pain signals to pass through. The gate could be closed again if stimulation of the large touch fibers was renewed. According to the theory, myelinated nerve fibers labeled A delta and B delta, which carry tactile information such as touch and pressure, override the slower-conducting pain information sent by the small-diameter myelinated and unmyelinated C fibers. Myelin serves as an electrical insulator to the nerve and increases the speed of transmission of an impulse. Therefore rubbing a painful knee can reduce the sensation of pain, and the gate is closed. However, when the intense pain stimulus continues, the gate can reopen. Reactivation of the large-diameter tactile fibers would be necessary to reclose the gate.

Melzack proposed that the individual's interpretation of pain was influenced by several internal and external factors. Therefore he suggested that external factors could be used to modulate pain. The gate control mechanism would then benefit from distracting methods such as music, social support, relaxation strategies, and other noninvasive interventions (McCaffrey, Frock, & Garguilo, 2003).

This theory has undergone periodic revision. According to the latest version, the gate control system is also influenced by natural analgesic inhibitory mechanisms involving the midbrain, medulla, and spinal cord. Attention, memory, anticipation, emotions, and release of chemicals by the nerve fibers in the dorsal horn of the spinal cord can serve as facilitating or inhibiting factors in the

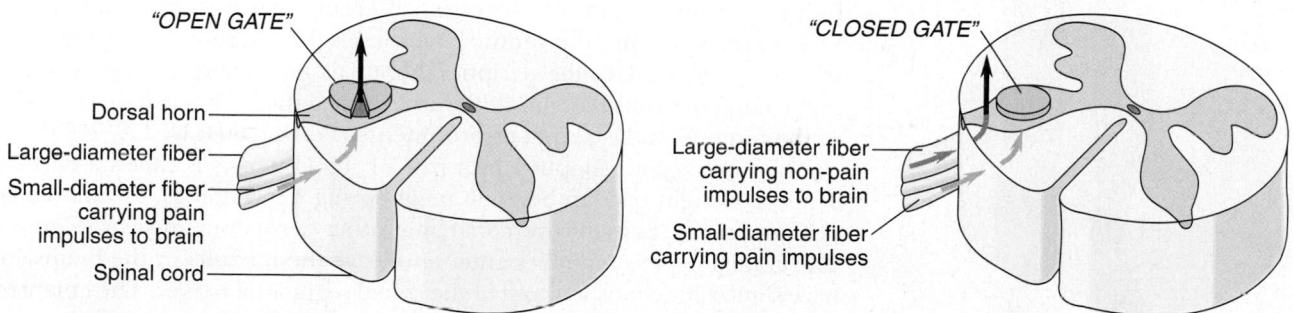

Figure 16-1 Gate control theory: Blocking the transmission of pain.

perception of pain signals. The introduction of this theory ushered in an era of advanced international pain research that has continued over the past 40 years (American Pain Foundation, 2004; Porth, 2004). Scientists now believe that the gate control mechanism is located at several levels of the central nervous system. Much of the information in the following section on the physiology of pain was gained through research based on the gate control theory.

Melzack, a professor at McGill University, developed the long-form McGill pain questionnaire (MPQ-LF). This tool includes a series of 20 descriptive categories to identify the sensory and affective characteristics and intensity of pain. The person may describe a pain as burning, scalding, or searing for the "hot" category or use the words *itchy, smarting,* or *stinging* in the "tingling" category. Affective categories include terms such *as tiring, sickening, fearful, punishing,* and *wretched.* Each of the terms within a category is rated according to its intensity. The questionnaire includes an anterior and posterior diagram of the body for identifying the location of the pain. A short form of 15 items (the MPQ-SF) was later designed to gain patient information when time is limited. This form includes 15 words related to sensory and affective categories. The person is asked to rate a type of pain as mild, moderate, or severe. The person also rates the overall intensity of pain on a visual-analogue scale from 1 (no pain) to 10 (severe pain) (McCaffrey, Frock, & Garguilo 2003).

THE PATHOPHYSIOLOGY OF PAIN

The complex mechanisms of the pain experience have been identified as: transduction, transmission, modulation, and perception. The term **transduction** refers to the initiation of electrical activity due to the impact of a noxious, painful, or unpleasant stimulus. The process of carrying the pain information along the axon of a sensory nerve to the spinal cord and various brain centers is called **transmission. Modulation**, or alteration, of the pain sensation occurs via a variety of physiological mechanisms and is an influencing factor in the perception of pain. The individual's perception, or attached meaning of the pain, is multifaceted, involving sensory input to several areas of the cerebral cortex.

This entire process involves the peripheral and central nervous systems. The peripheral nervous system (PNS) comprises the 12 pairs of cranial nerves and the 31 or 32 pairs of spinal nerves. The central nervous system (CNS) includes the cell bodies of neurons, axons, and dendrites of the brain and spinal cord.

Peripheral Nervous System

The paired sensory and motor spinal nerves of the PNS are arranged in a segmental pattern that corresponds with the segments of the vertebrae. Each spinal nerve enters the spinal canal through an intervertebral foramen, an opening between the vertebrae, and subsequently divides into two roots or branches. The dorsal root carries the afferent (sensory) information from the body to the CNS; and the ventral root carries the efferent (motor) information from the CNS back to the peripheral body tissues. There is a network of interconnecting neurons that modulate and control the body's responses to changes in the internal and external environments (Porth, 2004; UCLA, 2004).

The body region supplied by a pair of spinal nerves is called a **dermatome.** There is a slight overlap between neighboring dermatomes, so that damage to one area can be partially overcome by another dermatome nearby (Figure 16-2). The cranial nerve's branches enter and leave the medulla in the brainstem and have similar functions to those of the spinal segmental nerves. The enlarged dorsal horn of the medulla is able to process a great deal of information that traverses the nerves.

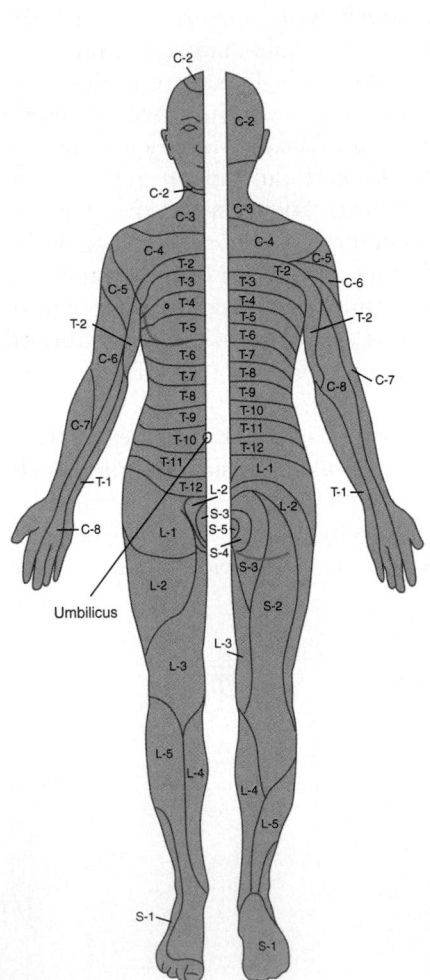

Figure 16-2 Dermatomes.

Fast Forward ▶▶▶

Brain Patterns During Pain

Physicians at the University of New Mexico noticed changes in brain patterns as a person experienced pain during a brain scan. The pain had triggered a large release of glutamine and glutamate, chemicals that assist in sending signals through the brain. This discovery will help in research on painful diseases and could lead to better pain-fighting techniques (Vorenberg, 2005).

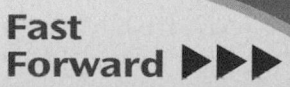

A **nociceptor** is a free nerve ending that is a receptor for painful (noxious) stimuli. The protective role of pain does not permit the nerve endings to adapt to repeated painful stimuli. In fact, repeated stimulation increases their sensitivity to pain. The sensitized nociceptors may continue to transmit the pain message even after the stimulus is removed. This hypersensitivity is termed **hyperalgesia (allodynia)**, a state where a slight or nonpainful stimulus, such as the touch of clothing, can be interpreted as very painful (Yezierski, Radsson, & Vanderah 2004). Cutaneous sensations such as touching, itching, tickling, temperature changes, and pain are transmitted to the CNS by nerve axons of other designated sensory nerve endings (Figure 16-3) located near to the body surface or the dermatomal areas. Nerve endings located in deeper tissues—including bone, muscle, tendons, and the smooth muscles of arterial walls—pick up messages from these tissues. Some nerve endings contribute to awareness of position (**proprioception**); of coordination of the body, head, and limbs; and of movement (**kinesthesia**).

Central Nervous System

Sensations of touch, pain, temperature, body movement, and position changes are separate from the special senses of vision, hearing, smell, and taste. The 2 to 3 million sensory neurons in the skin and other body tissues steadily deliver encoded information to the CNS. However, the person is aware of only a small proportion of this information, all of which is essential to the maintenance of numerous autonomic functions and of life itself.

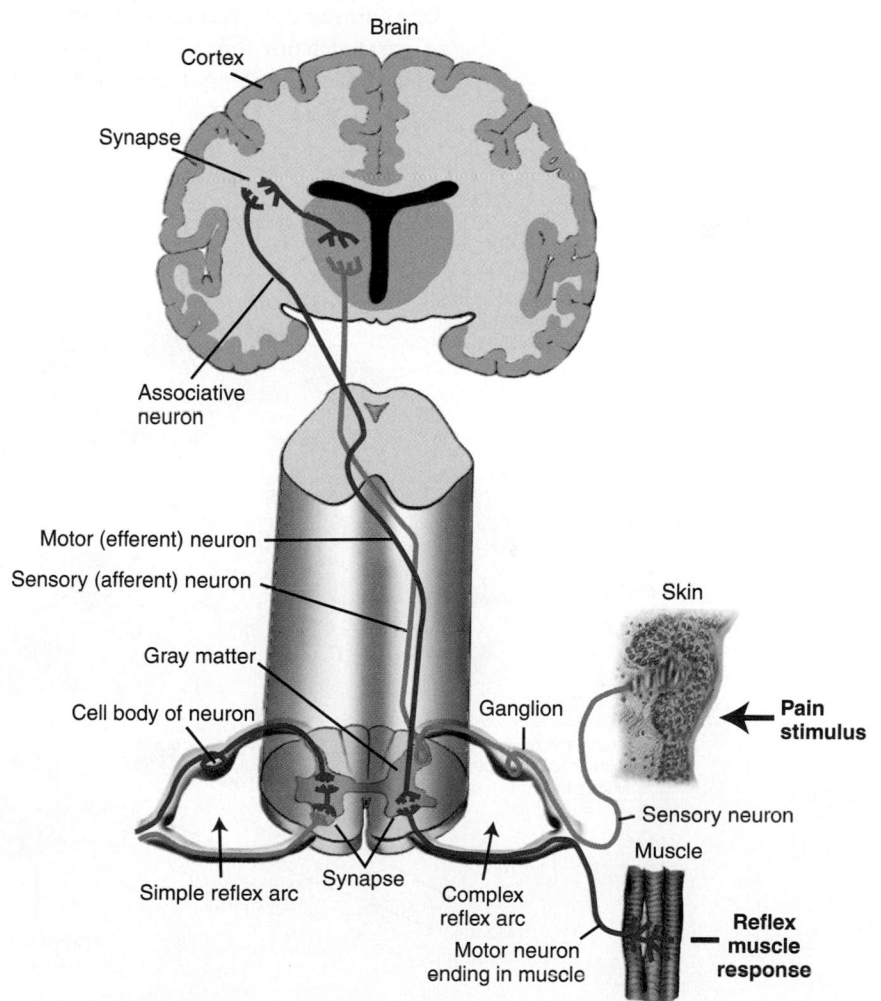

Figure 16-3 Reflex arcs.

All sensory information except for olfactory stimuli passes through the thalamus, which is located in the diencephalon of the brain. This vital area processes and coordinates the information before it is relayed to other destinations, such as the somatosensory cortex, which is located in the parietal lobe of the cerebrum of the brain. It receives the primary, or raw, sensory messages (Figure 16-4). The somatosensory association areas lie directly behind the cortex, where much of the **somesthesia,** the personal awareness of one's body, and body sensations are perceived. Here, along with input from the thalamus, the primary information is interpreted via the individual's memory, associated with the sensation and the current sensory experience. Interpretation of any stimulus depends on optimal functioning of all components of the transmission process.

The Autonomic Nervous System

The autonomic nervous system (ANS) is a major part of the CNS that continually regulates **homeostasis,** or equilibrium of the body's internal environment, and involuntary processes such as breathing, blood flow, pulse rate, and elimination. The two divisions of the ANS are the parasympathetic and the sympathetic systems, which have opposing or antagonistic actions. The parasympathetic division is involved in conserving energy and maintaining organ function during normal or minimal activity. Activation of the sympathetic system prepares the body for the "fight or flight" survival response in emergencies and stressful situations such as the pain experience. In response to pain and stress, the sympathetic system signals the release of epinephrine (adrenaline) and other hormones, resulting in increases in blood pressure, heart rate, and respiration. Activation of the hypothalamic-pituitary-adrenal (HPA) axis results in the release of cortisol from the adrenal glands and also places the person on alert. The release of these stress hormones can lead to anxiety and depression as well as

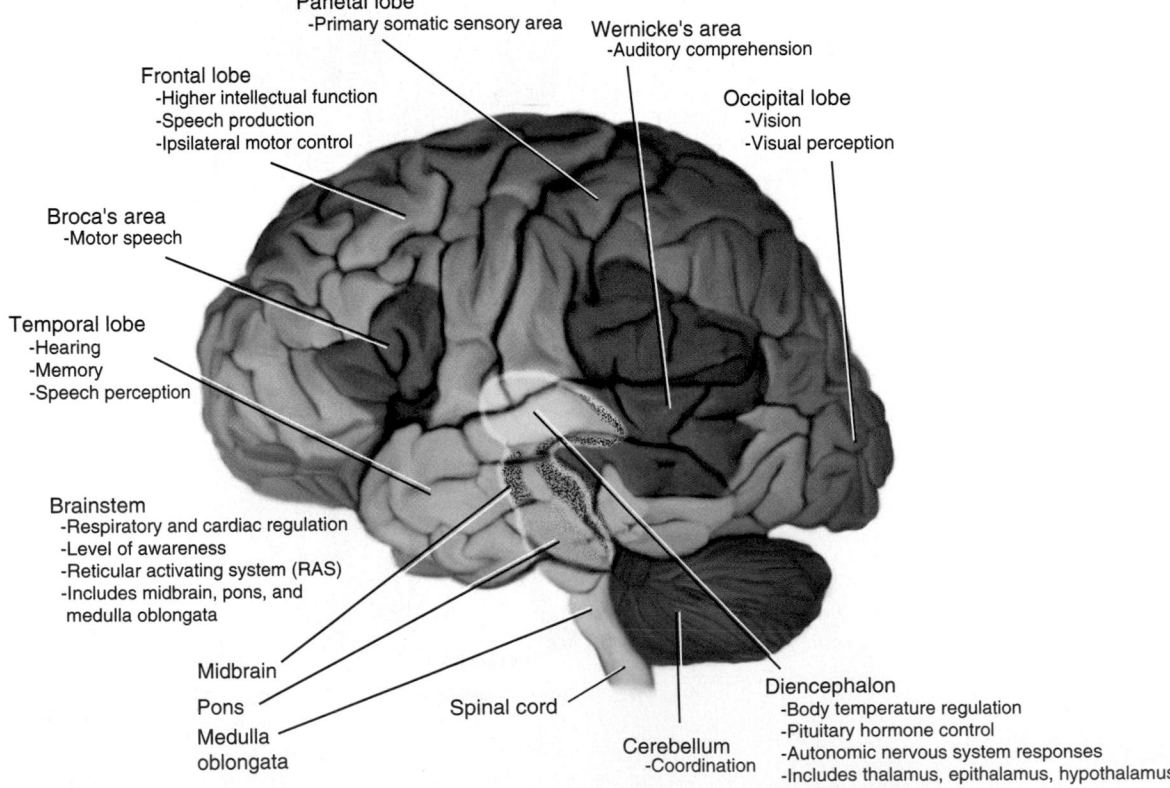

Parietal lobe
-Primary somatic sensory area

Wernicke's area
-Auditory comprehension

Frontal lobe
-Higher intellectual function
-Speech production
-Ipsilateral motor control

Occipital lobe
-Vision
-Visual perception

Broca's area
-Motor speech

Temporal lobe
-Hearing
-Memory
-Speech perception

Brainstem
-Respiratory and cardiac regulation
-Level of awareness
-Reticular activating system (RAS)
-Includes midbrain, pons, and
  medulla oblongata

Midbrain
Pons
Medulla
oblongata

Spinal cord

Cerebellum
-Coordination

Diencephalon
-Body temperature regulation
-Pituitary hormone control
-Autonomic nervous system responses
-Includes thalamus, epithalamus, hypothalamus

Figure 16-4 The locations and functions of the cerebral lobes, diencephalon, cerebellum, and brainstem.

contributing to the sensitization, or heightened response, of nociceptors to a stimulus (Curtis, Kolytolo, & Broome 2004).

PAIN MECHANISMS AND PATHWAYS

There are specific mechanisms of definite physiological pathways for pain transmission. The nociceptors, or receptors that have a very low threshold for responding to pain, are located in almost every body tissue. The nociceptors react to changes only in the tissues near them.

Transduction

Transduction is the response of these nociceptors to a noxious stimulus, which may be a chemical or electrical change (ischemia or substances released from injured tissue), a mechanical stimulus (effects of pressure or stretching of organs), or thermal change (extremes of heat or cold). Some nociceptors are selective in their response to stimuli; others respond to several types of stimulation. The release of a variety of inflammatory chemicals from damaged tissue cells plays a significant role in stimulating the pain process. These chemical substances include prostaglandins, histamine, bradykinin, serotonin, and substance P (an amino acid peptide thought to be an important neurotransmitter of pain), acids, proteolytic enzymes, and acetylcholine (Yezierski, et al., 2004). Several pharmacological and other therapeutic interventions can help alleviate the impact of these pain mediators; they are discussed later in this chapter.

Transmission

The transmission process of carrying the electrical impulse or pain information to the various brain centers involves several intervening mechanisms. The incoming messages activate the spinal cord transmission cells (T cells) that carry the messages to the brain centers. There is no actual "pain" until the interpretive process has been completed. The quality of pain depends upon the site of stimulation and the nature of fibers that transmit the sensation. **Fast pain,** or rapid pain, originates in the nociceptors of the large myelinated nerve fibers located in the skin, which respond to strong pressure, a cut, or high temperature, eliciting the withdrawal reflex. Examples include the sharp pain from a pinprick or pinch or brief exposure to well-localized heat; the pain stops when the initiating stimulus is stopped.

A fast pain message travels very quickly up the ascending spinothalamic tract to the thalamus. The message is immediately sent to areas in the brain that interpret it, and a return message is sent back, signaling muscles to contract. A fast pain message occurs at approximately 0.1 second following a painful stimulus (UCSD, 2004).

Slow pain originates in the nociceptors of the smaller, unmyelinated nerve fibers and has a longer throbbing or aching quality. The spinoreticular tract, an alternative pathway, is used for transmission and modulation of duller or more persistent pain. The pain message enters the dorsal horn of the spinal cord; then it is transferred to the other side of the cord and travels along a series of interconnected neurons terminating in the thalamus. The thalamus sends the message along its way to the cerebral cortex. A slow pain message begins approximately 1.0 or more seconds following a painful stimulus and can slowly increase in intensity. Two other ascending tracts are also involved in transmitting nociceptor messages. The spinoreticular tract passes through the area of the reticular formation and ends in the thalamus. The spinomesencephalic tract carries the message to the midbrain's periaqueductal gray (PAG) area and then on to the somatosensory cortex. The PAG is responsible for strong inhibitory responses to the transmission of pain.

Modulation

The physiological pain modulation system is composed of mechanisms that influence a person's perception of pain. These mechanisms include (1) the processing of sensory impulses by the ventral and dorsal horns in the spinal cord; (2) the natural, or endogenous, chemicals secreted by the CNS; and (3) the chemicals transmitted by the descending pathways from the brain to the dorsal horn. The dorsal horn houses a complex exchange of multiple biochemicals that can transmit and modulate sensory input.

The body also has a natural analgesic system composed of neuroreceptors (located in the CNS and various body tissues) and their opioid peptides, which are synthesized in the CNS. A neuroreceptor is a cell component that combines with a drug, hormone, or chemical to alter the cell's function. The opioid peptides are a group of 15 natural substances in the brain, certain endocrine glands, and the gastrointestinal tract that have morphine-like analgesic properties. The opioid peptides are called endorphins, enkephalins, and dynorphin. The bonding of these peptides to the specific receptors can be likened to the exact fit between a lock and a key. The interaction mimics the effects of morphine in the CNS and PNS and the central effects of other exogenous opioids. The endorphins are located primarily in the brainstem structures. The enkephalins are prevalent in the PAG area of the midbrain, limbic system, basal ganglia, hypothalamus, and the sympathetic nervous system. Additional biochemicals (monoamines), such as norepinephrine and serotonin, released via the medulla to the spinal cord's descending pathway, have profound modulating effects on pain sensations. Studies have indicated that stimulation of the brainstem centers can produce anesthetic effects that may last for an extended period. This discovery opened the way for the development of new strategies for relieving pain (Spee & Floyd, 2005).

Perception

Although many studies have been done, there is still much to learn and understand about the transmission of pain and its interpretation or meaning. The experience of pain is influenced by a great number of dynamic, ever-changing, and interacting physiological, biochemical, psychological, social, cultural, and emotional factors.

Pain Threshold and Pain Tolerance

Some people may have a higher or lower **pain threshold** than others, which is defined as the lowest intensity of a painful stimulus that the individual perceives as pain. The pain threshold can be influenced by inflammation at the injury site and other physiological factors including nausea, fatigue, and lack of sleep. The person's previous experience with pain, the anticipation that the pain will become worse, or a recurrence of pain in the same area may also lower the pain threshold. An individual's need for pain relief can also fluctuate. The effectiveness of physiological mechanisms in modulating pain can vary at different times of the day, thus allowing a lower pain threshold to prevail later in the day than in the morning.

Pain tolerance, or the amount of pain a person is willing to endure, is another major factor in the perception of pain. Pain tolerance can vary for the same person at different times and in different situations. The nurse must be cognizant of the numerous factors—such as genetics, culture, environmental influences, family structure, and relationships, and mental attitudes—that can affect the person's tolerance level.

RESPONSES TO PAIN

A person's perception and response to the pain experience can also be strongly influenced by factors such as fear, anxiety, depression, the situation in which the pain occurs, age, and gender. The location of pain can also affect perception. If pain, such as a headache, affects the person's ability to concentrate or interferes with his or her daily routines, its intensity may be rated as severe. Consider the varied responses a woman might have in facing the outcome of abdominal surgery for cancer and the outcome for a woman of the same age who has had a cesarean section.

Social-Cultural Influences

Stoicism is valued in many cultures, whereas in others individuals are expected to cope with pain by expressing or exaggerating their distress. Pain can be viewed as punishment for sins, so that the person is expected to tolerate pain without complaint in order to atone for his or her past wrongdoing. Individuals may believe that illness and pain is due to an imbalance in the environment, and that only the restoration of that balance will relieve the pain. The nurse's own culture, attitudes, and biases, based on preconceived ideas, can influence the way a patient's pain is assessed and managed. Responses to pain must be considered according to the person's perception of pain and to its meaning to the individual and family. Nurses must be cautioned not to stereotype individuals from any culture or age group, since each individual will cope uniquely and in a variety of ways (Spector, 2004).

Age

Children learn directly and indirectly from their parents or other care providers about how to respond to pain. The child discovers what level of pain justifies a complaint, how to express the complaint, how and when to stop complaining, and whom to approach for relief of pain. It is currently believed that the socialization of children influences the way in which they will respond to pain as adults (Stanley, Blair, & Beare, 2004).

Chronic pain is considered a common experience for most elderly persons. Approximately 80 percent of elderly persons have at least one chronic health problem associated with moderate to severe pain. Yet, the elderly often hesitate to report their pain because of the belief that pain is a normal part of aging and therefore to be endured, or they may fear their expressions of pain will not be believed. They may also be fearful of drug side effects and the potential for addiction to pain medications. Many elderly persons have been "conditioned" to tolerate pain (AMA, 2003). Approximately 40 percent of all patients with cancer are over 65 years of age. Adequate pain control is lacking for this population. Approximately 20 percent of the elderly population takes pain-relieving medications several times a week. However, as many as 80 percent of the elderly living in nursing homes who experience pain are undertreated. Such beliefs as that children feel less pain than adults and that the elderly do not feel pain as intensely as younger adults are misconceptions and now outdated.

Gender

Gender is another major influencing factor on responses to pain. Most cultures expect little boys and men to minimize outward expressions of pain, whereas it is appropriate for little girls and women to acknowledge pain openly. Prior to 1994, much of the research on pain medication was conducted with male sub-

---

Respecting Our Differences

Age Differences and the Pain Experience

- Health care providers should realize that pain in the absence of disease is not a normal part of aging.
- More than half of the people over 65 years of age have arthritis pain.
- Recognizing the prevalence of pain in the elderly is of prime importance because the fastest-growing segment of the U.S. population comprises those of age 85 and above. This number is predicted to grow to 7.5 million by 2020 and to 14 million by 2040.
- There is a mild age-related increase in pain threshold. However, this is not an indication that the older person experiences less pain when he or she actually reports it.
- Pain symptoms may not be typical for the elderly for myocardial conditions, intra-abdominal infections, various types of cancer, and some acute inflammatory conditions.
- Regular use of standardized tools and consistent documentation are the most important elements in pain assessment.

Source: Hanks-Bell, M., Halvey, K., & Paice, J. (2004). Pain assessment and management in aging. Online Journals in Nursing, 9(3), 1–18.

Fast Forward ▶▶▶

Pain Control

Acute and chronic pain control is a worldwide challenge for nurses. Strategies for change are:

- Increased knowledge and understanding of pain—the causes, sensations, and therapeutic interventions
- Changing beliefs that pain is an unavoidable result of illness, health care procedures, and aging
- Establishing policies that promote evidence-based pain management interventions

Source: Prevost, S. (2004). Improve pain management. In S. Hegyvary (Ed.), Working Paper on Grand Challenges in Improving Global Health. Journal of Nursing Scholarship, 36(2), 96–101.

jects; in that year, however, the National Institutes of Health (NIH) mandated that women and minorities must be included in clinical trials, especially in pharmacological studies. Scientists soon discovered that differences in gender biology affect pain perception and response. Studies indicated that women believed their emotions of fear and anxiety to affect their perception of pain adversely, whereas men focused more on the physical aspects. Women have a lower pain threshold and pain tolerance and seek medical help more readily than men; moreover, women's responses to opioids and other analgesics also vary from men's responses. Heart attack is now the number-one health threat to women. However, because they do not display the typical symptoms and type of pain, women who have had heart attacks are not hospitalized or treated as aggressively as men (Criste, 2002). A recent study also indicates gender differences in the metabolism of aspirin. Although a low-dose aspirin lowers the risk of a primary myocardial infarction in men, there were no significant effects in decreasing this risk in women (Ridker, et al., 2005).

The most prevalent painful disorders among women that are seen in both genders include fibromyalgia, Raynaud's disease, rheumatoid arthritis, multiple sclerosis, headaches, and facial pain, especially temporomandibular joint disorder (TMJ). It is thought that some autoimmune diseases such as systemic lupus erythematosus in younger women may be associated with hormonal factors. More "male-occupational" diseases may be seen in women as they assume formerly male-dominated occupations. The prevalent painful disorders for men that are seen in both genders include pancreatitis, duodenal ulcer, and ankylosing spondylitis. Men also have a higher incidence of injuries related to sports and motor vehicle accidents.

TYPES OF PAIN

There are two major classifications of pain, nociceptive and neuropathic pain, which is also called pathological pain.

Nociceptive Pain

Nociceptive pain occurs when the pain impulse is processed normally over intact nerves; that is, when there is no injury or malfunction of the neuronal transmission process. Nociceptive pain that originates from the bone, joints, muscles, skin, or connective tissue is termed **somatic pain;** pain arising from the body organs or gastrointestinal tract is referred to as **visceral pain.** Nociceptive somatic pain can be either cutaneous (from the skin or body surface) or deep pain involving tissues such as tendons, joints, bone, and nerves. Examples are pain due to rheumatoid arthritis and osteomyelitis. The term *visceral* refers to any of the large organs within a body cavity, i.e., the thoracic, abdominal, pelvic, or cranial cavity. Visceral pain is associated with acute appendicitis, cholecystitis, renal and ureteral colic, biliary and pancreatic tract inflammation, gastroduodenal disease, cardiovascular disease, and pleurisy. **Referred pain** is the result of the transfer of visceral pain sensations and deep somatic pain via the autonomic nervous system to a body surface at a distance from the actual origin (Figure 16-5). It is difficult for the brain to identify the exact origin of the pain, since both the body surface area and the deeper tissues are innervated by the same spinal nerve segment. Consider that the pain associated with myocardial infarction is commonly referred to the left arm, neck, and chest (Curtis, Kolytolo, & Broome 2004).

Neuropathic Pain

Pain that results from injury to a nerve, malfunction of the neuronal transmission process, or impaired regulation is called neuropathic pain, neuralgia, or pathological pain, which is frequently described as paroxysmal (a sudden

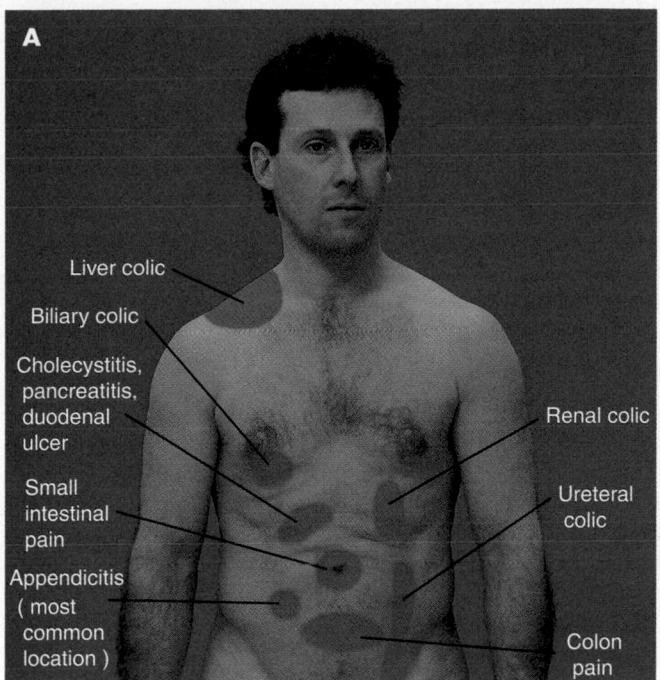 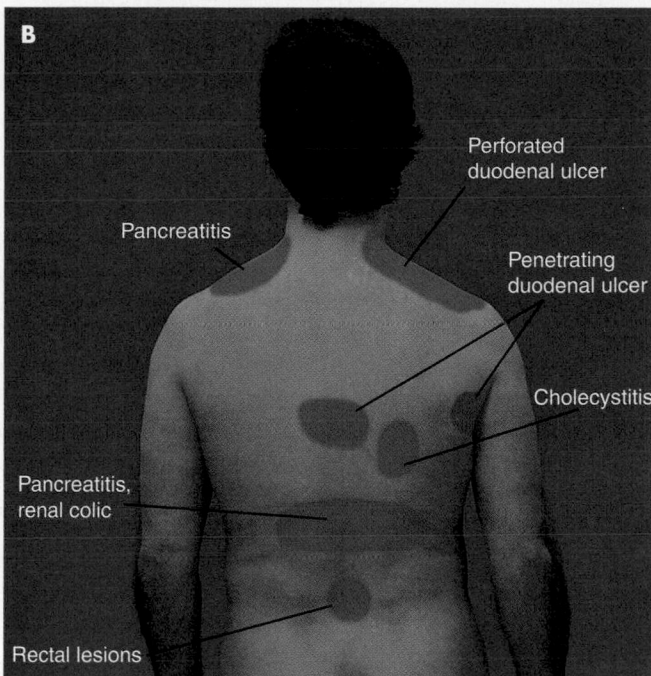

Figure 16-5 Areas of referred pain: A. Anterior view, B. Posterior view.

spasm-like pain) occurring along the branches of a nerve (Box 16-1). Causes include trauma, disease such as diabetes mellitus, herpes zoster, late stages of cancer, chemicals (i.e., drugs), and amputation (including mastectomy). Neuropathic pain that persists beyond the period of normal healing is associated with sensitization of the peripheral and central nervous systems. Examples include pain associated with trigeminal neuralgia, postherpetic neuralgia, and diabetic peripheral neuropathy (Hader & Guy, 2004; Loftus, 2005).

Pain presents itself in many different forms. The area of the body affected determines the area where signs and symptoms appear. In addition, the types of sensation are varied (Table 16-1).

Acute Pain

Acute pain is generally associated with an illness, injury, or surgery that results in tissue damage anywhere in the body, such as a burn, muscle injury, fractured bone or surgical wound. Americans spend more than $20 billion annually for treatment of lower back pain, one of the most common causes of acute and chronic pain. Acute pain is a common experience for the majority of hospitalized patients. It is also a warning sign that something is wrong; persistent acute pain may also interfere with the healing process. The pain of myocardial infarction or postoperative pain may cause a series of autonomic responses that prevent optimal function of the heart and lungs as well as other essential body systems. Remember that some of the clinical manifestations due to stimulation of the sympathetic nervous system (SNS) include increased heart rate and increased blood pressure (Vallerand, Reily-Doucet, Hasenau, & Templin, 2004).

Acute pain usually subsides following medication and treatment and goes away when healing takes place. When pain persists beyond the expected time required for healing of an injury or after the expected course of an acute disease, it is considered chronic. Therefore effective pain management is essential to avoid many complications such as delays in recovery, prolonged hospital stays, depression and anxiety, and development of the chronic pain syndrome.

BOX 16-1

PAIN DESCRIPTIONS

Nociceptive pain involves stimulation by chemical, mechanical, or noxious source (e.g., heat, cold). The pain occurs when there is normal processing of the pain impulse over intact nerves and no injury to or malfunction of the neuronal transmission process.

1. Cutaneous or superficial pain can be readily localized and the person can indicate where the pain is located.
2. Somatic pain (from body wall, muscles and bone) is less localized and can be described as aching or throbbing. It may be accompanied by nausea, sweating, bradycardia, and hypotension due to the autonomic nervous system response. Pain may radiate from the primary site, as seen in lumbar disc pain, which often radiates down the sciatic nerve. Arthritis is a type of chronic somatic pain.
3. Visceral, or splanchnic, pain is poorly localized and described as dull, colic-like, or cramping. It is often accompanied by diarrhea, sweating, and hypertension, since the pain is transmitted by small unmyelinated fibers that travel along with the sympathetic nerves to the spinal cord. Cancer pain and chronic pancreatitis are examples.
4. Referred pain can be severe at the body surface although there is minimal or no pain at the primary site of injury, since both the body surface area and the deeper tissues are innervated by the same spinal nerve segment.

Pathological Pain Syndromes

Neuropathic pain occurs as result of damage at any point in the pain pathway (e.g., to peripheral nerves, the spinal cord, brainstem, thalamus, or cerebral areas). It is described as a burning or severe shooting electrical pain sensation that frequently travels down a nerve to the dermatome associated with the peripheral nerve. It is also referred to as a stabbing pain or a "pins and needles" sensation. Examples include diabetic neuropathy, postherpetic neuralgia, and phantom limb pain.

1. Bone and muscular pain (includes ligaments, joint capsules, fascia, and tendons) usually occurs following stretching, ischemia, or forceful/sustained contractile activity. Injury causes a release of lactic acid and other substances that increase pain intensity. Such pain often radiates into surrounding tissues. Tension headaches are often due to tense neck and scalp muscles. Muscle ischemia due to intermittent claudication (a spasm in the extremities during walking) can result from occlusive vascular disease; the pain of coronary occlusion is also due to ischemia.
2. Vascular pain may be due to a pathological condition of the vessels or surrounding tissues, such as mixed vascular and neuropathic complications related to chronic diabetes mellitus. Other examples include migraine headaches and headaches associated with hypertension, brain tumors, and increased cranial pressure.
3. Pain due to inflammation occurs from infection or trauma and the subsequent release of acidic chemicals and distension of tissues.
4. Central pain results from injury to the CNS due to tumors, disease, stroke, or damage to the spinal cord. Such pain can be severe and constant. Brain masses can involve the cerebral cortex and elicit central pain in the opposite side of the body.
5. Thalamic pain is the perception of pain in one half of the body following injury to the thalamus. This type of pain is rare.
6. Back pain is very common and usually occurs in the cervical or lumbar regions. It is generally due to spinal disc injury or herniation of the nucleus pulposus, the cushioning substance between the intervertebral discs. Sensory and motor nerve damage may occur.

Peripheral and Mixed Central/Peripheral Pathological Pain

1. Causalgia from peripheral nerve injury such as damage to the brachial plexus or the median and sciatic nerves. When such pain is severe and persistent (intractable pain that is resistant to treatment), it can lead to depression and suicide. Any stimulus can initiate paroxysms of excruciating pain.
2. The pain of trigeminal neuralgia (tic douloureux) occurs along the mixed trigeminal cranial nerve. Severe facial pain results from minimal stimuli, including brushing the teeth, chewing or talking, a being touched by a draft of cold air, and so on.
3. Phantom pain following amputation of a body part consists of sensations that the part is still present. More severe pain is described as throbbing, burning, stabbing, or vise-like. Stump, or residual limb, pain may be caused by a neuroma at the amputation site.
4. Intracranial headache has many causes including changes in intracranial pressure, hypertension, hypoxia, medications, infection, and hemorrhage. The most common intracranial pain is due to migraine. Headaches of extracranial origin also have many causes. The most common problems include muscle tension, TMJ syndrome, and problems related to the eyes, sinuses, teeth, and ears.

Continued

BOX 16-1—cont'd

5. Cancer, or malignant, pain is commonly due to pressure or displacement of nerves by a growing tumor, interference with the blood supply, muscle spasms, pathological bone fractures, and the result of treatments.
6. Pain associated with HIV frequently occurs in the gastrointestinal tract, from herpes and cytomegalovirus infection, peripheral neuropathy, headache, and lesions of Kaposi's sarcoma that obstruct the lymph system.
7. Psychogenic pain is pain that is primarily due to emotional factors. The pain is initially physiological and is then exacerbated by stress, anxiety, and fear or anger. This type of pain is very real to the patient. Chronic muscle tension can lead to tension headache, backache, or visceral changes. Such conditions are often referred to as somatoform disorders and necessitate identification of the cause and appropriate treatment.
8. Pain of psychological origin is seen when an individual seeks treatment for pain when no actual pain exists. Some patients are very much aware that they are using this strategy as an excuse to avoid a responsibility, to obtain drugs, to gain sympathy or attention, or to claim an injury in order to receive compensation. This is also referred to as malingering or pretending; however, it should never be assumed that pain does not exist. A through assessment and accurate diagnosis are needed to rule out an actual physiological problem.

Adapted from Loftus, 2005; Curtis, Kolytolo, & Broome, 2004; McCaffrey, Frock, & Garguilo, 2003; UCSD, 2003.

TABLE 16-1 Body Surface Areas Related to Visceral Pain

AREA OF PAIN ORIGIN	BODY SURFACE	TYPE OF PAIN SENSATION
Lung	Anterior and posterior neck and upper chest. Pain may be unilateral or referred to the shoulder and the throat via the phrenic nerve.	Dyspnea, cough. Feeling of pressure, constriction/tightness. Identified as aching, sharp, burning, a "stitch."
Stomach	Right or midepigastric. Referred pain to posterior thorax.	Gastric ulcer—pressure, burning, heaviness, hunger. Food may cause pain that can be relieved by vomiting.
Pancreas	Left upper quadrant of abdomen with radiation to midline upper back or left shoulder.	Acute: Intense—unrelieved by antacids; usually accompanied by nausea and vomiting. Pain in acute episodes of chronic pancreatitis may not resolve with opiates.
Liver	Right upper quadrant or epigastric area—radiation to upper posterior chest	Discomfort/pressure. If abdomen is distended by ascites, patient may have difficulty breathing.
Kidney	Posterior costovertebral angle below 12th rib. Can be referred or localized. May radiate to lower abdomen and inguinal area.	Constant dull ache. Ureteral pain is severe and colicky.
Bladder	Suprapubic area with radiation to urethra.	Sharp, burning. Pain intensifies with urination.
Duodenum/jejunum	Midepigastric or periumbilical—may radiate to back midline between 6th and 10th vertebrae.	Aching, burning, cramp-like, gnawing; related to empty stomach; may be relieved by food or antacids.
Colon	Pelvic area. Often poorly localized. Characteristics of pain related to involved area and disease process.	Pain may be accompanied by rigidity of abdominal muscles and increases with pressure or motion. Pain may be intermittent or be a constant aching, cramping. Can mimic appendicitis pain
Esophagus	Left thoracic area with radiation to neck and upper shoulder.	Constant or occurs with swallowing (odynophagia). Sharp, constricting, sticking, crushing, stabbing or knife-like, "heartburn." Can be confused with anginal pain

Adapted from Curtis, Kolytolo, and Broome, 2004.

Chronic Pain

Chronic pain is defined as a sudden or slow onset of mild to severe pain. It can be constant or recurring without an anticipated or predictable end and usually lasts longer than 6 months. Because the etiology may not be apparent, chronic pain is considered to be a separate disease entity. Chronic pain is debilitating and has no useful purpose (Yezierski, et al., 2004). Migraine headaches and sickle cell crisis are often placed in this category; however, these problems can recur, and the acuteness of the "returning" pain requires very careful assessment and treatment. Recurrent pain can also be seen in patients with tension headaches, dysmenorrhea, inflammatory bowel disease, arthritis, and musculoskeletal disorders. Common disease conditions associated with chronic pain include osteoarthritis, rheumatoid arthritis, fibromyalgia, headache, backache, cancer pain, postherpetic neuralgia, trigeminal neuralgia (tic douloureux), chronic renal failure, chronic pancreatitis, chronic pulmonary diseases, phantom pain following amputation of a body part, and psychogenic pain that includes both a physiological basis and emotional elements, such as repeated episodes of severe stress. "Chronic pain can produce feelings of anxiety, despair, hopelessness and helplessness that exacerbate pain perception" (McCaffrey, et al., 2003, p. 281).

Additional disease conditions associated with chronic pain include nonmalignant progressive diseases such as AIDS, hemophilia, and connective tissue diseases; severe osteoporosis; painful polyneuropathy; and pelvic pain of

Fast Forward ▶▶▶

New Surgical Procedures for Chronic Back Pain Relief

More than 10 million Americans (men and women) have osteoporosis. Approximately 50 percent of women over 50 years of age suffer osteoporotic fractures; 700,000 of these are vertebral fractures. Some 30 to 40 percent of cancers metastasize to the spine, thus producing pain and weakening of the spinal structure. Sixty-eight percent of Americans experience episodes of low back pain due to degenerative discs, resulting in a loss of $24 billion in work time and an additional $27 billion in productivity and compensation. Chronic back problems have great potential for producing pain, deformity, and neurological damage. New procedures have been introduced to provide stability to the spine, reduce pain, and promote a better quality of life.

- Kyphoplasty is a procedure whereby a balloon is inserted through a needle to the fractured vertebra. The balloon is carefully inflated to create a cavity that moves the vertebra into its original position. A special type of cement (used in total hip and knee replacement) is instilled into this cavity, thus restoring stability and height to the spine.
- Vertebroplasty is a similar procedure; it also involves the injection of cement but without the use of a balloon. Both procedures can be done under local anesthesia on an outpatient basis. More than one vertebral fracture can be treated at a time. There are few risks and recovery time is short.
- Intradiscal electrothermal annuloplasty (IDET) is a minimally invasive procedure for the repair of a herniated cervical or lumbar disc. Heat is applied to close tears of the annulus (outer covering) of the disc.
- Total disc replacement is a revolutionary surgery replacing the traditional method of spinal fusion. An artificial disc is inserted to restore the damaged disc to its normal position and preserve spinal motion. The patient undergoing this procedure can return to an active life within a short time. Eligibility criteria exclude those who have osteoporosis, a previous fusion, scoliosis, or spondylolisthesis (forward slipping of a vertebra).
- The SB Charite artificial disc was developed in Europe. The two endplates are made of a cobalt-chromium alloy such as that used in total knee replacements. The inner core is made of polyethylene. Surgeries for replacement of several damaged discs at a time have been performed in Germany and France for quite some time. Clinical trials are under way in the United States with a view to obtaining FDA approval.

These experimental procedures are costly, and most are not currently covered by health insurance; however, the shorter hospital stay, briefer recovery period, and less potential need for further treatment may change this policy (Medline Plus, 2005b).

Fast Forward ▶▶▶

Vaccine for Herpes Zoster

Herpes zoster (shingles) is an adult-onset disease caused by reactivation of the varicella zoster virus in people who had chickenpox as children. The virus remains dormant in the body for many years and frequently reemerges in persons over 60 years of age who have a weakened immune system. Painful blisters form on the skin along a nerve pathway—usually on one side of the body trunk or the head and neck, with a high-risk of ocular involvement. The acute phase lasts 2 to 4 weeks. Many people experience postherpetic neuralgia, a severely painful neuropathic condition that may last for months or years.

A recent national clinical trial was conducted to test the effectiveness of Zostavax, an experimental high-dose version of the chickenpox vaccine, in stimulating an immune response among older adults. Findings indicated that (1) persons receiving the vaccine had fewer cases of herpes zoster; (2) those who did develop shingles had milder cases, (3) and fewer (66 percent) incidences of postherpetic neuralgia occurred among those who were vaccinated than among study participants who did not receive the vaccine.

These study findings hold great promise for many of the older population. Scientists have applied to the FDA for approval to make the vaccine available as a preventive measure. Approval is pending from the FDA.

Source: Oxman, M., Levin, M., Johnson, G., Schmader, K., Straus, S., Gelb, L., et al. (2005). A vaccine to prevent herpes zoster and post-herpetic neuralgia in older adults. New England Journal of Medicine, 352, 2271–2284.

DOLLARS AND SENSE

Financial Costs of Pain

Chronic pain is the most commonly cited cause of disability in the United States. Approximately 50 percent of the persons who seek medical help do so because of the primary complaint of pain. Each year 155 million persons experience at least one episode of acute pain, and one-third that number report that their pain is severe. An estimated 700 million workdays, at a cost of $60 billion, are lost annually in the United States. because of chronic pain (American Chronic Pain Association, 2003).

unknown etiology. Pain that is due to a known cause—such as malignancy, nerve compression or entrapment, phantom limb pain, spinal cord damage, and myofascial syndromes—and is resistant to therapy is referred to as chronic intractable pain (ACPA, 2003).

Cancer Pain

The multiple causes of cancer pain, or pain of malignancy, include the cancer itself; side effects of treatment; compression of bones, nerves, or body organs; poor blood circulation; blockage of an organ; metastasis; infection; and inflammation (ACPA, 2003). Radiation or chemotherapy can cause accumulation of fluid (edema), irritate or destroy healthy tissue, and sensitize nerve endings. Cancer pain has two components: persistent and breakthrough pain.

Persistent Pain

Persistent pain lasts for 12 hours or longer each day and is often referred to as background or baseline pain. The type of pain and its intensity often change throughout the various stages of the disease. Management of persistent pain is more difficult due to the variety of its causes. However, approximately 95 percent of cancer pain can be successfully controlled with drug and nondrug therapies. Flexibility in assessment and patient involvement in the plan of care are of prime importance because of the variations in diagnosis, the stage of the disease process, and the individual's responses to both the pain and therapeutic interventions. Patients may have personal preferences regarding pain management.

Uncovering the Evidence

Survey of Americans Living with Pain

Discussion: To determine the current awareness and understanding of pain and pain management issues among the general population of the United States, a random digit dialing system including all household telephone numbers (listed and unlisted) in the United States was used in 2002 to collect data. Data were collected through 800 telephone interviews with adults experiencing chronic pain.

The findings revealed the following:

- Seventy-two percent of respondents experiencing chronic pain had lived with it for more than 3 years; 34 percent had lived with pain for more than a decade.
- Seventy-eight percent of respondents believed that treatment with narcotic medications would cause addiction.
- Most respondents thought the typical person living with chronic pain was an adult at or above 65 years of age.
- A majority agreed that some people tend to exaggerate their pain to gain attention, avoid work, or to obtain painkillers. (More of the youngest respondents answered "strongly agree" to this statement.)
- One-third of respondents reported living with ongoing pain.
- Workplace Issues:
  1. Forty-one percent of employed persons who had chronic pain stated that it affected their ability to work a full day.
  2. Twenty-seven percent stated that the pain affected their ability to get to work.
  3. Sixteen percent stated that chronic pain affected their opportunities for career advancement.
- Pain Management:
  1. Eighty-one percent reported satisfaction with their prescribed plan of medical treatment.
  2. Eight-six percent of those taking prescription medications also reported using alternative treatments, including physical therapy (58 percent) massage (39 percent), and meditation (23 percent).
  3. Sixty-four percent of those who used over-the-counter (OTC) medications were satisfied with their relief of pain.
- Economic Fears: Three of ten persons were unable to have a prescription filled because of its cost or the lack of health insurance; they also felt it would become more difficult to obtain the needed medication in the future.

Implications for Practice: Patient education in the many pain-relieving modalities available and encouraging patients and their families to become a principal part of the treatment team are very important aspects of good pain management.

Source: American Chronic Pain Association (ACPA). (2004). Nurses' pain awareness kit. Retrieved from http://www.theacpa.org.

Breakthrough Pain

Breakthrough pain (BTP), or episodic pain, consists of acute flares of pain when medication or therapy does not relieve all of the cancer pain or other background pain of a severe illness. BTP is commonly seen in the more advanced stages of cancer and late-stage diseases such as AIDS. BTP can be spontaneous and unpredictable (**idiopathic pain**) or initiated by certain activities, such as walking, sitting, or coughing, and is often referred to as incidental pain. Severe BTP can last for a few minutes up to 30 minutes or an hour. The episodes may occur several times a day even though the person is on a regular analgesic schedule. BTP can also occur close to the next scheduled dose of an analgesic medication. If the episodes occur four or more times a day, the dosage of the regularly scheduled drug may have to be adjusted. BTP is treated with "rescue medications," such as immediate-release morphine, transmucosal fentanyl citrate, or ketamine, which work quickly and have a shorter stay in the body, thus producing fewer side effects. Other immediate-action medications are being developed.

Rhiner and coworkers (2004) reviewed three case studies of patients with cancer who experienced breakthrough pain while taking opioid medication around the clock for background pain. All experienced severe breakthrough pain that was not controlled by the commonly prescribed medications (short-acting morphine, hydromorphone, and oxycodone) or adjuvant medications;

the adverse side effects (such as nausea, gastric irritation, constipation, sedation or drowsiness, and confusion) interfered with activities of daily living and quality of life. "One patient's description of her pain stated: My pain is deep and constant, but throughout the day, there is a pain that comes on without warning, and it takes my breath away." A comprehensive physical examination was performed and an individualized pain management program devised for managing these patients' breakthrough pain with individualized titrated doses of fentanyl citrate. Each patient reported greater satisfaction with pain relief and fewer side effects. The review of these case studies demonstrates that breakthrough pain is not well understood and often not managed effectively. Pain management begins with a thorough understanding of all the components of pain. Assessment and management of breakthrough pain should be integrated into daily nursing practice. The patient's self-report is still the best evaluation of the quality of the pain, since there is no validated assessment for episodic pain. A comprehensive pain assessment must be done in order to provide the best pain relief (World Health Organization [WHO], 2004a).

Intractable Pain

Intractable pain is pain that is refractory or resistant to some or all forms of treatment. Many physicians hesitate to prescribe opioid drugs for noncancer intractable pain owing to concerns that their patients may become dependent or addicted to such drugs. The usual treatment consists of a combination of drugs and other therapies. Several states have developed policies and guidelines for treating intractable pain and to ensure protection for physicians against legal action for "overprescribing" opioid drugs. The guidelines state that the diagnosis should be made by two physicians based on the patient's history, physical examination findings, and empirical data. A medical plan of care must be established and careful monitoring must be included (American Pain Foundation, 2005).

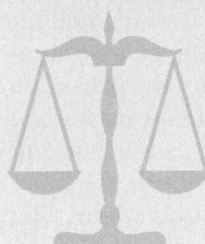

LAW IN PRACTICE

Medical Marijuana

Marijuana for medical purposes has been approved in 10 states. The FDA has classified it as a schedule 1 drug, which means that it has a high potential for abuse. It has not been approved by the FDA owing to the lack of evidence from controlled clinical trials regarding its effectiveness as a pain reliever; however, there is great interest in its use by individuals who have not had pain relief from other therapies. It has been used to treat glaucoma, AIDS wasting, neuropathic pain, spasticity of multiple sclerosis, and chemotherapy-induced nausea. Dronabinol (Marinol) is a drug with characteristics similar to those of marijuana; it has FDA approval for controlling nausea and vomiting due to AIDS and chemotherapy-induced nausea.

The U.S. Supreme Court (June 7, 2005) ruled that the federal government can overrule state laws and prosecute seriously ill individuals who continue to use marijuana even when they are doing so under doctor's orders.

Source: McDonald, J. (2005, June 7). Supreme Court decision trumps California law. San Diego Union Tribune. pp. A-1, 8.

Methadone, a drug developed prior to World War II, was originally used to treat withdrawal symptoms arising in the course of the detoxification process for persons addicted to heroin. It was also used to help these individuals abstain from the use of heroin. A social stigma of associating methadone with addiction to narcotics is a barrier to its beneficial use for other purposes. Currently, some hospices and other palliative care agencies have introduced methadone as a highly effective analgesic for patients who experience severe intractable pain. It is unique in its effectiveness for treating both nociceptive and neuropathic pain. Anecdotal reports have indicated it may decrease the need for antidepressants because it increases the release of serotonin and norepinephrine and their pain-modulating effects through the descending pathway of the CNS. Additional advantages include an administration schedule calling for one dose every 12 hours. Finally, it is an inexpensive drug. However, it has a long half-life and should not be used for intermittent pain, and it does cause respiratory depression. There is a complex process for switching the patient from other opioids to methadone (Westerbrook, 2005).

ASSESSING THE CLINICAL MANIFESTATIONS OF PAIN

A comprehensive assessment incorporates communication between the nurse and patient and development of a trusting relationship. The assessment begins with a pain history; its description, onset, duration, and frequency; information on exacerbating and alleviating factors; its impact on activities of daily living and diet; and the use of all current medication including OTC drugs and supplements. The history also includes questions about social, cultural, and spiritual influences on the pain experience. A focused physical assessment is done to identify the potential sources of pain (Kim et al., 2005).

Continuous reassessment is an essential component of pain management; however, it is often neglected. Its value lies in determining whether the management plan is effective or whether changes need to be made. Reassessment should be done and documented after each intervention. The nurse should also be aware that some patients do not request medication until their pain is severe; this complicates the pain control process. Often, the question "Are you in pain?" is an effective means for beginning the assessment and for educating the patient about the pain management process (Hader & Guy, 2004).

As mentioned previously, the autonomic nervous system regulates involuntary processes such as breathing, blood flow, pulse rate, digestion, and elimination, continually adjusting these activities to changing body needs. Sympathetic responses to mild to moderate pain can include pallor, increased blood pressure, increased heart rate and respirations (sometimes hyperventilation occurs), dilated pupils, diaphoresis, muscle tension, and anxiety. Symptoms often associated with pain include nausea, loss of appetite, restlessness, and insomnia or excessive sleeping. Parasympathetic responses are seen as the patient experiences severe pain. The symptoms include decreased blood pressure and pulse, nausea and vomiting, weakness, and prostration; loss of consciousness may ensue as the body's defenses collapse. Typical behavioral responses to acute pain are assuming a posture that minimizes pain or protects the injured part, withdrawing from touch, tensed muscles, crying or moaning, or appearing frightened (Hanks-Bell, et al., 2004). Typical behavioral responses to chronic pain—such as the person's total preoccupation with pain, anxiety, anger, depression, and fatigue—often complicate the assessment process.

Consistent use of assessment tools is the standard for determining the patient's subjective pain experience and for documenting and comparing those ratings over time. Four common tools for acute and chronic pain are: (1) the numerical rating scale, (2) the Wong-Baker Faces Scale, (3) the Verbal

---

Skills 360°

Systematic Pain Assessment

Steps for Systematic Pain Assessment

- **A:** Ask about pain regularly. Assess systematically.
- **B:** Believe the patient's and family's reports about pain.
- **C:** Choose pain control options appropriate to the patient, the family and setting.
- **D:** Deliver interventions in a timely, logical, coordinated fashion.
- **E:** Empower patients and families. Enable them to control their course to the greatest extent possible.

Source: Guidelines for Assessment and Management of Chronic Pain (ACPA, 2004).

Skills 360°

Pain Assessment Tools

1. Numerical Rating Scale. The patient is asked to rate the pain intensity on a scale from 0 to 10, with 0 indicating "no pain" and 10 indicating the "worst possible pain." The scale can also be simplified by using a scale of 0 to 5.
2. Wong-Baker Faces Scale. The patient uses faces to help describe the intensity of pain. This is particularly useful for pediatric patients and patients who cannot read or have a language problem. An explanation must be given to the patient regarding the meaning of each face. Example: A rank of 0 means "This face is happy—no pain." A rank of 10 indicates that "This face means as much as you can imagine—but you don't have to be crying to feel this bad."
3. Verbal Graphic Rating Scale. Words are used along a continuum that describes the intensity of pain. ("no pain" to "worst possible pain"). The scale can be modified using words that are better understood by the patient.
4. PAINAID Scale. This scale rates breathing, negative vocalizations, facial expression, body language, and comfort. This is especially useful in assessing the pain of patients with dementia.

Source: Hader, C., & Guy, J. (2004). Your hand in pain management. Nursing Management, 35(11), 21–27.

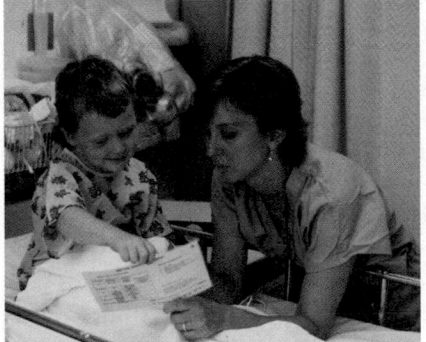

Figure 16-6 Nurse and child review a pain rating scale before the child experiences the pain.

Graphic Rating Scale, and (4) PAINAID Scale (Figure 16-6). The scales are user-friendly and some are written in different languages. The patient should be educated regarding the use of the tool and the same tool should be used each time. This will facilitate an accurate assessment and documentation. A description of each tool is in the pain assessment tools box.

The original COMFORT Behavior Scale was developed for use with pediatric patients in intensive care units by Ambuel and colleagues in 1992, and it has been modified for use in several settings (Ambuel, Hamlett, Marx, & Blumer, 1992). The tool is especially useful for assessing the behavior of infants, children, and adults who are unable to respond to pain measurement scales. The dimensions of the scale evaluate alertness, calmness, respiratory distress, crying levels, physical movement, muscle tone, facial tension, and comparison of current blood pressure and heart rate with baseline measures. A value of 1 to 5 is given for each dimension. A visual analogue scale is used to indicate how much pain the assessor thinks the patient has "at this very moment." Treatment details and information on the patient's condition are documented on the form. The health care team and family can, then, determine the appropriate interventions to the response of total assessment scores on the scale. The standard assessment or assessments before or after medication are also documented. Standard assessment can be made at the beginning of each shift or every 2 hours after major surgery for the first 24 hours. Additional assessment and documentation of patient responses to analgesic medication can be done before or after painful treatment procedures (van Dijk, Peters & Van Deventer, 2005; Ambuel, et al., 1992).

Barriers to Pain Assessment and Pain Management

Multiple complex and poorly defined barriers continue to have an impact on the assessment and management of pain for the health care system, the health care professional, and the patient (McCaffrey & Pasero, 2004). The traditional

Skills 360°

Quality of Life Scale: A Measure of Function for People with Pain

The Quality of Life Scale published by the American Chronic Pain Association (2003) is used to measure a person's ability to function. Functional activities are ranked from 0 (nonfunctioning) to 10 (normal quality of life).

0 = Staying in bed all day, feeling hopeless and helpless about life

10 = Normal daily activities each day. Having a social life outside of work/home. Taking an active part in family life.

Skills 360°

OLD CART Breakthrough Pain Assessment Tool

The OLD CART acronym is a useful pain assessment tool and is described as follows:

Onset of pain

Location(s) of pain

Duration of pain (constant or intermittent)

Characteristics (sharp, dull, throbbing, electric shock, tingling, pins and needles)

Aggravating factors (walking, sitting, lying down, other movement)

Relieving factors (medication, cold/warm applications, positioning)

Time factor (time of day or night at which pain is worse or better)

Source: Rhiner, M., Palos, G., & Termini, M. (2004). Managing breakthrough pain: A clinical review with three case studies using oral transmucosal fentanyl citrate. Clinical Journal of Oncology Nursing, 8(5), 507–512.

method of pain management consisted of administering analgesic medications only when a patient requested medication if the request was made within a strictly scheduled time frame, such as every 3 to 4 hours. This practice was based on the belief that the patient might become addicted or physically dependent on opioid (narcotic) drugs if the medications were given too often. The focus was on the biological causes of pain and ignored the psychological, emotional, and cultural needs of the person (McCaffrey, Frock, & Garguilo, 2003).

The health care professional may have inadequate knowledge of pain management or may perform an inadequate pain assessment owing to lack of knowledge. A survey of baccalaureate nursing programs revealed that less than 4 hours was specifically allocated to education on pain management (McCaffrey & Passero, 2004). The American Medical Association (AMA, 2003) also reported that health professionals are not well informed about analgesic pharmacology and pain therapy, have poor pain assessment practices, and ungrounded concern over regulatory oversight. A patient's pain should not be based on the professional's own beliefs and values or the misconception that a patient's lack of the typical expressions of pain indicates that no pain exists. Physiologically, the body adapts to pain after a time and vital signs normalize, therefore preventing further physical harm and prolonged stress on the body. On the other hand, prolonged exposure to pain does not produce tolerance to pain. In fact, tolerance is often decreased the longer a person experiences pain. Pain becomes an overwhelming experience involving every aspect of daily life. All pain does not have an identifiable physiological cause, and a particular noxious stimulus does not produce the same level of pain for everyone. Each individual responds in a unique manner.

The patient may be reluctant to report pain or to take pain medications because of fear of drug side effects or addiction, or due to lack of funds and access to medications. The patient may believe that pain indicates that the disease is worse, and that taking medications would delay or prevent further treat-

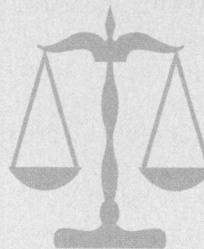

ETHICS IN PRACTICE

Ethical Considerations in Using Pain-Relieving Medications

It was not that long ago that health care students were actually taught that the first dose of morphine should also be the last and that no one ever died from pain, they just wished that they could. At least three generations of physicians, nurses, and pharmacists were taught to fear pain-relieving medications derived from opium (opioids).

Undertreatment of pain continues to be a major concern. Access to pain management services are lacking for many, including: people of color, the poor, and those living in rural areas. Protocols have been developed to permit people with terminal illnesses to die with comfort and dignity. However, the field of pain management is still young and evolving. It is essential for health care personnel to have the skills needed appropriate pain care management. Nurses must also be committed to educating consumers to the facts that pain is often treatable and nearly always manageable.

Source: Cole, E. (2005). The Last Word. U.S. Food, and Drug Administration. Retrieved March 10, 2005, from www.fda.gov.

ment of the underlying cause. The patient may also want to be perceived as a "good patient" or may try to be stoic in the face of pain. The patient may become too exhausted to mount a vigorous response to pain.

Other factors include the inability to communicate a description of pain or discomfort, as in the case of patients who are intubated or have an altered level of consciousness or aphasia. A language barrier between the nurse and patient may prohibit clear communication. The nurse must be knowledgeable about the patient's pain-associated behavior. The patient's family can be an excellent resource regarding behavioral clues for assessment purposes. All of these factors and the personal life experiences (of everyone involved) play a major role in facilitating and inhibiting the pain management process (ACPA, 2004; Hader & Guy, 2004).

NURSING DIAGNOSES

Based on the information gathered, examples of nursing diagnoses in the patient with pain may include the following:

- Ineffective coping related to anxiety, lower activity level, and the inability to perform normal activities of daily living
- Fear and anxiety related to actual/potential lifestyle changes
- Spiritual distress related to pain
- Deficient diversional activity related to pain

PLANNING AND IMPLEMENTATION

"Identifying the type of pain a patient experiences leads not only to an appropriate diagnosis, but assists with developing a pain management plan that meets the individual patient's needs" (Hader & Guy, 2004, p. 23). The current emphasis is on implementing an appropriate schedule for administering analgesic medications, providing physical comfort measures, and implementing complementary therapies to aid in alleviating the contributing factors to pain, such as anxiety, fear, hopelessness, depression, and inadequate coping strategies.

The specifically designed care strategies also provide a framework for evaluating therapeutic interventions. The "five Cs" of pain management include:

(1) comprehensive assessment,
(2) consistent use of assessment tools,
(3) continuous reassessment,
(4) a customized plan of care, and
(5) a collaborative or multidisciplinary approach, using both analgesic medications and nonpharmacological interventions.

Effective pain management also requires the continued support of the team to address all the strategic elements and promote positive outcomes.

Contemporary Pain Management Measures

Congress declared the calendar years 2001 to 2010 as the decade of pain control and research. In this connection, Representative Mike Rogers (Michigan) recently reintroduced the National Pain Care Policy Act—HB 1020 (American Chronic Pain Association, [ACPA], 2005). In addition, pain management guidelines have been established by the Joint Commission on Accreditation of Healthcare Organizations (JCAHO) and are supported by the National Pharmaceutical Council and other national pain organizations (JCAHO, 2003).

The major purposes of the guidelines are to (1) establish measurement as the key for improvement, (2) dispel false beliefs about pain and treatment, and (3) provide objective data to gain support for establishing policies, procedures, and educational programs to promote effective pain management. In addition to the general guidelines, specific guidelines have been established for the various types of pain. Health care organizations have developed new policies and procedures to implement these guidelines and to educate personnel as well as patients and their families. According to Hader and Guy (2004) and Chavis and Duncan (2003), the cornerstone of effective pain management is patient and family education.

Interventions for the Management of Acute Pain

Acute pain is managed by diagnosing the underlying cause and attempting to remove it or decrease its intensity and by the use of analgesic drugs appropriate for the severity and type of pain. For example, narrowed and constricted arteries may be the underlying cause of angina pectoris; vasodilators aid in relieving the associated pain. Working in partnership with the patient, the nurse and other members of the health care team should explore other methods to relieve or eliminate the pain. The measures may include providing physical care; teaching the patient to use pain assessment tools and to "splint" the area when moving or coughing; and using noninvasive measures such as the application of heat, cold, or transcutaneous electrical nerve stimulation (TENS). Distractive measures such as music, art, and movies or television have also been helpful in alleviating acute pain. Relaxation therapy to relieve anxiety, biofeedback, and other alternative therapies can be used to help prevent the development of chronic pain at this stage.

It is best to administer analgesic medications around the clock rather than as needed. Patients should be awakened when the analgesic dose is due; how-

Uncovering the Evidence

Pain Management for Surgical Patients

Discussion: Pain management methods were fragmented and inconsistent among several surgical departments within a two-hospital and outpatient services health care system. This research program implemented a team approach, reviewed current practices, and devised a more efficient program throughout the system. A needs assessment was conducted regarding the competencies of staff members as well as a review of patient records and a 12-month medication utilization review for surgeons and anesthesiologists. Key problems were identified, including inconsistencies in (1) documentation; (2) education for staff members, patients and families; (3) physician orders and protocols; and (4) physician education and clinical practice.

Documentation forms were standardized for all phases of perioperative care including pain measurement scales, preoperative anxiety, pain management strategies, and patient satisfaction.

Educational materials for patient and family members were revised and a new pamphlet entitled *Instructions for Comfort and Pain Management* was developed.

Education needs of staff members were identified by survey and used as the basis for the education program. A variety of initial and ongoing education methods were implemented. Anesthesia care providers agreed to select medications from a set of preformatted standing orders appropriate to each patient, including postoperative measures for oxygen, glucose monitoring, and so on in the postanesthesia care unit. Physician education consisted of consultations with clinical pharmacists, who encouraged the use of newly developed postoperative standing orders.

Implications for Practice: An organized pain management program was established throughout the health care system. Evaluation measures identified a more efficient pain management program, greater patient satisfaction, and support from staff members and physicians for implementing the changes and an ongoing monitoring process.

Source: Chavis, S., & Duncan, L. (2003). Pain management continuum of care for surgical patients. AORN, 78(3), 382–399.

PATIENT PLAYBOOK

Coping with Chronic Pain

The patient is not always able to communicate the total impact of chronic pain on functional activities or the quality of life. The family often provides an inappropriate pain assessment due to their inadequate knowledge about the management of chronic pain. Therefore you should teach the patient and family to:

- Learn all they can about the physical condition and understand that there may be no current cure.
- Become actively involved in the customized health care plan.
- Learn to set priorities regarding the activities can help the patient to have a more active life and to set realistic goals appropriate for pain management.
- Understand medication protocol and how to use nonpharmacological interventions, including stress management.
- Recognize when to seek assistance from members of the health care team.
- Recognize that emotions directly affect physical health. Learn how to deal with feelings and ultimately lessen the level of pain.
- Identify a modest and safe exercise program to build strength and tone muscles.
- Recognize that a combination of medical treatment, good coping skills, and peer support are the keystones in living a more productive, satisfying life.

Source: Hader & Guy, 2004; American Chronic Pain Association, 2003.

ever, they may refuse the medication at any time. It is important to determine the rationale for refusing the dose. Disturbing side effects such as nausea, constipation, dizziness, or sleepiness may be the reasons for refusal, and appropriate measures can be selected to minimize these effects (Manias, et al., 2005).

Interventions for the Management of Chronic Pain

The nurse cannot adhere to the acute pain model to guide assessment, for there will be instances when the patient's behavior and physical signs do not correlate with the patient's report of pain. The descriptor triad for chronic pain is "suffering, sleeplessness, and sadness." The signs of chronic pain include fatigue, anxiety, sleep disturbance, irritability, appetite disturbance, constipation, psychomotor retardation, decreased pain tolerance, social withdrawal, and mental depression. Assessment may be complicated by the presence of more than one chronic health problem. The McGill-Melzack pain questionnaire is particularly useful for assessing chronic pain. The management of chronic pain is similar to that of acute pain, with the additional goals of prevention and early management of adverse side effects and the enhancement of quality of life. The patient should be encouraged concerning the eventual success of the therapy, but at the same time realistic therapeutic goals should be set. The patient should also be informed that some pain is likely to continue.

Scientists continue to explore why chronic pain develops. It is known that the longer pain stimuli act on the CNS, the greater the probability that chronic pain will occur. Therefore early recognition and treatment of acute pain is of prime importance. If a patient is already experiencing chronic pain, the assessment and treatment are directed toward possible underlying causes and the management of the clinical symptoms. The perspective that chronic pain is an illness in itself rather than a symptom focuses attention on the factors of pathophysiology, psychology, and mind-body connection. A multidisciplinary approach is particularly beneficial in providing an objective and systematic management of chronic pain. The multimodal approach, or a combination of medications that allows the use of lower doses of each drug, and around-the-clock dosing are particularly useful in managing chronic pain.

In managing progressive pain, such as cancer pain and end-of-life pain, the nurse must help patients and their families understand that an increase in pain intensity may require an increase in dosage of the medication in order to manage the pain symptoms and provide the highest quality of remaining life. The American Nurses Association (ANA, 2003c) has issued a position statement that increasing the titration of a medication to achieve symptom control is ethically justified. Complementary/alternative therapies and other comfort measures should also be considered as mainstays in the plan of care (Yezierski, et al., 2004; Nicholson, 2003).

Physical Care of Patients with Pain

The patient's skin should be protected from irritants such as chemicals, mechanical injuries, and extremes of heat or cold, which lower pain tolerance. The nurse should handle sensitive or injured tissue carefully and assess for pressure areas, edema, distension of the bowel or bladder, changes in wounds, and any further damage to damaged tissue. Painful procedures should be performed when the analgesic medications have reached their peak effect (Hollinworth, 2005). Any drainage tubes should be checked frequently to make sure that they are patent and positioned correctly. Nonpharmacological interventions such as applications of heat and cold have been useful for localized pain related to a spasm, itching, joint pain, or headache. Close monitoring of the skin and circulation to the application area is required.

Safety First

Cautionary Warnings for New Pain-Relieving Medications

Recently (2005) there has been some controversy about the use of prostaglandin synthetase inhibitor (COX-2 inhibitor) drugs such as Celebrex, Vioxx, and Bextra, which have been very popular new analgesic medications particularly for patients with arthritis. Clinical trials revealed that cardiovascular risks, including heart attacks and strokes, as well as skin diseases such as the rare and potentially fatal Stevens-Johnson syndrome outweighed the benefits of the drugs. Vioxx and Bextra have been recalled from U.S. markets; Celebrex should be used with caution. Side effects of the OTC NSAID medications can also be harmful. The U.S. Food and Drug Administration (FDA) will require that all NSAID container labels include warnings.

The nurse should instruct patients to contact their health care providers regarding their pain management program and to educate themselves on how to regain control over their pain (FDA, 2006).

The patient should also be protected from fatigue, with sufficient rest and sleep periods. Changing positions frequently can help prevent ischemia due to immobilization. Correct body alignment can help prevent painful muscle contractures; elevating an edematous painful part may help to reduce pain. The patient should be informed about what the nurse intends to do before his or her position is changed. Allow the patient to assist in the process whenever possible. Family and other caregivers should also be educated about providing effective physical care.

Pharmacology

There are three major types of analgesics: nonopioids, opioids (narcotics), and adjuvants. The WHO has established a three-step ladder of cancer pain relief as a standard to follow. "This three-step approach of administering the right drug in the right dose at the right time is inexpensive and 80–90 percent effective. Surgical intervention on appropriate nerves may provide further pain relief if drugs are not wholly effective" (American Pain Foundation, 2004).

Nonopioid Analgesics

The nonopioid drugs are divided into two categories: acetaminophen and nonsteroidal anti-inflammatory drugs (NSAIDs). These drugs are most effective for mild to moderate pain involving the peripheral nervous system. Acetaminophen is useful in relieving pain and reducing fever; however, it provides very little anti-inflammatory effect. It is generally well tolerated. Adverse effects do occur when it is taken in high doses or for a prolonged time. An overdose can be fatal, as its metabolites bind with liver tissue, leading to hepatoxicity. Prolonged use can also cause renal damage.

There are eight groups of NSAIDs, each having its own unique qualities. Each has a different half-life, and some are available as OTC drugs while others are available only by prescription. The combination of two NSAIDs does not increase the effectiveness of either drug. NSAIDs reduce inflammation by blocking prostaglandin synthesis and by diminishing the activation of peripheral pain sensors, thus preventing the transmission of pain impulses. However, these drugs inhibit platelet aggregation and increase the risk of gastric bleeding and ulcers. These drugs should be taken with food or with a full glass of fluid.

Aspirin is the prototype of the salicylate drugs and has a variety of therapeutic uses, such as relieving mild to moderate pain of headache, neuralgia, myalgia, dental pain, and other nociceptive pain (Box 16-2). It is also used in small daily doses in preventing myocardial infarction (MI) and recurrent transient ischemic attacks (TIAs) because of its anti–platelet aggregation and anti-inflammatory effects. Aspirin can also cause kidney and liver problems when taken for an extended period. Hypersensitivity to aspirin or an overdose may produce tinnitus, vertigo, bronchospasm, or urticaria. Persons with asthma or a hypersensitivity to aspirin may also be sensitive to other NSAIDs. Aspirin should not be given to children younger than 12 years of age for any reason because of the risk of Reye's syndrome (a neurological problem associated with viral infections such as chickenpox and influenza that are treated with salicylates). Some analgesics are a combination of opioids and NSAIDs. Examples are: acetaminophen with codeine and oxycodone with aspirin (Percodan). Celecoxib (Celebrex), a selective COX-2 inhibitor, is a popular drug of choice for severe arthritis pain requiring high doses of an anti-inflammatory drug. However, adverse side effects include gastric bleeding, ulcers, and cardiovascular risks.

Proton pump inhibitors (PPIs) such as omeprazole (Prilosec) and lansoprazole (Prevacid) are often prescribed to lower the risk of gastric irritation. Misoprostol (Cytotec) is a synthetic prostaglandin E_1 analogue that also inhibits gastric acid secretion.

BOX 16-2

GROUPS OF NSAID DRUGS

Prostaglandin Inhibitors

1. Salicylates: acetylsalicylic acid (aspirin and related drugs such as diflunisal (Dolobid) and choline salicylate (Arthropan).
2. Para-chlorobenzoic acid derivatives or indoles: indomethacin (Indocin), sulindac (Clinoril), and tolmetin (Tolectin). Highly protein-bound drugs displace other protein-bound drugs, posing a high risk of toxicity. These drugs may decrease blood pressure and cause sodium and water retention.
3. Pyrazolone derivatives: phenylbutazone (Butazolidin). Has a long half-life. Adverse reactions are blood dyscrasias (agranulocytosis and aplastic anemia). These drugs should be reserved for severe inflammatory conditions and arthritis.
4. Propionic acid derivatives: ibuprofen (Motrin), fenoprofen calcium (Nalfon), naproxen (Naprosyn), suprofen (Profenal), ketoprofen (Orudis), and flurbiprofen (Ansaid). Ibuprofen can increase effects of warfarin (Coumadin), sulfonamides, some cephalosporins, and phenytonin. Analgesic effects can be decreased when taken with aspirin. Hypoglycemia may result when taken with insulin or an oral hypoglycemic. There is a high risk of toxicity when taken concurrently with calcium channel blockers.
5. Fenamates: meclofenamate sodium monohydrate (Meclomen) mefenamic acid (Ponstel). Potent drugs for acute and chronic arthritis. These have side effects similar to those of other NSAIDs.
6. Oxicams: piroxicam (Feldene). Used for long-term arthritic conditions. Is associated with a lower incidence of gastric distress and ulceration. Is highly protein-bound and should not be given with another protein-bound drug.
7. Phenylacetic acids: diclofenac sodium (Volatren), ketorolac (Toradol injectable).
8. Selective COX-2 inhibitors: celecoxib (Celebrex). Adverse reactions are gastric bleeding, ulcers, and cardiovascular events. It should not be used by persons with asthma or sensitivity to sulfa or aspirin.

Drugs under development include etoricoxib, parecoxib (may be used for parenteral administration), lumiracoxib. Persons at greatest risk for adverse reactions to NSAIDs include those who are over 65 years of age, have a history of gastric ulcer, have cardiovascular problems, or are taking concurrent drugs such as warfarin, corticosteroids, or multiple NSAIDs.

Adapted from Wilson, Shannon, & Stang, 2005.

Opioid Analgesics

The opioids (narcotics) such as morphine, fentanyl, and hydromorphone are called agonists because they bind to specific CNS receptors and mimic the regulatory function of the body's receptors. Opioids are effective in relieving all types of pain, especially acute and malignant nociceptive pain. Opioids can also provide pain relief for some patients with chronic nonmalignant pain and help to raise the pain threshold. They are not as effective in relieving neuropathic pain. In addition to pain relief, these drugs can produce an emotional high, an effect that can be addictive. A new drug, ziconotide (Prialt), has been introduced as the first in a new class of drugs known as N-type calcium channel blockers intended specifically to treat severe neuropathic pain. It selectively blocks the afferent nerve transmission channels, thus decreasing sensitivity to pain. It is given intrathecally (into the cerebrospinal fluid). This drug is considered only after other analgesics have been ineffective in providing pain relief. It should be used with caution, especially in elderly patients, because of potential adverse psychological side effects and interaction with CNS depressants (LexiComp, 2005).

Physical dependence on opioids is an involuntary altered physiological state that is produced by repeated administration of a medication. Physical dependence can develop when a person receives several doses a day of an opioid medication for 2 weeks or more. The medication is gradually withdrawn to avoid withdrawal symptoms. Physical dependence is not the same as **addiction,** which is defined as a compulsive disorder in which an individual becomes preoccupied with obtaining and using a substance even though its continued use results in a decreased quality of life. **Tolerance** to opioids occurs when a higher dose of a drug is required to achieve the desired effect (Jarzyna, 2005).

Meperidine (Demerol) is a synthetic morphine-like compound. It is primarily used for preoperative and postoperative medication and for obstetric anesthesia because it does not decrease uterine contractions and has a less depressive effect on neonatal respiration than morphine. Meperidine is no longer a major drug for acute or chronic pain owing to its short duration of action of 2 to 3 hours and the potential for cumulative toxic effects of normeperidine, its metabolite. The effects are not reversed by naloxone, an opioid antagonist. It is not recommended for patients with renal insufficiency, severe liver dysfunction, or dysfunction of the cardiovascular or respiratory systems. A decrease in blood pressure is a major side effect, especially in the elderly patient. Large doses can lead to neurotoxicity and seizures in the elderly and in patients with advanced cancer (McCaffrey & Pasero, 2004).

Mixed agonist-antagonist medications, a combination of the opioid and an opioid antagonist such as naloxone hydrochloride (Narcan), have been in use for the past 20 years to relieve moderate to severe pain. They were designed to help reduce opioid drug abuse. Examples include pentazocine (Talwin), butorphanol tartrate (Stadol), buprenorphine (Buprenex), and nalbuphine hydrochloride (Nubain). Reports indicate that drug dependence can occur (Jarzyna, 2005).

Adjuvant Medications

Adjuvant medications are often added to the analgesics. Anticonvulsants (such as gabapentin and tiagabine) and tricyclic antidepressants (such as amitriptyline, doxepin, and imipramine) aid in relieving neuropathic pain. Newer antidepressants such as fluoxetine (Prozac), paroxetine (Paxil), and sertraline (Zoloft) have fewer side effects than the tricyclics; however, there is less clinical evidence of their effectiveness. Selective serotonin reuptake inhibitors may also help to reduce neuropathic pain. Currently, a multimodal approach, a combination of opiate and NSAID medications, is used in order to alleviate peripheral and central pain. Combining medications from the different groups allows the use of lower doses of both types of drugs and a lower incidence of side effects (Hader & Guy, 2004; World Health Organization, 2004a).

Corticosteroids are given as anti-inflammatory medications. Muscle relaxants such as baclofen (Lioresal) can be used to provide systematic relief of spasms. Benzodiazepines (diazepam, midazolam, and others) are used as anxiolytics and also decrease skeletal muscle activity. The sedative-hypnotic/anxiolytic drugs (barbiturates, benzodiazepines, and nonbarbiturates) are primarily prescribed to promote sleep. A topical agent such as capsaicin is sometimes prescribed for neuropathic pain. However, because it causes a significant burning sensation, the patient may not be able to tolerate it. The lidocaine 5% patch, which has been used effectively in managing postherpetic neuralgia, is being tested in clinical studies to determine whether its effectiveness can be extended to manage pain of neuropathic and nociceptive origin, including musculoskeletal and arthritic pain. The patch is easy to use as a once-a-day application, thus facilitating compliance with long-term therapy. It can be used alone or in combination with other analgesic and adjuvant drugs. More than one patch can be applied at a time. There are minimal risks for systemic adverse reactions with other drugs. It may take several days before maximum effectiveness is achieved. A survey of patients with the mean age of 75 years reported satisfaction with using one to five patches a day for several years. "Sixty percent of the patients reported using the patch alone, while the others reported concomitant use of opioids, tricyclics, anticonvulsants, corticosteroids or acetaminophen" (Davies & Galer, 2004, p. 944).

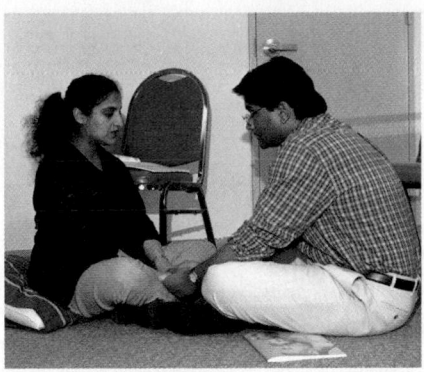

Figure 16-7 Childbirth preparation classes are a nonpharmacological way of treating pain; such classes often include techniques whereby the partner helps the expectant mother to relax, focus, and breathe deeply.

Drug Forms and Routes of Administration of Analgesics

Most drugs are available in multiple forms to allow delivery by a variety of methods. The three primary routes for drug administration are the enteral (gastrointestinal) route, the parenteral (subcutaneous, intramuscular, intravenous, epidural, intrathecal, and intracerebral) routes, and topical administration. The intramuscular route is seldom used for administering analgesics. Sometimes oral medicines are delivered via nasogastric or gastrostomy tube. At times drug solutions are administered intradermally or instilled into the cerebrospinal fluid, such as anesthetics (including patient-controlled anesthesia); or they may be injected into a joint (antibiotic or corticosteroid). The intra-arterial route can be used for delivering undiluted chemotherapy directly to the artery leading to a tumor. Implantable devices are now available for the ongoing management of pain. Areas for topical application include the skin and mucous membranes of the eyes, nose, ears, lungs, vagina, and rectum (Hader & Guy, 2004).

A common route for delivering analgesic medication for the hospitalized patient with acute pain is by the intravenous route. Advantages include prompt onset of action and bypassing the gastrointestinal tract. An infusion pump provides a consistent level of comfort. Patient-controlled analgesia (PCA) is a preferred option for many patients. Small pre-measured amounts of medication can be administered by bolus when the patient determines the need for additional medication. The nurse must continue to monitor the effects of the medication (Figure 16-7) (Table 16-2).

Changes in medication and delivery methods occur at various stages of the treatment process, as when (1) switching the delivery method, (2) substituting a different drug to avoid the adverse effects of another drug, (3) substituting a combination drug, (4) adding an adjuvant drug to avoid using a higher dose of an analgesic drug, (5) or transferring a patient from one level of care to another, such as discharge from the health care setting to home. When any of these changes occur and the patient still experiences pain, the goal is to provide **equianalgesia** (Table 16-3), the equal analgesic effects with the new medication or delivery method. The nurse should understand the concept of equianalgesia and how to interpret an equianalgesia chart.

Potential and Actual Side Effects of Opioid Analgesics

Ongoing assessment and management of potential and actual side effects of opioid analgesic medications such as constipation, nausea and vomiting, sedation and depressed respirations, circulatory depression, rashes and pruritus (itching) are important aspects of care. Constipation is an inevitable side effect of opioid analgesics. Individuals receiving analgesics on a long-term basis should be placed on a bowel management regimen. Treatment often consists of a high-fiber diet, fluids, and stool-softening medications such as Colace or Docusate. Bulk-forming laxatives (Fibercon, Metamucil), stimulating cathartics (bisacodyl), and suppositories (glycerin, Fleet Babylax) are sometimes prescribed. Antiemetic drugs such as the phenothiazines or metoclopramide (Clopra, Maxeran) are used to treat nausea and vomiting. In some instances, the patient may be able to tolerate another effective analgesic drug that does not produce the same side effects.

Sedation and respiratory depression are not always drug dose–related and can be related to individual differences among patients or their type of pain. Appropriate safety measures should be taken to prevent patient injuries due to sedation. Respiratory depression usually occurs within 15 minutes of intravenous administration and within 30 to 60 minutes following an oral dose. Drug overdose usually occurs in patients who have not received opioids previously or when there is an accumulation of doses due to renal or liver mal-

TABLE 16-2 Summary of Selected Analgesic Medications

DRUG	ROUTE OF ADMINISTRATION	SELECTED INDICATIONS
Nonopioid Analgesics: Acetaminophen and Selected NSAIDs		
Acetaminophen (Tylenol and others)	Oral	Mild to moderate nociceptive pain
Aspirin	Oral	Mild to moderate nociceptive pain Inflammation, anti–platelet aggregation
Ibuprofen (Motrin, Advil, others)	Oral	Mild to moderate nociceptive pain, chronic pain. Inflammation
Celecoxib, a COX-2 inhibitor (Celebrex)	Oral	Chronic pain—arthritis (under investigation for adverse side effects)
Mu Opioid Agonist Analgesics		
Morphine (Roxanol)	Oral, intramuscular, intravenous	Moderate to severe acute and chronic pain
Oxycodone (Roxicodone), opioid and NSAID, oxycodone and aspirin (Percodan), oxycodone and acetaminophen (Percocet)	Oral	Moderate to moderately severe pain
Fentanyl (Sublimaze)	Intramuscular/intravenous/ oral—transmucosal (fentanyl citrate—OTFC) Transdermal (Duragesic)	OTFC for breakthrough cancer pain
Methadone (Dolophine)	Oral	Severe pain (and as detoxification agent)
Moderate Opioid Analgesics		
Codeine	Oral, intramuscular	Mild to moderate pain. Antitussive (cough suppressant)
Agonist-antagonist Opioids		
Pentazocine (Talwin, Talacen)	Oral, intravenous	Moderate to severe pain. Adjunct to anesthesia
Buprenorphine (Buprenex)	Intravenous, epidural, intramuscular	Moderate to severe postoperative pain. Cancer and trigeminal neuralgia, trauma, ureteral calculi, M.I.
Adjuvant Medications		
Anticonvulsant Gabapentin (Neurontin)	Oral	Effective in treatment of neuropathic pain
Antidepressants Amitriptyline (Elavil) Fluoxetine (Prozac)	Oral	Effective in treatment of neuropathic pain, depression, insomnia
Anxiolytics Benzodiazepines: Diazepam (Valium) Alprazolam (Xanax) Buspirone (BuSpar) Lorazepam (Ativan)	Oral	Muscle spasms, insomnia. Also for anxiolysis
Corticosteroid Dexamethasone (Decadron)	Oral Some may be given intravenously or intramuscularly	Inflammatory pain

Adapted from Nurseweek pain charts, 2004; ACPA, 2004.

TABLE 16-3	Examples of Equianalgesia Medications	
DRUG	**PARENTERAL ROUTE**	**ORAL ROUTE**
Mu Opioid		
Morphine	10 mg	30 mg
Agonist-antagonist Opioid		
Pentazocine (Talwin)	60 mg	180 mg
Nonopioids		
Acetaminophen		650 mg
Aspirin		650 mg

function. Overdose can also occur when doses are far above the therapeutic level. Pupil constriction is a sign of drug toxicity. The nurse should make a careful ongoing assessment of the patient's responses (Brown & McCormack, 2005). Arousing the patient and establishing a patent airway may be all that is necessary. An antidote or opioid antagonist (naloxone) is given in small titrated amounts to reverse life-threatening opioid-induced respiratory depression. The antagonist has a greater affinity to the CNS opiate receptor site than the opioid has; therefore it displaces the opioid and blocks its action. The side effect of circulatory depression, or orthostatic hypotension, commonly occurs as the patient changes from a supine position to an upright one. The patient should be taught to avoid abrupt changes in position. The patient may need assistance when he or she is ambulating.

Rashes, pruritus, hives, redness, and swelling can be due to hypersensitivity or allergy reactions. Hypersensitivity is an exaggerated body response to the foreign substance. A drug allergy reaction is due to an altered physiological immune system response due to a previous exposure to the drug or a drug component. Idiosyncratic responses are unusual individual responses such as excitability in response to a sedative drug.

Additional side effects of opioids include dry mouth, urinary retention (particularly in the elderly), altered cognitive function and mood changes, sleep disturbances, and sexual dysfunction. Fluids, mouth rinses, and lozenges can help moisturize the oral mucosa. In urinary retention, the kidney continues to produce the normal amount of urine, but it is not voided. The bladder is raised above the pubic symphysis and is sometimes displaced to the side. The patient may be restless and diaphoretic. Placing the patient in an upright sitting or standing position, warming the bedpan, and providing privacy may help the patient to void. Pouring warm water over the perineum or giving the patient a warm bath will promote muscle relaxation. Gently stroking the patient's inner thigh may stimulate the micturition reflex. Other stress-reducing measures can be used. Catheterization may be necessary.

Examples of withdrawal symptoms include myoclonus (twitching or spasm of muscles that can also occur due to a drug), restlessness, irritability, and an increase in pulse rate and blood pressure. Applications of heat or cold may help to reduce the muscle activity. The patient should be assessed for skin damage and circulatory impairment from the applications. Anxiolytic drugs may also be prescribed.

All analgesic drugs have potentially significant end-organ toxicity. Drugs accumulate in the body whenever the dosage exceeds the amount that can be eliminated through excretion. The potential for toxicity is dependent on an

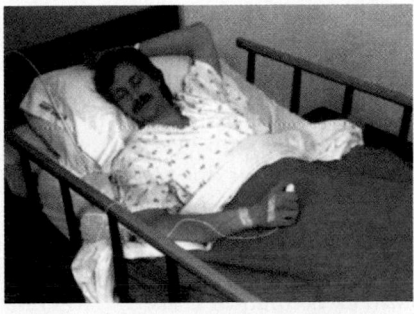

Figure 16-8 A patient using patient-controlled analgesia (PCA).

organ's capacity, regenerating ability, and reserves. The most serious toxicities affect the liver, kidneys, heart, and CNS. This is of particular concern in caring for elderly patients. Many elderly people take several medications for their health problems and are at risk for drug interactions and undesirable side effects. Drugs such as meperidine (Demerol), petazocine (Talwin), and propoxyphene (Darvon) can have greater toxic effects in the elderly. Smaller doses of opioids are not always the answer. The nurse must monitor the elderly patient very carefully (Shaw, 2006).

A reassessment should be conducted after every new pain management therapy is introduced. Usually a new analgesic is introduced at a "starter dose" and the dose is slowly increased until the pain level is stabilized. The assessment may be done on a regular basis such as every shift for hospitalized patients, every week for home care patients, and every few weeks or months for patients with long-term chronic pain. The drug therapy is considered effective if the pain is controlled at a level acceptable to the patient.

The nurse should also be aware of the interaction between drugs the patient may be taking and the course of the illness and the related signs and symptoms. Discrepancies can be noted between the patient's behavior and the report of pain. The patient may deny that pain exists, yet nonverbal signs may indicate severe pain. These differences can be due to fear, anxiety, or misconceptions about pain management. The nurse should explore the patient's interpretation of the pain experience and discuss appropriate pain management strategies. The nurse should also check for tolerance and/or physical dependence.

Geriatric Considerations

There are three age classifications of the older adult population; the young old (ages 65 to 75); the older old (ages 75 to 85); and the "elite old" (over age 85). However, the age classifications do not include the person's mental and physiological health. Those among the elderly who are frail, are cognitively impaired, or who have a history of alcohol and drug abuse are at higher risk for underreporting pain. Many older adults have coexisting diseases, take several prescribed and OTC medications, and are cared for by family members at home. Many older people have pain due to degenerative problems involving the vertebrae, joints, and legs. Osteoarthritis and rheumatoid arthritis are common problems.

Physiological changes of organs, such as the liver and kidneys, begin around age 30 and continue up to 85 years of age, when the decline accelerates. These changes will alter drug absorption, distribution, and metabolism. The older adult taking NSAIDs over a period of time is at greater risk for a gastrointestinal bleeding. The analgesic drug of choice is morphine; however, elimination of the drug will be longer. Therefore the drug dose may have to be adjusted. Most adjuvant medications have short half-lives and can be of benefit to the older person with minimal side effects. Most analgesic medications are started at a low dose and gradually increased as necessary. The oral route is preferred, as it is the least expensive, most convenient, and also safe. Rectal and transdermal routes can be appropriate if the patient cannot take the medication orally. The intravenous and subcutaneous routes are used for patients who need long-term opioid therapy. The intramuscular route should not be used because older people have some muscle wasting and less fatty tissue (Daniels, 2004).

For the geriatric patient, use caution or avoid use of drugs with long half-lives, such as the NSAID piroxicam (Feldene); opioids: methadone (Dolophine, levorphanol (Levo-Dromoran), and the benzodiazepine diazepam (Valium). All opioids can produce serious side effects in the geriatric patient due to renal insufficiency and the toxic effects of metabolites of drugs such as meperidine (Demerol) and propoxyphene (Darvon, Darvocet). Side effects can include drowsiness, dizziness, tiredness, confusion or cognitive changes (delirium), somnolence, psychomotor agitation, nausea, and dry mouth. Constipation is also a particular concern.

PATIENT PLAYBOOK

Administering Opioid Analgesics

The nurse should consider the following when administering opioid analgesics:

- Conduct an initial pain assessment including vital signs to establish baseline data.
- Determine what has helped to relieve the patient's previous pain experiences.
- Obtain a complete medication profile including over-the-counter (OTC) medications, vitamins, and herbal remedies that the patient is taking.
- Inform the patient of the necessity to report pain before it becomes severe or unbearable.
- Discuss the rationale of pain control with the patient and family so that all may be involved in the plan of care.
- Provide accurate information to reduce the fear of addiction to pain medication.
- Provide appropriate written information about the medication protocol.
- Reassess the patient's comfort level after providing medication.
- Avoid planning painful treatments/procedures or activities prior to mealtimes.
- Adjust the use of assessment tools as needed.
- Inquire about the patient's coping skills.
- Educate the patient regarding the potential side effects and adverse reactions specific to their medications

Contraindications for Administration of Opioid Analgesics

Opioid analgesics are contraindicated in patients with head injuries. The respiratory depressive effects of these medications can lead to the accumulation of carbon dioxide. Cerebral blood vessels will dilate and cause intracranial pressure. The opioid medications can be detrimental for persons with a respiratory disorder, decreasing the respiratory drive and increasing airway resistance. These analgesics can also cause hypotension and should not be given to patients in shock. The opioids are also contraindicated for alcoholic patients as well as those with renal or hepatic disease and should be given with caution. (see Patient Playbook feature).

Alternative Therapy

Complementary therapies have been used for centuries, primarily in countries other than the United States. These therapies are the mainstays of health care for an estimated 70 to 90 percent of persons worldwide. They have currently become major topics of discussion and debate in the United States. Surveys have indicated that 42 percent of the adults questioned have used one or more complementary therapies, such as meditation, massage, acupuncture, imagery, herbal substances, and others. Yet our current health care system is slow to accept anecdotal reports as evidence of effectiveness. It is essential that health care providers be cognizant of the therapies being used and how they can influence the plan of care.

In the 1950s, scientists expressed a greater interest in exploring the influence of environmental and situational stressors and other factors on human behavioral responses to illness and disease. At that time several theories, including the gate control theory and stress theories, were developed. These theories provided the basis for numerous studies related to illness, pain, and stress. Interest also focused on psychological effects on the neurological and immune systems. Then scientists began to explore some of the ancient Oriental healing arts and how they are used.

The National Center for Complementary and Alternative Medicine (NCCAM), established in 1998, has defined these therapies as mind-body medicine (MBT) involving behavioral, psychological, social, and spiritual approaches that are not commonly used in western health care. The NCCAM was established to investigate these therapies through scientific randomized trials (Spee & Floyd, 2005).

Astin and colleagues (2004) conducted a meta-analysis of several research studies related to complementary therapies for the management of pain due to arthritis, fibromyalgia, headache, backache, and chronic and acute pain. They also studied the use of complementary therapies for childbirth and recovery from surgical and other invasive procedures in both children and adults and ways to help cancer patients reduce the physical pain associated with treatment. Although many of these studies did not meet the criteria for scientific research, the findings did indicate that several of the MBTs may be considered adjunctive therapies to conventional medical pain management.

Astin also reported that the psychological and emotional stress that commonly accompanies chronic pain conditions can actually exacerbate pain and other symptoms. MBTs may reduce the effects of stress in several ways. Teaching coping skills and increasing the individual's awareness of thoughts and emotional patterns and the habitual ways of reacting to daily stressors may facilitate the development of greater control and mastery. Stress-reducing strategies may also reduce the physiological effects of stress and aid in restoring balance to the body system. The "relaxation response" resulting from the practice of different MBTs may also serve to decrease pain. Mindful meditation can provide a more objective perspective, and a "deconditioning" of the alarm-reactive response, resulting in less suffering and distress.

Psychological counseling, support groups, exercise and physical therapy can be important elements of a pain management program (Yezierski, et al., 2004). These findings are supported by nursing's core values of meeting the mind-body-spiritual needs of individuals. Nightingale (1859) advocated environmental changes that would facilitate the patient's well-being and cautioned that disease was not always the cause of suffering. She mentioned how the mind is adversely affected because of a physical illness. She also encouraged the use of music, pets, flowers, reading, and a view of the outside world as measures to improve the patient's mental, spiritual, and physical health.

Therapeutic touch (TT) is one type of alternative therapy; it is a noncontact technique derived from the "laying on of hands" associated with Far Eastern, European, and other religious philosophies. This method is based on a theory that the release of excess energy from the healer assists the ill person in the healing process. The basic principles can be learned, and workshops have been offered throughout the country. Healing touch is a similar technique and has become a certificate program of the American Holistic Nurses' Association in 1993 (Spee & Floyd, 2005).

"Energy field disturbance" is a recent nursing diagnosis defined as a disruption of the flow of energy surrounding a person's being, which results in disharmony of the mind, body, and/or spirit. Related factors include illness, injury, and situational factors such as pain, fear, anxiety, crisis, and maturational or age-related developmental difficulties. Therapeutic touch can be considered as a beneficial adjuvant nursing intervention. Guided imagery is often included in the therapy as well. Refer to chapters 10 and 14 for detailed information on stress and the various complementary methods.

EVALUATION OF OUTCOMES

Potential patient outcomes for each of the example nursing diagnoses for the patient with pain are:

- Ineffective coping related to anxiety, a lower activity level, and the inability to perform normal activities of daily living: The patient identifies his or her own maladaptive coping behaviors, available resources, and support systems, describes/initiates alternative coping strategies, and describes positive results from new behaviors.
- Fear and anxiety related to actual/potential lifestyle changes: The patient should be able to recognize the signs of anxiety, demonstrate positive coping mechanisms, and describe a reduction in the level of anxiety experienced.
- Spiritual distress related to pain: The patient describes his or her spiritual belief system positively, expresses personal feelings related to changes in beliefs, and expresses the desire to perform religious/spiritual practices.
- Deficient diversional activity related to pain: The patient's attention is diverted to other interests than illness and the clinical manifestation of pain.

KEY CONCEPTS

- Clinical manifestation of pain is a major health, economic, and social issue.
- Pain is an unpleasant sensory and emotional experience arising from actual or potential tissue damage or is described in terms related to the damage.

- Pain is a subjective experience and is "what the person says it is and exists when the person says it does."
- Pain is currently considered the fifth vital sign that should be included in the routine assessment.
- Nurses play a pivotal role in assessing and implementing interventions that promote effective pain relief.

Continued

KEY CONCEPTS—cont'd

- The pain experience is influenced by a great number of dynamic and ever-changing, interacting physiological, psychological, emotional, social, and cultural factors.
- Consistent use of assessment tools is the standard for determining the person's subjective pain and for documenting and comparing those ratings over time.
- Several barriers to pain management exist that include the values and beliefs of the health care system, the health care professional, and the patient.
- Contemporary pain management measures have been designed to meet standard guidelines, and policies in that regard have been established.

- A comprehensive knowledge of the pharmacological aspects of analgesic medications for effective pain management is essential.
- The nurse-patient relationship is a valuable component for establishing and maintaining a pain management plan.
- The cornerstone of effective pain management is patient and family education.
- Alternative therapies are particularly useful in reducing the stress associated with pain and for providing coping skills. These therapies are being integrated into the multidisciplinary plan of care.

REVIEW QUESTIONS

1. The purpose of myelinated nerve fibers is to:
   1. Speed pain sensations to the CNS for interpretation and response
   2. Slowly transmit touch and tickling sensations
   3. Strengthen the nerve fiber with a chemical compound
   4. Provide an electrical insulator to increase speed of transmission of an impulse

2. The latest version of the gate control theory suggests that:
   1. The control mechanism is in the dorsal horn of the spinal cord
   2. Strong pain sensations are not permitted to pass through the gate
   3. The control mechanism is influenced by internal analgesic substances
   4. It is not involved in pain reduction when exogenous analgesics are given

3. "Transduction of pain" refers to:
   1. Alteration of noxious sensations via perception feedback
   2. Initiation of an electrical activity due to the impact of noxious stimuli
   3. The pathway that carries pain information to the CNS
   4. The interaction between the PNS and CNS for interpreting the pain sensation

4. The term *allodynia* refers to:
   1. Personal awareness of body position
   2. Pain sensations arising from nerve ending in deeper body tissues

   3. Insensitivity to pain due to peripheral neuropathy or genetic factors
   4. Hypersensitivity to a noxious stimulus

5. The autonomic nervous system is a major part of the CNS that:
   1. Responds primarily to cognitive/thought stimulation
   2. Processes and coordinates incoming information to the CNS
   3. Regulates homeostasis or equilibrium of the body's internal environment
   4. Processes and coordinates all information sent from the CNS to the PNS

6. Endogenous opioid peptides are chemicals that are:
   1. Released as needed to assist in modulating pain sensations
   2. Easily broken down in the presence of opioid drugs
   3. Synthesized in the PNS to roam freely throughout the body systems
   4. Blocking the bond of exogenous analgesics and minimizing their effects

7. The best description for the cause of nociceptive pain is:
   1. When there is a disruption to the normal processing of the pain impulse
   2. Acute pain that is associated with injury or surgery resulting in tissue damage
   3. When there is no injury or malfunction of the nerve transmission process
   4. Pain with a sudden or slow onset that can build from mild to severe intensity

Continued

REVIEW QUESTIONS—cont'd

8. An example of neuropathic pain is:
   1. Pain from a torn ligament
   2. Lower back pain
   3. Cancer pain
   4. Phantom limb pain

9. Which of the following medications provide analgesia by blocking the production of prostaglandins?
   1. Opioids
   2. Anticonvulsants
   3. NSAIDs
   4. Tricyclic antidepressants

10. The cornerstone of effective pain management is:
    1. Interdisciplinary collaboration
    2. A standard care plan
    3. Patient and family education
    4. The combination of drug and nondrug therapy

REVIEW ACTIVITIES

1. Visit the Food and Drug Association Web site at: www.fda.gov
   a. Click on Consumer Education. Read the "Misuse of prescription pain relievers: The buzz that takes your breath away. Permanently."
   b. Read: "On the teen scene. Using over-the-counter medications wisely."
   c. Read "Managing chronic pain."
   d. Read: Clinical therapeutics continuing education (CE) article case study.
      Select two of the above topics and critique the information as a resource for patient education.

2. Visit the United Health Foundation Web site at http://UHFtips.org
   a. The purpose of this consumer Web site is "to provide support so people's health decisions are more informed and evidence based. The content can be used freely. Information is provided in English and Spanish. Examples include safe use of OTC pain relievers, safe use of daily aspirin, tips for parents, and how to read drug container labels. It also provides access to information for health professionals regarding evidence-based practice, located under "resources."
   b. Print out the patient medication record form. Use this to document the OTC medications taken by a geriatric person (over age 65) and instruct the person on the importance of updating the form as needed and to have it available in a wallet or purse to show to a health care provider. The form reminds the person to record pain, allergy, antacids, sleeping medications, laxatives, vitamins, and herbal remedies as well as prescribed medications. There is a place for the person's name and phone contact numbers on the form.
   c. Locate the brochures regarding communicating with the health care team. This includes the important questions the person should ask when a new medication is prescribed.
   d. Identify additional nursing diagnoses and potential outcomes that may be appropriate for the patient with (1) acute pain or (2) chronic pain. State specific nursing interventions that you believe to be appropriate

3. Access the Web site of the National Center for Complementary Alternative Medicine at http://nccam.nih.gov
   a. Select at least two categories of CAM methods and report the results of clinical trials of these methods.

4. Access the American Pain Foundation at: www.painfoundation.org. Click on publications from APF.
   a. Access the "Target Chronic Pain Notebook" Print it out. Use the brochure as a guide to assess the pain of five individuals and report your findings.
   b. Read the Patient Bill of Rights (related to pain). Print out the pain notebook. This is a tool patients can use to report their episodes of pain and their responses. Ask a person over age 65 who has pain to keep the log for a week. Go over the log with the person. Consider the nurse's role in using this as an assessment tool. Develop a written report of your findings.

Continued

REVIEW ACTIVITIES—cont'd

c. Read the various "Voices of People in Pain." Use the information provided in the personal comments to identify potential nursing diagnoses, potential patient outcomes, and possible nursing interventions.

d. View the audio/video series from *The Today Show* (2005) on *Easing Your Pain Today*. (Overview, medications, interventions, complementary approaches, and children and pain.) Identify five items of information that you learned from this series.

e. Read the teleconference archive comments *New Perspectives in Pain Management: Current Concerns and Safe New Directives* (3/30/05). Create a summary of at least two video presentations.

5. Access the American Chronic Pain Association at: http://www.theapca.org.
   a. Read and print out the "Nurses Pain Awareness Tool Kit."
   b. Read the "Ten Steps from Patient to Person" brochure.
   c. Read "It Takes Nerve"—information on neurological pain.
   d. Read "A Consumer Guide for Managing Chronic Pain" (PDF format).
   e. View the video clips on "What Is Chronic Pain?" "Is There Life with Pain?"
   f. Several other features on this Web site include articles from Partners for Understanding Pain; the news and features section, which includes "A Consumer's Guide for Managing Chronic Pain."

6. Access the U.S. government's report "Healthy People 2010" at: www.health.gov/healthypeople. There are 28 focus areas and 10 leading indicators.

a. Select topics related to pain. Develop a consumer's educational brochure for one of the topics.

b. Describe the role of the nurse in educating individuals on the prevention of health problems related to pain.

7. Access the online pain management series produced by the American Medical Association at: http://www.ama.cmeonline.com
   a. Review module 6 on pediatric pain management. Write a report outlining the responsibilities of the nurse in at least six pain management strategies for pediatric patients.

8. Access information at: http://www.pain.com to view an educational slide on the relationship of pain and mood/anxiety disorders. Other articles include information on breakthrough pain, cancer pain, and pain management for dying patients. Some assessment tools are presented.

9. Access the Nurseweek Web site at: www.nurseweek
   a. The course "A Nurse's Guide to Pain Management" is developed around a group of learning modules. It includes information on nonpharmacological pain relief measures. Links to other helpful resources are located here as well.
   b. Create a comprehensive list of nursing strategies that were presented.

10. Access http://www.genesishealth.com. This is a free download PDF file on pain management. Use the information in developing a care plan for
    a. a patient with acute pain
    b. a patient with chronic pain
    c. a patient with neuropathic pain.

Pharmacology: Nursing Management

Jane Harmon, PhD, MSN, CS-PMHNP

CHAPTER TOPICS

- Pharmacologic Principles of Drug Action

- Safe Medication Administration

- Anti-Infective Agents

- Cardiovascular Agents

- Drugs to Treat Circulatory Disorders

- Respiratory Agents

- Neurological and Neuromuscular Agents

- Gastrointestinal Agents

- Antidiabetic Agents

KEY TERMS

Absorption
Adverse effects
Bioavailability
Distribution
First pass effect
Metabolism or biotransformation
Peak drug level
Pharmaceutic
Pharmacodynamics
Pharmacokinetics
Pharmacology
Plasma half-life ($t_{1/2}$)
Polypharmacy
Protein binding
Receptor
Side effects
Therapeutic range
Trough drug level

Knowledge of pharmacology is essential to safe nursing practice. **Pharmacology** is defined as the scientific study of drugs and their origins, their actions on, and their interactions with living things through chemical processes. An accurate assessment of a patient depends on the nurse's ability to obtain a comprehensive drug history (Bullock & Manias, 2002). Nurses who know pharmacology are better prepared to fulfill their roles in managing patients' drug therapies and medication education. Consequently, they can anticipate and be more sensitive to patient needs (King, 2004). This chapter presents concise information about the pharmacological principles of selected medications as well as the nursing management of patients taking these. This chapter is not a substitution for a drug reference book. Information on prescribed drugs changes frequently as drugs are taken off the market and new ones become available. It is the responsibility of each practicing nurse to stay current on these new developments.

PHARMACOLOGICAL PRINCIPLES OF DRUG ACTION

The nurse must be aware of the effects of a medication from the time it is administered until it has been completely eliminated from the body. The practicing nurse can minimize the risk of making a serious medication error by knowing pharmacological principles and maintaining a broad base of knowledge about the medications that are administered, taking care not to administer any drug that is unfamiliar. It is the nurse's responsibility to recognize and question any inappropriate drug order that is written by the prescriber. Acting as a patient advocate, the nurse educates the patient about medication use and effects.

Pharmaceutic Phase

Oral medications must go through three phases: (a) pharmaceutic; (b) pharmacokinetic; and (c) pharmacodynamic before they can complete their desired task and are eliminated from the body. During the **pharmaceutic** phase an oral drug disintegrates and dissolves into particles that can cross the biological membrane for absorption into the body. Liquid medications are already in solution.

Pharmacokinetic Phase

Pharmacokinetics describes how the body acts on a drug. This phase describes the movement of a drug from the time it enters the body until it reaches its intended site of action, is chemically broken down, and excreted from the body. The action is divided into four processes: absorption, distribution, metabolism (biotransformation), and excretion.

Absorption is the stage that accounts for the movement of the drug from the site of administration into the bloodstream. To enter the blood stream, the drug must cross the plasma membrane. Without absorption, a drug cannot exert its effect. Absorption is the greatest determinant of the length of time it takes for a drug to begin its action. Factors that influence absorption include: (a) route of administration; (b) gastric motility; (c) pH (acid or alkaline); (d) blood flow to target site; and (e) lipid solubility. Intravenous (IV) drugs are absorbed at a faster rate than oral medications. Acidic drugs are more rapidly absorbed in an acidic environment, such as the stomach. Alkaline drugs are absorbed best in the alkaline environment of the small intestine. Changes in pH, either by the use of antacid medications or the aging process, alter the rate of absorption.

The lipid layer of most cell membranes permits lipid-soluble drugs to cross more easily. Drug-drug and drug-food interactions can affect absorption. For best absorption some drugs require a full stomach, and some require an empty stomach. A high-fat meal can slow stomach motility and decrease absorption. Drugs that stimulate intestinal motility can also decrease absorption. The nurse must be aware of these interactions and include this information in medication teaching.

Bioavailability is a subcategory of absorption and can be defined as the percentage of the drug within the systemic circulation that is available to achieve its intended effect in the body. Bioavailability is influenced by the same factors that affect absorption. Dosage forms from different drug manufacturers may have differences in their bioavailability.

Distribution is defined as the movement of the drug, after absorption into the bloodstream, to the site of its intended action. Blood flow determines the efficiency of this process. The organs of the body receiving the most blood supply are the heart, liver, kidneys, and brain. Because of lower circulating blood to the skin, bone, and adipose tissue, it is more difficult to deliver high concentrations of drugs to these areas.

Not all drug molecules in the circulating fluid will reach their target cells because of protein binding. Once in the bloodstream, the drug may attach itself to a protein molecule (usually albumin), forming a drug-protein complex. This process is termed **protein binding** and significantly impacts how much drug is available to the site of action. Drugs bound to protein circulate in the plasma until they are released or displaced from the drug-protein complex. Only the unbound portion of the drug is available to deliver its effect within the body. The unbound portion of the drug is called the free or active drug.

Drugs and other chemicals compete for the protein-binding sites. Drug-drug and drug-food interactions may occur when they compete for the same protein-binding sites. The result is fewer protein-binding sites and more circulating free drug. When free drug levels increase, there are greater risks of serious adverse effects and toxicity. One example of this is the drug warfarin (Coumadin). Coumadin is 99 percent protein-bound The antifungal Monistat, even with intravaginal use, and the sulfonamide anti-infective agents displace warfarin from protein-binding sites. As a result, warfarin levels are increased, and the patient is at greater risk for bleeding. It is the nurse's responsibility to know the protein-binding percentage for each drug administered. When giving multiple drugs that are highly protein-bound, the patient should be monitored closely for adverse effects. **Adverse effects** described as unwanted, negative responses to a drug, and these can range in severity from mild to life-threatening. The nurse should also monitor the patient's plasma protein and albumin levels. Low levels in both of these can increase the amount of free drug and increase the risk of toxicity.

Following absorption and distribution, drugs must be detoxified or broken down to a form that can be eliminated. This process is called **metabolism** or **biotransformation.** The liver is the primary organ of metabolism in the body, though the kidneys and the cells of the gastrointestinal (GI) tract also have high metabolic rates. Enzymes produced in the liver are responsible for this chemical change. The system in the liver responsible for this activity is the hepatic microsomal enzyme system. This system is also called the P-450 system, named after cytochrome P-450, which is the major component of the system. Not all drugs metabolized in the liver become inactive; some form active metabolites that may be more potent than the original drug. Consult a drug reference manual for information about P-450 metabolism before administering a drug. Drug-drug interactions and drug-food interactions occur. When a patient is taking more than one medication, a drug may induce metabolism by the P-450 system. This results in diminished drug availability. The other drug may inhibit hepatic enzyme production that decreases metabolism and results in more of the drug being available. Because many medications have a narrow margin of safety, it is extremely important to monitor serum blood levels carefully.

When drugs are administered by the oral route, they are absorbed directly into the hepatic portal circulation, which circulates blood to the liver before entering the general circulation and becoming available to body tissues. As the blood passes through the liver, some drugs are completely metabolized to an inactive form. This process is termed the **first pass effect.** Sublingual, rectal, and parenteral routes of drug administration should be used for those drugs that undergo extensive first-pass metabolism. Some examples of drugs that undergo extensive first-pass metabolism are the antianginal drug nitroglycerin and the antidiabetic agent insulin. Nitroglycerin is administered by sublingual or transdermal route. Insulin is administered by the subcutaneous or parenteral routes.

Drugs that have been metabolized then undergo the process of excretion, which is defined as the process in which a drug is removed from the body. The primary organ of excretion is the kidney, although drugs are excreted through the lungs, bowel, and exocrine glands as well. The chemical structure of the drug determines the organ of excretion. Gaseous and volatile compounds, such as nitrous oxide and alcohol, are removed through the lungs. Encouraging the patient to cough and breathe deeply following surgery facilitates the elimination of anesthetic agents more rapidly. Exocrine glands excrete lipid-soluble medication. This glandular elimination of medications accounts for the strange taste that some patients experience with some IV medications. When medications exit through sweat glands, the skin can become irritated. The nurse should implement strategies to protect skin integrity and maintain cleanliness.

The rate at which drugs are excreted determines their concentration in the bloodstream and in the tissues. Free drugs, water-soluble agents, electrolytes, and small molecules are easily filtered through the glomerulus. Proteins, bloods cells, products of metabolism (conjugates), and drug-protein complexes are not filtered because of their large size. Once filtered through the glomerulus, drugs and chemicals are reabsorbed into the renal tubule. Nonionized and lipid-soluble drugs cross the renal tubular membranes and return to the circulation; ionized and water-soluble drugs remain in the urine for removal. The nurse can encourage fluids to assist with proper elimination of medications.

Certain drugs may be excreted more rapidly if the pH of the urine changes. Weak acids, such as aspirin, are eliminated faster in alkaline urine, a weak base. The reason is that aspirin is ionized in an alkaline environment. A drug that is a weak base, such as diazepam (Valium), is eliminated more quickly in an acidic environment. This is helpful in cases of overdose. The nurse can administer sodium bicarbonate to raise the pH of the urine to be more alkaline to accelerate the excretion of an acid drug in case of overdose. Ammonium chloride acidifies the urine and helps to excrete alkaline drugs more quickly.

Altered kidney function results in the decreased ability to excrete medications. Careful monitoring of the patient's kidney function is a priority nursing responsibility. The nurse must take extra caution when administering drugs that are known to be nephrotoxic or in drugs that are known to have a narrow margin of safety. The best indicator of kidney function is the creatinine clearance. Other laboratory values to monitor include the blood urea nitrogen (BUN) and electrolytes. The nurse understands that inadequate elimination of a drug puts the patient at risk for adverse effects and toxicity.

Drug concentration determines the ability of a drug to exert a therapeutic effect. The effective dose is the minimum amount of a drug needed to produce a therapeutic effect. Toxic concentration is that level that would produce serious adverse effects. The **therapeutic range** is defined as the level between the minimum effective dose and the toxic concentration. The level of a medication must be maintained within this range to achieve desired effects and avoid symptoms of toxicity.

Plasma half-life ($t_{1/2}$) is the time it takes for half of the drug administered to be eliminated or the serum concentration to be decreased by half. Drugs with short half-lives must be administered more frequently, and drugs with longer half-lives can be given once daily (or longer duration). This can influence the pharmacological picture for a patient in many ways. Longer half-lives may improve patient compliance if patients do not need to interrupt daily activities to take their medication. However, for the patients experiencing bothersome side effects, the longer half-life drug will cause them discomfort for a longer period of time, because it takes longer to be eliminated.

Usually, several doses are required to achieve a therapeutic level. Resource reports vary, but it is generally accepted that it takes three to five half-lives to reach equilibrium, or steady state. Equilibrium is the point when the amount of drug entering the system is equal to the amount being eliminated. When it is necessary or desired to reach this level more quickly, a loading dose may be ordered. The loading dose is a one- or two-time order to administer a medication in a dose that is larger than the regular maintenance dose. Examples of drugs that are sometimes ordered in this manner are digoxin, glucocorticoid (Decadron), or heparin (anticoagulant). The nurse needs to remember that drugs must be given on a fixed regular schedule to maintain therapeutic level.

Pharmacodynamic Phase

Pharmacodynamics describes the biological and physiological effects the drug has on the body. Pharmacodynamic processes include the mechanism of action (how and where the drug exerts its effect) and the relationship between drug concentration and desired response. When drugs are being tested, data is gathered to determine the therapeutic index. The therapeutic index value is calculated by dividing the median lethal dose (LD) in 50 percent of the animals tested by the median effective dose (ED) in 50 percent of people or animals. The therapeutic index measures the safety margin of a drug. Drugs with a higher therapeutic index have a greater margin of safety. As values near one (1), there is greater risk for toxicity. Drugs with a narrow margin of safety require frequent and careful monitoring of serum drug levels to avoid symptoms of toxicity. The therapeutic index value formula is:

$$\text{Therapeutic Index} = \frac{\text{Median LD}_{50}}{\text{Median ED}_{50}}$$

Receptors are defined as the site on the cell membrane that can be occupied by a drug to cause an effect within the body. The theory that drugs bind to receptors on cells explains how drugs produce their effects. When a drug binds to a receptor, a specific activity of the cell can be enhanced or inhibited. An agonist is a drug that produces the same type of response as the original substance in the body. A drug that blocks the activity of the original substance is called an antagonist.

Pharmacology reference manuals contain valuable information. The nurse must understand the terminology to understand the significance. Knowing that pharmacokinetics is concerned with how the body acts on the drug, the nurse will include in the nursing assessment factors that may interfere with a drug's absorption, distribution, metabolism, or excretion. Knowledge of pharmacodynamics supplies the nurse with valuable information to include in medication teaching to ensure that the patient receives benefit from the medication.

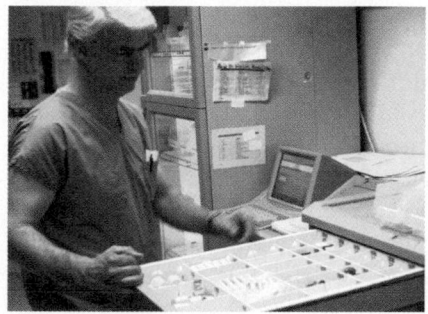

Figure 17-1 Prepare oral medications following the five rights: patient, time, medication, dose, and route.

SAFE MEDICATION ADMINISTRATION

Medication errors are a major problem in the health care industry. MEDMARX, the U.S. Pharmacopeia's voluntary medication error tracking system, received reports of 192,477 incidents in 2002. Computerized order entry is one effort being developed to reduce the incidence of errors (Lafleur, 2004). Patient safety is the number one consideration in medication administration. The goal for implementation of safe medication practices is to limit the number and severity of adverse drug effects. Technology may reduce errors, but diligent nursing care is still required. Nursing education programs go to great lengths to ensure that nursing students understand the Five Rights of Medication Administration (or some sources state six) (Figure 17-1). When tracking medication errors in health care facilities, the primary cause is a deviation or failure to adhere to these five rights (Box 17-1). Professional nurses can advocate for patient safety by maintaining a continued awareness of, and adherence to, the principles learned in nursing school.

Five Rights and Three Checks

The first of the five rights of medication administration is the need to select the right patient. Nurses must correctly identify the patient for which the drug is intended. Consistently matching the medication administration record (MAR) to the patient's identification armband is one way. Asking patients their names is not sufficient. The Joint Commission on Accreditation of Healthcare Organizations (JCAHO) is requiring health care facilities to implement policies that require two forms of identification. This includes matching two pieces of information, such as the patient's name and his or her date of birth with what is printed on the armband, then comparing the MAR to the armband. In the absence of an armband, the nurse should verify the patient's identity by requesting picture identification or by asking the patient for two identifying pieces of information (date of birth and address). The nurse should place the armband as soon as identity is confirmed.

The nurse must ensure that the right drug is being administered. Three checks can be implemented at this time. The steps involved include: (a) check the drug against the MAR when removing it from the storage location; (b) check the label against the MAR when preparing it for administration; and (c) check again immediately prior to administering the drug.

The nurse must ensure that the right dose is being administered. Several changes have occurred in the recent past to ensure that patients receive the right drug and the right dose. Physician orders are being sent directly to the pharmacy for interpretation. The vast majority of drugs are available by unit dose, and there is a movement to have electronic dispensing of medications. The nurse is responsible and accountable for using the resources available to know what dosages are appropriate and those that should be questioned. Another safe practice is to bring the MAR to the bedside with the medications in sealed packages. This plan offers yet another opportunity to compare the medication with MAR for accuracy.

The nurse must ensure that the medication is administered the right route. The nurse must apply the correct techniques required for the specific route of administration. To administer intramuscular medications, the nurse must identify the correct and most appropriate site for the medication being given. Oral medications may be given with or without food. Some medications cannot be crushed (Table 17-1).

The nurse must ensure that the medication is being given at the right time. Time will depend on the pharmacokinetic properties, particularly absorption and pharmacodynamics of the prescribed drug. If the physician does not specify times, it is important to refer to a reputable drug reference. Table 17-2 provides a list of common abbreviations used in scheduling medications. After careful tracking of medication errors, some abbreviations showed patterns of misunderstanding that resulted in errors. To prevent further misunderstanding the JCAHO published a "*Do Not Use*" abbreviation list (Table 17-2.)

The nurse must complete the right documentation. This is sometimes referred to as the sixth right to safe medication administration. Failure to document can result in serious medication errors. Charting a medication prior to its being administered may result in a patient not receiving a critical dose. Both constitute medication errors. Documenting goes beyond charting the medication time. Documentation should include pertinent assessment information, and in the case of as needed (PRN) medications, should include a follow-up assessment to determine if the medication achieved its desired effects.

Other rights have been described in the literature. Seen on the Patient Bill of Rights in many health care institutions is the following: the right for the patient to refuse medication. Based on the ethical principle of autonomy, the patient who is capable of making competent decisions can, when presented with all the information, make an informed decision to refuse medication. It is important that there is documentation that the patient understands the consequences of the decision. To give informed consent, the patient has a right to receive medication teaching. Patient teaching is a primary responsibility of the nurse. When providing medication instructions, the teaching plan should include the following information: the reason for taking the drug and the expected outcomes; the **side effects,** which are physiological effects the patient may experience that are not directly related to the desired effect of the drug,

TABLE 17-1 Routes of Administration

ROUTE OF ADMINISTRATION	ADVANTAGES	DISADVANTAGES
Oral	Patient comfort Economical Ease of administration Medications can produce either local or systemic effects	Avoid when patient is experiencing nausea or vomiting, has impaired gastric motility, or is postoperative surgical resection of the GI tract Gastric secretions delay some medications Contraindicated in patients with dysphagia May irritate the lining of the GI tract, discolor teeth, or have an unpleasant taste Cannot be given when patient has gastric suction. May need to be held if patient has nothing by mouth for a test. Check with health care provider
Parenteral routes: Subcutaneous Intramuscular IV Intradermal	Alternative to oral route More rapid absorption	Increased risk of infection because of break in protective skin barrier Avoid in patients with decreased clotting times (or taking anticoagulants) Greater risk due to faster absorption rates Can cause anxiety in some patients
Skin topical	Provide primarily local effects Usually painless Minimal risk of side effects	Risk for systemic effects because of rapid absorption in patients with skin abrasions Burning may occur
Transdermal	Provide prolonged systemic effects, with limited side effects	Leaves an oily or pasty substance on the skin; may soil clothing May not stay in place if the patient is diaphoretic; medication patch may to be reapplied (increased cost).
Mucous membranes: Eyes, ears, nose, vagina, rectum, and ostomy	Permits local application of medication Aqueous solutions are readily absorbed; capable of producing systemic effects Alternative route to oral	Mucous membranes are sensitive Rectal and vaginal insertion can be embarrassing for the patient Ear irrigation is contraindicated if eardrum is ruptured Rectal suppositories are contraindicated if the patient is neutropenic or has thrombocytopia or has had rectal surgery, has active rectal bleeding, or has a closed head injury
Inhalation	Provides rapid relief for local respiratory problems Easy access	Some local agents can cause serious systemic effects

Adapted from Broyles, B. E., Reiss, B. S., & Evans, M. E. (2007). Pharmacological aspects of nursing care (7th ed.). New York: Thomson Delmar Learning.

and how to manage them; adverse effects, which need to be reported to the health care provider; instructions for medication self-administration; and other special monitoring requirements that the specific drug may necessitate. The nurse should adapt education materials to the patient's level of understanding and evaluate understanding at the end of each education session. Providing written materials can be reminders and reinforcements of information.

TABLE 17-2 **Table of Common Abbreviations and JCAHO List of Abbreviations Not to Be Used**

COMMON ABBREVIATIONS

AC	Before meals
Ad Lib	As desired
AM	In the morning
BID	Twice daily
Cap	Capsule
Gtt	Drop
H/Hr	Hour
HS	Bedtime
PC	After meals
PM	In the evening
PRN	As needed
QID	Four times daily
STAT	Give immediately
Tab	Tablet
TID	Three times daily

JCAHO "Do Not Use" Abbreviation List

PROHIBITED ENTRY AND EXPLANATION	PREFERRED USAGE
Q.D. (once a day) and Q.O.D. (every other day) can be confused with one another	Daily and every other day
Trailing zero after a decimal point (e.g., 4.0) makes it easy to overlook the decimal point	Use a zero before a decimal point (e.g., 0.4 mg) but never after
MS, MSO_4, and $MGSO_4$ can be read as morphine sulfate or magnesium sulfate	Morphine sulfate or magnesium sulfate
U (unit) can be mistaken for a zero	Unit
IU (international unit) can be misread as IV or as 10	International unit

Adapted from Joint Commission on Accreditation of Healthcare Organizations. (2004). 2004 national patient safety goals. Retrieved February 7, 2005, from http://jcaho.org.

Geriatric Considerations

The elderly population occupies a large proportion of inpatient hospital beds. It is important for the nurse to take into consideration the changes in geriatric physiology that impact this group's response to drug therapy (Figure 17-2). A major problem identified in the geriatric population is polypharmacy. **Polypharmacy** can be defined as the situation in which multiple drugs are prescribed to treat a variety of conditions. With knowledge of pharmacokinetics, the nurse realizes that taking many drugs creates the possibility of drug-drug interactions, variable levels of medication, and increased risks for adverse

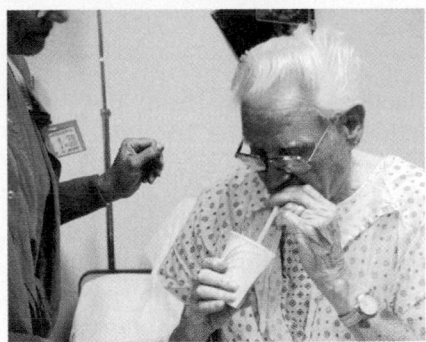

Figure 17-2 Elderly patients require special considerations when taking medications.

effects. It is important that the primary health care provider be aware of all the medications a person is taking so that the risk can be minimized.

The aging process can alter the pharmacokinetic process. Absorption is altered because of a change in gastric pH and peristalsis. Gastric pH becomes more alkaline (pH increases), and peristalsis tends to slow down. Both factors affect absorption. Laxative use, a common practice of the elderly, can cause medications to be eliminated before they provide a benefit.

The aging cardiovascular system with decreased cardiac output and less efficient blood circulation can slow drug distribution. Generally, medication must be started in lower doses and slowly increased to a safe, effective dose. Metabolism is altered because of changes in liver function. Liver enzyme production decreases making it more difficult to detoxify or break down drugs. The aging liver also produces fewer albumins that decrease the number of protein-binding sites available. The result is increased levels of free (active) drugs in the circulating fluids and greater risk of toxicity and drug-drug interactions.

Excretion is impacted by decreased blood flow to the kidney and decreased nephron function or filtration. Without being able to eliminate drugs efficiently, blood concentrations of drugs tend to rise and cause toxicity. Percentage of body water decreases, and the geriatric patient is particularly vulnerable to dehydration. Levels of some drugs are increased by fluid volume deficit. The ratio of body fat to water increases, which enhances the storage of fat-soluble drugs and vitamins. The ratio of fat to muscle increases, which decreases metabolism. A more general concern is that immune function tends to decrease with age, so the elderly patient is at greater risk for autoimmune diseases and infections. The nurse should advocate for routine immunizations, such as influenza and pneumonia, for the elderly.

Pharmacological Resources Available to the Practicing Nurse

Drug information is readily available to the practicing nurse. JCAHO requires that up-to-date drug reference books be located on each hospital unit. Hospital pharmacists are a phone call away. The Internet provides immediate access to current information on medications for both professionals and the lay person. The disadvantage of Internet resources is that one must be discriminating about the source of the information. Many drug references written for nurses are now available with versions that can be downloaded onto a personal digital assistant (PDA) A partial list of available resources for current drug information include: (a) United States Pharmacopeia, (b) Davis Drug Guide for Nurses, (c) Mosby's Drug Guide, (d) Lexi-Comps Drug Information Handbook for Nursing, (e) Epocrates, and (f) PEPID RN.

Ethical Considerations

Providing medication information that enables the patient to make decisions about pharmacotherapy regimens reflects ethical practice and support for the ethical principle autonomy. The nurse practice act of each state defines the role of the nurse in relation to drug administration. The administration of medications by the nurse includes several aspects of legal liability. The nurse cannot give medications without a complete written order (Box 17-2). Nurses are responsible for their actions even with a written order. It is the nurse's responsibility to question any order that appears inappropriate. Because lack of knowledge about medications is a cause for errors, the nurse must stay current in pharmacotherapeutics. The nurse must never give a medication without knowing what it is, what it is for, and what to evaluate. To give a medication without knowing these points is unsafe practice.

BOX 17-2

COMPONENTS OF A COMPLETE DRUG ORDER

- Full name of the patient
- Date and time the drug order was written
- Name of the drug to be given to the patient
- Dosage of the drug to be administered
- Frequency of administration
- Route of drug administration
- Signature of person writing the order

ANTI-INFECTIVE AGENTS

Anti-infective drugs are used to treat infections resulting from the rapid growth of invading pathogens. These pathogens may be bacteria, fungi, viruses, protozoa, or rickettsiae. Laboratory tests, such as a culture and sensitivity, should be done before initiating antibiotic treatment. The culture identifies the organism, and the sensitivity determines the antibiotic that would be most effective against the infecting microorganism. Indiscriminate use of broad-spectrum antibiotics without laboratory identification of the pathogen is a leading factor in the development antibiotic resistance. The nurse must remember that a culture must be collected before administering the first dose of an antibiotic. In this discussion, the terms antibacterial, antimicrobial, and antibiotics are used interchangeably.

Bacteria are single-cell organisms without a nucleus capable of reproducing every 20 minutes. Bacteria create toxins that cause cell death. Bacteria can be classified by the structure of the cell wall. Under a microscope, a crystal violet gram stain is applied. The bacteria that maintain the violet stain have a thick cell wall and are called gram-positive bacteria. Examples of gram-positive bacteria are staphylococci, streptococci, and enterococci. Bacteria with a thinner cell wall lose the violet color and are called gram-negative. Examples of gram-negative bacteria are *Escherichia coli, Klebsiella, Pseudomonas,* and *Salmonella.*

Shape of the cellular wall is a second means of classifying bacteria. Rod shapes are called bacilli, spherical shapes are called cocci, and spirals are called spirilla. A third factor used to classify bacteria is their ability to use oxygen. The bacteria that thrive on oxygen are called aerobic; those that grow best without oxygen are called anaerobic.

Anti-infectives can be bacteriostatic or bactericidal. Bacteriostatic drugs inhibit the growth of the offending organism and depend on the host's body defenses to destroy the bacteria. Bactericidal drugs kill the offending organism. Depending on the drug dose and serum blood level, some anti-infectives can do both. Body defenses, which affect the host's ability to fight infection, include: (a) age; (b) nutrition; (c) immune system function; (d) levels of white blood cells; (e) organ function; and (f) circulation. Three major adverse reactions associated with anti-infective therapy are hypersensitivity reaction, superinfection, and organ toxicity.

Anti-infectives are grouped into classifications by their chemical structure or therapeutic properties. Anti-infectives belonging to the same chemical groups have similar antimicrobial properties and similar side effects. Another way to classify these drugs is by mechanism of action. Examples include: inhibition of cell wall synthesis, alteration in membrane permeability, inhibition of protein synthesis, inhibition of synthesis of bacterial RNA and DNA, and interference with metabolism within the cell.

To be effective, the drug must have an affinity to the binding sites on the cell wall and must penetrate the bacterial cell wall at a high enough concentration to disrupt or destroy the bacteria. The longer the drug stays bound to the cell, the better the action. The drug must be maintained at a minimum effective concentration (MEC) to be effective. Nursing implications are that anti-infectives are scheduled over 24 hours, and timing of administration is important.

Penicillins and Cephalosporins

Penicillin drugs kill bacteria by disrupting their cell walls. The portion of the chemical structure of penicillin that is responsible for its antibacterial effects is the beta-lactam ring. This ring inhibits the bacterial enzyme needed for cell division and cellular synthesis. When penicillin binds to penicillin binding protein located on the bacterial cell wall, the cell wall is weakened, and water enters the cell. The result is cell death. The action of penicillin is most efficient during cell division. Some bacteria secrete the beta-lactamase enzyme. The beta-lactamase enzyme that attacks and inactivates penicillin and other beta lactam antibiotics called penicillinase.

Cephalosporins, like penicillins, contain a beta-lactam ring that accounts for their antimicrobial properties. Because of their similarity, patients who are allergic to penicillins may also be allergic to cephalosporins. This is known as cross-sensitivity. The mechanism of action of cephalosporins is the same as that of the penicillins. There are four generations of cephalosporins. The first through third generations demonstrate increased activity against gram-negative organisms and anaerobes and less activity against gram-positive organisms. First generation does not enter the cerebrospinal fluid and is less effective against aerobic gram-negative organisms such as *E. coli* and *Klebsiella pneumoniae*. Fourth generation has increased activity against gram-positive cocci and gram-negative bacilli (Broyles, Reiss, & Evans, 2007).

Indications

Aminopenicillins are broad-spectrum antibiotics that are effective against both gram-positive and gram-negative bacteria. They are used to treat upper respiratory tract infections, pneumonia, otitis media, sinusitis, sexually transmitted diseases ([STDs] not including gonorrhea), wound infections and urinary tract infections (UTIs), meningitis, skin, bone, and joint infections, stomach infections, blood and valve infections, gas gangrene, tetanus, anthrax, and sickle cell anemia. Additionally, penicillins are frequently ordered prophylactically to prevent endocarditis in patients undergoing dental, GI, and pulmonary procedures.

Extended-spectrum penicillins (antipseudomonal penicillins) are effective in treating gram-negative organisms such as *Pseudomonas aeruginosa*. These penicillins are called beta-lactamase inhibitors and exert their effect by inhibiting the bacterial beta-lactamase enzyme. The combination of broad-spectrum penicillin with a beta-lactamase inhibitor has proven to be more effective in treating bacterial infections and extends the antimicrobial effects. Augmentin is an example of this combination: amoxicillin plus clavulanic acid.

Third generation cephalosporins are used to treat cervicitis, urethritis, pharyngitis, and proctitis caused by *Neisseria gonorrhoeae*. These antimicrobial agents are effective in treating upper respiratory tract infections, such as bronchitis, pharyngitis, otitis media, sinusitis, and pneumonia. They are also used to treat UTIs, skin and tissue infections, and Lyme disease.

Pharmacokinetics

It is important to refer to a reputable nursing drug reference for the pharmacokinetic properties of the specific prescribed drug. Oral dosing of penicillin should be three to four times greater than the parenteral dose because of extensive first-pass effect and the instability of penicillin in the acid environment of the stomach. Absorption is unpredictable when given intramuscularly because of irritability of the tissues. When given intravenously, it should be administered slowly over 12 to 15 seconds to minimize discomfort and prevent needle obstruction. Some preparations, such as Pen V, amoxicillin, and Augmentin, need to be given with food to minimize GI upset. Others need to be taken with a full glass of water and one hour before or two hours after meals to increase absorption.

Cephalosporins are generally well absorbed. Food can delay absorption, but bioavailability is not affected. To promote absorption, the nurse needs to schedule oral administration of antacids, histamine H_2 blockers, iron supplements, and foods fortified with iron two hours before or after oral administration of cephalosporins.

Pharmacodynamics

Beta-lactam antibiotics exert bactericidal effects when used in therapeutic dosages and are administered by the appropriate route. Drug administration should be continued for at least 10 days to decrease the risk of rheumatic fever in beta-hemolytic streptococcal bacterial infections, such as strep throat. Glomerulonephritis can become a sequela of this infection if treatment is inadequate.

Laboratory Monitoring

Monitor complete blood count (CBC with white blood cell count with differential). Penicillins can cause increased bleeding; therefore, it is necessary to monitor prothrombin time (PT) and international normalized ratio (INR) if patient is on oral anticoagulants and activated partial thromboplastin time (aPTT) if on a parenteral anticoagulant. The nurse should monitor liver function tests, such as alanine aminotransferase (ALT), aspartate aminotransferase (AST), bilirubin, and alkaline phosphatase. An elevated aPTT may require the administration of the antagonist protamine sulfate. If the PT is prolonged, the nurse needs to be prepared to administer vitamin K. The nurse should monitor electrolytes, especially potassium and sodium. The penicillins are structured with a sodium or potassium salt. When a high sodium penicillin is administered, serum sodium may be elevated, which often causes a decrease in potassium. With parenteral administration or prolonged administration, renal function needs to be monitored by checking BUN and serum creatinine and doing a urinalysis.

Side Effects and Adverse Effects

Central nervous system (CNS) side effects that may occur include lethargy, hallucinations, anxiety, depression, twitching, convulsions, and coma. GI side effects include nausea and vomiting, diarrhea, abdominal cramps, increased liver function tests, and colitis. Hematological side effects include anemia, increased bleeding time, bone marrow depression, and granulocytopenia. Metabolic side effects include hyperkalemia, hypokalemia, and alkalosis. The medications may cause taste alterations, sore mouth, dark, discolored tongue, hives, pruritus, rash, and edema. Side effects tend to be mild unless the patient is allergic. Patients complain of GI side effects, such as nausea and vomiting, most frequently.

The most serious adverse effect is anaphylactic, which is often fatal if not treated immediately. Symptoms include: (a) nausea and vomiting; (b) urticaria, pruritus; (c) severe dyspnea, stridor, tachycardia, and hypotension; and (d) diaphoresis, vertigo, loss of consciousness, and circulatory collapse. It is important to remember there is a cross-sensitivity between penicillin and cephalosporin drugs.

Other serious adverse effects that may occur are a serum sickness–like reaction that is evidenced by skin rash, pain in the joints, elevated temperature, exfoliative dermatitis, blood dyscrasias, and superinfections. Pseudomembranous colitis, often caused by *Clostridium difficile,* is a superinfection in which the normal flora of the intestine has been altered, and severe diarrhea develops. If this occurs, a change in antibiotics is required. Patients being treated with cephalosporins may develop seizures. By discontinuing the cephalosporin agent, the problem should resolve.

Nursing Management

There are many interventions to be employed when taking penicillins and cephalosporins. The patient needs to be provided with specific drug information and instructed to take the complete course of treatment. Teaching should emphasize drinking adequate fluids and maintain nutrition, especially protein, to ensure adequate protein binding for the drug and efficacy of action. Oral penicillin G should be taken with water, because acidic fruit juice can inactivate the drug's antibacterial activity. The patient should schedule dosages over 24 hours to maintain adequate levels. In general, the patient should report signs of hypersensitivity or superinfections to the health care provider. (Note: eating cultured dairy products will help discourage superinfections.) (see Red Flag.)

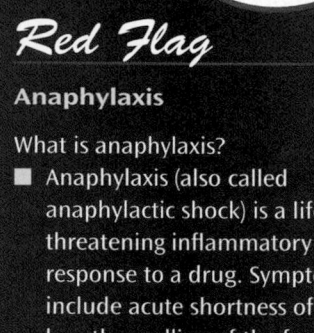

Red Flag

Anaphylaxis

What is anaphylaxis?
- Anaphylaxis (also called anaphylactic shock) is a life-threatening inflammatory response to a drug. Symptoms include acute shortness of breath, swelling of the face and throat, hypotension, and tachycardia. Without rapid intervention, cardiac arrest and death can occur.

How is anaphylaxis treated?
- Remember your ABCs: Maintain the patient's airway, breathing, and circulation.
- Epinephrine, the drug of choice, will be administered intravenously or subcutaneously depending on the severity of the reaction and the physician order.
- Another antihistamine, such as diphenhydramine (Benadryl), may be given to prevent further anti-inflammatory response.
- Provide supplemental oxygen.
- Monitor blood pressure and pulse until stabilized and returned to normal (Hathaway, 2004)

Nursing Management

There are a wide variety of nursing strategies to be used for patients who are taking penicillins and cephalosporins. Examples of these management approaches are shown in Box 17-3.

Macrolides, Tetracyclines, Aminoglycosides, and Fluoroquinolones

Though different in structure, these drugs are grouped together, because they are similar in spectrums of antibiotic effectiveness to penicillin and are used for people who are allergic to penicillin. The macrolides (erythromycin, clarithromycin, azithromycin, and dirithromycin) and tetracyclines are primarily bacteriostatic but can be bactericidal depending on the dose and the pathogen. Aminoglycosides and fluoroquinolones are bactericidal drugs.

Macrolides, so called because of their large size, are safe alternatives to penicillin. The macrolide antibiotics inhibit bacterial protein synthesis. They are bacteriostatic or bactericidal depending on dose and target organism. Salts are added to erythromycins to decrease their dissolution in the stomach. Erythromycin is prescribed frequently as an alternative for people allergic to penicillin.

Tetracyclines were the first broad-spectrum antibiotic effective against both gram-positive and gram-negative bacteria and many other organisms, such as mycobacteria, rickettsiae, spirochetes, and chlamydiae. They work by inhibiting bacterial protein synthesis and are bacteriostatic. Bacterial resistance has resulted from continuous use of these drugs.

Aminoglycosides are bactericidal, inhibiting bacterial protein synthesis by causing synthesis of abnormal proteins. Because this group of antibiotics is more toxic that others, their use is limited to serious gram-negative bacteria (*E. coli,* proteus, *Klebsiella,* and *Pseudomonas*), mycobacteria, and some protozoans.

Fluoroquinolones is the newest class of broad-spectrum bactericidal antibiotics. They affect deoxyribonucleic acid (DNA) synthesis by inhibiting two bac-

---

BOX 17-3

NURSING STRATEGIES FOR ADMINISTERING PENICILLINS AND CEPHALOSPORINS

- Assessing the patient for allergies. Remember, if a patient has experienced a previous hypersensitivity reaction to penicillins, cephalosporins should be avoided due to the risk for cross-sensitivity.
- Obtaining culture and sensitivity prior to initiating antibiotic therapy.
- Collecting vital signs and laboratory testing (CBC, electrolytes, and renal and liver function) prior and during treatment.
- Monitoring response to therapy: reduced fever, white blood cell decrease, absence of presenting symptoms, and improved appetite.
- After parenteral administration of penicillin, monitoring the patient for at least 30 minutes, especially after the first dose.
- Monitoring for superinfections (with *C. difficile,* antibiotic therapy should be discontinued and steps taken to ensure adequate fluid or electrolyte replacement).
- Assessing for bleeding disorders in the patient receiving cephalosporins, because these drugs may reduce PT levels through interference with vitamin K metabolism. Liver function is an important consideration, because it is important in the production of vitamin K.

terial enzymes: DNA gyrase and topoisomerase IV. The fluoroquinolones are effective against both gram-positive and gram-negative organisms.

Indications

Macrolides are used to treat upper and lower respiratory tract infections, GI tract infections, skin and soft tissue infections caused by *Streptococcus* or *Haemophilus* organisms, and otitis media. They are also used to treat syphilis, gonorrhea, chlamydia, Lyme disease, and *Mycoplasma, Listeria* and *Corynebacterium* infections. Clarithromycin (Biaxin) is used with omeprazole (Prilosec) to treat *Helicobacter pylori* associated with peptic ulcer disease (PUD).

Because the large number of resistant bacterial strains to tetracyclines, their use is limited to a few diseases, such as: Rocky Mountain spotted fever, typhus, cholera, Lyme disease, ulcers caused by *H. pylori,* and chlamydial infections. Because tetracyclines bind metal ions such as iron and calcium, tetracycline absorption can be reduced by as much as 50 percent if taken with milk or iron.

Aminoglycosides are for serious infections. Streptomycin sulfate was the first aminoglycoside available for use and was used to treat tuberculosis. It is not used as much today because of its ototoxicity and the bacterial resistance that can develop. Streptomycin is still the drug of choice to treat tularemia and bubonic forms of plague. Aminoglycosides are poorly absorbed through the GI tract, so they are usually administered intramuscularly or intravenously with the exception of Neomycin that is given orally to decrease bacteria and other organisms in the bowel prior to surgery.

Fluoroquinolones are used to treat UTIs, bone and joint infections, bronchitis, pneumonia, gastroenteritis, and gonorrhea.

Pharmacokinetics

Macrolides and fluoroquinolones have many potential drug-drug interactions, because they are highly protein-bound. Drugs such as carbamazepine, warfarin, or theophylline may have increased effects when given concurrently with macrolides. Zithromax has a longer half-life with less frequent dosing and fewer or less intense GI side effects. The acid in the stomach inactivates erythromycin, so it is administered as coated tablets or capsules intended to dissolve in the small intestine. Aminoglycosides are generally given intramuscularly or intravenously, because they cannot be absorbed through the GI tract and do not cross into the cerebrospinal fluid.

Oral antacids, iron, zinc preparations, and sucralfate reduce the absorption of fluoroquinolones. Caffeine elimination with ciprofloxacin (Cipro) is decreased. Use of nonsteroidal anti-inflammatory drugs (NSAIDs) with levofloxacin (Levaquin) increases CNS stimulation, including seizures; levofloxacin may also increase or decrease blood glucose in conjunction with oral antidiabetic agents. With oral anticoagulants, bleeding may increase because the antibiotics alter intestinal flora and interfere with synthesis of vitamin K.

Pharmacodynamics

Onset of action and duration is dependent on the preparation route of administration. Please refer to a current drug reference manual for this information. A general principle is that drugs administered intravenously will have a more rapid onset of action.

Laboratory Monitoring

It is important to check the white blood cell count with differential to determine therapeutic response. Neutrophils and immature neutrophils, called stabs or bands, are increased in acute bacterial infections. In addition liver function tests should be conducted to assess for early signs of hepatotoxicity. Serum creatinine, BUN, creatinine clearance, and urinalysis should be checked for signs of nephrotoxicity. With streptomycin therapy, caloric tests are assessed for baseline data and to monitor for vestibular toxicity. Peak and trough drug levels are drawn on patients receiving aminoglycosides. The **peak drug level** is defined as the time it takes for a drug to reach its highest concentration in the blood. It is drawn 15 to 30 minutes following IV infusion of an aminoglycoside to determine that toxic levels do not occur. If the peak is too high, the dosage may need to be decreased. The **trough drug level** is defined as the minimum blood serum level of a drug reached immediately before the next scheduled dose. It is drawn immediately before the next scheduled IV infusion to determine that therapeutic levels of the drug are maintained between administrations. If the level is low, the dosage or the frequency of administration may need to be increased.

Side Effects and Adverse Effects

Macrolides stimulate smooth muscle and increase GI motility resulting in diarrhea. These antibiotics can exacerbate existing cardiac pathology that is evidenced by palpitations and chest pain. The patient may experience CNS side effects, including hearing loss preceded by tinnitus and GI symptoms, such as stomatitis, flatulence, epigastric distress, anorexia, nausea and vomiting, and an abnormal taste. Skin side effects that may appear are jaundice, rash, pruritus, and urticaria. Thrombophlebitis at the peripheral IV site may develop because local irritation during infusions. (See Uncovering the Evidence.)

Photosensitivity is a side effect of tetracyclines, which may lead to tingling and burning of the skin, similar to sunburn. They are also known to interfere with the effectiveness of oral contraceptives, and women need to use alternative methods of contraception while taking this drug. Neuromuscular function may be impaired in patients receiving aminoglycosides. Patients with neuromuscular disorders, such as myasthenia gravis and Parkinson's disease, may

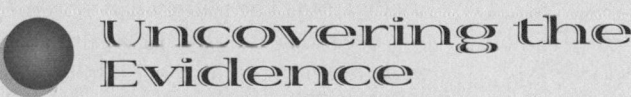

Uncovering the Evidence

Oral Erythromycin Risks

Discussion: In a recent study involving 1,476 cases of confirmed cardiac deaths, researchers documented that patients concurrently taking erythromycin and other drugs that inhibit the enzyme CYP3A of the cytochrome P-450 system were five times more likely to experience sudden death than patients not on erythromycin and other CYP3A inhibitors. When erythromycin is taken alone the low risk of cardiac death is doubled. The researchers studied the medical records of Medicaid patients from Tennessee who died of cardiac arrest between 1988 and 1993 to compare the outcomes for patients taking erythromycin or amoxicillin. Erythromycin prolongs cardiac repolarization and amoxicillin does not. The researchers also looked for other drugs that inhibit erythromycin metabolism.

The results showed that those who took erythromycin along with drugs, such as calcium channel blockers, which are known to inhibit its metabolism, are five times more likely to develop ventricular dysrhythmias and sudden death.

Implications for Practice: The researchers from this study urge prescribers to select another anti-infective, such as amoxicillin, for patients taking CYP3A inhibitors. Different anti-infective agents will potentially have better results for patients.

Source: Ray, W. A., Murray, K. T., Meredith, S., Narasimhulu, S. S., Hall, K., & Stein, C. M. (2004). Oral erythromycin and the risk of sudden death from cardiac causes. New England Journal of Medicine, 351(11), 1089.

experience greater muscle weakness. Other side effects include headache, paresthesia, skin rash, and fever.

The fluoroquinolones can produce CNS effects, such as headache, dizziness, fatigue, lethargy, insomnia, depression, restlessness, confusion, and convulsions; GI side effects; skin side effects, such as photosensitivity, blurred vision, and tinnitus. Macrolides can cause hepatotoxicity, nephrotoxicity, ototoxicity (erythromycin), and superinfections. See Uncovering the Evidence for the new findings that taking erythromycin with other drugs that inhibit enzyme CYP3A can increase the risk of sudden cardiac death. Aminoglycosides are most known for their toxic effects on the kidneys and vestibular apparatus. Risk of ototoxicity is increased when aminoglycosides are administered concurrently with other nephrotoxic drugs or other ototoxic drugs, such as furosemide and vancomycin.

Nursing Management

Education is a vital component when caring for patients taking macrolides, tetracyclines, aminoglycosides, and fluoroquinolones. The patient needs to be provided with specific drug information (e.g., name, dose, and schedule). The patient needs to be instructed to report signs and symptoms of increasing infection and to report signs and symptoms of superinfection. Patients must be reminded to complete the full course of treatment and to schedule doses over a 24-hour period to maintain a therapeutic level. Education to include protein in the diet is reinforced, because these drugs are highly protein-bound and need protein for improved action. In general, photosensitivity precautions are suggested and tetracyclines are not to be taken with milk products, iron supplements, magnesium-containing laxatives, or antacids. Patients must be taught that alkaline foods (e.g., dairy products, vegetables, and legumes) can decrease the pH of the stomach and inhibit absorption of the fluoroquinolone antibiotics. The patient taking aminoglycosides is taught to increase fluid intake, unless contraindicated by the health care provider, to promote excretion of the medication. The patient can be reminded that macrolides can exacerbate existing heart disease, and the health care provider should get baseline hearing tests and monitor for hearing loss from macrolides (erythromycin) and aminoglycosides. The patient should also be monitored for nephrotoxicity, as tetracyclines are contraindicated for patients with renal disease. Patients should be taught that they need to monitor for ototoxicity. Also, tetracyclines decrease the effectiveness of oral contraceptives, so females should be instructed to use alternative forms of birth control while taking these medications.

Sulfonamides

Sulfonamides are the oldest antibacterial agents. They were first isolated from coal tar derivative in the early 1900s and first used for coccal infections in 1935. Sulfonamides have broad-spectrum activity and are effective against both gram-positive and gram-negative bacteria. They are bacteriostatic, and they act to suppress bacterial cell growth by inhibiting bacterial synthesis of folic acid (folate).

Indications

Sulfonamides are used to treat UTIs, especially *E. coli,* the most common cause of cystitis, *Chlamydia trachomatis* causing blindness, pneumonia, brain abscesses, mild to moderate ulcerative colitis, active Crohn's disease, and rheumatoid arthritis. Pyrimethamine is the only effective drug treatment for toxoplasmosis and is the drug of choice for the treatment of nocardiosis.

Pharmacokinetics

Sulfonamides are classified by their rate of absorption and excretion. Many drug-drug interactions are potentially problematic when administered with sulfonamide drugs. Bleeding times may be increase for patients taking anticoagulants (warfarin). The combination of sulfonamides with oral hypoglycemic agents may lead to excessive drops in blood glucose. There is a cross-sensitivity with diuretics, such as acetazolamide, and the thiazides, and with sulfonylurea antidiabetic agents. Use of these agents in patients with previous hypersensitivity to sulfonamides can induce a skin abnormality called Stevens-Johnson syndrome. Patients who are stabilized on phenytoin (Dilantin) may experience signs of phenytoin toxicity (e.g., nystagmus or ataxia). The combination of trimethoprim and sulfamethoxazole (Bactrim) combines a sulfonamide with a folic acid antagonist. This results in a synergistic effect against certain bacteria.

Common classifications of sulfonamides include: (a) short acting (e.g., Gantrisin or sulfadiazine); (b) intermediate-acting (e.g., Gantanol); (c) poor absorption (e.g., sulfasalazine); and (d) ultra-long acting (e.g., sulfadoxine).

Laboratory Monitoring

To assess and monitor renal function the nurse should obtain creatinine, BUN, creatinine clearance, and urinalysis. It is necessary to monitor liver function tests including the ALT, AST, bilirubin, and alkaline phosphatase throughout treatment for hepatic function. The nurse should check the CBC and white blood cell count with differential to determine response to therapy and for early detection of any blood dyscrasias.

Side Effects and Adverse Effects

The most common side effect of sulfonamides may include an allergic response, such as skin rash and itching. Though uncommon, blood disorders may develop with prolonged use and high doses. GI disorders may also occur. The early sulfonamides were insoluble in acid urine; thus crystalluria and hematuria were common problems. Photosensitivity can occur. Cross-sensitivity can occur between other sulfonamides but does not occur with other antibacterial drugs.

Sulfonamides are generally safe drugs but can cause some potentially serious adverse effects. Serious adverse effects include hypersensitivity reactions and potentially fatal blood abnormalities. Aplastic anemia or agranulocytosis may occur because of the direct toxic effect on the bone marrow. Acute hemolytic anemia may occur in those patients whose red blood cells are sensitized due to a G6PD enzyme deficiency. These reactions are uncommon, but when they do occur the drug must promptly be discontinued. The most serious form of skin hypersensitivity is the Stevens-Johnson syndrome, consisting of redness and ulceration of the mucous membranes of the eyes, mouth, and urethra. This resembles the appearance of second-degree burns and has been described with all sulfonamides.

Nursing Management

The patient taking sulfonamides can be taught to complete the full course of treatment and create a schedule over a 24-hour time period to maintain therapeutic level. The patient must take the medication with a full glass of water and take it with food, if not contraindicated, to minimize GI upset. In addition, the patient should be taught to eat small, frequent meals with at least 2,500 to 3,000 mL fluid intake per day. The nurse should instruct the patient to take safety precautions if experiencing dizziness, disturbed equilibrium, or seizures and to avoid direct exposure to sunlight, use sunscreen, and wear protective clothing to decrease effects of photosensitivity.

CARDIOVASCULAR AGENTS

Many drugs affect the cardiovascular system. This section will discuss cardiac glycosides, antianginal, and antidysrhythmic drugs. Drugs that stimulate the autonomic nervous system influence heart contractions. Drugs that stimulate the sympathetic nervous system increase the heart rate, whereas drugs that stimulate the parasympathetic nervous system slow the heart rate.

Cardiac Glycosides

Digitalis is one of the oldest drugs, with documented use since 1200 A.D. It is obtained from the purple and white foxglove plant. Digitalis preparations are used to treat congestive heart failure (CHF). The American Heart Association (AHA) defines heart failure as a complex clinical syndrome that impairs the ability of the ventricles to fill with or eject blood. The myocardium is weakened and enlarged and can no longer pump the blood into the systemic circulation in an effective manner. As a result there is insufficient oxygen available to the tissues in the body. The patient can experience right- or left-sided failure. In right-sided failure the heart does not pump returning (unoxygenated) blood into the right atrium from the systemic circulation. The result is blood and fluid buildup in peripheral tissues (peripheral edema). The patient with right-sided heart failure exhibits jugular venous distension, liver engorgement, ascites, and sacral, pretibial and pedal edema (Riggs, 2004). In left-sided failure the left ventricle does not contract forcefully enough to pump blood from the left atrium and lungs into the aorta. This causes excessive amounts of blood to stay in the lung tissue, causing crackles in posterior lung fields. The patient may have a rapid heart rate, as well as rapid and labored breathing, and pulse oximetry may indicate low O_2 saturation. One type of heart failure can lead to another.

Cardiac glycosides act by inhibiting the sodium-potassium pump. As sodium accumulates, calcium ions are released from their storage areas in the cell. The release of calcium ions causes a more forceful contraction of the myocardial fibers (positive inotropic action). By increasing myocardial contractility, cardiac output is increased, which results in improvement of all symptoms of CHF. A drug's ability to change the heart rate is termed a chronotropic effect. When a drug influences the speed of conduction, this is termed a dromotropic effect. Digitalis preparations have both a negative chronotropic action (a decrease in heart rate) and a negative dromotropic action (suppression of the sinoatrial [SA] node and slowing of the conduction velocity through the atrioventricular [AV] node).

Indications

Cardiac glycosides are used to treat heart failure. The two primary cardiac glycosides are digoxin and digitoxin. Both are effective. The primary difference is that digitoxin has a longer half-life. Digitalis has a narrow margin of safety. Serious adverse effects may result from unmonitored treatment.

Cardiac glycosides are also used to treat atrial fibrillation (a cardiac dysrhythmia with rapid uncoordinated contractions of the atrial myocardium) and atrial flutter (a cardiac dysrhythmia with rapid contractions of 200 to 300 beats per minute [BPM]). This is accomplished through the negative chronotropic and negative dromotropic actions of the digitalis preparation.

Pharmacokinetics

Digoxin in oral tablet form has greater than 70 percent absorption. The rate is 90 percent in liquid form and 90 to 100 percent in capsule form. The protein-binding power for digoxin is low (25 percent), but the half-life is long (30 to 45 hours). Because of its long half life, drug accumulation can occur. The liver metabolizes 30 percent of digoxin and the kidneys eliminate roughly 70 percent. Kidney dysfunction can affect excretion of digoxin, and thyroid dysfunction can alter the metabolism. Digitoxin is a potent cardiac glycoside that has a long half-life and is highly protein-bound It is seldom prescribed, but similarities between the names digoxin and digitoxin require that the nurse exercise extreme caution to administer the correct drug.

Laboratory Monitoring

Before initiating digoxin therapy, the nurse needs to draw a baseline serum digoxin level and baseline levels of potassium, magnesium, and calcium. Serum digoxin levels should be drawn periodically during therapy and at any time the patient exhibits signs of toxicity (Table 17-3). The blood sample should be drawn at least six hours after the daily dose and preferably just before the next daily dose. The therapeutic range of serum digoxin is 0.7 to 2 mcg/mL, and the toxic level is greater than 2 mcg/mL. Elderly are at greater risk for toxicity because of impaired renal function and decreased albumin.

Side Effects and Adverse Effects

The most common side effects of digoxin are nausea, loss of usual appetite, and headache. More serious side effects that can also indicate toxicity include vomiting, diarrhea, shortness of breath, and leg muscle cramps. The most serious adverse effect of digoxin is its ability to cause dysrhythmias, particularly in patients who have low potassium levels. Complaints of visual disturbances such as seeing halos, a yellow or green tinge, or blurring should signal the need for a serum digoxin level to determine that the drug is within therapeutic range. Digoxin toxicity may go unrecognized, because it may look like the flu.

Nursing Management

There are many interventions when administering cardiac glycosides. The patient should be taught to count pulse for one full minute prior to taking digoxin. If the pulse falls below 60 BPM or rises above 110 BPM or if skipped beats are present, the patient should be instructed to call his or her health care provider. In addition, the patient is encouraged to report signs of toxicity (e.g.,

TABLE 17-3 **Digoxin Toxicity**	
Clinical manifestations	Treatment
Anorexia	Because of long half-life, treatment is geared to removal of the drug. Acute toxicity can be treated with gastric lavage, activated charcoal to limit absorption, or administration of digoxin-Fab fragments (Digibind), which is an antidote. Patients are admitted to an intensive care unit for cardiac monitoring.
Diarrhea	
Nausea and vomiting	
Bradycardia (pulse less than 60 BPM)	
Premature ventricular contractions (PVCs)	
Cardiac dysrhythmias	
Headaches	
Malaise	
Blurred vision	
Visual change	Prevention
Halos or rings of light around objects	Assess drug-drug interactions
Seeing lights or bright spots	Assess for toxicity
Changes in color perception, especially yellow green	Assess electrolytes (K, Mg)
Blind spots in vision	Push IV digoxin over five full minutes
Confusion	Check digoxin levels
Delirium	

Adapted from Broyles, B. E., Reiss, B. S., & Evans, M. E. (2007). Pharmacological aspects of nursing care (7th ed.). New York: Thomson Delmar Learning.

nausea, vomiting, and decreased appetite) and to hold his or her next scheduled medication. The patient is educated to avoid over-the-counter (OTC) medications or herbal preparations, such as ginseng, which can increase the risk of digoxin toxicity. Ma-huang and ephedra may cause dysrhythmias. A baseline and ongoing physical assessments need to be taken, including neurological, heart rate, blood pressure, and cardiac rhythm. Advise patients to eat foods high in potassium, such as oranges, bananas, fruit juices, vegetables, and potatoes, if taking loop diuretics. The intake and output need to be monitored, and the patient must be weighed daily and assessed for clinical manifestations of heart failure.

Antianginal Agents

Antianginal agents are used to treat angina pectoris. Angina is defined as acute cardiac pain caused by inadequate oxygen reaching the myocardium. Over six million Americans have angina pectoris, with over 350,000 new cases each year. It is more prevalent in people over 55 years of age. There are three types of angina. When the anginal pain is predictable in frequency, intensity, and duration, it is called classic or stable angina. The second type of angina is known as atypical or variant angina (Prinzmetal's) angina. It is caused by spasms of the coronary arteries and tends to occur at the same time of night during rest or sleep. A third type is called unstable (preinfarction) angina. More than eight million patients with chest pain who visit an emergency department each year, 1.4 million have unstable angina. Up to half of these patients will develop a myocardial infarction within hours of arriving at the emergency department. Unstable angina is chest pain that occurs more often and with less exertion than stable angina and possibly even when the patient is at rest (Metules & Bauer, 2005). The goals of pharmacological intervention are to reduce the frequency of angina episodes and to terminate an incident of acute anginal pain once it is in progress. The antianginal drugs increase blood flow either by increasing oxygen supply (nitrates) or by decreasing myocardial demand (beta blockers). Angina is treated with three classes of drugs: (a) nitrates; (b) beta blockers; and (c) calcium channel blockers. Nitrates are used for stable angina, because they offer rapid pain relief. Nitrates and calcium channel blockers relax both the arterial and venous smooth muscle. This relaxation decreases the workload of the heart and promotes vasodilation. Beta blockers decrease the heart rate and contractility, which decreases oxygen demand.

Indications

Nitrates are used to treat both classic (stable) and variant (vasospastic or Prinzmetal) angina. Beta blockers are prescribed to manage symptoms of classic angina. They are also used to manage hypertension, acute myocardial infarction, and supraventricular tachycardia. Because of their ability to slow the heart rate (negative chronotropic effect) and reduce contractility (negative inotropic effect), beta blockers have been useful in reducing the frequency of anginal attacks caused by exertion. They are sometimes considered a first-line drug for chronic angina. Calcium channel blockers are Class IV antiarrhythmic drugs that inhibit the influx of calcium ions through slow channels into the cells of myocardial and arterial smooth muscle. The antianginal effect is achieved by dilating coronary arteries and arterioles to improve oxygen delivery to the myocardium. Calcium channel blockers are used to manage both classic and activity-induced variant angina, essential hypertension, and dysrhythmias.

Pharmacokinetics

Nitroglycerin, taken sublingual (SL), is absorbed rapidly and directly into the internal jugular vein and right atrium (Figure 17-3). The nitroglycerin in Nitro-bid ointment and in the Transderm-Nitro patch is absorbed slowly

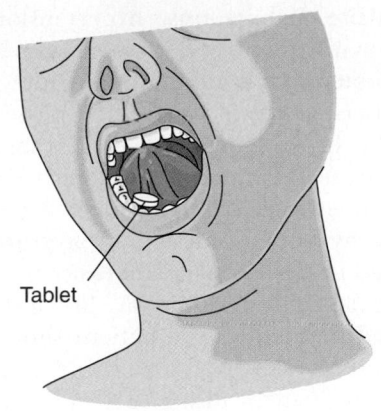

Figure 17-3 Sublingual administration of a nitroglycerin tablet.

through the skin and is excreted primarily in the urine. Beta blockers block the $beta_1$ receptor site. They block the release of epinephrine and norepinephrine at beta receptors in the arteries and the heart, thereby preventing vasoconstriction and tachycardia (Riggs, 2004). The result is a slower heart rate and decreased blood pressure. Nonselective beta blockers decrease the pulse rate and can cause bronchoconstriction. Cardioselective beta blockers act more strongly on the $beta_1$ receptors, thus decreasing pulse rate but have less risk of bronchoconstriction because they do not affect $beta_2$ receptors. These drugs are well absorbed orally. Propranolol and metoprolol are metabolized and excreted by the liver. Half of atenolol is excreted unchanged by the kidneys, and half is excreted unabsorbed in the feces. Calcium channel blockers are 80 to 90 percent absorbed through the GI mucosa. All are highly protein-bound. The effect of first-pass metabolism varies by drug.

Laboratory Monitoring

Nitroglycerin may cause a false report of decrease in serum cholesterol. Beta blockers may induce false-negative test results in exercise tolerance electrocardiogram (ECG). Patients taking calcium channel blockers should have baseline and periodic tests of hepatic and renal function. Both beta blockers and calcium channel blockers can affect blood glucose so diabetics should be monitored closely.

Side Effects and Adverse Effects

Nitrates cause headaches in 50 percent of people taking the drug. Other side effects include postural hypotension, dizziness, weakness, and faintness. When nitroglycerin ointment or transdermal patches are discontinued, the dose should be tapered slowly to avoid a rebound effect of severe pain. Reflex tachycardia may occur if the nitrate is given too rapidly. The adverse effects of treatment with beta blockers that need attention and intervention can be grouped into four categories; fluid retention, fatigue, bradycardia and heart block, and hypotension. Fluid retention may be indicative of worsening CHF. When fatigue inhibits functioning, the health care provider is encouraged to lower the dosage or stop completely if there is evidence of peripheral hypoperfusion. Both nonselective and selective beta blockers cause a decrease in pulse rate and blood pressure. For nonselective beta blockers, bronchospasm, behavioral or psychotic response, and impotence are potential adverse reactions. Vital signs should be monitored closely when treatment is initiated. Beta blockers should not be discontinued abruptly; to do so can precipitate reflex tachycardia or life-threatening dysrhythmias.

Calcium channel blockers may cause headache, hypotension (more common with nifedipine and less common with diltiazem), dizziness, and flushing of the skin. Constipation is a concern, especially with oral and sustained-release forms. Calcium channel blockers can cause changes in liver and kidney function. Nifedipine (immediate release) has been associated with an increased incidence of sudden cardiac death. All forms of nitroglycerin can cause dizziness and headache; after sublingual use, rest for 15 minutes to avoid dizziness. If pain persists after three nitroglycerin tablets (or sprays) at five-minute intervals, call 911 and go to the hospital. This could be a sign of an impending myocardial infarction. The patient should take a sublingual or spray nitroglycerin before an event that might cause angina, such climbing stairs, exercise, or sexual intercourse. A sublingual nitroglycerin tablet may be taken, even if the patient is wearing a nitroglycerin patch. IV nitroglycerine must be diluted in 5% dextrose or 0.9% NaCl solution. Never give IV push, as IV nitroglycerin must be delivered by infusion pump. Monitor blood pressure and heart rate every 5 to 10 minutes while titrating the infusion.

Beta blockers can cause both pulse and blood pressure changes. The patient should be instructed to not stop taking this medication. Abrupt withdrawal of the medication can lead to severe rebound reactions including sweating, shakiness, severe headache, malaise, palpitations, hypertension, myocardial infarction, and life-threatening dysrhythmias. The patient should change positions slowly to avoid postural hypotension. In addition, encourage the patient to stop smoking as smoking increases hepatic metabolism of beta blocker medications, leading to unpredictable or lesser response. Assess thoroughly for history of asthma, allergies, or chronic obstructive pulmonary disease (COPD); beta blockers may lead to bronchospasm. Patients receiving IV beta blockers should be monitored for ECG rhythm and rate, blood pressure; reduction of sympathetic stimulation can lead to cardiac standstill.

Calcium channel blockers can cause irregular or slower than baseline level. Therefore, the vital signs must be monitored frequently. The patient should change position slowly to avoid postural hypotension, stop smoking, and avoid alcohol consumption. The patient should report any bruising, petechiae, or unexplained bleeding. Advise patient to report gradual weight gain and evidence of edema, as it may indicate onset of CHF.

Antidysrhythmics

A cardiac dysrhythmia (arrhythmia) is defined as an abnormal heart rate or pattern. Sinus tachycardia is defined as a heart rate that is between 100 and 180 beats per minutes with a normal P wave and QRS complex. Sinus bradycardia is a heart rate that is less than 60 beats per minute with a normal P wave and QRS complex (Brown, 2003). The ECG identifies the type of irregularity. Cardiac dysrhythmias frequently occur following a myocardial infarction but may also be caused by hypoxia, hypercapnia, excess catecholamines, or alterations in electrolytes.

The desired effect of antidysrhythmic medications is to restore normal cardiac rhythm. Antidysrhythmic drugs accomplish this task by altering electrical conduction properties of the heart. This alteration can be the result of: (a) blocking adrenergic stimulation of the heart; (b) depressing myocardial excitability; (c) decreasing conduction velocity in cardiac tissue; (d) increasing recovery time (repolarization) of the myocardium; or (e) suppressing automaticity (spontaneous depolarization to initiate beats). Antidysrhythmic drug are grouped into four classes: (a) fast sodium channel blockers 1A, 1B, and 1C; (b) beta blockers; (c) potassium channel blockers; and (d) slow (calcium) channel blockers. Drugs that affect the electrical properties of the heart have a narrow margin of safety. They have the ability to correct a dysrhythmia as well as the ability to worsen or create new dysrhythmias.

Indications

- Class I: Fast-acting sodium channel blockers are divided into three subcategories based on subtle differences in their actions. Class 1A drugs are used to treat atrial and ventricular dysrhythmias, paroxysmal atrial tachycardia (PAT), and supraventricular dysrhythmias. They are also used to prevent PVCs and ventricular tachycardia that are not severe enough to require cardioversion. Quinidine, a drug in this class, is known as a chemical cardioversion agent useful to convert atrial fibrillation to normal sinus rhythm. These drugs slow conduction and prolong repolarization. When sodium ion release is blocked, depolarization is prevented. Class 1B drugs (lidocaine) slow conduction and shorten repolarization. These drugs are used in acute ventricular dysrhythmias. Class 1C drugs prolong conduction with little to no effect on repolarization. These are used to treat life-threatening ventricular dysrhythmias.
- Class II: Beta blockers (Inderal) reduce calcium entry; decrease conduction velocity, automaticity, and recovery time. As stated in the discussion of antianginal agents, beta blockers block beta$_1$ receptors when given in therapeutic doses. In higher doses they can block beta$_2$ receptors in the lungs, leading to increased risk of bronchospasm, especially for people with a history of asthma or COPD. Blocking beta receptors reduces renin activity that suppresses the renin-angiotensin-aldosterone system. The effect of

depressing this system is reduction in the systolic and diastolic blood pressure, decrease in force of contraction, and decrease in heart rate. The results of blocking beta receptor stimulation are myocardial irritability and decrease in heart rate and force of contraction, depression of automaticity of the sinus node, and reduction of conduction velocity. Beta blockers are used to treat atrial flutter and fibrillation, tachydysrhythmias, and ventricular and supraventricular dysrhythmias (Brown, 2003).

- Class III: Potassium channel blockers prolong repolarization and are used in the emergency treatment of ventricular dysrhythmias when other antidysrhythmics are ineffective. These drugs, bretylium and amiodarone, increase the refractory period and decrease intraventricular conduction.
- Class IV: Calcium channel blockers block the influx of calcium ions, thereby decreasing the excitability and contractility of the myocardium. These drugs slow conduction velocity and increase the refractory period of the AV node, resulting in a lower heart rate and decreased strength of the heart muscle contraction. They are prescribed for patients with supraventricular tachydysrhythmias and are also used to prevent paroxysmal supraventricular tachycardia.

Pharmacokinetics

The 1A blockers are rapidly absorbed from the GI mucosa. Food and pH change the absorption rate. Protein binding varies with specific drug. See the discussion in the anginal section for beta blockers and calcium channel blockers. A thorough drug history should be obtained as these drugs interact with a number of other drugs including cardiac glycosides, cimetidine, anticonvulsants, nifedipine, and warfarin. Class III drugs have extremely long half-lives (10 to 55 days).

Laboratory Monitoring

The nurse should monitor baseline as well as periodic renal and hepatic function tests. Blood glucose and serum potassium need to be checked. Any electrolyte imbalance must be corrected before beginning therapy. The ECG should be monitored closely. Beta blockers can alter glycogenolysis causing an increased incidence of hypoglycemia in type 1 diabetes. Patients taking class III medications need to have thyroid and pulmonary function tests in addition to an evaluation of arterial blood gases.

Side Effects and Adverse Effects

Class IA antidysrhythmics, such as procainamide, can cause hypotension, GI disturbances, headache, rash, insomnia, dizziness, ataxia, hallucinations, and weakness. The side effects of class IB drugs, such as lidocaine, are blurred vision, tinnitus, drowsiness, nausea and vomiting, lightheadedness, confusion, hypotension, and AV block. Beta blockers and calcium channel blockers cause bradycardia and hypotension. Severe hypotension is the most serious adverse effect for beta blockers. Class III drugs, bretylium and amiodarone, can cause nausea, vomiting, hypotension, and neurological problems. Class III drugs have many possible adverse effects that the nurse must watch for. CNS alterations include peripheral neuropathy, abnormal gait, and paresthesia. Bradycardia, cardiogenic shock, CHF, and heart block are cardiovascular adverse effects. Corneal microdeposits, blurred vision, optic neuritis, optic neuropathy, blindness, corneal degeneration, macular degeneration, and photosensitivity may result. The skin can develop a slate blue pigmentation and a rash (Hogan, 2005). Even with appropriate treatment, all antidysrhythmic drugs can precipitate life-threatening dysrhythmias. Patients should be carefully monitored when treatment is initiated.

Nursing Management

The nursing management for administering antidysrhythmics begins with teaching the patient about the necessity to not skip doses and not taking two doses at once if a dose is missed. In addition, the patient must avoid the use of alcohol, caffeine, and tobacco. Prior to taking a beta blocker or calcium channel blocker take pulse and report pulse rate of below 60 BPM to the health care provider. The patient also is instructed to report shortness of breath, postural hypotension, signs of bleeding, excessive bruising, fever, nausea, persistent headache, changes to vision or hearing, diarrhea, or dizziness (class 1). The class III medications may cause vision changes, so the patient should be informed of the need to have regular eye exams. In addition, the patient should avoid prolonged sun exposure when taking class III medications and wear dark glasses to ease photophobia. Class III medications may cause GI upset, so inform the patient to take medication with food or a small snack and to be aware that constipation is a common problem of these drugs, so there is a need to eat foods high in fiber. The nurse must assess the patient for heart block, severe bradycardia, AV block, and asthma. Monitor laboratory reports for liver, lung, thyroid, stomach, and neurological dysfunction.

Diuretics

A diuretic is a drug that increases urine output by inhibiting sodium and water reabsorption from the kidney tubules. Diuretics are used to decrease hypertension and to reduce edema (peripheral and pulmonary) in patients with CHF and renal or liver disorders. The antihypertensive effect is obtained by promoting sodium and water loss by blocking sodium and chloride reabsorption. This causes a decrease in fluid volume and lowering of blood pressure. With fluid loss, edema should decrease. When sodium is retained, water is also retained, and blood pressure increases. Diuretics may cause the loss of other electrolytes, including potassium, magnesium, chloride, and bicarbonate. Diuretics are classified as: (a) thiazide and thiazide-like; (b) loop or high ceiling; (c) osmotic; (d) carbonic anhydrase inhibitor; and (e) potassium sparing.

Indications

Thiazide and thiazide-like diuretics act on the distal convoluted renal tubule, beyond the loop of Henle, to block sodium reabsorption and increase potassium and water excretion. Thiazides are used to treat mild to moderate hypertension and peripheral edema in people who have normal kidney function. Their hypotensive effect may be due to direct arteriolar vasodilation. Excretion of sodium chloride and water causes a decrease in vascular fluid, and the result is a decrease in cardiac output and a decrease in blood pressure. Sodium, potassium, and magnesium are excreted along with water, but calcium is reabsorbed creating a risk for hypercalcemia.

The loop or high-ceiling diuretics act on the ascending loop of Henle by inhibiting chloride transport of sodium into the circulation. Sodium and water are lost along with potassium, calcium, and magnesium. The loop diuretics increase sodium excretion up to 20 to 25 percent of the functional load of sodium, enhance free water clearance, and maintain their efficacy unless renal function is severely impaired. Loop diuretics do not affect blood sugar, but uric acid does increase. These are potent diuretics and cause immediate, rapid diuresis. They exert their antihypertensive affect by dilating the renal vessels to allow a temporary increase in glomerular filtration rate (GFR) and a decrease in peripheral vascular resistance. They can increase renal blood flow up to 40 percent. Because of their rapid action, loop diuretics are used to treat patients with edema, pulmonary edema, CHF, chronic renal failure, and hepatic cirrhosis.

Osmotic diuretics increase the osmolality (concentration) of the plasma and fluid in the renal tubules. Sodium, chloride, potassium, to a less degree, and water are excreted. These drugs are used to prevent renal failure, decrease intracranial pressure, and to diminish intraocular pressure.

The carbonic anhydrase inhibitors block the action of the enzyme carbonic anhydrase, which is needed to maintain the acid-base balance. When this enzyme is inhibited, sodium, potassium, and bicarbonate are excreted. This group of drugs is used primarily to decrease intraocular pressure in patients with open angle glaucoma.

Potassium-sparing diuretics, weaker than thiazide or loop diuretics, are used as mild diuretics or in combination with another diuretic. They act directly on the distal convoluted tubule to increase sodium excretion and decrease potassium excretion. Potassium-sparing diuretics are used to decrease blood pressure and decrease edema associated with heart failure. The nurse should not administer a potassium supplement with these diuretics, because hyperkalemia can result.

Pharmacokinetics

Thiazides are well absorbed through the GI tract and have a longer half-life than the loop diuretics. They should be taken early in the day to avoid nocturia. Thiazide diuretics are ineffective if creatinine clearance level is less than 30 mL/minute. Allow two to four weeks for the maximum antihypertensive effect. The GI tract readily absorbs loop diuretics. They are highly protein-bound drugs that have half-lives that vary from 30 minutes to one-and-a-half hours. Osmotic diuretics are administered by slow IV infusion. Crystallization of mannitol in the vial may occur when the drug is exposed to low temperatures. The nurse should warm the vial to dissolve crystals prior to administration.

Laboratory Monitoring

The nurse should obtain baseline lab tests, such as CBC, electrolytes (especially sodium and potassium), BUN, creatinine, uric acid, and blood sugar. Hemoglobin (Hgb) and hematocrit (Hct) need to be checked as these may be increased because of hemoconcentration. The nurse should monitor for blood dyscrasias or liver or kidney damage. Blood sugar and lipids need to be evaluated for possible drug interactions. Also platelet and CBC should be checked prior to and periodically throughout therapy for patients taking carbonic anhydrase inhibitors (Daniels, 2003).

Side Effects and Adverse Effects

The principle adverse effects of diuretics include electrolyte depletion as well as hyponatremia and azotemia. The serum chemistry and electrolyte abnormalities of thiazide diuretics include hypokalemia, hypomagnesemia, and bicarbonate loss, hyperglycemia, hyperuricemia, and hyperlipidemia. Other thiazide side effects include dizziness, headaches, nausea and vomiting, and constipation. Toxic adverse effects of thiazide diuretics include renal failure, aplastic anemia, agranulocytosis, thrombocytopenia, and anaphylactic reaction.

Loop diuretics can cause CNS effects of dizziness, headache, orthostatic hypotension, or weakness; GI effects, such as nausea, vomiting, abdominal pain, elevated lipids with decreasing high-density lipoproteins (HDLs), pancreatitis, anorexia, and constipation; genitourinary effects of excessive urination, nocturia, and urinary bladder spasms; photosensitivity, sulfonamide allergy, and ototoxicity, which is evidenced by tinnitus, hearing impairment, deafness, vertigo, and a sense of fullness in the ears; and, skin effects of dermatitis, urticaria, pruritus, and muscle spasm. Adverse effects include electrolyte imbalances, such as hyponatremia, hypochloremia, hypokalemia, hypomagnesemia, hypocalcemia, and hyperuricemia. Thrombocytopenia, systemic vasculitis, interstitial nephritis, thrombophlebitis, agranulocytosis, and aplastic anemia have been reported.

The side effects and adverse reactions of mannitol include fluid and electrolyte imbalances, pulmonary edema from rapids shifts of fluids, CHF, seizures, nausea, vomiting, tachycardia from rapid fluid loss, and acidosis. In addition to electrolyte imbalances, the carbonic anhydrase inhibitors can cause the following: (a) confusion; (b) drowsiness and paresthesias; (c) hearing dysfunction; (d) GI upset; (e) polyuria; and (f) transient myopia. Adverse effects that have been reported are metabolic alkalosis, anaphylaxis, and bone marrow depression.

The main side effect of potassium-sparing diuretics is hyperkalemia. If a potassium-sparing diuretic is given with an angiotensin-converting enzyme (ACE) inhibitor, hyperkalemia could become severe or life-threatening because both drugs retain potassium. GI disturbances of anorexia, nausea, vomiting, and diarrhea can occur.

Nursing Management

The nursing management for the administration of diuretics is similar across the various categories of diuretics. The nurse must monitor vital signs for hypotension and tachycardia, and check serum electrolytes, calcium, and uric acid levels. (Note: uric acid buildup can cause gout, which causes tenderness or swelling of the joints.) The thiazide diuretics need to be taken early in the day to avoid nocturia. For any of the diuretics, the nurse must monitor blood pressure on a regular basis and withhold the diuretic if the blood pressure is too low. The patient should be weighed every two to three days and report changes of more than two pounds. Patients are at risk for the development of dehydration with diuretic administration and must be monitored in this regard. The nurse must observe for hypokalemia with non–potassium-sparing medications. In contrast, the patient must be monitored for hyperkalemia (nausea, diarrhea, abdominal cramps, and tachycardia followed by bradycardia) in potassium-sparing diuretics. Sodium levels must also be monitored by avoiding food high in sodium that can make the diuretic ineffective. In addition, sodium imbalances can cause hypotension and dizziness. The nurse should encourage the patient to report ringing in the ears immediately, particularly with loop diuretics. Also, the nurse must monitor serum glucose, because thiazides alter carbohydrate metabolism, which results in hyperglycemia.

Antihypertensive Agents

The latest statistics estimate that 50 million Americans have hypertension, and because of the absence of symptoms, as many as 30 percent do not know it (Woods, 2004). The latest guidelines from the Joint National Committee on Prevention, Detection, Evaluation, and Treatment of High Blood Pressure (JNC7) defines normal blood pressure as systolic blood pressure less than 120 mm Hg and blood pressure less than 80 mm Hg. Hypertension is defined as a blood pressure such that the systolic pressure is greater than 140 mm Hg, and the diastolic pressure is greater than 90 mm Hg. Those people having a systolic pressure of 120 to 139 mm Hg or a diastolic blood pressure of 80 to 89 are described as prehypertensive. People with prehypertension are twice as likely to develop hypertension as those who blood pressure is normal. Hypertension having no specific cause is called primary, idiopathic, or essential. Essential hypertension is the most common type of hypertension, accounting for 90 percent of all cases. Secondary hypertension is caused by identifiable factors, such as excessive secretion of epinephrine by the adrenal glands or by narrowing of the renal arteries.

Because hypertension is often a silent condition with no recognizable symptoms, patients do not heed warnings to control their diet, stop smoking, drink in moderation, and control their stress. Other risk factors include being of African American descent, having a positive family history, having diabetes, or having hyperlipidemia. Untreated or uncontrolled hypertension can lead to an increased workload for the heart that can cause the heart to fail and fluid to back up into the lungs, which is a condition called heart failure. Vessels providing blood and oxygen to the brain can suffer damage, resulting in transient ischemic attacks, cerebrovascular accidents (CVAs), or strokes.

A cluster of neurons located in the medulla oblongata, called the vasomotor center, regulates blood pressure. Nerves travel from the vasomotor center to the arteries where smooth muscle is directed to constrict, which raises blood pressure, or dilate, which lowers blood pressure. The vasomotor center is provided with information from the baroreceptors in the aorta and internal carotid artery. The baroreceptors provide information about the vascular system. Baroreceptors sense pressure within the large vessels. Chemoreceptors recognize levels of oxygen, carbon dioxide, and the pH in the blood. The vasomotor center reacts to the information it receives by raising or lowering the blood pressure accordingly.

Hormones affect blood pressure. Norepinephrine and antidiuretic hormone (ADH) are potent vasoconstrictors that raise blood pressure. The renin-angiotensin system of the kidneys plays a significant role in regulation of blood pressure. Renin stimulates production of angiotensin II, a vasoconstrictor, which causes the release of aldosterone. Aldosterone promotes sodium and water retention. Retention of sodium and water increases fluid volume that then increases blood pressure.

Treatment of hypertension includes reduction of risk factors and medication. The types of drugs used to treat hypertension include diuretics, calcium channel blockers, and agents affecting the renin-angiotensin system, beta-adrenergic agents, and direct acting vasodilators.

Diuretics reduce blood pressure and edema by increasing urine production and enhancing water and sodium excretion. Diuretics are used as first-line drugs in treating mild hypertension, except for patients with diabetes. For those patients an ACE inhibitor should be used as the first-line drug (Woods, 2004). Hydrochlorothiazide, a thiazide, is the most frequently prescribed diuretic for mild hypertension.

The sympatholytics comprise five groups of drugs: (a) beta blockers; (b) centrally acting; (c) alpha blockers; (d) peripherally acting; and (e) alpha$_1$ blockers and beta$_1$ blockers. Beta blockers reduce blood pressure by blocking stimulation of the beta receptors in the heart by epinephrine and norepinephrine, thus decreasing heart rate and cardiac output. They also interfere with the release of renin by the kidneys to decrease the renin-angiotensin mechanism, leading to a decrease in blood pressure. Beta blockers tend to be more effective in lowering blood pressure of those patients with higher renin levels.

Centrally acting sympatholytics decrease the sympathetic response (inhibit the sympathetic cardio-accelerator and vasoconstrictor centers) from the brainstem to the peripheral vessels, resulting in less vascular resistance and a resulting decrease in blood pressure. They have minimal effect on cardiac output or blood flow to the kidneys. Methyldopa (Aldomet) and clonidine (Catapres) are examples of drugs from this group.

Alpha-adrenergic blocking agents decrease vasomotor tone to cause vasodilation, which results in a decreased blood pressure. They help maintain renal blood flow rate. Peripherally acting sympatholytics (adrenergic neuron blockers) block norepinephrine release from the sympathetic nerve endings, causing a decrease in norepinephrine release that results in lowering of the blood pressure. There is a decrease in both cardiac output and peripheral resistance. Examples of drugs in this group are reserpine and guanethidine. Both are potent antihypertensive agents and are used to control severe hypertension.

Alpha and beta blockers block both the alpha$_1$ and beta$_1$ receptors. Labetalol (Normodyne) and carteolol (Cartrol) are examples of drugs from this group. Dilation of the arterioles is the result of blocking alpha$_1$. The effect on the alpha receptor is stronger than the effect on the beta receptor; therefore, blood pressure is lowered and pulse rate is moderately decreased.

Direct-acting arteriolar vasodilators relax the smooth muscles of the blood vessels, mainly the arteries, causing vasodilation. Vasodilators cause an increased blood flow to the brain and kidneys. With vasodilation, blood pressure decreases, and sodium and water are retained causing peripheral edema. Diuretics can be given to reduce edema.

ACE inhibitors inhibit ACE, which in turn inhibits the formation of the vasoconstrictor angiotensin II, which blocks the release of aldosterone. The reduction in aldosterone limits sodium and water retention by the kidneys

Safety First

Beta Blockers

The alpha-beta-adrenergic blocker labetalol can be ordered for a patient in hypertensive crisis. The nurse must be careful to administer the dose per protocol. With an incorrect method of IV administration, the patient can go into cardiac arrest. When ordered to treat hypertensive crisis, the starting dose should be administered slowly over two minutes to prevent a sudden drop in blood pressure. Terms such as *IV push* or *bolus* are inappropriate, because they imply giving the drug quickly. Implementing the following safety measures can prevent similar errors:

- Clarify any order with inappropriate terms, such as IV push for labetalol.
- Obtain IV push guidelines from the pharmacy, including safe injection times for various medications. Post the guidelines in medication use areas and ask the pharmacy to add alerts to labels of all medications that require slow administration.
- Use the lowest available concentration of intravenous drugs to avoid administering them too rapidly or dilute if not contraindicated. If possible, use a syringe pump to administer medications that may cause adverse effects if given too rapidly.

Adapted from Cohen, M. R. (2005). Labetalol crisis: Speed kills. Nursing, 35(2), 18.

---

while retaining potassium. Also ACE inhibitors inhibit the degradation of bradykinin, which may cause a dry, hacking cough for some patients. ACE inhibitors cause little effect on cardiac output or heart rate, and they lower vascular resistance. ACE inhibitors are first-line treatments with hypertension and diabetes, heart failure, and impaired renal function (Woods, 2004).

Angiotensin II receptor antagonists (AII blockers) are a new group of antihypertensives. Their action is similar to ACE inhibitors, to block the release of aldosterone. They differ in that they block angiotensin II from the angiotensin I receptors found in many tissues. AII blockers cause vasodilation and decrease peripheral resistance. Losartan (Cozaar) and valsartan (Diovan) are drugs in this class.

Calcium channel blockers decrease heart rate and contractility and help prevent vasospasm by blocking slow-moving calcium channels in the heart myocardium and vascular smooth muscle. These should be used with caution in patients with heart failure, because myocardial contractility is already compromised (Woods, 2004). Verapamil (Calan) and nifedipine (Procardia) are drugs in this class.

Indications

All the drugs discussed previously are used for treating hypertension. More specific indications for drug groups will be discussed further in this section. Alpha blockers are used to treat peripheral vascular disorders, hypertension, and benign prostatic hypertrophy (BPH). The alpha blockers are useful in treating hypertension in patients with lipid abnormalities. They decrease the very low-density lipoproteins (VLDLs) and the low-density lipoproteins (LDLs) that are responsible for the buildup of fatty plaques in the arteries. In addition, they increase the HDLs. Because they do not affect glucose metabolism or respiratory function, they are safe for patients with diabetes or asthma. Prazosin is an example of an alpha-adrenergic blocker.

Direct-acting vasodilators (hydralazine and minoxidil) are potent antihypertensive agents used for moderate to severe hypertension. Nitroprusside and diazoxide are used for acute hypertensive crisis.

ACE inhibitors are used primarily to treat hypertension. Some of the agents are also effective in treating heart failure. As a rule, these drugs are not first-line antihypertensive agents; however, they are the preferred antihypertensive drug for patients with diabetic neuropathy. African Americans and older adults do not respond with the desired reduction in blood pressure unless these medications are combined with a diuretic. Alpha$_2$ blockers are approved for the treatment of hypertension. Like ACE inhibitors, AII blockers are less effective in African Americans (see Respecting our Differences).

Laboratory Monitoring

The nurse should obtain bilirubin and BUN to assess liver function, CBC, blood glucose, serum uric acid and creatinine to assess renal function, electrolytes, and ECG. Be alert to electrolyte imbalances, such as increased potassium and decreased sodium levels. When prescribed ACE inhibitors, the patient should also be checked for agranulocytosis indicated by a decrease in platelets and bone marrow depression. With angiotensin II antagonists, the nurse should monitor white blood cell count for neutropenia and electrolytes for hyperkalemia.

The groups of drugs that target angiotensin I and II receptors have common side effects, such as orthostatic hypotension, CNS stimulation, and the potential for both hyperkalemia and altered glucose metabolism. Each of these drugs carries the risk to develop adverse effects that include blood dyscrasias, cardiac dysrhythmias, and unwanted blood pressure changes.

Nursing Management

The administration of antihypertensive medications affects the cardiovascular system in many ways. The nurse must take the vital signs regularly and observe for cardiac output changes. The patient must be assessed for clinical manifestations of postural hypotension, heart failure, peripheral edema, and syncope. The patient should be monitored for their blood glucose levels and blood pressure more frequently if taking insulin or oral antidiabetic medications. Antihypertensives need to be taken for three to four weeks to achieve therapeutic effects and should not be stopped abruptly. Specific medications can cause side affects that need to be monitored individually (e.g., ACE inhibitors can cause infections, facial swelling, loss of taste, difficulty breathing, and dry cough). The patient should be advised to use alternative birth control methods instead of oral contraceptives when taking alpha$_2$ antagonists. In general, the patient should be encouraged to avoid alcohol use, excessive exercise, prolonged standing, and exposure to heat that may increase risk for developing side effects (Box 17-4). And, the nurse must instruct the patient to avoid long-term NSAID therapy because NSAIDs decrease the effectiveness of the ACE inhibitor. NSAIDs inhibit formation of prostaglandin, which is needed to maintain renal function. In the presence of NSAIDs, the kidneys will retain sodium and water, increasing hypertension and worsening heart failure (Woods, 2004).

MEDICATIONS TO TREAT CIRCULATORY DISORDERS

Hemostasis, or stopping of the blood flow, is the result of a complex coagulation mechanism in the body that protects the body from both internal and external injury. It consists of vasoconstriction, platelet aggregation, and thrombin and fibrin synthesis. Drugs can change hemostasis by four basic mechanisms: (a) prevention of clot formation through inhibition of the release of certain clotting factors with anticoagulants; (b) prevention of the formation of clots by inhibiting platelet aggregation using anticoagulant or antiplatelet; (c) removal of an existing clot by dissolving the clot using a thrombolytic; or (d) promotion of clot formation by inhibiting the destruction of fibrin with an antifibrinolytic. Anticoagulants are the most frequently prescribed hemostasis modifier. Regardless of mechanism, all anticoagulants will prolong the time it takes for the body to form clots.

Anticoagulants

Anticoagulants are drugs that prolong bleeding time in an effort to prevent the formation of thrombi (clots). The drugs are normally classified as parenteral (Heparin) or oral (Coumadin) and are widely used in the treatment of thromboembolic disease. Drugs from both groups are used to treat venous conditions such as deep-vein thrombosis (DVT) and pulmonary embolism (PE). Arterial conditions, such as coronary artery disease (CAD), rheumatic heart disease, and atrial fibrillation, alone or in combination with valve disease, atrial fibrillation before and after cardioversion, postsurgical valve replacements, and cerebral vascular disorders are also treated with anticoagulants. Arterial disorders, however, are more responsive to antiplatelet agents. Anticoagulants are also used prophylactically for patients on extended periods of bedrest, postoperative patients, and those patients with a history of previous clotting disorders.

The presence of thrombi in the body can be life-threatening. To achieve a rapid response, anticoagulant therapy is usually initiated by IV infusion. Once stabilized the patient is placed on an oral anticoagulant. Careful monitoring of coagulation studies is needed throughout anticoagulation therapy.

Indications

The parenteral anticoagulants include heparin and the low molecular weight heparins, such as enoxaparin (Lovenox) and dalteparin (Fragmin). Heparin plays an active role in the intrinsic pathway, which is the pathway in which fibrin formation occurs. Heparin combines with a plasma heparin cofactor named antithrombin III (ATIII), and this complex causes inactivation of specific clotting factors (IIa, Xa, XIIa, XIa, and IXa) to prevent the fibrinogen from changing to fibrin in the clotting cascade. The heparin/ATIII complex has a strong anticoagulant effect that inhibits conversion of fibrinogen to fibrin, prevents formation of a fibrin clot, and inhibits thrombin. Because of its immediate effect, heparin is the treatment of choice for patients having DVT, PE, and embolism as a result of atrial fibrillation. The low molecular weight heparins have a similar mechanism of action to heparin. They bind with antithrombin III, which inhibits the synthesis of factor Xa and the formation of thrombin. Because they produce a more stable response than heparin, there are fewer follow-up lab tests required, and family members can be taught to give the necessary injections at home. These have become the drug of choice for a number of clotting disorders, including the prevention of postoperative complication and DVT.

The oral anticoagulant warfarin (Coumadin) inhibits clot formation by interfering with the hepatic synthesis of vitamin K–dependent clotting factors, including factors II (prothrombin), VII, IX, and X. Warfarin competes for vitamin K, making it unavailable for synthesis of the clotting factors. Vitamin K plays an active role in the extrinsic pathway, a pathway that forms fibrin and acts within seconds, in the clotting cascade. Oral anticoagulants are used for the management of patients with actual, potential, and recurrent health problems, such as DVT, PE, acute myocardial infarction, heart valve replacement, atrial fibrillation, and antiphospholipid syndrome.

Pharmacokinetics

Because of its large molecular size, heparin has poor penetration into the CNS and breast milk and it cannot cross the placental barrier. It is highly protein-bound. Heparin is metabolized in the liver by a heparin-inactivating enzyme called heparinase, and inactivated metabolites are excreted in the urine.

Unlike heparin, warfarin does cross the placental barrier and enters breast milk. It is highly protein-bound, most notably to albumin, and it is metabolized in the liver. Warfarin has a narrow therapeutic range and must be carefully monitored. It has a high potential for drug-drug and food-drug interactions related to hepatic metabolism (P-450) that can lead to ineffective therapy or toxicity. It has a slow onset of action and may take up to one full week to exert its full anticoagulant effect. It is not uncommon to have patients begin warfarin therapy while they are still on a heparin infusion. The heparin infusion is tapered off as the PT/INR tests reach appropriate levels.

Laboratory Monitoring

APTT is a diagnostic blood test that determines intrinsic clotting response and is measured in seconds; it is used to monitor the patient receiving heparin therapy. To be effective, APTT levels should be stabilized at one-and-a-half to two times the control value. Protamine sulfate is the antidote that reverses the action of heparin. The dose will depend on both the amount of heparin that is given and the time period following administration. The nurse should never give more than 50 mg in a 10-minute period (administered IV push).

PT, a diagnostic blood test used to measure extrinsic clotting response, and the INR, a standard reference range used to establish consistency in reporting PT levels, are both used to monitor the patient's response to therapy; the two are used in conjunction because of the variation of the individual dose response. Depending on the indication for use, the desired range of the PT and INR will vary. A PT level one-and-a-half to two-and-a-half times the control value is considered effective. INR levels range from a usual 2 to 3 range to a higher level of 3 to 4.5 if the patient has a mechanical cardiac valve replacement. Vitamin K is the antidote that reverses the action of warfarin (Daniels, 2003).

Side Effects and Adverse Effects

Side effects of heparin include hemorrhage, hematuria, epistaxis, bleeding gums, and thrombocytopenia (decrease in platelets). A serious adverse effect is a severe form of thrombocytopenia called heparin-induced platelet aggregation (HITT), or white clot syndrome. This can be fatal if not treated aggressively. Thrombocytopenia is more pronounced (less than 100,000/mm) and begins between 3 and 12 days following the start of heparin therapy. Osteoporosis may develop in patients receiving long-term heparin therapy.

Side effects of warfarin include ecchymosis of the skin, bleeding from any tissue or organ, GI and dermatological problems, hypotension, and thrombocytopenia. The most serious adverse effect of warfarin therapy is bleeding and is usually seen at the higher doses. At toxic levels the patient may experience GI symptoms (nausea, diarrhea, intestinal obstruction, anorexia, and abdominal cramping), dermatological manifestations (rash, urticaria, and purple toe syndrome, which is a discoloration caused by decreased perfusion due to the release of microembolism), increased serum transaminase levels, hepatitis, jaundice, burning sensation in the feet, and transient hair loss.

Nursing Management

To care for patients taking heparin and warfarin, inform the patient that frequent blood testing is required to make sure that effective anticoagulation is achieved. The patient should be instructed to report signs of bleeding, such as bleeding gums, bruises, hematuria, nosebleeds, blood in the stool, hematemesis, and petechiae. And the patient should use a soft toothbrush and electric razor to minimize even mild trauma that could lead to bleeding. Review the patient's medication history and dietary intake to determine potential drug-food interactions. The nurse must remember to ask about food and herbal supplements. Specific to warfarin, the patient should avoid foods high in vitamin K and take the medication daily in the evening. The patient should not stop taking the warfarin unless instructed to do so by the health care provider or the patient experiences a bleeding episode. The nurse must monitor the patient's baseline labs with regard to initiation and continuation of therapy (PT/INR). Vitamin K may be ordered to reverse the action of warfarin depending on results of the PT and INR. Because warfarin competes for binding sites in the liver, there is high potential for drug interactions relative to enzyme inhibitors and enzyme inducers; these chemical reactions will affect the serum concentration level of warfarin.

The nursing management for the administration of heparin begins with monitoring the patient's baseline labs. The heparin should be titrated according to protocol with reference to APTT results and administered via continuous infusion. APTT is commonly measured every six hours. When levels are extremely high, the heparin infusion is stopped for one or more hours, and the APTT is measured in two to three hours. The patient should have a monitoring of daily weight for patients on weight-based heparin protocol. The patient should be observed for signs of bleeding, have a thorough skin assessment, hemoccult all stools, and evaluate pertinent labs. The nurse should verify with pharmacy or with another registered nurse (RN) the correct dose of heparin before administering or adjusting the heparin infusion. The nurse must evaluate dosage for safety and therapeutic range based on normal adult dosage range of 20,000 to 40,000 units per 24 hours. Heparin is usually administered in units per hour. The nurse should have an antidote available (e.g., protamine sulfate). In addition, the nurse must be sure to carefully identify strengths on product label, as several concentrations of heparin are available.

Antilipemics

Antilipemics lower abnormal blood lipid levels. Lipids composed of cholesterol, triglycerides, and phospholipids are transported in the body bound to protein in various amounts. Triglycerides form a large family of different lipids that contain three fatty acids attached to glycerol. They store most of the fat in the body and serve as important energy sources. Triglycerides account for 90 percent of total lipids. Phospholipids are formed when a phosphorous group replaces one of the fatty acids in the triglyceride. This class is essential to building plasma membranes. The third class of lipids is the steroid group, so named because it contains the sterol nucleus. Cholesterol is the most well-known of the steroid lipid. Cholesterol serves as a building block for a number of essential biochemicals, including vitamin D, bile acids, cortisol, estrogen, and testosterone. The body, however, needs only a small amount. Because the liver can synthesize cholesterol from other chemicals, dietary cholesterol is unnecessary.

Because of their insolubility, lipids must attach to a protein for transport through the body. This lipid-protein complex is called an apoprotein. These are classified chylomicrons, VLDLs, LDLs, and HDLs. The HDL lipoprotein is known as the good lipoprotein. HDLs have a higher percentage of protein and fewer lipids and serve to remove cholesterol from the blood stream and deliver it to the liver. The main components of the other lipoproteins are cholesterol and triglycerides, which are known to contribute to atherosclerotic plaque in the blood vessels. Elevated cholesterol, triglycerides, and LDL place the patient at a higher risk for coronary artery disease. The total cholesterol should be below 200 mg/dL, LDL-cholesterol levels be 100 mg/dL or lower, HDL levels be above 40 mg/dL, and triglycerides should stay below 200 mg/dL.

Nonpharmacological interventions should be initiated before antilipemics are prescribed. These measures include dietary modification (decreasing intake of cholesterol and saturated fats), exercise, smoking cessation, and weight loss. Antilipemics are prescribed when hyperlipidemia remains even after nonpharmacological measures are implemented. There are four classes of drugs used to treat hyperlipidemia: HMG-CoA reductase inhibitors (statins); bile acid resins; fibric acid agents; and nicotinic acid (niacin or vitamin B_3).

Indications

The HMG-CoA reductase inhibitors (statins) inhibit the enzyme HMG-CoA reductase in cholesterol biosynthesis. Inhibition of hepatic synthesis of cholesterol results in a lowering of serum cholesterol. It is most effective in decreasing LDL and slightly increases HDL. Reduction in cholesterol levels can be seen in lab results as soon as two weeks. Research is ongoing to find other uses for the statin drugs. Statins block the vasoconstrictive effect of the A-beta protein, a significant protein involved in Alzheimer's disease. Preliminary research suggests that use of statins may protect against dementia by inhibiting the protein and thus slowing dementia caused by blood vessel constriction.

Bile acids are a group of nonabsorbable amine compounds that work in the GI tract to bind with bile acids. Bile acid resins bind bile acids that contain high concentrations of cholesterol. Because of their large size, resins are not absorbable from the small intestine. The bound bile acids and cholesterol are eliminated in the feces. The liver responds to the loss of cholesterol by making more LDL receptors, which removes even more cholesterol from the blood in a mechanism similar to that of the statin drugs. These medications have more frequent side effects than the statin drugs.

Clofibrate and gemfibrozil are fibric acid derivatives that are effective in reducing triglyceride and VLDL levels that have not responded to dietary management. Nicotinic acid is a vitamin that is occasionally used to lower lipid levels. It is the active form of vitamin B_3 (niacin) in the body and is water-soluble. Nicotinic acid lowers most lipoprotein levels (total cholesterol, LDL, triglyceride, and lipoproteins) and increases HDL levels. The dosage required to achieve lipid lowering is significantly higher (1 g three times per day) than vitamin replacement doses (25 mg per day). Though effective at decreasing LDL cholesterol by as much as 20 percent, nicotinic acid produces far more side effects than the statins. Because of its ability to produce vasodilation, niacin can also be used to treat peripheral vascular disease. Pellagra (dermatitis, diarrhea, and dementia) is the clinical deficiency of niacin.

Pharmacokinetics

Bile acid resins have the potential to bind to many other medications, such as thyroxine, digoxin, diuretics, antibiotics and warfarin; because of this, the medication should not be given concurrently with other medications. Fibric acid derivatives are highly protein-bound and should not be taken with anticoagulants, because they compete for protein sites.

Laboratory Monitoring

The nurse should monitor baseline labs for cholesterol and triglyceride levels before and throughout therapy with any lipid-lowering drug. These tests are necessary to determine effectiveness.

Statins are metabolized by the liver and have been know to cause elevation in liver function tests. Baseline measurements should be obtained before starting therapy. Because of drug-drug interaction, patients taking digoxin concurrently should have regular digoxin levels drawn, as they may need to decrease their dose. Creatinine phosphokinase (CPK) levels should be obtained if muscle myopathy is suspected. Elevation of the CPK is reason to discontinue therapy.

The nurse should monitor serum potassium, because fibric acid derivatives have been known to cause hypokalemia. The CBC should be checked, because decreased Hgb, Hct, and white blood cells may be seen with use of gemfibrozil. Nicotinic acid leads to increases in blood glucose, uric acid, and serum transaminase levels (Daniels, 2003).

Side Effects and Adverse Effects

Side effects of the statins include GI disturbances (nausea, vomiting, heartburn, dyspepsia, flatulence, and diarrhea), pain and myalgias, headache, rash, dizziness, and sinusitis. Adverse effects are related to altered liver function (elevated serum transaminase). Liver function tests should be monitored closely. A serious skeletal muscle adverse effect, known as rhabdomyolysis, has been reported with the use of statin drugs.

Because bile acid resins act in the GI tract and are not absorbed, they have no systemic side effects. They can, however, cause significant GI effects, such as constipation, abdominal pain, bloating, nausea and vomiting, diarrhea, and steatorrhea. Increasing fluid intake and foods high in fiber can decrease constipation. Bile resins may worsen symptoms in person with PUD, hemorrhoids, inflammatory bowel disease, or chronic constipation. Early signs of peptic ulcer are nausea, abdominal pain, and distension. Vitamin deficiencies (A, D, and K) are associated with use of these drugs. Skin rash and irritations of the tongue and perianal area have been reported. Adverse effects include hypoprothrombinemia and decreased erythrocyte folate levels.

Side effects of fibric acid derivatives include abdominal or epigastric pain, jaundice, headache, blurred vision, and depression. Rash, dermatitis, and pruritus have been reported with gemfibrozil. Back pain, muscle cramps, myalgia, and swollen joints may occur. Patients taking these drugs may develop gallbladder disease and acute appendicitis. Other adverse effects that may develop are eosinophilia and hypokalemia.

Common side effects that may occur with use of nicotinic acid are flushing caused by prostaglandin release, postural hypotension, vasovagal attacks, pruritus, increased sebaceous gland activity, dyspepsia, epigastric pain, and nausea. Megadose therapy has been associated with liver damage, hyperglycemia, hyperuricemia, and cardiac dysrhythmias. In patients predisposed to gout, an increase in uric acid levels may precipitate a gout attack.

Nursing Management

With all lipid-lowering drugs, lab work will be ongoing in nature to determine patient response and to evaluate for potential side effects. For the statins, the nurse must encourage the patient to take the medication with the evening meal to coincide with the body's timing of cholesterol production. In addition, statins may be taken with or without food. Instruct patient to report unexplained muscle pain, tenderness, jaundice, or loss of appetite.

When the nurse administers bile acid resins, the patient should be instructed to increase high bulk diet with adequate fluid intake and report side effects immediately (e.g., constipation). Also, the patient should take vitamin supplements to replace folic acid, fat-soluble vitamins, and vitamin K. Colestipol tablets should not be crushed, chewed, or cut and should be taken with adequate fluids. Vitamin deficiencies may require supplementation or discontinuation of the drug. When administering fibric acid derivatives, the patient must report unexplained bleeding, and the nurse should encourage the patient to restrict carbohydrate and alcohol intake. The patient must be monitored closely for right upper quadrant abdominal pain or vomiting. In the administration of nicotinic acid, the patient is encouraged to change positions slowly to avoid sudden drops in blood pressure, and to avoid direct exposure to sunlight. In addition, flushing in face, neck and ears may occur within two hours after oral ingestion and immediately after IV administration and may last several hours. Taking one aspirin 30 minutes prior to nicotinic acid dose will help decrease this effect. It should be taken with cold water because hot water increases flushing. In addition, alcohol intake may increase flushing, and nicotinic acid may decrease glycemic control in non–insulin-dependent diabetic patients. The nurse must monitor blood sugar levels more frequently until effects of nicotinic acid are known.

RESPIRATORY AGENTS

The respiratory system offers a rapid and efficient mechanism for delivering drugs. The large surface area of the bronchioles and alveoli and the rich blood supply to these areas result in almost instant onset of action for inhaled substances. Several types of devices are used to deliver inhaled medications. Nebulizers are small machines that vaporize a liquid medication into a fine mist that can be inhaled. If the drug is a solid, it may be administered using a dry powder inhaler (DPI). A DPI is a small device that is activated by the process of inhalation to deliver fine powder directly into the bronchial tree. Turbohalers and rotahalers are types of DPIs. Metered dose inhalers (MDIs) are a third type of device. MDIs use a propellant to deliver a measured dose of drugs to the lungs during each breath. The patient times the inhalation to the puffs of drug emitted from the MDI (Figure 17-4).

There are many disadvantages to administering medications via the inhaled route. The exact dose that the patient receives is dependent on the patient's breathing pattern and correct use of the device. Even under ideal situations, only 10 to 50 percent of the drug actually reaches the bronchial tree. To reduce oral absorption of inhaled medications, patients should be instructed to rinse their mouths thoroughly after each treatment.

COPD and restrictive pulmonary disease are the two major categories of lower respiratory tract disorders. Four major pulmonary disorders cause COPD: (a) chronic bronchitis; (b) bronchiectasis; (c) emphysema; and (d) asthma. Restrictive lung disease is a decrease in total lung capacity as a result of fluid accumulation or loss of elasticity of the lung. Conditions that result in restrictive lungs disease are PE, pulmonary fibrosis, pneumonitis, lung tumors, thoracic deformities, and disorders affecting muscular wall, such as myasthenia gravis. Bronchodilators, inhaled corticosteroids, and leukotriene modifiers are used in the management of these disorders. Bronchodilators are used to open narrowed airways, glucocorticoids are used to decrease inflammation, and leukotriene modifiers reduce inflammation in the lung. Cromolyn and nedocromil act as anti-inflammatory agents by suppressing the release of histamine and other mediators from the mast cells.

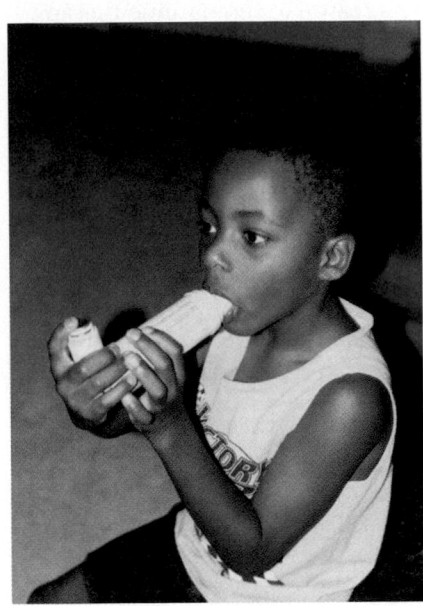

Figure 17-4 Child using an MDI with a spacer and mouthpiece.

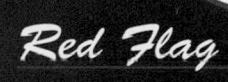

Bronchodilators

Beta-adrenergic agonists (sympathomimetics) are drugs of choice in the treatment of acute bronchoconstriction. Sympathomimetic agents that are specific for beta$_2$ receptors in the lung are preferred over the older nonselective agent epinephrine, because they produce fewer cardiac side effects. They act by increasing intracellular levels of cyclic adenosine monophosphate (cAMP) that relaxes bronchial smooth muscle and dilates constricted bronchi and bronchioles. These actions decrease airway resistance so that the patient can breathe more easily. Medications can have alpha, beta$_1$ or beta$_2$ activities. Beta-adrenergic receptors increase heart rate and force of myocardial contraction.

Methylxanthines are a group of bronchodilators that are chemically similar to caffeine. Theophylline and aminophylline were the drugs of choice for bronchoconstriction 20 years ago, but their narrow margin of safety and high potential for drug-drug interactions limit their use today (Adams, Josephson, & Holland, 2005). There are several explanations for how methylxanthines work. The original thoughts were that they inhibited phosphodiesterases (PDE), the enzyme that breaks down cAMP, thus increasing intracellular cAMP. Bronchodilation is a result of increased levels of cAMP. Methylxanthines cause the release of endogenous catecholamines, which causes sympathetic stimulation, and subsequent relaxation of airway smooth muscle. Theophylline exerts an anti-inflammatory action by inhibiting both prostaglandin synthesis and the release of bronchoconstrictive substances from leukocytes and mast cells (Broyles, et al., 2007). With bronchodilation, cilia in the airways can more effectively clear mucus.

Indications

Bronchodilators improve forced expiratory volume (FEV) by altering airway smooth-muscle tone rather than by changing lung elastic recoil. These drugs improve lung emptying, tend to reduce dynamic hyperinflation, and increase exercise performance.

Because beta-adrenergic agents produce rapid airway dilation, they are used to relieve the shortness of breath and wheezing caused by bronchospasm in an acute asthma attack. They are also used in the treatment of emphysema, acute and chronic bronchitis, and relief of bronchospasm. Alpha-adrenergic stimulators can act as decongestants for constricted blood vessels in the nasal cavity. Selective beta$_2$ agonists are the preferred drugs for bronchial smooth muscle dilation because they produce fewer cardiac side effects. A practical method to classify beta-adrenergic agonists is by their duration of action. The ultrashort-acting drugs, such as isoproterenol (Isuprel) and isoetharine (Bronkosol), produce bronchodilation immediately, but duration of action is only 2 to 3 hours. Short-acting agents such as metaproterenol (Metaprel) and terbutaline (Brethine), also act quickly but last 5 to 6 hours. Intermediate-acting sympathomimetics, such as albuterol (Proventil) and levalbuterol (Xopenex), last about 8 hours. The longest acting agent is salmeterol (Serevent), which exerts effects for up to 12 hours.

Methylxanthines stimulate the CNS and respiration, dilate coronary and pulmonary vessels, and cause diuresis. This group of drugs is used to treat bronchoconstriction associated with COPD (diseases such as chronic bronchitis, asthma, and emphysema). Because of their slow onset of action, their use is primarily prevention of asthma attacks. Theophylline administered by IV infusion is a treatment of status asthmaticus to relieve symptoms that have not responded to faster acting beta agonists. Methylxanthines can also be used in the treatment of pulmonary edema by the action of decreasing vascular permeability and paroxysmal nocturnal dyspnea (PND). The use of xanthine derivatives has declined, because of the side effect profile of these drugs. Because methylxanthines are nonspecific inhibitors of all subsets of phosphodiesterase enzymes, they have a wide range of negative effects. Low doses of theophylline are much safer than higher doses and appear to have additional effects on the airway than bronchodilation, including anti-inflammatory and immunomodulatory effects (Broyles, et al., 2007).

Pharmacokinetics

Theophylline is metabolized in the liver and excreted in the kidneys. Cigarette smoking enhances metabolism of theophylline, so drug dosage may need to be increased. Theophylline dosages should be based on lean body weight because theophylline does not enter the adipose tissue. There is greater risk for theophylline toxicity in patients with liver disease, CHF, and acute viral infections because of impaired metabolism. When the $beta_2$ agonist is delivered by a MDI or DPI, the patient must be instructed in the correct use of the device. If the patient does use the device correctly, medication may be trapped in the upper airways. Mouth dryness and throat irritation can result. Excessive use of the aerosol drug can result in tolerance and loss of effectiveness. On occasion, severe paradoxical airway resistance (bronchoconstriction) can develop due to excessive use of sympathomimetic oral inhalation. Frequent dosing can cause tremors, nervousness, and increased heart rate.

Laboratory Monitoring

The monitoring of these medications is specific to the individual medication. For example, the nurse must monitor blood sugar, because use of sympathomimetics stimulates liver production of glucose. Thyroid function is monitored because sympathomimetics can exacerbate the symptoms of hyperthyroidism. When administering theophylline, the nurse must obtain serum blood levels, which have a therapeutic range of 1 to 20 mcg/mL. Adverse effects are more frequently seen when levels are above 30 mcg/mL. Seizures have been reported when levels exceed 40 mcg/mL.

Side Effects and Adverse Effects

Though each agent has its own particular side effects, side effects common to adrenergic bronchodilators are nervousness, tremor, cardiac stimulation, and increased blood pressure. Other side effects may include hypokalemia, hyperglycemia, nausea, vomiting, chest pain, and cardiac dysrhythmias. Paradoxic bronchospasm and urinary retention may also occur.

Methylxanthines have many side effects that include: (a) GI upset (nausea, vomiting, anorexia, and gastroesophageal reflux during sleep); (b) cardiac dysrhythmias (sinus tachycardia, extra systole, palpitations, and ventricular dysrhythmias); (c) hyperglycemia; and (d) transient increased urination. Signs of CNS stimulation, including tremors, dizziness, hallucinations, restlessness, agitation, headache, insomnia, and cardiac stimulation evidence signs of serious adverse effects and toxicity.

Nursing Management

The nurse must monitor vital signs, especially heart rate and blood pressure related to cardiovascular effects. The nurse must monitor blood glucose levels carefully in diabetic patients; hypoglycemic agents may need to be adjusted. The nurse must immediately assess dyspnea, chest pain, palpitations, seizures, headaches, hallucinations, or vision changes. The patient is instructed to not take more than the prescribed dose because of risk of hypertension, tachycardia, dysrhythmias, and angina. In addition, the nurse teaches the patient to use the inhaler properly and has the patient demonstrate the technique. The patient should wait one to three minutes between inhalations of aerosol medications and avoid eye contact with inhaler spray. The absence of wheezing and shortness of breath is the desired outcome of treatment. In addition, the nurse can increase fluids to help decrease the viscosity of respiratory secretions if not contraindicated. To aid in the prevention of complications, the nurse must recognize early signs of respiratory problems so that intervention can begin as soon as possible. The nurse must note amount, color, and character of sputum, as well as monitor baseline pulmonary function tests and recheck periodically throughout treatment. The nurse will monitor blood levels of methylxanthines and give them at regularly scheduled intervals to maintain therapeutic blood levels. Methylxanthines can cause irritation of the upper airways that may result in coughing, dry mucous membranes, and a bitter taste. To help with dry mouth and bitterness, patients can rinse their mouths frequently or use sugarless hard candy. Use proper diluent with parenteral administration. The nurse must also remember that aminophylline is administered at a rate no faster than 25 mg/minute because of the risk of cardiovascular collapse.

Inhaled Corticosteroids

Regular treatment with inhaled corticosteroids does not prevent disease progression in patients with COPD; however, regular use of an inhaled steroid can reduce the frequency of exacerbations and improve their health status. Glucocorticoids are the most effective drugs available for the prevention of acute asthmatic episodes. Their exact mechanism of action is uncertain, but it is known that they suppress inflammation. It is thought that inhaled glucocorticoids stabilize the membranes of cells that release bronchoconstricting substances, such as histamine. The cell membranes of neutrophils, the white blood cell that increase in concentration in response to inflammation, are stabilized. Inflammation causing substances are not released, and as a result, inflammation is decreased and bronchodilation occurs. With reduced inflammation and decreased production of mucous secretions, bronchoconstriction is lessened. Inhaled glucocorticoids may have a role in increasing the responsiveness of bronchial smooth muscle to the effects of beta agonists.

Indications

Glucocorticoids are used prophylactically in chronic asthma to decrease inflammation and, therefore, lessen airway obstruction (Pruitt & Jacobs, 2005). Oral glucocorticoids may be used for the short-term management of acute asthma. They are also used to treat chronic bronchitis, COPD and cystic fibrosis, and bronchospastic disorders that do not respond sufficiently to bronchodilators.

Pharmacokinetics

The chemical structures of inhaled glucocorticoids have been slightly altered, so there is less systemic absorption and, therefore, fewer side effects. When an inhaled glucocorticoid is added to the regimen, the dose of an oral glucocorticoid may need to be decreased.

Laboratory Monitoring

The patient is monitored carefully when taking inhaled corticosteroids. These medications decrease the response to skin test antigens, and the nurse must postpone skin testing until completion of glucocorticoid therapy. In addition, the medication increases blood glucose levels, and therefore, blood sugar levels must be monitored frequently. Corticosteroids mask the usual signs of inflammation, which makes the nurse need to carefully assess for signs of infections.

Side Effects and Adverse Effects

With inhaled glucocorticoids, side effects consist primarily of irritation of the upper respiratory system with symptoms, such as pharyngeal irritation and sore throat, coughing, dry mouth, oral fungal infections, and sinusitis. If absorbed systemically, serious adverse effects, such as adrenocortical insufficiency, fluid and electrolyte imbalances, nervous system effects, and endocrine effects, may occur. Patients on these drugs are more susceptible to dermatological effects and osteoporosis. Rhinitis, or inflammation of the nasal mucous membranes, menstrual disturbances, and palpitations have been reported.

Nursing Management

Corticosteroid administration requires the nurse to provide many instructions to the patient because of the many side affects of these medications. In general, the patient needs to be instructed to carefully follow the prescribed methods of administration and to not overuse them. In general, corticosteroids must not be stopped abruptly. They should be tapered slowly over a two-week period under the direction of a health care provider. The patient should know the symptoms of steroid use, including moon face, acne, increased fat pads, increased edema and should be instructed to notify the health care provider if these symptoms occur. In addition, the patient should report a weight gain of more than five pounds in one week. The nurse can also teach the patient that inhaled glucocorticoids are to be used as maintenance drugs and are ineffective in acute bronchospasm. The nurse can teach the patient about the early signs of respiratory difficulty, such as activity intolerance and nighttime awakening with asthma symptoms. Chronic use of inhaled glucocorticoids can predispose the patient to osteoporosis, which should be remembered when working with the elderly. Also, the nurse can instruct the patient to rinse their mouth after use of medication, because oral candidiasis and hoarseness may occur.

ANTISEIZURE MEDICATIONS

Drugs used to treat seizures are considered CNS depressants. Seizures are sudden, transient episodes of exaggerated motor activity or abnormal behavior caused by excessive electrical discharge of cerebral neurons. Epilepsy is diagnosed when seizures recur spontaneously over time.

Seizures are considered a symptom of an underlying disorder. Etiologies are varied. In 50 percent of patients, seizures are primary, or idiopathic (of unknown cause). In the other 50 percent of patients with seizures, the cause may be trauma, infectious diseases, metabolic disorders, vascular diseases, or neoplastic disease. Epilepsy is a chronic seizure disorder. Pregnancy is a major concern for patients with epilepsy, because some antiseizure medications decrease the effectiveness of oral contraceptives. Women who take antiseizure medications need to be instructed to use additional barrier methods of birth control. Most antiseizure drugs are pregnancy category D and should not be used during pregnancy. Individual antiseizure medications can cause a folate deficiency that has been linked to neural tube defects. Antiseizure agents are prescribed specific to the type of seizure that the patient exhibits.

Antiseizure drugs suppress abnormal electrical impulses from the seizure focus to other cortical areas. They stop the seizure but do not eliminate the cause of the seizure. Antiseizure medications are generally taken throughout a patient's lifetime. There are many types of antiseizure drugs used to treat epilepsy, including the hydantoins (phenytoin, mephenytoin, or ethotoin), long-acting barbiturates (phenobarbital, mephobarbital, or primidone), succinimides (ethosuximide), oxazolidine (trimethadione), benzodiazepines (diazepam or clonazepam), carbamazepine, and valproic acid (Depakene).

Antiseizure drugs affect the movement of electrolytes across neuronal membranes and alter the balance of neurotransmitters. In a resting state, neurons are normally surrounded by a higher concentration of sodium, calcium, and chloride ions. Potassium levels are higher inside the cell. An influx of sodium or calcium into the neuron enhances neuronal activity, whereas an influx of chloride ion suppresses neuronal activity. The goal of the antiseizure pharmacotherapy is to suppress neuronal activity just enough to prevent abnormal firing. They exert their effects by three general mechanisms: (a) stimulating an influx of chloride ion, an effect associated with the neurotransmitter, gamma-aminobutyric acid (GABA); (b) delaying an influx of sodium; and (c) delaying and influx of calcium. There are four major chemical classes of antiseizure medications: hydantoins, benzodiazepines, succinimides, and barbiturates.

Indications

Phenytoin, a hydantoin, is the first antiseizure drug used to treat seizures. Discovered in 1938, it is still the most commonly used drug for controlling seizures. It reduces motor cortex activity by suppressing the influx of sodium. Phenytoin is a broad-spectrum drug that is useful in treating all types of seizures except absence seizures.

Benzodiazepines are widely prescribed drugs used not only to control seizures but also for anxiety, skeletal muscle spasms, and alcohol withdrawal symptoms. They achieve seizure control by stimulating the release of GABA by the GABA nucleus, which provides a generalized CNS depressant effect. Clonazepam is effective in controlling absence seizures. Absence seizures are generalized seizures because neural impulses travel bilaterally and symmetrically through the brain. Absence seizures last only a few seconds and usually involve staring and loss of responsiveness. There, however, may be slight motor activity with eyelid fluttering or myoclonic jerks. Clorazepate dipotassium is often used in adjunctive therapy for treating partial seizures. In partial (focal) seizures only a portion of the brain is involved. The neuronal impulse starts on one side and travels only a short distance. Simple partial seizures have a small focus, which may be limited to a slight twitching of the arms, legs or face; a sudden burst of emotions; altered sensory responses, such as smelling odors that are not present or hearing and seeing things that are not there; or they may progress to a generalized seizure. IV diazepam is primarily used to terminate status epilepticus, a medical emergency of continuously recurring seizure activity. Continuous tonic-clonic seizure activity results in hypoxia, hypoglycemia, acidosis, and hypothermia because of increased metabolic needs, lactic acid production, and heat loss during contraction. Without treatment, status epilepticus leads to brain damage and death (Adams, et al., 2005). With benzodiazepines, tolerance develops after only a few months, and dosages need to be adjusted. Benzodiazepines are not usually used alone in seizure management.

The succinimide drug group is used primarily to treat absence (previously called petit mal) seizures. Ethosuximide (Zarontin) is the succinimide of choice in this group (Broyles, et al., 2007). Seizure control is achieved by suppressing the influx of calcium ions that has the effect of increasing the seizure threshold. With less calcium in the neuron, it is less likely that the neuron will reach an action potential to generate an impulse. This results in suppression of abnormal foci.

The long-acting barbiturate, phenobarbital, is prescribed to treat the generalized tonic-clonic seizures and acute episodes of status epilepticus seizures. Tonic-clonic seizures are described as episodes of intense muscle contractions followed by muscle relaxation. The seizure may be preceded by an aura described as a sensory warning, which may be a smell, a spiritual feeling, or vision. In addition the tonic-clonic muscle activity, the patient may be incontinent of urine and feces and breathing may become shallow or stop momentarily. A postictal state follows the seizure. During this time the patient is drowsy, confused, and may sleep soundly. Barbiturates enhance the inhibitory action of GABA by stimulating the influx of chloride ions, decreasing impulse transmission to the cerebral cortex.

Other drugs used to prevent seizures are carbamazepine (Tegretol) and valproic acid (Depakote). Carbamazepine is effective in treating refractory seizure disorders that have not responded to other antiseizure drugs. It is used to control generalized tonic-clonic seizures and partial seizures, as well as a combination of these seizures. Other uses for carbamazepine include the treatment of bipolar disease, for pain relief in trigeminal neuralgia, and for alcohol withdrawal. Carbamazepine inhibits nerve impulses by limiting influx of sodium ions across cell membranes in the motor cortex. Valproic acid has been prescribed for absence, generalized, and mixed types of seizures. Additionally, valproic acid has been approved by the FDA for management of manic episodes in patients with bipolar disorder and is used in the treatment of migraine headaches. Valproic acid depresses CNS activity by slowing the influx of sodium ions across neuronal membranes.

Pharmacokinetics

Phenytoin is slowly absorbed in the small intestine. It is highly protein-bound; a decrease in serum protein or albumin can increase free phenytoin serum level. The liver excretes inactive metabolites in the urine.

Laboratory Monitoring

The monitoring of antiseizure medications begins with their serum drug levels. The following are three examples of blood levels for antiseizure medications: (a) Phenytoin: 10 to 20 mcg/mL; (b) carbamazepine: 5 to12 mcg/mL; and (c) Depakote: 40 to 100 mcg/mL. The nurse must obtain baseline and ongoing tests of renal and liver function that include AST, ALT, bilirubin, BUN, and creatinine. In addition, the nurse must obtain baseline and ongoing CBC, Hct, and Hgb to detect serious blood dyscrasias. The patient's baseline and ongoing blood glucose levels are to be monitored. The patient's urine must be assessed for hematuria and valproic acid can increase the risk of false-positive for ketones in the urine, as well as interfering with thyroid function tests. Antiseizure drugs can increase alkaline phosphatase.

Side Effects and Adverse Effects

The severe side effects of hydantoins include gingival hyperplasia, overgrowth of the gum tissues (reddened gums that bleed); neurological and psychiatric effects, such as slurred speech, confusion, depression, and thrombocytopenia (low platelet count); and leukopenia (low white count). Toxic effects include bone marrow depression and cardiovascular collapse. Long-term use of hydantoins may result in hyperglycemia because of inhibition of the release of insulin. Less severe side effects include GI effects (nausea, vomiting, and constipation), CNS effects (drowsiness or headaches), skin effects (rash lupus erythematosus, alopecia, and hirsutism), visual changes (nystagmus, blurred vision, and diplopia) and hypocalcemia. Urine may be discolored to pink, red, or brown.

Side effects of benzodiazepines include CNS effects (dizziness, drowsiness, confusion, headache, and fatigue), orthostatic hypotension, blurred vision, and constipation, dry mouth, rash, and itching. Adverse effects and signs of toxicity include neutropenia, respiratory depression, ECG changes, and tachycardia.

The side effects of succinimides include CNS effects, such as drowsiness, dizziness, fatigue, euphoria, and lethargy; GI effects of nausea, vomiting, heartburn, or anorexia; pink urine; skin effects including urticaria and pruritic erythema; and vision changes, such as myopia and blurred vision. Adverse effects that may develop are agranulocytosis, aplastic anemia, thrombocytopenia, leukocytosis, eosinophilia, pancytopenia, and Stevens-Johnson syndrome. Psychosis or extreme mood swings, including depression with overt suicidal intent can occur (Adams, et al., 2005). Toxic effects similar to hydantoins are bone marrow depression and cardiovascular collapse.

The most common side effects of barbiturates are lethargy, sedation, hyperactivity (in children and the elderly), cognition slowing, and ataxia (Cross, 2004). Adverse effects include coma, Stevens-Johnson syndrome, angioedema, and thrombophlebitis. In addition to common CNS side effects, carbamazepine can increase PT and cause syndrome of inappropriate antidiuretic hormone (SIADH). Life-threatening adverse effects include blood dyscrasias, paralysis, hepatitis, Stevens-Johnson syndrome, hypertension, CHF, dysrhythmias, and AV block.

Side effects of valproic acid include sedation, drowsiness, GI side effects, and a rash. The most serious adverse effect is hepatotoxicity. The nurse should monitor for blood dyscrasias, pancreatitis, and toxic hepatitis.

The efficacy of birth control pills is decreased by the use of enzyme-inducing antiseizure drugs, such as carbamazepine, phenytoin, and phenobarbital. Women should be instructed to use a second method of birth control. Women of childbearing age should take at least 1 mg of folic acid to decrease the rate of neural tube defect in the fetus.

Nursing Management

The administration of antiseizure medications involves the individual assessment of each medication. For example, benzodiazepines require the assessment of orthostatic blood pressures, and the nurse must hold the medication if the blood pressure drops significantly. In the administration of succinimides, the nurse must monitor renal studies (e.g., urinalysis, BUN, and creatinine). In addition, the nurse must obtain CBC, Hct, Hgb, and reticulocyte counts every week for four weeks. Also, the nurse must monitor hepatic studies (e.g., AST, ALT, and bilirubin). The nurse must assess the patient for allergic reactions, such as red, raised rash, or exfoliative dermatitis. And, the nurse must monitor the patient for blood dyscrasias, fever, sore throat, bruising, rash, or jaundice.

The nurse must monitor barbiturates for respiratory status and assess results of blood studies, renal and liver function, and blood dyscrasias. In the administration of carbamazepine, the nurse must observe for allergic reactions, including purpura or red raised rash. These medications have oral forms which may be given with food or milk to reduce GI symptoms. The chewable pills must be chewed or crushed and should not be swallowed whole. The patient must be instructed that grapefruit juice may increase peak concentrations. When administering Depakote, the nurse must monitor blood, hepatic and renal studies, including red blood cells, Hct, Hgb, serum folate, PT, platelets, vitamin D, reticulocyte count, AST, ALT, bilirubin, urinalysis, BUN, and creatinine. When hydantoins are administered, the nurse must brush the patient's teeth with soft toothbrush, gently floss to prevent gingival hyperplasia, and instruct the patient to have regular dental checkups.

When administering antiseizure medications, the patient must avoid other CNS depressants, including alcohol, because of additive effects, including increased sedation. In addition, the patient must use alternate barrier methods of birth control because antiseizure drugs may decrease the effectiveness of oral contraceptives. Patients on antiseizure medications can be encouraged to carry an ID card or medical alert bracelet.

ANTIULCER AGENTS

Ulcers can occur in the esophagus, the stomach, or the duodenum within the upper GI tract. Their name is derived by the location. Duodenal ulcers occur 10 times more often than gastric or esophageal ulcers. The release of hydrochloric acid (HCL) from the parietal cells of the stomach is influenced by histamine, gastrin, and acetylcholine. Peptic ulcers occur when there is a hypersecretion of hydrochloric acid and pepsin that erode the GI mucosal lining.

The predisposing risk factors for developing PUD include the following: a family history of PUD; blood group type O; cigarette smoking; intake of foods and beverages containing caffeine; drugs, particularly glucocorticoids, aspirin, and NSAIDS; stress; and infection with *H. pylori*. The characteristic symptom of duodenal ulcer is a gnawing or burning abdominal pain that occurs one to three hours after meals. The pain goes away when the patient eats. Nighttime pain, nausea, or vomiting is not typical. If the erosion progresses more deeply into the mucosa, bleeding may occur and is evidenced by bright red blood in emesis or black, tarry stools. Gastric ulcers are less common and have different symptoms.

Red Flag

Keeping the Patient Safe During a Seizure

If a patient has a seizure in the nurse's presence, position patient to prevent injury. If in bed, the nurse should put him or her on the side to allow drainage of secretion and put bed in flat position. If not in bed, the nurse should position the patient on the floor with a pillow under the head. The nurse should not put anything in the patient's mouth, but should have suction equipment and oxygen available. The nurse should time the duration of the seizure. If the seizure continues longer than three minutes, the nurse should make sure the patient has a patent airway. If the nurse is unable to establish IV access, medication may need rectal administration. When the seizure ends, the nurse should draw blood for routine lab to determine cause. The nurse must monitor vital signs and cardiac status and stay with the patient. The nurse should chart the characteristics and duration of the seizure as level of consciousness and note the loss of consciousness. In addition, the nurse must implement seizure precautions per agency protocol.

Adapted from Broyles, B. E., Reiss, B. S., & Evans, M. E. (2007). Pharmacological aspects of nursing care (7th ed.). New York: Thomson Delmar Learning.

While relieved by food intake, the pain may continue for several hours after a meal. Loss of appetite as well as weight loss and vomiting are more common.

Pharmacotherapy for treating PUD includes OTC and prescription drugs from the following five classes: H_2 receptor antagonists, proton pump inhibitors, antacids, antibiotics, and miscellaneous drugs. Patients are encouraged to change lifestyle factors that contribute to PUD, such as eliminating smoking, decreasing alcohol intake, and reducing stress.

Histamine$_2$ Antagonists and Proton Pump Inhibitors

Histamine has two types of receptors: H_1 and H_2. The activation of H_1 receptors on the parietal cells in the stomach produces classic symptoms of allergy, whereas activation of H_2 receptors produces hydrochloric acid. Histamine H_2 antagonists are effective in suppressing both the volume and acidity of stomach acid (Broyles, et al., 2007).

Proton pump inhibitors (PPIs) bind to the enzyme $H+$ (a proton) and $K+$-ATPase in the stomach. This enzyme acts as a pump to release acid (also $H+$ or protons) in the parietal cells of the stomach onto the surface of the GI mucosa. When this enzyme is blocked, acid secretion is decreased. PPIs are able to inhibit gastric acid secretion up to 90 percent more than the H_2 blockers

Indications

H_2 antagonists are used to treat duodenal ulcers, gastric ulcers, hypersecretory conditions, such as Zollinger-Ellison syndrome, and gastric reflux disease. They are also used for prevention of stress ulcers in critically ill patients and in combination therapy to treat *H. pylori.*

PPIs are used to treat erosive or ulcerative gastroesophageal reflux disease (GERD) or duodenal ulcers, active benign gastric ulcers, and NSAID-associated gastric ulcers on a short-term basis. They are also used for healing and for maintenance to reduce the return rates of heartburn symptoms in erosive or ulcerative GERD.

Pharmacokinetics

The first H_2 blocker was cimetidine (Tagamet). Cimetidine, which has a short half-life and short duration of action, blocks about 70 percent of acid secretion for about four hours. Good kidney function is important because 50 to 80 percent of the drug is excreted in the urine unchanged. If antacids are given at the same time, the effectiveness of the H_2 blocker is decreased. Cimetidine is used less frequently than other H_2 antagonists because of its numerous drug-drug interactions due to its C-450 system inhibition and because it must be taken up to four times a day. Three other H_2 antagonists, ranitidine, famotidine, and nizatidine, are more potent than cimetidine. In addition to blocking gastric acid secretions, they also promote healing of the ulcer by eliminating the cause. Their duration of action is longer; therefore, less frequent dosing is needed. They also have fewer side effects.

PPIs have a short half-life and are highly protein-bound. They should be taken before meals. Caution should be used in patients with liver impairment. (See Uncovering the Evidence.)

Laboratory Monitoring

Patients taking histamine$_2$ antagonists and PPIs should be monitored for renal and hepatic function. In addition, their CBC should be monitored to evaluate for anemia. Several individual medications have their own considerations as they are assessed. For example, ranitidine (Zantac) can cause a false-positive urine prolactin; cimetidine (Tagamet) can cause a false-negative reading on

---

PATIENT PLAYBOOK

Histamine$_2$ Antagonists and PPIs

The nurse can instruct the patient taking histamine$_2$ antagonists and PPIs to:

- Stop smoking because smoking causes gastric stimulation.
- Avoid use of antacids within one hour of dose. (H_2 antagonists)
- Take medication as directed.
- Once-a-day dosing should be taken at bedtime; if prescribed more than once daily, take before meals.
- Avoid gastric irritants, such as alcohol, aspirin, or NSAIDS.

Adapted from Broyles, B. E., Reiss, B. S., & Evans, M. E. (2007). Pharmacological aspects of nursing care (7th ed.). New York: Thomson Delmar Learning.

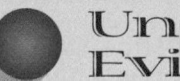

Uncovering the Evidence

Risk of Community-Acquired Pneumonia (CAP)

Discussion: Drugs that reduce gastric acid secretion can increase a person's risk of pneumonia, according to the results of a study involving more than 300,000 people. People taking PPIs, such as esomeprazole (Nexium), lansoprazole (Prevacid), and omeprazole (Prilosec), had almost twice the risk of developing community-acquired pneumonia (CAP) as former users of these drugs. Researchers theorize that by reducing germ-killing stomach acid, these drugs allow pathogens from the upper GI tract to colonize the respiratory tract. Researchers reviewed the medical records of 364,683 patients and identified 5,551 cases of pneumonia. One hundred eighty-five of the cases of pneumonia occurred in patients taking acid-suppressing drugs. Histamine$_2$ receptor antagonists also raised the risk, but not as much.

Implications for Practice: Nurses can assess patients taking acid-suppressing medications for respiratory complications. The complications for patients can potentially be minimized with this additional nursing management strategy.

Source: Laheij, R. J., Sturkenboom, M. C., Hassing, R., Dieleman, J., Stricker, H. C., Jansen, J. (2004). Risk of community-acquired pneumonia and use of gastric acid-suppressive drugs. JAMA, 292, 1955–1960.

allergen skin test, increase prolactin, alkaline phosphatase and creatinine levels and may alter gastroccult testing caused by blue dye used in testing tablets; famotidine (Pepcid) may cause increased liver function enzymes levels; and nizatidine (Axid) can cause a false-positive urobilinogen.

Side Effects and Adverse Effects

CNS side effects, such as dizziness, drowsiness, confusion, and headache, are more likely to occur in the elderly. GI side effects that may occur are altered taste, diarrhea, constipation, and dry mouth. IV cimetidine has been known to cause dysrhythmias and hypotension. Though rare, these drugs can cause hepatotoxicity. Long-term use of H$_2$ antagonists may lead to vitamin B$_{12}$ deficiencies, because they decrease absorption of the vitamin.

PPIs will affect the absorption of medications, vitamins, and minerals that need an acidic environment in the stomach. Adverse effects include dizziness, headache, abdominal pain, diarrhea, and rash. Adverse effects that have been reported include pancreatitis, liver necrosis, hepatic failure, toxic epidermal necrolysis, and Stevens-Johnson syndrome. Patient should be monitored for agranulocytosis, myocardial infarction, shock, and CVA.

Nursing Management

When administering antiulcer medications, the nurse can explain to the patient that reduced doses are required for patients with hepatic or renal impairment. In addition, the patient should be assessed for medication interactions. The patient can be monitored for the laboratory tests including liver function test, CBC, and renal function (BUN and creatinine). Protonix and AcipHex must be swallowed whole, and IV Protonix should be administered over a period of 15 minutes at a rate not greater than 3 mg/minute (7 mL/min). An in-line filter should be used.

ANTIDIABETIC AGENTS

Diabetes mellitus (DM), a chronic disease resulting from deficient glucose metabolism, is caused by insufficient insulin secretion from the beta cells (refer to chapter 57). This results in high blood glucose levels (hyperglycemia). The classic clinical symptoms of diabetes are increased frequency of urination (polyuria), increased thirst and fluid intake (polydipsia), and as the disease progresses, weight loss despite increased hunger and food intake (polyphagia). Untreated diabetes produces long-term damage to arteries that leads to heart disease, stroke, kidney disease, and blindness. Patients with diabetes who require medications are classically treated with either insulin or oral hypoglycemic agents.

Insulin

Available since 1922, insulin is used for the treatment of type 1 diabetes mellitus. Type 1 DM is characterized by elevated blood glucose levels caused by a lack of insulin secretion in the pancreas. A plan that includes meal planning and exercise, in addition to insulin, is required to control blood glucose levels. The treatment goal with insulin therapy is to maintain blood glucose levels within strict, normal limits to prevent the many complications of this disease. Insulin restores the ability of cells to use glucose as an energy source. Several types of insulin are available, differing in their onset and duration of action. Almost all insulin today is human insulin obtained from recombinant DNA technology. While some patients still use pork or beef insulin, human insulin is more effective, causes fewer allergies, and has a lower incidence of insulin resistance. Insulin is administered subcutaneously. Doses are individualized for each patient's needs. Two different compatible insulins may be mixed to obtain a desired effect. Regular insulin, which is clear, is always drawn up in the syringe first, followed by the cloudy insulin (see Fast Forward).

Indications

Insulin is used to treat both type 1 and type 2 DM and diabetic ketoacidosis (DKA). Insulin also lowers plasma potassium levels and is used as emergency treatment of hyperkalemia.

Pharmacokinetics

Regular and NPH insulins are well absorbed with all routes of administration. Both insulins can be administered subcutaneously, but only regular insulin can be given intravenously. The half-life varies. Insulin is metabolized by the liver and is excreted in the urine.

Laboratory Monitoring

The patient who is receiving antidiabetic agents is primarily monitored with blood glucose testing (Figure 17-5). In addition, the patient is monitored with a fasting blood glucose, a glucose tolerance test, and glycosylated HgbA$_{1c}$, which is a blood test representative of the average blood glucose level over the past several weeks. In addition, the patient can be monitored by obtaining a urinalysis and check for glucose and ketones, as well as monitoring serum electrolytes.

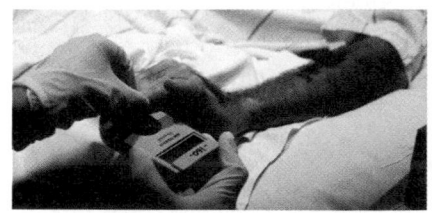
Figure 17-5 Blood glucose monitoring.

Side Effects and Adverse Effects

The most serious adverse effect of insulin therapy is hypoglycemia. Hypoglycemia occurs when blood glucose levels drop below 50 mg/dL. Hypoglycemia can be the result of taking too much insulin, not getting food soon enough after taking insulin, or skipping meals. Signs of hypoglycemia include tachycardia, nervousness, trembling, headache, confusion, lack of coordination, and cold and clammy skin. Without prompt treatment with glucose seizures, coma, and death may follow.

Insulin Management

The nurse can instruct the patient to do the following in their management of diabetes:

- Instruct the patient regarding the signs of hypoglycemia and hyperglycemia.
- Inform the patient that hypoglycemic reactions are more likely to occur when insulin reaches its peak effect, during exercise and during acute illness.
- Administer glucagons by injection as taught if there is a hypoglycemic reaction.
- Do not drink sugar-containing liquids.
- Self-monitor blood glucose (SMBG) as per protocol, particularly when engaging in regular exercise.
- Follow dietary restrictions for weight control and consult with the dietitian.
- Wear a medical alert tag or bracelet.

Adapted from Broyles, B. E., Reiss, B. S., & Evans, M. E. (2007). Pharmacological aspects of nursing care (7th ed.). New York: Thomson Delmar Learning.

Hyperglycemia (DKA) occurs when blood sugar is elevated to a level greater than 300 mg/dL. With inadequate amount of insulin, the sugar cannot be metabolized and fat catabolism occurs. The use of fatty acids (ketones) for energy causes ketoacidosis. Unlike the rapid onset of hypoglycemia, symptoms of hyperglycemia usually develop over a few days. Symptoms of ketoacidosis include extreme thirst, polyuria, fruity breath odor, Kussmaul breathing (deep, rapid, labored, distressing, dyspnea), rapid pulse, and dry mucous membranes.

Nursing Management

General nursing strategies for patients with diabetes who are being managed with insulin are to assess for clinical manifestations of the complications associated with diabetes (e.g., DKA or hypoglycemia). In addition, the continued effectiveness of the insulin therapy is evaluated by assessing the patient with diabetes for long-term complications related to acceleration of atherosclerosis (hypertension, heart disease, and stroke); retinopathy leading to possible blindness; nephropathy leading to possible renal failure; neuropathy leading to lower limb ulcerations and amputation, impotence, and gastroparesis. The patient should also be given specific parameters for his or her insulin administration when there is insufficient food intake or during times of changes in activity levels.

Oral Hypoglycemic Agents

In type 2 DM insufficient amounts of insulin are secreted to meet metabolic needs or there is a lack of sensitivity of insulin receptors. Type 2 DM is usually controlled with oral hypoglycemic (antidiabetic) agents, which are prescribed after diet and exercise have failed to reduce blood glucose to normal levels. All oral antidiabetic agents lower blood glucose levels. They are classified based on their chemical structures and mechanisms of action. The sulfonylureas were the first oral antidiabetic agents available and are divided into first and second generation categories. Though both are effective, second generation drugs have fewer drug-drug interactions. Sulfonylureas act by stimulating the release of insulin from islet cells and by increasing the sensitivity of insulin receptors on target cells. The most common adverse effect of sulfonylureas is hypoglycemia, which is caused by taking too much medication or not eating enough food.

The biguanides, such as metformin (Glucophage), act by decreasing the hepatic production of glucose and reducing insulin resistance. Biguanides alone do not cause hypoglycemia or weight gain. Because of the risk of lactic acidosis, metformin is contraindicated for patients receiving dialysis (Leydig, 2005). The alpha-glucosidase inhibitors, such as acarbose (Precose), lower blood glucose by delaying the absorption of dietary carbohydrates in the small intestine. These agents are well tolerated and have minimal side effects. When taking this drug, the patient's diet should consist of reduced complex carbohydrates. When used with insulin or another sulfonylurea, hypoglycemia may occur.

Indications

The thiazolidinediones, or glitazones, reduce blood glucose by decreasing insulin resistance and inhibiting hepatic gluconeogenesis. The meglitinides are the newest class of oral hypoglycemics that act by stimulating the release of insulin from the islet cells. They demonstrate the same efficacy as the sulfonylureas and are well tolerated. The patients must be monitored closely for hypoglycemia.

Pharmacokinetics

The sulfonylurea, acetohexamide (Dymelor), is well absorbed by the GI tract and is highly protein-bound. Less than 2 percent of acarbose (Precose) is absorbed intact from the GI tract. The liver metabolizes acetohexamide, with 50 percent converted to metabolite. There are two half-lives: the half-life of the drug metabolite is three times as long as that of the pure drug. The $t_{1/2}$ life of acarbose is two hours. The kidneys excrete acetohexamide unchanged in the urine. Because of acarbose's poor absorption, 50 percent is excreted in the feces and 35 percent is excreted in the urine.

Laboratory Monitoring

The patient receiving oral hypoglycemics for insulin dysfunction is monitored closely with laboratory tests. The continued SMBG testing can be performed by the patient to ensure a balance of the blood glucose. In addition, the patient can be monitored with a CBC with differential, platelet counts, and a baseline and ongoing liver function tests.

Side Effects and Adverse Effects

The sulfonylureas are generally well tolerated. Hypoglycemia related to drug overdosage, drug-drug interactions, altered drug metabolism, or inadequate food intake may occur. Adverse reactions are those of hematological disorders including aplastic anemia, leucopenia, and thrombocytopenia. When taken with alcohol a disulfiram-like reaction may occur causing flushing, palpitations, and nausea.

Biguanides may cause decreased appetite, nausea, and diarrhea that usually subside over time. They also increase the absorption of B_{12} and folic acid. Alpha-glucosidase inhibitors cause flatulence, cramps, abdominal distension, and diarrhea. They may decrease the absorption of iron over time, leading to anemia.

Nursing Management

The general nursing strategies for management when receiving hypoglycemics is similar to that of receiving insulin therapy (see chapter 57 for more specific information). The hypoglycemics should be taken 30 minutes before breakfast or as directed by the health care provider. The patient should take missed doses as soon as remembered unless close to next dose and should be instructed to not double-up on the dose. As stated, the patient should continue to carefully monitor the blood glucose levels with SMBG testing. The nurse must instruct the patient to monitor nutrition and exercise carefully and consistently. In addition, the patient can take the hypoglycemics with food if there are GI clinical manifestations. The patient should recognize symptoms of hypoglycemia (e.g., tachycardia, nervousness, sweating, headache, and confusion). The patient should always carry a source of simple sugar for use if this occurs. As a cautionary measure the patient should be educated to swallow tablets whole and not crush sustained-release tablets.

KEY CONCEPTS

- Pharmacokinetics describes the actions the body has on a drug. The four pharmacokinetic processes are absorption, distribution, metabolism, and excretion.
- Careful adherence to the principles of safe medication administration is necessary to provide for patient safety.
- Monitor all persons on anti-infective agents for allergy or history of hypersensitivity, possible drug-drug interactions, side effects, adverse effects, and effectiveness of therapy.

- The cardiac glycoside, digoxin, is used to treat CHF. Digoxin has the chronotropic effect of slowing the heart rate and the positive inotropic effect of increasing the force of contraction of myocardial fibers.
- Four classes of antidysrhythmic drugs are used to restore normal cardiac rhythms. These are: (a) fast sodium channel blockers 1A, 1B, and 1C; (b) beta blockers; (c) potassium channel blockers, and (d) slow calcium channel blockers.

Continued

KEY CONCEPTS—cont'd

- Diuretics are used to treat hypertension and to reduce both pulmonary and peripheral edema in people with CHF and renal or liver disorders.
- ACE inhibitors decrease blood pressure by inhibiting ACE that acts to inhibit the formation of angiotensin II that is a vasoconstrictor.
- Anticoagulants prolong bleeding time in an effort to prevent the formation of thrombi (clots). Heparin is for parenteral administration, and warfarin (Coumadin) is the oral form.
- Antilipemics are drugs that lower abnormal blood lipids. These drugs are divided into classes that include HMG-CoA reductase inhibitors (statins), bile acids, fibric acid derivatives, and nicotinic acid.
- Inhaled glucocorticoids are the most effective drugs available for prevention of acute asthmatic episodes. The most frequently occurring side effects of inhaled corticosteroids are related to irritation of the upper airway.

- Antiseizure medications suppress abnormal electrical impulses from the seizure focus to other areas in the brain. Seizures are classified as partial, generalized, and special epileptic syndromes.
- Antiulcer drugs include histamine$_2$ blockers and PPIs. They act to decrease acid in the stomach and as a result relieve the symptoms of PUD, GERD, and hypersecretory disorders.
- Insulin is used to treat both type 1 and type 2 DM. The goal of insulin therapy is to maintain blood glucose levels in a normal range between 60 and 100 mg/dL.
- Oral hypoglycemic agents are prescribed for patients with type 2 DM when diet and exercise have failed to decrease blood glucose levels.

REVIEW QUESTIONS

1. A patient who is taking NPH insulin every morning reports feeling weak and tremulous in the midafternoon. Which of these actions should the nurse take?
   1. Take the patient's blood pressure
   2. Give a PRN dose of regular insulin
   3. Check the patient's blood sugar
   4. Have patient lie down

2. The health care provider has prescribed the oral hypoglycemic agent glyburide for a patient with type 2 DM Before administering this drug, the nurse should assess the patient for:
   1. Penicillin allergy
   2. Cephalosporin allergy
   3. Shellfish allergy
   4. Sulfonamide allergy

3. Anticoagulants would be contraindicated for a patient with a recent history of:
   1. Atrial fibrillation
   2. Gastric ulcers
   3. Presence of mechanical heart valves
   4. DVT

4. Which of the following should be included in a teaching plan for patients who receive lipid-lowering agents, such as simvastatin (Zocor)?
   1. Dietary fat intake need not be limited.
   2. The drug increases risk of coronary or lung disease.

   3. You will need periodic evaluation of liver function.
   4. You will notice a decrease in exercise tolerance.

5. The desired outcome of therapy with a methylxanthine derivative, such as theophylline (Theo-Dur) is:
   1. Deceased wheezing
   2. Decreased platelet clumping or aggregation
   3. Increased cardiac heart rate
   4. Increased urine output

6. Cimetidine (Tagamet) and ranitidine (Zantac) both block H$_2$ receptors to:
   1. Decrease the respiratory rate
   2. Increase gastric motility
   3. Decrease gastric acid secretion
   4. Cause contraction of smooth muscle in the bronchial tree

7. The nurse monitors the patient taking digoxin for sign of toxicity. Which of the following indicate a need to check the digoxin level?
   1. Double vision
   2. Gastric upset
   3. Lower extremity edema
   4. Slowed capillary refill

Continued

REVIEW QUESTIONS—cont'd

8. Medication teaching for a patient who has been prescribed sublingual nitroglycerin tablets for treatment of angina should include to:
   1. Dissolve tablets in water before swallowing
   2. Take only one tablet per hour
   3. Report side effects of hypotension, flushing, and headache
   4. Call 911 if pain persists after three doses at five-minute intervals

9. Patients receiving the diuretic furosemide (Lasix) are often prescribed which of the following to prevent a common side effect of the drug:
   1. An antidepressant
   2. A potassium supplement
   3. Folic acid
   4. Vitamin K

10. You are preparing to administer morphine sulfate to your patient. Which route would be affected by the first-pass effect?
    1. IV
    2. Sublingual
    3. Oral
    4. Rectal suppository

11. Drug half-life (t $_{1/2}$) is defined as the amount of time required for 50 percent of a drug to:
    1. Be absorbed by the body
    2. Reach a therapeutic level
    3. Exert a physiological response
    4. Be eliminated from the body

12. The criteria for determining drug dosages in the elderly should be based on:
    1. More on age than height or weight
    2. More on weight that age
    3. On the total body water (TBW) content
    4. Overall renal and hepatic function

13. Which of the following is a serious side effect of aminoglycoside antibiotic therapy?
    1. Excessive thirst
    2. Decreased hearing
    3. Jaundice
    4. Increased urine output

14. After receiving ampicillin (Amoxicillin) for five days, the patient complains of mouth sores, diarrhea, and vaginal itching. The nurse knows that these symptoms indicate:
    1. Anaphylactic reaction to drug
    2. Ineffectiveness of drug therapy
    3. Spread of her infection
    4. Superinfection

REVIEW ACTIVITIES

1. Select a sample of frequently administered medications. Look up in drug reference book. Have students discuss pharmacokinetic risks with each of the drugs.

2. Develop a nursing care plan for a patient with emphasis on pharmacological interventions. Ask students to present the signs and symptoms of a medical disorder, selected medication, baseline laboratory monitoring, informed consent and medication teaching, first dose monitoring, and evaluation.

3. Role-play principles of safe medication administration.

4. Discuss the differences between side effects and adverse effects.

5. Student assignment: Browse selected nursing journals for examples of medication errors. Discuss ways to prevent.

6. Discuss: Your patient is taking two highly protein bound drugs. What measures can you take to ensure patient safety? Give examples.

7. What measures can you take to minimize the risk of or promptly intervene in the life-threatening adverse effect of anaphylactic shock?

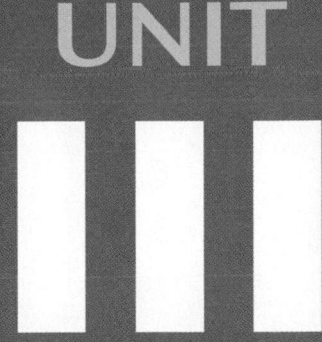

UNIT

III

Settings for Nursing Care

Health Care Agencies

Frances Vlasses, PhD, RN

Laura M. Rogers, RNC, MSN

KEY TERMS

Access
Adult daycare
Assisted living
Continuing care
Critical access hospital (CAH)
Gross domestic product (GDP)
Health insurance
Health maintenance organizations (HMOs)
Hospice
Integrated care delivery system
Length of stay (LOS)
Long-term care
Managed care organizations (MCOs)
Medicaid
Medicare
Outcome variables
Preferred provider organization (PPO)
Preventive care
Primary care
Process variables
Restorative care
Structural variables
Synergy model
Tertiary care
Total quality management (TQM)

CHAPTER TOPICS

- Health Care Cost and Financing
- Access to Health Care
- Health Care Quality
- Classifications of Health Care Agencies
- The Future of Health Care
- Practice Model
- Nurse's Role in Health Care Agencies

Health care systems consist of all the people and actions whose primary purpose is to promote, restore, or maintain health. A systems framework incorporates the components of input, such as resources, output, and feedback interacting to create an interdependent mechanism for achieving common goals. This framework is a helpful backdrop to understanding how all the parts or agencies work together to create a health care system. After centuries as small-scale largely private or charitable entities, our current health care systems have grown in this century as knowledge has been gained and applied. They have contributed enormously to better health. Figure 18-1 describes the interrelation of health care organizations in the United States.

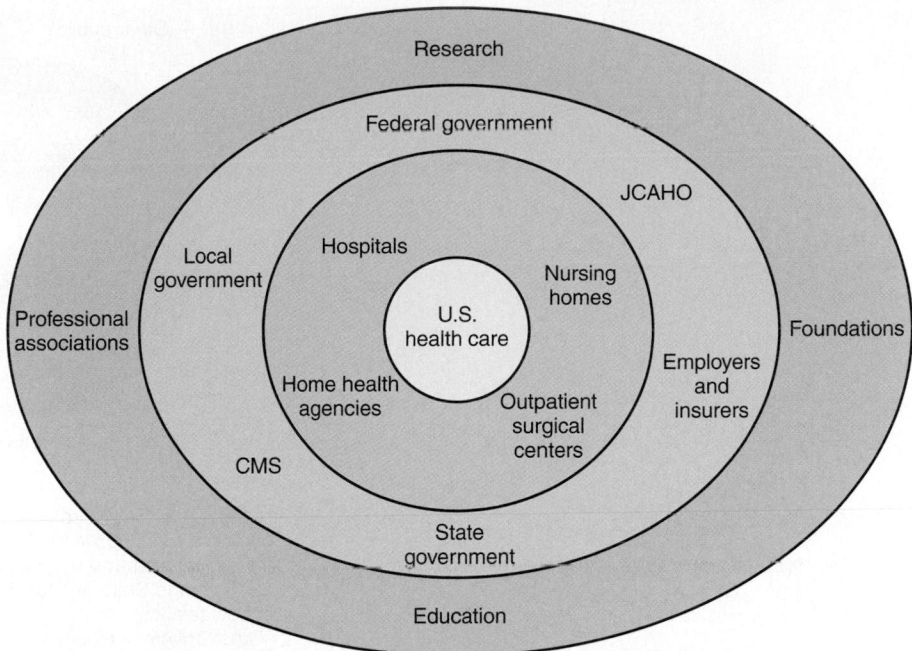

Figure 18-1 Interrelation of U.S. health care agencies. *Adapted from Shortell, S., & Kaluzny, A. (2006).* Health care management: Organization design and behavior (5th ed.). *New York: Thomson Delmar Learning.*

HEALTH CARE COST AND FINANCING

The goal of an excellent health care delivery system is to deliver high-quality, cost-effective care to all citizens. To accomplish such a goal, core values of cost, access, and quality must be intrinsic to the health care system. It seems, however, that these three factors provide more paradox than foundation, because it is difficult to balance cost with quality.

The U.S. **gross domestic product (GDP)** is the total value of final goods and services produced in a year in the United States. The U.S. health care system is often criticized as highly fragmented, yet in 2004 about 16 percent of the GDP was dedicated to health care, more than was dedicated to any other GDP category. In fact, Americans spent $1.9 trillion, more than $6,000 per person, on health care in 2004.

It is reported that over 48.1 million Americans are uninsured, and this number is expected to grow. Most health care services are provided through employment-based insurance. **Health insurance,** payment for benefits of a covered sickness or injury, relates to the financing of health care. Figure 18-2 shows how insurance breaks down between private and public funds. Thus, multiple payers function as intermediaries between the financing and the delivery of health care services.

Public financing includes the Military Health Services System (MHSS), the Department of Veterans Affairs (VA), the Indian Health Service (IHS), Medicare, Medicaid, and the State Children's Health Insurance Program (SCHIP). Private insurance includes self-insurance, commercial insurance, and **managed care organizations (MCOs)** that implement health care using managed care concepts. MCOs include **health maintenance organizations (HMOs),** which focus on covering care that keeps people well, and **preferred provider organizations (PPOs),** a type of managed care plan in which members receive more coverage if they choose to pay higher premiums. **Access** to health care services, the ability to obtain affordable health care when needed, is determined largely by insurance.

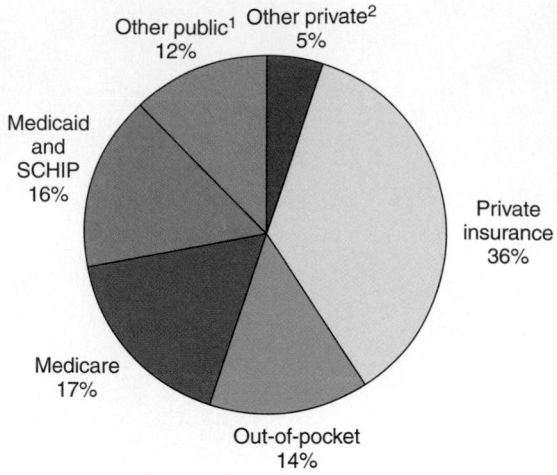

Other public[1]
12%

Other private[2]
5%

Medicaid
and
SCHIP
16%

Private
insurance
36%

Medicare
17%

Out-of-pocket
14%

[1]"Other public" includes programs such as workers'
compensation, public health activity, Department of
Defense, Department fo Veterans Affairs, Indian Health
Service, and State and local hospital subsidies and
school health.
[2]"Other private" includes industrial in-plant, privately
funded construction, and nonpatient revenues, including
philanthropy.

Figure 18-2 Sources of health care insurance. *Adapted from Centers for Medicare and Medicaid Services. (n.d.).* Statistics and data. *Retrieved August 30, 2005, from http://www.cms.hhs.gov.*

DOLLARS AND SENSE

An Innovative Alternative to Agency Staffing

Costly measures are needed to maintain staffing levels in times of nursing short-age. One such measure is the use of temporary staff from external agencies. Organizations that provide temporary nursing staff demand premium fees, which can present a financial burden for the department of nursing. Nurses employed by hospitals that use agency nurses then find themselves in situations where they are working side by side with professionals earning much higher hourly rates and who, although well-intentioned, may not be working to capacity because of unfamiliarity with patients or organizational procedures. Such situations can lead to morale problems and salary dissatisfaction.

Jones (2005) reports an innovative approach to nurse staffing that provides monetary rewards to nurses at the point-of-care in return for their commitment to the department's monetary guidelines. In her example, nursing staff take responsibility for staffing decisions. They are given complete information on staffing requirements based on patient data along with the necessary professional development to support their decision making. The incentive to share in any budget surplus that might result energizes the staff. The first department that achieves its budgetary goals places half of their budget surplus in an educational fund that they manage and split the remaining funds among all team members. The project is now in its fourth year of implementation. Beyond the obvious financial benefit, this innovation advanced additional positive outcomes. As a result of their autonomy in decision making, staff state that they feel more empowered and retention is improved, both essential components of a healthy work environment.

Respecting Our Differences

Although we strive to deliver quality care to all patients, to eliminate health care disparities nurses must set goals to move beyond personal cultural beliefs and patterns. This requires a willingness to develop awareness through individual reflection and cultural assessments and to participate in professional development to gain understanding of the values, health needs, and health beliefs of diverse ethnic populations. In this way nurses can incorporate clinical outcome data that accurately reflect the populations they serve. Through assessing the needs of their service community nurses can help design and advocate for service delivery changes that are culturally appropriate. Further, all nurses can participate in developing work teams that are culturally competent by welcoming individuals who have the talents and gifts to address the needs of the populations they serve. The Office of Minority Health and the Standards for Culturally and Linguistically Appropriate Health Care Services (CLAS) provide the roadmaps that health care providers and administrators can use to build delivery systems that are inclusive. Nurses have a responsibility to familiarize themselves with these resources to deliver care that will yield quality patient outcomes.

ACCESS TO HEALTH CARE

American health care is not considered the best in the world by many. According to the *Health, United States, 2005* report from CMS (2006) the United States is ranked 28th in infant mortality, the number of infant deaths per 1,000 live births, and the World Health Organization (WHO) ranks the U.S. 37th in overall health system performance (CMS, 2005). Inherent to the WHO rankings is the concept of access. Access to care can be defined as an important determinant of health status comprised of five components: availability, accessibility, accommodation, affordability, and acceptability. Measures associated with access to care can effectively assess the delivery of health care services and its public health policies within the United States. A national health promotion disease prevention initiative is called *Healthy People*. The mission of this monumental initiative is to increase the quality and years of healthy lives. *Healthy People 2010* (2004) seeks to measure, and thus improve, access to health care services as shown in Figure 18-3.

HEALTH CARE QUALITY

Addressing quality within health care was catapulted into national headlines when the Institute of Medicine report (2000), *To Err is Human,* was released. This report quantified deaths resulting from errors in health care at 98,000 per year. Subsequently, *Crossing the Quality Chasm* outlined steps to focus health care enterprises on quality (Institute of Medicine, 2001). Quality concerns led to heightened interest in establishing mechanisms for measuring and ultimately ensuring quality in health care.

The classic model for the evaluation of quality (Donabedian, 1998) provides for the measurement of structure, process, and outcome variables. **Structural variables** are defined as characteristics of the work force and work environment, such as certification, licensure, and nurse-patient ratios. **Process variables** are defined as operational features, including computerized health care provider order entry and evidence-based practice. **Outcome variables** are defined as consequences of care delivery and are often categorized as humanistic, financial, and clinical. An example of a humanistic outcome is patient satisfaction. **Length of stay (LOS),** the length of time a patient remains hospitalized, is a process

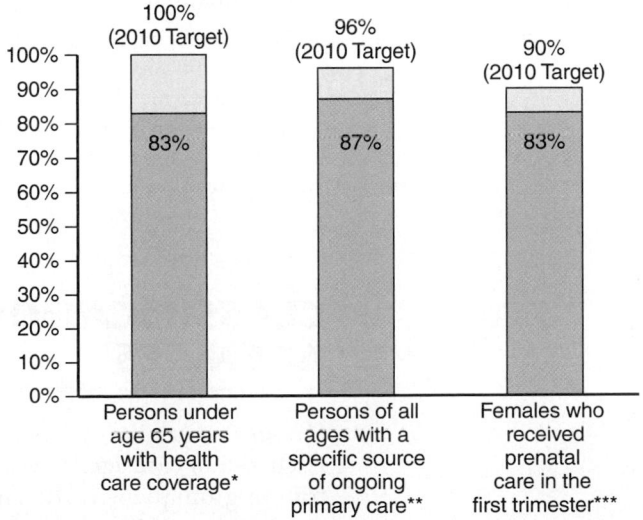

Figure 18-3 Access to health care. Sources: Centers for Disease Control and Prevention, National Center for Health Statistics. National Health Interview Survey. *1997 and **1998. Centers for Disease Control and Prevention, National Center for Health Statistics. National Vital Statistics System. *** 1998. *Adapted from* Healthy People 2010. *(2004).* About healthy people 2010. *Retrieved May 14, 2005, from http://www.healthypeople.gov.*

outcome and readmission rates are considered financial outcomes. Clinical outcomes include mortality, morbidity, and infection rates. Critical access hospitals (CAHs) are small rural hospitals that provide health care services in partnership with an acute care hospital in exchange for a higher payment schedule than that approved for other hospitals.

Currently, the health care industry has moved toward **total quality management (TQM),** a systematic approach to planning and implementing continuous improvement in quality that integrates continually assessing for improvements with achieved outcomes to enhance quality and performance through the measurement of data. The purpose of data is to understand, control, and improve the processes and structures within enterprises to achieve better outcomes. Data are essential for establishing baselines, comparisons, or benchmarking and measuring improvement.

The use of payment and public dissemination of cost information are strategies used to leverage greater change. The Centers for Medicare and Medicaid Services (CMS) has instituted a payment strategy based on the national quality measures (2004). In this strategy, Medicare funds can be withheld from hospitals if the hospital's outcomes of care for treatments associated with community acquired pneumonia, acute myocardial infarction, and congestive heart failure do not meet benchmark standards. *Hospital Compare* (2005) is a public reporting strategy wherein the results of an institution's national quality measures are publicly displayed on the Internet. Insurers, both private and public, have become value-based purchasers of health care. Value-based purchasing includes several strategies directed at improving the quality of care, encouraging the efficient use of resources, and improving information to consumers to assist them in making choices.

Groups such as the National Quality Forum (NQF) and the Agency for Healthcare Research and Quality (AHRQ) are leading national efforts to quantify health care services. These national health care organizations are challenging policy makers, such as CMS and the Joint Commission on Accreditation of Healthcare Organizations (JCAHO) to review and update their standards to ensure alignment with improving the quality of health care services. Unfortunately, quality gaps prevail, especially between the best and worst hospitals. Recently, HealthGrades, 2005 reported a 20 percent increase in hospital-acquired infections. In a study published in the *Journal of the American Medical Association,* Koppel et al. (2005) report how a computerized physician order entry (CPOE) facilitates medication errors. To sum up the quality quandary:

> Medicine being a compendium of successive and contradictory mistakes of medical practitioners, when we summon the wisest of them to our aid, the chances are that we may be relying on a scientific truth the error of which will be recognized in a few years' time. So that to believe in medicine would be the height of folly, if not to believe in it were not greater folly still, for from this mass of errors, there have emerged in the course of time many truths.

> Marcel Proust, *The Guermantes Way* (2002 [1920])

CLASSIFICATION OF HEALTH CARE AGENCIES

Currently a myriad of health care agencies exist in the U.S. health care system. Each health care agency is distinct, with its own mission, values, and goals contributing uniquely to the larger health care system. However, both gaps and overlaps in mission and services exist, implying the need for connectivity, synergy, and means for safe passage for patients between the various agencies across the overall health care system. The concepts of connectivity, synergy, and safe passage are integral responsibilities of the nurse's role and are discussed in depth in the section on Practice Model.

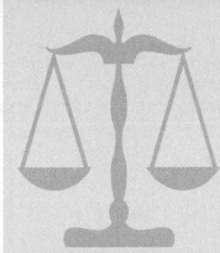

ETHICS IN PRACTICE

Hospital Report Cards

Richard Umbdenstock, Chairman of the American Hospital Association, believes that the public sharing of information and outcomes will have only positive effects on the relationship between hospitals and communities (Grayson, 2004). Hospitals may have as many as 5 to 10 mandatory state and federal reporting initiatives and multiple opportunities for voluntary reporting as well. These initiatives may be under the auspices of employer coalitions, consumer groups, or health care regulatory bodies, such as JCAHO (National Committee for Quality Healthcare, n.d).

Although there appears to be some disagreement on approach, many states have moved forward with legislation providing for hospital report cards. Illinois served as an early adopter implementing their requirements in January 2004. The Illinois legislation requires public access to nurse staffing and patient outcome information. It includes specific language requiring the reporting of nosocomial infections. Further, it guarantees whistle blower protection. Collecting and analyzing the data and preparing it in useful formats for health care consumers continues to be challenging. However, providing public access to performance information is considered a successful strategy for strengthening quality improvement initiatives (National Committee for Quality Healthcare, n.d).

Differing categories of health care agencies have been developed to identify the levels of care that span the continuum from preventive services to technologically complex care and continue through long-term care to hospice and palliative care. Figure 18-4 provides a useful framework for discussion of health care agencies based on the level of care an agency provides. This framework is also useful in representing how agencies may relate to each other. Throughout the framework the important concepts of cost, access, and quality are included in relation to how they are being addressed within particular health care agencies.

Although we are considering agencies by care levels, services for several levels of care are often provided within a single agency. For example, a school-based health center may provide primary care to its community, as well as preventive services to the student population. Another example is that emergency department nurses working in a high-tech tertiary care agency may participate in injury prevention outreach programs in the community. Further, in an attempt to become a more economically responsible health care system, agencies often join together formally to offer comprehensive services addressing many levels of care with efficiency. These unions, which may be affiliations or integrated delivery networks, may comprise hospitals, group practices that include nurses, nurse practitioners, and physicians from a variety of specialties and health plans.

Preventive Care Agencies

Preventive care can be described as care that focuses on health promotion, including educational and preventive programs that are designed to promote healthy lifestyles. Many agencies and services include preventive health care as

LEVEL:	Preventive care	Primary care	Secondary care	Tertiary care	Quaternary care	Restorative care	Continuing care

TYPE:	Education
	Innoculation
	Healthy lifestyle
		Diagnostics
		Routine treatment:
		  Medical
		  Surgical
		  Behavioral
		Stabilization and
		  transfer
			Diagnostics
			Emergent
			  treatment
			Intermediate care
				Diagnostics
				High tech
				  treatment
				Critical care
					Diagnostics
					Highly focused:
					  Complex
					    treatment
						Rehabilitation:
						  Physical
						    therapy
						  Occupational
						    therapy
						  Speech therapy
						Blind center:
						  Cane walking
						  Braille
						Intermediate
						  postoperative
						  treatment
							Chronic care
							Palliative care
							Comfort care
							End of life care

AGENCY:	Public health
	  agency
	Primary provider
	  office:
	    Multiple
	    disciplines
	Clinic
	Academic health
	  service
		Practitioner office:
		  Physician
		  Nurse
		    practitioner
		  Multiple
		    disciplines
		Clinic
		Academic health
		  service
			Hospital:
			  Acute care
			  Specialty care
				Hospital:
				  Acute care
				  Specialty care
					Hospital:
					  Specialty care
						Hospital
						  rehabilitation
						Home Health
							Adult daycare
							Long-term care
							Hospice

NOTE: Levels may be skipped or repeated

Figure 18-4 Continuum of care across agencies.

part of their mission including ambulatory care centers, public health clinics, school-based health centers, occupational health centers in industry, and corporations and associations representing the concerns of special interest groups. As our health care system continues to move to a health promotion model insurers and health plans that have economic interests in keeping people healthy have developed programs to educate their members about illness and accident prevention. Health promotion is not new to the nursing profession. As a result, nurses can be found employed in a variety of agencies lending nursing expertise about areas of need identification, educational resources, design, and of course, direct patient education.

The American Lung Association (ALA) is an example of a preventive health care agency providing programs to prevent lung disease and promote lung health. The ALA is the oldest voluntary health organization in the United States with a national office and constituent and affiliate associations around the country. Founded in 1904 to fight tuberculosis, the ALA today fights lung disease in all its forms, with special emphasis on asthma, tobacco control, and environmental health.

Preventive Care Costs and Financing

Costs associated with preventive care services are usually nominal to participants. The ALA is funded by contributions from the public, along with gifts and grants from corporations, foundations, and government agencies. By focusing on health promotion strategies these programs, in fact, lower health care costs by reducing the incidence of disease, thus reducing the need to use expensive health care resources.

Access to Preventive Care

Access to preventive care programs depends on a network of interdependent health care agencies promoting these services. Preventive care agencies depend on word of mouth, advertising, community activism, and social structures, such as churches and schools to help them educate the public. The ALA informs and educates the public about the impact and prevention of lung disease in a variety of ways. This information is disseminated through many channels, including its Web site, public service announcements, news releases and conferences, and spokespersons who can address lung disease issues via print, broadcast, and electronic media.

Preventive Care Quality

Quality associated with preventive care services is related to successful prevention of disease and the promotion of health within communities. By focusing on asthma education, tobacco control, research and professional education, and advocacy programs, the ALA has developed many programs and strategies for fighting lung disease. "Open Airways for Schools" is the ALA's elementary school education program for children with asthma. "Open Airways" teaches children with asthma to understand and manage their illness so they can lead more normal lives. An important part of this program is the facilitation of asthma care partnerships with school nurses and teachers, as well as health care providers, families, and ALA volunteers (American Lung Association, n.d.b).

Smoking control and prevention programs are offered by the ALA. "Teens against Tobacco Use" (TATU) is a peer-teaching tobacco control program aimed at deterring youngsters from taking up smoking (American Lung Association, n.d.d). For people who already smoke, the ALA offers its "Freedom from Smoking" program, a peer-support smoking cessation program (American Lung Association, n.d.a).

The ALA is active in the pollution control arena and has become the leading public advocate for clean air, as well as the chief source of information and public education on the health hazards of air pollution. The ALA has published a number of special reports on air pollution, the most popular being the *American Lung Association State of the Air* report. This report presents information on air pollution on a state by state, county by county basis, using the latest data available for nationwide comparisons (American Lung Association, n.d.c).

A broad program of grants and awards designed to further both basic and applied research in lung function, and lung disease is funded by the ALA. This funding has led to such major breakthroughs as the use of lifesaving surfactant therapy for thousands of premature infants with respiratory distress syndrome (RDS).

The ALA's advocacy programs influence the development and enforcement of laws and regulations related to lung health at the national, state, and local levels. The ALA played a major role in the passage of the landmark federal Clean Air Act, as well as the law prohibiting smoking on domestic passenger airline flights. As a result of an ALA lawsuit filed in 1993, the Environmental Protection Agency established revised, stricter air quality standards for smog and soot.

Primary Care Agencies

Primary care is the basic and routine health care that is provided in an office or clinic by a health care provider, such as a physician or nurse for both adults and children. These services are often provided in outpatient care or ambulatory care settings that may include private practice, free-standing facilities, mobile health agencies, and public health centers. Physicians, psychologists, and advance practice nurses may combine services in group practices to provide comprehensive primary care to patients. Freestanding facilities include walk-in clinics, surgi-centers, and urgent care centers. Mobile health units provide primary, episodic, and emergent care to citizens at risk, such as the homeless or those who are rurally isolated. Public health agencies provide primary care services, such as screening and treatments for sexually transmitted diseases and tuberculosis, as well as mental health services. In areas where health care services are scarce, rural hospitals are an example of a primary care agency.

Nurses and nurse practitioners play significant roles in primary care, often taking responsibility for early assessment, risk identification, anticipatory guidance, health screenings, immunizations, and treatment of nonacute illnesses. In rural hospitals, nurses and nurse practitioners must function with a great deal of autonomy, often being the most accessible health care provider. In such cases nursing expertise is needed to assess, stabilize, and transfer based on patient need. Nurses in these situations are critical to maintaining continuity of care across agencies.

Primary Care Costs and Financing

Rural hospitals are also known as **critical access hospitals (CAHs),** a category of hospital certification established by Congress in Section 4201 (Medicare Rural Hospital Flexibility Program) of the Balanced Budget Act of 1997 and amended by the Balanced Budget Refinement Act of 1999 (BBRA); the Medicare, Medicaid, and SCHIP Benefits Improvement and Protection Act of 2000 (BIPA); and the Medicare Prescription Drug, Improvement, and Modernization Act of 2003. CAHs provide outpatient, emergency, and inpatient services and are reimbursed at 101 percent of reasonable costs for inpatient services so as to attract and retain skilled care providers and to achieve adequate support to survive financially. The facility has a choice of cost-based or all-inclusive rates for outpatient services (AdminaStar Federal, 2003).

Access to Primary Care

Small rural hospitals with no more than 25 total beds where patients are hospitalized 96 hours or less are designated as a CAH by an appropriate state agency. CAHs must provide health care services usually at least 35 miles away from any other hospital and must be affiliated with a rural health network. Rural health networks can be described as organizations consisting of at least one CAH and one hospital that furnish acute care services through an agreement covering patient referral and transfer and the provision of emergency and nonemergency transportation between the CAH and the hospital. As of March 2003, there were 850 CAHs in the United States (Mantone, 2005). BBRA also allows "state-designated" hospitals that closed in the last 10 years to convert to CAHs.

Primary Care Quality

A quality indicator associated with health care agencies relates to the accreditation process. The accreditation process validates health care agencies based on national safety and quality standards established by CMS. In fact, the required agreement between the CAH and the network hospital expands and ensures regulatory compliance. In 2002, CMS permitted JCAHO the ability to conduct both the initial survey to become a CAH and recertification surveys. CAHs are exempt from the requirement to transmit data via a performance measurement system to JCAHO but are required to select and use six performance measures relevant to the services they provide and the patients they serve (JCAHO, n.d.). Information about the JCAHO is available at www.jcaho.org.

Secondary Care Agencies

Secondary care includes routine hospitalizations or surgeries hallmarked by short lengths of stay that involve more complex diagnostics and procedures. Secondary care agencies also include specialty hospitals that focus on pediatric, behavioral health, and rehabilitation services. Nurses providing secondary care are skilled in inpatient care delivery, including preparation and assisting in such areas as diagnostic testing, medication administration, nutritional support, postsurgical care, and many others. Nurses working in secondary care often develop areas of intellectual competence and expertise related to their area of specialty. Of course, all levels of inpatient care require nurses who are skilled communicators to effectively work with interdisciplinary teams and the patient's family and visitors.

Wills Eye in Philadelphia, Pennsylvania is an example of a secondary care specialty hospital providing health care services including nine subspecialties from common eye problems to rare sight-threatening diseases.

Secondary Care Costs and Financing

Since its founding, Wills Eye has been treating anyone needing ophthalmic care without regard to creed, color, gender, or financial status. Although financial health care costs are reimbursed through Medicare, Medicaid, or private insurers, Wills Eye provides care regardless of a patient's financial status or ability to pay. Annually, Wills Eye serves numerous patients with limited financial resources at a cost of nearly $5 million (Wills Eye, n.d.). Charitable giving has been the driving force behind Wills' mission to improve and preserve sight. Through generous donations, patients receive screenings and exams, eyeglasses, and critical medical and surgical care without regard to their ability to pay.

Access to Secondary Care

The board of directors of city trusts governs Wills Eye, established in 1832 through a bequest of Quaker merchant James Wills to the City of Philadelphia. It is a nonprofit specialty institution with such clinical expertise and sophistication of diagnostic and treatment procedures that it is a worldwide referral center. Wills Eye has also branched into the community with a network of same-day surgery centers throughout Pennsylvania, New Jersey, and Delaware. Wills Eye provides laser vision correction at its center in downtown Philadelphia and centers throughout the tri-state region. Wills Eye maintains free public eye screening that has been held in the Wills Eye building every spring since 1980 for members of the community. Adults and children over the age of three are screened for various eye problems by members of the Wills Eye staff who volunteer their time. The visual acuity of screening participants is provided by Wills Eye ophthalmic technicians.

Secondary Care Quality

Wills Eye has consistently been ranked as one of the best hospitals in the United States by *U.S. News & World Report* since the survey's inception in 1990. Many of the special instruments and techniques that are commonplace in ophthalmology were invented or developed at Wills Eye. The implantation of an artificial intraocular lens to replace a clouded lens due to a cataract was pioneered in the United States in 1952 by Warren Reese, M.D. and Turgut Hamdi, M.D., both Wills Eye health care providers. A vitrectomy machine, now widely used for eye microsurgery, was invented in 1972 by Wills Eye physician Jay L. Federman, M.D (Wills Eye, n.d.). Today, research at Wills Eye is carried out in the hospital's research department, the hospital's subspecialty services, and in cooperative efforts involving both ophthalmologists and laboratory scientists within Wills Eye, as well as through government agencies like the National Eye Institute.

Tertiary Care Agencies

Tertiary care is specialized consultative care often initiated by referral from a primary or secondary health care provider. Tertiary care is necessary for individuals requiring acute and complex interventions, such as high-risk cardiac surgery, organ transplant, or trauma services. Academic health science centers provide tertiary care. The Johns Hopkins Hospital in Baltimore, Maryland, is an example of a tertiary care agency.

Nurses working in tertiary care agencies are skilled in complex inpatient care delivery with special focus on managing individuals with multiple system problems and needs. Such patients have a high degree of dependence that requires a high degree of surveillance and swift intervention. The complex care requirements exhibited by tertiary facility patients require nurses to have more in depth knowledge, critical thinking and problem-solving ability, and sophisticated technological skill. Patients usually have multiple providers and consultants as required by their multiple and diverse needs for care.

Therefore, nursing in tertiary level agencies is expected to be part of large and often complex multidisciplinary team. By nature, tertiary care centers are important sites for educating and training future health care professionals so nurses also interact with students from various disciplines. In a tertiary setting, clear communication and assertive advocacy is vital to ensure safe passage and care continuity for the patient and family.

Tertiary Care Costs and Financing

The Johns Hopkins health care system delivers tertiary services throughout the Maryland area. These world-renowned facilities attract patients from across the state, across the country, and around the world. Out-of-state patients accounted for 22.4 percent of Johns Hopkins Hospital billings in 2002 with patients utilizing private and public financing for their tertiary care services. The Johns Hopkins Hospitals also treat Maryland patients who cannot afford to pay, providing $144.3 million in uncompensated care in 2002 (Johns Hopkins Institutes, 2003).

The State of Maryland and Johns Hopkins are tightly linked as partners in economic development. During a 10-year period, state contributions to the Johns Hopkins Institutes were $102.8 million and private grants and contributions exceeded $142 million. Additionally, Johns Hopkins is the leading recipient of research funds from the National Institutes of Health (NIH).

Access to Tertiary Care

To avoid situations in which those carrying private insurance might enjoy superior primary care to those who are either publicly insured or not insured at all, the Johns Hopkins Institutes actively strategize programs and policies to address disparities associated with access to health care services. Johns Hopkins Hospital, the flagship of the Hopkins Health System, provides 977 acute care beds. The Hopkins Health System includes three hospitals and an extensive network of outpatient locations in Baltimore, Carroll, Frederick, Harford, Howard, Montgomery, Prince George's, and Washington counties that provide access to the hospitals. The Johns Hopkins facilities house critical care centers vital to the statewide trauma system, including adult trauma, eye trauma, and pediatric trauma centers at the Johns Hopkins Hospital, as well as the adult trauma center and the Baltimore Regional Burn Center at the Johns Hopkins Bayview Medical Center.

Tertiary Care Quality

For the 16th year in a row, the Johns Hopkins Hospital has topped the *U.S. News & World Report's* annual rankings of American hospitals. Johns Hopkins is a leader in health care quality as demonstrated by its handling of the death of Josie King, an 18-month-old girl admitted in 2001 after suffering from second-degree burns from a bathtub accident. Josie died from dehydration three weeks after being admitted to the Johns Hopkins Bayview Center. Josie's parents settled out of court, but since then have worked tirelessly to educate health care providers on safety and quality issues by telling their story and initiating the Josie King Patient Safety Program. Josie's mother, who stayed by her daughter's side day and night and witnessed her daughter's death, has traveled to medical conferences in Boston, New Orleans, Washington, and Chicago and was invited to speak in Mexico and the Netherlands. She has addressed medical students at Hopkins and launched a Web site, www.josieking.org.

Care Costs and Financing

The Shrine of North America is an international fraternity of approximately 500,000 members whose official philanthropic mission is to their children's hospitals (Shriners' Hospitals of North America, n.d.). Shriners' Hospitals are open to all children without regard to race, religion or relationship to a Shriner. There is never a charge to the patient or parents for any health care services provided at a Shriners' Hospital. The gift of free health care is made possible by the generosity of many donations. Donations go to the Shriners' Hospitals Endowment Fund, which supports all 22 Shriner's Hospitals for Children. If a patient referred to a Shriners' Hospital requires services the hospital does not provide, such as urology or outpatient physical therapy, Shriners' Hospitals for Children assists the family in obtaining insurance coverage for the required services.

Access to Care

Any child may be eligible for care at a Shriners' Hospital if the child is under the age of 18, and there is a reasonable possibility the child's condition can be helped. A Shriner's hospital can be reached by calling 1-800-237-5055 in the United States. In an emergency the referring physician treating the burned child should telephone the chief of staff at one of the Shriners' Burn Centers.

Care Quality

Shriners' hospitals have been involved in clinical research since the early 1920s. Since opening the Shriners' Burn Centers the survival rate for children with burns over 50 percent of their total body surface area has doubled. Today these specialized hospitals are saving the lives of children with burns over more than 90 percent of body surface area.

Restorative Care Agencies

Restorative care includes follow-up care after surgery, home care, and rehabilitation. The need for restorative care may result from an acute illness episode, surgery, exacerbation of a chronic illness, or from a disability. The goal of restorative care is to assist the patient to regain an optimal level of functioning following these events. Restorative care agencies may include rehabilitation hospitals or services, home care agencies, and skilled nursing facilities. Nurses in these agencies must possess excellent medical-surgical skills. However, these settings also require a long-term view of how the admitting incident may affect the patient's quality of life. Because the patient's LOS is longer in these agencies, nurses have opportunities to develop strong therapeutic relationships with the patients that help individualize treatment plans and reinforce lifestyle changes. Along with physicians, physical and occupational therapists, social workers, and other members of the interdisciplinary team, nurses in restorative care agencies strive to help patients set and achieve their goals for recovery.

An example of restorative care is the Rehabilitation Institute of Chicago (RIC). Founded in 1954, RIC has earned a worldwide reputation as being a leader in patient care, advocacy, research, and educating health professionals in physical medicine and rehabilitation. People from around the world choose RIC because of its expertise in treating a range of conditions from the most complex (cerebral palsy, spinal cord injury, stroke, and traumatic brain injury) to more common arthritis, chronic pain, and sports injuries. It is estimated that 19.3 percent of the U.S. population, or 49.7 million Americans, report having disabilities. If the prevalence of major chronic conditions remains unchanged, the number of Americans with functional limitations will rise by more than 300 percent by 2049 (Reis, Breslin, Lezzoni, & Kirschner, 2004). Recent studies indicate that people with disabilities share these common characteristics:

- A significantly higher use of health care services.
- Frequent expressions of dissatisfaction with their care.
- Susceptibility to disparities in health care.
- Experiences of widespread lack of appropriate accommodations.

Restorative Care Costs and Financing

The landmark 1990 Americans with Disabilities Act (ADA) and its predecessor law, Section 504 of the Rehabilitation Act of 1973, created a comprehensive national mandate that prohibits disability-based discrimination. Together, these laws call for public and private health care services, programs, and providers to treat people with disabilities in a nondiscriminatory and integrated manner and to ensure that they have an equal opportunity to participate in, and benefit from, health care services.

In 1997, of the 41 million low-income people Medicaid covers, nearly 7 million qualified based on disability. In 1998, about one in four nonelderly people with disabilities who were eligible for Medicaid was enrolled in Medicaid managed care plan. Thus, the principles of the ADA and Section 504 are important tools for shaping the way care is delivered by private and public health plans.

Access to Restorative Care

RIC has over 30 locations in the Chicago area and Southern Illinois, including alliances with Illinois Masonic Medical Center, Alexian Brothers Medical Center, Riverside Medical Center, Southern Illinois Healthcare, and RML Specialty Hospital. RIC offers programs and services through its advocacy and community outreach efforts to improve the quality of life for people with physical disabilities. Programs include the Center for Health and Fitness, Vocational Rehabilitation, Health Resource Center for Women with Disabilities, and an Injury Prevention Program that educates children and adults on preventing disabling injuries.

Restorative Care Quality

In 2005 RIC was ranked "Best Rehabilitation Hospital in America" for the 15th year in a row by *U.S. News & World Report* (Rehabilitation Institute of Chicago, 2005). RIC is the home of the Northwestern University Feinberg School of Medicine's Department of Physical Medicine and Rehabilitation, and operates one of the largest psychiatrist programs in the United States. Additionally, RIC offers more than 100 continuing education courses every year, attracting more than 7,000 health care professionals, worldwide.

The Searle Research Center at RIC is one of the nation's largest programs of its kind in the country. With more than $6 million in federal and private grants, the goal of scientists at the Searle Center is to provide practical solutions for people with physical disabilities. RIC is the only federally funded stroke rehabilitation research and training center in the country. Research teams are involved in more than 50 projects including:

- Cutting-edge studies with the Lokomat, a robot that may help paralyzed people walk.
- Brain mapping to determine how the brain activity changes after strokes.
- Creating a "cyborg" that connects animal brain cells and a robot in the quest for more functional artificial limbs.

RIC is also the recipient of a $3.5 million grant awarded by the U.S. Department of Education's National Institute on Disability and Rehabilitation Research (NIDRR) to research measures in rehabilitation outcomes and effectiveness (Rehabilitation Institute of Chicago, n.d.).

Two key agencies play central roles through accreditation and related services in improving the safety and quality of the restorative health care provided to the public. In 2002, RIC was accredited by both JCAHO and the Commission on Accreditation of Rehabilitation Facilities (CARF).

Continuing Care Agencies

Many individuals require ongoing care for disabilities, chronic diseases, or permanent changes in functional level following an acute disease episode or trauma. This level of care is referred to as **continuing care**. **Long-term care** can be described as extended assistance for the chronically ill, mentally ill, or disabled with a focus on assistance with carrying out basic activities of daily living that may be provided in private homes or public facilities.

Types of community-based long-term care agencies include adult daycare, homemaker services, and hospice. **Adult daycare** facilities provide health, social, and recreational services to adults who require supervision and care while their family members are otherwise engaged with work responsibilities. **Hospice** includes palliative and end-of-life care for patients and their families. Types of institutional long-term care facilities include assisted living, skilled nursing, and subacute care. **Assisted living** facilities provide personal care services, 24 hour supervision, social activities, and health care services. Examples of continuing care agencies are nursing homes that provide skilled nursing services and subacute care such as wound care, feeding tubes, injections, and ventilator care.

Continuing Care Costs and Financing

It is estimated that approximately 40 percent of our current population will require long-term care. Health insurance plans may cover some of the skilled health care services required after an illness or injury but usually for a limited period and only as long as health conditions show an improvement. Health plans typically do not cover ongoing chronic care, such as an extended stay in an assisted living facility or a continuing need for assistance. Unfortunately, no health insurance plan will cover all long-term care needs.

Medicaid is a state-based program supplemented by federal funds that acts as a safety net to provide health services to the indigent. Medicaid covers long-term care services and might cover care if the person requiring continuing care services meets the state's poverty criteria. Usually this means expending all but $2,000 of assets and savings (except for one's house and car). It also means receiving care from a limited number of state-approved providers, most often institutions, such as nursing homes that are willing to accept Medicaid payments. Medicaid is the number one provider for nursing home care costs.

Medicare is a National health insurance program for people age 65 years and older, people under aged 65 with disabilities, and people with end-stage renal disease. Medicare provides coverage to approximately 40 million Americans. Medicare will cover the first 100 days of continuing care in a nursing home if the services are skilled and required after a hospital stay of at least 3 days or within 30 days of being discharged from that specific hospital stay. Additionally, Medicare may require some deductibles and copays. Medicare also covers limited home visits for skilled care.

Long-term care insurance is now available to provide coverage of persons requiring long-term care services. This type of insurance helps pay for long-term care services, such as home care or care in a nursing home or assisted living facility.

Access to Continuing Care

A determinant for receiving continuing care services is the private or public funding available to people requiring long-term care. About three million elderly and disabled Americans receive care in our nation's nearly 17,000 Medicare and Medicaid certified nursing homes (Centers for Medicare and Medicaid Services, n.d.). Slightly more than half of these are long-term nursing home residents, but nearly as many have shorter stays for rehabilitation care after an acute hospitalization. About 75 percent are age 75 or older. The care of nursing home residents is a high priority for the Bush administration, the Department of Health and Human Services (DHHS), and the CMS. CMS began enforcing new nursing home regulations as an outgrowth of the Omnibus Budget Reconciliation Act (OBRA) of 1987.

Continuing Care Quality

In November 2001, HHS Secretary Tommy G. Thompson announced the Nursing Home Quality Initiative to continue to improve quality of care in nursing homes. The quality initiative, an important component of CMS's comprehensive strategy to improve the quality of care provided by America's nursing homes, is a four-prong effort that consists of:

- Regulation and enforcement efforts conducted by state survey agencies and CMS.
- Improved consumer information on the quality of care in nursing homes.
- Continual, community-based quality improvement programs designed for nursing homes to improve their quality of care.
- Collaboration and partnership to leverage knowledge and resources.

CMS designed regulation and enforcement activities to ensure the public that Medicare and Medicaid nursing homes comply with regulatory requirements for patient health, safety, and quality of care. CMS monitors data that nursing homes report through two data sets: the Minimum Data Set (MDS) and administrative data from the Online Survey, Certification, and Reporting System (OSCAR). CMS uses these aggregated data sets to provide a comprehensive view of the individual receiving care in the nursing home. State survey and certification agencies focus on the quality of care furnished to residents as measured by indicators of medical, nursing, rehabilitative, dietary, and nutritional care services, activities and social participation, as well as sanitation, infection control, and the physical environment (Box 18-1). Surveys also include a review of compliance with residents' rights, written plans of care, and an audit of the residents' assessment.

Indian Health Services

The Indian Health Service (IHS), an agency within the DHHS, is responsible for providing federal health services to American Indians and Alaska Natives (AI/AN). IHS includes health care agencies that provide care at many of the levels already discussed but with a more specific population purpose and

---

BOX 18-1

NATIONAL NURSING HOME PERFORMANCE MEASURES

The core of the nursing home survey process is a four- to five-day on-site visit to see that a nursing home is meeting federal health and safety requirements. The standard survey takes a snapshot of the care given to beneficiaries at the time of the survey. Nursing home surveys are unannounced, and by law, must take place based on a statewide average of once every 12 months but not longer than once every 15 months. The survey process also requires states to conduct surveys within prescribed time frames any time a serious problem is alleged. The survey includes these national performance measures:

- Percent of residents whose need for help with daily activities has increased.
- Percent of residents who have moderate to severe pain.
- Percent of residents who were physically restrained.
- Percent of residents who spent most of their time in bed or in a chair.
- Percent of residents whose ability to move about in and around their room got worse.
- Percent of residents with a urinary tract infection.
- Percent of residents who have become more depressed or anxious.
- Percent of high-risk residents who have pressure sores.
- Percent of low-risk residents who have pressure sores.
- Percent of low-risk residents who lose control of their bowels or bladder.
- Percent of residents who have a catheter inserted and left in their bladder.
- Percent of residents who lose too much weight.

Information from these measures, survey results, and complaint data are for public use and are available at www.medicare.gov/NHCompare.

mission. The provision of health services to members of federally recognized tribes grew out of a special government to government relationship between the federal government and Indian tribes. This relationship, established in 1787, is based on Article I, Section 8 of the Constitution and has been supported by numerous treaties, laws, Supreme Court decisions, and executive orders. The IHS currently provides health services to approximately 1.5 million AI/AN belonging to more than 557 federally recognized tribes (Indian Health Services, n.d.).

IHS Costs and Financing

The U.S. government began appropriating federal funds specifically for IHS in 1925. The IHS, a partnership of federal, tribal, and urban Native American operated health care programs, is the primary source of health care services for many AI/AN. Federal funding for IHS is not an entitlement, like Medicare and Medicaid. The IHS programs depend on annual discretionary appropriations. Unlike entitlement programs or privately purchased health insurance plans, a defined package of health care services is not ensured to eligible Native Americans who need services. Consequently, the level of services provided by IHS varies depending on available federal funding. Most of the IHS budget pays for personal health care services, such as diagnostic examinations, medications, and outpatient services similar to those in a mainstream health plan. Portions of IHS appropriations go to public health functions like sanitation facilities for clean water and waste disposal (Indian Health Service, n.d.). The federal appropriation only provides about 59 percent of the necessary funding to IHS for health care services similarly found in a mainstream health plan.

Access to IHS

To receive IHS health care benefits tribe members must go to the registration office of the local IHS facility in person and present proof of enrollment as a member of a federally recognized tribe. IHS services are provided directly and through tribally contracted and operated health programs. Health services also include health care purchased from more than 9,000 private providers annually. The federal IHS health care system consists of 36 hospitals, 61 health centers, 49 health stations, and five residential treatment centers. In addition, 34 urban Indian health projects provide a variety of health and referral services. The IHS clinical staff consists of nurses, physicians, pharmacists, dentists, sanitarians, and physician assistants. The IHS also employs various allied health professionals, such as nutritionists, health administrators, engineers, and medical records administrators.

IHS Quality

IHS is the principal federal health care provider and health advocate, and its goal is to raise the health status to the highest possible level for the Native American people. Preventive measures involving environmental, educational, and outreach activities are combined with therapeutic measures into a single national health system. Within these broad categories are special initiatives in traditional medicine, elder care, women's health, children and adolescents, injury prevention, domestic violence and child abuse, health care financing, state health care, sanitation facilities, and oral health including Urban Indian Health Programs (UIHP) and UIHP Clinics.

However, the AI/AN population has long experienced health problems disproportionately compared with other Americans. Their life expectancy is still five years less than other Americans. They die at significantly higher rates than other Americans from alcoholism, tuberculosis, diabetes, accidents, suicide, pneumonia and influenza, and homicide. Native American families are much more likely than any other American families to live in homes that have sanitation facilities that do not meet modern standards.

The Veterans Affairs Health System

These agencies provide services across several levels of care and have a unique mission and purpose. The mission of the VA Health System is to serve the needs of America's veterans by providing primary care, specialized care, and social support services. To accomplish this mission the VA is a comprehensive, integrated health care system. During the last several years the VA has put its health care facilities under five networks that provide more health care services to more veterans and family members than at any time during VA's long history.

VA Health System Costs and Financing

Perhaps the most visible of all VA benefits and services is health care. The VA's health care system includes 157 medical centers, with at least one in each state, Puerto Rico, and the District of Columbia. The VA operates more than 1,300 sites of care, including 862 ambulatory care and community-based outpatient clinics, 134 nursing homes, 42 residential rehabilitation treatment programs, 207 Veterans Centers, and 88 comprehensive homecare programs.

Each year Congress establishes the budget allocation for the VA. When the budgeting process is not completed by the beginning of a fiscal year congress must extend the current budget for a stipulated interim. It is not unusual for several extensions to be declared and when the budgeting process is significantly slowed, selected indirect care providers may be furloughed or laid off pending budget approval. During a furlough, efforts are made to sustain direct patient care services. For 2005, President Bush sought $67.7 billion for the VA budget—a $5.6 billion increase over 2004, primarily for health care and disability compensation (VA Health System, n.d.).

Access to VA Health System

VA health care facilities provide a broad spectrum of medical, surgical, and rehabilitative care and engage in research that has resulted in significant advances in prosthetics and blind care. A unique system of five national residential sites for blind programs serves eligible nonveterans, as well as veterans. More than 4.8 million people received care in VA health care facilities in 2003. The VA is used annually by approximately 75 percent of all disabled and low-income veterans. In 2003, the VA treated 567,300 patients in VA hospitals and contract hospitals, 55,756 in nursing homes, and 25,314 in residential rehabilitation treatment programs. The VA's outpatient clinics registered approximately 49.8 million visits (Veterans Affairs, n.d.). The VA's health care system serves as a backup to the defense department during national emergencies and as a federal support organization during major disasters.

The VA has experienced unprecedented growth in the medical system workload over the past few years. The number of patients treated increased by 22 percent from 4.1 million in 2001 to more than 5 million in 2004. Of the 24.8 million veterans currently alive, nearly three quarters served during a war or an official period of conflict. About a quarter of the nation's population, approximately 63 million people, are potentially eligible for VA benefits and services, because they are veterans, family members, or survivors of veterans.

To receive VA health care benefits veterans must enroll. Enrollment criteria are numerous and complex. For instance, Congress stipulates by law the inclusion dates of military service and the income levels that qualify a veteran for enrollment. Only veterans who served during a conflict window stipulated by congress and whose income is below the maximum stipulated by congress are eligible to enroll. A sliding scale of needs-based fees guides the amount a veteran pays for services.

There are over 7.4 million veterans enrolled in the VA health care system. When they enroll, veterans are placed in priority groups or categories that help the VA manage health care services within budgetary constraints and ensure quality care for those enrolled. Veterans with service-connected disabilities receive priority access to care for hospitalization and outpatient care.

The VA provides health care and benefits to more than 100,000 homeless veterans each year. While the proportion of veterans among the homeless is declining, the VA actively engages veterans in outreach, benefits assistance and transitional housing. The VA has made more than 300 grants for transitional housing, service centers, and vans for outreach and transportation to state and local governments, tribal governments, and nonprofit community and faith-based service providers. Programs for alcoholism, drug addiction, and post-traumatic stress disorder have been expanded in recent years, along with attention to environmental hazards.

The VA Health System Quality

The National Center for Patient Safety (NCPS) embodies the VA's uncompromising commitment to reducing and preventing adverse events while enhancing care. The NCPS represents a unified and cohesive patient safety program with active participation by all of the VA hospitals supported by dedicated patient safety managers. In February 2002 the NCPS was awarded the John M. Eisenberg Patient Safety and Quality Award for developing and implementing a systems approach to error reduction within the VA's 163 health care facilities (VA National Center for Patient Safety, n.d.). The John M. Eisenberg Patient Safety and Quality Awards were established in 2002 by the National Quality Forum (NQF) and JCAHO.

In 2005, estimated funding for VA research was $402 million. Funding from non-VA sources such as the NIH and other government agencies and pharmaceutical companies will contribute another $800 million to VA research. The VA currently supports approximately 3,000 researchers at 115 VA health centers and its career development program provides young scientists an opportunity to develop skills as clinician-researchers.

VA researchers played important roles in developing the cardiac pacemaker, the computed tomography (CT) scan, radioimmunoassay, and improvements in artificial limbs. The first liver transplant in the world was performed by a VA surgeon-researcher. VA contributions to health care knowledge have won VA scientists many awards, including the Nobel Prize and the Lasker Award (VA Health Care, n.d.). In addition, the VA manages the largest medical education and health professions training program in the United States. VA facilities are affiliated with 107 medical schools, 55 dental schools, and more than 1,200 other schools across the country. More than half of the physicians practicing in the United States have received part of their professional education within the VA health care system.

THE FUTURE OF HEALTH CARE AGENCIES

An ideal health care system should provide the delivery of seamless care across health care agencies. New models of care delivery called **integrated care delivery systems,** a network of organizations that provide a coordinated continuum of services to a defined population, are evolving to meet this goal.

Kaiser Permanente, a nonprofit health plan, is an example of an integrated health care delivery system providing comprehensive services to the population served. This integrated system includes Permanente Medical Groups, a medical group foundation, and Kaiser Foundation Hospitals providing services in nine states and Washington, D.C. Over 8.2 million members of Kaiser Permanente can expect attention to issues, such as immunizations, health education, and screening, for early disease detection to maintain optimum health (Kaiser Permanent, n.d.). Because of their unique organizational structure that includes both acute care resources and a health plan, members can access the full range of sophisticated hospital and technical services under the Kaiser umbrella delivered by Kaiser-employed interdisciplinary teams.

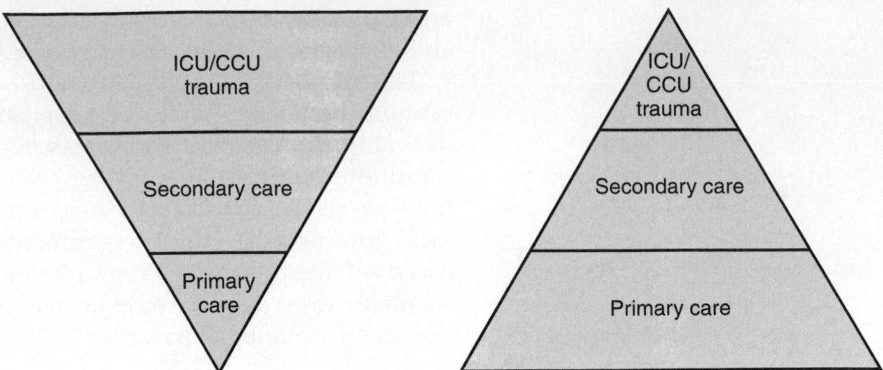

Figure 18-5 Conceptual model of a paradigm shift.

Purchasers of health care, both private and public, present a formidable driver for the development of new models of care. Key to their influence is the tracking of quality through measurement. Value-based purchasing, also known as pay for performance, is dependent on quality measurement for analyses. Quality measuring tools are specific to each agency and its constituency. Paying for performance is a powerful motivator for systems to improve the delivery of health care.

A dynamic effect of the interplay between cost, access, and quality is the paradigm shift from a medical model of care to a health model. The current focus on acute and high-tech interventions based on the medical model is necessary but does not address basic health needs or reform health policy for society. Future trends in health care services incorporate a health care delivery model wherein primary care is the foundation for health care services as modeled in Figure 18-5. This shift toward quality primary care, along with advances in technology and research has significantly contributed to the increasing life expectancy in the United States.

With over 20 different institutes and centers focusing on scientific research, the NIH conduct and fund research to uncover new knowledge and its applicability toward improving health care. Within the NIH is the National Institute of Nursing Research (NINR). Part of the mission of the NINR is to improve the clinical settings (agencies) in which health care services are provided. Nursing research involves clinical care in a variety of settings such as the community and home, as well as more traditional health care sites (National Institute of Nursing Research, nd.). Nursing research is critical to the creation of scientific advances, evidence-based practice, and their translation into providing cost-effective health care services that do not compromise quality.

PRACTICE MODEL

How does nursing fit into the current structure of the American health care system? The fit that excellent nursing practice seeks to achieve is not a match with the health care system but rather a synergistic interplay between the nurse's competencies and the patient's needs for nursing care. Is practice defined by location? The site of care may determine the type of diagnostic testing or sophisticated interventions available to the patient and to some degree a nurse's technical competencies are developed to support such interventions. However, the practice of nursing is ultimately defined only within a relationship with a patient. Through this relationship, patient needs are identified and nursing resources are applied.

Do changes in the system change professional practice and if so, how can professional standards be maintained? As systems change, opportunities for

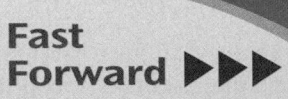

Fast Forward ▶▶▶

Minute Clinics

Nothing works better than innovation to jumpstart a lagging commercial market. Whether it's new technology or entrepreneurship health care, like any other business, health care, too, can benefit from innovation. As announced by major broadcast and print media, walk-in health care clinics are already available in some neighborhood food, drug, or retail stores. Need a blood pressure check for yourself or a throat culture for your child? Need groceries, too? Patients are given a pager to do their shopping while waiting their turn to be seen for health care evaluation. A nurse practitioner at the "Minute Clinic" can diagnose and treat many common ailments and write prescriptions at a fraction of the usual cost of an office visit; typically only $25 to $60. Approximately 250,000 people have been treated at Minute Clinics, offering convenience and economy for both the patient and the store.

changes in the nursing role develop. Because nursing is a profession and, as such, is self-governing, professional organizations such as the American Nurses Credentialing Center (2005) have evolved objective measurements and credentialing procedures that transcend the geographical site for care delivery. These credentialing processes serve as a guarantee of quality for the public. How can patients experience safety and continuity if practice is variable from agency to agency? If nurses continually define their services in relation to the patient's evolving needs, level of functioning and health goals, continuity in the patient's progress through the health care system can be ensured by the nurse providing safe passage.

In 1860 Florence Nightingale put forth the principle that nurses provide the environment for healing to take place (1969 [1860]). These words provide a mandate for nurses to design and support the development of a health care system in the United States that is both patient-centered and holistically focused. In 1966, Henderson's theory of nursing brought the significance of the nurse-patient relationship into clear focus. Later, Imogene King (1971) placed this relationship within the context of the environment. Following these traditions, Curley (1998) brought these same threads together in a model that has been shown to inform nurses' practice in any type of agency.

The work of Martha Curley (1998) and the American Association of Critical Care Nurses (AACCN) provide an approach for defining professional practice and the nurse's role in today's health care environment. A closer look at the synergy model they developed demonstrates the consistency and permanency of the nursing role, regardless of the setting. It provides a framework in which to consider professional practice and patient outcomes in a complex health care system.

Synergy Model

The **synergy model** can be defined by reviewing its main principles. Foundational to the framework is the assumption that *patient characteristics* and *nurse competencies* should match. When this occurs, synergy takes place. This synergy is the force that leads to positive patient outcomes and safe passage for patients.

Patient Characteristics

Every individual has a unique set of personal characteristics that transcend health and illness. These characteristics are based in a person's physical, emotional, spiritual, social, cultural, and economic background. According to the synergy model these characteristics include: stability, complexity, predictability, resiliency, vulnerability, participation in decision making and care, and resource availability. The individual's presentation in any illness episode reflects that individual's own personal constellation of characteristics at the current point on their health-illness continuum. Thus, the assessment of an individual's characteristics becomes the nursing care template for all practice interactions.

Nurse Competencies

A set of eight nurse competencies is also defined by the synergy model. Included are clinical judgment, advocacy and moral agency, caring practices, facilitation of learning, collaboration, systems thinking, diversity of responsiveness, and clinical inquiry. This assumes that these competencies encompass all areas of practice. These competencies also exist on a continuum and vary according to the expertise of the nurse and the care requirements of the patient. Early in a nursing career a nurse might have a minimum level of skill in each competency. However, the nurse's competencies strengthen through clinical experience and role maturation. The Real World Scenario highlights a challenge faced by a novice nurse that calls for several competencies identified in the synergy model.

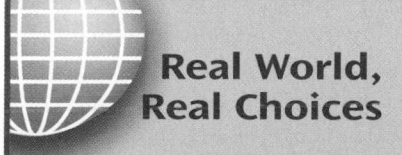

Real World, Real Choices

Workload Complaints: Are They Justifiable?

You have been on the job for about six months working the night shift on a busy medical-surgical unit. The nursing assistant comes to you to complain about her work load, again. You realize that this employee usually leaves parts of her assignment undone and is unpleasant to work with because her constant complaining. What do you do?

Skills 360°

Communication Skill: SBAR

JCAHO suggests that communication problems are a top contributor to sentinel events. A sentinel event is an unexpected occurrence involving death or serious physical or psychological injury. Such events are called *sentinel*, because they signal the need for immediate investigation and response. The AACCN *Standards for Establishing and Sustaining Healthy Work Environments* includes skilled communication, i.e., "nurses must be as proficient in communication as they are in clinical skills" as their number one standard. Developed by a team of health care providers at Kaiser Permanente, the SBAR communication technique is easy to use and easy to remember and appears in Table 18-1.

Excellent nursing care results when the nurse can tap into the appropriate level of skill and knowledge from each area of competence thereby individualizing care to each patient's specific characteristics and needs for nursing care. Excellent health care systems result when the care delivery environment of the agency enables the patient to be appropriately matched with the nurse.

Safe Passage

Fragmentation and errors are primary quality concerns in health care today. Safe passage, the final concept in the synergy model, addresses these issues. Nurses have a unique opportunity to implement and provide safe environments for patients in the health care system. Based on knowledge of the patient's unique characteristics the nurse provides safe passage by expertly navigating the complexities of the health care system for the patient. In fact, tending to the environment of health care is essential in providing safe passage and is inherent in nurse competencies. The idea of safe passage within a system requires values for patient safety, excellence in practice, and efficient care delivery systems. By ensuring safe passage, more positive patient outcomes can be achieved.

Outcomes

Government reports of medical errors, research evidence of links between systems failures and untoward clinical outcomes, and legislative actions to monitor and control practice are fueling a drive toward quality health care outcomes across all health care agencies. Curley (1998) suggests the adoption of the ANA *Nursing Care Report Card for Acute Care Settings* as a reasonable model for the delineation of outcomes. Outcomes emanate from the patient, the nurse, and the health care system.

Kerfoot (2004) provides evidence of the applicability of the synergy model to all areas of practice. The American Association of Colleges of Nursing (AACN) and others have adapted the synergy model to explicate competencies and professional development needs and to define leadership roles. Pacini (2004) discusses how the synergy model has been integrated into clinical education. She states that expectations related to leadership and expertise in assessment, curricular design, program management, [and] outcomes analysis have been easily incorporated into job descriptions. Pacini emphasizes that staff education programs start with assessments of the nurse as an individual with unique competencies as the basis for future growth and development.

The synergy model offers several important principles that enlighten our understanding of nursing responsibility within the health care system including:

1. The model defines practice in relation to patient need.
2. The model permits a focus on systems thinking as a nurse competency, bringing this often invisible, yet critical, aspect of nursing care to light.

TABLE 18-1	**SBAR Technique for Communication**
S	Situation—Identify the patient's name and problem, i.e., tachypnea, dropping B/P, and loss of consciousness (LOC).
B	Background—State pertinent background information, i.e., fractured hip.
A	Assessment—State concern, i.e. I think we may be dealing with a pulmonary embolism.
R	Recommendation—State what you want, i.e., oxygen and transfer to intensive care unit (ICU).

Source: SBAR technique for communication: A situational briefing model. *(2005).* Retrieved September 2, 2006, from www.ihi.org.

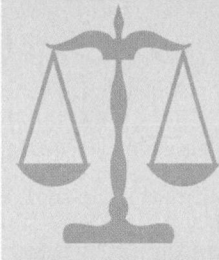

ETHICS IN PRACTICE

Nursing Ethics Forum of the Swedish Hospital in Chicago

Nurses' commitments encompass those to their profession, to the institutions that employ them, and most importantly, to their patients. These commitments are recognized in the American Nurse Association *Code of Ethics for Nurses*. The Nursing Ethics Forum of Swedish Covenant Hospital in Chicago was developed by nurses, for nurses, to empower them to identify, address, and resolve ethical issues in patient care and professional practice. The Forum also provides the structure and process to link the expression of ethical concerns with organizational resolution of such concerns. The Forum achieves its purpose through educational programs, case review, discussion of ethical dilemmas, and support of policy development and process improvement initiatives to enhance ethical nursing practice. Each representative plays a critical role in addressing ethical issues within his or her own patient care area, acting as a resource for nurse colleagues and for patients. All nurses and the hospital's ethicist are invited to attend. Future goals include implementation of the End of Life Nursing Education Consortium (ELNEC) program, the inclusion of an ethics assessment within the patient's health record, and partnering with nurse leaders from local nursing homes to address advanced care planning.

Source: DeLaune, S., & Ladner, P. (2006). Fundamentals of nursing *(3rd ed.). New York: Thomson Delmar Learning.*

3. The model highlights the importance of nurses' work in creating safe passage for patients across diverse health care agencies, achieving quality outcomes through continuity of care.
4. The model provides a mechanism to identify areas of practice specific to all types of patients along the health continuum.
5. The model defines nurse-sensitive outcomes and a method to identify them.

Overall, the synergy model provides a critical link between nursing services and health system planning. It provides a road map for the development of excellent nursing services within the health care delivery system, regardless of the health care agency or the system's design.

NURSE'S ROLE IN HEALTH CARE AGENCIES

The role of the nurse in health care agencies should be in accordance with the needs of the population served and the service focus of the agency. The health care agencies discussed utilize registered nurses, nurse practitioners, and nurses with advanced preparation in leadership in various positions based on competence levels. Professional nurses offer direct patient care services at both the generalist and advanced practice level, each developing specialist competencies based on areas of professional interest. However, the role responsibilities discussed in this section constitute core professional nursing responsibilities transcending specific role expectations.

Uncovering the Evidence

Association Between Nurse: Patient Ratio and Failure to Rescue

Discussion: The purpose of this study was to determine what association, if any, exists between nurse/patient ratio and patient mortality due to failure to rescue (deaths following complications) among postoperative surgical patients. This cross-sectional study surveyed 10,184 staff nurses and data from records of 232,342 general, orthopedic, and vascular surgery patients discharged over a 20-month period. Administrative data from 168 hospitals was also included in the analysis. Study measurements included risk-adjusted patient mortality and failure to rescue events within 30 days of admission, nurse-reported job satisfaction, and job-related burnout data. The investigators report a 7 percent increase in mortality within 30 days of admission, a 7 percent increase in failure to rescue rates, a 23 percent increase in the likelihood of nurse burnout, and a 15 percent increase in the likelihood of nurse dissatisfaction associated with each additional patient assigned to a nurse.

Implications for Practice: The quantity of patients for whom a nurse is simultaneously responsible carries significance for the safe and clinically positive outcome of the patient's care. Yet, determination of patient assignment must also take into consideration the synergy between the knowledge, skill, and experience of the nurse and the complexity and volume of the nursing diagnoses and interventions required by each patient. Together, these factors must inform the patient assignment determination to achieve safe, quality patient outcomes. This study represents a landmark investigation of the effects of nurse staffing and the educational preparation of the nurse on patient outcomes and the quality of care and has become an important part of the professional dialogue on patient safety.

Source: Aiken, L. H., Clarke, S. P., Sloane, D. M., Sochalski, J., & Silber, J. H. (2002). Hospital nurse staffing and patient mortality, nurse burnout, and job dissatisfaction. The Journal of the American Medical Association, 288(16), 1987–1993.

Assessment

Patient care is dependent on careful assessment of both the presenting health issue and life situation. Nurses are in an ideal position and have the necessary expertise to quickly develop the therapeutic interactions needed to care for patients often in the midst of crisis. Nurses' responsibility to understand the patient and family over and above the specific disease process provides an important context and template for continuing health interventions.

For example, an 18-year-old insured woman who is a college student, newly diagnosed with diabetes, can be directed to agencies, such as a student health clinic or to a private practice group for treatment, education, and direction. Contrast this situation with an 80-year-old man with poor vision, living alone with comorbid diagnoses of congestive heart failure and depression. In the latter case the types of support and services available are not as easily focused. These contrasting situations demonstrate how significant knowing the patient's characteristics in the context of their life can affect health care decisions.

The nurse's assessment of patient characteristics that are based in a person's physical, emotional, spiritual, social, cultural, and economic background provides the fundamental necessities for quality care. According to the synergy model these characteristics include: stability, complexity, predictability, resiliency, vulnerability, participation in decision making, and care and resource availability. This is the information that ultimately will determine the effectiveness or fit of the care plan to the patient's needs and situation. From this information, nurses can determine the competencies best suited to the patient's situation, generate referrals as needed, and ensure the appropriate level of care and agency.

Safe Passage

There is great complexity and therefore great potential for fragmentation in the health care system. Guiding patients to ensure appropriate care as they interact with providers is a critical nursing responsibility. The nurse's ability to provide safe passage can contribute immeasurably toward positive clinical outcomes.

Cost, Access, and Quality

Nurses' understanding of the patient's characteristics and health requirements, as well as the health care system, can open the appropriate doors to health care services. The nurse's ability to guide patients to the appropriate level of care ensures access and efficient use of resources. The nurse provides appropriate interventions and safe passage that contribute to improved outcomes at both the patient and system level. In these ways the nurse's role is essential in addressing the balance between cost, access, and quality.

KEY CONCEPTS

- Affordable cost, reasonable access, and ensured quality of outcomes are the values that are intrinsic to health care agency operations.
- The United States spends a greater proportion (16 percent) of its GDP on health care than on any other GDP category, yet the system is highly criticized as fragmented and inadequate.
- Health care agencies can be generally classified by the level of care provided: preventive, primary, secondary, tertiary, restorative, or continuing. Several levels of care may be provided simultaneously by a single health care agency.
- The VA health care system and the IHS are government programs that include health care agencies that provide care at many levels but only for specific populations whose members must prove their eligibility.

- CAHs are small rural hospitals that provide health care services in partnership with an acute care hospital in exchange for a higher payment schedule than that approved for similar services at other hospitals.
- Integrated care delivery systems are evolving to provide seamless, coordinated care for comprehensive disease management of a defined population across a network of affiliated health care agencies.
- Innovative responses to competition for patients is transforming retail businesses into agencies for provision of preventive health care.
- The synergy model provides a framework from which to examine the nurse-relationship relationship across all areas of practice and across all health care agencies. Components of the relationship are patient characteristics, nurse characteristics, and safe passage.

REVIEW QUESTIONS

1. Which of the following is not a component of Donabedian's framework for the evaluation of quality?
   1. Structural variables
   2. Outcome variable
   3. Process variable
   4. Patient satisfaction

2. Which of the following types of health care agencies would be considered part of a primary care delivery system?
   1. Hospitals
   2. Mobile mammography screening
   3. Helicopter transport
   4. Durgi-center

Continued

REVIEW QUESTIONS—cont'd

3. Identify the essential characteristic of the synergy model.
   1. Synergy occurs when nurse competencies match patient characteristics.
   2. Clinical judgment and caring practices form the basis for excellent care.
   3. Tending to the environment of health care is an important part of nursing.
   4. Curley suggests that outcomes should emanate from the nurse, the patient, and the health care system.

4. Medicare is:
   1. The national health insurance program for people age 65 years and older
   2. A program that pays for medical assistance for indigent individuals
   3. An insurance program administered by state government
   4. All of the above

5. What percentage of the gross national product was dedicated to health care in 2004?
   1. 15.6 percent
   2. 8.4 percent
   3. 16 percent
   4. 26.7 percent

6. Which of the following is not considered to be one of the major cornerstones of our current health care system?
   1. Prescription drug reimbursement for the elderly
   2. Cost of health care
   3. Access to quality health care
   4. Quality and safety

7. The hospital report card is an example of a quality measure used to evaluate what category of health care service?
   1. Primary care
   2. Continuing care
   3. Tertiary care
   4. Preventive care

8. In health care agencies nursing responsibilities are guided by:
   1. The board of trustees
   2. Patient needs
   3. JCAHO
   4. Positive clinical outcomes

9. Secondary care includes:
   1. Nursing homes
   2. Routine hospitalization
   3. Childhood immunizations
   4. Hospice

10. Medicaid is:
    1. The national health insurance program for people aged 65 years and older
    2. A program that pays for medical assistance for certain indigent individuals
    3. An insurance program administered by state government
    4. Not available to patients until they have exhausted all but $2,000 of their assets

REVIEW ACTIVITIES

1. Interview a family practice health care provider, an individual over the age of 65, and an individual who has had multiple experiences with a hospital or clinic, i.e., an individual with a chronic illness. Ask each of them to share their perceptions of how well the health care system functions to meet the needs of patients. If they could change one thing about the system what would it be?

2. To prepare yourself as a health care provider in a multicultural world, it is necessary to gain an understanding of the issues surrounding health and ethnicity. The community tool box offers a wealth of information and assistance in skill development. Go to the Web site and complete at least one activity. The examples below from the table of contents are great places to begin.
   a. Cultural Competence in a Multicultural World at: http://ctb.ku.edu/tools/en/chapter_1027.htm
   b. Building Culturally Competent Organizations at: http://ctb.ku.edu/tools/en/sub_section_tools_1176.htm#tool4

Continued

REVIEW ACTIVITIES—cont'd

3. Pick a health care agency in your community that you have never visited. Walk through the agency noting its sensual ambience, i.e., colors, odors, noise, light, etc. From your perceptions, what level of care do you surmise is provided?

4. Make an appointment to speak with the chief nursing officer of the previous agency. Discuss how synergistic care is provided in that agency.

5. Investigate what levels of care are available in health care agencies within a 10-mile radius of your home.

Visit the Contemporary Medical-Surgical Nursing online companion resource at www.delmarhealthcare.com for additional content and study aids. Click on Online Companions then select the Nursing discipline.

Critical Care

Sharon Little-Stoetzel, RN, MS

CHAPTER TOPICS

- Critical Care Unit
- Common Problems and Needs of the Critically Ill Patient
- Family Member Needs
- Hemodynamic Monitoring
- Cardiac Assist Devices

- Intracranial Pressure Monitoring
- Airway Assistance
- Mechanical Ventilation
- Nursing Management of Patients Requiring Mechanical Ventilation

Critical care units or intensive care units are specialized care areas for patients who are critically ill. Patients admitted to critical care units require concentrated nursing care as well as frequent monitoring of vital life functions. Critical care units may be either specialized or generalized. Generalized units admit a variety of critically ill patients regardless of their diagnosis or specialized units. Specialized intensive care units focus on specific areas of care, such as coronary, medical, surgical, trauma, neurological, pediatric, or neonatal.

CRITICAL CARE UNIT

The medical field experienced a great interest in open-chest and external defibrillation in the resuscitation of patients with myocardial infarction (MI) in the 1950s (Julian, 2001). During this time it became clear that patients could be successfully treated with cardiopulmonary resuscitation (CPR) when they experienced cardiopulmonary arrest. Cardiopulmonary resuscitation is more beneficial if started as soon as the patient experiences cardiac arrest. In the 1950s, patients who were at high risk for cardiac arrest were distributed throughout the hospital. Consequently, lifesaving treatment was delayed. In 1961, Dr. Desmond G. Julian recommended that all patients experiencing signs or symptoms of cardiac arrest be admitted to one ward with the capability of electrocardiograph (ECG) monitoring (Julian, 2001). Monitoring patients by ECG began in Sydney, Australia in 1962, and one of the first critical care units opened in the United States in Bethany Hospital located in Kansas City, Kansas, to ensure prompt treatment of cardiopulmonary arrest. The opening of this unit was necessary because of the lack of prompt treatment of cardiac arrest. Initially, resident physicians staffed intensive care units, but it was soon deemed necessary to utilize nurses for the monitoring of these patients. The role of the critical care nurse was developed with this realization.

The Critical Care Nurse

The American Association of Critical Care Nurses (AACN) defines critical care nursing as a nursing specialty that involves human responses to life-threatening conditions (AACN, 2002). Life-threatening conditions or a potential for life-threatening problems could include a wide range of concerns resulting from a MI to postoperative care following a liver transplant. The critical care nurse must be knowledgeable about pathological processes, while also recognizing the psychological impact those conditions may have on the patient. The critical care nurse must treat the whole patient. This encompasses the physical, psychological, spiritual, emotional, and social aspects of the patient and the impact of his or her illness on family members.

Critical care nurses can become certified in critical care nursing through AACN. The certification process is designed to validate a nurse's knowledge of caring for critically ill patients (AACN, 2003). Nurses who pass the examination may use the initials CCRN after their name indicating certification in critical care nursing. The AACN exam tests critical care knowledge utilizing application and analysis questions. In addition to passing the exam, the critical care nurse must spend a minimum number of hours in the critical care setting to become a certified critical care nurse. Nurses renew their critical care certification every three years and may become certified in adult, pediatric, or neonatal content areas. To patients, certification indicates that a nurse is qualified and competent and has passed meticulous requirements to obtain this credential (CCRN, 2003).

Nurse practitioners can become certified as a National Acute Care Nurse Practitioner by passing the American Nurses' Credentialing Center's certification examination (ACNP, 2003). Critical care clinical nurse specialists may become certified after passing an AACN exam (CCRN, 2003). Nurses must also show evidence of expertise in clinical knowledge, judgment, and skills to obtain the CCNS. Minimum requirements for obtaining a CCNS include a master's degree and completion of clinical practice hours for both certification exams. Critical care nurses maintain competency through annual review courses.

Registered nurses who work in intensive care units have additional preparation beyond their basic nursing education. Most hospitals that have intensive care units offer basic critical care courses for nurses who are new to the intensive care unit setting. The content in these courses typically consists of ventilator management, hemodynamic monitoring, shock management, intracranial pressure monitoring, specific intensive care assessments, and conditions of various body systems. Additional training in arrhythmia interpretation and management is included in the nurse's orientation.

Delivery of Nursing Care

As patient acuity is higher in the intensive care unit setting; nurse/patient ratios are lower than on general medical or surgical units. Typically the intensive care unit nurse cares for one to two patients per shift. The registered nurse is responsible for all aspects of patient care including hygiene and vital signs. This delivery system of nursing care is important for the critically ill patient. This total patient care modality allows for continuous expert care. Most intensive care units primarily utilize registered nurses, although many hire unlicensed assistive personnel to provide assistance with certain technical tasks.

The Critical Care Patient

Patients are admitted to the intensive care unit when they need continuous comprehensive observation and monitoring by professional nurses. They may be admitted following a procedure or by written order by an attending health care providers. See Box 19-1 for an example of admission criteria to the intensive care unit.

Once the critically ill patient has stabilized and no longer needs continuous observation by the critical care nurse, the patient is transferred to an intermediate care or general medical or surgical unit. Occasionally patients will be discharged to home from the intensive care unit, but usually patients from the critical care units require continued hospitalization (Box 19-2). Placement of patients after discharge from the intensive care unit will depend on the needs

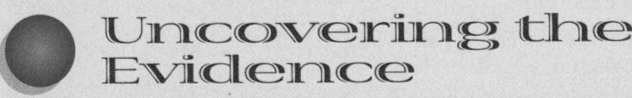

Uncovering the Evidence

Intensive Care Staffing and Patient Outcomes

Discussion: This retrospective review examined 2,606 patients who had abdominal aortic surgery in Maryland. Low-intensity staffing was considered a 1:3 ratio or greater during the day and night shifts, medium-intensity staffing was considered a 1:3 ratio or greater on either the day or night shift, and high-intensity staffing was considered a 1:2 ratio or fewer on the day and night shifts. Complications that were identified by a panel of four physicians included: (a) cardiac complications; (b) respiratory complications; (c) renal failure; (d) septicemia; and (e) platelet replacement. The researchers found that there was a statistically significant difference in the amount of complications associated with lower staffing levels. Patients cared for on units with low-intensity staffing were two times more likely to have respiratory complications than those cared for in high-intensity staffed units.

Implications for Practice: The implications of this study are important for administrators to consider when discussing the costs of quality patient care. The researchers also suggest that nurse managers may be able to use this evidence to advocate for increased technical support for RNs.

Source: Dang, D., Johantgen, M., Pronovost, P., Jenckes, M., & Bass, E. (2002). Postoperative complications: Does intensive care unit staff nursing make a difference? Heart and Lung, 31(3), 219–228.

BOX 19-1

INTENSIVE CARE UNIT ADMISSION CRITERIA

I. A patient may be admitted to the intensive care unit by order of the attending health care provider.

II. A seriously or critically ill patient who would benefit from intensive nursing care is eligible for admission. This patient would qualify by one or more of the following clinical findings:

A. Chest pain with one of the following:
1. ECG changes consistent with MI
2. Elevated cardiac enzymes consistent with MI
3. Unstable dysrhythmia
4. Requirement for IV nitroglycerin
5. Accompanied by heart failure

B. Hypertensive crisis with:
1. Dyspnea
2. Altered LOC or paresis
3. Blood urea nitrogen (BUN) greater than or equal to 45, creatinine greater than or equal to 3.
4. The need for intravenous Nipride

C. Respiratory distress associated with
1. Rales
2. Peripheral edema
3. Abnormal ABG
4. New onset of vital sign changes with circulatory or respiratory compromise:
5. Pulse less than or equal to 40 beats per minute or greater than or equal to 180 beats per minute
6. Respiration less than or equal to 8 or greater than or equal to 30
7. Systolic blood pressure less than or equal to 80 mm Hg, or greater than or equal to 200 mm Hg
8. Diastolic blood pressure greater than or equal to 120 mm Hg
9. Temperature less than or equal to 94° degrees Fahrenheit (34.4° Celsius) or greater than or equal to 105° Fahrenheit (40.5° Celsius)
10. Postural blood pressure decrease greater than or equal to 50 mm Hg

D. Newly discovered pulmonary edema, vessel occlusion, cardiac tamponade, hemothorax, or pneumothorax with circulatory or respiratory compromise, or pleural effusion with respiratory compromise.

E. Cardiac dysrhythmias including:
1. Sustained ventricular tachycardia
2. Sustained ventricular fibrillation
3. Torsades de pointes

4. Sustained supraventricular tachycardia with rate greater than or equal to 160 beats per minute and associated with chest pain or respiratory distress

F. Cardiac rhythms requiring use of a temporary transvenous pacemaker, which may include:
1. Third-degree heart block (complete heart block)
2. Second-degree heart block (Type II)
3. Sinus bradycardia with low systolic blood pressure

G. New onset of the following critical lab values:
1. Hematocrit less than or equal to 28 with angina
2. Creatinine phosphokinase (CK-MB) elevated and greater than 5 percent
3. Lactic dehydrogenase upper limits of normal with chest pain or ischemia on ECG
4. Serum sodium less than or equal to 115 or greater than or equal to 160
5. Serum potassium less than or equal to 2 or greater than or equal to 6
6. Serum calcium less than or equal to 7.5 with ECG changes consistent with hypocalcemia (ventricular dysrhythmias), or greater than or equal to 15
7. Serum magnesium less than or equal to 0.8

H. New onset of the following critical ABG values
1. PO_2 less than or equal to 50 on room air
2. PO_2 greater than or equal to 50 on room air
3. HCO_3 less than or equal to 16, or greater than or equal to 40
4. pH less than or equal to 7.3, or greater than or equal to 7.5

I. Patients requiring mechanical ventilation

J. Head trauma, intracranial bleed, or intracranial edema associated with any of the following:
1. Fluctuating LOC
2. Elevated blood pressure
3. Decreased pulse
4. Pupillary changes

K. Trauma associated with any of the following:
1. Multiple fractures
2. Flail chest
3. Cervical spine fracture
4. Spinal cord fracture or injury
5. Cardiac changes

L. Medically unstable operative patients

Continued

BOX 19-1—cont'd

INTENSIVE CARE UNIT ADMISSION CRITERIA

M. Actual or potential for airway obstruction

N. Continuous seizures

O. Hemorrhage from any site with hematocrit less than or equal to 21 with hemoglobin less than or equal to 7

P. Acute suicide attempt

Q. Hyperglycemia associated with acidosis or decreased LOC

R. Bilibor or multilobar pneumonia

S. Clinical conditions that indicate the need for

1. Invasive monitoring
2. IV cardiac inotropes
3. IV vasopressors
4. IV vasodilators
5. IV antiarrhythmics
6. IV thrombolytics
7. IV beta blockers
8. Titrating an IV insulin drip

T. During the hours when the recovery room is closed, a patient may be admitted for postanesthetic care until the patient is recovered.

BOX 19-2

INTENSIVE CARE UNIT DISCHARGE CRITERIA

I. When the patient's condition no longer indicates the need for intensive nursing care arrangements will be made for transfer to an appropriate nursing unit as soon as possible.

II. Guidelines for discharge

A. Absence of unstable dysrhythmia(s) for the previous 12 hours

B. Respiratory status stable for the previous 12 hours, as evidenced by:

1. Oxygen saturation of 90 percent or greater, or

2. Supplemental oxygen requirement of 40 percent or less in the chronically mechanically ventilated patient who is able to participate in the management of his or her ventilator.

C. Vital signs have been stable for the previous 12 hours.

D. Absence of the need for IV drugs to maintain cardiac status or blood pressure.

E. Absence of the need for invasive monitoring.

F. Chest pain controlled by oral, sublingual, or topical medications (nitroglycerin) for the previous 12 hours.

G. Terminally ill patients who will receive palliative care and aggressive treatment will be discontinued.

Source: Berardino, M., Morrone, O., Sciacca, P. F., Rosato, R., Ciccone, G., & Massaro, F. (2004). Discharge criteria from intensive care unit in brain injured patients. Acta Neurochir (Wein), 146(5), 453–456.

---

of the patient and the types of units available in the hospital. Intermediate care unit patient populations can vary widely. Some intermediate care units take patients who require mechanical ventilation but are hemodynamically stable. Other intermediate care units may not have the ability to manage patients requiring mechanical ventilation. Discharge criteria from the intensive care unit should meet the needs of the specific institution.

Optimal care of the critically ill patient admitted to a critical care unit includes input from a group of health care providers. The interdisciplinary team includes physicians, nurses, pharmacists, respiratory therapists, social workers, physical therapists, nutrition specialists, and chaplains. Registered nurses lead the team in patient care conferences about patients who are particularly challenging or require extensive stays in the intensive care unit. In addition to the interdisciplinary team that cares for the daily needs of the patient, an ethics committee may be asked to discuss a patient in the critical care unit. Ethical issues are common to the critical care environment. Life support technology is regularly used, and sometimes the decision to terminate lifesaving measures is unavoidable. The ethics committee discusses these cases individually with input from the interdisciplinary team and family members.

COMMON PROBLEMS OF THE CRITICALLY ILL PATIENT

In addition to their medical condition, patients in the critical care setting can face numerous physiological and psychological challenges. Critically ill patients are vulnerable to infection, poor nutrition, the effects of immobility, pain, anxiety, lack of sleep, and communication challenges.

Infection

Patients who are critically ill often become immunocompromised, increasing their susceptibility to infection. Most patients in the critical care setting have intravenous (IV) lines and invasive tubes that may unwittingly introduce infection. Nutritional deficits may also contribute to the patient's susceptibility to infection. The critical care nurse must be vigilant in protecting the patient from potentially infectious sources. Strict hand washing protocols should be a priority for nurses. Standard precautions should be used as well as adhering to additional precautions as patient conditions warrant. Changing IV lines according to protocol is also paramount in protecting the patient against infection. Important nursing functions for the patient who develops an infection include: (a) monitoring for signs and symptoms of infection; (b) culture and sensitivity results; and (c) administering appropriate antibiotics. The critical care nurse must monitor the immunocompromised patient closely as sepsis, septic shock, and multiple organ failure are life-threatening conditions.

Nutrition

Providing optimal nutrition to the critically ill patient can be a challenge for the critical care team. Critically ill patients are often in a hypermetabolic state resulting in increased caloric requirements. Patients are often unable to obtain the required calories because of their inability to eat normally. This prolonged inability may be because of anorexia, mechanical ventilation, altered mental state, or dysfunction of the gastrointestinal (GI) tract. The caloric requirements for each patient should be determined and will vary depending on age, activity level, actual illness, wound healing requirements, and prior nutritional status along. The critical care nurse, in conjunction with a nutrition support specialist and health care providers, is responsible for identifying patients at risk for malnutrition and communicating these needs appropriately. Critically ill patients are nourished by either enteral or parenteral feedings. Ongoing nutritional assessment is part of the critical care nurse's responsibility and includes monitoring weight, prealbumin, transferrin levels, and nitrogen balance (Sole, Lamborn, & Hartshorn, 2001).

Immobility

Critically ill patients frequently face immobility issues that present challenges to their physical condition and may increase their time in the intensive care unit. Patients with life-threatening conditions spend a significant amount of time lying in their hospital beds. Often, the medical equipment and the patient's physiological condition do not allow for normal mobility. Patients who are hemodynamically unstable are unable to turn or sit, because these activities induce hypotensive or hypoxemic episodes. Additionally, activity may cause drastic changes in heart rate. Patients with head or spinal injuries may be required to stay immobile to prevent further injury to the brain or spinal cord. However, the consequences of immobility are well-documented. Documented complications of immobility included pressure ulcers, deep vein thrombosis, pulmonary complications, and muscle wasting. Promoting the positive effects of mobility while trying to minimize the negative effects can be challenging for the critical care nurse. Patients who are hemodynamically stable obviously benefit from adhering to a strict repositioning schedule. Many intensive care units utilize continuous lateral rotation beds to turn patients who are hemodynamically unstable or have serious pulmonary conditions. Many of these beds have specialized mattresses that provide continuous rotation to prevent pressure ulcer formation (Martin, 2001). Some of the beds also provide chest physiotherapy. The critical care nurse must frequently assess the skin for areas of potential breakdown and treat accordingly. The critical care nurse often consults with a wound care nurse who specializes in pressure ulcer assessment and treatment. The critical care nurse must frequently assess the patient's pulmonary status. Atelectasis, an antecedent to pneumonia, may occur in patients who are immobile (Martin, 2001). Nosocomial infections, such as pneumonia, frequently occur in patients who require extended treatment in an intensive care unit. This complication may further prolong the patient's hospital stay, delay ventilator weaning, and contribute to mortality.

Pain

Most patients in the critical care setting experience pain with varying intensity. Discomfort, stress, and anxiety have adverse physiological effects. The patient experiencing pain from open-heart surgery is less likely to use an incentive spirometer or ambulate to the chair, thus compromising their postoperative recovery. Pain in critically ill patients can come from many sources, such as wounds, infections, inadequate tissue perfusion, and surgery (Stanik-Hutt, 2003). Medical and nursing procedures also contribute to distress in the critically ill patient. Common intensive care unit procedures, such as repositioning, central venous catheter placement, removal of wound drains, changing of dressings, tracheal suctioning, and removal of femoral sheaths, cause pain in these patients. Unfortunately, many patients do not receive analgesics prior to these procedures (Puntillo, et al., 2002). Unrelieved pain produces anxiety and affects the critical care patient's recovery period. Pain prevention and management should be a priority for every intensive care unit patient (Stanik-Hutt, 2003). Critical care nurses should request analgesics to be available 24 hours a day to prevent acute onsets of pain. Nurses should assess regularly for discomfort. Subjective descriptions are the most reliable measures of assessing the intensity of a patient's pain. When assessing a patient who is unable to vocalize, the use of visual adds, such as letters or numbers, are helpful to ascertain their discomfort level. Body language and physiological parameters may need to be utilized as assessment parameters for the patient with altered mental status.

Anxiety

Most patients in the intensive care unit experience feelings of anxiety. The intensive care unit can be a distressing environment because of the machines, noises, odors, and flow of strangers. This sensory overload can contribute to the anxiety the patient may already be experiencing. Critically ill patients may lack familiar stimuli. Sleeping in a strange bed, being deprived of personal surroundings, loss of daily routines, and limited contact with family members add to the patient's anxiety. Signs and symptoms of anxiety vary depending on

Skills 360°

The Laughter Cart

Motivated to find ways to meet the emotional and spiritual needs of her intensive care unit patients, Cindy Motley MSN, CCRN, developed the Laughter Cart to be used by nursing staff as a tool to facilitate therapeutic communication and interaction with critically ill patients and their families. The cart is stocked with comedy movies, puppets, bubble machines, and other props designed to make people laugh. Inspired by Universal Studio's 1998 movie, "Patch Adams," starring Academy Award winner Robin Williams, Motley uses the cart to bring laughter to the bedside and to create a sense of shared experience. In this way she provides an emotional outlet and coping mechanisms. The true Patch Adams (on whose life the movie was based) explains that laughter increases the release of catecholamines and endorphins, the body's natural "feel good" chemicals. Laughter also stimulates the immune system by causing a decrease in cortisol secretion and lowering sedimentation rate. A good laugh can improve tissue oxygenation, decrease residual air in the lungs, improve peripheral circulation, and create a relaxation response. Other examples of the use of humor and laughter for health promotion and healing include the Laughter Mobile Program, developed by Duke University Medical Center in Durham, North Carolina and Rx Laughter at UCLA's Jonsson Cancer Center.

the patient. The physical symptoms of anxiety may include: (a) tachycardia, (b) tachypnea, (c) restlessness, (d) inability to sleep, and (e) diaphoresis. The patient may be tearful, verbalize feelings of anxiety, experience angry outbursts, or need continuous attention by the nurse. Fear can progress to the point of agitation or even delirium. Antianxiety interventions are helpful for the intensive care unit patient (Frazier, et al., 2003). These interventions include: (a) administering anxiolytics, (b) encouraging unrestricted visitation by family members, (c) providing therapeutic communication, (d) ensuring adequate pain relief, (e) using guided imagery, (f) communicating the treatment plan, (g) offering music therapy, and (h) spending extra time with the patient. Nurses can also help control environmental noise by lowering alarm volumes when possible, keeping social conversation and laughter to a minimum, and decreasing telephone ring volumes.

Sleep

Sleep is physiologically and psychologically necessary for all individuals. Unfortunately, in the critical care setting, most patients experience disruptions in their normal sleep patterns. The disruptions include noise, constant exposure to bright light, pain, anxiety, and medications (Honkus, 2003). Frequent nursing assessments can also contribute to sleeplessness in critically ill patients. Lack of sleep can exacerbate delirium in some patients, and it can delay ventilator weaning in others. Critical care nurses must consider sleep as an important component in their patient's treatment plan. One of the first steps in promoting sleep is to make sure the patient is comfortable and has decreased anxiety. The nurse should minimize unnecessary noise and lights and recognize any important nighttime rituals, such as bathing or watching the nightly news. The patient will benefit from maintaining these rituals while in the hospital. The critical care nurse should perform necessary assessments and procedures while allowing a minimum of two hours of uninterrupted sleep (Honkus, 2003). Lastly, the critical care nurse should realize that some

Uncovering the Evidence

Patient Stress: Can They Sleep?

Discussion: Ninety-seven cardiac patients were assessed regarding noise and other environmental stressors while in the intensive care unit. All patients had coronary artery bypass surgery, valve replacement surgery, or both. The independent variables were assessed using Topf's 24-item disturbance due to hospital noise scale. Sleep was then evaluated with the Verran and Snyder-Halpern sleep scale.

Conclusions: The researchers concluded that noise, a different bed, pain, and anxiety accounted for significant variance in the quality of the patient's sleep.

Implications for Practice: Critical care nurses must realize that there are multiple factors surrounding a critically ill patient's inability to sleep and that these factors may be different for each patient. But certainly, noise, pain, and anxiety, in addition to an unfamiliar bed, are factors contributing to insomnia. If nurses are aware of these stressors, they can help to alleviate them and promote sleep in the patient.

Citation: Topf, M., & Thompson, S. (2001). Interactive relationships between hospital patients' noised-induced stress and other stress with sleep. Heart and Lung, 30(4), 237–243.

patients might benefit from sleep medications and should consult the appropriate health care provider.

Communication

Impaired communication may occur in the critical care patient because of endotracheal or tracheostomy tube placement, paralyzing and sedating medications, or altered mental status. It is important for the critical care nurse to recognize that the inability to communicate contributes to the stress of being critically ill. The patient may experience additional fear and anxiety as well as powerlessness. It is imperative that alternate methods of communication be provided to the patient. These modalities may include: (a) picture boards, (b) paper and pen, or (c) agreed on gestures or signals. Use of these alternative methods, explanations of procedures and equipment, the use of therapeutic touch, and reassurance in periods of increased anxiety are helpful tools for communicating with the critically patient and their family.

FAMILY MEMBER NEEDS

Critical care nurses care for family members as well as their patients. Families of critically ill patients experience a crisis with the admission of the patient to the intensive care unit. With admission to the critical care unit, families fear losing their family member. They face disruptions in every day life accompanied by potential financial concerns. Families may also have to make difficult decisions about their loved one's health care. The critical care setting is generally unfamiliar and intimidating to families.

Family members can impact the critically ill patient in many ways. They can help ease the patient's anxiety by providing familiarity. Families can help explain procedures and medications to the critically ill patient. Families can also provide more information about the patient to the health care team to ensure holistic care (Slota, Shearn, Potersnak, & Hass, 2003). Family members can also assist the patient with discharge instructions and requirements. However, if family members are anxious, their presence may not have a positive impact on the patient. Usually the benefits of family visitation far outweigh the negative effects. Pet visitation with strict enforcement of infection control measures may also be beneficial to the patient (Cullen, et al., 2003). Research is limited in this area because of the subjective nature of the effects, but anecdotal evidence suggests that visitation by a pet may encourage feelings of well-being. Pet visitation is a component in many critical care unit policies.

There have been numerous studies on the needs of families with critically ill patients. Leske (2002) suggests that there are five principal needs that are experienced by most families. These needs include: (a) reassurance, (b) flexible visitation, (c) information, (d) comfort, and (e) support. The first need is to receive reassurance. Families of the critically ill patient need to be reassured that there is hope and that their family member is receiving the best possible care available. The second identified need of families is to be near the patient as much as possible. This can be accomplished through flexible visitation. In the past, critical care units have had strict visiting policies. It was not uncommon for families to see their loved one once or twice daily for ten minutes at a time. As research on family needs of the critically ill have become available, intensive care unit staff have responded with more flexible visiting policies. Families require information about their loved one. Providing information to family members decreases their feelings of anxiety and powerlessness. Informed families feel supported when making important decisions about their loved one's care. The fourth need of families is to feel comfortable. Adequate space in waiting rooms assists with families' comfort. The nurse can also provide information on places to eat and where restrooms are located.

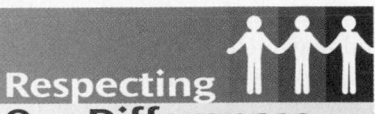

Respecting Our Differences

Families in the 21st Century

In today's society, family can be defined in many ways. Family includes couples without children, single parent-child combinations, couples living together, and homosexual couples. Leske (2002) states that it may be best to define family as any individual who considers himself or herself to be a family member. Cullen, Titler, and Drahozal (2003) define family as individuals whom patients have identified as having significant relationships with. Now, the family has a broader definition than it had in earlier years.

The fifth common need of families is the need to have support available. Various support measures are important and may include assistance from religious leaders, social services, or mental health experts.

HEMODYNAMIC MONITORING

Critically ill patients require intensive monitoring to maintain vital functions. In many patients, hemodynamic monitoring assists the health care team in deciding on the most beneficial forms of therapy. Hemodynamics is defined as the impact that certain forces have on blood circulation throughout the body. This monitoring evaluates cardiac function, tissue perfusion, blood volume, tissue oxygenation, and vascular tone (Swearingen & Keen, 2001). Nurses monitor hemodynamics while taking blood pressure. In the critical care setting, hemodynamics is typically monitored using invasive devices, although noninvasive devices are also used. The critical care nurse may monitor continuous systemic arterial pressures, pulmonary artery (PA) measurements, pulmonary artery wedge pressures (PAWP), cardiac output (CO), systemic vascular resistance (SVR), central venous pressure (CVP), left atrial pressure (LAP), and mixed venous oxygen saturation (SvO_2). When these parameters are combined with the physical exam, lab values, and other appropriate assessments, they can be essential in establishing or evaluating a patient's response to therapy. The most common complications of invasive monitoring are bleeding and infection.

Cardiac Output

Pulmonary artery (PA) catheters allow nurses to measure CO. **Cardiac output (CO)** is defined as the amount of blood ejected by the heart in one minute. CO is further explained by the equation $CO = HR \times SV$. Heart rate multiplied by stroke volume equals CO. Stroke volume is the amount of blood ejected by the heart during each cardiac cycle. CO can be an important parameter to measure in critically ill patients. Monitoring this parameter can help the nurse and health care providers determine adequacy of response from medications, fluid, or mechanical devices. Normal cardiac output is 4 to 8 L/minute. The wide variation in the normal value is because of the differences in body sizes of individuals. **Cardiac index** is a parameter that is frequently measured in addition to the cardiac output. Cardiac index is calculated by dividing the patient's cardiac output by the patient's body surface area (BSA). Because cardiac index is customized to the patient, it is considered to be a more accurate reflection of the patient's CO. A normal cardiac index is 2.5 to 4.2 L/minute/m^2. Abnormally low COs may result from various factors affecting heart rate or stroke volume. Extremely slow or fast heart rates can cause inadequate filling of the left ventricle and therefore, reduce CO. Conditions that affect contractility of the muscle fibers of the heart may cause a decrease in CO. Common causes of contractility problems include MI and cardiogenic shock. Patients can have lowered stroke volumes because of decreased preload or increased afterload. Abnormally high CO can occur in hypermetabolic states, such as fever or hyperthyroidism. High CO is also seen in episodes of increased physical activity and in early stages of septic shock.

Preload

Preload is characterized by the amount of cardiac muscle fiber stretch preceding each contraction. Preload is determined by the volume in the ventricles at the end of diastole (end diastolic volume). According to Frank-Starling's Law, in normal heart function, the greater the end diastolic volume or the more the myocardial fibers have stretched at the end of diastole, the stronger the ventricular contraction. Therefore, as preload increases, there will be a corresponding increase in the CO and cardiac index. Alternatively, when preload decreases, there is a corresponding decrease in force of contraction resulting in a decreased CO and cardiac index. In patients who are hypovolemic, preload can be increased with fluid or blood administration. In patients who are hypervolemic, preload may be reduced with diuretics. As venous return is a primary determinant of preload, medications that cause venous vasodilation also decrease preload. When a patient has a PA catheter in place, preload is measured by obtaining CVP (right-sided preload), PAWP, PA diastolic pressure, and LAP.

Afterload

Afterload is defined as the pressure and forces opposing ventricular contraction. If arterial blood pressure is elevated, the ventricles must generate more pressure to eject their volume. Pulmonary vascular resistance is the primary force opposing the right ventricle, and SVP and arterial blood pressure are the primary forces opposing the left ventricle. When the ventricles must generate higher pressure to accomplish systolic ejection, cardiac oxygen demand increases. This is especially concerning in the patient who has preexisting coronary artery disease or heart failure. Patients who have an abnormally high afterload will actually experience a decrease in CO and cardiac index. It is necessary to reduce afterload in these patients to raise their CO and cardiac index. Afterload reduction may be accomplished primarily by administering arteriole vasodilators. Afterload is increased in patients with hypertension, pulmonary hypertension, as well as in conditions, such as hypothermia that causes vasoconstriction. Afterload is decreased in conditions where there is vasodilation.

Contractility

The force of ventricular contraction will also have an affect on stroke volume and CO. **Contractility** (the force of ventricular contraction) is affected by preload and afterload. Contractility is also affected by factors that influence muscle contraction. The interaction of actin and myosin will certainly affect muscle contraction. Electrolytes, such as calcium and potassium, as well as sympathetic stimulation will affect cardiac muscle contraction. Additional increases in contractility can be achieved through administration of positive inotropic medications such as Inocor (Amrinone) or digoxin. Any increases in contractility will cause subsequent increases in myocardial oxygen demand. Acidemia and hypoxia will reduce contractility (Swearingen & Keen, 2001). Beta blockers and calcium channel blockers will also have negative inotropic effects and reduce myocardial oxygen demand.

Equipment for Hemodynamic Monitoring

The critical care nurse should be familiar with all the equipment necessary for the insertion of IV lines as well the needed supplies for monitoring the patient after the lines are inserted. All hemodynamic monitoring of patients will require four necessary pieces of equipment, including: (a) a monitor that records the appropriate waveform; (b) a transducer; (c) an amplifier; and (d) a combination pressure bag, fluid flush system, and tubing (Sole, et al., 2001).

The monitor records the appropriate waveform or value of the component being monitored. The waveform will usually be on continuous display and be located under the ECG recording on a multichannel bedside monitor. Waveforms are typically printed and interpreted in the patient's record at the beginning of the nurse's shift and as needed for changes in patient condition or evaluation of therapies (Figure 19-1).

The transducer is attached to the tubing and fluid flush system and is important for accurate monitoring. Transducers are capable of measuring

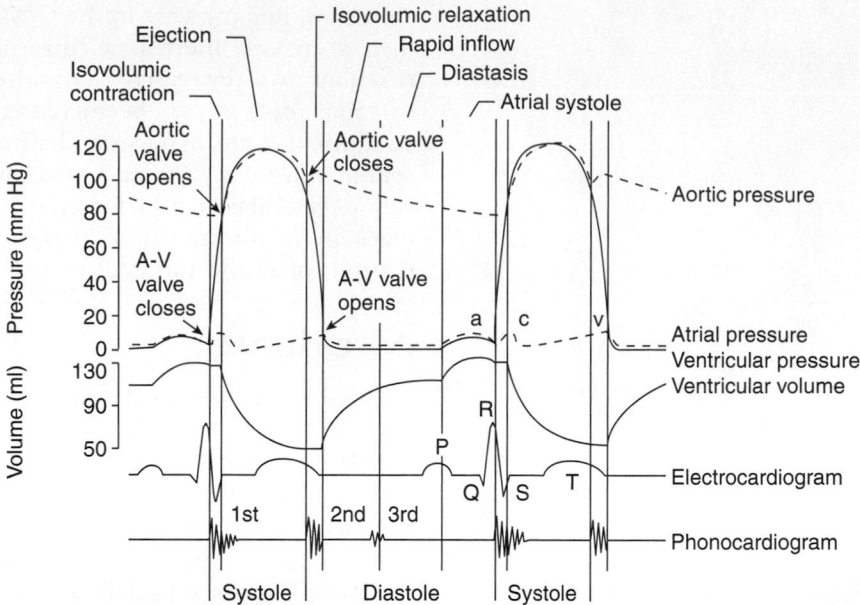

Figure 19-1 Events of the cardiac cycle.

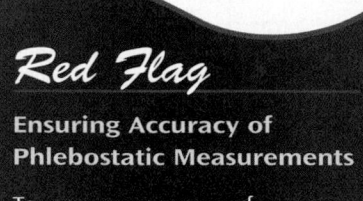

Ensuring Accuracy of Phlebostatic Measurements

To ensure accuracy of measurements, it is important to eliminate any effect that surrounding atmospheric pressure may have on the monitoring system. This effect is eliminated through zeroing the system. The nurse turns the stopcock off to the patient's pressures, removes the cap on the stopcock connection, and pushes the zero button on the monitor. When the value on the screen reflects zero pressure, zeroing the transducer is completed. The cap and stopcock are returned to their normal monitoring position. Zeroing of the transducer is routinely performed prior to insertion of the catheter, once or twice per shift, or whenever the system is disconnected, changed, or extremes in values are obtained.

flow, pressure, temperature, light intensity, and sound. These measurements are changed into electrical signals that can be displayed on the patient's monitor. The electrical signals are enhanced by the amplifier, which is connected to the transducer. Electrical signals are interpreted with more accuracy with use of the amplifier.

The fluid flush system tubing must be primed and connected to a pressure bag prior to insertion of the appropriate catheter. Once the appropriate catheter is inserted, the fluid flush system tubing is connected to the catheter for the purposes of flushing the system and preventing clot formation in the line and catheter. The solution is typically heparinized normal saline (NS) and delivers approximately 3 mL/hour. A rapid flush device is used to clear the line when blood samples have been obtained. An inflated pressure bag surrounds the solution to infuse small amounts of fluid through the line.

Measurement of Hemodynamic Parameters

As patient treatment decisions are made based, in part, on the values obtained during hemodynamic monitoring, it is vital that the nurse ensure accuracy of these values. Leveling the transducer to the patient's right atrium is necessary to ensure accurate readings. To level the transducer, the nurse must position the transducer at the patient's **phlebostatic axis.** To place the transducer at the level of the phlebostatic axis, the nurse must locate the midpoint of the anterior and posterior chest at the fourth intercostal space (McGhee & Bridges, 2002). Once this is located, the nurse places the transducer level at this position to obtain accurate readings. Once readings are obtained from this location, it is imperative that the phlebostatic axis is marked on the patient. This will ensure consistency in the measurements.

Air in the system will also affect accuracy of parameters measured. The critical care nurse should take care to remove all air bubbles during initial priming of the tubing and practice routine monitoring for air in the already established line. Five strategies are recommended to maintain an air-free system: (a) fast-flush the system after opening for zeroing or taking a blood sample, (b) routinely ensure that all connections and stopcocks are tight as this will help prevent air bubbles from occurring, (c) ensure there is a sufficient amount of the flush solution available and to maintain the pressure bag inflated to 300 mm Hg, (d) refrain from adding stopcocks or extensions to the line; and (e) periodically flick and flush the tubing system.

The critical care nurse must also ensure accuracy in the waveform patterns that are displayed on the monitoring device. Distortions in waveforms could produce inaccurate blood pressure and PA catheter values. The nurse should perform dynamic response testing every time the catheter is zeroed. To perform square wave testing the nurse rapidly initiates and releases the fast-flush device on the line while observing the monitor or printing a hard copy of the waveform. The system is optimally damped when the sharp upstroke produced by the flush ends in a flat line at the maximal indicator on the monitor or hard copy (Darovic, 2004). The flat line is immediately followed by a rapid downstroke in the waveform that extends below the baseline, then immediately returns to baseline after one or two quick oscillations. When the system is overdamped, the positive deflection in the square wave is indistinct. The downstroke does not go beyond the baseline. When overdamping occurs, the systolic pressure is incorrectly lower, and diastolic pressure is inaccurately higher. The waveform itself appears dampened. The nurse should investigate the system for these possible problems in the line, including: (a) blood clots, (b) kinks, (c) air bubbles, or (d) loose connections (Darovic, 2004). There will be many amplified oscillations after the downstroke of the square when the system is underdamped. The waveform will appear sharply exaggerated and will display a falsely high systolic pressure. To correct the system the nurse should remove all air bubbles, use a larger diameter tube, obtain shorter tubing, or use a damping device (Darovic, 2004).

Intra-Arterial Monitoring

Intra-arterial blood pressure monitoring is accomplished by inserting a catheter into the artery of a patient, attaching the catheter to a fluid flush system with a transducer, and attaching the transducer to a cable that is connected to a monitor. Intra-arterial monitoring allows for a continuous display of the patient's blood pressure that may be necessary in unstable patients. Noninvasive methods of obtaining blood pressure do not allow for continuous monitoring, and they are not accurate when blood pressures are at extreme levels. Another advantage of intra-arterial monitoring is the ability to obtain certain blood samples from patients without needle sticks. This is especially beneficial to the patient who requires frequent monitoring of blood samples.

Indications

Any patient who is hemodynamically unstable will likely require intra-arterial monitoring. Patients who require vasoactive IV medications to maintain a normal blood pressure will be candidates for intra-arterial monitoring. Vasoactive medications such as dopamine hydrochloride (Intropin), norepinephrine (Levophed), or nitroprusside sodium (Nipride) can cause rapid changes in blood pressure and continual monitoring of blood pressure is always indicated. Patients who require mechanical ventilation will also be candidates for intra-arterial monitoring. Patients who are placed on mechanical ventilation need to have frequent arterial blood gas (ABG) analysis to determine appropriate ventilator settings and evaluate treatment. Patients admitted to the intensive care unit in diabetic ketoacidosis will often have arterial lines because frequent monitoring of ABGs.

Procedure

Intra-arterial monitoring requires that a catheter be inserted into a patient's artery. Frequently the artery of choice is the radial artery and should be inserted only after a positive Allen's test is obtained. The brachial or femoral arteries may also be sites of catheter insertion depending on patient condition. The health care provider cannulates the artery using aseptic technique using a flexible plastic over the needle catheter that is longer than a regular IV catheter. The nurse should have the flush system primed with fluid. The pressure bag should be inflated to 300 mm Hg and attached to the cable and monitor prior to insertion. Once the artery is cannulated, the catheter is connected to the flush system tubing that contains the transducer. The arterial waveform should be present on the monitor. The transducer should then be zeroed to atmospheric pressure and leveled to the phlebostatic axis. The insertion site should be dressed and blood pressure values and waveform recordings documented.

It is essential that the critical care nurse recognize normal waveform patterns in the patient who has intra-arterial pressure monitoring. Normally there is a sharp uprising in the waveform during systole followed by a descending waveform during diastole. The dichotic notch on the descending waveform occurs because of the closure of the aortic valve. This closure occurs midway between systole and diastole. The mean arterial pressure (MAP) reflects the usual pressure systemically throughout the cardiac cycle. The MAP is continuously displayed for the nurse to monitor and record. To perfuse vital organs, the goal for hypotensive patients is a MAP of at least 60 mm Hg. The MAP can also be calculated by the following equation when necessary:

$$\frac{\text{systolic B/P} + (2 \times \text{diastolic B/P})}{3}$$

Complications

Complications associated with intra-arterial monitoring can be serious and include infection, hemorrhage, thrombosis, and embolism. Using aseptic technique during insertion, tubing changes, dressing changes, and blood sampling are vital to help prevent infection. Contaminated stopcock caps and syringe tips can be a potential source of infection in the patient who has multiple blood samples drawn. The nurse should change pressure line tubing in accordance with institutional policy.

Hemorrhage or acute blood loss can result from disconnected tubing or dislodgement of the catheter. Ensuring that all connections are tight will help to prevent disconnection of the tubing. It is also vital that the alarms are activated on the monitoring device. If the line becomes disconnected, the waveform on the monitor will be affected as the signal will be interrupted. Monitor alarms will sound if this occurs. Monitor alarms are also typically set to alarm at a lowered systolic or MAP, which will occur if the catheter becomes dislodged.

The nurse can help prevent an embolism from occurring by checking for and removing any air from the system. Thrombosis can be prevented by using heparin in the flush fluid and maintaining the fluid at a sufficient volume. The nurse should assess the appropriate extremity routinely for evidence of poor perfusion.

Pulmonary Artery Pressure Monitoring

PA pressure monitoring is accomplished by insertion of a long, pliable catheter into the vena cava that rests in the PA. This **pulmonary artery (PA) catheter** has the capability of monitoring different pressures in the heart because of its openings. The catheter is capable of monitoring right atrial pressure (RAP), sometimes referred to as CVP, pulmonary systolic and diastolic pressures, and PAWP. A thermistor is located on the tip of the distal port of the catheter and is used for measuring CO. The thermistor is also useful for continual measurement of body temperature. The port with the attached syringe inflates the balloon located on the distal lumen and is responsible for the obtaining the PAWP The PA catheter was first introduced by Swan and Ganz in the 1970s and is still sometimes referred to as the Swan-Ganz catheter.

There are different types of PA catheters that vary according to the number of lumens and functions. The thermistor, injective port, balloon inflation port, and distal port are common to all PA catheters. An additional port, a venous infusion port (VIP) is added to some PA catheters and allows for continuous infusion of fluids or medications. There are other PA catheters that are capable of transvenous pacing, continuous CO monitoring, and continuous (SvO$_2$) monitoring. Monitoring left ventricular function and fluid volume status are indications for PA catheter monitoring.

Procedure

The equipment needed for PA catheter insertion is usually kept in the critical care unit. Some intensive care units keep a rolling cart complete with supplies to bring to the patient's bedside. The insertion of a PA catheter is a sterile procedure, so most carts contain sterile drapes, sterile gowns and gloves, and masks. The kit used for insertion usually contains a disinfecting solution for the site and lidocaine to numb the insertion site. Insertion sites may include brachial, internal or external jugular, and subclavian locations. The pressure tubing that is needed for insertion is similar to the pressure tubing used for arterial lines. The typical tubing for the PA catheter will have two flush devices and transducers for continuous monitoring of both the PA and right atrial pressures. The pressure tubing is primed with heparinized saline prior to insertion. Two monitors will be required to continuously monitor the pulmonary artery and the right atrial waveforms. The appropriate CO monitor and solution will also be needed.

The critical care nurse has many responsibilities during the insertion of a PA catheter. After priming the tubing and gathering the needed monitoring equipment, the nurse should ensure proper functioning of monitors. During insertion, the catheter passes through the right atrium and right ventricle and rests in the pulmonary artery. The nurse should monitor and record pressures as the catheter passes through these chambers. The nurse should also record the PAWP as it is obtained during insertion. Recordings of waveforms should be documented in the patient's record as well as the recorded values. As the catheter passes through the right ventricle, the patient will likely experience ventricular arrhythmias. It is important for the nurse to have emergency medications available in case these arrhythmias persist. The nurse should note and record the centimeter marking present nearest the insertion site. This information will be important to monitor catheter movement. Lastly, the nurse's role during insertion, as with any procedure, is to reassure the patient. Patients are often apprehensive during this procedure and will require a comforting presence. Some patients may need anxiolytic or pain medication to rest comfortably during the insertion. Versed or morphine are medications that may be used. Once catheter insertion is completed, the nurse should prepare the patient for a chest X-ray (CXR) to verify catheter placement.

Pulmonary Artery Parameters

After insertion of the PA catheter, the nurse will monitor the right arterial pressure, PA systolic, PA diastolic, the pulmonary capillary wedge pressure, and CO at certain intervals throughout the shift and as needed to evaluate treatments (Figure 19-2). The right atrial or CVP measures right ventricular preload with a normal value of 0 to 8 mm Hg of mercury. The PA systolic pressure is the peak pressure with a normal value of 15 to 25 mm Hg. The PA diastolic pressure is the lowest pressure point with a normal value of 6 to 12 mm Hg. The PA diastolic may be elevated in pulmonary hypertension or fluid volume excess. The PA systolic pressure will be elevated in the patient who has pulmonary hypertension. The mean PA pressure reflects the average pressure with a normal value of around 15 mm Hg.

Measurement of right atrial pressure is completed on measurement of all other hemodynamic parameters. Right atrial pressure is measured with the proximal lumen of the PA catheter. A transducer and cable are attached to the proximal lumen and the right atrial waveform is recorded. Right atrial pressure is measured at end expiration to eliminate values associated with intrathoracic pressure

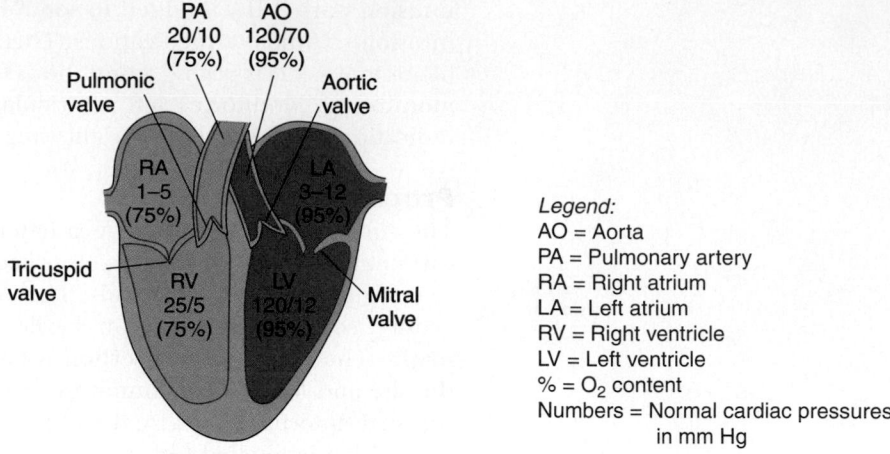

Figure 19-2 The configuration, normal pressures, and oxygen content of the heart chambers.

TABLE 19-1	Normal Values for PA Catheter Monitoring
MEASURE	**NORMAL RANGE**
RAP or CVP	0–8 mm Hg
Right ventricular (RV) pressures	Systolic 15–25 mm Hg
	Diastolic 0–8 mm Hg
PA pressures	Pulmonary artery systolic (PAS) 15–25 mm Hg
	Pulmonary artery diastolic (PAD) 6–12 mm Hg
PAWP	4–12 mm Hg
Pulmonary vascular resistance	20–120 dynes/sec/cm^{-5}
SVR	770–1500 dynes/sec/cm^{-5}
CO	4–8 L/min. average resting for adults
Cardiac index	2.5–4.2 L/min/m^2

Adapted from Darovic, G. (2004). Handbook of hemodynamic monitoring (2nd ed.). St. Louis, MO: Saunders.

changes. Elevated right atrial pressures may be because of right ventricular failure or volume overload. Abnormally low right atrial pressures may be because of hypovolemia. A single central venous IV catheter may be placed to measure right atrial pressure and administer fluids when a PA catheter is not indicated.

Pulmonary capillary wedge pressure is measured when the balloon on the tip of the catheter is slowly inflated and allowed to wedge into a branch of the PA. Once the balloon wedges, the catheter reads only pressure in front of the balloon. During diastole, the mitral valve is open reflecting left ventricular end diastolic pressure. Therefore, the PAWP is an indirect measurement of left ventricular function. The normal value for a PAWP is 4 to 12 mm Hg (Table 19-1). The wedge pressure is elevated in patients who have altered left ventricular function or elevations in blood volume. The PAWP will be abnormally low in patients who are hypovolemic from dehydration or hemorrhage. The nurse at the end of expiration must read all parameters as intrathoracic pressure will cause changes in the readings obtained from pulmonary artery catheter monitoring.

Complications

The complications associated with PA catheter monitoring can be serious and should be watched for by the critical care nurse. The catheter may be dislodged with patient movement, displacing the catheter into the right

Displacement of the PA Catheter into the Right Ventricle

Displacement of the PA catheter into the right ventricle will be evident by the waveform present on the monitor. The patient may experience frequent to sustained ventricular ectopy from this displacement. The balloon on the catheter should be inflated to the recommended volume (usually 1.5 mL). The health care providers should then redirect the catheter back into the PA (Darovic, 2004). If the patient is experiencing sustained ectopy causing hemodynamic instability, then the catheter should be pulled back into the right atrium with the balloon deflated. If the patient is still having symptomatic ectopy once the catheter is out of the ventricle, then the patient should be treated with synchronized cardioversion or medications as appropriate.

ventricle causing arrhythmias. The nurse should maintain continuous cardiac monitoring of the patient in addition to checking the centimeter marking for catheter movement. As with any invasive procedure, there is always a risk of infection. The nurse should monitor the insertion site for signs and symptoms of infection as well as adhere to institutional policy regarding pressure tubing changes. Aseptic technique should be used during dressing changes as well as when IV tubing is changed or added to the system. Bleeding is another complication that can occur with catheter insertion or unusual movement at the site. Normal bleeding times should be verified prior to insertion, and the site should be monitored routinely for evidence of bleeding or hematoma. Air embolism may occur if lines become disconnected or the balloon ruptures. An embolus may occur if nonheparinized saline is used. Maintaining adequate pressure on the solution will also help to maintain a patent catheter. Less commonly, a PA rupture could be caused by overinflation of the balloon or pulmonary infarction could occur as a result of leaving the balloon inflated. It is not recommended to inflate the balloon frequently or leave the balloon inflated for more than 10 to 20 seconds at a time.

CO measurements may be obtained in the patient who has a PA catheter in place. Monitoring CO and cardiac index in critically ill patients is important to determine how effective the heart is at meeting the demands of their body. Continuous CO monitoring is available with certain types of PA catheters which record an average value every 30 seconds (Swearingen & Keen, 2001). Continuous monitoring of CO would allow health care providers to evaluate treatment even more timely than the typical intermittent thermodilution technique. The intermittent thermodilution technique is still the most common method of obtaining a patient's CO. This technique involves injecting a solution (5 to 10 mL of dextrose 5% in water [D_5W] or NS) into the injective port of the PA catheter. The thermostat at the distal end of the catheter senses the change in temperature and the computer calculates a CO. The thermostat wire connector should be attached to the monitor prior to obtaining the measurement. IV solution of D5W or NS is attached to the tubing with the end secure into the injective port of the PA catheter. A sterile 5 to 10 mL syringe is attached for injection purposes. The nurse should inject the recommended volume of solution into the injective port steadily and rapidly as verified by the waveform recording on the monitor. Once three values that are similar are obtained, the average CO is calculated.

Once the vital signs, CO, right atrial pressure and PA pressures have been obtained, the nurse feeds all the values into the computer. The nurse can then validate other important parameters. SVR can be calculated once CO is obtained. SVR measures resistance or pressure (afterload) the left ventricle has to exceed to eject its volume. Normal systemic vascular resistance is 770 to 1,500 dynes/sec/cm-5 (Darovic, 2004). SVR is calculated by the formula (Swearingen & Keen, 2001):

$$SVR = \frac{(MAP - RAP)}{CO} \times 80$$

SVR will be elevated in conditions that cause vasoconstriction, like hypothermia or certain types of shock, which may be compensatory and not necessitate treatment. However, an elevated SVR creates a greater workload on the heart and may need to be lowered for patients with heart failure or MI. Typical treatment in those cases will consist of vasodilator medications to lower SVR. Vasodilation will occur with antihypertensive medications and distributive forms of shock (Figure 19-3).

Pulmonary vascular resistance measures afterload affecting the right ventricle. Pulmonary vascular resistance will be elevated in patients who suffer from pulmonary hypertension, hypoxemia, pulmonary embolism, or acidemia. Patients

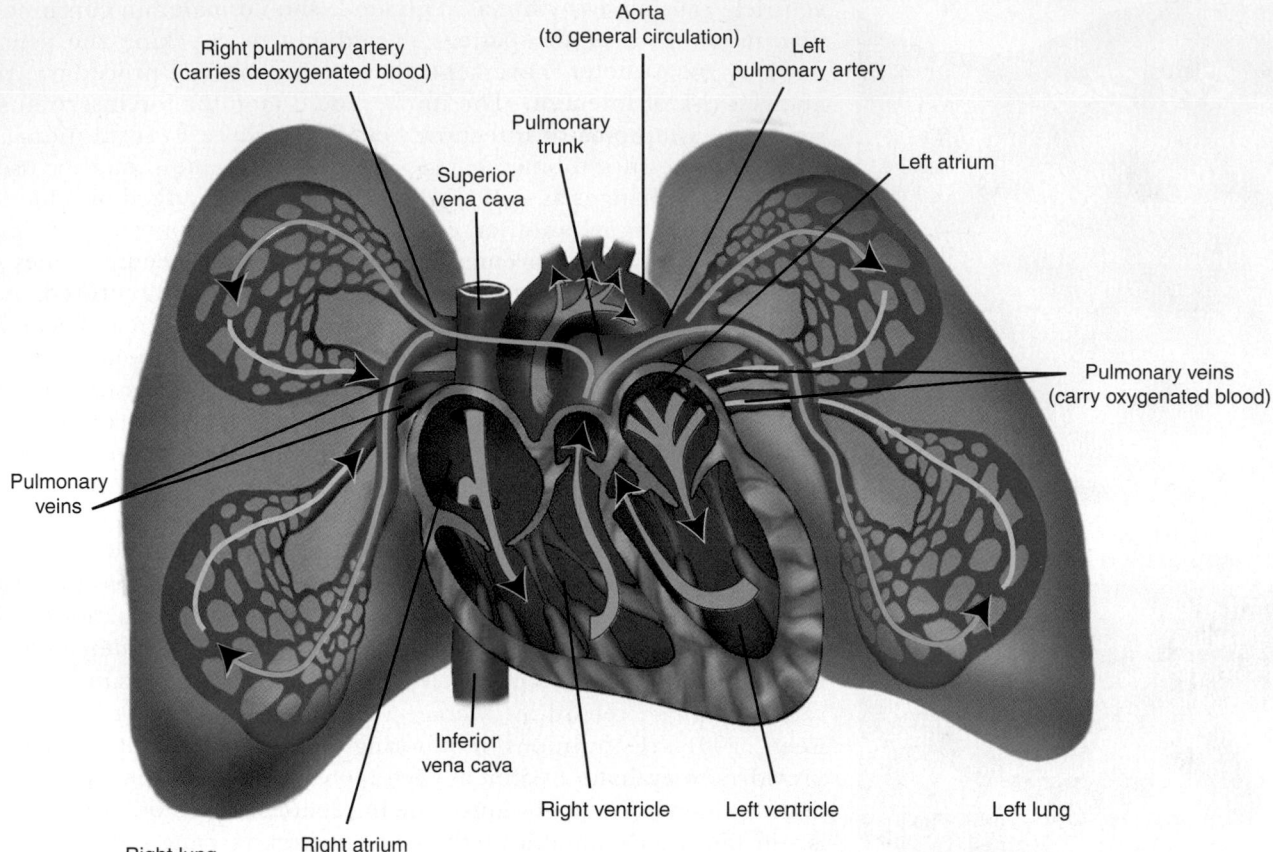

Figure 19-3 Major structures of the heart and pulmonary circulation.

who have chronic pulmonary hypertension ultimately suffer from right ventricular failure. The right ventricle fails because of its increased workload to overcome high pulmonary vascular resistance. Pulmonary vascular resistance will be decreased in conditions that cause vasodilation. Normal pulmonary vascular resistance is 20 to 120 dynes/sec/cm-5 (Darovic, 2004). The formula for pulmonary vascular resistance is (Swearingen & Keen, 2001):

$$PVR = \frac{(PAM - PAWP)}{CO} \times 80$$

Both systemic and pulmonary vascular resistance can be individualized for the patient by dividing the patient's body surface area into the resistance value obtained. These values are referred to as SVR index and pulmonary vascular resistance index respectively.

Left Atrial Pressure Monitoring

LAP monitoring is not as commonly performed as other methods of hemodynamic monitoring. However, it can give valuable information that may be warranted in the patient who has experienced cardiac surgery. A catheter is inserted into the left atrium during surgery and brought through the chest wall. Once this catheter is connected to a transducer and monitor, the nurse can continuously record pressure in the left atrium. When the mitral valve is open, LAP directly reflects left ventricular end diastolic pressure. Normal LAP is 8 to 12 mm Hg. LAP will be elevated in left ventricular dysfunction, mitral stenosis, or any condition causing hypervolemia. LAPs will be decreased in patients who are hypovolemic.

Patient position during hemodynamic measurements is important for the nurse to monitor, because changes in position during measurements may affect the values. The nurse should have assurance that changes in values are because of the patient's condition and not because of changes in patient position, air in the tubing, or malfunction of equipment. The supine position is the usual standard for measuring hemodynamic parameters. The patient's angle may vary from 0 to 60 degrees without considerably changing the values of the PA parameters (Darovic, 2004). Any time the patient's position must be changed beyond this angle, the nurse must relevel the transducer to the phlebostatic axis. Patient position should be documented clearly when hemodynamic parameters are measured so that there can be consistency in the manner values are obtained.

Mixed Venous Oxygen Saturation

Some PA catheters have the ability to continually monitor mixed venous oxygen saturation. **Mixed venous oxygen saturation (SvO$_2$)** is a measurement of the amount of hemoglobin saturated with oxygen compared to the total amount of hemoglobin in the PA (Darovic, 2004). It helps the practitioner determine whether the body's oxygen demand is being met by the oxygen supply. Because the blood sample taken is from the PA, it is a mixture of venous blood from all sites of the body. The normal value for a mixed venous oxygen sample is 60 to 80 percent. The PA catheters that measure SvO$_2$ contain fiber optics, which transmits light to red blood cells. The other fiber optic detects the amount of reflected light and transmits the amount to the computer. The computer continuously displays the average SvO$_2$ level for the nurse to monitor.

Decreases in SvO$_2$ can be the result of conditions that cause increases in oxygen demand or decreases in oxygen supply. Certain forms of shock, hypoxemia, anemia, shivering, pain, fever, or anxiety can cause the SvO$_2$ to be decreased. Nursing care activities can cause transient decreases in the SvO$_2$, such as turning, bathing, and suctioning.

Increases in the SvO$_2$ indicate a decrease in oxygen demand. The causes of increased SvO$_2$ include sepsis, cirrhosis, alkalosis, hypothermia, hypocarbia, or administration of large amounts of banked blood (Darovic, 2004). Other causes may also include polycythemia, neuromuscular blockers, or ethanol or cyanide toxicity. A wedged PA catheter will also give a high SvO$_2$ value. PA catheters that measure continuous SvO$_2$ must be calibrated routinely to ensure accuracy of values.

CARDIAC ASSIST DEVICES

The **intra-aortic balloon pump** is a catheter with an oblong balloon on the end. When attached to the pump helps to ease the workload on the patient's heart by decreasing afterload. The action of the balloon also helps to increase coronary blood flow. The balloon inflates and deflates according to the cardiac cycle and is a temporary method of therapy. An intra-aortic balloon pump is used for patients who are awaiting coronary artery bypass surgery, are post-coronary artery bypass surgery, have severe left ventricular failure, are experiencing cardiogenic shock, have cardiomyopathies, or are waiting for a heart transplant (Swearingen & Keen, 2001). Contraindications to the insertion of a balloon pump include: (a) severe peripheral vascular disease, (b) lack of femoral pulses, (c) coagulopathies, (d) extreme aortic insufficiency, (e) dissecting aneurysms, and (f) history of aortofemoral or aortoiliac bypass grafts (Comer, 2005).

Procedure

The intra-aortic balloon is inserted either at the patient's bedside in the intensive care unit emergently or in surgery. The balloon catheter is inserted into the femoral artery and advanced toward the heart until it rests in the descending thoracic aorta. Once inserted, the pump machine is attached and timing is determined. Helium or carbon dioxide (CO_2) is used to inflate the balloon during diastole and deflate the balloon during systole. This synchronization with the cardiac cycle is known as **counterpulsation.** The intra-aortic balloon pump assists the heart in essentially two ways. During diastole, the balloon inflates helping the blood move above and below the aorta. The heart benefits from better blood flow and perfusion when the balloon inflates. Other vital organs benefit from the antegrade movement of blood into the systemic circulation. The balloon deflates during ventricular systole. This deflation helps to decrease pressure in the aorta, which, in turn, helps to decrease afterload. Afterload reduction helps the left ventricle empty more completely and reduces its workload. Timing of inflation and deflation is determined by the patient's ECG tracing or arterial pressure waveform. Typically the pump to cardiac cycle is a 1:1 ratio, meaning the pump assists on the patient's every heart beat. When patients require long-term balloon counterpulsation, they need to be weaned off the pump. Weaning is performed by gradually decreasing the pump to cardiac cycle ratio. For example, the pump assists on every third to fourth cardiac cycle. The balloon pump may be discontinued once the patient can tolerate decreased assistance. In many intensive care units trained pump technicians assist with the technical aspects of the equipment. Nurses receive specialized training in the care of the patient requiring counterpulsation because of the complexity and complication potential (Table 19-2).

Complications

While the intra-aortic balloon pump can be a lifesaving device for many patients, there are several complications that may be associated with its use. Aortic dissection may occur with insertion and requires immediate surgery for repair. As with any invasive device, infection is a complication with intra-aortic balloon pumps. Nurses should monitor the femoral dressing for signs of infection as well as perform dressing changes according to policy. Signs and symptoms of infection from the balloon will require removal of the device. Thrombus formation may occur as well as impaired circulation to the extremity. At least hourly, the critical care nurse must be vigilant about assessing circulation to the affected extremity. Distal pulse checks, temperature, and color should be monitored and documented. Because of the risk of bleeding, especially in patients receiving heparin or anticoagulants, the insertion site must be monitored for bleeding. The patient should also be kept relatively flat during intra-aortic balloon pumping. Occlusion of the catheter could occur if the patient sits upright or is allowed to flex his or her hip. When kinking of the catheter occurs, breakage can be the result. Complications associated with immobility include: (a) pressure ulcers, (b) atelectasis, and (c) patient discomfort or pain. The balloon could become dislodged or develop a leak. Proper patient positioning should help to prevent dislodgement. If the balloon becomes dislodged into the subclavian, the patient will lose pulses in the upper extremities (Comer, 2005). The left arm may become cyanotic, cold, and mottled. If the renal artery becomes occluded because of migration of the balloon, the patient will have decreased urinary output. The balloon can also occlude the femoral artery. If this occurs, the patient's leg will be cold, mottled, cyanotic, and have absent pulses. If the balloon develops a leak or does become dislodged, it will need to be removed immediately.

Ventricular Assist Devices

The **ventricular assist device (VAD)** is a mechanical device designed to eliminate the workload required by the left ventricle and the right ventricle. The VAD is used for long-term therapy. Patients who have severe heart failure and are awaiting heart transplantation as well as patients who are unable to be weaned off cardiopulmonary bypass are likely candidates for a VAD. The VAD cannula is usually inserted in surgery and has three components, the cannula,

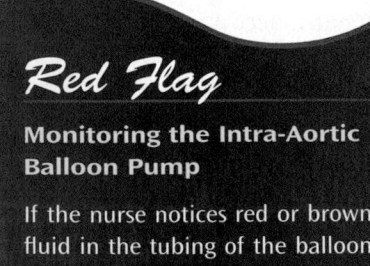

Red Flag

Monitoring the Intra-Aortic Balloon Pump

If the nurse notices red or brown fluid in the tubing of the balloon pump, the health care provider should be notified immediately. This means there is a break in the catheter and blood is entering the tubing. The nurse should prepare for immediate removal of the catheter.

TABLE 19-2 **Management of the Patient Requiring Intra-Aortic Balloon Pumping**

INTERVENTION	RATIONALE
1. Monitor vital signs frequently, every 15 to 30 minutes if unstable. Vital signs should be monitored at least every hour in stable patients.	Adjustments may need to be made in the timing of the balloon based on heart rate to ensure optimal effectiveness.
2. Monitor MAP at least every hour.	Helps to monitor for effectiveness of counterpulsation.
3. Monitor PA pressures every hour: systolic, diastolic, and wedge pressures.	Helps to monitor for effectiveness of counterpulsation.
4. Assess CO and cardiac index every hour until stable. Calculate SVR	Helps to monitor for the effectiveness of counterpulsation.
5. Monitor for malfunction of the pump. Refill the balloon with helium or CO_2 every two hours and as needed.	Helps to ensure optimal therapeutic effect of pump.
6. Monitor LOC and for neurological deficits.	Helps to monitor for adequate perfusion to brain tissue.
7. Monitor urine output hourly. Notify physician if less than 30 mL/hour or greater than 200 mL/hour (without the benefit of diuretics or fluid challenges).	This helps to monitor for adequate perfusion to the kidneys. Oliguria or anuria could occur with dislodgement of the balloon.
8. Monitor for adequate signs of circulation in appropriate extremity. Monitor color, temperature, pulse presence, and pain in affected extremity.	This action helps to monitor for dislodgement of the balloon.
9. Keep head of bed as flat as possible, less than 15 degrees. Do not allow flexion of involved leg.	This prevents the catheter from kinking and breaking.
10. Monitor insertion site for bleeding or hematoma formation.	Typical anticoagulation therapy may result in bleeding at catheter sites.
11. Explain all procedures and cares associated with counterpulsation.	Allows patient to make informed choices and increases compliance with therapy.
12. Assist with range of motion to unaffected extremity.	This helps to prevent complications related to immobility.
13. Monitor prothrombin time, activated partial thromboplastin time, international normalized ratio (INR), platelets and hemoglobin and hematocrit daily.	This helps to monitor for bleeding and identify patients at risk for potential bleeding.

Adapted from Comer, S. (2005). Delmar's critical care nursing care plans (2nd ed.). Clifton Park, NY: Thomson Delmar Learning.

the pump, and the external power source (McCafferty, Sorbellini, & Cianci, 2002). The VAD is either inserted into one or both ventricles depending on the patient need. The cannula delivers blood to the pump, and once it is full, blood is then sent back to the aorta or PA. The device enables blood to bypass the ventricle and allows the heart to rest or heal. VADs are external or implantable. Patients with a VAD experience greater mobility than patients with a balloon pump. However, patients who have a VAD are seriously ill and require more nursing support. General nursing care involves monitoring for infection, bleeding, vital signs, and hemodynamic parameters. Patients with VADs who are stable and are weaned from vasoactive drips may be transferred to telemetry units and discharged to home while awaiting a cardiac transplant (McCafferty, et al., 2002).

INTRACRANIAL PRESSURE MONITORING

Patients are often admitted to the intensive care unit when there are diagnoses of traumatic brain injury, stroke, intracranial hemorrhage, brain tumor, or infection and inflammation of brain tissue. Many of these patients are at great risk for developing increased intracranial pressure and need constant nursing care and monitoring. Prevention of increased intracranial pressure eliminates further damage to brain tissue and poor outcomes. Intracranial pressure monitoring is performed on patients who are at risk for developing increased intracranial pressure and will benefit from pressure-relieving interventions. Patients who have conditions that are irreversible will not likely be candidates for intracranial pressure monitoring.

The brain, blood, and cerebrospinal fluid are normally fixed inside the cranial vault. Under normal circumstances, when one of these elements increase, the other one or both must decrease in relation to the increase to prevent substantial increases in the intracranial pressure (modified Monro-Kellie doctrine as cited in Sole, et al., 2001). In the event the patient has a pathological brain condition, these compensatory mechanisms will not be effective. Therefore, even transient increases in intracranial pressure will be detrimental to the patient. While increases in intracranial pressure should be prevented in these patients, it is also important that the brain receive adequate blood supply. **Cerebral perfusion pressure,** the pressure at which cerebral tissue is perfused, should be maintained at greater than 70 mm Hg while maintaining intracranial pressure at less than 15 to 20 mm Hg (Swearingen & Keen, 2001). Cerebral perfusion pressure may be calculated by subtracting the intracranial pressure from the MAP.

Increases in intracranial pressure can occur any time there is a primary or secondary brain injury. As pressure in the intracranial vault increases, pressure is placed on the surrounding tissue and structures. The pressure is not equally distributed and may result in shifting of brain tissue from higher pressure to lower pressure. This herniation places pressure on structures that can cause brain damage and death.

There are several types of herniations that may occur. Cingulate herniation occurs as a result of increased intracranial pressure on one side that results in shifting to the opposite hemisphere causing compression of cerebral vessels and tissue (Swearingen & Keen, 2001). This herniation results in decreases in level of consciousness (LOC).

Uncal herniation occurs when the uncus of the temporal lobe passes through the tentorial notch causing compression of the oculomotor nerve and the posterior cerebral artery (Swearingen & Keen, 2001). The midbrain becomes compressed and can cause deteriorating levels of consciousness. Pupils are usually fixed and dilated on the side of the herniation. This emergent condition should be treated rapidly to avoid coma or death.

Central herniation usually is caused by massive cerebral edema that ultimately causes compression on the brainstem (Mayer & Chong, 2002). Signs and symptoms will include changes in LOC, alterations in pupil size, and changes in respiratory patterns. Decorticate posturing leading to decerebrate posturing and Cheyne-Stokes respirations are later signs (Sole, et al., 2001). These signs and symptoms may occur rapidly and even when promptly treated, often result in death.

The cerebellar tonsils can herniate through the foramen magnum and result in distortion and compression of the brainstem. Once this occurs, the respiratory and cardiac centers of the brainstem become damaged, resulting in death.

Types of Intracranial Pressure Monitoring

Intracranial pressure monitoring may be warranted on patients who have increased intracranial pressure or who are at significant risk for developing elevations in intracranial pressure. General criteria when contemplating invasive monitoring of intracranial pressure is indicated when patients meet three criteria (a) the patient is at risk for elevated intracranial pressure, (b) the patient is comatose with a Glasgow Coma Scale score equal to or less than 8, and (c) the patient has an abnormal computed tomography (CT) scan (Mayer & Chong, 2001). According to the prognosis, aggressive intensive care treatments may be warranted. As with any invasive lines and catheters, infection is always a consideration when contemplating this type of monitoring. The advantages and disadvantages of intracranial pressure monitoring must always be taken into consideration prior to its initiation. The patient must have thorough neurological assessments by the critical care nurse to accompany the intracranial pressure values. The combination of assessments is the most valuable to the health care team. There are four types of intracranial pressure monitoring tools.

The intraparenchymal probe is a small probe that is inserted into brain tissue. The fiber-optic probe is connected to a monitor that displays a pressure waveform. The transducer is located on the tip of the probe, so the nurse does not need to be concerned with the level of the transducer. This probe is relatively easy to insert and has a lower risk of infection. This probe does carry a risk of intracerebral bleeding. The catheter is typically fragile and may break causing the need for a replacement catheter. The equipment is expensive for these types of probes.

The epidural probe is placed in the epidural space between the skull and the dura mater (Sole, et al., 2001). Because of its location, this type of probe is easy to insert and has the lowest risk of intracerebral infection. In this system the values obtained may not be as reliable when intracranial pressure is elevated with type of system. Readings may be inaccurate after a few days as these catheters may easily become displaced and are prone to malfunction (Mayer & Chong, 2002). There is also no way to drain cerebrospinal fluid as with other systems.

The intraventricular catheter is placed in the lateral ventricle in the nondominant hemisphere via a burr hole. The catheter is connected to a fluid-filled system and is attached to a transducer connected to a monitor to view waveforms. This system has a chamber that allows for therapeutic drainage of cerebrospinal fluid. With this system the transducer must be leveled at the location of the foramen of Monro (the external auditory opening). These types of systems are considered to be accurate and allow for drainage and laboratory samples of cerebrospinal fluid as needed. There is a risk of infection as well as intracerebral bleeding associated with these systems. There is also the potential for difficult insertion of the catheter and a risk of rapid removal of cerebrospinal fluid.

The subarachnoid screw is placed in the subarachnoid space for pressure monitoring. Although there is risk of infection with this method, it is somewhat less likely than the risk associated with a catheter. Insertion is generally not difficult and cerebrospinal fluid pressure readings are considered to be reliable. This method is not useful for draining cerebrospinal fluid, and there is a risk of bleeding or hematoma during insertion.

Methods of monitoring that utilize the fluid-filled pressure tubing systems are maintained as closed systems to prevent infection. These systems must also be zeroed and balanced to ensure accuracy of the values. Intracranial pressure is measured as a mean pressure at the end of expiration. Tubing and dressing changes are performed according to institutional policy. The critical care nurse must be able to analyze waveforms to better assess the patient's intracranial pressure.

Intracranial Pressure Waveforms

The normal intracranial pressure waveform is similar to PA or arterial pressure tracings. When a tracing is recorded, the waveform corresponds to each heartbeat. Three types of abnormal waveforms have been identified.

A waves are also called plateau waves and are related to severe intracranial hypertension. These waves are seen with pressures of 50 to 100 mm Hg and may last for minutes to hours (Mayer & Chong, 2002). When intracranial pressure is this elevated, there is great risk of low cerebral perfusion pressure with resulting ischemia and herniation. Prompt treatment of these patients is required to prevent further brain injury and death.

B waves are seen in pressures at levels of 20 to 50 mm Hg. B waves will correspond with respiratory pattern and may occur every one to two minutes. These waves may serve as precursors of A waves and serve as a warning to the nurse that there is a possibility of increasing intracranial pressure.

C waves are small waves with pressures less than 20 mm Hg and their significance has not been determined. C waves may correspond with blood pressure and respirations.

Management of Patients with Increased Intracranial Pressure

Managing patients with increased intracranial pressure requires intensive monitoring and assessment by the nurse. In addition to intracranial pressure monitoring, the nurse must perform neurological assessments routinely to evaluate results of therapies. Signs and symptoms of increased intracranial pressure include decreased LOC and hypertension that may or may not be accompanied by bradycardia. These two signs are almost always present in patients who have increased intracranial pressure (Mayer & Chong, 2002). Patients may also have a headache, vomiting, papilledema, and changes in respiration. Patients will also require close monitoring of their hemodynamic and oxygenation status. The goals of therapy will include an intracranial pressure of less than 20 mm Hg and preservation of functional brain tissue by maintaining a cerebral perfusion pressure of greater than 70 mm Hg.

One intervention to lower intracranial pressure is to administer an osmotic diuretic such as mannitol (Guyton & Hall, 2001). Mannitol pulls fluid from brain tissue into the systemic circulation thereby reducing intracranial pressure. The fluid is then removed from circulation by the kidneys. While mannitol is the agent most commonly used, loop diuretics may also be considered. Furosemide (Lasix) is the loop diuretic most commonly used. When diuretics are utilized, the nurse must assess for excessive volume depletion that could lower cerebral perfusion pressure and lead to further cerebral ischemia. Hypotonic fluids, such as 5% dextrose or 0.45% sodium chloride should be avoided in these patients as their use could precipitate cerebral edema. Isotonic solutions should be utilized when there is difficulty maintaining cerebral perfusion pressure due to hypovolemia.

Maintaining proper patient positioning will also help prevent further increases in intracranial pressure. The head should be maintained in a midline position to facilitate venous drainage. This outflow of drainage is the primary determinant of intracranial pressure in adults who are healthy. Therefore, maintaining proper head alignment is of primary importance. The head of the bed should be maintained at about 30 to 45 degrees elevation. Elevating the head of the bed at a higher degree could lower cerebral perfusion pressure. Trendelenburg's position should never be used as this position could cause elevations in intracranial pressure. Care should be taken by the nurse to prevent tight securing of devices around the neck such as endotracheal (ET) tube holders and central line dressings.

Maintaining proper oxygenation and ventilation will be extremely important in patients with increased intracranial pressure. As other tissues in the body can go for minutes without oxygen due to anaerobic metabolism, the brain needs a constant supply of oxygen and glucose for its neuronal activity (Guyton & Hall, 2001). Often, the oxygen requirements of these patients will need to be met with intubation and mechanical ventilation. Most patients with increased intracranial pressure will suffer from altered LOC and need intubation to protect the airway. Ensuring protection of the airway and appropriate delivery of FiO_2 will help meet the patient's brain oxygen requirements. Oxygenation goals can be evaluated by ABG analysis and monitoring pulse oximetry. Hyperventilation of the patient may also be warranted. Lowered PCO_2 levels are associated with reductions in intracranial pressure by causing vasoconstriction. Carbon dioxide has a vasodilating effect on cerebral blood vessels. Lowering the level of carbon dioxide in the blood will cause vasoconstriction. Hyperventilation has been a common practice in the past. However, vasoconstriction of cerebral vessels also lowers perfusion. Decreased perfusion to the brain may also cause further injury. The critical care nurse should be aware that mechanically ventilated patients might need to be suctioned on occasion. The nurse should be certain that suctioning is warranted and that hyperoxygenation is performed prior to the procedure. Intracranial pressure rises with suctioning and coughing and should only be performed when absolutely necessary. It is usually necessary to sedate these patients.

Sedation of patients with increased intracranial pressure will help to prevent episodes of severe coughing and agitation as well as promote comfort in the patient. Narcotics, such as fentanyl, and anxiolytics, such as midazolam (Versed), may be used but may mask changes in the patient's LOC. Neuromuscular blockers in conjunction with sedatives may be used to promote ventilator compliance but may also mask neurological changes. Agents used for pain control and sedation should have short half-lives so that neurological status may be assessed when necessary.

The patient's room should be kept as quiet as possible to eliminate any unnecessary anxiety associated with environmental noises. Nursing activities should be spaced to allow adequate rest periods and prevent overstimulation. The patient's response to visitors should be evaluated and when necessary, visitors should be restricted. The lighting in the patient's room should be dimmed in most cases. The nurse should use a calm, soothing voice when explaining procedures or nursing activities. Reassurance should be provided to the patient even when the patient's LOC is diminished.

Additional treatment of patients with increased intracranial pressure includes accurate, frequent monitoring of temperature. Hyperthermia should be treated to avoid increasing cerebral metabolism. Acetaminophen and cooling blankets are the treatments of choice for fevers. The nurse must also be vigilant in monitoring the patient for seizure activity that could substantially increase intracranial pressure. Ideally, the patient will be on seizure prophylaxis by the administration of IV fosphenytoin (Cerebyx).

AIRWAY ASSISTANCE

An important nursing intervention is to help the patient maintain an open airway. Many patients need assistance maintaining an airway in the intensive care unit. Anesthesia, medications, and altered mental status are common causes of altered airways. One of the first interventions the intensive care unit nurse can perform is proper head positioning. The head-tilt, chin-lift method is taught by the American Heart Association to all health care providers in basic life support classes. The jaw thrust method is used for those individuals with possible spinal injuries. The critical care nurse can perform either of these methods on patients who are unable to maintain their open airway. Obviously, it would be difficult for the nurse to continuously help maintain an open airway in a patient utilizing only head positioning.

Oral Airways

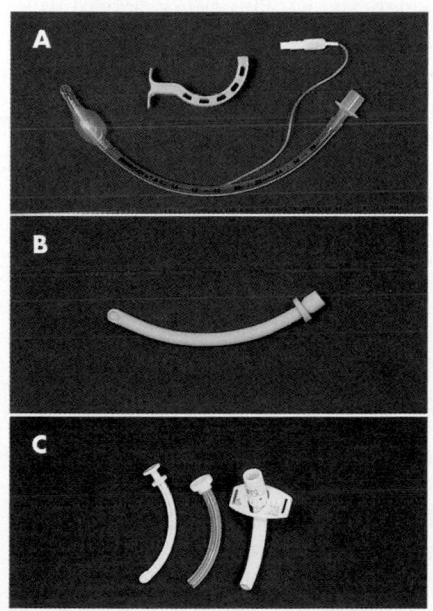

Figure 19-4 Types of artificial airways: A. Oral airway and ETT, B. Nasal trumpet, C. Tracheostomy tube.

Oral airways are stiff plastic tubes inserted into the patient's mouth to prevent the tongue from sliding back into the pharynx and blocking the airway (Figure 19-4). Oral airways are useful to help maintain an open airway in patients who have had anesthesia or have altered mental status. They may be used to maintain an open airway in patients having seizure activity. Oral airways are also useful to maintain an open airway in the patient needing support by a bag-valve-mask apparatus. They may also be used to prevent the patient who is orally intubated from biting the endotracheal tube. Oral airways are extremely uncomfortable and should be used primarily on patients who are sedated or have altered mental status and for a limited time.

It is important that the oral airway be inserted properly to prevent pushing the tongue back and blocking the airway. The nurse must first choose the proper size for the patient. The oral airway comes in several sizes and best fits the patient when it measures up from the corner of the patient's mouth to the tip of the ear lobe. Once the proper size is determined, the nurse explains the procedure to the patient and has suction equipment available. The airway is inserted into the patient's mouth upside down. Once the airway is to the back of the pharynx, the airway is rotated. Upon insertion, the nurse must verify that the airway is indeed open, and monitor the respiratory status of the patient. Proper head alignment and position should be maintained after insertion of the airway.

Nasal Airways

Nasal airways, also referred to as nasal trumpets, are soft, flexible tubes that are inserted into the nasal passage to maintain an open airway. The nasal airways are more comfortable for patients who are conscious. They are commonly used for patients who require frequent nasotracheal suctioning. As with the oral airway, the nurse must choose the appropriate size for the patient. To measure the oral airway measure from the nares to the tip of the ear lobe and then adding 1 inch. Once the proper size is determined, the nasal airway should be lubricated with a water-soluble lubricant. Once the procedure is explained to the patient, the airway is inserted gently into the nasal passage. The airway should be advanced to the medial side of the nasal passage while inserting downward. On insertion the nurse should assess patency and monitor for complications of the nasal airway. Some bleeding of the nasal passage is common. Excessive blood loss should be reported. If the nasal airway is left in place for long periods, then the patient may be at risk for sinusitis.

Endotracheal Intubation

Endotracheal intubation refers to the passage of a tube into the trachea through either the mouth or nares to maintain an open airway. The endotracheal tube (ETT) has an inflated balloon on the end to help aid ventilation of the patient. The adaptor on the opposite end is designed to fit an ambo-bag-valve device for ventilatory assistance or to attach it to a mechanical ventilator. Patients may be intubated emergently during a respiratory arrest or during a period of severe respiratory compromise. Patients are also intubated during general anesthesia or under other conditions where maintaining an open airway is difficult for the patient. Patients may also be intubated to facilitate copious secretion removal.

Health care providers, nurse anesthetists, some respiratory therapists, and paramedics are typically trained to perform endotracheal intubation. The critical care nurse assists with the procedure and has many responsibilities during the intubation. Once the decision has been made to intubate the patient, the nurse should obtain the necessary equipment. The equipment for intubation is usually kept on the crash cart inside the intensive care unit or in an intubation tray. The nurse will need to ensure that there is suction equipment at the bedside including a tonsil tip suction catheter. The ETT tray should include: (a) a laryngeal scope (curved or straight), (b) an ETT, (c) lubricant, (d) a stylet, (e) a syringe for balloon inflation, (f) an oral airway, and (g) Magill forceps. Personal protective eyewear and gloves should also be at the bedside for the health care team. Consent for the procedure should be obtained from the patient or the next of kin if the patient is unable. In the case of a respiratory arrest, the patient will need to be emergently intubated, and consent is implied.

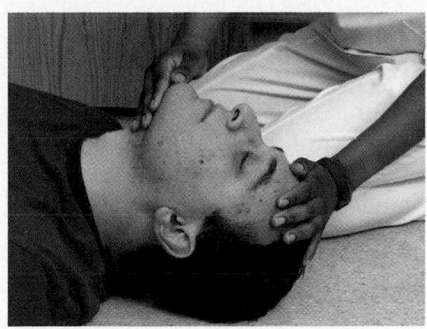

Figure 19-5 Head in sniffing position.

Once the equipment is at the patient's bedside the procedure for intubation will begin. Unless it is during a respiratory arrest, the patient will likely be given an anxiolytic (Versed or Ativan) or a paralytic agent. Often, the patient is also given an anesthetic agent at the back of the throat. All of these agents are designed to make the procedure more comfortable. The patient's head is place in the "sniffing" position to facilitate entry into the trachea (Figure 19-5). Prior to the insertion of the tube, the patient should be hyperoxygenated and hyperventilated with a bag-valve-mask device delivering 100 percent oxygen.

Once the patient has been oxygenated and ventilated and has received the appropriate medication, the individual performing the insertion places the laryngoscope into the mouth of the patient. The laryngoscope comes equipped with a light to better view the vocal cords. Typically suctioning of the oropharynx is required at this point to remove excess secretions or emesis. Aspiration is a frequent complication of endotracheal intubation and every effort should be made to prevent life-threatening aspiration of gastric contents. The ETT is lubricated with a topical ointment, and the stylet is placed in the center of the tube to ease insertion. Once the vocal cords come into view, the health care provider inserts the tube through the vocal cords and stops above the carina. The cuff is then inflated with the syringe.

If the health care provider is unable to insert the ETT into the proper position within 20 to 30 seconds, the patient should again receive supplemental oxygen and ventilation via the bag-valve-mask device. Often, the nurse is asked to place his or her fingers over the patient's Adam's apple to help with visualization. Once the tube is inserted the nurse, health care provider, or respiratory therapist auscultate bilateral lung fields to ensure proper placement of the tube. Stomach intubation can occur and can be verified by auscultating over the upper quadrants of the abdomen. An end tidal CO_2 detection device may also be placed on the end of the tube to detect for the presence of exhaled CO_2. If the tube is inserted too far, right mainstem bronchus intubation may occur and can be verified by CXR. All patients should receive a portable CXR after the procedure to verify appropriate placement. Once the tube is in position, the nurse or respiratory therapist secures the tube with tape or an ETT holder. The nurse should document the centimeter marking at the lip of the patient to monitor for tube movement.

Nasotracheal intubation may be performed instead of oral. The tube is passed through the nares until it is in the proper place. Nasotracheal intubation is only performed on patients who are capable of spontaneous respiration yet need intubation. The tube may also be passed during a bronchoscopy procedure. Once tube position is verified, the tube is taped and secured.

Tracheostomy

If a patient needs long-term artificial airway support, a tracheostomy may be required. A tracheostomy is placed by surgical incision in the trachea, either in the operating room or at the patient's bedside. A **tracheostomy tube** is placed and is secured by sutures. A tracheostomy will be required for all patients who require long-term ventilator support. Current recommendations related to tracheostomy placement and mechanical ventilation include: (a) patients who require high levels of sedation to tolerate the artificial airway; (b) patients with extremely weak respiratory muscles; (c) patients who might have psychological benefit from eating and speech; and (d) patients who may need more mobility to complement physical therapy (National Guideline Clearinghouse, 2002). There are different types of tracheostomy tubes that serve different purposes. Tubes that have an inner cannula and are cuffed are the most commonly used in the critical care setting.

BOX 19-3

INDICATIONS FOR MECHANICAL VENTILATION

- Decreased oxygen saturation or oxygen deficit
- Increased work of breathing and respiratory rate with impending respiratory failure
- Apnea
- Ventilatory failure as evidenced by rising $PaCO_2$
- Protection of airway with altered LOC
- Worsening CXR

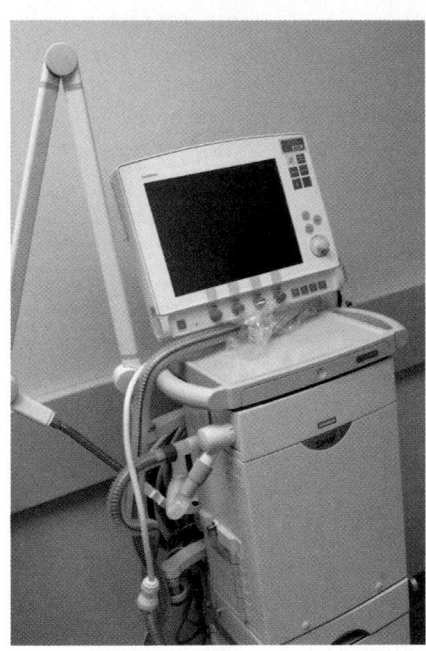

Figure 19-6 Example of a mechanical ventilator.

MECHANICAL VENTILATION

Many patients in the intensive care unit setting need ventilatory assistance through a mechanical device known as **mechanical ventilation** (Box 19-3). Patients who have impending or acute respiratory failure will be candidates for mechanical ventilation. Surgical patients who have underlying respiratory problems will often need ventilatory assistance after a major surgery. Possible reasons to place the patient on mechanical ventilation may include a worsening of ABGs, decreased oxygen saturation, increased respiratory rate and work of breathing, or worsening of CXR results. Many patients in the intensive care unit setting become well enough to have mechanical ventilation withdrawn. Occasionally, patients need longer term ventilatory support and when stable are transferred to another unit or discharged to home on a mechanical ventilator. There are essentially two types of mechanical ventilation, negative pressure ventilation, and positive pressure ventilation. Negative pressure ventilation includes the iron lung and does not require an artificial airway. Negative pressure ventilation is typically not used in the intensive care unit setting (Figure 19-6).

Positive Pressure Ventilation

The most common type of ventilatory support in the intensive care unit setting is positive pressure ventilation. Air is forced into the lungs via an artificial airway, an ETT, or tracheostomy. Positive pressure ventilators can deliver air according to a preset volume or a preset pressure. Common positive pressure ventilator modes include synchronized intermittent mandatory ventilation (SIMV) and continuous mandatory ventilation (CMV). These modes can be set to deliver air in a certain volume or deliver the air until a certain pressure is reached.

Continuous Mandatory Ventilation

Continuous mandatory ventilation (CMV) is a mode of ventilation that delivers a minimum preset respiratory rate to a patient. If the order is for the patient to have 12 breaths per minute, then the ventilator will deliver 12 breaths in that minute. When CMV is in the volume control mode an appropriate tidal volume will be ordered based on the patient's weight and will be delivered with each breath. Because a full breath will be delivered with minimal effort on the patient's part, this mode is good for patients who have minimal drive to breath or need to rest their respiratory muscles. This mode is frequently used for patients who have underlying chronic respiratory problems and come into the intensive care unit with an acute exacerbation.

Synchronized Intermittent Mandatory Ventilation

The **synchronized intermittent mandatory ventilation (SIMV)** mode of ventilation will deliver a preset tidal volume or pressure for every preset breath. The term synchronized means that the breaths are delivered according to the timing of the patient's own respiratory effort. The major difference between SIMV and CMV is the patient's inspiratory effort. When the patient on SIMV inspires independently the ventilator does not deliver the preset volume or pressure, instead the volume of air inspired is generated by the patient's own effort, and as a result SIMV may result in respiratory muscle fatigue. This mode is frequently used for patients being weaned from mechanical ventilation or for patients who require short-term ventilatory support and have no underlying lung disease.

Pressure Control Ventilation versus Volume Control Ventilation

Pressure control ventilation delivers breaths at a preset target pressure. During this mode of ventilation the inspiratory flow decreases as the alveolar pressure nears the pressure in the airway (Hess & Kacmarek, 2002). This mode of ventilation is used when the patient's condition warrants close monitoring of pressure. There is no set tidal volume because the air is delivered toward a preset pressure. The tidal volume is determined by the amount of air delivered prior to reaching the preset pressure. The nurse should monitor the tidal volumes while the patient is in this mode of ventilation. Once the preset pressure is reached the ventilator will stop pushing in air even if the patient has not received enough volume for gas exchange (Pruitt & Jacobs, 2004).

Volume control ventilation solves this volume for gas exchange problem. But, there are other concerns when a patient requires volume control ventilation. For instance, when the ventilator delivers a preset volume to a patient, there is always a risk that the inspiratory pressures may climb too high. When the patient has poor lung compliance, there is always a concern that the peak inspiratory pressure (PIP) may rise too high resulting in trauma to the patient's lungs (Pruitt & Jacobs, 2004) (Figure 19-7).

Ventilator Settings

Patients who are being mechanically ventilated have prescribed ventilator settings that are adjusted according to patient condition. Typically, the respiratory therapist works in conjunction with the nurse and health care provider to monitor and change the patient's ventilator settings as needed. The patient needs to have a preset fraction of inspired oxygen (FiO_2). The FiO_2 may be set anywhere from 21 to 100 percent. Initially, the patient should have a FiO_2 set at 100 percent (Hess & Kacmarek, 2002). After initial intubation and mechanical ventilation and once the patient is stable, the FiO_2 may be titrated according to the patient's pulse oximetry. The tidal volume (V_t) is set unless the patient is in pressure control mode. **Tidal volume** is the amount of air exchanged or delivered with each inspiration and expiration. The amount of V_t will be determined by the patient's weight. Typically, the V_t can range from 4 to 12 mL/kg depending on lung compliance and pathophysiology (Hess & Kacmarek, 2002). Patients who have restrictive lung disease have a lower V_t in contrast to those without an underlying lung disease. Those patients need tidal volumes set at 6 to 8 mL/kg (Pruitt & Jacobs, 2004). In additional to the V_t the respiratory rate is also set on the ventilator. The rate determines how many

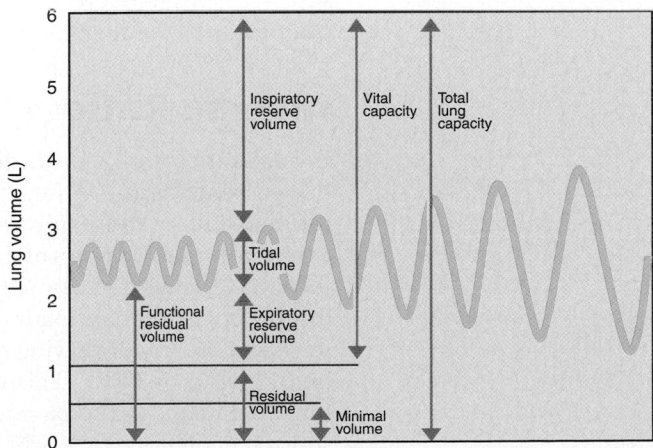

Figure 19-7 Graphic representation of lung volumes and capacities.

breaths per minute are delivered to the patient by the ventilator. Occasionally, patients are weaned from mechanical ventilation by gradually decreasing the number of breaths per minute. Positive end expiratory pressure (PEEP) is often initially set in the patient requiring mechanical ventilation to prevent atelectasis. Flow patterns, peak flow, inspiratory time, and sensitivity are initial settings for the patient requiring mechanical ventilation.

Additional Ventilator Settings and Modes

Positive end expiratory pressure (PEEP) is an additional ventilator setting, which adds pressure at the end of expiration on ventilator breaths. PEEP helps to keep alveoli open and available to participate in gas exchange. The end result is usually increased oxygenation. Most patients requiring mechanical ventilation will receive PEEP at around 5 cm H_2O routinely to keep normal functional residual capacity. The typical PEEP level in patients who require more than 5 cm H_20 is 5 to 20 cm H_2O. PEEP is added to the ventilator breaths to decrease the FiO_2. If a patient is unable to tolerate lowering the FiO_2 from 100 percent, PEEP is added to increase the oxygenation so the FiO_2 can be lowered. High levels of PEEP can cause pneumothorax or decreased venous return, compromising CO.

Continuous Positive Airway Pressure

Continuous positive airway pressure (CPAP) adds to the functional residual capacity in patients who are spontaneously breathing. CPAP may be delivered via mask or by a ventilator. CPAP masks are frequently used for patients who suffer from sleep apnea. CPAP may also be used to "buy time" prior to intubation and mechanical ventilation. CPAP is used for the patient on the ventilator when spontaneous breaths are taken. Positive airway pressure is maintained throughout the spontaneous breaths with CPAP. It helps to open alveoli allowing them to participate in gas exchange. CPAP may be used to augment spontaneous breaths that are taken during the weaning process.

Pressure Support Ventilation

Pressure support ventilation (PSV) is used to support the patient's breath and to help increase the patient's tidal volume. Pressure support ventilation (PSV) provides positive pressure as the patient is taking a breath that ultimately helps to reduce the work of breathing. Pressure support ventilation is often used as a weaning mode to help the patient overcome the dead space in the ventilator circuit during spontaneous inspiration. During the weaning process the level of pressure support is gradually decreased. Pressure support may also be used to augment the spontaneous breaths of patients who are on SIMV. Pressure support helps to decrease the work of breathing on those breaths and may be used routinely while patients are in that mode of ventilation.

Inverse Ratio Ventilation

Inverse ratio ventilation is delivered as a pressure controlled or volume controlled ventilation (White, 2005). **Inverse ratio ventilation** is a comparison of the inspiratory and expiratory times known as the I/E ratio (inspiration to expiration ratio). In normal breathing the expiratory time is longer than the inspiratory time. Occasionally, the patient's condition may require a longer inspiratory time than expiratory time. Patients who require a longer inspiratory time are usually having difficulty improving oxygenation with just increasing the FiO_2 or PEEP. This mode of ventilation may be quite uncomfortable for the patient; so the patient who requires a prolonged inspiratory time and shorter expiratory time will require sedation and perhaps paralysis (Hess & Kacmarek, 2002). Complications that may be associated with inverse ratio ventilation include air trapping causing elevated pressures and decreased venous return causing decreased CO.

Airway Pressure Release Ventilation

Airway pressure release ventilation (APRV) unites two levels of CPAP pressures (White, 2005). The high CPAP level, also referred to as P High (Frawley & Habashi, 2001) helps the patient increase lung volume during spontaneous breaths. The lower CPAP level, also referred to as P Low (Frawley & Habashi, 2001), allows for a reduction of the mean airway pressure. When this mode of ventilation is used, it is usually combined with an inverse I/E ratio. The mandatory breaths delivered by the ventilator are similar to pressure control ventilation when the patient has no spontaneous breathing. However, unlike traditional modes of ventilation, APRV allows for spontaneous breathing during any point of the respiratory cycle (Hess & Kacmarek, 2002). This method of mechanical ventilation may be helpful in preventing lung injury associated with mechanical ventilation (Frawley & Habashi, 2001). Other advantages of this type of ventilation include: (a) lower airway pressures, (b) lower minute ventilation, (c) spontaneous breathing, and (d) a decreased need for sedation or neuromuscular blockade.

Mandatory Minute Ventilation

In mandatory minute ventilation (MMV) a minimum desired minute ventilation is ordered (Pruitt & Jacobs, 2004). This setting instructs the ventilator to monitor the minute ventilation (V_e) and deliver additional breaths when the patient falls below the minimum minute ventilation during spontaneous breaths. The mandatory breaths that are used to assist the patient will be delivered according to a preset volume. The nurse may assist the patient by delivering increased pressure support to help during the weaning process (White, 2005).

Proportional Assist Ventilation

Proportional assist ventilation (PAV) is a mode that allows the ventilator to act in response to the patient's work of breathing on a breath-by-breath basis (White, 2005). The ventilator adjusts the support it provides depending on the patient's effort. Through microprocessors that utilize feedback mechanisms, ventilators are able to individualize the support provided to the patient (Table 19-3) (Pruitt & Jacobs, 2004).

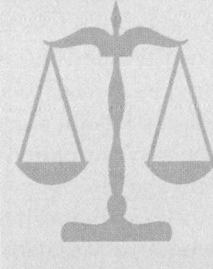

ETHICS IN PRACTICE

Providing Mechanical Ventilation Information

Prior to committing the patient to mechanical ventilatory support, deliberation should be made as to the likelihood that the disease could be reversed (Hess & Kacmarek, 2002). The patient should be informed of all potential benefits and risks that accompany mechanical ventilation as well as the potential length of time the patient will need the ventilatory support. The decision to place the patient on mechanical ventilation is ideally made prior to an emergent situation. Care should be taken to inform family members as appropriate. Any advanced directives the patient may have should be in place on the chart and documented in the patient's history. If the patient declines lifesaving mechanical ventilation, then the patient should be ensured that all comfort measures would be instituted.

TABLE 19-3	Commonly Used Mechanical Ventilation Abbreviations and Symbols
ABBREVIATION	**MEANING**
FiO_2	Fraction of inspired oxygen
V_t	Tidal volume
RR	Respiratory rate
CMV	Continuous mandatory ventilation
SIMV	Synchronized intermittent mandatory ventilation
APRV	Airway pressure release ventilation
V_e	Minute ventilation
PEEP	Positive end expiratory pressure
CPAP	Continuous positive airway pressure
PSV	Pressure support ventilation
I/E	Inspiratory time related to expiratory time
ABG	Arterial blood gas
PIP	Peak inspiratory pressure
ETT	Endotracheal tube
FRC	Function residual capacity

NURSING MANAGEMENT OF PATIENTS REQUIRING MECHANICAL VENTILATION

In addition to monitoring for, and preventing complications of, mechanical ventilation, the nurse has additional responsibilities when caring for patients who are mechanically ventilated (Table 19-4). The critical care nurse should ensure that all patients who are receiving mechanical ventilation have an Ambu bag connected to supplemental oxygen and suction equipment at the bedside. An Ambu bag is necessary to deliver manual breaths to the patient any time the ventilator malfunctions or there is loss of power to the ventilator. A mask should also be at the bedside in case of unplanned extubation by the patient. The ventilator alarms should be on at all times to alert the nurse when there are problems. High-pressure alarms are activated when the patient has a large amount of secretions, the patient is coughing, and the patient is biting on the tube. The alarms are also engaged when there are kinks in the ventilator circuit, pneumothorax, hemothorax, or bronchospasm. Low-pressure alarms are activated when the ventilator circuit is disconnected, with a leak in the ETT or tracheostomy cuff, or if the patient does not receive the prescribed amount of V_t. An apnea alarm will sound if the ventilator does not distinguish a breath within a certain time period. This alarm is especially important during patient weaning. The critical care nurse must respond to all ventilator alarms promptly to prevent catastrophic consequences. If the cause of the alarm is not rapidly apparent, the patient may be manually ventilated during the assessment. The respiratory therapist should be consulted when a malfunction of the ventilator is suspected.

The critical care nurse should ensure that patients receiving mechanical ventilation have continuous pulse oximetry monitoring and adequate measurements of ABGs ABG analysis allows the practitioner to analyze values for a given

TABLE 19-4 Nursing Management of Patients Requiring Mechanical Ventilation

INTERVENTION	RATIONALE
1. Secure artificial airway and monitor for tube movement.	This action helps to prevent unplanned extubation.
2. Auscultate lung field at least every four hours and as needed.	This action will help monitor for effectiveness of interventions.
3. Suction artificial airway as needed, hyperoxygenate prior to, during, and after procedure.	This action helps to prevent desaturation during suctioning of the patient.
4. Position patient in semi-Fowler's or high-Fowler's position if possible.	This position helps to facilitate lung expansion. This position helps to prevent aspiration of secretions.
5. Administer antibiotics and bronchodilators as ordered.	The bronchodilators help to promote secretion removal. Antibiotics will be appropriate for the patient with infection.
6. Monitor the patient's volume status and hydrate as appropriate.	This action will help to promote thinner secretions and aid in their removal.
7. Turn the patient every two hours and as appropriate.	This helps to facilitate secretion removal.
8. Maintain constant monitoring of pulse oximetry values. Document values on flow sheet.	Pulse oximetry monitoring helps to detect decreases in oxygen saturation. Documentation helps to identify changes in saturations in accordance with treatments and interventions.
9. Titrate FiO_2 according to SpO_2 values.	This action helps to prevent hypoxemia or oxygen toxicity.
10. Monitor ABG results and adjust ventilator settings accordingly.	This helps to maximize therapeutic effects of adjusted settings.
11. If necessary, apply soft wrist restraints patient.	This helps to prevent unplanned extubation.
12. If the patient is orally intubated, secure tube on alternating sides of the mouth daily. For example, left side on Day 1 then right side on Day 2.	This action helps to prevent ulcer generation and tissue necrosis from the pressure of the ETT.
13. Monitor ETT cuff pressure at least once per shift.	This action helps to prevent over-inflation of the ETT cuff and possible tissue necrosis.
14. Provide oral care at least every two hours and as needed.	To help prevent dryness and ulcer formation in the mouth.
15. Ensure appropriate ventilator alarm settings. Review meanings of high- and low-pressure alarms. Respond to ventilator alarms promptly.	These actions help to prevent further injury to the patient when complications occur or the patient becomes disconnected from life support.
16. Monitor ETT and ventilator circuits turning and repositioning patient.	Careful monitoring of tubing and ETT helps to prevent unplanned extubation.
17. Wash hands before and after any patient care activities.	Helps to prevent ventilator-associated pneumonia.
18. Explain all procedures to the patient and family.	This helps to ensure compliance with ventilator.
19. Administer antianxiety medication as ordered and required by the patient.	This action helps to promote ventilator compliance.
20. Provide alternative methods of communication.	This action helps to lessen feelings of powerlessness in the patient and helps to reduce anxiety.

Adapted from Comer, S. (2005). Delmar's critical care nursing care plans (2nd ed.). Clifton Park, NY: Thomson Delmar Learning.

point in time. Trends of blood gases are more helpful in determining patient care interventions as well as responses to treatments (Hess & Kacmarek, 2001). Normal PaO_2 of 80 to 100 mm Hg is normal in healthy individuals. A PaO_2 of greater than 60 mm Hg is generally acceptable in the mechanically ventilated critically ill patient (Hess & Kacmarek, 2001). This should produce an oxygen saturation level of greater than 90 percent. Normal $PaCO_2$ is 35 to 45 mm Hg and measures the adequacy of alveolar ventilation. Adjustments in the V_t and respiratory rate will normalize the $PaCO_2$. To preserve lower inspiratory pressures, the clinician may lower the V_t tidal volume and allow the $PaCO_2$ to rise beyond normal limits.

Continuous pulse oximetry (SpO_2) monitoring is a noninvasive method to monitor oxygenation saturation. SpO_2 monitoring allows for titration of the FiO_2 without performing more frequent ABG analysis. Continuous SpO_2 monitoring also allows the nurse to quickly detect episodes of hypoxia that may occur with weaning. Documentation of the SpO_2 value is usually completed every hour unless the patient's condition warrants more frequent assessment. Breath sounds should also be monitored and documented every two to four hours depending on the patient's condition. The critical care nurse is also responsible for making sure the patient receives ordered CXRs. Patients on mechanical ventilation have a daily CXR to monitor lung condition and tube placement.

The critical care nurse performs endotracheal suctioning on patients because they are not able to cough up secretions (Table 19-5). The patient may need suctioning when there are visible secretions, excessive coughing, frequent high-pressure alarms, or decreases in oxygen saturation. Restlessness may indicate hypoxemia, and the patient may require suctioning to clear the airway. Suctioning should last no longer than 10 to 15 seconds (Sole, et al., 2001). The nurse should only suction when necessary, because the patient may experience drastic drops in oxygen saturation, changes in vital signs, increased intracranial pressure, airway trauma, or infection with suctioning. To prevent oxygen desaturation, the nurse should hyperoxygenate the patient prior to suctioning. This may be done by delivering 100 percent FiO_2 for several breaths before and after suctioning. The nurse should monitor the patient's vital signs during suctioning and stop the procedure if the patient's heart rate or blood pressure indicates severe compromise. Prior to suctioning, the patient should receive an adequate explanation of the procedure (Figure 19-8).

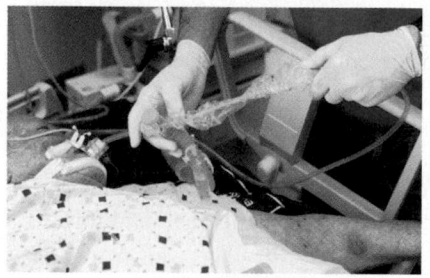

Figure 19-8 Endotracheal suctioning.

TABLE 19-5 General Guidelines for Endotracheal In-line Suctioning

Determine need for suctioning. (Assess the patient.)

Explain the procedure to the patient including rationale and benefits.

Gather equipment including personal protective devices. Wear gloves and goggles.

Hyperoxygenate the patient before, during, and after the procedure. Hyperventilate the patient if necessary (activate the manual sigh button on the ventilator).

Set the suction regulator between 80–140 mm Hg.

Insert the catheter without activating suction until resistance is met.

Withdraw the catheter while applying suction (depressing the white button on the connector end) intermittently. Do not apply suction for more than 10–15 seconds.

Ensure the catheter is completely withdrawn and assess the need for further suctioning.

When endotracheal suctioning is complete, rinse the catheter with sterile saline by instilling saline in the irrigation port while depressing the suction button.

Suction the patient orally with a Yankauer catheter if necessary. Turn off suction.

Document breath sounds before and after suctioning. Document amount, color, and consistency of secretions. Document and report how the patient tolerated the procedure.

During the procedure, continually assess for patient tolerance of the suctioning. Monitor for desaturation, changes in heart rate, or blood pressure.

Adapted from Daniels, R. (2004). Nursing fundamentals. Clifton Park, NY: Thomson Delmar Learning.

Complications of Intubation and Mechanical Ventilation

Common complications of intubation include ischemia and necrosis of the oral or nasal mucosa. For the patient who is nasally intubated, the nurse needs to monitor for skin breakdown in the nares. The tape around the tube in the nares also needs to be secure to prevent movement and subsequent further skin damage. The nurse should document skin assessment around the nares routinely. The oral mucosa needs to be assessed routinely for signs of impaired circulation. The nurse and respiratory therapist may help to prevent skin breakdown by moving the oral tube from one side to the other routinely. It is also important that the ETT holder be kept as dry as possible.

Tracheal Damage

The ETT and tracheostomy tube can cause laryngeal and tracheal damage. Most tubes have low-pressure cuffs that help to decrease the incidence of damage, but damage will occur in cuffs that have too much pressure or are in place for long periods of time. The amount of air or pressure in the cuff should be monitored and should range from 20 to 25 mm Hg (Hess & Kacmarek, 2002). The critical care nurse or respiratory therapist typically performs routine monitoring of cuff pressures. Cuff pressures should also not be allowed to become too low. Cuff leaks occasionally occur and can cause ventilation problems. If a cuff leak is serious enough to cause an inadequate a V_t in the patient, the patient will need reintubation with a new endotracheal tube.

Unplanned Extubation

Extubation before the patient is ready is a medical emergency. The cause of unplanned extubations depends on the circumstances. The ETT is uncomfortable and the patient may have a natural urge to pull the tube out. This can easily occur in the patient who is not kept comfortable with medication or is not physically restrained. Staff can accidentally pull the ETT out when turning the patient or adjusting the ventilator tubing. The ETT can also slip out if not securely restrained. When an unplanned extubation occurs, the nurse needs to ensure airway and breathing in the patient. If necessary, the patient should be ventilated with an Ambu bag-valve-mask device. If the patient is breathing, the patient should at least receive supplemental oxygen. The health care provider should be notified immediately and reintubation supplies should be brought to the bedside. Keeping the patient comfortable with sedation and keeping the patient physically restrained can prevent unplanned extubation. The ETT should be kept secure with tape or appropriate holder. The holder should not be allowed to become wet or loose. The nurse should monitor the centimeter markings on the tube for movement routinely. Care should always be taken when working with tubing or turning the patient requiring mechanical ventilation.

Because the ETT causes the glottis to remain open and prevents the natural cough and gag reflex, the risk of aspiration in mechanically ventilated patients is high. Upper airway secretions are commonly aspirated and can be the source of pneumonia in these patients. Mechanically ventilated patients also often require tube feedings that can be sources of aspiration. Aspiration frequently causes pneumonia, which contributes to the morbidity of the critically ill patient.

Ventilator-Associated Pneumonia

Ventilator-associated pneumonia (VAP) is a common complication in the mechanically ventilated patient and has a high mortality rate. Nurses must be vigilant about monitoring for and preventing VAP. Once the diagnosis of VAP is made, antibiotics will be prescribed. Hand washing is an important intervention for health care workers, especially during suctioning and oral care

Red Flag

Unplanned Extubation

As a critical nurse you should be prepared to manually ventilate the patient who has been inadvertently extubated. An Ambu bag valve mask apparatus connected to 100 percent FiO_2 should always be available at the bedside. Page a "Code Blue" in the absence of respirations to alert other members of the health care team. Intubation supplies need to be available at the bedside to reintubate the patient. If the patient is breathing, appropriate FiO_2 needs to be delivered via mask or cannula. Continuous SpO_2 monitoring should be performed in addition to ABG analysis.

with the mechanically ventilated patient. The importance of oral care in the prevention of VAP has been well documented. Oral care should be performed every two hours on mechanically ventilated patients unless otherwise indicated (Table 19-6). Unless specifically contraindicated, the patient's head of the bed should be elevated to 45 degrees to prevent aspiration of gastric secretions.

Aseptic technique with endotracheal suctioning should also be used to prevent VAP. A closed system of all ventilator tubing and suction catheters should be maintained as much as possible to prevent entry of bacteria. While turning the patient, care should be maintained to prevent water from the ventilator tubing entering the patient's airways. Suction equipment and catheters should be replaced per protocol of the institution. Saline lavage should not be used routinely during suctioning of the patient. Instillation of saline into the ETT may introduce bacteria and contribute to the development of VAP.

Careful monitoring of tube feedings in mechanically ventilated patients will also help to prevent aspiration of GI contents. Patients receiving tube feedings should have their head of the bed elevated at least 30 to 45 degrees at all times. The nurse should monitor for high gastric residuals at least every four to six hours. Tube feedings should be stopped in patients who have elevated residuals. The ETT cuff pressure should also be maintained above 20 mm Hg to prevent aspiration. Schleder (2003) recommends that respiratory therapists and nurses collaborate to promote strategies that prevent VAPs. Strategies to prevent VAP should be a part of every team member's orientation to the intensive care setting.

Barotrauma

Barotrauma can also occur with mechanical ventilation. Barotrauma most commonly occurs in the mechanically ventilated patient who is on excessive V_ts or elevated levels of PEEP or has existing chronic lung conditions that cause overdistension of alveoli. If enough air outside the alveoli travels into the pleural space, the end result could be a tension pneumothorax. A tension pneumothorax could be potentially life-threatening, requiring a needle thoracotomy or

---

TABLE 19-6 Oral Care for the Mechanically Ventilated Patient

ASSESS/DOCUMENT

1. Assess patient's mouth for dryness, inflammation, and the presence of crusting.

2. Document any skin or oral mucous membrane breakdown, if present.

3. Initiate wound care intervention in the nursing care plan for any breakdown found during the assessment of the patient's mouth.

CLEANSE

1. Provide mouth care by brushing teeth and cleansing mouth with appropriate solution at least every 2 hours to maintain oral health and prevent infection.

2. Suction will be utilized to prevent incidental aspiration of saliva, cleansing solution, and such when oral care performed.

3. All Yankauer suction handles are labeled with the date and time the package was opened. Suction handles will be discarded and replaced every 24 hours.

4. Mouth swabs will be discarded immediately after use. A new mouth swab will be used each time the patient's mouth is cleansed.

MAINTENANCE CARE

1. Apply nonpetroleum oral care emollient to maintain hydration and prevent dryness.

ETT REPOSITIONING

1. The patient's ETT will be repositioned by the respiratory therapist or RN at least every 24 hours. ETT placement will be documented every shift by the RN caring for the patient.

Adapted from Munro, C. L., & Grap, M. J. (2004). Oral health and care in the intensive care unit: State of the science. American Journal of Critical Care, 13(1), 25–33.

Uncovering the Evidence

The Effectiveness of Antibiotic Prophylaxis for Respiratory Tract Infections

Discussion: The researchers reviewed 36 randomized trials that involved 6,922 subjects. The selection criteria included randomized trials of antibiotic prophylaxis for respiratory tract infections among adult intensive care unit patients. Combinations of topical and systemic prophylactic antibiotics reduced respiratory tract infections and overall mortality in adult intensive care patients. Topical administration included the application of antibiotics to the oropharynx. Selective decontamination of the digestive tract was also used and involved eradicating and preventing the carriage of microorganisms from the oropharynx and GI tract.

Implications for Practice: Critical care nurses need to be vigilant about administering antibiotics prescribed to their patients and use measures that help prevent nosocomial pneumonia. Nurses should monitor culture and sensitivity results when available to ensure appropriate drug choices.

Source: Liberati, A., D'Amico, R., Pifferi, S., Torri, V., & Brazzi, L. (2004). Antibiotic prophylaxis to reduce respiratory tract infections and mortality in adults receiving intensive care (Cochrane Review). The Cochrane Database of Systematic Reviews, 3;(1):CD000022.

chest tube. The critical care nurse should assess for barotrauma by monitoring airway pressures. Peak alveolar pressure should be kept less than 30 cm H_2O (Hess & Kacmarek, 2002). Adjustments in ventilator settings should be made in patients whose peak airway pressures are rising. The critical care nurse should also auscultate lung sounds and respiratory rate frequently.

Stress Ulcers

Stress ulcers are also complications of mechanical ventilation and often occur within 72 hours of illness (Papadakis, 2006). Stress ulcers are ulcerations in the stomach of critically ill patients. These place the patient at great risk for developing GI bleeding. Patients who are on mechanical ventilation are especially at risk for the development of stress ulcers. Prevention of stress ulcers in the mechanically ventilated patient includes prophylactic administration of proton pump inhibitors, histamine (H_2) blockers, or sucralfate. There is a possibility that administration of proton pump inhibitors or H_2 blockers may raise the gastric pH that allows for increased growth of gram-negative bacteria. The gram-negative bacteria could therefore colonize the pharynx and eventually lead to the development of nosocomial pneumonia. Sucralfate may be the agent of choice for prevention of stress ulcers.

Communication

Because the ETT passes through the glottis, the patient who is intubated and mechanically ventilated will be unable to speak. This inability to communicate presents many challenges for the patient, the family, and the health care workers. It may also contribute to the patient's feelings of anxiety and powerlessness. To minimize patient anxiety, the nurse must learn to understand the patient who is unable to communicate. Picture and word boards can provide alternative forms of communication. The images contained on these boards depict feelings, such as anger and sadness, as well as basic needs, such as water and a blanket.

Word boards provide the alphabet for patients to spell and contain common words, such as pain and doctor. These boards should be easily accessible for the patient to use with family members and health care workers. Some patients prefer to write notes to communicate their needs. Providing the patient with a clipboard, paper, and pencil may facilitate this. The patient may need to be unrestrained while writing notes, so the nurse should be present during this period. If the patient is too weak to communicate through writing or communication boards, the nurse can develop other means of communication. Occasionally, it may be necessary for the nurse to ask yes or no questions and have the patient signal his response by nodding or tapping their finger. Sometimes patients can mouth words and use gestures that are understandable to the nurse, although the family may have difficulty comprehending these. In a study performed by Wojnicki-Johansson (2001) patients were asked to identify the method of communication they preferred. Fifty-four percent of the patients preferred body language, gestures, and touch, 32 percent of the patients preferred the paper and pen method, and 23 percent of the patients preferred yes-no questions. Combinations of various methods of communication were identified as favorable by 36 percent of the patients.

Anxiety

Anxiety is a common experience for mechanically ventilated patients. Anxiety is often increased, because the ETT is uncomfortable. Patients may also be apprehensive about their condition and being in the intensive care unit. The patient's room should be kept quiet and relaxing. The nurse may use therapeutic communication techniques to help identify major sources causing the anxiety. Therapeutic touch, when performing patient care, may be helpful. It is usually necessary for the patient to be on some form of antianxiety medication (Table 19-7). Benzodiazepines, such as midazolam or lorazepam, are commonly used. Diprivan is another medication that is commonly used for sedation in the mechanically ventilated patient. These medications may decrease feelings of anxiety and restlessness as well as promote ventilator compliance.

TABLE 19-7 Medications Commonly Used to Enhance Compliance with Mechanical Ventilation

DRUG NAME	CLASSIFICATION	EXPECTED ACTION	USUAL DOSAGE	NURSING IMPLICATIONS
Morphine sulfate	Strong opioid analgesic Schedule II narcotic	Activates mu receptors causing relief of pain, reduction in anxiety, and promoting sense of well-being.	Dosage for adults is 2–6 mg IV diluted in 4–5 mL of sterile water or saline every one to two hours as needed. Continuous drip may be used 1–5 mg/hr.	Monitor the patient for hypotension. Monitor bowel function (causes constipation). In case of overdose, Narcan may be administered.
Fentanyl	Strong opioid analgesic Schedule II narcotic	Activates mu receptors for effects much like morphine sulfate.	0.05–0.1 mg IV or intramuscularly. Give over 1–2 min.	Monitor patient's vital signs. Have Narcan for overdose. Protect drug from light.
Lorazepam (Ativan)	Benzodiazepines Anxiolytic	Has depressant action on the central nervous system (CNS). Depresses neuronal function in the CNS.	1–4 mg IV every 2–6 hours. Given sometimes in continuous drip of 1–4 mg/hr. Dilute IV in equal amounts of D₅W or NS. Do not exceed 2 mg/min IV.	Monitor vital signs (hypotension may occur) and LOC. May need to adjust dosage in renal or hepatic disease. May treat overdose with flumazenil (Romazicon).

Continued

TABLE 19-7 Medications Commonly Used to Enhance Compliance with Mechanical Ventilation—cont'd

DRUG NAME	CLASSIFICATION	EXPECTED ACTION	USUAL DOSAGE	NURSING IMPLICATIONS
Midazolam (Versed)	Benzodiazepines (Anxiolytic)	See Lorazepam	1–2.5 mg initially, after waiting two minutes may give an additional 1 mg in two-minute intervals up to 5 mg. May be given as a constant infusion of 1–5 mg/hr.	See Lorazepam. May cause arrhythmias when given IV, patient should be monitored. May cause pain at injection site.
Propofol (Diprivan)	Sedative-hypnotic Anesthetic	Exact mechanism of action unknown. Produces unconsciousness with 60 seconds.	Usual dosage is 25–75 mcg/kg/min constant infusion.	Can cause respiratory depression, and hypotension. Monitor blood pressure Bottle should be discarded after six hours. Rapidly eliminated on discontinuation, patient should wake up quickly.
Haloperidol (Haldol)	High-potency neuroleptic sedative	Blocks receptors for dopamine in the CNS.	2–5 mg IV push and may be given every hour up to total of 50 mg. May be given 5 mg/min. All IV doses are unlabeled.	Nurses should monitor for extrapyramidal symptoms. Monitor for hypotension and CNS depression. Provide frequent oral care.
Vecuronium (Norcuron)	Nondepolarizing neuromuscular blocker	Competes with acetylcholine at nicotinic mu receptors at myoneural junction. Causes relaxation of skeletal muscles.	Initial bolus given 0.08–0.1 mg/kg Continuous infusion to start at 1 mg/kg then adjust to patient response. Usual rate is 0.8–1.2 mcg/kg/min	Response to dosage needs to be monitored closely with nerve stimulator. Patient should receive supplemental medication for anxiety and pain. Have an anticholinesterase available to reverse effects. Monitor for malignant hyperthermia.
Atracurium (Tracrium)	See Vecuronium	See Vecuronium	Initial bolus 0.4–0.5 mg/kg Continuous of maintenance is generally 5–9 mcg/kg/min	See Vecuronium May be drug of choice for patients with renal or hepatic disease.
Pancuronium (Pavulon)	See Vecuronium	See Vecuronium	Bolus 0.06–0.1 mg/kg may be repeated every 20–60 minutes	See Vecuronium

Adapted from Gahart, B., & Nazareno, A. (2002). Intravenous Medications (18th ed.). St. Louis, MO: Mosby; Lehne, R. (2004). Pharmacology for nursing care. St. Louis, MO: W.B. Saunders; Sole, M., Lamborn, M., & Hartshorn, J. (2001). Introduction to critical care nursing. Philadelphia: W. B. Saunders Company; Spratto, G., & Woods, A. (2003). PDR nurses' drug handbook. Clifton Park, NY: Thomson Delmar Learning.

Dosages should be adjusted prior to weaning and extubation because these medications may cause respiratory depression.

Neuromuscular blockers may be required in patients who require paralysis. Paralysis may be necessary in patients whose condition necessitates minimal oxygen consumption. Neuromuscular blockers may be used to promote compliance with the ventilator in patients who require high-level ventilator settings. Neuromuscular blockers should always be used in conjunction with anxiolytic or analgesic, as these medications do not possess those properties. Patients

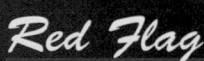

should have their level of paralysis monitored when on a neuromuscular blocker. Train of Four (TOF) is one method to determine level of paralysis. The electrodes are placed on the ulnar nerve and then a series of four impulses is delivered rapidly to the patient. If the patient has the appropriate level of paralysis his thumb will twitch one to two times out of the four impulses. The medication may need to be increased if more twitches are present and decreased if less are present. Typically, patients should have their medication lowered daily to assess neurological status. The most commonly used neuromuscular blockers are vecuronium, atracurium, and pancuronium. Succinylcholine is a short-acting neuromuscular blocker that is used for muscle relaxation during the intubation process.

Impaired Nutrition

Patients who are intubated and mechanically ventilated will be unable to eat normally. For patients who require mechanical ventilation for over 2 to 3 days, malnutrition can become an important issue for the patient. Unless contraindicated, enteral tube feedings are usually started on patients who require long-term ventilatory support. Total parenteral nutrition will be required when tube feedings are contraindicated. There is an important relationship between nutrition and respiration (Hess & Kacmarek, 2002). If the patient receives too few or too many calories, the end result can be respiratory failure. In the patient who already has a compromised respiratory status, poor nutrition can contribute to complications. One of the most profound effects that malnutrition can have is a weakening of the respiratory muscles. If patients have weakened respiratory muscles, they may be unable to be successfully weaned from the ventilator. Laboratory data will need to be monitored to follow the patient's nutritional status. Albumin levels may be monitored in patients but are not considered to be specific or timely because the half-life is approximately 20 days. Prealbumin is considered to be a better indicator of protein loss because its half-life is shorter, approximately 2 to 3 days. Low transferrin levels may be present in patients who are malnourished and should be monitored (Cavanaugh, 2003). One of the most accurate measures of nutritional status may be the evaluation of nitrogen balance. Nitrogen balance may be calculated by the following equation: Nitrogen balance equals protein intake (6.25 minus urinary urea nitrogen) plus 4 (Sole, et al., 2001). If the resulting value is negative, then protein catabolism is occurring, and the patient has poor nutrition. The patient's nutritional requirements may be calculated using a basal energy requirement calculation. It is important that the health care provider and nurse consult the nutrition support specialist for assessment of the patient's nutritional status.

Patients who require supplemental nutrition because of mechanical ventilation will require insertion of a nasogastric or oral gastric tube, a nasoduodenal tube, or a nasojejunal tube in which to deliver the enteral feedings. Enteral feedings are considered to be closer to normal eating when compared with parenteral nutrition. There are various types of formulas available, which contain anywhere from 1 cal/mL to 2 cal/mL. The health care provider, dietician, and nurse may collaborate to choose the formula that will best fit the patient's needs.

Total parenteral nutrition (TPN) is an alternative method of delivering nutrients to the mechanically ventilated patient when the GI tract cannot be used. There are various formulas that can be used based on the patient's needs. Formulas include glucose, amino acids, electrolytes, minerals, and lipids. Certain medications may be added including insulin if needed. TPN is typically delivered through a central line site due to the hyperosmolarity of the solution. Infection, hyperglycemia, and fluid and electrolyte imbalances are common complications of TPN. The critical care nurse is responsible for maintaining sterility of the system, monitoring for fluid and electrolyte imbalances, and monitoring finger stick blood sugars to help prevent these complications.

Patients may suffer from hypotension due to decreased CO when on mechanical ventilation. Intrathoracic pressure is increased when the patient is on mechanical ventilation causing a decrease in venous return. Decreased CO occurs most frequently when the patient is on higher levels of PEEP. The nurse must monitor the patient's blood pressure closely when levels of PEEP need to be increased. The patient may require infusion of fluids or vasopressors to maintain adequate MAPs Patients who have adult respiratory distress syndrome frequently need PEEP levels from 10 to 20 cm H_2O.

When the patient is mechanically ventilated there is increased pressure on the baroreceptors in the thoracic aorta (Swearingen & Keen, 2001). This pressure causes the body to respond as if it were volume-depleted. The body produces and releases more antidiuretic hormone in response to volume depletion. Antidiuretic hormone causes the kidneys to retain water. As a result, patients may become hypervolemic with an increase in generalized edema and pulmonary secretions. The patient's fluid volume may be monitored with CVP monitoring or PA pressure monitoring. Patients may need diuretic therapy if they experience adverse reactions to the retained fluid.

Patients requiring mechanical ventilation may also experience complications related to their ventilator settings. Oxygen toxicity may occur in patients who require high levels of oxygen to maintain adequate tissue oxygen saturation. When oxygen toxicity occurs, the lungs become more congested and atelectasis develops (Guyton, 2001). A patient's FiO_2 should be titrated to below 50 percent, if possible, to decrease the incidence of oxygen toxicity. When patients are on the CMV volume mode of ventilation, there is the potential for them to exhale too much carbon dioxide. When the patient starts to generate negative pressure by taking a breath, the ventilator gives the patient a full tidal volume of air. The ventilator will do this as many times a minute as the patient attempts to take a breath. This action causes the patient to blow off too much carbon dioxide and respiratory alkalosis ensues. Sedating the patient and decreasing the respiratory rate can help control the respiratory alkalosis.

Ventilator Weaning

Patients who are mechanically ventilated will have the ultimate goal of being able to sustain effective ventilations without the aid of the ventilator. Discontinuing mechanical ventilation should be accomplished when the patient is deemed able to sustain effective spontaneous respirations. Most patients require **ventilator weaning,** or a gradual lessening of ventilatory support to have mechanical ventilation successfully discontinued. In most patients successful weaning from mechanical ventilation occurs when the patient's physiological condition has significantly improved. For example, if the patient was intubated and placed on mechanical ventilation for pneumonia, when the pneumonia has cleared, the patient should be able to be extubated and mechanical ventilation discontinued. Patients who require longer term ventilatory support usually have a longer weaning process than those patients who are mechanically ventilated for just a few days. Often, patients who require longer term ventilatory support have more complex illnesses than those patients who are on short-term mechanical ventilation. Ventilator weaning will be more challenging in the former patients and will require assessment and planning by a multidisciplinary team (Henneman, Dracup, Ganz, Molayeme, & Cooper, 2002). Communication among all team members is essential in planning and implementing the weaning plan. Salipante (2002) suggests that members of the team include: (a) an experienced medical intensive care unit nurse as coordinator, (b) a pulmonary critical care health care provider, (c) a physical therapist, (d) a respiratory therapist, (e) a nutritionist, (f) a speech therapist, (g) a psychiatric clinical nurse specialist, and (h) a social worker. This team approach ensures holistic treatment in caring for the patient.

Protocols for weaning patients from mechanical ventilation may improve patient outcomes and decrease the costs for caring for critically ill patients (National Guideline Clearinghouse, 2002). Three studies show support for protocols that are designed for use by therapists and nurses to identify patients ready for spontaneous breathing trials. The studies included a large number of subjects, and the experimental groups in each study had less weaning time and lowered costs when compared to the control group that received standard medical care.

Indications

The patient who is ready to be weaned from mechanical ventilation should have several indicators present. The patient's illness should be reversed or markedly improved. The patient should have adequate nutritional status in addition to having normal electrolytes. The patient should not be hemodynamically unstable, as identified by the absence of myocardial ischemia and the lack or significance decrease of vasopressor therapy. There are also several indices that may be measured by the health care provider or respiratory therapist. Ventilatory muscle strength may be measured by vital capacity and maximum inspiratory pressure. The rapid-shallow breathing index is measured by dividing the respiratory rate by the V_t after one minute of discontinuation of oxygen and ventilatory support and may be the best predictor of success (Hess & Kacmarek, 2002).

Once the decision is made to start the weaning process, the method of weaning will then be determined. There are various methods available, and no one modality is superior. CPAP trials are the most common method of weaning. Pressure support trials are also used, and both involve a gradual decrease of the support they provide while the patient is still connected to the ventilator. During either of these trials the patient is spontaneously breathing, hence, the term weaning trial is considered to be synonymous with spontaneous breathing trials. SIMV may also be used as a weaning method. The respiratory rate is gradually decreased until the patient is extubated when SIMV is used. Regardless of the method used, the patient will need periods of rest. Discontinuation of mechanical ventilation will not be successful if the patient is exhausted from the weaning process. The patient who requires several days of weaning should be allowed to rest on full ventilatory support during the overnight hours.

Nursing Management

Weaning from mechanical ventilation can be a frightening experience, especially for the patient who has become dependent on the ventilator. Psychological support should be provided during the process of weaning and extubation. The process should be explained to the family and patient, and both should be kept informed of the patient's progress. Sedation should be decreased during the process of weaning to prevent hypoventilation. The patient may experience even more feelings of anxiety as anxiolytic dosages are diminished. The critical care nurse and family play major roles in providing support for the patient. Providing reassurance and making the patient as comfortable as possible will be helpful in ensuring a successful weaning trial.

The patient should be closely monitored for any evidence of respiratory compromise during the weaning trials. Typically, ABG analysis is performed after the trial has started and prior to its end. The patient should have continuous monitoring of SpO_2 during the process. Respiratory rate, blood pressure, and heart rate should also be continuously monitored during the weaning trial. Drops in SpO_2 or increases in respiratory rate, heart rate, and blood pressure, as well as arrhythmias, can indicate respiratory distress. Significant changes in these parameters would warrant discontinuation of the trial. The critical care nurse should be alert for accessory muscle use, diaphoresis, and relayed subjective feelings of shortness of breath. In most cases the nurse can also monitor for decreases in expired V_t, which might indicate excessive fatigue. The patient may need to be returned to the previous ventilator settings and his readiness to wean reevaluated. Patients who fail the spontaneous breathing trial should be assessed for the reason of failure. Once that reason is reversed, if the patient still meets criteria to start weaning, then the patient should start again on weaning trials. Patients should not be considered to be ventilator-dependent until three months of weaning attempts have failed.

The critical care nurse has many responsibilities once the patient is ready for extubation. The nurse should have oral suction available to suction the oropharynx and mouth just prior to extubation. The cuff should be deflated, and the tube removed promptly. The patient will generally experience coughing during this period and should be forewarned. The nurse should be ready with suction as the tube is removed, because patient will generally produce copious secretions. An oxygen mask or cannula should be ready prior to extubation and placed on the patient once the tube is removed. Respiratory assessment should be completed frequently after extubation including vital signs and auscultation of all lung fields. ABG analysis will generally be performed 30 to 60 minutes after extubation while SpO_2 monitoring should be continuous. The nurse should observe for signs of respiratory distress caused by tracheal or laryngeal edema, which may occur postextubation. The nurse should encourage deep breathing, coughing and turning frequently to facilitate movement of secretions.

Once extubation has occurred, the patient may experience temporary hoarseness and should be encouraged to limit conversation initially. Hoarseness should resolve completely within a few days. The patient may be allowed to have a few ice chips initially and then progress to a liquid diet once difficulties with swallowing have resolved. Oral care should be provided after extubation, and the male patient thoroughly shaved as appropriate. It is often soothing to patients to have their face washed and dried after removing the ETT holder.

Withdrawal of Life Support

Occasionally, the decision to withdraw life support may be appropriate when there is no hope the patient will recover. This decision may be made as a result of the patient's request and designated surrogates in conjunction with the health care team. There also may be a referral to an ethics committee to ensure alternatives and circumstances are explored prior to withdrawal of life support. When further intervention is deemed futile, the withdrawal of mechanical ventilation may be initiated. The critical care nurse will play an important role during this time. Analgesics and sedatives should be administered prior to extubation of the patient. These medications should be administered in sufficient dosages to prevent air hunger or distress. Morphine sulfate and fentanyl are often the drugs of choice for this purpose (Tierney, et al., 2004). Psychological support will be necessary for family during this difficult time. Continuing support and comfort measures for patients are crucial during this process. Information should be provided regarding expected course of events. Families are often anxious about the timing of death after extubation so nurses should remain with the patient and family as appropriate. Predicting the timing of death is difficult and may only serve to create more anxiety in family members when inaccurate. Open visitation by family members should be encouraged during this period of time. The nurse should receive assistance in caring for family members from social services or clergy as appropriate.

These circumstances may also be difficult for nurses themselves. Some nurses may find this process even more emotionally challenging if the patient has been in the intensive care unit for a long period of time. Nurses should understand that they are also vulnerable to experiencing feelings of loss and grief. Nurses must recognize when they are experiencing these feelings and be open to receiving assistance in managing them. The critical care nurse should seek emotional assistance and support from colleagues, clergy, and employee assistance as appropriate.

KEY CONCEPTS

- Critical care units were originally developed to group patients who were at risk of cardiopulmonary arrest in an effort to expedite their treatment.
- Critical care nursing is a nursing specialty that involves human responses to life-threatening illnesses.
- Registered nurses may become certified in critical care nursing by passing a certification examination and required clinical hours, which allows them to possess the CCRN title after their name.
- Patients will be discharged from the intensive care unit when the need for intensive nursing care no longer exists. Many acute care facilities have discharge criteria that must be met by the patient prior to transfer to a general floor or intermediate care unit.
- An interdisciplinary team is the best approach to providing optimal care of the critically ill patient.
- Family members may be experiencing a range of emotions related to the admission of a family member to the critical care unit.
- Critical care nurses may support families through the crisis of having a member in the intensive care unit by flexible visitation and open communication.
- Nursing management of the patient with a balloon pump includes monitoring of circulation in the affected extremity, monitoring for leaks in the balloon, proper patient positioning, and evaluating patient response to the device.
- The VAD is used to bypass one or both ventricles in a severely compromised heart. Bypassing the ventricle allows it to rest and potentially heal. The VAD may be used longer than the intra-aortic balloon pump.
- Complications of the VAD include bleeding, infection, and thrombosis.
- Several types of patients may be at risk for increased intracranial pressure on admission to the critical care unit. Brain injury, stroke, tumors, and infection can all cause the patient to be at risk for increased intracranial pressure.

- Patients with increased intracranial pressure are at risk for the development of herniation. Types of herniation include: cingulate, uncal, central, and tonsillar.
- Patients who are unable to maintain an open airway may be assisted in keeping their airway open by positioning, oral, nasal, endotracheal, and tracheal airways.
- Endotracheal intubation refers to the passage of a tube into the patient's airway through the mouth or nares. The tube may be attached to a mechanical ventilator or to an Ambu bag for assisting the patient with ventilation.
- Indications for mechanical ventilation include respiratory or ventilatory failure, worsening of ABGs, increase work of breathing or apnea, and worsening CXR.
- Patients should be suctioned on an as-needed basis to assist clearing the airway. Patients should be hyperoxygenated before and after suctioning. The procedure should last no longer than 10 to 15 seconds.
- Nursing care of mechanically ventilated patients should include prevention of unplanned extubation. Patients should be appropriately chemically or physically restrained.
- Health care team members may communicate with the mechanically ventilated patient by the use of picture boards, writing, gestures, and mouthing words.
- The nurse will need to assess the patient for respiratory distress immediately after extubation. Ongoing assessment of the patient is important to detect early signs of respiratory distress. Deep breathing combined with coughing and activity will help facilitate mobilization of secretions.
- Life support may be withdrawn on patients when there is no hope of recovery. This should be done in consultation with the patient, family, and members of the interdisciplinary health care team. Consultation with the ethics committee will be appropriate.

REVIEW QUESTIONS

1. Your trauma patient has the following blood gases: pH 7.60, PCO_2 = 28, PO_2 = 76, HCO_3 = 26. He is on the ventilator CMV = 12, V_t = 700, FiO_2 = 50 percent, PEEP = 5. His vital signs are as follows: blood pressure =110/50, pulse = 100, respiratory rate = 32, and temperature = 99.0° F (37.2° C). Your patient weighs 70 kg. The most appropriate treatment for this patient at this time is:
   1. Decrease his FiO_2 to 40 percent to decrease his oxygen delivery
   2. Give morphine or Versed
   3. Decrease the CMV rate to 6
   4. Decrease his V_t to 400

2. A patient is maintained on a mechanical, volume-controlled ventilator. He is requiring PEEP to maintain adequate oxygenation. What physiological events are associated with this treatment?
   1. Decreased CO, pneumothorax
   2. Increased CO, pulmonary edema
   3. Increased CO, decreased renal perfusion
   4. Increased venous return, pneumothorax

3. A patient is on CMV, positive pressure mechanical ventilation for respiratory failure. The ventilator alarm sounds with low exhaled tidal volume. The nurse should investigate this as a possible cause for the alarm:
   1. Tachypnea
   2. A leak in the endotracheal cuff tube
   3. Secretions in the airway
   4. Decreased lung compliance

4. The nurse is caring for a patient who is on positive pressure ventilation, the SIMV mode. The ventilator high pressure alarm sounds. The nurse enters the patient's room and should investigate for which of the possible causes of a high pressure alarm (select all that apply)?
   1. Tension pneumothorax
   2. Disconnection from the ventilator circuit
   3. Secretions in the airway
   4. The patient is coughing
   5. A leak in the endotracheal cuff tube
   6. Bronchospasm

5. Which of the following might delay ventilator weaning?
   1. PaO_2 of 50 on a FiO_2 of 60 percent
   2. A potassium level of 3.4 mEq/dL
   3. The requirement of morphine sulfate and Versed while on mechanical ventilation
   4. Intolerance to enteral feedings

6. Which patient would most need intra-arterial pressure monitoring? A patient admitted to the intensive care unit to start on nitroprusside drip for hypertensive crisis.
   1. A patient on TPN therapy who needs blood glucose monitoring
   2. The patient who has been weaned from mechanical ventilation
   3. The patient who had an MI two days ago

7. The intra-aortic balloon pump deflates at which point in the cardiac cycle?
   1. Systole
   2. Diastole
   3. Opening of the tricuspid and mitral valves
   4. During repolarization

8. The PA catheter passes through which valves of the heart upon insertion?
   1. The mitral then aortic
   2. The tricuspid then aortic
   3. The mitral then pulmonic
   4. The tricuspid then pulmonic

9. Your patient with heart failure requires afterload reduction. Which hemodynamic parameter would best assess a patient's response to afterload reduction?
   1. CO
   2. PAWP
   3. CVP
   4. SVR

10. A low CVP may indicate:
    1. Right heart failure
    2. Left heart failure
    3. Hypervolemia
    4. Hypovolemia

11. A PAWP of 25 may indicate:
    1. Left heart failure
    2. Right heart failure
    3. Hypovolemia
    4. Pulmonary hypertension

1. Your patient is currently on mechanical ventilation for exacerbation of chronic obstructive pulmonary disease (COPD) initiated by pneumonia. The patient's ventilator settings are as follows; CMV, volume control with a rate of 12 breaths per minute, FiO_2 of 70 percent, V_t of 800, and PEEP 5 cm H_2O. The patient weighs 65 kg. What complications associated with mechanical ventilation is your patient most at risk for? What are other complications of mechanical ventilation?

2. Your patient is on the current ventilator settings; CMV, volume control, 12 breaths per minute, FiO_2 of 70 percent, V_t of 800, and PEEP 5 cm H_2O. You patient's ABG analysis reveals the following results: pH 7.52, $PaCO_2$ 31, PaO_2 108, HCO_3 23. What is the interpretation of these ABG results? What ventilator settings might be appropriate for this patient?

3. Your patient has been admitted to the intensive care unit with a diagnosis of acute brain injury. The family is asking for information on the nursing care that will be provided for this patient. Identify all of the nursing interventions that you might utilize on this patient. What are the rationales for the interventions?

4. A 55-year-old white male car salesman is admitted to your unit with the diagnosis of left-sided cerebrovascular accident (CVA) with right hemiplegia. He is currently intubated with ventilator settings of CMV = 16, FiO_2 = 50, V_t = 800, and PEEP = 5. His vital signs are blood pressure: 210/140, temperature: 99.2° F (37.3° C), pulse: 120, and respiratory rate: 16. An arterial line is inserted along with a triple lumen catheter to start a Nitroprusside (Nipride) drip. On admission, the patient was unresponsive but has been starting to arouse. He has on bilateral wrist restraints. After insertion of the lines, his family requests to visit at the bedside. He is married with three children ages; 21, 18, and 15 years.

What do you anticipate will be the reactions or feelings of the family on the first visit? What interventions can you employ to help the family on the initial visit? On the patient's third intensive care unit day he is extubated and on 40 percent facemask. His right side is flaccid, and he has expressive aphasia. His family is in the room constantly and is quite tearful at times. His wife has mentioned many times that they have many bills, and she does not know what will happen to them now. What are some particular issues that are concerning the family at this point? What can you do to help them work through some of these issues? The patient is on his fifth hospital day and has transfer orders out to the regular floor. His wife has expressed concerns that he is too ill to be transferred out. The patient appears somewhat anxious about the move as well. What can you do to help relieve some of their anxiety? What issues might the patient or family be concerned with at this point in his recovery?

Continued

5. Your patient is a 45-year-old man who has been in a coma on life support for seven months after suffering from a traumatic brain injury. The patient's mother and wife approach you at the end of your shift. Both women appear to be upset. The mother asks you how long you think they should wait before withdrawing life support. How do you answer this question? What are the support services available for this family while making this decision? What is the nurse's role during this process?

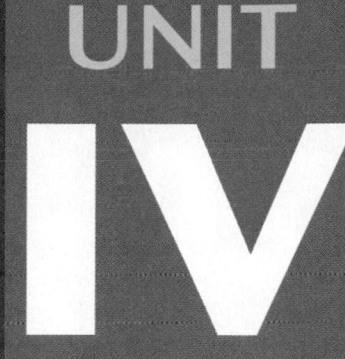

UNIT IV

Perioperative Patient Care

Preoperative Nursing Management

Corinne Grimes, RN, DNSc, AOCN

CHAPTER TOPICS

- Trends in Preoperative Care
- Preparing the Patient for Elective or Nonemergency Surgery
- Preparing the Patient for Unplanned or Emergency Surgery

Surgery is an important technique that is used to diagnose or to treat illness or injury with the goal of restoring patients to an acceptable state of health, or for cases in which disease is nonrecoverable, to alleviate distress. The term **perioperative** means around surgery, an inclusive term that denotes the **preoperative,** prior to the **intraoperative** (the operative period from entry into the operating suite through departure from the postanesthesia care unit [PACU]) period or events leading up to entry into the surgical suite, intraoperative, and **postoperative** periods (takes the patient from the time of departing from the surgical suite through the length of their hospital stay and beyond). The surgical journey begins when the patient first becomes aware of the need for surgery and ends when the patient is well enough to go home or to an intermediate care facility. The perioperative experience may be one of the most tension-producing periods of hospitalization. It is important for all nurses to be able to manage care effectively for patients during this most vulnerable and important period of the hospital stay. Patients and families may enter a state of heightened awareness. They may begin to take in everything about the atmosphere. The care nurse is a pivotal person in setting the style for all others in the preoperative period. Therefore, it is vitally important for the generalist nurses and adult care nurses in any setting to understand the perioperative experience. Readings within this chapter will help the nurse to understand, to explain, and deliver the best care. Preoperative care discriminates between elective surgery patients and nonelective patients. Nonelective patients are those who must undergo emergency surgery or who must enter surgery quickly. These patients will have few options other than to undergo surgery. In such cases, surgery is truly not elective. When the decision to have surgery is elective, there is often time to prepare thoroughly and to take advantage of all the specialized services provided by hospitals, clinics, and surgicenters. This chapter places the reader in a position to walk with the elective patient and the patient's family as they anticipate surgery, practice preoperative exercises, gain knowledge about the surgery, and perform immediate preoperative tasks. For the nonelective or emergency surgery patient, the reader follows along with the patient as preparations are made, and the patient progresses rapidly to the point at which surgery begins. Unlike the typical experience for the elective surgery patient, the emergency surgery patient may experience this time in life alone or without significant family members. In such cases, the nurse may have to act as the patient advocate, ombudsperson, and confidante. It is important that the generalist nurse, as well as the more specialized emergency care nurse, know the progression of care leading up to the moment when the emergency admission patient enters the surgical area. Whether the surgery is elective in nature with months to prepare, or unexpected with only a short period to get ready, nursing care will be highly instrumental in optimizing outcomes for the patient and family. This chapter ends with the patient and family at the door of the surgical suites. As the reader progresses through the chapter, it may be helpful to visualize each situation, both from the nursing point of view and that of the patient or family member. It may be helpful to picture the novice patient's worldview, as well as that of the seasoned, experienced surgical patient. What measures the nurse chooses will depend on how the nurse assesses patient needs.

HISTORY OF NURSING CONTRIBUTIONS IN OPERATIVE CARE

From earliest days, it is likely that people tried to repair themselves using surgical techniques. However, because a break in the body's skin or membranous surfaces constitutes a break in important (and the body's largest) lines of defense, these early attempts no doubt met with mixed success. These early patients' natural abilities to recover from even surface types of surgery would have been predictive of outcome. Nutrition, heredity, relative safety of the surgical setting, and the relative cleanliness of surgical tools would have had a bearing on which cell lines would go on to become our ancestors and which might end abruptly.

Although factors, such as general asepsis, or cleanliness, were discovered earlier, until the mid-1800s, there was a problem with performing deep surgical interventions. Not only was there tremendous pain involved in amputation of a leg or removal of an inflamed appendix, the muscle tissue surrounding the surgical site would not relax during surgery, even if the patient lost consciousness. Muscle spasm would increase the difficulty of visualizing and working with the tissues located deeply within the body. The early 19th-century surgeons would have had to rely on speed and sharp tools, as well as a team of husky individuals to hold the patient down.

Fortunately, in the mid-19th century in the United States, anesthesia via inhalation first became manageable. Although initially used by a country physician in the South, more formal techniques were perfected in the 1840s. This was a few years before the American Civil War and just in time for surgeons and nurses to be able to use more advanced surgical techniques to manage the wounded. Following the discovery of anesthetic agents, surgeons would no longer need speed to complete operations. No longer did the surgeon need a team of strong, dedicated, and single-minded individuals to hold the patient down, and the surgeon did not need to wrestle with tight musculature to accomplish what was surgically necessary. The most important effects of the discovery of general anesthesia were that survival rates rose dramatically, and patients could return to family and loved ones without the memory of having gone through the horrors of surgery without anesthesia. The amnesic effects of general anesthesia prevented recall of the surgical experience.

Modern nursing was coming of age during this same period. It was a distant foreign war that would enable Florence Nightingale to come to power and influence in her home country as well as the rest of the world. Florence Nightingale, Elizabeth Blackwell, and others would have a profound influence on the ways in which nursing, particularly perioperative nursing, would emerge to become what it is today.

Nightingale believed in placing the body in the best condition for nature to act on it (1860). Her views included the need for thorough training of nurses to be able to promote patient wellness through hygiene, nutrition, rest, and activities designed to build strength. This pattern, of considering all the patient's perioperative needs, has continued through today. Working well before the age of such wonders as penicillin, the array of other antibiotics, and even more recent modern miracles, such as hyperalimentation delivery systems, Nightingale was able to save many who might otherwise have perished. Her early work was conducted in and around the Crimean War of the decade before the U.S. Civil War. Thanks to some astounding publicity, a well-connected set of family and friends, and brilliant observational powers, Nightingale was able to train a generation of nurses to heal the entire body, rather than just the area of immediate surgical need. Her nurses were also excellent surgical nurses, but they were able to incorporate much more into their healing arts.

Nightingale was able to build a base for the modern ideas of nursing as a holistic profession. Her ability to focus on the whole patient, rather than solely the body part that was affected and in need of surgery, formed a basis for the modern perioperative nurse's focus on understanding the condition of the patient and family before, during, and following surgical intervention. Using statistics to generate pictures of measures that would improve outcomes for patients, Nightingale was able to convince legislators as well as lay people that such things as sociocultural measures could influence physical well-being.

Nightingale was one of the first nurse theorists to use what equates to the nursing metaparadigm of person, health, environment, and nursing as her basic tenets. This has led those who practice perioperative nursing to assess and to work with the patient as well as the environment in which the patient exists at any moment during the perioperative experience. In addition to her work as a holistic bedside nurse, a theorist, a statistician, and a politically astute nursing leader, Nightingale's work created a framework for development of the nurse as manager-administrator-trainer for all those who have a hand in patient care. The perioperative nurse works with leadership to evaluate and revise what nurses do before, during, and after the surgical event. The nurse is patient advocate, as well as one to whom the family turns for information and advice.

TRENDS

Recent trends in surgical intervention have included gene therapy delivered in utero in an effort to avoid surgical correction for a range of inherited diseases. In addition, the mapping of the human genome enabled recent attempts at correction of such hereditary problems as macular degeneration through the surgical passage of corrected gene sequences directly into the eye. Microsurgical approaches now hasten recovery from many types of abdominal surgery. No longer are incisions universally long, penetrating through all tissue layers to arrive at the organs to be altered. Through a series of small slits, the surgeon may now place fiber-optic visualization devices, lights, surgical instruments, and infusion devices that will allow air to separate organs for ease in visualization. Instead of recovering from major tissue disruption, the patient need only recover from the equivalent of a series of punctures. Time to recovery is vastly shortened.

Pain is one of the things that many people fear when surgery is considered. Thanks to small internal computers, patient-controlled analgesia devices allow patients recovering from surgery to pace the timing of their own medication delivery. The control and immediate relief from medications delivered instantly and intravenously have made a great difference in patient comfort and recovery times following surgery.

Efforts to involve the patient and family in the preparation and recovery process surrounding the actual surgical event have also evolved. For example, in the country's larger hospitals, those who will undergo hip replacement or knee replacement surgery will begin to practice mobility maneuvers long before the surgical event. Their families will assist throughout their recovery, having been taught to use somewhat complex medical devices and to perform detailed assessment. While there is some controversy as to whether this preoperative teaching makes a difference in overall outcome (McDonald, Hetrick, & Green, 2004), it may influence patient and family feelings of control.

In addition to technological and social changes surrounding perioperative care, there have been changes in the traditional makeup of the surgical team. Gone are the days when the office nurse and the health care provider worked side-by-side to care for patients, often performing office surgery or surgery in the home without benefit of other assistive personnel. The generalist natures of these earlier nurse-health care provider teams included tasks such as preparing medications, delivering anesthesia, and rolling cloth bandages as well as shepherding patients through an often prolonged postoperative period.

Today, in some of the nation's major health care facilities, there are preoperative preparation teams comprised of clinical nurse specialists, occupational and physical therapists, pharmacists, dietitians, and social workers that will ensure that patients and families will enter into the surgical experience fully prepared. These caregivers will teach patients and families what they need to do well before the surgical event. Surgeons, health care providers-in-training, nurses, and specially educated surgical assistants will inhabit the surgical suite as the patient undergoes the operative process. Anesthesia may be delivered by anesthetists, anesthesiologists, or certified registered nurse anesthetists. Those performing noncomplex surgery may be physicians, physicians' assistants, or nurse practitioners. The team clearly has a new face.

Monitoring the patient in the delicate, immediate, postoperative period falls to nurses who observe and intervene using a new generation of sophisticated devices. No longer is hypoxia, or the condition of lowered levels of oxygen in the bloodstream, noted through changes in skin and nailbed color. There are now portable and readily available pulse oximeters to quantify precisely the state of peripheral tissue oxygenation. These are easy to use and relatively foolproof.

Surgical tools continue to evolve. Some of the newest instruments are capable of staunching the flow of blood without damage to surrounding tissues. Visualization of even the deepest areas of the body is accomplished with relative ease without traumatizing muscles and other tissues. Recovery, following use of these procedures, can be a matter of hours rather than days.

One trend that has continued is that the nurse's focus remains all-inclusive. The nurse works with the whole patient, assessing for and influencing current status in relation to physiological, psychosocial, and spiritual realms. The surgeon focuses primarily on the physical area needing surgery and pays close attention to other needs during and around the surgical episode. The nurse works at the bedside 24 hours a day and 7 days a week, attending to expressed and unexpressed needs involving a range of body systems. The nurse also collaborates with all those who will influence the patient's recovery: family, friends, and fellow professionals. As in the days of Nightingale, the nurse's work is directed toward placing the patient in the best situation for nature to act in all phases of preparation for surgery, during the surgical event, and during recovery from surgery.

To understand the need for effective preparation for surgery, not only for the patient's swift and satisfactory recovery, but also to satisfy insurers and comply with government trends, it is necessary to examine the role of two recent developments: (a) the advent of diagnosis-related groups making lengths of recovery and acute care hospital stays predictable, and (b) clinical pathways as tools to assist nurses and others to track patients' progress along a continuum beginning with admission through the time of surgery or other treatment and culminating in readiness for discharge.

Pathways and Diagnosis-Related Groups

Clinical pathways and diagnosis-related groups (DRGs) legislation came about in the early 1980s (Baker, 2002). The DRG initiatives were designed to trim the costs of health care in the United States in general and had the effect of shortening patient hospital stays. Clinical pathways were devised so that individual hospitals could track intermediate steps in each patient's recovery process to determine if the patient was recovering according to expected milestones or if recovery was delayed. At the height of use of clinical pathways, delays in recovery would call for extensive paperwork to be forwarded explaining why the patient (by now termed an outlier) was not recovering at the expected speed. While this might seem cold-hearted at first glance, the idea was to analyze what might delay recovery in the aggregate. That is, were there hospital-based challenges that could set back recovery? In the end, some of the best current-day strategies and techniques came about from DRG and clinical pathway initiatives.

This spirit of trying to shorten hospital stays fostered advances in surgical techniques. There were also pioneering efforts designed to make the perioperative experience safer to prevent complications that would lead to more intensive, sometimes dangerous, and definitely expensive hospital stays. It was also felt that, in educating family members or others who might act as caregivers following earlier discharge from the hospital, the patient would enter a safer and more familiar realm for recovery much earlier than had been the case before the advent of DRG legislation.

This also meant that the nurse as educator would need to develop effective means of transmitting discharge information in a consistent manner. Discharge documentation would center on delivery of standardized printed materials along with return demonstrations by patients and home caregivers. Return demonstration was effective in showing that patients had learned the material and could carry on following earlier discharge from the hospital or clinic setting. Additional information on discharge teaching is provided in chapter 22.

Although DRG legislation was designed to save the government money, and thereby relieve taxpayer burden in the United States following a period of spiraling health care costs, the likelihood is that it stemmed the rising tide only slightly. However, it did have the unexpected effect of making surgery faster, safer, and, in most cases, less likely to lead to complications requiring prolonged treatment.

Short Stay Surgery

Short stay surgery is a term that came into wide use in the 1980s following DRG legislation. The term may be equated with such terms as ambulatory surgery, same day surgery, or outpatient surgery. There are even freestanding clinics, detached from the hospital proper and totally dedicated to surgery, known as surgical centers, or surgicenters. These were constructed specifically to meet the needs of the short stay surgical patient and the family. The idea with all of these is that the patient enters the facility on the day of surgery, and, if all goes well, is discharged on the same day, or, at the most, within 23 hours following admission. The patient will often have had preliminary laboratory studies and radiologic examination on an outpatient basis in the days leading up to surgery. This scheduling shortens the hospital stay. The postoperative nurses in short stay settings are educated in ensuring that patients and families will be able to carry on safely at home. They provide education about exercises, diet, relaxation and rest, self-assessment, complications to report, and how to gain immediate access to professional care should the need arise. Although it can be frightening for the patient to know that this early self-care is necessary, the skilled short stay surgery nurse will be able to discharge patients knowing that they possess the requisite skills to carry them safely through the postoperative period.

Finally, the skilled short stay surgery nurse will be able to detect even subtle changes in the patient's condition that signal the need for the patient to be admitted to the hospital setting. In such cases, the patient will not be discharged to a home setting within 23 hours but will stay in the care setting for a longer period to ensure safe recovery.

Remote Assessment

Another recent trend is that of **remote assessment.** When patients and health care providers are located in remote areas, there is sometimes a need to confer with specialists located in larger, urban population centers. This can now be accomplished remotely using satellite imagery. Real-time streaming video can be projected in both directions through the use of camera uplinks and downlinks. The injured or ill patient can be examined by the local physician with the examination transmitted almost instantaneously to the health care provider specialist located hundreds of miles away. In this way, patients can receive the best in health care with timely recommendations from specialists.

When used preoperatively, remote assessment helps the patient to decide whether or not to have surgery. If there is a need to travel to a larger population center for the procedure, this tool can assist with decision making related to timing and other needs. Under some circumstances video linkage has been used to guide remote care providers through the steps of surgery. Finally, remote assessment following surgery will guide postoperative personnel in making care decisions. Using the same uplinks and downlinks, postoperative physical examination can be transmitted via streaming video (motion picture) form to major medical centers. In that way the patient and care team can take advantage of up-to-date and specialized knowledge to assist in the recovery process.

Complementary Therapy

Complementary therapy, also known as alternative therapy, is a label that encompasses a wide range of treatments that fall outside traditional Western medical therapy. While modern medicine considers its practices to be grounded in science and, therefore, to represent the safest and best practices, complementary therapy has never been totally discarded by the Western world. There is thought to be a benefit to things that may not be measurable in purely scientific terms. Some patients, in concert with hospital-based care, use treatments such as acupuncture, massage therapy, and herbal therapy.

In a 2004 news item presented by the British Broadcasting Corporation, it was estimated that 25 percent of the British population used some type of complementary therapy each year (Price, 2004). However, because many who use complementary therapy will not disclose this information to health care providers or nurses, and many tend to use even the most unreliable Internet sources to gather information, it is important to advise patients and families to use caution in embracing these modalities.

When considering the influence of complementary therapy, the nurse who is gathering patient data must ask about the use of alternative therapy. Some of the more useful therapy accessible through the Internet are mind-body therapy such as relaxation and guided imagery (Weiger & Eisenberg, 2002). Others are acupuncture and massage therapy. In some cases, herbs or other practices may complement a course of hospital treatment. However, in other cases, the use of alternative treatments may interfere with health care provider-prescribed treatments or in the rare case, might lead to complications or even death. Sometimes, the nurse's careful noting and communication skills will make a difference in outcome for the patient by making the care team aware of possible influencing factors, such as the use of alternative therapy.

Whenever possible, the nurse should make every effort to learn about a patient's use of such things as relaxation therapy, self-hypnosis, or various sorts of teas or lotions to support those measures that will help the patient come through the hospital experience. For example, the presurgical patient who is able to relax and get a good night's sleep prior to surgery will, at the least, enter the next day's experience better rested and in a more positive frame of mind. The nurse who encourages the family to continue with measures that have been successful at home will be providing a link with past patient successes that may help to allay fears, promote confidence, and be of great psychosocial support during the naturally stressful surgical period.

As complementary theories are studied from a scientific perspective, support may be provided for the benefits of what might seem unorthodox at first to the Western mind. It is probable that as modern communication provides information about commonly used therapies from around the world, there will be renewed interest within the scientific community in exploring what works. For example, recent studies have shown that prayer may improve aspects of patients' reactions to surgery.

The Influence of Religious Faith on Operative Outcomes

Spirituality and religious faith can influence either the patient or their family's response to surgery. The perioperative nurse must be able to set aside personal beliefs and assist patients and their families to understand and cope with their fears and anxiety related to the stressors associated with surgery. An understanding of the components of spirituality and religious faith are essential.

Spirituality

There are many definitions of **spirituality** (using faith to assist patients through difficult or stressful experiences). Some are broad and others are specific. Clark, Drain, and Malone (2004) define spirituality as the attempt to attach meaning to experience, to maintain hope, and to search for transcendence. The elements of spirituality are listed as: religion, beliefs and values, intuition, knowledge from the unknown, a sense of belonging, and as a reverence for life.

Wright (2005) defines spirituality as the human desire for a sense of meaning, purpose, connection, and fulfillment through intimate relationships and life experiences. Spirituality is employed by some human beings to guide how they live their everyday lives. For others, it is a great comfort in times of deep tragedy. There has been renewed interest in spirituality in health care in recent years. Recent initiatives in the United States have been designed to examine the effects of alternative and complementary therapy in healing those who are sick. It is felt that sometimes immeasurable or indistinct entities may have an influence on health outcomes. Alternative practices may create a sense of peace or relaxation. The use of alternative health practices may, in some circumstances, help to restore a sense of individual control in the face of difficult circumstances.

Religious Faith

Religious faith is defined as a belief system involving a supreme being or beings with defined structural elements. The world's major religions, such as Christianity, Islam, Hinduism, Buddhism, and Taoism, are often used as support in times of illness by a variety of patients from many cultures.

The Joint Commission on the Accreditation of Health Care Organizations (JCAHO) is responsible for conducting periodic inspections of health care facilities in the United States. Based on JCAHO requirements, health agencies are required to attend to the emotional and spiritual needs of patients. From examination of JCAHO guidelines, a series of studies and recommendation have been constructed. For example, Clark et al. (2004) recommend that there be emphasis on empathy, the handling of needs in a timely and considerate way, and the development of secluded spaces within hospital walls. In addition, in hospitals of the future, bedside access to the Internet may help patients and families to have constant and familiar ways in which to contact others for worship.

Some religious groups have teachings that are specific and well-known in health care circles not for what they espouse but for what they recommend be omitted. The Christian Science religion teaches that people are capable of self-healing through individual faith. Some religious groups forbid the exchange of body fluids with others, such as receipt of blood transfusions. Even though it may be difficult for the individual nurse to support such practices, there are hospital or clinic guidelines that assist with decision making when these situations are encountered. The hospital's administrative structure is designed to ensure that the bedside care nurse has access to leaders who are well versed in making specific arrangements for patients and families whose religious faith is grounded in nonmainstream practices. Considering the stress encountered by those who are undergoing surgical intervention, the perioperative nurse should always have contact information for leadership and chaplain services readily available.

Electronic Trends

The use of computers in hospitals is now common. Computers analyze, store, and transmit admission information, health care provider notes, laboratory findings, radiologic findings, and past patient health records. Computers are involved in billing activities, room assignments, and levels of care. Some hospitals have invested in computer documentation systems designed to be used by nurses, the largest segment of workers within a hospital.

There are currently many clinics across the country in which health care providers respond to their patients' e-mails, make treatment decisions, and advise the patient, all without the need for an in-person clinic visit (Withrow, 2004). Such e-consults are bound to become popular. E-mail is sometimes more convenient, time-saving, timely, and cost-effective than are more traditional visits and phone calls. For surgical patients who arrive home and discover that pain medications are not fully effective, the system would create a choice of using the telephone or e-mailing for additional medication.

Another cutting-edge initiative will be the widespread use of portable electronic health records. The Fast Forward describes ways in which this technology will enhance patient safety and allow for effective treatment decisions even in unfavorable environments.

While advocates envision rapid diagnosis and effective treatment, there have always been concerns about privacy with such systems. Nurses across the country, and particularly perioperative nurses, will act as patient advocates when such prototypes begin to be tested in clinical settings. Although there will no doubt be built-in safeguards, the danger of personal information being discovered and misused is always a possibility.

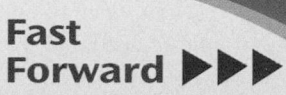

Fast Forward ▶▶▶

Use of Streaming Video for Emergency Preoperative Assessment

The latest generation of cameras capable of producing electronic streaming video images will revolutionize emergency care (Dennis, 2003; Sheehan, 2004). A minute-by-minute recording of conditions and the rescue efforts undertaken at accident scenes will allow care providers at the hospital, the patient's destination, to view patient status and traumatic events before the accident victim even arrives at the doors to the emergency department. For example, a motion picture record of the motor vehicle with the victim inside and the angle of stresses on the vehicle's metal parts will enable the emergency department team to visualize what types of injuries the patient has probably sustained. The emergency team at the hospital will know what type of trauma room to prepare and whether the patient will need immediate surgery or whether there will be time for stabilization. In addition, use of a global positioning system will enable ambulances to communicate in all weather conditions and even in rural areas (Sheehan, 2004). This will result in faster, more accurate treatment.

Fast Forward ▶▶▶

Portable Electronic Health Records

For years, patients have been able to wear a bracelet that alerts health care personnel to allergies or health conditions. Such bracelets allow for effective treatment even if the patient is unconscious or unable to relate such information. A newer initiative in electronic medical records involves the wearing or implanting of a patient's entire history on a microchip. In the case of the surgical patient, an entire health history, including allergies, medical conditions, past surgeries and outcomes, and current and past medications will be placed within a small computer chip. People will carry the chip, perhaps in the form of a bracelet or credit-card sized wallet feature, store it at home, and bring to the clinic or hospital. Hospital or clinic computers could then access the chip in time of need.

An additional device that is being contemplated for use by the military as well as hospitals across the country is the implantable chip (Feder & Zeller, 2004; Kanellos, 2004). Such a chip could be scanned by a handheld reader and would reveal a person's health history, allergies, current health status, and other details useful in developing appropriate treatment. This could be important in the case of disaster situations or with those who are unable to give medical information, such as those with neurological problems. A theater medical information program (TMIP) is being tested within the military (McGlinchey, 2004). Even military personnel in far-away duty stations could confer with health personnel using a laptop computer.

In addition to electronic medical history devices that use microchips and scanners, the video camera will be a useful tool for nurses within the decade. The earliest models are already in use in hospitals with active emergency departments.

For perioperative patients, the age of technology will mean greater safety, efficiency, and freedom from unnecessary anxiety. However, it will be more important than ever for the perioperative nurse to add the caring, humanistic, high-touch elements to this new high-technology health care world.

ELECTIVE AND NONEMERGENCY SURGERY

Elective surgery is usually not urgent, and the patient and family will have time to consider several factors and to prepare. Because it usually does not involve emergency situations or the need to do something rapidly, the patient and family may want to investigate settings, surgeons, and other factors before scheduling an elective surgical event. Insurers may also request that there be communication about the type of surgery, the surgeon, and the facility. These will be approved by the insurer and will result in full or partial insurance coverage.

The Decision to Undergo Surgical Intervention

There are a variety of factors that lead a person to seek medical advice. Some people routinely see health care providers at annual health examinations. Others visit the health care provider only when their health status changes, particularly if they are unable to continue with their usual daily routines. Nonemergency surgery occurs in situations in which the patient has choices: to have surgery, to delay surgery, or not to have surgery.

In addition to choosing to have surgery, the patient will also be selecting a surgeon, a facility in which to have surgery, and deciding when to have surgery. Each of these decisions is made during a period in which the patient may not be physically comfortable. Add to that the underlying fear that surgery may not accomplish all that the patient hopes, and it is easy to see that the preoperative time can be stressful.

Selecting a Surgeon

There are several ways in which a patient or family members can gather information about surgeons prior to making a decision as to which will be the right one to choose (Box 20-1). Physicians typically display diplomas that show from which universities their degrees were granted. The reference section of the local library, or if close to a university, one of the libraries there, will have materials with information about degree-granting institutions. One can then check to ensure that the surgeon graduated from a reputable school. If one recognizes the name of the institution without additional checks, this can mean a reputation for high-quality education, so it may be possible to skip the extra library reference check.

In addition, patients and family members may want to check that the surgeon is board certified. Board certification involves specialized study and testing following a surgeon's entry into practice. One should be sure that the board certification is in the area that pertains to the pending surgery. For example, one would not want a surgeon who is board certified in gastroenterology to perform orthopedic surgery.

There are also factors that are unwritten but that will assist patients with decisions when a choice must be made between several equally appropriate surgeons. Such things as personality or bedside manner can be important to patients and families. Another clue to having selected a fine surgeon will be waiting times for office visits. Most health care providers train office staff not to overbook. In the case of a surgeon, sometimes unexpected emergencies call the surgeon away from office hours. In such cases, the office staff should have been trained to let waiting patients know of any delays and offer the option of making an appointment on another day. If a patient finds the routine waiting room time to be hours to see the surgeon, it may be a sign that the surgeon is overcommitted.

In addition to credentials, it is important to note which local hospitals have granted the physician staff privileges. Most physicians are on the staffs of all of the major hospitals in the area. If the surgeon has limited privileges and can practice only in one facility, a patient needs to explore the reasons for this. Also, health insurers routinely send out, or provide access to, physician provider directories through Web sites. These directories list names, addresses, and staff privileges of physicians in the area. In addition, Web sites usually list physician publications and additional information about areas of individual expertise. In larger cities, there may be hospital consortia that are groups of hospitals managed by one umbrella organization. Health care provider listings will provide details of consortium affiliation.

Major hospitals and health care centers also maintain physician credential files. Fellow physicians maintain these for purposes of oversight. Should the physician practices ever have come under question, particularly within the confines of the hospital, it is likely that notes will have been placed within the files. Groups of senior physicians are able in this way to ensure that physicians practicing at a given institution have sufficient documentation to have privileges revoked should the need arise. Another point to check is whether or not the institution at which the physician has privileges is a participating institution within a patient's insurance plan. All these steps create confidence for the patient and family.

BOX 20-1

CHOOSING A SURGEON

- Trace degree-granting institutions: Universities attended
- Search for publications online
- Is the surgeon board certified?
- Is board certification in the appropriate specialty?
- Staff or admitting privileges: Consistency with insurances?
- Assess bedside manner
- Evaluate office waiting times
- Word of mouth: From trusted others

BOX 20-2

CHOOSING A HOSPITAL OR SURGICAL CENTER

- Preliminary steps: Does the surgeon have privileges?
- Preliminary steps: Will your insurance provide coverage at this facility?
- Size: 300 to 500 beds is usually adequate
- Emergency department: Level I is most experienced
- Is there an ICU in the hospital?
- Does the hospital have Magnet Status?
- Does the hospital have a national reputation?
- Does the advertising emphasis match your needs?
- Is the hospital affiliated with a university?
- Personal observations
- Experiences of acquaintances

Finally, as a last check, word of mouth never hurts. The patient may want to think about a surgeon who is recommended by a trusted other. Family or friends may have reliable information that will assist as the patient makes a decision. If there is a nurse that the patient knows, particularly a nurse educator, it might be time to check impressions with that person. Advocacy is an important part of what nurses do. Sometimes nurses can help form a connection between the patient and a physician.

Selecting a Health Care Facility

There are several types of facilities in which patients have surgery. The hospital is the one that will be most familiar to patients. Box 20-2 lists elements that will assist patients in choosing a health care facility.

In selecting a hospital at which to have surgery, it is usually quite safe for the patient to rely on the health care provider to make a choice. For example, the surgeon is familiar with strengths and weaknesses of local facilities as well as the patient's geographic location. When there are several hospitals from which to choose, the patient might want to examine the facilities individually before confirming the date for surgery with the health care provider. As a first step, perhaps the patient will want to consider the size and age of the facilities in the area. For example, hospitals of less than 100 beds, particularly when located in rural areas, may not have the caliber of resources available to larger hospitals. The financial situation of smaller hospitals is often not as secure as would be the case with larger institutions located in larger cities. However, for minor surgery it is definitely convenient for those in rural areas to rely on the services of their local facility.

At the other end of the continuum would be large hospitals, such as those with over 800 beds. These large hospitals tend to vary in quality. City or county hospitals must absorb the costs of treating the indigent and those without insurance. While this is often buffered by other incentives, it decreases the profit margin for the hospital. Therefore, the hospital may need to decrease expenditures for amenities, such as decorative touches or the ambience in family waiting areas. A patient or family might want to avoid such facilities under normal circumstances. However, the emergency departments of such facilities are usually Level I, or highly skilled at taking in emergency cases with a physician specialist on duty at all hours throughout the week. In comparison with Level II or III emergency departments, Level I centers have considerably more practice in early treatment of even the most seriously injured. This experience creates expertise. And the patient may want to bear in mind that it is the intensive care team or the emergency department team who will respond in case of a code or cardiac arrest in another area of the hospital. Training and experience count in such situations.

With larger hospitals or some of the famous medical centers, such as Sloan Kettering or MD Anderson, their large size is a mark of success. Such facilities often split their joined mini-hospitals but connect them in the same geographic location allowing services to roam and cover a wide range of patient needs.

For the patient's local area, usually a facility of 300 to 500 beds is a safe choice. The size means advantages in frills and services over the small facility. The hospital can afford to have efficient support services, such as sophisticated radiologic diagnostic areas and the best respiratory therapy services. In addition, this type of center usually is able to link in to the latest in care communication technology and changes in care delivery systems as these are developed.

Another factor in choosing a hospital is university affiliation. A landmark work, *Doing better and feeling worse,* says that university-affiliated hospitals that have training programs for interns and residents tend to stay abreast of even the most recent developments in medical care (Knowles, 1977). The care tends to be up-to-date, and patients have several layers of learned individuals reviewing their cases. The problem is that health care providers in training tend to be slightly less efficient at ordering the proper tests, making final decisions, and advising the patient. That is, the patient's hospital stay may be slightly longer. The patient who chooses the university-affiliated hospital should be prepared for some additional delays and perhaps a bit more testing than would routinely take place in another type of facility.

For final consideration, the patient should think about the hospital's focus for advertising. For example, some hospitals advertise their heart center or neuro trauma services. When a facility actually puts a main area forward, it tries to ensure that this service is, indeed, exceptional.

The granting of Magnet Status is another recent trend. The nursing service department of a hospital that has been granted Magnet Status tends toward excellence. In magnet facilities, nursing service attracts and retains the best nurses and practices in cutting-edge ways. For example, following the 1999 report from the Institute of Medicine on the dangers of hospital care in the United States, the Robert Wood Johnson Foundation funded the Transforming Care at the Bedside (RWJF-TCAB) initiative (Robert Wood Johnson Hospital, 2006). Beginning with three carefully selected hospitals, TCAB has now enlarged the base, bringing in dozens of facilities. All share knowledge gained from asking nurses to design changes that will ensure safety and efficacy for hospitalized patients and families. Some of the results are the creation of pocket devices on which nurses can send or receive information, new alerting signals for patients who might be at risk of falling, and the creation of bar code scanning systems to reduce medication errors. Magnet hospitals tend to attract such initiatives. Nursing service leaders want to remain trendsetters and to enhance the reputation of the facility. Therefore change is welcomed, and analysis of improvements is ongoing. The patient who is contemplating surgery may want to consider Magnet Status when choosing a facility.

The patient will often want to make some personal observations prior to selecting a hospital for perioperative care. Once some tentative decisions have been made, the patient may want to visit the hospital or hospitals in which surgery might be planned.

It is suggested that the patient and family take in the atmosphere of the hospital. Useful observations are noted in Box 20-3. They should visit the lobby. Many lobbies tend to be grand and to have a certain resemblance to the hotel lobbies found in larger cities. Is there an information desk? Do the people at the information desk tend to be helpful? Ask to be directed to the hospital cafeteria. Does it seem inviting? Does it offer a variety of foods and have plenty of waitpersons? Or does it resemble the place where you wait while having your car tuned up—some ripped plastic furniture and machines to dispense food and beverages? Even though cosmetic appeal is not everything when a patient and family are setting out to find a good hospital, sometimes, lack of attention to detail in these areas may represent lack of attention to detail in other areas.

The patient should try to take a look at the surgical admitting areas. Do personnel seem friendly and competent? Are there long waiting lines for service? Is there privacy for those who are responding to admission questions (often personal), and is there an attempt to maintain confidentiality in the admitting area? There should be individual cubicles or widely spaced desks at which patients sit to give information. The patient should beware of an admitting area that resembles a bank lobby with long lines and having to stand in front of a cage while giving information.

In relation to confidentiality, while touring the hospital (Box 20-4), the patient might want to look for staff that does not discuss patients among themselves, even in hospital elevators and the cafeteria. Perhaps the patient will want to ride a few elevators or have a snack in the cafeteria. Sit within earshot of a cluster of nurses. There are strict rules against the casual revealing of personal patient or family information. Should a patient or family member hear staff discussing such things, beware. A lack of attention to this on the part of the hospital may signal carelessness or lack of respect for patients in other areas as well.

BOX 20-3

OBSERVATIONS FOR HOSPITAL SELECTION

- Information desk located in lobby?
- Helpful information desk volunteers?
- Inviting cafeteria with selection of food choices?
- Long waiting lines for service?
- Privacy in the admitting area?
- Do personnel discuss patient matters in public areas?
- Are halls dark? Is there equipment cluttering the halls?
- Do staff personnel on hospital units seem rushed or angry?
- Are there dry hand cleaners in halls, and does the staff use them between patients?
- Are patient rooms and bathrooms clean?

BOX 20-4

TOURING A HEALTH CARE FACILITY
- Lobby atmosphere
- Information desk
- Hospital volunteers
- Character of the cafeteria
- Surgery admission areas: Check for long waits, discomfort, or abrupt intake personnel
- Confidentiality: Check elevators and cafeterias for violations
- Hallways: Darkness, clutter, excess noise may indicate problems
- Technology: Is it clean and is patient information protected
- Will you have a private room?
- Rooms: Ambience, a view, and is the bathroom clean?

The patient or family might want to examine the typical medical-surgical hospital unit. Do the hallways seem overly dark? Do the care personnel looked rushed or angry? Is there any shouting going on? Is there a jumble of equipment piled in the hallway? Is there modern dry hand cleaning devices scattered up and down the hallway walls? If the patient lingers in the hallway, will the patient see nurses using these to clean their hands between patients? Even though nurses may wash their hands at in-room sinks, occasional pauses by some of the personnel to use the hallway dispensers is something the casual observer should note. If the patient or family wishes to go to greater lengths, a look at the keyboards of the hallway computers and the telephone receiver sets will reveal whether the unit takes steps to maintain general cleanliness.

The patient should peek into a vacant patient room. Does the patient room seem crowded, or is the wall covering starting to peel? Are the patient rooms private or semiprivate? Many modern hospitals have only private rooms. The private room is generally preferred for obvious reasons. The patient in a private room knows that there will be no one snoring in the next bed and keeping one awake. There will be no concerns about another patient or the patient's visitors overhearing things best kept private. Also, there is no worry about a communicable disease wafting its way into the next bed. The patient should ask at the information desk in the lobby on the way out whether or not the hospital contains solely private rooms.

Next, the patient might want examine the bathroom area. Does the patient room have a clean bathroom area? The patient will want to examine the bathroom as one might at a fine hotel. The patient will want to look for darkness, dirt, or odd, unidentifiable aromas. Mold means problems, not only here, but possibly as a general hospital problem. Is there an easy-to-use emergency call bell anchored on the wall adjacent to the toilet? Does the room have a somewhat modern looking thermostat on the wall? Does it appear to have been taken off the wall a time or two? If so, the patient might anticipate room temperature problems.

Finally, the patient will want to ask friends and associates whether they have ever been patients at the hospital. In most cases, those who have actually spent time there will advise the patient well. Spending days in a hospital bed will make an observer and critic out of even the most even-tempered of individuals. If a friend or associate of the patient says it seemed fine, that is definitely a positive recommendation.

Box 20-4 is a checklist that could be adapted for use by patients or family members when touring a prospective hospital. Knowing of an excellent facility well in advance will be helpful in decreasing feelings of stress when the surgical event is imminent. It also helps the patient and family to prepare articles that might be useful during the hospital stay. The patient playbook feature contains guidelines that will also help when the patient is visualizing the setting. It describes what to bring to the hospital.

Although surgery can be a daunting experience for anyone, careful preparation is most helpful. Patients are advised to select a surgeon who is capable, and a hospital that possesses the right qualities. Planning ahead will give the patient and family confidence.

Categories of Surgical Procedures

Surgery may be categorized according to relative risk: minor or major (Price, 2004). **Major surgery** involves greater than minimal risk to life in some way, such as happens with surgeries involving multiple systems or that require long periods of time in the operating suite. **Minor surgery** involves minimal risk to life, one body system, and minimal incision length and depth. Surgery, major or minor, may also be described as elective surgery, urgent, or emergency surgery. Surgery may be curative or, when it is designed to make the patient more comfortable, palliative in nature. Surgery may be described by body location, as in abdominal surgery, brain surgery, lung surgery, or orthopedic surgery.

In the case of elective surgery, patients and family members have time to plan for the event in advance. In most cases, there is no rushed or urgent feel-

PATIENT PLAYBOOK

What to Bring to the Hospital or Surgicenter

The nurse can advise patients to bring the following with them prior to their surgery:

1. Wallet or purse items: Use these briefly for identification and intake purposes, then send them home with a trusted other while surgery is in progress. Plan to keep a small amount of money at hand for postoperative phases, but surrender it to family just before the surgical event.

2. Clothing: Take something comfortable to wear to and later from the hospital or surgical center, such as a sweat suit or jeans with comfortable shoes. Plan to change into a hospital gown prior to surgery. Do not plan to return to such things as personal pajamas or a nightgown immediately following surgery. If the patient stays in the hospital for a prolonged period, it is estimated that they may be free of bulky dressings, complex intravenous (IV) lines, and other tubes by postoperative day 3 or so. This will be the soonest that the patient would want to consider dispensing with hospital gowns and scrub pants, robe, and charming, skidless, footie slippers. For those having surgery in a short stay surgicenter, the patient will probably return home wearing comfortable, stretchy sweat pants and shirt that same day.

3. Recreational items: If the patient anticipates a hospital stay of greater than two days, plan to bring something relaxing and entertaining. Because the family pet will not be permitted, perhaps magazines or books, needlework, or a handheld electronic game might be nice. However, it may be inadvisable to consider work items as either recreational or relaxing. The laptop, a large sheaf of business documents, and two cell phones might hamper recovery if only through making the patient inaccessible to the nurses.

4. Business items: See # 3.

5. Cell phones: The use of cell phones in proximity to other electronic devices is a subject of rich and varied debate. As long as the patient is in an ordinary hospital room, it is considered safe to have a personal cell phone and a handheld personal data assistant (Grimes, 2005). Draping these things directly on the top of the patient's personal IV pump is not recommended, however. If the patient is in a room in the intensive care unit (ICU) or in a specialized cardiac unit, these devices should be turned off.

6. Jewelry and wristwatches: A good rule of thumb is not to take anything that would be dearly missed if it were lost. Check with the hospital in advance to see if the patient will be permitted to wear his or her wedding band to surgery.

7. A list of home medications (including complete dispensing information available on the labels) or the medications themselves *if* these can then be sent home promptly with a family member or trusted other.

Adapted from Daniels, R. (2004). *Nursing fundamentals: Caring and clinical decision making. New York: Thomson Delmar Learning.*

ing in the days leading to the time of surgery. Although there may be fears or tension, there is also time to adjust. Some of the vital elements of nursing care involve establishing rapport and familiarizing the patient and family with the setting, determining baseline patient status, analyzing internal studies, patient and family teaching, and other preparation, such as giving feedback for patient mastery of postoperative exercises.

Decision Strategies and Informed Consent

Sometimes the decision to undergo surgery is quick and relatively simple. The patient may have been considering the procedure for a time. Occasionally, there is no doubt in the patient's mind that this is the correct course of action to ensure a given state of health. In other cases, the decision is more difficult. Sometimes, it is unclear as to whether the patient possesses capacity to give permission for surgery. Or, the decision is difficult because of relative risk or doubt about the outcome. In any case, all hospitals and clinics should have protocols to ensure that a patient's rights to full information are not violated and to make sure that the patient's signature on the surgical consent form (Figure 20-1) represents full and free agreement rendered after full and free disclosure related to the surgery.

SAMPLE

Standard Consent to Surgery or Special Procedure

Patient Name _____

Attending Physician _____

Surgeon or Supervising Physician _____

1. (*Name of facility*) maintains personnel and facilities to assist your/the patient's physicians and surgeons in their performance of various surgical or other special diagnostic or therapeutic procedures. These operations and procedures may involve risks of unsuccessful results, complications, injury, or death, from known and/or unforeseen causes, and no warranty or guarantee is made as to results or cure.

   You have the right to be informed of such risks as well as the nature of the operation or procedure; the expected benefits of such; and any available alternatives and their risks and benefits. Except in case of emergency, operations or procedures are not performed until you have had the opportunity to receive this information and have given your consent. You have the right to consent or refuse any proposed operation or procedure any time prior to its performance.

2. Your/the patient's physician/surgeon has recommended the operation or procedure set forth below. Upon your authorization and consent, the operation or procedure set forth below, together with any different or further procedures which in the opinion of the supervising physician/surgeon may be indicated due to an emergency, will be performed on you/the patient. The operation or procedure will be performed by the supervising physician or surgeon named above (or in the event of an emergency causing his/her inability to complete the procedure, a qualified substitute supervising physician or surgeon), together with associates and assistants, including anesthesiologists, pathologists and radiologists from the medical staff of (*name of facility*) to whom the supervising physician or surgeon may assign designated responsibilities. The persons in attendance for the purpose of performing specialized medical services such as anesthesia, radiology, or pathology are not agents, servants, or employees of the facility and your/the patient's supervising physician or surgeon, but are independent contractors, and therefore your agents, servants, or employees.

3. The pathologist is hereby authorized to use his/her discretion in disposing any member, organ, or other tissue removed from your/the patient's person during the operation or procedure set forth below.

4. Your signature below constitutes your acknowledgment that: you have read and agree to the foregoing; that the operation or procedure set forth below has been adequately explained to you by the above named physician/surgeon and by your/the patient's anesthesiologist and that you have received all of the information that you desire concerning such operation or procedure; and that you authorize and consent to the performance of the operation or procedure.

Procedure: _____

_____

_____

Signature (Patient/Parent/Conservator/Guardian)   Relationship (if other than patient)

_____

Date   Time   Witness

I have been informed of the risks/benefits and alternatives of blood product infusions. I consent to the use of blood product infusions.

_____

Signature (Patient/Parent/Conservator/Guardian)   Relationship (if other than patient)

_____

Date   Time   Witness

(Name of Facility   (Patient Identification–Stamp)
Address of Facility)

Figure 20-1 Sample of a standard consent to surgery or special procedure form.

The physician is responsible for describing the need for surgery, the surgical procedure, and anticipated risks and recovery time to patients and families. The nurse may concurrently sign that he or she has witnessed a patient's signature on a formal consent form or may be a witness for the patient's signature later and closer to the time of surgery. The nurse will also answer questions and reinforce physician teaching. Figure 20-2 provides a sample of a preoperative checklist. In addition to witnessing the signature that indicates that consent for surgery has been given, the nurse will also assemble all pertinent records, lab and diagnostic results, and other written indicators of the patient's readiness for surgery, and will perform other measures leading to the time of transport to surgery. These are all indicated on a hospital's preoperative checklist.

In some cases, it is necessary for the nurse to act as patient advocate. The reader will note that nurse advocacy is important in the preoperative period. It has been noted that this is often a stressful period in which patients and family members are particularly vulnerable. As an example of a situation in which a nurse might be involved in advocacy, consider the following situation. Occasionally, a patient may have a change of heart and may want to alter a decision previously made to have surgery. The patient may have signed a consent form but now wants to refuse to have surgery. The nurse will often be first to know and to transmit this information to the surgical team. The patient should never be urged by the nursing staff to go forward with the surgery in such cases. The patient is in the midst of a particularly vulnerable time and will need the nurse to be a neutral party who can bring in additional expertise when such moments arise. The nurse is the first-line patient advocate.

In cases in which simple clarification is needed, the nurse provides additional information requested by the patient about the day of surgery or the aftermath of the event. Some patients will want intensive teaching about the actual events of the day of surgery while others will prefer to simply have it unfold. One of the nurse's jobs will be to carefully assess how much information is needed and wanted and how rapidly or deeply it should be delivered. Again, acting as advocate, the nurse will ensure that each patient has sufficient information but will not pelt the patient with more than is desired or than can be absorbed. Sometimes, the nurse will question whether or not a recently sedated patient is capable of giving informed, written consent. Or in the case of family members acting in a patient's interests, the nurse must mediate when there are conflicting views or emotions. In all of these, the nurse tries to act as an advocate for the patient.

In most cases, the decision to have surgery rests squarely with the patient. In cases in which the patient is not competent to make the decision, there are avenues for making this decision on the patient's behalf. The hospital's risk management team or ethics committee can be of assistance when there is doubt or when additional expertise is needed to determine proper guardianship or who should sign a consent form on the patient's behalf. Using the hospital's chain of command will ensure that the bedside care nurse has appropriate support when there are questions.

Time Frames and Tasks

In addition to making the decision to have elective surgery, there are other tasks for the patient and family in the time leading to the day of surgery. Sometimes these involve spiritual measures. At other times, there may be personal or legal matters to be taken care of prior to the day of surgery. Many patients want to have their affairs in order. This plan can relieve the patient and family of worry in the hours before surgery. The next sections describe some of the timing for preparation measures leading to the day of surgery.

If there is sufficient time, it is wise for the patient to adopt healthy dietary, rest, and exercise habits, even if these mean a change in lifestyle. However, it is questionable as to whether the patient who has spent a lifetime outside the bounds of moderation could or should try to rapidly turn around long-standing

	CK (✓)	COMMENTS	NURSE CK (✓)
COMPLETE NIGHT BEFORE SURGERY			
List allergies			
Procedure scheduled			
Surgical permit signed/witnessed			
History/physical on chart and/or dictated			
Preanesthetic evaluation done			
Able to state type and purpose			
Demonstrates ability to perform: Deep breathing, turning and coughing exercises			
Leg exercises			
P.M. care with shower or bath given			
Nail polish removed and makeup removed			
Old chart requested and obtained			
Type and crossmatch for _____ units of blood			
Blood consent signed and witnessed			
Labor work a. CBC _____ b. UA _____			
Tonsillectomy and adenoidectomy patients: a. ___PTT b. ___PT c. ___Platelets			
If ordered by MD: a. ECG ___ b. Chest X-ray ___			
Add other lab work ordered (specify)			
Notify surgeon of abnormal lab work			
New progress note and physician order sheet on chart			
Weight			
NPO after midnight (if applicable)			
Signature of Nurse _____		Date _____	
COMPLETE DAY OF SURGERY			
Jewelry removed and secured with responsible party			
Dental prosthesis and contact lenses removed			
Voided on call to surgery			
Indwelling catheter ordered and inserted			
Tampon removed			
Identiband and/or bloodband on/checked for accuracy			
Time _____ Pulse _____ Resp _____ B/P _____ Temp. _____			
Pre-op medicine given medication _____ Time _____ AM PM			
Siderails up and bed to lowest level			
Patient instructed not to get out of bed without nursing assistance			
Addressograph plate/MARs on chart			
VS 30 minutes after pre-op (if remains on unit)			
BP _____ P _____ R _____ T _____			
Old chart sent to surgery per request			
Surgical prep done and checked			
To surgery Time _____ Via _____			
Signature of Nurse _____		Date _____	
Holding Room Nurse Signature _____		Date _____	

Figure 20-2 Preoperative checklist.

habits. For example, the patient who is markedly overweight will want to eat nutritious meals but should not be advised to suddenly cut calories in an overly rigorous way. The patient who has spent a lifetime in sedentary activities should not be advised to suddenly take up jogging in the two days prior to surgery. Moderately healthy living, including rest, will be beneficial for those who are to undergo surgery.

Usually, whether the patient is admitted to the hospital prior to surgery or enters into the surgical situation as a short-stay patient, thorough health status information and health history will be gathered. The nurse will elicit information about each patient's medical diagnosis and the reason for surgery as well as what type of surgery is planned.

In addition, the nurse will obtain thorough information about complicating factors, such as past illnesses, injuries, congenital disorders, and past surgeries. Information about chronic metabolic disorders (diabetes, arthritis, or hypertension), the effects of aging in the individual, underweight or overweight problems, addiction, or psychiatric disorders will be necessary to safely guide the patient through surgery (Altman & Taylor, 2004). Information about food, airborne, and drug allergies should be elicited.

Of recent interest is the problem of latex allergy (Price, 2004). This is a reaction to proteins found within natural rubber and can have serious consequences. In fact, deaths have been attributed to allergic reactions to the latex in anesthesia equipment or other products located within the surgical suite. Such adverse occurrences were more prevalent prior to discovery of this type of reaction to even the latex proteins found in more traditional types of rubber gloves. The nurse should be vigilant about eliciting information about latex allergy.

Patients should be asked about previous adverse surgical events, such as reactions to anesthesia or particularly traumatic surgical experiences (Altman & Taylor, 2004). Of particular importance is prior cardiac disease, such as angina, heart attack, or congestive heart failure. Prior pulmonary problems, such as smoking history or chronic pulmonary disorders, also require special handling around the time of surgery. Patients and families should communicate this information in cases in which the initial screening activities were interrupted or whenever the presurgical interview is less than complete. The nurse should make every effort to set a tone of empowerment for the patient and the family. Patients should be given confidence that their views and their information are important to those who will care for them. In this way, the conveying of important information is unlikely to be quashed by patients who do not want to seem bothersome.

For those patients who are on medications for chronic problems, such as hypertension, hypercholesterolemia, diabetes mellitus, or arthritis, the medication regimen will usually remain unchanged prior to the day of surgery. Patients should plan to bring a complete listing of medications, including dosages, timing, and routes of administration with them to the initial interview or intake into the hospital. Another method of conveying complete information would be to bring the actual medication containers, complete with pharmacy labels, to the hospital or clinic for recording in the medical record prior to surgery (Figure 20-3).

As noted earlier in the chapter, it will be particularly important for the person who uses herbal remedies or nontraditional medicine to reveal similar information about types of remedies, amounts, timing, and routes of administration. Sometimes, patients do not think of herbal substances as having affects such as prescribed medications. But, the course of anesthesia and patient physiological responses during surgery may be influenced by alternative therapy. The nurse should ensure that the agency protocols include questions related to preoperative patients' use of nontraditional substances, such as herbal remedies.

Finally, the patient and family should consider whether or not they would want to donate blood designated for use by the patient during or following

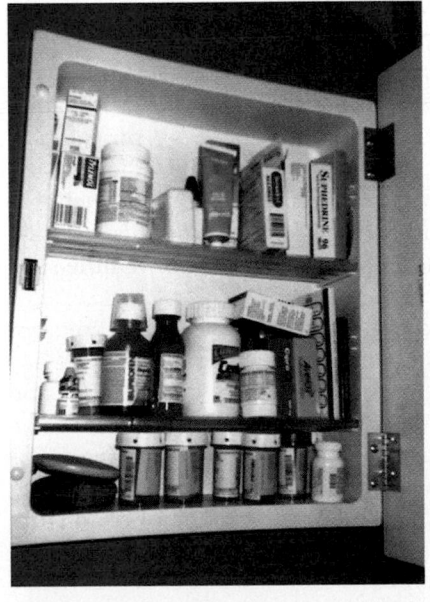

Figure 20-3 It is important to ask the patient which prescription and OTC medications are used.

Preoperative Telephone Contact

For patients and family members who are at home awaiting surgery, there are sometimes needs that arise during the evening or night hours. Patients should not hesitate to telephone when needs arise. To ensure that the call is a positive one and results in prompt meeting of a patient's needs, the following list may be helpful.

- The physician's telephone number will be listed on the physician's business card, the preoperative instruction sheets, or in the telephone book.
- A second telephone number should be that of a 24-hour pharmacy located near the patient's residence. This can be given to the physician to enhance communications.
- The patient should not fear that the actual surgeon will be awakened in the middle of the night. One of the physician team members who does not have surgery responsibilities the next day will be designated to respond to such calls.
- The patient will not need to try to meet somewhere to pick up prescriptions. The designated physician on call can telephone prescriptions for sleeping medications to a 24-hour pharmacy. Most physicians' offices also have electronic means of forwarding prescriptions to the pharmacy.
- The patient who needs to contact the physician's office should have allergy information readily at hand prior to making the call.

Adapted from Daniels, R. (2004). Nursing fundamentals: Caring and clinical decision making. New York: Thomson Delmar Learning; Estes, M. (2006). Health assessment and physical examination (3rd ed.). New York: Thomson Delmar Learning.

surgery. The patient may donate blood for later use, or family members may designate their donated blood for later use by the patient. The hospital or local blood bank has guidelines about timing prior to surgery and procedures for directed donation. They will be able to advise whether or not there is sufficient time for a patient to recover from blood donation by the day of surgery. The patient should not donate within 72 hours prior to surgery but may be able to donate as often as every three days prior to the 72-hour cutoff time. Some patients will need advice from their health care provider before donating. The patient and family will want to discuss preferences should predonated blood supplies be insufficient to meet needs. Again, nurses or blood bank personnel will be able to deliver information or refer the patient to those who can. A section within the informed consent documents will ask for patient preferences in relation to blood transfusion.

For certain types of surgery in which mobility will be affected or in which recovery will call for active and specialized participation by patients and families, education will be necessary. Examples of these types of surgery would be major orthopedic surgery, such as total hip replacement or total knee replacement, or organ transplantation in which survival depends on a strict postoperative regimen with exact compliance and relatively sophisticated, daily self-assessment. In these cases, the nurse and others will call patients and families in for educational sessions, often conducted with others who will be learning prior to their own pending surgeries.

Many disciplines use group educational sessions. For the orthopedic patient, the nurse will describe care centering on the surgical experience. Pain management techniques including use of patient controlled analgesia devices will be described. The nurse will have patients practice postoperative positioning and repositioning techniques designed to minimize discomfort. The nurse will discuss the usual timeline for anticipated recovery events or recovery trajectory. The physical and occupational therapists will demonstrate use of specialized orthopedic devices, such as pillows designed to maintain limbs in alignment following hip surgery or continuous passive motion machines to exercise knees following replacement of joints. Physical therapists and occupational therapists will have patients practice putting on shoes and socks without deep bending, and using appliances to pick up objects on the floor while recovery is in progress. Dietitians usually participate in these sessions by eliciting patient dietary preferences, advising on diet in the weeks leading to surgery, and encouraging family members to supply the patient with favorite foods once the immediate postoperative period allows.

For those who will undergo organ replacement, there are several visits to the medical center at which the surgery will take place. In addition to batteries of tests designed to map the patient's physical status and likely postsurgical needs, psychological evaluation plays an important role in predicting and managing the patient's course of recovery. The patient also practices analyzing daily lab results and making medication decisions based on this analysis. Patients are taught signs of crisis and measures to take to avert or handle such postprocedure emergencies.

For all patients who undergo surgery, a preliminary visit to the hospital or outpatient setting offers familiarization and comfort later. Nurses should make every effort to convey a sense of welcome and empowerment to patients and families. The feelings of security generated by early encounters will often improve the postoperative experience. In addition to gathering setting information prior to need, the family or patient should drive to the hospital or outpatient setting at the approximate time of day that will coincide with arrival purposes on the day of admission. Timing the trip, locating parking, and visualizing the journey will ease unnecessary anxiety when the actual day arrives.

In addition to familiarizing themselves with the hospital in general, patients and families should ask for directions to the cafeteria, gift shop, or chapel. They may want to visit the unit to which the patient will be transferred following release from the recovery room, also known as the PACU (pronounced pack-you). Locating the kitchenette, visitor lounge, soda machines, and even the restrooms will make orientation for the family much easier when the actual surgical date arrives. Rules are usually posted or can be obtained from the information desk if there will be children visiting the recovering patient.

Families should look for a posted listing titled, The Patient Bill of Rights. It lists all of the things that are to be expected within the walls of the hospital or outpatient setting, such as the right to information, the expectation of preservation of dignity, and the right to see and have explained all hospital billing charges.

Families are advised to check on other matters when visiting the setting in which surgery will be performed and recovery will take place. Whether the surgery is expected to be minor or major, recovery time rapid or prolonged, it is wise to make use of this visit to prepare. Making a list can help focus the patient during what may be an emotional time.

It is wise to find out where to wait for word that the surgery is complete. In some settings, there is a specially designated surgery waiting room. In other hospitals or clinics, the family is expected to wait in the patient's assigned room. Knowing the appropriate place will ensure that the health care provider will also be able to locate the family when the surgery is over. Visiting the appropriate room well ahead of the day of surgery will point the way to coming to the experience with adequate supplies and such things as family comfort foods or other things to occupy the waiting time.

The family should select a family spokesperson to receive information and convey it outward from the hospital to other family members not present. Sometimes two or more persons will be selected for support roles for the patient and for communication purposes. The centralized or one-person communication role is particularly important to ensure that nurses are able to devote maximum time to patient care. That is, nurses are easily able to give progress reports and bulletins to one or two family members, but they may encounter serious time drains if calls for information are too numerous or too frequent.

It is recommended that patients pack well in advance of the trip to the clinic or hospital. It is also recommended that the patient leave valuables at home or be prepared to give them to a trusted other rather than leave them in a bedside table or elsewhere in the hospital room. Patients should take only enough items for a short stay. Family or others will be able to retrieve additional necessities at a later time. In this way, should the patient be transferred, for example, to the ICU, in which personal belongings will not usually be permitted, the family need not take a large number of items home.

Whether the patient remains at home on the day before surgery or will be within hospital walls, it is important to recognize the need to carry through with preparations and to ensure adequate comfort and rest. Family members or close friends are often essential in fostering feelings of comfort on the day and evening before surgery. It makes sense for them to avoid certain topics of conversation and to restrict the number and duration of their visits. The 24-hour period before surgery is an excellent time to go over preparations for pet care or absence from work or other responsibilities. Reassurance that everything is covered will ease the minds of many patients. Reminiscing may also help during a time when patients' thoughts sometimes turn to worrying about what types of problems could occur.

In addition to psychosocial needs, patients are usually given instructions to perform certain tasks to help them prepare physically for surgery. Taking an evening shower with special soap or a mild and nonirritating soap is sometimes called for. In the past, when patients were all routinely hospitalized on the day before surgery, a technician would arrive in a hospital room to scrub and shave the patient in a wide swath encompassing the surgical area. More recently, such preparations have been shown to be unnecessary and even counterproductive. Thorough skin cleaning during a shower or at the sink with nonirritating soap solution is considered the best way to decrease microbial colony counts.

Because anesthesiologists and surgeons prefer to examine the patient and review preoperative laboratory results and other studies close to the time of surgery, they may routinely visit their hospitalized patients on the evening before surgery. Surgical consent forms are usually reviewed and signed at this time. Families and patients should know that there is a legal requirement for the physician to fully disclose the nature of the surgery and the risks involved with the patient's particular type of surgery. The same holds true for any anesthesia that may be used. Finally, the patient is presented with alternatives to surgery before the physician reaches the point at which a patient signature may be affixed to the surgical consent form. Often, it is the nurse who witnesses the patient's signature. The nurse as witness is noting that the patient is capable of giving consent at the time of signature and coercive measures have not been used to elicit consent.

The nurse's role as patient advocate is necessary during preoperative nursing management. Sometimes, surgeons believe that the surgery or other procedure is highly necessary for patient survival or quality of life. Or, perhaps the physician or surgeon will be trying to use well-practiced techniques for assuaging a patient's possible anxieties. An example would be the oncology, or cancer, specialist who truly believes that an experimental treatment will provide an extension of life of high quality for a potentially terminally ill patient. This health care provider may downplay the potential risks or miseries of undergoing the procedure. Usually, though, surgeries and special procedures fall into the category of routine.

Perhaps nothing is as unpopular with patients on the evening before surgery as the directive to eat a liquid supper or to have nothing by mouth (NPO) after midnight. A problem sometimes arises when the patient faithfully follows these instructions only to find that surgery will be delayed until the next afternoon or beyond. Understanding that this sometimes happens will help the patient and family not to feel quite so disappointed. Sometimes anxious patients and families construe these delays to mean problems with hospital operations or that the surgical services are second-rate. Usually, a postponement in surgery is related to a surgical emergency that cannot wait.

Although a surgery schedule will come out the day before surgery, and the approximate time of surgery may be derived from the schedule, it is important to interpret this information with a seasoned eye. Families should be made aware that the transporter will arrive at least an hour before the scheduled time of the surgery. Many a spouse or sibling has arrived in the patient's room at 6:45 a.m. for a procedure scheduled to start at 7:00 a.m., only to find that the patient was rolled to the surgery holding area at 6:00 a.m. It is important for the nurse to volunteer this information so that patients and families can prepare. To miss those last few moments together can be devastating for a family member or other visitor.

Another important preparation for those patients who are to undergo a procedure involving a particular side of the body, such as knee replacement, will be marking and confirming which side is to be the operative side. This should be done while the patient is alert and competent to confirm the location. If the patient is not competent, then a spouse, parent, guardian, or family designee will be consulted. When unsure of guardianship or the appropriateness of a family member in confirming location, the nurse will use the agency's chain of command to elicit the appropriate procedure to be followed.

Finally, patients and families should be aware that many patients are restless on the evening and night before surgery. The pending loss of control over one's physical self, perhaps combined with fear of death, will make even the most stoic individual unable to sleep well. Therefore, sleeping medications are routinely prescribed for most patients. Patients and families may be safely reassured that taking such a medication will not lead to addiction and that most do not have significant side effects, particularly when taken to deal with a specific episode. It should be kept in mind that sleeping medications, even those with which a repeat dose is prescribed, will usually not be permitted after 2:00 a.m. in most hospitals. However, should the patient be wide awake at 3:00 a.m. following only a few hours of sleep and with a 10:00 a.m. surgery time, the nurse will contact the physician on call to request a short-acting medication.

For those who might have trouble sleeping on the eve of surgery, many hospitals have invested in modified air flotation mattresses that can be set to perfectly comfort any aching joints or to cradle the preoperative patient. In addition, with the press of a button, the head and foot ends of hospital beds can be raised or lowered by the patient to achieve additional comfort. Should the patient or family member notice that the bed in their assigned room has an uncomfortable mattress, that individual should be encouraged to request a different mattress.

For those who will spend the evening before surgery at home, there should be no hesitation in calling the physician's office at any time of night. The Patient Playbook carries instructions maximizing the effectiveness of this type of preoperative communication.

On arrival, the patient's insurance and social information will be recorded, unless this has been done previously. A hospital name band will be placed around the patient's wrist. For those who have donated blood or who have designated donations from family, a special tag will usually have been given to the patient. Nursing personnel should note such an arrangement in the medical record when the patient arrives at the hospital or clinic room.

Intake personnel will want to know about advance directives or who might hold power of attorney to act on the patient's behalf. If the patient or family member has appropriate documents relating to such directives, these will be copied and placed in a prominent section of the medical record. The nurse should make an additional note that all previous documents are contained within the medical record or chart.

Patients are routinely placed on NPO status. This indicates that they are to have no food or water by mouth. There has been debate recently about how far in advance of scheduled surgery the patient is to be placed on NPO status. A discussion about recent evidence-based practice findings related to maintaining an empty stomach prior to surgery can be found in chapter 22.

Patients may be asked to take an additional shower on the morning of surgery. Patients will be asked to change into a hospital gown. The gowns are designed to allow easy access to various parts of the patient's body. Also, gowns are made of inert material, unlikely to react with substances found in the surgical suite and unlikely to produce local burns should current be used in the act of resuscitation.

The nurse in the hospital room or intake area will sometimes place an IV catheter into the patient's arm. Most nurses who prepare patients for surgery are experienced at starting these. In some cases, the intern or resident will do so once the patient reaches the preoperative area, known as the anteroom. Preoperative medications may later be given through the IV line. Sometimes, the surgeon will want a dose of an antibiotic to be given to prevent infection later on. Preoperative relaxant agents may be given through the IV line, as may preliminary anesthesia once the patient has been received in the surgical suite.

Meanwhile, prior to the time when the patient goes to surgery, the patient's name band will be checked and the patient may again be asked about allergies. In addition, the patient will be asked to remove jewelry. Some facilities will permit a taped-down wedding band to remain. Others do not. Depending on the surgical area, the patient may be asked to remove all underwear.

Close to the time of surgery, a bladder catheter may be inserted to continually drain the bladder during and after surgery. This may be done for the purposes of exact measurement of urinary output, because the lower abdominal area will be subject to swelling or pressure as the result of surgery, or because the surgeon wants to prevent undue pain for the patient who would otherwise have to frequently reposition to urinate following surgery. The nurse should remember that some patients are given the equivalent of a gallon or more of liquid intravenously during surgery. Bladder catheters can be helpful in the short term.

Once preparations are complete, the nurse leaves for a time and later returns to alert the patient that the operating room has called. This will be the time when the nurse will direct the uncatheterized patient to use the bathroom. The nurse ensures that this final bathroom trip takes place prior to the administration of any preoperative medication. Once the preoperative medication has been given, the nurse will instruct the patient to stay in bed. The call light will be placed within easy reach, and the patient will be instructed to use it to call the nurse should a need arise. Under no circumstances should the patient try to navigate around the hospital room following the administration of preoperative medications, because these are usually a powerful combination of analgesics and muscle relaxants.

Family may stay with the patient on the day of surgery until the patient arrives at the door to the surgical suites. In some hospitals a family member may be allowed to stay with the patient in the surgery anteroom. The nurse and transporter will know the time when the family member must be left behind. In the case of children, a parent will often stay with the child until the time when anesthesia is administered.

Planning and Implementation

The nurse's role in preparing any patient for surgery will involve a range of activities. These include:
- A keen awareness of safety considerations.
- Physical assessment of the patient.
- Assessment of the environment.
- An awareness of best practices.

The perioperative nurse's role extends to planning the activities involved in preparing the patient before surgery, supporting the patient during surgery, and assisting the patient in recovering from surgery. These nurses are accomplished specialists, who ensure that the surgery environment is safe and is ready to handle the particular types of surgery scheduled for the day. A member of the surgical nursing team will ensure that those who are to perform surgery that day are given the tools and environment that will foster successful outcomes for all patients. The perioperative nurse also performs checks to ensure that the environment remains safe throughout the day for each patient. The nurse may have met the patient and family during a preliminary visit to an outpatient center or same day surgery center. They may follow up after the surgical event with visits to the patient's room, if the patient must spend time in the hospital or may telephone to check personally with patient or family on the status of each surgical patient after discharge.

In cases in which surgical technicians perform some of the direct assistive activities in and around surgery, the nurse acts as manager and observer. It is the nurse's job to assess the environment, to ensure that supplies and personnel are ready and available, and to perform certain legally mandated activities. Descriptions of roles and associated tasks will be addressed more explicitly in chapter 21.

The patient and family will interact with others prior to the day of surgery. There will be a need for the health care provider or office staff to inform the hospital or clinic of pending surgery and for the facility's specialists to contact insurers to ascertain financial coverage for the surgery. When the government will be involved as insurer, such as with patients covered under Medicare or Medicaid, the hospital or clinic will be able to ensure coverage well before the day of surgery. Patients should be informed that this is being done and to call the hospital or clinic registration area should there be questions or any doubts about the process. Also, it may be helpful later, in the case of billing disputes or secondary insurers not being notified, for patients to know the name and telephone number of the manager of this area of the hospital or clinic. This will help with consistency should the patient need to telephone to correct any billing or insurance errors.

On the day of surgery or the day before, an intake specialist will prepare a one-page document that will list basic information about the patient, such as next of kin or religious preference. This one-page document will be placed at the front of the medical record for use during the time the patient is there. A medical record number will be assigned and an armband placed. The patient should check for correct spelling of name on the armband and that the band fits relatively comfortably before leaving the intake area of the facility. Another band can be produced within a short time if needed.

The next person who might be encountered will be a hospital or clinic volunteer. This person will escort the patient and family to the preoperative room. This is usually a private room or cubicle. In some instances, particularly with patients for whom only a short stay is anticipated, the volunteer will stop to weigh and measure the patient on the way to the room.

On entry into the preoperative room, a nurse or someone designated as an assistive person by the hospital or clinic will visit the patient. This person will take temperature and measure blood pressure and pulse. The assistive person may invite the patient to change into a hospital gown. The patient may or may not be instructed to remove jewelry or other foreign objects at this time.

When preoperative needs arise, the patient or family member may call on the correct person. Assistive personnel have a variety of titles. Training for such personnel varies from institution to institution. Assistive personnel may be called nursing assistants (NAs), clinical assistants (CAs), or unlicensed assistive personnel. Another title is that of technician, implying a greater degree of training and a skill level involving capability of using some of the more sophisticated types of equipment. But the person who interprets, analyzes, and acts based on findings from the assistive personnel is always the registered nurse (RN). State laws mandate that the nursing assessment and analysis take place within hours of admission to an acute care setting and that the assessment and analysis of findings be done by an RN, licensed to practice in the state.

Various specialists take on other preoperative roles and functions. For example, radiologic technicians perform chest X-rays. Venipuncture, or blood drawing, may be needed close to the time of surgery or may have been done within the recent past before admission to the hospital or clinic. Venipuncture may be performed by unlicensed assistive personnel connected with the intake unit, or by phlebotomists whose role is solely to draw blood. Other specialists might include the physical therapist who, in the case of pending orthopedic surgery, may assess and measure the patient for crutches. Members of the clergy might also want to visit, particularly if the patient expressed such an interest at intake time. Housekeeping staff frequently circulate through the hallways and enter the room to tidy up or clean.

A recent trend is that of keeping a log. Frequently family members pack a small notebook with the other things that will be taken to the hospital. This can serve several purposes. Should the family later want to thank certain personnel by name, they will be able to refer to the notebook for correct spelling or for the name of the nurse manager to whom they might write. In addition, some will record date and time of routine events that occur. This recording can be helpful, for instance, in the case of a new medication with an uncertain effect. The family can then consult notes to recall the name of the wonderful new medicine at a future time, or in another case, the terrible medicine that was given before the patient developed a rash. While patients will later have full access to their entire medical record from any hospitalization, sometimes it is helpful to refer to handwritten and familiar notes to supplement what is in the medical record. Patients and family members tend to keep more detailed notes or to notice events and atmosphere in a more riveting way than hospital or clinic personnel for whom things tend to fall into the category of familiar routine.

Nurses should not be offended by the note-taking family. Because dangers abound in modern hospitals, vigilance at the bedside is important. Most seasoned nurses welcome this extra layer of protection. Many nurses have been saved from folly by patient comments such as, "I thought the doctor said I'd be getting two little pills before I went down to surgery." The nurse should remind families and patients that they may ask for what is needed at any time. Should surgery be delayed, personnel can contact the surgical manager for updated forecasts, including probable time for surgery. The patient and family have every right to be informed about this important matter.

From the family's point of view, the role of all preoperative personnel will be to ensure safety, to eliminate unnecessary stress, to try to enhance the patient's ability to come through surgery successfully, and to make the patient and family feel welcome and well cared for, particularly during the initial intake period.

Developing a caring relationship with the patient is necessary. Surgery usually involves some degree of stress for the patient and family; therefore, it is important for the nurse to set a tone of competence and understanding. It is helpful for patient and family to know from the outset that the nurse will be there to support them and to ensure safety at all times. These functions begin with establishing initial rapport and continue through all of the events as the patient comes closer to the doors of the surgical suite.

There are many ways in which the nurse can maximize patient communication and feelings of comfort. One of the first is in observing and asking. The hospital or clinic nurse should look for signs of relaxation, or conversely, anxiety. It is important to validate this with the patient. If the patient confirms feelings of stress or anxiety, it is imperative to ascertain the source of the feelings.

There are several ways in which the nurse can foster effective communication with any patient, particularly with a patient on the verge of surgery. Smiling when first meeting the patient conveys a sense of openness and welcome. Of course, there will be situations in which this is unwise, such as in the presence of a patient in great pain. It is also prudent to maintain a certain distance when talking. The nurse should not touch the patient in an overly familiar way. The nurse should refrain from addressing patients or family members by their first names, as many people would feel disrespected. When in doubt, the nurse should be a little more conservative, or formal, in perioperative situations. The nurse should not take a chance on offending.

Finally, because some level of education and familiarization with the environment is necessary, the nurse should elicit information about the preoperative patient's readiness to learn. Readiness to learn is covered in greater depth in the perioperative teaching sections of chapter 22. Readiness to learn can be determined in several ways. The first is to ask the patient how much he or she already knows about the surgery, the agenda for the day of surgery, and the activities to be practiced for the time after surgery is complete. In this way, the nurse can determine appropriate level of teaching and how much detail will work best with each patient. This tailoring of information helps to individualize care and assist the patient in their care.

The nurse's job continues with assessment of the patient. First, the nurse will become familiar with the patient's past health history, including previous illnesses, previous surgeries, and the patient's current health problems. The health history may already be available in written form, sent from the health care provider's office or recorded in the clinic or outpatient setting at an earlier time, or as part of an intake interview with the patient or family. As part of the process of assessing past history, the nurse will determine how the patient and family feel about pending surgery. In cases in which there were any untoward occurrences from past medical or surgical treatment, the nurse should ensure that this is passed along so that the surgical team will be aware. In that way, the repeating of past unfortunate episodes can be avoided, and in cases in which complications might recur, preventive steps can be taken. Knowing the patient's and family's view will also help nursing staff to provide an extra measure of emotional support when needed.

As part of the health history, the nurse will ensure recording of any chronic diseases or other conditions that will have a bearing on ability to withstand the physical stresses of surgery. Careful recording of allergies to foods, drugs, or things inhaled will also ensure that a safe environment is provided for the patient. The nurse should assess for latex allergy. It is also important to record potentially complicating factors, such as diabetes, overweight or underweight, past or current alcohol or drug abuse, or past or current psychiatric disorders (Taylor & Altman, 2004).

As the nurse continues with the intake interview, it is wise to recall patient statements about past health matters. In this way, when the nurse physically examines the patient, there will be an opportunity pay closer attention to those body areas that are indicated by past history or patient statements about current difficulties. While the health history elicits areas for closer examination, the review of systems proceeds in a structured way to elicit information about current patient problem areas. Usually, the nurse proceeds in head-to-toe fashion, asking questions about status on day of surgery. Phrasing this in terms of what the patient said during the most recent review of systems will speed the process along. For example, the nurse might ask if there have been any changes in hearing or vision lately or anything to report from the latest time the patient was interviewed. The nurse would then ask the patient about any recent changes in sleeping patterns or attention span or the like. The nurse might then move on to the next head-neck area, and, in that way, proceed downward through the body, ending at the toes.

In conjunction with or following the review of systems, the nurse will continue to assess the patient. Physical assessment usually progresses in the same head-to-toe fashion, as did the review of systems. However, because this is a surgical patient, the nurse will direct the major part of assessment toward two areas: the part of the body on which surgery will be performed and any of the body systems that will be involved with anesthesia. In chapter 21, there will be a discussion of the types of anesthesia, including local anesthesia, regional anesthesia, spinal anesthesia, and general anesthesia. Prior to reporting in for surgery, most patients will have been told what type of anesthesia is planned. In the case of any surgery, however, there is the possibility that general anesthesia could be needed. Therefore, the nurse should carefully and specifically assess the cardiovascular and respiratory systems to establish a baseline for comparison should general anesthesia be required. The same is true for baseline cognition, memory, and neurosensory function.

It is important for the nurse to consider the family during the preoperative and intraoperative period. This section deals with the nurse's need to know the patient and the family along several dimensions: individual, social, cultural, in terms of family role relationships, and from the perspective of age.

Nurses often use an inclusive, holistic model of patient care. That is, nurses consider patients' responses to illness and always consider the individual to be more than the sum of atoms, molecules, or body systems. Depending on patients' needs, consideration may range from entire physical systems, such as circulatory or neurological; to tissue level, as when the nurse reads a histology report; or to cellular or even ionic level, as when the nurse examines potassium level. Nurses strive to understand the families within which their patients live. Nurses work with the societies that humanity builds, the sociocultural context in which people are found, and the summative properties of people as individuals.

The nurse working in the United States may be expected to work with a range of cultures (Estes, 2006). The nurse may work with the foreign visitor or with the Native American who adheres to a set of cultural mores far different

Respecting Our Differences

Preoperative Cultural Considerations

Leininger and McFarland (2006) noted that every society has certain values and norms. Values are things that are desirable. Norms are rules of behavior. That is, each culture has expected interpretations for ways in which people behave. The preoperative nurse will be able to develop trust and rapport through understanding and respecting a variety of cultural values and norms.

The preoperative nurse who ignores a culture's values and norms may inadvertently heighten a patient's feelings of uncertainty or stress during a naturally tense time. When the nurse makes assumptions about the sociocultural context in which a patient lives or works, they may also overlook important patient needs. For example, the nurse may be astonished that the kindly older patient with whom she developed such rapport and who has recently recovered from surgery has no clothes in the closet in the room. The nurse might later discover that the patient lives under one of the city's bridges, has to take a taxi to the bridge when discharged, and must be assisted to select used clothing from the closet maintained in the emergency department.

In another case, the nurse who is oblivious to signs of disrespect in any one of a number of Asian cultures may consistently loom over the patient in a way that denotes ignorance of height considerations as marks of respect. Another cultural consideration for an Asian patient is to point the toe at a treasured patient possession, such as a cherished pair of slippers, thereby demeaning the article. For a Western-educated nurse, this may mean little, but for the patient or family, it could mean a great deal.

---

from those of the European. The nurse may care for a child of an immigrant family or the senior member of an Asian-Pacific Islander family. The Respecting Our Differences provides examples of patients with specialized cultural needs or habits related to socioeconomic differences.

There have been a number of books written that explain the ways of other cultures. The preoperative nurse may want to become familiar with some of the basic tenets of acceptable behavior of those from other cultures (Cioffi, 2005). During times of tension in health care situations, such knowledge is invaluable.

The preoperative nurse should be familiar with the role the patient plays within the family circle. It takes only a short period of assessment to become familiar with the patient's immediate family and, therefore, the patient's concerns during a period of incapacitation. In Western culture, the father is expected to be strong and stoic. School-aged children visiting their hospitalized mother may dread the period during which their mother will be away. Or the mother may be troubled by feelings that all will not be well with her children.

While these things may seem obvious, it is surprising how often the busy nurse overlooks signs of discomfort stemming from the patient's worries about fulfilling an expected role within the family. Sometimes, when the nurse has an opportunity to make visiting family members feel more comfortable, ignoring their presence may inadvertently project signs of coldness to visiting family members. As society becomes more complex, the nurse who works around surgical cases will do well to tap into the varied electronic resources that assist in the development of a culturally appropriate and role-honoring persona that blends well with patient needs.

Preoperative nurses should be aware of changes throughout the life span. For the young patient who occasionally comes through surgical settings designed for adults, there is a need for the nurse to recognize comfort needs and age-related assessment and preparation requirements. When possible, children should remain with parents through the time of initiation of anesthesia. Parents may be encouraged to bring some familiar objects for the child who is awaiting surgery. Some hospitals encourage visits before the day of surgery so that the parents and child can visualize the setting. This is a good time to show the variety of toys and other amusements that are available in preoperative areas frequented by children.

In contrast, for elderly patients, pace is important. Although hospital personnel have a tendency to move quickly to be efficient, they should slow their pace when working with elderly patients. Positioning for comfort and attending to joint pains can be challenging as the preoperative waiting time stretches on. Sometimes, providing extra pillows can enhance comfort when using hospital beds or modified stretchers. Inviting family to walk around in nearby halls with patients can ease positional discomfort.

For those patients who are beyond child and teen years but have not yet reached retirement age, other factors may concern them. Those with children at home may have concerns over parenting while one parent is "out of action." For those who are employed outside the home, there is the nagging concern sometimes that the job needs the person, and that hospitalization is interrupting possibly in an irretrievable way.

The patients that are in the preoperative phase may have decisional conflict and disturbed sleep patterns preoperatively. A preoperative nursing-sensitive outcome that relates to death anxiety might be that the patient and family will express control related to thoughts of possible adverse consequences of surgery. In other words, although any human might fear what could happen physically during a time when total control of life and limb is surrendered to others, there is the thought that many are able, with family support, to hold that in abeyance in order to go through with the necessary surgical procedure. This is a nurse-sensitive outcome with which the nurse handling preoperative care can clearly have an impact. The nurse's knowledge, confidence, teaching expertise, body language, direct communication, and comforting skills may influence the patient's responses.

Nurse-sensitive indicators are helpful in evaluating how a nursing unit does over time in effectively preparing patients for surgery. Such results can be measured in the aggregate rather than by focusing on individual cases. Aggregate outcomes may be measured by means of patient satisfaction surveys, throughput times from start to finish of surgeries, down times between surgical cases (the business end of things), safety outcomes for a period of time, and, finally, and most importantly, the actual patient physiological outcomes compared with standard data from other institutions. In addition, evidence-based practice is a newer trend in preoperative nursing management designed to create teams of experts who evaluate research and make recommendations based on the weight of evidence to those nurses working directly with patients and families.

Environmental Safety

The preoperative nurse acts to provide both environmental safety, personal patient safety, and support of families. The environment through which the patient will pass in the preoperative, intraoperative, and postoperative periods is carefully set up to avoid some of the dangers that are an inherent part of providing anesthesia and performing surgery. The environment will also contain special features for rapidly handling crises should these arise. Support of the family includes instructions on what to expect the day of surgery, where to wait, and procedures for visiting their loved one in the recovery room.

The surgical suite can be a dangerous place for patients, the surgical team, and the support staff. Explosions or fires can occur when the volatile gases and sparks interact. Ambient room temperature can seriously impact surgical outcomes. The handling and disposal of sharp objects is another potential safety hazards. The perioperative nurse must act proactively to ensure environmental safety for the patient. In the early days of use of anesthetic gases, dating from the 1800s, hospital surgical suites were placed on the top floors of hospitals. In that way, in the case of the periodic explosion as the result of a spark interacting with flammable gases, the damage would be limited. Those people below the level of the explosion and subsequent fire would be safe in the case of limited structural damage or more easily able to escape without harm.

Today, surgical suites may be safely placed on the ground floor or below. Understanding of electrical discharge, flammability within the surgical area, and the institution of safety measures in all surgical areas across the country have made surgery a much safer process for patients and for personnel. Some of these measures are noted in chapter 21. Should the student observe a surgery, there will be an opportunity to put paper booties over shoes and to pass across a meter designed to anticipate and remove the possibility of shedding small sparks. Occasionally, accidents still happen but on a much smaller scale than what occurred in earlier times.

In addition to the possibility of explosion, anesthetic gases may have other untoward effects. Despite trying to contain anesthetic gases within confined containers and tubing leading to patient delivery systems, some gases manage to escape into the ambient air in surgical suites. These gases can have an effect on personnel. Some hospital operating rooms transfer pregnant employees to other units to guard against the teratogenic effects of some anesthetic gases. Even though the possibilities of effects on the developing fetus are remote, there is still a danger (Price, 2004).

Because air temperature has an effect on metabolism, and because hypothermia, or having a low body temperature, can have unfortunate consequences, the preoperative nurse will want to take steps to guard against patients developing low body temperatures. A normal oral body temperature ranges from 37.4° C (97.6° F) to 37.4° C (99.4° F). When using a centigrade system of measurement, the normal oral temperature is approximately 37° C (98.6° F). Hypothermia is a lower than normal temperature. When preventing hypothermia, a first step that the preoperative nurse may take would be to identify those at risk, such as the very old or very young, those who have heart disease or might be more at risk for same, those who might be expected to bleed more easily, and those will be undergoing more complex surgery or surgery in which larger areas of the body will be exposed to cool air temperatures.

Another aspect of danger for the patient undergoing surgery is the handling and disposal of sharp objects. Some patients will have received preoperative medication that will sometimes cause the patient not to notice that sharp objects are in the immediate environment or impinging on skin surfaces. In addition, sharp objects should be handled and placed carefully and discarded in specially designed containers. The presence of sharp objects always poses a risk for hospital personnel (Daniels, 2004).

Personal Patient Safety

One important task for the preoperative nurse is providing for the personal safety of the patient as they prepare for surgery. This includes filling out the preoperative checklist, confirmation of the surgical site, documenting any allergies, ensuring that all required laboratory and diagnostic results are noted, and consent checks.

The preoperative checklist provides a clear, one-page final clearance document for those going to surgery. It is prepared prior to the patient's transfer to the surgical anteroom. Many of the items on the checklist are completed prior to medicating the patient with any mind-altering substance, so that responses will be accurate and filled in by a patient with a relatively clear head. The patient must clearly be identified as the right patient (Figure 20-4). Other checklist items are completed by personnel preparing the patient and can be done close to the time of surgery. Examples of such items to be checked are confirmation that the surgical site is correct, and identification of allergies to

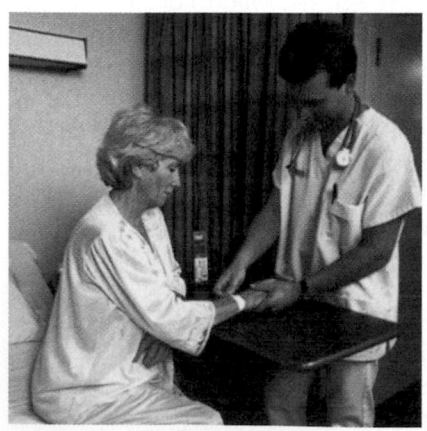

Figure 20-4 The nurse is checking this surgical patient to ensure the identification of the patient.

foods, medications, inhalants, or latex. Other elements are also checked, such as the recording of recent vital signs, method and completion of site preparation, accord that the consent form is in order, and the patient's wishes related to receiving blood products.

It might seem obvious that the site agreed on by the physician and patient would be readily recognized at the time of surgery. After all, the contract between a patient and physician often comes after years of the physician and patient interacting and after a thorough knowledge by the physician about the patient's needs. The surgeon would take great care to ensure that site identification is correct. This would seem to be common sense. It would appear that mistakes related to misidentification of the type of surgery or the site for performing surgery would be rare. However, errors do occur.

Following a number of tragic surgical mistakes, great pains are taken to ensure that the surgical site has been correctly identified. To educate the student or practitioner of the art of nursing, a synopsis of one such mistake is provided in the Safety First below.

Identification and communication about allergies is another vital personal safety element prior to the patient leaving the preoperative unit for the surgical anteroom. Surgical personnel in the anteroom will recheck allergy statements made while the patient is clearheaded. Because the patient will be heavily medicated or completely unconscious during surgery and immediately after, it is imperative that personnel know of substances that should not be given to the patient or that should not be circulating in the environment around the patient. Knowledge of food allergies, for example, might be important in eliminating an environmental substance commonly used perioperatively. For example, those with an allergy to shellfish may also be allergic to iodine products. Knowledge of the food allergy would cause the surgical team to select a skin-cleaning product without iodine just to be sure there were no reactions.

Latex allergy has led to deaths. Natural rubber latex contains proteins that are capable of stimulating an immune response in susceptible individuals. This

---

Safety First

Identifying the Correct Surgical Site

A tragic error concerned an elderly gentleman in Florida. This man was suffering from severe and irreparable damage to leg tissues as a result of chronic metabolic and vascular conditions. More conservative treatments would not have changed this grim situation. The patient agreed to a more drastic measure. It was deemed essential for surgeons to amputate his leg to save his life. Tragically, the wrong limb, the healthier limb, was amputated. The patient awoke from anesthesia to be greeted with news of the mistake in identifying the correct limb. A second surgery was performed to amputate the leg that had originally been intended. This patient now faced a life without either leg; something that would make recovery incomparably more difficult and that would negatively affect the patient's remaining quality of life. Beyond the physical effects of this error, such an error would cause any human being to live

the remainder of a lifetime with the thought of, "If only they hadn't made this mistake." The psychological toll must have been immense. Following a number of such incidents that culminated in the Florida episode, preoperative checklists have been modified and hospital identification procedures have been made more exact. The intended surgical site is marked with a water-soluble marker while the patient is awake and alert and able to validate that the side chosen will be correctly selected once sedation or anesthesia have begun. In addition, when limb surgery is to be performed, the modern surgical team now performs a procedure known as time out. Prior to initiating the incision, all members concentrate and focus on the surgical procedure to be performed. It is felt that this one extra step slows the pace at one of the most critical times for the surgical patient.

response may range from mild itching or ocular swelling to an anaphylactic reaction and possible death. The preoperative nurse, when gathering information from patients, needs to explore thoroughly any reports of allergies and should realize that repeated exposures to latex increase the probability that a patient may become latex sensitive. This information is particularly important in the case of the patient who will undergo surgery and anesthesia in which many of the routinely used pieces of equipment contain a substantial latex component. For this reason, major hospitals have constructed areas that are latex free, including designated surgical suites. In addition, special tags are placed to alert the surgical and recovery teams to the presence of patients at risk.

Careful preoperative history taking will reveal patients at risk so that steps can be taken to protect the patient through safeguarding the environment. Risk factors for latex allergy include: (a) multiple exposures to health care situations, perhaps beginning in childhood and spanning many years; (b) a history of allergies, including food allergies or eczema; and (c) perhaps a simple history of contact dermatitis.

Another important safety measure for preoperative patients is checking the results from laboratory and other diagnostic data. Some diagnostic procedures are performed before surgery and are designed to rule out physiological problems. In patients with a history of cardiovascular disorders, an electrocardiogram (ECG) is performed close to the time of surgery and is checked for the presence of unanticipated dysrhythmias, such as irregular heartbeats or conduction aberrations. Health care providers may want to examine a series of ECGs before making decisions about the patient's abilities to withstand the rigors of surgery. Serum electrolytes will be considered in pronouncing that it is safe to proceed with surgery. Of particular importance will be measurement of serum potassium, magnesium, and calcium, electrolytes that are involved with steady cardiac activity. Blood cell counts will reveal patients who are anemic or prone to bleeding or infection. Routine chest radiological exams or pulmonary function studies may be performed to identify severity of respiratory compromise in those patients who have a history or pulmonary problems or who fall into an age range in which identification of possible problems is essential.

Recording of all results should be accomplished by the time of transfer to the surgical anteroom. Tests ordered and completed should be listed on the preoperative checklist and compared with the health care provider's orders for completeness. All results should be placed within the chart. Most hospitals have policies dictating what tests should be performed under what circumstances and within what time frame prior to surgery. The nurse should be aware of the policies of the facility in which care is performed.

Consent forms leave little margin for error. In addition to sections that clearly name the nature of the planned surgery, there are checklist attachments outlining the facts of almost all common surgical procedures. The same is true for the type of anesthesia being planned. The descriptions of risks are highly useful. Checklist attachments to consent forms may encourage the patient to check to be sure that the surgeon or surgeon's representative fully explained risks, alternative procedures, and the details of the surgery to which the patient is agreeing.

There is a three checks system that nurses should routinely use when verifying the exact wording of verbal or telephoned physician orders. It is wise for the nurse preparing the patient for immediate surgery to perhaps perform a final check related to the patient's understanding about surgery. In addition, the final check about the surgical site creates confidence that the patient will have an error-free experience. The three checks involve a careful reading of the original physician's order for the wording of the consent form. The nurse might also want to check this against the physician's history and physical examination page and, finally, against the physician's progress notes. All should match. Following this first type of solitary scrutiny, the nurse can read the procedure's name from the consent form and ask the patient and family if that is correctly phrased. If the patient or family agrees, the nurse reads the procedure one more time. This constitutes the third check. Others will repeat the process in the surgery anteroom. However, there will come a point, sometimes on the releasing unit prior to transport to the surgery anteroom, when the patient will be medicated with a mind-altering substance for the purposes of relaxation and preanesthesia preparation. Validation should not be done after that point.

Finally, it has already been pointed out that, in cases involving a limb or an organ of which there are two, the preoperative nurse may want to have the patient point to the correct site. This identification should be in accord with what is on the consent. If there is any discrepancy, the surgical area should be called, and a physician involved in the case should come to the releasing unit to clarify and mark the appropriate site. Again, some facilities encourage nurses to mark the incorrect side or site with a symbol indicating not to touch that side or site. In each case, nurses should follow their hospital's policy.

The blood consent form will ensure that the patient has access to full information about risks, expected benefits, and alternatives related to receipt of transfusions. If time permits in the weeks or months leading up to elective surgery, patients and families may want to explore the possibilities of **autologous donation** (self-donation by the patient) or donation of units of blood designated by family members for use by the patient. These directed donations will be made available within the hospital around the time of surgery.

Support for Families

The nurse should go over the agenda for the evening before surgery and that of the day of surgery. It helps if patients and families can visualize settings in advance. For example, the nurse should consider walking the family to the surgical waiting area, or in hospitals in which the surgeon will expect the family to wait in the patient's room that should be made clear to family in advance. In this age of high tech, some hospitals provide videodisks for home viewing or may have these available for scrutiny by patients and families on admission. Such disks might cover orientation to the room, samples of postoperative exercises for patients and families to perform and practice at home, or even a tour of the surgery anteroom of PACU. There might be a filmed follow-through of the sights and sounds as patients are transferred within the hospital. While this preview was once thought to heighten anxiety, it is now recognized that it benefits some patients and reduces anxiety.

Some individuals prefer a maximum of information prior to and during a stressful encounter. People who tend to move in this direction are called "monitors." Others, termed "blunters," prefer to self-distract and not focus on the stressful moment. Miller devised an instrument capable of predicting whether monitoring or blunting is the preferred style of the individual.

The preoperative nurse should be aware that there are individual differences in style, not only on the part of the patient but also with family members. The nurse can plan to set up the environment, ensuring that necessary information is delivered but using methods that will fit with family members' preferred styles. For example, the spouse who is vigilant and wants timely information will appreciate the preoperative nurse's directions on how to obtain information while waiting in the designated waiting area. Or the vigilant spouse might benefit from knowing usual time frames, such as that it may take up to 30 minutes within the surgical suite to prep the site for surgery, including positioning and draping. For the vigilant person, detail is important. However, the preoperative nurse will want to focus attention on such a person's reactions to information to ensure that information is spaced well and that the person is not being overloaded.

For the family member who prefers distraction rather than a focus on immediate facts or surroundings, most waiting rooms have television, magazines, and

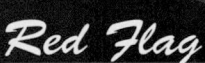

Red Flag

Obtaining Consent Via Telephone

Whenever emergency telephone permission must be elicited for consent purposes, the preoperative nurse will have a second licensed nurse listening on a telephone extension. It is best if the second nurse is one who operates in an administrative capacity within the hospital or clinic. The person giving consent should be made aware that the second person would acknowledge that consent is given and that it constituted informed consent. Although such cases are rare, problems with guardianship and consent do occur. The preoperative nurse who knows how to handle the situation will save time and decrease feelings of stress for all participants.

snacks readily available. The preoperative plan may involve mentioning items this family member might want to bring to the hospital for distraction purposes. In addition, the preoperative nurse might want to mention time frames for phases of surgery so that the family member can leave the waiting area for a time but be accessible by cell phone.

Many people possess characteristics of vigilance mixed with a need for distraction at tense moments. The preoperative nurse will want to match his or her style to that of the people with whom he or she is dealing. In addition, the nurse must know the information that must be delivered and understood regardless of a patient's or family member's personal style. Such things as informed consent to have surgery or to receive blood products require attention regardless of the patient or surrogate's personal style or feelings. If strong rapport and trust have been developed, there is little chance that the preoperative nurse will miscalculate what information to deliver when and thereby place an unnecessary burden on the patient or family member.

Pharmacology

Close to the time of surgery, there will be a need for the administration of preoperative medications. The nurse will notify the patient that the surgical transporter is coming to the room and will invite the patient to put on gown and remove all else. The patient will be asked to use the bathroom one more time before preoperative medication is given. Once the patient returns to bed, and preoperative medication is given, the patient is asked to remain in bed and request help to get up. This protocol is to prevent accidents resulting from effects of medication.

The types of preoperative medications are: (a) opioids, such as morphine sulfate; (b) amnesic muscle relaxants, such as Valium, Versed, or Ativan; (c) anticholinergics, such as atropine or scopolamine; and (d) antacids or hydrogen ion antagonists. Opioids provide analgesia, decrease anxiety, and provide sedation. Products such as Valium, Versed, or Ativan act as muscle relaxants or antianxiety medications. However, these are also amnesics, and in some patients the amnesic effect may be quite strong. With opioids in general, and the amnesics, the nurse should monitor closely for respiratory depression and lack of muscle coordination. Anticholinergics are given when the health care provider would like to reduce oral and respiratory tract secretions. These also may decrease chances of postsurgical vomiting and aspiration. The hydrogen ion antagonists (or proton pump inhibitors) reduce gastric acid. This can be important in the immediate perioperative period as well as in the days after surgery. It is felt that use of these products may reduce the occurrence of stress-induced gastritis and even gastric ulceration.

The preoperative nurse will also want to consider medications that the patient routinely takes on an outpatient basis. Anticoagulants prolong clotting time and may increase risks of hemorrhage. However, stopping or reducing dosage too aggressively in the preoperative period may precipitate problems from whatever condition necessitated their use. Antihypertensive medications may have an affect on intraoperative blood pressure. Diuretics used preoperatively may have the same effect and may also be associated with electrolyte imbalances (Broyles, Reiss, & Evans, 2007).

For obvious reasons, the nurse will ensure that any documents requiring a clear head will have been signed prior to administering preoperative medications. In addition, a final set of vital signs will have been taken just prior to administering medications. This data will serve as a baseline during and immediately after surgery.

Transfer Strategies

With young patients, a parent will frequently be allowed to carry the child to the surgical area and to remain until anesthesia is initiated. With those who are teens or adults, there is usually no reason why the parents, spouse, or another

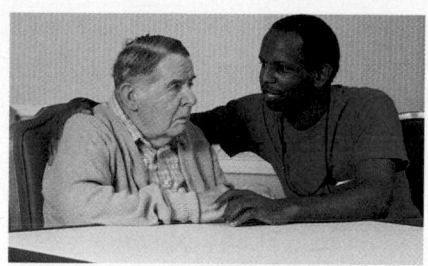

Figure 20-5 Nurse explaining upcoming surgical procedure to frail elderly.

BOX 20-5

COUPLES AT RISK: THE FRAIL ELDERLY

There is a particularly vulnerable type of preoperative patient; some have termed this the frail elder. When the frail elder and spouse or siblings live together, sometimes they depend on each other for daily existence. When one of the two must be hospitalized, it places both at risk. It is wise for the nurse to consider external but related sources of support in such cases. When the stress of pending surgery is added to the tensions of hospitalization, intervention may be necessary. Some questions that the nurse might ask are listed.

- Is there family who might become involved?
- Have the frail partners enlisted their help or is there reluctance?
- Will nursing intervention make the situation worse?
- How might a team be assembled to examine the problem? Who might be valuable members of such a team?

The nurse must use sensitivity in exploring the situation. Sometimes, the couple will have a trusted other who will assist with making difficult decisions. The more the nurse knows, the better the nurse is able to help.

may not go with the patient to the anteroom and remain until the patient is actually wheeled away into the surgical suite. The preferred method of transport for the adult will usually be the hospital stretcher. Stretchers, once called gurneys, are capable of handling oxygen, IV fluid bags and lines, urinary catheters, and other devices that may be affixed to the patient or accompanying the patient to the surgical area. The chart, or medical record, will also accompany the patient. Elastic stockings for use after surgery accompany the patient and will be placed immediately after the procedure. Patient and family should watch that someone rechecks the name band prior to transport.

For those who are to undergo major orthopedic procedures, the patient will often be transported in the hospital bed. As the patient undergoes surgery in one section of the surgical area, the bed will be prepared in another to include the positioning of specialized mobility devices or traction for use following surgery. It is possible to perform surgery while the patient remains in bed, but this is unlikely.

Population Based Care

In perioperative nursing, there are several populations that have specific concerns.

This section will examine the: (a) frail elderly, (b) person who have guardianship issues, (c) the obese, (d) persons who smoke, and (e) persons who consume alcohol or illicit drugs. First the frail elderly are often persons whom nurses will identify as being couples at risk (Figure 20-5). Sometimes those couples who have reached advanced age must be treated in special ways compared to those who are in their preretirement years. That is, those who are the frail elderly are sometimes less resilient. When a spouse or sibling comes into the hospital and is in frail condition, the other spouse or sibling may need to be considered in planning for the surgical experience. Some considerations for the nurse dealing with such situations are listed in Box 20-5.

Sometimes the physician and partners know the couple and their histories well and have made special provisions for this time, but sometimes the nurse will need to be the wise advocate. The most serious problems will arise when there are to be no family members involved or when permanent institutionalization against the couple's will is a possibility. When these issues include separation of the couple, the outcome for both will be something that neither partner desired.

In addition to the frail elderly, the perioperative setting often has populations with guardianship issues. Nurses should follow the hospital's chain of command when there are issues involving guardianship. That is, nursing administrators or their designees have received specialized training in issues of guardianship. Or in complex cases, the administration may want to confer with the hospital's legal or risk management team for a recommendation. Law in Practice provides examples of situations in which guardianship is in question.

The next population of persons who have specific needs as related to perioperative nursing are persons who are obese. To determine if a person is at an unusual weight for age and height, the nurse may want to rely on a nutrition textbook, a commonly available slide calculator, or a body mass index calculation. There are also specialized calipers that assist in this determination. Sometimes, the appearance of the patient will be an indication that the patient is thinner than average or heavier than average. Although the person who is thin, emaciated, and generally undernourished will present a certain set of difficulties, those who care for such a patient will be able to overcome nutritional deficiencies in the weeks prior to elective surgery through supplements delivered in a variety of ways, including directly into the vasculature. While this may not solve all problems, it offers the hope that surgical risks related to undernourishment can be minimized.

At the other end of the weight range are those who are defined as obese. While metabolic changes of aging often make for differences in body size and shape as people age, these must be managed during surgery. Although many

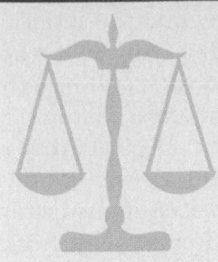

LAW IN PRACTICE

Guardianship

Examples of guardianship issues are the underage patient who requires surgery when a parent or guardian cannot be located. Another is the person with diminished capacity from brain injury or congenital defect that must have surgery. Or in some cases, patients are brought to the emergency department with indeterminate identification and the possibility of being underage for the purposes of consent. Sometimes patients and family disagree, particularly when the patient is a teenager seeking independence who may have a slightly different worldview from that of the parents. The nurse may then need to call in an expert in such issues to ensure that the rights of all are preserved while the most effective decisions are made.

Another guardianship issue arises when the patient has a long-standing court-appointed guardian who sent papers to ensure that consent was properly elicited. Sometimes the papers are misplaced, and there is a delay. This should be avoided whenever possible. The preoperative care nurse has access 24 hours a day to supervisory support, and through such support, a risk management team well versed in handling issues of consent. The team's representative will be able to offer decisions based on such factors as the state's legal age of consent or regulations permitting surgery in emergency circumstances. Using the health care agency's chain of command will result in an appropriate decision.

of those who are octogenarian and weigh more than 20 percent over what height and weight charts would find ideal, the surgical team is usually easily able to make successful adjustments. Such adjustments involve dosages of medications, amounts and mixtures of anesthetics and inhaled gases, and such things as positioning and lengths of time spent in unusual operative positions. The population may have heightened risks for immediate perioperative complications, such as atelectasis, aspiration, delayed return of full consciousness, and wound management problems. The surgical team will be able to factor in these elements, along with considerations related to patient age and past level of health. Other perioperative complications of a more serious nature are arrhythmia, heart failure, and acute pulmonary conditions.

A certain degree of being overweight for age and height is termed morbid obesity. This is defined as a weight that, over the long- or short-term, is incompatible with life. America is expected to have an epidemic of obesity throughout the 21st century, so it is reasonable to expect that all those who deliver perioperative care will deal with individuals who are profoundly overweight. The person who is profoundly overweight presents a unique set of challenges. The modern science of **bariatric therapy** involves dealing with specific problems of management of weight, management of physical spaces, and treatment of those who are greatly overweight. Government and insurance companies now provide coverage for bariatric treatment. Bariatric hospital units are being created across the country. These bariatric units deal with direct matters of safe weight management, including specialized surgical intervention to promote safe weight loss. Bariatric units also deal with management of the patient perioperatively whether the surgery is for weight control purposes or for other reasons. Those who are contemplating surgery might explore whether or not they meet criteria for admission to a bariatric unit. Perhaps the decision will be made to undergo surgery at a medical center that specialized in treating the particular condition rather than in routine management of persons with special weight needs. The patient and family may then have to ensure that provisions are made in advance of admission. This may be done by speaking to the hospital ombudsman. Failing that, the patient and family may want to consult a clinical nurse specialist who can assist the hospital with the necessary advance planning.

Some of the first challenges for the profoundly overweight individual are those of geography and physical spaces. The preoperative nurse and those who will care for the patient during and following surgery need to be prepared to deal with these issues. The patient who is morbidly obese faces beds, stretchers, and surgical tables that are designed for average-sized people. Even bathroom facilities are designed for those of average weight and height. In addition, the patient who is profoundly obese often suffers wider swings in fluid and electrolyte balance around the time of surgery, particularly if maintained on NPO status for prolonged periods of time.

The person who is profoundly obese is expected to have greater pulmonary alterations based on physiological inability of the diaphragm to descend as fully as that of the person of average weight. That is, inspiratory reserve volume and overall vital capacity may be less than in those whose weight is average. This decrease may result in diminished lung recovery capabilities, pneumonia, atelectasis, greater problems with aspiration, and problems with positioning on the side postoperatively. It is estimated that obese individuals must have additional blood vessels to support the maintenance of additional body cells and tissues. Consequently, the heart must work harder awake or sleeping to maintain strength. When the stress of surgery is added to an already taxed system, surgical risks increase.

Another population of people with specific perioperative needs is people who smoke. The preoperative nurse will want to estimate pack years when taking a health history related to smoking cigarettes. The number of packs per day is multiplied by the number of years the patient has smoked cigarettes. Or in cases in which the patient uses other nicotine-based products, it is important to note quantifying figures. Cigarette smoking alters the lining cells within the respiratory tree. The mucociliary elevator is no longer able to move secretions effectively. In addition, when cigarette smoking results in chronic obstructive pulmonary disease, secretions become thickened and the lung tissue changes. Even chest configuration is altered. It is anticipated that this will result in potentially greater difficulty during surgery and more sluggish respiratory system recovery after surgery.

Nicotine also has circulatory effects such as vasoconstriction or vasodilation that is unrelated to normal physiological needs. Some who have stopped smoking know the effects of nicotine withdrawal on alertness and concentration. Somnolence is prevalent during early withdrawal periods. Cravings for cigarettes intrude on thoughts as the person tries to complete short tasks. Those close to those who are withdrawing from nicotine also know the mood effects that ensue.

In addition to these physiological effects of nicotine and nicotine withdrawal, there are psychological effects. The patient who is a heavy smoker and is facing surgery as well as its aftermath in a smokeless hospital or clinic environment has concerns about nicotine withdrawal. Sometimes the use of nicotine patches and other products, such as Wellbutrin for mood control assistance, will help.

The last population of people with individual perioperative needs are those who consume alcohol or take illicit drugs. The person ready to undergo surgery that is dependent on alcohol or is addicted to drugs faces withdrawal.

Delirium tremens (DTs) is a feature of alcohol withdrawal in those who are alcoholics. DTs are characterized by neuromuscular alterations, hallucinations, often frightening for the patient, and deranged thought processes. The nurse caring for the patient postoperatively will find the care a challenging experience.

Those who are chronic alcoholics or who abuse drugs are often malnourished. They may suffer from liver damage or other chronic and untreated disorders. Their surgical course may be more unpredictable and their recovery more delayed than with those who do not have such addictions. The perioperative nurse may anticipate delayed wound healing from the effects of malnutrition or unpredictable reactions to medications ordered in the course of hospitalization.

It is important but sometimes difficult for the preoperative and postoperative nursing staff to remain nonjudgmental when working with these patients. The patient is sometimes far from compliant with the ordered or indicated regimen of treatment or care. Some patients become violent and abusive as part of the mental changes during the withdrawal period. In addition, should the patient need to be restrained to protect self or others, this action becomes an additional management difficulty for nurses and family members.

NONELECTIVE SURGERY

Nonelective surgery can be divided into two types. There is the emergency surgery that occurs when an accident or other form of injury occurs unexpectedly and without warning. An example would be a car crash or a fall from a ladder. Because the family and patient did not expect it to happen, they must adjust to the accident and the immediate need to give consent for surgery.

Another type of nonelective surgery entails a physiological condition that demands immediate surgery to prevent complications or death. An example would be the discovery of something creating pressure on the brain that, if unrelieved, would result in brain damage. Examples might be a rapidly expanding tumor or a leaking blood vessel.

In the case of nonelective or emergency surgery, there is an important set of differences. This section provides a discussion of some of the events that may precipitate nonelective surgery. There will be a consideration of methods the nurse may use to elicit vital information and to give the best care during these times of stress or urgent need. Preoperative principles connected with disaster management and inevitable mass casualties will be presented.

Preceding Events

Preceding events likely to lead to emergency surgery are accidents, including motor vehicle or motorcycle accidents. Bicycles or all-terrain vehicles are also frequently involved in accidents leading to emergency surgery. Gunshot wounds are common causes of emergency department visits and subsequent emergency surgery. Falls and work-related injuries, such as traumatic amputation, also require emergency surgery. Some of the types of preceding events are those in which preservation of life or prevention of vastly diminished quality of life leaves no choice other than immediate surgery. The surgery must even be performed without consent at times. Discussion of what the nurse will do in terms of advocacy in such situations is provided in the following section.

Urgent and Emergent Care

In cases of severe trauma, there may be a need for emergency surgery. Examples of events that may cause severe trauma are explosions and fires, building or parking garage collapse, motor vehicle accidents, and sports accidents. In addition to these events that could happen anywhere, each state in the United States also has types of traumatic events that relate particularly to that state. These are not unusual within a state's borders and are often connected to the ways in which citizens earn a living. In the state of Texas, for example, some of the most common causes of severe trauma are cattle ranching accidents, farming accidents, and oil rig mishaps. Some of the equipment used on farms, ranches, and rigs is particularly dangerous. In addition, near oil rigs, fire is an ever-present danger. It is not a coincidence that one of the largest burn centers in the nation is located in Texas.

In addition to these accidental types of injury, combat also causes severe trauma. In a previous era, combatants were engaged in fighting in formally declared wars. Today, civilian populations may be targets in undeclared wars. These wars know no borders. Risk may be present half a world away or within a small radius from where the nurse and other prospective casualties live and work. The nurse of the future will need to be adept at handling many types of trauma in many types of settings.

Another type of situation that may call for nonelective, or emergency, surgery involves physiological instability that is unrelated to direct trauma. In such cases, even though the cause is a physical illness rather than an accident, war injury, or the result of terrorism, the surgical team will have to act quickly. The surgical team will not have the luxury of waiting for full patient stabilization prior to surgical intervention. Examples are the appendix that is on the verge of rupture or fulminant or septic shock that arises from an infected central venous access device. In such cases, surgery must be performed without delay or the patient will die or will suffer grave and irreversible consequences.

In cases of urgent, emergency surgery, shortcuts are encouraged in making the patient ready for surgery. Time is critical, so while the need to be especially careful is paramount, delays are discouraged. As is always the case, the surgical nurse will join with the surgery team to promote patient well-being, including acting as an advocate, should the need arise.

The highest priority is given to preservation of life, unless there is an active, legal document that supersedes this rule, such as no code status or outside-the-hospital-do-not-resuscitate orders. In all other cases, attention will be given first to preserving life and function. Therefore, the emergency team will deal with physical status initially, leaving psychosocial and spiritual needs as close follow-ups. That is why, in popular shows in the media, there are scenes with emergency personnel gathering history and taking physical preservation steps first. Only later are patient and family psychological needs met.

In the case of the unaccompanied trauma victim, the team will make every effort to reach family. This is particularly important to gather history and to ensure that what is done is in accord with an unconscious patient's preexpressed wishes. In addition, should there be religious constraints in effect, it helps for the surgical team to be aware of these constraints. The receipt of blood products is contraindicated in the case of some religions. The hospital's risk management team may be best at handling such situations. For the nurse at the bedside, calling on the next person in the chain of command is vital. Nursing supervisors are available around the clock and are responsible for assisting when legal-ethical dilemmas arise. Most hospitals have written policies in effect that will guide hospital personnel. In addition, chaplain services are available around the clock on an on-call basis to respond to just such contingencies.

In the case of surgery needed immediately to preserve a patient's life, the team will go forward even though it means bypassing some of the preoperative teaching that would have taken place had there been more time. In addition, there is usually no time for the patient to practice such things as postoperative exercises through return demonstration. That will have to wait for the recovery period.

The preoperative nurse will ensure that routine laboratory findings are reported promptly to the rest of the surgical team. This is particularly critical with values such as serum electrolytes, complete blood count, and coagulation studies. Any abnormal results should be communicated immediately. Elicitation of allergy information is vital. For example, the patient who has latex allergy could be placed in danger should latex anesthesia equipment be used. Or the patient who is allergic to iodine might have difficulty handling contrast dye material. The surgical team needs this information.

In relation to protecting the patient who undergoes urgent or emergency surgery, the preoperative nurse also needs to ensure that the surgical team, particularly those who will be responsible for anesthesia and monitoring, are aware that an emergency patient is underweight or overweight. Patients who are smokers or who routinely or recently have used controlled substances will need to be handled with precision in the delivery of anesthesia and in recovering from its effects. While physical preparation often takes precedence with emergency surgery, the nurse needs to consider legal-ethical matters. The next section will illustrate some of the peculiar problems that may arise, and how best to handle these to ensure satisfactory outcomes.

Legal-Ethical Concerns and Need for Psychological Support

There may have been little time to consider and adjust to the situation for the patient, family, employer, or others. Those who would like to be at the patient's side may be far away or in transit when the surgical event begins. In addition, there is often no opportunity to have all the work, insurance, or notification and approval "ducks in a row," as would be the case with elective surgery.

In the short time from discovery of the need for surgery, there are sometimes extra and unanticipated feelings of guilt or uncertainty surrounding nonelective surgery. For the accident victim, there is always the question of prevention. Did someone else cause this event? Was carelessness to blame? Was drinking or the use of any one of a number of substances involved? Was age involved? Who else was around when it happened? In addition to the usual concerns present when surgery is elective, there are the additional psychosocial concerns when the surgery is nonelective. These concerns are even more pressing when the reason for surgery involves an accident and its aftermath.

The portable, computer-compatible, streaming, emergency vehicle video camera was mentioned earlier in the chapter in connection with rapid preparation needs for surgical emergencies. This direct visualization and recording assists the preoperative group with assessing the extent of an emergency patient's injuries. Not only will this transmit, in real time, the scene of the accident, including where the victims are found and what sort of trauma was likely, but also the process of removing, packaging, and transporting in the ambulance for the rapid ride to the hospital (Dennis, 2003; Sheehan, 2004). Through viewing these events prior to the patient's arrival, the emergency team at the hospital can anticipate equipment and other immediate patient needs as well as set up for rapid transport to surgery following sometimes foreshortened stabilization. This also has implications for the family who may be involved with moral-ethical or legal decision making at a later time.

The advent of such procedures also fits nicely with the camera-equipped trauma rooms in modern hospitals. Sometimes, these are helpful for the health care team for later review and training. In cases with legal-ethical questions at a later date, these provide valuable evidence. There may be times when these would even be used for the family to view at a later date. Wilson, Anderson, Toms, Fleetwood, and Phelps (2006) noted that the family who are able to witness pivotal moments in emergency care can be assisted in coming to terms with emotional sequelae.

Even when there has been no accident involved, the emotional fallout for the patient who undergoes urgent, nonelective surgery may be noticeable. The person for whom surgery is nonelective will be left with unanswerable questions. Should I have called the physician at the first sign? Should I have done better at annual checkups? Why did I continue to smoke cigarettes? Is God punishing me?

The urgent nature of the surgery and the shortened time to prepare may make everything seem more distressing in the case of nonelective surgery. However, there are rare exceptions. Sometimes, although urgent, the surgery is expected to have a happy outcome. One that comes to mind is childbirth procedures designed to decrease harm from unusual in utero baby positions. The outcome will be positive, even though the surgery is unexpected. Another possibility is the removal of a foreign object from the ear, nose, or another body orifice of the young child. Some of the uncertainty and lack of adjustment time will be offset by the expectation that results will be positive and the chances of harm minimal.

However, many cases will be less positive. There is a sense of urgency and an uncertain outcome in cases of motor vehicle accidents involving multiple systems trauma. Recent research has shown that it is a wise idea to allow family to be present under emergency circumstances prior to surgery, even when the possibility of death is present (Wilson, et al., 2006).

When a parent, guardian, spouse, or other individual is on the way but has not yet arrived, it may be a matter of urgency to begin surgery. In such cases, there are special provisions. The emergency department or preoperative care nurse will usually alert administrative personnel or follow carefully crafted guidelines. For the nurse in such situations, using the hospital or clinic chain of command is the best course of action. Often there is an individual who has received special training in what to do under such circumstances. A physician-specialist in emergency medicine usually knows the proper course of action, as does the nurse supervisor or the people on call for the risk management group. Legal counsel and chaplains are routinely called in, particularly with unusual cases, and are typically well versed in the proper ethical-legal steps when the situation is out of the ordinary.

Disasters

It is probable that there has been attention to disaster management ever since the days of the pioneers, who staved off starvation, floods, and occasional attacks from Native Americans. However, disaster management took on new importance following the events of September 11, 2001. The World Trade Center attack meant that, for the first time in U.S. history, other countries or representatives of disenchanted groups could attack our homeland directly and without warning. The resulting mass casualties, including primarily civilians, were unprecedented in the country's history. No longer would the soldier be the one attacked. It would appear now that civilians would be targeted in large numbers.

For that reason, the perioperative nurse needs to be aware of methods and resources for use in disaster situations. In addition to having a general awareness of national groups and initiatives, the preoperative nurse will routinely participate as each hospital holds periodic disaster drills. Sometimes, in the course of disaster training or even more immediately in the case of an actual disaster, an understanding of disaster terminology is needed.

There has always been an effort to be aware of and to have drills related to emergency situations prior to the events of September 11, 2001. However, the events of that day created national, state, and local initiatives aimed at training large numbers of personnel to cope with what might be the disaster situations of the future. Emergency departments, emergency medical service entities, such as vehicular and dispatch, fire departments, and government groups, as well as schools of nursing and medicine, have practiced coordinated drills since early in 2002. There are now training courses offered at universities. Of particular importance will be coordinated rescue, containment, and triage efforts post-disaster. Surgical arenas will assume importance and will become portable and high tech. The need for those who will extend health care provider services, such as nurses, nurse practitioners, certified registered nurse anesthetists (CRNAs), and advanced practice nurses (APNs) of all sorts will emerge early in this century.

The result of drills has also been identification of nurses who are prepared to assist in time of disaster, and databanks directing coordination efforts. For example, in the state of Texas, databanks identify nurses with needed skills in the event of disaster, including those who may perform minor surgery or diagnose and prescribe. In addition, Red Cross training is an essential element for those who are needed in a layperson's capacity to provide support services with mass casualties. For example, although a specially trained Red Cross nurse is required to open a field shelter, civilian volunteers largely staff the shelter on a 24-hour basis. In addition to the need for surgery to save lives, there will be a need to identify and track those who are injured. Again, special tagging and follow-up will be essential following disaster situations. Natural disasters present additional concerns. Sanitation and inaccessibility of the site to assistive personnel are two prime concerns.

Other Concerns

In addition to support in times of local or national disaster, there are a number of agencies that assist following the individual emergency or emergency surgery. Sometimes such cases will involve extensive and complex recovery periods. Families will sometimes exhaust traditional, shorter-term resources and will need long-term help and financial support. For example, for family members who provide full patient care for extended periods, there is often respite service to allow them to have personal times away. This rest and recovery are often essential for those who would otherwise become fatigued and discouraged.

KEY CONCEPTS

- The preoperative nurse acts as patient advocate.
- Preoperative nursing behaviors include attention to the psycho-social, cultural, and spiritual needs.
- Holism emphasizes assessment of the entire patient and family situation: body, mind, and spirit.
- The advent of DRGs has led to shorter hospital stays with an emphasis on the nursing role in preventing surgical complications.
- Inpatient units devoted to the short hospital stay or the detached surgical clinic are now common.
- It is imperative for health care providers to have a thorough knowledge of preoperative safety measures.
- The preoperative nurse acts as educator and coach.
- Specific areas of preoperative teaching include the agenda on the day of surgery, including respiratory exercises, pain management techniques, the possibility of drainage tubes, dressings, casts, IV lines, and monitoring or oxygen equipment.

- Patient assessment includes history taking, physical assessment, interpretation of laboratory studies, and familiarization with radiologic or other diagnostic tests.
- The operative consent is a specialized document that includes an area of agreement related to the surgery itself, as well as sections to request patient choices related to blood transfusion.
- Guardianship assurance is necessary for the incompetent or underage patient.
- The preoperative checklist is a specialized final check to ensure that all ordered preoperative measures have been performed.
- Surgery may be major or minor. Surgical nomenclature addresses the body area or body system that will be involved, the surgical approach, and the intended result.
- Preceding events likely to lead to emergency surgery are accidents, such as motor vehicle, bicycle or motorcycle accidents, gunshot or knife wounds, falls, and work-related injures.

Continued

KEY CONCEPTS—cont'd

■ Mass casualty and civilian disaster injuries are a special category of preceding event calling for emergency or urgent surgery.

■ The preoperative nurse should elicit information on code status in emergency cases.

■ In the case of the emergency preoperative patient, allergies, preexisting conditions, and even religious constraints may be discovered prior to surgery when the patient wears a medical alert bracelet.

REVIEW QUESTIONS

1. In responding to a preoperative patient's question about complementary therapy, which *initial* response by the nurse is most likely to be helpful?
   1. None of those therapies have been shown to have scientific merit.
   2. Tell me what you mean. Are you speaking about something like relaxation therapy or more along the lines of herbal remedies or something else?
   3. There has been a renewed interest in such things as acupuncture lately.
   4. Does your surgeon know of your interest?

2. In thinking about the distinctions between spirituality and religious faith, identify the patient statement that indicates a developing sense of spirituality in the hours before surgery.
   1. I think my need to have cardiac surgery may be a sort of wake-up call. I may need to take more time to stop and smell the roses after this.
   2. Will you pray with me?
   3. When my minister shows up, tell him I'll be right back.
   4. Will I have to stop eating and drinking tonight at midnight?

3. A hospital is holding a series of meetings to inform nurses of new technology in preoperative areas. Identify the technology use that the assembled nurses might want to question:
   1. More sophisticated lighting controls to be managed by patient voice requests
   2. A foot-of-the-bed scrolling screen on which the preoperative patient can view current vital signs and heart rhythm tracings
   3. A bedside computer on which the patient can dial up a series of preoperative teaching films
   4. An electronic voice-activated bedside system for patient use in making requests of the care team

4. Identify the most likely and most serious danger in the future use of implantable electronic chips for containing a patient's health history:
   1. The chip could be deactivated by such things as supermarket scanners.
   2. The wrong patient's records could be implanted.
   3. Unnecessary pain
   4. Violation of confidentiality

5. The nurse is instructing the preoperative patient on what items to bring to the hospital for an anticipated two-day stay. Identify the patient statement that indicates the need for additional teaching:
   1. I think I'll leave my rings and watch at home.
   2. Why don't I just copy my medication bottle labels onto a list and not bring in a bunch of medicine bottles for the nurses to check.
   3. My spouse is checking out five or six library books and will be ready to bring in a favorite if I'm feeling good after surgery.
   4. If I bring in my laptop computer, maybe I can catch up on some office work.

6. From the list, identify surgeries that would be classified as major:
   1. Laparoscopic cholecystectomy
   2. Pneumonectomy
   3. Incision and drainage of an axillary abscess
   4. Coronary artery bypass graft
   5. Total left hip replacement
   6. Appendectomy

7. The suffixes, *-ectomy* and *-ostomy/-otomy* refer to:
   1. Fusion and splinting
   2. Removal and opening into
   3. Stomach and GI tract
   4. Incision and drainage

Continued

8. Identify the case in which the preoperative nurse will notify the surgeon or surgical area and place a temporary hold on patient transport to surgery.
   1. The nurse inadvertently gave the patient a preoperative IV dose of morphine a few minutes before the consent was signed.
   2. The nurse assistant reports the patient has a 39.2° C (102.5° F) oral temperature.
   3. The patient states he is having second thoughts about surgery.
   4. All of the above

9. Identify the correct statement about prevention of wrong site surgery:
   1. Have the conscious patient identify the correct site with a visible mark
   2. Because the surgical permit lists the correct site, no additional measures are necessary beyond careful permit review.
   3. The nurse should verbally ask the alert patient to state the area to be operated on and should document the patient statement in the nursing notes.
   4. Knowing that the surgeon has carefully preplanned for the surgery, no additional checks are needed.

10. Which task may not be delegated by the preoperative nurse to unlicensed assistive personnel?
    1. Drawing blood for preoperative analysis
    2. Performing a bedside blood glucose check
    3. Performing initial physical assessment on patient entry into the hospital
    4. Orienting the patient to the hospital room

11. From the list provided, select patients who may be at greatest risk for instability in and around the time of surgery (select all that apply):

1. The 96-year-old retired person who will have repair of a right foot bunion
2. A 30-year-old cancer patient who is mildly immunosuppressed following a recent round of chemotherapy
3. The 61-year-old patient with a history of hypertension that is well controlled with medication
4. The 56-year-old patient with a 10-year history of emphysema
5. A 23-year-old who is 5′ 6″ tall and weighs 125 pounds

12. The term used to denote self-donation of blood products prior to the day of surgery is:
    1. Allogeneic
    2. Autonomous
    3. Autologous
    4. Alopecic

13. Identify the incorrect statement related to emergency surgery:
    1. The most common causes of emergency surgery include gunshot wounds, accidents, and combat injuries.
    2. The highest priority in the emergency department is given to preservation of life. There are no exceptions.
    3. The nurse will routinely perform physical assessment and lab draws as first priorities with the emergency patient likely to need surgery, even if it means decreased time for communicating with the family.
    4. In cases of emergency that involve life threat, formal consent procedures may be temporarily bypassed.

REVIEW ACTIVITIES

1. List three nursing diagnoses commonly associated with preoperative care.

2. Based on an understanding of historic trends and current realities, project realistic preoperative care trends for the early part of the 21st century.

Continued

REVIEW ACTIVITIES—cont'd

3. In relation to the response to activity 2, name two moral-ethical or legal problems that might arise.

4. Describe how the nurse might go about advising a patient or family on choosing a physician or hospital for surgical intervention.

5. Describe the differences between major and minor surgery. Identify some types of surgery that were once considered major and required extensive hospitalization that are now categorized as minor.

6. Name surgical procedures that are likely to require blood transfusion. Discuss teaching points that the preoperative nurse might use to assist the patient to make decisions related to transfusion in advance of surgery.

7. In teaching the patient and family about pending surgery, describe day-of-surgery preparation activities. Include what the timing of presurgical events is likely to be and what the off-unit areas may look like. Describe postoperative tubes, monitors, and other hardware the patient might encounter when initially recovering from the surgical experience. Describe two things to be taught in relation to postoperative pulmonary management.

8. Name three classifications of frequently used preoperative drugs.

9. Identify preexisting health conditions that would predispose to danger at the time of surgery or that might result in prolonged hospital stay.

Intraoperative Nursing Management

Kathryn Schroeter, PhD, RN, CNOR

CHAPTER TOPICS

- Role of Surgical Team Members
- Intraoperative Nursing Care
- Surgical Environment
- Anesthesia and Sedation
- Surgical Errors
- Ethics in Perioperative Practice

KEY TERMS

Anesthesia
Anesthesia care provider
Asepsis
Conscious sedation
Deep sedation/analgesia
Disseminated intravascular coagulation (DIC)
Hypothermia
Laminar airflow
Malignant hyperthermia (MH)
Minimal sedation (anxiolysis)
Perioperative
Prions
Sedation

The intraoperative phase of patient care refers to the time in which the patient is in the operating room. However, it also refers to the nursing care provided by the circulating nurse and the scrub nurse. This care actually begins before the patient enters the room with the circulator performing a preoperative patient assessment and then working with the scrub nurse to obtain the necessary supplies, equipment, and medications for the care of each specific patient during the intraoperative phase of hospitalization. The intraoperative nurse may also be called a **perioperative** nurse, meaning that care is provided to the patient before, during, and after the surgical procedure. Perioperative nursing is a specialized area of nursing practice.

THE ROLE OF THE PERIOPERATIVE NURSE

Perioperative nursing has evolved over more than 100 years, largely as a result of developments in surgical technique, technological advances, and changes in the role of women in society. The profession has evolved to focus primarily on how care is provided to surgical patients. Perioperative nurses work in environments that contain technological advances, pioneering surgical techniques, and increasing workplace pressures. Furthermore, recruiting nurses to work in this speciality is challenging. As a result, providing high-quality patient care is an increasingly complex task.

Role performance of perioperative nurses requires careful examination and explication. A philosophical shift must occur for nurses to understand and value their own therapeutic input into patient care. Nurses need to work toward defining their role more clearly, become more proactive, accept responsibility for the nursing role, develop programs of clinical supervision to monitor their own role performance, research the needs of patients undergoing surgery, and the effectiveness of nursing interventions on patient care and well-being. The ever burdening shortage of nursing specific to the perioperative setting mandates that educational programs be developed. It is difficult to educate new nurse for perioperative nursing, and there are an ever decreasing number of new graduates that enter into the field of perioperative nursing (Geslak, 2005). The perioperative nurses' role includes a specialized knowledge base and physical skills in the perioperative setting as identified in Box 21-1.

BOX 21-1

PERIOPERATIVE KNOWLEDGE AND SKILLS OF THE NURSE

The perioperative nurse can:
- Demonstrate a comprehensive knowledge and understanding of the perioperative nurse's role in the areas of: anesthetics, PACU, circulating or scrub roles, and RN first assistant
- Demonstrate competency in the clinical skills pertinent to the areas outlined above
- Apply principles of aseptic technique and explain how this knowledge applies in other areas within the operating suite
- Assess, plan, implement, and evaluate individualized nursing care plans for the surgical patient that takes into consideration life variables such as culture, ethnicity, socioeconomic status, sexuality, and religion
- Utilize advanced knowledge of the possible changes in anatomic and physiological functioning that may occur following surgical intervention to provide procedure specific preoperative education
- Use a systematic method of inquiry to identify minor and complex health problems that may have an impact on the patient's surgical experience
- Discuss the legal and ethical issues pertinent to caring for patients undergoing surgical intervention
- Participate and contribute effectively as a member of the multidisciplinary health care team
- Identify individual stressors in the surgical patient and develop an action plan that addresses these stressors and the perioperative nurse's response to them
- Identify trends influencing the role of the perioperative nurse through interpretation and discussions of current published records

Students observing in surgery are advised to eat before attempting to stand for long periods in rooms in which anesthetic gases are used. In addition, the student should be aware of other considerations that involve personal and patient safety (Box 21-2).

Perioperative nurses work closely with the surgical patient, family members, and other health care professionals to help plan, implement, and evaluate treatment. They implement the theory and principles of perioperative nursing in the performance of basic skills. They understand and practice the principles of asepsis, sterilization, disinfection, and infection prevention through the implementation of perioperative nursing care standards (e.g., preparing the patient and self for a surgical procedure). They utilize communication skills and apply the nursing process to the perioperative period, including admitting procedures. They also implement the principles of nursing care of patients during induction and emergence from anesthesia (McGarvey, Chambers, & Boore, 2004).

Perioperative nurses understand and promote the ethical, legal, and moral obligations inherent to their role. They utilize principles of postanesthesia nursing care and the safety practices and elements of surgical suite management. They know how to use and care for surgical instruments, sutures, and equipment. They are cognizant of emergency procedure protocols and are prepared to handle such instances as they arise in practice. They focus on the nursing actions to be taken during surgical procedures and the specialized care requirements of pediatric and geriatric patients.

BOX 21-2

TIPS FOR THE STUDENT WHEN OBSERVING IN OPERATING ROOM

1. Read about the area and the roles of personnel in advance. Be able to visualize what will perhaps happen next. Look at the world from the patient's point of view, particularly if the patient arrives in the surgical suite in a conscious state.
2. Wear comfortable shoes. You may be on your feet for hours.
3. Plan to eat breakfast. Although you may never eat breakfast under any circumstances, make an exception. The combination of a small amount of circulating ambient anesthetic gases and prolonged standing in one place may make you feel lightheaded, especially on an empty stomach.
4. Make sure that you know the dress code and are able to access the appropriate set of scrubs for your day of observation.
5. Bring nothing valuable with you to the setting. Although regular staff members have lockers to secure valuables, you will not.
6. Wear identification. If you are a student, make sure that everyone can see your nametag. The word *student* should be readable.
7. If you become lightheaded during observation you should do one of two things: (a) head for the door, go into the hallway, and then sit down before you faint or (b) if you cannot make it to the door, try for the wall (away from the surgical field). Slide down to a sitting position. Others will assist you soon afterward. You will recognize lightheadedness or feelings that you are going to faint by slight nausea, a feeling of darkness closing in from the sides of your vision, ringing in your ears, sweating, and rapid heart rate. Do not ignore the feeling, thinking that it will pass.
8. Before leaving, thank those who permitted you to observe in this setting. If you are following the patient through to the PACU, be vigilant in observing patient status and in alerting care personnel to changes.

Adapted from Price, P. (2004). Surgical technology for the surgical technologist (2nd ed.). New York: Thomson Delmar Learning.

THE SURGICAL TEAM

As a fundamental member of the surgical team, the perioperative registered nurse works in collaboration with other health care professionals, which may include the surgeon, circulating nurse, anesthesia care provider, surgical assistant, and other assistive personnel. The number of team members differs depending on type of surgery performed.

Surgeon

A surgeon has completed four years of medical school and has received further specialized training after medical school. Most surgeons have passed exams given by a national board of surgeons for the purpose of certification.

Anesthesiologist

An anesthesiologist has completed four years of postmedical school training in anesthesia, in addition to the required four years of medical school. Anesthesiologists usually further specialize in certain surgery specialties, such as pediatric anesthesia. The anesthesiologist is involved in all three phases of surgery: preoperative, intraoperative, and postoperative management.

Certified Registered Nurse Anesthetist

Nurse anesthetists take care of the patient before, during, and after surgical or obstetrical procedures. The certified registered nurse anesthetist (CRNA) constantly monitors every vital function of the patient and can modify the anesthetic to ensure maximum safety and comfort. A nurse anesthetist has a bachelor degree in nursing, followed by specialized training in anesthesia. Nurse anesthetists are required to pass a national certification exam to become CRNA prior to beginning practice.

Operating Room Nurse

Operating room (OR) nurses may be certified in the specialty of perioperative nursing practice. The credential for certification in perioperative nursing is the CNOR. Credentialing is provided for perioperative nurses through the Competency and Credentialing Institute (CCI). Credentialing represents a level of professional achievement and a demonstrated knowledge of clinical competence and practice standards and achieving a CNOR credential demonstrates proficiency in support of quality patient care and sets a standard of commitment to the profession of OR nursing. According to recent research on the value of certification obtaining the credential reflects a deep personal commitment and sense of accountability that are of intrinsic value to the certified perioperative nurse (Gaberson, Schroeter, Killen, & Valentine, 2003). There are other areas in which perioperative nurses may obtain certification in a variety of specialty surgical areas, examples being orthopedics, plastic, and reconstructive surgical nursing.

The perioperative nurse is a registered nurse (RN) who provides nursing care to surgical patients preoperatively, intraoperatively, and postoperatively. Perioperative nursing requires a unique, highly developed set of knowledge, skills, and attitudes. This nurse plans and directs nursing care for patients undergoing operative and other invasive procedures. Perioperative RNs work in all types of health care facilities, such as hospitals, ambulatory or outpatient surgery centers, and health care provider offices. Under the umbrella term of *perioperative nurse* there exist subcategories specific to the intraoperative phase of patient care, i.e. circulator, scrub, and registered nurse first assistant (RNFA) (Price, 2004).

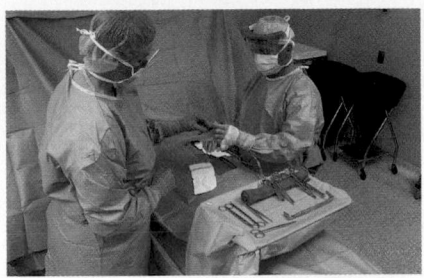

Figure 21-1 The scrub nurse passing an instrument to the surgeon.

Circulator/Circulating Nurse

Circulator nursing duties are performed outside the sterile field. The circulator is responsible for managing the nursing care of the patient within the OR and coordinating the needs of the surgical team with other care providers necessary for completion of surgery. This nurse utilizes critical thinking skills as he or she observes the surgery and the surgical team from a broad perspective and assists the team to create and maintain a safe and comfortable environment for the patient. The circulator assesses the patient's condition before, during, and after the operation to ensure an optimal outcome for the patient. In the OR, most patients are anesthetized or sedated and are powerless to make decisions on their own behalf during the intraoperative phase. The circulating nurse serves as the patient advocate while the patient is least able to care for himself or herself. The role of the circulator may not be delegated to unlicensed assistive personnel (UAP), Licensed Practice Nurse (LPN) or Licensed Vocational Nurse (LVN) (Daniels, 2004).

Scrub Nurse

Scrub nurses work directly with the surgeon within the sterile field, passing instruments, sponges, and other items needed during the procedure (Figure 21-1). Duties of the scrub nurse may be found in Box 21-3. The ster-

---

BOX 21-3

DUTIES OF THE SCRUB NURSE

Preoperative Case Management

- Don OR attire and PPE
- Gather necessary equipment and supplies
- Create and maintain the sterile field
- Scrub and don sterile gown and gloves
- Organize the sterile field for use
- Count necessary items
- Assist team members during entry of the sterile field
- Expose the operative site with sterile drapes

Intraoperative Case Management

- Maintain the sterile field
- Pass instrumentation, equipment, and supplies to the surgeon and surgical assistant(s) as needed
- Assess and predict (anticipate) the needs of the patient and surgeon and provide the necessary items in order of need
- Medication preparation and handling
- Count necessary items
- Specimen care
- Dressing application

Postoperative Case Management

- Maintenance of the sterile field until the patient is transported
- Removal of used instruments, equipment, and supplies from the OR
- Care and maintenance of instruments, equipment, and supplies following use
- Preparation of the OR for the next patient

Adapted from Price, P. (2004). Surgical technology for the surgical technologist (2nd ed.). New York: Thomson Delmar Learning; Rothrock, J., McEwen, D., & Smith, D. (Eds.). (2003). Alexander's care of the patient in surgery (12th ed.). St. Louis, MO: Elsevier

ile field is the area closely surrounding the OR table and instrument tray. Surgical team members who work within the sterile field have scrubbed their hands and arms with special disinfecting soap and generally wear surgical gowns, caps, eyewear, and gloves. This is a nursing role that may be delegated to UAPs, LPNs, or LVNs.

Registered Nurse First Assistant

The registered nurse first assistant (RNFA) has gone through additional extensive education and training to deliver surgical care. They directly assist the surgeon by controlling bleeding, using instruments and medical devices, handling and cutting tissue, and suturing during the procedure. The RNFA may also be involved with patient care before and after surgery. The RNFA is able to be certified in this specialty area of perioperative nursing, thus obtaining the credential CRNFA (Phillips, 2004).

Surgical Services Education Coordinator or OR Educator

This perioperative RN educator works with staff members and patients to promote education and competence. As a patient educator, this nurse assists the patients and their family members in providing information regarding surgical care and treatment. As a staff educator, these nurses design, coordinate, and implement orientation, staff development, and continuing education for the personnel who work in the surgical services department.

Director of Surgical Services/OR Director

The nursing director manages the business of the facility's operating rooms. The OR director oversees and is responsible for budgets, staffing, supplies, scheduling, and other areas that keep the OR running.

Surgical Technologist

A surgical technologist (ST) is an allied health professional who works as part of the surgical team to ensure that the operative procedure is conducted under optimal conditions. The ST is responsible for three phases of patient care, or surgical case management, with minimal direction or supervision from their surgical team members. To qualify to take the surgical technologist credentialing exam, an individual must be a graduate of a Commission on Accreditation of Allied Health Programs (CAAHEP) or an Accrediting Bureau for Health Education Schools (ABHES) accredited surgical technology program (or a currently or previously credentialed ST). The certified surgical technologist uses the CST credential (Phillips, 2004).

Surgical Specialties

All members of the surgical team must be able to work quickly and accurately, with a commitment to detail. A number of activities must be integrated according to priority when under pressure in stressful and emergency situations. Manual dexterity and physical stamina are vital. Sensitivity to the needs of the patient as well as other members of the surgical team must be demonstrated. Many different surgical specialties exist, including, but not limited to: cardiac, thoracic, vascular, general surgery, maxillofacial, neurosurgery, gynecological, ophthalmology, oral, plastic, orthopedic, otolaryngology, genitourinary, reconstructive, and urologic (Table 21-1).

TABLE 21-1	Classification of Surgical Procedures
High-risk	Major emergency operations
	Major aortic or vascular procedures
	Peripheral vascular procedures
Intermediate-risk	Carotid endarterectomy
	Head and neck procedures
	Intraperitoneal and intrathoracic procedures
	Orthopedic surgery
	Prostate surgery
Low-risk	Endoscopic procedures
	Skin and breast operations
	Cataract surgery

Adapted from Price, P. (2004). Surgical technology for the surgical technologist (2nd ed.). New York: Thomson Delmar Learning; Rothrock, J., McEwen, D., & Smith, D. (Eds.). (2003). Alexander's care of the patient in surgery (12th ed.). St. Louis, MO: Elsevier.

ANTICIPATED OUTCOMES OF NURSING CARE

The patient-nurse bond is founded on trust that the nurse will advocate for and safeguard the patient. The nurse strives to promote the patient's optimum operative outcome. Patient outcomes are observable, measurable physiological and psychological responses to any nursing intervention. A patient outcome model focuses practice on the high risks that patients in need of operative or other invasive procedures may encounter. In the OR environment, the high risks are injury and infection, so the focus areas for care team practice are based on freedom from infection and freedom from injury. All care team members contribute to these patient outcomes.

The sterile processing department members contribute when they decontaminate instruments as the first step in the sterilization process, and STs and scrub nurses contribute when they manage sterile fields. All activities of perioperative nurses contribute to keeping the surgical patient free from injury and infection. The nurse in the role of circulator performs the preoperative assessment, noting individual patient needs and risk factors; organizes and manages the OR care environment to promote freedom from infection and injury; and evaluates the care in terms of these outcomes (Daniels, 2004). In addition, during a baseline assessment, the OR nurse assesses a patient's risk factors and can thus advocate for the patient if he or she requires a special intraoperative pressure-relieving device. With such nursing interventions, intraoperative-related iatrogenic injuries, such as burns, nerve damage, deep tissue or skin surface trauma, should decrease, as should the subsequent chance of nosocomial infections.

Nursing Sensitive Outcomes or Indicators

The Association of periOperative Registered Nurses (AORN) has established the Perioperative Nursing Data Set (PNDS), which is used to describe the care interventions provided by perioperative nurses (AORN, 2005a). The PNDS is a standardized nursing vocabulary that addresses the perioperative patient experience from preadmission until discharge. As a nursing language, it is validated, reliable, and useful for clinical practice. It is the first, and to date the only, nursing language developed by a specialty organization that has been recognized by the American Nurses Association (ANA) as a data set useful for nursing practice.

The PNDS can serve many purposes including, providing a framework to standardize documentation; providing a universal language for perioperative nursing practice and education; assisting in the measurement and evaluation of patient care outcomes; and providing a foundation for perioperative nursing research and evaluation of patient outcomes (Box 21-4). The PNDS can also assist nurses with documentation, care plans, critical pathways, competency assessments, performance appraisals, policies and procedures, job descriptions, and educational programs for orientation and an academic program (Kleinbeck, 2002).

NANDA and the Nursing Process

Perioperative nurses utilize the same nursing process that all nurses use where they assess, diagnose, implement, and evaluate the patient care that they provide. Based on the information gathered, examples of nursing diagnoses for the perioperative patient may include the following: risk for infection; risk for impaired skin integrity related to positioning, immobilization, pressure, or shearing forces; risk of injury related to surgical environment, extraneous objects, and equipment (laser, electrical, and use of X-rays/radiation); and risk of hypothermia. Examples of potential outcomes for perioperative nursing diagnoses are:

- The patient is free of signs and symptoms of infection.
- The patient is free of signs and symptoms of physical injury.
- The patient is free from signs and symptoms of injury related to positioning.
- The patient is free from signs and symptoms of laser, electrical, and radiation injury.
- The patient is at or returning to normothermia.

The perioperative nurse follows the nursing process as well as the ANA code of ethics when providing nursing care to the surgical patient. Perioperative explications of the ANA code of ethics for nurses serves as the guideline for ethical patient care in the surgical setting (AORN, 2005a).

Pediatric Considerations

Perioperative nurses must be able to provide age-specific care for the pediatric patient. Children are more likely than adults to experience a variety of problems, including those related to pain management in the perioperative period. Many pediatric patients are recovered in a setting, such as the outpatient setting, that is principally oriented to the care of adults. To accommodate children, the department must have the necessary personnel and equipment, and the nurses must have knowledge of the procedures that are specifically oriented to the special needs of children. Nursing staff should be familiar with the care of children, e.g., pediatric airway management, cardiovascular physiology, pharmacology, and the developmental, behavioral, and emotional responses of pediatric patients (Potts & Mandleco, 2002).

The nurse is aware that preparation prior to a hospitalization or surgical intervention is important for children. All preoperative discussions should be age appropriate, use child-friendly language, and attempt to reduce the stresses that lead to fear and anxiety. Because no one can promise there will not be pain or discomfort for the pediatric patient, responding to questions in a straightforward manner will help promote the child's trust, which is also important. It is natural for children to fear the unknown, and hospitals look and smell different from any other place in the child's experience. Children feel less anxiety

---

BOX 21-4

PNDS: EXAMPLES OF INTRAOPERATIVE INTERVENTIONS

- Implements aseptic technique and assesses susceptibility for infection
- Performs skin preparations
- Monitors for signs and symptoms of infection, and administers prescribed prophylactic treatments
- Initiates traffic control
- Identifies physical alterations that may affect procedure-specific positioning and positions the patient
- Implements protective measures to prevent skin or tissue injury due to thermal, chemical, or mechanical sources and evaluates for signs and symptoms of injury to skin and tissue
- Uses supplies and equipment within safe parameters
- Performs required counts
- Implements thermoregulation measures

Adapted from Beyea, S. C. (Ed.). (2002). The perioperative nursing data set (2nd ed.). Denver: AORN, Inc.

if they have a chance to tour the hospital and the OR prior to admission. The perioperative nurse can help explain what will happen during the surgical procedure and any tests that the child will experience. Perioperative nurses encourage pediatric patients to bring a toy, stuffed animal, or other familiar object to the hospital so the child will feel more secure. It is also helpful to allow the parents to stay with their child as much as possible during a hospitalization and immediately preoperatively. Parents may want to make arrangements to remain with their child as long as possible prior to surgery and to be present in the recovery room as the child wakes up. This step may help a child be calmer and more compliant with necessary medical procedures.

Perioperative nurses need to address fluid and electrolyte management of the pediatric surgical patient. Having the appropriate size equipment and instrumentation is important in facilitating appropriate pediatric care. Having the correct size pediatric vascular access devices available, for example, will facilitate the process of establishing intravenous (IV) fluid and medication administration. The anesthesia provider will also have appropriate sized endotracheal tubes, along with any necessary modification of medication dosage and administration methods.

Pain Management in Pediatric Patients

Unfortunately pediatric pain has historically been undertreated because of health care providers' attitudes and myths; it has only been since the 1980s that pain in children has been treated aggressively (Potts & Mandleco, 2002). The most prominent myth is that infants and young children do not experience or remember pain; this is now known to be untrue. It has been argued that, while the risk in administering pain medication is understood, some health care providers are inadequately trained in the palliation of pain. This statement may be equally applicable to nurses.

Ideally, postoperative pain management begins in the OR. However, the most difficult aspect of pain management in children is adequate assessment of the severity of the pain, particularly in the preverbal child. If pain assessment is inadequate, the nurse may underestimate the child's pain with the outcome being one of unnecessary suffering. Inadequate pain control may also result in hypertension in children. The post anesthesia care unit (PACU) nurse must be familiar with pediatric vital sign norms and aberrations when monitoring patients. Behavioral assessment tools are often used for younger children, but visual scales (e.g., numbers or faces) should be used whenever possible in older children (Estes, 2006). Many health care providers are concerned that opioids will cause respiratory depression, but this is extremely uncommon in patients with ongoing pain if small doses are used and titrated to effect. Distraction techniques and parental presence may help pediatric patients as well.

It is the nurse's responsibility to recognize and respect those aspects of pain management that are unique to children. The nurse, caring for the pediatric patient, becomes the parental surrogate, advocating for the child, assessing pain, and providing timely and effective relief. The assessment and treatment of pain in children are important parts of nursing care, and failure to provide adequate control of pain amounts to substandard and unethical practice. Understanding pain management across the life span, therefore, becomes an integral part of the ethical practice of the perianesthesia nurse.

Geriatric Considerations

Advances in surgical and anesthetic techniques combined with sophisticated perioperative monitoring are factors that have contributed to an expanding number of older adults undergoing surgery. Preoperative assessment is useful to identify factors associated with increased risks of specific complications and to recommend a management plan that minimizes the risks. Each person should be assessed individually, and judgments should be based on an individual's problem and physiological status not on age alone. Older people often have multiple comorbid conditions that limit their functional capacity and recovery and increase the risk of death. An initial complication is much more likely to lead to other complications; failure of one organ to function adequately is more likely to lead to failure of other organs.

Advanced age, poor functional status at baseline, impaired cognition, and limited support at home are risk factors for adverse outcomes. However, when age and severity of illness are directly compared, severity of illness is a much better predictor of outcome compared to age. Emergency operations carry a greater risk compared to elective operations in all age-groups, particularly elderly people.

Cardiac complications are among the most common and most serious postoperative problems. The strongest predictors of adverse cardiac outcomes are recent myocardial infarction (MI), uncompensated heart failure (HF), unstable ischemic heart disease, and certain cardiac rhythm disorders. The major clinical predictors are unstable coronary syndromes, decompensated HF, significant arrhythmias, and severe valvular disease. Intermediate clinical predictors are mild angina pectoris, prior MI, compensated or prior HF, and diabetes mellitus. Minor clinical predictors are advanced age, abnormal electrocardiogram (ECG) findings, rhythm other than sinus, low functional capacity, history of stroke, and uncontrolled systemic hypertension. Elderly people can also have presbycardia (decreased function of cardiac muscle) and silent coronary artery disease even in the absence of cardiac risk factors (Price, 2004). HF is a significant risk factor associated with poorer outcomes. Identifying HF based on findings from a careful history and physical examination is important. HF and clinically significant arrhythmias require in-depth evaluation and control before elective, noncardiac surgery is performed. Uncontrolled preoperative arrhythmias are aggravated by the stress associated with the induction of anesthesia and intubation of the airway.

Diabetes mellitus can be an intermediate clinical predictor of perioperative myocardial ischemia not only because of the association between diabetes mellitus and coronary artery disease but also because of the increased incidence of other perioperative complications, including ketoacidosis, stroke, renal failure, and sepsis. Prevention of hyperglycemia during the perioperative period has been shown to improve wound healing, reduce the risk of infection, and reduce cerebral damage in the presence of a hypoxic event.

Pulmonary Disease in Geriatric Patients

Pulmonary disease increases the risk of postoperative complications, accounting for 40 percent of postoperative complications and 20 percent of deaths (Price, 2004). Age-related changes, such as increased closing volumes and decreased expiratory flow rates, predispose older people to pulmonary complications. The additive effect of supine position, general anesthesia, and abdominal incisions leads to a significant reduction in functional residual capacity and an associated increase in airway resistance. The combination of these effects can predispose patients to atelectasis, with the risks of hypoxemia and infection. Additionally, postoperative pain and use of analgesics contribute to a reduced tidal volume and impaired clearing of secretions dependent on adequate coughing and deep breathing.

The preoperative functional level has been shown to be a reliable predictor of pulmonary complications. Interventions, such as preoperative smoking cessation, antimicrobial therapy for bronchitis, perioperative bronchodilator therapy, optimization of therapy for uncompensated right HF, inhalation of humidified gas, postural drainage, and chest physiotherapy, can reduce pulmonary complications, lower mortality, and shorten hospital stays. Fatal pulmonary embolism accounts for a larger proportion of operative deaths in elderly people. An estimated 20 to 30 people of patients undergoing general surgery without prophylaxis develop deep vein thrombosis, and the incidence rate is as high as 40 percent in those undergoing hip and knee surgery, gynecological

Respecting Our Differences

Geriatric Patient Care

To care effectively for geriatric patients perioperative nurses need a working knowledge of the aging process and its effects on sensory systems and of data gathered preoperatively regarding patients' deficits, especially hearing and vision deficits. By using perioperative baseline data, nurses can reduce risk factors for communication problems and anticipate postoperative sequelae. The perianesthesia nurse and the perioperative nurse should maintain frequent communication during the operative procedure and immediately following the transfer of patients to the PACU.

Interventions related to vision and hearing, such as returning patients' glasses and hearing aids as soon as possible postoperatively, will help the PACU nurse's overall patient assessment. Some geriatric patients have increased pain thresholds; therefore, perianesthesia nurses should assess elderly patients' pain levels carefully. Increased pain threshold and decreased tactile sensation can cause elderly patients to be unaware of pressure areas that may have developed during the intraoperative phase of care. Consequently, the perianesthesia nurse must make a concerted effort to assess patients' skin as well as repositioning patients and padding bony prominences to avoid pressure-related injuries.

Cognitively impaired elderly patients may be at greatest risk for undertreatment of pain during the initial postoperative period. Acute confusion is a notable problem among older adults. It can diminish the geriatric patient's ability to localize, interpret, or communicate pain or discomfort to nurses. Acute confusion needs to be viewed as a priority problem for nurses when caring for elderly patients. The patient's self-report of pain may prove to be an unreliable indicator of discomfort if the patient is confused. Ethical practice includes the perianesthesia nurse acquiring and maintaining a knowledge base adequate to provide care to patients of all ages. Pain, being a subjective experience, is of special importance as the assessment of it often relies on objective signs in addition to the subjective reports from the patients themselves.

cancer operations, open prostatectomies, and major neurosurgical procedures. Perioperative interventions should focus on thrombosis prophylaxis, oxygen therapy, prevention and treatment of perioperative hypotension, and prompt identification and treatment of postoperative complications.

Patients with Parkinson disease require special attention during the perioperative period. Withholding medications in patients who are to have nothing by mouth (NPO) can cause significant worsening of symptoms. Patients may experience hypoxia from stiffening of chest wall muscles, dysphagia, and worsened tremor, which can cause increased pain at the operative site. If possible, a weighted feeding tube can be used to administer the medication at appropriate times.

Geriatric patients experience a variety of changes in sensory function. Decreased neuronal density and nerve conduction in the central nervous system contribute to overall sensory loss in elderly patients. While individuals age differently, the perioperative nurse must be aware of changes in vision, hearing, touch, and pain sensitivity as these will have an impact on the care provided.

THE SURGICAL ENVIRONMENT

The intraoperative environment is brightly lit, relatively quiet, and temperature and humidity controlled. The design of the environment focuses on the maintenance of surgical asepsis. To prevent patient infection, guidelines for

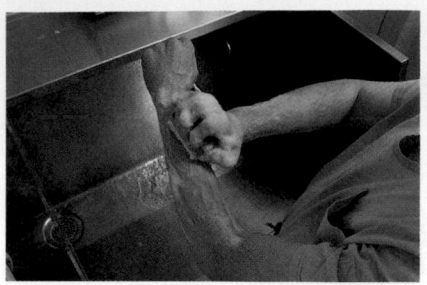

Figure 21-2 Nurse performing a surgical scrub using a counted brush stroke method.

asepsis are strictly adhered to by the surgical staff. Sterile technique is the term that describes the surgical team members' adherence to principles of asepsis in the operative setting. **Asepsis** refers to the absence of pathogenic organisms.

Asepsis and Sterility

An item that is to be considered sterile means that it is free from microorganisms. The process of sterilization kills all microorganisms and spores, whereas the process of disinfection kills organisms but does not kill the spores. All items or objects that are not sterile are considered unsterile or contaminated. Skin cannot be sterilized, but the number of microorganisms may be reduced through vigorous scrubbing (Figure 21-2). Microorganisms cannot penetrate dry cotton fabric and nonwoven paper or plastic wrappers. Intact skin helps to prevent the entry of microorganisms. Sterile technique takes into consideration the means by which microorganisms can be transmitted (e.g., direct contact, airborne droplets, fluids, or capillary action).

Traffic Control

To maintain environments with minimal exposure to microorganisms, the areas of the surgical suite are controlled for access by all types of personnel, (e.g., staff, visitors, and patients). The goal is to minimize microorganisms by monitoring and restricting the amount and type of people passing into, through, and out of the OR environment. Designated traffic patterns for personnel to follow assist with this goal. Increasing environmental controls and surgical attire as progression is made from unrestricted to restricted areas decreases the potential for cross-contamination. According to the AORN Recommended Standards and Practices (2006), traffic patterns should be designed to facilitate movement of patients and personnel into, through, and out of defined areas within the surgical suite. Signs should clearly indicate the appropriate environmental controls and surgical attire required (AORN, 2006).

Most surgical suites are divided into three designated areas that are defined by the physical activities performed in each area: the unrestricted area, the semirestricted area, and the restricted area. The unrestricted area includes a central control point that is established to monitor the entrance of patients, personnel, and materials. Street clothes are permitted in this area, and traffic is not limited. The semirestricted area includes the peripheral support areas of the surgical suite and has storage areas for clean and sterile supplies, work areas for storage and processing of instruments, and corridors leading to the restricted areas of the surgical suite. Traffic in this area is limited to authorized personnel and patients. People in this area should wear surgical attire to include long-sleeved jackets that are buttoned or snapped closed during use. All head and facial hair should be covered by a surgical cap or hood.

Sterile supplies may be stored in various areas in the department of surgical services. Some wrapped and sterilized sets and prepackaged supplies are kept in the sterile processing storage area. These items may also be kept in storage rooms within the surgical suite environment, such as designated semirestricted areas of the department.

The restricted area includes operating and procedure rooms, the clean core, and scrub sink areas. People in this area are required to wear full surgical attire and cover all head and facial hair, including sideburns and necklines. Nonscrubbed personnel should wear long-sleeved jackets that are buttoned or snapped closed during use. Masks are required where open sterile supplies or scrubbed persons are located (AORN, 2005a).

People from other departments entering the semirestricted or restricted areas of the surgical suite for a brief time for a specific purpose may don coverall suits designed to cover outside apparel totally. A transition zone exists where one can enter the area in street clothing and exit into the semirestricted or restricted zone in surgical attire. Locker rooms serve as a transition zone between the outside and inside of a surgical suite and may serve as a security point to monitor people admitted to the suite (AORN, 2005a). There are also substerile areas within the surgical environment. These areas are usually located attached to an OR and may contain scrub sinks and autoclaves.

Patients entering the surgical suite should wear clean gowns, be covered with clean linens, and have their hair covered. Clean gowns, linens, and hair coverings are worn by patients to minimize particulate shedding during surgical procedures (AORN, 2005b). Patients are not required to wear masks while in the surgical suite unless they are under respiratory precautions (for example, a patient with active pulmonary tuberculosis or other airborne respiratory disease). While in the restricted area, the mask could hinder access to the face and airway and might increase the patient's anxiety. Keeping the sterile field away from the head of the surgical bed until the patient is draped will minimize the possibility of contamination.

Movement of personnel should be kept to a minimum while invasive and noninvasive procedures are in progress (AORN, 2005b). Careful assessment and planning for patient care needs by surgical team members can reduce the need for excess movement or activity during procedures. Air currents are a potential source of microorganisms that can contaminate surgical wounds. Microbial shedding increases with activity, and greater amounts of airborne contamination can be expected with increased movement of surgical team members (Rothrock, McEwen, & Smith, 2003). Doors to the operating or procedure rooms should be closed except during movement of patients, personnel, supplies, and equipment. The air pressure within each operating or procedure room should be greater than in the semirestricted area. Leaving the door open can disrupt pressurization and cause turbulent airflow that could increase airborne contamination as well as affect the temperature and humidity levels in the room. Conversation and the number of people present should be minimized during procedures. An increase in airborne microorganisms can occur with an increased number of people present. Movement, talking, and uncovered skin areas can contribute to airborne contamination (AORN, 2005b).

The flow of clean and sterile supplies and equipment should be separated from contaminated supplies, equipment, and waste by space, time, or traffic patterns. Supplies prepared for surgical procedures outside the surgical suite (e.g., in sterile processing) should be transported to the surgical suite so as to maintain cleanliness and sterility and to prevent physical damage. Use of correct procedures for transporting items preserves the qualities of the sterile and clean environment (Rothrock, et al., 2003). Supplies and equipment should be removed from external shipping containers in the unrestricted area before transfer into the surgical suite. External shipping containers may collect dust, debris, and insects during shipment and may carry contaminants into the surgical suite.

The flow of supplies should be from the clean core through the operating or procedure room to the peripheral corridor. Soiled supplies, instruments, and equipment should not reenter the clean core area. They should be contained in closed or covered carts or containers for transport to a designated decontamination area. The decontamination area and soiled linen and trash collection areas should be separated from personnel and patient traffic areas. Separation of clean and sterile supplies and equipment from soiled materials by space, time, and traffic patterns decreases the risk of infection (AORN, 2005b).

Traffic patterns may be affected during construction, renovation, and maintenance. Specific traffic plans for construction personnel and movement of supplies, equipment, and debris should be developed and implemented. Policies and procedures should establish guidelines for quality assessment and improvement activities to be used when monitoring traffic control patterns in the surgical practice setting (AORN, 2005a).

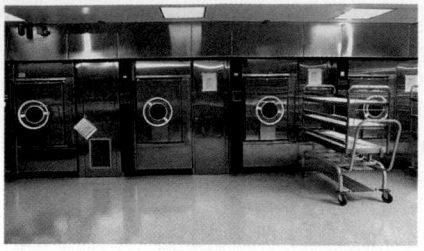

Figure 21-3 Steam sterilization area.

Methods of Sterilization

Some commonly used methods of sterilization are high pressure or temperature (e.g., autoclave) for items that can withstand high temperature (Figure 21-3). For items which are unable to withstand high temperatures and pressure, ethylene oxide gas is the preferred method of sterilization. Sometimes cold chemical sterilization may be used effectively for other items. Box 21-5 describes in detail the various sterilization methods.

BOX 21-5

STERILIZATION METHODS

- High pressure or temperature steam sterilization using an autoclave and appropriate monitoring systems to ensure sterility. An autoclave is a type of gravity displacement or prevacuum sterilizer. For sterilization to be effective, items being processed require exposure to direct steam contact at the required temperature and pressure for the specified time. Pressure serves as the means to obtain the high temperatures needed to kill microorganisms. High temperature of the steam, 121 to 132° C (250 to 270° F) kills microorganisms in 3 to 20 minutes, depending on the type of sterilizer and wrapping.

- Dry heat utilizes static air or forced air is used to sterilize items. A higher temperature is required for a dry heat unit than for a steam processor. For sterilization to occur, the cycle must be brought to correct temperature and then maintained at that temperature. Actual time needed to sterilize instruments will depend on the size and arrangement of the load, the type of wrapping material, and unit efficiency.

- Gas sterilization with ethylene oxide (ETO) or gas plasma using an approved gas sterilizer and appropriate monitoring systems are used to ensure sterility and personnel safety. All materials sterilized by ETO require safe aeration time. Instruments that cannot tolerate heat are processed with high level disinfectants or with low temperature sterilization, such as ETO gas or hydrogen peroxide gas plasma.

- Cold chemical sterilization is also used for some items. Effective and proper use of chemical sterilization is dependent on many factors, including the use of chemicals classified as sterilants. Those classified as disinfectants are not adequate. Items to be sterilized must be relatively smooth, impervious to moisture, and be a shape that permits all surfaces to be exposed to the chemical sterilant. The items being sterilized must be exposed (immersed) to the sterilant for the prescribed period of time. Rinsing chemically sterilized items prior to use in the surgical procedures is imperative. Instruments, implants, and tubing (both inside and out) must be rinsed with sterile saline or sterile water prior to use to avoid tissue damage. Only products classified as sterilants are to be used for sterilizing instruments and implants for surgery. These products must be used according to the manufacturer's recommendations to ensure adequate sterilization. Examples of sterilants are hydrogen peroxide, hydrogen peroxide/peracetic acid combinations, and glutaraldehyde. Glutaraldehyde exposure limits have been set by the OSHA guidelines.

Adapted from Association for the Advancement of Medical Instrumentation (AAMI). (2005). Standards. Sterilization in health care facilities (part 1) and sterilization equipment (part 2). *Arlington, VA: AAMI Publications; Price, P. (2004).* Surgical technology for the surgical technologist *(2nd ed.). New York: Thomson Delmar Learning.*

Sterilization of Supplies and Equipment

Many supplies, such as gloves, surgical blades, and suture materials, are commercially available in sterile, ready-to-use packs. However, it is frequently necessary to sterilize (in-house) items, such as surgical instruments, drapes, gauze, gowns, and catheters/devices for implant. When considering methods for sterilization, it is important to differentiate between sterilization and disinfection. Sterilization kills all viable microorganisms, while disinfection only reduces the number of viable microorganisms. High-level disinfection will kill most vegetative microorganisms, but will not kill the more resistant bacterial spores. Commonly used disinfectants, such as alcohol, iodophors, quaternary ammonium, and phenolic compounds, are not effective sterilants and therefore are not acceptable for the use on items intended to be used in survival surgical procedures.

The sterilization process itself is not the concern but rather how the entire process is performed. It is important to remember that sterilization is an event. It requires the maximum control of all variables so as to affect a minimum margin of doubt in the end result. Flash sterilization implies that we can achieve sterilization instantaneously. However, many factors can adversely affect the outcome of effective sterilization.

Flash sterilization can be performed in gravity displacement or prevacuum sterilizers that are equipped for such cycles. Perkins recommends minimum flash exposure times. All hinged instruments should be in the open position, multiple-part devices should be disassembled, and items with lumens should be flushed with sterile distilled water immediately before sterilization. Porous items include those items made of rubber, latex, silicone, and plastic.

The AORN Recommended Practices for Sterilization in the Practice Setting (2006) state that flash (steam) sterilization should be carefully selected to meet special clinical situations. Flash sterilization should be used only when there is insufficient time to sterilize an item by the preferred prepackaged method or

TABLE 21-2 Sterilization Terms and Definitions	
Sterilization	A process that will destroy all forms of life applied especially to microorganisms
Disinfection	The destruction or inhibition of most pathogenic agents on inanimate objects by chemical or physical means; disinfection cannot occur in the presence of organic debris
Levels of disinfection	Used for instruments, equipment, and surfaces that do not require sterility or cannot be practically sterilized
	There are three levels—high, intermediate, and low with the intended use for patient care determining the level of decontamination
Sanitization	The process of removing organic debris in order that disinfection can occur
Bacteriostatic	An agent that will inhibit increases in the number of bacteria
Bactericidal, fungicidal, and virucidal	An agent that will destroy (kill) bacteria, fungi, or viruses

Adapted from Price, P. (2004). Surgical technology for the surgical technologist (2nd ed.). New York: Thomson Delmar Learning; Rothrock, J., McEwen, D., & Smith, D. (Eds.). (2003). Alexander's care of the patient in surgery (12th ed.). St. Louis, MO: Elsevier.

TABLE 21-3	Spaulding Critical Items
Critical	Touches bone or penetrates soft tissue; must be sterilized
Semicritical	Touches mucous membranes but will not touch bone or penetrate soft tissue; sterilize or high-level disinfection if sterilization will alter the item
Noncritical	Has contact with intact skin; intermediate to low-level disinfection or simple cleaning

Adapted from Association for the Advancement of Medical Instrumentation (AAMI). (2005). Standards. Sterilization in health care facilities (part 1) and sterilization equipment (part 2). Arlington, VA: AAMI Publications.

when the surgical suite has been specifically designed to incorporate flash sterilization of instrumentation (e.g., sterilizer doors open into each room).

The Association for the Advancement of Medical Instrumentation (AAMI) (2005) recently outlined the steps necessary to ensure efficacy of the flash sterilization process. Two important steps in the process of sterilization are proper cleaning and the confinement and containment of the devices after sterilization to avoid any contamination.

Instrument Sterilization and Disinfection

The terms shown in Table 21-2 are used to describe processes that involve different levels of destruction of microorganisms to which surgical instruments and materials may be exposed.

The Spaulding system is a standard system of classification for sterilization and disinfection. It classifies instruments according to their use, which in turn determines how they will be decontaminated. This system is explained in Table 21-3.

Preparation for Instrument Sterilization and Disinfection

Instruments have to be cleaned prior to sterilization or disinfection to dislodge blood, saliva, and other debris, which may act as barriers to the sterilization or disinfection process. The principal objective in wrapping is to protect sterilized instruments from environmental contamination. The correct packaging for sterilization needs must be utilized. In many institutions the majority of surgical instrumentation is cleaned, wrapped, and sterilized for use in surgery by personnel in the sterile processing department.

Sterilization Monitoring

Failure to follow the manufacturer's instructions on equipment usage, improper wrapping, overloading or improper loading, or sterilizer malfunctions will impair the sterilization process (Rothrock, et al., 2003). Monitoring includes a combination of process parameters: mechanical, chemical, and biological. Mechanical is human observation that the sterilizer is working correctly. This includes observing and assessing the gauges on the sterilizer. Chemical indicators are generally part of the packaging or the tape and change color when a given parameter is reached (e.g., time, temperature, or pressure). These indicators do not guarantee that sterilization has taken place; only that the items have been exposed to conditions that are conducive to the sterilization process. Biological indicators are known as spore tests and are used to demonstrate that sterilization has occurred. These are the only accurate test for sterilization. Biological indicators are specific to the sterilization method used.

Soiled surgical instruments should be transported to the decontamination area in a manner that prevents contamination of the person transporting them and the environment. The area in which the instruments are decontaminated should be physically separated from the area in which the instruments are inspected and reassembled. Doors leading to the decontamination area should be kept closed. Personnel assigned to the decontamination area should wear personnel protective equipment ([PPE], e.g., head cover, shoe covers, impervious gown, gloves, and face and eye protection) when cleaning surgical instruments. All PPE should be removed and hands washed when leaving the decontamination area (AORN, 2005b).

Using enzymatic detergents aids in the decontamination process. All devices should be thoroughly cleaned and rinsed following the manufacturers' instructions. Proper cleaning agents are necessary to make the cleaning process more efficient and to protect the surgical instruments' finish. All detergents should be measured carefully and used in accordance with the manufacturers' instructions. Instruments with multiple parts should be disassembled for cleaning. Soft-bristled brushes should be used to clean the instruments, with particular attention paid to ratchets, serrations, and box locks (joints). Manual cleaning should be done while holding the instrument and the brush under the water level to prevent aerosolization of bacteria (AAMI, 2005).

Flash sterilization can be done with the device unwrapped or with a single wrapper. In addition, flash sterilization containers are available that totally contain the instrument during and after sterilization. The AAMI (2005) recommends that flash sterilization be tested in facility's sterilizers to validate that sterilization can be achieved when used in particular sterilizers. The process for container validation is described in the AAMI document. It is important that the manufacturer of the containers provide written, scientific documentation that sterilization containers are suitable for the flash sterilization process.

After decontamination, surgical instruments should be treated with a water-soluble lubricant often referred to as instrument "milk" because of the white color. This lubricant protects the instrument's surface and can prolong its life. Manufacturers' instructions must always be followed when using this product. This type of lubricant should be allowed to air dry. Items with multiple parts should be kept disassembled for sterilization to allow the steam to make contact with all instrument surfaces (AAMI, 2005).

Monitoring the Sterilization Cycle

All flash sterilization cycles should be monitored to validate the effectiveness of the process (AORN, 2005a). Administrative controls, such as charts, printouts, and gauges, should be monitored, interpreted and initialed by the sterilizer operator for correlation with the proper cycle times and temperatures for items being processed. Chemical indicators should be used in each cycle to verify that all sterilization parameters have been met.

Biological monitoring is recommended at least weekly and preferably daily. The organism used to test for steam sterilization is *Bacillus stearothermophilus*. The manufacturer of the biological monitor being used should provide documentation that the product has been tested and is indicated for flash sterilization cycles. Biological tests are available that provide a reading within one hour for flash cycles. All items that are flash sterilized should be documented on a flash sterilization log. A log should be maintained at each flash sterilizer and changed daily. The logs are necessary to meet the requirements to be able to trace items in the event of a sterilizer malfunction. All sterilization logs should be maintained with the charts or printouts for each day so they can be easily retrieved for reference. It is important that the flash sterilization process be monitored for improvements. All sterilizer operators should receive initial training and continuing education to ensure proper use of the sterilization equipment. All biological and chemical monitoring should be interpreted and verified before the instruments are used.

Ideally, surgical departments would contain sufficient surgical instrumentation to allow for proper decontamination and terminal sterilization. However, if flash sterilization must be performed, the proper protocols should be followed by all personnel. Practitioners must see that policies and procedures are developed to ensure that all steps in the flash sterilization process are followed correctly and that continuous quality improvement monitors are developed to verify the efficacy of the process.

OR Environment

There are certain conditions, such as temperature, humidity, and airflow, that are necessary in the OR to provide an optimal environment (Rothrock, et al., 2003). Strict control of the temperature in operating suites is mandatory. For adults, the critical ambient temperature desirable is 20 to 22° C (68 to 72° F. For infants and children this may be increased up to 24°C (74° F). **Laminar airflow** (filtered air circulating in parallel-flowing planes) is often used in operating suites to decrease the risk of infection (Price, 2004). However, a research team headed by surgeon Harvey R. Bernard at Barnes Hospital in St. Louis, Missouri, has found that surgeons, nurses, and patients themselves carry most of the dangerous germs, especially the resistant strains of staphylococci, into the OR. Relatively few organisms appear in the air, and it makes little difference whether the air is continually drawn fresh from outdoors, or whether it is recirculated after filtering.

It is the humidity that contributes most to the safety of the air. Germs such as staphylococcus thrive in dry air (relative humidity less than 35 percent) and in moist air (65 percent or over). The recommended operating room humidity level is 50 percent, a setting that is best for operating personnel, worst for germs, and moist enough to minimize the dangers from static electricity.

The Air Supply System

Surgical air handling systems need to respond to changes in the use of ORs that have been brought about by new technologies and new surgical procedure or by a renovation that increases the size of a particular OR or operating suite. Today's surgeries require larger rooms, with enough space for the significantly greater amount of equipment and number of people involved. The renovations needed to accomplish this often require modifications to large portions of the air handling system.

Sepsis after total joint replacement is related directly to environmental contamination. Some types of environmental control, such as laminar airflow or ultraviolet light, are the most helpful with greater than 90 percent reduction of airborne bacteria at the wound and 60 percent reduction of airborne bacteria in the OR. To reduce environmental bacteria contamination, the number of personnel in the OR and the length of time for the actual surgery should be reduced, because wound contamination occurs first by direct fallout from the environment and second by contaminated equipment and gloved hands that initially were contaminated by the environment.

ORs should be maintained at positive pressure with respect to corridors and adjacent areas. Positive pressure prevents airflow from less clean areas into clean areas. Conventional OR ventilation systems produce a minimum of about 15 air changes of filtered air per hour, and three (20 percent) of these air changes per hour must be fresh air. Air should be introduced at the ceiling and exhausted near the floor. Recommended ventilation parameters for ORs have been published by the American Institute of Architects, and the U.S. Department of Health and Human Service.

Laminar airflow is designed to move particle-free air (called ultra clean air) over the aseptic operating field at a uniform velocity to sweep away particles in its path. This airflow can be directed vertically or horizontally, and the air is usually passed through a high efficiency particulate air (HEPA) filter. In the surgical environment, air should be supplied at a lower velocity above the operating table and at a higher velocity at the perimeter of the operating table. The objective is to draw the low velocity air into the outer higher velocity air and then exhaust it. This arrangement removes most contaminants emitted at the table and provides a suitable clean environment in ORs.

STANDARD PRECAUTIONS IN THE SURGICAL ENVIRONMENT

Standard precautions are designed to reduce the risk of transmission of microorganisms from both recognized sources of infection in the hospital. Standard precautions protect both patients and employees. Standard precautions include treating blood and all body fluids (secretions, excretions [except sweat], nonintact skin, and mucous membranes) as infectious regardless of their source, hand washing before and after patient contact or contact with infectious substances, and using appropriate PPE when there is potential exposure to infectious substances (Mangram, et al., 2005).

All body substances, except sweat, are to be treated as infectious regardless of their source. Recognition of potential exposure risks is important. To reduce the likelihood of exposure when dealing with potentially infectious substances, it may be necessary to choose an alternative procedure, technique, or type of equipment.

Hand Washing

Hand washing is an important means of reducing the risks of transmitting microorganisms from one person to another or from one site to another on the same patient. The level of hand contamination is highest after contact with blood or body substances (Mangram, et al., 2005). Even if gloves have been worm, hands may become contaminated during glove removal. Wearing jewelry has been shown to increase the microbial load normally carried on hands. Therefore, excessive jewelry wearing is not recommended during patient care activities (AORN, 2005b). Hands must be washed before and after patient contact or contact with items contaminated with blood or body substances.

Personal Protective Equipment

Appropriate personal protective equipment (PPE) is to be worn when there is potential for exposure to infectious substances. PPE is comprised of gloves, protective face and eyewear, gowns, and other protective apparel (Daniels, 2004). Gloves provide a protective barrier and prevent gross contamination of the hands when touching potentially infectious substances. They reduce the likelihood that microorganisms present on the hands of personnel will be transmitted to patients during invasive or other patient-care procedures that involve touching a patient's mucous membranes and nonintact skin. Gloves protect the hands of personnel from becoming transiently colonized with microorganisms from a patient or object that can be transmitted to other patients. Gloves must be changed between patient contacts. Wearing gloves does not replace the need for hand washing because gloves may have defects or be torn during use, and hands can become contaminated during glove removal. Therefore, hands should be washed after gloves are removed. Gloves should be chosen to fit hand size, flexibility, and tactile sensitivity needed during the procedure(s), potential for exposure to blood and body fluids during the procedure(s) both in terms of the amount and the length of time exposed, and exposure to other substances that break down glove material, such as disinfectants and solvents. An assortment of disposable (single use) gloves is available in a variety of sizes and materials (e.g., latex, nonlatex, vinyl, or rubber). Health care workers and patients can have allergies to latex, which include latex gloves. Allergy histories should always be known before beginning a procedure so that appropriate precautions or preventive actions can be taken.

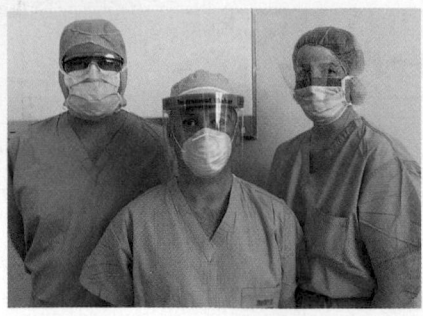

Figure 21-4 Examples of protective eyewear.

Masks, goggles, or face shields must be worn to provide protection of the mucous membranes of the eyes, nose, and mouth during procedures and patient-care activities that are likely to generate splashes or sprays of blood, body fluids, secretions, or excretions and to provide protection against the spread of infectious large particle droplets (Figure 21-4). Face shields that cover below chin level, wrap around to the ears, and allow for prescription glasses provide the best protection. Prescription glasses alone do not provide protection from splatter and splashes (Mangram, et al., 2005). Masks should be made of thick, sturdy cotton material to filter microorganisms. Gauze is not an acceptable material for a mask, because it is too loosely woven. Masks should be worn so that the mask fits snugly against the face, is secured along the sides of the face, and molded over the bridge of the nose. Air should not enter around the mask edges. Beards should be kept groomed so that the mask fits as closely to the face as possible. Masks should be changed between patients or if the mask gets wet. Masks should be removed as soon as the treatment is over and should not be kept dangling around the neck (AORN, 2005b).

Scrub clothing alone does not provide adequate protection from blood and body fluid exposure (AORN, 2005b). Various types of gowns and protective apparel must be worn to provide barrier protection and reduce opportunities for transmission of microorganisms. Gowns are worn to prevent contamination of clothing and to protect the skin from blood and body fluid exposures. Gowns and other appropriate protective apparel must always be worn when there is potential that an exposure will occur (Mangram, et al., 2005). Protective garments should fit staff members appropriately. There are types of scrub clothes that are designed for the activity and amount of fluid likely to be encountered. If the scrub clothes become soiled with blood or body fluids, health care providers need to glove and remove clothing immediately. Sterilized surgical gowns are considered sterile in front from the chest to the level of the sterile field. Sleeves are sterile from 5 cm above the elbow to the cuff. The neckline, shoulders, underarms, and back of the gown are considered to be unsterile. Gowns should be put on after surgical scrub and before gloving.

Specimens that are collected in surgery must be handled with gloved hands. All collected specimens must be labeled and contained in a plastic biohazard lab specimen bag. Health care organizations have policies and procedures in place to direct the care and handling of surgical specimens. Governmental guidelines and recommendations, such as OSHA and the Centers for Disease Control and Prevention (CDC), are also in place for this purpose.

Prion diseases, such as Creutzfeldt-Jakob disease (CJD), are a group of degenerative brain diseases that have received much attention during the past few years. They occur in animals (e.g., dogs, cows, and primates) as well as humans and are rapidly fatal once symptoms develop. In humans, CJD remains rare, with an incidence of less than one per million in the general population.

Prions, such as those found to cause CJD, pose a unique infection prevention problem because **prions,** which are protein-containing infectious agents, can survive recommended heat or high-pressure steam sterilization processes. In addition, chemical disinfectants, including sterilants, such as glutaraldehydes and formaldehyde, are not strong enough to eliminate prion infectivity on contaminated instruments and other items. Therefore, surgical instruments and other critical devices contaminated with high-risk tissue (e.g., brain, spinal cord, or eye tissue) from patients with known or suspected CJD require special treatment (Rutala & Weber, 2001). When an instrument requires sterilization or high-level disinfection, cannot withstand the rigors of this process repeatedly, and the cost is not inhibitive, it is then considered a disposable item.

Surgical Team Attire and Technique

During surgical procedures, both patients and providers are especially at risk of exposure to potentially infectious microorganisms. Along with the other elements of aseptic technique, proper surgical attire helps reduce the risk of post-

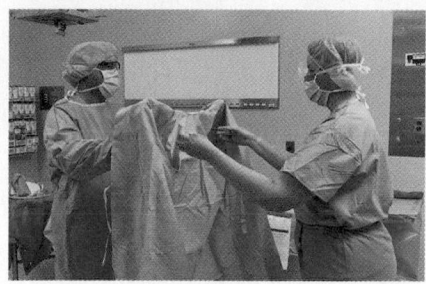

Figure 21-5 Assisting a team member with gowning.

procedure infections in patients by decreasing the likelihood that microorganisms will enter areas of the patient's body during procedures. Some elements of surgical attire are also designed to reduce the health care providers' risk of exposure to potentially infectious blood and tissue during surgical procedures.

Surgical attire includes gloves, caps, masks, gowns, protective eyewear, waterproof aprons, and sturdy footwear. Surgical staff members must be covered with a fluid-resistant gown when performing procedures with an increased risk of splashing of blood or body fluids. Proper surgical attire is worn in the OR during all surgeries except where institutional policies and procedures direct attire differently, such as for some clean procedures and scoping procedures. Surgical team members assist one another with the putting on gowns and gloves, being careful to maintain sterility (Figure 21-5).

Currently, surgical attire is the only available alternative to street clothes and should provide maximum comfort. Federal OSHA regulations consider an item of personal protection appropriate if it does not allow infectious materials to pass through to or reach the employee's work clothes or skin. Studies do not indicate that the use of a cover gown or shoe covers decreases surgical site infections (AORN, 2005b). In addition, hair is abundant with bacteria, and circulating staff members and anesthesiologists are in close proximity to sterile trays. Surgical caps should sufficiently cover the hair.

Scrub Clothes

There is some controversy regarding the need for OR staff to wear scrub clothes, including the need for members of the surgical team to wear scrub suits under their sterile gowns (Price, 2004). There is no scientific evidence to support the use of surgical scrub suits as a means of reducing infections. Decisions regarding the use of scrub clothes are usually made by each facility individually, after weighing the costs (e.g., supplies and laundry) and practicality (e.g., storage and availability of changing areas) against any potential benefit. Home laundering is not recommended by AORN, but some institutions have implemented this practice (AORN, 2005b).

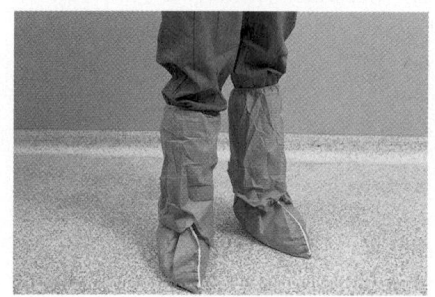

Figure 21-6 Impervious boot style shoe covers.

Sturdy footwear must be worn in the operating theater (Figure 21-6). Footwear protects the feet from direct exposure to blood and other body fluids and from injury from sharp or falling instruments and other items. There is no scientific evidence to support the use of shoe covers as a means of reducing the risk of infections in patients (AORN, 2005b). Staff members working in the surgical setting must be aware of the potential for contamination of their attire during operative procedures.

Scrub Technique

Appropriate scrub technique is an integral aspect of surgical asepsis. Aseptic technique also encompasses practices performed immediately before and during a surgical procedure to reduce postoperative infection. Antimicrobial agents are used for the health care provider's surgical scrubs, because they inhibit the growth and development of microorganisms and are safe for use on the skin. If an alcohol solution is used, it should be rubbed into the hands and fingernail areas and allowed to dry before resuming any activity as alcohol is flammable, and there exists the potential for fire when the electrosurgical unit or laser is activated. In addition, there are new brushless scrub products available that have decreased the hand scrub time to approximately one minute (AORN, 2005b).

Proper preparation of the patient's surgical site, using an antimicrobial cleansing product prior to surgery, is essential in reducing the number of microorganisms present on the patient's skin. The patient's surgical site should be thoroughly cleaned, and then an antiseptic is applied to the skin. Shaving is no longer recommended, because it causes small nicks and breaks in the skin where bacteria can grow and multiply; hair around the site may be clipped short if it might interfere with the procedure. Studies have demonstrated that patients who had not been shaved had significantly fewer postoperative infections than patients who had been shaved (AORN, 2005b).

Opening Sterile Supplies

The integrity of sterile packages should be preserved while being opened, dispensed, or transferred. Packaging integrity begins when the sterile instruments are packaged in the sterile processing area of the institution. When instrument sets are packaged in sterile canisters, special filters are inserted for use during the sterilization process. These filters must be inspected by the surgical staff members when the instrument canisters are opened in the surgical suite for set up purposes (AORN, 2005b).

Surgical staff members should recognize that a sterile or high-level disinfected (HLD) barrier that has been penetrated (e.g., moisture or tear) is considered to be contaminated. Perioperative staff members should also be aware of how they move within or around the sterile field in a way that maintains sterility during the entire perioperative process.

PATIENT SAFETY

Safe operative techniques can minimize the risk of infection. For example, intrauterine devices (IUDs) can be inserted without being handled by the provider if they are loaded into the inserter within their sterile packaging, thereby reducing the risk of contamination. Careful attention to bleeding and gentle tissue handling during surgery can further reduce the risk of infection. Surgical site infections may develop in a variety of ways and are usually observed post-procedurally, such as in tissue that has been damaged due to rough or excessive manipulation during surgery or when excessive bleeding occurs.

Laser

The word *laser* is an acronym for light amplification by the stimulated emission of radiation. Lasers are used in surgery to cut and coagulate tissue. The laser is, however, a complex piece of equipment that can cause fires and other damage if used incorrectly. There are four primary types of laser hazards: (a) optical radiation to the eye and skin, (b) electrical hazards, (c) chemical airborne contamination, and (d) miscellaneous ancillary hazards.

There needs to be a designated person available to operate the laser during surgical procedures. This person may be a specially trained nurse or technician. For safety purposes, the person designated as the laser operator should have no other duties during the surgical intervention (AORN, 2005a). Ocular and skin hazards associated with laser radiation receive the greatest attention, however, optical hazards in general are not potentially lethal, whereas electrocution and severe burns or skin damage are also possible under certain conditions. In the medical environment fluid spillage is possibly the major cause of an electrical hazard. This may be because of spillage into the equipment or by leaking coolant in some systems. Staff members should be educated to treat the laser like any other electrical or electronic equipment used in the OR environment.

When tissue is heated via coagulation there is often a resultant plume of smoke or related fumes that are emitted. The lung is the principle organ of the body susceptible to inhaled pollutants. Many of the inhaled fumes initiate an inflammatory response within the airways and alveolar areas of the lung. Small exposures over a period of years can lead to chronic airway narrowing and destruction of the alveolar area (e.g., emphysema). These changes in the alveolar area are characteristically produced by cigarette smoke. The laser, in addition to the electrosurgical units used intraoperatively, has the potential for the plume to carry viable organisms to unprotected OR personnel (AORN, 2005a). As a result, there is the need to use smoke evacuation equipment, smoke filters, and purpose-made laser face masks, designed to trap smoke particles. The smoke particles (carbon) can also block the OR suction system if they are not filtered from it.

Reflections and Nonreflective Instruments

Materials that do not appear specular or reflective (mirror-like) to the eye may be specular at the wavelengths provided by various lasers. Potential laser strikes on specular targets are to be avoided wherever possible. Instruments that absorb laser energy and get hot or reflect energy to adjacent tissue should be avoided during this type of surgery. Some surgical instruments are designed and manufactured specifically for use with the laser to diffuse the laser energy rather than absorb it ensuring that the density of the scattered reflected beam is low.

Fire and Explosion

Surgical lasers have the potential to set fire to flammable items in the OR, such as clothing and drapes. It is common practice to moisten sponges and other potentially flammable materials in the surgical site when using lasers. Red rubber or plastic endotracheal (ET) tubes are usually avoided when working in the airway with the laser as the oxygen-enriched anesthetic provides a combustible medium. Instead, metal ET tubes or foil wrappings of plastic endotracheal tubes are recommended.

If any alcohol-based preparations, such as a surgical skin prep solution, have been used on the surgical site, it is imperative that the solutions be allowed to dry thoroughly so as to avoid igniting when the laser is used. When working near the hairline, it is important that the patient has not used sprays or gels on the hair that may contain alcohols. The patient's bowel should be purged of methane before a gastroenterology laser procedure. The availability of a suitable fire extinguisher immediately accessible to the operative suite is recommended. Many scrub people will have a bowl of water kept on the surgical back table to reduce potential fire hazard.

Operating Protocol

The laser operator should always return the laser to a standby mode when not in use. This action prevents the inadvertent firing of the laser should the foot pedal be depressed accidentally. The use of a checklist is strongly recommended when using the surgical laser.

Surgical Fire

In addition to the surgical lasers, there are other pieces of surgical equipment that utilize electricity and heat. Heat, fuel, and oxygen, known together as the fire triangle, exist in ORs, raising the risk of surgical fires. Flammable materials common to the surgical environment include alcohol prepping agents, surgical gowns, drapes, hoods, and masks. These materials can be ignited by heat from surgical lasers, warming blankets, electrosurgical equipment, and high-intensity fiberoptic light sources. High concentrations of oxygen found in ORs serve as additional risk factors for surgical fires.

Technological advances in safety and the performance of electrosurgical units (ESUs) have made the ESU the most common piece of electrical equipment in the operating room. The constant presence of the ESU in the OR increases the potential for patient injury that is associated with the use of any piece of electrical equipment. To prevent injuries related to the use of an ESU, the perioperative nurse must understand the types of current used, types of ESUs available, and any potential complications and have a working knowledge of safe practices for using this piece of equipment in the perioperative setting.

Electrosurgery was engineered for broader surgical treatments and uses high-frequency current between two electrodes, one active electrode and one dispersive electrode, to cut, desiccate, or fulgurate tissue. The electrosurgical cut mode uses low voltage and high current flow. Cutting techniques require the active electrode tip to be in direct contact with the target tissue (Dennis, 2004). As the high-density current passes through the tissue, intracellular fluids are vaporized and the cell structure is destroyed. The current then takes the path of least resistance through the dispersive pad. Bipolar electrosurgery adheres to the same basic principles. The current is localized between the two electrodes on the target tissue. Delivery of current through bipolar modalities (e.g., forceps) uses lower voltage output than monopolar electrosurgery and is beneficial during delicate tissue procedures. Box 21-6 lists strategies for the nurse to implement in the OR.

Whenever electrical applications are used during surgical procedures, perioperative nurses must remain vigilant to ensure safe patient outcomes. The perioperative nurse must be knowledgeable in preventing electrical injury, applying principles of electrosurgical safety, and understanding potential risk factors. It is important to note that smoke from the electrosurgical unit is also potentially hazardous via inhalation.

Latex

Some children and adults have an allergy or sensitivity to latex. The powder from the inside or outside of latex gloves can contain the latex protein, which is the allergen factor for many individuals. When a person has contact with products that contain latex, he or she may exhibit watery or itchy eyes, wheezing, hives, flushing or a skin rash, itching, or swelling. In some cases, severe reactions, such as anaphylactic shock, can occur in which the person may have problems breathing, experience chest tightness, or have swelling of his or her throat or tongue. Severe reactions require prompt emergency treatment. Some people are more likely to become latex sensitive. These are people who have frequent exposure to latex from medical procedures. This group includes: children with spina bifida, children born with urological anomalies, and children or adults who have had many surgeries.

In rare cases, an allergic individual goes into shock when the blood pressure plummets and the airway becomes constricted. Without immediate treatment, the person will die. An injection of epinephrine—the same drug used to treat

---

BOX 21-6

ELECTROSURGICAL SAFETY STRATEGIES

- The electrosurgical unit (ESU) settings should always be confirmed verbally with the operator. Good practice is to always use the lowest possible power settings.
- Manufacturer's instructions should be followed and approved instruments or electrodes should be used.
- The ESU generator must be mounted securely on a cart or boom to prevent falling.
- Items should not be placed on top of the generator, especially potentially dangerous items, such as fluids.
- The ESU foot pedal should be kept in an impervious bag. Fluid from blood and irrigation solutions can cause a shock.
- Enforce cord and plug safety: The cord should be of adequate and plugs should never be yanked out of the outlet.
- Practice smart prepping. Care must be taken with types of prepping solutions that need to dry thoroughly.
- The ESU should not be used in the presence of flammable agents.
- Nurses should be able to assess the patient's skin integrity before, during, and after electrosurgery.

Adapted from AORN. (2005a). Recommended practices for electrosurgery. In Standards, recommended practices and guidelines *(pp. 248–250). Denver: Author.*

severe allergic reactions to bee stings—will counteract this life-threatening condition if administered immediately. There are many commonly used medical products that contain latex (e.g., rubber gloves, elastic bandages, adhesive tape, urinary catheters, electrode pads, protective sheets, or rubber tourniquets).

Cardiac Arrest

During the process of obtaining informed consent, the health care provider will discuss the risks and benefits of the surgical procedure according to the specific condition of each patient (Daniels, 2004). One of the risks of surgical intervention is the potential for cardiac arrest in the OR. A thorough history and physical should reveal this potential, and the surgical team can then modify the intraoperative care accordingly (e.g., bringing the code cart into the OR during the procedure).

The perioperative nurse must always be ready for possible emergencies in surgery as a cardiac arrest can result from a variety of sources, such as trauma or stress. The nurse should know the location of the code cart in the surgical suite area, and depending on the number of ORs in the institution, there may need to be multiple code carts available in the department at any time.

ANESTHESIA AND SEDATION

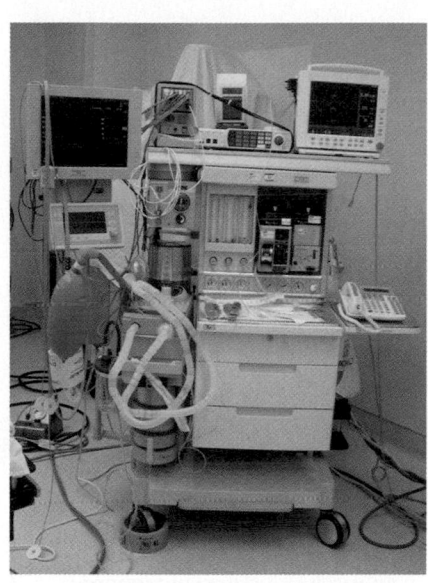

Figure 21-7 Anesthesia machine.

While the perioperative nurse is not directly responsible for the administration of anesthesia to the surgical patient, he or she is responsible for maintaining a knowledge base regarding anesthesia as well as being present to assist the anesthesiologist or CRNA with direct patient care during while the patient in being cared for in the surgical environment.

Types of Anesthesia

During surgery, patients are given some form of **anesthesia** (medicine for the relief or elimination of pain). Anesthesia refers to the loss of feeling or sensation or general insensibility to pain, induced by an anesthetic agent, such as medications or inhaled gases. General anesthesia causes loss of consciousness, relaxes the muscles, and produces amnesia. Local or regional anesthesia numbs only a specific area. The type and dosage of anesthesia is administered by the anesthesiologist or nurse anesthetist. The **anesthesia care provider** (e.g., anesthesiologist or nurse anesthetist who delivers anesthesia to patients in surgical settings) will have an anesthesia machine and an anesthesia cart for supplies and equipment necessary for the administration of anesthetic (Figure 21-7).

There are variations in the terms sedation and analgesia, and these terms are defined and clarified by the American Society of Anesthesiologists (ASA). The term **sedation** refers to the reduction of anxiety, stress, irritability, or excitement by the administration of a sedative agent or drug. **Minimal sedation (anxiolysis)** is a drug-induced state during which patients respond normally to verbal commands, and although cognitive function and coordination may be impaired, ventilatory and cardiovascular functions are unaffected (ASA, 2004). Moderate procedural sedation/analgesia, or **conscious sedation,** is a drug-induced depression of consciousness during which patients respond purposefully to verbal commands, either alone or accompanied by light tactile stimulation (Reeves, Havidich, & Tobin, 2004). **Deep sedation/analgesia** is a drug-induced depression of consciousness during which patients cannot be easily aroused but respond purposefully following repeated or painful stimulation. Reflex withdrawal from a painful stimulus is not considered a purposeful response. The ability to independently maintain ventilatory function may be impaired. Patients may require assistance in maintaining a patent airway, and spontaneous ventilation may be inadequate. Cardiovascular function is usually maintained (Fryer & McIntosh 2005).

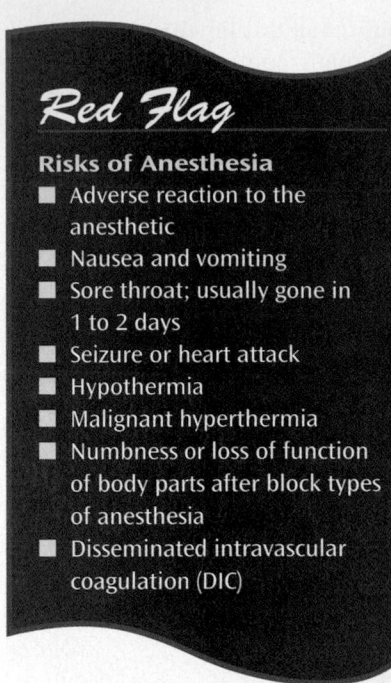

Red Flag

Risks of Anesthesia

- ■ Adverse reaction to the anesthetic
- ■ Nausea and vomiting
- ■ Sore throat; usually gone in 1 to 2 days
- ■ Seizure or heart attack
- ■ Hypothermia
- ■ Malignant hyperthermia
- ■ Numbness or loss of function of body parts after block types of anesthesia
- ■ Disseminated intravascular coagulation (DIC)

Because sedation is a continuum, it is not always possible to predict how an individual patient will respond. Practitioners intending to produce a given level of sedation should be able to rescue patients whose level of sedation becomes deeper than initially intended. Rescue of a patient from a deeper level of sedation than intended is an intervention by a practitioner proficient in airway management and advanced life support. The qualified practitioner corrects adverse physiological consequences of the deeper-than-intended level of sedation (e.g., hypoventilation, hypoxia, and hypotension) and returns the patient to the originally intended level of sedation (ASA, 2004). Monitored anesthesia care does not describe the continuum of depth of sedation, rather it describes a specific anesthesia service in which an anesthesiologist has been requested to participate in the care of a patient undergoing a diagnostic or therapeutic procedure (ASA, 2004).

There are various forms of anesthesia. The type of anesthesia provided depends on the type of surgery and the patient's medical condition. Usually, an anesthesiologist will administer a sedative in addition to the anesthetic. Different types of anesthesia are described in Box 21-7.

Risks of Anesthesia

There are risks with anesthesia. Some surgeries cannot be done at all if anesthesia is not an option (see Red Flag).

BOX 21-7

TYPES OF ANESTHESIA

- Local anesthesia is medicine given to temporarily stop the sensation of pain in a particular area of the body. A patient remains conscious during a local anesthetic. For minor surgery, a local anesthetic can be administered via injection to the site.
- Regional anesthesia means numbing only the portion of the body that will be operated on. Usually an injection of local anesthetic is given in the area of nerves that provide feeling to that part of the body.
- Spinal anesthesia often used for lower abdominal, pelvic, rectal, or lower extremity surgery. An anesthetic agent or medication is injected into the fluid in the spinal canal.
- Epidural anesthesia is similar to a spinal anesthetic and also is commonly used for surgery of the lower limbs. It is also administered as an anesthetic during labor. A thin catheter is placed in the epidural space, which is in the middle and lower back, just outside of the spinal space.
- General anesthesia causes a patient to be unconscious during surgery. The medicine is either inhaled through a breathing mask or tube or administered through an IV line. General anesthesia is a drug-induced loss of consciousness during which patients cannot be aroused, even by painful stimulation. The ability to independently maintain ventilatory function is often impaired. Patients often require assistance in maintaining a patent airway, and positive-pressure ventilation may be required because of depressed spontaneous ventilation or drug-induced depression of neuromuscular function. Cardiovascular function may be impaired.

Adapted from Broyles, B. E., Reiss, B. S., & Evans, M. E. (2007). Pharmacological aspects of nursing care (7th ed.). New York: Thomson Delmar Learning.

Disseminated Intravascular Coagulation

Disseminated intravascular coagulation (DIC) is the syndrome that occurs when the clotting cascade goes awry. This is a clotting and bleeding disorder that results from the generation of tissue factor activity within the blood. This trigger of the coagulation cascade quickly leads to significant thrombin production, which perpetuates its own formation. In little time, the existing regulatory factors, such as antithrombin III, protein C, and protein S, are consumed. As a result, large amounts of thrombin are generated, leading to a hypercoagulable state. In the normal physiological state, plasmin is responsible for breaking fibrin into fibrin split products, thereby limiting the amount of fibrin clot being formed. In DIC, the quantity of plasmin is increased leading to the generation of significant quantities of fibrin degradation products and this often results in bleeding. Some causes of DIC are: (a) complications of obstetrics in which uterine material with tissue factor activity gains access to the maternal circulation such as in abruptio placenta; (b) infection with gram-negative bacteria, which secrete an endotoxin that induces the generation of tissue factor; (c) malignancies, particularly adenocarcinoma of the pancreas or prostate as well as promyelocytic leukemia; and (d) head trauma (Littleton & Engebretson, 2002).

The underlying cause of DIC must be identified and treated, (e.g., uterine evacuation for abruptio placenta, broad-spectrum antibiotics for gram-negative sepsis, and replacement therapy with cryoprecipitate and platelets). This condition is a disorder of the clotting cascade. It results in depletion of clotting factors in the blood and occurs when the body's blood clotting mechanisms are activated throughout the body instead of being localized to an area of injury. Small blood clots form throughout the body, and eventually the blood clotting factors are used up and not available to form clots at sites of real tissue injury. Clot dissolving mechanisms are also increased. Tests used to identify DIC are: fibrinogen, serum fibrinogen, prothrombin time (PT), partial thromboplastin time (PTT), platelet count, and thrombin time test (Daniels, 2003).

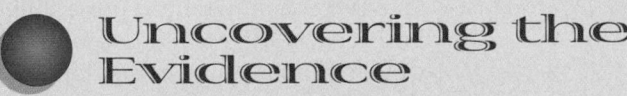

Uncovering the Evidence

Retained Objects in the Intraoperative Setting

Discussion: This study included 54 patients with a total of 61 retained foreign bodies (of which 69 percent were sponges and 31 percent instruments) and 235 control patients. Thirty-seven of the patients with retained foreign bodies (69 percent) required reoperation, and one died. Patients with retained foreign bodies were more likely than controls to have had emergency surgery (33 percent versus 7 percent, P<0.001) or an unexpected change in surgical procedure (34 percent versus 9 percent, P<0.001). Patients with retained foreign bodies also had a higher mean body mass index and were less likely to have had counts of sponges and instruments performed. The risk of retention of a foreign body after surgery significantly increases in emergencies, with unplanned changes in procedure and with higher body mass index.
Implications for Practice: The study encourages nurses and the health care team members in surgical settings to take precautions to prevent foreign bodies from being left in patients.

Source: Gawande, A., Studdert, D., Orav, E., Brennan, T., & Zinner, M. (2003). Risk factors for retained instruments and sponges after surgery. New England Journal of Medicine, 348, 229–235.

The goal is to determine the underlying cause of DIC and provide treatment for that identified cause. Replacement therapy of the coagulation factors is achieved by transfusion of fresh frozen plasma. Cryoprecipitates may also be used if fibrinogen is significantly low. Heparin, a medication used to prevent thrombosis, is sometimes used in combination with replacement therapy. The underlying disease that causes the disorder will usually predict the probable outcome. Complications of DIC include severe bleeding, stroke, and lack of blood flow to arms, legs, or organs.

INTRAOPERATIVE COMPLICATIONS

Intraoperative complications can often be prevented with prevention and careful surgical team members. However, when problems do occur, they may include foreign objects, such as instruments or needles, being retained inside the patient; hypothermia; or patient injury.

Retained Objects

Retained objects are considered a preventable occurrence, which careful counting and documentation can significantly reduce, if not eliminate. According to AORN, members of the entire surgical team can be held liable in litigation for retained foreign bodies (2005b). There is always a risk that an object used during the surgical procedure may inadvertently be left in the patient. To prevent this from occurring, perioperative nurses perform surgical counts or X-rays are taken of the patients' surgical sites postoperatively. In addition, other factors are being studied that can predict high risk patients or situations for retained objects in surgery (Gawande, Studdert, Orav, Brennan, & Zinner, 2003).

Surgical Counts

The recommended practice for sponge, sharp, and instrument counts developed by the AORN Recommended Practices Committee is intended as achievable recommendations representing what is believed to be an optimal level of practice (AORN, 2005b). Sponges should be counted on all procedures in which the possibility exists that a sponge could be retained. Sponge counts should be performed before the procedure to establish a baseline, before closure of a cavity within a cavity, before wound closure begins, at skin closure or end of procedure, and at the time of permanent relief of either the scrub person or the circulating nurse. Sponges should be separated, counted audibly, and concurrently viewed during the count procedure by two individuals, one of whom should be a RN circulator. When additional sponges are added to the field, they should be counted at that time and recorded as part of the count documentation (Price, 2004).

Sharps and other miscellaneous items should be counted on all procedures. Sharps and miscellaneous item counts should be done before the procedure to establish a baseline, before closure of a cavity within a cavity, before wound closure begins, at skin closure or end of procedure, and at the time of permanent relief of the scrub person and circulating nurse. Initial sharps counts should be performed and recorded on all procedures. Counting sharps and miscellaneous items is not only important in preventing foreign body retention; the continuous accounting for these items can lessen injuries to those scrubbed in the sterile field.

Instruments should be counted for all procedures in which the likelihood exists that an instrument could be retained. Instrument counts should be performed, before the procedure to establish a baseline, before wound closure, and when feasible, at the time of permanent relief of the scrub person or circulating nurse. Instrument counts protect the patient by reducing the likelihood that an instrument will be retained. Retention of surgical instruments accounts for approximately one third of retained item case reports. Additional measures for investigation, reconciliation, documentation, and prevention of incorrect surgical counts should be taken (Nursing Law's Regan Report, 2005). Sponge, sharp, and instrument counts should be documented on the patient's intraoperative record. Documentation of counts is illustrated in Box 21-8.

Hypothermia

Hypothermia is a condition where the body temperature falls between less than 36° C (96.8° F) (Price, 2004) and is classified as mild if not less than 32° C (89.6° F). Hypothermia may not be immediately resolved. Anesthesia can affect temperature in three stages. Induction of anesthesia causes vasodilation, which allows movement of heat from the center with no net loss of body heat to the environment. The greatest temperature drops may occur within the first 40 to 60 minutes of anesthesia and may also be related to patient exposure during skin preparation and positioning. Significant reductions in core temperature have also been noted at the end of orthopedic procedures after tourniquet deflation.

Hypothermia may be less likely to occur if regional anesthetic techniques are employed, perhaps because the hypothalamic thermoregulation remains intact. However, vasodilation may still occur so there may still be an impairment of shivering in the area of the block. It may be because of this usual absence of shivering that routine temperature monitoring is less likely to be carried out, resulting in hypothermia sometimes remaining undetected in these patients. If a combination of regional (epidural) and general anesthesia is used, the risk of hypothermia may be increased because of the combined effects on the thermoregulatory mechanisms (Evered, 2003).

Consequences of Hypothermia

Known and suspected adverse effects of hypothermia are diverse; variations in serum potassium levels, postoperative instability, an increased risk of myocardial ischemia in the first 24 hours following surgery, and increased mortality. Hypothermia can have an impact on arterial blood pressure and is associated with cardiovascular complications. Hypothermia is thought to affect protein metabolism and decrease subcutaneous oxygen tension. These effects on skin oxygen tension have also been shown to increase the incidence of surgical wound infection in patients having colorectal surgery. This link between intraoperative hypothermia and tissue viability can also be related to the development of pressure ulcers.

It has also been suggested that the development of hypothermia leads to a longer overall hospital stay. Furthermore, the incidence of perioperative morbid cardiac events was higher in hypothermic patients who were known to be at high risk of coronary disease and who had abdominal, thoracic, or vascular surgical procedures. It is also clear that patients having major surgery, especially if the abdominal cavity is opened or if there is extensive fluid irrigation or infusion, are particularly at risk of intraoperative hypothermia if no preventive action is taken.

Hypothermia impairs coagulation through inhibiting the series of enzymatic reactions of the coagulation cascade, which controls the hemostatic system. It is therefore a contributory factor to abnormal bleeding and the development of coagulopathy after shock, trauma, or massive transfusion. The body and its organs are designed to function at an optimal core temperature of 37° C (98.6° F), and there is evidence that hypothermia can be physiologically harmful. Although the use of intraoperative warming therapies is not always economically viable in patients who are young and healthy, the elderly and especially those with comorbidities, will certainly benefit (Carter-Templeton, 2005).

BOX 21-8

COUNT DOCUMENTATION

- Types of counts and number of counts
- Names and titles of personnel performing the counts
- Results of surgical item counts
- Notification of the surgeon
- Instruments intentionally remaining with the patient or sponges intentionally retained as packing
- Actions taken if count discrepancies occur
- Rationale if counts are not performed or completed as prescribed by policy

Adapted from Price, P. (2004). Surgical technology for the surgical technologist (2nd ed.). New York: Thomson Delmar Learning; Rothrock, J., McEwen, D., & Smith, D. (Eds.). (2003). Alexander's care of the patient in surgery (12th ed.). St. Louis, MO: Elsevier.

Patient Temperature Management

Body temperature should be monitored and maintained as close to normothermic as possible during the preoperative period. Overheating because of excessive use of warming devices and inappropriate monitoring of body core temperature can result in passive hyperthermia. Monitoring and maintaining body temperature during the preoperative phase has a significant impact on the patient's risk for the following: myocardial ischemia, cardiac morbidity, surgical site infection, surgical bleeding, and patient discomfort. Skin temperature monitoring has limitations. Core temperature monitoring, such as those utilizing the esophageal or tympanic membrane, is often a preferred measurement technique for anesthetized patients. Passive hyperthermia does not result from thermoregulatory intervention and can be treated easily by discontinuing active warming devices and removing excessive insulation on the patient.

Direct contact of the patient's skin with plastic surfaces should be avoided. When used, temperature-regulating devices should be placed in an effective and safe manner and monitored during the surgical procedure. Any heat-regulating device should be used according to the manufacturer's recommendations. Thermal burns or pressure necrosis may occur when using temperature-regulating devices. Unless temperature-regulating blankets are designed to be placed next to patients' skin, a thin cloth covering is needed to protect surgical patients.

Measures to prevent hypothermia should begin in the preoperative phase and continue into the postoperative phase. Perioperative nursing interventions include applying warm blankets on the patient's arrival in the surgical area and after sterile drapes are removed; limiting the amount of skin surface exposed during positioning and skin preparation; limiting time between prepping of the skin and draping; preventing surgical drapes from becoming wet; adjusting the room temperature; monitoring patient temperature to avoid overheating; using heat-maintenance devices (e.g., caps, blankets, leggings, or warming units); warming irrigation or infusion solutions; and humidifying the airway.

The anesthetized patient loses heat intraoperatively and is unable to restore body heat through the normal mechanism of shivering or increased muscle activity. Hypothermia occurs during the immediate preoperative phase and continues throughout the postoperative phase. Factors that contribute to perioperative hypothermia include, but are not limited to, decreased metabolic heat production, increased environmental heat loss, redistribution of heat within the body, patient's age, induced inhibition of thermoregulation during surgical procedures, patient's physical status, type of anesthesia used, body fat, and length and type of surgical procedure.

Preventive measures protect the patient from heat loss due to radiation, conduction, or evaporation. Skin integrity should be inspected before, periodically during (when possible), and after using devices such as ice packs, temperature-regulating blankets, and heat lamps. Individuals vary in their ability to tolerate heat and cold. Conditions that predispose patients to injury include age, immobility, body fat, open wounds, broken skin, edematous areas, abscesses, peripheral vascular disease, confusion or unconsciousness, nerve injuries, or regional anesthesia.

Intraoperative Fluid Management

The intraoperative management of fluid therapy has great potential for influencing intraoperative and postoperative morbidity and mortality. Awareness of preoperative hemodynamic status, particularly as it influences the preload/ventricular output relationship, is critical in avoiding serious cardiovascular complications early in the course of anesthetic induction and maintenance. The implications of anesthetic pharmacology, positioning, thermoregulation, ventilatory support, surgical manipulation, operative site, duration, tissue

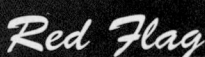

Red Flag

Symptoms of Malignant Hyperthermia

The health care team in the intraoperative arena must be aware of the following list of clinical manifestations of malignant hyperthermia (MH).

1. Masseter spasm: contracture of the chewing musculature of the jaw is a possible early sign.
2. Early manifestations of MH include: metabolic acidosis, elevated creatininase, varieties of arrhythmias, and tachycardia.
3. Possible differential diagnoses include: thyrotoxicosis, pheochromocytoma, porphyria, histamine liberation, hypovolemia, and hypoxia.
4. Fulminant MH crisis: early signs are: sinus tachycardia, rise of the end expiratory CO_2, metabolic acidosis, rigor of the muscles, hypoxemia, and flush of the skin.
5. Specific early changes are the raise of the end expiratory CO_2 together with the metabolic acidosis. Hyperthermia is a late sign. Rhabdomyolysis is a sign of the severity of the MH.

(Torpy, 2005)

trauma, and blood loss must be appreciated in determining how much fluid to be administered.

RNs keep track of irrigation fluids and other solutions used during surgery on the sterile field. They also position bloody sponges in clear canisters or bags for viewing by the anesthesiologist or CRNA to facilitate the patient's estimated blood loss during the procedure. Based on estimated patient fluid loss, replacement fluids may be administered during the procedure as needed.

Safety in Positioning

The goals of safe patient positioning are to keep the patients as comfortable possible, keep the operative area exposed as needed, ensure that the vascular supply is unobstructed and that there is not undue pressure on an body parts. The appropriate patient position must protect the nerves and not interfere with respiration. Gentle restraint must be applied with safety straps to ensure that the patients remain stable on the operating table. Patients can experience nerve damage to the extremities if the patient is positioned wrongly or if they are not padded appropriately. In addition, the eyes can dry out if not kept shut when appropriate, and the ears can be misshapen by lying wrong on them during the surgical event. In addition, circulation can be compromised and extremities and other parts of the body can be impaired with too little blood flow to an area from incorrect positioning. Special care must be taken when positioning children, elderly, frail, or obese patients. Bony prominences must be padded. Specialized padding material is available for use in surgery.

Malignant Hyperthermia

Malignant hyperthermia (MH) is a life-threatening, acute pharmacogenic disorder, developing during or after a general anesthesia. Both a genetic predisposition and one or more triggering agents are necessary to evoke MH. Triggering agents include all volatile anesthetics (chloroform, ether, halothane, enflurane, isoflurane, sevoflurane, and desflurane) and depolarizing muscle relaxants (suxamethonium). The classical MH crisis shows a hypermetabolic state, caused primarily by the muscles of the skeletal system. Besides this classical form of MH, there exist abortive forms with unspecific signs like tachycardia, arrhythmia, and a rise in temperature (Litman & Rosenberg, 2005). Improved monitoring, better knowledge of MH by the anesthesiologists, and the therapy using dantrolene have reduced the incidence of the classic MH crisis. Nevertheless, MH is a dangerous disease, and anyone who is involved with anesthesia and anesthetics should have up to date knowledge about diagnosis and therapy of MH (Carter-Templeton, 2005).

MH is an autosomal-dominant, inherited disorder. The incidence of the genetic MH predisposition is 1 in 10,000, the clinical incidence about 1 in 30,000. This means that not every patient with a genetic predisposition to MH develops a MH crisis during exposition to triggering agents (Litman & Rosenberg, 2005). Volatile anesthetics or suxamethonium cause a rise in the mycoplasmotic calcium concentration. Different mechanisms influencing the intracellular calcium concentration could be genetically determined. The rise in calcium concentration leads to an activation of actin and myosin filaments and explains the rigidity and the masseter spasm, one of the early signs of a MH. The raised calcium concentration leads further to a stimulation of the energy-consuming processes in the skeletal muscle, leading to a metabolic acidosis, and further if the CO_2 rises to a respiratory acidosis. The hypermetabolism seen in MH leads to several clinical signs like hypertonia, arrhythmia, tachycardia, and hyperthermia (Torpy, 2005). Laboratory signs are hyperkalemia, a raised creatininase, and myoglobinuria, caused by a damaged cell membrane (Daniels, 2003).

MANAGEMENT STRATEGIES OF MH

- Stop triggering (volatile anesthetics, anesthesia circuit change not necessary)
- Hyperventilate patient with 100 percent O_2
- Deepen anesthesia with opioids, benzodiazepines, barbiturates, or propofol
- Prepare dantrolene perfusion
- Adjust ventilation according to blood gas analysis and end expiratory CO_2
- Check immediately, after 30 minutes, 4 hours, 12 hours, 24 hours blood gases, electrolytes, creatininase, myoglobin, and lactate (arterial catheter)
- Stop surgery, if it is elective and if there are signs of masseter spasm or fulminant MH crisis
- Begin overall body cooling: for example ice water through a nasogastric tube
- Continue to do additional monitoring: arterial catheter, central venous catheter, swan-Ganz catheter, or urinary catheter

Adapted from Yoshitatsu, S., Sambuughin, N., and Muldoon, S. (2004). Malignant hyperthermia genetic testing in North America working group meeting. Anesthesiology, 100(2), 464–465.

MH is a heterogenetic disorder. Some MH families showed a defect on chromosome 19, on the ryanodine receptor gene. Ryanodine, an alkaloid, binds selectively to the ryanodine receptor, a calcium channel in the sarcoplasmatic reticulum. Other families with MH predisposition showed no ryanodine receptor defect. Because of the heterogenicity it is impossible to perform a MH test based on genetics. The clinical symptoms of MH are not uniform and that is why it is classified as a syndrome. The onset of the symptoms is also quite variable (Litman & Rosenberg, 2005).

There are a variety of strategies implemented with malignant hyperthermia. Box 21-9 lists actions for care of MH.

It is important for the surgical team to create strategies of preventing MH. During a preoperative visit, patients should be questioned regarding any unclear complications related to general anesthesia, muscle disorders within the family, myalgia, muscle cramps, and dark urine. In evaluating the serum laboratory studies, a persistent elevated creatininase could be a hint to a MH predisposition. When a patient is identified as a candidate for MH, preoperative medications that may be prescribed are the benzodiazepines (e.g., anxiolysis).

ETHICS IN PERIOPERATIVE PRACTICE

Ethical practice is paramount to any area of nursing care and the perioperative practice environment is no exception. Perioperative nurses need to be able to effectively deal with ethical issues in the surgical setting. Nurses are most often affected by ethical conflicts that involve the compromise of their personal beliefs and values and this may result in the violation of their professional and personal integrity, which can lead to moral distress and burnout (Corley, 2002). Prolonged moral distress will lead nurses to reconsider their current profession and may contribute to the shortage of nurses. Frustration, anger, and guilt are some of the manifestations of such moral distress and can actually lead nurses to avoid patients and give less than optimal care (Nelson, 2004).

Ethical issues in perioperative nursing include issues reflecting safety, as well as the resource allocation aspects of nursing: staff, surgical supplies, equipment, and OR time (Biton & Tabak, 2003). The OR is an area of nursing where the ratio of nurse to patient is 1:1, and the nurses in this study reported that they liked this feature of their environment. Perioperative nurses do have much patient contact, although the majority of it may occur when the patient is under anesthesia.

Ethics in perioperative practice has become especially prominent today, as a focus on patient safety has come to the forefront. Perioperative nurses have a historical tradition of promoting patient safety by intervening to minimize the risks related to surgical infection and injury (Beyea, 2002). The action of intervening in high-risk situations may be motivated by practice standards, professional duty, and ethical values and beliefs. When surgical errors happen, there also occurs the responsibility or duty to report the errors and that is where the ethical imperative enters into nursing practice. Ethical practice is important to nursing as it underpins the fiber of the practice itself by providing an action guide for nurses. With the increased awareness of medical malpractice in general, and surgical or perioperative errors in particular, it has become imperative for nurses to be able to speak out when errors, or the potential for errors, become evidenced.

The ANA Code of Ethics for Nurses with Interpretive Statements (2005) third provision asserts that the nurse promotes, advocates for, and strives to protect the health, safety, and rights of the patient. This provision specifically directs nurses to take some type of action to support the rights of their patients. The concept of ethics as an action guide is inherent in nursing practice and nursing practice involves nurses having the power and knowledge to competently care for patients (Kennedy, 2004).

Organ Donation

The Operating Room Staff Advisory Council was formed by the United Network for Organ Sharing (UNOS) in 2001 (Price, 2004). Since its inception in 1986, UNOS has joined with professional organizations to collaborate on educational initiatives regarding organ donation and transplantation. As a result of these efforts, tailored educational resources have been created for targeted professional groups. UNOS has historically formed advisory councils to initiate a dialogue among particular groups that has led to the creation of appropriate initiatives and resources.

The UNOS is a national nonprofit organization that under contract with the U.S. Department of Health and Human Services administers the national Organ Procurement and Transplantation Network (OPTN). As the OPTN, UNOS maintains the national list of patients awaiting solid organ transplants, operates the computer system for allocating organs to those on the waiting list, and gathers data to evaluate the clinical and scientific status of donation and

Uncovering the Evidence

Ethics in Perioperative Nursing

Discussion: As health care evolves, factors, such as patient safety, rising costs, rights and advocacy, resource allocation, and the increasing elderly population, have emerged as ethical issues that impact nursing practice. If the nurses perceive ethical issues as causing moral distress, they may choose to leave the nursing profession altogether. How nurses perceive ethical issues, however, may differ depending on various factors such as the nurse's practice environment or education and training.

The purpose of this qualitative study was to describe nurses' experiences of ethical situations in perioperative nursing practice, with the goal of gaining a more profound knowledge of the nature of their ethical perception and analysis. Participants (n=22) were adults of either gender, of any ethnic group, having worked in the OR environment for at least one year, and who spoke English. Study participation involved an audiotaped interview that focused on the ethical experiences of the participants in perioperative practice.

Results revealed that perioperative nurses perceived ethics in their practice as "doing the right thing" along with a strong patient advocacy component. The nurses were primarily concerned with patients' rights in a setting where patients cannot always speak for themselves. They strongly voiced concerns over respecting differences in patient values and beliefs; even if in conflict with their own personal beliefs and values. The nurses tended to rely on best interests standards when caring for patients in surgery, e.g., when the wishes of the patients were unknown to them.

Implications for Nursing: This study has prompted research other nursing specialty areas as well as patient responses and experiences of ethics in health care. It has promoted a work culture of support and empowerment. It encouraged the examination the impact of corporate compliance and harassment regulation on nursing practice. It has modified the way perioperative patients are processed. Technology may yield more ethical issues in perioperative practice. It promotes the continual ethics education in academia and on-the-job.

Source: Schroeter, K. (2003). Ethics in perioperative practice: Patient advocacy. AORN Journal, 75(6), 941–949.

transplantation in the United States. Equally important is the UNOS commitment to educate professional groups and the general public regarding donation- and transplantation-related issues.

Ethical issues are present in all specialty areas of nursing, and research has been done to better understand how nurses in perioperative practice perceive ethical issues in their work environment.

PATIENT SAFETY GOALS

The first National Patient Safety Goals were established by the Joint Commission on Accreditation of Hospital Organizations (JCAHO) in July 2002 to help accredited organizations address specific areas of concern about patient safety. Each year the goals and associated recommendations are reevaluated; some may continue while others will be replaced because of emerging new priorities. New goals and recommendations are announced in July and become effective January 1 of the following year. JCAHO's 2004 National Patient Safety Goals, addressed several areas of patient care with direct implications for OR care. The following are some of these goals: (a) improving the accuracy of patient identification; (b) improving the effectiveness of communication among caregivers; (c) improving the safety of high-alert medications; (d) eliminating wrong site, wrong patient, and wrong procedure surgery; (e) improving the safety of infusion pumps; (f) improving the effectiveness of clinical alarm systems; and (g) reducing the risk of health care–acquired infections. This goal requires compliance with current hand hygiene guidelines established by the CDC (JCAHO, 2004).

Transportation

Potential hazards associated with patient transport and transfer activities should be identified, and safe practices should be established. The patient always should be attended by appropriate personnel during transport and transfer. Patient needs should be assessed by an RN before transport to determine the necessary skill level of transport personnel. Many patient care problems can occur during transport. Observation and assessment by a registered professional nurse allows for identification of potential problems and implementation of appropriate interventions.

When selecting the appropriate transport vehicle, design features to be considered include, but are not limited to, locking devices on wheels; protective devices, such as safety straps and side rails and for cribs rails high enough to prevent a standing child from falling out; stable, adjustable IV poles or stands; holding devices for oxygen tanks; positioning capabilities; controls that are easy to operate and within reach of the operator; maneuverability; sufficient size; removable head and foot boards; mattress stabilizing devices; easily cleanable surfaces; and a rack or shelf to hold monitoring equipment. These design features promote safety and help prevent injury to patients and staff members during transport (Daniels, 2004).

An adequate number of staff members should be available to ensure patient and staff member safety during transport and transfer activities. Individual patient assessment will dictate the number of staff members needed. A minimum of four staff members is needed to move an adult who is unable to assist with transfer. To promote the safety of patients and staff members, patient movement devices may be useful. If mechanical devices are not available, extra personnel may be needed. Safety devices include, but are not limited to, roller devices, hoists, and slides. Specific needs of the patient should be assessed and appropriate interventions implemented during the transport phase. All health care providers must be aware of interventions to keep the patient safe, such as (a) locking wheels on the transport vehicle and the patient's bed during transfer activities; (b) elevating side rails and using safety straps; (c) hanging and securing IV containers away from the patient's head; (d) protecting the patient by giving special attention to the head, arms, and legs; (e) ensuring that one staff member remains at the head of the patient transport vehicle; so as to provide access to the patient's airway in case of respiratory distress or vomiting; and (f) pushing the transport vehicle with the patient's feet first, avoiding rapid movement through hallways and when turning corners.

KEY CONCEPTS

- The intraoperative phase refers to the time in which the patient is in the OR.
- The perioperative nurse is a RN who provides nursing care to surgical patients preoperatively, intraoperatively, and postoperatively.
- The circulator nursing duties are performed outside the sterile field.
- An ST is an allied health professional who works as part of the surgical team to ensure that the operative procedure is conducted under optimal conditions.
- The scrub nurse works directly with the surgeon within the sterile field, passing instruments, sponges, and other items needed during the procedure.
- There are many surgical specialties including: vascular, cardiac, thoracic, oral, maxillofacial, plastic, urologic, and orthopedic.
- The PNDS is organized terminology used to describe the care interventions provided by perioperative nurses.

- Standard precautions are designed to reduce the risk of transmission of microorganisms from recognized sources of infection in the hospital.
- Appropriate PPE is to be worn when there is potential for exposure to infectious substances.
- The powder from the inside or outside of latex gloves can contain the latex protein, which is the allergen factor for many individuals.
- Anesthesia refers to the loss of feeling or sensation or general insensibility to pain, induced by an anesthetic agent, such as medications or inhaled gases.
- DIC is the syndrome that occurs when the clotting cascade goes awry.
- Retained objects are considered a preventable occurrence, which careful counting and documentation can significantly reduce, if not eliminate.
- MH is a life-threatening, acute pharmacogenic disorder, developing during or after general anesthesia.
- Perioperative nurses need to be able to effectively deal with ethical issues in the surgical setting.

REVIEW QUESTIONS

1. Which of the following is within the sterile field?
   1. Items above the level of the draped patient
   2. Items below the level of the draped patient
   3. The gowned and gloved provider's back
   4. From the gowned and gloved provider's head to the chest

2. Which of the following is correct regarding surgical attire?
   1. If sturdy footwear that completely covers the foot and is worn only in the surgical area is available, shoe covers are not needed for infection prevention purposes.
   2. Sterile surgical gloves are considered sterile if gloved hands drop below the level of the waist.
   3. When removing surgical gloves, always remove the gloves simultaneously.
   4. Caps and masks worn in the OR should be sterile.

3. Which of the following is true regarding standard infection control precautions?
   1. Standard precautions are strategies used to reduce the risk of transmission of pathogens in the health care setting.
   2. Standard precautions should be used in caring for all patients, regardless of their infectious status.
   3. Expanded or transmission-based precautions are used beyond standard precautions to interrupt the spread of certain pathogens.
   4. Standard precautions apply to exposure to blood, all body fluids and secretions (except sweat), nonintact skin, and mucous membranes.
   5. All of the above

Continued

4. Hand hygiene refers to:
   1. Using plain soap and water
   2. Using an antiseptic hand rub (e.g., alcohol, chlorhexidine, or iodine)
   3. Using antimicrobial soap and water
   4. All of the above

5. Indications for hand washing include:
   1. When gloves are removed and before leaving the OR
   2. Before washing contaminated instruments
   3. When hands are visibly soiled
   4. Before patient care
   5. 1, 3, and 4 are correct.
   6. All of the above

6. Which of the following is not usually worn as PPE when anticipating spatter of blood or body fluids?
   1. Jacket with long sleeves
   2. Gloves
   3. Head covering
   4. Protective eyewear or face shield
   5. Face mask

7. Which of the following is not true regarding gloves?
   1. Certain hand lotions can affect the integrity of gloves.
   2. Wearing gloves replaces the need for hand washing.
   3. Sterile surgical gloves are recommended for surgical procedures.
   4. Certain gloves are latex-free.

8. Which of the following statements regarding processing of contaminated instruments is false?
   1. Instruments should be processed in an area separate from where clean instruments are stored.
   2. Personnel should wear latex-free utility gloves.
   3. Instruments only need cleaning if they have visible contamination.
   4. Cleaning an instrument precedes all sterilization and disinfection processes.

9. Which of the following statements is true regarding monitoring the correct functioning of a sterilizer?
   1. A chemical indicator should be placed in a visible area of the package before sterilization processing.
   2. A biological indicator spore test should be processed through a sterilizer cycle at least once a week.

3. A biological indicator control test matching the same lot of the spore test should be submitted with the sterilizer spore test.
   4. Mechanical assessments of sterilizer cycle time and temperature should be monitored.
   5. All of the above

10. The term *laser* is an acronym for:
    1. Lateral accumulation of serial emission of radiation
    2. Light accumulation of surface energy rays
    3. Light amplification by the stimulated emission of radiation
    4. Light amplification of supersonic electrical reams

11. What are the early signs of MH?
    1. Decreased core body temperature and decreased CO_2
    2. Bradycardia
    3. Flushed skin tone
    4. Tachycardia, arrhythmia, elevated CO_2, masseter spasm
    5. All of the above

12. What are the main steps in the emergency treatment of MH?
    1. Activate the emergency medical code team
    2. Stop triggering agents, hyperventilation with high O_2 flow, dantrolene intravenously
    3. Administer dantrolene subcutaneously
    4. Begin cardiopulmonary resuscitation (CPR)

13. What is the differential diagnosis of MH?
    1. External heating, septicemia, thyrotoxicosis, pheochromocytoma, anaphylaxis, respiratory problems, pulmonary emboli, and myopathy
    2. External heating only
    3. Elevated blood pressure and pulse
    4. Dizziness and blurred vision

14. What monitoring should one use for a general anesthesia in an individual suspected to have MH?
    1. ECG, blood pressure, CO_2 monitoring, and pulse oximeter
    2. Temperature, creatininase, electrolytes, and blood gas analysis
    3. 2 only
    4. 1 and 2 are correct.

REVIEW ACTIVITIES

1. List four nursing diagnoses commonly associated with intraoperative patient care. Identify two nursing interventions for each of your four nursing diagnoses.

2. Discuss appropriate nursing interventions for the care of the patient with MH.

3. List four potential surgical errors. Discuss methods to prevent the four potential errors.

4. Discuss the factors associated with electrical safety in the OR.

5. Identify six principles of surgical asepsis. Discuss how the surgical team implements three of these principles.

6. Identify four factors that can contribute to perioperative hypothermia.

Visit the Contemporary Medical-Surgical Nursing online companion resource at www.delmarhealthcare.com for additional content and study aids. Click on Online Companions then select the Nursing discipline.

Postoperative Nursing Management

Corinne Grimes, RN, DNSc, AOCN

Darla Grimes, MS, RN

CHAPTER TOPICS

- Trends in Postoperative Nursing Management
- Nursing Care: The Day of Surgery
- Postoperative Recovery Milestones
- Home Management for the Postoperative Patient
- Future of Postoperative Nursing

KEY TERMS

Approximated
ASA scale
Compartment syndrome
Ectopy
Hematoma
Hemovac
Incentive spirometer
Major surgery
Minor surgery
Pain scales
Patient controlled analgesia (PCA)
Purulent
Thermoregulation

Postoperative care begins at the time the surgeon completes the work of surgery. From the surgical suite, the patient will travel to the post anesthesia care unit (PACU). This chapter will follow the patient from PACU through discharge from the hospital or clinic. The work of the postoperative nurse is performing care, ensuring safety, encouraging, supporting, and teaching of patients and families and is the focus of this chapter. Some patients return home shortly after their postoperative care, while others enter an intermediate care unit designed to strengthen them for a later return to their previous setting or to home. The postoperative period can be intense, both physically and psychologically, but the nurse is in a unique position to ensure the highest quality of care and the most desirable outcome, one patient at a time.

REVIEW OF TRENDS IN POSTOPERATIVE NURSING MANAGEMENT

Prior to the 20th century, there were large wards throughout hospitals, both in field situations during wartime and in the cities in more permanent structures. The patient who had completed surgery would be transferred directly back to the ward for recovery from surgery. Death rates following surgery were much higher than those of today. Today's successes in recovery from surgery are due, in part, to advances in surgical techniques as well as the advent of specialized areas in which patients might recover from the effects of surgery and anesthesia.

Following the 1900s, there was a trend toward ensuring recovery from surgery in specialized units. Recovery rooms became popular and were later renamed PACUs. These adjoined the surgical area and allowed ready access by the surgeon or anesthesia personnel should problems develop during the first minutes or hours following completion of surgery. This change improved outcomes to some extent. However, it was not until the time of World War II that the modern PACU was developed.

Capabilities for handling emergencies and more sophisticated technology were developed in the postwar years, and mortality and morbidity rates fell. The modern PACU allows convenient access for the surgical team, and therefore, shortens time from discovery of a problem to direct health care provider assistance. The PACU provides a centralized location, specific and specialized training for nursing personnel, and access to sophisticated equipment. Nurse staffing levels in the PACU allow for individualized attention and direct visualization of each patient at all times.

THE POST ANESTHESIA CARE UNIT

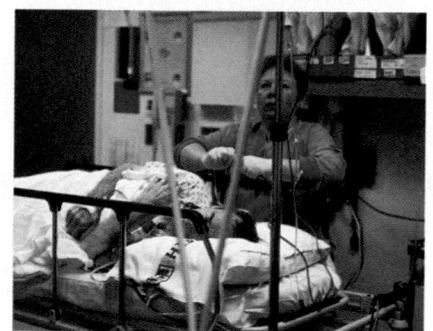

Figure 22-1 Nurse caring for patient in the PACU.

When the surgeon determines that the operation is complete, the team in the surgical suite completes last minute details and makes preparations to move the patient safely to the PACU (Figure 22-1). Most patients spend one to two hours in the PACU. From the time the patient is transferred out of the surgical suite until the time the patient is transferred from PACU to another unit, the patient is closely observed. There is one nurse caring for one to two patients. Within the PACU setting, the patient receives specialized care until cardiovascular status, respiratory status, consciousness, and activity levels are adequate (Barone, Pablo, & Barone, 2004). Some patients bypass PACU and go directly from surgery to the critical care unit (CCU). Therefore critical care nurses are also trained to care for those recovering from the immediate effects of surgery and anesthesia. Airway, breathing, and circulation are highly important during this most vulnerable period. The vigilant postoperative nurse protects the patient during a time in which the patient is unable to perform vital functions independently.

The PACU is the first of a series of postoperative destinations through which the patient will travel. When the PACU nurse assesses the patient for readiness for transport to another unit, it is considered a definite postoperative milestone. The patient's status is less dangerously dependent, and the patient and family begin to participate actively in the recovery process.

Recovery Factors

There are several areas of special concern when a patient is recovering from surgery. The initial decision involves whether to send the patient to PACU or directly to the CCU. Some considerations that may help to determine transfer directly from the surgical suite to the critical care setting are comorbidities that might threaten recovery, such as unstable diabetes mellitus, multiple trauma, or preexisting cardiac or respiratory pathology (Aragon, Ring, & Covelli, 2003). Other deciding factors might be a difficult surgical course, whether the patient had major surgery or minor surgery, and continuity of care for those patients who were in the critical care unit prior to surgery (Barone, et al., 2004). Chapter 21 describes surgical procedures deemed major and minor. **Major surgery** involves operations characterized by risk to life, such as those involving multiple systems or that require long periods in the surgical suite under anesthesia. The patient who spends many hours in surgery undergoing major, complex surgical procedures will be more likely to need the specialized nursing care available in the CCU. For the patient having **minor surgery** lasting under an hour, he or she will usually not need extensive recovery measures and may even be discharged on the day of surgery.

Regardless of destination, PACU or the CCU for these first few hours, immediate postoperative nursing care calls for specialized knowledge and vigilance on the part of the nurse. The nurse who cares for recovering patients needs to ensure that airway, breathing, and cardiovascular status are maintained. The nurse needs to be aware of the type of anesthesia used and anticipated time until the effect of anesthesia dissipates. Nursing assessment centers on internal and external measures of stability such as cardiorespiratory function and **thermoregulation** (a patient's status in relation to internal temperature control). In addition, the nurse must position the recovering patient safely in the immediate postoperative period.

Recovery from Anesthesia: The PACU

It is important for care nurses throughout the hospital to be able to visualize the PACU. This specialized unit is the setting in which the patient first awakens or first recovers full consciousness following surgery. There may be strong and sometimes disturbing memories associated with this unit for the patient and in some situations, for family members. The nurse who receives the patient within another unit following PACU routinely assesses memories and the emotions surrounding the PACU experience to assist patients and family members in recovering emotional equilibrium.

The PACU nurse recognizes that there are certain steps to be taken in a definite order to ensure patient safety and successful recovery from the effects of anesthesia and surgery. To ensure safety, members of the surgical team transport the patient to the PACU area. Observers of the PACU will detect a definite pace to patient admissions and discharges. Waves and fluctuations in patient arrivals are linked to the surgery schedule. Some of the busiest times for surgery and recovery are midweek. And the busiest times on these days occur from late morning until early evening. Most of the time, nurse staffing levels are predictable. However, all PACU areas have contingency plans for meeting unexpected emergency needs.

The PACU is usually a large room with an array of bays for surgical stretchers. The series of bays into which the patient is pushed are in two lines, usually, with a wide aisle between. Sometimes the room is long and in one direction, and sometimes it is right-angled. In smaller hospitals or clinics, it may be square. Nurses are able to visualize each bay and to maximize observation opportunities with each patient. Each bay also has a curtain for privacy.

There is an array of equipment at the head of each bay, as well as convenient ceiling hooks for hanging infusing fluids or other gear. At the head of the bay, there are outlets for oxygen delivery, suction, and delivery of air. There are manual blood pressure cuffs and electrical outlets, including those that continue to function should the hospital's power go out. There is a functioning cardiac monitor in most bays. The PACU nurses are familiar with multiple intravenous (IV) pump sets, often as combination machines. There is sufficient space for these in the bay. Some bays are wide enough to accept a standard hospital bed, often used for postorthopedic cases.

The patient's immediate surroundings in the recovery area begin with the surgical stretcher. Unlike the simple "cot with wheels" that one might visualize and that was prevalent in mid-20th century hospitals, the modern surgical stretcher is a more complex transport vehicle. It usually has a tray under the area on which the patient lies. This can be used to carry oxygen apparatus, documents, special appliances, or any number of needed supplies. Should a cardiac monitor-defibrillator accompany the patient, this may be placed at the foot of the stretcher. There are usually foot pedals that raise and lower any part of the stretcher or lock the wheels for safety. This is important for ergonomic reasons.

Ergonomics is the science of what makes the human body function without strain. For those who transport up to 20 patients per day, it is important to avoid strain on shoulders, back, or other sensitive areas. Pedals and handles that allow easy release or changing of patient position help to prevent injuries to transport personnel, nurses, and health care providers. The stretchers used to transport surgical patients must push freely. It is important to maintain surgical stretchers properly and to ensure a regular schedule of periodic maintenance.

Maintaining stretchers and purchasing up-to-date replacement stretchers is important to ensure the safety of patients and hospital personnel. There are state-of-the-art surgical beds or stretchers that are fully motorized and that with the push of a button, move the bed or stretcher forward. Similar to "dead man" switches on lawnmowers, there is a safety device that calls for the operator to be actively pushing a bar to engage the motor. If the bar is released, the bed or stretcher comes to a halt as the motor is disengaged. It is anticipated that these beds and stretchers will save transporters and patients from injury.

Attention is paid to ease in cleaning PACU surfaces. Sometimes, this results in a "surgical" appearance. The area may seem formidably sterile with tile floors, walls, and bare ceilings. The temperature in the surgical suites is often cool, as may be the temperature in PACU. When the patient is transferred to PACU, there may be difficulty in staying warm for both the patient and family, when a member is allowed to sit at the bedside. For the patient, there are warming blankets and other devices, but the family may need to bring along warm sweaters or jackets. Circumstances for family members in surgical waiting rooms are described in chapter 21. Often, after the patient is stable and the health care provider has briefed the family on the surgery and the patient's condition, one family member is given the opportunity to sit with the patient as the patient recovers.

However, for reasons centering on confidentiality rights, not all patients are able to have a family member sit at the PACU bedside during the recovery process. Some of the areas of concern in the Health Insurance Portability and Accountability Act (HIPAA) legislation are described in Ethics in Practice.

Hospital architecture has changed to support the heightened awareness of patient privacy needs that began with passage of the HIPAA. For example, because patient privacy must be protected, newer recovery areas have cubicles that are enclosed for the sake of privacy rather than large rooms with only a curtain separating patients. This redesign of recovery areas is especially important in the case of pediatric patients. It is important that the parent be in attendance in a private area for the sake of the child. The intent is that the child or infant will go to sleep with a parent in attendance and will wake with the parent at the bedside.

Some hospitals have designated surgical intensive care units, or SICUs, in which surgical cases will spend at least one night and perhaps more. Patients with specialized monitoring equipment, such as arterial lines, pulmonary-artery catheters, or intracranial pressure (ICP) monitors, are perhaps better placed in intensive care settings soon after the surgery is complete (Barone, et al., 2004). This is due to the need for staff with specialized training or the one-to-one continued labor-intensive requirements for observation beyond the initial surgery recovery period. In both settings, the nurse will have a similar focus in the first one to two hours following completion of surgery. This will continue until the

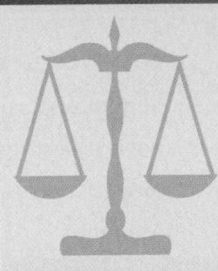

ETHICS IN PRACTICE

HIPAA: Implications for Perioperative Care

The intent of the HIPAA is to protect patient confidentiality while allowing access to patient information by those with a need to know. The following guidelines assist caregivers in protecting patient information.

- Information is shared among perioperative health care personnel on a need-to-know basis.
- Written information is to be covered so that casual observers cannot violate patient privacy. No open clipboards hanging around or placed on tables without blank cover sheets.
- No information is to be given over the telephone unless certain safeguards are in place and family and patient concur.
- Telephoned preoperative or postoperative reports are to be given over secure lines (usually land lines).
- Computer systems over which patient information travels are to be secure. Security should be sufficient so that those who do not have a direct need to know may not access patient information casually.

Adapted from Bergren, M. (2004). Information technology: HIPAA-FERPA revisited. Public Health Nursing, 20(2), 107–112.

effects of anesthesia have dissipated and the immediate hemodynamic effects of the surgical experience have passed.

Postoperative Physiological Stabilization

When receiving a patient, the nurse first assesses patient positioning based on type of surgery done. The nurse does a rapid head-to-toe visual assessment to include the surgical site and checks the patient's vital signs: blood pressure, heart rate, respiratory rate and quality, pulse oximetry, and body temperature. The nurse pays special attention to respiratory and circulatory stability. As the nurse checks the patient, he or she is receiving an initial patient report from the surgical team and supervising as the patient is being connected by the staff to equipment that will enable the nurse to monitor stability throughout the PACU stay. This all takes place within a matter of minutes. Steps taken are well choreographed, well rehearsed, and everyone knows his or her job. There are usually no wasted motions and little need for shouted reminders. With a well-trained PACU or critical care team, the scene flows in a similar quiet and confident fashion. It is the job of the experienced nurse manager to observe scenes such as this and to base future training on performance of the crew at such pivotal moments.

For assessment, a head-to-toe pattern is wise to follow. The most frequently checked areas are cardiac and respiratory stability. Table 22-1 indicates this prioritization. The receiving nurse is ruling out life-threatening complications initially. Assessment of the particular surgical site and any areas distal to the surgical site follows. Level of consciousness or return of regionally or centrally blocked areas is also vital in this immediate postoperative assessment.

Respiratory stability is determined through the use of pulse oximeters as well as through auscultating the chest and assessing respiratory rate and

TABLE 22-1 Possible Postoperative Complications

SYSTEM	COMPLICATIONS
Respiratory*	Respiratory depression
	Airway: Obstruction
	Airway: Spasms
	Aspiration
	Pneumonia
Cardiovascular*	Thrombi/emboli
	Hypervolemia: Fluid volume excess
	Hypovolemia: Fluid volume deficit
	Shock
	Complex dysrhythmias
	Tachycardia
	Bradycardia
Thermoregulation	Acute temperature alterations
Neurological	Altered mental status
	Pain
	Peripheral nerve trauma
GI	Nausea/vomiting
	Constipation
	Ascites
	Paralytic ileus
Genitourinary	Urinary retention
	Urinary tract infection
Integumentary	Infection
	Wound dehiscence
	Evisceration
	Decubiti
Musculoskeletal	Decreased range of motion
	Activity intolerance

*Highest priority assessment.
Adapted from Dixon, L. (2002). Postoperative complications and the older adult. Geriatric Nursing, 23(11), 203.

rhythm. The standard for a more routine surgical case is to obtain a full set of vital signs and to perform modified physical assessment at least every 15 minutes for at least the first hour of time spent in PACU. More frequent vital signs and overall physical assessment are done with less stable patients.

Postoperative patients require supplemental oxygen, at least for a short period of time after surgery, because they may still be retaining anesthetic gasses in their lungs. In addition, basic respiratory patterns may be altered by neurological changes from the anesthetic agent so that full saturation of circulating blood is supported via supplemental oxygen as the patient recovers. Finally, should the patient have had significant blood loss in surgery, numbers of circulating red blood cells may be decreased. Therefore, supplemental oxygen will help in the recovery of the patient.

In PACU, oxygen is usually delivered to the patient via facemask or a blow-by device. The blow-by is an oxygen delivery device that resembles a plastic half-mask. It sends richly oxygenated air to the patient's nose and mouth without touching the nose and mouth directly. It is popular for short-term use, because it can be less uncomfortable than a standard facemask when used for brief periods. It is often used in PACU with recovering patients. From a standard flow meter on the wall at the head of the bed, a rate of 10 liters per minute is set on arrival in PACU. An exception may be made for the patient with permanent carbon dioxide narcosis, such as one with chronic obstructive pulmonary disease (COPD) who has suffered from years of bronchitis, emphysema, or asthma. For these patients, the oxygen flow rate may be reduced to as little as 3 liters per minute because of such a patient's tendency to breathe at much too slow a rate when higher oxygen flow rates are set.

Some patients arrive from the surgical suite with an artificial airway in place. The artificial airway is a hollow, hard plastic tube that is passed through the mouth and just into the oropharynx. The artificial airway ensures that the tongue not occlude upper areas of the respiratory system in patients who may be neurologically compromised. Following deeper anesthesia, patients may be temporarily unable to keep the tongue from blocking the airway, and an artificial oral airway may be used. There is also a softer rubber nasal airway that passes through one nostril and down from the nasopharynx to the oropharynx. This device works in the same way, as does the oral artificial airway to ensure an open passage for air exchange. The nurse removes the airway once the patient becomes responsive and more consistently alert, or once the return of motor activity indicates that the patient is uncomfortable with the airway in place.

Concurrently with the establishment of respiratory stability, the nurse ensures hemodynamic stability. Heart sounds are assessed; the patient is attached to a cardiac monitor to follow heart rate and rhythm; and the nurse assesses apical-radial and peripheral pulses. Blood pressure is assessed by means of an electronic blood pressure cuff set to monitor frequently. In some patients who have undergone more serious cardiac surgery or who are expected to be hemodynamically unstable, central blood pressures is ascertained through a central line. The type of surgery will determine the hemodynamic monitoring criteria.

For most patients, blood pressure is maintained at a level within 30 mm Hg of their preoperative average. It is important for the patient to come to surgery with a full set of preoperative vital signs. The health care provider may order treatments to maintain the patient's vital signs within narrow parameters. This usually requires medication titration. The nurse will maintain or alter the flow rate of specifically ordered medications based on the individual patient's vital sign values throughout the stay in PACU.

As with any vital signs, if there are sudden changes or worsening trends in heart rate, respiratory rate, or blood pressure, the health care provider needs to be notified promptly. Experienced postoperative nurses are the first to spot significant changes in respiratory or hemodynamic status and to take action quickly. The PACU or critical care nurse also assesses for urinary output as a sign of hemodynamic stability as well as renal function. An early tendency toward fluid retention is not unusual because the body under siege tends to retain fluid for a period of time. The important thing is the maintenance of at least 30 mL of urinary output per hour in a catheterized patient. In the non-catheterized patient, assessment of urinary output will usually be done following transfer from PACU.

Following assessment of the respiratory and circulatory system, abdominal assessment should be done to determine the presence or absence of bowel sounds. Absence may be perfectly normal depending on the type of surgery done. With any type of surgery postwhich a large abdominal incision, one greater than a short stab wound, is made, the gastrointestinal (GI) system ceases functioning for a number of days (Mythen, 2004). With laparoscopic surgeries, in which retractors are seldom used and the series of small incisions do not signal assault to the body, the patient often does not have a decrease in or absence of bowel sounds. Such patients can be discharged from the hospital as early as the day of surgery.

In addition to noting presence or absence and quality of bowel sounds, abdominal character, such as any firmness or distension, should be noted. Palpation will determine comfort levels and may be done lightly once the patient is quite stable. In the case of abdominal surgery, the registered nurse (RN) should examine the skin, including any incisional sites, dressings, and drains that are present. The nurse checks for drainage each time vital signs are checked. In the case of those with casts or dressings placed over the incision, an inked circle is made periodically in the case of an expanding area of drainage.

Assessment of level of consciousness begins on arrival in PACU and continues as the patient recovers from the effects of anesthesia or sedation. It is not expected that the patient is fully conscious at the time of transport to PACU. However, anesthesia or sedation can start to wear off in as little as five minutes. The PACU nurse begins to communicate with the patient at this time. It is believed that position in space and receptivity to touch may return sooner than hearing in the unconscious patient. For this reason, the PACU nurse may choose to touch the patient lightly when communicating by voice. Once the patient is able to verbalize, short questions answerable with "yes" or "no" or with a name can be used to assess level of consciousness, as well as patient comfort. The nurse needs to address the patient by name at this time and to orient the individual to place and time. Repeating questions several times may be necessary before the patient is able to respond appropriately.

For some patients, anesthesia is spinal or regional (see chapter 21). In these cases, the nurse assesses for return of full consciousness from sedation and for return of sensation and motion in the upper or lower extremities. The return of voluntary motion is best accomplished by requesting that the patient move the affected part. Sensation may be assessed by the nurse's lightly touching distal areas and asking the patient with eyes closed to identify the area touched.

Another measure of immediate stabilization is thermoregulation. Following the surgical event, there will be a return of the ability of the body to regulate internal temperature. Soon after transport, the receiving nurse determines body temperature and makes every effort to combat hypothermia. Although there are individual variations, human temperature usually hovers within a degree of the accepted oral norm of 98.6° F (37° C). Hypothermia begins when the body's oral temperature is less than 96.8° F (37° C). Warmed blankets are often used, or, if needed, Bear Huggers. The Bear Hugger is a special type of blanket that uses pockets filled with circulating warm air. This device sustains a proper temperature for an extended period. When used in PACU, it ensures that normothermia is achieved quickly and safely. Should the patient experience chills and shaking, often termed rigors, an analgesic medication may stabilize the patient and end the episode.

Once the patient has been initially positioned and assessed, patient positioning needs to be addressed more fully. The surgical team will have paid special attention to those patients who might be in danger of compression of certain areas of the body during surgery. In PACU, a report is given on positioning. Patients generally come out of the surgical area in a supine position. Once the patient is considered stable, the head of the bed can be raised to 30 degrees for pulmonary safety. With operations involving any of the extremities, placing pillows for elevation can help to reduce postoperative swelling. For patients who have had lower back or spinal surgeries, positioning them on their side with a pillow between their knees, or on their back with a pillow under their knees helps reduce strain on the operative site. Some of the neurological surgeries require the patient to remain in a flat, supine position for a period of time following surgery.

If positioning is not addressed in the health care provider's orders, the transport team is able to advise the PACU nurse. Some types of positioning

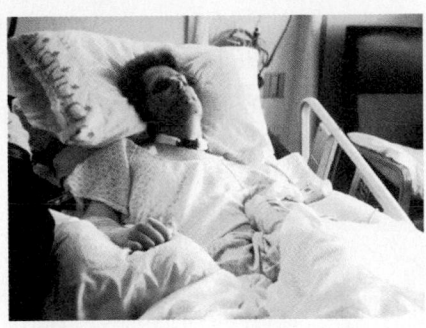

Figure 22-2 A turning schedule in the PACU helps to promote more compliance with preventive measures for providing care.

involving traction may not be initiated until the patient is released from PACU to the floor. Nurses may have to be creative with positioning from time to time, especially with patients who have multiple incisional areas (Figure 22-2). The novice PACU nurse should not hesitate to ask more experienced nurses for assistance. Some hospitals, clinics, or health care providers provide standardized order sheets that allow the surgeon to indicate those elements of postoperative care that apply to an individual patient. This allows the PACU and subsequent receiving unit to plan carefully to ensure consistency in care.

When the patient has been positioned, is hemodynamically stable, and the initial assessment is completed, a more extensive report is delivered by the person who administered anesthesia. This is a time when the PACU nurse ensures full understanding of the procedure that was done and how the patient reacted while in surgery. The report should include the patient's name, age, procedure, past medical history, allergies, volume infused, estimated blood loss (EBL), urine output, any medications received during the procedure, including antibiotics and anesthesia used, any dressings, splints, casts, or drains placed, positioning during the procedure, and length of the procedure. The anesthesia provider will remain until the PACU nurse formally accepts responsibility for the patient.

The patient in PACU is assessed continuously for overall stability and return to a preoperative level of consciousness. Even those patients who received spinal, regional, or local anesthesia may be heavily sedated at the time of arrival in PACU. For this reason, the vigilant nurse will focus on sustaining vital functions and ensuring a safe environment, including appropriate positioning, until the patient is able to do so unassisted.

If a family member is in attendance in PACU, the nurse may want to take this opportunity to assess the family member's knowledge and when necessary, educate about what is happening and how the family member might assist. This is particularly useful in the case of the family member who has not been exposed to surgical situations in the past.

Wound Stabilization

Patients normally arrive in PACU with a surgical dressing in place. The surgical wound area needs to be checked for visible bleeding. Rarely, there may be a large area of bruising that extends beyond the borders of the dressing. If the bruise is large and hot, it is referred to as **hematoma.** The problem with hematoma is that it may place pressure on the surgical incision and later, if it remains for several days, may provide a rich medium for microbial growth. The PACU nurse will report the presence of hematoma to the health care provider. In some cases, the surgeon will want to drain the hematoma. The PACU nurse also checks for the presence of drains that may have been placed by the surgeon, such as a penrose drain. A list of drains and characteristics of each appears in Table 22-2.

In the PACU, nurses may reinforce dressings but usually do not change the initial surgical dressing. It is an old tradition that the surgeon changes the initial surgical dressing. Because the surgeon placed drains, often intertwined with layers of dressing, and because the surgeon knows how much bleeding would be expected following surgery, it is the surgeon's prerogative to reserve the right to perform the first dressing change. Usually, this is not a problem for the PACU nurse. Charge nurses and bedside nurses in surgery receiving units beyond PACU usually are aware of individual health care provider preferences or they may be spelled out in standardized sets of orders that accompany the patient to the receiving unit.

If any drainage is showing on the dressing, the nurse circles the area and marks it with time and date. This provides a way to gauge how much seepage is occurring. When excessive bleeding or hematoma formation has occurred, the surgeon should be notified right away so that a wound site assessment can be performed. Sometimes, the outer layer of a routine surgical dressing is thick and waterproof. The nurse should slide the gloved hand under the

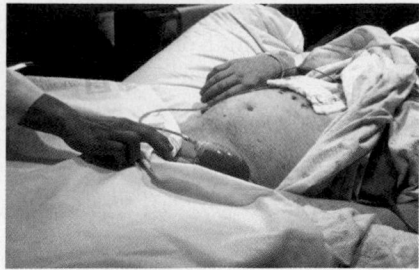

Figure 22-3 A hemovac drain site on a recovering postoperative surgery patient.

TABLE 22-2 **Wound Drains**		
COMMON NAME	**DESCRIPTION**	**CHARACTERISTICS**
Penrose drain	Floppy blue or cream colored; rests between layers of dressing	Short-term drain to give fluids under the wound a channel to drain to the surface; prevents pressure on suture lines
Davol	Drainage tubing connects to pie-plate shaped device	Same characteristic as JP, but collection container is round and flat; not as common as JP, but still occasional use
Hemovac	Thin clear tubing empties from under the wound surface to a clear, plastic, balloon-shaped collection container (Figure 22-3)	Contents of bulb are emptied and measured every eight hours; opening the small stopper on the bulb device, emptying, then compressing the bulb and restoring the stopper allow for slight negative pressure to help pull underlying contents to surface.

Adapted from Altman, G. (Ed.). (2004). Delmar's fundamental and advanced nursing skills (2nd ed.). New York: Thomson Delmar Learning.

"down" side of the patient: the area where drainage would flow as a result of the effects of gravity. In some cases, while the surface of the dressing is dry and intact, there may have been significant hidden bleeding between the patient and the mattress. The nurse should not disturb positioning requirements for the patient when performing this check. During the first days after surgery, the patient's dressings need to be changed. For more detailed information, nursing skills textbooks provide specific guidelines.

Casts are treated in similar fashion with a few additional assessment measures. In addition to placing the casted limb up on pillows, the nurse should be careful to use the palms of hands in maneuvering the wet or damp cast or to slide hands under supporting pillows to handle the damp cast. Complete drying of the freshly applied plaster cast takes at least two full days. Fiberglass casts take less time. Additional measures involving cast handling are noted in chapter 60, as well as descriptions of the types and locations for cast application.

The PACU nurse assesses for circulation, sensation, and motion distal to the cast in affected extremities. For a leg cast, the checks are performed at the foot or toes. Intact dorsi- and plantar-flexion, as well as identification of light touch are assessed. The toes should resemble the toes of the other foot and capillary refill should be less than three seconds (Estes, 2006). However, in many patients, the affected toes may be slightly swollen if the limb is not elevated. The nurse should be concerned about pale, cold toes without blanch. These findings may signal arterial problems and should be reported to the health care provider quickly. Estimated hospitalization times for various types of surgery are provided in Table 22-3.

TABLE 22-3	Estimated Hospitalization Times for Various Surgeries	
SURGERY	LENGTH OF PROCEDURE (EST.)	LENGTH OF HOSPITAL STAY (EST.)
Inguinal herniorrhaphy	1–1.5 hrs	Day surgery; 23 hour observation
Sigmoid colectomy	2.5–3 hrs	6–8 days
Thoracotomy	3–4 hrs	7–8 days
Cholecystectomy	1–1.5 hrs	Open: 3–5 days
Laparoscopic	Variable	12–23 hours
Mastectomy	1–1.5 hrs	24–48 hours
Small bowel resection	1–2 hrs	5–7 days
Cesarean delivery	1 hr	3–4 days
Vaginal hysterectomy	1–1.5 hrs	2–4 days
Total hip replacement	2–3 hrs	7–8 days
Craniotomy	2–3 hrs	Variable
Radical neck dissection	2–2.5 hrs	3–5 days
Arthroscopy of knee	1–2 hrs	4–6 hours
Coronary artery bypass graft	4–6 hrs	6–8 days
Retropubic prostatectomy	2–2.5 hrs	4–6 days

Postoperative Pain Management

Pain management has received increased attention with the movement toward patients' rights and the advent of more sophisticated means for delivery of pain medication. The rule of thumb about pain management is that pain is what the patient says it is. **Pain scales** are commonly used to quantify this subjective measure and to evaluate if the chosen intervention is effective at relieving the patient's pain. Ideally, the pain scale should be introduced to the patient prior to surgery with three pain scale points identified: what level the patient considers "adequate" pain control, what level the patient considers "uncomfortable" pain control, and what level the patient considers "unbearable." These points should then be charted for future nurses to use as guides in pain management with this patient. Chapter 16 includes a full discussion of the use of pain scales in all patient populations.

Type and site of surgery are predictors of severity and duration of acute pain. The degree of tissue trauma and the positioning of the patient are also factors that play a role. When surgery is the result of repair of acute traumatic injury, particularly when there are several sites involved in the trauma or subsequent repair, pain may be long term and more difficult to control.

There are many ways to manage pain in the postsurgical patient. Interventions used to alleviate pain generally fall into one of two categories: pharmacological management and nonpharmacological techniques. In the PACU setting, pharmacological management is most commonly used. Most medications are delivered through the IV route (Bush & Griffin-Sobel, 2003). Because of airway considerations, oral medications are generally not ordered for PACU patients at this time.

No matter what type of intervention is used, the goal of the PACU nurse in pain control is to make the patient as comfortable as possible without creating a situation in which the patient is overmedicated. The anesthesiologist often accompanies the patient to PACU and remains accessible in case of instability. The anesthesiologist often pays special attention to pain control needs. Additional details on pain management are provided in chapter 16.

PACU Discharge

The patient reaches a point, usually within 2 hours after arrival in PACU, when consciousness has returned, or in the case of the sedated patient with regional or spinal anesthesia, when sensation and motion have returned. Once the PACU team determines that the patient's level of consciousness is appropriate and that the patient is stable in terms of vital signs, assessment findings, wound, and pain control, the decision is made to transfer the patient to a next destination. Sometimes the patient goes to a routine postsurgical unit within the hospital. In the case of the short-stay patient, there may be a transfer to a short-stay postsurgical unit and then discharge home within 23 hours of arrival at the hospital or clinic. In other cases, the patient is transferred to the hospital's CCU.

Assessment Needs and Criteria for Discharge from PACU

The nurse in the PACU cares for the patient for one to two hours before noting a return to full consciousness, continued stability in vital signs, and adequate pain control. It is at this point that transfer out of PACU is considered. Immediately before patient transfer out of PACU, the nurse assesses carefully to see whether or not the patient meets criteria for discharge from PACU. A member of the anesthesia team usually writes or approves the discharge order. There is a set of transfer orders to be used by the receiving nurse, whether on a traditional medical-surgical unit or in the intensive care unit (ICU). The Aldrete System may be used to assess readiness for discharge from PACU (Table 22-4). This is a numeric scoring system that indicates stability across five measures: activity, respiration, circulation, consciousness, and oxygen saturation level.

The nurse carefully assesses airway, breathing, and circulation. The nurse observes for wound stability and internal temperature regulation. Assessment of GI function includes whether there are bowel sounds and whether the patient has nausea. Finally, neurological function is assessed once more prior to release. The Red Flag provides assessment parameters that would indicate a pending respiratory emergency if left untreated.

In relation to transport, the patient needs to be evaluated hemodynamically. Cardiovascular elements to be assessed prior to PACU discharge include: heart rate stability, blood pressure remaining close to the presurgical readings; palpable peripheral pulses; capillary refill less than three seconds in all extremities; EBL of concern; the latest hemoglobin and hematocrit levels; status of dressing or surgical area for hemorrhage; and the patient's return to level of consciousness consistent with the amount and type of anesthesia and analgesia. If the PACU nurse finds a need to retain the patient or to consider the patient to be less than fully stable, it will be his or her responsibility to notify the health care provider or surgical team immediately. Prompt action is indicated when there is any question about postoperative stability.

EBL figures will have been provided to the PACU nurse verbally as well as in the written operative record. This should be passed on to the receiving nurse prior to transporting the patient from PACU. Massive blood loss is considered to be loss of one third of circulating blood volume. That would be approximately 1,500 mL out of the five liters of circulating blood in the adult patient.

For the orthopedic patient, the same assessment should be done prior to discharge from PACU as that on arrival. Particular attention is paid to measures of adequate circulation, sensation, and motion. Sometimes, patients who have surgical repair of fractures also have a limb or limbs in traction. For those

TABLE 22-4	**The Aldrete System**	
Activity	Able to move all limbs voluntarily on command	2
	Able to move two limbs voluntarily on command	1
	Able to move no limbs voluntarily on command	0
Respirations	Able to deep breathe and cough freely	2
	Dyspnea or shallow, limited breathing	1
	Apneic, no spontaneous respirations	0
Circulation	Blood pressure ± 20 percent of preprocedure reading	2
	Blood pressure ± 20–49 percent of preprocedure reading	1
	Blood pressure ± 50 percent of preprocedure reading	0
Consciousness	Fully awake	2
	Arousable on calling	1
	Not responding	0
Color	Normal, Maintains greater than 92 percent saturation on room air	2
	Pale, dusky, blotchy, needs oxygen to maintain greater than 90 percent saturation on room air	1
	Cyanotic, oxygen less than 90 percent saturation even with oxygen	0

Adapted from Sloman, R., Rosen, G., Rom, M., & Shir, Y. (2005). Nurses' assessment of pain in surgical patients. Journal of Advanced Nursing, 52(2), 125–132.

in traction from the time of emerging from the surgical suite, the traction is maintained in a straight line of pull during the transport period. The patient remains in the same bed for the duration of the hospital stay. Neurosensory checks are similar to those for other patients.

The patient on the verge of being discharged from PACU does not have to be completely normothermic. If the patient feels cold and is still shivering despite the use of warming blankets, it may be wise to keep the patient in PACU, eliciting an order for a narcotic analgesic and observing its effects.

When reporting information to the receiving unit's nurse about pain levels, the PACU nurse should be sure to mention types of medication, routes, and times received. Routine use of one of the pain scales is recommended.

Transfer from PACU

The steps involved in transfer of the patient begin with a health care provider's order. The surgeon may come by personally to see the patient or may phone the transfer order to the PACU nurse based on his or her observations of relative patient stability. The surgeon may come out of surgery between cases to write orders. The surgeon often writes conditional orders. These will use wording indicating that, if certain criteria are met, the patient may be transferred. The surgeon will select the appropriate unit for care based on needed level of care. Because the nurse is with the patient from time of PACU admission, the nurse often provides data on which the health care provider will base destination and transfer orders. Therefore, the PACU nurse needs to be aware of which destinations will provide what services.

For those patients who will not be discharged directly to a short-stay unit and then to home within 24 hours, one way of looking at levels of care involves thinking of four basic areas for in-hospital care. The four levels are: (a) the postsurgical hospital unit; (b) the telemetry unit for those patients who are stable in all ways except hemodynamically; (c) the intermediate care unit; and (d) the ICU.

The first type of unit, the postsurgical or postoperative unit, is best for those patients who are stable within hours after surgery and will not require a great deal of one-on-one attention. The nurse-to-patient ratio on such a unit is usually 1:4 or 1:5 on day shift. This arrangement allows the nurse to focus efforts on patients who are freshly out of surgery. The nurse is also able to find time to teach family members how to support the patient in the earlier hours of postoperative care as well as later, closer to the day or time of discharge. Most modern postsurgical units have private rooms with ample space for visitors and equipment. There are accessible hallways for ambulation, comfortable chairs, an in-room phone and television, and the patient's bathroom. In addition, there are clinical assistants who are able to supply the patient and family with beverages or other things that will make recovery smoother.

The telemetry unit is best for those patients who are stable in all ways except for cardiovascular function. On such a unit, the patient has electrodes attached to the body. Small sticky pads on the skin surface (primarily over the chest) are connected to sheathed wires and a box of about the size of a television remote control device. This box may be worn in a pouch around the neck. When activated, the device sends signals to ceiling sensors and then along to a bank of cardiac monitors in a distant room or at the nurses' station. In some older hospitals, the bank of monitors is located in another wing or on another floor of the hospital. The bank of monitors, each representing an individual patient, is constantly observed. The use of the telemetry system allows specially trained personnel to scan heart rhythms of all telemetry patients continuously. The care nurse is notified whenever a patient's rhythm changes in a way that could indicate problems. The postoperative patient who is sent to the telemetry unit eventually is discharged to the postsurgical unit once cardiac rhythms are considered adequate and once overall hemodynamic indicators are stable. The decision to discharge is made by checking complete blood count (CBC) and electrolyte values, as well as overall vital signs and pulse oximetry. If enough days have passed for postsurgical stability, the patient may be discharged from the telemetry unit directly to the home setting.

Some hospitals have intermediate care units for surgical patients. These are designed for the patient who is not unstable to the point that full intensive care services are required but who is too sick for the regular hospital unit. Such patients may require smaller nurse-patient ratios, such as 1:3, to manage special needs or may need the type of equipment and monitoring that are generally more difficult to provide outside the intermediate care setting. There may be multiple body systems involved in the patient's recovery, but the patient is not unstable overall. Examples are patients in need of having vital signs assessed every two hours through the night based on past history or instability in PACU as well as those who are confused or whose serum electrolytes reflect the need for closer observation.

Those who are acutely and dangerously unstable at the time of PACU discharge are usually sent to the CCU. Patients whose surgeries were long or involved are also transported to the CCU for closer observation. Some hospitals have SICUs specifically for such situations. A common reason for transfer to such a unit is slowness in shaking off general anesthesia. For example, a patient with a respiratory rate of 8 breaths per minute, as compared to the adult normal of 12 to 20 breaths per minute when off ventilatory assist devices, might be a candidate for an overnight stay in the CCU. The anesthesia group might prefer that the patient remain intubated and on a ventilator until full control of respiratory function is possible for the patient. This is not an uncommon situation in older patients.

Another reason for a patient to go from PACU to the CCU is anticipated instability based on the magnitude of surgical disruption. Some surgeries are lengthy, requiring heavy levels of anesthesia for prolonged periods or higher levels of blood loss and tissue problems. These are followed by the need for close observation. For some patients, extensive GI surgery, such as the Whipple procedure, or cholecystectomy with the traditional long incision, will dictate the need to be placed in the SICU. These patients are in need of one-on-one care for a day or two.

Whether the patient is transferred to the postsurgical unit, telemetry, intermediate care, or CCU a set of orders accompanies the patient. A complete set of health care provider's orders are printed on paper designated for that purpose and include a stamped portion at the top delineating the patient's name, age, gender, health care provider, and medical record number. The health care provider must write the date at the beginning of the orders. It is best if the health care provider also includes the time, but this is not always done. Orders may be implemented without the time written by the health care provider. The health care provider's signature should be written at the end of the set of orders.

Those who move patients from PACU to another unit receive special training. If there is any doubt, the recovering nurse should accompany the patient to the next destination and ensure stability prior to the nurse's departure to return to PACU. In these cases, the portable monitor-defibrillator and supplemental oxygen devices are transported along with the patient on the stretcher. In cases in which the patient is considered stable, the transporter will have been trained to observe respiratory pattern and level of consciousness on the trip to the next unit. The transporter is usually a specialist in transferring the patient from stretcher to bed.

NURSING CARE DURING THE FIRST 24 HOURS POST-SURGERY

The first 24 hours post-surgery may include short-stay (also called 23-hour), surgical inpatient stay, or admission to a critical unit. No matter where the patient spends the first 24 hours, the nurse or family member will be monitoring the patient's recovery.

The Short-Stay Patient

It has been noted that, for some patients, a stay of less than 24 hours is probable. The **ASA scale** (evaluation method used by anesthesiologists to determine risk of patients undergoing surgical procedures), illustrates one phase of the decision-making related to postoperative destination (Table 22-5). A patient status of "1" or "2" is considered perfect for ambulatory surgery. These are patients who are either quite healthy prior to surgery, or those who have mild systemic disease. Perioperative needs are expected to be safely manageable within the short-stay setting. With additional evaluation, status 3 patients may also be considered acceptable for short-stay surgery in selected cases.

Insurers pay differentially for short-stay patients. There has been a trend toward building detached surgery centers for patients who may be safely discharged within this relatively short time frame. These are freestanding clinics with surgical suites that specialize in pretesting, surgery, and recovery for those patients who are expected to have uncomplicated recoveries and who will be discharged in under 24 hours or at most two days. Even though such clinics or freestanding surgery centers are often detached from hospitals and the specialized services that hospitals provide, they are usually a short helicopter ride away, should an emergency develop. Nurses are trained to know when this is necessary, and health care providers do not hesitate when the need for rapid transfer is indicated.

TABLE 22-5 ASA Physical Status Classification

SCORE	DEFINITION
1	Healthy patient
2	Mild systemic disease
3	Severe, mobility limiting systemic disease; disease is not incapacitating
4	Severe systemic disease involving life threat
5	Moribund
6	Brain dead or tissue donor

Adapted from Barone, C., Pablo, C., & Barone, G. (2004). Postanesthetic care in the critical care unit. Critical Care Nurse, *24(1), 38–45.*

Once the short-stay patient's surgery is complete and the patient is in the recovery room, the family is brought back to sit with the patient. The recovery room nurse will talk to all about what they can expect at home in terms of pain management, such as prescriptions and wound care. The nurse will also discuss any mobility issues, such as crutch walking. Return appointments are arranged, or the nurse provides a set of phone numbers for health care provider contact or appointments.

Details on assessing learning readiness and nursing measures that revolve around teaching are addressed later in this chapter. For the patient who leaves well in advance of 24 hours from the time of surgery, it is particularly important for the discharging nurse to describe signs and symptoms that warrant a call to the health care provider The nurse should make it clear that there is someone available 24 hours a day to receive such calls. There should be no hesitation on the part of patient or family. A list of matters that would require such a call is provided in the Health Care Provider Call Guidelines of the Patient Playbook.

The discharging nurse should provide written materials and supplies that might be needed in the immediate future, such as dressing materials and porous tape. The family is given the opportunity to demonstrate any care mea-

PATIENT PLAYBOOK

Health Care Provider Call Guidelines

In case of emergency following hospital or clinic discharge, the family or patient is to telephone emergency services (911) and follow instructions. It may be necessary to be transported to or report to the emergency department without delay. For less urgent matters, the patient and family should use the health care provider's telephone number provided at hospital or clinic discharge. Call in case of concern, or when there is inadequate relief of symptoms of discomfort. Instructions should be:

1. Do not hesitate to telephone the health care provider's office 24 hours a day and 7 days a week.
2. When a call is placed, there is a recording with a set of instructions or the call connects with an answering service that locates the health care provider on call for the group. This health care provider is to respond to calls at any time of the day or night.
3. The responding health care provider is responsible for having been briefed on your case and is prepared to advise, to telephone additional prescriptions to your preferred pharmacy or to answer questions. Be sure to have the telephone number of your preferred pharmacy on hand before placing a call to the health care provider.
4. Have a listing of allergies or other medications you are taking.

5. You should definitely telephone the health care provider if you have unrelieved pain, fever (consistent oral temperature ranges of 100 to 101.5° F [37.7° to 38.3° C] or more), or excessive bleeding or discharge. If you feel lightheaded or are having any mental changes (saying odd things or becoming somnolent), you need to telephone the health care provider or perhaps consider emergency services.
6. It is helpful to have an electronic blood pressure (sphygmomanometer) with pulse meter at your house. These are simple to use and are helpful in making a decision as to whether symptoms call for a visit to the emergency department immediately, rather than a simple call to the health care provider.
7. Be prepared to describe symptoms requiring intervention. For example, when did unrelieved pain begin and precisely where it is located. Is it crushing or sharp or burning in nature? Is it an ache? Does a certain position relieve it?
8. Be prepared to take notes in case the health care provider gives you instructions. Perhaps a family member can be on a telephone extension for that purpose.
9. Have a list of questions prepared should there be more than one area of concern.

sures that might be needed. Before leaving, the patient should be able to demonstrate the ability to sip drinks without nausea, vomiting, or choking. The discharging nurse should also ensure that the patient is urinating. Current standards are 200 mL of urine output within the first six to eight hours following the end of surgery.

The nurse instructs the patient and family about setting up the home with safety in mind. For example, for the patient who is crutch walking, there should be no loose throw rugs or furniture in the way of free ambulation throughout the house. If stairs are to be navigated, the physical therapy team will want a return demonstration of stair walking by the patient prior to discharge. Only noncomplex cases receive care in surgicenters, so the nurse anticipates the patient's safe return home on the day of surgery or by the following day. But, this outpatient treatment makes it imperative that there be a family member or other who is able to observe and assist should the patient become unwell during the immediate recovery period. For orthopedic cases, the nurse teaches cast handling. There should be pillows in the car for placement of the still-damp cast.

Finally, the nurse needs to teach the patient and family about filling prescriptions. Most surgicenters have in-house pharmacies that fill prescriptions. The nurse also should describe how to get a prescription changed without having to visit the health care provider. For example, if the patient finds that the prescribed pain medication is not effective, a call can be placed to the on-call health care provider. The patient or family member should know the phone number of a favorite pharmacy so that the health care provider can telephone a new order to be picked up by the family member.

The Patient Receiving Inpatient Care

In the case of the patient who is going from PACU in the hospital to a post-surgical unit, there is a need for safety in transfer. For the receiving nurse, the room setup becomes important, as does a thorough report on patient condition and immediate notification by the transporter or unit staff of the patient's arrival in the room.

Major surgical procedures often involve a stay as an inpatient. Prior to release from PACU, there is a telephoned exchange of information between the receiving nurse and the PACU nurse. In some more modern facilities, the releasing nurse records a full report over the telephone and calls the unit secretary with estimated arrival time (ETA) of the patient. The receiving nurse goes to a wall or pocket phone, dials in codes, and receives the recently recorded report, including contact information of the sending nurse, should there be questions.

The receiving nurse makes final preparations within the receiving room or arranges for this to be done by support personnel. Family members who may have been waiting in the room are told that the patient is returning. They are asked to vacate when they see the patient appearing. A family exit into the hallway makes space for the stretcher to enter the room. This is also a good time for one family member to greet the patient from the hallway. It can be reassuring to patients to know that family members are present to shepherd the patient through this period of recovery from surgery. It is also reassuring to the family to note that the patient does not appear excessively uncomfortable at this time. Instruction to family members on where to stand and what to do has a certain benefit for later in the recovery process. It sets up the idea that family members are invited to be active participants in the patient's recovery.

The receiving nurse signals additional personnel that the patient has arrived. The unit secretary is able to call nurses to have them gather. The receiving nurse will then direct personnel. Box 22-1 contains principles for safe patient transfer as well as tips to protect personnel during the transfer process from stretcher to bed. Details are tailored toward avoidance of common mistakes in the transfer process.

BOX 22-1

TRANSFER PRINCIPLES: BODY MECHANICS AND IMMEDIATE PATIENT COMFORT

1. Prearrange the receiving room: bed location, height, furniture, assessment instruments, and plastic ware. Get the excess furniture out of the room or move it into the bathroom alcove.
2. Pull the bed about a foot from the wall. Place it closer to the window side of the room but leave a space for transfer people to be able to stand.
3. Prepare the oxygen flow meter, suction apparatus, and IV equipment.
4. Give notice to unit personnel who will assist with the transfer that they will be needed and approximately when.
5. Use a padded transfer board unless the patient can scoot over with minimal assistance.
6. Have two on each side if a full transfer. The tallest go toward the head. If extra people are there, one can manage the feet and lower limbs. Place the odd-numbered person on the receiving side of the bed.
7. Ensure that both bed and stretcher wheels are locked.
8. Check bed's overall height and configuration. It should match that of the stretcher. Identify the leader or caller. Practice a slight knee bend or two to get your muscle memory going.
9. The first slide is to the edge. The leader will verify that the transfer team is in accord with this. When ready, the leader calls, "*Count of three,*" and the team follows up by slightly lifting and sliding the patient when the "*three*" is heard.
10. If it is to be a two-part maneuver, the leader again calls, "*Count of three.*" When "three" is heard, the team slightly lifts, slides, and sets the patient on the bed.
11. Ensure that the team participates in ensuring patient safety and comfort prior to all rushing out of the room. Be sure covers are in place.
12. Safety and comfort are ensured when side rails are up, patient positioning is correct and comfortable, linens are comfortable, the under linens have no wrinkles, the stretcher is out of the room, and the first set of vital signs have been done.
13. Instruct the family: when to leave the room, where to stand, when to come back in, how many initially, and they can greet the patient on the way to the room.
14. Place the nurse call light within easy reach. Instruct patient and family how to use.
15. When the patient shows signs of being more alert, have the patient perform a return demonstration of deep breathing or incentive spirometry use.

Adapted from Altman, G. (Ed.). (2004). Delmar's fundamental and advanced nursing skills (2nd ed.). New York: Thomson Delmar Learning.

The nurse may also want to use this time to let the family know of some of the things that will make the patient more comfortable during the recovery period (e.g., kitchenette use, ice machine location; visitor bathrooms, or tour of the unit's waiting area). It is also important to inform the family about desirable visitor ages and how many family members should visit at one time. In addition, the family needs to know how to detect that the patient is tired and needs to sleep. It is probable that one or two family members will want to remain at the bedside. Early briefing efforts will result in family confidence and a smoother experience for all.

Nursing Care Beyond Transfer

Most major hospitals have designated units that provide postoperative care. Nurses are specially trained and are able to handle the expected as well as the unanticipated. Postoperative nursing care continues on the surgical unit until discharge out of the hospital or until the patient becomes unstable in a way that requires transfer to a higher level of care, such as the CCU. Postsurgical nurses must be aware of patient factors that require transfer. In addition, these nurses recognize that the nursing supervisor is able to assist with making such decisions.

As good as postoperative care personnel are, it is even better to have many sets of eyes to watch over the postoperative patient. It is especially important to instruct family to watch respiratory rates and patterns or to let the nurse know of dramatic changes in the patient's condition. While this instruction might seem common sense to many, for the novice visitor, there may be a need for special instruction. For those patients who have no visitors at the bedside, be certain to devise a close observation system for those patients who are not fully alert or who might not be capable of signaling the nurse. For those patients who exhibit a low respiratory rate, it may be necessary to alert anesthesia and to be prepared to deliver a reversal agent at the bedside on the postoperative unit.

A recent national initiative is that of having a rapid response team arrive, whenever a patient is experiencing an episode of instability that may be predictive of adverse physiological outcome (Winters & Dorman, 2006). While in this situation it may be too early to call a code, the unit nurse may need the team of experts to advise on what to do: whether to prepare for transfer prior to a code or whether to take certain steps to guard against further deterioration in the patient's condition. While not all patients have access to the services of such a team, it is important for the postoperative nurse to be able to detect and manage instability in the first 24 hours.

As time passes, the patient will eventually experience postoperative day one (POD 1), a time that begins the day after the day of surgery (DOS), then POD 2, POD 3, and so forth. With each day that passes, the typical patient moves nearer to hospital discharge. Average length of hospital stay for many procedures is under four days. Some of the lengthier times involve complications or challenges to mobility, nutrition, or cardiorespiratory stability.

Ensuring the patient's safety on the surgical unit is important. Once the patient arrives in the room, the nurse usually assists the transporter in moving the patient. Some of the more modern hospitals are being constructed with ceiling-stored, pull-down devices designed to eliminate staff injury in patient movement and to protect patients during transfers and repositioning. For those who have not yet achieved this state-of-the-art room situation, there is a need to plan carefully prior to attempting the movement of the patient from stretcher to bed. Nursing skills textbooks provide additional details about body mechanics and the need for safety measures in assisted patient transfers.

Bedding that is not immediately needed should also be removed once patient transfer to the receiving bed is completed. Excess linens are sent outside with the transporter. The transporter should stay with the receiving nurse long enough for a brief examination of the patient and a set of vital signs to be taken. The nurse will note whether pulses are regular, whether skin is warm and dry, and whether capillary refill is adequate in all extremities. The medical record is given to the receiving nurse by the transporter or left at the central desk with the unit secretary or other support staff. Following departure of the transporter, the nurse performs an abbreviated head-to-toe assessment, if time permits, before other measures need to be done. The nurse then invites the family into the room. The nurse provides brief instruction after a few minutes on what family members can do to promote rest, comfort, and safety.

The receiving nurse has a set of initial priorities. For the patient, the nurse ensures physiological stability, comfort, and progress as gauged by typical recovery pathways for patients who have had similar surgeries. For the family, the situation will dictate the nurse's priorities. For some, ensuring readiness for assisting the patient is important. Or, in other cases, the nurse ensures that family members get some rest soon after the patient is stabilized on the postoperative unit. This is particularly important in the case of an older or infirm spouse or other family member. After the determined treatment and stabilization, the focus shifts to appropriate education prior to patient discharge. The receiving nurse first focuses on immediate patient needs.

Nurses should be familiar with basic principles approved by their hospital or clinic for general management of patients in the postoperative period. These are to be found in a manual on the unit or more frequently, on the unit's computer with other policies, procedures, and protocols. More specific management directives are to be found in the same locations or listed in the form of routine orders and instructions that the unit secretary will affix to the chart.

Postoperative care of the patient who has had cardiac catheterization and who has a particular surgeon or cardiologist will differ markedly from that of the patient who has returned from open reduction and internal fixation of a femur fracture and who has a different health care provider or orthopedic surgeon. Health care provider groups may have separate sets of routine orders, each differing from those of other groups. The receiving nurse should be guided by the standards of practice of the postoperative nursing unit as operationalized in the policies, procedure descriptions, and protocols as well as by the health care provider's orders for the particular patient.

For the patient who is allowed clear fluids by mouth, the nurse ensures that water and other favorite clear fluids, such as soda pop or juice, are at the bedside. If the health care provider's order permits advancing the diet beyond clear fluids, the nurse asks the unit secretary to order a dinner meal, perhaps of clear or full liquids. When the patient does not want the dinner tray, it can always be returned to the kitchen (Huckleberry, 2004).

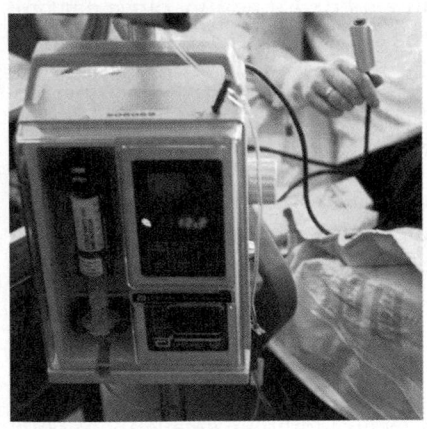

Figure 22-4 PCA pump.

The receiving care nurse needs to check patient comfort levels continually. In addition to using a pain scale to quantify pain or level of comfort, the nurse observes for grimacing, guarding of the operative area, or reluctance to move about in the bed. If there is a patient controlled analgesia (PCA) device settings and patient responses should be checked initially and every four hours with appropriate documentation. PCAs are being used often in the initial postoperative recovery period. **Patient controlled analgesia (PCA)** is a way to manage postoperative pain that helps the patient to maintain a sense of control (Figure 22-4). Most devices allow for a continuous rate of medication to be delivered each hour, with additional doses delivered on a "need" basis that is controlled by the patient. Studies have shown that this type of medication administration is more effective for controlling postoperative pain than other forms. The nurse still needs to be vigilant with assessing pain level, quality, and location. After surgery, education should be done with both the patient and family about the PCA, about the medication being delivered by the PCA, how it works, and how pain assessment is done using the pain scale. As part of this education, the nurse should remind the patient and the family to "hit the button" only when needed. There have been cases in the past in which patients have had issues with respiratory depression because of a well-meaning loved one pushing the button. By teaching families about pain assessment and having them to contact the nurse if the patient is not achieving adequate pain relief, safe interventions can be maintained and alternative therapy can be tried.

There is a time after the first 24 hours when the patient may not need the control provided by the PCA. Pain relief may then change to another administration route. Chapter 16 provides a comparison of several commonly used opioid analgesics. It is useful for nurses to be aware of equianalgesic considerations to recommend substitute dosages when moving, for example, from IV medications to an oral route. The intramuscular route is sometimes still used for pain relief for some patients, although more rarely with the advent of the

FACTORS ASSOCIATED WITH DELAYS OR IMPAIRMENT IN WOUND HEALING

- Crush injuries
- Foreign bodies
- Necrosis
- Repeated injury to the same site
- "Tense" closure sites (obese patients; lengthy incisions; incisions over skin folds, joints)
- Wound infection
- Irradiation
- Poor nutrition
- Steroid use
- Low oxygen levels: locally or systemically
- Persons who do not receive adequate overall rest
- Persons who do not rest the area of injury
- Older patients
- Those with: atherosclerotic disease, diabetes mellitus, thromboembolic disorders, chronic stress, cirrhosis, renal failure, or cancer

PCA device. However, the intramuscular route may provide longer, more sustained action. Nonpharmacological pain management includes techniques, such as guided imagery, controlled breathing, and stimulation, such as with trans-electrical neural stimulation (TENS) units. These are listed in chapter 16. Family support should be enlisted in alerting staff when the patient has uncontrolled pain. For family members who remain at the bedside, the care nurse needs to instruct them to notify the nurse if the patient seems uncomfortable (Frasco, Sprung, & Trentman, 2005).

The postoperative nurse checks drains for position and possible kinking or pulling. For drains with receptacles for fluid, drain fluid levels are checked every four to eight hours and recorded. Drain receptacles are usually emptied every eight hours and amounts and descriptions of drainage recorded. The hope is that wounds will heal by primary intention. Edges are brought together (approximated) by staples or sutures. Healing time can be as little as a day or so for small cuts or may take a week to 10 days for larger incisions. For wounds that are cavity-like defects or in which edges cannot be brought together, healing is by second intention. This type of closure is also known as granulation and is characterized by gradual filling from the deeper areas to the outer, skin surface of the wound. Healing often takes up to several months. A third type of healing is delayed closure. Heavy wound contamination or patient instability at the time of surgery is indicative of the need for the surgeon to allow the wound to remain open for several days before it is secured with sutures. Factors that may delay wound healing or that call for delayed closure are provided in Box 22-2.

Regular use of correct dressing and wound care terminology will make documentation more descriptive, succinct, and accurate. For example, **approximated** wound edges (also called borders, or margins) are well connected without gaps. This may be similar to a zipper effect with tightly connected tissue. Drainage that is serous is clear. Sanguinous drainage is bloody. Drainage that has characteristics of both is referred to as serosanguineous. Yellow or green drainage is considered **purulent** (containing the detritus of white blood cell activity within an infectious process usually). The amount of drainage may be scant, moderate, or heavy (copious). The drainage may have an odor, such as foul-smelling. It is important to document wound appearance, location, size, and the amount and type of drainage. In some facilities, photographs are routinely mounted in medical records to track progress with healing of problematic wounds and for use by caregivers to determine whether wound care measures are effective over time.

If leg compression devices or hosiery are ordered, these may already be in place when the patient returns from surgery. If not, the receiving nurse should place them. If the stockings or compression devices were not sent to the room with the patient, these may be ordered from the supply area. It is important to explain to the patient and family that the devices are preventive and need to be used while recovery is in progress. The patient and family need to be aware that stockings should be removed for at least an hour daily to inspect the skin, wash the feet and legs, and allow any areas of inadvertent pressure to be released.

The room within the postoperative unit will have been set up to include a urinal at the bedside for male patients who do not have an indwelling urinary catheter. The nurse may want to consider placement of a bedside commode for female patients who may be unable to walk to the bathroom. Meanwhile, a bedpan may be placed in the room's bathroom for in-bed use in the immediate recovery period. Recall that urinary output should be at least 30 mL per hour when the patient has a urinary catheter. The patient should void within four to six hours of arrival from PACU. Current standards are 200 mL of urine output within the first six to eight hours following the end of surgery. Sometimes, early urinary output is less than would be predicted from intake through IV fluids and the patient's oral intake. This decrease is because of the body's tendency to retain fluids during times of physiological stress. However, when the patient reaches the POD 1, this trend should disappear, and output will return to normal.

The receiving nurse ensures that all health care provider's orders are accurately transcribed. On some postoperative units, the unit secretary or ward clerk may have received training to enable transcription of orders onto the directions section of the chart known as the Kardex. To ensure timely implementation of all orders, the receiving nurse should have a copy of the health care provider's orders in hand while the unit secretary transcribes. The unit secretary may also transcribe medications onto the medication administration record, or MAR. But it is the receiving nurse's responsibility to promptly review and implement all orders, as well as to check for accuracy and to set up appropriate medication administration times on the MAR. The nurse pays particular attention to cross-checking the perioperative sheets prior to setting up medication times in case a first dose has been administered in PACU. The receiving nurse checks the perioperative or PACU records for the latest time the patient received pain medications, especially if there has been a time lag since verbal report was given. This information has been conveyed during verbal report, but a second check does no harm. The receiving nurse makes a special note of parameters for vital signs that require a phone call to the health care provider. If laboratory specimens, such as serum electrolytes or a CBC, are ordered, the receiving nurse ensures these are sent promptly and checks periodically for results, especially those that will require further management.

Once the patient is comfortable and stable, the receiving nurse makes sure that medications are on the way from pharmacy, that the appropriate diet is sent for the next meal, and that patient and family are aware of prescribed activity levels. The experienced perioperative nurse, working in tandem with an experienced nursing assistant or clinical assistant, should be able to perform initial assessment, institute safety and comfort measures, implement health care provider's orders, and return to the patient's bedside in time to check the vital signs at the 15-minute mark following the patient's arrival on the unit.

What the nurse does throughout the remainder of the shift depends on the patient's status and response to the surgery and to the nursing measures. At one of the early bedside checks, it is appropriate to instruct the family again and to answer any questions. Often at this time, the family will have made observations or will need some explanations or forecasting about what might occur next. For example, if the family notes that the patient is sleeping a lot, and if all else is stable, the nurse may safely reassure the family that this is an expected outcome from anesthesia and pain medications. The experienced nurse may even hazard an educated guess as to when this will subside and the patient might become more alert. However, false or ill-advised reassurance should never be given, such as in the case of the patient who is several hours out from surgery and shows signs that pain medication is ineffective. In such cases, the nurse will tell the patient and family what he or she intends to do and will follow up immediately to ensure adequate pain control.

To ensure the delivery of safe care for the recently transferred postoperative patient, the nurse should instruct the family to let the nurse know if there is evidence of uncontrolled pain; if there are breathing changes; or if the patient shows signs of needing assistance in changing position. The family should alert the nurse if the patient is nauseated or vomits. The nurse must alert the family not to touch settings on pumps. If alarms sound, the family is advised to let them go on sounding to alert care personnel to come in. Pain management needs to be sufficient for the patient to rest and to resume activities.

At the series of early checks, the nurse keeps the ABCs in mind: (a) airway; (b) breathing; and (c) circulation. The nurse checks vital signs centrally when listening to the chest with a stethoscope but also checks peripheral circulation with all patients: (a) extremity warmth; (b) color; (c) pulses; and (d) capillary refill. In addition, the nurse notes presence or absence of peripheral pain and the presence of edema. Level of consciousness and orientation to time, place,

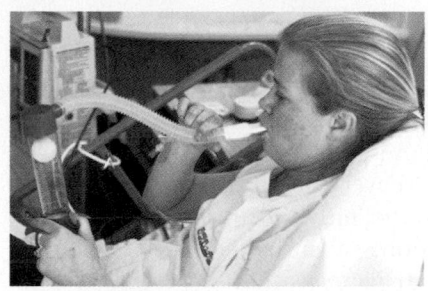

Figure 22-5 Using incentive spirometer.

person, situation, and the ability to remain awake are indications that central neurological function is intact. When something changes in this area, the nurse should keep in mind that it might be lingering effects of analgesia or anesthesia, or in another case, it might mean lack of oxygen to the central nervous system, electrolyte imbalance, or signs of being overmedicated. There are other possibilities, but the nurse should investigate likely possible causes first. If there is a suspicion that blood pressure and heart rate may be less than desirable, the nurse should personally recheck latest values manually. If there is a problematic trend, the health care provider or in some facilities, response team, is notified.

The patient should be reminded at hourly intervals to deep breathe and use the **incentive spirometer** (a machine used to allow patients a quantifiable aid in deep breathing postoperatively) (Figure 22-5). The family may need to prompt the patient. Leg exercises should be performed. It is helpful when the patient has been instructed and has had an opportunity to practice leg exercises prior to surgery. These consist of rotating ankles, dorsi- and plantar-flexion of feet and toes, and bending and extending legs. In addition, a maneuver called quadriceps setting may be performed while the patient is primarily in bed for the first 24 hours following surgery. This consists of straightening the legs and pressing the knee to the mattress. It is thought that this sometimes helps with overall leg strength and circulation when the patient first begins to get out of bed and ambulate following surgery.

Anticipating Complications

Despite the best nursing care and the most standardized and effective of surgical techniques, some patients experience complications. These may be manifested through any one of the body's physiological systems: cardiorespiratory, neurosensory, endocrine, GI, urinary tract, skin, or musculoskeletal system.

Respiratory system complications might be of an emergency nature. These would include severe respiratory depression, manifested through a slow respiratory rate, an irregular respiratory pattern, pulse oximetry readings below 90 percent, air hunger, or blood gases indicating respiratory acidosis or hypoxemia. The nurse should also be aware that air hunger may be a sign of airway closure related to early anaphylaxis.

Such occurrences as postoperative pneumonia are slower to develop but may be just as deadly. The signs and symptoms of pneumonia are listed in chapter 32, and should be studied by those who are caring for postoperative patients. Sometimes hypoventilation may be related to incisional pain. In this case, reinforcement of teaching, return demonstrations involving use of splinting maneuvers, and sufficient pain control will help to overcome the tendency to breathe in a shallow pattern. An illustration of splinting is provided in Figure 22-6.

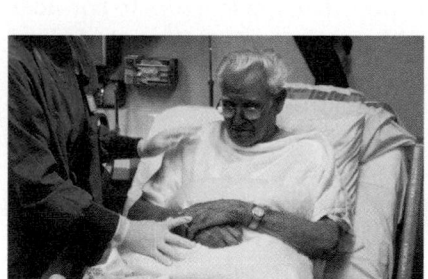

Figure 22-6 The patient holds a pillow over the chest or abdomen to splint himself while coughing.

Cardiovascular complications may be precipitated by severe blood loss. Blood loss may lead to low blood pressure as a result of physical shock. Dysrhythmia or **ectopy** (heartbeat arising from a location other than the sinoatrial node on a monitor screen) may signal also signal an irritable heart. Such complications may be precipitated by electrolyte imbalance, hypoxia, or any one of a number of other problems. There may be vascular problems distal to a surgical site or those that arise from inadequate exercise following surgery. Whether stationary or mobile, blood clots may result in life-threatening complications. Retained fluids may result in temporary heart failure.

Compartment syndrome may be a complication of orthopedic surgery or trauma caused by inadequate space for tissue swelling complication, which arises from swelling in the soft tissues and muscles that in turn causes compromised circulation to that area. This can occur especially if a limb is in a fixed cast, but the patient continues to swell because of injury. Treatment for this is commonly to remove the cast and perform a fasciotomy, with closure of the fasciotomy occurring approximately three days later. This is prevalent with limb trauma, and may result in permanent nerve damage and deformity.

With all complications, early discovery and rapid, definitive treatment have an effect on outcome. Those who are responders in crisis situations practice lifesaving measures within the walls of the hospital repeatedly. But it is up to the postoperative bedside care nurse to discover early indications of complications. Neurosensory complications may be either central or peripheral. Central nervous system signs of complications might be altered level of consciousness; mental status changes, vital sign patterns that indicate increased ICP, and changes in sensorium. Peripheral signs indicating complications might be pain, or lack of pain, peripheral deficits in sensation or motion, circulation changes, or edema around the ends of cast edges and the like. The tendency of a limb to assume a position of deformity or local tremors may also indicate a peripheral neurosensory complication if not discovered early.

In relation to GI or urinary function, more common complications include urinary tract infection, temporary GI slowdown related to abdominal surgery, a more serious paralytic ileus resulting from electrolyte imbalance or interruption in blood supply, and renal failure. Skin complications may be precipitated by pressure points, interruptions or delays in wound healing, or allergy to tapes or latex. Orthopedic devices, such as traction pins or casts, are particularly likely to foster irritation and skin breakdown.

A particularly rare but serious complication is wound dehiscence, or separation of the wound edges. A more extreme form is evisceration. This occurs when the contents of the abdominal cavity come through separated postsurgical muscle, fascia, and skin to emerge onto the surface of the body, or when the suture line separates down to the internal organ layer. The nurse discovering evisceration should cover the wound with sterile saline–soaked dressing material with a waterproof dressing or pad over the top. This is maintained until the patient is taken to surgery, usually within minutes.

Particularly with surgery that took place in regions close to exocrine or endocrine glands, electrolytes and hormonal delivery systems may have been temporarily disrupted. The nurse should be alert to wide fluctuations in vital signs, heart rhythms, or neuromuscular function. The nurse needs to consider metabolic antecedents in the postoperative patient with musculoskeletal tremors or conversely, the patient who does not show normal levels of reflexivity in these early hours. When there is any question, the health care provider is notified.

RECOVERY MILESTONES BEYOND THE DAY OF SURGERY

For the patient who may spend days recovering in the hospital, the patient and nurses will engage in daily mutual goal setting. This may involve pain control planning, ambulation progress, and improving appetite and energy level. Some facilities use wipe-off boards placed on the wall in an accessible location visible to the patient and family. Progress toward achievement of this short list of mutually agreed on goals will help the patient and family to see progress and will encourage the patient and family to take a measure of control prior to discharge from the hospital.

A good place to start in this mutual goal setting is with comfort. This is closely followed, in importance, by activity level. It is known that there can be severe complications of prolonged bed rest, such as pneumonia, thromboembolism, and other forms of hemodynamic instability. So it is important for postoperative care personnel to assist the patient in achieving the ordered levels of activity.

The patient and family will look forward to daily progress in the areas of activity, energy, nutrition, comfort, and healing. As the patient progresses, some of the equipment can be removed and other things used less often. As the patient's vital signs stabilize, assessment of vital signs and pulse oximetry readings is done less often, perhaps as little as once per waking shift. When the patient is able to consume sufficient nutrients and is no longer likely to be nauseated, IV fluids are stopped. Because the patient may need access, the peripheral IV site is usually retained through the 96-hour mark beyond insertion time. Sometimes the site is maintained to deliver periodic IV medications. As pain control becomes more certain, the intravenous PCA device is discontinued in favor of oral pain medications. Today, intramuscular medication delivery routes are out of favor because of possible tissue or nerve damage around the delivery site.

In the case of stomach or intestinal surgery, hospitalization may be prolonged. Bowel sounds typically return by POD 3 following stomach or intestinal surgery. This is a signal that the body will accept nutrients ingested by the patient. However, for those who have undergone extensive GI surgery, bowel sounds may not return for perhaps seven or eight days. In such cases, nutritional needs may be met for a period of time with supplements that bypass the GI system. Such things as hyperalimentation (HAL) or total peripheral nutrition (TPN) may be used to represent the delivery of proteins, fats, carbohydrates, fluids, and various vitamin and mineral supplements via the IV route. The postoperative nurse may be guided in safe delivery by skills textbooks and hospital policy.

Ambulation progresses as the patient continues to recover from surgery. Ambulation requires patient cooperation and often family support. The patient is aware that discomfort often accompanies early efforts to get out of bed. This awareness may result in early reluctance to get up and to walk. And, unlike the areas of hydration or assessment of overall stability, walking cannot be something performed solely by care personnel. The patient needs to take responsibility for activity levels in the early postoperative period. The nurse helps by reminding, physically assisting, ensuring adequate pain relief, and providing positive reinforcement.

The postoperative nurse knows approximate distances on his or her hospital unit to document progress with patient ambulation effectively. The nurse, for example, is able to say, on POD 3 that the patient ambulated 120 yards in the hallway with a steady gait, unassisted. Pointing out distances to an interested patient may provide motivation to progress. The patient and family who are able to track ambulation and strength-building milestones after surgery will feel a sense of satisfaction and progress. Both know that progress in these areas brings them closer to the time when discharge from the hospital is possible. Some common terms in use to describe postoperative ambulation are listed in Box 22-3. These can be utilized to document relative ease or difficulty for each patient.

Another sign of progress for the hospitalized patient is wound healing. After a certain period of time, the health care provider will determine that the wound may be left open to the air, or OTA. For those patients who were able to go home from the hospital or clinic within 23 hours from surgery, this usually happens at the first office visit. But in cases in which the patient experiences a longer hospital stay or delayed recovery, leaving the wound OTA may occur before the patient is discharged from the hospital. When a wound is left OTA, caregivers need to be vigilant in minimizing anything that could cause excessive pressure at or around the wound site. The nurse may want to instruct the patient to cover the wound when wearing clothing that might snag on staples or sutures. The nurse should also instruct the patient about what to do if signs of problems develop, such as redness around the incision area or slight dehiscence.

The patient and family are taught signs of complications prior to discharge. Numbness and tingling anywhere, shortness of breath, palpitations, elevated temperature, sudden increase in pain or change in the quality of pain, or mental status changes signal a need to inform health care personnel. In addition, troublesome signs and symptoms, such as constipation, urinary burning or retention, or itching, should be reported and managed promptly through testing, medication, or other means (Andersen, Kallehave, & Andersen, 2004).

BOX 22-3

TERMINOLOGY TO DESCRIBE AMBULATION

Level of Assistance

- Independent implies that the patient walks easily without the need to rely on people or devices.
- One-person assist means that the patient needs to rely on one other person to stand, sit, transfer, or walk. This may or may not be in addition to use of a device.
- Two-person assist (or more) usually means that the patient does not have the strength or coordination to transfer or ambulate without relying on other people. This often means that there is quite a bit of difficulty with even noncomplex maneuvers.

Device Support

The person documenting should also show that the patient walked with a device and how the patient performed. Commonly used devices and gaits are:
- Walker
- Rolling walker
- Tripod cane
- Cane

Crutches

When referring to crutch walking, there are some commonly used abbreviations. It is suggested that the agency's list of acceptable abbreviations be consulted before using these, however.
- CW is crutch walking
- TDWB is touch-down weight bearing
- NWB is non–weight bearing

In addition, there are other ways in which to describe crutch gaits. These are listed in the orthopedic chapter.

Quality of Stride or Gait

- Steady implies that balance and coordination are strong.
- Unsteady or poor balance would be noticeable particularly with turns or backing up to a chair.

Distance

To estimate distance in the absence of precisely measured intervals on the hospital unit, the nurse might want to measure the distance of stride. For the person with average foot length, with normal walking, each stride forward is around 12 inches or 1 foot in length. Then, to estimate distances around the hospital unit, the nurse will want to stride, perhaps, from a patient's room to the nurse's station or the end of the hall.

Adapted from Altman, G. (Ed.). (2004). Delmar's fundamental and advanced nursing skills (2nd ed.). New York: Thomson Delmar Learning.

Many patients ask about continuing with postoperative stockings or compression devices when home. Usually, patients do not continue to use sequential compression devices on their legs following hospital discharge. However, support stockings may be encouraged. The continued use of support stockings is recommended following some types of surgery, such as surgery that involves the areas of the body through which leg vasculature travels as it returns to the main vessels of the trunk. Such surgeries, as hip replacement, urinary surgery, or lower bowel surgery, may result in swelling that would impede blood return. The nurse can explain the purpose of the devices and advise the patient to ask the health care provider for recommendations at the first office visit. However, the nurse should also explain safety in use by teaching the patient and family to remove the stockings for at least an hour a day, perhaps morning and evening. The legs and feet may be washed at this time. However, while foot massage is helpful, the patient should be cautioned not to massage the legs or calves. If there is an area of stagnation in the vessels of the legs, it is felt to be best not to disrupt the tissues through massage during the months immediately following surgery.

Family and Cultural Aspects of Care

Because of the development of ways to eliminate information barriers in the Internet age, it is now easier than ever to learn about other cultures in our multicultural society. Many institutions include sections on admission and preoperative forms in which patients can comment on any specific cultural needs they may have during their hospital stay. If an institution does not do this, the postoperative nurse may simply ask the patient or the patient's family directly if there are any special needs that they may have.

Language barriers may be handled through a hospital's maintenance of an updated listing of translators. It is probable that, in a hospital of over 200 beds or so, there are trained translators available on a 24-hour-a-day, 7-days-a-week, around-the-clock basis. Another trend that is prevalent along the states that border Mexico is to require nursing students of larger schools to take a Spanish language course designed for those in the health care professions. These types of courses are particularly popular in a time of relaxation of restrictions to free travel between countries. Some patients in hospitals, particularly in border states, speak only Spanish. In view of changing demographics, it is wise for nurses to be able to interview and converse in at least two languages.

One of the first things the nurse might do in making those of other cultures feel welcome is to provide introductions. In addition to a verbal introduction, along with noting the time through which the nurse will care for the patient, the nurse can also list names of all personnel on a mounted in-room wipe-off board. This is helpful to those who use the Western alphabet but who do not speak English fluently. The nurse may want to identify a family member who can act as the family spokesperson. For those whose primary language is not English, this person is often one who can be contacted for translation. However, awareness of confidentiality principles, particularly HIPAA legislation, and the need for accurate translation of more complicated medical terms may mean that the nurse will summon a hospital translator in some cases rather than relying on the multilingual family member.

The Older Adult

Another family consideration involves fostering comfort for the elderly.

Family support may be critically important for the surgical patient. The nurse should make every effort to provide a welcoming atmosphere and to assist each family member with settling in. Encouragement of repeat visits enables the patient to have a sense of being cared for and about by the professionals as well as family. In some cases, the typical recovery and home planning period does not occur. For example, some patients have experienced adverse events. An unexpected death may, unfortunately, be a possibility. It is particularly important for the nurse to be able to act with sensitivity in such situations. Use of the chain of command enables the hospital-based nurse to summon assistance from those trained to act to support family and patient in such circumstances. Not only nursing supervisors, but also clergy or others

Respecting
Our Differences

Postoperative Considerations for the Older Adult

Whether it is the postoperative patient or a visitor, it is important to ensure comfortable places to sit, beverages, and room temperature adequacy for all. In addition, the nurse caring for the older person who is a patient should allow extra time to perform routine activities including walking and bathing. Care alterations for those who are beyond middle age might include:

1. Following the aging adult's needs for a slower pace.
2. Allowing rest periods during activities.
3. Not mistaking hearing or vision difficulties for confusion or slow-wittedness.
4. Showing respect and consideration through remembering to introduce self and others to the patient or family.
5. Maintaining awareness to the patients ability to adapt to room temperature changes, poor lighting, stressors, and rapid alterations in fluid or electrolyte status diminish as people age and ensuring adequate hydration, room temperature, lighting, and noise control for the aging adult.
6. Having respect for the autonomy of the older adult through being aware of situations that call for explanations or for asking permission.
7. Trying to avoid calling older people by first names because this may be interpreted in some cultures as denoting lack of respect.
8. Giving full attention and eye contact on greeting the patient.

may be able to assist when such events occur. Hospital chaplains have received training in how to meet spiritual as well as cultural needs of citizens of the world's countries and major religions.

When the patient suffers an adverse consequence around the postoperative period, it is often unanticipated. The family has not had a long period in which to adjust. A death may be completely unexpected. Emotions may be strong. The care nurse should not rely solely on himself or herself in these situations. The bedside care nurse does not always have the time or expertise to handle all matters of concern to the family. A death often means hours of support needs for the family before even basic decisions can be made. There is no simple way to hasten the initial part of the grieving process.

Fortunately, in most cases, the patient is discharged to the home setting, and the course of the hospital stay will have been uneventful. The postoperative nurses may take pride in a job well done and feel a sense of assurance that all is well with the patient and family. The team that anticipates a routine discharge for the patient will want to begin planning early for the time when the patient is able to leave the facility.

HOME PLANNING

For those who have an uneventful course of surgical recovery in the hospital as well as for those who spend a longer-than-anticipated period, there comes a time when discharge planning begins in earnest. It has been said that the nurse is the 24-hour-a-day generalist who observes all aspects of patient well-being. Whether the postoperative nurse organizes thinking around a body systems model or a response model, the nurse is the manager who puts it all together. Close to the time of discharge, the nurse and others must assess the patient's current level of function in all areas as well as evaluating the readiness of the home and family to receive and maintain the patient over the coming days and weeks. Typical patient needs involve pain control, activity and rest, nutrition, elimination, and wound management. Information on contacting professionals after discharge is also needed. Arranging return appointments for postoperative checkups is important as is instruction related to the schedule for return to work.

Discharge Planning

It has been said that discharge planning begins with admission to the hospital or clinic setting. This is especially so in the case of the surgical patient. At the time of admission, the nurse reviews the patient's history, current status, and home situation. The nurse may be the first person to identify patient and family needs that require special planning early in the stay with an eye to later discharge.

The nurse has access to resources perhaps unknown to the family and patient. For example, it is the job of the health care provider and nursing staff to gather together with family, perhaps the patient, and others to discuss discharge management. If the discharging unit engages in formal discharge planning rounds, others will often meet with nursing staff and health care provider to plan for special cases. A listing of those likely to be involved in discharge planning for the surgical patient includes nursing management, clinical nurse specialist, bedside care nurse, health care provider, social worker, dietitian, physical therapist, occupational therapist, home services representative, pharmacist, and clergy.

The health care provider may have known the family for many years and has a clear sense of what might be needed. The clergy, physical and occupational therapists, social workers, dietitians, and perhaps home health services have specialized knowledge and skills to assist with planning for posthospital recovery. Even in the hospital unit or clinic that does not conduct formal rounds, there is the possibility of nursing setting up a special meeting with those who have an interest or who need to be involved. Although the relatively healthy person may not need full, interdisciplinary discharge planning, there is other cases in which this is necessary.

Teaching/Learning Principles for the Postoperative Patient

Before the nurse begins to teach, it is important to assess two areas: current patient and family knowledge base and readiness to learn. In this way, the nurse can avoid frustrating the patient and family by teaching content that has been absorbed previously. Failure to take the time to assess prior learning and current knowledge base may also have the unfortunate consequence of making the patient or family mistrust the intelligence or competence of the nurse who makes this omission. In some cases, it may actually seem an insult to the patient. The patient may feel that the least the nurse can do is to become familiar with the patient's case.

In addition to assessing knowledge base, the nurse must assess readiness to learn. Certain conditions may interfere with a patient's or family's ability to absorb information. Issues such as pain, anxiety, or the wrong setting may be distracting, making it difficult to concentrate. Other stressful events going on in the patient's family or work roles, or even historic events, such as family members in dangerous situations in other countries, may mean that a patient or family members will have difficulty absorbing discharge information.

The length of time between notification and the need to absorb information may make it difficult for the people involved in discharge teaching to learn what needs to be learned. This problem is particularly difficult when the patient or family must absorb complex wound care or activity information in a short period. When home equipment or other special arrangements must be made quickly, just prior to discharge, the difficulty is compounded. Box 22-4 contains information about postoperative teaching.

Nurses need to examine their readiness to teach by taking a few minutes to "center" oneself, initiating a sense of calm and focusing on the task at hand. This may be particularly necessary in rushed or tense situations. These skills can enhance the ability of the nurse to appear competent and relaxed at the time of discharge teaching. Is the nurse familiar with the patient and family from a time before? Has the nurse taken the time to review the postsurgical history? Is the nurse able to visualize any obstacles or strengths that might have an impact on this stage? Is the nurse able to concentrate enough to assess or are there other tasks competing for attention?

The nurse usually has a preferred style of teaching, but the nurse must tailor the teaching mode to fit with the preferred learning style of the patient. For example, if the patient has been highly observant throughout the stay, often taking notes or anticipating next steps, the nurse may want to consider the person's strong cognitive style and frame discharge teaching within that context. The active learner may have different style needs from those of the more passive person.

There are three types of learning: cognitive, affective, and psychomotor. Cognitive learning is demonstrated by knowledge of facts. A learner is able to recite, to write, to list, to select something, or to describe. An example would

---

BOX 22-4

DISCHARGE TEACHING TIPS

Assessment of Readiness to Learn
- Timing: Can the patient and family focus at this time?
- History: Are there nonhealth distractions in the patient's life at this time?

Assessment of Current Knowledge Base and Learning Style
- Ask questions: What does the patient already know?
- Design teaching to match patient's preferred style of learning.

Timing
- Select intervals that match attention span.
- Will the patient be alert?
- Can the teacher eliminate interruptions?

Setting
- Most are comfortable with familiar surroundings.
- Is there peace and quiet for the session?

Tools
- Are written materials advisable?
- Are other materials needed?

Evaluation of Learning
- Is return demonstration possible?
- Can one evaluate affective, cognitive, and psychomotor realms?
- How and when the teacher evaluate?

Adapted from Ouellet, L., Hodgins, M., Pond, S., Knorr, S., & Geldart, G. (2003). Post-discharge telephone follow-up for orthopaedic surgical patients: A pilot study. Journal of Orthopaedic Nursing, 7(2), 87–93; Whitney, J., & Parkman, S. (2004). The effect of postoperative physical activity on tissue oxygen and wound healing. Biological Research in Nursing, 6(2), 79–89.

be a teenager who was able to list things to do to avoid skin problems prior to a summer vacation.

Affective learning pertains to emotions. This may happen when the learner invests in something or commits to acquiring information. The individual feels that the information is helpful. The opposite may happen when, emotionally, the learner is disinterested or even has an aversion to acquiring information or performing something. An example would be when a person makes an informed decision not to undergo genetic testing in light of the possibility that he or she might have an incurable hereditary disease. Although emotions may sometimes defy simple analysis, the individual may be making a choice that involves maintaining hope. Psychomotor learning has occurred when the individual is able to demonstrate, physically, the mastery of a task or a piece of learning. An example is the nursing student who practices how to give an injection until the task becomes automatic. The negative side of this might be the person who learned a task in youth, only to have to unlearn a poor way of performing and acquire the correct skill set.

Another consideration is that of group versus individual teaching format. In applying these to the postoperative patient, the nurse must consider whether the patient received group teaching in the weeks leading to surgery or whether strong, individualized teaching is needed just prior to patient discharge. This determination makes a difference in nursing approach. For example, it is now common in the more progressive hospitals around the country to bring in patients who is having major lower limb orthopedic surgery for a workshop or series of workshops. These are usually held within a month or two prior to the elective surgery. The patient brings a family member or friend to participate and to be a helper when later needs arise after the postoperative return home.

Some hospitals preteach the surgical patient and family member to recognize and use equipment that will be present following surgery. Emphasis is placed on pain management, positioning, personnel who assist patients following surgery, and how to meet daily needs. This is particularly important with mobility-limiting surgery. Physical therapy and occupational therapy personnel allow attendees at such sessions to practice with various devices, such as wheelchairs, shoe and sock assist devices, and Velcro fasteners. Things to do and not to do in terms of positioning are emphasized. Patients practice postoperative exercises and how to sit up or stand following surgery.

This preparation has a later bearing on the amount and type of discharge teaching that the discharging hospital unit needs to consider. For the patient and family who faithfully practiced requisite maneuvers and who are able to cite do's and do not's and who have home equipment and the home setting prepared, there is obviously less content for the discharging orthopedic or other postsurgical nurse to teach. The patient who has received only the briefest of one-on-one sessions the day before discharge needs more individual instruction from the nurse.

The benefits of individual, one-on-one teaching is ideal for teaching technical skills, for assessing mastery of steps in learning tasks, and for flexibility in taking advantage of teachable moments. When the nurse concentrates on a particular patient rather than a group, there is time for close observation as the patient practices a skill or technique. The nurse may also be able to divide teaching sessions to bring the patient along more slowly to mastery of steps in a complex technical procedure that need to be performed at home. For example, for the newly diagnosed insulin-dependent diabetic patient who is recovering from limb surgery, the act of safely drawing up and administering an injection may call for several sessions allowing mastery each day of each of the individual steps. Timing these sessions is important because the patient's physical therapy and occupational therapy sessions take place each day at prescheduled intervals.

In some situations, group teaching may be a better choice. Benefits of group teaching include economy (in a financial sense) and economy of effort on the part of the teacher or teaching team. In addition, bonding with other patients and families during group teaching sessions may assist preoperative or recovering patients. Mutual support and camaraderie can help ease anxiety. Finally, a third element in group teaching is the fostering of positive attitude. The patient may take cues from others and be able to overcome fear or other resistance factors through the sense of not being alone.

A final note about postoperative teaching principles is that those patients with low literacy should be identified and steps taken to ensure that their learning experience is successful. The incorporation of audio and visual aids enhance their education. For example, a short-filmed segment will show the viewer exactly how to perform a task. A videodisk can be sent home with the patient who owns a DVD player, or a printed diagram can refresh the memory at a later point. The nurse would be aware that those with decreased ability to read tend to speak articulately but may not ask many questions or inform the teacher that they cannot read. A tendency to have shorter attention spans and to rely more on visual cues is also a characteristic of this type of learner.

Prior to discharge, the nurse is involved in teaching wound care to the patient and family. The postoperative nurse assessing the acquisition of this content may want to look for outcomes across all three dimensions of learning mastery: cognitive, affective, and psychomotor. Beginning with the psychomotor aspects, return demonstration of dressing changes or handling of such things as hemovac devices show the discharging nurse that the patient will have no trouble with these at home. The nurse may also want to assess cognitive mastery in a number of ways. The nurse may simply ask whether there are questions, and leave it at that. Or, in another case, asking the patient or family, "What would you do if . . . ?" is another way in which understanding can be assessed. Finally, the nurse should be vigilant in relation to affective learning. Are the patient and family feeling that postoperative management at home is possible for them at this time? Are there fears?

It has been shown that the combination of verbal and written instruction is more successful in knowledge retention than is either one alone. At one and three months post-instruction, the groups that received both visual and auditory instruction, including typewritten copy to take home, fared better in retained knowledge. Many institutions have preprinted sheets that have both text and pictorial directions. These can be sent home with the patient. Some patients and family members use these as references once the discharge education period has faded.

It is also important to provide supplies or a listing of supplies that might be needed at home before the patient is discharged. Planning for prescriptions and for equipment chargeable to the insurance plan is also vital. Taking care of these needs in advance will ensure a smooth transition from hospital to home. Knowing that effective return demonstration of such techniques as dressing change or administration of medications may be complex tasks for the patient or family member, it is wise to begin teaching and "testing" early.

Patient and Family Teaching

Surgical units that perform similar types of surgery on a frequent basis may want to have preprinted instruction forms or discharge orders. These can be available in hard copy or on computer, as long as they are readily accessible at time of discharge. In addition, the nurse needs to take time to go over the discharge orders or instructions with the patient and family. There needs to be a relaxed atmosphere, which enhances the retention of information by the patient. If it is possible to elicit demonstration as a way of evaluating the learning, this mode is best.

Wound care is often the area of teaching most requested by the patient and family. It is one area with which the patient may have had no past experience. While the patient or family member may have had ample opportunity to observe the nurse performing wound care or changing dressings, there may be a need to have a practice session or two to build patient confidence and provide an opportunity for the nurse to assess wound care knowledge. Usually, the patient will go home with a simple wound dressing consisting of one or two layers of soft gauze bandage.

If the patient is to change the dressing at home, there is no need to wear gloves when the old dressing is removed. For others, if the wound continues to drain at home, the family member will perhaps want to don exam gloves to remove the old dressing. Clean hands usually suffice to apply the new dressing. The nurse may want to point out that hands should touch what is the outer surface of the dressing but not the underside that comes into direct contact with the wound. Once the new dressing has been placed over the wound, it should be left alone and not largely repositioned.

While the dressing is off the wound, it is wise to inspect for redness, swelling, or any pulling apart of the wound edges (Figure 22-7). Cleaning products are not usually recommended, because it has been shown that these do not hasten wound healing and may disrupt the natural healing process. Because gauze serves as a filter for germs but does not lock in moisture, it is wise for those using this dressing material to refrain from covering the entire surface with tape. Taping the edges of the dressing allows moisture to escape, provides a barrier against microbes, and protects the wound from being irritated by clothing. Although most wound care products are available at drug stores and in drug sections of supermarkets, the nurse may want to send an initial supply home with the patient to ensure a smooth first day or two at home.

It would be unusual for a patient to be sent home with a Penrose drain. If there are drains at the time the patient is discharged, they are usually those with receptacles, such as the hemovac. The patient or family member needs to demonstrate how, with clean hands and a supply of 30 mL plastic medicine cups or 240 mL marked plastic cups, the receptacle can be emptied and the vacuum reinstituted.

Pain control is another topic for discharge teaching. The nurse usually writes the names and dosage schedules on a discharge instruction sheet, along with the health care provider's phone number for use should the prescribed medications not be effective in controlling pain. The nurse once again compares the prescribed medications with the patient's identified allergies to be sure that there is no likelihood of allergic reaction. It is a good idea for the nurse to go over the written medication list to ensure that the patient has no questions and understands how to take these at home. The nurse gives written prescriptions to the patient or a family member. Should these be lost following discharge, the patient may refer to the written instruction sheet when calling the health care provider's office for a replacement set to be phoned in to the local pharmacy. The nurse also describes steps the patient should take if the medications are ineffective, as well as early signs of possible allergy or other undesirable effects.

Activity and rest are important topics for discharge teaching. Hospital discharge forms often have a summary phrase to describe such recommendations as usual activity levels, or no heavy activities, or the like. The nurse may want to discuss examples of what is meant by these phrases. For example, the nurse may recommend that the patient who has had GI surgery not reach up to shelves in the kitchen to pull objects down. The patient may be advised not to stretch when waking in the mornings until pain has diminished, and the wound is well healed. The patient with an abdominal incision might want to avoid sweeping or vacuuming for a time. Lifting anything should be done with caution or not at all. The nurse should stress that walking is important. It has been known statistically for many years that inactivity postoperatively may be associated with a number of complications.

In relation to hygiene, the surgeon will have instructed the patient about when showering is possible. Usually, tub baths must wait until the patient

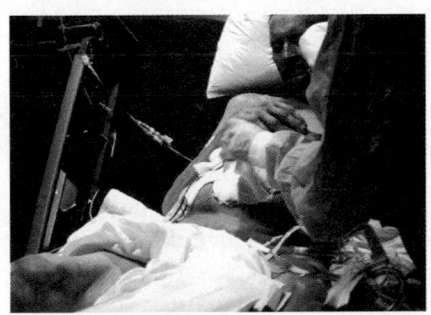

Figure 22-7 Removing the old dressing to inspect the wound.

receives permission at the first postoperative visit to the health care provider's office. Any dressing material is usually left in place when showering because the old dressing material helps to protect the wound from water pressure. Later, when staples or sutures are removed and the wound is closer to being fully healed, the area is left open to air. Until then, the protective "old" dressing is removed following showering and a fresh dressing applied.

Nutrition will usually be as it was before the surgery except in the case of special diets or supplementary programs necessitated by GI surgery or other medical conditions. Should persistent nausea and vomiting occur following discharge, these should be reported. Nausea and vomiting might be early signs of drug allergy or another postsurgical complication. The health care provider will order the patient's diet plan. Usually, "*as tolerated*" is indicated on the discharge teaching form. For some, liquid dietary supplements are needed.

Teaching about medications is important, including instructions to take the medication exactly as prescribed. That is, the patient will receive a supply of clearly labeled medication at the pharmacy after discharge. The pharmacist often goes over how and when to take the medication, as well as the side effects. The patient should not deviate from these instructions (either the verbal ones or those typed onto the medication container). If there is a reason to suspect a need to alter the timing or amount of medication, the patient may want to call the health care provider's office. Often, the office nurse is free to discuss the problem and advise the patient or will call back with new instructions once the health care provider has been informed. The patient should not stop the medication prior to completion of the full course of therapy.

The nurse should assess the impact of discharge teaching particularly as it relates to medications. The nurse may elicit cognitive understanding by asking for purposes of each of the medications in turn. It is particularly important for the nurse to elicit affective domain reactions: Does the patient seem willing to follow these directions at the time of discharge? If not, what is the patient's perception? What is the patient's attitude about taking medications? Careful documentation of understanding at the time of discharge provides a clear reference point should difficulties develop later.

Signs and symptoms of complications should be highlighted during discharge instruction sessions. One of the more important would be fever, often defined as an oral temperature greater than 100.5° F (38° C). In some institutions, the standard is that oral temperature will exceed 101° F (38.3° C) to be considered a reportable fever.

Another sign of possible complications is a dramatic or sudden change in pain level. Unusual discharge or bleeding from the surgical site or local redness or heat around the surgical area would also be noteworthy and reportable by the patient. Extension of an existing area of bruising or the development of new bruises is a concern the patient should report via telephone to the physician's office. In thinking about possible coagulation problems that might be initially noted through bruising, the patient and family should be alert to any changes in level of alertness, the onset of confusion, dizziness, or fainting. These might relate to bleeding internally or anemia related to hidden blood loss, or any one of a number of other problems. Even a persistent decline in energy levels between the time when the patient is discharged and the initial days at home is noteworthy and should probably be reported to the health care provider by the patient or family.

Unless the patient has had genitourinary surgery requiring specialized postoperative observation and care, urination should usually continue as it was prior to surgery. The patient should void at least every six to eight hours. Urine should not have sediment, blood streaks, clots, or be cloudy. Urination should not be painful, and the patient should not have difficulty in initiating urinary stream. In addition, the sudden onset of urinary frequency or urgency should be reported to the health care provider.

The patient should also be aware that pain medications and postoperative inactivity may predispose the patient to constipation. The patient should be guided by presurgical elimination patterns in deciding whether constipation is a problem. With certain types of surgery, such as GI surgery, there are special instructions related to bowel elimination. Again, both written and verbal instructions should be provided to patients at discharge.

In most cases, neurological function should return to preoperative levels immediately following in-hospital recovery from the effects of anesthesia. Exceptions occur whenever there was surgery involving the brain. Or sometimes, in the case of central neurological trauma or in-hospital stroke, the patient will have established a new baseline for neurological response prior to discharge. Deviation from this baseline may signal additional problems. The family needs to check with the health care provider or in some cases, report to the emergency department if sudden or dramatic changes occur.

Metabolic and endocrine concerns are another area for discussion as part of discharge teaching. The health care provider often orders blood sampling at the time of the first office visit. The sample will provide information about circulating electrolytes as well as a CBC. By studying this information, the clinic staff is able to determine whether the patient has fully recovered from the effects of surgery and its aftermath. However, prior to the time of the first office visit, the family and patient should be aware that failure to thrive at home, such as loss of appetite or a dramatic posthospital change in energy level, might be a signal that something is wrong.

The nurse must balance the time that is spent in teaching and the topics discussed. Sometimes, giving too much information all at once will confuse or distress the patient and family. The nurse must be careful to assess the patient's readiness to learn and must carefully plan how much information is too much. Providing too much verbal information about possible complications could set the normally recovering patient on a path of many a sleepless night spent worrying needlessly about whether symptoms indicate a need for concern. On the other hand, giving too little information could set the patient up for reacting slowly when faster action was necessary. Most hospital discharge forms contain sufficient information for the patient and family to carry on safely and effectively at home. The nurse will use a variety of skills in assessing, teaching, and evaluating in order to ensure an effective discharge and a successful course at home.

Electronic Resources for the Postoperative Patient

Because patients in the computer age are usually familiar with library resources and may own their own computer at home, it is also helpful for the nursing unit to provide a list of credible Web sites. As technology becomes more advanced, and more common, health care providers look for new and innovative ways to incorporate these new tools into patient care. One way this is being done is with patient education. HeartCare is an Internet-based postoperative teaching and support system used by post-CABG patients after discharge. This system is especially useful in extending how RNs can continue caring for patients even with the tendency for shorter patient hospital stays in today's managed care health system. One author points out that this system is useful to supplement nurses' traditional patient education role. The teaching role of nurses, then, is transformed from a single point in time to an ongoing, enduring, and patient controlled process. This creates a patient who takes an active role in self-management (McDonald, Hetrick, & Green, 2004). This type of technology can also be used to allow nurses and patients to better individualize postoperative care and teaching.

Another way technology is being used is with remote monitoring of patients in the hospital. Some large hospital systems are using remote systems to supplement staff in areas where patients can deteriorate rapidly, such as the CCU, or where nurses have large patient loads, such as postoperative floors. The nurses who staff the remote systems are able to monitor vital signs, such as blood pressure, pulse, respirations, pulse oximetry, temperature, and in critical care areas may include parameters, such as increased ICP and arterial pressure. The remote operator can then notify caregivers of any concerning trends in the patients vital signs. Early indications show that there may be a reduction in morbidity and mortality, as well as decreased length of patient stay in some units.

There are some concerns about using remote monitoring systems, however. One is that the nurses on these units will spend more time on the care of the machines rather than the patients, especially in the early stages before all the technological problems have been worked out. Another concern is that the remote monitoring systems may not be as effective as they can because of lack of proper training for staff. Finally, by using remote monitoring, there is a feeling that the patient and family may not have enough access to all of the caregivers if questions or concerns arise.

In addition to online resources, social service departments maintain current listings of local service groups. For example, if a patient lives alone and is unable to grocery shop or perform light housework for a number of weeks after surgery, the social service department may be able to make arrangements for in-home services. From a listing of all agencies available in the local area to help patients, social workers are able to make recommendations based on their experience and knowledge of insurance provisions and patient needs. They are able to make evaluative recommendations based on personal experience with local groups or agencies. Most nursing units that are located within cities have their own set of social workers who specialize in providing the appropriate follow-up care for patients who usually utilize the nursing unit. They can assist in preparation of a convenient set of access numbers, a manual of contact information for those who will need additional assistance after discharge, and online resources that are readily contactable prior to discharge. Once a family unit has tapped into the system, unnecessary worries tend to evaporate. There is still work to be done prior to discharge, but the in-hospital or in-clinic preplanning tends to place responsibility in the hands of those who will take over from the nursing staff.

In this age of clinical pathways, it is anticipated that most patients will recover in predictable ways and according to predictable timelines. For example, the surgical patient of lesser acuity with a small incision often returns home within 23 hours following surgery. Or the patient who may have comorbidities and an abdominal incision may spend a predictable three days in the hospital. While this is not always the case, such timelines help nurses and others to plan.

The system of diagnosis related groups (DRGs) is a listing of average lengths of stay within the hospital or acute care setting based on main diagnosis or on the procedure being done during a traditional hospital stay. The system takes into account comorbidities. Comorbidities are health problems that are a part of a patient's health or illness pattern when the patient is not in the hospital. For example, such ailments as chronic respiratory disorders (COPD), diabetes mellitus, or chronic heart failure (HF), would be comorbidities for the patient being admitted for orthopedic surgery.

To ensure that the hospital does not lose money in patient care, there is a strong focus on keeping patients within the usual and customary recovery trajectory, or pathway. In addition to financial aspects, it is considered safer for a patient to be out of the hospital and at home than it is to linger within the walls of an acute care facility. Psychologically, the patient and family may feel a sense of disappointment if discharge home is delayed beyond what they had come to expect. For these reasons, it is important for the nurse to be able to discover those for whom discharge delay is likely and to take steps to avert unplanned delays.

Delayed Recovery

Despite attention to detail and the best in care while a patient recovers in the hospital from surgery, there will always be individual circumstances and individual recovery rates that must be considered by the nurse who cares for postsurgical patients. It is helpful to consider how to predict cases in which the patient will spend a longer than average period recovering from surgery. If the nurse can predict, sometimes the nurse can help the patient or family to adapt when the delay occurs. Sometimes the nurse can take steps to prevent the patient from becoming what has come to be known as an "outlier." The outlier remains a hospital inpatient long beyond the time for which the family is prepared or for which insurance will pay.

Predicting and Preventing Outlier Situations

Under the DRG system, comorbidities are taken into account when projecting an individual patient's probable length of stay in an acute care facility, such as the hospital. The hospital is reimbursed for services for the individual patient based on the DRG system's estimate. Therefore, it is in an acute care facility's best interest to try to promote discharge readiness within the usual, customary length of time.

If a potential overstay situation can be discovered early in the surgical patient's hospital stay, or even prior to admission, then steps can be taken remove conditions that might delay discharge. If a patient has chronic conditions, such as diabetes mellitus or chronic lung disease, then the care nurse can anticipate and plan with the patient and family prior to surgery. For example, if a family member and the patient are aware of nothing by mouth (NPO) status prior to surgery, they and the nursing staff can be sure that the patient does not receive insulin or agents that might result in hypoglycemia. Because prolonged hospital stays may expose the patient to dangers, it is important for postoperative nurses to understand the latest findings in relation to recovery from surgery.

Despite reliance on the best practices that are known to exist, there are times when patients do not recover swiftly and uneventfully from surgery. There can be disappointment and some degree of uncertainty about the remainder of the recovery period for those surgical patients who must spend a longer than average time in the hospital. This can be even more difficult for the patient who is not discharged to the home setting but to a rehabilitative care setting.

Long-Term Recovery in Special Settings

In contrast to those patients who are able to go directly from hospital or clinic to their home setting, there is a group of patients who are not able to proceed directly home. This is the group of patients who must make a stop along the way for rehabilitative care. This care is designed to strengthen the patient's abilities, so that the patient is able to function successfully at home at a later date. Sometimes this step is necessary, because the patient cannot achieve sufficient mobility to be able to maneuver outside a special setting. Or, in other cases, it is because the patient has no live-in at-home support system or because the patient's at-home support system consists of frail or weakened individuals.

Patients who need specialized recovery care often experience a distressing emotional impact. It is usually disappointing for patients to learn of the need for care beyond their stay in the hospital setting. For example, for patients who have had such things as extensive limb surgery, there is recognition that recovery will require prolonged physical therapy and wound management. The use of specialized, nonportable, rehabilitative equipment mandates a stay in an extended care facility, often for months. But, despite recognition by the patient of this need for extended stay, there is the desire to be home as soon as physically possible. Even for patients and families who were educated prior to surgery to expect the need for staying in a rehabilitative or extended stay facility, it is emotionally distressing when the decision is actually made for this option. Some patients and families fear that the patient will not be able to progress. There is concern that the extended stay might turn into a lifetime stay far from the comforts of home.

Most people fear loss of control over the environment in such circumstances. One is not solely in charge of one's own diet or TV show choices, or even when to go to bed or to get up in the morning. There are the ever-present thoughts, "Will junk food be permitted? Do they allow wine with my dinner? Will I be there through the holidays? Can a family member come by and take me out to the movies or to a mall?" There is just something about going from hospital to an extended stay setting that carries with it a special set of concerns.

This concern is for self and one's own future and can be compounded, in the case of the frail elder, who must be home alone for the first time in years when the spouse or sister or brother is temporarily in an extended-stay setting. Perhaps physically stronger, more active family members were able to visit and support both frail people while the immediate postoperative period came and went. Now when faced with perhaps weeks of an extended care stay for one of the partners, the situation changes. The stronger, more physically able family members must now decide to return to their previous lifestyles and responsibilities. Decisions must be made prior to their departure. Will the sole household inhabitant be safe on his or her own? Will this person be able to manage physically? How is the memory? Will medications be taken appropriately? What about food shopping or communications? This is a time of great uncertainty for the entire family.

Preservation of the patient's right to choose and to be returned to the home setting as soon as possible is everyone's goal. Not only does this make sense from a humanitarian standpoint, but it also makes sense from a purely economic standpoint. Safe home recovery allows for home visits to ensure progress, as well as for the patient and family to resume autonomy and preferred lifestyles as soon as possible.

To use a hypothetical case, let us say that this older couple is able to return to life as usual once the husband has recovered from orthopedic surgery involving one lower limb. It is reassuring to know that the loved one will spend only an extra four days in a specialized facility and that arrangements have been made to have specialized equipment delivered to and set up in the home. There will be bathroom grab bars, a toilet extension that will raise the height of the toilet and make sitting and standing easier, and a rolling walker. In such a hypothetical scenario, the family will also be relieved to know that once the time in the extended care facility is over and the patient returns home, the physical therapist will visit weekdays in the morning and afternoon for continued gait training and strengthening; that the visiting nurse will assess the wound daily and do specialized dressing care daily for the first week home; and that the patient will have the rented motorized scooter available until the middle of next month for those forays outside the house. The visiting nurse has already assessed household safety and made recommendations to the visiting family members. The departing family members will take the visiting nurse's suggestions. They will use blocks to raise the heights of the bed and favorite chairs, remove and store the throw rugs, and ensure that the medical supply house has delivered the small reaching, gripping, and zipping tools that this couple will need.

How does the nursing staff identify those in probable need of an intermediate care facility prior to a return home? Typically, people who have sustained orthopedic or neurological problems as a result of accident or disease are in need of more time to recover. Severe, lingering deficits with mobility or communication usually require extended care away from home. For example, those who have had total hip replacement or total knee replacement, and are unable to achieve a steady gait after four days in the hospital, or who become extremely fatigued with even a trip into the adjoining bathroom are candidates for intermediate care. Another example is the patient who had surgery to relieve central nervous system pressure following a motor vehicle accident. While the patient is stable in terms of basic body system functions, there are lingering communication and judgment deficits as well as an inability to recall how to use the walker from day to day. The health care provider feels that some of these deficits will resolve with time. The family may be unable to manage the patient until the person can get around more easily. Consequently, this individual would need an extended care facility.

Another consideration for those who have recovered beyond the point of needing to be in residence at an extended stay facility might be a day service. This type of service is covered under most insurance plans or through federally funded programs. Such a service provides those with specialized training who come to the home. Others provide a day facility at which the family can drop the patient for periods during the day. In that way, patients know that the home setting is there for them, but that during their extended recovery period, there is a site conveniently located to access special services.

THE FUTURE OF POSTOPERATIVE NURSING

Recent trends in postoperative nursing means safer, more effective care for surgical patients. The reliance on evidence-based practice is possible now because electronic access to a variety of databases by those of all ages. Some ways in which this will have an impact on postoperative nursing are expected to be safer practices resulting in fewer avoidable errors, sophisticated methods for ensuring rapid recovery from surgery, and the ability to detect subtle patient changes in a timely way. The development of highly visual teaching/learning methods will result in smoother hospital-to-home transitions and perhaps decreased feelings of stress for patients and families.

A recent example of hospital-to-home transition improvement is the introduction of a nurse-led telephone service for those who have been discharged from an emergency assessment area (Lee, 2004). There are indications that telephone followup by nurses may improve discharge practices as well as patient confidence at home regardless of the area of the hospital from which the patient is discharged.

Even more futuristic is the possibility of remote assessment from the comfort of home. The Fast Forward describes some of the possibilities for technology to enhance analysis of patients outside the walls of hospitals and clinics.

Postoperative nursing will continue to develop new ways in which to ensure that "high tech" is not all that the patient experiences. High touch has always been an acknowledged need within health care, and there is no reason to think that this trend will not continue. Sometimes, high touch means comfort in traditional ways, such as simple nurse presence at the bedside or using soothing voice tones. Nursing staff used to ensure that all hospitalized patients received back massage each evening just before bedtime and if music was also provided, so much the better. This could be brought forward to the present in a variety of ways. For example, much of what physical therapists do relies on knowing the motion of the body's joints and the body's responses to such things as heat or massage. To relieve physical discomfort or stress before or after surgical intervention, nursing and physical therapy could form partnerships to design new systems. Such systems might even follow patients home. It might be possible to design devices that could be programmed to deliver a prescribed course of temperature therapy, massage, or other form of relaxation therapy. These simple measures might be designed to decrease stress within the hospital and other health care settings, with or without the presence of a human operator during the course of the intervention. In addition to designing measures of this sort that will alter physical responses to the surgical experience, it may be possible to design and test measures to carry the patient and family through the entire perioperative experience in a more relaxed frame of mind. It is probable that future surveys will reveal ways in which nursing can remove stress points or alter their impact.

Finally, there have been predictions that the most difficult health care needs will revolve around the social problems engendered by poverty, emotional illness, and fragmented societies. It is probable that the types of surgical intervention and the settings in which surgery is performed will be different in the decades to come. As global societies become the norm, the United States may see a day when it is called on to deal with world health problems using unprecedented combinations of inventiveness and caring. The nurse has always been capable of being comfortable in high technology and high caring situations. It may fall to nursing to prepare for this new world.

KEY CONCEPTS

- PACU has led to decreased morbidity, mortality, and shortened hospital stays.
- Use of modern technology to monitor and treat complications, unexpected postoperative events preserves patient integrity, and ensures positive outcomes.
- High touch nursing care using holistic principles is necessary within modern high technology health care settings.
- The short-stay unit allows recovering patients with minor surgical interventions to complete the recovery process at home.
- The PACU nurse assesses the patient in the immediate postoperative period with respiratory and cardiovascular systems being priority.
- The postoperative nurse will assess level of consciousness or return of sensation and motion to extremities in the case of spinal or regional anesthetic blocks.
- HIPAA mandates special techniques to ensure adherence to patient's confidentiality rights.
- Beyond the initial 24 hours, patient progress depends on resumption of activity levels.

- Respiratory and cardiovascular function is promoted through ambulation, return to healthy lifestyle habits, and deep breathing to promote efficient air exchange.
- Freedom from potential adverse events will center on effective initial care and later teaching by the nursing team.
- Because family or the patient will take up care on discharge, the nursing team continues teaching efforts as the patient nears discharge time.
- The nurse will try to provide both verbal and written forms of teaching, as well as allowing sufficient time for return demonstration.
- Return demonstration is an effective means of evaluating postoperative discharge teaching effectiveness.
- The family and patient will be instructed in home safety.
- Verbal and written instructions on health care provider contact will be given to the patient and family at discharge.
- Recent trends in postoperative nursing means safer, more effective care for surgical patients.

REVIEW QUESTIONS

1. Which of the following actions by a postoperative nurse reflects incomplete understanding of patient confidentiality needs under HIPAA?
   1. Sharing information with health care personnel on a need-to-know basis
   2. Discussing patient recovery times with an unidentified caller
   3. Using a cover sheet on clipboard
   4. Stopping unidentified personnel from looking through a patient's chart
   5. Selecting family spokesperson to relay information to family and friends of patient

2. Which of the following should the PACU nurse assess as a priority on arrival of the patient from the operating room?
   1. Cardiorespiratory
   2. Integumentary
   3. Patient anxiety
   4. Level of consciousness

3. During the first 24 hours after surgery, which of the following indicators would need immediate follow-up?
   1. Patient states "My pain is 3/10."
   2. Patient's blood pressure is 130/85.

Continued

3. Patient reports pain when coughing.
4. Patient states, "I like having this dog here keeping me company."

4. The patient's respiratory rate is eight breaths per minute upon arrival on the postsurgical floor from PACU. What should be the first course of action?
   1. Stimulate the patient using voice and touch to encourage increased respirations
   2. Call the anesthesiologist to come to the unit to reverse anesthesia
   3. Give no pain medication until respiratory rate improves
   4. Take no action; this is within normal parameters for an adult patient

5. Identify wound findings that would require action on the part of nurse:
   1. Dime-sized area of drainage on exterior of soft gauze dressing
   2. A 5-cm area of hot, darkened skin visible at distal end of dressing
   3. Total of 3 mL of drainage taken from hemovac every shift
   4. Approximated wound edges

6. Mr. Smith arrived on your unit 40 minutes ago from PACU. Report stated that patient received morphine 2 mg intravenously an hour ago. Mr. Smith states that the pain is again 8/10. Mr. Smith has a respiratory rate of 18, BP is 145/85, and pulse is 90. What would the RN's best option be?
   1. It is too soon to medicate. Try using distraction techniques to help manage pain.
   2. Examine transfer orders and select appropriate pain mediation
   3. Reposition the patient
   4. Ensure the patient that deep breathing will help alleviate pain

7. The PACU report indicates that EBL during surgery was 1,000 mL. From the list, select the most important indicators for the care nurse to examine:
   1. Perform routine postoperative checks, because EBL is within normal limits for the type of surgery performed
   2. Assess vital signs and level of consciousness
   3. Assess the dressing for indications of hemorrhage
   4. Assess for return of bowel sounds

8. Following major abdominal surgery, when should the discharged patient definitely call the health care provider (select all that apply)?
   1. Oral temperature of 102° F (38.8° C)
   2. Persistent weakness and fatigue

3. Mental status changes
4. Decreased appetite
5. Noting that incisional pain feels worse just prior to bedtime

9. Identify the patient most likely to experience delayed wound healing:
   1. A 25-year-old patient who had right knee replacement and who consumes an 1,800 calorie/day diet
   2. An 86-year-old patient, post GI surgery who has seven hours of uninterrupted sleep per night
   3. A 31-year-old type 1 diabetic patient recovering from a skin graft to the right lower extremity
   4. A 23-year-old post-appendectomy patient who is returning to a presurgical routine of one mile per day as a bicycle workout

10. Which of the following indicates further teaching is needed about leg compression devices?
    1. The patient states that the compression stocking should be removed for one hour per day.
    2. The patient states that the compression stocking should continue to be worn routinely until the first followup visit to the health care provider.
    3. The patient states that the compression stocking should not be put back on once it is taken off.
    4. The patient states that the compression stocking can be worn under street clothing after discharge.

11. Which of the following indicates inadequate hydration?
    1. Seven hours after surgery, patient's urinary catheter contains 50 mL.
    2. Patient's mucous membranes are pink.
    3. Patient skin turgor has no indication of tenting.
    4. Patient's urinary catheter contains 350 mL seven hours after surgery.

12. Mr. Smith is experiencing POD 2 after abdominal surgery. His nasogastric tube was pulled yesterday. He has bowel sounds in four quadrants, is not passing flatus, and has had no bowel movement. Which of the previous data indicates that Mr. Smith is not ready for a full (regular) diet?
    1. Has not passed flatus
    2. Has not had a bowel movement
    3. Nasogastric tube was discontinued yesterday
    4. Has bowel sounds in all four quadrants

Continued

REVIEW QUESTIONS—cont'd

13. From the list provided, select the RN action that would be most *inappropriate* when dealing with Mr. Jones, an 86-year-old patient (POD 2) receiving dressing change instructions?
    1. The RN provides a written list of instructions, complete with diagrams.
    2. The RN has Mr. Jones perform a dressing change himself prior to discharge.
    3. The RN delivers the instructions while assisting Mr. Jones to the restroom.
    4. The RN delivers the teaching to both Mr. and Mrs. Jones.

14. Identify the most appropriate elements for ensuring the success of discharge teaching:
    1. Thorough assessment of the patient's readiness to learn
    2. Keeping all sessions less than 5 min in length to ensure patient attention
    3. Using solely written materials to ensure accuracy of information
    4. Using closed-ended questions to obtain feedback from patient about teaching

REVIEW ACTIVITIES

1. List five priorities for care within the PACU.

2. Based on care priorities for the patient who has been transferred from PACU to the postoperative care unit, discuss appropriate nursing interventions for the recovering patient.

3. When caring for the older patient, will your style of care change? If so, describe three ways in which you would choose to alter care routines.

4. List four possible complications for the patient recovering from surgery.

5. Select a typical postoperative ethical dilemma. Describe your initial handling of the situation. What resources can you draw on to assist you with this difficult situation?

6. List six nursing diagnoses commonly associated with the postoperative patient.

7. Describe wound care teaching for the patient recovering from abdominal surgery. The patient will be discharged with a **hemovac** (Jackson Pratt [JP]) with a need for a waterproof pad over soft gauze for the three days (twice a day changes) leading up to the first health care provider visit. Be detailed about general hygiene measures and imagine the patient asking you about such things as showering.

UNIT
V

Alterations in Cardiovascular and Hematological Function

Assessment of Cardiovascular and Hematological Function

Barbara Voshall, RN, MN

David Voshall, PhD, MD

CHAPTER TOPICS

- Anatomy/Physiology of the Hematological System

- Anatomy/Physiology of the Cardiovascular System

- Assessment and Diagnostic Tests of the Hematological System

- Assessment and Diagnostic Tests of the Cardiovascular System

The blood is a complex mixture of water, inorganic ions, simple and complex organic compounds, and cellular elements. The blood takes nutrients to the cells, and it removes products (both useful and waste) from the cells. It is the primary route that most compounds (hormones, fuels, and structural precursors) get moved through the body. In a sense, it is the essence of life. The blood vessels are the highway of life. Thus, an analysis of the blood provides information about many different organ systems and the overall functional status of the body. The blood is carried through the body in a closed system. The heart is the pump that propels the blood through a system of arteries, capillaries, and veins. Abnormalities in the system are evaluated by a series of noninvasive tests and invasive exams.

ANATOMY AND PHYSIOLOGY (HEMATOLOGICAL SYSTEM)

The hematological system is complex and essential to a wide variety of functions in the human body. In general, the hematological system is comprised of the circulating aspects of the blood products, such as the plasma. The various components that are circulated have many functions. For example, the white blood cells are vital to the immune response of the body. The products of the blood that make hemostasis possible are included in the anticoagulant capabilities of the hematological system (Rizzo, 2006).

Plasma

Water is the medium in which the other material including inorganic, organic, and biochemical molecules and cells are carried. Too much water causes the system to overflow, and when there is too little water, there is not enough volume to circulate to all the tissues. **Plasma** is the liquid portion of the circulation system that carries organic and inorganic elements. The electrolytes, for example, sodium, potassium, chloride, magnesium, calcium, and phosphate, are dissolved in the water. The body has many mechanisms to control these electrolytes within a narrow range, providing a stable bath for the cells.

Plasma also carries glucose to the cells in the blood. The concentration of glucose is kept fairly constant within the body. All of the tissues can take up glucose. The liver is unique in being the only organ that can release glucose into the blood. Other simple molecules commonly found in the blood include thyroid hormone, epinephrine, steroid hormones, and cholesterol.

More complicated macromolecules in the plasma include proenzymes or proteins that need to be changed to become enzymes; an example of a proenzyme is the clotting protein that circulates in the blood, which will be discussed later in the chapter. Antibodies provide one level of immune surveillance for the body. Albumin provides an amino acid pool that helps keep the water in the blood vessels that contributes to oncotic pressure. Polypeptide hormones help regulate the various processes in the body, like insulin, helping to control blood glucose. The complement proteins are proteins that can punch a hole in the bacterial cell wall or membrane, and they also circulate in the blood.

Normally, there is a slow rate of death of cells in the body. Some of the molecules that are contained in these cells are released into the blood as cellular degradation takes place. These markers, both enzyme and protein, can be measured and normal values established. When the cells become inflamed or dead, increased amounts of these compounds are released into the blood, and the increased levels of these enzymes can be measured. For example, troponin is a compound that is found in muscles. When there is damage to the heart muscle, it can release enzymes which become elevated.

The **cellular components** of the blood include the erythrocytes or red blood cells, the white blood cells, and the platelets (Figure 23-1). The erythrocytes deliver oxygen to the cells. The white blood cells are involved in the immune protection of the body. The platelets are the first responders when there is damage to the inner lining of a blood vessel. The cellular components of the blood are all derived from a stem cell. This stem cell can produce all the other cells, that is, the red blood cells, the white blood cells, and the platelets. The stem cell can make the platelets, red cells, and white cells—both lymphocyte and granulocyte series. The multipotent stem cell can differentiate into the progenitor cells. These progenitor cells can then reproduce themselves, or form the erythrocyte precursor cell (rubriblast), the granulocyte precursor cells, or the platelet precursor cells. One can harvest or collect the stem cells from a person and put them back into the same person or into a person who

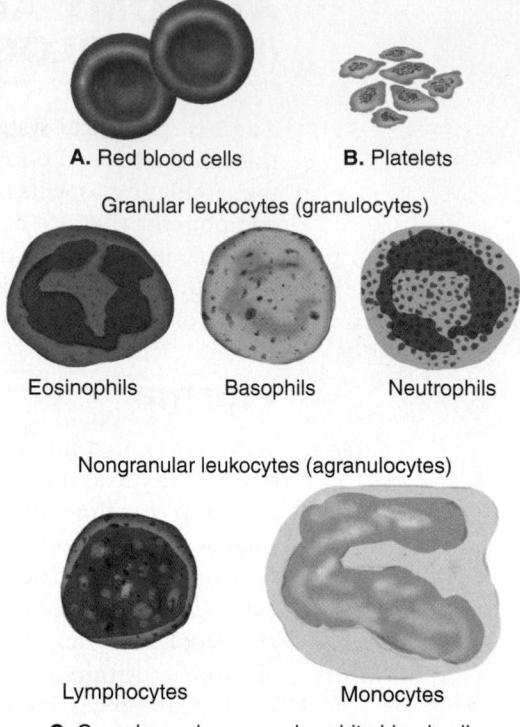

A. Red blood cells   **B.** Platelets

Granular leukocytes (granulocytes)

Eosinophils   Basophils   Neutrophils

Nongranular leukocytes (agranulocytes)

Lymphocytes   Monocytes

C. Granular and nongranular white blood cells

Figure 23-1 The cells in blood: A. Red blood cells (erythrocytes), B. Platelets (thrombocytopenia), C. White blood cells (leukocytes).

is compatible. This process is called a stem cell transplant. Once the stem cell is placed into the patient, it can reproduce all the cell types.

Erythrocytes

The production of the red blood cells occurs in the bone marrow. The bone marrow is found in the middle of the bones. The production of red blood cells is called erythropoiesis. Red blood cells have a life span of about 120 days. The process of erythropoiesis needs to replace this loss so the concentrate of red cells and hemoglobin in the body stays relatively constant. Erythrocyte production begins with the division of the common myeloid precursor under the influence of a polypeptide called erythropoietin. Erythropoietin is a growth factor that stimulates the erythroid precursors. The erythropoietin enters the process and causes the differentiation of the common myeloid precursor to the rubriblast, which is the first cell made in the erythrocyte series. The committed rubriblast can duplicate itself, or it can form rubricytes that are a little closer to the final product, the erythrocyte. During this period the nucleus shrinks and is then reabsorbed. The reticulocyte, the last cell type before the erythrocyte leaves the bone marrow and circulates in the blood for one to two days. The end result of the process is the formation of the erythrocyte. One rubriblast can form 14 to 16 erythrocytes, which is called **amplification.** Normally only about 1 percent of the erythrocytes mass in the body is formed in a day. The reticulocyte count is a useful clinical evaluation indicator of erythropoietic activity and indicates the formation of new red blood cells.

The erythrocyte is the final cell in the erythropoietic process. It does not reproduce itself, thus it does not have a nucleus. The earlier cells, however, do reproduce themselves and thus need to be able to make the chemicals necessary to make deoxyribonucleic acid (DNA), the genetic code, so that the daughter cells have the necessary information to reproduce themselves or make the next cells in the maturation process. All of the information necessary for the entire body is contained in this genetic DNA code, although only the information necessary for the formation of the erythrocyte is used. All the DNA in the nucleus must be replicated and a second copy made prior to cell division.

DNA consists of four bases. Two are called purines, adenine, and guanine, and two are called pyrimidine, cytosine, and thymine. These bases must be available when the DNA is replicating itself or the replication process stops. The production of the thymine is unique, because it requires a methyl transfer reaction. Methyl transfer reactions require vitamin B_{12} and folate. They hold and transfer the methyl group to be in adequate amounts for thymine synthesis to occur. While the molecular mechanism of this transfer is beyond the scope of this discussion, it is worth noting that a lack of adequate amounts of vitamin B_{12} or folic acid prevents the thymine from being produced. This inhibition will in turn block the process necessary to make the erythrocytes, and an anemia may result, called production failure.

The function of the erythrocyte is to transport oxygen from the lungs to the cells of the body. The erythrocyte has some basic requirements to meet to accomplish this function. First, the erythrocyte structure must be flexible to allow the bending and flexing necessary for the erythrocyte to survive the physical trauma of traversing the capillaries. Second, the erythrocyte has to maintain an internal environment that provides the energy necessary for the limited metabolic processes that occur, for example, keeping the iron in the hemoglobin in the ferrous form. Finally, the erythrocyte has to have some mechanism to move the necessary nutrients, for example glucose, from the plasma to the interior of the cell.

Between the outside of the erythrocyte and the inside of the erythrocyte is the cell membrane of the erythrocyte. While membranes are different between different organs or tissues, they have some similar characteristics (Berg, Tymoczko, & Stryer, 2002). Membranes are sheet-like structures, two molecules thick. Membranes are amphipathic, that is, they have a nonpolar side and a polar side. The polar side orients to the outside of the membrane in contact with the polar aqueous environment that is found on both sides of the membrane. A nonpolar water-avoiding (hydrophobic) side orients in the middle of the membrane. The hydrophobic core prevents polar molecules, like the ions sodium, potassium, calcium, chloride, or glucose, from passing randomly through the membrane. Noncovalent molecular forces hold the two layers of the membrane together.

Cholesterol is an important component of membranes. The cholesterol is distributed throughout the membrane and contributes to the flexibility of the membrane. Too much or too little cholesterol in the membrane will change the shape of the erythrocyte.

The erythrocyte membrane has a cytoskeleton. This is a series of proteins that interact with each other and with the membrane. This cytoskeleton creates the toughness the erythrocyte requires to squeeze through the small spaces in the capillaries. As it transfers through the capillaries it is bent and twisted into an elliptical shape. The cytoskeleton returns the erythrocyte to its original shape. The cytoskeleton also anchors various proteins that pass from the inside of the membrane to the outside of the membrane. One of these proteins makes up the ABO typing proteins. The proteins of the ABO blood types are a type of protein called glycoprotein. Glycoproteins are made up of amino acids and carbohydrates. In the case of the O blood type, the carbohydrates are the default type, that is, they are the same in all three blood types. In blood type A, a fifth carbohydrate called n-acetyl galactosamine is added. In the blood type B, a fifth carbohydrate named fructose is added.

Hemoglobin

Oxygen is picked up in the lungs and transported to the peripheral tissues. Hemoglobin is a complicated molecule that contains four protein chains, a porphyrin ring system, and iron. Hemoglobin is the molecule in the erythrocyte that binds the oxygen in the lungs and releases the oxygen in the tissues. The formation of the hemoglobin begins in the rubriblast stage and continues until the mature erythrocyte is formed. The concentration of the hemoglobin in the cell continues to increase through this process.

The protein chains of the hemoglobin are called globulins. Globulins are a particular type of protein. The body can make six different types of globulin chains that are found in hemoglobin at different stages of human development or in certain disease states. The chains are called alpha, beta, delta, epsilon, gamma, and zeta. The chains of the hemoglobin produced depend on the age of the person. The hemoglobin in a fetus has to pick up and deliver oxygen in a different setting than the hemoglobin of an adult. The hemoglobin structures are different to adapt to these different situations. In the adult, 95 percent of the hemoglobin contains two alpha protein chains and two beta protein chains (Hgb A). There is a smaller amount of Hgb A_2, which contains two alpha protein chains and two delta protein chains, and an even smaller amount of fetal hemoglobin, which contains two alpha protein chains and two gamma protein chains.

The second component of the hemoglobin molecule is a complicated ring system called a porphyrin. The ring system holds the iron in the middle of it, while the outer parts of the ring system, found around the edges, are anchored in the protein chains. There is one porphyrin ring in each of the protein chains, and four porphyrin rings per hemoglobin molecule. The body can produce the porphyrins and does so in the mitochondria. As noted earlier, the mitochondria disappear from the mature erythrocyte so all the production of the porphyrin occurs before the mature erythrocyte. The starting molecules for this complicated ring are simple enough, the amino acid glycine, and succinyl CoA (a molecule from the *Tri Carboxylic Acid* cycle).

The third component of the hemoglobin molecule is the iron. Iron exists as one of two ions, ferrous (Fe^{++}) and ferric (Fe^{+++}). The difference between these two ions is the number of electrons in the outer shell of the atom. Because the electron is negatively charged, the ferrous ion has one more electron, and hence a +2 charge instead of a +3 charge.

Iron is a fairly plentiful ion in the body. It is used in many different processes and is stored in many different types of cells for use. Too little iron causes many problems in the cells, but too much iron is also toxic to the cells **(hemosiderosis)**. Thus, the adsorption and transport of iron is a tightly controlled process. Iron is contained in the diet and is mostly in the ferric (+3) state. It is reduced to the ferrous state in the acidic environment of the stomach. The chemical reaction that occurs is called an oxidation-reduction reaction and involves the transfer of an electron to or from an ion. When an ion is reduced, it gains an electron (with a −1 charge). When an ion is oxidized it loses an electron, a positive ion will become more positive by one. Thus, when the iron ion goes from plus three to plus two, it is said to have been reduced. When the iron ion goes from +2 to +3 it has been oxidized. The ferrous ion is then absorbed in the small bowel. It moves into the cells, where it is oxidized to the ferric ion and is stored in association with a protein, apo-ferritin, to form ferritin. Ferritin is the common storage form of iron and can be found in many tissues. The iron can also bind to a transport protein called transferrin. In the formation of hemoglobin, iron is incorporated first into the porphyrin ring that is then the iron-porphyrin structure is incorporated into each of the protein chains. The iron ion is what actually holds the oxygen in the hemoglobin molecule. While there are four different binding sites for oxygen in the hemoglobin, they do not all bind the oxygen with the same strength.

Oxygen binds hemoglobin allosterically as opposed to linearly. When the first oxygen molecule binds to one of the hemoglobin chains, a shape change occurs in the corresponding protein. That shape change modifies the affinity, or the desire for oxygen. As each molecule of oxygen is added, the strength with which it is held decreases. This also affects the oxygen release. The linear model is straight-line relationship between the oxygen concentration and the percent of oxygen bound. The allosteric model is curved. You can see that the allosteric model binds more oxygen at a lower oxygen concentration. This curve is called the **oxyhemoglobin dissociation curve** (see chapter 30). When the oxygen concentration shifts to the right more oxygen is released. Some other factors that affect the dissociation curve are a rise in body temperature, an increase in hydrogen ions, that is a more acid environment, and a chemical called, 2,3 diphosphoglycerate (2,3 DPG). This allosteric binding works both ways for the hemoglobin. When the hemoglobin is binding oxygen, it does so more efficiently than expected. However, the opposite is also true. When the oxygen pressure drops as it does in the peripheral tissues, more oxygen is released by the hemoglobin for use by those tissues. Because the peripheral tissues have a lower oxygen concentration than the lung, this has some clear benefit by making the oxygen is made available to the tissues.

The peripheral tissues also have a lower pH, meaning they are more acidic, than the lungs. This is because of the acid production in the peripheral tissues and the ability of the lungs to blow off carbon dioxide that causes a rise in the pH. Not surprisingly, the pH also has an effect on the oxygen binding by the hemoglobin. As the pH goes up, the curve shifts to the left, and there is less oxygen released; as the pH goes down, the curve shifts to the right, more oxygen is released to the tissues. This results in significant changes in the release of oxygen, again consistent with the needs of the tissues.

Finally, 2,3 DPG can affect the binding of oxygen. This compound is derived from the metabolic pathways previously described. It normally binds to the hemoglobin molecule in low amounts. However, in hypoxemic, or low oxygen states, the cell will form more 2,3 DPG. This shifts the saturation curve to the right, and like the pH this action results in more oxygen being released for the same oxygen pressure, which is a good thing if the patient is having problems with hypoxemia.

The erythrocyte, even without the mitochondria, is metabolically active. It produces and uses adenosine triphosphate (ATP), which is the primary energy source for the whole body. It also produces a compound, called glutathione, which is important in protecting the cell from damage from oxygen. Oxygen can form hydrogen peroxide that damages the erythrocyte. The erythrocyte must also make the reduced form of nicotinamide adenine dinucleotide (NAD) represented as NADH, and nicotinamide adenine dinucleotide phosphate (NADP) represented as NADPH. These two compounds are required in many oxidation-reduction reactions in the erythrocyte. Glycolysis is instrumental to the physiological processes described in the activity of the use of erythrocytes. In glycolysis, glucose is catabolized, or broken down, into pyruvate. Because the erythrocyte does not have a mitochondria, the pyruvate is reduced to lactate, which is released into the blood. For the oxygen to be transported, the iron must stay in the ferrous state. The ferric state, oxidized or +3, cannot bind and transport oxygen. A disease state in which the iron of the hemoglobin is in the +3 is called methemoglobinemia. Thus, mechanisms must occur within the cell to keep the iron in the ferrous state, that is reduced or +2 form. There are two systems in the erythrocyte that do this. Both require a reduced form of a niacin derivative (NADH or NADPH) to work.

Aging of Erythrocytes

The red cells, like all other cells in the body, age. The life span of the red cells is about 120 days. Over time, for various reasons, the red cell loses it elasticity. At some point, it becomes so stiff that it is trapped by cells of the reticular endothelial system like the spleen and destroyed. The reticuloendothelial system (RES) removes about 1 percent of the red cells per day. New bone marrow cells replaced these old cells. The RES splits the hemoglobin molecule into its component parts, protein, porphyrin, and iron. The protein is broken down into the component amino acids. The iron is transferred back to the body stores using the protein transferrin. The porphyrin ring is broken down into bilirubin. Bilirubin is not a soluble molecule, so it is transferred back to the liver attached to albumin. This form of bilirubin is not measured directly in the lab and is called the indirect bilirubin. In the liver the bilirubin is conjugated, meaning joined, with another molecule that makes it more soluble and excreted into the bile. This form of bilirubin can be measured in the lab and is called the direct bilirubin. You measure the total bilirubin and the direct bilirubin, and then subtract the direct bilirubin from the total bilirubin to determine the indirect bilirubin.

White Blood Cells

In general, there are three types of cells in a human drop of blood. The most numerous have a red appearance and are the red blood cells, or erythrocytes. The largest cells, in terms of size, do not have this color, and are called the white blood cells. Finally, there are small cells that are the platelets. The white blood cells have specific patterns. These patterns, whether by staining techniques or more sophisticated methods, have led to the dividing of the white cells into the subgroups of granulocytes and lymphocytes.

The granulocytes include the neutrophils, eosinophils, and basophils. These cells, along with the lymphocytes, discussed below, interact to protect the body from infection and are involved in immunological and inflammatory responses in the body. The neutrophils come from the common stem cell. Recall that the common stem cell is the cell that produces the other components of the blood. The first cell produced from the common stem cell is called the common myeloid progenitor cell. This cell can then split into the precursor cells for neutrophils, eosinophils, or basophils. As the granulocytes are formed they respond to infections and inflammatory situations by going to the site of inflammation and releasing compounds that change the microenvironment and attract other cells to the site of the infections or inflammation.

The normal granulocyte concentration in the blood is 5,000 to 10,000 cell/mcg. Most of these cells, 55 to 65 percent, are neutrophils. However, the total number of granulocytes in the body is much higher because of the ability of the granulocytes to marginate, which is to move out of the circulation into the tissues. If one considers all granulocytes in all locations, the mass of these cells begins to equal that of the mass of the liver. The granulocytes can suddenly leave the peripheral tissues, which is a process called **demargination.** When this occurs, the concentration in the peripheral blood can double or even triple.

The granulocytes have a number of functions in the immune or inflammatory response. The first is sticking around or adherence. The neutrophils circulate and migrate in and around the tissues. When they come to an inflamed area, they stick to the vessel wall and begin to concentrate in the area. Then neutrophils will migrate into the tissues, a process called chemotaxis and begin to concentrate in the area of the inflammation or infection. Once involved, they can release a number of different chemicals, for example leukotrienes, prostaglandins, interleukins, and they can ingest, a process called phagocytosis, which will kill most bacteria.

Phagocytosis is the literal eating of a foreign substance. The energy for this process comes from glycolysis. The phagocytotic process is inhibited by malnutrition or high blood sugars. Basically, the granulocytes surround the foreign material, engulf it, surround it with a membrane, and then pinch off the membrane forming a small vesicle containing the foreign material. This complex is then moved inside the granulocyte. The granulocyte contains granules, hence the name. One group of these granules, the lysosome merges with the vesicle, and the lysosome releases its contents into the vesicle. The contents of the lysosome contain enzymes that will digest the material in the vesicle. The granulocytes also contain granules that are released into the inflamed or damaged area.

These granules contain a number of enzymes that will modify the site and ultimately allow the damaged or foreign material in the site to be removed.

The eosinophils are similar in function to the neutrophil but respond to a different set of stimuli. Whereas the neutrophil responds to the bacterial infections, eosinophils are more classically associated with infections from parasites. Eosinophils are also more involved in the reaction to allergies. The eosinophils release a number of enzymes into the tissue including various hydrolytic enzymes.

Basophils are the third cell in the granulocyte series. The basophils are produced in the bone marrow and in the peripheral blood and can migrate to the tissues. The basophils in the tissues are called mast cells. These cells are central in a number of inflammatory reactions. When the mast cells are activated, they release a number of substances into the area. The substances include cytokines that recruit other cells to the area, prostaglandins, leukotrienes, heparin, and histamine. The mast cells may contain immunoglobulin E (IgE) receptors and as such be involved in the allergy or asthma responses. The mast cells are mostly located near small blood vessels (Janeway, Travers, Walport, & Shlomchik, 2005).

There are two major types of lymphocytes, which are the cells that work in acquired immunity (see chapter 41). The lymphocytes are found in the lymphoid tissue, such as in the bone marrow, lymph nodes, gastrointestinal tract, and the spleen. There are two types of cells: the thymic derived cells, or T cells, that are responsible for cell-mediated immunity, and the bursa equivalent cells, or B cells, which are lymphocytes used for humoral, that is antibody mediated, immunity. The T lymphocytes comprise the majority of the circulating lymphocytes. The B cells are fewer in the plasma and are found mainly in the lymphoid tissues. The lymphocytes compromise 20 to 40 percent of the white cells found in the peripheral blood smears. A third type of lymphocyte, not shown in the graph, is called a natural killer (NK) cell. The NK cell is though to be important in recognizing and killing some types of tumor cells, and some of the cells that are infected with virus.

The Process of Hemostasis

Hemostasis is involved in stopping blood loss when the vessels are compromised (narrowing of the vessel and clot formation), and it arrests the clotting system when a clot has already formed. The components of hemostasis include the a part of the blood vessel wall, the endothelial lining, the platelets, fibrinogen (the protein precursor to fibrin), a complex cascade of enzymes, and enzymes that stop the continued formation of the clot. A cascade of enzymes is a series of proteins that circulate in an inactive or proenzyme state but are activated in the area of injury where clot formation is needed.

Platelets

Platelets are the cellular components of the hematopoietic system. They are derived (like all the other blood cells) from the bone marrow stem cell discussed earlier. The megakaryocyte is the largest cell in the hematopoietic system. The megakaryocyte fragments to form thousands of platelets, which do not have nuclei. The development of the megakaryocyte is unique in that it reproduces the nuclear material multiple times but does not divide. Consequently, a cell develops, which has multiple copies of the nuclear material, a state termed polyploidy.

Although small, the platelet has a active function. On the surface of the platelet are numerous receptors, places where things attach. Some of these receptors are responsible for making the platelet sticky, a process called activation. Other receptors are responsible for holding the platelets thus forming a platelet plug. The concentration of platelets in the blood runs between

150,000 to 350,000/mcg. The activated platelets are bound together through a fibrinogen bridge. The fibrinogen bridge binds to the Gp IIb-IIIa receptors between the platelets. This forms a platelet plug. Two important aspects of the platelet plug are the formation of a negatively charged surface and the activation of a receptor on the platelet that can bind products of the protein cascade, termed a procoagulant effect.

Another major component of the hemostasis system is the clotting cascade. The clotting cascade consists of a series of proteins that circulate in a pro-enzyme, or inactive state. The clotting cascade has two distinct sides: (a) the intrinsic side and b) the extrinsic side. The intrinsic side is activated by exposure to a negatively charged surface (for example, the membrane surface of the platelet plug). The extrinsic side is activated by the presence of a protein called thromboplastin that is released from injured tissue. The physical properties of each of the components, the clotting factors, and the coagulation cascade are shown in Table 23-1.

TABLE 23-1 Physical Properties of Coagulation Factors

FACTOR	CLOTTING PATHWAY	HALF-LIFE IN VIVO (HOURS)	PLASMA CONCENTRATION (MG/DL)	OTHER CHARACTERISTICS
I	Intrinsic, extrinsic, common pathway	90–150	200–400	Activity destroyed during coagulation process, present in absorbed plasma
II	Intrinsic, extrinsic, common pathway	50–100	10–15	Consumed during coagulation process
III	Extrinsic system only	n/a	0	Found in tissues
V	Intrinsic, extrinsic, common pathway	12–36	0.5–1.2	Activity destroyed during coagulation process, present in absorbed plasma
VII	Extrinsic system only	4–6	0.05–2.0	Present in serum
VIII/vWK	Intrinsic system only	8–12	0.001–0.1	Activity destroyed during coagulation process, present in absorbed plasma
IX	Intrinsic only	20–24	0.3–0.4	Present in serum
X	Intrinsic, extrinsic, common pathway	24–65	0.5–1	Present in serum
XI	Intrinsic only	40–80	0.5–12	Present in serum and absorbed plasma
XII	Intrinsic only	50–70	3–4	Present in serum and absorbed plasma
XIII	Intrinsic, extrinsic, common pathway	72–150	1–2.5	Activity destroyed during coagulation process, present in absorbed plasma
Prekallikrein (PK)	Intrinsic only	35	3–5	Present in serum and absorbed plasma
High molecular weight kininogen (HMWK)	Intrinsic only	150–160	6–9	Present in serum and absorbed plasma

Adapted from Hoffman, M., & Monroe, D. (2005). Rethinking the coagulation cascade. Current Hematology Reports, 4(5), 391–396; *Moran, T. A., & Viele, C. S. (2005). Normal clotting.* Seminars in Oncology Nursing, 21(4 Suppl 1), 1–11.

The three parts of hemostasis form a dynamic process that is best understood by going through the process as a whole. The endothelial wall of the blood vessel is structured to keep the platelets or other blood products from sticking. The endothelium is said to be thromboresistant and achieves this resistance through various mechanisms. One mechanism is to keep the blood flowing by releasing a vasodilator that is a substance that dilates blood vessels, called prostacyclin. The endothelium also secretes a substance that activates plasminogen that is a precursor to plasmin. Another clot preventing endothelial mechanism is the breakdown of the substances that would cause the platelets to activate.

However, when the endothelium is damaged, the clotting mechanisms activate to form a clot. The first thing that happens with an injury is the vasospasm of the blood vessels around the injury. This vasospasm accomplishes two things. First, it slows bleeding, and second, it creates a pooling or stasis of the blood in the immediate area that allows platelets to begin to accumulate and activate. The injury of the endothelium will expose collagen in the blood vessels walls to the platelets. Collagen is one of the molecules that can activate the platelets.

The platelet is the first step of clot formation. When a blood vessel is injured, the platelet adheres to the injured vessel wall. The activation of the platelets leads to the clumping of the platelets and an initial platelet plug. This process will start quickly after the injury. On exposure to the collagen, the platelet will degranulate activating other platelets. The platelet releases ADP, 5 hydroxytryptophan (5-HT), and other active compounds. The 5-HT will increase the vasoconstriction of the blood vessels. The ADP will activate other platelets. This degranulation will also activate the platelets. The activation of the platelet leads to a change in the shape of the platelet. This leads to the exposure of a receptor Gp IIb/IIIb that binds fibrinogen/fibrin forming the platelet plug. The cross bridging of the fibrinogen between the platelets forms a three-dimensional platelet clump that initially stops the bleeding.

The second part of hemostasis is the formation of the fibrin clot. This occurs by the activation of a protein cascade. The intrinsic pathway can be activated by the negative charges on the surface of platelet plug. The extrinsic pathway can be activated by the exposure to tissue thromboplastin. Both pathways, however, lead to the same endpoint, the conversion of fibrinogen to fibrin monomers. The fibrin monomers line up side-by-side and end-to-end. However, for the clot to remain, the fibrin needs to be cross-linked. This cross-linking is catalyzed by activated factor XIII that is XIIIa. It forms a covalent bond between fibrin monomers (an amide bond between glutamic acid on one chain and lysine on another) resulting in a stable clot.

It is clearly important to be able to stop bleeding by the formation of a clot as soon as possible. Less clear, but equally important is the ability to turn off the clotting mechanism. If this cessation were not to occur, after the first injury, probably being born, the entire vascular system would clot. The halting of the clotting process occurs via a system call fibrinolysis. Plasmin serves in this function. The plasmin destroys fibrin, fibrinogen, and some of the clotting factors. Plasmin will circulate and stay active until the liver destroys it. The products of plasmin action are called fibrin degradation products, or FDP, that can be measured in the blood. Some of the conditions that can cause an elevation of the FDP are extensive tissue damage, sepsis, shock, disseminated intravascular coagulation, blood transfusion reactions, thromboembolic states, cancer, and deep vein thrombosis (DVT) (Daniels, 2003).

A second system that inhibits clotting involves two commonly measured proteins, protein C and protein S. Protein C circulates in an inactive form. Thrombin, discussed previously, will activate protein C. The activated protein C then binds with protein S and this complex inactivates factors Va and factor VIIIa. Deficiencies of either of these proteins can lead to problems with excessive clotting, because they inhibit the clotting process.

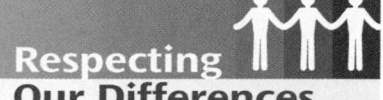

Respecting Our Differences

Age-Related Changes in the Hematological System

The age-related changes seen occur mostly from the percentage of the bone marrow that changes. This is usually not clinically significant, however, in illness the loss of hematopoietic tissue reduces the ability to replace red blood cells lost. The replacement of red blood cells may be inhibited because of iron deficiency. In an elderly patient, intestinal iron absorption may not be changed, but there is slower erythropoiesis that reduces the ability to get the iron into the red blood cells. Platelet counts are generally unchanged with aging; however there may be an increased platelet adhesion. There are also increased levels of factors V, VII, and IX, as well as fibrinogen, which increase the risk for the development of blood clots. Lymphocyte function decreases as well; there is decreased T cell function. These changes may contribute to the increase incidence of infections and malignancy in the elderly.

ASSESSMENT

Assessment of the hematological system begins with a personal and family history. The history may be significant for detecting hematological dysfunction. The patient's gender, age, family history, and personal history of blood problems are included. Women, in general, have a lower hemoglobin and hematocrit, especially during the reproductive years. Dysfunction of the hematological system may result in decreased energy and ability to complete activities of daily living. Fatigue may result from the decreased ability of the blood to carry oxygen from a decreased hemoglobin and hematocrit. Socioeconomic assessment assesses the availability of money for food, medication, and support services. A history of bleeding or coagulation disorders in a family member may point to a hereditary predisposition to the disorder. The nurse should ask the patient if there is a history of excessive bleeding after a dental or medical procedure, a cut, surgery, or childbirth. Abnormal bleeding from a platelet disorder may be localized to sites in the skin and mucous membranes. It occurs immediately after an

TABLE 23-2 Medications that Alter Coagulation		
	GENERIC NAME	**BRAND NAME**
Antiplatelets	Acetylsalicylic acid	Aspirin
	Dipyridamole	Persantine
	Clopidogrel	Plavix
	Aspirin/dipyridamole	Aggrenox
	Anagrelide	Agrylin
	Cilostazol	Pletal
	Tirofiban	Ticlid
	Eptifibatide	Integrilin
	Abciximab	ReoPro
Anticoagulants	Heparin	
	Warfarin	Coumadin
	Bivalirudin	Angiomax
	Fondaparinux	Arixtra
	Antithrombin III	ATnativ
	Dalteparin	Fragmin
	Tinzaparin	Innohep
	Enoxaparin	Lovenox
Thrombolytic	Urokinase	Abbokinase
	Alteplase	Activase
	Anistreplase	Eminase
	Streptokinase	Kabikinase
		Streptase
	Reteplase	Retavase
	Tenecteplase	TNKase

Adapted from Broyles, B. E., Reiss, B. S., & Evans, M. E. (2007). Pharmacological aspects of nursing care (7th ed.). New York: Thomson Delmar Learning.

injury and is treated with pressure. Bleeding from defects in the coagulation factors may be in deep tissues and is not stopped with pressure (Kasper, et al., 2005). A personal or family history of excessive formation of blood clots is also significant. This could be in the form of DVT, pulmonary infarction, myocardial infarction, and cerebral vascular accident just to name a few. The history also includes a medication history. Many medications and herbal compounds can have anticoagulant effects (Table 23-2).

Dietary history is significant in assessing for amount of iron, folic acid, and vitamin B_{12} in the diet. Consumption of too much alcohol can interfere with nutritional intake and can result in liver damage that can cause a decrease in the production of clotting factors. Table 23-3 summarizes possible objective assessment findings associated with abnormal hematological functioning.

DIAGNOSTIC TESTS

There are two primary methods by which blood is analyzed. Various anticoagulants, such as heparin, can be added to the collection tube so that the blood does not clot, and the plasma, which is the liquid part of blood, can be

---

TABLE 23-3 Physical Assessment for Hematological Problems

ASSESSMENT OF SYSTEM	FINDINGS	POSSIBLE CAUSES
Skin	Pallor	Decreased hemoglobin, hematocrit and red blood cells
	Purpura—Abnormal bleeding under the skin may be seen in elderly from blood leaking from capillaries from minor trauma	Trauma Steroid purpura Clotting disturbances; thrombocytopenia Abnormal platelet function Clotting factor defects Disseminated intravascular coagulation
	Petechiae—pinpoint hemorrhages under the skin, round, dark red or purple in color. The diameter is less than 2 mm	Thrombocytopenia, platelet disfunction, viruses, abnormal bleeding times from anticoagulants or trauma
	Ecchymosis—superficial bleeding under the mucous membrane or skin	Abnormal bleeding times from anticoagulants.
	Hematomas—deeper palpable bleeds under the skin	Trauma Abnormal bleeding times from anticoagulants
Head and neck	Assessment bleeding can cause compression of the airway Intracerebral hemorrhage is a possible cause of death from severe coagulation disorders	Abnormal coagulation may cause excessive bleeding especially after surgery to the neck, such as a thyroidectomy
Joints	Assessment of pain and discoloration of joints or joint deformities	Common in deficiencies of factors VIII and IX (hemophilias)
Abdomen	Assessment of pain retroperitoneal hematomas can cause femoral nerve compression	Subcutaneous administration of anticoagulants may be injected into an abdominal muscle that may cause hemorrhage
Renal—urinary tract	Blood may in urine	Abnormal bleeding from anticoagulants
Respiratory system	Difficulty breathing	Low hemoglobin

Adapted from Estes, M. (2006). Health assessment and physical examination (3rd ed.). New York: Thomson Delmar Learning.

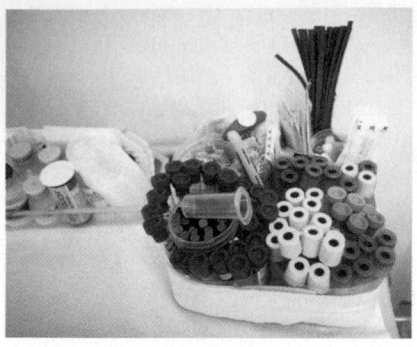

Figure 23-2 Vacutainer tubes used for collection of blood specimens.

analyzed (Figure 23-2). This method is necessary, for example, when analyzing the proteins in the clotting cascade. The other method is to draw the blood into a tube that does not have any anticoagulants in it. The blood will clot and the cellular material and clot will separate from the **serum,** which is the liquid part of blood after coagulation. This can be analyzed for various components.

When a tube of blood with an anticoagulant in it is drawn, the blood will separate into different layers. The top layer is the plasma; if the blood clots, this will be the serum. On the bottom is the erythrocyte layer, and in between is the **buffy coat,** an area that is lightly colored and contains mostly white blood cells. One of the early tests done on blood consisted of allowing this separation to occur and measuring the percentage of volume occupied by the red blood cells. This percentage is called the hematocrit (Daniels, 2003).

The process of drawing blood is determined by the protocol of the institution. Hematological studies can be performed on blood collected by venipuncture, which is blood collected from a vein. The blood is collected in tubes that are labeled by color for identification (Table 23-4).

The body reaches a steady state and thus can generate some normal levels. A normal level is defined as that found in 95 percent of an asymptomatic population. Thus, while there is no absolute normal level, there are absolute abnormal levels but rather a range within which the patient is considered normal. Remember however that these are relative. A patient's hemoglobin may have dropped by 2 grams and still be in the normal range, but the drop is abnormal for the patient.

The laboratory values associated with the erythrocyte will include the number, and size of the cell, the concentration of the cells in a column of blood, and hematocrit (Table 23-5). The hemoglobin concentration will also be reported. The iron metabolism can be measured with the iron concentration, ferritin, an iron storage protein, and the total iron binding capacity. The production of the erythrocytes will be reflected in the reticulocyte count. Finally, the breakdown of the erythrocyte will be reflected in the bilirubin level specifically the indirect.

The normal lab values for the granulocytic series include count of the leukocytes and the percentages of neutrophilic bands, neutrophils, basophils, and eosinophils seen in a peripheral smear. Classically, the technologist will count one hundred cells and count the number of each type, that number then being expressed as a percentage. In addition, there are a number of laboratory tests

TABLE 23-4	**Commonly Used Specimen Collection Tubes**	
TUBE COLOR	**TUBE CONTENTS**	**TYPICAL USE**
Lavender	EDTA	Complete blood count
Gold or marbled	Serum separator	Blood banking (serum); therapeutic drug monitoring
Red	None	Blood banking (serum); therapeutic drug monitoring
Blue	Citrate	Coagulation studies
Green	Heparin	Coagulation studies
Yellow	Acid citrate	HLA typing
Navy	Trace metal free	Trace metals (example, lead)

Adapted from Daniels, R. (2003). Delmar's manual of laboratory and diagnostic tests. *New York: Thomson Delmar Learning.*

TABLE 23-5 Common Laboratory Tests of the Red Cell System

LAB TEST	NORMAL RANGE
Erythrocyte count	Adult male: 3.8 to 6.1 million cells/mcg. Adult female slightly lower
Hemoglobin	Male: 14–17 g/dL
	Female: 12–16 g/dL
Hematocrit	Male 41–51 percent
	Female 36–47 percent
Mean corpuscular volume	80–100 fl
Mean corpuscular hemoglobin	28–32 pg
Iron	60–160 mcg/dL
Total iron binding capacity	250–460 mcg/dL
Ferritin	15–200 ng/mL
Reticulocyte count	0.5–1.5 percent
Absolute reticulocyte count	23,000–90,000/mcg
Bilirubin	Total 0.3–1.2 mg/dL
	Direct 0–0.3 mg/dL
	Indirect bilirubin 0.2–0.8 mg/dL

Adapted from Daniels, R. (2003). Delmar's manual of laboratory and diagnostic tests. New York: Thomson Delmar Learning.

TABLE 23-6 Laboratory Tests for Hemostasis

TEST	NORMAL RANGE	TEST FUNCTION
Thrombin time	15–22 sec	Measures the ability of thrombin to convert fibrinogen to fibrin
Prothrombin time	11–13 sec	Tests the extrinsic system generally expressed as international normalized ratio (INR)
Partial thromboplastin time	28–30 sec	Tests the intrinsic system
Fibrinogen level	150–350 mg/dL	Measures the level of fibrinogen
Bleeding time	Less than 10 minutes	Measures the time it takes for a standard skin incision to stop bleeding

Adapted from Daniels, R. (2003). Delmar's manual of laboratory and diagnostic tests. New York: Thomson Delmar Learning.

to evaluate the various parts of the hemostasis system (Table 23-6). And there is an expense associated with the procurement of these laboratory tests.

ANATOMY AND PHYSIOLOGY (CARDIOVASCULAR SYSTEM)

The circulatory system provides a means to pump blood throughout the body. The heart functions as two separate pumps. It has four chambers: the right and left atrium and the right and left ventricles (Figure 23-3). The right side of the heart pumps blood to the lungs, and the left side of the heart pumps blood out through the systemic circulation. The heart sits in the mediastinum, the space in the chest between the lungs. The rib cage provides anatomical landmarks

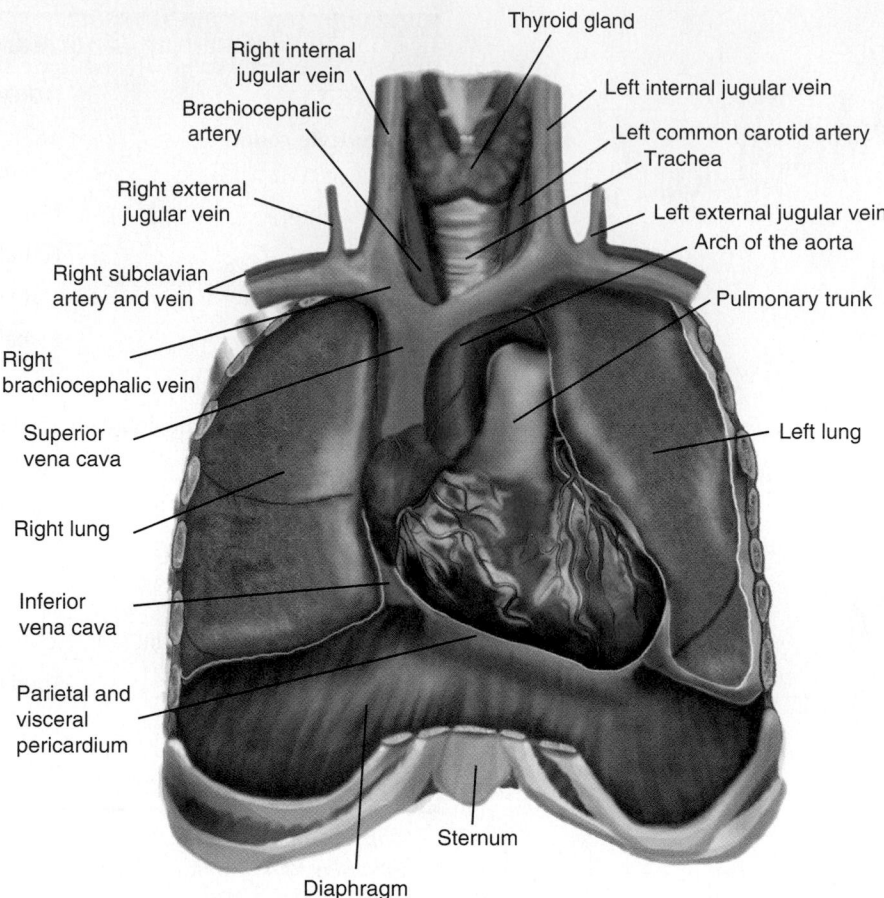

Right internal jugular vein
Brachiocephalic artery
Right external jugular vein
Right subclavian artery and vein
Right brachiocephalic vein
Superior vena cava
Right lung
Inferior vena cava
Parietal and visceral pericardium
Diaphragm
Sternum
Thyroid gland
Left internal jugular vein
Left common carotid artery
Trachea
Left external jugular vein
Arch of the aorta
Pulmonary trunk
Left lung

Figure 23-3 Position of the heart in the thoracic cavity.

that can be used to assess the cardiac function. The heart is generally positioned behind the sternum with the apex going toward the left at the fifth intercostal space (ICS) in the midclavicular line. The placement of the heart varies with body types. In the tall, slender person the heart may be positioned more vertically, whereas the heart of a short person may be more horizontally positioned. The heart is described as right- and left-sided. This description is helpful when considering the sides as separate pumps. The right side of the heart pumps the blood to the lungs, and the left side pumps the blood to the systemic circulation.

Pericardial Layers

The heart has three layers: the inner-most layer called the endocardium; the middle layer called the myocardium; and the outer-layer called the pericardial surface. The endocardial layer is continuous with the endothelial layer of the arteries, veins, and capillaries to form a continuous closed cardiovascular system. The myocardium, the center portion of the heart muscle, varies in thickness depending on the chamber. The heart is surrounded by the fibrous pericardium, also called the parietal layer, which surrounds the heart and attaches to the great vessels, which are several large blood vessels that return the blood to the heart. The parietal pericardium surrounds almost the entire ascending aorta and main pulmonary artery as well as portions of the inferior and superior venae cavae and the pulmonary veins (Fuster, Alexander, & O'Rourke, 2004). The inner lining of the pericardium is the visceral pericardium. It is the delicate inner lining of the parietal pericardium and is the outer lining of the great vessels. When this layer is over the heart, it is called the epicardium. The epicardium contains the epicardial coronary arteries and veins. There are also autonomic nerves, which function to change blood pressure and heart rate when stimulated. Lymphatics are also present to help prevent an abnormal accumulation of fluid, known as a pericardial effusion, in the pericardial space. There is also adipose tissue that may accumulate with age and obesity. The space between the layers of the pericardium contains approximately 10 to 30 mL of fluid and is called the pericardial cavity. The pericardial fluid provides lubrication for the surrounding membranes to provide smooth movement when the heart beats.

Fibrous Skeleton of the Heart

The four valves in the heart are anchored to their valve rings known as annuli. These rings are at the base of the heart and join to form the fibrous skeleton of the heart. The atrioventricular (AV) node passes through this fibrous skeleton. The tissue composition of the fibrous skeleton does not conduct the electrical impulse, so it works to isolate the electrical activity of the atria from the ventricles. So under normal circumstances for the impulse to travel from the atria to the ventricles is through the AV node (Fuster, et al., 2004). If there is a block in the AV node, electrical impulses cannot be conducted from the atrium to the ventricles, and the result is complete AV block.

Chambers of the Heart

The four chambers of the heart consist of the right and left atrium and the right and left ventricles. The atrium has a smaller muscle mass and has lower pressures than the ventricles. The blood flows into the heart from the venous system by way of the superior and inferior vena cava. Because there is not a valve between the vena cava and right atrium, there is a continuous flow of blood into the right atrium. The blood from the venous system is low in oxygen and high in carbon dioxide (Rizzo, 2006). The right and left atria have small appendages that are referred to as auricle appendages, which have the appearance of small flaps. When the atria are fibrillating, or a quivering type motion, blood clots may form in the right and left auricles. The blood normally remains in the atrium until the pressure in the atrium exceeds the right or left ventricular pressure. Under normal circumstances, the cardiac valves are competent, which means that blood does not pass through the valve until the pressure gradient is changed and the valve opens. When the valve opens, the blood enters into the right or left ventricle. The period of time in which blood enters the ventricles is referred to as diastole. During this time, blood goes into the ventricles by flowing from an area of higher pressure to an area of lower pressure. Near the end of diastole, the atrium contracts to increase the amount of blood that enters into the ventricle. When the pressure in the ventricle exceeds the atrial pressure the tricuspid valve closes.

Heart Valves

The tricuspid valve separates the right atrium from the right ventricle and allows blood to flow in one direction. The valve has three leaflets that are supported by the chordae tendineae. These structures hold the valve leaflets in place like the cords on a parachute. These are attached to the wall of the ventricle by the papillary muscle. When the ventricle contracts the valve leaflets are pulled into place to prevent a backflow of blood from the right ventricle into the right atrium. When the blood leaves the right ventricle, it enters the lungs via the pulmonary arteries through the pulmonic valve. When approximately 60 percent of the blood, ejection fraction, is emptied from the right ventricle, the pulmonic valve closes, which prevents the blood from regurgitating back into the right ventricle.

The pulmonic valve has two leaflets and separates the right ventricle from the pulmonary artery. In the lungs the blood goes through the pulmonary vasculature where it exchanges oxygen and carbon dioxide. It then returns to the left atrium of the heart through the pulmonary veins. These vessels return to the posterior surface of the heart. The blood is transported from the left atrium through the mitral valve. The time that the blood is entering into the left ventricle is the diastolic filling time. The mitral valve has two cusps. The valve functions as a one-way valve to prevent blood from flowing back into the atrium during left ventricular contraction. As with the tricuspid valve, the mitral valve is held in place by the chordae tendineae and papillary muscles. When the left ventricle contracts, the blood flows into the aorta over the aortic valve. The period when the blood is ejected from the ventricle is the systole. The aortic valve has three cusps and closes at the end of contraction to prevent blood from going back into the ventricle.

Systemic Circulation

When the blood is transported through the aorta, it goes to the systemic circulation. This system supplies blood to all organs except the lungs. The blood vessels branch into smaller and smaller arteries. The arteries have an elastic nature that allows them to stretch and relax to maintain blood pressure in the vessels. When the arteries are narrowed the action is called vasoconstriction, and when they dilate, it is referred to as vasodilation. As the arteries become smaller, they are termed arteriole when the diameter is less than 0.5 mm. The vessels then spread into a network of capillaries. The precapillary sphincters contract and relax to regulate blood flow into the capillaries. The capillary walls are thin enough to allow the transport of metabolites, oxygen, carbon dioxide, and other substances, such as hormones, to move between the vessels and tissue.

The blood travels from the capillary network into the venules and as the circulatory conduit becomes larger, venules are referred to as veins. Veins are more numerous than arteries and have thinner walls. Some of the veins, such as those in the lower extremities, have valves to keep the blood propelled toward the heart. When a person is upright, the muscles of the legs compress the veins to further assist the blood flow to the heart.

Coronary Artery Circulation

The heart is supplied with blood from blood vessels that originate at the base of the aorta. The vessels are termed right and left coronary arteries (Figure 23-4). There may be some variation of the placement of coronary arteries from person

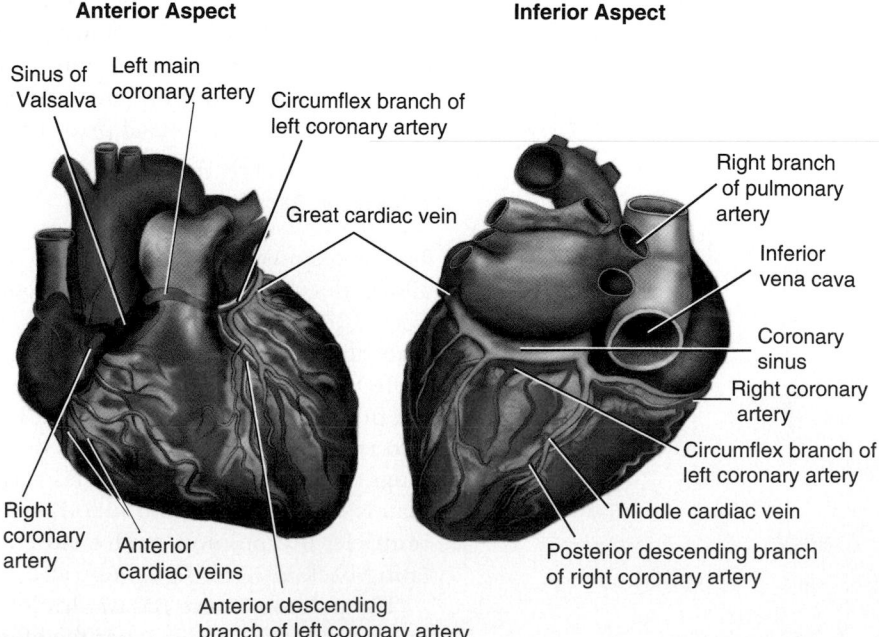

Anterior Aspect   **Inferior Aspect**

Sinus of Valsalva
Left main coronary artery
Circumflex branch of left coronary artery
Great cardiac vein
Right coronary artery
Anterior cardiac veins
Anterior descending branch of left coronary artery
Right branch of pulmonary artery
Inferior vena cava
Coronary sinus
Right coronary artery
Circumflex branch of left coronary artery
Middle cardiac vein
Posterior descending branch of right coronary artery

Figure 23-4 The coronary arteries and major veins of the heart (anterior and inferior view).

to person. The right coronary artery (RCA) arises from the right aorta at the aortic sinus. It then runs diagonally to the right side of the heart in the in the groove between the right atrium and the right ventricle. The RCA curves around the right side of the heart and runs along its posterior surface. The artery continues to supply the left atrium and inferior (lower) surface of the left ventricle. The marginal branch arises from the right coronary artery and supplies the right ventricle and the lateral walls of the right atrium and right ventricle. The left main coronary artery is larger in diameter than the right coronary artery. It arises from the left aortic sinus. It passes in front of the pulmonary artery and the left atrium and divides into two branches, the left anterior descending (LAD) artery and the circumflex branch. The LAD artery wraps around the cardiac apex and goes a variable distance toward the base of the heart. It has branches that supply the anterior septum. This artery supplies AV junction and part of the left bundle branch in the conduction system. The LAD also supplies the anterior wall of both ventricles. The circumflex artery runs posteriorly and supplies the lateral wall of the left ventricle and part of the mitral papillary muscle (Fuster, et al., 2004).

Factors Affecting Blood Flow

Blood flow is regulated by factors that affect flow of fluid through a closed system. The property of pressure can be measured in millimeters of mercury (mm Hg). Fluid moves from higher pressure to lower pressure. In the vascular system the fluid moves from the higher pressure arterial system to the lower pressure venous system. Resistance also contributes to the blood flow. The length and diameter of the blood vessels contributes to resistance. The diameter of blood vessels can greatly affect the total peripheral resistance. The autonomic nervous system contributes to reflex control of total cardiac output (CO) and vascular resistance. The sympathetic stimulation of the arterioles and venules contributes to constriction and relaxation of the vessels. Sympathetic stimulation of the heart results in increased strength of contraction and faster heart rate. Parasympathetic stimulation of the heart results in a lower heart rate.

Baroreceptors are specialized stretch receptors that are located in the walls of the aorta and carotid arteries. In the carotid arteries the baroreceptors are in the carotid sinuses that are in the upper part of the neck. The thin walls of the carotid sinuses contain a large number of nerve endings that are sensitive to distortion or stretch. The baroreceptors in the aorta are located in the aortic arch. Stimulation of the baroreceptors from an increase in blood pressure results in an impulse traveling on the vagus nerve. This action causes a decrease in blood pressure by diminishing heart rate and peripheral resistance. When the blood pressure decreases, the impulses are transmitted to the vasoactive centers in the medulla to increase sympathetic activity resulting in an increased heart rate, cardiac force of contraction, and arterial and venous constriction. Consequently, blood pressure rises.

Cardiac Cycle

The cardiac cycle is representative of the contraction and relaxation of the ventricles and corresponds to the systolic and diastolic phases of the blood pressure. The maximum pressure in the arteries occurs during ventricular contraction. During this time blood is forced into the pulmonary arteries and aorta and is the systolic pressure. It corresponds to the closing of the tricuspid and mitral valves and opening of the pulmonic and aortic valves. When the ventricles have ejected their contents, the pressure in the pulmonic and aorta exceeds the ventricular pressures, and the pulmonic and aortic valves close. The tricuspid and mitral valves open to allow blood to enter the ventricles from the atria. This is the diastolic phase, also known as ventricular relaxation. During this time the pressure in the arterial system is the lowest. In the pulmonary system systolic pressure is about 25 mm Hg, and the normal diastolic pressure is about 8 mm Hg. In the systemic system the systolic pressure is about 120 mm Hg, and the diastolic pressure is about 80 mm Hg (Estes, 2006).

The pulmonary vascular system is a low-pressure system. The mean arterial pressure, which is calculated by taking the sum of twice the diastolic blood pressure plus the systolic blood pressure and dividing it by 3, is less than 15. The mean arterial pressure in the systemic vascular system is normally less than 100. A surge of blood entering the systemic vasculature causes the elastic arteries to increase in diameter rapidly resulting in expansion of an artery as the wave of blood goes through the vessel during systole. During diastole the pressure drops and the arterial walls relax. This rhythmic throbbing is palpated as a pulse over arteries that are close to the surface of the body. When the heart is electrically stimulated, it then responds by physically contracting to propel the blood into the blood vessels.

The contractile properties of the heart are dependent on the tension on the muscle at the beginning of the contraction. In the heart this is **preload,** which is the amount myocardial fibers are stretched immediately before contraction. This is the end-diastolic portion of the cardiac cycle. The amount of volume at the end of diastole determines preload. The more blood that returns from the venous system the higher the preload; this is known as the Frank Starling curve. To a degree, the higher the preload, the stronger the contractile force within the limits of the Frank Starling curve. There is a point when increased preload does not result in an increased CO. The degree of the fibers being stretched in the heart is a function of pressure that is generated by the amount of blood volume returning to the ventricle, and it is referred to as ventricular end-diastolic pressure (VEDP). Therefore, it reflects ventricular end-diastolic volume. There is a relationship between ventricular end-diastolic volume and pressure, if the ventricular end-diastolic volume increases or decreases, it would be expected that the pressure would change as well.

Ventricular **afterload** is reflected as the amount of pressure that the ventricle must generate to push its contents out into circulation. This is the amount of pressure in the vessel that is leading from the ventricle, so in the left ventricle it is the systolic pressure in the aorta. The higher the pressure, the more the workload is on the ventricle. Factors that increase afterload are the volume and viscosity of the blood that is being pumped out and the resistance in the peripheral vascular system.

Arterial **blood pressure** (a measurement of the pulsations on the arterial walls during systole and diastole) is regulated hemodynamically to maintain adequate tissue perfusion. Blood pressures changes continuously because of changes in positioning, muscular activity, and circulating blood volume. Antidiuretic hormone and the renin-angiotensin system also have major effects on blood pressure. Blood volume that is pumped out of the ventricle during each contraction is call stroke volume. Under normal circumstances, stroke volume ranges from 40 to 80 mL per contraction. In the clinical setting the ejection fraction is the most commonly used index of contractile function (Fuster, et al., 2004). **Ejection fraction (EF)** is the percentage of blood that is emptied from the ventricle during systole. An EF of 60 to 70 percent is the expected normal finding. Any condition that damages the contractile force of the heart, such as a myocardial infarction, may reduce the EF. The total amount of blood that is pumped from the heart in a minute is the CO. CO is figured by multiplying stroke volume (SV) by the one minute heart rate (HR). The formula is: $SV \times HR = CO$. In the normal physiological state, if CO increases, blood pressure will increase, and inversely, if CO decreases, blood pressure will also decrease. Total blood volume in the human body is approximately 5 liters. There are variations due to age, gender, and body size. Approximately 75 percent of the volume is in the systemic circulation (60 percent in the veins and 10 percent in the arteries), the heart accounts for 15 percent, and 10 percent is in the pulmonary vasculature.

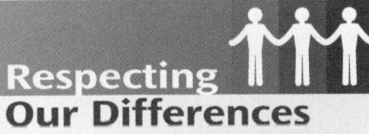

Respecting Our Differences

Age-Related Changes to the Cardiovascular System

The age-related changes in the cardiovascular system include decrease in the maximum heart rate in response to exercise. However the maximum stroke volume does not go down just as a consequence of aging. Heart disease can also have a profound effect on the stroke volume. The decreased ability for physical work with aging is probably a combination of decreased heart rate, deconditioning, and cardiovascular disease. The blood vessels in the arterial system may become more rigid. The loss of elasticity could increase afterload and increase the workload on the heart. When these conditions are combined with disease, the manifestations of symptoms are worsened. The nurse must carefully assess the elderly with the age-related changes in mind. In addition, the nurse must look for clinical manifestations of such pathologies as heart failure and cardiac output deficiencies when assessing the elderly.

Blood pressure can be measured invasively by placing a small tube called a catheter in an artery and connecting it to a recording device. This is a direct measure of the systemic blood pressure. The unit of measure used for blood pressure is millimeters of mercury (mm Hg). The expected blood pressure is 120/80. The higher number represents the systolic pressure, which is the pressure while the heart is beating, and the lower number represents the diastolic pressure, which is the pressure when the left ventricle is resting between beats.

ASSESSMENT

The landmarks for conducting a cardiovascular assessment are based on the bony structures of the chest: (a) the sternum, (b) the ribs, and (c) the clavicles. The underlying organs are visualized using these landmarks and are used to describe and document associated assessment findings. For cardiac assessment the anterior chest is visualized. There is a line that runs vertically down the middle of the sternum and is known as the midsternal line. To the left, half way across the clavicle is the left midclavicular line. The line that is at the distal end of the clavicle and in the fold of the axilla is the described as the anterior axillary line. The line that travels down the middle of the axilla is the midaxillary line, and the back of the axillary area is the posterior axillary line. The bony area where the manubrium and sternum come together can be palpated as a groove and is the angle of Louis. This area is used to identify the ICSs. Across from the angle of Louis is the second rib and directly below that is the second ICS (Daniels, 2004).

Subjective data is information that patients tell the examiner about their health status. This information can be obtained in an organized manner through a health history. The date and time of the health history is included, because the status of the patient may change over time. The nurse needs to be attentive to information that the patient may add in informal communications, such as conversations during a procedure. The health history for the cardiovascular system is focused to identify information relating to the heart and blood vessels. The history begins with biographical data. This includes gender, age, occupation, support system, and source of the information, such as patient or other reliable person. This information is used to begin assessing the patient's risk factors for heart disease. The risk factors that cannot be altered are age, gender, ethnicity, and family history. As a person ages the risk of atherosclerotic heart disease is increased. In general men have an increased risk for atherosclerotic heart disease at a younger age, however, after menopause heart disease is the leading cause of death in women. The reason for seeking care in the focused assessment of the cardiovascular system focuses on chest discomfort, awareness of the heart beating, such as racing or skipped beats, and shortness of air. The completeness of the health history depends on the acuity of the situation. If immediate interventions are required, the complete health history will be delayed. The history of symptoms includes chest discomfort. This may be manifested as pain, pressure, burning, fullness, or squeezing sensation. The discomfort or pain from myocardial ischemia most often is substernal and spreads to the neck, jaw, shoulder, or arms (Box 23-1). Women may not experience any chest discomfort or pain but may present with fatigue and shortness of breath.

Dyspnea is a sensation of difficulty breathing that is not appropriate for the level of exertion (Estes, 2006). Dyspnea may or may not be associated with a cough. This subjective finding may occur with decreased blood supply to the heart or left-sided heart failure. Other manifestations of difficulty breathing include orthopnea, or labored breathing, when lying flat. This is a classic symptom of left-sided heart failure but may be associated with pulmonary conditions as well. Palpitations are described as sensations of fast or irregular beating of the heart. These may be described as fluttering or throbbing sensations below

---

BOX 23-1

PAIN EVALUATION

- Evaluate pain on a scale of 1 to 10.
- Evaluate how long the pain has been present.
- Determine if the pain is located in one spot or if it radiates to any other areas.
- Ask whether there is any numbness, tingling, or weakness associated with the pain.
- Determine if the pain is recurrent determine the time of day when the pain is the worst.
- Determine if the pain or discomfort is related to activity, if so what activities influence it.
- Evaluate what the patient has used to treat the pain or discomfort.
- Evaluate if there are any other symptoms or signs associated with the pain, such as shortness of air or sweating.
- Note if the pain or discomfort is related to an injury or surgery to the affected area.

Adapted from Brill, J. (2004). Trends in pain syndrome diagostic technology. Practical Pain Management, 4(4), 12–19.

Skills 360°

Cardiovascular Assessment

The information that the nurse obtains during the evaluation of the signs and symptoms related to the cardiovascular system are communicated through written documentation and verbally. The documentation may be written in a narrative form or through a computerized documentation system. Health care systems may be using a standardized computer program to facilitate consistent and complete documentation throughout its system. It is imperative that the nurse be proficient in the skills of assessment of the patient and accurate in the documentation of the findings.

the sternum or in the neck. The palpitations may occur from premature beats, or a sustained tachycardia. These need to be evaluated by a heath care provider to determine the severity of the condition. Episodes of syncope are manifested as transient and may include sudden loss of consciousness. A slowing of the heart rate or neurological conditions may cause theses episodes. Edema is the accumulation of excess amounts fluid in the body tissues. If the excessive fluid is in the lungs, it can lead to difficulty breathing. Edema in the extremities leads to swelling in the most dependent areas. Fatigue is the sense of overwhelming tiredness. It can lead to the inability to complete activities of daily living and a decline in mental ability.

Chest pain can have many different causes (Table 23-7). The cause of the pain may result in different characteristics of pain and associated findings may be helpful in determining if the pain is from the heart or other causes.

Changes in the extremities that include paresthesia, numbness and tingling, color changes with position, or temperature changes are documented. Pain that occurs in the lower extremities with exercise is termed intermittent claudication and is indicative of decreased blood supply to the legs.

The past medical history is assessed to determine possible contributing factors for heart disease that may be present. Childhood diseases that may contribute to heart disease are rheumatic fever and congenital heart disease. Previous surgeries are assessed to determine if there were any related heart problems. Previous electrocardiograms (ECGs) need to be assessed to use as baselines for current recordings. The nurse should ask the patient if there is a history of chronic diseases, because these may increase the risk of heart disease. These include diabetes, hyperlipidemia, and hypertension. Other disorders that may contribute to a patient's health status are pulmonary and renal diseases. Family history is ascertained to see if there are familial conditions that may contribute to heart disease. A family history of this illness in close family members, such as parents, siblings, or children is a major risk factor. African Americans may have an increased risk of hypertension that could contribute to an increased risk of coronary artery disease. See Box 23-2 for questions that can be asked as part of the history taking process.

TABLE 23-7 **Differentiating Chest Pain**		
ETIOLOGY OF PAIN	**CHARACTERISTIC OF PAIN**	**ASSOCIATED FINDINGS**
Cardiac ischemia (also known as acute coronary syndrome)	Pain: Burning, squeezing or aching, heaviness, smothering	Not reproducible by palpation of the chest wall, may be relieved with rest, nitroglycerin, or oxygen, and may or may not be accompanied by ECG changes
Aortic dissection	Pain: Sudden sharp, and tearing, and radiates to shoulders, neck, back, and abdomen	Neurological complications: hemiplegia, sensory deficits secondary to carotid artery occlusion May present with a new murmur, bruits, and/or unequal blood pressure in upper extremities.
Pericarditis	Pain: Often severe; retrosternal; worsened with breathing, coughing, and change in position; radiates to the back; and may be accompanied by dyspnea	A pericardial friction rub and/or distended neck veins may be present
Pulmonary embolus	Pain: Sudden onset, sharp pleuritic type or stabbing, varies with respiration. Older adults may present with vague chest discomfort	The most frequent symptom is dyspnea and the most frequent sign is tachypnea; may have a cough and hemoptysis with a small embolism
Pneumothorax	Pain: Sudden onset, tearing or pleuritic, worsened by breathing	May also have dyspnea, tachycardia, decreased breath sounds, and a deviated trachea
Pneumonia	Pain: Sudden that is exacerbated by coughing and deep breathing	Present with fever (not always present in the elderly), chills, tachypnea, and a productive cough
Esophageal rupture	Pain: Associated with swallowing and is sudden in nature	May be from a penetrating trauma or a blow to the epigastric area
	May be constant and in the area behind the sternum in the epigastric area	Consider this if patient has a first or second rib fracture
Musculoskeletal—costochondritis	Usually affects the third, fourth and fifth costochondral joints. Onset of anterior chest pain may begin suddenly or gradually. May mimic cardiac pain. Pain may radiate to the arms or shoulders	Pain treated with anti-inflammatory drugs, analgesics and steroid injection
	Is aggravated by deep inspirations, twisting, sneezing, coughing, and deep inspirations.	

Adapted from Estes, M. (2006). Health assessment and physical examination (3rd ed.). New York: Thomson Delmar Learning.

Objective information for the cardiovascular system is gathered from the physical assessment and the use of diagnostic tests. The steps for the physical examination of the cardiovascular system are inspection, palpation, percussion, and auscultation. Inspection begins by assessing the patient's general appearance. While gathering the subjective information the nurse examines the patient's color, posturing, comfort level, and breathing pattern. It is expected that the patient's coloring be consistent with the ethnic background, and the breathing pattern be regular and without distress. The general contour of the chest is noted (Table 23-8). The expected finding is a 2:1 anteroposterior diameter. If there is a 1:1 ratio, the patient has a barrel chest configuration that may be associated with chronic obstructive pulmonary disease. Other chest abnormalities may include pectus excavatum, pectus carinatum kyphoscoliosis, and

---

BOX 23-2

HISTORY OF THE CARDIOVASCULAR SYSTEM

The nurse can ask the patient the following questions when assessing the cardiovascular system:

- Have you experienced fatigue or activity intolerance?
- Have you experienced a recent viral illness?
- Have you experienced a recent weight gain?
- Have you had any changes in skin texture, color, or temperature?
- Do you have any sores or ulcers that will not heal?
- Have you had any changes in your nail beds shape or color?
- Have you had episodes of headaches?
- Have you had any ringing in your ears?
- Have you had any nosebleeds?
- Have you had any difficulty breathing?
- Do you have a history of lung disease?
- Have you ever smoked or were you raised in a family that smoked?
- Are you postmenopausal?
- Do you use oral contraceptives or are you taking estrogen for hormone replacement therapy?
- Have you had any muscle weakness or leg cramps with exercise?
- Have you had any syncope, headaches, and behavioral changes, such as confusion or loss of memory?
- Do you have diabetes or thyroid disease?

TABLE 23-8 Physical Abnormalities of the Chest

CHEST ABNORMALITY	DESCRIPTION
Barrel chest	A chest that has an increased anteroposterior diameter to a 1:1 diameter.
Pectus excavatum (funnel chest)	A chest condition in which there is a depression of the inferior (lower) portion of the sternum. The sternum may compress on the heart and great vessels resulting in murmurs and decreased blood return to the heart that may result in decreased activity tolerance.
Pectus carinatum (pigeon chest)	The sternum is displaced outward and the costal cartilages around the sternum are depressed giving the appearance of a pigeon chest.

Adapted from Estes, M. (2006). Health assessment and physical examination (3rd ed.). New York: Thomson Delmar Learning.

---

ankylosing spondylitis. Any of these disorders may be related to abnormalities of the cardiac structures (Fuster, et al., 2004).

The skin color is assessed. In the Caucasian patient the skin is expected to have a pinkish coloration. A bluish discoloration of the skin and mucous membranes is called cyanosis. This cyanotic hue occurs because deoxygenated hemoglobin is in the skin capillaries, usually in the lips, nail bed, and mucous membranes. This is termed central cyanosis. Peripheral cyanosis is a bluish color in the fingers and toes. In dark-skinned persons cyanosis may be detected in the mucous membranes in the mouth and in the conjunctivae (Kasper, et al., 2004). Generally, cyanosis appears whenever the arterial blood contains more than 5 grams of hemoglobin is deoxygenated in each 100 mL of blood. A person with anemia almost never becomes cyanotic because there is not enough hemoglobin for 5 grams of it to be deoxygenated in the arterial blood. For a comparison a person with abnormally high hemoglobin may have an excessive amount of deoxygenated hemoglobin and may have cyanosis even with adequate amounts of oxygen available. To confirm adequate oxygenation, pulse oximetry or arterial blood gas analysis may be performed. Pallor is a pale discoloration of the skin and may be associated with decreased hemoglobin. To check for chronic hypoxia examine the patient for nail clubbing. Have the patient lift both hands and inspect them. Assess the color of the skin and the nail beds. Look for any skin lesions, edema, or clubbing of the fingers. The expected angle of the nail bed is 160 degrees. When chronic hypoxia is present the nail bed may flatten to an angle of 180 degrees. Capillary refill is checked to test the integrity of the peripheral circulation. It is done by applying pressure to the fingernail and then quickly releasing the pressure to the fingernail or toenail. The nail will initially lose its color and be blanched. The pink appearance is expected to return with two seconds or less. Taking three seconds or longer may indicate impaired blood flow to the extremity.

The nurse inspects the lower extremities by looking at skin color. The color would be expected to be consistent with the patient's race. The nurse should also note if there is a color change when the leg is in the dependent position. Hair distribution may be related to vascular flow. Decreased blood flow to the extremity may result in loss of hair. The dorsal surface of the toes can be examined for hair if the legs are shaved. Malnutrition may result in shiny skin. The presence of sores and ulceration may indicate arterial insufficiency or venous stasis. A brownish discoloration of the skin in the lower extremities may indicate venous insufficiency. Localized redness of an area may be from an infection or a DVT. The veins in the legs are normally flat and not prominent. The presence of varicose veins appears as a blue venous pattern and may be raised. Standing may make the varicose veins more prominent.

The jugular veins are inspected with the patient in a supine position and the head of the bed elevated to 30 to 45 degrees with a light showing across the neck. The internal jugular veins are deeper than the external jugular veins (Estes, 2006). A slight pulsation may be visible above the clavicle. Palpation of the extremities includes palpating and rating pulses on a scale of 0 to 4 (Box 23-3).

Other assessments of the extremities include: (a) skin changes, (b) vascular changes, (c) clubbing, (d) capillary refill, (e) skin turgor, and (f) peripheral edema. Inspection of the patient's precordium is carried out from patient's right side (Box 23-4). Compare the temperature of the extremity with the temperature of the patient's body. The temperature of the skin is noted using the dorsal surface of the examiners hand.

Palpation of the precordium includes assessing for the apical impulse, pulsations, and thrills that are abnormal tremors or vibrations from a cardiac murmur when felt in the precordium (Figure 23-5). A heave is described and is also called a lift which occurs when there is an enlarged and dilated left ventricle. The assessment for pulsations is carried out using the finger pads in the intercostal areas over the cardiac landmarks. Thrills are assessed using the palmar surface of the hand over the cardiac areas. When inspecting the aortic area no pulsations should be visible or palpated. If a pulsation is present, it may indicate that an aneurysm is present at the aortic root. If the patient has hypertension, the aneurysm may become bigger, and a rupture can occur at any time. The risk for rupture is greater when the aneurysm is greater than 5 cm in diameter (Estes, 2006).

The precordium is the area on the front surface of the chest that is over the heart, great vessels, pericardium, and some lung tissue. Assessment is carried out in a systematic manner. The aortic area is the second ICS to the right of the sternum. The pulmonic area is the second ICS on the left side of the sternum. Erb's point is assessed in the third ICS on the left side of the sternum. The tricuspid area is in the fifth ICS on the left side of the sternum. The mitral area in located in the fifth ICS at the midclavicular line on the left side of the precordium. This area is also known as the apical area. The landmarks for the cardiac valves are not where the valves are located but where the heart sounds

---

BOX 23-3

RATING PULSES IN THE EXTREMITIES

0	Absent or unable to palpate
1+	Diminished
2+	Brisk, expected for radial artery
3+	Increased
4+	Bounding

BOX 23-4

STEPS OF THE PRECORDIUM ASSESSMENT

1. Palpation of the precordium
2. Palpation of extremities: temperature, pulses
3. Percussion of the patient's precordium
4. Auscultation: stethoscope
5. Heart sounds: physiology, location, and timing

Adapted from Estes, M. (2006). Health assessment and physical examination (3rd ed.). New York: Thomson Delmar Learning.

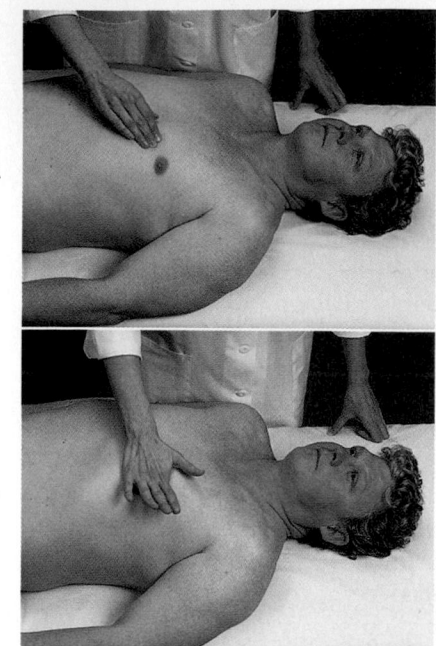

Figure 23-5 Palpating the heart: A. Pulsations, B. Thrills.

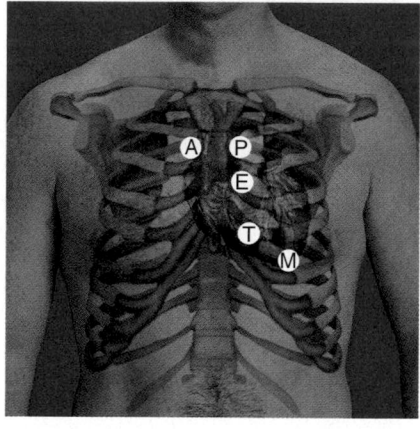

Figure 23-6 The cardiac landmarks for auscultation: A, aortic area; P, pulmonic area; E, Erb's point; T, tricuspid area; M, mitral area.

are heard best (Figure 23-6) (Estes, 2006). The aortic and pulmonic areas are located at the base of the heart, and the tricuspid and mitral areas are located at the apex of the heart.

Inspection of the precordium is performed from the patient's right side with the patient at a 45-degree angle with a light shining across the chest. Any movement of the precordium is noted. Each cardiac area is inspected and palpated individually. When visualizing the pulmonic area, no pulsations should be visible. A pulsation or bulge may be present if pulmonary stenosis is present and blood flow from the right ventricle into the pulmonary artery occurs resulting in right ventricular hypertrophy (Estes, 2006). Pulsations should not be visible or palpable in midsternal area to the left of the sternum, or in the tricuspid area. Right ventricular hypertrophy may result in a palpable right ventricular heave. Chronic right ventricular hypertrophy may result from recurrent, medium-sized pulmonary emboli that do not lyse, intravenous (IV) drug abuse, parasites, tumor tissue that travels to the pulmonary vascular bed, or primary pulmonary hypertension (Kasper, et al., 2004). Percussion of the precordium is of limited use. It can determine the borders of the heart but is less specific than use of precordial inspection and palpation. Therefore it is usually deferred in a cardiac assessment.

The mitral area may have a visible pulsation when the left ventricle lies close enough to the surface of the chest to see visible pulsations during systole. Present in about half the adult population, this occurs at the same time as the carotid pulse (Estes, 2006). When the pulsation occurs, it should be present in only the fifth ICS in the left midclavicular line. If left ventricular hypertrophy is present, a heave may be present that is visible and palpable in two or more ICSs in the mitral area. Left ventricular hypertrophy may occur as a result of long-term hypertension, cardiomyopathy, or left ventricular outflow obstruction.

Cardiac auscultation is completed in a systematic approach to assess the aortic, pulmonic, Erb's point, and tricuspid and mitral areas. The nurse should listen to a few cardiac cycles in each spot. The stethoscope is used over the cardiac auscultatory areas. The diaphragm of the stethoscope is used to hear high-pitched sounds, and the bell is used to listen for low-pitched sounds. When using the diaphragm, the stethoscope is placed firmly on the skin. The bell of the stethoscope is placed lightly on the skin making sure that all parts of the bell are touching the skin, but being careful not to apply too much pressure, which would cause the skin beneath the bell to stretch and transmit sounds like the diaphragm.

The first (S_1) and second heart (S_2) sounds are generated from closure of the cardiac valves. S_1 is produced when the valves between the atrium and ventricles close, which includes the tricuspid and mitral valves. The sound is produced by vibration of the valves, surrounding blood, great vessels, and ventricular wall. At the beginning of systole, the intraventricular pressure increases and results in backflow of blood against the mitral and tricuspid valves causing them to close. After the valves close, vibrations of the elastic valve leaflets and chordae tendineae occur (Estes, 2006).

The tricuspid component of S_1 is not normally heard, because the pressures are higher in the left side of the heart than in the right side of the heart. The mitral component of S_1 is best heard in the mitral area, which is in the fifth ICS in the left midclavicular line. The first heart sound is louder with increased exercise, increased metabolic states. S_1 may be soft in rheumatic fever, heart failure, and an acute myocardial infarction (Estes, 2006).

S_2 is primarily caused by closure of the aortic and pulmonic valves. At the end of systole the pressure in the ventricles is less than it is in the pulmonary artery and aorta. When this occurs, the pulmonic and aortic valves close and cause a vibration in the leaflets of the valves and the surrounding blood, blood vessels, and ventricular wall. S_2 is heard using the diaphragm of the stethoscope over the aortic, second ICS left sternal border, and pulmonic, second ICS right sternal border, areas. The aortic and pulmonic valves close together during expiration and the aortic component is the loudest. During inspiration there is increased venous return to the right side of the heart causing the pulmonic valve to close after the aortic valve resulting in a split S_2. This split sound should disappear on expiration. This pattern is called a physiological split of S_2.

The third and fourth heart sounds are low-pitched sounds that occur early and late in the diastolic filling portion of the cardiac cycle (Table 23-9). When they are heard in association with disease to the heart, they are called gallop sounds (Fuster, et al., 2004). If they are present they give information about the patient's ventricular function and compliance, which are related to the ventricle's ability to stretch to accommodate incoming blood.

The third heart sound (S_3) is heard during early diastole about a third of the way though. This sound occurs from blood rushing into the ventricles. It occurs when there is enough blood entering the ventricles to create reverberation from the elastic tension on the ventricular walls. The elasticity of the ventricular walls is necessary for stretching to occur to accommodate the inflow of blood. This is a low-pitched sound that cannot normally be heard with the stethoscope in the adult. In children, young adults, and high output states, such as pregnancy, an S_3 may be auscultated. This is a physiological S_3 and is rarely found in adults over the age of 40. It would be more commonly heard in a thin person. It is best heard in the apical position with the patient in the left lateral position.

In an adult it is more likely to be a pathological S_3 that is usually associated with ventricular dysfunction from heart failure and fluid overload (Estes, 2006). The sound occurs in this case from decreased rates of blood entering a ventricle that is overfilled with a large end-systolic volume, because the heart is too weak to empty its contents during systole. S_3 may also be called ventricular gallop, because it resembles the sound of a galloping horse. In nursing, a valuable assessment is to identify a patient who may be developing acute heart failure so collaborative care may be initiated early and possibly prevent complications or death.

During the cardiac assessment the bell of the stethoscope is placed on the chest lightly. If the right ventricle is affected the sound will be best heart in the tricuspid area, which is at the lower left sternal border. If the left ventricle is involved, the sound will be heard the loudest in the apical area, the fifth ICS, and left midclavicular line. Having the patient lie on the left side or having the patient lean forward to bring the heart closer to the chest wall may accentuate the sound.

The fourth heart sound (S_4) is associated with atrial contraction. It is associated with the blood rapidly entering the ventricle when the atria contract, which occurs in the last third of diastole. This sound is low-pitched and not normally audible with the stethoscope. S_4 sound may be audible when the blood is pushed

TABLE 23-9 Abnormal Heart Sounds

HEART SOUND	DESCRIPTION	POSSIBLE CAUSES
Third heart sound (S_3)	Low-pitched diastolic sound heard best with bell of the stethoscope	Normal in children; associated with heart failure in adult
	Also called ventricular gallop	
Fourth heart sound (S_4)	Low-pitched diastolic sound heard best with bell of the stethoscope	Associated with acute myocardial infarction and hypertension
	Also called atrial gallop. Associated with atrial contraction. Occurs in the last third of diastole	

Adapted from Estes, M. (2006). Health assessment and physical examination (3rd ed.). New York: Thomson Delmar Learning.

into a ventricle that is resistant to filling. Conditions that may cause this are acute myocardial infarction, long-standing hypertension, and aortic stenosis. When S_4 is present it is heard the best when the patient is turned in the left lateral position (Fuster, et al., 2004). Because the sound is associated with atrial contractions conditions in which atrial contraction is absent, such as atrial fibrillation will not have an S_4. The timing of S_4, which is the end of diastole, immediately precedes S_1, so it may sound like a split S_1. A way to distinguish between them is to note if the sound is heard with the diaphragm or bell of the stethoscope. Because S_4 is a low-pitched sound, it will be best heard with the bell.

Prosthetic heart valves produce a varied sound depending on the type of valve used. The sound location depends on which valve was placed. It may be in the aortic, pulmonic, tricuspid, or mitral area. Mechanical prosthetic valves that are a ball in cage design, bileaflet St. Jude valve, or a tilting disk, make a distinct clicking sound. Valves that are from human tissue (homograft) or animal tissue (heterograft) are more like the sounds of normal heart sounds (Fuster, et al, 2004).

A cardiac murmur is a sound that is an auditory vibration that varies in loudness, pitch, and duration of sound. The sound lasts longer than the heart sounds described thus far. The main contributing factor to heart murmurs is turbulence of blood flow. Normally the flow through the heart is smooth and sounds are not produced as the blood flows over the structures such as heart valves. Turbulence occurs when blood is pushed with a high velocity, and it is pushed through an opening that is irregularly shaped or narrowed such as occurs with damage to heart valves. Three main factors contribute heart murmurs. The first cause is a high flow rate when the blood is pushed through a normal or abnormal opening. The second is blood flowing normally, but the opening is narrowed or irregular. Third is if there is regurgitant, or backward, flow through a valve that is not able to close completely. This may also occur if there is a hole between the septum of the atrium or ventricles or a patent ductus arteriosus (Fuster, et al., 2004).

Heart murmurs may occur during systole or diastole depending on the cause. Heart murmurs are considered innocent, if they occur during systole and not related to structural defects in the heart. Pathological murmurs are associated with heart disease and may occur during systole or diastole (Box 23-5 and Table 23-10).

Murmurs are further evaluated using the terms quality, pitch, and configuration. In regard to quality, the terms that are used to describe the murmur are descriptive of the type of sound heard (e.g., harsh, blowing, hissing, or musical). The pitch of a murmur can be assessed by auscultating low-pitched murmurs with the bell of the stethoscope and these murmurs may occur when there is a lower pressure type of murmur (e.g., mitral stenosis when there is a stenotic valve). High-pitched murmurs are heard best with the diaphragm of the stethoscope. These may be associated in situations in which the blood is in a higher pressure situation, such as during systole when blood is being pushed over a stenotic aortic valve. In general, high-pitched murmurs are easier to hear. Last, the configuration when assessing a murmur is evaluating the pattern of the murmur by the pattern that is heard. Crescendo is used to describe a murmur that is soft and progressively becomes loader and then subsides (Figure 23-7). Decrescendo is when the murmur is louder in the beginning and then becomes softer until it is gone. Crescendo decrescendo is a murmur that begins soft, builds, and then tapers off. A heart murmur that is heard throughout systole is termed a pansystolic or holosystolic murmur.

The evaluation of a newly discovered or changing heart murmur may be evaluated as a collaborative problem. If the murmur is diastolic or continuous and associated with signs and symptoms of cardiac decompensation, it is treated as an emergency and would require echocardiography and cardiac catheterization if indicated. Further treatment would be determined at that time. A pericardial friction rub is due to inflammation of the pericardial sac in which fluid may or may not be present. It has a high-pitched quality and

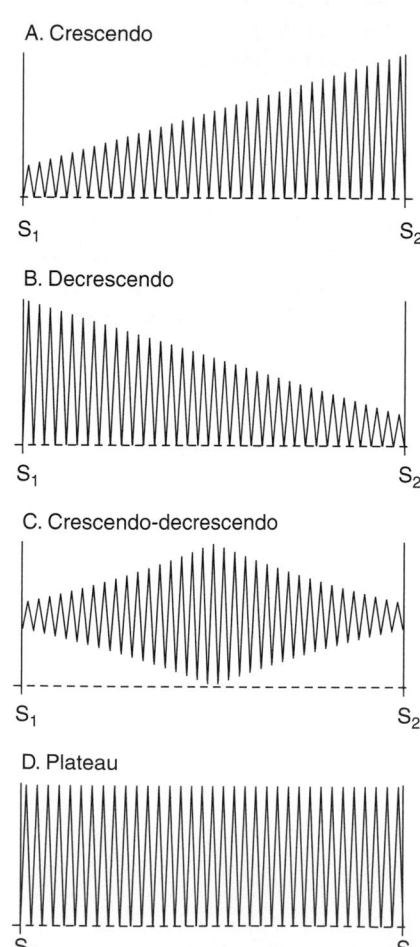

Figure 23-7 Characteristic patterns of murmurs.

BOX 23-5

ASSESSMENT OF HEART MURMUR

When assessing heart murmurs the following information is evaluated:

- Location: Note the area where the heart murmur is the loudest. The cardiac auscultation points are most often used; these are aortic, pulmonic, Erb's point, and tricuspid and mitral areas.
- Radiation: Note if the murmur is heard in surrounding areas. These areas of transmission often are related to the flow of the blood. For example, a murmur of aortic stenosis may radiate to the neck and a mitral regurgitation murmur may be transmitted to the axillary area.
- Timing: The murmur is evaluated in its timing in the cardiac cycle. A murmur that occurs between S_1 and S_2 is a systolic murmur, and if it occurs between S_2 and S_1, it is a diastolic murmur. When assessing the timing remember the S_1 is loudest in the tricuspid and mitral areas, and S_2 is loudest in the aortic and pulmonic areas. To distinguish the timing it may be helpful to palpate the carotid pulse and note that S_1 occurs simultaneously with the pulse.
- Intensity: A grading system that grades heart murmurs on a scale from I to VI is most frequently used. When using this system a murmur would be reported as the number that was appropriate and a VI scale; for example, a grade III murmur would be III/VI. So there is no confusion about which grading scale was used.

Adapted from Estes, M. (2006). Health assessment and physical examination (3rd ed.). New York: Thomson Delmar Learning.

TABLE 23-10 Grading of Heart Murmurs

Grade I	Faint on auscultation, not heard with every beat. Requires concentration and a high quality stethoscope.
Grade II	Heard with every beat, but a soft sound.
Grade III	A moderately loud sound. It is easily heard.
Grade IV	Very loud, the stethoscope must be completely touching the chest wall. It is usually associated with a thrill on palpation over the affected area.
Grade V	Extremely loud and can be heard with part of the stethoscope off the chest wall. It is associated with a thrill on palpation over the affected area.
Grade VI	This murmur is so loud, the stethoscope can be close to the chest to be heard. It too is associated with a thrill on palpation over the affected area.

Adapted from Estes, M. (2006). Health assessment and physical examination (3rd ed.). New York: Thomson Delmar Learning.

---

sounds like leather or hair being rubbed together and has a scratchy sound. It is heard best when the patient leans forward or has the knees up to the chest it can also be heard by having the patient hold his or her breath after blowing out as much air as possible. This sound is commonly heard for a few hours after an acute myocardial infarction. It may also be present with pericarditis and renal failure.

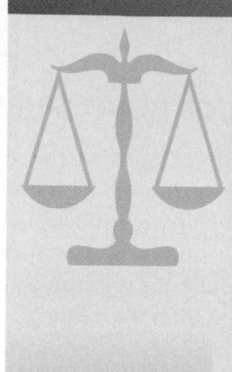

ETHICS IN PRACTICE

Delegation of Cardiovascular Assessment Skills

The National Council of State Boards of Nursing developed a tool to determine which nursing tasks may be delegated. It is important for the nurse to determine which parts of the cardiovascular assessment may be delegated to unlicensed assistive personnel. In the cardiovascular assessment, advanced cardiac care and vital sign monitoring are the responsibility of the registered nurse (Dochterman & Bulechek, 2004). Unlicensed personnel would need to carefully be educated regarding his or her responsibility in reporting specific manifestations to the nurse (e.g., hypertension, general skin pallor, or change in mentation).

DIAGNOSTIC TESTS

Noninvasive testing of the cardiovascular system includes evaluation of the blood pressure, ECG, and echocardiogram. Blood pressure is measured indirectly and reported in millimeters of mercury using a stethoscope and sphygmomanometer or a Doppler (an instrument that uses Doppler sound waves to determine blood pressure. This is useful when it is difficult to hear the Korotkoff sounds.

The **12-lead electrocardiogram (ECG)** is a standardized recording of the electrical activity of the heart. The ECG may be used to detect cardiac ischemia, enlargement of the chambers of the heart, and abnormal rhythms. Leads are placed on the extremities and chest to view the electrical activity from 12 different angles.

Exercise electrocardiography is useful as a noninvasive procedure for evaluating the patient with angina (see Box 23-5). The most common test for diagnosis of coronary artery disease and estimating survival is the exercise stress test (Box 23-6). In this procedure a 12-lead ECG is recorded before, during, and after exercise. The exercise is usually done on a treadmill. The test uses standardized protocol to increase the workload gradually by making the treadmill go at a faster rate and an increased grade. During this time the patient's heart rate, rhythm, blood pressure, and symptoms are monitored and recorded.

The stress test is usually stopped when the patient has symptoms. The patient is instructed to report chest discomfort, severe shortness of breath, dizziness, or extreme tiredness. These would indicate a need to stop the test and may show a possible relationship to cardiac disease. Objective data from the procedure would be heart rate, blood pressure, or ECG changes. The expected changes during the exercise test include the heart rate and the blood pressure increasing as the speed and grade of the treadmill are increased. The interpretation of the information is correlated between the objective and subjective data. This test may be associated with false-positive results, and therefore more testing may be necessary. If the patient is not able to reach a high enough heart rate, the findings may not be diagnostic.

The chest x-ray (CXR) provides information on the size of the heart and pulmonary circulation, lung disease, and abnormalities of the aorta. Patients have the procedure done in radiology unless their conditions prevents them from leaving the nursing unit, in which case a portable X-ray machine can be transported to the unit. The last time the patient had a CXR is determined and

Red Flag

Monitoring Blood Pressure

A patient was recovering from abdominal surgery. Her blood pressure at 0900 was 154/70. The patient complained of abdominal pain and pressure that felt like her catheter was infected. At 1230 the nurse evaluated her blood pressure and found that the blood pressure was 60/48. The patient was conscious and stated that her pain was decreased. The patient was then placed in a Trendelenburg position, and the health care provider was present and ordered an increase in IV fluids. The patient was transferred to the intensive care unit.

INDICATIONS FOR EXERCISE TESTING

The indications for exercise testing are:

- Validate the diagnosis of angina.
- Determine the severity of limitations to activity from angina.
- Assess the prognosis in patients with cardiac disease including cardiomyopathies, myocardial infarction, and coronary artery disease.
- Evaluate effectiveness of therapy for cardiac patients.
- Screen asymptomatic persons for silent heart disease. This is controversial because of the high number of false positive results.

Adapted from Tierney, L. M., McPhee, S. J., & Papdakis, M. A. (2004) Current medical diagnosis and treatment *(43rd ed.). New York: Lange Medical Books/McGraw-Hill.*

Fast Forward ▶▶▶

Specialized equipment for Procedures

Smaller equipment is becoming available that will make it possible for nuclear cardiology to be available in an office setting. At the present time most procedures are performed in a hospital setting. This increase in office-based practice may make it possible to have the equipment available in triage settings.

if the interpretation is available for comparison. Pregnancy is also assessed to prevent exposure to any fetus. The patient is instructed to remove all metal objects that could interfere with the cardiac and pulmonary images.

An **echocardiogram** is the evaluation of the heart's structure and function with images and recordings using ultrasound. Ultrasound is sonic, pertaining to sound, energy using a frequency that is above the range that the human ear can hear. When the signal travels through tissue, the beam will travel in a straight line. If the beam meets a structure of different acoustic impedance, part of the wave will be reflected, and the remaining signal will be transmitted. The reflected energy is known as an echo and is used to construct the image of the heart in echocardiography (Fuster, et al., 2004). Echocardiography is a noninvasive tool that can be performed at the patient's beside or in an outpatient setting. A transducer is used to transmit and receive the ultrasound signal. The heart valves, size of the ventricles, and regional wall motion can be assessed using this technique. Other abnormalities that are assessed using the echocardiogram are hypertrophic cardiomyopathy, mitral valve prolapse, pericardial effusion, vegetative growths on cardiac valves, and cardiac tumors (Tierney, McPhee, & Papdakis, 2004). Surface echocardiography may be performed by placing the transducer on the patient's chest and usually begins with the transducer in the left parasternal position. The patient lies quietly with the head of the bed at about 15 to 20 degrees. Transesophageal echocardiography may be used to improve the quality of the echocardiogram and to have a better view of posterior structures. This view shows atria and atrioventricular valves and prosthetic valves. It is better than surface echocardiography in diagnosing mitral regurgitation, especially with prosthetic valves, left atrial thrombi, and vegetations on valves. It also is sensitive in evaluating aortic dissection. When atrial thrombi are not identified in patients in atrial fibrillation, the patient is determined to be at low risk for embolization, and the patient may have earlier cardioversion (Tierney, et al., 2004). The transducer is attached to a gastroscope that is passed into the esophagus in a sedated patient. A signed consent form is needed before the procedure. Stress echocardiography is used in conjunction with the information from ECGs. An echocardiogram may be done during or immediately after exercise. If a patient is unable to exercise, dobutamine infusions can be used to stress the heart. If there is transient depression of ventricular wall motion, it may indicate that there is lack of oxygen to the heart muscle.

Myocardial nuclear perfusion imaging is performed by the department of nuclear medicine and includes different categories of procedures depending on the type of pathology that is suspected and the particular radionuclide that is used. The information that can be assessed with this procedure includes myocardial wall motion, EF, blood flow to the myocardium, the size of the ventricles, and integrity of the valves. Thallium chloride is used at rest and in conjunction with a stress test to assist in assessment of coronary artery disease and myocardial infarction. Another product that may be used is Cardiolite Technetium Tc99mm Sestamibi for injection (Broyles, Reiss, & Evans, 2007). This product, a radiopharmaceutical, is made up of a small protein that is marked with technetium Tc99mm sestamibi. The product is given intravenously and goes through the vascular system to the heart. For resting and stress examinations there are two injections, the first injection occurs when patient is at rest, and the second injection occurs when the patient is vigorously exercising. A scanning camera is used during each of the sessions to allow the visualization of the radioactive tracer in the heart. The pictures of the resting and stressed heart are compared to assess for changes. When there is narrowing of the coronary arteries, blood flow may be diminished, and subsequently the uptake of the radionuclide will be decreased. Exercise should result in increased blood flow to the myocardium, so if there is a narrowing, it may be detected with this test. If there is decreased flow to an area, the test shows as a "cold spot" on the radionuclide study. This test may be performed

Preparing the Patient for a Stress Test

The nurse can present the following instructions to prepare the patient for a stress exercise test:

- Wear comfortable clothing and supportive shoes for the procedure.
- You may be asked to remove clothing over the chest.
- You might be allowed to have a light meal preceding the exercise test.
- Please report any chest discomfort, dyspnea, leg cramps or soreness, and extreme fatigue.
- The length of the test varies, but will likely take between 20 and 50 minutes.
- You will be allowed enough time for preparation and adequate cool down after the test is concluded.
- The nurse will assist in prepping the skin, cleaning it, and shaving hair if necessary for good contact with the electrodes.
- You will be monitored throughout the procedure and after until all vital signs have returned to normal.

Adapted from Daniels, R. (2003). Delmar's manual of laboratory and diagnostic tests. New York: Thomson Delmar Learning.

on a patient with suspected coronary artery disease who may not be a candidate for a cardiac catheterization.

Cardiac catheterization and coronary angiography are procedures that can be performed either as outpatient or inpatient procedures depending on the condition of the patient. They are performed in a cardiac catheterization lab by specially trained cardiologists. In these procedures the right heart can be catheterized by accessing the venous system. A small catheter, which is radiographic, is inserted in a large vein and threaded through the vena cava, through the right atrium and into the right ventricle. To assess the left heart the catheter is inserted into the arterial system, usually the femoral artery and is threaded into the aorta and into the heart. Contrast material that is a radiographic dye outlines the heart and vessels. Pressure gradients across the valves may be measured to evaluate the functioning of the valves. Special catheters are used to inject dye into the right and left coronary arteries for visualization. This information is used to evaluate the filling of the coronary arteries.

Clinical implications for cardiac catheterization and coronary angiography are to diagnosis coronary artery disease and assess for atherosclerotic lesions. Left heart and right heart function may be evaluated including information about heart pressures and structural abnormalities, such as congenital abnormalities, defects in the heart valves, tumors in the heart, mural thrombi, septal defects, and aneurysms in the vessels or ventricular wall (Daniels, 2003).

An electrophysiological (EP) study of the heart is an invasive procedure that focuses on the electrical activity of specific tissues of the heart. This testing is done through the use of multiple electrode containing catheters. These are placed in various locations of the heart touching the endocardial surface of the heart. These give a view of ECGs from inside the heart. During EP studies the function of the SA node, AV node, and the bundle of His to the Purkinje system can be evaluated. The location of abnormal electrical activity can be diagnosed and, in some cases, treated.

Nursing Management

Patient teaching before the echocardiogram differs depending on the type of procedure done. For the resting surface echocardiogram, the patient needs to be informed that the procedure takes from 30 to 45 minutes and that there are not food or fluid restrictions. During the procedure the patient will be placed in various positions and asked to remain still, turn from side to side, and sit up during the procedure. Gel will be used for the transducer, and the instrument will moved to different positions. The echocardiogram will be displayed on a screen. The procedure is noninvasive and is not associated with pain or discomfort.

The transesophageal echocardiogram requires nursing care for a tube being placed in the esophagus. The patient is at increased risk for aspiration, because the patient is given an anesthetic for passage of the transducer into the esophagus. Anesthesia will be determined on an individual basis. The patient should be assessed for medications and if these are to be held or taken before the procedure. The patient is instructed not to have anything to eat or drink four to six hours before the procedure and to arrange to have someone drive home if this is an outpatient procedure. Any gastrointestinal problems are assessed, such as ulcer, hiatal hernia, or swallowing problems. During the echocardiogram, the patient will be taken to a special room where the procedure will be done. A spray will be used to anesthetize the throat, and conscious sedation may be performed. The patient will then be placed on his or her left side, and a lubricated tube will be placed in the esophagus. During this time the patient's vital signs are being monitored. The procedure usually takes from 20 to 40 minutes. After the procedure the patient continues to be monitored until vital signs are stable to prevent the risk for aspiration. Eating and drinking may be resumed when the throat is no longer numb and the gag reflex is intact

Nursing care before myocardial nuclear perfusion imaging includes teaching about the test procedure and the purpose of the test. The patient is not to have anything to eat or drink 4 to 5 hours before the procedure. Any substances that contain caffeine for 24 hours before the procedure or theophylline are to be avoided, because these can increase the heart rate. The nurse should assess the patient for pregnancy, lactation, and allergies to contrast medium. Baseline vital signs and neurological status need to be checked. During the procedure the patient is required to remain still during the duration of the scan. The procedure itself does not cause pain, but there may be discomfort for some patients from positioning. The patient should be instructed to void before the procedure and remove all jewelry and metal objects. The nurse administers sedative. The health care practitioner orders analgesics. The patient needs to fast 4 hours before the procedure (Daniels, 2003). During the procedure the patient is asked to report any chest, arm, or jaw discomfort leg cramps or pain, dizziness, or dyspnea. During the procedure, standard precautions are followed and the patient is assessed for allergic reactions to the contrast medium. After the test the patient and caregivers are instructed to wash their hands after bowel movements and voiding, because the urine and feces contain the excreted radionuclide.

If a patient cannot reach a high enough heart rate for diagnosis of heart disease using exercise protocol, pharmacological agents may be used. One class of agents is vasodilators. The two agents used for this are adenosine or dipyridamole. The medications provide a threefold to fivefold increase in coronary blood flow. Adenosine is used more often than dipyridamole because of its rapid onset and onset of peak effect. Medications that are classified as methylxanthines, which include caffeine or theophylline, block the adenosine binding and can eliminate the vasodilation of the coronary arteries. These may result in false-negative stress perfusion studies. It is recommended that patients not consume medications that contain theophylline and caffeine or beverages that may contain caffeine, such as coffee, soft drinks, and chocolate prior to the test. In some cases pharmacological stress protocols are combined with exercise testing (Fuster, et al., 2004).

Adenosine is infused and if the patient is able, he or she may be asked to walk slowly on a treadmill during the 5-minute injection. This may reduce the side effects of the medication and improve the quality of the test. Adenosine slows conduction through the AV node. Therefore, it is contraindicated in patients with greater than first-degree AV block or sick sinus syndrome. Another serious reaction to adenosine is bronchospasm. Therefore adenosine is contraindicated in patients with bronchospasm (Fuster, et al., 2004).

For patients with a history of asthma, chronic obstructive pulmonary disease with bronchospasm, or patients who have ingested caffeine, dobutamine stress test may be used. There is a lower pressure response and there are more side effects that include ventricular arrhythmias. Therefore, it is not preferred but is an alternative for patients who have contraindications to the vasodilator agents.

Cardiac catheterizations and angiography require the patient to sign an informed consent. The patient is instructed that the procedure is performed in a cardiac catheterization laboratory, and the individual should not have anything to eat or drink before the procedure. All metal objects, such as hair clips, glasses, and jewelry, are removed. The procedure is performed on a hard table that may change positions, and patients may be asked to hold their breath as the dye travels through the heart and lungs. When the dye is injected into the chambers of the heart, a hot sensation is felt throughout the body that lasts about 30 seconds. Assessment before the procedure includes allergies to contrast material, renal function because the dye may alter renal function, and if the patient is taking the diabetic medication metformin (Glucophage), it should be held for iodinated contrast studies. Also the nurse evaluates for anxiety and premedicates the patient as ordered 30 minutes before the procedure. Administration of the patient's medication is determined by the practitioner and institution protocol. During the cardiac catheterization/angiography, all team members follow standard precautions. The patient is assessed for allergic reactions to the dye. Vital signs and the patient's cardiac rhythm are monitored, because of the potential for life-threatening arrhythmias occurring during the procedure. The nurse may also assist the practitioner in medication administration and patient position changes during the procedure. After the test is completed, the arterial puncture site is compressed to stop bleeding. The site is monitored for a hematoma formation. Vital signs are monitored every 15 minutes until the patient is stable. The patient will be advised as to the length of immobilization of the extremity, based on the method used to stop the bleeding and the protocol of the institution. The nurse continues to monitor the patient for cardiac signs and symptoms and rhythm disorders. The pulses distal to the puncture site are monitored to assess for the possibility of a clot forming from the arterial puncture. If the patient develops pain, the leg becomes cold, and the pulses cannot be palpated an occlusion is suspected and the practitioner is notified immediately.

The EP procedure is similar to a patient having a cardiac catheterization. Beforehand the patient has nothing by mouth and the administration of medications is determined on an individual basis. The procedure may last for hours, so patient's comfort is a concern. The type of anesthesia is determined on an individual basis. The patient may have venous or arterial access (Bosen & Flemming, 2003). After the procedure the catheters are removed, and pressure is applied to the site. The patient is instructed to remain in bed for 2 to 3 hours for venous access and up to 6 hours if the artery is punctured. Exertion is to be avoided for 24 hours, and no lifting of items greater than 10 pounds is allowed for two to three days.

KEY CONCEPTS

- The objective evaluation of the hematological system includes the red blood cells, hemoglobin, hematocrit, and the white blood cells.
- The white blood cells include granulocytes, which include the neutrophil, eosinophils, and basophils, and the lymphocytes.
- The heart works as two pumps with the right side of the heart pumping blood to the lungs, and the left side pumping blood to the systemic circulation.
- Blood pressure is measured indirectly and the systolic and diastolic numbers are reported in millimeters of mercury.
- The systemic circulation supplies blood to the organs and tissues of the body.
- The heart is supplied by the right and left coronary arteries that originate at the base of the aorta.
- The cardiac cycle reflects the contraction and relaxation of the heart.

- EF is an index that estimates contractile function of the left ventricle.
- Past medical and family history is assessed to determine previous heart conditions and risk factors for heart disease.
- Heart sounds are assessed in the following positions: aortic, pulmonic, Erb's point, tricuspid, and mitral.
- Exercise or chemically induced stress electrocardiography is used to assess the function of the heart with an increased workload.
- Cardiac catheterization and coronary angiography is invasive. A catheter is placed in the vascular system and threaded to the heart where dye is injected to assess chamber function and visualize the coronary arteries.
- Nursing management for cardiac system diagnostic tests relies on patient education.

REVIEW QUESTIONS

1. Which of the following blood products or proteins are used in blood clotting?
   1. Platelets
   2. Fibrinogen
   3. Basophils
   4. Heparin

2. Which of the following areas are best used to assess the pallor due to anemia?
   1. Mucous membranes and conjunctivae
   2. Inner aspect of the forearm, fingernails, and lips
   3. Nasolabial fold, palpebral conjunctiva, and lips
   4. Lips, behind the ears, and fingernails

3. In general, which of the following causes the normal heart sounds?
   1. Blood filling the left ventricle
   2. Blood entering the left atrium
   3. Closing of the heart valves
   4. Opening of heart valves

4. What is the phase of the cardiac cycle during which the ventricles relax and the decreased intraventricular pressure causes the mitral valve to open?
   1. Systole
   2. P wave
   3. Diastole
   4. T wave

5. What is the extra heart sound, normal in some children and young adults, that occurs early in diastole during a period of rapid ventricular filling and which in the older adult signifies heart failure?
   1. S_1
   2. S_2
   3. S_3
   4. S_4

6. Which normal heart sound is produced when the pressure in the ventricle drops below aortic pressure and the aortic valve closes?
   1. S_1
   2. S_2
   3. S_3
   4. S_4

7. Which heart sound is produced when the ventricle contracts, and the ventricular pressure rapidly exceeds left atrial pressure causing the mitral valve to close?
   1. S_1
   2. S_2
   3. S_3
   4. S_4

8. A physiologically split S_2 sound is best auscultated over which area?
   1. The cardiac apex near the fifth and sixth ICS
   2. The area of apical impulse near the fifth ICS
   3. The cardiac apex near the second ICS
   4. The left second ICS close to the sternum

9. Which of the following is the approximate auscultation site for the mitral valve area in the adult?
   1. Second ICS to the left of the midsternal line
   2. Fourth ICS, 2 to 3 cm to the right of the midsternal line
   3. Fifth ICS, approximately at the left midclavicular line
   4. Third ICS at the left midsternal border

10. What is the scale used to assess heart murmurs?
    1. I to IV
    2. I to VI
    3. A to E
    4. I to III

REVIEW ACTIVITIES

1. What blood cells are derived from the stem cell in the bone marrow?

2. What are the characteristics of the red blood the allow them to carry oxygen?

3. What cells make up the white blood cells?

4. Which white blood cells fight infection, and what is their role?

Continued

REVIEW ACTIVITIES—cont'd

5. Where do platelets come from?

6. Trace the blood flow through the heart.

7. Listen to the heart sounds on a patient in the clinical setting and document the findings.

8. Complete a cardiovascular assessment in a clinical laboratory simulation.

Coronary Artery Dysfunction: Nursing Management

Sharon Narducci, MSN, RN, FNP-BC, CCRN

Kristi Bennett, RN, ANP, MS

CHAPTER TOPICS

- Coronary Artery Disease (CAD)
- Angina
- Acute Coronary Syndromes (ACS)

C oronary artery disease (CAD) is the leading cause of death in the United States and industrialized societies throughout the world. A decline in CAD-related deaths in the United States over the last decade is likely because of campaigns to increase awareness for early recognition and risk factor modification, as well as, advances in medical and surgical therapies. Large expenditures of time, energy, money, and resources are spent on saving and improving the quality of life of patients with CAD. Nurses play a pivotal role in the care of patients with this disease. This chapter will discuss the nurse's collaborative role in management of these patients.

KEY TERMS

Angina pectoris
Atherogenesis
Atherosclerosis
Cardiogenic shock
Coronary artery bypass grafting (CABG)
Dressler's syndrome
Foam cell
High-density lipoprotein (HDL)
Levine's sign
Low-density lipoprotein (LDL)
Myocardial infarction (MI)
Percutaneous coronary interventions (PCI)
Pericarditis
Pulsus alternans
Syndrome X

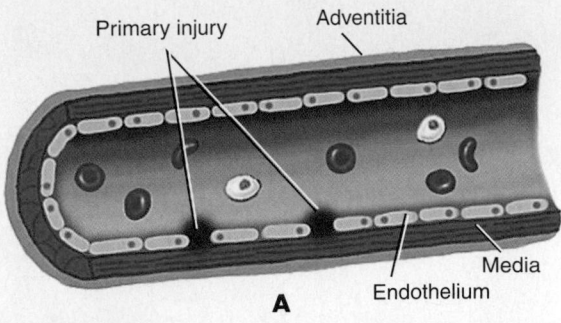

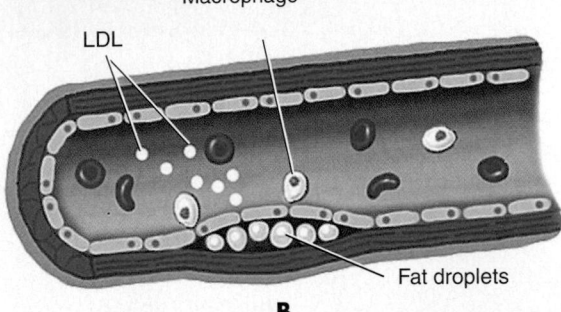

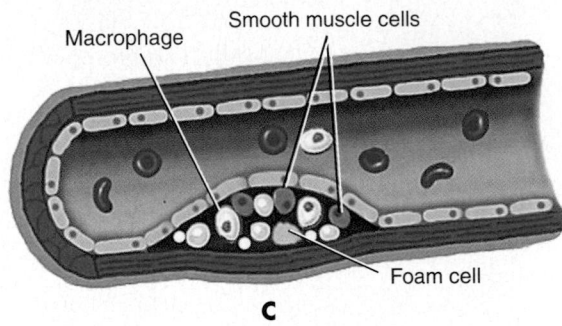

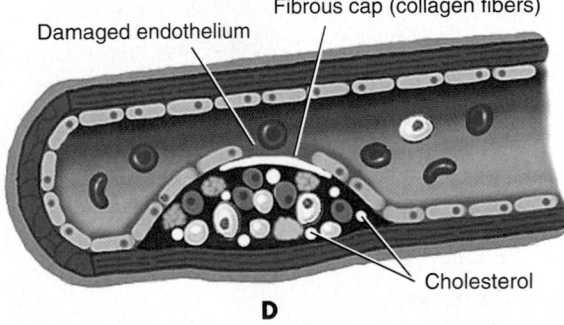

Figure 24-1 Atheroma formation: A. Endothelial injury, B. Influx of lipids, C. Accumulation of lipids, proliferation of smooth muscle cells, and accumulation of macrophages, D. Atheroma.

CORONARY ARTERY DISEASE

CAD, arteriosclerotic heart disease (ASHD), coronary heart disease (CHD), cardiovascular heart disease (CVHD), and ischemic heart disease (ICHD) are all interchangeable terms to describe the same disease. CAD is a blood vessel disease of the epicardial arteries responsible for supplying the myocardium with blood rich in oxygen and nutrients. The major contributor to CAD is **atherosclerosis** or hardening of the arteries. The cellular processes of atheroma formation are intricate and involve several progressive steps of formation (Figure 24-1). Atherosclerosis begins as fatty streaks of the arterial wall in adolescents, progressing to hard fatty plaques that narrow the arteries lumen in adulthood. These atherosclerotic plaques can rupture creating thrombotic occlusions. Ischemia occurs when reduced blood supply through narrowed arteries or thrombotic occlusion does not meet myocardial oxygen demand. Prolonged ischemia can lead to tissue death and **myocardial infarction (MI)** (prolonged ischemia, 20 minutes or more, results in myocardial cellular death). The clinical presentation of CAD varies widely from stable angina to MI and sudden death.

Epidemiology

According to the American Heart Association ([AHA], 2005), the prevalence of CAD in the United States is 13,000,000 people. In the United States, Caucasians have a higher rate of CAD than other races. However, African American males have a higher incidence of new MI or sudden death. Although the death rate in the United States has declined by 26.5 percent over the last decade, CAD remains the leading cause of death for men and women. CAD is responsible for one of every five deaths, with coronary events occurring every 26 seconds and death occurring every minute. Approximately 335,000 people a year die of CAD before arrival to the hospital or in the emergency department. Most of these deaths are due to sudden cardiac death (SCD). About 50 percent of men and 64 percent of women have no previous symptoms of CAD prior to sudden death. For people who survive a heart attack, there is an increased incidence of substantial illness and death including another heart attack, sudden death, heart failure, and stroke.

Etiology

A variety of factors are commonly associated with the risk of developing CAD. These CAD risk factors are classically categorized as nonmodifiable and modifiable. Nonmodifiable risk factors are age, gender, and family history. A report based on analysis of three large prospective studies defined the major CAD risk factors as hyperlipidemia, hypertension, smoking, and diabetes mellitus (Greenland, et al., 2003). In addition to these major modifiable risk factors, the AHA (2005) also includes obesity and sedentary lifestyle. Controlling these major modifiable risk factors can reduce the incidence of adverse coronary events. There are nine potentially modifiable risk factors that account for 90 percent of risk for an initial MI. This study has applicability worldwide, because the risk factors were consistent regardless of sex, race, and geographical location.

Chronic renal disease is now considered a CAD risk equivalent (Antman, et al., 2004). The way people deal with stress and anger has been linked to increased risk of CAD but requires further research to confirm these behavioral factors' significance. Other emerging risk factors for CAD under investigation include lipoprotein (a), C-reactive protein, and homocysteine levels (Daniels, 2003). For the purpose of this chapter CAD nonmodifiable risk factors are identified as age (older than 45 for males, older than 55 for females), gender (males at greater risk than females), and family history (CAD in first-degree relative; males younger than 55, females younger than 65). The major modifiable risk factors are hyperlipidemia, hypertension (blood pressure greater than 140/90 mm Hg), smoking, diabetes mellitus, obesity, and sedentary lifestyle.

Nonmodifiable Risk Factors

The nonmodifiable risk factors are age, gender, and family history. Patients cannot change these characteristics and health care providers are not focused on the management of these variables. The risk of CAD increases with age with 83 percent of deaths occurring over the age of 65. Females tend to lag behind males by 10 years with this difference decreasing with advancing age. In comparison to premenopausal women, rates of CAD are two to three times higher for postmenopausal women (AHA, 2005). Family history of premature cardiovascular disease is a significant risk factor especially for younger individuals (Lloyd-Jones, et al., 2004).

Modifiable Risk Factors

The risk of CAD increases with the presence of variables that can be changed by the patient. These variables are termed modifiable risk factors. Some sources will classify the modifiable risk factors into major and minor modifiable risk factors. The major modifiable risk factors are hyperlipidemia, hypertension (blood pressure greater than 140/90 mm Hg), cigarette smoking, diabetes mellitus, obesity, and sedentary lifestyle. In addition, the remaining modifiable risk factors include low daily fruit and vegetable intake, alcohol consumption, and psychosocial index (Wheaton & Pinkstaff, 2006).

Hyperlipidemia

Cholesterol and triglycerides are the major plasma lipids. These lipids are essential for cell membrane formation, hormone and steroid synthesis, and are precursors for free fatty acids. The two sources of serum cholesterol are ingested animal products that are absorbed from the intestine (exogenous) and cholesterol that is synthesized by the liver (endogenous). Seventy percent of plasma cholesterol is transported to the liver and other body tissues by **low-density lipoprotein (LDL)** or bad cholesterol. LDL is the main lipid component of the atherosclerotic plaque and is considered bad cholesterol, because increased levels reflect increased tendency to CAD. LDL is the main lipid component of the atherosclerotic plaque. There are many subtypes of LDL. The smaller denser particles, such as, very low density lipoproteins (VLDL) are considered more atherogenic and are more common in males and diabetics. **High-density lipoprotein (HDL)** or good cholesterol transports plasma cholesterol away from atherosclerotic plaques and to the liver for metabolism and excretion. HDL is considered good cholesterol, because increased levels decrease the tendency to CAD. As intake and synthesis of lipids exceed cellular metabolic needs or when too little is metabolized or excreted, an increase in lipid concentrations in the vascular space contributes to atherosclerosis development. Primary causes of hyperlipidemia include dietary sources and genetic disorders. Secondary causes of hyperlipidemia are due to hormone imbalances, liver and kidney dysfunction, alcohol consumption, and certain drugs such as beta blockers and cyclosporine (Rizzo, 2006).

Elevated total cholesterol, high LDL, low HDL, and high triglyceride levels are linked to increased CAD risk (Table 24-1) (Grundy, et al., 2004). Over

TABLE 24-1 Classification of Lipid Levels

CLASSIFICATION	TOTAL CHOLESTEROL (mg/dL)	LDL (mg/dL)	HDL (mg/dL)	TRIGLYCERIDE (mg/dL)
Optimal	Less than or equal to 200	Less than or equal to 100 (less than or equal to 70 in patients with CAD or equivalent)	Greater than or equal to 60 (counts as a negative risk factor)	Less than or equal to 150
Near optimal		100–129		
Borderline high	200–239	130–159		150–199
High	Greater than or equal to 240	160–189	Less than or equal to 40	200–499
Very high		Greater than or equal to 190		Greater than or equal to 500

Adapted from Rizzo, D. (2006). Fundamentals of anatomy and physiology (2nd ed.). New York: Thomson Delmar Learning.

50 percent of the U.S. population over the age of 20 have a total cholesterol level greater than 200 mg/dL, with Mexican-American males leading the pack. Over 45 percent have LDL levels greater than 130 mg/dL, 26 percent have HDL levels less than 40 mg/dL, and Caucasian males have the highest prevalence. Even more concerning is that 20 percent of adolescents have cholesterol levels greater than 200 mg/dL (AHA, 2005). Various studies confirm that therapy that lowers lipid levels can significantly reduce adverse cardiovascular events and is indicated for both primary and secondary prevention of CAD (Cannon, et al., 2004; Sever, et al., 2003).

Hypertension

Hypertension is defined as a blood pressure greater than 140/90 mmHg on two readings five minutes apart (Table 24-2) (Chobanian, Bakris, Black, & Cushman, 2003). Hypertension is a well-established risk factor for cardiovascular disease. CAD is the most common cause of death in hypertensive people. One in every three adults has hypertension, with men more likely to have it than women until the age of 55, then women are more likely than men to have it. Hypertension is more common in African American females and males than other races (AHA, 2005). The cause of hypertension in more than 90 percent of cases is called essential hypertension. Hypertension causes shearing force injury to the arterial intimal lining, proliferation of smooth muscles cells, enhancement of vascular calcium accumulation, and lipid infiltration contributing to the atherosclerotic changes of arteries. In addition, hypertension increases the workload of the heart by increasing afterload, causing left ventricular hypertrophy, and precedes the development of heart failure. Control of hypertension can significantly reduce cardiovascular events, most notably reducing heart failure by up to 50 percent.

Cigarette Smoking

There are 48 million cigarette smokers in the United States. Smokers usually start in adolescence, with 80 percent beginning before the age of 18. Cigarette smoking increases the risk of dying from CAD by 200 to 400 percent and is proportional to the number of cigarettes smoked per day. In addition, secondhand smoke exposure and pipe and cigar smokers as well as tobacco chewers have an increased risk of CAD (AHA, 2005). Carbon monoxide, the by-product of combustion, and nicotine contribute to CAD in several ways. Catecholamine release increases heart rate and blood pressure. This increases the workload of the heart and oxygen consumption. Carboxyhemoglobin pro-

TABLE 24-2	Blood Pressure Classification
BP CLASSIFICATION	**SBP mm Hg DBP mm Hg**
Normal	Less than or equal to120 and less than or equal to 80
Prehypertension	120–139 or 80–90
Stage I hypertension	140–159 or 90–99
Stage II hypertension	Less than or equal to 160 or less than or equal to 100

Adapted from Cuddy, M. (2005). Treatment of hypertension: Guidelines from JNC 7 (The Seventh Report of the Joint National Committee on Prevention, Detection, Evaluation, and Treatment of High Blood Pressure). Journal of Practical Nursing, *55(4), 17–23; Winegarden, C. (2005). From "prehypertension" to hypertension? Additional evidence.* Annals of Epidemiology, *15(9), 720–725.*

duction has a negative inotropic effect, reduces oxygen delivery, and lowers ventricular fibrillation threshold. The irritant effects of cigarette smoking cause injury to the endothelial lining, impairing function, and promoting atherosclerotic changes and platelet aggregation. Within one year of smoking cessation, the risk of CAD decreases by 50 percent, and former smokers' risk approaches nonsmokers within three years.

Diabetes Mellitus

Diabetes increases the death rate for patients with CAD by 200 to 400 percent. In addition, CAD is the leading cause of death for diabetics (AHA, 2005). Hyperglycemia, insulin resistance, hyperinsulinemia, and glucose intolerance all increase the risk of CAD. Diabetes alters lipid metabolism, causes subclinical inflammation, promotes a prothrombotic state, and impairs endothelial function, promoting **atherogenesis.** The metabolic syndrome, also called insulin resistance syndrome, is a constellation of disorders including abdominal obesity, hypertension, diabetes, and hyperlipidemia. This metabolic syndrome is significantly related to the development of CAD.

Physical Inactivity

Only 31 percent of adults in the United States participate in regular physical activity. Regular physical activity is more likely in college graduates and higher income brackets. Hispanic (American) adults are least likely to participate in regular physical activity. The risk of CAD associated with physical inactivity is comparable to hypertension, dyslipidemia, and cigarette smoking (AHA, 2005). Moderate intensity regular physical activity, such as walking, can reduce the risk. Regular exercise's beneficial effects are related to elevation in HDL, reduction in blood pressure, weight reduction, and decreasing insulin resistance.

Obesity

Overweight and obesity in adults is defined as a body mass index (BMI) equal to or greater than 25 and 30 kg/m², respectively. Overweight in children is defined as over the 95th percentile of the growth chart. Among adults in the United States, 65 percent are overweight and 30 percent are obese, with the highest prevalence in African American women. Most alarming is that an estimated 9 million children and adolescents, the majority Caucasians, are overweight or obese, and 10 percent of preschoolers are overweight (AHA, 2005). Obesity is associated with an increased risk of CAD and mortality. Obesity is also associated with other risk factors including hypertension, insulin resistance, glucose intolerance, hyperlipidemia, and inactivity. The distribution of fat in the abdominal area, or central obesity, is associated with the highest risk (Brunner, Thorogood, Rees, & Hewitt, 2006).

Pathophysiology

Endothelial cells of the arterial intimal layer form a permeable barrier and produce substances that inhibit platelet aggregation and promote vasodilatation. Atherosclerosis begins with injury to the endothelial lining that allows abnormal accumulation of lipids, progresses to development of fibrous plaques with lipid rich cores and hardening of the arterial wall, finally these plaques become complicated lesions that are stable or vulnerable. This process is the basis for the development of atherosclerotic lesions over time or atherogenesis.

Injury to the endothelial lining can occur through elevated plasma levels of lipids, increased shear forces as in hypertension, chemical toxins found in smoking, and infections like chlamydia. Endothelial injury allows entry of lipids, especially LDL, to the intima. LDL becomes biochemically modified by oxidation and glycation. These modified LDL particles recruit monocytes and promote expression of inflammatory mediators. Monocytes differentiate into macrophages that act as scavengers ingesting modified LDL in large quantities. These engorged lipid-laden macrophages, or **foam cells,** are the major component of the fatty streak. The fatty streak is the first visible sign of atherosclerosis and is found in coronary arteries usually by adolescence. The fatty streak appears flat and yellow. These lesions are benign and do not cause obstruction or symptoms.

Fatty streaks can progress to fibrous plaques. The foam cell stimulates the release of growth factors that promote intimal smooth muscle cell and connective tissue migration and proliferation. This fibroproliferative process is accelerated by the foam cells' chronic activation of platelets, growth factors, and inflammatory mediators. These lesions have a fibrous cap composed of smooth muscle cells surrounded by connective tissue with a core filled with lipids, fibrous tissue, and necrotic debris. The raised fibrous plaque begins to develop after the second or third decade of life and increases with age. The fibrous plaque appears as white or grayish and protrudes into the lumen of the artery. The borders may have smooth or rough edges and can form on one portion of the artery or circumferentially involve the whole lumen.

The final process of atherosclerotic plaque progression usually occurs after the third decade of life when the fibrous plaque becomes a complicated lesion. The foam cell increases in size, becomes increasingly calcified, rigid, and fragile. The intimal surface can ulcerate and disintegrate. Platelets and inflammatory factors are activated and thrombi accumulate, further increasing the size and instability of the plaque. The plaque becomes increasingly complex as the lesion hardens and enlarges, taking on further lipids, thrombi, damaged tissue, and calcium. As the plaque enlarges the artery may become partially or completely occluded. Over time a vulnerable or stable plaque develops.

Stable plaques usually have a thick fibrous cap protecting a small lipid core with high levels of smooth muscle and low levels of inflammatory cells. This lesion can produce significant arterial narrowing but is less likely to rupture. On the other hand, the vulnerable plaque has a thin fibrous cap protecting a large lipid core with high levels of inflammatory cells. Angiographically these lesions may appear insignificant but are more likely to rupture and produce an acute thrombotic event (Puddu, Cravero, Puddu, & Muscari, 2005).

Types of Angina

Angina pectoris means pain in the chest. The different types of angina (i.e., stable, unstable, Prinzmetal's variant angina, silent angina, and syndrome X) have varying presentations and are presented in this section. Stable angina is usually due to a stable, fixed, obstructive atheromatous plaque with a thick fibrous cap in one or more coronary arteries. Ischemic episodes are precipitated by factors that increase oxygen demand, for example, exercise, or reduce oxygen supply, for example anemia. Chest pain occurs predictably with the same onset, duration, and intensity and is relieved when the precipitating factor is removed or with nitroglycerin.

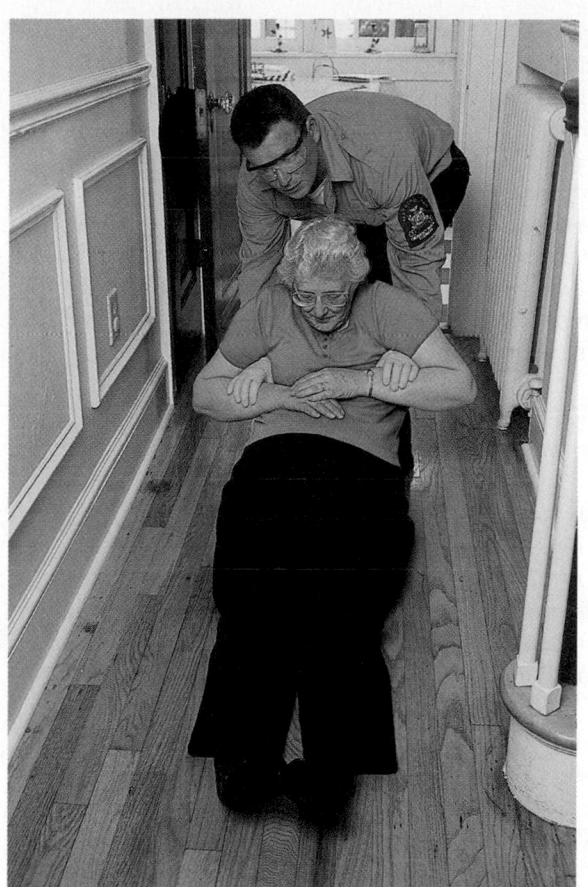

Figure 24-2 A paramedic moves a SCD patient to a large enough area to perform ACLS measures.

Unstable angina is typified by an increase in frequency, duration, and intensity of symptoms at lower levels of activity and even at rest. Unstable angina is often the precursor to MI. Unstable angina and MI are now classified as acute coronary syndrome (ACS). These syndromes are the result of rupture of an unstable or vulnerable plaque. Unlike a stable plaque, a vulnerable plaque has a thin fibrous cap and large lipid core. Rupture of the plaque results in platelet aggregation and thrombus. ACS will be discussed later in this chapter.

In the case of coronary artery spasm, also known as Prinzmetal's variant angina, underlying coronary artery stenosis may be absent. Ischemia occurs because of transient focal decreased oxygen supply unrelated to oxygen demand. The length of time the artery is in spasm determines the severity of ischemia and often occurs at rest.

Ischemia can occur with no pain at all and is referred to as silent angina. Silent angina is particularly common in diabetics, suggesting that pain receptors may be altered in this condition. An alarming 80 percent of patients have episodes of asymptomatic ischemia. Asymptomatic ischemia has the same prognosis as symptomatic patients.

Syndrome X refers to patients with classic angina symptoms without angiographic evidence of CAD. Evidence of ischemia is demonstrated on diagnostic evaluation such as stress electrocardiogram (ECG), nuclear scans, and echocardiogram. The etiology of this disorder is unknown. The hypothesis is that small vessels, too small to be visualized on angiogram, are unable to dilate effectively during episodes of increased myocardial oxygen demand (Asbury & Collins, 2005).

Assessment with Clinical Manifestations

Clinical manifestations of CAD include angina pectoris, ACS, and SCD (Figure 24-2). These manifestations develop when the myocardial demand for oxygen exceeds the coronary arteries ability to supply the heart with adequate oxygen to meet the demand. This results in myocardial ischemia. Myocardial oxygen supply is dependent on the blood's oxygen-carrying capacity and the rate of blood flow. Myocardial oxygen demand is dependent on ventricular wall stress, heart rate, and contractility. Ischemia can occur because of any factor or condition that disrupts the delicate balance between myocardial oxygen supply and demand (e.g., anemia, aortic stenosis, CAD, cardiomyopathy, cardiogenic shock, arrhythmias, or vasculitis).

The usual response to increased oxygen demand is increased oxygen supply through coronary artery dilation and increased blood flow rate. In CAD, the stenotic and hardened coronary arteries are unable to meet the increased oxygen demand. This is because of their inability to effectively dilate and because the artery beyond the obstruction is already chronically dilated. A coronary artery with a significant stenosis may be able to meet low oxygen demands at rest, but it is usually unable to meet any increase in oxygen demand caused by precipitating factors, such as exercise. A significant stenosis is defined as luminal narrowing greater than 70 percent for a major coronary artery or greater than 50 percent of the left main coronary artery. In addition, diseased hearts are unable to significantly increase the rate of blood flow.

At the cellular level, ischemic myocardial cells convert from aerobic to anaerobic metabolism. Anaerobic metabolism produces lactic acid and other by-products that accumulate. These factors are believed to stimulate peripheral pain receptors in the cervical and thoracic distribution accounting for typical anginal pain (Rizzo, 2006).

The health care provider must learn to assess patients with angina and to examine the variety of clinical manifestations exhibited with anginal episodes. There needs to be an expedient nature in this process because of the potential for deteriorating symptomology. The most important step in the evaluation of CAD is a detailed health history obtained from the patient. Angina is usually the first presenting symptom in patients with CAD. It is important to remember that women, diabetics, and elderly patients may not present with typical angina pain. The five assessment components of symptoms are quality, location, duration, factors that precipitate the symptoms, and factors that relieve the symptoms. The nurse asks open ended questions to assess angina symptoms. The following memory aid can be used to organize questions (Table 24-3).

Angina pain quality is typically described as pressure, heavy, squeezing, constrictive, suffocating, vise-like, or "like an elephant sitting on my chest." Angina is rarely described as pain. Episodes may vary from mild to severe. Several symptoms may accompany angina pain including nausea, diaphoresis, shortness of breath, fatigue, dizziness, weakness, and anxiety. Anginal pain is not stabbing or sharp and does not change with respirations, position change, or pressure applied to the chest wall. To demonstrate anginal pain, the patient may place a clenched fist over the sternum. This is referred to as the **Levine's sign,** the universal sign for angina.

The location of angina is usually substernal or on the left side of the chest. Radiation to the epigastrium, neck, jaw, shoulders, arms, or back is common. Indigestion-like pain and pain between the shoulder blades may be dismissed by the patient as not being cardiac in origin. Pain above the jaw, below the upper abdomen, and a small focal area in the chest is rarely angina.

Angina is precipitated by activity, emotional stress, cold weather, or a large meal. Stable angina is steady discomfort that lasts several minutes, not usually more than 5 to 10 minutes, and more than a second or two. Angina is usually relieved by rest or elimination of the event that precipitated the episode or with use of sublingual nitroglycerin. Pain that lasts for hours or days or is fleeting is rarely angina. The extent that angina effects patient's daily living activities is important for grading and risk stratification (Table 24-4). In addition to assessment of symptoms, careful history taking includes medical, surgical, family and social history, habits, current medications, allergies, and a thorough review of systems. The nurse probes for the presence of risk factors and educational opportunities.

The physical assessment includes examination, auscultation, palpation, and percussion of the chest, abdomen, skin, and extremities. Obtain a complete set of vital signs including temperature, blood pressure, heart rate, respiratory rate, ECG tracing, and oxygen saturation. If there is the opportunity to examine the patient during an episode of angina, transient signs of myocardial ischemia may be present. Observe the patient for signs of anxiety and pain.

TABLE 24-3 PQRST

P	Precipitating event	What brings on your discomfort? How far can you walk, climb stairs, or exercise before you have discomfort? What relieves your discomfort?
Q	Quality	What does the discomfort feel like? Are there any other associated symptoms?
R	Radiation	Where is the discomfort located? Does the discomfort go anywhere else on your body?
S	Severity	On a scale of 1–10, with 10 being the most severe discomfort, can you rate your discomfort?
T	Timing	When did the discomfort begin? How long did the discomfort last? Have you had this discomfort before? How has the discomfort changed over time?

Adapted from Estes, M. (2006). Health assessment and physical examination *(3rd ed.). New York: Thomson Delmar Learning.*

TABLE 24-4	**Grading of Angina Pectoris**
Class I	Ordinary physical activity does not cause angina, such as walking, climbing stairs. Angina with strenuous, rapid, or prolonged exertion at work or recreation.
Class II	Slight limitation of ordinary activity. Angina occurs on walking or climbing stairs rapidly, walking uphill, walking or stair climbing after meals, in cold, in wind, under emotional stress, or only during the few hours after awakening. Angina occurs on walking more than two blocks on the level and climbing more than one flight of ordinary stairs at a normal pace and in normal condition.
Class III	Marked limitation of ordinary physical activity. Angina occurs on walking one to two blocks on the level and climbing one flight of stairs in normal conditions at a normal pace.
Class IV	Inability to carry on any physical activity without discomfort. Angina symptoms may be present at rest.

Adapted from DeLaune, S., & Ladner, P. (2006). Fundamentals of nursing (3rd ed.). New York: Thomson Delmar Learning.

Increased heart rate, blood pressure, temperature, and diaphoresis reflect increased sympathetic response. Auscultation of heart tones may reveal an S_4 gallop due to decreased ventricular compliance. The patient may appear short of breath, auscultation of heart tones may reveal an S_3 gallop, and lungs may reveal bibasilar inspiratory crackles. These findings are due to an increase in end diastolic pressure from reduction in ventricular systolic contractility and diastolic relaxation leading to pulmonary congestion. Auscultation of a systolic murmur of mitral origin occurs with dysfunction of the papillary muscles. With decreased cardiac output because of cardiac ischemia, pale, cool, cyanotic skin; diminished pulses; fatigue; weakness; and confusion may be present.

Between episodes of angina, the physical examination may be completely normal. Clues to risk factors may be found, such as hypertension and hyperlipidemia xanthomas. Noncardiac sources of chest pain may become evident. For example, pain with palpation of the chest wall points to a musculoskeletal source of chest pain.

Diagnostic Tests

A variety of noninvasive and invasive tests are available to diagnose CAD and angina. Specificity and sensitivity for predicting CAD vary among tests and are used in conjunction with the patient's history, severity of symptoms, physical examination, and risk stratification to determine the next level of diagnostic testing and interventions. Nurses are instrumental in the collaborative management and patient education of patient's undergoing diagnostic testing.

Differential Diagnoses for Angina

Angina can be confused with other conditions and can be mimicked with the traditional discomfort of angina pectoris. Chest pain related to gastrointestinal (GI) disease is usually brought on by certain foods and unrelated to exercise. Musculoskeletal pain is usually described as a discreet spot on the chest wall, increases with palpation, varies with changes in position, and is relieved with nonsteroidal anti-inflammatory drugs (NSAIDs), not nitroglycerin. Pleuritic pain due to pericarditis or pulmonary disease is usually sharp, changes with respirations, and is associated with a friction rub. Careful assessment can help distinguish between myocardial ischemia pain and other disorders.

Electrocardiogram

The 12-lead ECG is a recording of the electrical activity of the heart. ECG recordings are one of the most useful tools to identify and locate areas of ischemia or infarction of the heart. During an episode of angina, T wave flattening or inversions and ST segment depression may be seen on the ECG due to subendocardial ischemia. When angina subsides, the ECG changes resolve.

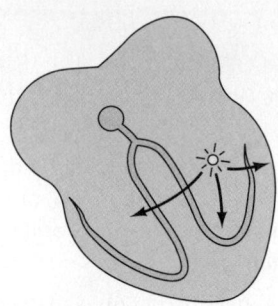

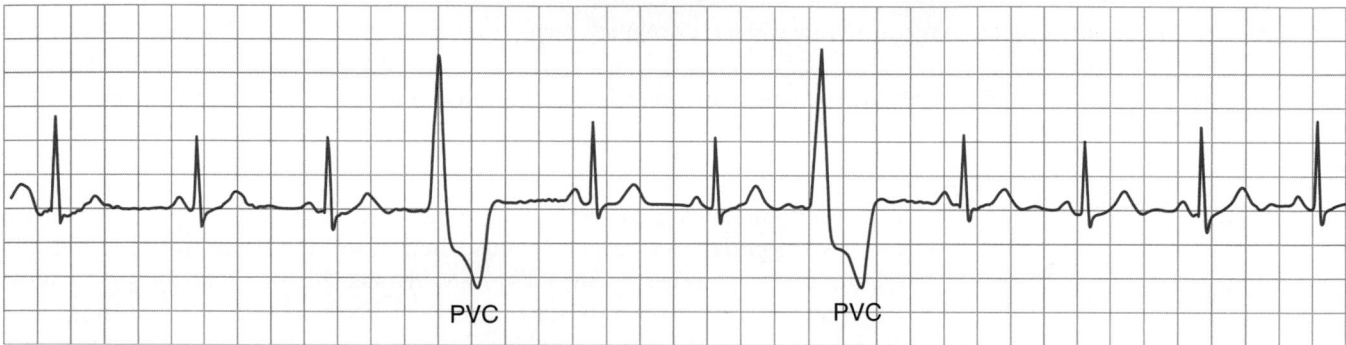

Figure 24-3 Premature ventricular contractions interrupting the normal sinus rhythm.

Between episodes of angina the ECG is usually normal or may reveal evidence of CAD or concomitant cardiac disease. For example, pathological Q waves indicate previous MI, the risk factor hypertension is indicated by left ventricular hypertrophy, and arrhythmias and bundle branch blocks may be related to CAD or other cardiac conditions. Another example of abnormal electrophysiology is the development of premature ventricular contractions that may indicate the patient's increasing abnormal electrical susceptibility, which could indicate pathology (Figure 24-3).

Holter Monitor

Continuous ambulatory ECG recordings with a Holter monitor can be used in the outpatient setting to capture ischemic episodes. The Holter monitor is a device that has ECG leads and a mechanical memory that records the ECG while the patient is participating in his or her normal daily activities. The patient can keep a journal of his or her activities, and the Holter monitor records the ECG. Then, the care provider examines the relationship between the activities and the ECG pattern to see if there is a positive correlation between the two variables. In addition, the monitor will detect the frequency of rhythms and the types of rhythms during the time of the Holter monitors' use (Stone, 2005).

Chest X-Ray

Although not diagnostic, the chest x-ray (CXR) can reveal clues to CAD, such as, heart enlargement, calcifications of the aorta, and pulmonary vascular congestion. CXR may also identify noncardiac causes of chest pain, for example rib fractures.

Laboratory Tests

A laboratory test to diagnose stable angina is not currently available. Cardiac markers can diagnose MI and are discussed later in this chapter. A CBC and chemistries are helpful in identifying other diseases in the differential diagnosis. Homocysteine and C-reactive protein levels may be elevated. Screening for risk factors may be indicated, such as lipid panel and glycohemoglobin.

ECG Stress Test

Because a rest ECG obtained during or between episodes of angina may be normal, an ECG exercise stress test is a valuable diagnostic tool for assessing presence and location of ischemia. The ECG stress test is a simple, cost-effective tool, with a high specificity to rule out patients with low risk or low likelihood of having CAD. This test is also used to evaluate effectiveness of therapy and determine need for referral for further more invasive and expensive testing. During this test, the patient is attached to an ECG monitor and exercises on a treadmill or stationary bicycle to progressively higher workloads. During the test, the patient is monitored for chest discomfort or dyspnea. Heart rate and ECG tracing are continuously recorded, and blood pressure is checked at regular intervals. The test is continued until the patient reaches 85 percent of age-predicted maximal heart rate. Interpretation of the test includes the patient's symptomatic response, exercise capacity, hemodynamic response, and ECG recordings. This test is considered positive if the patient's typical angina develops, or abnormalities consistent with ischemia develop on the ECG. Patients with markedly positive tests are more likely to have severe, multivessel coronary disease. Use of medications, such as beta blockers, calcium channel blockers, digoxin, and antihypertensive medications, may affect the test results. The health care provider may ask the patient to hold these medications before the test unless the purpose of the test is to evaluate the effectiveness of such therapy.

Stress Echocardiogram

Similar to ECG recordings, echocardiographic images between episodes of angina may be normal. Therefore the exercise stress echocardiogram is a useful tool to assess for the presence and location of ischemia demonstrated by wall motion abnormalities. First an echocardiogram is performed with the patient at rest. Like the stress ECG, the patient then exercises on a treadmill or stationary bike to progressively higher workloads. Immediately following exercise, an echocardiogram is repeated. Then the preexercise and postexercise echocardiographic images are compared. Ischemic areas of the heart are identified by regional wall motion and contractility abnormalities including hypokinesis (reduced wall motion), akinesis (absence of wall motion), dyskinesis (paradoxical wall motion), and absence of wall thickening during systole. Echocardiograms can identify additional evidence of ischemia, such as papillary muscle dysfunction, increased end diastolic pressures, and ventricular aneurysms with or without thrombus (Daniels, 2003).

Pharmacological Stress Tests

Pharmacological stress testing is used for patients unable to exercise and uses various agents to simulate the stress of exercise. Dobutamine, an inotrope, increases myocardial oxygen demand by stimulating the heart rate and force of contraction. Use of vasodilators, dipyridamole, or adenosine, are also used to increase myocardial oxygen demand. Dipyridamole blocks the cellular uptake of adenosine and thereby increases its circulating concentration. Vasodilation occurs when adenosine binds to its vascular receptors. As ischemic regions are already maximally dilated, the drug-induced vasodilation increases flow to the myocardium perfused by healthy coronary arteries and steals blood away from the diseased segments. ECG recordings and echocardiograms following injection of these pharmacological agents reveal areas of ischemia similar to the results achieved by exercising the patient (Daniels, 2003).

Nuclear Scans

Nuclear scans are used to assess for presence and location of ischemia, as well as, the extent of infarcted myocardium due to MI. A radioactive tracer is injected intravenously immediately following stress with exercise or pharmacological agents and followed by scanning. The scan follows the tracer as blood flows throughout the myocardium. Nuclear perfusion imaging displays ischemic myocardium as regions of relatively decreased perfusion called defects or cold spots. Scans can be repeated in 12 to 24 hours to evaluate if the defect is reversible (ischemic) or fixed (infarcted). Ischemic regions, or reversible defects, are reperfused and no longer appear as cold spots on repeat imaging. Fixed defects or infarcted areas do not reperfuse and continue to appear as cold spots on repeat imaging. This information is also used to determine areas of reversible ischemia or viable myocardium that is amendable to reperfusion interventions.

Coronary Angiography

Coronary angiogram, or heart catheterization, is an invasive procedure that is considered the gold standard for diagnosis of CAD. This procedure directly visualizes the coronary artery anatomy and assesses hemodynamic parameters and ventricular function. A right-sided heart catheterization involves a catheter placed through a vein, advanced to the heart, and injection of radiopaque contrast to evaluated hemodynamic parameters. A left-sided heart catheterization involves a catheter placed through an artery, advanced to the coronary arteries, and injection of radiopaque contrast to visualize coronary artery anatomy. During this procedure, a ventriculogram can be performed by injection of radiopaque dye into the left ventricle to assess function. Fluoroscopic visualization of the coronary arteries defines the location and severity of blockages. The ventriculogram identifies areas of wall motion and contractility abnormalities. Coronary angiogram is the only definitive test to diagnose coronary spasm or variant angina. Results of this study are used to determine treatment options and prognosis.

Other Diagnostic Studies

There are several emerging diagnostic studies on the horizon. Positron emission tomography (PET) is used to evaluate cardiac metabolism and to assess tissue perfusion. Magnetic resonance imaging (MRI) helps identify the site and extent of an MI, assess the effects of reperfusion therapy, and differentiate reversible and irreversible tissue injury. Electron beam computed tomography (EBCT) can identify patients at risk for developing CAD by revealing coronary plaque. The efficacy for routine use of these tests in diagnosis and treatment of CAD is not currently established.

Nursing Diagnoses

Based on the information gathered, examples of nursing diagnoses in the patient with CAD may include the following:
- Acute pain (angina) related to the imbalance between myocardial oxygen supply and demand.
- Ineffective tissue perfusion related to myocardial ischemia and decreased cardiac output.
- Anxiety related to pain, perceived threat of death, possible lifestyle changes, and diagnosis of CAD.
- Activity intolerance related to angina, pulmonary congestion, fatigue, and inadequate tissue perfusion.
- Ineffective therapeutic regimen management related to lack of knowledge related to disease process, prognosis, and treatment strategies.

Planning and Implementation

CAD is a multisystem dysfunction disorder and consequently requires prioritizing the care for patients with this pathology. The plan of care is complex, and the responses to the nursing care require nurses to use critical decision-making skills at their highest level.

Goals

Treatment of stable angina has two main goals. The first goal is to improve quality of life by decreasing episodes of angina and ischemia. The second goal is to increase quantity of life by preventing progression to MI and death.

Collaborative Management

Collaborative management with a multidisciplinary team approach is essential for the management of CAD. Treatment of stable angina focuses on use of medications, risk factor modification, and patient and family education. The nurse plays an active role in the collaborative management of patients with CAD. In addition, nurses play an active role in research to improve patient care. For example, a recent nursing research study focused on documenting the knowledge about cardiovascular disease and acute myocardial infarction (AMI) symptoms in older individuals with coronary heart disease. The study found that more than 95 percent of the older men and women knew typical symptoms of and AMI, such as jaw pain, pressure, shortness of breath, arm or shoulder pain, and sweating. Less than 75 percent of both men and women knew that symptoms such as neck pain, nausea or vomiting, back pain, heartburn, and jaw pain could be symptoms of AMI. The article concluded that education and counseling of older patients at high risk for heart disease should emphasize atypical symptoms (Tullman & Dracup, 2005).

Pharmacology

Three classifications of pharmacological agents are used to prevent angina: nitrates, beta-adrenergic blockers, and calcium channel blockers. These agents decrease the workload of the heart and increase myocardial perfusion. Three classifications of pharmacological agents are used to prevent MI and death: antiplatelets, angiotensin-converting enzyme (ACE) inhibitors, and therapy that lowers lipids levels (Table 24-5).

Cardiac medications potentially have serious consequences in their effects. The nurse must administer cardiac medications safely and realize the severe nature of the administration of this category of medications (see Safety First feature).

Nitrates increase oxygen delivery and reduce myocardial oxygen demand through reduction in preload and afterload while vasodilating coronary arteries. Nitrates dilate coronary arteries and collateral vessels increasing blood flow and oxygen delivery to the myocardium. In addition, nitrates cause venodilation, thus decreasing preload and the amount of blood returning to the heart, which in turn reduces myocardial workload. Finally, nitrates dilate peripheral arteries and reduce systemic blood pressure. This reduces systemic vascular resistance, the pressure the heart has to pump against, which in turn decreases myocardial workload. Reduction in myocardial workload translates to decreased oxygen demand.

Nitrates are available in various preparations for acute treatment and prevention of angina. Pills or sprays are used sublingually for immediate relief of angina during an acute episode (see Red Flag feature). These preparations may also be used as a preventive measure taken several minutes prior to an activity that typically triggers an angina attack. Long-acting preparations are used to prevent recurrence of angina and are available as oral and topical preparations. Nitrate tolerance is overcome with nitrate-free intervals daily. Common side effects include headache, hypotension, and palpitations from reflex tachycardia. Reflex tachycardia can be controlled with concomitant use of beta blockers.

Beta-adrenergic antagonists block the catecholamine stimulation of β_1 receptors in the heart responsible for increased inotropy (force of contraction) and chronotropy (heart rate). β_1 blockade decreases the force of myocardial contraction and slows the heart rate. In addition, beta blockers reduce

---

Red Flag

Patient Education for Anginal Episodes

- Stop activity, sit or lie down.
- Place one nitroglycerin tablet under the tongue and allow to dissolve. (Do not chew.)
- Tablet will cause a tingling sensation, heart pounding, flushing, and headache.
- Stay in resting position for 15 to 20 minutes and get up slowly after taking nitroglycerin to prevent fainting from postural hypotension.
- If angina is not relieved in five minutes, the dose may be repeated two times at five-minute intervals for a total of three doses.
- If angina is not relieved after three doses, seek immediate medical attention.
- Report angina that increases in frequency, lasts longer, limits previous level of activity, and occurs at rest.
- Carry tablets at all times.

Source: Broyles, B. E., Reiss, B. S., & Evans, M. E. (2007). Pharmacological aspects of nursing care (7th ed.). New York: Thomson Delmar Learning.

TABLE 24-5   Common Medications for the Treatment of CAD

DRUG	ACTION	NURSING CONSIDERATIONS
Nitrates Nitroglycerin (SL, PO, Spray, Patch, IV) Isosorbide dinitrate (Isordil) Isosorbide mononitrate (Imdur)	Vasodilation of coronary arteries Venodilation: decreases preload Arterial dilation: decrease afterload	Have patient lie down when taking SL form Monitor for hypotension Monitor for headaches Allow 8–12 hours drug free interval for PO/Top routes to prevent tolerance IV is titrated to effect and replaced with PO/Top usually if symptom free for 24 hours Topical nitrate application sites should be visible areas, hairless, and rotated. Clean excess from skin when patch removed. Wear gloves when contact with drug is anticipated Instruct patient to avoid use of phosphodiesterase inhibitors (Viagra/Cialis) within 24 hours of nitrate use due to severe hypotension reaction
Beta blockers Nonselective blocker β_1 and β_2: Atenolol (Tenormin) Selective blocker β_1: Metoprolol (Lopressor, Toprol XL):	Decrease inotropy and chronotropy Decrease afterload Increased diastolic time increases coronary perfusion	Titrated to target HR 50–60 Monitor for symptomatic bradycardia, hypotension, prolonged PR interval, high-degree heart blocks, heart failure Monitor for shortness of breath and wheezing Assess for noncompliance related to fatigue and sexual dysfunction
Calcium-channel blockers *Nondihydropyridines* Verapamil hydrochloride (Calan, Isoptin) Diltiazem hydrochloride (Cardizem) *Dihydropyridines* Amlodipine (Norvasc) Nifedipine (Procardia) Nicardipine (Cardene)	Decrease inotropy and chronotropy Decrease preload and afterload Coronary artery dilation Prevent vasospasm	Monitor for symptomatic bradycardia, hypotension, prolonged PR interval, high-degree heart blocks Monitor for edema Implement constipation prevention strategies (i.e., fiber, stool softeners)
Antiplatelet agents Aspirin 75–325 mg/day	Aspirin: inhibits thromboxane stimulated platelet aggregation Anti-inflammatory	Prevent gastric irritation: use enteric-coated or buffered preparations, give with food, monitor for GI bleeding Take for life
Angiotensin I converting enzyme inhibitors (ACEI) Captopril (Capoten) Benazepril (Lotensin) Enalapril (Vasotec) Fosinopril (Monopril) Lisinopril (Prinivil, Zestril) Ramipril (Altace)	Block the enzyme that converts angiotensin I to angiotensin II Decrease preload and afterload Promote endothelial vasodilatory and antithrombotic actions	Monitor for hypotension, hyperkalemia, and renal failure Cough is a common side effect
Lipid-altering agents *HMG CoA reductase inhibitors* (Statins) Atorvastatin (Lipitor) Fluvastatin (Lescol) Lovastatin (Mevacor) Pravastatin (Pravachol) Rosuvastatin (Crestor) Simvastatin (Zocor)	Improve endothelial function and stabilize plaque Block liver synthesis of cholesterol Decrease LDL 18–55 percent Increase HDL 5–15 percent Decrease TG 7–30 percent	Monitor liver function studies, eye exams for opacities, and evaluate for myopathy Take at bedtime when cholesterol is synthesized by liver

Continued

TABLE 24-5	**Common Medications for the Treatment of CAD—cont'd**	
DRUG	**ACTION**	**NURSING CONSIDERATIONS**
Bile acid sequestrants Cholestyramine (Questran) Colestipol (Colestid) Colesevelam (Welchol)	Bind bile acids in intestines: removal of lipids in feces Decrease LDL 15–30 percent Increase HDL 3–5 percent	Gritty taste GI disturbances common (nausea, dyspepsia, flatulence, constipation) Take 30 minutes before meals Interfere with absorption of other drugs. Take other drugs one hour before or four hours after
Niacin Nicotinic acid (Niacin, Niaspan, Slo-niacin)	Inhibits liver secretion of lipoproteins and decrease synthesis by decreasing release of free fatty acids from adipose tissue Decrease LDL 5–25 percent Increase HDL 15–35 percent Decrease TG 20–50 percent	Hot flashes and pruritus: Take aspirin 30 minutes to one hour before drug and after food GI disturbances (nausea, vomiting, diarrhea): take with food Monitor for gout, hyperglycemia, liver dysfunction Take at bedtime
Fibric acid derivatives Clofibrate (Atromid) Fenofibrate (Tricor) Gemfibrozil (Lopid)	Decrease liver synthesis and secretion of VLDL Decrease LDL 5–20 percent Increase HDL 10–35 percent Decrease TG 20–50 percent	Mild GI disturbances (nausea, diarrhea) Monitor for gallstones, myopathy (especially if combined with statins) Increases effects of anticoagulants and hypoglycemics
Cholesterol absorption inhibitor Ezetimibe (Zetia)	Inhibit intestinal absorption of cholesterol Decrease LDL 15–20 percent Increase HDL 4–9 percent Decrease TG 8 percent	Monitor for fatigue, headache, abdominal pain, and diarrhea Monitor for liver dysfunction especially if combined with statins

Adapted from Broyles, B. E., Reiss, B. S., & Evans, M. E. (2007). Pharmacological aspects of nursing care (7th ed.). New York: Thomson Delmar Learning.

blood pressure, decreasing afterload and myocardial oxygen demand. Reduction in myocardial contraction force also decreases myocardial oxygen demand. Slowing of the heart rate increases time in diastole when coronary perfusion occurs, thus improving oxygen supply.

Usually beta blockers are well-tolerated with few side effects. Beta blockers can cause varying degrees of heart block. Also beta blockers can blunt the usual tachycardia related to catecholamine-mediated triggers, such as exercise, fever, and hypoglycemia. Blockade of β_2 receptors of the bronchial tree can precipitate bronchospasm, especially in patients with pulmonary obstructive diseases. Fatigue and sexual dysfunction are common causes of noncompliance.

Calcium channel blockers reduce the influx of calcium through calcium channels of smooth muscle cells causing vasodilatation and cardiac depression. There are two classifications of calcium channel blockers, dihydropyridine or nondihydropyridine. Dihydropyridines are vasodilators that decrease oxygen demand by venodilation, decreasing preload and arterial dilation, decreasing afterload. Dihydropyridines increase oxygen supply by coronary artery dilatation. These agents are also used in the treatment of variant angina to prevent vasospasm. In addition to being vasodilators, nondihydropyridines reduce myocardial oxygen demand by decreasing force of contraction and slowing the heart rate (Broyles, Reiss, & Evans, 2007).

Short-acting and immediate-release calcium channel blockers increase the risk of adverse cardiac events. Therefore, only long-acting calcium channel blockers are recommended in the treatment of stable angina. Calcium channel blockers can be added to beta blockers when symptoms are not controlled with beta blockers alone or in place of beta blockers if adverse side effects develop. Combination

Safety First

Safely Administrating Cardiac Medications

A patient has the following medication order: Lopressor 50 mg PO BID hold for heart rate less than 60, systemic blood pressure less than 100. The following are steps to take to ensure patient safety?

1. **Five rights:** Begin administration using the five rights for medication administration (right patient, right medication, right dose, right time, and right route).

2. **Right parameter:** Know the ordered holding and administration parameters and contraindications to administering medications. For example, you would not administer an antihypertensive medication to a patient that is hypotensive even if a hold parameter was not ordered.

3. **Right response:** Did the patient respond to the medication they way you anticipated. For example, did the blood pressure maintain within goal, is it still too high, or did it drop too low? The nurse's role in administering medication is not over after the patient receives the medication. It is the role of the nurse to ensure that the patient does not suffer any adverse effects and goals are met as a result of the medication.

4. **Right of the patient to be educated:** All patients should be fully educated regarding their medications including the name, dosage, frequency, route, action, potential side effects to report, any ongoing monitoring that will be required, and applicable food and drug interactions. Tip: Teach or reinforce some information with each administration. Example, "Mr. Jones, this is your Lopressor 50 mg dose that you take in the morning and before bedtime. It is being used to treat your hypertension. I want to make sure your blood pressure does not go too low so I will be checking your blood pressure regularly. Checking your blood pressure regularly will also be important when you go home. Please let me know if you feel dizzy because that can be a sign your blood pressure is too low."

5. **Right documentation:** Document the drug administration, patient's response, reason held if applicable, health care provider communication, and patient education.

6. **Right reporting:** Report to health care provider and hospital reporting systems, when appropriate: inadequate patient response, side effects or adverse drug reactions, and medication errors. Reporting of adverse drug reactions and errors via appropriate systems is important to improve processes to reduce future adverse events.

Adapted from Broyles, B. E., Reiss, B. S., & Evans, M. E. (2007). Pharmacological aspects of nursing care *(7th ed.). New York: Thomson Delmar Learning; DeLaune, S., & Ladner, P. (2006).* Fundamentals of nursing *(3rd ed.). New York: Thomson Delmar Learning.*

of calcium channel blockers and beta blockers must be done with caution because of the negative chronotropic and inotropic effects that increase the risk of high degree heart block and precipitation of heart failure, respectively. Other side effects include edema, constipation, headache, and hypotension.

Aspirin is routinely used in the treatment of CAD and prevention of MI. Antithrombotic effects of aspirin are related to the irreversible inhibition of cyclooxygenase (COX) and synthesis of platelet thromboxane A_2 inhibiting platelet aggregation. This effect lasts for the life of the platelet. Additionally, aspirin's anti-inflammatory effects are believed to stabilize atherosclerotic plaque. Unless contraindicated, such as allergy or GI irritation, aspirin is continued indefinitely. In cases of aspirin intolerance or allergy, clopidogrel (Plavix) is an alternative antiplatelet therapy for stable angina. Clopidogrel blocks adenosine diphosphate (ADP)-mediated platelet aggregation.

ACE inhibitors block the enzyme responsible for converting angiotensin I to angiotensin II. This effect decreases preload and afterload reducing myocardial oxygen demand. In addition, ACE inhibition promotes endothelial vasodilatory and antithrombotic functions. Cough, renal failure, hyperkalemia, and hypotension are some side effects. Angiotensin receptor blockers (ARBs) are alternatives for patients with intolerance to ACE inhibitors due to persistent cough. ARBs block angiotensin receptors directly with a similar effect as ACE inhibitors on preload and afterload reduction. With the exception of cough, side effects are also similar.

Various studies have demonstrated that lipid lowering agents, especially statins, reduce adverse events and slow the progression of CAD. In addition to lipid lowering effects, statins have actions that improve endothelial function, stabilize atherosclerotic plaque, lower inflammatory markers, and alter thrombogenic mechanisms (Grundy, et al., 2004). Various lipid lowering agents are available. These agents are used alone or in combination to achieve goal lipid levels.

Initiation of beta blockade and ACE inhibitors within 72 hours of onset of an AMI reduces ventricular remodeling and mortality. These agents should be continued indefinitely unless the patient develops complications from the medications.

Surgery

There are a number of surgical interventions used in the treatment of CAD. Some are much less invasive and have quick recovery time, with few complications. Other surgical interventions require immediate care in the coronary care unit (CCU) and have a much greater percentage of patients who experience complications. The following section presents information from least invasive to most invasive in nature.

Percutaneous coronary interventions (PCI) are commonly used for the treatment of significant CAD and emergent treatment in AMI. The advantage of PCI includes low mortality and morbidity, minimal discomfort, short hospital stay, short recovery time, and early return to work. Percutaneous transluminal coronary angioplasty (PTCA) is performed during the heart catheterization procedure (Figure 24-4). Under fluoroscopy, a guidewire followed by a catheter is advanced into the stenotic section of the coronary artery. Then the balloon at the end of the catheter is inflated under high pressure. This compresses the plaque against the vessel wall increasing lumen size. The improvement in size of the coronary lumen increases coronary perfusion and myocardial oxygen supply. Additional PCI techniques to remove atheromatous material for specific lesions include use of rotating blades or burrs, transluminal extraction catheters (TEC), laser therapy, and directional coronary atherectomy (DCA). Unfortunately, PTCA has a restenosis rate of approximately 50 percent. However, new PCI catheters, guidewires, techniques, stents, and drug therapy are areas of aggressive research and continue to evolve as promising advances in the arena of PCI (Campbell & Torrance, 2005).

Due to a high restenosis rate, PTCA is rarely performed alone and frequently combined with stent placement. Stents are stainless steel mesh-like devices deployed at the site of stenosis with the balloon catheter. The stent acts like a scaffold to hold the artery open. Common medications to prevent acute restenosis include preprocedure aspirin and loading doses of platelet ADP-

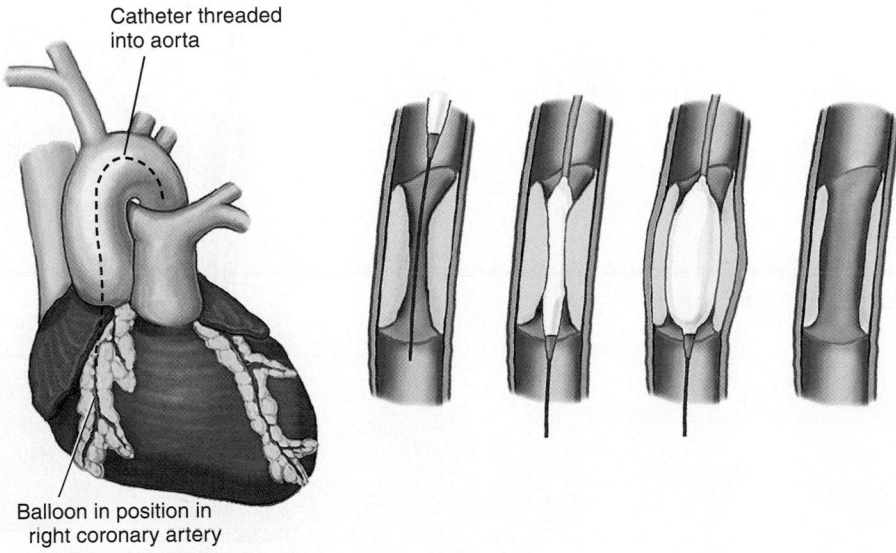

Catheter threaded into aorta

Balloon in position in right coronary artery

Figure 24-4 PTCA.

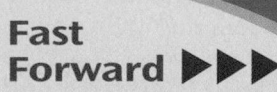

Fast Forward ▶▶▶

Gene Therapy

Gene therapy is an exciting new field of research for the treatment of CAD (Puddu, Cravero, Puddu, & Muscari, 2005). Gene transfer by direct intracoronary injection is intended to stimulate angiogenesis and development of collateral circulation. Results of preliminary studies show evidence of angina prevention measured by an increase in exercise tolerance and gene therapy appears to be safe.

receptor inhibitors (clopidogrel [Plavix]), heparin during the procedure, glycoprotein (GP) IIb/IIa receptor blockers (abciximab [ReoPro], eptifibatide [Integrilin], tirobifan [Aggrastat]) during and postprocedure, and long-term use of aspirin and ADP-receptor inhibitors. Use of drug-eluding stents has significantly decreased restenosis rates. Drug-eluding stents are coated with a drug, such as sirolimus, that reduce the intimal smooth muscle proliferation responsible for restenosis. Intracoronary radiation therapy (brachytherapy) is a promising PCI treatment for restenosis (Campbell & Torrance, 2005).

Patients undergoing PCI have preprocedure and postprocedure care similar to the diagnostic cardiac catheterization patient. Postprocedure care includes continuous ECG monitoring and frequent vital signs, access site checks, distal circulation evaluation, and pain assessment. Monitor closely for potential complications such as artery restenosis or dissection or rupture, access site bleeding or hematoma or pseudoaneurysms, retroperitoneal bleed, thromboembolism, contrast dye allergic reaction, and renal failure. Discharge teaching must include stressing the importance of continuing antiplatelet therapy with aspirin and ADP-inhibitor agent (clopidogrel) long term to prevent restenosis. Patients are usually discharged the day after PCI.

Coronary artery bypass grafting (CABG) is a surgical procedure in which veins and arteries are used as conduit to bypass the coronary artery stenosis. Common conduits harvested for bypass grafting are the internal mammary arteries (IMA) from the chest, radial arteries from the arms, and saphenous veins (SVG) from the legs (Figure 24-5). CABG is indicated for patients with, significant left main or left main equivalent disease (greater than 70 percent proximal left anterior descending and left circumflex artery), significant three vessel disease especially with reduced left ventricular ejection fraction, significant proximal left anterior descending with one or two vessel disease. Surgical revascularization is considered for patients based on factors such as surgical risk, location of significant lesions, extent of CAD, cardiac function, adequate targets for graft placement, availability of adequate conduit, and morbid conditions.

The CABG procedure is traditionally performed via a median sternotomy incision while the patient is on the cardiopulmonary bypass (CPB) machine. On entry to the operating room, the patient is anesthetized, intubated, prepped, and lined. The CPB machine is used to anticoagulate, cool, oxygenate, and circulate the blood while the heart is stopped for surgery. A cardioplegia solution, high in potassium, is used to perfuse the heart. This

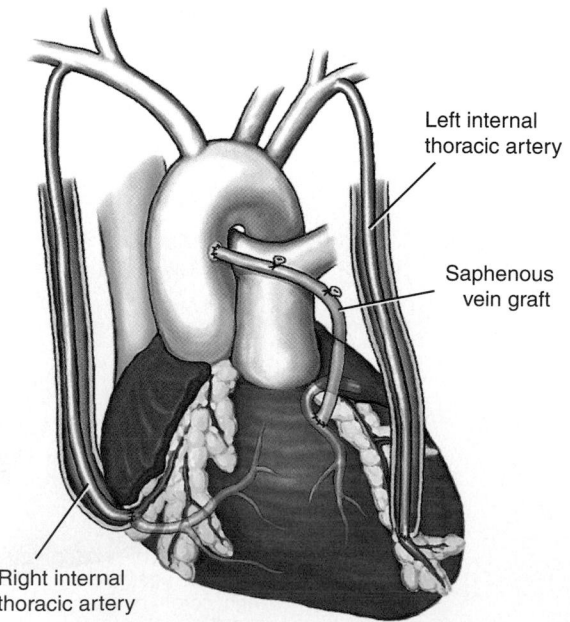

Left internal thoracic artery

Saphenous vein graft

Right internal thoracic artery

Figure 24-5 CABG: Internal mammary (thoracic) artery and saphenous vein anastomosed to coronary arteries.

Common Discharge Instructions Following CABG

The nurse can teach the patient to do the following after discharge of having a CABG:

- Do not lift, push, or pull anything greater than 5 to 10 pounds for four to six weeks.
- Do not drive for four to six weeks.
- Do not sit behind the air bag for four to six weeks.
- Return to work as prescribed by the health care provider usually in four to six weeks.
- Follow cardiac rehab instructions regarding walking (e.g., increasing walking time by 5 min/week until walking 20 to 30 min three to four times a week).
- Resume sexual activity when physical exercise is tolerated well (e.g., able to climb two flights of stairs comfortably).
- Monitor the incision for signs or symptoms of infection.
- The bulge at the top of the sternal incision is normal and will go away in four to six weeks.
- Do not soak in water until incision is completely healed; wash gently; do not apply creams or powder to incisions.
- Avoid hot water while showering, because it can make you dizzy.
- Continue prescribed medications, aspirin, beta blockers, statins, and ACE inhibitors, to reduce adverse events.
- Depression is common and usually resolves in four to six weeks.
- Call health care provider for signs of infection, recurrent angina, shortness of breath not relieved with rest, weight gain greater than 2 to 3 pounds for two to three days, severe fatigue for two to three days, fast or slow heart rate, pain that gets worse with deep breathing.

process reduces myocardial oxygen consumption and myocardial ischemia while stopping the heart to provide a still operative field. Conduit is harvested from the leg, arm, or chest. Veins from the leg are reversed to prevent flow obstruction from venous valves. Veins from the leg and arteries from the arm are grafted or anastomosed to the aorta proximally and below the coronary artery stenosis distally. The distal of the IMA end is dissected and anastomosed below the coronary artery stenosis. IMAs can also be used as free grafts. In this case IMAs are harvested and grafted like veins and arm arteries. These new conduits increase myocardial oxygen supply.

Following the grafting procedure, the patient is slowly rewarmed with the CPB machine. The cardioplegia solution is flushed from the heart, and the heart begins beating. Sometimes defibrillation is required to restore normal heart rhythm. The CPB machine is weaned, and the suture sites are observed for bleeding. Then the surgeon places temporary pacing wires and chest tubes. The sternum is wired closed, and the skin is sutured. Finally the patient is transported to the recovering unit.

Based on the patient's underlying condition, availability of equipment, and health care provider training, minimally invasive techniques may be part of the CABG procedure. These techniques include surgery on the beating heart without CPB or off pump (OPCAB), access through a small or alternative incision approach, such as a mini sternotomy or a thoracotomy (MIDCAB), using scopes and robotics. Minimally invasive techniques decrease pain, length of stay, incision size, complications, and recovery time. Routine preoperative, intraoperative, and postoperative management of the CABG patient incorporate national guideline recommendations and rapid recovery principles that improve quality, reduce complications, contain costs, and decrease length of stay. An example of a rapid recovery program is displayed in Box 24-1.

Throughout the hospitalization, the nurse supports the rapid recovery principles. Also the nurse monitors for, prevents, and manages potential complications following CABG such as, bleeding, cardiac tamponade, cardiogenic or hypovolemic shock, electrolyte imbalances, respiratory or any other organ failure, arrhythmias (atrial fibrillation is most common), pain, constipation, nausea, MI, encephalopathy or stroke, and infection.

Transmyocardial laser revascularization (TMR) is a procedure in which lasers are used to create channels in the left ventricle. These channels allow blood flow from the ventricular chamber to the myocardial microcirculation immediately improving oxygen delivery to ischemic areas. Additionally, blood flow through these channels stimulates angiogenesis and development of collateral circulation which takes about three to six months. TMR can be performed percutaneously or surgically through a median sternotomy or left thoracotomy approach. Postprocedure care includes monitoring the patient for complications, such as ventricular arrhythmias, cardiac tamponade, and heart failure.

Patient and Family Teaching

The nurse also plays an active role in the education of patients and family members who have CAD. Nurses provide extensive discharge instructions for the implementation of secondary prevention strategies after heart surgeries, MIs, and other cardiovascular crises. The Patient Playbook feature highlights common discharge instructions following CABG.

In addition to the education that patients need after cardiovascular surgeries, the nurse must provide teaching to patients regarding cardiovascular risk factors. Patients need to gain an understanding that their continuing improvement from their cardiovascular pathologies is dependent on how they modify their lifestyle (see Skills 360° feature).

Modifiable risk factors for cardiovascular disease need to be focused on by the nurse when caring for patients after their surgeries and after cardiovascular crises allow their discharge from acute care. Some of the modifiable risk factors are smoking, hypertension, hyperlipidemia (nutrition), physical inactivity, obesity, and diabetes mellitus (Table 24-6).

BOX 24-1

HIGHLIGHTS OF THE CARDIAC SURGERY RAPID RECOVERY PROGRAM

- Same day admission process for elective surgery
- Minimally invasive techniques for qualifying patients decrease pain, recovery time, scar size and complications.
- Research-based standardized orders and protocols including national guideline recommendations to improve short- and long-term outcomes.
- Bloodless surgery techniques include state-of-the-art diagnostic testing, blood salvage techniques, medications to increase red blood cell production, and predonation of patient's own blood in specific cases.
- Timely extubation or removal of the breathing tube for most patients on the same day of surgery. Many patients do not remember having the breathing tube due to the use of a medication with amnesic properties.
- Pain management is accomplished by using a variety of medications and relaxation techniques. A combination of pain medications are individualized to the patient's condition and include injections of local anesthetics in the operating room, narcotics given by patch, pills, and intravenously, NSAIDs (nonnarcotic), and use of splinting techniques.
- Alternative therapy (e.g., music therapy to provide distraction and decrease pain and anxiety).
- Control of nausea and constipation with a combination of preventive and treatment medications, a specialized diet, and activity program.
- Multifaceted incision care protocol to reduce surgical site infections including standardized preoperative and intraoperative preparation procedures, daily dressing changes, showers with antibacterial soap, preventive antibiotics, and tight control of blood sugars.
- Progressive activity begins with sitting up the night of surgery and progresses as tolerated by the patient to prevent complications and aid recovery. Physical therapy, occupational therapy, speech therapy, and a specialized nutritional support team are available to assist patients with reconditioning needs.
- Aggressive pulmonary exercises led by respiratory care practitioners using a variety of breathing devices and a heart-shaped coughing pillow to prevent lung complications.
- Education: Comprehensive instruction and materials are provided regarding disease process, surgery, the hospital stay, risk factor modification, medications, and discharge instructions.
- Follow-up includes early home phone calls to reinforce education and answer questions, cardiac rehabilitation referral, home health nursing as needed, and primary and specialty health care provider appointments within the first month of discharge.

Adapted from Harkness, K., Smith, K., Taraba, L., MacKenzie, C., Gunn, E., & Arthur, H. M. (2005). Effect of a postoperative telephone intervention on attendance at intake for cardiac rehabilitation after coronary artery bypass graft surgery. Heart and Lung, *34(3), 179–186; Tsai, S., Lin, Y., & Wu S. (2005). The effect of cardiac rehabilitation on recovery of heart rate over one minute after exercise in patients with coronary artery bypass graft surgery.* Clinical Rehabilitation, *19(8), 843–849.*

Skills 360°

Risk Factor Modification

Risk factor modification will require the patient to make therapeutic lifestyle changes (TLC) to reduce future risks of cardiovascular events. The nurse plays a pivotal role in patient education. The nurse first assesses the patient's learning style, current level of knowledge, and readiness to learn. Discussion begins with instruction regarding CAD, treatment and goals to control angina and prevent MI and death. Then the nurse works together with the patient to develop an individual and realistic plan emphasizing TLC. Education is reinforced with written materials and involvement of family members. The plan should focus on assisting the patient problem solve barriers. To provide long-term support, community resources are provided including cardiac rehabilitation programs, local support programs, and web sites. Finally reassess the patient's knowledge and ability to comply with the plan. Continue to reinforce information as needed.

TABLE 24-6 Teaching Guide for CAD Risk Factor Modification	
RISK FACTOR AND PRIMARY GOAL	**TEACHING POINTS**
Smoking Goal: Complete cessation	Counsel patient and family to quit smoking and to avoid secondhand smoke Provide contact information for local smoking cessation programs Explore pharmacological aids including nicotine replacement and bupropion Enlist family and friends to support efforts Identify daily routines that trigger the urge to smoke and develop a plan to change routines by substituting other activities for smoking, i.e., exercise, meditation Substitute sugarless hard candy, gum, and vegetable sticks for the act of smoking Avoid people who smoke and common smoking places
Hypertension Goal: BP less than or equal to 140/90	Check blood pressure regularly and keep a log to bring to health care provider appointments Take medications as prescribed Limit salt intake to 2,400 mg/day Do not add salt when cooking, keep salt shaker off the table, season with fresh herbs and spices Avoid processed, canned, pickled, and fast food Stop smoking Decrease alcohol intake Control or reduce weight Exercise regularly
Hyperlipidemia (nutrition) Goal: LDL less than or equal to 100 mg/dL (optional less equal to 70 with CAD equivalent) HDL greater than or equal to 40 mg/dL Triglyceride less than or equal to 150 mg/dL	Have lipid panel checked regularly Take medications as prescribed TLC diet: Total fat 25–30 percent, saturated fats to less than or equal to 7 percent, complex carbohydrates 50–60 percent, protein 15 percent of total daily calories and total cholesterol less than or equal to 200 mg/day, Fiber 25 g/day Steam, bake, broil, grill, or stir fry foods Avoid high fat foods like meat, avocados, olives, nuts, butter, salad dressing, organ meats and shrimp, egg yolks, palm and coconut oils, high fat dairy products, fried foods Choose fresh fruits and vegetables, egg substitutes or egg whites, lean meats, fish, vegetable oils, low fat dairy products Buy a heart-healthy cookbook Achieve and maintain a healthy weight Exercise regularly
Physical inactivity Goal: Minimum 30 minutes three to four times/week	After approval by the health care provider begin a regular exercise program Count pulse before, during, and after exercise. Stop and rest if pulse increases to more than 20 beats above resting pulse Warm up and cool down Walk for 5 to 10 minutes at a moderate pace. Increase by 1 to 2 minutes per session to each the goal of 30 to 45 minutes. Maintain pace that does not increase heart rate above 20 beats from baseline and ability to talk General guidelines: Carry nitroglycerin at all times Walk on level ground Avoid walking in temperatures hotter than 29°C (85°F), more than 75 percent humidity, cooler than 4°C (40°F) Wait one hour before or after meals Wear comfortable walking shoes and loose-fitting clothing Drink plenty of water and bring along Stop if heart rate more than 20 beats above baseline, angina, palpitations, short of breath, dizziness. Notify health care provider if symptoms do not resolve after 15 minutes

Continued

TABLE 24-6 **Teaching Guide for CAD Risk Factor Modification—cont'd**

RISK FACTOR AND PRIMARY GOAL	TEACHING POINTS
Obesity	
Goal: BMI less than or equal to 25 kg/m²	Follow calorie-restricted diet: Avoid fad and crash diets
	Provide community contact information for weight reduction programs
Waist circumference less than or equal to 40 inches for males, less than 35 inches for females	Exercise regularly
Diabetes mellitus	
Goal: HbA$_{1c}$ less than or equal to 7 percent	Follow calorie-restricted diet
	Monitor glucose levels regularly and keep a log to bring to health care provider appointments
	Take medications as prescribed
	Control or reduce weight
	Exercise regularly

Adapted from Brunner, E., Thorogood, M., Rees, K., & Hewitt, G. (2006). Dietary advice for reducing cardiovascular risk. The Cochrane Database Systematic Reviews (1), CD002128; DeLaune, S., & Ladner, P. (2006). Fundamentals of nursing (3rd ed.). New York: Thomson Delmar Learning; Roth, R. (2007). Nutrition and diet therapy (9th ed.). New York: Thomson Delmar Learning.

Evaluation of Outcomes

Potential patient outcomes for each of the example nursing diagnoses for the patient with CAD are:

- Acute pain (angina) related to the imbalance between myocardial oxygen supply and demand. Verbalize relief of chest pain and demonstrate ability to manage chest pain that is not relieved.
- Ineffective tissue perfusion related to myocardial ischemia and decreased cardiac output. Maintain adequate tissue perfusion to all organ systems and extremities including stable vital signs, pulses, oxygenation, and ECG tracings.
- Anxiety related to pain, perceived threat of death, possible lifestyle changes and diagnosis of CAD. Demonstrate effective coping strategies and verbalize reduced anxiety.
- Activity intolerance related to angina, pulmonary congestion, fatigue, and inadequate tissue perfusion. Return to baseline level of activity.
- Ineffective therapeutic regimen management related to lack of knowledge related to disease process, prognosis, and treatment strategies. Verbalize understanding of disease process, prognosis, and complies with treatment strategies.

ACUTE CORONARY SYNDROME

ACS includes life-threatening conditions that can occur at any time in patients with CAD. ACS encompasses a continuum that ranges from an unstable pattern of angina to the most severe form of AMI, the condition of irreversible necrosis of heart muscle.

Although the exact incidence is difficult to ascertain, using first listed and secondary hospital discharge data, there were 1,680,000 unique discharges for ACS in 2001. Despite the daunting statistics, there has been a continuous decline in the mortality rate associated ACS because of advances in treatment and preventive measures (Antman, et al., 2004).

Pathophysiology

The majority of ACS results from disruption of an atherosclerotic plaque with platelet aggregation and formation of an intracoronary thrombus. The thrombus turns an area of plaque narrowing into one of severe or complete occlusion, and the decreased blood flow through the involved artery causes a severe imbalance between myocardial oxygen supply and demand. The degree of ACS that develops depends on the amount of coronary obstruction and associated ischemia. A partially occlusive thrombus is the typical cause of the unstable angina and non-ST segment elevation myocardial infarction (NSTEMI). If the coronary artery is completely occluded by the thrombus, it results in severe ischemia with accompanying necrosis causing a more severe form of ACS, a ST segment elevation myocardial infarction (STEMI). The thrombus responsible for causing the symptoms associated with ACS is generated by interactions with the atherosclerotic plaque, the coronary endothelium, circulating platelets, and the vasomotor tone of the vascular wall. Prolonged ischemia, 20 minutes or more, results in myocardial death (Topol, 2005).

Complications

There are a number of complications of ACS, any of which if untreated can result in death (e.g., arrhythmias, congestive heart failure [CHF], cardiogenic shock, papillary muscle dysfunction, ventricular aneurysm, pericarditis, or SCD). Therefore, the nurse must practice astute assessment skills and be observant to detect the beginning clinical manifestations of any of the following complications.

The most common complication after an AMI is arrhythmias, which occur in 80 percent of AMI patients and include tachycardia, bradycardia, heart block, and atrial or ventricular fibrillation. Ventricular fibrillation is the most common cause of sudden death in patients in the prehospital period. Continuous ECG monitoring is essential. Arrhythmias may require the use of antiarrhythmia medications and temporary pacing devices for symptomatic patients.

CHF is a complication that occurs when the contracting power of the heart has decreased (systolic dysfunction) or myocardium becomes stiff (diastolic dysfunction). CHF begins with subtle signs, such as slight dyspnea, restlessness, agitation, or slight tachycardia. Jugular vein distension, crackles heard in the lungs, and the presence of an S_3 or S_4 heart sounds may indicate the onset of CHF.

The complication of **cardiogenic shock** occurs when inadequate oxygen and nutrients are supplied to the tissues because of severe left ventricular failure. Cardiogenic shock often requires aggressive support of contractility and blood pressure with the use of inotropic and vasoactive drugs. Intra-aortic balloon pump therapy may be required to stabilize the patient before and after revascularization procedures. Cardiogenic shock in patients with AMI has a mortality rate higher than 70 percent.

Another complication of ACS is a ventricular aneurysm that occurs when the infarcted myocardial wall becomes thinned and bulges out during contraction. A large aneurysm reduces cardiac function and is prone to thrombus development and ventricular arrhythmias.

Patients with ACS may experience the complication of papillary muscle dysfunction if the area of infarction includes or is adjacent to these structures. Papillary muscle dysfunction causes mitral valve regurgitation detected by a systolic murmur at the cardiac apex radiating toward the maxilla. Severe papillary muscle dysfunction can present with symptoms similar to heart failure.

Another complication of ACS is **pericarditis,** which is an inflammation of the pericardium and can cause compression of the myocardium leading to decreased filling and emptying of the ventricles. This compression can result in a tamponade effect causing cardiac failure. Pericarditis chest pain varies from mild to severe and is typically aggravated by coughing, inspiration, and movement of the upper body. The pain is usually different from pain associated with MI. **Dressler's syndrome** is a pericarditis that develops 2 to 10 weeks after an MI. The inflammatory response is believed to be the result of an autoimmune reaction to myocardial neoantigens.

The most serious complication of ACS is SCD, which is unexpected death from cardiac causes. With SCD there is a sudden disruption in cardiac function commonly caused by ventricular fibrillation, producing an abrupt loss in blood flow. Death usually occurs within one hour of onset of acute symptoms. Sudden death from cardiac causes is estimated to account for about 50 percent of all deaths from cardiovascular causes. In 25 percent of people who die of sudden cardiac death, this is their first manifestation of CAD.

Assessment with Clinical Manifestations

The assessment of the patient is extremely important in the management of the patient with ACS. The nurse must know what to examine regarding both subjective and objective data.

The subjective data if obtained from a reliable source is just as important as a good physical examination. The history of present illness reveals the location, severity, intensity, quality, duration of chest pain, as well as the time of onset. Pain may radiate down the left arm or both arms, upward to the neck or jaw, or backward to the scapular region. The pain may be described as crushing, squeezing, or the worst pain ever experienced. Inquire about precipitating factors, such as exercise, smoking, or stress. Find out what measures were used to attempt to control symptoms, such as rest, nitroglycerin, or using antacids and if any of the measures worked. It is important to collect a past health history related to previous history of MI, angina, aortic stenosis, cardiomyopathy, hypertension, diabetes mellitus, anemia, lung disease, and hyperlipidemia. Inquire about use of medications including nitrates, calcium channel blockers, beta blockers, antihypertensive drugs, antilipidemic drugs, and blood thinners. Use of phosphodiesterase inhibitors; such as Viagra and Cialis, have been shown to cause severe hypotension and cardiovascular collapse if administered within 24 hours of a nitrate. Establish if there is a family history of CAD and inquire about other risk factors for CAD, such as lipid profile, tobacco use, stress levels, and exercise patterns.

The nurse performs a physical examination of the patient experiencing ACS by observing the patient for anxiety, fear, and restlessness. In addition, the nurse examines the patient for posturing that indicates the presence of chest pain (e.g., clutching or rubbing chest, leaning forward). Other clues indicating ischemia include:

- Integumentary: Cool, clammy, pale skin.
- Neurological: Altered level of consciousness, syncope.
- Respiratory: Dyspnea, or shortness of breath, crackles, and tachypnea.
- Cardiovascular: Tachycardia, bradycardia, **pulsus alternans** (alternating weak and strong heart beats) arrhythmias, S_3, S_4, hypotension, hypertension, or murmur.
- GI: Vomiting.
- Genitourinary: Decreased urine output.

Diagnostic Tests

Common diagnostic studies used to determine whether a person has sustained an AMI include an ECG and serum cardiac markers. Additional diagnostic testing after a MI are the same as those described for CAD.

Serial ECGs are needed to rule out or confirm an AMI. Changes in the QRS complex, ST segment, and T wave caused by ischemia and infarction can develop quickly after an AMI. During myocardial ischemia, ST segment and T wave changes often appear. Acute ischemia usually results in transient horizontal or downsloping ST segment depression and T wave flattening or inversions. Occasionally, ST segment elevations are seen; this is suggestive of more

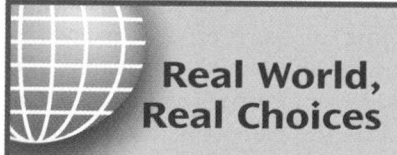

Real World, Real Choices

The Nurse Role in an ACS Patient

Mr. Jones is a 56-year-old male entering the emergency department with the chief complaint of chest pain. The midsternal chest pressure is rated at 8/10, radiates to his left arm, began following intercourse, was unrelieved with rest, and was associated with diaphoresis. He offered that he took 325 mg of aspirin prior to leaving his home.

What should the nurses do as Mr. Jones comes to the emergency department?

severe transmural myocardial ischemia. For diagnostic and treatment purposes, it is important to distinguish between STEMI and NSTEMI. Patients with STEMI tend to have a more extensive MI that occurs more quickly than NSTEMI and is associated with prolonged and complete coronary thrombosis. Patients with NSTEMI usually have transient thrombosis or incomplete coronary artery occlusion.

Serial ECGs are important for diagnosis of AMI, because the ECG may be normal on initial presentation. As cellular damage interrupts the normal electrical depolarization, subsequent changes on the ECG may develop on subsequent ECGs. Typically ECGs are performed on admission and repeated in six and eight hours. Diagnosis is made on the evaluation of serial studies.

Certain proteins, called serum cardiac markers, are released into the blood in measurable quantities from necrotic heart muscle after an ischemic event. When cardiac cells die, their cellular enzymes are released into the circulation. Release of intracellular macromolecules from injured myocytes provides information regarding the extent of myocardial damage. The most common markers used in the diagnosis of AMI are the creatine kinase (CK) MB band and troponin. Total CK is a nonspecific marker of muscle damage. The CK enzymes are fractionated into bands, including the MB band. The MB band is specific to the myocardial cells and can be used to quantify the extent of myocardial damage. After an AMI, CK levels begin to rise approximately 3 to 12 hours, peak in 24 hours, and return to baseline within two to three days.

Troponin is a myocardial muscle protein released into the circulation with myocardial injury. In the heart there are two subtypes, troponin T and troponin I. Cardiac specific troponin T and cardiac specific troponin I have different amino acid sequences than skeletal muscle forms of these proteins. Therefore these markers are highly specific indicators of cardiac damage following an MI. These markers have a greater sensitivity and specificity for myocardial injury than CK MB. Troponin rises as quickly as CK and remains elevated for two weeks. Troponin levels increase 3 to 12 hours after the onset of MI, peak at 24 to 48 hours, and return to baseline over 5 to 14 days (Topol, 2005).

Echocardiography is useful in assessing the ability of the heart walls to contract and relax. Following an AMI, an echocardiogram can identify wall motion abnormality from infarction or ischemia. For further discussion of this diagnostic test see the section on CAD.

Other health conditions that mimic ACS include gastroesophageal reflux, esophageal spasm, biliary pain, acute cholecystitis, pericarditis, aortic dissection, pulmonary embolism, pneumonia, pneumothorax, and musculoskeletal conditions, such as chest wall pain, spinal osteoarthritis, and cervical radiculitis. Careful history, physical examination, and diagnostic tests are used to diagnose ACS.

Nursing Diagnoses

Based on the information gathered, examples of nursing diagnoses in the patient with ACS may include the following:

- Acute pain related to myocardial ischemia and decreased myocardial oxygen supply as manifested by severe chest pain and tightness, radiation of pain to neck and arms.
- Ineffective tissue perfusion (cardiac) related to myocardial injury and potential pulmonary congestion as manifested by decrease in blood pressure, dyspnea, arrhythmias, peripheral edema, and oliguria.
- Anxiety related to perceived or actual threat of death, pain, possible lifestyle changes as manifested by restlessness, agitation, and verbalization of concern over lifestyle changes and prognosis as evidenced by statements concerning death and dying.

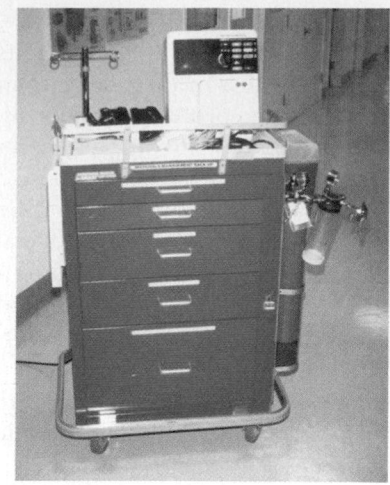

Figure 24-6 Crash cart (emergency resuscitation cart).

- Activity intolerance related to fatigue secondary to decreased cardiac output and poor lung and tissue perfusion as manifested by fatigue with minimal activity, inability to care for self without dyspnea, and increased heart rate.
- Ineffective therapeutic regimen management related to lack of knowledge of disease process, rehabilitation, home activities, and medication as manifested by frequent questioning about illness, management, and care after discharge.

Planning and Implementation

There are a wide variety of nursing interventions to enact for patients with AMI. The major goals of care for patients with AMI are to limit myocardial damage and prevent complications and recurrent events. Often a code is initiated to use advanced cardiac life support (ACLS) measures in an attempt to reverse the processes of the AMI. A crash cart is used by ACLS certified personnel to resuscitate the patient (Figure 24-6).

Patients with manifestations of ACS must receive immediate treatment. Delays may increase myocardial damage and decrease the chance of survival. Treatment starts before the patient arrives at the hospital. When a patient or family calls 911, they will be instructed to have the patient chew an aspirin. This action alone reduces mortality by 23 percent. The patient experiencing acute symptoms needs immediate transportation to a hospital, with a CCU if possible.

Although the treatment of ACS patients overlaps, there are some critical differences between the initial treatment of STEMI and NSTEMI patients. Patients with STEMI benefit from immediate thrombolysis or PCI, whereas patients with NSTSEMI do not have the same benefit. The goal of treatment of STEMI is door-to-needle (thrombolytics) in less than 30 minutes or door-to-balloon (PCI) in less than 90 minutes.

The first 24 hours after an AMI is the time of highest risk for sudden death. There is a significant benefit if treatment is administered within the first hour of onset of symptoms. The first hour after the onset of pain is a crucial time frame for salvage of the myocardium. Therefore efforts continue to decrease the time for initial treatment (Antman, et al., 2004).

Pain control is a priority. Pain stimulates a sympathetic response that increases myocardial oxygen demand. Oxygen therapy is applied to improve oxygen delivery. In addition to nitroglycerin, pain is treated with IV morphine sulfate (MS). MS reduces pain, as well as reduces myocardial oxygen demand, by decreasing the sympathetic response of pain. Also, MS reduces myocardial oxygen demand by vasodilating arteries and veins, decreasing afterload and preload, respectively. MS is given IV in 2 to 5 mg increments. The patient is monitored closely for respiratory depression and hypotension. Continued pain is an indicator of continued myocardial ischemia.

Pharmacology

The pharmacological treatment for improved perfusion following an AMI focuses on anti-ischemic and antithrombotic therapies. Anti-ischemic therapy usually consists of beta blockade and IV nitroglycerin. Antithrombolytic therapy is initiated with the administration of antiplatelet medication (aspirin) if the patient had not taken one before reaching the emergency department.

Fibrinolytic therapy offers the advantage of availability and rapid administration. Fibrinolytic therapy has evolved to actually stopping the infarction process instead of just treating symptoms. Mortality rates have decreased 2.5 percent to 5 percent with fibrinolytic treatment. Treatment of the AMI is geared toward quickly dissolving the thrombus and reperfusing the myocardium before cellular death occurs. To be of most benefit, fibrinolytic therapy must be given as soon as possible, ideally within the first hour of onset of symptoms and preferably within the first six hours of onset of symptoms. Commonly used fibrinolytics are recombinant plasminogen activator (reteplase, Retavase), streptokinase

LAW IN PRACTICE

The Liability of the Nurse in the Administration of Analgesics

Can a nurse be sued if a patient's pain is not adequately controlled? The answer is yes. Recent court cases illustrate that they are willing to take on pain treatment issues. A California jury awarded a family $1.5 million to an 85-year-old-man who had experienced severe pain before he died. The nurse caring for the patient continued to document the patient's pain as 7/10 despite pain medication. The health care provider who undertreated that patient's pain was found liable. The nursing staff settled before trial.

To protect oneself legally, make sure that nursing practice reflects the Joint Commission on Accreditation of Healthcare Organization's (JCAHO) pain management standards. Patients have a right to adequate pain relief and rely on nurses to act as their advocates. Always remember to document the patient's pain level, action taken, reassessment, as well as follow-up action if the pain remains uncontrolled (D'arcy, 2005).

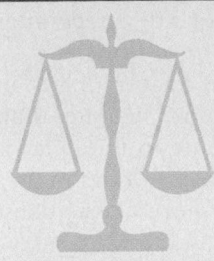

Respecting Our Differences

Women and CAD

CAD has traditionally been viewed as a disease of men, when in fact CAD is the number one killer of American women. Heart disease kills almost 10 times more women than breast cancer. Cardiovascular disease causes more deaths in women than men. Women tend to manifest the symptoms of CAD 10 years later than men and typically have symptoms of angina rather than MI. Women also have a much higher mortality and reinfarction rate within one year following MI than men. Diabetes mellitus has been found to be the most powerful predictor of CAD in women. Women with diabetes have five to seven times the risk for developing CAD when compared to nondiabetic women. Because CAD in women manifests with angina and women have a poorer prognosis following acute MI, aggressive teaching about the reduction of risk factors and counseling about lifestyle modifications should be implemented after the diagnosis if CAD to prevent MI.

(Streptase), and tissue plasminogen activator (tPA, alteplase, Activase). Choice of thrombolytic therapy is guided by considerations of cost, ease of administration, and efficacy. Patient selection is important, because the person receiving fibrinolytic therapy may have a minor or major bleeding episode as a consequence of therapy. Absolute contraindications include active internal bleeding, active inflammatory bowel disease, active peptic ulcer disease, active pericarditis, defective homeostasis, GI or genitourinary bleeding less than six months previous, history of hemorrhagic stroke, known bleeding disorders, neurological procedure less than two months previous, pregnancy, recent surgery or trauma less than two months previous, suspected aortic dissection, and uncontrolled hypertension (Lapointe & Haines, 2006).

Prior to administration of fibrinolytics, the nurse screens patients for bleeding risks, obtains baseline vital signs and physical assessment. Monitor patient for resolution or recurrence of chest pain, resolution or return of ST abnormalities, and early peak of cardiac biomarkers signifying successful reperfusion. Assess for evidence of bleeding. Provide simple explanations for the patient and family and offer realistic reassurances.

Anticoagulation therapy is frequently used in patients with ACS. Unfractionated heparin or low molecular weight heparin inhibit thrombin or factor Xa respectively. Anticoagulation therapy prevents propagation of the thrombus.

GP IIb/IIIa receptor inhibitors bind to the GP IIb/IIIa receptor on the platelet, which prevents the binding of fibrinogen and platelet aggregation. Common GPIIb/III, as used in ACS, include abciximab (ReoPro), eptifibatide (Integrilin), and tirofiban (Aggrastat).

Population-Based Care

There are several populations that experience ACS at an increased amount. For example, women are seen to have increasing difficulties with ACS (see Respecting Our Differences feature). In addition, the aging process greatly increases the correlation with the development of ACS. The following section elaborates more specifically populations that experience ACS.

The incidence of CAD increases with advancing age. The elderly typically present with atypical signs and symptoms, which may cause a delay in seeking care. Older patients often experience silent MIs and come to the emergency department with shortness of breath, heart failure, or pulmonary edema but without chest pain. Absence of chest pain as a classic symptom often impedes recognition of the fact that the older person is experiencing MI. Nurses should

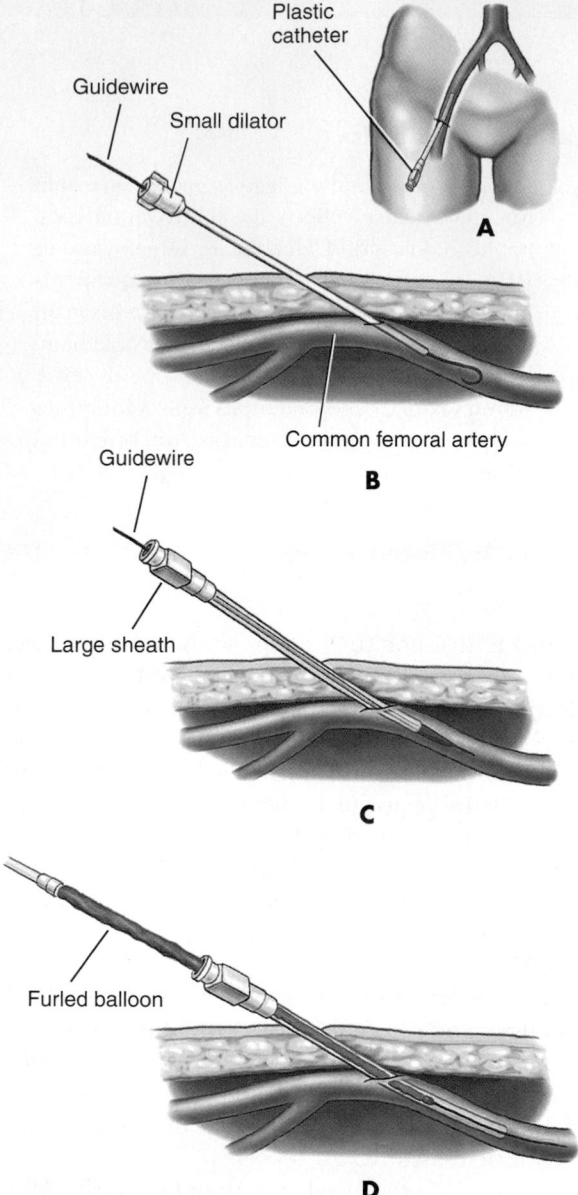

Figure 24-7 Intra-aortic balloon pump insertion: A. Needle cannula assembly is inserted into femoral artery, B. Small dilator is threaded over guidewire, C. Large sheath is inserted over guidewire, D. Balloon is inserted into sheath.

also be aware that older adults may be more sensitive to medications and should monitor them closely for side effects after administration.

African Americans typically experience longer delays in seeking treatment for MI and have higher mortality rates than Caucasians. One factor believed to contribute to the delay is that African Americans have a greater incidence of dyspnea as an acute symptom of MI rather than the more classic chest discomfort.

Surgery

In hospitals with PCI available, this is the treatment of choice for STEMI. PCI includes PTCA, a procedure performed under fluoroscopy in which a balloon-tipped catheter is inserted through a peripheral artery and maneuvered into the stenotic segment of the coronary vessel. The balloon is inflated under pressure, and the plaque is compressed against the wall of the artery. The improvement in the size of the coronary artery lumen increases coronary perfusion and myocardial oxygen supply stopping the ischemic event and preventing necrosis.

Patients experiencing ACS with hemodynamic instability may benefit from placement of an intra-aortic balloon pump (IABP). The IABP, inserted into the descending thoracic aorta, inflates during diastole, augmenting early diastolic pressure and coronary artery perfusion. The balloon deflates rapidly at the end of diastole, decreasing afterload, resulting in an increase in cardiac output (Figures 24-7 and 24-8).

Alternative Therapy

Many people choose to utilize alternative therapy for treatment of CAD or in conjunction with standard medical therapy. There has been an increased interest in specific foods and their bioactive constituents as a therapeutic approach to treating or preventing CAD. These foods are often termed functional foods or nutraceuticals, and are defined by the American Dietetic Association (ADA) as whole, fortified, enriched, or enhanced foods that have a potential beneficial effect on health when consumed as part of a varied diet on a regular basis, at effective levels. The National Cholesterol Education Program has recognized two functional foods, plant sterols and stanols and soluble fiber, as approved therapies in managing hyperlipidemia. Other dietary therapies available for the treatment and prevention of CAD are antioxidants. Antioxidant nutrients have shown promise in reducing risk factors for cardiovascular disease such as platelet aggregation (Carson, Burke, & Hark, 2004).

Additional therapies can help in reducing the patient's anxiety. Techniques such as progressive muscle relaxation, guided imagery, and music therapy have been shown to decrease anxiety, reduce depression, and increase compliance with activity and exercise regimens.

Patient and Family Teaching

Patient and family teaching should begin the minute the patient arrives to the emergency department and continue through discharge. By the time the patient is ready for discharge, he or she should have an understanding of his or her cardiac condition, chest pain management, activity, medications, risk factor modification, diet restrictions, and signs and symptoms to report to a health care provider (Table 24-7).

Cardiac rehabilitation combines exercise training with coronary risk factor modification in patients with established heart disease. The goals of cardiac rehabilitation are to improve functional capacity, alleviate or lessen activity-related symptoms, reduce disability, and identify and modify coronary risk factors in an attempt to reduce subsequent morbidity and mortality due to cardiovascular illness. The ultimate goal of cardiac rehabilitation is to restore and maintain an individual's optimal physiological, psychological, social, and vocational status. The following section identifies four phases of cardiac rehabilitation.

Phase I of cardiac rehabilitation takes place in the hospital after a heart attack. At this time the staff will determine how well patients can care for themselves (bathing, dressing, and grooming) and measure the patient's ability to exercise. Patients and their families will be provided education about important lifestyle changes that will need to be made. Patients will typically begin a light exercise program of walking while they are still in the hospital. Referral is made for outpatient follow-up.

Phase II of cardiac rehabilitation is the transitional phase of cardiac rehabilitation after the patient leaves the hospital and centers around recovery at home. Phase II focuses on increasing activity. The exercise program is usually low intensity to prepare for a more moderate to high intensity program in the next phase of rehab.

Phase III of cardiac rehabilitation refers to the outpatient cardiac rehabilitation programs, which are the third step in rehabilitation following a heart attack. Phase III includes supervised exercise and a variety of measurements and assessments. In addition to restoring physical function, phase III focuses on reducing the risk of future heart conditions through TLC counseling, education, and reinforcement of secondary prevention pharmacological therapy.

Phase IV of cardiac rehabilitation is often referred to as the maintenance phase of cardiac rehabilitation, because it emphasizes long-term lifestyle changes, such as a regular exercise program. Phase IV programs are usually held at a community facility or at home and will be tailored to the patient's specific needs.

The AHA is an excellent source for patient education and professional service referrals for the patient with CAD, including various cookbooks. For patients that require CABG, the Mended Heart is a nationwide program with local chapters that provide education and support for patients and their families. Investigate locally for programs for smoking cessation, weight reduction, and cardiac rehabilitation that may or may not be connected to local hospitals.

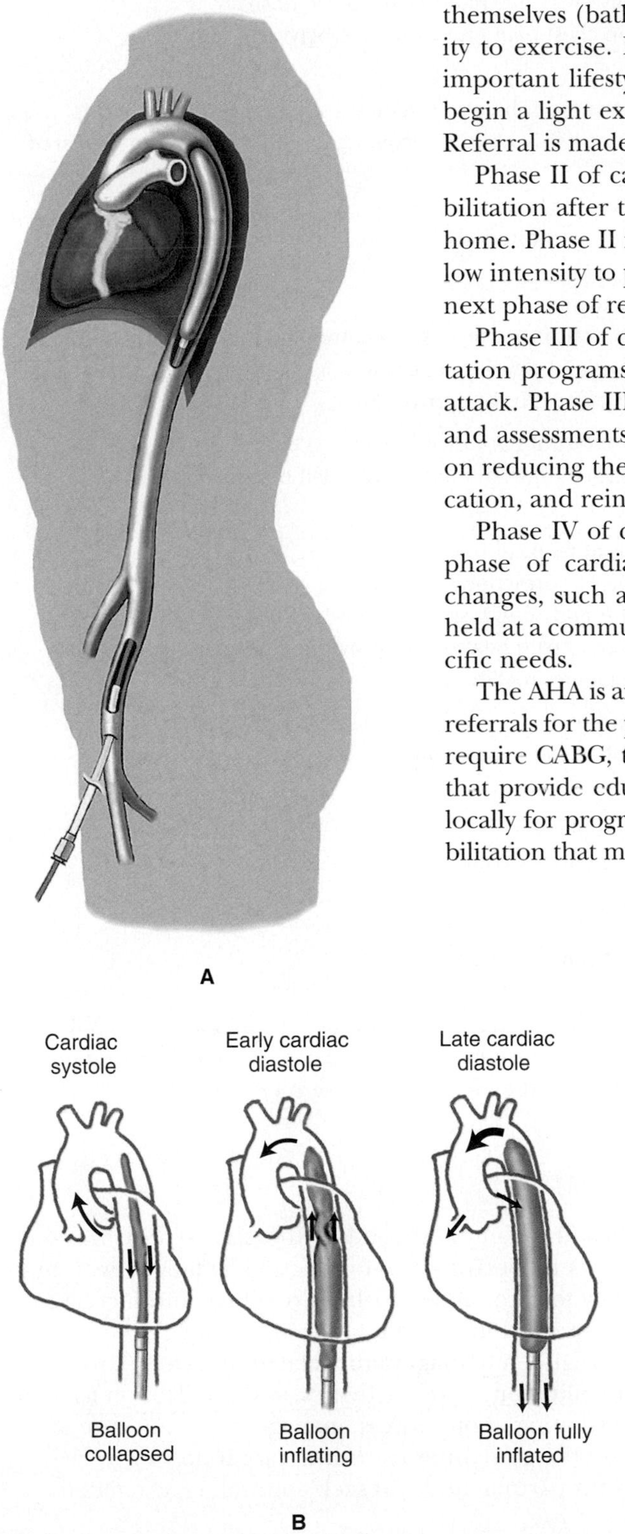

Evaluation of Outcomes

Potential patient outcomes for each of the example nursing diagnoses for the patient with ACS are:

- Acute pain related to myocardial ischemia and decreased myocardial oxygen supply as manifested by severe chest pain and tightness, radiation of pain to neck and arms. State that the chest pain is alleviated, appear comfortable, and have resolution of ST segment and T wave changes.

- Ineffective tissue perfusion (cardiac) related to myocardial injury and potential pulmonary congestion as manifested by decrease in blood pressure, dyspnea, arrhythmias, peripheral edema, and oliguria: Remain hemodynamically stable: maintain a stable rhythm, maintain a blood pressure within acceptable range, adequate urine output, mental alertness, palpable pedal pulses, and clear lungs on auscultation.

- Anxiety related to perceived or actual threat of death, pain, possible lifestyle changes as manifested by restlessness, agitation, and verbalization of concern over lifestyle changes and prognosis as evidenced by statements concerning death and dying. Indicated decreased anxiety.

A

Cardiac systole	Early cardiac diastole	Late cardiac diastole
Balloon collapsed	Balloon inflating	Balloon fully inflated

B

Figure 24-8 IABP mechanics: A. The balloon is situated in the descending aorta, B. The balloon is deflated during cardiac systole and inflated during diastole.

TABLE 24-7	**Discharge Instructions After AMI**
Understanding of cardiac condition	Explain basic cardiac anatomy and physiology Describe in simple terms the differences among coronary artery disease, angina, and MI Discuss how the heart heals after an MI
Chest pain management	Stop activity and rest Take nitroglycerin sublingually every five minutes for three doses Call 911 if no improvement in chest pain after three nitroglycerin tablets
Activity	Increase activity levels gradually Stop activity if chest pain, shortness of breath, dizziness, or extreme fatigue occurs Avoid lifting, pulling, or pushing heavy objects (weighing 10 to 20 pounds until cleared by health care provider) Avoid straining to have a bowel movement Ensure adequate sleep with daily rest periods Avoid extremes in temperature Avoid tension and stressful activities Resume sexual relations with health care provider recommendation and when able to climb two flights of stairs without developing chest pain or shortness of breath Return to work when cleared by health care provider
Medications	State purpose, dose and side effect of each drug Design a routine with daily structure when medications will be remembered
Risk factors	Avoid smoking Practice appropriate methods of relaxation daily Follow low-fat, low-sodium diet as prescribed Maintain ideal body weight for body build, size and gender Control associate health problems with health care provider coverage: hypertension, hypercholesterolemia, or diabetes mellitus
Diet	Consult dietician to review and reinforce prescribed heart healthy diet Ensure the primary caregiver has diet instructions
Signs and symptoms to report to a health care provider	Increased shortness of breath Increased swelling of feet and ankles. Rapid weight gain (i.e., 2 to 4 pounds in one day) Unusual fatigue Dizziness or fainting Palpations or unusually fast or slow heart beat Side effects of medication

Adapted from Carson, J. S., Burke, F. M., & Hark, L. A. (2004). Cardiovascular nutrition: Disease management and prevention. Chicago: American Dietetic Association; Topol, E. J. (2005). Acute coronary syndrome. New York: Marcel Dekker.

- Activity intolerance related to fatigue secondary to decreased cardiac output and poor lung and tissue perfusion as manifested by fatigue with minimal activity, and inability to care for self without dyspnea, and increased heart rate. Will tolerate gradual increasing levels of activity.
- Ineffective therapeutic regimen management related to lack of knowledge of disease process, rehabilitation, home activities, and medication as manifested by frequent questioning about illness, management, and care after discharge. Will verbalize the guidelines for home care following an MI, will discuss concerns with partner, and will seek counseling as needed.

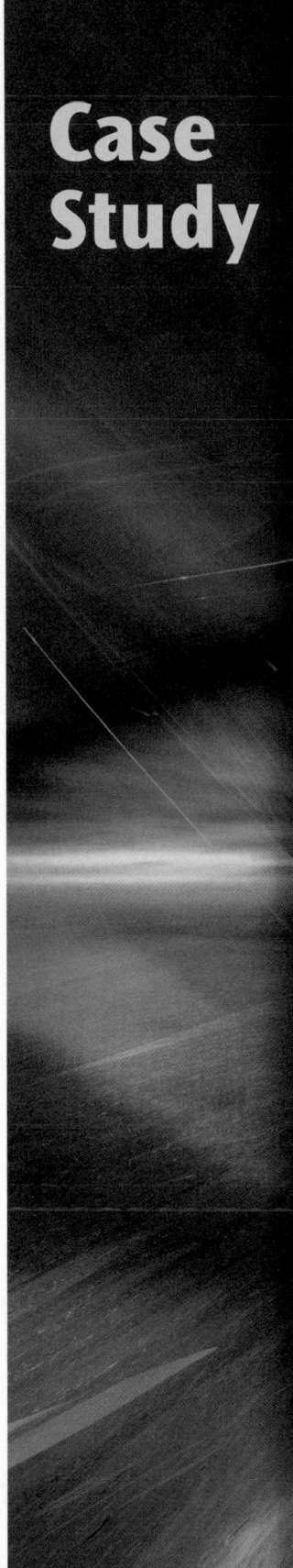

Case Study

Nursing Care Plan

Mr. Brody came to the emergency department complaining of chest pain unrelieved by nitroglycerin (NTG) and rest. He was admitted to the coronary care unit with a diagnosis of unstable angina and mild CHF. During the physical assessment, the nurse discovers that Mr. Brody has a history of MI with a coronary artery bypass graft surgery four years ago. Over the past year, he has had increasing shortness of breath, intermittent chest pain relieved with rest, and generalized fatigue. He complains of being unable to work the long days he used to as a carpenter and requires several 15–20-minute rest periods throughout the day. His physical examination reveals diminished breath sounds in the bases of his lungs, mild tachycardia, diaphoresis, and capillary refill greater than 3 seconds.

Assessment

This patient has a history of cardiac disease with an increase in chest pain, fatigue, and shortness of breath. The results of the physical examination (diminished breath sounds in the lungs, tachycardia, and decreased capillary refill) indicate problems with oxygenation and tissue perfusion. The patient's expressed concern about fatigue and frequent rest periods indicate a need for conservation measures. Levine's Theory of Conservation will be a good fit as a plan of care is implemented.

Nursing Diagnosis #1: Activity intolerance as related to CHF as evidenced by complaints of shortness of breath, chest pain, and the need for frequent rest periods during activities.

Expected Outcomes

The patient will:
1. No longer complain of shortness of breath.
2. Have no episodes of chest pain on discharge to home.

Planning/Intervention/Rationale

1. Review therapeutic regimen with patient (e.g., medications, activities, and rest periods). Following therapeutic regimen, such as taking medications to improve cardiac function and increase urinary output, decreasing and eliminating shortness of breath and chest pain. *Preserves structural integrity.*
2. Assist patient in planning rest periods during periods of physical activity, such as construction work. *Allows for conservation of energy to complete activities with decreased stress and anxiety.*

Evaluation

Patient experienced no shortness of breath or chest pain and is following therapeutic regimen at home. Patient took rest periods at least every three to four hours and was able to complete his day of work without as much fatigue within three weeks of being discharged.

Nursing Diagnosis #2: Fatigue as related to CHF as evidenced by complaints of inability to complete a day of work without fatigue and continued shortness of breath.

Case Study

Expected Outcomes

The patient will:

1. State his energy levels are greater in one week and will be able to complete normal days of construction work within three weeks.
2. Does not experience tachycardia or shortness of breath after returning to work and normal activities of daily living.

Planning/Interventions/Rationale

1. Teach energy saving techniques for construction work and activities of daily living. *Conservation of energy allows patient to complete activities with decreased anxiety and allow consideration for other activities of life.*
2. Teach self-monitoring of pulse rates, educate spouse as to the clinical manifestations of decreased perfusion and cardiac performance, and plan activities that the patient can participate in with decreased energy expenditure. *Encourages self-efficacy and increases family involvement as a support system for patient.*

Evaluation

Patient completed his days of work with scheduled rest periods within one week of discharge and states his energy level is higher than when first discharged home. Spouse verbalized the methods of assessing her husband as related to cardiac efficiency and developed daily routines with husband that kept him from being fatigued.

KEY CONCEPTS

- Atherosclerosis is the major contributor to CAD, the blood vessel disease of the epicardial arteries supplying oxygen and nutrients to the myocardium.
- Atherosclerosis begins as fatty streaks of the arterial wall in adolescents, progressing to hard fatty plaques that narrow the artery lumen in adulthood and can rupture creating thrombotic occlusions that cause ischemia.
- There are several risk factors associated with the development of CAD including age, sex, family history, hyperlipidemia, hypertension, cigarette smoking, diabetes mellitus, obesity, and sedentary lifestyle.
- CAD presents as stable angina and ACS.

- The goals of angina treatment are to improve quality of life by decreasing episodes of angina and ischemia and increase the quantity of life by preventing progression to MI and death.
- Treatment of angina includes the use of medications, therapeutic lifestyle changes, percutaneous interventions, and surgery.
- The goals of ACS treatment are to limit myocardial damage and prevent complications and recurrent events.
- Treatment of ACS includes initiating prompt care, managing acute pain, reperfusing the myocardium, preventing complications, preventing myocardial remodeling and heart failure, rehabilitation, and patient education.

REVIEW QUESTIONS

1. Which of the following are risk factors for CAD?
   1. Obesity
   2. Hyperlipidemia
   3. Cigarette smoking
   4. All of the above

2. Typical stable angina symptoms include all of the following except?
   1. Chest pressure occurring with activity
   2. Chest pressure relieved with rest or nitroglycerin
   3. Chest pressure lasting greater than 20 minutes not relieved by rest
   4. Chest pressure that occurs with the same onset, duration, and intensity

3. The clinical spectrum of ACS includes:
   1. Stable angina and STEMI
   2. Stable angina and NSTEMI
   3. Unstable angina and SCD
   4. Unstable angina, STEMI, and NSTEMI

4. The atherogenesis of CAD begins with all of the following except:
   1. Fatty streak
   2. Unstable plaque
   3. Injury to the endothelial lining of the artery wall
   4. Adolescence

5. Initial diagnostic studies in the setting of an acute MI include an ECG and:
   1. Cardiac enzymes
   2. Exercise stress test
   3. Nuclear stress test
   4. MRI

6. The following are common medications used for CAD and ACS:
   1. Aspirin
   2. Beta blockers
   3. Nitroglycerin
   4. All of the above

7. Identify at least three nursing diagnoses for patients with angina and MI.

8. List the five components of patient education for patients with stable angina.

9. The goals of therapy for stable angina are to improve the _____ of life by _____ and _____ of life by _____.

10. The goals of therapy for acute MI are to _____ and prevent _____.

REVIEW ACTIVITIES

1. Describe briefly what you believe to be happening to Mr. Anthony from a pathophysiological perspective in the following scenario. Mr. Anthony is a 66-year-old Caucasian male admitted yesterday with the chief complaint of chest pain. He describes his pain as midsternal pressure radiating to his left arm, associated with shortness of breath when running and relieved with rest. He has been fairly sedentary for the last five years and recently started running a week ago. The pain has recurred with each attempt to run so he presented to the emergency department. He ruled out for MI by serum markers and ECG. He is pain free since admission. He is scheduled for a treadmill stress test later in the day. Mr. Anthony has a positive history for hypertension for 10 years, he has smoked one pack of cigarettes a day for 40 years, and his father died of MI at age 50. His physical examination is normal, including vital signs, and his lipid panel is pending. Current medications include Lopressor 50 mg PO BID, aspirin 325 mg PO daily, Imdur 30 mg PO daily, lisinopril 5 mg PO daily, and nitroglycerin SL prn chest pain.

Continued

REVIEW ACTIVITIES—cont'd

2. Read patient educational materials available at your clinical site for CAD, MI, stress testing, cardiac catheterization, PCI, and coronary artery bypass surgery. After reading the material, present your findings to your clinical group of peer nursing students.

3. Describe the nursing interventions following one of the following diagnostic tests performed for cardiovascular patients: 12-lead ECG, cardiac catheterization, PTCA, or exercise stress test.

4. Locate local programs for smoking cessation, weight reduction, and cardiac rehabilitation. Then, communicate your findings to your nursing peers and instructors.

5. If available at your clinical site, arrange to follow the clinical specialist, clinical case manager, or nurse practitioner for cardiac patients. Observe these advanced care providers and keep a journal of their nursing interventions. Then, share your findings with your peers in a clinical seminar.

Heart Failure and Inflammatory Dysfunction: Nursing Management

Amy Goodwin, RN, MSN, APRN, BC

Julie S. Williard, RN, MS, NP-C

CHAPTER TOPICS

- Heart Failure

- Heart Muscle Disease and Inflammation Dysfunction

- Valvular Dysfunction and Disease

KEY TERMS

Carditis
Contractility
Endocarditis
Endocardium
Hypertrophy
Idiopathic
Mitral facies
Myectomy
Myocarditis
Pericarditis
Pericardium
Petechiae
Prophylactic
Sequela
Valvular regurgitation
Valvular stenosis
Valvuloplasty

The cardiovascular system is one of the most important body systems. There are many research studies validating the relationship between the science of nursing and the positive outcomes that nurses have on patients with disorders of the cardiovascular system. This chapter will present specific information on several major dysfunctions of the heart, including heart failure, heart muscle disease and inflammation, and valvular dysfunction and disease.

HEART FAILURE

According to the National Heart, Lung, and Blood Institute (2006b), heart failure is a condition in which the heart cannot pump enough blood throughout the body. It does not indicate that the heart has failed to beat, but rather that it is not pumping effectively. More specifically, it means that the heart cannot fill with enough blood and pump with enough force.

Heart failure, also known as cardiac failure or congestive heart failure (CHF), may occur when any one of the processes of the circulatory or vascular systems fails and is unable to maintain circulation of blood adequate to meet the metabolic or volumetric needs of the body. Heart failure stems from the inability of the right ventricle to pump blood into the lungs or from the inability of the left ventricle to pump blood into the systemic circulation. CHF is the phrase used to describe the congestion that results from the heart's inability to pump blood efficiently. CHF is not the same as a myocardial infarction ([MI] heart attack), in which a coronary artery is blocked, and is not the same as cardiac arrest, in which the heart actually stops beating.

Epidemiology

Heart failure affects almost five million people in the United States, and the number is steadily increasing. The number of new cases of heart failure each year has reached 550,000 with an estimated 300,000 deaths each year caused by heart failure (National Heart, Lung, and Blood Institute, 2006b). Between 40 to 75 years of age, more men than women will be diagnosed with heart failure. After the age of 75, both sexes are equally affected. According to the American Heart Association (2006b), heart failure is associated with a poor prognosis; one in five people with heart failure will die within one year of diagnosis.

Etiology

The National Heart and Blood Institute classifies heart failure into two categories: diastolic and systolic heart failures. Systolic heart failure occurs when there is an inability of the ventricles to contract and pump blood adequately. This inability can be caused by an insult to the heart or by the normal processes of aging. The aging process often results in stiffness in the vasculature of the heart due to a loss of elastin, increase in collagen deposits, and thickening of smooth muscle layers in the arteries. The heart muscle responds similarly to aging by becoming stiffer because of an increase in connective tissue mass and a change in the function of calcium in the heart muscle cells, resulting in ventricular **hypertrophy** (abnormal enlargement, increase in size and mass, of a body part or organ). Cardiac stiffness and altered calcium handling leaves the heart unable to fully contract (Deaton, Bennett, & Riegel, 2004).

Diastolic heart failure occurs because of the heart's inability to relax; this inability results in a decrease in ventricular filling. Diastolic failure, also a response to a change in the function of calcium in the heart muscle cells, leads to impaired diastolic filling of the left ventricle (Zevitz, 2004).

Pathophysiology

Systolic and diastolic heart failure lead to a decreased amount of blood being circulated to the body. The heart attempts to compensate for its inability to pump efficiently by increasing the rate of the contractions (increased heart rate), by attempting to force blood out of the ventricle by increasing the size and strength of the ventricular muscle (ventricular hypertrophy), and by increasing the volume of blood that is pumped by increasing the capacity of the ventricle (ventricular dilation). These compensatory mechanisms are considered pathology of the heart, or cardiomyopathy. Hypertrophic cardiomyopathy (HCM) is the thickening of the ventricle wall. Dilated cardiomyopathy is described as thinning and stretching of the affected ventricle.

Episodes of acute heart failure affect the sympathetic nervous system and renin-angiotensin system. These two systems act to maintain flow and pressure to the vital organs. Increased neurohormonal activity results in increased myocardial **contractility** (the capability of muscle fibers to shrink), selective peripheral vasoconstriction, salt and fluid retention, and blood pressure maintenance. As a chronic state of failure ensues, these same mechanisms cause adverse effects (Satou & Herzbert, 2004). This neurohormonal response is what guides the treatment of heart failure.

Another classification of heart failure commonly referred to in the literature is right-sided and left-sided heart failure. When the right ventricle fails, the appropriate terms used are right-sided heart failure or right ventricular heart failure. Failure of the left ventricle is also referred to as left-sided heart failure or left ventricular heart failure. When one of the ventricles fail, it is almost inevitable that if left untreated, the other side of the heart will be affected, leading to a complete failure of the heart.

Right-sided heart failure can occur as a result of chronic lung diseases, congenital heart disease, primary pulmonary hypertension, heart valve disease, and left-sided heart failure. In right-sided heart failure, the right ventricle loses its ability to pump efficiently causing blood that would normally be pumped through the heart into the lungs, back up into the systemic circulation. This backup of blood causes congestion that can affect the liver, the gastrointestinal (GI) tract, and the periphery (arms and legs) (Hart, 2004). Patients with right-sided heart failure will often experience varying degrees of dependent edema, which reflects the inadequate pumping action and force of the right side of the heart. The edema is noticeable first in the feet (Figure 25-1), then the ankles, and a progressive increase of fluid will move in a proximal direction in the legs.

Left-sided heart failure can occur as a result of chronic coronary artery blockage, high blood pressure, excessive alcohol consumption, MI, valvular insufficiency, hypothyroidism, heart defects, heart valve anomalies, abnormal blood vessel connections, and heart muscle infection and disease. In left-sided heart failure the left ventricle loses its ability to effectively pump oxygenated blood into the systemic circulation leaving the body starving for oxygen and nutrients (Kang, 2004).

Heart failure is most commonly considered a chronic health condition. Acute heart failure, also known as pulmonary edema, is heart failure that occurs as a result of a relatively quick insult to the heart. This acute form of heart failure occurs as a result of a MI, liver failure, kidney failure, hematologic conditions that cause hemodynamic imbalance, and as a result of an exacerbation of chronic heart failure.

Characteristic of acute heart failure is an abnormal accumulation of fluid in the lungs. This fluid disperses into all available lung spaces, even those that are used for oxygen exchange. This alteration in the ability of the lungs to perform their oxygenation function results in a rapid onset of symptoms such as panic, anxiety, shortness of breath, cough, and restlessness. Shortly, the pulse increases in an effort to pump oxygen into the body, but it will be weak and ineffective. A backup of blood will ensue, and the jugular neck veins will distend. The decrease in peripheral oxygenation will reveal ashen skin, cyanotic nail beds, and circumoral pallor. Eventually, the heart will not receive enough oxygen to function properly. The oxygen saturation levels in the blood will begin to decline. The lung sounds and breath sounds will become moist and noisy with frothy (sometimes pink)

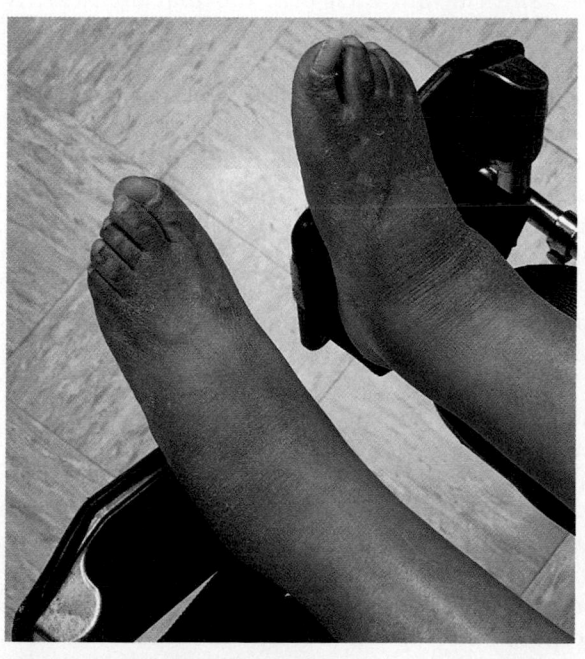

Figure 25-1 Edema is often a prominent sign in right-sided heart failure.

sputum. The patient may manifest signs of confusion. These symptoms are ominous and require immediate intervention.

Assessment with Clinical Manifestations

Assessment of heart failure is best accomplished through a holistic approach of gathering data from a health history, a thorough physical examination with attention paid to the cardiovascular and pulmonary systems, and objective measurement of various body parts and function.

A health history is useful in exploring the patient's experience with illness and elements of life that affect his or her response to illness. Particular attention is paid to, although not limited to, ailments related to heart failure. Questions about sleep are appropriate. Inquiry should be made about the patient's need for use of increasing numbers of pillows. The more pillows needed for ease of orthopnea often indicates a worsening of the heart failure condition. Sleep disturbances, particularly when the patient is awakened with shortness of breath, can indicate an increase in severity of conditions.

A health history is useful in describing the patient's ability to tolerate activities of daily living. Inquiry about causes of shortness of breath is important. Good questions for patients might include: What makes the symptoms worse? What makes the symptoms better?

A health history is an appropriate time to inquire about the patient's emotional response to CHF as a chronic illness. Questions about coping and family dynamics give a holistic picture of the patient. Inquiry about coping, loss, and grief concerning alteration in health status can spark important family and provider discussions. These are the types of discussions that direct the prioritization and planning of care of the patient.

Assessment of the cardiovascular system begins with inspection and palpation. Minimal information is gained with these methods concerning heart failure. Auscultation provides the most information about heart failure. Blood pressure, heart rate, and heart rhythm are assessed. An increase in blood pressure and a rapid heart rate indicates that the workload of the left ventricle is increasing. A rapid rate also indicates that the stroke volume has decreased and that the ventricle has less time to fill, which inhibits the heart's ability to maintain an adequate cardiac output. An auscultated S_3 is a sign that increased blood volume remains in the ventricle with each beat and that the heart is beginning to fail.

Assessment of heart failure includes the pulmonary system that begins with inspection. Oxygenation measures, respiratory effort, rate, and depth of respiration on exertion and at rest provides significant information about patients with heart failure. Oxygenation can be determined through measuring the percentage of hemoglobin saturated with oxygen in the blood. This is accomplished noninvasively by using a pulse oximeter or by performing an arterial puncture and to obtain blood gas levels. Decreased levels of oxygen in the blood can indicate a problem in the pulmonary system. An increase in the work of breathing, an increase in the rate of respirations, and an increase in the depth of respiration all indicate strain on the system. Palpation and percussion can reveal extensive pulmonary congestion. Auscultation of anterior, posterior, and lateral lung sounds bilaterally are recommended to detect an increase of fluid and pulmonary congestion. Increased fluid in the lungs is evident when wheezes and crackles are heard in the lung bases. Treatment of heart failure often eliminates the wheezes and crackles. Treatment, accomplished through administration of diuretics, is evaluated by reassessing the lung sounds. Successful treatment is achieved when there is a decrease or elimination of pulmonary crackles.

Further assessment can point to other signs and symptoms of heart failure. A decreased level of consciousness because of a decreased amount of oxygen provided to the brain can be indicative of CHF. Jugular neck vein distension is

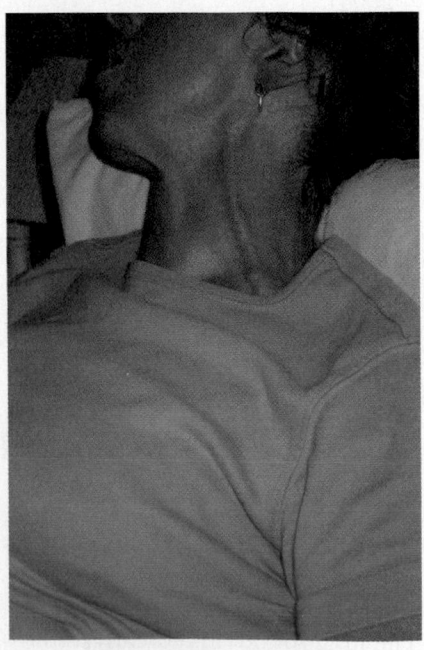

Figure 25-2 Jugular neck vein distension.

BOX 25-1

SYMPTOMS OF RIGHT-SIDED HEART FAILURE

- Swelling of feet and ankles.
- Frequent nocturnal urination.
- Pronounced neck veins.
- Palpitations.
- Irregular or rapid heartbeat.
- Fatigue.
- Weakness.
- Faintness.

considered abnormal and can be an indication of increased volume and pressure in the heart (Figure 25-2). The lower extremities may show signs of decreased perfusion with a palpable coolness, paleness, cyanosis, edema, and poorly healing wounds. Examination of the liver can reveal an increased venous pressure of the hepatojugular reflux. Right-sided heart failure may present with the symptoms shown in Box 25-1.

Conditions that may precipitate pronounced symptoms in those who are predisposed to heart failure include increased activity, increased intake of fluids or salt, fever, infection, anemia, arrhythmias, hyperthyroidism, and kidney disease. Physical examination reveals the signs displayed in Box 25-2.

Diagnostic Tests

When heart failure symptoms and physical assessment reveals signs of heart failure, the following diagnostic tests may give more insight into the patient's condition. An electrocardiogram (ECG) can show signs of thickening of the heart muscle and dysrhythmias. An echocardiogram (an ultrasound of the heart) may show heart enlargement, decreased cardiac function, and heart abnormalities. A multiple gated acquisition (MUGA) scan is a useful noninvasive tool for assessing the function of the heart and can evaluate the ejection fraction (Daniels, 2003). A chest X-ray (CXR) may show enlargement of the heart and will also give information about abnormalities in the lungs.

Stress tests, also called treadmill tests or exercise tests, show how the heart functions when it is working hard and when it is stressed or exercised. The more pumping and harder the heart works, the more oxygen that is required for the body to continue working hard. A stress test shows if there is a decrease in the amount of blood that is supplied to the arteries. A stress test gives information about the amount of work that the heart can tolerate and still be able to supply the body with oxygenation demands. Stress tests are used to evaluate for coronary artery disease (CAD), which may be the cause of heart failure.

Tracer studies or radioactive imaging is a means of assessing the heart through introducing low-dose radioactive tracers that are injected into the blood stream and are visualized going to the heart. These studies can give information about perfusion defects and metabolic abnormalities of the myocardium (Czernin, Gambhir, Brunken, & Schelbert, 2004).

Laboratory tests may also be performed to confirm presence of heart failure. A CBC can give information about the oxygen carrying capacity of the blood. Imbalances of potassium, sodium, and calcium are especially important indicators of the pumping ability of the heart. Fluid and electrolytes levels can explain peripheral edema, vascular congestion, and kidney disease. Urinalysis sodium and specific gravity levels are useful in diagnosing the urine concentrations indicate kidney failure. A brain natriuretic peptide (BNP), a hormone found in the left ventricle, is used to help diagnose and grade the severity of heart failure (Daniels, 2003). Thyroid function and iron level tests are used to rule out disorders whose signs and symptoms mimic heart failure. These are treatable causes of heart failure.

Serum inflammatory markers, such as serum interleukin-6 (IL-6), C-reactive protein (CRP), and spontaneous production of tumor necrosis factor-alpha (TNF-α), have been shown to be associated with an increased risk of CHF. (Cesari, 2003). The TNF detected in heart failure patients has two functions; to reduce vascular smooth muscle tone and myocardial contractility and to correlate with clinical severity. IL-6 is a cytokine protein that assists in regulation of the immune system. CRP is a measure of inflammation and is part of the immune reaction that protects the body from infection in the face of injury. These lab values indicate the inflammation that affects the coronary arteries. Inflammation of the coronary arteries may lead to narrowing of the coronary arteries, which in turn increases the risk of heart failure.

HEART FAILURE CLINICAL MANIFESTATIONS

Right-Sided Heart Failure

- Palpable dysrhythmia.
- Auscultated dysrhythmia.
- Weight gain.
- Distended neck veins.
- Enlarged liver.
- Ankle edema.

Left-Sided Heart Failure

- Shortness of breath, paroxysmal nocturnal dyspnea.
- Palpitations, tachycardia.
- Cough with frothy, blood-tinged mucus.
- Fatigue, weakness.
- Syncope.
- Weight gain, fluid retention.
- Oliguria.
- Dysrhythmic heart rate, heart murmurs, extra heart sounds.
- Lung crackles, decreased basilar lung sounds.

Source: Hart, J. A. (2004). Right-sided heart failure. *Retrieved June 24, 2006, from http://www.nlm.nih.gov; Kang, S. (2004).* Left-sided heart failure. *Retrieved June 24, 2006, from http://www.nlm.nih.gov.*

Cardiac catheterization is a procedure used to help identify causes and degree of heart failure. The procedure is performed by placing a catheter through a vein that leads to the heart. An angiogram, also called a left heart catheterization, is a procedure in which the arterial system is accessed. An X-ray is taken during a cardiac catheterization procedure to allow visualization of the internal anatomy of the heart and blood vessels after the intravascular introduction of radiopaque contrast medium (dye) and can assist in measurement of pulmonary artery pressure (Murthy, 2004). Sometimes a dye can be injected into the veins, which allows a real-time movie-type visualization of the heart while it is functioning. Cardiac catheterization is most useful in diagnosing the pressure of the heart's chambers, thus identifying the amount the heart is experiencing and degree to which they are able to pump blood.

Myocardial biopsy tests for cardiomyopathy. Myocardial biopsy, performed during the cardiac catheterization procedure, is the retrieval of a part of the heart muscle that is sent for laboratory testing. The heart muscle is examined for inflammatory markers that would indicate an infection or enlargement.

Magnetic resonance imaging (MRI) is a noninvasive, still image test used to examine the heart muscle. Instead of using an X-ray, MRIs use radio waves and a magnet to display multiple cross-sectional images of the heart giving a three-dimensional picture of the heart. Using this sophisticated technology, it is possible for MRIs to detect enlargement of the heart or decreased heart functioning.

Nursing Diagnoses

Based on the information gathered, examples of nursing diagnoses in the patient with heart failure may include the following:
- Activity intolerance related to compromised oxygen transport system secondary to heart failure.
- Risk for ineffective breathing pattern related to excessive secretions secondary to cardiopulmonary dysfunction.
- Anxiety related to actual threat to biological integrity secondary to heart failure and death.

Planning and Implementation

Heart failure occurs in the presence of an overworking heart muscle that causes respiratory difficulty and multiple cardiac and respiratory signs and symptoms. The cause of the heart failure and its stage are the primary factors used in determining the most appropriate treatments. The goal of the treatment of heart failure is aimed at decreasing the cardiac workload to improve the cardiac function and control symptoms. Nursing management of heart failure is varied and depends on the severity of patient symptoms. Nursing management of heart failure largely depends on assessing and evaluating the effectiveness of medical and multidisciplinary management of the patient. Research has shown that nurses who are specially trained in the care of patients with heart failure can improve hospitalized patient outcomes.

Treatment for mild symptoms includes controlling volume overload through monitoring sodium and fluid intake. Dietary restrictions of salt are recommended. Fluid intake may also be restricted. These restrictions, whether recommended in isolation or with other treatments, make up the most basic concept of volume control in the treatment of heart failure.

Treatment of acute heart failure consists of pharmacological therapy, such as morphine, diuretics, and cardiovascular support medications that are often administered intravenously for quick administration. Respiratory support consists of nonrebreathing oxygen by mask to relieve hypoxemia and dyspnea. Respiratory support may evolve into intubation and mechanical ventilation with positive end-expiratory pressure (PEEP). Nursing management includes

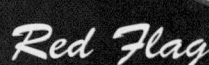

Red Flag

Acute Pulmonary Edema

Acute pulmonary edema is the condition of fluid accumulating in the lungs in a matter of minutes. The patient will have labored and rapid breathing; frothy, bloody fluid containing pus coughed from the lungs (sputum); tachycardia and possibly serious disturbances in the heart's rhythm; cold, clammy, sweaty, and bluish skin; and a drop in blood pressure resulting in a thready pulse.

The nurse should plan to place the patient in a sitting position, administer high concentrations of oxygen, assist with administering drug therapy, and assist with mechanical ventilation.

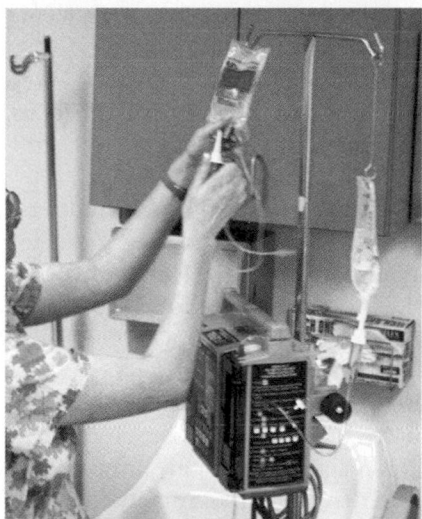

Figure 25-3 Multiple medications are common in the treatment of heart failure.

assessment of symptoms, administration and monitoring of therapeutic regimen, measuring treatment effectiveness, and providing physiological and psychological support.

Monitoring of oxygenation via pulse oximetry and arterial blood gases is one of the more important of nursing management activities. Positioning the patient for maximum cardiovascular functioning is also important. If possible, patients should dangle legs to decrease the venous return to the heart. The head of the bed should remain elevated so that there is a decrease in the amount of lung surface area affected by the increased fluid volume. Also important in nursing management of patients with CHF is reassurance and anxiety reduction. At a time when the heart is working its hardest, anxiety can cause more work for the heart.

Collaborative Management

It is clear that management of heart failure requires knowledge, dedication, and consultation of several disciplines. Physical therapists can help recommend and encourage physical exercise and troubleshoot physical limitations. Respiratory therapists can assist in evaluating and maintaining the optimal pulmonary function of patients with CHF. Nutritionists can assist in the dietary management of the heart failure. Psychologists can help in the psychosocial aspects of depression and anxiety. Social workers can assist with the psychosocial aspects that interfere with maintaining a health home life and health care network. It takes many disciplines to implement an effective therapeutic regimen. Randomized prospective clinical trials of inpatient multifaceted programs targeted at reducing morbidity associated with heart failure found that multidisciplinary interventions can reduce hospitalization readmission rates and length of stay.

Pharmacology

Treatment for moderate heart failure symptoms includes introducing a medicine regimen. There are many medications found to benefit patients by reducing the heart's workload (Figure 25-3). Angiotensin converting enzymes (ACE) inhibitors (e.g., captopril, enalapril), angiotensin receptor blockers (e.g., bisoprolol, carvedilol), vasodilators, nitrates, beta blockers, diuretics (e.g., furosemide, torsemide), hormones, digitalis, and aspirin are all used for treatment of heart failure (Broyles, Reiss, & Evans, 2007).

ACE inhibitors work by decreasing the pressure the heart must overcome to eject blood from the heart by interfering with the renin-angiotensin-aldosterone system. This interference results blocking the conversion of angiotensin I to angiotensin II in the kidney, causing a decreased aldosterone, increased sodium excretion, and in peripheral vasodilatation that allows for decreased pressure-causing volume in the heart and a decrease in blood pressure (Jessup & Brozena, 2003). Clinical research in the form of random controlled trials has found that when compared with placebos, ACE inhibitors significantly reduce ischemic events, mortality, and hospital admissions for heart failure patients. In addition to promoting vasodilation and reducing aldosterone secretion, ACE inhibitors can enhance the action of the cardio-protective effects of bradykinin and work to modify cardiac remodeling an apoptosis (cellular suicide). For those patients who are asymptomatic for heart failure, ACE inhibitors can delay the onset of symptoms and reduce major cardiovascular events (McKelvie, 2003).

Angiotensin receptor blockers (ARBs) work similarly to ACE inhibitors by decreasing the pressure the heart must overcome to eject blood from the heart by interfering with the renin-angiotensin-aldosterone system. ARBs are typically used when ACE inhibitors are not tolerated by the patient. ARBs have not been shown to be more effective than ACE inhibitors for the treatment of heart failure (Jong, Demers, McKelvie, & Liu, 2002).

Skills 360°

Nursing Management for Patients with Heart Failure

Patients with heart failure are often faced with lifestyle changes that become obstacles to attaining optimum health. In this case, the role of the nurse becomes that of a partner in health where the nurse assists the patient in motivating them toward healthy behaviors. Foremost among the interventions are seeking to understand the person's frame of reference, particularly via reflective listening, expressing acceptance, and affirmation, eliciting and selectively reinforcing the patient's own self-motivational statements, expressions of problem recognition, concern, desire and intention to change, and ability to change; monitoring the patient's degree of readiness to change; and ensuring that resistance is not generated by jumping ahead of the patient.

Anticoagulants and antiplatelet medications are not typically used as a primary treatment for heart failure, but are commonly prescribed for concurrent problems in patients with heart failure. Anticoagulants and antiplatelet agents are used to prevent cardiac events (cerebral vascular accidents and MIs) in patients at risk of developing blood clots. One of the functions of anticoagulants and antiplatelet agents is to ensure the integrity of the vascular system by keeping the blood free of clots. Maintaining vascularity is one of the solutions in the management and symptom control of heart failure patients. Research has found a reduction in mortality and cardiovascular events with use of anticoagulants in patients with heart failure, who have concomitant disease processes that require use of such agents. Research does not yet support routine use of anticoagulants in heart failure patients who remain in sinus rhythm.

Beta blockers are medications that block the uptake of norepinephrine throughout the body. Some beta blockers are formulated to work specifically to block the beta receptors of the heart. Beta receptors can be found many places in the body like the heart, lung, arteries, brain, and uterus. Beta blockers work like a lock and key. The beta blocker fits chemically into beta receptors, which prevents the body's normally produced norepinephrine from binding to the receptors. Norepinephrine that is left unblocked causes the fight or flight response. Reduction of the fight or flight response allows the heart to relax (Uren, Odbert, & Davey, 2002). In addition, a significant increase in the left ventricular ejection fraction occurs after treatment with beta blockers.

Digoxin (digitalis), classified as a cardiac glycoside, is used to increase the heart's contractility. Although the exact action of cardiac glycosides is known, it is commonly agreed that increased glycoside concentrations lead to increased myocardial cell contraction. Digitalis is prescribed to increase the ability of the heart to contract, thus enhancing the pumping function during atrial fibrillation, a common arrhythmia of right-sided heart failure (Hart, 2004). Digoxin is use in patients who have symptomatic CHF and are often used in conjunction with other medications, such as ACE inhibitors, diuretics, and beta blockers. In patients who have normal sinus rhythm, research indicates that digitalis has a useful role in the treatment of CHF.

Diuretics help the body to dispose of volume overload. Fluid and salts are excreted to reduce pressure that too much volume places on the heart. Any patient taking diuretics should be closely monitored for dehydration, hyponatremia, and hypokalemia. Diuretics have been shown to reduce the risk of worsening heart failure, improve exercise capacity, and reduce the risk of death related to heart failure (Faris, et al., 2002).

Antihyperlipidemics are not typically used as primary treatment of heart failure but are commonly used in heart failure patients for concurrent problems. Antihyperlipidemics are agents that lower lipids, which are used to prevent cardiac events (cerebral vascular accidents and MIs) in patients with hyperlipidemia. One of the functions of antihyperlipidemic agents is to ensure the integrity of the vascular system by lowering plasma cholesterol. Maintaining vascularity is one of the solutions in the management and symptom control of heart failure patients.

Nitrates function to increase venous capacity, reduce the resistance in the circulation, and dilate coronary arteries. These actions allow blood to circulate more freely and decrease the blood volume responsible for the increased pressure and strain on the heart muscle.

Vasodilators work similarly to ACE inhibitors and ARBs to decrease blood pressure by dilating vessels to decrease the circulating volume of blood that the heart must pump. Vasodilators, however, act directly on muscles in the blood vessel, rather than interfering with the renin-angiotensin-aldosterone system.

Medications that have been found to be contraindicated in patients with CHF are listed in Table 25-1.

TABLE 25-1 Recommended and Contraindicated Medications in Heart Failure	
RECOMMENDED MEDICATIONS FOR HEART FAILURE THERAPY	**CONTRAINDICATED MEDICATIONS FOR HEART FAILURE PATIENTS**
Loop diuretics for volume overload	Alcohol
ACE inhibitors (titrate upward to optimal dose)	Cocaine
Beta blockers (titrate upward to optimal dose with support and monitoring)	Antiarrhythmic agents except amiodarone
	Calcium channel blockers except amlodipine
Digitalis	NSAIDs (associated with development of CHF and interact with ACE inhibitors)
Spironolactone for advanced heart failure (with optimal doses of ACE inhibitors and beta blockers. Monitor for complications such as hyperkalemia)	
	Thiazolidinediones (may cause fluid retention)
	Metformin
ARBs if ACE inhibitors are not tolerated	

Source: Deaton, C., Bennett, J. A., & Riegel, B. (2004). State of the science for care of older adults with heart disease. Nursing Clinics of North America, 39(3), 495–528; Masoudi, F. A., & Krumholz, H. M. (2003). Polypharmacy and comorbidity in heart failure. British Journal of Medicine, 327(7414), 513–514.

Surgery

Severe heart failure requires a more aggressive regimen. Although not considered treatment of heart failure, surgical interventions are recommended when there are conditions contributing to the severity of heart failure. Surgery may be an option when there is a valvular disease, valvular dysfunction, or rhythm dysfunction. Heart failure caused by a valvular disorder often results in a need for heart valve replacement. Intermittent ventricular fibrillations often require implantation of a cardiac defibrillator.

Coronary artery bypass graft (CABG) surgery, frequently termed cabbage surgery from the acronym, is a type of open-heart surgery in which the heart is accessed through the sternum. In CABG, blood is bypassed around the arteries that are clogged by plaque, fat, and cholesterol to restore optimal blood flow of oxygenated blood to the heart. Patients are admitted from their CABG directly into a coronary care unit (CCU) (Figure 25-4) until they are stable enough to be transferred to a telemetry unit or cardiac recovery unit.

Valve surgery, also called valve replacement, valve repair, and heart valve prosthesis, is the treatment for heart failure when the problem derrives from a valvular dysfunction or disease. The heart's valves are designed to provide one-way flow of blood through the heart. The opening and closing of the heart valves produce the sound of the heartbeat. Valves may be replaced or simply repaired. Heart valve surgery is done while the patient is under general anesthesia. The procedure begins with an incision made through the sternum, making it an open-heart surgery. Incoming blood is directed away from the heart into a heart-lung bypass machine (Figure 25-5). This machine performs as the body would by oxygenating the blood and pumping it throughout the body during the operation. (Daller, 2004).

Evaluation of Outcomes

Potential patient outcomes for each of the example nursing diagnoses for the patient with heart failure are:

- Activity intolerance related to compromised oxygen transport system secondary to heart failure. The patient maintains activity level within capabilities, as evidenced by normal heart rate and blood pressure during activity, as well as absence of shortness of breath, weakness, and fatigue.

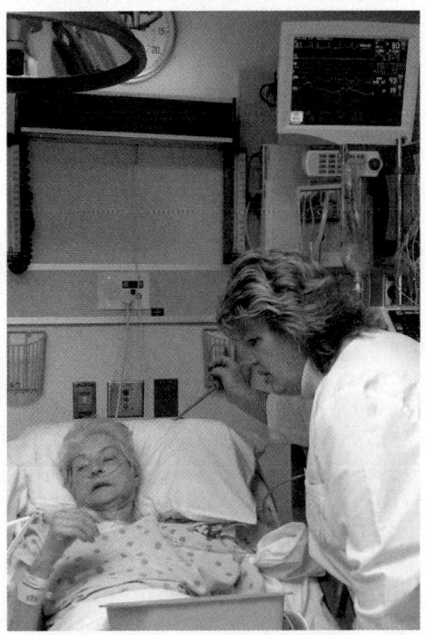

Figure 25-4 Patient in CCU on her second day postoperative CABG.

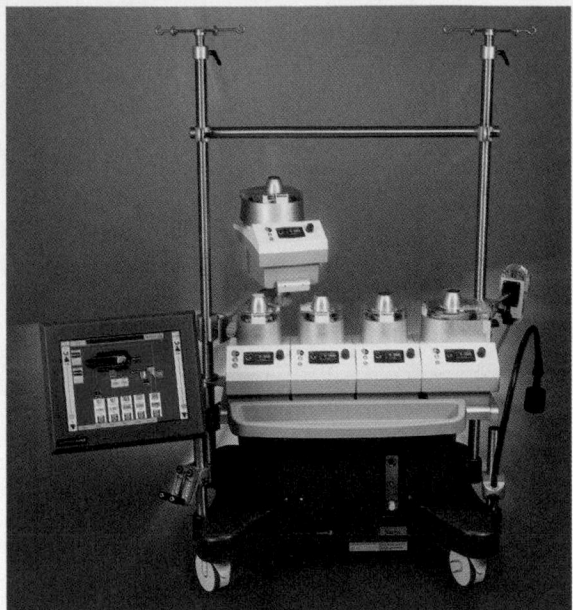

Figure 25-5 Terumo, advanced perfusion system 1 (Courtesy of Teromo Cardiovascular Systems Corporation).

Fast Forward ▶▶▶

Treatment for Heart Failure in the Future

The heart failure treatment timeline has been described as following:

Prior to 2000, treatment was mostly nonpharmalogical (bed rest, inactivity, and fluid restriction) and pharmacological interventions (digitalis, diuretics, vasodilators, inotropes, and neurohormones). Current technology brings more device-laden interventions, such as cardiac resynchronization therapy (CRT), implantable cardiac defibrillators (ICD), and left ventricular assist devices (LAVD). The future decades are predicted to have cellular and genetic treatment options such as gene therapy, cell implantation and regeneration, and xenotransplantation (Staylor, 2005).

- Risk for ineffective breathing pattern. The patient's breathing pattern is maintained by eupnea, normal skin color, and regular respiratory rate or pattern.
- Anxiety related to actual threat to biological integrity secondary to heart failure and death. The patient should be able to recognize the signs of anxiety, demonstrate positive coping mechanisms, and describe a reduction in the level of anxiety experienced.

HEART MUSCLE DISEASE AND INFLAMMATION DYSFUNCTION

Heart muscle disease is called cardiomyopathy and is a problem with the physical shape of the muscle. Heart muscle inflammatory dysfunction is called **carditis** (an inflammation of the heart muscle). Both cardiomyopathy and carditis can cause a problem with the heart's ability to function.

Cardiomyopathy is a disease of the heart muscle; often its origin is unknown. Cardiomyopathy is a serious condition that can lead to heart failure, dysrhythmia, and death. Diseased heart muscle is unable to function correctly, which results in decreased functioning of the heart. A decreased functioning of the heart results in an impaired cardiac output, decreased stroke volume, stimulation of the sympathetic nervous system, stimulation of the renin-angiotensin-aldosterone response, increased systemic vascular resistance, increased sodium and fluid retention, and increased workload of the heart, which eventually leads to heart failure. The Cardiomyopathy Association (2004) currently recognizes four types of cardiomyopathy: dilated, hypertrophic, arrhythmogenic right ventricular, and restrictive.

Dilated Cardiomyopathy

Dilated cardiomyopathy (DCM), a disease of the heart muscle, results in a dilated heart chamber, which expands much the way a balloon expands. DCM results in a decreased ability for the heart to pump strongly and forcefully. DCM is associated with coronary heart disease (CHD), hypertension, and heart valve disease. Risk factors attributed to DCM are family members with DCM, a history of Coxsackie B viral infection, autoimmune disease, toxins (alcohol, chemotherapeutics), and pregnancy. DCM leads to a weakened, thin heart muscle wall that is unable to pump blood efficiently throughout the body, causing heart failure.

Assessment with Clinical Manifestations

Assessment includes noting the common signs and symptoms of DCM. Signs and symptoms include shortness of breath due to congestion of the lungs and dependent edema, which is the accumulation of fluid in body parts below the heart that indicates an inability of the heart to effectively pump fluid throughout the body. Other signs and symptoms of DCM include tiredness, palpitations, syncope, and chest pain (The Cardiomyopathy Association, 2004).

Nursing Diagnoses

Based on the information gathered, examples of nursing diagnoses in the patient with DCM may include the following:
- Activity intolerance related to compromised oxygen transport system secondary to heart muscle dysfunction.

- Risk for ineffective breathing pattern related to decreased respiratory depth secondary to pain.
- Pain related to friction rub and inflammatory process.

Planning and Implementation

When additional information is needed to make a definitive diagnosis, other tests and studies may be required. These may include cardiac catheterization, biopsy of heart tissue, study of the electrical activity of the heart, and radioactivity studies to assess the heart's contractility (The Cardiomyopathy Association, 2004). Planning and organizing the timing of testing and care of the patient is an important step in caring for the patient. Nursing management of patients with DCM includes assessment of the patient's family and support systems. DCM often runs in families. Therefore, it is important to encourage the family members to have diagnostic testing for DCM for prevention of further disease processes. DCM is associated with anxiety and depression (The Cardiomyopathy Association, 2004). These associated symptoms can be as important to the quality of life for DCM patients as other treatment of the disease. Assessment of associated anxiety and depression are integral in the nursing management of DCM patients. Referral to support groups and national DCM organizations is important. Anticipating and answering frequently asked questions is important. Unlike valvular disorders, DCM does not require **prophylactic** (preventing or contributing to the prevention of disease) antibiotic use prior to dental and other invasive procedures unless the patient has an associated valvular problem.

Pharmacology

Medical management of DCM consists of minimizing symptoms and making the patient comfortable. ACE inhibitors are used to prevent further dilation of the heart. Beta blockers are used to reduce the strain that heart failure has on the heart when heart failure is present. Diuretics are used to decrease the amount of fluid that the heart has to pump. Anticoagulants are used to decrease blood clots that affect circulation. Antiarrhythmics are used to maintain the most effective electrical stimulation that maintains the efficiency of the heart.

Surgery

When medical treatments are ineffective, other treatments are necessary. Cardioversion, heart transplantation, pacemaker insertion, and implantable defibrillators are necessary to maintain effective heart functioning (The Cardiomyopathy Association, 2004).

Evaluation of Outcomes

Potential patient outcomes for each of the example nursing diagnoses for the patient with DCM are (Box 25-3):
- Activity intolerance related to compromised oxygen transport system secondary to heart muscle dysfunction. The patient maintains activity level within capabilities, as evidenced by normal heart rate and blood pressure during activity, as well as absence of shortness of breath, weakness, and fatigue.
- Risk for ineffective breathing pattern. The patient's breathing pattern is maintained by eupnea, normal skin color, and regular respiratory rate or pattern.
- Pain related to friction rub and inflammatory process. The patient should verbalize an adequate relief of pain along with the ability to realistically cope with the pain if it is not completely relieved.

Hypertrophic Cardiomyopathy

HCM is an increase in the size and thickness of the heart muscle. The cause of HCM is not clear, although a strong familial link has been shown. Otherwise, HCM is considered **idiopathic** (a disease state that arises from an

---

BOX 25-3

NIC/NOC FOR HEART MUSCLE DYSFUNCTION

NIC

Activity Intolerance
- Oxygen therapy
- Respiratory monitoring
- Vital signs monitoring

Risk for Ineffective Breathing Pattern
- Medication management
- Oxygen therapy
- Teaching: disease processes

Pain
- Pain management
- Medication management
- Positioning

NOC

Activity Intolerance
- Self-care status
- Activity tolerance
- Physical fitness

Risk for Ineffective Breathing Pattern
- Endurance
- Positioning
- Circulation status

Pain
- Medication response
- Comfort level
- Pain control

unknown cause). The sheer size of the hypertrophic heart muscle decreases the volume of blood that can be accommodated in the heart's chambers (Figure 25-6). Likewise, the size and thickness of the hypertrophic heart muscle disallows timely cardiac relaxation that is necessary for quick blood filling of the heart chambers. The heart tries to compensate for the lack of ventricular filling by having the atria pump more forcefully to maintain the necessary volume of oxygenated blood needed for body system survival.

Assessment with Clinical Manifestations

Assessment of HCM may reveal an asymptomatic patient, or include shortness of breath, chest pain, palpitations, light-headedness, and blackouts. Physical examination may reveal a palpably forceful apical pulse and heart murmur. Suspicious signs and symptoms would prompt inquiry into their findings. Often an abnormal ECG result is found in HCM patients. Definitive diagnosis of HCM is dependent on visualization of excessive thickness of the heart muscle as seen on an echocardiogram.

Nursing Diagnoses

Based on the information gathered, examples of nursing diagnoses in the patient with HCM may include the following:

- Activity intolerance related to compromised oxygen transport system secondary to heart muscle dysfunction.
- Risk for ineffective breathing pattern related to decreased respiratory depth secondary to pain.
- Pain related to friction rub and inflammatory process.

Planning and Implementation

Often, additional information is needed to plan the care of a patient with HCM. Other diagnostic tests, such as cardiac catheterization, coronary angiography, electrophysiology studies, exercise testing, Holter monitoring, and radionuclide studies, may be used to provide additional information and determine extent of disease (The Cardiomyopathy Association, 2004). An ECG allows for visualization and evaluation the dysrhythmic changes consistent with left ventricular hypertrophy. The cardiac catheterization allows the health care provider to rule out CAD as a causative factor.

Nursing management for HCM involves educating the patient about his or her individualized physical exertion recommendations. Nursing management of patients with HCM also includes assessment of the patient's family and support systems. HCM often runs in families. Therefore, it is important to encourage the family members to have diagnostic testing for HCM for prevention of further disease processes. Weight reduction is suggested for those obese HCM patients, moderation in alcohol intake is suggested, and flu vaccination is considered. HCM patients are encouraged to avoid overexertion, acute loss of body fluid volume, situations that may predispose one to fainting, hot showers or water immersion, and medication that quickly drops blood pressure. Any of the following symptoms are to be reported to the patient's health care provider immediately: sudden loss of consciousness, episodes of rapid palpitation, onset of central chest pain, and unexplained breathlessness.

Pharmacology

Medical management is aimed at treating symptoms, as no cure is known for HCM. Medical treatment includes use of beta blockers when heart failure is present, to reduce the strain on the heart. Calcium channel blockers are effective in reducing the stiffness of the myocardium to improve the chamber filling. Antiarrhythmics are used to maintain the most effective electrical stimulation that maintains the efficiency of the heart. Diuretics are used to decrease the amount of fluid that the heart has to pump. Anticoagulants are used to

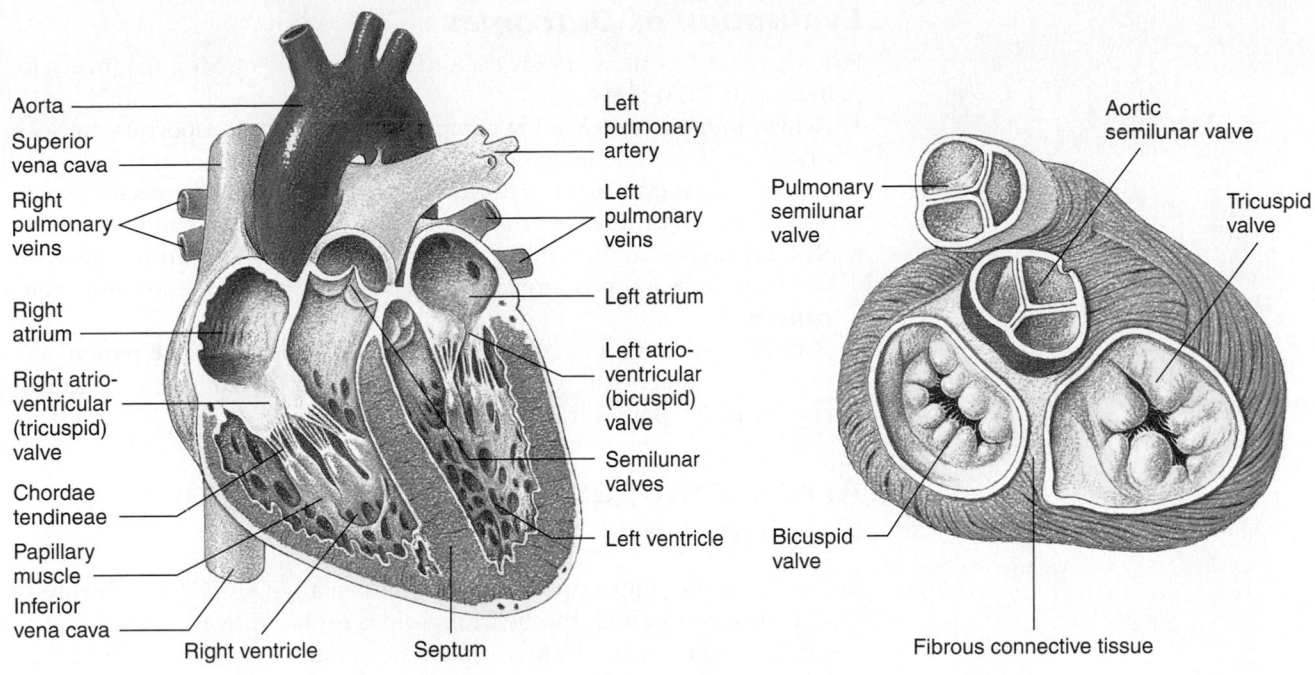

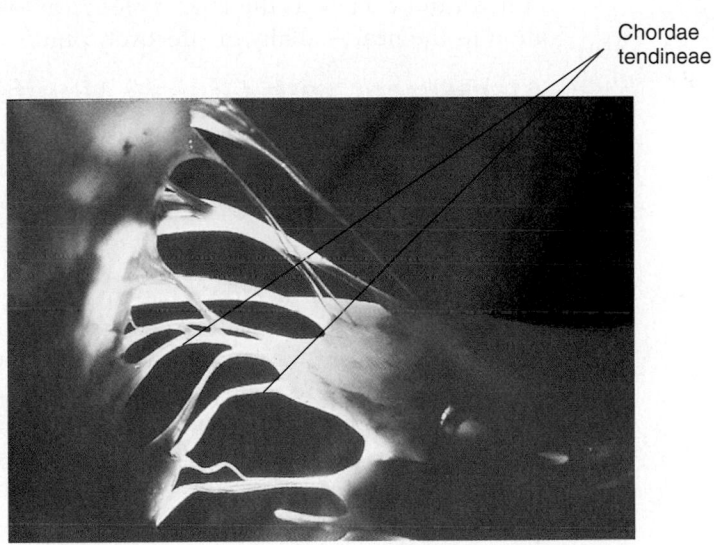

Figure 25-6 The heart and its valves.

decrease blood clots that affect circulation. Although **endocarditis** (inflammation of the endocardium) is rare, people who have turbulent blood flow in the left ventricular outflow tract or across the mitral valve should receive antibiotic prophylaxis prior to dental procedures and any other situations, in which there is an increased risk of bacteria entering the bloodstream (The Cardiomyopathy Association, 2004).

Surgery

When these medical treatments are ineffective, other treatments are necessary. Surgical management for those patients who do not receive relief from symptoms with medical management may include a **myectomy** (removal of the offending muscle). Heart transplantation is necessary for some who have severe alteration in the heart's ability to pump effectively. Still other possible treatments include electrical cardioversion, pacemaker insertion, and implantable defibrillator.

Evaluation of Outcomes

Potential patient outcomes for each of the example nursing diagnoses for the patient with HCM are:

- Activity intolerance related to compromised oxygen transport system secondary to heart muscle dysfunction. The patient maintains activity level within capabilities, as evidenced by normal heart rate and blood pressure during activity, as well as absence of shortness of breath, weakness, and fatigue.
- Risk for ineffective breathing pattern. The patient's breathing pattern is maintained by eupnea, normal skin color, and regular respiratory rate or pattern.
- Pain related to friction rub and inflammatory process. The patient should verbalize an adequate relief of pain along with the ability to realistically cope with the pain if it is not completely relieved.

Arrhythmogenic Right Ventricular Cardiomyopathy

Arrhythmogenic right ventricular cardiomyopathy (ARVC) is a disease of the cardiac muscle in which the heart muscle is replaced by fibrous scar and fatty tissue. The right ventricle more likely to be affected. The cause of ARVC is unknown; however, it is thought to be genetically linked. The progressive loss of heart muscle affects the heart's electrical functioning, which leads to alteration in the heart's ability to effectively pump.

Assessment with Clinical Manifestations

Assessment of ARVC may reveal an asymptomatic patient, or the patient may complain of palpitations, light-headedness, fatigue, fainting, syncope, and signs and symptoms of heart failure.

Diagnostic Tests

Diagnostic tests may include a patient's history and such tests as an ECG, a Holter monitor, an exercise test, an echocardiogram, and blood testing. With this information in hand, the health care provider is able to rule out other causes of heart failure and cardiomyopathy, allowing for a diagnosis of exclusion. Other diagnostic tests, such as MRI, cardiac catheterization, and biopsy studies, may be used to provide additional information and determine extent of disease. An ECG allows for visualization and evaluation the dysrhythmic changes consistent with left ventricular hypertrophy. The cardiac catheterization allows the practitioner to rule out CAD as a causative factor. A biopsy of the heart tissue allows for analysis of myocardial tissue cells.

Nursing Diagnoses

Based on the information gathered, examples of nursing diagnoses in the patient with ARVC may include the following:

- Activity intolerance related to compromised oxygen transport system secondary to heart muscle dysfunction.
- Risk for ineffective breathing pattern related to decreased respiratory depth secondary to pain.
- Pain related to friction rub and inflammatory process.

Planning and Implementation

Management of ARVC consists of minimizing symptoms and controlling any resultant arrhythmias. When these medical treatments are ineffective, other treatments are necessary (e.g., pharmacology, surgery). Nursing management includes lifestyle advice. ARVC patients should refrain from overexertion and should report any cardiomyopathic symptoms to their health care provider. Nursing management of patients with ARVC also includes assessment of the patient's family and support systems. ARVC often runs in families. Therefore, it is important to encourage the family members to have diagnostic testing for ARVC for prevention of further disease processes. Weight reduction is suggested for those obese ARVC patients, moderation in alcohol intake is suggested, and flu vaccination is considered. Any of the following symptoms are to be reported to the patient's health care provider immediately: sudden loss of consciousness, episodes of rapid palpitation, onset of central chest pain, and unexplained breathlessness.

Pharmacology

Antiarrhythmics are used to maintain the most effective electrical stimulation that maintains the efficiency of the heart. ACE inhibitors are used to prevent further dilation of the heart. Diuretics are used to decrease the amount of fluid that the heart has to pump. Anticoagulants are used to decrease blood clots that affect circulation. Prophylactic antibiotics are used only in patients who have concomitant valvular disease.

Surgery

Cardioversion, ablation therapy, heart transplantation, pacemaker insertion, and implantable defibrillators are necessary to maintain effective heart functioning.

Evaluation of Outcomes

Potential patient outcomes for each of the example nursing diagnoses for the patient with ARVC are:
- Activity intolerance related to compromised oxygen transport system secondary to heart muscle dysfunction. The patient maintains activity level within capabilities, as evidenced by normal heart rate and blood pressure during activity, as well as absence of shortness of breath, weakness, and fatigue.
- Risk for ineffective breathing pattern. The patient's breathing pattern is maintained by eupnea, normal skin color, and regular respiratory rate or pattern.
- Pain related to friction rub and inflammatory process. The patient should verbalize an adequate relief of pain along with the ability to realistically cope with the pain if it is not completely relieved.

Restrictive Cardiomyopathy

Restrictive cardiomyopathy (RCM) is a disease of the ventricular heart muscle in which the muscle walls become stiff, but not necessarily thickened. The cause is not known; however, metabolic disorders, **sequela** (any abnormality following or resulting from a disease or injury or treatment) of radiation therapy, and family history of cardiomyopathy have been identified as causes in some people.

Pathophysiology

The stiffness of the heart wall muscle causes a resistance against which the atria have to pump blood. Blood may back up into the lungs and major veins of the neck and liver. The heart tries to compensate for the ventricular resistance by having the atria pump more forcefully to maintain the necessary volume of oxygenated blood needed for body system survival. The result of ineffective compensation is heart failure.

Assessment with Clinical Manifestations

Assessment of RCM reveals symptomatic and asymptomatic patients. Symptomatic patients present with heart failure in the following clinical manifestations: crackles on pulmonary auscultation, jugular vein distension, pitting edema of dependent body parts, and enlarged liver, fatigue, and shortness of breath.

Diagnostic Tests

Diagnosis of RCM requires physical examination, ECG, and an echocardiogram. With this information in hand, the health care provider is able to rule out other causes of heart failure and cardiomyopathy, allowing for a diagnosis of exclusion. Other diagnostic tests, such as MRI, cardiac catheterization, and biopsy studies, may be used to provide additional information and determine extent of disease. An ECG allows for visualization and evaluation the dysrhythmic changes consistent with left ventricular hypertrophy. The cardiac catheterization allows the health care provider to rule out CAD as a causative factor. A biopsy of the heart tissue allows for analysis of myocardial tissue cells.

Nursing Diagnoses

Based on the information gathered, examples of nursing diagnoses in the patient with RCM may include the following:
* Activity intolerance related to compromised oxygen transport system secondary to heart muscle dysfunction.
* Risk for ineffective breathing pattern related to decreased respiratory depth secondary to pain.
* Pain related to friction rub and inflammatory process.

Planning and Implementation

Medical management includes treatment of symptoms and sequela. Severe cases may require heart transplantation. Nursing management of patients with RCM includes assessment of the patient's family and support systems. RCM can be genetically linked, therefore it is important to encourage the family members to have diagnostic testing for RCM for prevention of further disease processes.

Evaluation of Outcomes

Potential patient outcomes for each of the example nursing diagnoses for the patient with RCM are:
* Activity intolerance related to compromised oxygen transport system secondary to heart muscle dysfunction. The patient maintains activity level within capabilities, as evidenced by normal heart rate and blood pressure during activity, as well as absence of shortness of breath, weakness, and fatigue.
* Risk for ineffective breathing pattern. The patient's breathing pattern is maintained by eupnea, normal skin color, and regular respiratory rate or pattern.
* Pain related to friction rub and inflammatory process. The patient should verbalize an adequate relief of pain along with the ability to realistically cope with the pain if it is not completely relieved.

Carditis

Inflammation of the heart or heart valves is termed carditis. The three types of carditis are endocarditis, myocarditis, and **pericarditis** (inflammation of the pericardium). Rheumatic endocarditis, a type of bacterial endocarditis, has had a higher incidence in developing countries because of poorer recognition and treatment of streptococcal infection, which is the causative agent in rheumatic endocarditis (Saver, Hodgson, Van Norman, & Bahler, 2004).

Bacterial Endocarditis

Bacterial endocarditis is an infection of the heart's inner lining (**endocardium**) or the heart valves. Certain types of bacteria can damage and destroy the heart's endocardium and heart valves. Bacteria travel to the heart via the bloodstream. Bacteria can enter the bloodstream during medical procedures, such as professional teeth cleaning; tonsillectomy or adenoidectomy; examination of the respiratory passageways with an instrument known as a rigid bronchoscope; certain types of surgery on the respiratory passageways, the GI tract, or the urinary tract; or gallbladder or prostate surgery. It is not common that these procedures will cause endocarditis in healthy people. People with one or more of the following are at greater risk of contracting endocarditis: an artificial (prosthetic) heart valve, a history of previous endocarditis, heart valves damaged (scarred) by conditions, such as rheumatic fever, congenital heart, heart valve defects, or HCM (American Heart Association, 2006b).

Pathophysiology

Once in the bloodstream, bacteria travel through the heart, and they attach to any insult that the heart may already have encountered, for example, valvular problems, structural abnormalities, or scar tissue. Bacteria such as streptococci, enterococci, pneumococci, staphylococci, fungi, and rickettsiae invade the endocardium and proceed to destroy it.

It is important to note that a common cause of sore throat, group A beta-hemolytic streptococcal pharyngitis, can lead to a condition known as rheumatic fever. Rheumatic fever can lead to rheumatic heart disease, a bacterial endocarditis. Prompt treatment of strep throat with the appropriate antibiotic can prevent the advancement of the streptococcal infection into a cardiac debilitating disease. Rheumatic endocarditis is debilitating because of the destruction of the heart's valves. Rheumatic endocarditis causes **valvular regurgitation** (backward flow of blood through a heart valve) and **valvular stenosis** (a narrowing or constriction of the diameter of a bodily passage or orifice).

Assessment with Clinical Manifestations

Assessment of the patient with endocarditis may reveal vague signs and symptoms of infection including malaise, anorexia, weight loss, cough, back pain, and joint pain. Auscultation of the heart may reveal heart murmurs from damage to heart valves. Janeway lesions are seen in patients with acute bacterial endocarditis. The lesions appear as flat, painless, red to bluish-red spots on the palms and soles. Eye examination may show retinal hemorrhages with a central area of clearing (called Roth's spots), and **petechiae** (small, pinpoint hemorrhages) may be detected in the conjunctiva. The fingertips may become enlarged, and the nails may curve (clubbing) (Wener, 2004). The patient's history may reveal a new onset of headaches or transient ischemic attacks due to emboli that have traveled to the cerebral arteries.

Diagnostic Tests

Definitive diagnosis of bacterial endocarditis is made after obtaining serial blood culture results that are positive for the offending microorganism. It is important to note that negative blood cultures do not rule out infective endocarditis. An echocardiogram may be useful in the diagnosis of infective endocarditis by showing structural changes and onset of heart failure.

Nursing Diagnoses

Based on the information gathered, examples of nursing diagnoses in the patient with bacterial endocarditis may include the following:
- Activity intolerance related to compromised oxygen transport system secondary to heart muscle dysfunction.
- Risk for ineffective breathing pattern related to decreased respiratory depth secondary to pain.
- Pain related to friction rub and inflammatory process.

Planning and Implementation

Management of bacterial endocarditis hinges on prevention of infectious endocarditis. If prevention fails, microorganism eradication is the goal of treatment. Nursing management involves assessing and monitoring patients with infective endocarditis. Assessing and monitoring for signs and symptoms of heart murmurs, embolism, increased infection, and heart failure. Assessment to evaluate the effectiveness of treatment is also important. Antibiotic therapy will include ensuring appropriate infusion site and tolerance to medication. Assessment of potential side effects and complications is important. Nursing management must include patient education and identification of patient and family coping mechanisms.

Pharmacology

Antibiotic therapy for endocarditis often includes long-term intravenous (IV) therapy with periodic blood cultures drawn to evaluate therapy effectiveness.

Surgery

Surgical management is required after eradication of bacteria is demonstrated. Surgical valve repair of replacement is often necessary for treatment of damaged heart valves.

Evaluation of Outcomes

Potential patient outcomes for each of the example nursing diagnoses for the patient with bacterial endocarditis are:

- Activity intolerance related to compromised oxygen transport system secondary to heart muscle dysfunction. The patient maintains activity level within capabilities, as evidenced by normal heart rate and blood pressure during activity, as well as absence of shortness of breath, weakness, and fatigue.
- Risk for ineffective breathing pattern. The patient's breathing pattern is maintained by eupnea, normal skin color, and regular respiratory rate or pattern.
- Pain related to friction rub and inflammatory process. The patient should verbalize an adequate relief of pain along with the ability to realistically cope with the pain if it is not completely relieved.

Myocarditis

Myocarditis is an inflammation of the myocardium, the middle muscular layer of the heart. Myocarditis may result from an infections agents (virus, bacteria, or fungus), parasitic agents (parasites, protozoa, or spirochetes), or toxic agents (poison, allergens, or immunosuppressants). Myocarditis can cause dilation of the heart, thrombi on the heart wall, infiltration of circulation blood cells around the coronary vessels, and degeneration of the muscle fibers themselves.

Assessment with Clinical Manifestations

Assessment of the patient with myocarditis may reveal an absence of symptoms or symptoms such as fatigue, dyspnea, palpitations, chest discomfort, and abdominal discomfort. Auscultation of the heart may reveal heart murmurs from damage to heart valves or an irregular rhythm.

Nursing Diagnoses

Based on the information gathered, examples of nursing diagnoses in the patient with myocarditis may include the following:

- Activity intolerance related to compromised oxygen transport system secondary to heart muscle dysfunction.
- Risk for ineffective breathing pattern related to decreased respiratory depth secondary to pain.
- Pain related to friction rub and inflammatory process.

Planning and Implementation

Management hinges on prevention of myocarditis. This may be accomplished by maintaining an up-to-date immunization record related to influenza and hepatitis immunizations. If prevention fails, prompt treatment is suggested that aims at reducing the heart's workload, treating the causative infections, and at treating the symptoms and resultant heart failure.

Nursing management involves assessing and monitoring patients with myocarditis. Assessing and monitoring for signs and symptoms of heart murmurs and heart failure. Assessment of potential complications and increased symptoms is important. Nursing management must include patient education and identification of patient and family coping mechanisms.

Evaluation of Outcomes

Potential patient outcomes for each of the example nursing diagnoses for the patient with myocarditis are:

* Activity intolerance related to compromised oxygen transport system secondary to heart muscle dysfunction. The patient maintains activity level within capabilities, as evidenced by normal heart rate and blood pressure during activity, as well as absence of shortness of breath, weakness, and fatigue.
* Risk for ineffective breathing pattern. The patient's breathing pattern is maintained by eupnea, normal skin color, and regular respiratory rate or pattern.
* Pain related to friction rub and inflammatory process. The patient should verbalize an adequate relief of pain along with the ability to realistically cope with the pain if it is not completely relieved.

Pericarditis

Pericarditis is an inflammation of the **pericardium** (the thin membrane that surrounds the heart). The membrane surrounding the heart contains fluid that also becomes inflamed with pericarditis and puts pressure on the heart. Causes of pericarditis may include a viral, bacterial, fungal infection; parasitic organism; idiopathic, autoimmune diseases; hypothyroidism; renal failure; MI; neoplasm from nearby tumor in the lung, breast, or the blood; irradiation; drugs; injury and trauma; or surgery (Gentlesk & McCabe, 2004).

Assessment with Clinical Manifestations

Assessment of pericarditis may reveal chest pain that is different from angina in that it is sharp and stabbing rather than a feeling of pressure. Signs of fever, dyspnea, and abdominal pain may be found. Physical assessment may reveal tachypnea, tachycardia, febrile state, the Beck triad (hypotension, elevated jugular pressure, and muffled heart sounds), and pulsus paradoxus (Gentlesk & McCabe, 2004).

Diagnostic Tests

Diagnosis of pericarditis requires gathering many lab studies (CBC, erythrocyte sedimentation rate, CRP, blood urea nitrogen [BUN], creatinine, cardiac enzymes, blood cultures, rheumatoid factors, antinuclear antibodies, and tuberculin testing) and imaging studies (CXR, echocardiography, computed tomography, MRI, and ECG) (Gentlesk & McCabe, 2004).

Nursing Diagnoses

Based on the information gathered, examples of nursing diagnoses in the patient with pericarditis may include the following:

* Activity intolerance related to compromised oxygen transport system secondary to heart muscle dysfunction.
* Risk for ineffective breathing pattern related to decreased respiratory depth secondary to pain.
* Pain related to friction rub and inflammatory process.

Planning and Implementation

Management requires gathering many lab studies (CBC erythrocyte sedimentation rate, CRP, BUN, creatinine, cardiac enzymes, blood cultures, rheumatoid factors, antinuclear antibodies, and tuberculin testing) and imaging studies (CXR, echocardiography, computed tomography, MRI, and ECG) to rule out of other disease processes (Gentlesk & McCabe, 2004). Oxygen and telemetry should be applied and monitored. The progression of disease state and the exacerbation of signs and symptoms should be monitored.

Nursing management includes constant assessment, reassessment, and monitoring of disease process and treatments. It is important to avoid non-steroidal anti-inflammatory drugs (NSAIDs) and corticosteroids in acute MI-related pericarditis due to the healing and remodeling of the muscle.

Evaluation of Outcomes

Potential patient outcomes for each of the example nursing diagnoses for the patient with pericarditis are:

- Activity intolerance related to compromised oxygen transport system secondary to heart muscle dysfunction. The patient maintains activity level within capabilities, as evidenced by normal heart rate and blood pressure during activity, as well as absence of shortness of breath, weakness, and fatigue.
- Risk for ineffective breathing pattern. The patient's breathing pattern is maintained by eupnea, normal skin color, and regular respiratory rate or pattern.
- Pain related to friction rub and inflammatory process. The patient should verbalize an adequate relief of pain along with the ability to realistically cope with the pain if it is not completely relieved.

VALVULAR DYSFUNCTION AND DISEASE

The gatekeepers of the heart are the valves that allow and restrict blood flow in to and out of the heart's chambers and into the pulmonary artery and aorta. Heart valves are made of thin, strong tissue that controls blood flow in response to pressure changes in the heart's chambers during systole and diastole of the cardiac cycle.

The different types of valves include the atrioventricular valves and the semilunar valves. Atrioventricular valves, as the name suggests, are found between the atria and the ventricles. The right side of the heart houses the tricuspid atrioventricular valve, which has three leaflets. The left side of the heart houses the bicuspid (or mitral) atrioventricular valve, which has two leaflets. Both of these atrioventricular valves are anchored by chordae tendineae, which connect them to the papillary muscles and ventricular wall.

The semilunar valves are found between the ventricles and the arteries that direct blood out of the heart. The right ventricle pumps blood into the pulmonary artery through the pulmonic valve. The left ventricle pumps blood into the aorta through the aortic valve. During systole, the heart's ventricles contract, causing increased pressure in the ventricles, which forces blood into the corresponding arteries. The valves open to allow blood flow into the arteries and function to disallow backflow (or regurgitation) of blood from the arteries back into the ventricles.

Pathophysiology

Heart valves function much like full-length one-directional swinging western-style bar room doors work. They allow free flow of blood in one direction. Regurgitation occurs when the valves are unable to close appropriately because of continued pressure in the ventricles, improper fitting of the valve's leaflets due to inflammation, weakness of the valves from illness, improperly shaped leaflets because of infection, and degeneration of the surface of the leaflets. Regurgitation allows some of the blood to flow back through the valve, in the opposite direction of the way the blood is meant to flow. The term stenosis is used to describe the valve's inability to properly open. This dilemma causes a reduction in the amount of blood that is allowed through the valves and a resultant increase in blood volume that remains in the heart chamber.

Heart valve diseases are typically more serious when the left side of the heart is affected. The left side of the heart is the major pump for the cardiovascular system. Based on its location in the heart, the mitral valve has perhaps the most important job of all. Understanding of its common disorders is essential in the study of heart valve dysfunction.

Mitral Valve Prolapse

Mitral valve prolapse (MVP) is usually an asymptomatic condition in which the mitral valve leaflets stretch into the atria during systole. Long-term stretching of leaflets can cause the leaflet to be unable to effectively close during systole, which allows blood to be pumped back into the left atrium from the left ventricle.

When considering the prevalence of MVP, it is important to note that is dependent on the consistency of diagnostic criteria, which is not always clearly defined. Approximately 20 to 60 per 1,000 people have MVP. It can occur at any age however, patients above 45 years of age face a greater likelihood of complications. Prevalence is greater in females and diagnosed earlier than in males; however, men older than the age 50 are at the highest risk of complications. Genetic links have been found (Jones, Hodgson, Bahler, & Orford, 2004).

While most cases of MVP remains asymptomatic, some patients have symptoms such as fatigue, shortness of breath, light-headedness, dizziness, syncope, palpitations, chest pain, and anxiety. In extreme cases, the stretching of the leaflet can expand too far, and the result is sudden death.

Assessment with Clinical Manifestations

Assessment of the mitral valve is accomplished through auscultation of the heart. A systolic click is an early sign that a valve leaflet is ballooning into the left atrium. Considering the physiology of MVP, it might also be possible to auscultate a regurgitation of blood. Transesophageal echocardiography (TEE) is useful in the assessment of cardiac murmurs, stenosis, and regurgitation of all four cardiac valves, prosthetic valve function, and patients with infective endocarditis.

Nursing Diagnoses

Based on the information gathered, examples of nursing diagnoses in the patient with MVP may include the following:
- Excess fluid volume related to decreased cardiac output secondary to valvular disease.
- Activity intolerance related to compromised oxygen transport system secondary to valvular disease.
- Risk for infection related to compromised host defenses.
- Fear related to present status and unknown future.

Planning and Implementation

Medical management of MVP is not a curative venture. Symptoms of MVP may be treated through use of antiarrhythmic medications. Chest pain that is associated with MVP may be treated with beta blockers or calcium channel blockers. Advanced stages of MVP may result in the need for surgical repair or replacement of the mitral valve itself. Patients with bothersome symptoms of MVP are encouraged to avoid caffeine, alcohol, smoking, ephedrine, and epinephrine.

Nursing management of MVP is largely focused on patient education. For those patients who are asymptomatic, patient education is mainly focused on having the patients identify the symptoms of MVP and report new symptoms to their health care provider. Management of symptoms is also a nursing focus. Nursing management involves helping patients minimize palpitations, chest

Respecting Our Differences

Gender Ratio of MVP

MVP, unlike other disorders, does not differentiate between one's nationality and race. It does differentiate between the sexes and age ranges. The female/male MVP ratio is approximately 3:1, with females being three times more likely to have MVP than males. Although MVP is considered a congenital disorder, the echocardiographic findings are often absent in newborns. The age of onset is typically between 10 and 16 years of age (Plewa & Worthington, 2004).

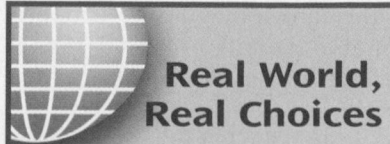

Real World, Real Choices

Diagnosing MVP in the Emergency Department

A 16-year-old patient presents to the emergency department complaining of new-onset heart palpitations. After obtaining the patient's history, the triage nurse finds out that the patient has a history of MVP. The prudent nurse knows that 40 percent of MVP patients have heart palpitations (Plewa & Worthington, 2004). A physical examination reveals an S_2 murmur. What is the next thing the nurse should do?

Choices:

A. Prioritize the patient third after the 2-year-old (with a fever of 38.9° C [102° F] and a systolic murmur) and the 78-year-old (who states, "I feel fine, but the volunteer at the Wellness Fair said that I have an extra S_3 heart sound, so I came to the emergency department immediately.")

B. Inquire about the patient's social habits.

---

pain, fatigue, or autonomic dysfunction. For patients with anxiety, provide reassurance about the benign prognosis of the condition in the large majority of cases. Patient education entails teaching about the need for antibiotic prophylaxis prior to undergoing dental, oral, respiratory tract, or esophageal procedures (Jones, et al., 2004).

Patients with mild cases of MVP can safely engage in any sport or exercise. Those patients with serious arrhythmias, significant mitral regurgitation, a prolonged QT interval, unexplained syncope, aortic root enlargement, or a family history of sudden death due to MVP should avoid high-intensity, competitive sports (Jones, et al., 2004).

Other nursing considerations include attention paid to lifestyle, diet, and exercise. Patients with palpitations may benefit from avoiding caffeine, alcohol, and tobacco. Weight loss should also be encouraged in overweight patients. Those with hypotension should increase salt and fluid intake. Patients with a history of focal neurological events and who are in sinus rhythm should avoid smoking cigarettes and taking oral contraceptives. Nearly all patients should be encouraged to exercise (Jones, et al., 2004).

Evaluation of Outcomes

Potential patient outcomes for each of the example nursing diagnoses for the patient with MVP are:

- Excess fluid volume related to decreased cardiac output secondary to valvular disease. The patient maintains adequate fluid volume and electrolyte balance as evidenced by vital signs within normal limits, clear lung sounds, pulmonary congestion absent on X-ray, and resolution of edema.
- Activity intolerance related to compromised oxygen transport system secondary to valvular disease. The patient maintains activity level within capabilities, as evidenced by normal heart rate and blood pressure during activity, as well as absence of shortness of breath, weakness, and fatigue.
- Risk for infection related to compromised host defenses. The patient remains free of infection, as evidenced by normal vital signs and absence of purulent drainage from wounds, incisions, and tubes. Infection is recognized early to allow for prompt treatment.
- Fear related to present status and unknown future. The patient should manifest positive coping behaviors and verbalize a reduction in the amount of fear of having this disease.

Mitral Regurgitation

Mitral regurgitation is a disorder of the mitral heart valve in which blood is erroneously pumped from the left ventricle into the left atrium during systole. The cause of mitral regurgitation stems from a dysfunction or disorder of the valve leaflets, the chordae tendineae, the annulus, or the papillary muscles. Some group A streptococcal infections can cause rheumatic heart infections that are most often implicated as a cause of acquired mitral regurgitation (Horenstein, Pettersen, & Walters, 2002).

The blood that backflows from the left ventricle competes for space in the left atrium with the blood that comes from the lungs. This causes an increased volume of blood in the left atrium, resulting in an increase of pressure on the walls of the left atrium. Increased atrial wall pressure causes dilation of the atrium, and it also causes the atrial walls to work harder to pump the extra blood down into the left ventricle. This increase of work, results in an increased muscle wall thickness, called hypertrophy. The increased pressure in the left atrium also means that the lungs have more resistance when working to pump blood into the left atrium through the pulmonary vein. The lungs are unable to sustain working against an ever increasingly hypertrophic and dilated left atrium. The resistance is overwhelming, and the blood backs up into the lungs, resulting in pulmonary edema.

Assessment with Clinical Manifestations

Assessment of mitral regurgitation often results in the patient remaining asymptomatic. When symptoms do occur, they are often vague and nonspecific and can present as fatigue, generalized weakness, dyspnea with or without exertion, palpitations, and cough. Auscultation of the heart may reveal a systolic murmur. Palpation of the pulse may reveal an irregular rhythm. Acute heart damage, such as MI, can cause mitral regurgitation, which often presents as CHF.

Nursing Diagnoses

Based on the information gathered, examples of nursing diagnoses in the patient with mitral regurgitation may include the following:
- Excess fluid volume related to decreased cardiac output secondary to valvular disease.
- Activity intolerance related to compromised oxygen transport system secondary to valvular disease.
- Risk for infection related to compromised host defenses.
- Fear related to present status and unknown future.

Planning and Implementation

Medical management of mitral regurgitation requires an echocardiogram for definitive diagnosis. Treatment is the same as treatment of CHF. If surgical treatment is required, a mitral valve replacement or **valvuloplasty** (plastic surgery performed to repair a valve in the body) will be necessary.

Evaluation of Outcomes

Potential patient outcomes for each of the example nursing diagnoses for the patient with mitral regurgitation are:
- Excess fluid volume related to decreased cardiac output secondary to valvular disease. The patient maintains adequate fluid volume and electrolyte balance as evidenced by vital signs within normal limits, clear lung sounds, pulmonary congestion absent on X-ray, and resolution of edema.
- Activity intolerance related to compromised oxygen transport system secondary to valvular disease. The patient maintains activity level within capabilities, as evidenced by normal heart rate and blood pressure during activity, as well as absence of shortness of breath, weakness, and fatigue.
- Risk for infection related to compromised host defenses. The patient remains free of infection, as evidenced by normal vital signs and absence of purulent drainage from wounds, incisions, and tubes. Infection is recognized early to allow for prompt treatment.
- Fear related to present status and unknown future. The patient should manifest positive coping behaviors and verbalize a reduction in the amount of fear of the having this disease.

Mitral Stenosis

Mitral stenosis, a narrowing or constriction of the diameter of the mitral valve opening, is most commonly caused by rheumatic heart disease, and if untreated, it can lead to pulmonary hypertension and death. Approximately two thirds of mitral stenosis cases occur in women, and it has been found that there is a genetic or familial incidence of rheumatic fever. Mitral stenosis progresses over time, and there is no known medical treatment, apart from prevention of recurrent rheumatic fever (Saver, et al., 2004).

Mitral stenosis narrowing can be caused by a fusion of the mitral valve leaflets or a thickening of the mitral valve leaflets, which results in the obstruction of blood flow from the left atrium in to the left ventricle. Increased resistance of the mitral valve causes increased pressure in the atrium. To continue pumping the same volume of blood into the left ventricle, the left atrium will attempt to compensate. As the atrium works harder, dilation of the atrium occurs. In the same way it compensates in mitral regurgitation, the atrium's increase in work in mitral stenosis results in an increased muscle wall thickness, called hypertrophy. The increased pressure in the left atrium also means that the lungs have more resistance when working to pump blood into the left atrium through the pulmonary vein. The lungs are unable to sustain working against an ever increasingly hypertrophic and dilated left atrium. The resistance is overwhelming, and the blood backs up into the lungs, resulting in CHF. Pulse may be irregular, and 30 to 40 percent of patients with symptomatic mitral stenosis develop atrial fibrillation, which increases the patient's risk of embolism if he or she is over 25 years of age (Saver, et al., 2004).

Assessment with Clinical Manifestations

Assessment of a mitral stenosis patient may reveal no symptoms or may reveal dyspnea on exertion, fatigue, and cough with hemoptysis. History often reveals chest pain, rheumatic fever, and dysphasia. Inspection may reveal a prominent wave in the jugular venous pulse, and in late stages, signs of peripheral edema, enlarged liver, ascites, and **mitral facies** (a florid appearance with cyanosed cheeks) if pulmonary hypertension has developed. Palpation may reveal a displaced apex beat due to the enlarged right ventricle with a right ventricular heave. Auscultation of the heart may reveal a diastolic murmur and a displaced apex beat. Palpation of the pulse may reveal an irregular rhythm (Saver, et al., 2004).

Nursing Diagnoses

Based on the information gathered, examples of nursing diagnoses in the patient with mitral stenosis may include the following:
- Excess fluid volume related to decreased cardiac output secondary to valvular disease.
- Activity intolerance related to compromised oxygen transport system secondary to valvular disease.
- Risk for infection related to compromised host defenses.
- Fear related to present status and unknown future.

Planning and Implementation

Medical management of mitral stenosis requires an echocardiogram for definitive diagnosis. The extent of disease is determined through use of an echocardiogram and cardiac catheterization with angiography. Medical treatment consists of prevention of recurrence, exacerbation, and treatment of symptoms (the same as with CHF). Surgical treatment requires valvuloplasty and valvular defusion. Prophylaxis to prevent recurrent rheumatic fever, as with endocarditis, is important (Saver, et al., 2004).

Nursing management of mitral stenosis is largely focused on assessment and patient teaching. It is important for the nurse to evaluate patient knowledge related to decreasing salt intake, avoiding strenuous exercise, and use of antibiotics for prophylaxis of recurrence and prevention of infection.

Evaluation of Outcomes

Potential patient outcomes for each of the example nursing diagnoses for the patient with mitral stenosis are:
- Excess fluid volume related to decreased cardiac output secondary to valvular disease. The patient maintains adequate fluid volume and electrolyte balance as evidenced by vital signs within normal limits, clear lung sounds, pulmonary congestion absent on X-ray, and resolution of edema.
- Activity intolerance related to compromised oxygen transport system secondary to valvular disease. The patient maintains activity level within capabilities, as evidenced by normal heart rate and blood pressure during activity, as well as absence of shortness of breath, weakness, and fatigue.

- Risk for infection related to compromised host defenses. The patient remains free of infection, as evidenced by normal vital signs and absence of purulent drainage from wounds, incisions, and tubes. Infection is recognized early to allow for prompt treatment.
- Fear related to present status and unknown future. The patient should manifest positive coping behaviors and verbalize a reduction in the amount of fear of the having this disease.

Aortic Regurgitation

Aortic regurgitation, like mitral regurgitation, may result from inflammatory diseases of the heart or congenital conditions. Aortic regurgitation is found in 13 percent of men and 8.5 percent of women. It is more common in adults; age of onset depends on underlying cause. Three quarters of patients with pure or predominant aortic regurgitation are male. There is some evidence of a genetic or familial link of aortic regurgitation, and it is more common with rheumatic fever (Scherger, et al., 2004).

Pathophysiology

Aortic regurgitation is a disorder of the aortic heart valve in which blood erroneously returns back through the aortic valve into the left ventricle during diastole. This occurs after systole, in which the left ventricle correctly pumped blood from the left ventricle through the aortic valve, into the aorta. This extra blood in the left ventricle, along with the blood that correctly came from the left atrium, increases the volume of blood in the left ventricle. The left ventricle attempts to compensate for this volume and increase of pressure on the walls of the ventricle through dilation of the ventricle. The compensation causes the ventricle walls to work harder to pump the extra blood into the aorta. This increase results in an increased muscle wall thickness and an increase in the force needed to expel the blood from the ventricle into the aorta, causing an increase in the systolic blood pressure. Conversely, the diastolic blood pressure decreases as the arteries compensate for the high systolic pressure by inducing a vasodilation, in which the peripheral arterioles relax and allow blood to divert to the peripheral body parts.

Assessment with Clinical Manifestations

Assessment of aortic regurgitation often reveals an asymptomatic patient. A patient history may reveal increased dyspnea on exertion, fatigue, and paroxysmal nocturnal dyspnea. Some patients may state an awareness of forceful pulsations in the upper thorax and head regions due to an increased force with which the left ventricle is required to perform. Cardiac auscultation may reveal a diastolic murmur. After palpation, the nurse may be able to palpate the increase in intensity of carotid and temporal pulses. A hallmark sign of aortic regurgitation is a palpable pulse that is intense and then quickly weakens. The pulse pressure, the difference between the systolic blood pressure and diastolic blood pressure, described above, widens (Singh, Sharma, Nanda, Reddy, & Strom, 2004).

Nursing Diagnoses

Based on the information gathered, examples of nursing diagnoses in the patient with aortic regurgitation may include the following:

- Excess fluid volume related to decreased cardiac output secondary to valvular disease.
- Activity intolerance related to compromised oxygen transport system secondary to valvular disease.
- Risk for infection related to compromised host defenses.
- Fear related to present status and unknown future.

Planning and Implementation

Medical management of aortic regurgitation requires an echocardiogram, radionuclide imaging, ECG or Holter monitoring, MRI, or cardiac catheterization for definitive diagnosis. Medical treatment consists of prevention of recurrence, reduction of symptoms, and initiation of surgical treatment (Singh, et al., 2004). Surgical treatment, recommended before heart failure occurs, consists of valvuloplasty or valve replacement. Prevention of recurrence and exacerbation involves prophylactic use of antibiotics to prevent infection and further injury to the heart valves.

Nursing management of aortic regurgitation is largely focused on assessment and patient teaching. It is important for the nurse to evaluate patient knowledge related to use of antibiotics for prophylaxis of recurrence and exacerbation of infection.

Evaluation of Outcomes

Potential patient outcomes for each of the example nursing diagnoses for the patient with aortic regurgitation are:

- Excess fluid volume related to decreased cardiac output secondary to valvular disease. The patient maintains adequate fluid volume and electrolyte balance as evidenced by vital signs within normal limits, clear lung sounds, pulmonary congestion absent on X-ray, and resolution of edema.
- Activity intolerance related to compromised oxygen transport system secondary to valvular disease. The patient maintains activity level within capabilities, as evidenced by normal heart rate and blood pressure during activity, as well as absence of shortness of breath, weakness, and fatigue.
- Risk for infection related to compromised host defenses. The patient remains free of infection, as evidenced by normal vital signs and absence of purulent drainage from wounds, incisions, and tubes. Infection is recognized early to allow for prompt treatment.
- Fear related to present status and unknown future. The patient should manifest positive coping behaviors and verbalize a reduction in the amount of fear of the having this disease.

Aortic Stenosis

Aortic stenosis is a narrowing or constriction of the diameter of the orifice between the left ventricle and the aorta. Aortic stenosis is the most common valvular heart disease, with a characteristic harsh systolic murmur, occasionally with a thrill along the left sternal border, often radiating to the neck (Pearson, Kabongo, Ejnes, & Bahler, 2004).

Epidemiology

Aortic stenosis is three to four times more frequent in men than in women, with no clear genetic or familial link. Approximately 25 percent of patients over the age of 65 and 35 percent of those patients over the age of 70 have echocardiographic evidence of sclerosis. In addition, 2 to 3 percent of these elderly patients exhibit hemodynamic evidence of stenosis (Pearson, et al., 2004).

Etiology

Causes of aortic stenosis may include congenital unicuspid or bicuspid valve rather than the expected tricuspid formation of the valve. Also implicated in the cause of aortic stenosis are rheumatic fever, cusp calcification, leaflet fusion, and degenerative changes of the aortic valve.

Pathophysiology

Narrowing and constriction causes the left ventricle to compensate for the increased resistance by pumping slower than normal, but with more force. The ventricle's increase in work with aortic stenosis results in an increased ventricular muscle wall thickness. Hypertrophy of the left ventricle requires the heart to work harder and energy expenditure to perform the pumping responsibilities required by it.

Assessment with Clinical Manifestations

Assessment of aortic stenosis often reveals an absence of symptoms, whereas advanced aortic stenosis, characterized by a decrease in blood flow to the brain, results in multiple assessment findings. Dyspnea upon exertion is common. Dizziness, syncope, and angina are frequently found when oxygen supplies have decreased in aortic stenosis patients. Auscultation reveals a systolic murmur, while palpation reveals a thrill.

The common aortic stenosis triad of symptoms are chest pain, heart failure, and syncope.

Nursing Diagnoses

Based on the information gathered, examples of nursing diagnoses in the patient with aortic stenosis may include the following:
- Excess fluid volume related to decreased cardiac output secondary to valvular disease.
- Activity intolerance related to compromised oxygen transport system secondary to valvular disease.
- Risk for infection related to compromised host defenses.
- Fear related to present status and unknown future.

Planning and Implementation

Medical management of aortic stenosis requires an echocardiogram, CXR, and an ECG for definitive diagnosis of the associated left ventricular hypertrophy. Medical treatment consists of prevention of recurrence and exacerbation of disease and relief of symptoms (angina, syncope, and atrial fibrillation). In the absence of response to medical management, surgical repair of the aortic valve is recommended. Nursing management of aortic stenosis is largely focused on assessment and patient teaching. Patients should be able to identify new symptoms and know to report them. It is important for the nurse to evaluate patient knowledge related to use of antibiotics for prophylaxis of recurrence and exacerbation of infection.

Surgery

Surgical management of heart valve repair (see section on valve repair) and replacement (see section on valve replacement) surgery consists of ensuring that there is minimal risk for bleeding, thromboembolism, infection, CHF, hypertension, dysrhythmias, hemolysis, and valve obstruction.

Evaluation of Outcomes

Potential patient outcomes for each of the example nursing diagnoses for the patient with aortic regurgitation are:
- Excess fluid volume related to decreased cardiac output secondary to valvular disease. The patient maintains adequate fluid volume and electrolyte balance as evidenced by vital signs within normal limits, clear lung sounds, pulmonary congestion absent on X-ray, and resolution of edema.
- Activity intolerance related to compromised oxygen transport system secondary to valvular disease. The patient maintains activity level within capabilities, as evidenced by normal heart rate and blood pressure during activity, as well as absence of shortness of breath, weakness, and fatigue.
- Risk for infection related to compromised host defenses. The patient remains free of infection, as evidenced by normal vital signs and absence of purulent drainage from wounds, incisions, and tubes. Infection is recognized early to allow for prompt treatment.

- Fear related to present status and unknown future. The patient should manifest positive coping behaviors and verbalize a reduction in the amount of fear of the having this disease.

Valvular Surgery

Heart valve repair and replacement surgery consists of ensuring that there is minimal risk for bleeding, thromboembolism, infection, CHF, hypertension, dysrhythmias, hemolysis, and valve obstruction.

Valve repair (valvuloplasty) is considered when the valves of the heart become stenotic to the point that constriction of the heart valve obstructs or diverts the normal flow of blood. Valvuloplasty can be performed under general anesthesia in the surgical setting or with local anesthetics and mild sedation in the cardiac catheterization laboratory. Occasionally, cardiopulmonary bypass, the process of using a machine to act as the heart and lungs, may be used when a patient is under general anesthesia.

Determining the type of valvuloplasty that is performed depends on the location and extent of defect with which the patient presents. There are three main types of procedures: commissurotomy, annuloplasty, and chordoplasty. Commissurotomy, a common form of valvuloplasty, is the procedure used to separate fused valve leaflets by cutting or manually pulling apart the leaflets. Benefits of the procedure are the immediate positive results and that general anesthesia and bypass are not required.

Balloon valvuloplasty, a type of commissurotomy, is a cardiac catheterization laboratory procedure in which a catheter, with a small deflated balloon at the tip, is inserted into the femoral vein or artery and threaded through the artery to the opening of the narrowed heart valve. The balloon is inflated, which stretches the valve open and separates the fused leaflets. Then the balloon is deflated and removed.

Annuloplasty is a procedure used to strengthen the junction of the leaflets to the heart muscle (Figure 25-7). In this procedure, general anesthesia and bypass are required. There are two types of annuloplasty: a ring procedure and a leaflet repair. In the ring procedure, the surgeon places a ring at the junction of the valve leaflets and the heart muscle. The ring acts as a surrogate annulus, ensuring that the annulus is the desired size to prevent regurgitation. Leaflet repair is considered when the leaflets are elongated or ballooning. In the leaflet repair, the extra tissue of the leaflet is removed. Chordoplasty is the repair of the chordae tendineae of the mitral valve. This involves repairing the defect in the shape of the chordae tendineae that causes regurgitation.

Valve replacement is recommended instead of valvular repair when leaflets are calcified or irreparable (Figure 25-8). Valve replacement requires general anesthesia with cardiopulmonary bypass. Valve replacement consists of removing the diseased valve and replacing it with a donor valve (prosthesis). There are two types of prostheses: mechanical made from metal and biological made from bovine, porcine, and cadaver donors (Daller, 2004). The mechanical valve requires long-term anticoagulation (warfarin [Coumadin]) therapy to prevent risk of thromboembolism (Daller, 2004).

Nursing Diagnoses

Based on the information gathered, examples of nursing diagnoses in the patient with valve replacement may include the following:

- Excess fluid volume related to decreased cardiac output secondary to valvular disease.
- Activity intolerance related to compromised oxygen transport system secondary to valvular disease.

PATIENT PLAYBOOK

Preoperative Teaching

Patients should be taught the following prior to their heart valve replacement surgery:

- Information about the events on the day of surgery.
- Orientation to the intensive care unit.
- Monitors.
- IV lines.
- Drainage tubes.
- Breathing tube.
- Ventilator.
- Expectations of activity levels.
- Expectations of exercises.
- Expectations of pain management.
- Dietary changes.

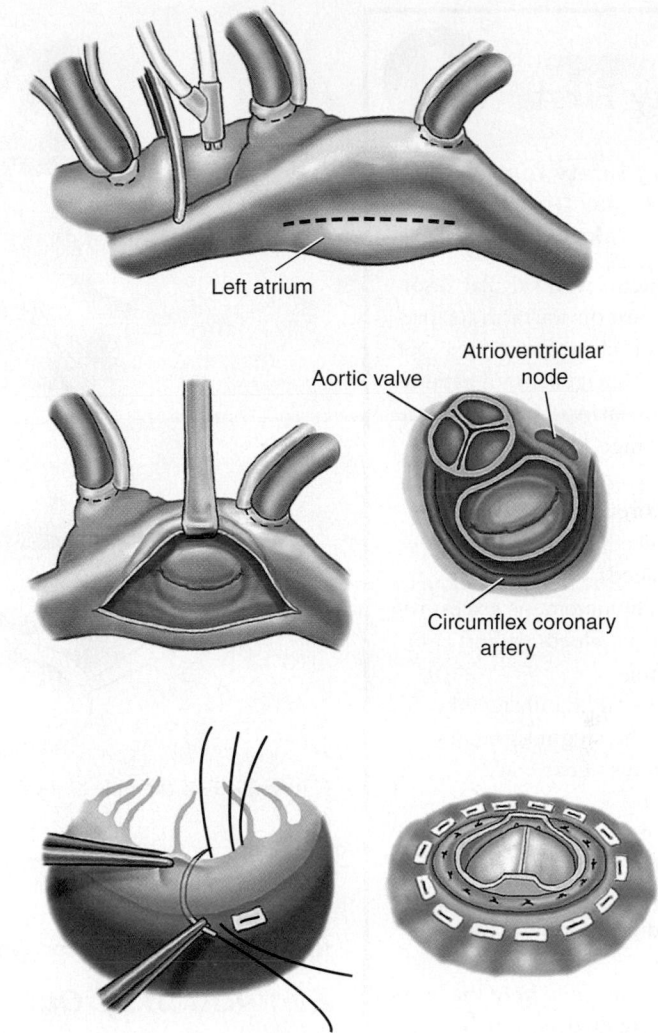

Figure 25-7 Mitral valve annuloplasty.

- Risk for infection related to compromised host defenses.
- Fear related to present status and unknown future.

Planning and Implementation

Medical management of heart valve repair and replacement surgery consists of ensuring that there is minimal risk for bleeding, thromboembolism, infection, CHF, hypertension, dysrhythmias, hemolysis, and valve obstruction.

Nursing management of the heart valve repair or replacement surgical patient occurs in a critical care unit. Management consists of hemodynamic monitoring, anesthesia recovery, wound care, and patient teaching.

Hemodynamic monitoring involves maintaining blood pressure through administration of IV fluids and hemodynamic medications. Also important to hemodynamic monitoring is the monitoring and treatment of cardiac dysrhythmias. Anesthesia recovery involves assessment of the neurological, respiratory, and cardiovascular systems. Wound assessment and management are also important.

Patient teaching requires a simple explanation of the anatomy of heart, the functioning of coronary arteries, and explanation of surgery. Surgical teaching is shown in the patient playbook.

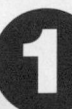

Safety First ❶

Ensuring Safety for Patients with Valvular Disorders Who Are Taking Warfarin

Many patients with valvular disorders who are on warfarin for prevention of clots are at risk for bleeding. Management of patients taking warfarin should include the following:

- These patients should be monitored for hematuria, excessive bruising, petechiae, nosebleeds, melena, tarry stools, hematemesis, excessive menstrual bleeding, and gum bleeding.
- Patients and family members should be taught signs and symptoms of excessive bleeding.
- Patients should be taught the importance of following the prescribed dosage and attending follow-up appointments.

Also important is to note that warfarin has many drug interactions, and over-the-counter (OTC) medications should be approved by the practitioner or the pharmacist.

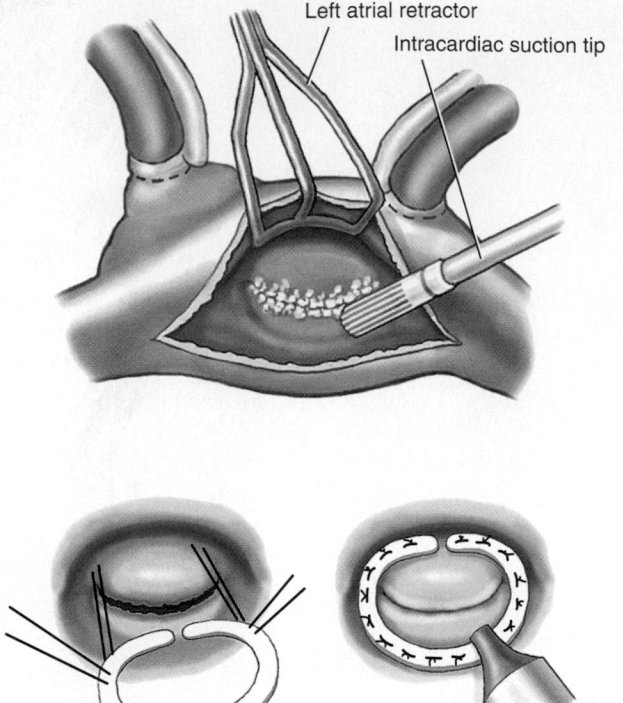

Figure 25-8 An example of a valve surgery: Mitral valve replacement.

Purpose of medications and side effects are also important for educating the patient. Clear explanations of the purpose for long-term anticoagulant therapy and antibiotic prophylaxis are necessary.

Evaluation of Outcomes

Potential patient outcomes for each of the example nursing diagnoses for the patient with valve replacement are:

- Excess fluid volume related to decreased cardiac output secondary to valvular disease. The patient maintains adequate fluid volume and electrolyte balance as evidenced by vital signs within normal limits, clear lung sounds, pulmonary congestion absent on X-ray, and resolution of edema.
- Activity intolerance related to compromised oxygen transport system secondary to valvular disease. The patient maintains activity level within capabilities, as evidenced by normal heart rate and blood pressure during activity, as well as absence of shortness of breath, weakness, and fatigue.
- Risk for infection related to compromised host defenses. The patient remains free of infection, as evidenced by normal vital signs and absence of purulent drainage from wounds, incisions, and tubes. Infection is recognized early to allow for prompt treatment.

KEY CONCEPTS

- Heart failure is a condition in which the heart is physiologically unable to meet the metabolic demands of the tissues.
- Conditions that can produce heart failure are valvular problems, cardiomyopathies, cardiac inflammatory disease, and trauma to the cardiac tissue.

- Initially the heart attempts to compensate by increasing the heart rate and force of contraction.
- Long-term compensation by the heart causes a negative result—the heart works harder, which in turn worsens the degree of heart failure.

Continued

KEY CONCEPTS—cont'd

- Heart failure is classified in different ways: the cause of the failure, the symptoms it causes, the side of the heart that is affected, and whether the problem is a problem with the muscle's pumping or relaxing.
- DCM is a condition of the left ventricle having a larger volume to hold with a thinner muscle wall with which to pump.
- HCM is a condition of the ventricle having a thickened muscle which reduces the volume it can hold and reduces its ability to relax.
- RCM is a condition of the wall of the ventricle being restricted from movement.
- Carditis is an inflammation of the heart.
- Carditis is treated with antibiotics and pain medication.

- Ideally, the blood flows in one direction through the heart.
- Regurgitation causes the direction of some of the blood flow to change, which results in higher volume of blood in areas that are not prepared to handle it.
- Direction changes in the blood flow cause the heart to work harder to compensate for the increase in volume of blood.
- Stenosis hinders the momentum of the blood flow.
- Decreased momentum of blood flow results in blood to gather with higher prevalence of clotting and a change in the heart muscle to ensure peripheral perfusion.

REVIEW QUESTIONS

1. Which of the following statements most accurately describes a cardiac catheterization?
   1. A procedure that requires general anesthesia
   2. A noninvasive procedure
   3. Provides visualization of the heart by injecting radiopaque dye into the vessels
   4. Is the retrieval of a part of the heart muscle that is sent for laboratory testing

2. Which of the following would the nurse expect to find in the assessment of a patient with heart failure?
   1. Murmur
   2. Strong, bounding pulses
   3. Bradycardia
   4. Ease of respirations

3. Which of the following symptoms is seen with pulmonary venous congestion or left-sided heart failure?
   1. Peripheral edema
   2. Tachypnea and dyspnea
   3. Neck vein distension
   4. Weight gain

4. Which of the following statements is true about giving oxygen to a patient with heart failure? Oxygen is:
   1. Administered via mechanical ventilation only
   2. Contraindicated in heart failure
   3. Useful mostly for the purpose of reducing anxiety
   4. Prescribed to decrease the work of breathing

5. An ACE inhibitor causes which of the following to occur?
   1. Increased vascular resistance
   2. Vasoconstriction
   3. Increase in cardiac volume and cardiac pressure
   4. Increased sodium excretion

6. Which of the following disorders is jugular neck vein distension most prominent?
   1. Heart failure
   2. HCM
   3. Carditis
   4. MVP

7. Which of the following is not important in teaching a patient about HCM?
   1. Importance of flu vaccine and avoidance of overexertion
   2. Moderation of alcohol intake and avoidance of acute loss of body fluid volume
   3. Weight reduction and avoidance of hot showers
   4. Importance of increased caloric intake and sublingual nitroglycerin

8. Which of the following denotes a disease of the heart muscle?
   1. Cardiomyopathy
   2. MVP
   3. CHF
   4. Pericarditis

Continued

REVIEW QUESTIONS—cont'd

9. In a patient with cardiomyopathy whose treatment has failed, what is the next course of treatment?
   1. Heart transplantation
   2. Valve replacement
   3. Valve repair
   4. CABG

10. A patient presents with pink, frothy sputum. What is the most appropriate nursing action?
    1. Hold the next routine dose of diuretic
    2. Call the physician stat
    3. Insert an IV line
    4. Insert a nasogastric tube

REVIEW ACTIVITIES

1. Describe the pathophysiology involved in valvular disorders.

2. Compare and contrast signs and symptoms of each valvular disorder.

3. Describe various procedures used to correct valvular problems.

4. Describe the care of the patient after interventions for vascular disease.

5. Describe the recommended dietary treatments for patients with heart failure.

6. Describe how nursing should teach and monitor positioning affects oxygenation in a patient with heart failure.

7. Discuss the nursing management (domains of nursing) of caring for a patient with heart failure.

8. Compare and contrast the four different types of cardiomyopathy and interventions required.

9. Prioritize the following nursing diagnoses based on Maslow's Hierarchy of Needs for patients with heart failure:
   ____ Activity intolerance related to insufficient knowledge of adaptive techniques needed secondary to impaired cardiac function.
   ____ Risk for ineffective respiratory function related to excessive secretions secondary to cardiopulmonary dysfunction.
   ____ Anxiety related to powerlessness and vulnerability.

10. Prioritize the following nursing diagnoses based on Maslow's Hierarchy of Needs for a patient with cardiomyopathy:
    ____ Activity intolerance related to insufficient knowledge of adaptive techniques needed secondary to impaired cardiac function.
    ____ Risk for ineffective respiratory function related to decreased respiratory depth.
    ____ Pain related to friction rub and inflammatory process.

Arrhythmias: Nursing Management

Sharon Little-Stoetzel, RN, MS

Barbara Voshall, RN, MN

CHAPTER TOPICS

- Conduction System of the Heart and Electrophysiology

- ECG Monitoring

- Sinus Arrhythmias

- Atrial Arrhythmias

- Junctional Arrhythmias

- Heart Blocks

- Ventricular Arrhythmias

- Management of Arrhythmias

- Basic and Advanced Cardiac Life Support

KEY TERMS

12-lead electrocardiogram (ECG)
Arrhythmias
Automaticity
Axis
Conductivity
Contractility
Defibrillation
Depolarization
Dysrhythmia
Excitability
P wave
PR interval
Purkinje fibers
QRS complex
QT interval
Repolarization
SA node
Synchronized cardioversion
T wave

Interpretation of **arrhythmias,** which means deviations from normal cardiac rhythms, is an important skill for nurses in caring for patients. This is especially true for nurses who work with patients on telemetry units, intensive care settings, postanesthesia care units, emergency departments, and other settings where cardiac monitoring is utilized. Patients on medical-surgical units often need **12-lead electrocardiograms (ECGs),** which is a diagnostic tool that evaluates the electrical activity of the heart by utilizing 12 views; the ability of the nurse to interpret these ECGs is also essential. Students will often find the terms arrhythmia and dysrhythmia used interchangeably. Arrhythmia means a deviation from normal rhythm, and **dysrhythmia** means a disturbance in rhythm. Both terms may be utilized when discussing cardiac rhythms, as either term is appropriate. Arrhythmias occur in many populations of patients. The patient with cardiac disease, electrolyte disturbances, myocardial infarction, respiratory disorders, as well as other illnesses and medications have the potential to affect disturbance normal cardiac rhythm. The ability of the nurse to interpret arrhythmias while simultaneously assessing the patient's response to arrhythmias is crucial to the care of the patient. Some arrhythmias will have serious effects on cardiac output while others will be less detrimental. The nurse must able to differentiate between origin and conduction of rhythm disorders. Therefore, the goals of this chapter are to provide a brief review of the cardiac conduction system and cardiac electrophysiology, provide a step-by-step method of interpreting arrhythmias, discuss current treatment of arrhythmias, and review steps of basic life support (BLS) and algorithms from advanced cardiac life support (ACLS).

ANATOMY AND PHYSIOLOGY

The cardiac conduction system is a pathway of specialized cells that are capable of transmitting the electrical impulse of the heart throughout itself. It is because of this pathway that the four chambers of the heart function together to supply blood throughout the body. The electrical impulse spreads throughout the heart much like ripples that are created when a rock is dropped into water. Defects in this conduction system can cause arrhythmias.

Sinoatrial Node

In normal cardiac anatomy, the sinoatrial node (**SA node**) is the primary pacemaker of the heart that has an inherent rate of 60 to 100 beats per minute. It is located at the junction of the superior vena cava and the right atrium (Kasper, et al., 2005). Normally, the SA node discharges electrical impulses at a rate of 60 to 100 times per minute. Because this rate is faster than other areas in the heart, the SA node is referred to as the dominant pacemaker of the heart. The SA node is about 2 to 3 millimeters wide and about 1.5 cm long. Blood is supplied to the SA node by the sinus node artery. The sinus node artery branches off the right coronary artery in about 60 percent of the population and comes off the circumflex coronary artery in approximately 40 percent of the population. The sinus node responds to impulses from the autonomic nervous system that results in accelerating or slowing down the heart rate. Once the impulse leaves the SA node, it spreads through the atria and travels down to the atrioventricular (AV) node.

AV Node

In the normal heart, the electrical impulse must enter the ventricles through the AV junction that consists of the AV node and superior portion of the bundle of His. The AV node is located above the tricuspid annulus, anterior to the coronary sinus, and at the base of the interatrial septum. In the majority of the population the AV node receives its blood supply from the posterior descending coronary artery. A major function of the AV node is to slow the electrical impulse between the atria and ventricles to give time for the atria to contract and empty their contents into the ventricles (Kasper, et al., 2005). Another function of the AV node is to serve as a secondary pacemaker in case the SA node fails to fire. The intrinsic rate of the AV node 40 to 60 beats per minute.

The bundle of His is a continuation of the AV node that allows the impulses to enter into the ventricles. It is located across the interventricular septum and has a blood supply from a branch of the anterior descending artery in addition to the AV nodal artery. The bundle of His then divides into the left and right bundle branches. The left bundle branch divides into two fascicles while the right bundle contains only one fascicle.

Purkinje Fibers

Once the impulse has traveled through the bundle branches, the impulse enters the endocardium via conductive fibers, known as the **Purkinje fibers,** which are conductive fibers that help to spread the electrical impulse throughout the ventricular muscle. Because of the velocity of the impulse and the location of the fibers, the impulse is spread throughout the ventricles. The Purkinje fibers serve as backup pacemakers in the heart in case the SA node and AV node fail to fire. The Purkinje fibers have an inherent firing rate of 15 to 40 times per minute. This rate is typically not fast enough to maintain adequate cardiac output.

Electrophysiology

The electrical stimulation of the heart occurs at the cellular level by a process called an electrical impulse. The electrical charge on the inside of the cell is negative when compared to the outside of the cell. The electrical charge inside the cardiac cell measures approximately -80 to -90 mV. This is called the resting membrane potential and is maintained "primarily by the concentration gradient of potassium across the cell membrane" (Kasper, et al., 2005, p. 1333). When cardiac cells are electrically stimulated, depolarization occurs. **Depolarization** is the electrical change in the interior of an excitable cell from negative to positive, which results in an action potential. The shape of the action potential varies depending on which part of the conduction system is being represented.

The action potential of the His-Purkinje system is representative of the following phases. Phase 0 occurs when the rapid depolarizing current occurs from a swift entry of sodium into the myocardial cells causing the charge to become more positive. This is followed by a slower entry of calcium. The entry of calcium is followed by the recovery phase that is called **repolarization,** which is defined as an electrical change in the interior of an excitable cell following depolarization in which the inside of the cell becomes more negatively charged. The repolarization phases are referred to as phases 1, 2, and 3. These phases occur as a result of an outward flux of potassium. Phase 4 occurs when the normal resting membrane potential is reached. Electrolytes return to their normal resting state via the sodium-potassium pump.

During the action potential there are periods when the cells cannot be stimulated by other electrical stimuli. This time frame is referred to the refractory period. During this time cardiac tissue resists being depolarized; therefore, no action potential happens until the cells have recovered. During this refractory period, a stimulus that is greater than normal may have a propagated response, but this occurs more slowly than expected (Kasper, et al., 2005).

Depolarization and repolarization refer to the electrical activity of the cardiac cells. The mechanical activity of the heart, or muscle contraction, follows the electrical activity. Both the electrical and mechanical activities combine to form the cardiac cycle. Depolarization occurs in the cells of the heart, and when the cells are stimulated, there will be a mechanical contraction of the cells. Repolarization follows, and then the cardiac muscle cells relax, and the heart enters diastole. The electrical activity of the heart is traced when the patient is being monitored for arrhythmias. In most circumstances the assumption is made that systole and diastole, or contraction and relaxation, of the cardiac muscle are occurring, but the patient's pulse can be checked to confirm this.

Automaticity occurs when a group of cells has the ability to generate an electrical impulse spontaneously. The resting membrane potential (phase 4) in these cells automatically reaches the rate of discharge. The SA node is normally the dominant pacemaker of the heart, because it has the highest preset rate of discharge. This is an example of normal automaticity. Abnormal automaticity occurs when cells outside the SA node cause depolarization and start to serve as the dominant pacemaker or cause irregularities in rhythm. Causes of abnormal automaticity are various and can include; medical interventions, such as pacemaker insertion, hypoxemia, cardiac disease, medications, electrolyte imbalances, stress, and stimulants.

All cardiac cells have the property of excitability. **Excitability** of a cell means the capacity of the cardiac cell to depolarize in response to an electrical impulse. Because all cells have the property of excitability, all cardiac cells have the potential to possess the property of self-excitation (Rizzo, 2006). Self-excitation refers to the capacity for automaticity.

Conductivity is the ability of cardiac cells to transmit an impulse. All cardiac cells have the property of conductivity. This allows the electrical impulse that is generated in the SA node to be conducted throughout the entire conduction system.

The myocardium is able to produce a contraction after being stimulated. **Contractility** is the ability of the cardiac muscle in response to a stimulus to shorten to produce systole. Because of this property, when the electrical activity is visualized on the monitor it is assumed that the mechanical contraction follows the electrical activity.

ECG MONITORING

The heart has an electrical force that runs through it. The electrical current passes into the surrounding tissue, and a small portion of the current reaches the external surface of the body. The electrical waves can be recorded by placing electrodes on the skin on the opposite sides of the heart. An ECG records the electrical waves as they travel through the body.

The 12-lead ECG is the most commonly used evaluation procedure to diagnose heart disease. This test is frequently done with the patient at rest. It may also be used in a stress test (see chapter 24). Interpreting the data obtained requires special training. It is used to evaluate for cardiac disease and may reflect anatomic abnormalities, molecular and electrolyte problems, signs of decreased oxygen to the cardiac muscle, and drug-induced problems with the heart (Fuster, Alexander, & O'Rourke, 2004).

Leads are placed on the body in various positions to view the electrical activity of the heart. An imaginary line is drawn between the two electrodes of the positive and negative leads in a bipolar lead and between the positive electrode and the reference point in a unipolar lead. This line is called the **axis.** The electrical current flow through the heart is reflected in the recording of the ECG. When there is no electrical activity in the heart because of the resting or polarized state, the electrical activity is weak, or it is not in a plane that a particular lead can record, the ECG records a straight line. This line is called the isoelectric line.

When depolarization occurs or when positive charges precede negative charges, the wave moves through the heart and cells change from negative to positive as sodium ions enter into the cell (Fuster, et al., 2004). As the positive depolarization wave travels toward a positive electrode of the ECG, a positive (upward) deflection is recorded. As the electrical current travels away from the positive electrode, the waveform is mostly a negative (downward) deflection. When the electrical current is perpendicular to the lead, the electrical waveform may be isoelectric or biphasic, which means the waveform has both an upward and downward deflection.

During the process of repolarization or the phase when the cell is returning to the resting or polarized state, the negative charges precede the positive charges. When this occurs, a positive or upright deflection, the T wave, is registered in the positive lead of the ECG that is recording over that area of the heart (Fuster, et al., 2004).

The arms and the legs are linear extensions of the heart's electrical field. Bipolar leads are electrodes of opposite polarity that are placed on the arms and legs. A unipolar biphasic lead is one electrode placed at reference points on the precordium. The electrical force is amplified and recorded on special ruled paper or displayed on an oscilloscope. The instrument that records the electrical activity of the heart is the electrocardiograph. The recording of the electrical activity of the heart is the ECG.

The standard ECG has 12 electrode leads. The electrodes are connected to the arms and legs and precordial leads are placed on the chest wall. This placement gives the examiner twelve different views of the heart. An advantage to using the precordial leads is that some abnormalities are not apparent in every lead of the heart. A single monitoring lead can be helpful when evaluating the patient's heart rate and rhythm, but it may not detect abnormalities, such as ischemia or differentiation of blocks in the conduction systems and ectopic focus of the generation of complexes.

The frontal leads record information about the current of flow through the heart and reflect electrical activity in the right, left, inferior (bottom), and superior (top) portions. The frontal leads are leads I, II, III, aV_R, aV_L, and aV_F. The horizontal plane records information about the electrical flow that is right, left, anterior, or posterior areas of the heart. This information is recorded on the precordial leads V_1–V_6.

The leads that are placed on the extremities are called limb leads, and they record the electrical activity in the frontal plane of the heart. The bipolar leads have positive and negative electrodes that are about the same distance from the heart. These leads are leads I, II, and III. The currents recorded from these leads are the axis of the heart. The unipolar leads are augmented leads. The letter *a* stands for augmented. In this type of recording, two of the limbs are connected through electrical resistances to the negative terminal of the electrical resistances to the negative terminal of the electrocardiograph, and the third limb is connected to the positive terminal. When the lead is on the right arm, it is aV_R, when it is on the left arm it is aV_L, and aV_F is on the left leg.

The precordial leads are unipolar leads that are placed on the chest. These leads are preceded by the letter *v*, which indicates a unipolar lead. The electrical axis of the precordial leads records electrical activity from the anterior, posterior, right, and left. This is determined by proper placement of the ECG leads. The numbers V_1–V_6 are used for standard placement of electrodes on a patient's chest. The lead placement is the same for men and women. The chest landmarks are used for placement of the electrodes. Steps included in placing the leads include identifying the second intercostal space and moving the fourth intercostal space to place V_1 on the right side of the sternum. V_2 is then placed over the fourth intercostal space on the left side of the sternum. Lead V_4 is then placed in the fifth intercostal space in the midclavicular line, and V_3 is placed halfway between V_2 and V_4. The placement of V_5 is in the fifth intercostal space in the anterior axillary line, and V_6 is in the same intercostal space in the midaxillary line.

The precordial leads reflect electrical activity to the following areas of the heart: (a) lead V_1 the right ventricle; (b) lead V_2 and V_3 interventricular septum; (c) lead V_4 over the apex of the left ventricle; and (d) V_5–V_6 the lateral wall of the left ventricle. The equipment that is needed to perform a standardized 12-lead ECG include the ECG machine, cables, leads, electrical paper for the machine, and disposable electrodes. Skin preparation items include a cleaning solution and a specialized rough patch or a dry wash cloth to rub on the skin to remove dead skin cells and improve the electrodes' contact with the skin. Because hair may interfere with the contact of the electrode with the skin, it may need to be shaved.

Specially trained technicians or nurses may conduct an ECG. Patients are informed that no electrical current will pass from the machine to them. Patients should also be told that some hair may need to be shaved, and they will need to expose their chest, arms, and legs. During the procedure they need to lay still, not talk, and breathe normally to decrease the likelihood of electrical interference on the recording. The nurse should instruct a patient to report any episodes of chest discomfort, shortness of breath, or palpitations.

Monitoring Leads

Continuous cardiac monitoring is used to monitor a patient's heart rate and rhythm for an extended period of time. In a critical care or telemetry unit the patient is usually monitored during the entire stay on the unit. In an outpatient

BOX 26-1

PREPARING FOR PLACEMENT OF LEADS

Preparation of the skin prior to the placement of the electrodes is important to ensure optimal ECG tracings. Lack of appropriate preparation often results in increased artifact and decreased transmission of the accurate electrical activity of the heart. It is the nurse's responsibility to complete adequate preparation of the skin, as follows. The skin should be clean and dry; use rough patch on back of monitor electrode to remove dead cells; if possible, place the electrode over an area with the least amount of hair, shave hair if necessary; check for adequate gel on the electrode, do not use dry electrodes; and assess the patient's skin at regular intervals for redness and irritation. Use alternate type of pad if skin allergy exists.

BOX 26-2

STEPS TO SET UP TELEMETRY ECG MONITORING

- Insert the appropriate battery into the telemetry transmitter. Follow the instructions from the manufacturing company.
- Connect the lead wire system into the transmitter, making sure there is a proper connection.
- Prepare the skin as necessary.
- Attach the cable (lead wires) to the electrodes.
- Remove the backing from the electrode, and check for gel that is moist.
- Apply the electrodes to the chest firmly checking that the electrode is making good contact.

setting, such as cardiopulmonary rehabilitation, the patient is monitored while in an exercise session, which may last from one to two hours.

The monitoring may be on a hardwired system or a telemetry system. When using a hardwire monitoring cardiac monitors are connected to a permanently mounted system. There is usually a monitor at the bedside and at the nurse's station to monitor the patient's heart continuously. Some units are equipped for multiple purposes and can assess blood pressure, pulse oximetry, and hemodynamic status (see chapter 24). The advantage to this system is that the nurse can monitor the rhythm at the bedside. It is useful for units where the patient is confined to a small area. The disadvantage is that the patient has limited mobility and must be attached to the system.

Telemetry systems use a transmitter to carry signals to antenna that are strategically placed around a unit to provide continuous monitoring, even when the patient is ambulatory. This allows the patient to move about a unit and still be monitored. The patient has electrodes placed on the chest (Box 26-1). These are attached to wires that are connected to a battery powered transmitter box. This system is useful for telemetry units in a hospital and for cardiopulmonary rehabilitation units. A disadvantage is that the oscilloscope may be in a different location. In a hospital setting the monitoring stations are located in a central area and may have units mounted in the hallway. Many units come with a portable oscilloscope that can be placed at a patient's bedside as needed. The patient needs to be instructed to keep the transmitter dry.

Monitoring leads are bipolar leads. Bipolar leads have a positive and negative electrode and a third electrode, or ground, which is placed on the patient to decrease electrical interference on the ECG tracing. Systems are available to monitor single or multiple leads. With placement of the leads it is possible to record the 12-lead ECG using electrodes placed on the patient's chest.

The placement of leads for the monitoring system follows the same principles as the standard 12-lead ECG. But instead of putting the electrodes on the arms and legs, all of the leads are placed on the patient's chest. This positioning results in less movement and prevents artifact on the monitor that distorts the waveform and makes interpretation difficult.

Monitoring units may use three, four, or five electrodes. Each system has specific instructions for placing the positive, negative, and ground electrodes. When a system uses three electrodes, the patient should be monitored in lead II. When lead II is monitored, the positive electrode is placed on the lower left chest, and the negative electrode is placed just below the clavicle on the right side of the chest. The ground electrode may be placed below the clavicle on the left side of the chest. Because the positive electrode is on the lower left chest, the atrial and ventricular depolarization wave travels directly toward the recording electrode. This usually results in an upright P wave from atrial depolarization and an upright QRS complex from ventricular depolarization.

Utilizing a three-lead system, it is also possible to monitor in a modified chest lead 1 (MCL_1). The MCL_1 positive electrode is placed in the equivalent position of V_1, which is the fourth intercostal space on the left side of the sternum. The negative electrode is placed at the left shoulder and the ground at the right shoulder. The expected complex is a biphasic P wave, a small R wave (first upright deflection), and a large S wave (the downward deflection following the R wave). This lead is helpful in evaluating conduction defects, such as right bundle branch block.

A five-lead wire system is used in many hospital settings. This system utilizes electrode placement that has the capability of running a 12-lead ECG by using an exploratory chest lead as well as the standard limb leads. The leads are color coded with manufacturer's instructions on placing the lead electrodes following manufacture's recommendations for ECG monitoring using telemetry (Box 26-2).

Troubleshooting Cardiac Monitoring Problems

For accurate interpretation of cardiac monitor strips, it is important to recognize factors that distort the pattern on the cardiac monitor or the recording on paper (Table 26-1). Artifact on the monitor can be from electrical interference, excessive body movement, and poor electrode contact with the skin. A dry electrode causes poor contact with the skin. Sixty-cycle interference is also called electrical interference and causes a wide distortion of the waveform on the ECG. A wavy baseline of the waveform may be from chest wall movement, a lost electrode from excessive perspiration, or lead placement that is exaggerated by patient movement. Equipment that is not functioning properly may also distort the complex. Another problem is a faulty battery in a telemetry unit. This malfunction causes a wide baseline. Excessive wear on electrode wires may also cause interference. To keep equipment in good working order, proper care is imperative. Keeping the unit dry and free from damage will ensure that it records accurately.

A flat rhythm strip may occur because of low voltage in the monitored lead, and it may be necessary to monitor the patient in a different lead that will record a larger waveform. A flat strip may also be the result of dry electrodes, absent electrodes, or equipment failure. Abnormal waveforms may simulate a life threatening arrhythmia, such as ventricular fibrillation or asystole, when in fact these are simply a monitoring problem. The first step in treatment is to assess and treat the patient.

THE NORMAL ECG COMPLEX

The nurse must be able to recognize normal ECG complexes to better interpret rhythms that are abnormal. The normal ECG tracing contains complexes composed of the P wave, QRS complex, and T wave. In addition, the cardiac cycle also corresponds to specific components of the electrophysiological conduction cycle (Figure 26-1). It is important for the nurse to determine the amount of time it takes for the electrical impulse to travel normally through the heart. This timing will be determined by measuring the PR interval and QRS interval, which can be obtained from the normal ECG tracing. The isoelectric line will help the nurse determine whether the waveforms are positive, or those above the isoelectric line or waveforms that are negative, or those falling below the isoelectric line. Many times these will be determined by lead placement. The nurse must also be able to determine how many times the complexes occur in one minute as well as the regularity of those complexes.

Calculating Heart Rate

The paper used in heart monitor recording devices is standard throughout all institutions. To calculate heart rate from a patient's ECG recording the nurse must record a rhythm strip. The graph paper is divided into small and large squares. Horizontally, those squares represent time. Each small square equals 0.04 seconds of time. Each large square represents 0.20 seconds in time. Each large square contains five small squares that total 0.20 seconds. Five large boxes equal one second in time and 15 boxes represents three seconds in time. The graph paper will include hash marks at the top or bottom of the graph at various points in time, every one or three seconds. Most frequently, graph paper will display a hash mark every 15 large boxes or every three seconds. These marks help to distinguish three seconds in time. Once a recording has been obtained, there are various methods for determining the patient's heart rate.

One method of calculating ventricular heart rate is to count the number of small squares between two QRS complexes. The tallest peak of the QRS

TABLE 26-1 Troubleshooting Cardiac Monitor Problems

MONITOR PROBLEM	CAUSE	POSSIBLE REMEDY FOR PROBLEM
Artifact causing waveform distortion from muscle contraction	Patient movement	Check patient to assess if they have chills and warm room if necessary.
	Respiratory movement	Ensure that electrode is applied to a flat non-muscular part of the torso.
	Tremors	
	Chills	Check electrode making sure that the electrodes are in contact with skin and reapply if necessary.
	Seizures	
	Bad connections between the electrode and connector	Dry skin and reapply electrode if the patient is diaphoretic.
	Diaphoresis	
Alarm for false high rate	Gain set too high for lead placement, and monitor is double reading the QRS complexes	Assess patient's potassium level for T wave, taller than expected.
		Reset gain on monitor.
Weak signal from telemetry monitor	Patient too far away from the antenna system for telemetry	Return patient to specified antenna coverage area
		If patient is in the specified area, move the transmitter for better coverage.
QRS complex is too small to register by the telemetry unit	Lead may be isoelectric and not have enough voltage to be registered by the unit	Check leads for proper placement.
	Electrodes placed in improper positions	Try another lead for monitoring patient.
	Cable or wire damage	Check for damaged wires or cables.
Baseline wander	Movement of patient	Reapply electrodes to nonmuscular areas, checking for contact with the skin.
	Electrodes placed over moving muscle	
	Respiratory movement	
Electrical interference	Malfunction of electrodes	Reapply electrodes.
60-cycle (AC) Interference	Electrical equipment around bed	Check electrical equipment for proper grounding.
Baseline flat	Dry electrode	Change electrodes
	Patient disconnected from monitor	Check patient connection to monitor
	Cable or wire malfunction	Change wire or cable if this is determined to be the cause.
Wide distortion of monitor pattern	Dead battery	Change battery in telemetry unit.

Adapted from Grauer, K., & Ruskin, J. (2004, February). Palpitations and arrhythmias: Benign or threatening? Patient Care, 30–36.

complex (the R wave) is determined, and then the small boxes between are counted. Once the number of small boxes is obtained, then that number is divided into 1,500. This method of calculating heart rate is considered to be reliable only if the heart rhythm is regular. Small boxes between two consecutive P waves would determine the atrial rate. A similar method would be to count the number of large boxes between consecutive P waves or R waves and divide that number by 300. This method is reliable only if the heart rhythm is regular. When a heart rate ruler is used, the rhythm again needs to be regular to ensure accuracy of the rate.

Another way of determining heart rate is to record a six-second strip of the patient's heart rate and then count the number of complexes recorded in a six-second period. After obtaining this number multiply it by 10 to

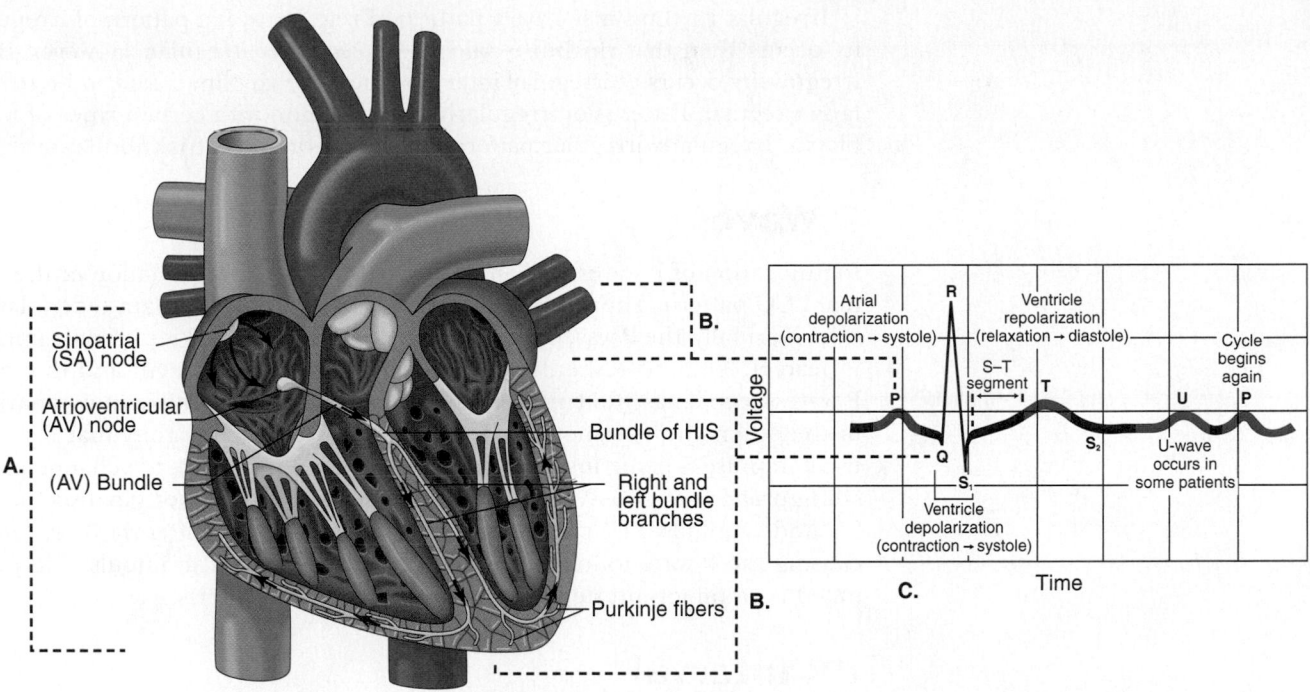

Figure 26-1 A. Conduction system of the heart, B. Relationship of the conduction system to an EKG strip, C. Relationship of S_1 and S_2 heart sounds to an ECG strip.

calculate the heart rate per minute. This is the most common method used to calculate heart rate, because it is the quickest method and can be used when the heart rhythm is irregular. Additionally, a longer rhythm strip may be run when the rhythm is irregular or the patient's apical pulse is counted for a full minute.

The vertical boxes on the graph paper measure the height of the ECG complex. Each vertical small square represent one millimeter. In a standardized ECG the increased height of the complexes may reflect hypertrophy of the cardiac chambers. In some electrical disturbances increased height may be present. Hypertrophy of the atria and ventricles may only be confirmed by utilizing the tracings from a standardized 12-lead ECG.

Determining Rhythm

Once the nurse has determined heart rate, the regularity of the beats should be assessed. Determining rhythmicity of the P waves assesses the regularity of the atrial rhythm. The rhythmicity of the QRS complexes determines the regularity of the ventricular rhythm.

Regularity of atrial rhythm is easily determined once a rhythm strip has been obtained. The nurse should place one point of the calipers on one P wave and then spread the calipers out until the other point is touching the next corresponding P wave. Once that P wave is located, the tip of the calipers remains on that P wave and the calipers are flipped over to the next consecutive P wave. If the distance between the P waves is equal, then the atrial rhythm is regular. If the distance between the P waves is different, then the rhythm is irregular. The same method is done using the R waves to determine ventricular rhythmicity.

A similar method can be used without the aid of calipers. The nurse places a blank sheet of paper under the complexes of the ECG recorded strip. A mark is made on the paper that corresponds to the appropriate wave. The next mark is placed under the next consecutive P or R wave. Then, much like flipping the calipers, the paper is moved to the next consecutive P or R wave. If the intervals in the P or R waves stay consistent, then the rhythm is regular. If the intervals are not equal, then the rhythm is irregular.

Irregular rhythms may have a pattern of regularity. If a pattern of irregularity occurs then that rhythm is said to be regularly irregular. However, if an irregularity occurs at irregular intervals, then the rhythm is said to be irregularly irregular. Patterns of irregularity are common with certain types of heart blocks. Irregularly irregular patterns are common with atrial fibrillation.

P Waves

Identification of P waves is an important step in the interpretation of the normal ECG pattern. The **P wave** is a graphic representation of atrial depolarization. Normally, the P wave is a small rounded complex and is normally upright in lead II. The nurse should identify that P waves are present and that each P wave precedes a QRS complex. All P waves should look alike in comparison to the others in the same lead. P waves that are present signify that the electrical impulse is being initiated in the SA node. When there is a change in the configuration of the P wave, the impulse may not be originating in the SA node. Impulses may originate from other areas of the atria or AV node causing the P wave to look different. Identifying where an impulse has originated is an important step in interpretation of arrhythmias.

PR Interval

Once P waves have been identified the nurse should next determine the PR interval. The **PR interval** is an estimate of the amount of time it takes the impulse to travel from the SA node through the AV node, the bundle of His, and the main part of the left bundle branch (Fuster, et al., 2004). The PR interval is measured by counting the small boxes from the beginning of the P wave to the beginning of the QRS complex. The normal PR interval measures from 0.12 seconds to 0.20 seconds in heart rates of 60 to 100 beats per minute. So the normal PR interval will be between three to five small boxes. If the PR interval is longer than 0.20 seconds, then the impulse is traveling slower than normal or is delayed. If the PR interval is shorter than 0.12 seconds then the impulse is traveling faster than normal, or the impulse has not originated in the SA node.

QRS Complex

The **QRS complex** is a graphic representation of ventricular depolarization, which represents the amount of time for the impulse to travel from the left bundle branch and traverse the rest of the ventricle through the remainder of the conduction system. The three waveforms that comprise the complex can vary in appearance depending on lead placement, normal alterations, or pathology.

In situations where the Q wave is present, it is the first negative deflection of the complex and reflects ventricular depolarization. The R wave is defined as the first positive, upward deflection following the P wave. The R wave is positive in lead II. It is usually tall and upright. The Q wave may or may not precede the R wave. Large deep Q waves may indicate necrosis of myocardial tissue. The S wave is the first negative deflection following the R wave. As stated earlier, QRS complexes can vary in configuration and may be normal variations.

QRS Interval

The QRS interval is measured from the beginning of the complex, the first deflection after the P wave to the end of the complex. The end of the complex is measured where the last wave returns to baseline. The QRS complex represents the amount of time it takes for the electrical impulse to travel from the bundle of His, down the right and left bundle branches, to the Purkinje fibers.

The normal QRS interval measures from 0.04 to 0.10 seconds. When the QRS interval is longer than normal, there is a delay in the conduction of the impulse. Delays in conduction through the ventricles are usually caused by blocks in the bundle branches or impulses generated from an ectopic focus in the ventricle. When the delay is because of a block in the bundle branches, the patient is said to have a bundle branch block. An ectopic focus is defined as an impulse that is generated outside the SA node. In these situations, the QRS will appear wider than normal and may have a different configuration. Diagnosing a right versus a left bundle branch block is best done with a 12-lead ECG.

T Wave

The **T wave** is a graphic representation of ventricular repolarization. One can assume that atrial repolarization occurs but is hidden by the QRS complex. The T wave follows the QRS complex and is larger in size than the P wave. Usually the T wave is deflected in the same direction of the QRS complex. While not usually part of the basic arrhythmia interpretation process, it is important to note that changes can occur with the T wave. Changes in the T wave amplitude or configuration can occur with myocardial ischemia, infarction, or electrolyte disturbances, such as hypokalemia or hyperkalemia.

QT Interval

The **QT interval** is the graphic representation of the amount of time it takes for ventricular depolarization and repolarization. It is measured from the beginning of the QRS complex to the end of the T wave. The normal QT interval depends on the heart rate. Obviously, the faster heart rate, the shorter the QT interval. Formulas are available to calculate the QT interval in relation to the heart rate, defined as the corrected QT interval or QTc. Generally, with a heart rate of 60 beats per minute the expected QT interval is 0.40 to 0.44 seconds (Fuster, et al., 2004). Certain medications and electrolyte disturbances may abnormally prolong the QT interval. These causes would be important for the nurse to note as prolongation of the QT interval could lead to serious and possibly fatal arrhythmias.

Systematic Approach to Arrhythmia Interpretation

To interpret arrhythmias, the nurse must use a systematic approach to ensure an accurate diagnosis (Box 26-3). The first step in diagnosing a rhythm is to calculate the heart rate. A normal heart rate is from 60 to 100 beats per minute. This is the normal intrinsic rate of the SA node. The second step is to determine whether the rhythm is regular or irregular. Once the first two steps are completed, the third step is to determine whether or not P waves are present. P waves should be identified during this step in addition to observing the configuration. The nurse should determine if all the P waves look alike and if QRS complexes follow each P wave. After evaluating the P waves and the QRS complexes, the PR interval should be determined. The QRS interval and QT intervals should then be calculated respectively.

CAUSES OF ARRHYTHMIAS

When patients are evaluated for abnormal heart function, frequently the cause is abnormal conduction of electrical impulses that result in malfunction of the heart muscle. Arrhythmias occur commonly and some may be considered benign, but others are considered to be potentially life-threatening. Arrhythmias are considered to be potentially dangerous when they cause hemodynamic

---

BOX 26-3

SYSTEMATIC APPROACH TO ARRHYTHMIA INTERPRETATION

Step 1: Determine rate
Step 2: Determine rhythmicity
Step 3: Determine P waves
Step 4: Determine PR interval
Step 5: Determine QRS interval
Step 6: Determine QT interval

compromise. When the arrhythmia affects cardiac output to the degree that the patient experiences signs and symptoms, such as hypotension, syncope, chest pain, shortness of breath, altered level of consciousness, nausea and vomiting, and diaphoresis along with other signs of decreased cardiac output, then treatment should be initiated. There are various physiological mechanisms by which most arrhythmias occur. These mechanisms generally can be divided into two major categories. These are abnormalities that occur with the conduction system that include heart blocks and reentry and abnormal impulse generation that includes problems with automaticity or triggered activity.

Reentry

Reentry occurs when fibers in the heart are reactivated by the same electrical impulse instead of the impulse traveling down the normal conduction system. This condition occurs when the progression of the electrical impulse is delayed or blocked. The delayed electrical impulse prematurely depolarizes neighboring cardiac cells once they have repolarized. The impulse then may travel up (antegrade) in the conduction system, then down (retrograde) causing a circuit of electrical impulse migration. A reentry circuit typically causes a tachycardia. Paroxysmal atrial and junctional tachycardias occur frequently because of a reentry mechanism.

Enhanced Automaticity

All cardiac cells have the potential to generate an electrical impulse. The sinus node, AV node, and Purkinje fibers are the locations of the cells that normally possess the property of automaticity. Arrhythmias occur when these normal pacemakers generate impulses greater than their intrinsic rates. Enhanced automaticity can occur not only with the normal pacemakers of the heart but also with other cardiac cells. In certain situations, cardiac cells can spontaneously depolarize and generate an impulse that is conducted throughout the heart. These ectopic foci may replace the SA node, the dominant pacemaker, if impulses are generated at a faster rate. Enhanced automaticity occurs for various reasons. Medications, especially those that increase heart rate are capable of causing enhanced automaticity. Digitalis toxicity, electrolyte disturbances, and myocardial ischemia or infarction are also causes. Hypoxemia is also a common cause of enhanced automaticity.

Triggered Activity

Triggered activity occurs due to afterdepolarizations. When a cell is depolarized, it may depolarize again depending on the situation. When this occurs, atrial or ventricular ectopic beats are generated. Triggered activity results in premature beats and other tachyarrhythmias. Early afterdepolarizations alter the sodium and potassium currents during repolarization and result in a prolonged QT interval placing the patient at risk for developing torsades de pointes. Causes of triggered activity include increased circulating catecholamines, digitalis toxicity, hypoxemia, electrolyte disturbances, myocardial ischemia or infarction, QT-prolonging drugs, and abnormal stretching of the myocardium.

SINUS RHYTHMS

Many types of arrhythmias are presented in this chapter. Though sinus rhythm is not an arrhythmia, it is presented as the overall goal of arrhythmia treatment. There are arrhythmias that occur as a result of malfunction of the sinoatrial node, such as sinus bradycardia, sinus tachycardia, sinus arrhythmia, and sinus arrest and exit block. The atrial arrhythmias include atrial tachycardia, premature atrial contractions, atrial flutter, and atrial fibrillation. The junctional arrhythmias presented are premature junctional contractions, junctional rhythms, and junctional tachycardia. Delays or blocks in the conduction system cause the common types of heart blocks that are presented. Lastly, ventricular arrhythmias including premature ventricular complexes, ventricular tachycardia, ventricular fibrillation, and idioventricular rhythms are presented.

Normal Sinus Rhythm

Normal sinus rhythm (NSR) is the goal of all treatment for arrhythmias (Figure 26-2). NSR has a rate from 60 to 100 beats per minute with a regular rhythm. The P waves are easily identified, and they all look alike in the same lead. There is a P wave for every QRS complex. Additionally, the P waves are small and rounded. The PR interval is between 0.12 to 0.20 seconds and remains constant from complex to complex. The QRS interval is of normal duration. The QT is considered normal. When a patient displays a normal sinus rhythm, the nurse can assume that all impulses originate in the sinus node, and the electrical impulses are traveling down the normal conduction pathway of the heart. Normal sinus rhythm needs no treatment.

Sinus Bradycardia

A bradycardia is defined as a heart rate slower than normal. Sinus bradycardia is a heart rate slower than 60 beats per minute initiated by the SA node (Figure 26-3). Sinus bradycardia can be easily interpreted by using the systematic approach to arrhythmia interpretation. The heart rate will be less than 60 beats per minute. The rhythm in sinus bradycardia is regular. P waves will be present and will precede each QRS. P waves will be upright in lead II. The PR interval will be a 0.12 to 0.20 in duration and constant from beat to beat. The QRS complex will be less than 0.10.

The causes of sinus bradycardia are varied. For many athletes, sinus bradycardia is a normal rhythm and is of no concern. Many cardiac medications, such as beta blockers, can contribute to a slowing of the SA node. Certain pathological states, such as acute myocardial infarction, increase parasympathetic tone that may result in a bradycardia. Hypothyroidism can also cause a

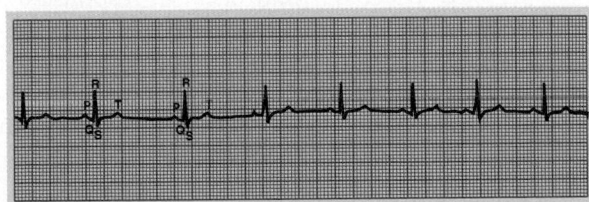

Figure 26-2 Normal sinus rhythm.

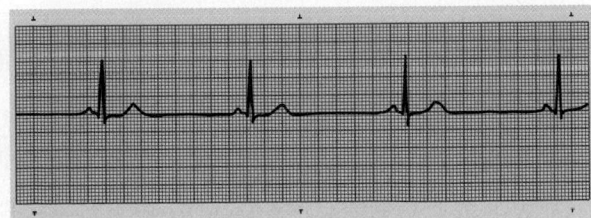

Figure 26-3 Sinus bradycardia.

sinus bradycardia. Vagal stimulation that occurs with vomiting, Valsalva maneuvers or carotid sinus massage can also cause sinus bradycardia.

The most important consideration when treating any arrhythmia is the patient's response to the arrhythmia. The nurse must assess whether or not the patient is hemodynamically compromised from the rhythm. In sinus bradycardia, the slow heart rate should be treated when the patient becomes hypotensive. Treatment should also be considered when the patient complains of chest pain, syncope, or shortness of breath associated with the bradycardia.

Atropine sulfate may be the drug of choice if the patient requires treatment. Atropine can temporarily increase the heart rate. If the bradycardia requires long-term treatment, a pacemaker may be inserted.

Sinus Tachycardia

A tachycardia is defined as a heart rate that is faster than normal. Sinus tachycardia occurs when the SA node fires at a rate faster that 100 beats per minute but the impulses subsequently travel down the normal conduction pathway (Figure 26-4). Typical rates of sinus tachycardia are 100 to 180 beats per minute. The rhythm is usually regular but may be slightly irregular depending on the rate. P waves are present and are upright in lead II. There is a P wave preceding every QRS complex. The PR and QRS intervals are of normal duration and remain consistent from beat to beat.

There are many potential reasons for developing sinus tachycardia. Pain, fever, and exertion are three common causes of sinus tachycardia. In addition, stress and anxiety may produce a rapid heart rate. Certain prescribed medications as well as stimulants, like caffeine and nicotine, may induce a tachycardia. Pathological states, such as hypovolemia, hypoxemia, hyperthyroidism, or inflammatory processes, can cause sinus tachycardia. A thorough assessment is necessary to be able to effectively treat the tachycardia. Sinus tachycardia can be problematic if it occurs in patients recently diagnosed with myocardial infarction. Tachycardias cause increased workload on the heart that may lead to more injury in the infarcted area of the heart. The most appropriate treatment of sinus tachycardia is to address the underlying cause.

Sinus Arrhythmia

Sinus arrhythmia is a common type of arrhythmia, occurring in healthy children and young adults, as well as in some elderly individuals. This arrhythmia may occur in response to changes in vagal tone during respirations. Typically the heart rate increases during inspiration and decreases on expiration. There is some speculation that this arrhythmia could have a positive effect on gas exchange by providing more efficiency in ventilation-perfusion matching. In the elderly, this rhythm may be due to coronary artery disease or myocardial infarction. Patients taking digitalis may also develop this rhythm. The typical heart rate of sinus arrhythmia is 60 to 100 beats per minute but may decrease below 60 beats per minute during intermittent episodes of bradycardia or increase above 100 beats per minute during episodes of tachycardia. All

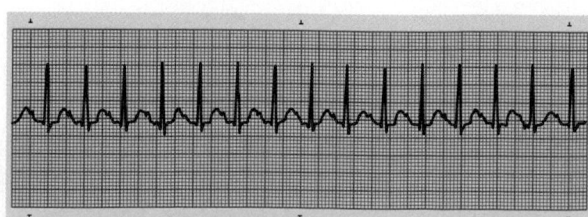

Figure 26-4 Sinus tachycardia.

impulses are generated by the SA node and travel down the normal conduction pathway. The rhythm is irregular, but when affected by breathing, the pattern will be regularly irregular. P waves will be present and will occur prior to each QRS complex. The PR interval will be 0.12 to 0.20 seconds and slight variation may occur with changing heart rates. The QRS will be less than 0.10 seconds.

Treatment for sinus arrhythmia will depend on the hemodynamic status of the patient. If the patient is hemodynamically stable and otherwise asymptomatic, the rhythm requires no treatment. If the patient is symptomatic during periods of bradycardia, then the patient will be treated with atropine sulfate or pacemaker insertion.

Sinus Arrest and Sinus Exit Block

A sinus arrest occurs when the SA node fails to generate an electrical impulse, and therefore, no P wave is present. A sinus exit block occurs when the SA node generates an electrical impulse, but it gets blocked in the conduction system before it spreads to the atria. In both arrhythmias, the P wave does not occur when it is next expected. The heart rate in individuals with either arrhythmia is usually around 60 beats per minute but will be slower during the episodes of sinus exit block or arrest. The rhythm in both arrhythmias is irregular. When P waves occur, they will look normal and will precede the QRS complex. The PR interval and QRS intervals are of normal duration. On occasion, it will be difficult to distinguish between the sinus arrest and sinus exit block, but differentiating the two can be accomplished by examining the rhythm. When sinus arrest occurs the SA node has not fired. When the rhythm starts again, the next P wave and QRS complex timing will be independent of the P wave and QRS complex that occurred before the arrest. In a sinus exit block the SA node fires, but the impulse is blocked. Because the SA node fires, the next occurring P wave and QRS complex that occur after the block will be timed in accordance with the P wave and QRS complex that occurred before the block. If the underlying rhythm were sinus rhythm, then appropriate interpretation would be sinus rhythm with sinus exit block or sinus rhythm with sinus arrest.

Causes of sinus arrest and sinus exit block can include medications, such as beta blockers, digitalis, and calcium blockers. Pathological conditions such as myocardial infarction and sick sinus syndrome can also cause these arrhythmias. Any conditions that cause an increase in vagal tone on the SA node can cause sinus arrest or sinus exit block to occur. The patient will be treated if symptoms occur or if the patient becomes hemodynamically unstable. Temporary treatment will consist of administering atropine sulfate IV push. If the arrhythmia continues, a permanent pacemaker will be indicated.

ATRIAL ARRHYTHMIAS

Atrial arrhythmias are most frequently caused by enhanced automaticity of the atrial tissue. Enhanced automaticity may occur as a result of stress, hypoxia, electrolyte abnormalities, digoxin toxicity, hyperthyroidism, or injury to the atrium.

Premature Atrial Complexes (Contractions)

A premature atrial complex ([PAC] contraction) occurs when an electrical impulse is generated in an area of the atria outside of the SA node. The electrical impulse then travels down to the AV node, where it could be blocked, transmitted normally to the ventricles, or transmitted abnormally to the ventricles. Premature atrial complexes can occur with many underlying rhythms. In addition to diagnosing the premature atrial complexes, the underlying rhythm must also be evaluated by the nurse. If the underlying rhythm is sinus rhythm, then the heart rate will be between 60 to 100 beats per minute. The rhythm will be irregular, as the premature atrial complexes will occur earlier than the expected complexes in a regular rhythm. P waves will be present, but those P waves that occur with the premature atrial complex will look different. This variance is because the P waves on the premature complexes do not originate from the SA node. Typically the PR interval will be 0.12 to 0.20 seconds, but the PR interval on the PACs may be different from the underlying rhythm. The QRS interval will be less than 0.10.

PACs result from various causes. Tobacco and caffeine can precipitate formation of premature atrial complexes. Sympathetic stimulation and alcohol intake can also cause the formation of these complexes. Certain medications, myocardial ischemia, mitral stenosis, and atrial septal defects may be the underlying reasons for PACs. PACs may also be seen in patients with chronic obstructive lung disease. Treatment of PACs will consist of treating the underlying cause. Treatment may consist of avoiding precipitating elements, such as caffeine or tobacco. If the cause of the PAC is the patient's medications, then the medications may need to be adjusted.

Atrial Tachycardia

Three or more premature atrial complexes that occur consecutively are considered to be atrial tachycardia. Atrial tachycardia occurs as a result of impulses originating in the atrial tissue outside of the SA node. The impulses can originate in one location in the atria, the focus. Multiple areas can generate impulses in which the plural form foci would be used. When there are multiple sites in the atria with impulses causing a tachycardia, the rhythm is interpreted as multifocal atrial tachycardia. When the atrial tachycardia is sustained, the rate is generally from 130 to 180 beats per minute. The rhythm may be regular if there is one ectopic focus generating impulses. The rhythm may be irregular if there is more than one ectopic foci. P waves will be present and precede all QRS complexes. The P waves will look different from the underlying rhythm, and the shape of the P wave will depend on the ectopic site in the atrium. The PR interval will generally be of normal duration, but the PR intervals may be different from the PR interval of the underlying rhythm. The QRS interval is generally less than 0.10 unless it is associated with a bundle branch block.

Digitalis intoxication may cause atrial tachycardia especially if the patient is also hypokalemic. Patients who have myocardial ischemia or dilated cardiomyopathy may also be at risk for developing atrial tachycardia. Patients suffering from chronic obstructive lung diseases, in particular, are at risk for developing multifocal atrial tachycardia because of their chronic state of hypoxemia. Cardiac tumors may also cause the development of atrial tachycardia. Rapid rates in atrial tachycardia need to be treated promptly. The patient will likely be symptomatic as the rate becomes faster. As the filling time for the ventricles (diastole) decreases, the patient will become hypotensive and will experience episodes of syncope. Patients may need to be treated promptly with synchronized cardioversion. Radio frequency ablation therapy may also be an option for some patients. Digitalis levels and electrolyte status should be evaluated in appropriate patients and corrected if they are abnormal.

Atrial Flutter

Atrial flutter occurs as a result of an ectopic focus in the atrial tissue that generates an impulse at such a high speed that it becomes the dominant pacemaker (Figure 26-5). Usually that focus is located lower in the atria near the AV node. The impulse spreads throughout the atria in a retrograde manner. The atrial rate can vary from 240 to 340 beats per minute. Because of the atrial rate and abnormal impulse condition, the cardiac output of the patient may be compromised. Just prior to ventricular systole, the atria normally squeeze

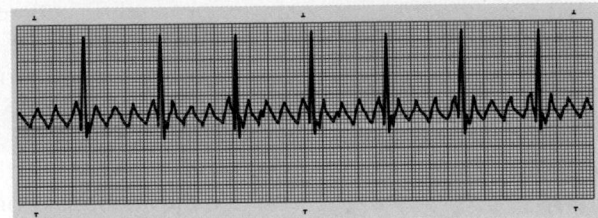

Figure 26-5 Atrial flutter.

the remainder of their volume into the ventricles. This "atrial kick" represents any where from 20 to 30 percent of the total cardiac output. Loss of atrial kick could cause the patient to be symptomatic with this arrhythmia. Atrial flutter is characterized by F waves that occur in a characteristic sawtooth pattern. The ventricular rate can vary depending on how many electrical impulses are blocked at the AV node. Generally, for every two impulses that occur, one is prevented from entering the ventricle. This pattern is called a 2:1 conduction pattern and can be visualized on the rhythm strip as two F waves for every QRS complex. Therefore, the ventricular rate is usually 150 to 170 beats per minute. The atrial rhythm is usually regular. The ventricular rhythm will either be regular or irregular depending on the rhythm with which the impulses are blocked. As stated previously, typical P waves will not be present as the SA node is not the dominant pacemaker. F waves will be the primary atrial activity. The QRS complex will usually have an interval that is less than 0.10 unless there is a bundle branch block.

Atrial flutter can be caused by various pathological conditions. Any chronic conditions that cause right atrial or right ventricular hypertrophy can precipitate atrial flutter. Patients who have undergone open-heart surgery or are experiencing congestive heart failure may be prone to the development of atrial flutter. Any conditions that may cause damage to the SA node, such as myocardial infarction or pericarditis, could lead to atrial flutter. Hyperthyroidism could also cause the development of atrial flutter.

Treatment of atrial flutter will depend in part on how symptomatic the patient becomes. The patient may be symptomatic from the loss of atrial kick or the rate of the ventricular response. Ventricular response may be controlled with the administration of calcium channel blockers or beta blockers. When patients are experiencing hypotension, syncope, chest pain, or other symptoms from a rapid heart rate, they may be treated with synchronized cardioversion to terminate the arrhythmia quickly. Adenosine may be injected intravenously to terminate the atrial flutter and restore the patient to a normal rhythm. Radio frequency ablation of the accessory pathway may also be used in patients to terminate the arrhythmia.

Atrial Fibrillation

Atrial fibrillation is caused by multiple ectopic foci in the atria that generate electrical impulses at a rate of greater than 400 beats per minute (Figure 26-6). On a rhythm strip, the atrial activity is characterized by coarse or fine fibrillatory

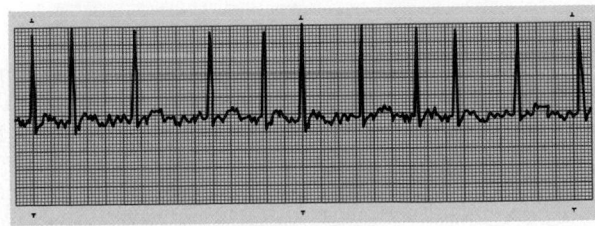

Figure 26-6 Atrial fibrillation.

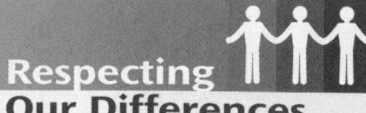

Respecting Our Differences

Atrial Fibrillation in the Elderly

Atrial fibrillation is a common complication following open-heart surgery. Studies have found that atrial fibrillation occurs more commonly in elderly individuals following coronary artery bypass surgery. Contributing factors as to why the elderly are more vulnerable to developing atrial fibrillation following surgery are increased wear and tear and increased stretching of the tissue of the atrium, increased interstitial collagen, and increased fatty infiltrate. Nurses should be aware that elderly patients are more at risk for developing atrial fibrillation. Continuous telemetry monitoring may be required for some patients. The nurse should report irregularities in pulse or apical heart rate in patients who are not monitored. The nurse may also prepare and administer Amiodarone for rhythm conversion or Diltiazem for rate control in the patient who has developed atrial fibrillation (Kern, 2004).

waves. The baseline between the QRS complexes may look rough and uneven. The ventricular response is usually rapid and can vary from 100 to 180 beats per minute. The rhythm in atrial fibrillation is characterized by its irregularly irregular pattern. Because the SA node is not the dominant pacemaker, there are no identifiable P waves. A PR interval cannot be determined. QRS complexes are usually 0.10 or less unless the impulses are aberrantly conducted.

Atrial fibrillation is commonly associated with conditions, such as coronary heart disease with or without an acute myocardial infarction. Heart failure and rheumatic heart disease along with open-heart surgery can also lead to the development of atrial fibrillation. Atrial enlargement, mitral stenosis, pericarditis, alcoholism, and hyperthyroidism are also conditions that can cause atrial fibrillation.

Signs and symptoms associated with atrial fibrillation occur because of the rapid ventricular response and loss of atrial kick. Patients may experience symptoms associated with low cardiac output. Rapid ventricular response may be controlled by the administration of calcium channel blockers and beta blockers. Synchronized cardioversion may also be used, especially when the patient is experiencing extremes of heart rate necessitating rapid termination of the rhythm after adequate anticoagulation or after presence of atrial thrombi have been considered. Radio frequency ablation may also be used in certain patients to treat atrial fibrillation.

Patients who have frequent episodes or chronic atrial fibrillation may be prone to the development of thrombi in the atria. As the atria are unable to produce an effective contraction, blood pools in the atria leading to the development of clots. Thrombus formation could lead to the development of a cerebrovascular accident (CVA) or pulmonary embolism. These patients may need to be treated with heparin sodium while in the acute care setting. Warfarin (Coumadin) may be prescribed for the patient for prevention of thrombi on a long-term basis.

Supraventricular Tachycardia

A supraventricular tachycardia is defined as any tachycardia in which electrical impulse occurs in supraventricular tissue (Fuster, et al., 2004). The term supraventricular means located above the ventricles. The term tachycardia means these rhythms will exceed rates of 100 beats per minute. This umbrella term is used to describe such rhythms as atrial tachycardia, atrial fibrillation, atrial flutter, and junctional tachycardia.

JUNCTIONAL RHYTHMS

Junctional rhythms are arrhythmias that originate in the AV node located between the atria and ventricles. The tissue around the AV node is referred to as junctional tissue. Students may hear both junctional and nodal terms used interchangeably to refer to these arrhythmias. Causes of junctional arrhythmias are primarily either enhanced automaticity or conditions like heart block, where the junctional tissue needs to take over as the primary pacemaker of the heart.

Premature Junctional Complexes

Premature junctional complexes occur when there is an ectopic focus in the AV junction that generates an electrical impulse that travels down to the ventricles with backward (retrograde) conduction through the atria. As their name implies, these beats occur early or prior to the next expected beat. The rate depends on the rate of the underlying rhythm. If the underlying rhythm is normal sinus rhythm, the rate will be 60 to 100 beats per minute. The underlying rhythm may be regular, but the premature junctional complexes make the overall rhythm irregular. P waves will be present if the underlying rhythm is sinus rhythm. The P waves of the premature junctional contraction could have one of several possibilities. The P waves may be negatively deflected or appear inverted in leads II, III, and aV_F. They may occur right before, during or just after the next consecutive QRS complex. If the P waves occur during the QRS complex, they will appear to be absent. If the P wave occurs before the QRS complex, the PR interval will be less than 0.12 seconds. If the underlying rhythm is normal, then the PR interval and QRS complex will be of normal duration.

The most common cause of premature junctional complexes is digitalis toxicity. Administration of other cardiac drugs, such as procainamide or excessive administration of epinephrine or norepinephrine, can also lead to the development of premature junctional complexes. Patients with congestive heart failure or those who have had myocardial infarction can also have premature junctional complexes. Any other conditions that lead to enhanced automaticity of the AV junction can cause premature junctional complexes. There is usually no treatment required for premature junctional complexes unless the patient becomes symptomatic. Withholding digitalis or decreasing the dosage may be indicated to prevent worsening of the arrhythmia.

Junctional Escape Rhythm

A junctional escape rhythm occurs when the SA node fails to fire, and the AV node takes over as the dominant pacemaker in the heart. The rate of this rhythm is from 40 to 60 beats per minute because that is the inherent rate of the AV junction. The rhythm is usually regular. P waves may be present before, during, or after the QRS complexes. The P waves may also appear inverted. If P waves are present before the QRS complex, the PR interval will be less than 0.12 seconds. The QRS complex is typically less than 0.10 seconds.

Junctional escape rhythms may occur in patients who have had myocardial infarction with subsequent damage to the SA node. Damage to the SA node may cause sinus arrest necessitating the AV node to replace the SA node. Patients will require treatment of the junctional escape rhythm if they become symptomatic from the bradycardia. Hypotension, syncopal episodes, chest pain, and other symptoms of compromised cardiac output may occur. Treatment usually consists of emergent transvenous or transcutaneous pacing.

Junctional Tachycardia

Junctional tachycardia occurs when the AV node replaces the dominant pacemaker of the heart. This rhythm can occur when there is enhanced automaticity of the AV nodal tissue. The heart rate can be from 70 to 140 beats per minute. The rhythm is referred as an accelerated junctional rhythm when the rate is from 70 to 100 beats per minute. When the rate is above 100 beats per minute, the rhythm is called a junctional tachycardia. Junctional tachycardia is usually regular in rhythm. P waves may be present before, during or after the QRS complex. P waves could also be inverted. The QRS complex is typically less than 0.10 seconds.

The most common cause of junctional tachycardia is digitalis toxicity. Myocardial infarction, especially when there is damage to the AV node, can also precipitate junctional tachycardia. Patients with acute rheumatic fever or myocarditis could also develop this arrhythmia. Excessive administration of sympathomimetic medications as well as low potassium levels can also cause junctional tachycardia.

Withholding digitalis is necessary for the patient who has digitalis toxicity. Administration of Digibind may be necessary in patients who have extremely elevated digitalis levels. Other treatment may be considered, especially if the ventricular rate is rapid enough to diminish cardiac output. Cardiac output may also be reduced by lack of an atrial kick.

HEART BLOCKS

Arrhythmias may be caused by defects in the conduction system. Impulses may be generated normally but become delayed or lost at various points of the conduction system. In the normal heart the AV node sends the impulses through the ventricles without difficulty. When there are defects in the conduction system including the AV node, impulses may be delayed or completely blocked. This is what occurs in the varying degrees of heart block.

First-Degree Heart Block

First-degree AV block occurs when there is a delay in the impulse transmission at the AV node (Figure 26-7). This delay usually occurs with every impulse and can be seen on every beat on the recorded rhythm strip. In this arrhythmia, the impulse is generated by the SA node at its usual inherent rate of 60 to 100 beats per minute. The rhythm is usually regular. P waves are visualized and precede each QRS complex. All P waves look a similar. The PR interval is the identifying factor in this rhythm. Because the impulse is delayed in the AV node, the PR interval will be prolonged, longer than 0.20 seconds. The QRS complex duration will be less than 0.10 seconds.

First-degree AV block occurs frequently in association with inferior myocardial infarction. Digitalis toxicity can also cause first-degree AV block to form. Treatment is usually not needed, as the patient is typically asymptomatic. Continued monitoring in these patients may be indicated to observe for worsening forms of heart block. This vigilance is especially important in the patient immediately after a myocardial infarction.

Second-Degree AV Block Type I

Second-degree AV block type I (Wenckebach phenomenon) occurs when there is a progressive delay of the electrical impulse at the AV node with each consecutive heartbeat. This delay continues from beat to beat until an impulse is completely blocked at the AV node. Once a beat is blocked, the progressive delay starts all over again. This usually occurs in a pattern that is characteristic of second-degree type I AV block. The rate in this arrhythmia is generally from 60 to 100 beats per minute. The rhythm is regularly irregular because the arrhythmia typically follows a pattern. P waves are present at the usual rate of the SA node. They all look alike as the impulse is generated in the SA node. There is a P wave for every QRS complex until the delay progresses to a dropped QRS following one P wave. The PR interval gradually lengthens in consecutive beats until the QRS is dropped. The PR interval following the dropped beat shortens, and then the PR interval starts to lengthen again in the next pattern of beats. QRS complexes are generally measured at 0.10 seconds or less.

An inferior myocardial infarction is a common cause of second-degree AV block type I. Digitalis administration and myocardial ischemia are other causes of this arrhythmia. The nurse should continue to monitor the patient for signs of worsening heart block. Treatment may not be necessary unless the patient's ventricular rate becomes too low to maintain sufficient cardiac output. If the patient becomes symptomatic, a pacemaker needs to be inserted. If the cause

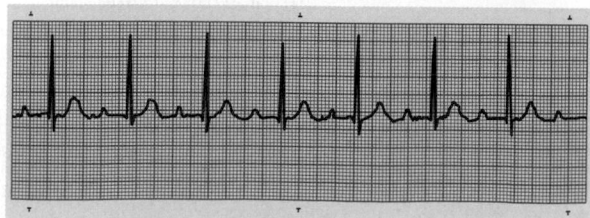

Figure 26-7 First-degree heart block.

is from vagal stimulation, atropine 0.5 to 1 mg intravenously is recommended (ACLS protocol). Second-degree AV block type I is also referred to as Mobitz type I second-degree AV block.

Second-Degree AV Block Type II

Second-degree AV block type II occurs when impulses generated in the SA node are selectively blocked in the AV junction. This type of arrhythmia occurs frequently in conjunction with a bundle branch block. This type of block is considered to be a more serious block than second-degree AV block type I. This block is also called Mobitz type II (Figure 26-8). Typically, the atrial rate will be from 60 to 100 beats per minute. The ventricular rate will depend on the number of impulses relayed to the ventricles. The rhythm is usually irregular. The P waves typically look alike as the impulses originate in the SA node. The number of P waves in relation to the number of QRS complexes will vary depending on the number of impulses conducted. This is usually expressed in a ratio, for example, 2:1 or 3:1. There may be 2 P waves for every QRS or 3 P waves for every QRS respectively. The PR interval on conducted impulses will typically be between 0.12 to 0.20 seconds and will remain constant. The QRS complex may be of normal duration or may be prolonged depending on the presence of a bundle branch block.

The most common cause of second-degree AV heart block type II is myocardial infarction. Digitalis toxicity may also result in second-degree AV heart block. Beta blockers and calcium channel blockers can also cause second-degree AV heart blocks, type I or type II. Patients who have second-degree AV heart block type II are usually symptomatic if they become bradycardic. Patients may complain of chest pain or shortness of breath. They may become hypotensive, diaphoretic, and experience episodes of nausea and vomiting. Treatment will almost always consist of a pacemaker insertion. An external pacemaker may be applied in an acute situation. Atropine sulfate may be considered emergently to speed up the heart rate temporarily while obtaining pacemaker insertion supplies. Second-degree AV heart block type II will occasionally progress to complete heart block.

Complete Heart Block (Third-Degree Heart Block)

Complete heart block occurs when the impulses generated by the SA node are not conducted to the ventricles (Figure 26-9). There is essentially no communication between the atria and ventricles as they are each beating independently of each other. Because none of the SA node impulses reach the ventricles, the AV

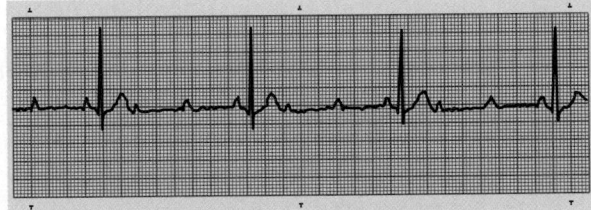

Figure 26-8 Second-degree AV block: Mobitz type II.

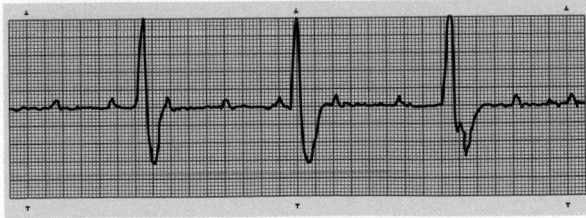

Figure 26-9 Complete heart block.

node or Purkinje fibers take over impulse generation for the ventricles. The atrial rate in this rhythm is typically between 60 to 100 beats per minute. The ventricular rate will depend on the site of the escape pacemaker. If the site of the pacemaker is the AV junction, the ventricular rate is generally from 40 to 60 beats per minute. If the impulse is being generated from the Purkinje fibers, the ventricular rate will be from 10 to 40 beats per minute. The rhythm in complete heart block is generally irregular. P waves will be present but will have no association with the QRS complexes. Measurement of the PR interval is not indicated, as there is no relationship between the P wave and the next occurring R wave. If the ventricular impulse is generated in the AV junction, then the QRS interval will be less than 0.10 seconds. If the impulse is generated below the AV junction, then the QRS complex will be greater than 0.10 seconds.

Complete heart block can occur commonly with digitalis toxicity and myocardial infarction. Other causes may be myocarditis or rheumatic heart disease. Certain medications, such as calcium channel blockers and beta blockers, can also cause complete heart block. Most patients are symptomatic and require a pacemaker insertion. Symptoms are characteristic of low cardiac output.

VENTRICULAR ARRHYTHMIAS

Ventricular arrhythmias occur as a result of an ectopic focus located in the ventricles, which generates an electrical impulse. This impulse is conducted throughout the ventricles following an abnormal conduction pathway. Because the QRS complex represents ventricular depolarization, ventricular arrhythmias will be observed in the changes that occur within the QRS complex.

Premature Ventricular Complexes

Premature ventricular complexes (PVCs) are beats that occur earlier than the expected beat from an impulse generated in the ventricle (Figure 26-10). PVCs are generally followed by a compensatory pause. A compensatory pause occurs when the distance between the R wave preceding the PVC and the following R wave is equal to the distance between three R-to-R intervals. If the underlying rhythm is sinus rhythm, the heart rate will be 60 to 100 beats per minute. The underlying rhythm may be regular, but when PVCs occur, the underlying rhythm will be irregular. P waves will be seen on a normal underlying rhythm, however, there will not be P waves related to the PVC. PR intervals should be of normal duration in the underlying rhythm. When the PVC occurs, the QRS complex will be characteristically wide and bizarre. The QRS interval will measure greater than 0.10 and be in opposite deflection of the normal looking QRS complex. The PVC will occur prematurely in relation to the normal rhythm and have increased amplitude. The T wave almost always occurs in the opposite direction of the last part of the QRS complex.

Occasionally, there is more than one ectopic focus in the ventricles generating impulses that spread throughout the ventricles. When this is occurring,

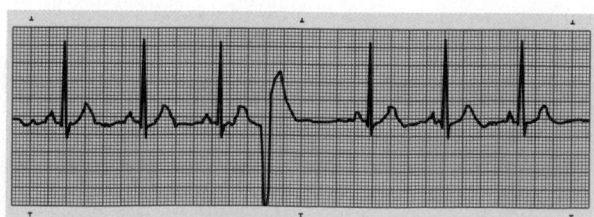

Figure 26-10 Premature ventricular complexes.

the PVCs will look different from one another. These PVCs will be called multiformed PVCs. When PVCs that are occurring look similar, the term uniformed PVCs is used.

There are many causes of PVCs. Hypokalemia, medications, and hypoxemia are common causes. Other causes may include myocardial ischemia, infection, hypovolemia, increased sympathetic activity, hypercalcemia, and ingestion of stimulants or alcohol. The asymptomatic patient will not need treatment. In conditions of hypokalemia or hypoxemia, treatment of the underlying cause will diminish the occurrence of PVCs. The nurse should monitor for occurrences of consecutive PVCs occurring together.

Ventricular Tachycardia

Ventricular tachycardia occurs when the patient experiences sustained, consecutive PVCs (Figure 26-11). Patients may occasionally experience runs of three to five concurrent complexes, which may not have a negative affect on cardiac output. It is when the patient experiences a sustained run of complexes at a rate greater than 100 beats per minute that cardiac output is usually affected. At this point ventricular tachycardia is a medical emergency, and the patient should be promptly treated to prevent death.

The ventricular rate is greater than 100 beats per minute and generally between 110 and 250 beats per minute. The rhythm is generally regular but it may be slightly irregular. There may be sporadic P waves throughout the arrhythmia. These may occur as a result of retrograde conduction or from firing of the SA node. The P waves that occur are dissociated from the QRS complexes. The QRS complex is usually wider than 0.12 seconds.

Ventricular tachycardia may occur as a result of myocardial infarction, cardiomyopathy, congenital, or valvular heart disease. Potassium imbalances and drug toxicities may also cause ventricular tachycardia. Left ventricular hypertrophy and congestive heart failure may also precipitate the formation of ventricular tachycardia.

Treatment of patients with ventricular tachycardia is paramount. If the patient becomes unresponsive and has no pulse, the rhythm is treated identical to ventricular fibrillation. The patient should be immediately defibrillated with 200 joules with increasing energy levels in up to three consecutive shocks.

The patient may have a pulse present with ventricular tachycardia but be experiencing symptoms of decreased cardiac output. The patient may be hypotensive, diaphoretic, pale, and having episodes of syncope. The patient may also experience chest pain and shortness of breath. These patients also need prompt treatment to prevent further compromise of cardiac output. The patient will benefit from synchronized cardioversion starting at 50 to 100 joules. In the conscious patient, a sedative is usually given prior to cardioversion to facilitate comfort.

Medications are usually first-line treatments in the patient with ventricular tachycardia who is relatively asymptomatic. In the patient who is normotensive and awake, intravenous (IV) amiodarone is the treatment of choice. Obviously, if the patient who experiences episodes of ventricular tachycardia is not being

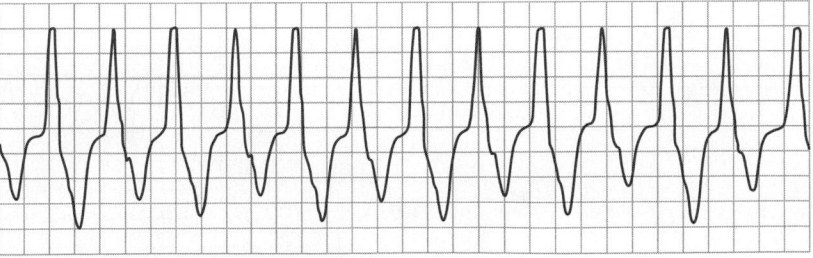

Figure 26-11 Ventricular tachycardia.

cared for in the ICU, that patient needs to be transferred to the ICU for close observation and continuous cardiac monitoring.

Torsades de Pointes

Torsades de pointes is a type of ventricular tachycardia with a unique, characteristic pattern. The term is French meaning "twisting of the points," which describes the pattern of the arrhythmia. The QRS complexes are in a characteristically wide-to-narrow pattern that resembles end-to-end hourglasses placed on their sides. This arrhythmia occurs in association with a prolonged QT interval. There are many factors that may predispose the patient to the development of long QT syndrome (LQTS). LQTS can occur as a result of a congenital abnormality, or it may be acquired in the adult from medications, cardiac or cerebral disease, or electrolyte disturbances. Drug-induced causes are more common that congenital causes of torsades de pointes (Fuster, et al., 2004).

The patient with torsades de pointes will experience syncopal episodes that may self-terminate. The rate of this rhythm can vary from 250 to 350 beats per minute. The patient will experience no effective cardiac output with the rapid rate, so this arrhythmia is considered to be life-threatening.

Treatment of the patient with nonsustained torsades de pointes would include identification and discontinuation of the medications associated with prolonged QT interval. Identification and correction of electrolyte abnormalities, such as magnesium and potassium, are also priorities in treatment. When the torsades de pointes is refractory and does not respond to magnesium sulfate, isoproterenol may be used in a mix of 1 mg in 250 mL of normal saline, lactated Ringer's solution, or D$_5$W (Cummins, 2003). Sustained torsades de pointes without a pulse should be treated promptly and includes defibrillation at 200 joules with increasing energy in three consecutive shocks. The ventricular tachycardia without a pulse algorithm that is followed in ACLS is also used in this situation.

VENTRICULAR FIBRILLATION

Ventricular fibrillation occurs as a result of multiple ectopic foci that originate in the ventricles (Figure 26-12). The rhythm is chaotic and is characterized by a coarse wavy baseline. Because there are multiple ectopic foci firing chaotically in the ventricle, the ventricles are unable to perform an effective contraction. Therefore, ventricular fibrillation produces no cardiac output, and the patient does not have a pulse.

Ventricular fibrillation occurs as a result of myocardial infarction, potassium imbalances, and as the result of certain drug toxicities. Ventricular fibrillation can also occur as the result of acidosis and extreme hypoxemia. Electrocution

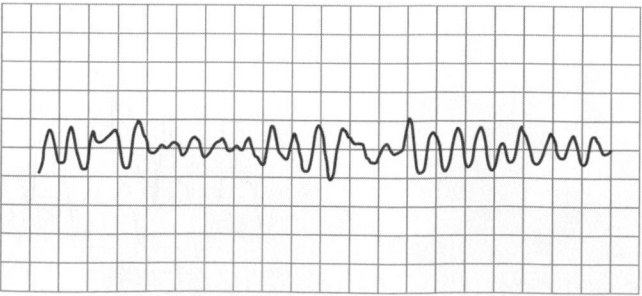

Figure 26-12 Ventricular fibrillation.

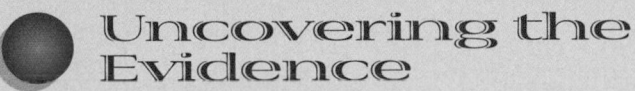

Uncovering the Evidence

Ventricular Tachycardias

Discussion: The researchers studied records of 340 men and 59 women who had known coronary artery disease and who had also received an implantable cardioverter-defibrillator. The purpose of the retrospective study was to compare differences between gender in occurrence of ventricular tachycardia or fibrillation. Patients who had an implantable cardioverter-defibrillator had documented episodes, which made them candidates for the study. Subjects were controlled by type of device. The results of the study showed that women were less likely to experience sustained ventricular tachycardia or fibrillation especially in patients who experienced a sustained monomorphic ventricular tachycardia.

Implications for Practice: Nurses should recognize that men are at greater risk of developing sudden cardiac death than women even in the presence of coronary disease. Male patients should be educated about their risks and taught measures to reduce those risks. Because of the increased risk in males, nurses should be vigilant in exploring unique ways to teach the male patient.

Source: Lampert, R., McPherson, C., Clancy, J., Caulin-Glaser, T., Rosenfeld, L., & Batsford, W. (2004). Gender differences in ventricular arrhythmia recurrence in patients with coronary artery disease and implantable cardioverter-defibrillators. Journal of the American College of Cardiology, 43*(12), 2293–2299.*

can cause ventricular fibrillation. It can also occur following procedures of the heart, such as cardiac catheterization or pacemaker insertion.

Ventricular fibrillation is a medical emergency and must be successfully treated immediately to prevent death. Treatment consists of immediate defibrillation starting at 200 joules with increasing energy in up to three consecutive shocks. If a defibrillator is not available, cardiopulmonary resuscitation (CPR) should be performed until a defibrillator arrives. If the patient's ventricular fibrillation cannot be terminated, then ultimately, the patient will become asystolic.

Idioventricular Rhythm

An idioventricular rhythm also called ventricular escape rhythm occurs when the SA node stops being the dominant pacemaker, and the AV node fails. The Purkinje fibers take over as the dominant pacemaker of the heart in an idioventricular rhythm. The typical rate in this rhythm is between 15 and 40 beats per minute. In an accelerated idioventricular rhythm, the heart rate is generally between 40 and 100 beats per minute. The atrial rate is not measurable. The rhythm is generally regular. P waves are not present in this rhythm, so there is no measurable PR interval. The QRS complex is generally wider than 0.10 seconds.

Digitalis toxicity or an acute myocardial infarction can precipitate an idioventricular rhythm. Other situations where an idioventricular rhythm can be observed are in cases of sinus arrest or complete heart block where the AV node does not replace the SA node as the dominant pacemaker. The patient will likely be symptomatic with this rhythm unless the ventricular rate is over 60 beats per minute. The patient will be hypotensive with other accompanying symptoms of decreased cardiac output. The treatment goal of the idioventric-

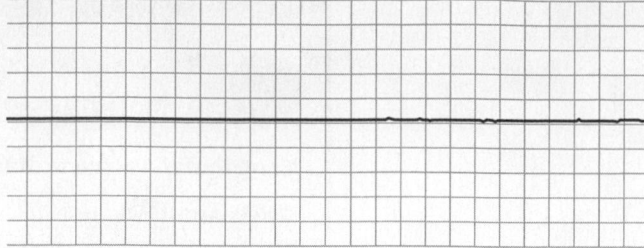

Figure 26-13 Asystole.

ular rhythm is to speed up the heart rate. This may be done temporarily by the IV administration of atropine sulfate. A transcutaneous pacemaker should also be used emergently in an attempt to increase the heart rate. This rhythm needs to be treated promptly as it can deteriorate rapidly into asystole. Other possible treatments for severe bradycardia are isoproterenol and epinephrine.

Asystole

Asystole occurs when there is an absence of any electrical activity in the ventricle (Figure 26-13). In the absence of electrical activity, no mechanical contraction occurs. Therefore, the patient has no pulse, and there is no cardiac output. The rhythm strip will look like a straight line or wavy line on the monitor. The patient is monitored in more than one lead to confirm asystole (Cummins, 2003). The patient requires immediate treatment according to ACLS protocol. CPR should be performed immediately. Intubation and IV access should be established to administer medications. Atropine sulfate and epinephrine are considered to be first-line medications in the treatment of asystole. Patients who go into asystole often have a poor prognosis, and termination of efforts to revive the patient should be considered as appropriate.

Pulseless Electrical Activity

Pulseless electrical activity (PEA) occurs when there is electrical activity being generated in the heart without the corresponding mechanical activity. The monitor will show an electrical rhythm that may even resemble normal sinus rhythm. Without the mechanical activity though, the heart does not contract and the patient has no pulse. The presence of PEA often results in a poor prognosis. PEA can occur following many pathophysiological states. The mnemonic consisting of five H's and five T's will help the health care provider to remember all potential causes of PEA. The five H's stand for hypovolemia, hypoxia, hydrogen ion (acidosis), hyperkalemia/hypokalemia, and hypothermia. The five T's stand for tablets (drug overdose or ingestions), tamponade (cardiac), tension pneumothorax, thrombosis (coronary), and thrombosis (pulmonary) (Cummins, 2003). Treatment of PEA should start with immediate CPR and attempted correction of the precipitating cause. Epinephrine is the initial medication of choice during CPR when an IV line has been established and the patient has been intubated.

MANAGEMENT STRATEGIES

There are many options when considering treatment for the patient who is experiencing arrhythmias (Table 26-2). When patients are experiencing arrhythmias that are considered to be benign, treatment may only be supportive in nature. Obviously, when a patient is experiencing life-threatening arrhythmias, treatment will be instituted emergently. Ideally, a complete his-

TABLE 26-2	Nursing Management for the Patient with Arrhythmias
NURSING MANAGEMENT	**RATIONALE**
Provide continuous ECG monitoring	To detect rapidly the occurrence of arrhythmias
Maintain heart rate alarms at appropriate limits	To detect bradycardia or tachycardia promptly
Administer antiarrhythmic medications per protocol or as ordered	To maintain therapeutic blood levels of appropriate medications
Administer CPR or defibrillation as appropriate for life-threatening arrhythmias	To restore perfusion or terminate ventricular fibrillation promptly
Maintain SpO$_2$ levels greater than 90 percent with supplemental O$_2$ if needed	To prevent hypoxia-induced arrhythmias
Monitor electrolyte levels and replace as necessary	Abnormally high or low potassium and low magnesium levels can precipitate arrhythmias
Maintain at least one patent IV site	To be able to administer emergency medications when needed
Monitor serum levels of antiarrhythmic medications	To prevent toxicity of medications and to maintain therapeutic blood levels
Provide information to the patient regarding disease process, procedures, and medications	To allay patient anxiety and promote compliance with medical and nursing regimens
Teach patient regarding symptoms of arrhythmias, such as chest pain, syncope, weakness, and fatigue	So patient can identify arrhythmias and seek early treatment
Teach patient to take own pulse	To monitor for side effects of medications or to detect arrhythmias
Teach patient to avoid proarrhythmic substances	Patient should avoid caffeine and recreational drugs that may be proarrhythmic

Adapted from Comer, S. (2005). Delmar's critical care nursing care plans (2nd ed.). Clifton Park, NY: Thomson Delmar Learning.

tory and assessment should be obtained from the patient prior to the decision to institute treatment. Patients should be evaluated for symptoms associated with the arrhythmia, such as chest pain, syncopal episodes, dyspnea, or fatigue. A complete medication history should also be obtained from the patient. Over-the-counter (OTC) medications as well as herbal and recreational products can induce palpitations and arrhythmias. There are many substances that have the potential for causing arrhythmias or palpitations. Some of these are alcohol, amphetamines, caffeine, bronchodilators, digitalis, ephedra, opiates, and antibiotics (Grauer & Ruskin, 2004). In addition to medication history, the patient's past medical and family history should also be evaluated. A 12-lead ECG should be performed on the patient in addition to 24-hour Holter monitoring. Echocardiogram and laboratory studies may also be helpful in evaluating arrhythmias for treatment.

Pharmacology

Treating arrhythmias with medications can be a paradox for health care providers. There are various effective antiarrhythmic medications that can be used in patient treatment however; most antiarrhythmic medications can also cause arrhythmias to occur. When medications are identified as causing arrhythmias, the term proarrhythmia is used to describe those medications. The benefits of pharmacological treatment should always outweigh the risks, and when patients are treated with medications, they should have frequent follow up by health care providers for side effects, compliance, and complications. Antiarrhythmic medications are classified by their actions on electrolyte movement during fast and slow cardiac action potentials according to the Vaughan Williams classification scheme.

Class I antiarrhythmic medications consist of those medicines that block sodium channels. When sodium channels are blocked, the electrical impulse becomes slowed in the atria, AV junction, and ventricles. These medications are helpful for tachyarrhythmias and ventricular ectopy. This class constitutes the biggest group of antiarrhythmic medications and is further broken down into groups identified as IA (e.g., procainamide and quinidine sulfate), IB (e.g., phenytoin), and IC (e.g., propafenone) (Broyles, Reiss, & Evans, 2007).

Class II antiarrhythmic medications consist of the beta blockers (e.g., esmolol and propranolol). Beta blockers block the beta receptors in the heart. When beta$_1$ receptors are blocked, the effects are decreases in cardiac contractility and a slowed heart rate. Beta blockers are helpful in treating tachyarrhythmias that are of ventricular or atrial in origin.

The Class III antiarrhythmic medications include those medications that have the action of blocking potassium channels (e.g., amiodarone, bretylium tosylate, and sotalol). Because these medications block potassium channels, they have the effect of delaying repolarization. These drugs are given primarily for treatment of ventricular arrhythmias, including ventricular tachycardia and ventricular fibrillation.

The Class IV antiarrhythmic medications are the calcium channel blockers. The only two calcium channel blockers that exert their effect on calcium channels in the heart are verapamil and diltiazem. These drugs are given primarily to slow ventricular rate in atrial fibrillation and discontinue supraventricular tachycardia.

The last group of antiarrhythmic medications includes adenosine, digoxin, and ibutilide (Corvert). These medications act by various mechanisms that do not fit under the other classes of antiarrhythmic medications. Adenosine has an extremely short half-life and is therefore given IV push and is used primarily to abruptly stop supraventricular tachycardias. Digitalis slows conduction through the AV node and is given primarily to slow ventricular rate in atrial fibrillation and flutter. Ibutilide is also given for the treatment of atrial fibrillation and atrial flutter.

The pharmacological management of cardiovascular arrhythmias can be expensive. Many patients do not have health insurance or cannot afford the tremendous costs of these medications. The increasing complexity of the health care system is beyond the budget constraints of many people, particularly in the management of patients with a wide variety of arrhythmias.

Defibrillation

Defibrillation is defined as the delivery of an electrical shock to the heart so that it completely depolarizes cardiac cells in an effort to terminate ventricular fibrillation. Defibrillation is performed by attaching specialized electrode pads or paddles to the patient's chest and delivering an electrical shock starting at 200 watts/second. It may be performed in the hospital setting by specially trained health care providers. Paramedics and emergency medical technicians carry defibrillators when responding to emergencies in the general public. Automatic defibrillators are being placed in public areas, such as airports and shopping malls, for use by minimally trained bystanders. Defibrillation is the most vital intervention in treating ventricular fibrillation and ventricular tachycardia without a pulse. Because resumption of normal activity of the heart requires adequate stores of high-energy phosphates that are rapidly used up in ventricular fibrillation, early defibrillation is crucial to increase the chances of a successful outcome (Cummins, 2003).

There are various brands of defibrillators utilized in all settings. Nurses must be familiar with the operation of the defibrillator used in their health care setting. Nurses must also participate in the maintenance checks and balances that should be performed on all defibrillators to maintain proper functioning. Knowledge of pad or paddle placement should also be reviewed when maintenance checks are performed. The cables and connectors should be inspected for cracks or broken wires. The defibrillator unit should be clean and unobstructed. There should be an ample supply of ECG paper and fully charged batteries. The unit should come on when the power button is depressed and should charge to the appropriate level on testing. The electric current should never be discharged by placing the paddles together or discharging them into the air (Cook, 2003). When they are floated to unfamiliar areas in the hospital, nurses should also identify the location of the defibrillator.

Patient should receive immediate defibrillation when they are found to be in ventricular fibrillation or ventricular tachycardia without a pulse present. The patient will be unresponsive, breathless, and pulseless. The nurse should call for help on finding an unresponsive patient. The individual should be defibrillated as soon as the machine arrives at the patient's bedside. Cardiopulmonary resuscitation should be initiated before the defibrillator arrives. Electrode pads for defibrillation should be placed appropriately on the patient's chest to ensure direction of current flow (Figure 26-14). If the paddles are used, approximately 20 to 25 pounds of pressure should be applied when defibrillating the patient. All health care personnel should be clear from the immediate area when defibrillating the patient so they are not shocked also. Once all personnel are clear, the operator depresses both discharge buttons simultaneously. Recommended energy levels for ventricular fibrillation and ventricular tachycardia without a pulse are 200 joules, 300 joules, and 360 joules respectively in three successive shocks (Cummins, 2003). After each shock, health care providers should confirm the continued presence of the rhythm before delivering the next consecutive shock.

Synchronized Cardioversion

Synchronized cardioversion is indicated for the presence of ventricular, supraventricular tachycardias, atrial flutter, and fibrillation. **Synchronized cardioversion** is delivering an electrical shock to the heart that is synchronized with the patient's R wave. Ventricular tachycardia that is faster than 150 beats per minute should be immediately cardioverted (Cummins, 2003). The supraventricular tachycardia and atrial flutter and fibrillation should be cardioverted when patients are experiencing hemodynamic instability related to the rhythm. Recommendations for energy levels by the American Heart Association (AHA) are lower for synchronized cardioversion than for defibrillation. They recommend a standard sequence of energy levels starting from 100 joules to 200 joules to 300 joules to 360 joules. Atrial flutter may respond to an energy level of 50 joules. The first step in cardioversion should be to consider whether or not to sedate the patient. This will depend in part on the patient's vital signs and consciousness. The steps in synchronized cardioversion are similar to those in defibrillation.

Implantable Cardioverter-Defibrillator

Implantable cardioverter-defibrillators (ICD) are placed in patients who have recurrent ventricular arrhythmias and are at risk for sudden cardiac death (SCD). Within these devices, the functions are controlled by a microcomputer inside the pulse generator that has been programmed with certain instructions. These devices are surgically implanted with the generator generally being implanted in the front left shoulder. There are two leads coming off the generator that are placed in the atria and the ventricle respectively. Additional

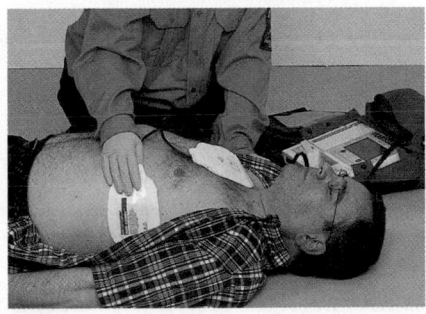

Figure 26-14 Placement of electrode pads for defibrillation.

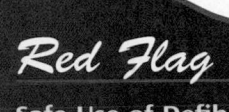

Safe Use of Defibrillator Pads

Defibrillator pads or paddles should never be placed over monitoring electrodes or implanted devices, such as permanent pacemakers. Pads or paddles should be at least 1 inch away from these to prevent damaging the device. Any transdermal medication patches should also be removed from the patient's chest prior to defibrillation (Cook, 2003).

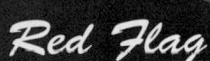

Red Flag

External Defibrillation

Do not delay external defibrillation for the patient in ventricular fibrillation who also has an implantable cardioverter-defibrillator if the device has failed to fire (Cook, 2003). Prepare for immediate external defibrillation. Then investigate as to the cause of the malfunction.

electrodes capable of delivering a high-energy shock are placed in the ventricle. There are additional electrodes in the superior vena cava and a generator that completes the circuit. When the generator senses ventricular fibrillation or ventricular tachycardia, an internal shock is delivered to the patient's myocardium. If the rhythm is unchanged, then the internal defibrillator is capable of delivering shocks of higher energy. The implantable cardioverter-defibrillators are also capable of delivering a synchronized cardioversion at a decreased energy level. Newer models of these devices are also capable of sensing a bradyarrhythmia or tachyarrhythmia and will start pacing or overdrive pacing the myocardium if needed.

Patients who require the ICD are not only at physical risk because of their cardiovascular disease, but also experience a wide range of psychosocial issues, which may have a strong impact on their quality of life. For many patients, having the ICD means the difference between living and dying. It is not uncommon for patients to experience conflicting emotions. Patients often live in fear of the times that the ICD will discharge.

Patients are also fearful that the ICD will not discharge when required to do so. Eckert and Jones (2002) found that patients experience profound feelings of anxiety and fear related to their lack of control over the timing of the activation of the device. Many patients also experience changes in their lifestyle. Patients are often restricted in their driving habits. This restriction may lead to isolation and lack of independence. Patients who need the insertion of an ICD need a good deal of education and support. Family support is often critical for these patients as well. There are many areas that have support groups for patients with ICDs.

Pacemakers

An artificial pacemaker is a device that sends an artificial stimulus to the heart to generate the electrical impulse. This is an especially important intervention when the heart rate is too slow. While pacemakers were originally designed to be lifesaving devices, they now are known to be lifesavers but also to improve quality of life. Nurses play an important role in the maintenance of pacemakers and patient safety (Box 26-4). The generator of the pacemaker sends regular stimuli to the myocardial tissue and depolarizes, or captures, the tissue. The electrical stimulus is then conducted throughout the entire myocardium. While

Fast Forward ▶▶▶

Growing use of ICDs

It has been predicted that the frequency of ICD implantation will continue to grow. The use of ICDs for the prevention of SCD will grow as at risk patients are better identified. The price of ICDs may decline because of the flexible purchase options available. Patients may purchase a basic package initially and add programmable options as the need arises. ICDs have also been predicted to become even more reliable and safe for patient use as improvements in lead technology are made (Fuster, et al., 2004).

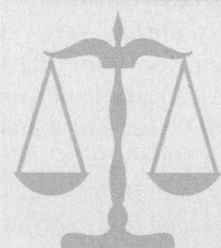

ETHICS IN PRACTICE

Patient Consent for Cardioverter-Defibrillation

Patients must consent to having an ICD implanted or a permanent pacemaker inserted. This should be thoroughly discussed with the patient who has an advanced directive. Patients may also request to have their ICD or permanent pacemaker support withdrawn when life-sustaining treatments are no longer warranted or desired (Mueller, Hook, & Hayes, 2003). It is likely that health care providers will care for a larger population of elderly patients who have permanent pacemakers or ICDs. As life-sustaining mechanical ventilation may be withdrawn under appropriate circumstances, ICD or permanent pacemaker support may also be withdrawn.

INTERVENTIONS FOR PATIENT WITH PACEMAKER INSERTION

1. Monitor ECG for the presence of arrhythmias and pacemaker malfunction. Post rhythm strip every four hours and as needed.
2. Monitor vital signs every 15 minutes after the procedure until stable or per protocol. Monitor every hour for at least four hours.
3. Monitor dressing or surgical site for evidence of bleeding.
4. Restrict movement of affected extremity after the procedure.
5. Monitor the patient for muscle twitching or hiccoughs.
6. Auscultate for muffled heart sounds or pericardial friction rub.
7. Assess for and report sudden episodes of chest pain.
8. Monitor for syncope, dizziness, weakness, or extreme fatigue.

Adapted from Comer, S. (2005). Delmar's critical care nursing care plans (2nd ed.). Clifton Park, NY: Thomson Delmar Learning.

pacemakers are utilized frequently to treat bradyarrhythmias, the rate of the pacemaker may be adjusted to override a tachyarrhythmia and slow it down.

There are two types of pacemakers: those that function according to a fixed rate and those that are demand pacemakers. Fixed-rate pacemakers send an electrical stimulus to the heart regardless of the patient's inherent heart rate. Demand pacemakers are designed to be sensitive of the patient's own intrinsic heart rate. These pacemakers sense the patient's own electrical activity and only send an electrical stimulus when they sense the patient's heart rate has decreased below a preset level. The pacemaker paces only when it is needed. Pacemakers may be either single- or dual-chamber pacemakers. Single-chamber pacemakers pace either the atria or ventricles. Dual-chamber pacemakers pace both the atria and ventricles. There are three different methods of instituting pacemaker therapy. The first is external pacing, which is used primarily in emergent situations, temporary pacing that is frequently used for short-term situations, and permanent pacing.

External Pacemaker

External pacing or transcutaneous pacing is accomplished by placing pacing electrodes on the patient and delivering a stimulus through the skin to the myocardium. External pacing is done primarily in emergent situations when the patient suddenly experiences extreme bradycardia or during asystole. The external pacemaker is used only on a short-term basis and is often employed only until a transvenous pacemaker can be inserted. In most health care facilities, the defibrillator or monitors that are on the crash carts have the capability of externally pacing a patient. The nurse should be familiar with how to work the external pacer so that when its use is called upon in an emergency, the nurse can operate the pacemaker easily.

The pacing pads are placed on the patient anteriorly and posteriorly. The anterior electrode is placed to the left of the sternum, and the posterior electrode is placed on the back behind the anterior electrode to the left of the thoracic spinal column (Cummins, 2003). This positioning of the electrodes sandwiches the heart to increase the chances of successful pacing. There should be good skin contact with the pacing electrodes. The patient's chest should be shaved if necessary. The ECG electrodes and leads from the pacing machine should be attached to the patient in addition to the pacing electrodes.

Once the pacing and ECG electrodes are in place, the pacemaker device should be turned on. The pacemaker rate should be adjusted to the prescribed level and then the current to be delivered should be adjusted until capture is achieved. Generally, all pacemaker devices deliver currents from 0 to 200 milliamps and allow rate adjustment from 30 to 180 beats per minute (Cummins, 2003). Once a paced beat is visualized on the monitor, the nurse should check the patient's pulse to ensure good hemodynamic response. The patient will need to be informed of the potential for pain related to the delivered milliamps. Sedation with a benzodiazepine or narcotic may be appropriate for the conscious patient.

Temporary Pacing

A transvenous pacemaker may also be inserted during emergent situations when the patient is experiencing extreme episodes of bradycardia, tachycardia, or heart block. Insertion of the transvenous pacemaker consists of inserting a wire with a pacing electrode into the right ventricle by entering the subclavian vein. The pacing wire is connected to an external generator where the rate and milliamp are controlled. Transvenous pacemakers are temporary treatments and may be inserted prior to a scheduled permanent pacemaker insertion. Epicardial pacing is accomplished by attaching electrodes to the patient's epicardium during open-heart surgery and attaching the leads to an external generator. Epicardial pacing is also a form of temporary pacing.

Permanent Pacing

Permanent pacemakers are implanted and used as a permanent pacemaking source. When it has been determined that the patient will need lifelong assistance from an artificial pacemaker, a permanent device is inserted. A permanent pacemaker may be inserted in similar manner to a transvenous pacemaker under local anesthesia. The generator is usually placed just under the skin anteriorly on the right side of the chest. The lead wires are placed in the right atrium or right ventricle. This procedure may be done in the operating room or in a cardiac catheterization lab under fluoroscopy. The patient should have continuous ECG monitoring during recovery to detect any initial pacemaker malfunctions. The pacemaker stimulus looks like a spike on the ECG recording. The pacer spike may be deflected positively, negatively, or biphasic depending primarily on lead placement. If the atria are being paced, then there will be a pacer spike just prior to the P wave. If the ventricles are being paced, there will be a pacer spike just prior to the QRS complex. Because the electrical stimulus is being produced from an alternate site, the impulse will be conducted outside of the normal pathway. Because of this alternate pathway, the QRS complex will be wider than normal, producing a QRS interval that is greater than 0.12 seconds. Correct interpretation of the patient's rhythm is usually identified by the amount of time the patient is being paced. The patient may have 60 paced beats in a heart rate that is 80 per minute. That patient is usually said to be paced approximately 80 percent of the time.

Permanent pacemakers have many capabilities that may be programmed to meet the needs of the particular patient. Pacemakers may sense and pace the atrium, the ventricle, or both. Pacemakers may be programmed to increase the heart rate appropriately, for example, when the patient is exercising and decrease it appropriately when the patient is sleeping. The nurse should make note of the type of pacemaker that is inserted and should know which chambers are sensed and paced. Pacemakers are categorized according to a five-letter code created by the Inter-Society Commission for Heart Disease in which the letters used when describing the pacemaker denote the chamber paced, the chamber sensed, response to sensing, programmable functions, and anti-tachyarrhythmia functions (Comer, 2005). The set rate of the pacemaker should also be known and documented on the patient's record.

Once a permanent pacemaker has been inserted, the operative site should be monitored for infection. Patients will usually be on an antibiotic prophylactically to prevent the occurrence of infection. Patients will also be instructed to limit mobility of their right arm for at least 12 hours after the procedure. Complications associated with permanent pacemaker insertion are uncommon but can include infection, bleeding, pneumothorax, arrhythmias, cardiac tamponade, pulmonary embolism, and electrical microshock (Comer, 2005). Malfunctions with the pacemaker can occur and should be monitored after the procedure.

Pacemaker Malfunction

Malfunction of pacemakers may be identified when the patient's rhythm is being monitored. Malfunctions may be related to lead placement, voltage, or battery life. The most common malfunctions are a failure to sense or capture. Failure to sense is an inability of the pacemaker to sense the patient's own inherent electrical activity. This malfunction causes the electrical impulses to compete for nondepolarized cardiac tissue. This may be identified on the monitor by observing pacemaker spikes occurring before, during, and even after the P wave and QRS complex. Ultimately, the patient could have arrhythmias related to the malfunction. Of particular concern would be an electrical impulse that occurs during the relative refractory period and causes the R on T phenomenon. This, in turn, could cause the patient to go into ventricular fibrillation. The sensitivity on the pacemaker needs to be adjusted to correct this problem.

Failure to capture occurs when the electrical impulse of the pacemaker fails to capture cardiac tissue. This situation may be identified on the monitor by observing the pacemaker spike with no corresponding P wave or QRS complex. Obviously, failure to capture is a concern if the patient requires the pacemaker for impulse formation the majority of the time. Usually, failure to capture occurs because the current output on the pacemaker is too low and needs to be increased.

Ablation Therapy

Ablation therapy can be used to eliminate many forms of supraventricular tachycardia and ventricular tachycardias (Grauer & Ruskin, 2004). Radio frequency catheter ablation is defined as the deliberate destruction of arrhythmogenic myocardial tissue or parts of the conduction system to control cardiac arrhythmias (Scheinman, et al., 2003). The offending tissue is previously identified by electrophysiologic studies. The destruction of the tissue is accomplished primarily by the delivery of thermal energy. Conditions that are treated with ablation therapy are accessory pathways that contribute to reentry arrhythmias, patient's reentry AV nodal reentrant tachycardia, atrial flutter, atrial fibrillation, and ventricular tachycardia (Fuster, et al., 2004). Patients who are candidates for radio frequency ablation are those who do not get a good response with antiarrhythmic therapy, have untoward side effects, or who do not want to take the medications on a long-term basis.

Complications have been reported depending on the type of ablation and the experience of the operator. Major complications include pericardial effusion, transient ischemic attack, and cardiac tamponade (Stabile, et al., 2003). Other complications that the nurse should monitor for after the procedure are hemorrhage, thromboembolism, hematoma formation, phlebitis, infection, and phrenic nerve paralysis that may decrease the expansion of the lung (Fuster, et al., 2004).

BASIC LIFE SUPPORT

All health care providers should be well trained and knowledgeable about the steps of basic life support (BLS). Advanced technology and medications are futile in the event of cardiopulmonary arrest without efficient, effective CPR. Cardiopulmonary arrest can occur in any setting, but it is extremely common in hospital settings. Nurses, health care providers, respiratory therapists, nursing technicians, pharmacists, and other ancillary staff should all be able to perform CPR in the event of an arrest. Nurses and health care providers should also be trained in ACLS to be able to facilitate successful outcomes of patients using a combination of medications, procedures, and basic CPR.

CPR is the process of artificially supporting a patient's breathing and heartbeat when respirations and pulse have ceased. Once a patient becomes apneic, there is a time period of approximately four to six minutes before the brain becomes severely anoxic. Artificially breathing for the patient helps the person maintain a limited supply of oxygen until the patient can receive more advanced life-support measures, in particular, defibrillation. Cardiac arrest victims are twice as likely as those victims who do not receive CPR to survive cardiac arrest if given CPR by bystanders. (Figure 26-15). Artificial respirations can be performed for the patient using mouth-to-mouth resuscitation, mouth-to-mask, mouth-to-nose, or mouth-to-stoma. In the health care setting, bag-mask ventilation may be performed by providers who have received specialized training. Rescue breathing is performed only after the airway has been opened by the head tilt-chin lift or jaw-thrust maneuver. The jaw-thrust maneuver is used for patients with suspected trauma including head and spinal cord injuries (AHA, 2006a).

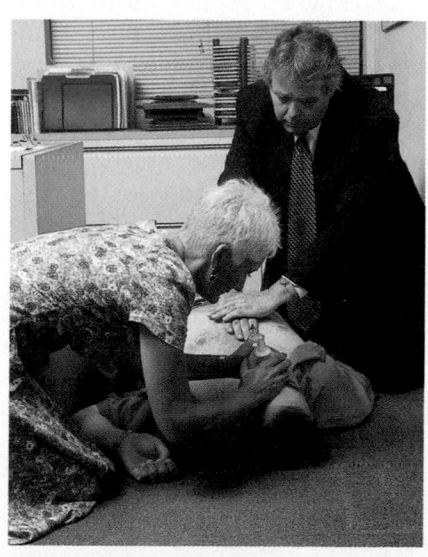

Figure 26-15 Early CPR by bystanders increases the survival rate of patients with a cardiac arrest.

External compressions are performed when the patient is pulseless. External compressions are performed to simulate contraction of the heart. The hands of the rescuer perform rhythmic compressions over the lower half of the sternum to press on the heart and create cardiac output. Even when compressions are performed correctly and at a rate of 100 times per minute, cardiac output is much lower than normal. Therefore, CPR should be viewed as a bridge to support a patient until health care providers trained in advanced life support techniques can provide more advanced strategies to facilitate patient survival. Health care personnel should receive initial training and become certified in CPR upon employment and receive appropriate updates and training at least every two years.

Steps in Basic Adult CPR

When the nurse discovers a patient who is suspected to have suffered a cardiopulmonary arrest, the first step is to always determine patient responsiveness. Gently shaking or tapping the patient and shouting "Are you okay?" will help to determine responsiveness (AHA, 2006a). This action should be enough to awaken the patient who has just fallen asleep. If the patient does not respond, the nurse should get help with the patient immediately. This may require yelling for other staff, dialing the emergency hospital line, or activating an emergency button. Once help is on the way, the nurse should roll the patient to his back and detect for absence of breathing. The nurse should open the airway by the head tilt-chin lift method and listen and feel for the presence of breathing. The nurse should also watch for rising and falling of the chest. In the absence of detectable breathing, the nurse should give two slow rescue breaths.

The nurse should perform rescue breathing by pinching the patient's nose and placing his or her mouth around the patient's mouth and blowing. Ideally, a barrier device or facemask should be used by the nurse when delivering rescue breathing. Face shields are clear silicon or plastic sheets that are placed over the patient's mouth and act as barriers between the nurse and patient's mouth (AHA, 2006a). There is an opening in the middle of the shield that allows air to flow into the patient. A facemask can be used to perform rescue breathing if available. A facemask is a hard plastic device that fits directly over the patient's mouth and nose with an opening to blow air into the patient's airway. The delivery of air into the patient's airway may also be accomplished by attaching the mask to an Ambu bag that is attached to an oxygen source. Aside from intubation and mechanical ventilation, bag-mask ventilation would be the preferred method in the hospital setting. This method requires training and practice to ventilate the patient effectively. Any time a facemask is used to ventilate the patient, the nurse should ensure a tight seal around the patient's mouth and nose. When performing rescue breathing, the nurse should observe for the chest to rise each time a breath is delivered and deliver each breath in one second.

Once two rescue breaths have been delivered, the nurse should assess the patient for signs of circulation. Signs of circulation may include breathing in response to the rescue breaths, movement, coughing, or the presence of a pulse (AHA, 2006a). If the nurse detects no signs of circulation, external chest compressions should be performed. Chest compressions are performed by placing the heel of one hand at the center of the chest between the nipples. Next, the nurse should place his or her other hand over the first. The nurse should be able to see the patient's chest while performing compressions. To be effective compressions should depress the sternum 1.5 to 2 inches on an adult. And, recently, the emphasis has been placed on push hard, push fast (e.g., delivering a faster rate of compressions as compared to a few years ago) to ensure enough oxygen delivery to the cells. Once other health care providers are present, pulse checks may be performed by palpating the femoral or carotid pulse to determine effectiveness of compressions. When available a backboard should be under the patient available to facilitate compression effectiveness. The nurse should perform compressions while positioned on the patient's side on his or her knees. Thirty compressions should be performed at a rate of 100 per minute. Once the first 30 compressions have been delivered, the patient should receive two ventilations at a rate of approximately 10 to 12 breaths per minute in the adult (12 to 20 breaths per minute in the infant and child). The cycle of 2 breaths and 30 compressions should continue without any interruptions that last longer than 10 seconds.

Airway Obstruction

If the health care provider is unable to provide effective ventilations, the patient may be suffering from an airway obstruction. The most common cause of airway obstruction in an unconscious victim is the tongue that falls back and blocks the airway. Any time the health care provider has difficulty providing effective ventilations, the patient's head should be repositioned and airway reopened to prevent obstruction by the tongue. Once repositioning has been performed, and if effective ventilations cannot be delivered, the nurse must suspect an airway obstruction because of a foreign substance. If the patient is already unconscious, the nurse must perform abdominal thrusts (also known as the Heimlich maneuver). This maneuver is performed by delivering five abdominal thrusts with the hands located just above the umbilicus (AHA, 2006a). Once these abdominal thrusts have been performed, the nurse should then attempt rescue breathing. The patient's head should be repositioned if the breath is ineffective on the first attempt. The nurse should continue abdominal thrusts and attempt ventilations until the obstruction is removed.

Nurses should also be able to perform the abdominal thrusts on conscious victims. Patients at risk for choking include those who have had a CVA or have altered mental status from medications or disease processes. Patients who attempt to eat without elevation of the head of the bed in hospitals are also at risk for choking. The nurse must be able to recognize signs of severe airway obstruction in the conscious patient. These signs include the inability to speak, poor cough effort, stridor during inhalation, or cyanosis. The patient will appear severely distressed and may grab his or her throat. Once the patient is choking, the nurse should stand behind the patient and place the fist above the umbilicus and grab the fist with the other hand. Abdominal thrusts should be administered until the obstruction is relieved, or the patient becomes unconscious (AHA, 2006a).

Automatic External Defibrillators

An automatic external defibrillator (AED) is a computerized defibrillator that analyzes heart rhythms and tells the operator when to perform defibrillation. AEDs have become commonplace in general public arenas and are available for use in large-volume areas, such as airports, amusement parks, and shopping malls. Public access defibrillation was designed to provide early defibrillation to victims of cardiac arrest. While AEDs are not typically used in the hospital setting, nurses should be trained on their use to operate one should the occasion arise (AHA, 2006a).

Once a victim is identified as being unresponsive, breathless, and pulseless, the AED should be activated. The electrodes should be attached to the monitor and placed on the patient's chest. These electrodes should be placed in the same position as those used with a regular defibrillator. The AED will analyze the rhythm once the electrodes are in place. During the time the monitor is analyzing the rhythm, the patient should not be touched so as not to induce artifact on the monitor. CPR should be stopped during this time. The computerized voice will announce when the rhythm is being analyzed as well as when it is being flashed on the screen.

Once it is determined that a shock is necessary, the computerized voice will announce that a shock is advised. The AED will start to charge to the appropriate energy level. Once a shock is advised, the operator of the AED should ensure that there are no individuals touching the patient by shouting "all clear" loudly. Once everyone is clear, the operator should push the shock button to deliver the current. Once the shock is delivered, the monitor will analyze the rhythm again. The analyze shock sequence will continue as determined by the manufacturer (AHA, 2006a).

If the AED does not recognize a shockable rhythm, it will inform the care provider that electrical shock is not advised. In this instance, the operator should check for a patient's pulse and if none present, should begin rescue breathing and external chest compressions. If the patient has a pulse but is not breathing, rescue breathing should be performed at a rate of 12 to 20 breaths per minute for the adult and 8 to 10 breaths per minute for the infant and child (AHA, 2006a) (Box 26-5).

ADVANCED CARDIAC LIFE SUPPORT

Advanced cardiac life support (ACLS) incorporates advanced lifesaving techniques, medications, and interventions in addition to BLS during a cardiopulmonary arrest. Prior the development of ACLS, a cardiopulmonary arrest in the hospital setting was a chaotic situation (AHA, 2006a). ACLS was developed to facilitate an orderly, systematic way of treating the patient in a cardiopulmonary arrest. As more hospital personnel such as nurses, physicians, respiratory therapists, and such become familiar with the algorithms associated with ACLS, the more coordinated the effort becomes to resuscitate the patient. When nurses become certified in ACLS, they are more able to anticipate medications and interventions that will be required in each patient scenario. Cardiopulmonary arrest situations can be extremely stressful for health care providers as patient's lives are at stake. When the nurse takes an ACLS course, cardiopulmonary arrest situations and their corresponding interventions are reviewed and practiced. This gives the nurse more confidence when encountering the real life-threatening situations in hospitalized patients.

Primary Survey

The basis for ACLS starts with the primary and secondary surveys. The primary survey is recalled by the letters A, B, C, and D. Recalling A reminds the health care provider to assess and manage the airway with noninvasive techniques (AHA, 2006a). B stands for assessing and managing breathing by using positive pressure ventilations. C is a reminder to assess and manage circulation by performing CPR until a defibrillator arrives on the scene. D reminds the health care provider to assess and manage any defibrillation needs by assessing the cardiac rhythm and defibrillating ventricular fibrillation or ventricular tachycardia without a pulse.

Secondary Survey

Conducting the secondary survey should include advanced and invasive techniques with the goal of resuscitation, stabilization, and transfer of care to the next highest level. The letters A, B, C, and D are also used to remind the health care provider of the appropriate priorities in managing care. Advanced airway devices, such as endotracheal intubation or emergent tracheostomy, may need to be performed to manage a compromised airway.

Assessing breathing may be done, in part, by assessing the placement of the artificial airway. This may be done by auscultation of breath sounds and measurement of carbon dioxide on exhalation. Once the appropriate placement of the artificial airway has been determined, the airway should be promptly secured. Adequacy of breathing may be assessed by measuring oxygen saturation and observing the rise and fall of the chest.

Circulation may be assessed and managed by a number of methods. Cardiac arrhythmias should be interpreted and treated. Circulation may be restored by defibrillation, cardioversion, and transcutaneous pacing. IV lines should be started to deliver emergency medications. Medications to terminate arrhythmias should be administered once an IV line has been established. Medications to support or treat blood pressure should be instituted.

The letter D in the secondary survey stands for differential diagnosis (AHA, 2006a). This means that the provider should identify and treat reversible causes of the patient's cardiopulmonary arrest.

VENTRICULAR FIBRILLATION/PULSELESS VENTRICULAR TACHYCARDIA

The ventricular fibrillation/pulseless ventricular tachycardia algorithm is the most important for health care providers to learn because most individuals who go into cardiopulmonary arrest are in ventricular fibrillation. The primary survey in this algorithm includes the same basic steps as any cardiopulmonary arrest. The patient should be assessed for responsiveness, and a defibrillator should be requested. The airway should be opened, and rescue breathing should be instituted. External chest compressions should be started while waiting for the defibrillator.

Once the defibrillator has arrived, the patient should be attached to the defibrillator pads, and the rhythm should be assessed. Once it has been determined that the patient is in ventricular fibrillation or pulseless ventricular tachycardia, the defibrillator should be charged to 200 joules. Once the initial shock is delivered, the patient should be assessed for continuation of the arrhythmia. Previously, three shocks in succession were delivered, but research has shown that there was too much delay in treatment, and in 2005, the AHA changed to delivering one shock and immediately following with the next stage of intervention (e.g., CPR and medications). As for the shock energies, a monophasic defibrillator requires all shocks to be 360 joules if the rhythm has not been terminated. A biphasic defibrillator is set at 200 joules in the first delivery and an equal or higher dose in subsequent deliveries (AHA, 2006a).

If the patient continues to be in ventricular fibrillation, the health care provider proceeds to the secondary survey. The patient should intubated with an endotracheal tube and have its placement confirmed. Effective oxygenation should also be confirmed. CPR should be continued, and the patient should have an IV line started. Epinephrine 1 mg IV push or 40 units of vasopressin should be given initially. The epinephrine dose may be given in 3- to 5-minute intervals while the vasopressin should be given once only. The patient should have a repeated defibrillation attempt within 30 to 60 seconds. The ventricular fibrillation/pulseless ventricular tachycardia algorithm then continues with CPR, medications, and repeated attempts to defibrillate at 360 joules. Other medications that may be considered are amiodarone, lidocaine, or magnesium if the patient is known to have low magnesium, or procainamide (Broyles, et al., 2007).

BRADYCARDIA ALGORITHM

The bradycardia algorithm emphasizes the importance of treating only the symptomatic bradycardias. Determining whether the patient needs treatment requires the nurse to combine the monitor and the patient assessment. This is ideal under every circumstance for arrhythmia management. Signs and symptoms that may be accompanied by a bradycardia include chest pain and shortness of breath, hypotension, altered level of consciousness, weakness and fatigue, diaphoresis, and nausea (Cummins, 2003). The primary survey should include assessment of the A, B, and C, and attachment of a monitor to determine the patient's rhythm. A patient in a bradycardia should never be defibrillated.

The secondary survey should include ensuring adequate oxygenation and establishing an IV line to give emergent medications or IV fluids (Cummins, 2003). A 12-lead ECG should be obtained while monitoring vital signs frequently. The cause for the bradycardia should be contemplated while treating the arrhythmia. If the patient has a new onset of bradycardia but is not experiencing signs and symptoms, the patient should be initially ECG monitored. If the patient is experiencing serious signs and symptoms, the patient's bradycardia should be promptly treated. Initially, atropine should be administered 0.5 to 1 mg IV push. Transcutaneous pacing, dopamine, epinephrine, and isoproterenol should all be considered as potential treatments for symptomatic bradycardia. If the patient's rhythm is type II second-degree or third-degree AV block, the nurse should prepare the patient for transcutaneous pacing with eventual transvenous pacing.

UNSTABLE AND STABLE TACHYCARDIA

There is also an algorithm is prepared to assist the health care provider in identifying patients at risk with unstable tachycardias. The patient who is unstable will exhibit signs and symptoms including shortness of breath, chest pain, altered level of consciousness, hypotension, pulmonary edema, and ischemia. Patients who present with an unstable tachycardia especially with a ventricular rate of more than 150 beats per minute will require synchronized cardioversion. The patient should have supplemental oxygen and an IV line on cardioversion. Emergency intubation equipment should also be at the bedside. The patient should be premedicated with a benzodiazepine or narcotic when ever possible.

Stable tachycardia refers to a heart rate of greater than 100 beats per minute that causes no major hemodynamic changes in the patient (Cummins, 2003). The rhythm is caused by an electrical disturbance in the heart and can include atrial fibrillation or flutter, other supraventricular tachycardias, or stable wide QRS complex tachycardias (ventricular or supraventricular in origin). If the tachycardia is determined to be ventricular in origin, then the ventricular tachycardia algorithm should be followed. When the patient has a stable tachycardia there is a little more time to try to diagnose the cause of the problem as long as the patient's airway, breathing, and circulation are addressed. A 12-lead ECG may be obtained along with appropriate lab studies and history. Vagal maneuvers may be attempted to slow the heart rate down. Carotid massage may be performed by the health care provider to slow the heart rate. The patient may be asked to cough or "bear down" to illicit a vagal response. Adenosine may be given to stop the heart to allow the SA node to take over pacemaker capabilities. If the patient is in atrial fibrillation or atrial flutter with a rapid ventricular response, a calcium channel blocker or beta blocker may be given to control the rate. In some patients, anticoagulation and synchronized cardioversion may be appropriate treatment for atrial fibrillation and flutter.

Nurses should seek out opportunities to learn more about arrhythmia recognition and treatment. This specialized knowledge is especially helpful in cardiopulmonary arrest situations. With certification in ACLS, the nurse can anticipate and participate in the treatments required at the time of arrest.

KEY CONCEPTS

- The conduction system in the heart is made up of specialized cells that generate and transmit electrical impulses.
- Depolarization and repolarization followed by the mechanical contraction and relaxation of the cardiac muscle constitute one complete cardiac cycle.
- Patients may require continuous cardiac monitoring while in the acute care setting.
- Arrhythmias are a common occurrence and vary from causing no symptoms to being life-threatening.
- Normal sinus rhythm has a rate of 60 to 100 beats per minute with a regular rhythm.
- Ventricular arrhythmias can be detected by changes in the QRS complexes and are the most serious of the arrhythmias.
- Benefits of using anti-arrhythmic medications should outweigh the risk for the patient to be started on medication.
- Defibrillation depolarizes the heart so that there is a short period of asystole in an effort to stop the arrhythmia and allow the heart to resume normal activity.

- Synchronized cardioversion is the delivery of energy to the heart synchronized on the patient's R wave.
- CPR is the process of artificially supporting a patient's breathing and heartbeat when respirations and pulse have ceased.
- An automatic external defibrillator analyzes heart rhythms and tells the operator when to perform defibrillation.
- ACLS incorporates advanced lifesaving techniques, medications, and interventions in addition to BLS during a cardiopulmonary arrest.
- Ventricular fibrillation and pulseless ventricular tachycardia should be treated with immediate defibrillation.
- The bradycardia algorithm emphasizes the importance of treating only the symptomatic bradycardias.
- There is also an algorithm is prepared to assist the health care provider in identifying patients at risk with unstable tachycardias

REVIEW QUESTIONS

1. During an analysis of an ECG strip, the critical care nurse assesses heart rate. If the rhythm is irregular, which is the best way to calculate heart rate per minute from a rhythm strip?
   1. Count the number of tiny boxes between two R waves and divide by 1,500
   2. Count the number of QRS complexes in a three-second strip and multiply by 25
   3. Count the number of QRS complexes in a six-second strip and multiply by 10
   4. Count the number of large boxes between two R waves and divide by 300.

2. Phase zero (depolarization) of the action potential begins when _____ ions move into the cardiac cell.
   1. Sodium
   2. Potassium
   3. Magnesium
   4. Chloride

3. The nurse responds to a telemetry alarm that shows a patient to be asystole. What should be his or her first action?
   1. Defibrillate
   2. Initiate cardiac pacing

   3. Begin CPR
   4. Establish unresponsiveness

4. A 50-year-old male patient displays a supraventricular tachycardia with a heart rate of 180 beats per minute. He complains of dizziness, nausea, and chest pain. The patient's blood pressure is 90/60. The nurse knows that the most appropriate intervention for this patient is to:
   1. Defibrillate
   2. Administer an angiotensin-converting enzyme (ACE) inhibitor
   3. Start a dopamine drip
   4. Ask the patient to cough

5. Your patient suddenly becomes unresponsive and pulseless and displays this rhythm on the monitor. The best initial intervention by the nurse is:
   1. CPR
   2. Defibrillation
   3. Amiodarone
   4. Transvenous pacing

Continued

6. A patient is exhibiting the following rhythm with a blood pressure of 100/58. He denies chest pain or dyspnea at this time. The most appropriate intervention at this time is:
   1. Transcutaneous pacing
   2. Atropine
   3. Isuprel
   4. To continue to monitor the patient

7. Treatment for ventricular tachycardia with a pulse could include these interventions (select all that apply):
   1. Defibrillation
   2. Amiodarone
   3. Vasopressin
   4. Synchronized cardioversion
   5. Lidocaine hydrochloride
   6. Epinephrine

8. The most appropriate treatment for ventricular fibrillation after defibrillation attempts is:
   1. Three more defibrillation attempts
   2. Epinephrine
   3. Atropine
   4. Synchronized cardioversion

9. Ventricular arrhythmias will be interpreted on the rhythm strip by primarily analyzing the:
   1. T wave
   2. P wave
   3. PR interval
   4. QRS complex

10. Which of the following is true concerning the primary survey associated with ACLS?
    1. Advanced airway devices, such as endotracheal intubation or emergent tracheostomy, are used.
    2. IV lines should be started to deliver emergency medications.
    3. The letter D in the secondary survey stands for defibrillation.
    4. The health care provider assesses and manages breathing by using positive-pressure ventilations.

REVIEW ACTIVITIES

1. Identify where the crash cart and defibrillator are located in your acute care setting. Perform a defibrillator check according to the institution's protocol. Identify the steps to take when defibrillating a patient who is in ventricular fibrillation. Locate the IV supplies and emergency medications on the crash cart.

2. You are receiving report from the night shift nurse at 0700. Your patient is starting on postoperative day 1 following an open reduction internal fixation of the right hip. The patient is 65 years old. The nurse reports that the patient has been sleeping since 0500 his heart rate on the monitor has been increasing throughout that time. The nurse points out that his heart rate has gone from 90 beats per minute to 126 beats per minute. You correctly interpret the rhythm on the patient's monitor as sinus tachycardia. What are the possible causes for this change in the patient's heart rate? What is the treatment for the sinus tachycardia?

REVIEW ACTIVITIES—cont'd

3. Go to a telemetry or cardiac care unit in your clinical agency. Run a rhythm strip of a patient and analyze the rhythm strip. What are the steps to interpretation? Were you able to successfully interpret the rhythm strip?

4. Go to a telemetry or cardiac care unit in your clinical agency. Run off at least three rhythm strips with patterns of activity that you recognize as arrhythmias. Identify the atrial and ventricular responses on the strips and label them on each strip.

5. In general, are atrial or ventricular arrhythmias more of a concern for a patient? Why?

Vascular Dysfunction: Nursing Management

Mary J. Yoho, PhD, RN

CHAPTER

27

KEY TERMS

Aneurysm
Anticoagulant
Aphonia
Arteriosclerosis
Atherosclerosis
Bruit
Buerger's disease
Debridement
Homans' sign
Hyperlipidemia
Raynaud's disease
Subclavian steal syndrome
Thrombophlebitis
Varicose veins
Venous stasis ulcer

CHAPTER TOPICS

- Atherosclerosis
- Peripheral Arterial Occlusive Disease
- Aneurysms
- Thrombophlebitis
- Buerger's Disease
- Subclavian Steal Syndrome
- Raynaud's Disease
- Varicose Veins
- Venous Stasis Ulcers

Diseases related to vascular dysfunction lead the causes of death in the United States, with 1 of every 2.6 deaths attributed to heart and blood vessels ailments (American Heart Association [AHA], 2004a). Common diseases include arteriosclerosis, atherosclerosis, peripheral vascular disease, and aortic aneurysms. According to the AHA, one in five people have some form of vascular disease. With the aging population of 65 and over reaching 40 million by 2010, the assumption can be made that the incidence of vascular disease will be on a continual rise.

ARTERIOSCLEROSIS AND ATHEROSCLEROSIS

Arteriosclerosis is also known as hardening of the arteries and is defined as a thickening and solidifying of the endothelial lining of the walls in small arteries and arterioles. **Atherosclerosis** is the development of plaques in the intimal layer of larger arteries, eventually developing blockage of the vessel lumen (Figure 27-1).

Epidemiology

Nearly one million people in the United States annually die of heart and blood vessel disease (National Heart, Lung, and Blood Institute, 2004a). Atherosclerosis usually affects people who are age 60 or older, because it accompanies the process of aging. Symptoms usually do not occur until at least 60 percent of the vessel lumen is occluded. Atherosclerosis has a common relationship with cardiovascular disease and cerebrovascular disease, indicating that people with atherosclerosis are more at risk for developing one or both of the associated diseases.

Etiology

There are numerous risk factors associated with the long-term development of arteriosclerosis and atherosclerosis, which are direct precursors of cardiovascular disease (CVD). Nonmodifiable risk factors include age, gender, and ethnicity. Women experience their first major incident 10 years later than men (AHA, 2004), though African American and Mexican American women have a higher incidence of CVD than Caucasian women of similar socioeconomic status.

Modifiable risk factors include hypertension, high cholesterol, physical inactivity, obesity, stress, and diabetes mellitus. Tobacco use is toxic to the endothelium and has been directly related to initiating vascular disease (American Cancer Society, 2006b). Decreasing modifiable risk factors can indirectly modify genetic risk factors. In addition, lifestyle risk factors can be positively correlated with the modifiable and almost all of the risk factors.

Pathophysiology

Arteriosclerosis and atherosclerosis occur as an accrual of lipids, calcium, blood, carbohydrates, and fibrous tissue located on the vessel intimal layer. The buildup of these products leads to the development of plaques, which causes narrowing of the vessel lumen, also known as vessel stenosis. As the lumen of the vessel constricts, complete obstruction may occur by formation of thrombosis, development of an aneurysm, or actual rupture of the vessel wall.

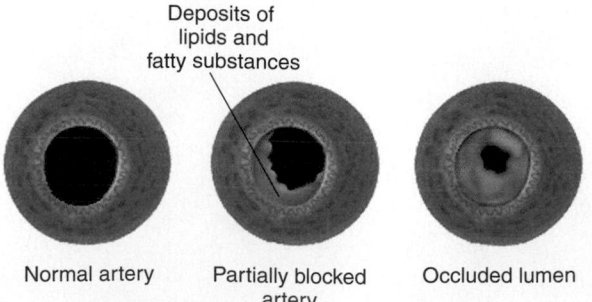

Deposits of lipids and fatty substances

Normal artery   Partially blocked artery   Occluded lumen

Figure 27-1 Progression of atherosclerosis.

Multiple theories have been developed to describe the development of arteriosclerosis and atherosclerosis. The reaction-to-injury, lipid hypothesis, and platelet aggregation theories are most generally accepted. According to the reaction-to injury theory, endothelial cells sustain injury due to prolonged hemodynamic forces such as shearing stress, chemical exposure, irradiation, and chronic hyperlipidemia. Lipid hypothesis relates to the accumulation of lipids after an intimal injury, which occludes blood flow. The platelet aggregation theory is the formation of a platelet cluster after an intimal tear, which produces a peptide that stimulates the proliferation of the smooth muscle cells in the intima. The general belief is that not one single mechanism is responsible, but multiple forms of the disease progression occur. Ultimately, these vascular lesions are composed of either fatty streaks or fibrous plaques.

Fatty streaks project into the vessel lumen, are smooth, found in people of all ages, and do not cause clinical symptoms. In contrast, fibrous plaques project into the vessel wall and often occlude the lumen. This irreversible plaque causes symptoms of decreased blood flow in the coronary arteries, as well as carotid and popliteal arteries, the bifurcations of the abdominal aorta, the common iliac arteries, and smaller arterial branches.

Genetics

Because aging is a risk factor in acquiring atherosclerosis, the prediction is that more people will notice it while experience symptoms of vascular insufficiency. Clinical trials continue examining the effectiveness of gene therapy in the treatment of vascular disease, and the use of vascular endothelial growth factor (VEGF) to stimulate new vessel growth. VEGF will be most useful in patients with end-stage peripheral disease, enhancing circulation and thereby reducing pain and increasing exercise tolerance.

Assessment with Clinical Manifestations

Hypertension and heart disease are often identified in people who develop arteriosclerosis and atherosclerosis within the arterial system (Figure 27-2). Vital sign assessment should include bilateral blood pressure readings and the assessment of both apical and radial pulses.

Further assessment includes the palpation of pulses at the femoral, popliteal, and pedal pulse sites. Prolonged capillary filling signifies poor blood flow to areas distal to the pulse and is identified as abnormal when the capillary refill is greater than three seconds. Capillary refill in the elderly has a different norm of greater than five seconds being significant. Temperature differences of extremities should be noted, in which cool or cold extremities often relate to inadequate circulation. Carotid pulses should also be assessed for the presence and quality of pulses and **bruits** (an adventitious sound of venous or arterial origin heard after auscultation or continuous wave Doppler).

Diagnostic Tests

Screening for elevated serum cholesterol levels should be routine for all patients with arteriosclerosis and atherosclerosis. Current criteria are established by the AHA (2004), and the recommendations are identified in Table 27-1. Homocystine, a sulfur-based amino acid, is often monitored to evaluate the patient's risk for the development of coronary artery and peripheral disease. A level greater than 15 μmol/L indicates a greater risk for the development of coronary artery disease (CAD) and peripheral disease. Coagulation studies are routinely performed for those taking **anticoagulant** medications (pharmaceuticals that prevent further clot formation in the body), as described later in this chapter.

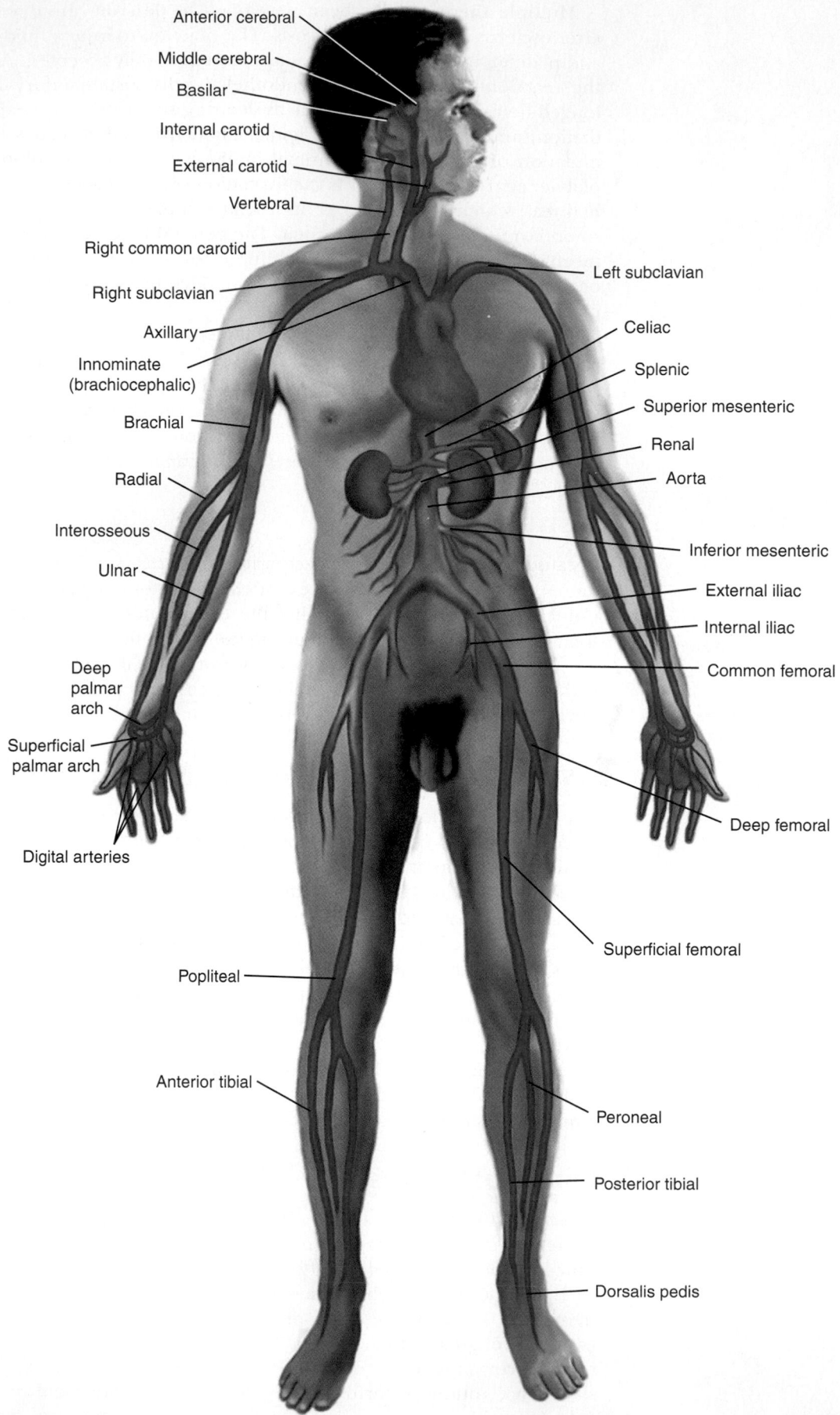

Figure 27-2 Arterial system anatomy.

TABLE 27-1	Laboratory Tests: Recommended Cholesterol Screening Levels for Patients with Arteriosclerosis and Atherosclerosis
CHOLESTEROL SCREENING LAB	**RECOMMENDED LEVEL**
Serum cholesterol	Less than or equal to 200 mg/dL
LDL	Less than or equal to 100 mg/dL
HDL	Less than or equal to 35 mg/dL
Triglycerides	Less than or equal to 200 mg/dL

Source: Daniels, R. (2003). Delmar's manual of laboratory and diagnostic tests. *New York: Thomson Delmar Learning.*

After the initial diagnosis is established, arteriography and magnetic resonance angiography may be utilized to evaluate the extent of disease and to support recommended interventions (Daniels, 2003). Medical and surgical recommendations are often derived from the results of radiographic diagnostic testing.

Nursing Diagnoses

Based on the information gathered, examples of nursing diagnoses in the patient with atherosclerosis may be found in Box 27-1.

Planning and Implementation

Arteriosclerosis and atherosclerosis are long-term chronic disease processes that are often not recognized until clinical manifestations occur. Conservative therapy is initiated, with invasive and surgical interventions reserved as treatment for the more severe symptomatic disease processes.

Goals

The goals for patients with arteriosclerosis and atherosclerosis are disease prevention and controlling the advancement of the disease process. Risk factor management in patients with arteriosclerosis and atherosclerosis involves therapy centered around nutrition and diet, smoking cessation, exercise, and pharmaceutical support.

Evidenced-Based Care

Risk factor management in patients with arteriosclerosis and atherosclerosis involves therapeutic changes in nutritional management and diet, smoking cessation, and pharmaceutical support. Exercise prescriptions are also agreed upon, which helps to decrease blood viscosity and improves muscle oxidative capacity (Zepf, 2003). Multiple studies have been conducted to support the effectiveness of implementing these strategies to control and prevent peripheral vascular disease. Nurses have provided research, which focuses on how to employ these strategies and keep patients actively involved in their own personal well-being. Integrating education and positive reinforcement are known to be a dynamic combination in assisting patients to achieve their goal of achieving lower lipid and cholesterol levels.

Nutrition

Cholesterol is located in animal sources, such as meat and eggs, and is the main contributor to **hyperlipidemia,** which is defined as elevated blood cholesterol levels. Diets limited to 30 percent or less in saturated fat content are

BOX 27-1

NURSING DIAGNOSES

- Ineffective peripheral tissue perfusion related to impaired circulation.
- Pain related to decreased oxygen supply to tissues.
- Risk for impaired skin integrity related to compromised tissue perfusion.
- Fear and anxiety related to actual or potential lifestyle changes.
- Knowledge deficit related to self-care and risk prevention.

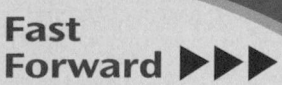

recommended by the National Cholesterol Education Program (2004), with suggested daily cholesterol intake to be less than 300 mg/day.

Patient education begins with the awareness of the amount of saturated fat and cholesterol consumed daily. A more structured meal plan may be needed to attain the objective of decreasing saturated fat and cholesterol, and if needed, achieve weight loss. The nurse educates the patient on the nutrients that various foods contain and collaborates with the dietitian for diet restrictions and daily nutritional interventions. Often family instruction is needed if the patient purchases his or her own food or prepares his or her own meals. A low-fat, low-cholesterol diet can greatly improve the patient's cholesterol, low-density lipoprotein (LDL), high-density lipoprotein (HDL), and triglyceride levels.

Pharmacology

Hyperlipidemia is an increase of lipids in the blood, and is a risk factor for the development of peripheral vascular disease. Treatment of hyperlipidemia includes the implementation of diet therapy, exercise, and agents that lower lipid levels to decrease the serum levels of cholesterol and lipids. The triglyceride level may be the factor that determines the drug chosen for therapy, and medications are sometimes given in combination with another drug that lowers lipids.

Drug types include bile acid sequestrants, hydroxymethylglutaryl-coenzyme A (HMG-CoA) inhibitors, fibrates, and nicotinic acid. Bile acid sequestrants bind with bile acids, which contain large levels of cholesterol, and lead to excretion in the feces. HMG-CoA inhibitors block the enzyme HMG-CoA reductase, which is the final step in the synthesis of cellular cholesterol. Fibrates, derivatives of fibric acid, stimulate the breakdown of lipoproteins and nicotinic acid, lower LDL and cholesterol levels, and increase HDL levels. Patients who incorporate drug therapy, exercise, and dietary restrictions but who do not achieve desirable LDL and cholesterol levels, may be placed on more than one agent that lowers lipids. Caution is used when combining agents, as severe side effects are more likely to occur than when using only one medication for lipid and cholesterol control.

Other pharmaceutical agents may be utilized to decrease the symptoms and increase the quality of life. These include medications to supply more blood to the muscles by reducing blood viscosity and increase vasodilation (Broyles, Reiss, & Evans, 2007). See Table 27-2 for pharmaceutical therapies that assist in the management of arteriosclerosis and atherosclerosis.

Health Care Resources

The disease processes associated with atherosclerosis are extremely expensive because of the tremendous implications on the health care system. Patients are not able to afford all of the treatment modalities that are available. In addition,

---

TABLE 27-2   Pharmacology Facts: Pharmaceutical Therapy for Management of Arteriosclerosis and Atherosclerosis

CLASSIFICATIONS	DRUGS	INDICATIONS
LMWH	Enoxaparin (Lovenox) Ardeparin (Normiflo) Dalteparin (Fragmin) Danaparoid (Orgaran)	Prevention of vascular claudication and DVT
Xanthines	Pentoxifylline (Trental)	Increases erythrocyte mobility and thereby reduces blood viscosity
Antiplatelet aggregating agents	Aspirin Clopidogrel (Plavix) Ticlopidine (Ticlid)	Inhibit platelet adhesion and aggregation, thereby preventing the formation of blood clots

Source: Broyles, B., Reiss, B., & Evans, M. (2007). Pharmacological aspects of nursing care (3rd ed.). New York: Thomson Delmar Learning.

DOLLARS AND SENSE

Controlling the Costs of CVD

The AHA (2004) estimates the direct and indirect costs relating to cardiovascular diseases at $368.4 billion. The direct costs include health care provider fees, hospital and long-term care, home health, durable medical equipment, and pharmaceuticals. Indirect costs relate to the patient's inability to work and include loss of productivity of both the patient and family members.

Nursing case management and the implementation of critical pathways have been proven to assist in controlling costs by managing the patient's plan of care while in the hospital. A wide variety of health care providers, including nursing, pharmacy, laboratory, radiology, physical and occupational therapists take part in the plan to provide the highest quality of care while implementing cost-reducing strategies. This strategy also assists in decreasing the length of hospital stay and evaluating the use of home care support.

Controlling risk factors is the most cost-effective method of managing diseases, which cause vascular dysfunction. Patients must not only be managed medically but also monetarily assessed to prevent noncompliance because of financial barriers. Medications, diet, treatments, and therapies can be cost-prohibitive for many patients on fixed incomes, and the nurse must collaborate with social services to obtain resources. Both federal and local resources may be available to assist in meeting the patient's financial needs and providing support to the patient.

third-party payment continues to increase its costs for the care that is provided for patients with atherosclerotic-related diseases. A continued controversy exists regarding the forms of management that should be expected as a patient's right to health care versus the reality of the expenses of the health care. Consequently, many patients do not have the financial capability of receiving all of the potential diagnostic tests or treatments for their disorders. The legal-ethical implications of the costs of care are complex and require continued problem solving within the health care delivery system. Controlling risk factors and emphasizing the prevention of CVD is also an important potential direction to pursue toward addressing the issues of cost containment in these patients (see Dollars and Sense feature).

Alternative Therapy

Alternative therapy may be included to assist patients in decreasing and ceasing their smoking and controlling their intake of fatty foods. These therapies include, but are not limited to hypnosis, acupuncture, biofeedback, and imagery. Gene therapy continues to be researched in the effort to validate its effectiveness in both identifying and preventing vascular plaques.

Patient and Family Teaching

Educating the patient and family members is a critical role of the nurse. Instruction is central to promoting vasodilatation and prevention of complications. Compliancy of diet therapy, smoking cessation, medication, and exercise regimens are crucial aspects in the prevention of atherosclerotic plaques. Multiple allied health personnel are often included in supporting the patient's care, including dietitians, cardiac rehabilitation staff, psychologists, pharmacists, and occupational therapists to assist with activities of daily living (ADL). Additional resources and Web sites related to patient education include the AHA, National Heart, Lung, and Blood Institute, Health Information Center, and the Vascular Disease Foundation. There are specific instructions that should be given to patients and their families to promote safety and quality of life as shown in Patient Playbook feature.

Cigarette smoking, as well as secondhand smoke, contributes to severe adversities. The nurse's role is to advise the patient to stop smoking and

Patient and Family Teaching Related to the Prevention of Atherosclerotic Plaques

The patient should be taught to:

- Avoid extreme cold, which promotes vasoconstriction.
- Avoid extreme heat, which places the patient at risk for injury.
- Not wear constrictive clothing, which impedes circulation.
- Position the extremity below the level of the heart to promote blood flow to extremities. Legs should not be crossed.

assess for the most effective way to provide support. Willingness to stop smoking and change behavior is a priority concern of the nurse's assessment. The nurse must provide education, as an example, and inform the patient that cigarette smoking lowers HDL levels and increases the risk for atherosclerosis, and the nurse must recommend strategies for overall improvement in their smoking cessation status (Daniels, 2004). Both oral and topical patch medications are available to assist the patient to stop smoking completely as shown in Table 27-3. In addition, nurses can refer patients to smoking cessation programs and encourage the patient regarding participating in these programs.

Exercise programs are recommended for prevention of vascular disease. The recommendation is 30 minutes of moderate exercise (e.g., walking, jogging, playing tennis, or biking) three to four times a week. Exercises can lead to a decrease in atherosclerotic plaques, an increase in collateral circulation, and assist in lowering lipid levels. It is recommended that patients are evaluated prior to initiating an exercise program with a physical examination and stress test.

Evaluation of Outcomes

Potential patient outcomes for each of the example nursing diagnoses for the patient with atherosclerosis are:

- Ineffective peripheral tissue perfusion related to impaired circulation. The patient should maintain optimal tissue perfusion to the periphery, as evidenced by strong peripheral pulses, good capillary refill, and good movement.
- Pain related to decreased oxygen supply to tissues. The patient should verbalize an adequate relief of pain along with the ability to realistically cope with the pain if it is not completely relieved.
- Risk for impaired skin integrity related to compromised tissue perfusion. The condition of the skin should be improved as evidenced by decreased redness, swelling, and pain.
- Fear and anxiety related to actual or potential lifestyle changes. The patient should be able to recognize the signs of anxiety, demonstrate positive coping mechanisms, and describe a reduction in the level of anxiety experienced.
- Knowledge deficit related to self-care and risk prevention. The patient should demonstrate motivation to learn, identify perceived learning needs, and verbalize an understanding of desired content.

TABLE 27-3 **Pharmacology Facts: Pharmaceutical Therapy for Smoking Cessation**

CLASSIFICATION	DRUGS	INDICATIONS
Transdermal nicotine	Habitrol Nicoderm Nicotrol Prostep	Provide nicotine without carcinogens in tobacco
Nicotine Polacrilex (gum)	Nicoderm	Provide nicotine without carcinogens in tobacco
Antidepressant	Bupropion (Zyban)	Nicotine-free nicotine withdrawal support

Source: Broyles, B., Reiss, B., & Evans, M. (2007). Pharmacological aspects of nursing care (3rd ed.). New York: Thomson Delmar Learning.

PERIPHERAL ARTERIAL OCCLUSIVE DISEASE

Though it may take years to develop, peripheral arterial occlusive disease can occur suddenly and severely. More common in lower extremities, the patient develops a decreased ability to ambulate certain distances due to arterial insufficiency. Ischemia of the distal extremities is demonstrated by persistent, increased pain, which is often worse at night and accompanied by cramping and fatigue. Nonmodifiable risk factors include age, gender (males are more at risk), and family history. Modifiable risk factors are considered a history of smoking, hypertension, hyperlipidemia, obesity, stress, and decreased activity. Peripheral artery occlusive disease is commonly seen in patients with diabetes mellitus.

Upper extremity arterial occlusive disease occurs less frequently and is most commonly due to a mass, trauma, or atherosclerosis. Arterial stenosis may be located at the base of the vertebral artery, producing symptoms similar to those identified in **subclavian steal syndrome,** which is further discussed in this chapter.

Epidemiology

Approximately 8 to 10 million people are treated annually for symptoms of chronic peripheral vascular disease. Men over the age of 50 and postmenopausal women are most frequently affected. Chronic and severe peripheral arterial occlusive disease can lead to disability and death.

Etiology

The age of onset and the severity are often determined by the number of risk factors. The threat of developing obstructive lesions also increases with advancing age and in patients with diabetes mellitus. Other risk factors include hypertension, hyperlipidemia, obesity, smoking, and familiar predisposition.

Pathophysiology

Embolus, often originating from the heart, is the most common cause of peripheral arterial occlusion. Intermittent claudication is a common characteristic, whereas plaques form on the arterial walls, trapping emboli, and causing blood flow to cease distally. Obstructions most often occur in the aorta below the renal arteries, and in the popliteal arteries.

Assessment with Clinical Manifestations

The affected extremity is frequently described by the six P's: pulseless, pain, pallor, paresthesia, paralysis, and poikilocythemia (Estes, 2006). Symptoms often occur unilaterally and lead to one extremity being diagnosed with peripheral arterial disease. Pain occurs both with activity and at rest and is decreased by placing the extremity in a dependent position, often hanging the legs over the bed or chair. Skin may be mottled, have evidence of ulcerations and muscle atrophy, and toes may turn black or gangrenous. The extremity may also exhibit numbness and feel colder to touch than the other extremity. Thickened nails and sparse hair also indicate decreased arterial circulation. Pulse assessment in lower extremities include the femoral, popliteal, pedal, and dorsalis pedis, all of which may be severely decreased or absent.

Diagnostic Tests

If pulses are not accessible by palpation, a stethoscope or Doppler (Figure 27-3) may be used to assess for blood flow. The ankle-brachial index (ABI) may also be incorporated to measure the ratio of the lower to the upper extremity blood

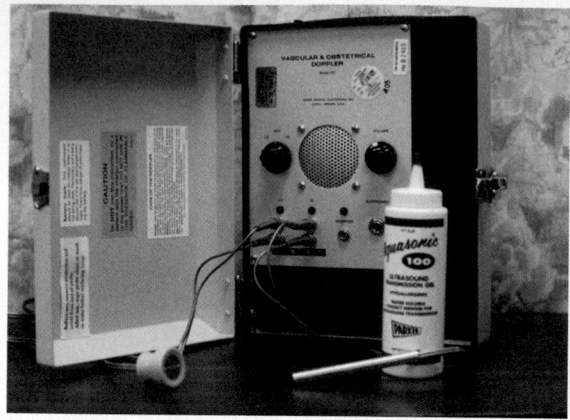

Figure 27-3 Doppler ultrasonography equipment.

pressure. Peripheral arterial occlusive disease is often classified by stages utilizing the Fontaine Staging System. Staging classifications are I through IV and identify the severity of the disease process. Patients may also undergo treadmill testing, ultrasound, or arterio-angiograms to identify the advancement and location of claudication.

Nursing Diagnoses

Based on the information gathered, examples of nursing diagnoses in the patient with peripheral arterial occlusive disease may include the following:

- Ineffective peripheral tissue perfusion related to impaired arterial circulation.
- Pain related to decreased oxygen supply to tissues.
- Risk for impaired skin integrity related to compromised tissue perfusion.
- Fear and anxiety related to actual or potential lifestyle changes.

Planning and Implementation

Though peripheral artery occlusive disease is a long-term chronic disease process, the claudication is extremely disabling. The general heath of the patient must be taken into consideration when deciding on a treatment plan. Palliative therapy may be considered if the patient cannot tolerate invasive or surgical intervention.

Goals

Risk factor management is the preventive goal, though peripheral arterial occlusions are often not identified until symptoms become consistent and intolerable. When an arterial clot is formed, restoration of circulation is the immediate goal.

Evidence-Based Care

Approximately 18 percent of patients diagnosed with peripheral arterial occlusive disease are over the age of 70 and have comorbid diseases including CAD, cerebrovascular disease, and carotid artery stenosis. In assessing the patients with symptoms related to arterial occlusions, the nurse should be aware that a history associated with symptoms of other related diseases needs to be reported to the health care provider. Utilizing the nursing process steps of

Skills 360°

Nurses Are Recognized for Their Honesty and Ethics

According to The Gallup Organization (2006) the annual survey on the honesty and ethical standards of various professions once again found the nursing profession at the top of the list. Nurses have been recognized in this number one position every year since 1999, except once, when they were first added to the poll. In 2001, after the September 11th terrorists attack, nurses came in second behind firefighters. By maintaining professional values and abiding by the American Nurse Association Code of Ethics (2001), nurses have been able to demonstrate a level of integrity unmatched by other professions.

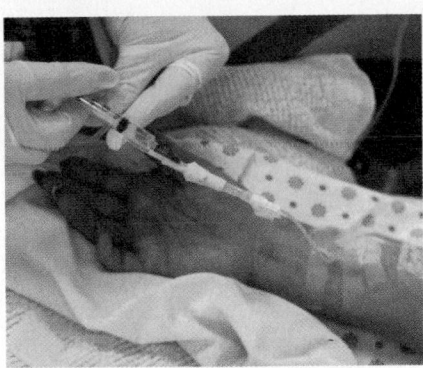

Figure 27-4 Administering a heparin bolus in patient with acute peripheral arterial occlusion.

assessment and analysis, can lead to accurate planning of care and early intervention for the patient who may be experiencing multiple disease-related health problems.

Pharmacology

In the treatment of acute peripheral arterial occlusion, intravenous (IV) anticoagulants are usually the first intervention. Heparin therapy is implemented to decrease the clot formation, and may be given in a bolus of up to 10,000 units (Figure 27-4). Patients are often placed on a heparin therapy protocol until the blood clot is dissolved. Discharge planning will include maintaining the patient on a low molecular weight heparin (LMWH) or an antiplatelet aggregating agent.

The use of thrombolytic drug therapy may also be recommended to dissolve an acute thrombus. These potent drugs are given in a monitored setting where the patient can be continuously evaluated for side effects, which include bleeding, hematoma at infusion site, and bruising. Hemoglobin, hematocrit, and platelet counts are frequently calculated to further assess and monitor for blood loss.

Health Care Resources

Pharmaceutical therapy, especially the utilization of thrombolytic therapy, is quite expensive. Hospital admission is required for patients who undergo IV anticoagulant or thrombolytic therapy. Invasive and surgical intervention may be indicated, and a nurse case manager often provides arrangements for home care postprocedure or postsurgery.

Surgery

Patients with severe symptoms related to the development of peripheral arterial occlusive disease may need to undergo either invasive or surgical procedures. Percutaneous transluminal angioplasty (PTA) is an invasive, nonsurgical procedure that is performed under radiology. Stenosed and occluded arteries are identified, which cause decreased circulation to the areas distal to the occlusion. A balloon catheter is advanced through the vessel to the diseased area and then inflated to decrease the level of occlusion and allow blood to pass though the vessel. Often a coil-like device, known as a stent, is guided by a catheter and placed over the previously occluded area to assist in maintaining patency of the vessel. A successful PTA and stent placement will prevent more invasive surgical procedures. Patients must be evaluated for this procedure, as many of these patients are not surgical candidates and this procedure is the only opportunity to provide relief extremity pain and loss of function. Bleeding at the catheter insertion site and reocclusion of the vessel are adverse reactions that may be experienced by some patients and must be monitored by the nurse.

For plaques, which are hard and do not respond to PTA, laser-assisted angioplasty and atherectomy are two other nonsurgical invasive techniques that may be utilized to attack firm, immovable arterial plaques. In laser-assisted therapy, a laser probe is advanced through the vessel to the side of the occlusion, and the heat emitted from the laser vaporizes the plaque and reopens the occluded artery. In atherectomy procedures, a mechanical rotation device, known as a Rotablator, scrapes the plaque for the vessel surface.

Surgical procedures are indicated for patients who have not responded to other forms of treatment, continue to have severe symptoms, and are at risk for limb amputation. An endarterectomy may be the procedure of choice, which involves making a surgical incision and removing the obstructing plaque. The artery is then sutured together, and blood is free to flow distally.

Bypass grafts are another surgical consideration to allow blood to flow around diseased vessels. Grafts can be either synthetic, man-made products, such as GorTex and Dacron, or autologous, utilizing a vein for another area of the patient. Both grafts require patency distal to where the graft will be surgically joined to the native vessel, known as the anastomosis site. Graft procedures are identified by the preanastomosis and postanastomosis vessels, for example axillo-femoral, aorto-iliac, aorto-femoral, and femoral-popliteal bypass procedures. Amputation of the extremity below the claudication must be considered if other interventions are not successful (Price, 2004).

Patient and Family Teaching

Discharge planning includes the control of modifiable risk factors, and encouraging lifestyle changes that support healthy living habits. Evaluation of the patient and family's knowledge of postoperative complications is essential. Physical and emotional support is often required to assist the patient with progression to independent ADL. The inclusion of home health nursing in the plan of care will provide essential support for both the patient and family during the postoperative period.

Evaluation of Outcomes

Potential patient outcomes for each of the example nursing diagnoses for the patient with peripheral arterial occlusive disease are:
- Ineffective peripheral tissue perfusion related to impaired arterial circulation. The patient should maintain optimal tissue perfusion to the periphery, as evidenced by strong peripheral pulses, good capillary refill, and good movement
- Pain related to decreased oxygen supply to tissues. The patient should verbalize an adequate relief of pain along with the ability to realistically cope with the pain if it is not completely relieved.
- Risk for impaired skin integrity related to compromised tissue perfusion. The condition of the skin should be improved as evidenced by decreased redness, swelling, and pain.
- Fear and anxiety related to actual or potential lifestyle changes. The patient should be able to recognize the signs of anxiety, demonstrate positive coping mechanisms, and describe a reduction in the level of anxiety experienced (Box 27-2).

BOX 27-2

POSTINTERVENTION CARE FOR PATIENTS WITH PERIPHERAL ARTERIAL OCCLUSIVE DISEASE

The nurse should assess for:
- Pulse presence and strength.
- Temperature of extremity.
- Capillary refill less than or equal to three seconds.
- Decreased sensation.
- Muscle movement and motor function.
- Signs and symptoms of bleeding.
- Increased edema.
- Pain not relieved with drug interventions.

ANEURYSMS AND AORTIC DISSECTIONS

An **aneurysm** is described as a permanent bulging and stretching of an artery, in which the dilation is two times or greater the size of the artery. This localized abnormality develops a weakness in the arterial wall and puts the patient at risk for serious complications.

Epidemiology

A wide variety of persons are at risk for the development of aneurysms. Cardiovascular and circulatory disorders are extremely prevalent in the population with multiple causes of aneurysm formation (e.g., arteriosclerosis, hypertension, trauma, cigarette smoking, and congenital weakness). Aneurysms occur at specific anatomic sites, most commonly at the aortic arch, thoracic aorta, and abdominal aorta. Men acquire aneurysms more frequently than women, and the risk of occurrence increases with age.

Etiology

Aneurysms are described by etiology and type. There are seven etiology classification aneurysms. Congenital aneurysms are related to several syndromes including Marfan's, Turner's, Ehler's-Danlos, and Menkes'. Tuberculosis sclerosis and syphilis have also contributed to the development of arterial aneurysms (Beese-Bjustrom, 2004). Mechanical, or hemodynamic, aneurysms are poststenotic, or related to arterio-venous fistulas, and amputations. Inflammatory, or mycotic aneurysms, refer to bacterial, fungal, or spirochetal infections as the underlying cause of the aneurysm formation. Traumatic or pseudoaneurysm is caused by either blunt or penetrating trauma to the artery. Aneurysms located at a graft suture line and the artery are classified as anastomotic or postarteriotomy. The origin of pregnancy-related degenerative aneurysms is often an inflammatory process.

Aneurysms are also described by type (Figure 27-5) because of their characteristics in the following manner:

- False aneurysm: Pulsating hematoma on all three layers of the artery, usually related to injury or trauma with blood clot formed on the exterior vessel wall.
- True aneurysm: Involvement of one, two, or all three layers of the artery.
- Fusiform aneurysm: Symmetric and diffuse involvement of the entire vessel.
- Saccular aneurysm: One-sided protrusion or out-poaching of one distinct area of the vessel.
- Dissecting aneurysm: Also known as dissecting hematomas, which splits the layers of the vessel wall and forms a hematoma.

Aortic dissection is a sudden tear in the intima of the aorta, where blood can enter into the vascular wall separation. The dissection of the aorta can advance above or below the tear and occlude any branching vessels supplying the gastrointestinal (GI) tract, kidneys, spinal cord, and lower extremities. Dissections may enter the pericardium, producing a hemopericardium, and causing a severe decrease in cardiac output. Symptoms are usually abrupt with severe pain and may extend to the back, shoulders, and abdomen. The aortic dissection is a surgical emergency, as the patient quickly deteriorates into hypovolemic or cardiogenic shock.

Pathophysiology

Because of one of the etiological causes, damage occurs to the middle (media) layer of the artery wall and then affects the inner (intima) layer. Aneurysm formation most frequently occurs in the abdominal aorta and the thoracic aorta, which could involve the descending, ascending, and transverse sections. The artery begins to stretch, is at risk for dissection, and can thereby also involve

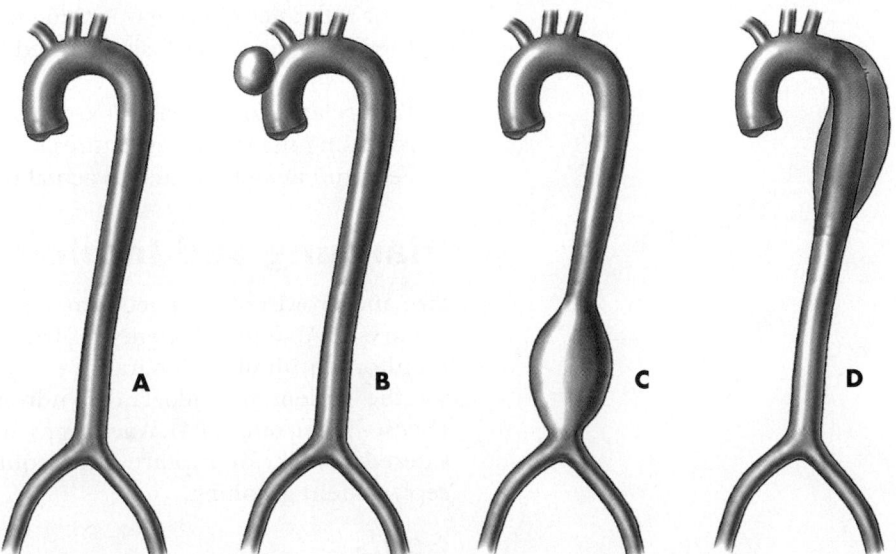

Figure 27-5 Various forms of aneurysms: A. Normal aorta, B. Saccular aneurysm, C. Fusiform aneurysm, D. Dissecting aneurysm.

other arteries, which branch off the affected section of the aorta. Tearing and rupture at the site of weakness are life-threatening complications, causing substantial hemorrhage leading to hypovolemic shock and requiring immediate surgical intervention.

Assessment with Clinical Manifestations

Awareness of symptoms indicating the presence of an aneurysm is critical in the nursing assessment. Though some aneurysms are asymptomatic, there are several symptoms, which when presented and identified, require immediate primary care provider notification.

Patients with abdominal aortic aneurysms (AAA) often present with nausea and vomiting from pressure applied to the intestines, back pain due to pressure to the spinal nerves, or a pulsation in the upper abdominal midline. The nurse may auscultate a bruit at the site of the aneurysm, but must avoid palpation of the site because of the risk of rupture. If circulation is impaired, the affected tissues may exhibit a decreased blood flow and appear bluish in color. Involvement of the nephrotic arteries will diminish blood flow to the kidneys, causing decreased kidney function and lead to kidney shutdown.

Aneurysms of the thoracic aorta can also cause severe back pain due to compression of surrounding tissues and structures. Bronchial obstruction, dyspnea, and dysphasia may occur depending on the location of the aneurysm. The patient may also experience hoarseness and **aphonia** (loss of voice) related to pressure on the laryngeal nerve. A pulsating mass above the suprasternal notch may be observed when assessing the patient.

Diagnostic Tests

Anterior-posterior and lateral X-rays are taken to identify the location of the mass, followed by computerized tomography (CT), and duplex ultrasonography. Transesophageal echocardiography may be utilized for thoracic aneurysms not easily seen with other diagnostic tests. Occasionally, a patient will have an aneurysm diagnosed while the patient is having diagnostic examinations for other disorders.

Nursing Diagnoses

Based on the information gathered, examples of nursing diagnoses in the patient with aneurysms may include the following:
- Ineffective tissue perfusion related to diminished circulation at and distal to the aneurysm.
- Pain related to decreased oxygen supply to tissues or pressure on surrounding tissues and structures.
- Fear and anxiety related to actual or potential serious complications.

Planning and Implementation

Size and growth of the aneurysm are the determining factors of managing an aneurysm. Abdominal aneurysms less than 6 cm (2.5 inches) in width are often monitored with ultrasonography every six months. Elective surgery is planned for the patient with Marfan's syndrome when the aneurysm reaches 5 cm. (Beese-Bjurstrom, 2004). Aneurysms of greater size or rapidly growing are considered at risk for rupture and require surgical repair of either bypass or replacement graphing.

Goals

The identification and prevention of risk factors for aneurysm development are the primary goals for the management of aneurysms. Once an aneurysm is identified and located, nursing management is focused on the reduction of complications. For example, the nurse can assist in controlling hypertension by decreasing stressful situations and keeping activity to a minimum. In addition, the education related to diagnostic and surgical procedures will assist the patient and family in understanding the disease process and interventions needed to repair the aneurysm. Furthermore, the nurse should inform the patient that straining during defecation, coughing, and ambulation are to be avoided. The monitoring of blood pressure, pulse, respirations, fluid intake and output, and level of consciousness are essential in identifying shock, hemorrhage, or dissection.

Evidence-Based Care

Cigarette smoking has been identified as a risk factor for diseases of both the peripheral vessels and the larger arteries, including the aorta. Health care providers educate patients on the risks related to smoking, but patients respond to being told to not smoke in many different ways. A qualitative study conducted by Pilnick and Coleman (2003) found that patients did not respond to the advice of smoking cessation by their general practitioners when the advice was linked to present health problems. Often there was an increase in defensive behavior and minimization of the smoking habit. Patient's responses to preventive health or health promotion advice on smoking cessation depend heavily on the patient-provider relationship. By building effective relationships with patients, health care providers may increase their success in facilitating patient's smoking cessation. Effective relationships between patients and their health care providers should be further studied to potentially create continued positive results for the patient.

Nutrition

A diet that is low in fat and cholesterol is advised for all patients but particularly those who are at risk for the development of vascular diseases. A low-fat, low-cholesterol diet can greatly improve the patient's cholesterol, LDL,

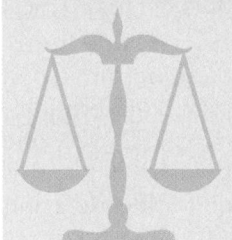

LAW IN PRACTICE

Drug Classifications Are a Life and Death Situation

The following is an actual legal case. A nurse working in an emergency department admitted a patient with symptoms of a respiratory infection. The patient informed the nurse she was allergic to Claforan and had an anaphylactic reaction to the drug in the past. This information was then documented in the allergy column of the emergency department patient's admission form. The nurse informed the health care provider of the patient's symptoms and drug allergy, and the health care provider ordered Rocephin. The nurse administered the Rocephin, the patient had a severe anaphylactic reaction, and died. What the health care provider and nurse did not consider is that Claforan and Rocephin are both third-generation cephalosporins.

Is the health care provider or the nurse responsible for the death of the patient? The pro-

fessional licenses of both the health care provider and the nurse were revoked by the state of Texas. Though the physician ordered the Rocephin administration, the nurse was found guilty of administering a drug that was related to a drug to which the patient had stated a severe allergy. The court felt the nurse was trained in pharmacology, had knowledge of drug classifications, and had access to drug information at the work site.

When you hear phrases such as "nurses have patient's lives in their hands," this account demonstrates the risky and unfortunate side of drug administration. Nurses must be 100 percent confident of their knowledge in the administration of drugs and question health care provider orders if not positive all the rights of drug administration are met.

Source: Ritchey C. (2005). Advice of counsel. Documentation puts nurse on solid legal ground. RN, 68(2), 21, 46, 58–59.

HDL, and triglyceride levels, minimizing the risk for the formation of aneurysms.

Pharmacology

Hypertension is a leading risk factor in the development of aneurysms. Pharmaceutical therapy includes antihypertensive drugs to keep the blood pressure in a safe range and decrease the risk of rupture. Antihypertensive medications require the nurse to administer them with great attention to detail because of the many potential side effects and adverse reactions of these classifications of medications.

Surgery

Prior to surgery, the patient's blood pressure and peripheral pulses should be evaluated as a baseline for postoperative assessment. A patient with a ruptured aneurysm is immediately taken to the operating room for surgical repair, but because of the severe loss of blood, the mortality is much greater than for those who have the repair electively.

The surgical procedure for aneurysm repair involves the placement of a Dacron graft above and below the proximal and distal aspects of the aneurysm. Patients who undergo surgical repair have potential complications for bleeding, hematoma, leaking at the site of the graft anastomosis, and wound infections. Respiratory depression, hypovolemia, renal failure, paralytic ileus, and cardiac changes need to be frequently assessed for the first 48 hours after surgery. The potential for graft occlusion, leakage, and rupture includes assessment of pulses distal to the surgical repair. Any changes in pulse strength, increase in coolness of extremities below the graft, color changes that include blue or white coloration of the abdomen or extremities, abdominal distension, or severe pain may also indicate the graph is not functioning or allowing blood to flow through the operative area.

For the first several postoperative days, the patient will have continuous IV fluids for hydration and an indwelling urinary catheter to monitor output, which should be no less than 30 to 50 mL/hr. A nasogastric tube to low intermittent suction eliminates gastric secretions and is removed after bowel sounds are audible. Lab values, which need daily monitoring include hemoglobin, hematocrit (28 percent or greater), electrolytes, creatinine, and blood urea nitrogen (BUN). To decrease the risk for respiratory complications, deep-breathing, turning, and incentive spirometry are encouraged every one to two hours. Ambulation usually begins the first postoperative day and is increased daily as tolerated. The surgical incision is observed for bleeding and signs of infection.

Patient and Family Teaching

Activity restrictions include not lifting heavy objects (limit 15 to 20 pounds) and activity restrictions for the first six to eight weeks after surgical repair. The patient will need wound care instructions and must notify the physician if redness of the wound site and drainage occur. Pain is managed with oral analgesics and using a pillow for support when coughing. Driving may be restricted for several weeks, and community support should be anticipated for transportation to physician appointments, grocery, and pharmacy. Home health and home care aides services are excellent support for patients who lack family support.

Evaluation of Outcomes

Potential patient outcomes for each of the example nursing diagnoses for the patient with aneurysms are:

- Ineffective tissue perfusion related to diminished circulation at and distal to the aneurysm. The patient should maintain optimal tissue perfusion to the periphery, as evidenced by strong peripheral pulses, good capillary refill, and good movement.

Red Flag

Detecting an Aortic Dissection

According to Beese-Bjurstrom (2004) the first priority for a patient who is diagnosed with an aortic dissection is to lower the patient's systemic arterial pressure and reduce cardiac contractility. Systolic blood pressure may be reduced to 70–80 mm Hg to accomplish pain relief, with morphine being the choice drug for aortic dissection. Antianxiety medication may be prescribed as needed. Monitor for cerebral and renal perfusion as the systolic blood pressure decreases. Continue to watch for complications, which include MI, neurological effects, bowel ischemia, and diminished peripheral pulses.

BOX 27-3

ASSESSMENTS DURING THE POSTOPERATIVE PERIOD

The nurse should assess for the following:

- Temperature and color of skin at and below the graft anastomosis.
- Abdominal distension.
- Blood pressure stability.
- Adequate urinary output.
- Signs and symptoms of internal bleeding.
- Surgical wound healing.
- Lab values within normal limits.
- Pain not relieved with drug interventions.

- Pain related to decreased oxygen supply to tissues or pressure on surrounding tissues and structures. The patient should verbalize an adequate relief of pain along with the ability to realistically cope with the pain if it is not completely relieved.
- Fear and anxiety related to actual or potential serious complications. The patient should be able to recognize the signs of anxiety, demonstrate positive coping mechanisms, and describe a reduction in the level of anxiety experienced (Box 27-3).

THROMBOPHLEBITIS

Thrombophlebitis is the inflammation of a vein accompanied by the formation of thrombus (blood clot), which can be dislodged and lead to pulmonary emboli. Deep vein thrombosis (DVT) is a term often used for this venous complication, which most commonly occurs in the deep veins of the lower extremities.

Epidemiology

DVT accounts for 600,000 hospitalizations annually in the United States. Pulmonary embolism resulting from DVTs causes 25 percent of hospital deaths (Andrews & Fleischer, 2005). Approximately 80 percent of DVTs originate in the calf and often migrate to the popliteal or femoral veins.

Etiology

Several conditions have been identified that have a tendency for the development of thrombophlebitis and clot formation. These causes are postsurgical procedures, pregnancy, ulcerative colitis, trauma, fractures, heart failure, and shock. Due to the reduction of muscle contraction, immobility and paralysis of the lower extremities also expose patients to the risk. IV therapy and medications, infections, and trauma also are causes of thrombophlebitis.

Pathophysiology

Predisposition to thrombophlebitis is not completely known, but a three factor development, known as Virchow's triad, has been associated with the creation of venous thrombosis. These factors include venous stasis, vessel wall injury, and alteration of blood coagulation. When the inner lining of the venous wall is injured or irritated, a clot is formed. The clot diminishes blood flow distal to the clot, causing venous congestion. Waste products accumulate in the blocked area, initiating the inflammatory response. Leukocytes and lymphocytes form at the clot site, platelet formation occurs, which preludes to a thrombus, and can break off and travel through the venous system to the pulmonary system.

Assessment with Clinical Manifestations

Thrombophlebitis is identified by pain, warmth, redness, and swelling (i.e., nonspecific immune response) at the site of the thrombus. Fever, malaise, and fatigue are often described by many patients. The extremity becomes edematous, is functionally impaired, and is measured against the nonaffected extremity. A small percentage of patients may exhibit a positive **Homans' sign** (dorsiflexing the foot, causing pain in the calf), and therefore is not an indicative sign of DVT.

Diagnostic Tests

In most incidences, the clinical findings, along with recognized risk factors, support the diagnosis of thrombophlebitis and DVT. A venogram, which uses radiopaque dye instilled into the venous system, may be used to identify the

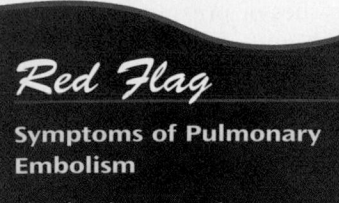

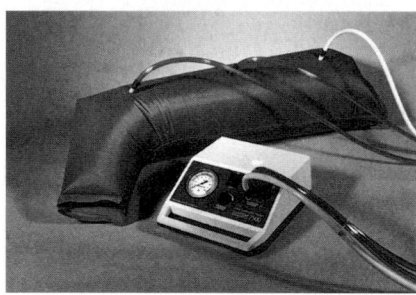

Figure 27-6 Alternating pneumatic compression device helps prevent thrombi formation (Courtesy of Beifersdorf-Jobst, Inc. Charlotte, NC).

direct location of the clot. Venograms are invasive tests, are painful, and have the potential to dislodge the clot. Duplex ultrasound scanning and Doppler flow studies, which are noninvasive, have less risk but may be difficult to interpret. Impedance plethysmography (IPG) is a more accurate diagnostic test to locate DVTs. IPGs use a sensor to record the blood flow before and after inflating a blood pressure cuff to impede venous flow. The presence of a clot is discovered when the blood flow is the same.

Nursing Diagnoses

Based on the information gathered, examples of nursing diagnoses in the patient with thrombophlebitis may include the following:
- Pain related to inflammation of the affected extremity.
- Altered tissue perfusion related to diminished blood flow.
- Knowledge deficit related to self-care and risk prevention.

Planning and Implementation

Phlebitis and DVT are short-term acute processes that are often identified by the presence of risk factors and occurrence of symptoms. Bed rest and anticoagulant therapy are initiated, and the patient is monitored for symptoms of pulmonary embolism.

Goals

Prevention of risk factors for development thrombophlebitis and DVT is the primary goal. Nurses assist in the prevention of venous stasis by promoting activities that prevent clot formation. Early postoperative ambulation is imperative in the preclusion of thrombus. Patients inactive or on bed rest need knee- or thigh-high elastic stocking, or use an alternating pneumonic pressure device that systematically inflates to promote venous circulation (Figure 27-6). Assisting the patient to change positions every two hours and promoting leg exercises are excellent nursing interventions in the prevention of venous thrombosis.

Evidence-Based Care

Traveling for long distances or sitting for extended periods of time promotes venous restriction and obstructs blood flow. Using the nursing process, the nurse should assess for symptoms and associated risk factors, lists nursing diagnoses, then develop a plan of care using concept mapping. Frequent evaluation is required to identify if the plan is working to progress the patient to wellness.

Pharmacology

Pharmacological management of thrombophlebitis and DVT begins with anticoagulant therapy to inhibit thrombus and clot. Heparin sodium (Hepalean) blocks the conversion of thrombin and fibrinogen to fibrin, thereby preventing further clot formation in the body. Heparin does not affect the existing clot, which is eventually absorbed by the body. Baseline prothrombin time (PT), international normalized ratio (INR), and blood and platelet counts are required prior to initial administration of IV anticoagulant therapy. Heparin therapy is weight-based and initiated with an IV bolus of approximately 100 units/kg of body weight. Continuous IV infusion is started, and the partial thromboplastin time (PTT) is monitored and maintained at one to two times the normal levels, thereby being therapeutic for the prevention of clot formation.

LMWH, for example, Lovenox, is given subcutaneously, has a longer half-life than heparin, and doses are adjusted according to the patient's weight. Dosing is usually scheduled daily or twice daily depending on the type to be administered. The patient can be taught self-administration for home management.

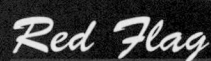

Red Flag

Complications of Heparin Therapy

During continuous IV heparin administration, the patient is continually observed for symptoms of bleeding, which includes frank bleeding, hematuria, occult blood in the stool, bruising, or petechiae. Platelet and blood counts are also screened during the five to seven days of infusion and are abruptly discontinued if complications or extremely prolonged PTT or INR results greater than 3. Protamine sulfate is the heparin antagonist used for excessive bleeding.

Warfarin (Coumadin) is oral anticoagulant therapy implemented four to five days prior to the discontinuation of heparin or LMWH. It is started at a low dose of 5 mg, then adjusted according to the patient's INR results. It is common for warfarin therapy to last three to six months after the incidence of DVT. Vitamin K, the antagonist for warfarin, can be administered for excessive bleeding.

Thrombolytic therapy is used to completely dissolve clots and must be initiated within three to five days of symptom onset. Streptokinase, recombinant tissue plasminogen activator (t-PA), and platelet inhibitors like abciximab (ReoPro) must be closely monitored for signs and symptoms of bleeding, as they have three times a greater incidence of bleeding than heparin. Pain is managed with oral nonnarcotic analgesics. Great care must be taken to administer and document anticoagulants as reflected in the Safety First feature.

Health Care Resources

Case management should be implemented while the patient is hospitalized, to assess for support once the patient is discharged from the hospital. Resources need to be appraised, as patients may need to be taught self-administration of LMWH for home management. Patients also must have routine lab (INR) while on anticoagulants, and transportation may be needed for physician and lab appointments. Community services need should be assessed, as the patient may qualify for these services.

Patient and Family Teaching

Prevention of further episodes of thrombophlebitis should include the avoidance of long periods of inactivity and sitting, use of support stockings, and liberal fluid intake. Anticoagulant therapy education is initiated by the nurse. Lab monitoring is scheduled on a routine basis and must be adhered to to maintain the highest level of effectiveness. Alcohol use decreases the effectiveness of anticoagulants, and this information needs to be included in the discharge planning.

Bleeding is the most severe complication of anticoagulant therapy. Bleeding from the nose or gums, rectal bleeding, bruising without cause, or prolonged

---

Safety First

Quality Documentation Can Reflect Safe Patient Care

Why is careful documentation of anticoagulants and their affects so important? Because accurate documentation is a professional standard required by nurses and acts as a tracking system of a patient's condition and as a way that nurses demonstrate the quality of care the patient is receiving.

There are many methods of charting used to demonstrate safe and effective nursing care, and often with mnemonics such as P.I.E, S.O.A.P, and D.A.R. There is one charting system that provides a record reflecting legal and safe patient care. The mnemonic, painter, is a reminder to document the following:

P: Plan of care and problems, and adjust the plan to reflect the patient's change in condition.
A: Assessment, which must be complete, accurate, timely, holistic, and systematic.
I: Interventions, which includes nursing care.
N: Notification, and collaborations with physicians and other health car providers
T: Teaching, and record all instructions given to the parent and family members.
E: Evaluation of the patient's response to care.
R: Record, of all medications and treatments, and refusals of care.

Adapted from: Daniels, R. (2004). Nursing fundamentals: Caring and clinical decision making. *New York: Thomson Delmar Learning.*

wound bleeding may indicate impaired clotting, and needs immediate medical attention (Box 27-4).

Evaluation of Outcomes

Potential patient outcomes for each of the example nursing diagnoses for the patient with the thrombophlebitis are:

- Pain related to inflammation of the affected extremity. The patient should verbalize an adequate relief of pain along with the ability to realistically cope with the pain if it is not completely relieved.
- Altered tissue perfusion related to diminished blood flow. The patient should maintain optimal tissue perfusion to the periphery, as evidenced by strong peripheral pulses, good capillary refill, and good movement
- Knowledge deficit related to self-care and risk prevention. The patient should demonstrate motivation to learn, identify perceived learning needs, and verbalize an understanding of desired content.

BUERGER'S DISEASE

Also known as thromboangiitis obliterans, **Buerger's disease** is an occlusive disease mostly located in small to medium-sized arteries and less frequently in veins. Though commonly found in the upper and lower distal extremities, Buerger's disease is associated with clot formation and fibrosis of the vessel wall. In prolonged cases, large extremities vessels may be affected.

Epidemiology

Buerger's disease is a rare disorder with an incidence of 1 in 8,000 people, and it is much more common in men than in women. It appears to be more common in Asians and in the Middle East, is rare among African Americans, and is rare in children.

Etiology

Buerger's disease is more prevalent in young adult males who smoke. Smoking cessation will halt the disease progress, but continuation of smoking will exacerbate the progression of the disease. Buerger's disease has also been identified as having a genetic predisposition and a correlation with autoimmune causation.

Pathophysiology

Inflammation occurs, and the vessels are prone to spasms and constriction. Inflammatory lesions appear in healthy isolated segments of normal vessels walls, which often occlude blood flow. Scarring, fibrosis, and thrombophlebitis occur, which develops into adhering of the vessels and nerves. Soft tissue and skin cells experience hypoxia, which leads to anoxia and tissue necrosis. Nail beds thicken, and peripheral pulses become weak and thready. As Buerger's disease progresses, pain occurs due to tissue death. Skin sloughs, ulcers form, and the extremity is at risk for gangrene.

Genetics

Though strongly associated with tobacco use, a familial predisposition and autoimmune etiological factors have been seen in patients diagnosed with Buerger's disease.

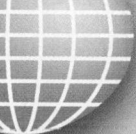

Real World, Real Choices

Sometimes the Nurse Must Suspect the System

Handwritten health care provider orders continue to be a the origin of many drug errors. Eighty-six-year-old Mary Rickers was admitted to the medical-surgical unit with symptoms related to her peripheral vascular disease, and was ordered 1.0 mg. of the opioid analgesic morphine sulfate, intravenous push, every four hours as needed for pain. The medication administration (MAR), which was computer-generated from the pharmacy, came to the unit, and the order read "10 mg. Morphine Sulfate, IVP, q. 4 h prn pain". The nurse administered the dose, which was written on the MAR. Thirty minutes after the morphine sulfate administration, the nurse returned to the room to assess Mrs. Rickers' pain. She found her patient unconscious and in severe respiratory depression. What should the nurse do?

Assessment with Clinical Manifestations

Extreme sensitivity to heat and cold, and pain in the digits due to ischemia are often early symptoms of impending tissue damage because of Buerger's disease. Affected tissues appear cyanotic and ruddy. Nail beds thicken, peripheral pulses become weak and thready, and skin may have blackish ulcerations. Intermittent claudication is a hallmark symptom, identified by cramps in the legs after exercise. The patient may complain of severe attacks, followed by remissions. Severe tissue impairment will cause pain in extremities at rest.

Diagnostic Tests

Plethysmographic studies of the digits may identify early stages of Buerger's disease. Doppler ultrasound and IPG are often used to discover the location of diminished blood flow. Arteriograms identify the extent of the disease process.

Nursing Diagnoses

Based on the information gathered, examples of nursing diagnoses in the patient with Buerger's disease may include the following:
- Ineffective peripheral tissue perfusion related to impaired circulation.
- Pain related to diminished oxygen flow to the affected extremity.
- Fear and anxiety related to actual or potential serious complications.

Planning and Implementation

Tobacco in any form must be restricted for both the symptoms and the Buerger's disease process to subside. The patient is informed to avoid long exposure to cold, thereby preventing further vasoconstriction. Patients are instructed to perform Buerger-Allen exercises to promote collateral circulation.

Pharmacology

Analgesics are used for pain relief associated with Buerger's disease, and vasodilators to increase tissue perfusion. If wound care is required, topical antibiotics are applied with dressing changes. Enzymatic debridement agents may be used as a replacement to surgical debridement.

PATIENT PLAYBOOK

Patient Teaching for Patients with Buerger's Disease

Instruct the patient to do the following several times a day:
- Lie flat on a bed with both legs elevated above the level of the heart for two to three minutes.
- Next sit on the edge of the bed with the legs dependent for three minutes.
- Then exercise the feet and toes by moving them up, down, inward, then outward.
- Lastly, return to the first position and hold for five minutes.

Surgery

In severe situations, surgical intervention may be considered. Sympathectomy, which involves the interruption of selected sections of the sympathetic nervous pathway, is used to treat vasospasms. Ulcerations may require debridement and possible skin grafting. In extreme disease progression of Buerger's disease there is circulation impairment, and amputation of digits or extremity may be needed.

Evaluation of Outcomes

Potential patient outcomes for each of the example nursing diagnoses for the patient with the Buerger's disease are:

- Ineffective peripheral tissue perfusion related to impaired circulation. The patient should maintain optimal tissue perfusion to the periphery, as evidenced by strong peripheral pulses, good capillary refill, and good movement.
- Pain related to diminished oxygen flow to the affected extremity. The patient should verbalize an adequate relief of pain along with the ability to realistically cope with the pain if it is not completely relieved.
- Fear and anxiety related to actual or potential serious complications. The patient should be able to recognize the signs of anxiety, demonstrate positive coping mechanisms, and describe a reduction in the level of anxiety experienced.

SUBCLAVIAN STEAL SYNDROME

Subclavian steal syndrome occurs when the subclavian artery is occluded, and blood flow is diminished, or obstructed, to the upper extremities. The arms experience ischemia, associated with pain and weakness during and after exercise. Atherosclerosis is a risk factor for the subclavian steal development. Blood clots form and eventually occlude the artery.

Etiology

Though there is no defined age identified with patients diagnosed with subclavian steal syndrome, it is more commonly seen in patients with risk factors related to atherosclerosis.

Assessment with Clinical Manifestations

In conjunction with pain and weakness, patients describe paresthesia of the affected arms. Bilateral blood pressures are taken, and it is considered significant is the difference is greater than 20 mm Hg. A subclavian bruit is an important diagnostic discovery. Brachial and radial pulses may also be diminished, and the extremity appears cyanotic.

Diagnostic Tests

Upon initial assessment, if discrepancies are noticed in bilateral blood pressures and pulse palpation, the health care provider must be notified so further studies may be considered. Doppler ultrasound and arteriogram are diagnostic tests to identify the location and severity of the claudication.

Nursing Diagnoses

Based on the information gathered, examples of nursing diagnoses in the patient with subclavian steal syndrome may include the following:

- Ineffective upper extremity tissue perfusion related to impaired circulation.
- Pain related to decreased oxygen supply to tissues.

- Risk for impaired skin integrity related to compromised tissue perfusion.
- Fear and anxiety related to actual or potential lifestyle changes.

Planning and Implementation

Patients who experience pain and diminished blood flow are considered for surgical intervention. Depending on the extent of the atherosclerosis, several options may be considered including subclavian artery endarterectomy, carotid-to-subclavian graft bypass, or subclavian artery angioplasty with stent placement. The nurses will monitor the surgical site for bleeding, including the formation of hematomas, and note the pulse, color, and temperature of the affected arm.

Evaluation of Outcomes

- Ineffective upper extremity tissue perfusion related to impaired circulation. The patient should maintain optimal tissue perfusion to the periphery, as evidenced by strong peripheral pulses, good capillary refill, and good movement.
- Pain related to decreased oxygen supply to tissues. The patient should verbalize an adequate relief of pain along with the ability to realistically cope with the pain if it is not completely relieved.
- Risk for impaired skin integrity related to compromised tissue perfusion. The condition of the skin should be improved as evidenced by decreased redness, swelling and pain.
- Fear and anxiety related to actual or potential lifestyle changes. The patient should be able to recognize the signs of anxiety, demonstrate positive coping mechanisms, and describe a reduction in the level of anxiety experienced.

RAYNAUD'S PHENOMENON

Raynaud's phenomenon is caused by unilateral vasospasm of the upper and lower extremities. Bilateral vasospasm is identified as **Raynaud's disease.** There are few identifiable differences between Raynaud's phenomenon and Raynaud's disease, and most practitioners would treat the two disorders as one disease process. Raynaud's phenomenon usually occurs in the age-group over 30 and is equally distributed between genders. Raynaud's disease has been seen in ages 17 to 50 and is more common in females (Sibell, Colantonio, & Stacey, 2005).

Epidemiology

Raynaud's disease affects approximately 4 in every 10,000 people. People who have atherosclerosis, rheumatoid arthritis, scleroderma or Sjögren's syndrome are more likely to develop Raynaud's phenomenon.

Etiology

The etiology of Raynaud's disease is unknown for either entity, but it has been related to diseases such as systemic lupus erythematosus, progressive systemic sclerosis, and several systemic connective tissue diseases. Episodes of exacerbation can be generated by stress and cold.

Assessment with Clinical Manifestations

Venospasms cause blood flow restriction, pain, and cyanosis, followed by redness. Pain is intermittent, extremities are numb and cold, and may exhibit swelling, and even ulcerations. Gangrene occurs when the disease progresses in severity (Figure 27-7).

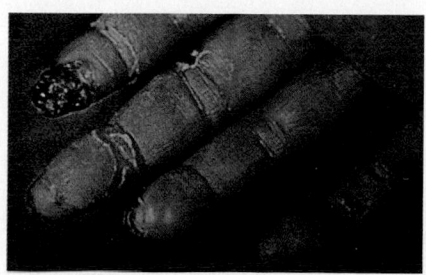

Figure 27-7 Raynaud's disease (Courtesy of Marvin Ackerman, M.D., Scarsdale, NY).

Diagnostic Tests

Doppler ultrasound is a noninvasive test used to measure blood flow. No specific lab tests are utilized to diagnose Raynaud's disease, but lab tests are often ordered to rule out connective tissue disorders.

Nursing Diagnoses

Based on the information gathered, examples of nursing diagnoses in the patient with Raynaud's disease may include the following:
- Ineffective upper or lower extremity tissue perfusion related to impaired circulation.
- Pain related to decreased oxygen supply to tissues.
- Risk for impaired skin integrity related to compromised tissue perfusion.
- Fear and anxiety related to actual or potential lifestyle changes.

Planning and Implementation

Patient education includes symptom control, including the identification of situations that exacerbate these indicators. A warm environment is essential, along with stress reduction. Interventions such as wearing warm clothing and gloves may be effective. If symptoms are not relieved, a lumbar sympathectomy may be performed. This is most commonly used in patients who experience severe foot pain. Patients may prescribe medicines that relax the walls of the blood vessels, or other medicines if the patient's condition is connected with another disease such as scleroderma (Box 27-5).

Pharmacology

Analgesics are used for pain relief, though they may not be effective. Vasodilators are prescribed to increase tissue perfusion, thereby decreasing symptoms.

Evaluation of Outcomes

Potential patient outcomes for each of the example nursing diagnoses for the patient with the Raynaud's disease are:
- Ineffective upper or lower extremity tissue perfusion related to impaired circulation. The patient should maintain optimal tissue perfusion to the periphery, as evidenced by strong peripheral pulses, good capillary refill, and good movement.
- Pain related to decreased oxygen supply to tissues. The patient should verbalize an adequate relief of pain along with the ability to realistically cope with the pain if it is not completely relieved.
- Risk for impaired skin integrity related to compromised tissue perfusion. The condition of the skin should be improved as evidenced by decreased redness, swelling, and pain.
- Fear and anxiety related to actual or potential lifestyle changes. The patient should be able to recognize the signs of anxiety, demonstrate positive coping mechanisms, and describe a reduction in the level of anxiety experienced.

VARICOSE VEINS

Varicose veins are torturous varicosities, in which the veins are dilated and lack surrounding muscle support. Though the saphenous veins of the legs are most commonly affected, hemorrhoids and esophageal varices are also in this category.

BOX 27-5

CARING FOR PATIENTS WITH RAYNAUD'S DISEASE

The nurse should assist the patient by the:
- Management of risk-management.
- Smoking cessation.
- Safety with sharp objects.
- Maintain extremity warmth.
- Stress management.
- Monitor for symptoms of gangrene.
- Medication compliance and monitor for drug interactions.
- Monitor vital signs, particularly blood pressure, due to risk for postural hypotension.
- Avoidance of situations that aggravate condition, such as extremely cold temperatures and prolonged ambulation.
- Assessed for home health and community-based support to promote the highest level of function and quality of life.

Epidemiology

Approximately 60 percent of the adult population in the United States are affected with varicose veins. They are found more commonly in Caucasians than in the African Americans and in people over the age of 30.

Etiology

There is a familial tendency, as the valves of the veins become incompetent and ineffective. Thrombophlebitis, obesity, and prolonged standing are risk factors. Abdominal pressure caused by pregnancy or dysfunction of the liver or pancreas are also known to contribute to varicose vein formation.

Pathophysiology

Incompetent venous valves lead to venous congestion and decreased venous return. The situation becomes chronic, and fluid seeps into the interstitial spaces, causing localized edema and impaired circulation. Surrounding tissue can become ulcerated and infected.

Assessment with Clinical Manifestations

The varicose veins appear distended, torturous, and bluish-purple in color. Patients state a heaviness in the legs exists, and the pain is often relieved when the lower limbs are elevated. Capillary refill is often prolonged, the skin may be discolored, and ulcers may form.

Diagnostic Tests

Ultrasounds and venograms may be used to identify venous status. The Brodie-Trendelenburg test is often performed to confirm the diagnosis of venous varicosities. A tourniquet is placed on the upper thigh while the patient is lying flat. The patient stands, and if the blood flows from the upper part of the leg into the superficial veins after the tourniquet is released, the venous valves of the superficial veins are identified as incompetent.

Nursing Diagnoses

Based on the information gathered, examples of nursing diagnoses in the patient with varicose veins may include the following:
- Ineffective lower extremity tissue perfusion related to impaired circulation.
- Pain related to decreased oxygen supply to tissues.
- Risk for impaired skin integrity related to compromised tissue perfusion.
- Anxiety related to possible career or lifestyle changes

Planning and Implementation

Management for varicose veins includes such things as weight loss for the obese patient, exercise, support hose, and avoidance of standing or sitting for long periods of time, which can impede blood flow. Veins can be chemically sclerosed, causing venous wall inflammation and eventual destruction of the vein.

Surgery

For multiple and severe varicosities, surgical interventions include vein ligation and vein stripping. Ligation involves tying-off the vein, stripping removes the vein. Postsurgical care involves wrapping the involved leg in bandages, which need inspecting for bleeding or dehiscence. The legs are elevated, the patient is instructed on contraction and relaxation exercises, and postoperative ambulation is encouraged. Support stockings are placed on the patient after bleeding has ceased. Patients are instructed to avoid constrictive clothing, to not cross their knees, and to participate in active or isometric exercises.

Patient and Family Teaching

Patients with varicose veins should be educated in a variety of areas. The patients should be encouraged to avoid strenuous physical activity, avoid constrictive clothing, and increase their participation in exercise, particularly walking and swimming. In addition, if the patient is overweight, he or she should be educated regarding a weight reduction plan and potentially using support stockings. As patients develop further problems with their varicose veins, they should be assessed for the need for medical management and then prepared for venous ligation or stripping.

Evaluation of Outcomes

Potential patient outcomes for each of the example nursing diagnoses for the patient with the varicose veins are:
- Ineffective lower extremity tissue perfusion related to impaired circulation. The patient should maintain optimal tissue perfusion to the periphery, as evidenced by strong peripheral pulses, good capillary refill, and good movement.
- Pain related to decreased oxygen supply to tissues. The patient should verbalize an adequate relief of pain along with the ability to realistically cope with the pain if it is not completely relieved.
- Risk for impaired skin integrity related to compromised tissue perfusion. The condition of the skin should be improved as evidenced by decreased redness, swelling, and pain.
- Anxiety related to possible career or lifestyle changes. The patient should be able to recognize the signs of anxiety, demonstrate positive coping mechanisms, and describe a reduction in the level of anxiety experienced.

VENOUS STASIS ULCER

Most commonly found on the lower extremities, **venous stasis ulcers** appear as an erosion of the skin. This leads to skin necrosis, open wounds, and black, hardened skin known as eschar.

Epidemiology

Approximately 75 percent of venous stasis ulcers occur with chronic venous insufficiency. The remaining 25 percent are attributed to burns, sickle cell disease, and arterial insufficiency.

Etiology

Chronic venous insufficiency causes 75 percent of these venous stasis ulcers. Other disease process contributing to the formation of venous stasis ulcers include diabetes, arterial insufficiency, burns, injuries, neuropathy, and blood disorders. Elderly patients are more at risk for ulcer development because of their prevalence to contract multiple chronic comorbidities.

Pathophysiology

The process of venous insufficiency begins as a decrease in the blood flow to the lower extremities. Lack of oxygen and nutrients to the tissues causes delayed cell metabolism, and over time, tissue death. Skin inflammation leads

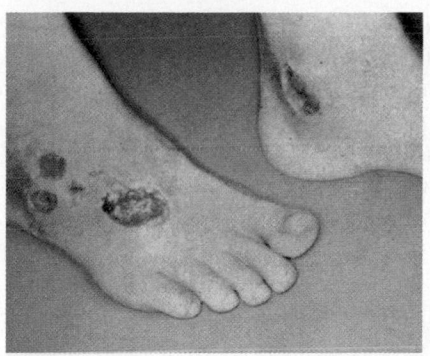

Figure 27-8 Venous ulcerations.

to ulcerations and open wounds, which drain. Venous stasis ulcers are an excellent media for organisms, inviting infection and possibly sepsis (Figure 27-8)

Assessment with Clinical Manifestations

Unless caused by neuropathy, the venous stasis ulcers are painful to touch, pressure, and when open to air. Fluid seeps into the interstitial tissues, causing edema of the foot and ankle. Femoral, popliteal, posterior tibial, and dorsalis pedis pulses are assessed to identify the possibility of arterial insufficiency.

Nutritional assessment should be completed after admission to the hospital. The expertise of a dietitian may be called upon to provide the patient with a diet high in protein and nutrients to support wound healing. Patient and family education are required to provide food selections and meal planning that encourage active participation of their care.

Diagnostic Tests

Doppler, angiogram, and venogram studies are often required to identify the underlying cause and construct a definitive diagnosis for venous stasis ulcers. Draining wounds should be cultured so appropriate pharmaceutical intervention can be implemented. Wound therapy may be initiated to treat infection.

Nursing Diagnoses

Based on the information gathered, examples of nursing diagnoses in the patient with chronic venous insufficiency may include the following:
• Impaired tissue integrity related to vascular insufficiency.
• Impaired physical mobility related to functional limitations and pain.
• Nutrition imbalance, less than body requirements, related to increased need for nutrients to promote wound healing.
• Knowledge deficit, related to the care and healing of lower extremity wounds.

Planning and Implementation

Dressings provide a moist, clean environment and are often combined with wound care routines and debridement. If an infection develops, venous stasis ulcers are also managed with oral antibiotics. Hydrocolloids are included in wound therapy to promote the formation of granulation tissue. **Debridement,** which is a mechanical method of eliminating necrotic tissue, serves as a healing process for infected and progressive wounds. Several methods may be used including surgically incising the nonviable tissue, and debridement with dry dressings, enzyme applications, and debridement agents. Pain management is often necessary prior to performing debridement procedures.

Evaluation of Outcomes

Potential patient outcomes for each of the example nursing diagnoses for the patient with chronic venous insufficiency are:
• Impaired tissue integrity related to vascular insufficiency. The condition of the skin should be improved as evidenced by decreased redness, swelling, and pain.
• Impaired physical mobility related to functional limitations and pain. The patient should perform physical activity independently or with assistive devices as needed. In addition, the patient should be free of complications of immobility, as evidenced by intact skin, absence of thrombophlebitis, and normal bowel patterns.

- Nutrition imbalance, less than body requirements, related to increased need for nutrients to promote wound healing. The patient verbalizes and demonstrates selection of foods or meals that will achieve a well-balanced diet intake to enhance wound healing potential.
- Knowledge deficit, related to the care and healing of lower extremity wounds. The patient should demonstrate motivation to learn, identify perceived learning needs, and verbalize an understanding of desired content.

KEY CONCEPTS

- Vascular dysfunction is often associated with common diseases including arteriosclerosis, atherosclerosis, peripheral vascular disease, and aortic aneurysms.
- Arteriosclerosis, also known as hardening of the arteries, is a thickening and solidifying of the endothelial lining of the walls in small arteries and arterioles, causing a diminished blood flow.
- Atherosclerosis is the development of plaques in the intimal layer of larger arteries, eventually developing blockage of the vessel lumen.
- There are numerous risk factors associated with the long-term development of arteriosclerosis and atherosclerosis, which is a direct precursor of CVD.
- Health care goals for patients diagnosed with arteriosclerosis and atherosclerosis include disease prevention and controlling the advancement of the disease process.
- Peripheral occlusive disease may take years to develop and can occur suddenly and severely. More common in lower extremities, the patient develops decreased ability to ambulate in certain distances due to arterial insufficiency.
- An aneurysm is a permanent, localized bulging and stretching of an artery. It must be identified and treated at early stage, or it may lead to serious complications.
- Vascular dysfunction can cause other diseases including Buerger's disease, subclavian steal syndrome, Raynaud's disease, thrombophlebitis, varicose veins, and venous stasis ulcers.

REVIEW QUESTIONS

1. Your patient is newly diagnosed with DVT of the right calf. The patient is also has a bleeding disorder. As the nurse, you know:
   1. Anticoagulant therapy may be contraindicated in patients with bleeding disorders.
   2. Anticoagulant therapy may be administered at half the usual dose.
   3. Anticoagulant therapy may be administered at two times the usual dose.
   4. Anticoagulant therapy may be administered at two times the usual rate.

2. A patient comes to the emergency center with symptoms of hoarseness, dysphagia, and tracheal displacement. You know these symptoms are most frequently related to:
   1. Cerebral aneurysm
   2. Aortic-renal aneurysm
   3. Thoracic-aortic aneurysm
   4. Abdominal-aortic aneurysm

3. Your patient, who takes warfarin (Coumadin) daily, is being discharged from the hospital today. As a part of your discharge teaching plan, you inform the patient he needs to immediately notify his health care provider if the following occurs:
   1. Consumes a serving of spinach, which contains Vitamin K
   2. Bleeding that continues longer than 10 minutes after pressure has been applied
   3. Receives a notice from the lab that his INR is 1.8
   4. Ate a spicy meal, then took an antacid after his noon meal to resolve indigestion

4. When a patient is being discharged on warfarin (Coumadin) therapy, which of the following statements is evidence that the patient understands the discharge teaching?
   1. Regular blood monitoring is needed.
   2. Moderate amounts of alcohol are OK.
   3. Aspirin can be used for joint pain.
   4. More spinach or broccoli is needed in diet.

Continued

REVIEW QUESTIONS—cont'd

5. Your patient is receiving warfarin (Coumadin) for treatment of a DVT. When you enter the patient's room you observe ecchymotic areas on his extremities, and he states his gums have been bleeding. Which nursing action is most appropriate?
   1. Administer his daily dose of warfarin, then notify the health care provider of the patient's status
   2. Administer the daily dose of warfarin. These are expected side effects.
   3. Hold the warfarin and notify the health care provider of the assessment findings
   4. Teach the patient to use a soft toothbrush and avoid injuries

6. The health care provider begins an IV infusion of t-PA. The nurse will be assessing for:
   1. Epistaxis
   2. Decreased pulse rate
   3. Increased blood pressure and restlessness
   4. Ankle edema

7. A patient is admitted to your unit with a diagnosis of DVT of the left leg and is on IV heparin. The nurse knows heparin is often used to treat DVT because it:
   1. Has an immediate effect and can be quickly reversed if needed
   2. Enhances clot formation caused by platelet aggregation in the arterial system
   3. Breaks down the clots formed in the venous circulation by stimulating fibrinolysis
   4. Suppresses the synthesis of the vitamin K dependent clotting factors preventing further clotting

8. Your patient has a venous ulcer. Which statement indicates the assessment data associated with these ulcers?
   1. Edema and pigmentation changes are not usually present around the area of the ulcer.
   2. Ulcers are characterized by irregular margins, ulcer beds are pink, and there is edema and swelling.
   3. Peripheral pulses are absent, edema is infrequent, and the ulcer is pink in color.
   4. Very painful necrotic, pale gray base and located in the heel, toes, or lateral malleolus

9. Which of the following signs and symptoms would be consistent with a diagnosis of pulmonary embolism?
   1. Fever, abdominal pain, and dyspnea
   2. Hypertension, chills, and painful cough
   3. Pleuritic chest pain, hemoptysis, and tachypnea
   4. Crackles in lungs, diminished heart sounds, and lethargy

10. Your patient had been diagnosed with several peripheral vascular diseases. Which of the following nursing diagnoses would be most appropriate for this patient?
    1. Sexual dysfunction
    2. Fluid volume deficit
    3. Ineffective airway clearance
    4. High risk for infections

REVIEW ACTIVITIES

1. According to Schuster (2002), concept maps are an innovative approach to care planning. It is essentially a map that assists the nurse to plan the care of the patient by diagramming the problems and interventions. It is a succinct visualizing process involving critical thinking, organization of data, and prioritization. All built on previous knowledge, the concept map is a holistic view of the patient and his or her situation. For this activity, develop a concept map for a patient admitted to your nursing unit with an AAA.

Continued

REVIEW ACTIVITIES—cont'd

2. List five to six characteristics of decreased oxygen, related to peripheral vascular disease.

3. When assessing a patient for readiness to be discharged home, what should be included in the nurse's assessment of the patient?

4. Develop a teaching plan for warfarin (Coumadin) administration.

5. List three NOC goals related to the following nursing diagnosis.

Hypertension: Nursing Management

Doris Denison, MSN, APRN, BC, CCRN

CHAPTER TOPICS

- Hypertension
- Risk Factors for Hypertension
- Management of Hypertension

Hypertension (elevated blood pressure) is a common chronic disorder that affects 65 million Americans. When left untreated, hypertension can lead to heart disease, kidney disease, and stroke. There is no cure; therefore lifestyle modifications and pharmacological therapy are necessary for **blood pressure** (the pressure against the flow of blood to or from the arteries or veins outside the chest) control. Treatment of hypertension must continue throughout life, making noncompliance a significant problem.

HYPERTENSION

Hypertension (high blood pressure) is a sustained elevation of systemic blood pressure to a level that places the patient at increased risk for target organ damage. These target organs include the eyes, brain, heart, kidneys, and great vessels. Hypertension has been called the silent disease, because there may be no initial symptoms. Patients may not be aware of their hypertension until it is identified on a routine assessment. However, many patients do not regularly see a health care provider and remain unaware of the dangers of untreated hypertension (Izzo & Black, 2003).

Epidemiology

Thirty percent of the U.S. population has hypertension (Fields, et al., 2004). This is a 23 percent increase from the year 2000. Worldwide, it is estimated, that as many as 1 billion individuals are living with hypertension, and 7.1 million deaths per year may be attributable to hypertension. In the United States 60 percent of the patients with a diagnosis of hypertension are being treated, but only approximately 35 percent are controlled at recommended levels. Much of the increased number of patients with hypertension can be attributed to the increasing problems of obesity and an aging population.

Etiology

Hypertension is characterized by type, cause, and severity. There are two major types of hypertension: primary (also called essential or idiopathic) and secondary. Approximately 90 percent of all the patients with hypertension have the primary type. The exact cause is unknown. The remaining 10 percent have the secondary type, which is related to or secondary to another disease. Some of the causes of secondary hypertension include renal artery narrowing, chronic kidney disease, hyperaldosteronism, pregnancy, and pheochromocytoma. Once the disease causing the hypertension is identified and treated successfully, the problem of hypertension is eliminated. Box 28-1 lists other potential causes of secondary hypertension (Woods, 2004).

Risk Factors

Primary hypertension results from a variety of nonmodifiable and modifiable risk factors. Nonmodifiable risk factors include family history, age, gender, and ethnicity. Modifiable risk factors include obesity, substance abuse, stress, diet, and sedentary lifestyle (see chapter 24). In general, the more risk factors a patient has, the greater the odds that they will be diagnosed with high blood pressure at some time during their life.

Nonmodifiable Risk Factors

There are several nonmodifiable risk factors (i.e., family history, age, gender, ethnicity) for developing hypertension. As the label implies, these are the variables that a person cannot change. Therefore, the nursing management related to these risk factors is to inform the patient of their relationship to hypertension. Because the patient can not change or modify their hypertension, these variables should not be emphasized.

Hypertension tends to run in families. If one parent has hypertension, there is a 25 percent chance of a patient developing it during his or her lifetime. When both parents have hypertension, the risk increases to 60 percent. Multiple studies have shown a genetic component in some families. However, the presence of hypertension in a family does not mean that all members will develop the disease. Even in families in which high blood pressure is prevalent, some blood relatives never develop hypertension. This may be because of environmental, lifestyle, or other factors, not yet identified (Berry & Shooner, 2004).

BOX 28-1

POTENTIAL CAUSES OF SECONDARY HYPERTENSION

Kidney
- Renal artery stenosis
- Chronic kidney disease
- Obstructive uropathy

Cardiac
- Congenital narrowing of the aorta

Endocrine
- Cushing syndrome
- Thyroid dysfunction
- Parathyroid disease
- Hyperaldosteronism
- Pheochromocytoma

Neurological
- Head trauma
- Brain tumor
- Spinal cord injury

Medications
- Sympathetic stimulants
- Monoamine oxidase inhibitors
- Estrogen therapy
- Nonsteroidal anti-inflammatory drugs (NSAIDs)

Sleep apnea

Pregnancy-induced hypertension

Detailed family histories can provide valuable evidence for familial transmission of high blood pressure. This information can aid in the diagnosis of the disease and the identification of other family members who may be at risk. For many patients and their relatives, lifestyle changes may make the difference between health and chronic illness. The stimulus to change behavior may be more powerful when people learn that they have a genetic susceptibility.

Blood pressure tends to rise with age. Primary hypertension typically appears between the ages of 30 and 50. Among all Americans age 65 and older, more than half have hypertension. Isolated systolic hypertension (ISH) occurs when the systolic blood pressure is 140 mm Hg or higher, but the diastolic blood pressure remains less than 90 mm Hg. The likelihood of developing ISH increases with advancing age. ISH occurs primarily in patients older than 50, with about one in four patients affected by age 80. The cause is believed to be loss of elasticity in the large arteries from atherosclerosis.

Among young- and middle-aged adults, men are more likely to have hypertension than women. After age 55, when most women are beyond menopause, high blood pressure is more common in women than in men.

Hypertension occurs more frequently in patients of African American descent than any other ethnic group in the United States. Among Americans age 18 and older, 32 percent of African Americans versus 23 percent of Caucasians have high blood pressure. The highest rates of hypertension in the United States occur among African Americans living in southeastern states. High blood pressure in African Americans generally develops at an earlier age, is more pronounced, and tends to progress more rapidly. Hispanic (Americans) and Native Americans develop hypertension at approximately the same rate as Caucasians.

Modifiable Risk Factors

There are a variety of modifiable risk factors for persons to develop hypertension (i.e., obesity, substance abuse, stress, diet, and sedentary lifestyle). These variables are the focus of patient teaching as related to controlling hypertension, as these factors can be modified by the patient.

Being overweight increases the risk for development of hypertension. There is a strong correlation between a gradual increase in body weight over a period of years and a concurrent increase in blood pressure. Body type strongly correlates with the development of hypertension. Upper body obesity (giving an apple shape) with increased amounts of subcutaneous fat about the midriff, waist, and abdomen, is associated with the development of high blood pressure. Patients who are overweight but carry the majority of the excess fat in the buttocks, hips, and thighs (giving them a pear shape) are at a lower risk for development of hypertension secondary to increased weight alone (Figure 28-1). Many times a loss of excess weight alone can return a slightly elevated blood pressure to normal.

Fat cells are the reason body shape makes a difference. Abdominal fat cells are larger than those deposited in the buttocks and thighs. The abdominal fat cells are more efficient at breaking down lipids into fatty acids. These fatty acids can travel directly along the portal vein to the liver. The flood of circulating fatty acids has many consequences. These include suppression of insulin breakdown, stimulation of the liver to release triglycerides, leading to atherosclerosis, and increased arterial sensitivity to the hormones that mediate blood vessel contractility, such as epinephrine.

Tobacco, caffeine, alcohol, and illicit drug use all have a negative impact on the development of hypertension. The chemicals in tobacco can damage the lining of the artery walls, making them more prone to the accumulation of plaques. Nicotine makes the heart work harder by temporarily constricting blood

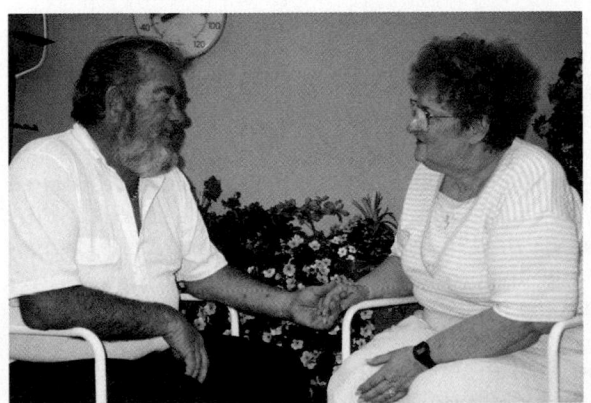

Figure 28-1 Two overweight persons who are at risk for developing hypertension.

Uncovering the Evidence

Obesity in America

Discussion: Evaluation of data gathered by the Centers for Disease Control and Prevention in the continuous survey known as the National Health and Nutrition Examination Survey (NHANES). The NHANES is a cross-sectional survey of civilian noninstitutionalized U.S. population using a complex, stratified, multistage probability cluster sampling design. There were 4,115 adult men and women involved in the study.

From 1988 to 1994, there were 97 million overweight adults in the United States. In the time period between 1999 and 2000, there were 120 million overweight adults. This is approximately a 24 percent increase in 10 years. The rates for being overweight and obese have increased for both genders, all age-groups, and all ethnic groups.

Study Purpose: To examine trends and prevalences of overweight and obesity, using measured height and weight data.

Implications for Practice: Excess weight is second only to smoking as a leading cause of preventable death in the United States. About 300,000 deaths per year are associated with excess weight and 430,000 deaths per year are associated with cigarette smoking. The increasing prevalence of obesity calls for more efficient prevention and treatment to become a high priority in public health.

Source: Flegal, K., Carroll, M., Ogden, C., & Johnson, C. (2002). Prevalence and trends in obesity among US adults, 1999–2000. Journal of the American Medical Association, 288, 1723–1727.

---

vessels and increasing heart rate and blood pressure. These effects are due to increased levels of epinephrine (adrenaline) during tobacco use. In addition, carbon monoxide in tobacco smoke, replaces the oxygen in the blood, forcing the heart to work harder to supply oxygen to the organs and tissues (Bialous & Sarna, 2004).

Caffeine intake raises blood pressure initially but adaptation by the body to its effects occurs quickly. Clinical trials lasting an average of 56 weeks have demonstrated a persistent relationship between caffeine intake and an increase in blood pressure. In other clinical trials with patients known to have hypertension, cessation of caffeine intake lowers blood pressure.

Excessive alcohol consumption contributes to as much as 20 percent of all the cases of high blood pressure. Consuming three or more alcoholic drinks a day doubles the risk of developing hypertension. The exact mechanism is not fully understood, but it is known that heavy drinking can damage the heart and other organs. The end organ damage from excessive alcohol intake puts the patient at risk for development of hypertension.

Illicit drug use, such as cocaine and amphetamines, increases the risk of developing hypertension. The use of such drugs narrows the arteries that supply blood to the heart, increasing the heart rate and damaging the heart muscle.

Stress does not cause high blood pressure, but a continuous high level of stress can dramatically increase it. If the stress continues at a high level for a long time, damage to the blood vessels, heart, and kidneys can occur. Stress can influence behavior by causing the development of unhealthy habits such as tobacco use, excessive alcohol intake, overeating, or illicit drug use. The physiological response to stress is an increase in **peripheral vascular resistance** (**[PVR]** the pressure against the flow of blood to or from the arteries or veins outside the chest), increased cardiac output, and stimulation of the sympathetic nervous system. Over time hypertension can develop.

The typical diet throughout the industrialized nations of the world contains too much fat and salt. The advent of convenience foods and fast foods over the last 50 plus years has played a large part in the calorie-rich, nutrition-poor dietary intake of the average person in the United States. These foods contain high levels of refined carbohydrates and elevated saturated fat. This is what makes them taste good. Cholesterol is one of the saturated fats. It is both manufactured by your body and a part of the typical American diet. Cholesterol is absolutely essential for a healthy body. It is necessary for cellular membrane synthesis and the building of essential hormones in the body. However, elevated levels of cholesterol promote the development of plaques in the arteries (atherosclerosis), causing them to narrow and be less able to dilate. These changes can increase the blood pressure (Champagne, 2006). When exposed to high sodium levels, not all people develop hypertension, only about half of the population. The human body needs a certain amount of sodium to maintain proper cell chemistry. People who are sodium sensitive and retain sodium more easily have problems because retaining sodium leads to fluid retention and elevated blood pressure.

Long work hours, modern conveniences, and a shortage of leisure time are a few of the reasons that Americans have become increasingly sedentary. According to the American Heart Association, only 27 percent of the population age 18 or older exercise enough for cardiovascular fitness. Physical activity is critical to controlling hypertension, because it makes the heart stronger. A stronger heart is able to pump more blood with less effort. Regular physical activity can lower blood pressure by 5 to 10 mm Hg.

Pathophysiology

The pressure required to move blood throughout the body, per minute is provided by the pumping action of the heart muscle, known as **cardiac output (CO)** and the PVR. Several body systems assist with controlling blood pressure by keeping it from rising too high or falling too low. These systems include: cardiovascular, renal, endocrine, and nervous.

When the heart releases blood into the main artery (aorta), the surge of blood creates pressure against the vessel walls. The harder the heart muscle has to work, the greater the pressure exerted on the artery walls. The blood pressure measured at the moment of contraction is the **systolic blood pressure.** The pressure measured when the ventricles are relaxed is called **diastolic blood pressure. Pulse pressure** is the difference between the systolic and diastolic pressures. A blood pressure of 122/78 has a pulse pressure of 44.

Blood pressure in the arteries closest to the heart is greatest and gradually decreases as the blood travels further away from the heart. The arteries are lined with smooth muscle that allows for expansion and contraction as the blood moves through them. The more elastic the arteries are, the less resistant they are to the flow of blood, and therefore less force is exerted on the walls. When arteries lose their elasticity or they become narrowed, resistance to blood flow increases and additional force is needed to push the blood through the vessels. The increased force can contribute to the development of hypertension.

The blood carries the accumulated cellular waste to the kidneys, where the nephrons filter out what can be recycled and dispose of the unwanted waste. The kidneys filter approximately one and one-half quarts per minute. Larger blood cells (red and white cells) and large chemical compounds are not filtered. Once waste products are filtered, the recyclable materials are reabsorbed. This includes 99 percent of the desired water, sodium, and other vital body elements. The whole process requires sufficient pressure to force the fluid through the filtering system. When blood pressure falls, the glomerular filtration rate (GFR) falls as well, and promotes the retention of sodium, chloride, and water. Sodium and water retention increases the blood volume and venous return to the heart, causing an increased CO and raising the systemic blood pressure (Rizzo, 2006).

To maintain adequate glomerular filtering pressure, the kidney has a backup system. The renin-angiotensin-aldosterone system is part of the hormonal control of blood pressure. The juxtaglomerular cells of the kidney release renin in response to reduced GFR, reduced blood volume, reduced blood pressure, and stimulation of β_1-adrenergic receptors on the cell surface.

Once renin is released it promotes the conversion of angiotensinogen to angiotensin I, a weak vasoconstrictor. Then, angiotensin-converting enzyme (ACE) acts on angiotensin I to form angiotensin II, a potent systemic vasoconstrictor, thus increasing blood pressure and PVR. Constriction of the renal blood vessels elevates blood pressure by reducing the GFR, which causes the retention of salt and water. Angiotensin II also causes the release of aldosterone, which acts on the kidneys to further increase retention of sodium and water (Rizzo, 2006).

An increase in the blood sodium osmolarity level stimulates the release of antidiuretic hormone (ADH) from the posterior pituitary gland. Antidiuretic hormone increases the extracellular fluid volume by promoting the reabsorption of water in the distal and collecting tubules of the kidneys. This causes an increase in blood volume and can cause elevated blood pressure.

Stimulation of the sympathetic nervous system results in the release of epinephrine (adrenaline) along with a small amount of norepinephrine by the adrenal medulla. Epinephrine increases cardiac output by raising the heart rate and increasing cardiac contractility. It activates the β_2 receptors of the skeletal muscle, causing vasodilation and the α_1 receptors of the skin and kidneys, causing vasoconstriction.

Within the walls of the heart, carotid arteries, and aortic arch are tiny node-like structures called baroreceptors. These structures continuously monitor the pressure in the arteries and veins. When a change in pressure is sensed, a signal is sent to the brain to either slow down or speed up the heart rate or dilate or constrict the blood vessels to keep the blood pressure within a normal range. The baroreceptors have an important role in the maintenance of blood pressure stability during normal activities. The walls of the arteries and veins have a single cell layer called the endothelium. By excreting vasoactive substances and growth factors that cause the blood vessels to constrict or dilate, the endothelium plays a crucial role in regulating blood pressure. A gas, called nitric oxide, present in arteries and blood, can also affect blood pressure. It signals the blood vessels to expand or vasodilate.

In the healthy person, the regulatory mechanisms function in response to the demands of the body. When hypertension develops, one or more of the blood pressure regulating mechanisms are malfunctioning. There is no way of predicting which patients will develop hypertension, but it is easy to detect high blood pressure. The major emphasis in the control of hypertension should be on early detection and effective treatment.

Assessment with Clinical Manifestations

Hypertension has been called the silent killer, because often the patient remains without symptoms until the blood pressure is severely elevated and target organ damage has already occurred. When symptoms do develop, they are secondary to damage of the blood vessels, various organs, and tissues or due to the increased workload on the heart. Secondary symptoms include fatigue, dizziness, angina, palpitations, and dyspnea. Some individuals with high blood pressure do not experience any clinical manifestations. Headache is the most commonly reported symptom. With elevated blood pressure, the headaches become more frequently reported as present on waking. The headache is felt in the back of the head, may or may not be reported as throbbing, and often last for only a few hours even when no analgesics are taken. One theory related to these headaches is that many patients with hypertension also suffer from sleep apnea, so early morning headaches may reflect nocturnal hypoxia and not high blood pressure.

The Joint National Committee on Prevention, Detection, Evaluation, and Treatment of High Blood Pressure (JNC VII) issued new guidelines, for the classification of hypertension, in 2003. The classification is based on the average of two or more properly measured, seated blood pressure readings on each of two

TABLE 28-1 JNV VII Classification of Blood Pressure in Adults

CLASSIFICATION	SYSTOLIC PRESSURE	DIASTOLIC PRESSURE
Normal	Less than or equal to 120 mm Hg	Less than or equal to 80 mm Hg
Prehypertension	120–139 mm Hg	80–90 mm Hg
Stage 1 hypertension	140–159 mm Hg	90–99 mm Hg
Stage 2 hypertension	Greater than or equal to 160 mm Hg	Greater than or equal to 100 mg Hg

Source: Cuddy, M. (2005). Treatment of hypertension: Guidelines from JNC 7 (The Seventh Report of the Joint National Committee on Prevention, Detection, Evaluation, and Treatment of High Blood Pressure). Journal of Practical Nursing, 55(4), 1–23.

or more separate occasions. Normal blood pressure is defined as systolic blood pressure less than 120 mm Hg and diastolic blood pressure less than 80 mm Hg (Table 28-1). Hypertension is a systolic blood pressure of 140 mm Hg or more and diastolic blood pressure of 90 mm Hg or more. Prehypertension is a new designation used to identify individuals at high risk for the development of hypertension. These individuals should be strongly advised to implement healthy lifestyle modifications to reduce the risk of developing high blood pressure in the future. The classification system does not address the presence or absence of risk factors or target organ damage (Cuddy, 2005).

The health history should include patient's health history, family history, risk factors, dietary intake, and psychosocial characteristics that might influence their response to hypertension or its treatment. A careful family history can provide valuable information related to family members with hypertension or end organ damage from hypertension. The nurse should review all of the risk factors for hypertension with the patient. A thorough dietary review includes assessing for adequate sodium, potassium, and calcium intake. This is also an ideal method of assessing for some lifestyle habits pertinent to diet. A diet that has several meals a week that are fast food or convenience foods may be a reflection of a highly stressful job or long hours at work.

Medications for the treatment of other complaints may negatively influence blood pressure. A thorough list of both prescription and over-the-counter (OTC) medicines should be obtained, including dose, frequency, and length of time using.

When reviewing the patient's psychosocial history, the nurse may be able to identify any lifestyle factors that may interfere with effective disease management. A job that requires travel or shift work may make compliance with a treatment regimen difficult. The presence or absence of a strong support system should also be assessed. Cultural or religious beliefs can also make it difficult to implement lifestyle changes. Some patients may have difficulty coping with the lifestyle changes needed to control high blood pressure. The nurse should assess the patient's past coping strategies.

Financial limitations can adversely affect treatment plans. If the patient must choose between eating and paying for medications, prescriptions may not be filled in a timely manner. A referral to social work for assistance options may assist with this. The education level can affect the patient's ability to understand his or her disease or follow a treatment plan. The nurse should assess the patient's ability to learn and retain information and tailor teaching to his or her specific needs (Box 28-2).

The physical examination of the patient should include an assessment of the patient's overall appearance. Measurement of height, weight, and waist circumference can assist in diagnosing hypertension. Obese patients have an

---

BOX 28-2

HYPERTENSION ASSESSMENT

The nurse can ask the following questions to query the patient for hypertension:

- Have you ever been told that your blood pressure was elevated? When?
- Have you ever been told that you have heart disease? When? What type?
- Are there any problems with your kidneys?
- Have you been told that you have thyroid disease? Diabetes? Pituitary problems?
- Do you use nicotine products? How much? How long?
- Do you consume alcohol products? How much? How long?
- Have you ever used any recreational drugs (cocaine, marijuana, crack, or heroin)?
- Are you currently taking medication to control your blood pressure? If yes, what?
- Have you taken blood pressure medications in the past? If yes, what? Why did you stop?
- Do any other members of your family have a history of hypertension or heart disease?
- Do you experience frequent fatigue or nosebleeds?
- Recall the last 24-hour dietary intake for sodium, potassium, and fat content.
- Have you recently gained or lost weight?
- Do you get short of breath or have a rapid heart rate with exertion?
- Have you ever had a headache behind your eyes (especially in the morning)?
- Do you ever experience dizziness, blurred vision, or numbness or tingling in your hands or feet?

---

increased risk of hypertension, and those with abdominal obesity have a greater risk than those with excess fat in their hips and thighs. As the nurse continues, the physical examination should include vital signs (temperature, pulse, and respiratory rate), neurological status, head and neck (retina, neck, and thyroid), heart, lungs, abdomen, extremities, and peripheral pulses. A full physical assessment is useful in detecting several conditions that produce secondary hypertension (Estes, 2006). There are many factors that can distort blood pressure readings (Table 28-2). In addition, the nurse should always take blood pressure measurements following the fundamental steps to ensure accurate readings (Artinian, 2004).

Diagnostic Tests

Basic laboratory and diagnostic studies do not detect hypertension, but they are useful for identifying the systemic effects of elevated blood pressure and any secondary causes.

Table 28-3 lists the tests and potential end organ damage. Serum electrolyte levels, especially sodium and potassium, are important as a baseline to assist with diagnosis and follow-up during treatment. Low serum potassium may indicate hyperaldosteronism. High potassium may indicate kidney damage. Blood glucose levels should be evaluated for possible diabetes mellitus. A fasting lipid profile may indicate hyperlipidemia, which can lead to arterial atherosclerosis and plaque formation. Serum creatinine and blood urea nitrogen (BUN) tests can help in the identification of kidney damage. About 50 percent of the patients with hypertension have normal plasma renin activity. Measurement of plasma renin activity can assist in the identification of kidney dysfunction. Routine urinalysis for albuminuria can assist in the identification of kidney damage or diabetes mellitus (Daniels, 2003).

Nursing Diagnoses

Based on the information gathered, examples of nursing diagnoses in the patient with hypertension may include the following:

- Altered health maintenance R/T lack of knowledge of pathology, complications, and management of hypertension.
- Fatigue R/T altered body chemistry (medications).

TABLE 28-2 **Factors Causing False Blood Pressure Readings**

PATIENT	EXAMINER
Arrhythmias	Hearing impairment
Anxiety	Vision impairment
Full urinary bladder	Knowledge of previous reading
Conversation	Knowledge of treatment
Pain	Procedural error
Medications	**EQUIPMENT**
Posture	
Time of day	Incorrect cuff size
Recent tobacco use	Inflation system leak
Recent physical activity	Defective stethoscope
Recent consumption of large meal	Won Velcro closing system
Recent consumption of caffeine	Ripped cuff fabric

ENVIRONMENT

Cold room
Excessively warm room
Load noises
Repetitive noises

Adapted from Artinian, N. (2004). Innovations in blood pressure monitoring. American Journal of Nursing, 104(8), 52–59; Estes, M. (2006). Health assessment and physical examination (3rd ed.). New York: Thomson Delmar Learning.

TABLE 28-3 **Screening Tests for Secondary Hypertension**

TEST	POTENTIAL DIAGNOSIS
Estimated GFR	Chronic kidney disease
Doppler flow study, MRA	Renal artery stenosis
CT angiography	Congenital narrowing of the aorta
Dexamethasone suppression test	Cushing syndrome
24-hour urinary metanephrine	Pheochromocytoma
24-hour urinary aldosterone	Primary aldosteronism
TSH	Thyroid dysfunction
PTH	Parathyroid disease
Drug screening	Medication induced
Sleep study with O_2 saturation	Sleep apnea

Adapted from Daniels, R. (2003). Delmar's manual of laboratory and diagnostic tests. New York: Thomson Delmar Learning.

- Ineffective coping R/T effects of chronic illness and major changes in lifestyle.
- Ineffective sexuality patterns related to side effects of medications.
- Risk for ineffective therapeutic regimen management R/T noncompliance with treatment.

Planning and Implementation

There are a wide variety of nursing measures to implement in the control of hypertension. Nurses must work together with the interdisciplinary health care team to decrease the hypertension problems of their patients. In the acute care settings, there are often many crises related to hypertension and early interventions that may decrease further development of critical problems associated with uncontrolled hypertension (e.g., cerebrovascular accidents, aneurysm ruptures, or renal pathology).

Evidence-Based Care

There are a number of nursing measures for controlling hypertension that are supported strongly in the literature. These measures can be labeled lifestyle modifications and have positive correlations with reducing hypertension in patients. These modifications include weight reduction; moderating alcohol, caffeine, and sodium intake; smoking cessation; stress reduction; and regular exercise.

Weight loss of as little as 10 pounds has been shown to reduce blood pressure or prevent hypertension in many overweight individuals. The ideal is to maintain normal body weight. Maintaining a normal body mass index is associated with reduced blood pressure. **Body mass index (BMI)** is a formula using weight and height to determine the percentage of total body fat. The formula does not differentiate between men and women. A BMI of 18.5 to 24.9 is considered healthy. A BMI of 25 to 29.9 indicates the patient is overweight, and a BMI of 30 or more indicates obesity. Waist circumference, used in combination with the patient's BMI

Skills 360°

Behaviors to Help with Achieving and Maintaining Weight Loss

- Make a commitment. There needs to be a strong motivation to lose weight. Seek out support from health care providers, family, and friends.
- Think positively. Concentrate on the positive successes, not on slip-ups. Avoid negative reenforcement situations.
- Get priorities straight. It takes a lot of mental and physical energy to change lifelong habits. Do not try losing weight if distracted by other major problems such as financial difficulties, death of family members, or marriage difficulties.
- Set realistic goals. Set weekly or monthly goals that allow for frequent monitoring of progress. A good weight loss plan generally involves losing no more than one to two pounds per week. Aim for a weight loss that improves blood pressure, blood sugar, and blood cholesterol levels.
- Know personal habits. Keep a log of emotions or situations that cause overeating. List what is eaten, when it is eaten, and reason for eating. A review of the information may identify relationships or patterns of overeating.
- Substitute healthy behaviors. Before eating impulsively, ask if the item is really wanted. Learn to say no without feeling guilty. Stay committed to the long-term weight loss goal. Use distraction as a means of avoiding impulse eating. When feeling stressed or angry, redirect the energy into something constructive (take a walk or clean a closet.).
- Change gradually. Change one behavior at a time. Practice the new behavior until it becomes a habit. After successfully changing that behavior, move on to another.
- Do not starve. Extremely low-calorie diets and special food combinations are not the answer to long-term weight control. The best way to lose weight is to eat nutritious foods and change eating habits.

is another important component for evaluating weight. As previously discussed, abdominal fat is associated with an increased risk of hypertension. To measure waist circumference, locate the highest point on both hip bones, and measure the abdomen just above these points (Janssen, Katzmarzyk, & Ross, 2004). A measurement of more than 40 inches (102 centimeters) in men and 35 inches (88 centimeters) in women significantly increases the risk of hypertension. A BMI of 25 to 29.9 and a waist circumference equal to or exceeding the guidelines indicates a need to lose weight. If the BMI is 30 or more, losing weight will not only improve health, but it will also reduce the risk of future illness. Many books, products, and programs promise to help individuals to lose weight. The best way to lose weight and keep it off is through lifestyle changes. Behaviors to help with achieving and maintaining weight loss are shown in the Skills 360° feature.

The JNC VII strongly recommends adopting the dietary approaches to stop hypertension (DASH) eating plan (Table 28-4). The DASH diet is rich in grains, fruits, vegetables, and low-fat dairy products. The plan limits fat, satu-

TABLE 28-4   Dietary Approaches to Stop Hypertension (DASH)

FOOD	DAILY SERVINGS	SERVING EXAMPLES
Grains	7 to 8	½ cup (3 oz/90 g) cooked cereal, rice, or pasta ½ cup (1 oz/30 g) ready-to-eat cereal 1 slice whole-wheat sandwich bread ½ bagel or English muffin
Fruits and vegetables	8 to 10	¼ cup (1½ oz/45 g) raisins or dried fruit ¾ cup (6 fl oz/180 mL) 100 percent fruit or vegetable juice 12 grapes 1 medium apple or banana ½ cup fresh, frozen, or canned fruit 1 cup (2 oz/60 g) raw leafy green vegetables ½ cup (3 oz/90 g) cooked vegetables 1 medium potato
Dairy products	2 to 3	1 cup (8 fl oz/250 ml) 1 percent or fat-free milk 1 cup (8 oz/250 g) low-fat yogurt 2 cups (16 oz/500 g) 2 percent or fat-free cottage cheese 1½ oz (45 g) reduced-fat or fat-free cheese
Meat, poultry, and fish	2 or fewer	2 to 3 oz (60 to 90 g) cooked skinless poultry, seafood, or lean meat
Fats	2½	1 tsp oil, butter, margarine, or mayonnaise 1 tbsp regular salad dressing 2 tbsp light salad dressing
	WEEKLY SERVINGS	
Nuts, seeds, or legumes	4 to 5	⅓ cup (1 oz/30 g) nuts or legumes ¼ cup (1 oz/30 g) seeds ⅓ cup (3 1/2 oz/105 g) cooked legumes 3 oz (90 g) tofu
Sweets	4 to 5	1 tbsp sugar 1 tbsp jam or jelly ½ oz jelly beans 8 oz lemonade

Adapted from Champagne, C. (2006). Dietary interventions on blood pressure: The Dietary Approaches to Stop Hypertension (DASH) Trials. Prevention of Nutrition-Related Chronic Diseases: Scientific Foundations and Community Interventions. Fifth Nestle Nutrition Conference, Mexico City, Mexico, October 7–8, 2004. Nutrition Reviews, 64(2 Part 2), S53–56; Roth, R. (2007). Nutrition and diet therapy (9th ed.). New York: Thomson Delmar Learning.

rated fat, and cholesterol while providing plentiful amounts of fiber, potassium, calcium, and magnesium. Multiple research studies have shown a reduction in blood pressure of 8 to 14 mm Hg in patients with hypertension, who follow the DASH diet.

Excessive alcohol intake increases blood pressure, and the calories have no nutritional value. Moderation is the best method for controlling alcohol intake. Alcohol reduces blood glucose levels in patients with diabetes mellitus and increases lipid levels in patients with cardiovascular disease. Recent research studies have shown that one to two glasses of red wine per day may protect the heart. An average-weight man should drink no more than 1 ounce of ethanol per day. That means 24 ounces of beer, 10 ounces of wine, or 3 ounces of 80-proof whiskey. Women and underweight men are more susceptible to the effects of alcohol and therefore, should restrict their intake to half of the amount recommended for the average-weight man.

Caffeine consumption is another negative variable in the development of hypertension. Reducing caffeine intake starts with knowledge of where and how much caffeine is being consumed. Table 28-5 identifies multiple sources and the amount of caffeine they contain. Individuals with high blood pressure should limit caffeine to about 200 mg on a daily basis. When reducing caffeine

TABLE 28-5 **Caffeine Sources**	
SOURCE AMOUNT	
Coffee ¾ cup (6 fl oz/180 mL)	
Brewed, drip	103 mg
Instant	57 mg
Decaffeinated	2 mg
Espresso (single shot)	
Regular	100 mg
Decaffeinated	5 mg
Tea ¾ cup (6 fl oz/180 mL)	
Black (brewed 3 minutes)	40 mg
Instant	30 mg
Decaffeinated	1 mg
Soft drinks 1½ cups (12 fl oz/360 mL)	
Cola (regular and diet)	31 to 70 mg
Noncola	0 to 55 mg
Chocolate	
Cocoa powder 1 tbsp	10 mg
Baking chocolate 1 oz (30 g)	25 mg
Chocolate milk 1 cup (8 fl oz/250 ml)	10 mg
Milk chocolate bar 1½ oz (45 g)	10 mg
Medications	
Fiorinal	40 to 80 mg
Excedrin Migraine	65 to 130 mg
Midol	60 to 120 mg
Vanquish	33 to 66 mg
Vivarin	200 mg

Adapted from Roth, R. (2007). Nutrition and diet therapy (9th ed.). New York: Thomson Delmar Learning.

BOX 28-3

SOURCES OF SODIUM

- Drinking water: 1 percent.
- Cooking salt and salt added at the table: 11 percent.
- Naturally found in food: 11 percent.
- Commercially processed foods: 75 percent.

intake, the best method is to taper the amount over several weeks. This helps to avoid headaches and other side effect that can happen with sudden withdrawal.

Sodium consumption is positively correlated with hypertension. The majority of sodium intake is from food, and many foods naturally contain some sodium. Most sodium ingestion comes from commercially processed foods and meal preparation at home (Box 28-3).

Human beings need about one-fourth teaspoon (500 mg) of sodium each day. It has been estimated that the average daily intake of sodium for individuals in the United States is between 4,000 and 6,000 mg. The kidneys usually control the amount of sodium in the body, but when there is kidney dysfunction, sodium accumulates, attracts water, increases the blood volume, and raises the blood pressure. Sodium restriction may be enough to control hypertension in many patients. Patients with low renin activity, such as African Americans and older adults, may be salt sensitive. These patients may benefit the most from restriction of sodium intake. Patients should consume less than 2,400 mg of sodium per day. The best method to help patients reduce their sodium intake is to remove the salt shaker from the table and the stove and learn to read the food labels for sodium content (Jurgens & Graudal, 2006). Table 28-6 describes sodium-based food additives.

Tobacco intake is positively linked to hypertension. Approximately 30 percent of patients with hypertension smoke cigarettes or use other tobacco products (chewing tobacco and snuff). Patients with high blood pressure, who also use tobacco products, are two to three times more likely to develop cardiovascular disease. They have an increased risk of dying from myocardial infarction (MI), heart failure, or stroke. Exposure to secondhand smoke, also called environmental tobacco smoke, is also a serious health hazard. In the United States, more than 50,000 nonsmokers die of cardiovascular disease caused by secondhand smoke each year.

Stopping the use of tobacco products may only reduce blood pressure by a small amount. Smoking cessation is important for several reasons: prevention of interference with some blood pressure medications and decreasing the risk of developing cardiovascular disease. By the end of one year of not smoking, the risk of MI is reduced by 50 percent and after 5 years, the risk is the same as individuals who have never smoked. After 10 to 15 years, the risk of cancer (lung and others) is the same as the nonsmoking population (Mitchell & Parish, 2005).

The most effective smoking cessation program combines education, counseling, social support, and medications. Education comes in many ways for smok-

TABLE 28-6 Sodium-Based Food Additives

ADDITIVE	USES	SOURCES
Salt (sodium chloride)	Cooking, canning, preserving	"At the table"
Monosodium glutamate (MSG)	Flavor enhancer	Home and restaurant cooking; canned or frozen food
Baking soda (sodium bicarbonate)	Leavening agent for bread or cakes	Alkalizer for indigestion
Baking powder	Mixture of baking soda, starch, and acid	Quick breads and cakes
Disodium phosphate	Quick cooking cereals	Processed cheeses
Sodium alginate	Used as an emulsifier	Chocolate milk and ice cream
Sodium benzoate	Used as a preservative	Relishes; sauces; salad dressings
Sodium hydroxide	Used in food processing	Ripe olives, fruits, vegetables
Sodium nitrate	Used as a preservative	Cured meats; sausages
Sodium propionate	Used as a mold inhibitor	Pasteurized cheese; breads; cakes
Sodium sulfite	Used to bleach fruits	Artificial coloring; preservative in some dried fruits

Adapted from Roth, R. (2007). Nutrition and diet therapy (9th ed.). New York: Thomson Delmar Learning.

ing cessation. The media (magazines, television, and radio) contain frequent advertisements giving rationale for smoking cessation. Information can also be found on the Internet. Hospitals, clinics, and the offices of health care providers have pamphlets and other printed materials encouraging smoking cessation.

Counseling should be included in every encounter with a health care provider. Social support from family and friends can be of great benefit to patients attempting to stop smoking. Formal support groups are often helpful. Medication has proven to be effective in helping patients to stop smoking. There are two classes of medications, nicotine-replacement therapy and smoking cessation aids, used to treat tobacco dependence (Table 28-7).

Common nicotine withdrawal symptoms include cravings, weight gain, insomnia, irritability, depression, frustration, anger, anxiety, difficulty concentrating, and restlessness. The symptoms are most intense during the first 24 to 48 hours and gradually decline over two to three weeks. However, the desire to smoke may persist for months or years. Remission and relapse are common, and smoking cessation may require multiple attempts (Prochazka, Kick, Steinbrunn, Miyoshi & Fryer, 2004).

Stress is another variable that has a positive correlation on the development of hypertension. The lower the stress level the less likely patients are to overeat, use tobacco, and drink alcohol excessively; these are all factors known to cause hypertension. A variety of relaxation techniques are available. Some require nothing more than the desire to find new methods of relaxing. Other strategies may require the assistance or teaching by a professional. Some of these techniques include exercise programs, meditation, yoga, Tai chi, progressive muscle relaxation, deep breathing, biofeedback, massage, guided imagery, and music therapy (Figure 28-2). Exercise programs such as walking, swimming, or riding a bike are useful in reducing stress. Meditation involves concentrated attention focused on one's inner state. Yoga is an ancient philosophy of the mind, body, and soul striving to be in harmony. Yoga therapy uses specific postures and sequences of postures to stretch or block areas of the body not in harmony. Tai chi involves almost weightless, fluid movements, with a focus on breathing, balance, and the concepts of empty and full. Progressive muscle relaxation involves the intentional tensing and relaxing of successive

TABLE 28-7 Medications for Smoking Cessation

FORM	SOURCE	ADVERSE EFFECT
Nicotine Replacement Therapy		
Gum Nicorette	OTC	Tachycardia; mild headache, sore mouth and throat; dyspepsia; nausea; hiccups; GI distress
Patches	Rx and OTC	Insomnia; abnormal dreams; pruritus; erythema; headache; nausea; vertigo
NicoDerm, Nicotrol nasal spray	Rx only	Insomnia; abnormal dreams; erythema; pruritus; headache; nausea; vertigo
Nicotrol inhalers	Rx only	Insomnia; abnormal dreams; pruritus; erythema; headache; nausea; vertigo
Nicotrol lozenges Commit	OTC	Tachycardia; mild headache; sore mouth and throat; dyspepsia; nausea; hiccups; GI distress
Smoking Cessation Aids		
Tricyclic antidepressants		
Bupropion (Zyban)	Rx only	Dizziness; headache; insomnia; nausea; sore mouth and throat
Nortriptyline (Pamelor)	Rx only	Dry mouth; sedation; constipation; tachycardia; insomnia; rash; GI distress

Adapted from Broyles, B. E., Reiss, B. S., & Evans, M. E. (2007). Pharmacological aspects of nursing care (7th ed.). New York: Thomson Delmar Learning; Spratto, G. R., & Woods, A. L. (2007). 2007 PDR nurse's drug handbook. New York: Thomson Delmar Learning.

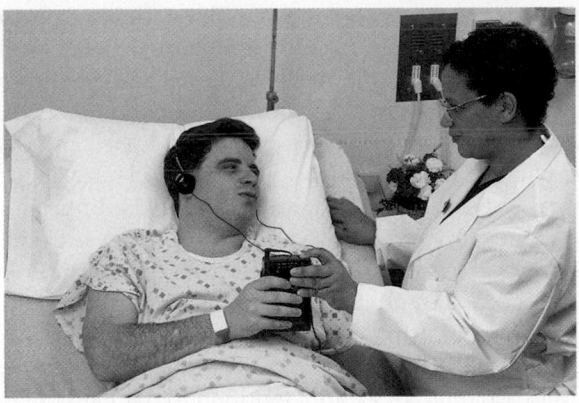

Figure 28-2 To help relieve the patient's stress and potentially lower his blood pressure, the nurse is providing him with music with which to listen.

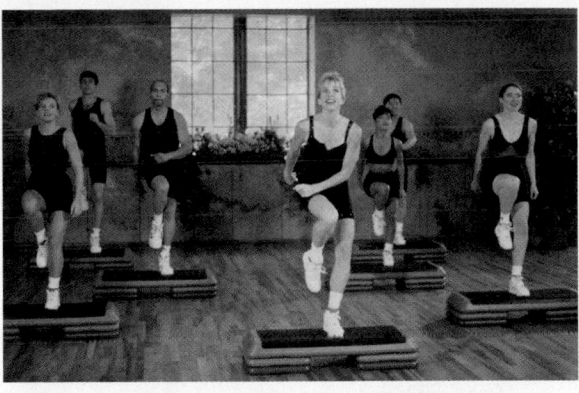

Figure 28-3 Exercise provides physiological and psychological benefits to individuals. Fitness centers are common places for persons to participate in organized aerobic activities. Courtesy of Photodisc.

muscle groups to promote relaxation and decrease anxiety. Deep breathing (also called diaphragmatic breathing) exercises have the individual focus on inhaling slowly until the lungs feel full, hold for six seconds, and exhale slowly. This increases mental alertness and reduces anxiety. Biofeedback involves applying physiological monitoring equipment, teaching the patient about muscle tension and its connection with peripheral blood flow, and training the patient to relax muscles in response to the machines feedback. Massage is the purposeful stroking and kneading of muscles to promote relaxation. Guided imagery involves experiencing a pleasant and peaceful setting or past event, while remaining still. All of these techniques can be recommended to help patients with life-stress management.

The JNC VII advises all patients who are physically able to participate in regular aerobic physical activity for at least 30 minutes a day, most days of the week (Figure 28-3). Exercise strengthens muscles and at the same time opens up arteries to allow for more nutrients and oxygen to flow into the tissues. The combination of a stronger, more efficient heart and blood vessels that are more open, leads to lower blood pressure (Cuddy, 2005).

It is not necessary to become an elite athlete to lower blood pressure. Moderate physical activities are beneficial to blood pressure and overall health, when done on a regular basis. Regular physical activity can lower blood pressure by 5 to 10 mm Hg. Regular exercise makes the heart stronger, allowing it to pump blood with less effort, this reduces the force exerted on the artery walls, and helps with weight loss. In addition to helping control blood pressure, regular exercise reduces the risk of MI, cerebrovascular accident (stroke), high cholesterol, diabetes, osteoporosis, and some cancers. The Department of Health and Human Services offers guidelines urging all Americans to become involved in regular physical activities. The federal guidelines recommend, as a minimum:

- Thirty to 60 minutes of moderate physical activity on at least five days a week.

  or

- Twenty minutes of vigorous physical activity at least three times a week.

There are three components to total fitness: aerobic activity, flexibility exercises, and strengthening exercises. Aerobic activities improve the heart and lung capacity. Flexibility exercises improve the elasticity of the joints. Strengthening exercises improve and maintain strong bones and muscle mass.

Aerobic activity has the greatest effect on controlling blood pressure. There are many aerobic activities (e.g., lawn mowing, climbing stairs, swimming, jogging, group sports). All patients with hypertension should request the approval from their primary health care provider before starting a regular exercise program. Begin the program at a lower level of intensity and gradually increase as

Staying Healthy in an Exercise Program

The nurse can instruct the patient to do the following to stay healthy while adhering to an exercise program:

- Drink plenty of water.
- Dress in loose fitting, comfortable clothing.
- Warm up before and cool down after exercise.
- Keep a regular routine for exercise.
- Avoid start-and-stop activities.
- Avoid the physical and emotional intensity of competitive sports.
- Wait two to three hours after a large meal before starting to exercise.
- Adapt activity to weather conditions.
- Avoid breathing carbon monoxide from heavy automobile traffic.
- Know the warning signs of MI and temperature-related illness.

Adapted from Daniels, R. (2004). Nursing fundamentals: Caring and clinical decision making. New York: Thomson Delmar Learning.

the body becomes more conditioned. Many individuals rush to start exercise programs, start at the maximum pace, and become injured or ill. Some activities may necessitate special equipment. Walking and jogging requires good shoes that support the feet. Bicycling requires a dependable bike, safety helmet, and pads for knees and elbows. There are a variety of exercise machines to help build aerobic capacity. These include stationary bicycle, rowing machine, treadmill, stair climber, cross-country skiing machine, and elliptical machines.

Getting started on an exercise program is the biggest challenge. Planning ahead makes starting easier. There several steps that help with planning, including setting simple goals, assembling any needed equipment, stretching before and after exercise, focusing on aerobic fitness, mixing activities, being flexible, building strength, and finding ways to stay motivated. Some things to help with staying healthy and avoiding injury are identified in the Patient Playbook feature.

Walking is a great exercise. It can be done at any time of day, it requires minimal equipment, and there are a wide variety of places to walk. If walking is not the activity of choice, the nurse can suggest many other activities (e.g., squash, racquetball, handball, judo, karate, rowing, soccer, rugby, or cricket). The specific exercise does not matter; it is the getting off the couch and doing regular exercise.

Collaborative Management

The goal for the collaborative management of high blood pressure is to prevent death and complications by achieving and maintaining a blood pressure of 140/90 or less. The optimal management plan should be inexpensive, simple, and cause the least amount of disruption in the patient's life. The JNC VII report recommends starting with nonpharmacological (lifestyle changes) methods and treat to goal. If the treatment goal is not reached, then pharmacological (medication) treatment should be started and titrated to goal. Management of high blood pressure begins with identification of the cause of the patient's hypertension (if possible) and its effect on the patient. A thorough history and physical examination is necessary. The health care provider needs to ask specific questions concerning blood pressure and any symptoms (as described in the Patient Playbook previously featured). Diagnostic studies should be done to rule out secondary causes of hypertension. Ultimately the goal for the treatment of hypertension is to reduce cardiovascular and renal morbidity and mortality. To achieve this goal the JNC VII has published clinical guidelines for the identification and management of hypertension (Table 28-8).

Pharmacology

When nonpharmacological management does not reduce the patient's blood pressure to goal, the health care provider may begin antihypertensive medications. The drugs currently available for treatment of hypertension work in one of two ways, reduction of the systemic vascular resistance (SVR) or decrease the volume of circulating blood. Diuretics promote the excretion of water (decrease the blood volume) and electrolytes by increasing the renal GFR. Vasodilating

TABLE 28-8	**Hypertension Identification and Follow-up**	
INITIAL BLOOD PRESSURE	**RECOMMENDED FOLLOW-UP**	**TREATMENT RECOMMENDATIONS**
Normal	Recheck in two years	None
Prehypertension	Recheck in one year	Lifestyle modifications
Stage 1 hypertension	Confirm within two months	Lifestyle modifications
Stage 2 hypertension	Re-evaluate in one month	Begin medications

Source: Cuddy, M. (2005). Treatment of hypertension: Guidelines from JNC 7 (The Seventh Report of the Joint National Committee on Prevention, Detection, Evaluation, and Treatment of High Blood Pressure). Journal of Practical Nursing, 55(4), 17–23.

drugs increase the diameter of the arterioles (reduce the SVR), by various mechanisms. More than two thirds of the patients with high blood pressure cannot be controlled by one drug and require two or more agents selected from different drug classes. The different classes of antihypertensive medications, their mechanism of action, and side effects, are described in Table 28-9.

Pharmacological therapy usually begins with a diuretic. Diuretics are divided into several classes: loop, potassium sparing, thiazide, and thiazide-like. Each class has a different mechanism of action. In 2002, the antihypertensive and lipid-lowering treatment to prevent heart attack trial (ALLHAT) study found that thiazide diuretics decreased morbidity and mortality better than ACE inhibitors or calcium channel blockers. Diuretics are the preferred treatment for isolated systolic hypertension in older adults (Kostis, et al., 2005). Aldosterone receptor blockers (such as spironolactone) prevent the effects of aldosterone on the kidneys. This allows the kidneys to remove the extra sodium and water.

TABLE 28-9 Pharmacologic Management of Hypertension

DRUG	ACTION	SIDE EFFECTS
Diuretics		
Thiazides		
Chlorthalidone (Hygroton)	Inhibits reabsorption of Na and Cl in proximal distal tubes	Low: K, Mgn, Na
Hydrochlorothiazide (Esidrix, HCTX)		High: Ca, glucose
Metolazone (Zaroxolyn)		Gout, hypotension, fatigue, $\downarrow$ libido
Chlorthalidone (Hygroton)		GI upset
Loops		
Furosemide (Lasix)	Inhibits reabsorption of Na and Cl in proximal distal tubes and the loop of Henle	Orthostatic hypotension
Bumetanide (Bumex)		Low: K, Mgn, Na, Ca
Torsemide (Demadex)		High: glucose
Ethacrynic acid (Edecrin)		gout, fatigue, $\downarrow$ libido
Potassium-sparing		
Spironolactone (Aldactone)	Inhibits aldosterone in distal tubules. Increases excretion of Na and H_2O. Decreases excretion of K+	Hyperkalemia; lethargy; hypotension, urticaria, agranulocytosis, $\downarrow$ libido
Triamterene (Dyrenium)		
Amiloride (Midamor)		
Aldosterone receptor blockers		
Eplerenone (Inspra)	Blocks the actions of ADH in the distal nephron; promotes renal excretion of sodium and water	Hyperkalemia; $\downarrow$ libido
Spironolactone (Aldactone)		
Sympatholytics		
Centrally acting α_2-agonists		
Methyldopa (Aldomet)	Suppresses CNS sympathetic outflow of the heart and blood vessels. Produces systemic vasodilation. $\downarrow$ SVR and BP	Dry mouth; sedation; rebound HTN; hemolytic anemia; liver disorders; sexual dysfunction
Clonidine (Catapres)		
Adrenergic neuron blockers		
Guanethidine (Ismelin)	Decreases SNS stimulation of the heart and blood vessels by inhibiting the release of norepinephrine	Severe orthostatic hypotension; dry mouth; rebound HTN; sedation; depression
Guanadrel (Hylorel)		
Reserpine (Serpasil)	Decreases SNS stimulation of the heart and blood vessels by depletion of norepinephrine	Depression; dry mouth; rebound HTN; sedation; nasal stuffiness
α_1 blockers		
Prazosin (Minipress)	Blocks α_1 receptors, causing peripheral vasodilation	Orthostatic hypotension; reflect tachycardia; nasal congestion; sodium and water retention; sexual dysfunction
Terazosin (Hytrin)		
Doxazosin (Cardura)	Thus $\downarrow$ BP and $\downarrow$ SVR	

Continued

TABLE 28-9	Pharmacologic Management of Hypertension—cont'd	
DRUG	**ACTION**	**SIDE EFFECTS**
Sympatholytics—cont'd		
Beta blockers		
Atenolol (Tenormin) Metoprolol (Lopressor) Nadolol (Corgard) Propranolol (Inderal) Timolol (Blocadren)	Beta blockade: ↓ HR, ↓ CO, ↓ SVR, and blocks renin release by the kidney	Bronchospasms; AV block; depression; bizarre dreams; insomnia; sexual dysfunction
Combined alpha and beta blockers		
Carvedilol (Coreg) Labetalol (Normodyne; Trandate)	Alpha blockade causes peripheral vasodilation; beta blockade ↓ HR and contractility	Postural hypotension; nasal congestions; bradycardia; ↓ CO; bronchospasms; insomnia; depression; impotence
Direct vasodilators		
Hydralazine (Apresoline) Minoxidil (Loniten)	Relaxation of arterial smooth muscles, thus ↓ BP and SVR	Tachycardia; sodium and water retention; SLE-like syndrome; headache; dizziness
Angiotensin Inhibitors		
ACE inhibitors		
Benazepril (Lotensin) Captopril (Capoten) Enalapril (Vasotec) Fosinopril (Monopril) Lisinopril (Prinivil; Zestril) Moexipril (Univasc) Perindopril (Aceon) Quinapril (Accupril)	Inhibit angiotensin-converting enzyme; prevent formation of angiotensin II; cause peripheral vasodilation; and suppress the effect of aldosterone	First-dose hypotension; rash; persistent dry cough; headache; angioedema; hyperkalemia; change in taste
Angiotensin II receptor blockers		
Candesartan (Atacard) Eprosartan (Teveten) Irbesartan (Avapro) Losartan (Cozaar) Olmesartan (Benicar) Telmisartan (Micardis) Valsartan (Diovan)	Directly block the action of angiotensin II; produces peripheral vasodilatation; decreases release of aldosterone	Headache; dizziness
Calcium Channel Blockers		
Dihydropyridines		
Amlodipine (Norvasc) Felodipine (Plendil) Isradipine (DynaCirc) Nifedipine (Procardia) Nisoldipine (Sular)	Blocks calcium movement into the cells; causes vascular dilatation, and reducing blood pressure	Reflex tachycardia; dizziness; flushing; headache; peripheral edema; gingival hyperplasia
Nondihydropyridines		
Diltiazem (Cardizem) Verapamil (Calan; Isoptin)	Blocks calcium movement into the cells; causing vasodilation, reducing blood pressure, and increasing coronary perfusion	Constipation; dizziness; facial flushing; headache; peripheral edema; gingival hyperplasia

Adapted from Broyles, B. E., Reiss, B. S., & Evans, M. E. (2007). Pharmacological aspects of nursing care (7th ed.). New York: Thomson Delmar Learning; Spratto, G. R., & Woods, A. L. (2007). 2007 PDR nurse's drug handbook. New York: Thomson Delmar Learning.

The sympatholytics (such as alpha and beta blockers) inhibit the sympathetic nervous system effects that elevate blood pressure. These drugs act either centrally on the vasomotor center, peripherally to inhibit norepinephrine release, or by blocking the receptors on the blood vessels.

Direct vasodilators relax the smooth muscle layer of the vessels, which reduces the SVR. Angiotensin inhibitors generally cause peripheral vasodilatation and suppress the effect of aldosterone. Specifically the ACE inhibitors block angiotensin-converting enzyme that prevents the formation of angiotensin II, causing the vasodilatation.

The angiotensin II receptor blockers (ARBs) directly block angiotensin II at the cellular receptor sites, causing vasodilatation. Calcium channel blockers vasodilate the arteries by interfering with the movement of extracellular calcium into the cells.

Patient and Family Teaching

The role of the nurse in blood pressure management is assessment, education, and supporting the needs of the patient. Assessment begins with the initial screening and documentation of elevated blood pressure. Taking a thorough health history and performing a complete physical examination help with the identification of concurrent diseases and risk factors specific to the patient. The nurse needs to teach the patient and family members the pathophysiology of hypertension, what tests will be performed to assist with the diagnosis, and interpret the test results. If the patient is identified as having normal blood pressure or prehypertension, teaching of lifestyle changes may help prevent or delay the development of hypertension. Patients can be taught to observe for changes in their blood pressure, such as **orthostatic hypotension** (hypotension occurring when changing position from supine to upright) and **pulsus paradoxus** (pathological decrease in systolic blood pressure by 10 mm Hg or more on inspiration) and to report those changes to their health care providers.

Once a diagnosis of hypertension is made, and lifestyle changes do not keep the patients blood pressure below 140/90, medications are usually started. The nurse plays an important role by teaching the medication regimen including the name of all medications, the mechanism of action, ongoing monitoring, and any potential side effects (Figure 28-4). The use of handouts or pamphlets gives the patient and family materials they can refer to if there are further questions. Teaching should include how to measure their blood pressure and pulse at least once a week and to keep a record for follow-up appointments. Instruct the patient to inform his or her health care provider of sudden changes in either blood pressure or pulse. In addition, patients need to be taught that they cannot suddenly stop taking their antihypertensive medications, or they run the risk of developing **rebound hypertension** (rapid increase in blood pressure after abrupt stopping of medication). Also, patients must be taught to not take too much of their antihypertensive medications or the complication of **hypotension** is likely to occur (blood pressure lower than needed for adequate tissue perfusion and oxygenation).

Whether the patient is newly diagnosed with hypertension or has been treated for an extended period, emotional support is extremely important. The nurse needs to educate and support the patient and family as they adjust to the lifestyle changes that are required. Teaching should address the physical, emotional, and social aspects of the disease. Depression is often a side effect of chronic diseases, such as hypertension. Referral to appropriate counseling may be required.

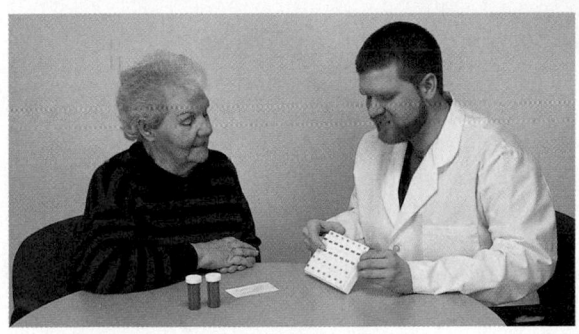

Figure 28-4 This nurse is teaching the patient regarding the antihypertensive medications recently prescribed.

Evaluation of Outcomes

Potential patient outcomes for each of the example nursing diagnoses for the patient with hypertension are:

- Altered health maintenance R/T lack of knowledge of pathology, complications, and management of hypertension. Patient identifies own unhealthy behaviors, seeks information about disease pathology and complications, develops realistic disease management goals, and identifies strengths and weaknesses for maintaining health.
- Fatigue R/T altered body chemistry (medications). Patient identifies energy patterns, implements energy conservation techniques, and shares perceived changes in lifestyle, role responsibilities, and relationships with family members.
- Ineffective coping R/T effects of chronic illness and major changes in lifestyle. Patient identifies own maladaptive coping behaviors, available resources and support systems, describes or initiates alternative coping strategies, and describes positive results from new behaviors.
- Ineffective sexuality patterns related to side effects of medications. Patient acknowledges changes in sexual functioning, identifies and implements pattern modifications with partner, and reports satisfying sexual activity.
- Risk for ineffective therapeutic regimen management R/T noncompliance with treatment. Patient identifies factors that impede effective management, implement strategies to assist with healthy lifestyle behaviors, and reduction of anxiety.

KEY CONCEPTS

- Hypertension (elevated blood pressure) is a common chronic disorder.
- Types of hypertension are primary (idiopathic) or secondary (related to another disease).
- High blood pressure results from a variety of known risk factors.
- Blood pressure = CO × PVR.
- The cardiovascular, renal, endocrine, and nervous systems all play a role in maintaining blood pressure.
- The JNC VII issues guidelines for the classification of hypertension.
- Health history, physical examination, and diagnostic studies are useful for identifying potential end organ damage and any secondary causes of high blood pressure.
- Lifestyle modifications include weight reduction, moderating alcohol, caffeine, and sodium intake, smoking cessation, stress reduction, and regular exercise.

- The DASH diet is rich in grains, fruits, vegetables, and low-fat dairy products and is recommended by the JNC VII for weight reduction.
- Individuals should limit caffeine intake to about 200 mg a day.
- Sodium restriction may be enough to control hypertension in many patients.
- Tobacco is the single greatest cause of disease and premature death in the United States.
- A variety of relaxation techniques are available and recommended to help patients with life-stress management.
- When lifestyle changes do not sufficiently reduce blood pressure, medications may be required.
- The drugs currently available for treatment of hypertension work in one of two ways, reduction of the SVR or decreasing the volume of circulating blood.
- The role of the nurse in blood pressure management is in assessment, education, and supporting the needs of the patient.

REVIEW QUESTIONS

1. Target organ damage that can occur from uncontrolled hypertension includes:
   1. Headache and dizziness
   2. Retinopathy and diabetes
   3. Dyslipidemia and kidney dysfunction
   4. Kidney dysfunction and left ventricular hypertrophy

2. When teaching a patient how to control hypertension, the nurse must recognize that:
   1. All patients with elevated blood pressure require medication.
   2. It is not necessary to limit salt intake if taking a diuretic.
   3. Lifestyle modifications are indicated for all patients with hypertension.
   4. If overweight, the patient must achieve a normal weight to lower their blood pressure.

3. Renin is secreted into the blood by the kidney structure known as the:
   1. Distal convoluted tubule
   2. Juxtaglomerular apparatus
   3. Loop of Henle
   4. Proximal convoluted tubule

4. The secretion of antidiuretic hormone (ADH) is stimulated by:
   1. Decreased venous return
   2. Hypervolemia
   3. Hypertension
   4. Decreased plasma osmolality

5. A patient with a blood pressure of 200/141 mm Hg would have:
   1. Primary hypertension
   2. Secondary hypertension
   3. Hypertensive emergency
   4. Hypertensive urgency

6. Patient teaching for modifiable risk factor reduction should include:
   1. Dietary factors
   2. Ethnicity
   3. Gender
   4. Family history

7. ACE inhibitors, such as captopril (Capoten) and enalapril (Vasotec), decrease both blood pressure and PVR by which mechanism?
   1. Direct arterial vasodilation
   2. Blocks the conversion of angiotensin I to angiotensin II
   3. Increasing the fluid excretion at the loop of Henle
   4. Peripheral vasoconstriction and central vasodilation

8. The interval between the first and second heart sounds is ventricular:
   1. Diastole
   2. Systole
   3. Presystole
   4. Protodiastole

9. The force that the left ventricle must generate to eject its blood volume is called:
   1. PVR
   2. Preload
   3. Afterload
   4. Cardiac index

10. Pulsus paradoxus is a sign of:
    1. Cardiac tamponade
    2. Prinzmetal's angina
    3. Acute bacterial endocarditis
    4. Left ventricular failure

11. Which medication is a non–nicotine-containing therapy used to support smoking cessation?
    1. Clonidine
    2. Bupropion
    3. Fluoxetine
    4. Venlafaxine

12. Which blood pressure measurement is considered normal according to the JNC VII guidelines?
    1. 118/78
    2. 128/85
    3. 130/85
    4. 140/90

13. A cause of secondary hypertension is:
    1. Hypoaldosteronism
    2. Hypothyroidism
    3. Patent foramen ovale
    4. Interstitial cystitis

REVIEW ACTIVITIES

1. Answer the following questions based on the following information.

   Fred Greene is a 38-year-old engineer having a regular health check-up. He is 6'1" tall and weighs 240 pounds. His blood pressure is 135/85 mm Hg, and his heart rate is 84 beats per minute with a regular rhythm. The health care provider notices that he has gained 22 pounds in the last year. Mr. Greene says that he was promoted at work, and his stress level has increased with the new responsibilities. He has started smoking again, and his job requires him to entertain two to three nights a week. Physical examination finds no other abnormalities. Laboratory tests are unremarkable except for:
   Fasting glucose 129 mg/dL
   Total cholesterol 224 mg/dL
   High-density lipoprotein (HDL) 30 mg/dL
   Triglycerides 326 mg/dL

   a. Based on the physical findings and lab studies, identify the lifestyle changes that you would suggest to Mr. Greene.
   b. What would you teach Mr. Greene?
   c. Identify three actual and two potential nursing diagnoses with identifying factors.

2. Identify the subjective and objective data that you would use when assessing the patient with hypertension.

Subjective Data	Objective Data
a. _____	1._____
b. _____	2._____
c. _____	3._____

3. List three causes of secondary hypertension and the diagnostic test used to identify it.

4. Provide patient education for a patient in the clinical setting who has hypertension. What types of instruction and education would you give the patient?

5. Describe the typical beginning of the pharmacological management for hypertension?

Hematological Dysfunction: Nursing Management

Rick Daniels, RN, PhD

CHAPTER TOPICS

- Anemias

- Platelet and Coagulation Disorders

- Polycythemias

- Neutropenia

- Mononucleosis

- Leukemias

- Multiple Myeloma

- Malignant Lymphomas

KEY TERMS

Agranulocytosis
Allogeneic transplantation
Autologous transplantation
Cheilosis
Erythromelalgia
Heinz bodies
Hemarthrosis
Hematopoiesis
Hemoglobinuria
Hemolysis
Leukopenia
Lymphadenopathy
Neutropenia
Petechiae
Pica
Plasmapheresis
Schistocytes

Hematology, the study of blood and its components, is a growing science. It is a system that encompasses the whole body and influences all other body systems. Hematology patients are increasing in number as the population ages. The patients can be challenging for professional nurses as many of their symptoms are hidden for years. When symptoms do arise, the patients tend to have significant laboratory changes and shifts in their homeostasis leading to exacerbation of the disease processes. This chapter will provide the professional nurse will an understanding of the hematology body system, explain laboratory findings, and assist in the assessment and management of these complicated patients.

ANEMIAS

There are a number of anemias that are relatively common blood disorders. Actually, anemias are a symptom of an underlying dysfunction and occur from a variety of etiologies. Anemia is defined as a condition in which the hemoglobin concentration is lower than normal, which means that there are fewer red blood cells (RBCs) circulating within the plasma. One marked result is the lack of oxygen to the cells and the consequences that follow.

Epidemiology

A wide variety of people are at risk for the anemias. It is more logical to consider the individual disorders as risks for the specific type of anemia. However, the following is a list of people at risk for having anemia: (a) those who have any type of iron deficiency from poor nutrition or other reasons; (b) females who have menorrhagia resulting from menstrual pathology; (c) alterations of erythropoiesis (e.g., thalassemia, sickle cell anemia); (d) trauma that results in excessive bleeding, either losing blood from the body or a shift of circulating plasma within the body compartments; (e) immunosuppression from a number of oncological disorders (e.g., leukemia, lymphoma); and (f) medication therapy that depresses bone marrow activity.

Etiology

There are many causes for anemia, which can be divided into three main categories. The first cause is a loss of RBCs due to bleeding from any source, such as a wound or trauma, the nose, or the gastrointestinal (GI) system. The second cause is a decreased production of RBCs, which can be from disorders such as bone marrow suppression, a lack of erythropoietin from renal diseases, or a deficiency of substances that are coproducers of RBCs (e.g., folic acid, vitamin B_{12}, iron). The third case is an increased destruction of RBCs, which can result from abnormal RBC structures (sickle cell anemia) or hypersplenism.

Pathophysiology

One method of identifying the pathophysiology for anemias is to examine the classifications for anemias. The three primary classes for anemias are (a) bleeding that results in RBC loss; (b) hemolytic anemia, which is caused by RBC destruction; and (c) hypoproliferative that results from defective RBC production. Each of these classifications are described.

There are many causes for bleeding and subsequent RBC loss. Regardless of the cause, the result is less circulating plasma and RBCs, which decreases the oxygen-carrying capacity to the cells and thus results in an anemic condition, which is fatiguing (Figure 29-1). The person with blood loss anemia can restore his or her own fluids if the initial loss is not severe. However, if too much blood and fluids are lost, the person must be transfused with some combination of blood and blood products.

Hemolytic anemias are caused by a premature destruction of the RBCs, and there is a release of hemoglobin from the RBC into the circulating plasma. This RBC destruction causes tissue hypoxia and stimulates erythropoietin production. In addition, there is an increased reticulocyte count, because the bone marrow is attempting to make up for the loss of RBCs. Bilirubin levels rise from the released hemoglobin, and **hemolysis** (destruction of RBCs) can result.

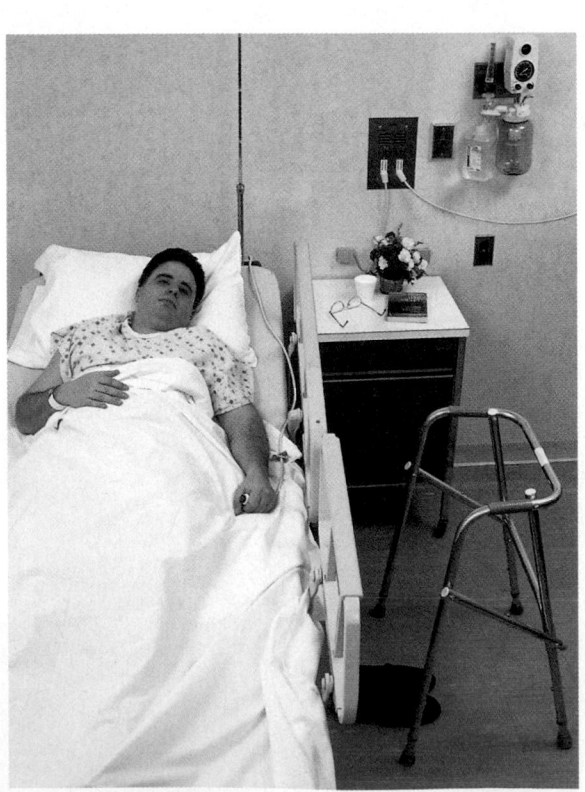

Figure 29-1 Patient is fatigued from condition of anemia.

In hypoproliferative anemia, the RBCs are decreased in number because of a low production by the bone marrow and show a low reticulocyte count. The dysfunction of the bone marrow is often due to medication damage, lack of factors that are normally necessary for RBC production (e.g., iron, folic acid, erythropoietin), or various chemicals.

Assessment with Clinical Manifestations

The anemic condition varies in severity from mild symptoms to life-threatening manifestations. In general, the more quickly the anemia has developed, the more serious the condition of anemia. A person who has slowly become anemic may adapt to relatively low hemoglobin levels and remain asymptomatic or have few symptoms of adaptation (e.g., tachycardia, decreased activity levels).

The nurse must assess the patient for typical symptoms of anemia, such as fatigue, weakness, generalized malaise, skin pallor, tachycardia, and shortness of breath. If the patient is experiencing severe anemia, the nurse must carefully consider the potential cardiovascular implications for the patient. The patient may be at risk for the heart to pump faster and harder in an attempt to make up for the decreased oxygen-carrying capacity during the anemic condition (overcompensation).

Patients who develop an anemic disorder and are typically active, such as a person in a labor-intensive vocation, will show pronounced clinical manifestations (e.g., shortness of breath, fatigue, or chest pain). On the other hand, the elderly person with anemia who has a decreased level of mobility and little exercise or activity may not show many signs or symptoms.

Also, patients with disorders that result in anemia may have other characteristic manifestations, which are more peculiar to the disorder than just the isolated manifestation of anemia, such as trauma victims. For example, the victim of a motor vehicle crash may have pain and sensory involvement that far exceeds their perception of problems with the anemia from fluid loss. The fluid loss would then need to be corrected with transfusion of intravenous (IV) fluids (Figure 29-2).

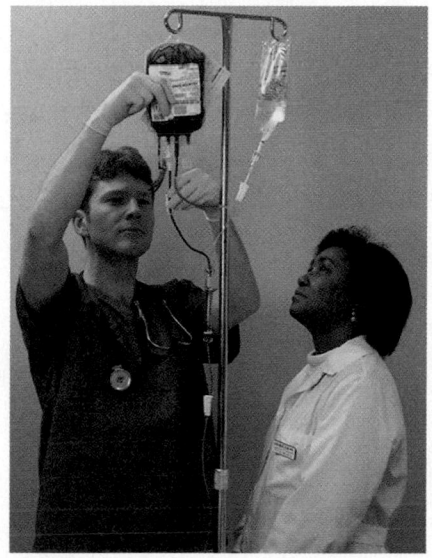

Figure 29-2 Blood product administration for the management of anemia.

Diagnostic Tests

There are many diagnostic tests that can be performed in patients with different anemic conditions. In the beginning stages of assessment, the hemoglobin, hematocrit, RBC indices, reticulocyte count, iron studies, and serum vitamin B_{12} are evaluated. In addition, other diagnostics are haptoglobin, erythropoietin, and CBC values. As a patient is continued to be examined, other tests may be bone marrow aspiration to evaluate the potential presence of malignancy, other sources of blood loss, or other chronic illnesses.

Nursing Diagnoses

Based on the information gathered, examples of nursing diagnoses in the patient with anemia are:
- Ineffective peripheral tissue perfusion related to impaired circulation.
- Activity intolerance related to fatigue.
- Pain related to decreased oxygen supply to tissues.
- Ineffective coping related to anxiety, lower activity level and the inability to perform normal activities of daily living.
- Pain related to decreased oxygen supply to tissues.

Planning and Implementation

The wide variety of anemias also mandates management strategies that are individual to the etiology of each anemia. In general, the careful assessment of the patient with anemia and monitoring the continued pathology is essential

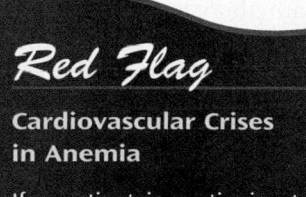

Red Flag

Cardiovascular Crises in Anemia

If a patient is continuing to lose body fluids either within or without the body system, the nurse must quickly assess the implications on the cardiovascular system. Electrophysiologic changes may occur, putting the patient at risk for a cardiac arrest.

Adapted from DeLaune, S., & Ladner, P. (2006). Fundamentals of nursing (3rd ed.). New York: Thomson Delmar Learning.

for each type of anemia. Determining whether the patient is at risk for cardiovascular system pathology, or arrhythmias is an example of a crisis that can result from many of the specific anemia conditions. Hypovolemic shock is another syndrome and type of crisis that can exhibit itself when an anemic condition continues to deteriorate. Management strategies across the anemia conditions can include such interventions as administration of oxygen, blood and blood products, careful hemodynamic monitoring, and the assessment of fluid homeostasis. More detailed and specific management implementation is seen in the following variety of anemia conditions.

Evaluation of Outcomes

Potential patient outcomes for each of the example nursing diagnoses for the patient with anemia are:

- Ineffective peripheral tissue perfusion related to impaired circulation. The patient should maintain optimal tissue perfusion to the periphery, as evidenced by strong peripheral pulses, good capillary refill, and good movement.
- Activity intolerance related to fatigue. The patient maintains activity level within capabilities, as evidenced by normal heart rate and blood pressure during activity, as well as absence of shortness of breath, weakness, and fatigue.
- Ineffective coping related to anxiety, lower activity level and the inability to perform normal activities of daily living. The patient identifies own maladaptive coping behaviors, available resources and support systems, describes or initiates alternative coping strategies, and describes positive results from new behaviors.
- Pain related to decreased oxygen supply to tissues. The patient should verbalize an adequate relief of pain along with the ability to realistically cope with the pain if it is not completely relieved.

HEMOLYTIC ANEMIAS

There are a number of hemolytic anemia conditions that are known to cause hemolysis of red blood cells. Acquired hemolytic anemia is that type of anemia that occurs outside the RBC. In addition, many of the hemolytic anemias are caused by genetic defects and may be associated with abnormalities that interrupt metabolic processes and prevent the normal biochemical actions within the cell, changes in the hemoglobin structure, or have plasma membrane defects.

Acquired Hemolytic Anemia

Acquired hemolytic anemia is caused by any number of factors that result in hemolysis outside the RBC. Etiological events that can result in acquired hemolytic anemia are trauma to RBCs produced by burns, radiation, or hemodialysis, drugs, toxins, autoimmune diseases, transfusion reactions, and bacterial infections.

The primary clinical manifestations of acquired hemolytic anemia vary from mild to severe, depending on the nature of the etiology of the anemia. The hemolysis that has caused the RBC destruction causes the patient to have an enlarged spleen from the increased burden of removing damaged RBCs. In addition, as the condition exacerbates, the liver is also challenged beyond its capability and can result in increased bilirubin levels and jaundice. In the most severe cases of acquired hemolytic anemia, the bone marrow expands, and the bones themselves may develop pathological fractures. In addition, the patient may develop the generalized symptomology of decreased oxygen-carrying capability and have manifestations of deoxygenation (e.g., skin pallor, tachycardia, or postural hypotension).

Thalassemia

Thalassemia is an inherited disease whereby hemoglobin synthesis is missing either the alpha or beta chains of the hemoglobin molecule. Consequently, hemoglobin production is deficient and weak microcytic, hypochromic RBCs are formed and labeled target cells because of their characteristic bull's eye appearance.

Epidemiology

Thalassemia affects certain groups of persons. Populations of Asians, particularly from China, the Philippines, and Thailand more often have alpha-defect thalassemia. Populations of Mediterranean ancestry (Greece and Southern Italy) are more likely to have beta-defect thalassemia (also called Mediterranean or Cooley's anemia). African Americans and Africans are more likely to have both alpha- and beta-defect thalassemia. Those children who have thalassemia rarely live to adulthood.

Pathophysiology

As stated, there are the two primary forms of thalassemia, alpha defect and beta defect. In addition, similar to sickle-cell anemia, only one deficient beta-chain–forming gene may be present, which is labeled beta thalassemia minor. Four genes cause alpha chain formation, and either one, two, three, or all four may cause the thalassemic condition. When all four genes are defective, it is labeled alpha thalassemia major and it is fatal and most commonly in utero.

Assessment with Clinical Manifestations

People with thalassemia minor are usually asymptomatic with some manifestations related to the defective hemoglobin. The signs and symptoms include mild to moderate anemia, bone marrow hyperplasia, mild splenomegaly, and bronze skin coloring. The more serious thalassemia will result in heart failure, liver and spleen dysfunction from increased RBC destruction, and severe anemia. Fractures of the long bones, ribs, and vertebrae may occur from bone marrow dysfunction and increased **hematopoiesis.** In addition, iron builds up in the heart, liver, and pancreas after repeated transfusions, which often leads to organic failure.

Planning and Implementation

The nurse develops a plan of care based on the individual progression of the disease. The depth of the anemia, RBC destruction, and complications such as heart failure require the nurse to be flexible and adaptive to meet the individual needs of the patient.

From a broader perspective, the nurse must remember to refer the patient for genetic counseling and be sensitive in this regard. The potential consequences for offspring and pregnancies make caring for the patient a delicate matter.

Glucose-6-Phosphate Dehydrogenase Anemia

Glucose-6-phosphate dehydrogenase anemia (G6PD) is a form of anemia caused by a genetic defect in RBC metabolism. Some patients develop the disease from a chronic genetic defect, but most contract the disorder when highly stressed with something like an inflammatory disorder or more likely the use of certain medications. This disorder occurs from many variations of the genetic makeup. The defective gene lies on the X chromosome and therefore affects more males than females. G6PD is somewhat common in African and Mediterranean persons. Usually the Mediterranean people develop more severe forms of the disease than the African populations. About 12 percent of African American males are affected with this disorder. This disease was first identified when researchers in World War II witnessed soldiers who developed hemolysis when being treated with primaquine for their malaria.

Assessment with Clinical Manifestations

Patients with G6PD are usually asymptomatic, having normal hemoglobin and reticulocyte levels. Certain medications cause hemolytic effects for patients with G6PD. These patients may develop jaundice, skin pallor, and **hemoglobinuria** (hemoglobin in the urine). In addition, reticulocyte levels then rise and manifestations of hemolysis occur. There may be **Heinz bodies** (degraded hemoglobin) in the RBCs. In more severe cases, recovery may not occur and continued transfusion may be needed.

Diagnostic Tests

G6PD is diagnosed with a screening test or by a quantitative assay of G6PD. Otherwise, the aforementioned Heinz bodies may be identified, as well as the hemoglobinuria.

Planning and Implementation

If the disease of G6PD has been initiated by a certain medication, then stopping that medication is essential to recovery. Transfusions are given in serious instances of the disease. Nursing care can include supportive measures during the hemolysis conditions. As a preventive measure, patients can be given a list of medications to avoid (Box 29-1). Otherwise, nursing interventions are the same measures as for any other types of hemolysis.

Hereditary Spherocytosis

Hereditary spherocytosis, also known as congenital hemolytic anemia, is the most common of the hemolytic disorders. There is no abnormality of the hemoglobin and it is found in 1 in 5,000 persons.

Pathophysiology

Hereditary spherocytosis is an autosomal dominant disorder and is presumed to mutate about 25 percent of the time. The hereditary defect is theorized to be caused by an abnormality of the erythrocyte membrane. This change causes the cells to develop into a spherical shape. In addition, they circulate in the blood of the spleen where they are prematurely destroyed.

Assessment with Clinical Manifestations

This disorder begins in utero or early infancy and exhibits itself with anemia and hyperbilirubinemia. The severity of the anemia varies as does the jaundiced appearance. There is usually splenomegaly and gallstones develop as early as four to five years of age. Aplastic crises are the most serious of the complications.

Diagnostic Tests

Diagnosis is made with family history, studies of osmotic fragility, blood smear, and autohemolysis. There is not one single test for identifying hereditary spherocytosis.

Planning and Implementation

The care for this child often involves removal of the spleen, which produces a clinical cure and is the primary treatment of this disorder. The nursing care involves normal postoperative care for a splenectomy.

Sickle Cell Anemia

Sickle cell anemia is a heredity disorder of an autosomal recessive defect and a type of chronic hemolytic anemia. The disease is known for its abnormally crescent-shaped RBCs. The genetic defect causes synthesis of an abnormal form of hemoglobin (HbS) within the red blood cells.

BOX 29-1

MEDICATIONS THAT HEIGHTEN THE HEMOLYTIC AFFECTS OF G6PD

- Antimalarial drugs (e.g., chloroquine)
- Common coal tar analgesics (including ASA)
- Nitrofurantoin
- Oral hypoglycemics
- Sulfonamides
- Thiazide diuretics
- Vitamin K

Adapted from Spratto, G. R., & Woods, A. L. (2007). 2007 PDR nurse's drug handbook. New York: Thomson Delmar Learning.

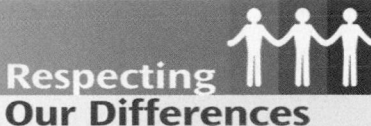

Respecting Our Differences

Exploring Sickle Cell Anemia in Ethnic Groups

The nurse must be sure to assess the potential of sickle cell anemia in the at-risk ethnic populations. Therapeutic communication techniques must be adhered to, for the patient to not be offended, and to realize the intent of the nurse in the interview process. African American patients should always be assessed for the potential clinical manifestations of sickle cell anemia because of the prevalence in this population.

Epidemiology

Sickle cell anemia is seen most in people whose origins are in equatorial countries, particularly of African descent. In addition, people from the Near East, the Mediterranean, and Central and South America also may have the disease. In the United States, 7 to 13 percent of African Americans carry the defective gene, having inherited it from one parent.

Etiology

The gene for sickle cell anemia is transmitted in an autosomal recessive pattern from parent to offspring. A parent with one HbS has a 50 percent chance of transmitting the gene to each child. If both parents carry the gene, each child has a 25 percent risk of inheriting the gene from both parents. A person who carries both HbS genes is likely to develop the sickle cell disorder.

Pathophysiology

Deoxygenation is the most important variable in determining the occurrence of the sickling disorder. The degree of deoxygenation is varied with the percentage of HbS in the cells. Sickled erythrocytes are stiff and cannot change their shape as easily as normal cells, which causes pathology. Anemia follows the sickle cell damage, and the disease process is intermittent in its progression. Once sickling occurs it tends to perpetuate itself and the extent, severity, and associated clinical manifestations depend on the percentage of hemoglobin that is HbS.

Assessment with Clinical Manifestations

In sickle cell disease, the general clinical manifestations are those of hemolytic anemia: fatigue, pallor, jaundice, and irritability. Excessive sickling processes can precipitate a crisis because of occluded circulation, sequestering of large amounts of blood in the liver or spleen, and impaired erythropoiesis.

Diagnostic Tests

The history of the parents and clinical manifestations are important in determining sickle cell disease. However, hematological tests are necessary for diagnosis. A sickle solubility test confirms the presence of HbS in peripheral blood, and hemoglobin electrophoresis provides information about the amount of HbS in the erythrocytes. Prenatal diagnosis can be made after chorionic villus sampling or with amniotic fluid analysis.

Nursing Diagnoses

Based on the information gathered, examples of nursing diagnoses in the patient with sickle cell anemia are synonymous with those for anemia listed earlier.

Planning and Implementation

The morbidity and mortality rates in children over the past 25 years have greatly decreased. Advanced management of fever, early diagnosis of sickle cell complications, aggressive use of transfusions, and management of pain have improved the patient's conditions. Immediate correction of acid-base imbalances and dehydration with IV fluids is essential. Infections are treated with antibiotic therapy. Bone marrow transplantation is the most definitive approach to treating the sickle cell disease, and a splenectomy may be performed in cases of certain hemolytic sequestration crises. Genetic counseling needs to be offered for people at risk for the disorder.

Pharmacology

Oxygen is administered as the sickle cell process affects oxygenation. Therapeutic use of antisickling agents, such as urea, cyanate, and carbamoyl phosphate are administered. Folic acid supplements may be given to meet the demands of the RBC production. Blood transfusions are often necessary during times of crisis.

Evaluation of Outcomes

Potential patient outcomes for each of the example nursing diagnoses for the patient with sickle cell anemia are:

- Ineffective peripheral tissue perfusion related to impaired circulation. The patient should maintain optimal tissue perfusion to the periphery, as evidenced by strong peripheral pulses, good capillary refill, and good movement.
- Activity intolerance related to fatigue. The patient maintains activity level within capabilities, as evidenced by normal heart rate and blood pressure during activity, as well as absence of shortness of breath, weakness, and fatigue.
- Ineffective coping related to anxiety, lower activity level and the inability to perform normal activities of daily living. The patient identifies own maladaptive coping behaviors, available resources, and support systems, describes or initiates alternative coping strategies, and describes positive results from new behaviors.
- Pain related to decreased oxygen supply to tissues. The patient should verbalize an adequate relief of pain along with the ability to realistically cope with the pain if it is not completely relieved.

NUTRITIONAL ANEMIAS

There are anemias that are caused by nutritional deficiencies that affect erythropoiesis (RBC production). These anemias may be caused by a lack of dietary intake, an increased need for the nutrients, or malabsorption problems. Vitamin B_{12} and folic acid anemias are also labeled megaloblastic anemias.

Iron Deficiency Anemia

Iron deficiency anemia develops when there is a loss of iron that becomes inadequate for RBC production. It is the most common type of anemia and is particularly common in the elderly.

Epidemiology

Adult females with menstrual bleeding are the most common patients with iron deficiency anemia. In addition, the elderly have increased bleeding tendencies related to hemorrhoids, GI bleeding, and cancer. There is also the potential lack of dietary consumption of iron from limited fresh foods because of lower socioeconomic status, lack of transportation, or uninformed people.

Etiology

There are many causes for iron deficiency anemia. Chronic bleeding for whatever reason is the normal pathology, for example, upper GI bleeding from peptic ulcerations, prolonged menstrual bleeding (the most common cause), and pregnancy.

Pathophysiology

Iron is found in hemoglobin, myoglobin, oxidative enzymes, and respiratory chain proteins, and is therefore essential for oxidative energy production. All levels of iron deficiency adversely influence tissue oxidative capacity, and severe reductions in hemoglobin causing anemia disturb oxygen carrying capacity (Bodnar, Cogswell, & McDonald, 2005).

Assessment with Clinical Manifestations

The patient with iron deficiency anemia has the general manifestations of anemia. In addition, the patient has chronic anemia and may develop brittle spoon-shaped nails, **cheilosis** (small fissures at the corners of the mouth), **pica** (craving for substances other than food, such as dirt, clay, starch, or ice cubes), and a smooth, painful tongue.

Nursing Diagnoses

Based on the information gathered, examples of nursing diagnoses in the patient with iron deficiency anemia are:
- Ineffective peripheral tissue perfusion related to impaired circulation.
- Activity intolerance related to fatigue.
- Pain related to decreased oxygen supply to tissues.
- Ineffective coping related to anxiety, lower activity level, and the inability to perform normal activities of daily living.
- Pain related to decreased oxygen supply to tissues.

Planning and Implementation

The most typical management for patients with iron deficiency anemia is to replace the dietary intake of iron-rich foods, along with oral or parenteral iron supplements.

Evaluation of Outcomes

Potential patient outcomes for each of the example nursing diagnoses for the patient with iron deficiency anemia are:
- Ineffective peripheral tissue perfusion related to impaired circulation. The patient should maintain optimal tissue perfusion to the periphery, as evidenced by strong peripheral pulses, good capillary refill, and good movement.
- Activity intolerance related to fatigue. The patient maintains activity level within capabilities, as evidenced by normal heart rate and blood pressure during activity, as well as absence of shortness of breath, weakness, and fatigue.
- Ineffective coping related to anxiety, lower activity level, and the inability to perform normal activities of daily living. The patient identifies own maladaptive coping behaviors, available resources, and support systems, describes or initiates alternative coping strategies, and describes positive results from new behaviors.
- Pain related to decreased oxygen supply to tissues. The patient should verbalize an adequate relief of pain along with the ability to realistically cope with the pain if it is not completely relieved.

Folic Acid Deficiency Anemia

Folic acid deficiency anemia results from a lack of folic acid. Folic acid is a vitamin that is necessary for RBC synthesis. Normally, folic acid is obtained in green leafy vegetables, liver, fruits, and cereals.

Epidemiology

Folic acid deficiency anemia is found in the chronically undernourished, such as alcoholics, drug abusers, and the elderly. Consumption of alcohol increases folic acid requirements. In addition, pregnancy increases the need for folic acid.

Pathophysiology

Basically, the same pathophysiology as for iron deficiency anemia. The missing folic acid levels adversely influence tissue oxidative capacity, and severe reductions in hemoglobin cause anemia, which disturbs oxygen-carrying capacity.

Assessment with Clinical Manifestations

The patient with folic acid anemia has the general manifestations of anemia. There are no neurological symptoms associated with iron deficiency anemia, which is in contrast to vitamin B$_{12}$ anemia.

Nursing Diagnoses

Based on the information gathered, examples of nursing diagnoses in the patient with folic acid deficiency anemia are:
- Ineffective peripheral tissue perfusion related to impaired circulation.
- Activity intolerance related to fatigue.
- Pain related to decreased oxygen supply to tissues.
- Ineffective coping related to anxiety, lower activity level, and the inability to perform normal activities of daily living.
- Pain related to decreased oxygen supply to tissues.

Planning and Implementation

The most typical management for patients with iron deficiency anemia is to replace the dietary intake of iron-rich foods, along with oral or parenteral iron supplements. There is also the need to identify the at-risk patients and encourage their iron replacement therapies, such as the prenatal vitamins that are iron fortified. The additional intake of iron may only be necessary for short periods of time in some populations.

Evaluation of Outcomes

Potential patient outcomes for each of the example nursing diagnoses for the patient with folic acid deficiency anemia are:
- Ineffective peripheral tissue perfusion related to impaired circulation. The patient should maintain optimal tissue perfusion to the periphery, as evidenced by strong peripheral pulses, good capillary refill, and good movement.
- Activity intolerance related to fatigue. The patient maintains activity level within capabilities, as evidenced by normal heart rate and blood pressure during activity, as well as absence of shortness of breath, weakness, and fatigue.
- Ineffective coping related to anxiety, lower activity level, and the inability to perform normal activities of daily living. The patient identifies own maladaptive coping behaviors, available resources, and support systems, describes or initiates alternative coping strategies, and describes positive results from new behaviors.
- Pain related to decreased oxygen supply to tissues. The patient should verbalize an adequate relief of pain along with the ability to realistically cope with the pain if it is not completely relieved.

Vitamin B$_{12}$ Deficiency Anemia

Vitamin B$_{12}$ deficiency anemia (cobalamin deficiency) occurs from either a lack of intake or in conditions of malabsorption (e.g., Crohn's disease), which is more common. In addition, the inability to absorb vitamin B$_{12}$ also exists with the lack of intrinsic factor seen in pernicious anemia (Andres, et al., 2006).

Epidemiology

Epidemiological studies show a prevalence of vitamin B$_{12}$ deficiency of around 20 percent in the general population of industrialized countries. Some studies have demonstrated a prevalence of 30 to 40 percent among elderly people living in the community, particularly those who are in institutions or who are sick. In addition, vitamin B$_{12}$ deficiency appears to be more common among patients who have a variety of chronic neurological conditions (e.g., dementia, Alzheimer's disease, stroke, Parkinson's disease)

Etiology

In elderly patients, vitamin B_{12} deficiency is caused primarily by food-cobalamin malabsorption and pernicious anemia. Deficiency caused by dietary deficiency or malabsorption is rarer. Other causes included dietary deficiency (less than 5 percent), malabsorption (less than 5 percent), and hereditary vitamin B_{12} metabolism diseases. Pernicious anemia, or Biermer's disease, is a classic cause of vitamin B_{12} deficiency and one of the most frequent among elderly patients (Andres, et al., 2004).

Pathophysiology

Primarily the resulting consequences from vitamin B_{12} deficiency is similar to anemia in general. Some differences exist in patients with pernicious anemia, which is an autoimmune disease characterized by the destruction of the gastric mucosa, especially fundal mucosa, by a primarily cell-mediated process. The lack of intrinsic factor, normally secreted by the gastric mucosa, which binds with the dietary vitamin B_{12} to assist in its absorption, causes the deficiency.

Assessment with Clinical Manifestations

Vitamin B_{12} deficiency occurs frequently among elderly patients, but it is often unrecognized or not investigated because the clinical manifestations are subtle. And, the body normally has large stores of vitamin B_{12}, and consequently it may take years for the deficiency to occur. However, the potential seriousness of the complications (particularly neuropsychiatric and hematological) requires investigation of all patients who present with vitamin or nutritional deficiency.

Among the classic manifestations are Hunter's glossitis, which causes the lingual papillae to atrophy, making the tongue look smooth and shiny, and neuroanemic syndrome. This syndrome includes combined sclerosis of the spinal cord and megaloblastic anemia with subacute combined degeneration of the spinal cord, which causes sensory disturbances and pyramidal motor disturbances. Typical neurological manifestations include polyneuritis, ataxia, and positive Babinski reflexes.

Nursing Diagnoses

Based on the information gathered, examples of nursing diagnoses in the patient with vitamin B_{12} deficiency anemia are:
- Ineffective peripheral tissue perfusion related to impaired circulation.
- Activity intolerance related to fatigue.
- Pain related to decreased oxygen supply to tissues.
- Ineffective coping related to anxiety, lower activity level and the inability to perform normal activities of daily living.
- Pain related to decreased oxygen supply to tissues.

Diagnostic Tests

The prominent diagnostic test for vitamin B_{12} deficiency is the Schilling test, which involves radioactive testing for the absorption capabilities of the body to vitamin B_{12}. In addition, an intrinsic factor serum test can be performed, but it is not specific to diagnosing pernicious anemia.

Planning and Implementation

The classic treatment of vitamin B_{12} deficiency, particularly when the cause is not a dietary deficiency, has been parenteral administration usually by intramuscular injection of the vitamin.

Evaluation of Outcomes

Potential patient outcomes for each of the example nursing diagnoses for the patient with vitamin B_{12} deficiency anemia are:

- Ineffective peripheral tissue perfusion related to impaired circulation. The patient should maintain optimal tissue perfusion to the periphery, as evidenced by strong peripheral pulses, good capillary refill, and good movement.
- Activity intolerance related to fatigue. The patient maintains activity level within capabilities, as evidenced by normal heart rate and blood pressure during activity, as well as absence of shortness of breath, weakness, and fatigue.
- Ineffective coping related to anxiety, lower activity level and the inability to perform normal activities of daily living. The patient identifies own maladaptive coping behaviors, available resources and support systems, describes or initiates alternative coping strategies, and describes positive results from new behaviors.
- Pain related to decreased oxygen supply to tissues. The patient should verbalize an adequate relief of pain along with the ability to realistically cope with the pain if it is not completely relieved.

PLATELET AND COAGULATION DISORDERS

There are normal coagulation factors that when pathology occurs result in various bleeding disorders. Normally, the vessels constrict and platelets aggregate to the site of bleeding where fibrin assists coagulation of the site. In addition, the platelets are controlled by thrombopoietin, a protein produced by the liver, kidney, bone marrow, and smooth muscle. Overall, the process of hemostasis, or blood coagulation, involves multiple stages (Box 29-2), and when it dysfunctions, various bleeding disorders result.

Thrombocytopenia

Thrombocytopenia is identified as a platelet count of less than 100,000/mL of blood. The bleeding is related to the lack of circulating platelets, which usually occurs in small vessels. A platelet count of less than 20,000/mL can cause spontaneous bleeding and bleeding from various locations in the body (e.g., nose, mouth, or GI tract).

Pathophysiology

There are three mechanisms for thrombocytopenia: (a) decreased production of platelets, (b) increased sequestration in the spleen, and (c) accelerated destruction of the platelets. In addition, there are two specific types of primary thrombocytopenia: (a) immune thrombocytopenia purpura (ITP) and (b) thrombotic thrombocytopenic purpura (TTP). A secondary thrombocytopenia may be caused by aplastic anemia, bone marrow cancer, radiation therapy, disseminated intravascular coagulation (DIC), or drug therapy.

ITP, which is also known as idiopathic thrombocytopenia purpura, is an autoimmune disorder with platelet destruction. Acute ITP is more common in children and chronic ITP is found in persons between ages 20 and 40, with women more affected than men. In ITP, proteins on the platelet cell stimulate autoantibody production. These autoantibodies adhere to the platelet membrane are seen by the spleen as foreign. The altered platelets are destroyed after one to three days of circulation. The clinical manifestations of ITP are described below.

TTP is a rare disease in which thrombi occlude arterioles and capillaries. It affects much of the body system and is unknown in its etiology. Acute TTP may

---

BOX 29-2

STAGES OF COAGULATION

Coagulation, or clotting, is a complex process that transforms blood from a liquid to a solid gel. Clotting is commonly described in three stages (Figure 29-3):

1. The formation of prothrombinase. This is achieved when two mechanisms of clotting, the extrinsic and intrinsic pathways, initiate the formation of prothrombin activator. Within these pathways, specific factors (designated by Roman numerals) and other chemicals found in the blood participate in the clotting process.
2. The conversion of prothrombin into the enzyme thrombin.
3. The conversion of soluble fibrinogen into insoluble fibrin.

Source: Robinson P. (2005). Is surgery safe for a patient with hemophilia? Nursing, 35(5), 1–3.

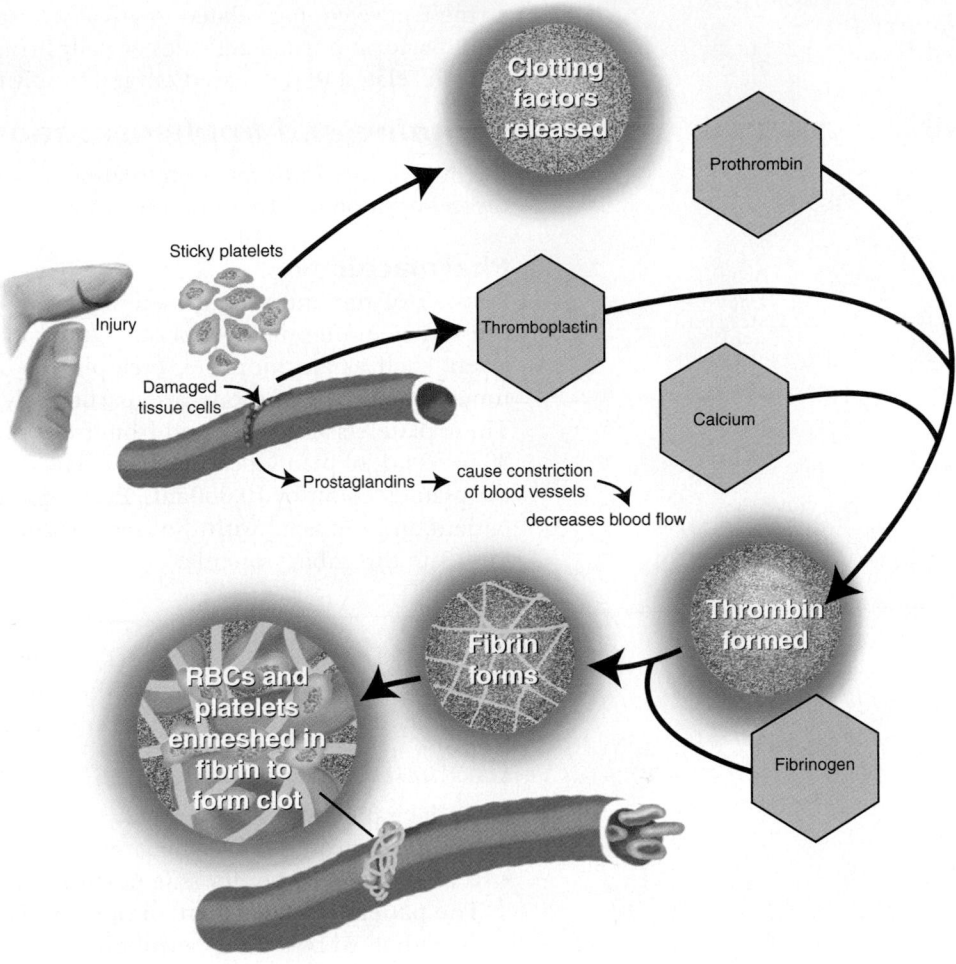

Figure 29-3 Process of clot formation.

be fatal within months with severe manifestations of bleeding, leading to seizure activity and a coma state.

Assessment with Clinical Manifestations

Thrombocytopenia causes subjective symptoms of bruising without specific trauma, bleeding gums, black or tarry stools (test positive with occult blood), hematemesis, headache, fever, nosebleed, recent weight loss, neurological symptoms, and prolonged menstrual periods. Objective signs of thrombocytopenia may be **petechiae** (small red or purple spots that do not blanch with pressure), purpura, bruises, and decreased platelet counts.

Diagnostic Tests

The diagnosis of thrombocytopenia is made from the following diagnostic tests: CBC; decreased platelet count; antinuclear antibodies (ANA) to assess autoantibodies; serological studies for cytomegalovirus (CMV), Epstein-Barr, hepatitis, toxoplasmosis, and HIV; and bone marrow examination (confirms aplastic anemia and megakaryocyte production).

Nursing Diagnoses

Based on the information gathered, examples of nursing diagnoses in the patient with thrombocytopenia are synonymous with those for anemia listed earlier.

- Ineffective peripheral tissue perfusion related to impaired circulation.
- Activity intolerance related to fatigue.
- Pain related to decreased oxygen supply to tissues.

- Ineffective coping related to anxiety, lower activity level, and the inability to perform normal activities of daily living.
- Pain related to decreased oxygen supply to tissues.

Planning and Implementation

The health care must focus on treating or removing the causative agents of the thrombocytopenia. Treatment measures are largely medicinal or surgical.

Pharmacology

Because of the autoimmune etiology, corticosteroids are prescribed to suppress the autoimmune process. Other immunosuppressive drugs may be given, such as azathioprine, cyclophosphamide, and cyclosporine. In addition, platelet transfusions are particularly helpful during an acute crisis. These platelets are developed from fresh whole blood, and one unit contains 30 to 60 mL of platelet concentrate. The first unit of platelets should increase the platelet count by 10,000 mL. **Plasmapheresis** (plasma is removed from the patient and replaced with the fresh frozen plasma) is the primary treatment for acute thrombocytopenia.

Surgery

When the patient with ITP relapses, a splenectomy is the treatment of choice. The rationale is that the spleen is where the platelets are destroyed and where antibodies are produced. This surgery often cures the disorder.

Evaluation of Outcomes

Potential patient outcomes for each of the example nursing diagnoses for the patient with thrombocytopenia are:

- Ineffective peripheral tissue perfusion related to impaired circulation. The patient should maintain optimal tissue perfusion to the periphery, as evidenced by strong peripheral pulses, good capillary refill, and good movement.
- Activity intolerance related to fatigue. The patient maintains activity level within capabilities, as evidenced by normal heart rate and blood pressure during activity, as well as absence of shortness of breath, weakness, and fatigue.
- Ineffective coping related to anxiety, lower activity level, and the inability to perform normal activities of daily living. The patient identifies own maladaptive coping behaviors, available resources, and support systems, describes or initiates alternative coping strategies, and describes positive results from new behaviors.
- Pain related to decreased oxygen supply to tissues. The patient should verbalize an adequate relief of pain along with the ability to realistically cope with the pain if it is not completely relieved.

Disseminated Intravascular Coagulation

DIC is not a disease but rather the sign of an underlying condition. DIC is a disruption of the hematological system that is characterized by widespread intravascular clotting and bleeding. It ranges from mild cases to being life threatening.

Etiology

There are many disorders that result in DIC. Anything that causes prolonged bleeding or intensive volumes of blood loss is commonly associated with DIC. Examples include aortic aneurysm, hemolytic uremic syndrome, burns, gunshot wounds, obstetric complications (e.g., septic abortion, amniotic fluid embolus, or abruption placenta), bacterial infections, sepsis, and viral infections.

Pathophysiology

DIC is caused by abnormal clotting processes in which a massive amount of tiny clots form in the microcirculation. At first this is a normal process of clotting, but as prolonged excessive clotting occurs, clotting factors are consumed faster than they can be replaced. The clotting activates fibrinolytic processes, which begin to break down the clots, and the fibrin degradation products are released, which contributes to bleeding. A vicious cycle is begun, and the ability to form clots is lost and hemorrhaging occurs.

Assessment with Clinical Manifestations

Initially, nurses must be aware of patients who are at risk for DIC. Then the patients need to be assessed frequently for manifestations of thrombi and bleeding. The patients with DIC will exhibit bleeding from such places as petechiae, bruising, GI and urinary tract bleeding, bleeding from venipuncture sites, frank oozing from incision sites, symptoms of the shock syndrome (tachycardia, pallor, or deoxygenation), cyanosis of extremities, and mental status changes.

Diagnostic Tests

The types of diagnostic tests to confirm DIC are CBC, platelet count, **schistocytes** (fragmented RBCs), prolonged coagulation studies (prothrombin time [PT], partial thromboplastin time [PTT], thrombin time), and increased fibrin degradation products.

Nursing Diagnoses

Based on the information gathered, examples of nursing diagnoses in the patient with DIC may include the following:
- Impaired gas exchange related to ventilation-perfusion inequality.
- Ineffective tissue perfusion related to the DIC.
- Anxiety related to the crisis of the DIC.

Planning and Implementation

Often, patients with DIC are in critical condition, which means they will have multiple system challenges. If the patient is experiencing septic shock, then the nursing care will be implemented with antishock measures. Patients will be assessed with a variety of body monitoring equipment (e.g., arterial blood gases [ABGs], pulse oximetry, or electrocardiogram [ECG]).

Goals

The major patient goals will include maintenance of hemodynamic status, intact mucous membranes, maintenance of fluid balance, maintenance of tissue perfusion, and having an absence of complications.

Pharmacology

The medical management for patients with DIC are restoration of the blood products, specifically fresh frozen plasma and platelet concentrates. The administration of heparin is somewhat controversial but may be given for its interference with the clotting processes and the chance of preventing further overuse of clotting factors. Heparin is usually only used when other methods of management are failing. Long-term heparin therapy may be used in patients with chronic DIC.

Evaluation of Outcomes

Potential patient outcomes for each of the example nursing diagnoses for the patient with DIC are:
- Impaired gas exchange related to ventilation-perfusion inequality. The patient maintains optimal gas exchange as evidenced by normal ABGs and alert responsive mentation or no further reduction in mental status.

- Ineffective tissue perfusion related to the DIC. The patient should maintain optimal tissue perfusion to the periphery, as evidenced by strong peripheral pulses, good capillary refill, and good movement.
- Anxiety related to the crisis of the DIC. The patient should be able to recognize the signs of anxiety, demonstrate positive coping mechanisms, and describe a reduction in the level of anxiety experienced.

Hemophilia

Hemophilia is a group of hereditary bleeding disorders that results from the deficiency of clotting factors. Depletion of factors VIII, IX, and X collectively makes up 90 to 95 percent of the bleeding disorders (Rizzo, 2006).

Pathophysiology

There are actually four different bleeding disorders that can be considered types of hemophilia. Each one exists because genetically it is deficient in regard to one or more clotting factors.

Hemophilia A (classic hemophilia), a factor VIII deficiency affects 1 in 10,000 males. It is transmitted to the offspring as a cross-linked recessive disorder from mothers to sons. The defect of hemophilia A on the X chromosome could cause the deficiency of factor VIII or its production. Factor VIII activity in hemophilia A is divided into three categories and is shown in Box 29-3.

Hemophilia B, or Christmas disease, signals a factor IX deficiency and affects 1 in approximately 40,000 males. Hemophilia B, like hemophilia A, is transmitted from mother to son as a cross-linked recessive disease. Although hemophilia A and B are clinically indistinguishable, identifying the specific deficient factor is necessary to determine appropriate treatment (Robinson, 2005).

Hemophilia C, also known as a factor XI deficiency, is also an autosomal recessive disorder. It primarily affects the population of Ashkenazi Jewish people and is somewhat rare based on that narrow population. The clinical manifestations are related to the prolonged partial thromboplastin time and are basically the same as for the previously described forms of hemophilia (see assessment with clinical manifestations section). Often these patients are identified in the perioperative arena with prolonged bleeding during or after surgery.

Von Willebrand's disease is a hereditary disorder that is often considered to be a type of hemophilia. It exists because of decreases in the quantity of von Willebrand's factor, categorized as Type I (mild) and Type III (severe) von Willebrand's disease, or qualitative defects of von Willebrand's factor (Type II). In hereditary platelet function disorders, the bleeding tendency is associated with abnormalities in platelet function rather than decreases in platelet count. Von Willebrand's disease is prevalent in approximately 1 percent of the general population (Philipp, et al., 2005).

The pathology for Von Willebrand's disease is slightly different from the other forms of hemophilia. The difference lies in the manner in which the effect of the clotting factor deficiency takes place at the site of the injury in Von Willebrand's disease, rather than more specifically in the formation process of the clot itself as seen in the other forms of hemophilia.

Assessment with Clinical Manifestations

The clinical features of hemophilia include joint and muscle hemorrhages, easy bruising, and prolonged, potentially fatal hemorrhage after trauma or surgery. The weight-bearing joints are most frequently affected. Untreated bleeding into the joint (**hemarthrosis**) can cause permanent damage and severely limit the range of motion to the affected areas. Even after the bleed-

---

BOX 29-3

THREE CATEGORIES OF HEMOPHILIA A

1. Severe hemophilia, indicating a factor VIII concentration of less than 1 percent of normal, causes frequent bleeding, even in the absence of trauma.

2. Moderate hemophilia signifies a factor VIII concentration of 1 to 5 percent. The patient will experience less bleeding than someone with severe hemophilia.

3. Mild hemophilia signifies a factor VIII concentration of 5 to 35 percent, which typically causes bleeding only after obvious trauma. Some people with mild hemophilia have a normal APTT result.

ing is controlled, joint inflammation leads to synovitis and may precipitate more bleeding into an already compromised joint. Eventually, the loss of cartilage causes hemophilic arthropathy with narrowing of the joint space, small bone pseudotumors, and limited range of motion, leading to permanent deformity and disability.

Diagnostic Tests

Serum studies will identify hemophilia by determining which clotting factors are deficient. Specific factors include serum platelets levels, factor assay tests, coagulation serum tests (e.g., PT, activated partial thromboplastin time [APTT], bleeding time), and amniocentesis or chorionic villus sampling to detect the genetic abnormality in utero (Robinson, 2005).

Ongoing factor assays will use a PTT testing to determine the correct dose of factor VIII replacement for preoperative and postoperative care. Normal plasma activity of factor VIII is designated at 50 to 150 percent, but a concentration of 35 percent is adequate for hemostasis. As a rule of thumb, the APTT test is prolonged when factor VIII activity is 25 percent below normal.

Nursing Diagnoses

Based on the information gathered, examples of nursing diagnoses in the patient with hemophilia are:
- Ineffective peripheral tissue perfusion related to impaired circulation.
- Activity intolerance related to fatigue.
- Pain related to decreased oxygen supply to tissues.
- Ineffective coping related to anxiety, lower activity level, and the inability to perform normal activities of daily living.
- Pain related to decreased oxygen supply to tissues.

Planning and Implementation

Delivering the best standard of care to a patient with hemophilia requires cooperation between a hematologist and nurses who are educated in caring for someone with hemophilia. Nurses must remember to network with the

---

BOX 29-4

NURSING MEASURES FOR HEMOPHILIA

These nursing measures will help prevent problems or detect them early if they develop in a patient with hemophilia:
- Frequently assess patient's vital signs, looking for signs of possible bleeding, such as hypotension and tachycardia.
- Monitor clotting factors as ordered and immediately report any abnormalities.
- Administer replacement therapy and blood transfusions as ordered.
- Avoid administering drugs that interfere with platelet aggregation
- Monitor for signs and symptoms of hypersensitivity reactions to factor replacement, including chest tightness, urticaria, and hypotension.
- Monitor stools for occult blood.
- Postoperatively, assess the surgical site for active bleeding and for signs and symptoms of hematoma formation and avoid any procedure that could trigger hemorrhage.

Adapted from Dunn, L. (2005). New blood. Nursing Standard, *20(4), 69; Robinson, P. (2005). Is surgery safe for a patient with hemophilia?* Nursing, *35(5),* Hospital Nursing, *1–3.*

TABLE 29-1	Pharmacology Management of the Types of Hemophilia
TYPE OF HEMOPHILIA	**MEDICATION**
Hemophilia A	Heat treated factor VIII concentrate or cryoprecipitate
Mild hemophilia A	Desmopressin acetate (DDAVP, Stimate)
Hemophilia B	Factor IX (IV); fresh frozen plasma when necessary
Hemophilia C (factor XI deficiency)	Fresh frozen plasma
von Willebrand's disease	Cryoprecipitate and DDAVP

Adapted from Broyles, B. E., Reiss, B. S., & Evans, M. E. (2007). Pharmacological aspects of nursing care (7th ed.). New York: Thomson Delmar Learning; Robinson P. (2005). Is surgery safe for a patient with hemophilia? Nursing, 35(5), Hospital Nursing, 1–3.

nursing coordinator in the local hemophilia treatment center to gain valuable information and insight into caring for the patient with hemophilia. Specifically, careful monitoring of the clotting factor levels and appropriate replacement therapy can help decrease crisis conditions for the patient, such as preventing excessive bleeding related to surgery. Box 29-4 identifies further nursing measures for the patient with hemophilia.

Pharmacology

Treatment of hemophilia with fresh frozen plasma, factor VIII or IX concentrates, and cryoprecipitates must be individualized for each patient and for each bleeding episode (Table 29-1). In years past, various replacement therapies were derived from animal and human blood. Each had disadvantages, including severe allergic reactions, transmission of HIV and hepatitis, and the need to infuse large amounts of fluids to adequately replace coagulation factors. However, in 1994, the development of recombinant factor VIII, a genetically engineered replacement factor, introduced a safer vehicle that minimizes the risk of transmitting viral infection. However, the preparation is expensive and may trigger antibody production (Philipp, et. al., 2005), as well as other risks (e.g., thrombosis) with recurrent use.

If the patient with hemophilia needs alternative therapy because inhibitors are present in his or her blood, he or she may receive prothrombin complex or activated prothrombin complex concentrates. Both products achieve hemostasis in the presence of inhibitors by activating the coagulation system through alternative routes. The drawback is that these concentrates may not control bleeding as effectively as recombinant factors.

Evaluation of Outcomes

Potential patient outcomes for each of the example nursing diagnoses for the patient with hemophilia are:
- Ineffective peripheral tissue perfusion related to impaired circulation. The patient should maintain optimal tissue perfusion to the periphery, as evidenced by strong peripheral pulses, good capillary refill, and good movement.
- Activity intolerance related to fatigue. The patient maintains activity level within capabilities, as evidenced by normal heart rate and blood pressure during activity, as well as absence of shortness of breath, weakness, and fatigue.
- Ineffective coping related to anxiety, lower activity level, and the inability to perform normal activities of daily living. The patient identifies own maladaptive coping behaviors, available resources, and support systems, describes or initiates alternative coping strategies, and describes positive results from new behaviors.

- Pain related to decreased oxygen supply to tissues. The patient should verbalize an adequate relief of pain along with the ability to realistically cope with the pain if it is not completely relieved.

POLYCYTHEMIAS

Polycythemia is an increased amount of red blood cells with a hematocrit level elevated to more than 55 percent in males and more than 50 percent in females. There are two major types of polycythemia: primary and secondary. In addition, some sources describe a third type of polycythemia, which is relative polycythemia. This third polycythemia (relative polycythemia) is caused by fluid loss, which causes an elevated hematocrit. It is managed with fluid restoration and will not be discussed further.

Primary Polycythemia (Polycythemia Vera)

Primary polycythemia is a neoplastic stem cell disorder that is somewhat rare. The myeloid stem cells proliferate and there is an increased amount of RBCs, white blood cells (WBCs), and platelet counts. The RBC is most focused on because of the extreme elevations that are seen. In addition, this condition can last for years, which also causes such things as splenomegaly and changes in the function of the bone marrow. This disorder is more common in European Jewish persons between the ages of 40 and 70.

Assessment with Clinical Manifestations

The patient with primary polycythemia may initially be asymptomatic, with increasing symptoms as the disease progresses. Patients will display manifestations based on the increased blood volume, such as hypertension, dizziness, fatigue, headache, paresthesias, and blurred vision. Venous stasis reveals a ruddy, red-colored complexion of the face, hands, feet, and mucous membranes. The patient can also develop cardiovascular system manifestations of angina, claudication, and dyspnea (Estes, 2006). There is often uncomfortable itching of the skin from the increased histamine response due to increased basophils. Hypermetabolism occurs also, which causes weight loss and night sweats. There may also be **erythromelalgia,** which is a burning sensation in the digits of the extremities.

Diagnostic Tests

Examination of RBCs, serum WBC levels, and platelet counts assist with the diagnosis of primary polycythemia. In addition there can be elevated serum erythropoietin, and bone marrow studies can reveal red stem cell hyperplasia.

Planning and Implementation

The nursing care is focused on prevention and education. Patients who are at risk for thrombosis should be assessed, and children, teens, and others should continue to be educated as to the risks of smoking. In addition, addressing cardiovascular risk factors also assists with preventing complications of primary polycythemia. Overall, the nursing measures are aimed at the specific manifestations of the patient. For example, if itching exists, the patient can be encouraged to take tepid or cool water baths, along with applications of bath products that have cocoa butter–based lotions and avoid anything that predisposes the individual to allergen responses (e.g., flowers, or perfumes).

A primary treatment measure is to perform phlebotomy by removing 300–500 mL of blood. This is done to keep the hematocrit within normal levels and may be done one to two times a week. This treatment depletes the iron stores and keeps the patient from producing the excess RBCs.

Pharmacology

Patients are told to avoid iron supplements or multivitamins. The use of aspirin therapy is controversial, but low-dose aspirin therapy may control thrombosis and still avoid the risk of bleeding. Antihistamines can be used for the pruritus, along with the other treatment measures described previously, and chemotherapeutic agents (e.g., hydroxyurea) may be used to suppress bone marrow function (Broyles, Reiss, & Evans, 2007). The risk of the chemotherapy is the development of leukemia, which will be addressed later in this chapter.

Secondary Polycythemia

Secondary polycythemia is increased numbers of RBCs in response to a reduced amount of oxygen or an excess of erythropoietin secretion. Secondary polycythemia is caused by things that cause an elevated erythropoietin level. Usually, the response is compensating for hypoxia as seen in chronic pulmonary disorders, smoking, and high altitudes. Also, secondary polycythemia can be caused by neoplasms, such as renal cell cancer, which stimulates the erythropoietin production.

Assessment with Clinical Manifestations

The clinical manifestations are similar to those of primary polycythemia. However, splenomegaly does not normally occur. The initial symptoms are masked by the manifestations of the diseases that are leading to the secondary polycythemia.

Planning and Implementation

Management of secondary polycythemia focuses on the main cause of the condition. There may also be the need for phlebotomy and patient education for the cessation of smoking if that is a cause for the secondary polycythemia.

NEUTROPENIA

Neutropenia is a decreased number of circulating neutrophils, usually less than 1,500 cells/mm³. **Agranulocytosis** is severe neutropenia, with less than 200 cells/mm³. At this level of crisis the patient is highly at risk and requires immediate health care attention. Neutrophils are the component of the WBCs that are affected most often in pathology (note: **Leukopenia** is a decrease in the total circulating WBCs). Neutrophils are a valuable part of the immune response, and when they are decreased it is normally related to either congenital or acquired conditions. The common causes for neutropenia are hematological disorders, starvation, prolonged infection or inflammation, and autoimmune disorders.

Assessment with Clinical Manifestations

The clinical manifestations for neutropenia are obviously specific to the cause of the neutropenia, but in addition, some generalized symptomologies are: opportunistic infections located in many parts of the body (e.g., oral mucosa, GI tract, or respiratory tract), malaise, chills, fever, weakness, and severe fatigue.

Planning and Implementation

The management of neutropenia is supportive care of the patient while affected by his or her pathology. Nurses must adapt their care to protect the patient from infection. Patient education is invaluable, particularly for the patient's discharge from the acute care setting. In addition, hematopoietic growth factors such as granulocyte-macrophage colony-stimulating factor (GM-SCF) can be given to stimulate granulocyte growth. Antibiotic therapy is typically a common therapy for the variety of infections that cause the neutropenia.

MONONUCLEOSIS

Mononucleosis (infectious mononucleosis) is caused by B cells in the oropharyngeal lymphoid tissues that result from Epstein-Barr virus (EBV). Mononucleosis most often is seen in young adults (ages 15–30) and is normally spontaneous and resolves itself within 90 days. The primary mode of transmission is via saliva and consequently used to be labeled the kissing disease.

Pathophysiology

Mononucleosis begins with a virus that invades the patient. The B cells produce antibodies in response to the viral antigen, and T cells are formed in response against the virus. The infected B cells and T cells, along with the destroyed leukocytes, are the causative agents for the enlarged lymphoid tissues.

Assessment with Clinical Manifestations

There is an incubation period for four to eight weeks. During this time the symptomology varies but can include fatigue, mild headache, fever, pharyngitis, and lymph node enlargement. In addition, some patients with prolonged infectious conditions will also develop splenomegaly. Recovery usually occurs within two to three weeks, but the patient may continue to have fatigue that has remissions and exacerbations for up to three months.

Diagnostic Tests

A WBC count identifies the increased lymphocytes and monocytes after the disease has invaded for the first four to eight weeks. These cells are partially malformed and atypical in nature. Also, the history of the patient is supportive of the diagnosis.

Planning and Implementation

The care for patients with mononucleosis is supportive of the individual clinical manifestations. Nurses can encourage the patient to take frequent rest periods (or bedrest), take over-the-counter (OTC) analgesics, and to avoid strenuous activities. In addition, preventing contamination with good hygienic practices is encouraged so that the disease spread is avoided.

LEUKEMIA

Each year, about 31,000 Americans are diagnosed with leukemia, a complex and relatively rare cancer of the blood. Four main types of leukemia differ greatly in presentation, timing, clinical signs, and symptoms at various stages. Understanding the types and treatments of the different leukemias will prepare the nurse to help patients confront the burdens associated with this disease.

Leukemia, a malignancy of bone marrow cells, occurs when cells arising from stem cells lose the ability to differentiate into WBCs, RBCs, and platelets. Instead, one type of abnormal WBC prevails, and normal cell line development declines.

Epidemiology

Acute leukemia is characterized by abrupt onset and rapid progression. Acute myeloid leukemia (AML) affects people of all ages, with the incidence rising sharply at age 60. Acute lymphocytic leukemia (ALL) most commonly affects children under 15, with the highest incidence before age 5. The cure rate for childhood ALL is 85 percent.

Chronic leukemia has a gradual onset, a prolonged clinical course, and relatively long survival. Chronic myeloid leukemia (CML) affects people at all ages, but the incidence rises sharply at age 45 to 50. Chronic lymphocytic leukemia (CLL) rarely strikes before age 45; most victims are over 65. Unlike the other leukemias, CLL can cause few or no symptoms for years and may be discovered during routine blood work (Rogers, 2005).

Etiology

No single factor has been pinpointed as a cause of leukemia, although genetics, drugs, and environmental and occupational exposures have been implicated. There are risk factors that exist for the leukemias, such as radiation exposure, chemicals (e.g., benzene found in gasoline and cigarette smoke), and retrovirus of human T-cell leukemia or lymphoma virus.

Pathophysiology

All blood cells begin as stem cells in the bone marrow, then follow one of two routes. Myeloid cells become RBCs, granulocytes (consisting of neutrophils, eosinophils, and basophils), monocytes, and platelets. Lymphocytic cells become T lymphocytes, B lymphocytes, and natural killer cells. Leukemia develops when blood cell development goes awry. Either the bone marrow produces too many immature WBCs, or WBCs in the blood are not destroyed in their normal processes of destruction.

Acute and chronic leukemias are classified as lymphocytic or myelogenous according to the predominant cell type. Biphenotypic leukemia is a name given to acute leukemia with both lymphocytic and myelogenous features. There are four general types of leukemia as follows: ALL, AML, CLL, and CML. There are more definitive systems for classifying leukemias that further differentiates acute leukemias, which are defined by the predominant cell that is involved (Rogers, 2005).

Assessment with Clinical Manifestations

There are a wide variety of clinical manifestations seen in patients with leukemia. The leukemic cells crowd out normal WBCs, RBCs, and platelets, causing anemia with fatigue, dyspnea, and pallor; frequent infections and flu-like symptoms; enlarged lymph nodes and spleen; bleeding, bruising, and petechiae; and bone and joint pain as leukemic cells increase pressure in the bone marrow.

Diagnostic Tests

In most cases, signs of leukemia are evident in CBC results and platelet counts, but a bone marrow biopsy is necessary for a definitive diagnosis. The bone marrow examination determines the cell type, the type of erythropoiesis, and the maturity of the leukopoietic and erythropoietic cells. A physical examination will often reveal lymph node enlargement, and the history of the patient will support the diagnosis with specific manifestations of the particular type of leukemia present in the patient (D'Antonio, 2004).

Nursing Diagnoses

Based on the information gathered, examples of nursing diagnoses in the patient with the different types of leukemia may include the following:
- Risk for infection related to leukemia.
- Fear and anxiety related to actual or potential lifestyle changes from leukemia.
- Ineffective coping related to leukemia.
- Knowledge deficit related to self-care and risk prevention.
- Nutrition imbalance, less than body requirements, related to nausea.
- Activity intolerance related to fatigue.
- Risk for imbalanced body temperature related to leukemia.

Planning and Implementation

A patient typically gets a leukemia diagnosis after having a physical examination, blood work, and a bone marrow biopsy. The nurse will care for the patient by keeping the patient comfortable during diagnostic procedures and offer emotional support during this initial time of diagnosis. Initially, the patient may be confused about treatment options and whether to seek a second opinion. Even after making critical health care decisions, the patient may have lingering practical concerns about family, work, and finances. The nurse will encourage communication between the patient, family, and the health care team and potentially refer the patient to organizations such as The Leukemia and Lymphoma Society for guidance.

A patient recently diagnosed with leukemia has much to learn about the disease. Thus, patient education for newly diagnosed patients with leukemia is essential. The nurse may encourage the patient to take a friend or family member to appointments with the oncologist and to take notes or tape record the visits. Also, the nurse may inform the patient to write down questions beforehand so he or she does not forget to ask something during the visit. The nurse can urge the patient to ask the oncologist to enumerate the risks and benefits of treatment options so the patient can list them for comparison before deciding. In addition, there is a tremendous workload issue for nurses caring for patients with the leukemias, as there are for many of the other hematological or oncological disorders (see Uncovering the Evidence feature).

There are a great variety of interventions for patients (Box 29-5) with leukemia and more information in this regard is provided within the descriptions of each of the four major types of leukemia.

Radiation

Radiation therapy is a valuable management strategy used in the treatment options for leukemia. The radiation is destructive to cellular DNA and therefore does damage to the quickly dividing cancer cells. Normal cells are also affected and consequently cause a variety of side affects when the radiation is applied. The types of delivery, effects, and care for patients receiving radiation therapy are further discussed in chapter 15.

Surgery

The primary forms of surgical treatment for the leukemias are stem cell transplantation and bone marrow transplantation. The decision of which treatment to use is specific to the patient and the type of leukemia present.

The options for postinduction therapy (consolidation) are more standard dose chemotherapy or a transplant of the patient's own stem cells (**autologous transplantation**) or stem cells from a sibling or unrelated donor with matching human-leukocyte-antigens (HLA) (**allogeneic transplantation**). Whether allogenic stem cell transplant (ASCT) improves the rate of long-term remission is

Uncovering the Evidence

Measuring the Time for Nursing Care on a Hematology Oncology Unit

Discussion: The study purpose was to develop a tool that could assist nurse managers in planning nurse staffing levels and assessing workload in hematology oncology units. A task-oriented method based on a time-and-motion study was used. Three general nursing procedures and seven specific oncological and hematological activities were observed, and the total amount of time needed for each patient was calculated. The sample was taken from patients with on of five categories of hematology or oncology disorders (i.e., autologous stem cell transplantation, allogeneic stem cell transplantation, graft versus host reaction, leukemia treatment, chemotherapy for solid neoplasm). The results showed a high variance in the more complex activities (e.g., changing infusion lines or applying dressings to Hickman catheters). A high standard deviation was also seen in administering blood transfusions. On the other side, well-standardized activities, such as patient monitoring, mouth cleaning, and medication administration had small standard deviation. Overall, the findings revealed precise estimations of the amount of time needed for the selected procedures.

Implications for Practice: The study clearly identifies different categories for hematology and oncology patients. This can assist nurses to more specifically label the types of patients on these patient arenas with high acuity levels. In addition, identifying specific nursing activities, which require more nursing work hours, could continue to aid nurse managers in making appropriate patient assignments for the nursing staff. The outcome is a better workload distribution and ultimately better nursing practice and better patient outcomes.

Source: Colombo, A., Solberg, B., Vanderhoeft, E., Ramsay, G., & Schouten, H. (2005). Measurement of nursing care time of specific interventions on a hematology-oncology unit related to diagnostic categories. Cancer Nursing, 28(6), 476–480.

Red Flag

Graft-Versus-Host Disease (GVHD)

After receiving the donor's stem cells, the recipient may develop (25–60 percent develop this rejection) a condition of GVHD, in which the recipient has a severe reaction to the new cells. The recipient will have fever, diarrhea, nausea, skin rashes, GI bleeding, and potentially liver damage. The recipient is critically ill and can remain in critical care for six to eight weeks during this time.

unclear. Allogeneic transplants from HLA-matched donors have produced a cure in 50 to 60 percent of patients in consolidation therapy. The regimen that precedes allogeneic transplant is so harsh that this option is usually reserved for patients younger than 55 years, who are more likely to survive the adverse effects of treatment.

The donors for a stem cell transplant must have tissue that is closely matched with that of the recipient. Hematopoietic growth factor is given to the donor for four to five days prior to harvesting the stem cells. The growth factor increases the concentration of the stem cells. The recipient of the stem cell transplant is given high doses of chemotherapy and radiation prior to the transplant to destroy the leukemic cells. Then the donor marrow is infused into the recipient, and the goal is for the transfusion to allow healthy cells to replace the leukemic cells. To prevent infection, the recipient is placed under neutropenic precautions until the WBC count rises to an acceptable level. The recipient is usually critically ill following the stem cell transplant and suffers the risk for infection and rejection of the transplanted cells (Nowlin, 2005).

Postremission therapy includes intensive consolidation treatment with either high-dose cytarabine or allogenic or autologous bone marrow transplantation (BMT). Disease-free survivals are comparable with any of these approaches. The major criticism of BMT in first remission is that although it is effective therapy, it is toxic, expensive, and not necessarily better than conventional treatment. In addition, only 30 percent of younger patients have an HLA-compatible donor. Allogeneic BMT is considered more effective than autologous BMT because some data suggest that part of the immunological effect of the graft may translate to antileukemic activity, resulting in lower relapse rates in patients with allogenic transplant. The risks and complications for BMT are similar to those for stem cell transplantation, including the GVHD (Nowlin, 2005).

BOX 29-5

GENERAL NURSING CARE FOR PATIENTS WITH LEUKEMIA

Anyone with lymphoma or leukemia requires skilled nursing care to cope with the diagnosis and to minimize adverse reactions to treatment. Remind the patient that most adverse effects of therapy can be managed and that many people continue working during treatment. To help the patient manage immediate and long-term problems, teach them about the following effects of his illness and therapy:

- Emotional issues. Encourage the patient to discuss feelings; provide reassurance and support. Teach the patient relaxation techniques and encourage the patient to seek help through a support group or counselor. If the patient is taking prednisone, advise to take it with breakfast or lunch to prevent insomnia and to notify the care provider if there are mood changes, which can occur with prednisone therapy.
- Infection. Teach the patient about infection risks. Review the signs and symptoms of infections and tell the patient to contact the care provider they develop any signs of infection.
- Hair loss and skin changes. Inform the patient about the potential for hair loss and explain that the hair will probably grow back after finishing chemotherapy. Encourage the patient to purchase a wig or hat before the first chemotherapy infusion. Tell the patient that the skin may dry and become more sensitive to sunlight so they may need to apply sunblock and wear protective clothing in the sunshine. The patient should also be told they may also notice changes in his nails.
- Fatigue. Encourage the patient to pace activities, rest frequently, and get help with activities of daily living (Figure 29-4).

- Reproductive issues. Discuss the potential for chemotherapy-induced sterility. For a male, review the need to prevent pregnancy in his partner because chromosome damage to sperm can negatively affect the fetus. Discuss sperm banking and provide resource information if he chooses this option. Teach a female patient that treatment can cause menstrual changes and menopause-like symptoms and make her susceptible to vaginal infections.
- Stomatitis. Encourage the patient to see a dentist before starting chemotherapy. Teach the patient to rinse his mouth with a solution of salt and baking soda in water to prevent infection and advise to avoid drinking alcohol. Inform the patient to call the health care provider if he or she develops mouth sores.
- Bladder and bowel changes. Advise the patient to drink plenty of fluids and to void frequently to prevent cystitis. Teach the patient to check the urine for blood and to call the health care provider if he or she develops frequency or discomfort with urination. The nurse should teach the patient to include fiber in the diet and encourage the use of a laxative if unable to have a bowel movement every two days. Tell the patient to call the health care provider if diarrhea develops. Monitor the response to antidiarrheal medication and assess for dehydration.
- Gastric irritation. If the patient takes prednisone, teach the patient to take it with food or milk. If the patient reports midepigastric distress, ask the care provider to prescribe medication to prevent gastrointestinal irritation.

Adapted from D'Antonio J. (2004). You can lessen leukemia's toll. Nursing, 34(7), Hospital Nursing, 1–4; DeLaune, S., & Ladner, P. (2006). Fundamentals of nursing (3rd ed.). New York: Thomson Delmar Learning.

Evaluation of Outcomes

Potential patient outcomes for each of the example nursing diagnoses for the patient with the different types of leukemia are:

- Risk for infection related to leukemia. The patient remains free of infection, as evidenced by normal vital signs and absence of purulent drainage from wounds, incisions, and tubes. Infection is recognized early to allow for prompt treatment.
- Fear and anxiety related to actual or potential lifestyle changes from leukemia. The patient should be able to recognize the signs of anxiety and describe a reduction in the level of anxiety experienced.
- Ineffective coping related to leukemia. The patient should demonstrate positive coping mechanisms and develop acceptance of the disorder.

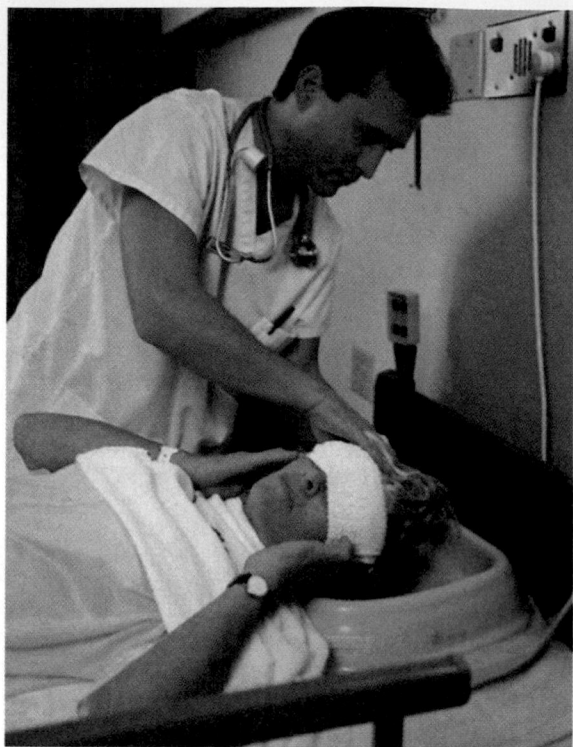

Figure 29-4 Shampooing a patient in bed who is fatigued from her leukemia.

- Knowledge deficit related to self-care and risk prevention. The patient should demonstrate motivation to learn, identify perceived learning needs, and verbalize an understanding of desired content.
- Nutrition imbalance, less than body requirements, related to nausea. The patient verbalizes and demonstrates selection of foods or meals that will achieve a cessation of weight loss and weighs within 10 percent of ideal body weight.
- Activity intolerance related to fatigue. The patient maintains activity level within capabilities, as evidenced by normal heart rate and blood pressure during activity, as well as absence of shortness of breath, weakness, and fatigue.
- Risk for imbalanced body temperature related to leukemia. The patient maintains body temperature within a normal range.

Acute Leukemias

A patient with ALL or AML must be hospitalized as soon as possible to start induction therapy, which is aimed to destroy all visible leukemic cells in the bone marrow and blood. The patients will receive a variety of different chemotherapy drugs, probably through an indwelling central venous access device. Patient education related to chemotherapy adverse reactions are an essential component of the management of the acute leukemias.

After induction therapy, residual leukemia cells are inevitable, so the patient will likely need further postremission chemotherapy. Some patients who qualify may then undergo stem cell transplantation. Acute leukemias progress rapidly and are characterized by ineffective, immature cells in the bone marrow crowding out and preventing development of normal cells. AML accounts for most acute leukemias in adults; ALL is more common in children (McKenzie, 2005).

Some initial signs and symptoms of acute leukemia are nonspecific. Rising numbers of immature cells can affect all the blood cell lines (e.g., RBCs, WBCs, platelets). Therefore, signs and symptoms are related to anemia, neutropenia, and thrombocytopenia. Further manifestations include pallor, headache, fatigue, malaise, loss of appetite, weight loss, tachycardia, shortness of breath, petechiae, ecchymoses, and splenomegaly. Bleeding or easy bruis-

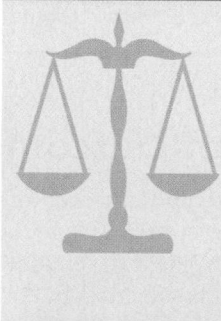

ETHICS IN PRACTICE

Stem Cell Research

There is currently much controversy over the use of stem cells obtained from fetal tissue. The use of federal funding is questioned and currently not allowed. The crux of the argument is whether obtaining fetal tissue is a breech of life and whether obtaining the stem cells is an ethical procedure. The issue is complicated, because right-to-life proponents argue that the fetus is a living human being and that doing research on fetal tissue can potentially create situations for obtaining fetal tissue from aborted fetus. Undoubtedly, this issue will remain for discussion and debate, both within and without the health care community.

ing after minor trauma, a characteristic sign of leukemia, stems from thrombocytopenia. Bone tenderness of the long bones, ribs, and sternum also may occur as leukemic cells expand the intramedullary space or invade the periosteum. Many clinical manifestations overlap with the chronic leukemias and can be referred to in the upcoming section that focuses on the chronic leukemia types.

Acute Lymphoblastic Leukemia

ALL is a stem cell disorder characterized by an overproduction of lymphoblasts in the bone marrow that eventually spill into circulation, producing lymphocytosis. As with the other acute leukemias, the most common symptoms experienced by patients include fatigue, bleeding, and recurrent infections resulting from the suppression of normal hematopoiesis in the bone marrow by the accumulating blasts. ALL primarily affects children and exhibits the best response to standard chemotherapy as compared to AML (Randolph, 2004).

Epidemiology

ALL represents 12 percent of all leukemia cases, with a worldwide incidence projected to be 1–4.75 per 100,000 people. Italy, the United States, Switzerland, and Costa Rica are the countries with the highest incidence of ALL. Hereditary link, genetic defects, and possibly radiation or chemical exposures are listed amongst the most significant risk factors. ALL is predominantly a disease of childhood, but it affects adults as well. It accounts for 80 percent of all leukemia cases in children. The incidence is slightly higher in men than in women and greater in Caucasians people than in African Americans. See chapter 15 for the types of causation factors that exist for generalized cancer pathologies.

Pathophysiology

Rapidly developing immature lymphocytes crowding out normal cells indicate ALL. In adults with ALL, the Philadelphia chromosome, the hallmark of CML, is the most common chromosome abnormality detected.

Diagnostic Tests

Refer to the diagnostic testing section in the introduction section of leukemia. In addition, the following are diagnostic testing information for ALL. Cytogenic testing on the bone marrow specimen identifies this marker. Poor prognostic factors for ALL include a high WBC count (25,000/mm^3 or greater) at presentation, presence of the Philadelphia chromosome, age over 50 years, and slow first remission (longer than four weeks) (Redaelli, Laskin, Stephens, Botteman, & Pashos, 2005).

Planning and Implementation

There are a wide variety of interventions and management strategies for the treatment of ALL. Refer to the general interventions shown in the beginning section of leukemia.

Pharmacology

The primary goal of ALL therapy is complete remission with restoration of normal hematopoiesis. Induction chemotherapy is administered in two phases. The first consists of daunorubicin, vincristine, and prednisone with L-asparaginase. The second phase, administered soon after the first, includes cyclophosphamide, cytarabine, and 6-mercaptopurine and prophylaxis with intrathecal methotrexate or cytosine arabinoside. Maintenance therapy must follow induction to prevent relapse. Several alternating regimens may be used for up to 36 months. The patient's risk factors determine the duration of treatment.

In adults, ALL does not respond to treatment as favorably as in children. The complete remission rates are comparable at 80 to 95 percent, but most adult patients relapse. The five-year survival rate is 20 to 30 percent in adults and 70 percent in children. The treatment in all age-groups consists of four phases: induction, consolidation, maintenance, and central nervous system (CNS) prophylaxis. Multiple chemotherapeutic agents are used, including vincristine, anthracycline, steroids, asparaginase, cytarabine, methotrexate, and mercaptopurine. The folate antimetabolites are not used until consolidation or maintenance therapy. Allogeneic BMT is necessary for cure in patients younger than 55 years with poor-risk disease or on relapse.

Acute Myeloid Leukemia

The past three decades have seen considerable advances in the understanding of the underlying mechanisms of AML and dramatic improvements in treatment. At present, decisions about therapy are largely based on prognostic factors identified at the time of diagnosis or shortly thereafter. These features include age, the karyotype of the leukemic clone, the initial leukocyte count, and the response to induction chemotherapy. Karyotypic analysis is particularly important, because it not only provides a vital prognostic indicator but also serves to identify biologically distinct subgroups of AML, which in some instances require specific types of treatment.

Epidemiology
The incidence of AML increases with age, peaking in the sixth decade of life. In the United States, there are about 10,000 new cases of AML and 7,000 deaths in those with an AML diagnosis per year. Current molecular studies of AML demonstrate that it is a heterogeneous disorder of the myeloid cell lineage. See chapter 15 for the types of causation factors that exist for generalized cancer pathologies.

Pathophysiology
AML is a malignant neoplasm of hematopoietic cells characterized by an abnormal proliferation of myeloid precursor cells, decreased rate of self-destruction, and an arrest in cellular differentiation. The leukemic cells have an abnormal survival advantage. Thus, the bone marrow and peripheral blood are characterized by leukocytosis with a predominance of immature cells, primarily blasts. As the immature cells accumulate in the bone marrow, they replace the normal myelocytic cells, megakaryocytes, and erythrocytic cells. This leads to a loss of normal bone marrow function and associated complications of bleeding, anemia, and infection. Stem cells destined to develop in the myelogenous line of cells normally mature into neutrophils, monocytes, eosinophils, RBCs, and platelets. But when these cells overwhelmingly commit to one type, most commonly neutrophils, AML develops (Valk, et al., 2004).

Assessment with Clinical Manifestations
Refer to general information on leukemias in this section. In addition, several clinical characteristics of AML influence prognosis. Factors in the patient's favor are age under 60 years, spontaneous rather than secondary leukemia, a WBC count less than 10,000/mm³, and the achievement of complete remission with one cycle of chemotherapy.

Diagnostic Tests
Refer to the diagnostic testing section of the introduction to leukemia. In addition, bone marrow biopsy is necessary to make the diagnosis.

Planning and Implementation
There are a wide variety of interventions and management strategies for the treatment of AML. Refer to the general interventions shown in the beginning section of leukemia.

Pharmacology

Treatment for AML consists of chemotherapy; specifically, induction and maintenance therapy. Induction chemotherapy usually consists of cytosine arabinoside and an anthracycline. The goal of induction therapy is to attain complete remission by eliminating leukemic cells from the bone marrow. Postinduction therapy (consolidation) is necessary to prevent relapse after remission. However, the optimal regimen has not yet been determined. From 25 to 35 percent of patients have a long-term remission after postinduction chemotherapy. Therapy with high-dose cytarabine has improved the duration of first remission in most young patients with AML. This is because most patients with AML are symptomatic at presentation and require immediate treatment with cytarabine. Response rates in newly diagnosed patients are 50 to 75 percent. Recently, dose intensification schemes with higher cytarabine doses have produced similar remission rates but longer disease-free survivals, at the expense of greater toxicity (McKenzie, 2005).

Chronic Leukemia

Chronic leukemias progress more slowly and rarely affect people under age 20. Allowing development of more normal cells, chronic leukemia may not affect the patient's health as severely until the advanced stages. CML typically strikes between ages 40 and 50, with slightly more men affected than women. CLL typically develops after age 40 and is most common in older men.

Although stem cell transplantation offers people with CML the only sure chance of cure, there continue to be forms of chemotherapy with excellent results (e.g., imatinib [Gleevec]), a drug approved in 2001.

Ironically, achieving remission from leukemia can cause the patient to have some ambivalence and uncertainty. Uneasy about losing the close monitoring, the patient may focus on minor health problems that are probably unrelated to leukemia. If the patient has a relapse, he or she may become even more distressed about the additional treatments that lay ahead.

If treatment fails and the hope of remission fades, the patient may have intense feelings of denial, depression, and fear. Encourage the patient to express negative emotions and to validate self-worth, social connectedness, and spirituality. More than ever, the patient needs compassion, caring, and respect. Refer the patient for hospice or palliative care so the patient and family can get support and education and learn how to manage symptoms. They also need support in confronting issues such as advance directives. See chapter 15 for the types of causation factors that exist for generalized cancer pathologies.

Assessment with Clinical Manifestations

Refer to the assessment information related to general leukemias. In addition, Box 29-6 indicates common problems to assess for and monitor in chronic leukemia, as well as the corresponding interventions.

Planning and Implementation

There are a wide variety of interventions and management strategies for the treatment of chronic leukemia. Refer to the general interventions shown in the beginning section on leukemia and in the assessment with clinical manifestation above.

Chronic Lymphocytic Leukemia

CLL is the most common leukemia, with an annual incidence of 1.8 to 3.0 per 100,000 people in the United States. Unlike acute leukemias and CML, CLL is not considered curable, but it may follow an indolent clinical course for many years. Many patients have no complaints at diagnosis and have only peripheral

BOX 29-6

COMMON PROBLEMS IN CHRONIC LEUKEMIA WITH CORRESPONDING INTERVENTIONS

- Myelosuppression caused by chemotherapy, which leads to anemia, thrombocytopenia, and neutropenia. Monitor and report the patient's lab results and teach the signs and symptoms of myelosuppression (e.g., fatigue, shortness of breath, bleeding, chills, fever, cough, or poor wound healing). Teach patient good mouth care and aseptic technique to prevent infection.
- Altered body image and mood. Before starting chemotherapy, encourage the patient to get a short haircut or purchase a wig. Short hair makes wig fitting easier and helps make eventual hair loss less traumatic. Encourage the patient to engage in meditation, hobbies, and similar activities and to stay as involved as possible in the usual routine.
- Sexual concerns. The care provider should discuss potential problems such as premature menopause, lack of interest in sex, and infertility with the patient and partner. Explaining that low libido due to treatment is usually temporary and reassure them. Someone concerned about fertility may choose to bank ova or sperm.

- Shifting roles and responsibilities. The patient and family should try to keep things as normal as possible, but he or she may need to reallocate responsibilities. Hiring help might be one solution.
- Loss of social contacts. Friends and extended family members may want to help, but not know how. Feeling awkward, they may shy away, increasing the patient's sense of isolation. Encourage the patient and family to pursue social contacts and to ask for others' help, rather than waiting for them to offer.
- Children feeling left out. Children can become anxious if they do not receive age-appropriate information about a family member who is ill. Along with their usual discipline and guidance, they need extra doses of reassurance and love, if necessary, from other relatives or friends.
- Fostering communication between the patient and family, health care providers, friends, and neighbors is a high priority. Assist patients and family members to find the right words and ask the right questions and refer them to a support group or counseling.

Source: D'Antonio J. (2004). You can lessen leukemia's toll. Nursing, 34(7), *Hospital Nursing, 1–4.*

lymphadenopathy or splenomegaly as a presenting feature. Treatment is not advocated in early asymptomatic stages, because the course of the disease is varied and there are no data supporting improvement in survival with early intervention. When therapy is indicated, first-line interventions usually include either chlorambucil (Leukeran) or a purine analog such as fludarabine phosphate (Fludara). The disease can be controllable for many years.

Epidemiology

CLL represents 22 to 30 percent of all leukemia cases with a worldwide incidence projected to be between less than 1 and 5.5 per 100,000 people. Australia, the United States, Ireland, and Italy have the highest CLL incidence rates. CLL presents in adults, at higher rates in males than in females and in Caucasians than in African Americans. Median age at diagnosis is between 64 and 70. Five-year survival rate in the United States is 83 percent for those younger than 65 years old and 68 percent for those 65 and older. As no cure is yet available, a strong unmet medical need exists for innovative new therapies. Experimental treatments under development include allogeneic stem cell transplant, miniallogenic transplants, and monoclonal antibodies.

Etiology

See chapter 15 for the types of causation factors that exist for generalized cancer pathologies. In addition, hereditary and genetic links have been noted. Persons with close relatives who have CLL have an increased risk of developing it themselves. No single environmental risk factor has been found to be predictive for CLL.

Pathophysiology

CLL is a monoclonal disorder with expansion of small lymphocytes of B cell (95 percent) or T cell (5 percent) lineage. CLL cells accumulate in blood, bone marrow, lymph nodes, and spleen, causing enlargement of these organs and decreased bone marrow function. The course of CLL depends on the disease stage. Median survival ranges from less than 19 months for patients with advanced disease to more than 10 years for those with the early stage of the disease. An indolent disease characterized by lymphocytosis, lymphadenopathy, and hepatosplenomegaly, CLL eventually poses a risk of death from recurrent bacterial and viral infections as the disease advances (Redaelli, et al., 2004).

Assessment with Clinical Manifestations

Refer to general assessment information in the leukemia information. In addition, patients are usually diagnosed at routine health care visits because of elevated lymphocyte counts. The most common presenting symptom of CLL is lymphadenopathy, while difficulty exercising and fatigue are common complaints. Most patients do not receive treatment after initial diagnosis unless presenting with clear pathological conditions.

Planning and Implementation

There are a wide variety of interventions and management strategies for the treatment of CLL. Refer to the general interventions shown in the beginning section of leukemia and in the preceding assessment with clinical manifestation section.

For CLL, oncologists commonly follow a watch-and-wait protocol, monitoring the patient for signs and symptoms of disease before initiating treatment. This approach may make the patient especially anxious, so teach the patient and his or her family about the disease's nonaggressive nature and reassure them. Also teach them what signs and symptoms to look for and when to report to the health care practitioner. When treatment becomes necessary, they may receive chemotherapy or a monoclonal antibody. A young person with CLL might undergo a stem cell transplant.

Pharmacology

Treatment of CLL with standard chemotherapy can produce remissions but cannot cure the disease. Because CLL is not curable and therapy may cause harsh adverse reactions, treatment is usually delayed until the patient develops signs and symptoms. The chemotherapy options include the alkylating agent chlorambucil with or without prednisone, the antimetabolite fludarabine, which may be the most effective single drug treatment currently available, and combined chemotherapy such as cyclophosphamide/vincristine/prednisolone (CVP). Rituximab is frequently combined with chemotherapy to enhance the response. The patient also may receive radiation therapy to sites of bulky lymphadenopathy (Broyles, et al., 2007).

Chronic Myelogenous Leukemia

Since the 1970s, it has been known that CML is associated with the Philadelphia chromosome. The Philadelphia chromosome is present in 95 percent of patients with CML, and it is an important diagnostic parameter. Its eradication is also an indicator of treatment response. The disease is characterized by progressive replacement of the normal elements of the marrow with mature myeloid cells no longer responsive to mechanisms that govern proliferation of normal myeloid cells. This results in an ever-increasing ratio of leukemic to normal myeloid cells (D'Antonio, 2005). See chapter 15 for the types of causation factors that exist for generalized cancer pathologies.

Pathophysiology

CML can be subdivided into three clinical phases: chronic, accelerated, and acute blastic phase. Patients usually present with fatigue, low-grade fever, and night sweats. CML is characterized by the presence of the Philadelphia chromosome and development of too many neutrophils, CML consists of three clinical phases shown in Box 29-7.

Diagnostic Tests

Refer to the diagnostic testing section of the introduction to leukemia. In addition, the diagnosis of CML is based on leukocytosis of up to 700,000 leukocytes/mm³ and basophilia. Bone marrow examination reveals hypercellularity with a left shift in myelopoiesis. The acquisition of additional chromosomal aberrations such as an extra Philadelphia chromosome decreases the ability for cell maturation, which terminates in blastic crisis (blast counts in the bone marrow greater than 30 percent). At this stage, all body organs are infiltrated by blasts and the patient dies of bleeding, infection, or thrombosis in organs such as the lungs or brain. The median time to blastic crisis is about four years.

Planning and Implementation

There are a wide variety of interventions and management strategies for the treatment of CLL. Refer to the general interventions at the beginning section of leukemia.

Pharmacology

The kinase inhibitor imatinib (Gleevec) is the current treatment of choice for CML. Most effective at inducing remission in the early stages, it is also well tolerated. Trials are under way to combine imatinib with other agents to enhance the response rate and duration.

Other agents used to treat patients with CML include interferon alpha, which has been shown to reduce growth and division of leukemia cells in 55 to 60 percent of treated patients. Because interferon alpha causes major adverse reactions, it is no longer the drug of choice to combat CML. Another agent, hydroxyurea, may prolong the chronic phase of CML but has not been shown to affect cell growth and development.

Surgery

Stem cell transplant from a compatible donor achieves long-term survival in many patients, but the risk of dying during the first 100 days is 20 percent. This intervention is most successful early in the chronic phase of CML. Allogenic

---

BOX 29-7

CLINICAL PHASES OF CML

The following are the three phases of CML:

1. The chronic phase follows an indolent course during which the patient may have mild symptoms and respond to standard treatments. The percentage of blasts in bone marrow is usually less than 10 percent.
2. The accelerated phase is characterized by spleen enlargement and progressive signs and symptoms, such as intermittent fevers, night sweats, and unexplained weight loss. The typical patient does not respond to treatment as readily, and bone marrow contains 10 to 30 percent blasts and promyelocytes. The accelerated phase typically lasts 6 to 12 months.
3. The blast phase indicates a transformation to an aggressive acute leukemia. The bone marrow contains more than 30 percent blasts, and promyelocytes and blasts commonly spread to other tissues and organs. Most patients die when CML reaches this phase.

Adapted from D'Antonio, J. (2005). Chronic myelogenous leukemia. Clinical Journal of Oncology Nursing, 9(5), 535–538, *561–563; Menzin, J., Lang, K., Earle, C., & Glendenning, A. (2004). Treatment patterns, outcomes and costs among elderly patients with chronic myeloid leukemia: A population-based analysis.* Drugs and Aging, 21(11), 737–746.

bone marrow transplantation in the chronic phase of CML can induce cures in 50 percent of patients, especially if it occurs within the first year of diagnosis before any evidence of disease progression from the chronic phase, and if previous busulfan therapy has been avoided

MULTIPLE MYELOMA

Multiple myeloma is the cancer of plasma cells. It is due to the unregulated proliferation of monoclonal plasma cells that are ineffective, accumulate in the bone marrow, and secrete monoclonal immunoglobulins and cytokines. The monoclonal immunoglobulins and cytokines that are produced from the plasma cells lead to decreased bone marrow function and destruction of bone tissue. Multiple myeloma is often identified in the primary care setting. Up to 30 percent of patients are diagnosed incidentally while being evaluated for unrelated problems. Its clinical presentation varies, but the most common clinical features include anemia, bone pain, lytic lesions, recurrent infections, renal insufficiency, and hypercalcemia. It is important for the health care provider to recognize its clinical features, perform the appropriate screening studies, make appropriate referrals to and coordinate care with oncologists, and arrange for emergency therapies if indicated (Mangan, 2005).

Epidemiology

Multiple myeloma accounts for 10 percent of all hematologic cancers. It is also the second most common hematologic malignancy after non-Hodgkin's lymphoma (NHL), with 15,270 new cases predicted in 2004 in the United States. It is estimated that approximately 11,070 people died of myeloma in 2004. The incidence of myeloma is rare in people under the age of 40 years. The median age of diagnosis is 65 years, with a slight male predominance. This rise in incidence may be related to such factors as early detection and diagnosis by clinicians, the improving life expectancy, the aging of the general population, and chronic exposure to environmental pollutants.

African Americans are twice as likely to develop the disease as are other Americans. In fact, multiple myeloma is the most common hematologic malignancy in African Americans. It accounts for only one to two cases per 100,000 of people of Asian descent. The reason for this racial disparity remains unclear. In a study conducted at the National Cancer Institute in 2000, it was found that the risk of multiple myeloma increased with decreased socioeconomic status in both African Americans and Caucasians. Socioeconomic status measurement included occupation, income, and education. Low social class may be a surrogate for a set of negative environmental characteristics such as poor housing, dangerous jobs that may result in differential exposure to occupational carcinogens, unemployment, lack of access to medical care, stressful home or work environments, poor nutrition, and exposure to infectious agents. There was a higher percentage of African Americans in the lower socioeconomic level than Caucasians, which may help to explain the higher incidence of the disease in African Americans (Mangan, 2005).

Etiology

The exact cause of myeloma is unknown. Environmental exposure to radiation and chemicals has been associated with an increased incidence of myeloma. The incidence of multiple myeloma is higher among those who are directly exposed to pesticides, herbicides, or ionizing radiation. Chronic immune stimulation and autoimmune disorders may also play a role in the pathogenesis of the disease.

Pathophysiology

Normally, mature plasma cells make up less than 5 percent of the bone marrow cellularity. Their precursors are plasmablasts, or B lymphocytes that migrate to the marrow from the lymph nodes after being stimulated by antigens and cytokines from the helper T cells in the lymph node. Once activated, they migrate to the bone marrow, where they stop proliferating and begin to differentiate to mature plasma cells. Healthy plasma cells produce the antibodies or immunoglobulins that are essential to our humoral immunity. These immunoglobulins are released in response to foreign antigen exposure. These immunoglobulins are IgG, IgA, IgM, IgD, and IgE.

An unregulated, progressive proliferation of monoclonal plasma cells accumulates in the marrow space and leads to secretion of cytokines by the tumor cells. The microenvironment of the bone marrow is thought to play an important role in the ability of myeloma to live and replicate. Included in this environment is interleukin-6, which is an essential cytokine for the survival and growth of myeloma cells. Interleukin-6 is also thought to mediate many of the abnormalities associated with myeloma, including anemia and hypoalbuminemia.

Assessment with Clinical Manifestations

The clinical presentation of multiple myeloma is changing, most likely as a result of diagnostic testing that detects the disease in earlier stages. Approximately 20 percent of all patients are without symptoms at the time of diagnosis. Clinical features of overt myeloma commonly include fatigue, anemia, bone pain and pathological fractures, recurrent bacterial infections, and renal dysfunction. Less common presentations include hypercalcemia and hyperviscosity syndrome. The presence of one or more of these symptoms is often the first clue of the diagnosis of myeloma. At the time of diagnosis, two thirds of patients will have anemia. Patients with myeloma commonly present with low back pain. Skeletal involvement, particularly the spine, accounts for the principle morbidity in the disease. More than one half of cases are diagnosed while evaluating a patient for bone or back pain. One third of patients are diagnosed following a pathological fracture. Bone pain is not only the most common presenting symptom; it can occur at any time during the course of the disease. This skeletal involvement and associated pain may interfere with functional ability and overall quality of life.

Renal insufficiency occurs in more than 30 percent of all individuals diagnosed with myeloma, and it is considered a poor prognostic factor, because it is associated with shortened survival. It is second only to infection as a leading cause of death for individuals with multiple myeloma. Causes include dehydration, infection, nephrotoxins, hypercalcemia, nephrocalcinosis, hyperuricemia, and urate nephropathy

Diagnostic Tests

The classic definition of multiple myeloma is characterized by a bone marrow infiltrated with 10 percent or greater plasma cells, the presence of monoclonal protein in the serum or urine, and evidence of systemic disease. Myeloma should be suspected in anyone over the age of 40 years; presenting with unexplained bone pain or fracture, osteoporosis, osteolytic lesions, anemia, renal failure, or recurrent infections. Initial workup of suspected myeloma involves laboratory testing of patient's blood and urine, radiographic evaluations, and bone marrow biopsy. The diagnosis of bone lesions is best done using skeletal surveys. Skeletal lesions are observed on simple radiographs in 80 percent of the cases.

Laboratory evaluation, including CBC and serum chemistries, may reveal anemia, hypercalcemia, and elevated serum total protein. Serum and urine electrophoresis with immunofixation (SPEP and UPEP) are completed to confirm the presence of the monoclonal protein. In less than 5 percent of all cases of myeloma, monoclonal proteins are not detected. This type of myeloma is known as nonsecretory myeloma.

Nursing Diagnoses

Based on the information gathered, examples of nursing diagnoses in the patient with multiple myeloma may include the following:
- Acute pain as related to bone involvement in multiple myeloma.
- Fear in response to the diagnosis of multiple myeloma.
- Ineffective coping related to anxiety, lower activity level, and the inability to perform normal activities of daily living.
- Activity intolerance related to fatigue.

Planning and Implementation

The decision to initiate therapy versus active observation depends on patient symptoms, age, and performance status, as well as the number of negative prognostic factors. Many patients with low-stage disease have an indolent course for many years without the need of therapy before the disease progresses. These patients should initiate a period of active observation, including close monitoring with blood work and radiographic studies, while avoiding the potential side effects associated with antimyeloma therapies. Encouraging adequate oral hydration and avoiding potentially renal toxic agents like IV contrast dyes, certain antibiotics, and other medications including nonsteroidal anti-inflammatory agents, is helpful in preventing renal insufficiency. Educating patients on the awareness of their urinary output and monitoring their weight daily can also detect a change in their disease status. Back braces can be helpful for vertebral compression fractures. Because of the increased incidence of infection in myeloma patients throughout their disease course, quick evaluation and treatment of infections are essential (Mangan, 2005).

Pharmacology

Present treatments for bone disease associated with myeloma include conservative measures such as nonsteroidal anti-inflammatory drugs (NSAIDs), opiates, gabapentin (Neurontin), and tricyclic antidepressants for analgesia. Local radiation therapy, decompression surgery, and glucocorticoid therapy may be necessary to treat lytic bone lesions; particularly those involving the spine with spinal cord compression.

With more advanced or higher stage disease, primary therapy has significantly improved the median survival from 7 to 24 to 30 months. Chemotherapy with antineoplastic agents for myeloma includes an induction therapy, which is designed to decrease the burden of the disease. High-dose therapy with stem cell support has become the standard postinduction therapy with some form of maintenance therapy following transplant, to help maintain remission duration.

Surgery

Autologous stem cell transplantation has become the standard of care as postinduction therapy in most patients under the age of 75 years. This procedure consists of patients, at the time of maximum response to induction therapy, undergoing peripheral stem cell collections after stimulation with granulocyte colony-stimulating factor (G-CSF), with or without a dose of mobilization chemotherapy. Once adequate stems cells are collected, high-dose melphalan is administered, followed by the infusion of the previously harvested stem cells. In general, high-dose therapy with autologous transplant nearly doubles median survival for newly diagnosed patients and is now considered standard of care for upfront therapy, particularly for those 70 years of age or younger.

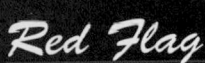

Red Flag

Calcium Imbalances in Multiple Myeloma

The incidence of hypercalcemia in patients with myeloma is approximately 25 percent. If the serum calcium level rises slowly, a patient can remain relatively asymptomatic for a period of time. If the rise is sudden, a hypercalcemic crisis can occur and result in coma, renal failure, or cardiac arrest. Prompt recognition and treatment of this disorder can result in the reversal of a life-threatening condition. Calcium is a critical regulator of many cellular processes that affect many organ systems, including GI, cardiac, renal, and neuromuscular. Early symptoms include fatigue, nausea, vomiting, anorexia, polydipsia, dry mucous membranes, or constipation. As the imbalance worsens, one may detect dehydration, confusion, loss of deep tendon reflexes, ECG changes, and orthostatic hypotension.

Mortality is low, less than 3 percent in patients younger than 65 years of age, and 5 to 8 percent in patients older than 65 years of age.

Allogeneic transplantation, using an HLA-identical donor stem cell as the rescue source following high-dose therapy, has shown encouraging results when undertaken early in the disease course in young patients. Allogeneic transplantation offers two advantages: the absence of tumor-contaminated grafts and the benefit of a graft-versus-myeloma effect. Approximately one third of patients remain disease-free for at least four years.

Maintenance therapies are long-term, low-dose therapies designed to prolong the duration of remission. Agents that have been used for patients with myeloma in remission have included alpha interferon, thalidomide, and pulse steroids such as prednisone and dexamethasone (Decadron). Maintenance therapy with interferon has yielded inconsistent results.

Evaluation of Outcomes

Potential patient outcomes for each of the example nursing diagnoses for the patient with multiple myeloma are:

- Acute pain as related to bone involvement in multiple myeloma. The patient should verbalize an adequate relief of pain along with the ability to realistically cope with the pain if it is not completely relieved.
- Fear in response to the diagnosis of multiple myeloma. The patient should manifest positive coping behaviors and verbalize a reduction in the amount of fear of the having this disease.
- Ineffective coping related to anxiety, lower activity level and the inability to perform normal activities of daily living. The patient identifies own maladaptive coping behaviors, available resources and support systems, describes or initiates alternative coping strategies, and describes positive results from new behaviors.
- Activity intolerance related to fatigue. The patient maintains activity level within capabilities, as evidenced by normal heart rate and blood pressure during activity, as well as absence of shortness of breath, weakness, and fatigue.

MALIGNANT LYMPHOMAS

Lymphomas are malignancies of the lymph tissue. The primary two types of lymphomas are labeled Hodgkin's disease and NHL. Lymphomas are defined by their increased levels of lymphocytes, histocytes, and their precursors. The lymphomas are the sixth leading cause of death and have increased in number tremendously in the past 35 years.

The cause of lymphomas is unknown, but there are identifiable correlates for these disorders. HIV disease and immunosuppression from drug therapy following organ transplantation increases the tendency to develop NHL. In addition, EBV and various chemicals in the environment increase the risk of contracting the lymphomas.

Hodgkin's Disease

Spread through the lymphatic system, Hodgkin's disease accounts for about 12 percent of lymphomas. Its etiology is unknown, but reduced immunity and infection with certain viral diseases have been implicated. The overall survival rate 10 years after diagnosis of Hodgkin's disease is 77 percent.

Epidemiology

Hodgkin's disease is 2.6 per 100,000 men and 2.2 per 100,000 women. Recently there has been a decline in Hodgkin's disease, particularly among the elderly. This is attributed to earlier diagnosis improvements. Hodgkin's disease occurs in a bipolar distribution, with the incidence being greatest between the ages of 15 and 35 and in patients over 50 years of age. In addition, this disorder is higher in Caucasians than African Americans. Worldwide, there is a higher number of persons with Hodgkin's disease in the United States, Netherlands, and Denmark; Japan and Australia have lower incidence rates (Pavlovsky & Lastiri, 2004).

Pathophysiology

Hodgkin's disease is a lymphatic cancer that develops in a single lymph node or a chain of nodes spreading throughout the lymph system (Figure 29-5). The lymph nodes that are invaded contain Reed-Sternberg, cells which are surrounded by host inflammatory cells. They may infect nearly any cells of the body. The stages for labeling Hodgkin's disease and NHL is shown in Box 29-8 (Cole & Dunne, 2004).

Assessment with Clinical Manifestations

Overall, the patient with Hodgkin's disease has one or more painless lymph node enlargements from obstruction and pressure (**lymphadenopathy**). The cervical or subclavicular areas are most common. These enlarged nodes are

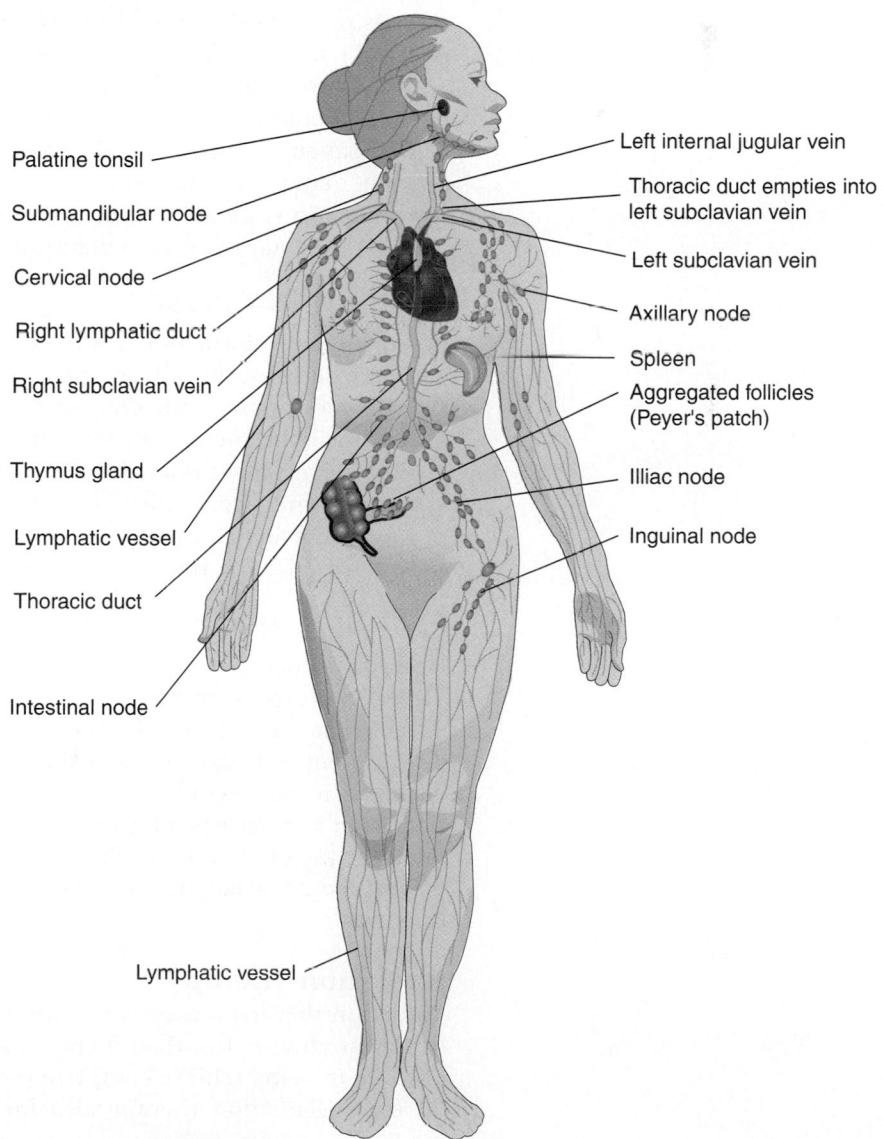

Palatine tonsil

Submandibular node

Cervical node

Right lymphatic duct

Right subclavian vein

Thymus gland

Lymphatic vessel

Thoracic duct

Intestinal node

Left internal jugular vein

Thoracic duct empties into left subclavian vein

Left subclavian vein

Axillary node

Spleen

Aggregated follicles (Peyer's patch)

Illiac node

Inguinal node

Lymphatic vessel

Figure 29-5 The lymph system.

often firm to palpation, and the patient may simply notice their presence on one side of the neck. As the disease progresses there are systemic manifestations, such as fever, weight loss, night sweats, pruritus, and generalized malaise. Herpes zoster conditions are sometimes seen. The CNS can also become involved and be evidenced by headaches, mental changes, cranial nerve or peripheral nerve involvement, and seizure activity. In addition, a mediastinal mass seen on routine chest X-ray (CXR) is somewhat common in Hodgkin's disease. More rarely, there can be secondary involvement of the trachea, bronchi, pleura, or lungs that could result in a cough and pulmonary effusions. There can be hepatic involvement and subsequent jaundice, along with hepatomegaly. And, there can be splenomegaly with accompanying abdominal pain (Louw & Pinkerton, 2005).

Diagnostic Tests

Biopsy of an enlarged lymph node establishes the diagnosis. When biopsy shows the presence of Reed-Sternberg cells, distinctive giant cells with one or two large nuclei, the diagnosis is Hodgkin's disease. Once diagnosed with Hodgkin's disease or NHL, the patient undergoes further diagnostic tests to stage the disease. Lymphoma is further identified as A (no symptoms) or B (the patient has such signs and symptoms as fever, chills, night sweats, and weight loss) (Peck, 2005).

Tests performed to stage lymphoma include CXR and computed tomography (CT) scans of the head and neck, chest, abdomen, and pelvis. Positron emission tomography (PET) of the entire body may help the clinician identify hypermetabolic areas that suggest malignancy and assist staging.

The patient's blood work will probably include a CBC to assess for anemia, a sedimentation rate, and a microglobulin level. He may also have a bone marrow biopsy to stage the disease. Lactate dehydrogenase levels are nonspecific markers that may be used to determine prognosis in NHL (Rogers, 2005).

Nursing Diagnoses

Based on the information gathered, examples of nursing diagnoses in the patient with Hodgkin's disease may include the following:
- Fear in response to the diagnosis of Hodgkin's disease.
- Risk for imbalanced body temperature.
- Ineffective coping related to anxiety, lower activity level, and the inability to perform normal activities of daily living.
- Knowledge deficit related to self-care and risk prevention.
- Risk for infection related to chemotherapy administration.

Planning and Implementation

Hodgkin's disease is treated with radiation therapy, chemotherapy, or both. There are also bone marrow and stem cell transplants as treatments (see section in leukemia), along with the use of monoclonal antibodies to the lymphoma cells. Patient education is essential in the treatments for Hodgkin's disease. The patient that receives radiation or chemotherapy for Hodgkin's disease increases the risk of another type of lymphoma, so they will continue to need encouragement for the monitoring of their manifestations after finishing treatment. The patient should be taught that after five disease-free years, the risk becomes close to normal.

Radiation Therapy

Radiation therapy is a common treatment choice for patients with stage IA or IIA nonbulky (less than 9 cm) Hodgkin's disease. More than 95 percent of these patients achieve complete remission, and 90 percent survive beyond 20 years. Radiation therapy also increases the risk of developing a solid malignancy, such as a breast or lung tumor, or thyroid disease if the radiation field during treatment included these regions.

Chemotherapy

Chemotherapy is appropriate for anyone with more advanced stage IIIB or IV disease, bulky disease (involving a large part of the chest and mediastinum), four or more sites of involvement, or extranodal disease. The standard regimen, known as ABVD, includes Adriamycin (doxorubicin), bleomycin, vinblastine, and dacarbazine. A patient who achieves a partial response with chemotherapy may have a complete response after undergoing radiation therapy to sites of residual disease.

Twenty to 30 percent of patients with Hodgkin's disease never achieve complete remission (all signs and symptoms eliminated) or partial remission (cancer shrinking but not disappearing). Another 20 to 30 percent achieve complete remission and then have a relapse. If a patient requires a second round of therapy, the duration of his or her response to initial therapy helps determine what he or she will receive next.

If Hodgkin's disease recurs within 12 months of initial therapy, the patient is more likely to have a poor outcome. Someone with a relapse more than 12 months after initial therapy can generally be treated successfully with combination chemotherapy. A patient who has a relapse after receiving radiation therapy alone has a 50 to 80 percent likelihood of long-term disease-free survival if he receives chemotherapy with ABVD for the recurrence. In someone who relapses after responding to chemotherapy, the clinician will consider high-dose therapy with autologous bone marrow or peripheral blood stem cell support.

Adverse reactions to chemotherapy for Hodgkin's disease and other malignancies depend on the regimen. The nurse's responsibility when administering chemotherapy is complex and demands that the nurse stay current with the evidence to support management strategies (Table 29-2). Therapy with ABVD may cause infertility, especially in males, although this is a smaller risk than with earlier regimens such as MOPP (mechlorethamine, Oncovin [vincristine], procarbazine, and prednisone). Chemotherapy also can cause sperm abnormalities and birth defects, so talk with the patient about the need to prevent pregnancy and the option of banking sperm or ova before starting treatment. Oncologists generally recommend that women avoid pregnancy for two years, and men should use contraception for six months after treatment (Max, et al., 2003).

Evaluation of Outcomes

- Fear in response to the diagnosis of Hodgkin's disease. The patient should manifest positive coping behaviors and verbalize a reduction in the amount of fear of the having this disease.
- Risk for imbalanced body temperature. The patient maintains body temperature within a normal range.
- Ineffective coping related to anxiety, lower activity level, and the inability to perform normal activities of daily living. The patient identifies own maladaptive coping behaviors, available resources, and support systems, describes or initiates alternative coping strategies, and describes positive results from new behaviors.
- Knowledge deficit related to self-care and risk prevention. The patient should demonstrate motivation to learn, identify perceived learning needs, and verbalize an understanding of desired content.
- Risk for infection related to chemotherapy administration. The patient remains free of infection, as evidenced by normal vital signs and absence of purulent drainage from wounds, incisions, and tubes. Infection is recognized early to allow for prompt treatment.

TABLE 29-2 Managing Problems Associated with Chemotherapy

THE NURSE CAN FOLLOW THESE GUIDELINES TO HELP THE PATIENT OVERCOME ADVERSE REACTIONS:

Myelosuppression

- Monitor CBC before each treatment.
- Administer packed RBCs as ordered.
- Administer growth factors as prescribed, granulocyte colony-stimulating factor, to decrease duration of nadir and epoetin alfa (Procrit) or darbepoetin alfa (Aranesp) to increase RBC production.
- Assess the patient for signs and symptoms of infection. Educate about decreased absolute neutrophil count and infection risk. Wear appropriate isolation clothing when caring for patient (Figure 29-6).
- Monitor temperature daily. Call the oncologist or hematologist if the patient's oral temperature exceeds 38°C (100.5°F).

Pulmonary Toxicity

- Obtain baseline pulmonary function tests.
- Assess the patient's pulmonary status before each infusion.
- Teach the patient to report cough, dyspnea, or shortness of breath.
- Hold bleomycin if the patient reports any symptoms of altered pulmonary status.

Cardiac Toxicity

- Make sure that the patient undergoes a MUGA (multiple-gated acquisition) scan or an echocardiogram to determine adequate left ventricular ejection fraction before the first chemotherapy dose.
- Teach the patient to report shortness of breath or palpitations.
- Monitor the total doxorubicin dose.
- Perform ongoing assessments for signs and symptoms of heart failure, including dyspnea on exertion, orthopnea, paroxysmal nocturnal dyspnea, and fatigue.

Nausea and Vomiting

- Administer antiemetics before administering chemotherapy.
- Assess the patient's level of nausea and vomiting with each treatment and modify the antiemetic regimen as indicated.
- Teach the patient how to use the prescribed antiemetic to prevent or treat delayed nausea and vomiting.

Extravasation

- Assess your patient's veins before and during each chemotherapy infusion.
- Teach the patient about the benefits of a central venous access device if peripheral access is poor.
- Assess blood return frequently during administration of vesicants such as doxorubicin, vinblastine, and dacarbazine.
- Treat extravasation promptly, according to facility policy.

Hypersensitivity Reactions

- Assess your patient's baseline vital signs. Bleomycin in particular can cause fever.
- Administer premedications such as acetaminophen and steroids before therapy and have emergency equipment readily available in case of anaphylactic or anaphylactoid reaction.
- Teach the patient to promptly report any unusual symptoms such as dizziness, itching, or pain.
- Monitor the vital signs throughout the infusion. Increase the infusion rate every 30 minutes only if the vital signs remain stable and he or she does not develop signs of an adverse reaction.
- Stop the infusion if he or she develops a reaction.

Neuropathy

- Assess the patient for sensory and perceptual changes before each treatment.
- Notify the oncologist of any changes (peripheral, gastrointestinal) that develop after the patient receives vinca alkaloids.

Pain at Injection Site: ABVD

- Administer dacarbazine in 100 to 250 mL of IV fluid and infuse slowly over one hour.
- Apply heat or ice above the injection site.

Flu-like Syndrome

- Premedicate with acetaminophen.
- Encourage the patient to drink plenty of fluids.

Hyperglycemia

- Monitor his serum glucose level.
- Increase monitoring frequency if the patient has diabetes. The prescriber may need to modify his or her antihyperglycemic therapy.

Adapted from Hennessy, B. T., Hanrahan, E. O., & Daly, P. A. (2004). Non-Hodgkin lymphoma: An update. Lancet Oncology, 5(6), 341–353; Rogers, B. (2005). Looking at lymphoma & leukemia. Nursing, 35(7), 56–64.

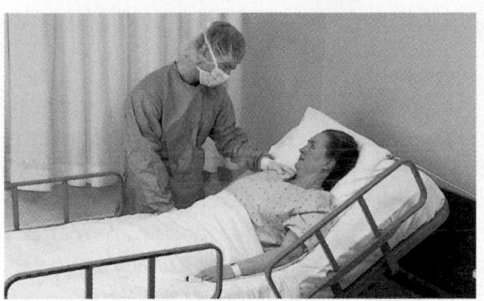

Figure 29-6 Nurse in isolation clothing working with patient who is immunosuppressed.

Non-Hodgkin's Lymphoma

NHL is a label for a group of disorders that are characterized by the malignant mutations of the lymphoid system not microscopically identified by the Reed-Sternberg cells and cellular anomalies seen in Hodgkin's disease.

Epidemiology

Scientists do not understand how NHL begins, but they do know that the incidence has increased about 7 percent annually over the past 20 years, primarily in older adults. The rate of occurrence is about 8 per 100,000 men and 6 per 100,000 women. NHL is multicentric in its beginnings with an early propensity to spread widely.

Etiology

What causes NHL is unclear, but factors that increase risk are long-term immunosuppressant therapy, bone marrow transplantation, inherited immune defects, rheumatoid arthritis, and previous treatment for Hodgkin's disease. Lymphoma related to HIV, now recognized as a separate entity, is treated differently than other types of NHL.

Pathophysiology

Spread through the bloodstream, NHL is classified as aggressive or indolent. Aggressive NHL is fast growing, so patients typically are sicker at diagnosis. Because the disease is discovered in the early stages, a cure is more likely. Aggressive NHL is divided into intermediate and high grades; although treated differently, both are curable. Indolent NHL is slow growing and poses more of a challenge to cure. Also known as low-grade NHL, the disease progresses slowly, so it is typically widely disseminated before being discovered. Even after treatment, most patients with indolent NHL have relapses.

Assessment with Clinical Manifestations

The clinical manifestations seen in NHL are similar to Hodgkin's disease. The changes seen in NHL are either local or systemic, with the cervical, axillary, inguinal, and femoral lymph node chains enlarging. As with Hodgkin's disease, the lymph enlargement is generally pain free and can occur over months and even years. However, in NHL there are more multiple peripheral nodal sites than in Hodgkin's disease, which more often localizes to single axial groups of nodes. Some people have extranodal areas of involvement in the nasopharynx, GI system, bone, thyroid, testes and soft tissue. In addition, some people have involvement that develops retroperitoneal and abdominal masses. In NHL, there is more of a noncontiguous involvement of the affected nodes, where in Hodgkin's disease there is a more organized spread with contiguity. NHL is also more widely spread than Hodgkin's disease (Evans & Hancock, 2003).

Diagnostic Tests

See the diagnostic tests section in the Hodgkin's disease section. Also, the diagnosis is NHL when biopsy shows infiltration of malignant B cells or T cells in the lymph system.

Nursing Diagnoses

See the nursing diagnoses in the Hodgkin's disease section. In addition, refer to chapter 15 for general management strategies and nursing diagnoses for patients with oncological disorders. The entire body system is often affected by NHL, and the resulting nursing diagnoses are varied and yet individual to the patient with NHL.

Planning and Implementation

When treatment for low-grade NHL is necessary, numerous options include single or combination alkylating agents and the addition of an anthracycline (an anticancer antibiotic, such as doxorubicin), radiation therapy, or biological agents (such as monoclonal antibodies). The choice depends on the extent of disease, the patient's signs and symptoms, and major organ dysfunction due to other medical conditions. Because biological agents produce a slower response, the patient may need chemotherapy for significant symptoms. Adding biological agents to various chemotherapy regimens may enhance the response (Luo, 2005).

Generally, a shorter initial response to chemotherapy means shorter survival. After subsequent treatments, each remission is typically shorter and of less quality than the preceding one. Although the histological features of disease at relapse are typically the same as at diagnosis, the disease could transform into a more aggressive type. High-dose chemotherapy with ASCT is a treatment option for someone with a recurrence. Considered a bone marrow rescue, ASCT is a standard approach to treating patients with relapsed disease who previously responded to chemotherapy. Allogeneic bone marrow transplant may be an option for someone with more resistant disease (Joo, et al., 2004).

A patient with NHL may receive radiation, chemotherapy, or both, depending on the disease grade and stage. Monoclonal antibodies such as rituximab (Rituxan) may be used to enhance the effects of chemotherapy. For someone with recurrent NHL, stem cell transplantation may be an option.

Chemotherapy

The standard treatment for intermediate-grade NHL has been CHOP (cyclophosphamide, hydroxydaunomycin, Oncovin [vincristine], and prednisone) chemotherapy, producing a cure in about 40 percent of patients treated. Recent data show that 60 percent of patients who also receive rituximab have long-term survival without relapse, so adding rituximab to the regimen (CHOP-R) has become the standard of care. The patient may receive radiation therapy, too, if he has only a partial response to chemotherapy or to prevent recurrence at sites of previous bulky disease (Hennessy, Hanrahan, & Daly, 2004).

Radiation

Typically, a patient with high-grade NHL requires combination chemotherapy, but radiation also plays a role in combating this disease. Studies suggest that receiving fewer chemotherapy treatments and radiation can be equally effective and less toxic than more courses of chemotherapy alone. Someone with clinical stage I high-grade NHL has a greater than 80 percent chance of cure with radiation to either the involved field or an extended field.

If the patient has localized low-grade NHL, radiation therapy alone offers a 60 to 80 percent chance of 10 years' survival and possibly a full cure. However, in disseminated low-grade NHL, early intervention does not appear to prolong survival, so watch-and-wait is an acceptable approach. The reason to delay is that the patient may remain stable for years without treatments that could cause adverse reactions and decrease quality of life.

If the patient chooses to watch and wait, the practitioner will monitor him or her and prescribe therapy if adenopathy and disease-related symptoms increase or if he or she develops organ compromise or bone marrow suppression. Multiple chemotherapy options are available if they want a more aggressive approach (Noga, 2004).

Evaluation of Outcomes

See the evaluation of outcomes in the Hodgkin's disease section. In addition, refer to chapter 15 for the evaluation of outcomes as related to general nursing diagnoses that patients have with oncological disorders. The nurse must adapt to a wide variety of complications and apply individual plans of care to the specific nursing diagnoses that accompany the patient's with NHL.

KEY CONCEPTS

■ The hematology system is different from all other systems within the human body, because it is in a liquid state and is comprised of bone marrow, blood cells, plasma, and the reticuloendothelial system (RES).

■ Anemia is a condition where the hemoglobin concentration is lower than normal, and there are fewer RBCs circulating within the plasma.

■ There are anemias that are caused by nutritional deficiencies which affect erythropoiesis.

■ The process of hemostasis, or blood coagulation, involves multiple stages, and when it dysfunctions, various bleeding disorders result.

■ Hemophilia is a group of hereditary bleeding disorders that results from the deficiency of clotting factors.

■ Polycythemia is an increased amount of RBCs with a hematocrit level elevated to more than 55 percent in males and more than 50 percent in females.

■ Neutropenia is a decreased number of circulating neutrophils, usually less than 1,500 cells/mm^3.

■ Mononucleosis (infectious mononucleosis) is caused by B cells in the oropharyngeal lymphoid tissues that result from EBV.

■ There are four main types of leukemia (cancer of the blood) that differ greatly in presentation, timing, and clinical signs and symptoms.

■ A patient with ALL or AML must be hospitalized as soon as possible to start induction therapy, with the goal to destroy all visible leukemic cells.

■ Chronic leukemias, CML and CLL, progress more slowly than the acute leukemias and rarely affect people under age 20 and may not affect the patient's health as severely until the advanced stages.

■ Multiple myeloma is cancer of plasma cells and is due to the unregulated, proliferation of monoclonal plasma cells that are ineffective.

■ Lymphomas are malignancies of the lymph tissue and the two primary types are labeled Hodgkin's disease and NHL.

REVIEW QUESTIONS

1. The hematology system is comprised of:
   1. Bone marrow, blood cells, and plasma
   2. Blood cells, interstitial fluid, and bone marrow
   3. Plasma, sugars, and blood cells
   4. Bone marrow, tissue, and plasma

2. Which of the following is not one of the three main categories of anemia?
   1. A loss of RBCs from any source of bleeding
   2. A decreased production of oxygen particles within the RBC
   3. An increased destruction of RBCs
   4. A decreased production of RBCs

3. Which of the following is true concerning thalassemia?
   1. It is caused by any number of factors that result in hemolysis outside the RBC.
   2. It affects certain groups of persons from specific geographical regions.
   3. It is a form of anemia caused by a genetic defect in RBC metabolism.
   4. It is the most common of the hemolytic disorders and there is no abnormality of the hemoglobin.

4. Which type of anemia is labeled a cobalamin deficiency?
   1. Folic acid deficiency anemia
   2. Hemolytic anemia
   3. Vitamin B$_{12}$ deficiency
   4. Iron deficiency anemia

5. Plasmapheresis is the primary treatment for:
   1. Thrombocytopenia
   2. TTP
   3. ITP
   4. Aplastic anemia

6. The clotting disorder that consumes the clotting factors and causes the patient to have tremendous clotting difficulties is:
   1. Hemophilia
   2. Acquired hemolytic anemia
   3. DIC
   4. Von Willebrand's disease

7. The type of polycythemia that is more common in European Jewish persons is:
   1. Secondary polycythemia
   2. Neutropenia
   3. Leukopenia
   4. Primary polycythemia

Continued

REVIEW QUESTIONS—cont'd

8. Which of the following describes acute myelogenous leukemia?
   1. It most commonly affects children.
   2. It affects people of all ages.
   3. It has its highest incidence in Italy, the United States, Switzerland, and Costa Rica.
   4. It typically develops after age 40 and is most common in older men.

9. CML is characterized by the presence of which of the following chromosomes?
   1. The Seattle chromosome
   2. The Gpa6 chromosome
   3. The Philadelphia chromosome
   4. The leukopenia chromosome

10. Multiple myeloma is similar to other cancers of the hematologic system. What distinguishes it the most from the other types of cancer?
    1. The low white blood cell count
    2. The bone pain
    3. The known cause being genetic
    4. The fact that Caucasians are five times as likely to get the disease

REVIEW ACTIVITIES

1. Describe the difference between iron deficiency anemia and folic acid deficiency anemia?

2. Find a patient who has DIC in the clinical setting and list the diagnostic tests for the DIC.

3. Compare and contrast hemophilia A and hemophilia C.

4. Compare and contrast acute and chronic leukemia.

5. Describe autologous stem cell transplantation.

6. Evaluate the effects of chemotherapy on a patient with either of the malignant lymphoma disorder.

Alterations in Respiratory Function

Assessment of Respiratory Function

Linda L. Morris, PhD, APN, CCNS

Elizabeth D. Archer, MS, DSN, PhD, APRN, BC, CS, ANP, CRRN, CNRN

KEY TERMS

Acidemia
Alkalemia
Apneustic breathing
Biot's (ataxic) breathing
Bradypnea
Bronchophony
Cheyne-Stokes breathing
Clubbing
Compliance
Dead space
Dyspnea
Egophony
Eupnea
Expiratory reserve volume (ERV)
Fremitus
Hemoptysis
Hypercapnia
Hypocapnia
Hypoxemia
Hypoxia
Inspiratory reserve volume (IRV)
Kussmaul breathing
Kyphoscoliosis
Kyphosis
Perfusion
Residual volume (RV)
Rhonchi
Scoliosis
Shunting
Stridor
Tachypnea
Tidal volume (Vt)
Ventilation
Vital capacity (VC)
Wheezes

CHAPTER TOPICS

- Anatomy and Physiology of the Respiratory System

- Respiratory Assessment

- Diagnostic Tests

R apidly expanding technology has not changed the need for astute clinical assessment skills as the hallmark quality of an expert nurse. As the learner gains clinical judgment, he or she will be able to reconsider each clinical situation from a perspective of increased complexity and move from novice to expert. It is the intent of this chapter on respiratory assessment to provide the framework from which the novice can begin and develop focused expertise through continued clinical involvement.

This chapter has three sections. The first section reviews anatomy and physiology of the respiratory system to provide a framework for clinical assessment. The second section is the assessment section, which begins with a focused history taking to identify areas of concern and follows with the four maneuvers of inspection, palpation, percussion, and auscultation. These skills are presented in that order to provide a comprehensive approach as well as guide the clinician in identifying specific issues. The third section presents specific diagnostic tests along with nursing implications of these tests.

ANATOMY OF THE RESPIRATORY SYSTEM

The respiratory system is divided into upper and lower tracts. The upper respiratory system includes the nose, pharynx, larynx, and upper trachea. The lower respiratory tract includes the lower trachea and the lungs. The entire system extends from the nose to the alveoli. Assessment of the respiratory system includes the use of various techniques in which inspection, auscultation, palpation, and percussion are used extensively to disclose normal and abnormal conditions. The essential function of the respiratory system is gas exchange, which is the delivery of oxygen to the tissues and removal of carbon dioxide. The two lungs lie on either side of the thoracic cavity and are separated by the heart, great vessels, and other structures of the mediastinum.

Thorax

There are 12 sets of ribs, the first seven ribs are labeled the true ribs because they are connected directly to the sternum through the costal cartilage. Ribs 8 through 10 are not directly connected to the sternum but connect indirectly to the rib above through the costal cartilage. The 11th and 12th ribs are called floating ribs, as they have no attachment to the sternum. The thoracic cage is a rigid but flexible structure that functions as both protection for the lungs and mechanical support for allowing the movements associated with ventilation. The thoracic cage houses the lungs and muscles of respiration. It consists of a cone-shaped bony structure, which is broader at the base and narrower at the top. On the anterior surface, the bony sternum with the attached rib cage forms the chest cavity from the 12 sets of ribs. At the base of the thoracic cavity, the convex surface of the muscular diaphragm separates the thoracic cavity from the abdominal cavity. The diaphragm aids in respiration by moving up and down. During inspiration, the diaphragm moves down and increases the volume of the thoracic cavity; during expiration, the diaphragm moves up and thereby decreases the volume. The costochondral junctions are the nonpalpable points at which the ribs join the cartilages. The suprasternal notch is a hollow U-shaped depression, or hollow, anterior to the sternum and lays between the clavicles (Estes, 2006).

The sternum is composed of three distinct parts: the manubrium at the superior position; the body of the sternum, which is centrally located; and the xiphoid with its distinct process palpable at the base. The angle of Louis, or the manubriosternal angle, is located at the articulation of the body of the sternum and the manubrium at the second rib (Estes, 2006). This is a landmark used to palpate ribs for placement of the diaphragm of the stethoscope to auscultate the anterior chest wall for respiratory findings. Each area between the ribs is called an intercostal space and is numbered by the rib above it. By starting with the angle of Louis as number one and palpating down to the second rib, one locates the second intercostal space. By moving the fingertips laterally to the midclavicular area, one is able to palpate each rib and intercostal space down to the tenth rib. The angle of Louis also delineates the location of the tracheal bifurcation into the left and right branches. The upper border of the atria relates to this landmark and coincides with the fourth thoracic vertebra on the posterior surface. The accessory respiratory muscles are used to accommodate increased oxygen demand. Pathology, such as that in asthma, may lead to the use of accessory muscles. The accessory muscles may also be used during exercise to accommodate a sudden demand in oxygenation.

The abdominal rectus, scalene, trapezius, and sternocleidomastoid are the accessory respiratory muscles (Estes, 2006). The last prominent landmark on the anterior surface, the costal angle or area between the left and right margins of the rib cage is identified as a depression immediately superior to the gastric area when the patient is in a supine position. The angle increases in the presence of chronic hyperinflation, such as in chronic obstructive pulmonary disease (COPD). Reference lines on the anterior surface include the midsternal and the midclavicular positions that enable rapid identification of physical findings at specific vertical locations. The midsternal line is exactly midway between the nipples and extends from the angle of Louis through the costal angle. The midclavicular line runs from the midpoint of each clavicle that lies between the acromioclavicular and sternoclavicular joints and extends vertically from the superior thoracic through the lower abdominal cavity.

On the posterior surface, the vertebra prominens is easily palpated at the base of the neck on the spinal column and is characteristically palpable by running the fingertip down over the most prominent bony spur that projects from the base of the neck. Spinous processes are also identified by palpating the bony prominences moving downward on the spinal column. The spinous processes match with the corresponding numbered rib down to the fourth thoracic vertebrae (T4). There, the spinous processes angle down from their vertebral body and overlie the vertebral body and rib below. The scapulae are located in each hemithorax at symmetrical positions and articulate with the clavicles at the proximal borders. They extend down to the seventh or eighth ribs. Reference lines on the posterior surface include the posterior axillary, midaxillary vertebral, and scapular lines. The posterior axillary and midaxillary lines identify lateral areas on the left and right sides of the patient, with the midaxillary being the most central reference point between the parallel anterior and posterior surfaces from the apex of the axilla downward. The scapular line extends from the inferior angle of the scapula downward.

Lungs

The lungs lie within the bony structure of the thorax. They are conical in shape, spongy in texture, and act as a "bellows" by moving air in and out of the respiratory tract (Figure 30-1). The apices of the lung lie at the uppermost portion of the thorax, the bases of the lung at the lowermost portion, and the apices rise above the clavicle.

The lungs are the main organs of respiration and prominently occupy the lateral chamber of the thoracic cavity. The lungs lie against the ribs anteriorly and posteriorly and meet the convexity of the diaphragm with a concave formation at the lower outer surface or base. The left lung is nearly 2.5 cm longer than the right lung because of the position the liver occupies below the diaphragm. The right lung is broader than the left because of the position occupied by the heart in the thoracic cavity. The right lung consists of three lobes (upper, middle, and lower) while the left lung has two lobes (upper and lower) (Estes, 2006). The apex or top of the lung extends to 2.54 cm to the inner one third of the clavicles and on the posterior surface; the apices border the 1st thoracic vertebrae (T1) process. The lower lung borders may extend to the 12th thoracic vertebrae (T12) on deep inspiration and to the 10th thoracic vertebrae (T10) on deep expiration. Fissures separate the lobes of the lungs. On the anterior surface and a left lateral view, the left upper lobe is separated by the horizontal fissure, which is located at the fifth rib, midaxillary line; the lower lobes (LL) are separated by the left and right oblique fissures. On a right lateral view, the right middle lobe lies between the fourth and sixth ribs and has the fifth rib at the midaxillary line as a posterior border. A posterior view reveals the spinous process of the 3rd thoracic vertebrae (T3) as the upper borders for the lower lungs and the lower borders for both upper lungs.

Figure 30-1 illustrates that the lungs are further divided into lobes by fissures. The left lung has two lobes, and the right lung has three lobes. The lobes are further subdivided into segments, resulting in a total of 18 segments, 10 in the right lung and 8 in the left lung.

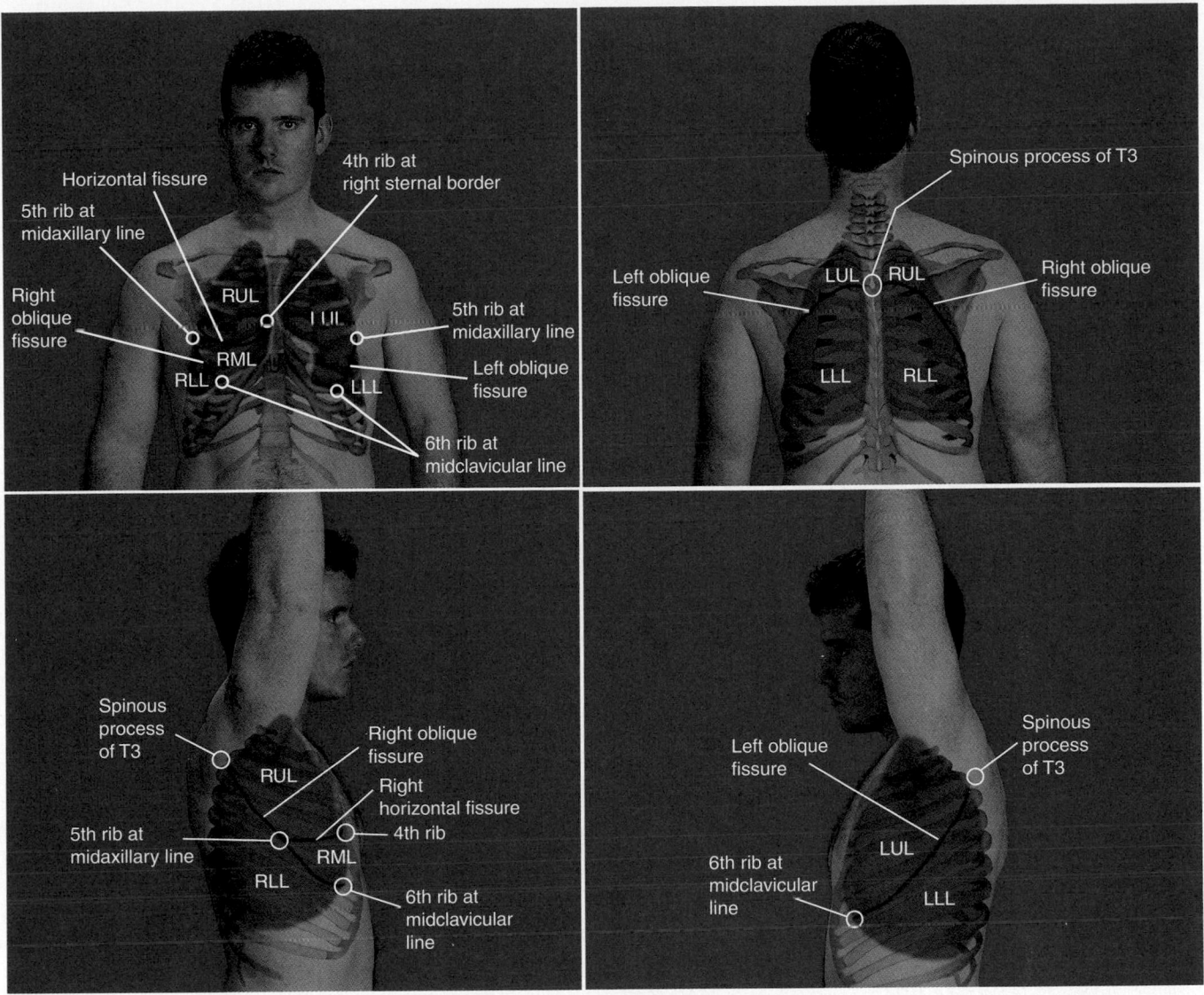

Figure 30-1 Lung fissures.

There is only a small portion of the lower lobes exposed anteriorly. Most of the anterior lung tissue is comprised of the left and right upper lobe. The right middle lobe is only evident anteriorly and laterally; it is not exposed posteriorly. The majority of the lung tissue posteriorly is the left and right lower lobes. The upper lobes are apparent posteriorly above the level of the third spinous process.

While examining the chest, it is often helpful to pinpoint locations and document them. The ribs and intercostals spaces serve as good horizontal landmarks. In addition, there are several vertical landmarks to be aware of; these are called reference lines (Figure 30-2).

The reference lines are imaginary lines that run vertically along the patient's chest. The midsternal line bisects the sternum. The midclavicular lines bisect the clavicle on the left and the right. The vertebral line is also called the midspinal line and bisects the vertebral column. The midscapular lines bisect the scapulae on the left and the right. There are three axillary lines. The anterior axillary line runs down the anterior axillary fold. The anterior axillary line is determined by holding the patient's arm in a neutral position, or as if the patient's arm were hanging down. The anterior axillary fold creates the path for the anterior axillary line. The posterior fold creates the path for the posterior axillary line, and the midaxillary line bisects the axilla.

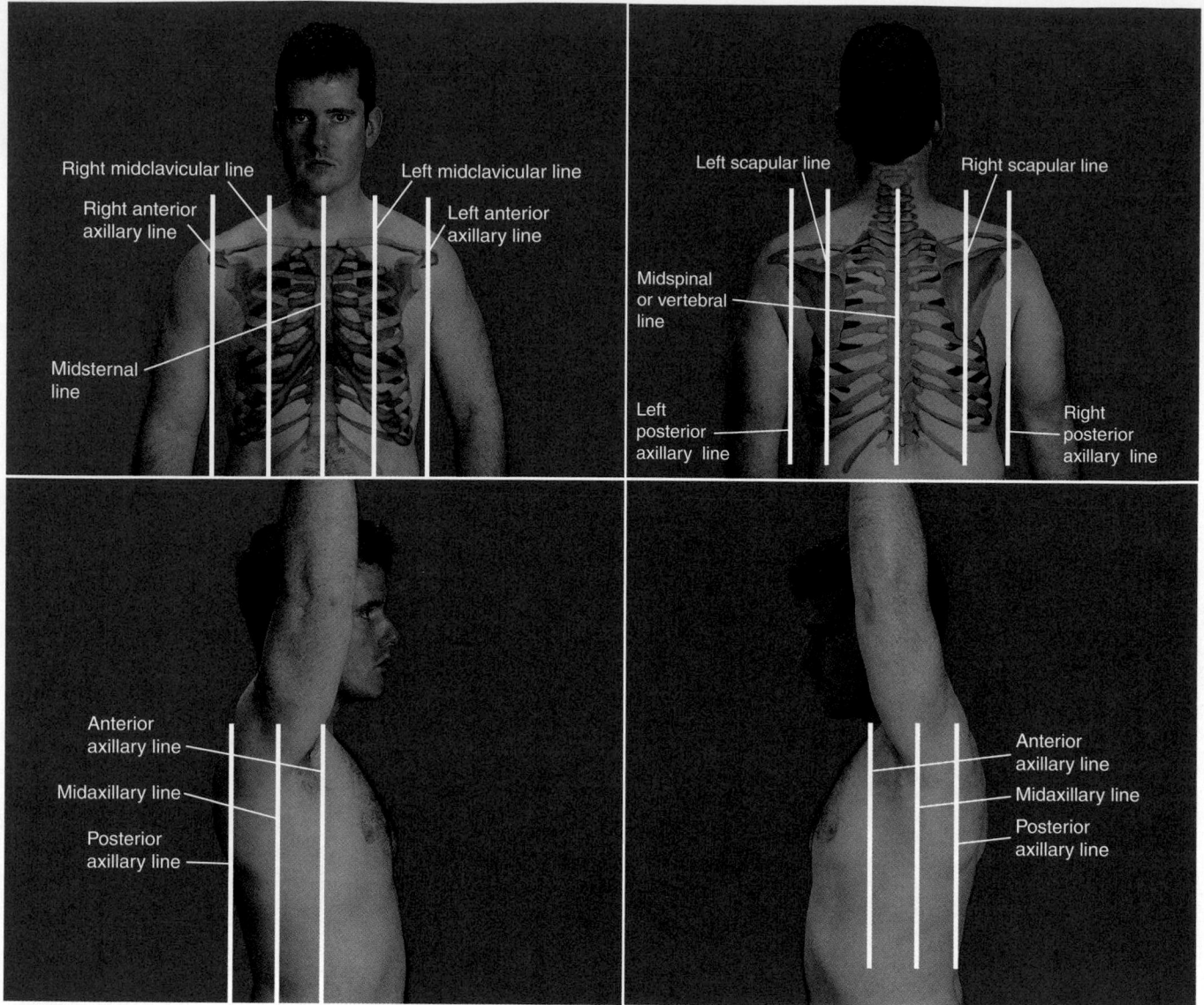

Figure 30-2 Imaginary thoracic lines.

When used with the ribs and intercostals spaces as horizontal landmarks, the vertical reference lines are useful tools to pinpoint the exact location of abnormal findings on the chest.

Each lung is encased in a thin, slippery, pleura, or serous sac. The chest wall and superior surface of the diaphragm forms the base of the thoracic cavity. This area is covered inside with parietal pleural tissue and is continuous with visceral pleura tissue that lines the outside of the lungs and extends into the fissures. The serous sac usually contains a few millimeters of fluid that acts as a lubricating cushion. The pleural cavity exerts a negative pressure that retains the lungs securely against the chest wall. Because of the small amount of fluid supplied by the pleura, the lungs move silently and smoothly in the chest cavity sliding up and down during respiration. The costodiaphragmatic recess is a small, potential reservoir that exists at the base of the lungs and is made up of pleural tissue. The pleura extend slightly below the level of the lungs, creating this reservoir, which has the potential for developing abnormal collections of air or fluid. If fluid or air accumulates in the reservoir, respirations will be impaired.

The mediastinum, or interpleural space, extends from the sternum to the spinal column between the right and left lungs and houses the heart, major vessels, trachea, esophagus, and lymph vessels. The trachea lies anterior to the esophagus and is 10–11 cm long in the adult (Estes, 2006). The trachea begins at the cricoid cartilage and bifurcates into the left and right branches just below the sternal angle at the level of the fourth or fifth vertebral process. Anatomically, the right bronchus is wider, shorter, and more vertical; hence it is more susceptible to aspiration and endotracheal intubation. The mainstem bronchi further divide into lobar or secondary bronchi. Both the trachea and the bronchi transport gases between the environment and the lung parenchyma that form the lung **dead space.** This space is that portion of ventilation that does not participate in gas exchange. The dead space is filled with air and is not used in gas exchanges with the environment. The bronchi also trap foreign particles that are inhaled from the environment, swept up by the bronchial cilia, and trapped by mucus produced by the goblet cells that line the bronchus. These particulate matter are usually expelled through sneezing, coughing, or swallowing.

The alveoli in which gas exchange occurs are the smallest functional units of the respiratory system. The number of alveoli, approximately 300 million in each lung, possesses an aerating surface area that is extremely large and provides working space for gas exchange that is equivalent to over 8, 400 square feet. Each alveolus is supplied with its own blood supply and lymph drainage system. Branches of the pulmonary artery carry blood to the capillaries surrounding the alveoli to be oxygenated. Branches of the pulmonary vein carry oxygenated blood from the alveoli to the heart (Estes, 2006).

The diaphragm is a dome-shaped muscle that forms the inferior border of the thorax. It is the primary muscle of respiration and is innervated by the phrenic nerve. The liver lies below the right margin of the diaphragm and causes a palpable border elevation.

Upper Respiratory Tract

The upper airway tract consists of the nose, turbinates, pharynx, tonsils, adenoids, epiglottis, trachea, and carina (Figure 30-3). The lower airway tract consists of the bronchi, hilum, bronchioles, cilia, and alveoli. The respiratory system is a continuous unit; however, the upper and lower airway tracts have some fundamental differences in purpose.

The upper airways function to warm or cool, humidify, and filter air. Air enters the respiratory system through the nose and mouth. The turbinates are roughened, bony structures that form the anterior portion of the nose and function to warm and humidify air. In addition, the inside of the nose is lined with hairs and mucous membrane that have a role in filtration of air by trapping foreign particles.

The trachea and bronchi have primarily cartilage in their walls and relatively little smooth muscle. They are lined by mucus and serous epithelial tissue as well as cilia. The pharynx consists of the nasopharynx, the oropharynx, and the laryngopharynx. The nasopharynx consists of the nose and adenoids, and further connects to the middle ear. The oropharynx contains the throat, tongue, and tonsils. The laryngopharynx contains the trachea and epiglottis. The epiglottis is a flexible cartilaginous flap that functions to protect the airway during swallowing. It closes over the trachea during swallowing to prevent food and liquid from being aspirated into the lower airway tract.

The larynx has several specific functions: to conduct air from the upper to the lower airway, to protect the lower airway from aspiration of foreign substances, to participate in the coughing mechanism, and to participate in phonation. The larynx consists of several cartilages connected to each other. The thyroid cartilage, or Adam's apple, is the largest of these cartilages. Below the thyroid cartilage lies the cricoid cartilage. This cricoid cartilage is the only one that forms a complete ring around the trachea. The vibrating portion of the larynx is the vocal cords. Each vocal cord is stretched between the thyroid cartilage and the arytenoid cartilage.

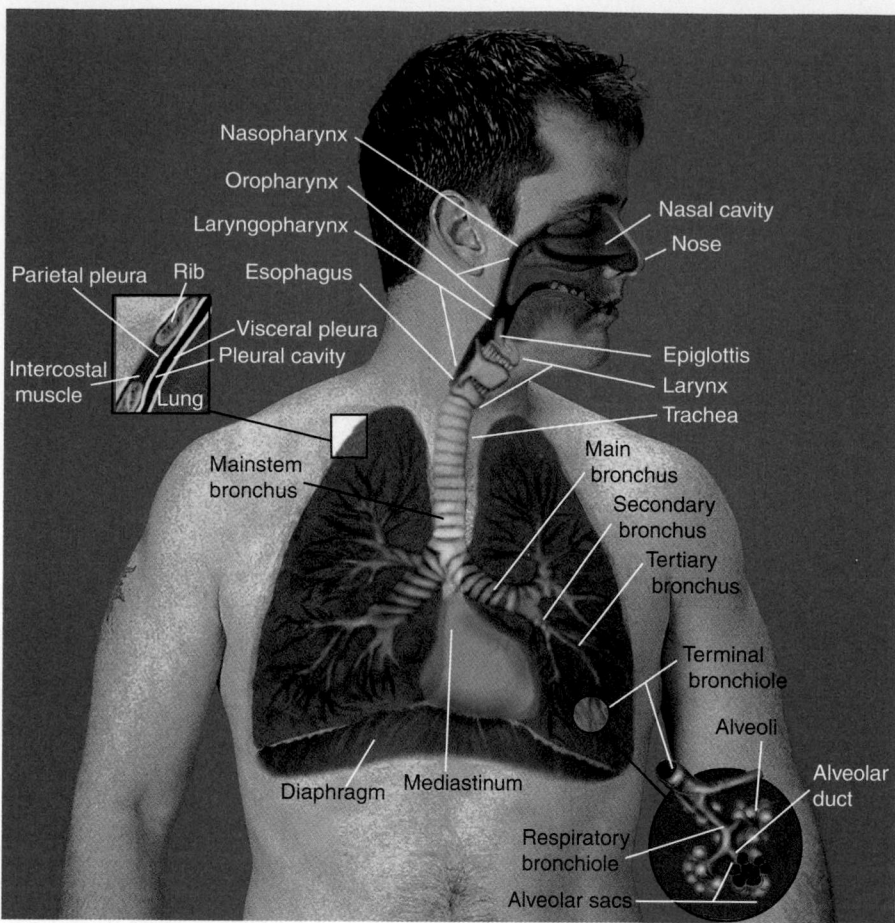

Figure 30-3 The respiratory tract.

Lower Respiratory Tract

The lower respiratory tract consists of the bronchi, bronchioles, and alveoli. At the level of the second intercostal space to either side of the sternum, the trachea bifurcates into the left and right mainstem bronchi. Breath sounds are typically loudest in this area. The base of the bifurcation of the trachea is the carina. If an endotracheal tube is inserted too far into the trachea, it is more likely that the tube will enter the right mainstem bronchus because of the gentler angle on the right compared to the more acute angle on the left.

The bronchi and bronchioles are innervated by the autonomic nervous system. Discharge of the receptors causes bronchoconstriction of the smooth muscle within the bronchi and bronchioles. This smooth muscle aids in respiration, because the bronchi dilate during inspiration and constrict during expiration.

There are 23 generations of airways in the entire lower respiratory tract. Each of the upper generations (0–16) consists only of air conducting passages. The lower generations (17–23) consist of a bronchiole and a group of alveoli. The fundamental respiratory unit is an alveolus with an adjacent capillary. It is within this fundamental unit where the exchange of oxygen and carbon dioxide occurs. There are over three million alveoli in the body that are composed of several types of pneumocytes. The surface area of a normal lung is large enough to cover a football field, indicating the enormous ability of the lung tissue to diffuse gas.

The alveoli are lined with two types of cells: Type I and Type II pneumocytes. Type I cells are flat and are the primary type of cells lining the alveoli. Type II cells are thicker and secrete a substance called surfactant. The alveoli have a natural tendency to collapse on expiration. Surfactant is a lipid and protein substance that decreases surface tension and functions to keep the alveoli open. Loss of surfactant is seen in a variety of pulmonary diseases, as well as smoking, and can result in alveolar collapse. Widespread alveolar collapse results in atelectasis and increased work of breathing.

Pulmonary Mechanics and Musculature

The pleura are membranes that protect the lung. There are two types of pleural membranes. The visceral pleura line the outer portion of the lung itself; the parietal pleura line the inner portion of the thorax. Normally, there is a thin film of fluid in the intrapleural space that allows increased cohesion between these layers as well as lubrication, allowing the pleura to glide smoothly against each other during breathing.

Several sets of muscles also play a role in the mechanics of breathing. Innervated by the phrenic nerve, the major muscle of breathing is the diaphragm. The diaphragm handles 80 percent of the work of breathing. Normally, the diaphragm is a convex muscle; however, on inspiration, the diaphragm contracts and flattens out. The diaphragm can move as much as 7 cm with deep inspiration. The downward movement of the diaphragm pushes on the abdominal contents, moving the abdomen outward. During normal respiration, the thorax and the abdomen move in concert with one another. With inspiration, the thorax and abdomen move outward together and with expiration, they passively recoil inward. With respiratory distress, however, the abdominal muscles sometimes contract paradoxically in an effort to assist with breathing efforts. This mechanism is called abdominal paradox.

There are several other sets of muscles that are involved in breathing. The external intercostal muscles and the parasternal muscles help to lift the rib cage during normal respiration. Inspiration is an active process. The accessory muscles include the scalene, sternocleidomastoid, trapezius, and pectoralis muscles. These muscles do not normally get involved in normal respiration; they are called into play only during respiratory distress.

Expiration is normally a passive process with recoil from the inspiratory effort. During times of respiratory distress, however, sometimes the abdominal muscles get involved. These muscles include the rectus abdominis, internal and external oblique, and the transverse abdominis. Contraction of these muscles increases intra-abdominal pressure and forces the diaphragm up.

Compliance of the lung describes its elasticity or distensibility. A lung with poor compliance is less distensible and may be due to a number of factors, including restrictive lung disease or a decrease in surfactant. Increased compliance can be seen in conditions that destroy alveolar walls and stretch tissues, such as emphysema.

Respiratory Defense Mechanisms

There are several mechanisms involved in protection of the respiratory system. The bone marrow produces macrophages and monocytes that are released into the blood stream and move into the pulmonary capillary circulation, the interstitial space, and the alveoli. They function to destroy invading organisms through phagocytosis and microbicidal activity.

The hairs within the nose strain large particles, but one of the primary defense mechanisms of the lung is the mucous blanket, also called the mucociliary escalator. The epithelial cells of the respiratory tract are lined with numerous mucous glands called goblet cells that become enlarged and inflamed with irritation. These glands produce approximately 100 mL of mucus per day. Mucus is composed primarily of water, with some glycoprotein, carbohydrate, and lipid. Within the mucous blanket and lining the surface of the epithelium are hair-like projections called cilia that beat upward, trapping foreign particles and pushing them toward the larynx in a continuously flowing sheet. These cilia beat at a rate of 1,000–1,500 cycles per minute and can move particles at a rate of 16 mm per minute. Defects in ciliary motility can lead to chronic sinusitis, recurrent lung infections, and bronchiectasis (Ganong, 2005).

The cough reflex is another primary defense mechanism. There are several factors involved for an effective cough. The cough reflex involves a large inspiration of air, closure of the epiglottis, closure of the vocal cords, contraction of the abdominal muscles, followed by explosive opening of the epiglottis and vocal cords, resulting in air pushed outward under pressure. Forced expiration against a closed glottis increases intrapleural pressure to 100 mm Hg or more. Sudden opening of the glottis produces an outflow of air at a rate of up to 600 miles per hour. The sneeze reflex is similar to the cough except that it involves only the nasal passages, and the glottis remains continuously open.

A hiccough is a spasmodic contraction of the diaphragm that produces an inspiration with glottic closure. The physiological basis of the yawn is uncertain as it also has an infectious nature; however, it has been suggested that deep inspiration stretches underventilated alveoli and prevents atelectasis. Yawning also increases venous return to the heart (Ganong, 2005).

PHYSIOLOGY OF RESPIRATION

The physiology of the respiratory system is multivaried and complex. The integration of other body systems (e.g., cardiovascular, neurological) with the respiratory system is essential to understand. In addition, there are numerous complicated factors responsible for respiration, which are discussed in detail in the following section.

Ventilation and Perfusion

Ventilation is the movement of air in and out of the lungs. **Perfusion** is the exchange of oxygen and carbon dioxide at the alveolar-capillary level. Air moves in and out of the lungs because of the difference in intrapulmonary pressure and atmospheric pressure. Movement of air into the lungs is called inhalation or inspiration; movement of air out of the lungs is called exhalation or expiration. Gas flows from an area of higher pressure to an area of lower pressure. Because of the movement of air from higher to lower pressure areas, the pressure within the lungs must be less than atmospheric pressure for inspiration to occur. Pressure in the lungs becomes less than atmospheric pressure when the diaphragm and other muscles of respiration contract, which enlarges the thoracic cavity. At this time intrathoracic pressure becomes less than atmospheric pressure, and air flows into the lungs.

The primary control of ventilation is regulated in the brain. The medulla and pons in the brainstem regulate automatic ventilation; however, the cerebral cortex allows voluntary ventilation to override automatic ventilation.

There are also chemoreceptors that function to regulate ventilation. Central chemoreceptors are located in the medulla and respond to changes in pH. When hydrogen ion concentration rises (acid), ventilation increases. When hydrogen ion concentration falls, ventilation decreases. Similarly, chemoreceptors respond to changes in $PaCO_2$ by moving carbon dioxide into the cerebrospinal fluid, which stimulates movement of hydrogen ions. Next chemoreceptors are innervated, which increases ventilation. Increased ventilation causes carbon dioxide to be blown off, drops the $PaCO_2$, and returns to normal ventilation.

There are peripheral chemoreceptors located at the aortic arch that respond to changes in PaO_2. Hyperventilation is the first response to hypoxemia and is controlled by this mechanism. Alveolar ventilation is normally

4 liters per minute, and pulmonary capillary perfusion (cardiac output) is approximately 5 liters per minute. This results in a ventilation/perfusion (V/Q) ratio of 4:5, or 0.8.

Each area of the lung has different ventilation and perfusion rates. For example, the apices of the lungs normally have increased ventilation to perfusion; while the bases of the lungs have increased perfusion to ventilation. The overall ratio is 0.8; however, this ventilation-perfusion rate is influenced by factors such as position, gravity, and underlying lung disease. A change in this ratio of ventilation to perfusion is termed ventilation-perfusion mismatch.

The transport of oxygen and carbon dioxide are controlled by the process of diffusion, the movement of particles from an area of higher concentration to an area of lower concentration. Perfusion is the exchange of oxygen and carbon dioxide at the alveolar level. Ambient air is composed of oxygen (21%), nitrogen (nearly 79%), and traces of water vapor and carbon dioxide. The concentrations are also shown in the alveoli, the venous side of the capillary, and the arterial side of the capillary to show the movement of these particles.

Dalton's law states that the total pressure of a gas is equal to the sum of the partial pressures of the gases that comprise it. The total pressure of room air is 760 mm Hg, or 1 torr. Notice that the concentration of carbon dioxide is increased on the venous side and is diffused into the alveolus. Also, notice that the concentration of oxygen in the venous side of the capillary is low, so oxygen moves out of the alveolus and is equalized on the arterial side.

Oxygenation status is accurately measured by pulse oximetry only when a patient is on room air. When a patient is on supplemental oxygen, the nitrogen washes out and is replaced by oxygen. Patients on supplemental oxygen can be significantly hypoxemic even though their pulse oximeter reading is within normal limits. For this reason, while pulse oximetry is a useful clinical measurement, it cannot be replaced by arterial PaO_2 measurements. The clinical measure of oxygenation status is PaO_2; the clinical measure of ventilation status is $PaCO_2$.

Respiration is a general term that includes all the processes associated with getting oxygen into the lungs and removing carbon dioxide. The efficiency of respiration is primarily dependent on two factors: the availability of the alveolus for gas exchange and the integrity of the adjacent capillary supplying the alveolus.

Ventilation-Perfusion Dysfunction

There are complex relationships of ventilation to perfusion and ventilation-perfusion defects. One must keep in mind that throughout an abnormal lung there may be a variety of areas of underperfusion or underventilation, and the patient will show signs of decompensation. There are essentially two types ventilation-perfusion mismatch. First, there is decreased ventilation related to perfusion, called **shunting.** This is the portion of the cardiac output that does not exchange with alveolar air. Normally people have 2 to 5 percent shunting, in which this small portion of the cardiac output returns to the heart unventilated. Clinical examples of shunting include vascular lung tumors, congenital heart disease, intrapulmonary fistulas, pneumothorax, hemothorax, pleural effusion, or obstruction of the bronchi or bronchioles. In shunting, the PaO_2 falls because less oxygen is delivered and the $PaCO_2$ increases because less CO_2 is expired (Ganong, 2005).

Another type of ventilation-perfusion mismatch is decreased perfusion related to ventilation, called dead space. Dead space is the portion of ventilation that does not exchange with an intact capillary, also called wasted ventilation. Anatomic dead space is that portion of ventilation that is within the upper airways, not in contact with a capillary. Alveolar dead space is the volume that is within the alveoli; however, there is no blood flow adjacent to it. A classic clinical example of dead space is pulmonary embolus, in which there is no problem with ventilation, but blood flow is prevented from reaching the alveolus. In the case of significant dead space, the $PaCO_2$ falls because less CO_2 is delivered and the PaO_2 increases, because less oxygen enters the blood (Ganong, 2005).

Hypoxemia versus Hypoxia

The definition of **hypoxemia** is a decreased level of oxygen in the arterial blood as measured by the PaO_2. The definition of **hypoxia** is a bit more general in that it refers to a state of decreased perfusion of oxygen to the tissues and is measured by pulse oximetry. The relationship of these two values to each other, the arterial oxygen tension to oxygen saturation, is expressed in the oxygen-hemoglobin dissociation curve.

Hypercapnia versus Hypocapnia

The clinical measure of ventilation is the $PaCO_2$. The normal range of arterial $PaCO_2$ is 35 to 45, with a mean of 40. **Hypercapnia** is defined as a $PaCO_2$ above 45; while **hypocapnia** is defined as a $PaCO_2$ below 35. Hypercapnia indicates that ventilation is inadequate, and measures must be taken to improve ventilation to reach normocapnia. Hypocapnia indicates there is too much ventilation (hyperventilation), and measures must be taken to decrease ventilation and return to normocapnia.

Oxygen Transport

Oxygen is transported in the body in two ways: (a) dissolved in the plasma and (b) attached to hemoglobin. The clinical measure of the dissolved oxygen is the PaO_2, and it accounts for only 3 percent of the oxygen that is transported in the body. The other way that oxygen is transported in the body is attached to hemoglobin (oxyhemoglobin), and this accounts for the remaining 97 percent of the oxygen that is transported throughout the body. The clinical measure of this oxygen attached to hemoglobin is the oxygen saturation (SaO_2, SpO_2). Each molecule of hemoglobin can carry four atoms of oxygen. When it does, it is labeled fully saturated. Clinically, fully saturated blood is seen when there is a SpO_2 of greater than 92 percent. When all of the sites do not have an atom of oxygen attached to it, it is desaturated. Desaturated blood is seen when there is a SpO_2 of less than 92 percent. Desaturation can result from numerous processes; however, oxygen has a certain affinity for the hemoglobin molecule.

Oxygen-Hemoglobin Dissociation Curve

The oxyhemoglobin dissociation curve seen in Figure 30-4 illustrates the relationship between the PaO_2 and the SaO_2 and also illustrates conditions that change the affinity of oxygen for hemoglobin.

Hemoglobin can be considered an oxygen magnet, or a sponge for oxygen. As is shown in the curve, the relationship between the PaO_2 and the SaO_2 is S-shaped. In other words, the curve has two parts, a flat part and a steep part. On the steep part of the curve, a relatively large change in PaO_2 causes relatively little change in the SaO_2. If a patient's PaO_2 drops from 100 to 60, there is relatively little change in the SaO_2 (from 97 to 90 percent). This is because the patient remains on the flat part of the curve.

On the steep part of the curve, however, the relationship between PaO_2 and SaO_2 is more fragile. In the steep part of the curve there is a relatively small change in the PaO_2, which will cause the patient's oxygen saturation to drop. The drop in oxygen saturation greatly affects oxygen delivery to the tissues. If the patient's PaO_2 drops from 60 to 40, this represents desaturation from 90

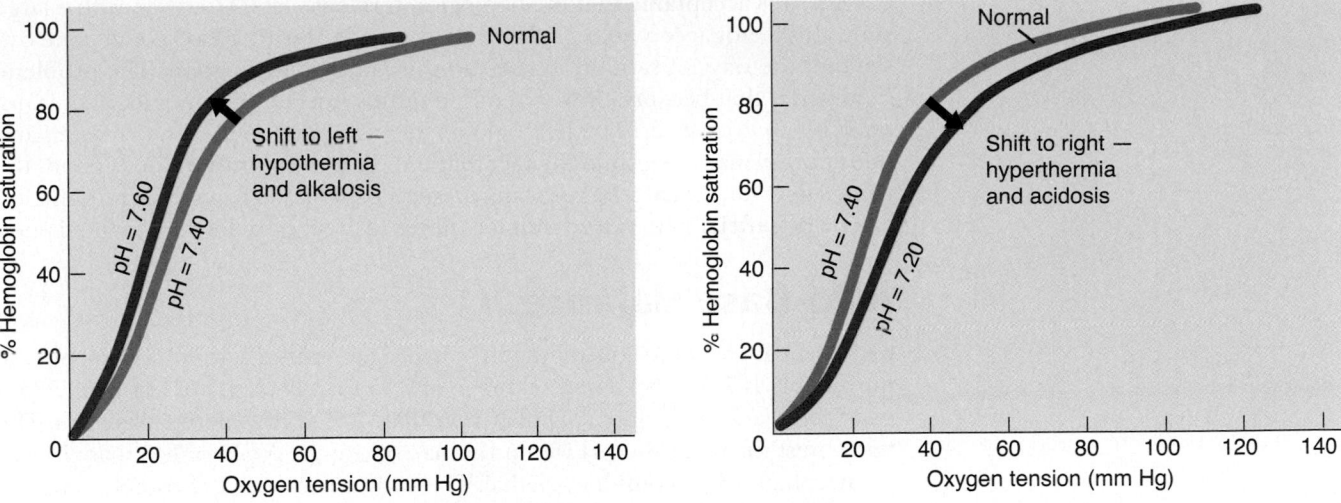

Figure 30-4 The oxygen-hemoglobin dissociation curve.

to 70 percent. The drop in oxygen saturation means that only 70 percent of sites on the hemoglobin molecule have an atom of oxygen attached to them, representing significant desaturation and significantly affects oxygen delivery to the tissues.

For the majority of patients, it is beneficial to be on the flat part of the curve, where changes in PaO_2 do not greatly affect oxygen saturation. The exception to this is the COPD patient, who frequently has PaO_2 values of 60 or less. These patients breathe on their hypoxic drive, and if their hypoxemia is corrected, they may have no stimulus to breathe and can develop ventilatory failure.

The affinity between oxygen and hemoglobin is not fixed and can change in response to a number of factors that change the affinity of oxygen for hemoglobin. These factors will change the curve and shift it either to the left or to the right.

Factors that cause decreased affinity of oxygen for hemoglobin will shift the oxyhemoglobin dissociation curve to the right. Oxygen will not be tightly bound to hemoglobin and more readily available for the tissues. These factors cause **acidemia,** which is a decreased arterial pH, less than 7.35, an increased $PaCO_2$, hyperthermia, and increased levels of 2,3-diphosphoglycerate (2,3-DPG). 2,3-DPG is a substance present in whole blood, which becomes depleted during the process of storage. Levels of 2,3-DPG are increased in anemia or other conditions of chronic hypoxia (Ganong, 2005).

The beneficial effect of a shift to the right in the oxyhemoglobin dissociation curve is that because oxygen is not as tightly bound to the hemoglobin, it is more likely to be released to the tissues and vital organs where it is needed. In the case of a febrile patient, the metabolic rate and oxygen demands are such that it is helpful to have the oxygen readily available for the tissues. With a small shift to the right, there is more availability of oxygen; however, this is not the case for a large shift. If the patient has a PaO_2 of 60 and a shift to the right, the oxygen saturation drops significantly, so there is desaturation of the arterial blood and decreased oxygen delivery. Therefore, small shifts to the right of the oxyhemoglobin dissociation curve can be beneficial, because it aids in oxygen unloading without greatly affecting oxygen delivery. However, large shifts to the right result in desaturation and are not beneficial.

Factors that cause increased affinity of oxygen for hemoglobin will shift the oxyhemoglobin dissociation curve to the left. These factors include **alkalemia,** which is an increased arterial pH more than 7.45, a decreased $PaCO_2$, and hypothermia. In the case of a hypothermic or alkalemic patient, metabolism and oxygen needs are diminished. Because the tissues do not need as much oxygen, it is acceptable that the hemoglobin release less. However, with a large shift, this is not acceptable. In this case, the patient with a PaO_2 of 60, one can see that the oxygen saturation rises, so the value appears good. The problem, however, is that because the oxygen is so tightly bound to hemoglobin, it is not available to the tissues. The hemoglobin acts as a magnet to attract oxygen and does not release it. Despite the fact that the oxygen saturation looks good, the tissues may not actually be receiving enough oxygen. So a small shift to the left can be beneficial, but a large shift interferes with oxygen delivery to the tissues.

Acid-Base Balance

pH is a measure of the concentration of hydrogen ions in a liquid. For blood, the normal pH is 7.40, with a normal range of 7.35 to 7.45. A pH of less than 7.35 is considered acidemia, and a pH of greater than 7.45 is considered alkalemia. The body must maintain the pH within this narrow range. A pH of less than 7.00 or greater than 7.80 is considered lethal. The body is composed of complex enzyme systems that regulate metabolism, and they are active only at a very narrow range of pH. Therefore, dramatic alterations in pH impair metabolism.

The Henderson-Hasselbalch equation is essential to understanding acid-base balance. This equation expresses the biological acid-base relationship of the body by looking at the relationship of carbonic acid to bicarbonate ion.

$$pH = pK\ (6.1) = \log \frac{[HCO_3^-]}{[H_2CO_3]} \quad \text{or} \quad \frac{\text{Kidneys}}{\text{Lungs}}$$

It is not as important to remember the exact equation as it is to remember the relationship of the lungs to the kidneys in the regulation of pH. This is because the kidneys are responsible for the regulation of bicarbonate in the serum. The normal range for bicarbonate in the blood is 22 to 26 mEq/L, with a mean of 24 mEq/L.

The lungs are responsible for the regulation of carbonic acid by adjusting $PaCO_2$ levels. The normal range for $PaCO_2$ is 35 to 46 mm Hg, with a mean of 40 mm Hg. The carbonic acid level equals the $PaCO_2$ times the solubility constant of 0.03. The normal carbonic acid level is 1.2 mEq/L.

$$40\ (\text{normal } PaCO_2) \times 0.03 = 1.2\ (\text{normal carbonic acid level})$$

The relationship of bicarbonate to carbonic acid is approximately 20:1. In other words, there is normally 20 times more bicarbonate than carbonic acid.

$$pH = 6.1 + \log \frac{24}{1.2} = \frac{20}{1}$$

For the pH to be normal, the ratio between bicarbonate and carbonic acid must remain 20:1. If the ratio drops, the pH will drop, causing acidemia. Consider the patient who goes into acute ventilatory failure, and $PaCO_2$ accumulates. If his $PaCO_2$ doubles to 80, see what happens to the 20:1 ratio. First, calculate the carbonic acid level:

$$80 \times 0.03 = 2.4\ (\text{carbonic acid})$$

Then find the ratio of bicarbonate to carbonic acid:

$$\frac{24\ (\text{bicarbonate})}{2.4\ (\text{carbonic acid})} = \frac{10}{1}$$

Because this ratio is smaller than 20:1, the pH will drop, causing acidemia. In considering the same patient, over time, his kidneys will retain bicarbonate. The bicarbonate level rises from 24 to 48 mEq/L. Now see what happens to the ratio:

$$\frac{48\ (\text{bicarbonate})}{2.4\ (\text{carbonic acid})} = \frac{20}{1}$$

Despite the fact that both the bicarbonate level and the $PaCO_2$ levels are abnormal, the 20:1 relationship has been preserved, and the pH will be normal. This is called compensation. In this example, the kidneys have compensated for the elevated $PaCO_2$ level by retaining bicarbonate.

Compensatory Mechanisms

There are three mechanisms that the body uses to maintain pH: the buffer system, the pulmonary system, and the renal system. The buffer system acts immediately and responds to moment-to-moment changes in pH that are of small magnitude. The pulmonary system acts within two to three hours, and the renal system responds within two to three days. In addition, there are two buffer systems, extracellular and intracellular.

The extracellular buffers are bicarbonate, phosphate, and plasma proteins that circulate in the serum and can buffer the blood by accepting a hydrogen ion. Intracellular buffering occurs within the red blood cells, which can also accept hydrogen ions. This buffer system has limited capacity and cannot compensate for large changes in pH. Therefore, the lungs are the next compensatory system that gets called into play.

The lungs begin to act within 10 to 30 minutes. They regulate pH by adjusting the level of ventilation, which changes the $PaCO_2$. When ventilation is increased, more CO_2 will be blown off, and this will cause the pH to rise. The opposite happens when ventilation decreases. The lungs will regulate pH only for moderate changes in pH. For large changes, the kidneys will also compensate.

The kidneys have a delayed response to changes in pH, and this may take several days. However, the kidneys are the most powerful system and have the potential to fully compensate for acid-base imbalances. The kidneys regulate pH by excreting hydrogen ions in exchange for sodium, reabsorbing bicarbonate, or excreting phosphates and ammonia.

BOX 30-1

POLK METHOD OF INTERPRETING ABGs

P = pH
O = oxygenation
L = lungs
K = kidneys

Arterial Blood Gas Analysis

Analysis of arterial blood gases (ABGs) is essential to our understanding of acid-base balance and oxygenation status. There are many methods of ABG interpretation. One of the simplest methods is called the POLK method, which is interpreted in Box 30-1.

The POLK method of ABG interpretation uses four values: pH, PaO_2, $PaCO_2$ (regulated by the lungs), and bicarbonate (HCO_3, regulated by the kidneys). These values tell information about two things: (a) the PaO_2 tells about the oxygenation status, and (b) the interaction between the pH, $PaCO_2$, and HCO_3 tells about the acid-base status.

Remember that the lungs control the $PaCO_2$ by blowing off or retaining CO_2 with ventilation, and the kidneys control the HCO_3 by striving to maintain the 20:1 relationship between carbonic acid and bicarbonate. CO_2 functions as an acid, and HCO_3 functions as a base (alkaline). However, remember that within their narrow normal ranges, both $PaCO_2$ and HCO_3 are acid-base balanced (Figures 30-5, 30-6, and 30-7).

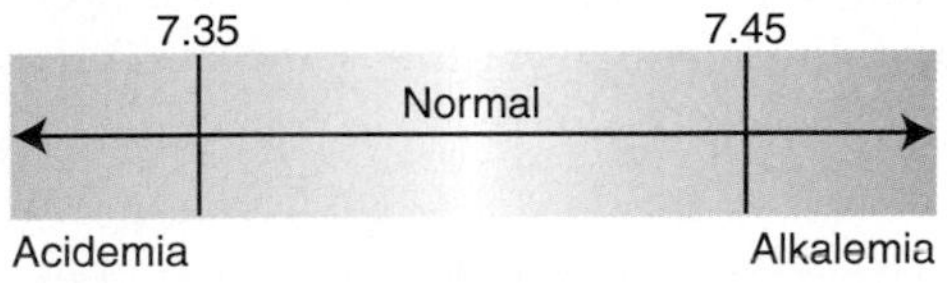

The normal values are (Figure 30-8):

pH: 7.35–7.45
PaO_2:   80–100 mm Hg
$PaCO_2$:   35–45 mm Hg
HCO_3:   22–26 mm Hg

A patient has the following blood gas results on room air (Figure 30-9):

pH: 7.52
PaO_2:   92
$PaCO_2$:   44
HCO_3:   37

The pH of 7.52 is higher than normal, indicating an alkalemia. The PaO_2 is within normal limits, so there is no problem with oxygenation. The $PaCO_2$ is 44, which is within normal range, however, the bicarbonate

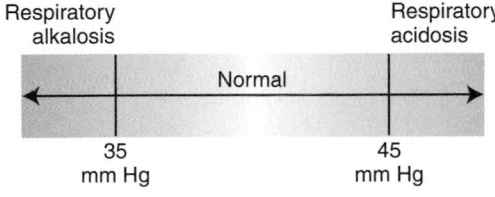

Figure 30-5 pH and acid-base balance; note normal range of pH as well as acidemia and alkalemia.

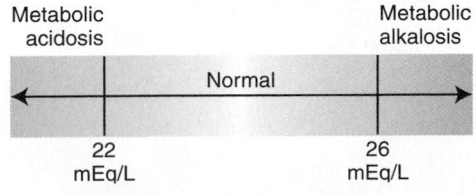

Figure 30-6 $PaCO_2$ and acid-base balance; note normal range of $PaCO_2$ as well as respiratory acidosis and respiratory alkalosis.

Figure 30-7 HCO_3 and acid-base balance; note normal range of HCO_3 as well as metabolic alkalosis and metabolic acidosis.

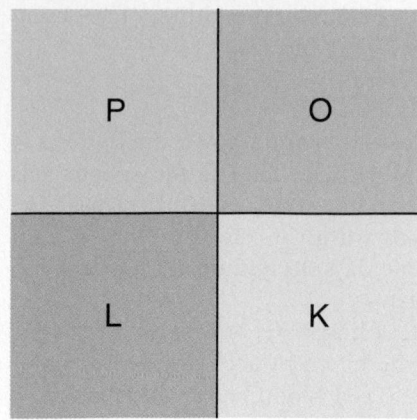

Figure 30-8 The POLK method of blood gas interpretation.

is too high at 37. So this patient has only the abnormality with the bicarbonate, which is too high. Therefore, a high bicarbonate level in and of itself is a metabolic alkalosis, which corresponds to a pH that is also too high. The interpretation for this set of ABGs is a simple (pure) metabolic alkalosis.

Common causes of metabolic alkalosis include vomiting, diarrhea, and nasogastric suctioning (Table 30-1). Other causes include conditions associated with decreased potassium and chloride. A common cause of metabolic alkalosis in the intensive care unit involves overuse of diuretics. This condition is called contraction alkalosis.

Another example of ABGs (Figure 30-10):

pH:	7.03
PaO_2:	60
$PaCO_2$:	100
HCO_3:	25

The severely low pH indicates a severe acidemia. The PaO_2 of 60 indicates a significant hypoxemia. The $PaCO_2$ of 100 is severely elevated, indicating a respiratory acidosis, and the HCO_3 is normal. So the interpretation for this set of ABGs is simple (but severe) respiratory acidosis with significant hypoxemia.

The next set of example ABGs is a bit different (Figure 30-11):

pH:	7.10
PaO_2:	99
$PaCO_2$:	12
HCO_3:	4

The low pH indicates a significant acidemia. The PaO_2 is normal; and both the $PaCO_2$ and the HCO_3 are significantly low. So we need to identify the primary cause of the acidemia. Can a low amount of respiratory acid ($PaCO_2$) contribute to this acidemia? Can a low amount of metabolic base contribute to this acidemia? Here we have abnormalities in both the respiratory and metabolic systems. When we have abnormalities going in the same direction

↑ 7.52	92
44	37 ↑

Figure 30-9 Simple (pure) metabolic alkalosis.

↑ 7.03	60 ↓
↑ 100	25

Figure 30-10 Severe respiratory acidosis with hypoxemia.

TABLE 30-1	**Causes of Acid-Base Imbalances**	
METABOLIC ACIDOSIS		**METABOLIC ALKALOSIS**
Diabetic ketoacidosis		Vomiting
Diarrhea		Overuse of diuretics
Lactic acidosis		Vomiting
Renal failure		Nasogastric suctioning
Extended use of TPN		
Ostomy drainage		
Respiratory acidosis		Respiratory alkalosis
Chronic lung disease		Hypoxia
Oversedation		Increased minute ventilation
Neuromuscular disease		Hyperventilation
Acute and impending respiratory failure		Pregnancy
		Fever
		Pain
		Severe anemia

Adapted from DeLaune, S., & Ladner, P. (2006). Fundamentals of nursing (3rd ed.). New York: Thomson Delmar Learning.

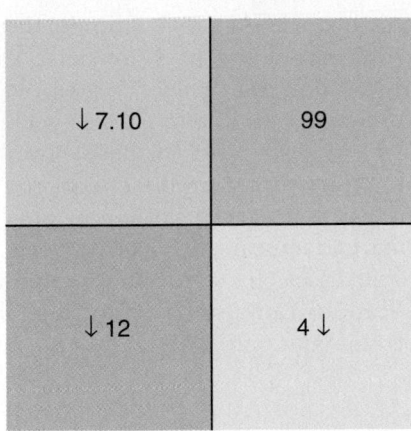

Figure 30-11 Partially compensated metabolic acidosis.

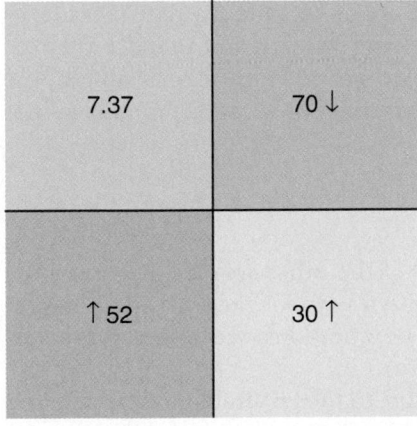

Figure 30-12 Fully compensated respiratory acidosis (or metabolic alkalosis) with hypoxemia.

(elevation or depression), there is compensation involved. If that is the case, we must identify the primary cause of the abnormality and determine whether the other system has partially or completely compensated for the abnormality. We can see that a low amount of respiratory acid cannot possibly create this severe acidemia, but a low amount of metabolic base has indeed created this acidemia. So the primary problem is metabolic acidosis. However, the lungs have begun to compensate by blowing off CO_2. We can see by the pH of 7.10 that the lungs have not yet been able to completely return the pH to normal, so the interpretation for this set of ABGs is partially compensated metabolic acidosis (McDaniel, 2005).

Common causes of metabolic acidosis include diabetic ketoacidosis, diarrhea, lactic acidosis, renal failure, prolonged use of total parenteral nutrition, and ostomy drainage (see Table 30-1).

Here is an example of full compensation in which the pH is completely normal (Figure 30-12).

pH:	7.37
PaO_2:	70
$PaCO_2$:	52
HCO_3:	30

In this case, the pH is normal; however, there is significant hypoxemia, and the $PaCO_2$ and HCO_3 are both elevated in the same direction. Because of this, there is compensation involved. And, the problem has been fully compensated as seen by the normal pH. To provide an accurate interpretation with a case of full compensation, more clinical information is needed; such as a trend of recent ABG results or some patient history. Otherwise, based on the values themselves it could be a fully compensated respiratory acidosis with hypoxemia or a fully compensated metabolic acidosis with hypoxemia. If the patient had a history of COPD, we might expect these results, because in COPD the problem is CO_2 retention and hypoxemia; yet the kidneys have completely compensated over time.

Respiratory Adjustments during Exercise, Hypoxia, and in High Altitude

There are a variety of variables that affect the adjustments a body must undergo to maintain good respiratory efforts. The variables addressed in this section are exercise, hypoxia, and high altitude. Each variable affects the body system differently, and the body adapts in different methods.

During exercise, there is extra heat, and CO_2 is removed. There is increased blood flow to the muscles, an increase in extraction of oxygen from the blood, an increase in ventilation that provides extra O_2, eliminates extra CO_2, and eliminates some of the heat that is generated. Blood flow can be increased from the normal of 5 liters per minute up to as much as 35 liters per minute. The increase in oxygen uptake is proportionate to the workload, but only to a maximal point. Beyond this point, oxygen consumption levels off and lactate from the muscles (a product of anaerobic metabolism) begins to accumulate in the blood. This is also called oxygen debt.

During exercise, there is also an increase in minute ventilation, which is respiratory rate multiplied times tidal volume. The respiratory rate increases, and there is also an increase in the depth of respiration. Body temperature also increases during exercise. After exercise, respiratory rate does not reach normal levels until the oxygen debt has been paid. This may take as long as 90 minutes after exercise has ceased. After exercise, the continued stimulus for ventilation is the elevated H^+ levels due to the lactic academia (Ganong, 2005).

Hypoxia affects brain tissue before the other tissues in the body. Initial symptoms of hypoxia include drowsiness, dulled sensations, disorientation, or headache. Other symptoms include anorexia, nausea, vomiting, and tachycardia. High altitude creates a problem of hypoxic hypoxia. At a high altitude, the composition of air remains the same, but the barometric pressure falls. At 10,000 feet, the alveolar PO_2 falls to nearly 60 mm Hg, which creates the hypoxic stimulation of the chemoreceptors to increase ventilation. This hyperventilation will also decrease PCO_2, resulting in respiratory alkalosis. Over time, people will acclimate to this condition by increasing production of red blood cells and erythropoietin, which will increase the overall oxygen-carrying capacity. In the meantime, however, symptoms can appear, such as irritability, insomnia, nausea, and vomiting. In extreme cases, high-altitude cerebral edema and high-altitude pulmonary complications can also develop. This is treated by return to lower altitude and a diuretic (Ganong, 2005).

ASSESSMENT

Despite all of the new technology available today, assessment of the thorax and lungs is a skill that is vital to nurses. Assessment is more than just listening to the chest with the stethoscope. There are many techniques that provide us with a wealth of information if we take the time to learn and practice them.

The purpose of respiratory assessment is to provide a basic screening of the patient's respiratory status, to establish a baseline, or to detect abnormalities from that baseline.

History Taking

Respiratory assessment, as with assessment of the other systems, begins with a complete history. It is important to begin with a series of general questions and depending on the patient's answers to those questions, move into more specific questions (see Patient Playbook feature).

Once the nurse learns the patient's answers to the general questions in a respiratory assessment, the nurse can focus on specific patient symptoms. Some of the most common respiratory symptoms include dyspnea, cough, wheeze, and chest pain. **Dyspnea** is defined as difficulty breathing. This is a descriptive term used to describe the patient's subjective feeling of shortness of breath. Dyspnea is the most important symptom of respiratory insufficiency, so it is important to ask the patient specific questions about his or her difficulty breathing.

Dyspnea is often effort dependent, but the presence of dyspnea in the absence of effort is characteristic of asthma, pulmonary embolism, or myocardial ischemia. There may be associated symptoms, such as wheezing or chest pain; however, it is important to ask specific questions about the dyspnea itself, as shown in the Patient Playbook feature.

Another respiratory symptom is cough. Asking a few questions about the patient's cough can provide a wealth of information to assist in treatment, such as When do you cough? During the day? At night? Do you bring up mucus? What color is it? Consistency? How much? and Do you have any spells when you can't stop coughing?

An acute cough can be associated with a viral upper respiratory infection or with other bronchopulmonary infections. It can also be seen during inhalation of an irritating or an allergenic substance.

Chronic cough can be associated with asthma, chronic bronchitis, gastroesophageal reflux, bronchiectasis, tuberculosis, or bronchogenic carcinoma. A productive cough implies an underlying infection (Table 30-2); a nonproductive cough implies a mechanical process, such as irritation.

Table 30-2 shows some of the common characteristics of sputum and associated conditions. Asking the patient some specific information about the sputum can be helpful in determining the problem. Color of sputum can be helpful in differentiating the problem. Bloody or rust-colored sputum can be seen in lobar pneumonia. Rust-colored or prune juice–colored sputum is a classic sign of pneumococcal pneumonia.

PATIENT PLAYBOOK

The Patient with Dyspnea

For the purposes of patient education, the nurse should ask the following types of questions to a patient with dyspnea:

1. When do you experience shortness of breath? At rest? When you lie flat? When you walk on level ground? Upstairs?
2. How far can you walk before you feel breathless? What symptoms make you stop walking?
3. How long have you noticed that you become short of breath?
4. Is it better or worse now than before?
5. Does this breathlessness wake you up from sleep? (Dyspnea that wakes patients up from sleep is called paroxysmal nocturnal dyspnea. It is often seen in patients with left ventricular failure or in COPD because of pooling of secretions and positional decrease in lung volume or changes in airway resistance during sleep.)
6. Is it the same, better or worse when you lie down? (Orthopnea is the term for dyspnea that occurs in the supine position and can be seen in heart disease or chronic lung disease.)

TABLE 30-2 Sputum in Pulmonary Conditions

SPUTUM QUALITY	ASSOCIATED CONDITION
Bloody, rusty-colored	Lobar pneumonia
Rust colored or prune juice colored	Pneumococcal pneumonia
Red or pink, frothy	Pulmonary edema
Red, bloody	Left heart failure, mitral stenosis, trauma to airway
Grayish-white, mucoid	Emphysema, tuberculosis
Large volumes of sputum that separates into layers; intermitted blood streaking	Bronchiectasis
Yellow or green	Bronchopulmonary infection
Foul smelling	Anaerobic infection such as lung abscess or necrotizing pneumonia
Musty odor, greenish sputum	*Pseudomonas* infection
Sweet odor, pinkish sputum	Serratia infection

Adapted from Estes, M. (2006). Health assessment and physical examination (3rd ed.). New York: Thomson Delmar Learning.

Red, bloody sputum can be seen in left heart failure, mitral stenosis, or trauma to the airway. **Hemoptysis** indicates either the presence of frank blood or blood-streaked sputum and is also classically seen in bronchitis, bronchiectasis, or neoplasm.

Grayish-white mucoid sputum can be associated with tuberculosis or emphysema. A large volume of sputum that separates into layers, with streaks of blood is characteristic for bronchiectasis.

Green or yellow sputum is often due to bronchopulmonary infection. Some types of organisms also have a characteristic odor. Greenish sputum with an offensive musty odor is characteristic of *Pseudomonas* infection. Pinkish sputum with a sweet odor can be due to infection with *Serratia*. Foul-smelling sputum is due to infection with an anaerobic organism and can be found in lung abscess or necrotizing pneumonia.

If a patient has chest pain, it is sometimes difficult to differentiate whether the pain originates with the respiratory or cardiac system. Generally speaking, respiratory muscular chest pain does not radiate, and there is often tenderness to palpation. Some of these questions may help to distinguish the pain, but if there is any doubt about the origin, do not rule out cardiac pain.

Patients with pleurisy also experience dyspnea, because their increased pain on inspiration makes them aware of every breath. Acute pleuritic pain is seen in patients with spontaneous pneumothorax, pulmonary embolism, and pneumococcal pneumonia. A more gradual onset of pleuritic pain is seen in tuberculosis and malignancy.

Myocardial ischemic type of pain is due to an imbalance in the supply and demand of oxygen in the heart muscle. The pain typical of angina can be brought on by a heavy meal, exercise, or emotional stress. This pain is classically described as pressure or squeezing in the center of the chest, sometimes with radiation to the jaw or one or both arms. However, the pattern of chest pain is often different in women. The chest pain of myocardial ischemia is often responsive to vasodilators, such as nitroglycerin and rest.

Inflammation to the joints and muscles of the thoracic cage can also be a cause of chest pain. This can also be associated with tenderness to touch over

Respiratory Muscular Chest Pain

For the purposes of patient education, you can ask the following questions regarding chest pain caused by respiratory effort:

1. Describe the pain. Rate the pain from 0 to 10.
2. Show me where the pain is located. (Pain that is localized on one side can be the result of pleurisy or inflammation of the pleural surface.)
3. It is constant or intermittent?
4. Does it hurt to touch your chest? Does it hurt to take a deep breath? Pain that increases with a deep breath or with a change in body position can be due to pleurisy
5. What brings on the pain? Pain after heavy meals, emotional upsets, or exercise can be due to angina.
6. Have you injured your chest recently?

the affected area. There are other general questions regarding the patient's history that may be helpful to ask:

1. Have you unintentionally gained or lost weight recently? How much?
2. Have you noticed a change in your voice recently?
3. Do your ankles swell? When?
4. Have you or any of your family members had a history of chest infections? If so, how have they been treated?
5. Have you been unusually tired lately?
6. Have you ever been told that you have asthma, bronchitis, allergies, cancer, tuberculosis? Anyone in your family?
7. Have you ever had a job that exposed you to dust, fumes, asbestos, or chemicals?
8. Have you traveled recently? Where?

If the patient responds positively to any of these questions, it is important to gather more information about those symptoms and focus part of your examination in those areas. In addition to a general survey, it is also important to ask about the patient's past health history and current level of functional ability. Ask about the patient's occupational history, looking for exposure to toxic chemicals or products, such as asbestos, coal dust, mold, etc. Ask about recent travel to foreign countries or military service. Ask about the patient's activities of daily living. Is the patient able to care for himself of herself? Has he or she noticed a change in his or her level of physical ability, such as ability to do housework, gardening, or walking from place to place? Has he or she noticed that he or she must stop and rest more frequently?

It is also important to ask about family history and its relation to the patient's current status. Ask about a family history of heart disease, lung disease, or chronic disease of any kind. Assessing the health history of family members is important not only genetically, but also from a perspective of social support. As more and more family members are participating in the role of a caregiver for a loved one, this has the potential to create numerous health and emotional issues for that person.

The health history accompanies the health assessment and is primarily employed to gather subjective data that is the patient's stated recollection of their past respiratory health experiences and conditions. In some situations, the patient may not be able to accurately recall events and conditions. In those cases, it is beneficial to consult another source whose reliability can be ensured. Additionally, the patient may be dyspneic and may require rest periods during the history portion of the examination. In all cases, an attempt should be made to discover previous conditions and treatments of the patient. If the condition of the patient is questionable, old medical records may be viewed, family members may be questioned, or records from physician's offices may be reviewed.

Respiratory Assessment in the Elderly

In addition to the usual health assessment questions, older adults should also be questioned about shortness of breath or fatigue with daily activities. Because many individuals experience a gradual slowing of physical activities, they are unaware that their overall respiratory status has decreased over time; hence they do not mention decreased activity tolerance as a concern. During normal aging, less pulmonary surface area is available for gas exchange, so even though the older adult may be able to maintain their usual functions, they may have longer periods of rest or require more frequent rest periods at the conclusion of those activities. By questioning the older adult about their usual level of activity and what tasks they engage in, you may be able to determine if they are having functional difficulties based on their pulmonary status (Delaune & Ladner, 2006).

Older adults with chronic respiratory diseases, including COPD, an acute disease including lung cancer, or tuberculosis, should be questioned about their ability to function daily at his or her usual level. Amount of weight changes should be determined at least every three months. Frequently, older adults with respiratory diseases find eating a difficult task and become dyspneic during meals. Consequently, they may fail to consume adequate calories because they are too short of breath or fatigued from the activity of eating. Assessment of weight and exploration of changes will provide useful information that will detect early weight losses related to inadequate nutritional intake. Questioning about the older adult's energy level and stamina is important because maintenance of activity level is an important consideration in planning care. An individual who notices that he or she tires more easily may experience coping problems related to management of their disease. Coping problems related to respiratory disease may require interdisciplinary team collaboration to identify and implement strategies that will address areas of care that require development of new strategies.

Functional status is often a reliable indicator of progressive losses. It is important to understand if the older adult's respiratory condition is having an adverse effect on his or her work or home life. Questions should focus on ability to complete specific tasks or activities in each setting. Questions should also probe the duration of time the patient has been experiencing symptoms. By asking her or him to rate his or her current activity level and compare it to the same time last year, the older adult may be able to pinpoint a time when deterioration seemed to begin. Additionally, consider the possibility that activities that cause shortness of breath or pain may be long-standing and may be perceived by the older adult as a condition that cannot be addressed. The patient may have little expectation that his or her condition can be improved, so he or she may be reluctant to indicate the severity of his or her respiratory-related symptoms. This case may be especially true in secondhand cigarette smoke in which the patient may reside with a smoker or have a history of previous passive exposure to tobacco. Emphysema and COPD may manifest so gradually that the older adult is unaware of the activity-limiting effects. Further, the older adult may believe that he or she is powerless to change his or her living condition and insist that his or her residence be free from smoke at all times.

The respiratory system is vulnerable to age-associated changes that contribute to overall decreased functioning and reserve. Inefficiencies in pulmonary functioning may contribute to increase susceptibility to disease because of ineffective clearance of the bronchopulmonary tree because of decreased ciliary activity and cumulative effects of chronic processes such as those of COPD or asthma (Estes, 2006). Normal aging changes associated with the immune system also predispose the older adult to development of acute respiratory diseases, because immunity is slower to react and initiate the inflammatory response with phagocytosis aimed at bacterial invaders. Hence, older adults are particularly susceptible to bacterial pneumonia, influenza, and tuberculosis. These acute processes are among the leading causes of mortality in older adults and have the potential for rapid transmission among this group in places of congregate living. For this reason, immunizations in this population are essential and should be addressed during the health history phase of the examination. Other age-related respiratory changes will be discussed in the assessment portion of this chapter.

Inspection

The respiratory system extends from the nose to the alveoli. Assessment of the respiratory system includes use of various techniques where inspection, auscultation, palpation, and percussion are used extensively to disclose normal and abnormal conditions. The purpose of inspection is to assess the configuration of the thorax, rate and pattern of breathing, movement of the thorax during respiration, and nonrespiratory movements within the chest.

Skeletal Deformities

There are several skeletal deformities that may have an effect on the function of the respiratory system. Figure 30-13 illustrates the common skeletal deformities of the thorax. **Kyphosis** is an exaggeration of thoracic spine convexity. Often this is due to osteoporosis secondary to aging, but other causes include Paget's disease of the bone and ankylosing spondylitis.

Scoliosis is an abnormal lateral deviation of the spine. Often this is a result of abnormal growth of the spine in childhood or as a result of polio or other musculoskeletal disorders. **Kyphoscoliosis** is a combination of kyphosis and scoliosis, which manifests itself as a hunchback appearance. It can be a result of severe unilateral lung disease or bone or muscle disorders. Because of the marked reduction in lung volumes, these patients often develop respiratory and cardiac disorders.

Barrel chest is seen in increased anterior-posterior to lateral diameter. In addition, the ribs often widen out and wing out horizontally, creating the appearance of the staves of a barrel. It is often seen in chronic emphysema as a result of long-term air trapping. It is also commonly seen in normal elderly persons.

Funnel chest (pectus excavatum) is a congenital disorder of abnormal depression of the sternum. It occurs in 1 in 300 live births, affecting boys more fre-

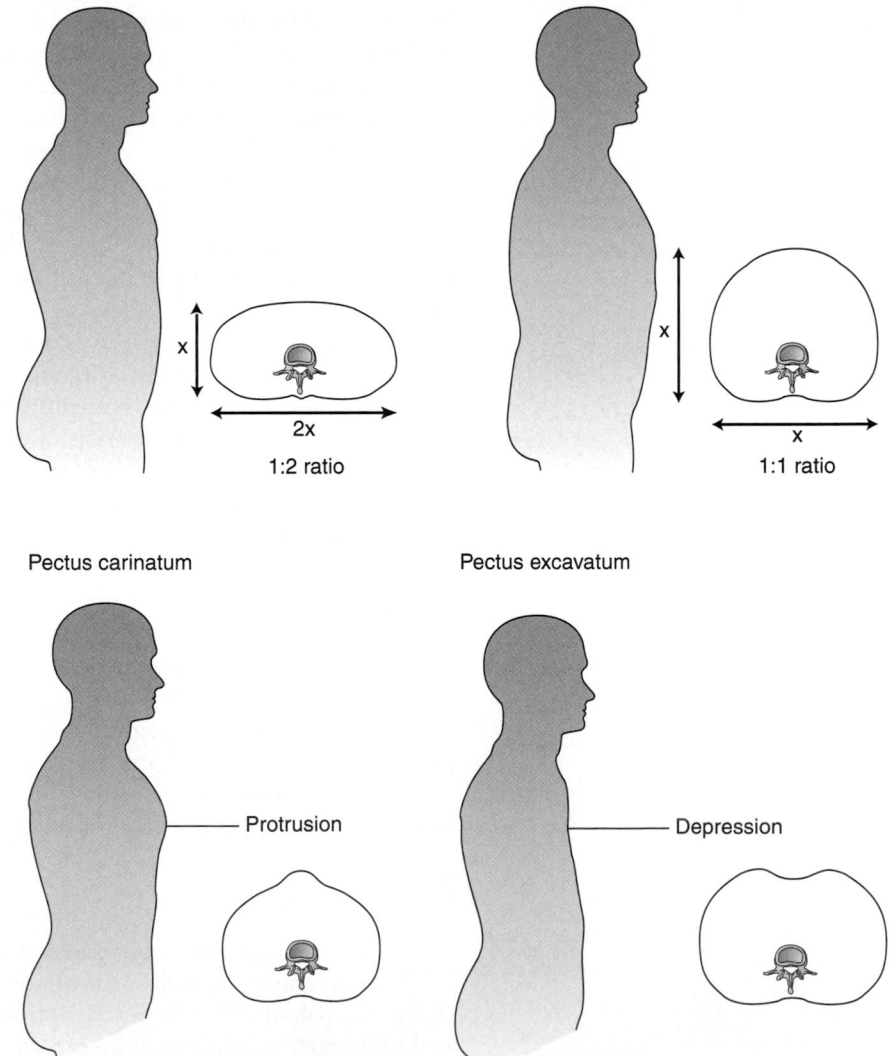

Figure 30-13 Common skeletal configurations of the thorax.

quently. It was also called cobbler's chest as a result of the chronic pressure that would be placed against the sternum during the shoemaking process. This condition can occur with rickets, Marfan's syndrome, mitral valve prolapse, arrhythmias, and systolic ejection murmurs frequently (Baron & Schwartzstein, 2004).

Pigeon chest (pectus carinatum) is an abnormal protuberance of the sternum and costal cartilages, which often manifests itself during the teenage growth spurt, seen more often in boys. This condition can occur in association with congenital heart disease (Estes, 2006).

Mouth, Nose, and Neck

The nose is one of the upper respiratory organs. Assess for patency by occluding first one nostril and then the other. Occlusion of the nostrils can occur in the presence of an upper respiratory infection, foreign body, nasal polyps, or allergies. Position the patient with the head in an extended position. Using the thumb, lift the tip of the nose. Inspect for color and patency of the mucosal membranes for color and discharge. Inspect the middle and inferior turbinates and middle meatus for color, swelling, drainage, lesions, and polyps. The nasal mucosa should appear pink or dull red without swelling or polyps. The septum should be at the midline without perforation, lesions, or bleeding (Estes, 2006). Normally, there will be a small mount of clear, watery discharge.

The mouth and pharynx are also included with the organs of the upper respiratory system. Inspection should reveal buccal mucosa that is moist, smooth, and without lesions. Color may vary based on race. Freckle-like macules may be normally present on the mucosa. Color of the mucosa may vary according to race. Gum tissue should be well-defined with no pockets between teeth and gum tissue (Estes, 2006). No swelling or bleeding should be visible. Teeth should be firmly surrounded by gum tissue.

With the patient's head tilted back and the mouth open widely, first observe if the pharynx is midline. Ask the patient to say "ah." The uvula should rise symmetrically. Observe the position, size, color, and general appearance of the tonsils. With a bright light, observe the throat. It is normally pink and vascular without swelling, exudates, or lesions. Note if redness, exudates, swelling, or patches are present on the posterior pharynx. Note the size of the tonsils, pillars, and uvula. Tonsils should be graded: 1+ means that tonsils are visible; 2+ tonsils are between the pillars and the uvula; 3+ tonsils are touching the uvula; and 4+ one or both tonsils occupy the space to the midline or beyond. Note the quality of the voice; normally no hoarseness will be evident. Causes of hoarseness include infection of viral or bacterial causes, tumors compressing the vocal cords, lesions of the larynx, overuse of the voice, or enlargement of the thyroid gland.

The neck should be supple and without tenderness to palpation. No use of accessory breathing muscles should be noted at the sternocleidomastoid, trapezius, or omohyoid muscles. Using the finger tips, palpate the lymph nodes of the neck. Palpate the lymph nodes including the deep cervical chain, posterior cervical chain, and the supraclavicular nodes. Normal findings should reveal no palpable nodes. Palpable lymph nodes should be explored by checking the path of lymph drainage.

Rate of Breathing

Another part of inspection is to assess the respiratory rate. Many textbooks quote a respiratory rate of 16 to 24 breaths per minute; however, the normal rate of breathing, or **eupnea,** for most adults at rest is actually slower at 12 to 20 breaths per minute. **Tachypnea** is a general term for breathing that is rapid and shallow. It can be a sign of hypoxemia or associated with pain, fever, or neurological problems. **Bradypnea** is the general term for slow breathing that is often associated with head injury, oversedation, or other drug overdose. The respiratory rate and the pattern of breathing can provide important information about the patient's underlying status.

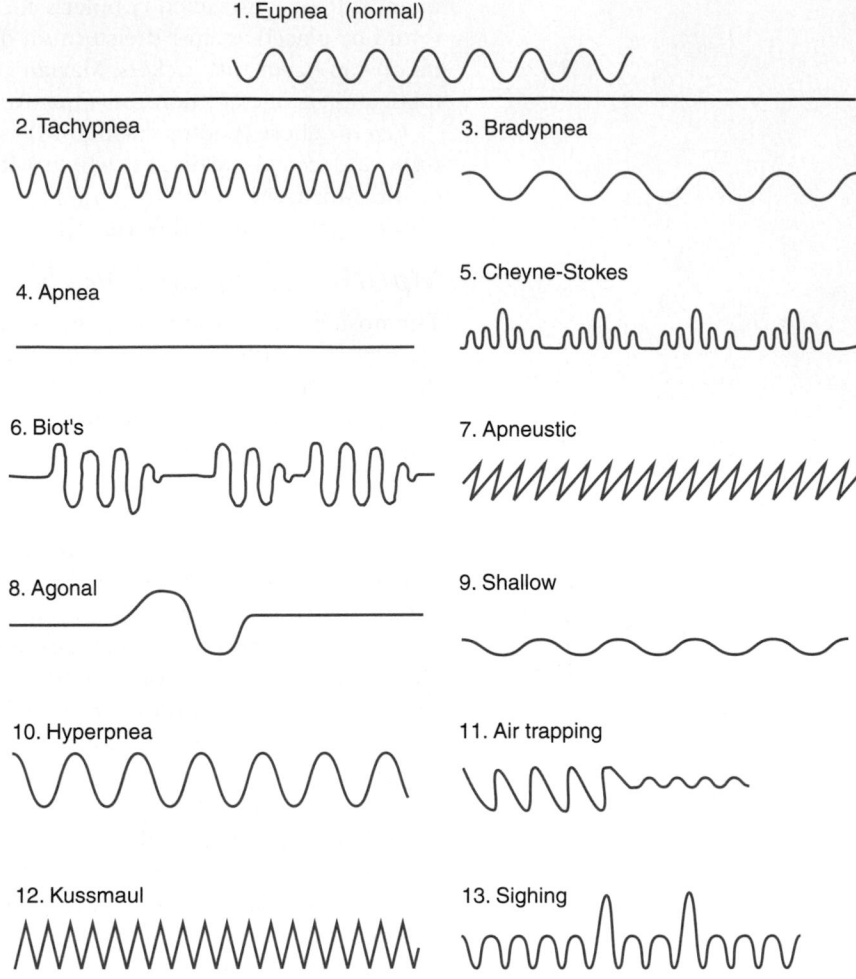

Figure 30-14 Rhythms of breathing.

Rhythms of Breathing

Figure 30-14 illustrates the rhythms of breathing as compared with a normal rhythm of breathing. **Kussmaul breathing** is rapid and deep breathing, often associated with an acetone odor as in diabetic ketoacidosis. **Biot's (ataxic) breathing** is a type of periodic breathing that is irregular in depth and rhythm and also has periods of apnea. This type of breathing often indicates increased intracranial pressure. **Cheyne-Stokes breathing** is another type of periodic breathing, in which there is a pattern of crescendo-decrescendo breathing with periods of apnea. Cheyne-Stokes respirations can be seen in a type of sleep apnea that is associated with heart failure, encephalopathy, or stroke (Chalela & Kasner, 2004). **Apneustic breathing** is prolonged inspiration and indicates neurological damage in the respiratory center of the brain.

Clubbing

Chronic hypoxia produces significant visible changes in the fingers, such as **clubbing,** which is an abnormal enlargement of the distal phalanges. Clubbing is often associated with cyanotic heart disease or advanced chronic pulmonary disease. The mechanism whereby diminished oxygen tension in the blood causes clubbing is of unknown etiology. Clubbing occurs in all digits but is most easily seen in the fingers. Clubbing is present if the transverse diameter of the base of the fingernail is greater than the transverse diameter of the most distal joint of the digit. The affected phalanx is full, fleshy, and notably vascular; the skin might be excoriated. It occurs first in the thumb and index finger.

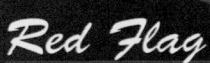

Normally the angle of the nail bed (x-axis) to the cuticle (y-angle) is approximately 160°. When this angle flattens out, this is also a sign of clubbing. It can also be detected by palpating a soft and spongy nail bed. The most obvious sign of clubbing is seen in fingertips that appear bulbous. In other words, the distal phalangeal depth is greater than the interphalangeal depth. Clubbing has also been associated with a variety of other disorders. These disorders include bronchogenic carcinoma, cystic fibrosis, bronchiectasis, empyema, lung abscess, HIV in children, and patients with cyanotic congenital heart disease.

Signs of Respiratory Distress

In addition to assessment of the shape of the thorax, the rate and rhythms of breathing, and the presence of clubbing, the nurse should also assess the patient for other signs of respiratory distress. Observe the mouth for the presence of cyanosis or pursed-lip breathing, the latter of which is seen in obstructive lung disease in an attempt to prolong expiration and keep the airways open. Observe the nares for signs of inspiratory flaring. Assess the accessory muscles of respiration: the intercostals, the sternocleidomastoid, and the abdominal muscles that come into play during distress.

It is important for the nurse to assess the early signs of hypoxemia before it progresses to respiratory distress (see Skills 360° feature). Early signs of hypoxia are change in mental status (e.g., confusion, restlessness, drowsy), change in vital signs (e.g., respiratory rate, heart rate), and headache. Late signs of hypoxemia are: arrhythmias, hypotension, cyanosis, and coma.

Early signs of hypoxemia are often quite subtle, but must be detected as soon as possible (see Red Flag feature). The earliest sign of hypoxia is a change in mental status. Often patients will manifest acute confusion or restlessness before a change in vital signs is noted. If possible, it is often recommended to immediately draw a set of blood gases to determine the arterial oxygen and carbon dioxide levels. If these levels are normal, a neurological explanation for this change in mental status can be explored.

It is not always necessary to wait for blood gases to be drawn before placing a patient on a mechanical ventilator. If a patient manifests an acute change in mental status, they will often require an endotracheal tube based on this sign alone. The diagnosis of acute ventilatory failure is defined as a $PaCO_2$ value of 60 mm Hg or greater. However, the diagnosis of impending ventilatory failure is made on the basis of the clinical signs: a change in mental status, an increase in respiratory rate, use of accessory muscles, abdominal paradox, or change in heart rate or blood pressure (Box 30-2).

Palpation

The purpose of palpation is to determine the movement of the chest and the consistency of the tissues underlying the hands of the examiner. Respiratory excursion is assessed by observing the movement of the chest during normal respiration. Place the hands on either side of the patient's thorax with the thumbs pointing to each other. Ask the patient to take a deep breath and watch the movement of the thumbs. The thumbs should move equally away from each other, then back toward each other. If one side of the chest is motionless, it could indicate pneumonectomy or any condition that prevents or restricts full ventilation of the lung.

Tracheal deviation can also be assessed by palpation. The trachea is part of the mediastinum that lies in the middle of the chest. The mediastinum includes the heart and great vessels, the esophagus, trachea, hilum, thymus gland, and numerous nerves. Deviation of the trachea can be caused by changes in intrapleural pressures. The trachea can be easily palpated by placing the fingers on either side of the suprasternal notch and pressing inward. If the trachea is not midline, it can be pulled toward the affected (abnormal) side in the case of massive atelectasis, unilateral pulmonary fibrosis, pneu-

Red Flag

Preventing Aspiration

Aspiration is the passage of fluid and solid particles into the lung. It tends to occur in individuals whose normal swallowing mechanism and cough reflex are impaired. Individuals at greatest risk for this dangerous disorder are those with a decreased level of consciousness or central nervous system abnormality. Those with substance abuse, sedation, anesthesia, seizure disorders, acute stroke, and Guillain-Barré syndrome should never be left without adequate supervision to ensure airway patency. Suction should be immediately available at all times. The head of the bed should be elevated at least 30° at all times, or the patient should be positioned on their left side to promote airway safety.

BOX 30-2

INDICATIONS FOR INTUBATION

The indications for intubation can be summarized in the mnemonic VOPS.

Ventilation: acute ventilatory failure: $PaCO_2$ 60 mm Hg or greater

 Impending ventilatory failure: change in mental status, increased respiratory rate, use of accessory muscles, increase in respiratory rate, abdominal paradox, or change in heart rate or blood pressure

Obstruction: any evidence of obstruction of the airway. Could be because of swelling, tumor, or foreign body impeding the flow of air

Protection: any evidence of the patient's inability to protect the airway. The primary protective mechanisms are the ability to swallow and the ability to cough.

Secretions: any evidence that the patient is unable to manage their own secretions

If the patient manifests any evidence of problems with ventilation, obstruction, protection, or secretions, the patient should have an artificial airway placed (endotracheal tube or tracheostomy) immediately.

---

monectomy, or diaphragmatic paralysis. The trachea can be pulled toward the unaffected (normal) side in neck tumors, thyroid enlargement, mediastinal mass, massive pleural effusion, or tension pneumothorax.

Fremitus

Fremitus is the feeling of vibration on the chest wall. Usually fremitus is assessed by asking the patient to say something with a low and deep resonating sound, such as 99, while the examiner places his or her hand on the patient's thorax in a side-to-side motion. The outer aspect of the palm is the most sensitive area to vibrations. Compare the vibrations from one side to the other. Fremitus may be increased or decreased, depending on the underlying condition. Conditions associated with increased fremitus are pleural effusion, pneumothorax, bronchial obstruction, pleural tumor, emphysema, and pneumonectomy. Conditions associated with decreased fremitus are pneumonia, compressed lung, atelectasis, lung tumors, pulmonary infarction, and pulmonary fibrosis (Daniels, 2004).

 Increased vocal fremitus will be present in any condition that favors the transmission of vibrations from the larynx to the chest wall. One principle to remember is that the presence of liquid or solid transmits sound more effectively than air-filled spaces. Therefore, vocal fremitus will be increased in conditions where the alveoli have been replaced by fluid or consolidation of lung tissue.

Percussion

The purpose of percussion is to set in motion the chest wall and underlying tissues to produce audible sounds. Percussion helps to determine whether the underlying tissues are air-filled or filled with fluid or solid. Percussion can penetrate tissues lying 5 to 7 cm below the surface. The proper technique for percussion is required to elicit meaningful information, remembering that the goal is to create a loud sound. To do this, one's fingernails must be short, and one must use the hands as a hammer and nail, striking one against the other to create a sound. First, press the middle finger, sometimes called the pleximeter finger, of the nondominant hand firmly and flatly over the intercostal space

TABLE 30-3	Percussion Notes and Associated Conditions	
CONDITION	**PERCUSSION NOTES**	**CONDITION**
Totally air-filled	Tympany	Gastric air bubble, large pneumothorax, pneumonectomy
More air-filled	Hyperresonant	COPD, asthma, small pneumothorax
Standard for comparison	Resonant	Normal lung
More dense	Dullness	Organs such as liver, heart, spleen, diaphragm, pneumonia, atelectasis, pulmonary edema, pulmonary fibrosis, lung and pleural tumors, pericardial effusion
Completely dense, solid	Flatness	Bone or solid tissue, massive pleural effusion or massive atelectasis

Adapted from Estes, M. (2006). Health assessment and physical examination (3rd ed.). New York: Thomson Delmar Learning.

(Estes, 2006). Use the tip of the middle finger of the dominant hand to strike sharply against the pleximeter finger, aiming squarely between the joints of the finger planted on the chest.

The quality and the pitch of the percussion note elicited can provide important information about the condition of the patient. There are five percussion notes, each one reflecting a difference in density from normal lung tissue, which has a resonant note, the standard for comparison. Table 30-3 illustrates the percussion notes, their qualities, and associated conditions.

A hyperresonant note is slightly less musical and slightly lower in pitch. It is normally heard on deep inspiration in children or in adults with a thin chest wall. Otherwise, it is an abnormal finding and may be heard in COPD patients, a small pneumothorax, or during an acute asthma attack. A tympanic note is musical and high in pitch. It is normal only over the gastric air bubble, but it can be mimicked by inflating the cheek with air and percussing over it. A dull note is muffled or thud-like. A dull note will be elicited over dense tissue, such as over a pleural effusion or muscle. A dull note will be heard when determining the level of the diaphragm. It will also be heard when assessing the borders of the liver, heart, or spleen. In addition, dull notes may also be heard in conditions such as pneumonia, atelectasis, pulmonary edema, pulmonary fibrosis, lung and mediastinal tumors, paralyzed diaphragm, and pericardial effusion. A flat note is not really a note. It is high in pitch and short in duration. A flat note indicates little or no air but rather solid tissue such as the liver or bone. It can be mimicked by percussing over the thigh or a bone. It may also be heard in massive pleural effusion or atelectasis. Percussion notes may vary within the same person, depending on the thickness of the underlying skin and subcutaneous tissue, breast tissue, and muscle.

Auscultation

Auscultation is the act of listening through a stethoscope. In respiratory assessment, the purpose of auscultation is to assess airflow through the tracheobronchial tree, to detect the presence of mucus, fluid, or obstruction in the air passages, and to assess the condition of the surround lungs and pleural space (Box 30-3).

Normal Breath Sounds

Breath sounds are best assessed by asking the patient to breathe with his or her mouth open and listening through the stethoscope from side to side. There are three types of breath sounds that are heard normally through the chest (i.e., vesicular, bronchial, or bronchovesicular) (Table 30-4). Generally speaking, the sounds that a nurse will hear depend on the area of the chest being listened to.

BOX 30-3

AUSCULTATING LUNG SOUNDS

When assessing your patients' lung sounds, ask them to breathe with their mouth fully open. When patients breathe through their nose, the sounds may be distorted because of the turbulence of the air moving through the smaller nasal passages.

TABLE 30-4	**Normal Breath Sounds**		
TYPE OF SOUND	**CHARACTER**	**SOUNDS LIKE**	**WHERE HEARD**
Vesicular	Inspiration: Expiration: 3:1 No pause between inspiration and expiration. Inspiration louder and higher pitched	Ocean Wind through the trees Soft and sighing May be inaudible if mouth is not open	Over entire lung, except major airways. Louder in children and adults with thin chest wall. Diminished in obese, elderly, or muscular persons
Bronchial	Loud, harsh, tubular Tubular, high-pitched Exhalation longer than inspiration Short pause between inspiration and expiration	Hollow Wind through tunnel	Over trachea
Bronchovesicular	Combination of vesicular and bronchial Inspiration = expiration No pause between inspiration and expiration	Muffled Blowing Combination	Over major airways Anteriorly: either side of upper portion of sternum Posteriorly: between scapulae
Absent or muffled	No sound Diminished sound	No sound Diminished sound	Throughout lung fields

Adapted from Estes, M. (2006). Health assessment and physical examination (3rd ed.). New York: Thomson Delmar Learning.

Vesicular sounds are those normal breath sounds that are heard over most of the chest. They are light and breezy in quality. Inspiration is somewhat longer and louder, with no pause between inspiration and expiration. They are the sound of alveoli opening and closing as air passes in and out. The predominance of the inspiratory phase is thought to be because of the laminar quality of the airflow in the smaller airways.

Bronchial or tubular sounds are only normally heard over the trachea. They are loud and harsh in quality, high-pitched, and sound hollow. There is a pause between inspiration and expiration, and the expiratory phase predominates. If they are heard when listening over the lung area, they result in abnormal sound transmission where liquid or solid has replaced normal lung tissue. This may occur in atelectasis, pneumonia, or lung tumors. The predominance of the expiratory phase in bronchial breath sounds is thought to be because of the turbulent nature of gas flow in the larger airways (Estes, 2006).

Bronchovesicular sounds are lung sounds that are relatively loud and medium in pitch. They are the sound of air as it passes through the larger airways, so they are best heard over the major airways. The best place to hear these sounds is where the trachea bifurcates to the left and right mainstem bronchi, at the level of the second intercostal space to either side of the sternum, or between the scapulae. The quality is a muffled and blowing sound, with no pause between inspiration and expiration.

Absent breath sounds may occur with tumor, foreign body, pneumonectomy, or malposition of an endotracheal tube. Breath sounds may be diminished in obese or in muscular individuals, where there is much more tissue through which the sound must be transmitted.

Adventitious Breath Sounds

Adventitious breath sounds are additional sounds that are superimposed on the normal breath sounds. Table 30-5 illustrates the various types of adventitious sounds, their character, and associated conditions.

TABLE 30-5	Adventitious Breath Sounds			
	CRACKLES (RALES)	**RHONCHI**	**WHEEZES**	**PLEURAL FRICTION RUBS**

Character	Intermittent
	High-pitched
	Heard at end of
	   inspiration
	Will not clear with
	   cough or suction
		Intermittent
		Loud
		Bubbling, gurgling
		May clear or change
		   quality with cough
		   or suction
			Continuous
			Dry
			Musical
			Most often heard on
			   expiration, more
			   severe on inspiration
				Interrupted
				Jerky
				Heard mainly at height
				   of inspiration
				No change with cough

Sounds Like	Crackling cellophane
	Little pops
	Rubbing hair next
	   to ear
	Milk poured over
	   Rice Krispies
		Blowing through
		   thick soup with
		   straw
			Musical
			Squeaking
				Grating, scraping
				Wet leather squeaking together
				Door creaking shut
				Rocking chair on wood floor

Indicates	Separation of alveoli
	   that have been stuck
	   together by fluid
	Always means excess
	   fluid in alveoli
		Fluid in larger
		   airways
			Air passing through
			   narrowed airways
			Vibration of swollen
			   membranes or thick
			   mucus
				Inflamed pleura rubbing
				   together
				Loss of lubricating fluid

Pathology	Pneumonia
	Pulmonary edema
	Diffuse interstitial
	   disease
	Bronchitis
	Fluid overload
		Bronchiectasis
		Bronchitis
		Pneumonia
		Poor mobilization
		   of secretions
			Asthma
			Bronchitis
			Poor mobilization of
			   secretions
			Pulmonary edema
			Foreign bodies
				Pleural infection
				Pulmonary emboli
				Fractured ribs
				Post lung surgery

Adapted from Estes, M. (2006). Health assessment and physical examination (3rd ed.). New York: Thomson Delmar Learning.

Crackles (formerly called rales in the United States and still called rales in the United Kingdom) are discontinuous crackling sounds, which are usually heard at the end of inspiration. They are thought to be because of delayed reopening of previously deflated alveoli that are partially filled with fluid. They can be mimicked by rubbing together a few strands of human hair. They can be heard in congestive heart failure, bronchitis, pneumonia, pulmonary fibrosis, or simply fluid that has accumulated in the lungs. They are often heard in smokers at the lung bases. They are often position-dependent and do not clear with coughing or suctioning.

Rhonchi are continuous sounds with a bubbling or gurgling quality. They may be inspiratory or expiratory and indicate a partial obstruction to airflow in airways that are narrowed by secretions or swelling. Because they result from fluid in the larger airways, they will disappear or change quality when the patient coughs or is suctioned.

Wheezes are high-pitched squeaking sounds that are produced by air passing through larger but narrowed airways. They are often heard on expiration; but if heard on inspiration, they are often indicative of more severe respiratory distress. Inspiratory wheezing is referred to as **stridor.** Wheezes are not affected by coughing and are commonly heard in asthma attacks and bronchitis. Stridor occurs in croup, laryngitis, epiglottitis, vocal cord dysfunction, and tracheal tumors, tracheal stenosis, and tracheomalacia (Savoy, 2005).

Pleural friction rubs are those sounds caused by an inflammation of the pleural space that is usually filled with a small amount of serous fluid that facilitates the pleura from passing smoothly over each other. The rub is heard loudest when the pleura are in closest proximity to each other, which is at the height of inspiration and the beginning of expiration. Pleural friction rubs are loud, grating, and discontinuous sounds that sound like two pieces of wet leather rubbing together or like a rocking chair on a wooden floor. It may sometimes be difficult to determine the difference between a pleural friction rub and a pericardial friction rub as the sounds can be similar. If that is the case, ask the patient to hold his or her breath. When the patient holds his or her breath, a pleural friction rub will not be heard, but a pericardial friction rub will remain.

Voice Sounds

Voice sounds are used to detect areas of consolidation of lung tissue. The presence of these sounds support the principle that sound is transmitted better through fluid or solid than through normal lung tissue. Normally, voice sounds are indistinct or muffled, but the sound will be much more distinct over areas of the lung that have been replaced with fluid or solid.

Voice sounds are elicited by asking the patient to speak while the nurse puts the stethoscope on the chest and listens from side to side. **Bronchophony** is the presence of distinct, clear, and relatively loud sounds heard over areas of the lung in which the normal alveoli are filled with fluid or replaced by solid tissue. They are elicited by asking the patient to say, one, two, three. They are present in the same conditions that caused increased tactile fremitus and bronchial breath sounds, including pneumonia, atelectasis, pulmonary infarction, and lung tumors.

Whispered pectoriloquy is similar to bronchophony, except the vocal cords are bypassed when the patient whispers, one, two, three. When present, they are clear, distinct, intelligible sounds. They indicate that areas of the lung have been replaced by fluid or solid tissue.

Egophony is the presence of loud, nasal, and bleating sounds heard when auscultating the lungs and is often heard just above a pleural effusion. They are elicited by asking the patient to say eeee. Normally, the examiner will hear the same sound through the stethoscope. However, in the presence of egophony, the examiner will hear a nasal and bleating aayy sound.

The presence of bronchophony, whispered pectoriloquy, or egophony indicates a type of consolidation of lung tissue, because liquids and solids transmit sound better than air-filled lung tissue.

Age-Related Changes in the Respiratory System

There are several factors to consider when evaluating age-related changes of the respiratory system. Changes may be structural in nature relating to the thorax, ribs, lungs, diaphragm, spine, or upper airways, or may occur from functional origins reflecting altered potential, oxygenation, vital capacity, excursion, or sustained performance. Typically, the respiratory system matures by age 20 with gradually diminishing efficiency occurring within five years (Ebersole, Hess, & Luggen, 2004). In normal aging, respiratory efficiency continues to decrease gradually throughout the life span. The capacity to inhale, hold, and exhale air decreases with age. The normal vital capacity at age 85 is only 50 to 65 percent of that of a 30 year old. Additionally, the older adult has difficulty taking oxygen from the atmosphere and delivering it to internal organs and tissues.

The respiratory system ages in conjunction with all other body systems. Elastin and collagen changes cause loss of elasticity of lung tissues. As aging continues, lungs remain hyperinflated even on exhalation and the proportion of dead space increases. This process is manifested in hyperresonance on auscultation. The respiratory system is dependent on the musculoskeletal system for normal functioning. The ribs and spine encase the lungs and are in close proximity to pulmonary tissue; hence they affect pulmonary performance. The musculoskeletal system is particularly vulnerable to aging processes, including osteoporosis. In aging, intercostal cartilage calcifies and causes the chest walls to stiffen, thereby making inspiration more difficult. Arthritis may develop in the costovertebral joints. Consequently, intercostal muscles atrophy, and the diaphragm flattens. Increased exertion by the older patient is required to fully expand the lungs as the chest walls stiffen.

As the spine ages and kyphoscoliosis develops, the ability to expand the chest is further limited by mechanical means because of decreasing ability to maintain a fully erect posture. A barrel chest may develop as a consequence to normal aging. Respiratory muscles weaken as a result of consistently less respiratory effort and increasing loss of mobility in the chest wall. Decreased strength of intercostal muscles, other muscles of respiration, and the diaphragm impair breathing. While the resting respiratory effort may be essentially adequate to meet metabolic demands, it is quickly overcome with any challenges compared to respiratory reserves of younger adults. Respiratory efforts during strenuous work or in stressful situations are not as successful in meeting basic metabolic demands; therefore shortness of breath may develop quickly, resolve more slowly, and produce marked overall fatigue once activity ceases. Moreover, decreased oxygen uptake and decreased elastic recoil of lung parenchyma also contribute to reduced endurance and increase the time required to recover after exercise or prolonged stress. Further age-associated changes to the respiratory system include decreased resistance to infection cause by a lowered immune system response and less effective self-cleaning action of the respiratory cilia (Ebersole, Hess, & Luggen, 2004).

Normal physiological changes may resemble pathology. Lungs of older non-smokers may reveal small areas of patchy lung tissue damage that mimics changes caused by emphysema. The extent of the age-related change is essential in determining if the condition is normal or disease-related. The **residual volume (RV)** is the amount of air remaining in the lungs at the end of a forced exhalation. The exchange of carbon dioxide and oxygen within the alveoli and capillaries decreases as a part of aging progression.

Other challenges, such as environmental pollutants including silicon, dust, particulate, asbestos, spray paint, products of internal combustion, and allergens, such as pollen and dust mites, add to the daily challenges that confront aging lungs. Despite these changes, elders without additional pathology breathe sufficiently well to meet their continuing metabolic demands.

In addition to musculoskeletal changes that occur in aging, additional changes limit respiratory function. Pain during breathing may substantially limit respiratory effort. There are several sources of pain that may limit respiratory efforts. One cause may be noncardiac sources of pain including those with origins in the cervical spine. Commonly first diagnosed in old age, arthritis may be a source of pain that adversely affects the chest wall and effectively limits breathing efforts. Spondylitis, which is an inflammation of the vertebrae, may also be a source of pain in older patients and may manifest as chest or chest wall pain. Herniated or bulging discs in the cervical or thoracic areas may result in chest pain that limits respiratory excursion. Some patients with metastatic disease may experience chest wall pain that limits their ability to breathe freely. Women with chest pain may or may not have coronary heart disease, and their symptoms of chest wall pain may not mirror symptoms men experience.

Other noncardiac sources of pain may originate from muscle sources within the chest wall, including costalgia, costochondritis, or intercostal neuralgia, that may manifest from intercostal muscles or cartilage between the ribs. These conditions are typically painful and limit the older patient's respiratory efforts. Pectoral myositis and spasm may be a source of pain with inflammation radiating across the anterior chest. An additional source of chest wall pain that may limit respiratory efforts is thrombophlebitis.

Pulmonary sources may cause chest wall pain including pain from pleurisy. Pleurisy is an inflammation of the parietal pleura of the lungs characterized by dyspnea and stabbing pain that leads to restriction of ordinary breathing with spasms of the chest on the affected side. Some older adults may feel pleuritic pain less intensely than younger individuals, but the condition is identical in severity.

Development of a pneumothorax may cause sudden, sharp chest pain that is immediately followed by difficult, rapid breathing and an absence of normal chest wall movement on the affected side. Pneumothorax is an abnormal collection of air or gas in the pleural space that causes collapse of the lung. It may develop without known causes or it may result from forceful coughing or a penetrating chest wound.

Pneumonia may also cause chest pain that is noncardiac in nature. Chest wall pain, accompanied by coughing, chills, and a high fever, is a sign of this acute, inflammatory condition of the lungs. Pneumonia is a frequently seen condition in elderly individuals who have not been previously immunized. Those with sedentary lifestyles and those who are bedridden are at increased risk of pneumonia and other respiratory dysfunction.

Pulmonary embolism is a serious source of chest pain that may present with symptoms similar to a myocardial infarction. It is often sudden in onset, accompanied by severe dyspnea, shock, and cyanosis, and may result in mortality if the embolism is extensive. Additional sources of chest pain include disorders of the gastrointestinal (GI) system, the vasculature of the abdominal aorta, and psychogenic causes include anxiety and depression.

DIAGNOSTIC TESTS

There are a variety of diagnostic tests and laboratory studies that are used to determine type and extent of lung disease or lung function. They are discussed in this section in the categories of laboratory tests, radiographic tests, and bedside monitoring. Information regarding the nursing management of each diagnostic test is included as appropriate.

Laboratory Diagnostic Tests

Laboratory tests of the pulmonary system reveal accurate data to evaluate the function of the pulmonary body system. The laboratory tests described in this section include ABGs, calculation of the PaO_2/FiO_2 ratio, and sputum studies. The nursing management involved with these diagnostic tests is minimal, aside from the actual skill involved in obtaining the body substances.

ABG Sampling

ABGs are obtained from an arterial puncture, usually done in the radial artery. The patient should be informed that the procedure may be uncomfortable, and for this reason, local anesthesia is often recommended. The skin is prepped with povidone-iodine and alcohol, and the artery is palpated with a gloved finger. A heparin-coated syringe is used to draw up the sample to prevent clotting of the blood. The needle is inserted, with the bevel up, at a 45° angle until a flash of bright red arterial blood is seen. Aspiration is seldom required as the force of the patient's blood pressure is usually adequate to fill the syringe. Two milliliters is enough for ABG analysis; however, if other lab tests are desired, more blood may be required. The needle is removed, and direct pressure is held over the site for a minimum 10 minutes to prevent extravasation of arterial blood. If the patient has an arterial catheter, at least 2 milliliters of fluid within the catheter must be withdrawn and wasted before obtaining the arterial sample. All air bubbles from the sample must be removed and the tip of the syringe sealed to prevent gas equilibration between the air and the blood, which will falsely increase the PaO_2 and lower the $PaCO_2$. If there is a delay in transport and analysis of the sample, it must be packed in ice to slow metabolism (Gammon, 2004).

PaO$_2$/FiO$_2$ Ratio

One simple test to measure effectiveness of gas exchange is the PaO$_2$/FiO$_2$ ratio, also called the P/F ratio. With normal lungs, one would expect a high number because the PaO$_2$ should rise significantly with a rising FiO$_2$. The lower the number, however, the more severe is the disease. In fact, acute lung injury is described as a P/F ratio of less than 300, and acute respiratory distress syndrome is described as a P/F ratio of less than 200. Both PaO$_2$ and FiO$_2$ are easy to obtain. The PaO$_2$ is collected as an ABG, and the FiO$_2$ is a pulmonary function test.

Sputum Studies

Collection of sputum is often necessary to determine the etiology of disease, determine type of organism, determine sensitivity of antibiotics, and determine whether malignant cells are present. Serial sputum studies may be necessary to determine response to treatment, such as those patients receiving antibiotics, steroids, or immunosuppressant drugs.

Proper technique during collection of the specimen helps to ensure quality results. Patients who are cooperative can be instructed to expectorate into a sterile container only after a deep cough. Expectoration of secretions from the mouth will result in inaccurate results. Ideally, the sputum specimen should be obtained prior to antibiotic treatment, rinsing the mouth with water or brushing the teeth prior to expectoration, and no food or fluids prior to expectoration (Boruchoff & Weinstein, 2004; Daniels, 2003). However, it is often not possible to adhere to these ideals.

Patients who are unable to cough can be suctioned to obtain a sterile specimen; however, one must remember that the suction catheter must pass through a sterile passage and exit into the area to be suctioned. Because of this, one cannot obtain a sterile specimen through an oral or a nasal airway. An endotracheal tube or a tracheostomy does provide a sterile passageway through which a sterile suction catheter can be inserted. When a collection device is attached to the suction catheter, the patient is suctioned, and the secretions are trapped within the collection chamber. If sterile saline is used to flush the secretions from the catheter, it must be nonbacteriostatic to prevent interference with the interpretation of results.

Bronchoscopy can provide an alternative method of obtaining secretions. However, it must be kept in mind that there is inevitable contamination of the lower respiratory tract by the oral flora on introduction of the instrument into the airways. This problem can be overcome with the use of a protected brush catheter.

Transtracheal aspiration is another method of obtaining sputum in those patients who are unable to cough up their secretions. In transtracheal needle aspiration, a needle-over-catheter is inserted directly into the trachea. A small amount of fluid is injected through the catheter, called a tickle tube, and the patient is allowed to cough. Fluid may also be aspirated through this catheter and sent for analysis (Christopher, 2003).

Radiographic Diagnostic Tests

Radiographic testing of the pulmonary system includes pulmonary angiography, chest X-ray (CXR), CT scanning, ventilation-perfusion scanning, and positron emission tomography (PET scanning). Several of these tests require expensive equipment, and interpretation is performed by a radiologist. The nursing management includes patient education regarding the upcoming test and physical support during the time of the diagnostic study.

Pulmonary Angiography

Angiography is an invasive test in which dye is injected into the pulmonary arterial system to detect the blood flow. It remains the most sensitive and specific test to diagnose even the smallest of pulmonary emboli. An arterial

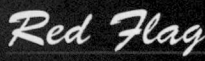

catheter is placed most often into the femoral artery. Contrast material is injected into a branch of the pulmonary artery. Risks of the procedure include problems related to insertion of the pulmonary arterial catheter itself, such as arrhythmias, ischemia, or hemorrhage. Other complications include contrast reactions or respiratory insufficiency (Thompson & Hales, 2004).

Nursing Management

The nurse explains the test procedure and that there may be potential allergies to the contrast medium. Then baselines of vital signs and a neurological assessment are determined. In addition, report any recent use of anticoagulants. After the angiography, the nurse monitors the patient's vital signs and continues to assess for a potential allergic reaction.

Chest X-Ray

Chest radiography is an important diagnostic test for any patient with pulmonary disease. Obviously, the CXR is noninvasive and can be applied across a range of almost any patient. For best results, CXRs are often taken as P-A and lateral, meaning that the beam is directed from the posterior aspect toward the anterior aspect of the patient's chest, as well as a separate lateral view. A-P (anterior to posterior) views are used when the patient is unable to stand and are often the only type of CXR done on patients in the critical care unit. A-P views provide more magnification and less sharp images, and therefore the P-A approach is usually preferred, when possible.

Fundamental skills in assessment of CXRs can be a useful skill for the nurse. Bones should be intact and symmetrical, with no evidence of fracture. Ribs should be equal distance apart. A good inspiratory film consists of the visualization of at least eight to nine ribs. The trachea and all structures in the mediastinum should be midline. Conditions which shift the mediastinum include pneumothorax and pleural effusion. The diaphragm should be clearly visible, with sharp costophrenic angles. Blunting of the costophrenic angles can occur in a variety of conditions, including pleural effusion, pneumothorax, and phrenic nerve injury. The lung tissue should be examined for any increase or decrease in density. Increased density can occur with an accumulation of blood, fluid, pus, or collapse of lung tissue. Decreased density can occur with anything that causes increased air in the lungs, such as COPD or pneumothorax.

The presence of tubes and lines can also be determined from examination of the CXR. Proper placement of endotracheal tubes, gastric tubes, or enteral feeding tubes should be confirmed by the physician; however, the nurse should become familiar with some of the basic skills of CXR interpretation (Daniels, 2003). In addition, the majority of nursing care associated with the CXR is related to the correct positioning and shielding of the patient during the X-ray.

Computed Tomography

Computed tomography (CT) provides a diagnostic method of evaluating the lungs in successive layers or slices. CT scanning incorporates a computer to perform complex calculations that determine the extent to which a variety of tissues absorb X-ray beams. It is superior to chest radiographs in its ability to detect fine differences in tissue densities. Contrast material can be injected that will increase the ability to detect subtle differences in density. There are over 1,000 specific protocols for CT scanning, so the indication for the test is an important consideration to determine the proper protocol for the test, and whether or not injection of contrast material is necessary. Contrast material usually improves visualization of structures. There are several methods of CT scanning of the lung. CT angiography is broad term for a specific technique in which contrast material is injected and images are taken in a specific timing sequence. CT angiography allows the vascular system to be viewed in three dimensions without visualizing overlying structures.

Helical CT scanning, also called spiral CT, was developed to overcome many false-negative results of conventional CT scanning because of motion artifact, or superimposed pixels producing different qualities in visualization of structures. Spiral CT scanning incorporates a continuous corkscrew scan that produces three-dimensional data. Helical CT scanning is performed with a sustained breath hold and therefore has several advantages over conventional CT scanning, including absence of respiratory motion and improved analysis of nodules. Patients must be able to hold their breath for 20 to 25 seconds with this test.

Spiral CT scanning is taking a series of images from different angles and manipulating them to create a three-dimensional image, as a helix. Helical CT scanning has also been shown to be useful in the diagnosis of pulmonary emboli, with a sensitivity ranging from 66 to 93 percent and a specificity ranging from 89 to 97 percent (Eng, et al., 2004).

Nursing Management

Major nursing considerations for CT scanning of the lung include radiation exposure and renal function whenever contrast material is involved. Patients should be assessed for renal function, diabetes, and pregnancy prior to the test. Radiation exposure is significant in young females of childbearing age as CT scanning of the chest involves relatively large doses of radiation, which may play a role in increasing the risk of breast cancer. Breastfeeding women are instructed not to breastfeed for a period of time after the test to prevent transmission of radioactive contrast material to the newborn. Nursing assessment is vital in screening patients for CT scanning. Patients must be assessed for kidney function and allergies to contrast material and iodine. Contrast material can be nephrotoxic. Another nursing consideration is screening patients for diabetes. If patients are taking the antihyperglycemic medication metformin, they must hold the drug for a period of time before and after the test, because it interacts with the contrast material and can cause acute renal insufficiency.

It is important for the nurse to understand general principles of nuclear medicine technology to help educate patients. Nuclear medicine tests study a function of an organ system, as opposed to other diagnostic imaging tests that visualize anatomic structures. A pharmaceutical is labeled with a radioactive isotope, which emits gamma and positron rays. This radiopharmaceutical is administered, and there may be a delay for it to reach the target organ. The organ is then imaged with a gamma camera that visualizes the distribution of the particular radiopharmaceutical, with hot spots or cold spots of activity showing an abnormality. Hot spots show increased uptake in diseased tissue, and cold spots show decreased uptake.

Gamma cameras are used to provide either static images, dynamic images, or single photon emission computed tomography (SPECT). Dynamic imaging allows visualization of blood flow associated with a particular organ. Static imaging, also known as planar imaging, acquires one two-dimensional image at a time. Whole body imaging is two-dimensional and acquires anterior and posterior sweeps of the patient's whole body. SPECT technology has revolutionized nuclear imaging because it provides three dimensions of data (Daniels, 2003).

Before a nuclear medicine procedure, the patient may need to follow a specific preparatory regimen, including NPO, no caffeine, hydration, or bowel preparation. The radiopharmaceutical may be administered by one of several routes: oral, intravenous (IV), intramuscular, intrathecal, or intraperitoneal. Depending on the target area, there may be a time delay after injection until the images are obtained.

Risks for the procedure include hematoma at the IV injection site, reactions to the radiopharmaceutical (e.g., rash, itching, bronchospasm, or anaphylaxis). Patients should be aware that the radiation exposure is minimal for these tests; however, depending on the type of radioisotope, it will be retained within their body for a period of time after the test, but it decays over time. Some of the isotope will be excreted in the urine, feces, or other body fluids (Daniels, 2003).

Patients must be cautioned and educated appropriately before the test. Pregnancy is a contraindication for most nuclear imaging tests. Lactating women are advised to stop breastfeeding for one to three days after the test as most radiopharmaceuticals are excreted in breast milk. The presence of any prosthesis within the body may shield the gamma rays from imaging. Age and current weight are important for accurate dosing of the radiopharmaceutical. It is also important to ascertain whether or not the patient has allergies especially to iodine or to contrast substances.

During the procedure, the patient may experience warmth, flushing of the face, salty taste, or nausea with injection of the contrast material, and this may be alleviated by slow, deep breaths. If patients develop respiratory distress, heavy sweating, numbness, palpitations, the nurse must be aware that these may be early signs of anaphylactic reaction. Routine disposal of body fluids and excretions is appropriate after most diagnostic procedures. Inspect the injection site for signs of bruising, hematoma, infection, or irritation (Daniels, 2003).

Ventilation-Perfusion Scan

The purpose of a ventilation-perfusion lung scan is to diagnose and locate pulmonary emboli, to determine the percentage of the lung that is functioning normally, and to assess the pulmonary vascular supply by estimating regional pulmonary blood flow. It is also helpful in diagnosing bronchitis, asthma, pneumonia, COPD, and cancer.

A ventilation-perfusion scan is actually two separate tests: a ventilation scan and a perfusion scan. It involves injection of a radioactive isotope into the vein to measure perfusion and the inhalation of a radioactive gas to measure ventilation. The patient should be instructed that the ventilation portion of the test requires breath holding for a brief period of time. The images are then examined to identify areas of the lung that are not well-ventilated or well-perfused. When used to diagnose pulmonary embolism, there will be ventilation in a particular area but no perfusion.

A normal perfusion lung scan can exclude the diagnosis of pulmonary embolus. A high probability lung scan indicates a high likelihood of the presence of pulmonary embolus. An intermediate probability scan indicates the need for further testing. The primary risk of the procedure is reaction to the contrast material.

Positron Emission Tomography

Positron emission tomography (PET) is a newer technique that allows the imaging of structures by their ability to concentrate specific molecules that have been chemically tagged with a positron-emitting isotope. It combines the use of positron-emitting nuclides and emission CT. PET generates high-resolution molecular-level images of physiological function, including glucose metabolism, oxygen utilization, blood flow, and tissue perfusion.

In PET scanning, a glucose analog molecule is tagged with a positron-emitting isotope of fluorine. Malignant cells utilize glucose more than other tissues and take up this isotope more actively. When this isotope comes in contact with an electron, energy in the form of gamma rays is released and images are recorded. Many studies involving PET scanning have found a sensitivity of 95 percent and specificity of 70 percent in detecting malignancy; however, the use and implications of PET scanning have yet to be fully explored. Currently, PET scanning has utility in oncology, cardiology, and neurology. It can determine the degree of operability in metastatic carcinoma. It can also measure the degree of myocardial blood flow and perfusion in coronary artery disease. PET scanning is also being used to diagnose a wide variety of dementias, including Alzheimer's disease, which shows a distinct pattern of glucose consumption. Patients should be instructed that the actual imaging time for a PET scan is one to two hours.

Actual time may be several hours between injection and completion of imaging (Daniels, 2003; Stark, 2004).

Bedside Monitoring Diagnostic Tests

There are several noninvasive monitoring techniques for pulmonary status available at the bedside. These diagnostic tests include capnography, oximetry, and polysomnography.

Capnography

Capnography and capnometry are noninvasive measures of exhaled carbon dioxide. Capnometry uses a continuous numeric display of carbon dioxide levels, and a capnograph uses a graphic display of a waveform. A sensor is connected to source, and the level of carbon dioxide is measured as end-tidal CO_2, or $P_{ET}CO_2$. Measurement of end-tidal CO_2 is clinically useful in many areas.

Capnography has many uses. Capnometers provide a continuous reading of the end-tidal CO_2 value, and calorimetric devices can be used intermittently to provide validation of the presence of CO_2, rather than a specific value. When placed correctly, these calorimetric devices show a change in color with each breath. This can be useful when confirming placement of an endotracheal tube, as long as continuous monitoring is not necessary. Capnography can also be used to confirm placement of a nasogastric tube with the absence of CO_2, to estimate the arterial $PaCO_2$, and to detect changes in pulmonary blood flow or dead space ventilation, warn of ventilator disconnection, predict survival during cardiac arrest, and identify end-expiration, which may be useful during hemodynamic monitoring. A significant difference between the $PaCO_2$ and the capnographic measure of CO_2 is considered to be diagnostic for dead space (Ahrens & Sona, 2003).

Oximetry

Oximetry has become a standard method of assessment of oxygenation in health care. Pulse oximetry compares the absorption of light in the capillary bed by using two wavelengths of light: red and infrared wavelengths of light (Jubran, 2004). Pulse oximetry is quick and easy to use; however, there are certain conditions in which light is absorbed at a frequency that is different from these two wavelengths, and therefore, the readings can be inaccurate. These conditions of inaccurate oximetry readings include carboxyhemoglobinemia and methemoglobinemia. If these conditions are suspected, cooximetry should be used, which provides six different wavelengths of light absorption and compares the amount of hemoglobin that is saturated with the amount of hemoglobin that is capable of being saturated (Mechem, 2004).

The accuracy of pulse oximeters depends on many factors. One must be cautious not to rely too heavily on pulse oximetry because patients can have a significant desaturation before it is detected with the oximeter. This is especially true of patients using supplemental oxygen. Factors that affect accuracy of the pulse oximeter include bright ambient light, low perfusion state, such as shock or hypothermia, IV dyes, such as methylene blue, skin pigmentation, or nail polish that is blue, black, or green. Location of the probe does not seem to be a factor. In most cases, the probe is located on the finger; however, accurate readings have also been used on the nose, ear, and forehead (Jubran, 2004). The nurse must realize that pulse oximetry does not assess ventilation status. If hypoventilation is suspected, one can clinically measure ventilation by measuring blood gases, specifically the $PaCO_2$, or by the use of capnography.

Polysomnography

Polysomnography has become more widely used in the past several years. It is a recording of sleep and breathing and is used to diagnose types of sleep apnea. Patients in the sleep laboratory are monitored for sleep stages, respiratory effort, airflow, oxygen saturation, arrhythmias, body position, and limb movements.

Sleep stages are monitored by using an electroencephalogram to monitor brain waves and an electrooculogram to monitor eye movements. Time in each of the sleep stages is determined, and total sleep time can be determined by adding the time in each stage. Light sleep occurs during stages 1 and 2; deep sleep is considered to be during stages 3 and 4, and REM (rapid eye movement) sleep is a separate stage. Sleep studies are most often done at night, but are best done when consistent with the sleep-wake cycles of the patient. Sleep studies monitor sleep stages as well as number of arousals and periods of apnea. Both of these measures can contribute to quality of sleep. Periodic limb movements can be counted as isolated events or in association with arousals.

Monitoring of respiratory effort and airflow is important, because apnea of a central origin shows a total absence of respiratory effort. In obstructive apnea, there is respiratory effort, but no inspiratory airflow, and in a mixed apnea, there is an initial absence of airflow, but an obstructive pattern develops. The presence, amount, and intensity of snoring during sleep can be determined with a sound monitor. A snoring index can be calculated, which represents the number of snores per total sleep time (Millman & Kramer, 2004).

A negative polysomnogram does not exclude the diagnosis of sleep apnea, because the quality of the polysomnogram is dependent on many factors. These factors include degree of nasal patency, body position, disruptive environmental factors, all of which may contribute to variability of the test.

Other Diagnostic Tests

Other diagnostic tests of the pulmonary system include bronchoscopy, bronchoalveolar lavage, lung biopsy, transbronchial or transtracheal needle aspiration, thoracentesis, thoracoscopy, and pulmonary function testing. These are valuable diagnostic tests that have great importance in pulmonary assessment.

Bronchoscopy

Insertion of a bronchoscope into the upper airways allows the clinician the benefit of direct assessment of the airways to evaluate lesions, investigate unexplained symptoms, remove foreign bodies or inspissated secretions, assess airway patency, and evaluate problems with endotracheal tubes. A rigid bronchoscope is often preferred in children in which there is suspected foreign body aspiration; however, flexible bronchoscopes have essentially replaced rigid bronchoscopy primarily because of their expanded capabilities.

Prior to the procedure, the patient should have eaten or drank nothing and should have a prior CXR. The procedure should be explained in detail and informed consent obtained. In addition to local anesthesia of the oropharynx or nasopharynx, the patient will require moderate sedation, so vigilant monitoring is essential. Atropine is often used to dry secretions, facilitate effectiveness of topical anesthetics, and inhibit bronchospasm.

A brush biopsy can also be performed during a bronchoscopy. During the brush biopsy a sheathed cytology brush is inserted through the bronchoscope and passed over a visible lesion, trapping bits of tissue within the bristles. Forceps can also be inserted through the bronchoscope and bits of tissue removed in that way. The tissue is then examined for pathology.

Bronchoalveolar Lavage

Bronchoalveolar lavage (BAL) involves the instillation of sterile saline into subsegments of the lung through a bronchoscope with subsequent aspiration and collection of this fluid. The fluid is instilled in aliquots of 20 to 60 mL, retrieved, and then processed, and cells are examined and counted. BAL is a useful procedure to assist with diagnosis of diffuse lung disease. Nurses assisting with this procedure must be aware that the volume of fluid recovered is influenced by the patient's smoking history. The average BAL fluid volume recovered in healthy nonsmokers is 50–80 percent of the instilled volume, compared with 20 to 30 percent in healthy smokers. The procedure should be terminated if the patient experiences respiratory distress or falling oxygen saturation. Risks of BAL include all of those for bronchoscopy, such as aspiration, oversedation, and bronchospasm, so the patient must not have eaten or drank anything prior to the procedure and be monitored closely during the procedure.

Lung Biopsy

A lung biopsy is the collection of a piece of lung tissue via bronchoscopy, open thoracotomy, or video-assisted thorascopic lung surgery (VATS). Lung biopsy is helpful to make a specific diagnosis, to assess active disease, or to exclude a neoplastic or infectious process. The transbronchial approach is often the initial method lung biopsy, especially when diffuse lung disease or infection is suspected. This approach involves passing a forceps or a biopsy needle through the bronchoscope. The specimen is then aspirated or obtained with forceps and sent to the laboratory for analysis.

VATS is the preferred method of lung biopsy in the operating room, because it is thought to be associated with less morbidity. Contraindications to surgical lung biopsy are diffuse end-stage lung disease, serious cardiovascular disease, pulmonary dysfunction, advanced age, and other major risks for surgery or general anesthesia. The number, size, and location of lung biopsies are determined by clinical suspicion (King, 2004).

Transbronchial Needle Aspiration

Transbronchial needle aspiration is a procedure used to obtain tissue for biopsy, most often in the staging of cancer or in the identification of pulmonary nodules. In the case of transbronchial needle aspiration, the bronchoscope is used to visualize the airway, and tissue is removed through the biopsy lumen. Tissue may be taken directly from the paratracheal, hilar, or subcarinal areas. Transbronchial needle aspiration includes all of the risks associated with bronchoscopy, including aspiration, and oversedate. Because of this the patient must not have eaten or drank anything prior and be monitored closely for signs of bronchospasm or oversedation.

Pulmonary Function Testing

Evaluation of pulmonary function is important for patients who have a history of lung disease or for those who have significant risk factors for developing lung disease. These include those who have restrictive or obstructive processes or air trapping, to detect response to treatment such as chemotherapy or surgery, to determine the presence of underventilated lung, or to assess chronic disease affecting the lung (Daniels, 2004). Numerous specific tests are included as part of comprehensive testing of pulmonary function, and they fall within three categories: airway flow rates, lung volumes and capacities, and gas exchange. The major tests included within pulmonary function testing include spirometry, measurement of lung volumes, diffusing capacity, measurement of flow rates, and respiratory pressures (Enright, 2004).

Spirometry is the most commonly performed tests of all of the pulmonary function tests. Accuracy depends on patient cooperation because the patient is asked to inspire maximally and exhale forcefully. This is called the forced vital capacity (FVC). When plotted against time, this forced expiratory volume can be measured at one second (FEV_1), two seconds (FEV_2), and three seconds (FEV_3) (Delaune & Ladner, 2006).

Tidal volume (Vt) is the amount of air in and out of the lung with a normal breath. Each tidal volume has two components: the volume of alveolar air that directly takes place in gas exchange (called alveolar volume) and the volume of air that does not take place in gas exchange (called dead space volume). Dead space volume is normally approximately 30 percent of the total Vt.

Inspiratory reserve volume (IRV) is the maximal amount of gas that can be inspired at the end of a normal inspiration. **Expiratory reserve volume (ERV)** is the maximal amount of gas that can be expired at the end of a normal exhalation. Residual volume is the amount remaining in the lungs and airways after a maximal expiration; in other words, the amount that cannot be exhaled (Estes, 2006).

From time to time, normal, healthy individuals take a larger than normal breath and may triple or quadruple their tidal volume. These larger than normal breaths are called sighs and occur up to 10 times per hour. A normal tidal volume is approximately 10–15 mL/kg of body weight.

Vital capacity (VC) is the volume of air in and out of the lung with maximal inspiratory effort and maximal expiratory effort. Measurement of VC requires patient cooperation to get meaningful results. Because it requires maximal inspiration and forceful expiration, vital capacity is an important measurement in assessing the patient's ability to cough and protect his airway. Vital capacity should be at least 15 mL/kg body weight (Lim & Morgenthaler, 2005).

Thoracentesis

Thoracentesis is another valuable pulmonary diagnostic test that involves the drainage of fluid from the pleural space. It can be used to determine the cause of a pleural effusion but is not usually required for a small collection of fluid. Thoracentesis can be done with needle aspiration and is often followed by insertion of a chest tube for a large collection of fluid (Daniels, 2003).

Nursing Management

The patient is placed in the upright position, and the needle is inserted one to two interspaces below the level where the percussion note becomes dull. Prior to insertion, the nurse teaches the patient regarding the local anesthetic that is used and the position in which the patient will be placed. At the beginning of the thoracentesis, the area is infiltrated with local anesthetic to minimize pain and prepped with povidone-iodine solution to facilitate sterile technique. The most common complication from a thoracentesis is pneumothorax, so the patient should have a CXR following this procedure to rule out pneumothorax (Sahn, 2004). If a large volume of fluid is removed, the patient should be able to breathe easier, so monitor the respiratory rate.

Thoracoscopy

A thoracoscopy is a pulmonary diagnostic test that involves passage of an endoscope through the chest wall to visualize structures and collect samples from the pleura. It is often done under local anesthesia or moderate sedation, but it also may be done in the operating room. If it is done in the operating room under general anesthesia, the surgeon uses the thorascope to perform a minimally invasive procedure, VATS. VATS procedures include lobectomy or pneumonectomy, pericardial window, repair of bronchopleural fistula, resection of lung nodules, and lung biopsy.

Nursing Management

Prior to the procedure, skin is prepped and the site is draped in the lateral decubitus position. During the procedure, the patient should be monitored with continuous electrocardiogram (ECG) recording and continuous pulse oximetry. At the completion of the procedure, a chest tube must be placed for removal of air and fluid. The chest tube should remain in place until any air leak has resolved, and the patient should be monitored with daily chest radiographs to assess chest tube position and lung reexpansion (Mathur, 2004). The nursing management prior to the thoracoscopy involves patient education regarding the procedure and placing emphasis on the chest tube that is left in place after the procedure.

Oxygen Delivery Systems

There are three primary indications for use of oxygen: decreased alveolar oxygen, conditions in which hypoxemia causes increased work of breathing, and conditions in which hypoxemia causes increased the workload of the heart. Any of these conditions can benefit from use of oxygen therapy. Oxygen is considered a drug and therefore, should be administered with care. Oxygen is administered or doses of oxygen are delivered in terms of its fraction of inspired oxygen (FiO_2). The FiO_2 of room air at sea level is 21 percent. Oxygen may be administered in a variety of ways. The best way to administer oxygen is determined by the minimum FiO_2 that is required to produce acceptable oxygen tension in the blood.

There are two broad categories of oxygen delivery systems: low-flow systems and high-flow systems. Low-flow systems should not be confused with low oxygen concentration. High-flow systems are defined as those that can meet all the inspiratory demands and can deliver a consistent flow rate. In high-flow systems, as minute ventilation increases (RR × TV), peak flow rate increases. Peak flow should be four times that of minute ventilation to prevent rebreathing of expired air rich in carbon dioxide. Examples of high-flow systems are Venturi masks, nonrebreathing masks, aerosol masks, and t-pieces. High-flow systems have the advantage of consistent FiO_2 delivery as well as the ability to control temperature and humidity because the entire inspiratory atmosphere is provided.

Low-flow systems do not meet all the inspiratory demands and do not deliver a consistent flow rate. Therefore, part of the tidal volume must be supplied with room air. Low-flow systems use entrainment of room air with a flow of oxygen into a reservoir. In low-flow systems, as the minute ventilation increases, there will be increased entrainment of room air, which will, in turn, lower the net FiO_2. Examples of low-flow systems include the nasal cannula, which uses the nasopharynx as the reservoir and the simple facemask, which uses both the oropharynx and nasopharynx as the reservoir. Other examples of low-flow oxygen delivery systems are partial rebreathing mask and the tracheostomy collar. The nurse must be aware that with low-flow systems, the FiO_2 can vary greatly with changes in tidal volume, respiratory rate, minute volume, and ventilatory pattern. In a low-flow system, the faster the respiratory rate or the larger the tidal volume, the lower the FiO_2. The converse is also true; the slower the respiratory rate or the smaller the tidal volume, the higher the FiO_2. Generally speaking, low-flow systems can be used with patients who are clinically stable, have a reasonable minute volume, and normal ventilatory pattern. A high-flow system may be necessary in those who do not meet those criteria.

Oxygen may also be administered through a catheter placed directly into the trachea, called transtracheal oxygenation (TTO). For patients who require chronic administration of oxygen, TTO can provide a beneficial alternative. A catheter tract is made surgically into the trachea, allowed to heal, and a soft flexible catheter is placed into the tract. Oxygen is then administered directly into the trachea. Reported benefits of TTO include improved compliance because of increased comfort and improved self-image, decreased cost, and greater exercise tolerance (Christopher, 2003).

Nursing Management

As with any medication, oxygen requires the nurse to monitor the patient during its administration. Occasional blood gases should be drawn to assess arterial oxygenation. Use of oximetry as a method of assessing oxygenation is useful only in those patients on room air. When patients are given any type of supplemental oxygen, the pulse oximeter reading is not an accurate reflection of true arterial oxygenation because of displacement of nitrogen in the alveolus.

KEY CONCEPTS

- Anatomy of thorax, lungs, and upper and lower respiratory tracts.
- Physiology of respiration, including medullary control, chemoreceptors, and ventilation versus perfusion.
- Transport of oxygen and carbon dioxide.
- Hypoxemia versus hypoxia.
- Acid-base balance, common imbalances, and interpretation of ABGs.
- Respiratory adjustments during exercise, during hypoxia, and in high altitude.
- Common respiratory symptoms, including dyspnea, cough, chest pain, and hypoxemia.
- Inspection for skeletal abnormalities, rate and rhythm of breathing, and clubbing.
- Palpation for tracheal deviation, respiratory excursion, and fremitus.

- Percussion technique and percussion notes.
- Auscultation for normal breath sounds, adventitious sounds, and voice sounds.
- Laboratory tests of the respiratory system, including blood gas sampling, P/F ratio, and sputum studies.
- Radiographic tests of the respiratory system, including CXR, pulmonary angiography, CT, ventilation-perfusion testing, and PET scanning.
- Bedside monitoring of the respiratory system, including oximetry, capnography, and polysomnography.
- Other diagnostic tests, including bronchoscopy, BAL, lung biopsy, transbronchial or transtracheal aspiration, thoracentesis, and pulmonary function testing.
- Oxygen delivery devices.

REVIEW QUESTIONS

1. Adventitious breath sounds that do not clear with coughing and reflect fluid deep within the alveoli are:
   1. Pleural friction rubs
   2. Crackles
   3. Rhonchi
   4. Wheezes

2. Your patient is on supplemental oxygen with an FiO_2 of 40 percent per Venti-mask. Lungs sound congested. His SpO_2 has been consistently reading 98 to 99 percent earlier in the day, but you notice that it is now 92 percent. Which of the following is *not* an appropriate response?
   1. Check blood gases to determine the cause of the apparent hypoxemia
   2. Suction the patient
   3. Continue to observe the patient, as the normal SpO_2 requires no intervention at this time
   4. Assess mental status, work of breathing, and change in respiratory rate

3. Clinical signs and symptoms of impending respiratory failure include:
   a. Increased respiratory rate
   b. Agitation
   c. Unresponsiveness
   d. Subjective feeling of difficulty breathing
   1. a, b
   2. a, d
   3. a, b, d
   4. a, b, c, d

4. Your patient has a large pleural effusion on the left side, with some compression of the lung tissue above the effusion. You would expect to find the following signs on examination of the chest.
   a. Diminished breath sounds on the affected side
   b. Slightly decreased respiratory rate
   c. Increased tactile fremitus on the left
   d. Presence of an E to A change on the left
   1. a, b, d
   2. b, c, d
   3. a, c, d
   4. a, b, c, d

5. For a patient on supplemental oxygen, the best method of assessing oxygenation status is:
   1. Pulse oximeter
   2. Cooximeter
   3. PaO_2
   4. Capnography

6. Shunting is:
   1. Normal ventilation with no perfusion
   2. Normal perfusion with no ventilation
   3. Normal ventilation with normal perfusion
   4. No ventilation with no perfusion

7. A patient has the following blood gases: pH: 7.26, $PaCO_2$: 72; PaO_2: 98; HCO_3: 26. What is the correct interpretation of these values?
   1. Respiratory acidosis
   2. Metabolic acidosis
   3. Respiratory alkalosis
   4. Metabolic alkalosis

Continued

REVIEW QUESTIONS—cont'd

8. A barrel chest can be seen in:
   a. Chronic obstructive lung disease
   b. Normal aging
   c. Tension pneumothorax
   d. Short term oxygen therapy
   1. a, b
   2. a, c
   3. a, d
   4. b, c

9. Low-flow oxygen delivery systems:
   a. Use entrainment of room air
   b. Use the mouth and nose as a reservoir
   c. Can deliver a consistent FiO_2
   d. Meet all of the patient's inspiratory demands
   1. a, b
   2. a, c
   3. a, d
   4. b, c

10. When eliciting a respiratory health history from an older adult, what data are vital to determining prior existing conditions despite current employment status?
    1. History of cystic fibrosis
    2. Employment history and occupational exposure
    3. History of childhood immunizations
    4. History of contact with poison ivy

11. Vesicular breathing occurs most frequently in which of the following conditions?
    1. Pneumonia
    2. Chronic airflow limitation from bronchitis
    3. Usual and normal breathing
    4. Apnea

12. Your patient experiences a drop in blood pressure on inspiration. This condition is most likely related to:
    1. Cor pulmonale
    2. Acute intrinsic asthma
    3. Pulsus paradoxus
    4. Hypotension

REVIEW ACTIVITIES

1. Your patient, Mrs. Hastings, an 82-year-old woman with pneumonia, asks you what she should expect in terms of her recovery after a recent bout of pneumonia. She admits that she is weakened and a little fearful of being alone. Although she has family nearby, they work outside the home; further, Mrs. Hastings is anxious to preserve her independence. What information will you share in your patient teaching? What concerns do you have about the likelihood of her experiencing problems at home? What are some reliable strategies to prevent a recurrence of pneumonia? What referrals will be helpful in identifying supports that will promote her independence?

2. Mr. Meyers, your patient with COPD, has a long history of secondhand cigarette exposure. His wife is not currently interested in smoking cessation and has always smoked at home. During a home health visit, you notice that Mr. Meyers has increasing dyspnea and coughing when his wife smokes in the living room where they sit together to watch TV. What can you tell the patient and his wife about secondhand cigarette smoke? What types of functional limitations are likely to occur if the current situation remains unchanged? What additional concerns do you have about Mr. and Mrs. Meyer's health in the upcoming cold months? What is your plan for patient teaching for this couple?

3. Mr. Myers is frail and has early cataracts. He is not strong enough to prepare his medications every day. Mrs. Meyers must be taught how to administer her husband's medicines. In planning teaching activities for the above couple, you notice that Mrs. Meyers watches television while you are discussing times to return to her home to visit. You also notice that she is easily distracted and seems preoccupied when you are discussing Mr. Meyer's medications with her. She sometimes responds correctly to your questions, but more often she seems confused and lost if there are more than two to three words in your directions. The television playing in the background makes your instructions difficult for her to understand. At times, she stares at her reflection in the window of the living room. Once, you noticed her waving to her reflection. You are concerned that Mrs. Meyers may not be the best person to learn Mr. Meyer's drug regimen. What other problems might Mrs. Meyers have with learning new information?

Continued

REVIEW ACTIVITIES—cont'd

4. In teaching Irma, your new 45-year-old patient with asthma, about exposure to and avoidance of environmental pollutants and allergens, you ask her to think about the various places she goes every week where she may be encountering environmental allergies that are triggers to asthma. She responds with the following information: she visits her adult daughter at her home in the country, shops in the local grocery store, rides a train weekly to the city to visit the library and the recently remodeled resale shop, she shops at the farm market near her home, works in her green house several time each week, drives her car to church, drops off items at the dry cleaners, exercises at the health club, and stops at the pet groomers to pick up her dog. In analyzing this list, you note some sources of possible irritation. What are these sources? How would you advise Irma to handle these necessary errands? What concerns do you have about her treatment regimen?

5. In auscultating the heart tones of Mr. Jeffers, your 29-year-old patient with acute bronchial pneumonia, you find it difficult to separate out the tones of the lungs from the tones. What maneuver do you employ to listen more closely to the cardiac sounds?

Upper Airway Dysfunction: Nursing Management

Julie S. Williard, RN, MS, NP-C

Amy Goodwin, RN, MSN, APRN, BC

CHAPTER TOPICS

- Allergic Rhinitis
- Viral Rhinitis
- Acute Sinusitis
- Chronic Sinusitis
- Acute Pharyngitis
- Tonsillitis and Adenoiditis
- Peritonsillar Abscess

- Acute and Chronic Laryngitis
- Obstruction during Sleep
- Epistaxis
- Fractures of the Nose
- Nasal Obstruction
- Laryngeal Obstruction
- Cancer of the Larynx

KEY TERMS

Alaryngeal voice
Cor pulmonale
Dyscrasia
Hematomas
Hemoptysis
Hypertrophic
Hypoxia
Immunotherapy
Mucositis
Odynophagia
Rhinitis
Rhinitis medicamentosa
Rhinorrhea
Somnolence
Stridor
Tracheostomy
Xerostomia

Upper respiratory infections (URIs) are the most common illnesses for which individuals seek outpatient medical care in the United States. They can be acute, self-limiting infections, or in some instances chronic, with symptoms that persist for a long period of time or that are recurrent. Epidemiological data concludes that this group of illnesses accounts annually for at least 20 million absences from work and 22 million absences from school. It is estimated that the general population spends two to three billion dollars annually on over-the-counter (OTC) medications to treat the symptoms of URIs (Anzueto & Niederman, 2003). Most URIs can be managed at home and rarely require hospitalization. However, many patients may be hospitalized with other acute or chronic illnesses or diseases, and URIs may be occurring concurrently and need to be managed by the nurse. Nurses may also encounter patients with URIs in the community setting or in long-term facilities. Nurses need to be able to recognize the signs and symptoms of URIs to provide appropriate care.

ALLERGIC RHINITIS

Rhinitis is a term used to describe a group of disorders that is characterized by inflammation and irritation of the nasal mucosa (Figure 31-1). These disorders may be classified as infectious or noninfectious. Infectious rhinitis is also termed viral rhinitis, better known as the common cold. Noninfectious rhinitis is divided into allergic and nonallergic. Allergic rhinitis can be seasonal, perennial, or occupational. It is estimated that allergic rhinitis affects approximately 40 million Americans (Mastin, 2003). Nonallergic rhinitis is a termed given to a group of syndromes that produce the symptoms of rhinitis but are nonimmunoglobulin E-(IgE) mediated (Mastin, 2003). Some conditions that may precipitate nonallergic rhinitis include changes in temperature or humidity, drugs (such as inhaling cocaine), pregnancy, stages of the menstrual cycle, or emotional factors.

Allergic rhinitis is defined clinically as a symptomatic disorder of the nose that is induced by an Ig-E mediated inflammatory response (Sheikh & Panesar, 2003). More women than men are affected and incidence rises with increasing age. There is a familial component to allergic rhinitis (Ferri, et al., 2004). Genetic predisposition to specific allergens has been shown to be as high as 50 percent in the general population (Price & Wilson, 2003).

Pathophysiology

On exposure to the sensitizing agent, the body initiates the inflammatory response by releasing histamines and leukotrienes. The blood vessels of the nasal mucosa begin to vasodilate with increased capillary permeability. These two factors cause swelling and congestion of the nasal mucous membranes. This inflammation causes increased production of mucus within the nasal cavity. The most common aggravating factors are foods, pollen, and animal dander (Table 31-1).

Assessment with Clinical Manifestations

Signs and symptoms of allergic rhinitis are the same regardless of the triggering event. Common clinical manifestations include the presence of **rhinorrhea** (thin, watery discharge from the nose), nasal congestion and obstruction, nasal itchiness, and sneezing. Headache and cough may also be present.

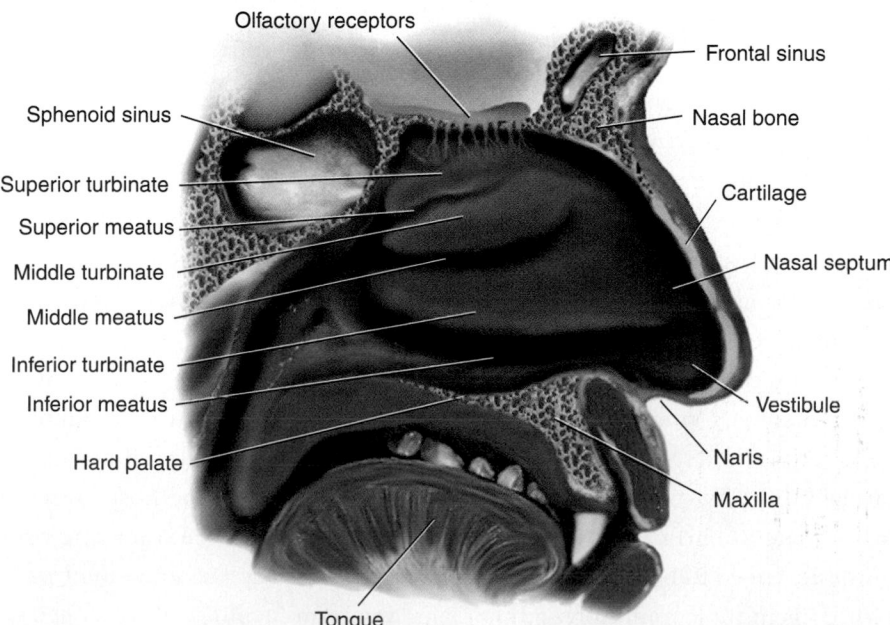

Figure 31-1 Lateral cross-section of the nose.

TABLE 31-1 Types of Allergic Rhinitis

	DEFINITION	COMMON TRIGGERS	NONPHARMACOLOGICAL TREATMENTS
Seasonal allergic rhinitis (SAR)	Signs and symptoms of allergic rhinitis (AR) that occur during a specific season. SAR is an IgE-mediated response to an allergen, often times pollen and molds	Tree/flower pollen, grass, or weeds	Reduce exposure Keep windows and door closed Air conditioning (for climate control: closed vents) Limited outdoor activity on sunny, windy, and humid days Shower or bathe after outdoor activity
Perennial allergic rhinitis (PAR)	An IgE-mediated response to environmental allergens including dust mites, mold, and animal dander that is present throughout the year and is usually indoors	Cockroaches, perennial molds, dust mites, or cat or dog dander	Clean sink, showers, window and garbage pails with Clorox or Lysol Use dehumidifier in damp area, removing stagnant water quickly Avoid carpeting, especially in damp areas Clean house while allergic patient is not home Encase bedding and pillow in hypoallergenic materials Wash bedding and clothes in hot water at least every two weeks
Occupational allergic rhinitis	AR that results from airborne substances in the workplace. This reaction may be mediated by allergic and nonallergic factors, such as laboratory animal antigens, grain, wood dust, and chemicals	Irritants, such as smoke, cold air, formaldehyde, hairspray, coffee beans, or latex	Avoidance of the allergen Using/wearing filter masks Limit exposure time

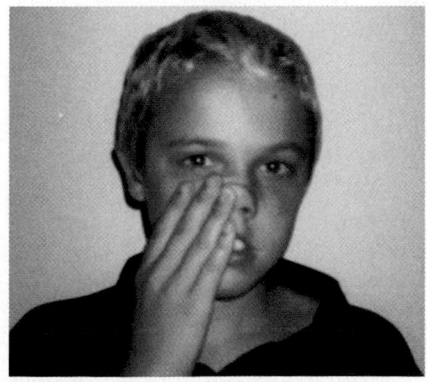

Figure 31-2 Illustration of the allergic salute.

Physical appearance of the patient will reveal a great deal of information. This is particularly helpful in children with severe allergic rhinitis (Figure 31-2). Children with allergic rhinitis exhibit a triad of signs: the allergic shiner, a darkening of the lower eyelid because of suborbital edema; the allergic crease, a transverse line above the tip and below the bridge of the nose; and the allergic salute, frequent wiping of the nose with the palm of the hand (Mastin, 2003). Other signs commonly present are a nasal quality to the voice, constant coughing from a postnasal drip, chapped lips, and a dry mouth from mouth breathing.

Examination of the nose may reveal edematous, pale, or blue-tinged nasal mucosa (Ferri, et al., 2004). Thin, watery discharge is present. Further abnormal assessment findings will depend on the presenting symptoms. These include, but are not limited to, irritated sclera, tenderness to palpation over the sinus cavities, serous otitis media, postnasal drip, redness of the pharynx, and enlarged lymph nodes in the head and neck region.

Diagnostic Tests

Careful history and physical examination provide the basis of diagnosis for rhinitis. Nasal smears may be taken to examine for the presence of eosinophils, indicating the cause of rhinitis is because of an allergen response. A board certified allergist may perform allergy testing for an individual who exhibits recurrent symptoms. Allergy testing may be done with a skin prick test or intradermal skin test. A skin prick test entails introducing a series of the most common allergens one by one into the skin via a needle prick. Intradermal testing consists of introducing allergens one by one under the skin by a subcutaneous injection. The allergens tested should be tailored to the patient's history. A positive skin test is demonstrated by local edema and redness at the site of injection. This indicates the presence of IgE antibodies that react with specific substances to produce an allergic response.

Nursing Diagnoses

Based on the information gathered, examples of nursing diagnoses in the patient with allergic rhinitis may include the following:
* Activity intolerance
* Ineffective airway clearance
* Acute pain
* Deficient knowledge

Goals

Patients need to receive instructions about the importance of environmental control at home, work, and school (Box 31-1).

Evidence-Based Care

Research findings provide the basis for evidence-based care. A variety of criteria have been developed to evaluate research findings and determine their appropriateness for patient care. Table 31-2 lists criteria that have been developed by the American Academy of Family Physicians for evaluating research evidence.

The following evidence-based care is from the First Consult Web site available at www.firstconsult.com:
* Numerous randomized controlled trials (RCTs) have shown that the oral antihistamines cetirizine, loratadine, and fexofenadine improve the symptoms of seasonal allergic rhinitis compared with placebo.
* Eight RCTs have shown that pseudoephedrine, in combination with a second-generation antihistamine, gives better symptom control than pseudoephedrine alone, an antihistamine alone, or placebo.
* There is no convincing evidence for the efficacy of intranasal azelastine in improving symptoms in seasonal allergic rhinitis.
* There is evidence that montelukast alone or in combination with loratadine is significantly better at improving nasal symptoms compared with placebo.
* The benefits of allergen specific **immunotherapy** (the process of introducing allergens to the body by injection for the purpose of increasing immunity) need to be balanced against the risks of serious adverse effects and death associated with giving large doses of allergens (Ferri, et al., 2004)

Nursing management of allergic rhinitis depends on the cause, which may be identified by obtaining a thorough history and physical examination. A careful history will reveal exposure to allergens, genetic predisposition, and aggravating factors. Prevention of allergic rhinitis focuses on educating patients about allergen avoidance and modification of their environment. Treatment for allergic rhinitis focuses on alleviating or reducing the symptoms.

BOX 31-1

ALLERGY AVOIDANCE MEASURES

House Dust Mites

- Enclose mattresses, box springs, and pillows in zippered, dust proof encasings
- Wash bed linens weekly in hot water (54° C [130° F])
- Reduce humidity to 50 percent
- Remove carpeting
- Replace feather or down-filled covers and pillows with synthetic items

Pollens

- Avoid freshly cut grass; do not mow the lawn
- Keep windows and door closed during allergy season
- Use central air conditioning to reduce pollen and humidity
- Shower after outdoor activities to remove pollen from clothing and skin

Molds

- Clean damp areas frequently, at least once a week, with a chlorine bleach solution
- Ventilate areas well (bathrooms, kitchens, and basement)
- Consider a dehumidifier if living in a humid climate

Pets

- Remove pet from home, if possible
- If unable to remove pet, keep it out of the bedroom and keep the doors and heating ducts closed
- Reduce cat allergen by bathing the cat every two weeks

Irritants

- Avoid cigarette smoke, perfumes, aerosol sprays, strong cleaning products, and dusty or polluted environments

---

TABLE 31-2 Evaluation of Evidence

To indicate the strength of the supporting evidence, each summary statement is accorded one of three levels.

LEVEL	CRITERIA
Level A	Systematic reviews of randomized controlled trials, including meta-analyses
	Good-quality randomized controlled trials
Level B	Good-quality nonrandomized clinical trials
	Systematic reviews not in Level A
	Lower quality randomized controlled trials not in Level A
	Other types of investigations: case-control studies, clinical cohort studies, cross-sectional studies, retrospective studies, and uncontrolled studies
Level C	Evidence-based consensus statements and expert guidelines

Pharmacology

Antihistamines are the mainstay of treatment in allergic rhinitis. The mechanism of action is to block the IgE-mediated response to the allergen. Blocking this response helps to reduce inflammation and swelling of the nasal mucosa, which in turn relieves the itching, sneezing, and runny nose. First-generation antihistamines are available as OTC medications. However, these medications generally produce sedation and cholinergic side effects. Newer second-generation antihistamines, available by prescription, have fewer side effects. Health care providers may prescribe a decongestant along with an antihistamine to help with the congestion that occurs with perennial rhinitis. Intranasal corticosteroids may be used as adjunct therapy to reduce swelling and allergic response for individuals who do not respond to oral medications. Nasal sprays are generally well tolerated with minimal, if any, side effects. Ophthalmic agents may be used to relieve itchiness, irritation, or redness of the eyes (Table 31-3).

Saline nose sprays may be helpful to alleviate irritation of the nasal mucosa and soften dry nasal secretions. Intranasal steroids may help reduce inflammation of the mucous membranes of the nose.

The nurse should review with the patient the proper technique for using nasal sprays. The following instructions should be included when teaching a patient the proper use of nasal sprays. Proper dosing and technique will increase the effectiveness of the spray and decrease potential side effects.

TABLE 31-3 **Medications Used in Treatment of Rhinitis**

CLASSIFICATION OF DRUG	DOSAGE	SIDE EFFECTS	EVIDENCE-BASED MEDICINE
Oral Preparations Antihistamines			
First-generation OTC			
Chlorpheniramine maleate (Chlor-Trimeton)	2-4 mg, TID or QID	Sedation, headache, dizziness, agitation, and urinary retention	No evidence that meets criteria
Clemastine (Tavist)	1.34 mg BID		
Diphenhydramine (Benadryl)	25–50 mg every 4–6 hours		
Second generation		Less sedation than first generation	
		Headache, urinary retention, dry mouth, and dyspepsia	
Cetirizine (Zyrtec)	10 mg daily		
Fexofenadine (Allegra)	60 mg BID or 180 mg daily		
Loratadine (OTC) (Claritin)	10 mg daily		Random controlled trials found montelukast plus loratadine to be superior in relieving daytime symptoms of seasonal allergic rhinitis than either medication alone. Level A
Decongestants			
Pseudoephedrine OTC (Sudafed)	30–60 mg QID	Caution use in hypertension Tachycardia, anxiety, dizziness, and drowsiness	In combination with second-generation antihistamines found to give better symptom control then either alone or placebo. Level A
Leukotriene Receptor Antagonists		Headache, nausea, infection, and diarrhea	
Montelukast (Singular)	10 mg at bedtime		
Zafirlukast (Accolate)	20 mg at bedtime		

Continued

TABLE 31-3   Medications Used in Treatment of Rhinitis—cont'd

CLASSIFICATION OF DRUG	DOSAGE	SIDE EFFECTS	EVIDENCE-BASED MEDICINE
Intranasal Sprays Antihistamines			
Azelastine (Astelin)	Two sprays each nostril BID	Headache, dizziness, nasal burning, and dry mouth	Random controlled trials found no convincing evidence of efficacy of Astelin in improving symptoms or improving quality of life with seasonal allergic rhinitis. Level A
Steroids			Meta-analysis found intra-nasal steroids to be more effective in relieving nasal congestion, discharge, sneezing, postnasal drip, and nasal itch than antihistamines. Level B
Beclomethasone dipropionate (Beconase)	1–2 sprays each nostril daily	Epistaxis, pharyngitis, broncho-spasm, headache, and light-headedness	
Budesonide (Rhinocort)	2–4 sprays each nostril daily		
Fluticasone propionate (Flonase)	1–2 sprays each nostril daily		

Adapted from Ferri, F. F., Saver, D. F., Mugge, R. E., Leickly, F. E., Millman, B., & Fox, R. (2004, August). Allergic rhinitis. Retrieved December 17, 2004, from http://www.firstconsult.com.

Patient teaching for proper technique for instillation of nasal spray is presented in the Patient Playbook.

Patient teaching includes reviewing the proper dosing of medications and their side effects. In the elderly and other high-risk populations, the nurse reviews the importance of receiving an annual influenza vaccination to reduce susceptibility to infections.

Evaluation of Outcomes

Potential patient outcomes for each of the example nursing diagnoses for the patient with allergic rhinitis are:
- Activity intolerance. The patient will perform activities of daily living with ease.
- Ineffective airway clearance. The patient will breathe with ease, moving sputum out of airway.
- Acute pain-physical well-being, symptom control, and be comfortable in the physical surroundings
- Deficient knowledge. The patient will provide a description of behaviors that promote health, description prevention and control of infection, description of managing medications safely

Complications

The recurrent nature of rhinitis is a problem for many individuals. The health care team must work together to ensure adequate patient teaching in avoidance of triggers, environmental control, and medication administration. It is important to inform the patient that allergic rhinitis can be recurrent and often chronic. The goal of treatment is to optimize symptom control. Patients whose symptoms worsen despite adequate therapy should be referred to an allergist for immunotherapy.

Patients with rhinitis are at risk for otitis media, sinusitis, nasal speech, epistaxis, and laryngeal edema (Ferri, et al., 2004). Inadequate control of symptoms may exacerbate asthma in some individuals.

VIRAL RHINITIS

Viral rhinitis is rhinitis with an infectious component. Often called the common cold, it is a self-limiting syndrome of the upper respiratory tract caused by a viral infection. Symptoms include general malaise, nasal congestion, rhinorrhea, sneezing, and sore or scratchy throat. The term common cold, or acute coryza, refers to an acute, usually afebrile viral infection of the respiratory tract, with inflammation in any or all parts of the airway, including the nose, paranasal sinuses, throat, larynx, and sometimes the trachea or bronchi. Colds are extremely contagious, because the virus begins to shed approximately 24 to 72 hours before the onset of symptoms. Onset of symptoms is usually abrupt and begins with a burning sensation in the nose or throat, followed by sneezing, malaise, and rhinorrhea (Beers & Berkow, 2004). Children usually have five to eight colds per calendar year. It is estimated that adults average two to four colds per year, presumably because immunity develops against organisms associated with respiratory infections (Anzueto & Niederman, 2003).

Epidemiology

Six classifications of viruses are known to cause the common cold. These are rhinovirus, coronavirus, influenza, parainfluenza, respiratory syncytial virus (RSV), and adenovirus. Within each class there exist many different strains of the virus. Rhinoviruses, for instance, account for 30 to 50 percent of all colds and produce more than 100 strains (Beers & Berkow, 2004). It is a commonly held myth that exposure to cold increases a person's susceptibility to develop rhinitis, but research findings do not support this claim (Ferri, et al., 2004).

Assessment with Clinical Manifestations

Clinical signs and symptoms that occur with viral rhinitis may manifest in any combination in individuals. Nasal congestion, runny nose, sneezing, nasal itching, general malaise, and scratchy throat are common. Headache, conjunctivitis, hoarseness, and cough may present. Cough is usually mild but could last for two weeks. Fever, if present, is usually low grade. When symptoms last for more than two weeks with worsening of fever or onset of systemic manifestations, the illness is no longer rhinitis but one of an acute upper airway tract infection.

Nursing Diagnoses

Based on the information gathered, examples of nursing diagnoses in the patient with viral rhinitis may include the following:
- Activity intolerance
- Ineffective airway clearance

Planning and Implementation

There is no cure for the common cold. Treatment is aimed at decreasing the impact of the symptoms and preventing secondary bacterial infection. Symptomatic treatment includes drinking adequate fluid, getting rest, and preventing chills. Antihistamines relieve sneezing, rhinorrhea, and nasal congestion. Topical (nasal) decongestants may provide rapid relief from nasal congestion but should not be used for more than three to five consecutive days. Overuse of decongestant nasal sprays can lead to rebound nasal congestion, which is also called **rhinitis medicamentosa,** and is often worse than the original symptoms. Warm saline gargles and lozenges provide relief from sore throat. Alleviation of cough should be sought only if it is severe, painful, or interferes with the ability to sleep and can be obtained by using OTC cough suppressants that contain dextromethorphan.

Herbal and complementary medicines are widely used for treatment and prevention but have not been shown to reduce the incidence or length of the illness. Common remedies include zinc lozenges, high dose vitamin C, and Echinacea. There is no role for antibiotics in the treatment of the common cold (Douglas, Chalker, & Treacy, 2004). Acetaminophen or nonsteroidal anti-inflammatory drugs (NSAIDs) are useful to help with fever, aches, and pain.

Evaluation of Outcomes

Potential patient outcomes for each of the example nursing diagnoses for the patient with viral rhinitis are:
- Activity intolerance. The patient will perform activities of daily living with ease.
- Ineffective airway clearance. The patient will breathe with ease, moving sputum out of airway.

ACUTE SINUSITIS

Prolonged nasal congestion and inflammation often leads to acute sinusitis. A general consensus has been that acute sinusitis signifies a bacterial invasion of the sinuses, but recent research shows that most viral infections also involve the sinuses. Individuals with allergic rhinitis are predisposed to developing sinusitis because of the constant inflammation within the sinus cavities. Structural problems of the nose, such as narrowed passages, a deviated septum, tumors, or polyps may be other causes of sinusitis.

Thirty-seven million Americans reportedly develop sinusitis every year, resulting in 16 million office visits per year (Davidoff & Cunningham, 2004). Americans spend over two billion dollars a year on OTC medications (Davidoff & Cunningham, 2004).

Acute sinusitis is an infection of the parasinuses. Four pair of parasinuses are located in the skull. These air-filled cavities decrease the weight of the skull and act as resonance chambers during speech (Krantz & Varon-Thomas, 2004). These cavities are lined with ciliated mucous membranes that trap debris.

Etiology

Predisposing factors for the development of sinusitis include allergic rhinitis, vasomotor rhinitis, rhinitis medicamentosa, upper respiratory tract infections, nasal polyps, immunodeficiency factors, and environmental factors, such as air pollution (Saver, Ferri, Murray & Demetroulakos, 2004). Smoking or living with someone who smokes also predisposes an individual to infection of the sinuses.

Pathophysiology

Most sinus infections begin as an unresolved upper respiratory tract infection of 7 to 10 days duration. Unresolved inflammation and edema of the nasal passageways often lead to obstruction of the sinuses with overproduction of secretions.

Impairment of the ciliated mucous membranes of the sinus cavity traps mucus. Infection within the sinus cavities can be viral or bacterial. The most common bacterial organisms that cause sinusitis are *Streptococcus pneumoniae, Haemophilus influenzae,* and *Moraxella catarrhalis* (Saver, Ferri, et al., 2004).

Complications for acute sinusitis are rare. Spread of infection can cause otitis media, mastoiditis, orbital cellulitis, osteomyelitis, bacterial meningitis, or a brain abscess. The presence of orbital cellulitis can lead to loss of vision and requires immediate referral for evaluation and treatment (Saver, Ferri, et al., 2004). See Table 31-4 for comparison of symptoms of sinusitis, allergy, and cold.

Assessment with Clinical Manifestations

To rule out spread of infection beyond the sinus cavities, assess the patient's head and neck thoroughly. Often symptoms are vague and nonspecific. Physical findings that are suggestive of sinusitis include:

- Purulent nasal secretions
- Increased posterior pharyngeal secretions
- Mucosal erythema
- Periorbital edema
- Tenderness overlying sinuses
- Air-fluid levels on transillumination of the sinuses, this test may produce numerous false-positive and false-negative results (Davidoff & Cunningham, 2004).

Patients often complain of unilateral face pain (on side of infection or inflammation), purulent nasal discharge, pain during mastication, anosmia (absence of smell), and headache. Less common symptoms include fever, nasal congestion, halitosis, toothache, metallic taste, or cough (Davidoff & Cunningham, 2004).

Diagnostic Tests

Imaging studies may be necessary when symptoms are vague, physical findings are undiagnostic, or if the patient has a less than favorable response to conventional treatment. An X-ray of the sinuses, called Water's view, can be done to detect congestion in the maxillary sinus cavities. A computed tomography (CT) scan is useful in visualizing both the soft tissue structures and the bony anatomy of the face and skull. Magnetic resonance imaging (MRI) is of limited

TABLE 31-4 Comparison of Symptoms

SIGN/SYMPTOM	SINUSITIS	ALLERGY	COLD
Facial pain/pressure	Yes	Sometimes	Sometimes
Duration of illness	At least 10–14 days	Varies	Under 10 days
Nasal discharge	Thick, yellow-green	Clear, thin, watery	Thick, whitish or thin
Fever	Sometimes	No	Sometimes
Headache	Sometimes	Sometimes	Sometimes
Pain in upper teeth	Sometimes	No	No
Bad breath	Sometimes	No	No
Coughing	Sometimes	Sometimes	Yes
Nasal congestion	Yes	Sometimes	Yes
Sneezing	No	Sometimes	Yes

value except for differentiating soft tissue changes associated with fungal sinusitis or to identify the presence of a tumor.

Nursing Diagnoses

Based on the information gathered, examples of nursing diagnoses in the patient with sinusitis may include the following:
- Acute pain
- Activity intolerance related to fatigue

Planning and Implementation

The nurse's goal in treating patients with acute sinusitis is to teach them the importance of self-care and prevention. The nurse emphasizes the importance of completing the entire course of antibiotics to prevent bacterial resistance and to assist in eradicating the infection. Side effects of medication need to be discussed with the patient. The nurse can suggest nonpharmacological therapies, such as applying warm compresses to the sinus area, humidifying the air with steam or a vaporizer, maintaining adequate hydration, and smoking cessation. When using a pan of water to obtain steam, the patient should be instructed to remove the pan from the burner before placing the face over it. To reduce the risk of inhaling bacteria or fungus from the steam, humidifiers or vaporizers must be cleansed daily and used only when a filter is in place.

Evidence-Based Care

Antibiotics are effective in radiologically or bacteriologically confirmed sinusitis, although the benefits are modest.
- There is limited evidence that antibiotics (including amoxicillin, cephalosporins, and macrolides) for 7 to 10 days are effective in the treatment of radiologically or bacteriologically confirmed acute maxillary sinusitis. Nevertheless, the moderate benefits of antibiotic treatment should be weighed against the potential for adverse effects.
- However, one randomized controlled trial of amoxicillin versus placebo for 10 days did not find any difference between treatments in patients with clinically diagnosed sinusitis.
- A systematic review of RCTs that compared antibiotics verus placebo or standard therapy in children with rhinosinusitis found that antibiotics, including amoxicillin, trimethoprim-sulfamethoxazole, and erythromycin, for 10 days reduces the probability of persistent symptoms. Erythromycin may be associated with more clinical failures than amoxicillin and trimethoprim-sulfamethoxazole. Again, the benefits are modest, and the risk of side effects should be considered (Saver, Ferri, et al., 2004).

Treatment of acute sinusitis focuses on eradicating the infection, shrinking the nasal mucosa, and reducing pain. Evidence-based medical research has shown the limited efficacy of antibiotic use in eradicating infection. This is in part because of their overuse resulting in subsequent bacterial organism resistance.

Pharmacology

When antibiotics are warranted for the eradication of a bacterial infection, first-line drugs of choice are amoxicillin (Amoxil), trimethoprim/sulfamethoxazole (Bactrim), and erythromycin (Davidoff & Cunningham, 2004). Second-line therapy includes the second-generation cephalosporins, such as cefprozil (Cefzil), cefuroxime (Ceftin), and cefpodoxime (Vantin) or amoxicillin/clavulanic acid (Augmentin). Newer broad-spectrum antibiotics that have been shown to be effective in treating sinusitis include the macrolides, azithromycin (Zithromax) and clarithromycin (Biaxin). Quinolones, such as ciprofloxacin (Cipro) and levofloxacin (Levaquin), can be used in individuals

DOLLARS AND SENSE

Price Comparison for Antibiotics Used to Treat Sinusitis for 14 days

DRUG/DOSAGE (MG)	NUMBER OF TABLETS	COST
Amoxil 500	30	$7.90–$11.99
Augmentin 500/125	30	$121.59–$123.39
Bactrim DS 800/160	30	$44.99
Cefzil 250	30	$131.49
Cefzil 500	30	$262.70
Vantin 200	30	$171.09
Zithromax 500	18	$272.25
Cipro 500	30	$153.07–$160.99
Levaquin	20	$186.32–$189.98

Adapted from Price compare: Antibiotics. *(2006). Retrieved August 13, 2006, from www.destinationrx.com/.*

allergic to penicillin or those patients that have not demonstrated improvement with first-line therapy (Davidoff & Cunningham, 2004). Quinolones are contraindicated in children less than 17 years of age. These newer drugs are more costly, and studies have not demonstrated superiority of one antibiotic over another in eradicating infection. However, the amount of organism resistance in a certain geographical area must be considered when selecting an antibiotic. The benefits of antibiotic therapy must be weighed against the potential for adverse effects. A 14-day course of antibiotics is recommended for all agents (Saver, et al., 2004).

Oral or topical decongestants may be employed to reduce swelling of the nasal mucosa by constricting blood vessels and reducing the blood supply to nasal mucous membranes. Topical steroids may also be used to reduce the size of nasal polyps and help shrink swollen nasal turbinates. OTC or homemade saline nose drops may soothe irritated nasal passages. Antihistamines have not been shown to be of benefit in reducing the symptoms of acute sinusitis. Their propensity to dry secretions may worsen the symptoms and delay drainage of the sinus cavity. There is insufficient evidence to support the role of wetting agents, mucolytics, or expectorants in treating sinusitis (American Academy of Allergy, Asthma, and Immunology, 2002). Pain relief can be accomplished with acetaminophen or ibuprofen.

Population-Based Care

According to the American Association of Otolaryngology–Head and Neck Surgery (AAO-HNS), children who do not respond to amoxicillin are unlikely to respond to trimethoprim/sulfamethoxazole (Bactrim) or erythromycin/sulfisoxazole (Pediazole), because bacteria are resistant to many of the older antibiotics. Children who fail two courses of antibiotics should be recommended for one of the following treatments: receive an extended dose and length of treatment, receive intravenous (IV) antibiotics, or a referral to an ear, nose, throat specialist (AAO-HNS, 2002a).

Evaluation of Outcomes

Potential patient outcomes for each of the example nursing diagnoses for the patient with sinusitis are:

- Acute pain: The patient should verbalize an adequate relief of pain along with the ability to realistically cope with the pain if it is not completely relieved.
- Activity intolerance related to fatigue: The patient maintains activity level within capabilities, as evidenced by normal heart rate and blood pressure during activity, as well as absence of shortness of breath, weakness, and fatigue.

CHRONIC SINUSITIS

Chronic sinusitis is an inflammation of the sinus cavities that persists for three to eight weeks but can continue for months or even years (NIAID, 2002). Data from the National Institute of Allergy and Infectious Diseases (2002) indicate that health care workers report 33 million cases of chronic sinusitis to the U.S. Centers for Disease Control and Prevention (CDC) on an annual basis. Americans spend an average of $5 billion yearly in treatment with an additional $60 billion in surgical treatment (Razek & Poe, 2004). Sinusitis is rarely life-threatening, but serious complications can occur because of its proximity to the orbital and cranial cavities. Chronic sinusitis is more frequent in the pediatric population because of the more frequent episodes of URIs (Razek & Poe, 2004).

Pathophysiology

Normal sinus function depends on an intact mucociliary transport system within the sinus cavity. Ciliary transport moves mucus along the sinus tract into the ostia and then into the nasopharynx for removal. Inflammation or obstruction that prevents the normal progression of drainage from the sinus cavities can lead to chronic sinusitis. Stagnation of secretions can be the result of an allergic disease, asthma, or untreated infectious process. Blockage of the nasal passages can occur from nasal polyps, tumors, or a deviated nasal septum.

Organisms producing chronic sinusitis are the same as those that cause acute episodes of sinusitis. Immunologically compromised individuals, such as those infected with human immunodeficiency virus (HIV), can have serious and often fatal infections of the sinuses with fungal or bacterial organisms. *Aspergillus fumigatus* is the most common organism associated with fungal sinusitis (Ramadan, 2004).

Complications

Complications from chronic sinusitis are uncommon. However, because of the proximity of the sinus cavities to the oral and cranial structures, thorough and adequate treatment should be instituted promptly to avoid occurrence of potential problems. Complications include periorbital cellulitis, subperiosteal abscess, cavernous sinus thrombosis, dental abscess, meningitis, and encephalitis (Razek & Poe, 2004).

Assessment with Clinical Manifestations

Clinical manifestations of chronic sinusitis include stasis of secretions, swollen nasal passages, and thick, bad tasting postnasal drainage. Postnasal drainage, coupled with inflammation, alters ventilation and produces a persistent cough, which worsens when the individual is in a recumbent position. Complaints of facial pain and swelling are usually more pronounced in the morning. Bending over can exacerbate facial pain. Headache, toothache, and fatigue are also common findings. Often patients will state that they experience changes in taste and smell. Fever and chills suggest that the infection has spread beyond the sinuses.

Physical examination of the sinus cavity reveals reddened mucous membranes with diffuse and purulent discharge that varies from yellow to green in color. Palpation over the infected sinus cavity may reveal tenderness and pain. Transillumination will reveal absence of a glow from the light source because of congestion and purulent fluid in the cavity.

Diagnostic Tests

A careful and complete assessment should be performed on any patient with complaints of facial pain or headache. A nasal swab with culture is helpful in determining the best antibiotic to initiate. Nasal endoscopy with aspiration of tissue will provide additional evidence of the causative factors, such as fungus, bacteria, or tumor origin. Sinus X-rays reveal areas of opacities where swelling and retained mucus is present. A CT scan provides better definition of the extent of the sinusitis. This is also a useful tool in guiding the surgeon if surgical aspiration of the infection or correction of the blockage is indicated.

Nursing Diagnoses

Based on the information gathered, examples of nursing diagnoses in the patient with chronic sinusitis may include the following:

- Ineffective airway clearance
- Acute pain
- Deficient fluid volume
- Deficient knowledge

Planning and Implementation

Every attempt is made to eliminate the aggravating factors that are causing the inflammation or obstruction. Underlying problems, such as vasomotor instability, mucociliary dysfunction, immune deficiencies, allergies, or asthma, must be controlled. (Razek & Poe, 2004). Several modalities are useful in treating chronic sinusitis.

Pharmacology

Antibiotics should be broad spectrum and given for four to six weeks without interruption. First-line antibiotics of choice include amoxicillin-clavulanate (Augmentin), second-generation cephalosporin (Ceftin), or erythromycin-sulfisoxazole (Pediazole). Macrolides, such as clarithromycin (Biaxin) or azithromycin (Zithromax), can be used for more resistant infections. Criteria for antibiotic selection include: (a) current sinus puncture study results demonstrating bacteriologic response; (b) knowledge of changing antimicrobial resistance in a community; (c) history of medication allergy, especially the sulfa drugs and cephalosporins; (d) adverse effect profile of the medication; (e) cost of the medication and the economic status of the patient; and (f) other factors that affect compliance, such as dosing and formulation (Razek & Poe, 2004).

Decongestants, either oral or topical, are helpful in reducing inflammation within the nasal passages thus facilitating drainage of stagnant mucus. Decongestant nasal sprays should be used sparingly and for no more than three to five days because of the risk of tolerance, rhinitis medicamentosa, or rebound congestion. Intranasal steroids are extremely helpful in reducing local inflammation without producing systemic side effects. Oral corticosteroids may be prescribed in severe, unresponsive cases. Antihistamines, cromolyn sodium, and topical corticosteroid nasal sprays may be helpful in controlling the allergic component that often provides the initial inflammation (Mayo Clinic, 2004).

Adjunct Therapy

Other measures useful in treating uncomfortable symptoms include breathing in warm, moist air from a vaporizer, applying warm packs over the sinus area, or washing the sinus cavity with warm saline solution. Remind the patient of the need for safety when using steam or a humidifier or vaporizer.

The majority of patients with chronic sinusitis are managed on an outpatient basis. Nursing management entails teaching the patient how to prevent recurrence of their symptoms by avoiding known allergens, ceasing to smoke, and foregoing air travel during a cold, allergy, or bout of sinusitis. During an episode of a cold, drinking plenty of fluids will help to keep mucus thin. Decongestants will help reduce inflammation and help facilitate drainage. It is important to reinforce recognition of sinus infection symptoms, necessity of completing all medications, and preventive measures.

Population-Based Care

In the aging population, the physiology and structure of the nose changes. The nose lengthens and the tip begins to droop. These alterations can cause a restriction of airflow. Narrowing in this region results in complaints of nasal obstruction, often referred to as geriatric rhinitis (AAO-HNS, 2002b). This syndrome produces many of the same complaints as chronic sinusitis and requires a thorough history and physical assessment for accurate diagnosis and treatment.

Surgery

If conservative treatment with antibiotics and decongestants fails, the patient may require allergy testing desensitization, or surgical intervention to drain the sinus cavity of infection or relieve obstruction (AAO-HNS, 2002c). Newer endoscopic sinus surgery is the most commonly performed sinus surgery. It is less invasive than conventional sinus surgery, with the added benefits of decreased of normal tissue and fewer complications.

Moreover, this procedure can most often be performed on an outpatient basis (AAO-HNS, 2002c). During endoscopy, the surgeon can correct structural abnormalities, remove polyps or other tumors, and wash away mucus and other debris. If fungus is present, aggressive surgery for removal of its debris and irrigation of the sinus cavity is necessary. When chronic sinusitis is caused by altered ability of the ciliary system to adequately drain mucus, an opening or window is created to allow for improved drainage. This procedure is called a Caldwell-Luc operation, named after the two health care providers who developed the procedure. This is most often performed when a malignancy is present in the sinus cavity (AAO-HNS, 2002c).

Evaluation of Outcomes

Potential patient outcomes for each of the example nursing diagnoses for the patient with chronic sinusitis are:

- Ineffective airway clearance. The patient maintains a patent airway by managing secretion.
- Acute pain. The patient reports feeling more comfortable. Uses comfort measures such as analgesics, hot packs, gargles, and rest.
- Deficient fluid volume. The patient maintains adequate fluid intake.
- Deficient knowledge. The patient demonstrates an adequate level of knowledge and performs self-care appropriately.

ACUTE PHARYNGITIS

Acute pharyngitis is an inflammation of the throat primarily caused by infection. In the United States, more than 10 million people are diagnosed with pharyngitis every year. Over half of all cases of pharyngitis are caused by viral infections (Thomas & Powers, 2002). Several bacterial species are capable of producing infection, most notably group A beta-hemolytic streptococci (GABHS [*Streptococcus pyogenes*]).

Epidemiology

Pharyngitis caused by *S. pyogenes* has a worldwide distribution. It is common all year but has a peak occurrence in late winter and early spring in temperate climates.

Etiology

No ethnic or racial etiology has been found to occur with GABHS. However, prevalence is higher in the pediatric population because of the more frequent occurrence of URIs. The peak incidence is between 5 to 15 years of age, which accounts for approximately 30 percent of all GABHS cases (Thomas & Powers, 2002). It is uncommon for children under the age of two to be infected with GABHS. By adulthood, the prevalence of GABHS falls to 5 to 15 percent of all cases (Thomas & Powers, 2002).

Pathophysiology

Large respiratory droplets containing the virus or bacteria are easily spread from person to person. Transmission is more likely to occur in crowded conditions, such as daycare facilities, schools, dormitories, or military barracks. Food- and water-borne outbreaks have been reported (Thomas & Powers, 2002). The incubation phase for GABHS is two to five days after exposure to the organism. Communicability of the disease is greatest during the acute infection phase.

Complications

With adequate teaching and understanding of instructions, patients with pharyngitis recover with no sequela. In the event that a streptococcal pharyngitis infection is inadequately treated or treatment is delayed, suppurative and nonsuppurative complications can occur. Suppurative complications are the result of infection spread beyond the pharynx and include (Thomas & Powers, 2002):

- Peritonsillar cellulitis
- Peritonsillar abscess
- Retropharyngeal abscess
- Parapharyngeal abscess
- Otitis media
- Sinusitis
- Mastoiditis
- Intracranial venous sinus thrombosis
- Pneumonia

Nonsuppurative complications include acute rheumatic fever and glomerulonephritis and are caused by autoimmune responses. Scarlet fever, which produces a scarlatina rash, is commonly seen, and is the result of the production of an endotoxin by certain strains of the *S. pyogenes* organism.

Assessment with Clinical Manifestations

Differentiating viral from bacterial pharyngitis on the basis of symptoms and physical examination is difficult. The presenting symptom in pharyngitis is a complaint of sore throat and pain with swallowing. The pharynx and tonsils may be mildly irritated or fiery red and covered with a purulent exudate. Fever and cervical adenopathy are generally more pronounced in streptococcal pharyngitis.

Several clinical algorithms have been devised to improve the diagnostic accuracy of streptococcal pharyngitis. The most reliable predictors include tonsillar exudates, tender anterior cervical lymph nodes, history of fever, and absence of cough. The presence of three to four of these criteria has a sensitivity and specificity of approximately 75 percent (Graham, 2002).

Diagnostic Tests

Diagnosis of streptococcal pharyngitis is made on the basis of either a rapid antigen testing (RAT) or the standard throat culture. The advantage to the RAT is that results are available in five to seven minutes and treatment can begin immediately. Because RAT is less sensitive than a throat culture, it is recommended to perform a standard throat culture on children and adolescents in the event of a negative RAT (Bisno, Gerber, Gwaltney, Kaplan, & Schwartz, 2002). The disadvantages to using standard throat cultures are that they are unable to distinguish active infection from the carrier state and exhibit unpredictability between lab and user. In addition results are rarely available in time to decrease symptoms. Serum antibody testing has no role in diagnosis or treatment of acute infections of streptococcal pharyngitis.

Nursing Diagnoses

Based on the information gathered, examples of nursing diagnoses in the patient with pharyngitis may include the following:
- Acute pain
- Deficient fluid volume
- Deficient knowledge

Planning and Implementation

Viral pharyngitis is treated with analgesics, antipyretics, and supportive care. Warm liquids will ease throat discomfort. Patients are encouraged to rest during the acute phase of the illness. Antibiotics have no role in the treatment of viral infections and may add to the increase of antibiotic resistance in the general population.

Of those individuals that meet the criteria for GABHS, intramuscular benzathine penicillin G remains the antibiotic treatment of choice (Thomas & Powers, 2002). This one-time dosing can be given immediately, is less costly, and eliminates patient noncompliance with finishing the complete oral regimen. Oral penicillin V is administered two to three times daily for 10 days. Alternatives for an individual who is allergic to penicillin include erythromycin or a first-generation cephalosporin, such as cephalexin or cefadroxil. Erythromycin is not as widely used as in the past because of the patient must take it three to four times per day. In addition, it has a bad taste and uncomfortable gastrointestinal (GI) side effects, including nausea, vomiting, and diarrhea.

Shorter dosing patterns of azithromycin (Zithromax) and cefdinir (Omnicef) have been used successfully in treating streptococcal pharyngitis. These drugs are administered one to two times a day for five days, which greatly enhances patient compliance.

Nursing management includes instructing the patient about the importance of finishing all antibiotics to properly eradicate the infection and to reduce antibiotic resistance of the bacteria. Instructions should be provided on how to take acetaminophen (Tylenol) or ibuprofen (Advil) for symptomatic relief of fever and discomfort of sore throat. Other measures that can ease the pain of a viral or bacterial sore throat are presented in the Patient Playbook.

Patients should be instructed on signs and symptom that need to be reported to their health care provider. Hospitalization is rarely necessary unless hydration or airway management becomes compromised.

PATIENT PLAYBOOK

Easing Sore Throat Pain

You can teach your patient these simple, but effective interventions for easing the pain of a sore throat:
- Gargle with warm salt water (1 teaspoon of salt per 8 ounce glass of water).
- Suck on throat lozenges or hard candy.
- Suck on flavored frozen desserts, such as Popsicles.
- Use a humidifier in your bedroom or other rooms where you spend a lot of time
- Drink lots of liquids.

Evaluation of Outcomes

Potential patient outcomes for each of the example nursing diagnoses for the patient with acute pharyngitis are:
- Acute pain. The patient reports feeling more comfortable. Uses comfort measures such as analgesics, hot packs, gargles, and rest.
- Deficient fluid volume. The patient maintains adequate fluid intake.
- Deficient knowledge. The patient demonstrates an adequate level of knowledge and performs self-care appropriately.

TONSILLITIS AND ADENOIDITIS

Tonsils are masses of lymphoid tissue found in the back of the throat on either side of the oropharynx. Adenoids are high in the throat behind the nose and the roof of the mouth (AAO-HNS, 2004d). Because of their location, both tonsils and adenoids are prone to infection from viruses or bacteria that attempt to invade the lower respiratory system. Tonsillitis and adenoiditis refer to inflammation of these tissues. Infection of these tissues can be viral or bacterial. The most common bacteria to invade the tonsils and adenoids is GABHS (Figure 31-3).

Etiology

Tonsillitis caused by the *Streptococcus* species most commonly occurs in children between the ages of 5 to15, whereas viral infections are more common in younger children. It is rare for tonsillitis to occur in children under the age of 2 years. Nearly all the children in the United States experience at least one episode of tonsillitis. Recurrent tonsillitis is diagnosed when an individual has seven episodes in one calendar year, five infections in two consecutive years, or three infections each year for three years consecutively.

Assessment with Clinical Manifestations

The symptoms of tonsillitis include sore throat, fever, snoring, change in voice or loss of voice (laryngitis), and uncomfortable or painful swallowing. Enlarged adenoids may cause mouth breathing, noisy breathing during the day, snoring, recurrent ear infections, foul breath, and change in voice quality. Because of the location of the adenoids, inflammation may cause blockage of the nasal passages. Infection can travel into the eustachian tubes and cause acute otitis media with possible rupture of the eardrum and permanent hearing loss. Physical examination may reveal redder than normal tonsils, a white or yellow coating on the tonsils, and swollen, tender lymph nodes in the neck.

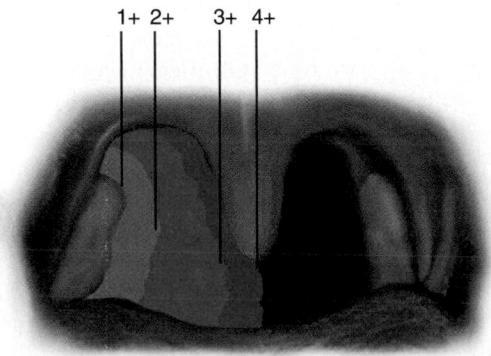

Figure 31-3 Grading of tonsils: 1+ tonsils are visible, 2+ tonsils are between the pillars of the uvula, 3+ tonsils are touching the uvula, 4+ one or both tonsils extend to the midline of the oropharynx.

Diagnostic Tests

Tonsils are cultured to determine if a bacterial infection is present. Serum mono spot, complete blood count (CBC), and serum electrolytes may be useful if systemic infection is suspected. If infection has spread into the neck region, radiologic films or a CT scan is indicated. In adenoiditis, if recurrent episodes of otitis media with effusion produce hearing loss, the patient should be referred for comprehensive audiometric testing.

Nursing Diagnoses

Based on the information gathered, examples of nursing diagnoses in the patient with tonsillitis and adenoiditis may include the following:
- Ineffective airway clearance
- Acute pain
- Deficient fluid volume
- Deficient knowledge

Planning and Implementation

Acute episodes of tonsillitis are treated as in pharyngitis with rest, fluids, warm liquids, and antibiotics if a bacterial organism is isolated. The most commonly used antibiotic is oral penicillin, which is taken for seven days. A short course of oral corticosteroids (three to five days duration) may help reduce the swelling of the tonsils or adenoids.

Surgery

Tonsillectomy is performed in cases of recurrent infection when treatment is unsuccessful, and there exists severe tonsillar hypertrophy. Adenoid tissue will be removed at the same time if it is also swollen and inflamed. Other indications for tonsillectomy include hearing loss secondary to frequent bouts of purulent serous otitis media, obstruction of the airway causing sleep apnea, severe dysphagia, and peritonsillar abscess. Although not performed as frequently as it once was, tonsillectomy is still among the most common surgical procedures performed on children in the United States (Drake & Carr, 2003).

Patients are treated with appropriate antibiotic therapy prior to surgery. The most common antibiotic used is oral penicillin, taken for seven days prior to surgery, or an intramuscular injection of Bicillin 100,000 units. Surgery is usually performed on an outpatient basis with the patient returning home the same day. In rare cases, such as severe bleeding or pain, the patient will remain in the hospital overnight for observation and pain control.

Priority nursing management of the patient recovering from a tonsillectomy or adenoidectomy includes monitoring for complications and providing pain relief. Appropriate nursing care requires continuous observation for signs of hemorrhage in the immediate postoperative period. Signs of postoperative bleeding include a drop in blood pressure, rapid pulse, emesis of blood, and pallor.

Pain can be managed both by nonpharmacological and pharmacological interventions. Nonpharmacological interventions include positioning the patient for comfort, usually in the prone position with the head turned to the side or the lateral position. Both of these positions allow for drainage of oral secretions until the patient is fully conscious and the gag and swallowing reflexes have returned. An ice collar is applied to the neck, and a basin and tissues provide the patient with a means to expectorate secretions. Once the patient is a fully awake, ice chip or sips of cool liquids can provide soothing relief of throat discomfort. Medicinal pain relief is most often achieved with acetaminophen (Tylenol) with or without codeine.

Because tonsillectomy is most often performed on an outpatient basis, it is important for the nurse to provide the patient and family with instructions for self-care and the understanding of the signs and symptoms of hemorrhage that must be reported to the health care provider. Postoperative bleeding occurs in 2 to 4 percent of cases within the first 12 to 24 hours after surgery. Much more common than immediate postoperative bleeding is secondary bleeding which can occur five to eight days postoperatively (Tierney, McPhee, & Papadakis, 2004). The patient is instructed to report frank bleeding. Other symptoms that should be reported to the health care provider includes: extreme nausea and vomiting, fever greater than 38.5°C (101.3°F), excessive swallowing or coughing, or pain not relieved by medication.

The patient should be instructed to maintain good hydration, start with soft foods for the first few days, take antibiotics as instructed, avoid smoking, and avoid heavy lifting for 10 days (Drake & Carr, 2003). Warm saline solutions instilled into the oral cavity may help with thick secretions but the patient should be warned against gargling because of the risk of hemorrhage at the surgical site.

Evaluation of Outcomes

Potential patient outcomes for each of the example nursing diagnoses for the patient with tonsillitis and adenoiditis are:
- Ineffective airway clearance. The patient maintains a patent airway by managing secretions.
- Acute pain. The patient reports feeling more comfortable. Uses comfort measures such as analgesics, hot packs, gargles, and rest.
- Deficient fluid volume The patient maintains adequate fluid intake.
- Deficient knowledge. The patient demonstrates an adequate level of knowledge and performs self-care appropriately.

PERITONSILLAR ABSCESS

A peritonsillar abscess (PTA), also known as quinsy, is a localized accumulation of pus in the peritonsillar tissues that forms as a result of suppurative tonsillitis (Gosselin, 2004). This complication of acute tonsillitis is more common in teenagers and young adults. Highest incidence is in the 15- to 35-year age-group (Gosselin, 2004).

Assessment with Clinical Manifestations

Common manifestations are sore throat, painful swallowing (dysphagia), fever, torticollis, and trismus (difficulty fully opening the mouth). The patient may also complain of severe headache, neck pain, or ear pain, and demonstrate a plumy or "hot potato" voice (Kazzi & Sheeks, 2004). Dehydration may be present because of the patient's reluctance to swallow food or fluids secondary to pain.

Physical examination reveals a displaced tonsil toward the center of the throat by the abscess, the soft palate is erythematous and swollen, and the uvula is edematous and displaced to the opposite side (Beers & Berkow, 2004).

Complications of PTA include recurrent tonsillitis or abscess, airway obstruction, aspiration pneumonia, or pneumonitis

Diagnostic Tests

Needle aspiration is performed to make the appropriate diagnosis. Aspirate is sent for Gram stain and culture. Most aspirates reveal a mix of aerobic and anaerobic organisms. The most common aerobic organism is *S. pyogenes,* which is reported in 30 percent of patients (Kazzi & Sheeks, 2004). A CT scan may be done if the patient cannot open his or her mouth. No radiographic studies are indicated.

Nursing Diagnoses

Based on the information gathered, examples of nursing diagnoses in the patient with a peritonsillar abscess may include the following:

- Ineffective airway clearance
- Acute pain
- Deficient fluid volume
- Deficient knowledge

Planning and Implementation

Because of streptococcal resistance of more than 30 percent and infection with mixed bacterial flora, many practitioners recommend combination therapy of a penicillin and metronidazole (Flagyl) (Kazzi & Sheeks, 2004). A short course of corticosteroids may be helpful in reducing edema and inflammation.

Surgery

Incision and drainage (I&D) was formerly the treatment of choice. However, it has fallen out of favor because of the risk of aspiration of purulent material and bleeding. Needle aspiration of the purulent material offers less risk to the patient, faster recovery, and results in resolution of the abscess in 90 to 95 percent of cases (Kazzi & Sheeks, 2004). Emergent tonsillectomy has not been shown to be desirable because of the increased risk of bleeding and higher cost of the procedure compared with more conservative and equally effective treatments (Kazzi & Sheeks, 2004). However, with repeated episodes of peritonsillar abscess, tonsillectomy three to four weeks after the disappearance of swelling and symptoms is the recommended treatment of choice (Tierney, et al., 2004).

Palliative relief can be obtained by offering the patient frequent sips of cool liquids, mouthwashes or gargles, mouth irrigations, or topical anesthetics. The nurse needs to remind the patient to perform irrigations or gargles every 1 to 2 hours for 24 to 36 hours.

Evaluation of Outcomes

Potential patient outcomes for each of the example nursing diagnoses for the patient with peritonsillar abscess are:

- Ineffective airway clearance. The patient maintains a patent airway by managing secretion.
- Acute pain. The patient reports feeling more comfortable. Uses comfort measures such as analgesics, hot packs, gargles, and rest.
- Deficient fluid volume. The patient maintains adequate fluid intake.
- Deficient knowledge. The patient demonstrates an adequate level of knowledge and performs self-care appropriately.

ACUTE AND CHRONIC LARYNGITIS

Laryngitis, an inflammation of the larynx, occurs as a result of infection and is classified as acute or chronic. Acute laryngitis has an abrupt onset and is self-limiting. If symptoms persist for more than three weeks, the laryngitis is classified as chronic.

Pathophysiology

The acute form of laryngitis is a result of voice misuse, environmental pollutants, or exposure to noxious agents. Infectious agents are most often viral with an occasional bacterial component. It may also occur as part of a common cold, bronchitis, flu, or pneumonia.

Chronic laryngitis takes longer to develop, and the duration is therefore longer. Chronic laryngitis may be caused by environmental factors, such as inhalation of cigarette smoke or polluted air (i.e., gaseous chemicals), irritation from asthma inhalers, vocal misuse (i.e., prolonged vocal use at abnormal loudness or pitch), or GI esophageal reflux (Shah & Shapshay, 2003).

Assessment with Clinical Manifestations

The underlying inflammation of the larynx produces a hoarseness or dysphonia (complete loss of voice) and severe cough. Symptoms usually last for 7 to 10 days. If symptoms persist for more than three weeks, a workup for chronic laryngitis should be undertaken. The patient may manifest symptoms of URI including sore throat, rhinorrhea, fever, congestion, postnasal discharge, fatigue, and malaise.

Planning and Implementation

If the laryngitis is part of a bacterial infection, antibiotics are started. The same antibiotics that are used to treat pharyngitis and sinusitis are used in treating laryngitis. Again, the increasing resistance of organisms to older antibiotics must be taken into consideration when choosing appropriate therapy. Prevailing evidence does not support the use of decongestants, antihistamines, or steroids. These agents may aggravate the symptoms because of their drying effect on the mucous membranes.

In cases where laryngitis is caused by an underlying disease process, such as asthma or gastroesophageal reflux, the health care provider must aim treatment at the underlying cause.

The nurse should reinforce the importance of voice rest, cessation of smoking, avoidance of environmental irritants, and rest. The nurse can suggest that patients increase their intake of cool liquids and use a humidifier or vaporizer to thin secretions and soothe the airway.

OBSTRUCTION DURING SLEEP

According to the American Sleep Apnea Association (ASAA), sleep apnea affects approximately 12 million Americans, most of whom are undiagnosed. The Greek word *apnea* literally means "without breath." People with sleep apnea may experience hundreds of episodes a night lasting from 10 seconds to over a minute with each episode (ASAA, 2004).

Etiology

Obstructive sleep apnea is more prevalent in men than women and in obese individuals (Rowley & Lorenzo, 2004). Although it has been diagnosed in children, obstructive sleep apnea is most often diagnosed in the third through sixth decades of life. Prevalence in the young African American population (less than 25 years of age) is greater than in the young Caucasian population (Rowley & Lorenzo, 2004). Obstructive sleep apnea tends to be more severe in the African American population as well (Rowley & Lorenzo, 2004). Risk factors include a family history of sleep apnea, hypothyroidism, recessed chin, large neck, cigarette smoking, and alcohol or sedative use.

Pathophysiology

There are three types of sleep apnea: obstructive, central, and mixed. Obstructive sleep apnea (OSA) is the most common type and involves the upper respiratory tract. With obstructive sleep apnea, obstruction of the airway occurs at either the soft palate (nasopharynx) or at the level of the tongue (oropharynx) (Rowley &

Lorenzo, 2004). In central sleep apnea, the brain fails to trigger the muscles of respiration. Mixed sleep apnea is a combination of these two types. Blood oxygen levels drop with each apneic episode in all types of sleep apnea.

Complications

Without treatment, individuals with OSA are at risk for severe and life-threatening complications of the heart and lungs. Secondary health problems include hypertension, dysrhythmias, myocardial infarction, stroke, **hypoxia** (reduced oxygen content or tension), and hypercapnia (abnormally increased arterial carbon dioxide tension), pulmonary hypertension, or **cor pulmonale** (hypertrophy or failure of the right ventricle resulting from disorders of the lungs, pulmonary vessels, or chest wall). It has been estimated that up to 50 percent of people with sleep apnea have hypertension (National Sleep Foundation, 2004). OSA can cause job-related and motor vehicle accidents.

Assessment with Clinical Manifestations

Physical examination of the individual with OSA may reveal the presence of a narrowed oropharynx, enlarged tonsils or uvula, or prominent tongue. Nasal obstruction by a deviated septum may be present (Tierney, et al., 2004).

During episodes of apnea, loud snoring or snorting is present. Bed partners are typically the ones to report this sign, because the affected individual is unaware of the snoring and may deny its existence. Other symptoms frequently reported are morning headaches, daytime **somnolence** (prolonged drowsiness or sleepiness), memory problems, personality changes, gastric reflux, sore throat, impotence, and fatigue.

Diagnostic Tests

Lab studies include a CBC, arterial blood gases (ABGs), and a thyroid stimulating hormone (TSH) level. Polysomnography is used to diagnose OSA. This test involves observation and measurement of the patient during sleep. The sleep technician performing the test monitors the patient's respiratory rate and effort, heart rate, airflow, blood oxygen levels, brain activity, eye movement, and muscle activity. The test may be performed either in the hospital setting or a sleep center.

Nursing Diagnoses

Based on the information gathered, examples of nursing diagnoses in the patient with obstruction or trauma to the upper airway may include the following:
- Ineffective airway clearance
- Ineffective breathing pattern
- Acute pain
- Deficient knowledge

Planning and Implementation

Patients usually seek treatment at the insistence of their partners because of loud snoring or excessive or inappropriate sleepiness. Several treatments exist based on the severity of the sleep apnea.

Obese individuals are encouraged to lose weight by dieting and physical exercise programs. Refraining from alcohol and sedatives is a vital aspect of treatment. Some individuals may need to change their sleep position to avoid lying on the back.

The standard treatment for OSA in a patient whose main symptoms are snoring with daytime somnolence is continuous positive airway pressure (CPAP) via nasal cannula or mask. This can be provided to the patient with or without supplemental oxygen. This treatment administers air or oxygen under pressure to prevent the soft tissues in the upper airway from collapsing during sleep (National Sleep Foundation, 2004).

Surgery

In severe instances of OSA, surgery may be needed to remove excess tissue or correct anatomical malformations. Tonsillectomy or uvulopalatopharyngoplasty (resection of the uvula and soft palate) may be indicated for individuals with enlargement of these tissues. Cranial reconstruction may be performed to correct malformations. **Tracheostomy** (operation of cutting into the trachea usually for insertion of a tube to overcome tracheal obstruction) provides definitive correction, because it bypasses the obstruction. This should be reserved for individuals with severe OSA or those that cannot tolerate CPAP therapy.

Nurses are instrumental in providing support to the patient by encouraging successful weight loss, a medically approved diet (such as the dietary approaches to stop hypertension [DASH] diet), and cessation of smoking and alcohol consumption. Teaching the patient and family how to manage CPAP or what to expect from surgical procedures requires collaboration by the nurse and the respiratory therapist.

Evaluation of Outcomes

Potential interventions and patient outcomes for each of the example nursing diagnoses for the patient with obstruction or upper airway trauma may include the following:

- Ineffective airway clearance. The patient will resume normal respiratory status ventilation and gas exchange.
- Acute pain. The patient will control comfort level, pain control, anxiety level.
- Deficient knowledge. The patient will participate in activities that are health promoting and illness preventing.

EPISTAXIS

Epistaxis is defined as an acute hemorrhage from the nasal cavity, nostrils, or nasopharynx (Rothenhaus, 2003). It is a frequent emergency department complaint that can most often be treated on an outpatient basis.

Epistaxis is classified on the basis of the primary bleeding site as anterior or posterior. Hemorrhage is most commonly anterior, originating from the nasal septum. A common source of anterior epistaxis is Kiesselbach plexus, a network of vessels on the anterior portion of the septum just superior to the posterior end of the nasal vestibule. Posterior hemorrhage originates in the posterior nasal cavity or nasopharynx, usually below the posterior half of the inferior turbinate or roof of the nasal cavity (Rothenhaus, 2003).

Etiology

The most common cause of nosebleeds is dryness or picking of the nose. Other causes include URIs, such as rhinitis and sinusitis, allergies, facial trauma, foreign body obstruction, nasal tumors or polyps, blood **dyscrasia** (nonspecific term for blood disease), vascular abnormalities, hypertension, and inhalation of illicit drugs, such as cocaine.

Planning and Implementation

Management of nosebleeds depends on the location of the bleeding site. A nasal speculum is used to access the location of the bleeding. For nosebleeds originating from the anterior portion of the nose, direct pressure may be the only treatment that is needed. The patient is shown how to lean forward slightly while pinching the soft outer portion of the nose against the nasal septum for about 5 to 10 minutes continuously. If this proves unsuccessful, additional treatment is indicted. If the source of bleeding can be visualized, an application of silver nitrate may help to stop the bleeding. Cotton pledgets soaked in 4% topical cocaine solution or a solution of 4% lidocaine and topical epinephrine (1:10,000) can be placed into the nasal cavity (Rothenhaus, 2003). They should remain in place for 10 to 15 minutes.

If bleeding is occurring from the posterior portion of the nasal cavity, packing must be used to stop the bleeding. Commonly used treatments include traditional nasal packing, nasal tampons or balloons, or prefabricated nasal sponges (Rothenhaus, 2003). Nasal packing may be left in place for two to five days. Oral antibiotics and analgesics may be prescribed.

Nurses should educate patients on how to prevent and treat nosebleeds. Children and adults should be taught the importance of not picking their nose. Petroleum jelly (Vaseline) can be used to lubricate the nares and prevent dryness. Humidifiers can be used at night to keep mucous membranes moist. Cigarette smokers are discouraged from exhaling smoke through their nares. Patients who experience frequent nosebleeds should be advised not to blow their nose forcefully, to avoid bending over or straining, and stay away from high altitudes. After control of epistaxis, a patient should avoid strenuous exercise for several days. Hot or spicy foods may cause vasodilation of the blood vessels, precipitating another episode of epistaxis. If recurrent epistaxis cannot be controlled within 15 minutes, the patient should be instructed to seek medical advice.

FRACTURES OF THE NOSE

The location of the nose makes it particularly susceptible to fracture. It is the most commonly broken bone in the human body. If a broken nose is left untreated, it can result in unfavorable appearance and function (Smith & Perez, 2004). Fractures of the nose should be suspected with any blunt trauma to the face.

Assessment with Clinical Manifestations

Bleeding and pain are the most common findings with a fracture of the nose. Soft tissue **hematomas** (swelling noted in tissue caused by extravasated blood) or a black eye may also be seen (Tierney, et al., 2004). Palpating the dorsum (bridge) of the nose for deformity, instability, crepitus, and point tenderness confirm the diagnosis (Beers & Berkow, 2004) X-rays may be needed to confirm the diagnosis and rule out involvement of other structures of the face.

Planning and Implementation

Controlling the bleeding and preventing excessive swelling are priorities with fractures of the nose. Ice packs or cold compresses can be applied to the nose. The nose is assessed for symmetry. Referral for surgical correction may be necessary.

The patient who experiences a fracture of the nose because of injury may be frightened or anxious. The nurse can help allay anxiety by explaining procedures. Applying ice packs to the nose and giving analgesics help reduce swelling and pain. The nose is often packed to stop the bleeding, forcing the patient to breathe through the mouth. Oral rinses can help reduce mouth dryness and remove dried blood.

NASAL OBSTRUCTION

Obstruction of the nose can be from nonanatomic or anatomic causes. Nonanatomic causes include chronic sinusitis, allergies, overuse of nasal sprays (rhinitis medicamentosa), birth control pills, hypertension, and, thyroid abnormality. Common anatomical causes include a deviated septum, nasal

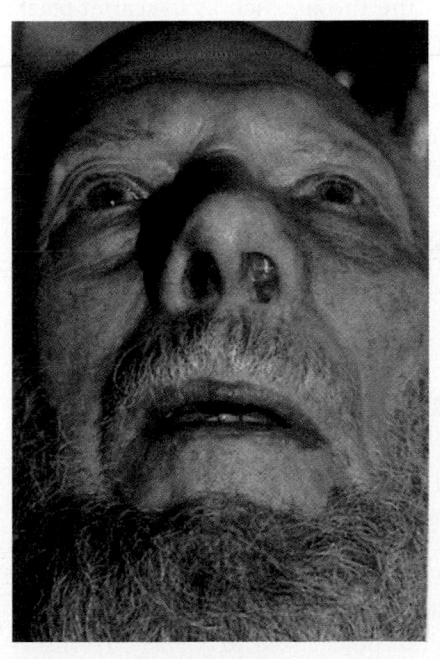

Figure 31-4 Nasal polyp.

polyps, enlarged adenoids, nasal foreign body, and **hypertrophic** nasal turbinates. Hypertrophic refers to an increase in size of an organ or structure secondary to inflammation or overgrowth of cells which is not related to tumor formation (Figure 31-4).

Planning and Implementation

The treatment of nasal obstruction requires removal of the obstruction. With nonanatomical obstructions, treatment of the underlying cause usually relieves the resistance to airflow.

If the patient has a deviated nasal septum, surgery is indicated to reshape the cartilage or bone. This operation is called a septoplasty or submucous resection (Watson & Rivkin, 2004).

Nasal polyps are grape-like, inflammatory swellings of the nasal and sinus linings. Polyps are treated initially with a short course of corticosteroids to determine if any shrinkage has occurred. If satisfactory shrinkage has not occurred or the patient does not obtain adequate relief, a polypectomy is performed. Most patients obtain improvement in their breathing after removal of the polyps, but they should be aware that polyps could reoccur.

Hypertrophied turbinates may also cause nasal obstruction. Depending on the severity of the swelling, the health care provider preference, and the impact on the patient's well-being, hypertrophied turbinates may be injected with steroids, cauterized, lasered, or trimmed.

Rarely is an individual hospitalized for nasal obstruction. Surgery can be performed on an outpatient basis. Nursing care includes managing postoperative pain, elevating the head of the bed to maintain a patent airway and reduce airway swelling. Frequent oral hygiene helps to overcome the dryness experienced from breathing through the nose.

LARYNGEAL OBSTRUCTION

Obstruction of the larynx may occur with an acute infectious process, such as in laryngitis, anaphylaxis, or with aspiration of a foreign body. No matter what the cause, obstruction can be serious and often fatal. Swelling of the mucous membranes within the larynx can close off the opening and lead to suffocation. Swelling of the larynx rarely occurs with acute laryngitis but is more often seen with epiglottitis and inflammation of the throat, such as in scarlet fever. In cases of a severe allergic reaction (anaphylaxis), the edema can close of the airway, leading to death if not reversed.

Aspiration of a foreign body causes a twofold problem. First, it obstructs the airways and makes breathing difficult. Later, the object can enter the bronchus and lead to irritation within the lower airways. If aspiration of a foreign body only partially obstructs the airway, it may go undetected producing a myriad of symptoms, such as cough, wheeze, **stridor** (a high-pitched, harsh sound during inspiration, caused by swelling or obstruction of the larynx), dyspnea, or cyanosis. Continuous irritation from the object may lead to edema and further obstruction.

Planning and Implementation

A bronchoscopy may be performed to visualize and extract the aspirated object. If unsuccessful, surgical removal is necessary. In cases of laryngeal edema, epinephrine or steroids are used to decrease the swelling and improve respiratory effort. An ice pack applied to the neck area may also alleviate the swelling.

In cases of aspiration of a foreign body into the larynx or trachea, the abdominal thrust is used to attempt to dislodge the object (see Red Flag). If unsuccessful, an emergency tracheostomy is performed to establish a patent airway.

Red Flag

Abdominal Thrusts: Technique for Relieving an Obstructed Airway

When a patient is choking on a foreign body, the abdominal thrust (also called the Heimlich maneuver) is used to relieve the obstruction. The nurse or other trained provider may institute these steps:

1. Stand behind the person who is choking.
2. Wrap both arms around the person's waist.
3. Place one fist, thumb side, against the person's abdomen, just above the umbilicus.
4. Grasp the fist with the other hand.
5. Deliver quick, upward thrusts with the fist against the abdomen, placing pressure against the diaphragm.
6. Continue until the object is expelled or the person becomes unconscious.
7. If the person is obese or pregnant, perform chest thrusts in the same manner.

These maneuvers help to lift the diaphragm and force enough air from the lungs to create an artificial cough. The cough is intended to move the object up into the mouth for expulsion. Each thrust should be given with the intent of dislodging the object.

If obstruction cannot be relieved, an emergency tracheostomy must be performed to bypass obstruction and restore oxygenation to organs and tissue.

CANCER OF THE LARYNX

Cancer of the larynx can occur in any of the three areas of the larynx: the supraglottic area (above glottis or vocal cords, includes the epiglottis, and false vocal cords), the glottic area (includes the true vocal cords and anterior and posterior commissures), and the subglottic area (below the glottis and extends to the lower border of the cricoid cartilage to the first tracheal ring) (National Cancer Institute, 2003b). The true vocal cords and the epiglottis are the most common sites for laryngeal cancer and account for greater than 95 percent of all laryngeal cancers (National Cancer Institute, 2003c). Laryngeal cancer makes up 1 to 2 percent of all malignancies worldwide. The incidence of the disease varies greatly from country to country. Spain has one of the highest rates in the world, with an incidence approaching 20 cases per 100,000 persons in some regions. Poland, France, and Italy also have high rates of the disease (Snyder & Lydiatt, 2003). Laryngeal cancer in the glottic and subglottic areas has a greater cure rate if detected early, because there is little lymphatic drainage in this area. Supraglottic cancers, however, tend to produce few symptoms and because of their rich lymph drainage, metastasis is common on diagnosis. Subglottic cancers account for only about 1 percent of all laryngeal cancers (Figure 31-5).

Epidemiology

The American Cancer Society (2003) estimates that in 2004, about 10,270 people in the United States will be found to have laryngeal cancer, and about 3,830 will die of this disease. The incidence is four times greater in men than in women. However, even though the incidence of laryngeal cancer is declining, it is on the rise for women. Most cancers of the larynx arise in the fifth and sixth decades of life (Saver, Demetroulakos, Groves, Millman & Mugge, 2004).

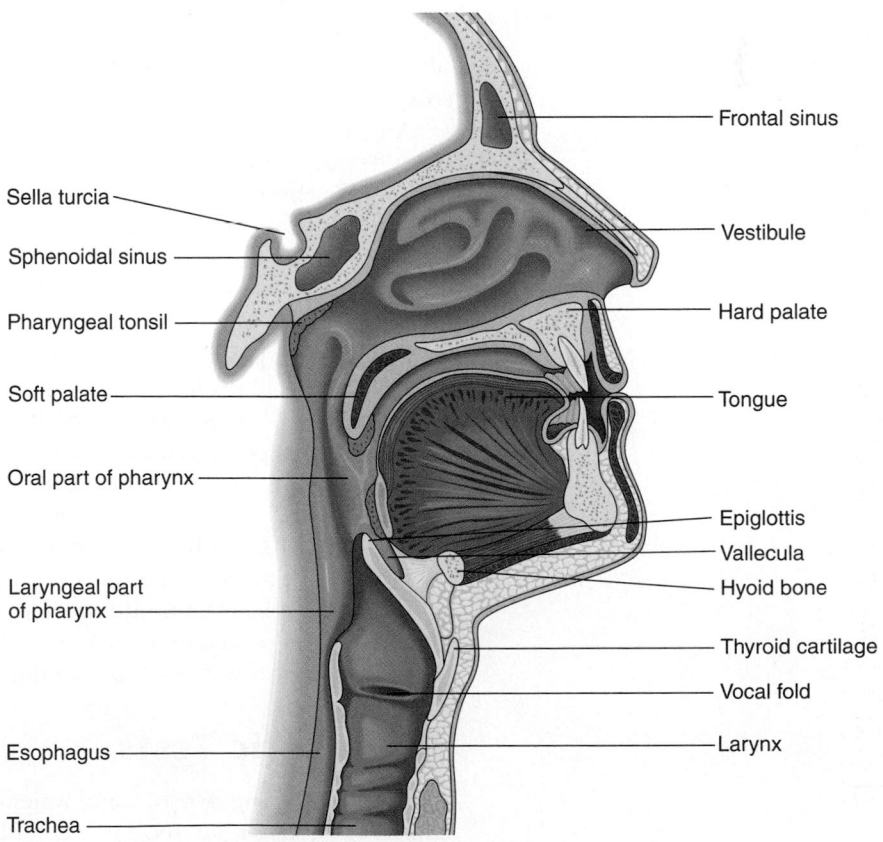

Figure 31-5 Sagittal section of the upper airway.

The incidence of laryngeal cancer is greater in African Americans than in Caucasians.

Etiology

A clear association has been made between smoking, excess alcohol ingestion, and the development of laryngeal cancer. A direct correlation exists between the amount of smoking and the chance of developing laryngeal cancer. Alcohol has been found to be a synergistic agent with smoking, increasing the risk 100-fold over individuals who are nonsmokers and nondrinkers (Snyder & Lydiatt, 2003). Other carcinogens associated with the risk of laryngeal cancer include exposure to wood dust, paint fumes, mustard gas, tar products, leather, asbestos, and metals. Other contributing factors in the development of laryngeal cancer include a weak immune system (such as in acquired immune deficiency syndrome [AIDS]), human papillomavirus (HPV), nutritional deficiencies (such as vitamins B and A and retinoids), and gastroesophageal reflux disease (GERD) (Saver, Demetroulakos, et al., 2004).

Assessment with Clinical Manifestations

Cancer of the vocal cords (glottis) is often found at an early stage because the patient complains of hoarseness. A health care provider should evaluate hoarseness that persists longer than two weeks, especially in individuals who are at high risk for laryngeal cancer. Tumor impingement on the vocal cords prevents vocal cord vibration, changes the quality of speech, and may affect speech production. The voice may become raspy, harsh, or lower in pitch and volume. Cancers arising in the supraglottic or subglottic areas are typically diagnosed at later stages because of the vagueness of symptoms. The patient may complain of a sore throat, cough, pain, or difficulty swallowing (Saver, Demetroulakos, et al., 2004). Hoarseness usually occurs only after these tumors have locally extended to the vocal cords or surrounding tissue. A lump or mass in the neck region may be present. As the tumor grows, the patient may experience persistent ear pain, dyspnea, dysphagia, **odynophagia** (severe pain on swallowing because of a disorder of the esophagus), weight loss, halitosis, frequent choking on food, or **hemoptysis** (expectoration of blood arising from the larynx, trachea, bronchus, or lung).

An initial assessment of the patient with suspected cancer of the larynx includes a complete history and careful assessment of the head and neck. This includes gathering information about the onset of symptoms, risk factors, family history, and coexisting medical conditions.

Direct questions that should be asked of a patient who presents with complaints of hoarseness should include:
- Is your voice hoarse?
- Is it hard or painful to swallow?
- Does it feel like a lump is in your throat?
- Does your neck or throat hurt? Where is the discomfort?
- Have you been coughing up blood or have you lost weight?
- Do you have an earache? Where else does it hurt?
- Do you smoke? How much per day?
- Do you drink alcohol? How much per day?
- How long have you had the symptoms?
- What previous treatment have you had?
- What is you occupation (to assess for environmental exposure to chemicals)?
- Have you ever noticed food coming back up into your throat (e.g., GERD)?

Diagnostic Tests

An indirect laryngoscopy, using a flexible or rigid endoscope, allows for visualization of the pharynx, larynx, and surrounding tissues. Mobilization, or movement, of the vocal cords is assessed. Failure to visualize any structure, changes in or lack of movement of the vocal cords, or any suspicious finding requires additional diagnostic procedures.

If a tumor is suspected, a direct laryngoscopy is performed. This procedure is performed with the patient under general anesthesia by an otolaryngologist or head and neck surgeon. This procedure allows for improved visualization of the entire larynx and surrounding structures for masses, mucosal irregularities, and asymmetry. A biopsy of suspicious tissue may be collected for histological evaluation. CT and MRI scans are useful to determine the extent of the tumor and soft tissue or lymph node involvement.

Squamous cell carcinoma is the most common malignancy in the larynx, accounting for more than 95 percent of all cases (Saver, Demetroulakos, et al., 2004). The staging system, developed by the American Joint Committee on Cancer, is the widely accepted method for classification of tumors or the head and neck. See Box 31-2 for the classification. This system classifies tumors based on location, lymph node involvement, and distance metastasis. It usefulness is in determining which treatment modalities will yield the best outcome for the patient.

Nursing Diagnoses

Based on the information gathered, examples of nursing diagnoses in the patient with cancer of the larynx may include the following:
- Ineffective airway clearance
- Impaired verbal communication
- Imbalanced nutrition, less than body requirements
- Risk for infection
- Risk for ineffective sexual patterns
- Risk for self-care deficit

Planning and Implementation

Treatment of laryngeal cancer depends on the staging of the tumor, which involves the location, size, and histology of the tumor, and the presence and extent of lymph node involvement. Prognosis depends on the size of the tumor, the location, and the degree of metastasis. Prognosis for small laryngeal cancers that have not spread to lymph nodes is good, with cure rates of 75 to 95 percent. Randomized, prospective trials have yet to demonstrate a benefit in either disease-free or overall survival for patients receiving chemotherapy (Saver, Demetroulakos, et al., 2004).

Evidence supports the use of endoscopic transoral laser surgery for tumor stage I glottic cancer (Saver, Demetroulakos, et al., 2004). It has also been used successfully to help with the symptoms of bleeding or obstruction when other therapies have failed or the tumor cannot be cured. During this procedure, an endoscope is inserted via the mouth to allow the surgeon to visualize the tumor. The tumor is then removed or diminished in size by a CO_2 laser. This procedure is less invasive than conventional surgery with most patients spending only a day in the hospital. Recovery time is shortened and speech is well-preserved.

Radiation can be used in laryngeal cancer to eradicate the tumor, preserve function, control local or distant spread of the tumor, and prevent metastasis. Most tumors that are stage I and II can be cured by radiation. Radiation alone is successful in treating 80 to 90 percent of patients with stage I laryngeal cancer and 70 to 80 percent of stage II patients (American Cancer Society, 2003). However, this cure rate varies depending on the location of the tumor. Radiation in combination with chemotherapy is often used for tumors of stages III and IV. Radiation can also be used in patients whose overall health status prevents the use of more invasive therapy. Radiation aids in shrinking tumors preoperatively before surgery. It can be beneficial in helping to control symptoms, such as bleeding, pain, or difficulty swallowing (American Cancer Society, 2003).

BOX 31-2

STAGING SYSTEM FOR CANCER OF THE LARYNX-TUMOR-NODE-METASTASIS (TNM)

According to the staging system, a tumor is graded on factors related to the location of the primary tumor and assigned a value ranging from T1 to T4. Depending on whether or not there is evidence of cancer spread to the lymph nodes of the neck (regional metastases), the cancer is staged N0 to N2. Distant metastatic spread of the cancer to other organs can occur, most commonly to the lungs, liver, and bone. If there are distant metastases present the patient is staged M1; if not, the stage is M0.

Laryngeal Cancer T staging

Glottic Cancers
- T1a: Tumor is confined to one vocal cord with normal mobility
- T1b: Tumor involves both vocal cords but mobility is normal
- T2: Extension of the tumor from the vocal cords to the supraglottic or subglottic larynx or impaired vocal cord mobility
- T3: Tumor is confined to the larynx but there is fixation of the vocal cord
- T4: There is invasion through thyroid cartilage and/or other tissues beyond larynx (e.g., trachea, thyroid, pharynx, and soft tissue of neck)

Supraglottic Cancers
- T1: Tumor is confined to one subsite of the supraglottic larynx and there is normal vocal cord mobility
- T2: Tumor invades mucosa of more than one adjacent subsite of supraglottis but vocal cord mobility remains normal
- T3: Tumor is limited to the larynx with vocal cord fixation and/or extension to postcricoid area or preepiglottic tissues
- T4: Tumor invades through thyroid cartilage, and/or extends into soft tissues of the neck, thyroid, or esophagus

Staging of Regional Metastases is as Follows

- N0: No evidence of regional metastases to cervical lymph nodes
- N1: Single neck node up to 3 cm in greatest dimension
- N2: Single node greater than 3 cm (but less than 6 cm), or multiple lymph nodes
- N3: Any node greater than 6 cm in greatest dimension

The Stage Is Then Assigned According to the Following Scheme

TNM Stage
- T1 N0 M0 I
- T2 N0 M0 II
- T3 N0 M0 III
- T1-3 N1 M0 III
- T4, N0-N1 M0 IVA
- T1-4, N2 M0 IVA
- T1-4, N3 M0 IVB
- T1-4, N0-3, M1 IVC

In general, the more advanced the overall stage the worse the prognosis. Prognosis is best for those who have no regional metastases (N0) and worst for those who have distant metastases (M1). Cancers of the supraglottic larynx are more likely to have regional neck metastases than are cancers of the glottic larynx.

Side effects from radiation are the result of external radiation to the head and neck. The parotid glands are particularly sensitive to radiation and respond by decreasing mucous production. Patients often experience **mucositis** (inflammation of a mucous membrane), ulceration of the mucous membranes, **xerostomia** (dry mouth), decreased sense of taste, dysphagia, sore throat, fatigue, and skin irritations.

Goals

The goal for the patient with a total laryngectomy is to learn to communicate by using an **alaryngeal voice** (alternative methods of speaking that does not include the larynx; method used by patients who have their larynx removed). Success of voice restoration depends on patient motivation, expectation, and the support network. The extent of the tumor and postoperative complications will affect the quality of speech (Carding, Welch, Owen, & Stafford, 2001). Three methods of voice restoration are available: esophageal speech, tracheoesophageal speech production, and the artificial speech aid or electrolarynx. No matter which method is chosen, the patient needs reassurance that perfecting alaryngeal communication takes time and practice.

Esophageal speech involves the patient being able to take air into the mouth and swallow or force the air into the esophagus by locking the tongue to the roof of the mouth (American Cancer Society, 2003). Forcing the air into the esophagus causes the walls of the esophagus and pharynx, as well as the returning air, to vibrate, producing a low-pitched sound. The tongue, lips, and mouth then form this sound into words. The advantage to this method is that the sound is more normal than speech produced by mechanical devices. It is less costly than other methods, because there is no equipment to buy. A disadvantage to this method it that it is more difficult to learn than speech produced with special devices, and it may be harder to understand. It is important to remind the patient that it can take months to perfect this form of artificial speech.

Tracheoesophageal speech is similar to esophageal speech, but a valve is placed in the tracheal stoma to divert the air into the esophagus. The procedure is called a tracheoesophageal puncture (TEP) and may be performed at the same time as the laryngectomy. The procedure creates an opening between the trachea and the esophagus. A one-way valve is inserted into the stoma and allows air to pass from the trachea into the esophagus, while preventing food from entering the trachea. To produce speech, the patient covers the opening and forces the air into the esophagus and out of the mouth. This allows the patient to produce sound in the same way as esophageal speech, but the sound produced is much more like natural speech. Tracheoesophageal speech is successful in 80 to 90 percent of patients and is a widely accepted form of alaryngeal communication, because it is fairly easy to learn.

Mechanical speech may be used while the patient is learning esophageal speech or tracheoesophageal speech or if the patient has been unsuccessful at either of these methods. Speech production occurs by means of a mechanical device that is powered by batteries (electrolarynx) or by air (pneumatic larynx). The electrolarynx is a handheld device, that when placed against the neck, causes sound to travel through the neck into the mouth. A pneumatic larynx is held over the stoma and uses air instead of batteries to make it vibrate. The sound travels to the mouth through a plastic tube. Both methods produce a mechanical sounding voice that may be difficult to understand. The advantage to mechanical speech is that communication is relatively easy.

Surgery

Surgery, once the mainstay of treatment for cancer of the larynx, is now reserved for advanced tumors with infiltration to the surrounding tissue or for tumors that have not been successfully treated with chemotherapy or radiation

(Ferlito, et al., 2000). The surgical procedure varies depending on tumor size, location, spread to the lymph system, or whether metastasis has occurred. A multidisciplinary team approach that involves health care providers, nurses, speech pathologist, dietitian, and psychologist are necessary to help the patient deal with the multitude of lifestyle changes that accompany surgery. Depending on the location and staging of the tumor, four types of laryngectomy are considered.

Partial laryngectomy is recommended in the early stages of glottic cancer when only one of the vocal cords is involved. It is often performed when radiation therapy alone fails to reduce or remove the entire tumor. Because only part of the larynx and only one vocal cord is removed, speech is preserved. The voice may change, and the patient may experience some degree of permanent hoarseness.

Supraglottic laryngectomy involves the removal of the hyoid bone, glottis, and false vocal cords. The true vocal cords, cricoid cartilage, and trachea remain intact. This surgery is required to manage stage I and stage II supraglottic tumors. During surgery, a radical neck dissection is performed with removal of the involved lymph nodes. The patient requires a tracheostomy tube until a stable airway can be maintained. The advantage of this procedure is that speech is preserved, because the true vocal cords are not removed. However, the quality of the patient's voice may change. Swallowing is grossly impaired and will require postoperative rehabilitation.

Hemilaryngectomy is performed if the tumor involves only one of the true vocal cords but is limited to the subglottic area. The one true vocal cord and one false vocal cord on the affected side are removed. The thyroid tissue on the affected side is also removed. The patient will require a tracheostomy tube and a nasogastric tube for 10 to 14 days postoperatively, until a stable airway can be maintained. The patient is at risk for aspiration following surgery. Speech is preserved, but patients may notice changes in their voice, such as hoarseness, roughness, or decreased force of speech. Again, swallowing will be impaired and require postoperative rehabilitation.

With invasive or infiltrating tumors such as those of stage III or VI, the entire larynx is often removed. Tumors in these stages have extended beyond the border of the larynx to the surrounding structures, tissues, and lymph nodes. With a *total laryngectomy*, the entire larynx, along with the hyoid bone, epiglottis, cricoid cartilage, and two or three rings of the trachea are removed. The manner in which a patient breathes and speaks is permanently altered. A total laryngectomy results in permanent loss of speech and a change in the airway. Without complications and with proper rehabilitation, the patient is able to resume normal swallowing.

Often a radial neck dissection is performed along with a total laryngectomy, because metastasis to the cervical lymph nodes is common. More advanced cancers may require excision of the sternocleidomastoid and strap muscles, as well as, the venous supply to the area. With or without neck dissection the patient will require a permanent tracheal stoma, because the larynx no longer provides the protective sphincter against aspiration. A tracheal stoma will offer protection against aspiration of food and fluid into the lower respiratory tract. Because airflow through the nose and mouth is minimal, a patient with a stoma loses the ability to warm and moisten the air that flows into the lungs. With air flowing into the lungs from the stoma, the patient may experience dryness of the mucous membranes and be prone to lung infections. Other complications include a salivary leak, development of a pharyngocutaneous fistula, and stenosis of the stoma. Difficulty swallowing can occur secondary to the development of esophageal or cervical stricture.

Speech Therapy

Speech therapy for a patient undergoing a total laryngectomy must begin before surgery. The patient and the family must be well informed of the available options and must be active partners in the decision-making process. The speech pathologist helps to educate the patient and family make the best choice for surgical voice replacement depending on the patient's age and personal preference. In the immediate postoperative period, an alternative form of communication must be used until the stoma is well healed and a permanent method of speech employed. Alternative methods of communication that can be used include writing, lip speaking, or using a keyboard, computer, or picture board. An artificial speech aid may be employed during this time to help with artificial speech. Once the patient is taking oral fluids, usually one to two weeks post-surgery, a permanent form of speech can be initiated.

Nutrition

Postoperatively, patients who undergo a laryngectomy are unable to take nutrition orally for about 10 to 14 days. During this time a patient will receive nutrition via IV fluids, enteral feedings through a nasogastric tube, or parenteral nutrition.

Once oral feedings can be resumed, the nurse needs to instruct the patient on the importance of thickening liquids to make them easier to swallow. Sweet foods should be avoided, because they cause increase salivation and decrease the appetite. The diet is advanced to solid food as tolerated. The nurse instructs the patient to eat slowly, chew food well before swallowing, and consume small amounts of food frequently. Following total laryngectomy, the larynx has been resected or removed. The airway is diverted from the esophagus and separated. Patients who are status post total laryngectomy cannot aspirate unless there is some form of medical complication, such as fistula. Laryngectomized patients who have had trachesophageal (TE) puncture may aspirate secretions or food only if the puncture site is not adequately stented with a catheter or prosthesis (e-mail correspondence, Jan Lewin, September 29, 2004).

It is important to remind the patient that the sense of smell and taste will be altered for a period of time after surgery. Alteration in the airflow directly into the tracheostomy causes the loss of smell that normally occurs as air flows over the olfactory end organs and the nose. The nurse needs to reassure the patient that over time interest in food will return.

Food high in protein and calories is important to help the patient regain strength and rebuild healthy tissue. The nurse or dietitian can help the patient choose foods for meals and snacks that are high in these factors. Adequate hydration is important to keep secretions loose and ease their expectoration from the lungs.

Patient and Family Teaching

Both the patient and the family need thorough and accurate teaching to manage the multitude of changes that occur after a laryngectomy. Physical, social, psychological, and spiritual needs should be included in discharge planning. Verbal and written instructions are necessary to ensure adequate information has been given. A homecare checklist can help to ensure all aspects of teaching have been covered (Box 31-3).

Evaluation of Outcomes

Potential patient outcomes for each of the example nursing diagnoses for the patient with laryngeal cancer are:
- Anxiety. The patient controls anxiety and information processing.
- Ineffective airway clearance. The patient prevents aspiration and maintains airway patency
- Impaired verbal communication. The patient is satisfied with communication.
- Imbalanced nutrition, less than body requirements. The patient shows an increased appetite and nutrition intake.
- Risk for infection. The patient prevents aspiration prevention and promotes wound healing.

BOX 31-3

HOME CARE CHECKLIST FOR THE PATIENT WITH A LARYNGECTOMY

On completion of the home care instruction the patient and the caregiver will be able to verbalize understanding of:	Patient	Caregiver	Date of Instruction
Clearing the airway and handling of secretions			
Cleaning of the tracheostomy tube and stoma			
Care of the skin around the stoma			
Reasons for wearing a protective cloth or shield over the stoma			
Need for humidification of inspired air			
Need for adequate hydration and nutrition			
Signs and symptoms of infection and when to notify the health care provider			
Emergency airway management			
Necessity of wearing a medical alert bracelet			
Alterative communication methods			
Availability of support groups			
Importance of regular scheduled followup appointments			

- Risk for ineffective sexual patterns. The patient has a good body image and self-esteem
- Risk for self-care deficit. The patient participates in self-care activities of daily living, and energy conservation.

Prognosis for laryngeal cancer depends on the staging, which includes tumor size, degree of infiltration, and distant metastasis. The earlier the tumor is found and the lesser the degree of infiltration, the better the outcome for the patient. The most adverse prognostic factors for laryngeal cancers include increasing T stage and N stage. Other factors that affect prognosis include patient age, sex, and characteristics of the tumor.

Individuals treated for laryngeal cancer have the greatest risk of recurrence within the first two to three years. Recurrences after five years are rare and usually represent new primary malignancies. If a patient continues to smoke and drink alcohol, the likelihood that the initial cancer will be cured, by any means, is diminished, and the risk of a second tumor is enhanced. Secondary tumor has been reported in the digestive tract in 25 percent of the patients whose primary tumor is controlled.

KEY CONCEPTS

- Common clinical manifestations of rhinitis include the presence of rhinorrhea, nasal congestion and obstruction, nasal itchiness, and sneezing.
- Medications for rhinitis focus on alleviating or reducing the symptoms.
- Avoidance of triggers is the most important factor in treating rhinitis.
- Careful attention should be made to complaints of chronic congestion in the elderly population, because it is often the result of structural changes because of the aging process and not chronic infection.
- *S. pyogenes* is the most common bacterial organism that produces streptococcus pharyngitis (strep throat).
- Acute and chronic laryngitis are a result of voice misuse, environmental pollutants, or exposure to noxious agents.
- With OSA, obstruction of the airway occurs at either the soft palate (nasopharynx) or at the level of the tongue (oropharynx).
- Epistaxis is most commonly anterior, originating from the nasal septum.

- Having the patient lean forward slightly while pinching the soft outer portion of the nose against the nasal septum for about 5 to 10 minutes continuously most often controls anterior nosebleeds.
- Obstruction of the larynx may occur with an acute infectious process, as in laryngitis, anaphylaxis, or with aspiration of a foreign body.
- Cancer of the larynx can occur in any of the three regions: supraglottic area, glottic area, or subglottic area.
- Although the incidence of laryngeal cancer is declining, it is on the rise for women.
- The greatest risk factor for developing laryngeal cancer is smoking.
- Individuals treated for laryngeal cancer have the greatest risk of recurrence within the first two to three years. Recurrences after five years are rare and usually represent new primary malignancies.
- Communication after a total laryngectomy remains one of the most difficult aspects of care.

REVIEW QUESTIONS

1. What should the nurse include about prevention of exacerbations with allergic rhinitis when giving discharge instructions to a newly diagnosed patient?
   1. Drink plenty of fluids
   2. Monitor for elevated temperature
   3. Avoidance of triggers
   4. Get adequate amounts of sleep

2. Which of these are common clinical manifestations of rhinitis?
   1. Nasal congestion, headache, and sore throat
   2. Nasal congestion, pyrexia, and rhinorrhea
   3. Headache, sore throat, and rhinorrhea
   4. Nasal congestion, rhinorrhea, and sneezing

3. In which of the following disorders should the nurse question an order to give the patient cetirizine (Zyrtec) because of the side effect profile?
   1. Essential hypertension
   2. Prostatic hypertrophy
   3. Pulmonary fibrosis
   4. Diabetes mellitus

4. Which statement is accurate when instructing a patient about the proper use of intranasal sprays?
   1. Tilt the head slightly forward and angle the bottle toward the side of the nostril

2. Blow the nose after spraying to prevent medication from entering the throat
3. Finish instillation of spray in to one nostril before spraying into the other
4. Inhale quickly to prevent irritation of the mucous membranes

5. A patient asks the nurse about using decongestant nasal sprays. Which of the following statements by the nurse is correct regarding administration?
   1. "They have to be used for several days before any effect on congestion is noted."
   2. "They should be used along with corticosteroid nasals sprays for maximum benefit."
   3. "They should not be used for more than three days because of they can worsen congestion."
   4. "They should be used sparingly because they can exacerbate a cough."

6. The nurse is caring for a patient with complaints of unilateral facial pain, stuffy nose, and headache. The nurse calls the health care provider to obtain an order for which of the following medications?
   1. Antihistamine
   2. Antibiotic
   3. Guaifenesin
   4. Decongestant

Continued

7. The nurse is obtaining a history of present illness on a patient who complains of facial pain, toothache, and inability to taste food. Which data obtained would alert the nurse that the infection has spread?
   1. Headache and fever
   2. Fever and chills
   3. Yellow secretions and fever
   4. Facial swelling and headache

8. The patient with chronic sinusitis returns to the clinic with complaints of inability to clear secretions from the airway. Which of these should be included in teaching the patient about self-care?
   1. Drink plenty of fluids
   2. Take decongestants as ordered
   3. Apply warm packs over the inflamed sinuses
   4. Irrigate the sinus cavities with warm saline solution

9. A patient presents to the clinic with complaints of a sore throat and pain on swallowing. The addition of what clinical findings is the most reliable predictors to indicate that the sore throat is caused by *Streptococcus pyogenes*?
   1. Fever, cough, and cervical adenopathy
   2. Fever, cough, and beefy red tonsils
   3. Fever, beefy red tonsils, and absence of cough
   4. Fever, cervical adenopathy, and tonsillar exudate

10. Discharge instructions for a patient status post-tonsillectomy should include which of the following?
    1. Use warm saline gargles to relieve sore throat pain
    2. Return to normal diet as soon as tolerated
    3. Be alert for excessive bleeding up to one week
    4. Encourage coughing to prevent aspiration of secretions

11. An adolescent presents to the community center with complaints of difficulty opening her mouth, pain on swallowing, and ear pain. On examination the nurse notices the uvula is deviated to the right and the left tonsil is swollen and red. The nurse recognizes this as symptoms of what upper airway disorder?
    1. Adenoiditis
    2. Severe pharyngitis
    3. Peritonsillar abscess
    4. Laryngitis

12. While performing a patient history, the nurse obtains information from the patient's spouse about frequent snoring and daytime sleepiness. Which action by the nurse is most appropriate?
    1. Obtain a pulse oximetry reading
    2. Perform an electrocardiogram (ECG)
    3. Assess for recent weight loss
    4. Assess for memory loss

13. What is the priority intervention for a patient that has sustained a fracture of the nose?
    1. Pain relief
    2. Prevention of aspiration
    3. Prevention of deformity
    4. Control of bleeding

14. What is the first symptom patients report with the presence of cancer of the glottis?
    1. Pain with swallowing
    2. Change in the voice
    3. Difficulty swallowing
    4. Persistent sore throat

15. The nurse is caring for a patient who is receiving radiation for treatment of a laryngeal tumor. The onset of xerostomia is because of what physiological change?
    1. Decreased activity of the thyroid gland
    2. Increased activity of the thyroid gland
    3. Decreased activity of the parotid gland
    4. Increased activity of the parotid gland

REVIEW ACTIVITIES

1. List four nursing diagnoses commonly associated with infections of the upper respiratory tract.

2. Discuss appropriate nursing interventions (NIC) associated with upper respiratory tract disorders.

Continued

REVIEW ACTIVITIES—cont'd

3. Discuss the pros and cons to using antibiotics in sinusitis.

4. Describe the problems associated with the use of the standard throat culture for diagnosing streptococcus pharyngitis and why rapid antigen testing is more efficacious.

5. Compare and contrast the management of epistaxis in the anterior and posterior regions of the nose.

6. List the risk factors associated with the development of cancer of the larynx.

7. Compare the alaryngeal communication techniques with respect to ease of use, cost, and mechanism of voice production.

Visit the Contemporary Medical-Surgical Nursing online companion resource at www.delmarhealthcare.com for additional content and study aids. Click on Online Companions then select the Nursing discipline.

Lower Airway Dysfunction: Nursing Management

Beth Strauss, MS, RN, APRN, BC

CHAPTER TOPICS

- Pneumonia
- Extra and Intrapulmonary Restrictive Lung Disorders
- Tuberculosis
- Pulmonary Fungal Infections
- Bronchiolectasis
- Lung Abscess
- Lung Cancer
- Pneumothorax
- Fractured Rib
- Flail Chest
- Pulmonary Hypertension
- Cor Pulmonale

KEY TERMS

Abscess
Cor pulmonale
Cough
Dimorphic
Disseminated
Dyspnea
Endemic
Granulomas
Hemoptysis
Idiopathic
Metastasis
Opportunistic
Pleuritic chest pain
Pneumothorax
Polycythemia
Purulent sputum
Tubercles

Lower airway disease and thoracic trauma pose many challenges for nurses. They can easily mimic other diseases, are often insidious in nature, and when symptoms do develop, the disease process may be in an advanced state. As a result, the nurse caring for people with lower airway dysfunction and thoracic injury must be vigilant to minute changes in a patient's condition. People with airway disease and trauma often face issues of pain control, potential or perceived loss of quality of life, ineffective airway clearance, alterations in health maintenance, and activity intolerance. Understanding the lower airway disease process can assist the nurse to anticipate slight changes in a patient's condition, define collaborative care, and offer nursing support and interventions. Three hallmark symptoms of pulmonary disease and thoracic injuries for which people seek medical treatment include dyspnea, cough, and hemoptysis. The first hallmark symptom, **dyspnea,** or shortness of breath, is caused by variety of disease processes, including asthma, metabolic acidosis, and acute respiratory distress syndrome (ARDS). The second hallmark symptom, **cough,** a sudden forceful expulsion of air, is a defense mechanism used by the body to rid the pulmonary tract of irritates or fluid and can be defined as acute or chronic. An acute cough is defined as a cough lasting three weeks or less while a chronic cough is a cough lasting more than three weeks. Eighty five percent of people affected with the common cold will cough within 2 days after exposure, 26 percent will still cough after 14 days, and a few are still coughing at six to eight weeks (Tierney, McPhee, & Papadakis, 2003). Gastroesophageal reflux disease (GERD) and other disease processes can also cause coughing as a result of the acid irritation of the pharynx. The third hallmark symptom, **hemoptysis,** is blood noted in the sputum, usually indicating an irritation of the lung fields. Common causes of hemoptysis include bronchitis, mitral stenosis, bronchiolectasis, lung cancer, pneumonia, pulmonary embolism (PE), and thoracic trauma. Blood in the sputum always necessitates an extensive diagnostic evaluation to rule out severe or life-threatening illness or injury. A person presenting with pulmonary infection and blood-tinged sputum may not need further evaluation if the bleeding stops once resolution of infection occurs, and the patient is otherwise healthy as well as a nonsmoker.

PNEUMONIA

Pneumonia is an acute or chronic infection of one or both lungs caused by microorganisms, such as viruses, bacteria, or chemical irritants. It is the fifth leading cause of death in the United States among people 65 and older. In 2001, 8 percent of hospital inpatient deaths were attributed to pneumonia (National Center of Health Statistics, 2002), and in 2002 the average length of stay (LOS) for person with pneumonia was 5.7 days. Pneumonia can affect anyone, but those at greatest risk are people less than 2 years of age or over the age 65 and the immunocompromised patient. Risk factors for mortality in pneumonia include increased age, alcoholism, active malignancies, immunosuppression, neurological disease, congestive heart failure, and diabetes.

Epidemiology

The bacterium *Streptococcus pneumoniae* accounts for 25 to 35 percent of all community-acquired pneumonias (CAPs) (American Lung Association, 2003b). In addition, bacterial pneumonia is often associated with concurrent viral infection that may suppress the immune system and disrupt the respiratory tract mucosa (Uphold & Graham, 2003). Symptoms may be insidious as a gradual decline in health following a cold to a sudden respiratory event, such as aspiration, or following an invasive procedure. Symptoms can mimic other disease processes and include fever, shaking chills, minor or severe **pleuritic chest pain** (pain that occurs with respirations), cough that produces rust-colored or greenish mucus, increased pulse, and bluish coloring of the lips and nails.

Viral pneumonia is more commonly seen in the younger population but may occur in the adult population and can be fatal in the most severe cases. Half of all pneumonias are caused by a virus and can be fatal in the most severe cases (Mayhall, 2004). Viral pneumonia has the same symptoms of bacterial pneumonia but with rapidly worsening symptoms within a 12- to 36-hour-period and may be further complicated by a bacterial infection, heart disease, lung disease, or pregnancy.

Mycoplasma pneumoniae, or atypical pneumonia, is caused by an unknown virus and was first identified in World War II. This type of pneumonia carries characteristics of both viral and bacterial organisms and occurs more frequently in the older child and young adult (Mayhall, 2004). Unlike viral and bacterial pneumonia, cough of patients infected with *M. pneumoniae* tends to come in violent attacks with only sparse white mucus preceded by early symptoms of fever and chills. **Opportunistic** pneumonias (organism-causing disease in a host whose resistance to fight infection is diminished) consist of *Pneumocystis carinii,* cytomegalovirus, and tuberculosis (TB).

Pneumocystis carinii pneumonia, (PCP) is a type of fungal infection that usually affects individuals infected with human immunodeficiency virus (HIV) or other immunocompromised patients, such as cancer patients receiving radiation or chemotherapy, transplant recipients, and individuals requiring prolonged use of corticosteroids. Healthy individuals with intact immune systems are usually not affected by this organism, because the immune system is able to combat the infection. Signs and symptoms of PCP can be insidious or sudden and may consist of: (a) fever; (b) tachypnea; (c) dyspnea; (d) nonproductive cough; and (e) hypoxemia. The diagnosis of PCP is confirmed by chest X-ray (CXR) and bronchoalveolar lavage, which collects organisms from the lungs by washing with repeated injections of water and removal of solution with suction. Unfortunately, there is no vaccine for PCP, and in the immunocompromised patient, PCP can be a deadly disease.

Pathophysiology

In pneumonia some or all of the alveoli, interstitial tissue, and bronchioles become filled with fluid or blood as a result of the inflammatory process of infection or chemical irritants. The warm moist pulmonary tissue provides an excellent medium for bacterial growth. On entry into the lung, the invading organism starts changing epithelial or surface cells in the alveoli, allowing the bacterial agent to adhere to the alveoli. The attached bacterium then destroys the defensive macrophages, or white blood cells, producing a further inflammatory response and infective state. Diminished lung ventilation occurs as a result of congestive areas in the lung.

Pneumonias are classified by the organism involved, location of infection, and origin of aspiration. Organisms causing pneumonia can be bacterial, viral, or chemical and may be of an intrapulmonary or extrapulmonary origin. Intrapulmonary origins include any disease process that originates within the lung fields. Extrapulmonary origin is any disease process that includes any abnormality of the chest wall, pleura, respiratory muscle, or when the pulmonary disease process has moved to another body system. Intrapulmonary and extrapulmonary diseases are discussed in this chapter.

Pneumonia organisms can be acquired either in the community or during an inpatient admission and can affect multiple sites in the pulmonary system. CAP is present in patients who are not residents of a long-term facility, usually occurs less than 48 hours after admission, and accounts for 40,000 deaths per year (American Lung Association, 2003a). Hospital-acquired pneumonia (HAP) usually occurs 48 hours or more after admission and is typically caused from artificial sources, such as aspirations, invasive procedures, or mechanical ventilation (Figure 32-1). Aspirations may be a witnessed or silent event that can occur over several days. High-risk patient groups for aspiration include the following: (a) receiving enteral feedings; (b) decreased level of consciousness (LOC); (c) requiring ventilator support; (d) underlying chronic lung disease; (e) a history of multiple or inappropriate antibiotic usage; (f) endotracheal intubation; and (g) invasive procedures.

Ventilator-associated pneumonia (VAP) is defined as pneumonia in a patient on mechanical ventilator support for more than 48 hours (Mayhall, 2004). Evidenced-based research has shown that the use of oral-tracheal versus a naso-tracheal tube for ventilation has resulted in fewer VAP cases (Tablan, Anderson, Besser, Bridges, & Hajjeh, 2004). Lobar pneumonia affects only a lobe of the lung, whereas bronchial pneumonia infects multiple areas throughout both lungs. Walking pneumonia is a nonmedical term used to describe pneumonia that does not require hospitalization.

Pneumonia bacteria usually found in the oropharynx and nasopharynx gains entry into the lungs by aspiration of secretions. It is estimated that 70

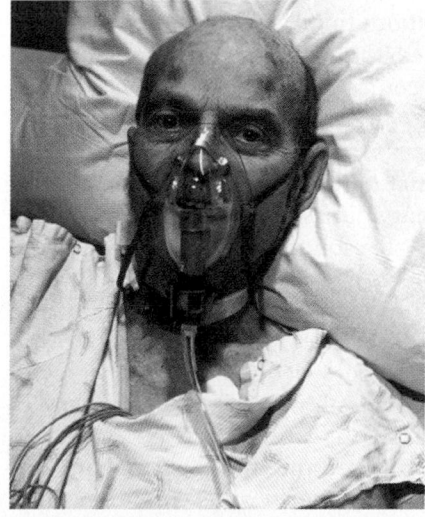

Figure 32-1 A patient with hospital-acquired pneumonia (HAP) being managed with oxygen therapy.

HIGH-RISK INDICATORS FOR ACQUIRING PNEUMONIA

- Chronic illness of the heart, lung, or kidney including asthma
- Diabetes
- Sickle cell anemia
- Congestive heart failure (CHF)
- People residing in a group or nursing home
- People over 50 years of age
- Infants between 6 and 23 months
- Women who are pregnant during the flu session
- People with weakened immune systems
- Long-term treatment with steroids
- Cancer treatment or chemotherapy
- Children or teens on long-term aspirin therapy
- Smokers

percent of healthy people have pneumococcus bacterium at any time in either the nose or throat, and approximately 50 percent of all adults aspirate small amounts of oropharyngeal secretions during sleep. The elderly are at risk for aspiration due to a slower swallowing ability. This ability to swallow is not impaired but slowed because of the normal aging process. High-risk indicators for acquiring pneumonia are listed in Box 32-1.

Assessment with Clinical Manifestations

Nurses are able to assist patients to resolve disease or improve function throughout the nursing process: assessment, diagnosis, planning, implementation, and evaluation of outcomes. The nurse must be precise, in the clinical assessment and data collection of the patient, to avoid misdiagnosis or incorrect interventions that can lead to negative patient outcomes. Clinical tools are provided to assist health care providers to make effective clinical decisions possible. One such tool, the pneumonia severity index (PSI), identifies patients with CAP who are at low risk for morbidity and mortality and who may be candidates for outpatient treatment versus inpatient treatment. Developed in 1997 the PSI places patients into five severity categories using a two-step process that evaluates the following factors: (a) age; (b) physical history; (c) comorbidity; (d) radiographic; and (e) laboratory results.

Mortality rates, among the four PSI classes, according to the class level. In class I mortality rates range from 0.1 to 0.4 percent. In class II mortality rates range form 0.6 to 0.7 percent. In class III the mortality range increases to 0.9 to 2.8 percent. Finally, class IV patients had a mortality rate of 27 to 31.1 percent. Those patients in class I or II may be treated as an outpatient, and people in class III or IV could be considered for hospitalization. The PSI has been a helpful and beneficial tool to assist health care providers. It is important to note that while tools exist, no tool or diagnostic test should be used as the sole predictor of illness, instead it should be part of the total clinical assessment.

Specific symptoms suggestive of pneumonia include: (a) fever; (b) chills or rigors; (c) sweats; (d) new cough (with or without sputum production); (e) pleuritic chest pain; and (f) dyspnea. In patients with a chronic cough change in sputum color requires further diagnostic workup. Pneumonia also can have nonspecific symptoms including: (a) malaise; (b) fatigue; (c) abdominal pain; (d) headaches; (e) anorexia; and (f) worsening of an underlying chronic illness. A thorough clinical and symptom history is vital to assist the health care provider correctly diagnose pneumonia from differential or other disease processes.

During the patient interview the nurse should not only look for the obvious symptoms of pneumonia but also inquire about nonspecific symptoms as well. The nurse should ask the patient to describe the cough, including amount, color, and consistency. Inquiring about recent illness in the household or at work will assist the nurse in developing a clinical picture. It is important to include past medical history risk factors for morbidity, such as amount of alcohol or drugs consumed, smoking habits, including pack per day calculations, and asthma or chronic obstructive pulmonary disease (COPD).

Physical examination findings may show a respiratory rate of greater than 20 as more oxygen is needed because the congestion of the alveoli. Fever above 37.8° C (100.0° F) is common as the body works harder to fight the infection. Other symptoms are tachycardia caused by the heart moving macrophages to the site of infection and increased oxygen needs, crackles heard on auscultation and dyspnea due to congestion of the alveoli, and pleuritic chest pain. When assessing lung sounds the nurse must be careful to record not only location, type of lung sound, when the sound occurs, but also an absence of lung sounds, which may signal another serious condition, such as pneumothorax, which is discussed further in this chapter. Crackles may be heard throughout all lung fields, or in one segment of the lung, signaling a lobar or bilateral lung field infection.

Diagnostic Tests

A CXR is recommended to confirm a diagnosis of pneumonia. Routine laboratory tests include complete blood count (CBC), glucose, serum electrolytes, hepatic enzymes, renal function, and sputum gram stain. Patients with diabetes who have an active infection and or dehydration will have an elevated glucose level. Serum electrolytes will assess fluid balance, and renal tests will show how effective the kidneys are working. Pulse goniometry may be used for those patients with chronic heart or lung conditions, because findings can tell the clinical picture of low oxygen before onset of symptoms. The nurse must be careful in assessment of pulse goniometry results, because processes such as peripheral vascular disease, anemia, and dehydration may falsify results. Pulmonary function tests may be used to rule out other disease processes. Purified protein derivative (PPD) of tuberculin tests will rule out tuberculosis. Tests for TB will also be discussed in this chapter.

Differential diagnosis are diseases or conditions that mimic the symptoms of pneumonia and include: (a) chronic pulmonary diseases; (b) atelectasis (absence of gas in the lungs due to a failure of expansion or reassertion of gas form the alveoli); (c) lung abscess; (d) PE; (e) pulmonary injury; (f) neoplasms; and (g) sarcoidosis, which is a liver disease of unknown origin marked by formation of lesions in the liver.

Nursing Diagnoses

Based on the evidence gathered, examples of nursing diagnoses for the patient with pneumonia may include the following:
- Ineffective airway clearance related to inability to remove airway secretions
- Impaired gas exchange related to congestion of alveoli
- Activity intolerance related to increased metabolic demands
- Fatigue related to hypermetabolic state and inadequate tissue oxygenation

Planning and Implementation

Prevention of pneumonia becomes the first priority for management, because aspiration of oropharyngeal secretions is the primary reason for pneumonia infections. Patients should be instructed to perform frequent oral hygiene and use good hand washing technique to avoid the spread of infection. In the hospital patients should perform oral hygiene at least every two to three hours. Patients needing ventilator support or unable to breath through the nose should have oral hygiene every one to two hours and as needed to maintain a moist mucosa. Nurses, being the frontline provider, have a responsibility to not only advocate for patients and ensure timely effective delivery of care interventions but also to provide best practice to promote positive patient outcomes. A recommendation for nursing practice is to change oxygen tubing, including nasal prongs or masks, when the tubing becomes contaminated. Most patients will develop nasal or oral residual on oxygen tubing when worn over time so the nurse must make sure to change any contaminated tubing. Oxygen masks can be cleaned with soap and water or changed according to organization policy and procedures. The second recommendation is to always use sterile water to fill bubbling humidifiers, while using normal saline for handheld nebulizers. A nurse should never use normal saline, a salt solution, to fill bubbling humidifiers or electrical equipment, as the salt can clog the respiratory machine, resulting in ineffective use and can present a patient safety fire hazard. Normal saline solution (0.9 %) provides the closest solution comparable to normal body fluid and is used for delivery of direct patient interventions, such as medications and irrigations. The nurse should always follow standard precautions when handling oral or nasal secretions to avoid contamination and further spread of the pathogen to vulnerable patients.

Safety First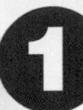

Oxygen Therapy

Oxygen therapy if not monitored closely can adversely affect patient outcomes. Patients who have COPD retain carbon dioxide (CO_2) as a result of the chronic effects of the disease. The body becomes acclimated to the retained CO_2, and the process becomes part of the normal respiratory process. Patients with COPD cannot tolerate high levels of oxygen, because the high level of oxygen can alter the CO_2 retention process, causing an acute respiratory event. A nurse can safely apply two liters of oxygen per nasal cannula on any patient in distress, including patients who retain CO_2; but the nurse must initiate an immediate pulmonary evaluation in the event higher amounts of oxygen are required (Figure 32-2). Patients needing more than two liters of oxygen require an immediate respiratory and pulmonologist evaluation.

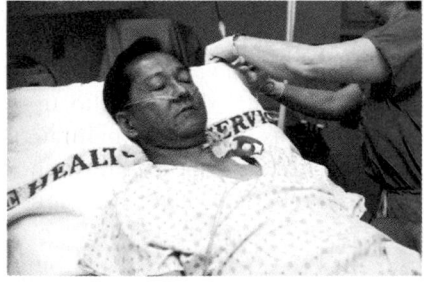

Figure 32-2 Oxygen delivered via a nasal cannula.

The Centers for Disease Control and Prevention (CDC) also recommends use of noninvasive positive-pressure ventilation delivered by face or nose mask instead of endotracheal intubation to prevent aspiration of patients needing ventilator support. When taking care of patients receiving enteral feedings keep the head of bed elevated at a 30- to 45-degree angle. Patients with a feeding tube placed into the small intestine have the same risk of aspiration as any patient with a feeding tube placed in the stomach, so any patient receiving enteral feedings must have the head of bed elevated at least 30 degrees. Elevated the head of the bed at a 90-degree angle for longer than 30 to 45 minutes can place pressure on the sacral tissue and cause skin breakdown. Adequate hydration will assist the body in fighting the infection as well as loosening secretions. The average adult requires 2 to 3 liters of fluid per day unless under a fluid restriction. When increasing hydration, fluids with caffeine (e.g., coffee, tea, and carbonated beverage) should be avoided as they have diuretic effects and can lead to dehydration.

Postural drainage and oxygen supplementation are used in the treatment of pneumonia. Postural drainage uses gravity to clear secretions, and chest percussion requires use of a cupped hand to hit the chest or back and loosen secretions. Oxygen may be administered by nasal prongs or face mask and should be administered to keep the oxygen saturation greater than or equal to 92 percent (see Safety First).

Patients having invasive procedures or surgery should be encouraged to take deep breaths and cough and ambulate as soon as possible after the procedure. Cough and deep breathing every one to two hours while awake provides expansion of the lung fields, allows oxygen to be delivered to tissues, and provides expulsion of secretions and infectious material. Use of incentive spirometry machine provides for the resistance needed to expand the lung fields and should be used on any high-risk patients at risk for acquiring pneumonia or those patients with pneumonia. Limiting activity and rest periods decrease oxygen demands of the body. Walking three to four times a day with rest periods of at least two hours can be an effective method to maintain mobility and provide rest. Pain medications should be given at least 30 to 45 minutes prior to any activity. Effective pain control will not only promote mobility but also allow more effective outcomes from chest physiotherapy that included using a cupped hand to strike the back to assist in losing secretions.

Evidence-Based Care

Research gives health care providers the prevailing indications ensuring the best care possible in being provided. Clinical research studies utilize human volunteers or subjects to find ways to improve patient outcomes. Other research studies are interventional trials that determine whether experimental treatments or new ways of using known therapies are safe and effective under controlled environments, and observational trials address health issues in large groups of people or populations in natural settings.

The Food and Drug Administration code of federal regulations define clinical trials as phase I, II, or III (Mayhall, 2004). Classification of phase number is based on the type of question that the particular study is attempting to answer (Table 32-1).

Pharmacology

As mentioned previously prevention of pneumonia is vital to improving patient outcomes. However, patients diagnosed with pneumonia require medical treatment to assist the body in fighting the infectious pathogen. It is important that the sputum cultures identify the correct organisms so that medications can target the specific pathogen. Unfortunately in CAP the pathogen causing the pneumonia is only identified in 40 to 50 percent of the time (Uphold & Graham, 2003). Antibiotics are used to treat existing infection should be as specific to the organism as possible to avoid resistant bacterium

TABLE 32-1	**Clinical Trial Phases**
Phase I	Researchers test a new drug or treatment in a small group of people (20 to 80) to evaluate its safety, determine a safe dosage range, and identify side effects.
Phase II	Researchers test a new drug or treatment to a larger group of people (100 to 300) to see if it is effective and to further evaluate its safety.
Phase III	Researchers test a new drug or treatment to groups of people (1,000 to 3,000) to confirm its effectiveness, monitor side effects, compare it to commonly used treatments, and collect information that will allow the drug or treatment to be used safely.

Adapted from Mayhall, G. C. (2004). Ventilator-associated pneumonia or not? Contemporary diagnosis. Emerging Infectious Disease Journal, 7(2), 11.

strains. Broad-spectrum antibiotics are helpful when the pathogen is not identified, and treatment needs to start immediately.

Oral antibiotics commonly used in the outpatient setting include azithromycin, levofloxacin, and doxycycline. Azithromycin is useful for younger and otherwise healthy people. Patients with existing cardiac or pulmonary disease may be prescribed oral doses of doxycycline or amoxicillin or clavulanate. Patients having a painful forceful cough may be prescribed cough mediations or narcotics. All patients receiving narcotics should be monitored closely for safety and potential respiratory side effects. Nebulizer treatments with bronchodilators, such as albuterol, help remove tenacious or sticky secretions.

Hospitalized patients usually receive antibiotic therapy via an intravenous (IV) line. Observation of the IV site should be completed prior, during, and after antibiotic therapy as these medications are irritating to the vein and may cause infiltration of medication into the body tissue. Close observation will allow the nurse to intervene before the medication causes harm. According to an American Medical Association (AMA) press release on March 22, 2004, antibiotics given to the elderly and high-risk patients with pneumonia within four hours after admission resulted in decreased LOS and mortality rates (AMA, 2004).

Multiple studies have been conducted addressing the topic of providing antibiotics within four hours of admission. Based on this combined research and other studies The Centers for Medicare/Medicaid Services (CMS), the regulatory body of Medicare and Medicaid administration, uses the antibiotic turnaround time as a quality indicator for appropriate and timely treatment of pneumonia. CMS list other quality indicators for the treatment of pneumonia including: (a) oxygenation assessment; (b) blood cultures obtained; (c) pneumococcal screening and vaccination; and (d) adult smoking cessation programs.

The implications of evidenced-based research are immense. Pneumonia can be a life-threatening illness that can result in positive patient outcomes and costs can be decreased by quick intervention. To provide the most effective practice, nurses treating patients with pneumonia must not only have precise assessments and accurate documentation, but they also must start pharmacological treatment quickly on admission to the hospital.

Pneumococcus vaccination is given to high-risk groups, such as people over 65 years of age and patients with chronic heart disease and asthma. Others receiving this preventive measure include health care workers and immunocompromised individuals. Vaccination is effective about 80 percent of the time with healthy adults and may be less effective with the extremely sick population (American Lung Association, 2003b). Medicare, as well as some state and private insurance companies, covers the cost of the vaccine. The vaccination may last up to 10 years and it is highly recommended for high-risk groups.

Uncovering the Evidence

Rapid Antibiotic Delivery and Appropriate Antibiotic Selection

Discussion: Using a retrospective chart review this research was undertaken to determine if three clinical variables in the treatment of pneumonia contributed to a decreased hospital stay for patients admitted with pneumonia. Three quality of care variables were measures: (a) site of antibiotic treatment in the emergency department versus inpatient initialization; (b) door to needle time or actual time before antibiotic therapy was initiated; and (c) appropriateness of antibiotic selection. Prolonged LOS was defined as greater than or equal to nine days. All subjects were older with a mean age of 67, and 57 percent of the subjects had a comorbid illness.

The results showed that the average door to needle time for the entire sample was 5.5 hours ± 3.5 hours. In the emergency department (ED) patients had a door to needle time of 3.5 hours ± 1.4 hours, and in the inpatient floor the door to needle time was 3 hours. Those patients with a longer door to needle time had a longer hospital stay. Research results also showed that only 56 percent of patients were treated with appropriate antibiotics. This research study is one example of the ongoing research looking at improving outcomes in an elderly patient admitted with CAP.

Implications for Practice: This study impacts nursing practice by exemplifying the need for nurses to administer antibiotic therapy in a timely fashion. Patients may benefit from decreasing the time it takes for antibiotics to be administered.

Source: Battleman, D. S., Callahan M., & Thaler, H. T. (2002). Rapid antibiotic delivery and appropriate antibiotic selection reduced length of hospital stay of patients with community acquired pneumonia. Archives of Internal Medicine, 167(6), 682–688.

Current studies are looking at the efficacy of recommending the vaccination to people 50 years of age, and many health care organizations have already made this recommendation a part of their preventive health care program (Sisk, Whang, Butler, Sneller, & Whitney, 2003). Unfortunately, in the first quarter of 2002 only 54 percent of adults over 65 received the vaccination (National Center for Health Statistics, 2002). Factors for low vaccination rates may be lack of knowledge regarding the importance or an inability to obtain the vaccination. Flu Mist, a new intranasal influenza vaccine, is a live virus vaccine intended only for healthy children and adults from 5 to 49 years of age and is currently available at health care organizations.

Patients with HIV and solid organ transplants are given preventive treatment to protect them from acquiring PCP. People with solid organ transplants are given preventive antibiotics after a transplant for up to six months. Blood and bone marrow transplant recipients receive treatment for one year as a result of increased immunosuppressant during periods of graft-versus-host disease (National Guideline Clearinghouse, 2004).

Patient and Family Teaching

Patient education for the patient with pneumonia includes good hygiene, importance of vaccination, and the recommendation to quit or decrease smoking. All patients should receive information on smoking cessation groups and therapy. To prevent relapse the patient needs a clear understanding of when to seek further treatment. Patient teaching about symptoms of illness would include increased difficulty in breathing, onset of rigors, increased fever or fever persisting longer than 48 hours, worsening cough, and medication intolerance. The onset of rigors in someone receiving antibiotics may signal a pending resistant organism or an ineffective medication regimen. The nurse taking care of people with pneumonia must be able to identify community versus acquired pneumonia, ensure timely delivery of antibiotic therapy, provide through patient education, and minimization of complications to sure patient outcomes of pneumonia prevention and resolution. If complications do occur they typically include worsening of pneumonia, bacterium, or meningitis. According to the National Center for Health Statistics (2002), 20 to 30 percent of the population over 65 with pneumonia will develop bacterial infection in the blood as a result of the primary infection.

Evaluation of Outcomes

Potential patient outcomes for each of the example nursing diagnosis for the patient with pneumonia are:
- Ineffective airway clearance. The patient will not aspirate, and there will continue to be airway patency.
- Impaired gas exchange. The patient will have adequate pulmonary tissue perfusion as manifested by normal arterial blood gas (ABG) results and normal CXR.
- Activity intolerance. The patient will perform activities of daily living and maintain endurance.
- Fatigue. The patient will have adequate comfort level, nutritional status, and energy.

EXTRAPULMONARY AND INTRAPULMONARY RESTRICTIVE LUNG DISORDER

Extrapulmonary refers to any disease that affects outside the lung fields and includes any abnormality of the chest wall, pleura, and respiratory muscles. It can also be applied to describe disseminating pulmonary disease, such as TB or lung cancer. Intrapulmonary refers to disease that originates and resides in the lung tissue. Restrictive disease is pulmonary disease that over time leads to a restriction of the respiratory mechanisms. Idiopathic restrictive disease is a term used when the exact cause is not known.

Pathophysiology

As a result of a chronic inflammatory stage the respiratory lung tissue becomes stiffer, requiring the respiratory muscles to work harder to obtain an adequate lung volume. This increased work of breathing requires more energy and oxygen so that a chronic hypoxia develops. Many times the disease process can go undetected until the lung tissue becomes so stiff that symptoms appear. By that time it may be difficult to reverse the damage to the lung fields (Table 32-2).

Assessment with Clinical Manifestations

Clinical presentation usually included dyspnea, lack of energy to complete activities of daily living, and hypoxemia. Because the disease process can mimic a variety of diseases the health care provider must slowly and methodically eliminate other disease processes. Treatment includes steroids to treat chronic inflammatory disease. Instruction in activates that conserve energy and supportive care, such as continuous positive airway pressure (CPAP), respirators, and portable

TABLE 32-2	Examples of Extrapulmonary and Intrapulmonary Restrictive Disease	
TYPE	**EXTRAPULMONARY RESTRICTIVE DISEASE**	**INTRAPULMONARY RESTRICTIVE DISEASE**
Location	Affects chest wall, pleura, and respiratory muscles—outside the lung but other organs not involved	Diseases of lung tissue Affects alveoli Located inside the lung
Examples	Pneumothorax	Pneumonia
	Lung cancer	COPD
	Cystic fibrosis	TB
	Flail chest	Asthma
	Rib fractures	Pulmonary hypertension

Adapted from Tablan, O. C., Anderson, L. J., Besser, R., Bridges, C., & Hajjeh, R. (2004). Guidelines for preventing health care-associated pneumonia 2003: Recommendations of CDC and the Healthcare Infection Control Practices Advisory Committee. Retrieved September 16, 2004, from http://www.cdc.gov/.

oxygen. The treatment goals include treatment of the primary condition, minimization of complications, and resolution of the disease process.

TUBERCULOSIS

Tuberculosis (TB), a chronic infection of the lung, caused by a mycobacterium resulting in the development of tubercles in the lungs. **Tubercles** are nodules or swelling of lymphocytes and epithelioid cells that form the lesions seen in TB. TB has caused disease in humans for thousands of years and may date from 5000 B.C. (Goldberg, 2004). To be infected with TB a person must be in repeated close contact with a person who has an active form of the disease. Currently one third of the world's population has been infected by tuberculosis mycobacterium. Worldwide two million deaths result form TB with 100,000 of the deaths occurring in children. TB deaths are most prevalent in the countries of Asia, Africa, and Latin America (Goldberg, 2004). In the United States TB infection rates steadily declined from 1992 through 2002, with 2002 being the first time in U.S. history that more foreign-born citizens developed TB than U.S.-born individuals (CDC, 2002b).

Epidemiology

According to the CDC (2002b), there was a 5.7 percent decline in cases from 2001 and a 43 percent decline from the peak of the TB resurgence in 1992.

TB remains on the rise because of the presence of HIV infections and increased travel or immigration from parts of the world where TB was never brought under control (Goldberg, 2004). It is estimated that nearly one billion people will become newly infected, over 150 million will become sick, and 36 million will die worldwide between now and 2020 if control is not further strengthened (American Lung Association, 2004). About 10 million Americans are affected with TB mycobacterium. Only about 10 percent will develop active disease in their lifetime. The other 90 percent will never get sick and develop latent TB. Extrapulmonary TB disease usually appears in isolation with one site or organ system involved.

Pathophysiology

Mycobacterium bacteria gain entrance to the body through droplets, which are inhaled into the alveoli. Macrophages are unable to successfully kill the mycobacterium organism, but they can develop giant cells to enclose the organism. T-lymphocytes work with the macrophages to form **granulomas** (mass of inflamed granulation tissue) that may kill the mycobacterium. The residual effect of the primary infection usually is a hard calcified lesion known as a Ghon complex. Latent tuberculosis infection (present or potential disease that is currently not active) occurs when a person exposed to the mycobacterium has a positive PPD test. This person is without an active clinical picture of disease with a normal CXR. This person has a 10 percent chance of developing TB if preventive pharmacological treatment is not initiated. Because treatment regimens have 60 to 90 percent effectiveness, the chances of acquiring active TB is low in healthy individuals. Upon exposure it typically takes six to eight weeks to convert to a positive PPD. Extrapulmonary TB can occur in patients with HIV infection. In extrapulmonary TB the mycobacterium is able to move from the lung to other body organs, causing disease. Extrapulmonary disease usually appears in isolation, with one site or organ system involved. Table 32-3 identifies common extrapulmonary TB infection sites and clinical presentations.

Most people acquiring new infection achieve immunological control and develop a latent TB infection. Secondary TB disease can present years after exposure when resistance is lowered. Occurrence of active disease is most often noticed in the first two to three years after infection. Patients present to the health care system with flu-like symptoms and believe they have a respiratory tract infection when in fact they have been infecting individuals with the Mycobacterium bacteria. There are a wide variety of pathological conditions that may increase the development of active TB from latent TB, such as HIV, substance abuse, recent infection of TB, diabetes mellitus

TABLE 32-3 Common Extrapulmonary TB Infections and Clinical Presentation	
SITE OF INFECTION	**CLINICAL PRESENTATION**
Lymphatic	Enlarged lymph nodes that persist for more than two to three weeks without any apparent explanation
Pleural	Usually unilateral
	May result from a pulmonary source during TB reactivation
	Many cases go undetected
Bone or Joint	Pott's disease (TB in the spine presents as back pain)
Genitourinary	Pyuria
	Hematuria
	Dysuria
	Focal pain or swelling
Meningeal	Affects children and those with HIV disease
	Develops gradually with fever, malaise, and irritability followed by more specific symptoms like back pain
Peritoneal, pericardial, and intestinal	Subacute symptoms with persistent pain

Adapted from Goldberg, S. (2004). Tuberculosis. Clinics in Family Practice, *6(1) 175.*

(DM), prolonged corticosteroid therapy, cancer of the head and neck, and end-stage renal disease.

Assessment with Clinical Manifestations

TB presents a broad clinical picture from no illness to end-stage disease. In the absence of clinical symptoms the illness is rarely infectious. However, TB should be suspected in a patient who presents with three or more weeks of cough, fever, or weight loss who is known to have TB infection or at risk for developing the disease (Goldberg, 2004). Weight loss over three pounds per week is considered significant, because healthy weight loss is one to two pounds per week. Night sweats, weakness, and chills may be present with progressive disease and hemoptysis.

Presenting symptoms of TB in adults are often vague and consist of a cough over three weeks duration, pleuritic chest pain, hemoptysis, fatigue, malaise, anorexia, night sweats, and periodic fevers. Symptoms of extrapulmonary disease depend on the site affected. As with pneumonia a thorough clinical history must be completed.

Diagnostic Tests

Tuberculin skin tests, using the Mantoux method, are used to evaluate the existence of infection or disease. A small amount of tuberculin is injected directly under the skin and the size of the induration is evalutated at 48 to 72 hours. Results are based on the amount of induration at the site and are reported as significant. When there is a five mm induration, it suggests the following: recent contact, an immunocompromised person, and an abnormal CXR. The patient may have a positive reaction to the TB test if he or she: (a) has been exposed to the Mycobacterium tuberculosis; (b) had TB previously which has been successfully treated; (c) has been immunized for TB with the BCG vaccine; or (d) is sick with TB.

CXR and sputum for smear and culture are other diagnostic tests for TB. Sputum for smear and culture must be collected on three different days to increase the chances of identifying the mycobacterium. If the sputum is collected at home, the specimen must be kept refrigerated (Daniels, 2003).

Nursing Diagnoses

Based on the evidence gathered, examples of nursing diagnoses for the patient with pneumonia may include the following:
- Ineffective airway clearance related to inability to remove airway secretions
- Impaired gas exchange related to active inflammatory process
- Activity intolerance related to increased metabolic demands
- Imbalanced nutrition, less than body requirements related to increased caloric requirements

Planning and Implementation

Research gives health care providers the prevailing indication to ensure that the best, more efficient care possible is being provided. Clinical research studies utilize human volunteers or subjects to find ways to improve patient outcomes. There are clinical research trials examining: the effectiveness of directly observed therapy in combined HIV and TB treatment in resource-limiting settings; daily isoniazid to prevent TB in infants born to mothers with HIV; moxifloxacin as part of a multidrug regimen for TB; and investigation vaccine for the prevention of **disseminated** (spread over a large area of the body, tissue, or organ) TB in people with HIV.

Respecting Our Differences

TB and Impartiality

TB can affect anyone who has close contact with a person with active TB. Prisoners, those of lower socioeconomic status, and substance abuse treatment program participants are some of the groups at high risk for acquiring the disease. The nurse must take caution to avoid labeling TB as a disease of the underserved or poor. Any person presenting to the hospital or clinics with a diagnosis of TB regardless of life circumstances and socioeconomic state should be treated with respect and dignity.

Goals

Preventing further spread to the community, deterring disease conversion, and resolving of active disease are the three main goals of treatment for TB. Treatment is also patient-centered based on both clinical and social factors and may include social support, treatment incentives, housing assistance, treatment of drug abuse, and coordination with provider and infectious disease team.

Pharmacology

Pharmacological treatment depends on cause and epidemiological factors. Four medications are used together for the immediate treatment of TB. Once the susceptible results are complete the treatment should be altered for the individual. Medications include isoniazid (INH), rifampin (RIF), ethambutol (EMB), and pyrazinamide (PZA) (Broyles, Reiss, & Evans, 2007). These four medications have proven effective in the treatment of TB. Several side effects can occur while completing the treatment regimen. A common patient compliant is gastrointestinal (GI) distress, including loss of appetite, nausea, vomiting, or stomach pain, during the first few weeks of treatment. Stomach irritation with TB treatment regimens becomes more prevalent as the medications must be given on an empty stomach or two hours after meals and may result in noncompliance with treatment regimen (Table 32-4).

The presence of minor side effects does not result in the discontinuation of medication, and patients are encouraged to continue treatment. A more severe side effect is mild to moderate hepatitis. Medications to treat TB are irritating to liver tissue. Over time the irritated tissue becomes inflamed, resulting in decreased liver functionality, which is manifested in elevated liver enzymes. If moderate hepatitis does occur, medication must be stopped to allow the irritated liver to heal (American Thoracic Society, Center for Disease Control, & Infectious Disease Society of America, 2003). Severe and fatal hepatitis can develop even after months of treatment. If needed, EMB or streptomycin, moxifloxacin, or levofloxan can be used until the cause of hepatitis is identified or the liver tissue heals. These medications are also given for those people who have first-line drug intolerance. Once the aspartate aminotransferase (AST) level has decreased to two times the upper limit of normal and symptoms have improved first-line medications may be restarted.

Recurrence of TB after treatment may occur within 6 to 12 months after the cessation of treatment. The most common reason for recurrence of disease is a noncompliance with the drug regimen. As mentioned previously common reasons for noncompliance with treatment regimens may be cost of treatment, inability to maintain follow-up visits, side effects, and length of treatment. Other factors in recurrence of disease are laboratory error, malabsorption of medication, inappropriate ordering of medications, and resistance to the medication (American Thoracic Society, et al., 2003). Laboratory error can result when the nurse provides a saliva sample instead of sputum. If the patient is unable to cough up secretions, the sample may be obtained through use of a suction catheter. Some patients may develop resistance to drug therapies or may not have received the correct medication regimen. Direct observation therapy (DOT) can minimize nonadherence and requires a health care provider to directly observe the complete administration of the medication. This method has been helpful to ensure compliance but can be difficult to manage.

Tuberculomas may present as solitary lung nodules and are usually resected during surgery for suspected lung cancer. The National Center for Infectious Diseases and the National Guideline Clearinghouse (2003) submitted the following educational and interventional recommendations for patient care:

- Counseling and testing for HIV for all patients with active TB.
- People traveling to countries with a high TB rate should obtain a PPD before they go and on return to the United States.

TABLE 32-4 **Treatment Regimens and Nursing Considerations for Tuberculosis**

DRUG	INDICATIONS FOR USE	DOSAGE	SIDE EFFECTS	NURSING CONSIDERATIONS
Isoniazid (INH)	Treatment of TB and prevention therapy	Preventive dose 300 mg/day For 6 months or 12 months with HIV	Numbness and tingling of hands and feet, loss of sensation, or unusual weakness Dark-colored urine Yellowing skin or eyes indicates liver irritability Report any persistent changes in patient condition; GI distress common with first dosing but should go away with treatment	Avoid in acute hepatic disease or if used in the past and developed hepatotoxicity Administer medication one to two hours before meals on an empty stomach Stains on clothing or contact lenses Complete entire course of therapy
Pyridoxine	Used as adjunct therapy to treat side effects of INH in people at risk for neuropathies or acute INH toxicity	10–50 mg per day	Toxicity can occur with doses 50 mg and over prolonged period of time	
Rifampin (RIF)	Management of active TB			Administer medication one to two hours before meals on an empty stomach Provide adequate hydration unless restricted (two to three liters per day). Increased risk of hepatotoxicity when used in conjunction with INH
Ethambutol (EMB)	Treatment of TB in conjunction with other medications; indicated when people are from areas where drug-resistant myotuberculosis is endemic, in HIV infected elderly, and when drug resistance is suspected	Options depend on individual disease states		Absorption increased when taken with aluminum salts Not recommended in children whose visual acuity cannot be monitored Periodic visual testing Monitor blood test kidney, liver, and bleeding tendencies Take as directed avoid missing doses

Adapted from Broyles, B. E., Reiss, B. S., & Evans, M. E. (2007). Pharmacological aspects of nursing care (7th ed.). New York: Thomson Delmar Learning.

Fast Forward ▶▶▶

TB Vaccine

BCG, or bacille Calmette-Guérin, is a vaccine for tuberculosis (TB) disease. BCG is used in many countries with a high prevalence of TB to prevent childhood tuberculous meningitis and miliary disease. However, BCG is not generally recommended for use in the United States because of the low risk of infection with *Mycobacterium tuberculosis*, the variable effectiveness of the vaccine against adult pulmonary TB, and the vaccine's potential interference with tuberculin skin test reactivity. The BCG vaccine should be considered only for very select persons who meet specific criteria and in consultation with a TB expert.

PATIENT PLAYBOOK

Patient Education for TB

The nurse can explain the following to the patient with TB:

- There are a variety of side affects with the medications that will be taken for the management of the TB, so inform the health care provider of anything unusual (e.g., nausea, GI problems, or fatigue).
- It is vital that patients be instructed that GI distress usually decreased after two to three weeks of treatment.
- Observe for the signs and symptoms of hepatitis (e.g., increased fatigue and weakness, malaise, anorexia, nausea or vomiting, or yellowing of the sclera).
- Periodic eye exams may be necessary if there are any visual problems.

- People with known TB should arrange private transportation. Those patients being treated for active TB should avoid airline contact for eight hours or more.

Patient and Family Teaching

Nursing interventions primarily include patient education on infection control techniques to minimize the risk of spreading the infection. Other instructions highlight side effects including hepatotoxicity, when to notify the health care provider, and importance of strict adherence to medication administration. The nurse should discuss the potential to develop resistance mycobacterium if the medication is not taken correctly to provide understanding and rationale for treatment. The patient is encouraged to maintain a good nutritional status so to improve the body's ability to combat disease.

Evaluation of Outcomes

Potential patient outcomes for each of the example nursing diagnoses for the patient with TB are:

- Ineffective airway clearance. The patient will not aspirate and there will continue to be airway patency.
- Impaired gas exchange related to active inflammatory process. The patient will have adequate pulmonary tissue perfusion as manifested by normal arterial blood gas (ABG) results and normal CXR.
- Activity intolerance related to increased metabolic demands. The patient will perform activities of daily living and maintain endurance.
- Imbalanced nutrition, less than body requirements related to increased caloric requirements. The patient verbalizes and demonstrates selection of foods or meals that will achieve a cessation of weight loss and weighs within 10 percent of ideal body weight.

PULMONARY FUNGAL INFECTION

Many fungi and mold are present in the everyday environment, such as soil, wild animals, and common mold spores. Pulmonary fungal infections are infections in the lungs caused by organisms of the fungi kingdom. Fungi lack chlorophyll and vascular tissue and can range from a single cell to a body mass. Most fungal infections are often localized to the skin or lungs, but they may become systemic. The majority of patients who become exposed to fungal organisms usually do not become ill. Fungal infections typically are more aggressive in the immunocompromised patient and can affect the central nervous system (CNS) bones, joints, or lymph nodes. Opportunistic fungal infections usually occur in patients with DM, alcohol abuse, neutropenia, corticosteroid therapy, and broad-spectrum antibiotic use. Pneumocystis pneumonia is a fungal infection found in the lungs of a variety of domesticated and wild animals and is distributed worldwide. Review the previous section on pneumonia for further review or information. Nonopportunistic infections usually occur in **endemic** (restricted to a particular region, community, or group of people) situations. This section will discuss four common pulmonary fungal infections: (a) blastomycosis; (b) coccidioidomycosis; (c) histoplasmosis; and (d) aspergillus.

Blastomycosis is a chronic fungal disease of the lungs caused by the fungus *Blastomycosis dermatitis*. Blastomycosis often mimics bacterial pneumonia or bronchogenic carcinoma and can be misdiagnosed leading to an unnecessary thoracotomy (Martynowicz & Prakash, 2002). This type of fungal infection is a rare but lethal disease in which symptoms can be asymptomatic, or it may move into a rapid fall of respiratory failure, extrapulmonary dissemination, and death.

Coccidioidomycosis is a pulmonary infection caused by the mold spore *Coccidioides immitis*. Coccidioidomycosis is widespread throughout Southern

California and the desert Southwest, Mexico, central and South America. An incubation period of 10 to 30 days is usually followed by respiratory tract infection with fever and occasional chills. Pleuritic pain is common compliant and can be mistaken for pneumonia. Symptoms may occur in only 40 percent of the cases (Tierney, et al., 2003). Nasopharyngitis may be followed by bronchitis that is accompanied by a dry or slightly productive cough. Extrapulmonary symptoms consist of arthralgia accompanied by periarticular swellings of the knees and ankles with meningitis occurring in 30 to 50 percent of cases of dissemination. Persistent pulmonary lesions occur in a small population and can vary from cavities, abscesses, or bronchiolectasis. It is estimated that 100,000 new infections occur each year (Chiller, Galgiani, & Stevens, 2003)

Histoplasmosis is a pulmonary infection caused by the inhalation of spores of *Histoplasma capsulatum* and most often does not produce symptoms. Histoplasmosis is a serous infection caused by soil-borne fungus, from bird droppings, and is prevalent in Ohio and the Mississippi river valley. Older people with chronic lung disease, infants, and young children are more at risk. Symptoms can be mistaken for pneumonia and include fever, cough, and mild central chest pain lasting one to five days. There are three types of infection: acute, progressive disseminated histoplasmosis, and chronic progressive pulmonary histoplasmosis. Disseminated diseases in profoundly immunocompromised host symptoms are fever and organ system involvement and may mimic septic shock if not treated quickly.

Aspergillosis is an inhaled pulmonary fungal infection caused by fungi of the genus. Allergic bronchopulmonary aspergillosis occurs in patients with preexisting asthma or CF and presents on CXR as fleeting pulmonary infiltrates accompanied by eosinophilia, increased levels of immunoglobulin E (IgE), and noted fungi in blood, which may result in saccular bronchiolectasis and end-stage fibrotic lung disease. Disease progression is a waxing and waning course with gradual improvement over time however, scaring can occur. Life-threatening invasive aspergillosis most commonly occurs in profoundly immunodeficient people, especially if combined with prolonged severe neutropenia. Colonization of preexisting pulmonary cavities may lead to the development of aspergilloma (Tierney, et al., 2003). Symptomatic aspergilloma is treated by surgical debridement.

Pathophysiology

There are approximately 50,000 different species of fungi, but only about a dozen cause 90 percent of all fungal infections. Fungi can grow into two forms of yeast or molds. Fungi may have **dimorphic** (existing in two shapes or forms) properties of yeast and molds. Infection is spread in one of three ways: (a) sensitivity to fungal antigens; (b) fungal toxicity; and (c) growth on host. A person can become sensitized to fungal antigens causing an allergic reaction that produces rhinitis, bronchial asthma, alveolitis, or pneumonitis. Fungi may produce toxic substances called mycotoxins that are harmful to humans. Fungi that grow on a host can produce an infection at the location of attachment. In healthy individuals the fungi growth can be successfully defected by the body defenses. As a result of a decreased ability to fight infection immunocompromised patients are at great risk for acquiring a fungal infection, becoming seriously ill, or even dying from the disease.

Assessment with Clinical Manifestations

As stated previously, most inhalation of fungal spores usually does not result in active disease. However a healthy person who inhales the fungal spores may develop active disease when that person becomes immunocompromised. It is important for the nurse to obtain a complete travel and work history including activities that may have resulted in exposure to soil disturbances, such as windstorms, bird droppings, such as cleaning of chicken coops or working by sea gulls, camping or hiking, causing exposure to dead wood or bird nests, and laboratory work or work on boats. Many of the symptoms of fungal infections can range from minor to full disseminated disease and can mimic other disease processes, such as lung cancer and pneumonia. Most fungal infections result in active disease present as flu-like symptoms that occur several weeks after exposure and usually last one to three weeks depending on the organism causing the infection. Flu-like symptoms may include fatigue, fever, cough, night sweats, and chills. Disseminated fungal disease in a profoundly immunocompromised host presents as fever, organ system involvement, and it may mimic septic shock if not treated quickly.

Diagnostic Tests

Several diagnostic tests are used to diagnose fungal infections. Sputum cultures are effective in defining organisms, but it may take up to five weeks to grow out the specific organisms. Wet smears and cytology examinations provide a quicker diagnosis. Serological assays are insensitive and not useful for diagnostic screening (Martynowicz & Prakash, 2002). Laboratory analyses show a moderate leukocytosis and eosinophilia, and CXR may pick up cavities or lesions. Increased levels of IgE demonstrate activation of an immediate hypersensitive or allergic reaction. Alkaline phosphates are used to evaluate bone involvement with extrapulmonary disease. Erythrocyte sedimentation rate (ESR) is elevated in inflammation or neoplasms.

Nursing Diagnoses

Based on the evidence gathered, examples of nursing diagnoses for the patient with a pulmonary fungal infection may include the following:
- Ineffective airway clearance related to inability to remove airway secretions
- Impaired gas exchange related to infection
- Activity intolerance related to increased metabolic demands
- Fatigue related to inadequate tissue oxygenation

Planning and Implementation

The management strategies for the treatment of the pulmonary fungal infections is similar to the previous section on respiratory disorders. Treating fungal infections remains the same as that for pneumonia and TB: resolution of disease and prevention of recurrence. Because immunocompromised patients are at greatest risk, prevention of recurrence is a primary goal along with resolution of disease without loss of life.

Evidence-Based Care

Much of the current research in fungal disease is evaluating pharmacological interventions and improvement of patient outcomes in the immunocompromised patient. The following are examples of clinical trials in relation to pulmonary fungal infections: several studies of itraconazole in the treatment and prevention of histoplasmosis, a fungal infection in patients with HIV; withdrawal of antifungal treatment for histoplasmosis in patients after improved immune response to anti-HIV drugs; and a pilot study of fluconazole treatment for histoplasmosis, blastomycosis, and sporotrichosis.

Pharmacology

Treatment of systematic disease usually consists of antifungal medications, such as itraconazole or fluconazole, or amphotericin. Oral itraconazole and fluconazole have been shown to have an overall response rat of 75 to 80 percent. Oral antifungal medications are an effective treatment, but therapy may continue for up to six months. Because disseminated or extrapulmonary disease can be a life-threatening condition in the immunocompromised individual, treatment may be a lifelong intervention (Tierney, et al., 2003). Amphotericin B is reserved for individuals who cannot take oral medications or who fail oral medication treatment. As with any medication the nurse must be aware of side effects.

IV fluconazole is reserved for those patients who are unable to take the oral form of medication or who are unable to tolerate amphotericin B. Rifampin, a medication used to treat TB, can decrease the effectiveness of fluconazole. Side effects of oral antifungal infections include: (a) headache; (b) seizures; (c) vertigo; (d) rash; (e) nausea; (f) vomiting; and (g) hepatitis. The nurse should monitor liver function and kidney function closely. A complete neurological and pulmonary assessment must be completed prior to initiation of antifungal medications. A baseline view of the overall patient condition will assist in assessment of changes.

Amphotericin B, given intravenously via a central line, must be administered according to established hospital protocol and monitored closely as the medication has the potential to cause acute renal dysfunction and is a caustic to skin. Caution should be taken to avoid the medication spilling on clothes or skin. Any spills must be cleansed up using hospital protocol for hazardous spills. During amphotericin B treatment encourage two to three liters of fluid per day to ensure adequate kidney function. Other side effects include muscle aches, dry mouth, nausea, vomiting anorexia, or hypotension. Collaborative interventions include providing analgesics for muscle aches and suggesting small, frequent meals to prevent or minimize GI distress. To moisten the mouth as well as enhancing salvia gland function the patient can suck hard candy or lemon wedges. The nurse can instruct the patient to avoid quick movements of the body or head and encourage assistance with mobility to minimize the hypertensive effects.

Evaluation of Outcomes

Potential patient outcomes for each of the example nursing diagnosis for the patient with pulmonary fungal infections are:
- Ineffective airway clearance. The patient will not aspirate and there will continue to be airway patency.
- Impaired gas exchange related to active inflammatory process. The patient will have adequate pulmonary tissue perfusion as manifested by normal ABG results and normal CXR
- Activity intolerance related to increased metabolic demands. The patient will perform activities of daily living and maintain endurance.
- Fatigue related to inadequate tissue perfusion. The patient maintains activity level within capabilities, as evidenced by normal heart rate and blood pressure during activity, as well as absence of shortness of breath, weakness, and fatigue.

BRONCHIOLECTASIS

Bronchiolectasis is an acquired or congenital disorder of the large bronchi in which chronic dilation of the bronchioles occurs over time, resulting in increased mucous formation and difficulty breathing. As with many of the diseases discussed in this chapter, the disease process may be diffused or localized. There are three types of bronchiolectasis based on the effects of the disease process: (a) cylindrical; (b) varicose; and (c) cystic (American Lung Association, 2003a). The first type of bronchiolectasis, cylindrical, is the mildest case that presents with only slight widening of the respiratory passages and may be a reversible condition. The second type is called varicose, in which air sacs fail in portions of the passages. The third type is cystic, the most severe type, involved ballooning or expansion of the air sacs. Bronchiolectasis is a disease caused by multiple insults of permanent dilation and destruction of the cartilage containing airways versus one episode.

Epidemiology

Congenital disorders that can lead to bronchiolectasis include cystic fibrosis (CF) and primary ciliary dyskinesia. Congenital disorders may have symptoms start as early as age 2 years. In the United States CF makes up about 50 percent of bronchiolectasis cases and will be discussed in detail in chapter 33 (American Lung Association, 2003a).

Etiology

Risk factors for acquiring bronchiolectasis include diseases or processes that permit chronic pulmonary insults. Smokers and people with pulmonary infections, such as fungal disease, are at risk because of the chronic irritation to the pulmonary system. Other patients at risk include those people with immunodeficiency states, such as acquired immune deficiency syndrome (AIDS), lymphoma, multiple myeloma, and leukemia. The final risk factors for acquiring bronchiolectasis include people with chronic liver or renal disease.

Pathophysiology

Bronchiolectasis is a vicious cycle of bacterial colonization, inflammatory change, increased production of mucus, scarring, and more bacterial colonization. Bacteria entering the respiratory tract leads to damage of the mucociliary mechanism. This damage in turn prevents bacterial clearance, enhancing inflammatory change, and intensifies production of mucus. Over time, stretching and enlargement of the respiratory passages occurs, resulting in scarring and deformity, which in turn permits more mucus and bacteria to build up and the cycle start over again.

Assessment with Clinical Manifestations

Symptoms of bronchiolectasis mimic many other lower airway diseases. One common symptom of bronchiolectasis is chronic cough, especially when lying down, that is productive of copious amounts of purulent sputum. **Purulent sputum** is a light green to yellowish white fluid formed in infected tissue and consists of white blood cells, cellular debris, and necrotic or dead tissue. Other manifestations are hemoptysis, hypoxemia with moderate and severe cases, weight loss, weakness, and dyspnea. Persistent crackles are heard at the base of the lung and clubbing of the fingers can occur in severe cases.

Diagnostic Tests

Diagnostic tests consist of CXR, sputum culture, computer tomography (CT) scan, and bronchoscopy. CXRs show peribronchial fibrosis and small cysts at the base of the lungs. High-resolution CT is the treatment of choice; and bronchoscopy is used to evaluate hemoptysis, remove secretions, and rule out obstructed airways. Auscultation identifies persistent crackles at lung bases (Estes, 2006).

Nursing Diagnoses

Based on the evidence gathered, examples of nursing diagnoses for the patient with bronchiolectasis may include the following:
- Ineffective airway clearance related to inability to remove airway secretions
- Impaired gas exchange related to production of copious amounts of mucus

- Activity intolerance related to increased metabolic demands
- Fatigue related to inadequate tissue oxygenation

Planning and Implementation

Treatment goals are to treat infection, minimize further damage, promote effective airway breathing, and remove secretions. This is accomplished by postural drainage, chest percussion, antibiotics, and inhaled bronchodilators. Oxygen may be administered by nasal prongs or face mask and should be administered to keep the oxygen saturation equal to or greater than 92 percent. Providing adequate hydration will liquefy secretions and make them easier to expectorate. Limiting activity and rest periods are interventions used to decrease the oxygen demands of the body. Walking three to four times a day with rest periods of at least two hours can be an effective method to maintain mobility and provide rest. Effective pain control will not only promote mobility but also increase patient outcomes from chest physiotherapy and cough and deep breathing exercises. Pain medication given 30 to 45 minutes before exercise is usually ineffective. Close monitoring of pain medications effects is required secondary to the CNS effects, including risk of falls and aspiration.

Cough and deep breathing exercises every one to two hours while awake will assist in the removal of organisms in the lungs. Chest physiotherapy and postural drainage use gravity to clear secretions while percussion uses vibration to loosen secretions. Oxygen is administered to aid in ensuring adequate ventilation and improving oxygen levels. Pulse oximetry will detect a change in condition before clinical symptoms are present. Abnormal readings on pulse oximetry can be a reflection of inaccurate date and not the true clinical picture, so the nurse should always assess the patient's condition whenever clinical data is collected. Lung resections, in the case of advanced disease or severe hemoptysis, are used only in a few patients who do not respond to treatment.

Evidence-Based Care

Research gives health care providers the prevailing indication to ensure the best care possible is being provided. Clinical research studies utilize human volunteers or subjects to find ways to improve patient outcomes. Current research is studying patients with CF and other pulmonary and pancreatic disorders. The purpose of this study is to provide information on the prognosis of the disease and recommendations for the management of CF. Because 50 percent of all bronchiolectasis cases in the United States are preventable, this research is important to assist in the prevention of bronchiolectasis.

Pharmacology

Antibiotics are given for 7 to 14 days and are selected depending on the organism involved. Amoxicillin, ampicillin, tetracycline, or sulfa medications are some of the antibiotics effective in treating acute episodes (Broyles, et al., 2007). Penicillins, such as amoxicillin, work by interfering with the bacterial cell wall synthesis or growth causing the cell wall of the bacteria organism to die. Amoxicillin is given by mouth in doses of 250 to 500 mg every eight hours or 500 to 875 mg twice daily. Patients with renal impairment may require a lower dose as this medication can be irritating to the kidney system. Oral suspensions remain stable for 7 days when at room temperature and 14 days when refrigerated. Amoxicillin side effects include: (a) hyperactivity; (b) insomnia; (c) rashes; (d) nausea; (e) vomiting; (f) diarrhea; (g) anemia; and (h) elevated liver function tests. Ampicillin may be given by mouth (PO), intramuscular (IM), or intravenously. Oral adult doses are 250 to 500 mg every six hours while IV doses are 500 mg to 3 g every four to six hours with a maximal dose of 12 g per day. In the hospital setting antibiotics are rarely given IM as this route can cause acute discomfort at the injection site with each dose given. If possible, oral or IV route of medication administration provides the best comfort to the patient. The nurse should closely monitor liver and renal function tests to ensure toxicity effects are not present. Bronchodilators are used to expand the bronchi, allowing removal of secretions through the use of an inhaled mist. A common bronchodilator medication used is albuterol. One effect of albuterol is tachycardia, so the nurse needs to assess pulse rate before and after administration to avoid a possible misinterpretation and or treatment of tachycardia with cardiac medications. The nurse must always know the baseline data and assessment of any patient.

Patient and Family Teaching

The nurse should provide education on smoking cessation programs as well as information on local support groups. Because the diagnosis of bronchiolectasis may result in a chronic disease state, it is important that patient and families have access to support groups. The American Lung Association is an excellent resource for education and treatment options. Other patient education emphasizes adequate hydration, activity as tolerated, and provision of rest periods after activity. The nurse also should discuss pain control and encourage patients to take pain medication when discomfort is first noted and not wait until pain is present to ensure effective pain control. Instruction on the side effects of medications and when to call the physician must be discussed to ensure quick access the health care system as well as patient safety.

Patient education should also recommend vaccinations against measles, pneumonia, and other infections to minimize the chronic effects of bronchiolectasis.

Evaluation of Outcomes

Potential patient outcomes for each of the example nursing diagnoses for the patient with bronchiolectasis are:

- Ineffective airway clearance. The patient will not aspirate and there will continue to be airway patency.
- Impaired gas exchange related to active inflammatory process. The patient will have adequate pulmonary tissue perfusion as manifested by normal ABG results and normal CXR
- Activity intolerance related to increased metabolic demands. The patient will perform activities of daily living and maintain endurance.
- Fatigue related to inadequate tissue perfusion. The patient maintains activity level within capabilities, as evidenced by normal heart rate and blood pressure during activity, as well as absence of shortness of breath, weakness, and fatigue.

LUNG ABSCESS

Acute inflammation can result in localized formation of an **abscess,** which is a collection or cavity of fluid or cellular debris as a result of necrosis. This cavity is often surrounded by infection as the body makes an attempt to destroy the abscess. Lung abscesses can be acute or chronic in nature. An acute lung abscess is one that is present less or equal to six weeks while a chronic lung abscess chronic is present more than six weeks.

Epidemiology

Lung abscesses can develop from pulmonary infections, such as pneumonia, mycobacterium tuberculosis, fungal infections, and bronchiolectasis. Aspiration of bacteria from the oral pharynx accounts for 60 to 75 percent of all lung abscess cases (Chaudhry, Capicatto, & O'Brien, 2002). Lung cancer can also cause lung abscesses as the cancer destroys pulmonary cells and forms a tumor.

Etiology

Two leading risk factors for aspiration include alcohol and mental status changes. Other risk factors for aspiration are dysphasia and oral pharyngeal dysfunction. Periodontal disease, an infection of the gums because decaying teeth, can allow bacteria from the infected gum to be introduced into the pulmonary tree, leading to an abscess formation. Lung abscesses are typically uncommon in people who wear dentures, and if it does occur, other sources for the infection must be sought out (Chaudhry, et al., 2002).

Pathophysiology

Lung abscesses start when a person has an impaired ability to clear bacteria from the pulmonary tract as a result of obstruction or tumor. The bacteria continue to reproduce and grow within the lung tissue, leading to a massive bacterial burden that causes tissue necrosis and formation of the lung abscess cavity, which may be filled with fluid or pus.

Assessment with Clinical Manifestations

Symptoms of lung abscesses mimic many of the other lower airway infections discussed in this chapter and include fever, chills, night sweats, productive cough of foul sputum, dyspnea, fatigue, weight loss, pleuritic chest pain, and hemoptysis. Patients with periodontal disease will often have foul-smelling breath. On auscultation of the lung fields, bronchial breath sounds are heard with percussion defining localized dullness over the involved lung. Clubbing of the fingers may also be present.

Diagnostic Tests

Laboratory tests consist of sputum samples and a CBC. Sputum samples will be evaluated using a gram-stain procedure and be examined for bacteria, mycobacterium, and fungal infections. A CBC will be used to identify infection type. The CXR will show a fluid-filled solitary cavity lesion surrounded by infection versus a solid nodule that is present with tumors. Because CXRs may not be conclusive or are suspicious for another disease process, a CT of the chest or bronchoscopy may be used to rule out conditions such as lung cancer.

Nursing Diagnoses

Based on the evidence gathered, examples of nursing diagnoses for the patient with lung abscess may include the following:
* Ineffective airway clearance related to inability to remove airway secretions
* Impaired gas exchange related to presence of cavity lesion
* Activity intolerance related to increased metabolic demands
* Acute pain related to muscle strain and effects of coughing

Planning and Implementation

Treatment goals for the patient with a lung abscess incorporate the same interventions for all lower airway pulmonary infections and include minimizing further tissue damage, promoting effective airway breathing, removal of secretions, and treatment of infection. This is accomplished by postural drainage, chest percussion, antibiotics, and inhaled bronchodilators. Oxygen may be administered by nasal prongs or face mask and should be administered to keep the oxygen saturation equal to or greater than 92 percent. Providing adequate hydration will liquefy secretions and make them easier to expectorate. Limiting activity and rest periods are interventions used to decrease the oxygen demands of the body. Walking three to four times a day with rest periods of at least two hours can be an effective method to maintain mobility and provide rest. Effective pain control will not only promote mobility but also increase patient outcomes from chest physiotherapy and cough and deep breathing exercises. Pain medication given 30 to 45 minutes before exercise is usually ineffective. Close monitoring of pain medications effects is required secondary to the CNS effects, including risk of falls and aspiration.

Cough and deep breathing exercises every one to two hours while awake will assist in the removal of organisms in the lungs. Chest physiotherapy and postural drainage use gravity to clear secretions while percussion uses vibration to loosen secretions. Oxygen is administered to aid in ensuring adequate ventilation and improving oxygen levels. Pulse oximetry will detect a change in condition before clinical symptoms are present. Abnormal readings on pulse oximetry can be a reflection of inaccurate data and not the true clinical picture, so the nurse should always assess the patient's condition whenever clinical data are collected. Lung resections, in the case of advanced disease or severe hemoptysis, are used only in a few patients who do not respond to treatment.

Pharmacology

Long-term antibiotic therapy is needed to accurately resolve a lung abscess. Penicillin interferes with growth of the bacterial cell wall causing the cell wall of the bacteria organism to die. An initial dose of penicillin is given intravenously, followed by subsequent IV doses of penicillin V 750 to 1,000 mg four times a day or clindamycin 600 mg every eight hours. When the patient is discharged home, dosing consists of clindamycin 300 mg by mouth four times a day for six weeks.

Metronidazole may be used as well, because up to one third of gram-negative anaerobes may produce β-lactamase. Clindamycin inhibits bacterial protein synthesis and is bacteriostatic or bactericidal depending on drug concentration, infection site, and organism (Broyles, et al., 2007). Patients allergic to penicillin are often given clindamycin, as the medication is not part of the penicillin family. The nurse must observe the patient for a potential cross-sensitivity reaction with clindamycin, especially in individuals allergic to penicillin. Cross-sensitivity reactions are allergic reactions that can occur when given the same class of medication. Any patient receiving an antibiotic should be monitored for an allergic reaction even if the person has been on a particular antibiotic before.

Patients with renal impairment may require a lower dose as these medications can be irritating to the renal system. In the hospital setting antibiotics are rarely given IM as this route can cause acute discomfort at the injection site with each dose given. If possible, oral or IV route of medication administration provides the best comfort to the patient. The nurse should closely monitor liver and renal function tests to ensure toxicity effects are not present. Bronchodilators are used to expand the bronchi allowing removal of secretions through the use of an inhaled mist. A common bronchodilator medication used is albuterol. One effect of albuterol is tachycardia, so the nurse needs to assess pulse rate before and after administration to avoid a possible misinterpretation and or treatment of tachycardia with cardiac medications. The nurse must always know the baseline data and assessment of any patient. He or she should also obtain a baseline blood pressure, pulse, respiratory rate, and notice of any rashes prior to administration of bronchodilators and antibiotics.

Patient and Family Teaching

Patient and family education include instruction of signs and symptoms of infection and when to call the health care provider including increase sputum or foul-smelling sputum, fever above 38.1° C (100.5° F). Patients should be instructed to rest prior to activity and to take frequent naps to allow the body to heal and decrease strain to the cardiac and pulmonary system. Instruction also includes increasing caloric intake and maintenance of a healthy diet to increase the body's immune system.

Evaluation of Outcomes

Potential patient outcomes for each of the example nursing diagnosis for the patient with lung abscess are:

- Ineffective airway clearance. The patient will not aspirate and there will continue to be airway patency.
- Impaired gas exchange related to active inflammatory process. The patient will have adequate pulmonary tissue perfusion as manifested by normal ABG results and normal CXR.
- Activity intolerance related to increased metabolic demands. The patient will perform activities of daily living (ADL) and maintain endurance.
- Acute pain related to muscle strain and effects of coughing. The patient should verbalize an adequate relief of pain along with the ability to realistically cope with the pain if it is not completely relieved.

LUNG CANCER

Cancer is caused by a variety of malignant neoplasms in which cells mutate and invade surrounding tissue and can travel via the lymphatic system or blood vessels to other secondary sites. Lung cancer is a term used to identify cancer in the lungs and can be primary or secondary. Primary cancer is the body system or site where the cancer was first observed. **Metastasis** is the transmission of cancer cells from the original site to one or more sites elsewhere in the body. For example, a person may have lung cancer as a primary site, but the cancer travels to the bone, causing bone cancer, which becomes the secondary site.

Epidemiology

One million patients worldwide die from lung cancer annually. Lung cancer remains the leading cause of cancer death in both men and women, with an estimated 347,000 people having lung cancer in the United States. The expected five-year survival rate for all people diagnosed with lung cancer is 16 percent compared to 63 percent for colon cancer, 88 percent for breast cancer, and 99 percent for prostate cancer. If lung cancer is caught in the early or localized stage survival jumps from 16 to 49 percent (American Lung Association Epidemiology and Statistic Unit Research and Scientific Affairs, 2004). While there have been improvements in treatment of lung cancer, those changes are relatively minor in relation to other cancer breakthroughs.

Etiology

Smoking is the number one risk factor in about 85 to 90 percent of those identified as having lung cancer. The pack per day or amount and years of smoking history has a direct relationship on the risk of acquiring lung cancer. The person who has smoked one pack per day over 10 years is at increased risk for having lung cancer over a person who has smoked half a pack per day for 8 years. However, if a person stops smoking, the lung tissue can heal over time and decreases the chance of acquiring lung cancer. Marijuana has more tar and also can cause cancers of the mouth and throat (American Lung Association Epidemiology and Statistic Unit Research and Scientific Affairs, 2004). Studies show that the lung cells of women are also more prone to the effects of smoking (American Cancer Society, 2004e). Secondhand smoke has also been shown to be more harmful than previous realized.

Another cause of lung cancer is asbestos exposure that starts in the pleura and develops into mesothelioma, a rare malignant form of lung cancer. Radon, a radioactive gas made by the natural breakdown of uranium, cannot be seen, smelled, or tasted. Smokers are sensitive to the effects of radon. TB

Respecting Our Differences

Smokers with Lung Cancer

Because the primary cause of lung cancer is smoking, people with lung cancer may be viewed as a person who caused their own illness by smoking. The nurse must remember that other factors, such as asbestos, can also cause lung cancer and should avoid labeling a patient as a smoker, because he or she has lung cancer. The patient who smoked and presents with lung cancer, as with all patients, must be treated with dignity and respect. Lung cancer patients are facing a life-threatening, scary, life-altering illness and need encouragement, support, and compassion without judgment or bias.

and pneumonia can leave scars on the lining of the lung, increasing the risk of lung cancer. Other risk factors for lung cancer include a diet low in fruits and vegetable, family history, and previous history of lung cancer.

Lung cancer classification depends on the size of the cell and includes small cell and large cell cancer. Small cell lung cancer (SCLC) makes up about 20 to 25 percent of all lung cancers and is almost always caused by smoking (American Cancer Society, 2004e). Non–small cell lung cancer (NSCLC) is further divided into three groups that are defined by location. The first group is squamous cell carcinoma centrally located near a bronchus. The second type of NSCLC, adenocarcinoma, which presents on the outer region of the lung. The third type of NSCLC is large cell carcinoma that can appear in any part of the lung, tends to grow quickly, and carries a poor prognosis. Another type of lung cancer called mesothelioma affects the cells of the pleura and is treated differently. Metastasis or secondary cancer is treated at the primary site.

Pathophysiology

Lung cancer starts in the lining of the bronchi when the cells mutate and develop over the course of several years. Changes in the lining allow new blood vessels to develop, which provide nourishment to the cancer cells. These cells continue to grow and develop into a mature cancer. Unfortunately symptoms usually do not appear until the cancer is well developed. Once the diagnosis of cancer is made the extent of the cancer is staged so that the right treatment plan can be initiated. Overall staging of cancer is also discussed in chapter 15. Most types of cancers are staged according to tumor size (T), lymph node involvement (N), and metastasis (M). SCLC has a staging system of limited and extensive. Limited SCLC implies only one lung and lymph nodes on the same side of one lung are affected. Extensive SCLC means that cancer has spread across both lungs, lymph nodes, fluid around lung, or distant organs. Once the stage grouping of TNM for NSCLC has been assigned, this information is combined an overall stage of using roman numbers 0 to IV. Patients with a lower stage have a more favorable outlook for survival (American Cancer Society, 2004e).

Assessment with Clinical Manifestations

Lung cancer symptoms usually appear when the cancer has become large enough to be seen on CXR. Lung cancer may be noticed on a sputum test in the early stages of the disease but is usually diagnosed when the cancer is big enough to be seen on CXR or a person presents in clinic with symptoms of metastasis to the breast, GI system, or prostate. Symptoms of lung cancer are diffuse and can mimic many of the diseases already discussed and include dyspnea, chronic cough with hemoptysis, enlarged lymph nodes, finger clubbing (a late sign of lung cancer), weight loss, bone pain, chest pain or tightness, and joint pain (U. S. National Library of Medicine & National Institutes of Health, 2004).

Diagnostic Tests

Tests to assist in the diagnosis of lung cancer include a multitude of procedures to determine a precise evaluation. These tests are shown in Box 32-2.

Nursing Diagnoses

Based on the evidence gathered, examples of nursing diagnosis for the patient with lung cancer may include the following:
- Impaired gas exchange related to compression of cancer tumor on pulmonary tissue
- Anxiety related to diagnosis of lung cancer

BOX 32-2

DIAGNOSTIC TESTS FOR LUNG CANCER

- CXR and sputum can be used for screening. However, this practice is not yet recommended as routine.
- Computed tomography (CT) provides information about size, shape, and tumor location.
- Low-dose CT (LDCT)—currently being studied as a screening mechanism in clinical trials (National Guideline Clearinghouse, 2003).
- Magnetic resonance imaging (MRI) is used to find cancer that has metastasized.
- Positive emission tomography (PET).
- Bone scan test to evaluate non–small cell lung cancer (American Cancer Society, 2004e).
- Sputum cytology sometimes can find cancers so small they cannot be seen on a CXR or a CT scan.
- Needle or open biopsy of the lung.
- Bronchoscopy assesses the lining of the airways.
- Thoracentesis and thoracoscopy assess the fluid around the lung.
- Bone marrow biopsy to assess for bone involvement.
- Blood tests, CBC, and sedimentation rate.

- Pain, acute and chronic related to effects of tumor expansion and compression of tissue
- Activity intolerance related to increased metabolic demands

Planning and Implementation

The overall management of lung cancer has treatment goals to maintain a good quality of life or cure cancer, if possible. There are treatment modalities in combinations of chemotherapy, radiation, and surgery. Improved techniques that allow faster sputum results also visualize cancer cells more clearly. As with any disease process, good nutrition helps combat disease while boosting the immune system. Increasing fruits and vegetables, whole grain foods, decreased alcohol consumption, and exercise when tolerated are all mechanisms to fight lung cancer. Treatment of lung cancer consists of chemotherapy, radiation, and surgical resection, which can be difficult for the patient to manage. Increasing calories to 2,500 daily will assist the body in combating the cancer and treatment regimen. The patient may find eating five or six small meals a day may be more easily tolerated and minimizes the nausea effects of chemotherapy. Many health care providers will recommend the unofficial C-diet. In this diet the patient is instructed to eat any food he or she wishes and not worry about calories. The nurse must monitor for fluid overload and especially for pleural effusions. Electrolytes and hydration must be assessed daily. A patient who has a thoracotomy should practice arm exercises to ensure continued mobility and promotion of lung expansion.

Confusion can occur as a result of the chemotherapy effects. It is important for the nurse to have a baseline assessment to obtain a full clinical picture of the patient's mental status. Patient safety is important to prevent falls that can occur as a result of medication side effects, pain, depression, and weakness. The nurse should make sure that the bathroom is accessible or that a commode is placed near the bed. Avoid clutter in the room or floor that the patient may have to step over and possibly trip.

Providing adequate hydration will liquefy secretions and make them easier to expectorate. Limiting activity and rest periods are interventions used to decrease the oxygen demands of the body. Walking three to four times a day with rest periods of at least two hours can be an effective method to maintain mobility and provide rest. Effective pain control will not only promote mobility but also increase patient outcomes from chest physiotherapy and cough and deep breathing exercises. Pain medication given 30 to 45 minutes before exercise is usually ineffective. Close monitoring of pain medications effects is required secondary to the CNS effects including risk of falls and aspiration.

Cough and deep breathing exercises every one to two hours while awake will assist in the removal of organisms in the lungs. Chest physiotherapy and postural drainage uses gravity to clear secretions while percussion uses vibration to loosen secretions. Oxygen is administered to aid in ensuring adequate ventilation and improving oxygen levels.

Evidence-Based Care

Research gives health care providers the prevailing indication to ensure that the best, most efficient care possible is being provided. There is extensive research being performed in the treatment of lung cancer and improvement of patient outcomes. Many of the studies are looking at effectiveness of chemotherapy agents and possible vaccine treatments. Further information on the research related to cancer is seen in chapter 15.

Pharmacology

Chemotherapy medications can cause side effects of hair loss, anorexia, and death of any healthy cells. Anemia may be a result of the destruction of red blood cells. The older a woman is, the more likely she will stop menstruating or lose her ability to become pregnant. Clinical trails of medications have found that erlotinib (Tarceva) prolonged survival in patients with advanced NSCLC who had progressed after standard therapy. Antianxiety medications, such as lorazepam, may be helpful in decreasing anxiety and allowing a restful sleep. Medications to relieve nausea include Zofran and ranitidine. Narcotic pain medications may be given by mouth under the tongue and may be sustained release or fast acting.

Radiation

Radiation can also be used in the treatment of lung cancer. External beam radiation is sometimes used as the main treatment of lung cancer to relieve such symptoms as pain, bleeding, or passages blocked by the cancer. External beam radiation is usually given in daily doses five days a week for six to eight weeks. Brachytherapy or internal radiation places radioactive material inside the lung but may lead to lung damage. Side effects of brain radiation usually become more serious one to two years after treatment and include headaches and trouble with thinking. Postoperative radiotherapy for NSCLC is detrimental to patients in the early stage and should not be used in the routine treatment of such patients (Cochrane Database of Systematic Reviews, 2004).

Surgery

Several surgical procedures may be performed. Lobectomy to remove a lobe or section of the lung or the entire lung can be removed in a pneumonectomy. Moderate pain occurs after surgery as the surgical incision is through the ribs. Dyspnea may occur after surgery, especially if the patient has bronchitis, asthma, or diseases of decreased lung tissue or capacity. If a person cannot tolerate surgery or the cancer is widespread, laser surgery may be used to treat the cancer or decrease side effects of tumor compression or metastasis. A newer surgical technique, called an embolization, selectively places a thin tube into the artery that supplies the tumor. Material is then injected into the tube blocking the blood flow and destroys the cancer cells. Alternative therapy is not recommended without the advice of the treatment team. Oxygen therapy is used to promote adequate oxygenation and provide comfort.

Patient and Family Teaching

Patient education includes preoperative patient education, diet recommendation, administration of medications, and importance of rest. Support groups such as the American Cancer Society, American Lung Association, and National Comprehensive Cancer Network are excellent sources of information and can assist the patient in finding a support group.

Evaluation of Outcomes

Potential patient outcomes for each of the nursing diagnoses for the patient with lung cancer are:

- Impaired gas exchange related to compression of cancer tumor on pulmonary tissue. The patient maintains optimal gas exchange as evidenced by normal ABGs and alert, responsive mentation or no further reduction in mental status.
- Anxiety related to diagnosis of lung cancer. The patient should manifest positive coping behaviors and verbalize a reduction in the amount of fear of the having this disease.
- Pain, acute and chronic related to effects of tumor expansion and compression of tissue. The patient should verbalize an adequate relief of pain along with the ability to realistically cope with the pain if it is not completely relieved.
- Activity intolerance related to increased metabolic demands. The patient maintains activity level within capabilities, as evidenced by normal heart rate and blood pressure during activity, as well as absence of shortness of breath, weakness, and fatigue.
- Adequate pulmonary tissue perfusion as manifested by normal ABG results and normal CXR.
- Activity intolerance related to increased metabolic demands. The patient will perform ADL and maintain endurance.
- Acute pain related to muscle strain and effects of coughing. The patient should verbalize an adequate relief of pain along with the ability to realistically cope with the pain if it is not completely relieved.

PNEUMOTHORAX

Pneumothorax is a collection of air in the pleural cavity that may occur as a result of trauma, TB, or chronic respiratory diseases. This collection of air between the lungs and the pleura (thin serous membrane that surrounds each lung) leads to a collapse of all or part of a lung.

Etiology

Risk factors for pneumothorax include: (a) smoking; (b) family history; (c) trauma; or (d) pulmonary disease affecting the pulmonary ability of the lungs to expand. There are four types of pneumothorax: (a) spontaneous; (b) traumatic; (c) iatrogenic; and (d) tension. As the name suggests, spontaneous pneumothorax occurs suddenly as a result of either a primary or secondary condition. An example of a primary condition is **idiopathic** (relating to a disease in which the cause is not identified) spontaneous pneumothorax that occurs in the absence of lung disease and mainly affects men between the ages of 20 and 40 years of age. The cause of the lung collapse is not known, but it is thought to occur from rupture of subpleural apical blebs in response to high negative intrapleural pressures, such as those produced with sport activities (Tierney, et al., 2003). Secondary spontaneous pneumothorax occurs as a complication of existing disease such as COPD, asthma, CF, TB, or pneumonia. In the case of a secondary spontaneous pneumothorax, the lungs are, through the effects of disease, unable to fully expand secondary to the congestion of the alveoli (in pneumonia) to fibrosis of lung tissue (in chronic pulmonary disease). This failure to expand builds up intrapleural pressure and places the person at risk for a collapsed lung.

Traumatic pneumothorax is a result of blunt physical trauma and can be further classified as penetrating or nonpenetrating. Penetrating traumatic pneumothorax is an injury that has open communication with the outside air caused by a sharp object that opens the chest cavity. A nonpenetrating traumatic pneumothorax is without communication with the outside air and occurs typically from the chest wall striking an object, such as a steering wheel during a motor vehicle accident (MVA).

Occult or hidden pneumothorax is defined as a lung collapse injury noted on CT scan but not detected on CXR. Iatrogenic pneumothorax occurs as a result of a procedure complication, such as thoracentesis, pleural biopsy, central line placement, or high positive-pressure ventilation settings.

Tension pneumothorax usually occurs in the presence of trauma, lung infection, cardiopulmonary resuscitation (CPR), or positive-pressure ventilation. The usual pressure of air in the pleural space exceeds the ambient pressure generated by the respiratory causing a tension pneumothorax to develop at anytime. The nurse taking care of any trauma patient must observe for a delayed tension pneumothorax.

Pathophysiology

Pneumothorax injury creates a one-way valve effect that causes air to continually collect within the pleural space. This trapped air leads to lung atelectasis, pulmonary collapse, and disturbances in ventilation. As a tension pneumothorax continues to develop, pressure is placed on the mediastinal structures, which in turn causes a shift of the trachea toward the unaffected side. This increased pressure on the mediastinum creates increased intra-aortic pressure resulting in a reduction in venous return. Pleural effusions occur as a result of the buildup of fluid in the lung. Pneumothorax can mimic cardiac tamponade, PE, or pneumonia.

Assessment with Clinical Manifestations

The nurse's assessment in respiratory emergencies must include airway, breathing, and circulation (ABCs) and basic life support techniques. Assessment and clinical manifestations of pneumothorax include pleuritic chest pain ranging from mild to severe on the affected side. Dyspnea, tachypnea, tachycardia, hypotension, and respiratory distress are common and can be a sudden or gradual event. In tension pneumothorax, air hunger or a gasping for breath may occur and tracheal deviation to the opposite side may be present with neck vein distension resulting from decreased venous return. Anxiety occurs due to inability to catch a breath, which is distressing and terrifying. Cough may or may not be present and may have hemoptysis. The severity of symptoms is a result of the size and involvement of the pneumothorax and lung involvement. On auscultation of the lung, breath sounds will be absent. The patient with a pneumothorax must receive treatment to remove the air or fluid to avoid pending respiratory failure, especially if there is an underlying COPD or asthma involvement.

Diagnostic Tests

ABGs reveal hypoxemia and respiratory alkalosis that results from abnormal loss of carbon dioxide due to hyperventilation. Electrocardiogram (ECG) changes reflect a left-side QRS axis and precordial T wave changes that may be misinterpreted as an acute myocardial infarction. CXR can see the pneumothorax, but it can only be seen on expiratory film (Daniels, 2003).

Nursing Diagnoses

Based on the evidence gathered, examples of nursing diagnoses for the patient with pneumothorax may include the following:

- Activity intolerance related to compromised oxygen transport system
- Anxiety related to actual or perceived threat to biological integrity
- Pain, acute related to lung collapse and placement of chest tube
- Ineffective breathing patterns related to collapse lung

Planning and Implementation

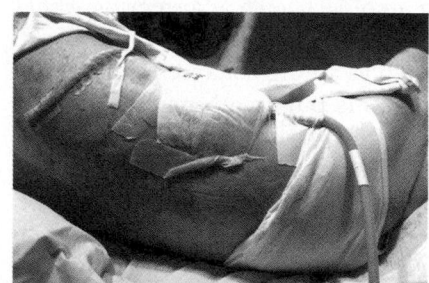

Figure 32-3 A patient with a chest tube that has been secured with bandages and tape to keep it from becoming dislodged.

Treatment goals for pneumothorax include: (a) removal of air and fluid from pleura space; (b) correction of acid-base imbalances; (c) minimizing further damage; and (d) reexpansion of the lung. To remove fluid or air from the pleural space, a chest tube must be inserted, using a large-bore needle, into the second intercostal space of the anterior midclavicular line. This creates a communication between the atmosphere and the pleural space, allowing the air or fluid to move out, which in turn, decompresses intrapleural pressure. After the needle decompression, a chest tube is inserted into the fifth intercostal space and connected to a chest drainage device (Figure 32-3). Oxygen may be administered by nasal prongs or face mask and should be administered to keep the oxygen saturation equal to or greater than 92 percent. Providing adequate hydration will liquefy secretions and make them easier to expectorate. Limiting activity and rest periods are interventions used to decrease the oxygen demands of the body. Walking three to four times a day with rest periods of at least two hours can be an effective method to maintain mobility and provide rest. Effective pain control will not only promote mobility but also increase patient outcomes from cough and deep breathing exercises. Pain medication given 30 to 45 minutes before exercise is usually ineffective. Close monitoring of the side effects of pain medication are required secondary to the CNS effects, including risk of falls and aspiration. Cough and deep breathing exercises every one to two hours while awake will assist in the removal of secretions in the lungs. Oxygen is administered to aid in ensuring adequate ventilation and improving oxygen levels.

Chest tubes can play a vital role in managing a pneumothorax. The purpose of any chest drainage system is to help reestablish normal vacuum pressures by removing air and fluid using a closed one-way method. Air and fluid goes out but is not exhaled into the thoracic cavity. Chest drainage is not only needed in the case of a pneumothorax but also following open-heart surgery, chest trauma, or pulmonary resections to drain accumulating fluid. Chest drainage systems are a one-piece design containing three chambers. These chambers provide separate functions of fluid collection, water seal, and suction control. Fluid drains into the fluid collection chamber from a long six-foot soft flexible tube. The nurse records this amount every shift by placing a pen mark, time, and date next to the current fluid level. This provides an accurate reflection of the patient's condition. The water seal collection chamber allows air to pass through fluid and bubble out but not return to the patient. The water seal column is calibrated and acts as a water manometer for measuring intrathoracic pressure. Suction, regulated by the control chamber, is used to help overcome an air leak by improving the rate of air and fluid flow out of the patient.

Patient and Family Teaching

Patients who have had a pneumothorax have a 50 percent chance of recurrence. Understanding when to call the health care provider is important, and the nurse should encourage the patient to have his or her health care provider or emergency numbers ready at all times. To minimize the risk of recurrence people should avoid smoking, high altitudes, flying in airplanes not pressurized, and scuba diving for six months.

Evaluation of Outcomes

Potential patient outcomes for each of the example nursing diagnoses for the patient with a pneumothorax are:

- Activity intolerance related to compromised oxygen transport system. The patient maintains activity level within capabilities, as evidenced by normal heart rate and blood pressure during activity, as well as absence of shortness of breath, weakness, and fatigue.
- Anxiety related to actual or perceived threat to biological integrity. The patient should be able to recognize the signs of anxiety, demonstrate positive coping mechanisms, and describe a reduction in the level of anxiety experienced.
- Pain, acute related to lung collapse and placement of chest tube. The patient should verbalize an adequate relief of pain along with the ability to realistically cope with the pain if it is not completely relieved.
- Ineffective breathing patterns related to collapse lung. The patient's breathing pattern is maintained by eupnea, normal skin color, and regular respiratory rate or pattern.

FRACTURED RIB

A fractured rib is a break or crack in the bone of one rib or multiple ribs supporting and protecting the chest cavity and organs within the chest. Broken ribs may occur from many causes such as a spontaneous pneumothorax, impact injury to the chest, or brittle bones.

Etiology

Rib fractures are one of the most common types of chest injury, are rarely seen in isolation, and usually emerge as part of the trauma picture. Studies have shown that the thorax may tolerate a 20 percent volume compression before rib fractures occur (Ullman, et al., 2003) Bone cancer, osteoporosis, and hyperparathyroidism make bone more brittle and increase the chance of sustaining a fracture. Stress fractures, or cracks in the rib bone, can occur as a result of weight lifting, rowing, and throwing sports (Perron, 2003) In athletes the middle ribs are most affected by acute trauma, with the fourth through ninth ribs being most prone to fracture.

Pathophysiology

Fractured ribs can cause a pneumothorax as the broken rib bones puncture the lung, and the sudden collapse of the lung and increased pressure of a tension pneumothorax may cause a stress fracture to the rib cage. Pneumothorax caused by rib fractures results in the stimulation of the sympathetic nervous system, causing hypotension to occur quickly (Dweyer & Uhl, 2003). Left-sided rib fractures can cause splenic injury, and right-sided fractures may cause hepatic injury. The elderly population with multiple rib fractures has an increased incidence of pneumonia and overall increased in mortality (Ullman, et al., 2003).

Assessment with Clinical Manifestations

People with rib fractures usually present with sharp, acute pain at the site of fracture (Figure 32-5). Pain can reproduced with palpation, deep inspiration, or cough if the patient is able to cough. Many times pain prevents the deep inspiration that patients need to cough. Bruising or muscle spasms may be seen at the

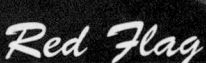

Red Flag

Ensuring Chest Tube Connections

It is vital that the nurse check to ensure that the connection between the chest tube and the collection device is attached and secure. Using plastic ties and securing with a binder, which is usually found in the operating room, will ensure the connection is safe. If this connection breaks you have a high risk of allowing air to move into the pleura space. It is also important for the nurse to replace the chest drainage system if it falls downs and the fluid output moves into other chambers. In case of accidental dislodging of the chest tube, cover site with occlusive Vaseline gauze and only tape on three sides to prevent tension pneumothorax from occurring (Figure 32-4). This dressing creates a one-way valve in which air can exit the pleural space on exhalation (Ullman, Donley, & Brady, 2003). If all four sides are taped, there is a risk of the complication of a tension pneumothorax.

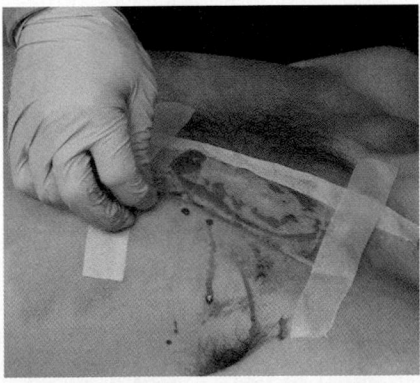

Figure 32-4 A chest wound is covered with a 4 by 4-inch dressing that is secured on three sides; the fourth side is left open as a vent.

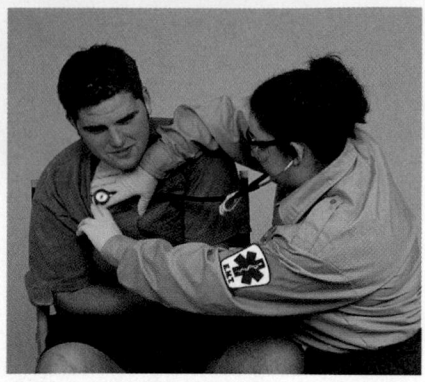

Figure 32-5 Breathing can be painful with a fractured rib.

injury site, and the patient may splint the side or take shallow breaths to avoid pain. Tachycardia usually occurs as the body reacts to injury stress.

Diagnostic confirmation is a result of a thorough event history, clinical findings, and CXR, which are successful at finding 50 percent of all rib fractures (Ullman, et al., 2003).

Nursing Diagnoses

Based on the evidence gathered, examples of nursing diagnoses for the patient with rib fractures may include the following:
- Ineffective breathing patterns related to rib pain
- Activity intolerance related to rib pain with movement
- Acute pain related to rib fracture

Planning and Implementation

Pain associated with rib fractures can interfere with everyday life and cause inactivity in normally active people. Atelectasis and pneumonia can be complications of rib fractures as a result of decreased expiration secondary to pain. As a result pain control remains the number one outcome for people with rib fractures. Other outcomes include stability of rib cage and prevention of hepatic, splenic, or pulmonary lung injury.

Pharmacology

Today's health care arena has more choice for pain control. Because opioids work in the CNS system and alter perception of pain, finding the right medication is crucial in effective pain control. Alternating opioids and nonsteroidal anti-inflammatory drugs (NSAIDs) remains an effective way to control pain. This combination works well as NSAIDs desensitize pain receptors in the CNS while opioids alter the perception of pain. During the acute phase of rib fractures, oral narcotics are rarely effective for pain control. The nurse must be careful to watch for pulmonary depression with IV narcotics. Direct intercostal nerve blockade can provide six hours of pain relief but must be reinserted every six hours for maximum pain control. A mixture of 2 percent lidocaine with bupivacaine is injected at the inferior border of the rib cage in question (Broyles, et al., 2007). Surgery may be needed in the case of organ injury or chest instability.

Patient and Family Teaching

Patient and family education must stress the importance of continuing activity as well as avoidance of driving, making decisions, and operating heavy machinery while on narcotic medications. Coughing and deep breathing needs to occur to prevent atelectasis and pneumonia. Recommend that all oral pain medications be given 30 minutes prior to exercise may decrease pain. Patients may return to activity when pain is under control; however, contact sports need to be avoided for four to six weeks.

Evaluation of Outcomes

Potential patient outcomes for each of the example nursing diagnoses for the patient with fractured ribs are:
- Ineffective breathing patterns related to rib pain. The patient's breathing pattern is maintained by eupnea, normal skin color, and regular respiratory rate or pattern.
- Activity intolerance related to rib pain with movement. The patient maintains activity level within capabilities, as evidenced by normal heart rate and blood pressure during activity, as well as absence of shortness of breath, weakness, and fatigue.

- Acute pain related to rib fracture. The patient should verbalize an adequate relief of pain along with the ability to realistically cope with the pain if it is not completely relieved.

FLAIL CHEST

Thoracic trauma can range from simple abrasions, contusions, rib fractures, and soft tissue injury to the thoracic organs themselves. Compression force is usually behind rib fractures in which the applied force exceeds the strength of the thoracic cage causing the fracture. Rib fractures can cause serious intrathoracic and abdominal injury, produce significant pain, and can place a person at risk for adverse patient outcomes. Flail chest occurs when three or more ribs are broken, leading to rib cage instability and resulting in a pulmonary emergency (Ullman, et al., 2003). Like rib fractures, flail chest is rarely seen in isolation but as a result of multiple injuries. Complications of flail chest include pneumonia, pulmonary contusion or bruising, and pneumothorax.

Assessment with Clinical Manifestations

Clinical assessment of flail chest is by observation. On inspiration the flail segment in pulled inward by the negative intrathoracic pressure and when the person exhales the positive-pressure forces the segment to protrude outward. Chest pain, dyspnea, tachypnea, and tachycardia are symptoms seen as well. The nurse caring for a patient with flail chest is working with a true pulmonary emergency that may result in death if not treated. Flail chest deaths increase with the age of the patient at time of injury.

Diagnostic Tests

Laboratory tests may include a CBC to check for infection and bleeding. A CXR may be ordered but may not show the true clinical picture. If the patient is stable, a CT scan may be ordered.

Nursing Diagnoses

Based on the evidence gathered, examples of nursing diagnoses for the patient with flail chest may include the following:
- Impaired gas exchange related to dysfunctional rib cage
- Acute pain related to flail chest
- Anxiety related to diagnosis of flail chest

Planning and Implementation

Treatment goals for the person with a flail chest include stability of life, repair of fracture, and adequate ventilation. Patients with flail chest will be intubated and require ventilator support to stabilize the broken thoracic cage. If long-term ventilation is needed, a temporary tracheostomy may be performed. Family education for the rationale and use of ventilator support must be completed in the initial acute phase of the flail injury. Families may be faced with the death of a loved one and need to have time to voice and share feelings. Clergy should be asked to further assist the family.

Surgery

Surgery may be indicated to correctly manage a flail chest condition. Internal fixtures maybe used, which are metal rods placed inside the body to support the thoracic cavity while external fixtures are placed on the outside. Internal fixtures tend to be permanent while external fixtures will be removed once the bone has healed. During the recovery from the surgical repair of the flail chest, the patient will continue to splint during respiratory efforts and potentially is at risk for pneumonia from a lack of depth of inspirations. During the recovery time, the patient is to be monitored for respiratory infections (e.g., shortness of breath, febrile, or productive cough).

Evaluation of Outcomes

Potential patient outcomes for each of the example nursing diagnoses for the patient with a flail chest are:

* Impaired gas exchange related to dysfunctional thoracic cage. The patient maintains optimal gas exchange as evidenced by normal ABGs or cardiac output, clinical manifestations, and alert responsive mentation or no further reduction in mental status.
* Acute pain related to rib fractures. The patient should verbalize an adequate relief of pain along with the ability to realistically cope with the pain if it is not completely relieved.
* Anxiety related to diagnosis of flail chest. The patient should be able to recognize the signs of anxiety, demonstrate positive coping mechanisms, and describe a reduction in the level of anxiety experienced.

PULMONARY ARTERIAL HYPERTENSION

Pulmonary arterial hypertension (PAH) is a rare disorder in which an elevated blood pressure exists in the pulmonary blood system. The average blood pressure in a normal pulmonary artery is about 14 mm Hg when the person is resting. In PAH the pulmonary arterial systolic pressure may be greater than 30 mm Hg with the mean pressure greater than 20 mm Hg. There is no cure for PAH, but several treatments are available.

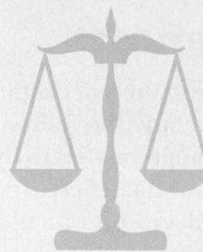

LAW IN PRACTICE

Appetite Suppressant Fen-Phen

The appetite suppressant Fen-Phen, a combination of phentermine and fenfluramine, was withdrawn from the market in 1997. Fen-Phen was associated with increased cases of cardiac valvular disease when the combination therapy was taken longer than 12 months. Patients who had taken the diet supplement Fen-Phen for longer than 3 months were associated with a 23-fold increase in the risk of developing primary pulmonary hypertension (PPH) (U.S. Food and Drug Administration, 1997). The resulting legal class action lawsuit resulted in a settlement trust against the manufacturers of the Fen-Phen product in relation to cardiac valvular disease. Because PPH is a slowly progressive disease in which symptoms may not be present for years, lawsuits are still pending in relation to diet suppressants and acquired PPH. The above case demonstrates the importance of the nurse documenting not only prescription medications but also any over-the-counter medications so that the health care provider has an accurate clinical picture of possible factors for disease.

BOX 32-3

RISK FACTORS FOR PULMONARY ARTERIAL HYPERTENSION

- Raynaud's disease
- Medications
  - Appetite suppressants such as Fen-Phen
  - Oral contraceptives
- Cocaine use
- Human immunodeficiency virus (HIV)
- Congenital heart defects
- Scleroderma (a congenital tissue disease)
- Liver disease
- Mitral valve or stenosis disease
- COPD, lung tumors, and chronic hypoxemia
- Sleep apnea
- Amyotrophic lateral sclerosis (ALS) (progressive neurological disease characterized by degeneration of motor neurons in the brain and spinal cord)

Epidemiology

The true incidence of PAH is unknown, but it is estimated that over 100,000 people in the United States are affected, with thousands more being diagnosed every year. PAH can develop at any age and affects any gender or ethic group. However, young and middle-age women between the ages of 20 and 40 have the highest incidence (American College of Rheumatology, 2004).

Etiology

According to the American Heart Association (AHA, 2004b), there are causes or risk factors that may predispose an individual to acquire PAH (Box 32-3). As shown, there are a wide variety of causes.

The two main types of PAH are primary and secondary. The cause of PPH is unknown and may have a familial cause in about 6 to 10 percent of cases (American Heart Association, 2004b). PPH is recognized by several different names including: (a) idiopathic pulmonary arterial hypertension (IPAH); (b) sporadic primary pulmonary hypertension; and (c) familial PPH. The cause of secondary PAH may not be known but usually present as a result of an underlying disease process. A complication of PAH is **cor pulmonale,** which is an acute strain of the right ventricle, caused by a disorder of the lungs or pulmonary blood vessels leading to right-sided heart failure. Cor pulmonale is described in detail later in this chapter.

An idiopathic cause and the rarity of the disease have made PAH difficult to study. However, it is thought that PPH starts with injury to the layer of cells lining the small blood vessels of the lungs called endothelial cells (National Heart, Lung, and Blood Institute, 2004b). This smooth muscle in the lungs contracts harder than normal, thereby narrowing or constructing the blood vessel. Over time this constriction leads to the development of increased tissue in the walls of the pulmonary arteries. In the disease process of PAH small arteries in the lungs consistently constrict causing an elevated blood pressure resulting in the right side of the heart pumping blood into the lungs against a higher resistance to flow. This resistance makes it difficult to pump the blood through the lungs when needed for exercise (Benisty, 2002). As a result, the amount of muscle increases in some arteries while muscle develops in other arteries that normally do not have muscle. Scarring or fibrosis occurs causing thickness and stiffness. Heart muscle increases as a result of the increased workload, and the right ventricle expands. Over time, the myocardium weakens from the overworking of the heart muscle and the effects of scarring or fibrosis; the right side of the heart fails, as the pumping of the heart grows weaker, which eventually leads to death.

Assessment with Clinical Manifestations

Clinical presentation is rarely picked up on physical examination until symptoms appear, and by the time symptoms occur the damage is already completed. Compounded with the insidious clinical symptoms, PAH may mimic other diseases such as congestive heart failure (CHF) and atrial fibrillation. The degree of symptoms also increases as the disease advances. Fatigue is often the first complaint; many individuals do not see a health care provider as they may think they are out of shape or simply overweight. Dyspnea, vertigo (dizziness), syncope (fainting spell), and bluish coloring of the lips and nails occur from hypoxemia and usually are a late sign of the disease. Peripheral edema present in the ankles or legs appears because of fluid accumulation secondary to the ineffectiveness of the heart pumping action. Palpitations (racing and a throbbing pulse) occur as the heart pumps faster and harder to accommodate the increased pulmonary pressure. Dull retrosternal chest pain resembling a myocardial infarction may be present as the heart muscle forcefully contracts.

Diagnostic Tests

Diagnostic testing is conducted to determine the pressure in the pulmonary artery, evaluate the effectiveness of heart and lung ability, and rules out any other conditions that may be causing disease symptoms. As with any lower airway disease, other disease processes must be ruled out so the correct diagnosis can be established. CXR shows heart enlargement and abnormal blood vessels and assists in ruling out the other disease processes such as COPD. ECG using sound waves can indirectly estimate the pressure in the lung vessels while an ECG records the electrical impulse of the heart. A stress test is completed to see the effects of exercise on the heart. Pulmonary function tests or spirometry may be done to look for other pulmonary causes or conditions but PAH itself may cause only a mild restriction of air movement.

Perfusion lung scan shows the pattern of blood flow in the lungs. CT scan of the chest shows abnormalities of the lung vessels and the condition inside the chest. Cardiac catheterization is performed to measure the pressure in the pulmonary artery and the right side of the heart. During the cardiac catheterization procedure, health care providers will evaluate the effects of vasodilating medications to identify the most effective treatment regimen (American Heart Association, 2004c). Routine blood tests, such as a CBC and hepatic and renal function tests are done to look for disease processes, such as lupus, scleroderma, cirrhosis, and HIV (National Heart, Lung, and Blood Institute, 2004b).

The diagnosis of PAH and the extent of the disease is rated by a classification system that uses four classes to identify the degree of symptoms. People affected with class I have no symptoms, and ordinary physical activity does not cause symptoms. In class II people are comfortable at rest but have symptoms with ordinary exercise. Class III encompasses people comfortable at rest but who have symptoms with less than ordinary physical activity. Finally class IV includes people who have symptoms at rest. In class III and IV the mean pulmonary arterial pressure is 50 mm Hg with the mean right atrial pressure is 10 mm Hg, and the cardiac index is approximately 2 L/min/m². Medical treatment effectiveness is calculated using the above measurements as a guide for clinical practice.

Nursing Diagnoses

Based on the evidence gathered, examples of nursing diagnoses for the patient with PAH may include the following:
- Ineffective breathing pattern related to PAH
- Impaired gas exchange related to active inflammatory process
- Activity intolerance related to increased metabolic demands
- Anxiety related to situational fears from PAH

Planning and Implementation

Treatment outcomes include reversal of any disease process, halting current disease, and maintaining an optimal quality of life. Because PAH is not curable, patient and families must have support systems in place to assist with the emotions of chronic life-threatening illness. Oxygen is needed to keep the O_2 saturation level above 90 percent to prevent further tissue damage. Some people require oxygen at all times and others only when exercising. Oxygen for 15 hours per day has been demonstrated to slow the progression of PAH in patients with hypoxemic COPD (Tierney, et al., 2003).

Evidence-Based Care

Research gives health care providers the prevailing indication to ensure that the best, most efficient care possible is being provided. Clinical research studies utilize human volunteers or subjects to find ways to improve patient outcomes. PAH, in relation to secondary disease and familial incidence, have been studied extensively to determine medication treatment effectiveness. There are clinical trials in relation to PAH as follows: secondary PAH in adults with sickle cell anemia; endothelial cell dysfunction in PAH; and genetic and environmental pathogenesis of PPH.

Pharmacology

Medications include use of diuretics make the right ventricle work more effectively by reducing the amount of water in the body. Vasodilators, or medications to expand the blood vessels, including angiotensin-converting enzymes (ACE) inhibitors, preventing the conversion of angiotensin I to angiotensin II, which is a potent vasodilator. Adenosine promotes coronary vasodilatation, which decreases vascular resistance and relaxes smooth muscles. This medication has a short half-life and is used in the assessment of PAH. Calcium channel blockers (CCBs) have been shown to be effective in one-fourth of all people with PAH but should be used with caution and under expert care (Badesch, et al., 2004). Verapamil should be avoided due to its negative inotropic effect. Diltiazem is used for relative tachycardia.

Anticoagulation therapy assists the right ventricle to work more efficiently. Warfarin (Coumadin) impacts the intrinsic pathway in the liver and is effective for PAH. The risk of GI bleeding may be higher in people with PAH in association with scleroderma, and the risk of hemoptysis increases in people with congenital heart disease (Badesch, et al., 2004)

Although epoprostenol has been available since 1995, decreased dosing has occurred over the years because of the overdosing patterns leading to increased cardiac output that exacerbates patient fatigue. Treprostinil is used and can cause pain at the IV site. Bosentan is the most common oral medication to treat PAH and is an endothelin receptor antagonist. There are several experimental drugs that show promise and may be used in the future. They include sitaxsentan and sildenafil (Badesch, et al., 2004).

Surgery

Transplantation is reserved for those who do not respond to therapy. Surgical procedures may include single or double lung transplantation and heart-lung transplantation. It is common to acquire bronchitis obliterans, an inflammation of the bronchioles after transplantation. Fewer complications occur when only one lung is transplanted. The rate of survival is with a 70 percent after one year, 60 percent after two years and 37 percent for five years (National Heart, Lung, and Blood Institute, 2004b). Listing of recipients of solid organs is complex, and selection criteria vary from center to center. Those people with end-stage lung disease without concomitant illness are a priority. The average person waits one-and-a-half to two years to obtain an organ transplant (Orens, 2004).

Patient and Family Teaching

Learning how to manage PAH is the primary education given to patients and families. There are several excellent support groups available to persons with PAH. The patient must be encouraged to exercise but not over exert. Instruction must be given on maintaining a proper fluid and nutritional intake. The patient should be taught to avoid dehydration and excessive heat as this raises the exertion of the heart. In addition, the patient should be informed of all medications and encouraged to take them as ordered. The patient should have a health care plan developed with the health care provider. Other precautions include: (a) bring supplemental oxygen with flights; (b) bring antibiotics for all respiratory tract infections; and (c) obtain the pneumococcal pneumonia vaccine every year.

Evaluation of Outcomes

Potential patient outcomes for each of the example nursing diagnoses for the patient with PAH are:

- Ineffective breathing pattern related to PAH. The patient's breathing pattern is maintained by eupnea, normal skin color, and regular respiratory rate or pattern.

- Impaired gas exchange related to active inflammatory process. The patient maintains optimal gas exchange as evidenced by normal ABGs and alert responsive mentation or no further reduction in mental status.
- Activity intolerance related to increased metabolic demands. The patient maintains activity level within capabilities, as evidenced by normal heart rate and blood pressure during activity, as well as absence of shortness of breath, weakness, and fatigue.
- Anxiety related to situational fears from PAH. The patient should be able to recognize the signs of anxiety, demonstrate positive coping mechanisms, and describe a reduction in the level of anxiety experienced.

COR PULMONALE

Cor pulmonale, right-sided heart failure, is an acute strain of the right ventricle caused by a disorder of the lungs or prolonged high blood pressure in the pulmonary artery. Over time this weakens the heart, leading to right-sided heart failure which in turn may lead to death. Right-sided heart failure can be acute or chronic. In an acute episode, dilation or overload of the right ventricle occurs as a result of a massive PE. Once the PE is resolved the injury should reverse. In chronic right-sided heart failure, growth and dilation of the right heart ventricle occur from diseases of the pulmonary vasculature. Muscle growth and dilation occur slowly over time and permanently alter the heart muscle.

Etiology

Almost any chronic lung disease causing prolonged low blood oxygen can lead to cor pulmonale (U.S. National Library of Medicine & National Institutes of Health, 2002). For example, the following are various causes of cor pulmonale: COPD, sleep apnea, chronic mountain sickness (an altitude illness that can occur at 8,000 feet or more), CF, PPH, chronic thromboembolic pulmonary disease, and pneumoconiosis, a chronic nonmalignant lung disease.

Assessment with Clinical Manifestations

Clinical symptoms come from the underlying disease process and may include chronic productive cough from the accumulation of fluid in the lungs. Dyspnea and cyanosis occur with exercise as the body fails in its attempt to move oxygen to the tissues. Hoarseness may occur due to the compression of the laryngeal nerve by enlarged pulmonary vessels. Chest pain may occur as a result of the pulmonary artery dilation and right ventricular cell death or ischemia. Severe symptoms of right-sided heart failure occur as fluid backs up in the lungs, and the heart is unable to move this fluid properly: (a) distension of the neck veins; (b) liver enlargement; (c) peripheral edema of the ankles; and (d) development of abnormal heart sounds, such as an S_3 ventricular or S_4 atrial gallop.

Diagnostic Tests

Diagnostic tests to assess right-sided heart failure include: (a) CBC; (b) ABGs; (c) CXR; (d) ECG; (e) CT scan; (f) pulmonary artery catheter placement to check pulmonary pressure; and (g) perfusion scans. A CBC may show **polycythemia,** an abnormal increase in the number of red blood cells. ABGs show the arterial oxygen saturation below 85 percent, and the Pco_2 (amount of carbon dioxide in the venous or arterial blood) may or may not be elevated. A CXR can show an enlarged right heart ventricle and pulmonary artery. The ECG results may mimic signs of a heart attack. Pulmonary function tests may show the underlying disease causing cor pulmonale. Cardiac catheterization will establish a definitive diagnosis.

Nursing Diagnoses

Based on the evidence gathered, examples of nursing diagnoses for the patient with cor pulmonale may include the following:
- Anxiety related to diagnosis of cor pulmonale
- Impaired gas exchange related to inability of the heart pumping mechanism and pulmonary edema
- Activity intolerance related to increased metabolic demands and inadequate tissue oxygenation

Planning and Implementation

Collaborative care of the patient with cor pulmonale is the same as in other chronic life-threatening diseases. Treatment outcomes include treatment of underlying disease, minimizing the effects of right-sided heart failure, and maintaining an optimal quality of life. The nurse must monitor for fluid overload and especially for signs of worsening right-sided heart failure and distress. Electrolytes and hydration must be assessed daily. Patient safety is important to prevent falls that can occur as a result of medication side effects, depression, fatigue, and weakness. The nurse should make sure that the bathroom is accessible or that a commode is placed near the bed. Avoid clutter in the room or floor that the patient may have to step over and possibly trip. Limiting activity and rest periods are interventions used to decrease the oxygen demands of the body. Walking three to four times a day with rest periods of at least two hours can be an effective method to maintain mobility and provide rest. Cough and deep breathing exercises every one to two hours while awake will assist in lung expansion and removal of lung secretions. Low-flow oxygen is administered via nasal cannula to aid in ensuring adequate ventilation and improving oxygen levels. Surgery may be needed to reverse heart defects causing cor pulmonale.

Nutrition

Nutrition is important to lower salt intake that can result in increased fluid retention. Dietary management includes the following:
- Limit salt intake. This includes avoiding smoked, cured, or canned meat products as they contain a high salt content.
- Eat high-fiber whole grains, bran, fruits, and vegetables.
- Consume foods high in potassium to replace potassium loss secondary to diuretic medication.
- Eat foods high in magnesium.
- Take a daily multivitamin.
- Restrict fluids.
- Increasing calories to 2,500 daily will assist the body in combating the effects of chronic pulmonary disease. The patient may find eating five or six small meals a day may be more easily tolerated and decrease dyspnea by avoiding excess stomach expansion that in turn can cause pressure on the diaphragm, decreasing the lungs' capacity to expand.

Pharmacology

Pharmacology for the treatment of cor pulmonale consists of removing excess fluid and treatment of underlying disease and consists of using diuretics, CCBs, bosentan, IV prostacyclin, and anticoagulants. Diuretics work by removing excess fluid through kidney excretion. Furosemide is a loop diuretic that is used to reduce excess fluid that results from heart failure. Any diuretic can cause electrolyte imbalances as water, sodium chloride, magnesium, and calcium are excreted with the excess fluid. Adverse reactions include orthostatic hypotension resulting from quick fluid loss, vertigo, blurred vision, parenthesis, pruritus, rash, hyperglycemia, or elevated glucose levels secondary to excess fluid loss, nausea and vomiting, and hearing loss with rapid IV infusions. Oral doses of diuretics usually start to work within 30 to 60 minutes while the IV route will take effect within five minutes. The medication has a duration of six to eight hours with oral doses and a two-hour duration with an IV dose. Routine oral doses are 20 to 80 mg every six to eight hours with the doses increasing by 20 mg until the desired effect is reached. IV dosages are usually 20 to 40 mg that may be repeated in 1 to 2 hours as needed an increased by 20 mg with each succeeding dose until the desired effect is reached. The total daily dose of furosemide is 1,000 mg/day (Broyles, et al., 2007). CCBs, such as diltiazem, are used to relax the smooth muscle and coronary vasodilation, thereby increasing oxygen delivery to the heart. Anticoagulants, such as heparin and warfarin (Coumadin), work to prevent the blood from clotting and are used in the treatment of thromboembolic disorders. When administering anticoagulants or monitoring a patient who is on anticoagulation therapy, the nurse must assess for signs and symptoms of bleeding. Signs of bleeding include bleeding gums, easy bruising, and elevated bleeding times as noted on blood chemistry.

Patient and Family Teaching

Patient education for the patient with cor pulmonale comprises teaching of the clinical manifestations and assessment needed to detect changes in the condition. When the patient is able to be discharged to the home setting, the patient can be instructed to call a health care provider when any of the following are noticed: a weight gain of two pounds in one day or five pounds in a week; increased swelling in the legs; respiratory infection or signs of infection (e.g., fever, increased cough, dyspnea, changes in sputum color); heart rate above 120 beats per minute; and chest pain or pain that lessens with rest (Cleveland Clinic, 2004).

Evaluation of Outcomes

Potential patient outcomes for each of the nursing diagnoses for the patient with cor pulmonale are:

- Anxiety related to diagnosis of cor pulmonale. The patient should be able to recognize the signs of anxiety, demonstrate positive coping mechanisms, and describe a reduction in the level of anxiety experienced.
- Impaired gas exchange related to inability of the heart pumping mechanism and pulmonary edema. The patient maintains optimal gas exchange as evidenced by normal ABGs and alert responsive mentation or no further reduction in mental status.
- Activity intolerance related to increased metabolic demands and inadequate tissue oxygenation. The patient maintains activity level within capabilities, as evidenced by normal heart rate and blood pressure during activity, as well as absence of shortness of breath, weakness, and fatigue.

Concept Map Case Study

Cristy Peters

Cristy Peters, aged 8, has been diagnosed with asthma, a chronic reactive airway disorder. She has been treated in the physician's office and the emergency department several times during the past five years for acute respiratory episodes, or asthma attacks. The primary causes for these episodes were infections and exposure to allergens. She has been hospitalized twice during the past two years. She is currently admitted to the hospital for an acute respiratory infection. Her temperature is 39.2° C (102.6° F); respirations are labored and rapid (30 to 40 per minute); pulse is 110; she has a productive cough of copious thick mucus, and expiratory wheezing is noted. Nasal flaring and intercostal retractions are noticed on inspiration. The physical assessment indicates that Cristy is small for her age; her chest is slightly barrel shaped; she appears fatigued and anxious. Her skin color is pale, lips and nail beds are cyanotic, and her breath sounds are diminished. The physician orders pulmonary function tests, pulse oximetry, and a sputum culture. Additional orders include: humidified oxygen via mask, respiratory therapy, and an intravenous line to be available for fluids and medications if needed. Medications include an aerosol bronchodilator, a systemic anti-inflammatory, and acetaminophen.

Cristy's parents appear anxious. Her father left the room to smoke a cigarette. He promised Cristy he would be right back. Mrs. Peters strokes Cristy's arm and speaks softly to her. She mentions that Cristy is worried about missing the school play that she has a part in tomorrow.

In this scenario, the family is your patient. Refer back to the sample concept map for assistance in designing a map for Cristy's case study. Add concepts where you believe they belong. (Some concepts may belong in more than one area.)

Current Nurses Drug Guide or Pharmacology Text

1. Why do you think the physician did not order an antibiotic for Cristy at this time? (What additional information would you like to have?)
2. How would you evaluate the effectiveness of each of her medications? Discuss the nurse's role in monitoring Cristy for drug-drug interactions.
3. List the nursing interventions you would use to:
    a. Facilitate easier breathing
    b. Promote decrease in Cristy's temperature
    c. Ensure adequate fluid balance
4. Identify the psychological needs of the family.
5. How would you cluster Cristy's symptoms or needs for the nursing diagnoses of impaired gas exchange and ineffective airway clearance?
6. Select at least two additional nursing diagnoses. What clusters of information in the case study will you use to support your selected diagnoses?
7. How would you evaluate the family's knowledge in using an incentive spirometer?
8. Prioritize the items to include in home care instructions for Cristy and her family.
9. Describe how you would communicate with the parents regarding stimuli, or triggers, in the environment that initiate Cristy's asthmatic episodes.
10. What would you include in an individual school health management plan for Cristy? (What measures would help to enhance Cristy's self-image?)

Suggested References: Ball, J., & Bindler, R. (2003). Pediatric nursing: Caring for children (3rd ed.) Reading, MA: Pearson Education.

KEY CONCEPTS

- Common clinical manifestations of lower airway disease include three hallmark symptoms: (a) cough; (b) dyspnea; and (c) hemoptysis.
- Community-acquired pneumonia (CAP) is present in patients who are not residents of a long-term facility and usually occurs less than 48 hours after admission to an inpatient unit.
- Hospital-acquired pneumonia (HAP) usually occurs 48 hours or more after admission and is typically caused from artificial sources, such as aspirations or mechanical ventilation.
- Extrapulmonary disease affects the chest wall, pleura (protective lining around the lungs), and respiratory muscles. Diseases such as TB can have an extrapulmonary spread to other organ systems.
- Intrapulmonary disease affects the lung tissue and alveoli located inside the lung.
- Currently TB is on the rise in the United States due to the presence of HIV infections and increased travel or immigration from parts of the world affected with uncontrolled TB infection.
- There are approximately 50,000 different types of fungi, but only about a dozen cause 90 percent of all fungal infections.
- Bronchiolectasis disease has a cycle of bacterial colonization, followed by inflammatory changes leading to increased production of mucus, resulting in scaring, which increases bacterial colonization and the cycle starts over.

- Lung abscesses can be acute or chronic in nature. An acute lung abscess is one that is present less or equal to six weeks, and a chronic lung abscess is present more than six weeks.
- Lung cancer is a term used to identify cancer in the lungs; it can be primary or secondary.
- There are four types of pneumothorax: (a) spontaneous; (b) traumatic; (c) iatrogenic; and (d) tension.
- Rib fractures are one of the most painful traumatic injuries possible.
- Flail chest occurs when three or more ribs are broken, leading to rib cage instability, resulting in a pulmonary emergency.
- The exact cause of pulmonary hypertension is unknown, but it can have a familial cause. Secondary hypertension may be a result of an underlying disease process.
- Cor pulmonale is an acute strain of the right ventricle caused by a disorder of the lungs or prolonged high blood pressure in the pulmonary artery.

REVIEW QUESTIONS

1. Which of the following is true concerning *Pneumocystis carinii* pneumonia?
   1. It is best labeled mycoplasma pneumonia.
   2. It is caused when patients are dependent on mechanical ventilators.
   3. It is usually found most commonly in pediatric patients.
   4. It is a type of fungal infection that often affects immunocompromised patients.

2. Which statement is accurate when describing patients with latent TB disease?
   1. Active disease with symptoms
   2. Positive PPD, no clinical picture of disease, and a normal CXR
   3. Extrapulmonary disease in the bones
   4. Inactive disease that is becoming active

3. Which of the following interventions are needed if the nurse becomes exposed to TB?
   1. PPD test six weeks after exposure
   2. Report to employee health
   3. Monitor for symptoms of active disease
   4. All of the above

4. Which of the following are true of lung abscesses?
   1. Two leading risk factors for aspiration include alcohol and mental status changes.
   2. The most common clinical manifestations are hypothermia and bradycardia.
   3. They are usually associated with pneumonia, tuberculosis, and cor pulmonale.
   4. The people normally affected are those with previous renal disorders and liver diseases.

Continued

5. A patient is admitted to your hospital unit with flail chest and placed in the intermediate care unit (IMC) for mechanical ventilation and naso-intestinal enteral feedings. The nurse should monitor for which of the following?
   1. TB because the patient will have prolonged close contact with other individuals.
   2. Chest tube placement because the lung has collapsed.
   3. Pneumonia because the patient is at high risk for acquiring infection.
   4. Cor pulmonale because the chest wall is unstable.

6. Which of the following interventions for monitoring of chest tubes and drainage systems should the nurse perform?
   1. Connections, suction control chamber, water seal, and breath sounds
   2. Drainage system operation, suction control chamber, water seal, and chest dressing secure
   3. Patient condition, drainage system operation, water seal, and suction control chamber
   4. Breath sounds, dressing intact, connections intact, and absence of breath sounds

7. Which of the following statement is true about chest tubes?
   1. Chest tubes allow movement of air to occur during expiration and inspiration, which expands the lung.
   2. Chest tubes are used only to expel air and should be clamped every four hours.
   3. If the chest tube pulls out the RN may replace the device making sure to clamp the tube for two hours after reinsertion.
   4. Chest tubes allow either air or fluid to leak out while acting as a one way valve to prevent further air from entering the pleural space.

8. A 20-year-old thin male presents to the clinic with sharp pain left side of his chest that is pleuritic in nature. He reports he was at a bar drinking when he noticed the pain. On auscultation you detect decreased breath sounds on the left. His vital signs are BP 150/90, pulse 100, respiratory ate shallow at 24, and patient is afebrile. Based on the clinical findings the nurse would suspect which of the following?
   1. Spontaneous pneumothorax
   2. Pneumonia
   3. Fractured ribs
   4. Tuberculosis

9. A 68-year-old patient presents to your emergency department after being in an automobile accident. She has sustained two fractured ribs, pulmonary contusion, and a scalp laceration. The nurse would immediately monitor for which of the following?
   1. Flail chest and immediate ventilation
   2. Pneumothorax
   3. Cor pulmonale
   4. Pneumonia

10. A 58-year-old patient presents to the clinic for routine visit for pulmonary hypertension. Recently he started using an epoprostenol pump infusion through a central line. He informs you that he will be traveling to London for three weeks. What patient education and nursing interventions would be appropriate?
    1. Instruction on actions to take if IV catheter breaks, emergency provider number, and how to access the emergency system in London
    2. Arrangement for extra supplies, medications, tubing, and pump
    3. Routine blood work completed several days before any trips
    4. All of the above

REVIEW ACTIVITIES

1. Select a patient in an acute care setting who has pneumonia and describe the management strategies that are used during his or her hospitalization.

2. Compare a patient who has a 5-mm induration size from a TB skin test, as contrasted with a patient who has a 10-mm induration.

Continued

REVIEW ACTIVITIES—cont'd

3. How are lung abscesses managed?

5. Compare the injury of fractured ribs with a flail chest.

4. Provide care for a patient with lung cancer caused from smoking. Evaluate yourself in regard to whether you are somewhat judgmental of the etiology for this condition. And, take measures to ensure that you can provide professional care to the patient.

Obstructive Pulmonary Disease: Nursing Management

Patricia Kelly, RN, MSN

Leslie H. Nicoll, PhD, MBA, RN, BC

May Mui, Pharm D, BCPS

CHAPTER TOPICS

- Chronic Obstructive Pulmonary Disease (COPD)

- Asthma

- Cystic Fibrosis (CF)

KEY TERMS

Atopy
Barotrauma
Bullae
Clubbing
Directed or controlled coughing
Dyspnea
Exacerbation
Hypoxemia
Polycythemia
Status asthmaticus
Triggers
Wheezing

L ower airway dysfunction is a leading cause of death and illness in the United States and throughout the world. From lost time on the job to the price of the care itself, the cost of these dysfunctions is staggering. Nurses care for patients with chronic obstructive pulmonary disease (COPD), asthma, or cystic fibrosis (CF) in the hospital and various outpatient settings, such as home care, pulmonary rehabilitation, and hospice settings. Patients with these lower airway dysfunctions may have changes within their lungs that lead to changes in the alveoli, a narrowing of the airways, or excess mucous secretion that lead to impaired gas exchange. Patients with CF also often develop restrictive lung disease because of the fibrosis, lung destruction, and thoracic wall changes associated with this disease. The nurse's role and collaborative management of the patient with these dysfunctions are discussed in this chapter.

CHRONIC OBSTRUCTIVE PULMONARY DISEASE

Chronic obstructive pulmonary disease (COPD) is a state characterized by airflow limitation that is not fully reversible. The airflow limitation is usually both progressive and associated with an abnormal inflammatory response of the lungs to noxious particles or gases. The cause of the irreversible airflow obstruction in COPD is the presence in the lungs of bronchiolitis, or small airway disease, and emphysema, which are present in a variable mix among patients (Snider, 2003).

Chronic bronchiolitis is a small airway disease of the lungs produced by an inflammatory process that causes structural changes in the small airways. Emphysema is a condition of the lungs characterized by abnormal, permanent enlargement of the alveoli distal to the terminal bronchioles accompanied by destruction of the alveolar walls and without obvious fibrosis. Many patients with COPD may also have chronic bronchitis.

Chronic bronchitis is the hypersecretion of mucus resulting in the presence of a productive cough lasting over three months and for more than two consecutive years (Chojnowski, 2003). Chronic bronchitis also results from an inflammatory condition in the lungs. Asthma with complete reversibility is not included in COPD, although there is a select group of patients with COPD who also have a component of asthma, diagnosed by characteristic inflammatory markers in their lungs from both disease processes (Snider, 2003).

Asthma is a chronic inflammatory disorder of the airways with bronchial hyperresponsiveness to a variety of stimuli and variable airflow obstruction and bronchospasm that is often reversible either spontaneously or with treatment. Asthma is discussed later in this chapter.

The symptoms of COPD can range from chronic cough and sputum production to wheezing and severe disabling shortness of breath. In some individuals, chronic cough and sputum production are the first signs that they are at risk for developing the airflow obstruction and shortness of breath that is characteristic of COPD. In others, shortness of breath may be the first indication of the disease (Chojnowski, 2003).

Epidemiology

According to the World Health Organization (WHO), COPD was the fourth leading cause of death worldwide in 2006. Almost 3 million people died from the disease in countries as diverse as Canada, Japan, China, Brazil, Great Britain, and France. In the United States, COPD is fourth in mortality and expected to move to third place by 2020. There are approximately 16 million adult Americans living with COPD. Many more may have COPD but do not know it, because they are not yet experiencing symptoms (Wisniewski, 2003).

Etiology

Cigarette smoking is, by far, the most important risk factor for COPD. Pipes, cigars, and other types of tobacco use, and passive exposure to smoke are also risk factors. Other risk factors for COPD that have been identified include, but are not limited to, the following: exposure to occupational dusts and chemicals, recurrent lung infections, airway hyperresponsiveness, low birth weight, and socioeconomic factors (e.g., exposure to outdoor and indoor air pollutants and poor nutrition).

The evidence that tobacco smoking is a major cause of lung disease is well documented; however, it is not the only significant cause of COPD. Monitoring of lung function reveals that substantial airflow obstruction because of an accelerated decline in lung function occurs in only a minority of cigarette smokers (approximately 15 percent of Caucasians and 5 percent of Asian

[Americans]). Patients with COPD typically show a decrease in both forced expiratory volume in one second (FEV_1) and forced vital capacity (FVC). In a normal adult, exhalation time should take four to six seconds. Patients with COPD need more time to exhale, which decreases FEV_1 and FVC. Lung volume measurements show a marked increase in residual volume and an increase in total lung capacity. This strongly suggests that genetic factors may determine which smokers will develop airflow limitation. It is inappropriate to state a clear etiology for COPD at this time (Snider, 2003).

Pathophysiology

COPD is characterized by a chronic inflammatory response throughout the airways, parenchyma (lung tissue), and pulmonary vasculature. With this chronic inflammatory response, macrophages, T-lymphocytes, and neutrophils are increased in various parts of the lung. Activated inflammatory cells release a variety of cell mediators, including leukotriene B4 (LTB4), interleukin-8 (IL-8), tumor necrosis factor-α (TNF-α), and others, capable of damaging lung structures, or sustaining neutrophilic inflammation. The inflammatory processes of COPD lead to repeated cycles of injury and repair of the airway wall. The repair process results in structural remodeling of the airway wall with increasing collagen content and scar tissue formation, which narrows the lumen and produces fixed airway obstruction. This is associated with such abnormal processes as airway edema, mucous hypersecretion, ciliary dysfunction, pulmonary hyperinflation, and cor pulmonale.

In COPD, there are airflow limitations that are progressive in nature. Recall that there are many types of conducting airways, that is, the trachea, bronchi, segmental bronchi, subsegmental bronchi, and nonrespiratory bronchioles. These conducting airways are anatomic dead space where no gas exchange occurs. No gas exchange occurs until after air flows from the nonrespiratory bronchioles, through the respiratory bronchioles and alveolar ducts, and enters the alveoli. The bronchioles are encircled by smooth muscle that constricts and dilates in response to various stimuli (bronchoconstriction and bronchodilation). Note that each bronchus has cartilage in its wall. In the main bronchi, the cartilage is less ring-shaped and more irregular, providing greater flexibility than that in the trachea. Each subsequent division of bronchi contains less cartilage, thus providing less structural support but more flexibility. These bronchi branch into smaller bronchioles that are without cartilage.

In COPD, there may be a breakdown of elastin, a protein in the connective tissue of the lungs. This connective tissue breakdown leads to destruction of the alveolar walls with airway obstruction, mucus accumulation in the inflamed bronchioles, air trapping in the alveoli as the alveolar walls collapse, and narrowing of the bronchioles. During inspiration, the bronchioles open, allowing gas to flow into the alveoli. During expiration, the bronchioles narrow, the alveoli collapse, and air is trapped. With this air trapping, hyperinflation and distension of the alveoli occurs and impairs the exchange of oxygen and carbon dioxide. Patients with COPD often have a barrel chest appearance as a result of hyperinflation, rib fixation in the inspiratory position, and excessive reliance on accessory muscles.

With air trapping, the stagnant air in the alveoli cannot supply adequate oxygen to the capillaries. This creates a fertile field for bacteria to grow. At the same time, carbon dioxide levels increase in the blood, causing fatigue, headache, and lethargy. If the patient also has bronchospasm or airway obstruction from other pulmonary diseases, this may further exacerbate the air trapping.

In addition to the inflammation and air trapping that occurs with COPD, an imbalance of proteinase and antiproteinase enzymes in the lungs may also occur. This imbalance and the presence of other inflammatory proteins and oxidative stress may further break down the connective tissue and damage the lungs. In response to nonspecific airway irritants, **atopy** (the hereditary tendency to develop immediate allergic reactions) and bronchoconstriction may also play a role in the development of COPD.

The changes seen with emphysema in COPD may be centrilobar or panlobar. In centrilobar emphysema, lung destruction begins in the central respiratory bronchioles and spreads outward toward the lung periphery. It involves dilation and destruction of the respiratory bronchioles. The lung destruction predominantly affects the upper lung zones and is associated with cigarette smoking. Centrilobar emphysema is a more common type of emphysema than panlobar emphysema.

In panlobar emphysema, lung destruction involves the entire lung. This type of emphysema is associated with a genetic alpha$_1$-antitrypsin enzyme deficiency. In panlobar emphysema, lung destruction involves the distal airway structures and alveolar sacs and often results in thin-walled larger air spaces. These air spaces are called blebs when they occur close to the visceral pleura. They are called bullae when they occur in the lung parenchyma.

Alpha$_1$-antitrypsin enzyme is a lung-protective protein produced by the liver. alpha$_1$-antitrypsin deficiency is responsible for about 5 percent of the cases (80,000 to 100,000) of emphysema in the United States. It is one of the most common genetically linked lethal diseases among Caucasians and affects approximately one in every 3,000 Americans. The genetically susceptible person is sensitive to environmental factors (e.g., smoking, air pollution, infectious agents, and allergens) and in time develops chronic obstructive pulmonary symptoms. This type of emphysema usually affects people of European descent and tends to appear in patients in their thirties. Blood testing can determine if the person is a carrier of the defective gene or alpha$_1$-antitrypsin deficient (Wisniewski, 2003). Genetic counseling is important and should be offered to people at risk. Alpha protease inhibitor replacement therapy, a costly treatment that slows the progression of the disease, can be ordered for patients with this genetic defect and for those with severe disease.

Regardless of the type, all patients with emphysema experience a reduction in elasticity of the lungs, an increase in pulmonary dead space, and an increased propensity of the airway to collapse during expiration, causing airway outflow obstruction. With the breakdown of the walls of the alveoli, the alveolar surface area in direct contact with the pulmonary capillaries continually decreases, causing an increase in dead space in the lung where no gas exchange can occur and oxygen diffusion is impaired. Recall that no gas exchange occurs in the conducting airways. Gas exchange occurs in the alveoli. This impaired gas exchange leads to **hypoxemia** (decrease in arterial oxygen in the blood). Later, carbon dioxide elimination is impaired, resulting in increased carbon dioxide tension or hypercapnia in arterial blood, causing respiratory acidosis.

As the alveolar walls continue to break down, the pulmonary capillary bed is further reduced. As a result, pulmonary blood flow is increased, forcing the right ventricle to maintain a higher blood pressure in the pulmonary artery. Over time, the vasoconstrictive effects of hypoxia result in pulmonary hypertension, leading to chronic pulmonary hypertension. This leads to right ventricular hypertrophy with eventual dilation and failure, resulting in cor pulmonale (see chapter 32). In addition, **polycythemia** is an increase in the number of red blood cells, usually above 55 percent. It occurs in COPD as the body attempts to increase the oxygen-carrying capacity of the blood in response to chronic lung disease and hypoxia.

Complications

Complications of COPD include pneumonia, atelectasis, pneumothorax, and cor pulmonale. Chronic hypoxemia may cause the pulmonary arteries to constrict, thus leading to pulmonary hypertension. Maintaining adequate oxygenation through an adequate hemoglobin level, improved ventilation or perfusion of the lungs, and continuous administration of supplemental oxygen, as needed, may help prevent pulmonary hypertension.

Viral infections pose a hazard to patients with COPD, because they are often followed by infections caused by bacterial organisms, such as *Streptococcus pneumoniae, Haemophilus influenzae,* or *Moraxella catarrhalis.* The nurse should encourage patients with COPD to be immunized against influenza and pneumococcus. It is also important to caution patients against going outdoors if the pollen count is too high or if there is significant air pollution.

Exacerbations of COPD may be caused by pulmonary embolism, pneumothorax, rib fractures or chest trauma, inappropriate use of a sedative, opioid, or beta blocker medication, and right- or left-sided heart failure. Any of these complications can be life-threatening in a patient who has minimal pulmonary reserve. They can lead to respiratory insufficiency and failure that may necessitate ventilator support until other acute complications, such as infection, can be treated.

Indications for noninvasive ventilator support with a mask, or invasive intubation with mechanical ventilation (Figure 33-1), for patients with respiratory failure include labored breathing with respiratory rates of more than 30 breaths per minute, restlessness, severe hypoxia, moderate to severe respiratory acidosis, decreased level of consciousness, respiratory arrest, and complicating conditions, such as shock, sepsis, and metabolic abnormalities. The goal of mechanical ventilation is to buy time for the treatments to take effect, rest the patient's respiratory muscles, and improve any gas exchange abnormality while avoiding ventilator complications. The nurse must review the patient's wish for mechanical ventilator support and the benefits and costs of care with the patient and family prior to the need for such care.

Assessment with Clinical Manifestations

Note that clinical findings may be completely absent early in the course of COPD. As the disease progresses, various symptom patterns and patient needs emerge as part of the history and physical findings of the patient (Table 33-1).

Symptom patterns may vary in the patient with COPD, depending on the underlying diseases present. Two of these diseases, emphysema and chronic bronchitis, have historically been referred to as pink puffers (emphysema) and blue bloaters (chronic bronchitis) (Tierney, McPhee, & Papakakais, 2004). This may be an oversimplification of COPD, but the terms continue to be used by clinicians.

Regardless of the lung disease predominating in the patient with COPD, the end result is that progressive airflow obstruction leads to a chronic ventilation–perfusion mismatch with blood flowing past the unaerated lung, resulting in hypoxia. Depending on the lung diseases present, various symptoms including barrel chest, cyanosis, and clubbing may occur. **Clubbing** is a bulbous enlargement of the distal fingers and nails associated with chronic cyanosis.

COPD is variable in its course. The severity of the disease depends on the degree of the symptoms and the airflow limitations. COPD is characterized by a history of three primary symptoms: cough, sputum production, and dyspnea on exertion and usually a history of exposure to risk factors for the disease. These symptoms and the patient's exercise tolerance often worsen over time. Chronic cough and sputum production can develop many years before the airflow limitation occurs (Chojnowski, 2003). The patient's chest is typically hyperresonant to percussion and may reveal wheezes or crackles. The patient may assume a tripod position, lean forward with the head tilted, and use the neck and chest muscles to breathe easier. Typically, there is a prolonged expiratory phase as the patient attempts to exhale against the chronic respiratory obstruction. A patient with severe COPD may have distant heart sounds and an ominously quiet chest because of the inability to move enough air for auscultation (Figure 33-2). The patient's **dyspnea** (labored or difficult breathing) may be severe, and it often interferes with normal daily activities.

Weight loss is common in some patients with COPD, because dyspnea interferes with eating. The work of breathing is energy depleting. Most patients are

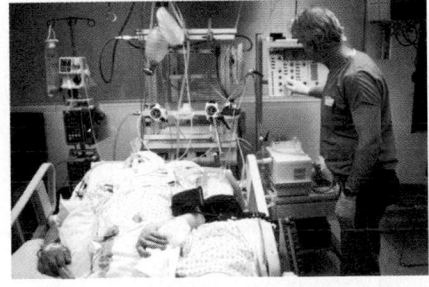

Figure 33-1 A patient with COPD on a mechanical ventilator because of the complication of hospital-acquired pneumonia.

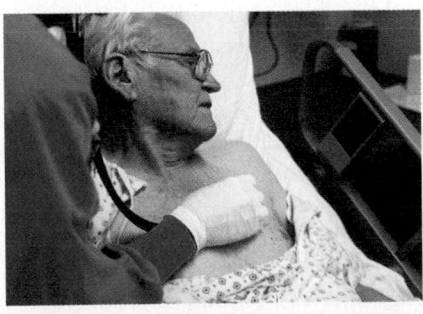

Figure 33-2 Auscultating the lungs of a patient with COPD.

TABLE 33-1 Assessment of the Patient with COPD

HISTORY	PHYSICAL FINDINGS	NEEDS
Patient and family history: Medications, allergy, diet, fluid intake, sinusitis, nasal polyps, low birth weight, depression, anxiety, and other diseases, especially lung and heart diseases	Shortness of breath rating scale	Teaching needs, e.g., disease, smoking cessation anxiety reduction, relaxation techniques, travel restrictions, and energy conservation
Alpha$_1$-antitrypsin deficiency	Abnormal temperature, pulse, respirations	Pulmonary rehabilitation, including nursing, respiratory, nutritional, sexual, occupational, or physical therapy referrals, as needed
Inhalation exposure: Smoking, cooking fuels, and other environmental, occupational, or recreational risk factors	Abnormal breath sounds	Information on community resources
Activities of daily living: Exercise tolerance, sleeping habits, and strength	Abnormal breathing pattern, e.g., pursed lip breathing, tripod position, use of abdominal muscles or accessory muscles of respiration	Home health assistance with oxygen, respiratory equipment, suction, ventilator
COPD and health-related quality of life	Dyspnea, cough, wheezing, and sputum production	
Family and social support systems	Abnormal blood pressure and weight	
Treatment compliance	Jugular vein distension, peripheral edema, and cyanosis; clubbing of the fingers; restlessness memory impairment or confusion; signs of pulmonary hypertension, cor pulmonale, polycythemia, respiratory infection or respiratory failure	

Adapted from Daniels, R. (2004). Nursing fundamentals. *New York: Thomson Delmar Learning; Estes, M. (2006).* Health assessment and physical examination *(3rd ed.). New York: Thomson Delmar Learning.*

fatigued and cannot participate in even mild exercise because of dyspnea. Patients with severe dyspnea often report a decrease in libido and state that they cannot even take a shower without running out of breath. As COPD progresses, dyspnea occurs even at rest, and the patient is at risk for respiratory insufficiency and respiratory infections, which in turn increase the risk for acute and chronic respiratory failure. Respiratory failure is discussed in chapter 65. The Global Initiative for Chronic Obstructive Lung Disease (GOLD) has classified COPD into four stages (Table 33-2).

Factors that determine the clinical course and survival of patients with COPD include history of cigarette smoking, passive smoking exposure, age, rate of decline of FEV_1 on pulmonary function spirometry measurement, hypoxemia, pulmonary artery pressure, resting heart rate, weight loss, and reversibility of airflow obstruction. Note that normal FEV_1 values vary with the height, weight, age, and sex of the patient. A normal FEV_1 is over 80 percent of predicted values for a patient's height, weight, age, and sex. See Table 33-3 for common pulmonary function measures.

TABLE 33-2 **Classification of Patients with COPD by Severity**	
Stage 0: At risk	Chronic cough and sputum production
	Lung function still normal on spirometry
Stage I: Mild COPD	Mild airflow limitation
	FEV$_1$/FVC less than 70 percent
	FEV$_1$ greater than or equal to 80 percent predicted and usually, but not always, chronic cough and sputum production
	At this stage, the patient may not be aware that lung function is abnormal
Stage II: Moderate COPD (Includes stage IIA and IIB)	Worsening airflow
	FEV$_1$/FVC less than 70 percent
	30 percent less than or equal to FEV$_1$, less than 80 percent predicted
	May have a progression of chronic symptoms of cough, sputum production, and dyspnea
	Stage IIA has 50 percent less than or equal to FEV$_1$, less than 80 percent predicted
	Stage IIB has 30 percent less than or equal to FEV$_1$, less than 50 percent predicted
Stage III: Severe COPD	Further worsening of airflow limitation
	FEV$_1$/FVC less than 70 percent
	FEV$_1$ less than 30 percent predicted or presence of respiratory failure or right heart failure
	At this stage, quality of life is very appreciably impaired and exacerbations may be life-threatening

Adapted from DeLaune, S., & Ladner, P. (2006). Fundamentals of nursing (3rd ed.). New York: Thomson Delmar Learning; Heffner, J. E. (2003). Chronic obstructive pulmonary disease: Translating new understanding into improved patient care. Respiratory Care, 48(12), 1184.

Diagnostic Tests

Diagnosis of COPD rests on a careful history and physical examination. Pulmonary function spirometry measures include FEV$_1$ and FVC. Screening for alpha$_1$-antitrypsin deficiency may be performed for patients who are age 45 or younger or for those with a strong family history of COPD. A bronchodilator reversibility test may be conducted to rule out asthma, determine the diagnosis, and guide treatment.

A chest X-ray (CXR) may be used to identify additional lung disorders, such as pneumonia and lung cancer. The CXR also reveals heart and lung size. In patients with emphysema, the diaphragm appears flattened and the lung fields are transparent, with marked, persistent, overdistension of the lungs and the presence of bullae. The pulmonary arteries appear enlarged and may indicate pulmonary hypertension.

Hyperinflation and parenchymal bullae or subpleural blebs may be apparent on thoracic computed tomography (CT) imaging. A thoracic CT is a noninvasive

TABLE 33-3   Pulmonary Function Spirometry Measures

Tidal volume (V_T)	Amount of air inhaled or exhaled with each breath during normal breathing; normal is 0.5 L
Minute volume (MV)	Amount of air breathed per minute
Inspiratory reserve volume (IRV)	Maximum amount of air inhaled forcefully after a normal inhalation; normal is 3 L
Expiratory reserve volume (ERV)	Maximum amount of air exhaled forcefully after a normal exhalation; normal is 1 L
Vital capacity (VC)	Maximum amount of air exhaled after maximum inspiration; normal is 4.5 L
Forced vital capacity (FVC)	Maximum volume of air forcibly exhaled from the point of maximal inhalation; normal is above 80 percent of predicted for patient's height, weight, age, and sex
Forced expiratory volume in one second (FEV_1)	Volume of air exhaled during the first second of the FVC; normal FEV_1 is above 80 percent of predicted values for a patient's height, weight, age, and sex; FEV_1 is reduced in airway obstruction
FEV_1/FVC: FEV_1 expressed as a percentage of the FVC	This ratio gives a clinically useful index of airflow limitation and helps differentiate obstructive versus restrictive pulmonary disease; normal value is above 80 percent of predicted for a patient's height, weight, age, and sex

Adapted from DeLaune, S., & Ladner, P. (2006). Fundamentals of nursing (3rd ed.). New York: Thomson Delmar Learning; Estes, M. (2006). Health assessment and physical examination (3rd ed.). New York: Thomson Delmar Learning.

computer imaging test that illustrates the lungs in a number of two-dimensional views. A CT is usually only done if the diagnosis is not clear or if a surgical procedure on a lung is being considered. Pulmonary artery pressure may be estimated on Doppler echocardiography if pulmonary hypertension is suspected (Tierney, et al., 2004).

An electrocardiogram (ECG) may be useful for the evaluation of ischemia, arrhythmias, and evidence of right ventricular hypertrophy or cor pulmonale. A right-sided heart catheterization may be indicated to evaluate right-sided heart pressures. A timed walking test, lung diffusion test, and an exercise stress test may also be used to gauge both heart and lung function.

Laboratory tests may include a theophylline level, if the patient is on theophylline to relieve bronchospasms, and a complete blood cell (CBC) count to check for polycythemia. Blood tests are often done to evaluate electrolytes, glucose, albumin, and pre-albumin and check the patient for any metabolic or nutritional disorders (Daniels, 2003).

Sputum cultures are not particularly useful and are not routinely recommended. The presence of purulent sputum may be sufficient evidence to start antibiotics empirically, based on the patient's symptoms. The common bacteria in COPD exacerbations include *S. pneumoniae*, *H. influenzae*, or *M. catarrhalis*. As COPD progresses, the patient's arterial blood gas (ABG) results will change. This reflects hypoxemia and carbon dioxide retention or hypercapnia.

Nursing Diagnoses

Based on the information gathered, examples of nursing diagnosis in the patient with COPD may include the following:

- Impaired gas exchange related to airflow obstruction from collapsed alveoli and narrow bronchioles
- Anxiety related to breathlessness, ineffective coping, and reduced socialization
- Ineffective breathing pattern related to increased mucous production and air trapping
- Activity intolerance related to fatigue and hypoxemia
- Nutrition imbalance, less than body requirements, related to increased energy expenditure from breathing difficulties

Planning and Implementation

After assessment and diagnosis, nursing management for patients with COPD includes planning, implementation, and medications designed to improve airflow and prevent disease progression. During this phase of the nursing process, nurses work with many members of the health care team to help patients cope, prevent COPD exacerbations, and manage their lifestyle and disease. All pulmonary irritants should be eliminated or reduced from the patient's environment. Controlled oxygen therapy may be needed, both in the hospital and at home. A major goal is patient achievement of a PaO_2 greater than 60 mm Hg or a pulse oximetry reading (SpO_2) of more than 90 percent.

It is important for the nurse and the health care team to work with the patient to improve airflow. The single most effective intervention to slow the progression of COPD is for the patient to quit smoking. Simply telling the patient to quit succeeds only 5 percent of the time. Smoking cessation is important because smoking impairs bronchial function by paralyzing ciliary action, increasing bronchial secretions, and causing inflammation of the mucous membranes, resulting in hyperplasia of the mucous glands. Recent surveys indicate that 25 percent of all American adults smoke. Patients may think it is too late to reverse the damage from years of smoking and that smoking cessation will not work. They must be informed that continuing to smoke slows down clearance of the airways and provides continued irritation. See Table 33-4 for the changes in physiological function after smoking cessation.

Factors that interfere with smoking cessation include the strength of the nicotine addiction, continued exposure to smoke at work or social situations, stress, depression, and habit. Continued smoking is also more prevalent among those with low income, lower levels of education, and psychosocial problems. Regardless of the setting (outpatient clinic, pulmonary rehabilitation, community, hospital, or the patient's home), the nurse has an opportunity to teach the patient about the risks of smoking and the benefits of smoking cessation.

Collaborative Management

Patients with COPD are often referred to a multidisciplinary pulmonary rehabilitation program to improve their airflow and optimize their functional status. In both randomized and nonrandomized clinical trials, pulmonary rehabilitation has been shown to improve exercise tolerance, reduce dyspnea, and increase health-related quality of life. Pulmonary rehabilitation is individualized for each patient and has educational, psychosocial, behavioral, and physical components. Topics addressed by the health care team in these programs may include pulmonary pathophysiology of COPD, medications, oxygen, nutrition, breathing exercises and retraining, respiratory treatments, lifestyle modifications for energy conservation, time management, symptom alleviation, smoking cessation, infection prevention, sexuality, and coping. The program often

TABLE 33-4 Changes in Physiological Function of Patients After Smoking Cessation

TIME ELAPSED SINCE SMOKING CESSATION	CHANGES
20 minutes	Temperature, pulse, and blood pressure return to normal
8 hours	Carbon monoxide blood levels drop
	Oxygen levels increase to normal
24 hours	Risk for myocardial infarction begins to decrease
48 hours	Nerve endings repair
	Ability to smell and taste is enhanced
2 weeks to 3 months	Circulation improves
	Walking becomes easier
	Lung function improves up to 30 percent
1 to 9 months	Coughing, sinus congestion, fatigue, and shortness of breath decrease
	Cilia in the lungs regenerate, improving handling of secretions
	Energy increases
1 year	Risk for coronary heart disease is half that of a smoker
2 years	Risk for coronary heart disease equals that of those who never smoked
5 years	Risk for lung cancer drops by half
	Stroke risk lessens
	Risk for cancer of the mouth and throat is half that of a smoker
10 years	Lung cancer death rate corresponds to that of nonsmokers
	Precancerous cells are replaced
	Risk for cancer of mouth, bladder, throat, kidney, and pancreas decreases
15 years	Risk for coronary heart disease equals that of a nonsmoker

Adapted from Daniels, R. (2004). Nursing fundamentals. New York: Thomson Delmar Learning; Karnath, B. (2002). Smoking cessation. American Journal of Medicine, 112(5), 399–405.

addresses communicating with the health care team, advance directives, living wills, and health care alternatives for the future as well.

Most outpatient pulmonary rehabilitation programs offer a 6- to 10-week program to those individuals affected by lung disease, such as emphysema, pulmonary fibrosis, asthma, and lung cancer. Through education and exercise, patients learn to better cope with their disease. The goal of the program is to help people lead a full, satisfying life and to restore them to their highest possible functional capacity. The education portion of the program focuses on classes to increase the patient's knowledge about lung disease and its management. Topics include pulmonary anatomy and physiology, respiratory and nonrespiratory medicines, stress reduction, nutrition, breathing retraining, bronchial hygiene, energy conservation, lifestyle modifications, and posture and body mechanics. These classes are taught by variety of disciplines, including registered nurses, respiratory therapists, occupational therapists, exercise physiologists, social workers, and physical therapists. All pulmonary rehabilitation programs have a medical director, usually a pulmonologist, as part of the team.

All patients entering pulmonary rehabilitation receive an evaluation. The patient's pulmonary muscle strength and lower limb strength are assessed. Precautions for physical activity, such as osteoporosis or musculoskeletal and neurological dysfunctions, such as poor balance or muscle weakness, which may limit a patient's ability to exercise, are identified. The program is then modified to allow the patient to exercise safely. The evaluation also helps to identify specific areas where a patient may need additional attention, such as a home exercise program to address these issues.

The exercise portion of the program focuses on improving the patient's strength and overall aerobic conditioning. The patient's heart rate, oxygen saturation, blood pressure, and in some programs, cardiac activity, are closely watched. Team members, including physical therapists, nurses, respiratory therapists, or exercise physiologists may monitor patients while they are exercising to make sure that they exercise safely and attain their maximum physical condition. Most patients work up to exercising for 20 minutes on the treadmill, stationary bike, upper body ergometer, and recumbent stepper. Patients also perform resistive strengthening exercises on free weights or machines to improve muscle strength and endurance.

Patient outcomes are monitored before and after a pulmonary rehabilitation program. Areas that are evaluated include a six-minute walk and questionnaires on shortness of breath and quality of life, as well as hospital admissions and hospital length of stays. Patients typically show improvement in all measured areas and dramatically decrease their admissions to the hospital.

The simplest improvements in a patient's life from pulmonary rehabilitation can have great impact. Patients often have difficulty doing the simplest activities of daily living. Showering is often an activity that can drain all of a patient's energy. With pulmonary rehabilitation conditioning and education, a patient can go from needing three breaks to take a shower to being able to shower in a shorter amount of time and with less exhaustion. It is not uncommon for a patient who could barely walk across a room at the beginning of the program to be able to walk 20 minutes or more on a treadmill in six weeks. The patients improve their quality of life and learn that they can still exercise, in spite of their lung disease. The pulmonary rehabilitation program is a rewarding place to work.

Pulmonary rehabilitation involving the collaborative management of the health care team helps the patient avoid hospitalizations and stay more active. When someone who is short of breath stops exercising, a spiral of inactivity begins that may result in the patient becoming housebound. Patients can identify pulmonary rehabilitation programs in their area by contacting the American Association of Cardiovascular and Pulmonary Rehabilitation or the American Lung Association.

Members of the health care team from nursing, medicine, physical therapy, and respiratory therapy use various strategies to improve airflow in patients with COPD. Postural drainage with chest percussion may be used because draining the lungs by gravity reduces the amount of secretions and the degree of potential infection (Figure 33-3). Note that some patients with COPD cannot tolerate the position changes required with postural drainage. Sometimes mucopurulent sputum must be removed by suction or bronchoscopy. Patients with COPD who cannot tolerate postural drainage may benefit from the Vest system. The Vest system uses high-frequency chest wall oscillation. The system has an inflatable vest connected by tubes to a generator. During therapy, the vest inflates and deflates rapidly, applying gentle pressure to the chest wall. This pressure works to loosen and thin mucus and to move it toward the larger airways, where it can be cleared by coughing or suctioning.

The breathing pattern of most people with COPD is shallow, rapid, and inefficient; the more severe the disease, the more inefficient the breathing. With practice, the patient can be taught to change the type of breathing to diaphragmatic breathing, which reduces the respiratory rate, increases alveolar ventilation, and helps expel as much air as possible during expiration. For diaphragmatic breathing, teach the patient to lie comfortably on the back with a pillow under the head. The knees should be bent to relax the stomach muscles. Instruct the patient to place one hand on the upper chest and the other on the abdomen and inhale slowly through the nose, using the stomach muscles. The

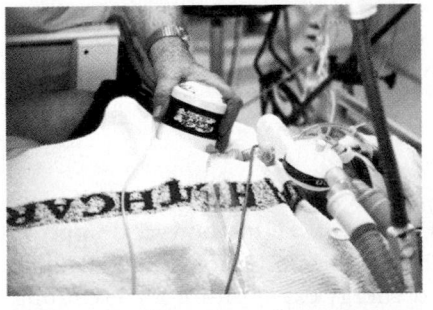

Figure 33-3 Physical therapist using a percussor for a patient with severe COPD.

patient should feel the hand on the abdomen rise during inspiration and fall during expiration, while the hand on the chest stays almost still (Estes, 2006).

Pursed-lip breathing helps prevent or reduce the air trapped in the lungs of patients with COPD. The patient is taught to breathe in slowly through the nose to prevent air gulping, then hold the breath for a count of three, purse the lips as if whistling, and then exhale for six slow counts. This method of breathing should be continued until the dyspnea subsides. If the recommended counting rhythm is uncomfortable for the patient, it can be changed to one that is more comfortable. Pursed-lip breathing also promotes relaxation, enabling the patient to reduce feelings of panic (Daniels, 2004). Patients who use pursed lip breathing can get their oxygen saturations to 93 percent or higher, with practice. Pulse oximeters are available from the pulmonologist or the health care supply store.

Directed or controlled coughing is a cough technique to expectorate sputum and avoid the fatigue associated with undirected, forceful coughing. Controlled coughing consists of slow, maximal inspiration followed by breath holding for several seconds and then two or three coughs. Some patients may benefit from huff coughing, which uses one or two forced exhalations, or "huffs," of air from low to medium lung volumes with the glottis open.

Other respiratory strategies can be used to improve the patient's breathing. Patients can use a flutter valve or a cappella device to provide positive end-expiratory pressure (PEEP) to their lungs. A flutter device helps clear mucus. It is a handheld pipe-like device with a plastic mouthpiece. The patient takes a slow deep breath, holds it for two to three seconds, and then exhales forcefully into the device as completely as possible. The stainless steel ball inside the device bounces during exhalation and causes vibrations that help to dislodge mucus from the airway. Many patients perform several breath cycles twice daily with the flutter device. The device helps improve bronchodilation when used with drug delivery via nebulizer or metered dose inhaler (MDI) with a spacer. It is contraindicated in patients with pneumothorax or right-sided failure (Daniels, 2004).

Ventilator support may be used for patient with stage III COPD to relieve symptoms and prolong quality of life. Ventilator support includes both noninvasive mechanical ventilation via mouthpiece, mask, or artificial airway, using either negative- or positive-pressure devices, and invasive mechanical ventilation by oro-naso-tracheal tube or tracheostomy. Either noninvasive or invasive ventilation can be done in both acute care and home health care settings to mobilize and clear retained secretions, deliver aerosolized medications, and improve ventilation and respiratory function, acid-base abnormalities, and altered mental status. It is contraindicated in patients with untreated pneumothorax, hemoptysis, active tuberculosis, or fractured ribs.

Nutrition

Nutritional and fluid assessment is an important aspect of care for the patient with COPD. Some patients with COPD are overweight; however, approximately 25 percent of patients with COPD may be undernourished. Patients may lose weight because of their increased energy expenditure for breathing. Patients who are overweight, possibly because of inactivity or medications, require a weight loss program. As a result of being overweight, these patients experience an increase in the work of breathing and shortness of breath.

Counseling about weight gain or loss, sodium restriction, food allergies, low-fat, complex carbohydrate diet, cholesterol reduction diet, reflux diet, diabetic training, treatment of osteoporosis, and alcohol restriction may be individualized to the patient's needs by the health care team. Meal planning and appropriate supplementation can help the patient with COPD maintain the strength needed to breathe. It is recommended that the patient eat three regular meals, although six smaller meals may be substituted if larger meals cause discomfort. The patient is also encouraged to increase fluid intake to 64 ounces of water daily, unless contraindicated, to help liquefy pulmonary secretions and make them easier to cough up.

Pharmacology

Several classes of medications are used to decrease symptoms and complications of COPD, although they have not been shown to modify the long-term decline in lung function of such patients. Medications commonly used include beta-adrenergic agonists (sympathomimetics), anticholinergics, corticosteroids, methylxanthines, and a combination of one or more of these drugs (Table 33-5).

Bronchodilators are the main pharmacotherapy for COPD. They relieve bronchospasm, reduce airway obstruction, and improve alveolar ventilation. Bronchodilators are generally used on a regular schedule, with additional doses given as needed. Bronchodilators may also be used before any activity likely to cause shortness of breath.

The most commonly used bronchodilators are inhaled anticholinergics and inhaled beta-adrenergic agonists. Inhaled anticholinergics are now considered first-line bronchodilators for patients with stable COPD. Ipratropium bromide (Atrovent), given as nebulizer or MDI, is a short-acting anticholinergic bronchodilator. Tiotropium bromide (Spiriva) is given as an inhalation powder through the HandiHaler. It is a long-acting inhaled anticholinergic that only needs to be given once a day.

For many years, beta-adrenergic agonists (sympathomimetics) have been the main pharmacotherapy for COPD. A number of sympathomimetics are currently available; however, there are considerable differences in route of administration, duration of action and $beta_2$ selectivity in these medications. The inhaled route, either by an inhaler or nebulizer, is preferred over the oral or parenteral systemic route, because inhalation delivers medication directly to the bronchi, has a quicker onset of effect, and lower potential for systemic toxicity as less medication is absorbed. Sympathomimetics with $beta_2$ selectivity, such as albuterol, bitolterol, pirbuterol, salmeterol, and formoterol are preferred over non–$beta_2$-selective sympathomimetics, such as metaproterenol because lower incidence of myocardial side effects.

TABLE 33-5 **Recommendations for Treatment of Patients with COPD**	
All stages	Avoid risk factors
	Encourage regular exercise and healthy lifestyle, begin smoking cessation program
	Vaccinate against influenza and pneumococcus
Stage I: Mild COPD	Short-acting bronchodilator, as needed
Stage II: Moderate COPD	Pulmonary rehabilitation
	Regular treatment with one or more bronchodilators
	Add inhaled corticosteroids if significant symptoms and lung response or if repeated exacerbations
Stage III: Severe COPD	Regular treatment with one or more bronchodilators; maximize therapy
	Add inhaled corticosteroids if significant symptoms and lung response or if repeated exacerbations
	Treat complications
	Pulmonary rehabilitation
	Long-term oxygen therapy if respiratory failure
	Consider surgical treatments

Adapted from Broyles, B. E., Reiss, B. S., & Evans, M. E. (2007). Pharmacological aspects of nursing care (7th ed.). New York: Thomson Delmar Learning.

Albuterol, given by MDI or nebulizer, is a short-acting beta$_2$-selective agonist that is especially useful for quick relief of symptoms. Salmeterol (Serevent), given by dry powder inhaler (DPI), is a long-acting beta$_2$-selective agonist used for chronic maintenance therapy. It is important to remember that long-acting agents should never be used as a rescue medication during acute episodes of bronchospasm.

Combination therapies use an anticholinergic and beta-adrenergic agonist medication. They have an additive effect beyond each medication alone. Methylxanthines, such as theophylline, were once used extensively for COPD. However, there has been much debate over their value in recent years. Theophylline is a modest bronchodilator. Although it has been shown to benefit some patients, it has many toxic side effects and numerous drug-drug interactions. All studies using theophylline were done with slow-release preparations. With the advent of inhaled long-acting beta$_2$-selective agonists and anticholinergics, theophylline in treatment of COPD is now limited.

While some patients with COPD do benefit from corticosteroids, the benefit is greater for patients with asthma. Routine use of corticosteroids should generally be avoided because of an unfavorable benefit to risk ratio. For some patients with COPD, inhaled corticosteroid therapy may improve airflow when added to existing bronchodilator therapy.

Long-term treatment with inhaled corticosteroids is usually reserved for those patients with severe disease, FEV$_1$ below 50 percent predicted, and repeated COPD exacerbations requiring treatment with antibiotics or oral corticosteroids. The inhaled route is preferred over systemic route because of the decreased risk of toxicity. For patients with an acute exacerbation of COPD, many practitioners recommend a short course of 7 to 14 days of systemic corticosteroids, either by the oral or parenteral route. There is mounting evidence, however, that a short course of systemic corticosteroids is a poor predictor of the long-term response to inhaled corticosteroids in COPD.

The use of mucus-clearing drugs, such as expectorants and mucolytics, has not demonstrated an improved outcome, although it does provide some symptom relief. Water remains the expectorant of choice. Patients with COPD should avoid regular use of antitussives to depress cough, because coughing has a significant protective role. Narcotics should be used with caution because of their respiratory depressant effect and potential to worsen hypercapnia.

Prolastin, a weekly infusion of alpha$_1$-antitrypsin, may be used for young patients with severe hereditary alpha$_1$-antitrypsin deficiency and some types of established emphysema. However, this therapy is expensive. Antioxidant agents, such as vitamins E, C, and beta carotene, and immunoregulator drugs, such as cilomilast and roflumilast, as well as new antiprotease medications, are currently being investigated for a possible role in COPD. Their routine use is not yet recommended.

Finally, all patients with COPD should receive an annual influenza vaccine and a pneumococcal vaccine. A second dose of pneumococcal vaccine is indicated if the patient received a dose more than 5 years ago and was younger than 65 years old at the time of vaccination.

Acute exacerbations of COPD are characterized by a sudden worsening of respiratory symptoms and impaired lung function. Exacerbations may result in significant morbidity and mortality. One of the most common triggers of an acute exacerbation of COPD is infection. Although a high percentage of these infections are of viral origin, bacterial infection may follow the initial viral infection. Effective antibiotic regimens have been shown to reduce symptoms and hospitalization. The use of antibiotics is indicated for patients with increased sputum purulence and volume, worsening cough, and dyspnea, as well as other signs of infection (e.g., fever, leukocytosis, and changes on CXR).

Therapy should be started within 24 hours of onset of symptoms to achieve the best outcome and is usually continued for at least 7 to 10 days.

Azithromycin (Zithromax) may be used for a shorter period of time because of its long half-life. It stays in the body system a few days after a short course of the medicine. Generally, antibiotics are given empirically to the patient with COPD based on the practitioner's judgment, experience, and the patient's clinical picture. The antibiotics used should be targeted toward bacteria most commonly responsible for infections in patients with COPD, that is, *S. pneumoniae, H. influenzae,* and *M. catarrhalis.* Examples of the antibiotics prescribed are: trimethoprim-sulfamethoxazole (Bactrim DS, Septra DS), amoxicillin (Amoxil), amoxicillin-clavulanate (Augmentin), ampicillin-sulbactam (Unasyn), and doxycycline (Vibramycin) (Broyles, Reiss, & Evans, 2007).

Many medications for COPD are given through MDI, DPI, or nebulizer. The MDI, the most widely used delivery system, is a pressurized canister containing medication that a patient may inhale into the lungs. Proper technique and the use of a spacer with the MDI improve drug delivery to the lungs and decrease drug deposition in the mouth. A variety of dry powder inhalers, such as Rotahaler and Diskhaler, have also been introduced. One major advantage of DPIs is that they are breath-actuated, so minimal hand-lung coordination is required for proper administration of the drug. Nebulizer therapy is reserved for acutely ill patients and those who cannot use inhalers because of difficulties with coordination or cooperation.

MDIs propelled by chlorofluorocarbons (CFC) have been the most widely used delivery system, but non-CFC propellant systems and DPIs are becoming more available. These alternatives are effective and well tolerated. As the patient improves, treatment will be decreased until the patient is receiving the correct dosage to manage symptoms and keep the treatment appropriate and the costs reasonable (see Dollars and Sense)

Oxygen Therapy

Oxygen delivery is actually considered a prescription therapy and is to be administered with great caution. In advanced COPD, the patient has severe and progressive hypoxemia because of limited airflow. Oxygen therapy for more than 15 hours per day has been shown to improve the patient's quality of life and survival. Long-term oxygen therapy is often introduced in stage III. Indications for oxygen supplementation include a PaO_2 at or below 55 mm Hg or a SaO_2 at or below 88 percent with or without hypercapnia or evidence of tissue hypoxia and organ damage, such as pulmonary hypertension, cor pulmonale, secondary polycythemia, congestive heart failure, or impaired mental status.

Oxygen is most commonly administered via nasal cannula. Oxygen is titrated to keep the patient with COPD relatively free of respiratory distress and maintain the oxygen saturation of hemoglobin level measured by pulse oximeter (SpO_2) at or above 90 percent. Follow these guidelines when using pulse oximetry (Figure 33-4):

PATIENT PLAYBOOK

General Directions for Using a DPI

The nurse should instruct the patient to do the following in self-administering a DPI:

- Remove the cap from the mouthpiece.
- Load the medicine into the inhaler. Hold the DPI sideways, horizontal, or upright while loading, as directed.
- Do not shake your DPI.
- Tilt your head back slightly and breathe out, getting as much air out of your lungs as you can. Do not breathe into your inhaler as this may affect the dose.
- Close your lips tightly around the mouthpiece of the inhaler.
- Breathe in deeply and quickly. This will ensure that the medicine moves deep into your lungs. You may or may not sense the medicine going into your lungs.
- Hold your breath for 10 seconds or as long as you can to disperse the medicine into your lungs. Repeat as directed.

DOLLARS AND SENSE

The Approximate Cost of Inhalers in Various Countries

MEDICATION	UNITED STATES	CANADA	MEXICO
Advair 250/50	$129.00	$103.00	$50.00
Flovent 110	$71.00	$49.00	$30.00
Combivent	$55.00	$34.00	$30.00

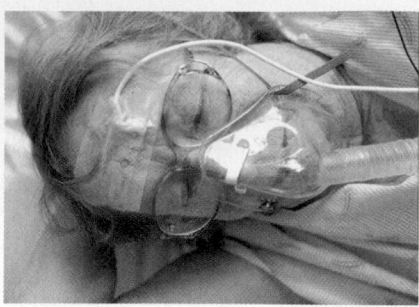

Figure 33-4 Pulse oximetry on the forehead and an oxygen mask used for a patient with COPD complications.

- Use pulse oximetry to obtain spot checks or continuous noninvasive readings of the patient's hemoglobin oxygen saturation. The SpO_2 measurement is done using a clip or probe attached to a sensor site (usually an earlobe or a fingertip). The pulse oximeter probe has a light source and a photodetector and measures the change in light absorption across a vascular bed during the arterial pulse.
- The pulse oximeter reviews the hemoglobin of each red blood cell in the cardiovascular system as it enters the capillaries of the finger, toe, or earlobe probe site.
- Avoid placing the sensor distal to arterial lines, blood pressure cuffs, and pressure dressings.
- Many factors can interfere with pulse oximeter accuracy. For example, an abnormal bilirubin level, abnormal carboxyhemoglobin or methemoglobin level, some lipid emulsions, and radiologic dyes can affect readings.
- Other factors interfering with pulse oximetry accuracy include excessive light from phototherapy or direct sunlight, abnormal hemoglobin, anemia, extremely dark skin pigments, excessive patient movement, excessive ear pigment, severe peripheral vascular disease, hypothermia, hypotension, vasoconstriction, acrylic nails, and dark nail polish.
- The patient's skin sampling area must have good circulation and be free of skin irritation to ensure accuracy.
- Normal pulse oximeter levels are 95 to 100 percent for adults.
- Be sure to correlate your pulse oximeter reading with the patient's overall status, that is, vital signs, respiratory assessment, dyspnea, breath sounds, color, restlessness, level of consciousness, and so on. When in doubt, check your patient's ABG reading and intervene to ensure your patient's oxygenation.

Oxygen supplied to the patient at home comes in compressed gas, liquid, or concentrator systems. Portable oxygen systems allow the patient to exercise, work, and travel. In patients with exercise-induced hypoxemia, oxygen supplementation during exercise can improve performance.

Surgery

Surgery is not frequently used for COPD, but it may be considered for carefully selected patients who continue to expectorate large amounts of sputum and have repeated bouts of pneumonia and hemoptysis despite treatment. If the patient still has some lung function, lung volume reduction surgery (LVRS) may be considered to improve dyspnea, diaphragmatic function, airflow, and exercise capacity. LVRS has been performed via median sternotomy and video-assisted thoracoscopy. In this procedure, 20 to 30 percent of each lung, the sections that are most filled with disease and no longer function, is surgically removed and the wound closed by stapling. This allows more space for the functioning sections of the lung to expand. The diaphragm goes back to its normal position so it can work more efficiently. LVRS also reduces the need for the accessory muscles of the neck and around the ribs to work so hard in the breathing effort. The cost of LVRS is between $33,000 and $70,000 for each procedure, and it may not be covered by insurance.

The National Emphysema Treatment Trial (NETT), supported by the National Heart, Lung, and Blood Institute (NHLBI), the Health Care Financing Administration (HCFA), and the Agency for Healthcare Research and Quality (AHRQ), is the first multicenter clinical trial designed to determine the role, safety, and effectiveness of bilateral LVRS in the treatment of emphysema. NETT researchers found that, on average, patients with severe emphysema who underwent LVRS with medical therapy were more likely to have improved function and did not face an increased risk of death, compared to those who received only medical therapy (Daniels, 2004). However, results for individual patients varied widely and LVRS is not yet recommended for widespread use.

Another surgical procedure used in carefully selected patients with COPD is a bullectomy. Some patients with emphysema develop **bullae** (enlarged airspaces

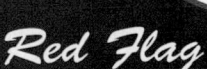

Red Flag

Response to Oxygen Therapy

Carefully monitor your patient's response to oxygen. Recall that the two chemoreceptors in the respiratory center that control the drive to breathe respond to carbon dioxide and oxygen. A $PaCO_2$ accumulation in the blood triggers the respiratory drive in healthy people. There has been concern that the patient with COPD could develop a tolerance for a high $PaCO_2$ level over time, as a result the patient's respiratory center may lose its sensitivity to the chronically elevated $PaCO_2$. Consequently, giving oxygen to this patient could depress the respiratory rate, leading to respiratory arrest. This concern must be balanced, however, with the important need that the hypoxic patient has for oxygen. While it is important to carefully monitor the effect of the oxygen on the patient's breathing and level of consciousness, it is also important to give enough oxygen to the patient who is hypoxic. Oxygen is given at the lowest rate needed to oxygenate the patient, as identified by the patient's clinical condition and ABGs. The patient is closely monitored, with frequent checks of vital signs, especially respiratory rate and effort, breath sounds, patient's shortness of breath rating, skin color, and level of consciousness, as well as pulse oximetry readings, and ABGs. The patient is taught to avoid increasing the flow of oxygen past the limit prescribed.

that do not contribute to ventilation but occupy space in the chest). They may rupture and lead to a pneumothorax. Sometimes they compress areas of the lung that do not have adequate gas exchange. Bullae may need to be removed surgically. A bullectomy may help reduce dyspnea and improve lung function.

A single or double lung transplant is also an option for patients whose disease is complicated by hypercapnia and pulmonary hypertension or when disease prognosis is worse than the survival rates of the surgical procedures. Some patients with COPD who have had a lung transplant more than 10 years ago are today enjoying life free of supplemental oxygen and are able to work and play. Patients should have this surgery performed at a facility where a large number of lung transplants are done annually (Box 33-1). For patients with the inherited form of emphysema, a liver transplant is also an option.

Not every patient will benefit from the surgical procedures. Specific criteria exist for referral for lung and liver transplantation. Organs are in short supply, and many patients die while waiting for a transplant. After organ transplantation, patients need to take immunosuppressant medications for the rest of their lives to prevent rejection of the transplanted organ. Antirejection drugs may increase susceptibility to the dangers of infection, so the patient should be taught to avoid large crowds or people who are coughing or sneezing. Patients should also self-monitor for any signs of infection and notify the practitioner as soon as possible if they are present.

Patient and Family Teaching

On discharge, the patient with COPD requires considerable patient and family teaching. A home visit is useful to help patients with COPD develop strategies to conserve energy and adopt a lifestyle of reduced activity. Patients do well in a climate with minimal shifts in temperature and humidity, and no extremes of heat and cold. Heat increases the body temperature, thereby raising oxygen requirements. Cold tends to promote bronchospasm. Air pollutants, such as fumes, cooking smoke, dust, and even talcum, lint, and aerosol sprays, may initiate bronchospasm. High altitudes aggravate hypoxemia. As much as possible, the patient should avoid emotional disturbances and stressful situations that might trigger a coughing episode.

Patients need assistance to increase their self-care activities and balance activity with rest. Members of the health care team teach the patient energy conservation, work simplification, and time management. The patient must coordinate breathing with physical activities, such as walking, bathing, bending, climbing stairs, and fitness exercises. The patient should bathe, dress, take short walks, and rest as needed to avoid fatigue and excessive dyspnea. Fluids should always be available and lightweight portable oxygen systems must be available for patients who require oxygen therapy during physical activity.

Note that any factor that interferes with normal breathing may induce anxiety, depression, mood changes and social isolation and lead to altered functioning. Many patients find the slightest exertion exhausting. Constant shortness of breath and fatigue may make the patient irritable and apprehensive to the point of panic. Restricted activity and loss of employment may cause the patient to react with anger, depression, and demanding behavior. The patient and family may need to be educated about many factors. The caregiver role for the patient with COPD can be difficult. The nurse will assess the patient's home environment and physical and psychological status to evaluate the patient's willingness and ability to cope with the plan of care. If the patient does not have access to a formal pulmonary rehabilitation program, it is important for the nurse to provide the education and breathing retraining necessary for the patient to improve quality of life. It is also useful to teach the patient how to prepare for visits to the health care provider, nurse, or other practitioner.

The patient and family can be taught to avoid environmental and occupational irritants, how to use respiratory devices (e.g., inhalers, peak flow meters, or nebulizers), and how to correctly use oxygen delivery systems. In addition, the patient can be instructed to have good nutrition and avoid excess weight gain or loss and to avoid substances, such as nicotine, alcohol, and drugs. The patient can be encouraged to seek assistance for adaptive home equipment, sexuality counseling, vocational retraining, and help with patient and caregiver relationships, and well spouse issues. Also, the patient can be reminded when to call for help or 911 and counseling for advance directives, living wills, and durable power of attorney for health care. The nurse may direct patients to community resources to help improve the patient's ability to cope with a chronic condition and give a sense of worth, hope, and well-being. In addition, the nurse should remind the patient and family about the importance of participating in general health promotion activities and health screening.

Evaluation of Outcomes

Potential patient outcomes for each of the example nursing diagnoses for the patient with COPD are:

- Impaired gas exchange related to airflow obstruction from collapsed alveoli and narrow bronchioles. The patient maintains optimal gas exchange as evidenced by normal ABGs and alert responsive mentation or no further reduction in mental status.
- Anxiety related to breathlessness, ineffective coping, and reduced socialization. The patient should be able to recognize the signs of anxiety, demonstrate positive coping mechanisms, and describe a reduction in the level of anxiety experienced.
- Ineffective breathing pattern related to increased mucous production and air trapping. The patient's breathing pattern is maintained by eupnea, normal skin color, and regular respiratory rate or pattern.
- Activity intolerance related to fatigue and hypoxemia. The patient maintains activity level within capabilities, as evidenced by normal heart rate and blood pressure during activity, as well as absence of shortness of breath, weakness, and fatigue.
- Nutrition imbalance, less than body requirements related to increased energy expenditure from breathing difficulties. The patient verbalizes and demonstrates selection of foods or meals that will achieve a cessation of weight loss and weighs within 10 percent of ideal body weight.

ASTHMA

Asthma is a chronic inflammatory disorder characterized by episodic exacerbations of acute inflammation of the airways. The airways may also be hyperresponsive to certain stimuli or triggers and can become obstructed via bronchoconstriction, mucous plugs, or increased inflammation when exposed (National Asthma Education and Prevention Program [NAEPP], 2002). Patients with asthma may experience symptom-free periods alternating with acute exacerbations. An **exacerbation** is a sudden increase in the seriousness of the disease with greater intensity in signs and symptoms, which lasts from minutes to hours or days. Most asthma attacks are short-lived, lasting minutes to hours, the patient seems to recover completely after each attack. There may be a phase of asthma in which the patient experiences some degree of airway obstruction daily. This phase can be mild, with or without superimposed severe episodes, or much more serious with severe obstruction persisting for days or weeks. The serious phase is known as status asthmaticus. In unusual circumstances, acute episodes of asthma can be fatal.

Epidemiology

Estimates show that nearly 16 million Americans have asthma and among the estimated 16 million U.S. adults with asthma, current asthma prevalence among racial and ethnic minority populations ranged from 3.1 to 14.5 percent, compared with 7.6 percent among Caucasians (Centers for Disease Control and Prevention [CDC], 2006b). Asthma can occur at any age and may interfere with school and work attendance, occupational choices, physical activity, and general quality of life. Billions of dollars are spent on inpatient and emergency management of acute asthma exacerbations. Hospitalization rates have been highest among African Americans and children. Despite increased understanding about the pathology of asthma and the development of better medications and management plans, the death rate from asthma continues to increase. It is consistently highest among African Americans ages 15 to 24 years old (Tierney, et al., 2004).

Etiology

Triggers cause the release of inflammatory mediators from the bronchial mast cells, macrophages, and epithelial cells and lead to recurrent episodes of wheezing, breathlessness, chest tightness, and coughing. Triggers can be grouped into several categories: allergenic, pharmacological, environmental, air pollution-related, occupational, infectious, exercise-related, and related to other health care conditions (Table 33-6).

Pathophysiology

The inflammatory response in asthma occurs in two phases: the early phase and the late phase (Schieken, 2002). In the early phase, approximately 90 minutes after exposure to a trigger, mediators are released from bronchial mast cells to begin a local inflammatory process. These mediators include histamine, leukotrienes (LTC_4, LTD_4, and LTE_4), bradykinin, and serotonin and lead to the development of cough, bronchial edema, and airway constriction.

TABLE 33-6 Asthma Triggers

TRIGGER	APPROACH
Allergens	Careful history
	Skin testing
	In vitro testing, as appropriate
	Avoid food additives, e.g., peanuts
	Avoid preservatives, e.g., sulfites
Pharmacology	Avoid NSAIDs, aspirin, beta blockers, piperazine, cimetidine, psyllium, rifampin, penicillin, tetracycline, and chemotherapeutic drugs
Environment (e.g., pets, cockroaches, mold, mildew, or dust mites)	Avoid pets and keep dust and moisture away from bedroom, carpets, and upholstery
	Avoid leaving food out and empty the garbage every night
	Exterminate your home with poison baits or traps rather than chemical agents
	Clean tubs, sinks, and showers regularly with a bleach-containing cleanser
	Dehumidify and avoid damp places, such as basements
	Clean and change heating and air conditioning ducts and filters regularly
	Use a high efficiency particulate air (HEPA) filter to remove almost all airborne particles
	Remove or replace worn carpet
	Encase mattress and pillows in an allergen-impermeable cover
	Wash sheets and blankets weekly in hot water of 130° F (54.4° C) or more
	Avoid lying down on a carpet, feather pillows, down comforters, or upholstery
	Use a dust mask while vacuuming or damp dusting

Continued

TABLE 33-6	Asthma Triggers—cont'd
TRIGGER	**APPROACH**
Air pollution (e.g., pollen, grass, cold or hot air, high humidity, smoke and chemical irritants)	Limit time spent outdoors during allergy season or extreme hot or cold season changes
	Use air-conditioning rather than open windows
	Stay inside during the midday and afternoon when the pollen count is highest
	Avoid hanging laundry outside to dry
	Start anti-inflammatory medications prior to allergy season
	Avoid indoor plants and flowers
	Limit use of wood burning stoves and fireplaces
	Avoid strong smelling products and perfumes
	Avoid tobacco, smoke, dust, fumes, other environmental chemicals, and food additives
	Avoid environmental change (new home, workplace or vacation lodgings)
Occupational exposure	Be aware of asthma triggers in workplace
	Maintain trigger avoidance with good ventilation and respiratory protection
	Avoid latex, glutaraldehyde (used in cold sterilization), isocyanate (used in orthopedic casting materials), and formaldehyde
	Avoid chemical smells (paint, chlorine, ammonia, and cleaning fumes)
	Avoid grain or wood dust, enzymes, dyes, nickel, platinum, and chromium salts
	Avoid pollens, gum arabic, synthetic dyes, rosin (soldering flux), inorganic chemicals (salts of nickel, platinum, and chromium), and various pharmaceutical agents
Infections	Use antibiotics as needed
	Take regular influenza and pneumonia vaccines
	Treat respiratory infections promptly
	Get culture and sensitivity of blood and sputum as needed
Exercise	Avoid exertion outdoors when levels of air pollution or pollen counts are high
	Consider premedication prior to exercise or exertion
Other conditions	Evaluate for presence of gastroesophageal reflux disease (GERD), sinusitis, rhinitis, viral respiratory infections, and food allergies
	Evaluate endocrine conditions (menses, pregnancy, or thyroid disease), as well as emotional disorders

Adapted from Roberts, K. (2003). Treating asthma in the zone. American Journal of Nursing, 103(11), 118–119; Sims, J. M. (2003). Guidelines for treating asthma. Dimensions of Critical Care Nursing, 22(6), 247–250.

The late phase begins within 3 to 10 hours of exposure to the trigger and may last for several hours to several days (Schieken, 2002). This phase begins as cellular components (including eosinophils, neutrophils, and macrophages) are activated, with degranulation of the mast cells and basophils and involvement of T lymphocytes and production of interleukins (Bukstein, Elder, Larsen, & Mellon, 2003). Airway obstruction and hyperresponsive airways develop, with inflammation, edema, increased mucous production, smooth muscle contraction, and hypertrophy.

Note that atopy, the genetic predisposition for the development of an immunoglobulin E (IgE)-mediated response to common airborne allergens, is a strong predisposing factor for developing asthma. Patients with atopic diseases, such as asthma, have an inherited predisposition for developing IgE antibody-mediated hypersensitivity to inhaled and ingested allergens that are harmless to people with no atopic disease. Atopic reactions have been noted with exposure to water-soluble proteins in latex products, such as rubber gloves, respiratory equipment, and catheters. Common reactions to latex are urticaria, angioedema, conjunctivitis, rhinitis, bronchospasm, and anaphylaxis.

Evidence indicates that subbasement membrane fibrosis may occur in some patients with asthma and that these changes contribute to persistent abnormalities in lung function. The importance of airway remodeling and the development of persistent airflow limitation needs further exploration and may have significant implications for the treatment of asthma.

The NAEPP (2002) has developed steps to classify asthma, which are useful in directing therapy and identifying patients at high risk of developing life-threatening asthma attacks. Patients are classified by their clinical features before treatment and the presence of only one of the severity features. Patients are classified by the most severe step in which any feature occurs (Table 33-7).

Complications

Complications of asthma may include airway obstruction, asphyxia, exhaustion, dehydration, atelectasis, pneumothorax, mediastinal and subcutaneous emphysema, cor pulmonale, infection, pneumonia, and status asthmaticus. Needleman, Buerhaus, Mattke, Steward, and Zelevinksy (2002) identify the importance of monitoring all patients for the incidence of nurse-sensitive

TABLE 33-7 Classification of Severity of Asthma in Adults

STEP	SYMPTOMS	NIGHTTIME SYMPTOMS	LUNG FUNCTION
Step 1: Mild intermittent	Symptoms up to twice a week	Up to twice a month	PEF greater than or equal to 80 percent predicted
	Asymptomatic and normal peak expiratory flow (PEF) between exacerbations		PEF variability less than 20 percent
Step 2: Mild persistent	Symptoms more than twice a week but less than once a day	More than twice a month	PEF greater than or equal to 80 percent predicted
	Exacerbation may affect activity		PEF variability 20 to 30 percent
Step 3: Moderate persistent	Daily symptoms	More than once a week	PEF greater than 60 percent to less than 80 percent predicted
	Daily use of inhaled short acting beta$_2$ agonist		PEF variability greater than 30 percent
	Exacerbations affect activity		
	Exacerbations at least twice a week and may last days		
Step 4: Severe persistent	Continual symptoms	Frequent	PEF less than 60 percent predicted
	Limited physical activity		PEF variability greater than 30 percent
	Frequent exacerbations		

Adapted from National Asthma Education and Prevention Program. (2002). Executive summary expert panel report: Guidelines for the diagnosis and treatment of asthma–update on select topics (No. 02-5075). Bethesda, MD: National Institutes of Health.

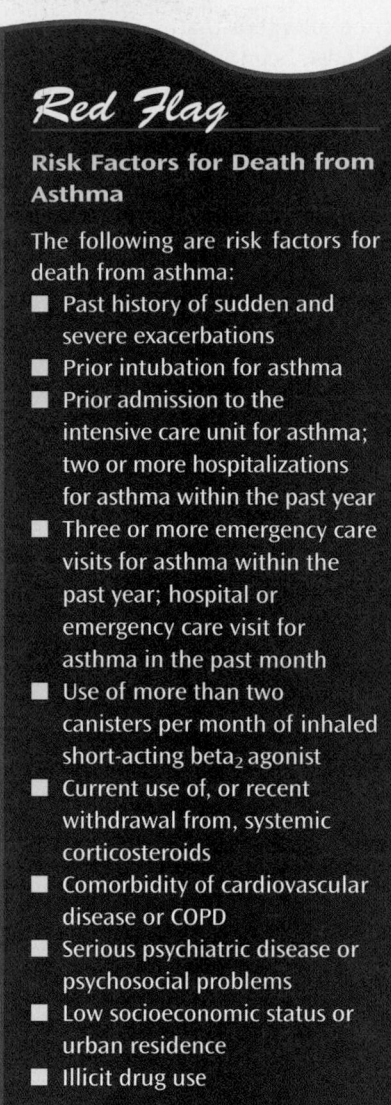

Risk Factors for Death from Asthma

The following are risk factors for death from asthma:

- Past history of sudden and severe exacerbations
- Prior intubation for asthma
- Prior admission to the intensive care unit for asthma; two or more hospitalizations for asthma within the past year
- Three or more emergency care visits for asthma within the past year; hospital or emergency care visit for asthma in the past month
- Use of more than two canisters per month of inhaled short-acting beta$_2$ agonist
- Current use of, or recent withdrawal from, systemic corticosteroids
- Comorbidity of cardiovascular disease or COPD
- Serious psychiatric disease or psychosocial problems
- Low socioeconomic status or urban residence
- Illicit drug use

patient outcomes, such as "failure to rescue" patients from death from pneumonia, shock or cardiac arrest, upper gastrointestinal (GI) bleeding, sepsis, or deep venous thrombosis, shock, sepsis, and pulmonary failure.

Despite the best care, some patients with asthma may have an exacerbation and require emergency or hospital care. **Status asthmaticus** is a severe asthma attack with bronchospasm that does not respond to conventional therapy. Acute hypercapnic and hypoxic respiratory failure occurs in severe states of the disease and may lead to death in minutes or hours. Many patients who die are found to have severe mucous impactions of their airways and marked inflammatory infiltration of their bronchial walls. Patients experiencing status asthmaticus or severe asthma exacerbation need to be evaluated immediately and receive prompt treatment. The goals of therapy are to reduce the airway obstruction by relaxing bronchial smooth muscles and reversing inflammation while supporting respiratory function. Treatment includes short-acting bronchodilators, systemic corticosteroids, and oxygen by nasal cannula.

Albuterol is the bronchodilator of choice because quick onset of action and beta$_2$ receptor selectivity. In the emergency setting, it is administered as an inhaler and most commonly as a nebulizer, at frequent intervals or continuously. The dose is titrated according to patient response to avoid the occurrence of adverse effects, such as tachycardia and tremors. Ipratropium may be used in combination if the patient does not respond to the beta$_2$-adrenergic agonist alone. High-dose systemic corticosteroids, administered by the parenteral or oral route, should be started early in therapy to reduce hospitalization and increase survival. They are usually given as a short course, with treatment duration depending on patient response and past history. Some patients with status asthmaticus will respond poorly to treatment. They can deteriorate rapidly and should be monitored in a critical care setting. Patients who develop altered mental status, acute CO_2 retention, poor response to treatment, or evidence of impending inspiratory muscle failure will require endotracheal intubation and mechanical ventilation. Intubation of an acutely ill asthma patient is technically difficult and is best done semielectively, before the crisis of a respiratory arrest. At the time of intubation, close attention should be given to maintaining an intravenous (IV) line and monitoring blood pressure and intravascular volume, as hypotension may accompany the administration of sedation. The main goal of mechanical ventilation is to ensure adequate oxygen while avoiding **barotrauma** (an injury to the lungs as a result of increased air pressure in the lungs that may occur as a result of increased air pressure in the lungs).

Assessment with Clinical Manifestations

Patient history often shows a pattern of asthma symptoms and a personal or family history of asthma, sinusitis, gastroesophageal reflux disease (GERD), rhinitis, nasal polyps, drug-induced asthma, and allergic skin conditions, including atopic dermatitis and eczema (Box 33-2). The airflow obstruction is at least partially reversible.

The most common indicators of asthma in adults include **wheezing** (high-pitched whistling sounds on expiration), cough, difficulty breathing, recurrent chest tightness, and history of obstructive symptoms that occur or worsen at night or in the presence of triggers. There may be breathlessness, increased respiration, tachycardia, pulsus paradoxus, hyperexpansion of the thorax, use of accessory muscles to breathe, appearance of hunched shoulders, chest deformity, increased nasal secretion, mucosal swelling, and nasal polyps. The patient may be cyanotic and use a tripod position to breathe.

Diagnostic Tests

Pulmonary function testing is needed to establish the diagnosis of asthma. The NAEPP (2002) expert panel recommends pulmonary function spirometry tests for asthma: (a) at the time of initial assessment, (b) after treatment is initiated

BOX 33-2

SAMPLE ROUTINE CLINICAL ASSESSMENT QUESTIONS

Monitoring Signs and Symptoms

Global Assessment

"Has your asthma been better or worse since your last visit?"

Recent Assessment

"In the past two weeks, how many days have you:

- Had problems with coughing, wheezing, shortness of breath, or chest tightness during the day?"
- Awakened at night from sleep because of coughing or other asthma symptoms?"
- Awakened in the morning with asthma symptoms that did not improve within 15 minutes of inhaling a short-acting inhaled beta$_2$ agonist?"

  Had symptoms while exercising or playing?"

Monitoring Pulmonary Function

Lung Function

"What is the highest and lowest your peak flow has been since your last visit?"

"Has your peak flow dropped below ___ L/min (80 percent of personal best) since your last visit?"

"What did you do when this occurred?"

Peak Flow Monitoring Technique

"Please show me how you measure your peak flow."

"When do you usually measure your peak flow?

Monitoring Quality of Life and Functional Status

"Since your last visit, how many days has your asthma caused you to:

- Miss work or school?"
- Reduce your activities?"
- (For caregivers) Change your activity because of your child's asthma?"

"Since your last visit, have you had any unscheduled or ED visits or hospital stays?"

Monitoring Exacerbation History

"Since your last visit, have you had any episodes or times when your asthma symptoms were a lot worse than usual?"

- If yes, "what do you think caused the symptoms to get worse?"

If yes, "what did you do to control the symptoms?"

"Have there been any changes in your home or work environment (e.g., new smokers or pets)?"

Monitoring Pharmacotherapy

Medications

"What medications are you taking?"

"How often do you take each medication?"

"How much do you take each time?"

"Have you missed or stopped taking any regular doses of your medications for any reason?"

"Have you had trouble filling your prescriptions (e.g., for financial reasons or not on formulary)?"

"How many puffs of your short-acting inhaled beta$_2$ agonist (quick-relief medicine) do you use per day?"

"How many [name short-acting inhaled beta$_2$ agonist] inhalers [or pumps] have you been through in the past month?"

"Have you tried any other medicines or remedies?"

Side Effects

"Has your asthma medicine caused you any problems?"

- Shakiness, nervousness, bad taste, sore throat, cough, upset stomach?"

Inhaler Technique

"Please show me how you use your inhaler."

Monitoring Patient-Provider Communication and Patient Satisfaction

"What questions have you had about your asthma daily self-management plan and action plan?"

"What problems have you had following your daily self-management plan? Your action plan?"

"Has anything prevented you from getting the treatment you need for your asthma from me or anyone else?"

"Have the costs of your asthma treatment interfered with your ability to get asthma care?"

"How satisfied are you with your asthma care?"

"How can we improve your asthma care?"

"Let's review some important information:"

- "When should you increase your medications?
- Which medication(s)?"
- "When should you call me [your physician or nurse practitioner]? Do you know the after-hours phone number?"
- "If you can't reach me, what ED would you go to?"

Adapted from Estes, M. (2006). **Health assessment and physical examination** *(3rd ed.). New York: Thomson Delmar Learning.*

and symptoms and peak expiratory flow (PEF) have stabilized to document attainment of near normal airway function, and (c) at least every one to two years to assess the maintenance of airway function.

Note that during an asthma exacerbation, the FEV_1 is markedly decreased but improves with bronchodilator administration. Spirometry measurements (FEV_1, FVC, and FEV_1/FVC) before and after using a short-acting inhaled beta$_2$ agonist helps determine whether there may be airflow obstruction (Daniels, 2003).

Patients with step 3 and step 4 asthma should be taught to monitor their symptoms and PEF regularly to identify exacerbations (NAEPP, 2002). Severe asthma is characterized by a PEF less than 120 L/min or less than 50 percent of flow predicted for the patient. Height, weight, sex, and age determine a patient's normal peak flow. Normal PEF is 80 to 100 percent of predicted flow (Sims, 2003). Pulmonary function is usually normal between exacerbations of asthma. PEF is generally lowest on first awakening and highest several hours before the midpoint of the waking day, between noon and 2 p.m. A 20 percent difference between morning and afternoon PEF measurement suggests asthma.

Additional pulmonary function studies, such as lung volumes, inspiratory, and expiratory flow volume loops, and a bronchoprovocation pulmonary function test with methacholine, histamine, or an exercise challenge may also be conducted. A diffusing capacity test may be helpful, along with assessment of diurnal variation in peak expiratory flow over one to two weeks.

CXRs of patients with asthma usually show hyperinflation, bronchial wall thickening, and diminished peripheral lung vascular shadows. CXRs are indicated when pneumonia, another disorder mimicking asthma, or a complication of asthma, such as pneumothorax, is suspected.

The diagnostic usefulness of serum measurements of biological markers of inflammation, such as cell counts and mediator titers in blood and sputum, is being investigated. Skin testing or in vitro testing to assess sensitivity to relevant environmental allergens may be useful in patients with persistent asthma. Evaluations for nasal polyps and sinus disease or gastroesophageal reflux may be considered in patients with pertinent symptoms and in those who have severe or refractory asthma.

During acute asthma episodes, sputum and CBC serum testing may disclose eosinophilia, (elevated levels of eosinophils), unless systemic corticosteroids have suppressed it. Elevated serum levels of IgE may be detected by in vitro methods, such as a radioallergosorbent test (RAST) (Daniels, 2003). Although they are sometimes used to establish a patient's atopic constitution, in vitro tests are expensive, are subject to laboratory error, and offer little advantage.

Hypoxemia during acute asthma attacks is revealed by ABG analysis and pulse oximetry. Initially, hypocapnia and respiratory alkalosis are present with asthma. As the patient's condition worsens and fatigue increases, the $PaCo_2$ level may rise. A normal $PaCo_2$ value may be a signal of impending respiratory failure. Other tests to detect hypoxemia include ECG and serum electrolyte and serum theophylline testing. A blood and sputum culture and sensitivity may be done if infection is suspected.

Nursing Diagnoses

Based on the information gathered, examples of nursing diagnoses in the patient with asthma may include the following:
- Ineffective airway clearance related to bronchospasm, mucosal edema, and increased mucous production
- Impaired gas exchange related to bronchospasm
- Ineffective breathing pattern related to bronchospasm
- Activity intolerance related to hypoxemia and fatigue
- Anxiety relating to illness, loss of control and nursing and medical interventions

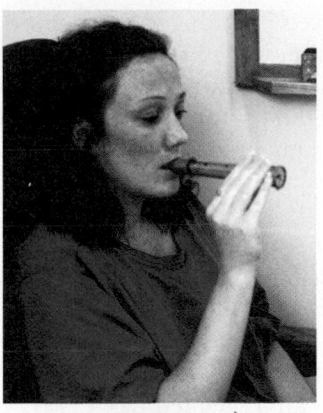

Figure 33-5 A peak flow meter used by this patient with asthma.

Planning and Implementation

Dyspnea may cause fear and anxiety for patient and family and exacerbate breathing difficulty with asthma. Nursing management of the patient requires a collaborative multidisciplinary team that uses a calm approach, friendly manner, and reassuring communication. The patient and family are taught an asthma action plan that includes symptom and peak flow monitoring, avoiding exposure to triggers, and taking prevention and control medications. An asthma action plan, along with an asthma diary, helps to guide the patient and family in self-management strategies in the event of an exacerbation. The plan also provides instructions regarding recognition of early warning signs of worsening asthma. Regular PEF monitoring is recommended for all patients with moderate or severe asthma, because it helps measure severity and, when added to symptom monitoring, indicates the current degree of asthma control (Figure 33-5). Once patients have found their personal best, the practitioner will set up three "zones" on the asthma action plan. These zones are based on percentages of the patient's personal best PEF and can be used as guidelines for managing asthma. The three zones are: (a) green zone: Good asthma control, 80 to 100 percent of personal best PEF; (b) yellow zone: Caution, 50 to 80 percent of personal best PEF; and (c) red zone: Health care alert, below 50 percent of personal best PEF.

Note that PEF shows diurnal variation and is measured with a PEF meter (see Patient Playbook). It is lowest on first awakening and highest several hours before midday. PEF should be measured in the morning before taking or using a bronchodilator and in the afternoon after bronchodilator use. A 20 percent change in PEF from morning to afternoon or from day to day suggests inadequately controlled asthma. A PEF value of less than 200 L/min indicates severe airflow obstruction. Based on their PEF measurement, patients must know whether to take their medication, call their health care provider, or go to the hospital (Tierney, et al., 2004). Patient self-management and early recognition of problems lead to more efficient communication with health care providers regarding asthma severity and appropriate intensification of therapy.

Pharmacology

Although the mainstay therapy for most patients is pharmacological, patient education, trigger avoidance, self-monitoring, and management skills are also important in the treatment of asthma. Current therapeutic guidelines include quick-relief and long-term control medications for the prevention of asthma symptoms. Quick-relief medications are used only during acute exacerbations and should not be used on a regular schedule. They promote prompt reversal of acute airflow obstruction and relief of accompanying symptoms by direct relaxation of bronchial smooth muscle. Frequent use of quick-relief medications indicates poor asthma control and the need to initiate or increase long-term control therapy.

Long-term therapy focuses on prevention and suppression of inflammation, which plays a vital role in the pathogenesis of asthma. Long-term control medications should be taken on a regular schedule (with or without symptoms) to achieve optimal control of persistent asthma. Daily inhaled corticosteroids are considered first-line therapy because of their effective anti-inflammatory properties. They have been shown to improve lung function, diminish symptoms, and decrease usage of $beta_2$-adrenergic agonists in patients with all levels of asthma severity. Use of a spacer device (such as Aerochamber or InspirEase) with inhaled corticosteroids may maximize medication delivery to the bronchi and minimize oropharyngeal deposition (Broyles, et al., 2007).

A long-acting inhaled $beta_2$-adrenergic agonist, such as salmeterol (Serevent), should be also used for patients with moderate persistent or severe asthma, in addition to inhaled corticosteroids. Inhaled mast cell stabilizers, such as cromolyn (Intal) and nedocromil (Tilade), can be used as alternatives for patients with mild persistent asthma or exercise-induced bronchospasm. Leukotriene modifiers, such as zileuton (Zyflo), montelukast (Singulair), zafirlukast (Accolate), and methylxanthine, can be used as additional agents for moderate persistent asthma. Leukotriene modifiers may also be useful for patients with aspirin or nonsteroidal anti-inflammatory drugs (NSAIDs) and exercise-induced bronchospasm or for those who are unable or unwilling to use an inhaler for mild persistent asthma.

All patients should have a quick-relief medication readily available for acute symptoms of bronchospasm. The drug of choice for acute symptom relief is a short-acting inhaled selective beta$_2$-adrenergic agonist, such as albuterol. An inhaled anticholinergic medication, such as ipratropium, can be used as an alternative for those who are intolerant to beta$_2$-adrendergic agonists. Short-acting bronchodilators should be used only on an as-needed basis.

The dose and frequency of medications used to control asthma depend on the type and severity of the disease. A stepwise approach for the management of acute or chronic asthma is recommended by the NAEPP (Table 33-8). Therapy should be initiated at a higher level than the patient's step of severity to establish prompt control of asthma. Therapy is than stepped down cautiously once symptom control is achieved and sustained.

The goal of therapy is to maintain adequate control with a minimal amount of medication. Regular follow-up visits with the practitioner at one- to six-month intervals are essential to maintain control and institute appropriate step-up or step-down therapy. If asthma control is not adequate, referral to a pulmonary specialist may occur at this time. As discussed earlier in this chapter, many asthma medications are administered orally or by inhalation via a nebulizer, MDI, or other inhalation device. Compared to systemic administration of the same drug, inhalation gives the advantage of delivery of high concentrations of medication directly to the lungs, as well as fewer systemic effects. Medications, including beta$_2$-adrenergic agonists, anticholinergics, methylxanthine, and corticosteroids, used in asthma are discussed in the COPD section of this chapter. Leukotriene modifiers and mast cell stabilizers are also medications given to modify the inflammatory response when managing asthma.

Population-Based Care

It is important to implement basic asthma care at the community level and include care that focuses on the needs not only of the patient currently suffering with asthma but also on the total population. Population-focused health care encompasses health care promotion, illness prevention, and community-based education about asthma for the public, patients, and family. Topics may include air quality, fitness, fluid intake and nutrition, self-care management, and smoking cessation, as well as asthma education programs for health care providers. Outpatient follow-up care needs to focus on ongoing, preventive asthma care versus acute episodic care. Patients with recurrent exacerbations may require a home visit to assess their environment for allergens. When needed, the nurse will refer the patient to community support groups.

Healthy People 2010 identified leading health indicators, which reflect the 10 major health concerns in the United States at the beginning of the 21st century and will be used to measure the health of the nation. Nurses are working with their communities and patients to decrease the incidence of diseases, such as asthma, by improving performance on the leading health indicators.

Patient and Family Teaching

Patient education is a critical component of asthma care. It requires an ongoing, age-specific patient, family, and practitioner partnership to help the patient avoid triggers, adhere to an asthma action plan, monitor symptoms and PEF, and take medications to achieve desired outcomes. The nurse may assist the patient in obtaining educational materials regarding asthma. Excellent materials are available from the NAEPP. Referral to a pulmonary rehabilitation program is useful for

TABLE 33-8 Management of Acute or Chronic Asthma

STEP	LONG-TERM CONTROL
Step 1: Mild intermittent	No daily medication needed
	Severe exacerbations may occur, separated by long periods of normal lung function and no symptoms; a course of systemic corticosteroids is recommended
Step 2: Mild persistent	Preferred treatment:
	Low-dose inhaled corticosteroids
	Alternative treatment:
	Cromolyn, leukotriene modifier, nedocromil, or sustained-release theophylline to serum concentration of 5 to 15 mcg/mL
Step 3: Moderate persistent	Preferred treatment:
	Low- to medium-dose inhaled corticosteroid
	Long-acting inhaled beta agonist
	Alternative treatment:
	Increase inhaled corticosteroids within medium-dose range
	Low- to medium-dose inhaled corticosteroids, and either leukotriene modifier or theophylline
	If needed, particularly in patient with recurring severe exacerbations,
	Preferred treatment:
	Increase inhaled corticosteroids with medium-dose range and add long-acting inhaled beta$_2$ agonists.
	Alternative treatment:
	Increase inhaled corticosteroids within medium-dose range and add either leukotriene modifier or theophylline
Step 4: Severe persistent	Preferred treatment:
	High-dose inhaled corticosteroid
	Long-acting inhaled beta$_2$ agonist
	Corticosteroid tablets or syrup long-term (2 mg/kg/day, generally not to exceed 60 mg/day). Make repeat attempts to reduce systemic corticosteroids and maintain control with high-dose inhaled corticosteroids
Quick relief: All patients	Short-acting bronchodilator; two to four puffs short-acting inhaled beta$_2$ agonist as needed for symptoms
	Intensity of treatment will depend on severity of exacerbation; up to three treatments at 20-minute intervals or a single nebulizer treatment as needed; course of systemic corticosteroids may be needed
	Note: Use of short-acting beta$_2$ agonists more than twice a week in intermittent asthma (daily or increasing use in persistent asthma) may indicate the need to initiate (or increase) long-term control therapy

Adapted from Broyles, B. E., Reiss, B. S., & Evans, M. E. (2007). Pharmacological aspects of nursing care *(7th ed.). New York: Thomson Delmar Learning; National Asthma Education and Prevention Program. (2002).* Executive summary expert panel report: Guidelines for the diagnosis and treatment of asthma–update on select topics *(No. 02-5075). Bethesda, MD: National Institutes of Health.*

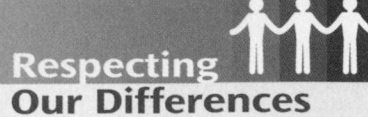

Respecting Our Differences

Hospitalization and Death Rates of Patients with Asthma

Hospitalization rates for asthma have been highest among African Americans and children. Death rates for asthma are consistently highest among African Americans ages 15 to 24 years old (Tierney, et al., 2004). As a professional, the nurse obviously needs to not discriminate, stereotype, or make judgments regarding the ethnicity of patients who have a higher incidence of a disorder such as asthma.

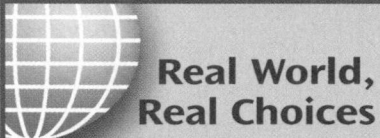

Real World, Real Choices

Delegating Safe Patient Transport

You are working in the ED and your patient with asthma has been dyspneic with cardiac irregularities for the last hour. A CXR looks suspicious, and the patient is scheduled for a CT scan. The CT department calls to say they are ready for the patient. Who will transport the patient to the department? Who will stay with the patient as the test is completed? What equipment should be available for the patient during this process?

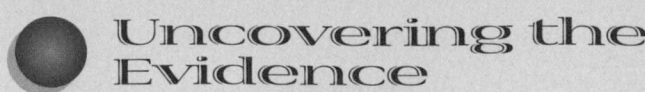

Uncovering the Evidence

Self-Management of Asthma

Discussion: This research study evaluated options for self-management education for adults with asthma. The authors searched the Cochrane Airways Group trials register and reference lists for randomized trials of asthma self-management education interventions in adults over 16 years of age. Fifteen trials met the inclusion criteria. Six studies compared self-management that allowed self-adjustment of medications according to an individualized written action plan with adjustment of medications by a physician. These two styles of asthma management gave equivalent effects for hospitalization, emergency department (ED) visits, unscheduled health care provider visits, and nocturnal asthma. In another six studies, self-management using a written action plan based on PEF was found to be equivalent to self-management using a symptom-based written action plan. Three studies compared self-management options. The first provided optimal therapy but tested the omission of regular review, which was associated with increased health center visits and sick days. The second showed that low intensity education was associated with more unscheduled physician visits than high-intensity education. The third study reported no difference between verbal instruction and written action plans regarding health care utilization or lung function.

Implications for Practice: Currently, it is recommended that all patients with step 3 or step 4 asthma use an asthma action plan with self-monitoring of PEF and symptoms.

Source: Powell, H., & Gibson, P. G. (2003). Options for self-management education for adults with asthma (Cochrane Review). In The Cochrane Database of Systematic Reviews (1), CD004107.

selected patients to improve their breathing and exercise activity. Some patients, especially those on systemic corticosteroids, may require a dietary evaluation.

Evaluation of Outcomes

Based on the information gathered, examples of nursing diagnoses in the patient with asthma may include the following:

- Ineffective airway clearance related to bronchospasm, mucosal edema, and increased mucous production. The patient maintains a patent airway and does not experience breathing difficulties.
- Impaired gas exchange related to bronchospasm. The patient maintains optimal gas exchange as evidenced by normal ABGs and alert responsive mentation or no further reduction in mental status.
- Ineffective breathing pattern related to bronchospasm. The patient's breathing pattern is maintained by eupnea, normal skin color, and regular respiratory rate or pattern.
- Activity intolerance related to hypoxemia and fatigue. The patient maintains activity level within capabilities, as evidenced by normal heart rate and blood pressure during activity, as well as absence of shortness of breath, weakness, and fatigue.
- Anxiety relating to illness, loss of control and nursing and medical interventions. The patient identifies own maladaptive coping behaviors, available resources, and support systems, describes or initiates alternative coping strategies, and describes positive results from new behaviors.

Uncovering the Evidence

Asthma Treatment Program

Discussion: The Harlem Children's Zone Asthma Initiative began in 2001 to screen children ages 12 and under for asthma in one of New York City's poorest neighborhoods. The initiative found that the rates of asthma were appallingly high: about one in four, or 26 percent compared to national rates between 5 and 7 percent according to the CDC. In two years, the initiative's team of nurses, health care providers, community workers, and health educators has screened 1,933 children. They found 580 children found to have asthma and gave them the option of joining an assessment, treatment, and prevention program. A comprehensive baseline assessment of each child includes an evaluation of the family health history, the child's home and external environments, use of medication and health care and emergency services, and school absences. Families learn about the disease and its treatments, and a team member assesses the home environment to help parents identify asthma triggers. Landlords are contacted to fix problems that affect the children's health, such as water leaks, which create mold, or construction, which causes dust and dirt. All families receive PEF meters, mite-proof bedding covers, high efficiency particulate air (HEPA) cleaners for the child's bedroom, HEPA filter vacuum cleaners, and information on asthma. Families are visited every three months by team members.

Implications for Practice: Nurses who work with patients with asthma must teach the patient and family how to improve their environment. Referral to a community or home health agency is often needed.

Source: Roberts, K. (2003). Treating asthma in the zone. American Journal of Nursing, 103(11), 118–119.

CYSTIC FIBROSIS

Cystic fibrosis (CF) is an inherited, autosomal recessive, chronic, progressive, and frequently fatal disease of the body's exocrine mucus-producing glands that primarily affects the respiratory, digestive, and intestinal systems and pancreas in children and young adults. This leads to lung infections, poor digestion, and poor food absorption. The sweat glands and the reproductive system are also usually involved.

Epidemiology

CF is the most common cause of severe chronic lung disease in young adults. It is usually diagnosed in infancy or early childhood, but patients, typically with chronic lung disease, may be diagnosed later in life. Approximately 38 percent of people living with the disease are 18 years of age or older. The median survival age for individuals with CF is 31 years of age, but survival past the age of 76 years has been documented. CF is one of the most common genetic diseases in Caucasians although it affects all races and ethnic groups. It is less common in African Americans, Hispanic (Americans), and Asian (Americans) (Gibson, Burns, & Ramsey, 2003). Individuals with CF must inherit one CF gene from each parent. More than 1,000 genetic mutations have been identified in CF, creating the innumerable variations in the clinical progression seen in this disease (Aronson & Marquis, 2004).

Pathophysiology

The biochemical abnormality in CF results from a mutation in a gene that produces a protein responsible for the movement of chloride and sodium ions through the cell membranes. The protein is called cystic fibrosis transmembrane conductance regulator (CFTR). CFTR is present in cells that line the passageways of the lungs, pancreas, colon, and genitourinary tract. When CFTR is abnormal, two of the hallmarks of CF result: blockage of the movement of chloride ions and water in the lung and other cells and the secretion of abnormal, thick mucus. People with CF lose excessive amounts of salt when they sweat, which can upset the balance of minerals in the blood and may cause abnormal heart rhythms or shock. The thick mucus secreted by CF patients accumulates in the intestines, lungs, pancreas, liver, and reproductive tract. This may result in frequent respiratory infections, lung disease, malnutrition, poor growth, diabetes, infertility, and various other health problems.

Assessment with Clinical Manifestations

Adults with CF may have a variety of pulmonary and nonpulmonary diseases characterized by airflow obstruction. Purulent secretions lead to bronchial plugging, and inflammation causes bronchial wall thickening and over time, airway destruction (Katkin, 2002). These conditions set up an excellent reservoir for continued bronchial infections.

Pulmonary signs of CF include a chronic or recurrent productive cough with sputum production, wheezing, dyspnea, recurrent infections, bronchiectasis, infiltrates, and scarring on CXR. Bronchiectasis is a congenital or acquired disorder of the large bronchi characterized by permanent abnormal dilation and destruction of the bronchial walls. Patients have an increased antero-posterior chest circumference, hyperresonance with percussion, and apical crackles on physical examination.

Other pulmonary conditions seen in the patient with CF include acute and chronic bronchitis, pneumonia, atelectasis, and peribronchial and parenchymal scarring. Pneumothorax and hemoptysis are common. Impaired gas exchange with hypoxemia, hypercapnia, and cor pulmonale occurs in advanced cases. Colonization of the airways with pathogenic bacteria usually occurs early in life.

Nonpulmonary signs of CF include sinusitis, nasal polyps, clubbing, abdominal problems, gassiness, rectal prolapse, liver disease, diabetes, pancreatic insufficiency, recurrent pancreatitis, distal intestinal obstruction syndrome, meconium ileus, steatorrhea, diarrhea, abdominal pain, nutritional deficiencies, biliary cirrhosis, gallstones, failure to thrive, abnormal sweat chloride concentrations, and urogenital abnormalities with infertility. Nearly all men with CF have congenital bilateral absence of the vas deferens with azoospermia. Patients with CF are at increased risk of developing malignancies of the GI tract, osteopenia, and arthropathies. Patients also often complain of decreased exercise tolerance, muscle weakness, recurrent infection, facial sinus tenderness, and purulent nasal discharge.

Diagnostic Tests

A diagnosis of CF is based on the result of a quantitative pilocarpine iontophoresis sweat test, which reveals elevated sodium and chloride levels, along with clinical signs and symptoms consistent with the disease. Repeated sweat chloride and sodium values of greater than 60 mEq/L or mutations in genes known to cause CF are present in most individuals with the disease. ABG studies often reveal hypoxemia and in advanced disease, a chronic, compensated respiratory acidosis. Pulmonary function studies show a mixed obstructive and restrictive pattern with reduced forced vital capacity and air trapping. A CT scan may show lung hyperinflation, pneumothorax, or bronchiectasis. Serum glucose levels may indicate hyperglycemia (Daniels, 2003).

Nursing Diagnoses

Based on the information gathered, examples of nursing diagnoses in the patient with CF may include the following:

- Ineffective airway clearance related to thick, tenacious mucus in airway
- Impaired gas exchange related to airway obstruction
- Nutritional imbalance, less than body requirements, and malabsorption of fats in the intestine, related to absence of pancreatic enzymes
- Deficient knowledge regarding self-care and medication management

Planning and Implementation

Early recognition and comprehensive multidisciplinary therapy improve symptom control of CF and the chances of survival. Referral to a regional CF center is strongly recommended. Conventional treatment programs focus on the following areas: clearance and reduction of lower airway secretions, prevention and treatment of respiratory tract infections, pancreatic enzyme replacement and adequate fluid and dietary intake, psychosocial support including patient and family teaching and genetic, nutritional, and occupational counseling, surgery, and medications.

Daily reduction of lower airway secretions is promoted by postural drainage, chest physical therapy, percussion and vibration techniques, strength and endurance training and exercise, PEEP or flutter valve breathing devices, directed cough, use of suction, active cycle of breathing techniques (ACTB), autogenic drainage, high-frequency chest compression, intrapulmonary percussive ventilator (IPV), and other breathing techniques (Lapin & Lapin, 2003). Note that exercise and breathing techniques promote coughing, which loosens respiratory secretions. These approaches are taught early to patients and their families individually or in pulmonary rehabilitation programs.

Supplemental oxygen is used to treat the progressive hypoxemia that occurs with CF. Oxygen may also help to minimize the pulmonary hypertension associated with chronic hypoxemia. Patients are taught to prevent respiratory tract infections by reducing exposure to crowds harboring possible infections and to people with known infections. The importance of good hand washing technique to prevent infection is stressed to patients and families. Early signs and symptoms of respiratory infection and disease progression are also taught, as well as when to notify a health care provider. Guidelines for infection control include the standard universal precautions and contact, droplet, or airborne precautions as appropriate, with documented or suspected infection with highly transmissible infectious bacteria (e.g., *Burkholderia cepacia* complex, multidrug-resistant *Pseudomonas aeruginosa*, methicillin-resistant *Staphylococcus aureus* [MRSA], or *Mycobacterium tuberculosis* (Saiman & Siegel, 2003). Patients with CF should also be warned to avoid areas undergoing building construction or renovation because of the risk of exposure to high aspergillus levels.

Sources of transmission that have been implicated in hospital outbreaks of CF-related pathogens include contaminated respiratory therapy equipment, multidose vials, home nebulizers, and tap water. All patients with CF who are infected or colonized with *B. cepacia* complex, MRSA, or vancomycin-resistant enterococcus (VRE) should be placed in private rooms (Saiman & Siegel, 2003).

The patient with CF needs to know the possible risks of close contact with other CF patients in nonhospital settings. Behaviors that increase the patient's risk for infection include physical intimacy, assisting with another patient's respiratory treatment, sharing personal items, being in a hot tub or whirlpool together, and sharing poorly ventilated areas, for example, in a bus or airplane.

Nutrition

The nurse needs to teach the patient the importance of pancreatic enzyme replacement and adequate fluid and dietary intake to promote removal of secretions and to ensure adequate nutrition (Box 33-3). Because CF is a lifelong

---

Fast Forward ▶▶▶

Genotyping and Gene Therapy

Genotyping or other diagnostic studies, such as measurement of nasal membrane potential difference, semen analysis, or assessment of pancreatic function, is performed if the patient's sweat test is repeatedly negative, but there is a high clinical suspicion of CF. Standard genotyping is a limited diagnostic tool, because it screens for only a fraction of the known CF mutations. Gene therapy is a promising approach to CF management, and many clinical trials are underway. Screening of family members and genetic counseling are suggested.

Source: National Cancer Institute. (2006). Gene therapy for cancer: Questions and answers. Retrieved August 25, 2006, from www.cancer.gov.

DOLLARS AND SENSE

Inhaled Medications

The cost of taking inhaled medications to treat CF can be high. For example, inhaled recombinant human deoxyribonuclease (rh DNase/Pulmozyme/Dornase alfa) can cost as much as $12,000 annually. This inhalant cleaves to extracellular DNA in sputum. When administered as inhalation (2.5 mg once or twice daily), it leads to improved FEV_1 and reduces the risk of CF-related respiratory exacerbations and the need for IV antibiotics. Pharyngitis, laryngitis, and voice alterations are common side effects (Tierney, et al., 2004).

disorder, patients learn early to modify their daily activities to accommodate their symptoms and treatment modalities.

Pharmacology

Management of the pulmonary component of CF involves anti-infective medications and respiratory therapy. The most prevalent microorganisms causing infections in the airways of patients with CF are *S. aureus* (including methicillin-resistant strains) and a mucoid variant of *P. aeruginosa*. *H. influenzae*, *Stenotrophomonas maltophilia*, and *B. cepacia* are occasionally isolated (Broyles, et al., 2007). Antibiotics are usually given when patients experience an increase in cough, sputum production, or shortness of breath. Antibiotic selection is based on the results of the culture and sensitivity testing of the sputum.

Common antibiotics used for respiratory infection in patients with CF include tobramycin (Nebcin), gentamicin, cefazolin (Ancef or Kefzol), vancomycin (Vancocin), linezolid (Zyvox), ceftazidime (Fortaz), piperacillin (Pipracil), piperacillin-tazobactam (Zosyn), imipenem-cilastatin (Primaxin), aztreonam (Azactam), cephalexin (Keflex), ciprofloxacin (Cipro), amoxicillin (Amoxil), amoxicillin-clavulanate (Augmentin), and TMP/SMX (Septra). Depending on the severity of the respiratory infection, oral or IV antibiotic therapy may be used. Multidrug-resistant bacteria are frequently present in patients with advanced disease who have received multiple courses of antibiotics. Combination antibiotics may be used for their synergistic effects. An alternative route of antibiotic administration is by inhalation of aerosolized antibiotic solution.

Tobramycin (TOBI) is an aerosolized medication and the best-studied antibiotic used to prevent or treat lower respiratory tract infections in patients with CF. The advantage of TOBI is that it is delivered to the actual site of infection, causing less systemic toxicity than the parenteral route. Concerns about aerosolized antibiotics include the potential emergence of drug-resistant organisms, equipment contamination with a drug-resistant organism, and the side effects of medications, such as bronchospasm.

Regular vaccination against pneumococcal infection and an annual influenza vaccination are advised for patients with CF. In addition, important therapies for CF include percussion and postural drainage, which help with the clearance of pulmonary mucus. Inhaled bronchodilators, such as albuterol, using two puffs every four hours as needed, should be considered in patients who demonstrate an increase of at least 12 percent in FEV_1 after inhaled bronchodilator treatment.

Several medications are used to manage CF. First, N-acetylcysteine (Mucomyst), given through nebulizer, may be used to decrease the viscosity of sputum and promote expectoration of secretions. However, there are no well-designed studies to show its benefit in patients with CF. It also has an unpleasant odor and taste. Second, dornase alfa (Pulmozyme) is a recombinant human deoxyribonuclease that has been approved for use in patients with CF. It is a mucolytic enzyme that reduces the viscosity of sputum, alleviates airway obstruction, and improves pulmonary function. It may also lower the incidence of respiratory infections, thus improving quality of life. Third, ibuprofen (Motrin) is an anti-inflammatory agent that may reduce the rate of deterioration in pediatric patients with mild disease. However, there is no proven efficacy to ibuprofen use in older populations. Last, routine use of systemic corticosteroids is not recommended because of the risk of long-term and short-term side effects. However, corticosteroids are often used in late-stage disease or during severe respiratory exacerbations to reduce inflammatory airway edema (Broyles, et al., 2007).

Surgery

Surgical lung transplantation is currently the only definitive treatment for advanced CF. Because there is a long waiting list for lung transplant recipients, many patients die while awaiting a transplant. Because of the chronically

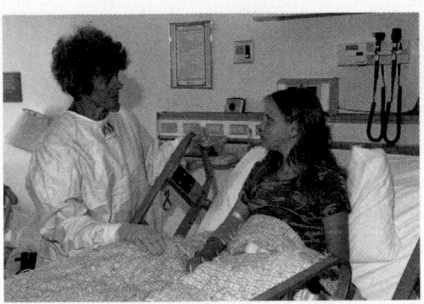

Figure 33-6 Patient education for CF should include the need for adequate nutrition, rest, and ongoing follow-up care.

PATIENT PLAYBOOK

Teaching Elements for the Patient and Family Living with CF

The nurse can instruct these elements to the patient and family with CF:

- Identify the age-specific training for patient and family related to the developmental stage of the patient
- Administer the medications as per order
- Carefully follow the nutritional evaluation and counseling advice
- Participate in strength and endurance training
- Take sodium and chloride replacement when exercising in the heat
- Use the controlled cough technique and postural drainage
- Refer to the CF Foundation and Web site

infected state of the lungs or heart and lung, double lung transplantation is required. A few transplant centers offer living lobar lung transplantation to selected patients. The three-year survival rate following lung transplantation is about 55 percent. A newer surgical procedure is the bilateral sequential transplant of a lower lobe from each of two living donors, who can be related or unrelated to the patient.

Patient and Family Teaching

Patient and family teaching and psychosocial support with genetic and occupational counseling is needed as CF progresses (Figure 33-6). Genetic counseling is offered to adults with a positive family history of CF and to partners of people with CF planning a pregnancy or seeking prenatal testing. Assessment of the home environment will identify modifications required to address changes in the patient's needs, increasing dyspnea, fatigue, and other nonpulmonary symptoms. For the patient whose disease is progressing and who is developing increasing hypoxemia, preferences for end-of-life care should be discussed. Patients and family members who need personal support as they plan for the future may be referred to the CF Foundation support groups at www.cff.org.

Evaluation of Outcomes

Potential patient outcomes for each of the example nursing diagnoses for the patient with CF are:

- Ineffective airway clearance related to thick, tenacious mucus in airway. The patient maintains a patent airway and does not experience breathing difficulties.
- Impaired gas exchange related to airway obstruction. The patient maintains optimal gas exchange as evidenced by normal ABGs and alert responsive mentation or no further reduction in mental status.
- Nutritional imbalance, less than body requirements, and malabsorption of fats in the intestine, related to absence of pancreatic enzymes. The patient verbalizes and demonstrates selection of foods or meals that will achieve a cessation of weight loss and weighs within 10 percent of ideal body weight.
- Deficient knowledge regarding self-care and medication management. The patient should demonstrate motivation to learn, identify perceived learning needs, and verbalize an understanding of desired content.

KEY CONCEPTS

- COPD is characterized by progressive airflow limitation that is not fully reversible. The airflow limitation is associated with an abnormal inflammatory response of the lungs to noxious particles or gases.
- Risk factors for COPD include a deficiency of alpha$_1$-antitrypsin enzyme, exposure to cigarette smoke, or other occupational or environmental air pollutants, and recurrent lung infections.

- Patients with COPD are often referred to a multidisciplinary pulmonary rehabilitation program to optimize their functional status.
- Surgical treatments for COPD include LVRS, bullectomy, and a single or double lung transplant.
- Asthma is a chronic inflammatory disorder of the airways.

Continued

KEY CONCEPTS—cont'd

- Diagnose asthma with history and physical, pulmonary function tests, and CXR.
- Keep airway support equipment accessible.
- Support and teach patient and family, as progressive dyspnea leads to increased anxiety and panic and aggravates a breathing problem.
- CF is a chronic, progressive, and frequently fatal autosomal recessive disease that primarily affects the respiratory and digestive systems and pancreas.
- Conventional treatment programs for CF focus on the following areas: clearance and reduction of

lower airway secretions, prevention and treatment of respiratory tract infections, pulmonary rehabilitation programs, pancreatic enzyme replacement, adequate fluid and dietary intake, psychosocial support, genetic and occupational counseling, and surgery.

- Early recognition of CF and comprehensive multidisciplinary therapy improve symptom control and the chances of survival.
- Referral of patients and their families to a regional CF center and the CF Foundation is strongly recommended.

REVIEW QUESTIONS

1. A patient with COPD who weighs 143 pounds is to receive 30 mg/kg of methylprednisolone (Medrol) IV. What is the correct dose in milligrams that the patient should receive?

2. The nurse is awaiting the arrival of a patient from the ED who is being admitted with COPD with cor pulmonale. In caring for this patient, the nurse should be alert to which of the following signs and symptoms of right-sided heart failure (select all that apply)?
   1. Jugular venous distension
   2. Hepatomegaly
   3. Dyspnea
   4. Crackles
   5. Tachycardia

3. Low-flow oxygen therapy is prescribed for your patient with COPD. What is the most essential action for the nurse to initiate?
   1. Anticipate the need for humidification
   2. Notify the practitioner that this order is contraindicated
   3. Place the patient in high-Fowler's position
   4. Schedule nursing care to allow frequent observations of the patient

4. Theophylline tablets are prescribed for a patient with COPD. A nurse instructs the patient about the medication. Which of the following nursing statements would not be a component of the teaching plan?
   1. Take the medication in an empty stomach
   2. Take the medication with food
   3. Continue to take the medication even if you are feeling better
   4. Periodic blood levels will need to be obtained

5. A nurse instructs a patient to use pursed-lip breathing. The patient asks the nurse about the purpose of this type of breathing. The nurse responds, knowing that the primary purpose of pursed-lip breathing is to:
   1. Promote oxygen intake
   2. Strengthen the diaphragm
   3. Strengthen the intercostal muscles
   4. Promote carbon dioxide elimination

6. A nurse is teaching a patient about the use of a respiratory inhaler. Which of the following would not be a component of the teaching plan?
   1. Remove the cap and shake the inhaler
   2. Press the canister down with your finger as you breathe in
   3. Inhale the mist and quickly exhale
   4. Wait one minute between puffs if more than one puff is prescribed

7. Which of the following is true of the pathophysiology of asthma?
   1. Asthma occurs in three phases: the early phase, the intermediate phase, and the late phase.
   2. The late phase begins within one to two days of exposure to the trigger and may last for up to approximately a week.
   3. The development of an IgE is a strong predisposing factor for developing asthma.
   4. Step 1 is the most severe classification category of acute asthma.

8. A patient with asthma is treated for acute exacerbation in the ED. A nurse reports which of the following, knowing that it is not an indication that the condition is improving?

Continued

REVIEW QUESTIONS—cont'd

1. Increased wheezing
2. Decreased wheezing
3. Warm, dry skin
4. A pulse rate of 80 beats per minute

9. A sweat test is performed on a child with a suspected diagnosis of CF. The nurse reviews the test results and determines that which of the following is a positive test result for CF?
   1. Chloride level of 20 mEq/L
   2. Chloride level of 30 mEq/L
   3. Chloride level of 40 mEq/L
   4. Chloride level of 70 mEq/L

10. Which of the following is true concerning CF?
    1. Tobramycin (TOBI) is an aerosolized medication and the best antibiotic used to treat lower respiratory tract infections in patients with CF.
    2. There are no regular vaccinations against pneumococcal infection associated with prevention for patients with CF.
    3. Patients with CF do not typically develop cancer disorders as a result of their respiratory disorder.
    4. Surgical lung transplantation is not currently a definitive treatment for advanced CF.

REVIEW ACTIVITIES

1. Identify what you would teach a patient with COPD who is worried about starting pulmonary rehabilitation. What can you tell the patient about the program to reduce his or her fears? What kind of classes and exercises can the patient expect to do? How can you measure outcomes?

2. Identify a pulmonary rehabilitation unit in your clinical agency. Answer the following questions: What types of patients are receiving care? Talk with a patient on the unit. How long has the patient been coming to the program? Has the patient noticed any improvement? How does the program measure patient improvement and outcomes?

3. Talk to a family of a patient with CF. Visit the Web site of the CF Foundation identified in Suggested Readings and Web Resources. Is there any information on this site that would be helpful for patient or families with CF?

4. Observe a patient with asthma on a patient care unit. Assess the management of the patient and evaluate the patient responses to the various strategies for care.

5. Arrange to make rounds with a respiratory therapist. Observe the kinds of treatments received by patients with COPD, asthma, and CF.

6. Go to the CF Foundation at http://www.cff.org. Explore the site, including the link to CF chapters and care centers and summarize the findings.

Visit the Contemporary Medical-Surgical Nursing online companion resource at www.delmarhealthcare.com for additional content and study aids. Click on Online Companions then select the Nursing discipline.

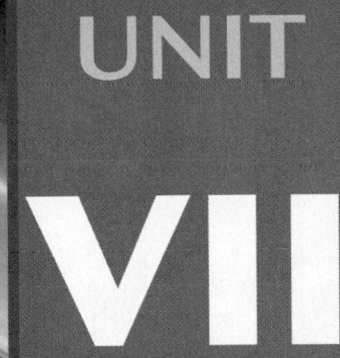

UNIT VII

Alterations in Neurological Function

Assessment of Neurological Function

Doris Denison, MSN, APRN, BC, CCRN

CHAPTER TOPICS

- Nervous System Cells
- Central Nervous System
- Peripheral Nervous System
- Autonomic Nervous System
- Neurological Assessment
- Neurodiagnostic Studies

The nervous system is a complex network of cells, tissues, and specialized organs. It is the center of thinking, judgment, memory, cognition, communication, behavior, emotion, sensation, and movement. There is both direct and indirect control of the body systems. For example, a stroke in the frontal lobe affecting the motor strip may result in seizures and loss of limb movement. The assessment of the nervous system is extremely important for the nurse to apply in the care of the patient in a wide variety of settings.

ANATOMY AND PHYSIOLOGY

The nervous system has two major divisions: the central nervous system (CNS), which consists of the brain and spinal cord, and the peripheral nervous system (PNS), which consists of the cranial nerves, the spinal nerves, and the autonomic nervous system (ANS). The entire nervous system is made up of two types of cells: neurons, which transmit or conduct nerve impulses, and neuroglial cells, which support the neurons.

Nervous System Cells

Neurons are the basic functional unit of the nervous system. They are specialized to gather, integrate, and respond to information from both the internal and external environment. Specialized cells called neuroglia support the neurons. The neuroglia have many functions: axonal insulation, removal of debris and dead cells, assisting with the circulation of cerebrospinal fluid (CSF), and they are a component of the blood-brain barrier.

Neurons

Each neuron consists of dendrites, a cell body, and an axon. The function of the neurons is to transmit impulses. Dendrites are short projections from the cell body that conduct impulses toward the cell body via afferent processes. Dendrites have varying numbers of branches, and each branch synapses with another cell body, axon, or dendrite. The cell body contains the nucleus and cytoplasm. It is the metabolic focal point of the neuron. Most of the cell bodies are found within the CNS. They are clustered together in ganglia or nuclei.

The axon is a long projection that conducts impulses away from the cell body via efferent processes. Axonal length varies from several micrometers to more than a meter, often branching near the end of the projection. The enlarged, distal end of each axon is called the synaptic, or terminal, knob. The synaptic knobs contain the mechanisms for manufacturing, storing, and releasing neurotransmitter substances. Each neuron produces one specific transmitter, capable of either enhancing or inhibiting the impulse.

Many axons, although not all, are covered with a myelin sheath, which is a white lipid substance. Myelinated axons are called white matter. Nonmyelinated axons are called gray matter. The myelin sheath is interrupted at intervals by the nodes of Ranvier. The nodes of Ranvier allow movement of ions between the axon and the extracellular fluid.

Characteristics of neurons include: excitability, conductivity, and the ability to influence other cells. Excitability is the ability to generate a nerve impulse. Conductivity is the ability to transmit impulses to other portions of the cell. Transmission of nerve impulses to other neurons, muscle cells, and glandular cells stimulate changes (Jenner & Olanow, 2006).

Nerve Impulses

The initiation of a nerve impulse involves the generation of an action potential. After the impulse is started, it travels along the axon as a series of action potentials. At the end of the nerve fiber, the impulse is transmitted across the synapse junction between the nerve cells by chemical mechanisms involving neurotransmitters. The nerve impulse moves from axon to axon until it reaches its destination.

Synapses

A synapse is the point where a nerve impulse is transmitted from neuron to neuron, neuron to muscle, or neuron to glandular tissue. The three components needed for transmission are a presynaptic terminal, a synaptic cleft, and a receptor site on the postsynaptic cell. When the nerve impulse reaches the presynaptic terminal, a neurotransmitter is released from tiny storage vesicles.

The neurotransmitter then crosses the synaptic cleft and attaches to receptor sites of the postsynaptic neuron. This alters the membrane permeability and causes a change in the electrical potential of the membrane.

Neurotransmitters

In the CNS, neurotransmitters are chemical substances that inhibit, excite, or modify the responses of another cell. In general, each neuron releases the same transmitter at all of its terminals. Over 30 neurotransmitters have been identified. The general chemical classes are amines (e.g., acetylcholine and serotonin), catecholamines (i.e., dopamine, epinephrine, and norepinephrine), amino acids (e.g., gamma aminobutyric acid [GABA], glutamic acid, glycine, and substance P), and polypeptides (e.g., endorphins and enkephalins). Table 34-1 summarizes the source and actions of the major neurotransmitters.

Neuroglia Cells

The second type of cells in the nervous system are neuroglia. They support the neurons by providing protection, structural support, and nutrition. In the CNS, there are four types of neuroglia: astrocytes, oligodendroglia, ependymal cells, and microglia. Clinically, astrocyte functions include: provision of nutrients, regulating synaptic connectivity, removal of cellular waste products, and control of molecular movement from blood to brain. Oligodendrocytes produce the myelin sheath that protects the neuron. Ependymal cells are found

TABLE 34-1 Neurotransmitters: Site and Action

TRANSMITTER	SITE	ACTION
Amines		
Acetylcholine	Brain, brainstem, basal ganglia, and autonomic nervous system	Usually excitatory Some inhibitory effects of parasympathetic nervous system (e.g., heart by vagus)
Serotonin	Medical brainstem, hypothalamus, and dorsal horn of spinal cord	Inhibits pain pathway of spinal cord Helps control mood and sleep
Catecholamines		
Dopamine	Substantia nigra to basal ganglia	Usually inhibitory
Norepinephrine	Brainstem, hypothalamus, and sympathetic nervous system	Usually excitatory, sometimes inhibitory Some excitatory, some inhibitory
Amino Acids		
Aspartate	Brain and spinal cord	Excitatory
Gamma aminobutyric acid (GABA)	Brain, basal ganglia, cerebellum, and spinal cord	Some excitatory; some inhibitory
Glutamic acid	Sensory pathways	Excitatory
Glycine	Spinal cord	Inhibitory
Substance P	Pain fibers of dorsal horns of spinal cord and hypothalamus	Excitatory
Polypeptides		
Endorphins	Pituitary gland, thalamus, spinal cord, and hypothalamus	Excitatory to systems that inhibit pain
Enkephalins	Spinal cord, brainstem, thalamus, and hypothalamus	Excitatory to systems that inhibit pain

Adapted from Scott, A., & Fong, E. (2004). Body structures and functions *(10th ed.). Clifton Park, NY: Thomson Delmar Learning.*

in the lining of the ventricular system, aid in the production of CSF, and act as a barrier to foreign substances. Microglia play a scavenger role by responding to infection or trauma to the CNS

Central Nervous System

The CNS has two major divisions: the brain and spinal cord. The brain is composed of the cerebrum, the brainstem, and the cerebellum. The spinal cord is the conduit for the ascending sensory and descending motor neurons. This is the pathway for two-way communication between the brain and the periphery. In addition, the spinal cord is the center for reflex action.

Bones

The bones of the skull and the vertebral column prevent injury to the brain and the spinal cord. The scalp moves freely and cushions the head from traumatic injury. The skull is the bony, rigid framework of the head. It is composed of the 14 bones of the face and the 8 bones of the cranium (Figure 34-1). Where the bones of the skull join, suture lines form. The four major suture lines are: sagittal, coronal, lambdoidal, and basilar.

The vertebral column is a flexible, stacked series of bones that support the head and trunk. There are 33 vertebrae: 7 cervical, 12 thoracic, 5 lumbar, 5 sacral fused into one, and 4 coccygeal fused into one (Figure 34-2).

Meninges

The brain and spinal cord are covered with a series of membranes called the meninges. These include: the dura mater, the arachnoid, and the pia mater. The dura mater is the tough, fibrous, outer layer, which lines the skull and vertebrae. The arachnoid is a thin, delicate middle membrane, where CSF is cir-

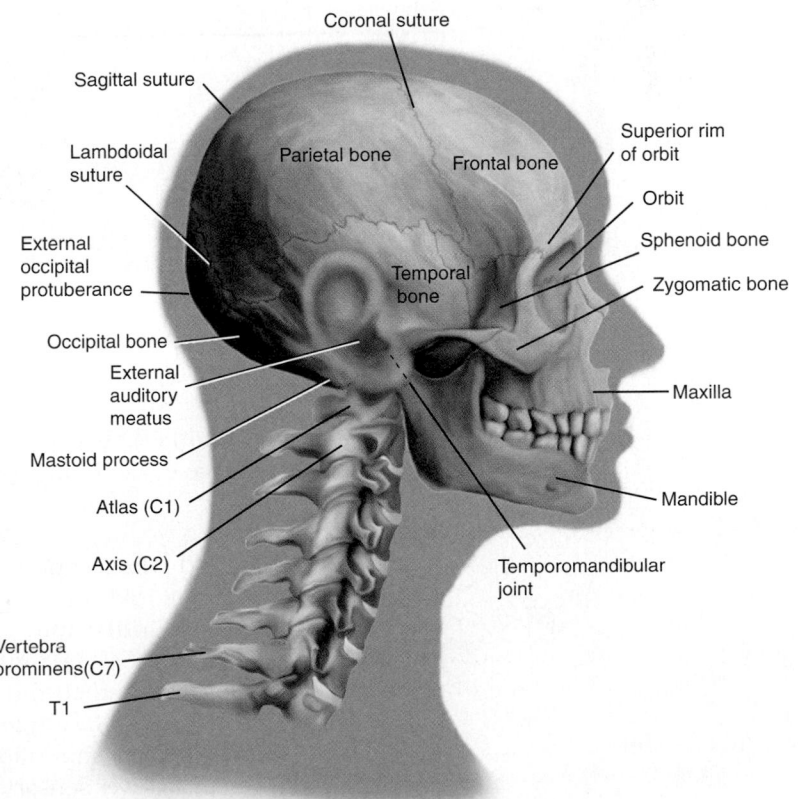

Figure 34-1 Bones of the face and skull (lateral view).

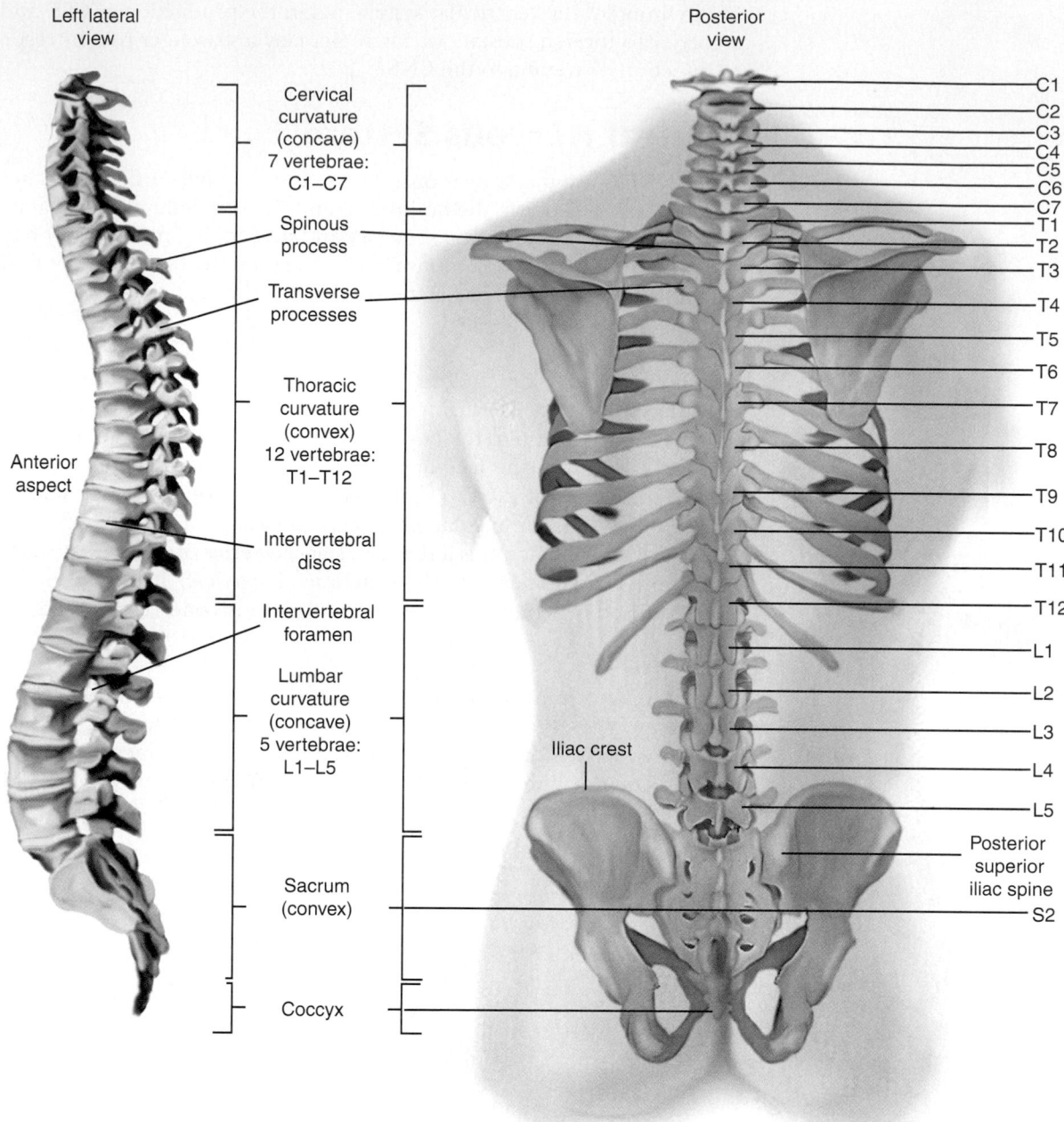

Left lateral
view

Posterior
view

Cervical
curvature
(concave)
7 vertebrae:
C1–C7

Spinous
process

Transverse
processes

Thoracic
curvature
(convex)
12 vertebrae:
T1–T12

Anterior
aspect

Intervertebral
discs

Intervertebral
foramen

Lumbar
curvature
(concave)
5 vertebrae:
L1–L5

Iliac crest

Sacrum
(convex)

Posterior
superior
iliac spine

Coccyx

C1
C2
C3
C4
C5
C6
C7
T1
T2
T3
T4
T5
T6
T7
T8
T9
T10
T11
T12
L1
L2
L3
L4
L5
S2

Figure 34-2 Bones of the spine.

culated and absorbed. The pia mater is the thin, vascular inner layer that covers the surface of the brain and spinal cord (Figure 34-3).

Brain

The cerebrum is the largest part of the brain. The surface of the cerebrum is covered by multiple folds or wrinkles, called gyri, which greatly increases the surface area. It is divided into two hemispheres, right and left, by a deep groove. Each hemisphere has an outer layer of neurons called the white matter and an inner layer called the gray matter. These two hemispheres of the cerebrum are connected by a thick band of white fibers called the corpus callosum. The corpus callosum allows the two hemispheres to communicate. Each hemisphere receives sensory and motor impulses from the opposite side of the body. The majority of people are left brain dominant. The left side controls language, while the right side controls perception (Figure 34-4).

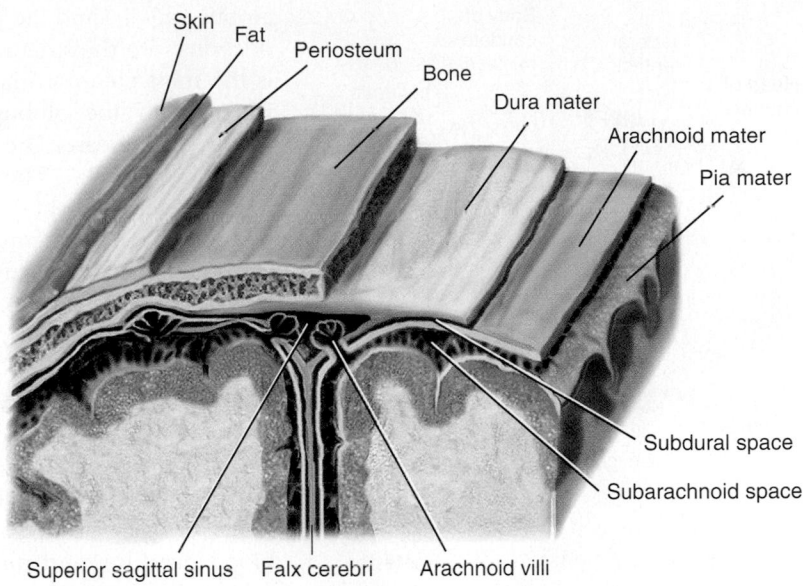

Figure 34-3 The meninges.

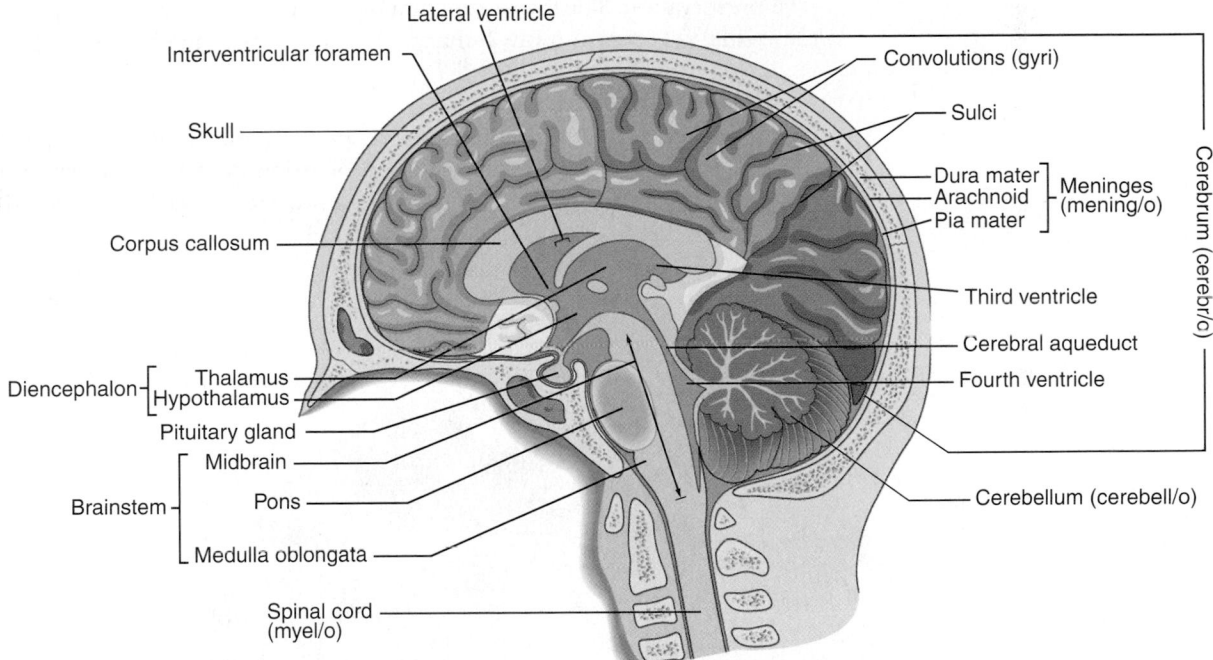

Figure 34-4 Cross-section of the brain.

Ventricles

There are four ventricles (or chambers) within the brain. These include: two lateral ventricles located within each hemisphere, the third ventricle and the fourth ventricle. The chambers are filled with CSF and are linked by ducts (also called foramen), which permit circulation. CSF is a clear, colorless fluid produced by the choroid plexus, located in the ventricles. It circulates through a closed system, which includes the four ventricles and area around the spinal cord. Reabsorption occurs via the arachnoid villi.

Basal Ganglia

The basal ganglia are found deep within the cerebral hemispheres. They consist of several collections of nuclei: the lenticular nucleus, the caudate nucleus, the amygdaloid body, and the claustrum. The lenticular nucleus is composed of the

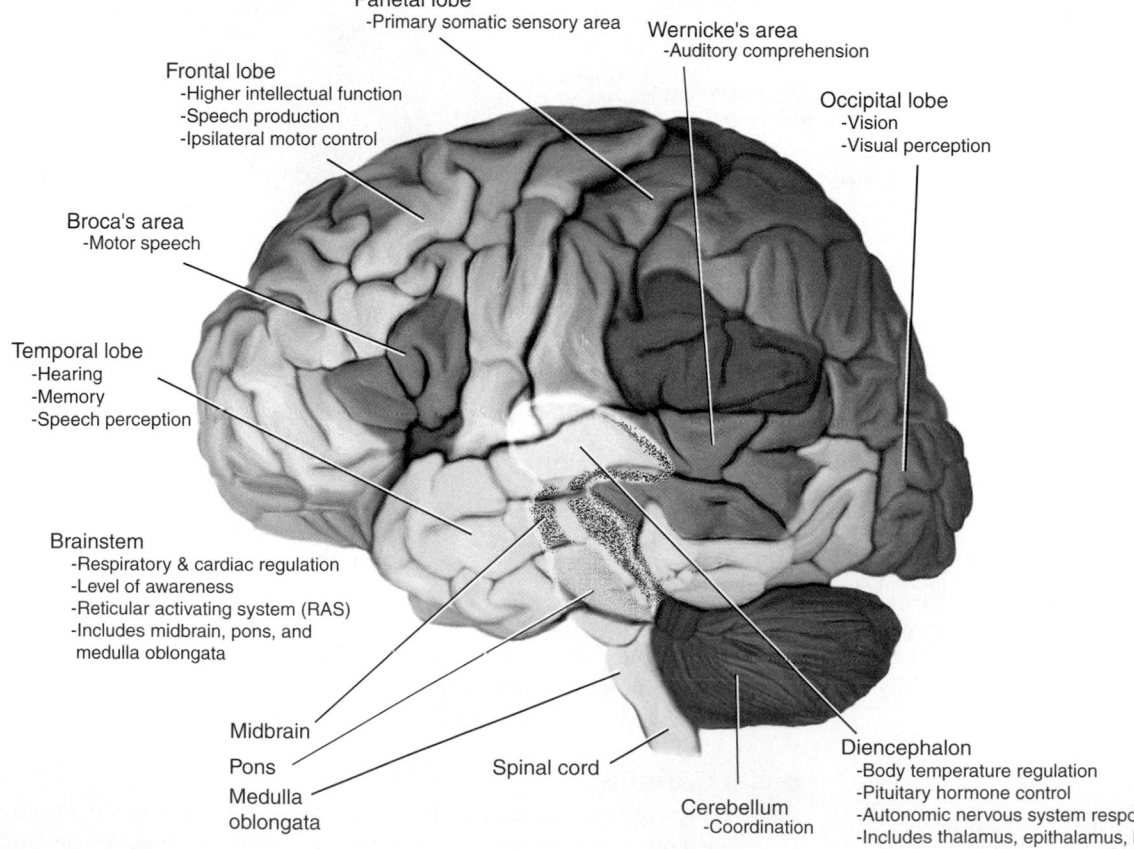

Head of caudate nucleus
Lateral ventricle
Body of caudate nucleus
Thalamus
Frontal lobe of cerebrum
Occipital lobe of cerebrum
Lenticular nucleus
Amygdaloid body
Tail of caudate nucleus
Anterior
Posterior

Figure 34-5 Basal ganglia.

globus pallidus and the putamen. The globus pallidus has extensive connections with the striatum, thalamus, and mesencephalon. The putamen is the most common site for intracerebral hemorrhage. Loss of cellular function in the globus pallidus and putamen is a component of Parkinson's disease. The amygdaloid body is an almond-shaped area near the temporal lobe. The claustrum is the barrier between the gray and white matter of the brain. The caudate nucleus is involved the origination of repetitive movements. The basal ganglia coordinate communication between the cerebral cortex and the cerebellum that controls motor activity (Figure 34-5). Lesions of the basal ganglia produce abnormal movements, including chorea, athetosis, hemiballismus, and dystonic posturing.

Lobes

The lobes of the cerebral hemispheres are: frontal, parietal, temporal, and occipital. Major functions of the frontal lobe include: high-level cognitive activities, information storage or memory, voluntary eye movement, basal motor control of breathing, gastrointestinal (GI) function, blood pressure, and motor control of speech in the dominant hemisphere. The parietal lobe is the primary sensory interpretation area. The temporal lobe is the primary auditory reception and interpretation area. Limbic area is part of the temporal lobe and is involved in emotional behavior and self-preservation. The major function of the occipital lobe is visual perception, some visual reflexes, and involuntary smooth eye movements (Figure 34-6).

Diencephalon

The diencephalon is composed of the thalamus, epithalamus, and hypothalamus. The thalamus is the initial processing area for sensory input. The epithalamus forms the roof of the third ventricle and the pineal gland. The hypo-

Parietal lobe
-Primary somatic sensory area
Wernicke's area
-Auditory comprehension
Frontal lobe
-Higher intellectual function
-Speech production
-Ipsilateral motor control
Occipital lobe
-Vision
-Visual perception
Broca's area
-Motor speech
Temporal lobe
-Hearing
-Memory
-Speech perception
Brainstem
-Respiratory & cardiac regulation
-Level of awareness
-Reticular activating system (RAS)
-Includes midbrain, pons, and medulla oblongata
Midbrain
Pons
Medulla oblongata
Spinal cord
Cerebellum
-Coordination
Diencephalon
-Body temperature regulation
-Pituitary hormone control
-Autonomic nervous system responses
-Includes thalamus, epithalamus, hypothalamus

Figure 34-6 The lobes of the brain.

thalamus regulates temperature, appetite, water metabolism, emotional expression, thirst, and a portion of the sleep-wake cycle.

Hypophysis

The hypophysis (pituitary gland) is connected to the hypothalamus by the hypophyseal stalk. There are two lobes, each releasing specific hormones into the systemic circulation. It is controlled by information processed by the hypothalamus. The function of the pituitary gland is discussed in depth in chapter 55.

Brainstem

The brainstem includes the midbrain, pons, and medulla. The midbrain is the center for auditory and visual reflexes. The pons controls respiration. The medulla plays a role in the control of heart rate, blood pressure, respirations, and swallowing.

Cerebellum

The cerebellum is located behind the brainstem and under the occipital lobe of the cerebrum. Functions of the cerebellum include: coordinate voluntary muscle movement, equilibrium, and maintenance of trunk stability. The cerebellum influences motor activity via its axonal connections to the motor cortex, brainstem nuclei, and descending pathways. Sensory information from the cerebral cortex, muscles, joints, and inner ear are used to refine the motor responses.

Cerebral Circulation

The source of blood to the brain occurs via the internal carotid arteries (anterior circulation) and the vertebral and basilar arteries (posterior circulation). These arteries join at the base of the brain to form the circle of Willis (cerebral arterial circle). The two anterior cerebral arteries (ACA) supply the medial portion on the frontal lobes. Two middle cerebral arteries (MCA) supply the outer portions of the frontal, parietal, and superior temporal lobes. The two posterior inferior cerebral arteries (PICA) supply the medial portions of the occipital and inferior temporal lobes. Venous blood drains from the brain via the dural sinuses that drain into the two jugular veins. Knowledge of the major arteries of the brain and the areas supplied is necessary for understanding and evaluating the signs and symptoms of brain tumors, cerebral vascular disease, and trauma. Cerebral aneurysms often occur at bifurcation points along the circle of Willis (Figure 34-7).

Blood-Brain Barrier

The blood-brain barrier maintains a functionally stable environment for the CNS. The barrier is composed of a network of endothelial cells surrounding specialized brain capillaries. This prevents the free movement of material from the bloodstream into the brain and protects the brain from toxic substances that may be circulating in the blood. While protecting the brain, it impairs the effectiveness of many drugs used to treat nervous system problems. For instance, dopamine must be administered in an inactive form (levodopa) and then converted to its active form before it can treat the tremor and rigidity of Parkinson's.

Spine

The spine is a flexible column formed by series of bones called vertebrae. The vertebrae serve multiple functions: protection the spinal cord, support the head, and provide spinal flexibility. Each vertebra consists of a body, arch, and foramen. The body is the anterior portion and contains a central foramen. The stacked vertebral foramina form the canal through which the spinal cord passes. The arch is the posterior segment and consists of two pedicles and two laminae, which support seven

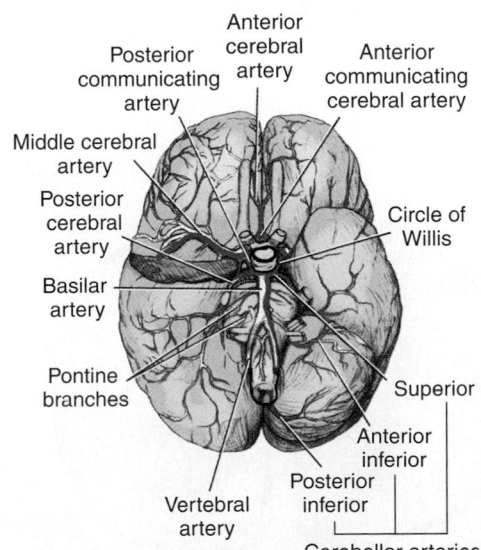

Figure 34-7 Circle of Willis.

processes. The pedicles form intervertebral notches through which the spinal nerves emerge. Processes provide spinal stability and points for attachment of muscles and ligaments.

The intervertebral discs are fibrocartilaginous structures located between the vertebral bodies. They vary is shape, thickness, and size at different levels of the spine. The function of these discs is to cushion movement. Aging, trauma, and poor posture are the most frequent causes of injury to the intervertebral discs.

Spinal Cord

The spinal cord extends from the medulla to the level of the first lumbar vertebrae. It exits the cranial cavity through the foramen magnum. A cross-section of the spinal cord reveals gray matter in an H pattern in the central portion (Figure 34-8). It is surrounded by white matter. The gray matter contains the cell bodies of the voluntary motor neurons, the preganglionic autonomic motor neurons, and interneurons. The white matter contains the axons ascending sensory and descending motor fibers. The myelin surrounding these fibers gives them their white appearance.

The ascending sensory tracts carry specific sensory information to the higher levels of the CNS. The information comes from specialized sensory receptors in the skin, muscles, joints, viscera, and blood vessels. Descending motor tracts carry impulses from the higher levels to the lower motor neurons. The lower motor neurons are the final step of the nerve impulse before stimulation of skeletal muscle. Upper motor neurons are located in the brainstem and cerebral cores and also influence skeletal muscle movement. Damage to the upper motor neurons, sometimes seen in multiple sclerosis (MS), may cause weakness, atrophy, hyperreflexia, or spasticity.

Spinal Cord Circulation

Circulation to the spinal cord comes from three sources: anterior spinal, two posterior spinal, and branches of the descending aorta. The anterior spinal artery comes from the vertebral arteries. The posterior inferior cerebellar or the vertebral arteries are the source of the two posterior spinal arteries. Venous return occurs via both intradural and extradural routes.

Peripheral Nervous System

The preceding part of the chapter discussed the CNS. The nervous system though has two parts. The second part is the PNS. The PNS is composed of the spinal nerves, cranial nerves, and the ANS.

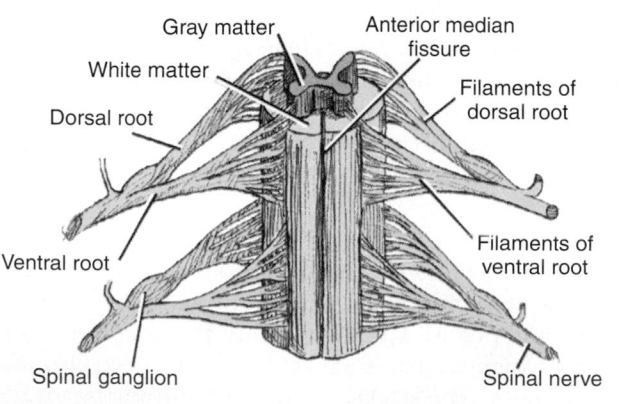

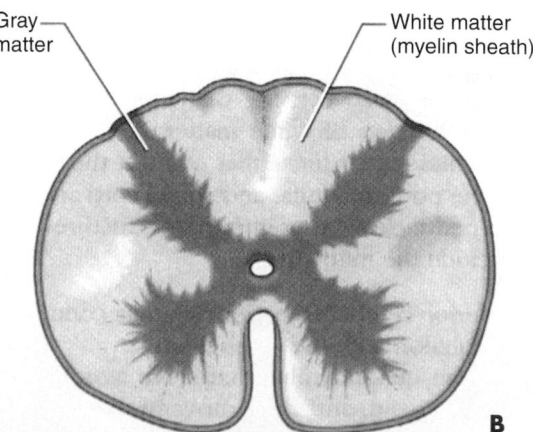

A   **B**

Figure 34-8 Spinal cord: A. Anterior view, B. Cross-section view—white and gray matter.

Spinal Nerves

The spinal nerves consist of 31 pairs exiting from the spinal cord. They include: 8 cervical, 12 thoracic, 5 lumbar, 5 sacral, and 1 coccygeal. Each spinal nerve has both a sensory and a motor component for a specific area of the body. The cervical and thoracic spinal nerves are near the areas they cover. The lumbar and sacral areas are farther away. The specific area for each spinal nerve is represented by a dermatome. For example, the patient with a lesion at L4 and L5 may complain of pain, numbness, or tingling of one or both lower legs, below the knee, including the great toes. When the discomfort is worse on the medial aspects of the legs, the lesion is at L4.

Sensory Receptors

Sensory input is collected throughout the body by receptors of pain, temperature, touch, vibration, pressure, visceral sensation, and proprioception. This information is transmitted to the cortex, along with input from the special senses: vision, taste, smell, and hearing.

Cranial Nerves

The cranial nerves provide both motor and sensory innervation for the head, neck, and viscera. Anatomically they begin in and emerge from the cranium (Figure 34-9). They are called cranial nerves as opposed to spinal nerves, which emerge from the spinal column. Individual nerves may be pure motor, pure sensory, or mixed. Two nerves, oculomotor (CN III) and vagus (CN X), include parasympathetic components. See Table 34-2 for specifics.

Autonomic Nervous System

The ANS has two, semi-independent components: sympathetic and parasympathetic. The two components function together to maintain homeostasis of the body's internal environment. The ANS is responsible for maintaining and regulating glandular function and the smooth muscles. The ANS also coordinates the functioning of the visceral organs. The sympathetic nervous system is responsible for initialing the protective mechanism, called the fight-or-flight response, whenever the body is exposed to stress. The parasympathetic system transmits impulses to the visceral organs and is responsible for those functions that are not under conscious control, called rest and repair or "general housekeeping." Table 34-3 lists the specific systemic responses of the sympathetic and parasympathetic systems to autonomic stimulation for each of the body systems.

Spinal Reflexes

A reflex is a response to a stimulus that occurs without conscious control. One way to classify reflexes is: stretch, cutaneous, and pathological. Muscle stretch reflexes are also called deep tendon reflexes (DTRs). Common DTRs are biceps, triceps, patellar, Achilles, and brachioradialis. Cutaneous reflexes are termed superficial reflexes. Superficial reflexes occur when noxious stimulation is applied to the skin. The response is withdrawal from the irritant. An example is contraction of the abdominal muscles when the skin is stroked. Pathological reflexes should not be present in healthy adults. Presence of a pathological reflex indicates interference with the normal CNS function. The upward movement of the great toe with flaring of the pedal digits is an example of a pathological reflex (Crimlisk & Grande, 2004).

The sensory input may come from muscles, tendons, skin, organs, and the special senses. Sensory information from the specific peripheral location is responsible for the motor impulses that return to the same peripheral location. This is called a reflex arc.

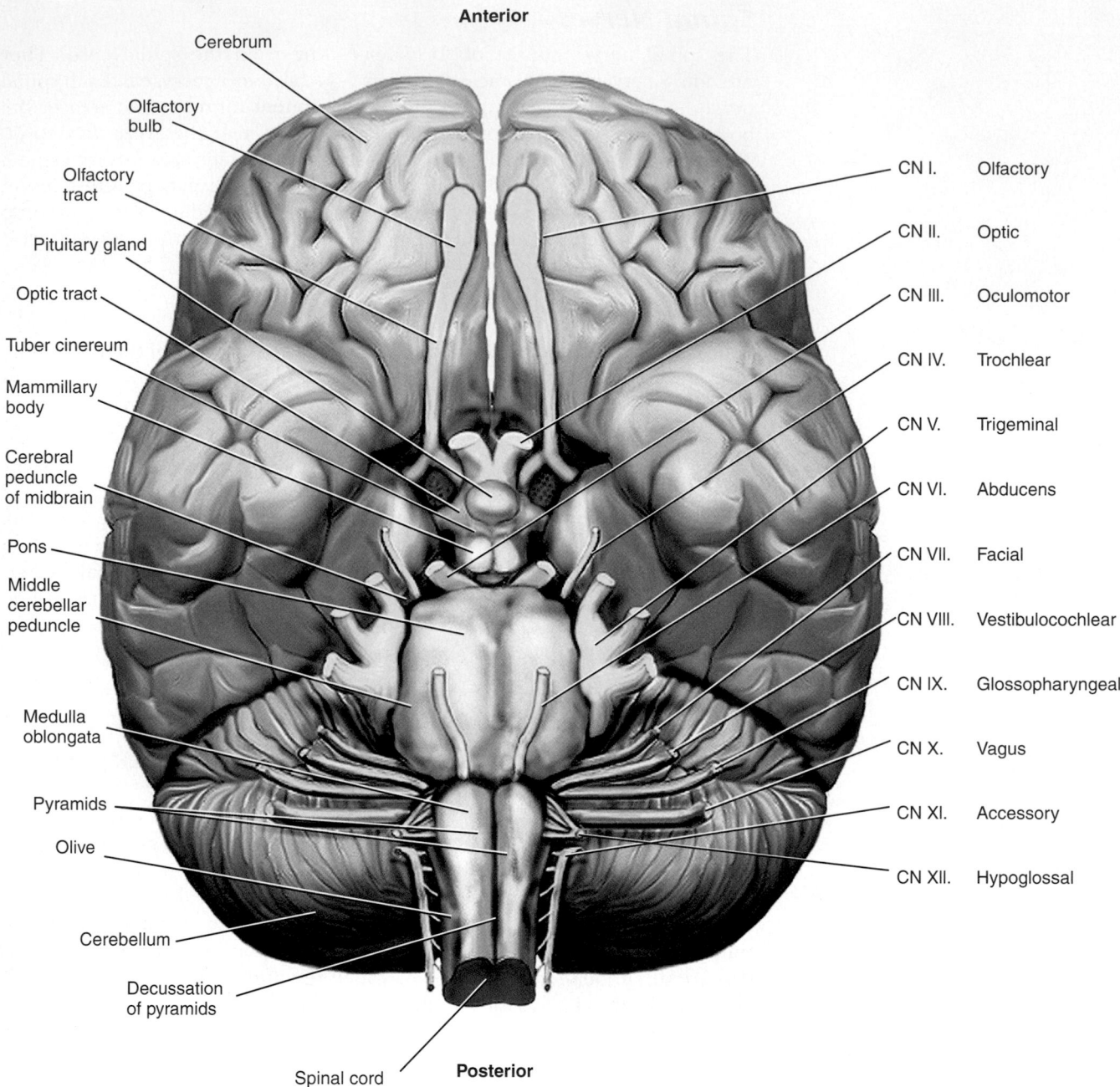

Anterior

Cerebrum

Olfactory bulb

Olfactory tract

Pituitary gland

Optic tract

Tuber cinereum

Mammillary body

Cerebral peduncle of midbrain

Pons

Middle cerebellar peduncle

Medulla oblongata

Pyramids

Olive

Cerebellum

Decussation of pyramids

Spinal cord

Posterior

CN I.   Olfactory

CN II.   Optic

CN III.   Oculomotor

CN IV.   Trochlear

CN V.   Trigeminal

CN VI.   Abducens

CN VII.   Facial

CN VIII.   Vestibulocochlear

CN IX.   Glossopharyngeal

CN X.   Vagus

CN XI.   Accessory

CN XII.   Hypoglossal

Figure 34-9 Cranial nerves and related structures.

Age-Related Changes

As the human body ages, patients begin to experience both motor and sensory changes. Chronic diseases of the bones, muscles, or joints can have a detrimental effect on the nerves motor function. With aging there is a decrease in both muscle bulk and nerve electrical activity. This causes diminished muscle strength and a decrease in reactions and movement time. Sensory function is diminished due to a decrease in total sensory receptors, decrease in electrical activity, and atrophy or degeneration of the taste buds, olfactory bulb, and vestibular system of the inner ear. Reflexes may diminish because of degeneration of the myelin sheath. Cognitive function continues at the same level as in younger years, unless disease impairs the brain. For example, arteriosclerosis and hypertension may lead to a cerebrovascular accident (CVA) that causes brain damage.

TABLE 34-2 Cranial Nerves

NERVE	FUNCTION
I. Olfactory	Sensory: Smell
II. Optic	Sensory: Sight
III. Oculomotor	Motor: Eye movements; contraction of iris
	Parasympathetic: Smooth muscles of eye socket
IV. Trochlear	Motor: Eye movement
V. Trigeminal	
Ophthalmic branch	Sensory: Forehead, eye, and superior nasal cavity
Maxillary	Sensory: Inferior nasal cavity, face, upper teeth, and superior mucosa of mouth
Mandibular	Sensory: Jaw surface, lower teeth, anterior tongue, and inferior mucosa of mouth
	Motor: Muscles for chewing
VI. Abducens	Sensory: Eye movement
VII. Facial	Motor: Muscles of expression, cheek muscle
	Sensory: Taste of anterior two thirds of tongue
VIII. Vestibulocochlear	
Vestibular	Sensory: Balance
Cochlear	Sensory: Hearing
IX. Glossopharyngeal	Sensory: Pharynx and posterior tongue (including taste)
	Motor: Superior pharyngeal muscles, swallowing
X. Vagus	Sensory: Viscera of chest and abdomen
	Motor: Larynx, middle and inferior pharyngeal muscles
	Parasympathetic: Heart, lungs, most of GI tract
XI. Accessory	Motor: Movement of neck muscles
XII. Hypoglossal	Motor: Movement of tongue

Adapted from Scott, A., & Fong, E. (2004). Body structures and functions (10th ed.). Clifton Park, NY: Thomson Delmar Learning.

ASSESSMENT

Knowledge of the anatomy and physiology discussed in the previous section helps the nurse with interpretation of his or her assessment findings. Assessment of the neurological system begins with the history. This interview collects subjective data. The second portion is the physical examination of the neurological system, which collects objective data.

History

A complete neurological health history assists the nurse to identify strengths and weaknesses and determine the extent of any problems involving the nervous system. The focus and extent of the examination is dependent on the patient's symptoms and the probable or actual diagnosis. Assessment begins with observation of the patient's level of consciousness (LOC). The nurse takes note of the patient's speech pattern, mental status, intellectual functioning, reasoning ability, and movement or lack of movement of all extremities while obtaining a health history. When the patient is alert, able to state his or her name, where he or she is, and what day it is, proceed with the health history.

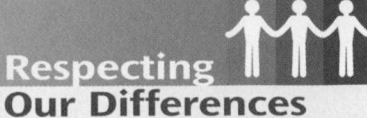

Respecting Our Differences

Patients with English as a Second Language

Assessment of patients for whom English is a second language is often difficult. The lack of the ability to communicate can lead to inaccurate assessments. The nurse may need to involve family or friends to assist with translating. The interpreter or family can assist with the orientation assessment. Orientation is a reflection of the patient's ability to correctly interpret and respond to stimuli. Many institutions keep a record of employees who can act as translators. There are also communication picture boards, which may be helpful.

TABLE 34-3 **Sympathetic versus Parasympathetic Response**

SYSTEM	SYMPATHETIC RESPONSE	PARASYMPATHETIC RESPONSE
Neurological	Pupils dilated	Pupils normal size
	Heightened awareness	
Cardiovascular	Increased heart rate	Decreased heart rate
	Increased myocardial contractility	Decreased myocardial contractility
	Increased blood pressure	
Respiratory	Increased respiratory rate	Bronchial constriction
	Increased respiratory depth	
	Bronchial dilation	
GI	Decreased gastric motility	Increased gastric motility
	Decreased gastric secretions	Increased gastric secretion
	Increased glycogenolysis	Sphincter dilation
	Decreased insulin production	
	Sphincter contraction	
Genitourinary	Decreased urine output	Normal urine output
	Decreased renal blood flow	

Adapted from Estes, M. (2006). Health assessment and physical examination (3rd ed.). New York: Thomson Delmar Learning.

If the patient is comatose or too lethargic to cooperate, the nurse must access secondary sources, such as family or significant others.

When assessing a patient with an altered LOC, use the Glasgow Coma Scale (Table 34-4). The Glasgow Coma Scale is the most widely recognized, standardized LOC assessment tool. The score is based on three categories: eye opening, verbal response, and best motor response. The best possible score is 15 and the lowest score is 3. A score of 8 or less generally indicates a significant alteration in LOC (Crimlisk & Grande, 2004).

Interview

The interview starts with the history of the present problem. The nurse needs to elicit the patient's description of the current problem as shown in the Skills 360°feature.

This information helps the nurse to focus the physical examination. A history of any past illnesses, surgeries, injuries, and medications that the patient is taking may identify related pathology. The social history may reveal exposure to toxic agents, such as viruses, alcohol, tobacco, drugs, or radiation. Family health history may help to identify genetic patterns of disease. For instance, parents or grandparents with chronic diseases or early demise may indicate the patient is also at risk. Prevention of diseases such as myocardial infarction (MI), diabetes mellitus (DM), or CVA may require early intervention by the health care team. Health history questions based on functional health patterns and specific to the neurological system are found in Box 34-1.

Physical Examination

The physical assessment examines in detail the function of the CNS. The examination evaluates six areas of neurological function: mental status, cranial nerves, motor, cerebellum, senses, and reflexes. Based on the health history,

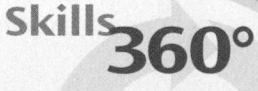

Skills 360°

Gathering a Patient History

The nurse asks the following:

Reason for seeking health care?

Symptoms?

When did problem start?

When is it worst?

What makes it worse?

What makes it better?

Associated symptoms?

TABLE 34-4 **Glasgow Coma Scale**

CATEGORY	RESPONSE	SCORE
Eyes open	Spontaneous—eyes open without verbal or noxious stimuli	4
	To speech—eyes open with verbal stimuli	3
	To pain—eyes open to noxious stimuli	2
	None—no eye opening with any form of stimuli	1
Verbal response	Oriented—aware of person, place, time, and personal data	5
	Confused—answers inappropriate, but language use correct	4
	Inappropriate words—disorganized, random speech	3
	Incomprehensible sounds—moans, groans, and mumbles	2
	None—no verbal response, even to noxious stimuli	1
Best motor response	Obeys commands—performs simple tasks and repeat on command	6
	Localizes pain—organized attempt to remove noxious stimuli	5
	Withdraws from pain—withdraws from source of noxious stimuli	4
	Abnormal flexion—occurs spontaneously or to noxious stimuli	3
	Abnormal extension—occurs spontaneously or to noxious stimuli	2
	None—no response to noxious stimuli; flaccid	1

Adapted from Estes, M. (2006). Health assessment and physical examination (3rd ed.). New York: Thomson Delmar Learning.

the nurse may decide to do a focused or a complete, baseline assessment. The baseline assessment data is useful for future comparison throughout the hospital course.

Mental Status

Subtle changes in mental status are one of the earliest indicators of a potential neurological event. The nurse needs a thorough baseline assessment for comparison, should changes occur. The components of the mental status examination include general appearance, behavior, speech, LOC, mentation, and cognitive function. Much of this information is gathered when doing the health history. When first introduced to the patient, the nurse should observe the patient's gait, posture, and general appearance. The patient's speech patterns, mood, and are evaluated throughout the interviewing and examining process. When assessing the LOC, use questions concerning the time, date or day of the week, location, and situation. To test memory, the nurse should ask questions that require specific answers. For example, "What is the name of the president?" or "What is the name of the last president?" Ask problem solving questions such as, "Subtract 7 from 100, and keep subtracting 7." The nurse should ask the patient to demonstrate simple requests. A simple request might be "Show me two fingers." Then ask the patient to do a more complicated task, such as, "Pick up your pen and write down a list of three words." Instruct the

BOX 34-1

NEUROLOGICAL ASSESSMENT QUESTIONS

Health Perception—Health Management Pattern

Have you ever been diagnosed with a neurologic illness? Seizures? Stroke? Brain or spinal cord injury? Infections of the brain or spinal cord? Brain or spinal cord tumors?

Have you ever been unable to move any body part? If yes, explain.

Any problem thinking clearly? If yes, explain.

Are you having any problems with your ability to see, hear, taste, or smell? If yes, explain.

Have you ever had any diagnostic tests for a neurological problem? If yes, explain.

Do you take any medications for a neurological problem? If yes, explain.

Do you use tobacco products or recreational drugs or drink alcohol? If yes, explain.

What safety practices do you use in a car? On a motorcycle? On a bicycle? Describe.

Nutrition—Metabolic Pattern

Describe your usual dietary intake for a 24-hour period.

Do you have difficulty chewing or swallowing your food?

Are you able to feed yourself? If no, explain.

Elimination Pattern

Has there been any change in your usual pattern of urinary or bowel elimination? If yes, explain.

Do you use laxatives, suppositories, or enemas to assist with bowel elimination? If yes, explain.

Are you able to go to the bathroom independently? If not, explain.

Do you postpone defecation? If yes, explain.

Has your doctor prescribed any medications to manage these problems? If yes, what?

Activity—Exercise Pattern

Describe your typical physical activities in a 24-hour period.

Do you have difficulty with balance, walking, or coordination? If yes, explain.

Do you use any assistive devices for ambulation? If yes, explain.

Do you have any weakness in your arms or legs? If yes, explain.

Do you trip or fall easily? If yes, explain.

Are you able to move all parts of your body? If no, explain.

If you have seizures, describe any precipitating factors, where it begins on your body, and how you feel afterward.

Have you ever experienced shakiness or tremors? If yes, explain.

Does this neurological problem prevent you from performing your activities of daily living? If yes, explain.

Sleep—Rest Pattern

Does your health problem interfere with your ability to sleep and rest? If yes, explain.

Do you take any medications to assist with falling asleep? If yes, what?

Do you ever have pain that awakens you at night? If yes, explain.

Describe your energy level.

Does sleep or rest restore your energy level? If no, explain.

Cognitive—Perceptual Pattern

Do you experience headaches? If yes, describe including frequency, type, location, and precipitating or relieving factors.

Do you ever feel dizzy or faint? If yes, explain.

Do you ever feel like the room is spinning? If yes, explain.

Do you ever experience burning, numbness, or tingling sensations? If yes, describe.

Do you ever experience blurring, double vision, or blind spots? If yes, describe.

Do you ever have problems with your hearing? If yes, explain.

Have you noticed a change in your ability to taste or smell? If yes, explain.

Do you ever have difficulty remembering things? If yes, explain.

Self-Perception—Self-Concept Pattern

How has this problem you are experiencing affected the way you feel about yourself? Describe.

Has the problem changed the way you feel about your life? If yes, explain.

How do you feel about any changes in your life because of this problem? Describe.

Role—Relationship Pattern

Is there a family history of neurological problems? If yes, explain.

Do you ever have difficulty expressing yourself and making others understand? If yes, explain.

How has having neurological problems affected your role in your family? Describe.

How has having neurological problems affected your interactions with family? With friends? At work? In social activities?

Has this problem affected your ability to work? If yes, explain.

Sexuality—Reproductive Pattern

Have your usual sexual activities been altered by this problem? If yes, explain.

Uncovering the Evidence

Evaluating Cognition in Patients

Discussion: The Mini-Mental State Examination (MMSE) is a useful tool for screening mental functioning. The tool measures orientation, immediate memory, short-term memory, and language functioning. There are some limitations to its use, because it is a verbal tool. People from different cultural groups or those with lower levels of education may score poorly.

Implications for Practice: The MMSE is a reliable clinical assessment tool that can be used for a rapid, screening evaluation of mental state or cognitive function. It takes approximately 10–15 minutes to administer. Scoring of points is 0–30. The lower the score, the more severe the alteration of mental state. This tool can be used to track changes over time.

Source: Folstein, M., Folstein, S., & McHugh, P. (1975). Mini-mental state: A practical method for grading the cognitive state of patients for the clinician. Journal of Psychiatric Research, 12(3), 189–198.

patient to remember the words, because you will ask him or her what they were in a few minutes. This is a simple way to test memory. Problems with the patient's ability to remember directions have implications for patient education (Crimlisk & Grande, 2004).

Cranial Nerves

Assessment of cranial nerve function is an essential component of the complete neurological examination. Because the cranial nerves are in pairs, each side must be evaluated separately. Findings from each side are then compared for symmetry.

CN I: Olfactory Nerve

This nerve should only be tested if the patient has indicated there is a problem. The sense of smell is tested by having the patient occlude one nostril and close his or her eyes. The examiner then takes a cotton ball soaked with a common, nonir-

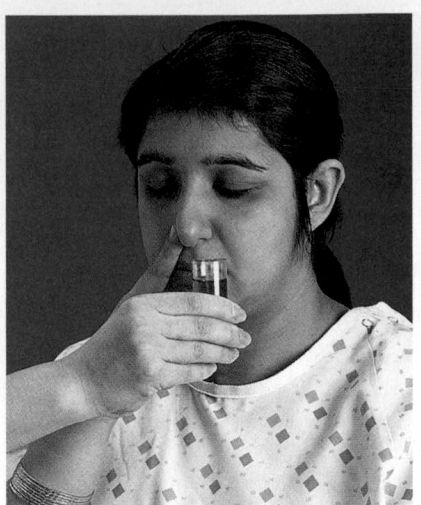

Figure 34-10 Testing of CN I (smell).

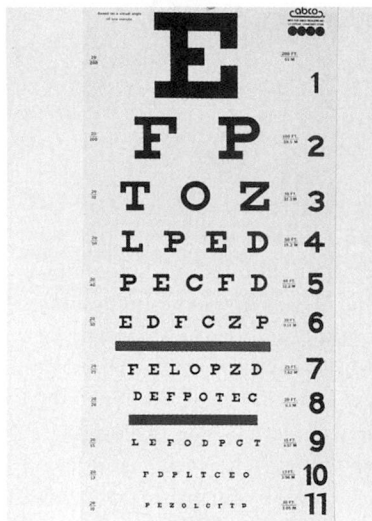

Figure 34-11 Snellen chart.

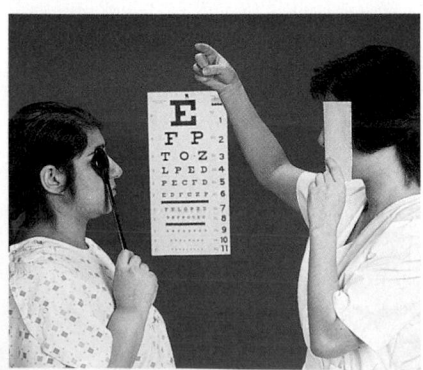

Figure 34-12 Testing visual fields by confrontation.

ritating substance and places it near the nonoccluded nostril (Figure 34-10). Repeat the process for the opposite side using a different scent.

Some common odors that patients should be able to identify if CN I is intact are: cloves, cinnamon, mint, citrus, or coffee. **Anosmia,** the loss or impairment of smell, can be seen with lesions of the frontal lobe or impaired blood flow to the MCA.

CN II: Optic Nerve

The optic nerve is the only cranial nerve that can be examined directly. Testing includes assessment of both visual acuity and visual fields. Each eye is examined separately while the patient covers the other one.

Visual acuity is tested by having the patient read a Snellen chart from 20 feet away (Figure 34-11). Have the patient start with one eye covered and read the lines from top to bottom (largest to smallest letters). Record the lowest line that the patient can read with 50 percent accuracy. Then have the patient cover the other eye and repeat the test. Lastly, have the patient read the chart using both eyes. You may test the patient who wears glasses with or without his or her glasses. The Rosenbaum pocket vision screener is a portable version of the Snellen chart. It is designed for bedside assessment of visual acuity. If these options are not available, have the patient randomly read from a newspaper or magazine. This will give you a gross evaluation of the patient's visual acuity.

Testing of the visual fields assesses the peripheral vision and functioning of the macula. One method of testing is called the confrontation test (Figure 34-12). In this test, the examiner stands or sits directly in front of the patient to be tested, at a distance of 18 to 24 inches. Eyes should be at the same level. Ask the patient to cover one eye. The examiner acts as a control and covers his or her opposite eye. Using a penlight, start at the periphery and move toward the center from right to left, above, below, and from the middle of each direction. Both the examiner and the patient should see the penlight move into his or her peripheral vision, at the same time (Estes, 2006). Abnormal findings of blindness or impaired vision in one or both eyes may be found in patients with transient ischemic attacks (TIA) or CVA.

Another assessment technique is called cardinal fields of vision or extraocular movements. For this test, the examiner stands facing the patient. Ask the patient to hold his or her head still and follow the penlight with his or her eyes only. Move the penlight through the six cardinal fields one at a time, returning to the central starting point before proceeding to the next field. Abnormal findings are failure of one or both eyes to follow the penlight in any direction may indicate weakness of the extraocular muscles. **Nystagmus** is an involuntary rhythmic movement of the eyes. It can be associated with neurological disorders or some medications.

CN III: Oculomotor Nerve, CN IV: Trochlear Nerve, and CN VI: Abducens Nerve

These cranial nerves are usually tested together, because they control the function of the extraocular eye muscles. The functions include: eyelid elevation, constriction of the pupils, and movement of the eye through the six cardinal directions. First observe how much of the iris is covered by the eyelid. Normally, about one third is covered. If more is covered, the patient has **ptosis** or drooping of the eyelid, usually from paralysis of CN III, myasthenia gravis (MG), or sympathetic innervation. Second, dim the room lights then assess the size, shape, and constriction of the pupils using a penlight. Have the patient focus on a distant object, hold the light about 8 inches from one eye in the patient's peripheral field of vision, and shine it directly into one of the pupils. Observe for constriction of the pupil in this eye, which is a direct reaction, and observe for constriction in the other eye, which is a consensual reaction. Both pupils should constrict at the same time. Note if the reaction is brisk (4+), less than brisk (3+), slow (2+), very sluggish (1+), or absent (0).

Repeat the assessment in the other eye. Third, test for convergence (eyes turning inward) and accommodation (pupils constricting with near vision). Hold a finger 8 to 12 inches from the bridge of the patient's nose. Instruct the patient to hold his or her head still, focus on a distant spot, and just move his or her eyes to the commands. Have the patient look at a finger, then the distant spot, and back again. Normally the pupils should constrict and converge equally. Normal findings for CN III, IV, and VI are documented as PERRLA which stands for pupils equal, round, and reactive to light and accommodation. Abnormal findings in patients reveal a dysfunction of these nerves causing them to complain of having difficulty climbing steps, because they are unable to look down or symptoms of **diplopia,** which is blurry or double vision (Almefty, Webber, & Arnautovic, 2006).

CN V: Trigeminal Nerve

The trigeminal nerve is the largest of the cranial nerves and has both motor and sensory components. Testing of the sensory component involves light touch and pinprick in each of the three divisions, ophthalmic, maxillary, and mandibular, of the nerve on both sides of the face. The patient should have his or her eyes closed during the testing procedure. Next, the motor component is evaluated. The strength of the mastication, masseter, and temporal muscles are evaluated by palpating them when the jaw is opened and then closed. The nurse should note differences in the tone or atrophy of the muscles bilaterally. Corneal reflexes, on the conscious patient, can be observed by having the examiner move his or her hand or a small object rapidly toward the patient's face. Observe for blinking. In the patient with a decreased LOC, testing of the corneal reflex involves the light touching of the cornea with a cotton wisp.

Abnormal findings reveal a loss of corneal reflexes indicates lesions of both CN V (sensory) and CN VIII (motor). Patients with lesions of CN V (motor), or after a CVA, may lose sensation or the ability to chew effectively. Severe facial pain is seen with trigeminal neuralgia (tic douloureux).

CN VII: Facial Nerve

The facial nerve is also a mixed cranial nerve with both sensory and motor components. The sensory component includes the sense of taste on the anterior two thirds of the tongue. The testing of the sensory component is often deferred, unless changes are noted in the health history interview. When tested, have the patient stick out his or her tongue and test each side separately. There are four classic modalities of taste: sweet (tip of tongue), sour (sides of tongue), salty (over most of tongue, but concentrated on the sides), and bitter (back of tongue, controlled by CN IX). A fifth taste modality (umami) has been known for approximately 100 years, but was recently added to the list once specific receptors were identified (Ganong, 2003). It is triggered by glutamate, specifically monosodium glutamate (MSG), which is used extensively in Asian cooking. The taste is sweet and pleasant, but different from the standard sweet taste. To test the patient, ask him or her to identify the different tastes as they are applied one at a time to the appropriate location on the tongue. Have the patient rinse his or her mouth with water between tests. Remember that a bitter taste is innervated by CN IX. Taste abnormalities include: **ageusia** (absence of the sense of taste), **hypogeusia** (diminished taste sensitivity), and **dysgeusia** (disturbed sense of taste). Many diseases and certain drugs can produce hypogeusia or dysgeusia (Zavarella, Leblebicioglu, Claman, & Tatakis, 2006).

When testing the motor component of the facial nerve, first observe the face for any asymmetry of the patient's features or facial movements. Observe for facial tics. Then, ask the patient to perform the following movements: raise his or her eyebrows, close his or her eyelids tightly, puff out his or her cheeks, smile, and frown. Observe for weakness or asymmetry of muscle movement. Abnormal findings of upper motor neuron lesions, lower motor neuron lesions, or a stroke can cause weakness or paralysis of the facial muscles (Crimlisk & Grande, 2004).

CN VIII: Acoustic Nerve

The acoustic nerve has two divisions: the cochlear and the vestibular. The cochlear division is involved in hearing. The vestibular division is involved in the sense of balance, which includes equilibrium, coordination, and orientation in space. First, examine the patient's ear canals for obvious blockages or malformations. Also check for excess cerumen (earwax), which may interfere with balance or hearing. Testing of the cochlear division is done by having the patient close his or her eyes and indicate when he or she hears the ticking of a watch or the rubbing of the examiner's fingers. Normal findings are when the patient can hear the watch or rustling 4 to 6 inches away. This test identifies only gross deficits, and deviations are indications for referral for a more comprehensive evaluation.

Next, check for lateralization and air and bone conduction. The Weber's test is used to evaluate lateralization, and the Rinne's test evaluates air-bone conduction. For the Weber's test, vibrate the tuning fork, place it at the center of the patient's forehead, and ask if the sound is heard equally in both ears. If not, ask the patient to describe the differences.

Normally, the sound is heard equally in both ears. In the Rinne test, both air conduction and bone conduction are tested. For the Rinne test, place the base of the lightly vibrating tuning fork firmly on the mastoid process. Ask the patient to note when the vibration is no longer felt. Quickly place the still vibrating tuning fork near the ear with the tines toward the ear. Ask the patient to note when the sound can no longer be heard. Normally, the sound should be heard longer through air than bone. Abnormal findings from either test are indications for further investigation. Testing of the vestibular portion of CN VIII is usually done during testing of the motor or cerebellar systems.

CN IX: Glossopharyngeal Nerve and CN X: Vagus Nerve

The glossopharyngeal and vagus nerves are usually tested together, because they innervate many of the same structures. In the pharynx, CN IX is primarily sensory, and CN X is mostly motor. First, take note of the patient's voice quality. If the patient is hoarse or has a nasal quality, he or she may have vocal cord lesions or paralysis. Second, observe the patient as he or she swallows a small amount of water. Ask if he or she frequently chokes on food or has trouble swallowing. **Dysphagia** (difficulty swallowing) can often be seen after neurosurgical procedures or CVA (stroke). Next, ask the patient to say "ah" and observe his or her uvula. It should move up and not deviate to the side. The palate should also move up when the patient opens his or her mouth. Observe for any asymmetrical movements. Lastly, tell the patient that the gag reflex will be checked next. Use a tongue blade to touch the back of the patient's throat lightly on each side. Loss of the gag reflex occurs with lesions of CN IX and CN X.

CN XI: Spinal Accessory Nerve

The spinal accessory nerve is tested in two segments: trapezius muscles and sternocleidomastoid muscles. Assessment of the trapezius is done by the examiner placing his or her hands on the patient's shoulders. Then, ask the patient to shrug his or her shoulders. Observe for strength and symmetry. The sternocleidomastoid muscles are assessed by the examiner placing his or her hand on one cheek and asking the patient to turn his or her head against a hand as the movement is resisted. (Figure 34-13). Again, observe for strength and symmetry. Repeat the test on the opposite side of the head. Abnormal findings are muscle weakness which can be seen with lower motor neuron disease or in some CVAs.

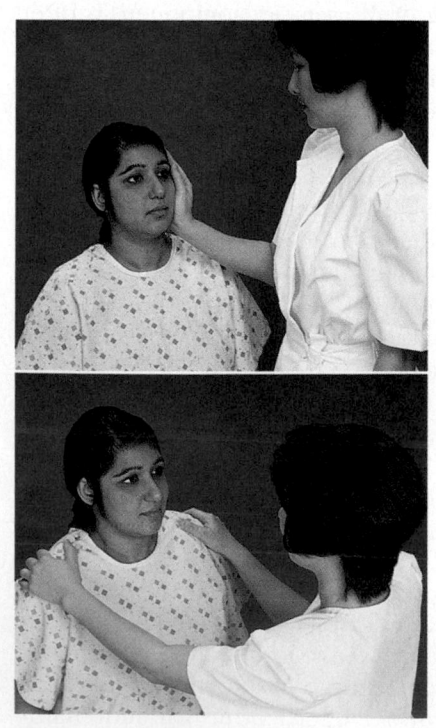

Figure 34-13 Testing CN XI.

CN XII: Hypoglossal Nerve

The hypoglossal nerve is tested by asking the patient to open his or her mouth, stick out his or her tongue, and wiggle it side to side. The tongue should be midline. Observe for asymmetry, atrophy, or fasciculations. Carotid endarterectomy is a common cause of dysfunction of CN XII. During the surgical procedure, the nerve can be stretched causing temporary weakness or severed causing permanent dysfunction.

Motor Function

The nerves of the motor system originate from the spinal cord and control muscle movement. The motor examination begins with the neck and proceeds from proximal to distal extremities. Major muscle groups are assessed for specific functions. Each muscle is evaluated for symmetry, size, tone, and strength. First, note the size and contour of each muscle or muscle group. Subtle differences may require measurement of the muscle pair and comparing for differences. Observe for any muscle wasting, atrophy, or hypertrophy. Muscle atrophy is seen with lower motor neuron lesions. Next, assess for tremors and fasciculations. Observe patient movements both at rest and with activity. With the patient relaxed, the examiner puts the joints through normal range of motion. Start with the shoulders and move systematically: elbow, wrist, fingers, hip, knee, and ankle. Compare assessment findings from both sides.

Abnormalities of muscle tone include spasticity, rigidity, and flaccidity. Spasticity, or hypertonia, refers to increased motor tone. The tone is greater with rapid movement than with slow movement. Spasticity is the result of injury to upper motor neurons. Rigidity is increased resistance that persists throughout movement and is related to lesions of the basal ganglia. Flaccidity, or hypotonia, refers to the decrease or loss of muscle tone. The muscle is weak, soft, and floppy. Flaccidity is due to lower motor lesions.

Muscle strength is assessed by having the patient move a specific muscle or group of muscles first against gravity then with resistance provided by the examiner. After each muscle group is assessed, it is graded according to the scale in Table 34-5. Findings are documented as a fraction with the numerator being the patient's score and the denominator as 5 for the maximum score possible.

Possible abnormal findings include weakness, hemiplegia, or paralysis. Weakness is seen with transient ischemic attacks (TIA) and some CVAs. Hemiplegia is found with CVAs. Paralysis is found in patients with MS, MG, and spinal cord injuries (SCI).

TABLE 34-5 Grading Scale for Muscle Strength	
GRADE	**STRENGTH**
5	Active movement against gravity; full resistance; normal muscle movement
4	Active movement against gravity; some resistance; examiner can overcome the patient's muscle resistance
3	Active movement against gravity
2	Active movement of body part when gravity eliminated
1	Weak palpated muscle contraction; no active movement noted
0	No muscle contraction noted

Adapted from Estes, M. (2006). Health assessment and physical examination (3rd ed.). New York: Thomson Delmar Learning.

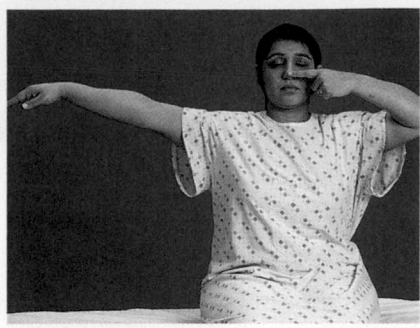

Figure 34-14 Testing coordination.

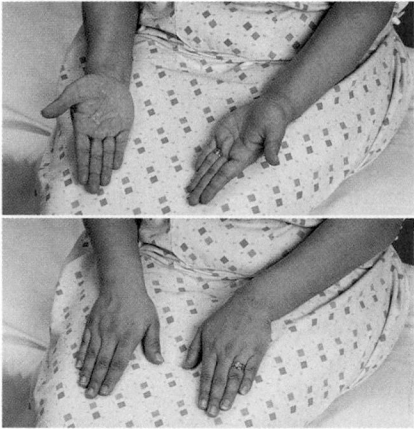

Figure 34-15 Rapid alternating movements.

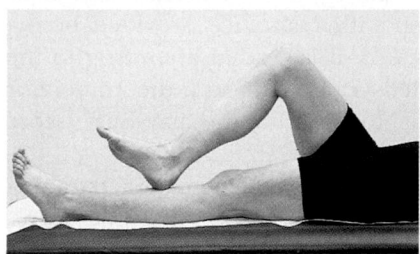

Figure 34-16 Heel slide.

Cerebellar Function

Evaluation of cerebellar function requires the assessment of coordination, balance, posture, and gait. Coordination involves the smooth, precise movement of multiple muscle groups. Testing can be done, using multiple techniques, with the patient sitting up. First, instruct the patient to sit with arms outstretched, eyes open, and facing the examiner. Ask the patient to touch his or her nose with one index finger, then the opposite finger. Have him or her rapidly alternate sides, and then close his or her eyes and continue to rapidly alternate sides (Figure 34-14). Observe for intention tremor or inability to accurately complete the task. Second, ask the patient to rapidly alternate patting his or her knees, first with the palms and then alternating palms with the backs of his or her hands (Figure 34-15). Third, finger coordination is tested by having the patient repeatedly touch his or her thumb to each finger sequentially. Repeat test with opposite fingers. Observe coordination and ability to perform tasks in rapid sequence. Fourth, with the patient either seated or supine, have him or her place one heel on the opposite shin, just below the knee, and slide the heel from the knee to the foot. Repeat on opposite heel (Figure 34-16). Observe leg coordination. Fifth, ask the patient to draw a circle or figure eight with his or her foot either on the floor or in the air. Repeat with the other foot (Figure 34-17). Observe for coordination and regularity of the drawing. Lastly, ask the patient to rapidly flex and extend the toes of one foot. Repeat on the opposite foot. Observe for rate rhythm, smoothness, and accuracy of the requested movements.

Abnormal Findings

Cerebellar disease is the cause of **dyssynergy,** which is a lack of coordinated muscle movement; **dysmetria,** which is impaired judgment of distance, range, speed, and force of movement; and **dysdiadochokinesia,** which is the inability to perform rapidly alternating movements.

The examiner tests balance by having the patient walk heel to toe along a line. Then have the patient walk on his or her toes, only. Follow with walking on his or her heels only. An alternative procedure is to have the patient hop on one foot and then the other. Protect the patient from falls.

Lesions of the cerebellar hemisphere (stroke or tumors) cause the patient to fall toward the affected side, and **ataxia,** a lack of muscle coordination, is observed. Midline cerebellar lesions cause a wide-based gait, and the patient is unable to perform tandem walking.

Posture and gait should be evaluated in ambulatory patients. Posture is the position or awareness of the body in space. Gait is the manner in which the patient walks. The examiner observes the patient walking and whether the patient uses assistive devices. This examination is made without shoes or socks, if possible. The nurse must be prepared to protect the patient from falls or injury. The nurse must ask the patient to walk back and forth in the examination area. Observe and note: gait, smooth or staggering, position of feet, normal or broad-based, symmetry of arm and leg movements, presence of uncoordinated movements or tremors, step height, normal, high, shuffling, and step length (normal, short, or long). Also, make note of the ease of turning and number of steps needed to turn.

Patients with Parkinson's disease stoop over while walking, shuffle their feet, and hold their arms close to their body. Patients with polyneuropathy walk on their heels and then their toes with the feet held wide apart. Often these patients stagger and watch the floor while walking, and their gait becomes worse when asked to close their eyes.

Romberg's Test

Ask the patient to stand erect, feet together, arms at his or her side, and eyes open. Stand close to the patient during the test to protect him or her, should he or she begin to fall. Repeat test with eyes closed. Observe for ability to main-

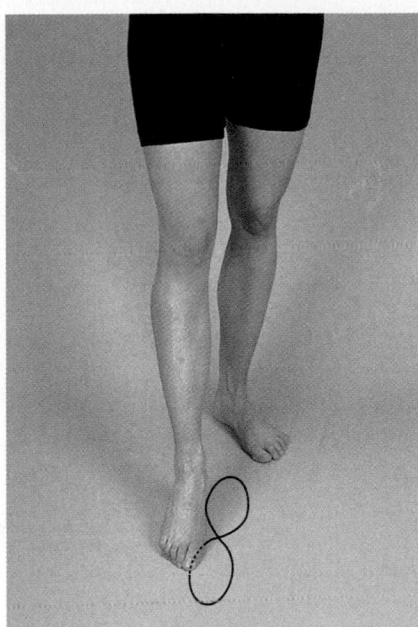

Figure 34-17 Testing coordination (Figure eight).

TABLE 34-6 Sensory Rating Scale	
RATING	**FINDINGS**
Normal	
Present, but diminished (abnormal)	
Absent	

Adapted from Estes, M. (2006). Health assessment and physical examination (3rd ed.). New York: Thomson Delmar Learning.

tain balance for 20 seconds with minimal swaying. Abnormal findings of cerebellar lesions (CVA or tumors) cause the unsteadiness.

Sensory Function

Evaluation of the sensory system tests the patient's ability to perceive various types of sensations. The body areas usually assessed are face, neck, deltoid regions, forearms, top part of the hands, chest, abdomen, thighs, lower legs, and top of the feet. See Table 34-6 for rating scale for sensory assessment.

Superficial sensation is tested using various modalities: light touch, pain, and temperature. First, ask the patient to close his or her eyes. The examiner uses a wisp of cotton to touch each of the assessment areas. Instruct the patient to indicate verbally when the stimulus is felt. Vary the stimulation sites to prevent the patient from anticipating subsequent areas. Compare both sides. Second, for assessment of pain use a disposable object (broken wooden applicator or open paperclip) to demonstrate sharp and dull sensations. Be sure to not use an item that will break or puncture the patient's skin. Dispose of your testing object when exam is completed. Ask the patient to close his or her eyes. Instruct the patient to indicate verbally when the stimulus is felt. Vary the stimulation sites to prevent the patient from anticipating subsequent areas. Compare both sides. Third, temperature is tested be using test tubes, one with warm water and one with cold water. Instruct the patient to indicate verbally when the stimulus is felt. Vary the stimulation sites to prevent the patient from anticipating the next area. Compare both sides. This portion of the sensory exam is normal when the patient is able to correctly identify light touch, superficial pain, and temperature accurately.

Abnormal findings of lesions of the peripheral nerves, brainstem, or spinal cord may cause **anesthesia** (absence of touch sensation), **hypesthesia** (diminished sense of touch), **paresthesia** (numbness, tingling, or prickling sensation), or **dysesthesia** (burning or tingling).

Lesions of the thalamus and peripheral nerves may cause: **analgesia** (insensitivity to pain), **hypalgesia** (diminished sensitivity to pain), or **hypergesia** (increased sensitivity to pain).

Deep sensation evaluates vibration, deep pressure pain, position, and discriminates fine touch. To test vibration a vibrating tuning fork is placed on the bony prominences (thumb and great toe). Instruct the patient to indicate verbally when the stimulus is first felt and again when it is no longer felt (Figure 34-18). Compare both sides. Normally, the patient should be able to sense vibration over the bony prominences.

Abnormal findings of some spinal cord lesions and polyneuropathies can cause loss of the vibratory sense. It is normally diminished in the elderly. When testing deep pressure pain the examiner squeezes the Achilles tendon, calf, and forearm muscle. Compare both sides. Note the patient's response. Next, the examiner tests position sense. Instruct the patient to close his or her eyes. Lightly grasp the patient's finger or great toe and gently move it up or down. Instruct the patient to indicate verbally which direction the digit is in. Vary the

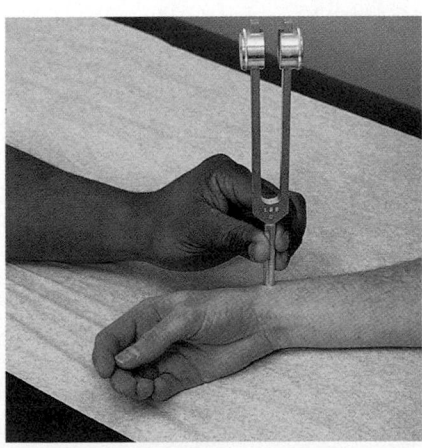

Figure 34-18 Sensory: vibration.

direction to prevent the patient from anticipating the digit location. Compare both sides. Abnormal findings of lesions of the posterior column of the spinal cord can affect the position sense.

Lastly, assessment of discriminate fine touch involves **stereognosis** (identify objects by touch) and **graphesthesia** (identify letters, numbers, or shapes drawn on hand). To test for stereognosis, ask the patient to close his or her eyes and place an object, such as a coin, paper clip, or key, into the patient's hand. Instruct the patient to feel the object. Ask the patient to name the object. Abnormal findings of dysfunction of the parietal lobe can cause **astereognosis** (lack of ability to identify objects by touch).

To test graphesthesia, first ask the patient to close his or her eyes. Then the examiner draws a letter, number, or shape in the patient's open hand. Repeat on the opposite side. Abnormal findings of lesions of the sensory cortex can cause a loss of the ability to identify letters or shapes when drawn on the palm.

Reflex Testing

Assessment of reflexes provides important information on the status of the CNS in both conscious and unconscious patients. Altered reflexes may be the earliest signs of a pathological condition. There are three categories of reflexes: deep tendon, cutaneous, and pathological. DTRs (muscle-stretch reflexes) occur in response to a sudden stimulus (e.g., tapping with a reflex hammer). It is important to use the correct technique to elicit the specific reflex. With the muscle relaxed and the joint in neutral position and supported by the examiner, the tendon is tapped directly with the reflex hammer. Normally the muscle contracts with a quick movement of the limb or structure. Both sides of the body are tested and assigned a score based on the scale in Table 34-7.

First, test the biceps reflex, by having the patient flex his or her arm slightly, with the palm up. Support the patient's arm at the elbow, with your thumb over the biceps tendon in the antecubital space. Strike your thumb with the reflex hammer. The biceps muscle should contract, and the arm should flex slightly. Repeat on the opposite side. To test the triceps tendon, support the patient's arm flexed at a 90-degree angle and strike the triceps tendon between the epicondyles just above the elbow. The muscle should contract and the elbow extends slightly. Repeat on the opposite side. Next, to test the brachioradialis reflex, support the patient's arm, flexed slightly with the palm down. Strike the radius, about two inches above the wrist. The forearm should rotate laterally and the palm turns upward. Repeat on the opposite side. For testing of the patellar reflex, the legs should be dangling. The examiner places his or

---

TABLE 34-7	**Deep Tendon Reflex Rating Scale**
RATING	**FINDINGS**
4+	Very brisk; hyperactive
3+	More brisk than normal
2+	Normal; average
1+	Diminished; sluggish; minimal
0	No response

Note: All reflexes are documented by a plus sign. There are no minuses used when rating DTRs.
Adapted from Estes, M. (2006). Health assessment and physical examination (3rd ed.). New York: Thomson Delmar Learning.

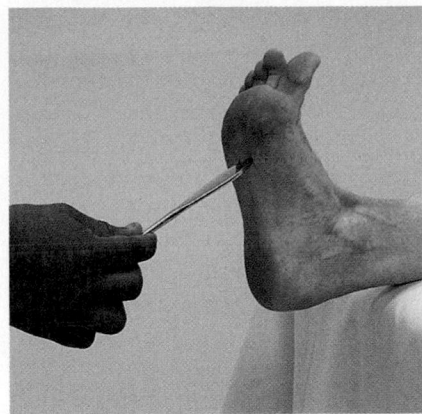

Figure 34-19 Testing of plantar reflex.

TABLE 34-8 **Pathological Reflexes**	
REFLEX	**TECHNIQUE**
Grasp	Stimulation of palm results in a grasp.
Snout	Stimulation of circumoral region results in puckering of lips.
Sucking	Stimulation of lips, tongue, or palate results in sucking movement.
Rooting	Stimulation of lips results in head moving toward stimulus.
Palmomental	Stimulation of palm results in contraction of the chin muscles.
Glabellar	Eyes blink each time the glabellar area (between eyes) is tapped. Normal: blinking stops after first few taps.

Adapted from Estes, M. (2006). Health assessment and physical examination (3rd ed.). New York: Thomson Delmar Learning.

her hand on the patient's thigh and strikes the distal patellar tendon just below the kneecap. The quadricep muscle contracts and the knee extends slightly. Repeat on the opposite side. When testing the Achilles tendon, the examiner supports the patient's foot, slightly dorsiflexed. Lightly strike the Achilles tendon behind the ankle. The foot should plantar flex. Repeat on the opposite side. The plantar reflex (also called Babinski's sign) is tested with the foot in the neutral position. With a moderately sharp object (key or the handle of a reflex hammer), stroke the lateral aspect of the sole from the heel to the ball of the foot, curving medially across the ball (Figure 34-19). Use the lightest stroke required for a response. Normal response is flexion of the toes. Abnormal findings of dorsiflexion of the great toe with fanning of the other toes can indicate upper motor neuron pathology.

Cutaneous reflexes are elicited by light, rapid stroking, or scratching of the tissue. The major reflexes tested are: corneal, gag, swallow, upper abdominal, lower abdominal, cremasteric, bulbocavernous, and perianal. Corneal reflexes (CN V or CN VII), gag, and swallow reflexes (CN IX or CN X), were discussed in assessment of the cranial nerves. The cremasteric, bulbocavernous, and perianal are not routinely checked. To test the abdominal reflexes, have the patient supine with clothing moved out of the testing area. Lightly but briskly stroke each assessment area using a tongue blade or warmed handle of reflex hammer. The grading of cutaneous reflexes differs from that used with DTRs. They are graded as either present (+) or absent (0). If present but weak, they are documented as weak. Abnormal findings of absent reflexes can indicate both upper and lower motor neuron pathology.

Pathological reflexes are also called primitive reflexes, because they are seen in infants and then disappear. If these reflexes reappear, they are found in patient's suffering from dementia syndromes or Parkinson's disease. Table 34-8 describes the assessment techniques. Grading of pathological reflexes is documented as presence (+) is abnormal and absence (−) is normal.

DIAGNOSTIC TESTS

Neurodiagnostic tests are performed as adjuncts to a complete history and physical examination. Health care providers can then correlate results from the neurodiagnostic tests with clinical effectiveness of various treatment modalities. Knowledge of the tests, pretest preparation, testing procedure, and necessary follow-up care will facilitate patient teaching by the nurse.

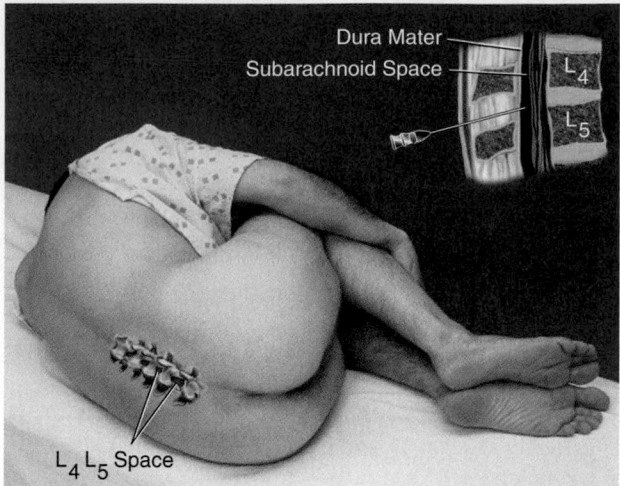

Dura Mater
Subarachnoid Space
L$_4$
L$_5$

L$_4$L$_5$ Space

Figure 34-20 Lumbar puncture.

Lumbar Puncture

A lumbar puncture (LP) is the most common method for obtaining CSF for analysis. This test is performed to examine the CSF for pathologies associated with specific diseases (Daniels, 2003).

Nursing Management

Explain the procedure to patient. Inform patient that the test is performed with he or she lying in the lateral recumbent position with knees flexed. Encourage oral fluid intake. Patient is to empty his or her bladder before the test starts. Baseline assessment includes vital signs and neurological status. Blood coagulation values should be checked before the test in all patients taking anticoagulation medications. Administer premedication if ordered.

The patient is placed in the lateral recumbent position with knees flexed (Figure 34-20). Using sterile technique, the practitioner inserts a hollow-core needle into the subarachnoid space, usually at L3–L4 or L4–L5. Once proper placement in the subarachnoid space is confirmed, instruct the patient to relax. Opening and closing pressure readings are documented. Three to five test tubes of CSF are usually collected and numbered sequentially. After the needle is withdrawn, pressure is held for one to two minutes, and a bandage strip applied to the insertion site. The tubes are sent to the laboratory for analysis. See Table 34-9 for a discussion of CSF analysis.

Maintain strict bed rest for a few hours as ordered. Encourage oral fluids. Monitor and compare vital sign and neurological assessment to baseline findings. Administer analgesia as needed.

Radiographic Studies

There are a variety of radiographic studies that are performed as diagnostic procedures. Radiological exams send radiation through the body to form a picture of the internal structures. X-rays turn film black, so areas that allow

TABLE 34-9 Cerebrospinal Fluid Analysis

PARAMETER	NORMAL VALUE	ANALYSIS OF ABNORMAL FINDINGS
Opening pressure	60–200 mm H$_2$O	Less than 60—dehydration; blocked CSF.
		Greater than 200—brain tumor, abscess, or cyst; subdural hematoma; hydrocephalus; cerebral edema.
Appearance	clear, colorless	Xanthochromia is often due to the breakdown of blood products. Turbidity or cloudiness is often due to increased white blood cells (WBCs), elevated protein levels, or infection.
Red blood cells (RBCs)	none	Cell count of RBCs indicates bleeding; serial reduction of RBCs in tubes sent from lumbar puncture (LP), may indicate a traumatic LP.
WBCs	0–8 μ/L	Elevations may indicate meningitis, tumors, and multiple sclerosis.
Protein	15–45 mg/dL	Elevations with infection, tumor, or hemorrhage.
Glucose	45–75 mg/dL	Elevations are not significant; a decrease indicates infection.
Microorganisms	none	
pH	7.35	
Specific gravity	1.007	

Adapted from Daniels, R. (2003). Delmar's manual of laboratory and diagnostic tests. *New York: Thomson Delmar Learning.*

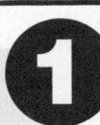

Safety First

Safety Precautions When Assisting with a Lumbar Puncture (LP)

When assisting the health care provider with a LP, the nurse needs to ensure the safety of the patient during the procedure. If the patient is unable to maintain a fetal position (knees held close to the chest by his or her arms), the nurse should assist the patient. The patient is positioned on the side, with his or her back close to the edge of the table. Standing on the opposite side of the table, facing the patient, the nurse should hold behind the patients bent knees and neck to gently maintain the examination position. It may be necessary to place a pillow under the patient's head or between his or her knees to maintain body alignment. If the patient is restless or unable to cooperate, two people may be needed to assist.

radiation to pass easily appear dark, while areas that block radiation appear white. Therefore, air-filled lungs appear blackish on X-ray, while bones appear white. X-rays are used in several basic ways; the most common are standard (plain) films, fluoroscopy, and tomography. In addition, when these studies include contrast mediums, they are more invasive. In general, these tests are invaluable to determining the presence of pathology and are often specific in terms of their ability to accurately diagnose a given disorder.

Radiological Examination of the Skull and Spine

Plain X-ray studies of the skull and spine are easy to obtain and noninvasive Damage to the nervous system may include bony fractures, bone erosion, curvature, dislocations, and calcification of soft tissue. Multiple views may be taken. These could include: anteroposterior (AP), lateral, oblique, special views of facial bones, and flexion-extension.

Nursing Management

There is usually no patient preparation needed. The nurse should explain that the X-ray procedure is similar to having a chest X-ray (CXR) done and that the exposure to radiation is minimal. Patients who are immobilized may require the nurse to accompany them to the radiology department. Impaired ambulation may require a stretcher for transport.

Once in the radiology department, the patient is directed to either lie on the examination table or stand, depending on the ordered studies. The patient is positioned for each of the desired views and instructed to not move during each X-ray. There is no required follow-up nursing care.

Computed Tomography

Computed axial tomography (CT scan) is considered one of the most accurate, quickest, easiest, and least expensive method of diagnosing neurologic problems. It combines X-rays with computer technology to produce a three-dimensional picture of thin cross-sections of the body. The X-ray beam rotates around the patient, and then the computer analyzes the data and creates a composite picture. The images may be enhanced by the use of contrast media. CT is sensitive to differences in tissue densities. This allows the neuroradiologist to identify any disease processes in the bones, soft tissue, or fluids. A limitation of the CT scanner is its inability to gather information about functional status.

Nursing Management

Teaching by the nurse should begin with a description of the CT scanner. When contrast media is planned, identification of any allergies to the media, shellfish, or iodine may require premedication. Instruct the patient regarding the need to lie still during the procedure. Identify any need for sedation because of anxiety. The patient is not usually kept to a nothing by mouth (NPO) order. A peripheral intravenous (IV) site may need to be implemented for contrast media injection.

The patient is placed flat on a movable table. His or her head is secured in a holding device. The table moves in and out of the cylindrical scanner. A non-contrast series of pictures is taken first. If contrast medium is ordered, it is administered intravenously, and the series is repeated. The entire procedure usually takes approximately 10–40 minutes.

If contrast agent is given, the nurse should monitor for any delayed reaction. When contrast agent is used, the diuresis that results may require replacement fluids.

Magnetic Resonance Imaging

Magnetic resonance imaging (MRI) is a computer-based imagining method that uses the body's own magnetic energy to visualize disease processes, such as strokes, tumors, trauma, seizures, edema, and brainstem herniation. The magnet causes changes in the radiofrequency signals produced by the body. These changes are detected and interpreted by the computer and then displayed as

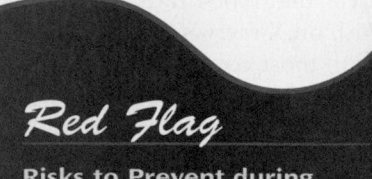

cross-sectional images. The procedure is noninvasive, unless contrast is required. When visualization needs to be enhanced, gadolinium, a non–iodine-based media, may be used (Daniels, 2003).

Nursing Management

The patient needs to be interviewed regarding any iron-based implanted objects (e.g., artificial joints, pacemakers, bullets or metal fragments, or clips or wires). The powerful magnetic field can cause such devices to move out of position, placing the patient at risk for hemorrhage or bleeding. The magnet can alter the internal settings for pacemakers. Make the patient aware that the procedure is noisy and earplugs are available. Patients who are claustrophobic may need to be sedated. Patients are not usually kept NPO.

The patient needs to remain motionless while enclosed in a tunnel containing the powerful magnet. A two-way intercom is available for the patient to communicate needs. First, a noncontrast series of pictures are taken. If contrast is ordered, it is administered intravenously, and the series is repeated. The procedure may take from 15–90 minutes to complete. If sedation is required, monitor the patient for return to baseline functioning. No further postprocedure nursing care is required.

Magnetic Resonance Angiography

Magnetic resonance angiography (MRA) uses the differential signal characteristics of blood flow to visualize the extracranial and intracranial blood vessels. The study provides both anatomic and hemodynamic information. It can be used in conjunction with contrast media (contrast-enhanced MRA [cMRA]). MRA is often used as a less invasive method of screening for and diagnosing cerebrovascular disease.

Nursing Management

The patient preparation for an MRA is essentially the same as the MRI. The time necessary to complete the procedure is about one to three hours to complete. In addition, the follow-up nursing care is also similar to the MRI. The patient should be assessed for boney prominences for pressure areas, and the patient must lie in the same position for most or all of the procedure.

Magnetic Resonance Spectroscopy

Magnetic resonance spectroscopy (MRS) provides information about the chemical composition of tissue. Chemical markers of neuronal integrity are evaluated using MRI techniques. This is often used to differentiate tumor versus abscess or infection versus autoimmune destruction. The patient preparation for MRS is essentially the same as the MRI.

Functional Magnetic Resonance Imaging

Functional magnetic resonance imaging (fMRI) is used to identify changes in cerebral metabolism or blood flow. It looks at chemical changes in response to specific tasks. These tasks consist of periods of activity and periods of rest. The result can functionally map the brain. The patient preparation for fMRI is essentially the same as the MRI.

Cerebral Angiography

Cerebral angiography (angiogram) is an invasive series of radiographic studies involving the injection of contrast medium. This allows the visualization of the intracranial and extracranial blood vessels. It is performed to detect vascular lesions such as, aneurysms, malformations, occlusion, and tumors of the brain.

Nursing Management

The nurse needs to describe what is involved and identify any allergies to shellfish or iodine. Explain that an IV catheter will be inserted using local anesthetic, usually in the femoral artery. A burning sensation, lasting 20 to 30 seconds, may occur when the contrast media is injected. This is to be expected. The patient needs to be NPO for approximately four to six hours prior to the procedure. IV hydration should be instituted when the patient is NPO. The initial assessment includes baseline vital signs, LOC, and evaluation of all peripheral pulses. Administer premedication when ordered.

The patient is taken to the angiography suite, placed on the examination table, and secured with straps. A headrest is used to immobilize the head. The radiologist locates and cleans the chosen puncture site and then threads the catheter into the artery. Once the catheter is placed, contrast media is injected and a series of radiographic images are obtained that outline the arterial and venous systems. After the catheter is removed, pressure is maintained for at least 5 to 10 minutes to prevent arterial bleeding.

After the procedure, bedrest needs to be maintained for 6 to 12 hours as ordered. Monitor the access site for signs of bleeding or formation of hematoma. A pressure dressing, sandbag, ice bag, or combination need to be maintained as ordered. Vital signs and neurovascular assessment of the area distal to the puncture site are compared to the baseline findings on a 15 minute to hourly routine as ordered. Instruct the patient to minimize movement of the involved limb and avoid flexion at the puncture site. LOC is also assessed for changes, which may indicate circulatory compromise, such as vasospasm, embolism, and thrombosis. Maintain hydration as the contrast media may result in increased osmotic diuresis and places the patient at risk for dehydration and renal tubular occlusion.

Digital Subtraction Angiography

Digital subtraction angiography (DSA) is the combination of X-ray films with computer enhancement to produce images of the cerebral circulation. The procedure is performed using the IV rather than the arterial route. It can be performed as an outpatient test and has few potential complications.

Nursing Management

The nurse needs to describe what is involved and identify any allergies to shellfish or iodine. Food is restricted for two hours before the test, but fluids are not. Instruct the patient to empty his or her bladder. Initial assessment includes baseline vital signs, LOC, and evaluation of peripheral pulses. Administer premedication when ordered.

The patient is taken to the neuroradiology suite, placed on an examination table, and secured with straps. The radiologist selects the puncture site, cleans it, and threads a large angiocatheter into the vein, usually, brachial. IV fluid is administered via a second IV catheter. A baseline X-ray is done to be used as a reference for the remainder of the films. The contrast media is injected, and serial films are compared to the baseline. The computer subtracts the baseline image and generates an angiographic image. DSA is less invasive, less costly, and more convenient for the patient than many other radiographic tests.

The nurse should monitor vital signs and neurovascular status every 15 minutes to hourly as ordered. Regularly evaluate the access site for bleeding. Encourage the patient to increase his or her oral intake for the next 24 hours. There are no activity restrictions.

Positron Emission Tomography

Positron emission tomography (PET) provides a three-dimensional structural and functional view of the brain. It combines CT with radioisotope scanning to measure the metabolic activity of the brain and assess for cell death or damage. The biggest limitation to PET scanning is the need for an on-site cyclotron to prepare the radioisotopes because of their short half-life.

Nursing Management

Explain the procedure to the patient. Instruct the patient to withhold caffeine, alcohol, and tobacco for 24 hours prior to the test. The patient is NPO for 6 to 12 hours before the test is scheduled. If the patient is diabetic, no

---

DOLLARS AND SENSE

Expenses of MRI Scans

With steadily rising health care costs, it is necessary to be aware of the cost of diagnostic tests. An MRI scan, when first available, cost between $2,000 and $5,000 per use. Now with increased use and availability, the cost of an MRI is between $300 to $1,000, depending on how many scans are done each year by the institution. The higher the volume of MRI scans, the lower the cost.

Fast Forward ▶▶▶

The Future of Functional Magnetic Resonance Imaging (fMRI)

Currently the standard test for language lateralization before surgeries planned for seizure disorders or neoplasm resection is the Wada test. This test involves a large medical team, iodinated contrast media, and radiation. It usually involves one to two hours of testing and four to six hours of patient recovery time. In the future, fMRI may replace the Wada test as the preoperative assessment tool for language lateralization. The fMRI usually requires 30–60 minutes of testing time and no postprocedure recovery time. The cost of the Wada test and fMRI were compared and substantial savings with the use of fMRI to evaluate language lateralization were found. Multiple studies have found the results of the fMRI to be equivalent to the Wada test.

antidiabetic medications, such as insulin or oral antiglycemics, are given before the test. Withhold glucose solutions or medications that alter glucose metabolism. Direct the patient to empty his or her bladder prior to the procedure. Instruct patient to not take sedatives or tranquilizers before the test.

The patient is placed on a stretcher and either inhales or is injected with a biologically active radioactive tagged compound made partially of water or glucose, and the mixture is then able to cross the blood-brain barrier. A computerized detector measures the radioactive uptake of these substances and produces a composite image. The areas where the radioactive material is located correspond to areas of cellular metabolism. The patient may be blindfolded if he or she desires and can have earplugs inserted for all or part of the test. The patient is asked to perform specific mental functions to activate different areas of the brain. The total procedure takes two to three hours.

The radioisotope is eliminated by the kidney and requires no special precautions. Encourage the patient to increase oral fluids.

Single-Photon Emission Computed Tomography

Single-photon emission computed tomography (SPECT) overcomes the limitations of PET scanning by using radionuclides that emit gamma rays. These compounds have longer half-lives; therefore they eliminate the need for an on-site cyclotron. The nursing management is essentially the same as for the PET scan.

Myelography

Myelography is an invasive procedure involving the injection of air or contrast media into the lumbar subarachnoid space via a lumbar puncture. After the medium is injected fluoroscopy, conventional radiographs or CT scans are used to visualize selected areas. The spinal subarachnoid space is assessed for obstructions, compression, or herniated intervertebral discs.

Nursing Management

Explain the procedure to patient. Inform patient that the test is performed with him or her lying on an examination table that tilts. Encourage oral fluid intake. Patient is to empty his or her bladder before the test starts. Baseline assessment includes vital signs and neurological status. Administer premedication as ordered.

The patient is placed in the lateral recumbent position with knees flexed. Using sterile technique, the practitioner inserts a hollow-core needle into the subarachnoid space usually at L3–L4 or L4–L5. The selected contrast medium (e.g., air, oil-based, or water-based) is injected. Images are generated by the selected scanner.

Maintain strict bedrest for a few hours as ordered. Encourage oral fluids. Monitor and compare vital sign and neurological assessment to baseline findings. Administer analgesia as needed (Daniels, 2004).

Electrographic Studies

There are several electrographic diagnostic studies that are valuable tests to explore the specific pathologies of diseases. These tests involve either magnetic fields or bioelectric waves produced in the body. The electromagnetic tests measure and record bioelectrical impulses in the body. The brain, heart, nerves, and muscles all produce electrical impulses that can be diagnostic for many different conditions. They prove to be important in the different choices that practitioners have in diagnosing disorders.

Electroencephalography

Electroencephalography (EEG) is a noninvasive method of evaluating the electrical activity of the cerebral hemispheres. This activity is measured be electrodes attached to the scalp. The EEG is used to identify areas of abnormal electrical discharge in the cerebral cortex. There are a wide variety of conditions that an abnormal EEG can identify, for example, seizure activity, tumors, cerebrovascular disease, degenerative brain disease, drug intoxication, or brain death (Ives, 2005).

Nursing Management

Inform the patient that the test is painless and there is no danger of electrical shock. Discuss the purpose and procedure of the test with the patient. Withhold caffeine, tobacco, and alcohol-containing products for 24 hours before the scheduled test. The patient is not to be NPO. Hair should be freshly shampooed, clean, and free of hairpins, sprays, or oils.

CNS depressants and stimulants should be withheld for 24 hours before the test. If a sleep deprived EEG is ordered, the patient should be kept awake from approximately 2 a.m. When anticonvulsants are to be held before the test, the nurse should monitor for any seizure activity.

Either a recliner-type chair or a bed is used to maximize patient comfort. This helps to reduce the need for position changes during testing. Patient movement can interfere with the EEG recording. Electrodes are applied to the patients scalp using a colloidal gel or paste. The patient must lie still during the baseline recording. The remainder of the test involves following directions for various activities: hyperventilation, photo stimulation, or sleep. Hyperventilation by the patient involves breathing deeply 20 to 30 times per minute, for three minutes. This causes cerebral vasoconstriction and alkalosis, which increases the possibility of seizure activity. Photo stimulation uses a strobe light. The patient looks directly at the light, which flashes with varying frequency (1 to 20 flashes per second). This is then repeated with the eyes closed. If the patient's seizures are triggered by changing light frequencies, the EEG will record the location of the activity. Sleep can be natural or induced by the administration of IV sedation. Temporal lobe epilepsy can be demonstrated best during sleep.

The standard test usually takes 40 to 60 minutes to complete. It is preferred that the test be done in the department where external stimuli can be controlled. During administration of the test, all patient movement is recorded, because this can affect the test results. The EEG can be done with portable machinery, but it is more difficult to control the external stimuli. Sleep study EEGs are usually in a video monitored, controlled environment. Instruct patient to wash hair to remove the electrode glue. Administer any medications that were held for the test. Sleep deprivation patients may require a nap.

Magnetoencephalography

Magnetoencephalography (MEG) is similar to an EEG but with the addition of a biomagnetometer. This highly sensitive machine has a passive sensor, which detects small magnetic fields generated by neural activity. It measures both extracranial and scalp electrical fields. It can accurately detect the location of a seizure, stroke, or injury. The nursing management for magnetoencephalography is essentially the same as for an EEG.

Electromyography

Electromyography (EMG) measures the electrical activity of the peripheral nerves by testing muscle activity. An EMG can be performed on specific areas of the muscles throughout the body. For example, an upper EMG would be implemented on the arms and could identify areas of decreased electrical activity associated with various neurological degenerative disorders.

Nursing Management

Explain the procedure to the patient. Inform him or her that there is slight discomfort associated with the insertion of needles into the skin where the test is performed. The patient does not need to be NPO. After making the patient comfortable, the technician cleans the body areas to be tested. Then he or she inserts sterile needles that measure the electrical activity of specific nerve pathways. No follow-up care is required.

Evoked Potentials

Evoked potential (EP) testing measures the electrical activity of nerve conduction along the sensory nerve pathways. Sensors are placed on the skin and scalp and then connected to a computer, which analyzes the incoming data and generates waveforms to depict the electrical activity (Table 34-10 for a description of each type of EPs). The nursing management EP testing is essentially the same as EEG.

Ultrasound

Ultrasound studies use sound waves to produce an image of internal organs, tissue, or fetuses. The sound waves are high frequency and inaudible to the human ear, with a frequency of higher than 20,000 cycles/second (normal human hearing is between 16,000 and 20,000 cycles/second). The ultrasound waves bounce back from the body tissues, producing echoes that the transducer records and displays on a monitor as a picture or into audible sound, which is known as the Doppler method. There are a wide variety of these types of tests and they are relatively noninvasive but are somewhat expensive in practice.

Carotid Duplex Studies

Carotid duplex scanning is a noninvasive method of evaluating for carotid occlusive disease. It is the combination of ultrasound with pulsed Doppler technology. The ultrasound signal is reflected off the moving blood cells and is registered as blood velocity. Stenosis of a blood vessel is indicated when there is increased velocity.

TABLE 34-10 Evoked Potential Types

TYPE	STIMULUS	PURPOSE
Visual		
Visual evoked potential (VEP)	Rapidly changing geometric designs or flashing lights	Locate lesion in visual pathway or visual cortex
Pattern reversal electrical potential (PREP)		
Visual electrical response (VER)		
Auditory		
Auditory evoked potential (AEP)	Multiple clicks to each ear via earphones	Locate lesion; evaluate the central auditory pathways of the brainstem; follow the course of recovery
Auditory brainstem evoked potential (ABEP)		
Somatosensory		
Somatosensory brainstem evoked potential (SBEP)	Electrical stimulation of selected peripheral nerves	Differentiate lesions of the peripheral nerve from those of subcortical or cortical central sensory pathways
Somatosensory evoked potential (SEP)		

Adapted from Daniels, R. (2003). Delmar's manual of laboratory and diagnostic tests. New York: Thomson Delmar Learning.

Nursing Management

Explain the procedure to patient. Patient does not need to be NPO. After the patient is taken to the testing area, he or she is made comfortable on a bed. The technician uses the ultrasound probe, placed on the carotid artery of either side of the neck, to evaluate the blood flow velocity of the blood vessels. A gel is used to enhance the sound. No specific follow-up care is required. The patient may want to wash his or her neck.

Transcranial Doppler Sonography

Transcranial Doppler (TCD) uses the same technology as carotid duplex studies. It records the velocities of the intracranial blood vessels. TCD is a noninvasive method of assessing: vasospasm associated with subarachnoid hemorrhage and altered intracranial blood flow dynamics related to occlusive vascular disease, cerebral autoregulation, the presence of emboli, and brain death.

Nursing Management

Explain the procedure to patient. Restriction of food or fluids is not required. The equipment is similar to the carotid Doppler. In this procedure, the probe is placed on the skin at various windows of the skull. These areas have a thin bony covering. The temporal, orbital, and suboccipital sites are used. The ultrasound signal is recorded as a wave velocities indicate narrowing or occlusion. A gel is used to enhance the signal. No specific follow-up care is required. The patient may want to wash off the gel residue.

KEY CONCEPTS

- The CNS consists of the brain and spinal cord.
- The PNS consists of the cranial nerves, the spinal nerves, and the ANS.
- Neurons transmit or conduct nerve impulses.
- The initiation of a nerve impulse involves the generation of an action potential.
- Neurotransmitters are chemical substances that inhibit, excite, or modify the responses.
- The brain is composed of the cerebrum, the brainstem, and the cerebellum.
- The spinal cord is the conduit for the ascending sensory and descending motor neurons.
- There are four ventricles (or chambers) within the brain and are filled with CSF and are linked by ducts that permit circulation.
- Functions of the cerebellum include coordinating voluntary muscle movement, equilibrium, and maintenance of trunk stability.
- The blood-brain barrier maintains a functionally stable environment for the CNS.
- The spinal cord extends from the medulla to the level of the first lumbar vertebrae.
- The PNS is composed of the spinal nerves, cranial nerves, and the ANS.

- The cranial nerves provide both motor and sensory innervation for the head, neck, and viscera.
- The ANS has two, semi-independent components: sympathetic and parasympathetic.
- Subtle changes in mental status are one of the earliest indicators of a potential neurological event.
- Evaluation of cerebellar function requires the assessment of coordination, balance, posture, and gait.
- Neurodiagnostic tests are performed as adjuncts to a complete history and physical examination.
- LP is the most common method for obtaining CSF.
- fMRI is used to identify changes in cerebral metabolism or blood flow.
- Cerebral angiography is an invasive series of radiographic studies involving the injection of contrast media.
- PET provides a three-dimensional structural and functional view of the brain.
- Myelogram is an invasive procedure involving the injection of air or contrast media into the lumbar subarachnoid space via a lumbar puncture.
- EMG measures the electrical activity of the peripheral nerves by testing muscle activity.

REVIEW QUESTIONS

1. When grading muscle strength, a score of 1 indicates:
   1. No muscle contraction
   2. Trace of contraction
   3. Active movement with gravity eliminated
   4. Normal strength

2. What instructions should the nurse give to the patient when performing the Romberg test?
   1. Close your eyes and remain still
   2. Place your index finger on your nose
   3. Jump in place
   4. Walk heel to toe

3. The patient who has difficulty choosing the right words and responds hesitantly is displaying symptoms of:
   1. Agnosia
   2. Homonymous hemianopsia
   3. Expressive aphasia
   4. Ataxia

4. When the nurse stimulates Babinski's sign in an adult, the big toe moves upward and the other toes fan out. This finding indicates:
   1. Normal neurological functioning
   2. Upper motor neuron disease
   3. Lower motor neuron disease
   4. Spinothalamic tract lesion

5. The ability to recognize an object's shape is known as:
   1. Graphesthesia
   2. Discrimination
   3. Stereognosis
   4. Visceroptosis

6. Paralysis of lateral gaze indicates a lesion of cranial nerve:
   1. II
   2. III
   3. IV
   4. VI

7. Stimulation of the parasympathetic nervous system results in:
   1. Dilation of skin blood vessels
   2. Decreased secretion of insulin
   3. Increased blood glucose levels
   4. Relaxation of the urinary sphincters

8. When preparing a patient for an EEG, the nurse should include which of the following statements?
   1. Do not take any food or fluids for six hours prior to the test.
   2. You must remain absolutely still during the test.
   3. Inform the technician if you are allergic to shellfish or iodine.
   4. Bright lights will be used during the procedure.

9. The consensual pupillary response is tested by:
   1. Asking the patient if he or she has trouble closing his or her eyes
   2. Directing a light toward one eye and observing the pupil on the opposite side
   3. Instructing the patient to cover one while you observe the opposite eye for extraocular movements
   4. Evaluating the ability of the patient's eyes to converge

10. One way to test the vestibular function of the acoustic nerve (CN VIII) is to:
    1. Check the auditory studies
    2. Ask if the patient experiences dizziness
    3. Have the patient shrug his or her shoulders
    4. Rub your fingers together near the patient's ears.

11. Which technique is recommended for eliciting a response to peripheral pain?
    1. Sternal rub
    2. Trapezius muscle squeeze
    3. Nail bed pressure
    4. Mandibular pressure

12. Cerebrospinal fluid (CSF) is reabsorbed into the venous system via the:
    1. Arachnoid villi
    2. Aqueduct of Sylvius
    3. Foramen of Monro
    4. Choroid plexuses

13. What is the significance of the blood-brain barrier?
    1. It is thought to result from increased capillary permeability.
    2. It allows drugs to diffuse freely from the interstitial space to the intravascular space.
    3. It limits the transmission of substances from the blood to the brain.
    4. Its disruption is rare in head-injured patients.

REVIEW ACTIVITIES

1. Identify the three neurotransmitters found in the basal ganglia and describe their impact on motor function.

2. Compare and contrast the sympathetic and parasympathetic divisions of the autonomic nervous system.

3. List the six major portions of the physical assessment of the neurological system.

4. Identify your priority nursing interventions when preparing your patient to have a CT scan.

5. Observe several neurological diagnostic studies in the practicum setting.

Dysfunction of the Brain: Nursing Management

CHAPTER 35

Beth Hickey, RN, MSN, CRRN, CNA

Carrie A. McCoy, PhD, MSPH, RN, CEN

CHAPTER TOPICS

- Cerebrovascular Accidents
- Brain Injuries
- Brain Tumors

The brain is the central processing unit of the body, similar to what is found in a computer. However, the brain works faster and better than any computer. It houses vast amounts of information throughout the life process. However, when there is a disruption in brain function, there are serious consequences. In this chapter, the nursing management of patients suffering from cerebrovascular accidents ([CVA] strokes), brain injuries, and brain tumors will be discussed.

KEY TERMS

Aneurysm
Aphasia
Cerebrovascular accident ([CVA] stroke)
Concussion
Contracture
Cushing response
Dysarthria
Dysphagia
Emboli
Expressive aphasia (Broca's aphasia)
Global aphasia
Hemiparesis
Hemiplegia
Hemorrhagic stroke
Homonymous hemianopsia
Intracranial pressure (ICP)
Ischemic stroke
Primary brain tumor
Receptive aphasia (Wernicke's aphasia)
Stereotactic radiotherapy (SRS)
Subarachnoid hemorrhage
Thrombus
Transient ischemic attack (TIA)

CEREBROVASCULAR ACCIDENTS OR STROKES

In the United States, every 45 seconds someone has a stroke, every three minutes someone dies from a stroke, and 700,000 new or recurrent strokes occur each year (American Heart Association [AHA], 2003). Strokes are the third leading cause of death in the United States, behind heart disease and cancer, and are the leading cause of long-term disability. Epidemiological studies have determined that 11 states in the Southeast (Alabama, Arkansas, Georgia, Indiana, Kentucky, Louisiana, Mississippi, North Carolina, South Carolina, Tennessee, and Virginia) have a 10 percent higher rate of stroke deaths than anywhere else in the United States (Steefel, 2004).

Epidemiology

Strokes also are a health concern worldwide. According to the World Health Organization ([WHO], 2004b), 5.5 million people died from a stroke, making strokes the second leading cause of death worldwide; the first is ischemic heart disease. In terms of disability, strokes rank seventh as a leading cause of disability worldwide and are estimated to move up to fourth by the year 2020 (WHO, 2004b). The countries with the highest mortality rate per 100,000 people are Russia, Romania, and Bulgaria (AHA, 2003).

A **cerebrovascular accident (CVA),** or **stroke,** occurs when a part of the brain is damaged due to a lack of blood flow. The term brain attack has recently been developed by the AHA in an effort to reinforce the importance of knowing the early warning signs (Box 35-1) and seeking medical attention quickly.

There are two main types of stroke, **ischemic stroke** (damage to the brain due to a clogged artery) and **hemorrhagic stroke** (when a blood vessel burst leaking blood into brain tissue or surrounding spaces). An ischemic stroke occurs when a blood vessel to the brain becomes clogged, and brain tissue supplied by that blood vessel begins to die. Approximately 88 percent of all strokes are ischemic in nature, and 8 to 12 percent of all patients die within 30 days of an ischemic stroke (AHA, 2003). Ischemic strokes are caused by either a **thrombus** (a blood clot that blocks a blood vessel) or an **emboli** (a blood clot or other particle plaque that breaks loose and blocks blood vessels). A blood clot may develop because of atherosclerosis, which is a buildup of plaque within a vessel wall. This affects blood flow and causes platelet aggregation, thus forming a clot. An embolic stroke occurs when a blood clot or other particle (e.g., atherosclerotic plaque) breaks loose from a vessel wall and occludes a smaller blood vessel in the brain.

A hemorrhagic stroke occurs when a blood vessel in the brain ruptures, leaking blood directly into the brain tissue or surrounding spaces. While only 12 percent of all strokes are hemorrhagic in nature, 38 percent of patients with hemorrhagic strokes die within 30 days (AHA, 2003). One type of hemorrhagic stroke is called a **subarachnoid hemorrhage** (blood that leaks into the subarachnoid space). This type of hemorrhage is caused by bleeding between the arachnoid meninges covering the brain and the skull, but blood does not invade the brain tissue. An intracerebral hemorrhage occurs when blood enters the brain tissue after a blood vessel ruptures. This can be caused by an **aneurysm** (a weakness in a blood vessel wall) or arteriovenous malformation (Soderman, Andersson, Karlsson, Wallace, & Edner, 2003). The different types of cerebral hemorrhage and management of cerebral hemorrhage will be discussed in greater detail in the section on head injuries.

BOX 35-1

MODIFIABLE RISK FACTORS FOR STROKE DEVELOPMENT

- Hypertension—this is determined by any consistent blood pressure reading above 140/90. Diet changes, medication, and stress management can affect hypertension.
- Hypercholesterolemia—high cholesterol is determined by a blood cholesterol level greater than 240 mg/dL. Dietary changes and medication can influence these levels. High cholesterol also can lead to atherosclerosis.
- Atherosclerosis—is a buildup of plaque in the walls of blood vessels. This plaque can break off, causing an embolic stroke or narrow a blood vessel leading to a thrombotic stroke.
- Atrial fibrillation—is when the upper chambers of the heart do not beat effectively. This causes blood to pool in the chambers and can lead to clot formation. These clots then are released into the blood system and can lead to a stroke. A person with atrial fibrillation is five times more likely to develop a stroke (AHA, 2003). A physician should evaluate atrial fibrillation for the appropriate treatment options. Medications, such as anticoagulants, can be used to decrease this risk factor.
- Obesity—being overweight places additional stress on the body and is usually associated with an inactive lifestyle. Getting into a regular exercise routine and eating properly can address this risk factor.
- Smoking—causes a decrease in oxygenation of the body. This can lead to damage to the blood vessel walls making a stroke more likely to occur.
- Drugs and alcohol—certain illegal drugs (e.g., cocaine and amphetamines), alcohol abuse, and prescribed medications (e.g., birth control pills) can increase the risk of a stroke. Birth control pills are especially risky if the person continues to smoke. Patients should be aware of any medication that may increase their risk of a stroke.
- Other health problems—diabetes and sickle cell anemia are also risk factors for stroke development. Diabetes is a consistent fasting blood sugar above 120 mg/dL. Diabetes affects the vascular system and can have devastating effects. It is important to assist patients with diabetes to properly manage their disease process. With sickle cell anemia, the red blood cells are shaped in the form of a sickle and are less able to carry oxygen to the tissues. These sickle cells can adhere to the lining of the blood vessel walls and form clots (AHA, 2003). Riddington & Wang (2002) reviewed studies evaluating the effectiveness of blood transfusions in the management of sickle cell anemia; they concluded that the risks associated with the blood transfusions caused concerns about the side effects outweighing the benefits of the treatment and noted further research was indicated.
- **Transient ischemic attacks (TIAs)**—are caused by a temporary loss of blood supply to a part of the brain that results in a temporary loss of function. These deficits resolve within 24 hours. They may also be called ministrokes and are a strong predictor of an impending stroke.

Etiology

There are many risk factors associated with a stroke. There are both modifiable and nonmodifiable risk factors (see chapter 24) (Box 35-2). In addition, the combination of these risk factors contributes greatly to the cause of CVAs.

Many people have multiple risk factors. This is why it is so important to educate patients about the risk factors that can be changed. The more risk factors

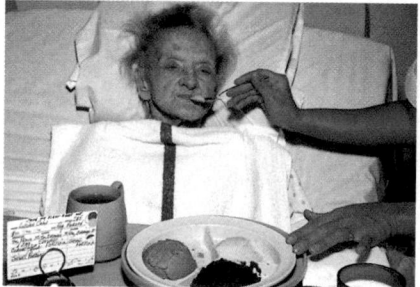

Figure 35-1 This patient with a stroke has multiple risk factors, which adds to her poor prognosis.

a patient has, the higher the likelihood that they will have a stroke in their lifetime (Figure 35-1).

Pathophysiology

To understand the effects of a stroke, it is important to understand what happens to the brain tissue when a stroke occurs. Normally the brain receives blood flow at 60 to 70 mL/100 g of brain tissue/minute, but when that rate is slowed to 25 mL, loss of function begins to occur due to lack of aerobic metabolism. If blood flow is not restored soon, cell death begins to occur. Within a few minutes of blood supply loss, a necrotic core develops. The necrotic core is tissue deprived of oxygen that is permanently damaged. The tissue surrounding the necrotic core, the ischemic penumbra, may continue to survive for a short time even though blood flow has been reduced. The focus of medical management is maintaining blood flow to the ischemic penumbra (Felberg & Naidech, 2003). The location of the tissue damage and the availability of collateral circulation help determine the patient's prognosis. For a more detailed description of the cellular changes that take place as brain tissue becomes anoxic, see the section on head injuries.

Assessment with Clinical Manifestations

The nurse must have keen assessment skills to appropriately assess and manage a stroke patient. The nurse should determine:
- Past medical history—this is important to determine if the patient might have any risk factors or other medical conditions that would affect treatment.
- Current medications—this is important if the patient is taking a medication that would interfere with treatment (e.g., anticoagulants).
- Symptom onset and progression—this is the most important factor, because it affects treatment options and is a factor in differentiating between an ischemic stroke and a hemorrhagic stroke. Patients with ischemic strokes may report a variety of symptoms depending on the location of the stroke; however, if a patient complains of a severe headache with rapid onset, this may be an indication of a hemorrhagic stroke. Some of the most common symptoms of ischemic stroke include weakness or paralysis on one side of the body, inability to maintain balance, blurred vision, dizziness, slurred speech, inability to concentrate, memory deficits, incontinence, fatigue, double vision, and headache. The nurse must remember that each patient may present with slightly different symptoms, because of the part of the brain that has been affected, but quick and effective management of a stroke can mean the difference between a patient returning to functional independence or lifelong disability or death.

Diagnostic Tests

Many diagnostic tools are available for patients suffering from a stroke. But many of these tools take time, which is critical when managing an acute stroke. The most common tool used to diagnose a stroke is a computed tomography (CT) scan. It is widely available in most hospitals and is an important tool to differentiate between ischemic strokes and hemorrhagic strokes. The CT scan can be read immediately, and treatment can begin quickly. The CT scan is done without contrast dye and does not require any preparation on the part of the patient (e.g., nothing by mouth [NPO] or intravenous [IV] access). A magnetic resonance imaging (MRI) may also be ordered, but MRI scans take longer, between 45 minutes and two hours. While an MRI allows the radiologist better imaging of blood vessels and brain tissue, it is contraindicated in patients with metal implants or pacemakers and patients who are claustrophobic.

Laboratory tests will be ordered to assist in diagnosis and to determine treatment options. The most common laboratory tests ordered will include: complete blood count (CBC), electrolytes, blood urea nitrogen (BUN), creatinine (Cr), prothrombin time (PT), and partial prothrombin time (PTT). Other tests may be ordered depending on other presenting symptoms. See Table 35-1 for a list of other tests that may be utilized in the diagnosis and treatment of a stroke.

Nursing Diagnoses

Based on the information gathered, examples of nursing diagnoses in the patient with a CVA may include the following:

- Impaired verbal communication related to different types of aphasia from the CVA.
- Disturbed sensory perception related to the neurological damage from the CVA.
- Impaired physical mobility related to the hemiparesis caused by the CVA.
- Risk for caregiver role strain related to the chronic nature of the resulting CVA.
- Risk for situational low self-esteem related to the variety of changes from the CVA.

Planning and Implementation

The goal of stroke management is to restore function and independence. This is done in with four different management areas: pharmacology, prevention, emergency management, and surgical intervention. The best outcome for

TABLE 35-1 Stroke Diagnostic Tests	
NAME OF TEST	**REASON**
Computerized tomography (CT) scan	Usually the first test done, because it can be done quickly and is readily accessible in most facilities.
	Used to differentiate between hemorrhagic and ischemic stroke
Magnetic resonance imaging (MRI)	Is more sensitive than a CT scan and is detailed in identifying small vessel strokes.
Magnetic resonance angiography (MRA)	Noninvasive test that allows imaging of the blood vessels.
	Especially helpful in determining collateral circulation.
Carotid ultrasound	Determines blood flow to the brain.
	Can detect atherosclerotic buildup.
Nuclear brain scan (cerebral angiography)	Areas of decreased blood flow will have less uptake of the radioactive dye and show damaged tissues.
Transcranial Doppler (TCD)	Noninvasive ultrasound, portable
	Assesses blood flow in cerebral vessels
Electroencephalogram (EEG)	If significant brain tissue involvement, may have little to no brain activity.
Evoked responses	In the area of the brain that is injured, the patient will have a decreased response to the stimuli.
Positive emission tomography (PET) scanning	Determines brain tissue functioning

Adapted from Stanford Stroke Awareness. (2002). Stroke awareness Part II: Diagnosis and treatment options. *Retrieved June 13, 2006, from www.stanford.edu.*

stroke management is not to have one. Prevention and early access to health care are vital to decreasing the number of strokes. In the Healthy People 2010 report (U.S. Department of Health and Human Services, 2002), one of the objectives is to decrease the number of stroke deaths and increase the public's awareness of the signs of a stroke. One of the biggest components to prevention is education. The AHA is playing an important role by having the warning signs of a stroke incorporated into all of their cardiopulmonary resuscitation (CPR) educational training. They have also associated the name stroke with brain attack; making it similar to a heart attack. This was done to encourage people to recognize the importance of seeking medical attention immediately. Many people still do not recognize the warning signs of a stroke and try to lie down, thinking that they will feel better when they get up. This is a serious problem, because delay in seeking health care can lead to devastating results.

Pharmacology

In addition to education, several medications are effective in preventing a stroke. These medications are anticoagulants, antiplatelets, and neuroprotective agents. Anticoagulants, usually heparin and warfarin (Coumadin), are given to prevent blood from clotting. Anticoagulation is especially important for patients with atrial fibrillation (King & LeMaire, 2002). According to the Agency for Health Care Policy and Research (Cohen & De LaMare, 2002), atrial fibrillation causes an estimated 80,000 strokes per year. The increased use of anticoagulant therapy, from 58 to 71 percent, has prevented 1,285 stokes. Antiplatelet medications are used to prevent platelets from clumping together, also known as platelet aggregation, and blocking blood vessels. When a blood vessel is injured, it is normal for the body to send platelets to an area to begin the healing process, but when too many platelets arrive, they can decrease blood flow to the tissues distal to the clot. Antiplatelet agents decrease the number of platelets in the blood stream. Antiplatelet medications include aspirin (acetsalicylic acid) and ticlopidine (Ticlid). Neuroprotective agents have been the focus of many clinical trials over the past few years. According to the National Stroke Association ([NSA], 2006), the objective of these drugs is to decrease the damage to the brain at the necrotic core caused by the ischemic cascade. However, there have been more than 49 different agents studied in over 114 trails without promising results (Murphy, 2003). Some drugs currently being investigated are glutamate antagonists, calcium antagonists, opiate antagonists, gamma-aminobutyric acid–A (GABA-A) agonists, calpain inhibitors, kinase inhibitors, and antioxidants (Beresford, Parsons, & Hunter 2003; Wahlgren & Ahmed, 2004). Investigation of neuroprotective agents will continue to be a focus of research in the future.

Emergency Management

In the emergent phase of a stroke it is important for the patient to seek health care attention immediately. Some hospitals have set up stroke teams or a stroke code, which alerts health care providers of a patient who is being admitted for a possible ischemic stroke. Having health care providers who are experts in the diagnosis and management of a stroke can help to expedite treatment and save valuable time, potentially improving patient outcome. It is also important to note that other neurological disorders, such as migraine headaches, epilepsy, syncope, peripheral nerve disorders, intracranial tumors or abscess, subdural hematoma, and metabolic disorders, such as hypoglycemia, may present with symptoms that are similar to those of a stroke. It is vital that the health care team be able to differentiate between these disorders and those of a stroke to accurately administer treatment (Adams, et al., 2003; Institute for Clinical Systems Improvement [ICSI], 2003).

According to the ICSI (2003), tissue plasminogen activator (tPA), which is a drug that helps to break up blood clots, should be administered to appropriate candidates within 60 minutes of the patient presenting to the ED. To achieve this goal, the health care team must work quickly and efficiently to appropriately diagnose the patient. The ED nurse should start the rapid triage protocol. Many hospitals may have a clinical pathway or care map (Figure 35-2) that can

Red Flag

The Priority Care for the Patient with an Acute Stroke Condition

Most stroke patients will be admitted through the emergency department (ED). In the acute phase, the nurse is responsible for management of the ABCs, (airway, breathing, and cardiopulmonary support). The patient may need to be assisted with airway management if his or her ability to swallow has been impaired, because he or she is at risk for aspiration of his or her saliva. Also, he or she will have a lot of anxiety and fear over his or her lack of ability to control his or her body. He or she may be confused or lethargic. Safety will be a major concern. The nurse should seek family support and involvement to stay with the patient to keep him or her calm. This also helps to decrease the family anxiety level if they can assist in care.

ST. JOSEPH'S HOSPITAL
E.D. DIAGNOSTIC & TREATMENT PROCESS FOR THROMBOLYTIC THERAPY FOR STROKE PATIENTS

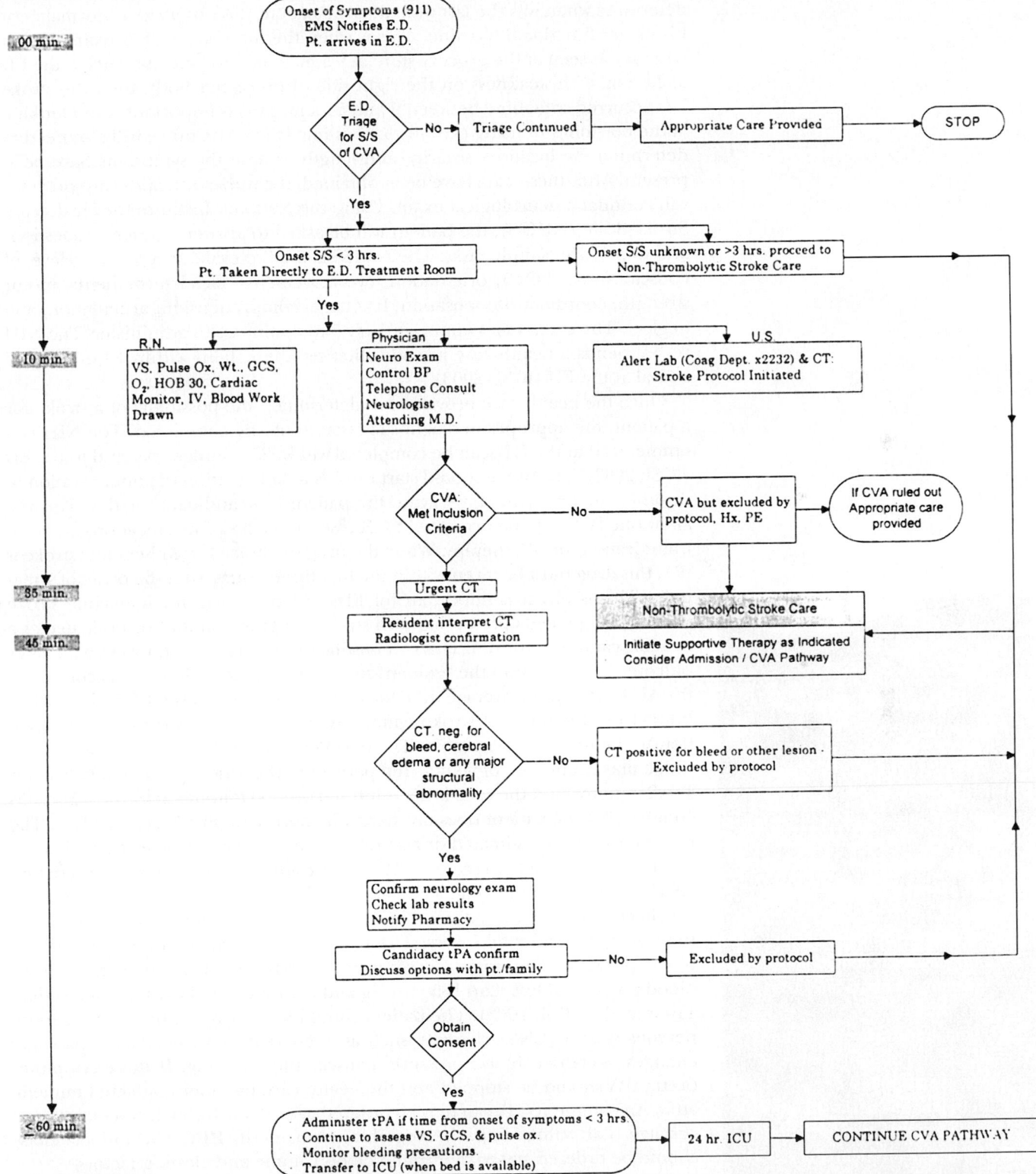

Figure 35-2 St. Joseph's Hospital emergency department diagnostic and treatment process for thrombolytic therapy for stroke patients care map. Courtesy of St. Joseph's Regional Medical Center.

be used to guide patient care in the ED. Patients that present to the ED within three hours of the onset of symptoms should be considered emergent, taken to a treatment room immediately, and the physician notified.

A history of when the symptoms began will be critical. The nurse should determine when was the last time that the patient was observed as normal or at his or her functional baseline. This is when the time begins. For example, if a patient was seen at the grocery store at 9 a.m. and he or she presents to the ED at 11 a.m. with weakness on the right side of his or her body, then the stroke has occurred sometime between 9 and 11 a.m. This is important when looking at the possibility of using certain clot busting drugs. The nurse will also need to determine the location, severity, and length of time the symptoms have been present. After these data have been obtained, the nurse or health care provider will conduct a neurological exam. Using the National Institute for Healthcare Stroke Scale (NIHSS), the patient will be asked to answer a series of questions and to perform simple tasks. The NIHSS is used to evaluate a patient's level of consciousness (LOC), orientation, eye movements, facial movements, motor strength, coordination, sensation, language, comprehension, articulation, and neglect. The exam takes approximately 5 to 8 minutes to administer. The NIH recommends a health care provider first see the patient within 10 minutes of arrival at the ED (ICSI, 2003).

Once the health care provider has determined the possibility of a stroke for a patient, the appropriate diagnostic tests should be completed. The NIH recommends that the CT scan be completed within 25 minutes of arrival to the ED (ICSI, 2003). The nurse should start two IVs in anticipation of administration of thromboembolytic therapy in case the patient is a candidate for tPA. This will allow one IV line to be dedicated to tPA. See Table 35-2 for indications and contraindication for tPA therapy. While the drug of choice for an ischemic stroke is tPA, this drug must be given within the first three hours from the onset of symptoms. This is why it is important for EDs to have a plan for managing stroke patients. All patients presenting with stroke symptoms should be evaluated as a possible candidate for tPA. This clot busting drug can greatly improve a patient's outcome if given within the "golden" three hour window. However, according to the AHA (2003), the average time for a patient to arrive in the ED is three to six hours from the onset of stroke symptoms. The goal of tPA is to restore blood flow to the ischemic penumbra. The dosing for tPA is 0.9 mg/kg intravenously, with a maximum dose of 90 mg. Ten percent of the dose is given in a bolus over 1 to 2 minutes, and the remainder is infused over 60 minutes after the CT results confirm that the patient does not have a hemorrhagic stroke (ICSI, 2003). The nurse must get an estimated or accurate weight to properly dose the patient.

After the patient has received tPA, they are admitted to an intensive care unit (ICU) for close monitoring. The patient will require vital signs and neurological checks every 15 minutes for 2 hours, then every 30 minutes for 6 hours, and then every hour for 24 hours. The nurse should also monitor the patient's blood pressure. The goal, according to the NIH, is to maintain the systolic blood pressure at less than 185 mm Hg and diastolic blood pressure at less than 110 mm Hg (ICSI, 2003). The patient should be closely monitored for central nervous system (CNS) changes, such as decreased LOC, headache, papillary changes, increased blood pressure, nausea, and vomiting. If these symptoms occur, tPA should be stopped and the health care provider contacted immediately. An emergent CT scan may be ordered to evaluate for an intracranial hemorrhage. Lab values (e.g., hemoglobin, hematocrit, PTT, PT, and platelets) should be ordered stat to determine blood volume and clotting factors.

For patients, with an ischemic stroke who are not candidates for tPA, aspirin should be given immediately, except when contraindicated (Klijn & Hankey, 2003). Heparin should be started at 800 to 1,200 units per hour to maintain a PTT between one-and-a-half to two times the patient's baseline.

All acute stroke patients should have close monitoring of blood pressure, hyperthermia, and glucose levels. The goal is to manage the blood pressure.

Red Flag

Nursing Care of a Patient Receiving tPA

A patient who has received tPA must be monitored closely and should be in an ICU or acute stroke unit. These patients are at high risk for intracerebral hemorrhage. Other important interventions are:

- No aspirin, antiplatelets, or anticoagulants should be given for 24 hours after tPA has infused.
- Avoid any invasive procedures (IC or intra-arterial devices or nasogastric tubes)
- Neurological checks should be done every 15 min for 2 hours
- If the patient's neurological status deteriorates, assume an intracranial bleed and notify a physician immediately

TABLE 35-2 Clinical Indications and Contraindications for tPA in Stroke Patients

Indications	Acute onset of neurological symptoms
	Onset less than three hours
	18 years or older
	No evidence of cerebral hemorrhage, sulcal edema, or swelling on CT scan
Clinical contraindications	Onset of stroke greater than three hours
	Rapid improvement of symptoms
	Mild stroke symptoms
	Obtunded or comatose state (involving middle cerebral artery stroke)
	Seizure activity at stroke onset or within three hour window prior to tPA
	Symptoms suggesting subarachnoid hemorrhage
	Uncontrolled hypertension (systolic blood pressure greater than 185 mm Hg or diastolic blood pressure greater than 110 mm Hg)
	Less than 18 years old
History contraindications	Minor ischemic stroke within 30 days
	Major ischemic stroke or head trauma within last three months
	History of intracerebral bleed
	Untreated cerebral aneurysm, arteriovenous malformation (AVM), or brain tumor
	GI or GU hemorrhage within last three weeks
	Lumbar puncture within last 3 days or arterial puncture (at noncompressible site) within last 7 days.
	Patients with international normalized ratio (INR) greater than 1.7 and taking oral anticoagulants
	Patients receiving heparin within last 48 hours and with elevated activated partial thromboplastin time (aPTT)
	Patients receiving low molecular weight heparin within last 24 hours
	Pregnant or anticipated pregnant female
	Known coagulation disorder
	Received tPA within last 7 days
Laboratory contraindications	Glucose less than 50 or greater than 400 mg/dL
	Platelet count less than 100,000 mm^3
	Prothrombin time greater than 15 or INR greater than 1.7
	Elevated APT
	Positive pregnancy test
Radiological contraindications	Intracranial hemorrhage
	Findings suggesting a new or evolving stroke
	Intracranial tumor, aneurysm, or AVM

Adapted from Institute for Clinical Systems Improvement. (2003). Diagnosis and initial treatment of ischemic stroke. Retrieved June 13, 2006, from www.guideline.gov.

The drugs of choice are labetalol (Normodyne) or enalapril (Vasotec). Based on current evidence-based practice, hyperthermia has been associated with poor outcomes in patients; therefore, the nurse should treat temperatures above 37.5° C (99.5° F) with Tylenol. For temperatures greater than 39.4° C (103° F), initiation of cooling blankets and ice packs should be warranted.

Managing hyperglycemia is also important. Avoid use of glucose in IV fluids and the use of corticosteroids, and monitor blood glucose levels frequently. Hyperglycemia should be treated with small dose subcutaneous insulin to prevent hypoglycemia (ICSI, 2003).

In the acute phase of stroke care, the nurse also initiates measures to prevent deep vein thrombosis (DVT) and other complications of immobility. Nursing care of the patient who has suffered a stroke will be discussed later in this chapter.

Surgery

For patients who have suffered an intracranial hemorrhage, the prognosis is generally poorer than that for patients who have sustained an ischemic stroke. Treatment for hemorrhagic stroke will depend on the location of the stroke and the blood vessels involved. Recent evidence suggests that in the case of hemorrhage into the ventricle of the brain, fibrinolytic agents injected into the ventricular system may dissolve the clot and improve outcomes (Lapointe & Haines, 2004). However this therapy still needs further investigation. Intraventricular bleeding can cause hydrocephalus, because the clot formed can block drainage of cerebrospinal fluid (CSF). When this complication occurs, a ventricular shunt is required to drain fluid. If the bleeding was caused by an aneurysm, a metal clip can be surgically inserted and placed over the aneurysm to prevent further bleeding. If the bleeding has formed a large clot (hematoma) that cannot be absorbed by the body,

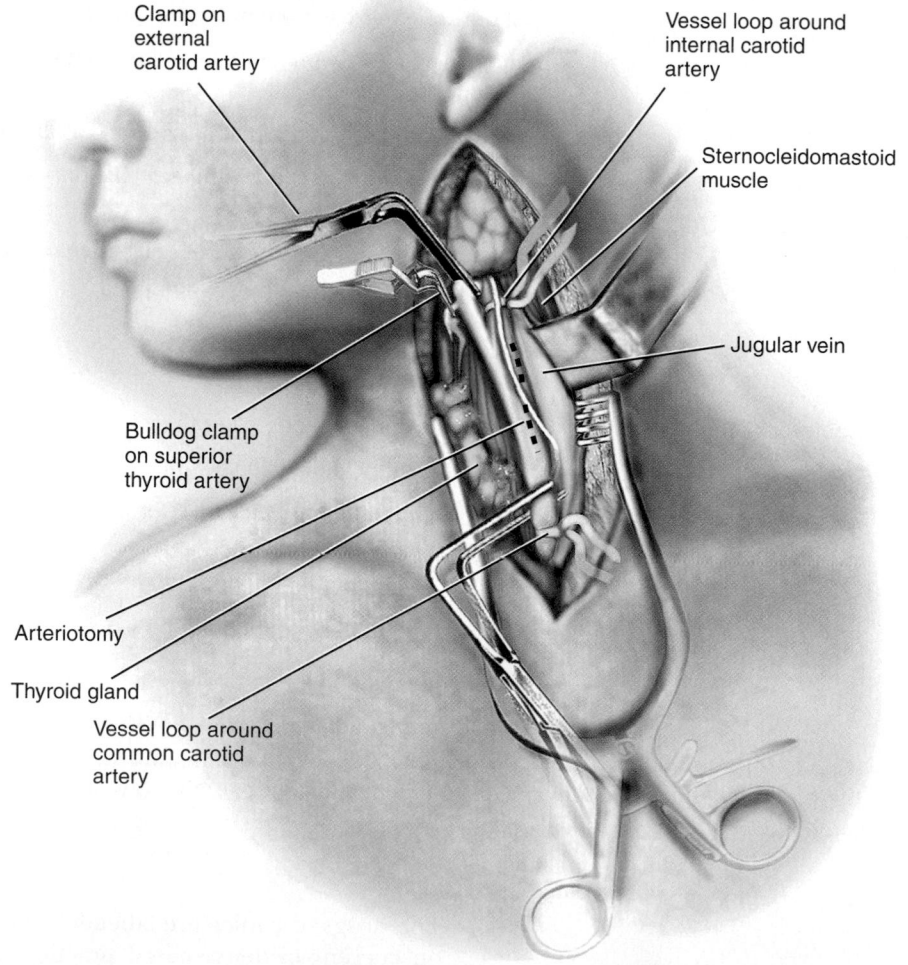

Figure 35-3 A carotid endarterectomy.

the patient may need to have the hematoma surgically removed. Some patients that develop hemorrhagic strokes have a condition called arteriovenous malformation (AVM). These are caused by errors in the development of the blood vessels in the brain that result in a localized arteriovenous shunt. About half of the patients with this condition are unaware that they have the condition until they have a hemorrhagic stroke. The risk of hemorrhage increases with the patient's age. AVMs are a significant risk factor for hemorrhagic strokes in young adults. Depending on the location and the size of the AVM, the patient may be a candidate for surgery, embolization, or radiosurgery (Soderman, et al., 2003).

Other surgical options include carotid endarterectomy to prevent stroke (Figure 35-3). Carotid endarterectomy is a surgical procedure that involves removing plaque from the carotid arteries. The surgeon creates an incision in the carotid artery and removes atherosclerotic plaque that has built up along the artery wall and impaired blood flow. In some cases, a stent is placed in the artery. Stenting is becoming a more popular option for patients with atherosclerotic buildup in the carotid arteries. While this procedure, also known as angioplasty with stent placement, has been done for many years in patients with coronary artery disease, it has only recently been approved for use in carotid arteries. Carotid stenting (Figure 35-4) involves placing a tiny balloon-tipped catheter into the carotid artery, inflating the balloon to improve blood flow, and then leaving a tiny mesh tube in place to keep the artery open (American Stroke Association, 2004; Coward, Featherstone, & Brown, 2004). With risks and complication rates similar to carotid endarterectomy, this procedure will most likely continue to gain popularity with health care providers and patients.

In patients who are ineligible for IV thrombolysis (tPA), catheter-based treatment may be an effective option. Catheter-based treatment involves local thrombolysis and or use of a balloon angioplasty or stenting (Ramee, Subramanian, Felberg, McKinley, Jenkins, Collins, et al., 2004). Ramee, et al. (2004) reported that 56 percent of patients in their study showed marked improvement in their NIHSS score, and 38 percent had independent survival at follow-up. This was a small study and needs further follow-up with larger clinical trials.

Evaluation of Outcomes

Potential patient outcomes for each of the example nursing diagnoses for the patient with the CVA are:

- Impaired verbal communication related to different types of aphasia from the CVA. The patient is able to use a form of communication to get needs met and to relate well with persons and environment.
- Disturbed sensory perception related to the neurological damage from the CVA. The patient achieves optimal functioning within the limits of physical impairments as evidenced by the ability to communicate effectively and to engage in meaningful activities.
- Impaired physical mobility related to the hemiparesis caused by the CVA. The patient performs physical activity independently or with whatever assistive devices are needed.
- Risk for caregiver role strain related to the chronic nature of the resulting CVA. The caregiver demonstrates competence and confidence in performing the caregiver role by meeting care that the patient requires.
- Risk for situational low self-esteem related to the variety of changes from the CVA. The patient recognizes, accepts, and verbalizes positive aspects of the self and his or her performance.

Following a stroke, patients may experience a vast array of complications. Following the initial ischemic episode cerebral hypoxia can result from poor

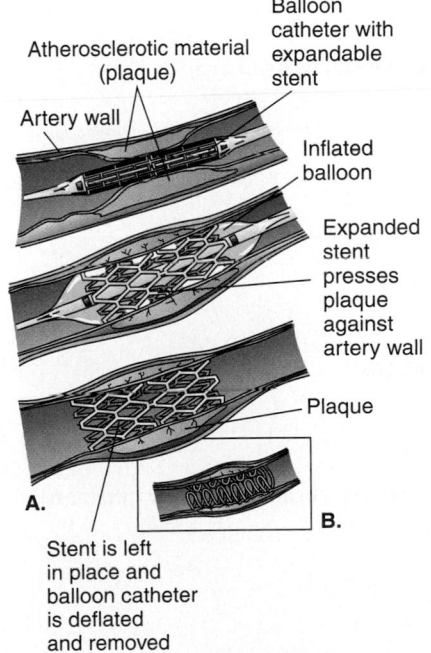

Atherosclerotic material (plaque)

Artery wall

Balloon catheter with expandable stent

Inflated balloon

Expanded stent presses plaque against artery wall

Plaque

A.

B.

Stent is left in place and balloon catheter is deflated and removed

Figure 35-4 Stenting and angioplasty.

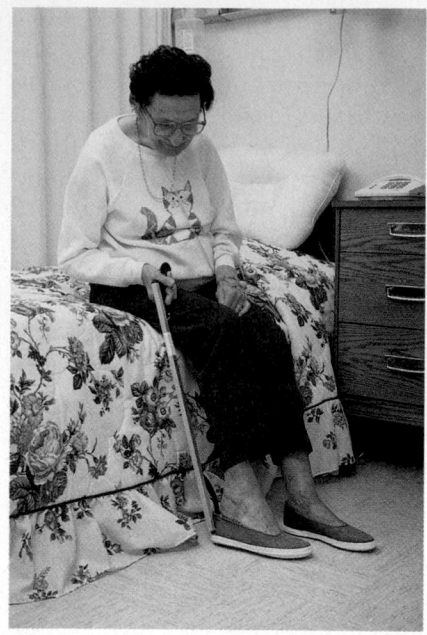

Figure 35-5 A patient in rehabilitation after having a stroke.

oxygenation, decreased cerebral perfusion, and vasospasm of cerebral vessels. The nurse plays a vital role in managing **intracranial pressure** ([ICP] the amount of pressure placed on the structures within the brain and promoting cerebral perfusion). In addition, the rehabilitation phase of care for the patient recovering from a stroke is complex (Figure 35-5). These issues will be discussed further in the brain-injured patient.

BRAIN INJURIES

According to the Centers for Disease Control and Prevention, 1.5 million individuals sustain brain injuries annually and another 5.3 million currently live with permanent disabilities associated with brain injuries. While it is estimated that only 74 percent of those with brain injuries are seen in a health care setting (e.g., hospital or clinic); the cost associated with mild brain injuries is estimated at $17 billion.

Epidemiology

The high-risk groups for brain injury are infants, young adolescents, adult males, and the elderly (Brain Injury Association of America [BIAA], 2006). See Table 35-3 for more information on specific behaviors that place these groups at increased risk for brain injury.

Etiology

The major causes of traumatic brain injury are motor vehicle crashes, followed by falls, assaults or firearms, and sports or recreation. Motor vehicle crashes account for 44 percent of traumatic brain injuries. Major contributing factors are not wearing seatbelts and driving while intoxicated. Alcohol intoxication

TABLE 35-3 Causes of Brain Injury by Age-Groups	
AGE-GROUP	**CAUSES**
Infants and young children	Shaken baby syndrome
	Falls (especially under 5 years of age)
	Motor vehicle crashes
	Abuse
	Firearms
Adolescents	Motor vehicle crashes
	Alcohol and drugs
	Inexperienced driving
	Poor use of seatbelts
	Speeding
	Underage drinking
	Illicit drugs (marijuana, cocaine, crack, or inhalants)
	Sports and recreation
Elderly	Falls
	Motor vehicle crashes

Adapted from Brain Injury Association of America. (2006). Retrieved June 13, 2006, from www.biausa.org.

alters perception and reaction time increasing the risk for a motor vehicle crash. Another factor is driver inexperience and high-risk behaviors, e.g., speeding. Several states have implemented a graduated driver licensing system for teen drivers to address the issue of inexperience.

Falls account for 26 percent of traumatic brain injuries. Falls are particularly problematic for the elderly. People over the age of 75 years often have sensory deficits (decreased vision or decreased hearing), generalized weakness, and slower reflexes. These factors contribute to a higher risk for falling. Also, some elderly take medications that can cause lightheadedness or dizziness and affect their balance.

Assaults and firearms accounted for 17 percent of all traumatic brain injuries (CDC, 2006c). Domestic abuse is a significant problem in our society. According to the BIAA, every nine seconds in the United States a woman is assaulted, and researchers have found the primary target for attack in women is the head, thus leading to head or brain injuries. Abuse is not limited to women, it also affects the elderly. In 2001, an estimated 33,000 people age 60 or older were treated in EDs for assault-related injuries (Mitchell, Hasbrouck, Ingram, Dunaway, & Annest, 2003). It is estimated that over half of all the homes in America have a firearm, and greater than 50 percent of firearm owners keep guns loaded and in an unlocked area.

Sports and recreation account for 13 percent of all traumatic brain injuries. Sports, such as boxing, football, soccer, baseball, horseback riding, all types of skating, and skiing, can place a person at risk for a head injury. Colliding with another player, getting hit in the head with a ball, and falling most often lead to mild brain injuries, or concussions; but some injuries lead to more serious brain injury requiring hospitalization.

Types of Brain Injuries

Trauma to the head may result in both primary and secondary injuries to the brain. A primary brain injury is one that is a result of a direct trauma to the brain (Celik, Aksoy, & Akyolcu, 2004). A secondary injury occurs as a result of an injury to the brain (hypoxia, cerebral edema, hypertension, increased ICP, or hypercapnia). A primary injury is called a traumatic brain injury (brain damage as a direct result of an external force). According to the BIAA, a traumatic brain injury is an insult to the brain, not of a degenerative or cognitive nature, caused by an external physical force, which may produce a diminished or altered state of consciousness, and results in an impairment of cognitive abilities or physical functioning. It can also result in the disturbance of behavioral or emotional functioning. These impairments may be either temporary or permanent and cause partial or total functional disability or psychological maladjustment (BIAA, 2004). In 1997, they came out with a definition for an acquired brain injury, stating it commonly results in a change in neural activity, which affects the physical integrity, the metabolic activity, or the functional ability of the cell. Secondary injuries can occur as a result of a primary injury.

Primary injuries to the brain may be classified as either open or closed injuries. An open injury occurs when there is a break in the skull (skull fracture). Skull fractures are caused by direct blows either from an object striking the skull (blunt instrument or projectile) or from the skull striking a surface. A depressed skull fracture results from a blow to the head that causes a part of the skull to be pushed inward, pressing on brain tissue. Patients with open injuries have an increased risk of infection because of the opening created by the fracture. One type of fracture, a basilar skull fracture, is often associated with CSF leakage from the ear or nose.

Closed injuries occur when there is no fracture to the skull but uncontrolled energy is transmitted to the underlying brain tissue causing damage. This damage can occur either at the site of the blow to the skull or to an area in the brain that is remote from the site of the injury. The brain is normally surrounded by CSF, which acts like a shock absorber during normal movement. The fluid protects the brain in the event of minor blows to the head. However, injury forces that cause rapid acceleration and deceleration (fall or motor vehicle crash) force the brain to move rapidly within the skull, causing it to strike rough surfaces that are opposite the site of direct injury. Injuries to sites remote from the impact are called contra-coup injuries.

The brain damage that occurs as a result of primary and secondary injury can be local or involve large portions of the brain. A contusion is a common local brain injury in which the brain tissue is bruised. Contusions can occur in any area of the brain but are most commonly seen in the frontal or temporal lobes of the brain. Diffuse axonal injury is a brain injury that results from rapid acceleration and deceleration forces. These forces produce shearing or tensile stresses that damage the axons of nerves (Smith, Meaney, & Shull, 2003). The damage can involve the brain stem and reticular activating system and result in prolonged coma. Patients with closed head injuries are at particular risk for secondary brain injury, which is brain damage caused by an internal force (e.g., swelling), because the bony skull in the adult is inelastic.

Secondary injuries occur hours to days after the initial injury as a result of the body's response to the initial brain injury. Factors that contribute to secondary brain injury include lack of oxygen, hypotension, or inflammatory processes that result in swelling of brain tissue and release of chemicals that damage healthy brain tissue (Celik, et al., 2004; Jeremitsky, Omert, Dunham, Protetch, & Rodriguez, 2003).

Pathophysiology

When the brain is injured, a number of pathological responses are set in motion. First the primary injury may injure blood vessels and disrupt the neuron axons and cell bodies. Damaged blood vessels, depending on the location of the injury, may bleed into the epidural area located between the skull and the outer covering of the brain, the subdural space, the subarachnoid space, or within the injured brain. Bleeding damages brain tissue by increasing ICP. Symptom onset is usually rapid if the bleeding is from an artery. However, symptoms resulting from venous bleeding can be delayed from hours to weeks.

Next a secondary process of auto destructive factors contributes to additional injury. Factors that have been identified as contributing to this process include: cellular anoxia and depletion of energy stores, cell membrane lipid metabolites, glutamatergic neurotransmission, intracellular calcium overload, release of free radicals, and inflammatory processes (Celik, et al., 2004). Energy is needed to maintain normal intracellular calcium levels. When energy supplies are low because of reduced blood flow and poor oxygenation, mechanisms that maintain normal intracellular calcium levels fail. Release of the neurotransmitter glutamate also leads to an influx of calcium into neurons and results in calcium-mediated cell death. Oxygen free radicals are thought to damage cells during reperfusion after a period of low flow causes ischemia. Oxygen free radicals can result in injury to cellular lipid membranes and damage of deoxyribonucleic acid (DNA), leading to cellular injury.

The normal relationship between brain glucose utilization and blood flow is also altered following head trauma. Directly injured tissue shows reduced glucose utilization, while adjacent uninjured tissue shows increased glucose utilization. The inflammatory processes and cellular edema lead to increased ICP from cerebral edema. The increased pressure results in compensatory mechanisms that raise blood pressure in an attempt to maintain blood flow to the brain. These compensatory mechanisms lead to further increases in cerebral pressure. The increased pressure leads to further injury through compression of brain structures in a closed head injury. As the pressure increases, downward pressure is placed on the brainstem, causing injury to brainstem structures. Pressure on the brainstem leads to damage of the third cranial nerve and results in pupil changes, which may be unilateral or bilateral, and in later stages may dilate pupils. Pressure on the respiratory center leads to changes in respiratory rate and rhythm and eventually leads to respiratory arrest. As pressure increases, other intracranial structures are affected, leading to inability to maintain temperature regulation and fluid balance.

Brain injuries are divided into three levels of severity, mild, moderate, and severe. A **concussion** is a mild form of brain trauma and accounts for 75 percent of all brain injuries (CDC, 2006c). Concussions are characterized by a brief loss of consciousness, period of a loss of memory for before and after the injury event (retrograde and antegrade amnesia), change in mental state (confusion), or change in neurological status (BIAA, 2004). The recovery from a mild brain injury is rapid with no permanent or lasting disability.

A moderate brain injury is characterized by loss of consciousness ranging from a few minutes to hours and days or weeks of confusion. The symptoms may last for months and may be permanent. Individuals with moderate injury usually have a complete recovery or are able to adapt to their disability (BIAA, 2004).

Severe brain injuries are characterized by prolonged loss of consciousness (days, weeks, or months) and severe neurological deficits. Recovery is limited and permanent disabilities are common (Table 35-4 discusses types of severe brain injury).

Complications

A number of complications may occur following brain injury. Hydrocephalus occurs when there is too much CSF in the ventricles. This leads to pressure on the brain tissue and deterioration in neurological status. The treatment is the removal of excess CSF fluid, and in some instances a shunt may need to be inserted (see brain tumors for more information on shunts).

TABLE 35-4	Types of Severe Brain Injury
TERM	**DEFINITION**
Coma	"State of unconsciousness from which the individual cannot be awakened"
	Little or no response to stimuli
	Does not initiate voluntary activities
	Can last for weeks, months, or years
Vegetative state	Can be awakened but is not aware of surroundings
	Eyes can open
	Responses to pain
Persistent vegetative state	A vegetative state that lasts longer than one month
Minimally responsive state	No longer in a coma or vegetative state
	Some basic reflexes
	Inconsistent in following directions
	Aware of surroundings
Locked-in syndrome	Rare neurological condition in which a person is conscious and able to think, but unable to move any part of their body except their eyes.
Brain death	The brain shows no sign of function

Adapted from Brain Injury Association of America. (2004). Support adequate finding of the traumatic brain injury act in FY 2005. *McLean, VA: Author.*

An infection related to a tear in the dura mater may occur. When a patient suffers an open brain injury or where there is a break in the continuity of the skull, the lining of the dura mater may tear, allowing bacteria to enter the brain. This is a serious complication and may lead to death unless the infection can be managed with antibiotics.

A stroke can occur secondary to intracranial hemorrhage associated with brain trauma or from a clot that develops because of the trauma and lodges in a small blood vessel. Depending on the nature and extent of the injury, a patient may be placed on anticoagulant therapy to prevent a thrombotic or embolic stroke.

Chronic headaches may be lasting sequelae of the brain trauma. A patient may complain of a headache for weeks or months after a brain injury. Treatment with analgesics and narcotics may be used cautiously as narcotics may mask neurological deficits. Also, some patients may experience long-term impairments in memory surrounding the events of the brain trauma.

According to the BIAA (2004), the development of Alzheimer's disease, Parkinson's disease, posttraumatic dementia, and chronic traumatic encephalopathy (dementia pugilistica) have been linked to traumatic brain injuries.

Assessment with Clinical Manifestations

The location and extent of a brain injury will determine the clinical presentation. Nurses must remember that there is no predictability with head injury patients. Patients that initially appear to have minor injuries may later become unconscious and rapidly deteriorate. Two patients presenting with the same mechanism of injury may present with different symptoms and have different outcomes. A patient presenting with a head injury may have all or some of the symptoms described below. It is important that any person with a suspected head injury seek medical attention immediately. Symptoms may occur immediately after injury or be initially absent or subtle with gradual onset occurring days after the initial injury. According to the BIAA (2004) and CDC (2006c), most head injury patients that sustain a brain injury will present with symptoms within three broad categories: physical, cognitive, and behavioral (Box 35-3).

The nursing assessment of the patient with a history of head injury begins with determining the mechanism of injury and whether the patient has a history of loss of consciousness or confusion. If the patient is unconscious on arrival at the hospital, determine if any of the following occurred: the patient was initially unconscious or became alert for a short period of time and then became unconscious again, which is a clue to an epidural hemorrhage (Table 35-5). There are several different locations that result in different clinical manifestations as there are neurological bleeds (Figure 35-6). Many patients with head injury have associated injuries of the neck. If the patient is conscious, ask about neck pain. If the patient is unconscious assume the patient has a neck injury until ruled out with diagnostic X-rays. Also, consider whether the patient might have sustained a neurological or cardiac event that contributed to the injury.

It is important to assess the airway and ventilation while maintaining cervical-spine (c-spine) immobility in the unconscious patient. Patients with brain injury and hypoxia have poorer outcomes. Patients with severe brain injuries will have changes in respirations. In addition, it is also important to assess circulation. Research evidence suggests that brain trauma patients with a history of hypotension have a poorer outcome than brain-injured patients without a history of hypotension (McDermott, Rosenfeld, Laidlaw, Cordner, & Tremayne, 2004; Vavilala, et al., 2003).

The nurse must next assess neurological function. The Glasgow Coma Scale score is used to assess LOC (see Table 34-4). The Glasgow Coma Scale must be obtained through interaction with the patient. A second measure of neurological function is pupil reaction. Assess pupils for pupillary light response,

---

BOX 35-3

CLINICAL MANIFESTATIONS OF BRAIN INJURY

Physical signs and symptoms include:

- Physical evidence of trauma: wounds, contusions, ecchymosis around the eyes (raccoon sign), or bruising behind the ear (battles sign). Raccoon eyes and battles sign are signs of basilar skull fracture.
- Impaired consciousness: may be brief with rapid recovery or a lengthy loss of consciousness, lethargy, or coma.
- Visual disturbances: blurring, photosensitivity (bright lights are painful), and loss of vision, or inability to move eyes. In addition, the pupillary changes can include: sluggish reaction to light, pupils do not react to light, or one pupil is larger than the other (Note: this is a sign of increasing intracranial pressure).
- Headache and neck pain.
- Leaking CSF from nose or ears: the fluid may appear clear but will have a positive reaction to glucose reagent strip due to high amount of glucose in CSF. If the drainage if bloody, place a drop on a white sheet, if a halo appears around the blood once it is dried, it is cerebrospinal fluid.
- Nausea and vomiting, which may be an early sign of increasing ICP.
- Respiratory distress: may have difficulty breathing and require ventilatory support. Slowing respirations are a sign of increased ICP.
- Dizziness, poor motor control, fatigue, inability to maintain balance, and ringing in the ears.
- **Hemiparesis** (weakness on one side of the body) or **hemiplegia** (inability to move of one side of the body).
- Seizures.
- Impaired speech: expressive or receptive **aphasia** (impairment in the ability to speak or comprehend) or **dysarthria** (difficulty in oral movement to form words).
- **Dysphagia** (inability to swallow).
- Sexual dysfunction.

Cognitive symptoms may include:

- Confusion, inability to concentrate, and shortened attention span
- Impairment in short-term and long-term memory; commonly seen with concussion.
- Difficulty reading and writing, and difficulty with problem solving and reasoning.
- Difficulty with planning, sequencing, impaired judgment, and slowed thought processes.

Behavioral symptoms may include:

- Agitation, irritability, and mood swings.
- Anxiety and restlessness.
- Delusions, paranoia, mania, and explosive behavior.
- Depression and decreased motivation.

---

size, and symmetry. A pupillary size greater than 4 mm is considered dilated. A measurement difference of more than 1 mm is defined as asymmetry.

The patient must also have an assessment of his or her temperature. Hypothermia has been associated with increased mortality in some studies (Jermitsky, et al, 2003). Hyperthermia may suggest injury to the hypothalamus or infection. Also, the patient must be assessed for other injuries. Patients that have sustained a severe head injury may have sustained other injuries that are overlooked because of the head injury.

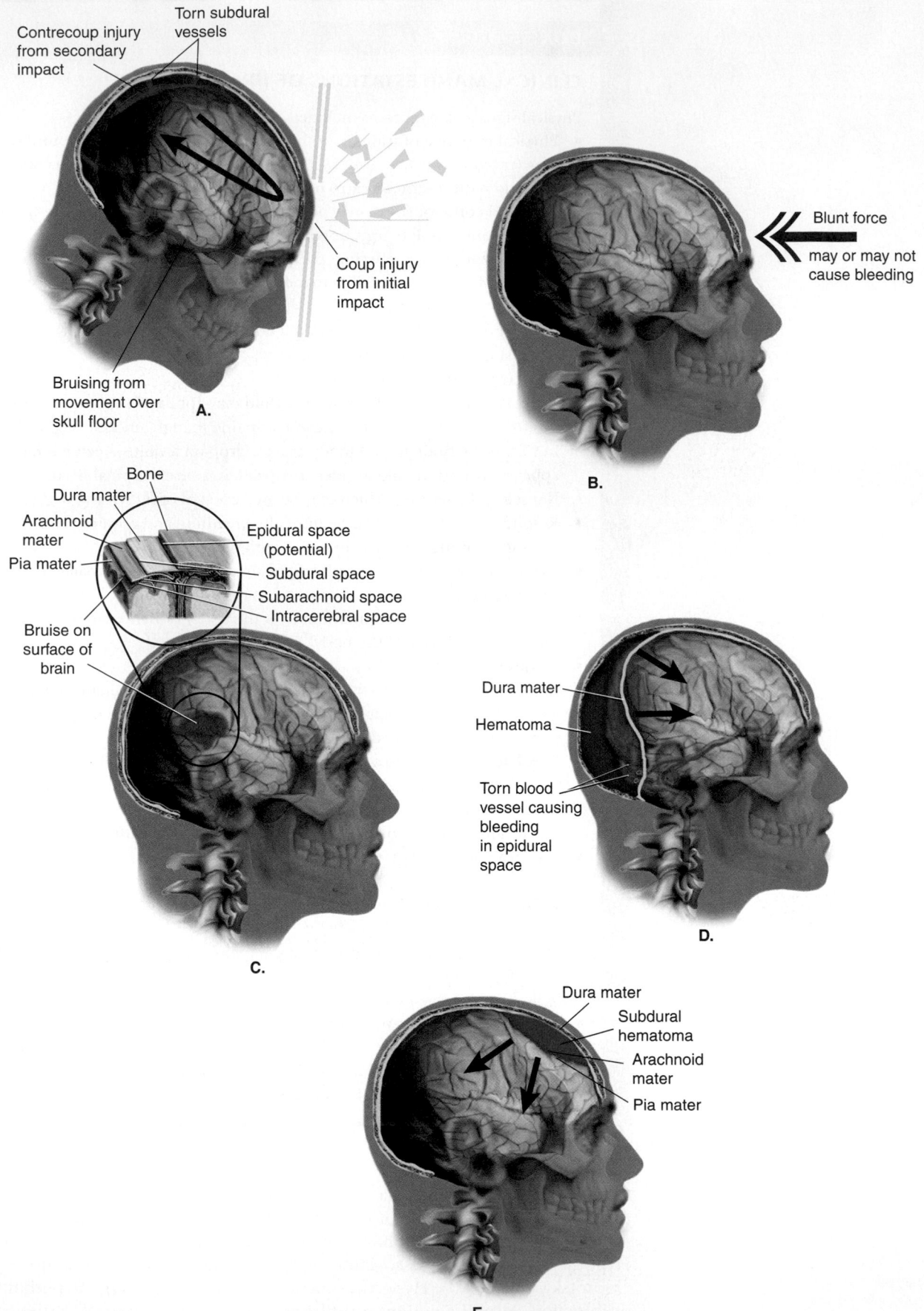

Figure 35-6 Brain injuries: A. Coup/Contracoup, B. Concussion, C. Contusion, D. Epidural hematoma, E. Subdural hematoma.

TABLE 35-5 Neurological Bleeds			
TYPE	**INCIDENCE OR CAUSE**	**SYMPTOMS**	**TREATMENT**
Acute subdural hematoma	5–25% of all severe TBI with contusion of laceration Venous blood between dura and brain	Coma Increased ICP	Surgical evacuation of blood Monitor ICP, neuro status, or cerebral perfusion
Subacute subdural hematoma	Higher incidence in elderly related to falls Venous bleed Develops into chronic subdural hematoma	Headache, confusion, aphasia, hemiplegia, seizures, or coma Can appear as late as 2 weeks May be mistaken for stroke	Decrease ICP Surgical evacuation of hematoma Seizure precautions
Epidural hematoma	Young adult males Arterial bleed usually caused by trauma	Brief loss of consciousness but resolves quickly, then a rapid decline in neuro status—nausea, vomiting, headache, seizures, hemiparesis, decreased level of consciousness, respiratory distress, or hypertension	Medical emergency Airway and respiratory management Decrease ICP and monitor cerebral perfusion Requires surgical intervention to remove clot and stop bleeding
Subarachnoid hemorrhage	Happens in males more than females 10–15% die before reaching hospital AVM aneurysm, trauma, drug abuse, or hypertension	Severe headache, decrease in level of consciousness, or neck stiffness	Surgery to repair aneurysm Control ICP Prevent seizures Monitor cerebral perfusion Prevent cerebral vasospasm

Adapted from Reddy, L. S. (2004). Heads upon cerebral bleeds. Nursing Made Incredibly Easy, 2(3), 8–16.

For the continued rehabilitation of the brain-injured patient, the Rancho Los Amigos Scale is often utilized to evaluate the patient's progress. However, overall nursing care will remain the same whether the patient has a head injury, stroke, or brain tumor.

Diagnostic Tests

Procedures used to diagnose brain injuries include neurological exams, neuro logical scales, radiological exams, and laboratory studies. During the neurological exam the health care provider will ask the patient some simple questions, ask him or her to follow simple directions, and assess functional ability. This allows the health care provider to determine the extent of the injury and the effect on the patient's ability to interact with the environment.

In the ED a CT will be ordered for all patients that have sustained a head injury. The CT scan will identify skull fractures, bleeding, and contusions of the brain. The CT scan is a screening tool, it cannot rule out some types of brain damage. For example, the CT scan does not provide information on diffusion axonal damage, which occurs at the cellular level, and the CT scan may also not initially detect small amounts of bleeding in the subarachnoid space. A second CT scan may be done later if no injury appears on the first CT scan. If a cerebral hemorrhage is noted on CT scan, an angiogram may be ordered to determine the exact location of the leakage within the vessel. Additional studies that may be ordered after initial treatment include an MRI. CT scans are more effective at detecting bleeding while MRI scans are more sensitive at detecting nonhemorrhagic injuries, such as diffuse axonal damage, cortical contusions, and brainstem injury (McElligott, Greewald, & Watanabe, 2003). A positive emission tomography (PET) scan or a single photon emitting computerized tomography (SPECT) scan may be performed to evaluate brain metabolism. The SPECT scan has the ability to provide a three-dimensional image of the brain.

Several additional imaging techniques are currently under investigation. Several of these techniques make use of the MRI. Diffuse-weighted imaging (DWI) uses MRI to detect subtle changes in the diffusion of water molecules in tissues. Perfusion MRI (pMRI) is used to examine blood flow. Perfusion MRI may be used in the future to determine whether altered consciousness is caused by vascular rather than metabolic, toxic, or infectious causes. Functional MRI (fMRI) measures changes in tissue perfusion based on tissue oxygenation. fMRI can be used to examine regional brain activity in response to sensory, motor, and cognitive stimulation. Proton magnetic resonance spectroscopy (MRS) uses MRI and available software to noninvasively assess brain biochemistry and may be useful in assessing severity of ischemia in traumatic brain injury (McElligott, et al., 2003).

Pulse oximetry is used to assess the patient's oxygen level, and if the patient requires mechanical ventilation, ABGs are ordered to monitor both oxygen and carbon dioxide levels. Depending on the severity of the head injury, and whether the patient also has associated injuries or other medical conditions, additional laboratory studies will be ordered. A CBC will be obtained to assess for infection and hemorrhage, and electrolytes will be obtained to monitor metabolic and renal status. If drug or alcohol intoxication is suspected, toxicology studies will be done, because ingestion of drugs and alcohol can mimic signs of brain trauma. Coagulation studies may be ordered for patients with a history of bleeding disorders or known to be on anticoagulants. Type and cross-matching of blood products may be ordered if the patient has evidence of additional trauma. In severe head injuries an electroencephalogram (EEG) may be ordered to evaluate the electrical activity of the brain. An EEG is one of the diagnostic tools used to evaluate brain death.

Nursing Diagnoses

Based on the information gathered, examples of nursing diagnoses in the patient with brain injuries may include the following:
- Acute confusion related to altered cerebral blood flow or cerebral edema.
- Disturbed sensory perception related to cerebral edema or injury.
- Fatigue related to cerebral edema or injury.
- Impaired memory, short-term or long-term, related to cerebral edema or injury.
- Impaired social interaction related to inappropriate behavior.
- Ineffective tissue perfusion, cerebral edema related to increased ICP.

Planning and Implementation

Head injuries can include patients that are mild to extremely severe in their consequences. On the one hand a patient can have a mild injury without consequences of any substance. On the other extreme a patient can have a head injury that results in increased ICP problems and have a high mortality rate with many complications. Nurses develop excellent methods of planning their care and setting goals, which optimizes the recovery of the patient regardless of the severity of his or her injuries.

Prevention

Most brain injuries can be prevented. Prevention activities include legislation, development of safer products, and education on proper use of safety devices by individuals. The implementation of airbags in vehicles can prevent a person from hitting the steering wheel; but without a seatbelt, the person can be tossed around the car and thrown from the vehicle, leading to a head injury. Legislation has been used to implement helmet and primary seatbelt laws and stricter driving under the influence (DUI) laws in many states. Federal laws have lead to safer automobiles. Education can be used to increase awareness of how alcohol and drug use affect the ability to drive vehicles and operate machinery. Teaching people the importance of wearing seatbelts and helmets is vital. The National Transportation Department and local law enforcement have various programs that educate people, especially teens, on these issues.

Completing a safety assessment of the home can prevent many falls. Removing throw rugs, providing adequate lighting (especially at night), and installing handrails in bathrooms and stairways and tub and shower rails can make for a safer home. Because the elderly are at higher risk for falls, they need to be encouraged to develop a regular exercise routine, such as walking and wearing nonslip, supportive shoes. Exercise keeps muscles and joints flexible and improves balance. Side effects of various medications (antihypertensives, sedatives, or narcotics) will place a patient at greater risk for falls. It is the nurse's responsibility to educate the patient about these side effects.

There are many programs available for people facing domestic violence issues. The nurse should assess all patients for domestic abuse and educate them about available community resources and make appropriate referrals. Many head injuries related to recreation and sports can be prevented though appropriate use of safety equipment. Adults who play sports should be taught the importance of wearing appropriate safety equipment. Properly worn helmets are one of the best ways to protect the head. There are three major programs that receive federal funding from this act. The CDC is responsible for research activities that monitor traumatic brain injuries in each state. They are also involved in community awareness, education, and outreach programs. The Health Resources and Services Administration (HRSA) state grant program works with individuals and their families who have suffered a brain injury, to provide them with services and community resources. The Protection and Advocacy Services State Grants for Individuals with Traumatic Brain Injury is involved in the legal representation and self-advocacy of people who have a traumatic brain injury. To increase community awareness, there are a number of events offered throughout the year related to brain injury safety. The month of October is National Brain Injury Awareness month, and December is National Drunk and Drugged Driving month. Keeping the public informed about the causes of brain injury and ways to prevent them is an important role for the nurse.

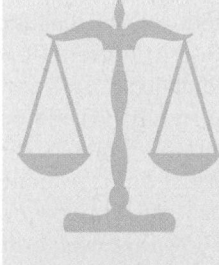

LAW IN PRACTICE

Traumatic Brain Injury Act

Because of the impact of traumatic brain injuries on society and the health care system, the federal government passed the Traumatic Brain Injury Act (P.L. 104-166) as part of the Children's Health Act of 2000 (BIA, 2004). This is the only federal legislation specifically designed for people with traumatic brain injury and is a foundation for coordinated and balanced public policy in prevention, education, research, and community living for people living with a traumatic brain injury and their families.

Goals

In general, the following are a variety of goals that nurses can have regarding the management and care of patients with head injuries. The nurse can prevent progression of secondary brain injury (e.g., hypoxia, hypotension, or changes in temperature). The patient can be monitored to ensure a safe environment and receive appropriate patient education in this regard. The patient can be returned to optimal functional status.

Collaborative Management

Patients with moderate to severe injuries will have their care managed either by a neurologist or a neurosurgeon. These are health care providers who specialize in caring for patients with neurological impairments. Other members of the health care team in addition to the physician and patient's nurse may include respiratory therapist, a dietitian, clinical pharmacist, and occupational and physical therapist. Until the patient's condition has stabilized, the patient will be cared for in an ICU. The patient may remain on a ventilator for respiratory support and on a cardiac monitor to evaluate his or her heart rate and watch for any cardiac arrhythmias. An endotracheal (ET) tube is used for short-term ventilation, but if the patient requires mechanical ventilation for an extended period of time, a tracheotomy tube will be inserted. If the patient has any swallowing difficulties, a nasogastric tube may be placed to provide nutritional support.

Management of Head Injury

Most brain injuries are considered mild. The patient will usually return home within 24 hours. Families are instructed to awaken the patient every 2 to 3 hours while sleeping to determine LOC. If the patient develops a headache that increases in severity, nausea or vomiting, visual changes, paralysis of a part of his or her body, or he or she becomes difficult to arouse, the family is instructed to return the patient to the ED or call 911. These symptoms may indicate delayed neurological injury, such as bleeding or developing cerebral edema. Patients who are discharged from the hospital should see their family health care provider for follow-up within a few days.

Care of the patient with a moderate to severe brain injury begins in the prehospital setting (Figure 35-7). Emergency medical personal provide initial airway, breathing, and circulatory management before the patient arrives at the hospital. In the ED airway and breathing management continue to have the highest priority, because some severely injured patients may not be able to breathe adequately on their own. Prepare to assist with intubation of the airway and mechanical ventilation if indicated. Place the patient on continuous pulse oximetry and monitor the patient frequently. The goal is to maintain oxygen saturation at 100 percent (Bader, Littlejohns, & March, 2003). Hypoxia below 90 percent, arterial hemoglobin saturation, is associated with poor outcomes.

The patient is placed on a cardiac monitor and any slowing of the heart rate or cardiac dysrhythmias is reported. IV access is needed to provide fluids and for administration of medications. An IV with an isotonic solution, such as normal saline, so as not to increase ICP is begun. In the instance of multiple trauma, the patient should have two IVs. The blood pressure is monitored closely. The mean arterial blood pressure should be maintained above 90 mm Hg. Episodes of hypotension are associated with poorer outcomes (Jeremitsky, et al., 2003). If the blood pressure falls below this level, notify the health care provider immediately and prepare to intervene with measures to prevent hypotension.

The patient's neurological status is monitored, and changes in the Glasgow Coma Scale score, changes in pupil response (e.g., asymmetry, sluggish response, or dilation), or a sudden increase in urinary output are also noted. These are all significant signs of increased ICP. Other signs are slowing respirations, slowing heart rate, and increasing blood pressure (**Cushing response**). Cushing response is a late sign of increasing ICP.

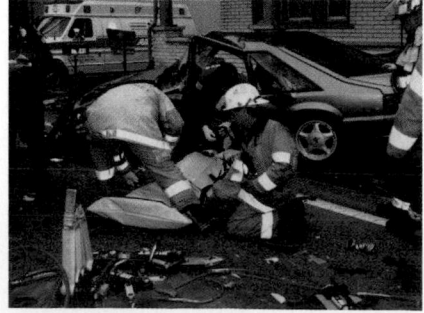

Figure 35-7 Motor vehicle collisions are the most common cause of traumatic brain injury. (Courtesy of David J. Reimer, Sr.)

The patient's body temperature is monitored, as damage to the hypothalamus may result in hyperthermia. Some patients may be placed on cooling blankets to lower overall body temperature. For every one degree centigrade that the body temperature rises, the metabolic rate in brain tissue and oxygen needs increases by 7 percent (Celik, et al., 2004). So by lowering the temperature of the body, the metabolic rate in the brain decreases; thus reducing metabolic demands, allowing the brain to begin to recover. Sedative or neuromuscular medications may be needed to prevent shivering and anxiety, which will increase body temperature. A recent study suggests that hypothermia may also be associated with poorer outcomes (Jeremitsky, et al., 2003).

Patients admitted to the critical unit may have a device inserted to monitor ICP. Monitoring ICP is important in the prevention of secondary brain injury. ICP is measured by placing a small tube in the ventricles of the brain. If the pressure gets too high, a ventricular drain (ventriculostomy) may be utilized to remove CSF. The fluid is then collected in a small bag at the bedside. In the past, one way to decrease ICP was through hyperventilation; however, current research now indicates aggressive hyperventilation may actually cause further brain damage by constricting blood vessels and further reducing blood flow to the brain tissue. Another treatment for increased ICP was barbiturate therapy. The use of barbiturates (pentobarbital and phenobarbital) was thought to decrease ICP by producing a sedative and hypnotic effect, but recent research has found that osmotic diuretics, increasing the head of the bed 30 degrees, and draining CSF to be just as effective (Celik, et al., 2004). The osmotic diuretic mannitol may be administered to help manage ICP.

In addition to ICP, the cerebral perfusion pressure (CPP) should be monitored. The CPP is the difference between the ICP and the mean arterial pressure (MAP). CPP is calculated by subtracting the ICP from the MAP. Normal CPP is 70 to 95 mm Hg. (Bretler, 2004). Cerebral blood flow (CBF) is also used to guide treatment in severe brain injury. Normal CBF is about 15 percent of the patient's cardiac output.

Methods are now available in the critical care setting to measure oxygen level in the brain. The goal is for the critical care team to balance the patient's ICP level with the brain oxygen level during the critical phase when the patient is at risk for secondary brain injury. The goal is to keep the oxygen saturation at 100 percent, the $PaCo_2$ between 35 and 40 mm Hg, the brain tissue oxygenation level at least 20 mm Hg, the ICP less than 20 mm Hg, and the CPP greater than 70 mm Hg. During the critical phase, the critical care nurse initiates changes to balance oxygen delivery to the brain and the ICP. This is the primary focus for the critical care nurse during the critical phase until brain swelling is reduced (Bader, et al., 2003).

The nurse plays a vital role in helping to prevent environmental stimuli that might cause an increase in ICP. Keeping lights on a low setting, keeping noise level at a minimum, and providing a calm and restful environment for the patient is important in the recovery process. Visitors may be limited to one or two people at a time for short visits. The family and friends need to be aware of the need to be quiet and not upset the patient. As with all patients who are immobile, the nurse must institute measures to promote healing and prevent complications. Patients with a brain injury should be turned every two hours to prevent skin breakdown. Special attention should be taken, because many patients will need to have the head of the bed at 30 degrees to decrease ICP. This places the coccyx and sacral areas at highest risk for skin breakdown. Also when positioning the patient, make sure to use pillows and support all extremities. Do not stress or hyperextend the neck, as this may increase ICP. Compression stockings or compression boots should be utilized to prevent DVT. The patient may also be placed on anticoagulant therapy to help prevent blood clots from forming.

Pharmacology

There are a variety of pharmacological therapy strategies for patients with head injuries. For example, patients with severe brain injuries are also at risk for seizures. Nursing measures should be implemented to reduce the potential for injury in the event of a posttraumatic seizure. Phenytoin, beginning with an IV loading dose may be ordered immediately after the injury and continued for the first seven days to reduce the incidence of posttraumatic seizures (Chang & Lowenstein, 2003).

Heightened alertness and anxiety will increase ICP, thus leading to secondary brain injuries. Antianxiety medication is given to manage nervousness; while antipyschotics are used to manage behavioral issues, such as combativeness, hostility, and hallucinations. However, some recent research investigating pharmacotherapy in behavior management suggests some evidence that beta blockers, such as propranolol (Inderal), pindolol (Visken), and metoprolol (Lopressor), anticonvulsants, such as carbamazepine (Tegretol), divalproex sodium (Depakote), and lamotrigine (Lamictal), and antidepressants, such as sertraline (Zoloft), fluoxetine (Prozac), and paroxetine (Paxil), in high doses may be effective in managing agitation and aggression (Deb & Crownshaw, 2004). However Deb and Crownshaw (2004) suggest further research should be done in this area. They also found some evidence to suggest that psychostimulants may be effective in managing apathy, inattention, and slowness in the brain-injured patient. Again, they suggest further research be conducted. In a study by Whyte, et al. (2004), methylphenidate (Ritalin) was found to be effective in patients with difficulty maintaining attention. They also suggest further research be done.

Surgery

In some cases, surgical intervention is required. A craniotomy may need to be performed to remove a large clot that is applying pressure to brain tissue. Craniotomy will be discussed in further detail with brain tumors. Burr holes may need to be drilled to relieve pressure within the skull cavity when pressure is rising rapidly. When the brain begins to swell after an injury, it only has a small area in which to expand. Burr holes allow the brain some additional room to swell but should be done with caution as this opens the brain up to the risk for infection. If the swelling continues, the brain may herniate (push down) into the brainstem. This is usually indicative of a poor prognosis, and many times the patient is never able to recover.

Patient and Family Teaching

Education of the family is an important role of the nurse in caring for a patient with a brain injury. The family may be experiencing a wide range of emotions. The intensive care unit can be an overwhelming and scary place for most families. Depending on the cause of the injury, they may feel guilt, anger, and frustration; but almost everyone will be anxious and fearful about the outcome of the injury. The nurse must be cognizant of what the family is experiencing and provide emotional support and encouragement. Keeping the family informed of the patient's condition and explaining procedures that are being done will help alleviate some anxiety. Because of patient confidentiality issues, the nurse should limit communication to one or two family members who have been identified as primary caregivers for the patient.

Evaluation of Outcomes

Potential patient outcomes for each of the example nursing diagnoses for the patient with a brain injury are:
- Acute confusion related to altered cerebral blood flow or cerebral edema. The patient will be conscious, oriented, and perform own self-care.
- Disturbed sensory perception related to cerebral edema or injury. The patient will have functional sensory status.

- Fatigue related to cerebral edema or injury. The patient will rest as needed and evidence endurance in their activities of daily living.
- Impaired Memory, short-term or long-term, related to cerebral edema or injury. The patient will recall events (both short- and long-term) accurately.
- Impaired social interaction related to inappropriate behavior. The patient will have control of their aggressive tendencies and participate in normal leisure activities.
- Ineffective tissue perfusion, cerebral edema related to increased ICP. The patient will display intracranial pressure within normal range.

BRAIN TUMORS

The National Institute for Neurological Disorders and Stroke (2006) estimates that in the United States, 40,000 people annually will develop a new brain tumor, and 25 percent of all patients with cancer will develop brain metastasis (where the cancer originates in one part of the body and spreads to another part of the body, as in this case the brain). The cancer usually originates in the lung and breast but can also start in the kidney, prostate, or as lymphoma or melanoma. While malignant brain tumors are only 1 percent of all cancers, they account for 2 percent of all cancer-related deaths (American Cancer Society [ACS] 2004g). While these statistics can appear rather grave, Jemal (2003) noted that patients are living longer with brain tumors than in the 1970s and 1980s.

Epidemiology

The incidence of brain tumors has increased during the past three decades. This is thought to be because of earlier diagnoses rather than an acute rise in actual incidence. There are approximately 17,000 new cases of brain tumors per year, of those, 9,600 are male and 7,400 are female (ACS, 2004g). Secondary brain tumors are more common and occur most frequently in the fifth, sixth, and seventh decades, with a slightly higher incidence in men.

Etiology

Brain tumors are an abnormal growth of cells within the brain tissue. The cause is unknown in many cases, but research is being done to investigate the correlation between exposures to radiation or cancer-causing chemicals. In some cases, genetics may be the cause, especially if the tumor develops in the brain or CNS first, such as neurofibromatosis or tuberous sclerosis.

Pathophysiology

There are several different classifications for brain tumors. Benign tumors are noncancerous and confined to one location or area. Benign tumors are usually slow-growing and usually do not cause much concern in other parts of the body. However because the brain is enclosed within the bony skull, expansion of any kind (tumors or edema) can place pressure on healthy brain tissue, thus leading to neurological compromise. A malignant tumor is cancerous, usually grows quickly, and can spread from one part of the body to another. A grading system has been developed to better understand the different types of malignancy with a grade I being the least malignant and grade IV being the most malignant (Brain Tumor Society, 2004). Use of this type of grading system is also important in determining the type of treatment and how quickly treatment should be initiated. A **primary brain tumor** means that the cancer originated in the brain tissue, however this is rare. A secondary brain tumor is one that started in another location in the body and spread to the brain or CNS.

PATIENT PLAYBOOK

Education Topics for a Patient with a Brain Injury

- Inform the patient to return to routine activities slowly and not to return to work too quickly.
- Tell the patient who has employment that requires the operation of heavy equipment that he or she must be given clearance before returning to work.
- Instruct the patient to prevent further injury to the head with the use of safety equipment (e.g., helmets).
- Discuss the importance of avoiding alcoholic beverages and illicit drug use.
- Educate the patient that he or she should inform the nurse of his or her use of any over-the-counter medications and any herbal remedies.
- Encourage the patient to eat a well-balanced diet for healing purposes.

Another term for secondary brain tumors is metastasis. Brain tumors are also termed for when they develop. Brain tumors present at birth are labeled congenital tumors, and tumors that develop after birth are called a neoplasm.

The most common type of brain tumor is a glioma. These tumors grow from glial cells and usually occur in the cerebral hemispheres of the brain. The most common type of gliomas is an astrocytoma. These tumors are usually seen in children, but if found in an adult, they are usually always malignant. While the choice of treatment is surgery for most astrocytomas, the location, size, and grade of a malignancy often determines the type of therapy. A study by Behin, Hoang-Xuan, Carpentier, & Delattre (2003) suggests that treatment for astrocytomas should only occur once the patient becomes symptomatic and then treatment should include surgery, radiotherapy, and chemotherapy (drugs used to kill cancer cells). While the median survival was only five to eight years, the study did not note any benefit to early treatment with chemotherapy.

Another type of brain tumor is a CNS lymphoma. This tumor develops from lymphocyte cells and is usually located in the cerebral hemisphere. This tumor disseminates tiny seeds throughout the brain and can infect the CSF, therefore diagnosis may involve a spinal tap (lumbar puncture) (Brain Tumor Society, 2004).

Meningiomas are tumors that arise form the covering of the brain and account for 25 percent of all brain tumors and are most common in people over the age of 40 years old. These tumors are slow-growing and nonmalignant, but they can reoccur. Adenomas, also known as pituitary tumors, originate in the pituitary gland and account for 10 percent of all brain tumors. These tumors are usually nonmalignant, curable, and found in younger adults. There are two types of pituitary tumors: nonsecreting and secreting. The secreting tumors cause the most problem by releasing high levels of pituitary hormones, which may lead to impotence, amenorrhea, abnormal body growth, hypertension, and hyperthyroidism. A tumor of the pineal gland accounts for 1 percent of all brain tumors. Primitive neuroectodermal tumors are most often found in children and young adults and are often malignant. Schwannomas are tumors found around nerve fibers and are usually benign. Schwannomas usually involve the eighth cranial nerve, affecting balance and hearing, and may also be called vestibular schwannomas or acoustic neuromas. Vascular tumors are rare and noncancerous, involving the blood vessels of the brain, with the most common being a hemangioblastoma (Brain Tumor Society, 2004).

One of the most common complications of cancer is metastasis to the brain. These cancers are called secondary brain tumors, and they occur in 20 to 40 percent of all oncology patients. The most common originating sites are the lung, breast, colon, kidney, and the skin from melanoma.

Assessment with Clinical Manifestations

The early symptoms of a brain tumor usually are rather subtle and are dependent on the location, size, and type of tumor. Symptoms will usually develop slowly and worsen over time, which is what causes patients to seek a health care provider. If a patient has an occipital tumor, the first symptoms may involve visual disturbances; whereas a patient with a tumor in the frontal lobe may experience personality and memory deficits. However, if the patient is experiencing an increase in ICP, the symptoms may be more generalized and less specific to a region of the brain, because of the fact that the entire brain is now compromised. This is why it is important to complete a thorough neurological assessment to determine the area of the brain being affected.

Headache is usually experienced by 50 percent of people with brain tumors. The pain may last for several minutes to several hours, but is usually more severe in the morning versus the afternoon; with coughing, sneezing, and posture changes are also problematic (Brain Tumor Society, 2004). Seizures may occur because of an interruption in the electrical activity in the brain. In a

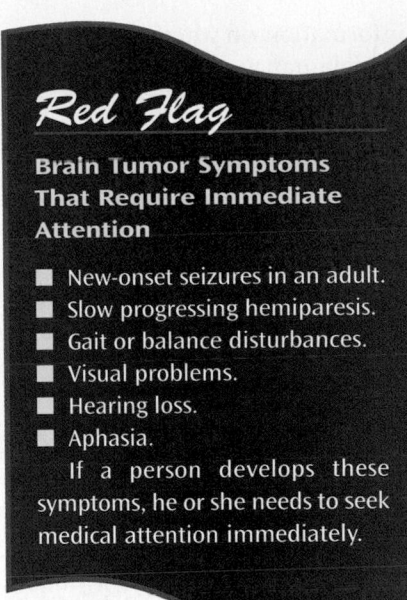

person without a previous head injury or illness, seizures are an important warning sign. Nausea and vomiting may or may not be associated with the headache, but nausea and vomiting can also be a symptom of increasing ICP. Visual deficits that may include blurred vision, double vision, or partial loss of vision may be related to increasing ICP that is causing reduced blood flow to the eye. Ringing or buzzing sounds in the ear may also be noted as well as balance problems, such as dizziness. Hemiplegia, hemiparesis, or general lack of coordinated movement may be associated with motor or sensory impairment. Behavioral and cognitive changes involving personality changes, inability to concentrate, poor memory, and communication deficits can all be associated with brain tumors.

Diagnostic Tests

While radiological exams are important in the diagnosis of brain tumors, an extensive physical exam also helps determine the area of the brain being affected and the extent to which the tumor is affecting healthy brain tissue. The physical exam focuses in on a neurological evaluation of the cranial nerves including: eye movement and reflexes, pupillary reaction, hearing, taste, smell, motor reflexes, strength and sensation, and balance and coordination (see chapter 34).

The most common radiological exams used in the diagnosis of a brain tumor are the CT scan and MRI. The CT scan can be used with or without contrast and is readily available in most hospitals. A CT scan can determine the location of the tumor and possibly the tumor type and can detect any associated cerebral edema and bleeding. A CT scan is often used to evaluate the effectiveness of treatment (decrease in tumor size) and whether a tumor is reoccurring. However, an MRI offers better imaging by distinguishing between healthy tissue and diseased tissue and is especially helpful when the tumor is near bone. MRS uses some of the same techniques as an MRI, but does not expose the patient to radiation. Instead, this exam detects the biochemical metabolism of the body and differentiates between healthy tissue and abnormal tissue (Brain Tumor Society, 2004). If the tumor is close to or invading blood vessels, an angiography may be needed. This study involves injecting a patient with dye and then obtaining images of the tumor, to identify the network of blood vessels supplying the tumor, and the blood vessels surrounding the tumor, especially if surgical removal is being considered. An angiography may also assist in determination of the tumor type. An EEG may be obtained to note an abnormal electrical activity in the brain, especially if the patient is having seizures (Daniels, 2003).

While these radiological tests are vital to determine the location and size of the tumor, treatment will depend on the tumor cell type. Determination of cell type is most often done through a biopsy. There are three different techniques used to obtain a biopsy: needle, stereotactic, and open biopsy (American Brain Tumor Association [ABTA, 2004a). A needle biopsy involves aspiration of tissue through a needle. A stereotactic biopsy is similar to a needle biopsy, but it uses the assistance of a computer to locate the tumor and guide the needle into a section of the tumor. Open biopsy involves making a surgical incision into the brain and removing a small piece of tumor tissue; this procedure is usually done during surgical removal of the tumor. The tissue sample is then sent to the pathology lab and evaluated by a pathologist, a health care provider who specializes in the identification of tissue types. Most pathology reports take approximately 24 hours to be completed, but in some cases a frozen section will be taken directly from the operating room and evaluated within 15 to 20 minutes. The pathology report is then given to the surgeon and a decision is made as to how to proceed with the surgical removal. Two of the most important components to the diagnosis of a brain tumor are determination of the origin of the cancer cell (primary site or secondary site) and the potential growth rate. The biopsy results will provide information on whether the tumor is benign or malignant and, if malignant, the malignancy grade. All this information is necessary for the health care provider to appropriately evaluate and develop a treatment plan for the patient.

Nursing Diagnoses

Based on the information gathered, examples of nursing diagnoses in the patient with a brain tumor may include the following:
- Impaired physical mobility related to weakness associated with the brain injuries.
- Risk for injury related to the physical difficulties of the brain injuries.
- Self-care deficit related to weakness or confusion from the brain injuries.

Planning and Implementation

There are three main types of treatment for patients with a brain tumor: surgery, radiation, and chemotherapy. Additional therapies are photodynamic and adjunctive medication therapy. The type of tumor and the grade of the tumor will help determine the course of treatment. In many cases, a patient will require more than one type of treatment (e.g., a patient will have partial surgical removal of the tumor, but need follow-up radiation to destroy the rest of the tumor). A patient's overall general health and past medical history also play a part in determining how the treatment plan will be pursued.

Selection of a health care provider may be one of the first things that a patient is confronted with after learning that they have a brain tumor. The nurse can encourage the patient to look for oncologists who have experience with his or her type of cancer and are willing to discuss all treatment options (including experimental treatments) clearly and fully and able to answer questions and concerns the patient may have. Hospitals affiliated with colleges or universities are more likely to have clinical research trials, if the patient is interested in experimental treatments. The nurse should also provide information on local support groups and community agencies that can provide additional information and services for the patient. Most patients will need a referral to a neurooncologist and possibly a neurosurgeon. A neurooncologist specializes in the management of patients with neurological disorders. Some treatments for cancer located elsewhere in the body are not appropriate for brain tumors. A neurooncologist is knowledgeable about what types of treatments can be used with specific types of brain tumors. A neurosurgeon specializes in surgical procedures involving the CNS.

Management of a patient in the acute phase of a brain tumor is similar to caring for a patient with a brain injury. Patients with brain tumors are at risk for increased ICP, seizures, and other postoperative complications (e.g., infection, pneumonia, or neurological compromise). However, the nurse must also assist in managing the side effects of radiation and chemotherapy (see chapter 15). One of the most frustrating side effects of both chemotherapy and radiation is fatigue. Patients complain that the fatigue is severe, persistent, and unpredictable. It is emotionally draining to be tired all the time. Sometimes the fatigue may have a clinical cause, such as anemia, which may be treated with medications such as epoetin (Procrit). Antiemetic drugs, such as, ondansetron (Zofran), trimethobenzamide (Tigan), or promethazine (Phenergan), may be needed to help control the nausea. These medications can be given before, during, and after the chemotherapy for prevention and management of nausea and vomiting. Patients should be instructed to avoid contact with people who are sick as their immune system has been suppressed by the chemotherapy agents. If a patient wants to become pregnant or becomes pregnant, she should consult her health care provider immediately, as some chemotherapeutic agents may affect her ability to conceive. Mouth and throat sores can be managed with antifungal

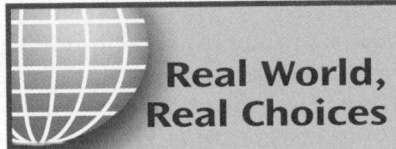

Real World, Real Choices

A Patient with Acute Neurological Clinical Manifestations

A 45-year-old office worker with a one-hour history of facial weakness, blurred vision, and left-sided hemiplegia is brought to the ED by life squad. The patient has a past medical history of atrial fibrillation, diabetes, and hypertension. He is a nonsmoker but works in a smoking environment. On assessment, his blood pressure is 210/95 mm Hg, pulse is 110 and irregular, and respirations are 20 per minute. He is anxious, because this is the first time he has been in a hospital. He also shares his concern about missing too much work and losing his job. How should the nurse best handle this situation?

agents, such as clotrimazole (Mycelex), and diet. Appetite changes may lead to significant weight loss; therefore foods should be visually appealing and focus on high caloric and high nutritional value but not large quantities. As with any treatment plan, the patient should be made aware of all the risks and benefits of each therapy and nursing interventions should be focused meeting patient needs.

For a patient who suffers from impaired memory, the nurse should provide orientation cues. Providing a clock and calendar will assist in orientation and provide security in being able to note the date and time. Compensatory strategies may be needed, such as making lists and having a scheduled routine to follow. Teaching should be kept simple and short and may need to involve the caregiver to reinforce learning when the nurse or therapist is not available.

A patient who has suffered brain damage may have deficits in problem solving and decision making. This may lead to problems with his or her ability to maintain a safe environment, manage finances, or keep a job. Strategies to facilitate problem solving need to be practical and applicable to everyday situations. Patients who have a brain tumor need to consider the use of advance directives and identifying a durable power of attorney for health care decisions. In the event that they are unable to make health care decisions for themselves, this person would know their wishes and be able to speak for them. For patients with a brain injury or stroke, the cognitive impairments usually occur quickly and there is no time for setting up a surrogate for health care decisions, but this may not be the case for patients with a brain tumor.

Impulsiveness involves the patient's desire to perform a task without planning the steps to accomplish the task. For example, a patient who has suffered a brain injury may decide that he or she wants to go to the bathroom but not realize that he or she is not strong enough to walk by himself or herself and not remember that he or she needs to put on his or her call light to request assistance. The patient will just act without thinking and place himself or herself at significant risk for injury. Impulsivity is often combined with a lack of judgment, which can lead to disastrous results. The nurse needs to be aware of these patient behaviors and provide a safe environment. The use of rewards or incentives may help to deter some of these behaviors.

Some patients with a brain dysfunction may exhibit explosive outbursts of anger and aggression. Dealing with these patients requires excellent communication skills and a caring attitude. In an effort to calm the patient, the nurse needs to speak in a soft, yet firm manner and attempt to redirect the behavior. The nurse also needs to conduct an environmental assessment to determine what triggered the behavior and, if possible, eliminate the contributing factor. Providing a calm, quiet place, such as the patient's room, may help to relax the patient and allow them to control his or her behavior. Patients may also benefit from a structured environment. Being assigned to the same group of nurses that understand the patient's routine will provide a sense of security and safety for the patient. Limiting the number of visitors, phone calls, and television may be necessary to prevent the patient from becoming overwhelmed. Also, providing frequent rest periods are necessary. While the patient may not have any visual physical impairments, the brain is still recovering. If needed, a medication regimen, including mood stabilizers, antipsychotics, and antidepressants may be helpful (Broyles, Reiss, & Evans, 2007). If the behavior cannot be managed, a patient may need to be enrolled in a structured day program or inpatient psychiatric care.

Most stroke patients will have some impairment in communication. Aphasia is when a person is unable to communicate verbally or understand what is being spoken or written. There are three types of aphasia: expressive, receptive, and global. **Expressive aphasia (Broca's aphasia)** is when a patient cannot express what he or she wants to say. The patient knows what he or she wants to say but cannot get the words to form. This type of aphasia may be associated with dysarthria, which is a slurring of speech due to weakness in the facial and oral muscles. **Receptive aphasia (Wernicke's aphasia)** is when a patient is unable to understand what is being said or what is written. It is a comprehension problem. The third type of aphasia is **global aphasia,** which is when a patient has both expressive and receptive aphasia. This type of aphasia is difficult to address because these patients cannot understand what is being said and cannot tell anyone what they need or want. A strategy in working with patients with global aphasia is to use of hand gestures and demonstration. Speech and language therapy will be an important part of a patient's recovery. When caring for patients with a communication deficit, the nurse will need to speak clearly and distinctly. The use of communication boards and gestures may be helpful for patients with severe expressive aphasia. For patients with receptive aphasia, the nurse may need to gesture or direct the patient to perform the task requested (e.g., brushing teeth or combing hair). The patient may be able to perform the task but unable to understand what the nurse is saying. Aphasia can be one of the most frustrating impairments in communication. The nurse must exhibit patience and allow time for the patient to express his or her needs, without jumping in to finish a sentence or help him or her find a word. Some patients may be able to write their needs, so having a pen and paper or chalkboard available will be helpful.

Mobility is one of the biggest concerns for a patient with brain dysfunction. Patients may experience mild weakness of an extremity to total immobility of all extremities. Hemiparesis is weakness on half of the body, while hemiplegia is paralysis (inability to move) on half of the body. Both hemiparesis and hemiplegia place a patient at high risk for falls and the complications associated with immobility. When a patient has hemiplegia or hemiparesis of an upper extremity, he or she is also at risk for subluxation of the shoulder. Subluxation is a partial dislocation of the joint; in most patients it is usually the shoulder. Because of the weight of the arm and his or her inability to move it, the arm tends to hang down pulling on the shoulder joint. This strains the shoulder muscles and over time will pull the shoulder partially out of socket. Some nursing strategies to address subluxation are to support the arm and shoulder with pillows while the patient is in bed and when up in a chair. When the patient ambulates, the use of a sling to support the arm and keep it in alignment with the body will be important. With weakness of the lower extremity, a patient may be in need of an ankle foot orthosis (AFO) or brace to support the ankle and prevent internal or external rotation. The nurse should encourage the patient to wear the AFO during all ambulation or transfers. Spasticity is when a muscle is has an increase in tone that causes an abnormal position or posture.

Spasticity occurs in 65 percent of stroke survivors and can affect activities of daily living, ambulation, and transfers (Ibrahim, Wurpel, & Gladson, 2003). Treatment usually involves stretching, strengthening, splinting, and cold therapy for vasoconstriction. Antispasticity drugs and physical therapy is vital in the management of spasticity. Some medications utilized for spasticity are botulinum toxin, dantrolene sodium, baclofen, diazepam (Valium), tizanidine, and clonidine. Current evidence-based research indicates that the use of intrathecal baclofen (ITB) is effective in the treatment of spasticity related to stroke. The pump is surgically implanted and delivers baclofen directly into the intrathecal space, thus allowing for smaller doses with increased effectiveness. The ITB also allows for frequent titration of the baclofen depending on the level of spasticity. Patients will also need assistive devices for ambulation and transfers. Walkers, canes, wheelchairs, and scooters are all used to assist the patient in mobility. A hemi-wheelchair has a hard seat, which promotes proper sitting posture. A hemi-cane and quad-can are used to help with stability. A walker is used for stability, but the patient must have the upper body strength to lift and maneuver the walker. A wheeled walker may be used, but the patient must be able to maintain some balance.

The nurse must also watch for spasticity, which may lead to the development of a **contracture** (muscle shortening). Contractures occur when a muscle has not been adequately stretched and becomes resistant to stretching. If not treated, contractures can become permanent and disabling to the patient. Nursing care should always include both active and passive range of motion for any patient with hemiparesis or hemiplegia. Edema may occur as a result of an extremity being dependent (hanging below the level of the heart). The nurse should take steps to support and position extremities to promote venous return. Some patients may also experience ataxia. Ataxia is when a person has an abnormal movement pattern. This pattern may appear uncoordinated or jerky. This again places the patient at risk for injury related to falls.

The patient with a brain tumor often has many difficulties with self-care and accomplishing the normal tasks of the activities of daily living. Simple forms of care, such as dressing and grooming, are not easily performed. Therefore, nursing care is needed to assist the patient with his or her daily care.

Sensory-perceptual deficits are in the patient's ability to sense (seeing and feeling) and interpret the data. There are several different types of sensory-perceptual impairments. **Homonymous hemianopsia** is when a patient has lost vision in half of one eye and the nasal half of the other eye. With this visual impairment, the patient is limited in his or her visual field and at risk for falls. Depth perception and a visual field cut may also be impaired, so that the patient does not see anything within that visual field. The patient may walk into a wall or only see the food on half of the plate. Unilateral neglect is when a person is not aware of one side of his or her body. This impairment may lead him or her to only dress one side of his or her body or forget about his or her arm, which is hanging off the chair. Nursing management involves reminding the patient to visually scan his or her environment constantly to watch for environmental hazards and to prevent injury.

Many stroke patients are diagnosed with dysphagia. Dysphagia is impairment in swallowing. It involves the oral and neck muscles and the gag reflex. A patient who cannot swallow properly is at significant risk for aspiration, dehydration, and malnutrition (Rodrigue, Cote, Kirsh, Germain, Couturier, & Fraser, 2002). When a patient with a brain dysfunction is admitted, nurses need to know how to perform a swallowing evaluation at the bedside to determine if further follow-up is needed by a speech therapist. The physician may order a barium swallow study to determine the severity of the dysphagia. Some patients may require a thickened diet, which involves the use of a cornstarch type mixture, to be placed in all their drinks, including water and coffee. The consistency may be like that of nectar or honey, depending on the amount of thickener used. It is important for the nurse to make mealtime as comfortable as possible. The dysphagic patient often has problems with self-concept because of spilling, drooling, and length of time it takes to eat. The nurse should provide a supportive environment by allowing the patient plenty of time to eat (this may entail reheating of foods) and trying to make the foods appealing. Some techniques to assist the patient with swallowing and prevent aspiration include having the patient tuck the chin with each swallow, turn the head toward the weak side to swallow, and hold the breath during a swallow and making sure the patient is in a proper sitting position (Mayer, 2004). For patients with severe dysphagia, enteral tube feeding may be required. The patient may have a nasogastric tube to temporarily provide nutrition with the hopes that the patient will regain some swallowing ability. However, if the patient shows little to no improvement, a gastrostomy tube may need to be placed for nutritional support. When a patient is NPO, it is extremely important to encourage good oral care but be careful of aspiration.

Incontinence is one of the major predictors of discharge disposition for most patients. This not only involves their ability to recognize the need to void or defecate, but also their ability to perform these functions independently. Some stroke patients are aware of the need to toilet but are not able to ambulate or transfer onto the commode without assistance. Also, the ability to manage clothing may be a problem for stroke patients. Making sure the bowel is empty is crucial. Administration of a stool softener and allowing for a regular routine to be established is important. Find out what the patient's routine was at home and then try to accommodate that schedule in the hospital. For bladder management, setting up a voiding schedule and avoiding fluids before bedtime may decrease incontinence. The nurse should also assess the patient for a urinary tract infection (UTI). If the patient had an indwelling catheter at all during his or her hospitalization, he or she is at higher risk for development of a UTI. For patients with a spastic bladder, antispasmodic medications may be helpful. While addressing incontinence, the nurse needs to pay particular attention to skin care issues. Patients who are incontinent are at greater risk for skin breakdown and infection.

Patients who have experienced a brain dysfunction may go through a myriad of emotions from anxiety about what is happening or going to happen to depression and hopelessness that life will never be the same again. In a study by Mukand, Guilmette, and Tran (2003), patients expressed anxiety about dying, changing relationships, loss of independence, change in roles and responsibilities, and financial issues. It is important for the nurse to be aware of all these issues to help the patient work through the emotions and understand how grieving these losses are an important part of the process. Allow the patient to talk about what has happened and how it has affected his or her life; then help the patient to talk about what he or she can do.

Motivation is an important factor in the recovery of any patient. Instead of focusing on what the patient is unable to do, the nurse needs to help him or her focus on what he or she can do. Coaching and encouragement should be a part of every aspect of care. Having the patient do as much as possible, independently, will help increase his or her self-esteem and decrease a sense of powerlessness. In a study by Robinson-Smith (2002), stroke patients who had a higher self-care self-efficacy had less depression. The nurse can help build confidence by helping the patient break the task down into smaller more manageable pieces and then giving them positive reinforcement during each step of the task.

While the stroke patient is struggling with what has happened in their life, the family or caregiver is struggling with change also. For many family members, a change in family roles and structure, financial concerns, time management issues, and dealing with behavior management issues will be a constant struggle. Clark and King (2003) noted that the family or caregiver will go through a sense of loss with a stroke, because their loved one has changed. Instead of the change being a slow and gradual process, such as with dementia, the family has suddenly been thrust into different roles with little to no time to adapt. Clark and King also found a higher level of depression among caregivers of stroke survivors than caregivers of patients with Alzheimer's disease.

They may not even want to assume this new role but are forced into it. It is important for the nurse watch for the signs of elder abuse. These signs may include: physical abuse, sexual assault, neglect, oversedation, or financial abuse (Allen, 2004). A great deal literature has been devoted to exploration of how caregivers are coping with caring for stroke survivors. In a study by O'Connell, Baker, and Prosser (2003), caregivers found the patient relying on them for all activities, including social interactions. The caregivers reported that they would have liked to have more information about the recovery process, emotional changes with the patient, and how to manage these changes. The nurse needs to help the family or caregiver recognizing the stress that a role change can bring and help to build on the strengths within the family unit (Bluvol, 2003). Caregivers are expected to learn a vast amount of information in a short period of time. It is easy for the nurse to overwhelm caregivers. Take time to talk with the family or caregiver to find out what he or she has the most concerns about and address those areas first.

While most patients will be discharged from an acute care or rehabilitation setting, caring for a patient with a brain dysfunction is far from over. With the shortening length of stay for many patients, nurses need to be aware of how to

Uncovering the Evidence

Family Caregivers of Patients with Strokes

Discussion: A study by Bakas, Austin, Jessup, Williams, & Oberst (2004) investigated what caregivers of patients, who had suffered a stroke, identified as the most time-consuming and difficult tasks. They found that while nurses might assume that the actual hands-on care would be the most difficult to master, caregivers felt that administering treatments and medications, providing personal care, running errands, and planning activities were their least difficult task. The most difficult tasks were managing behavioral issues, providing emotional support, carrying out household tasks, and managing finances. The most time-consuming tasks involved providing emotional support, providing transportation, managing finances, bills, health care forms, and doing household tasks. The least time-consuming tasks were finding eldercare, providing personal care, assisting with mobility and administration of treatments and medications, and communicating with the stroke survivor.

Implications for Practice: The implications for nursing care suggest that nurses should provide resources for caregivers to get assistance after discharge. Contacting a social worker or organization for referrals can do this. The nurse should also provide consistent follow-up to see how the caregiver is managing and, if symptoms of depression are noted, to seek psychological counseling. Having an understanding of what tasks are the most difficult and time-consuming for a caregiver will help the family prepare for the adjustments that will be needed once the patient goes home.

Source: Bakas, T., Austin, J. K., Jessup, S. L., Williams, L. S., & Obert, M. T. (2004). Time and difficulty of tasks provided by family caregivers of stroke survivors. Journal of Neuroscience Nursing, 36(2), 95–106.

assist these patients within the community. In 1988, the average patient suffering a stroke was in the hospital 11.1 days; in 2002 it has dropped to 5.3 days according to the 2002 National Hospital Discharge Survey (DeFrances, & Hall, 2004). That is a decrease of 5.8 days in the past 14 years. Based on this information, nurses will be caring for stroke patients in multiple health care settings. Some patients may be eligible for home rehabilitation or a type of day rehabilitation program, but insurance companies may not offer coverage for many of these services.

When preparing a patient for discharge to home, it is important to evaluate his or her home environment for safety concerns that were not present before the stroke. Looking at the entrance to the home, staircases, width of doors, and bathroom configurations are essential in helping to make a smooth transition. In some cases, a group of therapists may go into the home to evaluate and recommend modifications before discharge. Socialization is an important part of returning to the community. The patient should be encouraged to return to as many normal and routine activities as possible. The American with Disabilities Act has been instrumental in helping make most public buildings accessible to wheelchairs and other assistive devices. Involvement in support groups may help the patient and family continue to cope with ongoing issues of role change and stress. Support groups are an important part of any rehabilitation program. While these groups provide information on brain injuries and community services, they also give emotional support to family and friend to help them cope with life changes. Nurses should be aware of the resources available to families and of local support groups and encourage family involvement.

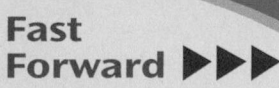

Fast Forward ▶▶▶

Gene Therapy in the Treatment of Brain Tumors

There are many therapies currently under investigation for patients with brain tumors. Gene therapy is investigating altering the genes in tissue cells and reprogramming them to self-destruct (suicide gene), slow the growth of the tumor, or to increase sensitivity to certain medications. These genes are injected into tumor cells with the hope that they will replicate and affect the tumor tissue (Castro, et al., 2003). There are studies that examine enhancing the body's own immune system to fight and destroy cancer cells. For example, an immune enhancer gene could be injected into a tumor to activate the patient's own immune response and cause the body to destroy the tumor. While research is promising in many areas of brain tumor management, it is important to note that all potential treatments must undergo extensive well-designed and carefully controlled clinical trials to evaluate the long-term effects on patients before any conclusions can be drawn.

Pharmacology

There are a number of medications used in the management of brain tumors. Corticosteroids are used to decrease cerebral edema and can be used in conjunction with other modalities, but these drugs may interfere with some chemotherapeutic agents. Anticonvulsants may be needed in the management or prevention of seizures, however because it may interfere with some chemotherapy agents, these drugs should not be used routinely (Behin, et al., 2003). Anticoagulants may be utilized to decrease the risk of thrombosis, and antidepressants may be effective in increasing neurological cognition in some patients with brain tumors.

Chemotherapy

Chemotherapy is the use of medications to kill tumor-causing cells, especially those tumors that are malignant. Chemotherapeutic agents may be used alone or in conjunction with radiation and surgery. The type of drug or drugs utilized will depend on the type of tumor, its location, and overall health of the patient. Some patients will receive chemotherapy everyday for weeks or months, and others will receive one dose every week for several weeks; the length and type of treatment will be determined by the oncology health care provider in conjunction with the patient and family. There is significant ongoing research in the development of new medications to treat brain tumors and various delivery methods that will target tumor cells without damaging healthy tissue. The specific drugs used in chemotherapy are divided into two main categories: cell-cycle specific drugs and non–cell-cycle specific drugs. Cell-cycle specific drugs are most effective during a certain part of the cell cycle. Non–cell-cycle specific drugs are effective at any point in the cell cycle (ABTA, 2004b). This is why it is important on biopsy to determine the specific cell type associated with the brain tumor so specific medications can be targeted to kill that cell type. Chemotherapeutic agents are also listed as being either cytotoxic or cytostatic. Cytotoxic drugs (e.g., cisplatin, methotrexate, or rapamycin) actually cause cell death, while cytostatic drugs (e.g., interferon or tyrosine kinase inhibitors) focus on stopping cell reproduction or alter the cell behavior (ABTA, 2004b).

One of the biggest obstacles for chemotherapeutic agents to overcome is attempting to cross the blood-brain barrier, because, while it was designed to prevent harmful agents from entering the CNS, it also prevents helpful medications from reaching the brain. Research is currently being conducted to find medications that can penetrate this barrier, but currently health care providers must use drugs, such as mannitol to help chemotherapeutic agents across the border. Some drugs that can cross the blood brain border include: BCNU (carmustine), CCNU (lomustine), procarbazine, and temozolomide (temdur) (ABTA, 2004b).

Specific information regarding the contraindications and complications in the administration of chemotherapy are described in chapter 15.

Photodynamic Therapy

Another therapy for brain tumor patients involves the use of light and light-sensitive drugs. Photodynamic therapy (PDT) differs from traditional chemotherapy in that it is not histologically cell specific; the treatment is localized (not systemic), and has little effect on healthy tissue. An intravenous photosensitive drug is used and within 48 hours the patient is taken into a surgical suite. In the operating room a laser may be inserted into the tumor tissue or into the cavity after the tumor has been removed. When the laser is turned on, the tumor cells appear to glow green, and the neurosurgeon is able to target the tumor cells with the laser to activate the drug and kill the tumor cells (ABTA, 2004a). Photodynamic therapy is limited to tumors that are visible, accessible, and sensitive to this type of therapy. As with any treatment modality, not all patients will respond to this therapy. Some important risk factors associated with photodynamic therapy include increased risk of cerebral edema, seizures, and extreme photosensitivity to light. The patient must be educated to wear protective clothing at all times, wear sunglasses, and avoid dental and visual exams for four weeks because of the intense exam lights utilized.

Surgery

Surgical removal is often the first line of treatment for brain tumors. The goal of surgery is to remove as much of the tumor as is possible without causing further damage to healthy brain tissue. This is often difficult when the tumor is malignant and surrounds or invades vital brain centers; however, some significant advances have been made in surgical intervention. If the tumor is because of cancer elsewhere in the body, the focus of treatment is on the primary site. Surgery may be utilized to assist with symptom management, but the original site of the cancer must be the focus to prevent further malignancy. Various surgical procedures may also be used to relieve pressure on brain tissue, to relieve seizures, to obtain a biopsy, or to allow direct access to the brain for treatment (ABTA, 2004c). While surgery may be the first line of treatment, some patients may not be good surgical candidates. The most common surgery is a craniotomy. A craniotomy involves removing a part of the skull bone to allow access to the brain tissue, and then the skull bone is replaced. A craniectomy is similar to a craniotomy, but the skull bone is not replaced, leaving a soft spot that will need to be protected (ABTA, 2004c). This type of surgery may be done to allow room for the brain to expand if edema is anticipated. Microsurgery involves the use of a microscope to visualize the surgical area, making it easier for the surgeon to remove the tumor tissue while limiting disruption to healthy tissue. Another type of surgery gaining in popularity is stereotactic surgery. This procedure uses computers to create a three-dimensional image of the brain and allows for precise location of the tumor. In some cases a frame is attached to the patient's skull at four points, and then an angiography is performed to create a picture of the tumor within the context of the frame. With a frameless surgery, tiny markers are taped or glued to the patient's head and then a scan is performed to produce a three-dimensional image. The surgeon uses a wand to touch the markers and then the computer can identify exactly where the surgical instrument is in relation to the brain tumor. While robotic surgery is currently in clinical trials, it is anticipated that this will soon be used to assist in neurosurgery. While embolization may not require a surgical incision, this technique has been useful in preventing blood flow from reaching a brain tumor, thus robbing it of nutrients (ABTA, 2004c). The tumor is then removed a few days later.

Shunts may be inserted in patients experiencing increased ICP due to an increase in CSF. A shunt is a flexible tube that is placed in a ventricle to drain excess CSF. The tube is then rerouted to the abdomen where the CSF empties into the peritoneal cavity. Ultrasonic aspirators use sound waves to vibrate the tumor, causing it to break into small pieces, which are removed with the use of a vacuum.

An important technique that is being used in conjunction with surgery is brain mapping. Brain mapping involves using various methods to draw a map or diagram of the brain. These procedures also may be referred to as stereotaxic procedures. Stereotaxic procedures are especially helpful when dealing with hard to reach tumors located deep in the cortex of the brain.

While surgical intervention is the treatment of choice in the management of brain tumors, it does involve significant risks and needs to be evaluated carefully. As with any brain surgery, patients are at risk for development of infection, hemorrhage, thrombosis, pneumonia, hydrocephalus, stroke, seizures, meningitis, and increased ICP. Goldhaber, Dunn, Gerhard-Herman, Park, and Black (2002) noted the venous thromboembolism (VTE) was the most frequent complication after a craniotomy, leading to DVT and pulmonary embolism. According to their study, enoxaparin or unfractionated heparin, compression stockings, and intermittent pneumatic compression use were found to prevent VTE. Surgical recovery will depend on the patient's general overall health status, age, and location of the tumor, and complexity of the surgical procedure performed.

Radiation Therapy

Radiation therapy uses a concentrated beam of energy to kill tumor cells. The goal of radiation therapy is to decrease the size of the tumor by slowing its growth and preventing tumors from reoccurring. The type and size of the tumor will determine the dose and type of radiation therapy used. Conventional radiation uses high energy X-rays or gamma rays to radiate an area. The dosage is usually the same for each treatment, and treatment lasts for six weeks. However, in the effort to kill tumor cells, healthy cells are also damaged by radiation. Interstitial brachytherapy has been largely replaced by stereotactic surgery, but it may be used in some cases. Interstitial brachytherapy involves surgical implantation of radioactive seeds directly into the brain tumor. It has been effective for recurrent tumors and when other therapy is not effective (Brain Tumor Society, 2004).

Stereotactic radiotherapy (SRS) uses radiation with or without invasive surgery to deliver a precise dose of radiation to a specific location within the brain. It is also called gamma knife, cyclotron, or Cyberknife and can be used for small benign tumors, highly vascular tumors, managing residual tumor that could not be removed surgically, and for recurrent tumors (Witt, Haas, Marrinan, & Brown, 2004). SRS limits damage to the surrounding brain tissue, thus decreasing the risk of posttreatment complications. Stereotactic radiotherapy should be considered for any tumor less than 30 to 35 mm in diameter, patients who are poor surgical candidates, and those who refuse surgery. SRS is most effective on AVM, acoustic neuromas, meningiomas, pituitary adenomas, and grade I and II malignant tumors. Before SRS can be initiated, significant brain mapping needs to occur to determine the exact location of the tumor within the brain and the dosage needed for treatment. After this information is obtained, the actual procedure can take up to four hours to complete. There are some side effects that nurses need to be aware of and are important in the education of the patient and family (e.g., headache, nausea and vomiting, diminished hearing). Two months after treatment an MRI is usually done to evaluate the efficacy of the treatment and determine the need for further management. Radiation therapy is an important tool in the treatment arsenal for brain tumors. Current evidence-based research suggests that patients with single brain metastasis, who have had complete surgical removal of the metastasis, should have follow up with whole brain radiotherapy to decrease the risk of tumor reoccurrence (Supportive Care Guidelines, 2004). Patients scheduled for stereotactic radiotherapy should be assessed for claustrophobia, especially if a frame is to be utilized, any allergy to IV dye, and their knowledge level and comfort with the procedure.

Rehabilitation

The rehabilitation phase begins when the patient arrives at the hospital. Rehabilitation is not a place within an institution; it is a philosophy. It can be done anywhere and anytime—on an acute care unit, in the ICU, clinic, school, and in home care. Nurses should always strive to promote the highest functional independence for a patient. Rehabilitation starts on admission and continues well beyond discharge. The goal of rehabilitation is to return the patient to the highest level of functional independence possible for that person. This will involve training the brain to work differently and adapting to new ways to perform routine activities. Each patient will be assigned specific team members for their unique needs. This team should include multidisciplinary specialists, such as health care providers, physical therapist, occupational therapist, speech-language pathologist, recreational therapist, vocational therapists, psychologists, dietitians, and nurses (Table 35-6). There are several different types of venues for rehabilitation. Acute rehabilitation is usually performed in a general hospital or free-standing rehabilitation hospital. The patient must require

TABLE 35-6	**Rehabilitation Team Members and Their Roles**
Physiatrist	Physician who specializes in rehabilitation medicine
Physical therapist	Focuses on mobility, balance, gait, strength, and coordination
Occupational therapist	Focuses on activities of daily living (bathing, dressing, etc.), home management
Speech-language pathologist	Focuses on communication (verbal and written), comprehension, memory, and dysphagia
Social worker	Focuses on discharge planning (support systems, financial resources, or community resources)
Psychologist	Focuses on cognitive and emotional status
Therapeutic recreational therapist	Focuses on leisure activities and resocialization
Vocational rehab counselor	Focuses on job retraining and adaptation
Biomedical/Rehab engineer	Focuses on designed adaptive equipment to assist with independence
Family physician	Manages other medical problems outside the realm of the physiatrist
Rehabilitation nurse	Focuses on promoting independence and coordinates follow-through for patient when not with other therapists (PT, OT, etc.)

3 hours of intensive therapy each day and be medically stable. A day treatment program is structured so patients are brought to the rehabilitation facility every day for a full day of therapeutic activities, but the patient returns home at night. Outpatient therapy is when the patient comes to the hospital, daily, for selected therapy times, but then returns home after the therapy sessions are finished. For patients who are homebound, various rehabilitation team members come to the patient's home and provide therapy. Community reentry focuses on helping the patient return to independent living and the possibility of returning to work. They also work with the patient on safety within the community and on financial and household management. Independent living programs help patients to regain as much independence as possible and then provide different levels of assistance as needed. These programs provide housing and a sense of community for patients with a brain injury.

Nurses are a vital component in the recovery process, because they are with the patient 24 hours a day, seven days a week. Patients sometimes feel that therapy stops when they leave the therapy department, however, it is important that therapy continues. It is the nurse's responsibility to make sure the patient continues to progress by following through on the activities he or she was doing in all other aspects of rehabilitation. Nursing care is focused on many different aspects for the patient. Depending on the area of the brain affected, the patient may have more impairment in one area and less in another. It is important for the nurse to understand where the injury occurred in the brain to be able to anticipate the care the patient might need, but remember that each patient is unique. The plan of care will need to be individualized for each patient based on his or her needs.

Evaluation of Outcomes

Potential patient outcomes for each of the example nursing diagnoses for the patient with brain injuries are:
- Impaired physical mobility related to weakness associated with the brain injuries. The patient should begin ambulating and increasing mobility status with success, as well as self-initiating correct body positioning.
- Risk for injury related to the physical difficulties of the brain injuries. The patient will practice fall prevention behaviors and not sustain any injuries.
- Self-care deficit related to weakness or confusion from the brain injuries. The patient will perform activity with coordinated movements and initiate self-care in performing activities of daily living.

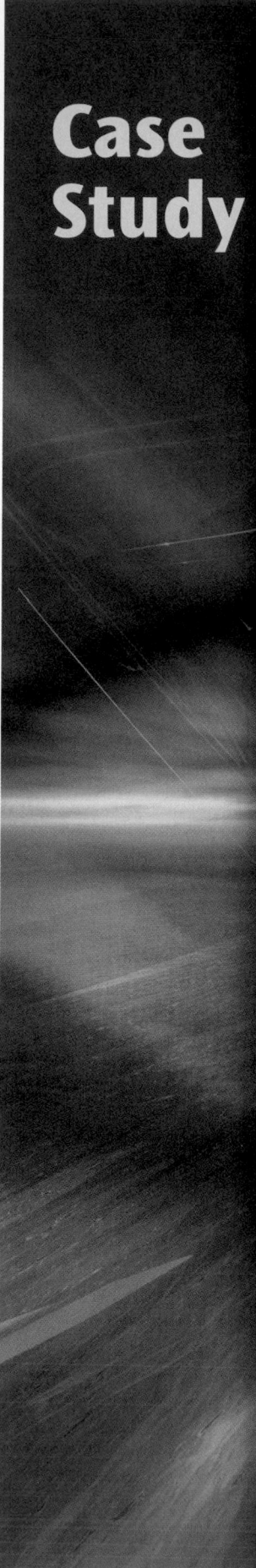

Case Study

Nursing Care Plan

Mrs. Lenier, age 77, was admitted yesterday after an ambulance transported her to the emergency department with left-sided hemiparesis. She was treated for a diagnosis of CVA after confirmation with a computed tomography (CT) scan. She was then admitted to the medical unit for follow-up care. Mrs. Lenier's assessment shows that she is normally left-handed and now has difficulty holding eating utensils. In addition, her left leg movements are weak, and her verbalizations are somewhat slow. Her history reveals that she resides in her home with her husband.

Assessment
- "I can't handle a milk carton with one hand."
- "I don't like to use a cane."
- Gait is unsteady and awkward
- Asymmetrical strength in arms and legs
- Unable to hold eating utensils in left hand

Nursing Diagnosis 1: Feeding self-care deficit related to weakness in left hand and inability to hold eating utensils.

NOC: Nutritional status: food and fluid intake

NIC: Nutrition management; Nutritional counseling

Expected Outcomes
The patient will:
1. Attend a teaching session on feeding herself with her left hand at 0930 on 6/15
2. Practice using adaptive spoon at 1330 on 6/15
3. Use adaptive spoon for meals beginning with breakfast on 6/16

Planning, Interventions, Rationales
1. Present a teaching session "feeding with nondominant hand at 0930 on 6/15." *For patients recovering from illness and injury, information about adapting to limitations fosters independence.*
2. Provide the patient with four foods of differing textures, adaptive utensils, and apron for a practice session at 1330 on 6/15. *Providing practice reinforces skills learned and fosters an improved confidence level in the learner.*
3. Notify the dietary department to include a right-hand adaptive spoon with breakfast tray on 6/16. *Using adaptive devices provides safety and promotes independence.*
4. Encourage patient to feed self independently at each meal, beginning on 6/16. *Recognizing and commending success promotes positive self-esteem.*

Evaluation
1. Mrs. Lenier attended the teaching session on 6/15, asked questions, and participated in the practice session.
2. Goal partially met. Mrs. Lenier practiced using eating utensils in left hand to feed self oatmeal, soup, peaches, and pudding on 6/15. Successful self-feeding with all foods except the soup. Continue practice and reevaluate on 6/22.
3. Goal partially met. On 6/16, fed self 80 percent of each meal, used adaptive utensils. Reevaluate on 6/19.

Nursing Diagnosis 1: Risk for injury: Falls related to unsteady, weak gait.

NOC: Risk control; Safety behavior: Home environment; Safety behavior: personal; Safety status: Falls occurrence; Safety status: Physical injury

Case Study

NIC: Health education; Behavior modification

Expected Outcomes

The patient will:
1. Participate in physical therapy evaluation of mobility strengths and weaknesses on 6/15 at 1100.
2. Attend a muscle strengthening class on 6/15 at 1500.
3. Perform all strengthening exercises prescribed twice a day at 1000 and 1600, beginning on 6/16.

Planning, Interventions, Rationales

1. Request physical therapy consultation for appropriate assistive devices, strengthening exercises, and gait training on 6/15. Collaboration with other health care providers provides the best care for the patient.
2. Escort patient to muscle-strengthening class on 6/15 at 1600. Provides safety and support as the patient begins to learn new skills.
3. Assigned caregivers will record each exercise, number of repetitions, and patient response twice daily Documenting patient progress toward the achievement of goals aids in outcome attainment and evaluation of care.

Evaluation

1. Goal met. Patient met with physical therapist on 6/15 and "listened well to the therapist."
2. Goal met. Patient attended muscle strengthening class on 6/15 at 1600 and participated fully.
3. Goal met. Patient attended muscle strengthening class and performed exercises as prescribed twice daily.

KEY CONCEPTS

- There are two main types of strokes (i.e., ischemic or hemorrhagic).
- The modifiable risk factors for a stroke include hypertension, hypercholesterolemia, atherosclerosis, atrial fibrillation, obesity, smoking, drugs, alcohol, and other health problems. Nonmodifiable risk factors include age, sex, family history, and past medical history.
- A CT scan is usually the first diagnostic test ordered for a patient suspected of having a stroke. Other tests include: laboratory tests, MRI, PET scan, EEG, and angiography.
- Medical treatment focuses on the ability to administer tPA.
- Complications of a stroke may include cerebral hypoxia related to poor oxygenation, decreased cerebral perfusion, and vasospasm.
- Brain injuries can occur as a direct blow to the brain (primary injury) or as a result of brain swelling, increased ICP, or cerebral hypoxia (secondary injury).

- There are three levels of brain injury, mild (concussion), moderate, and severe (coma).
- The most important signs and symptoms associated with brain injuries are impaired consciousness, visual disturbances and pupillary changes, headache, nausea or vomiting, and impaired cognition.
- Classifications of brain tumors include benign, malignant, primary, and secondary.
- The most common type of brain tumor is the glioma.
- Early symptoms of brain tumors are subtle and depend on the location, size, and type of tumor. The most common symptoms are headaches that get progressively worse as the day progresses, visual disturbances, seizures, weakness, and gait disturbances.
- Surgical intervention is the first treatment choice for most brain tumors. Radiation and chemotherapy may also be needed to prevent reoccurrence or to kill remaining tumor cells.

Continued

KEY CONCEPTS—cont'd

- Stereotactic radiotherapy is a new noninvasive procedure that targets tumor cells using a precise, focused beam.
- Nursing management involves assisting in relieving the symptoms of the tumor and the treatments: surgery (craniotomy), radiation, and chemotherapy.

- Caregiver role strain is a big concern. Nurses must understand the importance of providing caregivers with resources to prevent burnout while caring for their loved one.

REVIEW QUESTIONS

1. The type of CVA (stroke) that occurs when a blood vessel in the brain becomes clogged, usually by plaque buildup is a(n):
   1. Ischemic stroke
   2. Hemorrhagic stroke
   3. Aneurysm
   4. Subdural hematoma

2. Select a modifiable risk factor in the prevention of a stroke:
   1. Family history
   2. Sex
   3. Obesity
   4. Age

3. An important nursing intervention when caring for a patient receiving tPA is to:
   1. Complete neurological checks every 2 hours for the first 24 hours
   2. Change the IV site every shift
   3. Keep the diastolic blood pressure greater than 110 mm Hg
   4. Watch for decreased level of consciousness and increase in blood pressure

4. Usually this radiological test is the first one administered to a patient suspected of having a stroke:
   1. MRI
   2. CT scan
   3. PET scan
   4. EEG

5. A primary brain injury is caused by:
   1. ICP
   2. An external force
   3. An abnormal growth of brain tissue
   4. An internal force

6. A 16-year-old football player is confused after being struck in the head by another player. He states he does not remember much of what happened, just waking up in the hospital about two hours after being hit. This patient most likely is suffering from a:

   1. Concussion
   2. Moderate brain injury
   3. Severe brain injury
   4. Locked-in syndrome

7. The nurse is educating a group of 7-year-old children on preventing brain injury. One of the most important things to tell them is to:
   1. Always wear a helmet when riding your bike or skateboard or rollerblading
   2. Always wear knee and arm pads when riding your bike or skateboard or rollerblading
   3. Look both ways before crossing the street
   4. Always wear well-supported shoes when playing outdoors

8. A 67-year-old male is admitted to the intensive care unit following a fall down a flight of stairs. Upon assessment, the patient responds only to pain by withdrawing his hand and curses frequently. Using the Glasgow Coma Scale, the nurse rates this patient as a:
   1. 15
   2. 4
   3. 12
   4. 9

9. Your next door neighbor calls you (an RN) at 12 a.m. concerned about her 14-year-old son. She tells you that he fell while horseback riding around 4 p.m., and he struck his head on the ground, but did not lose consciousness. Now he is complaining of a severe headache and blurry vision. You should instruct your neighbor to:
   1. Let him rest until morning and then call the physician
   2. Give him ibuprofen for pain and some Benadryl for sleep
   3. Call 911 or take him to the emergency department
   4. Call your family physician and wait for a return call

REVIEW QUESTIONS—cont'd

10. A common medication given to help decrease ICP is:
    1. Aspirin
    2. Ibuprofen
    3. Lasix
    4. Mannitol

11. The most important nursing diagnosis when caring for a patient with an open skull fracture is:
    1. Risk for infection
    2. Risk for impaired skin integrity
    3. Risk for impaired swallowing: aspiration
    4. Risk for impaired physical mobility

12. A benign brain tumor is:
    1. Cancerous
    2. Noncancerous
    3. Fast-growing

13. A secondary brain tumor:
    1. Is only found in the brain or central nervous system
    2. Is benign and slow-growing
    3. Started somewhere else in the body and spread to the brain
    4. Started as a secondary brain injury

14. The most common form of brain tumor is a:
    1. Meningioma
    2. Glioma
    3. CNS lymphoma
    4. Adenoma

15. A patient is scheduled for stereotactic radiotherapy in the morning. The patient asks you about the procedure and what to expect. You tell him:
    1. It uses special drugs that are sensitive to light.
    2. It is effective on large brain tumors.
    3. It is a procedure that uses a precise beam of radiation therapy.
    4. It is best when used with malignant tumors.

REVIEW ACTIVITIES

1. A 57-year-old bus driver was recently diagnosed with a brain tumor. She has an appointment to talk with her physician tomorrow but is frightened and wants to know what questions she should ask her physician. Identify five important questions you should encourage your patient to ask her physician.

2. You are asked to speak to a group of teenagers about the prevention of brain injuries. What topics would you include in your presentation?

3. A caregiver is concerned about being able to care for her mother, who recently suffered a severe stroke in her home. What are some important nursing interventions to include in your education to this caregiver about caregiver role strain?

4. A 21-year-old patient with a brain injury is admitted to your rehabilitation unit. Identify some appropriate nursing interventions for this patient.

Continued

REVIEW ACTIVITIES—cont'd

5. Identify steps a patient could take to modify various risk factors for a stroke.

Dysfunction of the Spinal Cord and Peripheral Nervous System: Nursing Management

Constance J. Ayers, PhD, RN

KEY TERMS

Autonomic dysreflexia
Dermatome
Dysesthesias
Lancinating
Lower motor neurons
Neuralgia
Neuropathies
Paraplegia
Paresthesia
Quadriplegia (tetraplegia)
Spinal shock
Tic douloureux
Upper motor neurons

CHAPTER TOPICS

- Spinal Cord Injury
- Spinal Cord Tumors
- Peripheral Nervous Disorders

There are a number of central nervous system (CNS) disorders, which exhibit themselves in a variety of ways, often creating long-standing dysfunction. The primary dysfunctions of the CNS described in this chapter are spinal cord injuries (SCIs), spinal cord tumors, and peripheral nerve disturbances. Each disorder creates unique challenges, which affect motor and sensory functioning, and which usually result in long-term adaptation to changes in lifestyle and self-care abilities. A solid understanding of anatomy, physiology, and pathophysiology will contribute to a better understanding of each disorder and an ability to predict the occurrence of alterations, which will result in self-care challenges and painful syndromes. Unique challenges for patients and for their family members are characteristic of these disorders.

SPINAL CORD INJURY

Since 1995 when the actor Christopher Reeve was injured in a horse riding accident, the world has been able to put a "face" on SCIs. After his death in 2004, people became even more acquainted with his heroic activism to support research to find a cure for SCI, especially through stem cell research that has become promising. According to the Christopher Reeve Paralysis Foundation (CRPF), a person injures his or her spinal cord in the United States every 49 minutes. The typical person with SCI is male and between 16 and 30 years of age.

Epidemiology

The face of the person with an SCI has changed in recent years. With the aging of the population, the average age of the person with an SCI has risen from 28.6 in the decade of the 1970s to 38 years of age in 2000 (The University of Alabama National SCI Statistical Center, 2006). The number of people over age 60 who have an SCI has also increased, from 4.7 to 10.9 percent, attributable in part to improved accident response and thus survival rates. The overall incidence rate for SCI is 40 cases per one million people in the United States. This translates to more than 11,000 Americans injured each year. Currently, approximately 250,000 Americans are living with SCI and disability.

Etiology

The life expectancy of a person who has an SCI is somewhat lower than the general population and is increasingly less with higher levels of injury. Higher cervical injuries lead to shortened life expectancy, with ventilator-dependent patients experiencing significant losses to life expectancy. Prior to the 1970s renal failure was the primary cause of death for people with an SCI. Because of improved renal care, however, this is no longer the case. Primary causes of death for people with SCI that have the greatest affect on life expectancy are pneumonia, pulmonary emboli, and septicemia.

Most SCIs are caused by motor vehicle accidents, falls, violence, and sports accidents. Motor vehicle accidents account for 50.4 percent of injuries; falls are the second most common cause for SCI, followed by violence (primarily from gunshot wounds), and sports injuries as primary causes of SCI. Since 2000, SCIs resulting from violence and sports injuries have declined, while injuries from falls have increased.

Primary prevention of drug and alcohol related accidents is also a priority in prevention of SCI. Additionally, sports injuries, especially football injuries can cause SCI; therefore, continuing the education effort about prevention of SCI with the use of protective equipment in sports is warranted. The Think First National Prevention Foundation promotes education for the prevention of SCIs and provides an invaluable resource for nurses, health care providers, and the general public. Their efforts to promote airbags in automobiles have had a tremendous effect on the lowering of spinal injury and mortality rates from motor vehicle crashes.

Accidents are not the only culprits causing SCI. Osteoporosis is strongly linked to SCI in the elderly. In the elderly population, osteoporosis results in compression fractures of the vertebrae, leading to the risk and occurrence of SCI. Spinal tumors may also cause compression and injury of the spinal cord leading to loss of motor and sensory function below the level of the tumor. Other causes of spinal cord dysfunction include cervical spondylosis, myelitis, syringomyelia, and vascular diseases, which result in infarction or hemorrhage leading to spinal cord damage. It is important that nurses understand the leading causes of SCI, so that they can participate in prevention efforts to improve the health care outcomes attributable to SCI.

Safety First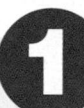

Prevention of SCIs

SCIs require the nurse to give serious consideration to primary prevention of accidents in the population, including continued teaching to the public about the use of seatbelts, and regarding the prevention of falls, especially in the elderly. Because falls from bicycles and horses are common causes of spinal injury, public education regarding the necessity of wearing helmets during these activities has helped the safety and prevention effort; however, the likelihood of SCI is not entirely preventable with helmets; the helmet effect is more attributable to the prevention of head injuries.

Pathophysiology

It is important to understand the structure and function of the spinal cord before considering the pathophysiology. Pathophysiological concepts are best understood in the context of the normal anatomy and physiology. Injury to the spinal cord leads to pathology that results because of interruption in the normal structure and functioning of the spinal cord.

One can envision the spinal cord as a power line delivering electricity along its route after leaving the power plant. If damage occurs to the power line, the circuit is broken, and power outages occur in the areas beyond the damaged line. Similarly, the spinal cord carries signals from the brain and CNS to the entire body. Damage or transection of the spinal cord causes loss of transmission of nerve signals beyond the injury resulting in loss of motor and sensory function.

The spinal cord is made up of white matter and gray matter (Figure 36-1). Gray matter is found in the inner areas of the spinal cord and comprises the anterior, lateral, and posterior horns. Sensory functioning arises from the dorsal half of the gray matter, and the ventral half of the gray matter is dedicated to motor functioning. Innervation of visceral and somatic regions of the body arises from the gray matter. Activation of the sympathetic and parasympathetic divisions of the autonomic nervous system occurs in the white and gray matter of the spinal cord.

The sympathetic nervous system is responsible for stimulating the adrenal glands to release epinephrine for the flight-or-fight response. This response will cause vasoconstriction, increased heart rate, and tachycardia. Ventilation and perfusion are also supported by the sympathetic nervous system, and sympathetic responses inhibit digestion and elimination. Sympathetic nervous system responses originate in the gray matter of the spinal cord and are transmitted from the first thoracic through second lumbar sections of the spinal cord. Damage to these areas of the spinal cord will affect the sympathetic nervous system response, causing acute and dangerous physiological issues for the patient.

The white matter of the spinal cord makes up the outer areas of the spinal cord (see Figure 36-1). The pathways for the ascending and descending spinal tracts are located in the white matter of the spinal cord and include the corticospinal tract, the spinothalamic tracts, and the posterior column. The corticospinal tract relays transmissions for motor activity. It originates in the brain, crosses over in the brainstem, and innervates the opposite side of the body. The spinothalamic tract originates in the spinal cord, crosses over within two spinal cord segments, and ascends to the thalamus. This tract transmits pain and tem-

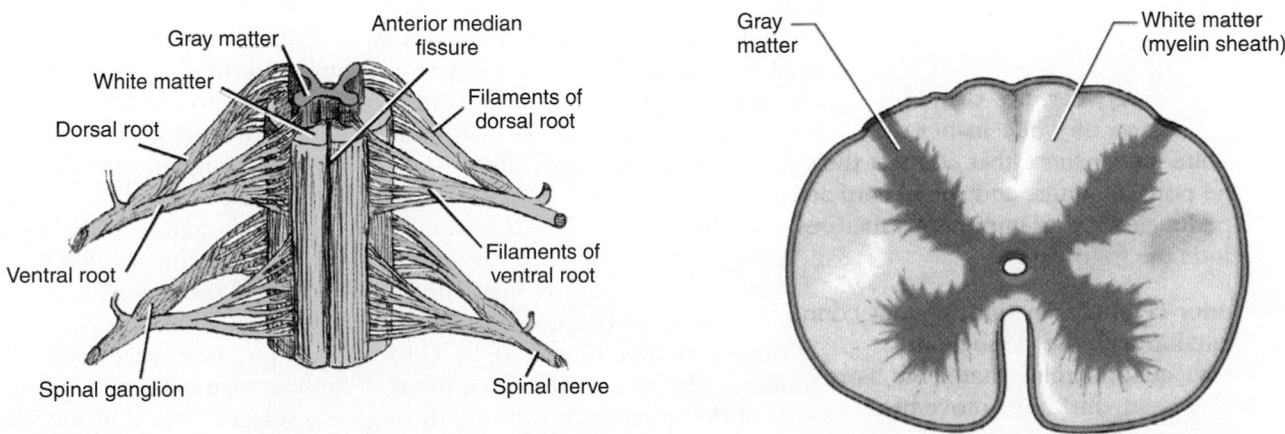

Figure 36-1 Spinal cord: A. Anterior view, B. Cross-sectional view—white and gray matter.

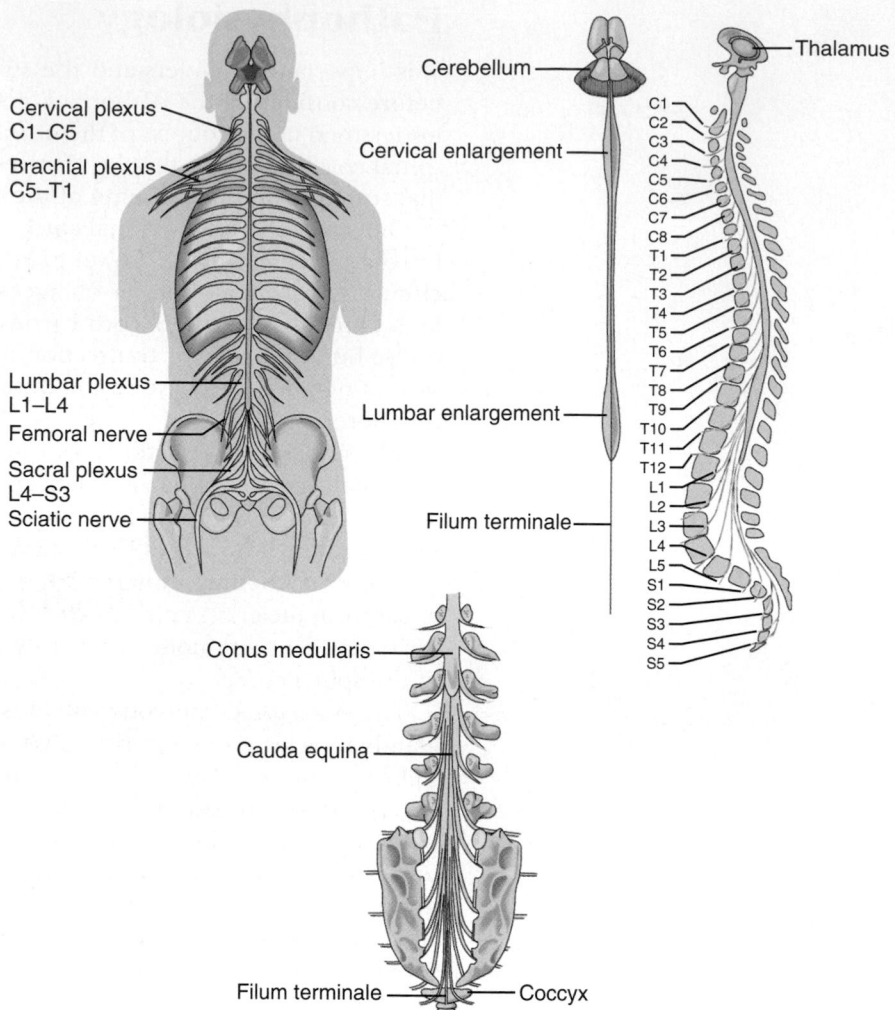

Figure 36-2 Spinal cord and spinal nerves.

perature sensation to the brain and thalamus. The posterior column relays position, vibration, and touch sensation from peripheral sensory neurons.

Activation of the parasympathetic nervous system occurs in the white matter, and originates in the brainstem and sacral areas of the spinal cord. Therefore, parasympathetic responses arise from the cranial nerves and from the sacral segments of the spinal cord. These responses contribute to digestion and elimination through innervation of the viscera, bowel, and bladder. Furthermore, these responses will decrease heart rate.

Spinal nerves corresponding to spinal and vertebral segments also exit the spinal cord. Dorsal roots transmit sensory input to the CNS while the ventral roots transmit motor impulses from the spinal cord to the body. The major plexuses or branches of nerves also innervate specific regions of the body. The cervical plexus innervates the neck and shoulders and houses the phrenic nerve (arising from C3 to C5), which innervates the diaphragm. Therefore, injury to this region of the spinal cord will lead to respiratory crisis if motor impulses from the phrenic nerve to the diaphragm are interrupted.

The vertebral column is made up of 7 cervical, 12 thoracic, 5 lumbar vertebrae, the sacrum, composed of 5 fused vertebrae, and the coccyx, composed of 4 fused vertebrae (Figure 36-2). Correspondingly, there are 8 cervical spinal segments, 12 thoracic spinal segments, 5 lumbar segments, and 5 sacral segments of the spinal cord running through the vertebral canal in the vertebral column beginning at the foramen magnum and ending at the first or second lumbar vertebrae.

Several anatomical mechanisms are present to protect against injury to the spinal cord, which is an extremely vulnerable area. The vertebrae are supported by anterior and posterior ligaments, providing stability to the vertebral column. Acting as cushions against injury are the intervertebral discs, which separate the vertebrae and shield the spinal cord from injury during movement. Even with this protection, because the vertebral column and the spinal cord are in close proximity to each other, injury to the vertebrae and the supportive soft tissue can result in disaster to the spinal cord.

Because the cervical vertebrae must allow for movement of the head and neck, they are innately unstable, thus making this the most vulnerable area of the spinal cord to injury. Logically, the cervical vertebrae are not fixed to the thoracic vertebrae to allow for this movement of the head and neck, but this leads to the danger of injury. Additionally, the mechanism for rotation of the head and neck are provide through the atlas and axis (C1 and C), which increase even more the risk of injury to this area of the spinal cord.

Damage to upper and lower motor neurons contribute to the degree and type of impairment in SCI. **Upper motor neurons,** the descending motor pathways, originate in the brain and synapse with lower motor neurons in the spinal cord. Upper motor neurons suppress firing of lower motor neurons. Without this suppression, lower motor neurons will fire spontaneously. This results in spasticity. Therefore, damage to upper motor neuron pathways will result in loss of control of reflex activity below the level of injury. The inhibition of reflex activity by the CNS by the upper motor neurons is essential in controlling primitive responses that can occur to local stimuli. Consequently, when upper motor neuron is lost through an SCI, spastic paralyses will result because of hyperactive responses to local stimuli.

Lower motor neurons (motor pathways that originate in the spinal cord and continue on as spinal nerves sending impulses to the peripheral areas of the body) originate in the spinal cord and continue on as spinal nerves sending impulses to the peripheral areas of the body. Impulses from stimuli from sites outside the spinal cord travel to the spinal cord and synapse with neurons to form responses back resulting in the classic reflex arc. Flaccid paralysis results from damage to lower motor neurons if interruption of this reflex arc occurs.

Clearly, with an understanding of the anatomy and the physiological functioning of the spinal cord and the CNS, the nurse will be able to anticipate that damage to certain areas of the spinal cord will contribute to or lead to dysfunction of the parasympathetic or sympathetic nervous system, alterations in pain, temperature, vibration, touch, position sense, and to loss of motor activity and sensation. It is possible for life-threatening alterations in ventilation and circulation to occur from an event that will cause interruption of nervous system responses. Furthermore, all systems of the body will be affected, so that nutrition and elimination are also affected, which will be discussed later in the chapter. Hallmarks of nursing care for SCI patients depend on a sound understanding of spinal cord anatomy and physiology.

Assessment with Clinical Manifestations

Assessment of SCI is dependent on an understanding of the manner in which SCIs are classified. Loss of motor and sensory functioning is consistent with the level of SCI, assessment of motor and sensory function will lead to an understanding of the level of SCI and the losses to functioning that may occur as a result. Classification of an SCI, along with the mechanisms of injury, is essential in the assessment of clinical manifestations of the injury. Also important to understanding the patient's situation and extent of injury will be the level of injury, which indicates the expectations for recovery, and the type of fracture that may or may not be present, which will indicate further damage associated with the injury.

Classification of SCI

SCI may be classified as complete or incomplete, depending on the degree of transection or injury to the spinal cord. Complete SCI occurs with complete transection of the spinal cord. This results in total loss of motor and sensory function below the level of injury. The neurological level of SCI is always designated as the lowest segment that has normal functioning. Therefore an injury at C3 indicates that C3 is the lowest segment with normal functioning. Functioning is lost below that level.

Because of the extent of loss of functioning and independence associated with an SCI, this is one of the most devastating types of injuries that a person can experience. Incomplete SCI occurs with partial transection of the spinal cord and results in loss of varying degrees of motor and sensory function below the level of injury. Sensory loss with an incomplete lesion generally follows the spinal tracts with corresponding loss of sensation according to the affected tract. SCI can also occur from an upper or lower motor neuron lesion. Each type of damage creates predictable responses, which require specific nursing care related to the type and level of damage.

Less permanent injury may occur as a contusion, which can cause edema of the affected area of the spinal cord, and results in significant dysfunction of the spinal cord. This usually resolves in days to weeks. Hemorrhage into the gray matter is often a more serious situation, and may create dysfunction consistent with a lower motor neuron lesion. Hemisection of the spinal cord will lead to Brown-Séquard syndrome (discussed later in the chapter).

Mechanism of SCI

Severe SCI occurs as a result of fracture-dislocation during injury. This causes compression, transection, or deformity of the spinal cord. Complete transection of the spinal cord results in immediate flaccid paralysis and loss of sensation below the level of the lesion. Loss of motor and sensory function below the level of injury is an indicator of an SCI that must be identified immediately by health care providers. In the period immediately after injury, reflex activity may be lost and urinary and fecal retention occur. As reflex activity returns, patients experience varying degrees of spasticity and flaccidity, depending on the involvement of upper or lower motor neurons. Spinal cord transection at the cervical cord level results in **quadriplegia (tetraplegia),** paralysis involving upper and lower extremities, whereas, injury of the spinal cord at the thoracic and lumbar areas results in **paraplegia,** paralysis involving the lower extremities (Tierney, McPhee, & Papadakis, 2004).

Lesser degrees of injury to the spinal cord are manifested by varying levels of weakness, urinary dysfunction, and loss of pain, temperature, and position sensation below the level of lesion. Spinal cord disturbances of these types include Brown-Séquard's syndrome, central cord syndrome, and anterior cord syndrome discussed later in this chapter.

Level of Injury

Injuries to the spinal cord can occur at the cervical, thoracic, lumbar, and to a lesser degree, coccygeal areas of the spine. Cervical injuries often result from motor vehicle accidents, football injuries, diving accidents, and falls, while thoracic and lumbar spine injuries may be more related to gunshot wounds as well as falls. In all cases, level of injury can be determined by the loss of motor or sensory functioning below the level of injury. Injury to the cervical spinal cord will result in quadriplegia; however, varying levels of motor and sensory functioning may be present in lower cervical injuries. High cervical injuries above C3 will result in loss of respiratory function and death unless ventilator support is immediately provided.

Cervical injuries result in quadriplegia and loss of movement and sensation below the level of injury, so that movement of the arms and hands are lost along with the potential for loss of head and neck control. C6 injuries are the most common cervical spine (c-spine) injuries because of the greatest mobil-

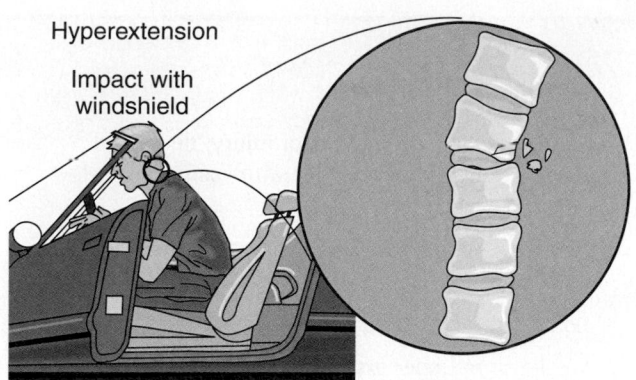

Hyperextension

Impact with windshield

Figure 36-3 Some spinal injuries cause damage to the spinal cord that is immediately evident.

ity of the neck at this area. Injuries at the thoracic level and below allow for movement of the arms and hands. Thoracic injuries allow for increasing abilities for self-care, while resulting in paraplegia. All levels of injury will result in varying losses of bowel and bladder functioning. The most common spinal cord injuries are to C1, C2, C4, C6, T11, and T12 because of the increased movement capabilities of those areas.

Types of Fractures Causing SCI

Because the cervical area is the most unstable area of the spinal cord, it is the most vulnerable area for injury. Cervical trauma results from flexion, hyperextension, and compression injuries and fractures. Hyperflexion injuries are the most common types of fractures, often resulting from motor vehicle crashes when a person's head hits the windshield with extreme force. This commonly occurs with a head-on collision of motor vehicles. Because the degree of hyperflexion is limited by the chin reaching the chest, the extent of injury is often not as great as with hyperextension injuries. Diving accidents may also result from hyperflexion injuries, generally causing damage at the level of C4 or C5. These injuries cause hyperflexion and dislocation of the vertebrae, with resulting tearing of the posterior ligament. The most common hyperflexion injuries occur at the level of C5 or C6 because of the greater degree of movement of this area of the c-spine.

Hyperextension injuries result from falls in which the patient strikes the face or chin during the fall resulting in hyperextension of the neck (Figure 36-3). This may also occur in a rear-end motor vehicle collision. In this situation the anterior ligament is torn along with vertebral fractures. Because a greater degree of movement of the neck is possible with this type of injury, complete transection of the spinal cord is more likely to occur in these types of injuries. In such cases, there is loss of movement and sensation below the level of injury. Hyperextension injuries may result in C4, C5, or C6 damage. Compression injuries occur from direct falls on the head, sacrum, or feet. As a result, the vertebrae fractured on impact compress the spinal cord. Diving accidents can be the main culprits in SCIs resulting from compression injuries.

Vertebral Injuries

The different vertebrae are injured in different ways. For example, the rib cage provides stability to the thoracic region of the spinal cord. Therefore, injuries to this region are not as common. Most injuries result from substantial impact to the thoracic spine. Compression injuries resulting from falls to the feet or buttocks may cause thoracic injuries as can a fall on the upper back. Gunshot wounds are also common culprits in thoracic injury. The most common thoracic injuries occur at T12 and L1. Second to cervical injuries, the lumbar area is a common site for SCI, also because it is less protected from injury. Extreme flexion of the spine in this area may cause injury. Sacral injuries are relatively common and are generally a result of falls. A common cause for sacral injuries is falls on the ice. The nerve roots from the lower spinal segments are susceptible to injury; however, the likelihood of permanent damage to this area is less than with vertebral fractures at other levels of the vertebrae.

Types of Incomplete SCI

Complete transection of the spinal cord results in flaccid paralysis and total loss of motor and sensory function below the level of the injury. Incomplete SCI results from partial transection of the spinal cord. With an incomplete lesion, some of the spinal tracts may be intact and loss of motor and sensory function will vary according to the level of the injury and the type of incomplete lesion. Four syndromes are associated with incomplete injury to the spinal cord and are: Central cord syndrome, anterior cord syndrome, Brown-Séquard syndrome, and posterior cord syndrome (Table 36-1).

TABLE 36-1	Syndromes of Incomplete Cord Injury	
SYNDROME	**TYPE OF INJURY**	**FUNCTIONAL DEFICIT**
Anterior cord	Flexion injury to cervical spinal cord	Motor paralysis below level of injury; decreased sensation, pain and temperature sensation below level of injury
Brown-Séquard	Penetrating injury (gunshot wound or knife wound) causes hemisection of the spinal cord	Ipsilateral motor paralysis and loss of vibration and position sense
		Contralateral loss of pain and temperature
Central cord	Hyperextension or hyperflexion injury damages cervical central cord; anterior horn is damaged	Weakness in upper extremities greater than weakness in lower extremities
Posterior cord	Cervical hyperextension injury damages posterior cervical spinal cord	Loss of position sense

Adapted from Jones, L., & Bagnall, A. (2004). *Spinal injuries centres (SICs) for acute traumatic spinal cord injury.* The Cochrane Database of Systematic Reviews (4), *CD:004442.*

Central cord syndrome occurs with hyperextension-hyperflexion injuries and causes damage to the central aspect of the cervical spinal cord. Central cord syndrome is characterized by microhemorrhages and edema in the central cord and compression of the anterior horn cells of the spinal cord. This syndrome causes weakness in the upper extremities to a greater degree than the weakness found in the lower extremities. Weakness is generally caused by edema and hemorrhage in the central area of the spinal cord. At this location of the spinal cord, nerve tracts travel to the hands and arms. Recovery usually depends on the resolution of the edema as early in the postinjury phase as possible. If spinal tracts are intact, the degree of loss of function will be less.

Anterior cord syndrome often results from a flexion injury that causes compression of the anterior two thirds of the spinal cord. A disc or bone fragment is generally the culprit in an anterior cord injury. This results in motor paralysis below the site of the injury. Decreased sensation, including pain and temperature sensation, also occur below the level of the injury. Because the posterior tracts of the spinal cord are not affected, touch, vibration, position, and motion sensation are not affected. Dorsal column function is also intact. Surgical treatment involves removal of bone fragments if the compression of the spinal cord is caused by fracture injury.

Brown-Séquard syndrome is often caused by a penetrating injury, such as a gunshot or knife wound. Ruptured discs may also cause this syndrome. Brown-Séquard syndrome is characterized by transection of half (also known as hemisection) of the spinal cord. As a result, ipsilateral (same side) motor paralysis and loss of vibration and position sense occur. Contralateral (opposite side) loss of pain and temperature also occur. Careful assessment can guide the diagnosis of this syndrome.

Cervical hyperextension injuries may result in posterior cord syndrome. As a result of this type of injury, compression of the posterior portion of the cervical spinal cord occurs. Dorsal columns of the spinal cord are injured resulting in loss of position sense (proprioception). Motor function, pain, and temperature sensation are salvaged with this type of injury.

Categorizing Incomplete SCIs

The American Spinal Injury Association (ASIA) Impairment Scale categorizes the degree of incomplete injury and expectations for functioning with each level of injury. Studies by the Model Spinal Cord Injury Systems (UAB) have gathered data related to neurological recovery from SCI over a 10-year period. The data reveal that improvements in ASIA motor score (and thus functioning) are related to the severity of injury. Patients with better ASIA grades after injury are more likely to have improvements in motor scores. Patients with motor score injuries at Grade B have a mixed prognosis; Grade A injuries have the worst prognosis for improvement (ASIA, 2004). Violent causes for injuries lead to a worse prognosis than nonviolent causes for injuries. Controversy still exists regarding how patients are classified with incomplete injuries, however, and there may be discrepancies in classification of patients. Nurses should be aware of this situation. These classification methods, though, are extremely useful to nurses and other health care providers in understanding the functional abilities of patients with spinal cord injuries and the degree to which improvement can be anticipated and supported.

Specific guidelines are provided by the ASIA to classify the level of SCI. These guidelines can be used by nurses and all health care providers to determine specific impairments related to the injury. Motor and sensory functioning should be tested along each nerve root to determine functioning or absence of functioning.

Damage to the spinal cord occurs as a result of the primary injury, as well as from the secondary effects of cellular and vascular changes that may occur after the primary injury. These secondary changes can occur from hemorrhage, edema, electrolyte imbalances, and release of catecholamines and toxic enzymes. These changes create a cascade of events that further lead to ischemia and hypoxia, and ultimately to further damage to the spinal cord. Consequently, early protective care and treatment are essential to halt this cascade of damaging events. Currently, there are a number of spinal cord centers in the United States meant to provide expert treatment for SCI. While research is considering whether the outcomes at the centers are better, it still is not known if the long-term outcomes are better if patients are immediately taken to one of these centers or cared for in a local hospital (Jones & Bagnall, 2004). Certainly, care within a few hours of injury is absolutely necessary to prevent long-term problems.

Nontraumatic SCIs

Several conditions may contribute to narrowing of the vertebral column and spinal canal thus contributing to the risk for SCI. Ankylosing spondylitis and rheumatoid arthritis may cause vertebral changes leading to SCI. Additionally, spinal tumors (discussed later in this chapter) may create space-occupying lesions, which compress the spinal cord and lead to SCI. In all these cases, traumatic injury to the spine may occur with resulting loss of motor or sensory function (Tierney, et al., 2004).

Diagnostic Tests

While there are newer diagnostic capabilities available for diagnosing SCI, the mainstay continues to be the X-ray. Cervical, thoracic, lumbar, and sacral X-rays provide important information about the presence of vertebral fractures. Direct supervision of radiologic tests is necessary to prevent further damage to the spinal cord (Figure 36-4). Protection of the patient from further injury during diagnostic testing is a nursing priority. Some manipulation of positioning under direction of the orthopod or neurologist may be necessary to visualize some cervical fractures and includes pulling the shoulders downward to visualize C7. It may also be difficult to visualize C1 and C2, leading to difficulty in diagnosing the injury.

Computed tomography (CT) and magnetic resonance imaging (MRI) scans may be used in the diagnostic process, but do not provide the essential diagnostic information. MRI scans will provide information about soft tissue injury,

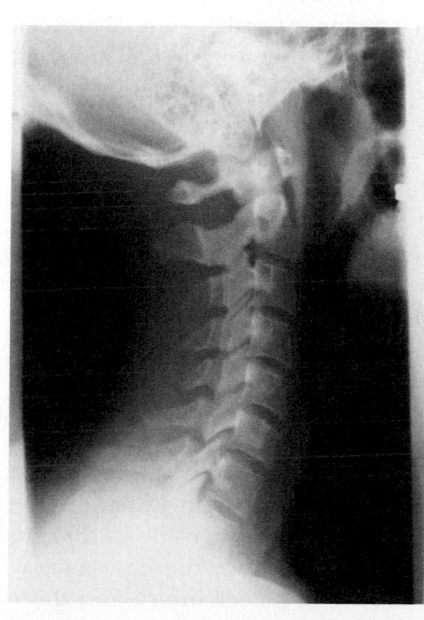

Figure 36-4 Radiological lateral cervical X-ray.

and CT scans will provide additional information about fracture and the extent of injury from fracture. Patient support by nurses in the diagnostic process will primarily include teaching about the need for remaining still and not movement. A nurse should be present to reinforce the need for keeping the patient immobile during this process.

Nursing Diagnoses

Based on the information gathered, examples of nursing diagnoses in the patient with SCI in the acute phases may include the following:

- Breathing pattern, ineffective
- Gas exchange, impaired
- Ineffective airway clearance
- Impaired physical mobility
- Elimination, impaired: bowel and bladder
- Risk for injury
- Self-care deficit: all levels
- Anxiety or fear related to the consequences of the SCI
- Ineffective coping related to the SCI

Planning and Implementation

Planning and implementation of nursing care during the acute phases of SCI are primarily related to maintenance of airway and breathing and prevention of further injury. The emergency care of the patient with an SCI must focus on airway, breathing, and circulation and then treatment to facilitate the best recovery from the injury, including pharmacological treatment in the early phase. At the scene of the accident, proper positioning or immobilization and support of ventilation will be the essential treatment modalities. In the emergency department, determination of the need for pharmacological intervention will be a priority, in addition to diagnostic testing to determine level of injury. Support for the patient and family during this crucial time will also be a priority for nursing care.

Acute Management of SCI

Complete spinal cord transection resulting from spinal trauma is always a possibility when injury to the back or neck occurs as in motor vehicle accidents and falls on the head, sacrum, or feet. Emergency treatment at the scene of an accident must take into consideration the possibility of spinal trauma. The likelihood of c-spine injury when a patient has experienced head trauma and is unconscious, is a possibility that must always be a priority assessment consideration. In those cases, immobilization of the head and neck will be essential to prevent further injury. If the patient has normal mental status, including no drug and alcohol impairment, and does not complain of neck pain, significant c-spine injury is unlikely. At the scene of an accident, immobilization of the head and neck and placement of the patient on a backboard for immobilization of the thoracic and lumbar spines is the standard of care. In addition, the patient must be suspected to have potential head injuries, which could also lead to increased intracranial pressure (Figure 36-5). Secondary prevention of further SCI is dependent on careful treatment with immobilization at the scene of the injury. Once a patient arrives at an emergency department, c-spine injury can generally be ruled out if all of the following criteria are met: the patient denies neck pain when asked; no neck tenderness is present on palpation; the patient did not lose consciousness, and there are no alterations in mental status from the injury or from alcohol or drug use. Furthermore, there is no paralysis or sensory changes, which might be indicative of a neck injury, and there are no other injuries, such as fractures in other locations, which could distract health care providers from identifying the presence of neck injury.

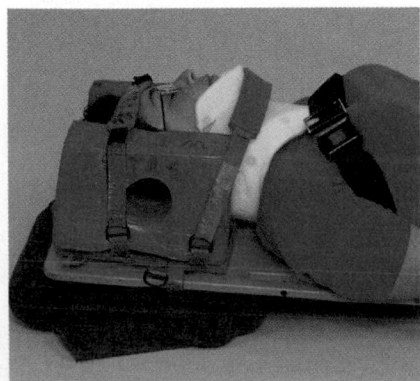

Figure 36-5 Acute management of SCI showing that a slight elevation of the patient's head can help decrease the intracranial pressure.

If any of the above is present, then the physician will order a cervical X-ray to determine if a c-spine injury has occurred. The likelihood of c-spine injury can be determined if there are vertebral fractures, if spinal processes are out of alignment, or if soft tissue swelling is present in the retropharyngeal area. In such cases, immobilization of the head and neck is maintained. It is imperative that nurses pay particular attention to these issues of immobilization of the head and neck to avoid serious and catastrophic consequences for the patient. Patients whose c-spine injuries were initially missed or had delayed diagnosis had a 10 times higher likelihood of serious secondary neurological damage of catastrophic proportions than patients who were initially correctly diagnosed (Jones & Bagnall, 2004).

For thoracic and lumbar spine injuries, complaints of pain and loss of a degree of motor and sensory function are indicators of potential SCIs In all cases, it is imperative that the patient is immobilized and medical care is sought immediately so that care can be taken to prevent further injury to the spinal cord.

It is crucial in the early stage of an SCI to stabilize the spinal cord to prevent further injury, align the spinal cord, and prevent deformities. Movement of the region surrounding the injury may lead to permanent injury, to paralysis, and to loss of function to an even greater degree than the initial injury itself. Patients involved in an accident who attempt to move to get away from a dangerous accident site may cause a worsening of the damage to the injured area leading to permanent damage to the spinal cord.

Controversy continues to exist about immobilization methods at the scene of a motor vehicle accident. Differences in opinion still exist with regard to whether to immobilize the head and neck in neutral position or to immobilize the head and neck in the position in which the patient is found. At the hospital, both surgical and manual techniques are used to stabilize an SCI. For patients who are helmeted, as in football, hockey, and motorcycle accidents, the patient's head and neck are immobilized with the helmet in place, because removal of the helmet may cause extension of spinal cord damage. This has been accepted as the standard of practice in sports medicine, and by the National Collegiate Athletic Association (NCAA). If the patient has arrested, respiratory support should be attempted with the chin-jaw thrust without movement of the head and neck. The safety of removal of the helmet when further airway support is needed has not been documented through research.

At the emergency department, the helmet and shoulder pads of a football player can be removed together at the same time, by a health care provider qualified to remove this equipment. However, football injuries generally do not involve high cervical injuries that produce respiratory arrest. Therefore, removal of the helmet for emergency respiratory support is not generally an issue. Football injuries to the spinal cord occur more often at the level of C5 or C7 because of the type of impact during play. With motorcycle accidents, the concern for additional injuries where there may be bleeding and hemorrhage may be a concern to health care providers and may therefore impair emergency treatment for the SCI. Only experienced and qualified practitioners in the emergency department should remove helmets in patients who potentially have SCI (Waninger, 2004).

Traction may be used as a method of treatment to achieve stability of the spine after SCI, although it is becoming less used with early surgical treatment for stabilization of the injury. Even though currently used in many cases, there is no evidence that spinal immobilization prevents adverse events in patients with spinal cord trauma. In fact, immobilization may lead to further damage to the airway and compromise pulmonary function (Bunn & Roberts, 2004). The debate about the use of traction details benefits and risks associated with each side of this argument. Immobilization is thought to prevent further damage. It is also thought that immobilization will cause airway compromise and lead to a life-threatening situation. Nurses should discuss the patient's treatment plan with the physician and collaborate on a detailed, individualized,

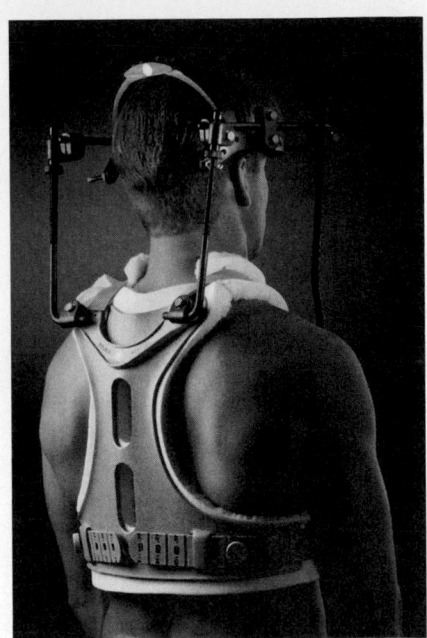

Figure 36-6 Halo vest (Courtesy of DePuy Acromed).

plan for each patient, understanding the specific restrictions and directions for the use of traction.

If used for cervical injuries, traction will support the process of realignment and will prevent mobility of an unstable area of the spinal column. Traction is not generally used for stability in thoracic or lumbar injuries. When used, cervical traction is usually accomplished with the use of Halo traction (described later). Cervical tongs, such as Crutchfield, Gardner-Wells, and Vinke, may be used; however, this type of traction is rapidly becoming obsolete. Tongs are attached by screws implanted in the patient's skull to accomplish reduction of the injury. Initially, five pounds of weight are applied per interspace beginning with C1 to the level of injury. Nurses should be aware of the fear associated with insertion of tongs and screws for attachment of Halo traction. Although not generally painful, the use of the drill for inserting tongs or screws in the skull creates anxiety in an already extremely anxious person. Care must be taken to ensure that weights (if used) hang freely and that tongs are secure as patients are turned in bed.

Currently, halo traction is the standard of care, and more frequently used than the cervical tongs either early in the treatment period or in the postoperative recovery period. The Halo traction brace also uses traction through the attachment of screws in the patient's skull. More movement is possible than with cervical tongs as the vest allows for the patient to be out of bed and contribute to personal care while continuing to stabilize the head and neck and thus the spinal cord (Figure 36-6).

During the period following surgery and if traction is used, the patient may be on bedrest. Sometimes a special bed, such as the Roto-Rest system may be used to promote circulation and prevent decubitus ulcers. However, patients may remain in a regular bed while cervical tongs are in place. Traction leading from the head of the bed must be evaluated periodically to ensure that weights are hanging free. Nurses must turn patients with assistance of additional personnel to prevent the dislodging of pins and prevent improper alignment of the patient.

For less serious injuries, hard and soft cervical collars may be used for head and neck immobilization. These collars allow for even more movement by the patient, however, they do not provide the degree of stability needed for an SCI. Whiplash injuries without damage to the spinal cord or stable c-spine fractures may provide enough stability and restriction of movement to allow for healing of inflammatory responses and strains of muscles in the head and neck area. At the scene of an accident, hard cervical collars along with sandbags may be used for immobilization of the spine for transport to an emergency center.

For thoracic and lumbar injuries, support braces (e.g., Clam-shell brace) may be used in combination with surgery for stabilization of the spine. Use of immobilization beds, such as a Roto-Rest, may be used in some circumstances depending on surgeon preference. These beds provide for stability, while also aimed at the prevention of the development of pressure ulcers. Halo vests may also be used in some circumstances to promote stabilization of the spinal cord and vertebral column.

Familiarity with Christopher Reeves' condition led to increased public awareness of the ventilation needs of patients with high cervical cord injuries. C3 or C5 innervation of the phrenic nerve is necessary for the innervation of the diaphragm, therefore, transection of the cord in high areas of the c-spine cause interruption of phrenic nerve innervation to the diaphragm resulting in the need for ventilatory support. The nurse should be aware that injury at the level of C4 or above will require mechanical ventilation. Patients should be on high-flow oxygen with pulse oximetry when they arrive at the emergency department until there is information about the level of the SCI.

Patients with high cervical injuries are not the only patients who experience respiratory-related problems and issues. Patients with T1 through T12 injuries will experience interruption of innervation of the intercostal muscles leading

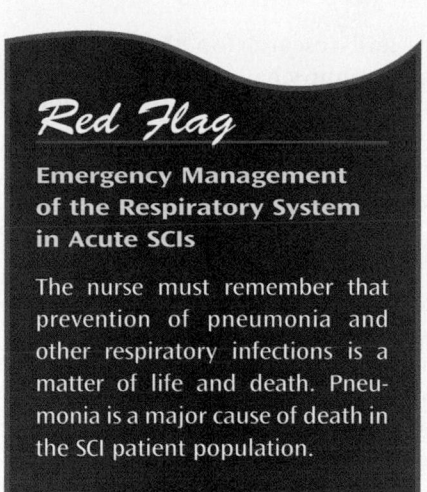

to inability to cough effectively and difficulty with inspiration and expiration. Additionally, tidal volume and vital capacity may diminish because of the loss of innervation of the intercostals muscles. During the rehabilitation period, tidal volume and vital capacity may increase as patients develop abilities to use accessory muscles.

Because of the interruption in chest muscle innervation, patients, particularly those patients with injuries at T7 and above, will need assistance with removal of secretions, especially during the acute phase of treatment. Attention to careful suctioning along with attention to patient responses to suctioning are crucial to prevent hypoxia and bradycardia. Patients with injuries at or above T12 are at risk for pneumonia and atelectasis. Therefore, vigorous pulmonary toileting is critical in the postinjury care of the SCI patient. Consultation with respiratory therapists will provide for care to decrease the risk of respiratory and pulmonary alterations, while maintaining safety. Careful attention to respiratory status and pulse oximetry readings, staying alert for readings less than 95 percent are necessary to prevent respiratory complications in this vulnerable patient.

Respiratory infections are also probable when compromised respiratory function is present as with these types of injuries. Attention to respiratory assessment, noting adventitious and abnormal breath sounds, will help to prevent the development of pneumonia and atelectasis. The age-old nursing standard of turning, coughing, and deep breathing is no more important in any patient population than in the SCI patient. The mechanics of accomplishing this standard, however, are fundamentally different because of the degree of nursing care assistance needed for the SCI patient during turning, coughing, and deep breathing.

Evidence-Based Care

Research has been ongoing for years to investigate and determine the potential for regeneration or repair of damaged spinal cord tissue. Patients are always extremely interested in current research that leads to hope for repair of the spinal cord for quadriplegia and paraplegia, so it is imperative that nurses who work with SCI patients have knowledge of the current research in this discipline. With today's technology, patients are readily able to access information and may need assistance in interpreting study results and information that is accessed. High-profile patients, like Christopher Reeve, sparked public interest in research to find a cure for SCI, and therefore most patients are informed, especially because of their personal stake in the success of scientific research (Estores, 2003). Therefore, staying aware of cutting-edge research on the nurse's part will engender confidence in nursing care and support for hope, as appropriate, on the part of the patient. It's important for nurses to remember that false hope for the possibility of walking again is different than placing hope in research to find a cure. Sometimes so much emphasis is placed on not supporting false hope that it is at the expense of a hopeful outlook on the part of the patient.

Studies that have focused on removal of myelin-producing cells, growth in the laboratory, and transplantation in injured areas of animals have shown promising results of growth of healthy myelin. Restoration of nerve transmissions in animals has already been shown. Current research is also examining the potential for bone marrow stem cells to repair damaged cells when transplanted into the cerebrospinal fluid (CSF) to migrate to injured areas in animals and is thus showing much promise. Mesenchymal stem cells have been found to migrate to injured thoracic spinal cord tissue, through injection into the subarachnoid space, providing a less invasive way to get stem cells to the site of injury. Stem cells have been shown to be effective in promoting recovery in stroke, through the prevention of cell death, and it is thought that this may be possible with SCIs as well, although this has not been shown yet.

Unfortunately, studies with human subjects have not been replicated yet; therefore, research still has much progress to make. Macrophages hold some

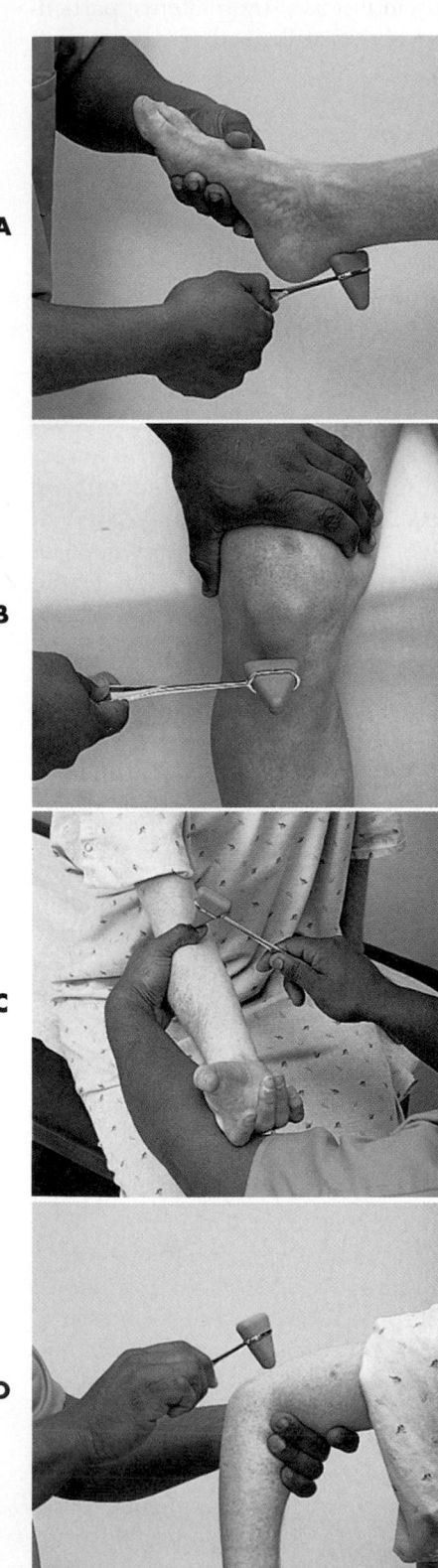

interest in promoting axon regeneration, and research on the concept of bridging across glial scar tissue at the site of the injury has also shown promise. The use of cAMP and Schwann cells are being studied to determine if these cells have a positive effect on axon regeneration. Gangliosides are also being studied because of their potentially positive effect on axon growth. Gangliosides have been shown to have promise in Parkinson's disease and for strokes, increasing the belief that they may also be useful in injured spinal cord tissue. Decreasing the damaging effects of chondroitin is also of interest. Chondroitin has an inhibitory effect on axon growth, and the administration of chondroitinase ABC degrades chondroitin promoting regeneration of tissue. Apparently, the make up of scar tissue with glial cells impairs the growth of other potentially useful cells. Developing circuits, which would allow for growth around the scar tissue (or a bridge), is holding much interest at this time too. Much interest exists in finding a successful treatment for SCI, which will lead to regeneration or repair of nerve cells in the spinal cord; this research is occurring around the world (Bunge & Pearse, 2003; Campos, et al., 2004; Chinnock & Roberts, 2004; Satake, Lou, & Lenke, 2004).

Current research has shown initial effectiveness of drug therapy in improving functional ability in SCI patients. Used for long-term treatment, patients with long-standing SCI have been treated with a new drug, 4-AP (4-aminopyridine). Those patients receiving this experimental treatment showed significant improvement in motor and sensory function when treated with the new drug as compared to patients in control groups. This shows promise especially for the potential of new drugs contributing to improvement of function in more than the first few hours post injury (Hinkle, 2004).

Landmark studies changed the standard of care for SCI several years ago when it was noted that secondary injury after the accident could be as much of the culprit for long-term loss of function as the primary injury. From that research came the standard of treatment with methylprednisolone administered intravenously within eight hours of injury (Bracken, 2004; Tierney, et al., 2004). More recently, magnesium sulfate at high doses is being studied for its inhibitory effect on excitotoxicity of the neural cells as a cause for secondary injury and resolution of secondary injury effects. This has shown the promising effects of neuroprotection in animal studies (Kaptanoglu, Beskonakli, Okutan, Surucu, & Taskin, 2003).

Accurate assessment is critical in all stages of care after SCI. In the early stages of injury, it may be difficult to assess motor and sensory function because of spinal shock. Continued assessment, however, provides a picture of effectiveness of medical treatment and nursing intervention. It will also help in determining realistic functional goals for rehabilitation and quality of life. Motor function is assessed as a part of the neurological assessment completed during the nursing assessment. Movement of extremities and movement against resistance should be included in the motor assessment along with flexion and extension of joints. Sensory assessment early in the treatment period after injury includes determination of sensation along dermatomes. Dermatome charts provide an idea of expected sensory function along sections of the body (dermatomes) innervated by spinal or cranial nerves (see dermatome chart). Spinothalamic tract sensation is tested by cotton swab, whereas pain sensation as a determination of posterior column function is tested by pin prick. Sensation alterations are determined as anesthesia, analgesia, hypoesthesia, and hyperesthesia. Proprioception (position sense) is tested by movement of the great toe upward or downward and asking the patient to confirm the direction.

Deep tendon reflexes (DTR) are tested to determine the presence of **spinal shock,** a loss of all motor and sensory function, generally occurring after SCI, or the degree of injury or impairment, complete or incomplete (Figure 36-7). The presence of DTRs indicates incomplete injury or resolution of spinal shock. During the phase of spinal shock, the patient has absent DTRs and a

Figure 36-7 Assessment of deep tendon reflexes: A. Achilles, B. Patellar, C. Biceps, D. Triceps.

flaccid paralysis. Presence of perineal reflexes may indicate the possibility that bowel and bladder training can be successful.

Understanding motor, sensory, and reflex activity will be beneficial in determining realistic functional goals with the patient. Rehabilitation, including bowel and bladder training, will depend greatly on the functional status of the patient. Taking into account the meaning of assessment data regarding motor, sensory, and reflex information will be beneficial in understanding the progress that the patient is making.

Pharmacology

Landmark studies just a few years ago were the first studies to really show that improvement could be achieved in neurological status after SCI. The introduction of pharmacological management was implemented. Little ground had been gained in the improvement of neurological status until these studies showed the effectiveness of methylprednisolone. Early treatment of spinal cord trauma with high doses of corticosteroids has been shown to be extremely effective in the prevention of spinal cord damage after trauma occurs. Currently, only treatment with the methylprednisolone protocol has shown effectiveness in the acute phase of SCI. Three clinical trials confirmed the effectiveness of methylprednisolone therapy. This research showed that intravenous (IV) administration of a 30 mg/kg bolus of methylprednisolone followed by 5.4 mg/kg/hr for 23 hours improves neurological recovery of function if administered within eight hours after injury (Tierney, et al., 2004).

Higher or lower doses of methylprednisolone have not been shown to be effective, and studies of doses begun after 8 hours post injury have had mixed results. Research continues to examine the promising effects of methylprednisolone and to identify other steroids that may be useful in the treatment of SCI. A recent study has shown that methylprednisolone given for an additional 24 hours (up to 48 hours) contributes to further improvement in function in those patients whose treatment was started 3 to 8 hours after injury (Bracken, 2004). Nurses must be particularly astute to the crucial need for methylprednisolone in the first hours after injury to provide patients with the best possible opportunity for improvement in motor and sensory function.

The improvement of neurological function after administration of methylprednisolone occurs because of the reduction of edema to the area of injury, but it is also thought to occur because of the effect of the methylprednisolone on the reduction of leukocytes to the area along with a decrease in free fatty acid production. Steroid treatment also inhibits breakdown of phospholipids, improving blood flow to the spinal cord, and stopping the inflammatory response, thereby avoiding further injury to the spinal cord. Methylprednisolone has been shown to counter many of the injury cascades that cause injury to the spinal cord.

When injury occurs, blood flow to the gray matter of the spinal cord is impaired. Several hours later, circulation to the white matter also diminishes. This disturbance of blood flow is related to several factors including edema, thrombi in the microcirculation, vasoconstriction from histamine release, and hypovolemia from spinal shock and hemorrhage. In addition, shifting of electrolytes to the extracellular compartments contributes to tissue damage, leading to necrosis. Movement of sodium in particular contributes to edema leading to further tissue damage. The gray matter is especially sensitive to hypoxia and as hemorrhage, edema, and thrombi accumulate, the cascade of injury sequelae is put into motion.

As the inflammatory response continues, edema begins to exert more pressure on the spinal cord, consequently damaging sensitive tissue. As the spinal edema progresses the swelling moves throughout the spinal cord. Keep in mind that these events are occurring within the immovable vertebral column; therefore, further damage to the spinal cord becomes even more likely. Finally, the release of free radicals exerts their neurotoxic effects. As this process proceeds, secondary injury following the primary injury leads to increasing damage from the initial injury. This cascade of events occurs within the first eight hours after injury. This cascade of events has been shown to be effectively halted by the administration of methylprednisolone, if given in this early stage.

Adverse effects of corticosteroid therapy may include delayed wound healing and hyperglycemia and should be assessed in patients receiving this therapy. This may mean that patients are more at risk for infection. Thus, patients may experience longer than necessary hospitalizations because of this risk for infection. Vigilant attention to assessment will serve to prevent infection or identify early signs of infection that can be treated immediately. Because of the effectiveness of corticosteroid therapy, nurses should be particularly attentive about the need for this treatment remembering that the medication's effectiveness has a small window of opportunity.

Attention to daily measurement of weight and to continuous neurological assessments is necessary to determine the effectiveness of the pharmacological therapy. Treatment after the initial stage of injury may consist of laminectomy and surgical fusion (especially if there is spinal cord compression), followed by traction, and treatment of spasticity, bladder and bowel dysfunction, and skin care for the long-term.

Surgery

Surgical treatment accomplishes stability of the spine through fusion of the vertebrae adjacent to the injury. Surgical instrumentation through the use of rods is used to improve stability of the thoracic spine. Often, cervical fusion will still be followed by traction postoperatively; however, cervical traction is used less frequently currently, depending on the stability after surgery and the potential for use of the more mobile halo traction. Fusion creates a stable spine without mobility after the operative procedure. Therefore, patients will need to be prepared for this change in function and mobility. This lack of potential for movement may require psychological adjustment by patients in the rehabilitation period. The operative procedure is generally performed with a posterior approach laminectomy in which rod instrumentation is used for stability or bone from the iliac crest used for the fusion. An anterior or lateral approach to the laminectomy can also be used for a spinal fusion.

Emergency Management of Complications of SCIs

There are several severe complications of SCIs. Spinal shock and neurogenic shock are forms of distributive shock that have high mortality rates and cause crises in the person with an SCI. The immediate response of the spinal cord to injury is spinal shock. This is a physiological response, as opposed to an anatomical response, which results in flaccid paralysis below the level of injury and a myriad of additional problems. Spinal shock results in complete loss of motor and sensory function including movement, bowel and bladder function, sexual functioning, autonomic responses, and reflex activity.

The pathophysiological response follows the damage of the sympathetic and parasympathetic nervous systems. If the injury is above T6, sympathetic innervation will be lost, and the heart, therefore will not receive input from the sympathetic innervation. At that level of injury, parasympathetic innervation will continue, and as a result bradycardia and vasodilation occur. Release of catecholamines occurs initially, which causes hypertension; but subsequently, hypotension occurs because of the impaired venous return. This situation results in hypotension and pooling of blood in extremities. Control by the hypothalamus will also be lost, resulting in loss of temperature control.

Patients with higher levels of injury (cervical injuries) experience the most life-threatening forms of spinal shock because of the effects on the autonomic nervous system. Because the autonomic response is not affected to the same degree in lower SCIs, patients with thoracic and lumbar injuries are not generally affected by spinal shock.

Spinal shock occurs soon after the injury, within the first week after injury, sometimes within 30 to 60 minutes of the injury and continues for up to six weeks or longer. Resolution of spinal shock is indicated by return of reflexes, replacement of flaccidity with hyperreflexes, and reflex emptying of the bladder. Appearance of Babinski's reflex is an indicator of returning reflexes. The bulbospongiosus reflex (also known as penile reflex) in male patients also appears at the resolution of spinal shock. Because of the effects of spinal shock, it is difficult, if not impossible to determine the level of injury and loss of function until spinal shock has resolved.

During the phase of spinal shock careful attention to fluid volume with administration of IV fluids is essential. Antiembolism stockings will prevent pooling of blood in extremities and will assist with circulation and prevention of formation of thrombi. Fluid overload may quickly cause congestive heart failure; therefore, astute assessment is always a priority.

There has been a tendency to view the prognosis for ambulation as related to the presence of spinal shock and the presence or absence of reflexes on the day of injury. This has been discounted by research, especially with regard to the recovery of reflexes in a caudal to rostral sequence, which has been the traditional view of recovery from spinal shock. Research now shows that reflexes reappear over several days following injury, and the pattern of recovery may be what is more related to the recovery of ambulation abilities (Table 36-2). Most often, the delayed Babinski response is the first reflex to recover followed by the cremasteric reflex. Deep tendon reflexes tend to recover in one to two weeks. Rehabilitation efforts may begin while the patient is still experiencing spinal shock.

As with spinal shock, neurogenic shock occurs more frequently in patients with SCI above the level of T6. Technically, neurogenic shock is included as an aspect of spinal shock, in patients with SCI only. Because of disruption of sympathetic input, decrease in vascular resistance and loss of vascular tone occurs from T1 and L2. Neurogenic shock is manifested by hypotension, bradycardia, and hypothermia. In this situation, the heart rate response to volume depletion or volume overload is lost; therefore, nurses must assess frequently for the signs of fluid overload or fluid volume deficit.

Autonomic dysreflexia, also known as autonomic hyperreflexia, is a life-threatening complication of SCI occurring as a disordered discharge of autonomic responses, which results in massive discharge of sympathetic responses. These sympathetic responses are triggered by input of noxious stimuli occurring below the level of injury. As a result, messages sent to the CNS are blocked at the level of injury. Patients with injuries above the level of T6 are at the greatest risk for this complication. Up to 85 percent of patients with injuries above the level of T6 experience autonomic dysreflexia after spinal shock has resolved. Most commonly, the noxious stimulus that triggers the autonomic response is a distended bladder or bowel or some other abnormality com-

TABLE 36-2 Assessment of Reflexes in Spinal Shock	
REFLEX	**ASSESSMENT**
Babinski reflex	Stimulation of the sole of the foot causes dorsiflexion of the great toe
Bulbospongiosus reflex	Tap to dorsal area of penis causes contraction of the bulbospongiosus muscle
Cremasteric reflex	Stimulation of inner aspect of thigh causes testes to retract on same side
Deep tendon reflex	Percussion and stretching of tendon causes contraction of muscle; includes biceps, triceps, quadriceps, and Achilles tendon reflexes

Adapted from Estes, M. (2006). Health assessment and physical examination *(3rd ed.). New York: Thomson Delmar Learning.*

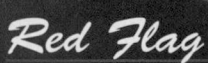

monly dealt with by people without injured spinal cords without a second thought. Spasms, abdominal pain, skin irritation, and pressure sores may also precipitate the response. As sympathetic nervous system activation occurs below the level of injury, vasoconstriction occurs along with a number of additional, sometimes life-threatening physiological responses.

Because the signal for a healthy physiological response to the noxious stimulus cannot transcend the level of the SCI and get through to the CNS, the sympathetic response from the level of injury will cause vasoconstriction of vessels below the injury. This ultimately results in severe, life-threatening hypertension. As a compensatory mechanism to lower the blood pressure, the parasympathetic nervous system produces vasodilatation above the level of the lesion. This results in bradycardia, but continued vasoconstriction in the lower body causes blood pressure to persist and ultimately to rise. The blood pressure may rise to 240/120 mm Hg, becoming a life-threatening situation. In this situation the priority for care is to identify and treat the condition immediately. Vasodilation of the vessels in the head and neck occur as well, creating flushing of the head and neck.

Unfortunately, the compensatory parasympathetic responses only occur above the level of injury, whereas, the sympathetic responses affect the entire body, causing the danger and life-threatening situation that arises. Ultimately, this scenario can lead to cerebral vascular accidents, renal failure, seizures, dysrhythmias, and death. Identifying and treating the stimulus for the response will correct these physiological responses to autonomic dysreflexia and is therefore a high priority for nursing care as well as for patient education. Nursing care focuses on assessment, identifying the source of the noxious stimulus, and treating or correcting the stimulus for the autonomic response. For example, a distended bladder can be caused by kinked tubing of the Foley catheter, triggering an autonomic response. Nursing care emphasizes checking the urinary drainage bag and tubing and teaching about the need to keep tubing unrestricted.

The following situations may trigger autonomic responses necessitating immediate treatment. The nurse must first identify the causative factor or triggering stimulus and remove the stimuli shown in Box 36-1. Guidelines for treatment of autonomic dysreflexia are outlined in the Skills 360° feature.

Teaching should emphasize to patients and their caregivers the need for identification of symptoms and assessment and treatment of stimuli for the autonomic responses. For example, if symptoms occur during digital stimulation, the caregiver must stop until the response has subsided. Autonomic dysreflexia as a result of skin irritation is usually alleviated by loosening clothing. This situation is especially dangerous, because the patient generally does not have the sensation to detect the problem; therefore, life-threatening hypertension may occur before it is detected. Caregivers need to pay particular attention to meticulous care, including proper position, proper fitting clothing, attention to bowel and bladder programs, and assessment for the potential for the development of autonomic dysreflexia.

To prevent serious consequences, pharmacological treatment of the physiological hypertension effect of autonomic dysreflexia must occur while the trigger for the response is being investigated. Vasodilators, such as nifedipine and nitrates, may be used to treat the hypertension resulting from autonomic dysreflexia. Phenoxybenzamine may also be used. Nifedipine will cause coronary and peripheral vasodilation; phenoxybenzamine will block catecholamines, while nitrates are coronary vasodilators. Phenoxybenzamine has also been shown to be effective for bladder spasms.

Teaching related to prevention of autonomic dysreflexia should include a discussion about the need to change positions in the wheel chair and bed at least every two hours. Vigilant attention to bowel and bladder programs will also result in prevention of the syndrome. Identification of symptoms of auto-

BOX 36-1

STIMULI THAT TRIGGER AUTONOMIC RESPONSES

The nurse should monitor the patient with an SCI for the following signs that are typical of stimuli for autonomic responses:

- Distended bladder
- Constipation or bowel impaction
- Pain
- Muscle spasms
- Sexual activity
- Labor (in females)
- Decubitus ulcers
- Urinary tract infections
- Tight clothing
- Ingrown toenails

Skills 360°

Management of Autonomic Dysreflexia

The nurse should monitor for the following clinical manifestations of autonomic dysreflexia:

- Recognize the signs and symptoms and continually monitor blood pressure and heart rate. Guidelines suggest every two to five minutes.
- Loosen any restrictive clothing or devices (urinary leg bag may be causing constriction).
- If the patient has an indwelling catheter, check for kinked tubing, and patency of system. Remove any kinks or obstructions. If the catheter is not draining, it should be irrigated with 10 to 15 mL of normal saline instilled at body temperature. Do not put pressure on the bladder. Guard against cold solutions, which may exacerbate the autonomic dysreflexia. If the catheter is still not draining, remove and replace the catheter, and consult the physician.
- Monitor the patient's blood pressure during drainage of urine by a urinary catheter. Drainage of large volumes of urine could cause hypotension.
- If symptoms persist, check for fecal impaction the second most common cause of this condition.
- Expect order for antihypertensive agent (e.g., nifedipine or nitrates) with rapid onset and short duration.
- For a pregnant woman who has signs of autonomic dysreflexia, refer the patient immediately for care by an obstetrical health care provider.
- After stabilization of the patient, provide teaching regarding the signs and symptoms of the disorder, and the need to seek immediate treatment.

nomic dysreflexia must be treated as a medical emergency, and once home, patients should be reminded to call 911 if symptoms occur, especially if not resolved by conventional treatment (removal of kinked catheter tubing, etc.). Patients and caregivers should also be prepared to explain to emergency and hospital personnel the probably nature of their condition, because many health care providers do not typically encounter autonomic dysreflexia.

The Paralyzed Veteran's of America Consortium for Spinal Cord Medicine also provides clinical guidelines for health care providers and for patients and caregivers to use in the identification and treatment of this disorder. These clinical guidelines have been adopted universally at spinal cord centers across the United States.

Nursing Management during the Rehabilitation Phase of Recovery

The patient with an SCI has nursing care and physical care needs for the rest of his or her life. Patients continue to be at risk for alterations in respiratory status: ventilation and gas exchange leading to risk for pneumonia, alterations in skin integrity and mobility, alterations in bowel and bladder elimination, altered circulation, alterations in neurological status, autonomic and spinal sensory and motor function, and numerous psychosocial and family related potential alterations. Essentially, the patient with an SCI has the potential for complications involving all aspects of the body, mind, and spirit.

Bowel and bladder dysfunctions are common complications of SCI, and most patients experience some degree of both bowel and bladder dysfunction because of loss of innervation of the bowel and bladder. During the phase of spinal shock, urinary retention occurs. During this phase, indwelling urinary catheterization is necessary, because the bladder is atonic and will become distended. On resolution of this phase, urinary output may stabilize, because reflex emptying may become possible as a result of decreasing inhibitory responses from the brain. At this time, patients can generally have intermittent catheterization, especially if they can tolerate increases in oral fluid intake. Patients should drink at least 3 liters of fluids per day to offset the potential for urinary tract infections (UTIs), a real risk at this stage and throughout the rest of the patient's life.

Paraplegic patients may be able to accomplish self-catheterization as a goal of the rehabilitation process. Quadriplegic patients will need caregiver support if intermittent catheterization is possible. In both cases, patients and caregivers will need to be taught aseptic technique for bladder and catheter care. Once an indwelling urinary catheter is discontinued, the nurse must assess regularly for urinary retention. Urinary retention will lead to UTI, so diligent assessment of urinary function is essential. Urinary retention will also lead to the development of urinary calculi, a somewhat common occurrence among patients with SCIs. Teaching regarding fluid needs is essential. The inclusion of cranberry juice in the fluid intake is controversial, because it has not been shown to decrease bacteriuria in patients with SCI (Waites, Canupp, Armstrong, & DeVivo, 2004). The use of cranberry juice does provide fluids and important nutrients, so is not detrimental. For patients with indwelling catheters, teaching regarding aseptic technique when changing and cleaning catheter bags, the use of leg bags, and nighttime catheter drainage management is important. Strict attention to proper catheter and urinary drainage bag care will decrease the potential for urinary tract infection.

Bowel elimination will also be affected by impaired reflex activity, which will lead to constipation and the possibility of impaction. It has also been found that colonic motility postprandially is diminished in patients with SCI (Korsten, et al., 2004). This will lead to even more difficulty with bowel elimination. A bowel training program must be implemented as soon as tolerated by the patient. Prevention of constipation and fecal impaction will be essential aspects of this bowel training program. During the rehabilitation phase of recovery, patients and caregivers are taught the digital dilation technique to facilitate bowel elimination. Stool softeners and assurance of dietary roughage and nutrients to support bowel elimination are essential. Adequate fluid intake will also support bowel elimination.

Bowel training is often assisted by consideration of time of day and timing of meals. Assisting the patient to the bathroom or commode soon after the morning meal, if that time is preferable, will promote bowel elimination. Establishing the routine, often with timing in relationship to meals will be beneficial to bowel elimination and to the regaining of a degree of normalcy in the patient's life.

Alterations in temperature regulation in patients with SCIs resulting from impaired autonomic nervous system responses makes the patient vulnerable to changes in environmental temperature. Hypothermia is a risk for patients, especially in the acute phase. Additionally, because of altered sensation that also occurs with the injury, patients should be taught not to use heating pads because of the risk for burns. Patients may also be in danger of frostbite, especially with loss of sensation and the vasodilation that accompanies spinal shock. These dangers may continue according to the level of SCI.

During all phases of the postinjury period and for the rest of the patient's life, the risk for decubitus ulcers is great because of the impact of an SCI on mobility. This was made real as it was identified as the initial culprit in the series of events that led to the death of Christopher Reeve in 2004. In the acute phase of the SCI, nurses must assess skin frequently and turn patients at least every two hours. This is a challenge when patients are in Halo traction or in cervical traction. Turning must be accomplished with at least two nurses, paying close attention to security of tongs if present.

The loss of innervation of the diaphragm and intercostal muscles leads to continued risk for pneumonia for the rest of the patient's life. The patient and family members must always be vigilant to the need for deep breathing, for activity, and for good pulmonary toilet. For many patients, the reality of an SCI is that the person with a c-spine injury will be dependent on a ventilator for the remainder of his or her life. This will require specialized nursing care, with teaching for family members and caregivers, along with home health nursing care. It will also require attention to maintenance of secretions and frequent auscultation of breath sounds to determine the possibility of the development of pneumonia, so that treatment can be instituted. Family members and caregivers will require instruction related to tracheostomy care, as the patient with a c-spine injury will have a tracheostomy for the purposes of ventilatory support and for suctioning to remove secretions.

Current research has identified the benefit of transcutaneous electric nerve stimulation (TENS) for stimulating the diaphragm to promote increased independence in ventilation and breathing. This research has been successful in allowing a degree of independence for short periods of time for patients who are dependent on a ventilator. Implanted TENS electrodes are providing a new source of ventilation support and lessening the risk of pneumonia and other hazards of loss of nerve innervation to the diaphragm and intercostals muscles.

Patients with cervical injuries and higher thoracic injuries who are not dependent on a ventilator will still need careful attention to pulmonary hygiene because of the loss of innervation of intercostal muscles. Paraplegics are not at risk to the degree that quadriplegics are with regard to respiratory status. They must still be aware of the need for respiratory care and the hazards of bedrest during times when they may need increased time in bed. In particular, because of the danger of decubitus ulcers, increased time in bed will bring with it increased risk for pneumonia (Winslow & Rozovsky, 2003).

Both quadriplegics and paraplegics will be confined to a wheelchair for the rest of their lives. Paraplegics and quadriplegics with lower cervical injuries will have the ability to manually power their wheelchairs. Quadriplegics with high injuries will need motorized wheelchairs with high back support and head support. The actuality of wheelchair confinement while out of bed means that patients are always at risk for development of decubitus ulcers at pressure points. Because patients have lost the sensation of pain that able-bodied patients have after sitting for extensive periods of time, they do not sense the need to change positions. Therefore, it is important to vary the times when in the wheelchair and in bed. Additionally, patients may be able to do lifting exercises periodically to relieve pressure on the sacrum. A turning schedule while in bed for quadriplegics is always a necessity for patients and their caregivers.

In reality, complications of decubitus ulcers are a serious threat to patients' well-being. Constant assessment by nurses during the hospitalization and rehabilitation phases and by caregivers in the home environment will help to identify early beginnings of pressure areas. Even with scrupulous nursing care and strict attention to turning and position changes, the chances of patients developing decubitus ulcers is great. Proper nutrition will promote skin integrity, and changing positions regularly will promote circulation in pressure areas. Consultation with Wound, Ostomy, Continence (WOC) nurses is helpful in determining strategies for preventing and for treating decubitus ulcers. Decubitus ulcers are difficult to treat once they are present. The dangers of infection become even higher once a patient has a decubitus ulcer. Currently, the best intervention for decubitus ulcers is prevention. Detailed individualized information regarding the prevention of decubitus ulcers is the best approach (Garber & Rintala, 2003).

A helpful tool for nursing staff and for caregivers of patients with SCI is a turning schedule. It is easy to develop a tool based on the patient's preferences for meals and other needs for supine position. Caregivers should develop some kind of method for remembering the turn schedule so that turning times are not missed. Because of the serious risk for decubitus ulcers, turning during the night is necessary. Caregivers will need support and assistance with turning a patient who is not able to assist. Patients who are paraplegic will be able to assist with turning and may become independent with turning. They will still need a turn schedule. The schedule provided above can be modified based on the patient's preferences, including time slots and being on the back and on a particular side at some times of the day. If, for instance, the patient's television is on the left side of the bed, the patient may have favorite programs that will necessitate turning to the left side at those times of the day. The schedule can be adjusted accordingly.

Patients who are quadriplegic will need complete assistance with transferring to the wheelchair and back to the bed. Nurses will need to be aware of proper transfer techniques and body mechanics to transfer patients. Rehabilitation facilities will assist patients and caregivers to learn the transfer techniques. Caregivers providing care for quadriplegic patients will need support of additional caregivers or family members in some circumstances.

A significant concern with immobility is the degree of atrophy of muscles that occurs. Range of motion exercises of all muscle groups is essential every day to maintain muscle tone, prevent the loss of muscle mass, and prevent contractures. Once patients are discharged from the hospital, caregivers will need to take over this activity and will need detailed teaching about this essential need that patients will have. Significant time is necessary for the level of exercise that patients will need, depending on level of injury.

Bone loss and the development of osteoporosis is also a concern in patients who have SCIs. Attention to calcium needs is necessary, within the specification of the total dietary prescription for the patient. Research has shown that patients with SCIs are more at risk for hip fractures than the general population because of increased bone loss. Bone loss also occurs at a faster rate in the knees. Based on this information, prevention efforts for fractures are a priority.

An upper motor neuron lesion will lead to spasticity, a common and disturbing situation that patients face. Spasticity often occurs on the resolution of spinal shock, which was characterized by complete suppression of reflexes, flaccidity, and loss of muscle tone. In contrast, after spinal shock resolves, a situation of hyperreflex activity often occurs. Spasticity may affect as many as two thirds of patients within the first year after SCI and is characterized by the involuntary uncontrolled movement of extremities associated with lower motor neuron lesions. Spasms interfere with positioning, with activities of daily living, and with most activities that could lead to any degree of independence. Furthermore, spasms can progress to becoming quite painful for patients.

Life for patients with SCIs changes in ways that most able-bodied people can never imagine. If physiological concerns were the only issues for nursing, providing care would certainly not be complicated. Major impacts on independence and body image occur no matter what the level of injury. Richmond and Thompson (2002) described psychosocial concerns for patients with SCIs as "devastating mental health issues with which the patient must deal" (p. 45). Varying degrees of dependence and loss of function create psychosocial responses that nurses must anticipate and support.

Because the SCI involves extreme overwhelming consequences and losses for patients, including losses to independence, to sexuality, to career, to lifestyle, and even to relationships, patients will experience significant grief and will move through the stages of grief for the losses as their recovery progresses. Early in the acute period after the injury, patients may focus on staying alive; but soon, their response may turn to denial and then anger as they experience the grief that accompanies this overwhelming situation. After the initial progression through the high acuity phase, patients realize how dependent they are on other people for the basic activities of daily living including bathing, eating, toileting, and elimination, along with all other activities. Realization of this level of dependence comes as a horrible blow and shock as they realize what has happened.

Initially, patients may emphasize their beliefs that they will be walking again and resuming their previous lifestyle. This may be a healthy outlook as the level of injury is still being determined. Later, this outlook may manifest as a denial of the extent of injury or of the lasting effects of the injury. Working through the grief associated with the injury may be a lifelong process for patients with SCIs.

Patients may be fearful of being dropped or injured while being turned or transferred. With the mechanics of traction and special beds, this is always a possibility and therefore not an unrealistic fear of patients. Furthermore, they may believe that their recovery is dependent on not being further injured. Making sure that two nurses are available for turning will reassure patients about their safety. Allowing the patient to work through the grief at his or her own rate will be necessary and will promote a healthy response to the process, which include viewing one's life in a positive way, a way in which the patient sees methods of contributing in spite of this overwhelming life change. Recent research has shown that some patients, even years after the injury, still mourn the losses associated with the injury and maintain a degree of anger and anxiety. These findings suggest that the process of acceptance and adjustment is a complex process not progressing in the same manner in all patients (Livneh & Martz, 2003). Nurses should not place expectations on patients and their psychosocial behavior at any point in time.

When adjustment or acceptance begins, patients start to look to the future and set goals for care and the future. At this stage, listening to stories from patients with SCI who have achieved levels of independence will be helpful to patients. Patients with similar injuries can have a profound positive effect on patients with more recent injuries. This is one reason that rehabilitation tends to be so successful. The development of camaraderie and friendships support the process of more than rehabilitation but also the movement through the stages of grief. During this stage, patients often start to find meaning in the experience and a purpose in life consistent with their new life experience.

Patients who have experienced an SCI are at more risk for suicide than the general population. Consultation with mental health professionals, including psychiatric mental health advanced practice nurses, will help nurses and family members to understand the patient's psychosocial responses to the injury and to identify meaningful ways to support the patient to progress in a mentally healthy manner while confronting and dealing with the injury, and to finding meaning in this life experience.

Extremes in patients' behavioral responses to the injury ranging from fear to sadness to anger may be seen in different patients. Responses to an SCI are not linear in the way in which they are lived. A caring approach with understanding of the extreme vulnerability and loss that the patient experiences will be effective in these circumstances. Generally, patients' responses to caring, involved nurses are not manipulative but rather appropriate and healing.

Evidence-Based Care

Treatment for spasticity has typically involved medication treatment. Baclofen has been the standard of treatment for years, with modest success. Other medications that may be useful include dantrolene, diazepam, and clonidine. Newer medications have become available, and newer modalities for administration of baclofen through the intrathecal route have become available. Individual studies have reported significant improvement in spasms for patients receiving baclofen by the intrathecal method (Taricco, Adone, Pagliacci, & Telaro, 2004). The use of valium has also been studied, and positive effects noted; however, the drowsiness associated with the use of valium is a limiting factor in its use. The current standard for treatment continues to be baclofen used alone or in combination with valium. In general, treatment for spasticity involves the use of baclofen and then using a decision tree to move upward to the addition of valium and then to intrathecal baclofen if patients become unresponsive to the previous therapy.

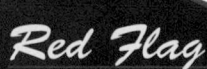

Risk for Disuse Syndrome and Hazards of Immobility

Vigilant scheduling of range of motion exercises and weight bearing exercises (as possible with assistance of physical therapists) for patients will prevent atrophy of muscles and the possibility of contractures of extremities. This is a real risk in patients with the realities of immobility that patients with SCIs face every day. Nurses and caregivers must pay particular attention to the need for a schedule for exercising the muscle groups every day.

Collaborative Management

SCIs create a nursing intensive situation for patients. It is one of few conditions where the need for nursing care is generally much greater than the medical care needs of patients after the acute phase of recovery. This means that nursing care can potentially have a much greater impact on the outcomes of care than medical care will have for this population of patients. In the acute phase of postinjury care, collaboration by members of the team will contribute to the greater positive outcomes. As the patient progresses, the care becomes much more nursing related while medical and other team members will contribute much less to the care of these patients. Therefore, the nurse has a great responsibility and a great opportunity to contribute to quality of life for patients who have experienced SCIs The challenges for nursing in caring for patients with SCIs relates to the comprehensive needs and the vulnerability of patients who are injured. The primary responsibility of nurses is in caring for the person in a holistic manner during the human response to injury, which epitomizes the core of nursing practice.

Because the effects of an SCI require lifelong adjustments and care, patients must be as knowledgeable as health care providers in the details of their care. This means that the health care team must emphasize inclusion of the patient in care throughout the entire recovery period. A primary nursing model of care will support the care of patients with SCIs in a much more thorough manner than other models of care. This is especially true during the rehabilitation phase of recovery; however, it is also beneficial in all phases of care. Because assignment of a primary nurse to the care of the patient with SCIs throughout the hospital and rehabilitation phases will ensure the development of a thorough nursing care plan with attention to interdisciplinary needs of the patient, this model will provide for the best nursing care outcomes.

An injury with significant consequences, such as an SCI, will result in a spiritual crisis for many patients, especially patients without strong spiritual development prior to the injury. Patients may question why this has happened to them, or why their God would allow something like this to happen. They may even feel like they are being punished for behavior that may have contributed to the event. In those cases, guilt may be a response that patients struggle to overcome. As patients progress through recovery, they may ask themselves questions about their purpose in life and why they are alive after such a horrendous accident. Patients may emerge from their recovery with a renewed sense of purpose in life, finding purpose in their place in life as a person who has an SCI and who can carry the message to others about finding themselves in the face of adversity. Patients are supported by the positive action of patients with SCIs who are role models as they advocate for research and improved care.

Nurses who are uncomfortable in caring for patients experiencing spiritual distress or spiritual crises will have difficulty caring for patients with SCI. Referral to a chaplain or religious leader of the patient's wishes will be helpful in the early stages of the injury and recovery. During this time, the life-threatening aspects of the injury will be more related to the spiritual needs than the questions that patients may have about spirituality. As the recovery progresses, questions of a spiritual nature and the meaning of their life in this new situation become more common. The ability to assess the need for spiritual care as a part of assessment of spiritual distress or spiritual crisis will be essential at this time.

Keeping in mind that a large majority of patients with SCI are young adult males, and the developmental tasks related to intimacy and isolation, sexuality issues are a major concern for recovery and rehabilitation. The nurse who is caring for the patient with SCI must have a thorough knowledge of level of injury and how the injury will affect sexual functioning. Unawareness of specific effects along with a lack of understanding of sexual issues for the patient with SCI will lead to distrust of the nurse and will inhibit the therapeutic relationship. Serious discussions at the request of the patient are necessary to promote understanding of the effects of the injury. The potential for alterations in sexual response, orgasm, erection in males, and fertility may all be possibil-

Respecting Our Differences

Cultural Considerations

Cultural issues will always be a factor to consider when providing care to patients with SCIs. Studies of young Hispanic (American) men who suffered an SCI found that family members, and even the fathers of young Hispanic (American) men, were involved in care, even though there is a degree of pride and a macho aura for males in this culture. Categorizing and stereotyping patients and families should be avoided. Assessment of cultural preferences and approaches to caring for family members must be performed and included in the plan of care. Because intimate care of a patient is a strong part of care of patients with SCI, close attention should be paid to the beliefs about intimate care in a particular culture, and nurses must support family members as they are faced with care that might be unfamiliar in their culture.

ities. No matter what the level of lesion, a lack of sensation in the perineal area and thus sensation during intercourse will occur.

If the patient has an upper motor neuron lesion, reflex sexual activity will be possible, and psychogenic erection may be possible for a patient with a lower motor neuron lesion. Reflex erection will not be possible for a patient with a lower motor neuron disorder. If it is possible, ejaculation may be retrograde into the bladder. Men with upper motor neuron lesions may be able to have erections as a result of external stimulation, and they may also have spontaneous erections, although these erections cannot be controlled or maintained.

Women with an SCI will not be able to have an orgasm, but they may remain fertile. Pregnancy and normal vaginal delivery is possible for women with SCIs. Nurses should assess for the presence or absence of menstrual periods since the injury. Generally, a professional with expertise should be available to discuss the details of sexuality after SCI. The nurse will still be asked questions from the patient and the significant other throughout the recovery period and will need to have an understanding of sexuality issues for the patient with an SCI. An honest, open approach is helpful for nursing care in this situation. A primary nursing model of care will enhance the development of a plan that can appropriately address sexuality for patients with SCIs.

Discussions among the nurse and the patient and significant other should emphasize the importance of open communication by partners. Respect for the religious and cultural backgrounds of the patient and significant other is essential during any discussions of sexuality. New families will experience grief over the loss of this aspect of their new lives; patients and spouses with longer term relationships will also experience significant loss, while perhaps being more comfortable with their lives together with this change for the future. Young men and women who have not established significant relationships yet will certainly experience sadness at the change in their sexuality.

Patients often have an indwelling urinary catheter, so teaching must emphasize the need to be mindful of this. For women, birth control methods, as appropriate, should be discussed. Autonomic dysreflexia may complicate what is believed to be a normal delivery if a woman does become pregnant. Sexual counseling may emphasize becoming aware of one's erogenous zones and learning to seek sexual pleasure from the partner's stimulation of these areas. Emphasis on the aspects of sexuality that remain and that can be maximized is important. Inclusion of the partner in discussions, if the patient is open to that, may be helpful.

Recent research has shown that the physical aspects of sexuality were not the most important factors in the quality of a relationship in a couple where one partner has experienced an SCI. Rather, it is the perception that the partner is happy and enjoys the experience. Psychosocial factors were more important than physical factors in contributing to a satisfying sexual relationship in these couples. Studies of the efficacy of sildenafil (Viagra) have also been undertaken in men with erectile dysfunction resulting from SCI. In men with injuries at the level of T6 through L5, a significant positive effect of the medication on satisfaction with the sexual experience was shown. Later studies have shown even more promise for the use of sildenafil in treating erectile dysfunction in men with SCIs. A significant number of patients with complete injuries benefited from the medication. This lends hope to the possibility of improving the quality of the sexual experience in men who have experienced SCIs.

Family members will also experience issues of coping with the injury, coping with changes in life and role changes that the patient experiences and role change for the family members as well. Spouses of patients with SCI will experience fears of the loss of independence, changes in levels of intimacy, and transition to the caregiver role. These changes will have a serious impact on family members, and they may experience the same movement through the stages of mourning as the patient does. Family members may experience denial and anger as the life of the entire family is transformed. Parents may care for adult children who had already left home, and spouses may be providing complete care for husbands and wives with SCI who once played a major role in the financial support of the family.

Nursing support to family members during this time should involve answering questions about the injury and level of function, care requirements, and referral sources. Family members will also need to understand their participation in the activities of daily living and the level of assistance needed. Social workers will be helpful with family members to determine the kinds of assistance with activities of daily living that can be provided when the patient goes home. Some patients may have resources for live-in help while many other families will plan on much more participation by family members in care depending on finances and resources available.

Evaluation of Outcomes

Presented below are the outcomes for care for the patient with an SCI presented according to nursing diagnosis. For alterations in neurological status the outcome of care will depend on the level of injury, and the nurse must look to the positive gains that can be made, such as head and shoulder movement and autonomic function not compromised, not to the outcomes that cannot be achieved, such as return of neurological function.

Because the patient with SCI experiences alterations in all areas of functioning, outcomes presented in Table 36-3 specify the expected outcomes for this patient. For example, it may not be possible to achieve independence in self-care abilities, but the nurse and patient can identify outcomes related to self-care that can be achieved. It is essential that the nurse identify the nursing diagnoses and outcomes that are the highest priority and ensure that the patient can achieve a lack of compromised status in those areas, such as tissue integrity and gas exchange.

SPINAL CORD TUMORS

The causes of spinal cord tumors are unknown. Spinal cord tumors can be classified as primary or metastatic tumors and may also be benign tumors. Most primary spinal cord tumors are benign, including the meningiomas and neurofibromas. The majority of spinal cord tumors are extramedullary (located outside the spinal cord) in origin and are classified as intradural or extradural tumors. Malignant metastatic tumors, lymphomas, and myelomas are generally extradural tumors. Primary extramedullary tumors, including neurofibromas and meningiomas, can be either intradural or extradural tumors.

Because of the location of spinal tumors, injury to the spinal cord occurs that causes spinal cord dysfunction the same as with SCI. The primary difference in effects is the gradualness of the dysfunction that occurs as opposed to the suddenness of SCI. The degree of magnitude of long-term sequelae depends on the extent of the tumor and the degree to which surgery removes the tumor and allows for normal spinal cord function.

Epidemiology

Only about 10 percent of spinal tumors are of the intramedullary type, which are located within the spinal cord itself. Ependymoma is the most common type of intramedullary tumor and occurs most often in the area of C6 through T2. The rest of the intramedullary tumors are gliomas and occur primarily in the cervical area of the spinal cord (Tierney, et al., 2004).

TABLE 36-3 **Outcomes of Care for Patient with SCIs**

Neurological status: Spinal sensory or motor function

Indicators:

Head and shoulder movement (as capable): Not compromised

Autonomic function: Not compromised

Deep tendon reflexes: Not compromised

Flaccidity: Not present: (as capable according to injury)

Neurological status: autonomic: Patient will be free of autonomic dysreflexia. Patient and family will verbalize signs of AD and appropriate actions to take.

Grief resolution: Patient and family members will exhibit movement through stages of grief.

Family normalization: Family members will verbalize return to preinjury lifestyle with modifications.

Depression: Patient will be free of depression.

Caregiver lifestyle disruption: Caregiver will identify methods for maintaining lifestyle within the new caregiver role.

Mobility level: Patient will achieve mobility with assistive person and device.

Nutritional status: Patient will consume nutrients adequate for body requirements.

Respiratory status: Gas exchange: lungs will be clear AP and laterally.

Self-care: Activities of daily living: Patient will accomplish activities of daily living with assistive person and devices.

Sexual functioning:

Indicators:

Adapts sexual technique as needed

Expresses ability to be intimate

Expresses ability to perform sexually despite physical imperfections

Expresses knowledge of personal sexual capabilities

Tissue integrity: Skin: Patient will be free of alterations in skin integrity. Skin will be pink, without evidence of development of ulcers.

Etiology

Metastatic tumors occur most frequently as a result of metastasis from the breast, kidneys, prostate, colon, and from lymphomas and multiple myeloma. Prostate tumors tend to metastasize to the thoracic region of the spinal cord, most commonly T8 through T10. Ovarian cancer usually metastasizes to the lumbosacral region of the spinal cord. Metastasis from other primary sites usually spread from the organ to the adjacent vertebral body. Multiple sites of the spinal cord may also be involved, especially with metastasis from the breast or prostate.

Pathophysiology

Pathophysiological changes that occur with a spinal cord tumor occur most often as a result of compression of the spinal cord at the level of the lesion. Compression of the spinal cord causes varying losses of motor and sensory function. Compression may also cause ischemia because of obstruction of

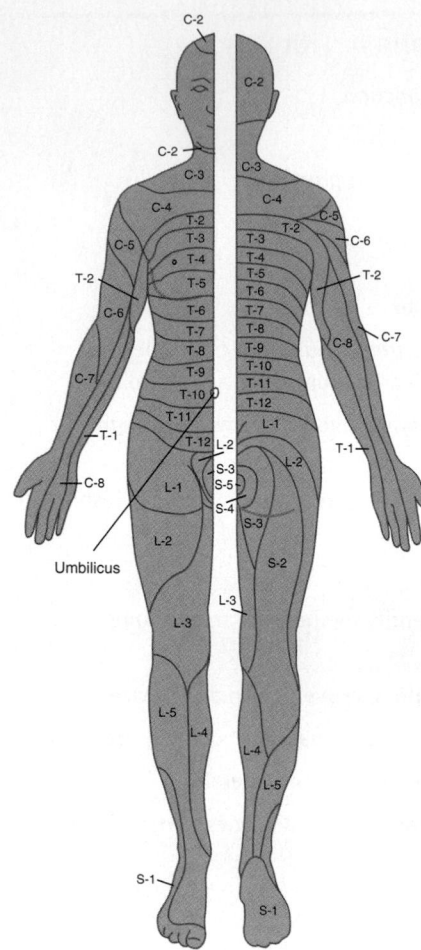

Figure 36-8 Anterior and posterior dermatomal distributions.

circulation. Edema may be present as injury to the spinal cord occurs and may ascend the spinal cord leading to death of tissue above the level of the tumor. Invasion of the spinal cord by tumors will cause loss of impulses and motor and sensory deficits, compression of spinal nerves, and alterations in reflex activity. Therefore, direct compression and ischemia, secondary to compression and culminating in arterial or venous obstruction, are the primary causes of spinal cord dysfunction associated with spinal cord tumors. In more rare circumstances, intramedullary tumors will cause symptoms from infiltration of spinal cord tissue.

The signs and symptoms of the tumor will lead to validation of the location of the spinal tumor, at the cervical, thoracic, lumbar, or sacral levels. It will be possible to map the sensory changes with the use of a **dermatome** (the area of skin innervated by a posterior spinal root) chart, which will show a correlation with the particular dermatome (Figure 36-8).

Assessment with Clinical Manifestations

Because spinal tumors often have gradual growth, symptoms may not be present until there is significant growth of the tumor. On the other hand, metastatic tumors may grow rapidly. Focal signs that may identify the location of the tumor include cranial nerve disturbances, respiratory difficulties, and **paresthesia** (abnormal numbness and tingling sensation). Commonly, pain is the earliest sign of metastasis to the vertebrae. Pain may also occur as a result of compression of a nerve root. Pain along with weakness and sensory changes are often identified. Patients may seek health care because of difficulties with bowel and bladder function, which become difficult to manage.

Motor deficits can occur for several pathophysiological reasons, as a result of upper and lower motor neuron lesions and from compression of spinal nerves. Loss of reflexes, weakness, and muscle wasting occur. An upper motor neuron lesion will result in spasticity and increased DTRs. Lower motor neuron lesions will result in weakness and flaccidity. Brown-Séquard syndrome (discussed previously in the chapter) may also occur. Sensation may be affected according to spinal tracts, which are compressed by the tumor. Unilateral compression by a tumor can cause contralateral and ipsilateral sensory affects because of its effect on the spinal tracts. Alterations in urinary elimination may progress to urinary retention, which signifies the need for urinary catheterization. Bowel elimination alterations may occur initially as constipation followed by increasing difficulty with bowel elimination.

The rate of growth of spinal cord tumors can ultimately be determined by neurological assessment. Patients tend to visit their health care provider as they identify changes in motor function and sensory function. Many spinal cord tumors are slow growing tumors, however, and may develop over a few years, with negligible neurological deficits for a significant period of time. If the tumor is a soft tumor, it may also conform somewhat to the space in the spinal column. However, a hard tumor will not conform as easily and will produce neurological deficits earlier.

Diagnostic Tests

Because progression of symptoms may be gradual, a detailed history and physical examination will be essential. Determining the progression of events through the history will be helpful in ascertaining how symptoms have occurred and increased and spread throughout the spinal cord over time. Additionally, neurological assessment will determine muscle weakness, sensory loss, pain, and altered DTRs.

Diagnosis of a spinal cord tumor will center on results of an MRI, so patients will initially undergo this procedure. Positron emission tomography (PET) images will also be performed to identify cancerous tissue. Physicians will perform an MRI and CT scan when patients seek treatment because of symptoms along with a history of known tumor elsewhere. In these situations, there is thus a potential for metastasis. Sometimes only the complaint of back pain, which is new in a patient with a history of cancer, will be the reason for diagnostic tests for spinal cord tumor. A myelogram will be performed to identify blockage of areas of the spinal cord. CSF analysis will also be performed at the time of myelogram (Daniels, 2003).

Nursing Diagnoses

Nursing diagnoses may be similar to the diagnoses for patients with SCI; however, degree of severity of neurological impairment will depend on progression of the tumor. It is important to identify symptoms early to prevent damage to the spinal cord. Based on the information gathered, examples of nursing diagnoses in the patient with spinal cord tumors may include the following:
- Pain related to compression of the spinal cord by the tumor.
- Neurovascular dysfunction related to growth of tumor compressing the spinal cord.
- Impaired elimination, bowel and bladder related to tumor growth and compression of the spinal cord.

Planning and Implementation

The initial focus of planning for the patient with a suspected spinal cord tumor will be to plan with the patient for the diagnostic tests, which will be performed to determine the etiology for the presenting symptoms. Patients will often arrive at the health care facility experiencing pain and loss of functioning, and if they have previously had a diagnosis of cancer, they may be quite fearful and anxious about the possibility of return of the malignancy. Once diagnosis is made, it is important to provide teaching to support the plan of medical care, which will usually include surgery. Preoperatively and postoperatively the patient will generally be receiving corticosteroid therapy for treatment of any edema related to the growth of the tumor. Postoperatively, the patient will participate in planning related to follow-up with chemotherapy and radiation therapy. Nursing care in all stages of medical and surgical treatment will include teaching related to the treatment modality and expected patient responses to the treatment modality.

Long-term planning and implementation will focus on assessment of neurological status and the potential for the patient to resume self-care activities. Treatment of pain will be a priority for nursing management throughout the course of the illness and treatment.

Pharmacology

There are a variety of pharmacological measures taken in the management of spinal cord tumors. The primary classifications of pharmacological treatments are in the forms of chemotherapy and the corticosteroids that are administered. Chemotherapy has limited application for treatment of spinal cord tumors. Chemotherapy may be useful for gliomas, lymphomas, and some lung and breast cancers. Adjuvant therapy, such as tamoxifen, may also be useful, when there is metastasis from the breast. Intrathecal chemotherapy is showing promise with the direct infusion of chemotherapy into the CSF from an Ommaya reservoir.

Dexamethasone at high doses is useful in treatment to decrease the edema associated with the spinal cord tumor. Ascending edema may be present, and the use of corticosteroids will be quite useful in these cases. This treatment in combination with radiation may provide relief of symptoms in patients with inoperable tumors. Patients must have antacids to protect the gastrointestinal (GI) tract when taking these corticosteroids (Broyles, Reiss, & Evans, 2007).

Surgery

For patients with epidural metastases, irradiation along with high doses of dexamethasone (25 mg four times daily) for three days and then in tapered doses is the usual treatment (Tierney, et al., 2004). This will result in reduction of edema and relief of pain. Surgery to remove the tumor in these patients is not usually performed unless irradiation and medical treatment is not successful, although there is controversy about the decision to do surgery in these patients. Radiation therapy tends to delay progression of symptoms. The prognosis in these patients is generally poor. For patients with most extramedullary intradural tumors, surgical removal of the tumor may be successful. Prognosis depends on the origin of the tumor and severity of compression and symptoms.

Emergency surgery is indicated when there is rapid progression of neurological symptoms. Sudden loss of motor and sensory function, including paralysis or loss of bowel and bladder function indicate a need for immediate surgery. This may maintain bowel and bladder function in patients with metastatic lesions and is an important quality of life consideration. Better neurological outcome is related to the degree of neurological deficit that is present. The greater the degree of neurological impairment, the poorer the prognosis. Paralysis is not reversible.

Extradural tumors often involve a less complicated surgery for removal. Such tumors as meningiomas may be completely removed. Intramedullary tumors are much more complicated and the chances for complete removal by surgery are less likely because of invasion of surrounding tissues. In these situations, surgery to accomplish decompression may be the primary goal.

Postoperative nursing care involves detailed neurological assessment along with treatment of pain and other complications. Motor and sensory function must be frequently assessed to identify the possibility of edema developing postoperatively. Complications that have been identified postoperatively in patients undergoing spinal cord tumor resection include the development of intracranial subdural hematomas, as unusual as this may seem. The development of a headache postoperatively should always be reported to the health care provider because of this possibility. It is thought that a puncture of the dura such as occurs with spinal surgery may cause the brain to be displaced downwardly, causing traction, laceration of vessels, and the collection of blood in the subdural space.

Newer techniques for surgery have become available. Laminectomies may still be performed to remove tumors. These surgeries may also involve spinal fusion. Laser surgery and microneurosurgical techniques are becoming available and improving outcomes in patients with spinal cord tumors. Microsurgical lasers make it possible to cut minute tissue bands and achieve immediate hemostasis, resulting in far fewer complications from bleeding and damage to the spinal cord.

During the surgical procedure, intraoperative monitoring of motor evoked potentials (MEPs) has become available to identify the possibility of motor impairment as a result of the surgical technique. Through the use of electrical stimulation these MEPs will provide information about the functioning of fibers in the spinal cord. These MEPs can be followed to determine functional integrity of the motor fibers, and when identified as lost, will be seen as damage to motor pathways. With these newer surgical techniques, surgery has become successful in treating spinal cord tumors.

Radiation Therapy

Radiation therapy is the primary treatment for metastatic spinal cord tumors. Primary spinal cord tumors may also be treated with irradiation. Because the spinal cord is more sensitive to radiation therapy than the brain, measures must be taken to protect the spinal cord from excess exposure. Radiation complications will cause a radiation damage manifested as sensory impairments occurring after the completion of the radiation treatment. This can progress to increasing neurological impairment, paralysis, and loss of bowel and bladder function.

Evaluation of Outcomes

Potential patient outcomes for each of the example nursing diagnoses for the patient with spinal cord tumors are:

- Pain related to compression of tumor, surgical treatment. The patient should verbalize an adequate relief of pain along with the ability to realistically cope with the pain if it is not completely relieved.
- Neurovascular dysfunction. The patient will demonstrate complete return of neurological functioning depending on prognosis.
- Impaired elimination, bowel and bladder. The patient will resume normal bowel and bladder function depending on prognosis.

PERIPHERAL NERVOUS SYSTEM DYSFUNCTION

Peripheral nervous system dysfunction is generally understood as **neuropathies** (dysfunctions of the peripheral nervous system). Neuropathies affecting the peripheral nervous system affect the cranial nerves, spinal nerves, peripheral nerves, and the autonomic nervous system innervation. Peripheral neuropathy results from altered structure or function of a peripheral nerve and may include motor, sensory, or autonomic impairments. Peripheral nerves innervate the extremities, and when damaged, result in motor and sensory impairments affecting the extremities. Peripheral nerves have motor and sensory components, with motor components originating in the lower motor neurons. Some nerves may be motor nerves, others are sensory nerves, and some are mixed in nature.

Etiology

Several etiologies exist for neuropathies, including disease and metabolic problems, drug induced causes, connective tissue causes, infections, trauma, neoplasms, entrapment syndromes, environmental exposure to toxins, and hereditary conditions. In addition to the above etiologies, injury can also cause neuropathy. Injuries to nerves often involve a plexus or injury to an extremity.

Pathophysiology

A thorough understanding of sensory dermatomes, reflexes, and muscle innervation will aid in understanding the signs and symptoms of neuropathies and nerve injuries. It will be possible to map neuropathies of sensory nerves through the use of a dermatome chart. Decreased or loss of sensation of light touch and pinprick will be noted along a particular dermatome. Patients generally complain of tingling, numbness, paresthesias (described by patients as pins and needles), and **dysesthesias** (described as a burning sensation). Pain is often a symptom accompanying nerve trauma and neuropathies, as is commonly seen in diabetic neuropathies (discussed in chapter 57) and trigeminal **neuralgia** (pain associated with peripheral nerves, and following the course of nerves).

There are many neuropathies; those caused by underlying disease, infections, and disorders, such as diabetes, uremia, alcoholism and nutritional deficiencies, acquired immune deficiency syndrome (AIDS), leprosy, sarcoidosis, are discussed elsewhere in this book. Neuropathies may also be caused by toxicities following exposure to industrial agents, pesticides, metals (mercury, thallium, and lead), and drugs, such as phenytoin, many of the neoplastic agents, and such drugs as isoniazid and pyridoxine used in high doses. Neuropathies may also occur as a complication of malignant disease, may occur before signs of the malignancy are apparent, or may occur after remissions and exacerbations. Careful assessment of occupational and health histories is necessary to reveal the possible etiologies for the onset of neuropathies.

Guillain-Barré Syndrome

An increasingly common peripheral nerve disorder is Guillain-Barré syndrome (GBS), which is characterized by acute neuropathy involving motor and sensory nerves throughout the peripheral nervous system.

Epidemiology

According to the Guillain-Barré Syndrome Foundation, the syndrome affects 1 or 2 people per 100,000 population in the United States. It is the most common cause of rapidly acquired paralysis in the United States (Blumenthal, Pria, Bon-Harlev, & Amir, 2004).

Etiology

GBS is an acute idiopathic polyneuropathy that often follows an infective illness. A flu-like illness caused by a variety of pathogens has been most often implicated as the instigating factor in GBS. Most frequently, *Campylobacter jejuni* has been associated with developed of the illness in adults, followed by cytomegalovirus, Epstein Barr, mycoplasma pneumonia, hepatitis A, and hepatitis B. It has also been associated with inoculations with vaccines for influenza, tetanus, hepatitis A, and hepatitis B, as well as with surgical procedures (Tierney, et al., 2004). Usually the acute infectious illness precedes the development of this syndrome by one to three weeks and is most often respiratory or GI in nature (Blumenthal, et al., 2004). The syndrome is thought to be an autoimmune disorder triggered by the infectious agent or event. Because of their decreased immune function, the elderly are more likely to develop GBS after one of these events (Kuwabara, 2004).

This neuropathy is a rapidly progressing disorder affecting primarily the motor components to the peripheral nerves involved. It is believed that the underlying illness triggers a demyelinization of the nerves leading to development of the neuropathy. This dysfunction is characterized by weakness that is generally proximal and symmetrical in distribution. Severity of the weakness varies widely across patients.

GBS usually begins in the legs and proceeds spreading to the arms, face, and sometimes to the muscles of respiration. Motor involvement is more common than sensory involvement; however, patients may experience peripheral paresthesias. Patients may also complain of neuropathic pain. Autonomic dysfunction is common in these patients and may include life-threatening tachycardias, hypotension hypertension, facial flushing, sweating abnormalities, pulmonary dysfunction, and impairments of sphincter control, similar to the autonomic dysfunction that can occur with SCIs.

Pathophysiology

GBS triggers an immune response, which causes destruction of the myelin sheaths of peripheral nerves. Because of the demyelination process, loss of nerve conduction occurs. This demyelination is generally patchy in its involvement. Edema and inflammation of nerves accompany the process leading to further impairment involving the nerves.

Assessment with Clinical Manifestations

Ascending GBS is the most common form of the disease and is characterized by a weakness that starts in the lower extremities and progresses to the trunk and arms, and finally to the cranial nerves affecting the head and neck. Motor deficits with this form of the disorder are symmetrical. DTRs are weak or absent, and sensory impairments of numbness is worse in the toes. Respiratory involvement occurs in 50 percent of patients with ascending GBS.

Descending GBS progresses from the brainstem downward with motor deficits occurring initially with the cranial nerves with progressing weakness downward. Respiratory involvement occurs rapidly in this form of the disease. DTRs are weak or absent. In most patients, GBS is usually seen as weakness of motor function progressing upward from the legs and involving the respiratory muscles in its progression up the trunk. Respiratory difficulties occur as the diaphragm and intercostal muscles become involved. Of the cranial nerves, the facial nerve (cranial nerve [CN] VII) is most frequently involved, although CN IX, X, XI, and XII may also be affected. Effects of cranial nerve involvement will be seen as dysphagia, paralysis of the vocal cords, and difficulty eating. If the vagus nerve is affected, autonomic nervous system signs will be apparent. Sensory involvement from GBS is characterized by pain and paresthesias affecting the hands and feet. Pain generally occurs in the extremities and more often during the night, which interrupts sleep patterns.

Assessment of occupational, infectious, and other exposure history is essential in the diagnostic phase of the illness. As the illness progresses, assessment of the extension of weakness, involvement of respiratory muscles, and the onset of respiratory dysfunction is essential. Assessment of the onset of autonomic symptoms is also a priority, especially the development of hypotension, which may become an emergency. Because patients may require care in critical care units, ongoing in-depth assessment should be done and recorded to note the progression, if any, of weakness. Neurological assessment should include assessment of paresthesias, dysesthesias, and paresis, along with any complaints of pain. Location and movement and progression of the paresis should be noted with each assessment. Vital signs should include any changes in respiratory status, the presence of hypotension or hypertension, and changes in heart rate, including tachycardia.

Detailed assessment of respiratory function is necessary throughout the stages of the disease. Assessment of respiratory rate, depth, and quality is essential at frequent intervals to detect what may seem to be minor changes in respiratory function. The nurse must also assess for signs of respiratory insufficiency, including signs of decreased oxygenation, such as cyanosis, diaphoresis, dyspnea, and anxiety. Pulse oximetry is necessary to maintain assessment of respiratory function. Oxygen will be administered as ordered.

Diagnostic Tests

Diagnosis is made through confirmation of the history of the patient and CSF analysis, which shows a high protein content. These changes may not occur at the same time as symptoms, because it takes two to three weeks to develop. Medical diagnosis will emphasize differential diagnosis, using a process of excluding other causes for the symptoms, which may include botulism, poliomyelitis, and exposure to heavy metals. The disease progresses over several months, however, most patients make a complete recovery. Ten to 20 percent of patients experience a permanent disability.

Nursing Diagnoses

Based on the information gathered, examples of nursing diagnoses in the patient with GBS may include the following:
- Ineffective breathing pattern
- Impaired gas exchange related to ventilation-perfusion inequality
- Ineffective coping related to anxiety, lower activity level and the inability to perform normal activities of daily living
- Knowledge deficit related to self-care and risk prevention

Planning and Implementation

Treatment of GBS is supportive in nature. Plasmapheresis has been shown to be effective, if instituted within three to four days of onset of the illness. It has also been shown to be effective for exacerbations that occur in chronic forms of the dysfunction. Treatment with prednisone is ineffective and actually has been shown to extend recovery time (Tierney, et al., 2004). Care focuses on support of respiratory function and the monitoring of pulmonary function tests to identify weakness of respiratory muscles and the need for critical care management. Management of hypotension is also a priority of care.

Prevention and treatment of respiratory failure is a priority of management. Common progression of the disease as it becomes more life-threatening and includes decreases in vital capacity, decreased ability to cough, and ineffective airway clearance. As vital capacity decreases, the atelectasis and hypoxemia become problematic. Additionally, increasing weakness occurs of the diaphragm and intercostal muscles occur as innervation decreases. At this point intubation and respiratory support may become necessary.

An additional concern for health care is the potential for autonomic dysfunction. Disturbances in cardiac rate and rhythm can occur, so cardiac monitoring is necessary in the critical stages of the illness. Additionally, paralytic ileus and urinary retention may occur as a result of autonomic dysfunction. A nasogastric tube may be necessary for gastric decompression. Intermittent catheterization or indwelling urinary catheter will be used for urinary retention.

Supportive and caring nursing interventions are essential because of the extremely frightening nature of this illness. Teaching about the effects of the illness and the usual self-limiting nature of the illness will provide realistic reassurance to patients. Providing answers to patient and family questions will be beneficial, as those answers are available. Because of the uncertain nature of the development of the illness, answers to the types of questions that patients have are not always available. The health care provider may provide information about the usual progression of the disease that occurs in a majority of patients.

Alterations in respiratory function comprise the priority nursing diagnoses. Patients may experience ineffective airway clearance and ineffective breathing patterns related to the weakness of respiratory muscles. Supportive respiratory care, along with suctioning if necessary to provide a clear airway, is essential in the critical stages of the illness. Instructions to cough and deep breathe, as the patient is able, will help to prevent the development of pneumonia. If respiratory function continues to decline, ventilatory support is necessary, and respiratory care by the nurse becomes the priority of care.

At this stage, patients may be frightened, fearing that they are dying. Because recovery statistics are currently optimistic, providing optimistic information about recovery potential will be helpful to patients. Caring and comforting presence by the nurses is essential in this stage of the illness. Patients are sometimes on ventilator support for months, so the optimism for positive outcome is difficult to maintain for many patients. Additionally, patients who are receiving ventilatory support will need assistance with communication, provided by the nurse.

Preventing alterations in skin integrity becomes a priority as weakness progresses, and independent movement and mobility is impaired. Turning the patient on a strict schedule is necessary to prevent the development of decubitus ulcers. Assessment of skin integrity is an essential component of nursing care contributing to the outcome of skin integrity for patients with GBS.

Of even greater concern related to immobility is the risk for deep vein thrombosis (DVT) and pulmonary embolism (PE). Prevention of DVT and PE is a priority and is achieved by administration of minidoses of heparin. Compression boots for prevention of DVT are not used because of the risk for damage to peripheral nerves with pressure from the boots (Green, Hartwig, Chen, Soltysik, & Yarnold, 2003).

Additionally, because of immobility, the risk for disuse syndrome is a potential issue. Range of motion to the extremities and all joints will prevent contractures as weakness develops in patients. Assistance with mobility and ambulation in many patients will be necessary as the rehabilitation stage progresses.

The progressing alterations in neurological status in patients with GBS mean that detailed neurological assessments are necessary in frequent intervals. Nurses must assess for progressing weaknesses affecting motor and sensory function as well as cranial nerve function. Neurological assessment is emphasized in early stages of the illness, but when respiratory function is affected, the priority for nursing care shifts to respiratory care, including maintenance of a patent airway and adequate respiration. Alterations in autonomic function frequently occur and can be dangerous in its effects. Nurses should be astutely aware of changes in blood pressure and heart rate. Most patients during this time will have hemodynamic monitoring with continuous electrocardiogram (ECG) monitoring to detect any dysrhythmias. Self-care abilities will vary with different patients and differing degrees of weakness. Support for eating, bathing, dressing, and all aspects of self-care are often necessary at some stages of the illness.

Pain becomes a serious concern as patients are recovering from GBS. This means that patients will need frequent assessment of pain and medications for the relief of pain. This may need to be accomplished by epidural infusions of narcotics, such as morphine. Pain will also interfere with sleep patterns, so relief of pain will also aid with sleep. As recovery progresses, an interdisciplinary approach to rehabilitation is most beneficial. Physical therapy will be necessary to help patients regain function and abilities.

Evaluation of Outcomes

Potential patient outcomes for each of the example nursing diagnoses for the patient with the GBS are:

- Ineffective breathing pattern. The patient's breathing pattern is maintained by eupnea, normal skin color, and regular respiratory rate or pattern.
- Impaired gas exchange related to ventilation-perfusion inequality. The patient maintains optimal gas exchange as evidenced by normal arterial blood gases (ABGs) and alert, responsive mentation or no further reduction in mental status.
- Ineffective coping related to anxiety, lower activity level and the inability to perform normal activities of daily living. The patient identifies own maladaptive coping behaviors, available resources, and support systems, describes or initiates alternative coping strategies and describes positive results from new behaviors.
- Knowledge deficit related to self-care and risk prevention. The patient should demonstrate motivation to learn, identify perceived learning needs, and verbalize an understanding of desired content.

Trigeminal Neuralgia

The cranial nerves are the peripheral nerves that originate from the brain. The 12 pairs of cranial nerves may be especially vulnerable to injury; some are more vulnerable to disease than others. The major cranial nerve dysfunctions discussed in this chapter are trigeminal neuralgia and Bell's palsy. An extremely painful condition, trigeminal neuralgia (also known as **tic douloureux**) affects the trigeminal nerve (CN V). This condition is characterized by extreme, intense pain affecting one or more branches of CN V. Unlike many other peripheral nerve conditions, there are no motor or sensory deficits associated with this condition. Patients describe the pain as sharp, stabbing, burning, and intense. This pain is so intense that it can become disabling. Pain is unilateral in location according to the affected nerve. The term tic refers to facial spasms that accompany episodes of the pain.

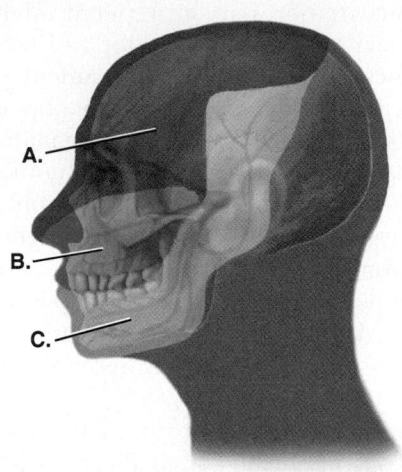

Figure 36-9 Areas of face innervated by the trigeminal nerve (CN-V): A. Ophthalmic, B. Maxillary; C. Mandibular.

CN V is the largest of the cranial nerves and has three divisions: the ophthalmic, maxillary, and mandibular (Figure 36-9). CN V has both motor and sensory components. The motor component innervates the temporal muscles, the muscles used for chewing (masseter), and sensory fibers relay pain, touch, and temperature sensation. The ophthalmic branch innervates the forehead, eyes, nose, temples, paranasal sinuses, and the nasal mucosa. The maxillary branch innervates the upper jaw, teeth, lip, cheeks, hard palate, maxillary sinus, and part of the nasal mucosa. The mandibular branch innervates the lower jaw, teeth, lip, buccal mucosa, tongue, part of the external ear, auditory meatus, and meninges. Trigeminal neuralgia generally affects the maxillary and mandibular branches and only rarely the ophthalmic branch of the nerve.

Epidemiology

Trigeminal neuralgia affects women more than men and generally occurs in middle and later years of life.

Etiology

Trigeminal neuralgia is believed to occur from pressure exerted by blood vessels on the fifth cranial nerve. This pressure eventually causes demyelination of the nerve resulting in severe pain (Brown, 2003).

Pathophysiology

The course of trigeminal neuralgia often includes remissions and exacerbations. Careful history will reveal periods of pain followed by remissions, which may last from days to years. As patients age, remissions tend to become shorter and less frequent. Characteristic of almost all cases of trigeminal neuralgia is a severe, almost disabling pain. Pain is described as a sudden, **lancinating** (stabbing or piercing) facial pain that originates near one side of the mouth and shoots toward the eye, ear, or nostril on the same side. The pain of trigeminal neuralgia may be triggered by touch, drafts of air, eating, and movement (Tierney, et al., 2004). Patients often try many ways to avoid pain, including not doing things that might trigger the pain, such as eating, talking, washing the face, brushing the teeth, or shaving. Therefore, patients may seek health care already being emaciated and disheveled in appearance. Patients may also attempt to talk without moving their face if this is known to trigger the pain.

The etiology of this disease is not known; however, infection (especially of teeth), and trauma have been associated with development of the disorder. Pressure by an artery next to the trigeminal nerve has been identified in many cases. Pressure may also be associated with a tumor or aneurysm, although intracranial tumor as a cause of trigeminal neuralgia is unlikely (Brown, 2003).

Assessment with Clinical Manifestations

Nurses should assess the location, intensity, quality, and characteristics of pain, including the patterns of occurrence, and aggravating and precipitating factors associated with trigeminal neuralgia. Nurses must assess the frequency of episodes of pain, the use of medications, and monitor lab values for side effects of the carbamazepine that involve liver function.

Diagnostic Tests

Diagnosis of trigeminal neuralgia is generally based on physical examination, which identifies the characteristic features of the pain following the pathway of the trigeminal nerve. CT scan is normal unless an underlying lesion or pathology exists. Multiple sclerosis as an underlying pathology has been identified in some cases, and should always be explored in younger patients with trigeminal neuralgia, even when there are no other neurological dysfunctions indicative of multiple sclerosis (Tierney, et al., 2004). Complaints of bilateral pain may also be associated with multiple sclerosis and should be evaluated (Brown, 2003). Occasionally, even when CT and MRI scans are negative, unsuccessful neurological treatment leads to further exploration, which will reveal structural cause for the dysfunction, such as pressure from an artery or vein on the nerve. In these cases, separation of the vessel from the nerve will lead to relief of symptoms. Trigeminal neuralgia is not generally caused by an intracranial mass. Surgical exploration is not used for patients with multiple sclerosis.

Nursing Diagnoses

Based on the information gathered, examples of nursing diagnoses in the patient with trigeminal neuralgia may include the following:
- Acute pain related to neurological impairment
- Alteration in nutritional status, less than body requirements related to pain associated with eating
- Social isolation related to pain
- Risk for loneliness related to pain and discomfort

Planning and Implementation

Medical treatment of trigeminal neuralgia is currently primarily comprised of pharmacological intervention. Other methods of treatment may include surgery and injections with alcohol, however alcohol injection and surgery are much less frequently recommended currently. The drug most commonly used for the treatment of trigeminal neuralgia is carbamazepine (Tegretol). Carbamazepine can also aid in diagnosis, because patients may respond immediately to this medication (Brown, 2003). Because this drug can be toxic to the liver and can also cause bone marrow depression, patients' laboratory values must be closely monitored while taking this medication. If patients cannot tolerate this medication, other choices include phenytoin (Dilantin), the second choice for pharmacological therapy. Gabapentin, baclofen, capsaicin, and amitriptyline may also be used for relief of symptoms if first-line therapy is not successful.

Medical treatment may become less effective over the long term, and surgical treatment may become necessary in some patients who have chronic trigeminal neuralgia. Neurodestructive procedures may be undertaken if medical treatment is not successful.

The primary concern of patients with trigeminal neuralgia is severe pain radiating along the nerve tract. Nursing care will focus on assisting patients to seek medical treatment for diagnosis, and supporting patients through exacerbation of the nerve dysfunction. This dysfunction becomes a chronic pain syndrome with the exacerbations and remissions associated with it. Even though carbamazepine has been useful in treating the dysfunction, it is not always effective, and its side effects may lead to the need to discontinue the medication. Pain and uncertainty about the medication regimen leads to psychosocial responses, including social isolation and loneliness. Malnutrition may occur because of the guarding by patients to prevent an episode of pain. Because patients do not want to get themselves in a situation where they may experience pain, they may isolate themselves socially, delay self-care activities of washing and brushing their teeth, and experience alterations in nutrition related to this fear of causing pain.

Assisting patients with nutrition, medication administration, assessment for side effects, and pain assessment and management are the primary nursing interventions for this dysfunction. Nursing interventions to assist patients to avoid the aggravating and precipitating factors may be helpful in preventing occurrences of the pain. Nutritional assessment and teaching regarding the necessity of a balanced diet, perhaps with the inclusion of soft foods will be helpful in maintaining nutritional status.

The social isolation that patients may experience because of the dysfunction can become quite severe. Identification of family members who are supportive of the patient in times of severe pain will be helpful in providing a safe and caring environment for the patient. Also, helping family members to understand the severity of the pain will bring a level of support to patients through the difficult painful episodes.

Evaluation of Outcomes

Potential patient outcomes for each of the example nursing diagnoses for the patient with trigeminal neuralgia are:

- Acute pain related to neurological impairment. The patient will report pain free status (0 on scale of 0 to 10). This may need to be adjusted depending on the success of treatment. The goal will be to maintain the patient in a pain-free state.
- Alteration in nutritional status, less than body requirements related to pain associated with eating. The patient will maintain nutritional status for body requirements.
- Social isolation related to pain. The patient will resume social activities once pain free.
- Risk for loneliness related to pain and discomfort. The patient will reconnect with friends and family and report a lower level of loneliness which is specifically related to the condition.

Bell's Palsy

Bell's palsy is a facial neuropathy that is characterized by paresis and pain. Considered an idiopathic neuropathy, patients complain of symptoms of paresis (weakness) initially, which worsen over the next few days. Pain often accompanies the paresis or may precede the symptoms of paresis. Generally the pain is self-limiting and may last for only a few days. Restriction of eye closure, stiffness of the face, and fine movement of the facial muscles occurs. Patients may also complain of alterations in taste.

Epidemiology

Bell's palsy is the most common cause of facial paralysis. Affecting men and women equally, approximately 40,000 people are diagnosed in the United States each year. Pregnant women are disproportionately affected.

Etiology

Bell's palsy is generally considered an inflammatory disorder and may be associated with reactivation of herpes simplex virus. Although this belief is controversial, it does have wide support as the cause (He, Zhou, Wu, Li, & Zhou, 2004). Increased support for the association of the herpes simplex virus and Bell's palsy is being reported (Doganci, Odabasi, & Turn, 2003).

Pathophysiology

Bell's palsy results from a lower motor neuron dysfunction causing a unilateral facial nerve (CN VII) paresis or paralysis on one side of the face.

Assessment with Clinical Manifestations

Characteristic symptoms of Bell's palsy initially include facial weakness (paresis), which begins abruptly and worsens over the following days. Pain accompanies the weakness but usually only lasts a few days. Patients complain of facial stiffness and may have limited eye closure and restricted movement of the facial muscles, which subsequently results in difficulty eating. Alterations in taste have also been known to occur.

Diagnostic Tests

Diagnosis of Bell's palsy is generally made after physical examination and careful assessment of cranial nerve function. The clinical picture of distorted face is a classic sign of Bell's palsy. Electromyography (EMG) may be performed to assess nerve damage, and MRI, CT scan, and X-ray will detect the presence of a tumor applying pressure on the facial nerve.

Nursing Diagnoses

Based on the information gathered, examples of nursing diagnoses in the patient with Bell's palsy may include the following:

- Acute pain
- Alteration in nutritional status, less than body requirements
- Disturbed sensory perception
- Disturbed body image
- Readiness for enhanced self-concept

Planning and Implementation

Because many of the cases recover without treatment, controversy exists regarding treatment of Bell's palsy. Only about 10 percent of patients experience long-term disability or disfigurement. In those patients, treatment is necessary to prevent disfigurement. In other patients, more than 80 percent have reported resolution of symptoms and recovery without treatment (He, et al., 2004). Poor prognosis for recovery is seen in patients who are elderly, who experience severe pain at onset, or who have degeneration of the facial nerve. Treatment for patients with severe pain consists of corticosteroids, generally prednisone 60 to 80 mg in divided doses for 4 to 5 days, with tapering doses over the next 7 to 10 days (Tierney, et al., 2004). Sometimes acyclovir is also prescribed for treatment because of the herpes virus association, although this is controversial. Studies have not shown the efficacy of acyclovir used alone as treatment. There is limited evidence that acyclovir used in combination with prednisone may result in improvement of symptoms.

Acupuncture as a complementary medical treatment has shown great promise in the treatment of Bell's palsy. Preliminary studies show significantly better responses in patients receiving acupuncture versus patients in a control group. However, these results are based on limited studies (He, et al., 2003).

Generally, assessment and teaching regarding the need to seek treatment early are the priority nursing interventions. Treatment should be started early after symptoms occur, within five days of onset to be effective, so early identification and referral for treatment is a necessity. For patients with restricted eyelid closure, instruction should be given to use eye drops to keep the eyes lubricated. If the patient cannot close the eye, an eye patch should be used to protect the eye or the patient should be taught to manually close the eye. Teaching regarding the use of corticosteroids should also be provided to patients.

Nutritional deficits occur with Bell's palsy because of the limitations on movement of the mouth on the affected side of the face. Frequent, small meals with soft foods are best tolerated by most patients. Sipping drinks through a straw and chewing on the affected side are often limited or impossible. Because of the difficulties with eating and the potential for disfigurement, emotional support is necessary during this time. Alterations in body image and self-concept occur because of the change in appearance. Emotional support provided by the nurse is necessary during this time. Reassurance that most patients recover completely is often difficult to understand when looking at oneself in the mirror and seeing a side of the face that sags and an eye that will not close.

Patients suggesting that they are interested in trying complementary or alternative therapy should be referred to their health care provider for further information. Nurses should become aware of the potential beneficial effects of complementary methods, such as acupuncture, and support patients in their attempts to find successful treatment for this condition. Sometimes, facial exercises and electrical nerve stimulation are suggested for treatment of Bell's palsy. Currently, there is no evidence that either treatment modality is efficacious. There is some evidence that electrical nerve stimulation may be helpful in treatment of long-term symptoms of Bell's palsy.

Evidence-Based Care

Recent research has shown that patients receiving the intranasal influenza vaccine used in Switzerland had an increased incidence of Bell's palsy. The intranasal influenza vaccine currently in use in the United States has not shown this association (Mutsch, et al., 2004).

Evaluation of Outcomes

Potential patient outcomes for each of the example nursing diagnoses for the patient with Bell's palsy are:

- Acute pain. The patient should verbalize an adequate relief of pain along with the ability to realistically cope with the pain if it is not completely relieved.
- Alteration in nutritional status, less than body requirements. The patient will maintain nutritional intake for body requirements.
- Disturbed sensory perception. The patient will report no numbness, tingling, or pain.
- Disturbed body image. The patient demonstrates enhanced body image and self-esteem as evidenced by ability to look at, touch, talk about, and care for actual or perceived altered body part or function.
- Readiness for enhanced self-concept. The patient will verbalize acceptance of self.

Ménière's Disease

Ménière's disease is a disorder thought to be caused by a range of inflammatory, traumatic, autoimmune, or idiopathic events leading to eventual dysfunction of the vestibulocochlear nerve (CN VIII) (Dieterich, 2004).

Epidemiology

Higher incidences of Ménière's disease have also been found in patients with herpes simplex virus (Vrabec, 2003). In addition, an association between Ménière's disease and the presence of hypothyroidism has also been investigated to determine if thyroid hormone supplements can be implicated in Ménière's disease (Brenner, Hoistad, & Hain, 2004). Research results indicate that the medication is probably not the underlying association, but rather it is believed that an autoimmune component can contribute to both hypothyroidism and Ménière's disease. This possibility is more likely in patients who are over 60 years of age.

Etiology

The etiology of Ménière's disease is not always certain, although two known infectious and traumatic causes of the disorder are syphilis and head trauma.

Pathophysiology

The events of inflammation, trauma, and autoimmune dysfunction are thought to cause one of the classic vertigo syndromes, which ultimately occur as a result of distension of the compartments in the inner ear leading to endolymphatic hydrops. Eventually rupture of the membranous labyrinth causes paralysis of the CN VIII (Dieterich, 2004).

Assessment with Clinical Manifestations

Ménière's disease is characterized by episodic vertigo along with a low-frequency sensorineural hearing loss, tinnitus, and a sense of pressure or fullness in the ear. Nystagmus is also present. Vertigo lasts from a few to several hours; however, symptoms progress in most patients to include a chronic tinnitus and hearing loss.

Diagnostic Tests

The diagnosis of Ménière's disease is made by the assessment of the several parameters that typically characterize the disease. Specific hearing tests to identify sensory or neural hearing loss will be undertaken initially, as will physical assessment to identify tinnitus and nystagmus. The caloric test will be done to assess for nystagmus, testing the vestibular system, and MRI may be performed to rule out tumor as the cause of symptoms. The caloric test is performed by irrigating the ear with cold water and observing the patient for rapid eye movements as a result. Hearing tests to identify sensory origin of hearing loss indicate an inner ear etiology for the hearing loss. Hearing tests which identify a neural etiology for the hearing loss will indicate CN VIII nerve damage. Electrocochleography may also be done to assess the electrical activity of the inner ear.

Nursing Diagnoses

Based on the information gathered, examples of nursing diagnoses in the patient with Ménière's disease may include the following:
- Risk for injury related to vertigo
- Nausea related to disturbance of the vestibular system
- Disturbed sensory perception, auditory

Planning and Implementation

Treatment for Ménière's disease is aimed at lowering pressure in the inner ear. Diuretics along with a low-sodium diet will relieve symptoms in many patients. Antibiotics may be used if infection is suspected as the underlying cause of symptoms. Ototoxic antibiotics, such as intratympanic gentamicin, may also be instilled in the ear; however, this is controversial as it has been shown to contribute to higher levels of hearing loss than in patients who had surgical section of the vestibular nerve (Hillman, Arriaga, & Chen, 2003; Hillman, Chen, & Arriaga, 2004). Surgical repairs may be performed but less frequently than medical treatment and with more danger of hearing loss.

Treatment of symptoms is important for patients because of the extreme discomfort caused by the vertigo, as well as the nausea and vomiting that often accompany the vertigo. Treatment with antiemetic medications is helpful to most patients. Bedrest may be the most promising and effective treatment for the vertigo associated with Ménière's disease. Medication treatment with antihistamines, using meclizine (Antivert) most commonly, has been successful in most patients. Histamines work by improving microcirculation. Corticosteroids have also been shown to have limited use when given over two to three weeks with tapering doses. Long-term therapy with corticosteroids may be used to maintain hearing and decrease the frequency of attacks (Dieterich, 2004).

Ménière's disease can be extremely disabling to patients because of the vertigo, nausea, and vomiting. The primary concern is the risk for injury from falls because of the vertigo. Teaching regarding safe activity and the need for bedrest should be provided to the patient. The degree of relief as a result of medications should be assessed periodically by the nurse. Additionally, assessment of hearing should also be performed periodically to determine if the disease is progressing and whether it has negative effect on the patient's hearing. Nausea is another disabling symptom of the disease. Assessment of the presence of nausea and teaching regarding the use of antiemetic medications is necessary with these patients.

Because experimental treatments exist for Ménière's disease, the nurse must be aware of current research that examines the different treatment for Ménière's disease and support the patient in talking with the health care provider to determine the best course of action. Emotional support is a primary intervention for patients with Ménière's disease. This can be a disabling disorder and can cause extreme distress. Frequently, the family members of a patient with Ménière's disease will not understand the disabling effect; therefore teaching for the family is essential.

Pharmacology

Recently, intratympanic steroids have been studied to determine their usefulness in the treatment of Ménière's disease. Because it is thought that there could be an autoimmune component to the disease, steroids, such as dexamethasone, could be useful for their anti-inflammatory effects. Current studies have shown promising results in restoring hearing loss in patients with endolymphatic hydrops associated with Ménière's disease (Hillman, Arriaga, & Chen, 2004). Administration of this medication is performed by the physician after anesthetization of the tympanic membrane.

Surgery

In those patients who are refractory to other methods of treatment for Ménière's disease surgery may become necessary. Surgery of the vestibular portion of the CN VIII is effective in these patients. Removal of the semicircle canals is also effective but not appropriate for patients whose hearing is not affected. Removal of semicircle canals is only used in patients with limited hearing in the affected ear.

Evaluation of Outcomes

Potential patient outcomes for each of the example nursing diagnoses for the patient with Ménière's disease are:
- Risk for injury related to vertigo. The patient will be free of fall or injury.
- Nausea related to vertigo. The patient will be free of nausea and vomiting.
- Disturbed sensory perception, auditory. Hearing status will be maintained at predisease level.

Peripheral Nerve Injuries

Injury to peripheral nerves can result from acute trauma or chronic entrapment syndromes. Motor vehicle accidents, falls, sports injuries, and occupational accidents may cause acute injuries. Impact from sharp objects may cause transection and laceration of nerves, and direct blows to nerves may cause injury by contusions to nerves. Traction on nerves through improper application of orthopedic traction or in motor vehicle accidents may also cause peripheral nerve injuries. Shoulder injuries are common nerve injuries resulting in motor vehicle accidents.

Pathophysiology

Trauma and injury often occurs in the plexuses. A plexus comprises a network of axons and may be vulnerable to injury. The brachial plexus is a common area of injury. Downward pressure on the shoulder may lead to upper brachial plexus injury, and a lower plexus injury results from traction and stretching of the arm. An upper plexus injury results in a functioning hand with a weak arm and shoulder, and a lower plexus injury results in a strong arm with a weak hand. Herniated discs and trauma are common causes of sciatic injury.

Assessment with Clinical Manifestations

The type and extent of injury will determine the signs and symptoms associated with the injury. Motor and sensory deficits along with autonomic affects may occur together or alone with injury. Signs and symptoms may include paralysis or paresis if some of the lower motor neurons are intact, muscular atrophy, absent DTRs, sensory losses, warm dry skin and trophic changes including cold, cyanotic skin.

Neurological assessment is an essential aspect of care of the patient with a peripheral nerve injury. Paresthesias, paralysis, paresis, and pain are common results of nerve injuries, and the degree of dysfunction associated with each of these findings will vary and may change according to the injury.

Diagnostic Tests

Most often, diagnosis is based on a history of injury along with a neurological examination. Neurological assessment will establish the motor and sensory components of the dysfunction and injury, including pain associated with the injury. CT, MRI, EMG, and nerve conduction velocity (NCV) studies are most useful in determining the type and extent of injury and nerve damage.

Nursing Diagnoses

Based on the information gathered, examples of nursing diagnoses in the patient with peripheral nerve injuries may include the following:
- Disturbed sensory perception related to nerve injury function
- Acute pain related to nerve injury
- Impaired physical mobility related to nerve injury
- Risk for injury related to casting or splinting
- Risk for altered tissue integrity related to casting or splinting
- Alteration in self-care related to nerve injury

Planning and Implementation

Treatment of peripheral nerve injuries may include surgical anastomosis of severed nerves. This is done soon after the injury to prevent further deformity. As the nerve shortens with surgery, contractions are at risk for occurrence. After surgery the limb is placed in a flexion position to compensate for the contraction. Physical therapy is essential to capitalize on the potential for regaining functionality of the extremities innervated by injured nerves. Pain associated with the injury should be treated with analgesics. It is important to identify and treat the pain, because pain will decrease the success of physical therapy and rehabilitation.

Pain management is essential, so in-depth pain assessment will be an ongoing nursing management issue. Determination and management of losses of motor and sensory function are the priorities for nursing care. Assessment of motor and sensory function along with color, warmth, and trophic changes of extremities are necessary. Because traumatic injuries, such as penetrating injuries, occurring with stab wounds can cause peripheral nerve injuries, it is important to assess neurological status of the peripheral nerves adjacent to the injured area when this type of injury occurs. Delay in treatment can mean significant loss of nerve function (Sunderamoorthy & Chaudhury, 2003).

If immobilization of the affected limb is ordered by the physician, the nurse will need to provide teaching regarding splint or cast care. Assessment by the nurse of circulation in the splinted or casted extremity will be a priority of care. The patient and family members should be taught to look for alterations in warmth, color, and the presence of tingling which are indicators of autonomic dysfunction and should be reported to the physician. The skin may be susceptible to breakdown and should be thoroughly assessed and cared for with lotion for dry skin. Lost sensory function will mean that patients will have disturbed sense of temperatures and should be careful with application of heat and cold because of the potential for injury to the extremity.

Evaluation of Outcomes

Potential patient outcomes for each of the example nursing diagnoses for the patient with a peripheral nerve injury are:
- Disturbed sensory perception related to nerve injury. The patient will report complete sensation without numbness or tingling in affected nerve areas, and will demonstrate motor functioning without restriction of movement in affected areas.

Safety First

IV Therapy and Peripheral Nerve Injury

It is important to note that damage to peripheral nerves can occur from insertion of IV cannulas into the cephalic vein. If patients complain of numbness or tingling on insertion of an IV cannula, the nurse should remove the cannula immediately. Measures to prevent injury to the superficial peripheral nerves, especially the superficial radial nerve include removing the cannula if the patient experiences paresthesias or numbness, and limiting probing when inserting an IV cannula. Peripheral nerve injury can be temporary or it may be permanent.

- Acute pain related to nerve injury. The patient should verbalize an adequate relief of pain along with the ability to realistically cope with the pain if it is not completely relieved.
- Risk for injury. The patient will identify signs of injury from cast or splinting and report to nurse or health care provider.
- Risk for tissue injury. The patient will identify signs of tissue injury from cast or splinting and report to nurse or health care provider.
- Self-care, activities of daily living, completely independent. The patient will complete activities of daily living without assistance.

Carpal Tunnel Syndrome

Carpal tunnel syndrome is considered an entrapment neuropathy in which compression of the median nerve occurs in the carpal tunnel, most often from pressure of the carpal ligament in the tunnel.

Epidemiology

Occupation-related history reveals the highest risk factors for development of the disorder, including repetitive movement of the wrists for prolonged periods of time. People at risk for development of carpal tunnel syndrome include computer keyboarders, typists, pianist, and construction workers who work with vibrating equipment. Women are affected more than men, perhaps because of the number of women in occupations where word processing is a dominant part of the job. Carpal tunnel syndrome has also been known to exist in athletes who are involved in repetitive digital flexion activities.

Etiology

Entrapment disorders occur from compression on the nerve from the anatomical structure. Ulnar nerve and radial nerve entrapment can also occur, although not as frequently as carpal tunnel syndrome.

Pathophysiology

The combination of a narrow channel along with edema, which may occur with trauma to tissues, results in pressure on the nerve in the structure resulting in entrapment. Carpal tunnel syndrome is characterized by pain of a burning and tingling nature. Patients may also complain of an aching pain that is exacerbated by activity, especially flexion and dorsiflexion of the wrist. The pain usually is worse at night. Distribution of pain along the median nerve is characteristic of the carpal tunnel syndrome and occurs as edema of tissue entraps the median nerve at the wrist a vulnerable area. The median nerve enters the carpal tunnel beneath the transverse carpal ligament. The tunnel comprises the transverse carpal ligaments superiorly and the carpal bones laterally and inferiorly. As the lumen of the tunnel narrows, movement of the nerve is compromised.

The resulting pain may radiate up the forearm and even to the shoulder and chest (Tierney, et al., 2004). Assessment reveals numbness and tingling when invoked by the carpal compression test, which involves pressure applied over the carpal tunnel. Muscle weakness appears later than the sensory disturbances.

Assessment with Clinical Manifestations

Symptoms of carpal tunnel syndrome include sensory and motor losses. Sensory losses follow the nerve track and include the palmar aspect of the first three fingers and half of the fourth fingers, and the dorsal aspects of the terminal phalanges of the second, third, and half of the fourth fingers. Patients complain of wrist pain, especially at night. Most pain is in the wrist and the areas innervated by the median nerve but may also radiate up the forearm. Pain is worse on wrist flexion. The patient also experiences weakness in areas of the hand, including difficulty with abduction of the thumb. As the condition progresses, wasting of the hand muscles can occur.

Diagnostic Tests

Diagnosis of carpal tunnel syndrome is made through the use of EMG and motor and sensory conduction delays determined through these tests. Physical assessment reveals positive Tinel's and Phalen's sign. Tinel's sign is elicited by tapping over the median nerve at the wrist and is positive if pain occurs. Phalen's sign is elicited by flexing the wrists at a right angle for one minute. Phalen's sign is positive if pain and tingling occur on flexion of the wrist.

Nursing Diagnoses

Based on the information gathered, examples of nursing diagnoses in the patient with carpal tunnel syndrome may include the following:
- Disturbed sensory perception related to carpal tunnel syndrome.
- Acute pain related to carpal tunnel syndrome.

Planning and Implementation

Nursing care of the patient with carpal tunnel syndrome primarily involves teaching about the use of the hand and wrist splint through limitation of movement to relieve pressure on the median nerve. Because many cases of carpal tunnel syndrome are occupational in origin, discussion of modifications to occupational activities may be necessary. Patients may have many concerns about work related activities, which should be referred to the health care provider. Physical therapy may be helpful in regaining activity after treatment concludes. Rest is important and limitation of movement is essential to prevent additional pressure on the median nerve.

Currently, the numbers of people affected by carpal tunnel syndrome is increasing because of word processing activities and keyboarding affecting many different types of workers. A thorough occupational history is necessary. Teaching about prevention of the syndrome includes proper positioning of wrists and hands at keyboards with wrists off the surface of the desk, or with support provided through gel type devices. For athletes experiencing symptoms, rest and immobilization will generally result in alleviation of symptoms. Nonsteroidal anti-inflammatory medications will also be of use in these patients. Surgery is usually not necessary for carpal tunnel caused by athletics.

Pharmacology

Treatment of carpal tunnel syndrome consists of relief of pressure on the median nerve through splinting of the hand and wrist for two to six weeks. Patients are taught to modify and limit their hand activities during this time. Nonsteroidal anti-inflammatory drugs may also be administered. Corticosteroid injections are used if there is no improvement with the traditional less invasive treatment.

Surgery

A surgical intervention which frees the median nerve may be a last resort in the treatment of carpal tunnel syndrome.

Evaluation of Outcomes

Potential patient outcomes for each of the example nursing diagnoses for the patient with carpal tunnel syndrome are:
- Disturbed sensory perception related to carpal tunnel syndrome. The patient's sensory motor functioning will not be compromised, as exhibited by freedom of movement and complete sensation in affected extremity. The patient will be free of numbness or tingling in affected extremity.
- Acute pain related to carpal tunnel syndrome. The patient should verbalize an adequate relief of pain along with the ability to realistically cope with the pain if it is not completely relieved.

KEY CONCEPTS

- Complete SCI results in loss of motor and sensory function below the level of injury.
- Spinal shock occurs immediately after injury and includes complete loss of motor and sensory functioning below the level of injury.
- Emergency treatment of SCI is essential to preserve functioning and to provide for improvement in the degree of neurological impairment.
- Understanding the anatomical and physiological effects of an SCI will provide an understanding of the neurological impairments that may be expected.
- Nursing management of the patient with an SCI in the acute phase will include assessment of respiratory and neurological impairment.
- Spinal cord tumors result from benign and metastatic tumors. Surgical removal of tumors is a priority; however, radiation and chemotherapy may be modes of treatment.

- Assessment of neurological status and loss of motor and sensory functioning is a priority for the patient with a spinal cord tumor.
- Peripheral nervous system disorders occur as a result of injury, disease, occupational exposures, infection, medications, as well as a myriad of other stimuli.
- Pain and sensory disturbances along with motor disturbances in some disorders are the primary symptoms of a peripheral nervous system disturbance.
- GBS often results from exposure to infectious organisms and progresses upward from the legs, causing paresis or paralysis of the diaphragm and intercostals muscles.
- Teaching regarding the effects and treatment of peripheral nervous system disorders is a hallmark of nursing care.

REVIEW QUESTIONS

1. The nurse is caring for a patient who has a C6 SCI. She anticipates that the patient understands the teaching about the long-term effects of the injury when the patient says:
   1. I will be able to transfer myself to the wheelchair and bed.
   2. I will be able to feed myself.
   3. I will be on a ventilator to support my breathing for the rest of my life.
   4. I will not need urinary catheterization after I am discharged from the hospital.

2. The patient has experienced an incomplete SCI resulting in Brown-Séquard syndrome. What abnormalities should the nurse expect the patient to experience (select all that apply)?
   1. Loss of pain and temperature sensation on the opposite side
   2. Loss of all motor and sensory function below the level of the injury
   3. Loss of motor function (paralysis) on the same side as the injury
   4. Loss of position sense and vibration on same side as the injury

3. What response would be the best response for a patient with a new SCI who asks if his current paralysis will be permanent?
   1. If there is a loss of function at the accident, it is not possible to regain motor functioning.

   2. There is often a period of spinal shock when it is difficult to determine if the paralysis will be permanent, and when it resolves there can be some regaining of abilities.
   3. You're experiencing spinal shock now; in three weeks you will regain your functioning when the spinal shock resolves.
   4. It's best to start trying to accept your limitations; it's unlikely that any improvement can occur.

4. A patient has been diagnosed with trigeminal neuralgia. Which medication is likely to be prescribed as a first choice for treatment?
   1. Phenytoin (Dilantin)
   2. Gabapentin
   3. Baclofen
   4. Carbamazepine (Tegretol)

5. Which of the following is not generally present in a patient with Ménière's disease?
   1. Hypothyroidism
   2. Nystagmus
   3. Tinnitus
   4. High-frequency hearing loss

6. The nurse is seeing a patient with Ménière's disease in the clinic for the first time; which of the following would the nurse do first:
   1. Assess for a history of taking thyroid supplements
   2. Teach about safety to prevent falls in patients experiencing vertigo

Continued

REVIEW QUESTIONS—cont'd

3. Refer to a health care provider for treatment of tinnitus
4. Instruct the patient about the need for bedrest

7. Which of the following is most indicative of pain associated with carpal tunnel syndrome?
   1. Burning, tingling pain, worse during the daytime when the patient is most active
   2. Burning, tingling pain that may be worse during the nighttime
   3. Throbbing pain that increases with extension of the wrist
   4. Throbbing pain that is worst with rest

8. Positive Phalen's sign for carpal tunnel syndrome is indicated by which of the following?
   1. Relief of pain on flexion of the wrist at a right angle for one minute
   2. Pain and tingling experienced on tapping over the median nerve at the wrist
   3. Relief of pain experienced upon tapping over the median nerve at the wrist
   4. Pain and tingling experienced on flexion of the wrist at a right angle for one minute

9. Emergency treatment with methylprednisolone for a patient with an SCI must be instituted in what time period?
   1. Within the first 8 hours after injury
   2. Within the first 24 hours after injury
   3. Within the first hour after injury
   4. Within 72 hours after injury

10. A patient with a cervical SCI has an upper motor neuron lesion. The nurse can anticipate that care will include which of the following?
    1. Administration of baclofen for spasticity
    2. Teaching regarding self-catheterization
    3. Teaching regarding ability to perform self-care dressing activities, including buttoning one's shirts and tying shoe laces
    4. Range of motion for flaccid extremities

11. The priority nursing action for a patient with an SCI experiencing a pounding headache and blood pressure of 220/120 indicating autonomic dysreflexia is to:
    1. Call the physician for order for antihypertensive medication
    2. Check for distended bladder or kinked catheter tubing
    3. Assess heart rate and skin temperature
    4. Check for fecal impaction
    5. Calcium channel blockers

REVIEW ACTIVITIES

1. Visit a rehabilitation facility and interview a patient with an SCI and family member to try to understand the physical and psychosocial issues faced by patients with SCI and their families. Ask about what changes are needed in the physical environment of the home of a patient with SCI. Ask about how family members have made changes in their lives.

2. Discuss the pathophysiological rationale for the use of methylprednisolone for SCI.

3. Develop a teaching plan for the prevention of carpal tunnel syndrome.

4. Discuss the postoperative care of the patient who has had surgical removal of a spinal cord tumor.

5. Explore the Christopher Reeve Paralysis Foundation Web site, and identify information provided for patients, for family members, and for health care professionals. Identify the newest research that is being reported on the Web site and consider how this research will impact nursing care of SCI patients.

Degenerative Neurological Dysfunction: Nursing Management

Doris Denison, MSN, APRN, BC, CCRN

CHAPTER TOPICS

- Headaches
- Seizures
- Multiple Sclerosis
- Parkinson's Disease

- Alzheimer's Disease
- Myasthenia Gravis
- Amyotrophic Lateral Sclerosis
- Huntington's Chorea

KEY TERMS

Akinesia
Aura
Bradykinesia
Cephalalgia
Chorea
Convulsion
Diplopia
Epilepsy
Plasmapheresis
Ptosis
Rhinorrhea
Seizure
Tremor

Chronic and degenerative neurological diseases can be both challenging and frustrating for patients, families, and health care providers. There is no known cure for these diseases. This chapter focuses on the management of chronic headache (cephalalgia), seizures, multiple sclerosis, Parkinson's disease, myasthenia gravis, amyotrophic lateral sclerosis, and Huntington's disease.

These neurological disorders involve either chronic disease or progressive deterioration of mental or physical function and can be devastating to both the patient and his or her family. The patient may become depressed, angry, fearful, or withdrawn when having to deal with the progression of the disease. Changes in body image, self-esteem, and lifestyle can enhance the emotional trauma of dealing with a progressively debilitating process. Families may experience despair, hope, love, resentment, guilt, and empathy for their family member. As the patient's condition continues to deteriorate, the family needs to deal with the emotional conflict precipitated by their sense of duty to the patient and the need to live their own lives. Health care providers are similarly frustrated by their wanting to alleviate the physical symptoms, prevent complications, maximize the patient's self-care abilities, and assist with lifestyle changes.

HEADACHE

Headache (**cephalalgia**) is the most common form of chronic pain and is responsible for an estimated 20 million visits to a health care provider every year. The National Headache Foundation estimates that more than 75 percent of Americans suffer from headaches, and of those, about 9 percent seek medical attention and 80 percent self-medicate. The cost of missed workdays and medical treatment is estimated to be about $50 billion annually. The level of dysfunction from headache varies with each person. For some patients, headache occurs occasionally and is relieved by an over-the-counter (OTC) analgesic. Others experience frequent and debilitating headaches that decrease their ability to work, interfere with personal relationships, alter family life, and decrease their quality of life. Headaches may also be a symptom of a more serious underlying condition that requires immediate intervention by a health care provider.

Headaches are generally classified as primary or secondary in nature. When no organic cause can be identified, it is considered a primary headache. Types of headaches include: tension-type, migraine, and cluster. The majority of headaches (90 to 98 percent) are primary. Secondary headaches have an underlying organic cause, such as aneurysm or tumor. Only primary headaches will be discussed in this chapter. Secondary headaches are discussed with the organic cause.

Tension-Type Headache

Tension-type headache is the most common type, accounting for 90 percent of primary headaches, and is considered the most difficult to treat. Tension-type headache is defined as intermittent with a variable duration.

 Uncovering the Evidence

Headache in the Workplace

Discussion: The purpose of this research was to study the impact of headaches on work attendance and its economic impact in two different workplaces. Questionnaires were sent to 800 employees in Sweden. Four hundred were privately employed, and 400 were employed at a public university hospital. The questionnaire addressed a variety of variables: number of headaches in a three-month period, duration of the headaches, decreased ability to work effectively, and number appointments with a health care provider for treatment of headache.

The prevalence of headache was 64 percent in the privately employed group and 78 percent in the hospital. Fifty percent of the subjects reported going to work despite their headache, and the mean number of days was 6.6 for the privately employed group and 6.1 days for the hospital employed group. A 25 percent decrease in work effectiveness was calculated. The economic impact was calculated as approximately 1.4 billion per year.

Implications for Practice: The economic impact of decreased workplace productivity is substantial, and the authors suggest that workplace-based treatment and prevention programs may be both financially and clinically advantageous.

Source: Raak, R., & Raak, A. (2003). Work attendance despite headache and its economic impact: A comparison between two workplaces. Headache, 43, 1097–1101.

Epidemiology

Prevalence of tension-type headaches has been reported as low as 30 percent and as high as 90 percent on a yearly basis. Lifetime prevalence is 78 percent, 63 percent for men, and 86 percent for women. Prevalence peaks between 40 and 50 years of age (International Headache Society, 2004).

Etiology

Etiology is multifactorial and may include:
- Sustained contraction of the pericranial muscles (muscle contraction headache).
- Referred pain from upper cervical joints, ligaments, and muscles.
- Prolonged peripheral pain may cause central sensitization.
- Physical or psychological stress, lack of sleep, anxiety, and depression.

Pathophysiology

Tension-type headache is caused by irritation of the pain-sensitive structures of the brain. The intracranial structures include portions of the trigeminal (cranial nerve 5 [CN V]), facial (cranial nerve 7 [CN VII]), glossopharyngeal (cranial nerve 9 [CN IX]), vagus (cranial nerve 10 [CN X]), and upper cervical nerves, the large arteries, and the venous sinuses. When the sensory receptors of the muscles, tendons, joints, and skin are stimulated, they transmit pain messages to the pain-sensitive areas of the brain. Tension-type headaches may be episodic or chronic (Table 37-1).

Assessment with Clinical Manifestations

Patients describe their headache as bilateral with a pressure or tightness sensation, becoming worse with physical activity, and a mild to moderately severe discomfort level. The headache does not involve vomiting, but there may be occasional feelings of nausea. Sensitivity to light (photophobia) or sound (phonophobia) may be reported. The headaches may occur over weeks, months, or years, and many patients can experience a combination of migraine and tension-type.

Identification of the headache's cause and its effect on the patient is the focus of collaborative care. A thorough history and physical examination is necessary. The health care provider needs to ask specific questions concerning the headache signs and symptoms (see the Patient Playbook). Diagnostic studies done to rule secondary causes of headache are summarized in Box 37-1. For complete discussion of these diagnostic studies, refer to chapter 34.

Diagnostic Tests

There are a variety of diagnostic tests that can be used in determining the type of headache that a patient suffers. These diagnostic studies could detect the cause of the headache and prevent the headache from progressing to a more severe problem (e.g., space-occupying tumor, malignant brain tumor). See Box 37-1 for a listing of the typical diagnostic studies used in assessing headaches.

BOX 37-1

HEADACHE DIAGNOSTIC STUDIES

Neurological examination (local infection; tenderness; swelling; bruits).

Routine laboratory studies (CBC; electrolytes; urinalysis).

CT (of sinuses).

Special studies (CT; EMG; EEG; MRI; MRA; angiography).

Legend: CBC, complete blood count; CT, computed tomography; EEG, electroencephalography; EMG, electromyography; MRI, magnetic resonance imaging; MRA, magnetic resonance angiography.

TABLE 37-1 Tension-Type Headache Comparison

	EPISODIC	CHRONIC
Duration	30 minutes to 7 days	minutes to hours
Frequency	10 episodes in six months	15 days/month for six months
Nausea or vomiting	none	possible nausea; no vomiting
Photophobia	sometimes	sometimes
Phonophobia	sometimes	sometimes

PATIENT PLAYBOOK

Questions Specific for Headache Assessment

The following are questions to ask patients when assessing their headaches:

Where does the headache hurt, and what were you doing when the headache started?

How long before the pain becomes severe? Slow? Fast?

How long do they usually last, and do the headaches recur (return within 24-hour period)?

How long have you had the headache?

Describe the pain and is the pain mild, moderate, or severe?

Rate your headache on a scale of 1 to 10 (10=worst; 1=least).

Do you have trouble with your vision before or during the headache?

Do you have any other symptoms with the headache?

What makes the headache worse and better?

How do the headaches affect your life?

Do you take any prescription, OTC medications, vitamins, or herbal supplements?

Have you seen doctors in the past concerning your headaches?

Have you been under more stress than usual lately?

Have you been depressed?

Do you have any family members with a history of headaches?

BOX 37-2

NURSING DIAGNOSES FOR HEADACHES

The following is a list of common nursing diagnoses for headaches:
- Acute pain related to headache, visual disturbances, and inability to perform job-related activities.
- Ineffective coping related to severe pain, stress, and changes in lifestyle.
- Disturbed sensory perception related to auditory, visual, and sensory alterations.
- Deficient knowledge related to lack of understanding about headaches and treatment regimen.
- Sleep deprivation related to pain, nausea, vomiting, and medication.
- Ineffective role performance related to pain and medication side effects.

Nursing Diagnoses

The nursing diagnoses for all of the headache types is displayed in Box 37-2.

Planning and Implementation

Nursing management of tension headaches focuses on patient teaching. Teaching should include medication regimen, nonpharmacological management, and stress reduction methods. The application of these management techniques can assist the patient treat their headaches and potentially alleviate the patient's pain (Frazel, 2004).

Pharmacology

Medication regimens commonly used for treatment of tension-type headaches are nonnarcotic analgesics, such as aspirin, acetaminophen, or ibuprofen. These may be combined with narcotics (codeine) or barbiturates (butalbital) for difficult to treat headaches. Patients should be cautioned about long-term use of aspirin because of its connection with gastric bleeding and coagulation alterations in susceptible patients. Long-term use of narcotics or barbiturates may be habit-forming. Chronic use of acetaminophen can lead to kidney damage and liver damage when combined with alcohol (Table 37-2).

Alternative Therapy

Nonpharmacological management includes techniques, such as application of heat or cold, biofeedback, acupuncture, acupressure, and hypnosis. Application of heat or cold reduces muscle tension and decreases pain. The nurse should teach the patient to use heat or cold for no more than 15 to 20 minutes for each application and to remove it from the skin between treatments. Biofeedback involves applying physiological monitoring equipment, teaching the patient about muscle tension and its connection with peripheral blood flow, and training the patient to relax muscles in response to the machines feedback.

Acupuncture involves the insertion of thin needles into specific areas of the body to modify physiological function. A provider trained in this ancient Chinese technique is required. Acupressure is an ancient Japanese and Chinese therapy that applies finger pressure to relieve pain, discomfort, and promote healing. This technique also requires a trained provider. Hypnosis is used to assist the patient to alter the pain perception of their headaches. Many patients who prefer to not take medications may be more comfortable with nonpharmacological treatment of their headaches.

Stress reduction methods may include exercise programs, meditation, yoga, or tai chi. Exercise programs, such as walking, swimming, or riding a bike, are

TABLE 37-2 Medications to Treat Headache

TENSION-TYPE HEADACHE	MIGRAINE HEADACHE	CLUSTER HEADACHE
Nonnarcotic Analgesics	*Nonnarcotic Analgesics*	*100 Percent O₂ Via Face Mask*
Aspirin	Aspirin	Ergot alkaloids
Acetaminophen (Tylenol)	Acetaminophen (Tylenol)	Dihydroergotamine (DHE)
Ibuprofen (Motrin Advil)	Ibuprofen (Motrin, Advil)	Ergotamine (Ergostat)
Caffeine	Naproxen (Aleve, Anaprox)	Triptans
Narcotic Combinations	*Narcotic Analgesics*	*Sumatriptan (Imitrex)*
Butalbital + aspirin (Fiorinal)	Codeine + acetaminophen (Tylenol #3 or #4)	Intranasal
Butalbital + acetaminophen (Fioricet)	Meperidine (Demerol)	Lidocaine
Caffeine + acetaminophen (Midol)	Butorphanol (Stadol)	Capsaicin
Antidepressants	*Triptans*	*Nonnarcotic Analgesics*
Sertraline (Zoloft)	Naratriptan (Amerge)	Indomethacin (Indocin)
Paroxetine (Paxil)	Sumatriptan (Imitrex)	
		Narcotic Analgesics
Amitriptyline (Elavil)	Almotriptan (Axert)	Butorphanol (Stadol)
Nortriptyline (Pamelor)	Frovatriptan (Frova)	Calcium channel blockers
	Rizatriptan (Maxalt)	Verapamil (Calan)
	Zolmitriptan (Zomig)	
	Ergot alkaloids	Lithium (Lithane, Eskalith)
	DHE	
	Ergotamine (Ergomar, Ergostat)	
Beta Blockers	*Beta Blockers*	*Corticosteroids*
Propranolol (Inderal)	Atenolol (Tenormin)	Prednisone
	Metoprolol (Lopressor)	
	Propranolol (Inderal)	*Anticonvulsants*
	Timolol (Blocadren)	Valproic acid (Depakote)
	Calcium channel blockers	
	Verapamil (Calan)	
	Nifedipine (Procardia)	
	Nimodipine (Nimotop)	
	Antidepressants	
	Amitriptyline (Elavil)	
	Imipramine (Tofranil)	

Adapted from Broyles, B. E., Reiss, B. S., & Evans, M. E. (2007). Pharmacological aspects of nursing care (7th ed.). New York: Thomson Delmar Learning.

useful in reducing stress. Meditation involves concentrated attention focused on one's inner state. Yoga is an ancient philosophy of the mind, body, and soul in harmony. Yoga therapy uses specific postures and sequences of postures to stretch or block areas of the body. Tai chi involves almost weightless, fluid movements, with a focus on breathing, balance, and the concepts of empty and full. All of these techniques can be recommended to help patients with life-stress management.

Evaluation of Outcomes

Potential patient outcomes for each of the example nursing diagnoses for the patient with tension-type headaches are:

- Acute pain related to tension-type headache. The patient should verbalize adequate pain relief and the ability to realistically cope with the pain if not completely relieved.
- Ineffective coping related to pain. The patient should verbalize feelings, identify personal strengths, and accept support.
- Disturbed sensory perception related to auditory, visual, and sensory alterations. The patient should verbalize decreased symptoms.
- Deficient knowledge related to lack of understanding. The patient should describe disease process, symptoms, and control measures.
- Sleep deprivation related to pain or medication side effects. The patient will report an optimal balance of rest and activity.
- Ineffective role performance related to pain and medication side effects. The patient should demonstrate healthy adaptation and coping skills.

Migraine Headache

Migraine headaches are common disorders. They are often self-treated; patients have their own interventions that they use, or nothing seems to decrease the headache and they just suffer with the pain. Migraine headaches affect patient's relationships, his or her employment, and often can be frustrating to live with the pain. Migraine headaches, along with cluster headaches, are considered a vascular headache.

Epidemiology

Migraine headache accounts for half of all patients with headache. It is estimated that 23 million Americans suffer from migraines, and more than 11 million experience significant headache related disability. Migraines affect 18 percent of women and 6 percent of men. Headaches may begin as early as 10 years of age with the highest incidence between 35 and 45 years and decreases with advancing age. The incidence of migraine is highest among Caucasians. Up to 65 percent of patients with a family history of headaches will also suffer from headaches. It is estimated that in the United States, $17 billion per year are related to diagnosis, treatment, and lost job productivity.

Etiology

Migraine headaches are the result of the interaction of various factors of varying importance in different individuals. Causative factors include:

- Genetic predisposition.
- Susceptibility to specific stimuli.
- Hormonal activity.
- Environmental triggers.
- Stress.

Pathophysiology

Migraines are characterized by vasodilation of the dural blood vessels, resulting in stimulation of the trigeminal nerve pain pathways. Then neuropeptides, involved in pain transmission, are released. The neuropeptides make the vasodilation worse and sensitize the brainstem, causing the associated symptoms of light, sound, movement, and odor sensitivity.

Assessment with Clinical Manifestations

The focus of care for the patient with a migraine is to identify the specific type of migraine and rule out any secondary causes. A thorough history and physical examination is necessary. The health care provider needs to ask specific questions concerning the headache signs and symptoms. Migraine headaches are characterized as episodic head pain, present on waking or occurring over a few minutes to hours while awake, and lasting from 4 to 72 hours. Approximately 98 percent of migraine patients experience moderate to severe pain during attacks and describe the pain as a steady ache to violent throbbing. They will identify the pain as being on one side of the head. The pain is made worse by physical activity. In addition, many migraine headaches are preceded with an **aura** (sensation that occurs immediately before a disorder, such as a migraine headache or a seizure). Associated aura symptoms include nausea, vomiting, and photophobia, phonophobia, and certain odors (osmophobia).

Diagnostic Tests

Diagnostic studies need to be done to rule out secondary causes of the headaches. They are summarized in Box 37-1.

Nursing Diagnoses

The nursing diagnoses for all of the headache types is displayed in Box 37-2.

Planning and Implementation

Nursing management of migraine headaches also focuses on patient teaching. Teaching should include medication regimen, trigger avoidance, nonpharmacological management, and stress reduction methods. Medication regimens commonly used for treatment of migraine headaches are based on severity of symptoms. For moderate pain relief, nonnarcotic analgesics may be sufficient. Symptom control for more severe headaches may include: alpha-adrenergic blockers, serotonin receptor agonists, vasoconstrictors, or corticosteroids (Glassroth, 2004). The nurse should teach the patient to avoid headache triggers. These triggers are listed in Table 37-3.

Evaluation of Outcomes

Potential patient outcomes for each of the example nursing diagnoses for the patient with migraine headache are:
- Acute pain related to migraine headache. The patient should verbalize an adequate relief of pain along with the ability to realistically cope with the pain if it is not completely relieved.
- Ineffective coping related to pain. The patient should verbalize feelings, identify personal strengths, and accept support.
- Disturbed sensory perception related to headache. The patient should verbalize decreased symptoms.
- Deficient knowledge related to lack of understanding. The patient should describe disease process, symptoms, and control measures.
- Sleep deprivation related to pain or medication side effects. The patient will report an optimal balance of rest and activity.
- Ineffective role performance related to pain and medication side effects. The patient should demonstrate healthy adaptation and coping skills.

Cluster Headache

Cluster headaches are a relatively uncommon type of headache. They can be as painful as a migraine headache and like the migraine are considered a vascular headache.

Epidemiology

Cluster headaches account for approximately 8 to 10 percent of all headache sufferers. Unlike migraine headaches, they occur more often in men than women. They do not occur in childhood but begin in patients between 30 and 60 years of age. Cluster headaches are not seen in first-degree relatives (parent, child).

TABLE 37-3	Migraine Headache Triggers

Foods Containing Amines
- Cheese
- Chocolate

Foods Containing Nitrates
- Processed lunch meat
- Hot dogs
- Smoked meats

Foods Containing
- Vinegar
- Onions
- Monosodium glutamate (MSG)

Fermented or Marinated Foods
- Caffeine
- Nicotine
- Ice cream
- Alcohol (specifically red wine)
- Emotional stress
- Fatigue

Drugs
- Ergot containing compounds
- Monoamine oxide (MAO) inhibitors

Etiology

Cluster headaches are believed to be a variant of migraine headaches. The cause is unknown, but a seasonal relationship is often noted in these patients. Patients are usually awoken at night without warning signs or aura.

Pathophysiology

The pathophysiology of the cluster headache is similar to a migraine headache; however, the triggers are different. The triggers include vasodilating agents (nitroglycerine), histamine, alcohol, and nicotine. Acetylcholine (ACh) is believed to play a role in the parasympathetic symptoms.

Assessment with Clinical Manifestations

The rapid onset of the pain with cluster headaches often wakes the patient from a sound sleep in the middle of the night. The pain is unilateral (one side of head), usually behind the eye, and so severe that the patient is unable to lie still, but paces the floor holding their head. Associated symptoms include nasal congestion, **rhinorrhea** (watery discharge from the nose), tearing, and redness of the eye on the affected side. Cluster headaches do not cause nausea and vomiting. They occur as a series of attacks. Each attack can last from 15 minutes to up to two hours. A cluster of attacks consists of one or more attacks everyday for 4 to 12 weeks. Then the patient usually has an attack free period lasting months to years.

Diagnostic Tests

Diagnostic studies need to be done to rule out secondary causes of the headaches. They are summarized in Box 37-1.

Nursing Diagnoses

The nursing diagnoses for all of the headache types is displayed in Box 37-2.

Planning and Implementation

The focus of collaborative care for the cluster headache patient is to rule out any secondary causes and prevention of attacks. A thorough history and physical examination is necessary. The health care provider needs to ask specific questions concerning the headache signs and symptoms. Diagnostic studies need to be done to rule secondary causes of the headaches. They are summarized in Box 37-1. In research studies, thermography has been used during an attack to demonstrate a cold spot above the eye, indicating reduced blood flow in that area.

Management of cluster headaches focuses on prevention. Teaching should include medication regimen and trigger avoidance. Medication regimens commonly used for treatment of cluster headaches are abortive and prophylactic drugs. Abortive therapy includes oxygen, subcutaneous or nasal sumatriptan, and topical lidocaine. Prophylactic therapy includes steroids, ergotamine preparations, lithium, calcium channel blockers, and anticonvulsants.

Evaluation of Outcomes

Potential patient outcomes for each of the example nursing diagnoses for the patient with cluster headaches are:

- Acute pain related to cluster headache. The patient should verbalize an adequate relief of pain along with the ability to realistically cope with the pain if it is not completely relieved.
- Ineffective coping related to pain. The patient should verbalize feelings, identify personal strengths, and accept support.
- Disturbed sensory perception related to headache pain. The patient should verbalize decreased symptoms.
- Deficient knowledge related to lack of understanding. The patient should describe disease process, symptoms, and control measures.

- Sleep deprivation related to pain or medication side effects. The patient will report an optimal balance of rest and activity.
- Ineffective role performance related to pain and medication side effects. The patient should demonstrate healthy adaptation and coping skills.

SEIZURES

A **seizure** is a sudden, uncontrolled discharge of electricity in the brain. Seizures are frequently a symptom of an underlying pathology. Seizures secondary to systemic or metabolic pathology are not considered epilepsy, if the seizures stop when the pathology is resolved. A **convulsion** is the abnormal motor response or jerking movements that occur during a seizure. **Epilepsy** involves spontaneously recurring seizures caused by chronic pathology. It is one of the most common neurological conditions (Gambrell & Flynn, 2004).

Epidemiology

About 2.5 million people in the United States have epilepsy with an increase of approximately 180,000 new patients each year. About 3 percent of people will receive a diagnosis of epilepsy at some time in their lives. The estimated annual cost of the diagnosis, treatment, and disability related to seizures is $12.5 billion. For hundreds of years, a diagnosis of seizures or epilepsy has carried a stigma. In recent years, Congress has allocated $4 million to epilepsy programs to support research, treatment, and public education.

Etiology

Seizures occur when there is an imbalance in the central nervous system (CNS). Individual susceptibility varies patient to patient. The episodic nature of seizures suggests triggers initiate the process. There are multiple causes for seizures (Table 37-4).

Pathophysiology

Seizure generation has two components: a seizure focus and the neuronal connections to that focus. The seizure focus is a group of hyperexcitable neurons. The area of the brain that is connected to the focus will determine the seizure manifestations. For example, a slow growing brain tumor near the in the frontal lobe will eventually cause a seizure to occur. The seizure focus is near the motor cortex, adjacent to the increasing tumor mass. When the hyperexcitable focus discharges, it is transmitted to the motor strip and a clonic seizure is the result. There are three global causes for seizures: physiological, iatrogenic, or idiopathic. Box 37-3 summarizes the causes of seizures. Environmental or physiological factors that can trigger a seizure are listed in Table 37-4.

Assessment with Clinical Manifestations

The clinical manifestations of a seizure are determined by the site of the disturbance (focus). The system of classification that has been used for 25 years is summarized in Table 37-5. In this system seizures are divided into three major classes: partial, generalized, and unclassified.

Phases of a seizure include the prodromal phase, the aural phase, the ictal phase, and the postictal phase. The prodromal phase is the signs or activity before the seizure, for example, a headache or feeling depressed. The aural phase is a sensation or warning that the patient remembers. An aura can be visual, auditory, gustatory, or visceral in nature, for example, an odor or flash-

TABLE 37-4 Seizure Causes

Physiological

CNS infections

Inborn errors of metabolism

Congenital malformations

Acquired metabolic disorders

- Hypoglycemia
- Uremia
- Hepatic encephalopathy
- Electrolyte disturbances
- Acid-base disturbances

Structural lesions

- Stroke
- Trauma
- Subarachnoid hemorrhage
- Subdural hematoma
- Tumors
- Scarring from old brain injuries

Iatrogenic

New medications or withdrawal from medications

Drug or alcohol use or withdrawal

Idiopathic

Common seizure triggers

- Fevers
- Menstrual cycle
- Flashing lights
- Fatigue
- Strong emotions
- Intense exercise
- Loud music

BOX 37-3

SEIZURE DIAGNOSTIC STUDIES

Neurological Examination

CT scan or MRI of the brain (rule out tumors, hemorrhage)

Routine laboratory studies: (CBC; electrolytes; LFTs, toxicology screen).

Skull X-rays (to rule out fractures, bone erosion, or separated sutures)

EEG (if no seizure activity on standard test, may require 24 hour continuous test).

Other: PET scan; SPECT scan

Legend: CBC, complete blood count; CT, computed tomography; LFTs, liver function tests; EEG, electroencephalography; MRI, magnetic resonance imaging; PET, positron emission tomography; SPECT, single-proton emission computerized tomography.

TABLE 37-5 Seizure Classification

Partial (Local, Focal) Seizures

Simple partial seizures (consciousness not impaired)
- With focal motor symptoms
- With somatosensory or special sensory symptoms
- With autonomic symptoms
- With disturbance of higher cerebral function

Complex Partial Seizures (Impaired Consciousness)

Begin as simple partial and progress to impaired consciousness
- With no other features
- With features of simple partial seizures
- With automatisms

Impairment of consciousness at onset
- With no other features
- With features of simple partial seizures
- With automatisms

Partial Seizures Evolving into Generalized Seizures
- Simple partial evolving to generalized
- Complex partial evolving to generalized
- Simple partial evolving to complex partial to generalized

Generalized Seizures (Bilaterally Symmetric, without Local Onset)
- Absence seizures
- Myoclonic seizures
- Clonic seizures
- Tonic seizures
- Tonic-clonic seizures
- Atonic seizures
- Unclassified epileptic seizures

Adapted from Commission on Classification and Terminology of the International League against Epilepsy. (1981). Proposal for revised clinical and electroencephalographic classification of epileptic seizures. Epilepsia, 22, 489–501.

ing lights. The ictal phase is the actual seizure. The postictal phase is the period immediately following the seizure. During this phase the patient is usually confused, disoriented, and does not remember the seizure. If left alone the patient may sleep deeply for several hours. A seizure may include some or all of the phases.

Additional clinical manifestations may include automatisms, clonus, autonomic symptoms, or Todd's paralysis. Automatisms are coordinated involuntary motor activities that occur during the seizure. Examples include lip smacking, chewing, fidgeting, and pacing. Clonus is the descriptive term for the pattern of spasm with muscle rigidity followed by muscle relaxation. Autonomic symptoms occur in response to stimulation of the autonomic nervous system. These symptoms include pallor, sweating, epigastric discomfort, flushing, piloerection, or dilation of pupils. Todd's paralysis is a temporary, focal weakness or paralysis following a seizure that can last up to 24 hours.

The focus of collaborative care for the patient with seizures is to obtain a comprehensive and accurate description of the seizures. A thorough health history and physical examination is necessary. The health care provider needs to ask specific questions concerning seizures (Box 37-4). Diagnostic studies need to be done to rule out secondary causes of the seizures. They are summarized in Box 37-3. Discussion of the specific tests can be found in chapter 34. The nurse needs to develop a comprehensive plan to help the patient deal with the psychosocial aspects of having a seizure disorder.

Generalized Seizures

Generalized seizures originate in all of the regions of the brain cortex. There is no aura or warning, but there is loss of consciousness. The seizure may last for a few seconds or several minutes.

- Absence seizures usually occur during childhood and last 5 to 10 seconds. If the seizure last for more than 10 seconds, there may be automatisms, such as eye blinking or lip smacking. They frequently occur in clusters and can occur dozens or even hundreds of times per day. The electroencephalogram (EEG) will show a 3 Hz (cycles per minute) spike and wave pattern, unique to this type of seizure.
- Atypical absence seizures usually begin before age 5 and are associated with mental retardation and a tendency for multiple seizure types. They last longer and are associated with muscle spasms.
- Myoclonic seizures are characterized by sudden, brief arm muscle contractions. Consciousness is usually not impaired.
- Clonic seizures demonstrate rhythmic, repetitive clonic movements of the arms, neck, and face. These movements are bilateral and symmetrical.
- Tonic-clonic (formerly called grand mal) seizures are the most common type of generalized seizure. The seizure will progress through all of the seizure phases and last two to three minutes. Because of the suddenness of this type of seizure, injuries, such as limb fractures, tongue biting, and head trauma, can occur. These seizures can occur any time of the day or night, whether the patient is awake or not. Seizure frequency is highly variable.
- Atonic seizures (drop attacks) are a sudden loss of muscle control, usually the legs, that results in falling to the floor, increasing the possibility of injury.

BOX 37-4

QUESTIONS SPECIFIC FOR SEIZURE ASSESSMENT

Have you ever had seizures before? What age?

Any trauma, tumors, or infections of the CNS?

Do you use nicotine products? How much? For how long?

Do you consume alcohol products? How much? For how long?

Any environmental exposure? Metals? Chemicals? Gases?

Do you use any recreational drugs?

Are you currently taking medication to prevent seizures? If yes, what?

Have you taken seizure medications in the past? If yes, what? Why did you stop?

Do any other members of your family have a history of seizures?

Any nausea, vomiting, or diarrhea recently?

Do you have headaches; muscle or abdominal pain; mood, behavior, or mentation changes before or after a seizure?

Do you have any numbness, tingling, or paralysis after a seizure?

Skills 360°

Nursing Assessment of the Seizing Patient

The nurse should evaluate the following activities during the seizure activity:

- Onset—Was it sudden? Was it preceded by an aura?
- Duration—When did it start? When did it stop? Any changes?
- Behaviors—Before, during, and after.
- Type of body movements. Describe in detail.
- Any loss of consciousness? How long?
- Incontinence—Bladder or bowel.
- Amnesia or confusion post seizure?

Partial Seizures

Partial seizures begin in a specific brain region and consciousness is usually not impaired. The clinical manifestations depend on the region of the brain where the seizure focus starts. There may be an aura or warning signs.

- Simple partial seizures are when consciousness is not lost. Depending on the seizure focus there may be motor, sensory, autonomic, or higher level cognitive clinical manifestations.
- Complex partial seizures are the most common type of epileptic seizure in adults. Consciousness and awareness of surroundings is lost. Automatisms may occur. The seizure typically lasts one to three minutes.

Status Epilepticus

Status epilepticus is defined as either continuous seizures lasting more than five minutes or two or more different seizures with incomplete recovery of consciousness between them. The most common cause of status epilepticus is abruptly stopping of antiepileptic drugs (AEDs). Status epilepticus can present clinically with tonic, clonic, or tonic-clonic movements. It is a medical emergency, because it is often accompanied by respiratory distress brought on by hypoxia or anoxia. Morbidity and mortality for status epilepticus is 20 percent. Subclinical status epilepticus is seen with partial seizures but can only be verified by EEG.

Diagnostic Tests

There are a variety of diagnostic tests that can be used in determining the origin and pathology of seizure activity. A list of these tests is shown in Box 37-3.

Nursing Diagnoses

Based on the information gathered, examples of nursing diagnoses in the patient with seizures may include the following:

- Risk for ineffective airway clearance related to obstructed airway during seizure activity.
- Risk for injury related to seizure activity and postictal weakness or paralysis.
- Anxiety related to changes in lifestyle, uncertainty, and changes in self-concept.
- Ineffective therapeutic regimen management related to lack of knowledge of seizure treatment.
- Ineffective coping related to chronic disease, altered self-concept, and social stigma.

Planning and Implementation

Prevention of seizures is the management goal. If the diagnostic testing reveals a treatable cause for the seizures, then it should be resolved. Epilepsy (recurrent seizures) is controlled in 70 percent of patients with antiepileptic medications (Table 37-6). A significant number of the remaining 30 percent may benefit from surgical intervention. Once the diagnosis of epilepsy is established, patient safety and health teaching by the nurse become the primary focus. The patient and their family need accurate information concerning the manifestations, etiology, and treatment of seizures. The nurse needs to educate and support the patient and family as they adjust to the lifestyle changes that are required. Teaching should address the physical, emotional, and social aspects of the disease. Actions and potential side effects of the medication regimen need to be taught, monitored, and adjusted to the desired patient response. Medications can only be effective if taken as prescribed. Seizure activity can be triggered if the patient suddenly stops or takes antiseizure medications sporadically.

The psychosocial affects may be more devastating to the patient and family than the seizures. During the period of adjustment, the patient may experi-

TABLE 37-6 Medications to Treat Seizures

FIRST-LINE DRUGS	SECOND-LINE DRUGS	STATUS EPILEPTICUS DRUGS
Phenytoin (Dilantin)	Ethosuximide (Zarontin)	Lorazepam (Ativan)
Valproate (Depakote	Methsuximide (Celontin)	Phenytoin (Dilantin)
Carbamazepine (Tegretol)	Clonazepam (Klonopin)	Fosphenytoin (Cerebyx)
Lamotrigine (Lamictal)	Topiramate (Topamax)	Phenobarbital (Luminal)
Phenobarbital (Luminal)	Gabapentin (Neurontin)	Midazolam (Versed)
	Primidone (Mysoline)	Propofol (Diprivan)
	Felbamate (Felbatol)	
	Levetiracetam (Keppra)	
	Zonisamide (Zonegran)	
	Oxcarbazepine (Trileptal)	

Adapted from Broyles, B. E., Reiss, B. S., & Evans, M. E. (2007). Pharmacological aspects of nursing care (7th ed.). New York: Thomson Delmar Learning.

ence problems at home, work, or with personal relationships. Safety precautions need to be implemented in the home and work environment. Fear of discrimination and social isolation may require counseling for both the patient and their family.

Pharmacology

The primary methods for treating seizure activity are pharmacological interventions. Many patients are treated successfully with their medication regimens, and the patients are able to live normal lives while adhering to the pharmacological interventions. A composite list of the medications commonly used is provided in Table 37-6.

Surgery

Surgical interventions for some patients with seizure activities is also a successful method of management. A surgical method of treatment is normally employed after other more conservative forms of management have been practiced. Table 37-7 provides the major surgical methods used to treat seizures.

Evaluation of Outcomes

Potential patient outcomes for each of the example nursing diagnoses for the patient with seizures:

- Risk for ineffective airway clearance related to seizure activity. The patient should not experience aspiration.
- Risk for injury related to seizure activity. The patient should not experience injury.
- Anxiety related to changes in lifestyle and self-concept. The patient should verbalize increased psychological and physiological comfort.
- Ineffective therapeutic regimen management related to lack of knowledge. The patient will verbalize understanding of disease process, etiology, and treatment measures.
- Ineffective individual coping related to chronic disease. The patient should verbalize feelings, identify personal strengths, and accept support.

TABLE 37-7	Surgical Treatment of Seizures
SURGERY	**PROCEDURE**
Temporal lobectomy	Removal of all or part of temporal lobe.
	Elimination of seizure focus.
Focal lesionectomy	Removal of scar tissue that is seizure focus.
Corpus callosotomy	Excision of the corpus callosotomy.
Hemispherectomy	Modified radical excision of temporal lobe in children with intractable seizures.
Vagus nerve stimulation	Placement of bipolar leads on vagus nerve and then attaching a programmable signal generator.

MULTIPLE SCLEROSIS

Multiple sclerosis (MS) is a chronic inflammatory disease of the CNS. MS is a relatively common neurological degenerative disorder and can be debilitating in some who are diagnosed with the disease. MS is known for its combination of remission times and its exacerbations of the disease symptomatology. Many people with multiple sclerosis live well with the disorder and learn to adapt well during the times of disease exacerbation. Typically, when a person is hospitalized for his or her MS disorder, the crisis is related to the secondary complications of the disease. For example, later in the disease process patients can become fatigued and are not able to be as mobile. One result of their fatigue and the degenerative nature of the disease are respiratory complications, which is common in the acute phase of MS.

Epidemiology

MS is the major cause of chronic disability in young adults. Onset of symptoms usually occurs between the ages of 20 and 40. MS occurs more frequently in Caucasian females than males (1.7:1). The ratio of Caucasian to non-Caucasian is 2:1. Geographically it is more common in the temperate and cold climates of the higher latitudes of the northern and southern hemispheres. There is some evidence that MS has a genetic connection. Incidence of MS in first-degree relatives is 20 times higher than in the general population. It is estimated that greater than 400,000 people are diagnosed with MS in the United States (Denis, et al., 2004).

Etiology

The cause of MS is not known. Current theories identify autoimmune-mediated inflammatory demyelination and axonal injury. No virus has been isolated. It is believed that two factors may initiate the inflammation: exposure to an environmental agent and genetic susceptibility. Research has demonstrated that multiple genetic factors are involved. Future research may identify how these genes operate and interact with the environment.

Pathophysiology

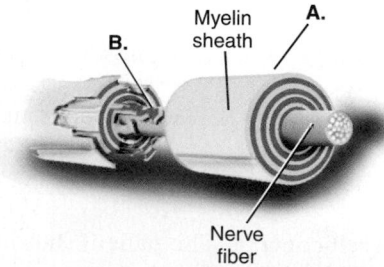

Figure 37-1 A. Normal nerve fiber and myelin sheath, B. MS destruction of myelin sheath.

MS involves the white matter of the CNS. Inflammatory cells (activated lymphocytes and monocytes) cross the blood-brain barrier, surround the blood vessels, and destroy the neuronal myelin sheath (Figure 37-1). Neurons and some axons are spared. The individual lesions are called plaques and may be as a few millimeters to as long as several centimeters. Because it acts like an insulator, loss of myelin and the subsequent degeneration and atrophy of the axons interrupts impulse transmission.

Assessment with Clinical Manifestations

The clinical course of MS has four categories: relapsing-remitting, secondary progressive, progressing-relapsing, and primary progressive. Relapsing-remitting disease is the most common form of the disease, seen in 80 percent of all cases. It is characterized by recurrent episodes of neurological dysfunction evolving over days or weeks. Recovery from each episode may be complete, partial, or with residual deficits occurring over weeks to months. Symptoms do not progress during remissions.

Secondary progressive disease is characterized by gradual deterioration with or without relapses, remissions, or plateaus. For many patients this is the second phase of the disease that started as relapsing-remitting. Progressing-relapsing disease starts with a gradual progression of disability without plateaus or remissions. Primary progressive disease is characterized by gradual neurological disability with noted relapses.

The clinical manifestations of MS may vary greatly among patients and can vary over time in the same patient. The most common presenting symptoms are: sensory loss (37 percent), optic neuritis (36 percent), weakness (35 percent), paresthesias (24 percent), diplopia (15 percent), ataxia (11 percent), and vertigo (6 percent). A summary of the clinical manifestations of MS can be found in Table 37-8. The clinical manifestations of MS can be exacerbated by being in a hot, humid environment or taking a hot bath.

TABLE 37-8 **Clinical Manifestations of MS**			
SENSORY	**MOTOR**	**CEREBELLAR**	**OTHER**
Numbness	Paresis	Loss of balance	Fatigue
Paresthesia	Paralysis	Loss of coordination	Optic neuritis
• Burning	Foot dragging	Ataxia	Impotence
• Tingling	Diplopia	Nystagmus	Sexual
• Prickling			dysfunction
Pain	Bowel/Bladder	Speech disturbances	Depression
Decreased	• Retention	• Dysarthria	Euphoria
perception	• Incontinence	• Dystonia	Visual loss
• Position		• Scanning speech	Trigeminal neuralgia
• Temperature		• Slurred speech	Facial palsy
• Depth		Tremor (dysmetria)	Heat intolerance
• Vibration		Vertigo	Nystagmus
Lhermitte's sign			Scotomas

Adapted from Denis, L., Namey, M., Costello, K., Frenette, J., Gagnon, N., Harris, C., et al. (2004). Long term treatment optimization in individuals with multiple sclerosis using disease-modifying therapies: A nursing approach. Journal of Neuroscience Nursing, 36(1), 10–22.

Diagnostic Tests

There is no single diagnostic test that confirms or rules out the diagnosis of MS. However, there are some specific tests that may assist with the diagnosis. A magnetic resonance imaging (MRI) of the brain and spinal cord with gadolinium infusion may identify bright lesions (T2-weighted images) in the corpus callosum and periventricular regions. A lesion larger than 5 mm helps to confirm the diagnosis.

Newer neuroimaging techniques such as fluid-attenuated-inversion-recovery (FLAIR) and magnetic resonance spectroscopy (MRS) have increased sensitivity and specificity for white matter abnormalities. FLAIR is able to detect two to three times the number of lesions seen on T2-weighted images. MRS looks at levels of N-acetylaspartate (NAA). Decreased NAA levels in MS plaques and apparently unaffected areas of white matter suggest the presence of axonal damage.

Lumbar puncture may be done to obtain cerebrospinal fluid (CSF) for analysis. Discussion of the procedure and CSF analysis is discussed in chapter 34. In MS, elevated immunoglobulin G (IgG) index, presence of oligoclonal bands (OCBs), and increased myelin basic protein in the CSF analysis helps to confirm the diagnosis. Oligoclonal bands are found in 85 to 90 percent of patients with MS but can also be found other inflammatory or infectious diseases.

Evoked potentials are also discussed in depth in chapter 34. Abnormal findings are demonstrated in more than 75 percent of patients with a diagnosis of MS. The test may be repeated to monitor for improvements related to medication regimens or disease progression. Neuropsychological screening also uses standardized tests to identify and quantify the cognitive, emotional, and behavioral abilities of the patient. The results can be used to help the patient

Skills 360°

Questions Specific to MS

The nurse should ask the patient the following questions as related to MS:

Have you experienced any recent of past viral infections? Vaccinations? Recent infections?

Do you live in a cold or temperate climate? Did you live there as a child? Adolescent?

Have you recently experienced increased emotional or physical stress? Pregnancy?

Is there any history of chronic fatigue or malaise in your family?

Have you recently lost or gained weight? How much? Was it a planned weight loss?

Do you have any problems with chewing or swallowing?

Have you experienced any problems with urination? If yes, describe.

Any problems or recent changes with bowel function? If yes, describe.

Have you experienced generalized muscle weakness or fatigue? Tingling? Numbness?

Do you experience tripping or stumbling while walking? If yes, describe episodes.

Have you experienced joint or muscle pain? Muscle spasms? If yes, describe.

Do you ever feel dizzy or like you are spinning? Describe.

Have you experienced any vision changes? Describe.

Do you have a constant ringing in your ears? Does it get better or worse? Describe.

Have you experienced any decrease in desire or performance of sexual activity?

Do you have any feelings of depression, anger, euphoria, or social isolation? Describe.

and their family understand the impact of the disease on the patients functional ability. Serial reassessment can track improvement or lack of progress.

Nursing Diagnoses

Based on the information gathered, examples of nursing diagnoses in the patient with MS may include the following:

- Impaired physical mobility related to muscle weakness, paralysis, or spasticity.
- Self-care deficit related to neuromuscular deficits.
- Impaired urinary elimination related to neuromuscular degeneration.
- Constipation related to inactivity and abdominal muscle weakness.
- Ineffective coping related to feelings of helplessness.
- Risk for impaired skin integrity related to decreased muscle strength and inactivity.
- Risk for ineffective airway clearance related to weak or ineffective cough effort.
- Risk for imbalanced nutrition: less than body requirement related to muscle weakness.

Planning and Implementation

The focus of collaborative care for the patient with MS is multifaceted and involves modification of the disease course, symptom management, prevention of complications, and management of psychosocial issues. A thorough health history and physical examination is necessary. Because there is no diagnostic test that specifically identifies MS, analysis of the history, physical examination, and diagnostic tests findings are needed to confirm the diagnosis.

A program of physical therapy using exercise and assistive devices can help the patient to maintain a high level of functioning. A daily exercise program should include range-of-motion and muscle-strengthening components. If assistive

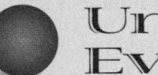

Uncovering the Evidence

Thalmic Stimulation for Tremor

Discussion: The purpose of this research is to study the long-term effect of deep brain stimulation (DBS) in patients with MS. The methods used are preoperative and postoperative evaluation of the study participants including MRI, the Extended Disability Status Scale (EDSS), the Bain-Finchley tremor scale, neuropsychological testing, and a patient self-assessment of the benefits of surgery.

The findings revealed the EDSS scores averaged 7.2 before surgery, 6.8 at six months postsurgery, and 7.8 at late follow-up. Tremor scores averaged 5.4 before surgery, 1.7 at six months postsurgery, and 2.1 at late follow-up. MRI scans did not show any new MS plaques related to the DBS probe. Neuropsychological testing showed mild to moderate decline in cognitive function related to disease progression.

Implications for Practice: Use of deep brain thalamic stimulation significantly reduced the tremor experienced by patients with MS but did not improve other objective measures of function. Surgical implantation of DBS for relief of tremors should only be considered in patients with stable disease and disabling upper extremity symptoms.

Source: Schulder, M., Sernas, T., & Karimi, R. (2003). Thalamic stimulation in patients with multiple sclerosis: Long-term follow-up. Stereotactic and Functional Neurosurgery, 80(1–4), 48–55.

TABLE 37-9 Drugs for Treatment of MS		
DRUG	**USES**	**SIDE EFFECTS**
Immunomodulating Drugs		
Interferon beta-1a (Avonex)	Slow disease progression Reduce relapse	Flu-like symptoms; mild anemia; elevated enzymes
Glatiramer acetate (Copaxone)	Slow disease progression	Flu-like symptoms; injection site reactions; chest pain; weakness
Immunosuppressant Drugs		
Mitoxantrone (Novantrone)	Slow disease progression Reduce relapse	Nausea; diarrhea; amenorrhea; alopecia; anemia; respiratory or urinary infections
Corticosteroid Drugs		
Corticotropin (ACTH)	Exacerbations	Edema; euphoria; weight gain; insomnia
Methylprednisolone (Solu-Medrol)	Exacerbations	Edema; euphoria; weight gain; insomnia; hypertension; acne
Prednisone (Deltasone)	Mild exacerbations	Edema; euphoria; weight gain; insomnia; hypertension
Muscle Relaxants		
Diazepam (Valium)	Spasticity	Fatigue; ataxia; drowsiness; depression; vertigo; diplopia; confusion
Baclofen (Lioresal)	Spasticity	Drowsiness; vertigo; dizziness; ataxia; insomnia; slurred speech
Antiepileptic Drugs		
Gabapentin (Neurontin)	Neuropathic pain	Somnolence; dizziness; ataxia; fatigue
Carbamazepine (Tegretol)	Neuropathic pain	Sedation; dizziness; fatigue; ataxia; fever; confusion
Antidepressants		
Amitriptyline (Elavil)	Neuropathic pain	Dry mouth; sedation; tachycardia; ataxia; confusion
Fluoxetine (Prozac)	Depression	Insomnia; headache; anxiety; dizziness
Stimulant Drugs		
Amantadine (Symmetrel)	Fatigue	Insomnia; depression; anxiety; ataxia; headache; fatigue; confusion
Modafinil (Provigil)	Fatigue	Headache; dizziness; depression; anxiety; insomnia; fever; confusion; ataxia
Cholinergic Drugs		
Bethanechol (Urecholine)	Urinary retention	Hypotension; bradycardia; drooling; diarrhea; bowel or bladder obstruction
Neostigmine (Prostigmin)	Urinary retention	GI upset; urinary urgency; bradycardia; sweating; increased salivation
Anticholinergic Drugs		
Probanthine (Pro-Banthine)	Urinary frequency	Dry mouth; blurred vision; photophobia; urinary retention; constipation; tachycardia
Oxybutynin (Ditropan)	Urinary frequency	Dry mouth; blurred vision; photophobia; urinary retention; constipation; tachycardia

Adapted from Broyles, B. E., Reiss, B. S., & Evans, M. E. (2007). Pharmacological aspects of nursing care (7th ed.). New York: Thomson Delmar Learning.

devices, such as a brace, cane, or walker, are needed to maintain independence, the health care provider needs to teach safe use and maintenance of the device. If mild spasticity develops, physical therapy can help by retraining alternative muscle groups. When there is severe spasticity, medications can be helpful.

Stress reduction methods may include exercise programs, meditation, yoga, or tai chi. All of these techniques can be recommended to help patients with life-stress management.

Pharmacology

The health care provider needs to ask specific questions related to MS and its clinical manifestations. Modification of disease progression can be accomplished by using medications. Symptom management involves a variety of medications and other forms of therapy (Table 37-9). The major disease symptoms include spasticity, tremors, pain, urinary problems, sensory problems, depression, and fatigue.

Surgery

When spasticity can no longer be managed with oral baclofen (Lioresal), the patient may be a candidate for intrathecal (area surrounding the spinal cord) medication delivery. First, the patient is evaluated by physical therapy for baseline functioning level. Then a test dose of Lioresal is given, and the patient is again evaluated for functional improvement. Improvement is a positive indicator for surgical implantation of the catheter (near the spinal cord) and pump. The pump is then programmed (similar to a pacemaker) to deliver the lowest dose of Lioresal needed to manage spasticity. The patient must follow up with the health care provider every three months.

Evaluation of Outcomes

Potential patient outcomes for each of the example nursing diagnoses for the patient with MS are:
- Impaired physical mobility related to neuromuscular degeneration. The patient will verbalize increased strength and endurance.
- Self-care deficit related to neuromuscular deficits. The patient will participate in activities of daily living as much as possible.
- Impaired urinary elimination related to neuromuscular degeneration. The patient will report none or decreased episodes of incontinence.
- Constipation related to inactivity. The patient will report regular bowel movements.
- Ineffective coping related to feelings of helplessness. The patient should verbalize feelings, identify personal strengths, and accept support.
- Risk for impaired skin integrity related to inactivity. The patient will maintain intact skin.
- Risk for ineffective airway clearance related to weak or ineffective cough effort. The patient should not experience aspiration.
- Risk for imbalanced nutrition: less than body requirement related to muscle weakness. The patient should demonstrate methods to increase appetite.

PARKINSON'S DISEASE

Parkinson's disease is a relatively common neurological degenerative disorder that was first discovered by Dr. James Parkinson in the 1800s. Among the several types of Parkinson's disease, the idiopathic or degenerative form is the most common. A wide variety of causes are associated with Parkinson's disease, including genetic, environmental, and medication regimens. Parkinson's disease can be slow in its progression, but it is a disorder that ultimately leads to disability.

Epidemiology

Parkinson's disease occurs worldwide with equal incidence between men and women. Disease symptoms usually begin between the ages of 40 and 70, with peak age at onset occurring in the sixth decade. In North America, there are approximately one million patients with Parkinson's disease. It is estimated that 1 percent of the population over age 65 is afflicted.

Etiology

The etiology of Parkinson's disease is unknown. Several factors may play a part in the causing the disease including hereditary predisposition, environmental toxins, and aging. Several studies have examined the possibility of a gene that can be linked to Parkinson's disease. There have been a few case reports of multiple cases within an extended family. The search for a specific gene responsible for Parkinson's disease continues.

Environmental toxin exposure has been identified as a potential cause. Chemicals such as carbon monoxide, carbon disulfide, cyanide, manganese, and methylphenyltetrahydropyridine (MPTP) have been linked to the development of Parkinson's disease. MPTP is a contaminant often found in illicit street drugs. Another environmental exposure connected to the development of Parkinson's disease is seen in welders, but the age of onset is earlier (30 to 40 years old).

Two theories are being examined concerning aging as a cause of Parkinson's disease. The first theory states that the disease is an accelerated form of aging. The second theory attributes the cause to some acute insult to the substantia nigra, followed by a slow loss of neurons, and development of symptoms in the sixth decade of life. Research continues in hopes of eventually identifying a specific cause for Parkinson's disease.

Pathophysiology

Parkinson's disease is a slowly progressive degenerative neurological disorder caused by the loss of nerve cell function in the basal ganglia. The basal ganglia includes several structures, the substantia nigra, striatum, globus pallidus, subthalamic nucleus, and the red nucleus. Loss of nerve cells in the substantia nigra causes a reduction of dopamine production. Dopamine is the neurotransmitter essential for such functions as control of posture, supporting the body in an upright position, and voluntary motions (Calne & Kumar, 2003).

Assessment with Clinical Manifestations

Parkinson's disease often begins with mild or intermittent symptoms. The patient or his or her family may notice that he or she is feeling more tired than usual, he or she may move slower than previously, or a slight tremor may occur. Often the symptoms are attributed to aging. Because the disease is progressive, eventually the patient's ability to function independently is impaired.

Tremor is defined as a rhythmic, purposeless, fine trembling, or quivering movement resulting from the involuntary alternating contraction and relaxation of opposing groups of skeletal muscles. Resting tremor (also called passive tremor) occurs while at rest. Intention tremor occurs with initiation of movement. Parkinson's disease tremor is most commonly seen in the fingers and hands but may involve the entire arm, lower extremity, or facial musculature. The tremor disappears with complete relaxation and often is reduced during voluntary movements. Hand tremors are often described as pill-rolling (rhythmic movement of the thumb across the palm of the hand).

Muscle rigidity is a stiffness seen with resistance to passive muscle stretching. Lead-pipe rigidity is stiffness and inflexibility that remains uniform through-

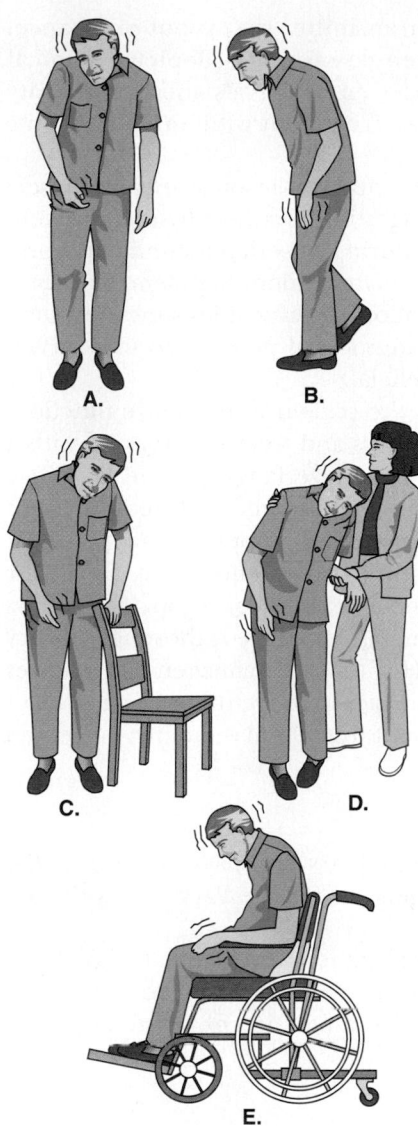

Figure 37-2 Progression of Parkinson's disease: A. Flexion of affected arm, B. Shuffling gait, C. Need for sources of support to prevent falling, D. Progression of weakness to point of needing assistance for ambulation, E. Profound weakness.

out the range of passive movement. Cogwheel rigidity is an abnormal rigor in muscle tissue characterized by jerky, ratchet-like movements when the limb is passively stretched. The rigidity is secondary to the depletion of dopamine causing a sustained contraction of the skeletal muscle groups. A common complaint is muscle soreness, a feeling of fatigue, achiness, and pain.

Akinesia (loss of movement) and **bradykinesia** (slowness of voluntary movement and speech) are responsible for the mask-like expression, difficulty swallowing, monotonous speech, and lack of arm swing. The patient has difficulty initiating movement, turning, or redirecting forward movement. Postural disturbances are secondary to the loss of postural reflexes and are characterized by stooped posture, shuffling gait, and broad-based turns. There is also a loss of the ability to protect oneself from harm. These voluntary movement changes put the patient at risk for injury from falls (Figure 37-2).

Common secondary manifestations of Parkinson's disease include: fine motor deficits, monotonic voice, mask-like face, generalized muscle fatigue, cognitive changes (e.g., impaired memory, visuospatial, depression), drooling, dysphagia, constipation, orthostatic hypotension, and urinary dysfunction. Many of the secondary manifestations can be exaggerated by the medications used to treat Parkinson's disease.

Diagnostic Tests

There are no specific diagnostic tests to confirm the diagnosis of Parkinson's disease. The diagnosis is based on history, physical examination, and presence of the major clinical manifestations. A conclusive diagnosis is possible only after all other potential causes have been ruled out. MRI and EEG may be normal. Magnetic resonance single-photo emission computed tomography (SPECT) has shown some promise in identifying the degeneration of the neurons in the substantia nigra. Positron emission tomography (PET) scanning can be done serially to identify the loss of dopamine producing cells in the brain. A full discussion of these tests can be found in chapter 34.

Nursing Diagnoses

Based on the information gathered, examples of nursing diagnoses in the patient with Parkinson's disease may include the following:
- Impaired physical mobility related to rigidity, bradykinesia, and akinesia.
- Impaired verbal communication related to dysarthria and tremor.
- Imbalanced nutrition: less than body requirements related to dysphagia.
- Self-care deficit related to inability to perform activities of daily living.
- Constipation related to immobility.
- Disturbed thought processes related to hallucinations and decreased cognitive abilities.
- Sleep deprivation related to rigidity and weakness.
- Risk for injury related to postural disturbances.

Planning and Implementation

Because of the chronic progressive nature of Parkinson's disease, the primary concern of the nurse caring for these patients is health teaching. In the early stages, the nurse needs to educate and support the patient and family as they adjust to the lifestyle changes that are required. Teaching should address the physical, emotional, and social aspects of the disease. In the beginning, actions and potential side effects of the medication regimen need to be taught, monitored, and adjusted to the desired patient response (Imke, 2003).

Maintaining a positive attitude can be difficult for both patients and their families. Short-term counseling with a capable psychotherapist can be helpful. Parkinson's disease is sometimes accompanied by depression and anxiety. Dopamine is not the only neurotransmitter that is out of balance. Serotonin is involved in mood, and when serotonin is depleted clinical depression can result. Depression decreases energy levels and productivity and interferes with personal relationships. Treatment with antidepressants can help to improve mood.

Nutrition is often a concern in patients with Parkinson's disease. Muscle weakness, tremor, and rigidity can make ingestion of a healthy diet difficult. Weight needs to be monitored. Serial monitoring of serum albumin and proteins levels can identify patients at risk for malnutrition. Supplemental feedings may be required. For patients with swallowing difficulties strategies, such as smaller, more frequent meals, adding commercial powders to thicken liquids, and upright positioning, may be beneficial.

Exercise and physical therapy can help the patient to maximize function. Regular moderate exercise can reduce stiffness and tremors. Working with a speech therapist can help the patient to maximize language and cognitive function. As the disease progresses, the patient and family will require more assistance with activities of daily living, emotional support, and potential financial concerns. Issues, such as admission to an extended care facility or hospice, need to be introduced early in the disease progression. This allows the patient to participate in the decision-making process. A thorough history and physical examination is necessary. Health care management involves the use of pharmacological therapy or surgical interventions. The goal of Parkinson's disease management is to prevent functional disability; however a cure is not currently possible.

Collaborative Management

Parkinson's disease demands the multidisciplinary approach to care of the patient. The focus of collaborative management for the Parkinson's disease patient is to:
- Decrease the severity of the clinical manifestations (symptomatic).
- Interfere with the pathological mechanisms of the disease (protective).
- Provide new neurons or stimulate growth and function of remaining cells (restorative).

Pharmacology

The goal of treatment is to control tremor and rigidity and to improve the patient's ability to carry out the activities of daily living. Replacing the dopamine deficit in the basal ganglia sounds simple. However, dopamine cannot be given orally as it is metabolized before reaching the brain.

Levodopa, a precursor of dopamine, can be given orally and then is converted to dopamine in the brain. Dopamine replacement is most effective in the first three to five years of use. Long-term use is associated with side effects, such as dyskinesias, hallucinations, and severe orthostatic hypotension. When anticholinergic drugs are given with the dopamine replacement, the effect of the dopamine is extended. The newer drugs, catechol-O-methyltransferase (COMT) inhibitors, block the enzyme that inactivates dopamine and increase the effectiveness of levodopa.

There are many medications used to treat Parkinson's disease, and examples of these medications are shown in Table 37-10.

Surgery

Some patients with Parkinson's disease respond differently to the pharmacological methods of treatment. Other patients have the potential for less conservative treatments in the form of surgical interventions. Some of these types of surgical management (Table 37-11) are relatively recent and have varying levels of success.

TABLE 37-10 Pharmacologic Management of Parkinson's Disease

DRUG	INDICATION	SIDE EFFECTS
Dopamine Precursors		
Carbidopa/levodopa (Sinemet)	Decrease rigidity; bradykinesia; tremors	Nausea; vomiting; orthostatic hypotension; dry mouth; constipation; dizziness; cough; sleep disturbances; hallucinations; confusion; dyskinesia
Dopamine Receptor Antagonists		
Bromocriptine (Parlodel)	Activation of dopamine receptors	Nausea; postural hypotension; sleep disturbances; confusion; agitation; hallucinations; dyskinesia
Pergolide (Permax)	Activation of dopamine receptors	Nausea; postural hypotension; sleep disturbances; confusion; agitation; hallucinations
Pramipexole (Mirapex)	Activation of dopamine receptors	Nausea; dizziness; somnolence; weakness; constipation; sleep attacks
Ropinirole (Requip)	Activation of dopamine receptors	Nausea; dizziness; somnolence; syncope; sleep attacks
Antiviral Agents		
Amantadine (Symmetrel)	Decrease rigidity and akinesia	Confusion; lightheadedness; anxiety; blurred vision; dry mouth; urinary retention; constipation
Anticholinergic Agents		
Benztropine (Cogentin)	Decrease tremors and rigidity	Dry mouth; blurred vision; urinary retention; photophobia; constipation; tachycardia; confusion; depression; hallucinations
Biperiden (Akineton)	Decrease tremors and rigidity	Same as Cogentin
Orphenadrine (Disipal)	Decrease tremors and rigidity	Same as Cogentin
Procyclidine (Kemadrin)	Decrease tremors and rigidity	Same as Cogentin
Trihexyphenidyl (Artane)	Decrease tremors and rigidity	Same as Cogentin
Monoamine Oxidase B (MAO-B) Inhibitor		
Selegiline (Eldepryl)	Delays disease progression	Malaise; dizziness; nausea; tremors; restlessness; increased bradykinesia; orthostatic hypotension; arrhythmias
COMT Inhibitors		
Tolcapone (Tasmar)	Improves motor function	Hepatic failure; dyskinesia; nausea; orthostatic hypotension; sleep disturbances; hallucinations
Entacapone (Comtan)	Improves motor function	Vomiting; diarrhea; constipation; dyskinesia; orthostatic hypotension; hallucinations; sleep disturbances

Note: When these drugs are used in combination the side effect profile is enhanced.
Adapted from Broyles, B. E., Reiss, B. S., & Evans, M. E. (2007). Pharmacological aspects of nursing care (7th ed.). New York: Thomson Delmar Learning.

TABLE 37-11 Surgical Management of Parkinson's Disease

SURGERY	PROCEDURE	OUTCOME
Thalamotomy	Lesion placed in the thalamus	Relief of tremors
Pallidotomy	Destruction of globus pallidus using electrical stimulation	Improved control of symptoms
Deep-brain stimulation	Placement of electrode(s) in the thalamus, then attaching to a pulse generator implanted in the infraclavicular region.	Relief of tremors
Experimental Treatments		
Adrenal tissue transplant	Provide viable dopamine producing cells into the caudate nucleus.	Long-term results have not been promising
Stem cell transplant	Provide viable dopamine producing cells into the caudate nucleus.	Long-term results have not been promising

Adapted from Lozano, A. (2003). *Surgery for Parkinson's disease the five W's: Why, who, what, where, and when.* Advances in Neurology, 91, 30–307.

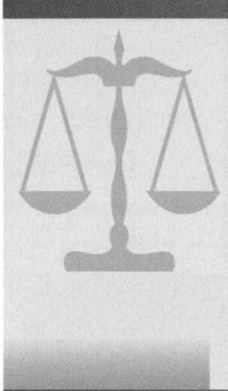

ETHICS IN PRACTICE

Stem Cell Controversy

Recent controversy has focused on the legal and ethical issues of using fetal tissue or stem cells obtained from cord blood. There is a continuing level of interest from specific research institutions and from specific lobbying groups to pursue the legalizing of stem cell harvesting. The future of this controversy is unfolding in continuing decisions at this time.

Evaluation of Outcomes

Potential patient outcomes for each of the example nursing diagnoses for the patient with Parkinson's disease are:

- Impaired physical mobility related to rigidity, bradykinesia, and akinesia. The patient will demonstrate increased strength and endurance.
- Impaired verbal communication related to dysarthria and tremor. The patient will demonstrate improved ability to express self.
- Imbalanced nutrition: less than body requirement related to dysphagia. The patient will demonstrate methods to assist with food intake.
- Self-care deficit related to inability to perform activities of daily living. The patient will participate in self-care activities as much as possible.
- Constipation related to immobility. The patient will report regular bowel movements.
- Disturbed thought process related to hallucinations. The patient will maintain reality orientation and communicate clearly with others.
- Sleep deprivation related to rigidity and weakness. The patient will report an optimal balance of rest and activity.
- Risk for injury related to postural disturbances. The patient will not experience injury.

Uncovering the Evidence

Immunization for Parkinson's Disease

Discussion: The purpose of this study was to evaluate the use of vaccine to activate immune cells in ways that are neuroprotective in a mouse model of Parkinson's disease. The methods involved the treatment of mice with Copaxone (copolymer-1), currently used to treat MS. The researchers then took immune cells from the immunized mice and injected them into mice which had received MPTP. MPTP causes Parkinson's-like neuronal degeneration in the brain. The findings revealed that mice treated with the Copaxone-treated immune cells had less degeneration of dopamine-producing neurons, lost fewer dopamine-transmitting nerve fibers, and had only a small decrease in dopamine production when compared to controls.

Implications for Practice: The use of vaccination for Parkinson's disease may serve as a method for arresting disease progression. More basic research needs to be done and to be approved by the Food and Drug Administration (FDA). Clinical trials must demonstrate both effectiveness and a low side effect profile.

Source: Benner, E., Mosley, R., Destache, C., Lewis, T., Jackson-Lewis, V., Gorantla, S., et al. (2004). Therapeutic immunization protects dopaminergic neurons in a mouse model of Parkinson's disease. Proceedings of the National Academy of Sciences of the USA, 101(25), 9435–9440.

ALZHEIMER'S DISEASE

Alzheimer's disease is the most common cause of dementia in Western countries, accounting for 70 percent of all cases. Alzheimer's disease is the fourth leading cause of death among the elderly. Alzheimer's disease has an incredible impact on the health care budget because of the chronic nature of the patients and their long-standing health care needs. Recently, the National Institutes of Health (NIH) has contributed greatly to the research funding for the study and interventions related to Alzheimer's disease. And, nursing as a profession has significantly impacted the methods of care for patients with this neurological degenerative disease.

Epidemiology

In the United States, it is estimated that four million people are diagnosed with Alzheimer's disease. And as the population ages, this number is expected to double by 2020. The financial burden on the patient, family, and society is estimated to exceed $100 billion per year. The incidence of Alzheimer's disease is slightly higher in Americans with African and Hispanic heritage. Women and men are affected equally.

Etiology

The exact etiology of Alzheimer's disease is unknown. However, risk factors for Alzheimer's disease include advancing age, family history, and possibly head injury. Advancing age is a major risk factor for developing Alzheimer's disease. It is not a normal part of the aging process. After age 65, the risk of Alzheimer's disease doubles every 10 years. Children of a parent diagnosed

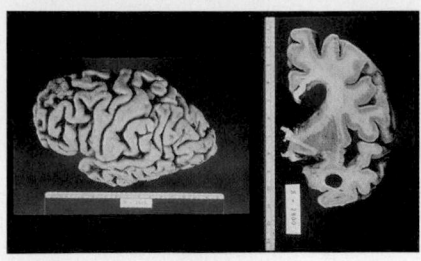

Figure 37-3 At autopsy, the cerebral cortex displays changes (white spots) caused by Alzheimer's disease (photo courtesy of the Alzheimer's Association).

with Alzheimer's disease have a 50 percent risk of developing the disease. Repeated head injury is thought to activate, by some unknown method, pre-existing risk factors.

Pathophysiology

While the exact cause of Alzheimer's disease is unknown, there are many pathophysiological findings that are understood. Several important findings are known, but how they are related is not yet understood. These findings include:

- Neuronal degeneration in the hippocampus (causing memory loss) and cerebral cortex (causing speech, reasoning, and higher function loss) (Figure 37-3).
- Neuritic plaques are spherical bodies, composed of protein fragments and remnants of axons and dendrites, which form outside of the neurons. They are considered a hallmark sign of Alzheimer's disease.
- Neurofibrillary tangles occur inside the neurons, when the normal microtubular arrangement become disrupted (tangled). They are considered another diagnostic sign of Alzheimer's disease.

The presence of neurofibrillary tangles and neuritic plaques has been suggested as a possible pathological mechanism. Whether or not the neuronal death is caused by a direct toxic effect or by predisposing the cells to injury remains to be determined. Neurotransmitter systems, such as ACh, serotonin, and norepinephrine, diminish over the course of the disease. Many of the clinical manifestations are related to the reduction or loss of these neurotransmitters in the brain (Eggenberger & Nelms, 2004).

Assessment with Clinical Manifestations

Alzheimer's disease is classified into three stages based on progression of clinical manifestations (Table 37-12). Disease progression is highly variable and may not follow the model exactly. In the early stage, cognitive deficits may not be recognized, family and friends may begin to identify subtle changes in memory and personality, and patients and families may compensate for the deficits. In the middle stage, continuing changes in memory, orientation, speech, and ability to perform the activities of daily living, may put the patient at risk for injury.

In the late stage, the patient is completely dependent on others for care. Common complications of the late stage of Alzheimer's disease include pneumonia, malnutrition, falls, dehydration, depression, delusions, and paranoid reactions.

Diagnostic Tests

Alzheimer's disease is diagnosed by ruling out other possible causes for the patient's symptoms. Currently the only method that can conclusively diagnose Alzheimer's disease is by finding pathological changes in brain tissue obtained by biopsy or autopsy. A dementia workup includes evaluation for delirium, depression, infections, thyroid dysfunction, nutritional deficits, heart failure, chronic pulmonary disease, arrhythmias, pain, and trauma. Laboratory studies should include complete blood count (CBC), electrolytes, renal, thyroid, and liver panels, and urinalysis. EEG, MRI, MRS, computed tomography (CT), SPECT, and PET scans may help to rule out other causes (discussed in chapter 34). Serial testing of memory and cognitive skill can be accomplished by using the Mini-Mental State Examination (MMSE) or other similar testing methods. Final diagnosis requires presence of dementia, disease onset between the ages of 40 and 90 years, and absence of other systemic system or CNS diseases.

TABLE 37-12	Stages of Alzheimer's Disease	
STAGE	**TIMEFRAME**	**CLINICAL MANIFESTATIONS**
Early	2–4 years	Forgetfulness; poor memory (may compensate by using notes)
		Declining interest in people, environment, and current events
		Impaired acquisition of new information
		Impaired judgment; mild cognitive changes
		Job performance declines; may lose job
		May be apathetic, irritable, or show signs of depression
		Normal EEG and CT
Middle	2–12 years	Progressive memory loss
		Disorientation to time, place, and events
		Impaired ability to follow simple directions or simple math
		Significant impairment of cognitive function and judgment
		Wanders at night due to sleep-wake cycle disturbance
		Neglects personal hygiene and activities of daily living
		Becomes increasingly irritable, evasive, and anxious
		May experience episodes of violent behavior
		EEG—slowing; CT—normal or dilated ventricles
Late	8–12 years	Extreme weight loss secondary to lack of eating
		Severe impairment of all cognitive functions
		Unable to communicate (verbal or written)
		Dependent on others for activities of daily living
		Incontinent of urine and feces
		Pathological reflexes can be elicited
		Motor skills are lost; becomes bedridden
		EEG—diffuse slowing
		CT—dilated ventricles and sulcal enlargement

Adapted from Larson, E., Shadlen, M., Wang, L., McCormick, W., Bowen, J., Teri, L., et al. (2004). Survival after initial diagnosis of Alzheimer's disease. Annals of Internal Medicine, 140(7), 501–509.

Nursing Diagnoses

Based on the information gathered, examples of nursing diagnoses in the patient with Alzheimer's disease may include the following:

- Self-care deficit related to inability to perform activities of daily living without assistance.
- Risk for injury related to impaired judgment, poor memory, and gait instability.
- Disturbed thought processes related to memory loss and cognitive deficits.
- Risk for ineffective coping related to disease progression.
- Impaired verbal communication related to cognitive decline.

Planning and Implementation

Because of the chronic progressive nature of Alzheimer's disease, a primary concern of the nurse caring for these patients is health teaching. In the early stages, the nurse needs to educate and support the patient and family as they adjust to the lifestyle changes that are required. Teaching should address the physical, emotional, and social aspects of the disease. In the beginning, actions and potential side effects of the medication regimen need to be taught, monitored, and adjusted to the desired patient response.

Nutrition is often a concern in patients with Alzheimer's disease. Muscle weakness and cognitive dysfunction may make ingestion of a healthy diet difficult. Weight needs to be monitored. Serial monitoring of serum albumin and proteins levels can identify patients at risk for malnutrition. Supplemental feedings may be required. For patients with swallowing difficulties strategies, such as smaller, more frequent meals, adding commercial powders to thicken liquids, and upright positioning, may be beneficial.

Exercise and physical therapy can help the patient to maximize function. Regular moderate exercise can reduce weakness and muscle atrophy. Working with a speech therapist can help the patient to maximize language and cognitive function. As the disease progresses, the patient and family will require more assistance with activities of daily living, emotional support, and potential financial concerns. Issues, such as admission to an extended care facility or hospice, need to be introduced early in the disease progression. This allows the patient to participate in the decision-making process.

Collaborative Management

The goal of collaborative management is to improve or slow the disease progression and maintain independent functioning for as long as possible. The health care team must work together with the patient and his or her caregiver(s) to support, educate, counsel, and provide strategies to assist with controlling the behavioral manifestations of the disease. Teaching for the patient and their family should include disease pathophysiology, medication actions and side effects, safety measures, and signs and symptoms of disease progression.

Pharmacology

Over the course of Alzheimer's disease there are many potential medications that a patient can be given. Cholinesterase inhibitors are given to enhance cognition and have a variety of successes in their treatment. In addition, a number of antidepressants may be given as the patients with Alzheimer's disease are often emotionally upset. There are even patients that have psychotic disturbances that can require medicinal therapy. A variety of medications can be given to patients with Alzheimer's disease. Examples are cholinesterase inhibitors to improve cognition (e.g., tacrine), serotonin reuptake inhibitors (e.g., citalopram, sertraline) to manage depression, tricyclic antidepressants (e.g., desipramine), and antipsychotics (e.g., haloperidol, risperidone) for the management of psychoses and behavioral disturbances.

Evaluation of Outcomes

Potential patient outcomes for each of the example nursing diagnoses for the patient with Alzheimer's disease are:
- Self-care deficit related to inability to perform activities of daily living. The patient will participate in self-care activities as much as possible.
- Risk for injury related to impaired judgment, poor memory, and gait instability. The patient will not experience injury.
- Disturbed thought process related to memory loss and cognitive deficits. The patient will maintain reality orientation and communicate clearly with others.

- Risk for ineffective coping related to disease progression. The family will acknowledge need for assistance.
- Impaired verbal communication related to cognitive decline. The patient will demonstrate improved ability to express self.

MYASTHENIA GRAVIS

Myasthenia gravis is a chronic, autoimmune, progressive neuromuscular disease characterized by abnormal weakness and fatigability of skeletal muscles. It is relatively rare compared to many of the other degenerative neurological disorders but is very affecting to those patients who contract the disease. It is typically a disorder that is not thought of when a patient first presents with clinical manifestations. Other diseases are ruled out, and then myasthenia gravis is confirmed by the history and physical, along with specific diagnostic tests that can be administered.

Epidemiology

Incidence rate is 5 per 100,000 people in the United States. More women than men (3:2) are diagnosed with myasthenia gravis. It can occur at any age but is most commonly seen between 10 and 65 years, with the peak age of onset between 20 and 30 years. Familial incidence is approximately 5 to 7 percent. Tumor of the thymus gland (thymoma) is present in up to 10 percent of myasthenia gravis patients. Thymoma is more common in patients over 30 years of age.

Etiology

Although the exact cause is unknown, it is believed to have an autoimmune etiology. Patients may seek health care providers for their fatigue and other somewhat vague symptoms, without suspecting a neurological disorder.

Pathophysiology

The autoimmune process destroys or blocks some of the ACh receptors at the postsynaptic muscle junction. There is a decrease in the number of available ACh receptor sites and concurrent structural change that diminishes ACh uptake. The end result is decreased strength of muscle contraction and with continued stimulation, profound fatigue. Usually the muscles innervated by the cranial nerves (face, lips, tongue, neck, and throat) are affected, but myasthenia gravis can affect any skeletal muscle group (Wakata, et al., 2004). There are three types of myasthenia gravis:

- Ocular—weakness of the eye and lid muscles only.
- Bulbar—involves breathing, swallowing, and speech (cranial nerves IX and XII) and.
- Generalized—involves the proximal muscles of the limbs and neck, usually with both ocular and bulbar manifestations.

Assessment with Clinical Manifestations

The onset of myasthenia gravis is usually gradual and extremely variable. The manifestations may fluctuate from hour to hour, from day to day, or over longer periods. They are made worse by exertion, exposure to temperature extremes, infections, menses, and excitement. Early findings in most patients are **ptosis** (drooping of eyelids) and **diplopia** (double vision). The ptosis may be unilateral or bilateral and becomes worse when the patient tries to look

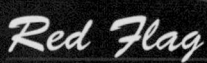
upward. The diplopia may be unilateral or bilateral. Pupillary response to light and accommodation remain normal. This progresses to weakness of other muscles innervated by the cranial nerves results in loss of facial expression, a smile that resembles a snarl, jaw drop, nasal regurgitation of liquids, choking on foods and secretions, and slurred, nasal speech.

Next, the muscles of the neck and extremities are affected. Problems with fine motor movements of the hands may include changes in handwriting patterns, difficulty in combing hair, repetitive movements, climbing stairs, walking, or running. Proximal limb muscles are more often affected than the distal muscles. As the disease continues to progress, weakness and fatigue can affect all muscle groups (Wakata, et al., 2004).

Diagnostic Tests

Diagnostic tests for myasthenia gravis include:
- Serum assay for circulating ACh receptor antibodies. If increased, it is confirmation of myasthenia gravis with a sensitivity of 80 to 90 percent.
- Electromyography (EMG)—there is a reduced response to electrical stimulation when myasthenia gravis is present. Refer to chapter 34 for a full discussion of this test.
- CT or MRI may be ordered to determine if the thymus gland is abnormal. Refer to chapter 34 for a full discussion of these tests.
- Tensilon test—the patient is injected (intravenously) with edrophonium chloride (Tensilon), a short-acting anticholinesterase agent. In patients with myasthenia gravis the response is rapid improvement of manifestations within 15 to 30 seconds and lasting approximately five minutes.

Nursing Diagnoses

Based on the information gathered, examples of nursing diagnoses in the patient with myasthenia gravis may include the following:
- Ineffective breathing pattern related to weakness of chest muscles and fatigue.
- Ineffective airway clearance related to chest muscle weakness and impaired cough and gag.
- Impaired verbal communication related to weakness of lips, mouth, pharynx, jaw, and larynx.
- Imbalanced nutrition: less than body requirements related to muscle weakness and dysphagia.
- Activity intolerance related to muscle weakness and fatigue.

Planning and Implementation

There is no cure for myasthenia gravis. The goal of treatment in patients with myasthenia gravis is to improve their muscle weakness and induce remission with minimal side effects. Treatment modalities include medications, plasmapheresis, and surgery. The most common management technique is the administration of anticholinesterases and immunosuppressive medications.

Once the diagnosis of myasthenia gravis is confirmed, patient safety and health teaching by the nurse become the primary focus. The patient and his or her family need accurate information concerning the manifestations, etiology, and treatment of myasthenia gravis. The nurse needs to educate and support the patient and family as they adjust to the lifestyle changes that are required. Teaching should address the physical, emotional, and social aspects of the disease. Actions and potential side effects of the medication regimen need to be taught, monitored, and adjusted to the desired patient response. Medications that may interfere with neuromuscular function should be avoided.

Activities of daily living are often compromised by the generalized muscle weakness and fatigue in patients with myasthenia gravis. Once the nurse establishes a baseline of functioning level for the patient, frequent monitoring of activities and assisting as needed, helps the patient to maintain as near normal a lifestyle as possible. Rest is critical, and the nurse should teach energy conservation measures to maximize function.

Communication may become difficult for the patient with myasthenia gravis. Dysarthria and nasal speech result from weakness of the muscles involved in speech. The speech dysfunction may make communication with others difficult. Alternative forms of communication, such as using yes or no questions, flash cards, pencil and paper, eye blinking, or communication boards, may reduce the patient's frustration.

Exacerbations of myasthenia gravis may be related to stress, comorbid diseases, hormonal fluctuations, trauma, medications, or extreme temperatures. Frequent assessment of respiratory function is necessary. Increasing muscle weakness often affects swallowing and breathing. This can result in aspiration, inability to clear secretions, or respiratory insufficiency. With severe respiratory dysfunction, the patient may require intubation, ventilatory support, and admission to an intensive care unit. Other causes for respiratory dysfunction are myasthenic crisis (severe muscle weakness due to stress or medicine) and cholinergic crisis (excess ACh).

When patients experience myasthenic crisis, **plasmapheresis** (removal of serum antibodies) may be used to stabilize their disease. It may also be used as a short-term treatment before the patient is scheduled for thymectomy surgery. Plasmapheresis is usually done at the bedside with a blood cell separator machine. The procedure takes approximately three to five hours and is repeated every two to three days for two weeks. Temporary improvement in muscle strength is seen after the first treatment.

Nutrition

Nutrition is often a concern in patients with myasthenia gravis. Muscle weakness and decreased ability to chew or swallow can make ingestion of a healthy diet difficult. Weight needs to be monitored. Serial monitoring of serum albumin and proteins levels can identify patients at risk for malnutrition. For patients with swallowing difficulties, strategies such as smaller, more frequent meals, high calorie snacks, adding commercial powders to thicken liquids, and upright positioning may improve nutritional intake.

Pharmacology

Pharmacological therapies constitute the primary methods of treatment for myasthenia gravis. Anticholinesterase agents (e.g., Mestinon, Prostigmin) are the first medications used to treat myasthenia gravis. Mestinon prevents the inactivation of ACh and enhances the stimulus transmission at the cholinergic junctions. When patients do not respond well to Mestinon, immunosuppressive agents may be tried (e.g., immune globulin, prednisone, Imuran). Prednisone is the drug of choice. Improvement or remission is seen in 70 to 80 percent of patients treated with glucocorticosteroids. Several types of medications (e.g., neuromuscular blocking agents, antiarrhythmic agents, beta blockers, or antibiotics) may increase the weakness experienced in myasthenia gravis, so this should be evaluated by the nurse.

Surgery

Surgical management for myasthenia gravis involves the removal of the thymus gland. For about 85 percent of patients with myasthenia gravis, surgery improves their clinical manifestations, and approximately 35 percent become drug free. Patients with pronounced respiratory weakness before surgery are at a higher risk for ventilator weaning difficulties after surgery.

Red Flag

Administration of Anticholinesterase Agents

Oral anticholinesterase agents must be administered on time or the patient may be too weak to swallow the pills. Mestinon's effect begins in 30 to 45 minutes, peaks in about two hours, and lasts three to six hours. The dosage schedule is usually individualized to produce maximal muscle strength for the patient.

Evaluation of Outcomes

Potential patient outcomes for each of the example nursing diagnoses for the patient with myasthenia gravis are:

- Ineffective breathing pattern related to weakness. The patient's breathing pattern is maintained as evidenced by eupnea, normal skin color, and regular respiratory rate and patterns.
- Ineffective airway clearance related to weakness, impaired cough, and impaired gag reflex. The patient will not experience aspiration.
- Impaired verbal communication related to muscle weakness. The patient will demonstrate improved ability to express self.
- Imbalanced nutrition: less than body requirements related to muscle weakness and dysphagia. The patient will ingest adequate nutrition.
- Activity intolerance related to muscle weakness and fatigue. The patient will identify methods to reduce activity intolerance.

AMYOTROPHIC LATERAL SCLEROSIS

Amyotrophic lateral sclerosis (ALS) is also called Lou Gehrig's disease, after the New York Yankee first baseman, who was diagnosed with the disease in 1939. ALS is a similar disorder to MS, but it is much faster in its progression, and its prognosis is much more severe.

Epidemiology

ALS is the most common motor neuron disease. Age of onset for the disease is between 40 and 60 years of age. It is more common in men than women by a ratio of 2:1. In the United States incidence is 5 per 100,000 people. Each year approximately 5,000 patients are diagnosed with the disease. There is an autosomal dominant component in 5 to 10 percent of all cases. ALS is a progressive disease that leads to death from respiratory arrest. Death usually occurs within 2 to 6 years.

Etiology

The exact cause of ALS is unknown. Several potential mechanisms have been suggested: a defect in glutamate metabolism, free radical damage, altered nucleic acid production by nerve fibers, and an autoimmune component. The excitotoxic hypothesis suggests that a defect in the metabolism, transport, and storage of glutamate (a neurotransmitter) may allow the toxic accumulation of glutamate to destroy the neurons. The second hypothesis states that accumulation of excess oxygen free radicals causes oxidative stress that destroys the motor neurons. The cytoskeletal hypothesis proposes that damage to the nerve fibers contributes to the motor neuron death. An autoimmune component has been reported in some patients. Current research focuses on identifying the disease mechanism and developing new treatments or potentially a cure in the future (Attarian, Vedel, Pouget, & Schmied, 2006).

Pathophysiology

ALS progressively demyelinates the motor neurons in the anterior horn of the spinal cord, brainstem, and cerebral cortex. It involves both upper and lower motor neurons. When upper motor function is lost, the affected muscles become spastic and weak, and deep tendon reflexes are increased. The loss of lower motor neuron innervation results in muscle flaccidity, weakness, atrophy, and paralysis. Intellectual ability, vision, hearing, and sensory function are not affected by the disease. Bowel and bladder function are usually spared until late in the disease (Attarian, et al., 2006).

Assessment with Clinical Manifestations

The initial manifestations of ALS can vary among patients, but usually weakness and wasting of the limbs are the first patient complaints. As the disease progresses other manifestations may be seen including:

- Muscle weakness, wasting, and atrophy, first in the hands, then in the shoulder and upper arm, and then in the lower limbs.
- Muscle spasticity and hyperreflexia.
- Muscle fasciculations (fine twitching).
- Atrophy of the tongue causing dysarthria and dysphagia.
- Dyspnea that can progress to respiratory failure.
- Fatigue.

Diagnostic Tests

There are no specific diagnostic studies or laboratory tests for confirmation of the diagnosis of ALS. An EMG may show abnormal electrical activity in the muscles. Nerve conduction studies may demonstrate abnormal responses to electrical stimuli. Muscle or nerve biopsy may demonstrate atrophy. CT, MRI, and EEG may be useful in ruling out other causes for the manifestations. A full discussion of these tests can be found on chapter 34.

Nursing Diagnoses

Based on the information gathered, examples of nursing diagnoses in the patient with ALS may include the following:

- Impaired mobility related to muscle wasting, weakness, and spasticity.
- Impaired communication related to impairment of the muscles of speech.
- High risk for aspiration related to impaired muscles of swallowing.
- Ineffective breathing pattern related to impaired muscles of breathing.

Planning and Implementation

Because of the progressive, degenerative nature of ALS, the primary concern of the nurse caring for these patients is health teaching. In the early stages, the nurse needs to educate and support the patient and family as they adjust to the lifestyle changes that are required. Teaching should address the physical, emotional, and social aspects of the disease. The actions and potential side effects of the medication regimen need to be taught, monitored, and adjusted to the desired patient response.

Exercise and physical therapy can help the patient to maximize function. Regular moderate exercise can reduce stiffness and spasticity. Working with a speech therapist can help the patient to maximize language function. As the disease progresses, the patient and family will require more assistance with activities of daily living, emotional support, and potential financial concerns. Issues, such as admission to an extended care facility or hospice, need to be introduced early in the disease progression. This allows the patient to participate in the decision-making process.

End-of-life issues need to be discussed with the patient and their family, early in the disease progression. When the patient is unable to chew or swallow the insertion of a gastrostomy will help to prevent aspiration pneumonia. Loss of the patient's ability to protect their airway may require the insertion of a tracheostomy and chronic mechanical ventilation that alters the patient's quality of life. These decisions need to be addressed before an emergency situation occurs.

Collaborative Management

Currently there is no cure for this disease. Treatment is supportive and requires a multidisciplinary approach, including medications, therapy (physical, occupational, speech, nutrition), teaching, counseling, and support. Physical ther-

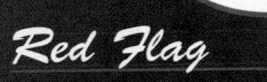

Red Flag

Locked-in Syndrome in ALS

The patient with ALS may develop locked-in syndrome as the disease progresses. Locked-in syndrome refers to a functional state where there is full consciousness and cognition, but severe paralysis makes communication and movement impossible. Lack of movement puts the patient at risk for complications, such as pressure sores, pneumonia, and sepsis. A regular schedule of preventive interventions needs to be implemented. Loss of the ability to speak can be devastating for the patient with intact cognition. A simple method of communication using eye blinking and vertical eye movements should be established. Currently there are computer-assisted methods of communication available. However, they are expensive and may pose a financial burden for the patient and his or her family.

apy should include a regular exercise regimen and supportive or assistive devices as needed. Occupational therapy can assist with adaptive devices to help with activities of daily living. Speech therapy can help the patient with improving or augmentation of altered speech patterns. Nutrition assessment and the eventual use of a gastrostomy tube for feeding may be necessary.

Nutrition

Nutrition is often a concern in patients with ALS. Muscle weakness, and decreased ability to chew or swallow can make ingestion of a healthy diet difficult. Weight needs to be monitored. Serial monitoring of serum albumin and proteins levels can identify patients at risk for malnutrition. Supplemental feedings and insertion of a feeding tube may be required. For patients with swallowing difficulties, strategies such as smaller, more frequent meals, adding commercial powders to thicken liquids, and upright positioning may be beneficial.

Pharmacology

Pharmacological management is used extensively in the treatment of ALS. Medications used for management of ALS include glutamate inhibitors (e.g., riluzole), benzodiazepines (e.g., diazepam), skeletal muscle relaxants (e.g., dantrolene), and antiarrhythmic agents (e.g., quinidine).

Evaluation of Outcomes

Potential patient outcomes for each of the example nursing diagnoses for the patient with ALS are:
- Impaired mobility related to muscle wasting, weakness, and spasticity. The patient will report increased strength and endurance.
- Impaired communication related to impairment of the muscles of speech. The patient will report improved ability to communicate.
- High risk for aspiration related to impaired muscles of swallowing. The patient will not experience aspiration.
- Ineffective breathing pattern related to impaired muscles of breathing. The patient's breathing pattern is maintained as evidenced by eupnea, normal skin color, and regular respiratory rate and patterns.

HUNTINGTON'S DISEASE (HUNTINGTON'S CHOREA)

Huntington's disease (also called Huntington's chorea) is a rare abnormal hereditary disorder of the CNS. It is characterized by chronic progressive **chorea** (involuntary purposeless, rapid movements) and mental deterioration that results in dementia.

Epidemiology

Men and women are affected equally, and the disease is more prevalent in patients of western European ancestry. The prevalence of Huntington's disease is estimated to be 5 to 10 per 100,000 people. In the United States, it is estimated that 30,000 individuals are affected and more than 125,000 at risk for developing the disease. The onset of Huntington's disease is usually between 30 and 50 years of age. Because of the late onset of the disease, transmission of the affected gene has often occurred years before the patient was diagnosed.

Etiology

Huntington's disease is genetic in its causation. This confirmed reason for Huntington's disease makes this a distinguishing characteristic among the other degenerative neurological diseases. More information regarding the genetic influences for Huntington's disease is enumerated in the Genetics section.

Pathophysiology

The pathological process of Huntington's disease is similar to Parkinson's disease. There is destruction of cells in the caudate nucleus and putamen areas of the basal ganglia and extrapyramidal motor system. Other areas of the brain may atrophy. The neurotransmitters, gamma-aminobutyric acid (GABA) and ACh are decreased. Dopamine is not affected, but the decrease of ACh causes a relative increase of dopamine in the basal ganglia. In Parkinson's the decreased dopamine causes slowing or loss of movement, but in Huntington's the excess dopamine causes uncontrolled movement.

Genetics

Huntington's disease is caused by autosomal dominant gene transmission. Offspring of a patient with Huntington's disease have a 50 percent chance of inheriting the gene. Identification of the gene responsible for Huntington's disease, which became available in 1993, allows the family members to be tested. This may be a difficult decision for the patient's family. If the test is positive, they will develop Huntington's disease. Family members who are asymptomatic may not want to know that they will develop the disease as they age (Etchegary, 2006).

Assessment with Clinical Manifestations

The hallmark clinical manifestations are intellectual decline and abnormal movements. Initially the patient may report feelings of restlessness, forgetfulness, clumsiness, frequent falls, and problems with speech, coordination, and balance. As the disease progresses, depression, memory loss, emotional lability, and impulsiveness may impair the patient's ability to work or maintain a normal routine. Motor manifestations include facial grimaces, protrusion of the tongue, jerky movements of the arms and legs, and gait disturbances. The gait changes put the patient at risk for falls. The disease progresses over a 10- to 20-year period until the patient is totally dependent. Death usually occurs because of aspiration pneumonia or sepsis.

Diagnostic Tests

Diagnosis of Huntington's disease involves a thorough history and physical examination. Genetic testing is done to identify the Huntington's trait. PET and SPECT studies may show evidence of decreased glucose metabolism. CT and MRI scans may identify gross wasting of the caudate nucleus and putamen and, in the late stages, atrophy of the lobes of the brain (Daniels, 2003). A full discussion of these tests can be found in chapter 34.

Nursing Diagnoses

Based on the information gathered, examples of nursing diagnoses in the patient with Huntington's disease may include the following:
- Risk for injury related to impaired motor function.
- Disturbed thought process: psychotic episodes related to lack of self-control and depression.
- Impaired nutrition: less than body requirements related to dysphagia.
- Impaired verbal communication related to cognitive deficits.
- Ineffective role performance related to disease process.

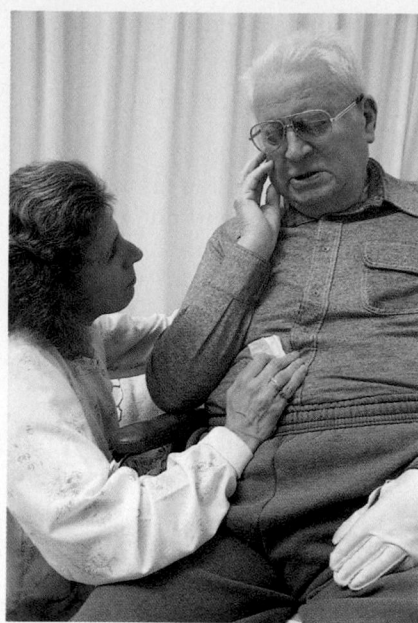

Figure 37-4 Nurse supporting and teaching patient with Huntington's disease in regard to the chronic debilitating nature of the disorder.

Planning and Implementation

There is no known cure for Huntington's disease at this time. Management is manifestation-based, supportive, and protective. Because of the chronic, progressive nature of Huntington's disease, the primary concern of the nursing caring for these patients is health teaching. In the early stages, the nurse needs to educate and support the patient and family as they adjust to the lifestyle changes that are required (Figure 37-4). Teaching should address the physical, emotional, genetic, and social aspects of the disease. The actions and potential side effects of the medication regimen need to be taught, monitored, and adjusted to the desired patient response.

Exercise and physical therapy can help the patient to maximize function. Regular moderate exercise can reduce stiffness and tremors. Working with a speech therapist can help the patient to maximize language and cognitive function. As the disease progresses, the patient and family will require more assistance with activities of daily living, emotional support, and potential financial concerns. Issues, such as admission to an extended care facility or hospice, need to be introduced early in the disease progression. This allows the patient to participate in the decision-making process.

Collaborative Management

Disease management includes rehabilitative therapy, teaching, counseling, and professional legal, financial, and estate planning advice. Support needs will increase as the patient's disease progresses. Families will require physical, emotional, and possible financial support, as a result of the patient's diagnosis.

Nutrition

Nutrition is often a concern in patients with Huntington's disease. Muscle weakness, tremor, and rigidity can make ingestion of a healthy diet difficult. Weight needs to be monitored. Serial monitoring of serum albumin and proteins levels can identify patients at risk for malnutrition. Supplemental feedings may be required. For patients with swallowing difficulties strategies, such as smaller, more frequent meals, adding commercial powders to thicken liquids, and upright positioning, may be beneficial.

Pharmacology

Pharmacological methods of treatment are carefully considered when treating Huntington's disease. Many medications can be used, and it is important to assess the combinations of medications that are used. Due to the organic nature of deterioration of the mental capabilities, there can be a tendency to overmedicate the patient with Huntington's disease. The care provider must assess the rationale for giving the medications and carefully administer these combinations of medication therapy. The common classifications of medications used in the treatment of Huntington's disease are shown in the Box 37-5.

Evaluation of Outcomes

Potential patient outcomes for each of the example nursing diagnoses for the patient with Huntington's disease:
- Risk for injury related to impaired motor function. The patient will not experience injury.
- Disturbed thought process related to psychotic episodes. The patient will maintain reality orientation and communicate clearly with others.
- Impaired nutrition: less than body requirements related to dysphagia. The patient will ingest adequate nutrition.
- Impaired verbal communication related to cognitive deficits. The patient will demonstrate improved ability to express self.
- Ineffective role performance related to disease progression. The patient will demonstrate healthy adaptation and coping skills.

BOX 37-5

MEDICATIONS ADMINISTERED TO MANAGE HUNTINGTON'S DISEASE

- Rilutek (riluzole) is currently being studied to decrease cognitive manifestations.
- Skeletal muscle relaxants to modify the choreiform movements.
- Antipsychotics to block the dopamine receptors in the brain.
- Antidepressants to help control the chorea, behavioral changes, and depression.

KEY CONCEPTS

- There is no known cure for chronic and degenerative neurologic diseases.
- Headache is the most common form of chronic pain.
- Types of headaches include tension-type, migraine, and cluster.
- Tension-type headache is caused by irritation of the pain-sensitive structures of the brain.
- Migraine is characterized by vasodilation of the dural blood vessels, resulting in stimulation of the trigeminal nerve pain pathways.
- Cluster headaches are believed to be a variant of migraine headaches.
- A seizure is a sudden, uncontrolled discharge of electricity in the brain.
- Seizures are divided into three major classes: partial, generalized, and unclassified.
- Generalized seizures originate in all of the regions of the brain cortex. There is no aura or warning, but there is loss of consciousness.
- Partial seizures begin in a specific brain region, and consciousness is usually not impaired.
- Status epilepticus is defined as either continuous seizures lasting more than five minutes on two or more different seizures with incomplete recovery of consciousness between them.

- MS is a chronic inflammatory disease of the CNS.
- There is no single diagnostic test that confirms or rules out the diagnosis of MS.
- Parkinson's disease is a slowly progressive degenerative neurological disorder caused by the loss of nerve cell function in the basal ganglia.
- Many of the secondary manifestations can be exaggerated by the medications used to treat Parkinson's disease.
- Alzheimer's disease is the most common cause of dementia in Western countries.
- Neuronal degeneration in the hippocampus and cerebral cortex, neurofibrillary tangles, and neuritic plaques have been suggested as a possible etiology of Alzheimer's disease.
- Myasthenia gravis is a chronic, autoimmune, progressive neuromuscular disease characterized by abnormal weakness and fatigability of skeletal muscles.
- ALS is a progressive disease that leads to death from respiratory arrest.
- Huntington's disease is characterized by chronic, progressive, involuntary, purposeless, rapid movements, and mental deterioration that results in dementia.
- Huntington's disease is caused by autosomal dominant gene transmission.

REVIEW QUESTIONS

1. A patient who has a migraine headache would be sensitive to:
   1. Touch
   2. Taste
   3. Humidity
   4. Sound

2. Nursing documentation of seizure activity should be:
   1. Brief and concise
   2. Highly descriptive and detailed
   3. In a flow sheet format
   4. Limited to the findings of the neurological examination

3. The teaching plan for a patient with epilepsy should include which of the following precautions?
   1. Warn your coworkers that you have a seizure disorder
   2. Wear a medical alert bracelet
   3. Lose weight to help control your seizures
   4. Avoid situations that are stressful

4. Eating which of the following food products is associated with migraine attacks?
   1. Dairy products
   2. Citrus juice
   3. Decaffeinated tea
   4. Coffee

5. Two distinguishing features of migraine are:
   1. Mood change and sharp pain between eyes
   2. Family history of headaches and headache-related disability
   3. Bilateral headache and rhinorrhea
   4. Insomnia and nausea

6. The most common sign or symptom reported by a patient with myasthenia gravis is:
   1. Early morning fatigability
   2. Pain that gets worse with position changes
   3. Weakness on exertion
   4. Fecal incontinence

Continued

REVIEW QUESTIONS—cont'd

7. Which of the following neurotransmitters is decreased in patients with Parkinson's disease?
   1. Acetylcholine
   2. Norepinephrine
   3. Serotonin
   4. Dopamine

8. Which of the following is the priority safety intervention when protecting the patient having a seizure?
   1. Placing a tongue blade between their teeth
   2. Ensure that the patient is restrained
   3. Position the patient to prevent aspiration of secretions
   4. Determine if the patient is incontinent

9. Which of the following drugs must be kept at the bedside of patient's with myasthenia gravis?
   1. Atropine
   2. Neostigmine
   3. Inderal
   4. Tensilon

10. An abnormal plantar reflex is commonly seen with:
    1. Cerebellar dysfunction
    2. Diffuse cerebral dysfunction
    3. Lower motor neuron lesions
    4. Upper motor neuron lesions

11. The brief sensory experience that occurs prior to the onset of seizure is called the:
    1. Prodromal phase
    2. Aura
    3. Epileptic cry
    4. Ictal phase

REVIEW ACTIVITIES

1. Discuss the differences in pathophysiology and treatment of tension-type, migraine, and cluster headaches.

2. Discuss the ethical issues related to withholding enteral feedings from a patient in a persistent vegetative state.

3. Describe the pathophysiology involved in the development of Parkinson's disease.

4. List four nursing interventions for the patient with myasthenia gravis and impaired swallowing.

5. Compare any three of the neurological degenerative disorders described in the chapter, as related to pathophysiology and clinical manifestations.

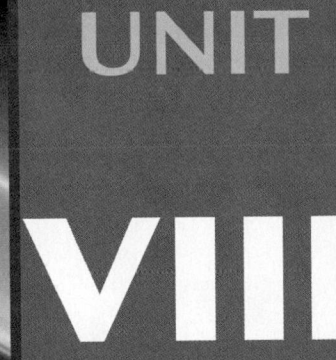

Alterations in Sensory Function

Assessment of Sensory Function

Crisamar J. Anunciado, MSN, FNP, RN

CHAPTER TOPICS

- Anatomy and Physiology of the Eye

- Anatomy and Physiology of the Ear

- Assessment of the Eye

- Assessment of the Ear

The visual and auditory senses have profound relationships to the function of the human body. The eyes are the windows to the soul is an often-quoted adage. It is through vision that an individual experiences the world around him or her. The ears provide senses for the person to have an awareness of his or her environment and an interpretation of the stimuli surrounding him or her. Both of these sensory organ systems are integral to the function and well-being of a person. When either or both of these organ systems have disorders, the person is affected greatly and can require assistance of many types from his or her health care providers.

In this section of this chapter, there will be a discussion of the anatomy and physiology of the eye, as well as important assessment components for a thorough assessment. This includes (a) review of related history, (b) test for visual acuity, (c) evaluation of visual fields, (d) testing ocular movements, (e) testing of cranial nerve reflexes, (f) external eye examination, and (g) ophthalmoscopic examination.

ANATOMY AND PHYSIOLOGY OF THE EYE

Disorders in vision may interfere with the individual's ability to function independently and affect his or her quality of life. The eyes are sensory organs, which receive visual stimuli that are transmitted to the brain for interpretation through the cranial nerve (optic nerve II). Approximately 70 percent of all sensory information reaches the brain through the eyes (Estes, 2006).

A thorough assessment of the eyes will reveal both local and systemic health, which in many cases may help the clinician identify eye and vision problems. It is important to note that the leading causes of blindness include diabetic retinopathy, glaucoma, cataracts, and age-related macular degeneration (Watkinson, 2005). Routine assessment of the eyes may help detect these and other problems early and prevent progression of these diseases that lead to vision problems and even blindness.

The structures and function of the eye are complex yet well understood. In this section are the identified anatomical structures of the eye. In addition, the physiology of each structural component of the eye is provided.

External Eye

The external eye comprises the orbital cavity, eyelashes, eyelids, extraocular muscles, lacrimal gland, and conjunctiva. The eye is an intricate body part and obviously vital to many functions in life.

Because the eyes are delicate organs, many protective structures surround it. The external parts of the eyes are protected from trauma by the bony structure of the orbital cavity. The eyelashes extend across the eyelids to protect the eyes from dust and foreign bodies. The eyelids (**palpebrae**) protect the eyes by covering the anterior aspect of the eyes, distributing tears and lubricating the eyes, protecting the eyes from foreign bodies, and limiting the amount of light that enters the eyes (Estes, 2006).

There are six extraocular muscles that hold the eyes stably in place and control eye movement (Figure 38-1). This includes two oblique muscles and four rectus muscles. These extraocular muscles are innervated by three cranial nerves, namely, oculomotor (cranial nerve III), trochlear (cranial nerve IV), and abducens (cranial nerve VI).

The lacrimal gland is part of the lacrimal apparatus. It is located in the temporal region of the superior eyelid. It moistens the eyes by producing and distributing tears across the conjunctiva and cornea.

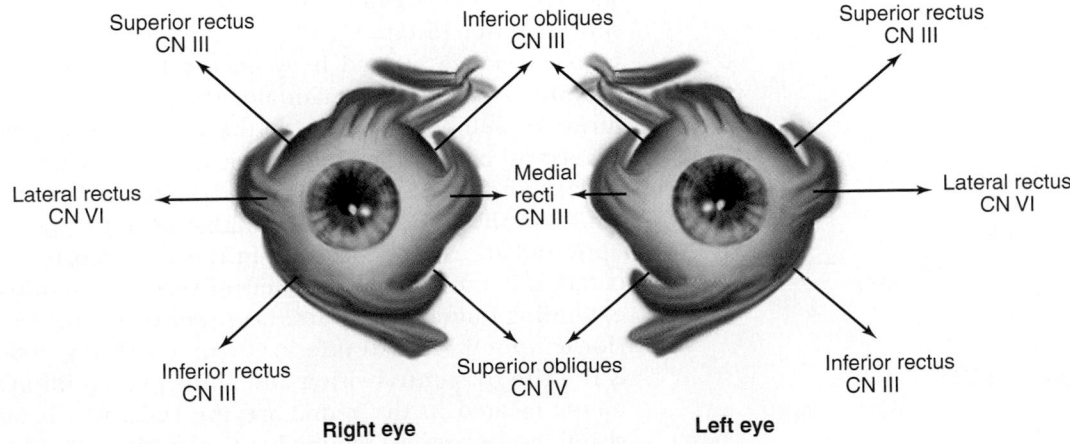

Figure 38-1 Direction of movement of extraocular muscles.

The conjunctiva is the uppermost layer that lines the eyelids and the anterior portion of the eyeball. This is divided into two portions: (a) the palpebral conjunctiva lines the eyelids, and (b) the bulbar conjunctiva covers the sclera. The conjunctiva protects the eyes from injury because of foreign bodies and desiccation.

Internal Eye

There are three coats, or tunics, comprising the internal structures of the eyes: (a) the outer fibrous coat include the sclera and the cornea; (b) the middle tunic includes the choroids, ciliary body, and iris; and (c) the inner nervous tunic is comprised of the retina and its structures.

The sclera appears as the white of the eye. It is a dense, avascular structure that supports the internal structure of the eye, maintaining its size and shape. The cornea is a smooth, avascular, and transparent tissue that is continuous with the sclera, replacing the sclera over the iris and the pupil. It separates the fluid in the aqueous chamber (anterior chamber) from the external environment. It retracts and permits light rays entering the eye through the lens to the retina. It has sensory innervation for pain as it is fed by the trigeminal nerve (cranial nerve V). Stimulation of this nerve causes the **corneal reflex,** a protective blink (Estes, 2006).

The choroids, located posteriorly, and ciliary body, located anteriorly near the iris, comprise the middle layers of the eye. The choroid contains small arteries and veins that provide blood supply to the eye (Estes, 2006). The iris is a circular, pigmented, and contractile muscular disc located at the center of the eye in front of the lens and behind the aqueous humor. The actions of the dilator and sphincter muscles of the iris, through the pupil as its central aperture, control the amount of light reaching the retina. This muscular activity is controlled by the parasympathetic (causes constriction) and sympathetic (causes dilation) nervous system. The **papillary reflex** causing direct and consensual reactions occur because of light stimulation. The optic nerve (cranial nerve II) transmits the stimulation to the brain, and the oculomotor nerve (cranial nerve III) transmits the reflex from the brain to both eyes. The lens is located immediately behind the iris at the papillary opening. It contains no blood vessels, nerves, or connective tissue. It is composed of transparent elastic fibers within the lens capsule. Contraction, or relaxation, of the ciliary bodies attached to the lens changes its thickness, thereby causing the lens to focus and refract light onto the retina (Estes, 2006).

The anterior chamber is located directly behind the cornea. It is filled with a clear, watery substance called aqueous humor, which is continuously produced by the ciliary body and drained through the Schlemm's canal. The movement of fluid in the anterior chamber maintains intraocular pressure of about 15 mm Hg $\pm$ 3 mm Hg. The vitreous humor is a clear gelatinous substance located between the lens and the retina in the posterior chamber of the eye. It maintains the placement of the retina and its structures, as well as the shape of the eyeball (Estes, 2006). The retina is the innermost coat of the eyeball. It is the sensory network of the eye, receiving visual stimuli, and transmitting images to the brain from the optic disc, traveling via the optic nerve, through the optic tract, and then through the optic radiation for processing in the visual cortex (Estes, 2006). Blood circulation is provided by four sets of vessels stemming for the optic disc and extending outward; they are: (a) superior nasal, (b) inferior nasal, (c) superior temporal, and (d) inferior temporal (Estes, 2006). The macula or fovea is the site for central vision and color perception. Other neurosensory elements located in the retina are the rods, which mediate black and white vision, and cones, which mediate color vision.

The nurse can ask the patient the following types of questions:

- Is there any presence of unilateral or bilateral eyelid involvement causing vision impairment (e.g., hordeola or **ptosis** [drooping of the eye])?
- Is there difficulty with vision with one or both eyes? Use of corrective lenses? Description of what type vision impairment, near or distant vision, presence of halos around lights, diplopia, cataract, and floaters.
- Are you having any pain? The nurse can use OLDCART as an acronym for assessing pain in the eye. O = Onset (when did the pain start?), L = Location (identify location of pain, e.g., outside or inside the eye), D = Duration (how long has the pain been going on? Is it continuous or intermittent?), C = Characteristics (what type of pain is it, e.g. sharp, dull, superficial, deep, burning itching?) A = Aggravating factors (what makes it worse?), R = Relieving factors (what makes it better?), and T = Treatment (any treatment done? If so, what type?).
- Do you have any secretions coming from your eye? (e.g., color [clear or yellow], consistency [watery, creamy, or foamy], presence or absence of tears, and conjunctival redness).

Adapted from Estes, M. (2006). Health assessment and physical examination (3rd ed.). New York: Thomson Delmar Learning; Hoyt, K. S., & Haley, R. J. (2005). Innovations in advanced practice: Assessment and management of eye emergencies. Topics in Emergency Medicine, 27(2), 101–117.

ASSESSMENT OF THE EYE

Assessment of the eye by necessity includes the need for obtaining a thorough health assessment. This health history will include such things as the present history of the current eye problem, as well as the past history of the eye. In addition, the family history and personal and social history is essential as well.

Present Eye Problem

The nurse should ask the patient a variety of questions that address the current condition of his or her eye disorders or disease (see Patient Playbook).

Past Medical History

In addition, to the current status of the eye, the nurse must gather information regarding the previous medical history specific to the eye. There are several areas of concern as demonstrated in Box 38-1.

Family History

It is important to determine what types of genetic disorders potentially influence the eyes of the patient. Some of these disorders are listed in Box 38-2.

Personal and Social History

A personal and social history may influence the function of the eyes. Therefore, the nurse must gather information specific to these areas of their patient's condition. The following are areas for the nurse to focus on:

- Employment and history of eye exposure to environment irritants.
- Activities that may cause harm to the eye (e.g., smoking, contact sport, fencing, squash, or motorcycle riding).
- Allergies including which type if it is seasonal, perennial, and other associated symptoms.
- Corrective lenses including which type, duration of use, adequacy of correction, and date of late eye exam.
- Use of protective devices at work, sports, or other activities, which may endanger the eye.

Examination and Findings

Systematic eye assessment includes inspecting and palpating the appendages or extraocular structures surrounding the eye to include the eyebrows and surrounding tissues, then moving inward to test for visual acuity, assessing extraocular eye muscle movement, and lastly, performing an ophthalmoscopic examination of the intraocular structures. The equipment the nurse needs to examine the eye is: cotton wisp, eye cover, ophthalmoscope, penlight, Rosenbaum near vision card, and a Snellen chart.

Inspection and palpation of the eye includes the following examination components: (a) testing for visual acuity; (b) inspection and palpation of external ocular structures; (c) testing for visual fields; (d) testing for extraocular muscle function; and (e) ophthalmoscopic examination.

Visual Acuity

Begin eye assessment by testing for visual acuity. Visual acuity testing is the test of central vision assessing the eye's ability to distinguish small and specific details, using the smallest identifiable object that can be seen at a specific distance

Adapted from Estes, M. (2006). Health assessment and physical examination (3rd ed.). New York: Thomson Delmar Learning; Kuehn, B. M. (2005). Inflammation suspected in eye disorders. Journal of the American Medical Association, 294(1), 31–32.

BOX 38-1

HISTORY OF THE EYE

- History of any trauma or injury to the eye as a whole or specific structure or supporting structure of the eye, description of event surrounding the injury, and attempts at correction and degree of success.
- History of any eye surgery, when it was done, why it was done, and what was the outcome.
- Other chronic illness, which may affect vision (e.g., diabetes, glaucoma, or hypertension)

BOX 38-2

EYE DISORDERS

- Any type of eye cancer (e.g., retinoblastoma)
- Cataracts, diabetes, macular degeneration, color blindness, allergies affecting the eye, and other types of illness that may affect vision
- Strabismus, myopia, and hyperopia, which are disorders of eye refraction

(usually 20 feet using the Snellen's chart or 16 inches using the Rosenbaum near vision card).

Using the Snellen's chart, have the patient stand 20 feet away from the chart. Make sure the room is well-lit. Test each eye individually by covering one eye at a time with gauze or eye cover. Avoid applying pressure to the covered eye. If testing with and without corrective lenses, test without corrective lenses first. With one eye covered, have the patient read the letters on one line moving progressively downward to increasingly smaller lines until the patient could no longer discern all the letters. Record the corresponding visual acuity designated for that line. Repeat test on the second eye and cover the first eye. Record visual acuity findings and analyze results. A measurement of 20/20 vision indicates normal visual acuity. The higher the number to the right of the line, the worse the vision (e.g., 20/100 is worse than 20/60).

If a Snellen's chart is not available, a Rosenbaum near vision chart may be used. Have the patient hold the card at a comfortable distance of about 14 to 16 inches away from his or her face. Test one eye at a time by covering one eye with an eye cover or gauze. Ask the patient to read the letters of the smallest line possible. Record findings and analyze data.

Visual Field Confrontation Test

A visual field confrontation test is used to grossly assess peripheral vision. The nurses uses his or her own normal visual fields to compare with the patient's visual fields. Sit or stand opposite the patient at eye level, about two feet away. Ask the patient to cover the left eye as the nurse covers his or her right eye, which is directly opposite the patient's covered left eye. Then stare at each other's uncovered eye. The nurse extends his or her arm midway between himself or herself and the patient. The nurse holds a small object in his or her hand, such as a pen or penlight, and gradually brings this object centrally from eight different directions: right, left, above, below, and midpoints between these directions. The patient tells the nurse each time when he or she sees the object. The nurse and patient should be able to see the object entering the field of vision at the same time. Repeat this test with the other eye. The confrontation test is crude and imprecise. It can only be considered significant if it is abnormal. For more accurate visual field testing, refer the patient to an eye specialist (Estes, 2006).

Test for Color Vision

Color vision testing of the eyes may be done using color plates or an Ishihara chart, which are available in numerals produced in primary colors (Estes, 2006). When the patient identifies all the colors on six plates, the patient has normal color vision. Red green color blindness is a genetic disease that occurs in men, almost exclusively. Other diseases may also cause color blindness, such as macular degeneration, nutritional deficiency, or pathology of the fovea centralis. For routine color vision testing, check the patient's ability to identify or appreciate primary colors (McCullough, 2005).

Extraocular Eye Examination

The nurse must assess and evaluate the patient's extraocular eye in regard to the location, eyebrows, extraocular structures, eyelids, conjunctiva, cornea, iris, and pupil. Begin the assessment by observing the placement of the eyes in relation to the patient's face. The eyes should be location a third of the way down from the scalp line and approximately one eye's width apart. Inspect the patient's eyebrows. Note their size, shape, extension, and hair texture. If the eyebrow hair is usually coarse or does not extend to the temporal canthus, suspect hypothyroidism. Inspect the surrounding orbital tissue for signs of flakiness, edema (periorbital edema is an abnormal finding possibly due to hypothyroidism or the presence of renal disease), redness (may be a sign of infection or irritation), and puffiness, which may indicate allergies. In addition

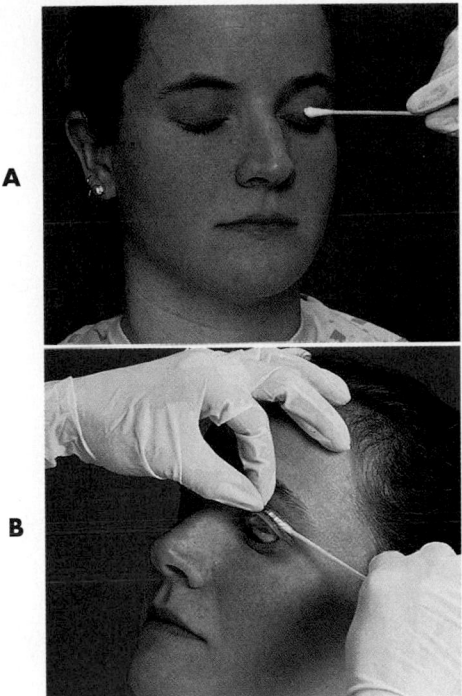

Figure 38-2 Assessing palpebral conjunctiva.

there may be lesions; such as **xanthelasma** (a yellow, lipid-rich plaque present on the eyelids), a **stye** or **hordeolum** (a localized inflammatory swelling of one or more of the glands of the eyelid), or sagging tissue below the orbit, which results from excessive tissue under the eyelid that may cause incomplete eyelid closure. To assess the eyelids, note the position of the globe of the eye (normal, prominent, or sunken). When the eye is open, the upper eyelids should partially cover part of the iris but not the pupil itself. If one eyelid covers the iris more than the other eyelid, consider ptosis, caused by a weakness of the levator muscle or paralysis of the oculomotor nerve (cranial nerve III). Observe the eyelids for excessive tearing or drying. The eyelashes should be turned upward and the eyelid margins should be pink. Also inspect the eyelids for inversion (when the lower lid is turned in toward the globe of the eye), called **entropion** or eversion (when the lower lid is turned away from the globe of the eye called **ectropion**).

Inspect both the bulbar and palpebral conjunctiva. To inspect the bulbar conjunctivae, gently pull the upper and lower eyelids apart without applying pressure to the globe of the eye. Ask the patient to look up, down, and to each side. The bulbar conjunctiva should be clear and free of erythema. Redness or erythema and the presence of cobblestone appearance may indicate allergies or infection (conjunctivitis). A common condition, called pterygium, is an abnormal growth of the conjunctiva extending over the cornea. It may interfere with vision if it crosses over the pupil. Inspect the palpebral conjunctivae (Figure 38-2). Ask the patient to look down. Lift the upper eyelids by holding the eyelashes against the eyebrows. The palpebral conjunctivae should be pink in appearance for Caucasians, red-orange in color for African Americans, and yellow-orange in color for Asian (Americans). Inspect the lid for color changes, erythema, edema, exudates, or foreign bodies (Estes, 2006).

Examine the cornea by shining a penlight tangentially (from both outer sides of the eye) and then directly into the cornea. The cornea should appear clear with no lesions. Test for corneal sensitivity, the trigeminal nerve (cranial nerve V), by touching a wisp of cotton on the cornea. The normal response is a blink, which indicates intact sensory and motor fibers trigeminal and facial nerve (cranial nerve VII), respectively. A condition called **arcus senilis** (lipid deposition on the periphery of the cornea) may be present in patients over the age of 60. This may indicate lipid disorder especially if it appears at a younger age.

Examine the iris pattern (it should be clear and flat), shape (round), size (regular and equal), and color bilaterally. In the presence of excessive pressure caused by acute-angle glaucoma, the iris may be pushed forward, causing the anterior chamber to appear small.

The nurse should test for direct and consensual pupillary response. Dim the lights in the examination room to allow the pupils to dilate. Shine the penlight (20 inches away) directly into one eye. Observe for pupillary constriction on the pupil being tested **(direct response)** and observe for pupillary constriction on the opposite pupil **(consensual response).** Pupillary constriction should be equal and simultaneous in both eyes. Note any inequality and sluggishness of response. Repeat the test on the other pupil. Test the pupils for accommodation by placing your finger approximately four inches from the bridge of the patient's nose. Ask the patient to look at a fixed object in the distance and then look at the nurse's finger. The patient's pupils should constrict when his or her eyes focus on the nurse's finger.

Extraocular Eye Muscle Movement

Assess for intact oculomotor (cranial nerve III), trochlear (cranial nerve IV), abducens (cranial nerve VI) nerves, and the six extraocular muscles (Miller & Newman, 2004). Test for the cardinal fields of gaze (Figure 38-3). Hold the patient's chin to stabilize the head and prevent movement. The nurse asks the patient to watch his or her finger as it moves through the six cardinal fields of gaze. Then he or she asks the patient to look to the extreme lateral or temporal

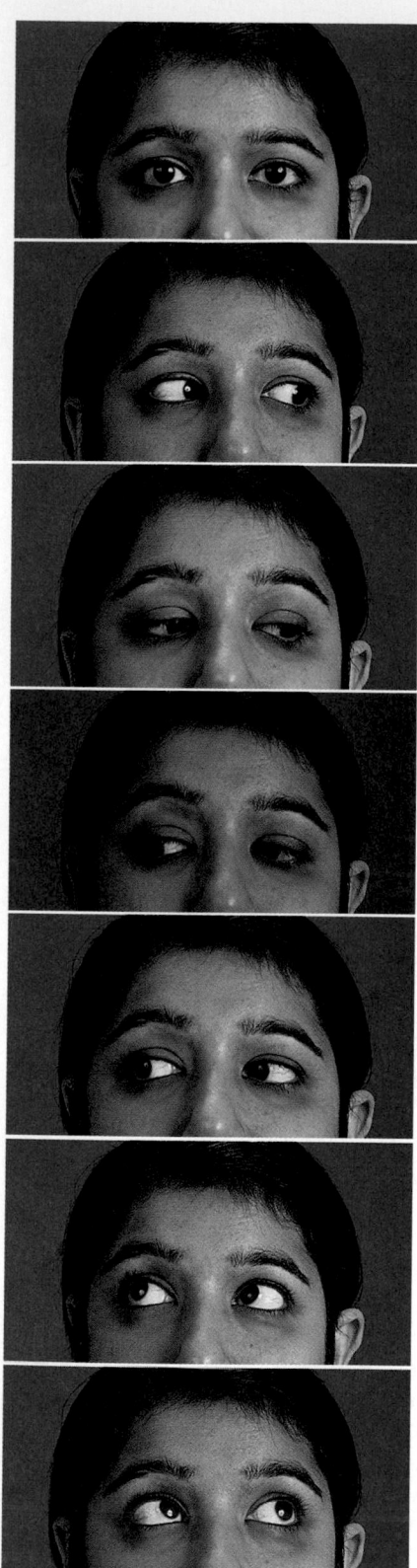

Figure 38-3 Cardinal fields of gaze.

field. Note any oscillating movement or back and forth movements of the eye, which is called **nystagmus.** A slight movement or nystagmus may present in the lateral gaze, but it is abnormal in any other fields of gaze.

Assess for corneal light reflex or Hirschberg test. Ask the patient to focus his or her gaze on a nearby object. Shine a penlight on the bridge of the patient's nose from about one foot away. Light should fall on the same place on the cornea bilaterally. If it does not, the patient may lack extraocular muscle coordination, which may be because of a condition called **strabismus (tropia)** (Estes, 2006).

Perform the cover, uncover test. You only perform this test when an abnormality is detected on one of the two previous tests. Ask the patient to look straight ahead at an object. Cover one eye with the eye cover. Observe the uncovered eye for any movement as it focuses on the object. Then, remove the cover on the other eye and observe any movement on this eye as it focuses on the object. Repeat this test on the other eye. Movement on the covered or uncovered eye may indicate convergent strabismus **(esotropia)** or divergent strabismus **(exotropia).**

Ophthalmoscopic Examination

An ophthalmoscopic examination can be helpful in identifying pathologies of the eye (Figure 38-4). This section describes the specific assessment techniques when using the ophthalmoscope.

Posterior Segment Structures

The funduscopic assessment (CN II) requires the use of a direct ophthalmoscope to assess the structures in the posterior segment of the eye. The ophthalmoscope consists of two parts: the head and the handle. To activate the light source in the head, depress the rheostat button and move it as far as possible. Move the aperture selector to produce the largest beam of light that can be visualized by focusing the beam of light on the palm of the hand. The larger beam is preferred when assessing an average-sized pupil, and the smaller beam makes assessment of a smaller pupil easier. Table 38-1 lists the various apertures of the ophthalmoscope and their uses. The lens selector allows you to choose lenses of varying power for different parts of the assessment. These lenses are marked with red and black numbers, signifying different focal lengths. The 0 lens sits between the red- and black-numbered lenses and has no correction. In some ophthalmoscopes, there is no color designation (red or black) and the lens power is signified by + or − signs in front of the numbers. A + sign is equivalent to black and focuses closer to the ophthalmoscope; a − sign is equivalent to red and focuses further from the instrument. These lenses compensate for the refractive error of both the patient and the nurse.

TABLE 38-1	Apertures of the Ophthalmoscope	
○	Small round light	Used to examine eyes with small, undilated pupils
◯	Large round light	Used for routine eye examinations and examination of dilated eyes
⊞	Grid	Used to assess size and location of funduscopic lesions
▯	Slit light	Assesses anterior eye and determines elevation of funduscopic lesions
●	Green light (red-free filter)	Used to assess retinal hemorrhages (which appear black) and small vessel changes

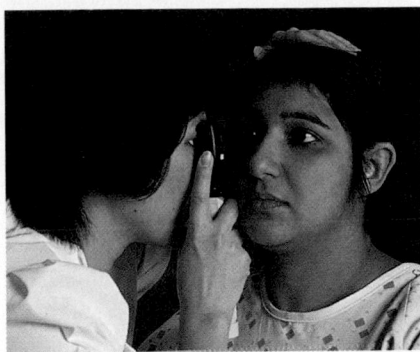

Figure 38-4 Examining with ophthalmoscope.

Retinal Structures

In a darkened room, ask the patient to remove eyeglasses; contact lenses may be left in place.

1. Instruct the patient to look at a distant object across the room. This will help to dilate the eyes.
2. Set the ophthalmoscope on the 0 lens and hold it in front of your right eye with your index finger on the lens selector.
3. From a distance of 8 to 12 inches from the patient and about 15° to the lateral side, shine the light into the patient's right pupil, eliciting a light reflection from the retina; this is called the red reflex.
4. While maintaining the red reflex in view, move closer to the patient and move the lens selector from 0 to the + or black numbers in order to focus on the anterior ocular structures.
5. For optimum visualization, keep the ophthalmoscope within an inch of the patient's eye.
6. At this point, move the lens selector from the + or black numbers, through 0, and into the − or red numbers in order to focus on structures progressively more posterior.
7. Focus on the optic disc at the nasal side of the retina by following any retinal vessels centrally (Figure 38-5).
8. You may need to reverse direction along the vessel if the disc does not appear.
9. Observe the retina for color and lesions, the retinal vessels for configuration and characteristics of their crossing, and the optic disc for color, shape, size, margins, and comparison of cup-to-disc ratio.
10. Describe the size, position, and location of any abnormality. Use the diameter of the disc (DD) as a guide to describe the distance of the abnormality from the optic disc. Use the optic disc as a clock face as a reference point to describe the location of the abnormality. Describe the size of the abnormality in relation to the size of the optic disc.
11. Repeat on the left eye.

Refer to Table 38-2. The red reflex is present. The optic disc is pinkish orange in color, with a yellow-white excavated center known as the physiological cup. The ratio of the cup diameter to that of the entire disc is 1:3. The border of the disc may range from a sharp, round demarcation from the surrounding retina to a more blended border but should be on the same plane as the retina. In general, there are four main vascular branches emanating from the disc, each branch consisting of an arteriole and a venule. The venules are approximately four times the size of the accompanying arterioles and are darker in color. Light

Skills 360°

Developing Skill with an Ophthalmoscope

The nurse practitioner student informs his preceptor that he is having difficulty using an ophthalmoscope. When he shined the light on the last patient's eyes, the appearance was more white than red. He asks you to help him improve his technique. How would you respond to the student?

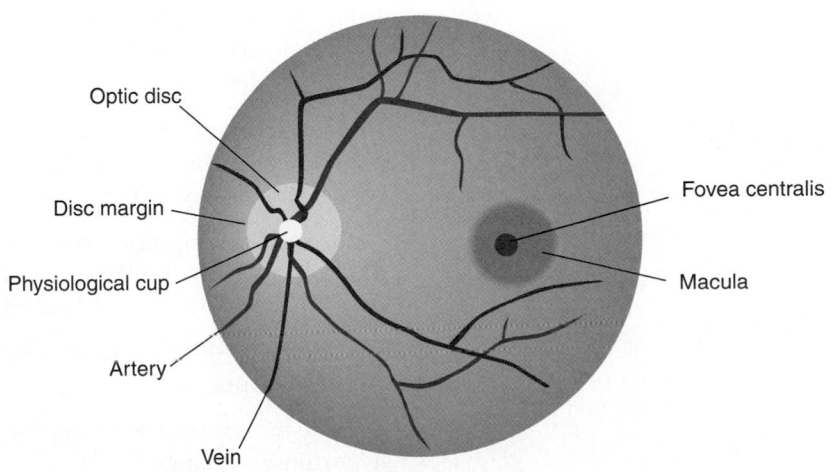

LEFT EYE

Figure 38-5 Optic disk.

TABLE 38-2 Retinal Color Variations	
FINDINGS	**CHARACTERISTICS**
Fair-skinned individual	Retina appears a lighter red-orange color Tessellated appearance of the fundi (pigment does not obscure the choroid vessels)
Dark-skinned individual	Fundi appear darker in color; grayish purple to brownish (from increased pigment in the choroid and retina) No tessellated appearance Choroidal vessels usually obscured
Aging individual	Vessels are straighter and narrower Choroidal vessels are easily visualized Retinal pigment epithelium atrophies and causes the retinal color to become paler

often produces a glistening "light reflex" from the arteriolar vessel. Normal arterial-to-venous width is a ratio of 2:3 or 4:5.

The red reflex is absent.

The presence of cataracts can prevent the red reflex from being observed due to the opacity of the lens.

The red reflex is absent and the pupil appears white.

Leukocoria, or white reflex, is found in retinoblastoma, congenital cataracts, and retinal detachment. This is often referred to as the cat's eye reflex.

The optic disc is pale.

Pallor is due to optic atrophy caused by increased intracranial pressure or from congenital syphilis; an intracranial space-occupying lesion, for example, meningioma; or end-stage glaucoma.

Optic atrophy is abnormal.

Optic atrophy occurs in retinitis pigmentosa. Arteriole narrowing and "bone spicule" are also noted on the fundus. There is a loss of central or peripheral vision, night blindness, and glare sensitivity in this familial condition.

The physiological cup exceeds the normal 1:3 ratio. The disc appears elevated above the plane of the surrounding retina.

Disc edema and loss of vision are caused by the papillitis resulting from optic neuritis. The disc is hyperemic, the margins are blurred, and the disc surface is elevated.

Disc edema and an elevated disc without loss of vision are found in papilledema, which is caused by increased intracranial pressure obstructing return blood flow from the eye. This is also called a "choked disc."

Glaucomatous cupping occurs due to increased intraocular pressure. The physiological cup is enlarged and may extend to the edge of the optic disc. Blood vessels are displaced nasally.

The normal white stripe of retinal arteries appears instead as a copper-colored stripe.

This is the copper wire appearance of retinal arteries characteristic of hypertensive changes.

At the crossing of retinal arteries over veins, the vein is not seen on either side of the overlying artery.

This finding is arteriovenous (A-V) nicking, a sign of retinal arteriolar sclerosis that occurs as the walls become thickened and obscure portions of the veins that lie underneath. This can also occur in hypertension.

Superficial retinal hemorrhages are flame-shaped hemorrhages found in the fundi or they may appear as red hemorrhages with white centers called Roth's spots. These hemorrhages form a pattern related to the nerve fibers that radiate from the optic disc.

These hemorrhages may be due to severe hypertension, occlusion of the central retinal vein, and papilledema. Roth's spots are sometimes associated with infective endocarditis.

Deep retinal hemorrhages, or dot hemorrhages, appear as small red dots or irregular spots in the deep layer of the retina.

Deep retinal hemorrhages can be associated with diabetes mellitus.

Diffuse preretinal hemorrhages occur in the small space between the vitreous and the retina.

Preretinal hemorrhages may occur in conjunction with a sudden increase in intracranial pressure.

Microaneurysms are tiny, round, red dots that can be seen in peripheral and macular areas of the retina.

These dots are small retinal vessels that dilate in diabetic retinopathy.

Neovascularization is the formation of new vessels that are very narrow and disorderly in appearance and may extend into the vitreous. These vessels may bleed, resulting in a loss of vision.

Neovascularization occurs in proliferative diabetic retinopathy.

Fluffy white or gray slightly irregular areas that appear on the retina and are ovoid in shape are abnormal.

Cotton wool spots represent microscopic infarcts of the nerve fiber layer and are due to diabetic or hypertensive retinopathy.

Drusen are small white dots in the fundus that are arranged in an irregular pattern. They may also occur on the optic disc, and may become shiny with calcification.

Drusen are findings of the normal aging process. They may cause loss of vision if they occur in the macular region.

Hard exudates are yellow with distinct borders, and are small unless they coalesce. They are arranged in round, linear, or star-shaped patterns.

Hard exudates are associated with diabetes mellitus or hypertension.

A cleft defect of the choroid and retina is abnormal. The size ranges from medium to large.

Coloboma is a congenital abnormality.

The red-orange retinal reflex is absent in the area of a retinal detachment. The area appears pearly gray and is elevated and wrinkled.

A detached retina may be associated with severe myopia, cataract surgery, or diabetic retinopathy, or it may be caused by trauma.

Fibrous white bands that obscure the retinal vessels are abnormal. Neovascularization may also be present.

These findings occur in proliferative diabetic retinopathy.

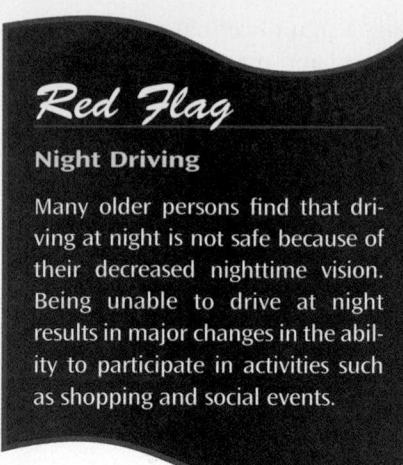

Macula

When the retinal structures and the optic disc have been assessed:

1. Move the ophthalmoscope approximately two disc diameters temporally to view the macula or ask the patient to look at the light. The red-free filter lens of the ophthalmoscope may also be helpful in assessing the macula. Because the macula is not clearly demarcated and because it is very light sensitive, you may have difficulty assessing it. The patient tends to turn away when the light strikes the fovea, making it difficult to assess details of the macular area.

2. Note the fovea centralis and observe for color, shape, and lesions.

3. Repeat with the other eye.

The macula is a darker, avascular area with a pinpoint reflective center known as the fovea centralis.

The retina is pale with the macular region appearing as a cherry-red spot.

This finding is central retinal artery occlusion, an indication of Tay-Sachs disease.

An enlarged macula is abnormal.

Respecting Our Differences

Gerontological Variations

Visual impairments are among the most prevalent chronic conditions in the older patient. Sight provides information to enable the patient to function safely in the environment. Prevention of sensory impairment and resulting handicaps are challenges for patients and health care providers.

During the aging process, the eye undergoes significant changes. First, by the age of 42, the lens cortex becomes more dense, compromising its ability to change shape and focus. This condition, presbyopia, is responsible for farsightedness and the need for bifocals. Next, there is a tendency for the lens to yellow and become cloudy. This change impairs a person's ability to discern various colors, especially blues and greens. In addition, pupils become smaller so that the amount of light reaching the retina is reduced. As a consequence, elderly individuals need more light to see and their eyes take longer to accommodate to darkness and glare. Finally, a decrease in tear production predisposes the individual to corneal irritation and conjunctivitis.

Cataracts, age-related macular degeneration, and glaucoma are the most common visual problems among elderly persons. Cataracts involve opacity and yellowing of the lens, which results in dimmed and blurred vision. Cataracts can be surgically removed.

Age-related macular degeneration is loss of central vision. Individuals experiencing this change require the use of magnification to compensate for visual loss. Systemic diseases that aggravate macular degeneration include diabetes mellitus and hypertension.

Glaucoma may cause total blindness if not treated. Increased intraocular pressure and inability of aqueous humor to flow out into collecting channels places pressure on the optic nerve. Early detection of glaucoma is critical; screening is recommended for all adults over age 40.

Inspection of the eyelids of the older individual often reveals slightly drooping upper and lower lids. The globe appears to be deeper in the socket, and the lacrimal gland may be visible because of lost subcutaneous fat around the eye (Watkinson, 2005).

Macular edema is caused by the leakage of fluid from retinal blood vessels. This can occur in diabetes mellitus, hypertension, age-related macular degeneration, and retinal blood vessel obstruction.

Sharply defined, small red spots are found in and around the macula.

These microaneurysms are pathognomonic of diabetes mellitus.

Macular borders are blurred, with a few spots of pigment near the macula; a hole may appear to be present in the center of the region, or a hemorrhage may have occurred.

This finding is characteristic of age-related macular degeneration. Hemorrhages, patches of retina atrophy, and pigmented areas may also be associated with this condition.

ANATOMY AND PHYSIOLOGY OF THE EAR

Ear

The ear has three sections: the external, the middle, and the inner ear.

External Ear

The external ear, which is also called the **auricle** or **pinna,** extends through the auditory canal to the tympanic membrane. The auricle receives sound waves and funnels them through the auditory canal to produce vibrations on the tympanic membrane. The auricle is composed of cartilage.

The external auditory canal is an S-shaped tube approximately 2.5 cm in length, with the outer third made up of cartilage and the remainder of bone covered by a thin layer of skin (Figure 38-6). The canal is lined with tiny hairs and modified sweat glands that secrete a thick, waxlike substance called **cerumen,**

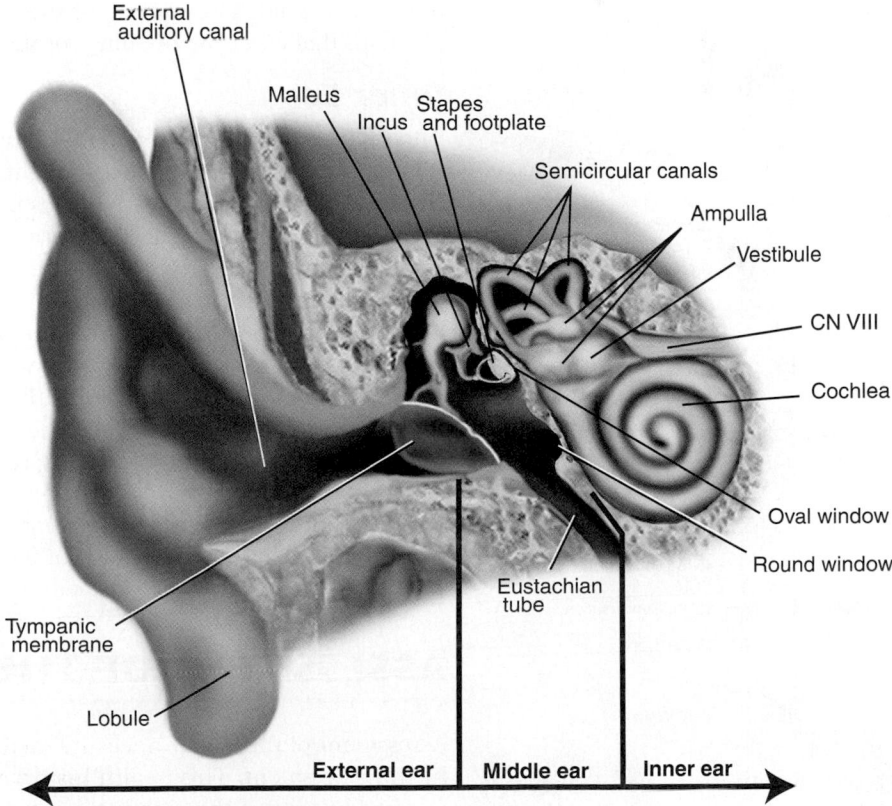

Figure 38-6 Cross-section of the ear.

which can vary in consistency from dry and flaky to wet and waxy. Cerumen ranges from a pale, honey color in light-skinned individuals to dark-brown or black in dark-skinned people.

Middle Ear

The middle ear is composed of the tympanic membrane, the ossicles, and the tympanic cavity. The cavity is an air-filled compartment that separates the external ear from the internal ear. The tympanic membrane, which is circular or oval and is about an inch in diameter, sits in an oblique position in the external canal so that it leans slightly forward. The rim of the tympanic membrane is called the annulus, the superior portion is the pars flaccida, and the tighter, largest area of the drum is the pars tensa.

The **ossicles** are three tiny bones—the malleus (hammer), the incus (anvil), and the stapes (stirrup)—that play a crucial role in the transmission of sound. The long handle, or manubrium, of the malleus extends downward from the short process and meets the tympanic membrane at the umbo. The stapes is held against the wall of the tympanic membrane at the oval window by tiny ligaments. The head of the malleus articulates with the incus, which in turn articulates with the stapes; they work as a unit when the tympanic membrane begins to vibrate. Vibrations set up in the tympanic membrane by sound waves reaching it through the external auditory canal are transmitted to the inner ear by rapid movement of the ossicles.

The tensor tympani and the stapedius are two tiny muscles involved in movement of the ossicles. The tensor tympani maintains the tension of the tympanic membrane and pulls the malleus inward when it contracts. The stapedius works in opposition by pulling the stapes outward. This coordinated movement is an important mechanism in reducing the intensity of loud sounds that might otherwise result in serious damage to hearing receptors in the inner ear.

The middle ear is connected to the nasopharynx by the auditory or **eustachian tube,** which serves as a channel through which air pressure within the cavity can be equalized with air pressure outside to maintain normal hearing. Equalization of pressure is aided by yawning or swallowing, which causes the opening of valve-like flaps that cover the openings of the eustachian tubes.

Inner Ear

The inner ear is a complex, closed, fluid-filled system of interconnecting tubes called the **labyrinth,** which is essential for hearing and equilibrium. The labyrinth has bony and membranous portions. The bony labyrinth is composed of the cochlea, the semicircular canals, and the vestibule. The vestibule is located between the cochlea and the semicircular canals and is important in both hearing and balance. The three semicircular canals located at right angles to each other provide balance and equilibrium for the body. The cochlea is a snail-shaped structure made up of three compartments. The first two compartments contain perilymph, and the third contains endolymph. As sound waves travel through the ear, they cause the perilymph and the endolymph to vibrate, stimulating the thousands of hearing-receptor cells of the organ of Corti. Nearby nerve fibers transmit impulses along the cochlear branch of the vestibulocochlear nerve to the brain, allowing us to hear. The human ear is capable of hearing within a frequency range of 20 to 20,000 Hz, and a decibel range of 0 to 140. Figure 38-7 illustrates the decibel levels of various commonly heard sounds.

ASSESSMENT OF THE EAR

Assessment of the ear by necessity includes the need for obtaining a thorough health assessment. This health history will include such things as the past and present history of the current ear problem, as well as, family, personal, and social history.

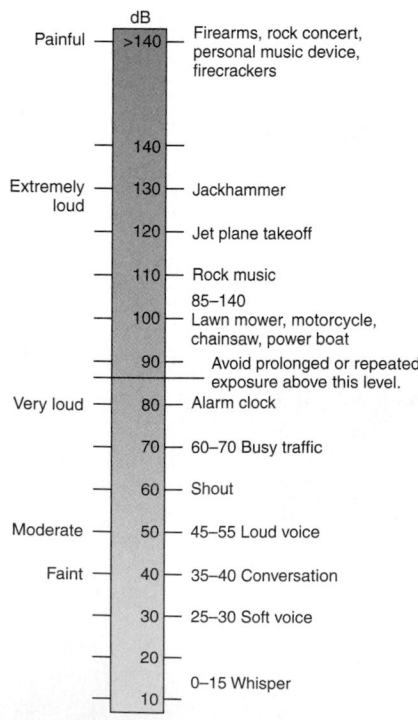

Figure 38-7 Decibel scale of frequently heard sounds. *Courtesy of Singular Publishing Group.*

Present History of Ear Problem

The most common complaints of long-term ear problems are because of hearing loss and tinnitus. Pain, discharge, and dizziness or vertigo are often short-term conditions (Estes, 2006). See the Patient Playbook for an assessment of the ear for potential disorders.

Past Medical History

In addition, to the current status of the ear, the nurse must gather information regarding the previous medical history specific to the ear. There are several areas of concern as demonstrated in Box 38-3.

Family History

It is important to determine what types of genetic disorders potentially influence the ears of the patient. Some of these disorders are hearing loss, Ménière's disease, allergies, or renal disease.

PATIENT PLAYBOOK

Assessing Ear Problems

The nurse can ask the following questions to further examine problems of the ear:

- Dizziness or vertigo
1. Assess for onset and duration of dizziness or vertigo.
2. Describe characteristics of dizziness to include type of motion, movement, changes in position, and body involvement (e.g., head or neck movement).
3. Ask patient if there are any associated symptoms (e.g., nausea, vomiting, ringing in the ears, unsteady gait, loss of balance, falling, vision changes, or hearing loss).
4. Ask patient any alleviating or relieving factors.
5. Note any medications taken, prescription and nonprescription medications, which may cause a side effect of dizziness or vertigo.
- Changes in or loss of hearing
1. Assess for onset and duration (constant hearing loss or intermittent).
2. Ask patient if it is it bilateral or unilateral, if the patient can hear loud or soft sounds, and if hearing loss is partial or complete.
3. Note any associated symptoms (i.e., ear pain, tinnitus, drainage, swelling, or fever).
4. Ask patient if he or she noted any alleviating or aggravating factors.

5. List any medications taken, prescription, and nonprescription medications, which may cause a side effect of changes in hearing or hearing loss.
- **Otorrhea** (liquid discharge or drainage from the ear)
1. Ask patient if the drainage is unilateral or bilateral.
2. Discuss characteristics of secretions (e.g., yellowish, purulent, bloody, foul odor, or watery).
3. Ask if there are any other associated symptoms (e.g., fever, headache, hearing loss, dizziness, or upper respiratory infections).
4. Discuss if any aggravating or alleviating factors.
5. Ask about timing, following trauma, and if it is constant or intermittent draining).
- **Otalgia** or ear pain
1. Ask patient about onset and duration of pain (i.e., constant, intermittent).
2. Note if pain is localized, unilateral or bilateral, and if it is radiating to the jaw or pinna region.
3. Ask about the type of pain (i.e., aching, dull, sharp, or stabbing).
4. Ask patient if there is any associated symptoms (e.g., hearing loss, fever, drainage, tinnitus, sore throat, dizziness, or fever).
5. Discuss any aggravating or relieving factors.

Adapted from: Estes, M. (2006). Health assessment and physical examination (3rd ed.). New York: Thomson Delmar Learning.

Skills 360°

The Patient with Decreased Hearing

Observe the patient for signs of hearing difficulty and deafness during the health history and physical exam. Turning the head to facilitate hearing, lip reading, speaking in a loud voice, or asking you to write words are signs of hearing difficulty. If the patient is wearing a hearing aid, ask if it is turned on, when the batteries were last changed, and if the device causes any irritation of the ear canal.

Personal and Social History

A personal and social history may influence the function of the ears. Therefore, the nurse must gather information specific to these areas of their patient's condition. In addition, the nurse can focus on employment and history of exposure to environment noise and use or lack of use of protective hearing devices.

Examination and Findings

Physical assessment of the ear consists of three parts:
1. Auditory screening (CN VIII)
2. Inspection and palpation of the external ear
3. Otoscopic assessment

Auditory Screening

Voice-Whisper Test

The following steps are necessary for a voice-whisper test:
1. Instruct the patient to occlude one ear with a finger.
2. Stand 2 feet behind the patient's other ear and whisper a two-syllable word or phrase that is evenly accented.
3. Ask the patient to repeat the word or phrase.
4. Repeat the test with the other ear.

The patient should be able to repeat words whispered from a distance of 2 feet.

The patient is unable to repeat the words correctly or states that he or she was unable to hear anything.

This indicates a hearing loss in the high-frequency range that may be caused by excessive exposure to loud noises (see Skills 360° feature).

Tuning Fork Tests

Weber and Rinne tests help to determine whether the type of hearing loss the patient is experiencing is conductive or sensorineural. In order to understand how these tests are evaluated, it is important to know the difference between air and bone conduction. Air conduction refers to the transmission of sound through the ear canal, tympanic membrane, and ossicular chain to the cochlea and auditory nerve. Bone conduction refers to the transmission of sound through the bones of the skull to the cochlea and auditory nerve.

Weber Test

To do a Weber test:
1. Hold the handle of a 512-Hz (vibrates 512 cycles per second to create a specific frequency) tuning fork and strike the tines on the ulnar border of the palm to activate it.
2. Place the stem of the fork firmly against the middle of the patient's forehead, on the top of the head at the midline, or on the front teeth (Figure 38-8).
3. Ask the patient if the sound is heard centrally or toward one side.

The patient should perceive the sound equally in both ears or "in the middle." No lateralization of sound is known as a negative Weber test.

The sound lateralizes to the affected ear.

This occurs with unilateral conductive hearing loss because the sound is being conducted directly through the bone to the ear. Conductive hearing loss occurs when there are external or middle ear disorders such as impacted cerumen, perforation of the tympanic membrane, serum or pus in the middle ear, or a fusion of the ossicles.

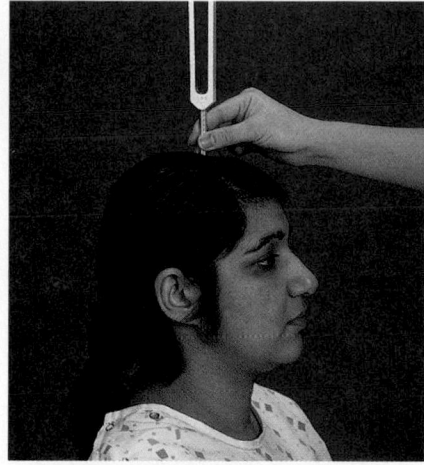

Figure 38-8 Weber test.

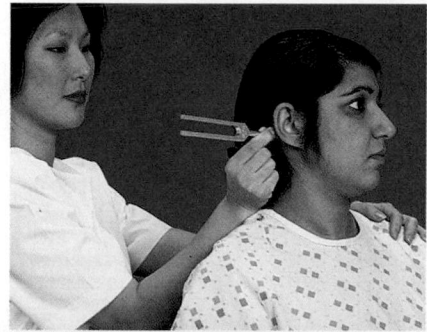

A

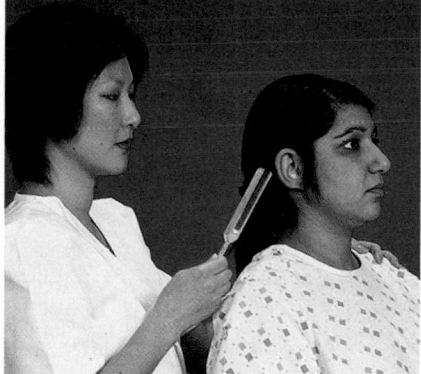

B

Figure 38-9 Rinne test.

The sound lateralizes to the unaffected ear.

This occurs with sensorineural loss related to nerve damage in the impaired ear. Sensorineural hearing loss occurs when there is a disorder in the inner ear, the auditory nerve, or the brain; disorders include congenital defects, effects of ototoxic drugs, and repeated or prolonged exposure to loud noise.

Rinne Test

To do a Rinne test:

1. Stand behind or to the side of the patient and strike the tuning fork.
2. Place the stem of the tuning fork against the patient's right mastoid process to test bone conduction (Figure 38-9A).
3. Instruct the patient to indicate if the sound is heard.
4. Ask the patient to tell you when the sound stops.
5. When the patient says that the sound has stopped, move the tuning fork, with the tines facing forward, in front of the right auditory meatus, and ask the patient if the sound is still heard. Note the length of time the patient hears the sound (testing air conduction) (Figure 38-9B).
6. Repeat the test on the left ear.

Air conduction is heard twice as long as bone conduction when the patient hears the sound through the external auditory canal (air) after it is no longer heard at the mastoid process (bone). This is denoted as AC>BC.

The patient reports hearing the sound longer through bone conduction; that is, bone conduction is equal to or greater than air conduction.

This occurs when there is a conductive hearing loss resulting from disease, obstruction, or damage to the outer or middle ear.

Bone conduction is prolonged in the context of a normal tympanic membrane, patent eustachian tube, and middle ear disease.

These findings are typical of otosclerosis.

External Ear

Inspection

To perform an inspection of the external ear:

1. Inspect the ears and note their position, color, size, and shape.
2. Note any deformities, nodules, inflammation, or lesions.
3. Note color, consistency, and amount of cerumen.

The ear should match the flesh color of the rest of the patient's skin and should be positioned centrally and in proportion to the head. The top of the ear should cross an imaginary line drawn from the outer canthus of the eye to the occiput. Cerumen should be moist and not obscure the tympanic membrane. There should be no foreign bodies, redness, drainage, deformities, nodules, or lesions.

The ears are pale, red, or cyanotic.

Vasomotor disorders, fevers, hypoxemia, and cold weather can account for various color changes.

The ears are abnormally large or small.

These abnormalities can be congenitally determined or the result of trauma. Frequently, this is accompanied by an absent external ear canal and middle ear, but an intact inner ear.

An ear that is grossly misshapen, damaged, or mutilated is abnormal.

Blunt trauma, such as in contact sports, to the side of the head is usually the cause.

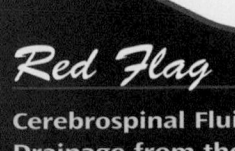

An external ear that is erythematous, edematous, warm to the touch, and painful is abnormal.

Perichondritis is an inflammation of the fibrous connective tissue that overlies the cartilage of the ear.

A tumor on the external ear is abnormal.

Basal cell and squamous cell carcinoma are the most common external ear tumors. Prolonged sunlight exposure is a predisposing factor for these tumors.

Purulent drainage is abnormal.

Purulent drainage usually indicates an infection.

Clear or bloody drainage is present (see Red Flag feature).

Clear or bloody drainage may be due to cerebrospinal fluid leaking as a result of head trauma or surgery.

A hematoma behind an ear over the mastoid bone is abnormal. This is called Battle's sign and indicates head trauma to the temporal bone of the skull.

A hard, painless, irregular-shaped nodule on the pinna is abnormal.

Tophi are uric acid nodules and may indicate the presence of gout. These are usually located near the helix. Many other nodules are benign fibromas.

Sebaceous cysts are abnormal.

Sebaceous cysts or retention cysts form as a result of the blockage of the ducts to the sebaceous gland.

Lymph nodes anterior to the tragus or overlying the mastoid are abnormal.

Lymph nodes may be enlarged due to a malignancy or an infection such as external otitis.

Palpation

To palpate the external ear:
1. Palpate the auricle between the thumb and the index finger, noting any tenderness or lesions. If the patient has ear pain, assess the unaffected ear first, then cautiously assess the affected ear.
2. Using the tips of the index and middle fingers, palpate the mastoid tip, noting any tenderness.
3. Using the tips of the index and middle fingers, press inward on the tragus, noting any tenderness.
4. Hold the auricle between the thumb and the index finger and gently pull up and down, noting any tenderness.

The patient should not complain of pain or tenderness during palpation.

Auricular pain or tenderness is noted.

Auricular pain is a common finding in external ear infection and is called acute otitis externa.

There is tenderness over the mastoid process.

Mastoid tenderness is associated with middle ear inflammation or mastoiditis.

The tragus is edematous or sensitive.

This finding may indicate inflammation of the external or middle ear.

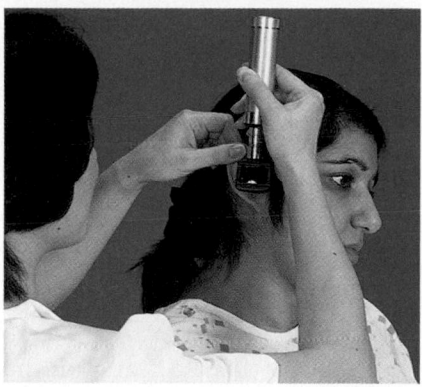

Figure 38-10 Assessment with otoscope.

Otoscopic Assessment

The steps in an otoscopic assessment are:

1. Ask the patient to tip the head away from the ear being assessed.
2. Select the largest speculum that will comfortably fit the patient.
3. Hold the otoscope securely in the dominant hand, with the head held downward and the handle held like a pencil between the thumb and the forefinger.
4. Rest the back of the dominant hand on the right side of the patient's head (Figure 38-10).
5. Use the ulnar aspect of the free hand to pull the right ear in a manner that will straighten the canal. In adults and in children over 3 years old, pull the ear up and back.
6. If hair obstructs visualization, moisten the speculum with water or a water-soluble lubricant.
7. If wax obstructs visualization, it should be removed only by a skilled practitioner, either by curettement (if the cerumen is soft or the tympanic membrane is ruptured) or by irrigation (if the cerumen is dry and hard and the tympanic membrane is intact).
8. Slowly insert the speculum into the canal, looking at the canal as the speculum passes.
9. Assess the canal for inflammation, exudates, lesions, and foreign bodies.
10. Continue to insert the speculum into the canal, following the path of the canal until the tympanic membrane is visualized.
11. If the tympanic membrane is not visible, gently pull the pinna slightly farther in order to straighten the canal to allow adequate visualization.
12. Identify the color, light reflex, umbo, the short process, and the long handle of the malleus. Note the presence of perforations, lesions, bulging or retraction of the tympanic membrane, dilatation of blood vessels, bubbles, or fluid.
13. Ask the patient to close the mouth, pinch the nose closed, and blow gently while you observe for movement of the tympanic membrane. A pneumatic attachment may be used to create this movement if one is available.
14. Gently withdraw the speculum and repeat the process with the left ear.

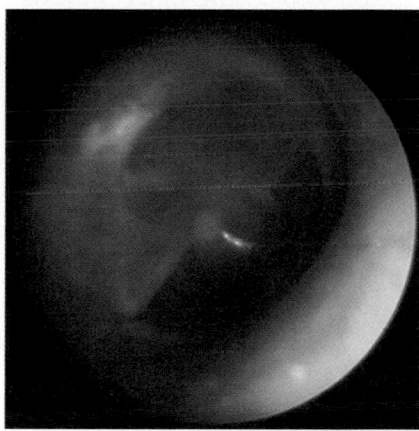

Figure 38-11 Normal tympanic membrane. *Courtesy of Singular Publishing Group, Inc.*

The ear canal should have no redness, swelling, tenderness, lesions, drainage, foreign bodies, or scaly surface areas. Cerumen varies in amount, consistency, and color. The tympanic membrane should be pearly gray with clearly defined landmarks and a distinct cone-shaped light reflex extending from the umbo toward the anteroinferior aspect of the membrane. This light reflex is seen at 5 o'clock in the right ear and at 7 o'clock in the left ear. Blood vessels should be visible only on the periphery, and the membrane should not bulge, be retracted, or have any evidence of fluid behind it (Figure 38-11). The tympanic membrane should move when the patient blows against resistance.

A foreign body in the external auditory canal (EAC) is abnormal.

Both adults and children can have foreign bodies in the EAC. Some objects are more difficult to remove than others; for instance, vegetables in the EAC can swell with time and make removal challenging.

Tympanostomy tubes, or PE tubes (pressure equalization) are surgically placed for prolonged otitis media with effusion (OME). The tubes allow drainage of the effusion, normal vibration of the ossicles, and equalization of pressures across the tympanic membrane. When a myringotomy has been performed with tympanostomy tube placement, the presence of the tubes (or lack of) needs to be documented.

A painful, boil-like pustule in the EAC is abnormal.

Furunculosis is an infection of a hair follicle. EAC edema and otorrhea may also be present.

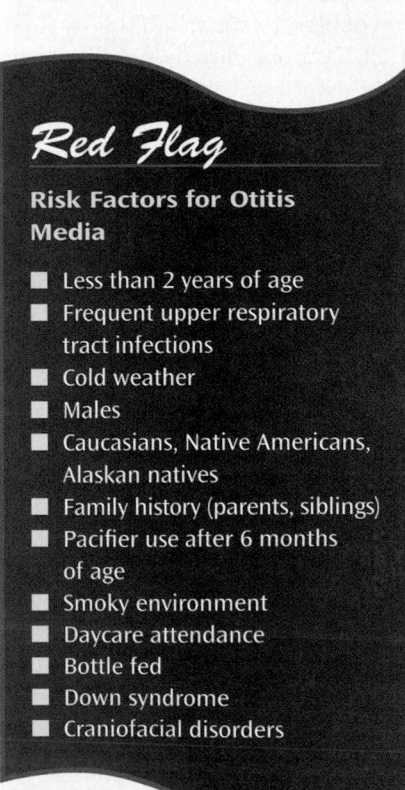

Black or brown spores, yellow or orange spores, or white fluffy hyphae in the EAC are abnormal.

Prolonged use of aural antibiotics can cause otomycosis, or a fungal infection, in the ear. Different strains of fungi cause the variations in appearance.

Bony, hard lesions in the deep EAC are abnormal.

These are exostoses. Patients who frequently participate in cold-water activities are at risk for developing them. If an exostosis becomes large enough, it can block the EAC and trap debris between it and the tympanic membrane. This can lead to infection.

Exquisite pain accompanied by erythema deep into the EAC and on the tympanic membrane, along with serous-filled blebs, is abnormal.

This describes viral bullous myringitis. This can easily be mistaken for acute otitis media.

The appearance of chalk patches on the tympanic membrane is abnormal.

These are calcifications found in myringosclerosis, which can occur after tympanic membrane surgery, infection, or inflammation. Myringosclerosis can be associated with a gradual hearing loss. Involvement of the entire tympanic membrane is called tympanosclerosis.

Air bubbles on the tympanic membrane are abnormal.

Conditions such as coryza and influenza and changes in extratympanic pressure (such as in scuba diving, airplane travel) can lead to eustachian tube failure.

The presence of blood in the middle ear is abnormal.

Hemotympanum occurs as a result of trauma to the head. The tympanic membrane can have a bluish hue or can be red in appearance.

A severely retracted tympanic membrane has exaggerated landmarks. Mobility of the tympanic membrane is decreased.

Retraction of the tympanic membrane can occur when the intratympanic membrane pressures are reduced, as in eustachian tube blockage caused by otitis media with effusion or allergies. Repeated negative pressure in the middle ear sucks in the tympanic membrane and leads to retractions. Over time, keratinized epithelial debris deposits itself in these retraction pockets and leads to ossicle fixation. This leads to cholesteatoma. A foul smelling ear discharge, as well as deafness, may accompany cholesteatoma.

There is redness, swelling, narrowing, and pain of the external ear. Drainage may be present.

Acute otitis externa is caused by infectious organisms or allergic reactions. Predisposing factors include excessive moisture in the ear related to swimming, trauma from cleansing the ears with a sharp instrument, or allergies to substances such as hairspray (see Skills 360° feature).

Hard, dry, and very dark yellow-brown cerumen is abnormal.

Old cerumen is harder and drier, and may become impacted if not removed.

The tympanic membrane is red, with decreased mobility and possible bulging (Figure 38-12).

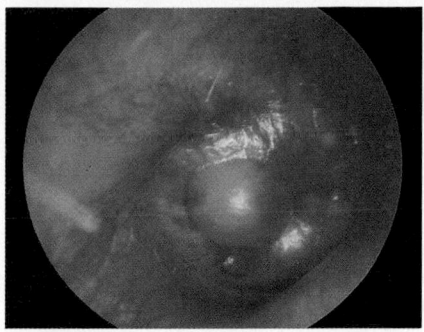

Figure 38-12 Acute otitis media. *Courtesy of Singular Publishing Group, Inc.*

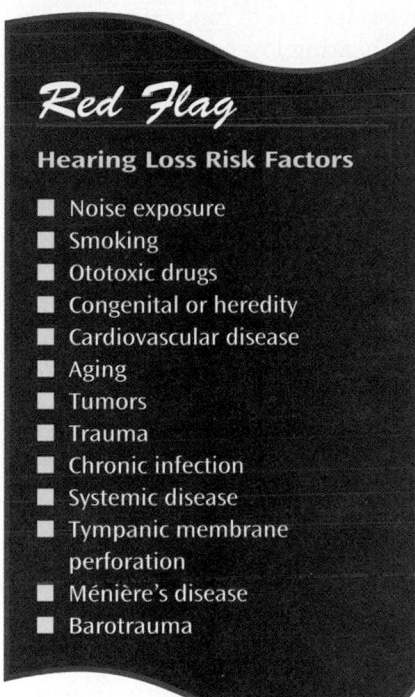

Red Flag

Hearing Loss Risk Factors

- Noise exposure
- Smoking
- Ototoxic drugs
- Congenital or heredity
- Cardiovascular disease
- Aging
- Tumors
- Trauma
- Chronic infection
- Systemic disease
- Tympanic membrane perforation
- Ménière's disease
- Barotrauma

This is acute otitis media (AOM), or an inflammation of the middle ear. Pain and fever may accompany the ear infection. Otalgia, fever, decreased hearing, irritability, disturbed sleep, and otorrhea may accompany the middle ear infection. *Streptococcus pneumoniae, Haemophilus influenzae,* and *Moraxella catarrhalis* are the major pathogens that cause AOM.

Along with a bulging eardrum and decreased mobility, the landmarks are diffuse, displaced, or absent (see Red Flag feature).

The late stage of acute otitis media causes landmarks to become progressively obscured.

Amber-yellow fluid on the tympanic membrane is abnormal. It may be accompanied by a fluid line or bubbles behind the membrane. Bulging may be present and mobility of the eardrum may be decreased. The patient may complain of ear popping, pain, and decreased hearing.

Otitis media with effusion, or serous otitis media, can be caused by allergies, infections, and a blocked eustachian tube. Table 38-3 compares AOM, OME, and otitis externa.

The tympanic membrane appears to have a darkened area or a hole.

A perforated eardrum is caused by untreated ear infection secondary to increasing pressure. Trauma to the ear canal can also cause a perforation (see Red Flag feature).

The tympanic membrane is pearly gray and has dark patches.

These patches are usually old perforations in the tympanic membrane.

The tympanic membrane is pearly gray and has dense white plaques.

These plaques represent calcific deposits of scarring of the tympanic membrane from frequent past episodes of otitis media.

TABLE 38-3 **Comparison of AOM, OME, and Otitis Externa**

	AOM	OME	OTITIS EXTERNA
TM color	Diffuse red, dilated peripheral vessels	Yellowish	WNL
TM appearance	Bulging	Bubbles, fluid line	WNL
TM landmarks	Decreased	Retracted with prominent malleus	WNL
Movement of tragus	Painless	Painless	Painful
Hearing	WNL/decreased	WNL/decreased	WNL
EAC	WNL	WNL	Erythematous, edematous

KEY CONCEPTS

- The eyes are sensory organs, which receive visual stimuli that are transmitted to the brain for interpretation through the cranial nerve (optic nerve II).
- The external parts of the eyes are protected from trauma by the bony structure of the orbital cavity.
- There are three coats or tunics comprising the internal structures of the eyes.
- The retina is the innermost coat of the eyeball, and it is the sensory network of the eye.
- The health history of the eye includes such things as the present history of the current eye problem, as well as the past history of the eye.
- In an assessment of the eye, it is important to determine what types of genetic disorders potentially influence the eyes of the patient.
- Systematic eye assessment includes inspecting and palpating the appendages or extraocular structures surrounding the eye.

- Visual acuity testing is the test of central vision assessing the eye's ability to distinguish small and specific details.
- A visual field confrontation test is used to grossly assess peripheral vision.
- Assessing extraocular eye muscle movement involves cranial nerves III, IV, and VI.
- An ophthalmoscopic examination can be helpful in identifying pathologies of the eye.
- The most common complaints of long-term ear problems are due to hearing loss and tinnitus. Pain, discharge, and dizziness or vertigo are often short-term conditions of the ear.
- The ossicles are three tiny bones that play a crucial role in the transmission of sound.
- Physical assessment of the ear consists of auditory screening, inspection, and palpation of the external ear and otoscopic assessment.

REVIEW QUESTIONS

1. Mr. Carter has a disorder of his palpebrae, which are his:
   1. Eyelashes
   2. Eyelids
   3. Conjunctiva
   4. Lacrimal glands

2. The extraocular muscles are innervated by which cranial nerves?
   1. Cranial nerves II, III, and VI
   2. Cranial nerves II, IV, and VI
   3. Cranial nerves III, IV, and VI
   4. Cranial nerves II, III, and IV

3. The parasympathetic nervous system causes the pupils to:
   1. Constrict
   2. Dilate
   3. Diverge
   4. Converge

4. Mrs. Johanson has a congenital defect that causes her to have color vision problems. This is due to a dysfunction of her:
   1. Rods
   2. Pupils
   3. Sclera
   4. Cones

5. The Snellen chart is responsible for testing:
   1. Pupil constriction
   2. Sensitivity to light
   3. Visual acuity
   4. Depth perception

6. Mr. Treat has recently experienced a yellow, lipid rich plaque lesion on the eyelid, which is labeled:
   1. Stye
   2. Xanthelasma
   3. Arcus senilis
   4. Entropion

7. After a head injury, Mr. Barnett experiences a left eye that does not constrict when light is shined in the right eye. This is labeled a problem associated with:
   1. Direct response
   2. Indirect response
   3. Consensual response
   4. Accommodation

8. When using the ophthalmoscope, the red numbers indicate:
   1. Anterior eye problems
   2. Posterior eye problems
   3. Glaucoma tendencies
   4. Pupil abnormalities

Continued

REVIEW QUESTIONS—cont'd

9. Mr. Lever has a purulent drainage coming from his left ear. This is described as:
   1. Otalgia
   2. Cerumen
   3. Vertigo
   4. Otorrhea

10. Mrs. Studer has a potential conduction problem of both ears. A test is performed that evaluates whether sounds are heard centrally or on one side. This is what type of test?
    1. Weber test
    2. Rinne test
    3. Voice-whisper test
    4. Otitis media

REVIEW ACTIVITIES

1. Select three to five patients and assess their eyes with an ophthalmoscope.

4. Perform nerve conduction testing with three patients' ears.

2. Compare and contrast four patients' pupil responses to both direct and indirect light stimulation.

5. Describe the shapes of four patients' ears.

3. Describe the red light reflex and the shape of the optic disk in an eye exam on a patient.

Visit the Contemporary Medical-Surgical Nursing online companion resource at www.delmarhealthcare.com for additional content and study aids. Click on Online Companions then select the Nursing discipline.

Visual Dysfunction: Nursing Management

Karen Wikoff, RN, DNS

CHAPTER TOPICS

- Ocular Movement Disorders
- Visual Acuity
- Refraction
- Presbyopia
- Color Perception

- Inflammatory and Infectious Ocular Diseases
- Ocular Disorders Resulting from Neurological Disorders
- Low Vision and Blindness

KEY TERMS

Amblyopia
Aphakic vision
Astigmatism
Blepharitis
Cryopexy
Diplopia
Emmetropia
Entropia
Enucleation
Exotropia (wall eyes)
Hyperopia (farsightedness)
Hypotany
Keratometry
Myopia (nearsightedness)
Nystagmus
Papilledema
Presbyopia
Ptosis
Strabismus

The eyes are complex organic structures and have a variety of intricate physiological elements (Figure 39-1). The visual fields of the eye are normally predictable and exist in specific pathways (Figure 39-2). Visual disturbances can range from minor disturbances easily managed with corrective lens to severe disturbances requiring complex interventions, including surgery. Whether the disturbances are minor, severe, or somewhere in between, the patient must adapt to the visual restrictions in activities of daily living. Dysfunction in vision can be the result of abnormalities in ocular movement, visual acuity, refraction, accommodation, color perception, and inflammatory and infectious diseases. Vision dysfunction may occur secondary to other pathological considerations, such as papilledema in neurological disorders and diabetic retinopathy.

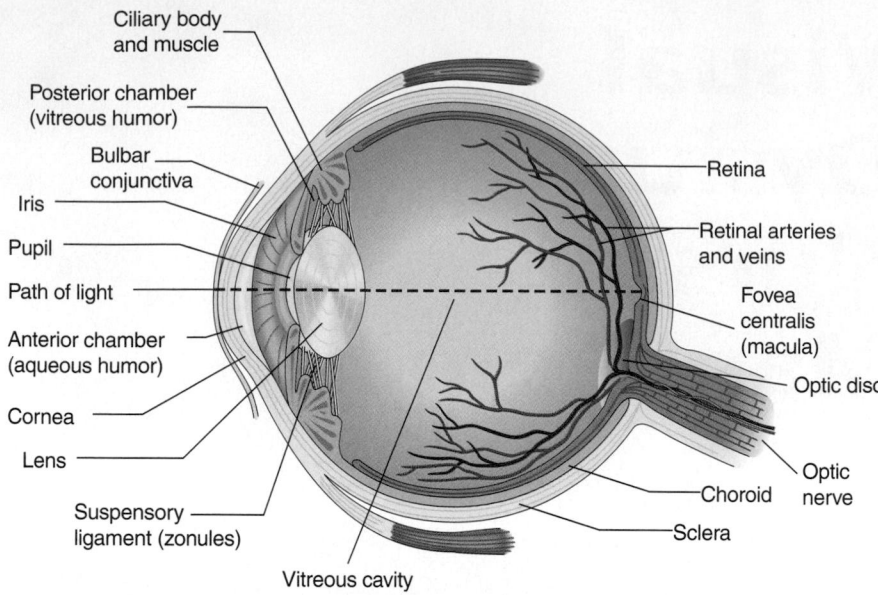

Figure 39-1 Lateral cross section of the interior eye.

OCULAR MOVEMENT DISORDERS

Ocular movement dysfunction can be the result of deviation in muscle movement from normal physiology (Figure 39-3), involuntary eye movement, or paralysis. There are three main ocular movement dysfunctions: (a) strabismus, (b) nystagmus, and (c) ocular muscle paralysis.

Strabismus

Ocular movement is controlled by the six extraocular muscles, four rectus and two oblique muscles (Riordan-Eva & Whitcher, 2004). **Strabismus** occurs when one muscle is weak and result in one eye deviating from the other when the eyes are focused on an object (Estes, 2006). Depending on the muscle or muscles involved the eye may deviate in an inward, upward, outward, or downward pattern. An eye that deviates outward is called **exotropia (wall eyes),** and an eye that deviates inward is known as **entropia. Diplopia,** or double vision, is the primary symptom of strabismus (Druz, 2005). **Amblyopia** is a reduction in visual acuity caused by cerebral blockage of visual stimuli, which can develop in the eye affected by strabismus. Causes of strabismus include weak ocular muscle tone, reduced visual acuity, or an oculomotor nerve lesion (Michelson, 2005).

Nystagmus

Nystagmus is an involuntary rhythmic movement of the eyes in a back and forth, or cyclical, movement. This can be caused by lesions in the labyrinth, vestibular nerve, cerebellum, and brainstem. Drug toxicities (e.g., phenytoin or alcohol), retinal disease, and diseases involving the cervical cord may, also, produce nystagmus.

Ocular Muscle Paralysis

Paralysis of ocular muscles may occur as a result of trauma or pressure on cranial nerves or diseases, such as diabetes mellitus (DM) or myasthenia gravis. This can result in limited abduction, abnormal closure of the lid, **ptosis** (drooping of the eyelid) or diplopia from unopposed muscle movement.

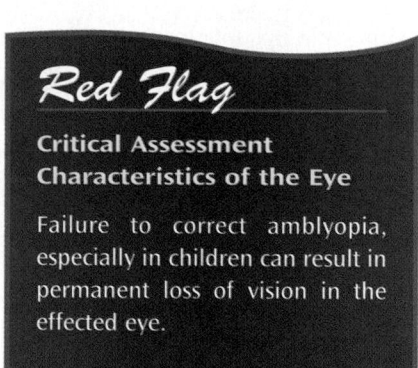

Red Flag

Critical Assessment Characteristics of the Eye

Failure to correct amblyopia, especially in children can result in permanent loss of vision in the effected eye.

LEFT VISUAL FIELD **RIGHT VISUAL FIELD**

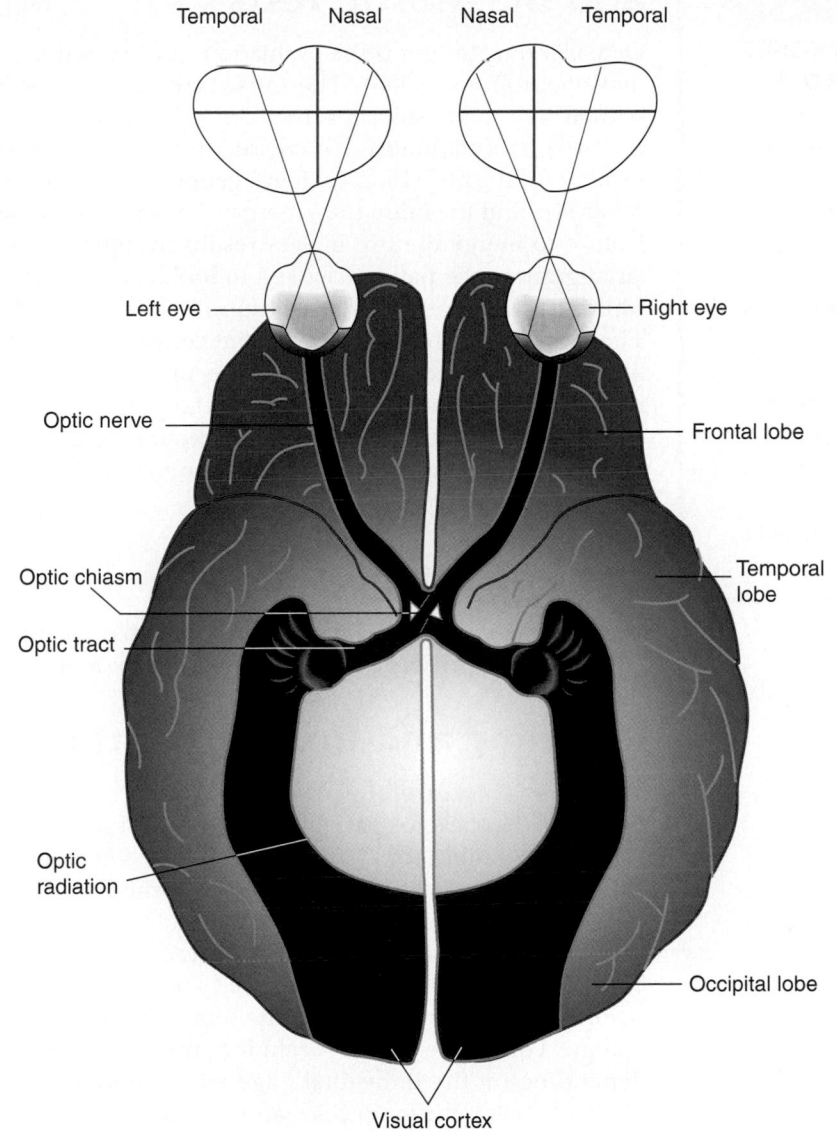

Figure 39-2 Visual pathway.

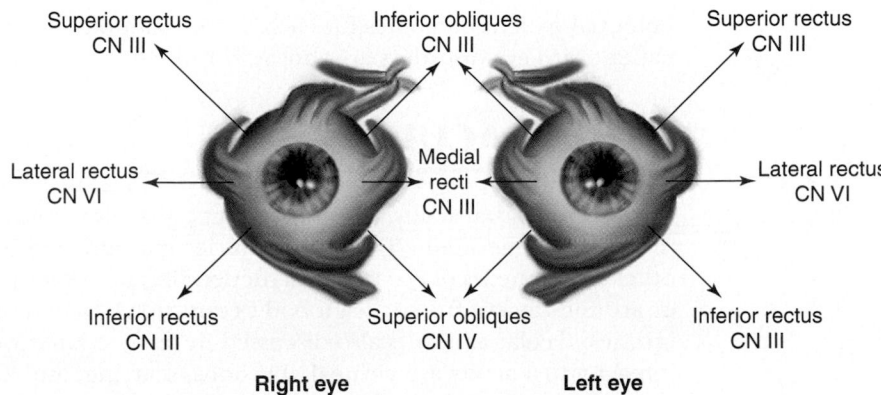

Figure 39-3 Direction of movement of extraocular muscles.

Assessment with Clinical Manifestations and Diagnostic Tests

Ocular motor testing is the evaluation of the alignment of the eyes and their movement (Estes, 2006). The nurse assesses the movement of the eyes on a regular basis and associates dysfunction with particular diseases and dysfunction (e.g., head injuries, increased intracranial pressure, or neurological insults). In normal vision each eye generates a visual image separate from the other eye, and the brain then merges the two images together into one image. Failure to merge the two images results in diplopia. To measure the binocular alignment the patient is asked to look at a penlight held several feet away while the nurse observes for location of the light reflection on the cornea. The light should be centered on the cornea, and any deviation suggests dysfunction of the ocular muscles. A second method of evaluating for ocular movement dysfunction is to instruct the patient to follow a target with both eyes as the target is moved in the direction of gaze. The nurse assesses the movement for speed, range, symmetry of movement, and fixation (Michelson, 2005).

Nursing Diagnoses

Based on the information gathered, examples of nursing diagnoses in the patient with eye disorders are included in Box 39-1.

Planning and Implementation

The nurse must carefully plan care for patients with oculomotor problems. Collaborative care for patients with ocular motor dysfunction includes monitoring the patient for changes in vision and correcting the muscle(s) surgically. Generally surgical intervention is a method of treatment used last and only when vision is impaired. Treatment of ocular motor problems usually starts with correction of refractive errors. In some situations the use of occlusion therapy may be effective. The nurse patches the eye to occlude vision either all or some of the time. In addition to adhesive patches, opaque contact lenses or occluders mounted on eyeglasses may be used depending on the individual's age and adherence to the medical regimen. Medical treatment for ptosis can include a pair of eyeglasses with a crutch made to hold up the eyelid; surgical repair can include adjustment of the one or more of the ocular motor muscles. In some situations correction of ptosis may be considered cosmetic and therefore not covered by traditional health insurance.

Evaluation of Outcomes

Potential patient outcomes for each of the example nursing diagnoses for the patient with eye disorders are shown in Box 39-2.

VISUAL ACUITY

Disorders of visual acuity include cataracts, glaucoma, retinal detachment, and macular degeneration. Traumatic injuries can affect visual acuity, as well as other components of eye function, depending on the location of the injury in or around the eye from foreign body, contusions, lacerations, and penetrating injuries. Ocular cancer is also discussed in this section. Corneal disorders that impact visual acuity are corneal abrasions, scarring, and keratoconus and are covered in this section.

BOX 39-2

EVALUATION OF OUTCOMES FOR PATIENTS WITH EYE DISORDERS

- Acute pain as related to pathophysiology of eye dysfunction. The patient should verbalize an adequate relief of pain along with the ability to realistically cope with the pain if it is not completely relieved.
- Anxiety related to possible vision loss. The patient should be able to recognize the signs of anxiety, demonstrate positive coping mechanisms, and describe a reduction in the level of anxiety experienced.
- Disturbed sensory perception related to visual impairment. The patient achieves optimal functioning within limits of visual impairment as evidenced by ability to care for self, to navigate

environmental safely, and to engage in meaningful activities.
- Ineffective health maintenance related to knowledge deficit. The patient describes positive health maintenance behaviors, such as keeping scheduled appointments, making diet and exercise changes, improving home environments, and following treatment regimens.
- Self-care deficit related to impaired vision. The patient safely performs (to maximum ability) self-care activities. Resources are identified that are useful in optimizing the autonomy and independence of the patient.

Cataracts

A cataract occurs as a part of the aging process for many individuals. In the United States, by the age of 80, more than half of the population will develop cataracts or have had cataract surgery. Cataracts occur simultaneously in both eyes yet the problem is often more acute in one eye than the other. Risk for the development of cataracts is seen in conjunction with disease (e.g., diabetes), personal behavior (e.g., smoking, alcohol use), medical treatment (e.g., side effect from use of steroids), and environment (e.g., exposure to sunlight).

Pathophysiology

Cataracts occur as the opacity of the lens becomes cloudy or turns a yellowish brown color, distorting the light passing through to the retina. The lens is made of water and protein; when the protein clumps together this produces the cloudiness. When the lens develops the yellowish brown color it often results in color distortion. Symptoms of cataracts include cloudiness or blurriness, reduced night vision, and color distortion or faded colors. Cataracts can also form after traumatic eye injury or secondarily to other eye problems, such as diabetes or surgery for glaucoma. Some children may be born with a congenital cataract that may or may not affect vision (McGwin, Hall, Searcey, Modjarrad, & Owsley, 2005).

Assessment with Clinical Manifestations and Diagnostic Tests

A visual acuity test such as use of the Snellen chart (Figure 39-4) is part of the assessment for vision impairment related to cataracts. A dilated eye examination will be performed to assist with diagnosis. Patients with cataracts usually notice no pain or discomfort (Estes, 2006).

Nursing Diagnoses

Based on the information gathered, examples of nursing diagnoses in the patient with cataracts are shown in Box 39-1.

Planning and Implementation

Management for patients with cataracts starts with adjusting corrective lens as frequently as necessary to ensure optimal vision. Surgical treatment for cataracts begins when vision is sufficiently impaired to interfere with activities of daily living.

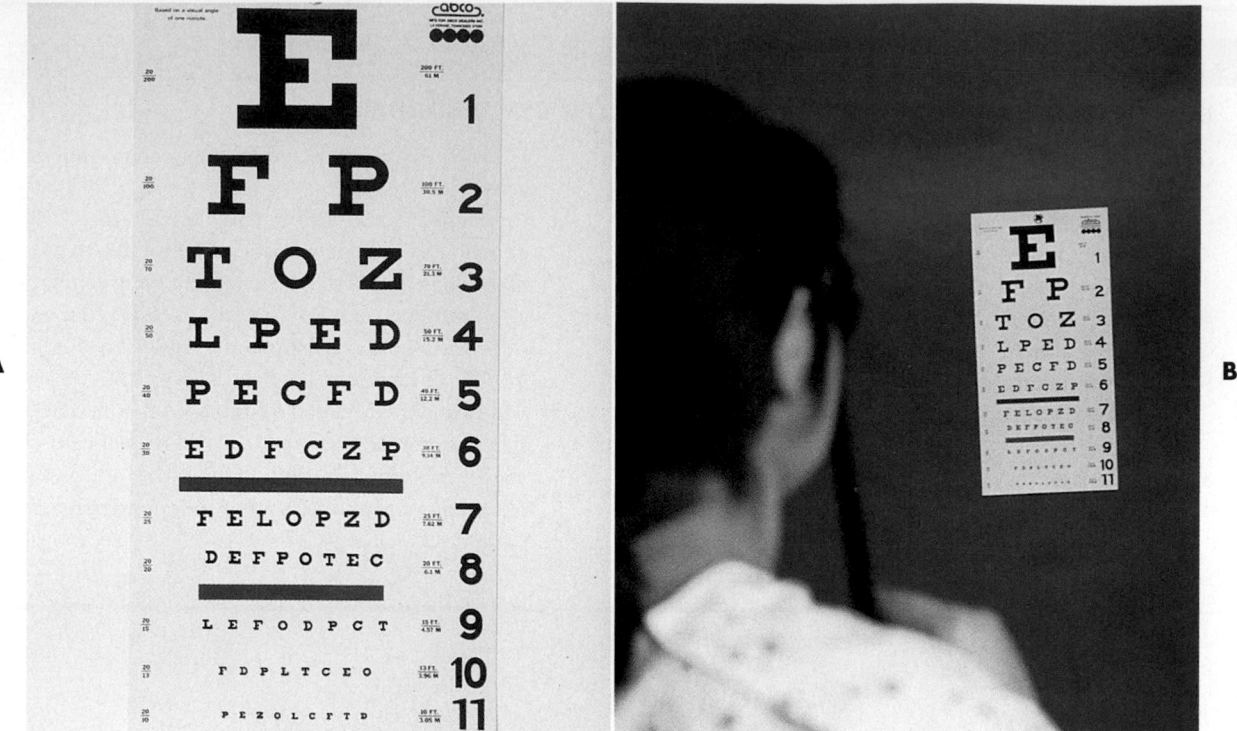

Figure 39-4 Visual acuity testing: A. Snellen vision chart, B. Assessing distance vision.

Surgery

There are two types of surgery phacoemulsification (phaco) or extracapsular surgery. In phaco an incision is made in the cornea, and a small probe is inserted into the eye. The device attached to the probe emits ultrasound waves that break up the lens, allowing for suction removal. In extracapsular surgery a slightly larger incision is made, and the lens is removed as a whole. An artificial intraocular lens (IOL) with corrective power is placed in the remaining posterior capsule of the eye. Following either surgery a patient may need glasses only for reading. When an IOL cannot be inserted, the eye is unable to accommodate resulting in **aphakic vision** (absence of the crystalline lens of the eye), which requires special corrective lenses (McGwin, et al., 2005).

Cataract surgery is done almost exclusively as an outpatient procedure. The patient will arrive in the morning and plan to be discharged by the afternoon. Preoperative nursing care includes preoperative history and physical, including medication usage, administration of eye drops to dilate the pupil and cause vasoconstriction, and patient education. Oral medications may be given in the preoperative phase to reduce intraocular pressure, such as acetazolamide (Diamox, Acetazolam). During the intraoperative procedure, the cataract is removed, and an IOL is placed in most patients.

Postoperative care usually includes use of eye drops including a steroid and antibiotic placed subconjunctivally. The eye is usually left unpatched, and the patient is discharged home. Patient education is extremely important in preparation of the patient prior to surgery and in the aftercare. Because many patients having cataract surgery are older, there is a need to emphasize the postoperative care of eye drop instillation. The postoperative period should be relatively free of complications, and pain or swelling are generally not expected. If pain with nausea and vomiting should occur, notify the ophthalmologist.

Evaluation of Outcomes

It is expected the patient will have improved vision from the preoperative assessment. Corrective lenses may or may not be necessary. Refer to Box 39-2 for evaluation of outcomes.

Glaucoma

Glaucoma is a group of diseases related to the amount of intraocular pressure in the eye occurring as a result of neurodegenerative processes. Increasing intraocular pressure can rapidly result in optic nerve damage causing a decrease in vision and blindness. There are two primary forms of glaucoma, closed angle and open angle. In addition, there is congenital, normal tension, and secondary forms, such as pigmentary and neovascular glaucoma. This section will cover the primary forms. After cataracts, glaucoma is the second leading cause of blindness worldwide. As the world population ages this will become an ever-increasing problem, because the blindness it causes is permanent. Open-angle glaucoma is more commonly seen in people of African or European decent, whereas individuals of Asian decent are more likely to develop closed-angle glaucoma (Katz, 2004).

Pathophysiology

In open-angle glaucoma the channels (trabecular meshwork or canal of Schlemm) that drain fluid within the eye become blocked, causing pressure to rise. This increased pressure pushes backward on to the vitreous humor, causing damage to the retina. Normal intraocular pressures (IOP) ranges from 10 to 21 mmHg, and as the pressure begins to rise it causes a gradual loss of vision. Because there are few symptoms, and vision loss is gradual, individuals may not notice for a long time that they are losing their sight. Closed–angle glaucoma occurs when there is a similar increase in IOP, but the onset is sudden, causing headaches, blurred vision, and pain in the eye (Katz, 2004).

Assessment with Clinical Manifestations and Diagnostic Tests

Glaucoma is determined through a comprehensive eye exam including a visual acuity test, visual fields test, dilated eye exam, and tonometry. Tonometry measures the pressure within the eye. Once it becomes apparent that there is a significant increase in IOP, it is important to take more than one measure of it. Several readings need to be taken throughout the day to establish a diurnal curve with the highest reading to be the treated pressure. The thickness or thinness of the cornea may give a false higher or lower IOP (Gray, 2005).

Nursing Diagnoses

Based on the information gathered, examples of nursing diagnoses in the patient with IOP are shown in Box 39-1.

Planning and Implementation

Glaucoma cannot be cured, and the damage is irreversible; nevertheless, the progression of the disease can be controlled with eye drops, oral medications, laser procedures, or surgery. These procedures and surgeries are done on an outpatient basis.

Pharmacology

All medications used to lower the IOP by either reducing aqueous inflow or increasing aqueous outflow with the goal of keeping the pressure in the mid to lower range (12 to 16 mmHg) of normal IOP. These drugs fall in the following categories: sympathomimetics, parasympathomimetics, beta-adrenergic antagonists, carbonic anhydrase inhibitors, and prostaglandin analogues. Each category has its advantages and disadvantages. The current gold standard for treatment of glaucoma is timolol.

Surgery

An increasingly popular choice of treatment is a trabeculoplasty, an argon laser procedure where the laser causes some of the areas of the drainage system to shrink, allowing for stretch opening of adjacent areas for increased outflow. This procedure often allows patients to reduce medications and avoid or delay further surgery.

The conventional surgery of choice is a trabeculectomy (creation of a fistula), where a small area of the trabecular meshwork is removed to allow the aqueous humor to drain. This procedure is done under local anesthetic, often with sedation. Follow-up includes an annual gonioscopy to inspect the anterior chamber of eye and for determining ocular motility and rotation. A gonioscopy is where a special lens with a mirror-like effect is placed on the eye to evaluate the trabecular meshwork through the slit lamp.

An area of increasing interest among ophthalmologists is use of surgically implanted drainage devices for patients with glaucoma resistant to eye drops (Gray, 2005). While these drainage devices are offering new alternatives, they are not without complications. Patients may develop **hypotany** (low intraocular pressure), inflammation, and excessive scar tissue formation.

Evaluation of Outcomes

The patient is followed regularly for progression of disease and changes in vision. With eye drops it is expected that the progression of disease will be greatly slowed, and there will be no loss of vision. Laser and surgical procedures should result in stabilization of vision and intraocular tension. Medications may or may not still be needed following laser or surgical intervention. Refer to Box 39-2 for evaluation of outcomes.

Retinal Detachment

Retinal detachment may also be called a detached retina or retinal tear. This occurs when the retina detaches by lifting or pulling away from its normal position. If not treated promptly, this can cause permanent vision loss. Retinal detachment can occur at any age, but it is more common in individuals over age 40. Other risk factors include extreme nearsightedness, previous history or family history of retinal detachment, previous cataract surgery, or a past eye injury.

Pathophysiology

The retina is composed of two layers; these layers can separate from each other or the wall of the eye. The more inner layer detects light, and the outer layer provides the support and nutrients to the retina. The nerve cells that detect light entering the eye then translate the information into nerve signals about what the eye sees. When the detachment occurs the retina no longer can process what it sees, which results in vision loss in that area. This vision loss can be minimal or severe depending on the size and location of the tear or detachment. There is always some vision loss after a retinal detachment (Wilkinson, 2005).

Assessment with Clinical Manifestations

The clinical manifestations of retinal detachment include floaters in the visual field and flashes of light or sparks when patients move their eyes or head. Floaters are like little cobwebs or specks that float in the visual field. The patient sees small dark shadowy shapes or crooked lines that move as his or her eye moves or drift when the eyes stop moving. They may be more annoying when looking at something bright like the sky or something white. Floaters are not usually treated unless they impair vision sufficiently to warrant treatment or cause retinal tears or detachment.

While floaters and flashes can occur for other reasons and do not signal retinal detachment, they may be a warning sign. The patient describes a shadow or curtain that has come down in the visual field and will not go away. Side vision is often affected and progresses over time (hours or days) as more of the retina separates from the wall. If the detachment involves the macula, vision loss can be severe or total in the affected eye. Retinal detachments rarely self-repair, and surgery is usually necessary (Wilkinson, 2005).

Diagnostic Tests

Retinal detachment is diagnosed through the medical history and an eye examination specifically through an ophthalmoscope (Figure 39-5). A tear or hole may be seen at the edge of the detachment.

Nursing Diagnoses

Based on the information gathered, examples of nursing diagnoses in the patient with retinal detachments are shown in Box 39-1.

Planning and Implementation

As stated in the Red Flag feature, retinal detachment is a medical emergency, and anyone experiencing the symptoms should see an eye care professional immediately. Retinal tears are evaluated for progression to detachment prior to initiating treatment. The treatment for a tear may be **cryopexy** (freezing of the retinal tear area) or laser photocoagulation performed in an outpatient surgery center or physician's office. The laser makes small burns around the tear to weld the retina back into place, where cryopexy freezes the area around the tear, and scar formation connects the tissues. Both of these procedures are done to keep the vitreous humor from passing through the tear and increasing the size of the detachment, thereby increasing the vision loss.

Surgery

Surgical options for retinal detachments include scleral buckling surgery, pneumatic retinopexy, or vitrectomy. A scleral buckle, the most common method of treatment, requires that a piece of silicone, rubber, or semihard plastic be placed against the outer surface of the eye and sutured into place. The piece pushes the sclera toward the middle of the eye, allowing the retina to settle back against the wall of the eye. The buckle may encircle the eye or just cover the area around the detachment. This surgery is usually performed in a hospital or outpatient surgical center under local or general anesthesia. Postoperative care includes monitoring for swelling, redness, tenderness, and pain management. This procedure has an 80 to 90 percent success rate. The scleral buckle can cause an increase in IOP, and the changes in the eye shape from buckle can result in a refractive error, affecting vision (Wilkinson, 2005).

When a pneumatic retinopexy is used to reattach the retina, the physician uses a bubble of gas to push the two layers back together again. This is usually done as an outpatient procedure under local anesthesia. Cryopexy or photocoagulation may be used to then seal the tear. The bubble is gradually absorbed over a week and keeps the tear closed and the retina flattened until a seal forms between the retina and the wall of the eye. This surgery takes about three weeks to achieve optimal healing. The patient may be expected to lie in a specific position for 16 to 21 hours per day to keep the bubble in the right location. Patients with confusion or attention problems would not be candidates for this type of procedure. The success rate is about 73 to 80 percent.

The third possible procedure is a vitrectomy, where the surgeon removes the vitreous fluid from the middle of the eye. The physician may then treat the retina with photocoagulation. At the end of surgery silicone oil or gas is injected into the eye to replace the vitreous fluid. This surgery may require an

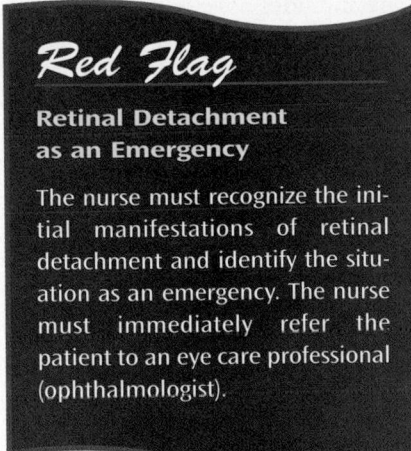

A

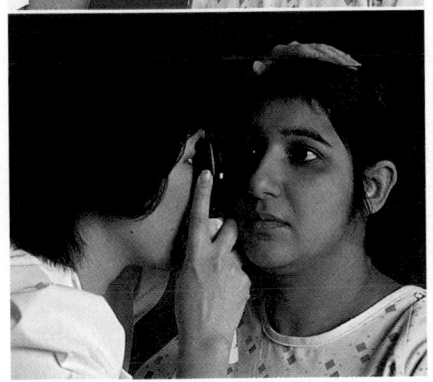

B

Figure 39-5 Examining retinal structures.

overnight hospital stay. The postoperative care includes assessment for bleeding into the vitreous area, further retinal detachment, fluid buildup in the clear cover of the eye (corneal edema), and increased IOP.

Evaluation of Outcomes

The expected outcome for a patient postprocedure for retinal detachment is that vision is optimized to its fullest potential. Patients may require new corrective lens after healing throughout the healing process. Refer to Box 39-2 for evaluation of outcomes.

Macular Degeneration

Recent statistics show approximately eight million individuals over the age of 55 have signs of early or intermediate age-related macular degeneration (AMD). Macular degeneration is largely an age-related disease process whereby central vision gradually deteriorates. Women are at greater risk of developing AMD, and Caucasians are more likely to develop the disease than African Americans. Family history and smoking are also significant risk factors.

Pathophysiology

Age-related macular degeneration is a painless disease where the macula gradually breaks down from the development of fatty, yellow, metabolic waste products, which accumulate in the retina. There are two forms of AMD, dry and wet. Dry (atrophic) AMD is the most common cause type, accounting for 90 percent of all people with AMD. This occurs because of a gradual deterioration of the macula from waste product buildup and lack of proper nutrition. The progress is slow and usually results in mild to moderate loss of sight; this usually does not cause a total loss of reading vision. Wet (neovascular) AMD is more devastating, because it can result in severe sight loss within a few short months. This type of AMD is caused by an abnormal growth of blood vessels in the macula, leaving the surface of the retina uneven (Wormald, Evans, Smeeth, & Henshaw, 2005).

Assessment with Clinical Manifestations

The most common early sign of dry AMD is blurred vision. As time progresses and fewer macular cells function, details become less clear with some improvement in brighter light. Continued degeneration can result in a small but growing blind spot in the middle of the visual field. As dry AMD worsens it can deteriorate into wet AMD because of the increased development of blood vessels in the area.

In wet AMD, instead of straight lines the patient sees wavy lines on the Amsler grid. As fluid leaks into the macular area from the increased blood vessels it lifts the macula causing a distorted vision. Central vision can also be lost as small blind spot may also begin to develop into wet AMD.

History of symptoms and complaints is important in the initial diagnosis. Determine whether the visual changes have an onset that was gradual or rapid, what is the duration of the symptoms and the degree of visual impairment, such as mild, moderate, or severe. Diagnosis is largely through the routine eye exam starting with use of the familiar Snellen chart where central vision is tested. Further testing includes dilating the pupil using a mydriatic to visualize the macula. A fundus examination is completed using direct ophthalmoscopy (Wormald, et al., 2005).

Diagnostic Tests

Diagnosis begins with an initial visual exam for specific signs of macular degeneration. Fluorescein angiography and indocyanine green angiography may be used to identify signs of macular degeneration.

Nursing Diagnoses

Based on the information gathered, examples of nursing diagnoses in the patient with AMD are shown in Box 39-1.

Planning and Implementation

Ongoing self-monitoring of vision is important in this disease. Patients can place an Amsler grid on the refrigerator and every morning assess for changes to vision. Diet supplements with vitamins, antioxidants, and zinc can have significant benefit in preventing disease progression. Patients may find the use of low vision aids, such as magnifiers for reading, telescopes to see into the distance, and talking watches supportive in maintaining quality of life.

The wet form of AMD may be treated with use of a laser, which may stop or lessen vision loss in the early stages. The laser destroys existing blood vessels, and the scar formation afterward may result in some permanent vision loss in the area of the retina affected. It is effective in about 50 percent of the cases. Photodynamic therapy using a light-activated drug given intravenously, and a laser beam can close the abnormal vessels while leaving the retina intact. Repeat treatment may be needed because closed vessels can reopen. Vitamins, antioxidants, and zinc arc useful in prevention as well as use of sunglasses that block ultraviolet sunrays from sun exposure. Currently there is no treatment for dry AMD (Wormald, ct al., 2005).

Evaluation of Outcomes

Patients rarely lose all their vision from macular degeneration. They are generally able to perform many normal daily activities even with poor central vision. Refer to Box 39-2 for evaluation of outcomes.

Traumatic Injuries

Traumatic injuries can occur at any age or at any time. The most common traumatic injuries include damage from penetration by foreign bodies, physical pressure resulting in a contusion, lacerations from sharp objects, and penetrating injuries.

Foreign Bodies

Forcign bodies in the eye are a common problem and can be the result of dust, dirt, eyelashes, or a fingernail. Because the cornea is an extremely sensitive area, a corneal abrasion may result. Corneal abrasions are often painful even when the scratch is relatively minor.

Planning and Implementation

It is important to seek health care immediately for any foreign body that is not removed by blinking. Fast-acting anesthetic agents can numb the area and allow a qualified health care professional to remove the object. Irrigation with normal saline can be used to rinse out loose particles of dust or dirt. Afterward antibiotic ointment may be used to prevent infection, and anti-inflammatory drops may be used to reduce discomfort until the cornea heals. An eye patch may be used to minimize movement of the eyelids during the healing process (Hoyt & Haley, 2005).

Evaluation of Outcomes

Successful removal of the foreign object, as well as return to normal eye function and sight, is the goal of removing an object from the eye. Refer to Box 39-2 for evaluation of outcomes.

Contusion

A periorbital contusion, or black eye, is a relatively common result of a traumatic injury to the face or head. Bleeding occurs in the area surrounding the eye; however, this may not be the extent of the injury. Often the eye globe is pushed back into the socket, stretching the surrounding muscles and soft tissues. This can result in the ocular muscle conditions and even rupture the globe. Pain and swelling are the most common clinical manifestations. Double

---

Red Flag

Impaled object in the Eye

The health care provider must treat the impaled object found in an eye by doing the following: (a) remember to assess the patient for priority injuries first, (b) leave the object in place and stabilize the patient's head, (c) place a cup over the impaled object and tape in place (Figure 39-6), and (d) transport the patient in a safe and efficient manner remembering to not allow the impaled object to move.

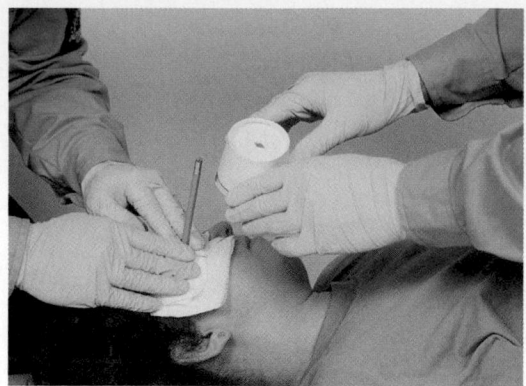

Figure 39-6 A cup helps hold an object impaled into the eye in place.

vision, loss of vision, loss of consciousness, inability to move the eye (look in different directions), and blood on the surface of the eye are signs of a more serious injury.

Planning and Implementation

Immediate health care attention should be sought for the above clinical manifestations. Initial treatment includes testing visual acuity and ophthalmoscopy. Additional testing may be performed depending on what was found, including X-rays to rule out orbital fractures. Rest and ice are the interventions for first aid. The ice should be wrapped in a cloth and applied to the effected area for 20 minutes an hour for every hour while awake for the first 24 hours. Avoid potential causes of injury until the eye has healed. Assessment by an ophthalmologist is necessary for injuries to the eye itself.

Evaluation of Outcomes

Return to normal eye function and sight with resolution of the excess fluid and swelling in the eye area are the desired results when treating a periorbital contusion. Refer to Box 39-2 for evaluation of outcomes.

Laceration and Penetrating Injuries

A full-thickness injury may occur to the cornea in the form of a puncture, or it may occur as a linear or irregular corneal laceration. The initial injury can cause complete or partial vision loss and put the patient is at risk for a secondary infection. Diagnosis is determined through the use of the standard Snellen chart and use of the slit lamp. Pressure on the globe should be avoided, the eye should be patched, and a patient with this condition should be referred to an ophthalmologist for a detailed examination.

Planning and Implementation

Every effort should be made to avoid any further injury by shielding the eye and elevating the head of the bed. The patient should be instructed not to touch the eye area and to rest until seen by the ophthalmologist. If there is a protruding body, do not remove it; the ophthalmologist should remove it. If the patient develops nausea and vomiting, antiemetics and NPO (nothing oral) status may be initiated. Broad-spectrum antibiotics should be started intravenously or orally after nausea and vomiting subside. Frequent eye examinations on follow-up are recommended for patients with lacerations or penetrating injuries because of an increased risk of traumatic cataracts and secondary glaucoma.

Evaluation of Outcomes

Rapid emergency treatment and referral to an ophthalmologist is the best option for minimal complications and vision loss. It is expected that vision loss will be related to the significance of the injury and damage to the cornea and other eye structures. Refer to Box 39-2 for evaluation of outcomes.

Ocular Cancer

Eye cancer can occur in nearly any anatomical structure of the eye, including the eyelid, the orbit, and conjunctiva. The most common ocular cancer is melanoma. A melanoma can develop in the ciliary body, conjunctiva, choroid, iris, and eyelid. A choroidal melanoma is the most common primary intraocular tumor.

Pathophysiology

Choroidal melanoma arises from melanocytes within the choroid. They may range from darkly pigmented to no coloration. As they grow choroidal melanomas can push against the retinal epithelium causing atrophy and decrease in normal choroidal circulation. These melanomas may progress silently until they produce noticeable vision loss. If the melanoma erodes into the blood vessels in adjacent areas, it can lead to vitreous hemorrhage. Metastases to distant locations are the generally the ultimate cause of death rather than local spread. The most common site of choroidal melanoma metastasis is the liver.

Assessment with Clinical Manifestations

Clinical manifestations can include ocular hypotension or hypertension and cataract if the tumor grows anteriorly. Patients may initially complain of blurred visual acuity and floaters. Severe ocular pain is rarely occurs and is related to the melanoma impinging on the posterior ciliary nerves or from increased intraocular pressure. Sunlight exposure is a likely contributor to the development of choroidal melanoma.

Diagnostic Tests

Ultrasound of the globe and orbit areas is useful in detecting tumors more than 2 to 3 mm thick. Computed tomograph (CT) scans and magnetic resonance imaging (MRIs) are less sensitive than ultrasound and more expensive. Other tests may be used to rule out metastases, such as chest radiograph and liver enzymes. Biopsy may be used only in cases in which it is difficult to distinguish whether the tumor is primary or metastatic.

Nursing Diagnoses

Based on the information gathered, examples of nursing diagnoses in the patient with ocular cancer are shown in Box 39-1. See also nursing diagnoses for patients with metastatic cancer in chapter 15.

Planning and Implementation

In the early stages of potential ocular cancer, the nurse must assess for abnormal ocular changes. The nurse must always refer the patient to ophthalmologists for further assessment and treatment plans. The majority of the management for patients with progressive or serious ocular cancers involves surgical interventions.

Surgery

The classic approach for large and complicated choroidal melanomas is the surgical removal of an eye, called **enucleation.** The reason for enucleation over globe sparing is to reduce the risk of metastatic spread. Enucleation may also be done in rare circumstances to relieve intolerable pain in a blind eye.

A medium-sized tumor is treated to plaque brachytherapy using iodine 125 because of its lower energy emission and good tissue penetration. The plaque is temporarily sutured to the sclera and limbus underlying the melanoma. Radioactive plaques are left in place for three to seven days. The goal of treatment is arrest of tumor growth or regression in size of the tumor. Complications of plaque brachytherapy include cataract, scleral necrosis, radiation retinopathy, and optic nerve damage. External beam irradiation using charged particles, such as protons, is an alternative to the brachytherapy.

Small tumors may be treated with a block incision, which is used hoping to salvage the eye, and many of these patients retain some useful vision. A block incision removes the tumor surrounding choroid, retina, sclera, and a 3-mm margin of health tissue. Complications include vitreous hemorrhage, retinal detachment, residual tumor, and cataract.

Postoperative care includes use of antibiotic, steroid, and cycloplegic eye drops. Patients may or may not have to wear and eye patch. In patients with enucleation postoperative care includes preparation for an artificial eye (ocular prosthesis) as a cosmetic substitute for the real eye.

Evaluation of Outcomes

Survival rates are 50 to 70 percent over 10 years for patients with choroidal cancer. The risk for metastases is great because of the often late diagnosis of the problem. Typical areas for metastases after the liver include lung, brain, and bones. Visual prognosis is poor, and patients require frequent follow-up eye examinations. Refer to Box 39-2 for evaluation of outcomes.

Corneal Disorders

Damage to the cornea can be painful and a serious dysfunction of the eye. Corneal disorders include corneal abrasions (one of the most common eye injuries), ulcerations, and keratoconus.

Abrasions

Corneal abrasions are one of the most common eye injuries and probably the most neglected. These injuries may result in permanent scarring and a loss of visual acuity and function. They occur as a disruption in the integrity of the corneal epithelium or because the corneal surface was denuded from physical external forces such as contact lenses or sports injuries. Many of these injuries are minor, but they can lead to blindness. These same injuries can place economic burdens on otherwise healthy people resulting in lost time at work or school. Corneal abrasions usually heal in two to three days without treatment; however, they can result in bacterial keratitis if the epithelium integrity is damaged or deteriorate into a corneal ulceration. Clinical manifestations include pain, watering, foreign body sensation, and photophobia. Treatment includes prophylactic antibiotics after trauma or surgery, cycloplegics for comfort, and an eye patch, which may or may not be worn (Calder, Balasubramanian, & Stiell, 2004).

Ulcerations

A corneal ulceration is considered an ophthalmologic emergency. Bacterial corneal ulcers usually occur from a traumatic break in the corneal epithelium allowing bacteria to enter. Other bacterial causes can include tear insufficiency, malnutrition, and contact lens use. Herpes simplex virus (HSV) is one of the most common causes of corneal ulceration. Visual acuity is affected based on location of the ulcer and whether inflammation is present in the cornea. Clinical manifestations include blurred vision, photophobia, pain, redness, and mucopurulent drainage. Emergent treatment includes an ophthalmologic consultation, cultures, and treatment with an antibiotic ointment to prevent vision loss.

Keratoconus

Keratoconus is a progressive, noninflammatory bilateral disease of the cornea characterized by thinning of the cornea layers leading to corneal surface distortion. The resulting visual loss is from irregular astigmatism, myopia, and secondarily from scarring. Risk factors for developing keratoconus include ocular allergies, rigid contact lens wear, and vigorous eye rubbing. It usually presents at puberty and progresses until the third or fourth decade of life; however, it can occur at any time.

Clinical manifestations include decreasing vision with distortion, glare, and diplopia. Patients often complain of difficulty in achieving satisfactory optimum vision with corrective lenses. Eyeglasses and soft contact lenses may be effective initially; however, as vision deteriorates rigid contact lenses may provide better vision. Diagnosis is determined through refraction, **keratometry** (measurement of the cornea), and use of the slit lamp. Primary treatment is rigid contact lenses. There is no direct pharmacological management of keratoconus; however, anti-inflammatory and antihistamine topical medications are sometimes helpful (Calder, et al., 2004).

Planning and Implementation

Corneal disorders of a serious nature are treated primarily with corneal transplantation. Corneal transplants are possible through the donation of cadaver corneas, letting family know of a person's wish to be a donor may improve the availability to corneas for transplant. Corneal transplants are done most often to treat vision loss as a result of disease, swelling, scarring, infection, or chemical burns. This is an outpatient surgical procedure lasting about an hour. Follow-up care includes the wearing of an eye shield for the prevention of injury during the healing process and antirejection eye drops.

Evaluation of Outcomes

Complete resolution of the corneal disturbances and no loss of visual acuity or function are desired outcomes. Refer to Box 39-2 for evaluation of outcomes.

REFRACTION

In normal vision, **emmetropia,** the light falls onto the retina without any distortion or abnormal bending of the light. In errors of visual refraction, which are the most common vision problems, the light passing through the layers of the eye to the retina is distorted. This can be caused by irregularities in the cornea, the focusing power of the lens, and the length of the eye (Huether, 2004).

Pathophysiology

There are three types of refraction error (Figure 39-7). **Myopia (nearsightedness)** occurs when the light passing through the eye is overbent or over-refracted. As a result the light rays are focused in front of the retina when viewing a distant object. Objects that are viewed up close are clear and distant objects are unclear. Myopia is treated with a corrective lens that redirects the light to the retina by changing the angle of the light. These corrective lenses are cut biconcave. **Hyperopia (farsightedness)** occurs when the light passing through the eye is focused behind the retina when looking a close objects. As a result, images up close are unclear, but images over 20 feet distant are clear. Hyperopia is treated with a convex corrective lens that redirects the light to the retina. The third refractive error is **astigmatism,** in which the light is spread over a diffuse area. Astigmatism occurs when there is an unequal curve of the cornea, and the light rays are bent unevenly. The exact cause of astigmatism is unknown, although there is some familial pattern. Astigmatism is treated with corrective lens in a cylindrical shape. It is not uncommon for refractive errors of myopia or hyperopia to coexist with astigmatism.

Nursing Diagnoses

Based on the information gathered, examples of nursing diagnoses in the patient with refraction problems are shown in Box 39-1.

Planning and Implementation

There are a variety of forms of management for refraction disorders. Several treatments are common (e.g., eyeglasses), and other dysfunctions require surgical intervention.

Eyeglasses

Refraction errors are treated with corrective lenses, such as eyeglasses or contact lenses. The strength of a pair of eyeglasses is determined by having a patient view through a number of different strength lenses until the patient

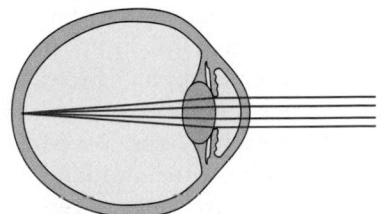

Normal eye
Light rays focus on the retina

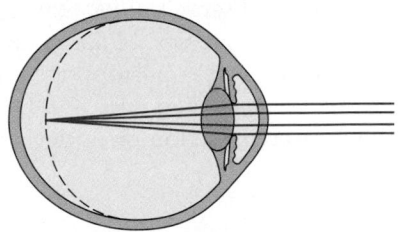

Myopia (nearsightedness)
Light rays focus in front
of the retina

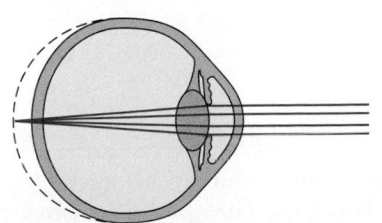

Hyperopia (farsightedness)
Light rays focus behind
the retina

Figure 39-7 Eye refraction.

identifies the best correction. Eyeglass prescriptions then have the lenses ground to achieve that strength.

Contact Lenses

Contact lenses provide similar vision correction to eyeglasses and are fit to the curvature of the cornea. The contact lenses float on the cornea using the normal eye secretions to maintain adequate moisture content. Dehydration can result in decreased visual acuity and direct contact with the cornea. There are currently two different types of contact lenses, hard and soft. Hard lenses have little flexibility and change the shape of the cornea was well as provide correction. Hard contact lenses require cleaning and can only be worn while awake. Soft contact lenses come in daily wear and extended wear options. The daily wear lenses are worn during the day hours and taken out at night and soaked in a cleaning solution. The extended wear option allows the user to wear the lenses even at night for up to a week without removal. The lenses are then either cleaned or disposed of depending on the type. Contact lenses can cause corneal abrasions and progress into corneal ulcerations if care is not adequate.

Surgery

Surgical treatment for refractive errors includes radial keratotomy (RK), laser vision correction, and Intacs. These procedures are done in physician offices or outpatient surgery centers. RK uses a diamond knife to make several incisions into the cornea in a circular rotation. This alters the mechanical structure of the cornea and changes its shape to correct nearsightedness. Results are rapid and patients see quite well within one to two days. Laser vision correction is done with photorefractive keratotomy (PRK) and laser in situ keratomileusis (LASIK). In PRK an excimer laser is used to reshape the surface of the cornea after the surface epithelial cells are removed. This differs from LASIK, in which a corneal flap is created and the laser is applied beneath. Rapid recovery is expected with PRK and LASIX procedures and a return to near normal vision without further correction. Intacs are a nonlaser procedure in which an intracorneal ring segment is placed under the cornea, which may be helpful for patients with low-level myopia. The benefits are they are removable and adjustable as eye changes occur.

Postoperative care includes use of antibiotic drops and steroid drops immediately after the procedure. Verification of flap placement, smoothness, and absence of debris are assessed. Patients may complain of scratchiness, tearing, burning, and sensitivity to light, which wane as time progresses. Makeup and swimming are contraindicated for the first one to two weeks postoperatively. Complications associated with these surgeries include dislodged flaps and flap folds, infection, refractive complications, such as overcorrection or undercorrection and dry eye syndrome.

Evaluation of Outcomes

It is expected with any of these procedures that optimal vision will be achieved. In most cases vision improvement is evident within one to two days. Refer to Box 39-2 for evaluation of outcomes.

PRESBYOPIA

Older adults begin to experience a loss of near acuity (near vision) as the lens loses its elasticity and accommodation of the lens fails. The condition, **presbyopia,** is evident as a patient will begin to hold reading material at a further and further distance from the eyes to establish focus. Treatment consists of using reading glasses or adjustments to glasses with a bifocal (two foci) or trifocal (three foci) in which the reading correction is in the lower portion of the lens.

COLOR PERCEPTION

Color perception determines much about how the world is perceived. The ability to distinguish color is composed of two stages; the first is through the light-sensitive receptors, and the second is through the neural components of processing, partitioning, and encoding information about wavelength that the photoreceptors collect. Hue is determined by the wavelength of content of colors that allows us to perceive colors. There are two separate and remarkably different systems for determining colors, the blue-yellow system and the red-green system. The blue-yellow system is more likely to be injured through toxic exposure, eye disease, or trauma, whereas the red-green system is more likely to be impaired because of congenital defects. These congenital defects rarely affect the blue-yellow system (Harper, Arsura, Bobba, Reddy, & Sawh, 2005).

Colorblindness

Colorblindness can be an acquired abnormality of color vision, such as with aging, when normal sensitivity to color gradually diminishes. It is thought to result from the progressive yellowing of the lens occurring with aging. While all colors become less intense, the ability to discriminate between blue and green is greatly affected. In patients with DM, color vision deteriorates more rapidly than in the general population (Harper, et al., 2005).

The genetic link to colorblindness is a cross-linked trait and occurs in about 8 percent of the male population. Among females colorblindness occurs in only about 0.5 percent of the population. The genetically linked colorblindness results in the inability to distinguish red from green. Testing for colorblindness is done with an Ishihara chart. There is currently no treatment for this visual dysfunction.

INFLAMMATORY AND INFECTIOUS EYE CONDITIONS

There are a number of intraocular and extraocular inflammatory and infectious conditions. The eye surface is a moist area rich in nutrients and subject to potential inflammation or infection, as are the areas around the eye. Blinking is one of the eye's protective mechanisms, with 12 to 20 blinks per minute the eye effectively brushes away most bacteria; furthermore, the natural tears are nutrient poor and contain antibacterial substances. Thus infectious conditions can occur as a result of the acquisition of a virulent microorganism or uncontrolled growth of an existing organism because of lowered resistance in the patient. The external conditions of hordeolum, chalazion, blepharitis, conjunctivitis, and keratitis are discussed. The internal structures of the eye are almost impenetrable; therefore, most internal infections are the result of trauma or surgical intervention (Kuehn, 2005).

Hordeolum

The sweat glands in and around the eyelid are at risk of inflammation or infection. When these inflamed sweat glands are reddened, swollen, and tender to touch they are called a hordeolum or stye.

Planning and Implementation

Management of inflammatory and infectious eye conditions includes the use of warm moist compresses and antibiotic ointment. In addition, the practice of good medical asepsis and avoiding touching the eye area are highly recommended.

Chalazion

A chalazion is a small benign tumor similar to a sebaceous cyst, hordeolum, or even a sebaceous carcinoma. To obtain a definitive diagnosis a biopsy is often necessary. Clinical manifestations include an initial redness and tenderness that progresses to swollen area without signs or symptoms of infection.

Planning and Implementation

Management of chalazion includes teaching good hand washing and avoiding touching the eye area with unclean hands. Antibiotic ointments may be applied, with warm moist compresses. Drainage and crusts are moistened with a wet cloth prior to removal. Surgical intervention may be indicated for chalazions that interfere with vision or are cosmetically displeasing.

Blepharitis

Inflammation of the hair follicles (cilia) and glands along the edges of the eyelids is called **blepharitis.** The eyelids become sore, red, and tender, with sticky exudates. The patient may complain of itchiness, watering eyes, and loss of eyelashes. Photophobia may also be a complaint. This is the most common infection seen by ophthalmologists (Kuehn, 2005).

Planning and Implementation

Blepharitis is most often a result of a staphylococcal infection and is treated with antibiotic eye ointment. Treatment should be vigorous to prevent development of hordeolum. Eyelid areas should be cleansed gently and patted dry frequently to minimize exudate developing crusts and hardening.

Conjunctivitis

Conjunctivitis, also called pink eye, can be the result of exposure to allergens or irritants and as such is not contagious. However, there is a bacterial or viral form known as infectious conjunctivitis and easily transmitted to others. Clinical manifestations are watery eyes, reddened appearance, itching, and burning-like pain.

Viral conjunctivitis may be caused by adenovirus, HSV, and rubella. In bacterial conjunctivitis the offending organisms include pneumococcus, streptococcus, staphylococcus, and gonococcus.

Parasitic infections can also occur such as *Chlamydia trachoma* or *Onchocerca volvos*. These infections while rarely occurring in the western countries are a leading cause of blindness in the world. Diagnosis is obtained through use of cultures and antigen detection assays (Kuehn, 2005).

Planning and Implementation

The care provided for conjunctivitis is focused on preventing spread and individual treatment. Good hand washing technique prior to touching the eye area and avoiding touching the eye and then handling other objects are good techniques for prevention. Health care workers should wear gloves when treating the eye. Allergen causes are treated with removal of the allergen if possible, rinsing with artificial tears, and use of topical medications, such as antihistamines and corticosteroids. Eye drops that treat the reddened appearance, such as vasoconstrictors may be cosmetically beneficial.

Care for bacterial or viral infections includes application of appropriate antibiotic ointments after a culture of the eye drainage is obtained. Oral antiviral agents, such as acyclovir or ganciclovir, may also be used. During the healing time makeup should be avoided and all old makeup replaced to prevent reinfection.

Patients with parasitic infections are treated with topical antibiotics or oral antibiotics (tetracycline or sulfonamides) depending on their exposure and recurrence.

Keratitis

Keratitis occurs when there is an inflammation and ulceration of the cornea. Because of the involvement of the cornea there is often a loss in visual acuity. The clinical manifestations include watery eyes, pain, and photophobia. Keratitis can be caused by drugs, vitamin A deficiency, sun exposure, trauma, immune-mediated response, or microorganisms. The most common viral cause is HSV and bacterial causes are *Staphylococcus aureus, Streptococcus pneumoniae, pseudomonas,* mycobacterium, and serratia. Patients wearing contact lens are at risk for bacterial infections and in particular those using extended wear contact lens.

Planning and Implementation

Therapy is directed at treating the underlying causes; for the bacterial causes antibiotic ointments are used if the epithelial layer remains intact. Systemic antibiotics maybe required for infections that leak into the cornea. HSV keratitis can result in retinitis or cataract, and if left untreated the virus may travel to the trigeminal ganglion and a latent infection is established.

Keratoconjunctivitis Sicca

Some individuals develop an inflammation of the cornea and conjunctiva known as keratoconjunctivitis sicca or dry eye syndrome. This occurs when the individual produces fewer tears and is more common in women, especially after menopause. Aging is also a risk factor, as people grow older they produce less lipids, which affects the tear film. With less oil to seal the water layer, the tears evaporate more quickly or rundown the cheek instead of staying in the eye to moisten it. Clinical manifestations include a scratchy or sandy feeling as though something was in the eye, irritation, burning, redness, and blurred vision that improves with blinking (Kuehn, 2005).

Planning and Implementation

The care goal is primarily to treat with artificial tears for lubricating the eyes. Closing the eye's drainage ducts with punctual plugs is an option for some patients, thereby keeping more fluid in the eye. One risk group are patients that are critically ill and in an intensive care unit often because of less blinking, potential for dehydration and dry conditions with in the unit. These patients require additional proactive care.

> ### PATIENT PLAYBOOK
>
> **Treatment of "Dry Eyes"**
>
> The nurse should instruct the patient to:
> - Drink 8 to 10 glasses of water daily.
> - Make a conscious effort to blink more frequently.
> - Avoid rubbing the eyes.
> - Inform the patient that high altitude, dry or winter climates may make the condition worse.

Iritis and Uveitis

Iritis is the inflammation of the iris, and uveitis is the inflammation of one or all parts of the uveal tract. The uveal tract includes the iris, the ciliary body, and the choroid. Currently uveitis is divided into four components: (a) anterior; (b) confined to the iris and the anterior chamber (iritis); (c) confined to the iris the anterior iris, the anterior chamber, and the ciliary body (iridocyclitis); and (d) posterior uveitis (choroiditis). Posterior uveitis is uncommon except in patients with AIDS that may develop cytomegalovirus retinitis. Uveitis can be acute and chronic (Kuehn, 2005).

Pathophysiology

While the exact pathophysiology is unknown, it is believed that uveitis is caused by an immune reaction. It is postulated the immune reaction is directed against foreign antigens. Uveitis is often associated with infections, such as HSV and autoimmune disorders, such as systemic lupus erythematosus and rheumatoid arthritis. Clinical manifestations include pain, eye redness, blurred vision, photophobia, and tearing. In posterior uveitis there may be floaters or occasional photophobia.

Assessment with Clinical Manifestations

A thorough ophthalmic assessment would include visual acuity, extraocular movement, ophthalmoscopy, measurement of IOP, and slit lamp examination. There is no laboratory or radiographic test that is generally performed except tests associated with the initial diagnosis of systemic disease.

Planning and Implementation

The first line of treatment is cycloplegic and steroidal ophthalmic drops. Patients may also receive oral steroids and immunosuppressive agents. Follow-up with an ophthalmologist is imperative. If vitreous hemorrhage occurs a vitrectomy may be used in patients who cannot take immunosuppressive agents.

OCULAR DISORDERS RESULTING FROM OTHER PHYSIOLOGICAL PROCESSES

While there are many other disorders that have ocular ramifications, this chapter will deal with the following three problems: (a) an ocular disorder occurring as a result of neurological dysfunction (papilledema); (b) diabetes retinitis related to DM; and (c) retinitis pigmentosa (RP) a genetic disorder.

Papilledema

When there is an increase in intracranial pressure as a result of trauma or other disease process a swelling of the optic disc **(papilledema)** may occur. Other causes include any tumors occupying space in the central nervous system, meningitis, and encephalitis. Papilledema usually occurs bilaterally and can develop rapidly or slowly over time depending on the underlying cause.

Pathophysiology

Because the subarachnoid space of the brain is continuous with the optic nerve sheath, as the cerebrospinal fluid pressure increases, the pressure is transmitted to the optic nerve. This results in swelling and inflammation of the optic nerve at the entrance to the retina. Clinical manifestations include headache, nausea, and vomiting. While visual symptoms may not occur, some patients develop graying of vision or transient flickering, blurry vision, and diplopia. Visual acuity is usually unaffected until the condition is quite advanced. In severe cases blindness can occur rapidly unless the pressure is relieved and the swelling decreases.

Planning and Implementation

Care is tailored to treat the underlying cause or causes. Efforts to reduce papilledema include carbonic anhydrase inhibitor diuretics, weight reduction in idiopathic intracranial hypertension, and corticosteroids for inflammatory causes. Surgical treatment may include removing the tumor, a ventriculoperitoneal shunt, or optic nerve sheath decompression.

Diabetic Retinopathy

Patients with DM are at risk of developing many different ophthalmic complications, including corneal abnormalities, glaucoma, cataracts, and neuropathies. However, the most common and potentially most blinding complication is diabetic retinopathy (see chapter 57).

Etiology

Risk factors include duration of diabetes, development of renal complications, systemic hypertension, and elevated serum lipids.

Pathophysiology

The exact mechanism by which diabetes causes retinopathy is unknown, however, there are several hypotheses. The first is that growth hormone may play a causative role, second is hematologic abnormalities in diabetes, such as erythrocyte aggregation, increased platelet aggregation, and sluggish circulation, may be factors. The third is related to the abnormal glucose metabolism where high levels of blood glucose are thought to have an affect on the retinal capillaries causing them to function poorly eventually leading to retinal hypoxia. About 8,000 eyes become blind each year from diabetes (Horowitz, Brennan, & Reinhardt, 2005).

Assessment with Clinical Manifestations and Diagnostic Tests

As with many eye disorders initial diagnosis may come with routine eye examination. To determine the extent of microvascular damage fluorescein angiography or ultrasound of the retina may be done.

Nursing Diagnoses

See Box 39-1. See also nursing diagnoses for patients with DM in chapter 57.

Planning and Implementation

The most important management of patients with DM is the management of glucose levels with the goal of intensive glucose control will decrease the incidence and progression of disease. The goal of the American Diabetic Association (ADA) to maintain a glycosylated hemoglobin level of less than 7 percent can help prevent or at least minimize the long-term complications of DM. Treatment with laser photocoagulation, vitrectomy, or cryotherapy has been successful in some patients in preserving vision. Patient education regarding glucose control, managing other complications well, and cessation of smoking have also proven beneficial.

Retinitis Pigmentosa

RP is the name given to a group of inherited diseases affecting the retina. Currently there are about 70 different genetic defects that have been identified.

Pathophysiology

RP is a progressive disease with a progressive loss of vision due to the loss of viable photoreceptors. In the progressive disease, central vision is spared the longest, with peripheral vision affected first. The individual may have either the rods or the cones affected. When the rods are primarily affected, it results in symptoms of night blindness and slow loss of peripheral vision, whereas the individual with cones primarily affected has decreasing visual acuity, development of color blindness, and day vision problems.

Assessment with Clinical Manifestations

History of loss of night vision and tunnel vision are often reported by patients. A complete history of vision changes is important as well as the adaptation to darkness. A complete ophthalmic examination is used to identify disease development or progression.

Nursing Diagnoses

Based on the information gathered, examples of nursing diagnoses in the patient with RP problems are shown in Box 39-1.

Planning and Implementation

There are multiple studies underway looking at methods of treatment and prevention; however there is no medical treatment currently. Today there is some recommendation for vitamin A supplementation. Treatment of symptoms may

BOX 39-3

CAUSES OF BLINDNESS

Cataracts 47.8 percent

Glaucoma 12.3 percent

Age-related macular degeneration 8.7 percent

Trachoma 3.6 percent

Corneal opacity 5.1 percent

Diabetic retinopathy 4.8 percent

be somewhat beneficial, such as cataract removal as cataracts develop; however, vision will still be affected by the development of RP, with possibly only central vision improvement. Future treatments may involve retinal transplants, artificial retinal implants, gene therapy, stem cells, nutritional supplements, and drug therapies.

LOW VISION AND BLINDNESS

Low vision is a general term used to describe a permanent functional vision loss that is not correctable by medication, surgery, or corrective lenses. Patients classified with low vision may have any one of a wide range of diseases. These individuals may find that their ability to perform activities of daily living, work, and pleasure are impaired. In addition to the traditional assessment for vision and visual acuity, consideration should be given to the individual's ability to cope with their limitations.

Legal blindness is defined as vision of 20/200 on a Snellen chart or less in the better eye with correction. Of the individuals in above classification about 10 percent are fully sightless. The rest have some vision, from light perception alone to relatively good acuity. Those who are not legally blind but have serious visual impairment possess low vision (Estes, 2006).

Epidemiology

The most common causes of blindness around the world, according to the World Health Organization, are shown in Box 39-3. Many of these diseases can be prevented through adequate nutrition and disease treatment, especially if treatment of infections is done in a timely manner.

Planning and Implementation

The care necessary for individuals with low vision and blindness is varied. Mobility is one of the greatest challenges for patients with these dysfunctions. In an era where individual transportation rather public transportation is the norm, the ability to get from place to place is greatly impeded in our social context. Patients can travel using a white cane, an international symbol of blindness, which when swung in a low sweeping motion across the intended path can detect obstacles. Individuals choosing to use guide dogs have been guaranteed access to public places as an individual personal right.

Assistive Devices

Patients with low vision have some options to help improve vision. Reading devices are available with a bifocal power of up to +5.00 diopters (D); however, this may distort vision for walking and other activities. Therefore, the patient may need a second pair of corrective lenses for other activities.

Microscope devices are used when the needed power is greater than 12 D. Because of the greatly reduced focal length, microscopes often are prescribed monocularly. Near telescopes, have a narrow field of view and can be designed for the individuals regular working distance.

Handheld magnifiers provide greater magnification than high-add readers and allow for a greater reading distance than microscopes, but they require good motor control. For this reason, handheld magnifiers are primarily used for short-term activities, such as shopping or using a phonebook. Stand magnifiers require less motor control and allow for a longer working distance. When illuminated, these magnifiers can increase the ease of readability for the patient.

Closed circuit televisions can provide a larger field of view than other forms of magnification. A handheld magnifier or camera is used to scan over the material that is projected onto the television monitor in an enlarged format.

Other adaptive equipment is available through multiple resources listed in the previous chapter. Large print newspapers and magazines are available in some communities. Dial markers can be used to dry gauges on ovens, dishwashers, washers, and dryers. Self-threading needles, books on tape, and talking clocks and watches are just some of the available adjuncts for patients.

HEALTH PROMOTION

It is the charge of health care workers to ensure that patients are educated regarding prevention of eye-related disease. Patients should be encouraged as part of their normal health promotion behaviors to see their eye care specialist on a regular basis. Because malnutrition is a cause of many eye conditions, patient education on adequate nutrition should be considered part of every episode of patient teaching.

Safety

In these same patients, safety should be an ongoing concern with patient education directed to methods to prevent injury to allow a patient the greatest freedoms without possible harm. Patients should be oriented to new environments, how to access care, or taught what to do in emergencies. In the health care setting, patients should be oriented to the individuals caring for them and the location of important items (e.g., call lights or bathrooms). At mealtime, patients need to be oriented to location of various eating utensils and foods on the tray. When ambulating a patient, the nurse should allow the patient to grasp his or her arm below the elbow and walk a half step ahead of the patient. Instruct the patient regarding any obstacles in the path and give notice to changes in direction. Safety precautions will make the patient more comfortable and ease the tradition from the home setting to the health care setting.

KEY CONCEPTS

- There are three main ocular movement dysfunctions: (a) strabismus, (b) nystagmus, and (c) ocular muscle paralysis.
- Ocular motor testing is the evaluation of the alignment of the eyes and their movement.
- Disorders of visual acuity include cataracts, glaucoma, retinal detachment, and macular degeneration.
- Glaucoma is a group of diseases related to the amount of IOP in the eye occurring as a result of neurodegenerative processes.
- Retinal detachment may also be called a detached retina or retinal tear.
- Macular degeneration is largely an age-related disease whereby central vision gradually deteriorates.
- The most common traumatic injuries of the eye include damage from penetration by foreign bodies, physical pressure resulting in a contusion, lacerations from sharp objects, and penetrating injuries.
- Eye cancer can occur in nearly any anatomical structure of the eye including the eyelid, the orbit, and conjunctiva.
- Corneal disorders include corneal abrasions, ulcerations, and keratoconus.
- In errors of visual refraction, which are the most common vision problems, the light passing through the layers of the eye to the retina is distorted.
- Older adults begin to experience a loss of near acuity (near vision) as the lens loses its elasticity and accommodation of the lens fails.
- The ability to distinguish color is composed of two stages, the first is through the light-sensitive receptors and the second is through the neural components of processing, partitioning, and encoding information about wavelength that the photoreceptors collect.
- Infections of the eye can occur as a result of the acquisition of a virulent microorganism or uncontrolled growth of an existing organism because of lowered resistance in the patient.

Continued

KEY CONCEPTS—cont'd

■ Conjunctivitis, also called pink eye, can be the result of exposure to allergens or irritants and as such is not contagious.

■ An ocular disorder occurring as a result of neurological dysfunction is papilledema.

■ RP is the name given to a group of inherited diseases affecting the retina.

■ Low vision is a general term used to describe a permanent functional vision loss that is not correctable by medication, surgery, or corrective lenses.

■ Patients should be encouraged as part of their normal health promotion behaviors to see their eye care specialist on a regular basis

REVIEW QUESTIONS

1. Which of the following is not one of the three main ocular movement dysfunctions?
   1. Strabismus
   2. Nystagmus
   3. Color blindness
   4. Ocular muscle paralysis

2. Mr. Jones has an abnormality of the eye in which both eyes are affected, yet the problem is often more acute in one eye than the other. This is most likely which condition?
   1. Cataract
   2. Keratoconus
   3. Glaucoma
   4. Retinal detachment

3. Mr. Bears has glaucoma, which was determined by testing the pressure within his eye. The diagnostic test revealing the presence of this eye pressure is:
   1. Intracranial pressure
   2. Ballottement
   3. Tonometry
   4. Trabeculectomy

4. Mrs. Carpenter, 83, has an eye condition where she has blurred vision and states it is better in bright light. In addition, she sees wavy lines on the Amsler grid (diagnostic test). This is most likely which condition?
   1. Glaucoma
   2. Diabetic retinopathy
   3. Age-related macular degeneration
   4. Strabismus

5. A patient is found after an accident with an impaled object in an eye. The nurse remembers to first do what?
   1. Place a cup over the impaled object and tape in place
   2. Remembers to assess the patient for priority injuries
   3. Pull out the object and observe for bleeding
   4. Turn the patient on their side, to prevent aspiration

6. What is the most common cause of ocular cancer?
   1. Melanoma
   2. Diabetes mellitus
   3. Intracranial pressure problems
   4. Hypertension

7. Mary has been rubbing her eye profusely for the past several weeks. Which of the following complications would she most likely be predisposed to from the rubbing action?
   1. Hyperopia
   2. Keratoconus
   3. Corneal ulceration
   4. Refraction

8. Mr. Clark has a visual problem that is correct with convex corrective lens. His problem is most likely what?
   1. Hyperopia
   2. Myopia
   3. Astigmatism
   4. Corneal abrasion

9. Mrs. Thomlin has an eye disorder in which there are inflamed sweat glands that are reddened, swollen, and tender to touch. This is:
   1. Uveitis
   2. Iritis
   3. Hordeolum
   4. Conjunctivitis

10. Mr. Evans has an inflammation of the cornea and conjunctiva known as keratoconjunctivitis sicca or dry eye syndrome. Which of the following is not an appropriate nursing intervention for this condition?
    1. Make a conscious effort to blink more frequently
    2. Avoid rubbing the eyes
    3. Inform the patient that high altitude, dry, or winter climates may make the condition worse
    4. Decrease daily intake of water

REVIEW ACTIVITIES

1. Assess six patients for ocular movement dysfunction by assessing their cranial nerves (CN) III, IV, and VI.

2. Evaluate four patients in regard to their visual acuity by administering a Snellen eye chart examination.

3. Examine three patients with an ophthalmoscope to specifically identify the retina and ask the patient questions specific to the condition of a retinal detachment.

4. Obtain permission to observe several specific eye diagnostic tests in either an acute care facility or clinic that performs eye tests.

5. Describe the emergency care for a patient with an object impaled in his or her eye.

6. Compare and contrast the three main types of refraction.

7. Compare and contrast two inflammatory and infectious eye conditions.

8. List at least five devices that can be used with patients who have low vision.

Auditory Dysfunction: Nursing Management

Diane Montgomery, PhD, RN

CHAPTER TOPICS

- Conductive Hearing Loss
- Sensorineural Hearing Loss
- Health Promotion
- Protective Devices
- Auditory Testing
- Communication Adaptation
- Hearing Aids

The ability to hear is one of the basic five senses in the body, which are considered necessary for an individual to communicate and interpret environment cues. With loss of normal hearing, the individual experiences decreased functional ability and social isolation. As an individual gets older, hearing begins to deteriorate. The ability to remain independent and maintain a healthy quality of life depends on the ability to function in society. Some hearing loss can be prevented while others who have already experienced profound loss may be helped with hearing devices.

AUDITORY DYSFUNCTION

Auditory (pertains to the sense of hearing) dysfunction affects an individual's ability to hear sounds. The degree and amount of dysfunction is associated with the affected location in the auditory system. This section of the chapter will discuss auditory dysfunction and its nursing management.

Epidemiology

Loss of hearing is the third leading cause of health problems in the United States affecting for the most part the elderly and young. Approximately 28 million Americans or roughly 1:10 have some degree of auditory dysfunction. One in four 65-year-olds and one in two 75-year-olds are hearing impaired. When hearing is diminished or lost, an individual has difficulty communicating with others and therefore must find alternative ways in which to exchange ideas. As the population ages so will the increase of hearing loss related to the aging process and prolonged excessive noise exposure. Research indicates that there is an increasing number of 46- to 64-year-olds with complaints of hearing loss secondary to repeated high noise exposure throughout their lifetimes (Bogardus, Yueh, & Shekelle, 2003; Brors & Bodmer, 2004; Rovig, 2004). Society has become more noise infested with new inventions to make tasks easier. Examples of excessive noise producers would include power tools, appliances, and other electronic devices. Excessive noise exposure has been linked to employment, loud music, high volume traffic, domestic appliances, and toys. The costs related to hearing loss are enormous and approximately $56 billion dollars per year are attributed to lost production, special education, and necessary medical care. Prevention is the first step in preserving hearing. Prevention begins with awareness of the level and type of noises throughout the environment and taking steps to decrease the amount that comes in contact with the inner ear. Depending on the cause and severity of loss, management can range from prevention to assistance with mechanical devices and cochlear implants to aural rehabilitation.

Etiology

Hearing loss can be caused by several factors including noise-induced exposures, disorders in the auditory system, and the normal aging process. The ability to perceive sound differs in degrees from the inability to understand certain words or certain sound's pitch to total deafness. Most people who have a hearing problem may not recognize that there is a problem until others mention the change in mannerisms. Although some are aware that they are experiencing a loss in hearing, they are often unwilling to tell anyone for fear of being stigmatized or being excluded from certain activities. A large number of individuals are too self-conscious and therefore not willing to reveal a weakness to others or show that they are aging. Hearing loss has long been considered an aging disease but can be associated with other factors.

Acquired Hearing Loss

Acquired hearing loss is caused by repeated damage to the auditory system. Besides noise pollution, head trauma, and infectious etiologies, such as otitis media and communicable diseases, can cause damage to the sensitive auditory system. Harm from noise can be related to a single loud blast or gradual repeated abuse throughout one's lifespan.

Ototoxic Medications and Auditory Dysfunction

Auditory dysfunction can also be caused by **ototoxic** (a substance that damages the acoustic nerve or hearing mechanism) medications, which include aminoglycoside antibiotics (gentamicin, tobramycin), loop diuretics (furosemide),

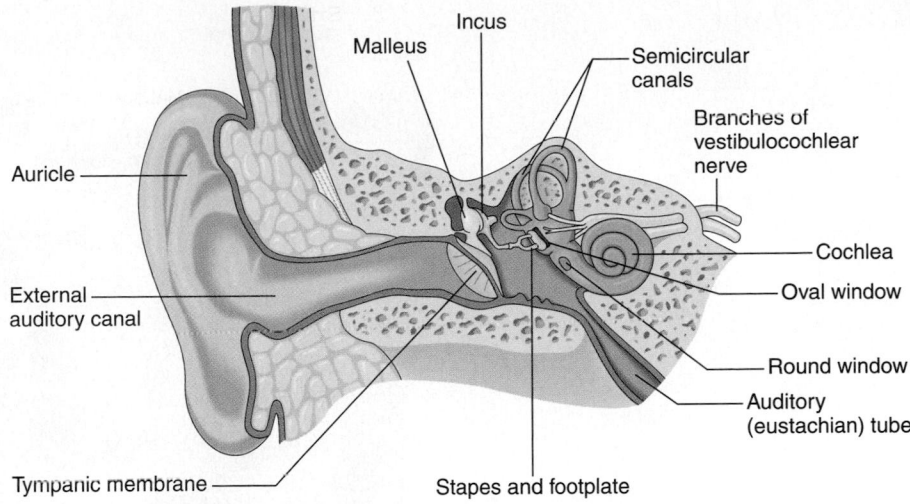

Figure 40-1 Ear structure.

antimalarial drugs (quinine sulfate, mefloquine), chemotherapy (cisplatin, carboplatin), and high-dose salicylates. Some of the medications cause temporary damage to the auditory system, in other words, when the medication is discontinued, the hearing will return to the previous state, while others cause permanent damage. Permanent damage is found to occur with aminoglycosides and chemotherapy drugs (Yueh, Shapiro, MacLean, & Shekelle, 2003). When a known ototoxic medication is prescribed, the risks and benefits to the patient should be considered. A baseline and follow up hearing test is recommended depending on the substance. There are over 200 different medications, which are labeled ototoxic, so the nurse needs to be diligent when administering medications. Being alert to the slightest change in the patient's hearing and investigating likely causes. Common symptoms experienced, include sensorineural hearing loss, tinnitus, and decreased equilibrium.

Head Trauma

Head trauma can also cause hearing loss, specifically injury to the temporal bone. The auditory receptors are located in the temporal region of the skull. Trauma to the area or an abrupt change in air pressure can cause a perforated tympanic membrane leading to the development of scar tissue and eventual hearing loss.

Pathophysiology

To understand the mechanism of hearing, the nurse must know the anatomy of the ear and how sound waves are transmitted, received, and interpreted. The ear has two main functions, hearing and maintaining balance equilibrium. The anatomy of the ear is such that it allows sound waves to be transmitted to the brain for interpretation from the outside world (Figure 40-1). Understanding the mechanism of how the ear functions is essential for the nurse to care for patients who experience hearing dysfunction. The responsibility of the nurse lies with preventing further damage to the auditory system, identifying the hearing loss, assisting the patient in adjusting to the degree of loss, and rehabilitation of auditory function when possible.

The ear is divided into three main sections: external ear, middle ear, and inner ear (Figure 40-2). The external canal extends from the external os or opening to the tympanic membrane. The middle ear is an air filled cavity, which contains the **ossicles** (the tiny bones located in the inner ear chamber: malleus, incus, and stapes), tiny bones that assist with transmitted sounds from the tympanic membrane to the inner ear. The inner ear provides the necessary

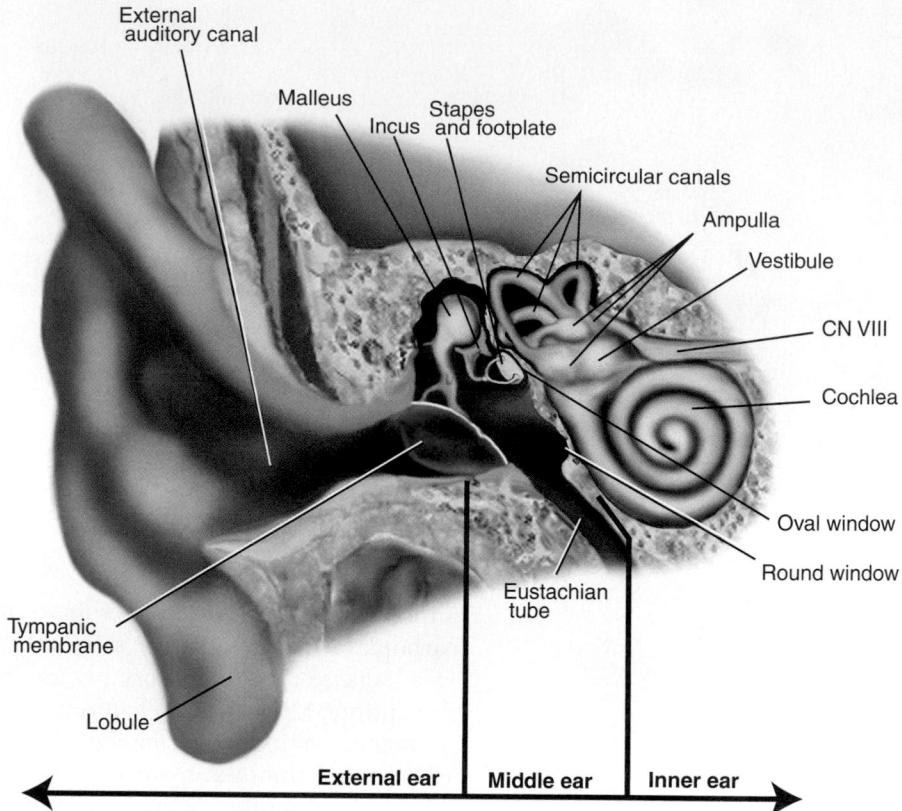

External
auditory canal

Malleus

Incus

Stapes
and footplate

Semicircular canals

Ampulla

Vestibule

CN VIII

Cochlea

Oval window

Round window

Eustachian
tube

Tympanic
membrane

Lobule

| External ear | Middle ear | Inner ear |

Figure 40-2 Cross-section of the ear showing the external, middle. and inner ear.

components for hearing and maintaining equilibrium, which begins with the oval window and contains the vestibule, semicircular canals, and cochlea. Inside the cochlea is the organ of Corti, responsible for transmitting sound to the acoustic nerve (eighth cranial nerve), which travels to the brain for interpretation. In other words, sound causes the tympanic membrane to vibrate, which results in movement of the ossicles; this movement travels through the oval window into the inner ear and disrupts the fragile hair lining of the Corti (end organ of hearing) located in the cochlea, sending an impulse to the acoustic nerve and then to the brain for interpretation.

The formation of the ear begins during the third week of gestation and continues through the first trimester of pregnancy, therefore any insults incurred during this most critical period of development can result in malformations of the ear. Depending on the extent and location of the abnormality, loss of hearing can occur.

Auditory dysfunction can occur at any age. As discussed above, hearing difficulties are related to several factors, including congenital malformations, noise level, and length of exposure, or acquired through infections or other pathology. The ability to learn speech, communicate and socialize depends on the capability to hear and interpret sounds.

Genetics

Congenital hearing loss can be derived from genetics, natal infections, or physical deformities of the ear. Inherited hearing loss can result from multiple of factors associated with autosomal dominant (50 percent chance), recessive (25 percent chance), or cross-linked (carried on the sex gene, male increased risk) chromosomal abnormalities. Certain conditions, such as

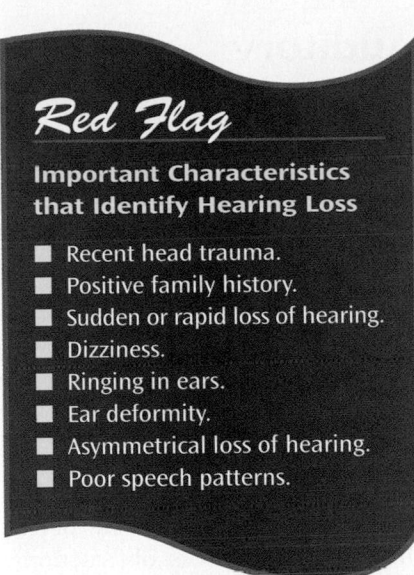

Down, Usher, and Treacher Collins syndromes, have known associated hearing impairments (Phillips, 2003). Other factors related to congenital hearing loss are ototoxic drugs administered before or after birth or maternal prenatal infections commonly associated with the TORCH infections (a set of infections which affect the growing fetus: toxoplasmosis, rubella, cytomegalovirus, and herpes-virus type 2 and other viruses, such as syphilis, HIV, hepatitis B, and human parvovirus).

Assessment with Clinical Manifestations

The history of a patient is the most important part of assessing a patient with hearing loss. It is necessary for the nurse to observe and assess for warning signs related to a loss of hearing while interviewing the patient. During the health history, the nurse should cover problems with balance, nutrition, such as any foods which affect hearing or cause ear discomfort, sleep disturbance-related to tinnitus or vertigo, functioning level, and allergies, which may affect the eustachian tube functioning.

Ascertaining an accurate health history is the initial way to identify a hearing problem and guide the physical exam to identifying the origin of the problem. Inquiring about any changes in hearing perception, balance, and physical signs of ear disorders are important factors to lead the focus of the physical exam. Included in the history should be items, such as pain or fullness in the ears, dizziness, or tinnitus. Has their communication style changed, are they more attuned to lip reading? Does the patient have any food allergies or taken any medicines that would be ototoxic? Have they had to alter their activities of daily living related to ear discomforts?

When performing a physical exam on a patient, a simple noninvasive way to test hearing would be the whisper test. Standing approximately two feet away from the patient and covering the opposite ear, the nurse whispers a word or phase to the patient and then has the patient repeat what was said. If the patient is unable to hear the word, it is repeated slightly louder until the patient can hear. Failure to repeat the correct word or phase or having to say the word in a normal or loud tone would indicate the need for formal audiometry testing.

Hearing loss is often subtle, and the individual learns to compensation to overcome the deficit. There are various degrees of loss of hearing that the individual can experience. The assortment includes missing some syllables or words, the inability to hear some tones or pitches, or profound deafness. The first clinical signs that emerge are when a person asks to have things repeated, asks others to speak louder, answers questions inappropriately, or does not respond to a question when asked. Common missed sounds are found in numbers, for example, the person misinterprets 50 for 15 or has difficulty distinguishing certain letters, such as th and s. Hearing impaired individuals often tilt their heads to listen or display unusual facies such as frowning when trying to listen to the conversation. Additional signs may include weariness or unexplained irritability. There is a misconception that people get used to the noise and therefore can tolerate higher degrees.

Degrees of hearing impairment are categorized into minimal, moderate, severe, and profound depending on the level of decibels (dB) of sound heard. Decibels are logarithmic units of measurement of sound intensities used to measure a person's hearing capabilities. Normal hearing is 0–15 dB; slight loss 16–25 dB; mild impairment 26–40 dB; moderate 41–55 dB; moderate severe 56–70 dB; severe 71–90 dB; profound greater than or equal to 91 dB (Bogardus, et al., 2003; Punch, Joseph, & Rakerd, 2004). Profound hearing loss is usually characteristic of a congenital abnormality. Individuals who are exposed to intensities greater than 80 dB on a regular basis are at increased risk of gradual irreversible hearing loss.

Three Classifications of Auditory Dysfunction

Auditory dysfunction is classified in three ways, conductive and sensorineural dysfunction and mixed. Loss of auditory function depends on the degree of loss, etiology, and location of damage in the auditory system.

Conductive Hearing Loss

Conductive hearing loss is generally treatable and is associated with an obstruction. Conductive hearing loss affects all pitches of sound waves and is associated with an obstruction in the external and middle sections of the ear. Because the patient appears to have loss of hearing in all frequencies levels, they tend to hear better in noisy situations. Speech patterns are appropriate, although they tend to speak softer because they have a tendency to perceive their own voice louder.

Conductive loss results in a blockage of sound waves in the external or middle portions of the ear. The loss results from insults from obstructions, infections, congenital deformities, and damage. The hearing loss is associated with anything that interferes with air conduction in the outer and middle ear chambers. This includes cerumen, foreign body, otitis externa, middle ear disease (e.g., otitis media with or without effusion), **otosclerosis** (a progressive hearing loss of predominately low tones), and stenosis of external auditory canal. Most of these conditions can be treated by medical or surgical management. Air conduction is decreased in conductive hearing loss, which is necessary for sound waves to be transmitted to the ossicles for vibrations and therefore be transmitted to the brain for interpretation. In conductive loss the sound is perceived as faint or distant but clear. Patients try to compensate by speaking softer because their own voice is perceived as louder. They have no added difficulty with hearing in a noisy environment. Conductive hearing loss can be differentiated from sensorineural by the loss of all frequencies as opposed to loss of the higher frequencies found in sensorineural loss.

Temporary causes of auditory dysfunction result from obstruction in the ear canal, which can be cerumen or foreign bodies lodged in the external canal. These substances obstruct the canal preventing sound from reaching the tympanic membrane, thereby preventing the vibratory movement necessary to initiate the sequence of hearing sound waves. The external canal can be visually inspected with an otoscope. By eliminating the obstruction, the patient can instantly hear as before. Another cause of conductive loss would be an external otitis media, which causes a narrowing of the canal leading to interference of sound waves hitting the tympanic membrane.

The most common cause of intermittent loss of conductive hearing is infections. Otitis infections include otitis media or otitis media with effusion. The infection decreases the vibratory movement of the tympanic membrane necessary for passing sound waves to the acoustic nerve to be interpreted by the brain. Repeated insults from recurrent otitis media may cause permanent hearing loss. Therefore, the nurse must be diligent in recognizing those at risk. Repeated damage to the tympanic membrane can cause scarring and thickening of the membrane, causing the vibratory response to be diminished and thereby affecting the ability to hear.

Conductive loss is also affected by injury to the middle ear, which would include the auditory ossicles. Pathology that would affect this region includes trauma, infections, and scar tissue. Adhesions from chronic otitis media can cause fibrous bands to interfere with movement of the ossicles causing a conductive hearing loss. Other conditions include otosclerosis, which is a progressive disorder that affects the ossicles and the stapes in particular (note: discussed in further detail later in the chapter).

Sensorineural Hearing Loss

Sensorineural hearing loss is caused by defects in the inner ear, in the acoustic nerve (eighth cranial nerve), or in areas of the brain. Congenital anomalies, systemic insults, and environmental factors fall into this category. The loss is noticed more in high-frequency pitches, and the patient appears to have more difficulty hearing in noisy environments, such as restaurants.

Sensorineural loss results from damage or deformities of the inner ear, the area where sound is identified by the cochlea and sent to the brain via the acoustic nerve. Sensorineural hearing loss is permanent and therefore cannot be corrected or treated, just managed. Sound is perceived as distorted. There is a greater loss in the higher frequency ranges, and therefore the patient has difficulty trying to understand conversations in a noisy crowed area. Specific conditions, which cause nerve damage would include noise pollution, presbycusis, congenital, environmental, infections, and various systemic conditions. In sensorineural hearing loss bone conduction is affected, which can be identified using the Rinne test.

Sensorineural hearing loss is the impaired function of the inner ear, which includes the auditory connections to the brain. The patient has the ability to hear sound but cannot understand speech. Causes of sensorineural hearing loss include congenital and hereditary factors, noise trauma, Menière's disease, and ototoxicity. Systemic infections such as tuberculosis, syphilis, Lyme disease, cytomegalovirus, human immunodeficiency virus (HIV), and Paget disease of bone can also lead to sensorineural hearing loss. Smoking has also been linked to sensorineural hearing loss from damage over the years to the fine ciliary hairs of the inner ear from both the smoker and secondhand smoke. Other disorders such as diabetes mellitus, bacterial meningitis, and trauma have been linked to sensorineural hearing loss (Yeuh, Shapiro, MacLean, & Shekelle, 2003).

Menière's Disease

Menière's disease is a degenerative condition of unknown etiology, which leads to progressive hearing loss predominately in middle age. Studies link the disease to excessive accumulation of fluid in the labyrinth or inner ear. Symptoms appear as dizziness, unilateral ringing in the ear, feeling of pressure or fullness in ear, and unilateral hearing loss. The patient experiences episodic attacks, which can render him or her debilitated and confined to bed for extended periods of time during the acute attack. The onset of the acute phase at times is so severe that the patient may drop to the floor. Menière's disease is a progressive chronic condition in which no cure is available. Approximately 50 percent of patients who have unilateral symptoms will develop signs in the unaffected ear over the course of the disease. Menière's disease usually affects patients between the ages of 30 and 60 years and tends to appear in families and is therefore thought to have a genetic component (Perez, Chen, & Nedzelski, 2004). When performing a physical examination, the neurological assessment is found to be within normal limits.

Pharmacology

Pharmacological management during the acute phase includes antihistamines, anticholinergic medications (antiemetic/antivertigo), and sedatives, which include benzodiazepines. Between attacks the patient should be placed on diuretics, medications with vasodilating properties, and antihistamines. Up to 85 percent of patients improve with medical management. Others may require surgical interventions.

Surgery

Surgery is indicated in patients who have frequent incapacitating attacks that interfere with activities of daily living. During surgery the vestibular nerve is resected to help relieve vertigo and stop further hearing loss. In perioperative teaching, the nurse provides safety and ways to minimize vertigo. The patient is instructed to call for assistance with ambulation and avoid sudden head movement and postural changes. Televisions, florescent bulbs, and flickering lights should also be avoided.

Patient and Family Teaching

After ruling out other central nervous system disorders, nurses should offer support, reassurances that Menière's disease is not life-threatening, and education on management, which includes special dietary intervention, the course of disease, and medication administration, which includes possible side effects. Patients are helped by initiating a low-salt diet and the elimination of all caffeine-containing products. These measures have been found to help decrease the symptoms. Patients should also stop smoking and avoid prolonged exposure to smoke. During the acute phase the patients are confined to bed rest and assistance with ambulation to prevent injury.

Labyrinthitis

Labyrinthitis is a rare disorder, which involves the inflammation of the labyrinth section of the inner ear caused by head trauma or various viral or bacterial infections. An organism enters into the inner ear chamber through the oval window causing the patient to experience sudden onset of vertigo, sensorineural hearing loss, horizontal nystagmus, and occasionally nausea and vomiting. The patient experiences a whirling vertigo with movement of the head. This condition generally affects healthy middle-aged adults and has a temporary self-limiting course. The disorder is usually preceded by an upper respiratory infection or an otitis media. Permanent hearing loss may occur if the organism damages the sensitive hairs of the inner ear. Safety of the patient should be a priority. Treatment includes administration of an anticholinergic medication, such as meclizine or prochlorperazine. The short course of the disease is helped by lying in a dark room with decreased stimuli. Antibiotics are prescribed if a bacterium is identified as the suspected organism. Although, many patients experience a single episode in their lifetimes, this can be a recurrent condition.

Vertigo

Vertigo (a sensation or feeling of a loss of equilibrium, sometimes referred spinning or whirling) is a condition that affects the equilibrium of a patient who experiences the feeling of motion while standing still. Vertigo is produced by an injury or lesion to the labyrinth or inner ear caused by various toxic substances, middle ear disease, postural hypotension, or occasionally as a complication to ear surgery. Patient's safety is of utmost importance. Patients are instructed to rise slowly and gradually increase their activity over time (Badke, Shea, Miedaner, & Grove, 2004).

Otalgia

Otalgia (pain in the ear) can occur with a variety of conditions from otitis infections, airplane rides, loud noise, trauma, or referred pain associated with dental conditions. The cause of the pain must be identified to be able to determine the appropriate management.

Mixed Conductive and Sensorineural Hearing Loss

Mixed conductive and sensorineural hearing loss occur when hearing loss results from a combination of both conductive and sensorineural factors. An example of mixed would be presbycusis, a progressive degenerative hearing loss associated with age caused by wear and tear on the inner ear over the years. This deterioration is from loud noise exposure of occupation and recreational environments and the aging process. Other causes would include inherent conditions from disease, dietary habits, and tobacco and alcohol ingestions.

Tinnitus (a ringing, buzzing, or jingling sound in the ear) is a symptom that is frequently reported and can be associated with both a conductive or sensorineural problem. The ringing, which can be disabling to some people, can be caused by something as simple as impacted cerumen or foreign bodies lodged in the external canal to a sign of Menière's disease or other pathology. Exposure in an area where a high level of noise is experienced for an extensive amount of time such as a rock concert can cause a temporary ringing in the ear, which should resolve within 48 hours after exposure (Folmer, Martin, & Shi, 2004).

When a patient presents with a complaint associated with the auditory system, the nurse takes a complete history to get a good picture of the lifestyle, habits, past and present medical history, and occupational and environmental risks. Items that must be included are occupations (current and past), hobbies, environmental living conditions, childhood illnesses, and family history including any genetic disorders known to have associated hearing deficits (Lang, 2004). Common symptoms that the patient presents to the office or clinic with are ear discharge, ear pain, ringing or other sounds in the ears, pressure or fullness, hearing loss, dizziness, or loss of balance. Obtaining the sequence of events will help to focus the physical exam assessment and lead to the diagnosis.

Mixed consists of a combination of both conductive and sensorineural properties. When the patient presents to the health care provider with mixed hearing loss, they exhibit signs and symptoms of both etiologies. A patient will experience properties of both bone and air conduction loss.

Changes with the Aging Process

Changes with the aging process have been associated with both conductive and sensorineural hearing loss. Alterations in the auditory system seen with aging include an increase in cerumen production, which appears to be drier (increasing the tendency to develop an impaction), an increase in the amount of hair growth in the external canal, and loss of elasticity in the lining of the canal leading to collapse. Atropic aging changes in the middle and inner ear lead to degeneration of neurons and decreased vascularity causing increased loss of hearing. The most common condition associated with aging is presbycusis, a degenerative loss of hearing related to constant insults to the fine hair lining of the cochlear over a lifetime. The exact cause is unknown. Loss of hearing associated with higher pitched sounds is most affected (Hietanen, Era, Sorri, & Heikkiness, 2004).

Etiologies of Conductive and Sensorineural Hearing Loss

There are a variety of causes for conductive and sensorineural hearing loss. Each of these etiologies has different clinical manifestations and effects on patients suffering from the different conditions.

Cerumen Production

The most common cause of conductive hearing loss is obstruction, which can be caused by a variety of reasons. The most common is impacted **cerumen** (a wax-like substance formed within the ear). Many people feel that it is necessary to use a cotton applicator to remove the wax or other debris from the canal and do not realize the ear is unique in that it cleans itself. By using the cotton-swab or other object the wax is merely pressed down contributing to impaction. Any object inserted into the canal has the potential to cause damage to both the canal and the tympanic membrane. The amount of cerumen production depends on the individual, and therefore it may be necessary to periodically have the ear canal irrigated to assist in the removal. Various otitic solutions are readily available and can be used to emulsify and disperse excess or impacted cerumen to also assist in removal (Rodgers, 2004).

Foreign Body

Anything that is abnormally found in the external ear canal is a foreign body. Cotton tips, which occasionally dislodge from cotton swab applicators, insects, or other objects, are just a few examples. Insects at times look for dark, moist areas and find their way into ear canals. If the patient presents with a buzzing or scratching sound in the ear, insects should be the first thought. If an insect is alive in the canal, the insect must be first killed before attempting to remove it. By instilling mineral oil or lidocaine, which kills the insect, makes the insect easier to be removed. Avoid placing water into the canal, which only makes the insect swell and thereby become lodged in the canal, making it more difficult to remove. Because the external ear canal is narrow and S-shaped, it makes many foreign bodies difficult to remove, and consequently the patient may need a referral to an otologist for removal.

Trauma

External ear trauma can result in accidental or induced injury, which often results in a perforated tympanic membrane or perichondrial hematoma. Etiologies of trauma range from abuse, sports or recreational injury, and industrial mishaps to accidents. External canal trauma can also be caused by insertion of objects in the canal. With a perforation, the patient experiences excruciating ear pain for a brief period of time and then relief in which they may then encounter a discharge. Any perforation of the tympanic membrane increases the risk of infections and decreases the ability to hear.

Eustachian Tube Dysfunction

For the auditory system to function properly, the eustachian tube must be fully open and functioning. The eustachian tube connects the middle ear with the nasopharynx, and its purpose is to equalize pressure and provide ventilation. When infectious processes cause inflammation or edema in the tube, it increases the risk of developing an otitis media. Common etiologies, which contribute to bilateral inflammation of the eustachian tube, are the common cold or upper respiratory infection and allergic rhinitis. The buildup of secretions and bacteria cause edema and obstruction of the tube. This creates decreased ventilation and the production of secretions leading to otitis media and decreased mobility of the tympanic membrane and thereby a decrease in hearing. When a unilateral eustachian tube obstruction is found, the patient should be evaluated for a tumor, which is a classic indication.

Ear Infections

The external otitis or what is commonly referred to as swimmers' ear affects the external ear canal, causing a narrowing and sometimes an occlusion to the canal. In this event sound waves cannot reach the tympanic membrane or just minimally reach the membrane decreasing the ability to hear sounds. Hearing loss is generally temporary and when the condition resolves hearing returns to normal. Prolonged moisture in the canal is the most common cause. External otitis can also be caused by foreign bodies in the ear, injury to the canal, and cerumen impaction. The most common offending organisms include corynebacterium, *Micrococcus* species, *Staphylococcus aureus,* and *Pseudomonas aeruginosa.* The classic symptom of external otitis is pain on movement of the ear lobe and the feeling of fullness. Prevention is the solution when considering external otitis.

Complications of Auditory Dysfunction

There are a wide variety of complications associated with auditory dysfunction. Among these are the common inflammation of the middle ear, otitis media, as well as perforated tympanic membrane, and other tympanic membrane anomalies, mastoiditis, masses in the external and middle ear, and otosclerosis. Each of these pathologies can cause hearing loss and have varying complications within the auditory system.

Otitis Media

Otitis media, an inflammation of the middle ear, is the most common cause of conductive hearing loss. The patient usually experiences allergies or an upper respiratory infection prior to developing an acute otitis media. Otitis media affects all age-groups but especially the young child. The most common organisms are *Streptococcus pneumoniae, Hemophilus influenzae, Moraxella Catarrhalis, Staphylococcus aureus,* and various other organisms to some degree. Acute otitis media can develop into otitis media with effusion, an accumulation of fluid behind the tympanic membrane with absence of infection. The fluid can be serous or mucoid consistency and can develop into a glue ear, which prevents the movement of the tympanic membrane. Decreased movement of the membrane prevents the ossicles from moving and thereby causes a temporary hearing loss. Once the fluid is dissolved, the hearing should return to normal.

Otitis media is diagnosed by history and physical examination and treated with antibiotics specific to the offending organism. The nurse educates the patient on management in the acute episodes stressing the importance of completing the course of antibiotics, common complications, such as perforation of the tympanic membrane, and when to seek medical care. Patients often experience ear pain, so nurses should evaluate the pain on a pain scale and discuss mild analgesics, which have been found to be helpful. Flying is not recommended until the infection is cleared. Instruct the patient to avoid water sports and to keep the ear dry during the acute phase. At the first sign of excruciating pain, the patient should be advised to seek medical care to rule out perforation of the tympanic membrane or other complications.

Perforated Tympanic Membrane

A complication of recurrent otitis media is a perforated tympanic membrane. Because the membrane is then unable to cause vibration of the ossicles, a conductive hearing loss is noted. The amount of loss is dependent on the size and location of the opening. A larger perforation that appears in the middle section of the membrane tends to cause the most hearing loss. Most perforations resolve spontaneously but can be repaired by grafting if persistent. The nurse needs to stress to the patient that no water or other substances should be placed into an ear that has a perforation unless directed by the health care provider.

When the patient presents frequently with otitis media, it may become unclear as to whether the previous infection had resolved or that a new one is now present. Chronic otitis media can cause persistent damage to the ossicles, which will result in sensorineural loss of hearing over time. Untreated chronic otitis media can lead to the spread of infection into the surrounding areas, such as brain abscess, meningitis, and mastoiditis.

Other Tympanic Membrane Disorders

Other complications of chronic otitis infections cause the tympanic membrane to retract, form adhesions, or develop necrosis of the tympanic membrane or ossicles. Scarring of the tympanic membrane decreases the movement or vibration of sound waves reaching the middle ear causing interference with the movement of the ossicles and thereby causing conductive hearing loss. Another complication of chronic otitis media is perforation of the tympanic membrane, which would also affect the patient's ability to hear sound waves by decreasing the vibratory movement of the ossicles.

Tympanic membrane abnormalities that interfere with the ability to hear include **tympanosclerosis** (formation of fibrous tissue around the ossicles preventing vibratory movement) and **bullous myringitis** (the presence of an infec-

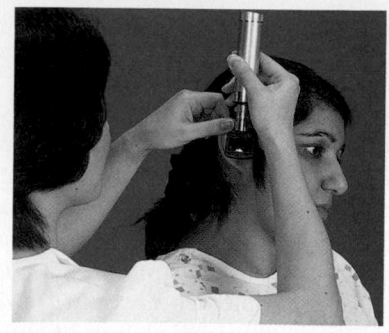

Figure 40-3 Position for otoscopic examination.

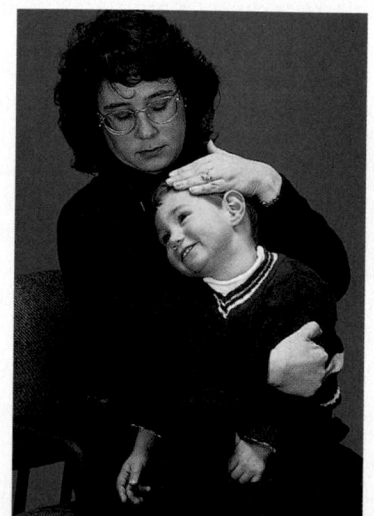

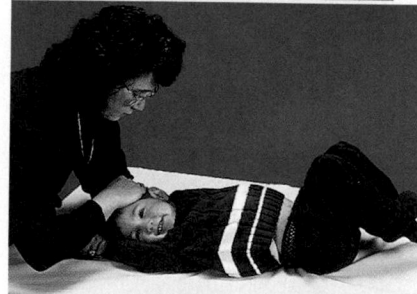

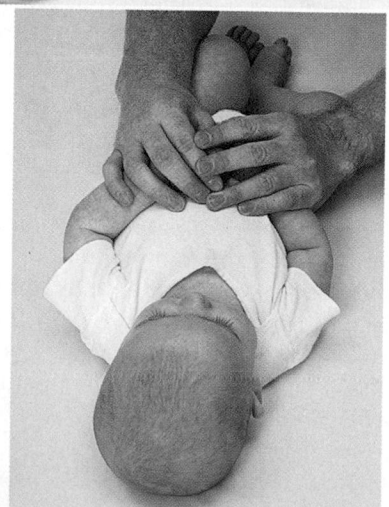

Figure 40-4 Positioning the child for the otoscopic examination.

tious vesicle and inflammation of the tympanic membrane caused by the organism *Mycoplasma pneumoniae*).

Mastoiditis

Mastoiditis (infectious process of the mastoid sinuses) interferes with bone conduction. The mastoid process is located directly behind the ear and connects temporal bone. Inflammation can occur with chronic middle ear infection. Signs and symptoms usually occur two to three weeks after an occurrence of otitis media and include pain and erythema to the site, fever, and protuberance of the auricle. Treatment of mastoiditis is a medical emergency.

Masses in the External and Middle Ear

Cholesteatoma is a cyst that contains an accumulation of squamous epithelium, keratin, and other debris and is associated with chronic otitis. As the lesion grows, it spreads into the middle and inner ear causing damage to the auditory structures and may continue to grow into surrounding areas and the brain tissue if not identified and removed in a timely manner. Damage to other cranial nerves that innervate the face can also lead to facial paralysis. Severe conductive hearing loss can result if damage occurs to the ossicles. Nursing management includes identification and monitoring patients at risk.

Other masses that cause a conductive hearing loss include benign (infectious polyp) or malignant tumors, which interfere with the ability of sound to reach the tympanic membrane or ossicles.

Otosclerosis

Otosclerosis is the most common cause of auditory loss in an individual from the age 15 to 50. Otosclerosis occurs as a result of the formation of spongy bone around the oval window, thus preventing movement of the stapes and causing atrophy of the organ of Corti. The ossicles become fused together and therefore are unable to vibrate and transmit sound waves to the acoustic nerve. Although the etiology is unknown, it has been linked genetically to certain families and is categorized as an autosomal dominant disorder. Otosclerosis generally presents in puberty and is more commonly seen in the Caucasian race, and females tend to be more prone to develop the condition. Pregnancy also appears to aggravate the condition.

Diagnostic Tests

The diagnosis of auditory dysfunctions should be investigated if the patient or the family report behavioral changes (speech too soft or too loud, repeats statements, or asks others to repeat phases frequently). Abnormal reports on hearing handicap inventory for adults and failed auditory testing should also be evaluated further. If the patient presents with a chief complaint of loss of hearing, it is important to ascertain if the condition appeared gradually or suddenly.

Otoscopic Examination and Tympanometry Testing

The use of the otoscope is a basic examination device used by the nurse in examining the inner ear. Correctly positioning the otoscope is essential and involves first placing the patient in a comfortable sitting position. Then the nurse holds the otoscope securely in the dominant hand and uses the other hand to correctly position the ear (Figure 40-3). A child can be allowed to lie down if they provide too much of a challenge to be in a sitting position (Figure 40-4). In addition, the nurse positions the ear differently in the infant than the adult (refer to a physical examination text for specific procedures).

While using the otoscope, **tympanometry** is a test performed (by the nurse) and is used to detect abnormalities in the middle ear such as fluid, eustachian tube dysfunction, or problems with the ossicles. The tip of the instrument is placed in the external os of the ear, a seal is established, and negative or

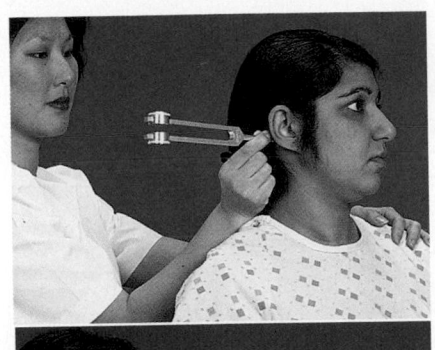

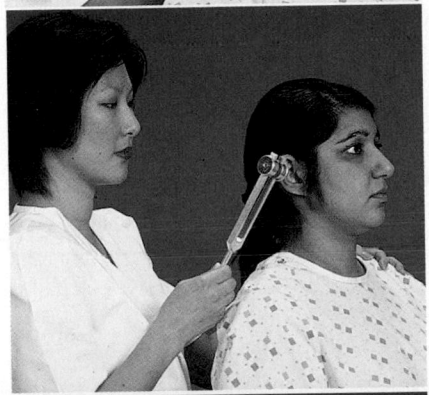

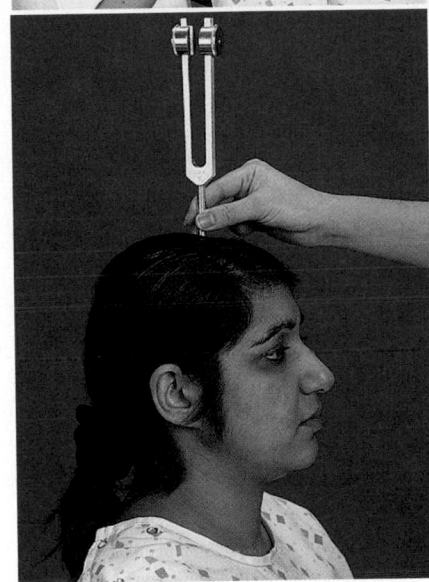

Figure 40-5 A. Rinne test, B. Weber test.

positive pressure is injected into the air to assess the movement of the tympanic membrane. The degree and direction of the movement will determine normality of the middle ear. The peak or lack of peak on the graph that is produced will indicate if there is an abnormality. Flat lines would indicate a perforated membrane, otitis media, or obstruction in the canal, such as cerumen or probe tip. The most important thing for the nurse to remember is to have a good seal; if there is a leak in the seal, air will escape around the probe tip and the pressure will not be sufficient to get an accurate test finding.

Rinne and Weber Tests

Specific tests performed to assess the patient's hearing would include the Rinne and Weber tests (Figure 40-5). By testing air conduction versus bone conduction of sounds, the examiner will be able to determine an auditory dysfunction. The Rinne test (tests air conduction) and the Weber tests (tests bone conduction) are performed using a tuning fork of 250, 500, or 1,000 Hz. To perform the Weber test, the nurse places the tuning fork on the front midportion of the patient's head and has the patient indicate if he or she hears the sounds equally in both ears testing for a unilateral deficit. The sound will be louder in the affected ear if it is a conductive loss and louder in the good ear if it is a sensorineural loss. The Rinne test, used to compare bone and air conduction, is performed by placing the tuning fork behind the ear on the mastoid process and having the patient say when the sound is no longer heard, the tuning fork is then moved to the front of the ear just outside the os, and the patient is then asked to indicate when sound is no longer heard. The Rinne test is normal is air conduction is twice as long as bone conduction (Estes, 2006).

Audiometer Test

The audiometer is the most common instrument in testing the hearing of individuals of all ages. The younger child who is unable to designate in which ear the sound is heard would not be able to perform this test and therefore other methods should be used. The audiometer emits specific sound pitches at different frequencies ranging from 125 Hz to 8,000 Hz (Punch, et al., 2004; Yueh, et al., 2003). Audiometric testing is performed on the patient by a specially trained nurse or audiologist. The patient is taken to a soundproof room (for best results) and tested on the different sound frequencies. The patient is asked to identify in which ear the tone is heard. A variety of sounds at different pitches is produced by the examiner, which tests the tone intensity of the hearing deficit. A printed audiogram is then obtained that notes the frequencies heard in each ear. Normal ranges are established nationally.

Brainstem Auditory Evoked Response Test

Brainstem auditory evoked responses (BAER or ABR) is another measuring device, which calculates the ability to hear in a patient who is unresponsive or incapable of performing an audiometer. The BAER measures the sound impulse needed to evoke a brain response, which will indicate the patient's ability to hear. This method is used mainly in patients who are unable to cooperate with standardized hearing testing, such as with auditory neuropathy, muscular dystrophy, psychiatric disorders, and abnormal brainstem disorder, such as stroke or other degenerative diseases. It is also widely used in newborns and young children who are unable to perform standard hearing tests. Because this machine utilizes high frequencies, adults over 70 years old are poor candidates for this method of testing because the aging process affects the ability to hear high-frequency sounds. The BAER is a painless test that produces clicks, which are introduced into the ear; on hearing these sounds the brain generates electrical impulses, which are then recorded (Box 40-1). The inability to initiate a brain response will indicate if the patient has a hearing deficit, an abnormality in the inner ear, eighth cranial nerve lesion, or other brainstem lesions. These abnormalities would then have to be further investigated (Johnson, Nicol, & Kraus, 2005; Sismanis, 2005).

BOX 40-1

ASSESSING A PATIENT WITH A HEARING DEFICIT

Questions to include in the history when trying to identify a hearing deficit should include:

- Are you able to hear a conversation in a crowded room or on the telephone?
- Do you have to turn the TV or radio up to hear the programming?
- Do you often get frustrated or argue when speaking with a family member or friend?
- Does hearing interfere with your social life?
- Do you avoid going to church, a movie, concert, or other activities because you cannot hear well?
- Do you have trouble understanding the conversation when in a noisy environment?

Nursing Diagnoses

Based on the information gathered, examples of nursing diagnoses in the patient with auditory dysfunction may include the following:
- Disturbed sensory perception, auditory, related to obstruction of ear canal, damage to inner ear.
- Anxiety related to inability to communicate.
- Knowledge deficit related to self-care and risk prevention.
- Impaired social interaction related to inability to hear others.

Planning and Implementation

Nursing care consists of educating the patient on proper care of the external ear. Avoid cleaning the ear canal with cotton tip applicators or other device, keeping it dry and free of debris. Cleaning increases the risk of tissue damage and interferes with the ear's normal process of cleansing. Once otitis externa develops, keep the patient comfortable with pain medication, treat the infection with topical antibiotics directed toward the most likely organisms (e.g., *Pseudomonas, S. aureus*), and reinforcing prevention.

Congenital and hereditary hearing loss can appear at any time in one's life span. Family patterns can be identified in most cases, but there are isolated cases as well. Hearing screening is now mandatory at birth to identify as many cases as early as possible to initiate interventions. In some cases the loss is gradual and does not present until later in life, or it may be an isolated case where no other family members are affected. Therefore, early identification using hearing screening devices should also be performed yearly at the annual medical maintenance visits.

Pharmacology

The administration of medications is dependent on the disease process and the organism involved. Antibiotics are used to treat infections of the ear specific to the suspected disease. Common organisms found in the ear are *S. pneumoniae, M. catarrhalis,* nontypeable *Haemophilus influenzae,* and *S. aureus.* The first line of treatment for acute otitis media is usually a course of amoxicillin when symptomatic (Broyles, Reiss, & Evans, 2007). Acute otitis media infection affects the pediatric patient more than the adult patient and is usually preceded with symptoms of upper respiratory disease, nasal congestion, cough, and sore throat. Other contributing factors would be environmental smoke, allergens, day care attendance, immune deficiencies, and hereditary factors.

Prevention of Otitis Externa

- Keep the ear canal dry.
- Dry the external canal immediately after water sports or bathing.
- Do not put anything into the ear canal.
- Use of drying agents such as 1:1 solutions of 2% boric acid and 70% ethyl alcohol or 1:1 solution of white vinegar and 70% ethyl alcohol helps dry the canal (place two to three drops into the ear canal before and after swimming).
- If otitis external present, stay out of the water until infection resolved.

Otitis media with effusion follows an episode of otitis media and is characteristic by fluid in the middle ear. Prolonged fluid in the middle ear leads to decreased hearing and may cause permanent damage if not resolved in a timely fashion. Chronic otitis media occurs when the individual experiences frequent ear infections that leads to repeated insults to the middle ear. This can lead to loss of hearing but also may lead to other complications such as mastoiditis. Mastoiditis requires immediate attention and initiation of parental antibiotics. Other findings that would affect the hearing would be a cholesteoma or a collection of proliferating epithelial cells, which if not treated would lead to other serious complications as discussed previously.

Ménière's disease can be managed with a low-salt diet. Medications found to be helpful are diuretics (such as furosemide and Diazide), vasodilators, antihistamines, anticholinergics, and sedatives (benzodiazepines). While experiencing extreme vertigo, diazepam (valium), and meclizine (Antivert) seem to manage the condition. There is no cure for the disease. The condition waxes and wanes through out the patient's life. Safety is a critical issue in the acute phase. Surgical intervention can be performed in patients with extreme vertigo (endolymphatic decompression) to relieve the pressure in the labyrinth (Perez, et al., 2004).

Surgery

On examination, increased vascularity is seen in tympanic membrane infections, such as otitis media, as indicated by a positive **Schwartze's sign** (rosy or reddish-blue color of the tympanic membrane related to vascular changes). An abnormal Rinne test indicates bone conduction to be equal or greater than air conduction. Surgical management has been found to be successful in improving approximately 90 percent of hearing in these patients. During the procedure a stapedectomy is performed whereby the stapes is removed and replaced with a prosthetic one. During surgery, the labyrinth and perilymph systems are disturbed, which can cause dizziness, nausea, vomiting, and nystagmus of the lateral gaze. Nursing care includes safety measures. The patient should be instructed to keep his or her head movement to a minimal and to avoid sudden head movement, coughing, sneezing, or straining. Nurses can also educate the patient on increasing the ingestion of vitamin D and calcium in his or her diet, which has been found to promote bone calcification in some studies.

Patients may choose to manage otosclerosis in a nonsurgical way, such as using amplifying devices or hearing aids. The nurse is in an ideal position to discuss all of the options with the patient in addition to reinforcing advantages and disadvantages presented by the surgeon, should the patient choose a stapedectomy with reconstruction. The nurse will also assist the patient in the referral process and be the main person to answer questions. Whether surgical repair is performed or not, safety is a concern, because the patient is probably experiencing decreased hearing and vertigo. Patients may also feel compelled to discuss the genetic component, because some patients may fear passing the condition on to the next generation.

Removing Foreign Bodies

Gentle irrigation performed in the medical clinic is effective in removing cerumen. The nurse instructs the patient about the procedure, gathers the equipment, and performs the irrigation. If patient has a perforated tympanic membrane, irrigation is contraindicated. Nausea, dizziness, or pain may be experienced during the procedure and should be reported. Documentation includes type and amount of solution and end results of what is obtained. The uses of cerumen curettes or spoons should only be done by specially trained medical personnel. Removing cerumen sometimes requires a wax emulsifier to dissolve the wax a few days before the irrigation (if the wax is hard and lodged into the canal).

Foreign body removal from ears involves manual removal with alligator forceps or curette. If a live insect is present in the canal, it must be killed before removing to make removal easier. Solutions used to kill the insect include placing a few drops of mineral oil or lidocaine into the canal.

Preoperative Care

Preparing a patient for surgery is an important part of nursing care. Preoperatively the nurse assesses the patient's baseline hearing abilities. If the degree of hearing will be affected during the procedure, the patient and nurse should discuss ways to communicate after surgery to aid in the patient's recovery process. With any surgery of the auditory system, the patient should be instructed not to do anything that will interfere with the eustachian tube function, such as blowing his or her nose, coughing, or sneezing, which may increase pressure in this area, leading to disturbance of the surgical site. It is important to explain this before the surgery, so that the patient understands what to expect after the procedure. This will also assist in communicating the directions to the patient if there is interference with his or her hearing after the procedure.

When preparing the patient for any auditory surgery, the nurse must address the patient's expectations and what he or she perceives are the end results. A complete history is performed reviewing past medical and surgical history. The patient should be assessed for the level of communication skills, so postoperatively the patient will be easier to converse with for postoperative instructions. During the interview, the nurse needs to talk in a slow, deliberate fashion, facing the patient and allowing for extra time if needed for understanding instructions. Try not to give lengthy instructions that the patient will have difficulty understanding. If the patient has hearing aids the nurse might suggest that the patient wear them into the surgical suite. All preoperative evaluations and laboratory testing is reviewed, the patient's functioning ability is evaluated, and the consent form is signed. As part of the preoperative workup, the patient should have baseline studies to compare postoperative hearing ability. The patient is assessed by using an audiogram and tympanometry to determine the etiology of dysfunction and baseline acuity.

Nurses are utilized in a variety of settings. The nurse in the physician's office assists with preparing the patient for surgery and what is expected postoperatively, obtaining a history, performing the auditory exam (if specially trained), and discussing what to expect immediately before and after the procedure. The patient is also prepared psychologically because feelings of grief may be experienced with any degree of hearing loss, and the sense of hearing is vital in communication. The patient also needs to know what the procedure entails.

Most often, local anesthesia is used with conscious sedation so the patient can be guided throughout the delicate process. The fact that the patient may be awake can be frightening to many patients; therefore the nurse needs to reassure the patient. Points to be discussed with patients undergoing any surgery would be steps of the procedure, postoperative expectations, alleviating the fear of unknown, and prevention of complications. The patient's compliance of preoperative and postoperative instructions leads to better patient outcomes.

A major concern of the patient would be complete loss of hearing after the procedure. Understanding and identifying realistic expectations of outcomes will help the patient throughout the surgical process. Postoperative pain management should be ordered for any discomfort the patient may feel. Common side effects of analgesic medications include dizziness or tinnitus, which may also be an effect of manipulating the components of the auditory system. The vertigo or tinnitus needs to be differentiated to identify common postoperative signs and symptoms following auditory procedures as opposed to complications.

Postoperative Care

Postoperative care of a patient who undergoes surgery to the auditory system, besides routine care of all patients having any surgical procedure, is preventing introduction of organisms or infection into the site, observing for excessive bleeding, or other possible complications. Vomiting may be a side effect from anesthesia and needs to be acted on immediately. Vomiting could cause damage to the surgical site. Patients who undergo auditory surgery should have their heads elevated, be monitored for vertigo, and avoid quick movements or turning of the head. The nurse needs to remember that the patient may have hearing loss in the operated ear and therefore should speak clearly in the unaffected ear or have a pad and pencil available for communication. When the patient is discharged from the hospital, instructions should be reiterated, such as avoiding sneezing, blowing nose, or other activities that could cause pressure in the middle ear. If the patient has to sneeze, he or she should do so with his or her mouth open. The patient should avoid showers, shampooing, or dipping head in water for at least one to two weeks or until the surgical site is healed. The surgical dressing should be kept in place, unless otherwise directed, and kept dry and clean. Part of discharge planning would also include the administration of medications, such as analgesics, antiemetics, antivertigo agents, and possibly antihistamines. Instructions on how to take the medications and what side effects to watch for should be included.

Instructions should also include positioning the patient on the opposite side away from the surgery. Lying on the operative side may affect the healing process and disrupt the graft (if one was used). The patient should avoid blowing his or her nose for at least one week, but if he or she finds it necessary to blow his or her nose, have the patient gently blow one nostril at a time. Likewise, if necessary to cough or sneeze, this should be done with the mouth open to avoid pressure on the ear. Physical exercise should be avoided for at least one week, after which time the patient can return to work unless contraindicated. If the patient works in a high noise environment, ear protection should be used.

Initially patients may have some dizziness or tinnitus and should be assisted with ambulation until this has resolved. Hearing may also initially be diminished in the operative ear but should return close to preoperative status depending on the type of procedure performed. After surgery, the patient should be assessed for cranial nerve functioning to note any deficits that might have occurred as a result of the surgical procedure. The cranial nerves most likely affected would be five, seven, eight, and nine, because they innervate many structures in this area. The patient can also exhibit some nystagmus especially when looking to the side.

In addition, care of the operative site would include noting the amount and type of drainage or bleeding, changing the dressing as directed (according to the surgeon), and teaching the patient or family on dressing changes after discharge if indicated. Depending on the procedure, little bleeding is expected after surgery. Some patients may have a small amount of serosanguineous discharge that can be easily absorbed by a cotton ball changed as often as necessary. Common postoperative findings include decreased hearing in the operative ear and various noises, such as snapping or crackling. Outcome goals include pain control, healing in a relatively short time, and as normal ear functioning as possible. A hearing test should be performed after the healing process has completed. Patients should avoid flying, water sports or underwater diving, physical activity, and heavy lifting for one to three weeks following surgery depending on the type of surgical procedure performed and based on the surgeon's recommendations.

Middle Ear and Mastoid Surgery

Myringotomy, or incision into the tympanic membrane, has been performed for years to promote drainage and relieve pressure. Before the invention of the tympanometry tubes, the physician, in the office, would make a small incision into the tympanic membrane if perforation was imminent or to identify the type of organism responsible for the otitis media when the antibiotic was not treating the infection. With any perforation of the tympanic membrane there is a chance of introducing an organism into the middle ear so the patient needs to be watched closely for signs and symptoms of otitis media, such as drainage from the ear canal, otalgia, and fever.

Myringoplasty (plastic surgery of the tympanic membrane) is performed in a patient who has a small perforated tympanic membrane that has failed to resolve or heal. The procedure involves placing a patch over the perforation. Chronic otitis media is a common cause. Following the procedure the patient is instructed to keep the canal dry and follow-up frequently in the office to assess the healing process. If the patch does not solve the problem or the hole gets bigger, a tympanoplasty must be performed. Repairing the tympanic membrane does not always improve the conductive hearing loss.

Stapedectomy or tympanoplasty is performed when reconstruction is necessary in the middle ear to improve conductive hearing loss. With the tympanoplasty a portion of the temporalis fascia is used to graft the affected portion of the middle ear. Care must be taken not to disturb the ossicles from their position. Risk factors that can occur after this type of surgery include increased pressure in the middle ear, displacement of the prosthesis of the ossicles, difficulties with balance, a risk of developing an infection, and postoperative pain.

A **stapedectomy** is a removal of the stapes and replaces the stapes with a prosthetic device, which is performed mainly in a patient with otosclerosis. A similar surgery, which is performed to repair one or more of the ossicles, is an ossiculoplasty. This procedure is also performed in a patient with otosclerosis. When the stapes becomes fused, it becomes necessary for the patient to undergo surgery for the insertion of a prosthetic replacement. This procedure has shown to increase the patient's ability to hear.

Mastoidectomy is an incision of the mastoid sinuses, which are located directly behind the ear. When a radical mastoidectomy is performed it involves the middle ear, and therefore is important to mention. The nurse is responsible for monitoring the patient postoperatively, watching for presence and amount of discharge or bleeding, fever, neck stiffness, limited neck range of motion, vomiting, dizzy, disorientation, headaches, or facial paralysis, all of which are complications that can occur following this type of surgery. When changing the dressing, aseptic technique must be used to avoid any infection. The mastoid bone is in direct contact with brain tissue, and therefore any infection can travel to the brain and cause further complications. Other complications include decreased muscle mass and disruption to hearing.

Other auditory surgery involves the removal of an acoustic neuroma, which is a benign tumor of cranial nerve VIII where the nerve enters the auditory canal or at the temporal bone. Early signs include a gradual unilateral hearing loss, tinnitus, intermittent episodes of mild vertigo, and decreased sensation in the canal. As the tumor grows and extends into the auditory system, the damage and hearing loss cannot be reversed. Treatment includes surgical removal of the tumor with as little damage to the surrounding tissues and cranial nerves. Facial paralysis is commonly coexists. Postoperative nursing management is similar to other auditory surgical procedures as previously discussed.

Repair of Inner Ear Disorders

Cochlear implant is commonly used in young children with congenital hearing loss but recently has also been used in older adults to assist with sensorineural hearing loss. The patient undergoes a surgical procedure to insert the device just behind the ear. The device is divided into three sections: a headpiece, speech processor, and receiver. The headpiece contains a microphone and transmitter, which picks up the sounds in the environment and sends them to the speech processor, which rearranges the sounds and sends them to the receiver, which is implanted behind the ear. The receiver then converts the sound waves to nerve impulses, which are sent to the brain for interpretation. Patients who receive the implant will be able to hear some sounds but will not have normal hearing. Studies have shown that individuals who receive cochlear implants have less depression, anxiety, and quality of life issues than those who chose not to have one (Birgen, Harris, Lindbaek, & Oslo, 2004; Cohen, Labadie, Dietrich, & Haynes, 2004). The best candidates for cochlear implants are patients who have established speech and language skills (Cullen, et al., 2004).

A great deal of controversy exists among the deaf community about the ethics of implanting cochlear implants in young children. The basis for this ethical dilemma stems from the beliefs that American Sign Language is a natural language and should remain as such. Leaders in the deaf community want to protect the deaf culture and therefore feel that children should be reared in that culture. It is believed that deaf individuals communicate and receive cues through visual images and live in a specialized culture similar to other cultures and encompass accepted values and beliefs. By implanting cochlear implants, which give the individual the ability to hear sounds, it alters the culture of the individual, which then contradicts the belief system in the deaf community. To compound the argument, studies show that children who are born deaf or who become deaf at an early age do not fair as well on language acquisition and still need the exposure of the deaf culture to exist. On the other hand, in research by Nicholas and Geers (2006), cochlear implants increased spoken language ability in profoundly hearing impaired children. The benefits of a cochlear implant to a hearing impaired child to achieve both speech and language skills comparable to a normal hearing child appears greater if the implant is placed when the child is a toddler as opposed to a preschooler. Adults and children who have had cochlear implants have been found to successfully integrate and function in a hearing society, but deaf community leaders feel they lose some of their cultural identity by doing so.

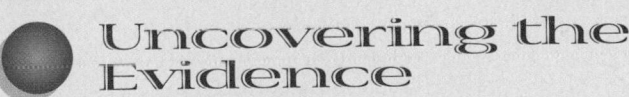

Uncovering the Evidence

Cochlear Implants in Children

Discussion: The purpose of this research project was to explore the results of improving hearing loss in 13 infants with profound hearing loss and had cochlear implants between the ages of 6 to 12 months of age. Infants were tested using two behavioral methodologies that have been successful for investigating speech perception and language skills in infants with normal hearing. The research involved using equipment that assessed infants' discrimination of speech sounds. In addition, the study was used to assess infants' ability to learn associations between speech sounds and objects. The findings revealed patterns of hearing associated with visual responses for the early implanted infants were similar to those of normal hearing infants. Also, the mothers' speech to infants with the implants was similar in pitch to infants with normal hearing who had the same duration of experience with sounds.

Implications for Practice: The nursing discipline can explore methods of patient education regarding the early identification of hearing impaired infants. The earlier the disorder is assessed, the potential increasing methods of treatment (e.g., cochlear implants) and the better the results for the patient. In addition, parents can be encouraged to stay in contact with their health care providers as related to questions or suspected concerns that are seen in their children.

Citation: Miyamoto, R., Houston, D., & Bergeson, T. (2005). Cochlear implantation in deaf infants. Laryngoscope, 115(8), 1376–1380.

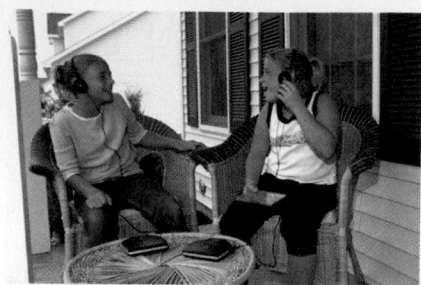

Figure 40-6 Hearing loss has been attributed to listening to loud music through earphones.

Patient and Family Teaching

Part of patient teaching involves preventive measures to assist the patient in maintaining an optimum quality of life. To do this, one looks to the levels of prevention. In caring for the patient, the nurse assists and discusses ways to prevent injury to the auditory system and to identify those at risk of developing an auditory dysfunction in every medical encounter. Other responsibilities include preventing further damage once loss occurs. Identification of patients with the greatest risk factors leads the preventive management.

Primary Prevention

The prevention model directs identification and management incorporating this into the nurse's role. Primary prevention speaks to minimizing risks in the environment. Primary prevention begins with educating and making the public aware of what constitutes dangerous noise. Any noise above 85 dB is considered dangerous, and prolonged exposure can cause damage to the sensitive auditory system. Areas found to be at the highest levels of noise pollution include various occupational and recreational activities. Occupations known to be at high risk include firefighters, police officers, airline personnel, and the military. Recreation also contributes to high noise levels whether as a participant or observer. Examples of high noise producing sports include hunting, car racing, and musicians. The obsession with rock concerts in teens and younger adults places the next generations at an increased risk of hearing loss, supporting recent studies indicating an increased prevalence of hearing loss found in the middle adult years (Figure 40-6). Preventive measures would also include the use of protective head gear, muffs, and hats to guard against head trauma, which inadvertently can cause auditory dysfunction.

Preventive measures should include educating the patient to become more aware of noise in the environment: turning down radio and television volumes; avoiding long periods in noisy surroundings, such as rock concerts; and wearing protective devices when indicated. When loud noise cannot be avoided, ear plugs or ear headphones should be used to decrease the amount of elevated sound levels that reach the inner ear. Included in the patient's education is the fact that the common practice of using plain cotton or cotton balls to decrease noise does not prevent the sound from reaching the inner ear and causing damage.

Environmental noise in the workforce is a serious problem and contributes to the increasing number of individuals who acquire hearing loss. To protect these workers the regulating body of OSHA (Occupational Safety and Health Administration) has specific guidelines that must be adhered to. OSHA supplies regulations associated with high noise levels in the workplace to prevent hearing loss associated with machinery or other equipment. Nurses who work in occupational nursing have stringent guidelines to follow established by OSHA. The occupational health nurse monitors the health status of each worker. As part of the nurse's responsibility he or she is specially trained in audiometric testing. In each clinic, a soundproof room is provided for the most accurate hearing assessment. All new employees are required to have a baseline hearing screening and yearly thereafter. Annual training and educational programs addressing noise pollution in the workplace are mandatory. Monitoring the noise levels in the workplace and keeping documentation of the levels are required to adhere to OSHA recommendations. In any work environment where the sound level measures greater than 90 dB, the employees must wear protective hearing equipment. A worker who is demonstrating changes in his or her hearing status in an environment that measures between 85 and 90 dB must also wear protective devices, because prolonged exposure to greater than 85 dB can cause permanent hearing loss.

Ear protection equipment comes in various forms.

- Ear plug are inserted into the ear canal and block the entire canal. Sound levels can be blocked from entering the ear by 15 to 30 dB if fitted properly. Commonly spongy type plugs, which easily mold to fit most auditory canals, are dispersed in many employee health clinics.
- Ear muffs fit snuggly over the entire external ear. Sound levels are also blocked by 15 to 30 dB.
- A combination of both ear plugs and the ear muff offers the most protection. The combination would be recommended in areas of extremely high noise level, for example airline runway workers.

Nurses have the responsibility to educate patients on the level of noise exposure in the household. Simply performing yard work puts the patient at risk of exposure greater than safe levels. Lawn mowers and leaf blowers emit noise levels greater than 90 dB. Most people are unaware of the level of noise that is produced by common household items. Patients should be instructed to spend shorter periods of time performing household tasks that use equipment that emits high levels of sound.

Secondary Prevention

Secondary prevention refers to the early detection (screening and referral). Everyone should have periodic hearing tests as part of their annual medical visits, especially if they work or live in an environment that has excessive noise levels. People are often unwilling to reveal a problem with their hearing, so this is an ideal time to discuss hearing and identify deficits. The earlier the loss is identified, the more quickly the management can be started.

Tertiary Prevention

Tertiary prevention is aimed at maintaining optimal functioning. Once the damage is done, it is important to maintain what hearing capabilities are left. Prevention of further damage is imperative, and education should be directed to decreasing sound insults by turning radio, television, and stereo volumes down to a safe level and taking breaks when using high level noise producing devices or using protective devices.

Noise Pollution

In the world today we are faced with noise pollution that leads to damage to the auditory system on a daily basis. Being more aware of the amount and type of noise in the environment is the starting point in prevention. The most effective preventive measure is controlling the noise exposure in the environment. Turn radio, television, and movie volume down to a safe level of less than 80 to 85 dB (Box 40-2). Other things that produce high noise emissions

---

BOX 40-2

COMMON SOUNDS AND ASSOCIATED DECIBELS LEVELS

- 20 dB   Whisper
- 60 dB   Conversation
- 70 dB   Vacuum cleaner, traffic noises
- 90 dB   Lawn mower, motorcycle, hair dryer
- 110 dB   Model airplane
- 120 dB   Chain saw, leaf blower, snowmobile, loud thunder clap
- 130 dB   Jack hammer, ambulance siren
- 140 dB   Jet engine, fire arms, firecrackers
- 150 dB   Rock concert

are firecrackers, machinery, gun shots, children's toys, and traffic. Hearing loss can also be caused by a sudden burst of sound, which causes an acute loss through trauma to the auditory mechanism, or it can be chronic with prolonged exposure to loud noises. Acute loss may be temporary with hearing returning in a couple of weeks.

Work environment provides a sustained high noise environment and protection is necessary. Protection of trauma to the ears can be achieved using various devices. When a worker, such as an air traffic controller, is exposed to extensive noise, ear muffs should be worn. Other devices to decrease sound trauma to the auditory system include ear plugs, which come in form fitting and premolded designed to fit a specific person's external ear canal. OSHA regulates the work environment and recommends that a hearing conservation program be in place for all industry, including monitoring of sound levels; annual hearing tests for all workers, including a baseline for comparison; mandatory annual training of all employees; hearing protective devices worn by every employee exposed to excessive noise levels; and accurate record keeping (Van Campen, et al., 2005).

Along with the workplace, recreational activities provide an enormous amount of sound and require protection. Hunting, skeet shooting, or target practice where a firearm is discharged are a few examples. Often not considered as noise producers, children's toys are found to have in some cases excessive levels of noise with the beeps, whistles, honks, and various other sounds. These are made to be amusing and entertaining for children, without consideration of the long-term consequences of the excessive noise levels and exposures.

Yard work is one of the biggest offenders of excessive noise pollution: the lawn mower, leaf blower, and other outdoor equipment emit a high level of noise at greater than 90 dB. Frequent breaks are recommended to eliminate prolonged exposure. Shorter periods of time spent with high frequency noise and wearing protective gear is less damaging and decreases long-term sequelae.

Studies show that the inability to hear disrupts normal routines, school and work performance, relationships, and activities of daily living. Warning signs of excessive noise exposure include having to raise your voice in normal conversation or the inability to hear a conversation approximately two feet away. After leaving a noisy area voices appear muffled or dull and frequently ringing of the ears is heard, or pain is experienced in the ears for short periods of time.

Communication Tools

As discussed previously, patients should be screened routinely for a hearing deficit when they present for their annual medical examinations. This gives the patient and medical provider a baseline and a way to monitor the pattern of hearing deficit expected over time. Because hearing loss is part of the aging process, it is expected to have some loss over a life span.

Once identifying a hearing deficit, it is important for the nurse to assist in establishing individual ways for the patient to communicate (see Skills 360° feature). Individuals with hearing loss tend to isolate themselves from others, so encouragement is needed for the patient to continue to be involved in outside activities and to not isolate himself or herself from previous enjoyable events. Understanding that everyone will experience some degree of hearing loss as part of the natural aging process may reassure some individuals. The patient needs to accept the fact that it is expected that some degree of loss will be experienced as he or she grows older. Offering ways for the patient to build confidence in communication and not be excluded in conversations is the responsibility of the nurse.

Individuals who have no hearing have access to various mechanisms in which to alert them to various sounds and therefore are able to function in a hearing world. These devices include items with flashing lights for door bells, telephones, alarms, and baby alerts. Some alarm clocks have flashing lights, and others have a vibratory mechanism to awaken the individual. Closed caption TV assists with keeping up with the latest in programming. Some telephones are set up to print out the message to communicate.

Skills 360°

Communicating with the Hearing Impaired

- Get the patient's attention.
- Face the individual directly.
- Ensure good lighting behind the patient.
- Can they read lips?
- Use simple clear sentences.
- When rephrasing the statement, change the wording.
- Keep hands or items away from your mouth while talking.
- Do not eat or chew gum when speaking.
- Be cognizant of facial expressions.
- Talk into the good ear (if one).
- Do not yell.
- Write things down for clarification.
- Use sign language.

Adapted from DeLaune, S., & Ladner, P. (2006). Fundamentals of nursing (3rd ed.). New York: Thomson Delmar Learning.

Lip reading is another way of communication that adds the ability to combine facial expressions and gestures to read words. Approximately 40 percent of people who have lost hearing understand spoken words and are able to learn to lip read. This also is found to be one of the first ways to communicate when hearing starts to diminish as compensation for the loss.

For patients who have an existing hearing impairment who use American Sign Language to communicate, learning sign language, as with any other foreign language, will facilitate communication. The nurse has an important role in patient care as the educator, mediator, and advocate. Without good communication the patient will not feel confident to raise questions and concerns for discussion. Also to be considered is the age at which the patient became impaired. If the patient has a congenital hearing loss or became deaf before acquiring language skills, he or she will communicate using both oral and sign language because he or she probably was raised with both. In contrast, a person who became deaf after acquiring spoken language, which is the case in the majority of hearing-impaired individuals, is reliant on verbal cues and will use amplification devices or lip reading for communication. No matter when the person lost his or her hearing, he or she will use other means of understanding what is being said, such as body language and facial expressions. The nurse needs to be cognizant of how he or she is expressing himself or herself so as not to be misinterpreted (Gates, Feeney, & Higdon, 2003)

Respecting Our Differences

Hearing Impairment in Different Ethnic Backgrounds

When the nurse is communicating with a patient who has hearing impairment from a different ethnicity, personal and cultural belief systems should be considered. Every patient comes with his or her own personal values, cultural variables, and cultural rules. Some patients may misinterpret gestures used to emphasize or to communicate a statement. Many gestures often have different meanings in the various cultures. So, the nurse needs to be careful and observant when using gestures in communication with the hearing impaired. Pointing, for example, is considered rude in some cultures.

Touch is also often used when trying to get a patient's attention, but in some cultures that may also be misinterpreted as offensive or a violation on the person. Another misinterpreted offensive act that needs to be kept in mind is closeness or getting too close to the patient to ensure that the patient can see what you are trying to convey. The nurse needs to recognize the patient's personal space and not get too close to communicate.

Another point to consider is direct eye contact; Americans place value on eye contact, while other cultures consider it rude to establish eye contact. The nurse needs to be cognizant of the patient's personal values when communicating and modify communication techniques with hearing impaired individuals from different cultures. Accepted length of silence also varies with different ethnicities. Allotting more time, not interrupting, and being prepared to repeat instructions will help with communication. Interrupting the patient is also often interpreted as rude or a loss of interest in what the patient is trying to convey. Understanding communication styles of different cultures is important but also avoiding stereotyping the patient at the same time.

Adapted from Daniels, R. (2004). Nursing fundamentals: Caring and clinical decision making. New York: Thomson Delmar Learning; DeLaune, S., & Ladner, P. (2006). Fundamentals of nursing (3rd ed.). New York: Thomson Delmar Learning.

Rehabilitation

In many cases the hearing deficit is permanent, and therefore the nurse must assist the patient in ways to compensate for the deficiency. One of the most important monitoring elements is obtaining a baseline hearing test and performing periodic screening tests throughout the patient's life span. Keeping abreast of the changes in loss of hearing over time will enable the nurse to adjust the patient teaching accordingly. Assisting the patient in accepting the loss and discussing ways to alter communication techniques are part of the nurse's responsibility, as well as providing the patient with preventive measures to avoid further loss. Patients who are computer literate can be given helpful resource Internet sites to obtain more information. Those who are not as computer savvy can be given contact numbers for additional information. Identifying support groups in the community for the patient to share similar characteristics have been helpful.

Patients who have a hearing deficit will isolate themselves from others. Encouraging participation is social activities is important. Patients can be offered activities that do not require a lot of conversation. Family members are a big part of the patient's life and need to be involved in the management and encouraged to include the patient in family gatherings. The focus for patients with hearing deficit should be on safety. Patients who are unable to hear the sounds around them are in danger of injury. The inability to hear a horn or siren puts them in arms way when crossing the street. At the same time, someone calling to them to avoid the dangerous situation is missed.

Hearing Aids

Hearing aids amplify sound, and therefore make it easier for patients with a hearing deficit to participate in conversations and activities. Whether or not a patient will wear a hearing aid depends on several factors. The patient's lifestyle and personality will influence this decision to some degree. A certain stigma is associated with a patient wearing a hearing aid, which prevents some patients from seeking the help they need. Other considerations are cosmetic, especially in the elder patient who does not want to appear old. Some patients are dissatisfied with the results, which stems from unrealistic expectations in the patient who feels the aid will return hearing to normal. Those who seek the assistance of hearing aids are usually motivated by difficulty hearing the television, radio, or other sounds, such as doorbell or telephone. Others seek assistance, because they feel left out of conversations. For stereo effect, hearing aids are fitted for both ears whether one or both ears have a deficiency.

Hearing aids are helpful in patients with auditory dysfunction where sound amplification is required. They all function about the same consisting of a microphone to pick up the sound, an amplifier to increase the intensity of sound, and receiver to deliver the sound to the inner ear. Hearing aids come in various shapes and sizes depending on a multitude of factors. Factors that contribute to the type of aid purchased are personal preference, particular auditory dysfunction, amplification, handling ease, design, and cost. Audiologists fit the patient with the most appropriate one for the patient. A period of adjustment is necessary initially.

At first the patient should try to adjust to the hearing aid by wearing it in a quiet environment with limited noise interference. Many older patients live in quiet households where this can easily be accomplished. Once becoming aware of noises in the home, the patient can venture out and listen to natural outdoor sounds and proceed to noisier environments, such as shopping areas. This gradual adjustment period allows the patient to adapt to the feel of wearing the instrument and learn to operate the controls thereby able to adjust the volume to a comfortable level. There are different types that the patient can purchase, which are described in the accompanying display (Box 40-3).

Some of the problems encountered by patients who are obtaining hearing aids are looks, cost, limited education, unrealistic expectations, difficulty in

---

BOX 40-3

TYPES OF HEARING AIDS

- In the canal and completely in the canal are the smallest available hearing aids. This type of aid fits completely in the ear canal, which allows the patient confidentiality and is cosmetically aesthetic. A patient with intact dexterity would be a candidate, because it is smaller than the others and more difficult to adjust volume or change batteries. As the patient ages, agility appears to decrease, so this would not be appropriate for an elderly patient who would have difficulty managing the small device.
- In ear hearing aids are fitted in the outer portion of the ear and molded to the patient. A slightly larger size allows the patient easier handling. This type of aid is given to a patient with mild to severe hearing loss.
- Behind the ear aid fits over the lobe of the ear, the mechanism sits in a case behind the ear and is connected to a molded ear piece. This type is more cumbersome but easier to manage in the older population and young children. Some patients do not have the dexterity to manage the in ear type and need one more bulky. Patients who benefit the most from this type would be those individuals with mild to profound hearing loss.

PATIENT PLAYBOOK

Care of Hearing Aids

- Change batteries immediately when not working.
  Batteries last approximately one week.
  Do not store batteries more than a month.
  Batteries are small, which makes them difficult to change and easily lost.
- Turn off the appliance when not in use.
  Leave the compartment open to reduce energy usage.
- Remove debris accumulated (directed by manufacturer).
  Clean ear molds at least once a week.
- Avoid hair products.
- Store in a cool dry place.
- Keep away from heat and moisture.
- Keep away from children and pets.

Adapted from Mueller, H., & Hawkins, D. (2006). Trouble-shooting hearing aid fitting issues: The case of the missing "ping." Hearing Journal, 59(1), 10, 12, 14–15.

care, and maintenance. A patient must accept the fact that they have a hearing problem and be optimistic about wearing the device to make it a successful venture. Nurses in a medical clinic or office come in contact with patients who wear a hearing aid and have questions about the device and therefore are often used as the resource individual. It is therefore important to know how to care for the apparatus.

There are two available types of hearing aids, analogue and digital, each with its own advantages and disadvantages. Analogue hearing aids come in two different forms. The basic analogue hearing aid is an amplifier of sounds programmed by the audiologist. The programmable analogue hearing aid has a microchip and is programmed to accommodate various environments. The digital hearing aid is more complex. It converts sound waves to digital signals and utilizes similar principles of the programmable analogue also adjusting to various conditions (Cohen, Labadie, Dietrich, & Haynes, 2004).

The patient needs a period of adjustment to be able to ignore background noises and focus on the conversation at hand. The background noise can be distracting and difficult to disregard. Programmable aids can be adjusted according to the deficiency and will filter out background noises to assist the patient in hearing the conversation. The patient must be aware that the hearing aid is just that an aid for participation in social situations where hearing is necessary not a cure for the disability, and it will it restore the patient's hearing to normal.

Although only one in five who would benefit with a hearing aid actually wear one, research has found that wearing hearing aids has positive effects on physical, psychological, and social functioning in patients with profound hearing loss. Patients who had assistance with hearing whether cochlear implants or hearing aids were also found to have better quality of life (Cohen, et al., 2004). Encouraging patients to obtain and utilize hearing aids can help to reduce the social isolation that individuals with hearing loss experience.

When communicating with a patient who has a hearing aid, look for ways to decrease background noises. Hearing aids amplify all sounds, and it is distracting for the patient when various alarms, conversations, and other sounds (e.g., telephones, pagers) are simultaneously heard. Take the patient into a quieter environment or private room if available to decrease as many extraneous noises as possible (Figure 40-7).

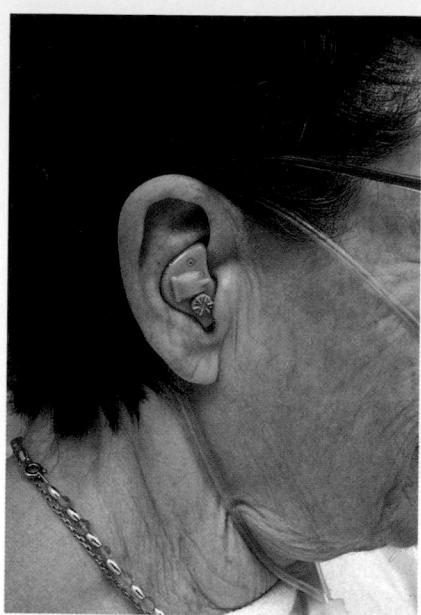

Figure 40-7 If a patient relies on hearing aids, make sure they are functioning before beginning the assessment examinations.

Other amplification devices assist the patient such as telephone amplification or typing machines are also available. These assist the patient in being able to communicate with others via telephone. The TDD (telecommunication device for the deaf) is a machine that allows the patient to type in a message, which is relayed to another individual with a similar piece of equipment or to an operator who then translates the calls. If the medical office sees a lot of patients who are hearing impaired, special telephone access should be available. Also, while in the hospital, the patient with a hearing impairment may need assistive devices on his or her telephones to communicate with family and friends to avoid feeling isolated.

External Otitis

External otitis, inflammation of auditory canal, results from moisture in the canal in most cases. The patient normally complains of pain and fullness in the canal demonstrated by moving the pinna of the ear. It is difficult to examine the canal, because edema is present that occludes or partially occludes the canal. Often a discharge is present. Treatment includes topical medications and mild pain relievers. Patient teaching includes instructions on techniques to maintain the integrity of the canal. Medical management depends on the identification of the organism to differentiate it from bacterial, viral, or fungal.

Often patients clean ear canals with anything that appears to be handy and do not realize that the canal should be left alone. Only the outer portion of the ear should be cleaned. By inserting different objects into the canal, injury to the tissue can occur, leading to a prime area for organisms to attack. Therefore, preventive patient teaching should include putting nothing smaller than your elbow into the ear, drying the canal after water sports or baths, and reporting any signs or symptoms of ear discomfort as soon as experienced.

Once external otitis appears, patient teaching should include instillation of the topical medication. As with all medications, it starts with washing hands. You may warm the drops by rubbing the bottle in your hands for a few minutes; never place it in a microwave because this causes uneven heating and an increased possibility of causing a burn. Have the patient tilt his or her head or lie on his or her side with the infected ear pointing to the ceiling; pull the pinna up and back, instill the drops, and have the patient remain in this position for approximately five minutes to ensure absorption. Until the canal is healed, water should be kept out of the ear. This can be accomplished by placing cotton in the os.

Otitis Media

Otitis media is infection of the middle ear common in children but can occur in any age. Treatment includes observation as well as the administration of appropriate antibiotics. With the increase of antibiotic resistance, if the patient is not acutely ill, it is now recommended to observe the patient for 48 to 72 hours to see if the condition resolves spontaneously. The nurse is important in maintaining contact with the patient and family for follow-up evaluation. If the patient is prescribed an antibiotic, the importance of completing the full course of medication is strongly encouraged. Other teaching topics include avoiding water sports, keeping the ear canal dry while bathing, and watching for changes in the patient's condition that may warrant follow-up before the recommended two to four week reevaluation. Chronic otitis media occurs when the patient has longstanding history of ear infections.

Overview of Nursing Care for Auditory Dysfunction

The nurse working with a patient who has hearing loss must understand the anatomy of the ear and the dynamics that cause the deficit. Loss that is attributed to obstruction is managed by removing or treating the blockage to allow sound waves to penetrate the inner chamber of the ear. The management of permanent loss is to supply the patient with assistive devices, such as hearing aids, telecommunication devices, and other signaling mechanisms. And lastly the patient must be taught communication skills, encouraged to participate in social engagements, and learn sign language or the technique of reading lips. Nurses look for measurable outcomes that indicate the patient is coping with the loss of hearing. A favorable outcome is when the patient has learned effective communication and participates in social activities. Effective communication is essential in patient teaching, to ensure the patient understands the diagnosis, etiology, management, and follow-up at every medical encounter.

Once the patient is diagnosed, the nurse can work with other health care providers to direct the best patient care for that patient. The nurse can assist the patient by educating the patient about the different disease processes, testing procedures, and follow-up expectations. Preparation of the patient aids in the progression of the disorder and the ability to work through the dysfunction. Some patients may require hospitalization until the acute phase is resolved.

Hearing loss is becoming an increasing problem and at a younger age. Loss of hearing is a societal burden that affects all aspects of an individual's life. Nurses need to start by becoming proactive in auditory health and restoration of auditory functioning by becoming sound aware. They need to promote appropriate precautions and protection for the patient's auditory system and promptly identify sudden hearing losses. Ways to decrease the amount of noise in the environment need to be emphasized to preserve as much hearing ability as possible before loss of functioning has occurred affecting the patient's quality of life.

What the future brings is promise in new technology for the hearing impaired, including devices to improve communication, understanding, and interpreting sound either implanted or external. Cochlear devices will be totally implanted with improved hearing and be undetectable to others. Improved oral-auditory educational programs to assist patients with hearing and interpreting cues for enhanced communication need to be developed. Nurses need continuing education in ways to communicate with the hearing impaired and remain strong advocates as the mediators between health care providers, patients, and social services to provide the best care for their patients.

Future research is looking at preserving the fine hair cells of the inner ear from damage received from high-intensity noise, ototoxic drugs, and other insults. Experimentation is being considered in replacing lost hair cells and developing more advanced devices to improve hearing (Brors & Bodmer, 2004). Nurses need to keep abreast of new discoveries to assist patients in decision making and appropriate patient care after the procedure is undertaken. Further research examining the ways to incorporate hearing assessment and ensure effective communication with patients to increase satisfaction and adherence to medical care should be developed. Quality of life should also be considered as new interventions are developed to identify which patients benefit most.

Evaluation of Outcomes

Potential patient outcomes for each of the example nursing diagnoses for the patient with the auditory dysfunction are:

- Disturbed sensory perception, auditory, related to obstruction of ear canal, damage to inner ear. The nurse will be able to assist in impacted cerumen with irrigation if the cause of the obstruction. If damage to the inner ear is present, the nurse gives support and perioperative instructions and assists the patient in obtaining auditory devices appropriate for the source.
- Anxiety related to inability to communicate. The patient should be able to recognize the signs of anxiety, demonstrate positive coping mechanisms, and describe a reduction in the level of anxiety experienced.

- Knowledge deficit related to self-care and risk prevention. The patient will demonstrate and report steps in the proper technique in handling and managing a hearing aid. He or she will have knowledge in volume control, storing when not in use, and cleaning the device appropriately.
- Impaired social interaction related to inability to hear others. The nurse will support and provide alternative ways to communicate and encourage the patient to participate in social activities. The patient will be willing to participate in one social event with family or friends.

KEY CONCEPTS

- The type of hearing loss depends on the affected location of the auditory system.
- The number of individuals with auditory dysfunction increases as environmental noise levels increase and the population ages.
- Permanent hearing loss is multifactorial.
- Prevention is the solution to preserving auditory function.
- Often the family member or friend identifies a hearing problem before the patient.
- Conductive hearing loss is differentiated from sensorineural by loss of all sound frequencies, not just higher frequencies.
- Meniére's disease is a chronic progressive condition for which no cure is currently available.
- A thorough history is necessary to identify causes of auditory complications.
- Insects found in the auditory canal should be killed before extracting. Never use water to kill the insect.

- Audiometer is used to test hearing in all ages and should be preformed annually.
- Nursing care consists of educating the patient on proper care of the external auditory canal.
- It is important to discuss postoperative expectations and communication methods before surgery for better patient understanding.
- Ear protection equipment is mandatory in occupations in which the sound levels measurement is greater than 90 dB.
- Frequent breaks are recommended when working with high noise producing equipment.
- Safety is of utmost importance in patients with hearing impairment.
- Effective communication is essential in patient teaching; poor communication leads to confusion, decreased satisfaction, and compliance.
- Always remember the patient cannot hear what is being said and include the patient in all aspects of care.

REVIEW QUESTIONS

1. A 70-year-old patient complains of difficulty hearing when out to dinner with his family. The type of hearing loss he most likely has is:
   1. Conductive hearing loss
   2. Sensorineural hearing loss
   3. Mixed hearing loss

2. A patient who has conductive hearing loss will have the following characteristics:
   1. Hearing loss is associated with higher pitch tones.
   2. Sound is perceived as distorted.
   3. Patient talks louder to hear better.
   4. Conversation can be heard in noisy environments.

3. You are taking care of a patient who just underwent a tympanoplasty. Which of the following interventions is appropriate?
   1. Place patient lying on operative side
   2. Encourage deep breathing and coughing
   3. Tell patient that hearing will return to normal immediately
   4. Assist patient with ambulation until vertigo resolved

Continued

REVIEW QUESTIONS—cont'd

4. A 65-year-old patient who is on high doses of aspirin to treat rheumatoid arthritis suddenly complains of tinnitus and difficulty hearing telephone conversations. The patient asks what can be done. The nurse responds by:
   1. Performing Rinne and Weber tests
   2. Informing the patient that tinnitus occurs with aging
   3. Instructing the patient that tinnitus is a side effect of aspirin
   4. Directing the patient increase the volume on the receiver

5. Signs and symptoms of Meniére's disease include all of the following *except:*:
   1. Tinnitus
   2. Severe vertigo
   3. Conductive hearing loss
   4. Sensorineural hearing loss

6. An adolescent comes in with complaint of hearing loss in the left ear. On examination with an otoscope the canal is found to be blocked with cerumen. What is the next course of action?
   1. Gently irrigate the canal
   2. Insert a cotton swab to remove debris
   3. Use an ear curette
   4. Refer to otologist for removal

7. A 65-year-old patient comes into the clinic with gradual onset of hearing loss. What are some ways to improve communication with the patient who has a hearing deficit?
   (select all that apply)
   1. Get the patient's attention before speaking
   2. Stand with the lighting behind you
   3. Speak very loud
   4. When asked to repeat, repeat same phase slower
   5. Keep hands away mouth while talking

8. A patient is diagnosed with a sensorineural hearing loss and asks if a hearing aid will help return his hearing to normal. Which statement about hearing aids is correct?

   1. Hearing aids only help patients with conductive hearing loss.
   2. Hearing aids increase volume but not clarity of sounds.
   3. Hearing aids will assist patient to hear sounds as normal.
   4. Hearing aids will eliminate background noises.

9. Degrees of hearing impairment are categorized according to sound intensity measurements or decibels. Normal hearing is measured at what range?
   1. 0–15 dB
   2. 16–25 dB
   3. 26–40 dB
   4. 41–55 dB

10. True or False: A patient who is exposed to a loud blast greater than 120 dB lasting 20 seconds can have permanent hearing loss.
    1. True
    2. False

11. Some work environments provide a sustained high noise setting and protection of employees hearing is therefore essential. The occupational nurse must follow OSHA guidelines, which include which of the following? (select all that apply)
    1. Baseline and annual hearing testing of all workers
    2. Monitoring sound levels in the workforce
    3. Biannual education and training of noise pollution
    4. Mandatory hearing protectors on all employees

12. A patient complains of frequent attacks of vertigo, tinnitus, nausea, vomiting, and intermittent hearing loss. These manifestations are characteristic of:
    1. Presbycusis
    2. Meniére's disease
    3. Otosclerosis
    4. Mastoiditis

REVIEW ACTIVITIES

1. You are the nurse taking care of a patient who is scheduled for a tympanoplasty. What are some of the things that you would tell this patient about the procedure to alleviate his or her fears of becoming totally deaf? What patient teaching would be important to include regarding the immediate postoperative period?

2. Identify resources in your clinical facility and community for patients with hearing loss. Choose a specific program and find out what is offered in ways to assist those with a hearing deficit. What does the program offer? Is the program easily accessible? Does the program monitor patient's progress?

3. Using the Internet, locate the different communication devices available for patients with a hearing deficit? Research the cost and available financial resources to assist the patient in obtaining these devices. What requirements or steps does the patient need to complete to obtain the pieces of equipment?

4. Make arrangements to visit an audiologist's office and become more familiar with the various types of hearing aids. Becoming more familiar will provide the students with a better understanding on ways to help the patient better adjust to his or her hearing aid.

5. Experience the sensation of hearing loss by wearing an ear muff and ear plugs. Have the other students practice different types of communication techniques. Discuss what works best and why.

Alterations in Immunological Function

Assessment of Immunological Function

Patrick Heyman, PhD, ARNP-BC

The immune system is tasked with three distinct and interrelated duties: (a) defense of the body from external invaders (pathogens and toxins); (b) surveillance in identifying the body's cells that have mutated and may become or have already become neoplasms (tumors); and (c) maintain homeostasis by removing cellular detritus from the system to ensure uniformity of cells and function (Price & Wilson, 2003). Traditionally, immunologists were only concerned with the first duty. It is only recently that the additional tasks of the immune system came to light. In many ways, the immune system can be thought of as the body's policy enforcers. It is responsible for making sure that the body's cells look sharp and do their jobs. Cells that slack or misbehave are destroyed, so not to affect the functioning of other cells. In its role of enforcer, the immune system also makes sure that the functioning of the body's cells is not impaired by foreign invaders. When the body is damaged, the immune system leads the way preparing the injured area for the healing and reparation process. With so much power over the functioning and viability of the body's cells, it is no coincidence that some of our worst diseases come about as a result of immune dysfunction.

Describing the immune system is a difficult task. Although there are relatively clear divisions in immune function, the components that make up these divisions have overlapping roles. Any general statement is sure to have two or three exceptions, and it is practically impossible to describe or define one part of the immune system without using terms that belong in another part and have not yet been defined. After a brief historical introduction, the approach of this text is to describe the overall interaction of the immune system, and then to discuss each of the components in greater detail, and then put the physiology together.

OVERVIEW OF IMMUNITY

Fast Forward ▶▶▶

Immune Function and Cardiovascular Health

It is known that the inflammatory part of the immune system plays a part in the formation of atherosclerosis (atherogenesis) in arteries for several years. In particular, it is known that macrophages ingested subendothelial cholesterol and became foam cells. In the past four years we have also learned that C-reactive protein (CRP) levels confirm that **inflammation** (a nonspecific response to any foreign invader involving the immune system) plays a part in atherogenesis and myocardial infarction (MI). It is thought that at least part of the antiatherosclerotic benefit of Statin cholesterol-lowering medications is because of their anti-inflammatory properties. But even more recently, it has been discovered that the specific (acquired) immune system plays a part in atherogenesis. Without lymphocytes, progression of an atherosclerotic plaque cannot occur. Natural killer (NK) cells are also implicated in atherogenesis (Linton, Major, & Fazio, 2004; Whitman, Rateri, Szilvassy, Yokoyama, & Daugherty, 2004). Essential enzymes in atherogenesis that interact with immune and inflammatory cells are being identified (Boehm, et al., 2004). Most of the experimental research is currently being conducted in animals because of the ethics involved, but human research is also taking place on a limited scale. In the future, assessing immune function will become part of assessing cardiovascular health.

The immune system is generally divided into two large categories, innate and acquired. **Innate immunity** (immunity that is inherent within a species and develops regardless of exposure), also called natural immunity, is present at birth and functions similarly regardless of the pathogen earning it the designation nonspecific. **Acquired immunity** refers to immunity that is not present at birth and develops either as a result of exposure or through an external source, such as colostrum or injection of immunoglobulin. Acquired immunity is also called adaptive or specific, because the immune response develops and changes in response to the specific pathogen. Adaptive immune responses are considered either humoral-mediated or cell-mediated. **Humoral-mediated immunity** refers to immunity that is mediated by B lymphocytes, plasma cells, and antibodies. **Cell-mediated immunity** refers to immunity that is mediated by T lymphocytes.

This simple division between types of immunity is muddied by the interactions between the innate (nonspecific) and adaptive immune systems. The adaptive immune system requires the innate immune system for initial activation. Once activated, however, much of its effector mechanisms (effectors are any cell or chemical that acts to eliminate invaders, as opposed to recognition) involve potentiating innate immune responses. Thus the innate system forms part of the adaptive system's response and vice versa. The innate immune system can eliminate some threats by itself, but many invaders either overwhelm it or evade detection by it. In these cases, the adaptive immune system is required. It takes 4 to 10 days for the adaptive immune system to mount its first response. Once developed, however, the adaptive immune system will retain some of its effector cells as memory cells. On subsequent exposures, the adaptive immune system can mount a response almost immediately.

The vital characteristics of both systems are recognition and effector mechanisms. Recognition mechanisms are the methods by which various immune system cells recognize invading cells and toxins or aberrant host cells. Effector mechanisms are the methods by which the immune system destroys and eliminates these threats.

The nonspecific immune system relies on receptors that detect common pathogenic features, such as bacterial cell wall polysaccharides. Most of these receptors are found on the surface of various white blood cells, but some of them are found on plasma proteins, such as complement C1q and CRP. A complement is a cascade of proteins in serum that, when activated, attract more leukocytes (white blood cells) to the site of activation, encourage phagocytosis, and lyse pathogen cell membranes. When one of the receptors is bound to its substrate, it activates a series of reactions that activates the nonspecific immune system and calls white blood cells to the site of injury. This process is called inflammation and will be discussed later in the chapter. The specific immune system also relies on receptors, but instead of relying on common pathogenic features, the receptors are designed to respond to only one feature, called an antigen. The two main receptors of the adaptive immune system are the T cell receptor (TCR) and antibodies. In a population of lymphocytes, there may be up to one million different receptors represented. When an invader is identified, only those lymphocytes whose receptors match the invader are activated (thus the specificity). Antibodies are released by B lymphocytes and contain the same receptors that the manufacturing cell featured. The B cell receptor is a membrane-bound antibody. The antibodies are plasma borne proteins that serve much the same purpose as the plasma proteins of the innate immune system, except that instead of recognizing common pathogenic features, antibody receptors recognize only their specific antigen.

Antigen

The term **antigen** originally referred to a molecule that caused antibodies to be generated, but it has now been refined to mean any molecule that can bind with a specific antibody. The term **immunogen** refers to any molecule that elicits an immune response. These may include viruses, bacteria, pollen, toxins, foods, transplanted organs, or transfused blood. There is a fine difference between immunogens and antigens, but for most purposes, they can be used interchangeably.

The bulk of an antigen's surface causes no immune response. Only certain portions of the surface are reactive. These reactive portions are called epitope (sometimes also called antigenic determinant). Most antigens have more than one kind of epitope and are called multivalent. Other antigens have repeated arrays of the same epitope. Antibodies are produced in response to epitope, not the antigen as a whole. Thus a multivalent antigen may react with more than one kind of antibody. A given epitope may be present on more than one antigen, so that one antibody may potentially react with more than one antigen.

The difference between immunogens and antigens is that all immunogens are antigens, but some antigens are not immunogens. That is, that some antigens by themselves do not elicit an immune response or antibodies. These are called **haptens.** For a hapten to elicit an immune response, it needs to be bound to carrier molecule at which point it becomes an immunogen. Two factors influence the ability of an antigen to elicit an immune response. One is the size or weight of the molecule. Smaller molecules tend to cause less reaction. The other factor is the concentration. Small quantities of an antigen may not cause an immune response. Haptens are clinically significant, because once bound to their carrier molecule, the immune system will produce three different kinds of antibodies against them. The first kind of antibody will react to the hapten regardless of whether it is bound or not. The second kind of antibody will react to the carrier molecule regardless of whether it is bound to the hapten or not. The third kind of antibody only reacts to the hapten-carrier complex. Hapten antibodies are important in immunology research, but they are also clinically significant as they form the physiological basis for penicillin allergy cross-reactivity with cephalosporins and other antibiotics. In clinical practice, immunogen and antigen are often used interchangeably, but a nurse should know the distinction.

Self versus Nonself

In all three of its roles, the immune system's essential requirement is the ability to distinguish between what is self and what is foreign (nonself). A group of genes responsible for the recognition of self is called major histocompatibility complex (MHC). The MHC manufactures two major types of MHC proteins that are essential in identifying the body's cells as self. Class I MHC proteins are present on the surface of the cell membrane of almost all host cells with a developed nucleus and platelets. They are also called **human leukocyte antigens (HLA),** because they were first identified on leukocytes. Substances lacking HLA are identified as nonself. Each person has an HLA that uniquely identifies him or her. As far as science can tell there are no two persons that have identical HLA, although twins may have similar HLA. MHC class II molecules are found mainly on immune system cells, but can be induced in other cells by interferons (proteins formed when cells are exposed to invaders, such as viruses that are able to activate other components of the immune system). Classes I and II MHC proteins also serve to present antigen to T cells.

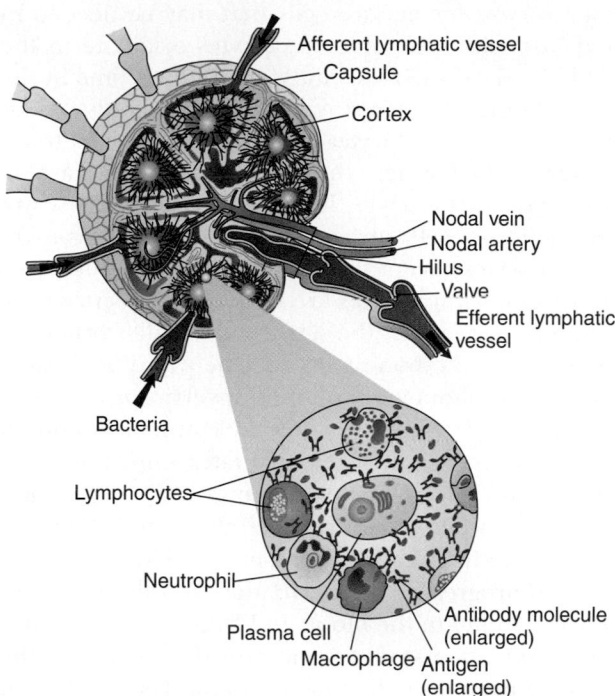

Figure 41-1 Cellular components of the immune system.

ANATOMY OF THE IMMUNE SYSTEM

The anatomy of the immune system is detailed and complex. There are many elements to consider within the immune system, and their interrelationships are complicated in nature. The structures of the immune system have been examined extensively within the field of biology and are well-defined. There are both larger anatomic organs and cellular components of a hematological nature comprising the immune system (Figure 41-1).

Physical Barriers

The human body is constantly surrounded by pathogens in the air, on solid surfaces, and in water. Pathogens are ingested with every meal and inspired with every breath. Before ever encountering an immune system cell, a pathogen must penetrate the body's outer defenses. These consist of barriers (e.g., mechanical, chemical, and microbial) that are considered to be part of the innate immune system. In addition to the barriers themselves, each of these areas is populated with members of the innate immune system and often with lymphoid tissue.

The most obvious physical barrier is the skin. The outermost layer consists of several layers of keratinized, water-resistant squamous cells. But skin is made even more formidable by secretions of lactose that lower the pH of skin, making it a less hospitable environment. Perspiration contains salt, which can be toxic to pathogens by hypertonic mechanism. Sebaceous glands secrete sebum that helps to trap invaders and actually inhibits some type of bacteria.

With regard to the digestive system, saliva in the mouth forms the first chemical barrier. The pH of saliva, combined with several enzymes, make it an unattractive place to live. The hydrochloric acid and pepsin of the stomach form the next inhospitable atmosphere that invaders will encounter. Bile salts, fatty acids, lysolipids, and other digestive enzymes are found in the small intestine. After making it through this gauntlet of digestive enzymes, the large intestines are thoroughly colonized with a wide array of flora, both bacterial and fungal. There are about 400 different kinds of bacteria in the intestines, weighing over a kilogram and outnumbering the body cells 10 to 1. These native flora make the intestines less hospitable to invaders through competition for space and nutrients.

The respiratory system begins with nasal hair and turbinates in combination with mucous secreting membranes, which all serve to trap invading pathogens and may contain immunoglobulin A (IgA) antibodies. Once in the bronchus, mucous secretions in combination with a cilia "elevator" serve to bring foreign particles to the carina, where the cough reflex helps to expel the invaders from the body. The epithelium of the lungs secretes two proteins called surfactants A and D, which coat pathogens making them more easily phagocytosed.

The eyes are protected by lashes and the blink reflex. Tears, which contain antimicrobial factors including IgA antibody, help to wash out pathogens that make it past the lids and lashes. The vagina is colonized with lactobacilli that secrete lactic acid, lowering the pH of the vagina and making it less hospitable. Yeast and lactobacillus compete with potential pathogens for nutrients, further preventing infection.

Leukocytes

The main cells of the immune system are white blood cells collectively referred to as **leukocytes.** Like all blood cells, leukocytes originate from the bone marrow. Stem cells (undifferentiated cells) in the marrow develop into the various white blood cells. In addition to serving as the birthplace for leukocytes, the bone marrow also acts as a reservoir for mature cells that may be needed in event of infection or blood loss. Although most leukocytes originate in the bone marrow along with red blood cells (RBCs), most spend little time in the blood. Leukocytes spend most of their time in storage, in lymphoid tissues, or dispersed throughout the host tissues. Leukocytes use blood mainly as a transport system to travel to areas of the body where they are needed. There are six families of leukocytes that have distinct roles in the body's defense. These are the monocyte-macrophages, dendritic cells, mast cells, granulocytes, lymphocytes, and NK cells. All the leukocytes except the lymphocytes are considered part of the innate immune system. Lymphocytes are the only leukocytes associated with the adaptive immune system. All the leukocyte families originally come from pluripotent stem cells in the bone marrow. The pluripotent stem cell differentiates into common lymphoid and common myeloid progenitors. All lymphocytes as well as NK cells are descended from the common lymphoid progenitor. The common myeloid progenitor differentiates into monocyte, dendritic cells, granulocyte, erythrocyte, and platelet precursors. The common lymphoid progenitor can also give rise to a dendritic cell that is indistinguishable from the dendritic cell derived from the myeloid.

It is imperative to understand progressive differentiation in order to understand leukocytes. The leukocytes found in the blood and lymph tissues are typically not fully differentiated. As a case study, monocytes descend from the common myeloid progenitor as previously discussed. Monocytes circulate in the blood until summoned to the tissues. At this time, they exit the blood vessels through specialized openings in the vessel wall and enter the tissue. Once in the tissue, monocytes differentiate yet again, maturing into macrophages, which usually live in the tissues until their death. Thus the macrophage is the final differentiation of a monocyte, and the monocyte is simply a relatively inert circulation form of the cell. Another way to think of progressive differentiation is to think of the monocyte as an observation form and the macrophage as the functional form. Most other leukocytes also undergo progressive differentiation. The exception is the granulocytes, which circulate in fully differentiated form.

Proliferation is the other concept necessary to understand white blood cells. Although lymphocytes originate in the bone marrow from stem cells, they are also able to reproduce within lymph tissue. When activated, lymphocytes will proliferate (reproduce) first and then differentiate into their final functioning form. This allows the few cells that are able to respond to a given invader to reproduce quickly without a corresponding increase in lymphocytes that are not needed for the present threat.

Monocyte-Macrophages

Monocytes are leukocytes found in relatively small quantities in the blood, because most of them are either in the tissues or stored in the bone marrow. Arising from the common myeloid progenitor, the majority of monocytes remain in the marrow, serving as a reservoir against infection. The immature stage is referred to as monocyte, while the fully differentiated stage is called a **macrophage.** Monocytes are continuously migrating to tissue and differentiating into tissue macrophages. Tissue macrophages are called different names, depending on the tissue in which they have differentiated. Tissue macrophages in the nervous system are called microglial cells, and macrophages in the liver are called Kupffer cells. No matter where they differentiate, tissue macrophages serve the same function, which is to monitor the surrounding tissue for invaders and foreign antigen. Collectively, they are sometimes referred to as mononuclear phagocytes.

Macrophages are one of three phagocytic cells (cells that engulf and destroy foreign pathogens, toxins, or other antigens) in the immune system. Having differentiated in tissues, macrophages are relatively immobile, monitoring the nearby tissue for invaders. Macrophages have receptors for a wide variety of common pathogen features, such as the glucan receptor and mannose receptor, scavenger receptor, which binds to negatively charged ligands that are components of many gram-positive bacterial cell walls, and the CD14 (LPS) receptor, which detects bacterial lipopolysaccharide. On detecting an invader, macrophages attempt to engulf the invader in an amoeboid-like process called **phagocytosis.** The cell membrane distorts and wraps around the particle until the two sides of the cell membrane touch. The cell membrane edges fuse themselves together, and the particle is encased in a vesicle made of membrane that was formerly part of the cell's outer membrane. This vesicle is called a phagosome or endocytic vacuole. Lysosomes containing destructive enzymes are then fused with the phagosome, and the enzymes are released into the phagosome. The phagosome-lysosome complex is called a phagolysome.

Macrophages are **antigen presenting cells (APCs)** and act as one of the first responders in the immune response process. Once activated, a macrophage releases cytokines and chemokines. **Cytokines** affect the way other cells act (*Cyto-* "cell" and *–kinein* "move"). **Chemokines** attract other leukocytes to the area to battle the invaders in a process called chemotaxis. See Table 41-1 for a list of selected cytokines released by macrophages and their effects. Because macrophage recognition of pathogens is so important, one of the main distinguishing features of pathogenic microbes (as opposed to nonpathogenic microbes) is the ability to overwhelm or evade macrophages and other segments of the innate immune system. For example, some bacteria coat themselves in a thick polysaccharide that is not recognized by macrophage or neutrophil receptors. Other pathogens, such as mycobacteria, can actually live and multiply inside of phagosomes by keeping the lysosomes from fusing with the phagosome.

One unique characteristic of macrophages is the ability to form giant multinucleated cells. When confronted with an overwhelming opponent, several macrophages can join together to form one large cell, the aforementioned giant multinucleated cells. This allows macrophages to engulf invaders that they other wise could not engulf.

Dendritic Cells

Dendritic cells are star-shaped cells that are so called because they resemble a neuron's dendrites. While we have been studying macrophages for more than 100 years, we have only known about dendritic cells for less than 35 years, and

TABLE 41-1	Important Cytokines Released by Macrophages and Their Effects	
CYTOKINE	**LOCAL EFFECT**	**SYSTEMIC EFFECT**
IL-1β	Activates endothelium Activates lymphocytes Local tissue destruction Increases access of effector cells	Fever Production of IL-6
TNF-α	Activates endothelium and increases vascular permeability, leading to increased entry of IgG, complement, and increased fluid drainage to lymph nodes.	Fever Mobilization of metabolites Shock
IL-6	Lymphocyte activation Increased antibody production	Fever Induces acute-phase protein production
CXCL8	Chemotactic factor recruits neutrophils, basophils, and T cells to site of infection	
IL-12	Activates NK cells Induces the differentiation of CD4 T cells into TH1 cells.	

Adapted from Janeway, C. A., Jr., Travers, P., Walport, M., & Shlomchik, M. J. (2004). Immunobiology, the immune system in health and disease *(6th ed.). New York: Garland Science Publishing.*

there is still much that we do not know about them. Their life cycle is more complicated than that of macrophages. The immature dendritic cells migrate to tissues, particularly the skin, airway, spleen, and lymph nodes. Like tissue macrophages, tissue dendritic cells are called different names depending on the tissue in which they live. Tissue dendritic cells that live in the skin are called Langerhans cells. Immature tissue dendritic cells are both phagocytic and macropinocytic; that is, they can ingest large amounts of surrounding interstitial fluid. Tissue dendritic cells break down proteins and display the ingested antigens on their cell membranes. At the end of their life cycle, they will migrate to lymph nodes and induce tolerance in lymphocytes, because they do not have costimulatory molecules in their immature stage. The signals for maturation are either direct contact with a pathogen or inflammatory cytokines. Pathogens are ingested when they are recognized by their common features as described above. Macropinocytosis allows the dendritic cell to ingest pathogens that have some mechanism to escape detection by phagocytic receptors. As the products are degraded inside the dendritic cell, they are able to recognize bacterial DNA, bacterial heat shock proteins, and viral double stranded RNA. Once activated, they differentiate into mature dendritic cells, develop costimulatory molecules, and migrate to the lymph nodes to activate the lymphocytes that migrate through the nodes (Vuckovic, et al., 2004).

Mature dendritic cells carry high levels of MHC on their cell membranes to present antigen to T lymphocytes. When the T cell with the right receptor recognizes the presented antigen, it proliferates and differentiates. The truly amazing thing about dendritic cells is that they are able to activate only the specific T lymphocytes that are needed to respond to a given invader, whether it is a virus, bacteria, or fungus. In some cases, this may mean activating just 1 in 10,000 or 1 in 1,000,000 T lymphocytes.

Fast Forward ▶▶▶

Dendritic Cell Research

Dendritic cells are seen as the missing key in many immunological disorders. Dendritic cell infection is crucial in defeating the body's defenses against several viruses, including Ebola and HIV (Geisbert, et al., 2003; Janeway, Travers, Walport, & Shlomchik, 2004). Both of these viruses neutralize dendritic cells keeping the body from mounting a defense against them. By the time the immune system is mobilized, it is often too late. It is hoped that understanding dendritic cells will aid in the treatment and possible vaccination against these diseases. Dendritic cells are also implicated in tumor formation, and research is being conducted to see if dendritic cells can be manipulated in a way as to be a kind of vaccine against cancer cells. In a cancer vaccine, dendritic cells would be harvested from the patient's body and cultured. Once a thriving culture has been established, tumor cells from the patient are introduced to the culture. The primed dendritic cells are then injected back into the patient where they initiate the immune response against the cancer. Trials are currently underway testing this technique in melanoma, lymphoma, prostate cancer, and colon cancer. Because of the large expense involved in developing a dendritic culture for each patient, additional research is being done to try and up-regulate dendritic cells in the body. In the opposite direction, research is being done in the areas of immune down-regulation. It is hoped that dendritic cell research will be able to provide effective cures for some autoimmune diseases and transplant rejection (Fecci, et al., 2003).

The dendritic cell's strength is also a vital weakness exploited by several viruses, such as human immunodeficiency virus (HIV) and measles. Instead of activating lymphocytes in lymph nodes against these viruses, the infected dendritic cell acts as a transportation system, allowing the virus to then infect the T lymphocytes.

Much of the extracellular debris that is ingested by dendritic cells is harmless, often by-products of dead body cells. Dendritic cells are essential in inducing and maintaining tolerance to these antigens, keeping the immune system from reacting to the body's antigens (Vuckovic, et.al., 2004). As T lymphocytes exit the thymus gland, dendritic cells are responsible for destroying cells that are reactive to self-antigens. This process is referred to as central tolerance and removes the majority of self-reactive T lymphocytes. Dendritic cells also induce peripheral tolerance, suppressing self-reactive lymphocytes that escaped central tolerance or cells that are reactive to antigens not expressed in the thymus.

Mast Cells

Mast cells are also descended from the common myeloid progenitor and differentiate in the tissues. Their blood borne precursor is currently unknown. Mast cells tend to live near the skin and connective of small blood vessels and contain granules with stored chemicals. When activated, they release substances within the granules (degranulate) that affect vascular permeability, particularly histamine. See Table 41-2 for a list of mast cell products. Mast cells are thought to play an important part in protecting mucosal surfaces from pathogens and help the inflammatory process to begin the process of healing damaged tissue, although they are primarily known for their role in immunoglobulin E (IgE)-mediated allergic reactions. In fact, mice that do not have fully differentiated mast cells cannot produce IgE-mediated inflammatory responses.

TABLE 41-2 Molecules Released by Mast Cells on Activation

CLASS OF PRODUCT	EXAMPLES	BIOLOGICAL EFFECTS
Enzyme	Tryptase, chymase, cathepsin G, carboxypeptidase	Remodel connective tissue matrix
Toxic mediator	Histamine, heparin	Toxic to parasites
		Increase vascular permeability
		Cause smooth muscle contraction
Cytokine	IL-4, IL-13	Stimulate and amplify TH2 cell response
Cytokine	IL-3, IL-5, GM-CSF	Promote eosinophil production and activation
Cytokine	TNF-α	Promotes inflammation, stimulates cytokine production by many cell types, activated endothelium
Chemokine	CCL3 (MIP-1α)	Attracts monocytes, macrophages, and neutrophils
Lipid mediator	Leukotrienes C4, D4, E4	Cause smooth muscle contraction
		Increase vascular permeability
		Stimulate mucous secretion
	Platelet-activating factor	Attracts leukocytes
		Amplifies production of lipid mediators
		Activates neutrophils, eosinophils, and platelets

Adapted from Janeway, C. A., Jr., Travers, P., Walport, M., & Shlomchik, M. J. (2004). Immunobiology, the immune system in health and disease *(6th ed.). New York: Garland Science Publishing.*

Granulocytes

The **granulocytes** are so called because when stained, they have granule-shaped objects visible within their cytoplasm, much like mast cells. They also have lobed irregular nuclei, earning the designation polymorphonuclear leukocytes (PMNs). The granules are lysosomes, which are vesicles filled with destructive enzymes. These enzymes are used to destroy invaders. **Neutrophils** are the most numerous granulocytes and thought to be the most important. Neutrophils are the third and final phagocytic cell in the immune system. On engulfing an invader, the granules are fused to the vesicle, and the enzymes are released into vesicle; where they may destroy the particle. Neutrophils are especially reactive to bacteria, and the number of circulating neutrophils greatly increases during bacterial infections. Neutrophils are the first responders to chemotaxis and are rarely found in healthy tissue. Neutrophils are relatively fragile compared to macrophages. They can only ingest a few bacteria before dying, but macrophages can ingest a hundred bacteria. Pus is mostly made up of bacteria and dead neutrophils. Because of their expendable nature, they appear in the blood in large numbers, with several times that number in reserve in the bone marrow. They are the most numerous granulocyte and often the most numerous leukocyte. Deficiency in neutrophils, called **neutropenia,** can cause overwhelming bacterial infection.

The other two classes of granulocyte cells are exocytic, meaning they produce their effects on outside cells as opposed to phagocytosed cells. **Eosinophils** are found in small quantities in the blood as most of them are distributed in the tissues. Their primary effector function is to release their highly toxic granules that can kill parasites and other microorganisms. They also produce cytokines, leukotrienes, and prostaglandins. Eosinophils are involved in defense against parasites and increase in numbers when the body has a parasitic infection. They are most well-known for their role in IgE-mediated allergic reactions and are often present in mucous secretions during allergic reactions.

Basophils, are the final and most inscrutable granulocyte. Not much is known about them, but they appear to have an effect against fungus and also play a role in inflammation. They behave similarly to eosinophils and are distributed throughout the tissues.

Natural Killer Cells

NK cells arise from the common lymphoid progenitor. They appear as large lymphocytes with cytoplasmic granules and circulate in the blood. Although lacking antigen-specific receptors, they are able to detect and attack a limited number of abnormal cells, such as tumor cells and cells infected with the herpes simplex virus (HSV). They are also able to kill cells that are coated in antibody, a process known as antibody-dependent cell-mediated cytotoxicity (ADCC), and are mediated by the Fc receptor (see antibody discussed later). NK cells are also activated by interferons and macrophage-derived cytokines.

Lymphocytes

There are two major types of lymphocytes, T lymphocytes and B lymphocytes, or simply T cells and B cells. All lymphocytes originally descend from the common lymphoid progenitor but differentiate differently depending on where they mature. Some lymphocytes mature in the bone marrow, while others migrate to the thymus for maturation. B lymphocytes are so called, because they mature to their intermediate stage in the bone marrow. When activated, B lymphocytes complete their differentiation process and become plasma cells, releasing antibodies. T lymphocytes are so called, because they mature in the thymus. T cell development is more complex than that of B cells. The first division of T cells is based on receptor chains. Most T cells have receptors consisting alpha (α) and beta (β) chains, but a second division T cells have receptors made of gamma (γ) and delta (δ) chains. These are called α:β and γ:δ T cells, respectively. The α:β T cells eventually become CD4 and CD8 T cells.

The function of γ:δ T cells is poorly understood, but they appear to function as innate immune cells, rather than adaptive immune cells.

Most inactivated lymphocytes are small and rather featureless with inactive nuclear chromatin. As late as the 1960s, many textbooks described these cells as having no known function. Indeed, lymphocytes do show little activity until activated by the presence of antigen and costimulatory molecules, usually presented by an APC, such as a macrophage or dendritic cell. On activation, lymphocytes differentiate into lymphoblasts, which undergo mitosis and then differentiate into the final activated phase taking on their specialized functions. Once the infection has been eradicated, most of the lymphocytes that were produced as a result of lymphoblast proliferation undergo apoptosis (programmed cell death); however, a few remain as memory cells enabling the body to respond rapidly to subsequent infections by the same pathogen.

The main functional characteristic of lymphocytes is the ability to mount specific immune responses against virtually any foreign antigen. All lymphocytes have a prototype receptor that changes during the intermediate maturation process so that taken as a whole, they are able to react with almost any possible antigen. The B cell and T cell receptors are closely related in structure, but they are different in function and will be discussed in more depth. The B cell receptor (BCR) actually consists of the antibody that the B cell will release when activated and can recognize only one specific antigen. BCRs (and antibodies) are only able to detect antigen that is in the extracellular fluid. The T cell antigen receptor (TCR) is structurally similar to the BCR, but does not recognize whole antigens. Rather it detects fragments of antigen that are displayed by MHC molecules on the surface of host cells. Thus the T cell, detects antigen within the host cells, such as viruses that have commandeered a cell's processes or a parasitic bacteria. Variability in the BCR and TCR is attained by mutation of the genes responsible for their production.

B Lymphocytes and Antibodies

B cells are lymphocytes that develop in the bone marrow. Their primary job on activation is to produce antibodies. B cells develop in the bone marrow until they express the immunoglobulin M (IgM) molecule on their cell surface. Once the IgM molecule is expressed the immature B cell undergoes self-tolerance testing and viability testing. The immature B cell migrates to the secondary lymph tissues, where it develops into a mature B cell, expressing both IgM and immunoglobulin D (IgD) molecules. Mature B cells, also called naïve B cells because they have not encountered their specific antigen yet, recirculate through the lymph tissues waiting to encounter their antigen and become activated. On activation, B cells proliferate and then become plasma cells, secreting antibodies.

The only immune function of the B cell is to release **antibodies** (proteins produced by plasma cells that recognize and bind to a specific antigen) when activated. Unlike T cells, which venture out of the lymph nodes when activated, plasma cells stay in the lymph node, secreting antibodies to be delivered to the systemic circulation. An antibody itself is a molecule composed of two segments, a recognition/binding segment and an effector segment. The recognition segment binds to the antigen, and the effector segment activates other components of the immune system. Thus antibodies may neutralize threats directly by physically binding to them and keeping them from damage. At the same time, antibodies recruit other components of the immune system to attack and destroy the threat.

Antibodies are a category of protein called **immunoglobulins (Ig).** All immunoglobulins share a similar structure. They are generally y-shaped molecules, with two recognition segments and one effector segment. The recognition segment is called the variable region or V region, because it changes from antibody to antibody to ensure that a wide range of antigens can be recognized. The different immunoglobulins perform different effector functions in the body.

B cells will be selected to secrete more of a given immunoglobulin depending on the type of immune response and the location in the body of the activated B cell. Immunoglobulin G (IgG) is the most abundant immunoglobulin in the body and is further divided into four subtypes (IgG1, IgG2, IgG3, and IgG4), where IgG1 is the most abundant in plasma and IgG4 is the least abundant. IgA is divided into two subtypes (IgA1 and IgA2). IgM and IgA can form polymers in the blood. IgM forms a pentameter, a molecule composed of five IgM antibodies joined by their C terminuses. IgA appears in the blood as both a monomer (single antibody) and a dimer (two antibodies joined at the C region).

Naïve B cells express both IgM and IgD on their surface. When activated, the B cell will produce IgM and IgD antibodies. However, later in the immune response, the B cell will change to producing IgG, IgA, or IgE by irreversibly recombining its DNA. At this point the cell can no longer produce IgM or IgD antibodies. The signal to switch antibody production is mediated by cytokines and T cells.

Antibodies work by four basic functions: neutralization, opsonization, activation of inflammation, and activation of complement. Neutralization is accomplished solely by the variable region of the antibody, and its effectiveness is determined by the antibody's affinity for the antigen. Its mechanism is the complete binding of an antigen by the antibody, so that there are no available binding sites, effectively rendering the invader inert. This process is especially important for bacterial toxins and viruses. A special case of neutralization is **agglutination.** This occurs when the arms of the antibody bind to the same epitope on different antigens. For example, the IgM pentameter has 10 binding sites and could theoretically bind 10 different bacteria that share the same epitope. This causes clumping, called agglutination. The second mechanism is called opsonization. When antibodies coat a bacteria or other pathogen, it can induce nearby macrophages to engulf the pathogen. This is especially important against bacteria that have natural defenses to keep macrophages from engulfing them. The third mechanism is the activation of inflammatory processes, including the activation of NK cells. The fourth mechanism is the activation of the complement cascade. Complement is a cascade of lytic proteins that are activated by antibodies. The activation of complement by itself can cause the death of some invaders, but it is always a signal to nearby phagocytic cells to attack the pathogen.

In an immune response IgM is the first antibody to be released. IgM has a fairly low binding affinity for epitope, and it is believed that the 10 binding sites of the pentameter provide a higher effective affinity for repetitive epitope, such as bacterial capsule molecules. Essentially it allows the IgM molecule to stick to an antigen longer until higher affinity antibodies can be manufactured. Although IgM appears in the blood as a flat pinwheel, on binding to an antigen, the other binding sites bend toward the antigen surface like spider legs. The pentameric nature of IgM also makes it a particularly potent activator of the complement cascade. Thus IgM is an excellent first responder.

IgG, IgA, and IgE are produced later in the immune response. They are smaller than IgM and can diffuse relatively easily out of the blood and into the tissues. IgG is the principal antibody found in the blood and tissues, while IgA is principally found in secretions, such as tears and saliva. IgG is an excellent opsonin, but IgA is not. This makes sense, as IgA works on epithelial surfaces that do not normally contain complement or phagocytes. These antibodies are produced and secreted close to where they will function. IgE is found only in low levels, but it has an extremely high affinity for mast cells and binds to mast cells even before it binds to antigen. Antigen binding to this mast cell–associated IgE triggers mast cells to degranulate and release their inflammatory mediators.

T Lymphocytes

T lymphocytes progenitors leave the bone marrow and migrate to the thymus gland, where they develop into T lymphocytes instead of B lymphocytes. Most of the T lymphocyte progenitors die in the thymus by apoptosis. T lymphocytes are divided early in development into α:b and γ:δ T cells. The α:β T cells later develop into CD4 and CD8 T cells. CD4 and CD8 are surface proteins on the membranes of T cells. For years, CD8 has marked **cytotoxic (killer) T cells,** and CD4 has marked **helper T cells,** which further differentiate into two subclasses, TH1 and TH2 cells.

During development, T lymphocytes go through two selection process. Positive selection encourages lymphocytes that bind weakly to self-antigens. While negative selection eliminates lymphocytes that bind strongly to self-proteins. The reason for this twofold process is that lymphocytes must be able to bind with MHC I and II (self-antigens) to generate an immune response, but lymphocytes that bind too strongly could possibly cause autoimmune disease. The MHC antigens that the T lymphocytes recognize as self are determined the by the MHC antigens present in the thymus gland.

Each naïve T lymphocyte can detect only one specific antigen, and it wanders the body's lymph nodes in search of its antigen. If it finds it, it proliferates and then differentiates into its active phase. It takes more than simply meeting its specific antigen to activate the naïve T cell. The T cell must meet its antigen while being displayed by an APC that also displays costimulatory molecules. Naïve CD8 T cells always differentiate into cytotoxic (killer) T cells, but they require more costimulation than CD4 cells to do so.

Primary Lymphoid Organs

Anatomically speaking, the immune system is largely identified with the lymphoid portion of the immune system. The primary lymphoid organs are the bone marrow and thymus gland, because lymphocytes develop and mature within them. The thymus gland is located superior to the heart. The thymus gland also serves as a reservoir for T lymphocytes. It is believed that the major function of the thymus gland is in the development of the immune system. It is larger in children than in adults. Removal of the thymus in children causes a reduction in the number of T lymphocytes and a higher number of granulocytes (Eysteinsdottir, et al., 2004). The effects of removing the thymus gland in adults are not well understood and only recently have begun to be studied. New evidence shows that the thymus is active in adults, and efforts should be made to preserve it during cardiothoracic surgery.

Secondary Lymphoid Tissue

Although lymphocytes are distributed throughout the body, they are concentrated in several tissues. The tissues where they aggregate and function are called secondary lymphoid tissues and include the spleen, lymph nodes, and epithelial lymphoid tissues. Secondary lymphoid tissues are strategically placed in the body so that invading pathogens will encounter them as early as possible, allowing the immune system to be activated before extensive damage can be done.

Spleen

The spleen is a fist-sized organ located on the left side of the body, behind the stomach. It acts as a filter, collecting antigen from the blood and destroying senescent RBCs. Most of the spleen is made up of tissue called red pulp, which primarily serves as the site of RBC destruction and also houses macrophages. Interspersed throughout the red pulp, lymphocytes surround arterioles forming pockets called white pulp. The organization of white pulp consists of two layers, the periarteriolar sheath, consisting mainly of T lymphocytes, and the B-cell corona, consisting of mainly B lymphocytes. The white pulp is responsible for generating immune responses to blood-borne immunogens and plays an important role in preventing septicemia. Removal of the spleen often results in life-threatening infections known as overwhelming postsplenectomy infections (OPSI) (Jirillo, et al., 2003).

Lymph Nodes

The lymph nodes are encapsulated lymphoid structures located throughout the lymphatic vascular system and provide the tissues and lymph with the same function that white pulp of the spleen provides for blood. Ranging in size from 1 to 20 mm, lymph nodes are responsible for generating immune responses to the immunogens in the lymph drainage and interstitial fluid that drains from local tissues into the lymph vessels. Lymph nodes are typically bean-shaped, with two layers, an outer cortex and an inner medulla. Several afferent lymphatic vessels enter into the cortex, which is separated into several compartments called follicles. Each follicle leads to the medulla, where the lymph fluid is consolidated, and one larger efferent lymphatic vessel exits from the medulla. The medulla is also associated with an artery and vein that is used for incoming naïve lymphocytes. The lymph nodes also act as a pump for lymph fluid, activated by random skeletal muscle contraction.

Lymph node follicles are divided into several distinct regions. The outer portion of the follicle is made up mostly of B cells. During an immune response, areas of intense B cell proliferation are called germinal centers. Follicles that do not contain germinal centers are called primary lymphoid follicles. Once a germinal center has been established, it is called a secondary lymphoid follicle. Primary follicles contain inactive B cells surrounding a specialized cell of uncertain origin, called a follicular dendritic cell (FDC). The FDC secretes chemokines that attract both inactive and active B cells. The next section of the cortex is called the paracortical area and is mostly made up of T lymphocytes. The third part of the cortex, which is closest to the medulla, is made up of macrophages and antibody-secreting plasma cells and is called the medullary cords.

Lymph nodes are designed so that APCs from the tissues will come into the lymph node through the afferent lymphatic vessel and encounter B lymphocytes first, then T lymphocytes, and will then take up residence in the medullary cords. This ensures that it will encounter both kinds of lymphocytes, and if the lymphocyte with the specific antigen it is presenting is not present, as that lymphocyte recirculates through the body, it will encounter it in the medullary cords. The recirculating naïve T lymphocytes enter the node through the arteriole using special adhesion molecules, called L-selectin, which allows them to stick to the artery's surface. Activated B cells remain in the lymph node and form germinal centers, but activated T lymphocytes need to travel to the site of infection. When T cells mature, they lose their L-selectin, so that they can no longer enter lymph nodes through the artery.

Epithelial Lymphoid Tissues

In addition to lymph nodes, there are also patches of unencapsulated lymphoid tissue located throughout the body in connective tissue. The gut-associated lymphoid tissues (GALT) include the tonsils, adenoids, Peyer's patches in the small intestine, and the appendix. GALT collects antigen from the surface of epithelial cells in the digestive tract. Peyer's patches are the most organized of the GALT and consist of a B cell center surrounded by smaller numbers of T cells. Specialized epithelial cells called multifenestrated cells collect the antigen from the lumen of the small intestine. Similarly, bronchial-associated lymphoid tissue (BALT) and mucosa-associated lymphoid tissue (MALT) provide the same functions in the bronchial tree and other mucosa.

Chemical Components

In addition to the leukocytes and antibodies, there are also a number of chemicals that make up the immune system. Many of these are secreted by leukocytes, but some are not. Chemical components serve several different functions. Two of these functions have already been discussed briefly in the leukocyte section; attracting cells and changing cell behavior. Chemicals that attract other leukocytes to the area are called chemokines. Chemicals that change the behavior of other cells are called cytokines. Some cytokines may induce vasodilation or increase vascular permeability. Other cytokines may activate leukocytes. The third function of chemical components is opsonization. A fourth function of chemical components is pathogen or toxin neutralization and direct destruction.

Cytokines

Cytokines are small proteins that affect the behavior of cells. The cytokines may act in an autocrine manner (affecting the cell that secreted it), paracrine manner (affecting adjacent cells), or even endocrine manner (affecting distant cells). The ability of a cytokine to act on distant cells depends on its ability to enter the blood and how long it stays in the blood (half-life). An important concept in understanding cytokines is that of kinases and kinase inhibitors. These enzymes destroy cytokine and preserve cytokine, respectively. Each cytokine has its own set of kinases and kinase inhibitors, which are important in the regulation of immune responses. Some diseases may not have anything to do with underproduction or overproduction of cytokines, but rather problems with these regulatory proteins. Too much kinase or too little kinase inhibitor will result in abbreviated immune response, while too little kinase or too much kinase inhibitor will result in prolonged immune response.

When cytokines were first being discovered, they were named **interleukins (IL),** to signify that they were secreted by a leukocyte. Over time, it became apparent that the cytokines are a diverse group of molecules structurally and behaviorally. Newer nomenclatures are being developed that group the cytokines according to their structure or function.

The **interferons (IFNs)** are a class of cytokine that was so named because it interfered with viral replication in cells that were previously uninfected. IFNs bind to nearby cells through an IFN receptor, which induces the cell to produce a variety of proteins that inhibit viral replication. In mice, the ability to manufacture the protein Mx in response to interferon confers immunity to influenza. In addition to this protein production, IFNs also stimulate the immune response to viruses by inducing the synthesis of MHC class I molecules on the surfaces of infected cells. Recall that the specific immune response to viruses depends on presenting antigen bound to MHC to T cells. Finally, IFNs activate NK cells to destroy viruses and virus-infected cells.

Chemokines

Chemokines are a subgroup of cytokines that attract other cells, a process called chemotaxis. They function mainly as chemoattractants, recruiting monocytes, neutrophils, and other leukocytes to the area; however, some chemokines also have roles in lymphocyte development and angiogenesis. Chemokines can be secreted by a wide variety of cells, including endothelial cells and keratinocytes (skin cells). They have been discovered fairly recently and originally shared the interleukin designation with cytokines. More recently, there has been as change in nomenclature to reflect their structure. The two main families of chemokines are called CC and CXC chemokines. The chemokine itself is designated by the letter l and a number, while the receptor is designated by the letter r and the same number. Thus, IL-8 became CXCL8 and binds to the CXCR8 receptor.

Complement

The **complement** system is a cascade of several lytic proteins that aid in pathogen destruction. They were first observed being activated by antibodies and enhancing the action of antibodies. Hence their discoverer called them antibody-complement proteins, which were later simplified to complement. The complement cascade consists of enzymes that aid in the destruction of pathogen membranes. To keep these enzymes from destroying host cells, they circulate in the blood as zymogens. To be activated, the zymogen is cleaved into two parts, freeing the active enzyme. An example of zymogens elsewhere in the body is pepsinogen, stored in stomach epithelial cells. Once secreted into the stomach, the hydrochloric acid cleaves pepsinogen into pepsin, which breaks down peptide bonds. This mechanism keeps pepsin from digesting the cell that stores it.

Complement proteins are designated by the letter *c* and then a number. The number does not represent the step in the cascade, but the order in which they were discovered. The complement cascade performs all four chemical component functions (cytokine, chemokine, opsonin, and effector). The three pathways for complement cascade activation are (a) the classical pathway, (b) mannose-binding lectin (MB-lectin) pathway, and (c) the alternative pathway. The classical pathway always begins with the binding of C1q to the pathogen surface. The MB-lectin pathway is initiated by the binding of MB-lectin to mannose containing carbohydrates in bacteria and viruses. MB-lectin is a serum protein that increases during inflammation. The alternative pathway can be initiated by the binding of spontaneously activated C3 in plasma to the surface of a pathogen.

PHYSIOLOGY OF THE IMMUNE SYSTEM

The physiology of the immune system is extremely complicated and complex. There continue to be many functions within the immune system that are not well understood and research exploring the immune system is extensive and ongoing.

Innate Immune Response

Innate immunity is dependent largely on the recognition of common pathogenic features, such as mannose and glucan found in bacterial cell walls. Because macrophages live in the tissues, they are usually the first immune system cell to encounter pathogens and typically begin the innate immune system response. When a macrophage recognizes an invader in addition to attempting to phagocytose the invader, it also releases cytokines and chemokines, thus inducing the inflammatory response. Inflammation plays three roles in the innate immune response. First, it brings more effector cells to the site and augments their killing ability. Second, it provides a physical barrier, through capillary coagulation, to keep the pathogens from spreading into the blood. Third, it prepares the tissues for healing. Inflammation is characterized by localized pain, erythema (redness), heat, and edema (swelling).

The first reaction to inflammatory chemokines and cytokines released by activated macrophages is local vasodilation, which causes the erythema and some of the heat. Vasodilation also serves to slow blood flow. The second reaction is the expression of adhesion molecules by the endothelium (inner layer of the arterial wall) to bind to circulating leukocytes. The combination of slowed blood and adhesion molecules allows leukocytes the time to migrate through the arterial wall into the tissues in a process called **extravasation.** The first leukocytes to migrate to the area are neutrophils, followed by monocytes, which differentiate into additional tissue macrophages. Later, eosinophils and basophils will migrate to the site (Janeway, et al., 2004).

The third reaction in the inflammatory process is increased vascular permeability. This allows fluid and plasma proteins to leak into the inflamed tissues, causing edema and pain. The plasma proteins, including complement and clotting factors, aid in the inflammatory process and immune response. For example, once the complement cascade is activated, C5a increases vascular permeability, induces adhesion molecules, and activates phagocytic cells and mast cells. Activated by C5a, the mast cells degranulate, releasing the inflammatory molecules histamine and tumor necrosis factor (TNF)-α.

This triggers the fourth reaction in the inflammatory process, causing blood clots to form, walling off the infected area from the blood supply. This allows the infectious antigens in the edematous fluid, usually inside a dendritic cell, time to travel through the lymph vessels to a lymph node where an adaptive immune response can begin. TNF-α is critical in the isolation of the infection from the rest of the body.

In addition to these local effects of inflammation, systemic effects are also evident. The release of TNF-α, IL-1β, and IL-6 (endogenous pyrogens) raise the body's temperature. Elevated temperature helps the body in a number of ways. It inhibits the growth of most pathogens, which tend to prefer lower temperatures; adaptive responses tend to be more effective; and increased temperature helps to protect the body from the harmful effects of TNF-α.

TNF-α is critical in the innate immune response, because it is so potent in vasodilation, increasing vascular permeability, and inducing clotting. These properties make it ideal for sending leukocytes to the site of infection and then walling it off. Unfortunately, if a pathogen does make it to the systemic circulation, these same qualities make TNF-α release backfire. When sepsis occurs, widespread systemic release of TNF-α occurs by macrophages in the spleen and liver. This systemic release causes systemic vasodilation leading to loss of blood pressure. At the same time, TNF-α also causes increased systemic vascular permeability leading to a loss of oncotic pressure and plasma, aggravating the drop in blood pressure caused by vasodilation. The clotting properties of TNF-α cause disseminated vascular coagulation throughout the systemic circulation, further impeding blood flow, while depleting the body's supply of clotting proteins, putting the patient at risk for hemorrhage. This condition is known as septic shock. It is the spleen's job to minimize systemic TNF-α release by filtering the blood and sequestering any pathogens.

TNF-α, IL-1β, and IL-6 also induce a response known as the acute phase response. The acute phase is characterized by a change in the proteins that the liver produces and secretes into the plasma. The proteins that are produced as a result of TNF-α, IL1β, and IL-6 are called acute-phase proteins. Some of the proteins act similar to antibodies, but rather than binding to specific antigens, they have broad-spectrum binding. Anything that triggers inflammation will trigger all of these proteins, so it is not a targeted response, as are antibodies. The first acute-phase protein is CRP. It has already been mentioned that CRP can activate complement. CRP binds to phosphocholine in bacterial and fungal cell walls and acts as an opsonin in its own right in addition to being able to activate complement. Another acute-phase protein is MB-lectin, which in addition to activating complement acts as an opsonin to monocytes, which unlike fully differentiated tissue macrophages, do not express a mannose receptor. The other two important acute-phase proteins are the lung surfactants SP-A and SP-D. These proteins bind to pathogens in the lung and act as opsonins for phagocytes.

The last systemic effect of inflammatory cytokines is **leukocytosis,** an increase in the numbers of circulating leukocytes, especially neutrophils. Additionally, TNF-α has a role in stimulating dendritic cells to migrate from the tissues in which they reside to lymph nodes. The systemic actions of the endogenous pyrogens (TNF-α, IL-1β, IL-6) are summarized in Table 41-3.

Adaptive Immunity

Adaptive immunity refers to the process whereby lymphocytes are activated against the specific invader that is threatening the body. It is also called specific, because only lymphocytes that are capable of countering the current pathogen are activated. The process of activation, proliferation, and differentiation takes four to seven days to occur. The end result of the process is destruction of the pathogen and the development of lymphocytes that are able to immediately respond to the same invader during subsequent infections.

TABLE 41-3   Systemic Effects of the Endogenous Pyrogens (TNF-α, IL-1β, and IL-6)

TISSUE AFFECTED	ACTION ON TISSUE	NET RESULT
Liver	Acute-phase protein production	Activation of complement
		Opsonization
Bone marrow, endothelium	Leukocytosis	Phagocytosis
Hypothalamus	Increased body temperature	Decreased viral and bacterial replication
Fat, muscle	Protein and energy mobilization to increase body temperature	Increased antigen processing
		Increased specific immune response
Dendritic cells	Migration to lymph nodes	Initiation of adaptive immune response

Adapted from Janeway, C. A., Jr., Travers, P., Walport, M., & Shlomchik, M. J. (2004). Immunobiology, the immune system in health and disease (6th ed.). New York: Garland Science Publishing.

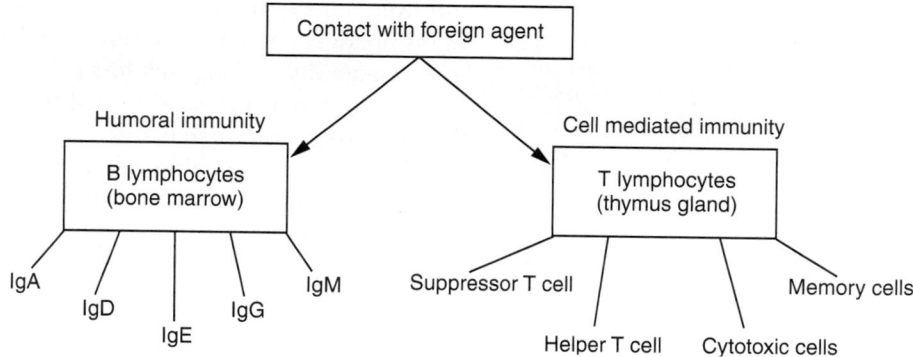

Figure 41-2 Humoral- and cell-mediated immunity in acquired immunity.

There are two basic pathways by which the adaptive immune system functions. These are termed humoral-mediated and cell-mediated immune responses (Figure 41-2). Both forms of immunity involve T cells and antibodies (produced by B cells), but the mechanism of activation is different.

Cell-Mediated Immune Response

Cell-mediated immunity refers to the activation of naïve T lymphocytes to proliferate and mature into armed effector T cells (Cytotoxic, TH1, and TH2 cells). A naïve T cell needs to have antigen presented to it by its appropriate MHC molecule. But this alone does not activate the naïve T cell. The T cell must also simultaneously receive a costimulatory signal. The only cells that are able to produce both classes of MHC and costimulatory molecules are dendritic cells, macrophages, and B cells. These are termed professional APCs and are the only cells that can activate or prime naïve T cells. Priming occurs in lymphoid tissues where naïve T cells are constantly recirculating.

When infection occurs, the innate immune system signals tissue dendritic cells to differentiate into mature dendritic cells that express costimulatory molecules. Cytokines also stimulate the dendritic cells to migrate into the lymph nodes. The vascular changes during inflammation serve to increase lymph drainage, which in turn speeds the dendritic cell's journey to the lymph nodes. There are resident macrophages in all the lymph nodes, and B cells are constantly recirculating through lymph nodes. In response to inflammatory cytokines, both can develop costimulatory molecules and thus be potentially able to prime T cells. Dendritic cells, however, are vastly more potent in priming T cells, and it is believed that in vivo, they are responsible for most if not all T cell activation.

As T cells migrate through lymph nodes, they transiently bind with every APC they meet. If the T cell recognizes its specific antigen in the presence of costimulatory molecules, the bond is strengthened and can last for days while the cell proliferates and differentiates into its active state. Its progeny, so far as space allows will also bind to the APC. The activated T cell will produce IL-2, which stimulates it and its progeny to proliferate and differentiate. Without the IL-2, the activated T cell will not proliferate. If a T cell recognizes its antigen, but costimulatory molecules are not present, the cell will go into an inactive state called anergy. Anergic cells cannot produce IL-2. Many transplant drugs that suppress the immune response to keep the body from rejecting the transplanted organ work by disrupting IL-2 from functioning normally.

After several days of proliferation, the activated T cells differentiate into mature effector cells that are able to produce all the effector molecules required in their roles as helper or cytotoxic T cells. These effector T cells no longer require costimulatory molecules to react to their specific antigen. They lose the adhesion receptors that allow them to recirculate in the lymph tissues and develop receptors that allow them to bind to the endothelium of infected tissue. This change ensures that they will be able to distribute to the infected tissues.

The case with naïve CD4 cells is a bit more complicated. Although, CD4 cells do not need large amounts of costimulation to activate, they must choose whether to become TH1 or TH2 cells. If TH1 cells are preferred, cell-mediated immunity will continue. If TH2 cells are preferred, humoral-mediated immunity will be stimulated. The difference can have profound consequences on the outcome. Bacteria such as *Mycobacterium tuberculosis* and *M. leprae* live inside of macrophages and other phagocytic cells. If TH1 cells are predominantly produced, there will be relatively small amounts of bacteria found, few antibodies, and the patient will most likely live a long time. If TH2 cells are predominantly produced, there will be large amounts of antibody produced, but because the bacteria are sequestered in macrophages, the antibody will not be able to reach them. The bacteria will multiply freely; the disease will be much more severe, and the patient will likely die soon.

Viral and other intracellular parasites cause activation of cytotoxic T cells, which are selective serial killers of other cells expressing the specific antigen. Cytotoxic cells kill host cells that are infected with pathogen. This accomplishes two things. It prevents more pathogen from multiplying inside the infected cell, and it allows the pathogen to be released into the extracellular fluid where it is susceptible to antibodies, macrophages, and other components of the immune system.

TH1 cells' main effector function is to activate macrophages. Most of the time, macrophages need no help from TH1 cells to destroy pathogens, but there are certain pathogens that live inside phagosomes and are able to prevent formation of the phagolysome. In addition to these macrophage parasites, other pathogens are not destroyed by macrophages unless the macrophage is activated. TH1 cells activate such macrophages to induce destruction of the already phagocytosed pathogen and to phagocytose extracellular pathogens. TH1 cells also activate B cells to produce certain classes of antibody.

The study of TH1 cells and macrophages has led to the conclusion that macrophages are naturally in an inactivated state and require two signals for activation. One of these signals is IFN-γ; the other signal can take a variety of forms. In TH1 cells, that second signal is provided by CD40 ligand (a membrane-associated protein). The IFN-γ can be produced by CD8 T cells, the TH1 cell itself, or NK cells. Activated macrophages also use a positive feedback mechanism, secreting IL-12, which induces the selective production of more TH1 cells. These mechanisms make activated macrophages extremely effective effector cells, but in addition to consuming large amounts of energy, their activation is associated with local tissue destruction because the proteases and oxides they release are equally destructive to host tissue.

In addition to the activation of macrophages, TH1 cells also express CD40 ligand and can kill infected macrophages. This may need to occur if the pathogens escape from the phagosome and enter the macrophage's cytoplasm. Both CD8 and TH1 cells can kill macrophages in this case. When the pathogens are released from the dead macrophages they can be killed directly by the TH1 cell or by CD8 T cells and are then susceptible to the antibody.

TH1 cells are also critical in recruitment of phagocytic cells to the site of infection. They produce IL-3 and granulocyte-macrophage colony-stimulating factor (GM-CSF), which stimulate neutrophil and macrophage production. They also produce the TNF-α and TNF-β, which continue the inflammatory process. They produce the chemokine CCL2, which attracts other T cells and macrophages to the site. Thus, although inflammation is considered part of the innate immune response, in its later stages, it is promulgated by the adaptive immune system. When pathogens are able to resist the efforts of the activated macrophages, chronic infection with inflammation occurs. This is often accompanied by a characteristic pattern in which macrophages envelop the area, T cells are present around the perimeter, and it is called a **granuloma.** Giant cells, previously described under the macrophages section, form in the center of the granuloma and attempt to sequester the pathogens. The purpose of a granuloma is to wall off the infection from the rest of the body, and it is sometimes surrounded with collagen tissue to aid in this purpose. The tissue in the center of the granuloma will die secondary to hypoxia and the effects of activated macrophages and is called caseation necrosis. If nothing else happens, eventually the infection will take over the entire body, but will take a fairly long time to do so. Acquired immunodeficiency syndrome (AIDS) patients are unable to form granulomas to sequester local infections and are susceptible to rapid fulminant forms of infections that would usually take years to kill most patients.

TH2 cell–mediated immunity will be discussed, because their primary function is to activate B cells, thus making them part of humoral immunity.

Humoral-Mediated Immune Response

Humoral-mediated immunity is the adaptive immunity pathway that was first discovered in the form of "antitoxins" in the blood against tetanus and diphtheria. Body fluids were once called humors, thus the term humoral immunity. All antibodies are produced by plasma cells that arise from the proliferation and differentiation of activated B lymphocytes. B lymphocytes typically require the help of a CD4 T lymphocyte, hence the designation helper T cells. Both TH1 and TH2 cells can activate B cells, but TH2 cells are more associated with humoral immunity.

The BCR has two functions in the naïve B cells; it serves to activate internal signals when bound to its specific antigen and also serves to bring the antigen inside the cell, where it is degraded and displayed on MHC class II molecules. The B cell does not typically proliferate until activated by a CD4 cell. Some pathogens, however, can directly induce B cell activation without T cell help, but the antibodies secreted will be limited in nature. Thus, just like the naïve T cell, the naïve B cell also requires costimulation. Protein antigens always require a T cell's costimulation, but many microbial constituents, such as bacterial polysaccharides and certain cell wall components, do not require T cell costimulation. This may be an added defense mechanism against autoimmunity, because bacteria do not produce protein, but host cells do. This relaxing of the costimulation requirement ensures quicker responses against bacterial antigens, while still protecting host cells from accidental activation against self-antigens.

Antibodies serve a variety of effector functions as described in B lymphocytes section, but the production of specific antibody classes is directed by T cells. IgM is the antibody class that will naturally be secreted by plasma cells, but makes up less than 10 percent of circulating antibody. CD4 T cells direct the change in antibody class production, a process called isotype switching. Cytokines are the driving factor in isotype switching, which involves recombining the DNA of the B cells, a usually irreversible process. Thus, a B cell that has switched from IgM production to IgA, IgG, or IgE cannot go back to making IgM.

Naïve B cells are continuously recirculating through the lymph nodes, much like naïve T cells. When they encounter their specific antigen, they are arrested in the lymph node at the B cell-T cell border by the development of adhesion molecules. Because they are trapped at the border or the T cell zone, it is likely that the APCs will also activate nearby specific T cells that can activate the B cell. Once activated, B cells travel to the medullary cords to proliferate and differentiate.

Next, B cell activation occurs, which is the formation of the germinal center as the proliferating T and B cells move to a primary follicle. B cells undergo somatic hypermutation with the goal of producing antibodies that have even more affinity for their specific antigen. Affinity maturation is the process whereby the B cells with the highest affinity are selected for survival. This process of affinity maturation also allows for progressively higher affinity antibodies to be produced over time. It will not be long, however, before T cells are activated and migrate to germinal centers to direct the humoral response. Non–T cell activation is important for immunity against encapsulated bacteria, such as *Haemophilus influenza* B (HIB), which can escape detection by phagocytic cells and hence activation of T cells.

The Total Immune Response

For a pathogen to invade the body, it must first pass the epithelial surfaces of the body (e.g., skin, mucous membranes, lungs) that have their own antimicrobial properties. Once past the epithelial surface, the pathogen will soon encounter tissue phagocytes (i.e., tissue macrophages, dendritic cells), which initiate the innate immune response and inflammation. It is unknown how many infections are cleared by the innate immune system alone, because such infections are likely to cause few if any symptoms. Moreover, deficiencies in innate immunity are rare, and when they are present, individuals succumb quickly to infection, unable to mount either an innate or an adaptive immune response.

Inflammation causes tissue dendritic cells to migrate to the lymph nodes, where it will activate the specific T lymphocytes that recognize its presented antigen. CD8 and CD4 T cells proliferate and differentiate into cytotoxic T cells and helper T cells. The helper T cells differentiate into TH1 and TH2 subclasses. The exact stimulus for preference of TH1 or TH2 is currently unknown but involves the nature of the presented antigen and cytokines. Cytotoxic cells destroy parasites and host cells infected with parasites. They also release cytokines that prevent uninfected cells from becoming infected and potentiate inflammation. TH1 cells activate macrophages and B cells. TH2 cells activate B cells to produce antibodies. Both TH1 and TH2 cells produce cytokines that affect inflammation. Effector cells of both the innate and adaptive immune system are guided to the site of infection by chemokines and adhesion molecules on the vascular endothelium. Antibody production takes place in the lymph nodes and are secreted into the blood. Memory T and B cells are produced and are ready to mount an accelerated immune response upon subsequent infection with the same pathogen (Fecci, et. al., 2003).

Immunological Memory

One of the main characteristics of the adaptive immune system is memory, the ability to remember past pathogens and mount an accelerated and heightened immune response against them. Memory responses are called secondary, tertiary, and so on. Memory is the property of the immune response that is exploited by immunization. Most memory cells are in a resting state, but a few are dividing at any given time. It is not known what the signal for memory cell division is. It is known that IL-7 maintains all memory T cells, and IL-15 maintains CD8 memory T cells. When an animal protein is injected, primed T cells are available almost immediately and are at maximum strength within five days. It takes a month before B cell and antibody production is at maximum capacity.

The responses of memory cells are different than primary immune responses. Memory T cells do not require costimulation, but on recognizing their antigen, they immediately begin proliferating. Memory B cells, already having been selected for their antibodies, produce primarily high-affinity IgG, IgA, and IgE as opposed to IgM. Memory B cells do not express IgM on their cell membranes, but whichever of the high-affinity isotopes they will produce, IgG, IgA, or IgE. The increased affinity of their receptor combined with increased ability to bind to T cells allows them to respond much quicker to infection than during the primary response. Memory cells also suppress the activation of naïve B and T cells. This effect is used therapeutically in mothers who are Rh− with Rh+ babies. Rh+ antibodies can be injected into the mother, which will suppress the production of Rh+ immune response.

Mechanisms of Immunization

The effector mechanisms of the immune response will depend on the infectious agent. The primary (initial) immune response is usually sufficient to clear the infection from the body, although some pathogens can evade the immune system and live in the body as long as the host lives. In some of these cases, protective immunity may be induced against the pathogens, preventing them from establishing a persistent presence in the first place. In the case of other pathogens, such as polio, even though the primary immune response clears the infection, the tissue damage is debilitating. Protective immunity involves two components. The first is antibodies, and the second is effector cells, such as primed T cells that can counter the infection. IgA antibodies are present in mucosal secretions and can keep some pathogens from ever entering the body, much less establishing a primary infection. This is the goal of immunization.

Immunization refers to the process first discovered by Edward Jenner 200 years ago. It involves the stimulation of the adaptive immune system so that when a person is exposed to the pathogen, his or her body has already developed immunity against it. In some cases, it is the toxin that a pathogen produces that is the true threat. This is the case with tetanus and diphtheria. In some cases, the toxic receptor-binding functions are located on separate portions of the toxin. In this case, it is possible to cleave the binding site from the toxin. This is called a **toxoid** and produces antibodies against the toxin but cannot harm the person. Toxoid immunizations can also take advantage of linked recognition of antigens. For example, once a baby has been immunized against the tetanus toxoid, it can be linked to HIB polysaccharides (Burns, Carroll, Drayson, Whitham, & Ring, 2003).

In cases where the toxin is extremely toxic or unusual, it may not be practical or possible to develop an immunization for human protection. Snake venom is an example of such a toxin. Snake toxin works too quickly for the adaptive immune system to be effective. Instead of immunizing a human, horses are immunized with the toxin. The horses produce antibodies against the venom, which are then separated and stored. These antivenom antibodies (antivenin) can then be injected into a snake bite victim. When the antibodies are against an organism, such as rabies or malaria, they are not called antivenin, but generically immunoglobulins. Antibodies have a limited half-life and confer immunity only for a limited time. Use of antibodies in this manner is called passive immunization (injection of antibodies to confer immunity rather than stimulating the body to produce its own antibodies).

Immunization against actual pathogens can be accomplished in one of four ways. First, a small amount of the pathogen, enough to cause an immune response but not enough to cause disease, can be inoculated. This depends on the virulence of the pathogen. Cholera needs several thousand cells to be ingested to cause disease, while Shigella can cause disease by ingesting as few as a dozen. The second option is for attenuated pathogen to be used; that is, using pathogen whose potency has somehow been altered so that it produces no or less severe disease. The oral polio vaccine is a live vaccine and occasionally caused polio instead of preventing it. The third option is to use dead pathogens that will produce an immune response despite not being alive. Some pathogens will not cause an immune response when inoculated in dead form. This could possibly be because of clearance of the dead pathogen by the innate immune system before activation of the adaptive immune system is possible. The fourth method is to use a surrogate nonpathogen. This is the technique used by Jenner for his first vaccine. The cowpox virus does not cause disease in humans, but it is close enough antigenically speaking to the smallpox virus to induce immunity to it.

Some immunizations are given as a series, usually about a month apart. This technique takes advantage of the germinal center's hypermutation. It takes about a month for germinal centers to become fully operational. Reimmunizing at this point, causes hypermutation to increase, causing a jump in the affinity of the antibodies produced. This is necessary for some dead pathogen vaccines, because it mimics what would naturally happen if there were dividing pathogens in the body. Without being able to reproduce, dead pathogens or antigens will be cleared relatively quickly, even by low-affinity antibody. Thus, reimmunization serves to boost the affinity as well as the amount of antibody produced against the antigen.

ASSESSMENT

Assessment of the immune system begins with a health history and physical exam, much like any other assessment. However, lab values play a larger part in immune assessment than some other areas. There is a tendency among some health care providers to focus only on the lab values, but the whole patient should be assessed, not only the lab tests. The history should include both past and present indicators and determinants of immune status. Areas to be considered include age; gender; infections and immunizations; allergies; disease states that affect immune status, such as autoimmune disorders, cancer, transplants, and diabetes; nutrition; surgeries; medications, and blood transfusions. The physical exam should include examination of skin and mucous membranes, lymph nodes and tonsils, respiratory, cardiovascular, genitourinary, and neurological systems.

Age and Developmental Considerations

Babies do not have a developed adaptive immune system. They receive much of their initial acquired immunity from their mothers in the form of colostrum during the first few days of breastfeeding and from immunizations. A health history of an infant or young child should include a breastfeeding history. As children develop and grow, their relatively naïve immune systems incline them to having more infections than adults. This is because of the relative lack of memory cells, which means that any infection that overwhelms the innate immune system will cause 4 to 10 days of illness, while the adaptive immune system is activated and mounts a response. As children grow older, the amount of infections should begin to plateau and level off as their repertoire of memory cells grows.

Young adulthood is typically a time of good health, but there are some areas of concern that should always be in the back of the nurse's mind. Many autoimmune diseases, including systemic lupus erythematosus (SLE) and multiple sclerosis (MS), tend to manifest in early adulthood. As the patient passes onto middle age and older, a variety of changes in the immune system make

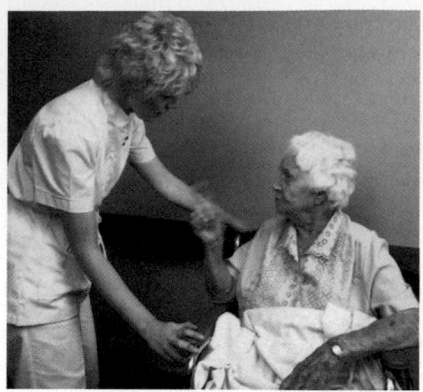

Figure 41-3 The aging process is a variable in this elderly woman's susceptibility to immune-related disease.

the body more susceptible to infections. Production and function of lymphocytes tends to decline. Response to APCs may also decrease, with fewer lymphocytes becoming activated in response to the innate immune system's activation. Autoimmune diseases continue to increase, although the exact etiology is unknown, because of decreased immune function and increased mutation, cancer incidence also increases.

Other physiological changes in combination with environmental factors and comorbidities also make older adults more susceptible to pathogens (Figure 41-3 and Table 41-4). As adults age, glomerular filtration tends to slow, causing a decrease in total urine production. At the same time, the bladder becomes less sensitive, even neurogenic, causing urine retention. In men, prostate hypertrophy can amplify this effect. The combination of less urine production and increased urine retention makes the bladder more susceptible to bacterial colonization, because ascending bacteria are not adequately

TABLE 41-4 Age-Related Changes in Immunological Function

BODY SYSTEM	CHANGES	CONSEQUENCES
Immune system	Impaired function of B and T lymphocytes	Suppressed responses to pathogenic organisms with increased risk for infection
	Failure of lymphocytes to recognize mutant or abnormal cells	Increased incidence of cancers
	Decreased antibody production	Anergy (lack of response to antigens applied to skin such as PPD)
	Failure of immune system to differentiate self from nonself	Increased incidence of autoimmune diseases
	Suppressed phagocytic immune response.	Absence of typical signs and symptoms of infection and inflammation
		Dissemination of organisms usually destroyed or suppressed by phagocytes (reactivation or spread of TB)
GI system	Decreased gastric secretions and motility	Proliferation of intestinal organisms resulting in gastroenteritis and diarrhea
	Decreased phagocytosis by liver Kupffer cells	Increased incidence and severity of hepatitis B, increased incidence of liver abscesses
	Altered nutritional intake with inadequate protein intake	Suppressed immune system
Urinary system	Decreased kidney function, hematuria, proteinuria, enlargement of prostate gland, neurogenic bladder, altered genitourinary tract flora	Urinary stasis and increased incidence of UTIs
Pulmonary system	Impaired ciliary action because of exposure to smoke and environmental toxins, reduced cough reflex	Impaired clearance of pulmonary secretions; increase incidence of respiratory infections
Integumentary system	Thinning of skin, loss of elasticity, loss of adipose tissue	Increased risk of injury, breakdown and infection
Circulatory system	Impaired microcirculation	Stasis and pressure ulcers; reduced healing of wounds
Neurologic function	Decreased sensation and slowing of reflexes	Increased risk of injury (ulcers, abrasions, burns, falls)

Adapted from DeLaune, S., & Ladner, P. (2006). Fundamentals of nursing (3rd ed.). New York: Thomson Delmar Learning; Martins, P., Pratschke, J., Pascher, A., Fritsche, L., Frei, U., Neuhaus, P., et al. (2005). Age and immune response in organ transplantation. Transplantation, 79(2), 127–132.

cleared on urination. Proteinuria and hematuria also increase with age, providing additional growth medium for bacteria in the bladder.

As skin ages, it begins to lose elasticity and subdermal fat, decreasing its strength. Concomitantly, many older adults have nutritional deficits, whether caused by diet or by malabsorption. Deficits in protein, vitamins, and minerals can cause delayed wound healing. The combination of thinner, brittle skin with impaired wound healing makes older adults more susceptible to infections. Peripheral neuropathies and peripheral arterial disease impair sensation and circulation, causing injuries to go unnoticed, and delaying healing further. Decreased mobility can lead to venous stasis ulcers and pressure ulcers.

Smoke and other particulate pollutants, which are omnipresent in industrial society, impair pulmonary function by damaging tissues. This results in increased mucous production and decreased elasticity secondary to scar tissue and can also lead to metaplasm and neoplasm. Concurrently, the cilia elevator and cough reflex decline in older adults, impairing their ability to clear the excess mucus. The mucus provides a growth medium for bacteria and enables inhaled toxins to remain in the lung, where they continue to damage lung tissue and may lead to cancer, fibrotic lung diseases, or emphysema.

Decreased gastric secretions and decreased gastric motility allow ingested and normal intestinal flora to proliferate, causing infections and opportunistic infections. Decreased motility also keeps pathogens in contact with the digestive mucosa longer, giving them more opportunity to penetrate the mucosa. Ulcers and colon polyps may cause gaps in healthy epithelial tissue, serving as an avenue for pathogen penetration.

Immunizations and Infections

Immunization is the most efficient way to prevent infectious diseases, but it is not without disadvantages. Immunization usually confers immunity only for a limited period of time. With newer immunizations, such as hepatitis B and varicella, the period of immunity is not well established. Vaccinations with live pathogens may potentially cause the disease they are meant to prevent. For example, the oral polio vaccine is no longer administered in the United States, because the virus is shed in the feces and a child in the house may contract polio. Moreover, many immunizations are produced using egg as a growth medium, and people with allergy to eggs may not tolerate many immunizations. Many immunizations need multiple inoculations to be effective, meaning the patient or the patient's parents must be responsible enough to return for the full immunization series. The childhood immunizations against tetanus, diphtheria, and pertussis (DPT) as well as the immunizations against polio and HIB require three to four inoculations. Additionally, tetanus and diphtheria require booster inoculations every 5 years (note: tetanus is sometimes given on a 10-year schedule; but if any puncture or impaling wounds are experienced, a booster should be given if the last tetanus immunization was more than 5 years ago).

The type and date of immunization should be documented as well as any booster immunizations. The time from immunization is important, as discussed previously. Recommended immunization schedules for childhood and adolescent immunizations can be obtained from the U. S. Centers for Disease Control and Prevention (CDC) either downloaded from their Web site (www.cdc.gov) or ordered by mail.

It is important to assess whether a patient has had an illness before administering an immunization. A patient who has had mumps or rubella does not need to be immunized against them. However, a patient who had unilateral mumps would benefit from immunization, as it may recur in the other salivary gland. Known exposures to diseases for which the patient has been immunized are important. Tuberculosis exsposure history and risk level assessment are important. People living in institutions, such as prisoners and hospital patients, are especially at risk. The last purified-protein derivative (PPD) tuberculosis test should be documented. A special case is the bacille Calmette-Guérin (BCG) vaccine against tuberculosis. This immunization was frequently given in third world countries, but its efficacy and duration are limited. However, patients who have received the BCG immunization will often show false-positives on PPD tuberculosis skin tests. Additionally, immunosuppression or immunodeficiency may cause PPDs to show false-negatives. In patients with history of BCG or with depressed immune systems, documentation of a chest X-ray (CXR), in addition to or lieu of the PPD, may be necessary.

Documenting past illness and infections is also important, especially for blood-borne pathogens, sexually transmitted diseases (STDs), and any treatments the patient may have undergone. The major blood-borne pathogens are hepatitis A, B, C, D, and E and HIV. Some blood-borne pathogens, particularly, hepatitis B and HIV, are also STDs and are often transmitted along with other STDs, such as HSV, humanpapilloma virus (HPV), syphilis, gonorrhea, and chlamydia. Many STDs also cause lesions that can serve as an entry point for other pathogens.

Patterns of illness may reveal either immune system dysfunction or an anatomic abnormality that predisposes the patient to a certain kind of infection. For example, patients with cystic fibrosis will have recurrent pulmonary infections as a result of inadequate mucous clearance, not because of immunosuppression. A thorough history will help to distinguish between causes of infections. History about persistent or recurrent infections and sores and lesions should be obtained.

Allergies

Ask the patient about any allergies that he or she may have to medications, food, or environmental factors. For all three causes of allergies, the source of the allergy, type and severity of reaction, the duration, treatment, resolution, and recurrence should be documented. If there have been recurrences, it should be noted whether the severity is increasing or decreasing. For severe allergies, or allergies that are increasing in severity, the nurse should inquire whether the patient has an emergency epinephrine injection system. Also document whether the patient has a Medicalert bracelet or necklace. The allergies should be documented on the history and placed on the front of the chart.

Allergies are inappropriate hypersensitivity immune reactions, and it is important to distinguish between true allergic reactions and other kinds of adverse drug reactions or unpleasant side effects. Amoxicillin can cause an amoxicillin rash in small children, which is harmless, transient, and does not indicate an allergy. This kind of rash should not be documented as an allergy to amoxicillin or penicillin. Nor should gastrointestinal (GI) bleeding secondary to nonsteroidal anti-inflammatory drug (NSAID) medications be documented as an allergy. True, it may be life-threatening, and is most likely a contraindication to future NSAID use, but it is not an allergy. Likewise, GI distress with erythromycin ethylstearate is not an allergy. Many patients will say they have allergies to medications simply because they do not like the side effects of the medication. However, there is a vast difference between having an allergy to a medication and simply, not tolerating the medication well. Being able to distinguish between the two is important in taking an allergic history. This is not to say that nonallergic adverse drug reactions are not significant, but mislabeling them as allergies is a significant error.

Food allergies are important to document, especially if the patient will be staying in a hospital, long-term care facility, or other overnight health care institution. Environmental allergies, such as to mold, dust, cosmetics, metals, or latex, are also important. If a patient has a latex allergy, care must be taken to ensure that all latex instruments, such as stethoscopes, are appropriately covered and that nonlatex gloves, dressings, and catheters are used. Allergies to adhesives can sometimes be worked around by using paper tape or skin

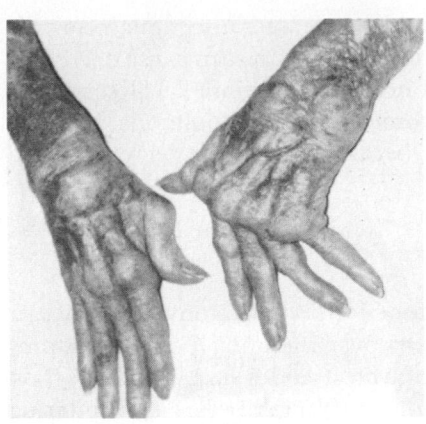

Figure 41-4 RA, an autoimmune disorder, may cause severe ulnar deformity.

prep, but sometimes reactions will still occur. In these cases, it should be considered as to how essential the adhesive is in the patient's treatment, how long the adhesive will be applied, and whether any antihistamines or other immunoactive medications will be administered.

The patient should also be asked about any history of atopic diseases, such as urticaria (hives), asthma, and atopic dermatitis. These diseases often accompany one another and are an indication of a hyperactive immune system. Patients with atopy are more likely to have other allergic problems.

Autoimmune Disorders

Ask the patient about any autoimmune diseases such as SLE, rheumatoid arthritis (RA), MS, and psoriasis (Figure 41-4). The onset, severity, duration, and treatments should be assessed. If the patient does not have any autoimmune disorders, the patient should be asked about family history. Family history of autoimmune disease strongly suggests a genetic predisposition to these kinds of disorders. Although autoimmune diseases are rare individually, collectively, they account for 5 percent of the U.S. population.

Generally speaking, autoimmune diseases affect more women than men. This difference is currently attributed to differences in sex hormones between men and women. Estrogen has shown an up-regulatory effect on immune function, while androgens have shown a suppressive effect on immune function. Estrogen increases the effects of T lymphocytes and decreases suppressors, while androgens preserve IL-2 and suppressor function. Estrogen also has an affect on the B-cell population expressing CD5 antigen that is associated with autoimmune disease.

Cancer

Personal and family history of cancer is obtained, including details of the date of diagnosis, type of cancer, method of diagnosis, and any treatments. Depending on the age, gender, and family history it may be appropriate to inquire about cancer screening, such as visual surveillance for skin cancer, testicular self-exam, last prostate exam, breast self-exam, last Pap smear, and colon cancer screening, such as hemoccult blood, sigmoidoscopy, barium enema, and colonoscopy. The patient should also be asked about any changes in their health. The acrostic caution is often used as a mnemonic:

C   change in bowel or bladder habits.

A   area (or sore) that does not heal.

U   unusual bleeding or discharge.

T   thickening or a lump in the breast, testicles, or elsewhere.

I   indigestion or difficulty swallowing.

O   obvious change in a wart or a mole.

N   nagging cough or hoarseness.

Chronic Illnesses

Assessment of chronic illnesses may also provide information about immune status. Many chronic diseases generate or depend on chronic states of inflammation for their progression. Atherosclerotic disease needs inflammation to progress, while osteoarthritis generates chronic local inflammation. Other diseases may depress the immune system. Chronic renal disease is associated with lower levels of erythropoietin and fewer numbers of all blood cells, including leukocytes. Additionally, remaining leukocytes may have altered function because of changes in blood pH and build up of uremic waste toxins.

Red Flag

Alcohol Consumption and Corticosteroids

If a patient has an autoimmune disorder, documenting alcohol consumption is important. High doses of corticosteroids and autoimmune diseases are associated with a condition called avascular necrosis (also called osteonecrosis ischemic necrosis) in which the marrow and eventually the trabecular bone die, leaving the bone weak and brittle. Corticosteroid use in patients who drink large amounts of alcohol is associated with an increased risk of avascular necrosis over corticosteroids alone. Patients who complain of bone pain may need to be referred for diagnostic magnetic resonance imaging (MRI) (Assouline-Dayan, Chang, Greenspan, Shoenfeld, & Gershwin, 2002).

Hyperglycemia in diabetes is associated with increased infections primarily because of neuropathy and arterial insufficiency, which in turn cause decreased awareness of injury and decreased wound healing. Additionally, glycosylation of leukocytes impairs their functions. Chronic obstructive pulmonary disease (COPD) can cause recurrent infections because increased secretions and decreased cilia elevator activity.

Surgery

Surgery can have an impact on immune function. Splenectomy in particular results in immunosuppression and leads to overwhelming postsplenectomy infections (see Spleen section). Removal of lymph nodes has a local effect on immune function, allowing pathogens to colonize longer before encountering the adaptive immune system. Removal of the thymus affects the maturation and function of T lymphocytes. Organ transplantation can affect immune function in several ways. Most transplanted organs will be attacked as nonself by the adaptive immune system. Immunosuppressive drugs are usually indicated throughout the rest of the patient's life, putting the patient at risk for both acquired infections and opportunistic infections. A transplanted kidney may actually aid immune function by increasing erythropoiesis, but this effect will most likely be negated by immunosuppressive therapy. Heart transplant patients receive a double hit to the immune system, because the thymus is usually removed along with the dysfunctional heart, and they receive immunosuppressive therapy. A special case is blood transfusion and use of other blood products, such as platelets and fresh frozen plasma. Transfused blood usually has antigens foreign to the patient's blood and may put them at risk for altered immune function. Moreover, there is a small chance that the patient may have been exposed to a blood-borne pathogen, such as HIV or hepatitis C. It is important to remember that although the blood supply is tested well for these common pathogens, lab errors do occur, and there may be new developing diseases that we have not yet identified (El-Alfy & El-Sayed, 2004).

Stress and Social Support

Stress, both real and perceived, can have a negative effect on immune function (Isowa, Ohira, & Murashima, 2004). Meanwhile, exercise, although stressful to the body, reduces perceived stress and in moderation can improve immune function (Glass, et al., 2004). It is currently unknown whether real or perceived stress has more influence on immune function, as studies often show conflicting results. It is currently believed that the brain influences the immune system via the limbic hypothalamus-pituitary-adrenal (HPA) cortex axis (Reiche, Nunes, & Morimoto, 2004). The limbic system is responsible for somatic effects of emotions. It is also believed that the immune system influences the HPA axis, a concept called bidirectional communication. This area is undergoing intense research at the moment in everything from exercise to biofeedback and prayer to meditation.

Patients should be asked about perceived stress in their lives as well as potentially stressful life events. Table 41-5 shows selected common life events and the average rank of how much stress they cause according the social readjustment rating scale (SRRS) (Holmes & Rahe, 1967). The patient is asked if any of the listed life events have occurred in the past 12 months. The associated scores are tabulated, and the sum is indicative of how much stress the patient is experiencing based on life events. Scores under 149 are considered low; scores of 150 to 200 are mild; scores of 201 to 299 are moderate; and scores above 300 are high. It is important to note that the SRRS was not developed simply as an indicator of stress but as an indicator of disease risk. It is important to keep in mind that the life events listed in the table are averages, and the actual stress caused by any one event may be greater or less than the

TABLE 41-5 Selected Stressful Life Events and Their Corresponding Life Change Units (LCU) from the Social Readjustment Rating Scale (SRRS)

LIFE EVENT	LCU
Death of spouse	100
Divorce	73
Marriage	63
Being fired from work	47
Reconciliation with spouse	45
Retirement	45
Outstanding personal achievement	28
Starting or ending school	26
Change in sleeping habits	16
Vacation	13

Adapted from Scully, J. A. (2000). Life event checklists: Revisiting the social readjustment rating scale after 30 years. Educational and Psychological Measurement, 60(6), 864–876.

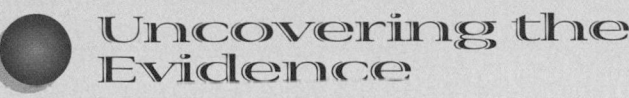

Uncovering the Evidence

Stress and Aging

Discussion: This study's purpose was to explore the effects of telomeres, which shorten as a person ages and then contribute to age-related dysfunction. The findings from this research study were that telomeres of monocytes in women who report the highest levels of stress showed an average of 10 years of aging when compared to women who reported low levels of stress. The important aspect to this study is that the cells assayed were immune cells, indicating the persons with higher levels of stress are more likely to experience age-related immune dysfunction. It is important to note that telomere length was affected by perceived stress regardless of actual stressful events.

Implications for Practice: The results of this study prompt the nurse to always remember to assess the stress levels of patients. And, to identify the amount of stress that patients are experiencing. In addition, this is extremely important for patients who are experiencing immunological disorders.

Source: Epel, E. S., Blackburn, E. H., Lin, J., Dhabhar, F. S., Adler, N. E., Morrow, J. D., et al. (2004). Accelerated telomere shortening in response to life stress. Proceedings of the National Academy of Science USA, 101*(49), 17312–17315.*

average. The nurse should also note that positive life events, such as a vacation, may be as stressful as negative life events.

Another area related to stress is social interaction. There are several studies that show that social isolation is associated with decreased immune functioning (Hawkley & Cacioppo, 2003). It is important to note that it is perceived social isolation (loneliness) that is associated with morbidity and mortality. Patients should be asked whether they feel lonely, isolated, or disconnected. In addition to stress and loneliness, sleep, energy level, and exercise should be assessed. The more normal a patient feels in daily life, the more likely he or she is to have a normally functioning immune system.

Pharmacology

A comprehensive list of medications should be obtained. The nurse should ask how long the patient has taken each medication and whether he or she is taking more or less than the prescribed dose. Many common medications, including NSAIDS, corticosteroids, cytotoxic agents, and anesthetics, can cause immune suppression in a variety of ways. Patients should also be asked if they have had an adverse event, such as leukopenia, in response to any medications.

In addition to medications, the nurse should also inquire about any herbal medications and over-the-counter (OTC) medications the patient is using. Tobacco, alcohol, and recreational drugs should be documented, as they can all have immune effects.

Lifestyle and Environmental Factors

The nurse should ask about any behaviors that may put the patient at risk for infections or altered immune function. These may include sexual behavior, travel history, and nutritional status. Occupational hazards may include inhaled toxins, such as coal dust or chemicals in factories. Other hazards may include being near radioactive substances or X-rays. Living near farms, factories, shipyards, and mines can put the patient at risk for decreased immune function. Exposure to sun and use of sunscreen is important in assessing risk for skin cancer.

Physical Examination

Vital signs should include age, temperature, blood pressure, and respirations. Temperature elevations may be suppressed in elderly patients and patients with immunodeficiency. The patient should be assessed for chills and perspiration. Examination of the skin and mucous membranes should include inspection for lesions, dermatitis, urticaria (hives), erythema, edema, discharge, and subcutaneous bleeding. The tonsils should be inspected, and the lymph nodes palpated in the face and neck, axilla, and groin. Nodes should be assessed for size, shape, consistency, and tenderness. The patient's respiratory cardiovascular, GI, genitourinary, and neural status should be evaluated, particularly paying attention to signs indicative of infection or signs that indicate increase risk of immune dysfunction. Hygiene and functional limitations should also be noted. Box 41-1 shows common physical signs associated with impaired immune function.

BOX 41-1

COMMON PHYSICAL SIGNS ASSOCIATED WITH IMPAIRED IMMUNE FUNCTION

Vital Signs

Elevated temperature
Changes in blood pressure
Changes in pulse
Changes in respiratory rate
Changes in weight

Constitutional

Chills
Night sweats

Respiratory System

Rhinitis
Cough (dry or productive)
Adventitious lung sounds (wheezing, crackles, rhonchi)
Bronchospasm

Cardiovascular System

Dysrhythmia
Vasculitis
Decreased peripheral pulses
Anemia

GI System

Hepatomegaly
Cirrhosis
Splenomegaly
Colitis
Vomiting
Diarrhea

Genitourinary System

Frequency and burning on urination
Hematuria
Proteinuria
Discharge

Skin

Dermatitis
Discharge
Lesions
Rashes
Hematoma or purpura
Edema
Urticaria (hives)
Inflammation

Neurosensory System

Cognitive dysfunction
Hearing loss
Visual loss or disturbance
Headaches
Ataxia
Tremor
Tetany
Decreased peripheral sensation

Adapted from Estes, M. (2006). Health assessment and physical examination (3rd ed.). New York: Thomson Delmar Learning.

Integumentary System

Skin should be examined for color, turgor, moisture, and temperature. Skin changes can often be indicators of immune dysfunction. Psoriasis manifests as scaly plaques. Patients with Sjögren's disease tend to have scaly skin and excessive perspiration. Patients with scleroderma have thick smooth skin. Patients with Grave's disease may have pretibial myxedema (thickening of the shin skin), fine, brittle hair, increased perspiration, and exophthalmus (bulging eyes). Elevated skin temperature may indicate inflammation, and cool skin temperature may indicate arterial insufficiency.

Skin lesions may also indicate immune status. Lesions and rashes should be characterized regarding their shape, configuration, and distribution. Any exudates or vesicles should also be noted. Rashes and lesions may indicate allergic disorders, such as urticaria (hives) or atopic dermatitis. Local maculopapular rashes with or without vesiculation are more indicative of a contact dermatitis or localized infection. Full body rashes are usually indicative of a systemic reaction. Dermographism is common in patients with chronic urticaria; dermographism means skin drawing and refers to an inflammatory response after lightly drawing on a patient's skin with a finger or other blunt instrument (note: dermographism should not be confused with the scratch test; see diagnostic tests). Moles should be carefully screened using the ABCD approach (asymmetry, border, color, and diameter). Suspicious lesions should be referred for biopsy. Kaposi's sarcoma is a usually rare skin cancer that occurs naturally but is fairly common in patients with HIV. Kaposi's sarcoma manifests as maculopapular lesions that range in color from pink to bluish-purple. Various infectious diseases cause rashes and lesions, including measles, herpes-zoster (chickenpox and shingles), HSV, and syphilis. Skin eruptions associated with viral infections are called viral exanthems. SLE is often associated with a malar rash, which is a red rash in the shape of a butterfly across the cheeks and nose. Patients with RA may have nodules and bony spurs in their finger joints. Their hands may become deformed from the disease. Many autoimmune diseases may cause alopecia. Alopecia is also associated with chemotherapy and radiation therapy.

Eyes, Ears, Nose, and Throat

Patients with allergies often have inflamed nasal turbinates and may have tender sinuses. They also tend to exhibit serous otitis media, visible as small air bubbles behind the tympanic membrane. Serous otitis media is caused by Eustachian tube inflammation, which does not allow mucosal secretions to drain. Patients may complain of headache, earache, vertigo, or lightheadedness associated with head movements. They may report exacerbation of any or all these symptoms when lowering the head such as when bending over.

The eyes may have dark circles underneath them, sometimes called allergic shiners, because of venous stasis. Patients with immune disorders or chronic allergies may have periorbital edema secondary to increased vascular permeability. The conjunctiva may be inflamed and can mimic infectious conjunctivitis.

The mouth may be dry from mouth-breathing because of chronic nasal obstruction. The throat may be inflamed from postnasal drip, and the tonsils may be enlarged. Patients with enlarged tonsils should be asked if that is a usual finding for them or a new finding. Exudates and lesions should be noted. Patients with immunosuppression may have thrush, an opportunistic candida infection, which appears as white patches throughout the mouth, throat, and tongue.

Lymph Nodes

Assessment of the lymph nodes includes inspection and palpation. The nodes of the head and neck and axillary and femoral nodes should be examined.

The location, size, shape, consistency, tenderness, and mobility should be noted. Having a few nontender, mobile, palpable nodes is usually a normal finding. Thinner patients tend to have more palpable nodes. Palpable supra-clavicular nodes should always be considered an abnormal finding and should be referred for further evaluation.

Respiratory System

Patients with allergies may also have respiratory symptoms. Recent studies have shown a link between allergic rhinitis in children and asthma. Patients with suppressed immune systems are at risk for pneumonia. Careful examination of the respiratory system is indicated. The skin and nails should be inspected for signs of cyanosis or clubbing. The chest should be observed for shape, breathing pattern, respiratory effort, and thoracic expansion. The lungs should be auscultated with attention paid to the breath sounds. Patients with allergies and acute bronchitis may wheeze. The nature of cough should be noted, and any sputum produced examined. Patients with comorbid conditions such as cancer or COPD should be evaluated in relation to their baseline.

Cardiovascular System

Much of the cardiovascular system can be evaluated while examining the skin. The temperature of extremities and the presence of hair on extremities give clues to peripheral arterial circulation. The nature of the pulses should be evaluated at least in the arms and feet. Weak or thready pulse may be associated with infections. Blood pressure may rise or fall in conjunction with infection. Absent foot pulses may also be a sign of arterial insufficiency. The heart sounds should be carefully noted. Murmurs may signify valve damage that makes the valves more susceptible to certain infections.

Neurological System

Many autoimmune diseases attack nervous tissue causing demyelination or other nerve damage. Nerves contain the CD4 antigen that HIV targets, making neurological dysfunction common in HIV and AIDS patients. Other diseases that decrease sensation such as Hansen's disease (leprosy) and diabetes mellitus increase the incidence of infections simply because the patient is not aware of any injury. Mental status, reflexes, sensation, deep tendon reflexes, and balance should be tested. Other signs of neurological dysfunction, such as tremor should also be noted.

DIAGNOSTIC TESTS

Most diagnostic tests for the immune system are blood tests. These hematological tests are identified and described in the section that follows. Other tests involve either biopsy of tissue or nuclear medicine tests.

Complete Blood Count with Differential

The most common laboratory test is the complete blood count (CBC) with differential. A normal CBC includes a gross leukocyte count, often abbreviated as WBCs (white blood cells). The differential breaks the WBCs into categories that usually include neutrophils, basophils, eosinophils, monocytes, and lymphocytes. Dendritic cells are not part of the CBC with differential (Box 41-2), and the differential does not distinguish between subtypes of lymphocytes.

To date, there has been no test to determine the status of dendritic cells. However, Vuckovic, et al. (2004) discovered a simple assay that allows for blood dendritic cell counts. In addition to total dendritic cells, it also allows for precise counting of five dendritic cell subsets. The researchers were able to use the new assay method to show that dendritic cells decrease in healthy individ-

---

BOX 41-2

CBC WITH DIFFERENTIAL

Differential values are usually reported as percentages of the total WBC count. Neutrophils are usually divided into two classes. Mature neutrophils are usually designated as segs (segmented cells). Immature neutrophils are designated bands, because their nuclei appear to have bands across them. Some labs will also report a value abbreviated as ANC (absolute neutrophil count). If the ANC is absent, it may be calculated by the nurse by adding the percentages of segs and bands and multiplying the sum by the WBC total. This number will give the total number of neutrophils in a cubic millimeter of blood. If the number is less than 1,000, the patient is considered to have immunosuppression. If the number is less than 500, the patient is considered to have severe immunosuppression. In addition to the segs and bands, occasionally, a patient may have a third category called blasts. Blasts are immature cells and should never be in circulation under normal circumstances. The most common reasons for blasts to appear are leukemia, rheumatic disease, or severe bone injury.

---

uals with age. They were also able to observe changes in various cell subsets with different cancers. It will take a few years for normal values to become established, but it is most likely that within the next 5 years dendritic cell testing will become common in immunological testing. In the next 10 to 15 years, it may become as routine as the CBC with differential.

Interpretation of CBC with differential can be straightforward or difficult. It is important that the nurse assess the whole patient and not simply the lab values. Nurses must always check the laboratory's normal ranges when interpreting a patient's lab tests. In general, neutrophil counts will increase during bacterial infections as the bone marrow releases some of its stores. If the percentage of segs increases more than the percentage of bands, it is called a shift to the right. If the bands increase more than segs, it is called a shift to the left and is usually indicative of either a more severe infection or an infection that has been going on longer.

Basophils typically do not increase or decrease in number in response to infections. However, they do increase in response to some inflammation and inflammatory diseases, such as Crohn's disease. They also increase in response to disorders involving the common myeloid precursor, such as polycythemia vera, myelofibrosis, and chronic myeloid leukemia. Hypothyroidism can also cause increases in basophils, and hyperthyroidism can cause decreases in basophils. Eosinophils typically increase during parasitic infections and during allergic reactions. Decreased eosinophils are usually not a cause for concern.

Mononuclear cells are relatively low in number, because most of them simply use the blood as a transport system before migrating to the tissues to differentiate into macrophages. As one of the first inflammatory responders, monocytes may increase or decrease in response to various conditions depending on the severity of the reaction, the duration of reaction, and the number of monocytes in the marrow reservoir.

Lymphocytes are the second most populous leukocyte in the blood. Increased lymphocytes may occur as an increase of absolute numbers lymphocytes or simply as a percentage of total leukocytes. There are a variety of disorders (Box 41-3) and medications that cause neutropenia. The most common medications that cause neutropenia are chemotherapeutic, thyroid inhibitors, and trimethoprim-sulfamethoxazole (Septra, Bactrim). In addition, many other medications cause neutropenia, such as antibiotics (e.g., penicillins,

ETIOLOGY FOR VARIOUS INFECTIONS THAT CAUSE NEUTROPENIA

Severe Neutropenia

Bacterial sepsis (especially gram-negative bacteria)
Infectious mononucleosis
Hepatitis B virus
HIV

Viral Infections

Infectious mononucleosis
Hepatitis B virus
HIV
Measles
Mumps
Rubella
Roseola
Malaria
Leishmaniasis
Cytomegalovirus
Colorado tick fever
Influenza
Dengue fever
Viral hepatitis
HSV
Parvovirus
Respiratory syncytial virus
Small pox
Varicella
Yellow fever

Bacterial Infections

Tuberculosis
Typhoid fever
Brucellosis
Tularemia
Rocky Mountain spotted fever

Fungal Infections

Histoplasmosis

Adapted from Janeway, C. A., Jr., Travers, P., Walport, M., & Shlomchik, M. J. (2004). Immunobiology, the immune system in health and disease (6th ed.). New York: Garland Science Publishing.

cephalosporins, and sulfonamides), cardiovascular medications (e.g., antiarrhythmics, antihypertensives), analgesics (e.g., NSAIDs, aspirin), antithyroids, antihistamines, and heavy metals (Broyles, Reiss, & Evans, 2007).

Radiological Tests

Radiological tests can also provide information about immune status. CXRs are often used to determine tuberculosis status and confirm pneumonia. MRIs, computed tomography (CT), and numerous nuclear medicine tests are used to screen for neoplasm.

Erythrocyte Sedimentation Rate

Blood is made up of RBCs and plasma. When still, the RBCs will settle to the bottom, and the plasma will float to the top. The erythrocyte sedimentation rate (ESR), sometimes called sed. rate, is simply a measure of how quickly the settling occurs. It is expressed in milliliters/hour. The normal ESR values change with age and gender and pregnancy. Elevated ESR is caused by acute inflammation phase reactants binding to red blood cells. ESR is used as a marker of tissue inflammation and is highly sensitive, but nonspecific (Daniels, 2003).

C-Reactive Protein

CRP is an acute-phase protein that is produced by the liver. It is one of the three binding mechanisms for C1q in the classical pathway for complement activation. It can be used to determine whether a disease is inflammatory or not. Examples include distinguishing type 1 from type 2 diabetes and distinguishing osteoarthritis from RA. CRP is nonspecific and is often ordered in conjunction with ESR. In recent years, subtypes of CRP have been discovered. Highly sensitive CRP (hsCRP) has been implicated as a marker for MI. The caveat is that hsCRP can help determine short-term risk for MI, but not long-term risk. In other words hsCRP is an indicator of atherosclerotic plaque rupture, but a link with atherosclerotic plaque formation has not been established.

Total Complement (CH50)

CH50 is a marker for the function of the entire complement cascade. It measures the ability of the sample to lyse IgG-coated RBCs. False readings can be obtained by delaying the test after obtaining the sample, so care must be taken to ensure that the sample is tested as soon as possible. Low complement levels indicate depletion or lack of production by the liver. The most common causes of depletion are the rheumatic diseases (e.g., SLE, vasculitis), septic shock, pancreatitis, severe burns. Lack of production may be caused by liver failure or severe malnutrition. Total complement is most useful in tracking the course of rheumatic diseases where a value of 20 percent below baseline indicates an exacerbation.

Complement C3

Because C3 convertase is the common link between all three complement activation pathways, it can serve as a marker for complement activation. The protein is measured by immunochemical assay. The interpretation is similar to total complement.

Complement C4

The C4 protein is involved only in the classical (intrinsic) pathway and can be used as an indicator of classical pathway complement activation. The protein is measured by immunochemical assay. The interpretation is similar to total complement.

Phagocytic Cell Function Tests

Despite the name, only the function of neutrophils and macrophages are tested, as dendritic cells are not found in high enough concentrations. The most basic phagocytic cell function test does not involve function at all, but is simply the sum of neutrophils and monocytes from the CBC with differential. The function assay evaluates the ability of phagocytic cells to recognize, ingest, degranulate (as appropriate), and otherwise destroy various pathogens.

Protein Electrophoresis

Electrophoresis takes two forms, but both involve putting a protein sample onto a gel and passing electrical current through the gel. The proteins will migrate to the other side of the gel. The distance various proteins travel is dependent on their size and electrical affinity. Some gels are uniform in their density, and protein distance will depend only on electrical affinity of the protein. Other gels are graded from less dense to more dense. These gradient gels will trap larger proteins, so that smaller proteins travel farther. Electrophoresis allows a sample of several kinds of proteins, such as serum, to be separated so that each kind of protein can be studied individually. Electrophoresis is used most commonly in immunological management of patients to evaluate serum proteins, such as albumin and globulins (alpha-, beta-, and gamma-globulins). They can also be used to screen for certain tumor proteins that are not secreted by normally functioning cells.

Immunoglobulin Electrophoresis

Immunoglobulin electrophoresis uses the same process as above, but in this case, the immunoglobulins are being separated and measured individually. Measuring the various immunoglobulins can aid in the diagnosis and management of several immunological and inflammatory disorders (Table 41-6).

Radioallergosorbent Test

IgE is usually present in serum in such small quantities that electrophoresis cannot accurately measure it. Radioallergosorbent test (RAST) is used to measure serum IgE. RAST is most often used in diagnosing allergies in combination with skin tests.

Antibody Screening Tests

Numerous tests are available that test for specific antibodies. Each antibody test is ordered individually and may test for antibodies against various bacteria, viruses, fungi, parasites, or cancers. Presence of the antibodies does not necessarily indicate that a patient has that particular disease.

Autoantibody Tests

Autoantibodies are antibodies that are produced against self and are always an abnormal finding. Autoantibodies attack and damage normal tissue and are responsible for some of the pathology of autoimmune diseases. One of the most common autoantibodies tested for are antinuclear antibodies (ANA), which attack the nuclei of cells. ANA is most commonly associated with SLE and other autoimmune disorders, but it can also be associated with various medications (Box 41-4). Another common autoantibody is rheumatoid factor (RF), which is commonly found in patients with rheumatoid diseases such as SLE and RA. Although usually an abnormal finding, both ANA and RF can be found in healthy older adults.

TABLE 41-6 **Diseases Commonly Associated with Abnormal Immunoglobulin Levels**

IMMUNOGLOBULIN	NORMAL RANGE	INCREASED LEVEL	DECREASED LEVEL
IgA	50–350 mg/dL	Lymphoproliferative disorders (e.g., multiple myeloma)	IgA
			Hypogammaglobulinemia
		Berger's disease (IgA nephropathy)	Protein losing enteropathy
		Chronic infection	Hereditary ataxia and telangiectasia
		Autoimmune disorders	Nephrotic syndrome
		SLE	
		Rheumatoid arthritis	
		Liver disease (e.g., portal cirrhosis)	
		Henoch Schonlein Purpura	
IgE	less than 25 g/dL	Allergic disorders	Congenital
		Asthma	Hypogammaglobulinemia
		Allergic rhinitis or hay fever	Acquired hypogammaglobulinemia
		Inhalant allergy	Sex-linked hypogammaglobulinemia
		Atopic rhinitis or sinusitis	Ataxia-telangiectasia
		Atopic dermatitis	IgE deficiency
		Urticaria	
		Bronchopulmonary *Aspergillus*	
		Hypersensitivity pneumonitis	
		Drug allergy	
		Food allergy	
		Parasitic infection	
		Ascariasis	
		Visceral larva	
		Migrans	
		Toxocara	
		Capillariasis	
		Echinococcosis	
		Hookworm (Necator)	
		Amebiasis	
		Immunological disorders	
		Hyper-IgE, recurrent pyoderma (Job-Buckley syndrome)	
		Thymic dysplasia or deficiency	
		Wiskott-Aldrich syndrome	
		Pemphigoid	
		Periarteritis nodosa	
		Hypereosinophilic syndrome	
		Neoplasm (i.e., IgE myeloma)	

Continued

TABLE 41-6 Diseases Commonly Associated with Abnormal Immunoglobulin Levels—cont'd

IMMUNOGLOBULIN	NORMAL RANGE	INCREASED LEVEL	DECREASED LEVEL
IgG	800–1,500 mg/dL	Chronic granulomatous infection	Hypo-IgG
		Inflammation	Protein-losing enteropathy
		Multiple myeloma	Nephrotic syndrome
		Liver disease	
		Infections	
		Autoimmune disease	
IgM	45–150 mg/dL	Liver disease	Hypo-IgM
		Primary biliary	Protein-losing enteropathy
		Cirrhosis	
		Early hepatitis	
		Waldenstrom's macroglobulinemia	
		Infection	
		Brucellosis	
		Malaria	
		Trypanosomiasis	
		Toxoplasmosis	

Adapted from Boehm, M., Olive, M., True, A. L., Crook, M. F., San, H., Qu, X., et al. (2004). Bone marrow-derived immune cells regulate vascular disease through a p27Kip1-dependent mechanism. Journal of Clinical Investigation, 114(3), 419-426; Janeway, C. A., Jr., Travers, P., Walport, M., & Shlomchik, M. J. (2004). Immunobiology, the immune system in health and disease (6th ed.). New York: Garland Science Publishing.

Antigen Tests

Antigen tests look for the presence of a specific antigen in the body. Commonly, antigen tests are used to determine the presence of a pathogen. Hepatitis B surface antigen (HBsAg) and Hepatitis B core antigen (HBcAg) tests can be used to determine whether a patient with hepatitis B antibodies has a chronic infection, has a latent infection, or has cleared the infection.

Other antigen tests look for antigens that the patient's body manufactures normally or abnormally. CD4 antigen can be used to measure the status of helper T cells in patients with HIV. Other CD4 antigens can be used to detect T cell leukemias and lymphomas or B cell tumors. Abnormal antigens include lupus erythematosus (LE) cell tests. LE cells are abnormal neutrophils that contain abnormal DNA and are present in two thirds of SLE patients. The indirect Coombs' test is used to determine erythrocyte antigens and help to determine blood type. The direct Coombs' test detects antibodies against RBCs and can help to diagnose hemolytic and autoimmune disorders.

Biopsy

A biopsy is simply a sample of living tissue. The biopsy is then examined for abnormalities. Examination may be histological (microscopic examination) or use a variety of previously described tests. Biopsies may be complete or partial. A complete biopsy completely removes the tissue being tested. Moles are often completely biopsied. Complete biopsies are sometimes considered curative if they remove all diseased tissue. Partial biopsies take only a portion of

---

BOX 41-4

DISEASES ASSOCIATED WITH ANTINUCLEAR ANTIBODIES (ANA)

Normal patient without underlying abnormality: 3–30% (More common in older women)

Rheumatoid Conditions

SLE
RA
Mixed connective tissue disease
Sjögren's syndrome
Necrotizing vasculitis

Infection

Tuberculosis
Chronic active hepatitis
Subacute bacterial endocarditis
HIV

Miscellaneous Conditions

Type 1 diabetes mellitus
MS
Pulmonary fibrosis
Silicone gel implants
Pregnant women
Elderly patients

Medications (Drug-Induced LE)

Phenytoin
Ethosuximide
Primidone
Methyldopa
Hydralazine
Penicillamine
Carbamazepine
Procainamide
Thiazides
Griseofulvin
Chlorpromazine
Isoniazid
Quinidine
Gold salts
Minocycline

Adapted from Broyles, B. E., Reiss, B. S., & Evans, M. E. (2007). Pharmacological aspects of nursing care *(7th ed.). New York: Thomson Delmar Learning; Janeway, C. A., Jr., Travers, P., Walport, M., & Shlomchik, M. J. (2004).* Immunobiology, the immune system in health and disease *(6th ed.). New York: Garland Science Publishing.*

---

the tissue and are considered diagnostic. Skin biopsies are used to screen and remove cancers or potentially cancerous lesions. Common biopsies of the skin include punch biopsy, incisional biopsy, excisional biopsy, and shave biopsy. Aspiration biopsy uses a needle to remove a portion of the tissue or fluid. Fine needle aspiration (FNA) biopsy is used to biopsy delicate internal organs. Liver, bone, and muscle biopsies all carry significant risk of infection and hemorrhage; all three usually require anesthesia.

Skin Tests

Skin tests test for an IgE-mediated hypersensitivity reaction to a specific substance. Skin tests usually take the form of patch tests, scratch tests, prick tests, or intradermal injection. In each case, the patient is exposed to a small amount of the substance to be tested. The exposed area is observed for reaction. In the patch test, the substance is simply placed against the skin. In the prick test, a needle with a small amount of the substance is used to prick the patient's skin. The scratch test is similar to the prick test, except that the patient's skin is scratched instead of pricked. The scratch test should not be confused with dermographism. A small amount of the substance is injected in the intradermal space in the intradermal test. The patch test is the least sensitive, while the intradermal test is the most sensitive. However, the more sensitive tests carry more risk of anaphylaxis and false-positives. The scratch test is the most likely to cause these adverse reactions and has been largely superseded by the prick test. The results of the prick test can be distorted by bleeding or by placing pricks to close together.

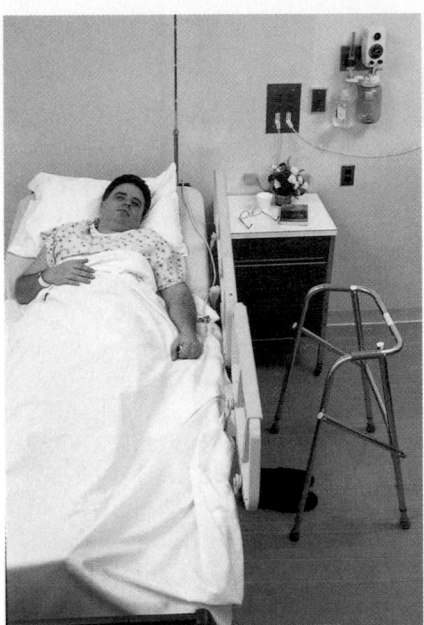

Figure 41-5 Stress management techniques will be important in the nursing considerations for this patient newly diagnosed with an STD.

Anergy Tests

Anergy tests inject a small amount of antigen into the intradermal space and the area is measured for induration at 48 to 72 hours. An induration of 5 mm or more is considered positive. The PPD used to screen for tuberculosis is an anergy test. Lack of induration is usually a sign that a patient has not contracted tuberculosis; however, false-negatives are common in patients with HIV, because their immune system is too suppressed to mount a reaction. This is referred to as anergy.

Anergy tests can also be used to screen for T cell immunodeficiency. A variety of antigens are injected in the intradermal space. Most healthy persons will display reaction to at least one of the antigens. Lack of reaction after 48 hours is considered a sign of immunodeficiency.

Nursing Management

Because so many immune function tests are blood tests, it is important that the nurse ensure that aseptic technique and appropriate wound care are maintained. This is especially important in patients who are or may be potentially immunosuppressed.

The primary nursing consideration in immune assessment is stress management (Figure 41-5). Patients who are hospitalized may benefit from stress reduction techniques, such as music, wearing their own clothes, exercise, and laughter. While assessment of immune function may occur as a routine procedure, such as determining whether a sore throat is streptococcus infection related, it is often associated with high stress situations. The fear of possibly having contracted an infectious disease such as HIV or herpes simplex virus can be more stressful than actual dealing with the disease (see Patient Playbook feature). The disease itself is bad enough, but social stigma that is carried for life can be worse in the patient's mind. Care must be taken to alleviate undue stress and fear when assessing the immune system. Because of the stressful nature of these kinds of assessments, patients may not understand instructions they are being given or may not remember. It is important not only to educate patients verbally, but to give them additional written education and instructions. One particular example is HIV testing. Because of the large social stigma and negative associations, federal law mandates that HIV test results can not be given out over the phone or mailed. Although patients sign a form stating that they understand this at the time they have blood drawn, many of them become upset when they call for their results and are told that they must come back into the clinic. Written instructions can help to allay this kind of situation.

It is also important not to prediagnose patients. Although a high ANA test is strongly associated with SLE, there are more than 15 other causes of elevated ANA, including various medications. In addition to fear of contracting a disease the uncertainty associated with not knowing what is wrong with one's body is also considerable. Many patients may be relieved to find out they have a disease, because it validates what they already suspected, which is that something was wrong with them. Some patients may actually become angry when they find out that diagnostic tests have returned negative. It is important to empathize with patients no matter which way their tests return.

Finally, patients should be educated on primary and secondary prevention of immune-related diseases. Immunizations, good hygiene, exercise, and stress management are all part of maintaining a healthy immune system. Patients should be educated about appropriate screening measures and symptom recognition for conditions they may be at risk for. This includes HIV and other STD tests for patients who engage in risky sex, regular PPDs for patients at risk for tuberculosis, and CBCs for patients with high risk for agranulocytosis or aplastic anemia.

KEY CONCEPTS

- The immune system is responsible not only for protecting the body against invading pathogens and toxins, but it is also responsible for removing extracellular detritus, protecting against cancer, and preparing damaged tissue for repair.
- The immune system is divided into two interacting systems called the innate and acquired immune system.
- Recognition of self and nonself is the most important aspect of the immune system's role, or else pathogens will be welcomed, and host cells will be destroyed.
- Antigens are substances that can bind with antibodies, and most antigens can bond with more than one kind of antibody.
- The sites where lymphocytes mature, bone marrow and thymus gland, are called primary lymphoid organs. The sites where lymphocytes aggregate to function are called secondary lymphoid tissues.
- B lymphocytes mature into plasma cells that secrete antibodies. There are five classes of antibodies that have distinct functions.
- IgM is the first antibody released. It forms a pentameter to effectively increase its affinity to antigen.
- B lymphocytes undergo mutations so that later antibodies have much higher affinity for their antigens.
- T lymphocytes mature into cytotoxic T cells and helper T cells, which further differentiate into TH1 and TH2 cells.
- The dendritic cell is the key to the activation of the immune system.

- The chemical components of the immune system act as cytokines, chemokines, opsonins, and effectors.
- The same properties that make TNF-α in isolating infections and activating the immune system make it deadly during sepsis.
- When the immune system is overwhelmed locally, it forms a granuloma to sequester the infection from the rest of the body.
- Active immunization creates memory B cells, which will quickly produce antibodies if the body is later infected with the pathogen.
- Passive immunization provides an infusion of antibodies that allow the body a reprieve to allow the body's own immune system a chance to activate.
- Vital assessment findings include age, gender, immunizations, medications, allergies, and past illnesses.
- Stress and social support can have a dramatic impact on immune function.
- Physical examination for immune assessment covers the entire body. The skin, mouth, and lymph nodes particularly tend to show early signs of immune changes.
- Laboratory tests should always be interpreted in light of the health history and physical examination.
- Aseptic technique and universal precautions should always be used when obtaining immune laboratory or diagnostic tests.
- Empathy and therapeutic listening can mitigate the stress of testing.

REVIEW QUESTIONS

1. Which of the following is not a role of the immune system?
   1. Defense of the body from external invaders
   2. Signal the body that bone marrow is suppressed
   3. Destruction of senescent erythrocytes and other cellular debris
   4. Surveillance against cancer

2. Which of the following are APCs? More than one answer may be possible.
   1. Neutrophils
   2. Dendritic cells
   3. Macrophages
   4. NK cells

3. What is the term for a substance that binds to a specific antibody? More than one answer may be correct.
   1. Hapten
   2. Antigen
   3. Immunogen
   4. Complement

4. Which of the following is a phagocytic cell?
   1. Neutrophils
   2. Basophils
   3. NK cells
   4. Plasma cells

Continued

REVIEW QUESTIONS—cont'd

5. What cell is the most potent activator of lymphocytes?
   1. Macrophages
   2. Neutrophils
   3. Mast cells
   4. Dendritic cells

6. Which of the following are primary lymphoid organs?
   1. Bone marrow
   2. Lymph nodes
   3. Spleen
   4. Thymus gland

7. Which of the following is a characteristic of innate immunity?
   1. Developed by colostrum
   2. Mediated T cells
   3. Has memory
   4. Initiates inflammation

8. When giving immunizations, which of the following assessments is not necessary?
   1. Allergy to eggs
   2. Family history of measles
   3. History of past immunizations
   4. History of past illnesses.

9. Which of the following reactions indicates a medication allergy?
   1. GI bleed with aspirin
   2. Nausea with azithromycin
   3. Diarrhea with tegaserod
   4. Angioedema with ramipril

10. Which surgery usually results in the destruction of a primary lymphoid organ?
    1. Cholecystectomy
    2. Splenectomy
    3. Tonsillectomy
    4. Heart transplant

11. Increased neutrophil count may be indicative of (more than one answer may be correct):
    1. Bacterial infection
    2. MI
    3. Inflammatory bowel disease
    4. Allergy

12. When assessing the immune system, which of the following provides the lens for interpretation of the assessment?
    1. Health history
    2. Physical examination
    3. Laboratory values
    4. Horoscope

REVIEW ACTIVITIES

1. Your patient, a 24-year-old Caucasian woman has been hospitalized with fever, fatigue, and weight loss and is awaiting results of diagnostic tests. She is afraid that she has SLE. What would you tell her regarding her lab tests?

2. Your patient is a 60-year-old Caucasian male who has been having increasing urinary tract infections (UTIs). What changes would put him at risk for increased UTIs? What additional things should be assessed?

Continued

REVIEW ACTIVITIES—cont'd

3. Your newly admitted patient has a latex allergy. What steps should be taken in their care?

4. Your patient is a 19-year-old student about to enter a nursing program. What immunizations should she need?

5. Your patient is a 32-year-old male and has come into the clinic for STD testing. What issues should you address with the patient regarding STD testing?

Visit the Contemporary Medical-Surgical Nursing online companion resource at www.delmarhealthcare.com for additional content and study aids. Click on Online Companions then select the Nursing discipline.

Immunodeficiency and HIV Infection/AIDS: Nursing Management

Ruth Grendell, MSN, RN

CHAPTER TOPICS

- The Protective Immune Response
- Immune Deficiency Disorders
- Hypersensitivity Disorders

- Autoimmune Disorders
- Collaborative Management of Patients with Immune Disorders
- Immunosuppressive Therapies

KEY TERMS

Allograft or homograft transplant
Antigen
Apheresis
Autoimmunity
Autologous transplant
Histocompatibility leukocyte antigens (HLA)
Immune response
Immunity
Immunodeficiency
Monoclonal antibodies
Plasmapheresis (plasma exchange)
Primary immune response
Secondary or specific antibody response
Syngeneic transplant

The immune system is vital to the human body as related to its processes for recognizing and protecting the body. There are many complex and intricate components to the immune system, which continue to be researched and understood. Recently, immunologists have recognized the immune system as a core control mechanism that is of equal importance as the neurological and endocrine control systems. It is important for the nurse to understand the numerous communication networks among these three systems and what happens when dysfunctions occur. In addition, the nurse must be knowledgeable about the guidelines and strategies developed by the health care system for a wide variety of immune system disorders that specifically involve nursing management. The focus of this chapter is to provide an overview of the immune response and its function in protecting the body and to discuss the collaborative and nursing management of individuals with immune deficiency disorders.

IMMUNODEFICIENCY

Immunodeficiency is the inability to produce a normal complement of antibodies or immunologically sensitized T cells (cell-mediated immunity) especially in response to specific antigens. The clinical hallmark is a propensity to unusual or recurrent severe infections. Most common infections from defects in the cell-mediated response are fungal and viral. Most common infections from defects in the humoral-mediated response are bacteria initiated. **Immunity** is the quality or state of being immune; a condition of being able to resist a particular disease through preventing development of a pathogenic microorganism or by counteracting the effects of its products. The **primary immune response** occurs when an antigen is initially introduced into the system. It involves both mast cell degranulation and activation of plasma proteins, i.e., complement, clotting factors, and kinin—polypeptides that increase blood flow and permeability of small blood capillaries. The **secondary or specific antibody response** includes the activation of B cells and the memory cells (IgG, IgM, IgA, and IgE); and activation of T cells, cytotoxic (killer) cells, lymphokine-producing cells, helper cells, and suppressor cells (humoral immunity) to a specific antigen. Common diagnostic studies related to the immunological disorders are listed in Box 42-1.

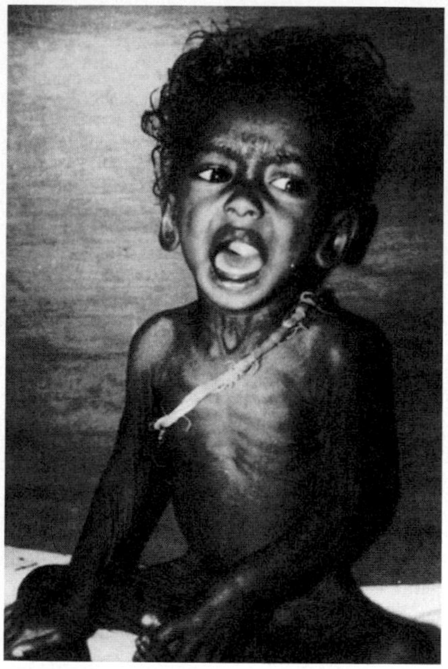

HUMAN IMMUNODEFICIENCY VIRUS INFECTION

One of the most recognized immunodeficiency diseases is human immunodeficiency virus (HIV) and the resulting acquired immunodeficiency syndrome (AIDS) diagnosis. By 2004, approximately 37.8 million people were documented as infected with HIV. This number included 35.7 million adults and 2.1 million children younger than 15 years of age known to be living with HIV/AIDS. The Centers for Disease Control and Prevention (CDC, 2005b) estimate that 850,000 to 950,000 U.S. residents are living with HIV infection; one fourth of these are unaware of their infection. Half of young people under 25 years of age acquired the infection through heterosexual sex; approximately two thirds of pediatric cases were acquired in utero from the infected mother. In 2003, the number of documented AIDS cases in the United States was 43,171 including 59 children under 13 (CDC, 2005b) (Figure 42-1). There is no cure or vaccine; however, technological advances in drug therapy have slowed the progression of the disease and increased life expectancy.

Figure 42-1 Child with HIV suffering with marasmus.

Epidemiology

HIV has become a worldwide disease with incredible negative affects on certain populations. The disorder was first named lymphadenopathy-associated virus (LAV) by French scientists in 1983. Later an American scientist labeled the virus as the human T cell lymphotropic virus. Three years later a different strain was discovered in Africa. This was the first clue that the virus could mutate quickly. There are two related but distinct types of HIV, HIV-1 and HIV-2. HIV-2, which is found primarily in Western Africa, comprises six distinct phylogenetic lineages designated as subtypes, or clades. Three groups of HIV-1 are currently recognized: M (major group), N (new or non-M, non-O), and O (outlier). The 11 subtypes of HIV-1 group M are identified as A–K. HIV-1 subtype B is primarily responsible for the epidemic in North America and Western Europe. Other subtypes, or clades, have been discovered in India, Africa, and Asia (Figure 42-2). This poses the great concern that new infections caused by these mutations will be evident worldwide as infected people travel from country to country (Bunnel, et. al., 2005).

BOX 42-1

CLASSIFICATION OF IMMUNOLOGICAL DISORDERS

Immunodeficient (Type I)

Acquired immunodeficiency syndrome (AIDS)
DiGeorge's syndrome—or anomaly: (Congenital absence of the thymus and parathyroids with loss of cellular immunity. Immunoglobulins are normal. Individual has facial abnormalities, congestive heart disease, decreased calcium, and increased susceptibility to infections—due to defect on chromosome 22.)

Autoimmune (Type II)

Myasthenia gravis
Ankylosing spondylitis (Marie-Strümpell disease)
Fibromyalgia
Polymyositis and dermatomyositis
RA* (classified as connective tissue disorder)
SLE* (vascular and connective tissue disorder)
Sjögren's syndrome
Vasculitis
Reiter's syndrome
Polymyalgia rheumatica and cranial arteritis.
Grave's disease* (unknown etiology, but autoimmune basis is suspected).
Hyperthyroidism with goiter (gland enlargement) and ophthalmopathy
Progressive systemic sclerosis (scleroderma)
*Includes disorders involving both the autoimmune and hypersensitive responses

Mixed Connective Tissue Disease

Lyme disease (rheumatic joint disease with a known cause, a tickborne spirochete).
Secondary arthritis (Whipple's disease)

Immunoproliferative (Type III)

a. Leukemia

Hypersensitive (Type IV)

Allergies
Asthma
Contact dermatitis
Note: List is not all inclusive.

Adapted from Porth, C. (2004). Pathophysiology: Concepts of altered health status (6th ed.). Philadelphia: Lippincott, Williams & Wilkins.

Etiology

Risk factors for HIV include unsafe sexual practices, rape, prostitution and multiple sexual partners, exposure to contaminated blood and contaminated needles, occupational exposure, and perinatal exposure (Jones, 2004). Perinatal exposure can occur during the pregnancy, during vaginal delivery, and through breastfeeding. Approximately 23 percent of babies born to HIV-infected women are infected. Additional contributing factors include genital lesions associated with other sexually transmitted diseases (STDs), unprotected anal intercourse, and sexual intercourse during menstruation. The risk

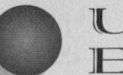

Uncovering the Evidence

HIV Transmission from Africa to the United States

Discussion: Increasing numbers of African immigrants have come to the United States in recent years. Several HIV-positive pregnant women from various African countries are seeking health care in city clinics. Health care personnel are unfamiliar with their particular needs and the cultural and structural barriers that African women encounter related to HIV prevention. A qualitative study conducted in a Philadelphia clinic identified barriers such as legal status, language problems, fear of the American health system, misunderstanding about HIV transmission, and lack of information about available antiretroviral treatment. Many of the infections are diagnosed later in their own countries, and because of the lack of knowledge about the disease they are slower to accept treatment. Other findings revealed that the male partner is excluded from treatment because of denial, refusal to be tested, or abandoning the family. Women are afraid to reveal their HIV positive status to family and friends; they hide their medications and use them inconsistently; they have little decision-making power about safe sexual practices (see Figure 42-2). Immigrants are ineligible for some of the health care benefits, because they cannot provide proof of residence and are unable to navigate the U. S. system, and many are too poor to afford medications.

Implications for Practice: There is a great need for developing culturally appropriate education about HIV prevention and treatment. Health care personnel need to know and understand the fears, experiences, and concerns of these populations.

Source: Foley, E. (2005). HIV/AIDS and African immigrant women in Philadelphia: Structural and cultural barriers to care. AIDS Care, 17(8), 1030–1043.

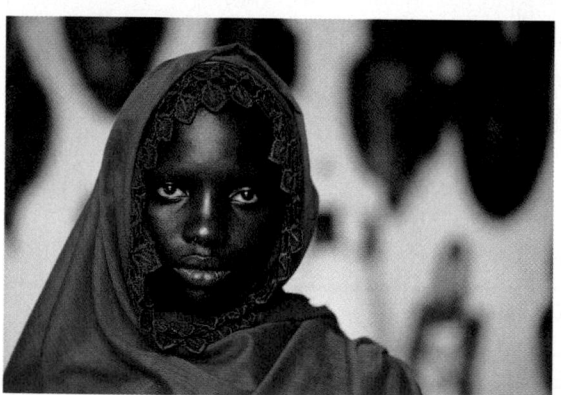

Figure 42-2 AIDS is continuing to rise in African women at alarming rates.

for infection is greater for the receiving partner because of the prolonged contact with the semen; however, the inserting partner may also be at risk. A recent survey indicated that young people are having casual sex at an earlier age and feel less guilt about it than previous generations (Figure 42-3). Sexual activity by teenagers is considered the norm. The availability of birth control, the acceptance of satisfying individual needs, and gender equality were cited as reasons for the cultural shift in behaviors. Oral sex has also become mainstream (Baker, 2005). HIV infection can be transmitted by blood, semen, vaginal or cervical secretions, and breast milk. The sero-conversion (the presence of antibodies in the blood) usually occurs in one to three months or up to six months after exposure. The infected individual is still infectious when no symptoms are present, and the ability to transmit infection is lifelong.

Occupational exposure as a risk factor is a concern for health care workers and for other service occupations, such as police and correction officers. Exposure to HIV infected blood via contaminated needle stick or sharp object, contact with infected breast milk, mucous secretions (vaginal, semen), and exposure to blood in the laboratory are the common sources. The actual risk is quite low; however the exposure risk increases (a) when there is visual blood on the instrument that causes the injury to the worker and (b) when the patient diagnosed with AIDS dies within 60 days of the worker's exposure because it is presumed that HIV concentrations were high at the time of the

Skills 360°

Transmission of HIV

The nurse should be aware of the following information. HIV is a fragile virus, which can be transmitted only under specific conditions that permit contact with infected body fluids. Transmission of HIV is similar to transmission of infection by other pathogenic microorganisms. Transmission of the HIV can then occur (a) within a short time frame after a person becomes infected with the HIV; (b) transmission is also dependent on a large amount of the virus entering the receiving body (host); (c) transmission is dependent on the potency, or virulence, and concentration of the virus; and (d) transmission is dependent on the immune status of the new host. HIV cannot be transmitted through casual contact, such as shaking hands, sharing eating utensils, using toilet seats, or working along side an HIV infected worker. The HIV is not transmitted through tears, saliva, urine, emesis, sputum, feces, or sweat.

Adapted from DeLaune, S., & Ladner, P. (2006). Fundamentals of nursing (3rd ed.). New York: Thomson Delmar Learning.

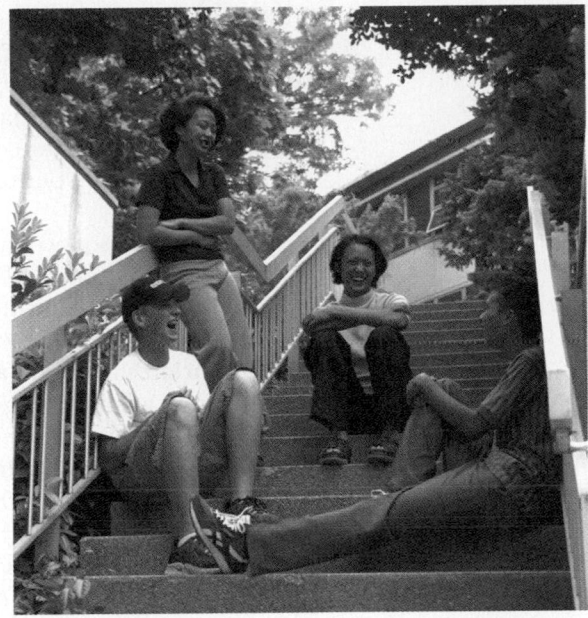

Figure 42-3 HIV in adolescents remains a risk because of the unsafe sexual practices in this population.

exposure. Workers at risk should follow the standard precautions when handling any body fluids and blood, and when performing procedures that place them at risk. Recommendations from the U.S. Public Health Service include at least a four-week prophylactic therapy with a combination of retroviral drugs. Transmission of HIV from an HIV-infected health care worker to a patient is also possible. Following standard precautions in all contacts with patients and administering prophylactic therapy to the patients should be followed.

Pathophysiology

The pathophysiology of HIV begins with several alterations of a limited number of cells that have CD4 receptors on their surfaces. Primary targets for the development of HIV because of these receptor sites are the CD4+ T cells (helper cells) that have more CD4 receptors. Other cells that have CD4 receptor sites include lymphocytes, monocytes, macrophages, astrocytes, and oligodendrocytes. The HIV retrovirus interacts specifically with the host cell receptors and uses the host cells for viral replication. HIV then interacts with the CD4 glycoprotein, which resides on the cell membranes, fuses itself to the cell, and injects itself into the cytoplasm where the viral ribonucleic acid (RNA) genome is then translated into deoxyribonucleic acid (DNA) by a retroviral enzyme-reverse transcriptase. The next step of the interaction involves a second DNA strand that is then formed as the cell's genetic material becomes partially viral. Normally, CD4+ T cells orchestrate the immune system process in responding to foreign antigens. An adult has approximately 800 to 1,200 of the T helper cells per μL of blood that have a lifespan of about 100 days; however an infected cell may die within 2 days, thus releasing the viral content (virions) into the blood stream to infect other cells. HIV replicates rapidly; sometimes more than 10 million virions are produced daily.

Significant loss of the CD4+ T cells results in the inability for the body to maintain homeostasis and increases susceptibility to opportunistic infections, or it can reactivate a latent disease process the individual previously experienced, such as the varicella zoster virus of chickenpox in childhood that can reemerge as shingles. Individual responses to the disease are varied; some individuals remain symptom free for many years; others succumb quickly. Even though an individual has no noticeable symptoms, the viral replication process continues.

In addition to damaging the immune system, HIV infection can cause damage to other parts of the body. Cranial and peripheral neuropathy, cardiomyopathy, pneumonitis, malabsorption in the small intestine, nephritis, cervicitis, arthritis, psoriasis, and gonad dysfunctions have all been directly associated with HIV infection. The results of damage to the hematological system are several types of anemia. It is sometimes categorized as a multisystem disease.

The criteria used to establish the diagnosis of AIDS are at least one of the following conditions: a CD4+ below 200 cells/μL; the development of one or more of fungal, viral, protozoal, or bacterial opportunistic infection(s); development of opportunistic cancers, such as invasive cervical cancer, Kaposi's sarcoma, Burkitt's lymphoma, immunoblastic lymphoma, or primary lymphoma of the brain; wasting syndrome defined by a loss of 10 percent or more of body mass; development of dementia.

Preexisting comorbidities, such as alcoholism, drug dependence, liver and kidney and other organ diseases, history of sexually transmitted diseases and psychiatric illnesses are additional influencing factors associated with the transmission and progress of HIV/AIDS. Early diagnosis, appropriate treatment with antiretroviral medications and medications to prevent opportunistic infections has increased survival rates.

Assessment with Clinical Manifestations

Early clinical manifestations of HIV disease resemble an acute mononucleosis-like syndrome, including chills and fever, myalgia, malaise, sort throat, nausea, photophobia, lymphadenopathy, maculopapular rash, and headache. Sometimes, there is a latent period of 10 years or more before other symptoms occur. Later clinical manifestations include chills and fever, night sweats, dry productive cough, dyspnea, lethargy, confusion, stiff neck, seizures, headache, malaise, fatigue, oral lesions, skin rash, abdominal discomfort, diarrhea, weight loss, sustained lymphadenopathy, and a wide variety of emotional responses, such as anger, fear, guilt, denial, depression, and suicidal tendencies.

As the immune system becomes overpowered, opportunistic infections or malignancy can occur. The most common infection is *Pneumocystis carinii* pneumonia (PCP). Additional respiratory infections include *Mycobacterium* tuberculosis, cytomegalovirus (CMV) infection, *Streptococcus* pneumonia, or pneumonias caused by multiple organisms. Kaposi's sarcoma (Figure 42-4), a vascular malignancy first noticed on the skin or mucous membranes, can also invade the lungs (Porth, 2004). Other systems that can be involved include vision disturbances or blindness because of CMV and herpes type 1 virus or varicella-zoster virus infections; adrenal insufficiency; gastrointestinal (GI) disturbances because of virus, yeast, protozoa, and bacteria infections or invasion of cancers; neurological disorders because of infection and the AIDS dementia complex; musculoskeletal arthralgia (joint pain) and weakness; and fluid and electrolyte imbalances.

Diagnostic Tests

During the initial infection, testing may reveal a high viral load and a dramatic drop in the CD4+ cell count. At this time antibodies are beginning to form and can be detected in approximately 4 to 12 weeks. However, the disease may not be detected in the early stages, because the person does not seek attention or inadequate history information is taken by the health care provider. If testing is performed too early, the report may be a false-negative result. Some HIV antibody tests such as the enzyme-linked immunosorbent assay (ELISA) results provide an indeterminate report. The Western blot test may not confirm the original immunoassay test. Repeated testing is recommended. Other testing

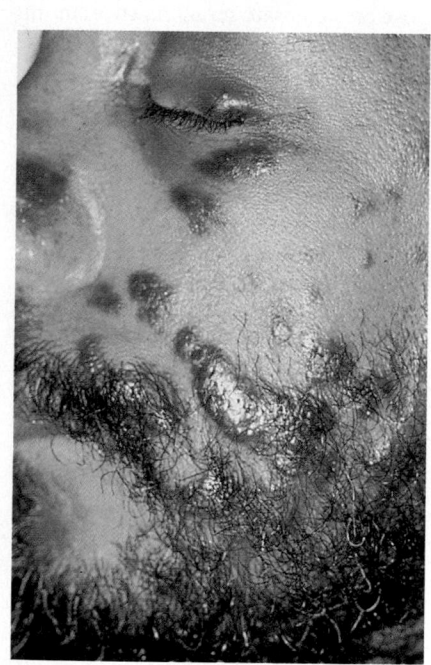

Figure 42-4 Kaposi's sarcoma. Courtesy of Robert A. Silverman, M.D., Clinical Associate Professor, Department of Pediatrics, Georgetown University.

methods include home test kits, salivary tests, and urine tests. However, the individual should not rely on the results without follow-up care with a health care provider. The current emphasis for monitoring is on evaluating the CD4+ cell counts (Daniels, 2003). The CDC has developed a classification system for HIV-infected adolescents and adults that emphasizes the importance of CD4+ testing in managing clinical manifestations.

A list of diagnostic tests and procedures is depicted in Box 42-2. Periodic testing is conducted to determine the patient's status and progress of the disease. Additional diagnostic tests would be performed to identify opportunistic infections. The individual may also have preexisting chronic disease conditions that require monitoring. The diagnostic findings are used to prescribe therapy. As new therapies are developed and individuals live longer with the disease, treatment will be required for many of the diseases that normally

---

BOX 42-2

DIAGNOSTIC STUDIES RELATED TO IMMUNOLOGICAL RESPONSE

Standard Blood Studies

- RBC count, hemoglobin/hematocrit, and reticulocyte count
- Sedimentation rate: The speed for RBCs to settle in a column of citrated blood per hour. Used in diagnosing progress of several abnormal conditions (such as chronic infections).
- WBC with differential count: Elevated in presence of infection.
- Lymphocytes: Cell markers: T cell, B cell, and so on.
- Platelet count: Involved in coagulation process.
- Proteins: Albumen, globulins, fibrinogen levels.
- C-reactive protein: Synthesized in liver; is a natural inhibitor of coagulation; deficiency in liver disease.
- Complement activity: System of 25 plasma proteins. When activated, a cascade of events mediates the defense against infection; facilitates phagocytosis, eliminates antigen-antibody complexes and destroys cell membrane of bacteria.

Additional Tests of Immunological Status

HIV Antibody Tests

- CD4 count: The hallmark of HIV infection—diminished or depleted T helper lymphocytes.
- CD4/CD8+ ratio: CD4+ lymphocytes are the primary target of the virus; therefore they decline, and there is a greater risk to develop opportunistic infections. The ratio to CD8+ lymphocytes is also low. CD8+ lymphocytes are suppressor-cytotoxic T lymphocytes.
- HIV-RNA concentration: Measures the amount of HIV in the blood—the viral load. The virus can be detected in the early stage of infection. The concentration level can be used as a baseline value. Changes in the virus count are important and are used to guide treatment strategies.

- ELISA: Detects HIV antibodies.
- Western blot test: Detects antibodies to specific viral proteins. This test is expensive and is often used as confirmation of a positive ELISA test.
- HIV antigen tests: Used for diagnosis in early stage of acute infection.
- DNA-PCR amplification: Detects the proviral DNA molecules in the infected nuclei of lymphocytes from the peripheral blood.

Immune Deficiency Disorders

- T and B lymphocyte assays: Increase in T lymphocytes is associated with acute lymphocytic leukemia, infectious mononucleosis, and multiple myeloma. Reduced levels may be due to AIDS, chronic lymphocytic leukemia, severe combined immunodeficiency disease (SCID) or long-term immunosuppressive therapy.
- Immunoglobulin assays: (Measures levels of IgG, IgA, IgM, IgD, and IgE. Increased levels of IgA and IgE may be seen in autoimmune and allergic disorders. Reduced levels of IgG, IgA, and IgM may be seen in lymphocytic leukemia.
- Bone marrow: Used to diagnose most blood dyscrasias, e.g., aplastic anemia, leukemias, pernicious anemia, thrombocytopenia.
- Lymphangiography: Visualization of the lymphatic system to detect primary malignancy (lymphoma) or metastatic disease. An oil-based dye is injected into the lymphatic system. X-ray studies are done.
- Allergy and autoimmune disorder testing: Includes skin testing for sensitivity to specific antigens and food allergies. Elimination diets are also used.

Note: The list is not inclusive.

Adapted from Daniels, R. (2003). Delmar's manual of laboratory and diagnostic tests. *New York: Thomson Delmar Learning.*

Patient, Family, and Caregiver Education

Patients, family, and personal caregivers should:

- Know the drugs being taken and how to take them (whether they should be taken with food or on an empty stomach; what time of day, and so on).
- The goal of retroviral therapy and importance of adhering to the prescribed regimen.
- Understand the interactions that can occur with other medications and herbal therapies.
- The importance of repeated testing and ongoing contact with the health care system.
- Recognize the potential side effects from the antiretroviral drugs and how to manage them (diarrhea, nausea, vomiting, gastric distress, headache, and so on).
- Know what social support and counseling services are available and how to access and use them.
- The changes in symptoms that should be reported immediately to the health care provider (fever, persistent shortness of breath, chest pain, dehydration, pain, watery diarrhea and abdominal pain, rectal bleeding, vision changes, onset of weakness, seizures, new oral lesions, rashes, severe depression, anxiety, hallucinations, exhibiting dangerous behavior toward self or others).

Adapted from DeLaune, S., & Ladner, P. (2006). Fundamentals of nursing (3rd ed.). New York: Thomson Delmar Learning.

occur in the aging population such as coronary artery disease, chronic obstructive lung disease, hypertension, and diabetes.

Nursing Diagnoses

A number of diagnoses related to HIV infection are used according to the stage of the disease, problems of the body system(s) involved and psycho-social factors. Based on the information gathered, examples of nursing diagnoses in the patient with HIV may include the following:

- Acute pain related to HIV.
- Fear in response to the diagnosis of HIV.
- Risk for infection related to HIV.
- Ineffective coping related to anxiety, lower activity level and the inability to perform normal activities of daily living related to HIV.
- Knowledge deficit related to self-care and risk prevention for HIV.

Planning and Implementation

The goals of nursing interventions are to improve the quality and quantity of the patient's life. Nurses use a holistic and individualized approach directed toward health promotion, prevention of infection, providing education related to safe sexual practices, identifying the risks of drug use, and decreasing the risk of perinatal transmission of HIV (Jones, 2004). Additional interventions include helping the patient to participate in self-care and to improve nutrition, to learn how to decrease fatigue, and to promote communication with the health care system and support network. Some of the greatest challenges are to assist the individual in coping with a chronic or life-threatening disease, overcoming fear, and minimizing spiritual distress.

In the advanced stages of the disease the goal of nursing care is to address the physical and emotional responses of the patient, whether potential or actual, which are related to the AIDS diagnosis. In many cases, the patient continues to receive care in the home except for crisis events. Home health care nurses must be alert for changes within the family structure as living with a chronic disease poses many stresses on the family unit including social isolation because of stigma associated with the disease, dependence, anger, frustration, economic concerns, feelings of powerlessness, and loss of control. Patients and families often need assistance in making treatment decisions and dealing with all the changes that transpire.

Terminal care can be especially stressful if the patient develops AIDS-dementia complex (ADC) because of HIV infection in the brain or by HIV associated central nervous system (CNS) problems. Cognitive, behavioral, and motor dysfunctions that occur include decreased concentration, depression, forgetfulness, social withdrawal, progression to dementia, paraplegia, incontinence, and coma. The focus of interventions is on maintaining a safe environment. Frequent reorientation and stress reduction methods assist in preventing confusion and disorientation. Support is given to the family and caregivers as they provide end-of-life care. Despite the many advances in HIV therapy, there still is no miracle cure. Nurses are a pivotal part in providing terminal care.

Collaborative Management

The goals of collaborative management are to initiate an effective antiretroviral treatment regimen, to promote health, and to prevent or treat opportunistic infections. The patient must assume a partnership role in the plan of care through making lifestyle changes, and adherence to the prescribed regimen. Education about the disease, modes of transmission, and how to improve personal health is of prime importance. The family and significant others who pro-

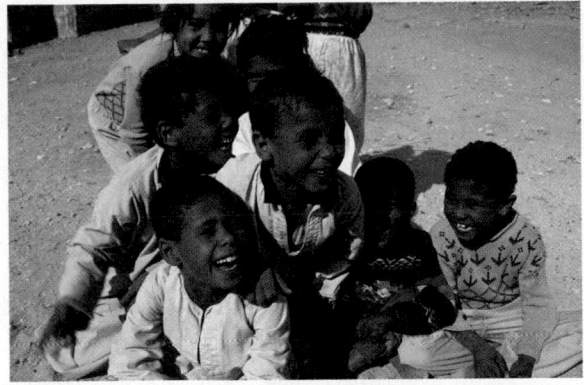

Figure 42-5 Organizations like UNICEF have initiated maternal and child health programs for diseases like AIDS to control the spread of the disease in countries like Africa.

vide social support should also be included in counseling and the plan of care. Collaborative management of the disease primarily takes place in the outpatient and community settings. The patient may be hospitalized for crisis events.

Pharmacology

Drug therapy is initiated as early as possible to reduce the HIV RNA (virion) levels in the blood and to maintain or increase the CD4+ levels to greater than 200 cells/μL and to delay the development of HIV-related symptoms and opportunistic infections. Highly active antiretroviral therapy (HAART) refers to a combination of antiretroviral drugs and is currently the preferred method to avoid development of viral resistance to the drugs. Resistance can also develop if the patient does not to adhere to the dose schedule for each drug. Each of the prescribed drugs is designed to target a specific phase of the viral cycle; therefore a missed or delayed dose permits the virus to continue to replicate itself. Several new drugs have been introduced that provide the opportunity to use more than one combination for individuals who do not respond to a specific group (Stenson, et. al., 2005).

Side effects include nausea and vomiting, anemia, leucopenia, myopathy, fatigue, headache, dizziness, and nasal congestion; dose-related peripheral neuropathy, hypersensitivity reaction, sore throat, rash, pruritus, cough, shortness of breath, and hepatitis. These drugs can also produce potentially lethal interactions with other drugs including over-the-counter (OTC) drugs and herbal therapies. The drugs are expensive, and many patients are not able to afford them, tolerate the side effects, or cannot adhere to the necessary scheduling and dietary changes. Children, especially, have difficulty with adherence to the therapy because of the numerous reactions, the aftertaste, and interactions with foods. Facilitating adherence requires educated and committed health care providers to work with the children and their caregivers (Pontali, 2005).

Long-term effects of HAART include hypertension, diabetes, osteopenia, and hyperlipidemia. Recent studies have indicated that suspending antiretroviral therapy for short intervals did lower triglycerides and blood pressure levels without decreasing the CD4+ blood levels. However, several of the study participants and health care providers opted to return to the antiretroviral therapy rather than risk further HIV complications (Casseb, Da Silva, & Alberto, 2005; Jacobs, Neil, & Aboulafia, 2005).

Three groups of drugs are currently approved as antiretroviral therapy: (Group 1) nucleoside reverse transcriptase inhibitors (NRTIs), nonnucleoside reverse transcriptase inhibitors (NNRTIs), and nucleotide reverse transcriptase inhibitors; (Group 2) protease inhibitors (PIs); and (Group 3) fusion inhibitors (Box 42-3). Scientists are continuing to research the possibility of developing a vaccine against HIV; however, one vaccine is not effective against the variety of HIV strains.

BOX 42-3

ANTIRETROVIRAL DRUG CLASSIFICATIONS

Nucleoside Reverse Transcriptase Inhibitors (NRTIs)

Zidovudine (AZT, ZDV, Retrovir)—the first developed drug
Didanosine (ddl, Videx)
Stavudine (d4T, Zerit)
Lamivudine (3TC, Epivir)
Abacavir (Ziagen)

Nucleotide Reverse Transcriptase Inhibitor

Tenofovir DF (Viread)

Nonnucleoside Reverse Transcriptase Inhibitors (NNRTIs)

Nevirapine (Viramune)
Delavirdine (Rescriptor)
Efavirenz (Sustival)

Protease Inhibitors (PIs)

Saquinavir (Fortovase
Indinavir (Crixivan
Ritonavir (Norvir)
Nelfinavir (Viracept
Amprenavir (Agenerase)
Kaletra (combination of lopinavir and ritonvir)

Fusion Inhibitor (Entry Inhibitor)

Enfuvirtide (Fuzeon)

Adapted from Broyles, B. E., Reiss, B. S., & Evans, M. E. (2007). Pharmacological aspects of nursing care *(7th ed.). New York: Thomson Delmar Learning.*

Evaluation of Outcomes

Potential patient outcomes for each of the example nursing diagnoses for the patient with HIV are:

- Acute pain related to HIV. The patient should verbalize an adequate relief of pain along with the ability to realistically cope with the pain if it is not completely relieved.
- Fear in response to the diagnosis of HIV. The patient should manifest positive coping behaviors and verbalize a reduction in the amount of fear of the having this disease.
- Risk for infection related to HIV. The patient remains free of infection, as evidenced by normal vital signs and absence of purulent drainage from wounds, incisions, and tubes. Infection is recognized early to allow for prompt treatment.
- Ineffective coping related to anxiety, lower activity level, and the inability to perform normal activities of daily living related to HIV. The patient identifies own maladaptive coping behaviors, available resources, and support systems, describes or initiates alternative coping strategies, and describes positive results from new behaviors.
- Knowledge deficit related to self-care and risk prevention for HIV. The patient should demonstrate motivation to learn, identify perceived learning needs, and verbalize an understanding of desired content.

IMMUNODEFICIENCY DISORDERS

Immunodeficiency disorders are due to dysfunction or impairment of one or more of the **immune response** (a body response to an antigen that occurs when lymphocytes identify the antigenic molecule as foreign and induce the formation of antibodies and lymphocytes capable of reacting with it and rendering it harmless) mechanisms. The mechanisms include phagocytosis, humoral response, B cell- and T cell-mediated response or combination, the complement system, and a combined cell and humoral response. The primary immunodeficiency disorders are associated with the various cell-mediated deficiencies. Examples of disorders include chronic granulomatous disease, DiGeorge syndrome, ataxia telangiectasia, selective IgA, IgM, or IgG deficiency, and graft-versus-host disease. Secondary immunodeficiency disorders can be treatment-related, such as radiation or surgery; drug-induced, such as chemotherapy and corticosteroids; infectious diseases including AIDS, chronic liver or renal disease, diabetes mellitus, malignancies, and systemic lupus erythematosus (SLE); and stress. SLE is also classified as an autoimmune disease.

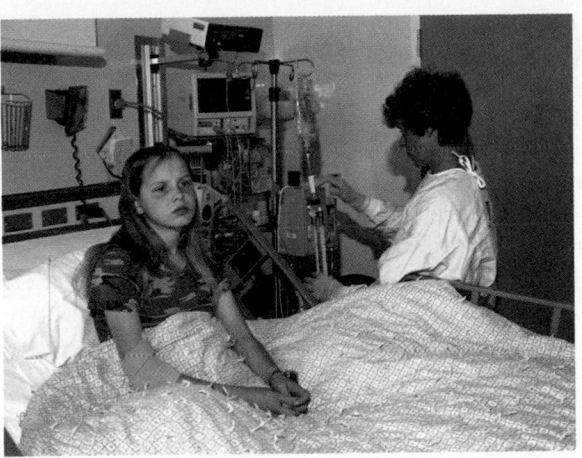

Figure 42-6 A child who is immunosuppressed from chemotherapy.

Young children and older people have suppressed immune systems and are more susceptible to infections than young and middle-aged adults because of a lack of sufficient immune resources (Figure 42-6). The destruction of lymphocytes by radiation or removal of lymph nodes, thymus, or spleen places the individual at high risk. Splenectomy is especially harmful for children. Cell-mediated immunity is greatly reduced in persons with Hodgkin's disease. Malnutrition also adversely affects cell-mediated immunity.

Graft-versus-Host Disease

Graft-versus-host (GVH) disease is the result of a transfusion of blood or a tissue transplant with cells that are incompatible with the host. It is hypothesized that lymphocyte T cells from the donor product attack and destroy the vulnerable cells of the host. The acute rejection response occurs approximately 7 to 30 days after the transplant. Target organs are the skin, lungs, the GI tract, and the liver. Clinical manifestations include maculopapular rash, pruritus, or pain; mild jaundice may be seen in liver disease along with elevated liver enzymes and possible hepatic coma; GI bleeding and malabsorption may occur in GI system disease. Bacterial and fungal infections are the greatest concern immediately after the transplant when granulocytopenia (great reduction in granulocytes) occurs. Interstitial pneumonitis is a common problem later in the rejection process. Corticosteroids are used to halt the rejection process; however, they, too, increase the individual's risk for infection.

Chronic GVH disease can appear approximately 100 days after the transplantation. Clinical manifestations resemble those of SLE. The skin has a scleroderma-like appearance, which is a taut, firm, hard, and edematous state; the lacrimal ducts and oral mucosa are dry.

Allograft or homograft transplant refers to cells and tissue obtained from the same species, as from a close relative or unrelated donor, who has a similar type of cell compatibility. The greatest success is with tissues from the cornea, bone marrow, artery, and cartilage. Sources for stem cells are peripheral blood, bone marrow, and umbilical cord blood. Histocompatibility testing is done to determine the similarities and differences in the complex set of proteins (**histocompatibility leukocyte antigens [HLA]** markers) on the surface membranes of all human nucleated cells, tissues, and blood cells, except red blood cells (RBCs). If the tissues of two people are histocompatible, there is less chance for the graft to be rejected. However, major incompatibility will trigger the immune response against the graft, and there is a greater chance for rejection. HLA gene markers on a cell to an antigen provide a biochemical profile unique as a fingerprint that is primarily determined by genetic factors. HLA genes take many forms and many combinations occur. Antigens located on a chromosome are inherited from each parent and the frequencies of HLAs vary considerably among the different races. There is a great need for donors from racial and ethnic groups (National Marrow Donor Program, 2005).

Bone marrow transplant (BMT) is currently used as treatment for a variety of hematological, malignant, and nonmalignant disorders, including immunodeficiency diseases and severe autoimmune diseases. A **syngeneic transplant** uses bone marrow cells donated by an identical twin with no detectable tissue incompatibility. An **autologous transplant** is the removal of bone marrow cells from the individual—treated and stored—then returned after the individual receives intensive chemotherapy or radiation. This process eliminates the GVHD response; however, a relapse may occur either because of contamination of the cells by malignant cells or failure of the chemotherapy or radiation to eradicate the malignant cells.

Immunosuppressive Therapy

Several immunosuppressive drugs have been designed to target specific phases of the immune response. Drugs are used in combination to permit lower doses of each drug and to minimize side effects. It is also important to use adequate drug doses that will suppress the immune response, yet retain enough immunity to prevent opportunistic infections and to prevent rejection of the transplant. The traditional therapy usually includes a calcineurin inhibitor (cyclosporine), a corticosteroid (prednisone; methylprednisolone), and mycophenolate mofetil (CellCept).

Monoclonal antibodies, genetically engineered immunosuppressive agents, are also used in combination with other drugs to prevent graft rejection. These agents hold great promise in the treatment of cancer, transplant rejection, and diagnosis of disease. Recombinant DNA technology, another form of genetic engineering, uses segments of DNA from one type of organism (e.g., *Escherichia coli,* yeast, or mammalian tissue) and combines it with genes of another organism to create large amounts of human proteins. The proteins include human insulin and cytokines, substances produced by white blood cells (WBCs) that assist in immunological cell growth, i.e., interlukin-2 and α-interferon. The cytokines function in both inflammation and the immune response (Janeway, Travers, Walport, & Shlomchik, 2004).

Apheresis is sometimes used for treating autoimmune diseases and other disorders. The procedure consists of withdrawal of blood from a donor, removal of one or more components (as plasma, blood platelets, or WBCs) from the blood, and transfusion into patients with low platelet or WBC counts; the remaining blood is transfused back into the donor. **Plasmapheresis,** or **plasma exchange,** is a process for removing plasma that contains components that are thought to be the cause of a disease, such as autoantibodies or antigen-antibody complexes. The plasma is usually replaced by normal saline, lactated Ringer's solution, frozen plasma, or albumen. The procedure involves removing whole blood through a needle inserted into one arm, circulating the blood through a cell separator where the blood is separated into plasma and the cellular components; the destructive components are removed, and the remainder of the contents is returned via a needle inserted in the opposite arm. The platelets, plasma proteins, WBCs, and RBCs can be selected separately. Side effects associated with the procedure are hypotension, probably because a vasovagal response or transitory volume changes, and citrate toxicity. Citrate, an anticoagulant, may cause hypocalcemia and result in headache, dizziness, and paresthesias (Broyles, Reiss, & Evans, 2007).

Hypersensitivity Disorders

Hypersensitivity to an allergen, or **antigen,** is because of a heightened immune response. The sensitization begins as an individual develops IgE antibodies to an antigen. The IgE antibodies adhere to the basophils and mast cells on the mucosal surfaces, the respiratory tract, and the GI tract. Reexposure to the antigen, or allergen, results in the hypersensitive responses, such as sneezing, asthma symptoms, and potential anaphylaxis. The responses are dependent on the host's defense mechanisms, the characteristics and concentration of the allergen, the route of entry, the amount of exposure, and the organ that is affected. Hypersensitivity disorders are more thoroughly discussed in chapter 43.

AUTOIMMUNE DISORDERS

Organs and tissues commonly affected by autoimmune disorders include blood components, such as RBCs, blood vessels, connective tissues, endocrine glands, such as the thyroid or pancreas, muscles, joints, and skin. Most of the autoimmune disorders are associated with the connective tissues of the body. Among the most common disorders are osteoarthritis, rheumatoid arthritis (RA), gout, SLE, progressive systemic sclerosis (scleroderma), and ankylosing spondylitis, which are all diseases that have common clinical manifestations of pain and impaired mobility.

Many factors are involved that cause the immune system to fail to recognize the body's normal tissue as self. Basically, these self-killing cells begin to break down normal cells in a particular area of the body resulting in the autoimmune disorder. Several theories have been proposed including genetic predisposition, infections, interaction of T and B cells, introduction of foreign tissue such as a blood transfusion or transplant tissue, and environmental factors. Viral infections have been linked to development of multiple sclerosis (MS) and type I diabetes mellitus. Rheumatic fever, caused by a streptococcal infection, has been linked to rheumatic heart disease. Drugs can be precipitating factors. Hormones have an effect on autoimmune diseases and more women have autoimmune disease than men. Autoimmune disorders and allergy are both caused by hypersensitivity reactions. It is believed that a history of allergies indicates increased risk of autoimmune disorders. Age is considered a factor because there is an increase of autoantibodies.

Much research has been conducted over the past 10 years to understand how the immune system works and to discover how the immune system may be enhanced to prevent these disorders or to promote healing. We do know that the immune system is sensitive to internal and external environmental factors. Nutrition has been found to play a vital role in the body's ability to fight infection and disease. Obesity may be a contributing factor to immune dysfunction. Depression has been identified as a factor that interferes with recovery, motivation, and compliance as well as decreasing energy and immune function.

Autoimmune disorders can involve a single organ or tissue that can result in local tissue damage, such as in Hashimoto's thyroiditis. The thyroid becomes enlarged and symptoms of hypothyroidism are present. Treatment is lifelong thyroid hormone replacement. Crohn's disease affects the GI system; MS affects the CNS. System-wide autoimmune disorders, such as SLE, involve the reaction of autoantibodies to almost every cell in the body. Goodpasture's syndrome is a disorder in which autoantibodies destroy the basement membrane of the lungs and kidneys. A person may experience a cluster of autoimmune diseases, e.g., RA and Addison's disease. As a result many outcomes may occur and encompass a multitude of autoimmune disorders. Some disorders have multiple interrelated causes.

Hormones or other substances normally produced by the affected organ may need to be supplemented. This may include thyroid supplements, vitamins, insulin injections, or other supplements. Disorders that affect the blood components may require blood transfusions. Measures to assist mobility or other function may be needed for disorders that affect the bones, joints, or muscles. **Autoimmunity** is controlled through balanced suppression of the immune system. The goal is to reduce the immune response against normal body tissue while leaving the immune response intact against microorganisms and abnormal tissues.

Rheumatoid Arthritis

RA is one of several inflammatory joint diseases that plague patients. The disease causes chronic inflammation in the connective tissue in the joints. RA can also cause systemic symptoms, such as "fever, malaise, rash, lymph node or spleen enlargement, and Raynaud phenomenon (transient lack of circulation to the fingertips and toes)" (Crowther & McCance, 2004, p. 1094). This is a debilitating chronic autoimmune disease that can be controlled and treated, but to date there is no known cure.

Epidemiology

Once thought of as an old person's disease, RA affects people from the young to the old. In the adult population the first symptoms of RA appear generally between the ages of 20 and 40, but can occur at any age (Hellman & Stone, 2004). RA occurs in 1 to 2 percent of adults and develops more in women to men (three to one ratio).

After the age of 55 it is estimated that RA occurs in 2 percent of men and 5 percent of women. A higher incidence is seen in North American Indians and Eskimos, which supports a genetic link. The onset of symptoms and speed with which the disease progresses, appears to also be linked to age and stressors. When RA develops at a younger age, the progress appears to be slow and insidious. In contrast, when the onset is after the age of 60, the patients develop symptoms that are acute and widespread but have a shorter duration and a better prognosis. On the other hand, with pregnancy, most women report an improvement in symptoms, but up to one third of women report no change in symptoms. Statistics related to RA include that 10 percent of patients will experience remission, 15 percent develop severe progressive and destructive symptoms, and 75 percent experience a slow progressing and gradually worsening course of symptoms.

Etiology

Despite years of research, the exact cause of RA remains elusive. It is thought to be a combination of genetic hormonal, environmental, and reproductive factors that lead to the development of the disease. Research has determined that most patients with RA have a Class Two HLA with an identified five amino acid sequence (Hellman & Stone, 2004).

Bacteria, mycoplasmas, and viruses may also be contributors to RA occurrences. The Epstein-Barr virus has been of particular interest to researchers in the cause of RA. Rheumatoid factors (RFs) develop as a result of prolonged or concentrated exposure to the organisms (an antigen-antibody response). RFs are immunoglobulins (Ig) that have become autoantibodies (IgG, IgM, and, occasionally IgA). The RF attacks the host tissue (self-antigens), specifically the synovial membrane, forming immune complexes (Crowther & McCance, 2004).

Pathophysiology

Joint deformity in RA is the result of repeated inflammation episodes (Figure 42-7). Damage occurs in four phases. (a) Initiation phase: some changes in the synovial lining of the joint are evident. (b) Immune response phase: A cascade of events begins as CD4 T cells stimulate the immune response; many leukocytes, macrophages, and fibroblasts migrate to the syn-

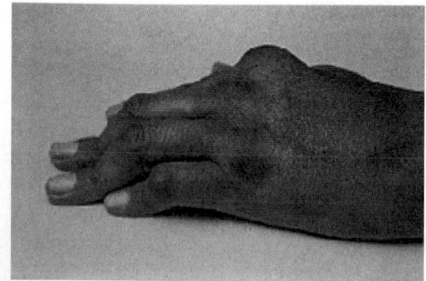

Figure 42-7 Arthritis is considered a chronic health problem. Courtesy of Arthritis Foundation.

ovial fluid; B lymphocytes arrive and release the IgM antibody that can be measured as rheumatoid factor (RF). Proinflammatory cytokines and enzymes begin the erosive tissue damage process; complement and other chemotaxins help to increase the inflammation; and the cytokines tumor necrosis factor-alpha (TNF-α) and interleukin-1 (IL-1) perpetuate the inflammatory process. (c) Inflammatory phase: Swelling caused by inflammation damages tiny blood vessels that contain the synovial fluid; the body releases arachidonic acid and lysosomal enzymes. Oxygen radicals develop. As the inflammation continues, the cells increase in size and become hyperactive stromal cells that thicken the synovial membrane. (d) The destruction phase: A thickened fibrous scar tissue (pannus) is formed and adheres to the articular (joint) surface of the cartilage. The fibrous tissue may become calcified; the joint becomes fused and results in permanent deformity. Joints commonly affected are the knees, ankles, shoulders, wrists, and proximal interphalangeal and metacarpophalangeal joints.

Assessment with Clinical Manifestations

Common early clinical manifestations include diffuse musculoskeletal pain, low-grade fever, possible anorexia, and loss of weight. Later, articular (within the joint) manifestations include synovitis (inflammation of the synovial capsule causing escape of synovial fluid into the synovial capsule). Subsequent hypertrophy and symmetrical joint deformity (particularly wrists, hands, or knees) occur. Pain; muscle spasm; and weakness, because of contractures of muscles, tendons, and ligaments; and muscle and soft tissue damage greatly impact the person's daily activities. Many times the shoulders are affected. Extra-articular manifestations that can occur at any time during the course of the disease include Sjögren's syndrome (chronic inflammatory eye disorder), pulmonary fibrosis, pericarditis, nerve compression, and vasculitis. Development of nontender rheumatoid nodules that are made up of granulation tissue surrounding a core of fibrous debris can occur in the subcutaneous tissue and even in visceral organs, such as the lungs and the heart. Sleep disturbances are common (Capriotti, 2004).

Stiffness and diminished function after prolonged activity especially on arising in the morning are hallmarks of the progressive severity of the disease (Figure 42-8). The person self-limits motion, usually by holding the extremity in a flexed position, which may result in contractures that further contribute to decreased joint function. At times, the individual may have a remission of symptoms for several months or years; however, remission seldom occurs if the joint damage extends beyond two years. Early diagnosis is important to prevent joint damage; however, erosion damage can be evident for 30 percent of those with an early diagnosis, and 60 percent have definite joint damage by two years. Diagnosis can be challenging because of the many clinical manifestations that mimic other syndromes (Capriotti, 2004).

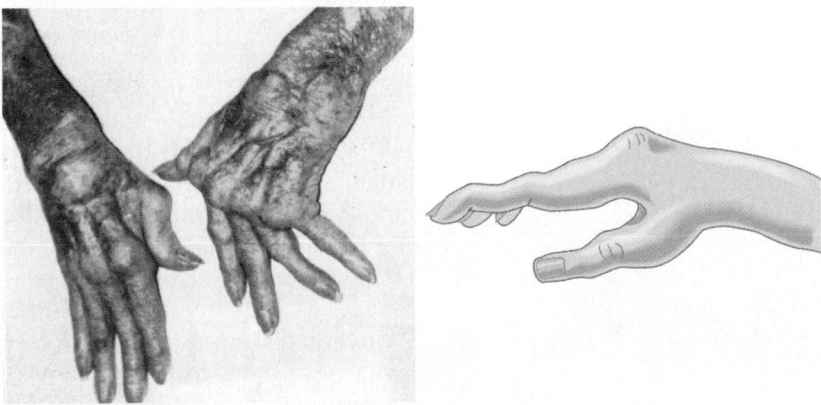

Figure 42-8 RA often results in ulnar deviation and swan neck deformity of the hand.

Skills 360°

Assessment of JRA

In 1975 a mysterious disease outbreak primarily affecting young people in Lyme, Connecticut, was misdiagnosed as JRA. Scientists discovered the disease was caused by the *Borrelia burgdorferi* (Bd), a spirochete bacteria. Lyme disease is usually transmitted by the deer tick, but a variety of other insects can be hosts. The disease can also be transmitted through sexual contact. The spirochete often embeds into multiple organs, tendons, muscles, the heart, and brain; it may lie dormant in cysts, and then reemerge at a later time. It is often resistant to drug therapy. Clinical manifestations mimic symptoms of several other diseases including Lou Gehrig's disease, chronic fatigue and fibromyalgia syndromes, irritable bowel syndrome, SLE, RA, and syphilis. ELISA and Western blot antibody test results may be inconclusive. Careful assessment and monitoring are essential.

Initial clinical manifestations include flu-like symptoms (headache, fever, and muscle aches); later manifestations include neck rigidity, jaw discomfort, muscle pain and stiffness, lymphadenopathy, burning sensations in lower extremities, and red eyes. Initial skin assessment may reveal a bull's eye mark and rash; however, different skin marks have been noted. Check for ticks on patients, especially on the lower extremities, who have been outside in high grassy areas, hiking, hunting, or camping in remote places. Ticks should be removed with tweezers without twisting. Provide education on preventive measures. The disease can also be transmitted through the placenta from mother to fetus and by blood transfusion.

Adapted from Sellman, S. (2005). Disease of disguise: Learning about Lyme. Canadian Journal of Health and Nutrition, 275(15), 76–78.

Juvenile Rheumatoid Arthritis

Juvenile idiopathic rheumatoid arthritis (JRA) is the most prevalent chronic disease in children under 16 years of age. Approximately 30,000 to 50,000 children in the United States have been diagnosed with the disease, and several cases have been reported worldwide. Onset usually occurs around 8 years of age with a later peak during puberty. Disease symptoms frequently mimic those of other diseases, and diagnostic tests can be inconclusive, resulting in misdiagnosis and a missed opportunity for early treatment. Initial symptoms are frequently called growing pains; however, enlarged knuckles that are warm to the touch complaints of pain in ankles, feet, or knees; and decreased range of motion should receive prompt attention (Myer, Brunner, Melson, Paterno, & Ford, 2005).

The chronic recurrent systemic and joint inflammation episodes restricts the child's ability to participate in physical activities, limits interaction with peers, frequently subjects them to taunting by other children, and affects the quality of life. Growth development is slowed, and because of the long-term articular and systemic effects of the disease and side affects of the immunosuppressive drugs, the child and family must face lifelong challenges. Children often have a better response to the drug methotrexate (MTX) than adults. Thalidomide, a drug once used as a sedative and antinauseate in the 1950s and 1960s, has been used in a six-month clinical trial with 13 children in the United States and Brazil. There was a positive response from 11 of the participants permitting a decreased use of steroids. Six individuals were able to discontinue steroid therapy. The participants agreed to use birth control precautions because of the teratogen side affects of the drug. Thalidomide is also

Uncovering the Evidence

Surgical Interventions for JRA

Discussion: To evaluate the outcome of surgery for children and adolescents who were followed for a minimum of 12 years postarthroplasty. Eight patients diagnosed with refractory JRA were evaluated preoperatively and postoperatively related to amount of pain, range of motion, walking ability, and radiological evaluation of alignment and component loosening (a total of 15 knees were evaluated).

Preoperatively, seven participants were in wheelchairs, and others had mobility dysfunction; postoperatively, six were able to walk and had a mean arc of motion from 36° to 79°. Twelve knees were pain free; radiographic evaluation indicated 13 of the 15 knees were in natural alignment and 2 were in valgus (bent outward). Three knees required further revision. All the participants were employed; all could function independently; four were married; and three had children.

Implications for Practice: Arthroplasty is a reasonable procedure for those who do not respond to the nonoperative procedures.

Source: Palmer, D., Mulhall, K., Thomson, C., Severson, E., Santos, E., & Saleh, K. (2005). Total knee arthroplasty in juvenile rheumatoid arthritis. Journal of Bone and Joint Surgery (Am), 87(7), 1510–1514.

used the cancer complications of HIV/AIDS in adults. Use of the drug must be carefully monitored (Pediatric Alert, 2004).

Diagnostic Tests

The most commonly used laboratory diagnostic test is that of serum RF. This factor is positive in approximately 80 percent of all patients with RA. Other laboratory findings (Box 42-4) that will show an elevation or be positive when RA is present are antimitochondrial antibody (AMA); antinuclear antibodies (ANA); antistreptolysin O (ASO); complement C3; C-reactive protein; lupus erythematosus cell preparation (LE prep); thyroid antibody (TA), and erythrocyte sedimentation rate (ESR). Slight anemia may be present. X-rays are useful when a series of films over time can be obtained. Comparison films allow monitoring of changes in the bony structure. Bone scans can detect early joint changes and confirm diagnosis of RA.

Samples of synovial fluid are assistive when confirming RA or differentiating diagnoses. Synovial fluid in early disease is straw-colored, slightly cloudy, and with many flecks of fibrin. The WBC count will be 3,500 to 25,000/mm^3.

Nursing Diagnoses

Based on the information gathered, examples of nursing diagnoses in the patient with RA may include those found in Table 42-1.

Planning and Implementation

Expected outcomes include preserving the individual's participation in daily activities, maintaining pain at a level that permits participation in self-care; to be able to balance rest and activity; to adhere to the therapeutic regimen; and to cope effectively with the numerous psycho-social-spiritual impact of the disease. The nurse is an integral part of the multidisciplinary team in coordinating the various activities that promote optimal outcomes. The nurse must, also, be knowledgeable of the latest drug safety information. Vigilant assessment of the patient's

---

BOX 42-4

THE AMERICAN COLLEGE OF RHEUMATOLOGY CRITERIA FOR DIAGNOSIS OF RA

- Morning stiffness lasting more than one hour
- Arthritis of three or more joint areas
- Arthritis of hand joints
- Symmetrical arthritis
- Rheumatoid nodules over extensor surfaces or bony prominences
- Serum rheumatoid factors
- Radiographic changes

Source: Janeway, C. A., Jr., Travers, P., Walport, M., & Shlomchik, M. J. (2004). Immunobiology: The immune system in health and disease (6th ed.). New York: Garland Science Publishing.

TABLE 42-1 **Nursing Diagnoses, Nursing Interventions Classifications and Nursing Outcomes for RA**

NURSING DIAGNOSIS	NURSING INTERVENTION CLASSIFICATIONS (NIC)	NURSING OUTCOMES CLASSIFICATIONS (NOC)
Pain, acute	Analgesic administration	Comfort level
	Pain management	Pain control
	Heat/cold application	Pain level
	Medication management	
	Transcutaneous	
	Electrical nerve stimulation (TENS)	
Pain, chronic	Analgesic administration	Comfort level
	Pain management	Pain control
	Heat/cold application	Pain: disruptive effects
	Medication management	Pain level
	Progressive muscle	
	Relaxation	
	Simple massage	
	Transcutaneous	
	Electrical nerve stimulation (TENS)	
Impaired physical mobility	Bed rest care	Coordinated movement
	Energy management	Joint movement: Active
	Exercise therapy: Ambulation	Mobility
	Exercise therapy: Joint mobility	Self-care: Activities of daily living
	Self-care assistance	Transfer performance
	Teaching: Prescribed activity/exercise	Knowledge: Prescribed activity
		Motivation
Activity intolerance	Activity therapy	Activity tolerance
	Energy management	Endurance
	Exercise promotion: Strength training	Energy conservation
	Teaching: Prescribed activity/exercise	
Self-care deficit:	Self-care assistance: Bathing/hygiene	Self-care: ADL
Bath/hygiene	Self-care assistance: Dressing/grooming	Self-care: Bathing
Dressing/grooming	Self-care assistance: Toileting	Self-care: Hygiene
		Self-care: Dressing
		Self-care: Grooming
		Self-care: Toileting

Adapted from DeLaune, S., & Ladner, P. (2006). Fundamentals of nursing (3rd ed.). New York: Thomson Delmar Learning; Janeway, C. A., Jr., Travers, P., Walport, M., & Shlomchik, M. J. (2004). Immunobiology, the immune system in health and disease (6th ed.). New York: Garland Science Publishing.

increased susceptibility to infections and toxic effects of immunosuppressive therapy to organs and tissues is essential. The nurse must be able to provide appropriate preoperative and postoperative care and participate in discharge education procedures to aid the patient and caregiver with skills and coping strategies to effectively manage living with a chronic disease. Particular attention should be given to social support and prevention of feelings of isolation.

The goals of treatment focus on pain management and reduction of inflammation, promoting remission, and increasing function abilities, and helping individuals to cope with the disabilities. Progression of the disease can be slowed with early aggressive treatment. Multidisciplinary approaches are used, including muscle strengthening, range of motion, and activities to prevent imbalance and the risk of further injury because of falls. Many people derive benefits from water exercise. Applications of heat or cold and use of analgesic ointments to the affected areas often provide pain relief; however actual massage can aggravate the inflammation in the acute inflamed joints. Immersion of the hands in warm paraffin baths followed by hand exercises has also been beneficial in relieving pain and stiffness. Transcutaneous electrical nerve stimulation (TENS) is commonly used for pain relief. Complementary or alternative therapy is a popular method with patients to integrate with the traditional medical methods. Acupuncture, yoga, massage, guided imagery, and therapeutic touch are examples. Surgeries, such as tendon transfer, surgical removal of the synovia in the affected joints, fusion of a joint, arthroplasty, and joint replacement have provided many individuals with freedom from pain, increased mobility, increased independence and quality of life (Price, 2004).

Nutrition

Although there is no specific nutritional therapy for the treatment of RA, it is important to employ the services of a dietitian. Weight loss is often associated with RA related to several factors: loss or change of appetite because of the stress of the disease or prescribed medications, inability to prepare meals secondary to loss of strength in hands or decreased stamina to prepare the meals; and depression because of the impact of a chronic and debilitating disease. Recommended nutritional intake is high in calories and vitamins (Crowther & McCance, 2004).

Pharmacology

Medications to manage RA include (a) selective and nonselective nonsteroidal anti-inflammatory drugs (NSAIDs); (b) synthetic and biological disease-modifying antirheumatic drugs (DMARDs); and (c) corticosteroids. Usually first-line nonselective NSAIDs that are available as OTC drugs and prescription NSAIDs are used to alleviate the symptoms of RA; however, they do not prevent the progress of the disease (OTC drugs are usually prescribed until a definite diagnosis of RA is made). Long-term use of NSAIDs can cause GI distress and bleeding and impaired renal function. Often a combination of drugs is used along with the NSAIDs. Prostaglandin analogues or proton pump inhibitors are used to protect the stomach mucosa. Until recently, COX-2 inhibitors (selective NSAIDs) were mainline drugs to reduce inflammation and to alleviate the pain and of arthritic disorders. However, FDA approval of Vioxx and Bextra has been withdrawn, and precautions have been issued for the use of Celebrex.

Aurothioglucose (goldthioglucose, Solganal) has sometimes been given intramuscularly to relieve the joint inflammation and to slow the progress of RA and JRA. It has been an adjunctive medication when symptoms have not responded to NSAIDs. There are several side affects, such as allergic reactions, skin rashes, nausea and vomiting, abdominal cramps, diarrhea, anorexia, and metallic taste. Currently the drug is rarely used (Spratto & Woods, 2007).

Currently, most individuals diagnosed with RA receive a combination therapy of MTX and a biological DMARD. Synthetic DMARDs include MTX, which has a potent immunosuppressant and anti-inflammatory effect. Infliximab (mAb) is a monoclonal antibody, which binds directly to the TNF-α and impairs its ability to bind to receptors on cell surfaces. It, also, has anti-inflammatory effects. Adalimumab, another genetically engineered IgG antibody drug, attaches to the TNF and impairs its ability to bind to cell surface receptors (Table 42-2).

TABLE 42-2 Examples of Drugs Used for RA Therapy

DRUG CLASSIFICATION	CHARACTERISTICS	SIDE EFFECTS	PRECAUTIONS/INTERVENTIONS
Nonselective NSAIDs Motrin, Advil (ibuprofen) Aleve (naproxen) Indocin (indomethacin Relafen (nabumetone) Feldene (piroxicam)	Provide pain and stiffness relief. Inhibit the cyclooxygenase pathways, which produce prostaglandins during inflammation cascade.	Esophagitis, gastritis, gastroduodenal ulceration.	Misoprostol (Cytotec) a prostaglandin analogue to protect gastric mucosa; Caution: not to be used in pregnant women, nursing mothers, and women planning pregnancy Prilosec (omeprazole) and other proton pump inhibitors to protect gastric mucosa
Selective NSAIDs COX-2 inhibitors	Reduce pain and inflammation. Most effective in combination with DMARDs	Gastric irritation (reduced in comparison to NSAIDs)	Proton pump inhibitors to reduce gastric side effects Some removed from market because of cardiovascular problems
Synthetic DMARDS Methotrexate (MTX) Infliximab Adalimumab	Diminish progression of RA	Bone marrow suppression, hepatotoxicity, pulmonary fibrosis, pneumonitis Hypersensitivity reactions	Vigilant monitoring of liver and renal function and symptoms of immunosuppression. CBC, CXRs. Teratogenic effects: not for pregnant women or women planning pregnancy. Alcohol abstinence.
Biological DMARDs TNF-α antagonists— Enbrel (etanercept) Remicade (infliximab) Humira (adalimumab) Adalimumab	Diminish cytokine response to inflammation; reduces damaging effects (erosion of bone) Safe for children over 4 years old with juvenile RA	Immunosuppression infliximab: Greater chance for developing lymphoma	Discontinue drug if infection occurs. Pregnancy safety is unknown. Children to have immunizations up to date.
Costimulatory blockers Abatacept (CTLA4Ig)	Inhibits stimulation of antigen-presenting cells in activation of T lymphocytes. Best results in combination with MTX.	Upper respiratory infection, GI distress, rash, dizziness	Monitor for adverse side effects.
Interleukin antagonists Kineret (anakinra)	Reduces erosive damage due to cytokines released by monocytes and macrophages.	Injection site reactions, headache, GI distress.	Not to be used in combination with TNF antagonists—increased risk of infection. Contraindicated for persons with active or chronic infections. No live vaccines to be given. Has not been tested in children, or for pregnancy safety.
Drugs under investigation Rituxan (rituximab) Genetically engineered monoclonal antibody.	Targets specific surface antigens on circulating B lymphocytes. Shows promise alone and in combination with MTX to reduce progress of RA	Immunosuppressant	

Adapted from Capriotti, T. (2004). The "alphabet" of rheumatoid arthritis therapy. Nursing, 13(6), 920–928.

"Abatacept (CTLA4Ig) is the first in a new class of biologic DMARDs known as co-stimulatory or second-signal blockers" (Capriotti, 2004, p. 425). Clinical trials have shown diminished inflammation and reduction in symptoms over a 12-month period. Kineret (anakinra), an interleukin antagonist, interferes with the proinflammatory effects of the body's cytokines.

Drugs under investigation include Rituxan (rituximab), a genetically engineered monoclonal antibody that targets specific surface antigens on circulating B lymphocytes. The drug has been used in treating lymphoma. A recent large investigation was conducted by the Arthritis Foundation to determine the effects of the rituximab in combination with MTX and cyclophosphamide. Findings demonstrated marked improvement in RA symptoms, but further research is needed (Capriotti, 2004; Chambers & Isenberg, 2005). Rituximab has also been used in combination with thalidomide for treatment of lymphoma and used alone or combination with other drugs to treat dermatomyositis, IgM-mediated neuropathies, Wegener's granulomatosis, Goodpasture's syndrome, myasthenia gravis, refractory pemphigus vulgaris, and idiopathic thrombocytopenia. The safety profile of rituximab indicates there are fewer adverse affects than other immunosuppressive agents. However, more research is needed because many of the studies have been small (Chambers & Isenberg, 2005).

Surgery

Most of the surgeries performed to correct the damage done by RA are joint replacements (arthroplasty). Most joints can be replaced with some degree of normal mobility returning to the joints. The most common joint replacements done are total hip and total knee replacements. These will be discussed in detail in the section on osteoarthritis. Finger, shoulder, elbow, and ankle joints can also be replaced.

Other surgeries done to repair RA damage are synovectomies (removal of the synovial membrane) joint fusions (total immobility of the affected joint), and tendon transfers to prevent deformities or relieve contractions.

Evaluation of Outcomes

Refer to Table 42-1 for the nursing diagnoses, nursing interventions classifications, and nursing outcomes displayed for RA.

Sjögrens's Syndrome

Sjögren's syndrome is a chronic inflammatory disorder involving the eyes that is primary problem or secondary to RA. There is a decrease in lacrimation and salivation due to obstruction of the secretory ducts by the immune complexes. Dry eyes (keratoconjunctivitis sicca) and dry mouth (xerostomia) are hallmarks of the disorder.

Manifestations include swelling of the lacrimal ducts and parotid glands and fatigue. The presence of RF, ANAs, and antiextractable nuclear antigen are revealed through diagnostic tests. Instillation of artificial tears helps to keep the eyes moist and to prevent corneal abrasions. Artificial saliva can also be used for the xerostomia. Untreated, the syndrome can result in visual problems, oral ulcerations, dental caries, and dysphagia. The presurgical procedure, nothing by mouth (NPO), is an uncomfortable experience for patients with this disorder. Artificial saliva should be used and ocular lubricants should also be instilled preoperatively.

Systemic Lupus Erythematosus

SLE is the most severe form of this autoimmune disorder and is classified as a multisystem disease. The discoid type is a milder form that affects the skin, primarily the face, neck, and upper chest. A third type of this disorder is a reversible form due to reactions to various medications, such as oral contraceptives, isoniazid, procainamide, and methyldopa, and others that are known to bind with the person's DNA. Another possibility is because of the correlation of the patient's genetic predisposition to SLE and how the medication is metabolized. SLE is a relatively rare condition that affects younger women between the ages of 15 and 40 years; therefore, this suggests a hormonal influence is involved. It is more commonly seen in African American, Hispanic (American), and Asian (American) women than in Caucasians. The incidence is higher in some families than in others. Pregnant women with SLE are more prone to spontaneous abortion and premature delivery. Close monitoring is needed (Alarcon-Segovia, et al., 2005).

Epidemiology

SLE is most prevalent among women and, in particular, those of African American, Asian (American), or Native American descent. The onset of SLE generally occurs between the ages of 15 and 45, with 80 percent of cases affecting women during their childbearing years. The incidence of SLE in the African American population is 1:250 versus 1:1000 in the Caucasian population (Trethewey, 2004).

Etiology

The etiology is unknown. Genetic predisposition, infection, environmental irritants, physical and emotional stress, and exposure to ultraviolet (UV) B radiation have been suggested as potential contributing factors.

Pathophysiology

A combination of factors is involved in the development of ANAs. The hyperactivity of B cells and a defect in the body's T suppressor cell that normally protects the body from developing ANAs triggers the inflammatory cascade of events that result in systemic tissue damage. The basement membrane of the kidneys is particularly vulnerable; deposits of the antibody complex can lead to glomerulonephritis. The ANAs that are produced in SLE are specifically directed at the cell nuclei (the cell command centers). When the cells die, the nuclei are released into the blood stream and bind with the ANAs and form a large complex that is deposited in the tissues. SLE complexes can affect any organ system, including the musculoskeletal system, the CNS, the heart, and blood vessels, causing vasculitis that results in a diminished supply of oxygen to the organs and tissues (Porth, 2004).

Assessment with Clinical Manifestations

Polyarthritis (involving many joints) and polyarthralgia (pain in many joints) are present in a majority of the cases. Pain is present in the small joints of the hands, feet, wrists, and knees. Extra-articular manifestations include lethargy, malaise, fever, and loss of weight. In the acute stages the patient may have a butterfly rash on the face that resembles the face of a wolf (Figure 42-9). The person may also develop pleural effusion and basilar pneumonia, generalized lymphadenopathy, pericarditis, hepatosplenomegaly. In severe cases delirium convulsions, psychosis, and coma may occur.

Manifestations of the chronic form are related to the organ or tissues involved. Fever, malaise, and weight loss may continue. The cutaneous lesions of the discoid type are evident as well as erythematosus (diffused redness) of exposed skin. Additional symptoms include generalized lymphadenopathy, severe hemolytic anemia, thrombocytopenic purpura, enlargement of the spleen, and cardiopulmonary problems, including pleural effusion, tachycardia, and peripheral vascular syndromes, i.e., Raynaud's phenomenon and gangrene. Ulcerative

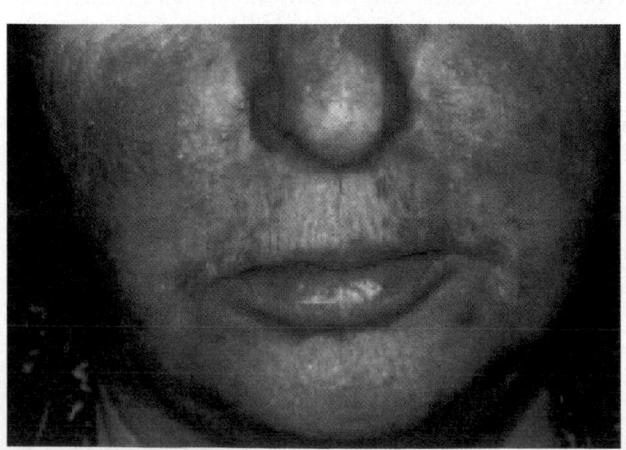

Figure 42-9 Butterfly rash seen in SLE. Courtesy of the American Academy of Dermatology.

mucous membrane lesions; GI disturbances, such as nausea, vomiting, bloody stools, and hepatic dysfunction; myalgia; and multiple neurological symptoms can occur. The disease is often called the great imitator and can be confused with RA because of the symmetrical joint involvement.

The course of the disease is variable. An acute episode can progress rapidly; however, the disease commonly develops into a chronic phase with remissions and exacerbations. The disease seems to be more severe when the onset occurs at a young age. Glomerulonephritis is the common cause of death. Cardiac and CNS problems are also major causes of morbidity. Recent developments in scientific technology has greatly improved survival rates and contributed to a better quality of life. However, the long-term survival rate is still unpredictable (NIAMS, 2005).

Diagnostic Tests

SLE should be suspected in patients with glomerulonephritis, photosensitivity, characteristic skin rashes, CNS disease, and various cytopenias, such as the Coombs'-positive anemia, hemolytic anemia, leukopenia, and thrombocytopenia. The ANA titer represents the most sensitive American College of Rheumatology (ACR) criteria (Gill, Quisel, Rocca, & Walters, 2003). More than 99 percent of patients with SLE demonstrate an elevated ANA titer at some point, although other situations, such as advancing age, infections, RA, and certain drugs, produce positive results. Testing for antibody to double-stranded DNA antigen (anti-dsDNA) and antibody to Sm nuclear antigen (anti-Sm) are specific to SLE and are therefore useful in differential diagnosis. Particularly in high titers, these tests demonstrate a high specificity for SLE, although their sensitivity is low, indicating that while these tests are useful in establishing a diagnosis of SLE, they should not be used to rule out SLE in the presence of a negative test result. A decrease in the complement factors C3 and C4, as well as an increase in their degradation products C3d/C4d, can be seen in active disease as a result of circulating immune complex disposition in tissues and activation of complement and are therefore useful in measuring disease activity.

Additional diagnostic tests may be warranted to rule out the presence of associated systemic complications. A kidney biopsy may be required if blood and urine evaluations indicate evidence of renal disease. In the presence of possible neuropsychiatric complications, a lumbar puncture may be performed to rule out infection. Magnetic resonance imaging (MRI) is the modality of choice for the identification of white matter lesions but may lack clarity in its ability to distinguish lesions from cerebral vasculitis. Psychometric testing may also be used. The presence of antiphospholipid antibodies and lupus anticoagulant are constitutive for antiphospholipid syndrome (Daniels, 2003).

Nursing Diagnoses

Refer to Table 42-1 for the nursing diagnoses, nursing interventions classifications, and nursing outcomes displayed for RA.

Planning and Implementation

A multidisciplinary approach is used to address the acute and chronic disease symptoms. The patient must be a partner in making treatment decision and in providing the health care team about the patterns of disease activity. The goals include prevention in progressive loss of organ function, reducing the possibility of exacerbation events, minimizing disability, and preventing complications of medication therapy. Medications include NSAIDs to reduce pain, inflammation, and fever. An antimalarial drug, such as hydroxychloroquine sulfate (Plaquenil), is sometimes used to control the fatigue, rash, cutaneous and musculoskeletal symptoms, and lung inflammation. Corticosteroids are used for initial symptoms and may be used periodically in low doses. Immunosuppressive drugs, such as cyclophosphamide, can be used.

A combination of rituximab, cyclophosphamide, and prednisolone was used in a study of five female patients with refractory SLE. All of the participants responded well to the therapy. Several small studies reported similar results. Consistent improvement in clinical manifestations and laboratory findings were reported (Chambers & Isenberg, 2005). Allogenic stem cell transplantation for patients with acute forms of SLE who have not responded to three or more months of medication therapy and immunosuppressive agents may prove to be a preferred treatment in the future. Current research activities are investigating the interaction between genes and environmental triggers and development of new drugs (NIAMS, 2005).

Nursing interventions will depend on the stage of the disease, the patient's response to the condition, and the severity and type of disease. Patient education is of prime importance throughout the course of the disease, including appropriate skin care, nutrition, and minimizing the risk of opportunistic infections. Because exposure to UV rays seems to exacerbate the disease process, it is imperative that the individual avoid sun exposure. The patient and caregiver must also be knowledgeable about the diagnosis and prognosis of the disease, the medication regimen, interactive effects with food and other medications, and the importance of communicating with the health care providers. Learning to cope with the disease, exacerbations, and prognosis involves psycho-social-spiritual support systems.

Evaluation of Outcomes

Refer to Table 42-1 for the nursing diagnoses, nursing interventions classifications, and nursing outcomes displayed for RA.

Progressive Systemic Sclerosis (Scleroderma)

Progressive systemic sclerosis is a rare connective tissue disease that involves excessive collagen deposition and changes in both the humoral and cellular immunity. Etiology is unknown. The localized form is less severe and primarily affects the skin. The morphea type skin lesions are hard, oval, and white with a purple ring surrounding them. Linear scleroderma has a lesion that is similar to a thick line of skin on the arms, legs, or forehead. That can become fixated to the subdermal structures, including the fascia that covers tendon sheaths and muscles.

Assessment with Clinical Manifestations

The generalized form involves the skin and many internal organs. Organs involved include the skin, the synovium, digital arteries, and parenchyma and small arteries in internal organs in the limited subcutaneous scleroderma form. The skin, muscles, joints, lungs, esophagus, heart, digestive system, and kidneys are often affected in the diffuse subcutaneous form, often termed as CREST. Clinical manifestations include:

- **C**alcinosis: The development of small white calcium deposits under the skin. A chalky fluid drains when the lumps break open.
- **R**aynaud's syndrome is prevalent in most patients with scleroderma. Spasms of arteries and arterioles occur spontaneously usually due to exposure to cold or emotional stress.
- **E**sophageal movement is decreased because of deposits of collagen and muscle atrophy.
- **S**clerodactyly of the fingers and toes.
- **T**elangiectasia: A permanent dilation of the capillaries, arterioles, and venules.

The localized form usually has a slow onset and clinical manifestations may not occur for 10 to 20 years. Clinical manifestations include pain, edema, calcification, and muscular atrophy. When the heart, lung, or kidney involvement is severe, it tends to occur early in the disease and often leads to high mortality.

Treatment is supportive and tailored to the clinical manifestations. The primary goal is to promote remission. Steroids and immunosuppressants in high doses are used. Nursing interventions include prevention of skin breakdown and ulceration. Patient education is directed toward proper skin care using gentle soaps and nonalchohol astringent lotions, and educating the patient how to manage the polyarthralgia and polyarthritis associated with Raynaud's phenomenon. Additional information includes avoiding activities that trigger pain, using protective joint strategies, avoiding extremes of cold, eliminating smoking, and resting the painful part during acute pain. Patients with esophageal dysfunction may require diet modifications. Ensuring that the patient continues follow-up care, and psycho-social-spiritual support is an important measure.

Case Study

Nursing Care Plan

Mrs. Donovan, has been HIV positive for nine years. She is in her primary health care provider's clinic complaining of intermittent nonbloody diarrhea and abdominal cramping that she has had for four weeks. In addition, she has a small burn wound on her right forearm that she states has not been healing well. She has lost 10 percent of her body weight in the past three weeks. She states, "I do not have the energy to eat or get dressed." On further questioning she said she has eaten primarily bread, cereal, milk, and potatoes.

Mrs. Donovan's vital signs are: blood pressure: 132/76; pulse: 78; respiration: 16; and temperature: 36.9° C (98.4° F). While at the clinic, Mrs. Donovan produces a stool specimen, and testing is performed for ova parasites, bacterial pathogens, *Clostridium difficile*, leukocytes, fecal fat, and D-xylose. Mrs. Donovan is educated as to appropriate nutritional habits and evaluated for dehydration symptomatology.

Assessment

Mrs. Donovan is a female patient with diarrhea, abdominal cramping, and a recent weight loss of 10 percent of her body weight. She has dry, scaly skin; pale conjunctiva; decreased hemoglobin, hematocrit, and mean corpuscular volume (MCV); decreased sodium, potassium, iron, and zinc; decreased serum albumin and transferrin; and a specific gravity of 1.028.

Nursing Diagnosis #1: Imbalanced Nutrition: Less than Body Requirements, related to inability to absorb nutrients because of HIV enteropathy.

NOC: Nutritional status; Nutritional status: Food and fluid intake; Nutritional status: Nutrient intake

NIC: Nutrition management; Electrolyte management; Enteral tube feeding; Nutrition therapy; Nutritional counseling; Nutritional monitoring; Weight gain assistance

Expected Outcomes

The patient will:
1. Receive adequate nutrients to meet metabolic needs.
2. Stabilize weight within 48 hours after initiation aids of nutrition support.

Case Study

3. Gain 0.25 to 0.5 kg/wk.
4. Select a diet high in calcium, iron, protein, and calories.

Planning/Interventions/Rationale

1. Weigh daily; record hourly intake and output (I & O); monitor blood pressure, pulse, and respiration rate every hour, breath sounds, edema. *Monitors overall health status for changes, balance of fluid intake and output, and signs of deterioration.*
2. Utilize a nocturnal tube feeding to deliver formula. *Antidiarrheal agents (antimotility drugs) can be very effective in reducing most diarrhea within 24 to 48 hours when administered correctly.*
3. Obtain food preferences from patient and offer smaller frequent meals. *Facilitates digestion and improves energy levels.*
4. Record percentage of meals consumed. *Monitors accurate consumption of nutrients.*
5. Coordinate medication administration with their absorptive characteristics. *To decrease malabsorption.*

Evaluation

1. Fluid intake and output balanced; diarrhea subsided in 24 hours; and afebrile.
2. Laboratory values within normal limits 48 hours postadmission.
3. Weight stabilized within 48 hours and patient tolerating small frequent meals.
4. The patient was able to select food items as prescribed by the nutritional support team and gained 0.45 kg in eight days.

Nursing Diagnosis #2: Diarrhea related to opportunistic enteric pathogens secondary to HIV.

NOC: Bowel elimination; Electrolyte and acid-base balance; Fluid balance; Hydration

NIC: Diarrhea management

Expected Outcomes:

The patient will:
1. Report less diarrhea within 24 to 48 hours.
2. Describe contributing factors to the diarrhea episodes.
3. Increase signs of rehydration within 24 to 48 hours (e.g., moist mucous membranes and skin turgor).

Planning/Interventions/Rationale

1. Monitor vital signs every four hours. *Severe dehydration causes a febrile response, and decreased fluids can cause hypotension.*
2. Increase oral intake to maintain a normal urine specific gravity or to approximate volume of diarrhea losses. *Good indicator of renal function and severity of dehydration.*
3. Encourage liquids (water, apple juice, or flat ginger ale) and discontinue solids.
4. Gradually add semisolids and solids (crackers, yogurt, rice, bananas, or applesauce) as diarrhea improves. *Absorption increases as diarrhea subsides.*

Evaluation

Patient will begin to show increased signs of hydration as diarrhea episodes decrease.

KEY CONCEPTS

■ The immune system is vital to the human body as related to its processes for recognizing and protecting the body.

■ The immune system provides the body with surveillance methods of protection against external threats to the body, such as viruses, bacteria, and other foreign substances, and to internal threats including abnormal tumor cells that develop.

■ Normally, CD4+ T cells orchestrate the immune system process in responding to foreign antigens.

■ The immune system may also have undesirable effects when the body recognizes allergens or self-tissue as abnormal or nonself.

■ Immunodeficiency disorders are due to dysfunction or impairment of one or more of the immune response mechanisms. The mechanisms include phagocytosis, humoral response, B cell- and T cell-mediated response or combination, the complement system, and a combined cell and humoral response.

■ The clinical hallmark of immune deficiency is a propensity to unusual or recurrent severe infections.

■ The etiology of many of the immune disorders is unknown. A complete history and physical examination are important components of the diagnostic process. A definitive diagnosis may take months to years as new symptoms appear.

■ Many factors are involved that cause the immune system to fail to recognize the body's normal tissue as self, including genetic predisposition, infections, interaction of T and B cells, introduction of foreign tissue, such as a blood transfusion or transplant tissue, and environmental factors.

■ Organs and tissues commonly affected by autoimmune disorders include blood components, such as RBCs, blood vessels, connective tissues, endocrine glands such as the thyroid or pancreas, muscles, joints, and skin. Most of the autoimmune disorders are associated with the connective tissues of the body.

■ The patient plays an important role in planning and adhering to the treatment regimen.

■ The goals in managing a chronic disease are to prevent or slow disease progression, managing existing comorbidity symptoms and complications, undergoing therapeutic procedures, rehabilitation activities, managing medications, and all the activities of daily living.

■ Some of the greatest challenges are to assist the individual in coping with a chronic and life-threatening disease, overcoming fear, and minimizing spiritual distress.

REVIEW QUESTIONS

1. During the early stages of a chronic disease, patients tend to focus on:
   1. Medication schedule
   2. Interpretation of symptoms
   3. Impact of lifestyle changes
   4. Understanding the disease process

2. The goal of HAART is to:
   1. Minimize side affects of the drugs
   2. Encourage patient compliance to the medication schedule
   3. Lower the CD4 cell levels
   4. Avoid viral resistance for each drug

3. Early clinical manifestations of GVHD include:
   1. Respiratory problems, i.e., interstitial pneumonitis
   2. Skin rash and pruritus
   3. Taut, firm, leather-like skin
   4. Dry lacrimal ducts and oral mucosa

4. Monoclonal antibodies are:
   1. B-cell antibodies developed against a foreign antigen
   2. Defective T-cell antibodies that do not recognize self tissue
   3. Genetically engineered immunosuppressant drugs
   4. Used in vaccines to assist in preventing infections

5. Hypersensitivity disorders are due to a (an):
   1. Immune deficiency disorder, such as HIV
   2. Autoimmune disorder, such as RA
   3. Heightened immune response to an antigen
   4. Desensitization of humoral immune components

Continued

REVIEW QUESTIONS—cont'd

6. The reversible form of SLE is due to reaction to drugs that are known to bind with the individual's DNA, such as:
   1. Beta blockers, such as Inderal
   2. Oral contraceptives, such as Levora
   3. Antibiotics, such as tetracycline
   4. Antimalarials, such as Plaquenil

7. Cell-mediated immunity is initiated by:
   1. Specific antigen recognition by T cells
   2. Nonspecific antigen recognition by B cells
   3. Release of complement cells into the blood stream
   4. Release of cytokines from white blood cells

8. Passive immunity involves:
   1. Transfer of antibodies through the heart of the mother to fetus
   2. Inoculation with vaccine containing live or killed infectious organisms
   3. Development of sensitized lymphocytes within the host body
   4. Response of memory cells to entry of an infectious organism

9. Sero-conversion is the presence of antibodies of HIV in the blood are detected by diagnostic studies with in:
   1. One to two weeks after exposure to HIV
   2. One to three months or more after exposure to HIV
   3. One month following the start of antiretroviral drug therapy
   4. Six months when immune-antibody complexes are formed

10. Criteria used to diagnose AIDS in an individual with HIV include at least one of the following conditions:
   1. CD4+ cell count above 200 cells/μL
   2. Anemia due to diminished RBC count
   3. Dysfunction of one or more organs
   4. Development of an opportunistic cancer

REVIEW ACTIVITIES

1. Review a case study related to HIV/AIDS. Role-play how you would assess a patient who is HIV positive on your assigned clinical unit. Formulate a nursing care plan and teaching plan for the patient in the case study.

2. Divide into small groups. Using a diagnostic studies text, research information and provide a report to entire group on the following tests: ELISA, Western blot technique, and T4 helper lymphocytes (CD4 cells). Include information that should be given to the patient and caregiver. Discuss the nurse's role regarding preparation for the procedure, in patient education, and in discussions with the health care team in planning interventions related to the diagnostic report.

3. Access the CDC National Prevention Information Network (NPIN) at: http://www.cdcnpin.org.
   Review the guidelines and recommendations for NIV/AIDS listed by category (community, counseling and testing, evaluation, patient care, prevention, surveillance, treatment and traveler's health). Write a report indicating what you see as the nurse's role in each of these categories.

4. Many patients with chronic immune diseases are perceived as demanding and manipulative. Consider some of the alternative measures (in addition to ones mentioned in the chapter) that can be used to help them cope with chronic pain and the disruption to their lives. Provide the rationale for their use.

5. Many persons diagnosed with an immune disorder continue to work, manage the household, care for children, or participate in social activities.
   a. Prepare information that contains guidelines for protection from infectious diseases.
   b. Locate the policy at your clinical facility regarding the procedures to follow when an employee is accidentally exposed to blood and other fluids of a person with HIV or AIDS diagnosis.

6. Research at least two immune disorders listed in Table 43-2 that have not been discussed in this chapter. Prepare a report that includes the etiology, clinical manifestations, collaborative, and nursing management. Document anticipated outcomes using the NOC classification system.

Allergic Dysfunction: Nursing Management

Linda Meuleveld, BA, RN, COHN-S, CCM, DABFN, VPS

CHAPTER TOPICS

- Immune System
- Allergic Dysfunction
- Pathophysiology of Allergic Reactions
- Types of Hypersensitivity
- Management of Patients with Allergic Disorders
- Atopic Asthma
- Prevention and Management of Anaphylaxis
- Allergic Disorders According to Type and Character

KEY TERMS

Allergen
Anaphylaxis
Angioneurotic edema
Antigen
Atopic dermatitis (AD)
Atopy
Autoantibody
Contact dermatitis
Hereditary angioedema (HAE)
Histamine
Hypersensitive response
Latex allergy
Pruritus
Serum sickness
Stridor
Urticaria
Wheezing

Diseases related to allergic dysfunction affect more than 50 million Americans. Common allergic diseases include allergic rhinitis, latex allergy, atopic dermatitis, food allergy, drug allergy, and allergy to venom of stinging insects. According to the National Institute of Allergy and Infectious diseases, allergies are the sixth leading cause of chronic disease in the United States, costing the health care system $18 billion annually. While the true number of deaths from drug reactions is unknown, anaphylactic reactions to penicillin occur in 32 of every 100,000 patients (American Academy of Allergy, Asthma, and Immunology, 2006).

ALLERGIC DYSFUNCTION

Allergic dysfunction is an altered response of the human body's natural defense against attack by microorganisms. When unfamiliar substances are identified and destroyed or inactivated, the body is performing a normal adaptive immune response. These immune responses fall into three categories shown in Table 43-1.

Immune responses are triggered when foreign substances called **antigens,** substances capable of stimulating an immune response, are identified by the immune system. The immune system has the ability to remember antigens from a primary immune response and respond quickly with a secondary response when the antigen is reintroduced. The immune system must also be able to distinguish between body proteins and foreign proteins to direct its attack toward the invading organism. The ability to recognize self from nonself is an important. Recognition is one of the four R's of immune response:

- Recognize self from nonself and triggering a response only when threatened by foreign invaders.
- Respond to nonself invaders by producing antibodies.
- Remember the invader so that there can be a quicker response if a subsequent invasion is detected.
- Regulate its action by turning on for the invader and turning off when the invader is destroyed.

Genetics

Genetics play a role in the way a person responds to invading organisms. **Atopy** is a personal or familial tendency to become sensitized and produce immunoglobulin E (IgE) antibodies in response to ordinary exposure to allergens. As a consequence, atopic individuals can be said to have a genetic predisposition to produce a prolonged IgE antibody response to allergens that are found in the general environment, such as pollens, dust mites, and molds. Atopy is a clinical definition that describes an IgE antibody high responder.

Pathophysiology

Most antigens are composed of proteins. All body cells have antigens on their surface. These antigens are unique to the individual and help the immune system differentiate between self and invader.

When a person is exposed to an **allergen,** a substance that induces an allergic reaction, for the first time, the immune system reacts protectively. The immune system initiates a series of biochemical and cellular events that translate into clinical symptoms. These events involve antigens, antibodies, release of **histamine** (a hormone that causes vasodilation and an increase in permeability of blood vessel walls), and varying response times, depending on the

Red Flag

Emphasize History of Allergies

When a patient mentions that he or she has allergies, the comment is a significant contribution to the medical history. It would be appropriate to discuss family history of allergies. Atopic individuals may have multiple allergies.

TABLE 43-1 Immune Responses

IMMUNE CATEGORY	RESPONSE/ACTION
Defense	Resisting invasion by foreign microorganisms
Homeostasis	Removing damaged cells
Surveillance	Recognizing and removing mutated cells

Adapted from Janeway, C. A., Jr., Travers, P., Walport, M., & Shlomchik, M. J. (2004). Immunobiology, the immune system in health and disease (6th ed.). New York: Garland Science Publishing.

person and the exposure. Histamine is a chemical produced by the body during allergic reactions (Janeway, Travers, Walport, & Shlomchik, 2004).

Antibodies circulate in the bloodstream and are present in almost all body fluids. When allergens first enter the body of a person predisposed to allergies, a series of reactions will occur that produce allergen-specific IgE antibodies. The IgE antibodies travel to cells, called mast cells, soon after they are produced. Large quantities of mast cells are found in the connective tissue of the nose, eyes, lungs, and gastrointestinal (GI) tract. IgE antibodies attach themselves to the mast cells and wait for their particular antigen to appear.

Primary and Second Response

The response to an allergen may be immediate or delayed. These responses are called the primary and secondary immune response (Figure 43-1). These two responses are immunoglobulin M (IgM) and immunoglobulin G (IgG). They are two classes of immunoglobulin the body produces in response to an antigen. IgM predominates in the primary phase, with IgG appearing later. On a subsequent exposure to the same antigen, in a secondary response, some IgM and large amounts of IgG are produced.

Antibodies are members of a class of proteins known as immunoglobulins, which are produced by B lymphocytes in response to an antigen. They are used by the immune system to neutralize foreign objects. Each antibody recognizes a specific antigen unique to its target. An antibody is specific to an antigen and is a primary immune defense.

IgE Response

After repeated low-dose exposure to allergens, atopic individuals develop specific IgE antibodies to the allergens. Subsequent exposure initiates a secondary humoral response. IgE molecules specific to an antigen attach to cell surface receptors on mast cells. The mast cell's response includes the release of histamine. The release of histamine creates the clinical manifestations of an allergic reaction.

Early Response

Within minutes after exposure of an allergic subject to antigen, an immediate (early) response follows. In the upper airway, the allergic individual begins to sneeze, which is followed closely by an increase in nasal secretions. After about five minutes mucosal swelling begins, leading to reduced airflow. These physiological changes are associated with increases in histamine, leukotrienes, prostaglandins, tryptase, and other proinflammatory mediators.

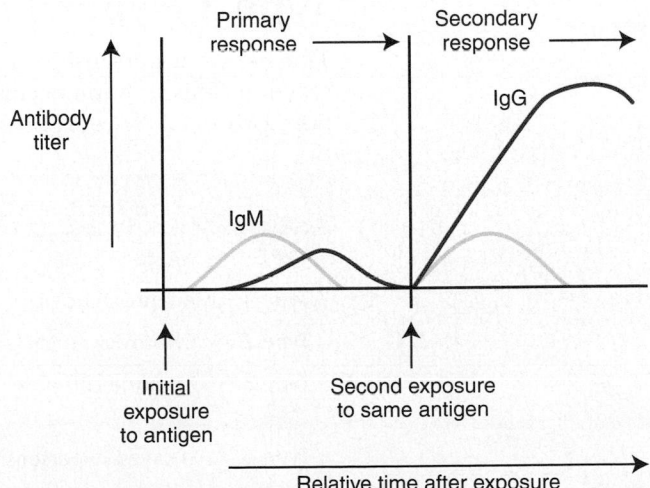

Figure 43-1 Primary and secondary immune responses. Following the initial exposure to a foreign antigen, the primary immune response, IgM, develops gradually. When the antigen is encountered a second time, it triggers a secondary response. In the secondary response large amounts of IgG are rapidly produced.

Late Response

Other than the immediate response to antigen, another response begins hours later. The late response does not occur in everyone. It appears to be dose related. The primary manifestation is airway obstruction.

Diagnostic Tests

The physicians most qualified to treat allergic diseases are allergists and immunologists. Diagnosis begins with a detailed medical history and physical examination. If indicated, a skin allergy test will be done, and blood testing may be done to determine the allergen causing the reaction. When the triggers are identified, a treatment program can be established. The first step in treatment is to minimize exposure to the identified allergen. Medications may be prescribed to reduce allergic symptoms and inflammation.

Nursing Diagnoses

This chapter will examine a variety of allergic disorders, and the specific treatment strategies for each will be presented. These sections will also include nursing diagnoses. However, the following are examples of general nursing diagnoses that are examples in the patient with allergic dysfunction and may include the following. (Note: the evaluation of outcomes will be presented as they apply in the diseases that follow in this chapter):
- Ineffective breathing pattern.
- Ineffective coping related to anxiety, lower activity level, and the inability to perform normal activities of daily living.
- Activity intolerance related to fatigue.
- Fear and anxiety related to actual or potential lifestyle changes.

TYPES OF HYPERSENSITIVITY

The immune system will normally react to protect people in the presence of a foreign antigen. The person with a hypersensitive reaction will have one of four types of reaction, as shown in Table 43-2.

An exaggerated or misdirected immune response to an allergen that results in tissue injury is called a **hypersensitive response.** These are classified in the Gell-Coombs spectrum of human hypersensitivity.

Type 1 Hypersensitivity

The type 1 hypersensitive reaction is an immediate type of hypersensitivity reaction. This reaction occurs when a specific antigen induces an allergic reaction, provoked by reexposure to the same antigen. The contact, inhalation,

TABLE 43-2	Hypersensitive Reactions: Gell Coombs Classification	
TYPE	**NAME**	**REACTION**
Type 1	Anaphylactic	Allergic rhinitis, asthma
Type 2	Cytotoxic	Transfusion reaction
Type 3	Immune complex	Systemic lupus erythematosus Rheumatoid arthritis
Type 4	Delayed hypersensitive	Transplant rejection reaction

Adapted from Janeway, C. A., Jr., Travers, P., Walport, M., Shlomchik, M. J. (2004). Immunobiology, the immune system in health and disease (6th ed.). New York: Garland Science Publishing.

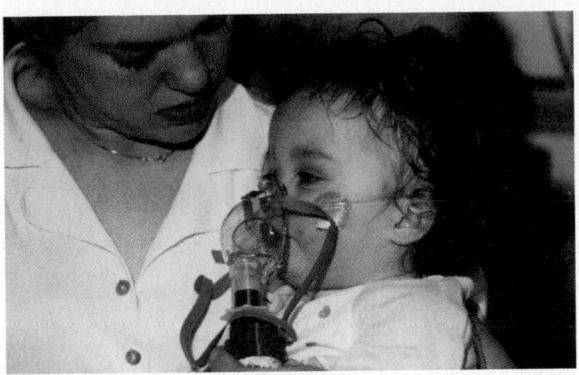

Figure 43-2 A child has experienced an allergenic crisis and is continuing to be treated with nebulizer medications via a mask to deliver the inhalants.

ingestion, or injection of the allergen creates an allergic reaction mediated by specific IgE antibodies, the cellular release of histamine, and other vasoactive mediators, resulting in an immediate local or systemic reaction (**anaphylaxis).**

The immediate type of hypersensitivity reaction may occur locally or systemically. The symptoms may range from mild to sudden death due to anaphylactic shock. Clinical examples include allergic rhinitis, allergic asthma, atopic dermatitis, and systemic anaphylaxis. When the patient has respiratory symptoms, there is a higher incidence of morbidity and mortality (Figure 43-2). Fatal and near fatal anaphylactic reactions can be traced to reexposure to foods, such as peanuts and drugs, such as penicillin or insulin. Hypersensitivity usually appears on repeated contact with the allergen (Box 43-1).

Type 2 Hypersensitivity

Type 2 hypersensitivity reactions are cytotoxic reactions where the antibody (IgG or IgM) is directed against antigen on an individual's own cells or against foreign antibody, such as that acquired after blood transfusion. This may lead to cytotoxic action by killer cells or to lysis mediated by the complement system. Cytotoxic reactions are serious and potentially life-threatening (Box 43-2).

Type 3 Hypersensitivity

Type 3 hypersensitivity reactions are immune complex reactions where immune complexes (antigen and usually IgG or IgM) are deposited in the tissue. The complement is activated causing local tissue damage and inflammation. The types of disease encountered are classified into acute and chronic serum sickness and local inflammatory response due to deposition of immune complexes in tissues (the Arthus reaction) (Box 43-3).

Type 4 Hypersensitivity

Type 4 hypersensitivity reactions are cell-mediated reactions, which are also called delayed hypersensitivity. Allergic contact dermatitis after exposure to ointments containing active drugs is the most frequent form of drug-mediated delayed hypersensitivity. Various forms of type 4 hypersensitivity are recognized: contact hypersensitivity, tuberculin-type hypersensitivity, and granulomatous hypersensitivity. Examples of diseases manifesting type 4 granulomatous hypersensitivity are Crohn's disease, leprosy, tuberculosis, sarcoidosis, and schistosomiasis.

Autoantibodies can also cause disease. An **autoantibody** is an antibody that reacts against a person's own tissue. They are organ specific. Systemic lupus erythematosus is an example of an autoimmune disease that is non–organ specific in that it is characterized by damage to multiple organs. Examples of diseases in humans caused by autoantibodies are autoimmune hemolytic anemia, autoimmune thrombocytopenic purpura, bulbous pemphigoid, glomerulonephritis (Goodpasture's syndrome), Graves' disease (hyperthyroidism), insulin-resistant diabetes mellitus, myasthenia gravis, pemphigus vulgaris, and pernicious anemia.

Atopy and allergy are not interchangeable terms. Atopy refers to an individual being prone to develop allergies because of a genetic state of hyperresponsiveness to sensitizing agents. It is associated with conditions such as asthma, allergic rhinitis (hay fever), and atopic dermatitis (allergic dermatitis). Allergy refers to the hypersensitivity that occurs on reexposure to a sensitizing allergen, causing the release of histamine and other inflammatory mediators.

Sensitizing agents can enter the body through various routes. They may be airborne and are breathed in; they may come in contact with the skin or

---

BOX 43-1

EXAMPLES OF TYPE 1 ALLERGIC REACTIONS

Anaphylaxis
Atopic asthma
Atopic eczema
Drug allergy
Hay fever

Adapted from Guillet, G., Guillet, M., & Dagregorio, G. (2005). Allergic contact dermatitis from natural rubber latex in atopic dermatitis and the risk of later type I allergy. Contact Dermatitis, 53(1), 46–51.

BOX 43-2

DISEASES MANIFESTING TYPE 2 HYPERSENSITIVITY

Autoimmune hemolytic anemia

Goodpasture's syndrome

Hemolytic disease of the newborn

Myasthenia gravis

Pemphigus

Adapted from Heidary, N., & Cohen, D. Hypersensitivity reactions to vaccine components. Dermatitis, 16(3), 115–120.

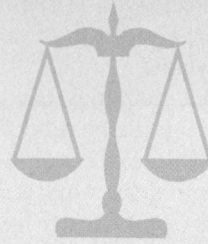

LAW IN PRACTICE

A Drug Side Effect or Hypersensitivity Reaction?

A 14-year-old girl was admitted for observation with the diagnosis of a rash related to antibiotic (amoxicillin) use. Three days earlier her parents had taken her to the doctor with complaints of a sore throat, cervical lymphadenopathy, and general malaise. The physician noted that the patient had a temperature elevation of 100.2° F (37.9°C). The patient was concerned that she would be too ill to take a trip a week away with her class during spring break. The physician responded to parental pressure by ordering amoxicillin. After three days, the parents brought their daughter to the emergency department with a rash covering most of her body. They were sure she was having a reaction to the oral penicillin she had been taking. The last dose of amoxicillin had been taken that morning.

The patient was diagnosed with mononucleosis (Epstein-Barr virus). The amoxicillin had been ordered to diminish the effects of a presumed bacterial infection. The patient was actually suffering from a viral infection that would not respond to an antibiotic.

The rash was not a symptom of penicillin allergy and did not indicate a future adverse reaction to penicillin. This fact was related to the patient by both the physician and the nurse assigned to the patient.

At a later date the patient was treated with penicillin for an infection and experienced an anaphylactic (type 1) reaction. She recovered,

but her family sued the physician for prescribing penicillin when the patient had a previous allergic reaction to penicillin. Because the nurse had explained to the family that the patient's rash was a side effect of amoxicillin, and not an allergic reaction to penicillin, she was also named in the suit. The case was settled out of court.

The earlier rash and the new penicillin allergy were not related. It is unfortunate for the patient that she developed an allergy to penicillin. The new drug allergy was not a consequence of the earlier rash. It is possible, however, for an atopic individual to be more prone to the development of allergies.

The nurse in this case delivered appropriate information to the patient and her family regarding the earlier rash and the amoxicillin. Nurses must be 100 percent confident of their knowledge when relaying information to patients and their families. Appropriate documentation of the conversation with the family by the nurse provided the only source of information regarding relay of information to the family and validated the nurses' comments.

Adapted from Janeway, C. A., Jr., Travers, P., Walport, M., & Shlomchik, M. J. (2004). Immunobiology, the immune system in health and disease *(6th ed.). New York: Garland Science Publishing.*

BOX 43-3

EXAMPLES OF HUMAN IMMUNE COMPLEX DISEASES

Polyarteritis nodosa

Poststreptococcal glomerulonephritis

Systemic lupus erythematosus

Adapted from Janeway, C. A., Jr., Travers, P., Walport, M., & Shlomchik, M. J. (2004). Immunobiology, the immune system in health and disease *(6th ed.). New York: Garland Science Publishing.*

mucous membranes. They may be swallowed and enter the GI system. They may enter the skin through injection or other means (Table 43-3).

Assessment with Clinical Manifestations

There are many elements of the nursing assessment in patients with allergic disorders. In addition, these patients also have many clinical manifestations. The nursing assessment is primarily divided into objective and subjective data as shown in Box 43-4.

Planning and Implementation

An altered immune system can manifest itself in many ways, but allergic, type 1 hypersensitive reactions (allergies), are the most common. Most of these allergies are chronic and are distinguished by remissions and exacerbations. Allergy treatment for chronic allergies focuses on a variety of issues. Initially, the nurse can help the patient make lifestyle changes to help the patient adjust to minimal allergen exposures. Next, the nurse should also reinforce the thought that medication and desensitization will only reduce the immune

TABLE 43-3 **Categories of Sensitizing Agents (Allergens)**

AIRBORNE (RESPIRATORY)	CONTACT (SKIN, MUCOUS MEMBRANE)	INGESTED (GI)	INJECTED (PERCUTANEOUS)
Pollens: plants, grasses, trees	Plants	Foods: egg, milk, peanut, shellfish, soy wheat, and nuts	Drugs
Pollens: plants, grasses, trees	Plants	Foods: soy wheat, and nuts	Drugs
Mold: fungal spores	Drugs	Drugs	Vaccines
Dust mites	Metals		Insect stings
Animal dander	Cosmetics		
House dust	Fibers, latex, chemicals		

Adapted from Janeway, C. A., Jr., Travers, P., Walport, M., & Shlomchik, M. J. (2004). Immunobiology, the immune system in health and disease *(6th ed.). New York: Garland Science Publishing; Mohapatra, S., Lockey, R., & Shirley, S. (2005).* Immunobiology of grass pollen allergens. Current Allergy and Asthma Reports, 5(5), 381–387.

Skills 360°

Prevention and Asthma

Asthma is a serious and growing health problem. An estimated 14.9 million people in the United States have asthma and are at risk for serious chronic or immediate illness. Asthma is responsible for about 500,000 hospitalizations, 5,000 deaths, and 134 million days of restricted activity a year. Yet most of the problems caused by asthma could be averted if people with asthma and their health care providers managed the disease according to established guidelines. These prevention efforts are essential to interrupt the progression from disease to functional limitation and disability and to improve the quality of life for people with asthma.

Adapted from Ait-Khaled, N., & Enarson, D. (2006). Management of asthma: The essentials of good clinical practice. International Journal of Tuberculosis and Lung Disease, 10(2), 133–137.

BOX 43-4

ASSESSMENT OF ALLERGIC DISORDERS

Objective Data
- Rash: location, symmetry, skin dryness, irritation, scratches, scaly skin, and urticaria (hives)
- Respiratory: wheezing or strider and shortness of breath
- Eyes: conjunctivitis, lacrimation, excessive rubbing, and blinking
- Ears: diminished hearing, immobile, or scarred tympanic membrane
- Nose: rhinitis, sniffling, sneezing, and swollen nasal passages
- Throat: continual throat clearing, red throat, swollen lips or tongue, or palpable lymph nodes in neck

Subjective Data
- Health information, health history, respiratory problems, seasonal exacerbations, and past allergies
- Medications: unusual reactions and OTC medications for allergies

Adapted from Estes, M. (2006). Health assessment and physical examination (3rd ed.). New York: Thomson Delmar Learning.

response to the allergen and help moderate the expectation of a symptom-free future. In addition, management of hypersensitivity reactions can include skin testing, and exploration of food allergies can also be identified though an elimination diet. Last, emotional stress and fatigue can intensify an allergic reaction. The nurse can be influential in helping the patient learn stress management and relaxation techniques, such as imagery and deep breathing.

ATOPIC ASTHMA

Asthma is a common inflammatory disease of the airways that causes airway hyperresponsiveness, mucous production, and mucosal edema. Asthma leads to recurrent episodes of clinical manifestations, such as cough, chest tightness,

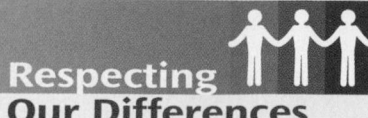

Respecting Our Differences

Ethnicity and Asthma Acute Care Admissions

Studies have shown that minority children (defined as African American and Hispanic [American]) have more hospitalizations and have more frequent emergency department visits than other groups. The study confirms that emergency departments serve as a safety net for children with asthma during exacerbations, particularly disadvantaged minorities. Evidence suggests that education and supportive programs can help improve outcomes for these children of different ethnic backgrounds.

Adapted from Ait-Khaled, N., & Enarson, D. (2006). Management of asthma: The essentials of good clinical practice. International Journal of Tuberculosis and Lung Disease, 10(2), 133–137; Boudreaus, E., Edmond, S., & Race (2003). Ethnicity and asthma among children presenting to the emergency department. Pediatrics III, (5), e615–e621.

respiratory wheezing, and dyspnea. Asthma differs from other obstructive disorders in that it is largely reversible, either with management or spontaneously.

Epidemiology

Atopic asthma is the most common form of asthma. According to the National Institute of Environmental Health Sciences, of the 17 million asthma sufferers in the United States, 10 million (approximately 60 percent) have atopic asthma. Three million are children, and 7 million are adults.

Etiology

Most patients with asthma also suffer from other allergic disorders. In fact, research from the World Health Organization shows that at least 70 percent of asthmatics also suffer from allergic rhinitis or hay fever. Nasal allergies and allergic asthma are both triggered by exposure to allergens, initiating a series of events that result in tightening of the airways, swelling of the lining of the airways, nose and eyes, and mucous production.

Atopic (extrinsic) asthma typically develops in childhood. Eighty percent of children with asthma have other allergies. Typically there is a family history of allergies. Other conditions, such as hay fever or eczema, are also present. Atopic asthma experienced in childhood often goes into remission in early adulthood, only to appear at a later age.

Pathophysiology

IgE plays a critical role in the allergic process. When an individual is sensitized to an allergen, such as pollen or animal dander, he or she produces an IgE antibody directed against that allergen. The IgE antibody attaches to mast cells. When the individual is exposed to that same allergen again, the allergen binds to the IgE on the mast cell causing it to release substances, such as histamine, prostaglandins, and leukotrienes, which cause symptoms, such as chest tightness, coughing and **wheezing** (a whistling sound when breathing out related to airway constriction).

Deaths from asthma have been declining in all categories but children younger than age 5. In this age range the asthma death rate has increased from 1.7 per million in 1999 to 2.1 per million in 2003.

Assessment with Clinical Manifestations

The clinical manifestations of atopic asthma include wheezing (rhinorrhea and rash [urticaria]). There will be a drop in the peak flow expiratory rate. When asthma symptoms are under control, the airways are open, and it is possible to force more air into the peak flow meter. When the airways are inflamed and constricted, it is not possible to blow as hard into the meter, making the peak flow rate lower.

Patients with allergic asthma may experience:
- Shortness of breath (SOB) with exertion or late at night.
- Coughing that may become chronic. It is usually worse at night, after exercise, or when breathing is exposed to cold, dry air.
- Chest tightness.

Prolonged attacks that don't respond to treatment with bronchodilators are a medical emergency and require emergency care. The nurse plays a vital role in evaluating patients for potential allergic reaction. A thorough nursing assessment should include discussion of subjective data such as:

Health information that discusses health history.

Respiratory problems, past allergies, and seasonal exacerbations.

Adapted from Broyles, B. E., Reiss, B. S., & Evans, M. E. (2007). Pharmacological aspects of nursing care (7th ed.). New York: Thomson Delmar Learning; DeLaune, S., & Ladner, P. (2006). Fundamentals of Nursing (3rd ed.). New York: Thomson Delmar Learning.

PATIENT PLAYBOOK

Triggers for Asthma

The nurse can instruct the patient to avoid triggers for asthma in the following ways:

- Pollen: Keep windows and doors closed, and use air conditioning to keep pollen out.
- Dust mites: Use special coverings for mattresses and pillows. Remove carpets, rugs and drapery in bedrooms. Wash bedding in hot water.
- Toys should not include stuffed animals.
- Keep humidity between 30 and 40 percent.
- Use a vacuum cleaner with a filter. Change filter and bag often.
- Animal hair and dander: Pet removal is best. If around pets, keep them out of bedrooms and off furniture.
- Mold: Try to eliminate mold in the environment. Dehumidifiers can help. Avoid freshly cut grass.
- Environment: Avoid cigarette smoke and all other types of smoke. When outdoor air quality is poor, stay indoors. Cover the nose and mouth during cold weather.
- Exercise: Perform slow warm-ups and cool-downs and be sure to use asthma medication approximately 10 minutes before beginning an exercise routine.

Skin rashes, past or present.

Unusual reactions to medications: OTC, medications for allergies and medications, vitamins, and health remedies taken over the previous two weeks.

Perceptions of health and family history.

Difficulties with malaise, fatigue, food intolerances, itching, or vomiting.

The physical exam with suspected allergic dysfunction should include observation of:

Skin: The presence of a rash should be noted, with a description that includes location, symmetry, skin dryness, irritation, scratches, scaly skin, urticaria (hives), or **pruritus** (itching).

Breathing: Listen for wheezing or stridor. Wheezing is the expiratory sound produced by the turbulent flow of air through constricted small airways (bronchioles). **Stridor** is the audible symptom produced by the rapid turbulent flow of air through a narrowed segment of the respiratory tract.

Eyes: Conjunctivitis, excessive rubbing and blinking, or lacrimation.

Ears: There may be complaints of diminished hearing and immobile or scarred tympanic membranes.

Nose: Rhinitis (inflammation of the mucous membrane that lines the nose) sneezing, sniffling, or swollen nasal passages.

Throat: Constant throat clearing, red throat, swollen lips or tongue, or palpable lymph nodes in the neck.

Diagnostic Tests

To determine presence of asthma, the clinician must determine that periodic problems with airway obstruction are present, that airflow is at least partially reversible, and that other etiologies have been ruled out. Family history, potential environmental factors (e.g., air pollution, high pollen counts, or molds) and comorbid factors (drug-induced asthma or gastroesophageal reflux) may accompany asthma. In addition the presence of various allergic reactions can be tied to asthma (eczema, rashes, or temporary edema). Any of the aforementioned variables may be used as diagnostic criteria for the presence of asthma.

Identification of the specific allergen provoking the reaction is pursued at some future point, when the allergic reaction is in remission. The gold standard for establishing allergen specific IgE antibodies is the skin-prick test (SPT). With this test a drop of allergen is applied to an intradermal prick. Positive results are indicated by a characteristic "wheal and flare" response. Use of certain medications can interfere with the validity of a skin-prick response. These include antihistamines, benzodiazepines, theophylline, and antidepressants. Corticosteroids have no effect on the SPT.

Nursing Diagnoses

Based on the information gathered, examples of nursing diagnoses in the patient with asthma may include the following:
- Ineffective breathing pattern related to SOB, mucus, and airway irritants.
- Impaired gas exchange related to ventilation-perfusion inequality.
- Ineffective coping related to anxiety, lower activity level, and the inability to perform normal activities of daily living.

Planning and Implementation

The management for asthma is heavily focused on patient education. Patient and family teaching is related to the prevention of asthmatic attacks through patient and family communication. The patient education includes a discussion of learning to anticipate triggers and practicing avoidance. Asthma triggers irritate the lungs and produce mucus, inflammation, and tightening of the bronchial tubes. Common triggers for asthma are shown in the patient playbook. In addition, there continue to be numerous research studies for the management of atopic asthma, and the future is promising for the continued advancement of the treatment of this condition (see Fast Forward feature).

The therapeutic management of asthma utilizes a balance among the diagnostic variables, the acute therapies for asthma, and the prevention or maintenance care of the patient (Table 43-4; Skills 360° feature).

PATIENT PLAYBOOK

Prevention of Serious Allergen Responses

The nurse can instruct the patient to prevent allergen responses by the following:

- The type of allergen influences the method of management needed.
- The nurse can help the patient, and other family members, to explore ways of avoiding allergen exposure by altering contact with specific allergens, such as pets, pollens, foods, or medications.
- The nurse can recommend the wearing of a medical alert bracelet.
- The nurse can make sure the allergen is listed prominently in all medical and dental records. The patient should also be encouraged to notify any other medical providers of the allergy

Adapted from Amado, M., & Portnoy, J. (2006). Recent advances in asthma management. Missouri Medicine, 103(1), 60–64.

TABLE 43-4 **Therapeutic Management of Asthma**

Diagnostic	Health history and physical exam
	Pulmonary function studies
	Bronchodilator therapy response
	Chest X-ray
	Pin prick test when indicated
	Sputum specimen (r/o bacterial infection)
	Blood level IgE, eosinophils
Treatment: Acute asthma	Inhaled beta-adrenergic drugs
	O_2 per mask or nasal prongs
	IV medications (e.g., corticosteroids, aminophylline)
	Nebulized or inhaled anticholinergic agents
	Increased fluid intake (oral plus IV to 3,000 mL
	Intubation and assisted ventilation, as indicated
Prevention and maintenance	Eliminate triggers
	Desensitization (if indicated)
	Follow prescribed drug regimen
	Trigger assessment of home and work
	Progressive plan for exercise

Adapted from Broyles, B. E., Reiss, B. S., & Evans, M. E. (2007). Pharmacological aspects of nursing care (7th ed.). New York: Thomson Delmar Learning.

Skills 360°

Health Promotion for Patients with Asthma

Health care management of illnesses focuses on diagnosis and treatment. This is an important component of the care plan for the patient experiencing an allergic reaction, such as allergic asthma. Treatment is directed toward reducing symptoms and regaining normal activities of daily living. This approach is necessary, but there is a new interest in creating and implementing effective health management and disease prevention programs, that would enable the patient with asthma to avoid becoming symptomatic. Research done by the Centers for Disease Control (CDC) indicates that an estimated 50 percent of an individual's health status is governed by lifestyle behaviors. Nurses play an important role in communicating to their patients' ways of pursuing healthy behaviors that will keep the patient's allergies from becoming symptomatic.

Adapted from Ait-Khaled, N., & Enarson, D. Management of asthma: The essentials of good clinical practice. International Journal of Tuberculosis and Lung Disease, 10(2), 133–137; Amado, M., & Portnoy, J. Recent advances in asthma management. Missouri Medicine, 103(1), 60–64.

Pharmacology

Medications are effective in managing asthma by reversing and treating bronchospasm, inflammation, and mucous clearance. A wide variety of medications arc uscd to treat asthma and are shown in Tables 43-5 and 43-6.

Drug therapy is an effective treatment for symptom relief. The major categories of drugs for symptom relief of chronic allergies include antihistamines, decongestants, multidose inhalants (Figure 43-3), corticosteroids, antipyretics, and mast cell stabilizers. The nurse can caution the patient about the many side effects associated with their use (Box 43-5).

Hyposensitization

When the allergen cannot be avoided and drug therapy is not effective, immunotherapy is recommended to reduce the level of sensitivity. It is a process in which small amounts of an allergen extract is administered in increasing dosages until hyposensitivity is achieved. Hyposensitization is indicated for individuals with anaphylactic reactions to insect venom (hymenoptera). Complete desensitization is not possible, and the nurse should instruct the patient to continue to avoid the offending allergen (Muller & Golden, 2004).

TABLE 43-5 **Pharmacology Facts: Pharmaceutical Therapy for Asthma**

CLASSIFICATION	DRUG	REACTION	COMMENT
Beta-adrenergic agonist Inhaled bronchodilator Systemic bronchodilator	Albuterol (Proventil, Ventolin), Metaproterenol (Alupent, Metaprel).	Relax bronchospasm bronchodilation Increases mucociliary clearance	Contraindicated with cardiac disorders Slow reaction
Corticosteroid Anti-inflammatory medications	Hydrocortisone (Solu-Cortef), Methylprednisolone (Medrol and Solu-Medrol), Prednisone	Reduce inflammation Decreases edema in bronchi Decrease mucous secretions	Side effects; skin changes, obesity, muscle weakness
Leukotriene modifier (a new class of anti-inflammatory recently FDA approved)	Zafirlukast (Accolate) Zileuton (Zyflo)	Inhibit the allergic process	Throat irritation Possible bronchospasm

Adapted from Broyles, B. E., Reiss, B. S., & Evans, M. E. (2007). Pharmacological aspects of nursing care (7th ed.). New York: Thomson Delmar Learning.

TABLE 43-6 **Pharmacology Facts: Pharmaceutical Therapy for Symptom Relief of Chronic Allergies**

CLASSIFICATION	DRUGS	INDICATIONS
Antihistamine	Coricidin, Seldane, Claritin	Allergic rhinitis, urticaria
Decongestant	Pseudoephedrine, Sudafed, Neo-Synephrine, Dristan	Nasal congestion
Corticosteroid	Flunisolide, Beconasc, and Nasalide	
Antipruritic	Calamine Lotion, and Tacaryl	Urticaria, pruritus
Mast cell stabilizer	Intal, NasalCrom, and Tilade	Allergic rhinitis and asthma symptoms

Adapted from Broyles, B. E., Reiss, B. S., & Evans, M. E. (2007). Pharmacological aspects of nursing care (7th ed.). New York: Thomson Delmar Learning.

BOX 43-5

PHARMACOLOGICAL MANAGEMENT FOR SYMPTOM RELIEF

Antihistamines, such as Coricidin, Seldane, and Claritin, are used for treatment of allergic rhinitis and urticaria. Their side effects include drowsiness, sedation, and poor coordination that could be hazardous when driving or operating machinery. These drugs can also cause GI upset, mouth dryness, blurred vision, and vertigo.

Decongestant (sympathomimetic) drugs such as pseudoephedrine, Sudafed, Neo-Synephrine, and Dristan are used in the management of chronic allergy patients. Because they are available OTC, they have a potential for misuse, resulting in the patient becoming overmedicated.

Corticosteroids are found in nasal inhalers such as Flunisolide, Beconase, and Nasalide.

Antipyretic drugs are applied topically in the form of Calamine lotion and Tacaryl.

Mast cell stabilizing drugs, such as Intal, NasalCrom, and Tilade, inhibit the release of histamines after antigen IgE interaction. They are available as a nasal spray, inhalant nebulizer solution, or oral tablet. They are often used to treat allergic rhinitis and asthma symptoms and have a low incidence of side effects.

Adapted from Ait-Khaled, N., & Enarson D. (2006). Management of asthma: The essentials of good clinical practice. International Journal of Tuberculosis and Lung Disease, 10(2), 133–137; Broyles, B. E., Reiss, B. S., & Evans, M. E. (2007). Pharmacological aspects of nursing care (7th ed.). New York: Thomson Delmar Learning.

Evaluation of Outcomes

Potential patient outcomes for each of the example nursing diagnoses for the patient with asthma are:

- Ineffective breathing pattern related to SOB, mucus, and airway irritants. The patient's breathing pattern is maintained by eupnea, normal skin color, and regular respiratory rate or pattern.
- Impaired gas exchange related to ventilation-perfusion inequality. The patient maintains optimal gas exchange as evidenced by normal arterial blood gases (ABGs) and alert responsive mentation or no further reduction in mental status.
- Ineffective coping related to anxiety, lower activity level, and the inability to perform normal activities of daily living. The patient identifies own maladaptive coping behaviors, available resources, and support systems, describes or initiates alternative coping strategies, and describes positive results from new behaviors.

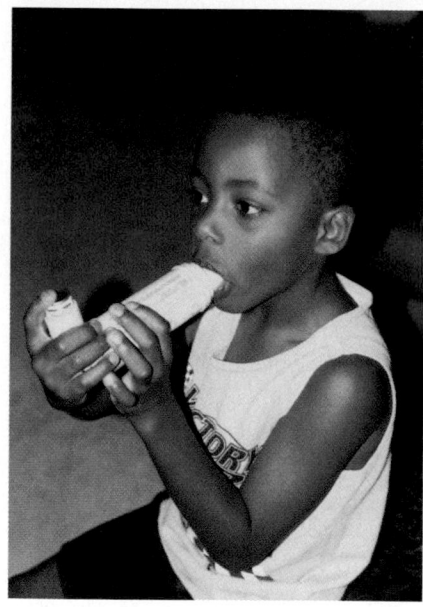

Figure 43-3 A child with an asthma attack using a metered-dose inhaler with a spacer and mouthpiece.

ANAPHYLAXIS

Anaphylaxis is an immediate, life-threatening hypersensitive allergic reaction (Gell and Coombs Type I: Immediate hypersensitivity reaction). This sudden and severe allergic reaction occurs within minutes of exposure in hypersensitive patients. It progresses rapidly and can result in anaphylactic shock and death within 15 minutes if medical intervention is not immediately pursued. Speed is the cardinal principal in therapeutic management of anaphylaxis. Anaphylaxis can be triggered by exposure to food (e.g., peanuts, wheat germ), medications (e.g., penicillin, morphine sulfate), insect venom (e.g., bee stings, spider bites), latex (e.g., gloves, equipment), exercise, or other diagnostic agents.

Epidemiology

Nearly 41 million people in the United States have sensitivities that put them at risk for anaphylaxis. It is estimated that 500 to 1,000 fatalities each year are related to anaphylaxis (Centers for Disease Control, 2002). The frequency of anaphylaxis is increasing, and this has been attributed to the increased number of potential allergens to which people are exposed. Unfortunately, in many patients being evaluated for anaphylaxis, no specific trigger can be identified.

Etiology

There are numerous risk factors associated with the incidence and prevalence of anaphylaxis. The nonmodifiable risk factors include age, gender, and race. Modifiable risk factors include the allergens route of entry, atopy, and exposure history (Box 43-6).

BOX 43-6

MODIFIABLE RISK FACTORS FOR ANAPHYLAXIS

Age

Adults have a higher reported rate of reactions to antibiotics, contrast media, anesthetic agents, and insect stings, whereas children have a higher rate of reported reactions to food antigens.

Gender

Anaphylaxis is more frequent in boys than girls under age 15, but among adults, women are more frequently affected than men. Women have a higher incidence of reactions to aspirin, muscle relaxants, contrast material, and latex, and men have a higher recorded incidence of anaphylaxis to insect sting venom. Women are also at higher risk for idiopathic anaphylaxis.

Race

No differences have been noted with race.

Route of Entry

Anaphylaxis can occur with all routes of administration, with episodes more frequent and severe if the offending antigen enters through the skin, (parenterally) rather than orally.

Atopy

The incidence of anaphylaxis to latex and foods is higher in atopic individuals. The data are conflicting regarding antibiotic reactions, with some studies finding anaphylaxis to penicillin more common in atopic patients and others finding no correlation between atopy and penicillin allergy, or even a lower risk for penicillin hypersensitivity with atopic individuals. Atopic people may be predisposed to anaphylactic or anaphylactoid reactions in general and atopy have been implicated as a risk factor for idiopathic anaphylaxis and exercise-induced anaphylaxis.

Exposure History

The likelihood of a repeat episode of anaphylaxis occurring decreases as the time interval between the original episode and subsequent reexposure increases. In addition, medications administered continuously are less likely to trigger a reaction than those given intermittently.

Adapted from Lebovidge, J., Stone, K., Twarog, F., Raiselis, S., Kalish, L., Bailey, E., et al. (2006). Development of a preliminary questionnaire to assess parental response to children's food allergies. Annals of Allergy, Asthma, and Immunology, 96(3), 472–477; Murphy, K., Hopp, R., Kittelson, E., Hansen, G., Windle, M., & Walburn J. (2006). Life-threatening asthma and anaphylaxis in schools: A treatment model for school-based programs. Annals of Allergy, Asthma, and Immunology, 96(3), 398–405.

Statistics issued by the CDC indicate that each year in the United States allergic reactions to bee stings, food allergy, latex allergy, drug allergy, and asthma result in anaphylactic reactions. Many of these reactions result in death due to anaphylactic shock, as illustrated in Box 43-7.

Pathophysiology

Anaphylaxis can be induced or aggravated by exercise, and some patients have recurrent symptoms for no identifiable reason. Histamine and other substances are generated or released when the antigen reacts with IgE on basophils and mast cells. These substances cause smooth muscle contraction (responsible for wheezing and GI symptoms) and vascular dilation and characterize anaphylaxis. Vasodilation and escape of plasma into the tissues causes urticaria and angioedema and result in a decrease in effective plasma volume, which is the major cause of shock. Fluid escapes into the lung alveoli and may produce pulmonary edema. Obstructive angioedema of the upper airway may also occur. Arrhythmias and cardiogenic shock may develop if the reaction is prolonged. Fluid escapes into the lung alveoli and may produce pulmonary edema. Obstructive angioedema of the upper airway may also occur. Arrhythmias and cardiogenic shock may develop if the reaction is prolonged.

Assessment with Clinical Manifestations

Patients with anaphylaxis have a wide variety of both local and systemic clinical manifestations. These reactions are depicted both in Figure 43-4 and Table 43-7.

Planning and Implementation

Anaphylactic reactions occur suddenly in hypersensitive patients following exposure to an offending allergen. The speed of response is the cardinal principal in therapeutic management of anaphylaxis. The following are four areas

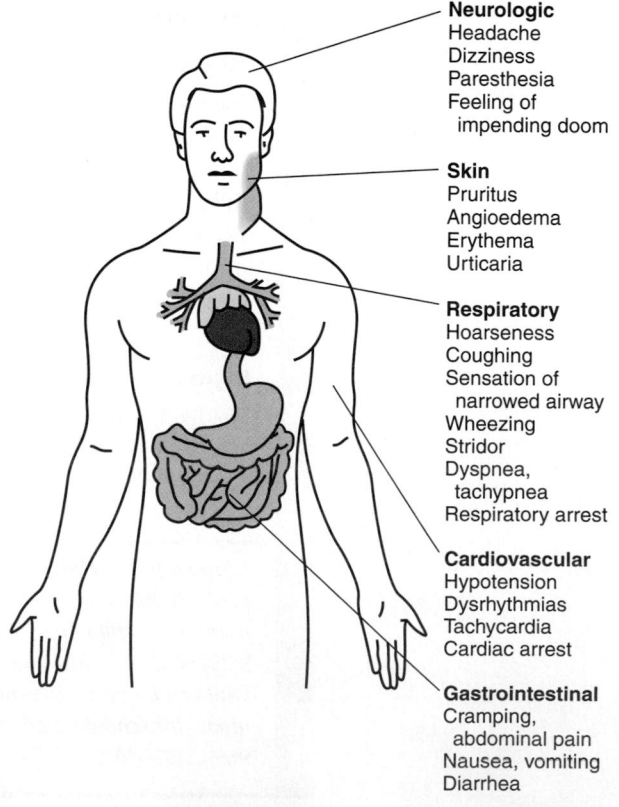

Figure 43-4 Clinical manifestations of a systemic anaphylactic reaction.

TABLE 43-7 **Clinical Manifestations of Anaphylaxis**

SYSTEM	SYMPTOM
Skin	Urticaria and angioedema, flushing, and pruritus
Respiratory	Dyspnea, wheezing, airway angioedema, and rhinitis
GI	Nausea, vomiting, diarrhea, cramping, and pain
Cardiovascular	Tachycardia, hypotension, cardiac arrest, and chest pain
Neurological	Headaches, dizziness, seizures, and sense of impending doom

Adapted from Lebovidge, J., Stone, K., Twarog, F., Raiselis, S., Kalish, L., Bailey, E., et al. (2006). Development of a preliminary questionnaire to assess parental response to children's food allergies. Annals of Allergy, Asthma, and Immunology, 96(3), 472–477.

TABLE 43-8 **Treatment of the Patient with Anaphylaxis**

INITIAL MEDICAL MANAGEMENT	MEDICAL THERAPY
Recumbent positioning	Epinephrine
Airway management Intubate if necessary	IV fluids
IV access	Histamine H_1 antagonists Histamine H_2 antagonists Steroids Inhaled/aerosolized beta-agonists

Adapted from Broyles, B. E., Reiss, B. S., & Evans, M. E. (2007). Pharmacological aspects of nursing care (7th ed.). New York: Thomson Delmar Learning; Murphy, K., Hopp, R., Kittelson, E., Hansen, G., Windle, M., & Walburn, J. (2006). Life-threatening asthma and anaphylaxis in schools: A treatment model for school-based programs. Annals of Allergy, Asthma, and Immunology, 96(3), 398–405.

of primary concern for the crisis management: (a) recognize the signs and symptoms, (b) maintain a patent airway, (c) prevent spread of the allergen by using a tourniquet when appropriate, and (d) administer appropriate drugs. In addition, the nurse must place the patient in a recumbent position, elevate the legs, keep the patient warm, and provide support for respirations with oxygen. The patient must have a maintained blood pressure with intravenous (IV) fluids. Hypovolemic shock may occur because of fluid moving from intravascular to interstitial spaces. Hypovolemic shock, if not treated early, leads to irreversible tissue damage and death (Pumphrey, 2003).

When an allergic disorder is diagnosed, treatment is aimed at reducing exposure, treating symptoms, and desensitizing the person through immunotherapy (Table 43-8). Adjuncts to therapy include medical alert bracelets, bee sting kits with an EpiPen, and education in emergency self-administration.

Pharmacology

Pharmaceutical management of anaphylaxis is necessary as an immediate treatment. Epinephrine is the most common medication given in acute care setting during the crisis of anaphylaxis, and Benadryl is likely the most typical nonprescription medication given to prevent anaphylaxis or to treat the early clinical manifestations of an allergenic reaction (Table 43-9).

TABLE 43-9   Pharmacology Facts: Pharmaceutical Therapy for Anaphylaxis

CLASSIFICATIONS	DRUGS	INDICATIONS
Parental adrenergic agents	Epinephrine (EpiPen, adrenalin)	Urticaria, angioedema, airway obstruction Bronchospasm
Inhaled beta-antagonists	Albuterol (Proventil, Ventolin)	Bronchospasm
H₁ receptor blockers (antihistamines)	Diphenhydramine (Benadryl)	Cutaneous lesions
H₂ receptor blockers (antihistamines)	Cimetidine (Tagamet)	Cutaneous lesions
Corticosteroids	Methylprednisone (Solu-Medrol, Depo-Medrol)	Bronchospasm, cutaneous lesions

Adapted from Broyles, B. E., Reiss, B. S., & Evans, M. E. (2007). Pharmacological aspects of nursing care (7th ed.). New York: Thomson Delmar Learning.

ALLERGIC CONDITIONS

An allergy is a specific immunological reaction to a normally harmless substance, one that does not bother most people. People who have allergies often are sensitive to more than one substance. Types of allergens that cause allergic reactions include pollens, dust particles, mold spores, food, latex, insect venom, or medicines.

Allergic Rhinitis (Hay Fever)

Pollen allergy, or hay fever, is one of the most common chronic diseases in the United States, with allergy to ragweed being the most common source of allergic rhinitis. Rhinitis is an inflammation of the nasal membranes and is characterized by a complex of symptoms that include sneezing, a stuffy or runny nose, itchy eyes, nose, and throat, and watery eyes. Allergic rhinitis symptoms are generated when the immune system encounters an allergen (pollen, mold, or dust) and a hypersensitive reaction causes the body to produce antibodies. Those antibodies combine with the allergen and produce histamine. The allergen is inhaled and causes a local inflammation or irritation of the mucous membranes that line the nose. Allergic rhinitis may be seasonal, reflecting an allergy to tree, grass, or weed pollens. Perennial allergic rhinitis can be the result of indoor allergens, such as feathers, mold spores, animal dander, or dust mites. Avoiding the allergen is the best treatment. Other treatments include treating the symptoms with antihistamines, decongestants, eye cleansing medications (Figure 43-5), and corticosteroids applied by nasal spray. Secondary infections indicated by facial pain or a greenish-yellow discharge may require antibiotic therapy.

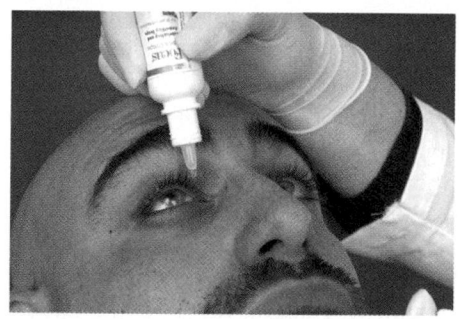

Figure 43-5 An eye cleansing medication being instilled via eye droplet.

Nursing Diagnoses

Based on the information gathered, examples of nursing diagnoses in the patient with allergic rhinitis may include the following:

- Risk for impaired membrane integrity related to inflamed mucous membranes.
- Deficient knowledge related to self-care and risk prevention.
- Fear and anxiety related to actual or potential lifestyle changes.
- Anxiety related to allergen avoidance.

Evaluation of Outcomes

Potential patient outcomes for each of the example nursing diagnoses for the patient with allergic rhinitis are:

- Risk for impaired membrane integrity related to irritation of the mucous membranes that line the nose. The patient has a resolution of the irritation of the nasal membranes.
- Deficient knowledge related to self-care and risk prevention. The patient should demonstrate motivation to learn, identify perceived learning needs, and verbalize an understanding of desired content. Knowledge of avoidance techniques should help avoid the risks and decrease anxiety.
- Fear and anxiety related to actual or potential lifestyle changes. The patient will be able to recognize the signs of anxiety, demonstrate positive coping mechanisms, and describe a reduction in the level of anxiety experienced.

Allergic Contact Dermatitis

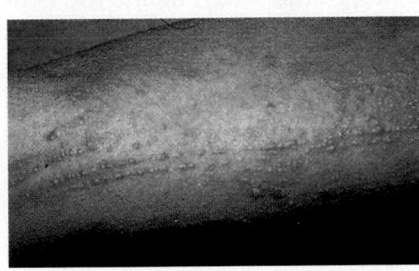

Figure 43-6 ACD note linear pattern to lesions. Courtesy of CDC.

Allergic contact dermatitis (ACD) is an inflammation of the skin caused by direct contact with an allergy causing substance. It is a type 4 allergic reaction, or delayed hypersensitivity reaction. The skin inflammation varies from mild irritation and redness to open sores, depending on the type of irritant, the body part affected, and the sensitivity of the individual. Irritants include water, soaps, detergents, solvents, acids, and alkalis. The rash is generally confined to the site of contact, but may be transmitted by the fingers to other sites (e.g., eyelids and genitals). Patients with atopic dermitis are particularly susceptible to developing ACD. There is typically a delay between the time of exposure and the onset of symptoms. Mild symptoms include itching, redness, swelling, and small blisters that may break, ooze, and crust over (Figure 43-6). More acute symptoms can occur with reexposure. These symptoms may involve respiratory symptoms, and rarely, symptoms may lead to respiratory collapse or shock. Latex allergy is a well-known example of ACD. Chemicals used in the harvesting and manufacture of latex can cause a cutaneous inflammatory condition similar to other sources of ACD reactions, such as poison ivy and nickel. A person wearing latex gloves may experience ACD. Treatment includes identification and avoidance of the allergen, moisturizing creams, topical steroid ointments, and antibiotics for secondary infection. Severe cases may require a short course of oral steroids.

Nursing Diagnoses

Based on the information gathered, examples of nursing diagnoses in the patient with ACD may include the following:

- Risk for impaired skin integrity related to urticaria and puritus.
- Deficient knowledge related to self-care and risk prevention.
- Fear and anxiety related to actual or potential lifestyle changes.

Evaluation of Outcomes

Potential patient outcomes for each of the example nursing diagnoses for the patient with ACD are:

- Risk for impaired skin integrity related to urticaria and pruritus. The patient's skin condition should be improved by decreased inflammation, urticaria, and pruritus.
- Deficient knowledge related to self-care and risk prevention. The patient should demonstrate motivation to learn, identify perceived learning needs, and verbalize an understanding of desired content.
- Fear and anxiety related to actual or potential lifestyle changes. The patient will be able to recognize the signs of anxiety, demonstrate positive coping mechanisms, and describe a reduction in the level of anxiety experienced.

Atopic Dermatitis

Atopic dermatitis (AD), also called atopic eczema or endogenous eczema, is a chronic disease that affects the dermis (skin). AD is linked to an exaggerated immune and inflammatory response that triggers elevated levels of (IgE. Studies done by the National Institute of Health indicate that 15 million people in the United States have symptoms of atopic dermatitis and that AD may develop at any age, but most often begins before the age of 5. AD is characterized by rashes and intense itching that may be accompanied by swelling, redness, blistering, oozing, crusting, and scales. The rashes are most commonly located on the face, inside the elbows, behind the knees, and on the hands and feet. The appearance of the skin depends on the amount of scratching and degree of secondary skin infection. The condition has periods of flare when symptoms exacerbate, and periods when the skin clears, and AD is in remission. Irritants found to be linked to flares of AD include wool and synthetic fibers in contact with the skin, certain soaps and detergents, solvents, dust, sand, and intermittent wetting and drying of the skin. The intense itching that is characteristic of AD provides a focus for nursing intervention. Scratching and rubbing in response to itching increases the inflammation and the possibility of secondary skin infections. Corticosteroid ointments and creams are used to treat AD. Antibiotics are added to the treatment plan as indicated.

Nursing Diagnoses

Based on the information gathered, examples of nursing diagnoses in the patient with AD may include the following:
- Risk for impaired skin integrity related to urticaria and pruritus.
- Deficient knowledge related to self-care and risk prevention.
- Fear and anxiety related to actual or potential lifestyle changes.

Evaluation of Outcomes

Potential patient outcomes for each of the example nursing diagnoses for the patient with AD are:
- Risk for impaired skin integrity related to urticaria and pruritus. The patient's skin condition should be improved by decreased inflammation, urticaria, and pruritus.
- Deficient knowledge related to self-care and risk prevention. The patient should demonstrate motivation to learn, identify perceived learning needs, and verbalize an understanding of desired content.
- Fear and anxiety related to actual or potential lifestyle changes. The patient will be able to recognize the signs of anxiety, demonstrate positive coping mechanisms, and describe a reduction in the level of anxiety experienced.

Urticaria

Urticaria (nettle-rash, hives, or wheals) is a hypersensitive dermatological manifestation in response to the release of histamine in an antigen-antibody reaction. This immune reaction causes vasodilation, skin eruptions, profound itching, and pain. The rash is composed of red circular, slightly elevated, or irregularly shaped eruptions and can appear on any part of the body. Each individual hive (or wheal) lasts a few hours and then fades away without a trace, as new hives appear. Urticaria may be localized in some patients, while others may have widespread eruptions. Many substances can trigger urticaria through an immediate hypersensitivity reaction (type 1). Urticaria is a symptom that can develop through exposure to a variety of things: viruses, medications, foods (most commonly nuts, chocolate, and fruits), parasites, chemicals (latex), physical stimulants (cold or pressure), and insect bites. In some cases the allergen

TABLE 43-10	**Pharmacology Facts: Pharmaceutical Therapy for Urticaria**	
CLASSIFICATIONS	**DRUGS**	**INDICATIONS**
Topical steroids	Triamcininolone (Aristocort)	Ointment used on dry or cracked skin, creams are used on inflamed skin or weeping lesions
Systemic steroids	Prednisone (Deltasone)	Severe cases involving more than 20 percent of total body surface (TBSA)
Antihistamines	Diphenhydramine (Benadryl) Hydroxyzine HCL (Atarax, Vistaril)	Used to relieve pruritus associated with contact dermatitis

Adapted from Broyles, B. E., Reiss, B. S., & Evans, M. E. (2007). Pharmacological aspects of nursing care (7th ed.). New York: Thomson Delmar Learning.

is idiopathic (no discernible cause). The acute form of urticaria lasts less than four to six weeks. Chronic hives is a case of hives that lasts longer than six weeks. Antihistamine medications are the primary treatment for urticaria (Table 43-10).

Nursing Diagnoses

Based on the information gathered, examples of nursing diagnoses in the patient with urticaria may include the following:

- Risk for impaired skin integrity related to urticaria and pruritus.
- Deficient knowledge related to self-care and risk prevention.
- Fear and anxiety related to actual or potential lifestyle changes.

Evaluation of Outcomes

Potential patient outcomes for each of the example nursing diagnoses for the patient with urticaria are:

- Risk for impaired skin integrity related to rash and itching. The patient's skin condition should be improved by decreased inflammation.
- Deficient knowledge related to self-care and risk prevention. The patient should demonstrate motivation to learn, identify perceived learning needs, and verbalize an understanding of desired content.
- Fear and anxiety related to actual or potential lifestyle changes. The patient will be able to recognize the signs of anxiety, demonstrate positive coping mechanisms, and describe a reduction in the level of anxiety experienced.

Angioneurotic Edema

Angioneurotic edema (also known as angioedema) is a condition that results from an allergic type reaction that involves histamine and the blood vessels in subdermal tissue. It is similar to hives, only the welts are larger, and it originates in a deeper layer of tissue. Angioedema may be caused by an allergic reaction to pollens, foods, medications, bee stings, cold, light, or exercise. Other types may be inherited or occur for idiopathic reasons. It is characterized by the appearance of large welts, usually appearing around the eyes and lips, but the welts may also occur on the hands, feet, and throat. Subdermal or submucosal edema may occur in other areas of the body, but when it occurs in the ear-nose-throat area, serious laryngeal swelling can be a hazard. Airway patency is a primary concern when a patient exhibits obvious edema of soft tissues of the face and neck. Airway intervention may be necessary. Angioedema may be progressive in nature and can be a prelude to anaphylaxis. Medications, such as epinephrine (EpiPen, Adrenaline), and antihistamines are directed toward blocking histamine that is producing the reaction.

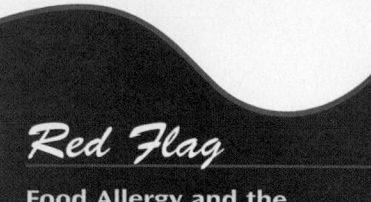

Red Flag

Food Allergy and the Impact of Ingredients

It is important for the nurse and the patient with a food allergy to become familiar with the composition of ingredients listed on food labels. A small amount of one ingredient has the ability to induce an allergic reaction. Here's an example:

Have you heard of casein? Casein is found in milk protein. It is an inactive ingredient sometimes added to products, like creamers and cheese, and may cause allergic reactions in patients with allergies to dairy products.

The Food and Drug Administration (FDA) received a report in which a child with a preexisting allergy to dairy products suffered a severe allergic reaction following ingestion of a chewable vitamin. The child was taken to the emergency department and recovered with treatment. The label on the vitamin indicated that the vitamin was free of starch, yeast, soy, wheat, dairy, gluten, egg, fragrance, artificial colors, and preservatives. However, the other ingredients section of the label listed sodium caseinate as an ingredient. The small amount of casein in one vitamin was sufficient to trigger child's allergic reaction.

Adapted from Janeway, C. A., Jr., Travers, P., Walport, M., & Shlomchik, M. J. (2004). Immunobiology, the immune system in health and disease (6th ed.). New York: Garland Science Publishing; Parker, E., Donato, L., Dalgleish, D. (2005). Effects of added sodium caseinate on the formation of particles in heated milk. Journal of Agricultural and Food Chemistry, 53(21), 8265–8272.

Nursing Diagnoses

Based on the information gathered, examples of nursing diagnoses in the patient with angioneurotic edema may include the following:
- Ineffective airway clearance related to soft tissue edema.
- Ineffective breathing pattern related to bronchospasm.
- Anxiety and agitation related to air hunger.
- Pain related to swelling of abdominal organs.
- Risk for impaired skin integrity related to urticaria and pruritus.
- Fear and anxiety related to the inability to control body response.

Evaluation of Outcomes

Potential patient outcomes for each of the example nursing diagnoses for the patient with angioedema are:
- Ineffective airway clearance related to soft tissue edema. The patient will maintain a patent airway as evidenced by unrestricted respirations.
- Ineffective breathing pattern related to bronchospasm. The patient will resume normal breathing patterns as evidenced by chest observation and auscultative chest sounds.
- Anxiety and agitation related to air hunger. The patient will demonstrate more relaxed postures as oxygen perfusion of tissues improves.
- Pain related to swelling of abdominal organs. The patient should verbalize an adequate relief of pain along with the ability to realistically cope with the pain if it is not completely relieved.
- Risk for impaired skin integrity related to urticaria and pruritus. The patient's skin condition should be improved by decreased inflammation, urticaria, and pruritus.
- Fear and anxiety related to the inability to control body response. The patient should be able to recognize the signs of anxiety and stress, demonstrate positive coping mechanisms, and describe a reduction in the level of anxiety experienced.

Food Allergy

A food allergy, or hypersensitivity, is an abnormal response to a food triggered by the body's immune system. The reaction to the food allergen may be either immediate or delayed. The patient may experience symptoms that range from GI distress to anaphylaxis. In adults, the foods that most often cause allergic reactions include shellfish, peanuts, walnuts, fish, and eggs. Children are often allergic to eggs, milk, and peanuts.

Some foods can cause severe illness and, in some cases, a life-threatening allergic reaction (anaphylaxis) that can constrict airways in the lungs, severely lower blood pressure, and cause suffocation by the swelling of the tongue or throat. Food allergens are proteins in a food that enters the bloodstream when the food is digested. The immune system produces IgE, a food specific antibody in people with inherited allergic tendencies.
- The first time a person with a specific food allergy eats the specific food, IgE specific to that food is released by the immune system.
- The second time that specific food is eaten, it interacts with the food-specific IgE and triggers the cells to release histamine.
- An allergic reaction to food can occur within minutes of eating the food. In other situations the allergic response may not occur for an hour.

When a person is allergic to a particular food, itching of the mouth may occur as they eat the food. If the food is digested, GI symptoms, such as vomiting, diarrhea, and cramping, may occur. When the allergens reach the bloodstream, there may be a drop in blood pressure. Hives and atopic eczema develop when the allergens reach the skin. As the reaction reaches the lungs, asthma may develop. A mild symptom such as a tingling in the mouth can progress rapidly to anaphylaxis requiring immediate assistance.

Eliminating foods that trigger an allergic reaction are identified through a process that eliminates suspect foods from the diet. The food is then reintroduced, and the result is evaluated. Treatment of food allergy consists of avoiding foods that trigger a reaction and treating symptoms during a reaction. Patients with known food allergies should wear a medical alert bracelet stating the food allergy. Many of these individuals also carry a syringe of epinephrine (EpiPen) and are prepared to inject themselves if they feel they are having an allergic reaction.

Nursing Diagnoses

Based on the information gathered, examples of nursing diagnoses in the patient with food allergies may include the following:
- Ineffective airway clearance related to soft tissue edema.
- Ineffective breathing pattern related to bronchospasm.
- Anxiety and agitation related to air hunger.
- Risk for impaired skin integrity related to urticaria and pruritus.
- Deficient knowledge related to self-care and risk prevention.
- Fear and anxiety related to actual or potential lifestyle changes.

Evaluation of Outcomes

Potential patient outcomes for each of the example nursing diagnoses for the patient with food allergies are:
- Ineffective airway clearance related to soft tissue edema. The patient will maintain a patent airway as evidenced by unrestricted respirations.
- Ineffective breathing pattern related to bronchospasm. The patient will resume normal breathing patterns as evidenced by chest observation and auscultative chest sounds.
- Anxiety and agitation related to air hunger. The patient will demonstrate more relaxed postures as oxygen perfusion of tissues improves.
- Risk for impaired skin integrity related to urticaria and pruritus. The patient's skin condition should be improved by decreased inflammation, urticaria, and pruritus.
- Deficient knowledge related to self-care and risk prevention. The patient should demonstrate motivation to learn, identify perceived learning needs, and verbalize an understanding of desired content
- Fear and anxiety related to actual or potential lifestyle changes. The patient will be able to recognize the signs of anxiety, demonstrate positive coping mechanisms, and describe a reduction in the level of anxiety experienced.

Latex Allergy

Latex allergy is a reaction to certain proteins in latex rubber. The amount of latex exposure needed to produce sensitization or an allergic reaction is unknown. Increasing the exposure to latex proteins increases the risk of developing allergic symptoms. In sensitized persons, symptoms usually begin within minutes of exposure, but they can occur hours later and can be quite varied. Mild reactions to latex involve skin redness, rash, hives, or itching. More severe reactions may involve respiratory symptoms, such as runny nose, sneezing, itchy eyes, scratchy throat, and wheezing. Anaphylaxis is a possibility. Health care providers wear latex gloves on a frequent basis and can become susceptible to latex allergy conditions.

Nursing Diagnoses

Based on the information gathered, examples of nursing diagnoses in the patient with latex allergies may include the following:
- Ineffective airway clearance related to soft tissue edema.
- Risk for impaired skin integrity related to urticaria and pruritus.

- Deficient knowledge related to self-care and prevention.
- Fear and anxiety related to actual or potential lifestyle changes.

Evaluation of Outcomes

Potential patient outcomes for each of the example nursing diagnoses for the patient with latex allergies are:

- Ineffective airway clearance related to soft tissue edema. The patient will maintain a patent airway as evidenced by unrestricted respirations.
- Risk for impaired skin integrity related to urticaria and pruritus. The patient's skin condition should be improved by decreased inflammation, urticaria, and pruritus.
- Deficient knowledge related to self-care and prevention. The patient should demonstrate motivation to learn, identify perceived learning needs, and verbalize an understanding of desired content.
- Fear and anxiety related to actual or potential lifestyle changes. The patient should be able to recognize the signs of anxiety, demonstrate positive coping mechanisms, and describe a reduction in the level of anxiety experienced.

Serum Sickness

Serum sickness is a type 3 hypersensitivity reaction that results from the injection of foreign protein or serum. The incidence of serum sickness is declining in the United States because of public health programs that have decreased the need for specific antitoxins, such as rabies and tetanus antitoxin. Primary serum sickness occurs 6 to 21 days after the administration of the antitoxin. Classic symptoms of serum sickness include pain and swelling at the injection site, followed by temperature elevation of 101 to 104° F (38.3 to 40° C), arthralgia, lymphadenopathy, and skin eruptions. Because it takes time for the body to produce antibodies to a new antigen, symptoms do not develop until 7 to 21 days after initial exposure to the antiserum. However, patients may develop symptoms in 1 to 3 days if they have previously been exposed to the offending agent. Exposure to certain medications (particularly penicillin) can cause a similar process. Unlike other drug allergies, which occur soon after receiving the medication for the second (or subsequent) time, serum sickness can develop 7 to 21 days after the first exposure to a medication. Blood products may also induce serum sickness. Other causes of serum sickness include serum used in the prophylaxis or treatment of botulism, diphtheria, gas gangrene, transplant rejection, and snake and spider bites. Treatment includes stopping the therapy that involves the suspected antigen and providing supportive therapy for the symptoms. Medications used to treat serum sickness include antihistamines and antipyretics. Corticosteroids agents help modify the immune response.

Nursing Diagnoses

Based on the information gathered, examples of nursing diagnoses in the patient with serum sickness may include the following:

- Risk for impaired skin integrity related to urticaria and pruritus.
- Risk for imbalanced body temperature. Fear and anxiety related to actual or potential health decline.
- Impaired physical mobility related to serum sickness.

Evaluation of Outcomes

Potential patient outcomes for each of the example nursing diagnoses for the patient with serum sickness are:

- Risk for impaired skin integrity related to urticaria and pruritus. The patient's skin condition should be improved by decreased inflammation, urticaria, and pruritus.

- Risk for imbalanced body temperature. The patient maintains body temperature within a normal range.
- Fear and anxiety related to actual or potential health decline. The patient should be able to recognize the signs of anxiety, demonstrate coping mechanisms, and describe a reduction in the level of anxiety experienced.
- Impaired physical mobility related to serum sickness. The patient should perform physical activity independently or with assistive devices as needed. In addition, the patient should be free of complication of immobility, as evidenced by intact skin, absence of thrombophlebitis, and normal bowel patterns.

Contact Dermatitis (Dermatitis Medicamentosa)

Contact dermatitis is an acute or chronic skin inflammation triggered in the epidermis by contact with a specific antigen or irritant. Primary irritant dermatitis results from direct allergen contact with the skin and usually produces discomfort immediately following exposure. ACD is a delayed hypersensitivity reaction requiring several hours for the reaction to become apparent. The skin inflammation and rash appear the same for both primary irritant dermatitis and allergic contact dermatitis. Affected individuals have abnormal redness of the skin (erythema) or itching (pruritus) following contact with various metal alloys (e.g., nickel), cements, and household cleaners. Strong irritants (e.g., acids, alkalis) can produce an immediate reaction that has the appearance of a thermal burn. The most common agents for allergic contact dermatitis are plants, such as poison ivy, poison oak, and poison sumac. Treatment of contact dermatitis depends on the type, extent, and area of skin lesions. Wet compresses, topical steroids, and systemic steroids (e.g., Prednisone) are used to treat severe cases involving 20 percent of total body surface.

Nursing Diagnoses

Based on the information gathered, examples of nursing diagnoses in the patient with contact dermatitis may include the following:
- Risk for impaired skin integrity related to urticaria and pruritus.
- Deficient knowledge related to self-care and risk prevention.
- Fear and anxiety related to actual or potential lifestyle changes.

Evaluation of Outcomes

Potential patient outcomes for each of the example nursing diagnoses for the patient with contact dermatitis are:
- Risk for impaired skin integrity related to urticaria and pruritus. The patient's skin condition should be improved by decreased inflammation, urticaria, and pruritus.
- Deficient knowledge related to self-care and risk prevention. The patient should demonstrate motivation to learn, identify perceived learning needs, and verbalize an understanding of desired content.
- Fear and anxiety related to actual or potential lifestyle changes. The patient will be able to recognize the signs of anxiety, demonstrate positive coping mechanisms, and describe a reduction in the level of anxiety experienced.

Hereditary Angioedema

Hereditary angioedema (HAE) is an inherited disorder of the immune system that causes painless swelling, particularly of the face, and abdominal cramping. HAE is a lifelong affliction that usually becomes apparent in adulthood. It is caused by low levels or improper function of a protein called C1 inhibitor. Patients with HAE are often found to be depleted of C1 inhibitor. This, in turn, affects blood vessels. People with HAE can develop rapid swelling in several prominent sites: subdermal tissues (face, hands, arms, legs, genitals, and buttocks); abdominal organs (stomach, intestines, and bladder), with a colicky pain in the abdomen that can mimic a surgical emergency; and the upper airway (larynx), which may result in laryngeal edema. Occasionally, erythema or mild urticarial eruptions may precede the edema. Precipitating factors of attacks may include trauma (particularly dental trauma), anxiety, and stress. Depending on the symptoms and the sites of the angioedema, intensive support may be necessary, including IV fluids. Intubation may be necessary in cases that are complicated by laryngeal edema.

Nursing Diagnoses

Based on the information gathered, examples of nursing diagnoses in the patient with HAE may include the following:
- Ineffective airway clearance related to soft tissue edema.
- Ineffective breathing pattern related to bronchospasm.
- Anxiety and agitation related to air hunger.
- Pain related to swelling of abdominal organs.
- Risk for impaired skin integrity related to urticaria and pruritus.
- Fear and anxiety related to the inability to control body response.

Evaluation of Outcomes

Potential patient outcomes for each of the example nursing diagnoses for the patient with HAE are:
- Ineffective airway clearance related to soft tissue edema. The patient will maintain a patent airway as evidenced by unrestricted respirations.
- Ineffective breathing pattern related to bronchospasm. The patient will resume normal breathing patterns as evidenced by chest observation and auscultative chest sounds.
- Anxiety and agitation related to air hunger. The patient will demonstrate more relaxed postures as oxygen perfusion of tissues improves.
- Pain related to swelling of abdominal organs. The patient should verbalize an adequate relief of pain along with the ability to realistically cope with the pain if it is not completely relieved.
- Risk for impaired skin integrity related to urticaria and pruritus. The patient's skin condition should be improved by decreased inflammation, urticaria, and pruritus.
- Fear and anxiety related to the inability to control body response. The patient should be able to recognize the signs of anxiety and stress, demonstrate positive coping mechanisms, and describe a reduction in the level of anxiety experienced.

KEY CONCEPTS

- Allergic diseases are common, affecting about 15 to 20 percent if the population.
- Immune response is triggered when the body recognizes and defends itself against allergens (microorganisms, viruses, and substances) recognized by the body as foreign and potentially harmful.
- Hyperresponsiveness is an overreaction of the body's immune response to allergens.
- Gcll and Coombs classifications are categories of immune response.

- Atopy is an inherited tendency for hyperproduction of IgE antibodies to common environmental allergens.
- Anaphylactic reactions are severe, life-threatening allergic reactions.
- Atopic asthma (allergic asthma) is a type 1 immune response to allergens.
- Hypersensitive reaction include other diseases and conditions, including food allergy, drug allergy, urticaria, latex allergy, drug allergy, and serum sickness.

REVIEW QUESTIONS

1. Your patient has a history of abdominal bloating, cramping, and loose stools and thinks that she has a food allergy. As a nurse, you know:
   1. Elimination and challenge diets form the basis for the diagnosis of food allergy.
   2. An SPT will help locate the problem.
   3. Blood testing will identify the food allergy.
   4. Hair sample testing will identify the food allergy.

2. A patient being treated for anaphylaxis will be given what drug by intramuscular injection?
   1. Hydrocortisone
   2. Epinephrine
   3. Theophylline
   4. Captopril

3. Your patient with a newly diagnosed latex allergy is being discharged from the hospital today. As part of your discharge teaching plan, you inform the patient that he needs to seek immediate medical attention if the following occurs:
   1. His medical alert bracelet falls off.
   2. He accidentally ingests sunflower seeds.
   3. He experiences swelling around the lips or eyes.
   4. He feels his heart pounding after strenuous exercise.

4. Atopic individuals have an inherited tendency to hyperproduce what type of antibodies in response to common environmental allergens?
   1. IgE
   2. Mast cells
   3. Histamine
   4. Prostaglandin

5. Hyposensitization (immunotherapy for a specific allergen) has been proven a benefit in which of the following conditions?
   1. Dust mite allergy
   2. Peanut allergy
   3. Wasp venom hypersensitivity
   4. Urticaria

6. A patient with an immediate type 1 hypersensitivity will respond to a SPT with the appropriate antigen by:
   1. A wheal and flare response immediately
   2. A wheal and flare response 48 hours later
   3. An increased susceptibility to herpes zoster
   4. A wheal and flare response within 5 to 10 minutes

7. You are covering for another nurse during lunch. You answer a call light for one of her patients. The patient is restless and complains of itching. The patient has an IV piggyback running. What first step should you take?
   1. Tell him you will get his nurse
   2. Take his blood pressure
   3. Shut off the IV piggyback and slow the IV to a keep open rate
   4. Give him a drink of water and turn on the call light

8. Which of the following signs and symptoms would be consistent with a diagnosis of atopic eczema in a 10-month-old infant?
   1. Webbing between the fingers and toes
   2. Lactose intolerance
   3. Dermatitis on face and flexural aspects of arms and legs
   4. Swollen eyes

9. Severe reactions to penicillin are more likely to happen when the medication is given by what route?
   1. Orally
   2. Intramuscular
   3. Through a nebulizer
   4. Parentally

10. Your patient is diagnosed with asthma. Which of the following nursing diagnoses would be most appropriate for this patient?
    1. High risk for infections
    2. Sexual dysfunction
    3. Ineffective airway clearance
    4. Fluid volume deficit

REVIEW ACTIVITIES

1. List four examples of hypersensitivity type 1 allergic reactions.

2. Develop a teaching plan for the family of a 14-month-old patient with newly diagnosed atopic asthma.

3. Name four categories of potential allergens that may cause anaphylaxis in hypersensitive patients.

4. Describe the best manner of diagnosing a food allergy.

5. What is the relationship of IgE and histamine in an allergic reaction?

6. What is the best treatment for hay fever (allergic rhinitis)?

7. Define atopy and discuss the impact it has on allergic reactions.

Visit the Contemporary Medical-Surgical Nursing online companion resource at www.delmarhealthcare.com for additional content and study aids. Click on Online Companions then select the Nursing discipline.

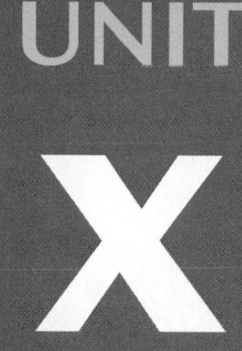

Alterations in Integumentary Function

Assessment of Integumentary Function

Cynthia A. Worley, BSN, RN, WOCN

CHAPTER TOPICS

- Anatomy and Physiology of the Integumentary System

- Factors Regulating Skin and Wound Repair

- Skin Changes throughout the Life Span

- Assessment of the Integumentary System

The skin is the largest organ of the body and is capable of regeneration and repair. If stretched flat, it wound measure about 3,000 square inches or almost two square meters. The skin weighs about six pounds, receives one third of the body's circulating blood volume and undergoes a seven-fold growth from birth to death. Its thickness ranges from 0.04 mm on the eyelids to 1.6 mm in soles of feet and palms of hands. The variations in thickness are also related to underlying structures and their protection (e.g., bones, muscles, or internal organs). Maintaining skin integrity is a complex process, and the skin is constantly exposed to a changing environment. The skin forms a protective barrier, assists in maintaining a homeostatic environment, and can resist limited physical, mechanical, and chemical assaults. The epidermal appendages, hair, nails, sweat, and sebaceous glands, which are also lined with epidermal cells, aid in repair and resurfacing in the event of skin injury (Johnstone, Farly & Henley, 2005).

ANATOMY AND PHYSIOLOGY

Human skin is divided into two layers, the epidermis (the outermost layer) and the dermis (the innermost layer) (Figure 44-1). Subcutaneous tissue lies below the dermis of the skin. Table 44-1 provides an overview of the structure, function, and clinical presentations of problems related to abnormal function of skin.

Epidermis

The epidermis is comprised of five layers of stratified squamous epithelial cells named (outer to inner) the stratum corneum, stratum lucidum, stratum granulosum, stratum spinosum, and stratum germinativum (Figure 44-2). Each layer has its own functions within the differentiation process. The epidermis is the thin, stratified outer skin layer that is in contact with the environment. It is avascular and without lymphatic channels or connective tissue. Therefore, the epidermis must derive its nourishment and blood supply from the underlying dermis (Johnstone, et al., 2005).

Epidermal tissue replenishes itself through a process called **keratinization.** Keratin is a highly insoluble, fibrous protein. During its lifecycle, the keratinocyte is first formed in the basal layer (stratum germinativum) and undergoes biochemical and morphological changes as it migrates from the innermost epidermal layer to the outermost epidermal layer. The epidermis is undergoing a constant turnover of new cells averaging every 26 to 42 days with complete renewal about every two months, a process called **differentiation.** The layers of the epidermis are named to reflect the changes occurring in the keratinocyte during differentiation. All layers of the epidermis consist of these types of peaks and valleys.

Cells in the Epidermis

Melanocytes are also present within the epidermis and are responsible for skin color or **pigmentation.** The normal number of melanocytes is nearly the same from person to person, regardless of skin color. It is the size and distribution of

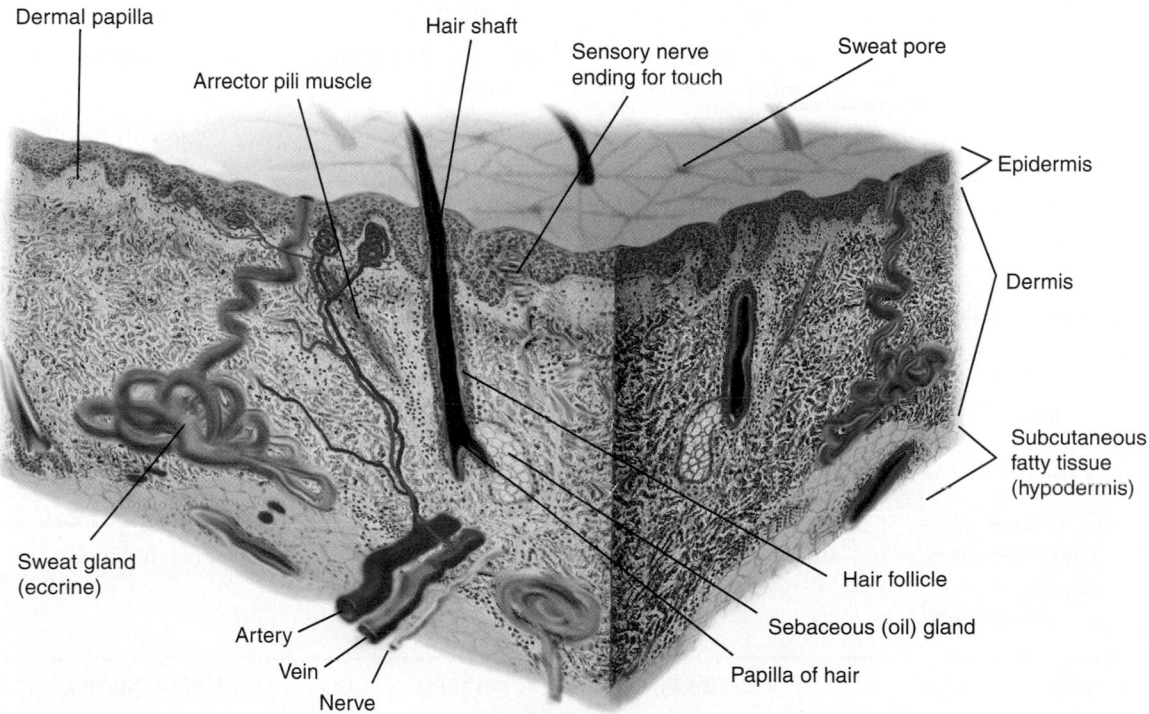

Dermal papilla

Hair shaft

Arrector pili muscle

Sensory nerve ending for touch

Sweat pore

Epidermis

Dermis

Subcutaneous fatty tissue (hypodermis)

Hair follicle

Sebaceous (oil) gland

Papilla of hair

Sweat gland (eccrine)

Artery

Vein

Nerve

Figure 44-1 Structures of the skin.

TABLE 44-1 Structures and Functions of the Skin

STRUCTURE	NORMAL FUNCTION	RESULT OF ABNORMAL FUNCTION	ABNORMAL CLINICAL PRESENTATIONS
Epidermis			
Stratum corneum	Protective barrier	Dryness, scaling, reduced barrier function	Psoriasis, eczema, pressure ulcers, burns (thermal or chemical)
Keratinocytes	Keratin synthesis, replenish stratum corneum	Reduced or impaired barrier function, abnormal transformation	Ichthyosis, actinic keratosis, skin cancers
Melanocytes	Skin pigmentation, melanin production	Increased or decreased skin color, malignant changes	Hyperpigmentation or hypopigmentation, suntan, malignant melanoma
Langerhans' cells	Immune response	Contact dermatitis	Rash, psoriasis
Basal cells	Replenish epidermal layers	Increased production, abnormal transformation	Basal cell carcinoma
Epidermal Appendages			
Apocrine gland	Apocrine sweat production	Odor, staining	Chromidrosis
Eccrine gland	Perspiration, thermoregulation	Fluid and electrolyte loss; reduced heat dissipation	Arrhythmia, heat stroke, heat exhaustion, anhidrosis
Sebaceous gland	Sebum production, lubrication, antimicrobial barrier	Obstruction of flow of sebum	Oily skin, acne
Hair follicle	Protection, appearance	Poor self-image	Alopecia, folliculitis, hirsutism
Nails	Protection, mechanical	Exposed nail bed, nail changes	Fungal infections, subungual problems, psoriasis
Dermis			
Macrophage	Immune response, chemotactic response	Poor inflammatory response, delay in healing	Job's syndrome
Mast cell	Histamine response, chemotactic response	Abnormal histamine release	Allergic responses, urticaria
Fibroblasts	Synthesis of collagen scaffold	Abnormal skin and wound tensile strength	Poor quality granulation tissue, fragile skin, scurvy, scleroderma, systemic lupus erythematosus
Endothelial cells	Neoangiogenesis: new vasculature (blood vessels)	Decreased blood flow, necrosis of tissue	Peripheral arterial and vascular disease
Lymphatic vessels	Removal of cellular debris and microorganisms	Poor interstitial fluid regulation	Edema, acute and chronic
Nerve fibers	Sensory perception	Inadequate tissue enervation, **pruritus** (itching)	Pruritus, atopic dermatitis, excoriation of skin
Subcutaneous tissue (below dermis-attaches skin to underlying tissues)	Protection of underlying structures, storage of energy and hormones	Atrophic changes, inadequate protection, malignant changes	Emaciation, obesity, malignant lipomatous tumors

Adapted from Johnstone, C., Farley, A., & Hendry, C. (2005). *The physiological basis of wound healing.* Nursing Standard, 19(43), 59–65.

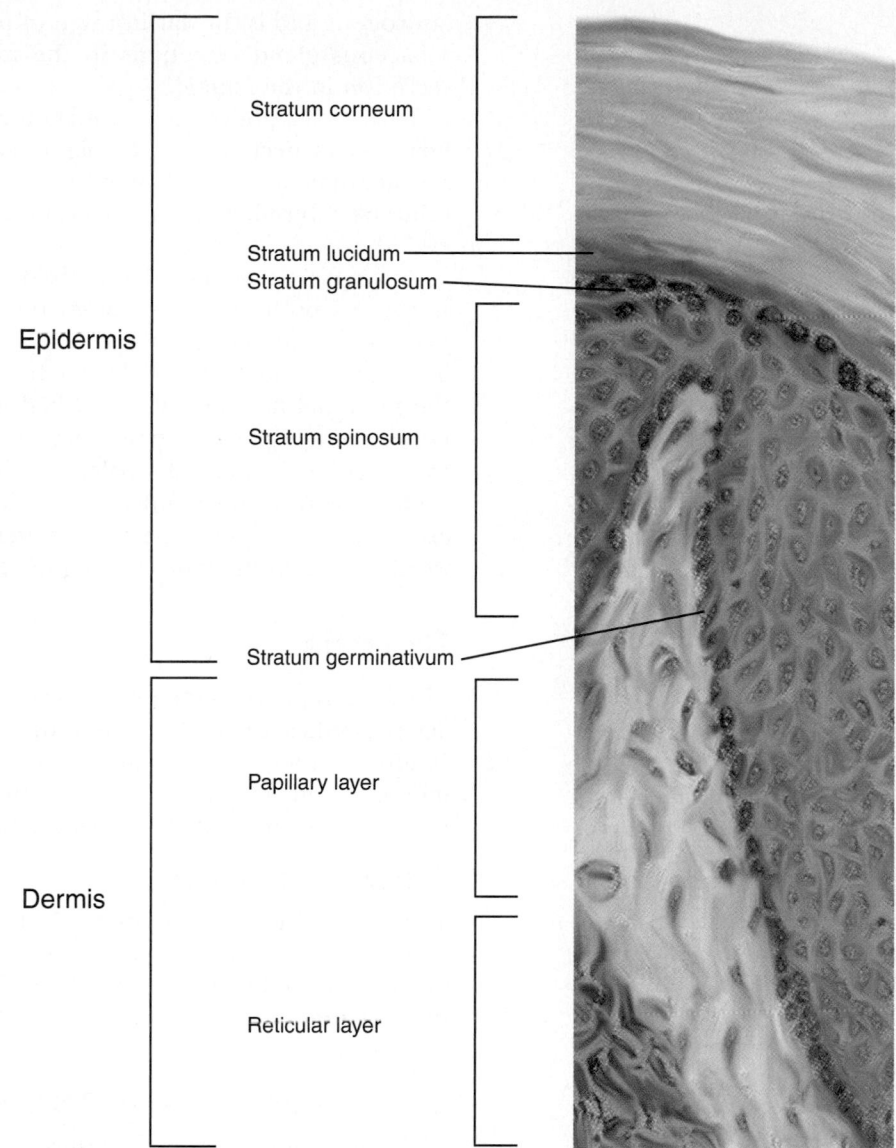

Epidermis

Stratum corneum

Stratum lucidum
Stratum granulosum

Stratum spinosum

Stratum germinativum

Dermis

Papillary layer

Reticular layer

Figure 44-2 Epidermal and dermal layers of skin.

melanosomes, the structures within melanocytes containing the melanin pigment, which differentiates lighter-skinned from darker-skinned individuals. Carotenoids are responsible for the yellow tone of the skin in some individuals.

Langerhans' cells originate in bone marrow and are antigen-presenting cells (APCs). They are responsible for foreign antigen recognition and provide immune protection. Langerhans' cells are found in several layers of the epidermis and are impaired by ultraviolet (UV) radiation. It is believed that Langerhans' cells are directly involved with allergic contact hypersensitivity.

Epidermal Appendages

The epidermal appendages are down-growths of the epidermis and extend into the dermis. They consist of exocrine, apocrine, and sebaceous glands, hair and hair follicles, and nails. The exocrine sweat glands play a role in thermoregulation; apocrine glands are located primarily in the axillae, breast areolae, and the anogenital area. These glands enlarge and become active because of reproductive hormones at puberty. Sebaceous glands are found throughout the skin except in the palms of the hands and soles and dorsum of the feet. Most sebaceous glands are associated with hair follicles (pilosebaceous unit). Sebaceous gland development is regulated by androgens and is the earliest sign of puberty. Testicular androgen regulates sebaceous gland secretions in the male and ovarian androgen regulates secretion in the female.

Hair serves physiological functions, such as insulation and prevention of heat loss, protection from UV light, tactile perception, and acts as social and sexual ornamentation. Most of the body is covered with fine or faint hair called vellus hair. Terminal hair is the coarser, darker hair of the scalp, eyebrows, and eyelashes.

The nails are layers of keratinized cells cemented together. The nail plate serves as a protective covering for the distal tips of the fingers and toes. The nail root lies posterior to the cuticle and is attached to the matrix. The matrix is undifferentiated epithelial tissue from which the nails arise and is located in the proximal nail bed. The nail bed is the vascular bed of the nail and lies under the nail plate. The periungual tissue surrounds the nail plate and the free edge of the nail. The pale, crescent-shaped area at the proximal end of each nail is the lunula. A damaged nail matrix produces a distorted nail. Nails are sensitive to physiological changes and will grow more slowly in cold weather and during illness (Doughty, 2004).

Dermis

The dermis provides the principle mass of the skin and mainly comprises collagen bundles usually 1 to 4 mm thick. Functions of the dermis include prevention of mechanical trauma, water storage, sensory enervation, and thermoregulation. The dermis contains macrophages, mast cells, fibroblasts, and lymphocytes, all of which play vital roles in wound healing.

Dermal Proteins

The essential proteins produced in the dermis are collagen, reticular fibers, and elastin. Collagen constitutes the majority of fibers in the dermis and is the major structural protein of the body. This protein is the most stress-resistant fiber of the dermis and provides tensile strength to the layer. Vitamin C is essential for production of collagen.

Components of the Dermis

The cells found within the dermis are important to tissue regeneration and repair. The macrophage is responsible for ingestion of bacteria and other substances and is the principle mediator of wound healing. Macrophages arise from the bone marrow and initially circulate in the blood as a monocyte. In the dermis the macrophage functions as part of the immune response and along with the Langerhans' cells, are capable of processing and presenting antigens to immuno-competent lymphocytes.

Endothelial cells are responsible for the formation of new blood vessel generation or **neoangiogenesis.** They reside in the lining of blood vessels and are activated shortly after injury to the vessel. Mast cells are responsible for histamine release in response to tissue injury and trigger the body's reaction to allergens. Fibroblasts are responsible for synthesis of collagen, elastin, reticular fibers, and ground substance (a viscoelastic substance that has the ability to mold to irregular objects and bind water). Fibroblasts are the principle cells of the dermis. Collagenase and gelatinase, the two enzymes produced by fibroblasts, also degrade collagen bundles. The dermis protects the epidermal appendages and supports a nerve and vascular network.

Lymphatic glands play a role in immune response by removing excess interstitial fluid and microbes. Blood vessels are responsible for perfusion and metabolic skin requirements and play a role in thermoregulation. Nerve fibers are responsible for perception of heat, cold, pain, itching, and pressure and also regulate vasoconstriction, vasodilation, and sweat secretion (Johnstone, et al., 2005).

Subcutaneous Tissue

The subcutaneous tissue consists of adipose or fat cells and lies below the dermis; however, it is not actually part of the skin. Collagen is also found in the subcutaneous layer. Thickness of this tissue varies throughout the body; it is nearly nonexistent in the eyelid, areolae, penis, scrotum, and anterior tibial region and is thickest in the waist area. The distribution of subcutaneous tissue is mediated by hormones, age, heredity, and eating habits. Subcutaneous tissue provides padding over bony prominences, joints, muscle, and internal organs, and serves as a shock absorber.

Protection

The skin provides an effective barrier against many forms of trauma, including mechanical, thermal, microbial, chemical, and radiant insults. The intact epidermis provides a physical barrier against microbial and chemical invasion. The natural biochemical barrier of the skin is called the acid mantle. The acid mantle consists of a mixture of lipoproteins (sebum) secreted by appendages in the epidermis and the acidity of this layer resists bacterial growth and invasion. Sebum has natural antibacterial substances that retard growth of microorganisms. Sebum and keratin also act as barriers against aqueous and chemical solutions. The mechanical strength of the skin comes from bonding of the structures in the epidermis and dermis. Subcutaneous tissue acts as a shock absorber, protecting underlying structures. Melanocytes, the pigment-producing cells of the epidermis screen and absorb UV radiation.

Homeostasis

Homeostasis refers to the fluid and electrolyte regulation function of the skin. Normal human skin breathes water off by the moisture vapor transport mechanism. Normal skin fluid loss is usually 200 g of water within 24 hours. The barrier properties of the skin prevent dehydration by controlled evaporation of internal fluids. The sweat glands open and close in response to external stimuli and to any changes in internal core temperature. The skin also limits absorption of external fluids and gases.

Excretion

The skin functions in the release of urea, bile, sweat, lactic acid, carbon dioxide, and sodium chloride. These functions are excretory in nature and eliminate substances that otherwise would be debilitating and toxic to the body. The renal and respiratory systems also excrete many of these substances.

Thermoregulation

Thermoregulation is the control of body temperature. The skin acts to control body temperature by conduction of heat through the skin for evaporation or absorption by other objects, radiation of heat from body surfaces, convection of heat by air currents, and evaporation of sweat. When the skin senses a warm external environment, the blood vessels dilate in response to promote heat loss. Conversely, the vessels constrict in a cool or cold environment to conserve the body's core temperature.

Synthesis

The skin synthesizes vitamin D by using UV light to convert 7-dehydrocholesterol in the epidermis. Vitamin D is important to calcium and phosphate metabolism and in the mineralization of bone.

Sensory Perception

The skin receptors function primarily in sensation of heat, cold, pain, light touch, itch, and pressure. Different nerves are responsible for each different stimulus and the concentration of nerve endings varies anatomically. Skin sensation is an integrated protective response to the external environment and an important protective mechanism of the skin. For example when a hand comes in contact with a hot object, one immediately pulls away from the heat source.

Psychosocial Function

The skin serves as an organ of communication and identification. The skin presents who we are to our external environment. Healthy skin provides a general sense of well-being and influences self-image. The increase in sebum production experienced during adolescence can trigger changes in the skin, such as acne. Severe cases of acne or cutaneous diseases will significantly alter a person's perception of self. Skin reactions to anger, anxiety, or fear may be manifested as sweating, pallor, or flushing. Reactions to a person's appearance indicate that the skin also serves the function of sexual attraction (Saunders & Edwards, 2004).

Healing

The skin can heal damage to its integrity by either a process of repair or regeneration. **Regeneration** is achieved by replacing damaged cells with the same cell type. Superficial damage to the epidermis is healed by resurfacing the wound with epidermal cells. Only the epidermis and superficial dermis are capable of regeneration, because epithelial, endothelial, and certain tissue substances can be reproduced. The skin repairs a dermal injury by filling the defect with dissimilar tissue because the dermis cannot be regenerated by the body (Johnstone, et al., 2005).

SKIN CHANGES THROUGHOUT THE LIFE SPAN

The skin undergoes numerous changes throughout the human lifecycle. Most of these changes are normal, harmless, and unchangeable. Changes, such as the damage caused by UV light exposure, can be minimized by appropriate preventive treatment (American Academy of Dermatology (AAD), 2006; Weil, 2005).

Newborn and infant skin is porous and easily damaged. The barrier function is not fully developed, the immune system immature, and the skin readily absorbs substances. Most dermatological products, with the exception of a few sun protection products, cannot be used on this age-group. During childhood the barrier and immunological functions of the skin mature. By 2 years of age barrier capability and immune functions are fully developed.

In the adolescent group hormonal secretion stimulates changes in hair follicles and sebaceous, eccrine, and apocrine glands. Hair follicle stimulation produces hair growth on the face in males and in the axilla and genital areas of both genders. This age-group is highly conscious of physical appearance, and the changes wrought by increased sebum production from the facial sebaceous glands resulting in acne can make teenagers self-conscious. Many dermatological pharmaceutical and over-the-counter preparation manufacturers target this audience with products designed to improve appearance (Frith, 2006).

During adulthood the evidence of sun exposure in younger years is seen as wrinkles; weathered-looking skin; age spots; **actinic keratoses** (premalignant lesions); and **telangiectasias** (dilatation of small blood vessels) (Figure 44-3) on the cheeks, nose, and ears, as well as pigmental changes, such as freckles

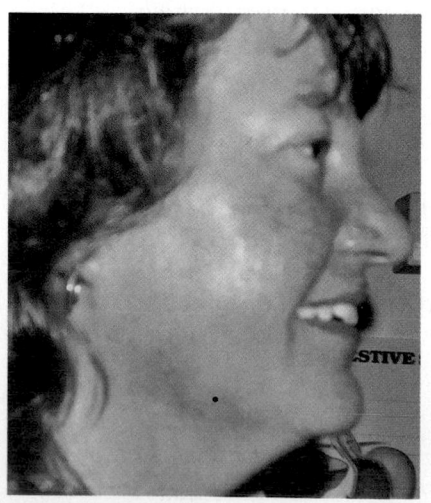

Figure 44-3 Telangiectasias.

and **lentigines** (flat brown spots seen on aged exposed skin). Non–sun-related changes include decreasing elasticity and immune responses and decreased healing rates. In the older adult there is a further decrease in the skin immune response, decreased rate of cellular repair, thinning skin, and a thinning and flattening of basement membrane resulting in an increased risk of skin damage from mechanical trauma. There is also a gradual loss of blood vessels resulting in decreased tissue perfusion and nourishment. Decreased vascularity in the skin of older adults results in diminished capacity to clear potent topical steroids, and therefore the use of such drugs ought to be avoided (AAD, 2006; Centers for Disease Control and Prevention [CDC], 2006d; Olson, 2004).

Cellular Effects of Aging on the Skin

Normal skin begins to show signs of aging by age 30 to 35 years. Sun exposure and burning in childhood, adolescence, and adulthood increases risk for malignant skin changes as people age. Continued sun exposure causes the skin to age more rapidly. Aged skin is thin, inelastic, and fragile. Normal aging should not be confused with photo-aging, because the two processes are biologically different. The difference can best be demonstrated by comparing the skin under the arm with the sun-exposed surface of the lower arm.

Changes in Epidermis

The epidermis becomes thin, and the rate of epidermal rejuvenation by keratinocytes in the basal layer decreases. Hair loss does not increase, but the hair follicles become less active and less dense. Decreased number of Langerhans' cells means a reduced immune response. Melanocytes in the hair bulb decrease production of melanin resulting in the loss of hair pigmentation. There is also a reduction in the density of sweat and sebaceous glands and blood vessels, which result in a decrease in skin hydration. Nails become more brittle and thicker. The number of mast cells decreases, resulting in a reduction in histamine release and inflammatory response. Macrophage differentiation rates are slower, and their functional capacity is diminished resulting in fewer available macrophages to marshal an immune response (Olson, 2004).

Changes in Dermis

The decrease in the number of elastin fiber bundles means that the skin becomes less tolerant of mechanical stressors and more prone to injury. Lymphatic glands decrease their efficiency at managing interstitial fluid levels. The number of blood vessels around glands and hair follicles decreases. Older patients experience a change in their degree of sensory perception and have a diminished capacity to sense pain, itching, heat, and cold. Fibroblasts produce less collagen, elastin, and reticular fibers, resulting in a decreased rate of granulation tissue formation and wound healing.

Changes in Subcutaneous Tissue

The skin becomes atrophic and fragile when subcutaneous tissue is lost. With this loss comes a decrease in the protective padding provided by this tissue layer, and the shock absorber function is reduced. Bony prominences, joints, bones, and internal organs are at increased risk for damage.

FACTORS REGULATING SKIN AND WOUND REPAIR

Many cellular substances control the healing pathway, because healing is a complex interaction between growth factors, cytokines, enzymes produced by cells throughout all phases of healing, and hormones. Growth factors are multichain protein molecules that control the proliferation and differentiation of

Uncovering the Evidence

Efficacy and Safety of Emollient Cream on Photo-Damaged Skin

Discussion: A two-year controlled study was conducted with 240 older adult participants to determine the efficacy and safety of Tretinoin emollient cream in the treatment of photo-damaged skin on the face. Tretinoin or a placebo product was applied once a day. Scheduled assessments were conducted over the study period. Findings indicated a significant improvement in the rough appearance, fine and coarse wrinkling, mottled hyperpigmentation, lentigines and sallowness of participants treated with tretinoin emollient. These findings suggest that tretinoin is an appropriate therapeutic treatment to use and test with a larger group of people with photo-damaged skin.

Implications for Practice: Health care providers can intervene in people at risk for potential photo-aging problems. The tretinoin medication can continue to be tested for its positive effects and application of it as a viable option for intervention.

Source: Kang, S., Bergfeld, W. Gottlieb, A., Hickman, J., Humeniuk, J., Kempers, S., et al. (2005). Long-term efficacy and safety of Tretinoin emollient cream 0.05% in treatment of photodamaged skin. American Journal of Clinical Dermatology, 6(4), 245–253.

cells. Growth factors function much like hormones in that they bind to certain sites on the membranes of cells and stimulate changes within those cells. Matrixmetalloproteases (MMPs) are collagenase, gelatinase, and stromelysin and are the most well-known MMPs. Hormones also participate in the regulation of wound healing. Metabolic conditions affecting regulation of hormones also contribute to problems in wound healing, particularly deficiencies in estrogen and insulin secretion and excess secretion of cortisol.

Healing is the restoration of structure and function of the skin after tissue damage. Injury precipitates a complex cascade of processes that are interdependent and interactive, the natural sequencing of which results in normal repair. Wounds that proceed normally through the repair process to healing are referred to as acute wounds. Recalcitrant or indolent wounds are wounds that fail to heal in the normal process and are referred to as chronic wounds. The understanding of wound repair is based on the acute wound model. The phases of wound healing are inflammation, proliferation, and maturation, and many factors are associated with impaired wound healing (Olsen, 2004).

ASSESSMENT

A thorough history will assist the health care provider to determine a correct diagnosis of skin and wound problems. The components of an adequate assessment are the history, chief complaint, past medical history, current medications, allergies, family history, psychosocial, and lifestyle history, including travel and occupational history and a review of systems. A thorough medication history is important to help determine if the skin disorder is related to drug side effects, such as vitamins, corticosteroids, antibiotics, hormones, and antimetabolites (antineoplastics used in cancer therapy). Chronic skin problems can affect an individual's self-image and confidence. People often spend large sums of money on products and cosmetic procedures to help erase the physical and psychosocial effects of their troubling skin conditions. People often must consider how much can be reasonably spent to improve skin appearance if it means that some basic necessities must be sacrificed (Doughty, 2004).

Review of Systems

The screening procedure includes a review of systems designed to identify problems of which the patient might have been unaware or did not previously mention in the history. Documentation of the general skin condition should be made. Specific problems of the skin should be described and noted with the appropriate biological system. The review of systems can be accomplished by means of a personal questionnaire or data can be collected through a direct interview as part of the history taking process. Refer to Table 44-2 for examples of information to include.

Assessment of the Skin

Overall skin color is noted. A generalized alteration in total body skin color and tone may indicate a systemic problem. Normal skin tone should be congruent with the patient's stated race (see Respecting Our Differences). Presence of a jaundiced skin tone indicates a hepatic or biliary pathology. Decreased generalized skin turgor suggests dehydration. Cyanosis and a cool temperature in an extremity suggest circulatory and vascular problems. There is a normal color vari-

TABLE 44-2 **Review of Systems Related to Skin Disorders**	
Personal perception of the skin problem	Description of daily hygiene practices
	Self-treatment or prescribed skin products for current or previous skin disorder.
	Description of onset, course, and treatment of current skin problem
	Contact with pets
Nutrition patterns	Recent changes in diet and food supplements
	Description of any changes in skin, hair, nails, mucous membranes, and healing of sores or lesions
Elimination patterns	Excessive sweating or dryness of skin
	Location of any swelling
Activities and exercise patterns	Use of protective skin preparations (some may be toxic)
	Fluid replacement practices
Sleep and rest patterns	Effects of skin problem on sleep and rest patterns.
Environmental changes	Change in laundry products, cosmetics, or other personal skin products
	Change in climate (heat, cold, or geographical changes because of travel)
	Stressful events
Self-concept Self-image	Emotional response and perception related to effects of skin problem on self-concept and self-image
	Impact on interrelationships
Coping strategies	Usual response to stress (effective or ineffective)
Cultural influences	Factors that may influence choice of treatment options.
	Beliefs or values that may influence feelings about the skin disorder

Adapted from Estes, M. (2006). Health assessment and physical examination (3rd ed.). New York: Thomson Delmar Learning.

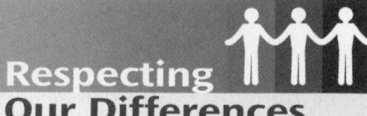

Respecting Our Differences

Skin of People of Color

Some skin conditions are misdiagnosed, such as psoriasis, eczema and atopic dermatitis. Darker spots may remain after a primary lesion heals. The skin is also prone to developing keloid scarring (a scar that continues to grow after healing takes place and invades normal tissue). It is also important to protect the darker skin from UV light.

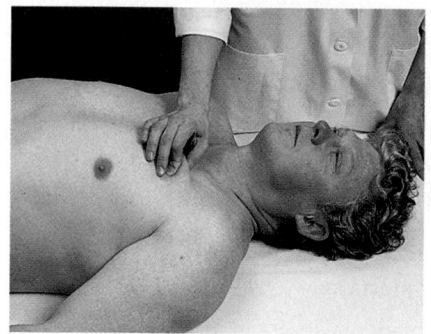

Figure 44-4 Nurse assessing skin turgor.

ation between sun-exposed areas and areas that generally remain covered or protected from the sun. However, the color should be uniform. Hyperpigmentation may indicate sun damaged areas (liver spots on the hands), and hypopigmented areas may indicate abnormal pigment or infectious processes.

Moisture

Moisture refers to the skin's level of hydration. The skin should feel supple and moist but not wet or clammy. Dryness, ichthyosis (dry, scaly skin), or **xerosis** (abnormal dryness of skin, mucous membranes, or conjunctiva) indicate a decreased level of naturally produced skin lubricants (sebaceous gland secretions). Relate findings of the examination to the patient's age to determine normal level of moisture. Skin that feels overly moist or cool is abnormal. **Diaphoresis** (profuse sweating) is abnormal and may indicate certain types of poisoning (e.g., alcohol), neurological problems, or endocrine problems.

Temperature

The temperature of the normal skin is uniformly warm and is a reflection of normal circulation. Excessive warmth indicates a higher core body temperature and is abnormal, possibly indicating an infectious process. Conversely, cooler skin temperatures usually indicate a circulatory problem (e.g., in emergent situations, cool skin indicates shock). Compare areas of temperature differences with the same area on the opposite side.

Texture

Texture refers to the general feel of the skin. Stroke the skin with the fingertips. Normal skin should feel smooth and resilient. Lumps or areas of unusual thickening or thinning (atrophy) are abnormal. Any raised or depressed areas should be noted and further evaluation is necessary.

Turgor

Turgor is the skin's elasticity, resilience, and hydration. It is measured by examining the amount of time required to return to normal after pinching the skin upward (Figure 44-4). The nurse gently pinches a fold of skin between thumb and forefinger; then releases the tented skin fold. If the skin remains elevated or tented for more than three seconds, turgor is decreased. Normal skin should return to its' usual contours within three seconds. As elasticity decreases with age, so does skin turgor.

Edema

Edema is an abnormal collection of fluid in the interstitial spaces between cells resulting in a lifting and separating of the layers of the skin. The nurse should assess for edema in any shiny, tight area of the skin noted on inspection. Severe edema can result in a blanching of the skin because of the pressure of the accumulated fluid. Palpate any edematous area for temperature changes, tenderness, and mobility. Press on the area for five seconds then release the area to assess for pitting edema. Depth of the residual indentation is measured in either millimeters or centimeters. Generalized edema or **anasarca** is associated with malnutrition, terminal illness, and metabolic fluid overload problems.

Tenderness

Tenderness is assessed by palpation and is an abnormal finding. Healthy skin palpation should not elicit any pain response unless injury is evident. Tenderness in a skin area may be indicative of infection, or related to a deep tissue problem. A classic symptom of tenderness is guarding, in which the patient protects the area from palpation by the health care provider.

Odor

Odor is a symptom of an underlying problem in healthy skin, with the exception of the axillae. Odor from open wounds usually represents bacterial or fungus colonization or may represent hygiene problems in skin folds or other areas of the body. Greenish-blue drainage with a musty odor indicates a possible *Pseudomonas* infection. Odor may also be indicative of a metabolic problem. A fruity odor of breath may indicate a serious metabolic disturbance of type 1 diabetes, called diabetic ketoacidosis, an emergent situation of overproduction of ketone bodies that results in metabolic acidosis.

Lesions

Lesions (altered areas of tissue) or wounds should be treated as abnormal findings and assessed and described in an orderly fashion. Location, distribution, size, arrangement, color, configuration, secondary changes, presence of drainage, contours, consistency, mobility, and tenderness must be documented (Figure 44-5). The names and descriptions of primary lesions (Figure 44-6) are summarized in Box 44-1.

Secondary lesions are the result of primary lesions, and include crusts, scales, fissures, erosions, excoriations, ulcerations, atrophy, scars, keloids, umbilicated (depressed like the umbilicus), and zosteriform, which is a linear arrangement such as seen in herpes zoster and keratosis follicularis (Figure 44-7).

Mobile lesions move freely when palpated; immobile lesions do not, indicating attachment to underlying tissue. Locations of lesions are described using position relative to anatomic landmarks. Size is measured in millimeters or centimeters. Distribution refers to the pattern of occurrence on the skin. Lesions may be localized, regional, or generalized. Arrangement refers to the pattern of nearby lesions (i.e., linear or satellite). Configuration relates to the shape of the lesion. Box 44-2 defines typical terminology used to describe the distribution and configuration of lesions.

Fast Forward ▶▶▶

Safety Measures to Prevent Untoward Events

For the past 10 years the Joint Commission on Accreditation of Healthcare Organizations (JCAHO) has required health care enterprises that seek JCAHO accreditation to provide written reports of untoward events and the actions being taken to prevent recurrence of such events. Accreditation can be withheld and monetary penalties can be incurred for failure to prevent such events. Increasing pressure to reduce health care costs and improve the quality of health care outcomes is beginning to generate closer examination of preventable conditions that are costly to treat. In the near future incidence of hospital-acquired skin problems; such as pressure ulcers, could result in denial of payment for care rendered.

BOX 44-1

PRIMARY LESIONS

- **Macules:** Flat circumscribed changes of the skin (flat nevi, café au lait spots, vitiligo, telangiectases, or capillary hemangiomas).
- **Papules:** Elevated circumscribed lesions (elevated nevi, verrucae, molluscum contagiosum, or individual lesions of lichen planus).
- **Nodules:** Circumscribed elevated, usually solid lesions (fibromas, neurofibromas, xanthomas, erythema nodosum, and various benign or malignant growths).
- **Plaques:** Elevated disc-shaped lesions (psoriasis, lichen simplex or chronicus neurodermatitis).
- **Tumors:** Larger and deeper circumscribed solid lesions—benign or malignant (lipomas, strawberry or cavernous hemangiomas, neoplasms).
- **Wheals:** Solid superficial elevations usually in response to pruritus conditions (insect bites, urticaria, or allergic reactions).
- **Vesicles:** Sharply circumscribed, elevated fluid-contain Vesicle lesions (herpes, dyshidrosis, pompholyx, varicella, or contact dermatitis).
- **Bullae:** Larger circumscribed, elevated fluid-containing lesions (burns, contact dermatitis, pemphigus, or epidermolysis bullosa).
- **Pustules:** Circumscribed elevations containing purulent exudates (pustular psoriasis, bromoderma, or smallpox)
- **Comedones:** Plugged secretions of horny material retain within a pilosebaceous follicle.
- **Burrows:** Linear lesions produced by tunneling of animal parasite (scabies).
- Telangiectasia: relatively permanent dilatation of superficial venules, capillaries, or arterioles (lupus erythematosus, dermatomyositis, or scleroderma).

Adapted from Estes, M. (2006). Health assessment and physical examination *(3rd ed.). New York: Thomson Delmar Learning.*

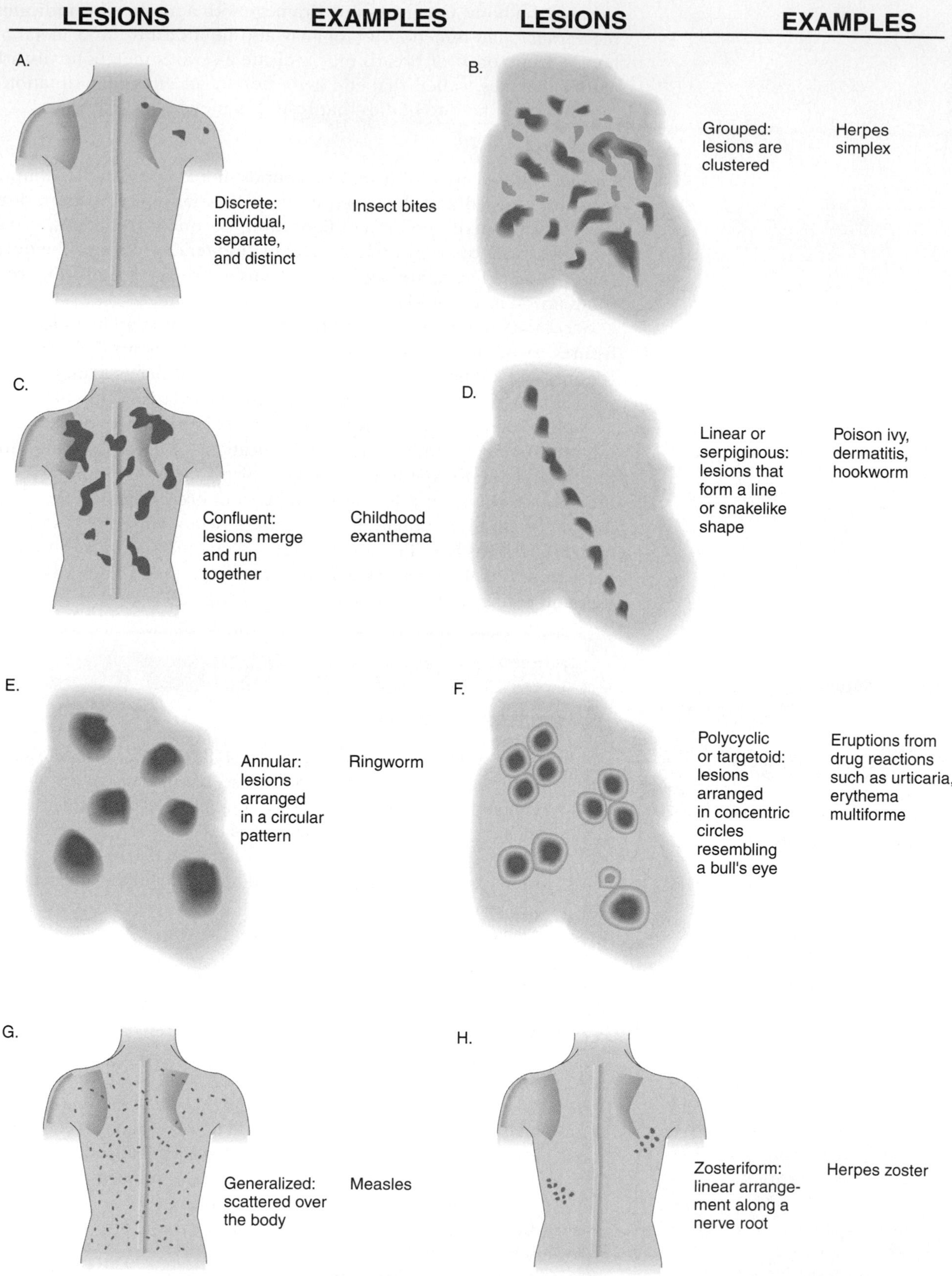

LESIONS	EXAMPLES	LESIONS	EXAMPLES

A.

Discrete: individual, separate, and distinct

Insect bites

B.

Grouped: lesions are clustered

Herpes simplex

C.

Confluent: lesions merge and run together

Childhood exanthema

D.

Linear or serpiginous: lesions that form a line or snakelike shape

Poison ivy, dermatitis, hookworm

E.

Annular: lesions arranged in a circular pattern

Ringworm

F.

Polycyclic or targetoid: lesions arranged in concentric circles resembling a bull's eye

Eruptions from drug reactions such as urticaria, erythema multiforme

G.

Generalized: scattered over the body

Measles

H.

Zosteriform: linear arrangement along a nerve root

Herpes zoster

Figure 44-5 Arrangement of lesions.

NONPALPABLE

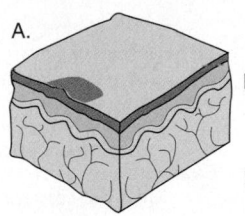

A.

Macule:
Localized changes in skin color of less than 1 cm in diameter
Example:
Freckle

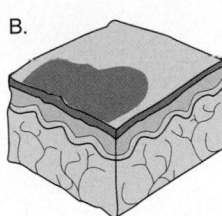

B.

Patch:
Localized changes in skin color of greater than 1 cm in diameter
Example:
Vitiligo, stage 1 of pressure ulcer

PALPABLE

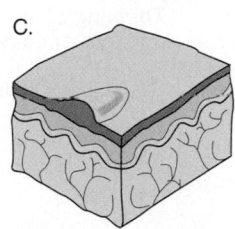

C.

Papule:
Solid, elevated lesion less than 0.5 cm in diameter
Example:
Warts, elevated nevi, seborrheic keratosis

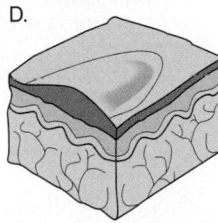

D.

Plaque:
Solid, elevated lesion greater than 0.5 cm in diameter
Example:
Psoriasis, eczema, pityriasis rosea

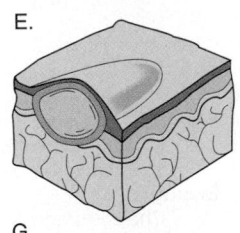

E.

Nodules:
Solid and elevated; however, they extend deeper than papules into the dermis or subcutaneous tissues, 0.5-2.0 cm
Example:
Lipoma, erythema nodosum, cyst, melanoma, hemangioma

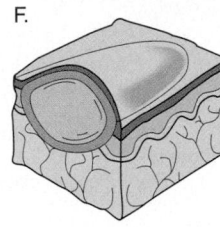

F.

Tumor:
The same as a nodule only greater than 2 cm

Example:
Carcinoma (such as advanced breast carcinoma); **not** basal cell or squamous cell of the skin

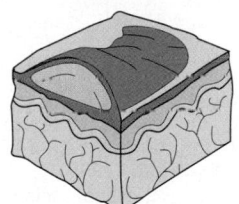

G.

Wheal:
Localized edema in the epidermis causing irregular elevation that may be red or pale
Example:
Insect bite, hive, angioedema

FLUID-FILLED CAVITIES WITHIN THE SKIN

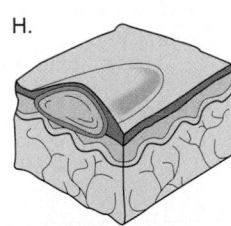

H.

Vesicle:
Accumulation of fluid between the upper layers of the skin; elevated mass containing serous fluid; less than 0.5 cm
Example:
Herpes simplex, herpes zoster, chickenpox, scabies

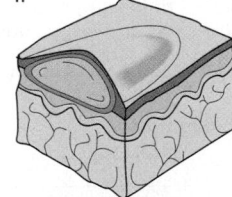

I.

Bullae:
Same as a vesicle only greater than 0.5 cm
Example:
Contact dermatitis, large second-degree burns, bullous impetigo, pemphigus

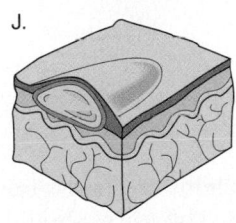

J.

Pustule:
Vesicles or bullae that become filled with pus, usually described as less than 0.5 cm in diameter
Example:
Acne, impetigo, furuncles, carbuncles, folliculitis

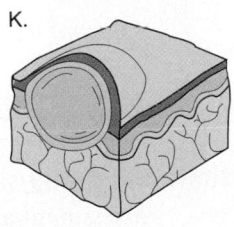

K.

Cyst:
Encapsulated fluid-filled or a semi-solid mass in the subcutaneous tissue or dermis
Example:
Sebaceous cyst, epidermoid cyst

Figure 44-6 Morphology of primary lesions.

ABOVE THE SKIN SURFACE

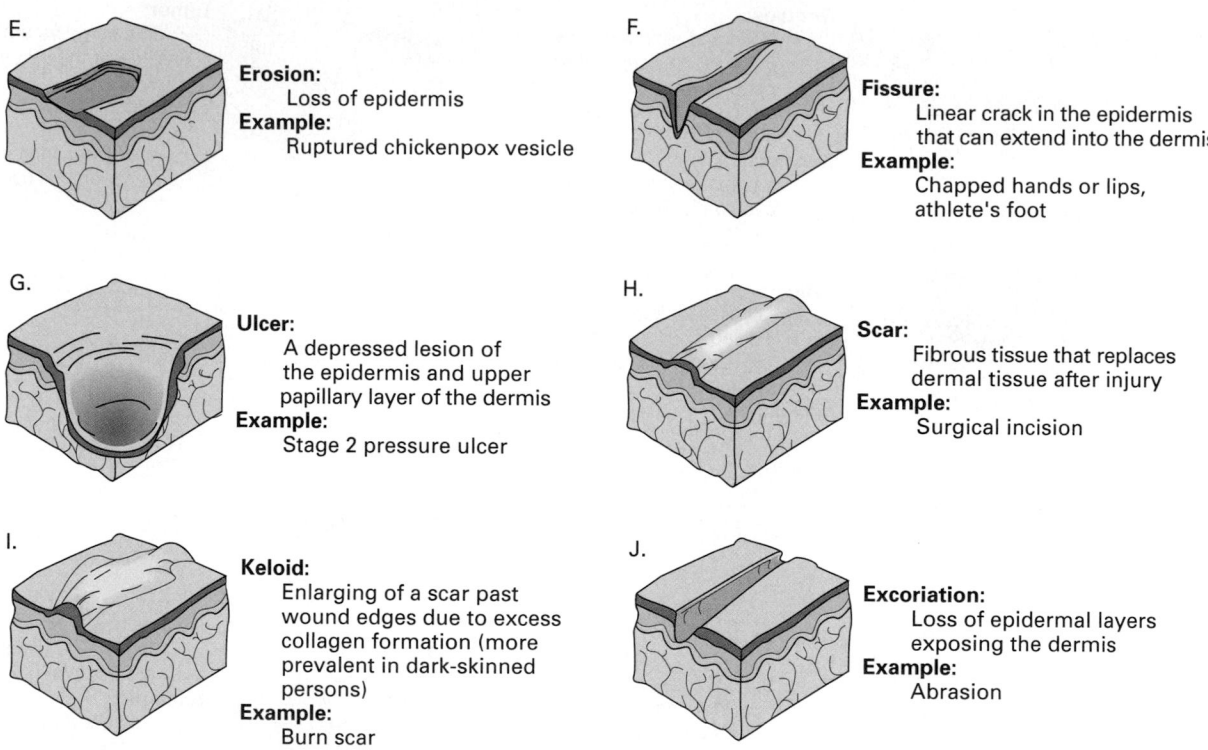

A.
Scales:
Flaking of the skin's surface
Example:
Dandruff, psoriasis, xerosis

B.
Lichenification:
Layers of skin become thickened and rough as a result of rubbing over a prolonged period of time
Example:
Chronic contact dermatitis

C.
Crust:
Dried serum, blood, or pus on the surface of the skin
Example:
Impetigo, acute eczematous inflammation

D.
Atrophy:
Thinning of the skin surface and loss of markings
Example:
Striae, aged skin

BELOW THE SKIN SURFACE

E.
Erosion:
Loss of epidermis
Example:
Ruptured chickenpox vesicle

F.
Fissure:
Linear crack in the epidermis that can extend into the dermis
Example:
Chapped hands or lips, athlete's foot

G.
Ulcer:
A depressed lesion of the epidermis and upper papillary layer of the dermis
Example:
Stage 2 pressure ulcer

H.
Scar:
Fibrous tissue that replaces dermal tissue after injury
Example:
Surgical incision

I.
Keloid:
Enlarging of a scar past wound edges due to excess collagen formation (more prevalent in dark-skinned persons)
Example:
Burn scar

J.
Excoriation:
Loss of epidermal layers exposing the dermis
Example:
Abrasion

Figure 44-7 Morphology of secondary lesions.

DIAGNOSTIC TESTS

Diagnostic tests for skin and wound care problems are based on a thorough assessment and documentation of the findings. The nurse should explain the procedure prior to starting the test and allow time for questions from the patient and any caregivers. A biopsy is usually taken from fresh, well-developed

---

BOX 44-2

DESCRIPTION AND CONFIGURATION OF SELECTED GROUP OF LESIONS

- **Annular:** Ring shaped (superficial fungal infections such as ring-worm, pityriasis rosea, seborrheic dermatitis, psoriasis, and others).
- **Dermatomal:** Localized into a dermatome supplied by one or more dorsal ganglia (herpes zoster and segmental vitiligo).
- **Eczematoid:** Suggest inflammation with tendency to thickening, oozing, vesiculation, or crusting (related to eczema).
- Iris lesions: Target-like concentric ringed lesions (erythema multiforme-Steven Johnson varieties).
- Keratosis: Circumscribed patches of horny thickening (seborrheic or actinic keratoses, chronic dermatitis and callus formation).
- Linear: Band-like configuration (nevi or scleroderma lichen striatus).
- Serpiginous: Serpent-shaped (lesions of cutaneous larva).

Adapted from Estes, M. (2006). Health assessment and physical examination (3rd ed.). New York: Thomson Delmar Learning.

---

lesions. The nurse should teach appropriate wound care of biopsy sites, possible side effects of tests, such as bleeding from sites or evidence of infection, and follow-up instructions. Mohs' micrographic surgery is a tissue-sparing method used to map tumors during frozen section (Daniels, 2003). For example, basal cell carcinomas spread finger-like projections into surrounding tissue that are not readily visible. Tissue is removed in thin layers and the edges are mapped to determine if the tumor has been completely removed or residual tumor still exists in the surgical site. Many of the skin disorders can result in additional hospital admissions and could be prevented with appropriate nursing management. There are many additional expenses to the health care system for continued skin breakdown issues (e.g., pressure ulcers or radiation burns).

Nursing Diagnoses

Based on the information gathered, examples of nursing diagnoses in the patient with disorders of the integument may include the following:
- Activity intolerance related to pain (or risk for activity intolerance)
- Anxiety related to the appearance of the integumentary disorder and its impact on interpersonal relationships
- Risk for infection related to a barrier break in the skin
- Disturbed sensory perception related to sensory nerve damage

The Health Care Team

A team of health care providers brings integrated expertise from multiple disciplines to the care of patients with integumentary system diagnoses. Both general practice and advance practice nurses, such as certified wound, ostomy, and continence therapists, may manage or provide the care. As appropriate, general and specialist health care providers, pharmacists, physical and occupational therapists, nutritionists, clergy, psychologists, and social workers may also collaborate on an integrated health care team. Some team members may provide care at community health care sites, and others may provide hospital-site care.

KEY CONCEPTS

- The epidermis is comprised of layers with unique functions and made up of stratified epithelial cells.
- The dermis provides the principle mass of the skin, and its functions include water storage, sensory enervation and thermoregulation and prevention of mechanical trauma.
- Functions of the skin include protection, homeostasis, regulation of fluid and electrolytes, excretion, thermoregulation, synthesis, sensory perception, psychosocial impression, and healing.
- Many of the skin changes that occur throughout the lifespan are normal, harmless and unchangeable. Normal skin begins to show signs of aging by ages 30 to 35.

- Acute wounds heal in an orderly manner in the healthy individual.
- Delayed healing occurs in chronic wounds to repeated or prolonged insults to tissues.
- A thorough history will assist the health care provider to determine a correct diagnosis of skin and wound problems.
- Assessment of the skin includes observation of color variations, moisture, temperature, texture, turgor, presence of edema, tenderness, odor, scars, and lesions.

REVIEW QUESTIONS

1. The epidermis replenishes itself by a process labeled as:
   1. Colonization
   2. Reconstruction
   3. Keratinization
   4. Differentiation

2. Cells that are responsible for skin pigmentation are:
   1. Langerhans' cells
   2. Fibroblasts
   3. Macrophages
   4. Melanocytes

3. Neoangiogenesis, a process during the wound healing process is the responsibility of:
   1. Mast cells
   2. Endothelial cells
   3. Fibroblasts
   4. Carotenoids

4. The major function of the subcutaneous tissue is to provide:
   1. Nutrients to the dermis and epidermis
   2. Padding over body joints and other internal structures
   3. Regulation of diffusion of oxygenation to tissues
   4. Maintenance of homeostasis and fluid and electrolyte balance.

5. Regeneration of skin is accomplished by replacing damaged tissue with:
   1. Dissimilar cell tissue
   2. A network of growth factor cells
   3. The same cell type
   4. Scar tissue

6. Repeated or prolonged insults to tissues can result in development of:
   1. Telangiectasia
   2. Capillary hemangiomas
   3. Dermatomal lesions
   4. Pressure sores.

7. The substances that control the proliferation and differentiation of cells are known as:
   1. Growth factors
   2. Tumors
   3. Burrows
   4. Bullae

8. In assessment of an edematous area, the nurse should palpate for:
   1. Hard nodules
   2. Temperature changes, tenderness, and mobility
   3. Keratosis
   4. Hypopigmentations and macular lesions

9. A teenager with severe acne decides that he does not want to participate in the swimming exercises that are part of the physical education course at his school. The nursing diagnosis that best describes this person's behavior is:
   1. Ineffective coping related to lack of social support
   2. Impaired skin integrity related to the skin lesions
   3. Social isolation related to anticipatory fear of rejection
   4. Anxiety related to lack of knowledge about his disease

Continued

REVIEW QUESTIONS—cont'd

10. Patient teaching for older adults should include information about avoiding the use of potent topical steroids because:
    1. Decreased vascularity in the skin decreases capacity to clear medications from the system.
    2. Thinning of skin increases risk of skin damage and bleeding when medication is applied.

3. Lentigines (flat brown spots) can become darker and increase absorption of skin products.
4. Presence of telangiectasias on the head and face delays absorption of topical skin products.

REVIEW ACTIVITIES

1. Develop an interview guide of questions to ask about skin problems. Interview at least three individuals from different cultures regarding their cultural beliefs about the etiology of skin disorders and the traditional remedies used. Compare your findings and provide a written report.

2. Develop a case study scenario for a 35-year-old person of color with psoriasis. Design a concept map outlining the various problems associated with the skin disorder. Develop a list of nursing diagnoses that can be applied in developing a plan of care for this person. (This may be a small group activity.)

3. Develop a teaching or learning plan for explaining how specific occupations (health care professionals, factory workers, plumbers, electricians,) and hobbies place persons at risk of contact dermatitis.

4. Design a check list for assessing the sun damage (photo damage) on an older person's skin. Which areas are at greatest risk of damage? Examine an older family member or a friend using this check

list. Prepare an informational brochure for that individual.

5. Access the American Academy of Dermatology Web site at: http://www.aad.org and click on Public Resource Center. Click on Skincarephysicians.com. Select one of the skin disorder links (acne, actinic keratosis, aging skin, eczema, psoriasis, rosea, or skin cancer). Review the information and develop an instruction pamphlet based on the answers to questions posed on the specific skin disorder.

6. Access the American Academy of Dermatology Web site at: http://www.aad.org and click on Public Resource Center. Click on Kids Connection. This is a special section for children age 8 to 12. Review the list of various skin disorders, such as relationship of diet to skin problem, or what causes hives or warts. Prepare a poster describing information about a selected skin disorder and share it with your class or share it with a group of children accompanied by a brief presentation.

Dermatological Dysfunction: Nursing Management

Cynthia A. Worley, BSN, RN, WOCN

CHAPTER TOPICS

- Guidelines for Nursing Management of Patients with Dermatological Dysfunction

- Debridement

- Methods of Treatment

- Common Skin Disorders

- Precancerous and Cancerous Conditions

The care of people with dermatological problems can be complex. In Western societies a person's physical appearance is highly valued, and a visible dermatological condition can be devastating psychologically and financially. Assessment of any skin condition requires knowledge of the anatomy and physiology of the skin, ability to determine the etiology of the problem, and critical thinking skills to determine the best of many effective methods of treatment. Some treatments are applicable across a wide variety of conditions; others are specific to certain conditions only. Before determining the appropriate treatment options for a variety of common dermatological conditions, the general guidelines for treatment must be considered.

KEY TERMS

Abscess
Acne
Anthropophilic
Atopic dermatitis
Autolytic debridement
Carbuncles
Cellulitis
Comedones
Contact dermatitis
Debridement
Enzymatic debridement
Folliculitis
Furuncles (boils)
Humectants
Lichenification
Mechanical debridement
Pediculosis
Pediculosis pubis
Photoaging
Photoallergic
Photochemotherapy
Phototherapy
Phototoxic
Pruritus
Psoriasis
Sycosis
Sycosis barbae
Tineas
Xerosis
Zoophilic

GENERAL GUIDELINES FOR MANAGEMENT OF PATIENTS WITH DERMATOLOGICAL DYSFUNCTION

Health care providers agree that the fundamental principles of wound healing and skin repair, must guide the health care provider assessing and diagnosing any skin problem or condition. The health care providers must first determine the etiology of the problem by taking a thorough history as discussed in chapter 44. Onset, duration, exacerbation, alleviation, and previous treatment must be examined. Without an accurate diagnosis of the cause of the skin or wound problem, appropriate treatment cannot be initiated. A patient with diabetes and a neuropathic ulcer on the plantar surface of the foot cannot be successfully treated without addressing the issue of glycemic control. Patients with a lower extremity ulcer must first be evaluated to determine if the ulcer is venous, arterial, or mixed before the appropriate medical or surgical intervention can be initiated.

On examination of the skin or wound problem the health care provider must eliminate or control infectious processes and remove any necrotic or devitalized tissue impeding healing. Initiating any treatment without first addressing these two critical issues may have disastrous consequences. Wound and skin lesions will not heal in the presence of heavy bacterial contamination. The body's immune response is concentrated on controlling the microbial burden rather than on initiating inflammation in the presence of infection or colonization. Necrotic tissue has been shown to harbor bacteria and interfere with wound healing and therefore must be removed for healing to begin. Infection is defined as the presence of 10^5 colony forming units (CFUs) identified on microscopic examination (Estes, 2006).

Next, the health care provider should identify any barriers to healing and correct those issues. The patient who is malnourished and trying to heal a large surface area burn or other type of skin condition will find that healing is frustrated by the nutritional problem. Adequate protein, vitamin, and mineral intake, as well as hydration are essential for healing. Patients with untreated or poorly controlled comorbidities, such as poor circulation or an impaired immune status, are at risk for impaired wound and skin healing by virtue of their chronic illness. The patient with an allogenic or matched-unrelated donor bone marrow transplant is immunologically at risk for any type of opportunistic infection as well as for graft-versus-host disease (GVHD), a risk factor in this type of transplant patient. The patient with GVHD of the skin is treated using steroids, and healing is impaired by the use of steroids. Therefore, during the GVHD treatment, breakdown of the patient's skin will be slow to resolve.

A moist wound environment must be provided and maintained for the wound to heal properly with a minimum of complications. Research has shown that wounds heal best in a moist environment; in other words, under some sort of dressing that prevents drying of the wound bed. If the wound is allowed to dry out, healing is delayed or halted, because the wound microenvironment is not conducive to cell proliferation and optimal cellular activity. White blood cells (WBCs), fibroblasts, macrophages, and endothelial cells all require moisture to migrate, divide, and perform their specific functions that facilitate healing. Finally, the health care provider knows that all of these guidelines for healing require that the patient understands the condition and participates fully in the treatment (Sheffield, Smith, & Fife, 2004).

DEBRIDEMENT

Debridement is the removal of necrotic tissue from a wound. Necrotic tissue is an impediment to wound and skin healing, and the necrotic tissue does not have to occur in large amounts to interfere with repair. A scab is not nature's

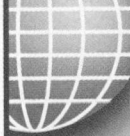

Real World, Real Choices

Sacral Pressure Lesion
Scenario

You are asked to evaluate the skin problem of an 89-year-old man with a history of a cerebrovascular accident (CVA) that has left him with right-sided weakness, dysphasia (difficulty swallowing), and aphasia (inability to speak). He is unable to provide you with a health history, but he is accompanied by a family member who is familiar with the patient's health history. Through your interview of this family member you learn that the patient has a history of hypertension and chronic atrial fibrillation. The patient resides in a skilled nursing facility and must rely on the nursing staff for all of his care. He is able to transfer from the bed to a wheelchair with assistance. The skin problem is a partial-thickness wound on the patient's sacrum that was discovered one week ago. There is an erythematous border around the wound and some bruising at the right edges. The base is pink and moist without odor. The family member reports that the facility's staff has been using a barrier ointment on the area. The patient is alert, cooperative, and afebrile.

Guideline 1: What is the etiology of the problem?

Guideline 2: How would you remove the necrotic tissue and what clinical manifestations would indicate an infection?

Guideline 3: What would be barriers and concerns for this patient?

Guideline 4: How and why would you maintain a moist wound dressing?

protective dressing; instead, a scab simply indicates that the wound bed has been allowed to dry. Even a paper cut will heal more rapidly with a topical antibiotic ointment and a cover dressing than when it is left open to dry.

There are four methods of debridement used to remove necrotic tissue from wounds. **Mechanical debridement** primarily makes use primarily of gauze dressings to remove necrotic or devitalized tissue from wounds. The gauze is moistened with saline or another solution, packed into the wound, and allowed to dry. Removal of the dry gauze mechanically lifts necrotic tissue from the wound. This is an inexpensive method of debridement. It is also painful to the patient and disruptive to both the new tissue bed being formed and to existing healthy tissue, which also adheres to the gauze and is torn away when the gauze is removed. It is not unusual for the wound bed to bleed when the gauze is removed, indicating a disruption of the new vascular network (Worley, 2004).

Enzymatic debridement is accomplished using a chemical debriding agent, usually an enzyme. Papain urea, either as a single ingredient or used in conjunction with a chlorophyll and copper complex and collagenase-based products are effective in liquefying necrotic tissue over time. Any enzymatic debriding agent requires a prescription and careful adherence to the directions for application. Most are rendered inactive in the presence of heavy metal ions, such as silver, or when the wound is treated with an antibiotic solution.

Autolytic debridement makes use of the normal phagocytic action of macrophages and leukocytes present in the wound. Moist wound dressings help the wound bed maintain a natural level of moisture, facilitating a normal inflammatory response. It is during inflammation that the macrophages and leukocytes establish control over bacteria present in the wound and provide the clean up service that removes cellular debris and devitalized or necrotic tissue. Debridement by autolysis is slower than enzymatic or sharp debridement, but it is the preferred method when the patient is immunocompromised or at risk for bleeding problems.

Sharp debridement is usually performed by a physician or specially trained nurse or other treatment team member. It can be done at the patient's bedside or take place in an operating room. Debridement is usually performed on deeper, chronic wounds, such as pressure ulcers and necrotic surgical wounds. The necrotic tissue is cut away from the wound using a cautery or scalpel. Sharp debridement is the quickest method used to remove devitalized tissue, but it is more costly when it must be done in the operating room under general anesthesia.

Conservative sharp debridement can be performed without anesthesia outside of the operating room when only superficial or loosely adherent tissue is removed. This method is rarely used alone, because not all the necrotic tissue can be readily removed. Usually an enzyme is used in conjunction with conservative debridement, especially if a series of debridements are required to remove all the necrotic tissue. The patient's condition must be thoroughly assessed prior to determining the most appropriate method of debridement (Worley, 2005).

METHODS OF TREATMENT

Topical therapy is used to perform a variety of functions in the treatment of dermatological problems. Lotions, solutions, and creams are used to restore normal skin hydration levels, reduce inflammation, relieve dermatological symptoms, act as a delivery system for other medications, reduce dryness and flaking, provide antimicrobial action, and cleanse and protect the skin. These types of medications are chosen for their active ingredient, the primary agent in the formula that treats the condition, or as a delivery system for the active ingredient to ensure that the active agent stays in contact with the skin. Table 45-1 lists common agents that are used to treat various skin conditions.

Topical vehicles used to deliver medications range from creams and ointments to aerosols and powders. Vehicles discussed in this section include creams, ointments, gels, aerosols, lotions, powders, and pastes. Most creams, by definition, are primarily water-based or oil-in-water-based emulsions with the water content 60 percent or less. The cream vehicle has the ability to provide lubrication to the skin and can be used almost anywhere on the body. They also are less occlusive and may increase dryness in some patients. Creams usually contain preservatives and can contain alcohol or propylene glycol, which can also cause dryness.

Ointments are similar to creams in that they are usually an oil-in-water emulsion, but the water content is 40 percent or less. Ointments are more occlusive and provide a better delivery vehicle because of their ability to trap the medication next to the affected area and increase absorption. Ointment preparations should not be used in situations of severe eczematous inflammation or in areas containing dense hair.

Gels are semisolid preparations, usually a combination of propylene glycol and water, which are most effectively used with inflammatory conditions that produce exudates. They make a good vehicle for medications effective for pruritic lesions, like poison ivy, because they have a drying and cooling effect. Some gels contain alcohol and can cause discomfort when used in dry, cracked, or eroded areas. Aerosols suspend the active ingredient in a base and deliver that ingredient under pressure. They are more drying and can be used to deliver medications to wet or hairy areas.

Lotions are powders suspended in a liquid, usually water, alcohol, or oil. The medications are delivered in a uniform residual film and have a cooling effect. Lotions can be used in hairy areas, such as the scalp, and have the

TABLE 45-1 Agents to Treat Skin Conditions

Topical Medications

MEDICATION	INGREDIENT OR TRADE NAME	NURSING MANAGEMENT
Antifungals	Nystatin (Mycostatin)	Drug chosen based on species of dermatophyte and severity and duration of infection
	Clotrimazole (Lotrimin)	
	Terbinafine HCL (Lamisil)	Review application and preapplication instructions
	Ketoconazole (Nizoral)	Possible side effects include skin irritation and overgrowth of fungus when occlusion is used
	Miconazole (Micatin)	
Antineoplastics	Imiquimod (Aldara)	Depending on whether lotion, cream, or solution usually applied once or twice daily
	Fluorouracil (Carac and Efudex)	
		Drug causes considerable inflammation and discomfort if large areas are treated
Antiparasitics	Permethrin (Nix and Elimite)	Infestations in home require entire family be treated as well as bedding, clothing, and carpets
	Lindane (Kwell)	
	Pyrethrin (RID)	Combs, brushes, curlers, head scarves or coverings, and hair clips must be washed in hot, soapy water
	Malathion (Ovide)	
	Ivermectin (Stromectol)	
Antipruritics	Lotions: Menthol (Eucerin itch relief)	May be applied frequently to relieve symptoms and discomfort unless contains an analgesic agent
	Camphor (Neutrogena anti-itch moisturizer)	
	Calamine lotion	Solutions containing analgesic agents should be applied as prescribed (two to four times daily)
	Oatmeal suspensions (Aveeno)	Observe for contact sensitivity
	Wraps: Boric acid (1 tbs/1 L H_2O)	
	Burrow's solution	
	Potassium permanganate	
	Alumen acetate	
Antiseptics	Chlorhexidine gluconate (Hibiclens)	May be used for irrigating and cleansing wounds but should not be used to moisten packing materials
	Iodine solutions	
	Hydrogen peroxide	Should not be used in healing well-granulated wounds
	Acetic acid	
	Buffered sodium hypochlorite (Dakin's solution)	Protect periwound skin from solutions
Antivirals	Docosanol (Abreva)	Apply as prescribed
	Penciclovir (Denavir)	May be oral medication or topical medication or both modalities may be used
	Famciclovir (Famvir)	
	Valacyclovir (Valtrex)	
	Acyclovir (Zovirax)	
Corticosteroids	Hydrocortisone (Westcort, Hydrocort, Hytone, etc)	Avoid use of strong formulation in treating face, neck, and intertriginous areas because increased side effects may result
	Triamcinolone (Kenalog and Aristocort)	
	Clobetasol dipropionate (Temovate)	Should be applied evenly over affected areas
	Fluocinonide (Lidex)	Should be applied only for prescribed time limit and monitored for side effects
	Desonide (DesOwen)	

Continued

TABLE 45-1 Agents to Treat Skin Conditions—cont'd

Topical Medications

MEDICATION	INGREDIENT OR TRADE NAME	NURSING MANAGEMENT
Immunomodulators (topical)	Pimecrolimus (Elidel)	Used to treat atopic dermatitis
	Protopic ointment (Tacrolimus)	May safely be used on face and around eyes
		Side effects are burning and stinging, increased risk of secondary infection and some risk of systemic absorption
Lubricating agents	Urea (Carmol)	Apply evenly and best applied immediately after bathing
	Lactic acid (Amlactin and Lac-Hydrin)	
	Petrolatum (Aquaphor and Eucerin)	
	Zinc oxide	
Psoriatic and seborrheic dermatitis shampoos	Chloroxine (Capitrol)	Side effects include skin irritation and dryness
	Pyrithione (Nizoral and Head & Shoulders)	
	Selenium (Selsun and Selsun Blue)	
	Tar solutions: Denorex, Ional T, Neutrogena T, and Tegrin Medicated	
	Sulfur/Salicylic acid: Ional Plus and Sebulex	
Psoriasis	Orals: Psoralens (Oxsoralen Ultra, 8-MOP, Trisoralen)	Side effects include nausea, insomnia, dizziness, headache, depression, and malaise
	Acitretin (Soriatane)	
	Methotrexate	Immunosuppressive, hepatic fibrosis
	Topical: Anthralin (Drithocreme, Psoriatec, ad Curastain)	Skin irritation and skin staining are primary side effects
	Tazorac	Mild irritant dermatitis
	Vitamin D_3 analogue (Dovonex)	Strong preparations should be washed out every morning with strong detergent (like Dawn liquid)
	Tars: Ichthyol, Mazon, PolyTar soap, Tegrin Medicated, and Fototar	
Rosacea medications	Metronidazole (Metro-Gel)	Preparations may sting or burn on application
	Sulfur/Na sulfacetamides (Avar, Clenia, and Sulfacet-R, Plexion)	Avoid triggers (sunlight, alcohol, and spicy foods)
	Azelaic acid (Finacea)	
Wart preparations	Cantharidin (Cantharone)	Protect normal skin from preparation
	Silver nitrate	Side effects include blister formation, skin irritation, pain, and dryness
	Salicylic acid (Compound W, etc.)	
	Podophyllin/podofilox (Condylox, Podocon, and Pododerm)	
	Interferon	
	Dichloroacetic acid	

Adapted from Broyles, B., Reiss, B., & Evans, M. (2007). Pharmacological aspects of nursing care (7th ed.). New York: Thomson Delmar Learning.

potential to absorb some moisture. They can cause drying because of the alcohol content, and the medication can wear off easily.

Powders are finely ground solid substances. They can be absorptive and can be used in hairy areas but can become caked in high-moisture areas, like the groin or perineum. Pastes are usually powders in ointments with water content of 50 percent or greater. They provide protection and decrease absorption. Zinc oxide is a commonly used paste. Most patients object to paste preparations, because they are messy and unsightly.

Both the active ingredient and the vehicle must be appropriate for the condition being treated. If the condition produces weeping blisters, a water-based preparation can provide a soothing, cooling, and drying effect. An ointment-based preparation provides the opposite effect; it increases the amount of moisture in the area and promotes lubrication. Inflamed skin absorbs substances more readily than noninflamed skin. When absorption of a medication needs to be increased, covering the area to be medicated with an occlusive dressing enhances the absorption rate (Broyles, Reiss, & Evans, 2007).

Topical Corticosteroids

Corticosteroids are the most commonly prescribed topical medications used to treat dermatological conditions. Steroids are used to decrease inflammation, relieve pruritus, and induce remission of certain cutaneous disorders. These drugs have a potency ranking of from I to VII. The least potent steroids, such as Hytone, fall into group VII and the most potent steroids, such as Cormax, fall into group I. Most dermatoses can be treated with steroids with a low to moderate potency. The best results are achieved when preparations of adequate strength are used for a specified length of time. Most of the group I steroids should never be used under occlusive dressings (Rudy & Parham-Vetter, 2003).

Side effects of steroids include atrophy of the treated area, telangiectasia, acneiform eruptions, burning and dryness, and bruising. It is rarely beneficial to apply a steroid cream more than twice daily, and the patient should be instructed to either follow-up with their health care provider or contact the office if and when the condition improves. As the condition improves, the frequency of application may be changed or the patient may be switched to a lower strength of steroid, another tar preparation, a moisturizer, or another topical preparation may be recommended. Table 45-2 provides information that is important for patients to understand. It is critical for the nurse to provide detailed patient education on the proper use and application of these potent drugs.

Topical Soaks and Wraps

Some dermatological conditions require soaks and wraps as standard treatment. Soaks and wraps can be performed in a variety of ways with a variety of solutions, the use of which will depend on the condition and goal of treatment. A wet environment will soften and loosen cellular skin debris, relieve pruritus, promote drying of moist dermatoses, decrease discomfort, and provide a cooling and soothing environment. Gradual evaporation of water provides the cooling effect to irritated or burning skin.

Soaks can be accomplished by either soaking or bathing the affected area in the solution or by moistening gauze and applying the gauze to the affected area as a dressing. The usual length of exposure is 15 to 20 minutes. Colloidal oatmeal (Aveeno) added to bath water is temporarily soothing but does nothing to increase skin hydration. Tar preparations will reduce inflammation and are helpful in scaling conditions, such as psoriasis or eczema.

Aluminum acetate solutions, such as Burrow's solution or Domeboro solution, a combination of aluminum sulfate and calcium acetate solution, have antimicrobial properties, but can be drying. A 1:40 Burrow's solution obtained

TABLE 45-2 What Every Patient Needs to Know About Topical Medications

PRINCIPLE	ACTION	RATIONAL
Accurate and appropriate use of product		
1. Review preapplication instructions.	1. Patients must clearly understand how to apply the medication, when to apply it, and where to apply it	1. Creams or ointments should be applied evenly and sparingly once or twice daily and only to the affected areas. Correct application will eliminate many potential problems
2. Instruct the patient in regard to appropriate application technique	2. Apply after bathing or cleansing the area.	2. Hydration of the area increases absorption of drug
3. Emphasize that medication is only to be used for the prescribed length of time and only on the area for which it is prescribed	3. Do not apply to face, perineal area or axillae unless otherwise directed by health care provider	3. Monitor areas closely if steroid is applied to these areas. Perineal and axillary areas are high-moisture areas, which will increase absorption.
4. Emphasize that overuse or misuse can result in serious cutaneous and systemic complications	4. Do not apply to broken or irritated skin	4. Absorption of the drug is increased in areas where skin is not intact.
5. Caution patient against lending medication to friends or relatives		
6. Instruct patient about who to call if any problems occur.		

Adapted from Broyles, B., Reiss, B., & Evans, M. (2007). Pharmacological aspects of nursing care (7th ed.). New York: Thomson Delmar Learning.

by mixing one packet in one pint of water can be used to moisten gauze dressings. The moistened gauze is then placed over the affected area and wrapped with dry gauze. Both tap water and saline can also be used in soaks and wraps. Potassium permanganate ($KMnO_4$) in a solution ranging from 0.25% to 0.5% has a cooling effect useful in relieving pruritus and removing cellular debris while providing an antimicrobial effect against *Pseudomonas aeruginosa*. Aluminum acetate solutions are useful in treating allergic conditions involving open, weeping blisters such as poison ivy, poison oak, or poison sumac.

Boric acid solutions can be used as mild bacteriostatic and fungistatic soaks to treat mild infectious processes. Bath oils are not recommended, because they provide a false lubricity to the skin and increase fall risk in the bathtub. As with any drug, patient education is critical to successful treatment.

Wraps are another method of delivering a solution to a target area. Wet wraps can be used immediately after soaking and will increase hydration and prolong the contact time of the solution with the affected area while providing a cooling and soothing effect. The location and severity of the condition will dictate how the wraps need to be applied.

In isolated areas such as forearms or lower extremities, a rolled gauze dressing, such as Kerlix or Kling, may be impregnated with the solution and wrapped around the affected area followed by a dry layer. When whole body treatments are required, wet pajamas or long underwear saturated with the solution and covered by a dry plastic sweat suit will accomplish the desired effect. Cotton gloves and socks can be used to deliver the solution to the hands and feet. The face can be dressed with a wet, then dry, layer of gauze with holes cut for the eyes, nose, and mouth. Moistening the dressings prior to removal reduces discomfort and tissue damage. As with any medication, the patient must be educated about the proper application techniques.

Moisture Retentive Dressings

Moisture retentive dressings are designed to maintain a moist wound environment. They are chosen based on the amount of drainage produced by the wound and the frequency with which they need to be changed. These dressings allow control of the affected skin's environment and provide a protective layer over wounds, ulcers, and refractory dermatoses. Modern-day wound dressings provide a protective barrier against dirt, added trauma, bacteria, and irritants. Moisture retentive dressings decrease discomfort, provide an optimal environment for healing and tissue regeneration, enhance absorption of topical medications, and have a longer wear time than more traditional treatment methods, such as Telfa or other types of gauze dressings (Altman, 2004).

Ranging from impregnated gauze wraps (Unna's boot or Vaseline gauze) to the more technologically advanced hydro fibers (Aquacel) and alginates (Sorbsan and Kaltostat), these dressings are usually easily applied and removed. Moisture retentive dressings can be used in a wide variety of dermatological conditions, from venous stasis ulcers and pressure ulcers to surgical and traumatic wounds. Selection of the most appropriate dressing is dependent on accurate diagnosis and wound assessment. For example, a hydrocolloid dressing will manage light to moderate drainage and has a wear time of up to seven days. However, a moderately draining lesion may overwhelm a hydrocolloid dressing before that seven-day period expires. A calcium alginate dressing is most appropriate for a heavily draining wound but requires a secondary or cover dressing to prevent desiccation of the dressing and the wound. Types of moisture retentive dressings include, but are not limited to, hydrocolloids, foams, hydro fibers, and transparent films.

Moisturizers and Lubricants

Products designed to hydrate the skin play an important role in the treatment of many pruritic, inflammatory, and zerotic skin conditions. In these conditions the goal is to eliminate drying agents from the treatment regimen. Perfumed soaps, lotions, and oils usually contain alcohol as the delivery vehicle for the fragrance and therefore should not be used in the treatment of dermatological conditions.

Skin is not dry because of a lack of oil but from a lack of water. Thus, the primary goal is to apply water to the skin and prevent its evaporation by occlusion. In other words, sealing the moisture into the skin allows hydration of the epidermis and retention of the moisture. Moisturizers and lubricants are designed to hydrate the epidermal layers of the skin. The excellent barrier properties of the skin prevent moisturizers and lubricants from penetrating beyond the epidermis. Regular usage of body moisturizers, particularly within three to five minutes of bathing or showering will aid in prevention of dry, flaking and itching skin.

If emollient products do not succeed in hydrating the skin, it may be necessary to prescribe more potent agents. **Humectants,** such as Aquacare/HP and Carmolare, are substances that promote moisture in skin. Urea and alpha-hydroxy acid are examples of humectants. Urea is a topical keratolytic, functioning to remove excess keratin and to soften and hydrate skin. Alpha-hydroxy acid products hold in skin moisture and decrease rough scale that creates the sensation of dryness. The most common alpha-hydroxy acids are lactic acid (LactiCare) and ammonium lactate (LacHydrin) (Broyles, et al., 2007).

Moisturizers and lotions containing aloe, vitamin E, jojoba, collagen, and elastin are also popular. Many people who use products containing these ingredients achieve the same results as if they used prescription-strength products containing urea or alpha-hydroxy acid. However, there is no scientific evidence showing that these ingredients have any intrinsic benefit beyond their minimal lubricating properties.

Phototherapy and Photochemotherapy

Sunlight has a profound effect on the skin and is associated with a variety of diseases. The skin of a person who has spent a significant amount of time outdoors or who has spent years achieving a healthy tan is thickened, wrinkled, and usually has darker pigmentation (Goldberg, 2004). Ultraviolet (UV) light from the sun causes the most skin reactions and conditions and is classified by the wavelength of the light: ultraviolet A (UVA), ultraviolet B (UVB), or ultraviolet C (UVC). UV light is beyond the spectrum of human vision, in the portion of the electromagnetic spectrum measuring 10 to 400 nanometers (nm) (Note: A nanometer is $1/10^7$ of a meter).

UVA light causes immediate and delayed skin pigment changes and does not contribute to burning and redness. However, the longer the light wavelength, the deeper the penetration into the skin and substructures. UVA can penetrate beyond the epidermis into the dermis and subcutaneous tissue. Chronic exposure to UVA results in the degenerative changes in connective tissue seen in **photoaging** (degenerative changes in connective tissue caused by chronic exposure to UVA), skin cancers, and immunosuppression. UVA can penetrate window glass and has **phototoxic** (rapidly developing nonimmunological skin reaction when exposed to light) and **photoallergic** (sensitivity to light that causes allergic reactions) effects. This type of light is consistent throughout the day and the year.

UVB light is far more damaging and produces the most harmful effects to the skin. This type of radiation is strongest in the summer when the earth is closest to the sun and is most intense between the hours of 10 am and 2 pm. Water, snow, and shiny surfaces reflect UVB radiation. The high amounts of radiation delivered by UVB produces the immediate skin changes associated with sun exposure: sunburn, tanning, inflammation, delayed erythema, and blistering and pigmentation changes. Chronic exposure to UVB also produces photoaging, photocarcinogenesis, and immunosuppression. Window glass absorbs UVB, and prior exposure to UVA enhances the sunburn reaction to UVB. UVC light is almost completely absorbed by the ozone layer and is transmitted only by artificial sources, such as germicidal lamps and mercury arc lamps.

Normal Aging versus Photoaging

Normal signs of aging begin to appear around age 30 to 35. However, unprotected, chronically exposed children can acquire significant sun-related skin changes by the time they reach the age of 15, and the effects of sun damage become apparent after the age of 20. Sun-damaged skin is characterized by thickened, yellowed, coarsening of the epidermis, irregular pigmentation, atrophy of subcutaneous tissue, telangiectasias, deep wrinkling, and other changes, including premalignant changes. UV light, produced naturally by the sun and artificially by other light sources, inhibits deoxyribonucleic acid (DNA) mitosis. UVA and UVB light are used in the treatment of dermatological diseases. UV light is also used to control pathogenic bacteria and viruses and is used in clean room technology where the sterility of the enclosed environment is critical. The differences between the normal aging process and aging related to sun damage are summarized in Table 45-3.

Phototherapy

Phototherapy is the treatment of certain dermatological conditions with artificially produced, nonionizing UV light. This type of therapy is useful in treating certain photobiological conditions, such as psoriasis, vitiligo, eczema, and

TABLE 45-3 Normal Aging versus Photoaging Skin	
NORMAL AGING SKIN	**PHOTOAGING SKIN**
Thin, fragile, and inelastic	Thickened, wrinkled, yellowish skin (solar elastose)
Thinning of epidermis	Thinning of skin, fine wrinkling (atrophy)
Gradual loss of blood vessels, dermal collagen, fat, and elastic fibers	Prominent blood vessels with easy bruising and tearing
Fine, shallow wrinkles that disappear with skin stretching	Deep wrinkles that do not disappear with skin stretching
	Diffuse erythema in fair-skinned persons
Decrease in density of hair follicles, sebaceous glands, sweat ducts, fine dryness of skin	Bleeding into skin following minor trauma (usually in sun exposed areas only—back of the neck, hands, arms), telangiectasias on cheeks, nose, and ears
	Freckles on face
Loss of subcutaneous tissue causes skin to become atrophic and fragile	Lentigo (large brown macules) on face, back of hands, arms, chest, upper back
Reduced elastin fibers result in decreased resilience of skin	Other pigmentation changes such as guttate hypermelanosis (discrete round, white macules) and irregular deep brown pigmented areas
	Seborrheic keratosis (superficial stuck on lesions, more numerous on sun-exposed areas)
	Actinic keratosis (localized thickening of epidermis)
	Comedones and cysts around the eyes

Adapted from Goldberg, D. (2004). Photodamaged skin. *New York: Marcel Dekker.*

cutaneous T cell lymphoma. UVB light is used in the treatment of photosensitive dermatoses and is contraindicated in patients with a history of previous nonmelanoma skin cancers or a family history of melanoma. Dosing of UVB is based on an estimation of the patient's ability to tolerate the treatment based on skin types I through VI and the minimal erythema dose, the smallest amount of UVB required to produce erythema. For example, patients with skin type I have a poor ability to tan, burn easily and severely, and then peel, whereas people with skin type VI are darkly pigmented and never burn. A genetic history is associated with each skin type. Skin type I people have fair skin; freckles; blue, green, or gray eye color; blonde, red, or light brown hair; and a northern European heritage. Skin type VI people have black skin and an African, American Indian, East Indian, or Hispanic (American) heritage (Goldberg, 2004).

A thorough history should be taken by the health care provider prior to initiation of any phototherapeutic regimen that includes skin malignancies, current medications, previous history of radiation exposure or therapy for cancer, and any medical conditions that can be stimulated by UV light, such as herpes simplex, cataracts, or lupus erythematosus. Ophthalmological assessment should be performed on any person displaying early cataract changes, a possible contraindication for photochemotherapeutic ultraviolet A light (PUVA). A variation of standard phototherapy, called the Goeckerman regimen, incorporates photosensitization with keratolytic agents and antipruritic properties of tar preparations. This therapy is used primarily for psoriasis vulgaris and atopic dermatitis. It is a labor-intensive process, requiring the patient to take tar preparation baths and after-bath topical tar medications followed several hours later by phototherapy.

Photochemotherapy

Photochemotherapy is UVA therapy combined with oral or topical 8-methoxypsoralen. This type of UV therapy is used to treat severe and unresponsive forms of psoriasis, atopic dermatitis, and cutaneous T cell lymphoma

(CTCL). The concept is that photosensitizing medications increase the skin sensitivity to the long-wave UVA light (Broyles, et al., 2007). These medications also induce repigmentation of skin in patients with vitiligo and have an antimitotic effect on psoriasis and CTCL. Dosage is established based on body weight, and the medication is taken with food one-and-a-half to two hours prior to treatment to minimize nausea. Topical preparations can be used to treat smaller areas or in patients for whom systemic administration is contraindicated. Phototherapy and photochemotherapy are long and sometimes complicated processes. Patients must be able to understand the treatment process and be willing to comply with the treatment regimen. A summary of important patient information can be found in the Patient Playbook.

COMMON SKIN DISORDERS

This section is by no means inclusive of the many types of dermatological problems encountered by patients and health care professionals. It will, however, serve as a framework with which to gain insight into the diagnosis and treatment of such conditions.

Acne

Acne is a papulopustular disorder of the pilosebaceous unit in which abnormally adherent keratinocytes cause plugging of the follicular duct, causing accumulation of sebum and keratinous debris. Onset can be from 8 to 10 years of age and continue until the late 20s or early 30s. It is the most common

---

PATIENT PLAYBOOK

Strategies for Management of Phototherapy and Photochemotherapy

The nurse should encourage the following as related to strategies for managing phototherapy and photochemotherapy:

- The nurse reviews pretreatment instructions with the patient, including when to take pretreatment medications.
- The patient and nurse should review the treatment schedule. Initial treatments are scheduled three times per week with rest periods.
- Psoralens should be taken with food one-and-a-half to two hours prior to photochemotherapy treatment to minimize nausea and ensure system absorption.
- Topical psoralens must be applied 30 minutes prior to beginning treatment.
- Assess patient prior to beginning treatment sessions. Ask patient about photosensitizing medications, over-the-counter (OTC) preparations, or other prescriptions.

- Skin needs to rest in between treatments, because erythema will manifest six to eight hours after exposure.
- Severe erythema that continues between rest periods may require a delay in treatment for a short time until erythema lessens and do not increase dosage if a treatment has been missed.
- Provide protective goggles to prevent eye damage from the light source.
- Arms and legs may require extra dosing; all other areas must be shielded.
- There is higher risk of burning with topical psoralens than with systemic medication. Absorption of drug is increased in areas where skin is not intact.
- Inform the patient that treatments will be delayed or stopped at their request.
- Caution patient against lending medication to friends or relatives
- Instruct patient about who to call if any problems occur.

Adapted from Altman, G. (2004). Delmar's fundamental and advanced nursing skills *(2nd ed.). New York: Thomson Delmar Learning; Broyles, B., Reiss, B., & Evans, M. (2007).* Pharmacological aspects of nursing care *(7th ed.). New York: Thomson Delmar Learning.*

dermatological problem in the pediatric and adolescent populations but can be seen in newborns (related to maternal androgens). Severity can range from mild to the severely scarring acne conglobata. About one in four people has acne significant enough to seek professional treatment. Acne is more prevalent in Western cultures and occurs in males and females equally, with the exception of acne conglobata, which occurs more in males (Liao, 2003).

Acne lesions can be inflammatory or noninflammatory and present as **comedones** (blackheads), papules, pustules, or nodules. Noninflammatory lesions are closed comedones and open comedones. Inflammatory papules, pustules, and nodules are classified as mild, moderate, or severe as shown in Table 45-4. Acne can have a profound psychological effect on people, yet it is often dismissed as merely a phase of the normal growth process and a minor affliction not worthy of treatment. Diagnosis is based on the physical appearance of the lesions.

Treatment of acne is based on the severity of the disease and includes cleansing with gentle surfactant products without abrasive soaps or other ingredients. Suppression of inflammation is important in the prevention of scarring. Benzoyl peroxide has a potent antimicrobial effect and will reduce the size and number of comedones and inhibit secretion of sebum. Topical antibiotics may also be prescribed to reduce bacteria associated with acne. Failure to respond to topical treatments indicates the need to evaluate the patient for systemic antibiotics, usually given over an extended period of time. Long-term usage of antibiotics may result in monilial vaginitis, thrush, and gastrointestinal (GI) symptoms (Spratto & Woods, 2007).

Hormone therapy may be indicated for severe cystic acne. Topical estrogens suppress sebaceous gland activity; estrogen therapy may need to be continued for three to four menstrual cycles. Severe disease may require the use of isotretinoin to inhibit inflammation. The dosage is determined by body weight, in divided doses, usually taken over several months. Comedonal acne responds slowly and several months of treatment are needed.

Mild inflammatory acne (defined as fewer than 20 pustules) is treated with benzoyl peroxide products, beginning with the lowest concentrations. Moderate to severe inflammatory acne is usually treated twice daily with benzoyl peroxide products, topical antibiotics, or a combination therapy of benzoyl peroxide, and sulfacetamide/sulfur products. Severe nodulocystic acne requires aggressive treatment, because the scarring can be severe. Oral antibiotics, conventional topical therapy, and periodic intralesional injections of Kenalog can keep this problem under control.

Atopic Dermatitis

Atopic dermatitis is a chronic, pruritic skin condition characterized by inflammation of the skin. The exact cause is unknown, but it does have a hereditary tendency. There is a cyclic pattern of exacerbation and remission that can continue throughout the patient's lifetime and a seasonal pattern may be demonstrated as

TABLE 45-4 **Severity Grading of Inflammatory Lesions**		
SEVERITY	**PAPULES/PUSTULES**	**NODULES**
Mild	Few to several	None
Moderate	Several to many	Few to several
Severe	Numerous or extensive	Many

Adapted from Estes, M. (2006). Health assessment and physical examination (3rd ed.). New York: Thomson Delmar Learning.

well. Health care providers believe that atopic dermatitis is a complex relationship between genetic, environmental, immunological, and pharmacological factors. Flares of the disease can be precipitated by stress, infection, seasonal climate changes, irritants, and allergens.

The disease usually begins in childhood and may stabilize as the patient ages. The prevalence of atopic dermatitis in children is currently estimated to be 7 to 17 percent having increased greatly since the 1960s. It is an increase that cannot be explained by genetics alone. Changes in lifestyle and environmental factors, as well as increased recognition, may be contributing to the increase. Diagnosis is based on the basic features of the disease and requires that patients exhibit three or more of these features: pruritus, typical morphology and distribution, chronic or chronically relapsing dermatitis, family history (asthma, allergic rhinitis, or atopic dermatitis), **lichenification** (thickening of the epidermis) in flexural areas in adults, and facial and extensor involvement in children.

Atopic dermatitis starts with itching that becomes a habitual itch-scratch cycle. Chronic dermatitis is the result of scratching over a long period of time that causes thickening of the skin. Acute inflammation begins with erythematous papules and erythema and may coalesce into dry, scaly patches. Distribution of the dermatitis tends to be symmetrical and is more pronounced in areas not covered by clothing. Patients with atopic dermatitis are susceptible to bacterial, viral, and fungal skin infections due primarily to a break in the integrity of the natural barrier properties of the skin. Secondary infections involving *S. aureus* are common.

Treatment of atopic dermatitis is aimed at relief of the dryness and pruritus and decreasing inflammation. The goal is to break the inflammatory cycles causing excess drying and cracking of the skin and the itching and scratching associated with the disease. Hydration of the skin is critical, and it is important to identify and control the triggers that cause the disease to flare. Occlusives, moisturizers, topical steroids, and tar preparations are used to control atopic dermatitis and are frequently used in combination. Occasionally, systemic antihistamines and antibiotics may be required. Systemic steroids are rarely used.

Cellulitis

Cellulitis is an infection of the skin characterized most commonly by redness, heat, pain, swelling and, occasionally, fever, malaise, chills, and headache (Figure 45-1). Abscess formation and tissue destruction usually follow if cellulitis is left untreated. Most health care professionals view cellulitis as a symptom rather than a disease and agree that the need to determine the cause is important. Typically, systemic antibiotics are used to treat cellulitis, but sometimes silver sulfadiazine creams are used. The patient is encouraged to refrain from weight bearing if the cellulitis is located in the lower extremities or foot because weight bearing can encourage more rapid spread of the infection either locally or to the bloodstream, causing septicemia. It is not uncommon to observe a generalized sloughing of epidermis in the involved area after resolution of the infection.

Contact Dermatitis

Contact dermatitis is categorized into two groups, irritant and allergic. Irritant contact dermatitis results when the skin comes in contact with a substance in the environment that acts as an irritant. It is a nonimmunological response to the irritant that is dependent on the person's ability to maintain the normal epidermal barrier. The extent of the dermatitis is related to the exposure time and concentration of the irritant. Characterized by erythema, blister formation, erosions, scaling, and drying and crusting of skin, irritant contact dermatitis damages the barrier component of the skin and can be either acute or

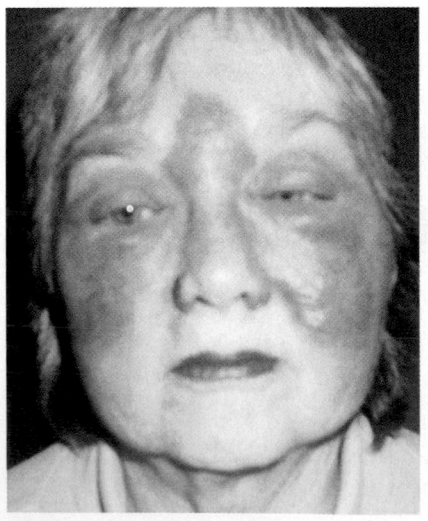

Figure 45-1 Cellulitis.

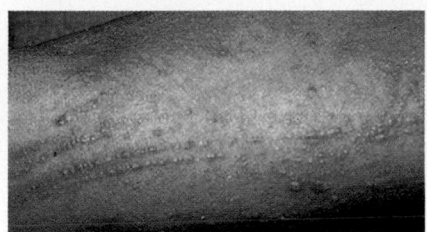

Figure 45-2 Allergic contact dermatitis. Courtesy of the Centers for Disease Control and Prevention.

chronic. Mild irritants cause drying, erythema, and fissuring. Chronic exposure to the irritant causes thickening of the epidermis and eczematous inflammation. Identification of the irritant is critical to treatment. Since the advent of universal precautions, many health care providers have developed this type of dermatitis in response to the latex in the gloves used for patient care or to the powder used inside the gloves to facilitate easy donning (Altman, 2004).

Allergic contact dermatitis is an inflammatory response to an antigen that follows absorption of that antigen into the skin; in other words, allergic contact dermatitis is a delayed hypersensitivity reaction (Figure 45-2). The person will not have a reaction with the first exposure, but their immune system will recognize the antigen during the sensitization phase and mark, or recruit, T lymphocytes within the body that will recognize the antigen with the next exposure. Reexposure to the antigen during the elicitation phase results in a skin response characterized by erythema, wheals and welt formation, blister formation, inflammation, papules, vesicles, scaling, fissures, and crusting. Examples of allergic contact dermatitis include adhesives allergies, cosmetics allergies (particularly around the eyes), plant allergies, such as poison ivy, poison oak or poison sumac, and metal allergies. Anyone can be allergic to any substance from skin care products, from deodorants to dyes used in shoemaking and the plastic earpieces on eyeglasses. Diagnosis is made through a careful history and examination of the skin condition, including any occupational or causal exposure to chemicals. Biopsy of the area is usually not helpful.

Treatment of irritant and contact dermatitis is dependent on identification of the sensitizing substance and controlling the symptoms. Patch testing is helpful in determining the cause of allergic contact dermatitis, but the health care professional needs to also test the patient's consumer products, such as soap, shampoo, and deodorant, as well as look for other possible causes. Patients need to read labels carefully, because many products contain sensitizing agents, such as lanolin, parabens, and fragrance.

It is important to minimize topical treatments and instruct the patient how to appropriately apply topical medications. Wet compresses can be used with solutions that provide a cooling effect. Topical corticosteroids are usually prescribed for application one to two times daily in chronic or recalcitrant cases. Usually removal of the causative substance will cause the condition to resolve. Antihistamines can be prescribed for pruritus. Severe plant reactions may require a short course of prednisone.

Folliculitis

Folliculitis is an acute inflammation of the hair follicle caused by physical irritation, infection, or chemical irritation. It is common and can be an associated symptom of a variety of inflammatory skin diseases. Removal of adhesive dressings, ostomy pouches and other adherent materials may trigger a follicular skin reaction. Superficial folliculitis is confined to the upper part of the hair follicle and presents as a nontender or tender pustule. Inflammation of the entire hair follicle, called **sycosis,** presents as a red, swollen mass that eventually turns into larger pustules. Deep, painful lesions may heal with scarring. The most common causes of folliculitis are bacterial *(S. aureus). Staphylococcus* folliculitis may occur on any body surface where the skin has been abraded or traumatized. **Sycosis barbae** is the inflammation of the entire hair follicle in an area that is traumatized through shaving it and begins with the development of papules or pustules that rapidly evolve into a more diffuse problem as shaving continues. Most infections are treated with oral antibiotics. Localized inflammations are treated topically with mupirocin (Bactroban). Extensive disease is treated with oral antibiotics (dicloxacillin or cephalexin) for at least two weeks until inflammation has cleared.

Shaving can also cause pseudofolliculitis barbae, a foreign body reaction to hair in individuals with a genetic inclination for curly, spiral shaped hair. This condition is commonly referred to as ingrown hair. In some instances, loops of hair can be seen imbedded in the skin and can be released by washing the beard for several minutes using a circular motion with a washcloth or toothbrush or using a syringe needle under the loop and firmly elevating the hair. Prevention requires that patients prone to this condition make certain that whiskers are softened prior to shaving, use a hair releasing technique, and avoid close shaving. Using a double or triple-bladed shaving system, alternately shaving with an electric razor, and avoiding the closest shave setting, helps to decrease the production of sharply-angled hair tips.

Fungal Infections

Fungal infections are also known as **tineas** and are perhaps the most common dermatological problems encountered by health care professionals. Dermatophytes comprise a large group of fungi that have the ability to invade and infect the skin, surviving on the dead keratinocytes found in the stratum. They can also survive on mucosal surfaces, such as mouth and vaginal areas where the keratin layer does not form, and can, in rare instances, invade deeper tissues. Normally, the acid mantle of the skin protects the epidermis from bacterial and dermatophyte invasion. Patients who are immunosuppressed, have a genetic susceptibility to dermatophyte infection, taking courses of antibiotics or chemotherapy, or engage in any activity that would cause a change in pH of the acid mantle including washing with harsh soaps or frequent showering are at risk for development for fungal infections.

Classification of dermatophytes occurs in several ways. Dermatophytes are classified by place of origin, type of inflammation and type of hair invasion. The origin may be an animal or **zoophilic** source; it may be a human or **anthropophilic** source; or it may emanate from an environmental or geophilic source. Anthropophilic dermatophytes are only found on human skin, hair, or nails. Zoophilic dermatophytes originate from animals but can be transferred to humans. Geophilic dermatophytes live in the soil but can infect humans.

Differences in types of fungal inflammations are evident in the severity of the inflammatory response. Animal and human infections result in a brisk inflammatory response. Environmentally sourced fungal infections usually produce a milder inflammation. Some species of dermatophytes invade the hair shaft. Microscopic examination of infected hair reveals spores either inside the shaft, or both inside the hair shaft and on the hair surface.

The most common fungal infections include tinea versicolor, candidiasis, tinea pedis, tinea cruris, tinea capitis, and tinea corporis. Tinea versicolor is a chronic infection seen on the trunk, arms, and neck. The organism causing this infection is the *Pityrosporum* species found in the normal flora of the skin in highest concentration in areas of increased oil production. Factors contributing to any fungal proliferation include heat and humidity, malnutrition, pregnancy, burns, steroid therapy, immunosuppression, and oral contraception. Lesions are circular and scaly, often appearing as white patches on tan skin. Diagnosis of tinea versicolor is made using a Wood's lamp and potassium hydroxide (KOH) stain (Figure 45-3). Cultures are rarely necessary. Treatment is selenium shampoos when the infection involves the scalp and hair. Other areas are treated with topical antifungal preparations and keratolytic soaps.

Candidiasis is perhaps the most common of all fungal infections and is caused by a proliferation of the normal yeast flora in the mouth, intestinal tract, or vaginal tract. Yeasts proliferate best in a warm, dark, and moist environment. Therefore yeast infections are usually confined to skin folds and creases or mucous membranes. Predisposing factors include immunosuppression, diabetes, oral contraceptives, antibiotic therapy, skin maceration, and topical steroid therapy. This form of yeast only affects the outer layers of epidermis and mucous membranes.

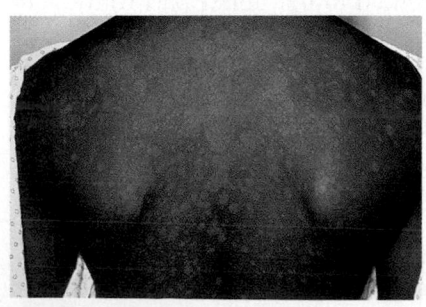

Figure 45-3 Tinea versicolor. Courtesy of Robert A. Silverman, M.D., Clinical Associate Professor, Department of Pediatrics, Georgetown University.

Monilial vulvovaginitis is the most common cause of vaginal discharge, itching, and odor. KOH wet mount examinations are routinely used to diagnosis this infection. Vaginal antifungals are effective in treating this type of yeast infection. However, the disease is considered recurrent if three or more episodes occur within one year.

Oral candidiasis is usually seen in infants resulting from passage through the birth canal, but it is also seen in adults. The infection involves the tongue and cheek lining causing a red, painful, fissured tongue surface with a white coating. The infection may then extend to the esophagus and trachea. An oral antifungal suspension is used to treat this infection in adults, and systemic antifungals may also be required. The solution is swished around in the mouth, then either spit out or swallowed, depending on whether there is esophageal involvement.

Tinea pedis is the most common infection of the feet. Like skin creases and folds, shoes provide a warm, moist environment for yeast growth. Tinea pedis is common in men, uncommon in women and, though uncommon, should be differentially diagnosed in prepubertal children with foot dermatitis. The locker room and communal bath areas of sports facilities is a prime source of this infection, hence the term "athlete's foot." Infections are found most commonly in the toe webs and soles of the foot. Toe webs can become macerated with scale, and the infection can spread out from the toe web if left untreated. Tinea pedis infections consist of erythematous, red macules, and pustules that become crusted. Itching is the most common complaint along with burning. Scratching the itch can result in secondary infections that compound treatment challenges (Carter, Dufour, & Ballard, 2004). Diagnosis is based on visual assessment of the lesions. OTC or prescription medications may be used to treat tinea pedis depending on the severity of the infection and whether it is acute or chronic.

Tinea cruris occurs in the groin and inner thigh areas, primarily during the summer months. Sweating and wearing wet clothing contribute to the development of the disease, again providing the warm, moist environment needed for yeast to proliferate. Men are affected far more frequently than women. The skin irritation caused either by skin or by clothing rubbing on the inner thigh surfaces can be misdiagnosed as a yeast rash. Also known as "jock itch" or "jock rot," tinea cruris lesions present in half-moon shapes and are usually bilateral with itching, burning, odor, and maceration of epidermis. As with most tinea infections, diagnosis is made based on presentation of rash and treatment can be either an OTC or a prescription antifungal.

Tinea capitis is a fungal infection involving the scalp that can extend onto the neck. The *Trichophyton* species is responsible for this infection that usually begins with several round patches of dryness or scale. Tinea capitis is common in urban areas, but it is also seen in impoverished areas where living conditions are crowded. Spores are shed in the area of people infected, and direct contact is not required for spread of the disease. Infection of the hair shaft is preceded by scalp infection, with the fungus growing through the stratum corneum and into the hair follicle below the area where the hair follicle is formed. The dermatophyte cannot cross the perifollicular stratum corneum into the hair but must burrow deep into the follicle to avoid the cuticle. This explains why topical antifungal agents are ineffective in treating this form of tinea.

Diagnosis of tinea capitis is based on the clinical presentation of lesions called kerions and patterns of hair loss. Clinically, these lesions present as boggy, indurated, tumor-like masses that are palpable in the scalp and exude pus. Four patterns of inflammation have been identified: (a) noninflammatory black dot pattern, a well-defined pattern of hair loss where the hair shafts are broken at the point where they exit the stratum corneum causing the appearance of a black dot; (b) inflammatory with a positive test for the presence of the *Trichophyton* antigen; (c) seborrheic with white flakes that resemble dandruff;

and (d) pustular with discrete pustules or scabbed areas without scaling or significant hair loss.

Occipital or cervical lymphadenopathy is usually present and lack thereof ought to cause the health care professional to question a tinea capitis diagnosis. Treatment includes oral antifungal medications and topical shampoos to reduce or control spore loads and treat asymptomatic carriers.

Tinea corporis involves the face, excluding the area of a beard in men, trunk, and limbs. This form of fungal infection has many manifestations with lesions varying in inflammation and depth of involvement. The classic presentation is a distinct, circular lesion with an advancing red, scaly border. Papules may be present. Itching, erythema, and follicular involvement are also common characteristics of the disease, which is also known as ringworm. Diagnosis and treatment is the same as for other tinea infections. It is important to minimize exposure of other people to the infection and begin treatment as soon as possible. Fortunately, treatment for fungal infections is readily available and effective.

Furuncles and Carbuncles

Localized bacterial infections can manifest as painful, indurated, or fluctuant, fluid-filled masses called **furuncles (boils).** Cellulitis can be prodromal or concurrent with the infection. An **abscess** is a cavity containing pus surrounded by inflamed tissue, the healing of which only begins after incision and drainage. *S. aureus* is the most common pathogen and furuncles occur primarily in areas of friction or minor trauma, such as beltlines, anterior thighs, neck area, axillae, and waistline. Deep red, firm, tender papules enlarge rapidly into a deep-seated nodule that remains stable and erythematous for days and then becomes fluid-filled. These painful lesions are most uncomfortable in constricted areas, such as the neck. The abscess either remains deep, is eventually reabsorbed, or it ruptures through the epidermis. Scarring is common when rupture occurs.

Carbuncles are aggregates of infected follicles originating deep in the dermis and subcutaneous tissue. Unlike furuncles, carbuncles form an erythematous, swollen, broad, and slowly evolving mass that can ulcerate and drain from multiple openings. This process is called pointing. Malaise, chills, and fevers, either precede or occur simultaneously with the infection. Sloughing and scarring are common. Several diseases can produce furuncles, the most common being a ruptured epidermal cyst or pilar cyst of the scalp. Warm compresses are used to provide comfort and draw the infection to the surface. Incision and drainage is the most rapid form of treatment. Once drained, the area should be packed to prevent closure of the skin before the abscess cavity heals outward. Oral antibiotics are prescribed for 5 to 10 days.

Herpes Infections

Herpes simplex viral infections are caused by two different viral types: herpes simplex virus-1 (HSV-1) and herpes simplex virus-2 (HSV-2). HSV-1 is generally associated with oral cold sores and fever blisters, and HSV-2 is associated with genital infections. Both types of infections are becoming more common and may be related to oral-genital sexual contact. Many of these infections are asymptomatic, and evidence of previous infection is determined by an immunoglobulin G (IgG) antibody titer.

HSV infections have two phases: the primary infection during which the virus becomes imbedded in the nerve ganglion and the secondary phase characterized by recurrent infections at the same site. Recurrence of genital herpes is six times more frequent than oral-labial occurrence. Infection can occur at any site on the skin, and infection in one area does not preclude subsequent infection at another site. The primary infection is usually asymptomatic. The severity of the disease increases with age and the virus can be spread through respiratory droplets, direct contact with infected people with active lesions, or contact with virus-containing fluid, such as saliva or cervical secretions.

Symptoms of primary infection occur three to seven days after exposure, beginning with sensitivity in the area; pain, tenderness, or burning. The lesions are grouped vesicles that are uniform in size on an erythematous base that heals as a tissue depression referred to as umbilicated. Crusts then form and usually heal without scarring. Secondary infection can be activated by local skin trauma, such as chapping or abrasion, or by a systemic response, such as fever or fatigue. The activated virus travels down the peripheral nerve to the site of the initial infection and causes the classic focal, recurrent infection. Prodromal symptoms last 2 to 24 hours, then the vesicles rapidly form on an erythematous base, becoming large, dome-shaped, fluid-filled lesions. They rupture and form erosions in the mouth or vaginal area or crusts on the lips and skin. The crusts are usually shed in about one week leaving pink, reepitheliazed skin. Secondary infections are less severe than primary infections. Diagnosis of HSV is done by assessment of the lesions and laboratory tests that depend on the stage of the disease for their sensitivity. Tzanck smear, Pap smear, viral culture, and serology for IgG antibody titer are common diagnostic tools. Treatment of HSV consists of cool, moist compresses of Burrow's solution, controlling secondary infections, and systemic or topical antivirals that may include Acyclovir, Famvir, or Valtrex.

Cutaneous Herpes Simplex

Cutaneous herpes simplex is a manifestation of HSV and mimics other vesicular eruptions. The most common forms are herpes whitlow, HSV of the buttocks or trunk, and herpes gladiatorum. Herpes whitlow usually occurs on the fingertips and can resemble a bacterial infection or warts. Health care professionals with frequent contact with oral secretions are particularly at risk. HSV of the buttocks is more common in women and the cause has not been identified. HSV of the trunk appears similar to herpes zoster, and diagnosis may only become apparent at the time of recurrence. Herpes gladiatorum is most frequently found in athletes who participate in contact sports. It is disseminated by direct skin-to-skin contact and early diagnosis is important to prevent further transmission.

Herpes Zoster

Herpes zoster, more commonly referred to as shingles, is a cutaneous infection caused by reactivation of the varicella chickenpox virus. As with HSV, the virus can become dormant along the skin of a dermatome, or nerve root ganglion, until conditions such as immunosuppression, emotional upsets, radiation, or lymphoma cause the virus to become active. The reactivated virus travels down the nerve, infecting the skin and giving this disease its classic asymmetrical appearance. Most commonly seen on the face, chest, and buttocks, any dermatome area of the body can be affected (Figure 45-4). Herpes zoster is less communicable than varicella, but people who have not had varicella may develop the disease after exposure to varicella. Prodromal symptoms include pain known as preherpetic neuralgia, itching, and burning generally localized to the dermatome area, and may precede eruption by four to five days.

The eruptions begin with red, swollen plaques that spread through the affected dermatome. Vesicles of varying sizes arise in the plaque and quickly become engorged with a milky fluid, usually three to four days following erythematous plaque formation. The disease is extremely painful, requiring significant amounts of narcotics and sometimes hospitalization. The patient has great difficulty tolerating dressings and clothing coming in contact with the affected area. Pain is neuropathic and results from altered central nervous system signal processing.

Diagnosis of herpes zoster is made by history and physical examination of the pattern and the character of the vesicles and surrounding skin. Treatment

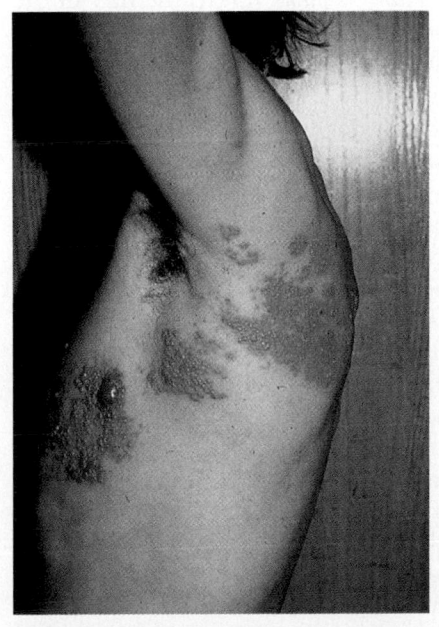

Figure 45-4 Herpes zoster. Courtesy of Robert A. Silverman, M.D., Clinical Associate Professor, Department of Pediatrics, Georgetown University.

of herpes zoster centers on pain control and antiviral therapy. Antiviral medications must be started within 72 hours of the onset of the rash or pain. Pain can be severe enough to require nerve blocks. Selection and dosage of medications is determined according to the needs of the individual patient. The same antiviral drugs used to treat HSV are used to treat herpes zoster.

Impetigo

Impetigo is a common, superficial skin infection beginning as a focal erythema and progressing to pruritic vesicles, erosions, and honey-colored crusts. Caused by staphylococci, streptococci, or both, these lesions can resemble infections, such as poison ivy. Clinical presentation begins with vesicle formation affecting only the stratum corneum. Diagnosis is based on history and appearance. Children in close physical contact with each other in school or in daycare have a higher rate of infection than the adult population. The disease is self-limiting but can last weeks without treatment. Lesions are usually confined in one area but can develop satellite lesions. The thin-roofed bullae collapse but may retain fluid for several days. A thin, varnish-like, honey-colored crust appears in the center of ruptured bullae. If the crust is removed a bright red, inflamed, moist base that oozes clear fluid is revealed. Serious secondary infections, including osteomyelitis, arthritis, and pneumonia, can follow seemingly superficial infections in infants. The skin around the nose, mouth, and limbs are the most common sites. Regional lymphadenopathy is common. Acute nephritis can occur when whole families are infected, usually developing one to three weeks after infection. Cultures are not routinely performed to confirm the diagnosis because its unique presentation confirms the diagnosis. Treatment of impetigo consists of oral antibiotics and topical mupirocin ointment (Carter, et al., 2004).

Pediculosis

Infestation with lice is called **pediculosis.** The louse, which is visible to the naked eye, is endemic all over the world and is estimated to cause 10 million cases in the United States annually. There are two species of lice that infect humans: the body louse, or *Pediculus humanus,* is the largest and infests the body and scalp; the smaller crab louse, or *Phthirus pubis,* infests the hair in the pubic area. Head lice can be found in all social and economic levels but are far more prevalent in people living in crowded conditions, and those living with poor hygiene conditions or practices.

The female louse lays eggs called nits each day for up to one month and then dies. The nits are firmly cemented to the base of a hair shaft close to the skin where adequate warmth will incubate them for 8 to 10 days and then they hatch. The louse will fully mature in 18 days. Nits are difficult to remove from the hair shaft. Head lice produce pruritic red papules and are most common in children. More girls than boys are affected, and head lice are found primarily at the back of the head and neck and behind the ears. The pruritus is worse at night.

Pediculosis pubis is a contagious, sexually transmitted disease (STD) and 30 percent of those persons infected with pediculosis pubis also have another STD. Pubic hair is the most common site, but the lice frequently spread to the perianal hair. The most common complaint is pruritus. Diagnosis is made by the presence of nits and pruritic rashes in a localized area. Combing will detect and remove live lice, both of which are easily visible under the microscope. Treatment of head lice consists of application of 1% permethrin lotion after a pretreatment shampoo. The lotion is allowed to remain on the hair for 10 minutes and then rinsed. Gamma benzene hexachloride available as 1% lindane or Kwell shampoo may be used, but it is less effective. Gloves must be worn when using Kwell shampoo, and the patient should avoid getting the shampoo on other body parts.

Pyrethrin, or RID, can be used for any type of pediculosis infection, but is less effective than other treatments. Treatment for pubic or body lice consists of lindane lotions or creams. Any treatment usually requires multiple applications. Bedding, head coverings, brushes, and combs must be dry cleaned or washed in hot, soapy water. Clothing of people with body lice may need to be ironed along each seam to remove oviposits.

Pemphigus

Pemphigus is a chronic problem resulting in the development of blisters. It is fairly uncommon in the general public, but incidence is increased in Mediterranean regions and Jewish peoples. Pemphigus is an epidermal autoimmune disease caused by circulating IgG autoantibodies that react with the intracellular cement that binds cells together. Bullae and blisters form, then rupture with crusting of the erosions. The bullae are flaccid, and the fluid released at the time of rupture smells foul. Treatment involves oral corticosteroids and other immunosuppressive medications, which controls but does not cure.

Pruritus

Itching, or **pruritus,** is one of the most common manifestations of dermatological problems. Even patients with normally healing wounds experience itching as part of the healing process. Most health care professionals involved in treating patients with dermatological problems agree that pruritus is a symptom not a disease. The cause of the itching needs to be determined and treated. In addition, the pruritus must be treated because the irritation leads to excoriation of the skin from scratching, and it is known that any break in the skin is an entrance for contaminants.

Pruritus can be a secondary symptom of conditions ranging from dry skin to cancer. Systemic diseases, such as herpes zoster, kidney failure resulting in uremia, drug reactions, hematological cancers, such as leukemia and lymphoma, liver diseases that increase bilirubin levels, and diabetes, can all have a pruritic component. Pruritus can also be caused by contact with chemical irritants, adhesives, plants, household chemicals, such as laundry products and other cleaning solutions, lawn care products, dyes, and fabric protection products. In other words, anything can cause a patient to itch. Skin tends to dry out more in the cold weather months than in warm weather months. Nonhummidified heat causes an increase in evaporation rates of the skin's natural water content. Perfumed soaps and lotions use alcohol as the vehicle for the fragrance and thus are drying agents. Universal precautions require health care professionals to wash their hands frequently and to wear gloves for patient care, contributing to drying the skin of their hands. Pruritus is also associated with allergic reactions to a variety of substances. People with hay fever or other environmental allergies complain of itching eyes. The determination of the cause of the pruritus is important to the treatment of the condition and alleviation of the itching.

Appropriate management of any skin condition requires accurate assessment and diagnosis of the problem. Dry skin may be the source of the pruritus or a contributing factor. Topical antihistamine creams and anesthetics are generally ineffective and should be avoided, because they can be potent sensitizers, particularly if used on inflamed skin. Elderly patients may have trouble following a regimen of frequent bathing or showering because of decreased mobility and increased fall risk. Application of more hydrating products is better in this situation but may require the assistance of other people. Antihistamine therapy should be used with caution in elderly patients, because these patients have a low tolerance and may experience enhancement of the usual side effects of antihistamine therapy.

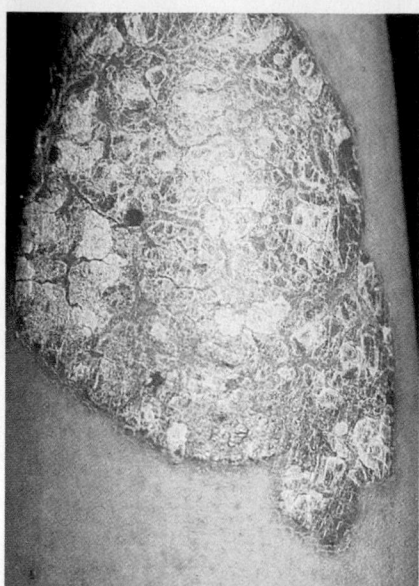

Figure 45-5 Psoriasis. Courtesy of Robert A. Silverman, M.D., Clinical Associate Professor, Department of Pediatrics, Georgetown University.

Psoriasis

Health care professionals estimate that 1 to 3 percent of the population has this genetically transmitted disease that crosses all racial groups. The origin is unknown, and the disease is lifelong, characterized by exacerbations and remissions that can be physically and emotionally debilitating. **Psoriasis** is a T cell mediated inflammatory disease characterized by epidermal hyperplasia (overproduction of epidermal tissue) usually localized in certain regions of the body. The prevalence of arthritis with psoriasis is higher than in the general population. Arthritis occurs in 5 to 42 percent of people with psoriasis. There have been several types of psoriasis identified. The most common forms are psoriasis vulgaris or classic plaque psoriasis, guttate psoriasis, and pustular psoriasis. Less frequently seen types include erythrodermic psoriasis, light-sensitive psoriasis, human immunodeficiency virus (HIV)-induced psoriasis, and Reiter's syndrome (Young, 2003).

Classic plaque psoriasis appears as well-defined plaques with a whitish or silvery appearance on a pink, violaceous or blue background (Figure 45-5). The borders or margins are raised and well-defined. The predominant locations of classic lesions are the scalp, elbows, knees, and lumbosacral areas. Smaller plaques tend to coalesce into larger ones.

Guttate psoriasis is less common comprising less than 2 percent of the psoriatic population. The onset of guttate psoriasis usually follows an upper respiratory infection caused by group-A B hemolytic streptococci *(Streptococcus pyogenes)* or a viral upper respiratory infection. This form usually presents two to three weeks after the infection and has a distinctive presentation. Scattered 1 to 10 mm droplike papules appear suddenly on the trunk and extremities, sparing the soles of the feet and palms of the hands. About 30 percent of people developing guttate psoriasis have their first episode before the age of 20; the disease may resolve spontaneously, is more responsive to treatment than the classic form, or it may evolve into chronic plaque psoriasis.

Generalized pustular psoriasis, also called von Zumbusch psoriasis, is the most common form of this version of psoriasis. Characterized by an explosive onset of burning erythema, it is a serious and sometimes fatal disease. Pustules form in an erythematous bed and coalesce into lakes of pus, appearing on the elbows, anal region, genitalia, and fleural areas of the axillae and knees. The patient is febrile, toxic, tachycardic, tachypneic, and has leukocytosis. Mortality rates can be as high as 30 percent without adequate treatment and relapses are common.

The diagnosis of psoriasis is made based on its visual presentation. The lesions of each of the three previously described types of psoriasis are distinctive, and biopsy is usually not necessary. In as high as 35 percent of cases other family members also have psoriasis, but the disease can skip generations. Pruritus is common in most forms of psoriasis. The severity of the disease is rated using the psoriasis activity and severity index (PASI). There are three steps involved when using the PASI to calculate the disease severity and the percentage of body involvement: (a) the overall severity of the lesion, (b) the psoriatic lesion signs, and (c) calculate the PASI (Young, 2003).

When using the PASI, the health care provider must first determine the degree of inflammation. Psoriatic plaques are successfully treated when the induration disappears. Residual skin that appears erythematous with hyperpigmentation or brown pigmentation is common when the plaque disappears and is often seen as a need to continue treatment when, in fact, use of the prescribed treatment should halt. When the plaque cannot be palpated, the treatment may be stopped. Treatment of psoriasis includes biological therapies, topical corticosteroids, UVB, and topical tar and anthralin preparations and is based on the percentage of the body surface involved. Topical and intralesional steroids, vitamin D analogues, tar and anthralin preparations, and UVB are recommended treatment options when less than 20 percent of the body surface is involved. Combination UVB and tar preparations, PUVA, methotrexate, cyclosporine, and the biological therapies are reserved for patients with more than 20 percent of body surface affected by the disease or the disease is recalcitrant. Patients often tell the health care provider that their mild psoriasis improves with exposure to natural sunlight. Steroids can be applied topically, administered by intralesional injection or taken orally. The treatment for psoriasis is usually lengthy and the cycle of exacerbation and remissions can last throughout the patient's lifetime.

Many topical and systemic treatments exist for psoriasis. Steroids can provide a rapid response and are usually given in pulse doses. UUV light therapy is used only on classic and guttate psoriasis. Tar and anthralin preparations are relatively inexpensive, but the staining effect is viewed negatively by many patients. Intralesional steroids can be used in limited areas only, because atrophy and telangiectasias occur at injection sites.

Rosacea

Rosacea is a chronic, inflammatory condition characterized by erythema, papules, pustules, and telangiectasis. Its etiology is unknown. The erythema is caused by atrophy of the papillary dermis and dilation of the superficial vasculature of the face. Commonly referred to as the rosacea mask, this condition affects the face and nose but can occur centrally in the T zone that includes the forehead. Blackhead formation is unusual. The condition has an insidious onset, usually developing between 30 and 50 years of age and affecting more women than men. It is more common in fair-skinned persons, predominantly of Celtic origin, with a history of flushing referred to as flushers and blushers. Factors affecting this condition include familial genetic predisposition, sun exposure, alcohol consumption, consumption of caffeine-containing products, extremes of temperature, spicy foods or beverages, and emotional stress. Sebaceous hyperplasia of the nose, termed rhinophyma, is seen more frequently in men and is associated with chronic rosacea. Commonly known as a W. C. Fields nose, sebaceous hyperplasia is often mistaken as an indication of excessive alcohol consumption. Eyelid inflammation and conjunctivitis can also occur.

Diagnosis of rosacea is based on the patient's history and clinical presentation. Treatment involves topical and sometimes systemic regimens. Avoidance of triggers, such as sunlight, alcohol, and spicy foods, may be enough to control mild rosacea. More severe cases require more persistent treatment. Topical retinoids, benzoyl peroxide, and topical antibiotics assist in controlling the severity of outbreaks.

Systemic therapy consists of oral antibiotics and retinoids. Oral contraceptives may also be used as adjunctive treatment and steroids may be required to treat severe, refractory cases. Patients should be cautioned not to over wash the face and to use only gentle cleansers. Avoid washcloths and sponges when cleansing the face, because fabrics can be abrasive. Prescribed medications should be applied to the entire face not just the affected areas, waiting 15 to 20 minutes after washing to apply medications.

Scabies

Scabies is a highly contagious, pruritic skin infection caused by a mite (*Sarcoptes scabiei*). Social and economic status has no bearing on the distribution of the disease, and it is prevalent throughout the world. Outbreaks usually occur in situations of close personal contact with the mite, gained through the sharing of inanimate objects, such as clothing or bedding with resultant transmission of the mite. Schools and skilled nursing facilities are common sites of infestation secondary to close contact and crowded sleeping areas.

Only the female mite causes the disease, burrowing under the stratum corneum to the stratum granulosum to lay eggs that hatch in 3 to 10 days. Both mites and eggs can exist outside the body. Either straight or serpentine burrows are visible on the skin and are anywhere from 5 to 20 mm in length. The burrows are pink-white and slightly elevated. Mites can often be seen at the end of the burrow, appearing in a vesicle or as a black dot. Vesicles are isolated and filled with a clear fluid rather than purulent material. These discrete lesions are a vital point in diagnosis. The most common areas of occurrence are the finger webs, buttocks, scrotum, penis, axillae, breasts, and the hands and soles of the feet in infants. Infants may have more widespread involvement. Severe itching is the most common complaint. Scratching will destroy the burrow and may make diagnosis difficult initially. Extensive involvement will result in erythema, scaling, and infection.

Diagnosis is based on the clinical presentation and the microscopic examination of scrapings of the involved areas. Mineral oil and potassium hydroxide wet mounts are used for diagnosis. A drop of mineral oil is placed over the suspected lesion then a scalpel blade is used to scrape off a sample of the affected area for examination under low power magnification. In the oil the skin scrapings adhere together while the mite moves freely and is readily identifiable. Potassium hydroxide mounts are performed in the same manner. Biopsy is rarely used.

The treatment of scabies is topical. Permethrin cream (Elimite) is the most effective medication. The cream is applied nightly for three nights, massaging the cream into the skin from the neck down. The cream is washed off in the morning. The patient needs to be cautioned that the product can stain clothing and bedding and that the odor can be objectionable. Gamma benzene hexachloride (Lindane and Kwell) may also be used, but it is not as effective as permethrin. All other people in the household or facility must also be treated to avoid recurrence. Clothing must be laundered in hot water or dry cleaned. All hard surfaces must be vacuumed, and the debris collected must be sealed in a plastic bag for disposal. Fabric articles that cannot be washed or dry cleaned should be placed in plastic bags and completely sealed for several weeks to avoid reinfestation.

Low dose steroids or antihistamines can be used to treat the pruritus. Hyperkeratotic plaques may form with continued scratching. Repetitive scratching causes excoriations in the skin, allowing entry of bacteria into the epidermis. If the bacteria enter the bloodstream, bacteremia and sepsis can result and be life-threatening.

The normal immune system will not affect the mite bio-burden. Immunosuppressed patients will not present with normal symptoms, will not have the normal itch-scratch cycle, and therefore may not seek early treatment. In this population the concentration of mites will be higher and such infestations may require prolonged treatment. Caregivers for these patients are also at risk for developing scabies because of the large numbers of mites.

Stasis Dermatitis

Stasis dermatitis is a condition that occurs on the lower extremities of patients with venous insufficiency and is exclusive to that disease. Cycles of inflammation, ulceration, and scarring result in brown-staining of the epidermis, induration, and sclerosing of the skin. Patients with stasis dermatitis have an increased propensity for developing allergies to topical agents. Inflammation may be chronic or acute. Pruritus, scaling, fissuring, weeping, and maceration are characteristics of stasis dermatitis. The scaling can become thick in chronic conditions, and fibrosis of the skin is common.

Diagnosis of stasis dermatitis is based on the clinical presentation, a careful history, and the other diagnostic methods for venous insufficiency previously discussed in chapter 27. Treatment of stasis dermatitis involves determining the etiology and hydrating the skin using topical steroids and wet dressings. Petrolatum products are usually contraindicated, because they will damage the rubber in compression wraps and stockings. Oral antibiotics may be given if the cellulitis is severe or bacterial overload is suspected. Wet dressings and compresses will soothe the area and suppress inflammation. Topical steroids should not be placed directly on ulcers, because they will stop the healing process.

Warts

Warts are benign epidermal growths caused by human papilloma virus (HPV). They are most common in children but can occur at any age. They are transmitted by touch; it is not uncommon to see additional lesions called kissing lesions in adjacent areas. The most common sites are the hands, fingers, periungual areas, and plantar surfaces. They can resolve spontaneously or require years of treatment. Warts obscure the normal lines in the skin and can be unsightly. Large collections can cause emotional problems in children when the perceptions of self-image are forming. They can also be erroneously perceived as a hygiene issue. Common warts *(Verruca vulgaris)* are elevated, well-circumscribed, irregularly shaped plaque-like projections with hyperkeratosis areas. Verruca plana, also known as plane warts, flat warts, or juvenile warts, are slightly raised, irregularly shaped, slightly keratotic lesions usually found on the dorsum of the hands and on the face. This type of wart is prevalent in patients with compromised immunity.

Diagnosis is based on the patient's history and visual inspection of the affected areas. Treatment of common warts includes topical salicylic acid preparations, liquid nitrogen, electrocautery, and blunt dissection for large lesions. Intralesional bleomycin sulfate is prescribed when other treatments fail. Treatment for plane warts includes retinoids, liquid nitrogen, cautery, and 5-fluorouracil cream.

Xerosis

Xerosis or severe dry skin can be either a result of dehydrated epidermis or be associated with a variety of dermatological conditions. Age-related xerosis results from a decrease in sebum production and water loss. Xerosis is more common in the winter months when it is referred to as winter itch and in dehumidified environments. The most severely affected skin appears criss-crossed with shallow, red fissures and that itch or burn, initiating an itch-scratch cycle. Xerosis may be treated by hydrating with an appropriate topical lotion after bathing. Severe cases may require a lactic acid lotion. As with other pruritic conditions, bathing or showering should be done with warm water and without scrubbing. Application of the lotion or cream should take place within three to five minutes after patting the skin dry.

PRECANCEROUS AND CANCEROUS CONDITIONS

Light-induced changes in the skin are dependent on the intensity and exposure of the skin to light as well as genetic factors. Tanning has a preventive aspect but by definition tanning is a sun-induced darkening of the pigment in the skin. The skin tans following moderate to intense exposure to the UVA of the sun. Research demonstrates that alternate UV light sources produce the same damage and photoaging as exposure to natural UV sources. In fact, the large amounts of UV radiation delivered to the skin from tanning bed sources can actually accelerate photoaging.

Sunburn

Sunburn is an overexposure to UVA that causes an inflammatory reaction of the skin. UV radiation changes skin cells histologically and has a cumulative effect over the lifespan. As with other burn classifications, sunburn is classified as first-, second-, or third-degree. First-degree sunburn produces mild, tender erythematous skin followed by desquamation. The skin heals without scarring. Second-degree sunburn is characterized by more tenderness and extreme erythema with edema and blister formation. The patient may peel more than once. There are no immediate curative treatments for sunburn. Topical aloe vera gels have gained favor in the last decade but only provide temporary relief from the burning or heat sensations. Topical anesthetics, such as Solarcaine, provide only temporary pain relief. Deep or third-degree sunburns are uncommon. They are induced by artificial means, such as sunlamps, tanning booths, or tanning lamps, that produce effects similar to third-degree thermal burns. Hospitalization is usually required for treatment of third-degree sunburn.

Sun Protection

Prevention of UV-induced skin damage to the dermal collagen and elastin fibers is best achieved by avoidance or at the least, the use of protective clothing and products with high sun protective factor (SPF). Remember, UV exposure has a cumulative effect. Approximately 43 percent of all Caucasian children in the United States experience one or more sunburns annually. Protection and good sun education needs to begin early. Unfortunately, many cultures view tanned skin as appealing and erroneously view the healthy tan as an indication of a more youthful mentality and physical appearance. In actuality, the more sun exposure people receive as children, adolescents and young adults, the faster signs of aging appear.

There are many methods for sun protection. To some extent the stratum corneum and melanin provide natural protection. Because sunburn is particularly harmful to the skin, causing precancerous and cancerous lesions, emphasis should be placed on prevention of the burn. Individuals who burn easily need to use sunscreens with an SPF of between 12 and 30. The more fair-skinned the person, the higher the SPF needs to be. It is safer to avoid exposure between the peak sunlight hours of 10 am to 3 pm. Even waterproof sunscreens should be reapplied every two hours and after exposure to water. For persons working out of doors, wearing dark, loose dry clothing with a tight weave will provide good protection. Long-sleeved shirts, hats, and long pants rather than shorts are best for individuals whose work requires exposure to the sun during peak hours. There is some evidence that antioxidant vitamin supplements will reduce sunburn erythema.

Sunscreens are designed to absorb, scatter, or diffuse UV radiation and visible light. Sunscreens should never be used as a means to lengthen the time an individual spends in the sun; this negates the beneficial action of the sunscreen. Titanium dioxide is an inorganic or nonchemical sunscreen that effectively blocks a wide spectrum of light. These products are thick pastes, some of which have colorful tints that children like for application to the nose and lips. Chemical sunscreens (PABA) absorb radiation, but can cause allergic reactions.

Malignant Skin Lesions

The most common form of photodermatosis is actinic keratosis (AK), an intraepidermal form of squamous cell skin cancer (Figure 45-6). It is more common in Caucasians and affects nearly 100 percent of elderly white persons. AK lesions appear in areas of chronic, high-intensity sun exposure and consist of aggregates of anaplastic keratinocytes that have undergone histological or morphological cell changes. Most actinic keratoses are seen on the face, scalp, and ears of men and on the arms. They can appear to spontaneously resolve, but new lesions frequently appear in the area. Left untreated, 10 to 20 percent of these lesions will invade the basement membrane of the epidermal-dermal junction and become invasive, more serious skin cancers.

Diagnosis is based on palpation and biopsy. The lesions are usually only a few millimeters to 1 to 2 centimeters in diameter and may range in number

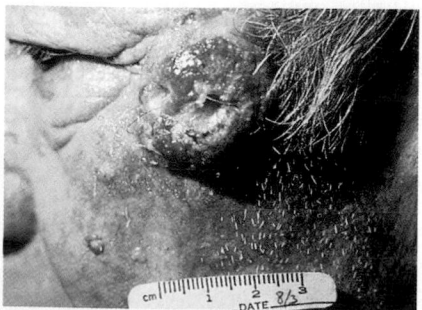

Figure 45-6 Squamous cell carcinoma. Courtesy of Robert A. Silverman, M.D., Clinical Associate Professor, Department of Pediatrics, Georgetown University.

from a few to hundreds. AKs range in color from a tan to a reddish tone but can also be the patient's normal skin color. The lesions are better recognized by palpation than by visualization. The epidermis is generally hyperkeratotic; the thicker the lesion, the more carefully it must be watched by the health care professional (American Academy of Dermatology, 2002).

Thickened AK lesions can progress to squamous cell cancer and be histologically indistinguishable from primary squamous cell skin cancer. Induration, inflammation, and oozing are suggestive of invasive malignant changes. Immunosuppression is a risk factor. Treatment of actinic keratoses can vary; cryotherapy, surgery, topical chemotherapy, and topical steroids are all methods to contain and control the disease.

Nonmelanoma Skin Cancers

The nonmelanoma skin cancers are the most common types of skin cancer in the United States. Over one million new cases were diagnosed in 2002, 70 percent of which were nonmelanoma cancers. The nonmelanoma skin cancers include basal cell carcinoma (BCC) and squamous cell carcinoma (SCC).

Basal Cell Carcinoma

Basal cell carcinoma (BCC) arises from the basement membrane at the epidermal-dermal junction. BCC results when basal cells fail to mature into the keratinocytes that normally become the stratum corneum and continue their mitotic activity beyond the basal layer. These growths result in bulky tumors that displace epidermis and dermis, eventually extending finger-like projections into other tissues including fascia, cartilage, and bone. BCC rarely metastasizes beyond the skin and, if present, is usually seen in patients with large primary tumors and tumors resistant to surgery and radiotherapy.

There are four types of BCC: nodular (most common); superficial (seen most frequently on the trunk and actinically damaged skin); morpheaform or sclerotic (more aggressive form producing more extension into surrounding tissue); and pigmented (seen in dark-complexioned persons). Each classification has distinctive characteristics:

- Nodular BCC appears as a pearly, translucent bump that bleeds easily and has telangiectasias within the lesion.
- Superficial BCC appears as a well-demarcated, erythematous, scaly patch that may form multiple sites with pearly, raised borders.
- Sclerotic BCC appears as pale yellow or white, flat or depressed, scar-like plaques that may remain undetected because of their appearance.
- Pigmented BCC lesions may appear blue, black, or brown with telangiectasias and a raised pearly border.

Diagnosis of BCC is determined by its appearance and also by biopsy. The pearly raised border is common in all types and is a valuable diagnostic tool for skin cancer.

Squamous Cell Carcinoma

Squamous cell carcinoma (SCC) is the most common skin cancer in the United States, comprising about 80 percent of all nonmelanoma skin cancers. This is a tumor consisting of keratinizing cells that can arise in the epidermis and proliferate indefinitely. SCC can occur anywhere on the skin and on mucous membranes. UVB in the form of exposure to sunlight during childhood, sunburns, ionizing radiation, outdoor occupations, freckling, facial telangiectasias, light skin, hazel or blue eyes, blonde or red hair, living in the southern parts of the United States and psoralen/PUVA treatment for psoriasis are all important in development of SCC.

SCC can spread by expansion and infiltration into surrounding tissues, shelving or skating, conduit, and infiltration and metastasis. Unlike BCC, SCC can initially spread to local lymph nodes and then on to the more distal lymph nodes via the lymphatic system. Metastasis occurs late in the course of the disease and only after the initial spread to subcutaneous and deeper facial lymph nodes. The rate of metastasis can be as high as 10 percent depending upon type, location, size, and underlying medical conditions. The lesions arising from AK will have a thick, adherent scale. The tumor is soft and easily movable within the skin and may have an inflamed, red base. The lesions are most commonly seen on the bald scalp, ears, forehead, and backs of the hands. SCCs not arising directly from AKs but from sun-damaged areas appear as firm, moveable, elevated masses with sharply defined borders and little surface scale.

Diagnosis is by the clinical presentation of the lesion and by biopsy. The health care provider needs to clearly differentiate between SCC and other processes producing similar lesions, such as Bowen's disease, leucoplakia, lichen sclerosis, atrophicus of the vulva, and cutaneous horn. Examples of treatment options are: cryotherapy (AK) liquid nitrogen, electrosurgery, surgical excision, topical chemotherapy, interferon, and biological modifiers.

Melanoma

Malignant melanoma is a serious tumor arising from abnormal melanocytes. Tumor cells grow rapidly and melanocytes are present in the skin, eyes, ears, GI tract, leptomeninges, and oral and genital mucous membranes. Melanoma has the ability to spread to any organ or tissue, including the brain and heart. Risk factors for the development of melanoma include UVB skin damage from sunburn, UVA radiation from tanning beds, a history of atypical moles, a family history of melanoma, and a previous history of nonmelanoma skin cancers, congenital giant nevus, immunosuppression or repeated blistering sunburns. Once a melanoma breaks through the basement membrane, the tumor has the ability to spread horizontally along the epidermal-dermal junction. Continued growth results in invasion of the dermis and substructures, signifying a vertical growth phase. Vertical growth carries a poorer prognosis (Ayers, 2004).

Recognition of melanoma in its early stages is important for treatment. The ABCDEs of melanoma are: *A*symmetry, *B*order irregularity, *C*olor variation, *D*iameter enlargement, and *E*levation. Changes in color and shape are always suspicious, because they are early signs of differentiation between nevi and melanomas. There are four subtypes of melanoma and each has a slightly differing presentation: Lentigo maligna melanoma is characterized by macular lesions with varied coloration and convoluted borders with notching; superficial spreading melanoma arises with a preexisting melanotic nevus and is 2.5 cm or less in size; nodular melanoma is elevated throughout the lesion resembling a blueberry and is associated with vertical growth; acral-lentiginous melanoma occurs on palms, soles, nail beds, mucocutaneous and mucosal surfaces, and varies in color from tan or brown to darkly pigmented lesions.

There are differing opinions as to whether melanoma in situ and amelanotic melanoma fit into these subtypes. Melanoma in situ presents with flat or raised lesions with histological features of melanoma but is confined to the dermis. Amelanotic melanoma is commonly nodular in nature and usually has an unpigmented pink color. Local recurrence is related to tumor depth and is defined as tumor growth near an original scar. Satellite lesions consist of small cutaneous tumors present in the dermis and subdermis located between the primary site and the lymphatic basin. Regional lymph node metastasis is predictive of visceral spread, and distant metastasis is more frequently to nonvisceral sites such as the skin, subcutaneous tissue, and distant lymph nodes. Late recurrence occurs 10 plus years after initial diagnosis and treatment. In about 2 to 6 percent of metastatic melanoma cases arise from an unknown primary site. Such melanomas are identified in lymph nodes. Survival rates are highest with cutaneous metastases and lowest with visceral metastases.

Diagnosis of the initial disease is based on its clinical presentation and biopsy. Ulceration is associated with tumor thickness and is significant.

Complaints of pruritus are also of concern. Lymphatic mapping with sentinel lymph node biopsy (SNB) is recommended for patients with regional lymph node metastases and is indicated in newly diagnosed invasive melanoma, for medium-thickness lesions or in thin lesions with a history of ulceration. Staging of disease is based on the TNM system (T, tumor; N, nodes; M, metastasis) used for most types of cancer staging. The treatment of malignant melanoma is summarized in Table 45-5.

Treatment consists of primary lesion excision for in situ disease and for lesions with a depth of 2 mm or less and margins of 2 cm margins or less. There

TABLE 45-5 Treatment of Malignant Melanoma

STAGE OF DISEASE	MEDICAL TREATMENT
Melanoma in situ	May have elective regional lymph node dissection (ERLND)
Excision with 0.5 cm margins	Some clinicians believe ERLND improves survival by removing occult nodal metastases before spreading to distant sites
<2 mm thick: 1 cm margins	Allows for adequate staging
≥2 mm thick: 2 cm margins	
Regional metastasis	Therapeutic lymph node dissection
	Possible adjuvant therapy
	Interferon
	Interferon alfa-2b and other trials
	Immunotherapy—parvum *(C. Parvum)*, transfer factor, immunomodulators
	Adjuvant chemotherapy and chemoimmunotherapy
	Excision of in-transit metastases
	Hyperthermic regional limb perfusion
	Adjuvant radiation therapy
	Adjuvant hormonal therapy
Stage III	Therapeutic lymph node dissection
	Other therapies as outlined above
Stage IV	Surgical management of isolated metastases
	Radiation therapy for palliation
	Hyperthermic perfusion
	Intralesional BCG
	Chemotherapy
	Dacarbazine (DTIC)
	Nitroureas
	Temozolomide
	Immunotherapy
	Interleukin 2 (experimental)
	Interferon (experimental)
	Monoclonal antibodies—immune response booster (experimental)
	Vaccine (experimental)—stimulate immune response to melanoma-associated antigens

Adapted from Broyles, B., Reiss, B., & Evans, M. (2007). Pharmacological aspects of nursing care (7th ed.). New York: Thomson Delmar Learning; Spratto, G., & Woods, A. (2007). 2007 PDR nurse's drug handbook. New York: Thomson Delmar Learning.

is some controversy among health care providers regarding elective regional lymph node dissection (ERLND) and its efficacy in treating localized disease. ERLND is the surgical excision of regional lymph nodes around the primary melanoma site when no nodes are palpable. The theory is based on the belief that disease will spread to the nodes initially before going to distant sites. ERLND does allow for adequate staging of the disease. Disease with regional lymph node involvement may be treated with multiple therapies including dissection, hyperthermic limb perfusion and possible adjuvant therapy in the form of biological response modifiers, such as interferon, chemotherapy, radiation therapy, and hormonal therapy. Adjuvant therapy is always recommended for patients who are free of disease but at high risk for recurrence and to complement excision in the management of metastasis to lymph nodes.

Limb isolation using a bypass circuit is used to deliver high-dose chemotherapy to an affected limb without risking systemic toxicity. Limb isolation is performed under general anesthesia. The main artery and vein of the affected extremity are connected to a bypass circuit to completely isolate the blood flow to and from the limb and a high dose of chemotherapy agent is administered into the perfusion circuit. Hyperthermic isolated limb perfusion is still used for intransient metastasis. The difference between these two isolated limb procedures is that in hyperthermic treatments the blood in the limb is heated prior to chemotherapy administration, because the heat is thought to increase effectiveness of the chemotherapy in advanced disease. Stage IV disease is not curable at this time, but several promising treatment regimens and experimental protocols are ongoing.

Nursing Management

Because of the advances in cancer treatment, cancer is now considered a chronic rather than fatal illness (see chapter 15). Patients are living for many years following cancer treatment. Patients with any cancer diagnosis may face psychological issues that are different from those experienced by the non–cancer population. For many years, the C word has struck fear into hearts and minds. Even in major cancer centers in this country some patients are concerned about their diagnosis becoming common knowledge. Family members ask health care professionals to not tell Mother or Dad about their cancer for fear of how the diagnosis might affect the patient. Others are deeply concerned about how a cancer diagnosis will affect their personal relationships with family, coworkers, and friends. In some cultures, a cancer diagnosis carries a social and economic stigma that results in isolation and shunning of the patient.

Skin cancers are visible, as is the treatment. A nurse may be in a unique position of being the first person to whom a patient voices fears about the diagnosis, treatment, and prognosis of the disease. The vast majority of patients want to know how the disease progresses, what to expect from treatment, how to prevent recurrence, and various other aspects of care and treatment. Nurses must implement strategies that help the patient maintain a healthy, natural skin barrier, if possible.

Cancer care is multidimensional, incorporating the skills and knowledge of a variety of health care professionals including social workers, nutritionists, chaplains, psychologists and other nursing and medical disciplines. Support groups, both hospital-based and national organizations, exist to provide information and a common experiential framework for patients and caregivers. The psychological impact of any disease has profound effects on the patient's life. Changes in body image, possible lifestyle changes because of time-consuming skin care regimens; concerns about disease progression, treatment failure or recurrence; and financial concerns will color the patient's perceptions and attitudes from the time of diagnosis forward. The nurse is often the first member of the health care team to whom the patient turns for information and support.

KEY CONCEPTS

- Care of persons with dermatological problems can be complex.
- Fundamental principles of wound healing and skin repair must guide the health care provider assessing and diagnosing any skin problem or condition.
- The health care provider should identify any barriers to healing and correct those issues.
- A moist wound environment must be provided and maintained for the wound to heal properly with a minimum of complications.
- Necrotic tissue is an impediment to wound and skin healing.
- Topical therapy is used to perform a variety of functions in the treatment of dermatological problems.
- Steroids are used to decrease inflammation, pruritus, and induce remission of certain cutaneous disorders.
- Moisture retentive dressings are designed to maintain a moist wound environment.
- Products designed to hydrate the skin play an important role in the treatment of many pruritic, inflammatory, and zerotic skin conditions.
- Sunlight has a profound effect on the skin and is associated with a variety of diseases and the effects of sun damage become apparent after the age of 20.
- Phototherapy is the treatment of certain dermatological conditions with artificially produced nonionizing UV light.

- There are many types of dermatological problems encountered by patients and health care professionals including acne, dermatitis, cellulitis, folliculitis, fungal infections, furuncles and carbuncles, herpes infections, impetigo, pediculosis, psoriasis, rosacea, scabies, warts, and xerosis.
- Sunburn is an overexposure to UVA that causes an inflammatory reaction of the skin.
- Prevention of UV-induced skin damage to the dermal collagen and elastin fibers is best achieved by avoidance.
- The most common form of malignant skin lesions are AK.
- Nonmelanoma skin cancers are the most common types of skin cancer in the United States, including BCC and SCC.
- Malignant melanoma is a serious tumor arising from abnormal melanocytes.
- Advances in cancer treatment in the last decade cancer, it is now considered a chronic rather than fatal illness.
- Radiation therapy is the prescribed treatment in greater than 50 percent of patients diagnosed with cancer and produces permanent skin changes in the irradiated area.

REVIEW QUESTIONS

1. The fundamental principles of wound healing and skin repair include:
   1. Clean the wound with an antibacterial substance, protect it with a dressing
   2. Clean the wound with an antiseptic substance, cover it with a sterile dressing
   3. Clean the wound with an antiseptic substance, leave it open to the air to heal
   4. Clean the wound, remove devitalized tissue, and apply moist sterile dressings

2. Commonly, treatments for dermatological dysfunctions are:
   1. Managed pharmacologically
   2. Managed with topical applications
   3. Managed by combining topical and systemic therapies
   4. Managed by removing the causative agent

3. Dermatological disorders are visually evident, therefore:
   1. Lesions are difficult to differentiate without microscopic diagnostic analysis.
   2. Lesions are readily identifiable.
   3. Lesions must be covered so as not to attract attention.
   4. Lesions can often be self-treated with OTC medications.

4. The etiology of dermatological dysfunctions may be:
   1. Bacterial, chemical, or endocrine
   2. Bacterial, viral, or fungal
   3. Allergenic, vascular, or genetic
   4. All of the above

Continued

5. Photoaging refers to:
   1. The facial age lines, which are evident in close-up photographs
   2. The facial age lines caused by prolonged exposure to ultraviolet B radiation
   3. The patches of discoloration caused by prolonged use of tanning beds
   4. The erythema caused by prolonged exposure to the sun

6. Which of the following is true concerning contact dermatitis?
   1. It is an infection of the skin characterized by redness, heat, pain, and swelling.
   2. It is usually diagnosed by biopsy.
   3. It is an acute inflammation of the hair follicle.
   4. It is treated on identification of the sensitizing substance and controlling the symptoms.

7. Most common dermatological problems encountered by health care professionals are:
   1. Tineas
   2. Staphylococcal infections
   3. Sexually transmitted infections
   4. Malignancies

8. Which of the following is true concerning rosacea?
   1. It is a highly contagious, pruritic skin infection caused by a mite.
   2. It has an insidious onset, develops between 30 and 50 years of age, affects more women than men, and is more common in fair-skinned persons.
   3. It is classified and evaluated by using the PASI method.
   4. It is a T cell-mediated inflammatory disease characterized by epidermal hyperplasia.

9. The ABCDEs of melanoma include:
   1. Altitude, brownness, circularity, diameter, and evolution
   2. Always, be, careful, to diagnose, early
   3. Asymmetry, border irregularity, color variation, diameter increase, and elevation
   4. Age, black coloration, dryness, and erythema

10. Pruritus:
    1. Is one of the most common dermatological diseases
    2. Is usually a sign that healing is underway
    3. Should alert the health care provider to change the wound dressing
    4. Can accompany malignant dermatological conditions

REVIEW ACTIVITIES

1. Arrange to spend a day observing patient care in a dermatology practice and note in a journal:
   - Types of complaints that motivate patients to seek care.
   - Questions that the health care providers usually asks the patient.
   - Diagnostic procedures, which are undertaken.
   - Length of time patients has been under care, for the same condition.
   - Types of treatment prescribed.
   - Questions that the patients usually ask the health care providers.
   - Extent to which the principles of wound healing and skin care are practiced.
   - Your impression of dermatological practice.

2. List three nursing diagnoses commonly associated with dermatological dysfunction. Identify two nursing interventions for each of your three nursing diagnoses.

Continued

REVIEW ACTIVITIES—cont'd

3. Discuss appropriate nursing interventions for the care of the patient with herpetic infections.

4. Evaluate the reasons that your peers believe that when they were adolescents they could have chosen to not protect themselves well from sunburn and develop strategies to encourage self-protection.

5. Examine warts that are present on your peers or patients and interview them regarding how they feel about having this condition. Explain the pathophysiology and strategies for treatment.

Burns: Nursing Management

Tanya D. Williams, RN, BSN, MSN, CCNS, APRN-BC

Tammy Coffee, MSN, RN, ACNP

Lynne Yurko, RN, BSN, CNA-BC

CHAPTER TOPICS

- Epidemiology, Etiology, and Pathophysiology of Burns

- Emergent Phase of Burns

- Acute Phase of Burns

- Rehabilitative Phase of Burns

KEY TERMS

Allograft
Autograft
Burn shock
Deep partial-thickness burn
Eschar
Escharotomy
Full-thickness burn
Heterograft (xenograft)
Homograft
Superficial burn
Superficial partial-thickness burn
Tumor necrosis factor
Zone of coagulation
Zone of hyperemia
Zone of stasis

Both physical and psychological healing subsequent to a major burn are prolonged processes. Both are accompanied by pain and drain energy. It is therefore easy for those recovering from a major burn to exist within a limited monotonous environment, slipping first into boredom, then into depression and desperation. Florence Nightingale recognized the critical responsibility nurses have for managing not only a patient's treatment regimen but also that patient's environment. Nightingale (1860) stated that fresh air, direct sunlight, elimination of unnecessary noise, variety of form, and brilliance of color are actual means of recovery, and what nurses must do is manage these aspects of the patient's environment so as to put the patient in the best condition for nature to act upon him or her.

BURNS

Burns are injuries to the skin and its underlying tissues caused by heat, chemicals, or electricity. Burn injuries are the second leading cause of accidental death in the United States. Approximately 80 percent of all burn injuries occur in the home with the remaining 20 percent occurring in industrial settings. Approximately 2.5 million people seek medical treatment for burns each year with 150,000 resulting in hospitalization and 10,000 resulting in death. When death occurs, it is either immediately after the injury or weeks later as a result of multisystem organ dysfunction (Stocking, 2005). The physical, psychological, and financial impact of the burn injury can be catastrophic and devastating to the patient and the patient's family.

Epidemiology

The skin is the largest human organ. A burn injury occurs when skin tissue is damaged. Causative agents include flame, scald, direct contact, chemicals, electrical current, and radiation (Figure 46-1). Commonly, burn events are associated with improper use of space heaters, fireplaces, and matches, as well as with ignition of clothing during cooking or smoking (Doe Report, 2005). Flame injuries are the most complicated and fatal burns with average hospital cost ranging from $36,000 to $117,000 (O'Conner & Besner, 2004). The larger the burn, the higher the cost, with additional expenses resulting from lost wages, property loss, and long-term care.

Etiology

Approximately 90 percent of burns are caused by household accidents. Scald burns occur more often in children age three and younger, and flame burns are more common with older children and adults (O'Conner & Besner, 2004). Over the past 40 years morbidity and mortality from burn injuries have decreased by 50 percent in the United States. During the 1960s burns covering

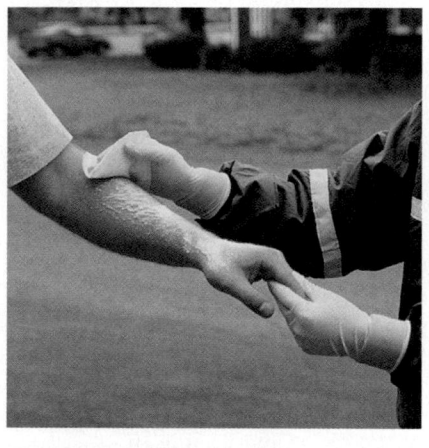

Figure 46-1 Dry chemicals should be brushed off first, and then large volumes of water used to rinse the residue off the patient.

DOLLARS AND SENSE

Blood Transfusion in Burns

Blood transfusions are a common practice for treating burn patients during the emergent and acute phases of recovery. Overall, approximately 11 million units of blood are transfused yearly in the United States. On average, each unit of blood costs $150. There are limited data to guide appropriate use of transfusions. In an effort to identify current burn center health care provider blood transfusion practices, a survey delineating transfusion practices was distributed to burn center directors across the country. They were asked to list factors affecting their blood transfusion thresholds and to provide their blood transfusion threshold based on patient age and percent of burn. The 2004 results of the survey reveal variable values in a variety of areas. For instance, one health care provider may interpret a hematocrit of 27 percent as need for blood, and a second health care provider may see no need for transfusion until the hematocrit falls to 22 percent. This 5 percent variability can have a significant impact on the cost of care. Without a standard practice guideline, cost of transfusions cannot be predicted or controlled. Prospective studies to establish safe, clinically effective, and cost effective guidelines are needed.

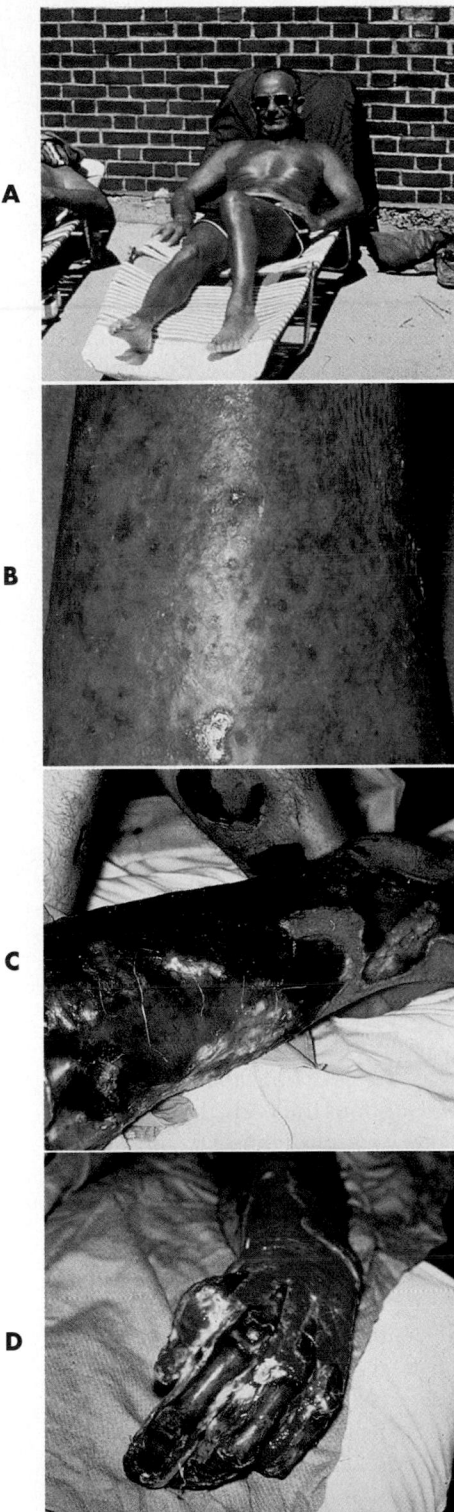

Figure 46-2 Types of burns. Courtesy of the Phoenix Society for Burn Survivors.

half the body were fatal. Today patients with burns covering 90 percent of the body can survive. This decline is because of successful prevention efforts and improved clinical management of people who sustain severe burns. Advances in treatment include an improved understanding of burn resuscitation, enhanced wound care treatments, appropriate infection control, improved treatment of inhalation injuries, and an improved approach to the hypermetabolic response to burn injuries.

Pathophysiology

The depth of a burn is dependent on the temperature of the burning agent and the length of time in which the agent is in contact with the skin. Early tissue damage may occur at temperatures of 104° F (40° C). Irreversible damage to the dermis occurs at temperatures of 158° F (70° C). Burn injuries are described as **superficial** (first-degree burns), **superficial partial-thickness** or **deep partial-thickness** (second-degree burns), and **full-thickness** (third- and fourth-degree burns). All are based on the degree of destruction of the epidermal and dermal layers of the skin (Figure 46-2).

Superficial burns involve only the protective outer epidermal layer of the skin that helps prevent injury, minimizes water loss, and regulates temperature. Sunburns are commonly superficial burns. Patients may have some areas of superficial burns surrounded by deeper burns. Partial-thickness burns are characterized by destruction of the epidermis and varying depths of the dermis, the second layer of skin that lies below the epidermis and above subcutaneous tissue. These burns are likely to be painful because nerve endings have been injured and exposed; but they have the ability to heal because portions of the epithelial cells are not destroyed. The presence of blisters often indicates a more superficial partial-thickness injury. Blisters may increase in size as the result of continuous exudation and collection of tissue fluid. During the healing phase of a partial-thickness burn, dryness and itching are common and are caused by increased vascularization of sebaceous glands, reduction of secretions, and decreased perspiration.

Full-thickness burns include destruction of the epidermis and the entire dermis, as well as possible damage to the subcutaneous layer, muscle, and bone. Nerve endings are destroyed, resulting in a painless wound. **Eschar,** is burned skin that is dead (denatured protein) and appears leathery that may form as the result of surface dehydration. Black networks of coagulated capillaries may be seen. Full-thickness burns require removal of the burned skin and grafting, because the destroyed tissue is unable to epithelialize. Often a deep partial-thickness burn may convert to a full-thickness burn because of infection, trauma, or decreased blood supply.

As a result of burns normal skin function is diminished, resulting in physiological alterations, including loss of protective barriers, escape of body fluids, lack of temperature control, destroyed sweat and sebaceous glands, and a diminished number of sensory receptors. The severity of these alterations depends on the extent of the burn and the depth of the damage.

Local Tissue Response

Damage to the skin from a thermal injury can result in immediate tissue changes. These changes, known as the zones of injury, were first described by Jackson in 1953. If the heat damage is severe enough, a **zone of coagulation** is formed. This is the area of the burn that has the most contact with the causative agent, causing the protein to coagulate. The damage is irreversible. Surrounding this area the blood vessels are damaged resulting in decreased perfusion to the area, or a **zone of stasis.** The cells in this area are still viable but because of poor blood flow and tissue edema are at risk for death over the next few hours or days. Other factors, such as dehydration and infection, may lead to further tissue necrosis in this area of stasis. Meticulous wound care, hydration, and prevention of infection are essential in limiting further destruction of this area. At the outer edge of the burn is a **zone of hyperemia,** or inflammation, characterized by viable cells with minimal injury. Blood flow is increased because of vasodilation from the release of vasoactive substances. This increased blood flow brings leukocytes and nutrients necessary to promote wound healing.

Systemic Tissue Response

A major burn injury is one of the most serious forms of trauma an individual can experience. Virtually every organ system is affected. Physiological changes are both local and systemic in nature. Systemic changes develop in a burn of greater than 25 percent of the total body surface area (TBSA). A shock state, known as **burn shock,** develops that is both a hypovolemic and a cellular shock. Burn shock involves massive fluid shifts of plasma, electrolytes, and proteins into the burn wound. This inflammatory response to the injury is necessary for healing, but excessive production causes cell damage. Tissue damage results from the release of many cellular mediators and vasoactive substances, such as histamine, serotonin, prostaglandins, and interleukin-1. These substances cause a systemic inflammatory response that affects multiple organ systems and causes increased vascular permeability, resulting in significant hypovolemia, an insufficient amount of circulating vascular volume, and edema. This phase begins at the time of burn injury, peaks in 12 to 24 hours, and lasts for 48 to 72 hours.

During the burn shock phase intravascular fluid is lost via evaporation through the wound and by edema formation. Vasodilation and increased capillary permeability results in the movement of fluid, electrolytes, and protein from the intravascular space to the interstitial space. Fluid movement is caused by both oncotic and osmotic forces. When capillary permeability reestablishes, this protein will be unable to move back into the intravascular space. The lymphatic system becomes overloaded and is unable to recirculate the protein. A significant hypoproteinemia, an abnormally low level of protein, ensues. The sodium level within the damaged tissue increases causing further movement of water from the intravascular space that potentiates wound edema and hypovolemia. Edema may be severe in highly vascular areas, such as the face. Patients with large surface area burns experience edema throughout the body that can impair peripheral circulation by compressing circulatory vessels in an extremity.

A generalized physiological response develops immediately after a burn injury. Initially a release of catecholamines (e.g., epinephrine and norepinephrine), vasopressin (antidiuretic hormone), and angiotensin II causes intense vasoconstriction and increased systemic vascular resistance. The blood pressure may be elevated, and the patient is tachycardic. This physiological response assists in the initial attempt to conserve fluid, but its increased capillary force also promotes burn edema. Cardiac output is decreased because of the release of these vasoconstrictive agents and its subsequent increased system vascular resistance and increased cardiac workload. Cardiac function continues to be depressed even after adequate fluid resuscitation pointing to the myocardial depressant effects of inflammatory mediators, such as **tumor necrosis factor** (an inflammatory biochemical), is released from the burn wound.

Pulmonary function may be affected even in the absence of an inhalation injury. More effort is required to breathe because of edema formation and from an increased pulmonary vascular resistance that develops from the release of mediators, such as serotonin. Also, the patient may be at risk for airway obstruction because of oropharyngeal swelling that increases once fluid resuscitation begins.

The kidneys, liver, and intestines are also affected during a major burn. Decreased blood flow to the kidneys as a result of hypovolemia and vasoconstriction and a significant release of antidiuretic hormone places the patient at risk for renal failure. Patients at greatest risk for renal failure have had a delay in their initial fluid resuscitation or develop sepsis. Hepatic perfusion is also compromised contributing to liver ischemia. Finally, the decreased bowel perfusion makes the patient prone to a paralytic ileus. Breakdown of the small intestine may occur, causing bacteria to move or translocate across the intestinal wall into the blood vessels, promoting the development of sepsis, an overwhelming bacterial infection of the blood and body organs.

Compromise of the immune system is the last significant effect of a burn injury. The break in skin integrity destroys the body's first line of defense. A complex change in the body's immune system results in bone marrow depression, immunosuppression, and a shorter life span of red blood cells. Damaged tissue triggers the release of the inflammatory cytokine cascade. The cascade is an inflammatory response designed to destroy microbes and potentiate tissue repair. Release of these cytokines (tumor necrosis factor and interleukins) impairs the function of lymphocytes, macrophages, and neutrophils, increasing the risk of infection. The nutritional deficit that occurs also decreases the burn patient's ability to fight infection. For the patient with a major burn injury, an infection that progresses to sepsis and multisystem organ dysfunction has serious consequences.

After the period of burn shock the patient remains acutely ill. This period is characterized by hypermetabolism (a higher than normal metabolic rate) and impaired nutrition. A negative nitrogen balance begins at the onset of the burn and is the result of tissue destruction, protein loss, and the stress response. It continues throughout the acute period and is secondary to continued loss of protein from the wound, tissue catabolism resulting from immobility, and an increased metabolic rate. Special attention to the nutritional needs of the patient is an integral part of the comprehensive care during this time. The patient is vulnerable to significant weight loss because of fluid evaporation from the wound and loss of solid body mass because of increased metabolism.

Complications of the gastrointestinal (GI) system occur frequently after thermal injury. Gastric and duodenal ulceration has been reported in severely burned patients. Bleeding is the major clinical problem for patients with these lesions. Treatment is aimed at prevention and is best accomplished by antacids, histamine-2 (H_2) blockers, and enteral feedings. Cholecystitis, pancreatitis, and hepatic dysfunction may also be seen as the result of tissue ischemia from hypoperfusion.

Planning and Implementation

Management of a person with a burn injury is extensive and costly. Discharge planning begins on admission using a multidisciplinary approach to ensure that quality and cost-effective care are provided. Three periods of treatment can be identified in the care of the seriously burned patient: the emergent, acute, and rehabilitation periods. The emergent period refers to the first 24 to 48 hours post-burn when the patient is admitted, the severity of the injury is determined, first aid and wound care are given, and burn shock is treated. The acute period of treatment begins at the end of the emergent period and lasts until all of the full-thickness wounds are covered with skin grafts or partial-thickness wounds are healed. The physical healing time is determined by the patient's medical condition, nutritional status, and ability to heal. A 40 percent injury requires approximately 40 days to heal. The rehabilitation period focuses on the patient returning to a useful place in society. Two areas of concern during the rehabilitation phase are (a) the restoration of function over joint surfaces that were scarred and (b) the emotional assistance that the patient and family will need.

The rehabilitation of the patient actually begins during early hospitalization and is addressed throughout the hospital stay. After the initial discharge, the patient may require emotional assistance and counseling, and many readmissions

BOX 46-1

PREHOSPITAL CARE OF MAJOR BURNS

- Remove victim form source of burn.
- Douse with water and remove nonadherent smoldering clothing to stop the burning process.
- If chemical burn, carefully remove clothing and flush wound with large amounts of water.
- If electrical burn and victim is still in contact with source, do not touch victim. Remove electrical source with dry nonconductive object.
- Establish patent airway and assess for inhalation injury. Give oxygen if available.
- Check peripheral pulse to assess circulatory status.
- Assess and initiate treatment for injuries requiring immediate attention.
- Remove tight-fitting jewelry and clothing.
- Cover burn with moist sterile or clean cover.
- Cover victim with warm, dry cover to prevent heat loss.
- Transport victim to nearest acute care facility.

Adapted from American Burn Association. (2005). Advanced burn life support course: Provider's manual. *Chicago: Author; Stocking, J. (2005).* Initial assessment and resuscitation. *Retrieved March 5, 2006, from http://www.astna.org.*

may be necessary for reconstructive procedures. Emotional and social healing depends on each patient's ability to cope with a new body image and society's acceptance of the change in the patient's physical appearance. Each of the three periods and the management required is discussed.

EMERGENT PHASE

The goals of management during the emergent period, the first 24 to 48 hours after a burn, are to secure the airway, support circulation by fluid replacement, keep the patient comfortable with analgesics, prevent infection through careful wound care, maintain body temperature, and provide emotional support. The nurse and physician work collaboratively to achieve these goals. The specific details of treatment are discussed under Nursing Management.

Prehospital Care and First Aid

At the scene of a burn injury, the first action should be to remove the victim from the hazardous environment. Removal may be accomplished by untrained witnesses to the injury or by trained emergency personnel. Length of exposure to the causative agent is directly related to the severity of the injury. Box 46-1 lists prehospital care priorities.

The most common causative agents for burn injury are scalding fluids, fire, chemicals, and electricity. Other types of injuries result from contact with hot surfaces. Regardless of the cause, the burning process must be stopped. Scald burns are the most common burn injury, particularly in children. Scald injury may be caused by steam or hot fluids and may affect a widespread area. Scald injury is related to the temperature of the liquid and length of exposure. Initial care consists of cooling the skin with cool water. First aid follows the same treatment plan as for all burns, that is, to stop the burning process.

Flame and flash injuries are the second most common types of burn injury and are commonly associated with an inhalation injury. These injuries may occur from house fires (caused by smoking in bed or children playing with matches) or ignited gasoline or propane. Injuries may be combined partial- and full-thickness burns. Duration of contact with the flame source will determine the depth of the injury. In the case of fire, flames should be extinguished, flammable or hot material removed from the victim, and the victim and rescuer removed from the unventilated or hazardous surroundings. If clothing is on fire, the victim's first reaction is to run, which only fans the flames. The best intervention is to stop the person, wrap him or her in a blanket, coat, sheet, or towel, and roll him or her on the ground to exclude oxygen and thereby put out the fire. The rule is stop, drop, and roll.

People who are confined to a wheelchair or limited in their movement because of a disability should learn to use a blanket or rug to smother a fire. The victim should drop to the ground and roll to smother all flames. The victim should never stand, because this will cause the flames and smoke to engulf the facial area, possibly igniting the hair and causing an inhalation injury. Any water source can be used to extinguish flames, cool the burn, or dilute the chemical unless the victim is still in contact with an electrical source. Once all the flame is extinguished, clothing (excepting clothing that adheres to the burned area), jewelry, and debris are carefully removed. Any clothing removed should be saved for possible analysis of flammability. Contact burns occur from direct contact with a hot substance, such as hot metal, stoves, tar, or irons. The area of burn is usually confined to the area where the substance came into contact with the skin. The treatment goal is to stop the burning process.

Currently there are more than 30,000 chemicals that are considered hazardous by regulatory agencies, and 2 percent of all burn unit admissions are chemical-related (American Burn Association, 2005). When chemical burns

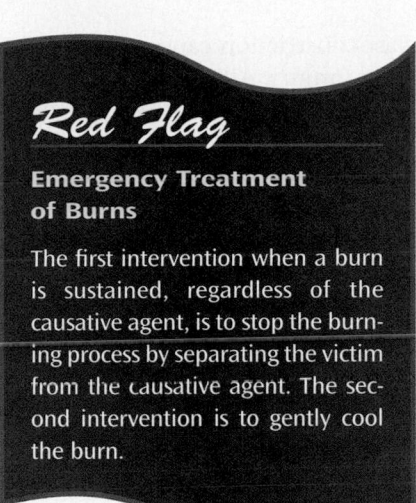

occur, they are usually acquired as a result of accidents in the home or an industrial setting. Household chemical burns may be caused by drain cleaners, disinfectants, and other chemicals used in the home. Industrial chemicals such as strong acids (hydrochloric), alkali and organic compounds, such as phenol, and petroleum products (gasoline) are common causes of chemical burns.

The severity of the injury is related to the chemical involved, its concentration, length of exposure, and the immediate treatment. Extent of penetration depends on the agent. Alkalis produce more tissue damage by a liquefaction necrosis process that loosens cellular tissue and allows deeper penetration. Acids cause protein coagulation necrosis that forms eschar that limits penetration (Collemer, 2004). Treatment should include irrigation of the area with copious amounts of water or saline, which will decrease the concentration, volume, duration of contact, and the mechanism of action.

Ocular chemical burns can occur from a ruptured airbag or whenever a chemical splashes onto the face. Treatment includes careful irrigation of the eye with water. Adequacy of the irrigation is determined by testing a sample of the irrigated fluid with litmus paper to test for the presence of acid or alkali. Ingestion of noxious chemicals may burn the upper GI tract. These burns are difficult to treat and frequently cause complications. If the chemical is a powder, the powder should be brushed off the skin prior to flushing the area (American Burn Association, 2005).

Hydrofluoric acid is used regularly in industrial settings. When skin comes into direct contact with the chemical, local tissue injury, systemic hypocalcemia, and potential arrhythmias can occur. Traditionally, treatment has been centered on the application of topical calcium gels or calcium gluconate injections, with intra-arterial infusions of calcium gluconate reserved for distal extremities and digits. New research indicates that facial hydrofluoric acid burns can be treated with a calcium gluconate infusion through the external carotid artery; a new option that has reportedly increased patient satisfaction when compared to the alternative forms of treatment (Nguyen, Mohr, Ahrenholz, & Solem, 2004).

Electrical burns account for approximately 3 percent of all burn unit admissions and approximately 1,000 deaths per year (American Burn Association, 2005). Electrical burns usually result from accidental contact with an exposed object that conducts electricity. Examples include electrical wiring, power transmission lines, and lighting. Damage depends on the intensity of the current. Voltage determines whether the current can enter the body or not. Low voltage cannot enter the body unless the skin is broken or moist. High voltage can enter the body and easily overcomes resistance. Electrical burns pose a special hazard to the victim because the total body surface area of the burn is not always apparent and is often internal. Dysrhythmias and neurological dysfunction are common. Extreme care must be taken when removing the victim from the electrical source to prevent a similar injury to the rescuer.

Initial management of all burn injuries follows the completion of the primary survey: airway, breathing, circulation, and presence of a neurological deficit. All are assessed and initial management begins. This includes the removal of the patient's clothing and a brief neurological exam. A secondary assessment is completed as long as the patient has no life-endangering injuries. The secondary assessment includes a more thorough head-to-toe assessment. A history is obtained, which includes the mechanism of injury, medical history (including allergies), and medications the patient is taking. During this assessment, the burn wound is evaluated and treated. Life-threatening conditions are always cared for before the burn wound. Standard precautions should be followed whenever there is a possibility of exposure to blood or other body fluids. This includes the wearing of gown, gloves, mask, and eye protection.

Burn wounds are covered with dressings dampened with normal saline or water, which eases the pain, reduces edema, and prevents evaporation of body water. The patient's entire body is wrapped in a dry cover to prevent heat loss.

BOX 46-2

BURN CENTER REFERRAL CRITERIA

A burn unit may treat adults or children or both. Burn injuries that should be referred to a burn unit include the following:

- Partial-thickness burns greater than 10 percent TBSA
- Burns that involve the face, hands, feet, genitalia, perineum, or major joints
- Third-degree burns in any group
- Electrical burns, including lightning injury
- Chemical burns
- Inhalation injury
- Burn injury in patients with preexisting medical disorders that could complicate management, prolong recovery, or affect mortality
- Any patient with burns and concomitant trauma (such as fractures) in which the burn injury poses the greatest risk of morbidity or mortality
- Burned children in hospitals without qualified personnel or equipment for the care of children
- Burn injury in patients who will require special social, emotional, or long-term rehabilitative intervention

Adapted from American Burn Association. (2005). Advanced burn life support course: Provider's manual. Chicago: Author; Stocking, J. (2005). Initial assessment and resuscitation. Retrieved March 5, 2006, from http://www.astna.org.

Ice should never be used, because sudden vasoconstriction causes severe shifting of body fluids and may increase the depth of injury. Although sterile dressings are preferred, clean dressings may be used because all dressings will be removed when the patient arrives at the medical facility. Oils, salves, and ointments should never be used on burns prior to evaluation at the hospital.

In the prehospital period pain in extensive burns is best controlled by gentle and minimal handling and by application of dressings to exclude air from burned surfaces. The degree of pain is usually inversely proportional to the depth of the burn injury. As mentioned earlier, full-thickness burns are usually painless, because nerve endings have been destroyed.

Burns are often more severe than they first appear to be; therefore even patients with burns that appear to be superficial should be seen by a health care provider. Patients with major burns should be transported to a regional burn center. According to the last recorded statistics developed by the Organization and Delivery of American Burn Association, there are 139 hospitals in the United States that have burn centers (Doe Report, 2005). These burn units are located throughout the country, and most are found in major medical centers in urban areas. Canada has 17 burn care centers. A hospital or burn center should be notified before a burn victim is transported so that they have time to prepare for the patient's arrival. Box 46-2 lists criteria for referral to a burn center.

Transfer of the patient should not be delayed because of difficulty in establishing an intravenous (IV) line. The American Burn Association teaches that an IV line is not necessary if the patient is less than 60 minutes from the hospital. When an IV line is established the recommended solution is Ringer's lactate infused at 500 mL/hour for an adult and 250 mL/hour for a child age 5 years or older.

For obviously small burns, fluids may be given by mouth with caution. Large burns may cause decreased peristalsis, and therefore nothing should be given by mouth. Patients with large burns, or who have inhaled smoke, may vomit and attention is needed to prevent them from aspirating vomitus.

To optimize burn care, the American Burn Association has created a national standard for voluntary review of burn centers according to a systematic approach to burn care. The verification is granted for a three-year period by the American Burn Association and the American College of Surgeons. Because of potential management problems, they recommend transfer of patients to a burn center based on burn size, depth, mechanism, and comorbid factors.

Emergency Department Management

Rapid and efficient care is essential in the emergency department management of the victim with a major burn. If any respiratory distress is present, an airway is established. Prophylactic intubation may be initiated if any heat or smoke has been inhaled, or if the head, neck, or face is involved. Inhalation injuries are best managed with controlled ventilation, because swelling of the upper airway can progress to obstruction. Endotracheal intubation is preferred over a tracheostomy. Edema of the respiratory passages frequently subsides within a few days after the initial injury; therefore surgery of the airway should be avoided. Depending on the severity of symptoms, emergency treatment may include oxygen, suctioning, and postural drainage.

After an airway has been established, circulatory support is addressed. Fluid is best replaced through two large caliber peripheral IV catheters. Placement of these catheters is preferred through an unburned site to prevent the introduction of infection. An indwelling urinary catheter is inserted to adequately monitor urine output. Hourly urine output measurements are used as a guide to the adequacy of fluid (plasma volume) replacement. Patients with burns more than 20 percent of TBSA are more prone to nausea, vomiting, and an ileus. Oral fluids are not recommended, because they create a threat of vomiting and aspiration. A nasogastric tube is inserted and attached to suction to prevent gastric distension (Doe Report, 2005).

Assessment with Clinical Manifestations

The professional burn care nurse understands the concepts that make the specialty of burn care unique. They develop a specialized knowledge base that accommodates every aspect of the patient's being and complements clinical nursing practice. Burn care nurses also participate in the advancement of burn care practice.

The assessment of the person who has sustained a severe burn focuses on the severity of the burn injury. Knowledge of circumstances surrounding the burn injury is extremely valuable in the management of a burn victim. This information can be obtained from either the burn victim or witnesses to the event. Data should include: (a) how the burn injury occurred; (b) when the burn injury occurred; (c) duration of contact with the burning agent; (d) location (enclosed area suggests possibility of smoke inhalation or carbon monoxide poisoning); and (e) presence of an explosion (suggests possibility of other injuries).

The burn victim's age and general health may modify treatment. Elderly patients and young patients have a higher mortality rate than a young adult with the same percentage of burn. Preexisting endocrine, pulmonary, cardiovascular, or renal disease or a history of drug abuse will decrease a victim's ability to cope with severe burns. Because most burn patients will require topical and systemic therapy with a number of drugs, allergies, and drug sensitivities must be determined and documented.

Many factors are considered in evaluating the severity of burn injury, including size and depth of the burn, the cause of the injury, and the patient's preinjury health status. Identification of known and unknown disorders may prevent fatal complications in the burn victim. A prior illness, such as diabetes or renal failure, may become acute during the postburn phase. The physiological stress of the burn experience may exacerbate a latent disease process or worsen an already active process and thus increase mortality. Diabetes and chronic obstructive pulmonary disease may be aggravated, or patients with atherosclerotic heart disease may develop a myocardial infarction.

For adults, the rule of nines is a tool used to estimate the percentage of the TBSA burned (Figure 46-3). The percentage of TBSA burned is estimated with the use of charts that depict anterior and posterior drawings of the body. In adults, the body is divided into areas equal to the multiples of 9 percent. In clinical practice the burned area is shaded in on the drawings and the amount of body surface burned is calculated from the shaded areas. Calculations are modified for infants and children younger than 10 years of age because of their relatively larger head and smaller body (consult a pediatric textbook for these figures).

The depth of the burn injury is evaluated on the basis of appearance, color, and sensation as shown in Table 46-1. The burn is classified as superficial (first-degree), superficial partial-thickness, or deep partial-thickness (second-degree), or full-thickness (third-degree). A laser Doppler is being used more frequently to evaluate the blood flow in the injured tissue to assist in definitive diagnosis of depth of injury.

The severity of a burn also depends on the age of the victim. Infants younger than 2 years of age and adults older than 60 years have a higher mortality rate than people in other age-groups with a similar size injury. The infant has a weak antibody response to infection, and in older victims the serious burn may aggravate the degenerative processes or exacerbate a preexisting health problem.

The body part involved is an important factor in evaluating the severity of a burn. The part of the body burned must be considered when the severity

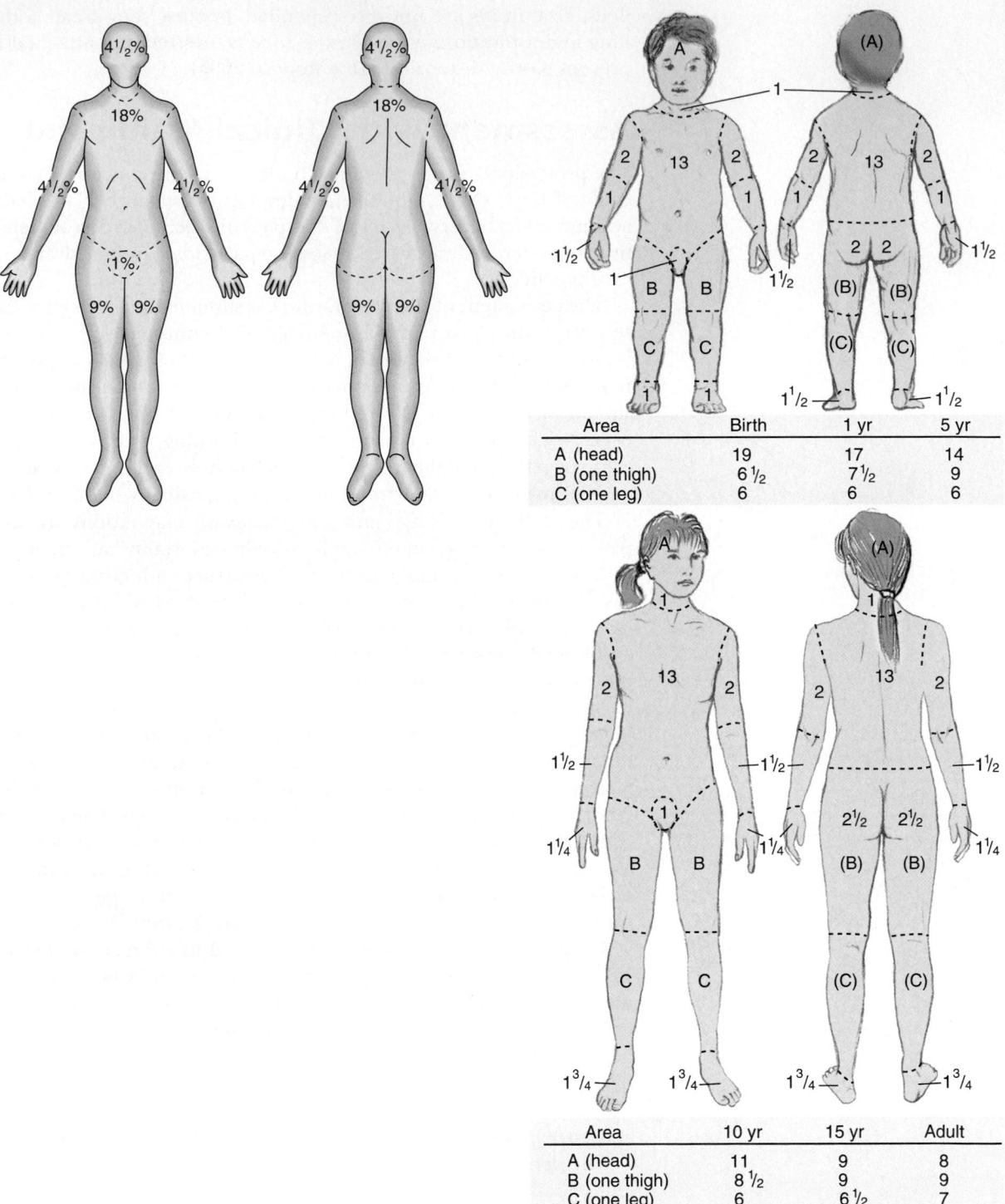

Area	Birth	1 yr	5 yr
A (head)	19	17	14
B (one thigh)	6 1/2	7 1/2	9
C (one leg)	6	6	6

Area	10 yr	15 yr	Adult
A (head)	11	9	8
B (one thigh)	8 1/2	9	9
C (one leg)	6	6 1/2	7

Figure 46-3 The rule of nines is used to estimate the percentage of body surface area burned.

of the burn is estimated. For example a 3 percent burn of the anterior surface of the thigh is not as serious as a 3 percent burn to the neck, face, or perineal area. Injuries that involve cosmetic and functional areas of the body require a longer period of recovery because of both physical and emotional reactions to the burn injury. A burn of the face, hands, and feet requires extensive, meticulous care, with extensive physical and occupational therapy. A burn of the head, neck, and chest may also involve injury to the respiratory tract and result in severe respiratory distress. Burns of the perineum are difficult to manage

TABLE 46-1	Characteristics the of Depth of a Burn Injury		
	SUPERFICIAL (FIRST-DEGREE)	**PARTIAL-THICKNESS (SECOND-DEGREE)**	**FULL-THICKNESS (THIRD-DEGREE)**
Skin depth	Epidermis	Entire epidermis; partial dermis; sweat glands; hair follicles intact	Epidermis, dermis; extends to subcutaneous tissue, possibly muscle and bone
Cause	Flash flame; ultraviolet light; sunburn	Contact with hot liquids or solids; flash flame to clothing; direct flames; chemicals; ultraviolet light	Contact with hot liquids or solids; flame; chemicals; electrical contact
Appearance	Dry, no blisters Minimal or no edema Blanches with fingertip pressure and color returns when pressure removed	Superficial partial injury Blisters that will increase in size; blanches with fingertip pressure and color returns when pressure returns; moist Deep partial injury Blisters present slower to increase in size; blanching decreased; less moisture	Dry with leathery eschar; charred vessels visible under eschar; blisters rare but thin-walled blisters that do not increase in size may be present; no blanching with pressure
Color	Increased redness	Superficial partial injury Pink Deep partial injury Pale, mottled with dull, white, tan, cherry red areas	White, charred, dark tan, black, dark red
Sensation	Painful	Painful	No pain; deep throbbing; nerve endings dead
Healing time	2 to 5 days with peeling; no scarring; may discolor	Superficial partial injury 5 to 21 days, no grafting Deep partial injury 21 to 35 days with out complications; may convert to full-thickness and require grafting	No healing potential; requires excision and grafting

Adapted from Doe Report. (2005). Burn injuries. The Doe report medical reference library. Retrieved March 1, 2006, from http://www.doeroport.com; O'Conner, A., & Besner, G. (2004). Burns a surgical perspective. Retrieved April 8, 2006, from www.emedicine.com.

because of the potential for contamination and infection. The circumferential or encircling burn of a limb, the neck, or the chest has serious consequences. This type of burn will cause constrictive contraction of the skin and produce a tourniquet effect that may impair breathing or circulation.

Identifying the causative agent is of prime importance, because the nature of the agent has a direct effect on prognosis and treatment. As mentioned previously, mechanisms of burn injury are flame and flash, contact, scald, chemical, and electric. The factors determining the severity of burns are: Size of burn, depth of burn, age of victim, body part involved, mechanism of injury, history of cardiac, pulmonary, renal, or hepatic disease, and injuries sustained at time of burn.

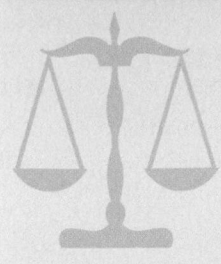

LAW IN PRACTICE

Burns as a Result of Abuse

Burns obtained as a result of child abuse are found in pediatric burn admissions. Common occurrences involve children 3 years of age and younger with either scald or contact burns. Socioeconomic status and single parent homes with more than two children have the highest incidences. Hospitalization is lengthy with a high rate of morbidity and mortality. When a child survives, the length of stay may be extended beyond recovery while a social worker, psychologist, and a child life specialist prepare the child for placement with other family members, or foster care. The Child Abuse Prevention and Treatment Act of 1974, requires all professionals to report suspected abuse or neglect (DeLaune & Ladner, 2006). Similarly, all professionals are required to report suspected abuse of elderly patients who may present with burns. Typical signs of abuse include: 12 or more hours delay in seeking treatment without a plausible reason, treatment sought by a nonrelation, parent of a pediatric patient or child of an elderly patient appears to be under the influence of drugs or alcohol, parent of a pediatric patient or child of an elderly patient is inattentive or lacks empathy, injury is inconsistent with description of the circumstances leading to the injury, and elderly patient sustains injuries ordinarily covered by clothing.

Nursing Diagnoses

Based on the information gathered, examples of nursing diagnoses in the patient in the emergent phase of burns may include the following:

- Ineffective airway clearance related to secretions, tracheobronchial edema, and obstruction.
- Deficient fluid volume related to intravascular fluid shift and evaporation.
- Hypothermia related to impaired temperature regulation and wound exposure.
- Risk for infection related to impaired skin integrity.
- Impaired skin integrity related to impaired perfusion and burn injured skin.
- Acute pain related to exposed nerve endings and associated trauma.
- Anxiety related to situational crises and threat of death.

Planning and Implementation

Nursing interventions include maintenance of a patent airway, adequate fluid volume, normothermia, initial wound care, comfort, emotional support, and patient and family education. People who are burned on the face and neck or those who have inhaled flame, steam, or smoke are observed closely for signs of laryngeal edema and airway obstruction. Data indicating potential or existing inhalation injury that is incurred from breathing in harmful gases, vapors, or particulate matter include: burns to face and neck, singed hairs (nasal, beard, or eyelashes), intraoral charcoal, especially on teeth and gums, brassy cough, hoarseness, copious sputum production, carbonaceous sputum, burn injury that has occurred in a closed space, smell of smoke on victim's clothes or on victim, and respiratory distress.

Adequate ventilation and oxygenation may be possible with the victim breathing room air; however, when any inhalation injury has occurred, it is best to give oxygen. When smoke is inhaled, carbon monoxide, which has an affinity for hemoglobin over 200 times as strong as that of oxygen, binds with hemoglobin, displacing oxygen. High carboxyhemoglobin (hemoglobin bound to carbon monoxide) levels impair tissue oxygenation resulting in tissue asphyxia. Providing the victim with 100 percent oxygen by mask will reverse this condition. If the victim is in respiratory distress or has a suspected inhalation injury endotracheal intubation may be necessary.

During fluid resuscitation, adequate volume is assessed by monitoring mental status, vital signs, peripheral perfusion, body weight, and urine output. A 15 to 20 percent weight gain in the first 72 hours of resuscitation is anticipated. Significant laboratory measurements include serum and urine electrolytes, serum and urine osmolality, and hematocrit. Hourly urine output is commonly used as a gauge for adequate fluid replacement. Fluid should be titrated to ensure an output of 0.5 mL/kg/hr or 30 to 50 mL/hour. The most common reasons for a urine output below 30 mL/hour, indicating insufficient fluid replacement, are that the calculated fluid replacement is behind schedule, and the patient's fluid requirements are greater than predicted. The urine is observed for color and analyzed for the presence of blood. The health care provider is notified if hematuria is present.

Other clinical criteria that indicate adequate resuscitation are pulse rate of 120 beats per minute or less, central venous pressure in the low to normal range, pulmonary artery end-diastolic pressure in the low to normal range, and mental lucidity. Signs of adequate fluid resuscitation include: pulse of 70 to 120 beats per minute; urine output of 30 to 50 mL/hour (adult); systolic blood pressure of 100 mm Hg; central venous pressure: 5 to 10 mm Hg; pulmonary capillary wedge pressure (PCWP): 5 to 15 mm Hg; and blood pH normal range: 7.35 to 7.45 and Base deficit greater than −6.

Acidosis indicates that fluids have not been given in sufficient quantities to maximize tissue perfusion. Anaerobic metabolism ensues when the metabolic tissue requirements are not met during resuscitation. Recent studies have indicated that presence of a base deficit, particularly less than −6 is a good indicator of the patient not having adequate fluid resuscitation.

After the first 48 to 72 hours, edema reabsorption begins. The urinary output increases dramatically and is no longer a reliable guide to fluid needs. Fluid needs are assessed by measuring serum and urine electrolyte levels. Fluid replacement, using 5 percent dextrose and water, is based on individual patient assessment. If dehydration occurs from diuresis, fluid replacement therapy is continued until blood volume is stabilized. Potassium may be added to the IV fluid because of potassium losses in the urine. The patient is monitored closely for signs of water intoxication pulmonary edema or congestive heart failure.

Patients may complain of moderate to severe thirst during this period. Aggressive oral hygiene may alleviate patient discomfort. If oral fluids are permitted, accurate recording of ingested fluids is important. Unlimited oral intake and failure to measure it may provide too much fluid in the circulating blood, resulting in water intoxication.

The loss of skin greatly decreases the severely burned patient's ability to regulate body temperature. The environment must be heat controlled and kept warmer than usual. Room temperature is maintained at 80 to 85° F (26.6 to 29.4° C) with humidity of 40 to 50 percent. Drafts must be eliminated. Fluid warmers, heat lamps, and warming blankets are used during burn shock. Prolonged exposure to air is avoided. Exposed areas of the body are covered with sterile sheets and blankets to decrease the loss of body heat through the open wounds while other areas of the burn are being cleansed.

Care of the burn wound can be delayed until all first aid measures have been initiated. Wound care should be carried out carefully and with as little discomfort to the patient as possible. One of the most important factors to be considered in wound care is that the patient has lost the ability to withstand infection in the area where the skin is damaged or destroyed. The goals of the initial wound care are as follows: (a) cleanse the wound to eliminate or decrease the dead tissue and debris that serve as the media for bacterial growth, (b) prevent further destruction of viable skin, and (c) provide for patient comfort.

During the admission procedure, the burn wound and the entire body are washed to remove dirt and debris as well as loose dead tissue on the burned areas. Detergents or antiseptic preparations are effective cleansing agents. Gentle cleansing with gauze is effective in removing dead tissue without causing further tissue damage. All hair in and around the burn wound is shaved and wiped off the skin, because hair attracts and shelters bacteria. Singed hair is clipped short to avoid bacterial contamination of the wound. Firm, intact blisters can remain undisturbed, because they are a natural protective and pain-free dressing. If the blisters are broken and the epidermis is separated, loose tissue must be debrided.

After the wound is cleaned and before a dressing is applied, cultures of the wound are obtained. Baseline cultures provide information about organisms present in the wounds at the time of admission. Prophylactic antibiotics are usually not indicated. Photographs are taken on admission and at intervals during the patient's hospitalization. These pictures provide a record of the appearance of the burn wound on admission, before the application of topical therapy, and during the healing process.

The constricting effect of nonviable tissue (eschar) from a full-thickness injury to the chest, neck, or extremities is an early complication. Edema forming rapidly under the constricting eschar will produce a tourniquet effect that causes occlusion of venous and arterial circulation and may result in ischemic necrosis, especially with unburned areas distal to the constrictive eschar. Frequent monitoring of distal pulses is part of an ongoing assessment to ensure uninterrupted vascular flow to all extremities. Extremities should be monitored for signs and symptoms of circulatory compromise, including diminished peripheral pulses, decreased capillary refill, paleness or cyanosis, temperature decrease, and increase in pain or paresthesia. It may be necessary to monitor circulation every 15 minutes.

Circumferential burns that go all the way around the neck or chest can lead to constriction of chest wall expansion and airway compromise, resulting in respiratory distress. Part of the respiratory assessment is monitoring chest excursions, respiratory rate, and ventilator settings, if the person is intubated, for high pressures and low tidal volume.

Pharmacology

Morphine sulfate is the drug of choice for pain relief and is given intravenously, in small increments (2 to 4 mg). A morphine drip can be used and titrated to the patient's pain. No medication of any kind should be given intramuscularly or subcutaneously, because it may pool and be absorbed later when cardiac output and blood pressure improve. Large doses of sedatives and analgesics are avoided because of the danger of respiratory depression and the potential for masking other symptoms (Broyles, Reiss, & Evans, 2007).

Tetanus prophylaxis is recommended by the American College of Surgeons. It is administered in the emergency department after determining the patient's immunization status. If the patient has been previously immunized but has not received tetanus toxoid in the preceding five years, the vaccine can be administered. If information about prior tetanus immunization is not known, treatment can be delayed for 72 hours until the status is determined or until a dose of human tetanus-immune globulin hormone can be administered with the initiation of an active tetanus immunization program.

BOX 46-3

INDICATIONS FOR FLUID RESUSCITATION

- Burns greater than 20 percent TBSA in adults
- Burns greater than 10 percent TBSA in children
- Patient older than 65 or younger than 2 years of age
- Patient with preexisting disease that would reduce normal compensatory responses to minor hypovolemia (i.e., cardiac or pulmonary disease or diabetes)

Adapted from American Burn Association. (2005). Advanced burn life support course: Provider's manual. *Chicago: Author.*

Respecting Our Differences

Refusal of Blood Products

Patient autonomy and the right to refuse treatment have long been subjects of controversy. Personal beliefs and lifestyles must be fully respected as treatment plans are developed and implemented, even when refusal of treatment puts the patient at risk for survival. The Jehovah's Witnesses religious community refuses transfusion of blood or blood components to remain faithful and obedient to God's law, as they perceive it (Karcioglu, Oskara, Civancr, & Ozucclik, 2003). The removal of such a critical and traditionally effective treatment is a challenge, particularly when the patient is fully competent and fully informed about the need to maintain circulating blood volume.

Replacing fluids and electrolytes (fluid resuscitation) is an essential part of the treatment of burn victims and is instituted as soon as the severity of the burn based on the parameters in Box 46-3 and the patient's condition are known. Ideally, fluid therapy is started within an hour after a severe burn to prevent the onset of hypovolemic shock. Insertion of two large-caliber peripheral catheters permits the rapid administration of fluids and electrolytes.

Fluids administered during the first 48 hours are given to maintain circulating blood volume. Traditional treatment of large burns includes blood transfusion. Whole blood is commonly administered during initial treatment. Additional fluids and electrolytes are added to replace losses from vomiting or from nasogastric drainage.

Two types of fluids are considered when calculating the needs of the patient: crystalloids and colloids. Crystalloids may be isotonic or hypertonic. Isotonic solutions, such as lactated Ringer's or physiological (0.9%) sodium chloride, do not generate a difference in osmotic pressure between the intravascular and interstitial spaces. Thus, large amounts of fluids are required to restore and maintain the intravascular volume. Hypertonic salt solutions have a milliosmolal content of 400 to 600 (280 to 300 mOsm is isotonic), thus creating an osmotic pull of fluid from the interstitial space back to the depleted intravascular space. The use of hypertonic solutions decreases the amount of fluid a patient needs during resuscitation, which helps decrease burn tissue edema and minimizes cardiopulmonary complications (pulmonary edema and congestive heart failure).

The consensus formula used to calculate the volume of IV fluid required for fluid resuscitation is based on the Parkland Formula (American Burn Association, 2005). Using this formula, the patient's fluid requirements for the first 24 hours post-injury are estimated. For adults the formula is: 2 to 4 mL of lactated Ringer's solution × body weight (in kg) × percent burn. Because blood volume falls rapidly, the first 48 hours is crucial as edema increases significantly. As edema increases, additional fluid is lost through the burn and the loss may be increased as high as 15 times normal. IV replacement is a must and is accomplished at a rapid rate. The time is calculated from the time of injury and not from the time the emergency care was initiated. The first one half of the total amount calculated is given in the first 8 hours after the injury. The second half is administered over the next subsequent 16 hours. For example, if a patient weighing 75 kg has a 70 percent TBSA burn, the fluid requirements are:

- 4 mL lactated Ringer's × 75 kg × 70 percent = 21,000 mL needed over the first 24 hours
- One half is needed in the first 8 hours, one half × 21,000 = 10, 500 mL in 8 hours, or 1,312 mL/hour.
- One half is needed in the next 16 hours, one half × 21,000 = 10, 500 mL in 16 hours, or 656 mL/hour.

Colloids may also be used to replace body fluids. The use of colloids is avoided in the first 12 hours post-burn. The capillary permeability caused by the burn injury begins to close at 12 hours. At this time patients may receive colloids, such as fresh frozen plasma, albumin, or dextran. The oncotic pressure generated by the colloids also helps pull fluid back into the intravascular space. In addition, fresh frozen plasma is beneficial in restoring lost clotting factors. Red blood cells are used only if the patient has had a significant loss or destruction of red cells. During the second 24 hours post-burn, one half to two thirds of the initial 24-hour volume is generally required. Also during this second 24-hour period, colloid solutions are used to replace intravascular volume once capillary permeability significantly decreases (Doe Report, 2005).

Surgery

Treatment of the constricting effects of the eschar by incising it is an **escharotomy,** which is performed on the burn unit. An escharotomy is a linear surgical incision through the burn eschar that releases the constriction

Safety First

Burn Prevention in the Community

Burn prevention informational health and safety fairs do not target audiences that involve children. Traditionally, trinkets, handouts, and posters are given away or are on display. To address this gap, the Central Ohio Burn Education Coalition, developed a television media Safety Day to provide a fun way for families to learn various child safety topics (DeLaune & Ladner, 2006). A wheel of safety similar to the Wheel of Fortune was used and each participant was asked to spin the wheel. Depending on what color the wheel stopped on, the player was asked an age-appropriate question about burn prevention. The youngest player was 3 years old. A correctly answered question afforded the player a visor imprinted with "Practice Your Plan." Incorrectly answered questions afforded the player an educational session that included information about home fire drills, before they received a visor. The wheel is mobile and has been used on college campuses and at the Ohio state fairs.

caused by the full-thickness injury. Patients have limited pain during an escharotomy, because the nerve endings have been damaged by the burn.

The patient is kept as comfortable as possible by gentle handling of the burn areas and by keeping the wounds covered so that air does not reach them. Small doses of morphine are given intravenously. Patients with significant burn injury receive a profound insult to their body and self-image. They are aware that they may not survive, which causes fear and helplessness. The shock and pain of the accident, the chaos and rush to the hospital, and the unknown surroundings and people all intensify the emotional stress. The nurse spends the most time with the patient and has a considerable influence on the patient's psychological adjustment.

Patient and Family Teaching

Nurses can help prevent accidental burns by participating in health education programs that stress fire prevention and the consequences of fires, such as burns, deformities, and death. Nurses also can promote legislation that would control hazardous practices and make working and living environments safer. Community health nurses are in an unusually advantageous position to recognize unsafe practices in the home and to help families develop safe habits of living. Nurses can raise the awareness of patients and the community to the burn problem with education and burn awareness campaigns.

Prevention programs can be developed to highlight seasonal activities that result in burn injuries. Approximately 80 percent of all accidental burns occur in the home and are caused primarily by ignorance, carelessness, and the curiosity of children. More than 35 percent of all fires and burn injuries involve children playing with matches and cigarette lighters. Prevention focuses on teaching parents and others caring for children to keep matches and cigarette lighters out of the reach of children. Some causes of seasonal burn injuries are barbecuing in the spring, sun exposure in the summer, yard clean-up in the fall, and holiday activities in the winter.

Smoke detectors are present in 13 of 14 homes. Data suggest that half of the home fires and three fifths of fire-related deaths occur in homes without smoke detectors. About one third of the homes with smoke detectors have hundreds of fire-related deaths, because the smoke detector does not work. Working smoke detectors wake people to the fire and allow them time to escape to safety. Prevention includes teaching the following: all homes should have working smoke detectors on each level of the home and in the hallway outside of the bedrooms, and batteries should be tested periodically and changed twice yearly in the spring and the fall.

In states and countries with time changes, such as the change between Eastern Standard and Daylight Savings times in the United States, battery changes can be timed to coordinate with these time changes. Batteries should never be removed for the reason that they go off during cooking as it is easy to forget to replace them. In most cities in the United States, the fire department will install smoke detectors free of charge to the elderly and others unable to do so for themselves. Fire departments in many communities have free smoke detectors for those unable to afford them. People who use home oxygen therapy should not smoke or be around flames. The oxygen should be at least 10 feet from an open flame (e.g., cigarettes, lighters, pilot lights, and candles). The high risk of burn injury can be reduced with patient and family education.

Burn injuries to adults are most often related to accidents while they are cooking, using microwave ovens, or smoking or otherwise using matches. Burns commonly occur when a person is distracted while cooking or falls asleep while smoking. Prevention centers on teaching persons of all ages to be especially careful of scald burns when using microwave ovens. Scald burns can occur when the power of the microwave is underestimated. All users need to be educated about the safe use of these ovens. Smokers need to be reminded to never smoke in bed, to be particularly careful about falling asleep while

Fast
Forward ▶▶▶

Burns and Dementia

New diagnostic and treatment regimens are resulting in prolonged life for both males and females. Longer life spans are associated with an increased incidence of dementia. More elderly patients with dementia are being admitted to burn units. The literature about dementia patients focuses on comorbid diseases and the association between dementia and incidence of burns in the elderly has not been studied in depth. Alden, Rabbits, and Yurt (2005) published a retrospective study of patients with dementia at a large urban burn center. Their data revealed that 22 percent of the study group required ventilatory support, 75 percent required intensive care, and 25 percent did not survive their burn. These staggering statistics suggest that a burn prevention program adapted to the elderly demented population is already overdue.

smoking and sitting in overstuffed furniture, and to be sure that cigarettes are completely extinguished, especially before going to bed. Elderly patients with dementia are at uniquely increased risk for severe burns.

The government's role in fire prevention centers around laws designed to protect the public. For example, rigid enforcement of laws requiring that industrial products be labeled when they are known to be flammable and that new products be tested carefully for their flammable qualities before being placed on the market is evidence of government efforts to protect the public from accident by fire. The surgeon general's report on goals to be achieved by 2010, include an increase in functioning residential smoke alarms and a reduction in residential fire deaths (Box 46-4) (USDHHS, 2000). These goals are particularly focused at high-risk groups: American Indian/Alaska natives and African Americans.

Industry can be made safer by constant vigilance of management in cooperation with fire safety officers and health care professionals to identify hazards and implement a safety program. All chemicals should be labeled, and antidotes should be identified and available. A core group of every workforce should be versed in emergency treatment of all types of burns for the protection of every employee.

Evaluation of Outcomes

Potential patient outcomes for each of the example nursing diagnoses for the patient in the emergent phase of burns are:

- Ineffective airway clearance related to secretions, tracheobronchial edema, and obstruction. The patient maintains a patent airway, adequate oxygenation, and ventilation and is free from strider and adventitious breath sounds.
- Deficient fluid volume related to intravascular fluid shift and evaporation. The patient experiences adequate fluid volume and electrolyte balance as evidenced by urine output greater than 30 mL/hour, normotensive blood pressure, heart rate 100 beats/minute, consistency of weight, and normal skin turgor.

BOX 46-4

HEALTHY PEOPLE 2010

The Surgeon General's goals for 2010 related to burn injury are focused on decreasing residential fire deaths through the presence of a functioning smoke alarm on every floor.

Goal # 1: Reduce the incidence of residential fires

    1998 baseline: 1.2 per 100,000 people
    2010 target: 0.2 per 100,000 people

Goal # 2: Increase total population living in residences with functioning smoke alarms on every floor

    1998 baseline: 88 percent
    2010 target: 100 percent

Goal #3: (Developmental) Increase the proportion of people who have access to responding prehospital emergency medical services

Adapted from United States Department of Health and Human Services (USDHHS). (2000). Healthy People 2010: Understanding and improving health. Retrieved May 5, 2006, from http://www.healthpeople.gov.

- Hypothermia related to impaired temperature regulation and wound exposure. The patient remains normothermic without clinical manifestations of infection.
- Risk for infection related to impaired skin integrity. The patient remains free of infection, as evidenced by normal vital signs and absence of purulent drainage from wounds, incisions, and tubes. Infection is recognized early to allow for prompt treatment.
- Impaired skin integrity related to impaired perfusion and burn-injured skin. The patient's skin condition should be improved as evidenced by decreased redness, swelling, and pain.
- Acute pain related to exposed nerve endings and associated trauma. The patient should verbalize an adequate relief of pain along with the ability to realistically cope with the pain if it is not completely relieved.
- Anxiety related to situational crises and threat of death. The patient should be able to recognize the signs of anxiety, demonstrate positive coping mechanisms, and describe a reduction in the level of anxiety experienced.

ACUTE PHASE

The acute period of treatment begins at the end of the emergent period and lasts until the burn wound is healed. The length of this period varies. If the burn is a partial-thickness injury, the acute period extends for 7 to 21 days; if the burn is a full-thickness injury over a large percentage of the body requiring surgery for skin grafting, the acute period may last for months. During this phase, a multidisciplinary approach to care is needed. During the acute period the two main principles of management are treatment of the burn wound and avoidance, detection, and treatment of complications. The most common complications are infection (septicemia and pneumonia), renal disease, and heart failure.

Diagnostic Tests

Laboratory testing during the acute period focuses on monitoring the patient's fluid and electrolyte balance. Chemistry profiles may be obtained once or twice daily during the patient's critical phase while fluid resuscitation is in progress. Complete blood counts are monitored to assess the patient's white blood cell count and hemoglobin and hematocrit values. Wound cultures are obtained once or twice weekly to track the bacterial colonization of the wounds. Ongoing surveillance of wound cultures is essential for early treatment of infection.

Evaluation of nutritional status is monitored through prealbumin levels and urine urea nitrogen. Patients who are intubated or have inhalation injuries require periodic chest X-rays. In addition, bronchoscopy is performed on patients with inhalation injuries to assess the degree of injury to the lungs.

Assessment with Clinical Manifestations

Burn patients are often frightened and anxious about their injury and the associated treatments. These responses can be compounded by the intensive care unit environment. Burn patients experience both physical and psychological pain. Physical pain is usually focused on specific activities, such as wound cleansing and debridement, dressing changes, and physical therapy. The nurse must assess the patient's reaction to pain and intervene appropriately.

A thorough head-to-toe assessment of the burn patient is performed every eight hours. Data includes mental status; vital signs; breath sounds; bowel sounds; dietary intake; motor ability; intake and output; weight pattern; circulatory assessment; and observation of burn wounds, grafts, and donor site. Purulent drainage, abnormal color, foul odor, redness or swelling in surrounding normal skin, or presence of healing should be noted. Changes in these parameters from shift to shift or from day to day make further investigation necessary.

Nursing Diagnoses

Based on the information gathered, examples of nursing diagnoses in the patient during the acute phase of burns may include the following:
- Impaired skin integrity related to burn injury and nutritional deficits.
- Risk for infection related to impaired skin integrity and altered immune response.
- Imbalanced nutrition: less than body requirements related to increased metabolic needs, protein loss, and decreased appetite.
- Acute pain related to exposed nerve endings and immobility.
- Deficient fluid volume related to increased insensible loss and evaporation.
- Impaired physical mobility related to decreased strength and endurance, activity intolerance, and depression.
- Disturbed body image related to altered body appearance or function.

Planning and Implementation

Nursing interventions for the care of the patient in the acute phase include promoting skin integrity, prevention of infection, providing nutrition, comfort and pain management, maintaining fluid balance, relieving anxiety, promoting activity, supporting and encouraging coping and self-care, and prevention of hypothermia. Healing of the burn wound is an essential component of care of the patient. Expert assessment skills are required to monitor the wound during healing and to detect any signs of infection. Wound care may be needed one to three times daily. Wound cleansing, debridement, and dressing application is accomplished during these treatments. The patient is adequately medicated prior to the procedure. Strict barrier precautions are maintained. Caregivers wear gowns, masks, eye protection, and gloves. The goals of wound care include prevention of infection, removal of devitalized tissue, prevention of further destruction of healthy tissue, and minimization of pain.

Hydrotherapy using a shower, tub, or spray table facilitates the removal of topical medications and loosens debris, sloughing eschar, and exudate. Wound care in a tub permits immersion of the patient into water or antimicrobial solutions. Soaking helps in the removal of topical agents and eschar and helps facilitate range of motion. Generally, tub therapy is limited to 30-minute intervals to prevent heat loss. Tub therapy is avoided in critically ill patients and those with a wound infection, because the infection may be transmitted to other areas of the body through the tub water. A spray table may be used for patients who are poorly mobile, have wound infections, or during their more critical phase. This method of hydrotherapy allows the patient to be recumbent, and water is provided through the use of temperature-controlled hoses. For patients who are mobile, a regular shower can be used. This method helps the patient resume activities of daily living.

Nonsurgical burn wound management involves removing exudates and necrotic tissue, cleaning the area, stimulating granulation and revascularization, and applying dressings. Restoring skin, whether by natural healing or grafting, starts with the removal of eschar and other cellular debris from the burn wound. This removal is called debridement and is an important part of wound healing. After removal of the gauze dressings, the wound is cleansed with a mild soap or noncytotoxic wound cleansing agent. Nonadherent exudate or debris is removed.

The burn patient is at tremendous risk for infection. Measures to prevent infection begin at the time the patient is admitted to the hospital and continue until healing is complete. Burn wound infection occurs through auto contamination, in which the patient's own normal flora overgrows and penetrates the internal environment. Burn wound infection also occurs through cross-contamination, in which organisms from elsewhere are transferred to the patient. Sources of infection may be endogenous or exogenous. Bacteria that survive in the hair follicles and glands are a source of endogenous infection. In addition, after burn injury, bacteria that normally live in the intestinal tract migrate or translocate across the intestinal wall and spread to the general circulation by way of the lymphatic system. Local and systemic infections (septicemia) are the most common complications of burns and are the major cause of death, particularly in burns covering more than 25 percent of the body. Therefore thorough wound cleansing is necessary to remove the debris that acts as a media for bacterial growth.

Organisms commonly causing burn wound infection include *Pseudomonas aeruginosa, Acinetobacter, enterococci,* and *Staphylococcus aureus (S. aureus).* These organisms are normally found on the skin or in the intestine and become a source of infection. Treatment of antimicrobial resistant organisms, such as methicillin-resistant *S. aureus,* vancomycin-resistant *enterococci,* and *aspergillosis,* is an increasingly difficult problem in burn centers (Havener, Roth, Arakere, and Barenfanger, 2005).

Fungal infections have an increased incidence in burn patients because of the use of broad-spectrum antibiotics. *Candida albicans,* which normally is found in the GI tract, accounts for the majority of the fungal infections. Cultures of the patient's wound may be taken on admission and at biweekly intervals to determine the presence of bacteria and their sensitivity to antibiotics.

Infection is commonly the cause of deterioration in the condition of a burn patient. Signs of infection include erythema and edema at the wound edges, increasing pain, odor, drainage, and decreasing function. The wound may show changes in color from red to violet, dark brown, or black and tissue necrosis may occur. Signs of sepsis in the burn patient are change in sensorium, fever, tachypnea, tachycardia, paralytic ileus (decreased tolerance of feedings), abdominal distension, and oliguria.

Drug therapy, isolation therapy, and environmental manipulation are strategies for preventing the introduction of exogenous organisms into the wound. Systemic antibiotics are used when burn patients have symptoms of an actual infection, including septicemia. Broad-spectrum antibiotics are given until the results of blood cultures and sensitivity status are available. At that time, more specific antibiotics, including the aminoglycosides, such as amikacin (Amikin) or gentamicin (Garamycin or Alcomicin) and cephalosporins, such as cephalothin (Keflin) or ceftriaxone (Rocephin), are used. Because of increased metabolism, burn patients generally require a larger than normal dose of these drugs to maintain therapeutic blood levels. If aminoglycosides are used, serial peak and trough blood levels are monitored to determine the efficacy of treatment and evaluate potential ear and kidney toxicity (Broyles, et al., 2007).

Placing the severely burned patient in a special burn unit can decrease the possibility of infection, because the unit environment is specifically equipped for infection control. If the patient is cared for in a general hospital unit, a private room is essential, and all equipment needed by the patient remains in the room. Some burn care philosophies state that isolation therapy effectively reduces cross-contamination. However, methods of isolation are varied and controversial. Some burn centers practice virtually no isolation, whereas others use near-total sterile conditions.

All isolation methods emphasize proper and consistent hand washing as the most effective technique for preventing infection transmission. All health care personnel wear gloves during all contact with open wounds. The use of sterile versus clean gloves for routine wound care varies by agency and is a matter of debate. Regardless of sterility, change gloves when handling wounds on different areas of the body and between handling old and new dressings.

The equipment on burn units is not shared among patients. Disposable items (e.g., pillows, syringes, and dishes) are used as much as possible. Assign any equipment used in daily routine care (e.g., thermometer, blood pressure cuff, and stethoscope) to that patient. Daily cleaning of the equipment and general housekeeping are essential for infection control. All equipment must be cleaned after use for one patient before it is used for another patient.

Because *Pseudomonas,* a gram-negative bacterium, has been shown to sequester in plants, the presence of plants and flowers is prohibited. Some burn units do not permit patients to eat raw foods (such as salads, fruit, and pepper) to reduce exposure to *Pseudomonas* organisms. Rugs and upholstered articles are difficult to clean and may harbor organisms, and their use is also restricted.

Visitors are restricted when the patient is immunosuppressed. People with upper respiratory infections or other illnesses and small children should not come into direct contact with the burn patient. Some burn units recommend that all visitors wear protective clothing (gowns, gloves, masks, and shoe and hair covers) in the room of the burn patient, but no data support the effectiveness of this approach.

Collaborative Care Management

Patients who suffer burn injuries require specialized care, which is best obtained in a burn unit. A multidisciplinary team including surgeons, nurses, physical and occupational therapists, social workers, microbiologists, clergy, child life workers, psychologists, volunteers, and other disciplines is involved in the approach to care. Referrals to other services are determined by the needs of the patient. For example, patients with other conditions, such as diabetes, may require consultation from an expert to assist in managing the diabetes during the acute period of their burn. Consultation with a psychiatrist may be indicated for patients whose burns were self-inflicted or for those who are having difficulty adjusting to their postburn appearance.

Nutrition

Metabolism can be increased by two or three times normal after moderate to severe burns because of stress, fluid loss, hypercatabolism, and immobility. Shivering and elevated levels of catecholamines, cortisol, and glucagon present after thermal injury increase oxygen consumption and heat production. In addition, there is depletion of liver and muscle glycogen and fat deposits, resulting in negative nitrogen balance and weight loss. Protein is broken down to provide amino acids for gluconeogenesis, preventing amino acids from incorporating into protein. This decreased rate of protein production prolongs wound healing and increases the patient's susceptibility to infection (Roth, 2007).

A burn patient remains catabolic until caloric intake exceeds caloric expenditure. This catabolic state may last for days or months depending on the severity of the burn. The patient's energy and protein requirements become those needed for normal homeostasis plus those required to offset the catabolic state and repair the burn injury.

Maintenance of a nutritional support program is critical to survival and is initiated on admission. The goals of the nutritional support program are to establish oral intake as soon as possible and to maintain sufficient caloric and protein intake to restore tissue loss. A team approach provides comprehensive input and integrates the efforts of the patient, health care provider, nurse, pharmacist, dietitian, and occupational and physical therapists.

A nutritional assessment is made during the first days of the burn injury and includes anthropometric measurements (to determine actual weight loss compared with ideal weight), indirect calorimetry, and laboratory studies (electrolytes, liver function tests, and urine). The admission assessment provides a baseline against which progress can be evaluated. Twenty-four-hour urine specimens and urea nitrogen tests may be obtained two to three times a week to evaluate the patient's nitrogen balance. Transferrin or prealbumin levels provide sensitive indicators of visceral protein status. Urinary nitrogen and serum albumin levels can be affected by insensible protein loss and hydration status.

Albumin's half-life of 20 days makes day-to-day evaluation of albumin difficult to interpret. On the other hand, prealbumin, which has a short half-life of 20 to 25 hours, provides a sensitive indicator of nutritional status and the patient's response to feeding.

Nutritional requirements for the burn patient are highly variable, depending on the extent and depth of injury and the patient's age, gender, preburn nutritional status, and preexisting diseases. Total caloric needs may be as high as 3,500 to 5,000 calories per day. Calories are provided to the patient as 20 percent protein, 50 percent carbohydrate, and 30 percent fat. Dietitians in burn centers most commonly use the Curreri formula and variations of the Harris-Benedict equation. These formulae are used as a guide to begin nutritional support (Roth, 2007).

Protein is essential to replace nitrogen loss through the wound and in urine and to promote tissue repair and healing. Protein needs in the adult increase from a normal of 0.8 g/kg of body weight to 1.5 to 3 g/kg. Protein calories must be dedicated to the wound and not used for energy needs. This is accomplished by providing the patient with sufficient carbohydrate and fat for energy use.

Increased carbohydrate and fat intake is provided to avoid protein catabolism and meet the patient's energy needs. Approximately 5 mg/kg/min of glucose are provided. Excessive carbohydrate administration is avoided to prevent increased carbon dioxide production and hyperglycemia. In addition to calories, fat provides fat-soluble vitamins and essential fatty acids. Calories provided by fat are limited to 30 percent because of the adverse effect that high fat levels have on the immune system.

Vitamin and mineral supplements are essential for optimal wound healing. Vitamins C and A, zinc, and iron are provided at doses higher than the recommended daily allowances. Vitamins A and C have roles as cellular antioxidants and are required for collagen synthesis. Patients may receive as much as 1,000 mg of vitamin C and 5,000 to 10,000 IU of vitamin A per day. Zinc levels decrease because of increased nitrogen excretion in the urine during the acute phase. Zinc is essential for wound healing and has a vital role in immune function. Patients receive supplementation of up to 220 mg/day. Iron may be supplied to treat anemia caused from blood loss after skin grafting. The use of anabolic steroids in combination with increased protein intake for the restoration of weight gain can be significantly increased post-burn (Demling, 2005).

Enteral feeding (oral or tube feeding) is the preferred method for the burn patient. A paralytic ileus or gastric dilation is frequently seen in the severely burned patient because of shock, stress, or sepsis. This may limit the patient's ability to tolerate gastric feedings for the first few weeks. Commonly, small-bore feeding tubes are inserted into the duodenum or endoscopically into the jejunum so that feedings may be initiated within the first 24 hours of injury. Early feeding decreases hypermetabolism, improves nitrogen balance, minimizes bacterial translocation from the gut secondary to muscle atrophy, and decreases diarrhea and hospital length of stay. Total parenteral nutrition is generally reserved for patients who are unable to tolerate enteral feeding.

Oral feeding is encouraged whenever possible. However, it is difficult for the patient to consume the number of calories needed from food alone because of pain and decreased gastric motility. Therefore, a combination of food by mouth, with supplements, such as milk shakes or commercially prepared products, and tube feedings may be necessary to meet the patient's nutritional requirements. The patient's food preferences are determined and the family is encouraged to bring favorite foods from home. Care is coordinated so that meal times are relaxed and not associated with other procedures, such as wound care. A social situation can be created by having burn patients eat together or with family members. Pain medication is provided so that the patient is comfortable at mealtime. Coordination with occupational therapy staff is essential if the patient needs assistive devices to hold utensils and cups.

Monitoring the patient's nutritional status is an ongoing process. Weight loss and gain are monitored daily during the critical phase and biweekly as the wounds heal. Initially, weight gain occurs because of fluid retention. As diuresis occurs, the patient's weight decreases because of fluid loss. Significant weight loss reflects protein loss and loss of fat reserves, as well as muscle mass. Prealbumin, urine urea nitrogen balance, and cholesterol levels are obtained to track nutritional status.

The patient's tolerance of feeding is monitored by evaluating bowel function. Diarrhea may be a problem for patients receiving antibiotics or tube feedings. Often burn patients have difficulties with constipation because of administration of opioids and decreased activity. Stool softeners, laxatives, and increased fluid intake may need to be provided.

Pharmacology

Administration of medications for the burn patient is supportive in nature. Analgesia is essential for pain control. The most commonly used agents are opioids, such as morphine sulfate, fentanyl, and codeine. Patients with major burns may require agents, such as ranitidine, famotidine, or sucralfate to prevent stress ulcers. Systemic antimicrobial agents are used only when evidence of infection is present. Topical antimicrobial agents are applied to the burn wounds based on depth of injury and wound culture results. Anabolic steroids, such as oxandrolone, have had positive effects in the recovery phase of a major burn. Anabolic steroids are used to attenuate the catabolic state, restore lean body mass, and promote wound healing (Demling, 2005). Current research is focused on the benefits of administration during the acute phase of injury. In addition, many burn patients have preexisting illnesses and require ongoing medication management of their current health problems.

There are a variety of topical medications that are used in the acute phase of burn therapy. For example, petroleum based antimicrobial ointments (bacitracin or Neosporin) are used for partial-thickness burns. Silver sulfadiazine (Silvadene) is a broad-spectrum cream which is used for deep partial- to full-thickness burns. Silvadene protects against gram-negative, gram-positive, and candida organisms. Mafenide acetate (Sulfamylon) is used to medicate deep partial- to full-thickness burns. It penetrates thick eschar and cartilage and inhibits epithelial tissue development. Silver nitrate is used to medicate deep partial- to full-thickness burns but penetrates eschar poorly. Other topical medications are collagenase, Acticoat, Xeroform, and Mepitel.

There are a variety of wound coverings used in the management of acute burns. For example, biosynthetic coverings are used for partial-thickness burns and wounds (e.g., Biobrane, TransCyte, and calcium alginate). Biological wound coverings for partial-thickness or excised wounds, flaps, or grafts are cadaver allograft, vacuum assisted closure dressings ([VAC] a negative-pressure wound dressing that promotes formation of granulation in tissue), pig skin (heterograft, xenograft), and PolyMem (Gottlieb & Furman, 2004; O'Conner & Besner, 2004).

Pain control is a major part of the burn patient's care. Uncontrolled pain affects all aspects of recovery, including tolerance of wound care, ability to eat, mobility, wound healing, and psychological adjustment. Acute pain is most successfully managed with narcotics. The methods and routes of administration are carefully evaluated on an individual basis. Attention is paid to pain management needs during dressing changes and other daily activities. During dressing changes, parenteral narcotics are given to achieve rapid onset of action. The use of agents such as ketamine, fentanyl, and self-administered nitrous oxide may be beneficial for some patients. Some methods for minimizing pain during dressing changes are to provide analgesic medications before dressing change, provide clear explanation to gain patient's cooperation, handle burned areas gently, encourage patient to participate in treatment whenever possible, and the use of distraction (DeLaune & Ladner, 2006).

Organization and planning for patient comfort from pain, itching, or general discomfort includes a plan for procedural, background, and breakthrough pain. The nursing assessment and plan of care and assessment include pain assessment with vital signs. An around-the-clock approach to pain management is essential for the burn patient. Undermedication may occur if the patient fears becoming addicted and fails to report pain or if the nurse fails to adequately evaluate the degree of pain. The use of a numerical analogue scale in which the patient rates the pain helps determine whether the pain is being adequately controlled. Providing medication at frequent intervals helps to maintain ongoing comfort. Time-released opioids and patient-controlled analgesia are also viable options. In addition, alternative methods of pain management can be used (e.g., music therapy, meditation, and diversional activities).

Surgery

Surgical management of burn wounds focuses on excision and wound covering. Skin grafts are applied to cover the burn wound and speed healing, to control contractures, and to shorten convalescence. Successful grafting reduces the patient's vulnerability to infection and prevents the loss of body heat and water vapor from the open wound. Grafting may be performed for cosmetic or functional purposes during the rehabilitative period. Procedures may be performed throughout the acute phase as burn wounds are made ready and donor sites are available.

Grafts may be permanent or only provide temporary coverage. An **autograft** is a permanent graft. The surgeon removes a piece of skin from a remote unburned area of the body and transplants it to cover the burn wound. A **homograft,** or cryo-preserved cadaveric **allograft** (skin graft), is a graft of skin obtained from a cadaver 6 to 24 hours after death that is used as a temporary graft. It can be used as fresh donor skin (stored in the refrigerator) or frozen donor skin obtained from a tissue bank. Disadvantages to the use of homografts are the high costs ($750 to $1,000 per square foot) and the risk of transmitting a blood-borne infection.

A **heterograft (xenograft)** is a graft of skin obtained from another species, such as a pig. Homografts and heterografts are both temporary skin coverings. Homografts, heterografts, synthetic substitutes, and biosynthetic dressings (Biobrane) are intended to provide temporary coverage while the burn wound heals. As the wound heals, these temporary coverings are gradually rejected and are easily removed from the newly healed skin. The advantage of a temporary graft is to reduce water, electrolyte, and protein losses at the burn surface. The covered wound is less painful and allows the patient freedom of movement. Temporary grafts act like human skin and may be used until the patient is ready for an autograft. Often, autografting is delayed as a result of complications, such as infection, pneumonia, or the critical status of the patient.

Dermal replacements or synthetic substitutes for skin are currently being developed and used in burn units throughout the United States. Integra, AlloDerm, and cultured epithelium are new products currently available. All of these products are expensive. The product alone may cost $20,000 or more per patient. Cost effectiveness is being evaluated, comparing costs and patient outcomes. The ultimate skin substitute should include the following properties: it would be inexpensive, nonantigenic, flexible and durable, prevent fluid loss, serve as a barrier to infection, adjust to the wound surface, grow with a child, not cause hypertrophic scarring, store easily with a long shelf-life, and be applied in one operation. There currently is not a perfect substitute for skin (Gottlieb & Furman, 2004).

Before the graft is placed on the wound, the surgical procedure of tangential excision or fascial excision is performed. In the tangential technique, the surgeon excises thin layers of the necrotic burn surface until bleeding tissue is encountered. Bleeding indicates that a bed of healthy dermis or subcutaneous fat has been reached.

In the fascial technique the surgeon excises the burn wound to the level of superficial fascia. Fascial excision usually is reserved for deep and extensive burns. Blood loss is minimal and grafting is usually successful. It is then covered with an autograft or skin substitute. The procedure is best performed between the second and fifth burn day.

Split-thickness skin grafts, full-thickness skin grafts, and primary closure are surgical techniques used to cover the burn wounds. Skin grafts are generally of split-thickness and include the upper layers of skin (epidermis) and part of the middle layer (dermis) causing a partial-thickness injury at the site of surgical removal (donor site). The grafts are removed with a dermatome blade from almost any unburned part of the body. The sizes of these grafts are determined by the sites available and the area to be covered.

Grafts may be used as sheets or are meshed. Meshing of the graft involves taking the sheet of skin after it is removed from the donor and feeding it into a meshing instrument that perforates the sheet with tiny slits. The meshing of the graft makes it more expandable so that it can be stretched to cover wider areas of the body surface. Healing time is slower for a meshed graft, because the skin must fill in open meshed areas (interstices), as well as attach to the granulation bed.

Sheet grafts are applied directly to the burn wound without meshing. They result in better functional and cosmetic outcomes and are used on the face, neck, hands, or around joints. Full-thickness grafts are composed of layers of skin down to the subcutaneous tissue. They are used if there is a well-defined area of a full-thickness burn, and it provides a better cosmetic appearance than split-thickness grafts when healed. Areas that benefit from full-thickness grafts are the hands, neck, and face. Full-thickness grafts can also be used in rehabilitative stages to restore body function and to release skin contractures.

Primary closure is another method of burn wound closure. It is used to close small burns by pulling the skin together and suturing the burn area together or by closing the area with local skin flaps. Graft sites require skilled nursing management. Autografts are secured in surgery with staples, dressings, and splints. Special precautions are taken to prevent sliding, slipping, or movement of the graft. The grafted area may be covered with a large, occlusive, bulky dressing to hold new skin securely in place. VAC dressings can be utilized during this time period. Splints applied in the operating room help to provide immobilization and maintain the position of the grafted areas.

The VAC device helps control wound drainage and enhances healing via a negative pressure dressing. Patients with compromised venous circulation or diabetic neuropathy sustaining a burn have been shown to benefit from use of this device. In addition, review of the literature suggests that this device has a positive impact on the length of hospital stay and thus on cost containment.

The dressing remains intact for 48 to 72 hours. Sheet grafts and full-thickness grafts are examined every 24 hours, because drainage or blood can accumulate under the graft. This fluid can be removed by aspiration with a needle, rolling the fluid with a cotton tip, or by cutting a small slit in the graft to drain the fluid. The graft dressings are removed slowly and carefully so that the graft is not disturbed.

The donor site represents a wound similar to that of a partial-thickness injury. Care of the donor site is as important as care of the graft itself, because donor sites that fail to heal result in an enlargement of the patient's open wound surface. Donor sites may be treated by a variety of methods. One method is covering the exposed surface with Xeroform and leaving it exposed to the air. Exposing the donor site to a heat lamp also promotes healing, because, as the drainage from the wound dries, it serves as a protective covering. The site usually heals within two weeks. Other methods include the use of Op-Site or Biobrane to the donor site. The area is kept wrapped and checked daily for drainage and healing (Figure 46-4). Many patients complain of severe pain in the donor site, and the nurse should not hesitate to give medications for pain. The pain should subside in 24 to 48 hours as the wound dries. The

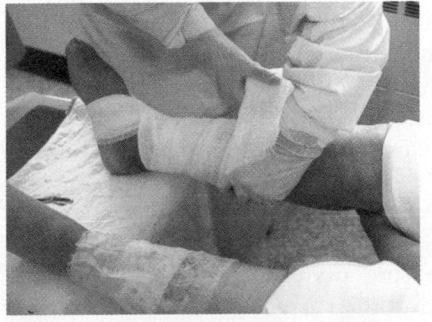

Figure 46-4 Nurse wrapping wet gauze with an external dressing of dry gauze bandages for a donor for burn tissue.

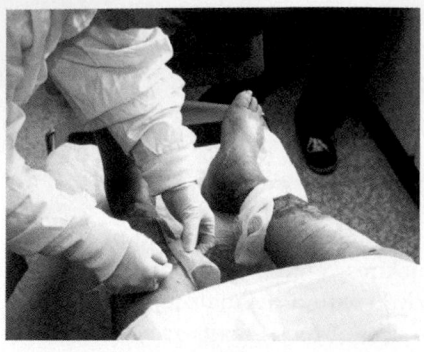

Figure 46-5 Nurse participating in mechanical debridement with burn patient.

wound is inspected daily for any signs of infection (erythema, purulent drainage, or foul odor). If infection develops, antibiotics may be administered, and the wound may be treated with wet dressings.

In deeper wounds in which eschar, or devitalized tissue, is present debridement may be required. Debridement may be surgical, enzymatic, or mechanical. Surgical debridement involves cutting the dead tissue away and is performed in the operating room with the patient under anesthesia. Enzymatic debridement involves the use of a topical enzyme that promotes separation of the eschar from the wound bed. During mechanical debridement, manual removal of eschar using gauze sponges, tweezers, scissors or other instruments is performed (Figure 46-5). As this is a painful procedure for patients, they must be adequately medicated. During this cleansing procedure, the wound is carefully assessed for signs of healing or infection.

Patient and Family Teaching

There are wide variety of patient and family teaching needs for the patient in the acute phase of burns. To begin, patients are taught the importance of maintaining fluid and electrolyte balance after discharge and the need to notify their health care provider immediately if they experience weight loss accompanied by headache, lightheadedness, fatigue, decreased urinary output, irritability, or rapid pulse, which are signs of fluid deficit. Patients also need to report signs of electrolyte imbalance, such as an increase in fatigue, abdominal distension, anorexia, vomiting, constipation, muscle cramps, paresthesia, or confusion. Patients are also taught to eat a well-balanced diet with sufficient fluid intake.

As the patient's wounds heal and pain is controlled, the patient needs to regain and maintain an optimal ability to move purposefully. Range-of-motion exercises are taught and performed actively at least three times a day. If the patient cannot move a joint actively, perform passive range-of-motion exercises. Burned hands require special attention. Encourage the patient to perform active range-of-motion exercises for the hand, thumb, and fingers every hour while awake. Ambulation is started as soon as possible after the fluid shifts have resolved. Patients with a variety of attached equipment (IV catheters, nasogastric tubes, electrocardiographic leads, and extensive dressings) can ambulate with preparation and assistance. Ambulation is performed two or three times a day and progresses in length each time. Regular physical activity inhibits the loss of bone density, strengthens muscles, stimulates immune function, promotes ventilation, and prevents many complications.

A burn injury is a sudden, unexpected event. Its impact on psychological well-being is enormous and promoting mental health is a major area of the burn patient's care. The psychological responses in the acute burn phase are related to the threat of survival. During the acute period, a variety of behaviors may be seen. The six most common reactions are withdrawal, denial, regression, anger and hostility, depression, and anxiety (Doe Report, 2005; Swartz, 2004). As the patient becomes aware of the extent of the injury and begins to evaluate its implications on his or her life, many problems may occur that affect the ability of both the patient and family to cope with the situation. During each of the psychological reactions, the patient may change their interactions with other people and exhibit a variety of behaviors that are somewhat dysfunctional. The nurse must adapt the care to accommodate these changes in behavior. The nurse plays a major role in maintaining and restoring the patient's mental health. Pain plays a significant role in the patient's level of anxiety and is commonly identified by patients as the worst part of their hospital stay. Controlling pain assists in decreasing anxiety. Ongoing education is imperative to assist the patient to understand the care given and to make realistic plans for the future. It is important for the patient to maintain a sense of hope for the future so that he or she can resume a normal life. Without hope, the patient will have less ability to cope, a sense of failure, and less gratifying interpersonal relationships. Emotional recovery from a burn injury is slower than physical recovery. Symptoms of psychological distress are present in a large number of patients up to one year after a burn injury. These symptoms include intrusive and distressing memories of the burn injury and avoidances of thoughts and feelings related to the burn. In addition, patients may experience increased irritability, anxiety, and sleep disturbances.

People with burn injuries are also at risk for the development of posttraumatic stress disorder (PTSD). In this condition symptoms occur after a psychologically traumatic event that would be considered outside the range of normal human experience (Swartz, 2004). The size and severity of burn and degree of disfigurement does not consistently predict the patient who will develop PTSD. Patients are more likely to develop PTSD if there is an actual or perceived lack of social support, the presence of a maladaptive coping style, or high emotional distress. Patients may be nonsymptomatic during hospitalization but develop PTSD after discharge. Therefore, ongoing psychological evaluation and intervention is necessary during hospitalization and during the months that follow.

The nurse needs to explore with the patient how she or he coped with stressful events in the past. It is important to remember that some patients were raised to be stoic when in pain or distress. Other patients were encouraged to express their feelings openly. Nurses should support the patient's coping style unless the patient indicates that he or she would be interested in exploring new methods of coping. Relaxation exercises, meditation, and music therapy may be useful in helping the patient cope with pain and other stressors. In some situations, hypnosis may be used with the goal of having the patient develop the ability to induce self-hypnosis during dressing changes and other stressful events. Patients are usually helped to cope if they are kept fully informed about what is planned for their care and what will be expected of them during various treatments. Then they are not forced to cope with unexpected events that can be upsetting, especially when they have had to give up most of their independence.

Families, like patients, cope best when they are kept fully informed and have a realistic understanding of what lies ahead for the patient. The family can be deeply disrupted by a serious burn to a family member. Initially, they are concerned about the patient's survival and need careful explanations of what is being done for the patient and why. The explanations may need to be repeated more than once, because the family members may be too distressed to comprehend what they are being told.

Social workers are helpful in exploring the family's concerns about role disruptions, plans for child care, financial concerns, and their own feelings of distress. Often the family members require considerable support from health professionals to work through their own feelings before they can be supportive to the patient. The burn team members meet to decide who will provide what support to the family. The family can best provide realistic support to the patient when they have accurate knowledge about what the patient will experience at each step in the recovery process. The family also needs information about community resources available to them and to the patient.

The patient is encouraged to express how he or she feels about the change in appearance. Individual counseling may be necessary for some patients as they integrate the change in their appearance into their self-concept. Other patients will benefit from being referred to a patient support group where they meet other patients in various stages of recovery. The patient is encouraged to participate as much as possible in his or her own care. Independence in the activities of daily living is supported. Some patients will require more encouragement than others in assisting with tasks, such as wound care. It is important that the patient be involved in developing a daily plan of care including meal selection, time of treatments, rest periods, therapy, and socialization.

Evaluation of Outcomes

Potential patient outcomes for each of the example nursing diagnoses for the patient with the acute phase of burns are:

- Impaired skin integrity related to burn injury and nutritional deficits. The patient's skin condition should be improved as evidenced by decreased redness, swelling, and pain.
- Risk for infection related to impaired skin integrity and altered immune response. The patient remains free of infection, as evidenced by normal vital signs and absence of purulent drainage from wounds, incisions, and tubes. Infection is recognized early to allow for prompt treatment.
- Imbalanced nutrition: less than body requirements related to increased metabolic needs, protein loss, and decreased appetite. The patient verbalizes and demonstrates selection of foods or meals that will achieve a cessation of weight loss and weighs within 10 percent of ideal body weight.
- Acute pain related to exposed nerve endings and immobility. The patient should verbalize an adequate relief of pain along with the ability to realistically cope with the pain if it is not completely relieved.
- Deficient fluid volume related to increased insensible loss and evaporation. The patient experiences adequate fluid volume and electrolyte balance as evidenced by urine output greater than 30 mL/hour, normotensive blood pressure, heart rate 100 beats/minute, consistency of weight, and normal skin turgor.
- Impaired physical mobility related to decreased strength and endurance, activity intolerance, and depression. The patient should perform physical activity independently or with assistive devices as needed. In addition, the patient should be free of complications of immobility, as evidenced by intact skin, absence of thrombophlebitis, and normal bowel patterns.
- Disturbed body image related to altered body appearance or function. The patient demonstrates enhanced body image and self-esteem as evidenced by ability to look at, touch, talk about, and care for actual or perceived altered body part or function.

REHABILITATION PHASE

Although rehabilitation efforts are started from the time of admission, the technical rehabilitative third stage begins with wound closure and ends when the patient returns to the highest possible level of functioning. The emphasis during this phase is the psychosocial adjustment of the patient, the prevention of scars and contractures, and the resumption of preburn activity, including work, family, and social roles. This phase may take years or even last a lifetime as patients adjust to permanent limitations that may not be apparent until long after the initial injury.

Diagnostic Tests

Specific diagnostic testing during the rehabilitation period depends on the patient's condition and progress toward goals. Overall, limited testing is required. Evaluation of nutritional status (prealbumin and urine urea nitrogen measurements) and the presence of infection (complete blood counts and wound or blood cultures) may be necessary (Daniels, 2003).

Assessment with Clinical Manifestations

Nursing management of the patient with burns during the rehabilitative phase includes continuous patient assessment, identification of nursing diagnoses, implementation of patient care interventions, and the evaluation of outcomes.

The patient must be helped to maintain range of joint motion to prevent scars from healing in positions that will result in deformity. Complaints of pain and pressure should not be overlooked, because neurological or circulatory damage may occur from an improperly applied splint or poor positioning. It is important that patients understand why ambulation or motion is necessary even though it may be painful.

The emotional impact of a severe burn is enormous. The psychological scars last forever and affect the victim and family for the rest of their lives. The extent to which the family unit adapts affects how the patient reacts to his or her new body image and feelings of self-worth. The hospital environment and hospital personnel influence the adaptation process. In the immediate post-burn period the nurse is primarily concerned with physiological survival of the patient. At the same time, the nurse must be able to identify psychological problems and coping mechanisms of the patient and family.

The nurse is responsible for assessing the patient's response to positioning, splinting, and exercise and the ability of the patient and family to perform daily wound care after discharge. Correct positioning must be maintained to avoid the development of contractures. The splinted limb is assessed for adequate circulation, cyanosis, and temperature, as well as the presence of adequate pulses. Exercise, activities of daily living, and ambulation must be continuously assessed for patient tolerance, both physically and emotionally. Complete and comprehensive instructions of wound and dressing care followed by return demonstrations are necessary before discharge.

Nursing Diagnoses

Based on the information gathered, examples of nursing diagnoses in the patient in the rehabilitative phase of burns may include the following:
- Impaired physical mobility related to pain, decreased strength and endurance, and contractures.
- Disturbed body image related to altered body function and visualization.
- Risk for impaired skin integrity related to nutritional deficit and fragile new tissue.
- Chronic pain related to joint and tissue contractures.
- Ineffective coping related to situational crises and ineffective support systems.

Planning and Implementation

Nursing interventions during rehabilitation of burns includes the promotion of mobility, self-care, a positive body image, skin integrity, comfort, and facilitation of patient and family coping through teaching. As the survival rate of patients with large and deeper burns increases, so does the challenge to maintain optimal functioning and cosmetic results. The percentage of patients with joint limitations increases as the degree and extent of burns increases. Although these patients may be critically ill, their rehabilitative needs must be addressed immediately. A comprehensive program of positioning, splinting, exercise, ambulation, and activities of daily living must begin on the first or second day post-burn and be carried through until after discharge. Any delays in initiating treatment will be detrimental to the patient's ultimate functional outcome.

Contractures are among the most serious long-term complications of burns. They result from muscle and joint stiffening, skin grafting, and prolonged bedrest. Although occupational and physical therapists are primarily responsible for addressing the patient's rehabilitation needs during all phases of the patient's recovery, the nurse is responsible for ensuring that all the recommendations of allied care providers are followed.

Therapeutic positioning is critical for patients with burn injuries, because the position of comfort for the patient is often one of joint flexion, which predisposes him or her to contracture development. Maintain the patient in a neutral body position with minimal flexion. Therapeutic positioning, placing body parts in antideformity positions, is vital to the prevention of burn contractures. The patient must be repositioned in bed (side-lying, supine, or prone) frequently and regularly around the clock. Correct positioning varies, depending on the area of the body burned. Maintaining appropriate positioning helps to maintain extremities and joints in the position of normal function and decrease contractures. Beds with pressure-reducing capability or low air loss may be necessary to limit skin pressure.

Prolonged rest in a semi-Fowler's position or with the pillow pushing the head forward must be avoided, even though many patients like this position, because it enables them to see about the room better. The bed can often be turned so that the patient can look about without having to assume positions that may lead to the formation of contractures. The bedside table may be changed from one side of the bed to the other at intervals to stimulate other body positions.

Splints prevent or correct contractures and immobilize joints after grafting. They are custom made and are often molded directly on the patient to ensure optimal conformity. It is the responsibility of the nurse to apply the splint properly and according to an established schedule. An improperly applied splint can promote contractures and lead to additional complications. The nurse assesses the splinted limb for adequate circulation, cyanosis, temperature, and the presence of pulses. Complaints of pain and pressure should be assessed, because damage may occur with an improperly applied splint. Some health care providers prefer to use the open method of treatment and use frequent exercise instead of splinting to prevent contractures.

Exercises and ambulation for prevention and correction of contractures are begun as soon as the patient is stable. Active exercises are preferred, although active assistance and gentle pressure exercises may be more realistic. Supervision by a physical or occupational therapist is desirable. Exercises may be performed more easily in water and may be done concurrently with dressing changes if the patient is able to tolerate the activity. Continuous passive pressure motion devices may be used to prevent contractures of affected joints. When burns are completely covered (by healing or by graft), exercises may be performed more easily in an occupational therapy or physical therapy department where the patient may also benefit from a change in environment.

Ambulation decreases the risk of thromboembolia and renal calculi, promotes optimal ventilation, helps maintain range of motion and strength in the lower extremities, orients the patient to the environment, and provides a sense of functional independence. Patients who have large burns have less ability to tolerate activity and will require a progressive approach to mobilization. Initially, the patient may need to be transferred with maximal assistance onto a stretcher chair and progress to a sitting position. Gradually, the patient may progress to a standing pivot transfer into a nearby chair and eventually ambulate with minimal assistance. Before getting out of bed, an elastic bandage support must be applied to the lower extremities to prevent venous stasis, edema, and orthostatic hypotension.

One of the ultimate goals in the rehabilitation of the burned patient is to maintain or restore the patient's independence in performing the activities of daily living. The occupational therapist aids in this process by selecting activities appropriate to the patient's medical, physical, and mental status. Activities that the nurse can encourage are self-feeding, communicating by telephone, reading mail, and assisting with grooming or burn wound management. The nurse supports the information taught by the physical and occupational therapists so that progress can be continued on the nursing unit, in the clinic, or in the home.

Regardless of its size, a burn injury represents a change in the individual's perception of self. As the burn heals, the patient must deal with a new appearance.

One specific area to address with the patient is the reaction of others to the sight of healing wounds and disfiguring scars. Patients with facial burns are especially subjected to stares and other reactions from the general public. Visits from friends and short public appearances before discharge may help the patient begin adjusting to this problem. Community reintegration programs can assist the psychosocial and physical recovery of the patient with serious burns.

The patient must have the opportunity to talk about concerns or fears. Some patients may be unable to discuss these with their family or significant others. The nurse must be prepared to listen actively and help the patient accept changes in appearance. The patient must be allowed to grieve for the loss of the former self. However, the patient should be encouraged to focus on the positive aspects of self.

To the adolescent, the thought of being different or conspicuous may be unbearable. If possible, the patient should see facial burns only after being prepared for the experience. The patient will need support and understanding to cope with his or her image in the mirror. The patient will exhibit readiness by asking to look in the mirror. Interaction with other burn patients who are further along in the healing process may help the patient feel that recovery is possible. In some cases, the recovery is good and although differences in skin pigmentation remain, the redness that accompanies healed burn wounds often fades considerably within a few months. Pigmentation problems are more acute for persons with brown or black skin. Their healed skin may be a different shade, freckled, or whitish. Commercial makeup products that help blend skin tones are available.

Whenever a wound of connective tissue heals, hypertrophic scarring will occur unless the skin adheres to the underlying structure. Hypertrophic scarring results from the overgrowth and overproduction of tissue. This occurs especially in areas of stress and movement, such as the hands, legs, and chest. The thickened rigid scar that results may later cause contractures. The application of controlled constant pressure to the surface of an immature scar will reduce the scar and leave smooth pliable tissue. If this pressure is applied to new healthy tissue, hypertrophic scarring decreases. These dressings also inhibit venous stasis and edema formation in areas with decreased lymphatic outflow. The pressure garments are constructed of a specially designed elastic woven material that provides tridimensional control. It is fitted to each patient individually and then custom made. Until the garment is completed, bandages can be used for a pressure dressing.

Even though pressure garments help decrease the formation of thick, disfiguring scars, patient acceptance is a problem. The garments are uncomfortable and make the patient warm, especially during hot weather. They must be tight enough to produce the 24 mm Hg of pressure required to exceed capillary pressure to be effective in reducing edema and scar formation. The patient must wear the garments 23 hours a day for six months to a year. A plan for exercise and splinting must be established before discharge. To prevent scar contracture, daily therapy sessions may be necessary for several weeks or months. The occupational therapist can develop aids to help with the activities of daily living.

Although less severe, pain remains a problem during the rehabilitation phase. Small areas of skin may remain open and continue to require dressing changes. In addition, newly healed skin is sensitive. Physical and occupational therapy and increasing activity may result in discomfort. Interventions are focused on administration of analgesics, diversional activities, relaxation techniques, and providing information about what the patient can expect. Daily hydrotherapy helps the patient relax tense muscles.

After discharge, the patient continues to adjust to temporary or permanent loss of function, cosmetic disfigurement, and the reactions of others. The ability to manage depends on coping mechanisms before the burn, the severity and site of the burn, and the reaction of others. The patient's adaptation to these changes can be evaluated during outpatient visits when the burn team and appropriate personnel are available.

Job retraining may be necessary if the burn injury caused loss of joint function or other physical limitations that prevent the patient from returning to former employment. The local office of the state labor and industry board can assign a vocational counselor to help the patient return to the workforce. Even if retraining cannot begin for several months, the contact with the vocational counselor and anticipation of retraining may help the patient look beyond immediate problems and think of the future.

Collaborative Care Management

Patients who are recovering from burn injuries require specialized rehabilitation care. A multidisciplinary team including physicians, nurses, physical and occupational therapists, social workers, clergy, child life workers, psychologists, volunteers, and other disciplines is involved in this approach to care. Nurses working in the rehabilitation unit need to provide care for patients of all age-groups and they must understand the rehabilitation requirements of burn patients. Community-based support services for patients are provided through rehabilitative and outpatient services. With patients being discharged earlier, education and wound care are generally completed after discharge. Treatment and teaching plans begin at admission and continue throughout the course of healing, regardless of the site for care. A multidisciplinary team of advanced burn care professionals is available and resources are provided to patients and families at different levels of healing. Support groups are available to assist patients with resocialization and coping with their burn injury for many years after discharge.

Nutrition

In the rehabilitative phase of burns, nutritional requirements continue to decrease. There is no longer the need for fluid resuscitation as an example. In addition, there is not the need for vitamin supplements. However, there is still a need to have a well-balanced diet with adequate fluid intake.

Pharmacology

The number of medications prescribed decreases as the patient progresses through the rehabilitation period. As wounds heal, less analgesia is required, and antimicrobial agents are prescribed only for documented infections. During the rehabilitative phase, the medications are needed primarily in a supportive fashion.

Surgery

Initial skin grafting is completed during the acute period. However, the patient may require reconstructive surgery to improve function and plastic surgery to reform ears, noses, or eyelids during the rehabilitation period. Scar tissue and contractures commonly occur one to two years post-burn and may require additional skin grafting. Therefore, surgical management continues to be a form of management as necessitated by the patient's condition as they recover.

Patient and Family Teaching

Before discharge, burn patients and their families have a great need for education so that they may take increasing responsibility for their own care. Discharge teaching involves the entire burn team, who work together to prepare the patient and family for discharge. Early discharge planning accomplishes two goals. First, it helps solve problems early. For example, if the

Fast
Forward ▶▶▶

Discharge Instructions using CD-ROM

Patient and family discharge instructions using a CD-ROM as adjuvant to written information is the wave of the future. Content of the CD-ROM can include:

- Description of the skin
- Depth of the burn
- Procedure for cleansing the burn
- Application of therapeutic garments
- Description and discussion of grafts and donor sites
- Care of healed skin
- Expectations as healing progresses

patient's house burned and needs to be repaired, the family may need to relocate. This could be done before discharge, thus preventing the added stress of moving after discharge. Second, early discharge planning emphasizes the future. If discharge is discussed, the patient and his or her family may realize more quickly that recovery and return to home are possible.

An effective, yet inexpensive, discharge education strategy is provision of written instructions. However, not all patients and their family members can read and complex procedures may be difficult to adequately illustrate in two dimensions. A CD-ROM can be inexpensively used and readily updated for individual or group viewing on home computers, DVD players, and some game systems.

Complete and comprehensive instructions followed by return demonstrations contribute to learning the necessary skills to be independent in self-care activities after discharge. Patients with a major burn should not be discharged from the hospital until they can care for themselves physically, with assistance if necessary, and are prepared to meet the stresses involved in returning to their former living patterns.

A major goal in discharge teaching is to prevent excessive scar formation by exercising, splinting, and applying pressure dressings. If these methods are not effective, reconstructive surgery may be necessary. A patient recovering from a major burn may need 12 to 18 months to achieve complete wound healing. Instructions should include how to care for the healed graft and nongrafted areas. Signs and symptoms of complications, including areas that may blister and break down, and signs of infection are also addressed. Written discharge instructions should include the name and phone number of a health care provider or nurse who the patient may call with questions or problems concerning follow-up care. A referral may be made to a home health agency that may be of assistance in dressing the patient's wounds at home.

Evaluation of Outcomes

Potential patient outcomes for each of the example nursing diagnoses for the patient in the rehabilitative phase of burns are:

- Impaired physical mobility related to pain, decreased strength and endurance, and contractures. The patient should perform physical activity independently or with assistive devices as needed. In addition, the patient should be free of complications of immobility, as evidenced by intact skin, absence of thrombophlebitis, and normal bowel patterns.
- Disturbed body image related to altered body function and visualization. The patient demonstrates enhanced body image and self-esteem as evidenced by ability to look at, touch, talk about, and care for actual or perceived altered body part or function.
- Risk for impaired skin integrity related to nutritional deficit and fragile new tissue. The patient's skin condition is improved as evidenced by decreased redness, swelling, and pain.
- Chronic pain related to joint and tissue contractures. The patient should verbalize an adequate relief of pain along with the ability to realistically cope with the pain if it is not completely relieved.
- Ineffective coping related to situational crises and ineffective support systems. The patient identifies own maladaptive coping behaviors, available resources and support systems, describes or initiates alternative coping strategies, and describes positive results from new behaviors.

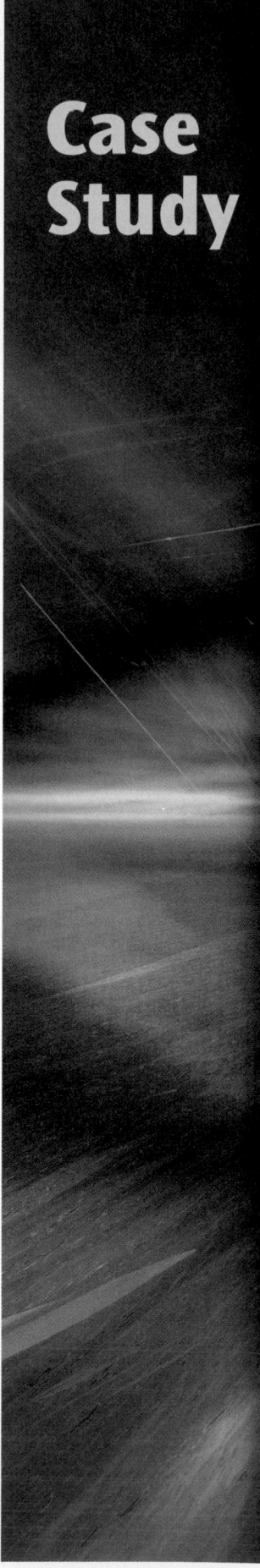

Case Study

Nursing Care Plan

Gary Bradburn, age 34, was admitted to the emergency department following a fire at a plywood mill where he worked. He had been exposed to the fumes from the burning materials and to the extreme heat and smoke of the fire. His face and surrounding hair, lower arms, and hands have first-, second-, and third-degree burns. His eyebrows and nasal hairs are singed, and his teeth have deposits of soot on them. To escape from the rear of the building, he had to make his way through the smoke and flames before reaching the outside. He rolled on the ground to extinguish the flames from his clothing. Gary is alert enough to answer questions.

One hundred percent oxygen is administered by mask. His neck is stabilized, and blood is drawn for baseline hematocrit, electrolyte, blood urea nitrogen (BUN), cyanide, and carboxyhemoglobin levels. Lactated Ringer's solution is started through a large-bore cannula in a peripheral vein. Pain medication is administered. The physician requests close monitoring for signs of impaired oxygenation (e.g., tachypnea, agitation or anxiety, and symptoms of upper airway obstruction, such as hoarseness, wheezing, or stridor). The emergency department nurse mentions that burns can result in multisystem damage; therefore, assessment of neurological and cardiovascular changes and symptoms of shock are also of prime importance. She comments that the first 24 to 36 hours are critical for burn patients and that early intubation may be necessary to avoid later difficulty because of edema of the larynx.

Assessment

According to the rule of nines assessment tool, a 34-year-old male suffering from first-, second-, and third-degree burns on approximately 27 percent of his body. The majority of the burns are superficial and first-degree in nature, but there is a potential of damage to the upper airway as evidenced by the nasal hairs and eyebrows being singed. In addition, the patient's oxygen saturation level is 92 percent, which is somewhat low for a man of this patient's age. The blood pressure, 138/86; pulse, 90; and respirations, 22. The patient's breath sounds are clear to auscultation and not diminished in the bases.

Nursing Diagnosis 1: Impaired gas exchange due to exposure to smoke poisoning and heat damage to lungs

NOC: Respiratory status: Impaired gas exchange and Impaired spontaneous ventilation; Ineffective tissue perfusion: Cardiopulmonary

NIC: Airway management; Oxygen therapy; Respiratory monitoring

Expected Outcomes

The patient will:
1. Demonstrate improved ventilation, adequate oxygenation as evidenced by an oxygen saturation level of at least 95 percent during his hospitalization.
2. Maintain clear lung fields and remain free of signs of respiratory distress during his hospitalization.

Planning, Interventions, Rationales

1. Monitor respiratory rate, depth, and effort including use of accessory muscles, nasal flaring, and abnormal breathing patterns. *These behaviors and a look of panic in the patient's expression may be indicators of hypoxia.*

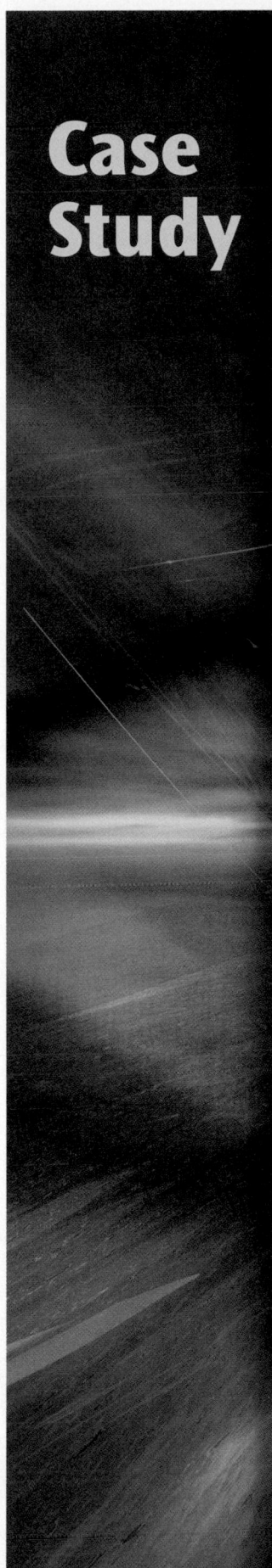

Case Study

2. Auscultate breath sounds every hour or more frequently as needed. *Crackles and wheezes may signify airway obstruction that can lead to or exacerbate existing hypoxia.*
3. Administer humidified oxygen through appropriate device. Monitor patient's behavior and mental status for onset of restlessness, agitation, or confusion. *Behavioral changes and mental status can be early signs of hypoventilation and impaired gas exchange.*
4. Monitor oxygen saturation continuously. Note blood gas results as available. O_2 *saturation of less than 90 percent or a partial pressure of O_2 of less than 80 indicates significant oxygenation problems.*
5. Position patient in semi-Fowler. Turn patient every two hours. Observe patient closely *following position changes. Turning critically ill patients with low hemoglobin levels or decreased cardiac output on either side can result in desaturation. Turn carefully and watch closely.*

Evaluation

Patient's oxygen saturation levels increased to 94 percent within 24 hours and to 96 percent and above within 48 hours. In addition, the patient's respiratory rate slowed to 16 to 20 breaths per minute within 24 hours, and the lungs were clear on auscultation throughout the acute hospitalization.

Nursing Diagnosis 2: Ineffective breathing pattern due to compensatory tachypnea

NOC: Respiratory status: Impaired spontaneous ventilation and Ineffective airway clearance

NIC: Airway management; Respiratory monitoring

Expected Outcomes

The patient will:
1. Return to a normal (regular) or effective breathing pattern.
2. Demonstrate an absence of cyanosis and other signs or symptoms of hypoxia.
3. Maintain arterial blood gases (ABGs) within an acceptable range.
4. Demonstrate appropriate coping behaviors related to breath control.

Planning, Interventions, Rationales

1. Observe rate and depth of respirations and breathing patterns and signs of cyanosis. Auscultate chest for presence of breath sounds and secretions. Monitor diagnostic test results. *Ongoing assessment provides basis for interventions to aid in restoring adequate breathing patterns and oxygenation.*
2. Observe for changes in emotional responses. *Dyspnea can have physiological or psychogenic causes. Fear, anger, and anxiety adversely influence breathing patterns (hyperventilation) and loss of sense of control.*
3. Medicate with analgesics as appropriate. *Promotes deeper respiration and ability to cough if necessary to clear airway (pain may be cause of hyperventilation).*
4. Suction airway as needed. *Removes obstructing secretions, clears airway for patient's who are unable to cough.*
5. Administer oxygen at lowest concentration prescribed. *Higher levels can inhibit patient's respiratory drive.*

Evaluation

Patient maintained a respiratory rate of 16 to 20 breaths per minute without any signs of cyanosis. He did not have any uncontrolled anxiety and was able to breathe in a controlled manner throughout this time of crisis. Analgesics were given periodically without affecting his rate and breathing pattern.

KEY CONCEPTS

■ Burn injuries can be traumatic, life-altering experiences for patients and their families.

■ Patient and family responses to a burn injury depend on age, culture, socioeconomic status, coping mechanisms, body image, family support, and previous experiences with pain.

■ The goals of management during the emergent period, the first 24 to 48 hours after a burn, are to secure the airway, support circulation by fluid replacement, keep the patient comfortable with analgesics, prevent infection through careful wound care, maintain body temperature, and provide emotional support.

■ The acute period of treatment begins at the end of the emergent period and lasts until the burn wound is healed.

■ Although rehabilitation efforts are started from the time of admission, the technical rehabilitative third stage begins with wound closure and ends when the patient returns to the highest possible level of functioning.

REVIEW QUESTIONS

1. Increased capillary permeability:
   1. Resolves within 12 hours
   2. Causes fluid to shift from the interstitial space to the intravascular space
   3. Only occurs with chemical burns to the skin
   4. May cause hypovolemic shock in large total body surface area burns

2. The rule of nines refers to a method:
   1. Used to estimate the total body surface burned
   2. Used to calculate fluid requirements
   3. Used to determine oxygen needs
   4. Used to estimate the depth of a burn

3. A superficial partial-thickness burn includes:
   1. Color pink, small thin-walled blisters
   2. Color pink, area moist, blisters large, pain sensation intact
   3. Color pink, area moist, will not blanch or refill, texture leathery
   4. Color pink, area moist, blanches with slow capillary refills no blisters

4. Factors that may contribute to insensible fluid loss in the burned patient include:
   1. Loss of protective covering of the skin
   2. Increased temperature
   3. Increased respirations
   4. All of the above

5. Wounds that appear moist and pale with sluggish capillary refill and white in color can be classified as:
   1. Deep partial
   2. Full-thickness
   3. Superficial-partial
   4. Partial

6. The fluid shift in burn shock is primarily:
   1. Water, electrolytes, and albumin
   2. Red blood cells, white blood cells, and water
   3. White blood cells, electrolytes, and globulin
   4. Water electrolytes and white blood cells

7. A 70-kg male patient sustains a full-thickness burn to his face, anterior trunk, and bilateral forearms. What is the total body surface area (TBSA) burned?
   1. 36 percent
   2. 32 percent
   3. 28 percent
   4. 24 percent

8. Calculate the fluid resuscitation requirement using the Parkland formula for the above patient.

9. What is the volume to be infused during the first eight hours (include hourly rate)?

10. What is the volume to be infused during the next 16 hours (include hourly rate)?

REVIEW ACTIVITIES

1. A married couple, both 30 years old is brought to the emergency department after burns from a house fire. The husband has a partial-thickness burn, and the wife has a full-thickness burn. What subjective data would help differentiate these two types of burns?

2. Incorporating general principles of psychological care, develop one nursing approach for each of the following patient responses to a severe burn: withdrawal; denial; regression; anger or hostility; and depression.

3. Describe the burn prevention teaching for a physically disabled 60-year-old man that lives alone?

4. Discuss the differences in priorities of care during the emergent and rehabilitative phases of burn injury.

5. You are caring for a 28-year-old male patient that does not understand why second-degree burns are categorized as superficial partial and deep partial. Describe how you would explain the categorized difference to him.

Alterations in Gastrointestinal Function

Assessment of Gastrointestinal Function

Elizabeth Torrence, RN, MN, EdD

CHAPTER TOPICS

- GI Tract Anatomy and Physiology

- Assessment of the GI Tract

- Clinical Manifestations of Pathology of the GI Tract

- Diarrhea

- Constipation

- Diagnostic Tests for the GI Tract

The gastrointestinal (GI) system functions in a fascinating relationship of various organs and biochemical systems working synergistically to provide nutrition to every cell in the body while assisting the body to rid itself of solid and semisolid waste and undigested food. When the learner studies the GI system, it is necessary to have knowledge of all other systems, because the GI system cannot be viewed unitarily as merely a hollow tube whose motility might change secondary to increased, decreased, or obstructive barriers. GI system dysfunction might be outside of the intestinal system yet influence GI function. GI dysfunction often presents as a complex of clinical signs and symptoms. The learner should approach the study of the GI system much as one would approach any ill individual. The patient must be viewed holistically and not as an isolated system. This chapter will detail selected problems associated with deregulation or dysfunction that might occur in the GI system regardless of etiology.

ANATOMY AND PHYSIOLOGY

The major organs of the GI tract include the intestinal tract (the hollow organs from the mouth to the anus) (Figure 47-1), the pancreas that through its exocrine function produces digestive enzymes, and the liver and biliary systems, which achieve important metabolic, digestive, and absorption functions. For this chapter, it is important to remember that the liver produces bile that aids in digestion and absorption of dietary fats and fat-soluble vitamins. Chapter 51 on liver dysfunction will detail other activities of the liver.

The GI tract has been called an integrated system in that its function is prescribed by neuronal control and endocrine functions. These controllers, aid in motility, digestion, absorption, and adjustment of nutrition intake (Keshav, 2004).

Mouth, Lips, Cheeks, Tongue, and Pharynx

The mouth, lips, cheeks, tongue, and pharynx aid in chewing, mastication, and moving food and fluid into the esophagus. Saliva, a product of exocrine glands in the oral cavity, lubricates the mouth and begins the digestive process. Approximately 1 to 2 liters of saliva are produced daily. Saliva serves to lubricate food in transit from the mouth, dissolves food in the mouth to enhance taste, contains alpha amylase (salivary amylase), which begins the digestion of carbohydrates, as well as antibacterial enzymes and immunoglobulins that are believed to protect an individual from serious infection.

The pharynx, controlled by the brainstem cranial nerves (glossopharyngeal and trigeminal nerves), participates with the tongue and other muscles of swal-

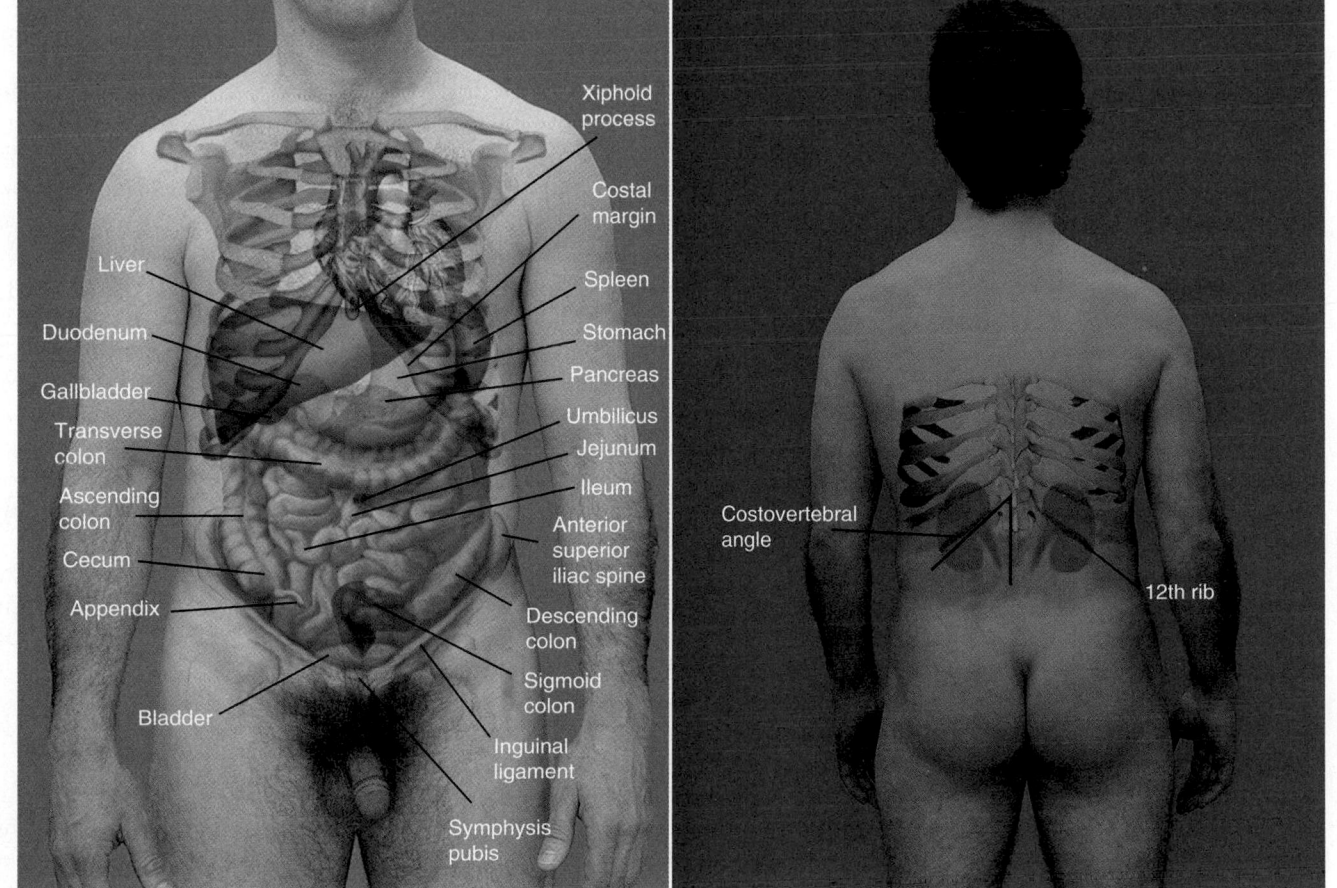

A

B

Figure 47-1 Digestive tract and structures of the abdomen: A. Anterior view, B. Posterior view.

lowing (pharyngeal, laryngeal, and esophageal). The process of swallowing, actively innervated, allows a bolus of food or fluids to enter through a relaxed esophageal sphincter into the esophagus.

Esophagus

The esophagus is a muscular hollow tube that moves food and fluid via peristaltic action toward the stomach. The esophagus is highly vascular and when compromised (e.g., ulceration or infection) can cause great irritation to the patient.

Stomach

Food enters the stomach, is mixed by the churning muscles of the stomach, and is moved along via the peristaltic activity of the stomach called the gastric slow wave. The gastric slow wave is three peristaltic waves per minute. When the contents of the stomach are semiliquid **(chyme),** the pyloric valve opens, and the chyme enters the duodenum of the small intestine.

When there is anticipation of food entering the stomach, the first phase of gastric secretion occurs (cephalic phase). Once food reaches the stomach, the gastric phase begins. The parietal cells under the influence of acetylcholine and histamine secrete HCl (hydrochloric acid). Gastrin produced by gastric G cells stimulates the parietal cells to secrete in response to food in the stomach. HCl in the stomach triggers pepsinogen, which generates pepsin. Pepsin begins the digestion of proteins in the food substrate. Within the stomach, intrinsic factor binds to vitamin B_{12}. This protects B_{12} from destruction as it is transported to the terminal ileum and absorbed. Gastroferrin in the stomach binds iron so that it can later be absorbed in the duodenum (Keshav, 2004).

Duodenum

The duodenum is the first part of the small intestine. The small intestine (duodenum, jejunum, and ileum) functions as the major digestive and absorptive area of the intestine. The duodenum collects pancreatic enzymes and alkaline bile via the ampulla of Vater. This serves to neutralize the acid environment from the stomach. The duodenal enterocytes release **enterokinase,** an enzyme that hastens effective digestion. Enterocytes from the brush border cells elaborate disaccharidases and peptidases that continue the digestive process. Because of the alkalinity, the bile salts emulsify fatty foods, which enhance the action of the digestive process. Fatty acids and cholesterol diffuse through the lipid membrane of the enterocytes, undergo complex transformation with apolipoproteins to produce chylomicrons, and are released. Transport proteins aid in absorption of sugars, amino acids, and electrolytes into the enterocytes. The duodenum selectively absorbs iron and calcium. Gallbladder contraction and pancreatic secretion are stimulated in response to duodenal secretion of cholecystokinin and secretin.

Interestingly, the small intestine is comparatively free of bacteria. Gastric acid, Brunner's glands, and Paneth cells in the small intestine aid the antimicrobial environment. Secretory dimeric immunoglobulins A (sIgA) also participate in maintaining the minimal antimicrobial setting (Keshav, 2004).

Pancreas

The pancreas is an essential organ of digestion. It produces copious amounts of the digestive enzymes trypsinogen, chymotrypsinogen, procarboxypeptidase A and B, pro-elastase, phospholipid A, pancreatic lipase, pancreatic amylase, ribonuclease, and deoxyribonuclease. The pancreas secretes these enzymes in response to the production of cholecystokinin. Additionally the pancreas produces 2 liters/day of a bicarbonate-rich alkaline liquid. This liquid neutralizes the acidic chyme entering the head of the duodenum. The alkaline environment thus enhances the action of the pancreatic enzymes.

Liver and Biliary Systems

The liver and biliary systems will be fully reviewed in chapter 51. Both systems are interrelated to the function of the GI system.

Jejunum and Ileum

The jejunum and ileum are the main areas for absorption of nutrients, vitamins, amino acids, sugars, and triglycerides. The jejunum and ileum together measure approximately 6 meters (19.5 feet) in length. Enzymes, such as disaccharidases and peptidases, are released from the mucosal cells. The jejunum acts on jejunal contents to absorb dietary folic acid.

Intrinsic factor is removed from vitamin B_{12} and absorbed in the terminal ileum. As fat is digested and absorbed in the terminal ileum, bile salts are reabsorbed and then recycled via entero-hepatic circulation. Another important difference in the ileum is the increase in lymphoid cells in the distal ileum. The distal ileum maintains a higher bacterial load. The lymphoid cells protect the terminal ileum in cases of Crohn's disease and bacterial infection.

Cecum and Appendix

The cecum is the first part of the large intestine. The appendix is a blind-ended tube-like structure exiting from the cecum. These structures have no function in the human. They are mentioned because of disorders that affect them, such as appendicitis and colorectal cancer.

Colon

The colon is the large intestine. It is approximately 1.5 meters in length. Its major function is to reabsorb liquid. The colon is rich in bacterial species. The majority of the bacteria are anaerobic bacteria. These bacteria are potentially pathogenic. The goblet cells of the large intestine generate large amounts of mucus. This coats and protects the epithelium from bacterial incursion.

Rectum and Anus

The rectum and anus act as a reservoirs and controllers of defecation. When the rectum is distended, the increased pressure stimulates peristalsis in the sigmoid colon and relaxation of the internal anal sphincter. The abdominal muscles contract and intra-abdominal pressure increases; if the external anal sphincter (under voluntary control) is relaxed, feces is expelled.

ASSESSMENT

The abdominal health history provides the nurse with important subjective information that assists in the physical assessment of the abdomen. Areas that the nurse needs to collect information from the patient in regards to GI abdominal health history are:

1. Family history. Does anyone in the family now have or have had GI problems, e.g., gallbladder disease, gall stones, liver dysfunction, jaundice, irritable bowel disorder, ulcerative colitis or Crohn's disease, stomach ulcers, hemorrhoids, any cancers of the GI tract (pancreas, liver, esophageal, stomach, colon, or rectal), gastroesophageal reflux disease (GERD), pancreatitis,

hernias (inguinal or other) hiatal, tubal pregnancy, ovarian cyst, uterine dysfunction, diarrheal conditions, or other chronic conditions that affected the GI system?

2. Past abdominal history and current problems. Has the patient ever experienced any of the conditions listed in number 1 or had any GI dysfunction? Does the patient have any current GI dysfunction? Has there been any recent weight gain or weight loss? Elicit details. Any GI surgery or other GI procedures? For what? Results? Has the patient been out of the country recently, if so, where?

3. Eating habits. Recall previous 24 hours; unusual eating requirements

   a. Appetite
   b. Food intolerance
   c. Bowel habits

4. Nutritional assessment. This is an excellent time to discuss health promotion activities, such as the food pyramid. The USDA Center for Nutrition Policy and Promotion released the latest food pyramid (Roth, 2007). It allows the consumer to select foods from various categories of the pyramid and monitor their own dietary and nutritional needs. Professionals are directed to explore this site to monitor dietary intake. Often during this part of the history, the nurse can ask about exercise and activity patterns.

5. Dysphagia or heartburn (pyrosis). Has the patient experienced any difficulty in swallowing? If so when did it begin? Have patient describe how often and circumstances when it occurs. Has the patient ever experienced burning in the throat or stomach? A feeling of fullness? At this point the nurse can ask about a chronic cough or recurrent upper respiratory infections. If the patient experiences any of these symptoms, what has the patient done to relieve these symptoms? What makes these symptoms worse?

6. Nausea/vomiting. How often? Describe the events before, during, and after the symptoms? Was there anything unusual about the vomitus, e.g., smell, color, presence of blood? Hematemesis caused from vomiting can occur with irritation or tears of esophagus, with stomach or duodenal ulcerations, and with esophageal varices. Careful questioning about the presence, amount, and circumstance is essential.

7. Abdominal pain. This is a vital symptom and can herald a variety of disorders. Acute pain in the abdomen is referred to as the acute abdomen. This requires urgency in assessment; early surgical intervention may be lifesaving.

   a. Ask the patient to point (with one finger) to the area that is painful.
   b. Is the pain just in this area or does it radiate (move around)? If so, where does it move? Is there anything that makes the pain better or worse?
   c. How long has the patient had the pain? Is the pain constant?
   d. Describe the character of the pain, e.g., dull, cramping, burning, stabbing, aching, or bloating type pain? On a scale of 1 to 10, with 10 as the worst pain the patient may have ever experienced, have the patient categorize the intensity of the pain.
   e. Is pain changed by food? Better or worse?
   f. What makes the pain worse (aggravating factors)?
   g. What things has the patient done to get pain relief (alleviating factors), e.g., antacids or other medications, rest, ice, heat, walking, lying still, other position(s)?

8. Medications. Because most medications are taken orally, it is essential to have the most up-to-date summary of all medications the patient takes. This includes all over-the-counter (OTC) medications and supplements. Included in this assessment should be the amount of alcohol the patient consumes. Skill in asking questions about medications is important, because patients often do not consider the nonsteroidal anti-inflammatory

drugs (NSAIDs), such as aspirin, acetaminophen, naproxen, ibuprofen, or any type of vitamin supplements as medications or that these may influence the GI system (Broyles, Reiss, & Evans, 2007).

GI Symptom Assessment

Because the GI system is responsible for the processing of ingested foods and fluids and the removal of waste products of digestion, any disruption in the processes that are responsible for these functions can lead to various symptoms. Nurses care for patients with GI dysfunction in the inpatient setting and in the clinic and outpatient or home environment. More than 50 percent of individuals with GI complaints have no physical findings, anatomical abnormality, or abnormal lab work (Giles, et al., 2005). This creates a conundrum when helping the individual understand the diagnostic and treatment parameters of a GI disorder.

Leading symptoms and complaints from patients with GI disorders include heartburn, **dysphagia** (difficulty in swallowing), dyspepsia, nausea and vomiting, gas, diarrhea, constipation, pain, and bleeding. Interestingly these symptoms may be associated with a GI problem but may also be associated with a separate and unconnected system disorder. Sometimes symptoms are minor and may require patient education in terms of diet change or lifestyle modification, but sometimes symptoms are indicative of a serious GI disorder.

In general, nurses should be familiar with GI symptoms and the approach needed for the patient. The nurse must know the inclusive history of the patient's symptom and listen carefully to how this symptom occurs in the patient's life. This will be valuable information as the diagnostic problem is differentiated, and a treatment protocol is put into place. The symptoms described are common GI symptoms that are important to know. These will be referred to in future chapters discussing various GI disorders.

Heartburn

Heartburn occurs daily in 7 to 10 percent of all Americans. **Heartburn (pyrosis)** is a substernal burning sensation often radiating to the neck experienced within one hour of eating or one to two hours after reclining. Ingesting foods that irritate the esophagus or decrease the esophageal sphincter pressure causes heartburn. Activities that increase intra-abdominal pressure (e.g., bending, lifting, exercise, straining at stool, or Valsalva maneuver) may also be related to heartburn. When assessing the patient for heartburn, the nurse should assess if the discomfort of heartburn changes with position, food, stress, or exercise.

When a patient describes this symptom, it is described as a burning in the throat, neck, and suprasternal or substernal area. Because of the current focus on GERD in the lay media, patients will often indicate that they have indigestion or acid reflux. Many times patients will have self-medicated with OTC preparations, such as antacids, acid blockers, or other similar available medications. It is important to elicit from the patient when this symptom is experienced. Because the cause of this symptom can be acid contents regurgitated into the esophagus, antacids improve the symptom. There are things that make heartburn worse—a late meal or snack, foods that are directly irritating to the mucosal surface of the esophagus or that lower esophageal sphincter tone, activity that raises intra-abdominal pressure (bending, lifting, and straining). If a patient has a chronic complaint of heartburn, the provider will do a workup for reflux disorder.

Painful Swallowing (Odynophagia)

Odynophagia (pain experienced when a person swallows) is associated with erosion of the esophagus. There are many cause of this pain. It is often linked with infections of the esophagus and subsequent inflammation (esophagitis) or esophageal erosion. Immunocompromised patients who have *Candida*, herpes, and cytomegalovirus infections (patients undergoing cancer chemotherapy or those with acquired immunodeficiency syndrome [AIDS] or human immunodeficiency virus [HIV]) may also develop painful swallowing. This can occur from esophagitis associated with certain medications, some antibiotics, tetracycline, doxycycline, and some antiviral agents.

Difficulty Swallowing (Dysphagia)

The patient will describe dysphagia as the food gets stuck or as a lump (globus) in his or her throat. Dysphagia is either oropharyngeal or esophageal (it is important to review the swallowing process and the afferent and efferent motor function provided by the cranial nerves [CN]). Oropharyngeal dysphagia is important to determine, especially if the patient is older or may have sustained a recent cerebrovascular accident. In addition, when a patient is in the hospital, it is important for the nurse to have any swallowing deficit assessed to determine interventions needed to prevent the patient from aspirating. Other neurological causes that interfere with motor control of the tongue or other oral structures are those that interrupt myoneural function. Afferent input to the swallowing center is through CN V, X, and XI; efferent motor response is mediated by CN V, VII, IX, X, and XII. Some examples of afferent input disorders are myasthenia gravis, certain neuropathies, multiple sclerosis, and Parkinson's disease. Structural abnormalities can also inhibit swallowing, such as oropharyngeal tumors, extrinsic pressure from an enlarged thyroid gland, or Zenker's diverticulum. Zenker's, or cricopharyngeal, diverticulum occurs from an abnormal cricopharyngeal sphincter. Upper esophageal sphincter (UES) dysfunction (cricopharyngeal achalasia) also contributes to oropharyngeal dysphagia. Either a motility disorder or a structural or mechanical process that impairs food moving through the esophageal lumen causes esophageal dysphagia. The patient will describe this sensation as food getting stuck.

The nurse should assess to determine if the dysphagia occurs with solids or liquids or both; whether the difficulty in swallowing is intermittent or getting progressively worse. This may be because of a mechanical or a motility disorder. Dysphagia associated with only solid food is suggestive of mechanical obstruction, (e.g., an esophageal ring—Schatzki's ring, which is a mucosal ring at the lower esophagus). The symptoms associated with an esophageal ring are often intermittent and long-standing. Progressive symptoms may be because of strictures from chronic reflux disease or carcinoma. If the patient is older, has a history of smoking, and ethel alcohol (ETOH) use, and has experienced weight loss, the patient may have an esophageal growth. Dysphagia associated with solids and liquids is suggestive of a problem with esophageal motility. Causes of this type of dysphagia may be esophageal spasms, achalasia, or scleroderma. If solid food is regurgitated, especially with coughing, **achalasia** (a motility disorder from failure of smooth muscle to relax or absence of muscular contraction of the lower esophagus) should be suspect.

Indigestion (Dyspepsia)

Indigestion, or **dyspepsia,** is an uncomfortable feeling in the upper abdominal region. This term is used to describe several imprecise complaints, such as epigastric pain, gnawing, bloating, fullness, early satiety, belching, heartburn, burning, and nausea. Dyspepsia is the most common symptom that patients complain about to their provider. It accounts for 70 percent of visits to a primary care provider. Twenty-five percent of adults have experienced some type of dyspepsia. Of those individuals who have undergone a diagnostic endoscopy for dyspepsia, about half will have normal results. Fifteen to 25 percent will be diagnosed with reflux disorder, and about 29 percent will have peptic ulcer disease. Patients over the age of 45 with dyspepsia often have weight loss, dysphagia, and recurrent vomiting. Alarm symptoms associated with dyspepsia include weight loss, anemia, bleeding, persistent vomiting, and dysphagia. One to 2 percent will have gastric cancer.

Dyspepsia is divided into nonulcer dyspepsia and dyspepsia secondary to peptic ulcer disease. Nonulcer dyspepsia is associated with GERD, problems with motility, gallbladder, liver, pancreatic dysfunction, medication-induced dyspepsia, dietary causes, ETOH ingestion, and endocrine or metabolic disorders, e.g., diabetes. Gallstones can cause severe indigestion, but the dyspepsia associated with gallstones or chronic cholecystitis is described as episodic. The dyspepsia and pain last a few hours and subside. *Helicobacter pylori* gastritis has been implicated in nonulcer dyspepsia but can lead to duodenal and gastric ulceration. *H. pylori* has been implicated in gastric cancer (Butcher, 2003).

Queasiness, Nausea, Regurgitation, and Vomiting

Nausea is a vague, unpleasant sensation of queasiness or feeling sick to the stomach, which may be accompanied by pallor, sweating, and increased saliva production. There is usually distaste for food, and the urge to vomit. Vomiting (emesis) or retching is the forceful expulsion (reverse peristalsis) of stomach contents through the mouth that involves the muscles of the chest and stomach (Table 47-1). Regurgitation is an effortless return of gastric contents into the mouth. Regurgitation can occur in the absence of vomiting and as a part reflux. Vomiting is centrally controlled and may be stimulated by afferent vagal fibers, the vestibular system, and the chemoreceptor trigger zone (CTZ). The causes of nausea and vomiting derive from various pathways and can be categorized into neurogenic, chemical, mechanical, infection, or irritation of the GI tract. More specifically, nausea and vomiting can be from medication, GI infection, food poisoning, intestinal obstruction, appendicitis, cholecystitis, systemic illnesses, pregnancy, or motion sickness or be self-induced. Mechanical complications can include rupture of the esophagus with subsequent mediastinitis (Boerhaave syndrome) or a Mallory-Weiss tear, which occurs at the esophagogastric junction.

Hiccups (Hiccoughs)

Hiccups are caused by sudden contraction of the diaphragm. Gastric distension can cause self-limiting hiccups. These occur from gastric distension with carbonated beverages, aerophagia (air swallowing), extreme hot or cold

---

TABLE 47-1 Act of Vomiting

Afferent Input

Afferent vagal fibers Splanchnic autonomic fibers from GI viscera	Serotonin 5-hydroxytryptamine (5-HT₃) receptors	*Stimulated by biliary or GI distension, mucosal or peritoneal irritation*
Vestibular system (CN VII)	Histamine H₁ and muscarinic cholinergic receptors	*Stimulated by motion, infection, vestibular neuronitis, acute labyrinthitis, Ménière's disease*
CNS centers—Vomiting center dorsal part of the medulla oblongata (main site of neural control of vomiting)		*Stimulated by sights, smells, or emotional (psychic) experiences*
Chemoreceptor trigger zone (CTZ) located in the floor of the 4th ventricle (outside of the blood-brain barrier)	Serotonin 5-HT₃ receptors Dopamine D₂ receptors	*Stimulated by drugs and chemotherapeutic agents, toxins, hypoxia, uremia, acidosis, and radiation*

Adapted from Rizzo, D. (2006). Fundamentals of anatomy and physiology (2nd ed.). New York: Thomson Delmar Learning.

liquids, or ETOH ingestion. Certain central nervous system disorders, psychogenic disorders, metabolic disorders, involvement or irritation of the vagus or phrenic nerve, and general anesthesia can also cause hiccups.

GI Gas

This is a general category of symptoms associated with belching, bloating, **borborygmus** (hyperactive bowel sounds), abdominal pain, cramps, and **flatulence** (gas formed within the GI tract and expelled via the rectum). The average adult swallows air into the upper GI tract, and most of the gas in the stomach is from this source. Air swallowing occurs after meals because of gastric distension and lower esophageal sphincter relaxation. Oxygen extracted from air is readily absorbed, but more than 78 percent of air is nitrogen that is only minimally absorbed. If excessive amounts of air are swallowed **(aerophagia),** abdominal distension and pain, belching, and flatulence may be experienced. Belching can be normal, but excessive belching is related to aerophagia. Minor behavioral modification can resolve this problem. Patients who experience severe belching from aerophagia can reduce this by eating slowly, not using a straw when drinking, not drinking carbonated beverages, not smoking, and not chewing gum. If belching is associated with other GI symptoms, more assessment that is complete must be done.

Normally between 500 and 1,500 mL of gas are expelled by the rectum per day. Flatus is produced from a combination of fermentation gases of carbohydrates and swallowed air. If flatulence is associated with a malabsorption disorder, that is, the patient is losing weight, has diarrhea, or may be anemic, a diagnostic workup may be necessary. Lactase deficiency is a cause of increased intestinal gas production. Reducing lactulose in the diet reduces these symptoms. Additionally, counseling the patient to reduce foods that produce gas during digestion is helpful. A trial eliminating or reducing various foodstuffs (e.g., beans, brussels sprouts, broccoli, cabbage, onions, foodstuffs containing high amounts of fructose, maltose, or lactulose) known to produce large amounts of gas during digestion should be recommended. If excessive flatulence persists, the patient may need further workup for a functional GI disorder; other causes of increased gas production are malabsorption syndromes or ingesting poorly absorbed carbohydrates (e.g., sorbitol, lactose, or lactulose).

Diarrhea

Diarrhea can be acute, self-limiting, a life-threatening event, or chronic. By definition **diarrhea** is an increase in the liquid state of the stool. There may also be an increase in frequency. Diarrhea is differentiated into acute and chronic. The World Gastroenterology Organization has practice guidelines for management of the patient with diarrhea. The causes of diarrhea are categorized into osmotic, secretory, mucosal injury, or normal volume.

Acute Diarrhea

Acute diarrhea is less than three weeks in duration and is divided into noninflammatory and inflammatory. In noninflammatory diarrhea, there is an absence of fever, blood in the stool, or fecal leukocytes; whereas in inflammatory diarrhea there are systemic aspects that include fever. An infectious or irritating agent in the bowel usually causes acute diarrhea, except in inflammatory bowel disease and radiation diarrhea. A good history is important in understanding the link of acute diarrhea with a cause.

Noninflammatory Diarrhea

Noninflammatory diarrhea is linked with cramps, bloating, nausea, or vomiting. Noninflammatory diarrhea may be from small intestinal enteritis that is produced by bacteria that produce toxins (e.g., *Staphylococcus aureus, Escherichia coli*, or *Clostridium*). These types of bacterial agents interfere with normal absorption in the small intestine.

Inflammatory Diarrhea

Inflammatory diarrhea is marked by fever and bloody diarrhea, and a health care provider should suspect tissue damage to the colon caused by invasion of an infectious agent. Examples are *Shigella, Salmonella, Campylobacter,* amoebic dysentery, or from a toxin produced by the invading organism (e.g., *Clostridium difficile, E. coli*).

The difference between these diarrheal disorders and inflammatory diarrhea, is that there is usually a smaller amount of diarrheal stool; the symptoms are left lower quadrant (LLQ) cramping, urgency, and tenesmus. Fecal leukocytes are present in infections with invasive organisms. *E. coli* is acquired from eating contaminated, improperly prepared meat. It results in severe, hemorrhagic colitis. It is the most common cause of bloody diarrhea in adults and hemolytic uremic syndrome in children (Friedman, McQuaid, & Grendell, 2003).

Chronic Diarrhea

Chronic diarrhea is greater than three weeks in duration. The causes of chronic diarrhea include osmotic, malabsorption syndromes, secretory and inflammatory conditions, and motility disorders, and chronic infections.

Constipation

Constipation is marked by straining at stool with the production of hard stools, decreased frequency, and a feeling of not completely evacuating the colon. The number of bowel movements a patient has is individual, but if a patient has fewer than three bowel movements per week or must vigorously strain, the patient is considered to have constipation. Constipation is a common complaint. Idiopathic constipation results from colonic inertia, which is a delay in transit time in the large bowel, pelvic floor dysfunction (e.g., dyschezia, anismus, or outlet obstruction), or constipation with normal transit time due to irritable bowel syndrome (Friedman, et al., 2003). It is an increasing complaint of patients as they age. It affects women more than men. It is due to sedentary lifestyle, poor diets (low in dietary fiber and fluid),and medications. In general, the causes of constipation can be categorized into lifestyle, medications, structural abnormalities, systemic diseases, and refractory constipation.

Abdominal Pain

Abdominal pain is separated into acute and chronic. Acute abdominal pain, often described as acute abdomen, can be a life-threatening problem. Most of the pain fibers supplying the abdominal viscera are C fibers; C nerve fibers generate dull, poorly localized pain. Abdominal pain is dull, gnawing, or burning and poorly localized. Pain fibers supplying the parietal peritoneum are both A-delta fibers (A-delta fibers generate distinct and localized pain response), and C fibers so that pain is more distinct and localized. A patient will experience abdominal pain when nerve fibers in the serosal, muscular, and mucosal layers are either mechanically (stretched or spasm) or chemically (inflammation, irritation, or ischemic) stimulated. In solid organs of the abdomen, pain is noted only when the capsule of the organ is stretched or invaded, e.g. obstruction, congestion, or a space-occupying lesion (Yamada, 2005). During the assessment of pain (see Skills 360° feature), the nurse should establish the location, quality (e.g., burning, throbbing, twisting, sharp, stabbing, knife-like, colicky, cramping, constricting, penetrating, boring, brief, or constant), intensity, onset, duration, chronology, alleviating and aggravating factors, such as position, movement, food, or liquids, associated symptoms, radiation sites, and behaviors that put the patient at risk (e.g., heavy ETOH intake, NSAIDs use).

Skills 360°

Pneumonic for the Nurse Assessing Pain: PQRST

Provokes: What provokes the pain?

Quality—What makes it better/worse? What does it feel like?

Radiation: Where is it? Where does it radiate?

Severity—Rate the pain on a scale of 1–10.

Time and **T**reatment: How long have you had it? What has been done already?

Adapted from Estes, M. (2006). Health assessment and physical examination (3rd ed.). New York: Thomson Delmar Learning.

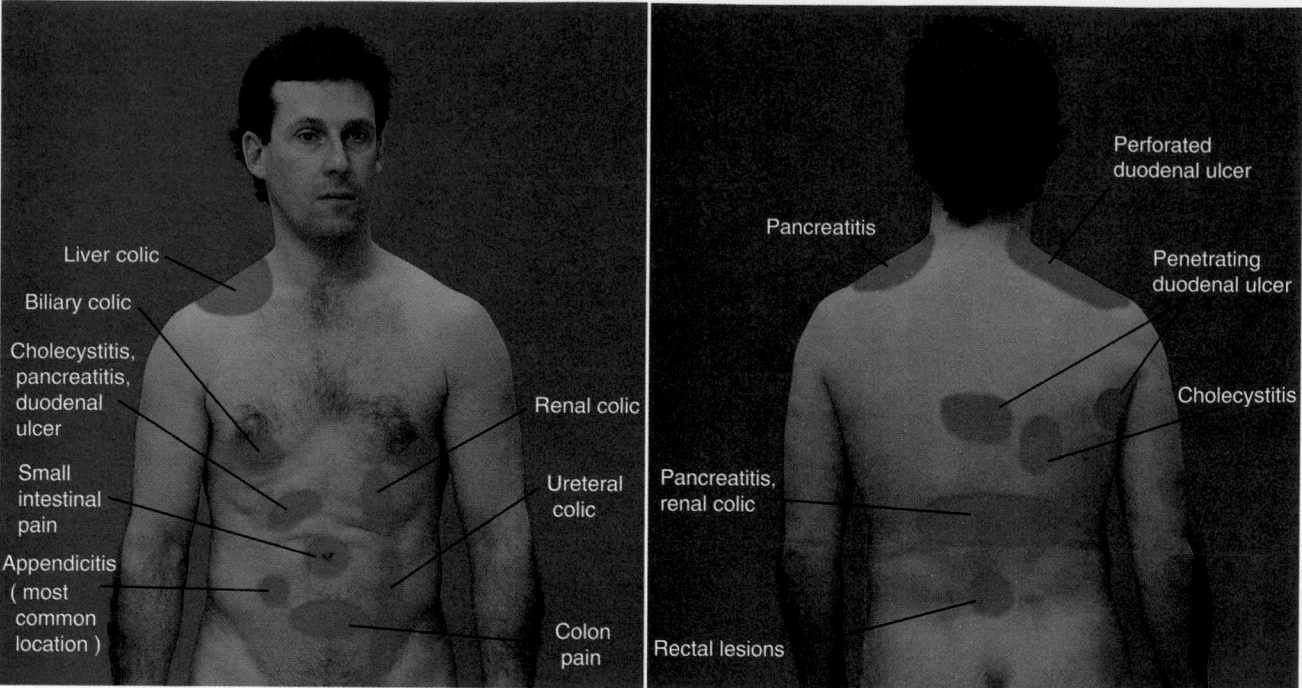

Figure 47-2 Areas of referred pain.

Referred Pain

Referred pain is noted in abdominal and GI disorders because of neuro-anatomic features (Figure 47-2) (Table 47-2). A single splanchnic nerve may provide sensory input from several abdominal organs and enter the spinal column at more than one level. Cutaneous and visceral afferent nerves end on the same secondary neuron in the dorsal horn of the spinal cord. This results in confusion by the brain of the place of the original stimulus (Friedman, et al., 2003).

Assessment

Although the GI tract begins in the mouth, the mouth and throat assessment is found in the chapters related to disorders of the head, eyes, ears, nose, and throat. When performing a GI assessment, the nurse uses all of the skills used in other types of assessments (Table 47-3).

Observation

When the nurse is looking, listening, thinking, and feeling, (those skills needed for good assessment) divide the abdomen into four quadrants and remember which organs are in each quadrant (Table 47-4). The four quadrants are right upper (RUQ), left upper (LUQ), right lower (RLQ), and left lower quadrant (LLQ).

As the nurse is performing the abdominal assessment, an organized approach to the patient is important. To perform the assessment, the patient should be lying supine. The abdomen should be exposed, the patient's head should be resting on a pillow (if the neck is flexed, the abdominal musculature may be contracted), and the knees should be bent to relax the abdomen. The room should be warm, and there should be suitable lighting. The nurse must note the appearance of the abdomen and describe whether it is flat, distended, enlarged, pulsatile, or symmetrical. The nurse can ask the patient to bear down to note any protrusion through weakened areas of the abdominal wall indicating potential ventral hernias. In addition, the nurse should note skin abnormalities and scars or the presence of jaundice, and cutaneous angiomas

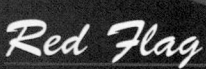

Serious Symptoms to Assess in an Abdominal Assessment

As an emergent condition associated with abdominal assessment, the nurse should observe how the patient is lying in the bed. If there is any guarding of the abdomen, there are serious conditions that should be considered (e.g., peritonitis, appendicitis). In addition, the nurse should note if the patient is lying still because of pain or if the patient is unable to find a position of comfort because of pain, which generally indicates a more serious condition.

Skills 360°

Skills the Nurse Demonstrates in Abdominal Assessment

Observation and inspection: looking with a careful eye in concert with cognitive thinking skills at the abdomen region.

Auscultation: occurs prior to palpation or percussion, because these techniques may alter normal bowel sounds. Auscultation uses a stethoscope to hear the sounds created by GI function.

Percussion: of the various structures to locate the organs beneath the abdominal wall, to establish the density of the various structures, and to check for swelling, fluid levels, or masses in the abdomen.

Palpation: When palpating the abdomen, the nurse must know both light and deep palpation. Palpation is performed to assess the size, location, and consistency of various structures in the abdomen (Figure 47-3).

Palpation and percussion: are also used to determine pain, tenderness, or masses in the abdominal cavity.

Adapted from Estes, M. (2006). Health assessment and physical examination (3rd ed.). New York: Thomson Delmar Learning.

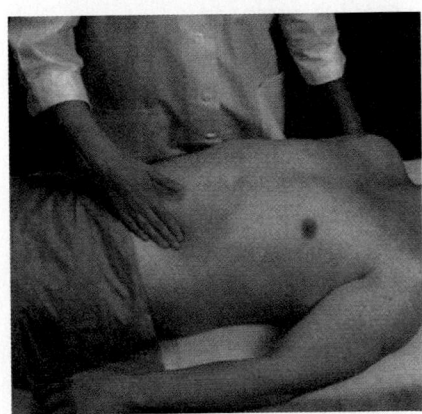

Figure 47-3 Light palpation of abdomen.

TABLE 47-2   Etiologies of Abdominal Pain: Anatomical Regions Where They Are Perceived

Right Upper Quadrant	Epigastrium	Left Upper Quadrant
Biliary stone	Abdominal aortic aneurysm	Gastric ulcer
Cholecystitis	Appendicitis (early)	Gastritis
Cholelithiasis	Biliary stone	Myocardial infarction
Duodenal ulcer	Cholecystitis	Pneumonia
Gastric ulcer	Diverticulitis	Splenic enlargement
Hepatic abscess	Gastroesophageal reflux disease	Splenic rupture
Hepatitis	Hiatal hernia	
Hepatomegaly		
Pancreatitis		
Pneumonia		

Periumbilical

Abdominal aortic aneurysm
Appendicitis (early)
Diverticulitis
Intestinal obstruction
Irritable bowel syndrome
Pancreatitis
Peptic ulcer
Recurrent abdominal pain (in children)
Volvulus

Right Lower Quadrant	Left Lower Quadrant
Appendicitis	Diverticulitis
Crohn's disease	Ectopic pregnancy (ruptured)
Diverticulitis	Endometriosis
Ectopic pregnancy (ruptured)	Hernia (strangulated)
Endometriosis	Irritable bowel syndrome
Hernia (strangulated)	Mittelschmerz
Irritable bowel syndrome	Ovarian cyst
Mittelschmerz	Pelvic inflammatory disease
Ovarian cyst	Renal calculi
Pelvic inflammatory disease	Salpingitis
Renal calculi	Ulcerative colitis
Salpingitis	

Diffuse

Gastroenteritis
Peritonitis

Adapted from Estes, M. (2006). Health assessment and physical examination (3rd ed.). New York: Thomson Delmar Learning.

(spider angiomas occur with portal hypertension). The nurse should note the umbilicus as to whether it is midline, inverted, or everted and whether there is any discoloration or inflammation or the presence of a hernia (note: Cullen's sign is a faint bluish color around the umbilicus secondary to hemoperitoneum [intra-abdominal bleeding]).

Auscultation

Auscultation is performed prior to palpation or percussion because touching the abdomen may change the tone of the bowel. The diaphragm of the stethoscope is used, and the nurse should warm the hands assessing the diaphragm

TABLE 47-3 Assessment of Abdomen: Normal and Key Findings

AREA OF ASSESSMENT/*NORMAL FINDINGS*	KEY FINDINGS
Abdomen: Inspect, Auscultate, Percuss, and Palpate	
Place patient in a supine position with knees flexed over a pillow, hands at sides or across chest. Undrape patient from xiphoid process to symphysis pubis to expose the abdomen.	Promotes relaxation of the abdominal muscles.

1. Stand at right side of patient.
   a. Inspect abdomen from rib margin to pubic bone. Note contour and symmetry (observing for peristalsis, pulsations, scars, striae, or masses).
   b. Inspect umbilicus for contour, location, signs of inflammation, or hernia.
   c. Observe for smooth, even respiratory movement.
   d. Observe for surface motion (visible peristalsis).
   e. Inspect epigastric area for pulsations. *Contour is flat or rounded and bilaterally symmetrical. Umbilicus is depressed and beneath the abdominal surface. Abdomen rises with inspirations and falls with expirations, free from respiratory retractions. Visible peristalsis slowly traverses the abdomen in a slanting downward movement as observed in thin patients. Pulsations of the abdominal aorta are visible in the epigastric area in thin patients.*

1. A convex symmetrical profile reveals either a protuberant abdomen (results of poor muscle tone from inadequate exercise or obesity) or distension (taut stretching of skin across abdominal wall). Asymmetry may indicate a mass, bowel obstruction, enlargement of abdominal organs, or scoliosis. Umbilicus bulging may indicate a hernia. Old scars are flat with a shiny appearance, blending with patient's pigmentation; new scars are raised and reddened. Atrophic lines or streaks reveal linea albicantes (striae) that occur with tumors, obesity, ascites, and pregnancy. Engorged or dilated veins around the umbilicus are associated with circulatory obstruction of superior or inferior vena cava. Uneven respiratory movement with retractions may indicate appendicitis. Strong peristaltic movement may indicate intestinal obstruction. Marked pulsations in epigastric area may indicate an aortic aneurysm.

2. Auscultate the abdominal quadrants for bowel sounds (high-pitched) using the diaphragm of the stethoscope.
   a. Begin by placing the diaphragm on the RLQ. Listen for a full minute to the frequency and character of the bowel sounds.
   b. Repeat Step a, proceeding in sequence to RUQ, LUQ, and LLQ.
   c. Listen at least 5 minutes before concluding the absence of bowel sounds. *High-pitched sounds, heard every 5 to 15 seconds as intermittent gurgling sounds in all four quadrants as a result of air and fluid movement in the gastrointestinal tract. Bowel sounds should always be heard at the ileocecal valve area.*

2. Hypoactive or diminished bowel sounds are soft and low and widely separated so that only one or two are heard in a 2-minute interval. Hypoactive is normal the first few hours after general anesthesia. Hypoactive sounds may indicate decreased motility of the bowel, such as occurs with peritoneal irritation or paralytic ileus. Absent bowels sounds (none heard for 3 to 5 minutes) may signal paralytic ileus, peritonitis, or an obstruction. Hyperactive (loud, audible, gurgling sounds similar to stomach growling; sounds also called borborygmi) may occur with diarrhea or hunger. Rushed, high-pitched, or tingling sounds suggest air or fluid under pressure; this may occur in the early stages of an intestinal blockage when heard in the portion of the bowel that precedes the obstruction (Estes, 2002).

3. Auscultate with bell of stethoscope over the aorta, epigastric area, renal arteries, and femoral arteries. Note bruits over each area. *Free from audible bruits.*

3. A bruit over an abdominal vessel reveals turbulent blood flow suggestive of an aortic aneurysm or partial obstruction (e.g., renal or femoral stenosis).

4. Percuss all quadrants in a systematic fashion. Begin percussion in RLQ, move upward to RUQ, cross over to LUQ, and down to LLQ. Note when tympany changes to dullness. *Tympany is heard because of air in the stomach and intestines. Dullness is heard over organs (e.g., the liver).*

4. Dullness over the stomach or intestines may indicate a mass or tumor, **ascites** (excessive fluid accumulation in the abdominal cavity), or full intestines.

5. Perform light palpation. Never palpate over areas where bruits are auscultated.
   a. Instruct patient to cough. If patient experiences a sharp twinge of pain in a quadrant, palpate that area last.
   b. With patient's hands and forearms on a horizontal plane, use fingerpads to depress the abdominal wall 1 cm in all four quadrants. Begin palpation in RLQ, move upward to RUQ, cross over to LUQ, and down to LLQ. Note texture and consistency of underlying tissue. *Should feel smooth with consistent softness.*

5. Tenderness and increased skin temperature may indicate inflammation. Large masses may be due to tumors, feces, or enlarged organs.

Adapted from Estes, M. (2006). Health assessment and physical examination (3rd ed.). New York: Thomson Delmar Learning.

Red Flag

Assessments for Acute Appendicitis

Rebound tenderness (Blumberg's sign): is a positive response, which may mean peritoneal irritation. The tips of the fingers are pressed gently into the abdominal wall and then suddenly withdrawn. A painful response is positive. Cutaneous hyperesthesia is elicited in the area of the skin over an appendix that is inflamed. Rebound tenderness is a classic sign of appendicitis (Figure 47-4).

Iliopsoas muscle test: The patient is asked to flex the right thigh (raises the right leg) against resistance (pushing down over the lower part of the thigh). The patient will experience pain in the pelvis because of irritation of the Iliopsoas muscle (Figure 47-5).

Obturator muscle test: The patient flexes the right thigh (raises the right leg) to 90 degrees. Holding the ankle, the leg is rotated internally and externally. If pelvic pain is produced is the muscle is inflamed (Figure 47-6).

TABLE 47-4 **The Four Quadrants of the Abdomen**

RUQ	LUQ
Liver	Stomach
Gallbladder	Spleen
Head of pancreas	Left lobe of liver
Right kidney and adrenal gland 1	Pancreas
Duodenum	Left kidney and adrenal gland
Hepatic flexure of colon	Splenic flexure of colon
Part of ascending and transverse colon	Part of transverse and descending colon
RLQ	**LLQ**
Cecum	Part of descending colon
Appendix	Sigmoid colon
Right ovary	Left ovary
Right ureter	Left ureter
Right spermatic cord	Left spermatic cord

Adapted from Estes, M. (2006). Health assessment and physical examination (3rd ed.). New York: Thomson Delmar Learning.

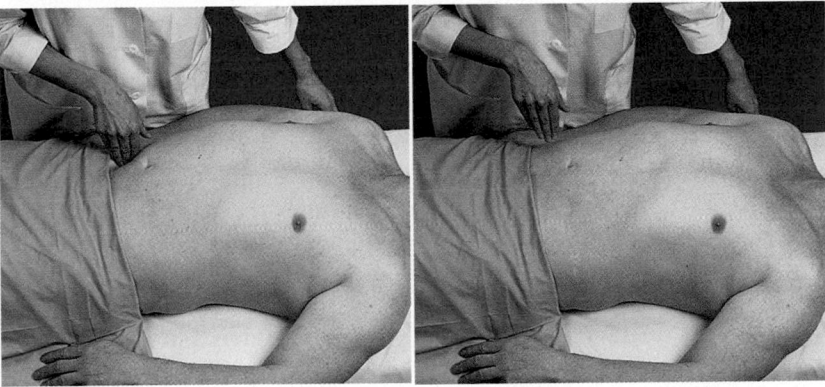

Figure 47-4 Rebound tenderness.

prior to placing on the abdomen. Then, the nurse listens in each of the four quadrants of the abdomen for approximately 20 seconds. Are bowel sounds (peristalsis) present? Describe the frequency and the quality of the sounds. Normally bowel sounds are usually heard every 2 to 5 seconds. Hyperactive bowel sounds are termed borborygmus; to declare absent bowel sound, then a nurse must listen for three to five minutes. In addition, the nurse must listen for vascular sounds; normally no vascular sounds or bruits are heard unless the patient has hypertension.

Percussion

The purpose of percussing the abdomen is to elicit either of two sounds: (a) tympanic (drum-like): this sound is produced over air filled structures; and (b) dull sounds: these sounds are produced over a solid structure (e.g., liver or a mass) or fluid (ascites or a full bladder). During percussion, notice if the patient experiences any pain as this may be a sign of peritoneal inflammation. Ordinarily you may not be able to percuss the liver, because it is not below the costal margin, although it may normally be 1 or 2 centimeters below the costal margin. In an individual with liver disease, you would be able to percuss as well as palpate the liver margins. The spleen is not normally percussed unless there is significant

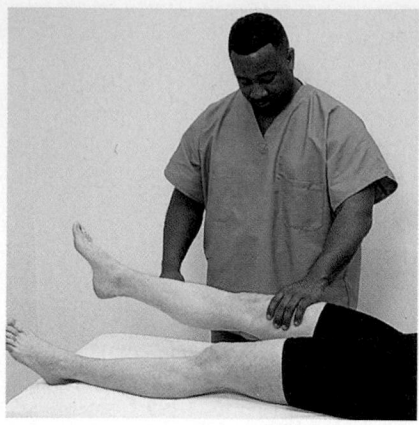

Figure 47-5 Iliopsoas muscle test.

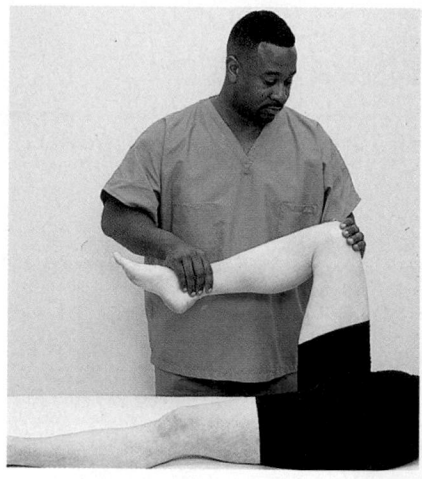

Figure 47-6 Obturator muscle test.

enlargement. Stomach contents often conceal the dull sound produced when percussing the spleen.

If the patient is suspected of having abdominal ascites, there are special maneuvers that the nurse can use to determine fluid in the abdomen. The first is the fluid wave. Shifting dullness is the second maneuver to test for ascites. With the patient lying supine, percuss over the top of the abdomen, this should elicit a tympany; moving down the side to the area of fluid should elicit a dull sound. Turn the patient onto his or her right side, the fluid will shift right. Percuss the upper left side of the abdomen, and tympany should be elicited; continue downward and the sound should change to dull at the level of the fluid shift.

Palpation

To assess the abdomen with palpation, first use light or gentle palpation. Assess each quadrant of the abdomen. This first pass is a scouting expedition that provides the nurse with information about any areas of tenderness or increased resistance.

Light Palpation

To perform light (gentle) palpation, place the palm of the hand lightly and firmly on the abdomen, gently press the fingers into the abdominal wall about 1 cm. If the patient is ticklish, have the patient place his or her fingers on top of your fingers. Often this reduces the ticklishness. Note any areas of tenderness. Areas of tenderness will require more careful assessment once the gentle palpation is completed.

Deep Palpation

Deep palpation involves using the pads and tips (most sensitive areas) of the index, middle, and ring fingers. The motion should be downward (depth of 4 to 5 cm), and the finger pads should move backward and forward to cause the abdominal wall to glide over the structures under the targeted area. To palpate the liver, bimanual palpitation is recommended. The right hand is inserted under the right rib margin. The left hand is placed under the right lower thorax. While the patient is taking a deep breath, the right hand is moved upward and inward. With the left hand move the right thorax upward. The lower margin of the liver will be palpated. It is unusual to be able to palpate the gallbladder. It lies on the posterior surface of the liver just right of the midclavicular line. When the gallbladder is inflamed, it is exquisitely tender. It is important to assess for Murphy's sign, where the patient is asked to breathe in while the examiners fingers are held under the liver border. This allows the gallbladder to descend. **Murphy's sign** is when the patient will guard the movement by an inspiratory arrest secondary to painful contact with the fingers, which confirms cholecystitis (inflamed gallbladder).

During the deep palpation, if any mass or enlargement is noted, the nurse should collect the following information: location, size, shape, surface, consistency (soft, hard, firm, spongy, or nodular), movement, pulsatile, pain, tenderness, and whether the mass is reducible.

Liver

Normally the liver does not descend beyond 1 to 2 cm of the costal margin and is not palpable. There are two methods to assess the liver. The nurse must use deep bimanual palpation to determine liver size. With the patient taking a deep breath, the nurse holds his or her fingers pointing up and parallel to the rectus muscles. The nurse pushes in and up toward the costal margin. The second method is for the nurse to place the right hand under the patient at about the 12th rib. With this hand, the nurse pushes upward. At the same time, the left hand is placed parallel to the rectus muscles with fingers pointing up toward the costal margin. The patient is asked to take a deep breath, and the nurse presses upward and inward. If the liver is palpable, the nurse will feel the liver roll (slip) under the palpating fingers.

Gallbladder

The gallbladder sits posterior to the liver. It is not palpable. Assessment of the gallbladder will be more appropriate taking an accurate history of the potential symptoms the patient has with dysfunction. For example, patients with gallbladder dysfunction may have upper epigastric pain, fatty food intolerance, and nausea.

Spleen

The spleen is not normally palpable. If the spleen is felt, it is softer than the liver. If it is enlarged, it must be measured in centimeters below the costal margin. Because a spleen can be damaged, especially if enlarged, the palpation should be done carefully. The nurse stands on the right side of the patient. With the left hand around the back of the patient, the nurse lifts the left rib cage to push the spleen forward. With the right hand, the nurse asks the patient to take in a deep breath and gently pushes in and up toward the left costal margin.

Pancreas

The pancreas is not palpable. Patients with dysfunction of the pancreas will likely have a supporting history of clinical manifestations related to the etiology of the disorder (e.g., alcoholism or cancer).

Kidneys and Urinary Bladder

To palpate the right kidney, the nurse places his or her left hand under the right flank while lifting forward in an attempt to push the kidney toward the anterior wall. With the right hand, the nurse deeply palpates the anterior wall just below the right costal margin while the patient takes a deep breath. The left kidney is rarely palpable but is palpated the same as the right kidney.

To assess the bladder, the patient should be asked to empty the bladder prior to the assessment. In addition, palpation is light in nature, and the nurse must pay attention to privacy and instruct the patient to relax during the assessment.

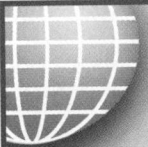

Real World, Real Choices

Abdominal Pain, Unknown Etiology

Mrs. Cynthia Reyes is a 56-year-old female, who is admitted to the medical floor due to blood in the stool and abdominal pain for three days. She is primarily going to be assessed with a variety of laboratory and diagnostic tests. A review of systems reveals bowel habit changes, loss of appetite, weight loss greater than 10 pounds, and fatigue for two months. Mrs. Reyes past medical history includes primary hypertension, obesity, GERD, and constipation. The patient's medications include hydrochlorothiazide (HCTZ) 25 mg by mouth every day, omeprazole 20 mg by mouth every day as needed, and Metamucil as needed. The patient's nutritional intake is usually high in fat, low in fiber, and less than two servings of fruits and vegetables per day. Her fluid intake consists primarily of sodas, tea or coffee, and possibly two cups of water per day. Mrs. Reyes' activity is sedentary, and her social history includes working as a clerical assistant for 25 years. She has been smoking cigarettes for 20 years,

has an occasional alcohol intake of two to three drinks per week, and denies the use of illicit drugs.

An assessment of Mrs. Reyes reveals that she has GI bleeding and recent history of abdominal pain. Her vital signs are: temperature 36.8° C (98.2° F), pulse 69, respiration 18, and blood pressure 112/56. Bowel sounds normal on four quadrants; tympanic to percussion; no costovertebral angle (CVA) tenderness; pain elicited on palpation of left lower quadrant; palpable mass noted on left lower quadrant area. Patient's skin color is pink and has good turgor. Rectal exam reveals 3-by-4-cm palpable lesion with stool positive for occult blood. Neurological system shows patient to be awake, alert, and oriented for three hours. A psychosocial assessment reveals her to appear nervous, crying, and fearful; patient states she has not been in the hospital since her husband died 10 years ago.

What would your nursing care plan be for Mrs. Reyes?

Umbilicus

Normally the umbilicus is midway between the xyphoid process and the pubis. During the assessment, the nurse should note the shape of the umbilicus. It can be round, oval, recessed, or protruding. An umbilical hernia will be noted during the assessment. With the patient lying supine, the nurse should ask him or her to raise his or her head and shoulder off the examining table. This maneuver contracts the rectus muscles. Normally the abdomen remains symmetrical. If a bulge appears in the midline, the patient may have diastasis recti, a separation of the layers of the muscle.

Referred Pain from Abdominal Structures

There is often pain that is referred from abdominal structures (see Figure 47-2). An assessment of the perianal area (anus and rectosigmoid structures) can reveal such pain. With the patient in a lateral position, a lithotomy (knee-chest) position, or standing position, the nurse visually inspects the area. Both the right and left buttocks are spread to observe the area. The skin around the anus is a dark reddish brown. Note if the skin is intact. Any abnormalities can be described using the face of a clock for location. The anal canal is 2.5 to 4 cm. long. It is surrounded by an external sphincter and internal sphincter. Visually inspect for any external hemorrhoids. Have the patient bear down. There should be no prolapse of any rectal tissue during this maneuver. The pilonidal area (sacrococcygeal) should be carefully inspected and palpated. There should be no edema, induration, or dimpling. With a gloved hand the nurse should place the lubricated finger against the anal verge. Apply firm pressure until you feel the rectal sphincter begin to relax. Slowly insert one finger in the direction of the umbilicus. Insert the pad of the finger first and rotate to introduce the tip of the finger. Continue to rotate the finger to assess the muscular ring of the anal canal. The mucosal surface should feel smooth. Palpate the anal canal and rectum up to about 8 to 10 cm. The nurse should explain to the patient that he or she may feel as if having a bowel movement.

DIAGNOSTIC TESTS

There are a wide variety of diagnostic tests performed for GI disorders. A wide variety of hematological blood tests can be used to confirm areas within the GI tract or accessory organs. These labs can be referred to in laboratory and diagnostic texts, such as that by Daniels (2003). The more common procedures will be covered, such as bowel preparations, nasogastric intubations, feeding tubes, and barium studies. Ensuring quality nursing care, following good nursing education principles, and applying therapeutic communication skills is essential for the patient undergoing diagnostic tests for the GI system (see Ethics in Practice feature).

In addition, when performing many GI procedures, it is standard that the patient is sedated. The technique used today is conscious sedation and is often managed by the nurse in the gastroenterology procedures lab. The nurse who manages conscious sedation has received additional education to manage the patient receiving these agents. These patients are at risk for cardiorespiratory complications from sedation that depresses the central cardiorespiratory center. Patients receiving conscious sedation are usually able to respond to verbal commands throughout the procedure. They can communicate discomfort, and they respond to light tactile stimulation. Airway patency is maintained, and spontaneous ventilation must be satisfactory to maintain adequate oxygenation. To ensure this patients are monitored with pulse oximetry (SpO_2—arterial oxyhemoglobin saturation), a necessary vital sign. The National Guidelines Clearinghouse has established guidelines for patients undergoing conscious sedation. A brief period of amnesia that erases any memory of the

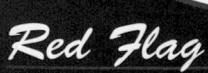

Red Flag

Enema Administration

Patients with severe abdominal pain, ulcerative colitis, or a history of megacolon should have a written order before enemas can be administered, because these conditions would normally prohibit the use of standard bowel preparation procedures, such as administration of laxatives and cleansing enemas.

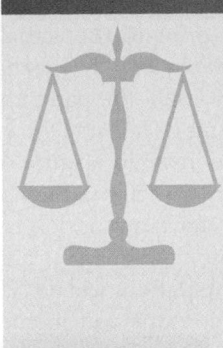

ETHICS IN PRACTICE

Hepatitis Risks

A 29-year-old man who recently emigrated from a third world country is seeking follow-up care for abdominal pain. On the first visit, you completed his health history and physical examination and obtained laboratory data. Your clinical suspicion is confirmed; the results of the lab tests show that he has hepatitis B. This man is sexually active with his wife. You inform him that it is important that his wife be clinically evaluated. He tells you that he will not have health care insurance for her through his job until next year, and it is too expensive for her to be seen until then. How would you respond? What information would you give to him?

procedure occurs with the use of conscious sedation. Patients should be made aware of this prior to the procedure.

Colonoscopy

Bowel cleansing is necessary for all colonoscopy procedures. The bowel preparation selected depends on the reasons for the procedure. It is important for the nurse to reinforce the importance of following the preparation as ordered by the provider. An adequate procedure cannot be done without adequate preparation of the bowel. The preparation procedure is rigorous, and the patient may have difficulty drinking the large amount of liquids necessary for a complete preparation, but it is essential.

If a clear view of the bowel mucosa is necessary, polyethylene glycol, an electrolyte solution (PEG-ES) is used. The patient is placed on a clear liquid diet for 24 hours prior to the procedure. The polyethylene glycol solution (GoLYTELY and CoLyte) is administered the day before the procedure. It is mixed in a one gallon container and refrigerated. An 8-ounce glass of the preparation is ingested rapidly every 10 minutes until the patient has taken the entire amount. Within about one hour of beginning the preparation, the patient will begin to have bowel movements. The stool will become watery, clear, and free of any solid material.

A second preparation material used is Fleet's phospho-soda. This preparation is also used for colonoscopy. The patient takes two 1.5-ounce doses of the laxative. The first dose is taken in the afternoon before the procedure, followed by 10 ounces of clear liquid and then three to five additional glasses of clear liquids prior to going to bed. Before bedtime, the patient should take the second 1.5 ounces of the Fleet's phospho-soda with the same amount of clear liquid or as directed.

Small-volume enemas may be necessary in the bowel preparation prior to the colonoscopy (or other diagnostic procedures of the bowel). The enema may be self-administered and is available OTC. Advise the patient to use the enema as the instructions on the package indicate.

A pill-based enema preparation is also available. Visicol (sodium phosphate monobasic monohydrate, USP; sodium phosphate dibasic anhydrous, USP). It is a laxative that is used for bowel preparation. Twenty pills are taken over a one-hour period the afternoon before the procedure. At bedtime, the physician may order up to eight more tablets, four at a time every 15 minutes with 8 ounces of water. Dulcolax (bisacodyl USP) tablets, a laxative, may be added to complete this regimen.

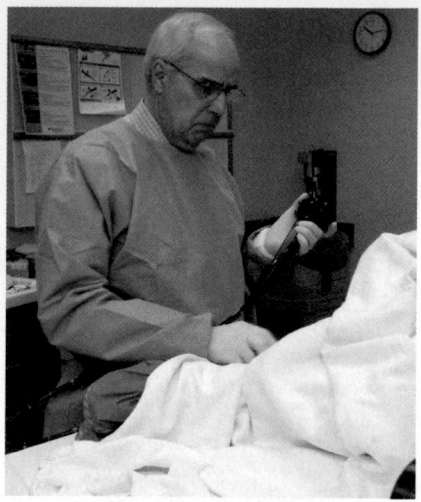

Figure 47-7 A colonoscopy in use to examine the bowel.

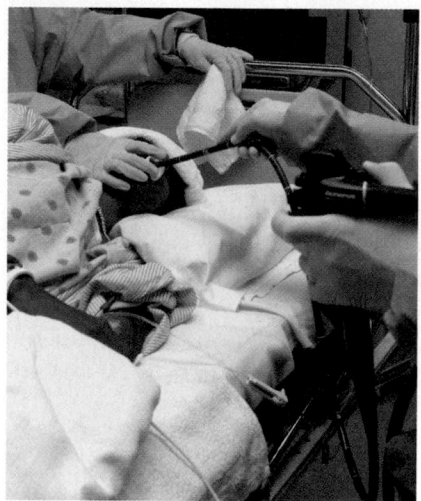

Figure 47-8 An upper endoscopy.

Continuing with bowel preparation, the patient should take nothing by mouth (NPO) for six hours prior to the actual procedure. Some medications may be taken with a sip of water, but the patient must confirm this with the provider. During the procedure itself, the patient may be consciously sedated. In addition, the patient is kept on his or her side during the procedure or positioned in a manner to keep the scope inserted (Figure 47-7). After the procedure, the patient is monitored for a return to a normal LOC and the ability to be discharged.

Patients may not have to undergo bowel preparation if they are being worked-up for chronic diarrhea. For an upper endoscopy, esophagogastroduodenoscopy (EGD), the patient will be NPO. If a patient is undergoing a 24-hour pH study of gastric contents, all medications that suppress gastric secretions would be stopped prior to the test. A patient who is undergoing capsule endoscopy is kept NPO just as with an EGD. During the procedure, the patient is usually managed with conscious sedation until it is finished (Figure 47-8). After the procedure, the patient is usually allowed liquids and food as tolerated.

Laparoscopy

Laparoscopy is a diagnostic procedure where the peritoneal cavity, pelvis and abdomen, is examined. This test is used to detect cysts, adhesions, fibroids, infections of the uterus, fallopian tubes, and ovaries; ectopic pregnancies, liver lacerations, and cirrhosis. The test may also be used for lysis of adhesions, ovarian biopsy, tubal sterilization, foreign body removal, and fulguration of endometriotic implants.

The patient is instructed on fast for eight hours before the surgery; the test is performed either with a local or general anesthetic agent, and the patient is placed in a lithotomy position. Then the patient is catheterized to ensure the bladder is empty, which avoids puncture of the bladder during the test with the laparoscope.

Proctosigmoidoscopy

This is a diagnostic test that takes three steps: (a) digital examination to dilate the anal sphincters to detect obstruction that might hinder passage of the endoscope, (b) a sigmoidoscope to examine the distal sigmoid colon and rectum, and (c) a proctoscope to examine the lower rectum and anal canal. The proctosigmoidoscopy is used to identify internal hemorrhoids, hypertrophic anal papillae, polyps, fissures, fistulae, and rectal and anal abscesses.

The patient is instructed on dietary restrictions and bowel preparations on an individual basis. If the patient has rectal inflammation, a local anesthetic agent is applied to decrease discomfort. Conscious sedation is often used. The patient is secured to a tilting table that rotates into horizontal and vertical positions.

Paracentesis

Paracentesis is the aspiration of fluid from the abdominal cavity. This test can either be diagnostic, therapeutic, or both. For instance, with end-stage liver or renal disease there is ascites (an accumulation of fluid in the abdomen). Pressure caused from the ascites can interfere with breathing and GI functioning. Aspiration in this instance is therapeutic. If a culture specimen is obtained, it is also diagnostic.

Have the patient void and obtain a body weight before the procedure. Place the patient in a high Fowler's position in a chair or sitting on the side of the bed. The skin is prepared, anesthetized, and punctured with a **trocar** (a large bored abdominal paracentesis needle). The trocar is held perpendicular to the abdominal wall and advanced into the peritoneal cavity. When fluid appears, the trocar is removed, leaving the inner catheter in place to drain the fluid. Observe the patient for pressure changes that can result from the rapid removal of fluid.

Postprocedure apply a sterile dressing to the puncture site. Monitor the patient for changes in vital signs and electrolytes. Instruct the patient to record the color, amount, and consistency of drainage on the dressing after discharge.

Nasogastric Tubes

A nasogastric tube can be inserted orally but is most often inserted nasally into the stomach. The size and type of tube selected is dependent on the indication. The tube is used for feeding or administration of medications, especially if the patient has impaired swallowing or is not able to ingest sufficient calories, secondary to neurological or other deficits impairing ability to ingest sufficient nutrition. A feeding tube may be placed distal to the pylorus or the ligament of Treitz (nasoduodenal or nasojejunal) if there is risk of gastroesophageal reflux, aspiration, gastroparesis, or other reasons to bypass the stomach.

In addition, a nasogastric tube provides a method for performing a **lavage** (the irrigation or washing out of the stomach contents). Patients may need to have this procedure performed after swallowing poisons, medications, and toxic substances.

Decompression of the stomach is performed to prevent vomiting or reduction of pancreatic or biliary stimulation especially if the patient has acute pancreatitis or if the patient persistently has gastric residual volumes greater 400 mL.

Esophageal Manometry

Esophageal manometry is a test that measures the pressure and activity of the esophagus in patients who exhibit esophageal motility problems. It is done with patients who have dysphagia, achalasia (cardiospasm), GERD, to exclude scleroderma, or for placement of a pH probe for 24-hour esophageal pH monitoring.

Secretin Testing

Secretin testing is used to determine if a patient has incipient chronic pancreatitis. It is indicated for patients with abdominal pain, weight loss, steatorrhea, or recurrent pancreatitis. The tube used is a Dreiling tube. It is a double-lumen tube with ports in the gastric and duodenal regions. The tube is inserted into the stomach and positioned so that the distal portion is past the ligament of Treitz. Once in place, aspirate is obtained from both the duodenal and gastric port. The pH of the gastric aspirate is checked. The gastric port is aspirated until there is no return of gastric contents. The duodenal aspirate is sent to the lab for cytology and HCO^-_3 levels. A test dose of secretin is administered intravenously to rule out an allergic response. If the allergic response is negative, the full dose is administered. Once the dose is administered, a duodenal aspirate is collected every 20 minutes for a total of four samples. A portion of the sample is placed into a collection tube for HCO^-_3 levels and placed on ice. The remaining fluid is pooled and sent for cytology.

The diagnostic results reveal cytology that should be negative. If positive, pancreatic cancer is suspected. If the HCO^-_3 is less than 90 mEq/L in all samples and the total volume is greater than or equal to 2 mL/kg the diagnosis is chronic pancreatitis.

Equipment for Gastric and Intestinal Intubation

The selection of the tube to use for oral and nasal gastric and intestinal intubation depends on the reason the patient needs the tube to be inserted. Other items needed are water and a straw to drink, emesis basin and towel, tongue blade, water-soluble lubricant and sometimes lidocaine jelly or atomized lidocaine to reduce pain during insertion, irrigating syringe, scissors, tape (Hy-

Tape, the original Pink Tape is recommended) or appropriate dressing to secure tube, and stethoscope to check for gastric insufflation.

Gastric decompression tubes (e.g., Salem Sump tube) are polyvinyl chloride tubes in both adult and pediatric sizes; measured in French diameters (10-, 12-, 14-, 16-Fr diameter). This tube has a double lumen; one is for suction of the gastric contents while the other is for the sump vent. The purpose of the sump vent is to allow air to prevent the main suction tube from adhering to the gastric mucosa or irritating the mucosal wall. This tube has a radiopaque line that allows for visualization of placement with a postplacement X-ray.

Gastric lavage tubes (e.g., Ewald) are large-bore 34-Fr outer diameter tubes used to irrigate the esophagus or the stomach with large volumes of irrigant solution. This tube is used when the aim is to remove particulate matter, e.g., bezoars, clots, or ingested toxins.

Intestinal decompression tubes (e.g., Andersen, Miller-Abbott) are tubes used to decompress the small intestine in the early management of mechanical obstruction without strangulation (Gowen, 2003). These tubes have a tungsten weighted inflatable latex balloon tip. The tubes have 24 aspiration ports designed to screen out material that could block the tubes. The tubes advance via peristaltic movement. Enough slack must be allowed so the tubes can advance. The tubes should not be fixed to the nostril until they have reached their placement point. There may be an order for a prokinetic medication, like metoclopramide or erythromycin, to enhance peristalsis. Distension of the stomach with injection of 350 to 1,000 mL of air can also enhance movement of the tubes.

Potentially these tubes can cause necrosis to the mucosal wall if they are not allowed to move with the peristaltic wave. These tubes are removed at 30-minute intervals, 30 cm at a time. Additionally the weighted tip can pass through the rectum. The capsule section is cut off, and the tube is removed according to instructions. Endoscopic placement is useful in any patient that has any problem that might obstruct easy access through the nasopharynx and esophagus into the stomach.

Wire-guided tube placement enhances the advancement of a nasogastric, nasoduodenal, or nasojejunal tube. A hazard of the wire-guided tube less than 4 mm is that it could potentially penetrate the trachea, perforate a bronchus, and enter the pleural space with minimal resistance. Feeding tubes with weighted tips have been used to enhance movement through the pylorus into the duodenum; however, evidence now indicates that a weighted tip is unnecessary (Marik & Zaloga, 2003).

Patient Preparation for Nasogastric and Nasointestinal Intubation

The nurse explains the procedure to the patient, why the tube is to be inserted, and how long it is anticipated that the tube will remain in place. The patient is kept NPO prior to the procedure (see Patient Playbook feature).

Contraindications and Complications

Contraindications for placement of nasogastric tubes are seen in patients with trauma to the maxillofacial structures or those suspected of possible basal skull fracture.

Complications for placement of nasogastric tubes include trauma that could occur during insertion or removal of the tube. This might be nasal, pharyngeal, laryngeal, esophageal, or gastric trauma or perforation. In the event a tube was inserted in a patient with maxillofacial trauma, intracranial penetration might occur.

In addition, while a nasogastric tube is in place patients might experience pulmonary aspiration, mucosal ulceration or irritation, and fluid and electrolyte imbalance.

PATIENT PLAYBOOK

Insertion of a Nasogastric Tube

- Ask the patient if he has ever had a nasogastric tube inserted before.
- Determine if there is any nasal obstruction or maxillofacial trauma.
- While holding closed one nostril, ask patient to inhale strongly through each nostril. Use the nostril that appears more patent.
- Check the gag reflex. A patient without a gag reflex is at risk for pulmonary aspiration.
- Procedure:
  - Have the patient sit upright (raise the head of the bed). If the patient is not able to cooperate, place the patient in a left lateral position. (This position decreases the risk of pulmonary aspiration.)
  - Placement of the tube depends on the purpose for the tube and the destination.
  - Estimate the length of tube to be inserted One formula suggested for determining length of insertion is the following formula which is $(NEX - 50)/2 + 50$ cm, where N is the shortest distance from the nose (N) to the earlobe (E) to the xyphoid (X) process. The insertion should be halfway between 50 cm and the xyphoid mark.
  - Lubricate the tube, have patient hold head down, insert tube horizontally to avoid abrading the turbinates. When the tip is at the pharyngeal wall, have patient sip water (dry swallow if NPO) as the tube is advanced. For the patient, this is the most uncomfortable part of the procedure. If the nurse meets resistance, withdraw the tube and retry. Do *not* force the tube. If the patient coughs, becomes cyanotic, or is unable to speak, remove the tube as it may have entered the trachea.
  - Steps to prevent the tube from entering the trachea must be taken in any situation where the patient cannot swallow on request, has an endotracheal tube in place, or a tracheostomy. These patients are at greater risk for inadvertent tracheal placement of the nasogastric tube. It has been reported that 2 percent of patients who have small-bore feeding tubes placed, enter the trachea with major complications occurring in 0.7 percent and death in 0.2 percent (Angus & Burakoff, 2003).
- While advancing the tube the nurse must observe for cough or hoarseness.
- Advance the tube to the predetermined length, checking periodically to see if the tube has coiled in the pharynx or mouth.
- To determine if the tube may have entered the trachea, place the end of the tube under water to observe for air bubbles. Another technique is to inject air into the port and auscultate the stomach to listen for the rush of air (gastric insufflation) into the stomach. A technique not often used is to sample for CO_2 from the tube. Unfortunately, these techniques are not as sensitive as endoscopic placement or radiographic guidance. If the tube is in the trachea, advancing the tube for proper stomach length 40 to 45 cm will cause lung injury.
- Confirm proper placement of the tube with a postinsertion X-ray. Aspirate the stomach contents and assess pH. A pH less than 4 indicates the aspirate is from stomach contents unless the patient is receiving proton-pump inhibitors.
- If the tube is to advance into the duodenum, the patient should be placed in the right decubitus position for several hours. Tape the tube with 20 to 30 cm of slack to allow for the tube to advance via peristalsis. If the tube is to advance to the jejunum, after the slack is gone, have patient lie on his or her back and then left decubitus position to encourage movement of the tube into the jejunum.
- If the position of the tube is assessed fluoroscopically, irrigate the tube to remove any contrast material and to maintain patency of the tube.

Adapted from Estes, M. (2006). Health assessment and physical examination *(3rd ed.). New York: Thomson Delmar Learning.*

Esophageal Dilation

Esophageal dilation is performed when a patient experiences peptic strictures often related to GERD. Another cause of esophageal stricture can be radiation, which is labeled Schatzki's ring. Treatment of these esophageal conditions is often an esophageal dilation procedure, which entails widening of the stricture with dilators, called bougies, of graded sizes (Price, 2004).

Preprocedure preparation includes NPO for six to eight hours. The patient may have conscious sedation, but most often only the pharynx is anesthetized with a topical agent. The procedure is usually done with three sequential dilators. The goal of the procedure is to relieve the difficulty the patient has with swallowing.

Feeding Tubes: Gastrostomy and Jejunostomy

Feeding tubes are placed when a patient is unable to manage his or her needed nutritional intake. Patients require 25 to 30 kcal/kg/day and 30 mL free water/kg/day. The American Society of Parenteral and Enteral Nutrition (ASPEN) maintains guidelines for the indications and use of feeding tubes. The National Guideline Clearinghouse maintains guidelines for the administration of specialized nutrition support as developed by ASPEN. The American Gastroenterological Association (AGA) endorses the use of percutaneous endoscopic gastrostomy tubes for prolonged tube feeding (more than 30 days) and nasogastric feeding when enteral feeding is needed for shorter time periods. The decision to use a nasoduodenal or nasojejunal tube is made if there is a risk of aspiration, GERD, or other reasons to bypass the stomach, e.g., acute pancreatitis. The route to use for enteral nutrition is based on the length of therapy as well as patient comfort.

Patient Preparation

If the feeding tube will be used for less than 30 days, select a nasogastric tube in the range of 8-Fr to 18-Fr. A larger bore nasogastric tube allows for suction if needed. Smaller tubes, 8-Fr to 12-Fr, are used for intestinal feeding (duodenal and jejunal). Whatever feeding tube is used, the nurse should read the package insert for the tube used and keep the insert in the patient's chart for reference for others. Complete documentation of time of placement and the length of tube inserted should be done. If the tube is advanced with peristalsis, each time the patient is assessed, the nurse should note the length of tube that is in the patient. A follow-up X-ray is done to check placement of the film and at 12-hour intervals to check for progression. The patient should be prepared by describing the reasons for the tube to be placed as well as the procedure for the intubation. There are times when the insertion of the tube must be done fluoroscopically. Once the tube is in place, it must be carefully taped, and the tube marked with a permanent marker in the event the tube slips out, it will be noted visually (Figure 47-9). Evidence has demonstrated that Hy-Tape, The Original Pink Tape, a unique water-resistant and washable tape is especially suited for securing feeding tubes.

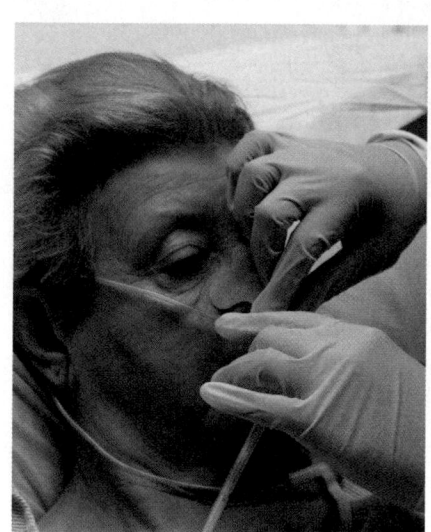

Figure 47-9 A nurse taping a nasogastric tube in place.

Patients with feeding tubes are at high risk for regurgitation and aspiration of gastric contents as well as oropharyngeal secretions. Other complications include bronchopulmonary injury from inadvertent placement of the feeding tube in the lung, perforation of the GI tract, erosion of the mucosal surface of the nasopharynx, and vocal cord paralysis. A small-bore tube tip can penetrate the brain, especially if the patient has a maxillofacial injury. These small-bore tubes can also knot in the stomach. When the tube is removed, the knot can damage the esophagus or nasopharynx (Noble, 2003).

Feeding tubes can become clogged. This occurs with the use of small-bore tubes, tubes made of silicone, medication that is not crushed sufficiently, medication and tube feeding formula incompatibility, formula and gastric acid precipitation, microbial contamination, and inadequate flushing of the tube. Evidence indicates the most effective method of maintaining patency of a feeding tube is routine flushing with water. To restore patency to a clogged tube it is recommended that pancreatic enzyme solutions be used (Keithley & Swanson, 2004).

Nasopharyngeal discomfort in patients with nasogastric or nasoenteric tubes can be mitigated by allowing the patient an occasional ice chip or using artificial saliva. If the patient needs a nasal tube for longer than 6 weeks, the tube should be replaced and the opposite nostril should be utilized for the replacement tube. To reduce mucosal damage and potential scarring and stricture, the smallest bore tube should be selected for the purpose.

Percutaneous Endoscopic Gastrostomy and Percutaneous Endoscopic Jejunostomy Tubes

A most important decision in determining whether a percutaneous endoscopic gastrostomy (PEG) or percutaneous endoscopic jejunostomy (PEJ) tube is inserted is to evaluate whether there is outcome data related to the underlying illness of the patient. Providers, other health care professionals, patients, and families should be knowledgeable of the benefits as well as the burdens associated with long-term enteral feeding (Calgary Health Region, 2004; Stroud, Duncan, & Nightingale, 2003). PEG tubes have become the procedure of choice for enteral nutrition in the United States. Recent recommendations are that PEG tubes should only be placed in conditions in which the patient can benefit (Plonk, 2005). These are limited and include early head and neck cancer, amyotrophic lateral sclerosis, malignant bowel obstruction with intractable vomiting, and acute stroke with dysphagia persisting for 30 days after hospital discharge.

Complications from the use of PEG or PEJ tubes include infection at the insertion site, fistula formation, peritonitis, sepsis, and necrotizing fasciitis. Of great concern is the high mortality rate, 20 to 40 percent, within one month of PEG or PEJ insertion (Stroud, et al., 2003).

With all enteral feeding, patients may experience nausea, abdominal bloating, and cramps from delayed gastric emptying. It is recommended that patients receive continuous feeding rather than bolus feedings. If needed, prokinetic agents (e.g., erythromycin or metoclopramide) are used to hasten gastric emptying and reduce GI discomfort.

Barium Studies

Barium (chalky white contrast medium) is an oral preparation that allows roentgenographic visualization of the internal structures of the digestive tract. The results of barium studies can reveal congenital abnormalities; lesions; spasm; reflux, stricture, and obstruction; inflammation; and ulceration; varices; and fistula. General patient preparation for barium studies should include:
- Placing the patient on NPO status after midnight.
- Administering a laxative the evening before and enemas the morning of the test.
- Forcing fluid postprocedure.
- Follow-up two to three days postprocedure to ensure the patient has had a normal brown stool.

Postprocedure barium will be expelled in the stool, making it milky white. Fluids are forced to help with the excretion of barium. If the barium is not completely excreted, it can cause intestinal obstruction.

Barium Swallow

Barium swallow (esophagraphy) is a fluoroscopic visualization of the esophagus following the ingestion of barium sulfate. Implement the nursing care discussed above for a patient with a barium study.

Skills 360°

Communication Regarding Ingestion of the Barium Sulfate

The oral solution of barium sulfate comes in flavored forms, and these have been improved as to their tastes over the past several years. The nurse must learn to communicate carefully that the solution is not as distasteful as it once was. However, the barium sulfate is still somewhat disliked by patients, but the nurse must learn to communicate the reality of the solution, while at the same time not being too negative about its taste.

Adapted from Daniels, R. (2003). Delmar's manual of laboratory and diagnostic tests. New York: Thomson Delmar Learning.

PATIENT PLAYBOOK

Instructions for a Barium Enema

The nurse instructs the patient:
- To eat a low-residue diet two days prior to the test.
- That during the procedure various positions will need to be assumed on the table to facilitate movement of the barium in the intestines.
- That the test will take about one hour.
- That the postprocedure cleansing enemas will be given to help remove the barium.

Adapted from Estes, M. (2006). Health assessment and physical examination (3rd ed.). New York: Thomson Delmar Learning.

Upper GI Study

Upper GI (UGI) is a fluoroscopic visualization of the stomach and small bowel following the ingestion of barium sulfate. In addition to the general preparation of the patient for a barium study, also instruct the patient that:

- He or she should not smoke for 24 hours prior to the procedure (smoking causes an increased production of gastric juices).
- During the procedure (which will last approximately two hours), pictures will be taken at 30-minute intervals with the patient in different positions.

Barium Enema

Barium enema (a rectal infusion of barium sulfate) is the roentgenographic study of the lower intestinal tract. The colon should be free of all fecal material to allow for maximum visualization (see Patient Playbook feature).

KEY CONCEPTS

- The major organs of the GI tract include the intestinal tract, the hollow organs from the mouth to the anus.
- The mouth, lips, cheeks, tongue, and pharynx aid in chewing, mastication and moving food and fluid into the esophagus.
- The abdominal health history provides the nurse with important subjective information that assists in the physical assessment of the abdomen.
- Leading symptoms and complaints from patients with GI disorders include heartburn, dysphagia (difficulty in swallowing), dyspepsia, nausea and vomiting, gas, diarrhea, constipation, pain, and bleeding.
- Dyspepsia is the most common symptom that patients complain about to their health care provider.
- Diarrhea can be acute, self-limiting, a life-threatening event, or chronic.
- Constipation is marked by straining at stool with the production of hard stools, decreased frequency, and a feeling of not completely evacuating the colon.

- Abdominal pain is separated into acute and chronic.
- There is often pain that is referred from abdominal structures and an assessment of the perianal area can reveal such pain.
- There are a wide variety of diagnostic tests performed for GI disorders.
- Adequate bowel preparation is necessary for all GI procedures.
- The laparoscopy is a diagnostic procedure in which the peritoneal cavity, pelvis and abdomen, is examined.
- Paracentesis is the aspiration of fluid from the abdominal cavity.
- Esophageal dilation is performed when a patient experiences peptic strictures often related to GERD.
- Barium (chalky white contrast medium) is an oral preparation that allows roentgenographic visualization of the internal structures of the digestive tract.

REVIEW QUESTIONS

1. What is a product of exocrine glands in the oral cavity that lubricates the mouth and begins the digestive process?
   1. Sweat
   2. Saliva
   3. Tears
   4. Stool

2. Which of the following organs would you expect to find in the left upper quadrant?
   1. Head of the pancreas
   2. Portions of the ascending and transverse colon

   3. Duodenum
   4. Spleen

3. What is acute pain in the abdomen labeled as?
   1. Hematoma
   2. Hypovolemic shock
   3. Acute abdomen
   4. Referred abdominal pain

4. The reason that auscultation is performed first when performing an abdominal assessment is:
   1. It is the quickest part of the assessment process.
   2. It is more convenient and causes less pain for the patient.

Continued

REVIEW QUESTIONS—cont'd

3. It is the easiest skill for the nurse to remember to perform.
4. It does not allow the sounds produced from percussion and palpation to alter what is auscultated.

5. Which of the following is true when assessing the liver?
   1. Normally the liver is easily palpated in adults.
   2. Normally the liver is percussed 4 to 6 cm above the costal margin.
   3. Normally the liver does not descend beyond 1 to 2 cm of the costal margin and is not palpable.
   4. Normally the liver sounds hollow on percussion.

6. Which of the following is true of conscious sedation?
   1. It is normally only performed for oral surgery.
   2. It is difficult to give to a majority of adults, due to the tremendous number of allergic reactions to the anesthesia.
   3. It allows patients to respond to verbal commands throughout the procedure.
   4. It is best delivered via the rectal route of administration to enhance its absorption.

7. Which of the following assessment techniques is not used to asses for ascites?
   1. Fluid wave
   2. Murphy's sign
   3. Shifting dullness
   4. Puddle sign

8. A positive Murphy's sign indicates an inflammatory process associated with:
   1. Ascites
   2. Appendicitis
   3. Cholecystitis
   4. Pelvic abscess

9. You have flexed the patient's right leg at the hip and the knee is at a right angle. You then internally and externally rotate the patient's leg and observe the patient's reaction. What is this assessment technique called?
   1. Iliopsoas muscle test
   2. Obturator muscle test
   3. Rovsing's sign
   4. Ballottement

10. What is the low-pitched sound that is auscultated in the abdomen and caused by turbulent blood flow?
    1. Borborygmi
    2. Venous hum
    3. Peritoneal friction rub
    4. Bruit

11. Secretin testing is used to determine if a patient has:
    1. Cholecystitis
    2. Gastritis
    3. Esophagitis
    4. Incipient chronic pancreatitis

REVIEW ACTIVITIES

1. State and describe the organs of the GI tract.
2. Perform a concise GI health history on an adult patient.
3. Describe the physiological processes involved during the act of vomiting.
4. Perform the physical assessment tests to determine if a patient has acute appendicitis.
5. Describe any two of the diagnostic tests used for the abdominal system.

Visit the Contemporary Medical-Surgical Nursing online companion resource at www.delmarhealthcare.com for additional content and study aids. Click on Online Companions then select the Nursing discipline.

Nutrition, Malnutrition, and Obesity: Nursing Management

Ellen K. Fleischman, MBA, RD, RN

CHAPTER TOPICS

- Normal Nutrition
- Nutrition Support
- Malnutrition
- Obesity

KEY TERMS

Anabolism
Catabolism
Chyme
Direct calorimetry
Disaccharides
Indirect calorimetry
Joint Commission on
  Accreditation of
  Hospitals (JCAHO)
Macronutrients
Metabolism
Monosaccharides
Peristalsis
Resting energy expenditure

During the 20th century, a shift occurred in the leading cause of death in the United States from infection to chronic disease. Chronic diseases are now responsible for 7 of 10 of the leading causes of death in the United States. The 3 leading causes of *preventable* death according to the Centers for Disease Control are tobacco use, improper diet, and physical inactivity. At least 70 percent of health care spending is on chronic diseases (MMWR, 2004). Nutrition plays a vital role in the prevention and management of chronic diseases, such as diabetes, cardiovascular disease, and cancer, as well as in the prevention of overweight and obesity. According to the American Cancer Society, one third of all cancer deaths in the United States could be prevented by eating a healthy, plant-based diet and maintaining a healthy weight. Nursing care of the medical-surgical patient requires a basic understanding of the physiology involved with nutrition and knowledge of an adequate diet and the interactions between foods and medications, as well as an understanding of the impact of proper nutrition and malnutrition on the health of the patient.

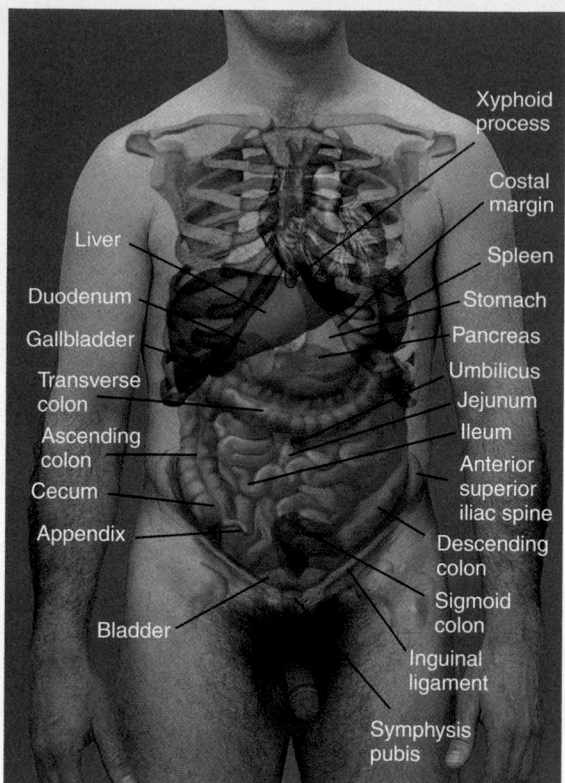

Figure 48-1 The gastrointestinal tract.

Labels on figure: Xyphoid process, Costal margin, Spleen, Stomach, Pancreas, Umbilicus, Jejunum, Ileum, Anterior superior iliac spine, Descending colon, Sigmoid colon, Inguinal ligament, Symphysis pubis, Liver, Duodenum, Gallbladder, Transverse colon, Ascending colon, Cecum, Appendix, Bladder

THE GASTROINTESTINAL TRACT AND NUTRITIONAL PROCESSES

The gastrointestinal (GI) tract plays a vital role in the nutritional aspects of a person's physiology. Anatomically, the GI tract begins with the mouth and ends with the anus. It includes the oropharyngeal structures, esophagus, stomach, pancreas, liver and gallbladder, small intestine, and large intestine (Figure 48-1). The GI tract is one of the largest organs in the body (Ganong, 2003).

The main functions of the GI tract are to extract and absorb nutrients from foods and beverages people consume, serve as a barrier to microorganisms, and excrete waste products. In addition, the GI tract participates in regulatory, immunological, and metabolic functions.

Processes of Digestion, Absorption, and Metabolism

To digest food and absorb the nutrients the body needs, a person must first process the food eaten. The GI tract converts large particles and molecules into smaller and more easily absorbed components and converts insoluble molecules into soluble ones. The resulting components plus vitamins, minerals, and water cross the intestinal mucosa and are absorbed into the lymph or blood, then delivered to the tissues. Food products end up being broken down into lipids (fats), carbohydrates, and protein. These nutrients are then utilized by the body through **metabolism,** meaning change, in which chemical and energy transformations occur. Nutrition is the source of exogenous compounds needed for metabolism (Ganong, 2003).

Digestion and Absorption

The process of digestion begins in the mouth. The chewing process reduces the size of food particles and saliva moistens the chewed food, preparing it for swallowing. Food and liquid travel from the mouth (oral cavity) down the esophagus to the stomach. In the stomach, food is mixed with acids and enzymes and, as a result, is converted into a liquid substance called **chyme,** as the process of digestion continues. The stomach mixes and churns food, releasing small amounts into the small intestine, where the majority of digestion takes place. The small intestine is divided into the duodenum, jejunum, and ileum. Most digestive processes take place in the duodenum and the upper jejunum, and by the time the food material reaches the middle of the jejunum, absorption of most nutrients has taken place. Starches are broken down to simple sugars by enzymes from the pancreas. Proteins are converted into amino acid chains and single amino acids. Fats are reduced to emulsions that are further broken down into smaller molecules. Secretions from the mouth, stomach, pancreas, small intestine, and gallbladder contribute fluid to the digested material. The majority of this fluid is reabsorbed by the small intestine, along with the remaining **macronutrients,** vitamins, minerals, and trace elements. Most of the remaining fluid is reabsorbed by the large intestine, along with electrolytes and vitamins produced by intestinal bacteria.

Digestion results from mechanical processes, such as teeth grinding and crushing food into small particles, as well as through chemical breakdown of food into molecules that can be absorbed. The process of **peristalsis** moves the food through the GI tract for further digestion and absorption. Absorption of nutrients is a highly complex process involving several mechanisms, including diffusion and active transport.

Carbohydrates

Carbohydrates are consumed in the form of starches; **monosaccharides** (simple sugar molecules) and **disaccharides** (two monosaccharides). The process of starch digestion begins in the mouth, where salivary amylase breaks small amounts of starch into smaller particles. Amylase is deactivated when it reaches the acidic environment of the stomach, and most carbohydrate digestion is completed in the small intestine. Pancreatic amylase breaks large starch molecules into smaller ones, and eventually starch is converted to glucose. Enzymes in the small intestine break down sugar molecules, such as disaccharides into monosaccharides. Monosaccharides are carried through the cells in the intestinal mucosa and into the bloodstream to the liver. Some glucose, a monosaccharide, is stored in the liver and muscles as glycogen, and the rest is carried from the liver to the tissues. Some carbohydrates, pectin, cellulose, hemicellulose, and fiber cannot be digested by the human body, because people are unable to break down certain linkages. These indigestible compounds provide bulk to the stool and assist in the process of elimination.

Proteins

Protein digestion begins in the stomach, where it is broken into smaller molecules called peptides. Further digestion of protein takes place in the small intestine, where peptides are hydrolyzed by enzymes into amino acids. Amino acids are absorbed via active transport and are carried to the liver for metabolism, then released into the circulation.

Lipids (Fats)

Lipids are consumed in the form of triglycerides, phospholipids, and cholesterol. Small amounts of lipids are digested in the mouth by an enzyme, called lingual lipase, and in the stomach by an enzyme, called gastric lipase. Most fat digestion takes place in the small intestine through the action of pancreatic lipase. Fat stimulates the release of hormones, such as cholecystokinin and enterogastrone, which inhibit gastric secretions and slow the motility of food from the stomach to the small intestine. In the small intestine peristalsis breaks large fat molecules into smaller ones, and bile, released by the gallbladder, helps to separate the fat molecules. Lipid molecules in various forms are transported by carrier proteins through the bloodstream to the adipose (fat) tissue, liver, and muscle.

Metabolism

Carbohydrates are transported to the liver in the form of glucose via the portal vein. This process stimulates insulin secretion from the pancreas. In a nondiabetic patient, insulin secretion is adequate to facilitate the process of glucose uptake into tissue cells. If carbohydrate intake is higher than what is needed for energy and storage in the liver and muscle, it is converted to fat for storage in the adipose tissue.

In healthy people, proteins in muscle and throughout the body are kept in balance as they are broken down and synthesized. Amino acids obtained through the digestion of protein intake replace protein stores, provide energy, and what is not needed is excreted in the urine, feces, and through the skin.

Fat is taken to the liver from various sources. The liver repackages the fat onto a carrier protein for transport. Cholesterol is used by cells as part of their cell membrane and by the liver to make bile acids. Fat is used to help hold body organs in place and protect them from trauma and also to insulate the body and thereby maintain body temperature. Fat is also used to transport digesting substances and fat-soluble vitamins, to aid absorption, and for energy. It is stored in the adipose tissue (Ganong, 2003).

COMPONENTS OF A NUTRITIONALLY ADEQUATE DIET

A nutritionally adequate diet is one that meets the needs of the individual at any particular stage of his or her life cycle. For example, a growing child will require more calories and different nutrients than an elderly person. In addition, a nutritionally adequate diet will support vital body systems, support a healthy weight and body composition, and help prevent chronic disease. According to the American Dietetic Association all foods can fit in a healthful diet if the portion sizes are appropriate, foods are consumed in moderation, and regular physical activity is maintained.

The first recommendations for nutrition were established by the Food and Nutrition Board of the National Academies in 1941. The recommended dietary allowances (RDAs) for vitamins, minerals, protein, and energy were developed because of wartime concern for adequate nutrition in military troops. Since that time, the RDAs have been used as a guide on which federal and state nutrition programs have been continually revised (Institute of Medicine [IOM], 2002). The U.S. Department of Health and Human Services (USDHHS) and the U.S. Department of Agriculture (USDA) publish dietary guidelines for Americans every five years. These guidelines were first published in 1980 and provide advice regarding dietary habits to promote health and prevent chronic disease for individuals two years old and older (U.S. Department of Health and Human Services, 2005; USDA, 2005).

The intent of the guidelines is to summarize current knowledge about nutrition into recommendations for the public. An example of an eating pattern that follows the dietary guidelines is the USDA food guide, called *My Pyramid,* displayed in Figure 48-2, which can be used as a teaching tool for patients. In 2004, My Pyramid replaced the former Food Guide Pyramid. The new pyramid symbolizes a personalized approach to healthy eating and physical activity, as well as the benefits of taking small steps toward a healthier lifestyle.

The body of current evidence regarding nutrition and chronic disease prevention led to the formation of a multidisciplinary expert panel from the National Institutes of Health (NIH), Health Canada, and the National Academy of Sciences IOM Food and Nutrition board. This panel was appointed by the USDHHS to review the scientific literature on macronutrients and energy and establish guidelines for intake to promote good nutrition and decrease the risk of chronic disease (Brooks, Butte, Rand, Flatt, & Caballero, 2004).

The panel published a report entitled *Dietary reference intakes for energy, carbohydrate, fiber, fat, fatty acids, cholesterol, protein, and amino acids* (IOM, 2002). This report is the sixth in a series, replacing and expanding the former RDAs with Dietary Reference Intakes (DRIs). This report focuses on carbohydrates, fat, protein, fiber, fatty acids, and cholesterol, as well as on calorie needs and physical activity.

To meet the body's nutritional needs while decreasing the risk for developing chronic disease, adults should get 45 to 65 percent of their calories from carbohydrates, 20 to 35 percent of calories from fat, and 10 to 35 percent of calories from protein. The guidelines for children are similar, except that infants and younger children need a higher proportion of fat, 25 to 40 percent.

Because exercise and nutrition go hand-in-hand to prevent chronic disease, the IOM panel found in their 2002 report that it would be necessary for most adults and children to participate in moderate physical activity for 60 minutes per day to make the transition from a sedentary lifestyle to an active one (Table 48-1). Although this exercise goal is higher than recommendations made in 1996 by the United States Surgeon General, the panel considered moderate physical activity to include routine daily activities, such

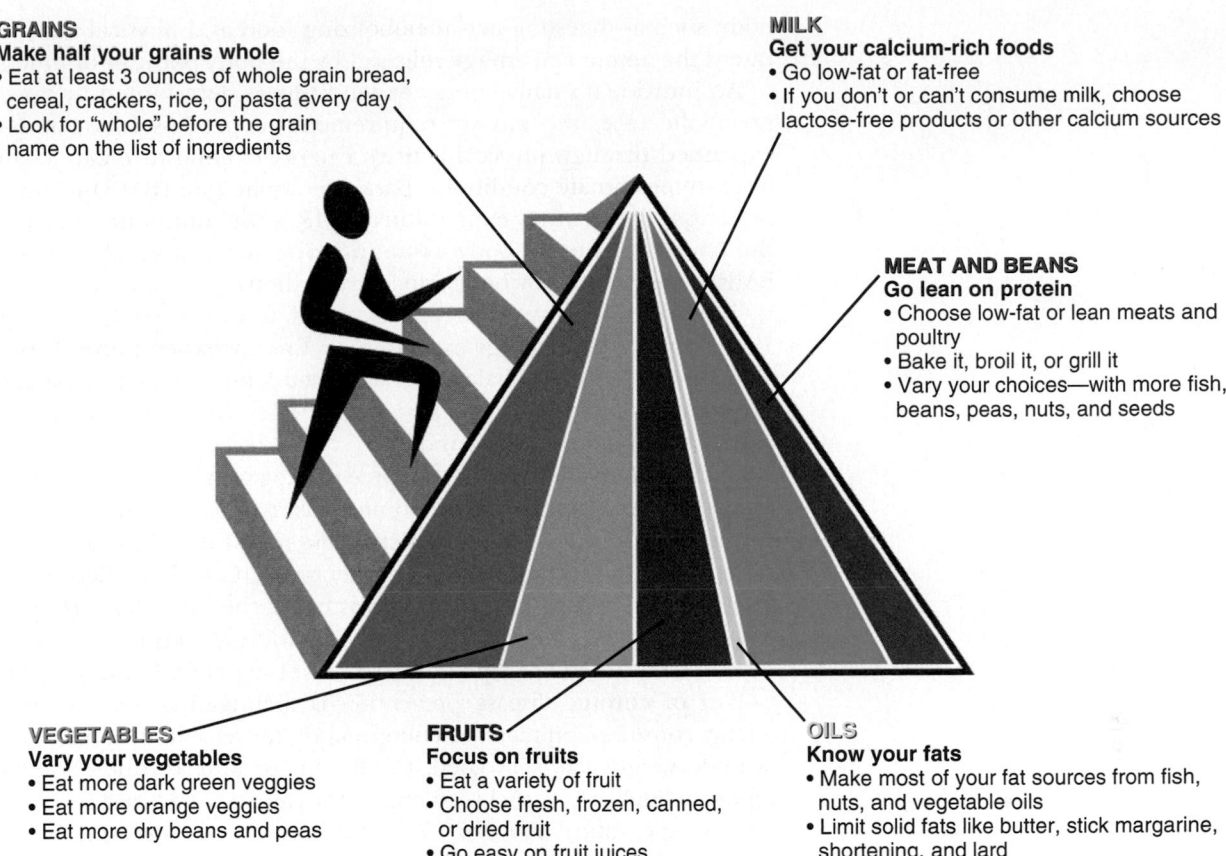

GRAINS
Make half your grains whole
• Eat at least 3 ounces of whole grain bread, cereal, crackers, rice, or pasta every day
• Look for "whole" before the grain name on the list of ingredients

MILK
Get your calcium-rich foods
• Go low-fat or fat-free
• If you don't or can't consume milk, choose lactose-free products or other calcium sources

MEAT AND BEANS
Go lean on protein
• Choose low-fat or lean meats and poultry
• Bake it, broil it, or grill it
• Vary your choices—with more fish, beans, peas, nuts, and seeds

VEGETABLES
Vary your vegetables
• Eat more dark green veggies
• Eat more orange veggies
• Eat more dry beans and peas

FRUITS
Focus on fruits
• Eat a variety of fruit
• Choose fresh, frozen, canned, or dried fruit
• Go easy on fruit juices

OILS
Know your fats
• Make most of your fat sources from fish, nuts, and vegetable oils
• Limit solid fats like butter, stick margarine, shortening, and lard

Figure 48-2 *My Pyramid* USDA Food Guide. (From Inside My Pyramid, by the U.S. Department of Agriculture, 2005.)

	GRAMS PER DAY OF CARBOHYDRATES	GRAMS PER DAY OF FAT	GRAMS PER DAY FROM PROTEIN
CALORIE LEVEL	**(45–65 PERCENT OF CALORIES)**	**(20–35 PERCENT OF CALORIES)**	**(10–35 PERCENT OF CALORIES)**
1,000	130–163[a]	22–39	25–88
1,200	135–195	27–47	30–105
1,500	168–243	33–58	38–131
1,800	202–292	40–70	45–157
2,000	225–325	44–78	50–175
2,200	247–357	49–86	55–192

TABLE 48-1 Macronutrient Recommendations

[a] *Minimum number of daily carbohydrate grams*
Source: Institute of Medicine. (2002). Dietary reference intakes for energy, carbohydrate, fiber, fat, fatty acids, cholesterol, protein, and amino acids. *Washington, DC: National Academy Press.*

as housekeeping, taking the stairs instead of the elevator, and walking the dog (Brooks, Butte, Rand, Flatt, & Caballero, 2004; IOM, 2002).

Metabolic Rate

In the normal human body, the processes of **anabolism** and **catabolism** are constantly taking place. Anabolic processes take up energy, and catabolic processes release energy. Energy released by catabolic processes supports functions of the body, such as digesting and metabolizing food and physical activity. Metabolic rate is the amount of energy released by the body per unit of time.

An individual's daily energy expenditure is determined by his or her basal metabolic rate, the energy requirement to process food, and the energy expended through physical activity. Energy expenditure can also be affected by extreme climate conditions. Basal metabolic rate (BMR) is the largest component of daily energy expenditure. BMR is the minimum work performed by the body to maintain body tissue integrity and a normal body temperature. BMR is determined by body size, composition, gender, and age.

The energy required to process food is estimated to be approximately 10 percent of daily energy expenditure. Energy expenditure through physical activity varies. Energy balance is achieved when there is a balance between caloric intake and energy expenditure. When an individual is in energy balance, body weight is maintained.

Energy can be defined as the force driving and sustaining mental activity or the capacity for doing work (Medline Plus, 2005a). The standard unit for measuring energy is the calorie, which is the amount of heat energy required to raise the temperature of 1 mL of water at 15° C by 1° C. Because the amount of calories used by the human body is large, the kilocalorie (kcal), equivalent to 1,000 calories, is used. Therefore, if an individual is in energy balance, kilocalories consumed are equal to kilocalories expended (Ganong, 2003).

Part of chronic disease prevention is maintaining energy balance so that energy consumption matches energy expenditure. With this balance, overweight or underweight can be avoided. The IOM Food and Nutrition board published a report in 2002, which included targets for calorie intake and recommended that energy expenditure be 1.6 to 1.7 times an individual's **resting energy expenditure** to maintain a healthy weight. Factors affecting resting energy expenditure include body size, composition, age, and gender (IOM, 2002).

In a research setting, **direct calorimetry** may be used to measure energy expenditure. The subject is enclosed in a chamber, and changes in the temperature of circulating air and water measure heat released by the subject. Heat released by the subject is a direct measure of energy expenditure. Because the subject is enclosed in a chamber and is isolated from caregivers, this method does not work well in the hospital setting.

Indirect calorimetry is therefore conducted in some hospital settings. There are many different methods of indirect calorimetry. Portable indirect calorimeters can be taken to the patient's bedside. They may be attached to the patient's ventilator, or a mask may be used for more stable patients. The machine measures the oxygen and carbon dioxide content of inspired and expired breath, as well as the volume expired by the lungs. Through measurements of gas exchange, energy expenditure is measured. In addition, because carbohydrate, protein, and fat metabolism each require a specific amount of oxygen and release a specific amount of carbon dioxide, this test can measure the amount of carbohydrate, protein, and fat utilized by the body. Because indirect calorimetry equipment is expensive, and the testing is labor intensive, not all facilities offer this service.

There are many methods of measuring and calculating energy expenditure or energy needs. Most calculations utilize factors such as height, weight, and age. In the hospital setting the guidelines and policies of the specific enterprise determine the calculations used. A consult for the clinical dietitian to assess a patient's nutritional needs can be ordered. The registered dietitian (RD) may estimate the patient's intake using the patient's 24-hour food recall or by asking the patient, family members, and health care providers about the amounts and types of foods consumed by the patient over the previous 24 hours. A calorie count may be ordered to compare the patient's intake to the individual's estimated needs. This usually involves recording the percentage intake of each item on the patient's menu for one to three days. A dietetic technician or RD will then summarize the results. This method of assessing a patient's intake is not precise in the hospital setting, however, because it relies on the consistent observation and recording by staff of actual foods eaten at all meals.

NUTRITION AND DRUG INTERACTIONS

The absorption, effectiveness, safety, and elimination of medications can be affected by food, and medications can have an impact on nutritional status. Foods can affect the absorption of medications and alter the pharmacokinetics of a medication. In the hospital setting, nurses need to be aware of potential food-drug interactions to avoid adverse drug events and to reinforce patient teaching (Figure 48-3). Although policies and practices vary, many health care enterprises have a process in place for identifying and monitoring potential food-drug interactions, as well as for teaching patients in preparation for discharge.

Although there are many potential food and drug interactions with which nurses need to be familiar, the interaction between grapefruit juice and certain medications is an interesting one. This interaction was identified accidentally in a study on alcohol consumption and a drug to lower blood pressure. When grapefruit juice was used to mask the taste of alcohol, more of the drug was absorbed than was expected. It was determined that compounds in grapefruit juice affect drug absorption in the small intestine.

Cytochrome P450

A group of enzymes called the cytochrome P450s are found in the liver and are involved with drug metabolism. The interaction between drugs and grapefruit juice involves cytochrome P450 3A and a protein in the small intestine, called P-glycoprotein, which affects the absorption of drugs. Cytochrome P450 3A metabolizes drugs so that they are more easily eliminated. Grapefruit juice can block P-glycoprotein and inactivate cytochrome P450 3A for up to 24 hours. Some of the medications affected by grapefruit juice are cyclosporine and felodipine. A total of 65 drug interactions were identified in the Thomson

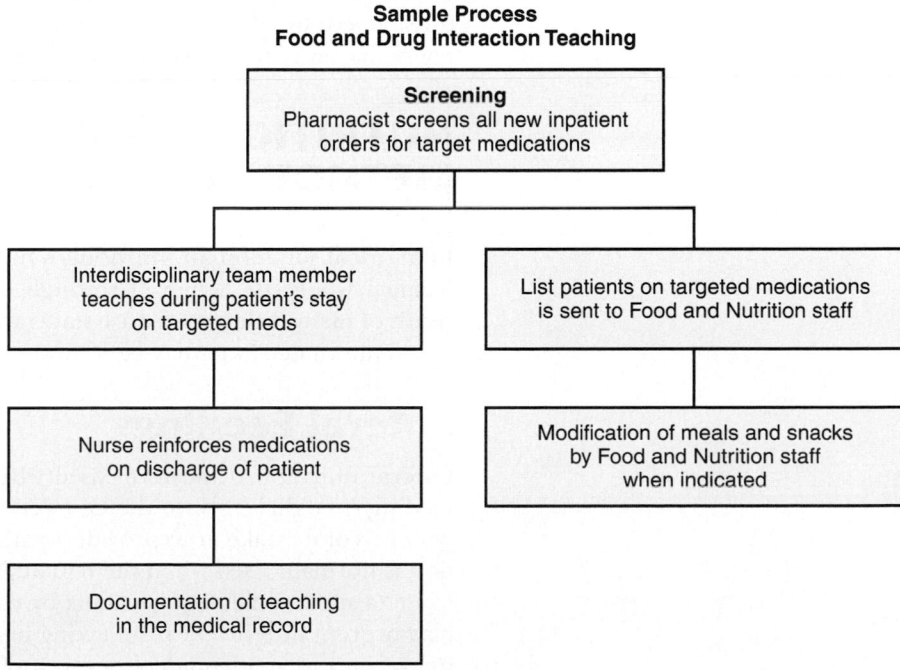

Figure 48-3 Sample process: Food and drug interaction teaching.

PATIENT PLAYBOOK

Teaching Points for Patients Taking Herbal Remedies

• Be aware that the word *natural* on a product label does not mean that a product is safe.

• Herbal products may interact with both over-the-counter (OTC) and prescription medications.

• Notify the health care provider and pharmacist of herbal products the patient is taking.

Micromedex database when grapefruit was entered as a search topic (Thomson Micromedex Healthcare Series, 2004).

Warfarin

Warfarin is a commonly used anticoagulant. Warfarin levels are measured through the international normalization ratio test (INR). Significant variation in the intake of foods high in vitamin K can disrupt the anticoagulation effect of warfarin. Foods high in vitamin K content include bananas, celery, and many other varieties of vegetables and fruits (Box 48-1). Therefore, nurses should advise their patients on warfarin to maintain a *consistent* intake of foods high in vitamin K after discharge to maximize the safety of warfarin therapy.

Natural Products

One area of potential food drug interactions has to do with so-called natural products. Herbal products and dietary supplements are considered by the general public to be safe and beneficial (Bailey & Dresser, 2004). In the 1999 to 2000 National Health and Nutrition Examination Study (NHANES), 52 percent of adults reported taking a dietary supplement in the previous month (Radimer, et al., 2004). Because herbal products and dietary supplements are classified as food supplements rather than medications, they are not regulated by the Food and Drug Administration (FDA). Patients often do not realize the importance of telling health care practitioners about the use of herbal products and dietary supplements, and significant interactions with medications have been documented.

Herbal products can mimic the actions, intensify, or oppose the effects of drugs. St. John's wort, an herbal product used to treat depression, increases the activity of cytochrome P350 A4 and, as a result, more of a drug is oxidized and is therefore less bioavailable. Patients should not mix St. John's wort with medications such as digoxin, theophylline, cyclosporin, and phenprocoumon, because the herb decreases the bioavailability of the medications. When St. John's wort is combined with cyclosporin it can result in organ rejection in post-transplant patients and increased human immunodeficiency virus (HIV) viral load in HIV-positive patients (Bailey & Dresser, 2004). The herb gingko biloba can interfere with warfarin and cause bleeding. Because of the potential interactions of herbal products and dietary supplements with other medications, the nurse needs to ask patients about the use of these herbal products, dietary supplements, and other OTC remedies when obtaining a medical history.

NUTRITION SUPPORT: ALTERNATIVE METHODS OF FEEDING PATIENTS

In an ideal situation an individual's nutrient needs would be met and energy balance would be achieved through eating a healthful diet. However, as a result of many different disease states and medical conditions, feeding patients via an alternate route may be indicated.

Enteral Feedings

Enteral nutrition is the term used when feeding a patient occurs through a feeding tube directly into the GI tract. It can be used either as an adjunct to a patient's oral intake or to provide a patient's complete nutrition. Enteral nutrition is normally used when the patient has a functioning GI tract but is unable to meet nutritional requirements by eating. The patient's medical condition may prevent him or her from taking in adequate food by mouth, or his or her intake may be inadequate as a result of acute illness or an inability to take in adequate nutrition due to mechanical problems, such as dysphagia.

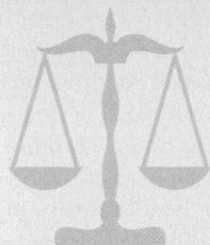

LAW IN PRACTICE

The Legal Implications of End-of-life Care

End-of-life medical treatment has been the subject of public debate since the case of Karen Ann Quinlan in 1975. Ms. Quinlan suffered respiratory arrest after drinking alcohol and possibly consuming the prescription medication, Valium. Karen suffered brain damage and was in a persistent vegetative state. After three months in the vegetative state, and with a poor prognosis, her family requested that she be taken off artificial life support. A legal battle ensued, and the Quinlans lost in a New Jersey Superior Court case. The decision was overturned by the New Jersey Supreme Court in January 1976. Karen was taken off the ventilator, but she continued to live in a persistent vegetative state until she died June 11, 1985. She had been unconscious for more than 10 years.

State laws and hospital policies related to end-of-life care vary; however, providing artificial fluids and nutrition via enteral feedings in patients can be considered medical treatment. The ideal situation is when a patient has expressed his or her wishes regarding end-of-life medical treatments (including providing artificial fluids and nutrition) in the form of an advanced directive. Hospitals accredited by the **Joint Commission on Accreditation of Hospitals (JCAHO)** are required to meet standard RI 2.80 on individual rights, which states that the hospital addresses the wishes of the patient regarding end-of-life decisions. Part of this standard requires providing patients with written information about their right to accept or refuse medical or surgical treatment, including forgoing or withdrawing life-sustaining treatment or withholding resuscitative services (2004).

Early enteral feeding has been demonstrated to improve wound healing, improve immune function, and reduce the length of hospital stay in the critically ill (Marik & Zaloga, 2003). When enteral nutrition is indicated the health care provider will order the enteral feeding product, the flow rate for the product to run on an enteral infusion device, and the route of enteral access. RDs in the hospital are an excellent resource to the health care provider and nurse for guidance about enteral feedings. They can assess the patient's nutritional needs, determine the optimal type of feeding and the flow rate to initiate and progress the feeding, establish the goal rate of enteral feeding, and monitor the patient's response to the feeding and ongoing nutrition status.

Before commercial enteral formulas were available, food was blenderized and thinned so that it could be passed down a tube. This practice is discouraged in the hospital setting because of the potential for bacterial contamination and the need to have the proper consistency of feeding. Enteral formulas can be delivered using an open or closed system. Canned enteral feeding products are emptied into a bag with the open system. The open system shown in Figure 48-4 is more labor-intensive for the nurse than the closed system and provides more opportunity for bacterial contamination. Closed system enteral formulas come in prefilled bottles. The formula bottle is spiked using a spike set, and the feeding flows through tubing to the patient. Hang-time of enteral

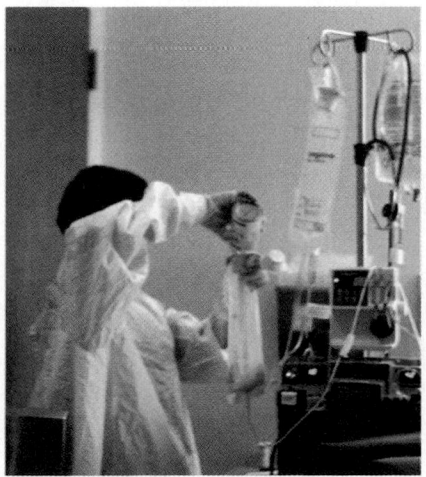

Figure 48-4 Open system gastrostomy feeding.

feedings will vary based on hospital guidelines and policy. However, because closed system products are sealed in the manufacturing process, they are sterile and can be hung over a longer period of time than open system products.

The choice of enteral feeding product is usually guided by the facility's enteral formulary (Table 48-2). The formulary normally includes a standard or house formula that is most commonly used. Specialty products, used for selected conditions, such as critically ill or immune-compromised patients, may also be available. Feedings vary in the amount and types of carbohydrate, protein or amino acids, fat, fiber, vitamins, minerals, and other components they contain. In addition, the osmolality of feedings will vary. Isotonic formulas simulate the osmolality of plasma (280–300 mOsm/kg) while hypertonic formulas have an osmolality higher than 300 mOsm/kg.

TABLE 48-2 Enteral Nutrition Formulary

CATEGORY	CAL/L	PRO (G/L)	FAT (G/L)	CHO (G/L)	INDICATIONS FOR USE
Group 1: Enteral Products That Meet the Needs of Most Patients					
Isotonic with Fiber	1,060	44 (17%)	35 (29%)	155 (54%)	Standard house with fiber formula for patients requiring fiber to maintain gut function
High Protein with Fiber	1,000	62 (25%)	29 (25%)	130 (50%)	Patients with protein losses from wounds, fistulas, trauma and hypercatabolic patients
CATEGORY	CAL/L	PRO (G/L)	FAT (G/L)	CHO (G/L)	INDICATIONS FOR USE
Group 2: Enteral Products with Specific Indications					
Isotonic, No Fiber	1,060	37 (14%)	35 (29%)	151 (57%)	Patients unable to tolerate fiber. Patients requiring restricted protein and/or electrolytes
1.2 Calorie/mL	1,200	53 (18%)	39 (29%)	160 (53%)	To provide adequate kcal without substantially increasing volume, such as with bolus and cyclic feedings
1.5 Calorie/mL	1,500	68 (18%)	65 (38%)	170 (44%)	Patients requiring fluid restricted, nutritionally dense formulas or with high caloric needs
2.0 Calorie/mL	2,000	84 (17%)	89 (40%)	216 (43%)	As above
Renal Failure	2,000	70 (14%)	96 (43%)	223 (44%)	Renal patients with electrolyte imbalances or requiring fluid restrictions. **Note other products may be more appropriate for patients on CRRT or dialysis with stable electrolytes
Hepatic Failure	1,500	40 (11%)	21 (12%)	290 (77%)	Protein-intolerant patients with hepatic encephalopathy
Uncontrolled Diabetes	1,060	45 (17%)	51 (43%)	119 (40%)	Patients unable to obtain glucose control on Group I formulas despite adequate glycemic management
Semi-Elemental, Low Fat, 1.0 Calorie/mL	1,000	63 (25%)	39 (33%)	105 (42%)	Patients requiring semi-elemental/low-fat formula due to GI dysfunction, pancreatitis, or intolerance to intact formulas
Semi-Elemental, High Protein, 1.5 Calorie/mL	1,500	94 (25%)	68 (39%)	135 (36%)	May be beneficial for patients with atypical non-healing wounds or those needing semi-elemental product with caloric density and high protein
Immune-Modulator	1,000	56 (22%)	28 (25%)	130 (53%)	May be useful for some patients needing immune-enhancing nutrients

Source: Used with permission by Sharp Healthcare, which retains all rights thereto.

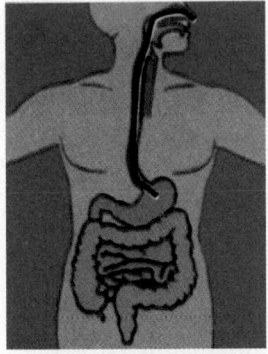
Nasogastric Route

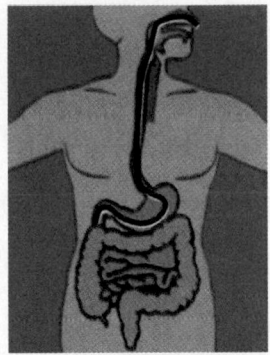
Nasoduodenal Route

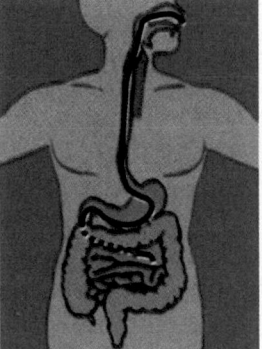
Nasojejunal Route

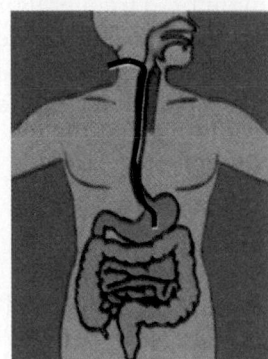
Esophagostomy Route

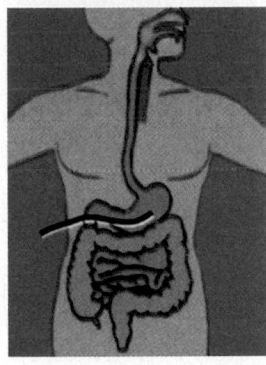
Gastrostomy Route

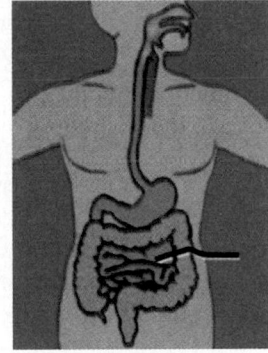
Jejunostomy Route

Figure 48-5 Enteral feeding routes.

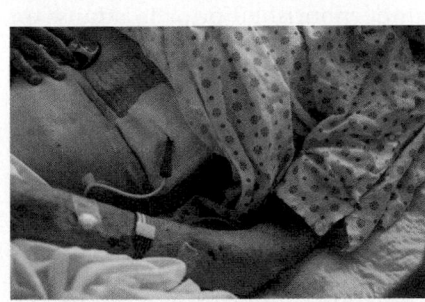

Figure 48-6 Gastrostomy feeding.

Enteral feedings may be administered continuously or intermittently. Continuous feeding is provided for most acute hospital patients using an enteral infusion device or pump running 24 hours a day. Feedings can be safely initiated in stable patients at a rate of 50 to 60 mL/hour and advanced by 10 to 25 mL/hour every four to six hours until the goal rate is achieved. Intermittent feedings are provided with different frequencies and volumes, depending on the needs of the patient. These feedings may be especially beneficial for patients receiving lengthy physical therapy or to mimic more normal eating patterns.

Enteral feeding tubes are made out of different types of material, such as silicone or polyurethane, and come in different sizes and lengths. The outer diameter is measured in French (F) units; one French unit is equal to 0.33 mL. The size of feeding tube selected depends on factors such as the product to be infused, location of the tube, and patient comfort. Feeding tubes generally have at least one port for feeding and one for flushing and will range in size from 5 F to 28 F. Feeding tube placement should be verified according to facility guidelines by air auscultation, chest x-ray (CXR), or through aspirating gastric secretions.

If a tube feeding is needed for less than six to eight weeks, it may be placed nasogastrically (NG) through the nose to the stomach or nasojejunally (NJ) through the nose to the small intestine. Placing a feeding tube into the stomach rather than the small intestine allows for easier tube placement and the use of larger bore tubes. Feeding tubes may also be placed into the distal duodenum or proximal jejunum and are referred to as postpyloric tubes. Nasogastric or nasoenteric feeding tubes may be contraindicated in patients with structural pathology in the head and neck or with facial fractures. In some cases an orogastric feeding tube may be used instead (Figure 48-5).

Gastrostomy Feedings

For longer term enteral feedings or when nasogastric or orogastric feedings are contraindicated, a more permanent feeding gastrostomy tube may be placed endoscopically or surgically through the abdominal wall. Various enteral feeding routes are shown in Figure 48-6. Although there are potential complications, such as infection or adverse reaction to anesthesia from the procedure of placing a gastrostomy tube, gastrostomy tubes are easier to maintain and replace than nasogastric or nasoenteric tubes and are more comfortable for the patient.

When a patient is receiving an enteral feeding, the nurse should pay careful attention to signs of possible complications and follow strict infection control practices. Signs of complications include nausea and vomiting, malabsorption, aspiration, abdominal distension, tube obstruction, diarrhea, and constipation. The head of the bed needs to be elevated 30 degrees during feedings and for one hour after a feeding has been discontinued to prevent aspiration. The nurse must ensure that the patient's medications can be safely passed through the feeding tube. Feeding tubes must be flushed before and after feeding and before and after medication administration to avoid tube obstruction. Because complications, such as nausea, vomiting, and diarrhea, can have other causes, it is important to assess for possible causes and notify the health care provider before assuming that the feeding is the cause.

Parenteral Nutrition

Parenteral nutrition (PN) is providing nutrients to a patient in an intravenous (IV) solution. This form of nutrition support is indicated when the patient is malnourished, has the potential for becoming malnourished, and is not a candidate for enteral feeding. PN can be provided through a peripheral vein at a low concentration or centrally through a large diameter vein, usually the superior vena cava.

PN formulations usually contain dextrose, amino acids, lipids, vitamins, minerals, and medications. Formulations must be carefully compounded under strict conditions in the pharmacy to prevent dangerous precipitation or infection. Complications of PN can be life-threatening and include GI atrophy, fluid overload, and sepsis.

Patients on PN should be monitored frequently. Some facilities have a nutrition support team for the daily management of enteral and PN. This team may include a health care provider, pharmacist, RD, and registered nurse (RN). This team can assist with the assessment and reassessment of patients on nutritional support.

MALNUTRITION

Malnutrition is a term that is used to describe an altered state of nutrition resulting from a deficiency, or excess, of one or more nutrients. Overnutrition is when a patient's intake is in excess of their need for one or more nutrients and undernutrition occurs when nutritional intake is insufficient. Malnutrition in hospitalized patients is generally a situation of undernutrition. When nutritional status declines in hospitalized patients it is usually associated with higher medical costs and increased likelihood of complications.

Epidemiology

Hospital personnel have been aware of the widespread presence of malnutrition in hospitalized patients since the 1970s when Butterworth published the famous article, "Skeletons in the Hospital Closet" in *Nutrition Today* (1974). Subsequent studies continue to highlight the prevalence and impact of malnutrition in hospitalized patients. The cost of hospital stays for patients who suffer declines in nutritional status, regardless of nutrition status on admission, is higher compared to patients who do not suffer declines in nutrition status.

Etiology

The etiology of malnutrition globally can be multifactorial and may include inadequate food intake because of poverty or isolation or frequent infections that lead to an inadequate intake of calories, protein, vitamins, and minerals. In the hospital setting the patient may be undernourished prior to admission or suffer a decline in nutritional status during the hospital stay. Causes of malnutrition prior to admission include financial constraints to consuming an adequate diet, pain from acute or chronic disease, inadequate intake resulting from medication side effects, and psychological factors, such as isolation and depression. During a hospital stay malnutrition may develop as a result of factors, such as disease state or inadequate food intake because of pain, nausea, and the difference of hospital food from their food preferences at home. The elderly are at high risk for malnutrition because of chronic medical problems, changes in taste and appetite, and social isolation. Other groups at risk for malnutrition include patients with cancer and acquired immunodeficiency syndrome (AIDS) because of the impact of the disease process and treatments on appetite and nutrient intake.

Assessment with Clinical Manifestations

Long-term undernutrition of protein and calories may be reflected in the form of marasmus, a condition resulting from inadequate intake of calories and protein to meet the body's needs. Severe tissue wasting, a decrease in lean body mass and subcutaneous fat stores, dehydration, and weight loss may be observed. The patient with marasmus has a cachectic appearance and may exhibit generalized weakness and a decrease in functioning (Hark & Morrison, 2003). Kwashiorkor is a state of protein depletion that may develop over a shorter period of time. Patients with kwashiorkor may appear weak, lethargic, edematous, and irritable (Hart & Morrison, 2003).

Diagnostic Tests

Laboratory diagnostic tests can be useful in the nutrition screening process to identify patients at risk, identify changes in nutrition status, and monitor the effectiveness of nutrition interventions. Nutrition-related laboratory tests include measures of visceral protein status, including the serum proteins, albumin, transferrin, prealbumin, and retinol binding protein shown in Table 48-3. Although albumin can be used to measure long-term changes in nutritional status, it is not the best indicator of nutritional status in hospitalized patients, because it has a half-life of approximately 21 days and is slow to respond to changes in nutritional status. Levels of less than 3 g/dL may indicate a problem. However, albumin levels in hospitalized patients may be decreased by factors other than malnutrition, such as fluid retention, liver damage, or renal disease.

Serum Transferrin

Serum transferrin can also be used to assess visceral protein stores, but its levels are not specific to nutritional status. Transferrin levels less than 100 mg/dL, 100 to 150 mg/dL, and 150 to 200 mg/dL may be an indicator of severely, moderately, and mildly depleted visceral protein stores, respectively, in patients with normal renal and hepatic function. The half-life of transferrin is eight days, so it is more sensitive than albumin, but not sensitive enough to use in daily monitoring of nutritional status. In addition, transferrin levels can be decreased by medications and medical conditions.

Prealbumin (Transthyretin)

Prealbumin, or transthyretin, has a half-life of 1.9 days and is a more sensitive indicator of nutritional status. It can be used to identify a decline in nutritional status as well as be used to monitor the effectiveness of nutrition interventions. Monitoring daily increases of 1 mg/dL may indicate a positive response to nutrition support; whereas increase of less than 2 mg/dL per week may indicate that nutrition support is inadequate or ineffective. Some medical conditions may alter prealbumin levels, but it is still a useful laboratory value for nutritional status.

Retinol Binding Protein

Retinol binding protein (RBP) has a half-life of 12 hours and can be used to monitor short term changes in nutritional status. RBP levels can be elevated by conditions such as renal disease.

Hemoglobin and Hematocrit

Anemia may occur in hospitalized patients and is defined as a decrease in red cell mass. Hemoglobin and hematocrit are the main measures used to indicate anemia. Iron deficiency may occur as a result of inadequate iron intake or a decrease in iron stores. Although some medical conditions may cause iron deficiency, the main cause of anemia is chronic blood loss. Once the cause of the iron deficiency anemia is identified, iron stores need to be replenished through iron supplementation. Improvement of iron deficiency through supplementation will take several weeks to appear in hemoglobin and hematocrit tests. Therefore, these tests are generally not useful measures of nutritional status.

TABLE 48-3   Laboratory Values Related to Nutrition Screening

TEST NAME	NORMAL VALUES FOR ADULTS
Albumin	3.5–5 g/dL
Transferrin	Adult male 215–365 mg/dL
	Adult female 250–380 mg/dL
Prealbumin	15–36 mg/dL or 150–360 mg/
Retinol binding protein	3–6 mg/dL

Adapted from Halas, M. (2004). Nutrition. In R. Daniels (Ed.), Nursing fundamentals: Caring and clinical decision making. New York: Thomson Delmar Learning.

Nursing Diagnoses

Based on the information gathered, examples of nursing diagnoses in the patient with malnutrition may include the following (Ackley & Ladwig, 2004):

- Adult failure to thrive.
- Deficient knowledge related to: Information misinterpretation or lack of exposure.
- Imbalanced nutrition: Less than body requirements.

Planning and Implementation

There are many interventions that can be employed for patients with malnutrition. The entire health care team must be utilized in both the planning and implementation phases of care.

Goals

The goal for the patient with malnutrition is to restore nutritional status as much as is possible given the patient's comorbid medical problems. This may involve supplementing the regular diet with high protein, providing high-calorie foods and beverages, adding vitamin and mineral supplements, or providing the patient with enteral or PN if he or she is unable to meet his or her nutritional needs with food.

Collaborative Management

The multidisciplinary team approach to improving nutritional status should include the physician, RN, nursing assistant, clinical dietitian, and may also include a pharmacist, social worker, discharge planner, occupational therapist, and other health care team members. The causes of inadequate food intake must be identified through history and physical examination. Modifiable factors must be corrected. This may include obtaining dentures from home for patients unable to chew hospital food, modifying diet textures, or making changes to medications that cause decreased appetite. Members of the multidisciplinary team need to review factors affecting the patient's nutritional status and modify the patient's treatment plan accordingly.

Pharmacology

Malnutrition may be related to medications that cause nausea, vomiting, diarrhea, or anorexia. Attempts must be made to identify the medications causing such side effects and either modify the doses or find a suitable substitute.

Health Care Resources

Malnourished patients who live alone or have limited incomes may benefit from obtaining meals from community services. Senior centers may offer meals at a reduced price. Agencies, such as Meals on Wheels, are available to deliver meals to those in need.

Patient and Family Teaching

Hospital-based RDs and the RN are excellent resources to educate the patient and family members about how to improve the patient's nutritional status. This education may include evaluating the patient's resources at home, referring them to appropriate community resources for meals at home, and reviewing general nutrition principles.

Evaluation of Outcomes

Potential patient outcomes for each of the example nursing diagnoses for the patient with malnutrition are:

- Adult failure to thrive. Patient will consume adequate fluid intake with no signs of dehydration.

- Deficient knowledge related to information misinterpretation or lack of exposure. Patient will list resources that can be used for support after discharge.
- Imbalanced nutrition: less than body requirements. Patient will consume adequate food and fluids to meet nutritional needs and be free of signs of malnutrition.

JCAHO Provision of Care, Treatment, and Services standards require that hospitals have written criteria for when a more in-depth assessment is completed (2004). JCAHO accredited hospitals have a process in place to screen patients for nutrition risk and refer at-risk patients for further assessment.

The Level II nutritional screening tool shown in Table 48-4 uses a point system to identify a patient's level of risk for malnutrition. Nutrition risk triggers

---

TABLE 48-4 Level II Nutrition Screening

Height: _____ cm/in   Weight: _____ kg/lb   BMI: _____   IBW: _____   UBW: _____
Diet Order: _____   Age _____   Male/Female
Food allergies/sensitivities noted: Y/N   Cultural/religious preferences noted: Y/N

RISK FACTOR	EVALUATION	POINT VALUE	TOTAL POINTS
Weight Status	Unintentional wt loss of 5% or more in past month	1 point	
	≤ 85% IBW	1 point	
	BMI ≥ 30 (obese)	1 point	
Medical Status/Condition	Comatose/unresponsive	1 point	
	Geriatric surgical (≥ 75 years old)	1 point	
	Nausea, vomiting, diarrhea, constipation for 3 days or more	1 point	
Eating Difficulties	Sore mouth	1 point	
	Chewing/Swallowing	1 point	
	Unable to feed self	1 point	
Recent Intake/Appetite (over past month)	Good (≥ 75%)	0 points	
	Fair (50-75%)	1 point	
	Poor (25-50%)	2 points	
	Minimal (< 25%)	3 points	
Skin	Pressure ulcer stage I	1 point	
	Pressure ulcer stage II, III, or IV	Automatic RD referral	
Labs	Albumin level _____	1 point if ≤ 3.0	
Education	If on a modified diet, does pt request or need a diet instruction? Y/N	Automatic RD referral for education if yes	
Risk Determination	CHOOSE ONE: 0-4 Low Nutritional Risk > 4 High Nutritional Risk (RD to follow)		TOTAL POINTS: _____ RD to follow: Y/N

COMMENTS:

_____

_____

_____

Signature _____ Date/time _____

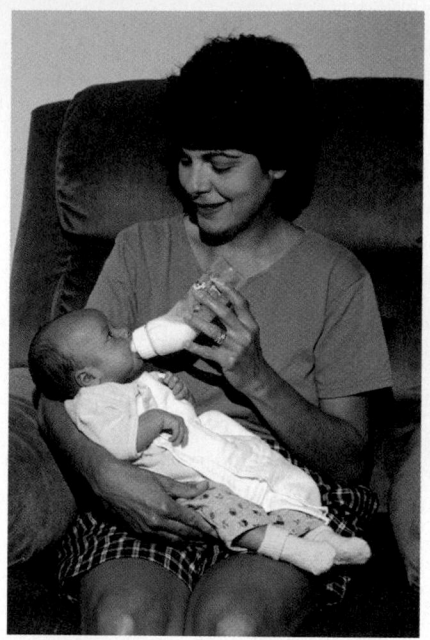

Figure 48-7 Visual assessment for nutritional risk.

may include factors, such as decreased food intake, weight loss, advanced age, and high risk medical diagnoses. Patients at nutrition risk are referred to an RD for further assessment and reassessment.

Taking a verbal diet history provides an opportunity to better assess knowledge and cultural impacts on the patient's nutritional habits. The probes, or questions, on the diet history form provided in Table 48-5 helps ensure that broad areas related to nutritional status are assessed. Yet, it is flexible enough to facilitate deeper exploration of troubling responses from the patient.

The nurse plays a vital role in the identification of patients at nutrition risk and in assisting family members to assess and meet the patient's nutritional needs (Figure 48-7) (Table 48-6). Patients may not initially meet nutrition risk criteria but may experience a decline in nutrition status during the hospital stay. Referring patients to dietetic technicians and dietitians when new nutrition risk factors, such as difficulty swallowing, decreased appetite, weight loss, and skin breakdown, develop can facilitate nutrition interventions. In addition, by ensuring that intake and output records and intake analysis or calorie counts are accurate, the nurse provides important data for the nutrition assessment.

TABLE 48-5 **Diet History**

Part 1: General Diet Information

Do you follow a particular diet?

What are your food likes and dislikes?

Do you have any especially strong cravings?

How often do you eat fast foods?

How often do you eat at restaurants?

Do you have adequate financial resources to purchase your food?

How do you obtain, store, and prepare your food?

Do you eat alone or with a family member or other person?

In the last 12 months have you

   experienced any change in weight?

   had a change in your appetite?

   had a change in your diet?

   experienced nausea, vomiting, or diarrhea from your diet?

   changed your diet because of difficulty in feeding yourself, eating, chewing, or swallowing?

Part 2: Food Intake History
      (24-Hour Recall, 3-Day Diary, Direct Observation)

Time	Food/Drink	Amount	Method of Preparation	Eating Location

TABLE 48-6 Comprehensive Nutrition History

Nutritional History

Physical Assessment

1. General appearance
2. Skin
3. Nails
4. Hair
5. Eyes
6. Mouth
7. Head and neck
8. Heart and peripheral vasculature
9. Abdomen
10. Musculosketal system
11. Neurological system
12. Female genitalia

Anthropometric Measurements

Height: _____ in or cm   % Weight Change: _____

Weight: _____ lbs or kg   Body Mass Index: _____

% Ideal Body Weight: _____   Waist/Hip Ratio: _____

% Usual Body Weight: _____   Triceps Skinfold: _____

Mid-Arm Circumference: _____ cm

Mid-Arm Muscle Circumference: _____ cm

Laboratory Data

Hematocrit (HCT): _____%   Hemoglobin (HGB): _____ g/dL

Cholesterol: _____ mg/dL   HDL: _____ mg/dL   LDL: _____ mg/dL

Triglycerides: _____ mg/dL

TIBC: _____ μg/dL

Transferrin: _____ mg/dL

Iron: _____ μg/dL

Total Lymphocyte Count: _____ cells/mm^3

Antigen Skin Testing: _____

Albumin: _____ g/dL

Glucose: _____ mg/dL

CHI: _____

Nitrogen Balance: _____ g

Diagnostic Data

X-rays _____

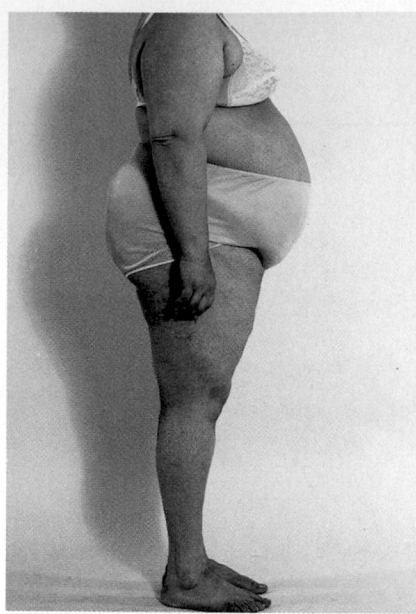

Figure 48-8 Obese adult. *Courtesy of the Armed Forces Institute of Pathology.*

BOX 48-2

CALCULATION OF BMI

The formula for calculating BMI is as follows:

$$BMI = \frac{Weight\ (kg)}{Height\ (m^2)}$$

BOX 48-3

BMI CATEGORIES

Underweight = less than 18.5

Normal weight = 18.5–24.9

Overweight = 25–29.9

Obesity = BMI of 30 or greater

Source: National Institutes of Health National Heart, Lung, and Blood Institute. (1998). Clinical guidelines on the identification, evaluation, and treatment of overweight and obesity in adults. The evidence report. *NIH Publication No. 98-4083, Bethesda, MD: Author.*

OBESITY

Obesity, as shown in Figure 48-8, continues to be a public health concern in the United States. In 2002 about 65.7 percent of Americans were overweight compared to 55.9 percent between 1988 and1994 (Headley, Ogden, Johnson, Carroll, Curtain, & Flegal, 2004). The causes of obesity appear to be multifactorial, including increased caloric consumption along with inadequate exercise (Goldberg, et al., 2004).

The body mass index (BMI) is a weight-stature index used as a measure of obesity and of malnutrition. The formula for determining BMI appears in Box 48-2. It is calculated using the body weight in kilograms divided by the square of the height in meters. Healthy weight is based on a BMI of 18.5–25. When a BMI reaches 25 to 29.9, it is considered overweight. The BMI of 25 was selected because research reveals increased mortality with BMIs above this level. Obesity is defined as a BMI greater than 30 (National Institutes of Health National Heart, Lung, and Blood Institute, 1998). The BMI categories are presented in Box 48-3.

Epidemiology

The incidence of overweight children and teenagers is on the rise. The rate of childhood obesity has tripled over the last 30 years in children ages 6–11, and doubled for ages 2 to 5 and 12 to 19. In a study of 11- to 13-year-old school children it was found that 35.3 percent had a BMI at or above the 85th percentile; and 17.4 percent of them had a BMI at or above the 95th percentile. BMI at or above 85 percent and less than 95 percent is considered at risk for overweight. Overweight is at or above the 95th percentile for gender-specific BMI charts for children. (Hedley, et al., 2004). A significant correlation between BMI, hours of television watched in the evening, and the amount of soft drinks consumed has been noted (Giammattei, Blix, Marshak, Wollitzer, & Pettitt, et al., 2003).

Etiology

Overweight children are at high risk for becoming overweight adults and are at risk for developing chronic diseases normally seen later in life. Overweight and obese adults are at increased risk for developing many serious health conditions, including hypertension, elevated blood lipid levels, type 2 diabetes, gallbladder disease, coronary artery disease, and certain types of cancer (Watkins, 2004).

The cause of type 1 diabetes is not known, but it is proposed that the body's immune system attacks itself, destroying the cells in the pancreas that produce insulin. As a result, type 1 diabetics must monitor their blood glucose regularly and use insulin. The incidence of type 2 diabetes mellitus is increasing significantly, not only in the United States but also in other industrialized societies. This increase is because of a sedentary lifestyle, increasing rates of obesity, and an aging population. Diabetes is the cause of many complications, such as end-stage renal disease and cardiovascular disease, both of which impact the patient's length of hospital stay, hospital costs, and mortality (MMWR, 2004; Winer & Sowers, 2004).

Assessment with Clinical Manifestations

There are many aspects to assessing patients who are obese. The first federal guidelines for identification, evaluation, and treatment of overweight and obesity were released in 1998 by the National Heart, Lung, and Blood Institute (NHLBI) in conjunction with the National Institute of Diabetes and Digestive

Kidney Diseases (NIDDKD). The guidelines were based on an extensive review of the research on overweight and obesity and were established for health care professionals to use in their practice.

The guidelines recommend that health care professionals measure the patient's BMI, evaluate the patient's risk factors, and measure waist circumference. Waist circumference of over 40 inches in men and over 35 inches in women indicates increased risk in patients with a BMI of 25 to 34.9.

Because it has been established that patients may enter the hospital in a state of poor nutrition and that the nutritional status of a well-nourished patient with acute medical problems may deteriorate during the hospital stay, it is critical that nutrition status be monitored throughout hospitalization. Changes in nutrition status may occur more slowly and be less noticeable than changes in medical status. Malnutrition may be identified via physical assessment and laboratory tests.

Physical assessment may be performed by the health care provider and other trained health professionals. A general survey may reveal muscle wasting and lethargy, which may indicate inadequate caloric intake. Increased temperature and respirations may indicate increased fluid and caloric needs. Signs of poor wound healing may indicate the need for increased protein and vitamins. Poor dental health may indicate an obstacle to adequate oral intake.

Nursing Diagnoses

Based on the information gathered, examples of nursing diagnoses in the patient with obesity may include the following (Ackley & Ladwig, 2004):
- Imbalanced nutrition: More than body requirements related to excessive intake in relation to metabolic need.
- Risk for imbalanced nutrition: More than body requirements.
- Disturbed body image.
- Anxiety related to change in lifestyle.

Planning and Implementation

The nurse is responsible for implementing a wide variety of nursing interventions for patients with obesity. Obesity causes many health problems. Therefore, weight loss is recommended to lower blood pressure, improve blood lipid levels, and lower elevated blood glucose. Strategies for successful weight loss include reducing caloric intake, increasing physical activity, and modifying behaviors to improve eating and exercise habits. The initial goal is to reduce body weight by 10 percent of baseline within six months of treatment through the loss of 1 to 2 pounds per week. A 10 percent weight loss in six months can be achieved by decreasing caloric intake by 300 to 500 calories per day for those with BMI between 27 and 35. For those with BMI greater than 35, it will require decreasing caloric intake by 500 to 1,000 calories per day to achieve a 10 percent decrease in weight in six months.

Collaborative Management with Multidisciplinary Team Approach

The nurse can play an important role in the nutritional status of the hospitalized patient by referring malnourished patients to the RD, alerting the health care provider regarding patients with swallowing difficulty or changes in nutritional and functional status, addressing the causes of mouth pain, and offering the patient supplemental foods and fluids allowed by the health care provider.

Pharmacology

Medications may be used to assist patients in their weight loss efforts; however, patients should try to modify their diet and lifestyle for at least six months before trying drug therapy prescribed by a health care provider. Weight loss

---

PATIENT PLAYBOOK

Patient and Family Teaching Related to the Management of Body Weight

The patient should be taught to decrease food intake through monitoring portion sizes:
- Read labels and serve a standard portion on a plate, rather than serving food out of a box or bag.
- Eat slowly so that the brain gets the message that the stomach is full.
- Take seconds of vegetables and salads instead of higher calorie foods.
- Try to eat three balanced meals at regular times.

medications can then be included in a weight loss program that includes dietary changes and physical activity. Patients should have BMI greater than or equal to 30 without additional risk factors, such as diabetes.

Surgery

Bariatric surgery for obesity has increased in popularity. The number of bariatric procedures has increased from 6,868 in 1996 to 45,473 in 2001 (Livingston, 2004). Weight loss surgery may be recommended for severely obese patients with BMI greater than or equal to 40 or BMI greater than or equal to 35 with comorbid conditions (i.e., diabetes, heart disease, or sleep apnea) when other methods of treatment have failed. Extremely obese patients are at high risk for premature death and do benefit from the conservative treatment of diet and lifestyle modification compared to patients who are less obese.

There are several types of bariatric surgical procedures. Some limit food intake but do not interfere with the digestive process. In adjustable gastric banding, a band of silicone rubber is placed around the upper part of the stomach creating a pouch and a narrow passage into the rest of the stomach. Vertical banded gastroplasty involves using a band and staples to create a stomach pouch. Although these procedures are easier to perform and may be safer than the procedures which impact the digestive process, the patients may lose less weight, they may suffer from vomiting as a result of the narrow passage into the stomach, and the band may break down.

Procedures that are used more commonly today restrict food intake and alter the digestive process. The Roux-en-Y gastric bypass is the most commonly performed procedure in the United States. A stomach pouch is created and connected to a Y-shaped section of the small intestine, thus bypassing absorption that would take place in the stomach and upper small intestine. Patients lose more weight and at a faster pace than with procedures, such as the adjustable gastric banding and the vertical banded gastroplasty. A disadvantage is that because of the altered digestion, long-term nutritional deficiencies may develop. To avoid nutritional problems, patients need to take vitamin and mineral supplements and ensure adequate protein intake. In addition, patients may suffer from dumping syndrome after consuming high-carbohydrate foods that result in stomach contents moving to the small intestine too quickly. The patient may suffer from nausea, abdominal pain, bloating, weakness, and diarrhea. Bariatric surgical procedures may be performed laparoscopically in some patients, and as a result will have smaller incisions (NIH, 2004).

Nursing care for patients on restricted diets in the hospital setting should be supportive. When conservative weight management is indicated, the nurse can help by gently reinforcing the rationale for weight reduction and assisting the patient with activity. The postoperative diets (Box 48-4) for bariatric surgery patients will be limited initially to facilitate digestion and prevent dumping syndrome.

BOX 48-4

POSTBARIATRIC SURGERY DIET PROGRESSION

First 1 to 2 Days While in the Hospital

- Ice chips
- Water or sugar-free, noncarbonated beverage, about 4 oz per hour

First Postoperative Visit with Surgeon, 5 to 12 Days Postoperatively

- Water
- Sugar-free, noncarbonated beverages
- Sugar free popsicles
- Diet Jell-O
- Decaffeinated coffee or tea
- Chicken or beef broth

Evaluation of Outcomes

Potential patient outcomes for each of the example nursing diagnoses for the patient with obesity are (Ackley & Ladwig, 2004):

- Imbalanced nutrition: More than body requirements. The patient will voice feelings about present weight. The patient will identify internal and external cues that increase food consumption.
- Risk for imbalanced nutrition: More than body requirements. The patient will compare current eating pattern with recommended eating patterns. The patient will explain the concept of a balanced diet.
- Disturbed body image. The patient will correctly estimate the relationship of body to environment.
- Anxiety related to change in lifestyle. The patient should be able to recognize the signs of anxiety, demonstrate positive coping mechanisms, and describe a reduction in the level of anxiety experienced.

NUTRITION AND AGING

There are many physical changes as a result of the aging process, as well as changes in nutrient needs. Older adults generally require fewer calories as they get older based on changes in body composition and decreased activity level. Older adults are more prone to dehydration, because they have decreased total body water as compared to younger people. In addition, their thirst mechanism may be altered and they may have inadequate fluid intake at home due to factors, such as difficulty obtaining groceries or GI problems. Older adults may have more indigestion or food intolerance than younger adults because of a decrease in gastric motility and gastric secretions, as well as delayed gastric emptying. In addition, constipation is a common problem as a result of medications, inactivity, and inadequate fluid and fiber intake.

Research on older individuals with healthy diets and active lifestyles indicates that many of the declines associated with aging can be counteracted by a healthy lifestyle. In a study of men and women 70 to 90 years old who followed a Mediterranean diet, did not smoke, were moderately active, and had moderate alcohol consumption, one third had lower mortality than individuals who had less healthful behaviors (Knoops, deGroot, Kromhout, et al., 2004). Although there are many countries bordering the Mediterranean Sea, common components of the Mediterranean diet include a high intake of fruits, vegetables, nuts, seeds, olive oil as a fat source, poultry, fish, minimal intake of red meat, and low to moderate intake of dairy products and wine (American Heart Association, 2001).

KEY CONCEPTS

- A nutritionally adequate diet plays a vital role in the prevention of chronic disease.
- There are many potential food and drug interactions with which the nurse must be familiar.
- Enteral or PN may be provided to patients unable to meet their nutritional needs through diet.
- Malnutrition in hospitalized patients increases complications, costs, and length of hospital stay.
- Obesity and type 2 diabetes are on the rise.
- The half-life of laboratory tests of nutrition status vary. Laboratory tests with a shorter half-life may be more valuable in the hospital setting.

REVIEW QUESTIONS

1. Nutrition research published in a report by the IOM Food and Nutrition Board recommended an ideal percentage intake of carbohydrates, protein, and fat to prevent chronic disease for adults. These percentages are:
   1. 20 to 30 percent of calories from carbohydrate, 30 to 40 percent from fat, and 40 percent from protein
   2. 45 to 65 percent of calories from carbohydrate, 20 to 35 percent from fat, and 10 to 35 percent of calories from protein
   3. 60 to 70 percent of calories from carbohydrate, 15 to 20 percent from fat, and 15 to 20 percent from protein
   4. None of the above

2. The nurse receives an order from the health care provider for indirect calorimetry. She knows that this is an order to:
   1. Record the patient's calorie count for three days
   2. Measure the amount of calories burned through a blood assay
   3. Estimate energy expenditure by measuring oxygen consumption and carbon dioxide production
   4. Collect accurate intake and output records

Continued

3. BMI is a weight-stature index used to classify obesity. You know your patient is considered obese if his or her BMI is greater than:
   1. 25
   2. 18
   3. 50
   4. 30

4. Your patient is being discharged on a medication called warfarin. In the discharge teaching for this patient, you should emphasize which of the following?
   1. Avoid food sources high in vitamin K to maintain INR levels
   2. Avoid foods high in vitamin C and iron because they will decrease the absorption of warfarin
   3. Maintain a consistent intake of foods high in vitamin K, such as dark leafy greens
   4. Increase your intake of foods high in vitamin K to reduce the dose of warfarin needed

5. Your patient's health care provider has just written an order for "NG" feeding. You know that this means the patient will be having:
   1. A feeding of special medicines for a nuclear gout study
   2. A nasogastric tube for feeding
   3. Oral medicines to prepare for a Niacin-globulin test
   4. A diet high in non-gas producing foods

6. Hospitalized patients may be fed enterally via a tube feeding. Which of the following statements about tube feedings is true?
   1. Because enteral feeding tubes can be uncomfortable for the patient, feeding via the parenteral route is a good alternative with less complications.
   2. To decrease the risk of aspiration, patients receiving continuous feedings should have the head of the bed elevated 30 degrees.
   3. Blenderizing foods and putting them through the patient's tube feeding is as beneficial as using commercial products and is much less expensive.
   4. When a patient has diarrhea, the tube feeding is always the cause.

7. The nurse should be alert to new nutrition risk factors, which can develop during the patient's hospital stay. These risk factors include:
   1. Chewing and swallowing difficulties
   2. Healing of skin breakdown
   3. Increased appetite
   4. Improved mental status

8. Which of the following lab results indications that your patient has decreased visceral protein stores and may be malnourished?
   1. Prealbumin 10 mg/dL
   2. Fasting blood glucose 135 mg/dL
   3. Total cholesterol 249
   4. Hemoglobin 5.2

9. In caring for an elderly patient, the nurse should be aware of the following aspects of aging on hydration:
   1. A decrease in total body fluids, increasing the risk for dehydration
   2. Elderly people are thirstier than younger people and may have fluid overload as a result of increased thirst.
   3. Adequate hydration is not a problem because the elderly usually have access to plenty of fluids.

10. Which of the following statements is true regarding nutrition and chronic disease?
    1. The incidence of obesity is stable; however, diabetes is on the rise.
    2. Poor nutrition is related to chronic disease, and chronic diseases are responsible for 7 of 10 leading causes of death.
    3. Nutrition plays less of a role in the development of type 2 diabetes than type 1 diabetes.
    4. Chronic diseases, such as diabetes, are caused by genetics rather than diet and lifestyle.

REVIEW ACTIVITIES

1. Your patient wants to know how to improve his diet. He is currently overweight and is concerned about getting diabetes because he has a positive family history. What general comments about an optimal diet would you offer and to which resources would you refer him?

2. Determine the BMI for a few friends or family members. Where do their results fall in the classification of normal versus overweight?

3. Review the list of sample tube feedings. Why would a patient need a formula higher in protein?

4. Ask nurses you know in your nearby hospital about their hospital's process for nutrition screening. What kinds of forms do they use, what nutrition risk factors are included, and what is their process?

5. What lifestyle factors are correlated with the rise in childhood obesity? What changes have you noticed during your lifetime regarding childhood obesity and the lifestyles of children today?

6. What are some interventions you can take with your elderly patients to help maintain their nutritional status?

Visit the Contemporary Medical-Surgical Nursing online companion resource at www.delmarhealthcare.com for additional content and study aids. Click on Online Companions then select the Nursing discipline.

Upper Gastrointestinal Tract Dysfunction: Nursing Management

Elizabeth Torrence, RN, MN, EdD

CHAPTER TOPICS

- Oral and Esophageal Disorders
- Nausea and Vomiting
- Gastroesophageal Reflux Disease
- Hiatal Hernia
- Dyspepsia
- Gastritis
- Stomach Cancer

KEY TERMS

Achalasia
Aphthous stomatitis
Apoptosis
Borborygmi sounds
Brash water
Dyspepsia
Dysphagia
Presbyphagia
Pyrosis
Sarcopenia

All illness results from the connection of genetics, environment, biology, and psychosocial variables. Especially in the approach to a patient with an upper gastrointestinal (GI) tract disorder the nurse must consider all of these variables. The degree of symptomatology associated with GI problems is not always explained by the diagnostic findings of endoscopy, manometry, or radiography. Emotional distress can influence individuals who have no history of GI dysfunction. During times of emotional upheaval, individuals may experience intense autonomic responses that can alter motility, vascularity, secretion, and pain perception. Likewise, GI dysfunction can affect areas of the brain, especially areas of the limbic system. This area of the brain is associated with the sleep-wake cycle, arousal, anxiety, and fear.

As with care for all patients, individuals with GI disorders should be listened to with empathy and be given reassurance and education. The nurse should ascertain the patient and family's expectations and concerns, ensure continuity of care through a collaborative care pathway, and support and encourage follow-up for health promotion activities.

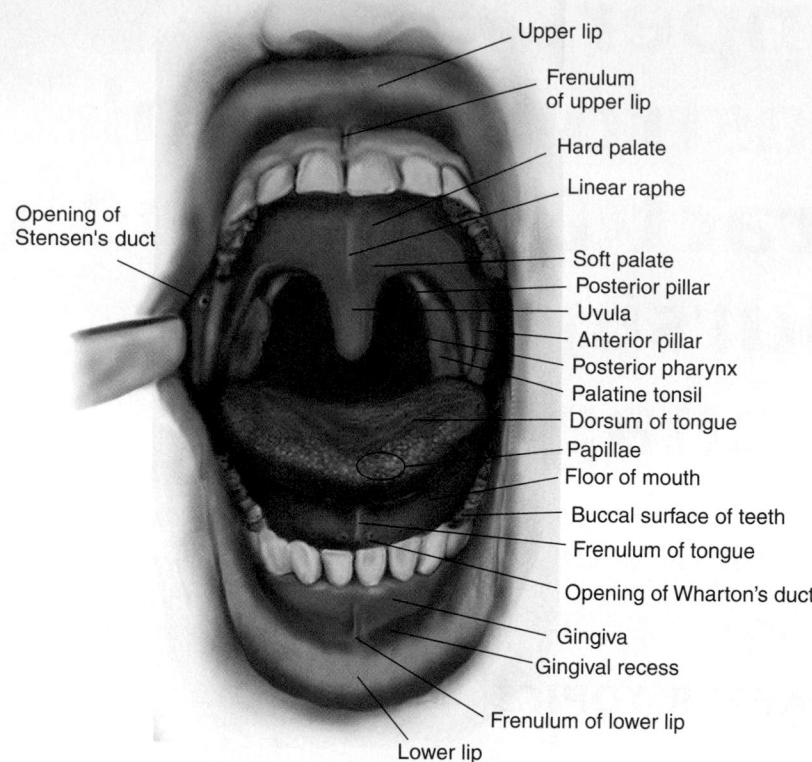

Figure 49-1 Structure of the mouth.

DISORDERS OF THE ORAL CAVITY

Ulcerative conditions of the gums and mucous membranes are labeled mouth ulcers (**aphthous stomatitis**) and occur in 20 percent of the population (Figure 49-1). Most mouth ulcers are minor and heal within 7 to 14 days. Herpetiform ulcers may take up to one month to heal. The causes of oral ulcerations can be found in the Table 49-1.

Etiology

More than 400,000 cancer patients experience oral problems, such as painful mouth ulcers, impaired taste, and dry mouth from salivary gland dysfunction. These individuals should receive dental assessment prior to beginning chemo or radiation therapy. If preexisting oral problems are resolved prior to cancer treatment, it may ameliorate complications and tissue damage. Patients who smoke have seven times the risk of developing gum disease. Nevertheless, any type of tobacco use, cigarettes, pipes, and smokeless tobacco raises the risk for gum disease, oral and throat cancers, as well as fungal infections (candidiasis). Heavy alcohol use also increases the risk of oral and throat cancer, especially if the individual also uses tobacco.

Planning and Implementation

Management of patients who have oral ulcers depends on the cause. Nurses must assess the mouth regularly, particularly when there are suspected complications associated with specific causes or problems (Figure 49-2). Rinsing the mouth with chlorhexidine may relieve the symptoms and reduce the healing time. Topical corticosteroids are also used to resolve these ulcers. Because eating may aggravate the discomfort the patient has with oral ulcer-

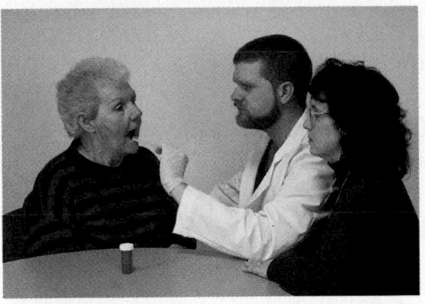

Figure 49-2 A nurse assessing the mouth of this patient with stomatitis with a concerned family member observing.

TABLE 49-1 Main Systemic and Iatrogenic Causes of Oral Ulcers	
Microbial Diseases	**Malignant Neoplasms**
• Herpetic stomatitis	**Blood Disorders**
• Chickenpox	
• Herpes zoster	• Anemia
• Hand, foot, and mouth disease	• Leukemia
• Herpangina	• Neutropenia
• Infectious mononucleosis	• Other white cell dyscrasias
• HIV infection	**GI Disease**
• Acute necrotizing gingivitis	
• Tuberculosis	• Coeliac disease
• Syphilis	• Crohn's disease
• Fungal infections	• Ulcerative colitis
Cutaneous Disease	**Rheumatoid Diseases**
• Lichen planus	• Lupus erythematosus
• Pemphigus	• Behçet's syndrome
• Pemphigoid	• Sweet's syndrome
• Erythema multiforme	• Reiter's disease
• Dermatitis herpetiformis	**Drugs**
• Linear IgA disease	
• Epidermolysis bullosa	• Cytotoxic agents
	• Nicorandil
Chronic Ulcerative Stomatitis	**Radiotherapy**
• Other dermatoses	

Adapted from Furlanetto, D., Crighton, A., & Topping, G. (2006). Differences in methodologies of measuring the prevalence of oral mucosal lesions in children and adolescents. International Journal of Pediatric Dentistry, 16(1), 31–39; Talhari, C., Angerstein, W., Becker, J., Ruzicka, T., & Megahed, M. (2005). Long-standing oral ulcers. Lancet, 365(9463), 1002.

ations, they may need mouth rinses that contain topical analgesics, such as viscous Xylocaine.

Nonulcerative Causes of Mouth Pain

Erythema migrans (benign migratory glossitis) is a nonulcerative inflammatory and sometimes painful condition of the tongue. It is characterized by multiple areas of erythema surrounded by yellowish-white borders. These lesions may be asymptomatic but often are painful. Because there is no effective treatment for this disorder, symptomatic relief is provided. Patients with particular systemic disorders may also experience oral glossitis. These include anemia, vitamin B deficiencies, oral lichen planus, aphthous ulcers, pemphigus, and syphilis.

Etiology

Causes of nonulcerative mouth pain can include:
• Infections, such as viral herpes simplex or bacterial infections;
• Mechanical injury from eating or drinking hot or spicy food or fluid.
• Irritants, such as alcohol, smoking and chewing tobacco.
• Trauma to the tongue, irregular areas of the teeth or dental appliances.
• Allergies and exposure to certain substances in toothpaste, mouthwash, breath fresheners, certain dyes in food, plastics in certain dental appliances (dentures or retainers), and some medications have been indicated, such as angiotensin-converting enzyme (ACE) inhibitors.

Oral Cancer Self-Assessment

The nurse should teach the patient the following as prevention of oral care of his or her face, lips, and oral cavity:

1. Look in the mirror at your face. Check for symmetry. Are there any lumps, swelling, or bumps that you notice on only one side of your face?
2. Assess the skin on you face. Is the texture the same throughout? Are there any moles, sores, or growths that have changed in size or color?
3. Check your neck and under your chin. Can you feel any lumps, tenderness or any area of swelling?
4. Assess your lips. Pull the lips up and down and look for any sores or color changes. Feel for any lumps, bumps, or change in the texture of normal mucous membrane.
5. With a flashlight, pull your cheek out so that you can look inside. Note any area of discoloration—extreme redness, white areas, or other discoloration. Check to see if there are any lumps, swelling, or bumps in either cheek. Is there any area of tenderness?
6. Are there any changes in the upper roof of your mouth, in texture, swelling, or color?
7. Look at all sides of your tongue. Are there any changes?
8. If you find anything that appears different or if you have any sores or areas in your mouth that do not heal within two weeks, call your dentist for follow-up.

Adapted from Estes, M. (2006). Health assessment and physical examination (3rd ed.). New York: Thomson Delmar Learning.

Nursing Diagnoses

Based on the information gathered, examples of nursing diagnoses in the patient with mouth pain may include the following:

- Impaired oral mucous membrane related to oral pain.
- Health-seeking behaviors related to oral pain.
- Risk for infection related to mouth pain.
- Risk for imbalanced nutrition, less than body requirements, related to oral pain.
- Impaired tissue integrity related to mouth pain.

Planning and Implementation

Once the cause of the disorder is determined, the plan of care can be formalized. During the diagnostic assessment, comfort measures and removal of known irritants should be initiated. Predisposing and contributing factors should be identified, and interventions to alter these factors should be part of the plan of care. Ulcerations should resolve in one week to 10 days once the contributing factors have been removed. Good oral hygiene is essential. Chlorhexidine 2% aqueous mouthwash is recommended. Topical pain relief can be provided with the use of oral mouthwash. Products such as benzydamine hydrochloride (Difflam) can be used. Topical corticosteroids can promote resolution of the ulcers. Products such as triamcinolone acetonide in cellulose paste are used. Any patient who has a mouth ulcer that lasts longer than three weeks should receive follow-up.

Evaluation of Outcomes

Potential patient outcomes for each of the example nursing diagnoses for the patient with mouth pain are:

- Impaired oral mucous membrane related to oral pain. The patient has intact oral mucosa.
- Health-seeking behaviors related to oral pain. The patient demonstrates appropriate oral hygiene.
- Risk for infection related to mouth pain. The patient remains free of infection, as evidenced by normal vital signs and absence of purulent drainage from wounds, incisions, and tubes. Infection is recognized early to allow for prompt treatment.
- Risk for imbalanced nutrition, less than body requirements, related to oral pain. The patient verbalizes and demonstrates selection of foods or meals that will achieve a cessation of weight loss and weighs within 10 percent of ideal body weight.
- Impaired tissue integrity related to mouth pain. The patient's skin condition should be improved as evidenced by decreased redness, swelling and pain.

Burning Mouth Syndrome

Burning mouth syndrome (oral dysesthesia, glossopyrosis, and glossodynia) is a constant burning sensation of the tongue seen in patients past middle age. It is thought to be a type of neuropathy. The discomfort is relieved by eating and drinking. There are many organic causes of this disorder, which include candidiasis, lichen planus, diabetes, xerostomia, ill-fitting denture, certain medications, and glossitis related to nutritional deficiencies such as vitamin B, folate, and iron. Patients with this syndrome should also be assessed for psychological dysfunction such as depression, cancer fears, or anxiety.

Planning and Implementation

In addition to gingival health, it is essential to assess the condition of the teeth. The nurse should determine if the patient has the ability to clean their teeth properly, note when the patient last visited a dentist for oral care, and determine if their dentition interferes with eating and nutritional intake. Oral care for the patient while hospitalized is essential (see Patient Playbook).

Dysphagia

Swallowing is a complex activity that begins in the mouth with adequate wetting and mastication of food and fluid. This requires good dentition, a healthy oropharynx, adequate salivation, and muscular strength. Because of the increasing numbers of older patients and limitations caused by age-related decreases in muscle mass **(sarcopenia)**, dysphagia in the elderly **(presbyphagia)** is underestimated. **Dysphagia** (difficulty swallowing) represents a major problem in the older adult and needs special attention to prevent aspiration pneumonitis or pneumonia, airway obstruction, malnutrition, and dehydration. Aspiration normally involves solid and liquid material entering the larynx below the true vocal cords. In addition, there is silent aspiration, which occurs without a cough response or voice change. Dysphagia must be recognized and assessed. Swallowing changes must be differentiated from age-related primary presbyphagia or secondary presbyphagia from other disorders (e.g., stroke, neuromuscular disorders). More than half of patients who experience a stroke demonstrate dysphagia dependent on when they are screened (Box 49-1).

Assessment with Clinical Manifestations

To prevent or decrease aspiration risk, screening must be done for all patients suspected of having swallowing problems or dysphagia especially patients who are at risk or have had a stroke (Box 49-2). Bedside assessment of aspiration risk is variable because of the increase in false-positive results. Interrater and intrarater reli-

---

BOX 49-1

DYSPHAGIA

Nurses are often the first health care provider who notices that the patient is experiencing chewing or swallowing problems. The estimates of dysphagia in health care facilities range from 25 to 45 percent. By the year 2010, the Agency for Health Care Research and Quality (AHRQ) predicts that because of our aging population more than 16,500,000 people will experience dysphagia and need care or intervention. Many disciplines are interested in the problem of swallowing. These include nurses, speech pathologist, occupational therapists, physical therapists, pulmonologists, respiratory therapists, otolaryngologists, and neurologists. Hence the nurse will be actively involved with the health care team in the assessment and management of patients with this disorder.

BOX 49-2

NORMAL SWALLOWING

Normal Swallowing Requires:

- Intact and integrated functioning of cranial nerves V, VII, IX, X, XI, and XII, nucleus of the medulla, and sensorimotor cortical system
- Coordination of sensory stimuli, motor function, and coordinated movements during the swallow.

Stages of Swallowing:

- Oral prep.
- Food and liquids placed in the mouth.
- Thorough biting, sucking, and sealing ingested material between lips and jaw.
- Oral contents are chewed and mixed with saliva, forming a bolus because of voluntary movements of the tongue, jaw, and floor of the mouth.
- Oral.
- Food or liquid directed posteriorly toward oropharynx via movement of tongue, palate, and facial muscles.
- Pharyngeal—swallowing.
- Bolus of oral contents moved through the faucial arches and squeezed through the pharynx via muscles of the pharynx and the base of the tongue.
- Nasopharynx closed by soft palate, larynx moves upward, the epiglottis tilts, the glottis, and supraglottis closes off using the true and false vocal cords.
- Cricopharyngeal sphincter relaxes and opens to allow the bolus to enter esophagus.
- Esophageal.
- Involuntary peristalsis advances the bolus through the esophagus into the stomach—sequential waves of muscular contractions.

Adapted from Estes, M. (2006). Health assessment and physical examination (3rd ed.). New York: Thomson Delmar Learning; Payton, C. (2005). Referral diagnosis and management of dysphagia. Pulse, 65(8), 64–65.

ability studies demonstrate inconsistency in assessment results. Nonetheless this assessment should be done, and if dysphagia is suspected, nursing measures to prevent aspiration should be put into place. Cervical auscultation is one method of determining if a patient is aspirating during swallowing. Cervical auscultation by a skilled clinician has produced significantly high false-positive results. Cervical auscultation is performed by listening with the bell of the stethoscope over the lateral area of thyroid cartilage produced during swallowing (Estes, 2006). Eighty percent of the time, people exhale after swallowing. In the elderly and dysphagic patients, inspiration was found to be more common (Smith & Connolly, 2003). It is not recommended as a stand alone method to determine aspiration.

Diagnostic Tests

Patients who have difficulty swallowing will often be scheduled for a barium swallow exam, an endoscopic evaluation, esophageal manometry, and possibly esophageal transit scintigraphy. The presence of a gag reflex has been used as an indicator of the patient's ability to prevent a silent aspiration, although studies with videofluoroscopy demonstrated aspiration in patients with an intact gag reflex (Higo, Tayama, Nitou, Watanabe, & Ugawa, 2003). Bedside water swallow tests produce subjective results and though done may not detect dysphagia. Despite overdiagnosing swallowing disorders, a most important part of the assessment of dysphagia remains a careful bedside assessment. The nurse should perform an in-depth history with careful questioning of the patient and the caregiver concerning problems associated with swallowing (Box 49-3). Investigators have suggested the use of a dysphagia checklist as a screening tool for all patients.

BOX 49-3

ASSESSMENT OF A PATIENT WHO IS EXPERIENCING DIFFICULTY SWALLOWING

Is the patient exhibiting any of the following symptoms?
- Difficulty swallowing liquids—may indicate a neurological disorder.
- Difficulty with voice (dysphonia) or speech (dysarthria, abnormal speech articulation)—may indicate motor dysfunction.
- Difficulty swallowing solids—may indicate a structural abnormality.
- Regurgitation—may indicate pharyngeal pouch.
- Progressive dysphagia—may indicate hypopharyngeal tumor. (Are there any indications of aspiration?)
- Wet voice quality, coughing after eating or drinking, recurrent pulmonary infections. (Is there pain or discomfort when swallowing?)
- Have patient describe what happens when he or she swallows.
- Does the patient have problems managing oral secretions? Do you assess that the patient drools?
- Are mealtimes prolonged? Is there difficulty with chewing? Does food feel like it sticks in the throat or chest?
- Has the patient lost any weight?
- How much is the patient drinking daily?
- Does the patient drink fluids during the meal?
- Has the patient noticed a change in eating habits?
- Are there any problems with the patient's dentition?
- When was the last time the patient had a dental check-up?
- With all of the questions related to symptoms the nurse should ask about the onset, duration, severity of the problem, and relieving or aggravating factors.

Adapted from Estes, M. (2006). Health assessment and physical examination (3rd ed.). New York: Thomson Delmar Learning.

Fiberoptic endoscopic examination of swallowing can be used but is poorly tolerated in frail elderly. The contraction of the pharynx blocks the view of the food or liquid in the pharynx and esophagus but after the swallow, what remains in the pharynx can be identified. Some investigators have proposed that the use of pulse oximetry with the water swallow screening test can be a sensitive predictor of dysphagia with aspiration (Smith & Connolly, 2003). With the water swallow screening test a 2 percent drop in baseline SaO_2 was able to demonstrate aspiration in over 81 percent of patients with dysphagia. This is an important assessment skill for the nurse to develop. In many institutions this assessment is performed by specially trained speech and language therapists.

Currently the gold standard for evaluation of dysphagia is videofluoroscopy (also known as modified barium swallow) with or without manometric evaluation. This assessment demonstrates the swallowing mechanism. It also provides information about maneuvers and positions that facilitate and improve swallowing, e.g., tucking the chin (neck flexion) or holding the breath before swallowing. This maneuver may decrease aspiration. Turning the patient's head to the weak side (affected side if the patient has had a stroke) may force the bolus of food toward the unaffected side of the pharynx and augment the swallowing effort. Videofluoroscopy can be poorly tolerated and unsuitable for patients who are frail, unable to follow instructions, or not able to sit. Equipment and trained personnel may not be available to provide the assessment.

Nursing Diagnoses

Based on the information gathered, examples of nursing diagnoses in the patient with dysphagia may include the following:

- Impaired swallowing.
- Risk for aspiration.
- Health-seeking behaviors.
- Risk for injury.
- Risk for nutrition imbalanced, less than body requirements, or readiness for enhanced nutrition.
- Chronic pain.
- Disturbed sensory perception.
- Impaired tissue integrity.

Planning and Implementation

Patients who are experiencing swallowing difficulties have as their primary problems risk for aspiration, impaired swallowing, nutritional imbalance, altered comfort, a need for therapeutic regimen management, and knowledge deficit. Because patients perceive that they experience difficulty in consuming swallowed material, solid or liquid, they are at high risk for many nutritional problems. The problems the patient experiences may be related to oropharyngeal dysfunction from cerebrovascular accidents, neuromuscular disorders, mucosal diseases like gastroesophageal reflux disease (GERD), radiation injury, or mediastinal diseases, such as tumors. Patients must be involved in the collaborative management and planning of their care as the diagnosis and treatment plan is put into place.

Presently there are many recommendations for managing patients with dysphagia, but the evidence for the most effective management of these patients is largely anecdotal. Results have been mixed in that the patient population has not been homogeneous, the protocols and interventions have not been consistent, and differing outcomes have been measured. Functional severity scales are subjective; hence it is difficult to objectively quantify the measurements. Investigators and practitioners draw conclusions that cannot statistically be generalized to larger populations (Hill, Hughes, & Milford, 2005). The first goal of treatment is to ensure treatment of any underlying disorders. The nurse must ensure that aspiration is reduced, and nutritional status must be optimized. Concurrently, individualized plans of care are devised. Interventions that become part of everyday practice and recommendations include dietary manipulation; altered swallowing techniques, referred to as compensatory maneuvers in the rehabilitation literature; surgery; and in some cases enteral feeding. The best therapy for an impaired functional activity is the activity itself.

Nutrition

Once aspiration status is assessed in relation to liquids and solids, a plan for dietary management should be established and the consistency of the food established. Some patients may be restricted to thickened foods (i.e., they cannot swallow liquids). Foods that are tough are difficult to swallow so a mechanical soft diet is ordered for the patient. Some patients may need a pureed diet, especially if their swallowing difficulty is with the oral phase. The dietician or nutritionist should be part of the team who is helping the patient and the family understand the nutritional and food preparation needs. For individuals who experience aspiration or regurgitation, there should be no eating at bedtime. Patients should be instructed to remain upright after eating and reduce the amount of liquid that they drink with meals.

Enteral feeding may be needed for some patients. The general guideline is any patient who cannot take in adequate nutrients and hydration by mouth or who has a functional bowel, must receive nutrients enterally. Patients who are initiated on early enteral nutrition have shorter hospital stays and better outcomes (Hildebrandt, Fracchia, Driscoll, & Giroux, 2003). The nasogastric feeding tube, the percutaneous endoscopic gastrostomy (PEG) tube, or the surgical gastrostomy are the choices available. Nasogastric tubes must be carefully selected for size and comfort as well as ease of insertion. Patients find these tubes uncomfortable. There is a high rate of these tubes being pulled out. Placement of these tubes must be checked radiographically prior to beginning the tube feeding. These tubes can be inadvertently inserted into the lung rather than the stomach or duodenum. The PEG is initially inserted by the physician or an advanced practitioner prepared to insert these tubes. These tubes are sutured in place or have a balloon inflated that prevents their removal. Complications associated with these tubes include bleeding or infection at the insertion site, peritonitis, and the potential for ascites, chest infections, and puncture of other abdominal organs during insertion. PEG feedings are associated with improved outcomes on measures of nutrition, weight, midarm circumference, and serum albumin as well as less treatment failures and fewer deaths.

Difficulty swallowing can be managed by speech pathologists and encouraged by nursing personnel. There are three types of swallowing therapy, compensatory, indirect, and direct therapy (Box 49-4).

Surgery

Tactile-thermal stimulation and electrical stimulation have been used. Results have shown that most patients responded to electrical stimulation. Swallowing function improved, and the treatment appeared to be safe. In addition, endoscopy can also be used to treat swallowing difficulties, as shown in Figure 49-3. Also, there are some patients that may need surgery. Surgery is needed when there is manometric evidence of obstruction to a bolus at the cricopharyngeal segment. The most common type of surgery is cricopharyngeal myotomy (CPM). The cricopharyngeus muscle is incised to reduce resistance to pharyngeal outflow. This surgery is accompanied by suspension of the thyroid cartilage. Alternatively some patients may be candidates for botulinum toxin injection into the pharyngoesophageal sphincter (PES). This procedure replaces the CPM. Other surgeries are available to patients dependent on the type of dysphagia the patient is experiencing.

ESOPHAGEAL DISORDERS

The lining of the esophagus is extremely vascular, and the esophagus itself is vital to nutritional balance. The more common disorders are elaborated on in this section, including achalasia, GERD, hiatal hernia, and esophageal cancer.

BOX 49-4

TECHNIQUES OF SWALLOWING THERAPY

1. Compensatory techniques—postural maneuvers such as proper positioning.
2. Indirect therapy—strengthening exercises to improve the swallowing muscles, such as lip, and tongue mobility exercises, active resistive exercise, vibratory inhibition, ice application, and stretching of oral structural muscles, repetitive head lift exercise to improve anterior excursion of the larynx and the cross-sectional area of the upper esophageal sphincter.
3. Direct therapy—exercises to strengthen the muscles while swallowing liquids and solids.

Adapted from Robbins, J., Gangnon, R., Theis, S., Kays, S., Hewitt, A., & Hind, J. (2005). The effects of lingual exercise on swallowing in older adults. Journal of American Geriatric Society, 53(9), 1483–1489.

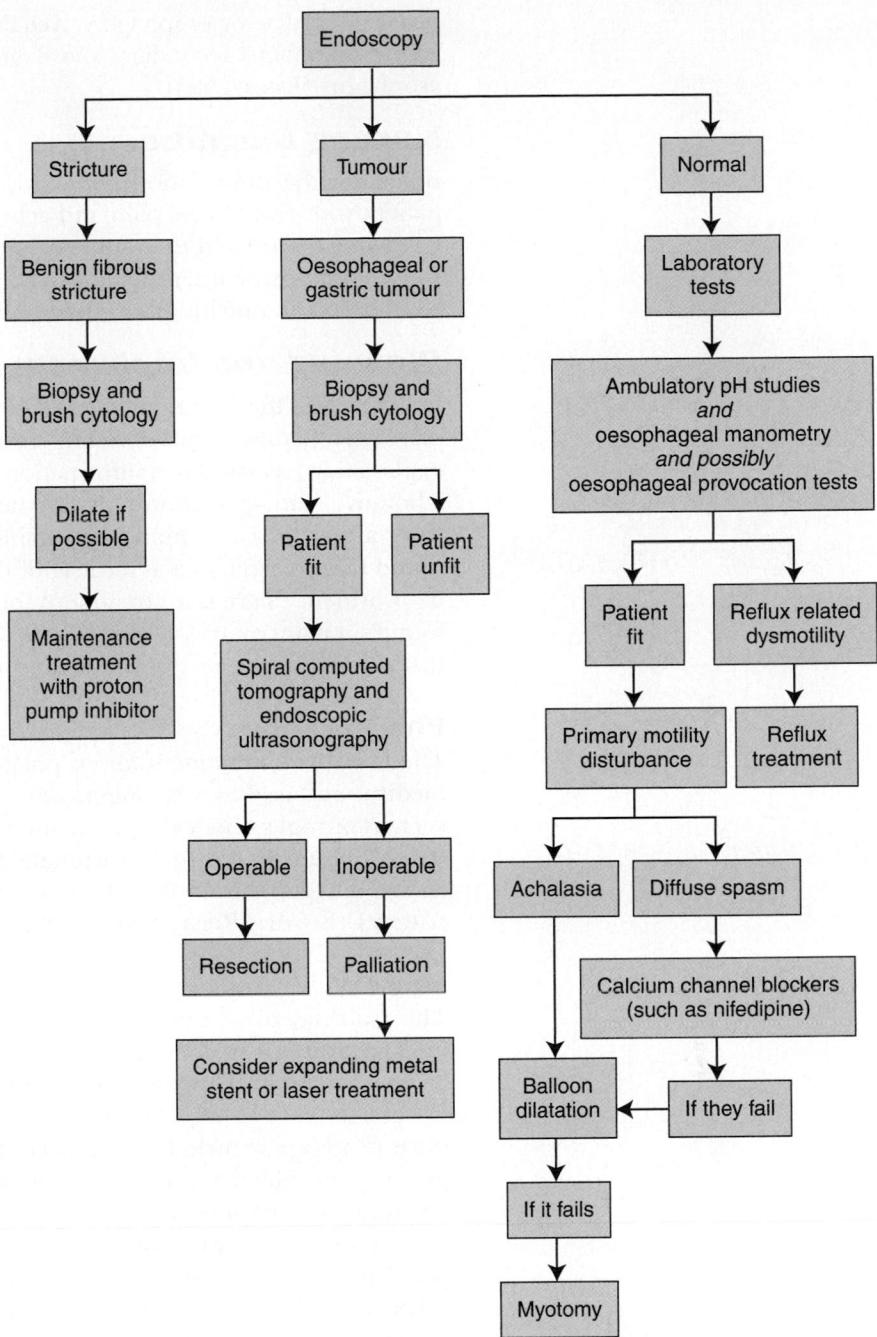

Figure 49-3 Algorithm for endoscopic management of dysphagia. Adapted from Hill, M., Hughes T., & Milford C. (2005). Treatment for swallowing difficulties (dysphagia) in chronic muscle disease. *The Cochrane Database of Systematic Reviews (Oxford)* (2), CD004303.

Esophageal Pain and Achalasia

Esophageal pain can be associated with dysphagia. It can be a result of irritation to the mucosal lining of the esophagus or mechanical distension of the esophagus. Because the pain associated with esophageal disorders is often the same as pain from cardiac origin, it is important to provide the patient reassurance as the diagnostic workup is performed. Esophageal pain is described as burning in the anterior chest. It is sensed in the throat and may radiate to the neck, back, or upper arms. This is similar to cardiac pain. Approximately 20 percent of the time that patients experience pain in the chest, shoulders, arms, neck, and back; it is impossible to differentiate the origin of the pain between cardiac or esophageal. **Achalasia** is a loss of peristalsis in the muscle of the esophagus secondary to a degeneration of neurons in the wall of the esophagus (Estes, 2006).

Nursing Diagnoses

Based on the information gathered, examples of nursing diagnoses in the patient with esophageal pain and achalasia may include the following:
- Acute pain related to esophageal pathology.
- Impaired tissue integrity related to achalasia.
- Imbalanced nutrition, less than body requirements, related to achalasia.

Planning and Implementation

Important in the management and plan of care for patients with esophageal pain is empathetic consideration during the medical workup. This includes explanation, reassurance, information sharing, teaching, and if necessary, collaborative management with psychotherapy. If the patient does have reflux disease, a plan of care should be established to manage this. If the patient is found to have achalasia as a cause of the esophageal pain, particular care will be provided. There is no treatment for peristaltic loss in the esophagus. If it is found on manometry that the lower esophageal sphincter (LES) fails to relax, the aim will be to relax or dilate the LES.

Pharmacology

The first line of treatment for esophageal pain and achalasia is often the same medications used to treat angina of cardiac origin. These include vasodilators, such as nitroglycerin, calcium channel blockers, such as verapamil, and isosorbide dinitrate (Isordil). Unfortunately the effect of these medications is not lasting and surgery is often the necessary next step of management for these patients (Broyles, Reiss, & Evans, 2007).

Surgery

The mainstay of treatment for achalasia is surgery or balloon dilation. This intervention is best for patients over 45 years of age. It is effective between 60 to 95 percent. Patients who have balloon dilatation (pneumatic dilation) are at risk for esophageal damage, tearing, or even rupture during the procedure (2 to 5 percent). The major complications of esophageal dilatation are perforation, bleeding, and bacteremia. Surgical intervention or esophageal myotomy may be selected in younger patients. The muscle fibers of LES are severed during this procedure. Ninety percent of patients experience an effective outcome, but they may also develop reflux disease. Another option to relax the LES and to reduce the symptoms is to inject the muscle with toxin (Botox). Currently the effectiveness of Botox injection is reported to be about 60 percent for about six months. At one year, only 32 percent continued to be symptom free. Although the patient undergoes endoscopy for this procedure, it is useful in patients who are at high risk for surgical intervention.

Evaluation of Outcomes

Potential patient outcomes for each of the example nursing diagnoses for the patient with esophageal pain and achalasia are:
- Acute pain related to esophageal pathology. The patient should verbalize an adequate relief of pain along with the ability to realistically cope with the pain if it is not completely relieved.
- Impaired tissue integrity related to achalasia. The patient will improve the condition of his or her impaired tissue integrity as evidenced by decreased redness, swelling, and pain.
- Imbalanced nutrition, less than body requirements, related to achalasia. The patient verbalizes and demonstrates selection of foods or meals that will achieve a cessation of weight loss and weighs within 10 percent of ideal body weight.

Gastroesophageal Reflux Disease

GERD refers to the backing up of gastric contents into the esophagus. As this happens, the patient experiences **pyrosis,** a substernal burning sensation often radiating to the neck, commonly called heartburn.

Epidemiology

GERD occurs in 15 to 20 percent of all adults. For many of these people, daily symptoms are common.

Etiology

There are several common problems that result in GERD. Causes of GERD are an incompetent LES, a motility disorder of the esophagus as previously described, and pyloric stenosis. In addition, the aging process correlates with an increased incidence of GERD.

Pathophysiology

During the swallowing process, the LES is normally closed. The backflow of gastric juices up into the esophagus is consequently prevented because of the difference in the pressure between the lower esophagus and the stomach. In GERD, the LES relaxes or is incompetent and the gastric contents are allowed to move upward during times of increased pressure. Examples of the pressure changes are when the stomach volume is increased, as after a meal or when the patient bends down.

The gastric contents are acidic and are made of pepsin and bile. These substances are irritating and over time the mucosa of the esophagus is affected by GERD, leading to esophagitis. Ulcerations may develop, which can result in bleeding, scarring, and strictures.

Assessment with Clinical Manifestations

The most common manifestation of GERD is pyrosis, particularly after eating when either bending over or lying down. The patient will experience a regurgitation of a bitter tasting solution in the mouth. This may lead to difficulty swallowing and pain from the irritation of the gastric juices. The patient may develop esophagitis, pharyngitis, or hoarseness. The complication of Barrett's esophagus can even lead to esophageal cancer, described in the next section.

Barrett's Esophagus

Barrett's esophagus was first identified in 1950 by Norman Barrett in a patient who had esophagitis with a peptic ulcer. Barrett's esophagus develops because of chronic reflux esophagitis (GERD), even though 25 percent of the population with Barrett's does not experience GERD. Current research is underway to consider the potential role of prostaglandins and leukotrienes in inducing inflammatory mediators that produce symptoms and promote disease advancement. As the disorder is progressing, chronic exposure of the esophagus to stomach acid damages the esophageal epithelium. Approximately 1 in 200 patients with Barrett's esophagus will develop adenocarcinoma. Even considering this information, there is no current evidence that screening the population for the presence of Barrett's esophagus will decrease the rate of adenocarcinoma of the esophagus. Nonetheless, the American Gastroenterology Association (AGA) recommends upper endoscopy with histological examination of esophageal biopsy for those individuals who have GERD symptoms. Additionally the patient may have a radiological exam, the barium swallow. The barium swallow may show thickening of the esophageal folds, ulcerations, and strictures as well as reflux of barium. Twenty-four hour ambulatory pH monitoring of the esophagus may also be performed as part of the assessment of the patient. Several variables are monitored with this procedure. The most clinically applicable result is the percent of time the pH remains below 4. Normally the pH is below 4 and less than 4.5% in a 24-hour period (1.1 hours out of 24).

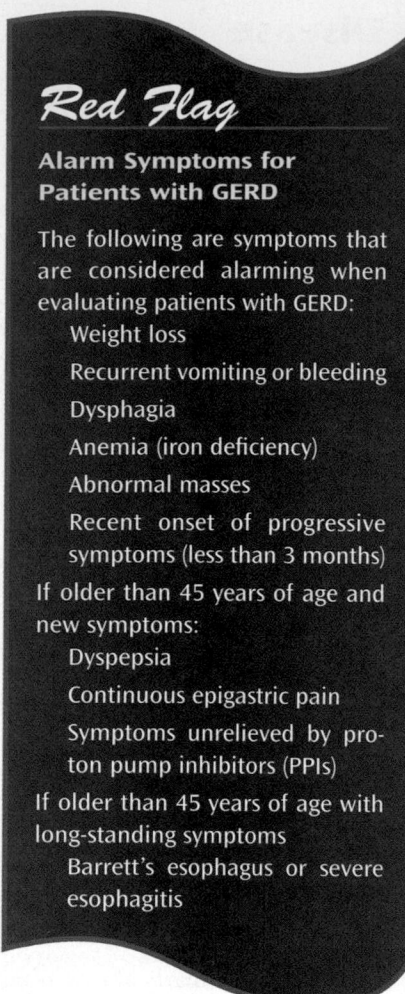

Patients with Barrett's esophagus present with the symptoms of reflux esophagitis because of the exposure of the esophagus to acidic gastric contents. The patient may describe heartburn or a burning taste in the back of the throat. At times patients may describe a sensation of saliva filling the mouth. This symptom is **brash water.** It occurs when the mouth suddenly fills with saliva secondary to reflex salivary secretion stimulated by acid back flow into the esophagus. Certain foods will also stimulate heartburn.

The aim of treatment for Barrett's esophagus is to decrease the reflux of acid into the esophagus until the symptoms of esophagitis are no longer evident. The American College of Gastroenterology updated their original guidelines for surveillance of individuals with Barrett's esophagus (DeVault & Castell, 2005; Inadomi, et al., 2003). These include two surveillance endoscopies with biopsies showing no dysplasia followed by surveillance every three years; treatment of GERD to reduce inflammation; and if dysplasia is present, confirmation by a second expert pathologist is needed. When a patient has low-grade dysplasia, annual surveillance endoscopies should be done; with high-grade dysplasia, the interval between endoscopies should be shortened, and surgical intervention should be planned. Antireflux surgery is controversial because outcomes of medication therapy (drugs to suppress acid release) when similarly stratified with surgical repair are the same. The management of patients with Barrett's esophagus is the same as for GERD.

Diagnostic Tests

The patient history is a primary method of suspecting GERD. After seeking health care, an upper endoscopy can reveal a reddened esophageal lining, which is indicative of GERD. Further tests can be a barium swallow, a 24-hour ambulatory pH monitoring, which detects the lowered pH levels commensurate with an acid environment, and esophageal manometry, which evaluates the pressures of the esophageal sphincters and esophageal peristalsis (Daniels, 2003).

Nursing Diagnoses

Based on the information gathered, examples of nursing diagnoses in the patient with GERD may include the following:

- Acute pain related to the gastric juices irritating the esophagus.
- Deficient knowledge related to self-care and risk prevention.
- Imbalanced nutrition, less than body requirements, related to the irritation of the esophagus.

Planning and Implementation

The management plan for GERD involves patient education regarding the noninvasive techniques for care (see Patient Playbook feature) and then common medication therapy. If the dysfunction is not able to be arrested, and the disorder continues, surgery may be indicated.

Pharmacology

The patient may initially self-administer antacids to decrease the esophageal pain. The antacids neutralize the gastric juices. If prescription medications are indicated, the patient may then be given histamine receptor blockers (e.g., Pepcid, Tagamet, or Zantac). These reduce the acid nature of the gastric fluids by blocking the histamine, which normally stimulates acid secretion. As GERD becomes more serious PPIs, medications that decrease release of acid may be given. The PPI (e.g., Prevacid, Prilosec) inhibit the hydrogen potassium pump, which reduces gastric acids. PPI allow the esophagus time to heal, as well as create a lesser acid environment.

Surgery

If medication strategies are not effective, surgery may be indicated as the GERD condition persists. Antireflux surgeries change the ability of the LES to inhibit gastric juices from reflux. There are laparoscopic surgeries, which can tighten the LES, and there is an open, more invasive surgery (Nissen fundoplication) which may be performed.

Evaluation of Outcomes

Potential patient outcomes for each of the example nursing diagnoses for the patient with GERD are:

- Acute pain related to the gastric juices irritating the esophagus. The patient should verbalize an adequate relief of pain along with the ability to realistically cope with the pain if it is not completely relieved.
- Deficient knowledge related to self-care and risk prevention. The patient should demonstrate motivation to learn, identify perceived learning needs, and verbalize an understanding of desired content.
- Imbalanced nutrition, less than body requirements, related to the irritation of the esophagus. The patient verbalizes and demonstrates selection of foods or meals that will achieve a cessation of weight loss and weighs within 10 percent of ideal body weight.

Hiatal Hernia

A hiatal hernia develops when there is a part of the stomach that protrudes through the esophageal hiatus. There are often no symptoms, but when it is evidenced the manifestations are similar to those in GERD.

Etiology

There is a correlation with age and hiatal hernia formation. Other causes are weakened esophageal diaphragm areas, increased intra-abdominal pressure (e.g., pregnancy), and shortening of the esophagus.

Pathophysiology

There are two primary types of hiatal hernias: (a) sliding hiatal hernia (type I), and (b) paraesophageal hiatal hernia (type II). In addition, there are types III, IV, and V, which are less common, and are differentiated by the amount of herniation. In a sliding hiatal hernia the upper stomach slides upward through the gastroesophageal junction. This type of hiatal hernia is often asymptomatic. The paraesophageal hiatal hernia results when a part of the stomach herniates through the esophageal hiatus. In this type of hiatal hernia blood flow can be constricted and patients can develop chronic or acute GI bleeding or gastritis.

Assessment with Clinical Manifestations

The symptomatology for hiatal hernias is similar to GERD, and many are asymptomatic. The manifestations are pyrosis, reflux, a feeling of satiation, dysphagia, bleeding, and substernal chest pain. The reflux symptoms are more common with a sliding hiatal hernia and fullness is more typical in the type II hiatal hernia. Potential complications of hiatal hernias are hemorrhaging, obstruction, and strangulation.

Diagnostic Tests

The presentation of the patient and their history often confirms the diagnosis. More definitive tests to diagnose a hiatal hernia are a barium swallow and an upper endoscopy.

Nursing Diagnoses

Based on the information gathered, examples of nursing diagnoses in the patient with hiatal hernia may include the following:

- Acute pain related to the gastric juices irritating the esophagus.
- Deficient knowledge related to self-care and risk prevention.
- Imbalanced nutrition, less than body requirements, related to the irritation of the esophagus.

Planning and Implementation

The nursing interventions and plan of care is similar for hiatal hernias as for GERD. This includes the potential surgeries and medications that are prescribed.

Evaluation of Outcomes

Potential patient outcomes for each of the example nursing diagnoses for the patient with hiatal hernia are:

- Acute pain related to the gastric juices irritating the esophagus. The patient should verbalize an adequate relief of pain along with the ability to realistically cope with the pain if it is not completely relieved.
- Deficient knowledge related to self-care care and risk prevention. The patient should demonstrate motivation to learn, identify perceived learning needs, and verbalize an understanding of desired content.
- Imbalanced nutrition, less than body requirements, related to the irritation of the esophagus. The patient verbalizes and demonstrates selection of foods or meals that will achieve a cessation of weight loss and weighs within 10 percent of ideal body weight.

Esophageal Cancer

Esophageal cancer, associated with the highest cancer mortality rate (five-year survival rate of 15 percent) is also one of the most rapidly increasing malignancies. This is a disease of older Caucasian males. The peak incidence is in patients 65 to 74 years old. Mortality rates are higher in patients from minority populations. Early detection through screening and surveillance is essential for any GI malignancy and even more so with cancers of the esophagus.

Epidemiology

There are two primary types of esophageal cancer: adenocarcinoma and squamous cell carcinoma. The risk factors for these types of cancer are listed in Table 49-2.

Lifestyle modification and chemoprevention for those individuals at high risk for the development of esophageal cancer is important. The nurse should assist patients to modify riskier behavior and select healthier lifestyles. It is imperative that nurses be involved in smoking cessation programs. Obesity is an important contributing factor in the epidemiology of esophageal cancer. Even though esophageal cancer rates are increasing, there is insufficient evi-

TABLE 49-2 **Primary Known Risk Factors for Esophageal Cancer**

ADENOCARCINOMA	SQUAMOUS CELL CARCINOMA
Smoking	Smoking
Chronic GERD	Alcohol ingestion
Barrett's esophagus	Exposure to nitrosamines
	Ingestion of lye
	Fanconi's anemia
	Achalasia
	Plummer-Vincent webs
	Tylosis

Adapted from Yang, C., Wang, H., Wang, Z., Du, H. Z., Tao, D., Mu, X., et al. (2005). Risk factors for esophageal cancer: A case-control study in South-western China. Asian Pacific Journal of Cancer Prevention, 6(1), 48–53.

dence that screening for esophageal cancer is effective except for those individuals with Barrett's esophagus (patients with Barrett's esophagus who have dysplasia are considered at risk and should be on a regular screening regimen dependent on the grade of the dysplasia), those with familial occurrence of adenocarcinoma, patients with tylosis, lye-induced strictures, and Fanconi's anemia (level III evidence). Respected experts suggest screening for patients who have been long-term tobacco users, alcoholics, and those diagnosed with achalasia. The degree of dysplasia found on the first screening will also dictate the screening endoscopy interval the patient will be asked to follow. Screening endoscopy may be recommended every three months for high-grade esophageal dysplasia or as infrequently as every five years if there is no dysplasia. Patients who have mucosal abnormalities should have biopsies and mucosal resection to determine if there is any malignancy present. Chemoprevention for patients at high risk should be implemented. This would include drugs to reduce acid—PPIs and nonsteroidal anti-inflammatory drugs (NSAIDs). NSAIDs seem to inhibit prostaglandin E_2 that decreases the production of the Barrett's epithelial cells (Homs, Steyerberg, Eijkenboom, & Siersema, 2006).

Pathophysiology

Cancer of the esophagus obviously is caused by malignant advancement into the esophageal areas. Once the malignancy penetrates the submucosa, the risk of metastasis as well as increase in mortality are substantial (Wang, Wongkeesong, & Buttar, 2005). Fifteen percent of esophageal cancers are in the upper one third of the esophagus; 50 percent in the middle one third of the esophagus, and 35 percent in the lower third at the gastroesophageal junction (GEJ). The major types of esophageal cancer are adenocarcinoma and squamous cell, as shown in the risk factor table. Identification of the stage of the esophageal cancer (by tissue examination) is necessary for the management of the cancer. Determining the stage of the disease is usually done with endoscopy and computed tomography (CT). Endoscopic ultrasound with fine needle aspiration may also be used. Also, refer to chapter 15 for more information on the theories of cancer cell development.

Assessment with Clinical Manifestations

Patients with esophageal cancer usually present with difficulty in swallowing. At this point, the esophagus is often 50 to 60 percent obstructed. This difficulty is progressive and leads to the second most common presentation pain, odynophagia (Friedman, McQuaid, & Grendell, 2003). Other symptoms often associated with esophageal cancer include anorexia, weight loss, hoarseness and voice change, aspiration, cough, and recurrent upper respiratory infections. Often the patient is anemic without over GI bleeding. As with all GI cancers, systematic staging of the disease is necessary to plan the most effective treatment.

Nursing Diagnoses

Based on the information gathered, examples of nursing diagnoses in the patient with esophageal cancer may include the following:
- Acute pain related to esophageal cancer.
- Anxiety related to diagnosis of esophageal cancer.
- Ineffective coping related to diagnosis of esophageal cancer.
- Imbalanced nutrition, less than body requirements.
- Anticipatory grieving related to diagnosis of esophageal cancer.
- Spiritual distress related to diagnosis of esophageal cancer.

Planning and Implementation

The aim of treatment will be palliative or curative based on the stage of the disease and the patient's health status. The collaborative team managing the patient's care should individualize the options and determine the most appropriate plan. General approaches to caring for patients with cancer are provided in chapter 15.

If the tumor is confined to the mucosa, the patient will undergo either an esophagectomy or endoscopic mucosal resection (Verschuur, et al., 2006). If the tumor penetrates through the submucosa, an esophagectomy is the treatment of choice. If the patient has evidence of metastasis to lymph nodes, chemotherapy and radiation are done prior to any surgical procedure (neoadjuvant therapy). If the cancer is advanced, palliative procedures may be done. The goals of palliative care are to alleviate pain and discomfort by alleviating difficulty in swallowing, to receive adequate nutrition, and to improve the quality of life. Prior to selection of any chemo or radiation therapy treatments, the patient should receive enteral nutritional support. It is recommended that esophageal stenting be selected to relieve symptomatology from tumor load. When a patient with esophageal cancer presents with persistent swallowing problems, anorexia, and weight loss, the cancer is at an advanced and often incurable stage. Hence, the plan for palliation is essential.

Evaluation of Outcomes

Potential patient outcomes for each of the example nursing diagnoses for the patient with esophageal cancer are:

- Acute pain related to esophageal cancer. The patient should verbalize an adequate relief of pain along with the ability to realistically cope with the pain if it is not completely relieved.
- Anxiety related to diagnosis of esophageal cancer. The patient should be able to recognize the signs of anxiety, demonstrate positive coping mechanisms, and describe a reduction in the level of anxiety experienced.
- Ineffective coping related to diagnosis of esophageal cancer. The patient identifies their own maladaptive coping behaviors and available resources and support systems. The patient also describes and initiates alternative coping strategies and the positive results from new behaviors.
- Imbalanced nutrition, less than body requirements. The patient verbalizes and demonstrates selection of foods or meals that will achieve a cessation of weight loss and weighs within 10 percent of ideal body weight.
- Anticipatory grieving related to diagnosis of esophageal cancer. The patient verbalizes feelings and establishes and maintains functional support systems.
- Spiritual distress related to diagnosis of esophageal cancer. The patient expresses hope in and value of his or her belief system and inner resources and expresses a sense of well-being.

Even though there have been significant improvements in diagnosis, surgical techniques, and neoadjuvant chemoradiation therapy, the overall five-year survival rate is less than 15 percent. Patients with a T1 or T2 disease stage have a five-year survival of 40 percent. Care of these patients and their families is a particular challenge to the entire health care team.

GI TRACT PAIN OF NONCARDIAC AND NONPHYSIOLOGICAL ORIGINS

There are several conditions seen in the upper GI tract that are somewhat different from the normal physiological causes. These conditions are noncardiac chest pain, which may have its etiology in the GI tract, panic disorders, and functional GI disorders (FGID).

Noncardiac Chest Pain

It is essential to discuss all patients who might experience noncardiac chest pain. The causes of this type of pain include patients with cardiac, GI, psychiatric, or musculoskeletal disorders. Accurately determining what the cause derives from may be challenging. Many patients have more than one disorder that can lead to chest pain, so decisional pathways (algorithms) have been used to assist in the diagnostic process.

GERD and esophageal motility disorders are discussed in this text, but it is important to discuss visceral hypersensitivity. Increased visceral hypersensitivity (heightened visceral nociception) is linked to patients with chest pain of unknown cause. It is seen with patients who have marked pain response to various visceral stimuli (e.g., distension, acid reflux, motility disorders). These patients must be managed so that any life-threatening disorder is ruled out secondary to cardiac ischemia. The common causes of this type of chest pain must be evaluated. This includes GERD and panic disorder while unusual causes of chest pain must also be examined. These unusual causes include costochondritis (inflammation of the costochondral cartilage), biliary colic, aortic aneurysm, and peptic ulcer disorder.

Panic Disorder

Panic disorder occurs in the same percentage of patients with chest pain as with GERD, 30 to 50 percent. If the diagnosis of panic disorder is suspected, a first step might be to use a panic assessment instrument to further assess the patient. Management of patients with panic disorder can be a challenge. Providing the patient and family with educational materials is important. This includes assisting the patient to understand that this disorder exists in 5 percent of the U.S. populace. Patients can be treated for this disorder with several types of medications and therapy. The most commonly used medications include antianxiety agents and antidepressants. Beta blocking agents are useful for those who also have autonomic symptoms, e.g., palpitations and tachyarrhythmias. Cognitive behavioral therapy that focuses on stress management and improving coping skills may be equal to pharmacotherapy for this disorder.

Functional Gastrointestinal Disorders

Before discussing those GI disorders, which are from organic or physiological changes, it is important for the nurse to be aware that many patients may have no physiological cause of their GI symptoms. Because of the brain-gut connection, patients who have FGID need a biopsychosocial approach. This includes an understanding of the patient's early life, life stress, physiology, and symptom control. As patients are being assessed for their GI symptoms, the workup will include a thorough history of the patient's background. This includes information related to whether the patient has ever experienced any previous psychiatric problems. Evidence demonstrates a high incidence of patients who present with dyspepsia and irritable bowel syndrome have previously experienced sexual abuse. Many patients with FGID have undue stress related to fear of a serious disorder, such as cancer. These patients need reassurance about the effect of stress on the GI tract. These patients experience more anxiety, depression, neuroticism, and somatic complaints. They need an understanding that stress releases neuro-hormones from the brain that have a direct effect on GI function. The question of whether the emotional response is a result of the symptoms must be assessed. Many of these patients are managed by primary care providers so the nurse may encounter these patients in outpatient clinics. These patients need a confident approach, a diagnosis that is realistic, and psychotherapy of the cognitive behavioral type. Placebo trials demonstrate the usual GI medications are not effective for these individuals (Yamada, 2005).

NONULCER DYSPEPSIA

Dyspepsia (indigestion) is a term is used to describe several complaints (e.g., epigastric pain, bloating, fullness, early satiety, belching, heartburn, and nausea). Dyspepsia is divided into nonulcer dyspepsia (NUD) or dyspepsia secondary to peptic ulcer disease (PUD). NUD is responsible for about 40 percent of all patients who complain of recurrent pain or discomfort in the epigastric region of the abdomen or retrosternal region. NUD can be caused by GERD, problems with motility, gallbladder, liver, and pancreatic dysfunction as well as medication-induced dyspepsia, dietary causes, and endocrine or metabolic disorders (e.g., diabetes). The symptoms of dyspepsia have been divided into ulcer-like, dysmotility-like, and unspecified (Logan & Delaney, 2005). Heartburn secondary to reflux (GERD) will not be discussed in this section.

Epidemiology

The health belief model supports the option patients choose to seek care when there is an assessment of a serious illness and the likelihood of cure. Studies have shown that patients with dyspepsia seek health care when there is a belief that lifestyle and stresses are related to the symptoms they are experiencing. Additionally there is a fear that the symptoms are a sign of a serious problem. Historically, a review of 36 studies in 1998 that looked at the results of esophagogastroduodenoscopy (EGD) in patients with dyspepsia, only 1.6 percent of the patients had cancer. In a later review of 17,792 patients who had an EGD, only 1.4 percent were diagnosed with a malignancy (Vakil, Talley, Moayyedi, & Fennerty, 2005).

Pathophysiology

The pathophysiology of dyspepsia is focused in several areas. These include medication side effects, some foods, and gastric sensory and motility dysfunction. Medication side effects are a major contribution to dyspepsia. The major drug groups associated with dyspepsia are NSAIDs, especially in individuals with arthritis, aspirin, potassium supplements, iron, antibiotics, steroids, ACE inhibitors, nitrates, levodopa, estrogen, and quinidine. There is evidence to demonstrate that if patients have to take NSAIDs, they should also take PPIs to protect the gastric mucosa. At times patients must be taken off of the offending medication to relieve the symptoms.

The link between gastric emptying and dyspepsia is controversial; the link between gastric hypersensitivity may be the dominant dysfunction (Talley, 2005). Gastric epithelium may be responsive to gastric acid. The data suggest that PPI therapy is helpful in functional dyspepsia. An older study demonstrated that gastric sensory and motor dysfunction may be linked to a central limbic processing abnormality associated with childhood abuse. A more recent study of patients with functional dyspepsia showed an association between childhood sexual abuse and gastroparesis and an association between adult psychological abuse and gastric hypersensitivity. Although a cause-and-effect relationship cannot be concluded, it continues to be an important relationship.

Assessment with Clinical Manifestations

Patients who present with NUD describe a variety of symptoms. These symptoms include epigastric pain, bloating, fullness, early satiety, belching, heartburn, and nausea.

Diagnostic Tests

Separating the clinical history and distinguishing organic dyspepsia from functional dyspepsia continues to be problematic. Nonetheless, patients worry about unexplained symptoms. The quality of life for individuals who have dyspepsia is compromised. Symptom relief could improve the quality of life and is an aim of care. Because there is a strong relationship between dyspepsia, PUD, and *Helicobacter pylori,* a controversy exists over the decision to evaluate the patient for *H. pylori* or to treat empirically. If PUD is diagnosed, the gastroscopist will obtain a biopsy for histology and urease testing.

Nursing Diagnoses

Based on the information gathered, examples of nursing diagnoses in the patient with NUD may include the following:

- Acute pain related to upper epigastric irritation.
- Imbalanced nutrition, less than body requirements, related to anorexia.
- Deficient knowledge deficit related to self-care and risk prevention.

Planning and Implementation

The approach to patients with NUD is complex. It is based on the dysfunction that causes the dyspepsia. Different studies predict different results. Nurses must be aware of the latest evidence and the recommendations for treatment. There are many questions that impact the management and prognosis of NUD. Gastroparesis continues to be looked at as part of the dysfunction. Gastric hypersensitivity remains under study and treatment for a certain set of patients. Because the association between symptoms and organic or functional causes of NUD are unclear, more assessment of causal relationship is needed. The American College of Gastroenterology endorses that in patients 45 to 50 years of age empiric treatment with acid suppressing agents are appropriate. For patients greater than 50 years of age, EGD is recommended.

Nurses need to be aware of the journey of patients who have dyspepsia. The pain, the uncertainty in diagnosis, the disease burden, the decisional conflict, and the therapeutic regimen cause continuous ambiguity for the patient. Patients need support and knowledge related to the selection of workup as well as the treatment selection.

Pharmacology

There management of NUD is often dependent on pharmacological therapies. For example, placebo response can be demonstrated but is not conclusive as an approach to the management of dyspepsia. Also, prokinetic agents can be useful because 5-hydroxytryptamine $(HT)_4$ receptors can relax the gastric fundus. Currently there are no substantive data to support its use in NUD. Gastric motility can also be addressed with erythromycin or azithromycin (motilin agonist). Stimulation of motilin receptors will hasten stomach emptying. Unfortunately these medications have side effects, which may prevent their use. Erythromycin is a powerful stimulant of motility in the antrum and fundus of the stomach. Fundal stimulation may worsen the dyspepsia. Additionally erythromycin produces conduction problems in the heart. It prolongs the Q-T interval and may cause sudden cardiac death. Azithromycin does not effect cardiac conduction time. Last, visceral analgesics are given, which include $5\text{-}HT_3$ antagonists (e.g., alosetron) and $5\text{-}HT_4$ agonists (e.g., octreotide) (Broyles, et al., 2007). The studies done using these agents did not have a placebo control, and therefore randomized controlled studies are needed.

Evaluation of Outcomes

Potential patient outcomes for each of the example nursing diagnoses for the patient with NUD are:

- Acute pain related to upper epigastric irritation. The patient should verbalize an adequate relief of pain along with the ability to realistically cope with the pain if it is not completely relieved.
- Imbalanced nutrition, less than body requirements, related to anorexia. The patient verbalizes and demonstrates selection of foods or meals that will achieve a cessation of weight loss and weighs within 10 percent of ideal body weight.
- Deficient knowledge related to self-care and risk prevention. The patient should demonstrate motivation to learn, identify perceived learning needs, and verbalize an understanding of desired content.

The outcome for patients with dyspepsia is not clear. Patients with dyspepsia must be followed up. Symptomatic treatment of these patients is appropriate when organic disease is ruled out. If the patient also has depression as a comorbidity, the outcome for improvement is poor. All relevant disorders must be considered and treated to optimize patient outcomes.

PEPTIC-ULCER DYSPEPSIA

PUD is one of the two types of dyspepsia. PUD is characterized by a loss of the mucosal lining of the stomach or duodenum. PUD has had a variety of therapies and strategies for treatment over the past several decades. There used to be an emphasis on bland diet medications and stress management to decrease the symptomology of PUD. More recently, recognition of the role of *H. pylori* in PUD greatly changed the management of this disorder.

Etiology

PUD is characterized by persistent pain, weight loss, poor appetite, bloating, nausea, and vomiting. The most common causative link to PUD is *H. pylori*. In the elderly, the prevalence of PUD is linked to the use of NSAIDs (e.g., aspirin, ibuprofen).

Epidemiology

There is also a familial link with the prevalence of PUD in first-degree relatives and monozygotic twins. Tobacco smokers are two times more likely to develop PUD than nonsmokers. *H. pylori* is a leading cause of gastritis, PUD, gastric cancer, and gastric lymphomas. The infection is transmitted by the fecal oral route, saliva, food, and water. If a patient is infected with *H. pylori*, it progresses from superficial chronic gastritis to atrophic gastritis. NSAIDs cause mucosal damage both by direct effect as well as systemic effects. NSAIDs damage epithelial cells and inhibit prostaglandin secretion, specifically COX inhibition, which reduces mucus and bicarbonate secretion, and hampers cell turnover because of reduced blood flow. Individuals with cystic fibrosis have an increased for PUD because of decrease in bicarbonate secretion.

Gastric epithelial cellular metaplasia leads to duodenal ulcer disease. The disease burden for PUD is high. The total direct cost of gastric and duodenal ulcers is estimated to be 3.3 billion dollars with a loss in productivity valued at 6.2 billion dollars (Yamada, 2005).

Pathophysiology

Most gastric ulcers are linked to *H. pylori* infection or NSAIDs. Three types develop as shown in Box 49-5.

Assessment with Clinical Manifestations

Abdominal pain is the major presenting symptom. The pain is described as burning, usually in the epigastric region, and is often relieved by food or antacids. A distinguishing symptom is that the patient will relate that the pain awaken them in the middle of the night. If the patient is less than 45 to 50 years of age, empiric antisecretory or acid suppression agents should be initiated unless there are red flag signs. If the patient is over the age of 50, they typically have warning signs or fail to respond to antisecretory or acid suppressing agents.

BOX 49-5

TYPES OF GASTRIC ULCERS

Type I—Ulcers in the gastric body (corpus) not associated with gastroduodenal disease.

Type II—Ulcers in the body (corpus) of the stomach but associated with gastroduodenal disease.

Type III—Ulcers in the prepyloric area.

Adapted from Yamada, Y. (2005). Handbook of gastroenterology (2nd ed.). Philadelphia: Lippincott, Williams & Wilkins.

Diagnostic Tests

When the history of the patient suggests PUD, patients should be tested for *H. pylori*. Then radiographic and endoscopic studies should be performed. And, if the patient demonstrates gastric ulceration on endoscopy, the exam should be repeated two months after medication therapy is initiated.

Nursing Diagnoses

Based on the information gathered, examples of nursing diagnoses in the patient with PUD may include the following:

- Acute pain related to upper epigastric irritation.
- Nutrition imbalance, less than body requirements, related to anorexia.
- Knowledge deficit related to self-care and risk prevention.

Planning and Implementation

Patients who are diagnosed with gastric or duodenal ulcers are treated in a similar manner as for nondyspepsia disorder. In addition, there are specific strategies using both pharmacological and surgical therapies.

About 10 percent of the time, patients are not responsive to ulcer treatment. If a patient has not responded to treatment in 12 weeks, a reevaluation of his or her treatment regimen should occur. It is sometimes found that the patient has not followed the regimen prescribed, has not discontinued the risk factors, such as smoking or the use of NSAIDs. If after evaluation, it is found that the patient has been conforming to his or her regimen, but ulcer disease persists, further endoscopic follow-up with multiple biopsies is required. Zollinger-Ellison syndrome (ZES) should be considered. This syndrome results from a gastric acid–secreting tumor, a gastrinoma. Approximately 90 percent of patients with ZES will develop PUD. The symptoms are refractory PUD, PUD with diarrhea, obstruction, perforation, or hemorrhage. ZES is diagnosed if fasting gastrin levels are greater than 1,000 pg/mL (normal is less than 150 pg/mL). Both medical and surgical treatment of ZES are available. Control of acid hypersecretion is important. PPIs are the most effective medication in the treatment of ZES. These medications inhibit acid secretion and promote ulcer healing. If the tumor has not metastasized, the gastrinoma should be resected. If curative resection is not an option, chemotherapy can be selected.

Pharmacology

There are specific medication categories with which PUD is managed. Overall, the types of medications that are used are: antacids, H_2 receptor antagonists, PPIs, and cytoprotective agents.

Over-the-counter (OTC) antacids are useful for the dyspepsia associated with PUD. The expected effects of these agents are to neutralize acid by cytoprotective activity (e.g., increased prostaglandin release, mucous production, and bicarbonate release), inhibition of pepsin, and binding of bile salts. Adverse effects may include hypercalcemia, metabolic alkalosis, renal problems, diarrhea or constipation, and sodium overload. These adverse effects depend on the formulation that is used (Broyles, et. al., 2007).

H_2 receptor antagonists are those medications that reduce acid secretion. Those that are approved for use are cimetidine, famotidine, nizatidine, and ranitidine. Once daily dosing of these agents is used to treat PUD.

PPIs are those agents that inhibit both basal and stimulated acid secretion. They are more effective in managing day time acid secretion than H_2 receptor antagonists. Patients should take these medications 30 minutes to one hour prior to meals.

Cytoprotective agents are those medications that bind to tissue proteins and form a protective barrier for the gastroduodenal epithelium. This protects from any erosive effects of acid, bile salts, and pepsin. Sucralfate is an example. Misoprostol is a cytoprotective agent that is a prostaglandin E_1 analogue. It inhibits gastric acid secretion and stimulates bicarbonate and mucous secretion. The limiting factors to all of these agents are the side effects. The nurse should be aware of other medications that the patient is receiving and knowledgeable of any untoward interaction. Patients need to know what side effects to be aware of and report these to their provider.

Complications of PUD and the Subsequent Therapy

Even though *H. pylori* causes PUD, the elimination of *H. pylori* is controversial for patients who have NUD. For patients who have *H. pylori*–related PUD, therapy to eliminate the infection is indicated. Because single-agent treatment regimens are ineffective, triple or quadruple therapy with antibiotics and PPIs is practiced. Additionally there is evidence that in *H. pylori* is eliminated in 80 to 95 percent of patients who receive two weeks of bismuth subsalicylate, metronidazole, and tetracycline plus an antisecretory agent. Follow-up is not necessary if the patient becomes asymptomatic although a one month follow-up to confirm *H. pylori* elimination should be considered. The rationale for treatment of patients with *H. pylori* infection is stunning. If *H. pylori* is eliminated, the recurrence rate of PUD is less than 10 percent; if *H. pylori* infection is not treated, the PUD recurrence rate is 50 to 100 percent.

For patients who have PUD that is linked to NSAIDs, the anti-inflammatory agent should be discontinued. Treatment would include the same regimen as for PUD secondary to *H. pylori* except for the antibiotic regimen. If NSAIDs must be continued, the use of PPIs have shown to heal both gastric and duodenal ulcers.

Surgery

Pharmacological management of PUD has been so effective that surgical management of PUD is infrequent. Whenever a patient has refractory PUD, gastric carcinoma must be ruled out. The operative solutions to the management of PUD are used only when the ulcer disease is intractable and the patient has persistent and severe symptoms (e.g., pain, blood loss). The procedures include vagotomy and drainage, highly selective vagotomy, vagotomy and antrectomy, and laparoscopic surgery. Highly selective vagotomy is the most widely used procedure for patients with duodenal ulcer. The vagal branches that serve the proximal stomach are ligated, which leaves the antral and pyloric portions of the vagus innervation to the stomach intact. This produces a 50 to 79 percent reduction in acid production. Antral resection of the stomach with a selective vagotomy and has the lowest ulcer recurrence rate. The type of surgery selected is dependent on the condition of the duodenum and the amount of stomach that must be resected. In the Billroth I anastomosis the duodenum is sewn to the stomach; in the Billroth II anastomosis, a gastrojejunostomy is performed and a blind duodenal limb is created.

If a patient experiences a perforated ulcer emergent surgery is indicated. If surgery is delayed, peritonitis and sepsis will result. Often the patient will have a gastric resection, which includes the ulcer. If the patient also experiences a hemorrhage with the perforation, the ulcer bed must be ligated or resected.

A complication seen after surgery for PUD is the dumping syndrome and accelerated gastric emptying occurs with truncal vagotomy and gastric drainage procedures. With the advent of highly selective vagotomy procedures the prevalence of dumping syndrome has declined. Early dumping syndrome occurs when hyperosmolar gastric contents rapidly pass into the intestines. This produces fluid shifts and the release of vasoactive hormones. Within 15 minutes to one hour the patient experiences diarrhea, pain, borborygmi, nausea, and vomiting as well as flushing, weakness, palpitations, diaphoresis, lightheadedness, and syncope. Late dumping syndrome occurs between two to four hours after a meal, and it is believed to be a result of excessive postprandial insulin release. The patient experiences reactive hypoglycemia. Management of dumping syndrome requires dietary modification. Patients should be instructed to eat low-carbohydrate meals and to limit fluid intake during meal time. Patients may also benefit from lying supine after a meal to delay gastric emptying.

Evaluation of Outcomes

Potential patient outcomes for each of the example nursing diagnoses for the patient with PUD are:

- Acute pain related to upper epigastric irritation. The patient should verbalize an adequate relief of pain along with the ability to realistically cope with the pain if it is not completely relieved.
- Nutrition imbalance, less than body requirements, related to anorexia. The patient verbalizes and demonstrates selection of foods or meals that will achieve a cessation of weight loss and weighs within 10 percent of ideal body weight.
- Knowledge deficit related to self-care and risk prevention. The patient should demonstrate motivation to learn, identify perceived learning needs, and verbalize an understanding of desired content.

In addition, medical management of PUD is extremely effective. Ninety to ninety-five percent of patients with PUD are treated successfully and do not require surgery. When surgery is needed, highly selective vagotomy and truncal vagotomy with antrectomy is preferred. The selection of Billroth I and II is dependent on the condition of the duodenum.

GASTRITIS, DUODENITIS, AND ASSOCIATED ULCERATIVE LESIONS

These conditions are not diseases. Gastritis has been classified into nonatrophic, atrophic, and special forms (note: the classification system for gastritis is the Updated Sydney System). Nonatrophic gastritis is caused by *H. pylori*. Atrophic gastritis is associated with *H. pylori* and with environmental factors, and special forms of gastritis include chemical, radiation, lymphocytic, noninfectious, and infections other than *H. pylori*. Gastritis can be acute or chronic. Acute gastritis presents as an acute upper GI blood loss, either a hemorrhagic blood loss or erosive. Chronic gastritis can be due to *H. pylori* without ulceration but with chronic superficial inflammation. Chemical gastritis is most often caused by NSAIDs and reflux of bile into the stomach. Atrophic gastritis is asymptomatic unless complications occur. Patients with autoimmune gastritis often present with anemia, either iron deficiency or pernicious. The patient will have the symptoms of vitamin B_{12} deficiency, which include red, smooth, sore tongue; anorexia; and numbness, paresthesia, weakness, and ataxia. Patients with gastritis are treated both symptomatically and as related to the causative factor. Peptic duodenitis is a direct result of chronic exposure to gastric acid. The epithelium of the duodenum is replaced with gastric mucous-secreting cells as an adaptive response to the acid exposure. These patients may have the same symptoms as patients with PUD. Patients with gastritis and duodenitis will require nursing management based on nursing diagnoses similar to most of the other GI disorders (Box 49-6).

STOMACH CANCER

Stomach cancer, also called gastric cancer, refers to the growth of a cancerous tumor in the stomach. It can develop in any part of the stomach and grow along the stomach wall into the esophagus or small intestine. Stomach cancer

BOX 49-6

NURSING DIAGNOSES FOR GASTRITIS, DUODENITIS, AND ASSOCIATED ULCERATIVE LESIONS

- Acute or chronic pain
- Fear
- Anxiety in response to an uncertain diagnosis
- Ineffective coping related to disease burden
- Deficient knowledge
- Decisional conflict
- Risk for injury, irritation to mucosa or muscular wall
- Imbalanced nutrition, less than body requirements
- Impaired tissue integrity

may extend through the stomach wall and spread to nearby lymph nodes and to organs, such as the liver, pancreas, and colon. Stomach cancer also may spread to distant organs, such as the lungs, the lymph nodes above the collar bone, and the ovaries. When stomach cancer spreads to an ovary, the tumor in the ovary is called a Krukenberg tumor. Stomach cancer is the second leading cause of cancer in the world.

Epidemiology

The American Cancer Society (2006a) estimates that 13,510 men and 8,350 women will be diagnosed with stomach cancer, and 11,550 men and women will die of cancer of the stomach in 2005. From 1998 to 2002, the median age at diagnosis for cancer of the stomach was 72 years of age. Approximately 0.1 percent were diagnosed under age 20; 1.6 percent between the ages of 20 and 34; 4.6 percent between the ages of 35 and 44; 10.3 percent between the ages of 45 and 54; 16.3 percent between the ages of 55 and 64; 26.3 percent between the ages of 65 and 74; 28.2 percent between the ages of 75 and 84; and 12.7 percent 85 and older.

Stomach cancer affects men twice as often as women, and is more common in African American people than in Caucasian people. Stomach cancer is more common in Japan, Korea, parts of Eastern Europe, and Latin America than in the United States. People in these areas eat many foods that are preserved by drying, smoking, salting, or pickling. Scientists believe that eating foods preserved in these ways may play a role in the development of stomach cancer. On the other hand, fresh foods (especially fresh fruits and vegetables and properly frozen or refrigerated fresh foods) may protect against this disease.

The overall five-year survival rate for people with stomach cancer in the United States is 22 percent. One reason for this is that most stomach cancers are found at an advanced stage. The outlook for survival is worse if the cancer is in the upper part of the stomach.

Etiology

Evidence is growing that in addition to genetic disposition, nutritional imbalance, consumption of certain foods, such as smoked foods, among other eating habits, hormonal and psychological factors, along with other immune suppressive factors play an important part in the development of GI cancer. Some studies suggest that a type of bacterium called *H. pylori,* which may cause stomach inflammation and ulcers, may be an important risk factor for this disease.

Pathophysiology

Stomach cancers are primarily adenocarcinomas and can be found in any part of the stomach. In stomach cancer patients, as in all cancer patients, the body's regulatory, repair, and immune mechanisms fail to prevent formation of a cancerous tumor. Some researchers call this failure a regulatory freeze or tolerance, which is because of a combination of causal factors that vary from one individual patient to another.

Cancer cells develop in every human being; however, not every newly produced cancer cell leads to a tumor. And, the body possesses a natural defense system in its intact immune system. In addition, an intact regulation of physiological cell death, called **apoptosis,** protects the organism from the development of a cancerous tumor. Therefore, it is of great importance to restore the natural regulatory, repair, and immune mechanisms, as a part of the healing strategy, or as prevention from the outbreak or progression of the disease.

Gastric Lymphoma

Gastric lymphoma is the second most common malignancy of the stomach. More than 90 percent of gastric B cell tumors (mucosa-associated lymphoid tissue or MALT) are associated with *H. pylori* infection. The nonspecific presentation of gastric lymphoma is similar to that of gastric adenocarcinoma. The physical assessment may demonstrate an abdominal mass or adenopathy. To stage this disease, laparotomy is needed. The Ann Arbor staging system is used to stage gastric lymphoma, and the treatment regimen is based on the stage. The prognosis for gastric lymphoma is encouraging. The five-year survival rate is 50 percent. Whereas the overall survival rate for gastric adenocarcinoma is less than 15 percent. Patients with the diagnosis of gastric cancer or lymphoma face a particularly uncertain future. Patients and families need a comprehensive plan of treatment.

Assessment with Clinical Manifestations

As with other forms of cancer, gastric cancer has a wide variety of symptoms. In the beginnings of the disorder, the patient may be asymptomatic. And, when manifestations do occur, they are usually not that specific in nature. The patient may have some mild abdominal pain, anorexia, indigestion, and other ulcer-like symptoms. As the disease progresses, later clinical manifestations are malnourishment, fatigue, and anemia problems associated with GI bleeding, and may have palpable masses. Patients may have referred pain from the stomach area to other body areas.

Diagnostic Tests

The patient history and physical examination are not that helpful in the diagnosis of stomach cancer, because gastric tumors are not palpable and manifestations not specific. The potential bleeding tendencies might show anemia as an indicator, and hematocrit and hemoglobin verify the severity of the anemic condition. Endoscopy, barium swallow, and cytologic washings are typical for more specific confirmation of the cancer. A tissue biopsy reveals the most definitive diagnosis of the cancer typology.

Nursing Diagnoses

Based on the information gathered, examples of nursing diagnoses in the patient with stomach cancer may include the following:
- Acute pain related to the pressure from tumor development.
- Risk for infection related to the immunosuppression of the chemotherapy and radiation.
- Fear.
- Anxiety related to the diagnosis of cancer.
- Imbalanced nutrition, less than body requirements, related to nausea from the administration of chemotherapy or surgical interventions.

Planning and Implementation

Patients with cancer of the stomach do not have one specific therapy that is a cure, except for surgical removal of the stomach. And, even then, the cancer may be metastatic in nature and other body systems may be affected. If there is metastasis, the goals for this patient become palliation and supportive management strategies.

Pharmacology

If surgery is not indicated or does not cure cancer of the stomach, then chemotherapeutic agents are recommended. In addition, chemotherapy may be used prior to surgery and there are positive correlations with this strategy.

EXAMPLES OF COMBINATION CHEMOTHERAPY USED IN TREATING STOMACH CANCER

FAM (5-FU, Adriamycin, mitomycin C)

5-FU plus methyl CCNU

5-FU plus Adriamycin

EAP (etoposide, Adriamycin, cisplatin)

FAP (5-FU, Adriamycin, cisplatin)

FAB (5-FU, Adriamycin, carmustine

Source: National Institute of Cancer. (2006). Stomach cancer: NIC drug dictionary. Retrieved June 25, 2006, from www.cancer.gov.

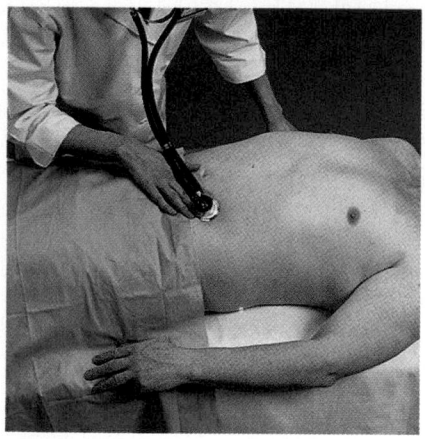

Figure 49-4 Nurse auscultating abdomen in presence of borborygmi sounds from dumping syndrome.

Commonly used chemotherapy for stomach cancer are combinations using 5-FU, Adriamycin, mitomycin C, cisplatin, and nitrosoureas (BCNU, CCNU) (Box 49-7).

Surgery

Surgery is the treatment of choice for stomach cancer, as long as adequate margins (5 to 6 cm) around the tumor can be obtained and regional lymph nodes are removed. Compared to subtotal or partial gastrectomy, total gastrectomy does not improve survival. There are a wide variety of surgical approaches to the treatment of stomach cancer. For example, a partial gastrectomy (e.g., Bilroth I, Bilroth II) may be performed. This surgery removes half to two thirds of the stomach. A total gastrectomy may be performed when there is cancer spread through the gastric tissue. There can also be a total gastrectomy accompanied with an esophagojejunostomy (construction of the esophagus to the duodenum or jejunum). In addition, an antrectomy can be performed, which is a partial resection of the stomach that may include part of the duodenum.

After gastric surgery, the patient may have a variety of complications and manifestations, which require specific nursing care. The management of pain, anxiety, patient education, restoration of general nutrition, and general nursing care for an abdominal surgery are indicated. The patient can have a problem with dumping syndrome, which occurs when there is too rapid filling of the small intestine. The patient has small gastric remains, which are connected to a larger opening into the intestine. The hypertonic intestinal contents draw fluid from the circulating plasma into the jejunum to dilute the high concentration of the fluid at that location. This causes the patient to have GI disorders (e.g., diarrhea, nausea or vomiting, epigastric pain, cramping, stimulated peristalsis, and increased motility). The patient may have unusual abdominal sounds with **borborygmi sounds** (loud, hyperactive bowel tones) (Figure 49-4). Dumping syndrome is treated with feeding with small, more frequent meals, taking liquids and solids at different times, and increasing proteins and fats, because they are eliminated more slowly than carbohydrates. After eating, the patient is encouraged to sit up to prevent reflux problems. Medications that can be prescribed are antacids, anticholinergics, sedatives, and antispasmodics.

The patient also may experience reflux of bile after the removal of the pylorus, which has similar treatments as those described in GERD situations. Also, patients may experience anemia from the lack of iron absorption (iron is normally absorbed in the duodenum and jejunum). In addition, intrinsic factor is decreased due to its production normally occurring in the stomach cells. Consequently, the patient may develop pernicious anemia, which is described in chapter 29.

Other malnutrition problems are somewhat common in gastric surgeries. Patients can develop folic acid deficiencies (refer to chapter 29), calcium absorption problems, and poor absorption of other nutrients from the removal of the stomach. And, the patient may continue to have problems of anorexia, which compromises his or her ability to consume normal meals and food intake. Nursing management is challenged with these types of nutritional problems, and referral to dietitians and counselors is often recommended.

Evaluations of Outcomes

Potential patient outcomes for each of the example nursing diagnoses for the patient with stomach cancer are:

- Acute pain related to the pressure from tumor development. The patient should verbalize an adequate relief of pain along with the ability to realistically cope with the pain if it is not completely relieved.
- Risk for infection related to the immunosuppression of the chemotherapy and radiation. The patient remains free of infection, as evidenced by nor-

mal vital signs and absence of purulent drainage from wounds, incisions, and tubes. Infection is recognized early to allow for prompt treatment.

- Fear related to the diagnosis of cancer; anxiety related to the diagnosis of cancer. The patient should be able to recognize the signs of anxiety, demonstrate positive coping mechanisms, and describe a reduction in the level of anxiety experienced.
- Imbalanced nutrition, less than body requirements, related to nausea from the administration of chemotherapy or surgical interventions. The patient verbalizes and demonstrates selection of foods or meals that will achieve a cessation of weight loss and weighs within 10 percent of ideal body weight.

KEY CONCEPTS

- Nurses are often the first health care provider who notices that the patient is experiencing chewing or dysphagia problems.
- Dyspepsia is the most common symptom that patients complain about to their provider.
- Ulcerative conditions of the gums and mucous membranes are labeled aphthous stomatitis and occur in 20 percent of the population.
- More than 400,000 cancer patients experience oral problems, such as painful mouth ulcers, impaired taste, and dry mouth from salivary gland dysfunction.
- Burning mouth syndrome is a constant burning sensation of the tongue seen in patients past middle age.
- Dysphagia represents a major problem in the older adult and needs special attention to prevent aspiration pneumonitis or pneumonia, airway obstruction, malnutrition, and dehydration.

- The more common esophageal disorders are achalasia, GERD, hiatal hernia, and esophageal cancer.
- The first line of treatment for esophageal pain and achalasia is often the same medications used to treat angina of cardiac origin.
- GERD occurs in 15 to 20 percent of all adults and daily symptoms are common.
- A hiatal hernia develops when there is a part of the stomach that protrudes through the esophageal hiatus, and there are often no symptoms.
- Esophageal cancer, associated with the highest cancer mortality rate, is also one of the most rapidly increasing malignancies.
- Stomach cancer may extend through the stomach wall and spread to nearby lymph nodes, the liver, pancreas, and colon, as well as spreading to distant organs (e.g., lungs, lymph nodes, ovaries).

REVIEW QUESTIONS

1. Mr. Jones has symptoms related to erosion of the esophagus. Which of the following is the correct label for his painful swallowing?
    1. Pyrosis
    2. Dysphagia
    3. Odynophagia
    4. Esophagitis

2. Mrs. Inez is having GI pain, which is specific to a region of her body. This is:
    1. Visceral pain
    2. Somatic pain
    3. Referred pain
    4. Abdominal pain

3. Mr. Steinway has burning mouth syndrome from candidiasis. Which of the following is true of this disorder?
    1. It is seldom seen in middle-aged adults.
    2. It is considered a mental health condition, often resulting from excessive anger.
    3. It is a constant burning sensation of the tongue.
    4. It is the most common GI disorder.

4. A PEG tube is:
    1. Synonymous with a nasogastric feeding tube
    2. Usually not used in the elderly population
    3. Typically inserted by a nurse in the patient's acute care room
    4. Sutured in place and has complications such as bleeding, infection, or peritonitis

Continued

REVIEW QUESTIONS—cont'd

5. Mr. Barnett has pain in the esophagus from esophagitis. This pain can be confused as:
   1. Dental disorders of the teeth
   2. Cardiac pain
   3. Appendicitis
   4. Acute bronchitis

6. Mrs. Tinen has been experiencing heartburn after meals and some regurgitation of fluids that taste foul when she is full, and she is often is not able to lie down comfortably just after eating. This is most likely:
   1. GERD
   2. Stomach cancer
   3. Achalasia
   4. Peptic ulceration

7. Mrs. Johanan is pregnant and experiencing pyrosis and regurgitation after eating her meals. This is most likely:
   1. Esophagitis
   2. Gastritis
   3. Hiatal hernia
   4. Aphagia

8. Mrs. Niyaki has a family history of stomach cancer. Which foods should her nurse instruct her to eat?
   1. Fresh fruits and vegetables
   2. Salted nuts
   3. Dried fish
   4. Smoked meats

9. Mrs. Garcia has recently has a gastric surgery. She is experiencing acute episodes of diarrhea that are sudden in occurrence, which is most likely:
   1. Borborygmi
   2. Flatus
   3. Dumping syndrome
   4. Apoptosis

REVIEW ACTIVITIES

1. Describe how you would instruct a patient to assess his or her oral cavity to detect early manifestations of cancer?

2. Observe a speech pathologist as he or she examines a patient in regard to his or her swallowing evaluation.

3. Ask for permission to observe an endoscopy performed in a special studies laboratory where you are enrolled in your clinical practicums.

4. Describe the patient education for GERD.

5. Describe the clinical manifestations experienced by a patient with peptic ulcer syndrome.

6. Describe how you would approach a patient with a new diagnosis of cancer of the stomach.

Lower Gastrointestinal Tract Dysfunction: Nursing Management

Milena Segatore, MScN, MNI-PG, CNRN

CHAPTER TOPICS

- Mal-absorption Conditions
- Acute Abdominal Pain
- Appendicitis
- Diverticulitis
- Bowel Obstructions
- Colorectal Cancer
- Irritable Bowel Syndrome
- Crohn's Disease
- Ulcerative Colitis

KEY TERMS

Acute abdomen
Adjuvant therapy
Anastomosis
Atresia
Borborygmi
Chyme
Colectomy
Diverticula
Diverticulosis
Fecalith
Fulguration
Hematochezia
Ileus
Intussusception
Laparoscopy
Laparotomy
Malrotation
Ostomy
Proctocolectomy
Referred pain
Somatic (parietal) pain
Steatorrhea
Tenesmus
Visceral pain
Volvulus

There are many disorders of the lower gastrointestinal (GI) tract, and patients in acute care settings have a wide variety of dysfunctions in the lower GI tract. The pathologies that exist within each organ are relatively common, and there are both medical and surgical approaches to providing treatment of the conditions of the lower GI tract. Nursing management carefully considers the disorders in the lower GI system and offers treatment and care that is essential to the patient. The types of conditions affect the patients and include, but are not limited to, acute inflammatory disorders, obstructive conditions, cancer within the region, and inflammatory bowel conditions.

SMALL INTESTINE

The small intestine, which is divided into the duodenum, the jejunum, and the ileum, is approximately 600 cm (6 meters, 240 inches, 20 feet, or approximately 6 yards) in length and 1 to 1.5 inches in diameter. The major role of the small intestine is the digestion and absorption of nutrients from the food and fluids ingested. The action of the columnar cells in the small intestine enhances the distribution of the products of digestion via the lymphatics and vascular system. Activity of the small intestine is a function of whether the intestine is in the fed state or the fasting state. **Chyme** (the semiliquid and partially digested stomach contents mixed with acids that enter the small intestine from the stomach) enters the duodenum. The motility of the small intestine mixes food with digestive enzymes. Transport and absorption of nutrients and electrolytes in the small intestine is dependent on nutrient status. Glucose and some amino acids (neutral) absorption are sodium dependent. The sodium/potassium (Na^+/K^+) pump enhances the movement and absorption of these nutrients into the blood. Lower in the colon and ileum, the Na^+/K^+-adenosinetriphosphatase (ATPase) pump enhances nutrient independent absorption of fluids and electrolytes. The hormone aldosterone also plays a role in this function.

Absorption of Nutrients

There are certain nutrients (i.e., vitamins, minerals, and electrolytes) that are absorbed in the GI tract that must be considered as a nurse is assessing the nutritional status of the patient when considering problems with digestion and absorption. During hydrolysis proteins are broken down into amino acids; polysaccharides into simple sugars; triglycerides into glycerol; and fatty acids and nucleic acids into substances more readily available for metabolism.

Folic Acid

Folic acid (folate) is an important water soluble B vitamin. It is essential in the production of red blood cells (RBCs), production of DNA, tissue growth, and cell function. Folic acid is needed for the production of certain digestive acids and to enhance the appetite. Folic acid is required by all childbearing women, as it is known to prevent neural-tube defect in the developing fetus. High total intake of folate has also been found to be inversely related to colon cancer. Usual food sources are beans, bananas, legumes, whole grains, dark green and leafy vegetables, poultry, pork, some shellfish, and liver. Only small amounts of folate are stored in the body so malnutrition can rapidly deplete body stores. Folic acid is absorbed via a Na^+-dependent carrier. Certain medications, like phenytoin (Dilantin) and sulfasalazine (Azulfidine), interfere with folic acid absorption. Folic acid deficiency can change the ability of the small intestine epithelium to absorb folic acid, hence the importance of a well-balanced diet high in folic acid as well as supplementation. Folic acid and B_{12} deficiency can lead to a megaloblastic anemia (Roth, 2007).

Cobalamin

Cobalamin (vitamin B_{12}) is essential to prevent pernicious anemia. Vitamin B_{12} is replaced in the diet by eating meat. Strict vegetarians will develop vitamin B_{12} deficiency unless they eat meat containing this vitamin or take a vitamin supplement. Because the body stores large amounts of B_{12} in the liver, the deficiency may not be readily seen for several years. In the duodenum, cobalamin combines with intrinsic factor (IF), which protects it from proteolysis, until it transits to the ileum where it is absorbed. Additionally pancreatic enzymes are necessary in this process. In summary, a functioning pancreas, the presence of IF, and a functional ileum are necessary to prevent cobalamin (vitamin B_{12})

deficiency. Mal-assimilation of iron may result in folate or vitamin B_{12} deficiency, which produces a megaloblastic red cell. Vitamin B_{12} deficiency produces neurological abnormalities, such as symmetrical paresthesias in the hands and feet, diminished vibratory and proprioceptive sense, ataxia, and spinal cord degeneration.

Iron

Iron (Fe) is essential to prevent anemia. Iron is present in both meat (heme iron) and vegetable (nonheme) sources. Heme iron is more readily absorbed than nonheme iron. Both types of iron are absorbed to a greater degree in the duodenum. Men need less dietary intake of iron (1 to 2 mg) than women (3 to 4 mg), especially menstruating women. The amount of iron absorbed is dependent on the total body iron content as well as the source of the iron. The absorption of nonheme iron can be reduced by the presence of certain food substances—plant phytates (soy beans), polyphenols (tea leaves, red wine), tea tannates, and even bran. Ascorbic acid (vitamin C) enhances the absorption of nonheme iron. Iron deficiency leads to hypochromic microcytic anemia. The patient with iron deficiency presents with pallor, atrophic tongue, koilonychias (spoon-shaped fingernails), cheilosis, or angular stomatitis (reddened lips with angular fissures).

Fat Soluble Vitamins

The fat soluble vitamins (A, D, E, and K) exist in large amounts, because there are large stores of these vitamins in the adipose tissue. Deficiencies are not apparent until there is long-standing mal-absorption or inadequate ingestion of these vitamins. Vitamin D deficiency can lead to many kinds of bone problems, i.e., osteomalacia, osteopenia, bone pain, cramps, and tetany. Vitamin K deficiency may lead to ecchymosis and easy bruising. Night blindness can be caused by a deficiency in vitamin A. Deficiency of vitamin E may lead to progressive demyelination in the central nervous system (CNS).

Hormones and Neurotransmitters

There are several hormones and neurotransmitters that enhance intestinal secretion. These include vasoactive intestinal peptides, bradykinin, prostaglandins, acetylcholine, serotonin, substance P (increases intestinal motility and vasodilatation), neurotensin, histamine, vasopressin, thyrocalcitonin, and others of which the mechanisms of action are unclear. These substances arise from the blood, nerve endings, endocrine cells in the intestinal epithelium, and intact enterocytes.

Substances that prevent secretion and promote absorption are the adrenal corticosteroids, somatostatins, the enkephalins, dopamine, and norepinephrine. The adrenal corticosteroids particularly the glucocorticoids increase absorption of electrolytes. Aldosterone also enhances intestinal absorption of electrolytes, especially sodium through the inhibition of the arachidonic acid cascade. Because the epithelium enterocytes are predominantly sympathetic sites, norepinephrine is the neurohormone elaborated. The effect is to inhibit electrolyte secretion and stimulate absorption. If a sympathectomy is performed, the individual will experience diarrhea. Patients with long-standing diabetes may also experience autonomic neuropathy and develop transient or persistent diarrhea.

Absorption of Fat

Absorption of fat occurs in stages. These are dependent on the function of the pancreas, liver, intestinal mucosa, and lymphatics. Dietary triglycerides must be broken down into glycerol and fatty acids. Disorders that impair lipolysis or fat solubilization could be rapid gastric emptying time with poor mixing of GI contents. This can result from a vagotomy or as part of the postgastrectomy syndrome. In Zollinger-Ellison syndrome, the pH of the duodenum is altered, which moderates the enzyme lipase. Decreased pancreatic function, cholestasis—liver disease, biliary obstruction, or alteration in enterohepatic circulation—may also inhibit fat absorption. Other disorders that will reduce fat absorption are celiac disease, Whipple's disease (chronic bacterial infection with *Tropheryma whippelii*), and lymphatic disorders, including lymphoma, short bowel syndrome (due to surgical removal or bypass of a large portion of the intestine, resulting in inadequate absorption of nutrients), and genetic defects that impair chylomicron formation. In fat mal-absorption, fatty acids bind calcium instead of oxalate. This leads to absorption of oxalate and may cause oxaluria and calcium oxalate kidney stones. Fat mal-assimilation results in diarrhea secondary to the irritant effect of fatty acids on the colon, weight loss, and malnutrition. A quantitative fecal fat determination is necessary to determine if the patient has **steatorrhea,** pale-yellow, greasy, fatty toll, or chronic watery diarrhea.

Absorption of Carbohydrates

Absorption of carbohydrates (CHO) is dependent on the action of enzymatic activity in the GI tract. Humans ingest CHOs in the form of starch, sucrose, and lactose. Digestion begins in the mouth with the action of ptyalin in saliva, which begins the digestive action of starch, an oligosaccharide. Sucrose and lactose are both disaccharides. Pancreatic enzymes and enzymes in the brush border of the intestine break down the oligosaccharides into disaccharides and further into monosaccharides for absorption into the mucosal cells and then into portal circulation.

Disorders that impair digestion and absorption of CHOs include pancreatic insufficiency, a deficiency of the enzymes along the brush border of the intestine, damage to the brush border, or enterocyte function secondary to disorders, such as gastroenteritis, celiac disease, sprue, or short bowel syndrome. These disorders injure the mucosal surface of the small intestine. If disaccharides reach the colon, increased intestinal gas is formed through colonic salvage of mal-absorbed CHOs in the small intestine. This has a salutary (beneficial) effect, because of the reduction in osmoles of the CHO, the fluid loss in feces is reduced. The intraluminal gases produced from the fermentation of the CHOs are carbon-dioxide (CO_2), hydrogen (H_2), and (CH_4) alkane/methane. The absorption of H_2 and then its subsequent exhalation through the lungs is the basis for the hydrogen breath test.

Of the types of enzyme deficiency that can occur, lactase deficiency is common. Lactase is located on the tip of the intestinal villi and is abundant in the jejunum. Intestinal disorders that damage enterocytes will increase symptomatology associated with lactase deficiency. Lactase is highest at birth and declines during the toddler years (three-and-a-half to five years of age). It decreases with age except in the Northern European population. An interesting cultural hypothesis has been proposed. Lactase persistence is common in regions where dairy farming prevails, but interestingly lactase is not induced with increased lactose intake (Box 50-1). Ingestion of small amounts of lactose usually does not produce symptoms even in individuals who are lactase deficient.

If CHO mal-assimilation persists, oxidative metabolism (catabolism) occurs, and fat and muscle (protein) are catabolized. The patient is weakened, with loss of muscle mass and mental slowing. The metabolic rate decreases because of decreased conversion of thyroid hormone, T_4 to T_3.

Absorption of Proteins

Most of protein digestion and absorption commences after pepsin acts on proteins in the stomach secondary to mixing in the stomach. Dietary protein is hydrolyzed by pancreatic protease action in the duodenum once enterokinase and trypsin catalyze (activate) the protease. This occurs in the first two thirds of the duodenum. Digestion occurs in the latter half of the duodenal lumen during sequential action of pancreatic endopeptidases and exopeptidases. The protein is further broken into peptides and amino acids. Cellular digestion of the peptides occurs at the brush border of the intestine. Considering this

---

BOX 50-1

EPIDEMIOLOGY OF LACTASE DEFICIENCY

It is important to emphasize with your patients that lactase deficiency is not a milk allergy. Lactase deficiency causes lactose mal-absorption. Lactase deficiency causes water to be drawn into the small bowel with a resulting osmotic diarrhea as well as the production of gas production causing flatulence, bloating, and cramping. The most common cause is idiopathic (without a recognizable cause). The incidence by ethnic group is as follows:

- Northern European: 2 to 15 percent
- Latino patients: 50 to 80 percent
- Ashkenazi Jews: 60 to 80 percent
- African American patients: 60 to 80 percent
- American Indians: 80 to 100 percent
- Asian (American): 95 to 100 percent

mechanism, mal-absorption of proteins can occur if there are any disorders that cause pancreatic insufficiency; enterocyte dysfunction, e.g., celiac disease, or loss of mucosal surface, short bowel syndrome. Protein mal-assimilation results in edema. Fluid leaks from the capillaries because of the drop in colloid osmotic pressure. The patient presents with diminished muscle because of the lack of protein. The absorption and assimilation of protein is necessary for most metabolic functions. The immune system is compromised in protein deficiency, which results in recurrent infections. Protein-calorie malnutrition is marasmus whereas protein energy malnutrition is kwashiorkor.

MAL-ASSIMILATION SYNDROMES

Optimal intake, digestion, absorption, and metabolism are necessary for healthy living. Because of the size (length, therefore surface area) of the GI tract there are many diseases that can impact nutrient digestion and absorption. Mal-assimilation occurs either by mal-digestion or mal-absorption.

Epidemiology

The epidemiology of mal-assimilation disorders as a single category is difficult to ascertain. It is important to know that specific risk factors associated with the GI system place individuals, groups, and even countries at risk for disease, disability, and death. In the poorest countries these include underweight, unsafe water and sanitation, diarrheal diseases, zinc deficiency, iron deficiency, vitamin A deficiency, and high serum cholesterol. In developed countries risk factors leading to disease, disability, or death related to the GI system are alcohol consumption, high serum cholesterol, high BMI, low fruit and vegetable intake, and iron deficiency. There are several systemic disorders associated with mal-absorption of nutrients shown in Table 50-1.

Pathophysiology

The two primary pathologies for mal-assimilation disorders are mal-digestion and mal-absorption. A brief description of each is presented.

Mal-Digestion Disorders

Mal-digestion disorders are intraluminal disorders often from impaired hydrolysis of intestinal contents. The major causes of mal-digestion include postgastrectomy dysfunction often referred to as a mixing disorder (see discussion on protein absorption), pancreatic insufficiency, a reduction in bile salt concentration

TABLE 50-1	Systemic Disorders Associated with Mal-absorption of Nutrients
ENDOCRINE DISEASES	**DIABETES, THYROID DISORDERS, ADDISON'S DISEASE, AND HYPOPARATHYROIDISM**
Collagen-vascular diseases	Scleroderma, vasculitis, systemic lupus erythematosus, polyarteritis nodosa
Amyloidosis	Abnormal production of immunoglobulins leading to inadequate absorption of nutrients from the gastrointestinal tract and gastroesophageal reflux disease
AIDS	Can lead to protein losing enteropathy especially albumin

Adapted from Roth, R. (2007). Nutrition and diet therapy (9th ed.). New York: Thomson Delmar Learning.

in the intestine, interruption in the entero-hepatic circulation of bile salts, and certain medications, e.g., neomycin, calcium carbonate, and cholestyramine.

Mal-Absorption Disorders

Mal-absorption disorders are those that impair transport of intestinal contents across the mucosal membrane of the lumen. The major causes of mal-absorption are a reduction in absorptive surface of the intestine secondary to resection or bypass; biochemical or genetic abnormalities, e.g., celiac disease, disaccharidase deficiency, hypogammaglobulinemia, or Hartnup disease (an inherited disorder that prevents the absorption of certain proteins leading to a deficiency of niacin and tryptophan, cystinuria, or monosaccharide mal-absorption); inflammatory or infiltrative disorders; and lymphatic obstruction.

Assessment with Clinical Manifestations

Assessment of mal-assimilation disorders is detailed as there are many changes that potentially can occur throughout much of the body. In general, it is important to assess the patient for weight loss, signs of vitamin and mineral deficiency (e.g., anemia, easy bruising), cheilosis (reddened lips and fissures at lip angles) or glossitis, various dermatitides, tetany, osteoporosis, ecchymosis, paresthesias, fatigue, weakness, muscle wasting, borborygmi and increased flatus (gas production), edema, and change in stools, especially steatorrhea.

Patients with pan-mal-absorption often complain of steatorrhea. Abdominal distension or bloating is caused by a fermentation process that occurs in the colon secondary to unabsorbed carbohydrates by colon bacteria. Anemia is noted as part of a broad array of abnormalities associated with vitamin and mineral deficiencies.

Diagnostic Tests

The patient who has a mal-assimilation disorder will present with a classic symptom array that may include a history of weight loss, change in eating and bowel habits, e.g., polyphagia, diarrhea, foul-smelling stools that float because of increased water and gas content, stools that may have a rancid odor and greasy character (occurs later), abdominal bloating, muscle wasting, bone pain, weakness, tetany, paresthesias, bleeding gums, and dermatological conditions, such as eczema. See Box 50-2 for routine lab tests for mal-assimilation disorders.

To further assess for intraluminal mal-digestion, assessment of biliary function is done. This includes liver biochemistry, abdominal ultrasound, and endoscopic cholangiography. Bile salts may fail to be reabsorbed if the patient has ileal disease. The patient will be evaluated for bacterial overgrowth syndrome (BOS), especially if the patient has a history of gastric or upper intestinal tract surgery. Twenty to 43 percent of diarrhea in patients with diabetes has BOS (Frye, Tamer, & Kunha, 2005).

Nursing Diagnoses

Based on the information gathered, examples of nursing diagnoses in the patient with mal-assimilation disorders may include the following:
- Imbalanced nutrition, less than body requirements secondary to mal-assimilation disorders.
- Risk for impaired skin integrity.
- Deficient knowledge related to diagnosis of mal-assimilation disorders.
- Diarrhea related to mal-assimilation disorders.

Planning and Implementation

Patients who have mal-assimilation disorders present with a variety of symptoms, diagnostic findings, and abnormal laboratory results. Once the site of the defect is established, treatment is instituted. If the problem (e.g., biliary obstruction) is

> **BOX 50-2**
>
> ### ROUTINE LAB TESTS FOR MAL-ASSIMILATION DISORDERS
>
> CBC with a peripheral smear to distinguish between a microcytic or microcytic anemia
>
> **Chemistry Screen:**
>
> Serum calcium, phosphorus, and alkaline phosphatase to detect osteopenia
>
> Serum electrolytes: Na^+, K^+, Cl^-, CO_2, Ca^{++}, and Mg^+.
>
> Serum albumin and total proteins to assess protein stores
>
> Serum cholesterol, carotene, and prothrombin time (vitamin K) indirectly gauges fat assimilation
>
> Liver profile AST (aspartate aminotransferase), ALT (alanine aminotransferase), and bilirubin
>
> Serum iron, total iron binding capacity (TIBC), and ferritin to evaluate proximal intestinal function
>
> Serum B_{12} level is indicative of the integrity of ileal function
>
> Red cell folate measures folate stores
>
> Shilling test with intrinsic factor suggests ileal dysfunction
>
> Stool pH tends to be low with CHO mal-absorption (less than 5.5)
>
> D-xylose test measures whether CHO is absorbed. If serum xylose levels are low after a test dose it is indicative of CHO mal-absorption.
>
> H_2 breath test assists in the evaluation of CHO absorption.
>
> Fecal fat measurement: fecal fat loss is about less than 5 percent of dietary intake. Elevation of fecal fat (steatorrhea) is an important diagnostic measurement to determine the presence of generalized mal-assimilation.
>
> *Source: Daniels, R. (2003).* Delmar's manual of laboratory and diagnostic tests. *New York: Thomson Delmar Learning.*

structural, surgery may be necessary. If the patient has pancreatic insufficiency, enzyme supplements will be administered, or if there is an obstructive lesion or neoplasm, insulin, dietary counseling, lifestyle modification, and surgery are options. If the intestinal mucosa is defective dietary modifications will be necessary (e.g., gluten withdrawal, nutritional supplements, antibiotics for BOS or Whipple's disease). If the lymphatics are the site of the problem, a low-fat diet will be suggested; the health care provider will perhaps suggest medium-chain triglycerides (MCTs), because these are more water soluble and as a result can be absorbed across the small intestinal wall into the blood more easily.

Replacement and or supplement therapy is instituted. This will include minerals, targeted vitamins and multiple vitamin therapy, folic acid, pancreatic supplements, bile salt binding agents, caloric supplements, and enteral supplements if needed.

Patient and Family Teaching

For patients with mal-assimilation disorders, lifestyle and nutritional management are essential. Patients and families will need to understand the basic pathology inherent in the disorder and management principles to maintain a normal adaptive life style.

Evaluation of Outcomes

Potential patient outcomes for each of the example nursing diagnoses for the patient with mal-assimilation disorders are:

- Imbalanced nutrition, less than body requirements secondary to mal-assimilation disorders. The patient verbalizes and demonstrates selection of foods or meals that will achieve a cessation of weight loss and weighs within 10 percent of ideal body weight.
- Risk for impaired skin integrity. The patient's skin condition should be improved as evidenced by decreased redness, swelling, and pain.
- Deficient knowledge related to diagnosis of mal-assimilation disorders. The patient should demonstrate motivation to learn, identify perceived learning needs, and verbalize an understanding of desired content.
- Diarrhea related to mal-assimilation disorders. The patient will pass formed stool no more than three times per day.

ACUTE ABDOMEN

Acute abdomen refers to a constellation of clinical signs and symptoms usually best treated by surgery. The term is nonetiologically specific and connotes a high degree of urgency and acuity. Acute abdomen has also been defined by its consequence, namely, the need for surgery. That is, it has been referred to as a surgical abdomen. Although the severity and pathology may mandate a surgical cure in some, a variety of medical emergencies may also cause acute abdomen, and medical remedies may be curative. By convention, acute abdomen caused by trauma is considered separately.

Epidemiology

Acute abdomen encompasses a spectrum of surgical, medical, and gynecological conditions, ranging from the mild to life-threatening, which require hospital admissions, investigation, and treatment, whereby the primary clinical symptom is abdominal pain. As such, it is seen in patients of every age and socioeconomic group. Acute abdominal pain is a ubiquitous disorder, accounting for 5 to 10 million patient encounters per year in the United States, and 5 to 10 percent of all emergency department (ED) visits. Ten percent of these patients require surgery, and the diagnosis is associated with 10 percent malpractice claims filed annually. The most commonly missed diagnoses are appendicitis and small bowel obstruction. It is estimated that at least half of general surgical admissions are emergent, and half of the admissions are for complaints of acute abdominal pain. In one pediatric study, one third of the children required surgery and in 90 percent of those cases, the diagnosis was appendicitis. Thirty-day mortality is estimated at 4 percent in those admitted with acute abdominal pain, and of those operated on, the rate rises to 8 percent. The highest mortality is associated with patients who require laparotomy for unresectable cancer, ruptured abdominal aortic aneurysm (AAA), and perforated peptic ulcer (Persiani, Biondi, Buccelletti, Rausei, & Silveri, 2006). Among patients 65 years and older, the fastest growing sector is 85 years and older, and the elderly have the highest mortality rates in the adult surgical population.

Generally morbidity, mortality, and diagnostic accuracy are worse for elderly patients with acute abdomen. This has been attributed to delays in diagnosis and treatment and the existence comorbidities Coexisting disease threatens physiological reserve and reduces the ability to cope with the stress of intercurrent acute events and its treatments. Atypical presentations are often related to the physiological effects of aging: For example diminished immunity impairs the ability to generate a febrile response to disease, and reduced neural sensitivity in the elderly may blunt their appreciation of pain, producing delays in presentation. Absence of typical signs and symptoms can be devastating. In acute appendicitis, it is thought to produce a higher rate of perforation. Biliary tract disease, the most common disorder requiring abdominal surgery in the elderly, typically produces right upper quadrant pain, but 25 percent have no significant pain, and fewer than one half will have a fever, leukocytosis, or vomiting. The situation is similar for diverticulitis and perforating ulcer disease. Rebound tenderness, classically the most reliable clinical sign of peritonitis, is normally absent in a large number of elderly. Meticulous perioperative management, use of minimally invasive surgical approaches, and percutaneous drainage of gallbladder and abscesses may help avoid major anesthetic and surgical stresses (Stain, 2005).

Etiology

Virtually all organs within the abdominal cavity are pain sensitive, and the etiology of abdominal pain is as varied as the contents of the abdominal cavity: Disorders affecting respiratory (e.g., pneumonia), vascular (e.g., myocardial infarction, aortic dissection), GI (e.g., appendicitis, cholecystitis), endocrine (e.g., pancreatitis), renal-urinary (e.g., renal lithiasis, pyelonephritis, ureteral obstruction), and reproductive organs (e.g., ectopic pregnancy, spermatic cord torsion, ovarian cyst rupture) can all cause acute abdomen. Common etiologies vary by age and cause can arise over again, or can arise as acute exacerbations of formerly stable chronic problem, e.g. bowel perforation during an exacerbation of inflammatory bowel disease.

Causes can be preliminarily organized as medical or surgical. Medical causes may arise from intra- or extra-abdominal pathology. For example, in the pediatric population, common nonsurgical diagnoses include constipation and pneumonia. Surgical causes can be organized by organ(s) involved and by the underlying pathology. An alternative classification categorizes etiologies into three general groups: vascular (e.g., ischemia, infarction, hemorrhage), obstruction of a lumen (e.g., adhesions, ectopic pregnancy, malignant bowel obstruction; ureteral or common bile duct stone), or perforation of a viscus (e.g., duodenal ulcer, gravid uterus). The most common cause of acute abdomen is appendicitis. In up to one third of cases, a clear diagnosis is never determined; a nonspecific pain is common in children.

Pathophysiology

Regardless of etiology, two major pathological processes, inflammation and obstruction, are implicated in acute abdomen. Inflammation may be infectious or noninfectious, but regardless of cause, the chain of pathological events is the same. Affected structures demonstrate reactive hyperemic, with exudation of fluid into tissues due to increased vascular permeability and an increase of filtration pressure.

Peritonitis is a general term denoting peritoneal inflammation; some authors use this term interchangeably with acute abdomen. Peritonitis can be generalized, or affect selected portions of visceral or parietal peritoneum (Estes, 2006). Consequences of peritoneal inflammation vary by the severity and duration of the underlying condition, the organ involved, patient age (physiological reserve), and comorbidities. Primary or spontaneous peritonitis occurs as a diffuse bacterial infection without an obvious intra-abdominal source of contamination. More common is secondary peritonitis, which occurs as a result of a primary event such as perforation, infection, or gangrene of an intra-abdominal organ. Leakage of GI and pancreatic secretions, bile, blood, urine, or meconium cause chemical peritonitis when they come into contact with the peritoneum. The inflammatory response increases blood supply and edema formation within the peritoneum. There is transudation of fluid into the peritoneal cavity and accumulation of protein rich exudates. Ongoing inflammation glues omentum lying over the affected structure to that structure and inhibits peristalsis, which limits the spread of infection or inflammation. Fluid accumulates within the lumen, causing the intravascular volume to fall and producing clinical signs of hypovolemia.

Intra-abdominal infection and peritonitis result in profound sepsis due to the bacterial content of the viscera and the huge surface area of the peritoneum. There is vast fluid loss, rapid bacterial absorption and endotoxin, and a marked systemic inflammatory response to the release of inflammatory mediators. This course of events sets off a complex septic cascade, which includes intravascular coagulation, circulatory failure, inadequate tissue oxygenation, and finally multiple organ dysfunctions. In the surgical setting, the most common cause of generalized peritonitis is perforation of an intra-abdominal viscus. Ischemia and infarction are potent triggers of inflammation; leakage of blood into the abdominal cavity from any sources tends to produce relatively few signs of inflammation.

Obstruction is the second pathological process. The colon normally generates intermittent contractions of low and high amplitude. Low amplitude, short duration bursts move luminal contents anterograde (frontward) and retrograde (backward), delaying colonic transit time, thus providing time for water and electrolyte absorption. High amplitude contractions create mass movement. In general colonic activation increases colonic motility (Bullard & Rothenberger, 2005). Vomiting develops early and in greater volumes when the level of obstruction in the gut is high, as swallowed air, food, secretions, and bile accumulate behind the site of obstruction and continue to distend the bowel lumen. When propulsive activity in the gut is impeded or blocked, a vicious cycle of distension and secretion is set in motion as the bowel continues to contract with increased, uncoordinated peristaltic activity (Ripamonte & Mercadante, 2004). Ischemia and increasing intraluminal pressures caused by unrelieved obstruction predispose the bowel to rupture.

Assessment with Clinical Manifestations

Given the spectrum of possible causes, a systematic approach is required for assessment and diagnosis. Efficient history taking and focused physical assessment require an appreciation of how pain is produced within the abdomen. Pain is of three types: somatic, visceral, or referred. **Somatic** or **parietal pain** is sharp or knife-like in character, usually precisely localized to the affected area. When visceral inflammation involves richly innervated parietal peritoneum, which is sensitive to mechanical, thermal, and chemical stimuli, sharp pain is felt at the site. In addition, there is reflex contraction of the corresponding segmental area of muscle, which causes rigidity of the abdominal wall (guarding) and hyperesthesia of the overlying skin.

Structurally, visceral peritoneum, which partially or totally invests the intra-abdominal viscera, is insensitive to mechanical, thermal, or chemical stimuli. **Visceral pain,** activated by traction on bowel mesentery, inflammation, ischemia, or distension of hollow or solid viscus is typically described as dull and deep-seated. Usually, it is vaguely localized to area occupied by the viscus during development. It is often associated with restless, diaphoresis, and nausea. Colic is considered a type of visceral pain, arises from hollow viscus with muscle in its walls (gut, gallbladder, or ureter), and results from excessive muscle contraction against an obstruction. Patients may be unable to remain still during the bout of colic but be pain free between attacks. The complex sensory innervation of abdominal cavity produces classical pain syndromes. For example, acute appendicitis typically begins with generalized periumbilical pain, which over time migrates to the right lower quadrant (RLQ).

Referred pain is pain perceived distant from its source. For example, small bowel distension radiates to the back and cholecystitis radiates to the inferior scapular border, reflecting embryological or dermatomal origins.

Skills 360°

History of Acute Abdominal Pain

A chief complaint of acute abdominal pain requires immediate focused evaluation: targeted history taking and a focused physical assessment. Physical exam lies at the heart of diagnosis and must be conducted to economically address the following questions:

- How severe is the physiological compromise?
- Is there a need for immediate resuscitation, urgent surgical consultation, and intervention?
- What diagnostic modalities will be most efficient and effective in determining the probable cause?

Pain assessment is the focus of the history; elements of the comprehensive pain history are summarized in Table 50-2. Beginning practitioners should be aware that even if they are unfamiliar with classical histories associated with specific pathological events, a comprehensive, systematic, and detailed history is invaluable to the consultants involved later in the care. Individual elements of the history can suggest a possible etiology or influence the degree of urgency appropriate to evaluating the problem. For example, the onset of pain suggests problem acuity: sudden, generalized, excruciating pain, with an onset under one hour suggests an intra-abdominal catastrophe, such as perforation of a viscus (e.g., ruptured ectopic pregnancy) or vascular catastrophe (e.g., bowel infarction or dissection) that may produce shock and require resuscitation and immediate, often life-saving surgery. Gradual onset suggests an inflammatory process.

Pain quality, or character, including any periodicity, is also suggestive. For example, colicky pain suggests an obstructive etiology, such as biliary, ureteric or intestinal colic and may be intense and severe. If colicky pain becomes continuous, significant inflammation should be suspected. Location is possibly the most valuable variable to the underlying diagnosis. For example, blood or pus below the left diaphragm can cause left shoulder pain. Migratory details are important to note; for example, if leaking duodenal contents reach the right paracolic gutter, the patient may complain of RLQ as well as epigastric pain. Late in the evolution of acute abdomen, pain may be generalized due to diffuse peritonitis.

Radiation away from the initial site signifies involvement of other structures: For example, pain from a duodenal ulcer radiating to the back suggests that inflammation has breached the wall and reached structures on the posterior abdominal wall. Radiation to the right scapula should raise the suspicion of gallbladder pathology; radiation into the ipsilateral groin and flank is suggestive of ureteral obstruction (e.g., kidney stones). A temporal course of the acute abdominal pain can further narrow the likely pathology and influence trajectory of care. Severe pain, lasting more than six hours and worsening over

TABLE 50-2 Pain Checklist	
Onset	Sudden versus duration (hours or days)
Character	Burning, cutting, boring, crampy, or colicky
Severity	0–10 scale
Location	Consider referred pain patterns
Radiation	Does the pain extend over a wide area?
Duration	Minutes to hours to days
Temporal course	Intermittent (waxing and waning) or continuous; is it getting better or worse?
Ameliorating factors	Is pain improved by changing positioning, food intake, or by medications?
Exacerbating factors	Is pain worse with movement?
Associated manifestations	Nausea, vomiting, changes in bowel habits or patterns; anorexia, rigors, shaking chills, fever, pulmonary, urinary, obstetric and gynecological symptoms (i.e., menstrual history; possible pregnancy), unintended recent weight loss, or drug use (e.g., steroids).

Adapted from Estes, M. (2006). Health assessment and physical examination (3rd ed.). New York: Thomson Delmar Learning.

time, increases the likelihood of surgery. If pain is subsiding, the probability of surgical disease falls.

Associated findings are more difficult to interpret. For example, vomiting may be attributable to pain severity or disease in the GI tract or self-induced, and can be bilious (small bowel obstruction) or nonbilious. Generally pain precedes vomiting in a surgical abdomen. This can be seen in appendicitis, cholecystitis, and small bowel obstruction. Vomiting followed by pain is suggestive of a medical cause. Diarrhea with pain is usually due to medical causes, with a few important exceptions. Obstruction causes classical clinical signs and symptoms; obstruction of a muscular viscus causes colicky pain, cresting and receding in waves, rather than the constant pain of inflammation, and tends to be worsened by general disturbance.

Focused history taking should occur simultaneously with inspection of the body habitus (physical appearance) and patient demeanor. It should be noted that the elderly and patients being treated with steroids may not report the same severity of pain as patients not on steroids or younger patients. The patient's overall appearance should be noted; for example, is the patient lying motionless or restless. A patient lying completely still is characteristic of peritonitis and should suggest serious intra-abdominal disease. Restlessness is associated with colicky pain. Dry mucous membranes might suggest dehydration.

The presence of tachypnea, tachycardia, hypotension, cold and clammy skin, altered mentation, low urine output, and fever suggest complicated disease with peritonitis and shock (Estes, 2006). If clinical signs suggestive of shock coexist with abdominal swelling or the patient is prostrate with board-like abdomen, the priority is immediate resuscitation and surgical consultation. Further deterioration may be averted if the patient is taken directly to surgery, where resuscitation and assessment can continue in conjunction with laparotomy.

Severe intravascular volume depletion or electrolyte abnormalities should be addressed immediately to preserve and support the vital functions and restore hemodynamic stability. Compromised renal perfusion raises the need for close monitoring of urinary output as volume resuscitation proceeds. High fever may be seen in abscess, pyelonephritis, septic cholangitis, or gynecological infections, such as salpingitis. However, absence of fever, particularly in the elderly, should never be relied on to exclude infectious intra-abdominal catastrophes. Abnormalities in cardiorespiratory parameters should raise questions about the need for enhanced monitoring and support—from continuous electrocardiographic and pulse oximetry to invasive hemodynamic monitoring, inotropic support, endotracheal intubation or mechanical ventilation. Adequate opioid analgesia should not be withheld during evaluation of the abdomen for fear of masking important clinical signs and delaying diagnosis. These strategies have been shown to be unfounded (Shabbir, et. al., 2004). Effective analgesia also facilitates patient cooperation during the examination.

Inspection should note the contour and color of the abdomen. Distension can suggest the presence of air, blood, or ascites, jaundice, or common bile duct obstruction (Estes, 2006). Cullen's sign, a bluish periumbilical discoloration, can occur with intra-abdominal bleeding; Grey Turner (tenderness) or Fox signs should be sought in the flank and inguinal area respectively. The location of hernia, mass, defects, and visible peristalsis and pulsatile masses should also be noted. Scars should be tested for the presence of herniation. Auscultation for bowel and vascular sounds (bruits, venous hums, or peristalsis) follows inspection. Absence of bowel sounds more than 30 minutes suggests peristalsis has ceased. Gurgles are produced by fluid-gas mixtures. A possibility of obstruction can be detected with absent bowel sounds, and **borborygmi** (a gurgling, splashing sound normally heard over large intestine). Palpation for masses, organomegaly (abnormal enlargement), and pain, and to confirm inspection and auscultatory findings should follow and should begin in areas distant from the pain (Estes, 2006). Every effort should be made to relax the patient. Guarding, or increased abdominal tone, is voluntary or involuntary, local or generalized. Involuntary guarding that fails to disappear during deep inhalation suggests underlying peritonitis.

The triad of generalized pain, board-like abdominal rigidity and rebound suggest peritonitis. Associated signs should be sought, such as Murphy's sign in acute cholecystitis or Rovsing's sign in appendicitis. Percussion concludes the exam, and is useful detecting the presence of air (tympanic) or fluid (fluid waves). Rebound tenderness is more accurately identified by percussion of the abdomen than by palpation with quick release (Estes, 2006). That is, rebound tenderness should be elicited by gently tapping the belly with the percussing finger. Maneuvers, such as the obturator and iliopsoas muscle tests, may be useful in detecting inflamed or perforated appendix. The examination should conclude with examination of the hernia orifices, genital, rectal, or vaginal examinations.

Diagnostic Tests

Laboratory, radiologic, and endoscopic diagnostics should not interfere with resuscitation and restoration of hemodynamic stability. They should complement the details of history and physical exam and are useful in supporting the diagnosis or narrowing the differential (Daniels, 2003). Laboratory findings, like signs and symptoms of shock, are nonspecific but can help focus attention on likely causes. Selection should be driven by historical and physical findings. Hematological investigations should minimally include CBC, with a differential and related tests, such as blood smear. Useful findings include leukocytosis, which suggest an infectious process (may be primary or secondary). Persistent elevation or rising white count suggests underlying inflammation or infection; a leukocytosis of 15,000 to 20,000 per mm^3 suggests bowel necrosis (Daniels, 2003). There can be a poor correlation with white blood cells (WBC) and intra-abdominal inflammation, so exclusions should not be made on the base of a normal WBC count. Abnormalities suggestive of a primary medical cause, such as sickling (sickle-shaped RBCs) that might have led to mesenteric ischemia or infarction may confirm clinical impression. Blood should also be sent for typing and cross-matching for patients who might require surgery or transfusion. A coagulation screen is required for any patient who might require surgery and to eliminate the presence of coagulopathy. Prolongations in international normalized ratio (INR) may require rapid correction prior to operation. Bleeding time may be requested by surgical consultants in specific instances. Prolonged clotting time or thrombocytopenia may suggest the possibility of hemorrhage as a primary or secondary etiology. Biochemistry studies should minimally include serum electrolytes, blood urea nitrogen (BUN), and creatinine as indices of renal function. Other assays should be selected on the basis of history or physical findings. For example, beta-hCG (human chorionic gonadotropin) in suspected pregnancy-related acute abdomen; liver function studies in acute hepatobiliary disease; and bilirubin, amylase, lipase, and calcium in acute pancreatitis; serum phosphate can be increased in mesenteric ischemia. Toxicology may be useful in selected cases (e.g., cocaine related). Microbiological testing (e.g., urine or blood cultures) ought to be considered in the presence of rigors and shaking chills, peritoneal signs, or history or clinical findings suggestive of an infectious etiology (e.g., pelvic inflammatory disease or septic ascending cholangitis) and dipstick-positive urine (for blood or WBC).

A 12 lead electrocardiogram (ECG) should be done in all surgical candidates to exclude acute myocardial ischemia or infarction and arrhythmias as cause of the pain. Presence of abnormalities may suggest the etiology of pain: For example, atrial fibrillation, in conjunction with abdominal pain may be indicative of mesenteric ischemia. Arterial blood gas analysis may be useful in ventilated patients, to assess the need for or adequacy of metabolic correction. Imaging should be selected for maximum yield in the shortest time; its purpose is pathological diagnosis. Common modalities are summarized in Table 50-3.

An upright chest X-ray (CXR) is the most appropriate means of detecting free intraperitoneal (pneumoperitoneum) gas under the diaphragm and should be done in cases of suspected perforation. It may also exclude respiratory causes of acute abdominal pain. The two most appropriate selections in a patient

TABLE 50-3 Imaging Modalities: Acute Abdomen

	ADVANTAGE	DISADVANTAGE	COMMENTS
CXR	Excludes some cardiorespiratory processes. Fast, inexpensive, noninvasive, minimal radiation exposure, portable.	None.	Identifies 50–90 percent of perforated viscus with pneumoperitoneum. Increased sensitivity with left lateral decubitus view.
Abdominal films	Fast, inexpensive, noninvasive, minimal radiation exposure, portable. Cross table lateral in left lateral position can detect as little 5–10 mL free air (e.g., air fluid levels in dilated loops of bowel [obstruction]); distended bowel (paralytic ileus), abnormal calcifications (gallstones, kidney stones, and some appendicoliths).	None.	75 percent of perforated duodenal ulcers have free air; colon, and stomach perforation can liberate large amounts of air.
Abdominal or pelvic ultrasound, (transabdominal or intravaginal)	Portable, safe, rapid, low cost, no radiation exposure. Visualizes gallbladder, biliary tree, liver, spleen, pancreas, appendix, ovaries, adnexa, and uterus.	Blind to many areas, especially in presence of large amounts bowel gas or free air. CT outperforms in combination of clinical evaluation and other modalities.	Yield high in those with palpable mass and suspected acute diverticulitis; Less useful if lab results are normal and clinical signs are nonspecific Routine use not associated with shorter LOS.
CT—abdomen and pelvis + IV or oral contrast	Gold standard for identifying disease processes. Work horse of acute abdomen evaluation.	Requires transport and support out of intensive care unit, ED, or operating room. Not as useful with hollow viscera pathology.	For patients who do not go to surgery, CT superior to clinical exam (90 percent versus 76 percent sensitivity) in diagnosing cause. Especially useful in patients without prior known abdominal disease.
Tc99m HMPAO [technetium-99m-hexamethyl propylene amin oxime] white cell labeled scanning	High sensitivity for IBD (91–96 percent).	Not as accurate as CT for abscess and fistulae (abnormal passage leading from an abscess to body surface).	Some role in elderly and appendicitis.

Adapted from Persiani, R., Biondi, A., Buccelletti, F., Rausei, S., & Silveri, N. (2006). Unusual acute abdomen: To operate or not to operate? Lancet, *367(9521), 1548; Raman, S., Somasekar, K., Winter, R. K., & Lewis, M. H. (2004). Are we overusing ultrasound in non-traumatic abdominal pain?* Postgraduate Medical Journal, *80, 177–179.*

with acute abdomen are plain films of the abdomen (two views) and computed tomography (CT) of the abdomen or pelvis, with or without intravenous (IV) and oral contrast. Rectal contrast may be indicated in selected patients. CT, which provides images with a high degree of anatomic detail, leads to pathological diagnosis in most cases. In one study, clinical examination accurately identified the anatomical lesion in 17.5 percent, and CT achieved (57.5 percent) greater than a threefold improvement. Ultrasound is particularly useful in gynecological and hepatobiliary disease. Angiography may be used when vascular etiologies are suspected (e.g., mesenteric ischemia, hemorrhage).

Consideration must be given to acute medical and surgical causes and prioritized by age. For example, among premature infants necrotizing enterocolitis is a not uncommon occurrence; but it is virtually unheard of among adults. Medical causes frequently produce a clinical picture that lacks specific localization and guarding. The broad differential reflects contents of abdomen represent every body system and can be intra- or extra-abdominal. Psychiatric discords, such as Munchausen's syndrome (fabrication of symptoms or self-mutilation to gain medical attention) or Munchausen's by proxy (faking another person's illness), should remain diagnoses of exclusion. Different classification schemes have been proposed; the variety includes genetic or developmental, infectious, vascular, neoplastic, infectious or inflammatory, and toxic or metabolic causes.

Nursing Diagnoses

Based on the information gathered, examples of nursing diagnoses in the patient with acute abdomen may include the following:
- Fear related to perioperative events.
- Deficient fluid volume related to intake less than body requirements.
- Acute pain related to acute abdomen.
- Risk of infection related to intra-abdominal processes and procedures.

Planning and Implementation

Goals of management are supportive and definitive. Definitive management of the underlying problem is as varied as the potential etiologies of acute abdomen. Supportive care runs the gamut from aggressive symptom palliative to resuscitation. Either may require immediate or delayed surgical intervention. Indications for admission to the hospital include surgical candidates, those who cannot eat or drink, febrile patients from infection, and those who have uncontrolled pain or require IV antibiotics.

Collaborative Management

Indications for adopting a nonsurgical approach include diagnostic uncertainty and equivocal physical findings. These patients should be admitted and closely monitored. Special attention should be paid to immunocompromised patients who may present atypically, and individuals who are unable to communicate. A period of close observation provides an opportunity to stabilize the vital functions, explore potential medical causes, and correct abnormalities. Patients with intra-abdominal sepsis may benefit from short-term, aggressive volume resuscitation and antibiotic therapy. Recent reviews of different antibiotic course of therapy (morbidity, mortality, cost, resource use) for the treatment of secondary peritonitis of GI origin suggested no specific benefit associated with any particular regimen (Wong, et al., 2005). Some potential surgical lesions might be managed initially by watchful waiting, such as a ruptured but contained duodenal ulcer.

Acute abdomen caused by medical conditions (e.g., sickle cell crisis, spontaneous bacterial peritonitis, *Clostridium difficile* pseudomembranous colitis, acute pancreatitis, acute hepatitis, acute salpingitis) require pathology specific management and involvement of appropriate consultants. Discovery of an abscess is not an automatic indication for open surgical management. Depending on location and patient status, percutaneous, fluoroscopy guided percutaneous drainage is often a viable option, sparing the patient urgent operation. For example, acute diverticulitis can often be managed medically with percutaneous drainage of abscesses, followed by elective surgery.

Surgery

There are a variety of potential surgical management strategies for patients with acute abdominal conditions. Surgical consultation should be sought for patients with severe or progressive pain, fecal vomiting, abdominal rigidity or guarding, rebound tenderness, hypertympanic (air-filled) abdomens, unclear etiology, or intra-abdominal fluid accumulation. Indications for operation include uncontrolled intra-abdominal hemorrhage (e.g., AAA in a viable patient), presence of peritoneal signs, pain with signs of sepsis without an obvious source, acute intestinal ischemia, and pneumo-peritoneum. An attitude of watchful waiting may be at adopted to give medical interventions an opportunity to create improvement, but this approach requires frequent and careful clinical monitoring. Surgical decision making about the approach, extent, whether or not to exteriorize the bowel, and how to close the wound are tailored to the specific cause (Golash & Willson, 2005).

Classically operative candidates undergo open **laparotomy,** a surgical incision into the wall of the abdomen, for definitive diagnosis and management. However, over the last decade, minimally invasive surgery, specifically, **laparoscopy,** a visual examination of the interior of the abdominal cavity, has played a growing role. A variety of operations are possible including diagnostic laparoscopy for critical patients with equivocal findings and definitive therapy for obstruction, diverticulitis, and acute appendix. When acute abdomen is caused by a medical problem, laparoscopy allows the surgeon to visualize large surface areas within pelvic and abdominal cavities, to biopsy suspicious areas, aspirate, culture, and ultrasound suspicious structures. Contraindications include hemodynamic instability, mechanical or paralytic ileus, coagulopathy, generalized peritonitis, severe cardiovascular disease, abdominal wall infection or marked distension, and multiple prior abdominal surgeries. Application is also limited by the availability of minimal invasive surgery (MIS) specialist general surgeons.

Laparoscopy is generally safe and well tolerated and can be performed under local anesthesia. Complications can occur during gas insufflation, trocar insertion, and the diagnostic exam; they include arrhythmias, bleeding, bile leak, perforation, laceration, vascular injury, and gas embolism. Postoperative concerns are the same as those associated with open procedures and include surveillance for hemorrhage and infection. Benefits are several; when CT and ultrasound findings are not definitive, laparoscopy provides a better evaluation of peritoneal cavity, paracolic gutters, and pelvic cavity than the standard laparotomy incision and improves diagnostic accuracy. Corrective surgery is often possible immediately following diagnosis. Patients report less pain, faster recovery, shorter stay, and fewer complications. The actual recovery period is related to the cause of the acute abdomen. Laparoscopic findings may necessitate open laparotomy for definitive correction (Majewski, 2005).

Preoperative management is directed at optimizing physical and psychosocial status of the patient. The vital functions require stabilization: systolic blood pressure should be restored to at least 100 mm Hg systolic, heart rate to under 100 beats per minute and adequate oxygenation. In the absence of central venous access, two large-bore IV catheters should be placed. Patients should be fasting (NPO) and may require antiemetics and a steroid bolus if the patient is steroid dependent, in addition to maintenance doses. Attention to glycemic control is indicated in diabetics. Nasogastric tube placement is invaluable for gastric decompression and provides some protection against macroaspiration. A bladder catheter should be placed to facilitate assessment of the adequacy of

Skills 360°

Adequate Analgesia

Adequate analgesia remains a significant problem in patients with acute abdominal pain. A recent review of 100 patients in EDs revealed the following disturbing findings. Overall wait time for analgesia ranged from 2 minutes to 14 hours. Patients with mild complaints waited longer than patients with severe pain (mean of 82 minutes). Females waited longer than men (mean 129 minutes versus 69 minutes). Patients transferred to wards fared far worse than those medicated in the ED (mean 5 hours versus ½ hour) (Shabbir, et. al., 2004).

intravascular volume replacement and hourly monitoring of output. Minimal urinary output is 0.5 mL/kg/hr. Preoperative antibiotic coverage is also indicated.

Pregnancy Considerations

Management of gravid women should be similar to that of nonpregnant patients. Like in the elderly, clinical presentation may be atypical, including the lack of peritoneal signs due to the distortion of the anterior abdominal wall and underlying organs. Laboratory findings may also be uncharacteristic. Severe disease, for example, can occur in the absence of leukocytosis. Both factors may delay diagnosis and definitive treatment. The diagnostic process is inherently more complex given the fact that it inescapably involves two patients, evaluation of the fetus, with at least fetal heart tone occurring simultaneously with evaluation of the mother. Evidence suggests that management of gravid women should include obstetrical consultation if surgery contemplated.

The two most common surgical emergencies in gravid women are acute appendicitis and cholecystitis requiring appendectomy in 1:200 to 1:6,000 pregnancies and cholecystectomy in 1:1,130 and 1:12,890 pregnancies. Obstetrical risks to the fetus are greatest in the first (fetal loss, spontaneous abortion) and third trimesters (premature labor, but not fetal loss). Despite improvements in surgical anesthesia, perinatal and perioperative care risks attend surgical intervention in pregnancy. The rate of fetal loss in gallstone pancreatitis is estimated at between 10 to 20 percent and as high as 20 to 30 percent in maternal intestinal obstruction. Ultrasonography is a safe and effective diagnostic modality, and exposure to radiation from a single diagnostic procedure does not result in harmful fetal effects. Magnetic resonance imaging (MRI) is to be avoided if at all possible during the first trimester. If possible, surgery should be deferred to the second trimester, the period of least risk. Laparoscopy, once contraindicated in this group, appears to be a safe alternative to open procedures in experienced hands. Advantages include less fetal depression. However, there is some concern that gas insufflations may elevate fetal risk. Pregnancy-specific recommendations should be incorporated into routine surgical care, such as the use of pneumatic compression devices, fetal monitoring, and careful positioning to relieve the vena cava of the pressure of the gravid uterus.

Evaluation of Outcomes

Potential patient outcomes for each of the example nursing diagnoses for the patient with acute abdomen are:

- Fear related to perioperative events. The patient should manifest positive coping behaviors and verbalize a reduction in the amount of fear of the having this disease.
- Deficient fluid volume related to intake less than body requirements. The patient experiences adequate fluid volume and electrolyte balance as evidenced by urine output greater than 30 mL/hr, normotensive blood pressure, heart rate 100 beats/min, consistency of weight, and normal skin turgor.
- Acute pain related to acute abdomen. The patient should verbalize an adequate relief of pain along with the ability to realistically cope with the pain if it is not completely relieved.
- Risk of infection related to intra-abdominal processes and procedures. The patient remains free of infection, as evidenced by normal vital signs and absence of purulent drainage from wounds, incisions, and tubes. Infection is recognized early to allow for prompt treatment.

Given the criticality of the pain history to the diagnosis of acute abdomen, inability to communicate, whether due to developmental level or diseases of mind and brain, elevates the degree of diagnostic difficulty. This may result in unnecessary hospitalizations and greater reliance on serial laboratory or imaging

DOLLARS AND SENSE

Costs of Diagnostics for Acute Abdominal Emergencies

Advances in imaging and widespread use American College of Radiology (ACR) guidelines appear to be influencing resource use. Use of CT imaging in one study improved diagnosis of appendicitis, and the authors estimated a net savings of $4,731 due to improved diagnostic accuracy. Use of CT is also thought to be financially valuable, reducing cost by reducing unnecessary admissions. The use of contrast highly increases spectrum of detectable pathology. Surgical approaches to the management of acute abdomen are believed to have profound impact on resource utilization. Currently, it is estimated that in acute abdominal emergencies, diagnosis is incorrect or too late in 5 to 20 percent of cases, resulting in increased morbidity, mortality, and costs. Laparoscopy may be one of the means of reducing delayed or inaccurate diagnosis (Daniels, 2003; Majewski, 2005).

testing; it may also have a direct impact on morbidity: Young children, unable to relate a detailed history are prey to nonspecific signs and symptoms and have a perforation rate as high as 50 percent.

Morbidity and mortality, readmission rates, and 30-day mortality rates are as varied as the causes of acute abdomen. The presence of comorbid conditions influences physiological reserve and response to stress of disease and trauma of medical, endoscopic, surgical, and anesthetic events.

The care of critically ill patients is labor-intensive, frequently requiring prolonged stays in the intensive care unit, participation of multiple consultants, and individualized nursing care. Pharmacological management of severe sepsis with recombinant activated protein C in early sepsis is expensive but shown to reduce 28-day mortality if used early (Broyles, Reiss, & Evans, 2007).

ACUTE INFLAMMATORY DISORDERS

There are two primary acute inflammatory disorders of the lower GI tract: (a) appendicitis and (b) diverticulitis. Each of these conditions involve inflammatory processes, which can be severe and have important ramifications as acute care pathologies.

Appendicitis

Appendicitis is an inflammation of the appendix organ, which is a small finger-like appendage just below the ileocecal valve. This is the most common emergency abdominal surgery in the United States.

Epidemiology

Appendicitis occurs in approximately 7 percent of the population and affects males more than females. It occurs more in teenagers than adults and most commonly between the ages of 10 and 30 years.

Pathophysiology

The function of the appendix is not completely known, but it does regularly fill with and empty digested food. When the appendix becomes inflamed, it often is obstructed in its proximal lumen, which is labeled **fecalith** (hard mass of fecal material). In addition, the inflamed appendix also includes such things as for-

TABLE 50-4	Classifications of Appendicitis
TYPE	**DESCRIPTION**
Simple	Appendix is inflamed but still intact.
Gangrenous	There is tissue necrosis and microscopic areas of perforation.
Perforation	There is large perforation, which involves contents flowing into the peritoneal cavity.

BOX 50-3

ROVSING'S SIGN FOR APPENDICITIS

The nurse can assess for appendicitis by first testing for McBurney's point (pain elicited in the RLQ when firm pressure is applied. Then, the nurse can further differentiate the diagnosis by assessing for Rovsing's sign as follows:

- Press deeply and evenly in the LLQ for five seconds.
- Note the patient's response.
- Abdominal pain when felt in the RLQ is a positive Rovsing's sign.

The Rovsing's sign is based on the concept that changes in the intraluminal pressure will be transmitted through the intestine when the ileocecal valve is competent. Pressing on the LLQ traps air within the large intestine and increases the pressure in the cecum. When the appendix is inflamed, this increase in pressure causes pain.

Adapted from Estes, M. (2006). Health assessment and physical examination *(3rd ed.). New York: Thomson Delmar Learning.*

---

eign bodies, tumors, calculi, and edema of lymph tissue. Appendicitis is classified into three different categories as shown in Table 50-4.

Assessment with Clinical Manifestations

The patient with appendicitis has relatively predictable clinical manifestations. There is periumbilical pain that may initially be vague and generally spread over the lower abdominal region. In time, the pain localizes to the RLQ and is often accompanied with a low-grade fever. During these beginning symptoms, the patient will also become nauseated and local tenderness can be stimulated at McBurney's point as shown chapter 47. In addition, an advanced technique for assessment is labeled Rovsing's sign (Box 50-3).

The different types of pain during appendicitis are somewhat dependent on the location of the inflammation. For example, pain on defecation likely means that the tip of the inflamed appendix is in the pelvis and is located against the rectum. Pain on urination probably means that the inflamed appendix is near the bladder. In addition, there may be some rigidity of the rectus muscles in the region. As the appendicitis condition worsens, and even perforates, the pain will become more acute, even with the patient remaining still. The patient often will draw their knees upward toward their chest in an attempt to decrease pressure from the tension of the abdominal muscles (see Red Flag Feature).

Diagnostic Tests

The patient's presenting symptomatology and history are the initial methods of diagnosing the condition of appendicitis. Then, the laboratory and X-ray diagnostics confirm the diagnosis. A CBC is obtained which reveals an elevated WBC ($10,000/mm^3$ to $20,000/mm^3$). In addition, abdominal X-rays, an abdominal

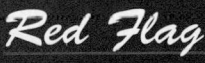

Red Flag

Peritonitis

The nurse must be aware of the potential complication of peritonitis in the patient with appendicitis, which may be fatal. Clinical manifestations for peritonitis are elevated WBC, high fever, severe and acute pain, drawing the knees up to the chest, tachycardia, and diaphoresis. These symptoms should be reported immediately to prevent untreated peritonitis.

ultrasound, and CT scans can be performed to detect the RLQ density of the inflamed area (Daniels, 2003). A urinalysis can be performed to rule out a urinary tract infection, and a pelvic examination on females is performed to rule out gynecological disorders.

Nursing Diagnoses

Based on the information gathered, examples of nursing diagnoses in the patient with appendicitis may include the following:
- Acute pain related to the appendicitis.
- Fear in response to the diagnosis of appendicitis.

Planning and Implementation

The care of the patient with appendicitis is focused first on supporting the patient during the acute pain and diagnosis of the condition. Then the nursing care turns to preparing the patient for the likely surgical management of the disorder. The goals are relieving the pain, reducing the anxiety and fears of the patient, preventing infection, decreasing the chances of dehydration, and preventing postoperative complications.

Pharmacology

Before the surgery, the patient will be started on IV fluids to maintain an adequate vascular volume. Antibiotic therapy is initiated prophylactically (e.g., third-generation cephalosporins) to prevent infection complications. Analgesics can be administered once the diagnosis is confirmed.

Surgery

An appendectomy (surgical removal of the appendix) is performed either with a laparoscopic approach or an open appendectomy. The former is less invasive, made through a smaller incision, and has fewer postoperative complications. During the surgery, there can be a removal of any contaminants from the region with an irrigation of the area with sterile normal saline. After the surgery, the patient is managed with normal postoperative care measures (e.g., ensuring good respiratory effort free of lung consolidation, frequent vital signs, maintaining IV fluids, assessing the wound, treatment for pain, preventing infection). The patient is placed in a semifowler's position to reduce the tension and pulling of tissue on the wound area. The patient will be given a diet as tolerated as they recover and are able to have a normal fluid intake. Discharge will likely occur within 24 hours, and the patient will be instructed to return for a follow-up visit to their surgeon for removal of the sutures within a week. The patient will also be advised to monitor their general activity level and to rest as needed. In addition, potential symptoms of infection and complications related to wound healing will be instructed with the patient education.

Evaluation of Outcomes

Potential patient outcomes for each of the example nursing diagnoses for the patient with appendicitis are:
- Acute pain related to the appendicitis. The patient should verbalize an adequate relief of pain along with the ability to realistically cope with the pain if it is not completely relieved.
- Fear in response to the diagnosis of appendicitis. The patient should manifest positive coping behaviors and verbalize a reduction in the amount of fear of the having this disease and the upcoming expected surgery.

Diverticulitis

Diverticula are sac-like outpouches of mucosa through the muscular layer of the bowel and may occur anywhere along the GI tract. The largest percentage, 90 to 95 percent are found in the sigmoid colon. When there are multiple diverticula and resulting pathology, the process is termed **diverticulosis.** And, diverticulitis results in disorders that progress to an inflammatory process of the diverticular sacs.

Epidemiology

Diverticula disorders increase with age, with only 5 percent having the disorder before age 40 and more than 50 percent of persons over age 80 develop this pathology. Higher incidences are seen in Australia, the United Kingdom, and the United States, and the disease is relatively rare in Africa and Asia.

Etiology

Diet is thought to play the most important role in the causation of diverticular disease. Specifically, diets that are high in fiber deficiencies and highly refined foods are more correlated with diverticular disease. In addition, other correlates with the disorder are decreased activity levels and constipation. The suggestion is that people with decreased blood supply or nutrients in the bowel are more susceptible to diverticular disease.

Pathophysiology

The formation of diverticula within the bowel is what eventually leads to diverticulitis. The muscles where there are diverticular areas thicken, and the lumen is narrowed, which increases intraluminal pressure. With a deficient fiber intake seen in diverticular disease, the bowel develops a higher pressure, and the mucosa herniates through the muscle wall, which forms the diverticulum. As the diverticulum increases in size, it obstructs the bowel area and causes irritability of the colon. Abscesses can form along with perforations, and the further complications of peritonitis and bleeding can occur.

Assessment with Clinical Manifestations

In diverticulosis, there may be a chronic asymptomatic condition with two thirds of the time. If there are manifestations, they would likely be constipation or diarrhea, lower abdominal pain in the left lower quadrant, irritable bowel syndrome (IBS) development, abdominal cramping, generalized fatigue, and low-grade fever. The patient with diverticulosis may have complications of bleeding and inflammation.

As diverticulitis develops, the patient has more acute symptomatology caused by the inflammatory processes in the colon. The most common manifestation is increasing pain levels that are on the left-side quadrant (LSQ) of the abdomen. During this condition, there is more likelihood of perforation of a diverticulum (Figure 50-1). The continued complications that are seen are bowel obstruction, hemorrhage, peritonitis, fistula formation, and adhesions of the inflamed tissue to the small bowel.

Diagnostic Tests

There are a variety of diagnostic tests that are used in diverticular disease. A CT scan is the best method of detecting abscesses and complications evidenced in diverticulitis. Serum studies, such as those in a CBC, will show increased infectious processes (e.g., leukocytosis, elevated sedimentation rate). In addition, bleeding can be evidenced by hemoccult testing and hemoglobin or hematocrit levels. A lower GI series (barium enema) can also confirm diverticular disease and would be contraindicated in acute diverticulitis due to the risk of contamination if there is an existing perforation. Last, abdominal X-rays can detect free abdominal air that is seen in diverticulitis and in perforations.

Nursing Diagnoses

Based on the information gathered, examples of nursing diagnoses in the patient with diverticular disease may include the following:

- Acute pain related to the diverticular disease.
- Fear in response to the diagnosis of diverticular disease.

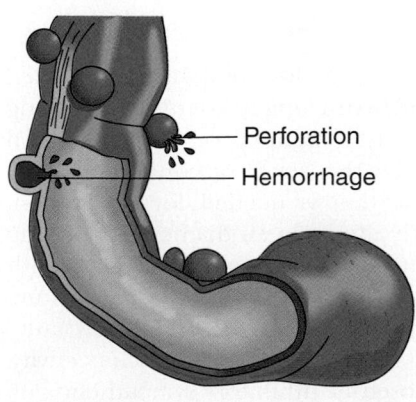

Perforation

Hemorrhage

Figure 50-1 Diverticula in the sigmoid colon.

Planning and Implementation

The prevention measures are of high priority for the diverticular disease processes. Nurses can perform patient education in the community related to the necessary dietary changes to include an increased fiber intake and teaching the early symptoms of diverticular disease. The elderly are more predisposed to this disorder, and therefore nurses must remember to address this population for the presence of diverticular disease.

As patients have acute diverticular disease, then their care strategies are dependent on whether they are treated with medications or surgery. Pain levels, anxiety, infections, and postoperative complications are the areas of greatest concern for the nurse. Continued dietary management strategies are employed.

Pharmacology

Broad-spectrum antibiotics are typically administered because of the inflammatory nature of diverticular disease, and specifically diverticulitis. Opioids are usually the analgesics of choice with severe pain; however, morphine is not the drug of choice as it causes increased intraluminal pressure. Stool softeners (Colace) and bulk-forming medications (Metamucil) are used to decreases the aggravation to the bowel area. In addition, antispasmodics (e.g., Pro-Banthine, Daricon) are administered for relief of abdominal cramping (Broyles, et al., 2007).

Surgery

When diverticulitis requires surgery, it is usually for peritonitis, an abscess, or continued hemorrhaging. The diseased portion of the bowel is resected and the remaining bowel is reanastomosed. There may also be a temporary ostomy (see ostomy section in this chapter) required to allow the area of the bowel to heal. The perioperative care is described in the colon cancer section described later in this chapter.

Evaluation of Outcomes

Potential patient outcomes for each of the example nursing diagnoses for the patient with diverticular disease are:

* Acute pain related to the diverticular disease. The patient should verbalize an adequate relief of pain along with the ability to realistically cope with the pain if it is not completely relieved.
* Fear in response to the diagnosis of diverticular disease. The patient should manifest positive coping behaviors and verbalize a reduction in the amount of fear of the having this disease and the upcoming expected surgery.

OBSTRUCTION

The GI tract, extending from mouth to anus, is a hollow food tube, specialized in structure and function for processing food, extracting nutrients, and passing wastes. Structurally, it is designed to generate movement of contents in a rostral (front) to caudal (back/tail) direction. Under the serosa or connective tissue lies a longitudinal layer of smooth muscle that is needed for propulsion. Beneath it lies a circular muscle layer, which alters lumen diameter, including the sphincters. Between them lies the myenteric plexus, which innervates both muscle layers. Lying beneath the muscle layers are submucosa and epithelium. Mucosa forms the lumen surface. Motility is principally generated by autonomic innervation, enteric nervous system, and smooth muscle activity. Stimulatory parasympathetic activity is opposed by inhibitory sympathetic outflow. Neural structures are accompanied on their course by parallel arteries and veins. Functionally, motility varies by region; for example, the colon lacks cyclic motor activity, but it generates low- and high-amplitude intermittent contractions. Low-amplitude, short-duration contractions delay colonic transit, allowing time for water and electrolyte absorption. Coordinated, high-amplitude contractions create mass movement. In general colonic activation increases colonic motility (Bullard & Rothenberger, 2005). Obstruction refers to the partial or complete impairment of the meandering course, innervation, structure, and the pathology involved. GI obstruction can be either mechanical (physical or structural) or functional. Most obstructions occur in the small intestine.

Ileus refers to intestinal obstruction due to partial or complete arrest of intestinal peristalsis and is also known as paralytic or adynamic ileus (Estes, 2006). In ileus, one or more nonmechanical factors interfere with the neuromuscular function of the bowel so as to impede the movement of the intraluminal contents. Acute colonic pseudo-obstruction (ACPO), also known as acute colonic ileus or Ogilvie's syndrome, is defined as a "functional disorder in which the colon becomes massively dilated in the absence of mechanical obstruction (Bullard, & Rothenberger, 2005, p. 1089).

Hindrance of the movement of intestinal contents may be due to physical or mechanical obstruction arising from within the lumen (e.g., malignant bowel obstruction) or bowel wall or by a lesion external to the bowel that compresses it externally. Interference may be partial or complete. Given that nutrient arteries and draining veins travel with neural elements to bowel segments, mechanical obstruction may also compromise supporting neurovascular structures. Obstruction can also be classified as simple or strangulated. Simple obstruction describes an obstruction in one site; closed loop obstructions are characterized by two sites of blockage. Strangulated obstruction is accompanied by vascular compromise of the segmental arterial supply and venous drainage. Strangulating obstruction occurs in nearly 25 percent of cases of small bowel obstruction and can progress to gangrene in as little as six hours. Although strangulation of the large bowel is rare, cecal perforation due to massive distension, or perforation of the bowel wall by tumor, or diverticulum may occur. Should these intra-abdominal catastrophes occur, signs of shock, often accompanied by signs of severe intravascular depletion, dominate the clinical picture and require prompt attention. The patient should be resuscitated and stabilized as described in acute abdomen. If not promptly recognized and relieved, these problems lead to significant morbidity and mortality.

Epidemiology

Patients who develop paralytic or mechanical obstruction span all ages and socioeconomic groups. The incidence of mechanical obstruction is related to the underlying cause. For example, malignant bowel obstruction is a common complication in patients with advanced abdominal or pelvic malignancies, notably colorectal, ovarian, and gastric cancers. Incidence in colorectal cancer (CRC) ranges from 4 to 24 percent and from 5 to 42 percent in ovarian cancer (Ripamonti & Mercadante, 2004). Other cancers (e.g., lung, breast) may also metastasize to the bowel. Small bowel obstruction (SBO) accounts for 20 percent of all acute surgical admissions. It is most commonly (60 percent) due to postoperative adhesions, fibrous bands within the peritoneum, which may compress bowel and cause obstruction, or be a focus for a **volvulus** (a twisting of the bowel on itself that causes obstruction). Prior abdominal surgery or sepsis (e.g., pelvic inflammatory disease, appendicitis) may cause adhesions. Surgeries most commonly associated with SBO are appendectomy, colorectal, and gynecological. Risk appears to be cumulative; gynecological surgery is associated with particularly high rates of adhesions and carries a mortality of 10 to 20 percent. Adhesions can produce SBO in as little as one month following surgery. SBO is associated with a mortality of 5.5 percent.

Ileus is common in medical and surgical populations, especially in bedridden patients, those with multiple comorbidities, and those being treated with opiates. In the intensive care setting, ileus is common in critically ill patients with sepsis, shock, respiratory pathology, and severe electrolyte abnormalities, especially hypokalemia (Bullard & Rothenberger, 2005).

Etiology

Paralytic ileus reflects altered neuromuscular function that impairs gut motility and has multiple potential causes. Ileus may reflect an imbalance between sympathetic and parasympathetic tone, disordered myenteric plexus activity (e.g., postoperative or a myopathy affecting gut muscular function). Medication use (e.g., some anesthetic agents, opiates) may contribute to this state of localized paralysis. Intraperitoneal and retroperitoneal infection, arterial or venous injury and metabolic derangements (e.g., hypokalemia) may also be associated with ileus.

Acute colonic pseudo-obstruction (ACPO) is most commonly associated with intra- or extra-peritoneal surgery. Multiple case reports and case series have linked this obstruction to adhesions that account for most postoperative instances. It is also associated with trauma (e.g., spinal cord injury) and medical conditions (age, sepsis, hypothyroidism; cardiorespiratory disorders, electrolyte abnormalities, i.e., hypocalcemia, hypokalemia, or hypomagnesemia) and medications (e.g., opioids, tricyclic antidepressant, and anesthetics. In the pediatric population large bowel obstruction may be congenital (Hirschsprung disease, aganglionic segment). Non-GI disease, e.g. diabetes mellitus or scleroderma, or idiopathic cases have been described as related causes (Bullard & Rothenberger, 2005).

Postoperative ileus (POI) is a common occurrence and has long been considered a potential and somewhat unavoidable consequence of surgical anesthesia. It prolongs hospitalization and increases costs. It typically leaves the small bowel largely unaffected, with function returning to normal within a few hours. Motility tends to return first to the cecum, then the sigmoid. The colon may remain inert for up to three days. There is no evidence that prophylactic nasogastric decompression after abdominal surgery hastens the return of bowel motility, prevents pulmonary complications, i.e., aspiration, reduces anastomotic leaks, increases patient comfort, or shortens length of stay (LOS). In this setting, nasogastric intubation should be selective rather than routine (Nelson, Edwards, & Tse, 2004). There is some evidence that use of thoracic epidural local anesthesia for patients undergoing laparotomy reduces GI paralysis compared with systemic or epidural opioids and achieves comparable pain relief. Nonsteroidal anti-inflammatory analgesia and laparoscopic procedures (versus open laparotomy) may similarly reduce the occurrence of POI.

Currently under review by the FDA is a novel agent, Alvimopan, (ADL 8-2698; Entereg), a peripherally selective opioid mu receptor antagonist, designed specifically to treat postoperative ileus. Concurrent administration of this GI-specific agent decreased the duration of POI without antagonizing the analgesic effectiveness of systemically administered opioids used ubiquitously to treat major surgical pain. It appears to be safe and well-tolerated when used for up to one week postoperatively. It has a relative contraindication in use with chronic opioid users, in whom it has precipitated local GI adverse effects. Due to minimal systemic absorption, dosage adjustments for renal, hepatic, and age–related impairment are not expected. Common side effects included nausea, vomiting, and hypotension. A detailed review of clinical trials and pharmacology are available elsewhere (Udeh, 2005). Common mechanical causes of SBO and large bowel obstruction (LBO) are summarized in Table 50-5.

The cecum, the widest part of colon with the thinnest muscular wall, is most vulnerable to perforation and least vulnerable to obstruction. By contrast, the sigmoid colon, though mobile, is the narrowest part of the large intestine and therefore, most susceptible to obstruction. Not surprisingly, diseases affecting the sigmoid are common causes of obstruction. In some cases, paralytic and

TABLE 50-5	Bowel Obstruction: Common Mechanical Causes
LOCATION	**COMMON CAUSES (IN DEVELOPED NATIONS)**
Small bowel	Adhesions (49–74 percent), tumors (~20 percent), hernia (~10 percent)
	Infants: **atresia** (absence or closure of a natural passage of the body, i.e., jejunoileal; duodenal, esophageal, or colonic), **malrotation** (failure during embryonic development of normal rotation of all or part of an organ or system), meconium ileus, volvulus, or **intussusception** (invagination, or telescoping, of one part of the intestine into itself).
Duodenum	Cancer (head of pancreas, duodenum)
Large bowel	Tumors (especially left sided lesions, e.g., CRC, ovarian cancer, diverticulitis (especially sigmoid), volvulus (especially sigmoid or cecum), or impaction.

Adapted from Bullard, K. M., & Rothenberger, D. A. (2005). Colon, rectum and anus. In F. C. Brunicardi (Ed.), Schwartz's principles of surgery (8th ed., pp. 1055–1117). New York: McGraw Hill; Shatnawi, N., & Bani-Hani, K. (2005). Unusual causes of mechanical small bowel obstruction. Saudi Medical Journal, 26(10), 1546–1550.

mechanical causes may coexist, i.e., in advanced colorectal cancer (Bullard & Rothenberger, 2005; Ripamonte & Mercadante, 2004).

Pathophysiology

In simple obstruction, ingested fluids, food, swallowed air, digestive juices or secretions, and gas accumulate behind the blockage. Distal bowel collapses and proximal loops dilate. Distension stimulates secretory activity, and the absorptive functions of mucous membranes fail. With increasing intraluminal pressures, mucosal veins and lymphatics become compressed, and the bowel wall becomes boggy and edematous. Active secretion and reduced absorption increase intraluminal fluid accumulation. Laplace's law proposes that increasing diameters accelerate the rise in tension experienced by the colon wall. That is, despite impeded or arrested forward transit of bowel contents, the bowel continues to contract with increased, uncoordinated peristaltic activity, leading to a vicious cycle of distension and secretion. Distension intensifies peristalsis and secretory derangements and increases the risks of dehydration, ischemia, perforation, peritonitis, and death. Bacteria content in stagnant bowel segments increases, and as obstruction progresses, may escape into the peritoneal cavity (Ripamonte & Mercadante, 2004).

Strangulation occurs when a loop of bowel is ensnared in a way that catches its vascular supply. Typically, strangulation begins with venous obstruction followed by arterial occlusion, resulting in rapid ischemia, infarction, gangrene and, ultimately, perforation. Treatment outcome reflects the interaction of a variety of factors, including the anatomic location and degree (partial or complete) of obstruction and whether or not the vascular supply is compromised. Whether or not decompression is accomplished before perforation and spillage of luminal contents into the peritoneal cavity occur and the prognosis of the underlying cause also affect outcome. Untreated, the mortality in strangulated SBO approaches 100 percent. Mortality falls dramatically with early surgical intervention.

Assessment with Clinical Manifestations

Assessment and clinical management vary by putative (supposed) cause, and location of the obstruction. SBO produces colicky, midabdominal pain often over a period of days. Vomiting occurs early in the course, especially with proximal simple obstruction. A change in the character of the pain (continuous, increasing severity) suggests the development of more ominous ischemic complications. Pain lasting several days, with progressive distension, suggests a more distal obstruction. Patients may also report constipation and the absence of flatus. A careful past medical history should note prior abdominal or pelvic surgery, history of malignancy (e.g., CRC), Crohn's disease, and drug exposure. LBO is unusual in patients under 50 years of age. Because the most common mechanical cause is CRC, enquiry about changes in bowel habits, stool caliber, unintended weight loss, and blood per rectum is essential. The history is one of gradual, then marked, distension, with lower colicky abdominal pain. Symptoms tend to develop more gradually than in SBO, and an acute onset should suggest an acute obstructive event, such as volvulus. Patients may report reduced to absent flatus for days preceding presentation and distension. If ileocecal valve incompetence allows reflux into small bowel, vomiting may occur.

Careful abdominal examination is necessary in suspected obstruction. Inspection may reveal scarring, which should suggest the possibility of adhesions. Distension, particularly in the flanks, may be prominent especially in LBO due to the distensibility of the colon. In combination with marked visible peristalsis, these findings should suggest intestinal obstruction. Auscultation typically reveals increased bowel sounds and high-pitched tinkling in early obstruction (Estes, 2006). Rushes of high-pitched peristalsis that coincide with cramping are typical. Hypoactive or decreased bowel sounds occur late in the clinical course. Should strangulation, infarction, and perforation occur, the belly may be silent. Auscultation is required for at least two minutes in a quiet abdomen. Paralytic ileus, intestinal obstruction due to partial or complete arrest of intestinal peristalsis, involving large and small bowel may produce abdominal distension, nausea, and vomiting. However, crampy pain is rare and bowel sounds may be preserved.

Percussion should follow auscultation: Gaseous distension typically produces tympanic percussion notes and is more marked in LBO (Estes, 2006). Palpation should follow percussion, and severe pain is unusual unless strangulation, ischemia or infarction, or perforation have occurred. In that case, there may be signs suggestive of peritonitis and acute abdomen, including guarding and rebound tenderness. A careful search for inguinal hernias, a rectal exam for masses (e.g., obturator hernia, CRC), and analysis of stool for occult blood conclude the abdominal assessment.

Diagnostic Tests

Diagnosis of obstruction is usually made on the basis of history and exam findings. However, electrolyte balance and CBC should be minimally assessed; the presence of fluid and electrolyte disorders is more common and more marked and SBO. Leukocytosis and the presence of metabolic acidosis should suggest ischemia or strangulation (Daniels, 2003).

Radiographic studies are intended to confirm diagnosis, distinguish between strangulating and simple obstruction, differentiate the causes, estimate the degree of obstruction, and exclude the possibility of colonic obstruction. Plain films of the chest and abdomen, supine and upright, are the primary studies used to demonstrate the presence of pneumo-peritoneum and air-fluid levels in loops of distended bowel respectively. Plain radiographs are diagnostically more accurate in cases of simple SBO. Cardinal signs of obstruction include absence of distal gas and air fluid levels, i.e. long air-fluid levels, classical step ladder pattern within a loop of bowel or an inverted U. ACPO classically reveals massive colon dilation in the absence of mechanical obstruction. Paralytic ileus produces distension of isolated segments of small and large bowel.

Evidence suggests that regional bowel distension that exceeds critical threshold diameters is positively correlated with the risk of perforation: Those critical diameters include 9 cm for the transverse colon (it is 9 cm), and 12 to 13 cm for the cecum. Should a watchful waiting approach be taken to management, successive measurements should be undertaken to track changes in lumen caliber.

Ultrasonography may reliably exclude SBO in up to 89 percent of patients and has a specificity of reportedly 100 percent. Enteroclysis (barium small bowel enema) or the intubation infusion method has improved preoperative diagnosis of lower grade SBO, but it requires naso-intestinal intubation that often requires conscious sedation and infusing the small bowel with barium liquid. CT enteroclysis, may be more reliable than CT alone in SBO. Enteroclysis is able to differentiate partial from complete obstruction, especially when clinical findings are nonspecific and plain films are normal. Enteroclysis should be avoided if perforation or ischemia are suspected. CT of abdomen and pelvis are indicated in symptomatic patients with indeterminate plain films, and is capable of visualizing varying diameters of bowel proximal and distal to the obstruction.

CT imaging is of growing importance when strangulated obstruction is suspected and demonstrated 81 percent sensitivity for high-grade obstruction. CT, with or without rectal contrast, is both more sensitive and specific for the obstruction than plain films (Aufort, Charra, Lesnik, Bruel, & Taourel, 2005). Contrast studies are secondarily indicated in suspected obstruction; although barium enema may rule out distal large bowel lesions, it should be preceded by endoscopic evaluation. Upper GI studies are contraindicated, because they may transform partial to complete obstruction or further complicate total obstruction.

Nursing Diagnoses

Based on the information gathered, examples of nursing diagnoses in the patient with obstruction may include the following:
- Fear related to perioperative events.
- Deficient fluid volume related to intake less than body requirements.
- Acute pain related to obstruction.
- Risk of infection related to intra-abdominal processes and procedures.

Planning and Implementation

Patients with suspected obstruction require hospitalization for diagnosis and treatment. Resuscitation and stabilization remain the first priorities of care and include reestablishment or support of hemodynamic stability, correction of fluid, electrolyte, and acid-base abnormalities, and transfusion support if indicated in the context of careful and frequent serial clinical and radiological examinations. Once stabilized, or concurrent with stabilization, decompression of the obstruction and definitive treatment of the underlying cause should be undertaken. Generally, mechanical causes should be excluded prior to medical or endoscopic intervention.

Pharmacology

In nonmechanical ileus with potentially reversible cause, the preferred initial management is conservative. Serial assessments to detect signs of peritonitis are recommended. Initially, radiographic evaluation should occur daily or more frequently. Monitoring should occur concurrently with the identification and correction or removal of contributory elements. Consultation with a pharmacist to review the patient's medication profile is often invaluable in identifying contributory drugs and recommending alternatives. Offending medications should be removed (e.g., opiates, anticholinergics). It should be noted that randomized clinical trial (RCT) evidence supports the efficacy of neostigmine use in ACPO; however, it has not been evaluated against endoscopic decompression. Strict bowel rest and careful attention to fluid replacement for loss as well as maintenance, with appropriate laboratory guided electrolyte supplementation (especially potassium), are indicated.

Commonly prescribed medications are: anticholinesterases (e.g., neostigmine), anticholinergics (e.g., scopolamine), antiemetics (e.g., chlorpromazine), antibiotics, and antisecretory medications (e.g., octreotide) (Broyles, et al., 2007). In addition, prokinetic agents should be avoided in mechanical obstruction, and unfortunately they have shown inconsistent results in ACPO. Antibiotics, typically second- or third-generation cephalosporins or broad-spectrum agents (e.g., meropenem), may be used to cover gram-negative bacteria and anaerobes. Selection varies with suspected diagnosis, clinical status of the patient, and institutional resistance patterns. Suspected sepsis should prompt appropriate microbiological cultures and parenteral antibiotic use. Pharmacological management of malignant obstruction often includes the use of analgesics, antispasmodics, anticholinergics, and possibly steroids.

Gastric Decompression

Decompression of SBO is intended to reduce or eliminate vomiting, protect the airway from macroaspiration, the bowel from perforation, and relieve pain. However, the means of decompression remains controversial; that is, whether to use nasogastric or naso-intestinal tubes. The effectiveness of decompression varies inversely with the distance between the tip of the tube and the site of blockage; thus in obstruction, a naso-intestinal, rather than a nasogastric, tube is considered the optimal method of decompression of the distended small bowel. Passage beyond the pylorus has the added advantage of relieving the colicky pain. The higher cost of a longer multipurpose tube, lack of familiarity, and need for two-stage use with initial gastric decompression, followed by advancement under fluoroscopic guidance into the proximal jejunum has been limited in use. In postoperative obstruction due to adhesions following gynecological surgery, gastric decompression successfully relieved SBO in approximately 80 percent of patients. Once bowel function returns, the nasogastric tube should be put to gravity drainage and then removed. Attempts to achieve decompression using a rectal tube are rarely effective, because obstruction is upstream from the site of decompression. However, it may be used with tap water enemas in ACPO in circumstances that cecal distension is not dangerously high or the pain severe. Patients are required to lie prone with hips elevated on pillow or knee chest with hips up, alternating right and elevated lateral decubitus positions hourly. This may be attempted for 24 to 48 hours depending on patient tolerance; failure should be followed by endoscopic intervention. The reported success of conservative management is highly variable, ranging from 20 to 92 percent.

Endoscopic Therapy

Endoscopic options may be appropriate for patients deteriorating with conservative management, who are continuing to progress in their symptomology or are considered inappropriate for a neostigmine trial. Although technically difficult and associated with risk of perforation, colonoscopic decompression may be attempted in ACPO. Success in experienced hands varies between 61 and 78 percent, with recurrence ranging from 18 to 33 percent. Perforation rate in colonoscopic decompression is as high as 3 percent (Bullard & Rothenberger, 2005).

Endoscopy is emerging as a useful modality for managing malignant obstruction. It may serve as a bridge to surgery when successful, providing an opportunity to stabilize the patient and evaluate the extent of disease. In operative candidates, it may avoid the need for diverting colostomy and a second operation for reanastomosis. **Anastomosis** is the surgical joining of the hollow tubular parts. Endoscopic laser therapy in malignant inoperable obstruction has been reported as a safe surgical alternative. Success been related to tumor size; treatment may require several sessions. Common complications include perforation, bleeding fistula, abscess, and pain (Davila, et al., 2005).

For patients with extensive tumor and multiple partial obstructions, endoscopic placement of self-expandable metal stents (SEMS) may be attempted. Location can be esophageal, gastroduodenal, or colorectal, and placement has a lower morbidity than surgery. Success rates are variable. Davila, et al. (2005) reported success in cancer palliation in 90 percent of 336 cases. Complications include perforation, bleeding, tumor ingrowth, overgrowth, and migration. Long-term outcomes, especially if stent placement is followed by chemotherapy or radiation, have not been studied well. Patients have been advised to follow a low-residue diet and use laxatives, stool softeners, or mineral oil to void impaction after SEMS placement. Endoscopic placement of a gastrostomy tube in a patient with malignant obstruction who is not a SEMS candidate may be used to reduce unabsorbed secretions, nausea, and vomiting. The patient may then be able to eat and drink because food drains directly out of the stomach.

Surgery

Definitive management of mechanical obstruction is surgical in most instances, typically by laparotomy or laparoscopic means. Surgery tends to be associated with a higher morbidity and mortality than medical or endoscopic procedures. Indications for urgent surgical consultation and management include a diagnosis of strangulated obstruction, or signs and symptoms of peritonitis, perforation, increasing leukocytosis, respiratory compromise, and fever. Elective laparotomy or laparoscopy should be considered in those whose ileus persists beyond a week, because in these instances the cause is usually mechanical. Patients with SBO who are managed with an initial nonoperative trial (usually a 48- to 72-hour trial) but fail the trial and proceed to surgery experience no apparent disadvantage. In malignant obstruction, contraindications include surgical evidence from past procedures of futility, reobstruction, presence of intra-abdominal carcinomatosis, diffuse intra-abdominal tumor burden or multiple palpable masses, poor performance status, large volume ascites, and patient refusal (Ripamonti & Mercadante, 2004). The choice of procedure is influenced by location and likely cause of obstruction; for example, a procedure by hernia repair might utilize a adhesiolysis in SBO, resection of CRC with anastomosis, or a diverting colostomy. In LBO, common procedures include right hemicolectomy for right-sided lesions and extended right hemicolectomy for lesions in the transverse colon. Other approaches may be diagnostic and palliative, such as the discovery of disseminated intraperitoneal cancer.

Laparoscopic approaches to obstruction, both diagnostic and definitive, are becoming more common and feasible. Evidence from small studies suggests that the minimally invasive approach is associated with more rapid return of GI function and shorter hospital LOS. Laparoscopy may not only be less likely to produce adhesions than laparotomy, but also feasible for lysing (release of) adhesions causing obstruction. However, some authors argue that laparoscopic adhesiolysis carries an unacceptably high risk of perforation and injury to organs caught in the adhesion bands; there is no clear evidence that minimal invasive surgery is superior to open surgical lysis of adhesions in terms of reforming of adhesions and subsequent obstruction (Golash & Willson, 2005).

Evaluation of Outcomes

Potential patient outcomes for each of the example nursing diagnoses for the patient with obstruction are:

- Fear related to perioperative events. The patient should manifest positive coping behaviors and verbalize a reduction in the amount of fear of the having this disease.
- Deficient fluid volume related to intake less than body requirements. The patient experiences adequate fluid volume and electrolyte balance as evidenced by urine output greater than 30 mL/hr, normotensive blood pressure, heart rate 100 beats/min, consistency of weight, and normal skin turgor.

COLORECTAL CANCER (CRC)

CRC is the fourth most common cancer worldwide; 1,025,152 new cases and 528,978 deaths a year are attributed to CRC. Fifty percent develop liver metastasis sometime in their course. On the European continent, there are 150,000 new cases annually, and 95,000 deaths. In the United States, CRC is the most common malignancy of the GI tract, with annual incidence of 145,000). Estimates for 2005 were 104,950 new cases (United States), with 56,290 dying from the disease. Approximately 40,000 patients will be diagnosed with rectal cancer in 2005. CRC is the fourth most common cancer in both men and women with a lifetime risk that approaches 6 percent (Leonard, Brenner, & Kemeny, 2005).

- Acute pain related to obstruction. The patient should verbalize an adequate relief of pain along with the ability to realistically cope with the pain if it is not completely relieved.
- Risk of infection related to intra-abdominal processes and procedures. The patient remains free of infection, as evidenced by normal vital signs and absence of purulent drainage from wounds, incisions, and tubes. Infection is recognized early to allow for prompt treatment.

COLORECTAL CANCER

As life expectancy across the globe continues to lengthen, and as other causes of mortality fall, cancer has become the second overall leading cause of death. Currently, it is the leading cause in women between the ages of 40 and 79 and men between the ages of 60 and 79 (Meric-Bernstam & Pollock, 2005) (Box 50-4). In part due to heightened understanding of etiology of many cancers, widespread public appreciation of preventive strategies (e.g., smoking cessation), increasing sensitivity of screening for early detection (e.g., mammography, colonoscopy), and advances in therapeutics, from 1992 to 1999 cancer death rates overall decreased by 1.5 percent in males and 0.6 percent in women. CRC refers to predominantly epithelial-derived tumors (e.g., adenomas and adenocarcinomas). Other colorectal tumors include carcinoid, lipoma, lymphoma, and leiomyoma (Bullard & Rothenberger, 2005).

Epidemiology

Over the past decade, incidence and mortality rates have remained stable or modestly decreased; likely due to improved screening, endoscopic removal of polyps, and modification of environmental factors (e.g., diet). Though highly treatable and often curative if found early, CRC is the second most lethal, accounting for about 55,000 to 56,000 deaths annually. Survival varies widely in the Western world and differences likely reflect different stage at diagnosis and therapy used to treat CRC. If diagnosed early, a five-year survival rate is approximately 90 percent; that percentage falls to 8 percent if diagnosed late. Racial differences in overall survival have been observed, without differences in disease-free survival. For example, mortality among African Americans remains higher than other ethnic and racial groups. More affluent patients appear to fare better than less affluent.

Etiology

One widely held opinion is that cancer "is a genetic disease that arises from an accumulation of mutations that leads to the selection of cells with increasingly aggressive behavior" (Bullard & Rothenberger, 2005, p. 260). Growing understanding of the human genome and its protein products and pathways suggest that virtually hundreds of genes and proteins are involved in the process of cell division and DNA replication. Gene mutations, which appear to be numerous and not uncommon, may activate oncogenes, inhibit tumor suppressor genes (e.g., APC gene), or disable mismatch repair genes. It appears that accumulation of mutations of various genes or proteins can sometimes lead to uncontrolled cancerous growth. A number of genes are being studied in CRC and are summarized in Table 50-6.

Seventy-five to 80 percent of CRC is sporadic or affects individuals of average risk. The remaining 20 to 25 percent report known risk factors. Hereditary CRC has two well-described forms and affects about 6 percent of the CRC population. Hereditary nonpolyposis colon cancer (HNPCC), or Lynch's syndrome, is a rare autosomal dominant disease, accounting for fewer than 5 percent of all CRC. As the most common hereditary CRC syndrome, it arises from

TABLE 50-6 **Genetics and Colon Cancer**		
SUPPRESSOR GENES (LOSS OF FUNCTION)	**ONCOGENES (AMPLIFIES FUNCTION)**	**FUNCTION AND ASSOCIATION**
	K-ras (proto-oncogene)	Perturbation of one allele disturbs cell cycle
		Induces cellular proliferation and inhibits apoptosis
DCC gene ("deleted" in colorectal carcinoma)		Loss of both required for malignant degradation
		May involve differentiation
p53 gene		Normally required for initiating apoptosis in cells with genetic damage
		Present in 75 percent of CRCs; present in multiple other cancers
DNA mismatch repair genes (e.g., *hMLH1, hMSH2*)		Normally identify and repair mismatched nucleotides in DNA or small insertion or deletion loops during DNA replication
		Nonrepaired replication errors lead to a damaged DNA
		HNPCC—defect in mismatch repair [caretaker] genes hMLH1, hMSH2, HPMS1-2

Adapted from Bullard, K. M., & Rothenberger, D. A. (2005). Colon, rectum and anus. In F. C. Brunicardi (Ed.), Schwartz's principles of surgery (8th ed., pp. 1055–1117). New York: McGraw Hill; Meric-Berstam, F., & Pollock, R. E. (2005). Oncology. In F. C. Brunicardi (Ed.), Schwartz's principles of surgery (8th ed., pp. 249–294). New York: McGraw Hill.

errors in mismatch repair. Type I confers a 50 percent risk in first-degree relatives; type 2 is associated with extracolonic malignancies, especially endometrial, ovarian, and cholangiocarcinoma. It is characterized by the development of early cancer (40 to 45 years of age) and is usually in proximal colon. It tends to have a favorable clinical course and respond better to 5-fluorouracil (5-FU) (Bullard & Rothenberger, 2005).

Familial adenomatous polyposis (FAP) is a rare autosomal dominant disorder, genetically related to mutations on the APC gene. Clinically, it is characterized by the development of hundreds, often, thousands of adenomatous polyps throughout the large bowel after puberty. Evolution to CRC is a certainty, occurring in the teens, most sometime during the 30's and inevitably by age 50. In 20 percent of patients, it is a new mutation. Patients may also develop cancers of the thyroid, gallbladder, adrenal glands, and brain (Bullard & Rothenberger, 2005). Individuals with a family history of CRC, but lacking identifiable hereditary syndromes or specific genetic abnormalities, are said to have familial colorectal cancer (FCC). FCC occurs in about 10 to 15 percent of patients; lifetime risk appears to increase with family history (FH). Diagnosis before age 50 is associated with higher incidence (Meric-Bernstam & Pollock, 2005).

Ethnic, racial, and migrant studies suggest important environmental influences in CRC. For example, Israel-, European-, and American-born male Jews are at a higher risk than those born in Africa and Asia; Japanese immigrants to America have a much higher rate than Japanese in Japan. CRC may be related then to a range of cultural, social, and lifestyle practices, and these may account for up to 70 to 80 percent of the cases. The implication is clearly that in many patients, CRC may be linked to modifiable risk factors and that management of risk behavior may have an impact on occurrence.

Validated nonmodifiable risk factors for CRC include age greater than 50 years, male, African American, history of adenomatous polyps, ulcerative colitis, or Crohn's disease, and first-degree relative with FAP, HNPCC, or history of breast, ovarian, or endometrial cancer. Genetics appear to affect the age of onset of CRC. Risk awareness is useful when it is useful in disease prevention, and the following factors have been linked to CRC.

Diet has a complex and poorly understood role in etiology of CRC. Numerous studies have often yielded contradictory results due to methodological limitations and the complexity of the subject itself. However, there appears to be weak but consistent evidence that dietary fat and meat (especially processed) intake is positively correlated with risk. Tumorigenesis appears to be enhanced as fat content increases, possibly by increasing bile acid concentration and altering interactions to amplify cell replication signals, and direct toxicity to gut mucosa, which may induce early changes (Bullard & Rothenberger, 2005). The interaction of dietary fat, protein, and caloric intake is also associated with CRC.

Fiber refers to a range of compounds (e.g., wheat, bran, cellulose, dried beans), and it appears that intake of foods rich in fiber is inversely related to CRC. Risk reduction may be selective for fiber source and may modify carcinogenesis by a number of mechanisms, including binding to bile acids, increasing fecal water, and diluting carcinogens. The selective value of fruit and vegetable fiber over cereal may reflect an association with other factors. There is no RCT evidence that increased dietary fiber intake reduces the incidence or recurrence of adenomatous polyps within a two-to-four-year period. The protective benefits of diets high in fruit and vegetables are equivocal at this time (Delaune & Ladner, 2006).

A recent meta-analysis (14 RCT) found no evidence that antioxidant vitamins confer protection against development CRC adenomas or cancer. The value of folic acid supplementation is being evaluated for its protective effects. There appears to be an inverse relationship between calcium intake and CRC risk. Calcium may bind to bile acids, thereby blocking their access to luminal epithelium or possess other protective effects.

Obesity and sedentary lifestyle increase cancer-related deaths, and in some studies obesity is associated with a twofold increase in CRC risk. The risk appears to increase with increasing body mass index (BMI) (Bullard & Rothenberger, 2005). Absence of a strong or consistent relationship of obesity and CRC may reflect differences in metabolic efficiency rather than simple overeating. Maintenance of a BMI of 18.5 to 25 kg/m^2 throughout life and 30 minutes of physical activity most days is intuitively sensible, though not associated with evidence of reduced risk. Moderate intensity activity (e.g., walking) may have an inverse association with large adenomas.

There is weak evidence that prolonged cigarette smoking (more than 35 years) increases the risk of adenomas and adenoma recurrence after polypectomy. There is only weak suggestion that in average risk individuals, use of NSAIDS, estrogen, folic acid, and calcium may be preventive.

Pathophysiology

Transformation from normal gut lumen epithelium to adenomatous polyp to carcinoma is a sequence of events is known as the adenoma-carcinoma sequence. A polyp is defined as any projection that protrudes from the surface of the intestinal mucosa into the lumen, regardless of histology (Figure 50-2). Pedunculated polyps have a stalk; sessile polyps lack years and, by definition, are dysplastic. The risk of transformation rises with lesion size. Inflammatory, hamartomatous, postsurgical, and other polyps are not associated with CRC. However, those that arise from abnormal mucosal maturation, due to proliferation or dysplasia, are recognized as cancer precursors. Although most polyps do not evolve to CRC, the fact that most CRC originates as polyp provides the

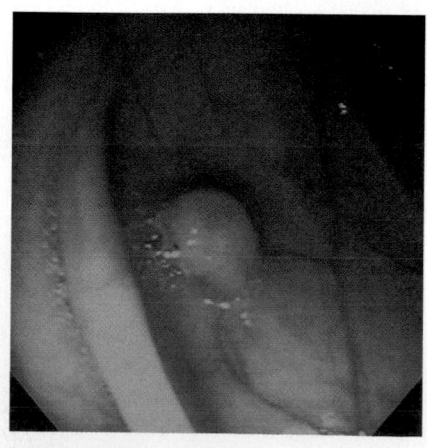

Figure 50-2 Colon polyp.

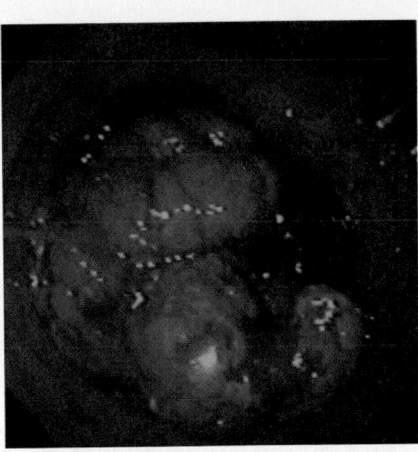

Figure 50-3 Colon cancer.

rationale for secondary prevention strategies and polypectomy before the lesion evolves into a CRC (Bullard & Rothenberger, 2005). Mutational events (activated oncogenes, deactivated suppressors) facilitate cell proliferation, and failure of repair lead to selection of growth advantage and progression to malignancy.

The lesion begins in mucosa and invades the bowel wall, involving adjacent viscera as it grows (Figure 50-3). It can grow to a size large enough to obstruct the gut lumen. Draining lymph nodes are the most common route of spread, and lymph node involvement precedes distant metastases or carcinomatosis. Depth of tumor invasion is the most significant predictor of lymph node spread; carcinoma in situ or high-grade dysplasia carries no risk of lymph node metastasis. The number of positive nodes found at operation correlates with the presence of distant disease and inversely with survival; four or more predict poor prognosis (Otchy, et. al., 2004).

Assessment with Clinical Manifestations

The history should include a detailed family history, including the number, degree of separation, age of onset, and presence of associated cancers that might suggest a familial syndrome. Questioning should address nonspecific complaints, such as fatigue, unintended weight loss, and anorexia. GI specific complaints, such as change in bowel habits, **tenesmus** (distressing, but ineffectual urge to evacuate the rectum), bloody stool, melena, and colicky abdominal pain should be noted (Estes, 2006). Alternating constipation and diarrhea in adults (older than 40 years of age) may be early signs of obstruction; and complaints or findings of blood in stool should never be dismissed as local disease (e.g., hemorrhoids), without excluding more proximal.

Findings are related to site of the lesion and the presence of complications (e.g., obstruction, perforation). Tumors in the cecum and ascending colon may become quite large without producing symptoms, because stool is liquid. Patients with lesions in the ascending colon often bleed chronically from ulcerations and present with anemia rather than prominent GI complaints. Development of microcytic anemia should prompt consideration for colonoscopy. Lesions in the transverse colon can produce cramping, occasional obstruction, and even perforation. Rectosigmoid masses are associated with tenesmus, narrow stools, and **hematochezia,** the passing of stools containing red blood rather than tarry stools. Abdominal exam may reveal visible or palpable masses, dull to percussion.

Diagnostic Tests

Screening for CRC lags far behind screening for other cancers. Screening may be practiced by about 20 percent of U.S. adults. In 1999, only 44 percent of adults underwent sigmoidoscopy or colonoscopy for screening or diagnosis; 40 percent had used fecal occult blood testing (FOBT) kits. Women more often had FOBT; more men had sigmoidoscopy. The most frequent reason for not being screened in one study was lack of recommendation by primary care physicians; other factors include fear or embarrassment, cost and reimbursement issues, and lack of access. There appears to be a real need to increase awareness and promote the use of regular screening as recommended. Current recommendations are summarized here and in Table 50-7. Screening is recommended to commence at age 50 in men and women, but no similar guidance is offered for when screening should cease; the impact of newer technologies, such as virtual colonoscopy is unclear at this time. Although the frequency and duration of screening has not been definitely established, all of the available methods reduce, to some degree, the risk of death from CRC.

TABLE 50-7 Screening and Detection: CRC

Average Risk Individuals

MODALITY	RECOMMENDATION	EVIDENCE
Digital rectal exam	None	Not recommended as an adequate screen, fewer 10 percent lesions within reach.
Fecal occult blood test (FOBT)	Annual Individuals older than 50 years of age.	Pros—Strong evidence for reduction in death ~16–23 percent (Levin, 2005) and incidence of CRC Sensitivity: 25–90 percent
		Rationale: most tumors and large polyps bleed intermittently. Trigger for other diagnostic testing.
		Cons—Large no. false positives
Flexible sigmoidoscopy	Every 5 years older than 50 years of age	Pro—Evidence decrease in deaths from CRC within reach; with FOBT increase sensitivity; detects 70–85 percent advanced lesions. Low-risk significant complications. Optimal screening interval not determined.
Barium enema (BE)—Air contrast	Every 5–10 years	No RCT evidence as screening test; less sensitive than colonoscopy detecting polyps. Perforation rare.
Colonoscopy	Every 10 years older than 50 years of age	Pro—Most sensitive and specific
		Con—Risk increases with diagnostic maneuvers; inconvenient, small risk complications including perforation (0.2–0.3 percent); costly.
		Frequency based on natural history of the adenoma-carcinoma sequence.
CT colonography Virtual colonoscopy	None	Pro—Noninvasive, short duration (10–15 minutes), requires mechanical bowel prep and air installation.
		High sensitivity and specificity in experienced hands: polyp detection (greater than 10 mm) approaches 90 percent
		Con—Clinical outcomes unknown; indirect evidence supports use of this modality; may be less cost-effective than colonoscopy.
CT	None	No screening indications
		Modality of choice for evaluation of distant metastases or synchronous lesions
Genetic screening	None	Not recommended for screening: rare incidence
		Con—Limited sensitivity, potentially misleading, not cost effective. Research context only
Carcino-embryonic antigen (CEA)	None	Origin—Embryonic endodermal epithelium.
		Not indicated for routine screening
		Nonspecific elevation in variety of malignant and nonmalignant conditions
High-risk groups		Depending on risk factor(s), begin at younger age, and occur more frequently
Genetic testing	Research and clinical decision making	Clinical application led to presymptomatic diagnosis in FAP and HNPCC; technically able to detect APC, *K-ras* mutations; studies in progress to compare these techniques with colonoscopy.
		Expensive; cost-effectiveness unproven
		FAP standard of care with genetic counseling, DNA testing for APC gene mutations: specificity is 100 percent; sensitivity 70–90 percent
		HNPCC tests not as sensitive; sequencing very expensive.

Continued

TABLE 50-7 Screening and Detection: CRC—*cont'd*

Average Risk Individuals

MODALITY	RECOMMENDATION	EVIDENCE
On the horizon	n/a	n/a
Stool based DNA		Screening effectiveness unknown
		Used in patients with known polyps or cancer
Positron emission tomography (PET)	Uses fluor-deoxyglucose (FDG)	Accuracy delineating metastatic from postoperative change; superior to CT for liver, intra-abdominal, and pelvic disease

Adapted from Daniels, R. (2003). Delmar's manual of laboratory and diagnostic tests. New York: Thomson Delmar Learning; Otchy, D., Hyman, N. H., Simmang, C., Anthony, T., Buie, W. D., & Cataldo P. (2004). Practice parameters for colon cancer. Diseases of the Colon and Rectum, 47(8), 1269–1284.

Nursing Diagnoses

Based on the information gathered, examples of nursing diagnoses in the patient with CRC may include the following:
- Chronic pain related to CRC.
- Fear in response to the diagnosis of CRC.
- Ineffective coping related to anxiety, lower activity level and the inability to perform normal activities of daily living.

Planning and Implementation

CRC has many implications for management strategies. There are a wide variety of manifestations that the patients will have and therefore many types of treatments. For slow development of the disease, less invasive therapies are encouraged, and surgeries are used for patients with more problematic cancer proliferation. See chapter 15 for further nursing implications when caring for patients with CRC.

Pharmacology

Cancer recurs in half of operated patients and is the most common cause of death. There is clear consensus that patients with metastatic CRC should be offered adjunctive chemotherapy (see chapter 15). The standard regimen for adjuvant therapy for CRC is not clear, but 5-FU, the sole agent with proven efficacy, has been joined by an array of new agents, combinations, schedules, and delivery modes. At the forefront of research are biological therapies, also known as immunotherapy, biotherapy, or biological response modifier therapy. Interacting with the body's immune system, they include interferons, interleukins, colony-stimulating factors, monoclonal antibodies (MOAB), vaccines, gene therapy, and nonspecific immunomodulating agents. MOAB antibodies can be designed to react with specific cancer cells, programmed to act against cell growth factors, and may be linked to anticancer radioisotopes to deliver these poisons direct to the tumor (Broyles, et al., 2007).

Radiation Therapy

Radiation therapy (RT) has little role in the treatment of colon cancer of any stage; its potential to injure abdominal viscera limits its usefulness. However RT has usefulness in preoperative and postoperative management of rectal cancer. Most trials of preoperative and postoperative monotherapy have shown a decrease in local recurrence, without a parallel improvement in survival.

Preoperative RT may convert a locally unresectable lesion to one amenable to operation; it favors preservation of the anal sphincter and may delay need for colostomy. The largest trial (Swedish) of preoperative RT reported a 61 percent decrease in local recurrence and overall improvement in survival; others have confirmed this finding in patients with advanced locoregional disease. Preoperative RT appears to be an acceptable alternative to standard practice of postoperative RT for patients with stage II and II resectable rectal cancer. RT followed by surgery has been shown to be more effective than operation alone in preventing local recurrence in patient with respectable rectal cancer and may improve survival. Patients who select preoperative RT should be aware that because staging is not definitive until after operation, they may derive little to no benefit from the intervention and at risk for the related morbidity.

Postoperative RT appears to be less effective, possibly because of rapid repopulation of tumor cells after surgery or relative hypoxia around the healing wound. Postoperative RT causes transient cystitis, diarrhea, and skin irradiation. Patients should be encouraged to consider participating in RCT to help define optimum treatment.

Combination Therapy: Chemotherapy and Radiation Therapy

The intent of preoperative combination therapy in rectal cancer is to maximize the likelihood of resection with clear margins and convert inoperable rectal cancer to an operable lesion. Regimens include 5-FU/leucovorin (LV) infusions, continuous 5-FU, or bolus. Capecitabine is being used. Fluorouracil may prime tumor cells and increase the cytotoxicity of RT, but its effect is unknown at this time.

Combination therapy is considered standard for patients with resected stages II and III rectal cancer. Evidence suggests that in this population, RT alone was superior to watchful waiting in local control of disease but there was no significant survival benefit. Chemotherapy produced a significant survival benefit over watchful waiting but no benefit in local control (Ozer & Diasio, 2004).

Surgery

Once a cancer has been found the major treatment is surgical resection. Endoscopic management at the time of diagnostic colonoscopy can be curative with polypectomy and is estimated to lower the incidence of CRC by 50 to 90 percent. Snare polypectomy is possible for pedunculated lesions; sessile polyps spreading over the mucosa present a greater technical challenge. Endoscopic mucosal resection (EMR) removes potentially malignant lesions or high-grade dysplasia by excising through mid-to-deep submucosa. Polypectomy is not benign and includes risks of perforation and bleeding. However, patients may heal and avoid surgery with bowel rest, close observation, and antibiotics. Every effort should be made to obtain tissue for pathological testing when polyps, masses, or strictures are seen. The optimal number of biopsies when removing polyps is undetermined. Highly suspicious but nondiagnostic lesions should be reviewed with a pathologist. Colonoscopy also allows marking malignant lesions (tattooing or metal clip placement) for subsequent identification during an open procedure and estimation of depth of invasion using endoscopic ultrasound (EUS) before EMR to determine depth of invasion and lymph node involvement. The inability to remove suspicious or cancerous polyps or confirmation of invasive CRC is indications for open or laparoscopic resections (Davila, et al., 2005).

There is weak RCT evidence for the benefit of preoperative mechanical bowel preparation of the bowel, but this practice remains a universal practice in North America. It may be easier to handle a prepared colon; the procedure is inexpensive and relatively safe. Patients can perform the prep at home the day before surgery; however, many present for operation dehydrated and require preoperative rehydration (Otchy, et al., 2004).

Prophylactic preoperative antibiotic coverage against anaerobes and aerobes decrease infection rate, mortality, and costs. Oral-parenteral combinations are common and need not be continued for longer than 24 hours when operation is elective. One large clinical trial demonstrated that a single preoperative dose of cefotaxime and metronidazole is as effective as three doses. Deep vein thrombosis (DVT) prophylaxis, using unfractionated heparin, low molecular weight heparin, or pneumatic calf compression has strong evidence of efficacy. Some surgeons use combinations of medication and mechanical prophylaxis in high-risk patients (Otchy, et al., 2004).

Patients should be screened for nutritional status, but routine supplementation is not indicated. Supplemental nutritional support is appropriate if the patient undergoing active treatment is malnourished or anticipated to be unable to ingest or absorb adequate nutrients for a prolonged period. Every effort should be made to obtain a fully informed consent prior to operation, including the purpose and extent of resection, outcomes, complications, alternatives to surgery proposed, and the prognosis (Ozer & Diasio, 2004).

Prior to definitive resection, it is imperative to visualize the entire colon and rectum to detect synchronous polyps or neoplasms. Preoperative evaluation should be prompt and include the elements in the following section. Preoperative identification of metastatic disease, especially in the lung and abdomen (liver) is not an absolute contraindication for surgery, but it may modify the approach. CT is the diagnostic modality of choice. The liver is the most common site of metastases via portal venous system. Patients with liver lesions who are surgical candidates have a chance of prolonged survival and cure (Leonard, Brenner, & Kemeny, 2005). Intraoperative ultrasound can be used if patients are taken to the operating room urgently. Alternatively, the liver can be scanned postoperatively. Preoperative CXR is common, but it has a yield as low as its cost and risk.

Patients with rectal lesions require preoperative endorectal ultrasonography (EUS) to evaluate lesion size and depth of invasion. This procedure has an accuracy of 82 to 93 percent; its ability to evaluate lymph node involvement is less accurate. Abdominal CT and EUS are the most cost-effective way of staging rectal cancer; pelvic CT and MRI are recommended to evaluate contiguous structures in the presence of large rectal tumors. The value of EUS after preoperative radiation therapy is not clear; accuracy falls due to inflammatory changes and its role is similarly unclear in postoperative surveillance for recurrence, which affects 10 to 30 percent of patients depending on stage and treatment (Davila, et al., 2005).

Carcinoembryonic antigen (CEA) can be used in preoperative elevation (more than 5 ng/mL) and is an independent predictor of poor outcome and increased risk of recurrence regardless of stage. Return to normal after surgery is associated with complete tumor resection and if it remains high, is associated with visible or residual disease (Otchy, et al., 2004). Periodic CEA assay is a cost-effective way of detecting recurrence or metastases and a means of monitoring treatment response in patients with metastatic disease. CEA testing is recommended every two to three months for two or more years (Meric-Bernstam & Pollock, 2005).

Resection of the Colon

Curative resection offers the greatest potential for cure in CRC. It results in 45 percent cure in rectal cancer. Surgery can be prophylactic, elective, or emergent depending on indication and patient presentation. It is usually offered to all new diagnosed patients unless life expectancy is short. Palliative resection in metastatic disease is advisable to halt further bleeding and avert eventual obstruction. A range of options are available for patients who by choice or by comorbidity are not surgical candidates. These options include laser photoablation or colonic stenting of malignant obstruction. In rectal cancer, **fulguration** (destruction of tissue using high-frequency electric sparks), laser photocoagulation, radiation therapy, and endostenting are possibilities. Aggressive preventive resection is advocated in some familial syndromes (Meric-Bernstam & Pollock, 2005). Total **proctocolectomy** (surgical removal of the rectum together with all or part of the colon) with J-pouch ileoanal anastomosis to prevent malignant transformation of the polyps has been advocated in FAP in patients as young as 20 to 25 years and creates the necessity to monitor the rectal stump if left behind. Others recommend abdominal **colectomy** (surgical operation to remove all or part of the colon) with ileorectal anastomosis. For patients with HNPCC found to be harboring adenoma or adenocarcinoma, total abdominal colectomy with ileorectal anastomosis is recommended. Women should consider total abdominal hysterectomy with bilateral salpingo-oophorectomy to avoid cancers of the reproductive organs.

Urgent or emergent surgery is required for CRC-related acute abdomen, suggested by signs of perforation, malignant obstruction or significant hemorrhage. LBO of the right or transverse colon requires right or extended right colectomy; left LBO has multiple options. Perforation requires resection, and peritonitis may be best managed with ileostomy. Management of CRC hemorrhage follows the same principles as elective resection, and failure to locate a site of bleeding should prompt a subtotal colectomy.

Surgical goals for CRC include complete tumor removal with its lymphovascular supply leaving margins of at least 5 cm; extended resections have not been shown to confer added survival benefit. Cancer attached to contiguous organs is technically challenging and requires en bloc resection (removal in a lump as a whole) to achieve a resection free of tumors. Use of no touch surgical technique, avoiding intraoperative manipulation that might shed tumor cells into portal circulation, though intuitively appealing, has no proven benefit to survival. Careful palpation of abdominal contents, with ultrasound examination of the liver during surgery is indicated: Presence of synchronous tumor (incidence 2 to 9 percent) may require total or subtotal colectomy; whether one or two procedures are required appears to make no difference in outcome or complication rates. Ten to twenty percent have liver metastasis at resection, and if the lesion(s) is amenable to resection, a single operation may suffice with a 25 to 40 percent five-year survival rate. Metastases to the ovary occur in 2 to 8 percent of the cases, and bilateral involvement may require bilateral oophorectomy (BSO). In postmenopausal women, consideration should be given due to combined risks of mircrometases and primary ovarian cancer. However, there is no proven benefit for prophylactic oophorectomy.

Palliative approaches usually involve placement of a proximal stoma, or a bypass colonic wall stenting may safely relieve acute malignant obstruction and permit subsequent resection. The comparative effectiveness of immediate resection versus stenting followed by surgery has not been determined.

Rectal Surgeries

Surgical goals in rectal cancer are to preserve the sphincter and avoid colostomy if at all possible; options are stage specific. Trans-anal local excision is possible in some instances with small, early stage tumor. The use of staples now allows end-to-end anastomoses by experienced surgeons with midrectal lesions and preservation of the sphincter with trans-anal or trans-coccygeal resection in some cases. The ideal margin in rectal cancer is 2 cm or more distal and 5 cm or more proximal. Abdomino-perineal resection (APR) with permanent sigmoid colostomy is the traditional operation for distal cancers and considered by most to be unavoidable if the cancer is within 5 to 6 cm of anal verge. Recurrence generally has a bad prognosis; patients may require pelvic exenteration.

Ostomy Conditions

As mentioned, the colorectal surgeries often result in the need for an ostomy. An intestinal ostomy is when a surgically created opening is made between the intestine and the abdominal wall (Figure 50-4). The opening at the skin surface exits is labeled the stoma. The actual name of the **ostomy** is individualized to the location of the stoma. Virtually any portion of the large and small intestine can be diverted or used to form a fecal reservoir. For example, an ileostomy is an ostomy made in the ileum. An ileostomy usually requires the

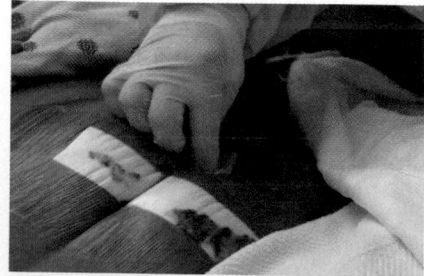

Figure 50-4 Sometimes a colon surgery results in an ostomy.

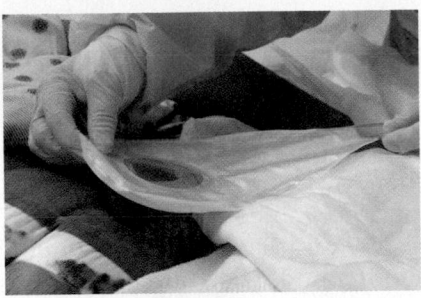

Figure 50-5 Providing ostomy care and applying new ostomy bag.

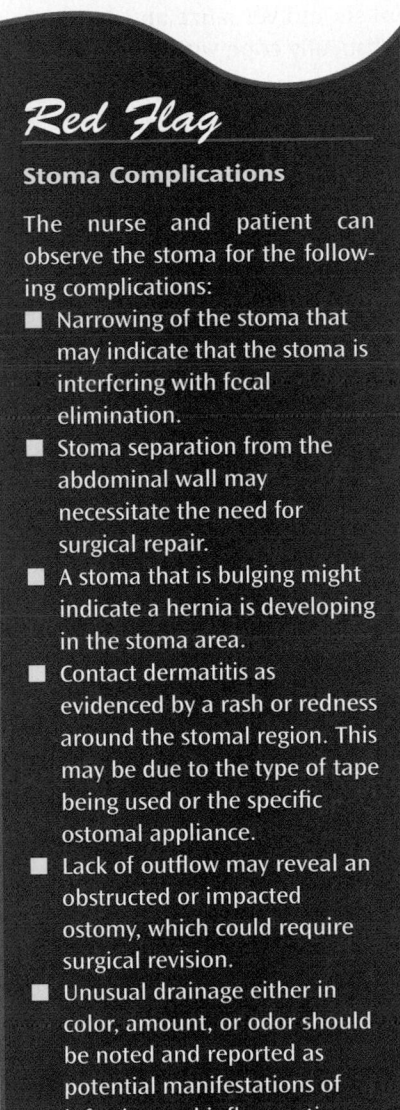

Red Flag

Stoma Complications

The nurse and patient can observe the stoma for the following complications:

- Narrowing of the stoma that may indicate that the stoma is interfering with fecal elimination.
- Stoma separation from the abdominal wall may necessitate the need for surgical repair.
- A stoma that is bulging might indicate a hernia is developing in the stoma area.
- Contact dermatitis as evidenced by a rash or redness around the stomal region. This may be due to the type of tape being used or the specific ostomal appliance.
- Lack of outflow may reveal an obstructed or impacted ostomy, which could require surgical revision.
- Unusual drainage either in color, amount, or odor should be noted and reported as potential manifestations of infection and inflammation.

complete removal of the colon, rectum, and anus. The anus is closed, and the end of the ileum is attached to the skin surface of the abdominal region to form the stoma. There are occasions where the ostomy is temporary (e.g., loop ostomy) to allow the tissues to heal in the area that is dysfunctional; such as diverticulitis or trauma. When the temporary ostomy is not needed, a follow-up surgery reattaches the bowel and restores fecal elimination. Another ostomy is a continent ileostomy (Kock's), whereby an intra-abdominal reservoir is made, and a valve is formed from the terminal ileum on its way to the abdominal wall. The feces collects in the internal pouch device, and the valve keeps fecal material from leaking through the stoma. In addition, a catheter is inserted into the pouch to drain the stool.

The fecal stream is diverted at the most distal point possible to maximize the absorption of the food, fluid, and electrolytes and to preserve continence. The ileostomy is more uncommon than it was during recent decades. A permanent ileostomy is typically reserved for patients with severe Crohn's colitis, familial adenomatous polyposis, or chronic ulcerative colitis. The temporary ileostomy may be created as one stage in an ileoanal reservoir procedure or as a staged procedure for the relief of obstruction of the ascending colon.

The nursing care for patients with ostomies begins preoperatively and follows the patient throughout the acute care experience. In addition, there are specific management strategies for the patient with an ostomy as he or she is discharged from the acute care setting and is going home or to another care facility. Preoperatively, the ostomy patient can be referred to an enterostomal therapist for patient education and thorough explanations of their upcoming surgery and ostomy appliance. In addition, the patient can be given information on the local chapter of the United Ostomy Association organization. This organization provides the patient the opportunity to meet members with ostomies and who can show the patient their ostomy and answer questions. Allowing the patient to ask questions and verbalize their fears and anxiety during this time is important. After the surgery, the postoperative care will include the mechanics of the application of the ostomy bag and devices (Figure 50-5). The patient should be encouraged to observe the nurses when the ostomy appliances are put on the stoma area. Specific instructions will be provided by the enterostomal therapist and as the patient condition improves, the patient and family will participate in the self-care of the ostomy device. An ongoing assessment of the stoma and the surrounding skin surfaces is necessary. The tape or application devices may cause sensitivity reactions or irritation and must be handled for with meticulous care (Estes, 2006). Complications of the ostomy are provided in the Red Flag feature.

As the patient continues to heal, they should be evaluated for continued positive adaptation to their ostomy. Nutrition imbalances, dehydration, electrolyte imbalances, and emotional disturbances, including body image difficulties, are all potential problems that the new ostomy patient may develop. Each of these problems needs to be recognized and then referred to the enterostomal therapist for resolution.

Staging and Prognosis

CRC prognosis is related to depth of tumor penetration (into bowel wall), presence or absence of lymph node involvement, and distant metastases. Staging systems are used to describe the anatomic extent of malignant process, and their accuracy is crucial to designing appropriate therapy. Postoperative staging is recommended for estimating prognosis and shaping decision making about **adjuvant therapy** (treatment given after the primary treatment) to increase the chances of a cure. Adjuvant therapy may include chemotherapy, radiation therapy, hormone therapy, or biological therapy (Germond, Figueredo, Taylor, Micucci, & Zwaal, 2004). The oldest and most frequently used system after resection is the DUKES, which has undergone several modifications. More recently, the Dukes scheme has been applied to the TNM classification (see chapter 15). The new, parallel scheme subdivides CRC into stages A through D, and because most recurrences are within the first three to four years, five-year survival rates are calculated. Five-year survival has improved for almost every stage over several decades. The reasons are early detection, more careful staging, and improvements in adjuvant therapy. The obvious limited success of surgery, chemotherapy, and radiation in advanced disease (stages C and D) underscore the criticality of early detection. In addition to stage, other indicators of poor prognosis include histology (poorly differentiated), high histologic grade, infiltration at margins, the young and old, males, persistently elevated serum CEA, tumor adherence to adjacent organs, bowel perforation, or colonic obstruction at time of diagnosis. In the future, DNA analysis may be used routinely to assess prognosis.

Evaluation of Outcomes

Potential patient outcomes for each of the example nursing diagnoses for the patient with CRC are:
- Chronic pain related to CRC. The patient should verbalize an adequate relief of pain along with the ability to realistically cope with the pain if it is not completely relieved.
- Fear in response to the diagnosis of CRC. The patient should manifest positive coping behaviors and verbalize a reduction in the amount of fear of the having this disease.
- Ineffective coping related to anxiety, lower activity level and the inability to perform normal activities of daily living. The patient identifies own maladaptive coping behaviors, available resources, and support systems, describes or initiates alternative coping strategies, and describes positive results from new behaviors.

IRRITABLE BOWEL SYNDROME

IBS is relatively common and is a motility disorder of the GI tract. IBS occurs in approximately one in six people, and is characterized with abdominal pain, diarrhea, constipation, or both. The cause of IBS is unknown, although there seems to be a genetic propensity to the disorder. In addition, stress exacerbates the manifestations, as does a diet high in fat, irritating foods, alcohol, and smoking.

Epidemiology

IBS occurs in up to 20 percent of the populations of regions in the Western hemisphere. It presents itself at a ratio of 3:1 women to men and occurs first in the second or third decade of life.

Pathophysiology

IBS is a disorder of intestinal motility. The changes seen are theorized to be caused by CNS alterations to the motor and sensory functions of the bowel. IBS caused an increased motor response in the small bowel and colon with heightened peristaltic intensity. There is also increased secretion of mucus in the colon, but there is not an inflammation of the tissue.

Assessment with Clinical Manifestations

Patients may initially seek health care for their symptomatology of increased abdominal pain or bouts of diarrhea or constipation. The patients may notice they have abdominal bloating and distension. The primary manifestations are the changes in bowel patterns, but otherwise there is a wide variety in the severity and symptoms of the disorder. Often, patients will describe their condition being stimulated when they eat certain foods (e.g., salads, fatty foods).

Diagnostic Tests

Diagnosis is not made with one single test. Usually, other GI tract disorders are also considered and eliminated with a variety of tests to allow the confirmation of the IBS diagnosis. Stool studies, visualization of the lower GI system (e.g., proctoscopy, sigmoidoscopy), manometry, and electromyography are performed. Also, serum studies, such as a CBC and erythrocyte sedimentation rate (ESR), are evaluated. An anemic condition can result from the potential blood loss and an elevated WBC, and ESR may result from a bacterial infection (Daniels, 2003).

Nursing Diagnoses

Based on the information gathered, examples of nursing diagnoses in the patient with IBS may include the following:
- Acute pain related to the IBS.
- Ineffective coping related to anxiety, lower activity level and the inability to perform normal activities of daily living.
- Diarrhea related to the altered GI motility.
- Constipation related to the altered GI motility.

Planning and Implementation

Patients with IBS are going to adapt to their disorder as they have compliance with the management of their disease. A careful assessment of what stimulates the condition is necessary to inform the patient in identifying these risk factors. A general assessment of the patient condition to detect complications, such as dehydration and stress, is important. Avoiding the irritating substances (e.g., alcohol, gas-forming foods, or sugars) is encouraged and referral to a dietitian may be indicated. A bulk-forming diet (e.g., bran) and water can reduce the occurrence of both diarrhea and constipation.

Pharmacology

There is no cure for the IBS condition, but there are several medications and herbal substances that can benefit the patient. Bulk-forming laxatives may reduce the pain and motility symptoms. Anticholinergics can interfere with parasympathetic nervous system innervation and decrease GI motility. Antidiarrheal agents (e.g., Imodium, Lomotil) can be given prophylactically or symptomatically on an as needed basis. Antidepressant drugs can assist in relieving the abdominal pain (Broyles, et al., 2007). There are herbal remedies with antispasmodic effects that can have benefits to the patient with IBS (e.g., anise, peppermint, sage).

Evaluation of Outcomes

Potential patient outcomes for each of the example nursing diagnoses for the patient with IBS are:
- Acute pain related to the IBS. The patient should verbalize an adequate relief of pain along with the ability to realistically cope with the pain if it is not completely relieved.
- Ineffective coping related to anxiety, lower activity level, and the inability to perform normal activities of daily living. The patient identifies own maladaptive coping behaviors, available resources, and support systems, describes or initiates alternative coping strategies, and describes positive results from new behaviors.

- Diarrhea related to the altered GI motility. The patient passes soft, formed stool no more than three times per day.
- Constipation related to the altered GI motility. The patient passes soft, formed stool at a frequency perceived as normal by the patient. The patient or caregiver verbalizes measures that will prevent recurrence of the constipation.

INFLAMMATORY BOWEL DISORDERS

There are two chronic inflammatory bowel disorders (IBD) that are similar but also have several differences: (a) Crohn's disease, and (b) ulcerative colitis. The cause of both diseases is unknown, but both have a hereditary implication and a geographical distribution. There may be autoimmune relationships to these disorders, but conclusive information has not been ascertained at this time.

Epidemiology

In general, IBD has a higher incidence in Caucasians and African Americans. In addition, there is a less incidence in Jewish populations on a percentage basis. Women are slightly more at risk for these disorders than men. And, persons from ages 10 to 30 are higher at risk. Patients with these pathologies have chronic conditions, typically managed with diet, medications, and even surgery.

Diagnostic Tests

In the early stages of IBD, making a definitive diagnosis can be challenging and difficult. The symptoms are nonspecific and may mimic other conditions. When a patient presents with symptoms, such as diarrhea, abdominal pain, or weight loss, IBD disease may be suspected. A thorough history is obtained, and a physical exam is completed. Initially, a proctosigmoidoscopy is performed to identify whether the bowel area is inflamed. A barium study will demonstrate the string sign, which reveals the constriction of a small intestine segment. The following blood and diagnostic tests are ordered: CBC, albumin, IBD serology panel (ANCA, IgG, ASCA IgG, and ASCA IgA), stool cultures, endoscopy (including video wireless capsule endoscopy), abdominal X-rays, small bowel series, and enteroclysis (Daniels, 2003; Jungles, 2004).

Nursing Diagnoses

Based on the information gathered, examples of nursing diagnoses in the patient with IBD may include the following:
- Chronic pain related to IBD.
- Diarrhea related to IBD.
- Nutrition imbalance, less than body requirements, related to IBD.
- Ineffective coping related to anxiety, lower activity level, and the inability to perform normal activities of daily living.
- Risk for impaired skin integrity related to compromised tissue perfusion.
- Fear and anxiety related to actual or potential lifestyle changes.

Planning and Implementation

There are varied care strategies for patients with IBD. There is not a cure for the disorder, and therefore supportive measures are the objective of care. A variety of medical treatments, surgeries, and nursing care is employed with an obvious need to involve the entire health care team in the care of patients with IBD.

The need for adequate nutrition in any chronic disease state is obvious, and even more so in IBD, in which patients are often malnourished and often highly catabolic, particularly during active disease stages. In children, exclusive nutritional therapy has been shown to be as efficacious as corticosteroids in induction of remission. The role of nutritional therapy in maintenance of remission in adult patients is less clear cut but nevertheless is still vital to the health of the patient.

Perhaps one of the simplest and most successful current therapeutic options in the maintenance of IBD is smoking cessation. Active smoking increases the risk of a disease flare by more than 50 percent compared with nonsmokers. There is a dose-dependent association between smoking and IBD activity, and this is particularly significant above 15 cigarettes smoked per day. Smoking is also associated with increased complication rates and lower scores about quality of life.

Pharmacology

The primary goals of medical therapy for IBD are to provide symptomatic relief, to reduce inflammation in the intestine, and to reduce the incidence of recurrent flares. Despite the variety of agents available for the treatment of IBD, none is ideal or accepted universally (Estiarte, Colome, Artes, & Jimenez, 2003). A combination of sedatives, antidiarrheal agents, and antiperistaltic medications are administered with a palliative goal. The use of corticosteroids in induction of remission of IBD has been shown to be highly effective and is well-established. Despite this, corticosteroids are ineffective in maintaining remission. The corticosteroids can be taken orally or parenterally in patients with acute exacerbations of IBD. Rectal corticosteroids are also given for patients to treat the distal colon disease.

Azathioprine (Imuran), an immunosuppressant and a thioguanine derivative, has become increasingly popular over the past 20 years and is now standard therapy in maintenance of IBD. Methotrexate has an established role in the treatment of active IBD and will induce remission in a significant proportion of patients with corticosteroid- and thiopurine-resistant IBD.

The role of antibacterials in IBD has mainly concentrated on treating active disease, but there is limited evidence for their use in maintenance of remission. Active IBD has been treated with oral metronidazole 200 to 400 mg three times daily, but this regimen is only marginally more effective than placebo. In addition, metronidazole appears to have an acceptable safety profile for use during pregnancy, although the efficacy of this agent in maintenance therapy of IBD has yet to be confirmed.

Surgery

When the nonsurgical methods of management fail, surgery is often recommended. More than half of the patients with IBD will have surgery during the course of their disease. A resection of the diseased portion of the colon is surgically removed, and because of the chronic nature of the disease, the patient may have multiple surgeries in their lifetime. Refer to the section on colon resection for specifics of the care of these surgical interventions. In addition, refer to the ostomy section in this chapter, as patients with IBD often require an ostomy intervention.

Evaluation of Outcomes

Potential patient outcomes for each of the example nursing diagnoses for the patient with IBD are:
- Chronic pain related to IBD. The patient should verbalize an adequate relief of pain along with the ability to realistically cope with the pain if it is not completely relieved.

Fast Forward ▶▶▶

Emerging Therapeutic Options for IBD

With the considerable advances in our understanding of the immunological mechanisms responsible for mucosal inflammation in IBD, an increasing number of therapeutic agents are being developed. These agents can be broadly divided into biological and nonbiological therapies. Of the nonbiological therapeutic agents, promising results have been offered by dietary manipulation, probiotics, and the newer immunomodulators. However, it is more difficult to discuss the maintenance role of some of the experimental biological therapies, as most trials in humans have concentrated initially on their role in active IBD.

- Diarrhea related to IBD. The patient passes soft, formed stool no more than three times per day.
- Nutrition imbalance, less than body requirements, related to IBD. The patient verbalizes and demonstrates selection of foods or meals that will achieve a cessation of weight loss and weighs within 10 percent of ideal body weight.
- Ineffective coping related to anxiety, lower activity level, and inability to perform normal activities of daily living. The patient identifies own maladaptive coping behaviors, available resources and support systems, describes or initiates alternative coping strategies, and describes positive results from new behaviors.
- Risk for impaired skin integrity related to compromised tissue perfusion. The patient's skin condition should be improved as evidenced by decreased redness, swelling, and pain.
- Fear and anxiety related to actual or potential lifestyle changes. The patient should be able to recognize the signs of anxiety, demonstrate positive coping mechanisms, and describe a reduction in the level of anxiety experienced.

Crohn's Disease

Crohn's disease is a chronic inflammatory bowel disorder with a relapsing and remitting course. Once remission is achieved, the main aim of the management of Crohn's disease is maintenance of that remission. Significant advances have been made into understanding the etiology and pathogenesis of inflammatory bowel disease. With these advances in understanding come increasing numbers of new agents and therapies, aimed both at active disease and the subsequent maintenance of remission in Crohn's disease.

Pathophysiology

Crohn's disease is a subacute and chronic inflammatory condition that usually begins with a small inflammatory lesion of the intestinal mucosa. Eventually, the inflammation continues and progression through all layers of tissue is seen. The deeper ulcerations, fissures, and granulomatous lesions persist into the deeper layers of the bowel wall. On examination, the affected bowel lumen has a cobblestone appearance with the inflamed areas surrounded by intact mucosa. These lesions are not continuous and are separated with normal tissue. As the disease progresses, the inflammation caused the bowel wall to thicken and become fibrotic and a narrowing of the intestinal lumen occurs. Fistulas are common between loops of bowel, as are adhesions of the diseased bowel areas. The absorption of nutrients is impaired as the jejunum and ileum are affected (Brookes & Green, 2004).

Assessment with Clinical Manifestations

The individual nature of the Crohn's disease allows for a wide variety of clinical manifestations. There is typically abdominal pain and tenderness that accompanies the disorder. Often the pain is relieved temporarily with defecation. In addition, eating can initiate the abdominal discomfort, and patients may consequently limit their food intake. This lends them to have nutritional deficits, weight loss, and experience malnutrition and even secondary conditions (e.g., anemia). Diarrhea is common and not necessarily positive for occult bleeding. There may be a palpable mass in the RLQ. Complications from Crohn's disease include ulcers, abscesses, fistulas, and intestinal obstruction. It can also affect other areas of the body including the joints, eyes, skin, and liver. A significant number of Crohn's patients undergo one or more surgical resections of the GI tract, causing disabilities and lifestyle changes.

Ulcerative Colitis

Ulcerative colitis is a chronic inflammatory bowel disorder that affects both the mucosa and submucosa of the colon and rectum. The patients with this disorder have exacerbations and remissions and have similar clinical presentation to Crohn's disease. The focus of care is supportive in nature; there is not a cure for ulcerative colitis.

Pathophysiology

The inflammatory process of ulcerative colitis begins at the rectosigmoid area of the anal canal. The disease destruction usually moves in a proximal direction but is often contained within the sigmoid and rectal areas. It is recurrent in its ulcerative and inflammatory nature, with abscesses in the submucosa, which spread and can lead to necrosis. Unlike Crohn's disease, the tissue inflammation and disease is continuous in nature as it affects the bowel. Eventually, the disease narrows the bowel with its inflammatory nature and shortens and thickens the bowel. The mucosa becomes reddened and ulcerated, bleeding easily and causing a loss of normal haustral movement (Brookes & Green, 2004).

Assessment with Clinical Manifestations

Ulcerative colitis is replete with exacerbations and remissions. The primary manifestations are diarrhea, abdominal pain in the left lower quadrant, and rectal bleeding. In mild cases, the diarrheal episodes may be fewer than five stools each day. As the disorder is more severe, the diarrhea may increase to as many as 10 to 20 bloody stools each day. The patient then is susceptible to a variety of complications that are secondary to bleeding and the nature of the inflammation. The chronic manifestations result in anemic symptoms, dehydration, fatigue, anorexia, weight loss, and generalized weakness.

Patients with continued ulcerative colitis may develop systemic manifestations, such as arthritis, skin and mucous membrane integrity debilitation, and uveitis or inflammation of the uvea. Patients may have problems with chronic clotting difficulties, which lead to thromboemboli formation.

The chronic loss of blood makes the patient at risk for chronic blood loss anemia (see chapter 29 for further descriptions of anemia). Therefore, the patient is monitored for tachycardia, hypotension, pallor, and follow-up on the level of serum indicators of blood loss (e.g., hemoglobin, hematocrit, or albumin).

The more severe complications of ulcerative colitis also include toxic megacolon and colon perforation. The toxic megacolon is a complication in which there is sudden motor paralysis and swelling of the colon that may affect all of the colon. The symptoms of toxic megacolon are fever, abdominal pain, nausea and vomiting, dehydration, and tachycardia. Perforation is associated with toxic megacolon and has a relatively high mortality rate from resulting peritonitis. In addition, there is an increased risk for CRC in patients with ulcerative colitis (refer to CRC section).

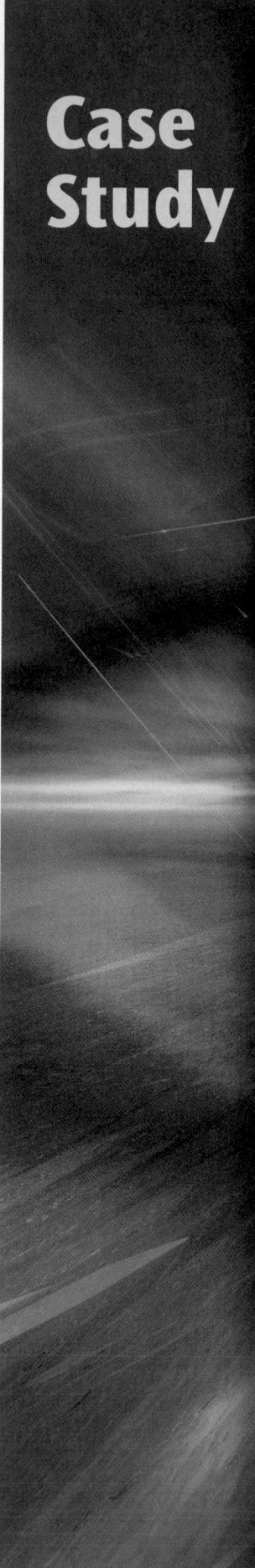

Case Study

Nursing Care Plan

Mr. Tony Gilliam is a 61-year-old old male who is admitted to the medical floor because of blood in the stool and abdominal pain for four days. He is going to be assessed primarily with a variety of laboratory and diagnostic tests. A review of systems reveals bowel habit changes, loss of appetite, weight loss greater than 10 pounds, and fatigue for nine weeks. Mr. Gilliam's past medical history includes primary hypertension, obesity, gastroesophageal reflux disease (GERD), and constipation. The patient's medications include HCTZ 25 mg by mouth every day, Omeprazole 20 mg by mouth every day as needed, and Metamucil as needed. The patient's nutritional intake is usually high in fat, low in fiber, and less than two servings of fruits and vegetables per day. His fluid intake consists primarily of sodas, tea, or coffee, and possibly two cups of water per day. Mr. Gilliam's activity is sedentary, and his social history includes working as a automotive mechanic for 31 years. He has been smoking cigarettes for 36 years, has an alcohol intake of four to six drinks per week, and denies the use of illicit drugs.

Assessment

Patient has gastrointestinal (GI) bleeding and recent history of abdominal pain. His vital signs are: temperature 36.9° C (98.4° F), pulse 74, respiration 18, and blood pressure 122/76. Bowel sounds normal on four quadrants; tympanic to percussion; no costovertebral angle (CVA) tenderness; pain elicited on palpation of left lower quadrant; palpable mass noted on left lower quadrant area. Patient's skin color is pink and has good turgor. Rectal exam reveals three-by-four-cm palpable lesion with stool positive for occult blood. Neurological system shows patient to be awake, alert, and oriented for three hours. A psychosocial assessment reveals him to appear nervous, quiet, and irritable; patient states he has not been in the hospital since his wife died 10 years ago.

Nursing Diagnosis: Acute pain related to colorectal mass.
NOC: Comfort level; medication response; pain control
NIC: Analgesic administration; conscious sedation; pain management; patient-controlled analgesia assistance

Expected Outcomes

The patient will:
1. Decrease pain level from 7 to 3 (on scale of 1 to 10) within 24 hours.
2. Relate an improvement of pain as evidenced by an increase in daily activities within 48 hours.

Planning/Interventions/Rationale

1. Evaluate pain frequently by asking patient to rate pain on scale of 1 to 10. *Provides ongoing assessment of pain that is measurable.*
2. Reduce or eliminate the factors that increase the pain experience. *Decreases overall pain response.*
3. Collaborate with patient to initiate noninvasive pain relief measures. *Broadens measures to decrease pain and incorporates nonmedication approaches to pain relief.*
4. Administer pain medications and assess response to the medications. *Provide optimal pain relief and reduces side effects.*

Evaluation

The patient verbalized that his pain was a 2 (scale of 1 to 10) within 24 hours. He took analgesics every four hours as ordered and had no side effects.

KEY CONCEPTS

- The small intestine (duodenum, jejunum, and ileum) functions as the major digestive and absorptive area of the intestine.
- The pancreas is an essential organ of digestion and produces copious amounts of digestive enzymes.
- The jejunum and ileum are the vital areas for absorption of nutrients: vitamins, amino acids, sugars, and triglycerides.
- The small intestine, which is divided into the duodenum, the jejunum, and the ileum, is approximately 600 cm in length and 1 to 1.5 inches in diameter.
- There are certain nutrients that are absorbed in the GI tract that must be considered as one is assessing the nutritional status of the patient when considering problems with digestion and absorption.
- The two primary pathologies for mal-assimilation disorders are mal-digestion and mal-absorption.

- Mal-digestion disorders are intraluminal disorders often from impaired hydrolysis of intestinal contents.
- Mal-absorption disorders are those which impair transport of intestinal contents across the mucosal membrane of the lumen.
- Describe the nursing management for a patient with an acute abdomen.
- Compare/contrast the acute inflammatory disorders of appendicitis and diverticulitis.
- Evaluate the management strategies of an obstruction of the lower GI system.
- Identify the interventions for patients with colorectal cancer.
- Describe the clinical manifestations of a patient with irritable bowel syndrome, and the associated treatments.
- Compare/contrast the inflammatory bowel disorders of Crohn's disease and ulcerative colitis.

REVIEW QUESTIONS

1. Intussusception that can lead to bowel obstruction is due to:
   1. Twisting of the bowel on itself
   2. A band of connective tissue compressing the bowel
   3. Telescoping of a loop of bowel into a lower loop of bowel
   4. Temporary paralysis of the bowel

2. Crohn's disease impairs the digestive process. Your assessment would include evidence of:
   1. Nausea and vomiting
   2. Weight loss and anemia
   3. Absence of bowel sounds
   4. Constipation and abdominal distension

3. Your teaching strategies for patients who have IBS would focus on:
   1. Lifestyle changes
   2. Bowel hygiene
   3. Dietary modifications
   4. Response to medications

4. IBS is best described as:
   1. A syndrome involving multisystems and many complaints.
   2. A cluster of vague abdominal complaints with no remission times.
   3. A functional bowel disorder with no signs of pathology present.
   4. The presence of diarrhea as the most prominent symptom.

5. Modifications in the daily diet to alleviate IBS symptoms include:
   1. A high soluble fiber diet.
   2. A diet low in fat.
   3. An increase in water intake.
   4. A high-protein diet.

6. An important change in lifestyle to aid in minimizing IBS symptoms is:
   1. Taking sips of cold drinks.
   2. Eating regular snacks.
   3. Drinking water with meals.
   4. Eating slowly.

7. The acidic chime from the stomach that flows into the duodenum is neutralized by the alkaline liquid secreted from the:
   1. Gallbladder
   2. Pancreas
   3. Jejunum cells
   4. Ileum cells

Continued

REVIEW QUESTIONS—cont'd

8. Which of the following neurochemical mediators has been implicated in the transmission of pain in the GI tract?
   1. Monoamine
   2. Epinephrine
   3. Serotonin
   4. Norepinephrine

9. In the United States and other developed countries, IBS is more prevalent in:
   1. Children
   2. Women
   3. Men
   4. The elderly

10. IBS symptoms can exacerbate following which of the events below?
    1. Anticholeric medications
    2. Weather changes
    3. Sexual activity
    4. Dietary intolerances

REVIEW ACTIVITIES

1. IBD has been linked to other illnesses such as multiple sclerosis, asthma, bronchitis, arthritis, and psoriasis. Access the MedicineNet.com at: http://www.medicinenet.com. (a) Review the information regarding the link of IBD to other illnesses; (b) review information on rectal bleeding, potential causes, location, and characteristics; and (c) prepare a brief patient teaching brochure.

2. Interview a nutritionist. Inquire what strategies are used to assist the individual diagnosed with Crohn's disease or IBS to modify the diet. Obtain a menu plan that outlines a typical daily diet. Use a cookbook to determine what recipes would be appropriate for the diet. Prepare a recipe pamphlet for the patient.

3. Develop a self-care teaching plan for a patient with a new colostomy. Discuss the various barriers that would affect the patient's and family members' learning to care for the colostomy. How would you determine whether they are coping with the changes in body function? What strategies can the nurse use to facilitate learning?

4. Research the etiology associated with peritonitis. Discuss the potential severe systemic effects and the usual clinical manifestations.

5. Research the etiology and risk factors for the development of herniations of the bowel. Develop a nursing care plan for a patient who has a surgical inguinal hernia repair.

6. Research information on the etiology and risk factors for development of hemorrhoids. What are the clinical manifestations?

Hepatic, Biliary Tract, and Pancreatic Dysfunction: Nursing Management

Valerie Lindquist Stalsbroten, RN, MC

CHAPTER TOPICS

- Hepatic System
- Hepatitis
- Hereditary Diseases of the Liver
- Cirrhosis
- Hepatic Abscesses
- Liver Trauma
- Cancer of the Liver
- Liver Transplantation
- Diseases of the Biliary Tract
- Pancreatitis

The hepatic, biliary tract, and pancreas are organ systems that have tremendous implications on the body. Each of these different organs has physiological functions that are vital to the body's health. If any of these organ structures is compromised, there are many consequences to the health of the individual.

KEY TERMS

Adducts
Ascending cholangitis
Ascites
Chemoembolization
Cholangitis
Cholecystitis
Cholelithiasis
Cholestasis
Gluconeogenesis
Glycogen hydrolysis
Glycogen synthesis
Gynecomastia
Hepatomegaly
Icterus
Jaundice
Kernicterus
Kupffer cells
Laparoscopic
    cholecystectomy
Liver lobule
Liver sweats
Refractory ascites
Sinusoids
Steatorrhea
Suppurative cholangitis

HEPATIC SYSTEM

The liver is the largest organ in the body. It is located directly beneath the diaphragm and is divided into the right and left lobes. The right lobe is the larger of the two. Directly below the liver are the stomach, pancreas, gallbladder, kidneys, and intestines. The liver is able to repair itself and regenerate damaged tissue to a certain extent. Although the liver is primarily considered when discussing the digestive tract, it is involved with over 400 metabolic functions necessary to a variety of pathways and is essential for life. Some of the vital processes of the liver are metabolism of proteins, carbohydrates, and fats; detoxification and filtering of foreign bodies, bacteria, and antigens; removal of old circulating red blood cells; synthesis of many substances (e.g., clotting factors, bilirubin, and cholesterol); and storage of substances (e.g., vitamins, minerals, and cholesterol).

The liver receives its blood supply from two sources. About 1,500 mL of blood travels through the liver each minute. The hepatic artery provides about one third of the incoming blood directly from the heart. This blood is well oxygenated. The portal vein supplies about two thirds of the incoming blood, carrying nutrient-rich but oxygen poor blood directly from the digestive tract. Blood in the portal vein is collected from the capillary beds, which drain the digestive organs (stomach, intestines, esophagus, spleen, and pancreas) and flows into the esophageal, splenic, pancreatic, mesenteric, epigastric, hemorrhoidal, and rectal veins. These veins are tributaries to the portal vein, which delivers the blood to the liver. Consequently, if blood flow is obstructed through the liver, these tributaries could also be congested. The portal vein is unique in its position between two capillary systems, collecting blood from the digestive organs and delivering it to the liver. If there is dysfunction of the portal vein, scarring or dysfunction of the liver or other impediments to blood flow, then the veins feeding into the portal vein can be affected.

The **liver lobule** is the functional unit of the liver. Each lobule consists of hepatocytes (liver cells) that are arranged in a hexagonal pattern around a central vein. Each hepatocyte has three surfaces: one faces the sinusoid or space of Disse, one faces the canaliculi, and one faces the other hepatocytes. **Sinusoids** are specialized capillaries found only in the liver and are identified by specific types of cells located there (Kupffer cells, hepatic stellate cells, and pit cells). Both the hepatic artery and the portal vein terminate in these sinusoid capillaries. **Kupffer cells** are specialized reticulo-endothelial cells of the liver and belong to the monocyte-macrophage system. They line the sinusoids, and their major responsibility is to phagocytize and filter bacteria, parasites, toxins, antigens, old blood cells, cellular debris, tumor cells, and foreign particles from the blood. As blood flows through the sinusoids, plasma moves into the space (space of Disse) between the sinusoids and the hepatocytes, generating significant portion of the body's lymph. The hepatic stellate cells, found in the space of Disse between the hepatocytes and the sinusoidal endothelial cells, are also known as Ito cells, lipocytes, and fat storing cells. Their major function is to process lipid molecules, especially retinoids. With injury, the hepatic stellate cells can relinquish their lipids and begin producing collagen. Blood flow and portal hypertension can be affected. Pit cells are highly mobile killer lymphocytes attached to the sinusoidal surface. They primarily eliminate tumor cells and virus-infected hepatocytes.

The liver is drained by two systems. A central vein carries blood from the liver lobules into increasingly larger veins. Blood that flows back to the heart from the liver is carried in the right and left hepatic veins. These veins join directly with the inferior vena cava (Figure 51-1).

The body needs available energy for biological processes and normal functioning. Carbohydrates in the form of glucose provide usable high-energy bonds for the liver and other organs. During the time of eating, nutrients can be distributed directly to the areas in the body requiring glucose. Some tissues,

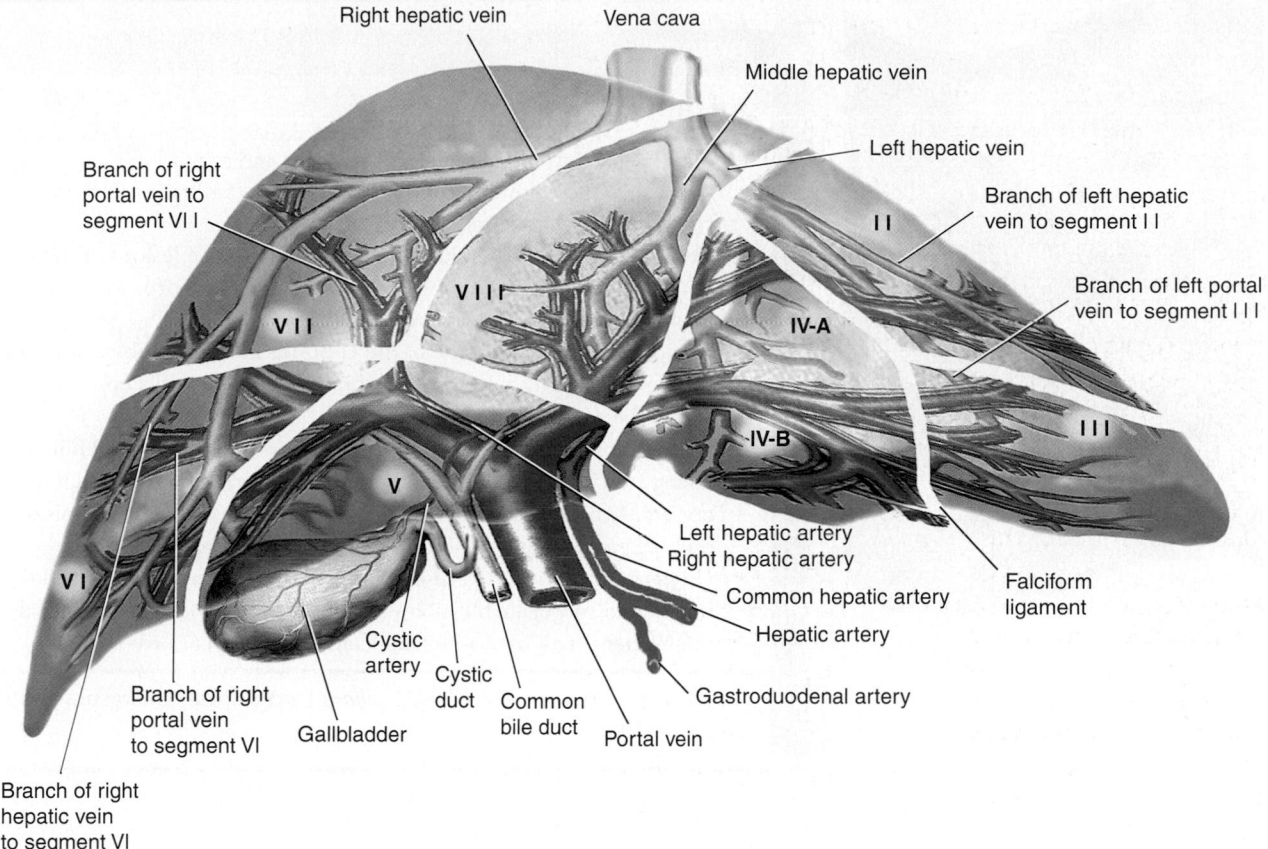

Figure 51-1 Segmental blood supply and ductal system of the liver.

such as muscle, can store limited supplies of fuel in the form of glycogen but only for future use by that organ. However, in the postabsorptive state and the fasting state, it is imperative that tissues have nutrients available for normal functioning. In particular, red blood cells and cells in the central nervous system require a constant level of glucose to function properly because these tissues are unable to store even small amounts of available energy supply.

When there is an abundance of glucose after a meal, the liver converts glucose to glycogen, which is stored in the liver, or to fatty acids, which are stored primarily in adipose tissue. A limited amount of fatty acids can be stored in the liver. During fasting this process is reversed, and the liver mobilizes the fatty acids, rendering them available as high-energy bonds in the form of glucose. **Gluconeogenesis** is the process of the liver converting predominant amino acids to glucose in the fasting state. Regulation of glucose metabolism in the liver is dependent on the concentration of glucose in blood coming into the sinusoids and the levels of insulin, catecholamines, and glucagons in the bloodstream. **Glycogen synthesis** is the conversion of glucose to glycogen, which can be stored in preparation of times of fasting, and **glycogen hydrolysis** is the conversion of stored glycogen into usable glucose to meet the immediate energy needs of the body.

There are a variety of substances that are metabolized in the liver. Each of these products has different effects on the body and is essential for their different functions. Bilirubin is a waste product of the breakdown of the hemoglobin molecule. Old red blood cells (senescent erythroid cells) are catabolized in the spleen, bone marrow, and liver. The hemoglobin molecule is further degraded, and the heme portion of the molecule is converted into bilirubin. Bilirubin binds loosely with albumin and is transported in the bloodstream to the liver, where the bilirubin is removed from the plasma. In the liver, the bilirubin is attached (conjugated) with another substance (glucuronide) so that it

Red Flag

High Bilirubin Levels

Bilirubin is an important indicator for liver and blood disorders (Box 51-1). High values of bilirubin cause jaundice, a yellowing of the skin and corneas. It is potentially damaging to neurological tissue and can cause encephalopathy and irreversible brain damage particularly in newborn infants with severe unconjugated hyper-bilirubinemia (Daniels, 2003).

BOX 51-1

BILIRUBIN LABELS

- **Jaundice:** Yellow pigmentation of the skin and sclera.
- **Icterus:** Yellow coloration in the sclera of the eye. It can be used synonymously with jaundice.
- **Kernicterus:** Yellow discoloration and degenerative lesions in the central nervous system (CNS) causing brain damage. Newborns with untreated jaundice may develop kernicterus.
- Phototherapy: Causes some of the H-bonds in the bilirubin molecule to become excited and this renders the molecule more water-soluble and able to be excreted.
- Encephalopathy: Can occur in newborns with unconjugated bilirubin of 20 mg/dL. The onset may be dramatic with refusal to feed, high-pitched cry, and hypertonicity. Survivors can suffer hearing loss, paralysis of upward gaze, mental retardation, and cerebral palsy.
- Crigler-Najjar disease: Recessive inherited disorder characterized by the inability to conjugate bilirubin. Patients display severe neurological impairments and have a life expectance of one year or less.

Adapted from Townes, D. A. (2004). Biliary tract disease. Emergency Medicine, *36(2), 17–19.*

---

can be excreted in the bile. It can be stored in the gallbladder or directly transported to the small intestine. Bacteria in the intestines breakdown the bilirubin into urobilin and is excreted in the feces. It is not uncommon for newborns to exhibit high bilirubin levels, because they lack the intestinal bacteria to adequately process the bilirubin in the gut or because of blood type incompatibilities and subsequent increased red blood cell destruction.

Conjugated bilirubin is also called direct bilirubin. Unconjugated bilirubin is not bound to another molecule and is referred to as indirect bilirubin. Total bilirubin lab tests reflect the amount of conjugated plus unconjugated bilirubin in the blood. In addition, bilirubin levels are particularly important when assessing newborns.

Bile contains bile salts, fatty acids, cholesterol, bilirubin, and other compounds. Albumin is a protein synthesized in the liver. It is the most abundant protein in the blood plasma and is responsible for transporting molecules, like bilirubin, and maintaining oncotic pressure in the intravascular space. Decreases in serum albumin indicate impaired liver activity or kidney disease, if the kidneys allow the protein to leak into the urine. Decreases in albumin could also reflect malnutrition or low protein intake, which may occur simultaneously with liver or kidney disease. When the oncotic pressure in the intravascular space in decreased, ascites and edema result. Cholesterol is a steroid that is primarily made in the liver, although some cholesterol is absorbed from the diet. It is important in the manufacture of estrogen and other hormones, cortisol, bile acids, and vitamin D. It is essential for the proper functioning of cell membranes. Estrogen is metabolized in the liver. When liver functioning is impaired, estrogen may not be removed from the bloodstream, exposing the body tissues to higher levels of this hormone. **Gynecomastia** (breast enlargement in men) can be a side effect of the buildup of estrogen.

Biliary Tract

The biliary tract is the other system serving the liver and is designed to drain bile. The production of bile is a major function of the hepatocytes. Bile is a fluid consisting of water, electrolytes, cholesterol, phospholipids, bile salts, and bilirubin. Bile is essential for fat emulsification and absorption. It is necessary for the digestion of fats and fat-soluble vitamins. Waste products may also be excreted in the bile fluid. Canaliculi are small, capillary-like structures that drain bile directly from the hepatocytes into increasingly larger bile ducts. Specialized cells lining the bile ducts are called cholangiocytes. The cholangiocytes can modify and reabsorb bile as well as secrete bicarbonate. Bile may be stored and concentrated in the gallbladder, which holds about 40 to 70 mL of bile. The gallbladder is drained by the cystic duct, which feeds into the common hepatic duct (which drains bile directly from the liver, bypassing the gallbladder). Together the cystic duct (from the gallbladder) and the common hepatic duct (from the liver) form the common bile duct, which carries bile that enters the small intestine at the sphincter of Oddi. Most of the bile salts are reabsorbed in the ileum and are, in turn, recirculated to the hepatocytes in the liver.

Pancreas

The pancreas is a long, thin glandular organ that is essential for digestion and metabolism. Two major types of cells are located in the pancreas: acini (exocrine cells) and islets of Langerhans (endocrine cells). Acini cells produce pancreatic enzymes that empty into ducts that feed into the duct of Wirsung. A second duct, the duct of Santorini may also be present. These pancreatic exocrine enzymes empty into the common bile duct through the ampulla of Vater, allowing them to enter the duodenum to aid in digestion. These enzymes are responsible for breaking down carbohydrates, fats, and proteins into smaller substances for absorption. The islets of Langerhans produce insulin (from the beta cells) and glucagon (from the alpha cells) and release these hormones directly into the bloodstream. These hormones are essential for regulating glucose metabolism (see chapter 57 for a discussion of insulin and glucagon). A third endocrine hormone has been identified. This is vasoactive intestinal polypeptide (VIP), and it affects gastrointestinal (GI) functioning.

The acinar cells of the pancreas produce enzymes that aid in the breakdown and absorption of proteins (proteases), lipids (lipase), and carbohydrates (amylase). Nucleases work on DNA and RNA. These enzymes are transported to the duodenum through the pancreatic duct. Because the primary goal is to break down tissues that are essentially the same as body tissues, protective measures are in place to protect the body from its own digestive juices. The acini package the proteases in an inactive precursor form (trypsinogen and chymotrypsinogen) and are activated by enzymes (enterokinase) in the intestinal mucosa. In addition, secretory vesicles in the pancreas have a trypsin inhibitor in case any digestive enzymes get prematurely converted to the active state and epithelial cells in the pancreatic duct secrete bicarbonate.

Diagnostic Tests

There are several ways to assess liver functioning. The nurse can physically palpate and percuss the liver as one method of assessing the size and location of the liver boundaries. In addition, serum tests are performed to screen patients with no symptoms (may be required for some insurance policy qualifications or prior to some procedures), detect disease, direct treatment, and monitor progress. Often liver enzyme assessments will be ordered before a patient is placed on certain medications that could be hepatotoxic. In addition to blood serum tests, bile fluid examinations, endoscopy, liver biopsies, ultrasound, computed tomography (CT), magnetic resonance imaging (MRI), nuclear medicine, angiography, and radiological tests can be performed (Nietsch & Kowdley, 2004).

Liver function tests (LFTs) are often ordered as a group. Usually these include albumin, total and direct bilirubin, alkaline phosphatase, aspartate transaminase (also known as AST or serum glutamic oxaloacetic transaminase [SGOT]), and

Skills 360°

Complications of a Liver Biopsy

Complications of a liver biopsy for the nurse to be aware of:
- Bleeding problems.
- Puncture of the kidney or intestines
- Puncture of lung with subsequent pneumothorax
- Puncture of the gallbladder
- Peritonitis

alanine transaminase (also known as ALT, glutamic pyruvate transaminase [GPT], or serum glutamic pyruvate transaminase [SGPT]). Further testing could include prothrombin time (PT) after receiving vitamin K, gamma glutamyl transpeptidase (GGT), ammonia (NH_3), amylase, viral studies for hepatitis antigens, isocitrate dehydrogenase (ICD), copper, and iron. Specific tests for genetic diseases may be available.

Liver enzymes can be elevated with conditions such as diabetes, obesity, autoimmune disorders, some viral infections (especially hepatitis), and some genetic diseases. Nonsteroidal anti-inflammatory drugs (NSAIDs), antibiotics, cholesterol-lowering medications, systemic acne medications, and antiseizure medications are some of the drugs that can alter liver enzymes. Alcohol is toxic to the liver and can initiate changes in the liver. The most helpful tests for the work-up of jaundice are alkaline phosphatase, AST, and ALT (Lam & Mobarhan, 2004).

The liver biopsy is used to procure a small sample of liver tissue to diagnose liver pathology. It is an invasive sterile procedure performed under local anesthetic. Ultrasound or CT scan may also be utilized at the same time to guide the practitioner in sampling the area of concern. A variety of disorders can be diagnosed, evaluated, or monitored with a liver biopsy, as identified in Box 51-2.

Nursing responsibilities require explaining the procedure to the patient, making sure that the patient has nothing by mouth (NPO) for 12 hours prior to the examination and making sure prothrombin and hemoglobin results are preformed and available before the test. Potential complications for the nurse to be aware of are listed in the Skills 360° feature.

The endoscopic retrograde cholangiopancreatography (ERCP) inspects the liver, gallbladder, and pancreas visually and radioscopically. A fiberoptic duodenoscope is inserted orally under general anesthesia into the duodenum. A small catheter is inserted into the common bile duct and pancreatic duct, and radiographic dye is introduced to visualize the liver, gallbladder, pancreas, and the different ducts. Bile sampling and interventions to remove stones from the ducts may be able to be performed at the time of the test. Potential complications of ERCP are perforation of the stomach, duodenum, and other ducts, pancreatitis, anaphylactic reaction to the contrast dye, aspiration of gastric contents, and reaction to anesthesia (Nietsch & Kowdley, 2004).

Nursing responsibilities include ensuring that the consent form, patent intravenous (IV) line, preoperative labs, and X-rays are available and instructing the patient to be NPO for 12 hours prior to the procedure. After the test, the patient remains NPO until the gag reflex returns. The nurse must continue to assess for signs of peritonitis, abdominal pain, nausea and vomiting, and septicemia.

Bile fluid can be procured by orally inserting a gastroduodenal tube into the duodenum. Fluoroscopic examination is used to confirm placement. Cholecystokinin is administered intravenously to make the gallbladder contract and release the bile, which is then sucked into a specimen trap. This test is done to assess cholecystitis, pancreatitis, parasites, and pancreatic carcinoma. Nursing care is similar to that for ERCP.

Bile salt absorption is a test that identifies unabsorbed bile salts in the feces and exhaled radioactive carbon dioxide in the breath after ingesting C-14 triolein. Presence of abnormal amounts of fecal fat indicates malabsorption of bile salts as well as diseases of the ileum or bacterial colonization in the gut.

Hepatobiliary scan utilizes radionucleotides, which are injected intravenously that are taken up in the bile. Sequential delayed imaging is necessary for 6 to 48 hours after initial injection. The patency of bile ducts is assessed as well as hepatocyte functioning. Acute and chronic cholecystitis, biliary obstruction, bile leak, and biliary atresia can be diagnosed.

The liver scan is a noninvasive test that utilizes IV radionucleotides and ultrasound. The ultrasound passes over the liver and spleen in the upper right quadrant, providing a three-dimensional picture. Hepatitis, cirrhosis, cysts, tumors, abscesses, trauma, and Hodgkin disease are some of the conditions that can be monitored by this technique.

A cholangiogram is an X-ray utilizing IV contrast materials to visualize the biliary ducts. IV cholangiography is being replaced by the ERCP. CT of the liver and biliary tracts may be used to visualize the ducts. Tumors, abscesses, iron overload, hepatitis, cirrhosis, radiation injury, and obstruction can be diagnosed.

Oral cholecystography is an X-ray that utilizes oral contrast material followed by X-ray. Gallstones and cystic duct patency can be assessed. This test has been replaced in some institutions by ultrasound.

Ultrasound of the gallbladder and biliary system is a noninvasive test to identify cholelithiasis and cholecystitis. If stones are seen, the patient may be asked to turn in various positions to ascertain if the stones are free-floating or obstructing ducts. Greater visualization is achieved with the patient fasting for 8 to 12 hours before the examination.

HEPATITIS

Hepatitis is inflammation of the liver. The most common cause of hepatitis is viral infection. Liver injury and subsequent inflammation can also occur from exposure to alcohol, drugs, toxins, and autoimmune conditions. Fatty liver can progress to hepatitis because of congestion creating inflammation (Ship, 2005).

Pathophysiology

There are three phases of hepatitis, which include preicteric, icteric, and posticteric (Box 51-3). The labels for these three phases are describing the level of jaundice seen in the patient.

Hepatitis can be either acute or chronic. Acute viral hepatitis occurs in the initial period after infection and symptoms are clinically similar for all viral types. Symptoms can range from subclinical asymptomatic infections to fatal acute infections. Traditionally chronic hepatitis has been considered to last greater than six months. Chronic hepatitis is identified by etiology, histology, and location. Only hepatitis B, C, and D are viruses responsible for chronic disease. It is not associated with hepatitis A or E. Other causes of chronic hepatitis include alcohol, liver-toxic substances (like carbon tetrachloride), prescribed medications (drug-induced), autoimmune diseases, and some hereditary diseases, such as Wilson's disease. Chronic active hepatitis (or chronic aggressive hepatitis) might occur after the acute viral hepatitis infection. Liver damage, patchy necrosis, and fibrosis contribute to liver failure and cirrhosis, and death often occurs within five years of onset. Fulminant hepatitis occurs in about 1 percent of infected people, mostly with hepatitis B virus (HBV) or HBV/hepatitis D virus (HDV) infection. This complication is characterized by aggressive progression of the disease, rapid deterioration, and marked liver necrosis. Acute liver failure ensues as the liver is unable to regenerate, and about 60 to 80 percent of these cases end in death (Soriano-Sarabia, et al., 2005).

Viral hepatitis is usually caused by RNA or DNA viruses identified as A to E. Other viruses that can cause hepatitis include non–A to E. Hepatitis F and G have been identified, but not much is known about them at this time. Hepatitis can also be caused by other viruses such as Epstein-Barr, yellow fever, herpes-simplex, varicella-zoster, and cytomegalovirus, although these are rare and are generally considered separate disorders. Table 51-1 offers information on the epidemiology and etiology of hepatitis.

Assessment with Clinical Manifestations

Nursing assessment should include extensive history taking. This would include asking about high risk behaviors, such as drug use, sexual behavior, sharing personal items, and living conditions. Other information should be ascertained, such as travel, exposure to possibly contaminated shellfish, restaurant patronage,

Text continues on p. 1708

BOX 51-3

PHASES OF HEPATITIS

- Preicteric (prodromal) phase is from the time of infection until the start of signs and symptoms, such as malaise, fever, nausea, and vomiting. Some smokers have an aversion to smoking as an initial sign. Joint pain and itching might also occur.
- Icteric phase is when jaundice sets in. Urine can be dark from increased bilirubin. Cholestasis may develop.
- Posticteric phase is the recovery phase when jaundice resolves and the liver starts to repair itself.

TABLE 51-1 Comparison of the Types of Hepatitis

VIRUS NAME TYPE OF VIRUS	SPREAD	PREVENTION/ VACCINATION/ GOOD HEALTH PRACTICES	WHO IS AT RISK	REPORTING PROCEDURES AND FOLLOW-UP	INCUBATION PERIOD AFTER EXPOSURE	SIGNS/SYMPTOMS AND DIAGNOSTIC TESTS	TREATMENT
Hepatitis A (HAV) RNA virus (picornavirus) of the enterovirus family	Fecal-oral route Close personal contact, including sex or sharing a household. Eating food or drinking water contaminated with HAV. Often shellfish caught in contaminated water could be the source. This is particularly possible when eating raw shellfish. HAV can be spread by food handlers infected with the virus.	Hepatitis A vaccine is available usually for people age 2 years and older. Always wash hands with soap and water after using the bathroom, after changing a diaper, before preparing food, and before eating. If hand washing facilities are not available, hand sanitizer should be used. Once infected with HAV, the person will be immune.	People living with infected people. Sex partners of infected persons. People traveling to other countries where HAV is common (everywhere except United States, Canada, Western Europe, Australia, New Zealand, and Japan).	Cases of acute HAV are reported to the public health authorities. Possible follow-up and screening can be done to prevent further infections from occurring.	15–50 days Average is 28 days	Usually the signs and symptoms are mild, viral flu-like symptoms. Some HAV can go undetected because the symptoms may be mild. Rare occasions, HAV can develop into fulminant hepatitis. People with chronic liver disease have a greater possibility of developing fulminating hepatitis. Jaundice is usually not evident. Anti-HAV is detected in serum to confirm diagnosis.	Immediately after exposure treatment is with immune globulin (IG). This is effective in about 85 percent of people if given within two weeks after exposure. After diagnosis, care is supportive, treating fever and flu-like symptoms. The disease usually resolves on its own. Avoiding alcohol is helpful because it can worsen liver disease. HAV has no known chronic carrier state and plays no role in the production of chronic hepatitis or cirrhosis.

Hepatitis B (HBV) or serum hepatitis. Double-shelled DNA virus. Virus has a core antigen (HBcAg) and a surface antigen (HBsAg).	HBV is transmitted through blood and body fluids (semen, saliva, or vaginal secretions) via skin and mucous membranes. Unprotected sex. Sharing needles and other drug paraphernalia. Mothers can inoculate the baby during the birth process. Accidental needle sticks.	United States strategy to prevent HBV infection is four-pronged: Prevent perinatal infection of infants born to HBsAg positive mothers. (This would require testing of mothers. This is recommended at the time that the pregnancy is confirmed. If this is not possible, then testing should be done at the time of delivery.) In addition, women who have clinically apparent hepatitis, multiple sexual partners, partners who are HBsAg positive, and women who have been treated for sexually transmitted diseases (STDs) or those who live in areas where there are high rates of HBV should also have	Health care workers and other persons in occupational groups that could be exposed to blood or body fluids. Inmates of long-term correctional facilities. Injection drug users. Sexually active men who have sex with men (MSM). Men and women who have more than one sexual partner in the last six months, have a history of sexually transmitted disease, or who have been treated in a STD clinic. Hemodialysis patients. Recipients of clotting factor concentrates. Long-term travelers. Patients and staff in institutions for the developmentally disabled.	Report all cases to the local health department. Partners of infected persons could be contacted and offered testing and treatment.	48–180 days The average incubation is 120 days. HBV is 100 times more infectious than human immunodeficiency virus (HIV) and 10 times more infectious that hepatitis C virus (HCV). Only about 30–50 percent develop acute HBV at the time of infection	Anorexia, nausea, vomiting, jaundice, fatigue, low-grade fever, arthralgias, rashes, light-colored stools, and dark urine are common. Infants often will have low birth weight, jaundice, lethargy, failure to thrive, abdominal distension, and clay-colored stools. Acute HBV may be mild or severe. About 15 percent of HBV infections progress to the chronic state. Liver biopsy may be done. Elevated aspartate aminotransferase (AST), alanine aminotransferase (ALT), bilirubin, PT, and LFTs are usually present. Usually HBsAg, Total anti-HBc, IgM anti-HBc, and Anti-HBs are tested to ascertain previous exposure to the virus or effective antibody	Immediate postexposure treatment Postexposure prevention with the HBV vaccine can be initiated within 12 to 24 hours with 70–90 percent success. Hepatitis B immune globulin (HBIG) can be administered within seven days of percutaneous exposure and two weeks after sexual exposure. Infants born to HBV-positive mothers should be given HBIG within 12 hours of birth, and hepatitis B vaccine should be administered before the child leaves the hospital and at one and six months after delivery. Testing for HBsAg and

Continued

TABLE 51-1 Comparison of the Types of Hepatitis—cont'd

VIRUS NAME TYPE OF VIRUS	SPREAD	PREVENTION/ VACCINATION/ GOOD HEALTH PRACTICES	WHO IS AT RISK	REPORTING PROCEDURES AND FOLLOW-UP	INCUBATION PERIOD AFTER EXPOSURE	SIGNS/SYMPTOMS AND DIAGNOSTIC TESTS	TREATMENT
Hepatitis B (HBV) or serum hepatitis Double-shelled DNA virus. Virus has a core antigen (HBcAg) and a surface antigen (HBsAg). —cont'd		their infants treated prophylactically. Vaccination of all newborns. Vaccination of all adolescents not previously vaccinated (usually required at the state level for all incoming middle-school–aged children). Vaccination of adults and adolescents in high-risk categories.	Babies born to HBsAg-positive mothers. Usually this happens during the birth process when the baby comes in contact with maternal secretions in the birth canal. Transmission across the placenta is unusual. Postpartum transmissions could occur through exposure to maternal blood, saliva, stool, urine, or breast milk. If a nursing mother has cracked nipples or other lesions on her breast, then HBV could be more likely to be transmitted.			response to vaccination. Another antigen, HBeAg, can reflect increased viral activity and subsequent increased infectivity. The presence of anti-HBe can indicate lower infectivity.	anti-HBs should be done between 12 and 15 months. In HBV endemic areas, prevention with HB vaccine should be standard practice for all newborns. After Diagnosis Interferon-alpha (injection three times a week) can decrease inflammation in 35–40 percent of patients. Lamivudine (orally daily) or adefovir dipivoxil (orally daily) may also be helpful, but further study is needed. Corticosteroids are contraindicated since viral replication is enhanced.

Virus	Transmission	Prevention	Risk Factors	Reporting	Incubation/Clinical Course	Diagnosis	Treatment
Hepatitis C (HCV) RNA virus.	Blood and plasma to skin and mucous membranes. Rarely it is spread by sexual contact. Rarely spread from HCV-positive mother to baby during the birth process.	No vaccine exists for HCV. Prevention efforts concentrate on standard precautions and infection control. Donor screening and product inactivation for blood and tissue products.	Intravenous (IV) drug users are at highest risk. People who received blood products or tissue transplants before 1992. Recipients of clotting factors before 1987. Tattoos and body piercings may be associated with increased infection, depending on sterilization practices of the practitioner.	All cases should be reported to the local health department.	14–180 days. Chronic infection occurs in about 85 percent of HCV-positive people. Chronic liver disease can develop in 70 percent of chronically infected people and can lead to cirrhosis, liver failure, and liver cancer.	Anti-HCV antibodies in serum. Influenza-type symptoms may be more severe than HAV.	Immune globulin is not proven effective immediately after exposure. After diagnosis, interferon, pegylated interferon, and ribavirin in combination are most effective. Hepatitis C patients with liver failure account for approximately 50 percent of all liver transplants.
Hepatitis D (HDV) RNA virus that needs the helper function of HBV to infect new hosts and replicate	Similar to HBV. IV drug users. Sexual partners of infected persons. People who have received blood products before July 1992 or clotting factors before 1987. It is possible for a mother to infect her baby during the birth process.	Preventing HBV also will prevent HDV. It is recommended that all persons be vaccinated. Standard precautions for all patients in the health care setting. Avoid contact with infected blood, contaminated needles, and an infected person's personal items.	See HBV list.	Report cases to the local health department.	14–56 days. Chronic hepatitis usually develops.	Coinfection symptoms are more severe than solitary HBV infection. Some patients are asymptomatic. Anti-HDV antibodies in serum.	Hepatitis preexposure or postexposure with hepatitis B immune globulin (HBIG) can be used. Chronic HDV is treated with alpha-interferon

Continued

TABLE 51-1   Comparison of the Types of Hepatitis—cont'd

VIRUS NAME TYPE OF VIRUS	SPREAD	PREVENTION/ VACCINATION/ GOOD HEALTH PRACTICES	WHO IS AT RISK	REPORTING PROCEDURES AND FOLLOW-UP	INCUBATION PERIOD AFTER EXPOSURE	SIGNS/SYMPTOMS AND DIAGNOSTIC TESTS	TREATMENT
Hepatitis D (HDV) RNA virus that needs the helper function of HBV to infect new hosts and replicate —cont'd	Coinfection is when HDV is acquired at the same time as the HBV. Super-infection is when chronic HBV patients acquire a subsequent HDV infection at a later date.						
Hepatitis E (HEV) RNA virus	Fecal-oral route. Most often associated with waterborne epidemics, especially in Asia, Middle East, Africa, and Central and South America. Eating food or drinking water contaminated with HEV. Often shellfish caught in contaminated water could be the source.	Hepatitis E vaccine is available usually for people age 2 years and older. Always wash hands with soap and water after using the bathroom, after changing a diaper, before preparing food, and before eating. If hand washing facilities are not available, hand sanitizer should be used. Once infected with HEV, the person will be immune.	People traveling to other countries where HEV is endemic (everywhere except United States, Canada, Western Europe, Australia, New Zealand, and Japan).	Cases of acute HEV are reported to the public health authorities. Possible follow-up and screening can be done to prevent further infections from occurring.	15–64 days.	The clinical course resembles that of HAV. Usually the signs and symptoms are mild, viral flu-like symptoms but can include jaundice, fatigue, abdominal pain, decreased appetite, nausea, vomiting, and dark urine. Some HEV can go undetected because the symptoms may be mild. Anti-HEV is detected in serum to confirm diagnosis.	Immediately after exposure treatment is with immune globulin (IG). This is effective in about 85 percent of people if given within two weeks after exposure. After diagnosis, care is supportive, treating fever and flu-like symptoms. Avoiding alcohol is helpful, because it can worsen liver disease.

	This is particularly possible when eating raw shellfish. HEV can spread by food handlers infected with the virus.						HEV has no known chronic carrier state and plays no role in the production of chronic hepatitis or cirrhosis. HEV is more severe in pregnant women, especially in the third trimester.
Hepatitis F (HCV) Hepatitis F (HFV) is possibly a variant of the HBV virus. Not much is known about the virus.							
Hepatitis G (HGV) or non-A–E hepatitis RNA flavivirus-like agent	Blood and plasma to skin and mucous membranes.	No vaccine exists for HGV. Prevention efforts concentrate on standard precautions and infection control.	IV drug users. Health care professionals and people who come in contact with infected blood products.	All cases should be reported to the local health department.	Chronic infection can occur.	Anti-HGV antibodies in serum. Influenza-type symptoms.	Supportive care after diagnosis Avoid alcohol because it exacerbates liver disease

recent body piercings and tattoos, occupational hazards, and alcohol consumption. Common diagnostic tests appear in Table 51-1.

Nursing Diagnoses

Based on the information gathered, examples of nursing diagnoses in the patient with hepatitis may include the following:
- Activity intolerance related to fatigue.
- Disturbed body image related to jaundice.
- Imbalanced nutrition: less than body requirements related to nausea.

Planning and Implementation

Many practices are in place to protect health care workers from various infections. Standard precautions must be practiced at all times. The ready availability of hand sanitizer in many settings helps decrease infection. The advent of needleless systems for administering IVs and medications has decreased needle sticks in hospitals and clinics. Requirements to have people vaccinated who have a high probability of being exposed to viral infection with hepatitis A (HAV) and HBV also prevent infection (Saldanha, Heath, Lelie, Pisani, & Yu, 2005).

Good health practices should be included in all patient education to prevent viral infection that could lead to the various types of hepatitis. This would include good hand washing after using the bathroom, before meal preparation, and before eating. Avoid raw shellfish. Avoid using anyone else's personal items like toothbrushes, razors, dental floss, nail clippers. Use condoms during sexual intercourse. Be sure of sterile practices before obtaining tattoos or piercings. If traveling, drink only water that is purified or treated. Peel fruits and vegetables before eating. Choose cooked food over raw vegetables. Be sure milk products are pasteurized. The patient should be encouraged to brush his or her teeth with bottled or purified water.

Treatment and nursing interventions focus on reducing the causative agent and addressing bothersome symptoms. For some virus-induced hepatitis, immune globulin or vaccination can be offered after immediate exposure. Other antivirals medications may be available. Promoting adequate physical and psychological rest is important. Diet therapy could limit fats and proteins. Often small, frequent meals are tolerated better than large meals, because hepatomegaly can reduce the capacity of the stomach. Increasing naturally occurring antioxidants in the diet is recommended. Vitamins and dietary supplements can improve nutrition. Often alcoholics eat sporadically, and their nutrition might be more compromised than people with nonalcohol-related hepatitis. Specific drug therapy is mentioned with the individual types of hepatitis. However supportive care can include antiemetics (however, prochlorperazine [Compazine] is avoided because of potential hepatotoxic effects). In all types of hepatitis, regardless of the cause, avoidance of alcohol is always helpful.

Evaluation of Outcomes

Potential patient outcomes for each of the example nursing diagnoses for the patient with hepatitis are:
- Activity intolerance related to fatigue. The patient maintains activity level within capabilities, as evidenced by normal heart rate and blood pressure during activity, as well as absence of shortness of breath, weakness, and fatigue.
- Disturbed body image related to jaundice. The patient demonstrates enhanced body image and self-esteem as evidenced by ability to look at, touch, talk about, and care for actual or perceived altered body part or function.

- Imbalanced nutrition: less than body requirements related to nausea. The patient verbalizes and demonstrates selection of foods or meals that will achieve a cessation of weight loss and weighs within 10 percent of ideal body weight.

Alcoholic Hepatitis

Inflammation of the liver can be caused by agents other than viruses. The most common nonviral source of inflammation is alcohol. Many factors work together in the presence of alcohol that can directly or indirectly cause inflammation to the liver.

Pathophysiology

The pathological factors that contribute to the development of alcoholic hepatitis are shown in Box 51-4.

Planning and Implementation

Treatment of alcoholic hepatitis can include corticosteroids to reduce inflammation; antioxidants to lessen the negative effects of free radicals; antibiotics to combat the increased permeability to intestinal bacteria; and vitamins and minerals to supplement the compromised functioning of the liver to synthesize and store needed materials.

BOX 51-4

PATHOLOGY OF ALCOHOLIC HEPATITIS

- Alcohol interferes with lipid metabolism, creating hyperlipidemia and fatty liver. This in turn can cause congestion and hypoxia, especially around the central veins.
- Long-term alcohol ingestion stimulates liver storage cells (stellate cells) to produce collagen, the protein that forms scar tissue, predisposing the person to fibrosis and resultant cirrhosis.
- Alcohol impairs the integrity of membranes surrounding the hepatocytes as well as membranes around organelles within the cells.
- In the presence of alcohol, prostaglandin and prostacyclin production is reduced. These molecules provide cell-protective functions in the healthy liver tissue, so cell defenses are decreased with alcohol.
- Production of thromboxane B_2 and leukotriene B_4 can increase. These molecules cause constriction of hepatic blood vessels and result in congestion and hypoxia, which leads to inflammation.
- Alcohol can cause an increase of cytokines, including tumor necrosis factor (TNF), which can cause damage to tissues directly and indirectly.
- Alcohol directly increases the permeability of bacteria and endotoxins in the intestine. Endotoxins are found on the outer membrane surface of some bacteria. Kupffer cells are activated by the endotoxins and in turn promote an inflammatory response, congestion, and hypoxia.
- Alcohol can increase the formation of free radicals, such as acetaldehyde. Some free radicals can bind closely with the patient's healthy tissues and create hybrid molecules called **adducts.** The body's own immune system might identify these newly formed molecules as foreign and subsequently launch an immune response to normal healthy tissue. These new hybrid molecules can also interfere with the normal functioning of hepatocytes. Normally, antioxidants in the body help to absorb or deactivate the free radicals, but antioxidants are reduced in the presence of alcohol.

Toxic and Drug-Induced Hepatitis

Inflammation of the liver can be caused by toxic substances and prescribed medications. Most hepatotoxins produce a dose-related effect of the liver, although other organs (especially the kidneys) might also be damaged. Substances that are toxic to the liver include carbon tetrachloride and other hydrocarbons and phosphorus. Amanita (psychotropic) mushrooms can be damaging. Medications that can have a negative impact on liver functioning are isoniazid, methyldopa, amiodarone, monoamine oxidase inhibitors, indomethacin, propylthiouracil, phenytoin, diclofenac, halothane (gas anesthetic), acetaminophen, and tetracycline (Broyles, Reiss, & Evans, 2007).

Autoimmune Hepatitis

Autoimmune hepatitis occurs when the body's natural immune defenses become sensitized to its own liver cells and start attacking hepatocytes and causing inflammation. This happens more to women (70 percent) than to men (30 percent). About half of those affected have other autoimmune disorders occurring, such as Grave's disease, ulcerative colitis, thyroiditis, proliferative glomerulonephritis, and autoimmune anemia.

Diagnosis can be with blood tests for antinuclear antibodies (ANA), antibodies against smooth muscle cells (SMA), and antiliver and antikidney microsomes (anti-LKM). Liver biopsy is definitive for autoimmune hepatitis.

Treatment focuses on slowing down the immune response with corticosteroids or azathioprine (Imuran). Other medications include mycophenolate mofetil, cyclosporine, or tacrolimus.

HEREDITARY DISEASES OF THE LIVER

Often, the many functions of the liver were identified when people presented with hereditary disorders that were traced to a defect or deficiency in liver metabolism. The following are some of the genetic disorders that emphasize the importance of the liver in bilirubin metabolism, copper and iron storage, enzyme production, and lipoprotein metabolism.

Crigler-Najjar disease, type I is a rare, recessive disorder characterized by the total inability to conjugate bilirubin. Most patients die within the first year of life.

Wilson's disease is an autosomal recessive disorder related to copper metabolism. Usually copper is secreted in the bile, but this is prevented in people with this disease. The copper accumulates over many years and is often diagnosed between the ages of 6 and 40. Excess copper can damage brain, eyes, kidneys, and red blood cells. Symptoms can include tremors, rigidity, inappropriate behavior, difficulty with speech, deterioration of work, and personality changes. Cirrhosis results from scarring of the liver. Those with this disease are at a greater risk for developing bone fractures, infection, and impaired kidney function. Some people may be diagnosed during an optical exam, if the examiner notices Kayser-Fleischer rings (brown, ring-shaped pigmentation) in the cornea. Blood and urine can be tested for ceruloplasmin, a protein that binds copper and is usually low in people with Wilson's disease. Liver biopsy would allow examination of liver tissue for copper accumulation.

Most people with Wilson's disease can be treated by avoiding foods high in copper (Box 51-5) and by taking metal-binding drugs (chelating agents). These include penicillamine (Cuprimine or Depen), and trientine (Syprine). Zinc acetate (Gatzin) helps interfere with copper absorption in the stomach and intestines. Liver transplantation is sometimes the only option left for treatment.

Hemochromatosis is the inherited tendency to extract excessive amounts of iron from food. The gene HFE is identified with this disorder. Eventually iron accumulates in the liver, heart, joints, testicles, and thyroid, creating problems such as cirrhosis, liver failure, liver cancer, congestive heart failure, cardiac arrhythmias, impotence, hypothyroidism, and diabetes. Initial complaints are vague, such as fatigue, decreased libido, amenorrhea, abdominal pain, and joint pain. Skin can become bronze or even grayish from the increased iron deposits in the skin. The iron can stimulate skin cells to produce more melanin.

A diagnosis of hemochromatosis can be made by assessing LFTs. When the LFTs are abnormal, the serum transferrin saturation (iron binds to the protein, transferring, in the blood) and serum ferritin (measures the amount of iron stored in the body) can be assayed. Liver biopsy can be used effectively for diagnosis. Several genes could be responsible for this disorder, although the presence of the defective gene is not a guarantee that the disease would be expressed. Genetic testing for the gene HFE is possible to identify the adult version of hemochromatosis. Juvenile hemochromatosis is caused by the gene called hemojuvelin. The cause of neonatal hemochromatosis is not yet known.

Treatment involves decreasing the iron load in the body by phlebotomy. Women often do not experience the effects of the disease until menopause sets in and the regular loss of blood stops. People should avoid foods high in iron, such as red meat, dried peas and lentils, and iron-enriched breads and pastas. Supplements with iron or vitamin C (this increases iron absorption) should be avoided. Discourage use of raw shellfish (increased possibility for infection) and alcohol (toxic to the liver).

Alpha-antitrypsin deficiency is an example of a genetic disorder that shed light on one of the many metabolic functions of the liver. This disorder affects the production of alpha-1 protein, which is produced in the liver and is then transported to the lungs. Its function is to neutralize enzymes that are released by white blood cells after pulmonary infection. If these enzymes are not neutralized, white blood cells continue to attack healthy tissue and destroy lung tissue after the infection is resolved. The alpha-1 antitrypsin deficiency creates problems in the liver, because the alpha protein is not utilized in the production of the alpha-trypsin. It then accumulates in the liver, causing congestion and can eventually lead to cirrhosis. Treatment is with alpha-1 proteinase inhibitor replacement therapy, Prolastin, which is administered intravenously on a weekly basis. However, the liver problems are still concerning, and patients need to practice good liver care by getting vaccinated for HBV and avoiding alcohol. In addition, they should avoid smoking to preserve lung integrity.

Abetalipoproteinemia is an autosomal recessive disorder of lipoprotein metabolism. People with this disease have difficulties absorbing fat from the gut, blood tests show absent low-density lipoproteins (LDL) and very low-density lipoproteins (VLDL) results, and triglycerides are almost undetectable. Total cholesterol is usually below 70 mg/dL. This presents problems with the utilization of fat-soluble vitamins but especially vitamin E, which is necessary for adequate neurological functioning. Red blood cells are deformed. Symptoms involve fatty stools, diarrhea, neurological dysfunction (ataxia, neuropathies, and other disorders), and failure to thrive in infants.

CIRRHOSIS

Cirrhosis of the liver is a chronic, progressive condition characterized by destruction of the liver cells and subsequent formation of fibrotic tissue that reconfigures normal, healthy liver tissue. This lack of elasticity causes blood, bile, and lymphatic systems to become congested and obstructed, and further damage is incurred. There are four major types of cirrhosis, which are differentiated by the underlying pathology. These include alcoholic cirrhosis (Laënnec's cirrhosis), postnecrotic cirrhosis (reflecting damage done by hepatitis infections in addition to toxic exposure), biliary cirrhosis, and cardiac cirrhosis. Alcoholic and postnecrotic cirrhosis account for the majority of people diagnosed with this disease.

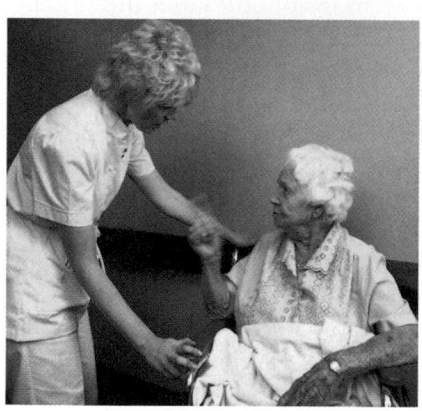

Figure 51-2 An elderly female is expressing hostility during a hallucination caused by alcohol withdrawal.

Alcoholic Cirrhosis

The destruction to the liver from alcohol often progresses from fatty liver to alcoholic hepatitis and culminates in alcoholic cirrhosis. However, some people develop cirrhosis without experiencing the other conditions. The effect of alcohol on the liver was outlined previously in this chapter. It should be noted that hypoxia, congestion, and inflammation provide conditions for fibrosis to occur. With infiltration by fat, leukocytes and lymphocytes, tumor necrosing factors, free radicals, and adducts further destruction is achieved (Kim, Wang, Jeong, Ahn, & Kim, 2005).

Epidemiology

Only about 50 percent of alcoholics develop cirrhosis. Hereditary, gender, and environmental factors influence development of serious disease (see Respecting Our Differences). Variations in different enzymes, such as alcohol dehydrogenase (ADH) and (ALDH), are implicated in some liver disease. ADH is primarily found in the liver, however, gastric ADH is also present to begin the digestion of alcohol when it is still in the stomach instead of absorbing the whole dose when it reaches the intestines. Genetic disorders coupled with heavy drinking can accelerate liver destruction.

Alcoholics with hepatitis C virus (HCV) develop alcoholic cirrhosis and liver problems at a younger age. Alcoholics who smoke greater than one pack per day have three times the rate of alcoholic cirrhosis. Interestingly, alcoholics who drink more than four cups of coffee per day have a fivefold lower incidence of alcoholic cirrhosis (Box 51-6). This is not because of the caffeine, because the same apparent protection does not hold true for equivalent forms of caffeine, such as tea (Rambaldi & Gluud, 2005). People suffering from alcoholism may experience a variety of mental health disturbances, such as clinical depression (Figure 51-3).

Postnecrotic Cirrhosis

Postnecrotic cirrhosis occurs most frequently in the wake of hepatitis infections. Hepatitis C is the predominant cause of viral-related cirrhosis, but often it takes several decades to develop. Chronic HBV and HDV can also cause cirrhosis. Autoimmune hepatitis, inherited diseases, and toxic or drug-induced liver damage can become necrotic and cause cirrhosis to develop.

Biliary Cirrhosis

Blocked bile ducts cause congestion, inflammation, and damage to the tissue in the liver. Some babies are born with biliary atresia, in which the bile ducts are absent or improperly formed, depriving the bile of avenues of exit from the liver and ultimately causing tissue damage. In adults, inflamed or blocked bile ducts can occur and scarring results. This can happen as a complication of surgery or trauma if the ducts are inadvertently injured.

Cardiac Cirrhosis

Cardiac or vascular cirrhosis occurs when blood flow out of the liver is restricted by severe right sided-sided failure. Tricuspid regurgitation can be associated with cardiac cirrhosis. Large amounts of blood are delivered to the liver each minute. When that blood is not able to exit at a predictable rate, liver engorgement occurs and the pressure in the liver vasculature increases, causing venous congestion, anoxia or hypoxia, and hepatic cell necrosis and subsequent fibrosis.

QUANTITY OF ALCOHOL CONSUMPTION

One drink is equivalent to:
- 12 oz beer
- 5 oz wine
- 1.5 oz distilled spirits or hard liquor

A heavy drinker would be one who consumes:
- 72 oz beer per day
- 1 liter of wine per day
- 8 oz distilled spirits per day

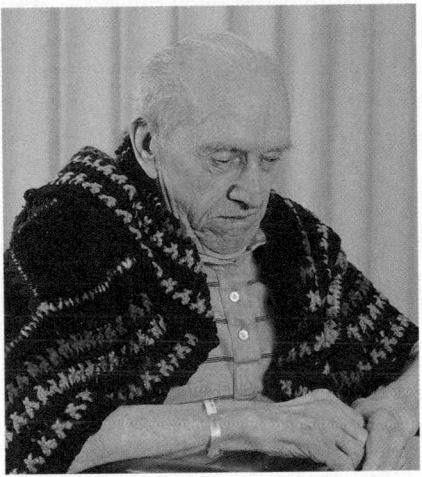

Figure 51-3 An elderly male suffering from alcoholism is clinically depressed.

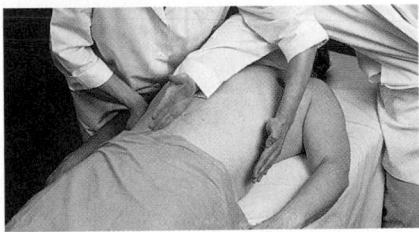

Figure 51-4 Assessing for ascites.

Pathophysiology

The pathophysiology of cirrhosis is multisystemic in its dysfunction. There are many complications evidenced in patients with cirrhosis. Some of the signs and symptoms that a patient has are irreversible, while other changes are reversible. The common complications of cirrhosis are discussed in the following section.

Ascites is the accumulation of fluid in the peritoneal cavity (Figure 51-4) and is seen as a common complication of cirrhosis. With the congestion of blood and lymph in the fibrotic liver, plasma can seep from the liver vasculature into the peritoneum. The term **liver sweats** refers to the movement of plasma from the lymphatic system into this potential space in the abdomen. When volume is decreased in the intravascular space because of plasma moving out, the body perceives this as low blood volume with the need to conserve water and sodium and makes the problem worse by increasing efforts to conserve blood volume (O'Brien, Chennubhotla, & Chennubhotla, (2005). **Refractory ascites** is that which cannot be effectively managed with normal therapies. Patients with refractory ascites are unresponsive to 400 mg of spironolactone (or 30 mg of amiloride) plus 120 mg of furosemide daily for two weeks. Refractory ascites could be caused by lack of compliance with the fluid or sodium restriction, spontaneous bacterial peritonitis, hepatocellular carcinoma, and renal failure.

When ascitic fluid becomes infected with bacteria in the absence of an obvious precipitating event, it is called spontaneous bacterial peritonitis (SBP). Increased fever or abdominal pain are typical, and polymorphonuclear (PMN) body count is greater than 250 cells/μL. It is possible for the peritoneal fluid to have negative bacterial cultures, and this is termed culture-negative neutrocytic ascites. Cefotaxime (Cefizox) is the antibiotic of choice.

With the destruction of liver tissue comes the impairment of the many metabolic functions performed by the liver. Some of the most important functions affected include:

- Storage of fat soluble vitamins. Vitamins A, D, E, and K are essential for many metabolic process that are compromised by decreased liver function.
- Synthesis of clotting factors (factors II, VII, IX, and X are all dependent of the fat-soluble vitamin K, which is not available with decreased liver function).
- Metabolism and transport of bilirubin is impaired. This negatively impacts digestion of fats.
- Regulation of gluconeogenesis, glycogen synthesis, and glycogen hydrolysis is compromised. Hypoglycemia and hyperglycemia can be serious.
- Cirrhosis causes resistance to insulin, and people develop type 2, insulin resistant diabetes.
- Ammonia metabolism where high levels of ammonia can have neurological symptoms. Portal-systemic encephalopathy can result.
- Lipid metabolism is impaired lipid and has a negative effect on cell membranes and organelle membranes. In particular, this can damage nerve cells.
- Albumin, the dominant plasma protein, is not adequately manufactured and can lead to fluid shifts and changes in oncotic pressure throughout the body and lead to renal vasoconstriction. Activation of the renin-angiotensin system causes more sodium and water retention, increasing general hypertension, exacerbating the original problem of portal hypertension and congestion. The problem of decreased plasma in the intravascular space can be a combined effect of mechanical issues. Blood is not able to move through the liver vasculature and squeezes plasma proteins into the peritoneal space. In addition, there are metabolic issues in which damaged liver cells have the decreased ability to synthesis albumin, the primary protein in blood responsible for maintaining oncotic pressure.

Assessment with Clinical Manifestations

Assessment is critical when caring for the person with liver disease. A constellation of signs and symptoms are listed in Box 51-7.

Planning and Implementation

Cirrhosis, along with the resulting ascites, can be treated with the following interventions: fluid restriction of 1,000 to1,500 mL per day, sodium restriction (limited to 200 to 500 mg per day), and diuretic therapy. Spironolactone (Aldactone) is the diuretic of choice because of its potassium-sparing properties. However, amiloride (Moduretic) or triamterene (Dyazide or Maxzide) may also be used. If the patient is compliant with the sodium and fluid restriction, furosemide (Lasix) may be added. Further management can be a paracentesis, peritoneovenous shunt, and transjugular intrahepatic portosystemic shunt. Paracentesis is the limited removal of fluid from the peritoneal cavity for diagnostic or therapeutic purposes. This can be performed at the bedside. It is most often used palliatively to reduce abdominal pressure, which can cause respiratory distress and abdominal pain. Fluid is removed slowly to avoid hypovolemic shock. The peritoneal fluid contains plasma proteins and electrolytes. Usually only 750 to 1,000 mL are removed at a time; however, larger volumes of 3 to 5 liters or more have been reported in the literature. Before the procedure, the nurse has the patient empty their bladder to decrease the

---

BOX 51-7

CLINICAL MANIFESTATIONS OF LIVER DISEASE

- Gastrointestinal (GI) findings include
  1. Abdominal discomfort, pain secondary to portal hypertension and ascites
  2. Anorexia and malnutrition
  3. Nausea and vomiting
  4. Clay-colored stools secondary to decreased bile formation or transportation
  5. Esophageal varices, hemorrhoids, and GI bleeding
  6. Fetor hepaticus (fruity-smelling breath)
  7. Gastritis
  8. Hepatomegaly
- Neurological findings include
  1. Asterixis
  2. Behavioral changes
  3. Changes in level of consciousness (LOC)
  4. Peripheral paresthesias
  5. Disturbed sleep patterns
- Cardiovascular findings include
  1. Cardiac arrhythmias
  2. Collateral circulation
- Pulmonary findings endocrine findings include
  1. Dyspnea
  2. Hyperventilation
  3. Hypoxemia
- Blood and immune system findings include
  1. Anemia
  2. Thrombocytopenia

  3. Splenomegaly
  4. Impaired coagulation
  5. Leukopenia
  6. Disseminated intravascular coagulation (DIC)
- Skin findings include
  1. Telangiectasias, spider angiomas on nose, cheeks, or torso
  2. Jaundice
  3. Palmar erythema
  4. Pruritus
  5. Caput medusae
  6. Increased skin pigmentation
  7. Petechiae
- Fluid and electrolytes findings include
  1. Ascites
  2. Edema
  3. Hypokalemia
  4. Hypocalcemia
  5. Hyponatremia
- Endocrine findings include
  1. Suppression of secondary sex characteristics in males, such as pectoral alopecia, changes in distribution of pubic and axillary hair
  2. Gynecomastia (in males)

possibility of injury to the bladder. Baseline vital signs, regularity of heartbeat (or electrocardiogram [ECG]), weight, level of consciousness (LOC), and abdominal girth need to be recorded. A consent form is required, so the nurse should allow for patient questions and ascertain the understanding of the procedure. During and after the procedure, the nurse needs to monitor the patient for hemodynamic changes, acid-base imbalances, and signs of electrolyte depletion. Cardiac arrhythmias may result from depletion of potassium or hypovolemia. Temperature is monitored to assess for infection, dressings are assessed for leakage, and urine is measured to ensure adequate output. The head of the bed can be kept at 30 degrees to allow for maximal respiratory expansion and minimize shortness of breath.

Surgery

When ascites continues to be a problem, a surgical shunt to divert excessive peritoneal fluid into the venous system may be attempted. A LeVeen peritoneovenous shunt (LPVS) diverts ascitic fluid via a pressure-sensitive one-way valve from the peritoneum to the internal jugular vein and ultimately into the superior vena cava. The movement of respiration helps to pump fluid through the valve. On inspiration, the diaphragm descends and increases pressure in the abdomen, allowing fluid to move toward the heart and reenter the vascular system. With the plasma proteins and electrolytes circulating, perfusion of the kidneys is improved, urinary output can increase, and there can be an increase in renal sodium excretion. Clinical improvements could include decreased abdominal girth, weight loss, and increased respiratory comfort.

The Denver peritoneovenous shunt (DPVS) is a variation of the LPVS in that it has a pump implanted subcutaneously, which can be manually compressed to open the unidirectional valve and allow for flushing of the tube connecting the peritoneum and jugular vein. This type of shunt did not improve the patency of the intrahepatic tubing. Unfortunately, patients with advanced liver disease and ascites are poor surgical candidates because of their increased abdominal pressure, potential to bleed, increased difficulties in metabolizing medications used in anesthesia, and their susceptibility for infection. Perioperatively, the patient may need antibiotics, blood products, vitamin K, and electrolytes.

Portal Hypertension

Portal hypertension is the constant pressure of the blood, bile, and lymphatics within the liver. This congestion can occur at the incoming sinusoid area (periportal or zone 1 of the liver), around the central vein that drains the blood from the hepatocytes (centrolobular area or Zone 3) or as it leaves the liver on the way to the inferior vena cava. When the blood meets with resistance, it tries to find other routes around the obstruction (collateral circulation). If this is not possible, all the vessels that bring blood to the liver are at risk for becoming engorged as well. It is this phenomenon that is responsible for other complications of cirrhosis such as:

- Esophageal varices—When the blood backs up, the vessels become distended, and in stretching, the walls become thinner and more friable. Varices can become life-threatening when these distended areas rupture and cause severe bleeding. Bleeding is usually caused by irritants (e.g., alcohol, gastric reflux, and some medications), mechanical insults (e.g., food, insertion of nasogastric tubes, or vomiting), and increased pressure or stretching caused by sneezing, vomiting, or physical exercise. It is possible for the patient to lose impressive amounts of blood when esophageal varices bleed. Hypovolemic shock is possible and constitutes a medical emergency.
- Splenomegaly.
- Hemorrhoids.

- Prominent abdominal veins (caput medusae).
- Bacterial translocation—When the veins serving the intestines become congested, there can be increased permeability of the membranes and bacteria may pass more freely into the bloodstream.

Nursing Diagnoses

Based on the information gathered, examples of nursing diagnoses in the patient with portal hypertension may include the following:
- Risk for infection related to portal hypertension.
- Activity intolerance related to portal hypertension.
- Risk for imbalanced fluid volume related to portal hypertension.

Planning and Implementation

There are many interventions for portal hypertension. In many instances, there is a need for surgical intervention as shown in the following section. Shunts to relieve the pressure in the portal vein created by cirrhosis were introduced as early as 1945. These original shunts diverted blood from the portal vein to the inferior vena cava, thus bypassing the fibrotic blockage that caused congestion in the liver. The portal tension was relieved, simultaneously relieving the pressure in the esophageal and gastric veins delivering blood to the portal vein. This was the first definitive surgical treatment for esophageal varices. The procedure fell out of favor in the 1970s because of an associated risk of encephalopathy and lack of clinical data that proved that survival rates were improved over nonsurgical therapy.

However, there were merits in relieving the pressure in the esophageal varices to prevent bleeding. The distal splenorenal shunt (DSRS) was designed to reroute blood only from the veins coming from the esophagus and stomach, while preserving the blood flow through the portal vein. The splenic vein was joined to the left kidney vein thereby selectively decompressing the esophageal and gastric varices. DSRS had a higher surgical mortality but less encephalopathy postoperatively. Patients with alcoholic cirrhosis do not do as well as those with nonalcoholic cirrhosis (Kim, et al., 2005).

A different shunting procedure is the transjugular intrahepatic portosystemic shunt (TIPS). A catheter is introduced by a radiologist into the jugular vein and advanced to the hepatic vein. The catheter is threaded into a large branch of the portal vein, and a stent is placed connecting the portal vein (bringing blood to the liver from the digestive tract) with the hepatic vein (returning blood from the liver to the heart). Advantages to this procedure include:
- Only a local anesthetic and mild sedation are used. (Many people with cirrhosis are unable to tolerate general anesthetics.)
- Major surgery is avoided. The TIPS procedure is tolerated better.
- TIPS reduces ascites in addition to relieving portal hypertension, but DSRS does not.

However, there are some disadvantages with this procedure as well.
- Encephalopathy is a postprocedure complication in about 25 percent of patients.
- If the patient is a candidate for liver transplant, this type of shunt can make transplant more difficult.

Sclerotherapy is the technique of injecting sclerosing drugs into the varices, causing a narrowing of the swollen veins, thus preventing bleeding and reducing swelling. This procedure is done endoscopically. If variceal bleeding reoccurs, the patient can still be offered a shunting procedure.

Evaluation of Outcomes

Potential patient outcomes for each of the example nursing diagnoses for the patient with portal hypertension are:
- Risk for infection. The patient remains free of infection, as evidenced by normal vital signs and absence of purulent drainage from wounds, incisions, and tubes. Infection is recognized early to allow for prompt treatment.

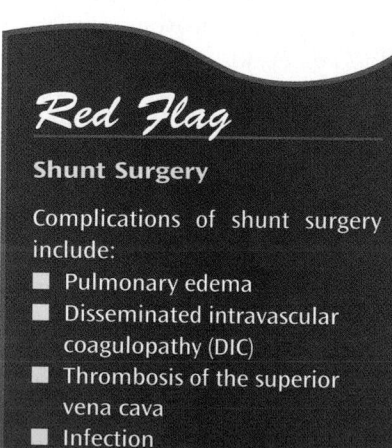

Red Flag

Shunt Surgery

Complications of shunt surgery include:
- Pulmonary edema
- Disseminated intravascular coagulopathy (DIC)
- Thrombosis of the superior vena cava
- Infection
- Blockage or dislodgement of the shunts

- Activity intolerance. The patient maintains activity level within capabilities, as evidenced by normal heart rate and blood pressure during activity, as well as absence of shortness of breath, weakness, and fatigue.
- Risk for excess fluid volume. The patient maintains adequate fluid volume and electrolyte balance as evidenced by vital signs within normal limits, clear lung sounds, pulmonary congestion absent on X-ray, and resolution of edema.

Hepatic Encephalopathy

Hepatic encephalopathy is also known as portal-systemic encephalopathy (PSE) or hepatic coma. This is a potentially reversible condition. Neurological symptoms include changes in LOC, slurred speech, behavioral changes and emotional lability, drowsiness, confusion, sleep disturbances, muscle twitching, progressing to rigidity, asterixis, and seizures.

Etiology

The causes of hepatic encephalopathy are from a combination of factors. Conditions that can precipitate hepatic encephalopathy include high levels of protein in the gut (both dietary and inadvertently through GI bleeding), hypovolemia, hypokalemia, constipation, and hepatotoxic medications.

Pathophysiology

It is already seen that impaired liver function can have a negative impact on the central nervous system by affecting the structure and functioning of cell membranes and glucose metabolism (with the consequences of interfering with cerebral energy utilization). When the liver is unable to perform its filtering and detoxifying functions, toxins can accumulate in the blood and eventually have an effect on the brain. However, hepatic encephalopathy is primarily linked to impaired metabolism of ammonia and other products of protein digestion. Protein is absorbed in the gut and intestines and transported to the liver, where it is catabolized into glutamine and ammonia. Ammonia is then used to form urea to be excreted by the kidneys. In addition, bacteria in the gut also produce ammonia. Increased membrane permeability makes it easier for products of digestion and bacterial endotoxins to cross into the portal vasculature. With compromised liver functioning, ammonia is not adequately converted to urea, and the levels of ammonia build up. Elevated ammonia levels are toxic to nerve tissue and cause the constellation of symptoms.

Planning and Implementation

Treatment for hepatic encephalopathy is focused on correcting the precipitating cause and reducing or eliminating dietary protein, preventing GI bleeding, and removing toxic enteric products in the intestines. Lactulose is a synthetic sugar that is used as a laxative. It works by pulling water into the gut to soften stool and increase peristalsis. It also helps to pull ammonia from the blood into the colon for expulsion. A range of two to four stools per day is recommended to treat high levels of ammonia. Oral neomycin can be administered to reduce the amounts of ammonia-producing bacteria in the intestines. IV antibiotics do not seem to have the same positive effect as the enteral route.

Hepatorenal Syndrome

Hepatorenal syndrome (HRS) is the evidence of progressive, irreversible renal failure in the presence of liver failure. Usually this is characterized by renal vasoconstriction and activation of the renin-angiotensin-aldosterone system (RAAS). In addition, there is a sudden decrease in perfusion of the kidneys and accompanying oliguria. The blood urea nitrogen (BUN) and creatinine levels can be elevated. It is not uncommon for serum ammonia and bilirubin to also be elevated. Two types of HRS have been identified. Type 1 is aggressive with rapid impairment of renal flow. Often this is associated with spontaneous bacterial peritonitis (SBP), even after infections appear to be resolved. Life expectancy after diagnosis is about 10 weeks. Type 2 HRS exhibits moderate, more predictable reduction of glomerular filtration. This condition has about a three- to six-month survival time (Gines, Guevara, Arroyo, & Rodes, 2003).

LECITHIN-CHOLESTEROL ACYLTRANSFERASE DEFICIENCIES

Lecithin-cholesterol acyltransferase (LCAT) is an enzyme that is synthesized only in the liver and is essential for cholesterol transport in the serum, lipoprotein metabolism, and lipoprotein structure. This enzyme has an influence on high-density lipoprotein (HDL), LDL, and VLDL levels, which impact cardiovascular functioning and subsequent disease. Diseases that affect the amounts of LCAT in the body have a profound influence on processes requiring lipoproteins. Hereditary disorders that caused the absence of LCAT helped to understand some pathways of lipid metabolism. People with familial LCAT deficiency are mostly of Norwegian descent and owe this condition to a recessive gene that, when expressed, manifests hypercholesterolemia, hyperphospholipidemia (high free cholesterol and phospholipids), and hypertriglyceridemia. Liver failure, renal failure, anemia corneal opacities, and atherosclerosis are common. Treatment is with fat-restricted diets.

FATTY LIVER (HEPATIC STEATOSIS)

The liver is the major organ for processing and storing fats (lipids). The three major types of lipids in the body are cholesterol, triglycerides, and phospholipids (the principle serum phospholipid is phosphatidylcholine, commonly known as lecithin). Lipids are usually hydrophobic (insoluble in water). The liver helps the lipids become modified with proteins to be more water-soluble for transportation in the blood. These new compounds are called lipoproteins. Lipoproteins are necessary for energy, membrane integrity, and synthesis of a variety of molecules needed in metabolic processes throughout the body.

There is a constant cycling of fatty acids between the liver and adipose tissue. As free fatty acid (FFA) concentrations in the blood increase, there is a similar increase of triglycerides synthesized in the liver. However, the liver has a limited capacity to oxidize and reesterify the fatty acids into triglycerides and VLDL, and when the capacity is exceeded and lipids account for more than 5 percent of liver weight, fatty liver results (Ristig, Drechsler, & Powderly, 2005).

Etiology

Certain conditions that can increase circulating fatty acids include obesity, pregnancy, poorly controlled diabetes, malnutrition or kwashiorkor, corticosteroids, prolonged treatment with total parenteral nutrition (TPN), as a side effect of some bariatric surgeries, and exposure to liver-toxic chemicals, such as carbon tetrachloride and yellow phosphorus. However, the most common cause of fatty liver is chronic alcohol ingestion.

Pathophysiology

Alcohol interferes with fat metabolism by causing lipidemia (especially triglycerides), stimulating lipolysis, and increasing the output of VLDL. Alcohol also can cause further damage through lipid peroxidation, which releases free radicals thereby impairing membrane integrity of organelles within the hepatocytes as well as the membrane surrounding the cell (Rambaldi & Gluud, 2005).

Assessment with Clinical Manifestations

Fatty liver can be categorized into two types, depending on the histology. Macrovesicular fatty liver exhibits large fat droplets that balloon the liver cell and push the nucleus to the periphery of the cell. The liver does not limit the amount of FFA it stores from the breakdown (lipolysis) of adipose tissue. Alcoholism, diabetes, and obesity are the most common causes of this type of fatty liver. In microvesicular fatty liver cells, small fat droplets fill the cells, the nuclei are not displaced, and the cells have a foamy appearance. Organelles (mitochondria, lysosomes, and endoplasmic reticulum) within the cells are negatively affected. This is most often seen with pregnancy, Reye's syndrome, and certain drug toxicities such as with valproic acid, tetracycline, and salicylate (Cua & George, 2005).

Macrovesicular fatty liver does not necessarily impair the overall functioning of the liver. It can be a reversible condition, if the cause can be eliminated. The most common finding of fatty liver is **hepatomegaly** (enlarged liver, palpated below the level of the ribs). Many people with this condition are asymptomatic, although some might experience right upper quadrant pain, tenderness, jaundice, and fatigue. Microvesicular fatty liver can be much more concerning clinically. In the early stages, patients can exhibit fatigue, nausea, and vomiting. Jaundice, hypoglycemia, coma, and DIC can result (Ristig, et al., 2005).

Diagnostic Tests

Diagnosis is confirmed by liver biopsy. In addition to specific serum tests, CT and ultrasound can also be ordered.

Planning and Implementation

Nursing care is supportive, depending on the symptoms. In addition, the patients should be taught to:
- Avoid alcohol.
- Follow low fat diet or the diet that is prescribed.
- Monitor signs and symptoms for new medications that might be ordered in place of medications that could exacerbate the fatty liver condition.

HEPATIC ABSCESSES

Hepatic abscess is an area of infection in the liver caused by bacteria, amoeba, or protozoa. This liver complication is relatively common, particularly in undeveloped countries.

Epidemiology

In the United States, Canada, and other developed Western countries the incidence is low, occurring in 8 to 16 people out of 100,000 and in men more than women by a ratio of 2:1. The vast majority of these cases is caused by bacterial infection and is referred to as pyogenic hepatic abscess. In the developing world, hepatic abscesses are much more common and are usually caused by amoeba and protozoa. Incidence is difficult to determine because of lack of access to health care and lack of systematic reporting and recordkeeping.

Etiology

The introduction of pyogenic bacteria into the liver is often (30 percent) secondary to extrahepatic biliary obstruction, such as cholangitis, choledocholithiasis, or biliary-enteric anastomosis, causing an ascending infection into the liver. Sometimes the infection can originate somewhere in the abdomen, with seeding of bacteria (e.g., *Escherichia coli, Klebsiella pneumoniae,* and streptococcal species) into the portal vein, which delivers blood from the digestive organs to the liver. Conditions predisposing to this include appendicitis, diverticulitis, inflammatory bowel disease, and proctitis. Systemic septicemia may be responsible for transporting an infectious agent to the liver via the hepatic artery (as in bacterial endocarditis), although this is rare. Injuries, such as stab wounds, blunt trauma or biopsies, can introduce infective agents directly into the liver. Even neonates have been known to develop hepatic abscesses following umbilical venous cannulation (Aggarwal, 2003).

Reports of hepatic abscesses attributable to *Mycobacterium tuberculosis* are rare. This type of infection probably occurs where milk is unpasteurized or if a tuberculosis patient swallows infected sputum into the GI tract. Infection by ameba and protozoa can present after amoebic dysentery. The causative agent is usually *Entamoeba histolytica.*

Pathophysiology

Obstructive liver disease and portal hypertension can increase the permeability of the membranes in the intestines, allowing infecting agents to enter the portal vein. Bacteria and amoeba enter the capillary system in the liver, where a local infection or abscess can flourish. Once established in the liver tissue, the infecting agent destroys liver tissue, creating a necrotic cavity filled with pus, leukocytes, and products of cell destruction.

Assessment with Clinical Manifestations

Signs and symptoms include fever and right upper quadrant pain. In addition, the patient may experience chills, malaise, pleuritic chest pain, right shoulder pain, anorexia, weight loss, hepatomegaly, and jaundice.

Diagnostic Tests

Lab work would include LFTs, complete blood count (CBC), PT, and blood cultures. Stool cultures identify amebic dysentery. Chest and abdominal X-rays can indicate the presence of gas and can help rule out other diagnoses. Radionucleotide (liver scan) studies can identify abscesses greater than 2 mm. Ultrasound and CT scans are helpful not only in initial diagnoses, but also with guided percutaneous drainage. Percutaneous drainage removes the fluid from the abscess. This fluid can be used to analyze the offending agent so more specific anti-infective treatment can be initiated.

Nursing Diagnoses

Based on the information gathered, examples of nursing diagnoses in the patient with hepatic abscesses may include the following:
• Acute pain related to hepatic abscesses.
• Hyperthermia to hepatic abscesses related to hepatic abscesses.
• Ineffective breathing pattern related to hepatic abscesses.
• Impaired gas exchange related to hepatic abscesses.

Planning and Implementation

Treatment employs anti-infective therapy and drainage of the abscess, either by percutaneous catheter (guided by CT or ultrasound) or surgery (which carries greater risk). Before blood and drainage cultures come back, patients may be started on metronidazole and clindamycin or Cipro. Third generation cephalosporins or aminoglycosides might be used. Percutaneous drainage works best when only one abscess exists. Multiple abscesses are more difficult to drain percutaneously. Left untreated, abscesses can rupture, causing 100 percent mortality rates. Surgical drainage would be performed if other abdominal surgery is required (such as appendectomy or cholecystectomy) or if the location of the abscess in inaccessible any other way.

Poor prognosis is associated with the patient being over 70 years old, having multiple abscesses, having more than one offending infective agent responsible for the abscesses, having malignant disease, and immunosuppression.

Nursing care focuses on ascertaining an accurate history from the patient, including travel history and alcohol use. Because the percutaneous drainage procedure can predispose the patient to pneumothorax, hemorrhage, and leakage into the abdominal cavity, the nurse must be alert to changes in the patient's condition that would indicate evolving problems. This would include changes in vital signs, difficulty breathing, and increased abdominal or chest pain.

Evaluation of Outcomes

Potential patient outcomes for each of the example nursing diagnoses for the patient with hepatic abscesses are:
- Acute pain related to hepatic abscesses. The patient should verbalize an adequate relief of pain along with the ability to realistically cope with the pain if it is not completely relieved.
- Hyperthermia to hepatic abscesses. The patient maintains body temperature below 39° C (102.2° F).
- Ineffective breathing pattern related to hepatic abscesses. The patient's breathing pattern is maintained by eupnea, normal skin color, and regular respiratory rate or pattern.
- Impaired gas exchange related to hepatic abscesses. The patient maintains optimal gas exchange as evidenced by normal arterial blood gases (ABGs) and alert responsive mentation or no further reduction in mental status.

LIVER TRAUMA

The liver is a large, solid organ fixed under the diaphragm. Because of its size, location, and vascularity damage can occur during blunt or penetrating trauma. It is second only to the spleen in being injured in blunt trauma to the abdomen. Most liver trauma in the United States is attributable to motor vehicle crashes and fighting. More men than women are affected.

Etiology

Liver trauma should be suspected if there is a history of the patient receiving an impact from the eighth rib to the middle of the abdomen. Steering wheels and seat belts can cause pressure on the abdomen during a motor vehicle accident (MVA). Often liver trauma occurs in conjunction with other abdominal trauma. About 45 percent of people with blunt liver trauma also have injury to the spleen, and rib fractures occur with 33 percent. Gunshots, stab wounds, shrapnel, and broken ribs can cause penetrating trauma.

Pathophysiology

The pathophysiology of liver trauma is that damage to the liver causes it to not function in its normal fashion. Consequently, liver trauma causes such things as changes in its metabolic functions, coagulation capabilities, and potential changes in the processes of gluconeogenesis. In addition, blunt the liver is so vascular, blunt and penetrating injuries can cause significant bleeding. It is possible for bile to leak into the peritoneal cavity and cause bile peritonitis.

Assessment with Clinical Manifestations

The patient will often feel right upper quadrant tenderness, pain, and nonspecific rebound tenderness. Clinical signs of blood loss and hypovolemic shock should be assessed at regular intervals. These signs include tachycardia, hypotension, tachypnea, diaphoresis, guarding of the abdomen, distension, rigidity, confusion, pallor, and cool, clammy skin. Some of these signs could also be seen with kidney or spleen trauma.

Diagnostic Tests

Lab tests may be nonspecific. Although LFTs could indicate liver damage, increased levels may just be indicative of previously undetected disease, such as fatty liver or alcoholic cirrhosis. An X-ray of the chest and abdomen could be ordered to assess for skeletal trauma, which could indicate associated liver trauma. CT scanning is extremely helpful in localizing site and extent of injury. It is possible to assess active bleeding and avoid unnecessary surgery. The iminodiacetic acid (IDA) radionucleotide study can assess for bile leaks. Angiography can also aid in evaluating vascular integrity.

Nursing Diagnoses

Based on the information gathered, examples of nursing diagnoses in the patient with liver trauma may include the following:
* Ineffective breathing pattern related to liver trauma.
* Acute pain as related to liver trauma.
* Deficient fluid volume as related to liver trauma.
* Ineffective tissue perfusion as related to liver trauma.

Planning and Implementation

Interventions for liver trauma include such things as IV fluid replacement and blood products. Bleeding may be stopped by introducing a catheter into the jugular vein, threading it to the liver, and placing a stent. Transcatheter embolization may also stem the bleeding. An exploratory laparotomy, suture placement, and liver resection might be necessary to stop bleeding. However, recent studies show that 86 percent of liver injuries have stopped bleeding by the time the patient reaches surgery. Treatment tends toward conservative clinical evaluation of hemodynamic status. Most people with liver trauma (80 percent in adults and 97 percent in children) are treated nonoperatively. Recovery may take 3 months for mild trauma to 15 months for more severe trauma.

Evaluation of Outcomes

Potential patient outcomes for each of the example nursing diagnoses for the patient with liver trauma are:
* Ineffective breathing pattern related to liver trauma. The patient's breathing pattern is maintained by eupnea, normal skin color, and regular respiratory rate or pattern.
* Acute pain as related to liver trauma. The patient should verbalize an adequate relief of pain along with the ability to realistically cope with the pain if it is not completely relieved.
* Deficient fluid volume as related to liver trauma. The patient experiences adequate fluid volume and electrolyte balance as evidenced by urine output greater than 30 mL/hour, normotensive blood pressure (BP), heart rate (HR) 100 beats/minute, consistency of weight, and normal skin turgor.
* Ineffective tissue perfusion as related to liver trauma. The patient should maintain optimal tissue perfusion to the periphery, as evidenced by strong peripheral pulses, good capillary refill, and good movement.

CANCER OF THE LIVER

Both benign and malignant tumors can form in the liver. The tumor is named based on the type of tissue from which it originates. In general, men experience more primary liver cancer than women. There is an increased incidence with chronic infections of HBV and HCV, cirrhosis, hemochromatosis, smoking, obesity, aflatoxins (fungal carcinogens found in peanuts, soy, wheat, corn, and rice), and inherited diseases, such as Wilson's disease and alpha-antitrypsin deficiency. Anabolic steroids also carry a risk of hepatocellular carcinoma.

Benign tumors do not metastasize. However, they may require surgical intervention, because they can compress other surrounding tissue or have the potential to burst and bleed. Hemangiomas begin in the blood vessels and hepatoadenomas start in the hepatocytes. Abdominal tenderness, liver mass, and bleeding can be evident. Focal nodular hyperplasia (FNH) can originate in bile duct cells, connective tissue, and hepatocytes.

Pathophysiology

There are two basic types of liver cancer: primary and secondary. These two type of cancer of the liver are described in the following section. Further specifics regarding the pathophysiology of cancer are provided in chapter 15.

Primary Liver Cancer

The most common type (75 percent) of malignant tumors in adults is hepatocellular carcinoma (HCC), also called hepatoma, because it originates in the hepatocytes. This is usually seen with multiple nodules in people with cirrhosis. People with cirrhosis have a 40 times greater risk of developing primary liver cancer than others without cirrhosis. HBV and HCV are also associated with increased incidence. Cholangiocarcinomas, or intrahepatic cholangiocarcinomas, account for 10 to 20 percent of primary liver cancers and begin in the small bile ducts located within the liver. Ascending inflammation from the gallbladder, ulcerative colitis, or chronic parasitic infection can predispose a person to this type of cancer. Angiosarcomas and hemangiosarcomas are the malignant cancers that form in the intrahepatic blood vessels, often as a result of the person being exposed to environmental carcinogens, such as vinyl chloride or Thorotrast. They grow rapidly and are frequently discovered at a point where therapy is ineffective. Hepatoblastoma is a cancer found in children under the age of 4. About 70 percent can be treated with surgery and chemotherapy with good results (90 percent survival with early diagnosis and treatment) (Toyoda, et al., 2005).

Secondary Liver Cancer

The liver is a major site for metastases, harboring and growing cancerous cells that originated in some other part of the body, such as the breast or colon. In most developed countries, this secondary type of liver cancer is more common than cancer that originates in the liver itself. This is not necessarily true for developing countries, where people may be more exposed to nutritional deficiencies, fungal infections, parasites, pesticides, and other carcinogenic agents (Kim, et al, 2005).

Assessment with Clinical Manifestations

Often patients present with epigastric pain, fatigue, anorexia, weight loss, and right upper quadrant pain. Jaundice, ascites, bleeding, and PSE can follow. Diagnosis can be made with ultrasound guided needle biopsy. A liver scan may be done first.

Nursing Diagnoses

Based on the information gathered, examples of nursing diagnoses in the patient with cancer of the liver may include the following:

- Anticipatory grieving related to the diagnosis of cancer.
- Caregiver role strain related to the disability associated with the liver cancer.
- Acute pain related to abdominal pressure.
- Imbalanced nutrition, less than body requirements related to anorexia, faulty absorption, and metabolism.

Planning and Implementation

Unfortunately, many primary liver cancers are fairly resistant to treatment. Often the disease has progressed far enough at the time of diagnosis that surgical resection is not helpful. However, techniques of ablation try to destroy the tumor without removing it. Usually, a thin catheter guided by ultrasound or CT is introduced into the tumor. Radiofrequency ablation (RFA) uses high energy radio waves and high-frequency alternating current to heat and destroy cancer cells. Percutaneous ethanol injection uses ethanol or alcohol to kill tumor cells. Cryosurgery freezes the tumors with liquid nitrogen and kills the cells.

Another technique to treat tumors that cannot be removed is to cut them off from their blood supply by injecting materials into the hepatic artery that causes it to block off. The hepatic artery apparently feeds most of the cancer sites. The healthy liver gets one third of its blood supply from the hepatic artery and two thirds from the portal vein. The catheter is introduced in the groin and threaded up to the hepatic artery via angiography. This procedure can be risky if infection or cirrhosis has already compromised liver circulation. Sometimes the embolizing drugs will be impregnated with chemotherapy drugs to deliver a concentrated dose directly to the area close to the tumor **(chemoembolization)** (Toyoda, et al., 2005).

Radiation

External beam radiation can be used to shrink the cancer, but this is often used palliatively to relieve pressure. More specific information regarding radiation therapy can be found in chapter 15.

Pharmacology

Doxorubicin (Adriamycin, Doxil, or Rubex) is the single most effective drug. Cisplatin (Platinol) and 5-fluorouracil (5FU) may also be added. Researchers are looking for more drugs that could be more targeted against liver cancer. Direct hepatic artery infusion (HAI) can deliver chemotherapy directly to the hepatic artery, allowing for the most concentrated doses to reach the tumor before the drug is detoxified by the liver.

Evaluation of Outcomes

Potential patient outcomes for each of the example nursing diagnoses for the patient with liver cancer are:

- Anticipatory grieving related to the diagnosis of cancer. The patient or family verbalizes feelings and establishes and maintains functional support systems.
- Caregiver role strain related to the disability associated with the liver cancer. The caregiver demonstrates competence and confidence in performing the caregiver role by meeting care recipient's physical and psychosocial needs.
- Acute pain related to abdominal pressure. The patient should verbalize an adequate relief of pain along with the ability to realistically cope with the pain if it is not completely relieved.

- Imbalanced nutrition, less than body requirements related to anorexia, faulty absorption, and metabolism. The patient verbalizes and demonstrates selection of foods or meals that will achieve a cessation of weight loss and weighs within 10 percent of ideal body weight.

LIVER TRANSPLANTATION

The first human liver transplant was performed in 1963, but the first successful liver transplant was done in 1967. With the development of newer immunosuppressive drugs to fight rejection of the implanted organ, liver transplantation has been considered standard practice since 1983. Liver survival rates depend on whether the recipient had an acute or chronic condition prior to the implant. Current survival rates for one year following surgery are 90 percent and for 5 years are 85 percent.

Etiology

There are many diseases and conditions that could be treated with a liver transplant, but the most common cause in the United States is cirrhosis due to hepatitis C. The most common reason for children to have a liver transplant is biliary atresia. In addition, reasons for treatment using liver transplantation are such things as alcoholic cirrhosis, cancer of the liver, ulcerative colitis, Crohn's disease, and various metabolic diseases. Over 17,000 people are on the waiting list to receive liver transplants at any one time.

Types of Liver Transplants

Two types of liver transplants can be performed, orthotopic and auxiliary. Orthotopic liver transplant, where the patient's own liver is removed entirely, is the most common type of transplant. This actually involves three operations:

- The removal of the donor liver, or in the case of a live donor, part of the liver. In the case of a cadaveric liver, the organ is usually removed at the institution where the donor died and is transported to the transplant center. For a living donor, the donor is usually in an adjacent operating suite. It is imperative to preserve the blood vessels and bile ducts to connect with the recipient's blood vessels and bile ducts. After removal, the liver is cooled, the blood is flushed out, and a preservative solution is instilled to replace the donor's blood. There can be ischemic damage to the donated liver during the cooling process.
- The removal of the recipient's liver is the most difficult operation of the three operations. People with liver disease needing transplant have difficulty with clotting, so they have a tendency to bleed. The portal hypertension and cirrhotic scarring makes dissection difficult.
- The implantation of the donated liver into the recipient. Once the blood vessels and bile ducts are connected the new liver should begin functioning. However, it is not unusual for there to be continued bleeding following surgery, and about 20 percent of patients need to be taken back to surgery to remove blood that has oozed into the abdominal cavity.

Auxiliary transplantation is a procedure that was developed in the 1980s and involves leaving part or all of the patient's liver in place and grafting in a healthy whole or partial liver, either from a cadaver or live donor. The auxiliary liver or liver segment regenerates and begins functioning. This type of surgery is used for patients who have genetic defects such as Crigler-Najjar syndrome and only one gene is unable to perform adequately, but that defect compromises the whole liver. In a syndrome such as this, the patient's own liver is able to function normally except for manufacturing the bilirubin gluconate, so problems with clotting factors and fibrosis are not present. The recipient is not totally dependent on the donated liver. Auxiliary transplantation can also be done in the event of major trauma to the liver, drug reactions, and fulminant liver failure, where there is a possibility for the patient's own liver to eventually recover. If the patient's own liver begins to work again, the transplant would not be necessary, and the patient would be able to stop the immunosuppressant drugs. It is technically difficult to attach the new liver to the patient's blood supply. And most postsurgical complications occur at the points of anastomosis.

Liver Donors

The live donor transplant program was developed in the late 1980s. There are several advantages. First it provides an organ for a specific individual. The operation can be planned for a time when both the donor and the recipient are in best health. The progression of liver disease and consequent deterioration may be avoided. The stress of waiting for an organ and living with the anticipation of sudden surgery is relieved. However, there are risks to being a living organ donor. The primary risks include the complications of surgery (Pierie, Muzikansky, Tanabe, & Ott, 2005).

Donor organs can be procured in one of two ways: (a) cadaveric organ, and (b) live donor. The specifics of both types of donor organs are provided in Box 51-8.

Liver Recipients

Criteria for receiving a donated liver is rigorously defined by the United Network for Organ Sharing (UNOS). This organization developed an online database, keeping track of all individuals waiting for any kind of transplant, matching donated organs to the list of waiting recipients, and managing time sensitive data. UNOS is a nationwide database that assists in the procurement of organs as well as the prioritization of patients around the United States. This prioritization utilizes the model for end-stage liver disease (MELD) and the pediatric end-stage liver disease (PELD) scores, which have replaced the older Child-Pugh score for predicting outcomes for survival after surgical procedures for end-stage liver disease (Ship, 2005). The conditions for prioritizing organ recipients are provided in Box 51-9.

When an appropriate match has been identified and offered to the institution where the transplant will take place, the institution has only one hour to accept the organ before it is offered to the next appropriate candidate on the waiting list. There is a great deal of stress and anticipation to being on the waiting list, and the nurse can assist the patient and family to deal with these issues during this time.

BOX 51-8

CADAVERIC AND LIVE DONOR METHODS OF PROCUREMENT

- Cadaveric organs come from people who have been declared brain dead, but other vital organs are healthy and have been adequately perfused. Sometimes the whole liver is transplanted into the recipient. However, the donor liver can be split, and the smaller left lobe implanted into a smaller person or child, and the larger right lobe would go to the larger recipient. Only about 4,000 cadaveric livers are available each year, so splitting the liver is beneficial for more patients but may be technically more difficult surgically.
- Live donor (living donor liver transplants [LDLT]) organs are usually donated to related family members (parents, siblings, or other relatives); however, organs can be donated by people who are not related, provided that the recipient is an appropriate match. The ability of the liver to regenerate makes it possible for the donor's and recipient's livers to grow to normal size after the transplantation surgery.

BOX 51-9

CONDITIONS TO PRIORITIZE ORGAN RECIPIENTS

- Appropriate parameters are met regarding size of the liver, ABO compatibility and MELD or PELD score.
- The amount of time spent on the waiting list.
- The degree of medical urgency.
  1. Candidates who have a life expectancy of less than seven days would include patients with fulminant liver failure.
  2. A person who has received a liver transplant in the last seven days, but the transplanted liver is nonfunctioning (defined as an aspartate aminotransferase (AST) greater than or equal to 5,000 and an international normalized ratio (INR) greater than 2.5 or acidosis with pH less than 7.3 or lactate of two times normal.
  3. Hepatic artery thrombosis in the first seven days of liver implant.
  4. Decompensated Wilson's disease.

Patients are asked to submit a complete list of pagers and telephone numbers to the transplant center so that individual can be notified in the event that a cadaveric liver becomes available. Patients also need to have travel plans worked out in advance in addition to how to pay for transportation. It is also important to keep as healthy as possible before transplant. This includes avoiding alcohol, eating a healthy diet, taking appropriate medications, avoiding recreational drugs, and following medical advice (Box 51-10). In addition, patients need to avoid other people with illnesses. Stress reduction and physical activity are also important (Pierie, et al., 2005).

Diagnostic Tests

All potential recipients and live donors undergo many tests, including psychological assessment to evaluate the decision to proceed with the transplant process. The living donor is evaluated for good general health, compatible blood type, and an altruistic motive for donating this gift of life. Tests for the donor include an abdominal ultrasound, MRI, blood tests, pulmonary function tests, ECG, and an exercise test.

Nursing Diagnoses

Based on the information gathered, examples of nursing diagnoses in the patient with liver transplantation may include the following:
- Risk for imbalanced body temperature related to complications of liver transplantation.
- Fear and anxiety related to actual or potential lifestyle changes.
- Knowledge deficit related to self-care and risk prevention.
- Ineffective coping related to anxiety, lower activity level and the inability to perform normal activities of daily living.

Planning and Implementation

The patient is notified when a liver becomes available. Usually the recipient carries a pager at all times so that the transplant center can notify the recipient of the new liver immediately. If the donated liver is from a live donor, both the donor and the recipient are in surgery at the same time. Usually the patient is in the hospital from one to three weeks.

Usually, the donor's first night after surgery is spent in the intensive care unit (ICU), then the donor is transferred to a specialized unit for recovery.

BOX 51-10

DISQUALIFICATION OF A TRANSPLANT RECIPIENT

Several conditions would eliminate or disqualify a person from being a transplant recipient. These include:
- Continuing to use alcohol or illegal drugs prior to surgery or being at high risk to begin engaging in these behaviors after surgery.
- Demonstrated noncompliance with previous medical care.
- Lack of support people to care for the patient after the operation.
- Advanced cancer of the liver or cancer that has metastasized to the liver. However, early discovery of primary liver cancer that is localized in the liver may be treated with transplantation.
- Advanced disease of the kidney, heart, vasculature, or lungs.
- Human immunodeficiency virus (HIV) or acquired immune deficiency syndrome (AIDS)

The usual hospital stay is four to seven days. Donors are usually recovered enough to go back to work in three to six weeks and are fully recovered in six to eight weeks. Expenses for the donor should be covered by the recipient's health insurance. Some complications that can occur after donation include unregulated proliferation of liver tissue and failure to regenerate new liver tissue, resulting in small for size syndrome.

Postoperative Care

In the postoperative period after transplantation, the most common problems include temporary decreased liver function, bleeding and hemorrhage, acute renal failure, bile leakage, hepatic artery thrombosis (HAT), fluid and electrolyte imbalances, infection and abscess formation, hepatitis recurrence, and acute graft rejection of the newly implanted organ.

Monitoring in the immediate postoperative period includes strict intake and output, paying special attention to measuring output from all drains placed during surgery. Abdominal ultrasound is performed often to assess for HAT, where a clot forms in the hepatic artery. These can be treated with medications or possibly surgery. A drainage catheter may be placed to manage bile drainage. Bacterial infection and the recurrence of HBV or HCV are other possible complications. While in the hospital, particular attention must be paid to vital signs for early signs of infection or rejection.

There is a high-risk period after transplantation that lasts for about three months. During this time it is important to avoid situations where the patient could be exposed to infection. This would include avoiding swimming in lakes and pools, avoid closed conditions, such as being in a movie theater, and avoiding adults and children who are sick or who have been immunized with live vaccine. The liver recipient is especially susceptible to infection because of the antirejections medications and because the liver is still establishing itself in the body. Throughout the rest of the recipient's life, the liver will be assessed for symptoms of graft rejection and the use of immunosuppressants will be continuous. It is imperative to abstain from alcohol. Recreational drug use should likewise be avoided. The patient should not self-medicate with over-the-counter drugs, because some of these could be hepatotoxic. Other long range problems can include diabetes, hypertension, and hypercholesterolemia. Usually the patient has monthly blood tests and assessment for organ rejection. Signs and symptoms of rejection include nausea, pain, fever, and jaundice.

Blood tests (serum bilirubin, transaminases, alkaline phosphatase, and prolonged PT) are usually ordered to assess liver function. A liver biopsy is necessary to determine if the liver is actively being rejected. If the liver was previously damaged from HCV or HBV, it is possible for the new liver to develop hepatitis C or B after the transplant. However, the HCV damage to the liver develops over a long period of time, and there are great benefits of having a transplanted liver (Pierie, et al., 2005).

Most patients can resume normal activity in 6 to 12 months. Women who have received liver transplants can become pregnant, but must be monitored closely, and the risk for premature birth is higher. Usually breast feeding is discouraged because the immunosuppressant medications can be transmitted to the baby through the breast milk.

Pharmacology

Immunosuppressive drugs used to decrease rejection of the new liver have problems with long-term use. In addition to the omnipresent threat of infection, these complications can include:

- Corticosteroids (prednisone) can predispose to osteoporosis, hyperglycemia, edema, and fluid and electrolyte problems.
- Cyclosporin (Neoral, Sandimmune, or Gengraf) can increase hypertension, growth of body hair, and kidney damage.
- FK-506 can produce headaches, tremors, diarrhea, nausea, kidney dysfunction, hyperglycemia, and hyperkalemia.

- Tacrolimus (Prograf) can cause seizures, GI bleeding, and anaphylaxis in addition to the side effects of ascites, hypertension, urinary tract infection, pruritus, rash, anemias, and generalized pain.
- Sirolimus (Rapamune) can cause leukopenia, thrombocytopenia, hyperlipidemia, arthralgias, and tremors.
- Mycophenolate mofetil (CellCept) can cause GI bleeding, diarrhea, vomiting, leukopenia, and sepsis.
- Basiliximab (Simulect) problems include heart failure, anaphylaxis, and wound complications.
- Daclizumab (Zenapax) can cause pulmonary edema.
- Azathioprine (Imuran) is related to serum sickness and can cause the patient to experience fever and chills, nausea, vomiting, anorexia, and pancreatitis.

Evaluation of Outcomes

Potential patient outcomes for each of the example nursing diagnoses for the patient with liver transplantation are:
- Risk for imbalanced body temperature related to complications of liver transplantation. The patient maintains body temperature within a normal range.
- Fear and anxiety related to actual or potential lifestyle changes. The patient should be able to recognize the signs of anxiety, demonstrate positive coping mechanisms, and describe a reduction in the level of anxiety experienced.
- Knowledge deficit related to self-care and risk prevention. The patient should demonstrate motivation to learn, identify perceived learning needs, and verbalize an understanding of desired content.
- Ineffective coping related to anxiety, lower activity level and the inability to perform normal activities of daily living. Patient identifies own maladaptive coping behaviors, available resources, and support systems, describes or initiates alternative coping strategies, and describes positive results from new behaviors.

DISEASES OF THE BILIARY TRACT

The biliary tract is devoted to transporting bile through the liver into the gallbladder and continuing on into the digestive tract. **Cholestasis** is any condition that impedes bile flowing freely through the bile ducts. This failure of bile flow can originate within the liver (intrahepatic) or beyond the liver (extrahepatic). When the bile is not flowing normally, patients usually exhibit:
- Clay-colored stools (because the bile does not reach the intestines where it is converted to urobilinogen, which normally gives feces the typical brown color).
- Dark urine (because an excess of bilirubin is in the circulation and is excreted through the kidneys).
- Jaundice (yellow skin and mucous membranes) and icterus (yellow sclera) also result from the increase in serum bilirubin.

Cholelithiasis

Cholelithiasis or gallstones, is a common problem, affecting about 16 to 20 million people in the United States, or 20 percent of the population. At least one million are diagnosed each year.

Epidemiology

Cholelithiasis is more common in people of northern European descent. Interestingly, 75 percent of elderly Pima Indians have evidence of gallstones.

Etiology

Cholelithiasis is more common in women, and the incidence is related to levels of estrogen. There are more reports of this condition with women on hormone (estrogen) replacement therapy (HRT or ERT) and those who are pregnant. The older, higher dose estrogen birth control pill had a higher incidence of gallstones associated with it. Medications that lower serum cholesterol can increase the occurrence of cholelithiasis. There can be familial tendencies for this condition, but this could also reflect a common diet, lifestyle, and genetics. Obesity is also related to cholelithiasis (Townes, 2004).

Pathophysiology

The most common gallstones are formed from cholesterol, which is a major component of bile. Stones may also be attributed to the calcification of bile pigments, but this is not as common. Stones can block or partially block the outlet of the gallbladder or move through the cystic duct into the common bile duct. **Cholangitis** is the inflammation of the bile duct and is usually attributable to the presence of gallstones. When the bile ducts become inflamed, there is increased edema, which, in turn, affects the circulation to the gallbladder by putting mechanical pressure on the capillaries. Increased edema can increase the permeability of the cell membranes and predispose the tissues to infection from bacteria from the gut. When intestinal bacteria infiltrates the gallbladder and ducts, an infection can be established. If the infection moves in the direction of the liver, it is called **ascending cholangitis.** If pus is produced in the biliary tract, it is called **suppurative cholangitis** (Townes, 2004).

Assessment with Clinical Manifestations

Most often the patient presents with complaints of pain in the midepigastric area, which can radiate to the right scapular region, anorexia, nausea, and vomiting. However, many people are asymptomatic, and the diagnosis of cholelithiasis is made incidentally when the patient has other tests performed. Fever, tachycardia, and hypotension can indicate the presence of infection, which can make the condition more serious.

Diagnostic Tests

The LFTs are often normal. Stones do show up on X-rays. Ultrasound is the most useful diagnostic test because the presence of stones, the motility of the stones, and the thickness of the gallbladder wall can all be assessed. This helps to determine if there is blockage in the biliary tract and if there is inflammation of the gallbladder secondary to the irritation of the stones.

Nursing Diagnoses

Based on the information gathered, examples of nursing diagnoses in the patient with cholelithiasis may include the following:
- Acute pain secondary to biliary obstruction.
- Ineffective coping related to nausea.
- Deficient knowledge related to diagnosis of cholelithiasis.

Planning and Implementation

The primary methods of treating cholelithiasis are surgery and medications. In addition, recommended nutritional programs with a low-fat diet, exercise, and follow-up with patients who have biliary tract manifestations are implemented.

Surgery

The treatment of choice is **laparoscopic cholecystectomy,** which is a surgical procedure using laparoscopy to remove the gallbladder. This operation was introduced in 1988, has a faster recovery time, fewer complications, and fewer bile duct injuries than the open cholecystectomy. In this operation, a small incision is made at the umbilicus plus three other puncture sites. Carbon dioxide gas may be pumped into the abdominal cavity to help to separate the organs, or there may be lifting and spreading devices that achieve the same effect without the gas. A laparoscope with video camera and laser technology is introduced. The gallbladder is dissected from the surrounding organs, drained of fluid and stones, and removed through the incision at the umbilicus. Only about 5 percent of laparoscopic attempts fail and culminate in open cholecystectomy. This happens when the gallbladder is anatomically inaccessible, the dissection to separate it from the surrounding organs is unsuccessful, or the surgeon is unable to remove the stones from the biliary tract. It should be noted that even after cholecystectomy, gallstones can still form in the biliary tree (Lledo, et al., 2005).

The open cholecystectomy can be performed when the laparoscopic technique fails, there are stones that are inaccessible to the laparoscope (Figure 51-5), or other surgeries are required at the same time (as in treating trauma). The surgeon makes an incision in the upper right quadrant beneath the ribs. Often the bile ducts and other abdominal organs will be explored. The gallbladder is dissected and removed, the cystic duct is ligated and a T-tube is inserted into the common bile duct to keep it patent. A Jackson-Pratt (JP) tube can be left in at the surgical site to drain fluid from around the area that housed the gallbladder.

Pharmacology

Nonsurgical treatment is possible utilizing bile salts, which help to dissolve the stones and get them back in circulation. This option is not popular, because it takes a long time to dissolve the stones, and there is more of a possibility that the problem will return. The drugs used in bile acid therapy are ursodeoxycholic acid (URSO, ursodiol, or Actigall) alone or in combination with chenodeoxycholic

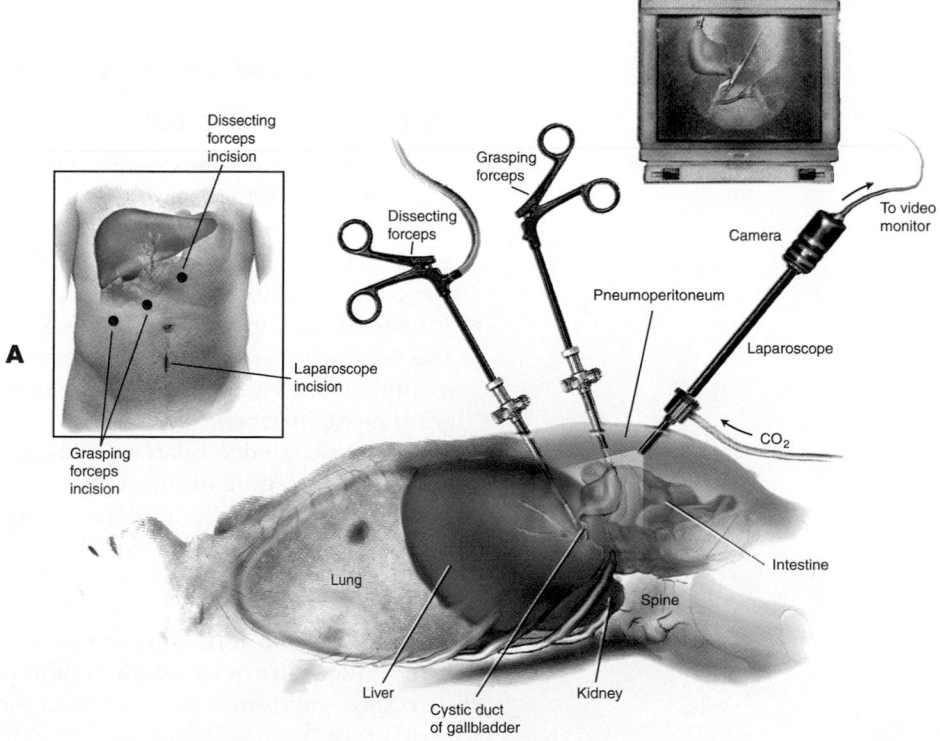

Figure 51-5 Laparoscopic cholecystectomy: A. Lateral view.

Continued

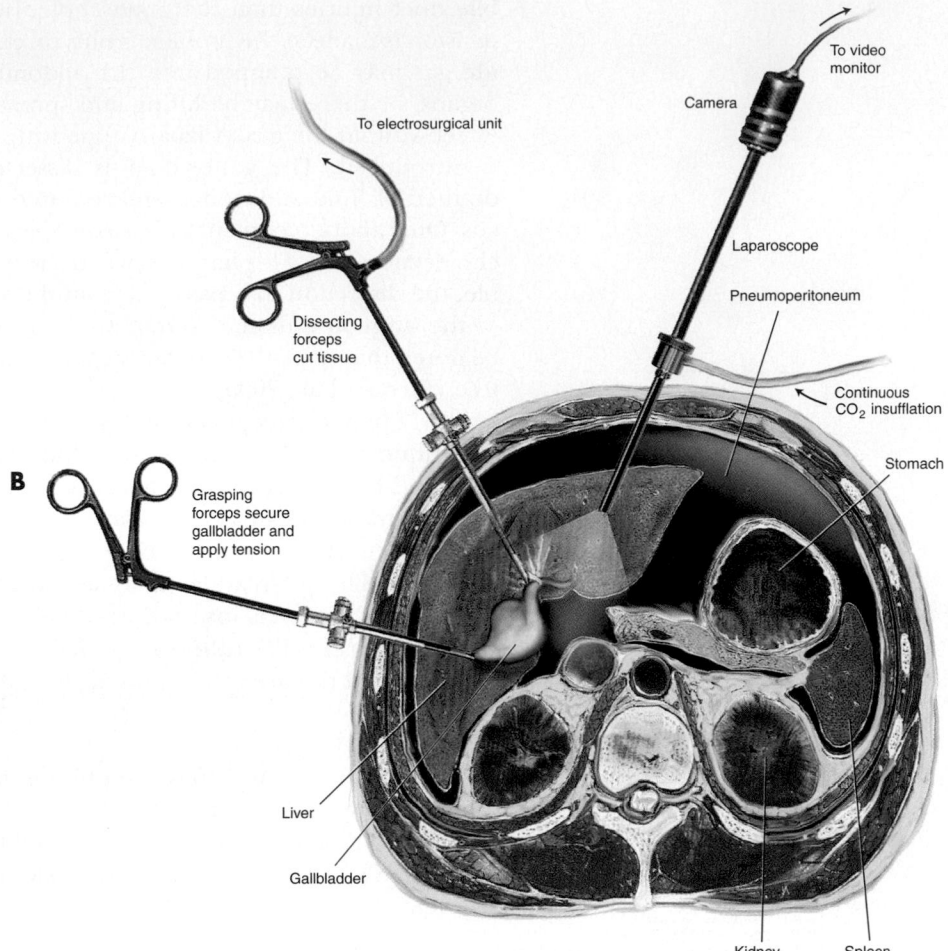

Figure 51-5—cont'd Laparoscopic cholecystectomy: B. Cross-sectional view.

acid (chenodiol, Chenix, or CDCA). Ursodiol may be used to prevent gallstones in people with a higher propensity for developing the condition.

Evaluation of Outcomes

Potential patient outcomes for each of the example nursing diagnoses for the patient with cholelithiasis are:

- Acute pain secondary to biliary obstruction. The patient should verbalize an adequate relief of pain along with the ability to realistically cope with the pain if it is not completely relieved.
- Ineffective coping related to nausea. The patient identifies own maladaptive coping behaviors, available resources and support systems, describes or initiates alternative coping strategies, and describes positive results from new behaviors.
- Deficient knowledge related to diagnosis of cholelithiasis. The patient should demonstrate motivation to learn, identify perceived learning needs, and verbalize an understanding of desired content.

Cholecystitis

Cholecystitis is the inflammation of the gallbladder. This can be acute or chronic and occurs in about 20 million people in the United States. In acute cholecystitis, gallstones are most commonly implicated, but bacteria can also cause the gallbladder wall to become irritated, a condition that is exacerbated by the increased presence of bile. Swelling and edema restricts the outflow of bile, which causes the distension of the gallbladder. Increased distension can alter the integrity and microcirculation of the gallbladder wall, causing sloughing, and possibly necrosis and gangrene. Perforation, rupture and peritonitis are possibilities. Chronic cholecystitis advances from the acute phase where the gallbladder is irritated and inflamed to the establishment of fibrotic tissue and contracted, inflexible capacity of the organ. This can be attributed to:

- Stones causing irritation and obstruction.
- Bacterial infection.
- Circulatory problems secondary to trauma, tumor impingement, shock, surgery, or dehydration.
- Pancreatitis (inflammation of the pancreas) can result if the biliary tract becomes inflamed, and the circulation or emptying of the pancreas is affected.

The epidemiology, etiology, pathophysiology, diagnostic tests, and nursing diagnoses are the same for cholecystitis as for cholelethiasis.

Assessment with Clinical Manifestations

Acute cholecystitis usually presents with pain and abdominal discomfort, which may be referred to the right shoulder. Because bile obstruction is not common, jaundice is not usually present. With chronic cholecystitis, inflammation of the organ is followed by fibrosis. Bile obstruction is more common and can result in inflammation of the bile ducts (cholangitis), the pancreas (pancreatitis), and jaundice. Increased bile salts lead to pruritus (itching).

The nurse should assess for history of pain and dietary discomforts, sleep patterns, and exercise routines. ERT and other medicines need to be assessed. The physical examination often reveals abdominal tenderness on palpation with rebound tenderness. **Steatorrhea** (fatty stools that float) may also be present along with the other classic cholestatic signs. In addition, nursing measures and evaluation of outcomes are the same as for cholelithiasis.

Primary Sclerosing Cholangitis

Primary sclerosing cholangitis (PSC) is of autoimmune etiology. Bile ducts within and outside the liver become inflamed and develop scar tissue. This results in the obstruction of bile flow. PSC is associated with ulcerative colitis and Crohn's disease and may share a common autoimmune mechanism. The incidence is greater with men than women. PSC often develops the fibrotic changes characteristic of cirrhosis. In addition to autoimmune causes, toxins and viruses are also being researched. Initial presentation of the problem includes jaundice and itching. Malabsorption of fats is evident by steatorrhea and a decrease in fat-soluble vitamins. Infection can set in from bacteria ascending the bile ducts from the intestines. Diagnosis is primarily by ERCP. MRI can also be helpful. LFTs, renal panel, and electrolytes would be ordered. The fat content in feces may be assessed. Medical treatment usually includes ursodiol, antipruritics, antibiotics, and fat-soluble vitamin supplements. Liver transplant is the only surgical option.

Primary Biliary Cirrhosis

Primary biliary cirrhosis (PBC) is characterized by inflammation and subsequent destruction of the bile ducts. Nine out of 10 cases are middle-aged women, although the incidence is low (10 to 12 cases in one million diagnosed

---

Skills 360°

Clinical Manifestations of Primary Biliary Cirrhosis

The nurse should observe the patient with complications of primary biliary cirrhosis for the following manifestations:

- Cholangitis with fever, chills, and pain.
- Ascending bacterial cholangitis.
- Septic shock is possible.
- Cholelithiasis is frequent.
- Problems related to fat metabolism and fat soluble vitamin deficiencies. Osteopenia and osteoporosis may occur, possibly due to vitamin D deficiency. About 12 percent of patients have vitamin D deficiency. Increased bleeding problems are associated with decreased vitamin K. Vitamin A may also be low, but overreplacement can also lead to problems with liver toxicity.

Adapted from Townes, D. A. (2004). Biliary tract disease. Emergency Medicine, 36(2), 17–19.

per year). Effects of hereditary factors, hormones, and the immune system are implicated in the incidence of PBC, because the occurrence of PBC is greater with people who have osteoporosis, arthritis, or thyroid problems. Although the disease is rare, it is more likely to occur in families where one relative has already been diagnosed (Prince, Christensen, & Gluud, 2005).

Pathophysiology

Pathology of primary biliary cirrhosis seems to involve the immune system, although the exact mechanism is unknown. Autoimmune factors can cause progressive inflammation. Destruction of the bile ducts predisposes to impaired transportation of bile from the liver. This congestion of bile creates cholestasis (decreased or inability for bile to flow through the bile ducts in the liver), which causes further hepatic injury and fibrosis.

Assessment with Clinical Manifestations

Patients are often asymptomatic in the early stages, but can exhibit increased alkaline phosphatase levels during routine screening tests for physicals. The most common complaints are fatigue and pruritus. Fever, abdominal pain, hepatomegaly, splenomegaly, and hyperpigmentation may also be present. Jaundice, variceal bleeding ascites, and encephalopathy are possible in the later course of the disease. At the time of diagnosis, many people do not have disease that has progressed to the cirrhosis stage, although untreated, destruction of the cells in the bile ducts will progress to fibrosis, and cirrhosis is evident.

Diagnostic Tests

Diagnostic tests include LFTs (especially alkaline phosphatase), PT, and antimitochondrial antibodies (AMA), all of which can be increased. Ultrasound and or CT scan are done to rule out biliary obstruction, and liver biopsy can be done to confirm the diagnosis. Magnetic resonance cholangiography may be employed. The ERCP is more definitive in diagnosing this condition, but it may be technically difficult to perform this test because of the sclerosing of the biliary ducts. Nursing diagnoses and evaluation of outcomes are the same as cholangitis.

Planning and Implementation

Complications include cholangitis with accompanying fever, chills, and pain. Septic shock could result. Aggressive antibiotic therapy would be required to treat this condition. Biliary tree strictures can be treated with cholangiography with balloon dilation of the narrowed duct. Biliary stone disease is possible. If the stones are only found in the gallbladder, the gallbladder can be removed. It may be necessary to remove the stone through sphincterotomy. Cholangiocarcinoma develops in about 10 to 15 percent of people with primary sclerosing cholangitis.

Pharmacology

Even if a patient is asymptomatic, it is important to treat the condition so that disease progression is arrested. Drug treatment focuses on reducing the immune response, modifying cholestasis, treating bacterial infections, controlling symptoms, and decreasing fibrogenesis. The medications to manage primary biliary cirrhosis are ursodeoxycholic acid (URSO, Ursodiol, or Actigall), which is a naturally occurring bile acid that can help to decrease the amounts of other more toxic bile acids; corticosteroids, which can be helpful in decreasing the autoimmune activity; cyclosporin, which is an antirejection drug, but can cause hypertension and kidney dysfunction; immunosuppressants (e.g., methotrexate, chlorambucil), which may be offered, but these can be damaging to the bone marrow; colchicine, an antigout agent, which interferes with white blood cells in initiating and perpetuating the immune response; aggressive antibiotic therapy; cholestyramine (Questran), which is usually recommended to control itching; and antiretroviral therapy (lamivudine or Combivir), which may be effective in arresting the disease (Broyles, et al., 2007).

Surgery

Surgical treatment for primary biliary cirrhosis could include:

- Cholangiography with balloon dilation of narrowed ducts
- Cholecystectomy
- Removal of gallstones through sphincterectomy
- Liver transplantation, which may be the only option for definitive treatment of end-stage disease (Allen, 2005)

Alternative Therapy

Alternative therapy for PBC can include treatment with silymarin. Silymarin is the active ingredient in milk thistle *(Silybum marianum)*. It is thought to protect the liver from toxic substances.

Cancer of the Gallbladder and Bile Ducts

Cancer of the gallbladder is rare. Incidence is higher with people who experience cholelithiasis, which is higher in Native American and Hispanic populations.

Epidemiology

Risk factors for cancer of the gallbladder include age (usually people are over age 60 when diagnosed with gallbladder cancer), bile duct abnormalities (this can predispose to increased irritation of the organs that come in contact with the toxins from the liver), cigarette smoke, chemicals (especially asbestos and azotoluene), and obesity. Women are twice as likely as men to get gallbladder cancer.

Cancer of the biliary ducts is also rare. Risk factors include primary sclerosing cholangitis (cholangiocarcinoma develops in about 10 to 15 percent of people with primary sclerosing cholangitis), ulcerative colitis, congenital abnormalities of the biliary tract (such as biliary atresia), gallstones in the bile ducts, parasitic infections, and toxic materials. In contrast to gallbladder cancer, men are slightly more likely to develop cancer of the bile ducts than women.

Assessment with Clinical Manifestations

Clinical manifestations for cancer of the gallbladder are varied. In addition, the symptomatology may be minimal to severe. Some of the manifestations may be: abdominal pain, especially in the upper right quadrant, anorexia, weight loss, nausea and vomiting, jaundice, pruritus, and an enlarged gallbladder.

Pathophysiology

Cancers within the gallbladder usually begin in the lining of the wall and are adenocarcinomas. Cancers that start in the bile ducts are cholangiocarcinomas. It is thought that the cells in the gallbladder and bile ducts can be damaged by toxins that come from the liver. Cholelithiasis and cholestasis may establish conditions that make these toxins more irritating, progressing to cancer.

Diagnostic Tests

Diagnostic tests include LFTs, ultrasound, CT scan, MRI, and ERCP. Laparoscopy and biopsies may be performed. However, many cancers are diagnosed after the gallbladder has already been removed for treatment of cholelithiasis. The nursing diagnoses and evaluation of outcomes is the same as those for cholangitis.

If the gallbladder has not been removed prior to diagnosing, the cancer may be designated as:

- Resectable, which means that the cancer is contained within the walls of the organ and has not invaded surrounding organs or traveled in the lymph to the nodes.
- Unresectable, which indicates that the cancer has spread to other organs, such as the liver stomach, pancreas, or intestines, and surgical removal would not be beneficial. The cancer could also invade the lymph system.
- Recurrent, which refers to cancer that has been treated or resected but reoccurs at a later time in other tissue.

Planning and Implementation

Treatment is generally by surgery. In addition to removing the areas of cancerous growth, stents can be placed as a palliative measure to keep the biliary tract open. When the tumor is too close to other blood vessels or vital organs, bypass surgeries may help to alleviate some symptoms but are not curative. Radiation and chemotherapy do not have a lot to offer at this time (Allen, 2005).

PANCREATITIS

Pancreatitis is the inflammation of the pancreas, a specialized digestive gland that has both endocrine and exocrine functions. Pancreatitis can take two forms, acute and chronic. Both disorders of the pancreas can be complicating to patients who have these conditions. There are complications for both anomalies of the pancreas and can provide a challenge to the health care providers as management strategies are performed.

Acute Pancreatitis

Acute pancreatitis is a serious but reversible condition that may become chronic if permanent scarring and damage to the pancreatic tissue occurs. It affects about 80,000 people each year in the United States. Mild cases of acute pancreatitis can resolve with resting the gut (NPO), IV hydration and electrolyte replacement, pain control, and bed rest. However, in about 20 percent of cases, serious problems can develop and involve local and systemic damage to tissues. There is a 5 to 10 percent mortality rate in hospitalized patients.

Etiology

Pancreatitis has many causes and a wide variety of resulting complications. The major causes of pancreatitis include: gallstone disease, alcoholism, infections (e.g., ascariasis, clonorchiasis, mumps, toxoplasmosis, coxsackievirus, cytomegalovirus, or tuberculosis), medications (e.g., azathioprine, mercaptopurine, sulfonamides, salicylates, furosemide, or methyldopa), trauma, obstruction, duodenal diseases, toxins, and genetic diseases that predispose the patient to cholelithiasis and obstruction of the biliary ducts, and cystic fibrosis.

Pathophysiology

The pathophysiology for pancreatitis relates to either the presence of gallstones or alcoholism. However, in about 10 to 30 percent of cases, no cause can be identified and is considered idiopathic. Whatever the initial cause of the inflammation, the exocrine enzymes that are produced in the acinar cells of the pancreas and help with digesting protein, carbohydrates, and fats can be prematurely activated, exacerbating the process leading to autodigestion of the surrounding tissues and more inflammation, edema, and ultimately necrosis. The edema compromises the microcirculation of the pancreas and initiates the release of cytokines, such as tumor necrosis factor (TNF), interleukin-1, and platelet-activating factor, all of which contribute to further damage in the pancreas and in other tissues.

Assessment with Clinical Manifestations

With the release of these cytokines and the exocrine and endocrine (insulin, glucagon, and VIP) enzymes into the bloodstream, systemic complications can quickly escalate. Some systemic complications include atelectasis, pleural effusion, acute respiratory distress syndrome (ARDS), respiratory failure, cardiovascular problems with hypovolemia, hypotension and shock, renal failure, coagulation complications, metabolic complications (e.g., hypocalcemia or hyperglycemia), GI problems, encephalopathy, and peripheral fat necrosis.

Clinical manifestations of pancreatitis include abdominal pain that radiates to the back, guarding and rebound tenderness, nausea and vomiting, and abdominal distension. Depending on some of the underlying problems, fever, tachycardia, tachypnea, and hypotension may also be present.

Diagnostic Tests

Laboratory tests include serum amylase and lipase. Both of these are increased with acute pancreatitis. An increased ALT can be indicative of gallstones, which could be associated with pancreatitis. CT scanning is the most useful test for determining the presence of pancreatitis as differentiated from other abdominal issues. Ultrasound can help diagnose the presence of gallstones.

Nursing Diagnoses

Based on the information gathered, examples of nursing diagnoses in the patient with acute pancreatitis may include the following:
* Activity intolerance related to fatigue.
* Acute pain as related to pancreatitis.
* Fear in response to the diagnosis of pancreatitis.
* Ineffective coping related to the diagnosis of pancreatitis.

Planning and Implementation

The goals for mild acute pancreatitis is to rest the gut, provide supportive care to treat symptoms, identify systemic complications early, and decrease pancreatic inflammation. Treatment includes bed rest, vigorous intravenous hydration, electrolyte replacement, pain control, and keeping the patient NPO. Patient controlled analgesia is effective, however morphine potentially causes the sphincter of Oddi to constrict and create more pain, so Demerol is recommended, but hydromorphone (Dilaudid) or other analgesics may be used. Decompression of the stomach by nasal gastric suction can relieve some of the nausea, vomiting, and abdominal distension. Patients may be treated conservatively until they are stable enough to have surgery to remove the gallstones. If a patient requires prolonged IV intervention, total parenteral nutrition (TPN) would be required. If infection is evident, aggressive antibiotic therapy would be used. Surgery may also be needed to treat extensive infections. It is possible for the autodigestion process to involve the circulation to the pancreas. This is a crisis situation that would necessitate surgery to stop the bleeding. Complications with kidney failure are possible and dialysis may be required. Acute pancreatitis can resolve with medical treatment. When the patients are released to home, they are instructed to refrain from drinking alcohol, because of its toxic effects on the pancreas and surrounding organs. Eating smaller, more frequent meals is also advisable.

Evaluation of Outcomes

Potential patient outcomes for each of the example nursing diagnoses for the patient with acute pancreatitis are:
* Activity intolerance related to fatigue. The patient maintains activity level within capabilities, as evidenced by normal heart rate and blood pressure during activity, as well as absence of shortness of breath, weakness, and fatigue.

Skills 360°

Nursing Care for Acute Pancreatitis

The nurse should perform the following measures in the management of acute pancreatitis:
* Strict intake and output and being alert for signs and symptoms of kidney failure.
* Monitor vital signs and be aware of early signs of internal bleeding, infection, and respiratory distress.
* Pain control.
* Assessment of all systems, but especially GI, respiratory, and cardiovascular.
* Blood glucose monitoring.
* Providing information about disease, diagnostic tests, and treatment.
* Provide information concerning alcohol reduction and elimination.

- Acute pain as related to pancreatitis. The patient should verbalize an adequate relief of pain along with the ability to realistically cope with the pain if it is not completely relieved.
- Fear in response to the diagnosis of pancreatitis. The patient should manifest positive coping behaviors and verbalize a reduction in the amount of fear of the having this disease.
- Ineffective coping related to the diagnosis of pancreatitis. Patient identifies own maladaptive coping behaviors, available resources, and support systems, describes or initiates alternative coping strategies, and describes positive results from new behaviors.

Chronic Pancreatitis

Chronic pancreatitis occurs when there is irreversible damage to the pancreatic acini, ducts, nerves, and islet cells because of continued irritation and injury. Pancreatic calcifications or dilated pancreatic ducts may be present. Digestive enzymes from the pancreas can irritate nearby tissue and cause scarring and further impede flow of enzymes, blood, and bile. Patients may present with the typical picture for acute pancreatitis or complain of diabetes symptoms or steatorrhea.

Epidemiology

Chronic alcoholism is implicated in about 70 percent of all chronic pancreatitis cases. Men between the ages of 30 and 40 are more likely affected than women. People may not seek treatment for pancreatitis, but on autopsy, pancreatitis is 50 times more prevalent in alcoholics than nondrinkers. In other cases, flow of exocrine enzymes can be affected by trauma, tumor, or pseudocysts. In 10 to 30 percent of patients, there may be no identifiable cause for the pancreatitis and is considered idiopathic.

Etiology

Chronic pancreatitis has a variety of causes. Hyperlipidemia and hypertriglyceridemia can be implicated. Autoimmune factors could also be at fault. Tropical pancreatitis is associated with people who live within 30 degrees of the equator. Symptoms can begin in childhood. Diabetes, malnutrition, and pancreatic calcifications are present. Environmental toxins, pathogenic agents, and toxic products that could be in the diet (cassava or sorghum) are all being investigated.

Pathophysiology

Chronic pancreatitis can be caused by alcoholism. In addition, chronic pancreatitis can be caused by actual physical trauma or cancer of the organ.

Genetics

The congenital abnormality pancreas divisum is the failure of the pancreatic ducts to fuse during embryonic development, leaving two separate (the dorsal and ventral ducts) to drain the different parts of the pancreas. Pancreas divisum may occur in 7 percent of the population, although those who go on to develop pancreatitis are few. Hereditary illnesses, such as cystic fibrosis and familial pancreatitis (mutations for the trypsinogen and the trypsin-inactivating genes), can illuminate other mechanisms at work. Cystic fibrosis is the most common cause of pancreatitis in children, because of the protein plugs within the ducts, causing reduced flow of pancreatic enzymes. In hereditary (familial) pancreatitis, the patient usually has two or more close relatives in the same generation with the same affliction. It is thought to be autosomal dominant and can be associated with increased pancreatic cancer.

Assessment with Clinical Manifestations

Chronic pancreatitis is characterized by pain, malabsorption, and diabetes mellitus. Pain can be acute or dull and constant. It may be referred to the back and be exacerbated with eating. Chronic irritation over many years may cause the pain to subside. In about 15 percent of patients, pain never develops. Pancreatitis affects digestion and absorption by decreasing the delivery of digestive enzymes to the gut and reducing the secretion of bicarbonate from the pancreatic ducts, lowering the duodenal pH. Weight loss and vitamin deficiency may be evident. Osteopenia and osteoporosis may occur because of decreased vitamin D. Diabetes mellitus occurs in 30 percent of patients with chronic pancreatitis. The inability to mobilize glucagons to maintain blood glucose levels can also be evident.

Diagnostic Tests

Diagnosis of chronic pancreatitis is divided into big duct disease and small duct disease. Big duct chronic pancreatitis indicates a dilation of the main pancreatic ducts and is common in alcoholic pancreatitis. Interventions for big duct disease can include endoscopic or surgical intervention. Small duct disease is more likely to be idiopathic and less responsive to surgical treatment, so emphasis would be on aggressive medical intervention.

Serum lipase and amylase are often normal in chronic pancreatitis. Serum glucose is helpful in diagnosing diabetes, but not in identifying the cause. Decreased serum trypsin, below 20 mg/dL in the presence of steatorrhea, is specific for chronic pancreatitis. Measuring fecal fat and fecal elastase could be important in diagnosing advanced disease (Daniels, 2003).

Abdominal X-ray and ultrasound can indicate pancreatic calcification. Diffuse calcification is seen in advanced pancreatic disease. This can help to differentiate chronic pancreatitis from tumors and focal trauma. Ultrasound can identify pancreatic atrophy or dilated pancreatic ducts. Gas in the bowel can obstruct the view. CT scan is most sensitive for identifying diffuse calcification and the dilation of ducts in big duct and small duct disease. Endoscopic ultrasonography (EUS) combines an ultrasound probe on the end of an endoscope and can contribute a clearer picture of the problem. Another endoscopic examination uses a collection tube in the duodenum, which collects pancreatic secretions when the pancreas is stimulated by the hormones secretin and secretin-cholecystokinin. This test is not available in all treatment centers. MRI and magnetic resonance cholangiopancreatography (MRCP) is useful in diagnosing biliary tract disease and less advanced chronic pancreatitis. The ERCP is probably the most sensitive test, but it carries the most risk and financial burden of all the tests. The ERCP can identify dilation or strictures in ducts, pseudocysts, and anatomical abnormalities. Biopsies can be taken at the time of ERCP to help differentiate between chronic pancreatitis and carcinoma of the pancreas. ERCP is most accurate in advanced disease, but less advanced disease remains much more difficult to diagnose.

Nursing Diagnoses

Based on the information gathered, examples of nursing diagnoses in the patient with chronic pancreatitis may include the following:
- Chronic pain related to chronic pancreatitis.
- Nutrition imbalance, less than body requirements, related to chronic pancreatitis.
- Knowledge deficit related to chronic pancreatitis.

Planning and Implementation

Digestive enzymes can be given orally. Lipase is the most variable enzyme, because it is dependent on the amount of fat in the meal. Lipase preparations need a higher pH than what is found in the stomach to have the most efficacy.

With pancreatitis, the bicarbonate is not secreted from the ducts, and the pH may be lower than usual in the intestine because of the bicarbonate deficiency. Diet should contain a moderate amount of fat (30 percent), high protein (24 percent), and low carbohydrates (24 percent). Diabetic diets can be helpful. Abstaining from alcohol is important, because the alcohol can cause more irritation, pain, and other problems. In addition, patients with chronic pancreatitis have difficulty in regulating blood glucose, because insulin and glucagons may be in short supply. Tight control of blood sugar can predispose the patient to hypoglycemia.

Pharmacology

Pain control often starts with the least potent medication, such as Darvocet-N or tramadol. Narcotic addiction can occur in 20 percent of patients. Tricyclic antidepressants can potentiate the effect of narcotics. Selective serotonin reuptake inhibitors (SSRIs) may also be helpful to treat pain and assist with rest. Pancreatic enzymes can provide some pain relief for people primarily with small duct pancreatitis by addressing some of the causes behind the pain. Gastric acid suppressors can also be used to decrease stomach acid. Antidiarrheals, such as octreotide (Sandostatin), have been beneficial in treating GI endocrine tumors, such as VIP tumors (VIPomas), and controlling the flushing and diarrhea that accompanies them. Antioxidants may also contribute to pain reduction.

Surgery

Surgical interventions for pain reduction can include ablation of the celiac plexus by analgesics guided by radiological means, laparoscopic stenting to keep the ducts open, dilation of strictures, removal of calculi, and drainage of pseudocysts. Open surgeries (nonlaparoscopic) may be used to visualize the pancreas, resect what is necessary, and ablate the nerves, which leads to the organ that conveys so much pain (Figure 51-6).

Evaluation of Outcomes

Potential patient outcomes for each of the example nursing diagnoses for the patient with chronic pancreatitis are:

- Chronic pain related to chronic pancreatitis. The patient should verbalize an adequate relief of pain along with the ability to realistically cope with the pain if it is not completely relieved.

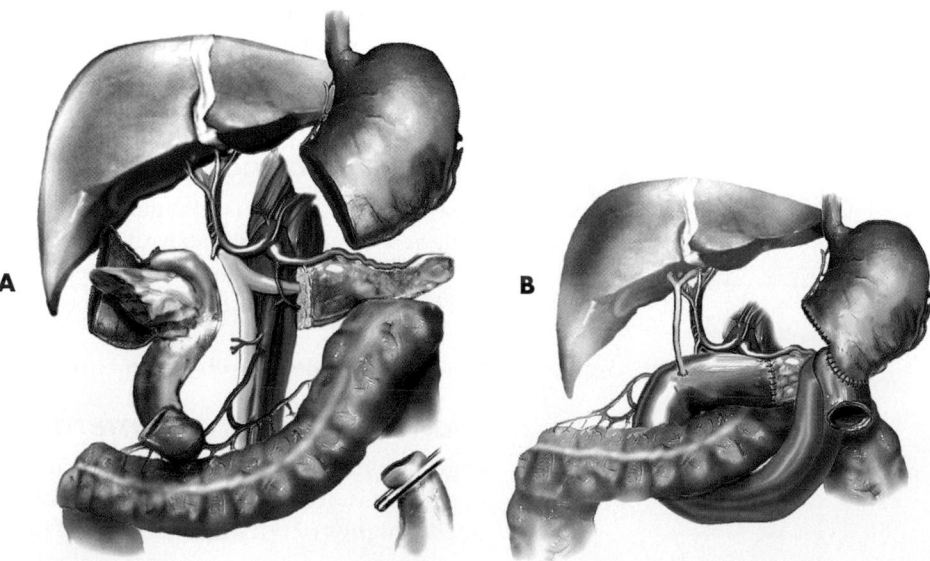

Figure 51-6 Whipple procedure (pancreatectomy): A. Resection, B. Reconstruction.

- Nutrition imbalance, less than body requirements, related to chronic pancreatitis. The patient verbalizes and demonstrates selection of foods or meals that will achieve a cessation of weight loss and weighs within 10 percent of ideal body weight.
- Knowledge deficit related to chronic pancreatitis. The patient should demonstrate motivation to learn, identify perceived learning needs, and verbalize an understanding of desired content.

KEY CONCEPTS

- Bilirubin is an important indicator for liver and blood disorders.
- The biliary tract serves the liver and is designed to drain bile.
- The most common cause of hepatitis is viral infection.
- HAV is transmitted by the fecal-oral route, and HBV is transmitted via blood and body fluids.
- The genetic disorders of the liver involve bilirubin metabolism, copper and iron storage, enzyme production, and lipoprotein metabolism.
- The destruction to the liver from alcohol often progresses from fatty liver to alcoholic hepatitis and culminates in alcoholic cirrhosis.
- Hepatic abscess is an area of infection in the liver caused by bacteria, amoebas, or protozoas.

- The liver is large and because of its size, location, and vascularity damage can occur during blunt or penetrating trauma.
- Liver cancer is named based on the type of tissue from which it originates and in general, men experience more primary liver cancer than women.
- Liver transplantation has been considered standard practice since 1983, with the development of newer immunosuppressive drugs to fight rejection of the implanted organ.
- Cholelithiasis (gallstones) is a common problem, affecting about 16 to 20 million people in the United States.
- The treatment of choice for an inflamed gallbladder is laparoscopic cholecystectomy, which is a surgical procedure using laparoscopy to remove the gallbladder.

REVIEW QUESTIONS

1. The liver has many complicated functions. Which of the following is the definition of gluconeogenesis?
   1. It is the conversion of glucose to glycogen, which can be stored in preparation of times of fasting.
   2. It is the conversion of stored glycogen into usable glucose to meet the immediate energy needs of the body.
   3. It is the synthesis of glucose from amino acids during times of fasting.
   4. It is the production of amino acids and bile.

2. Mr. Portier has an endoscopic retrograde cholangiopancreatography (ERCP). Which of the following organs does this diagnostic test not inspect?
   1. The liver
   2. The thymus
   3. The gallbladder
   4. The pancreas

3. Mr. Victorini has hepatitis A. Which of the following are true of this disorder?
   1. It is blood borne, causes fatigue, and has an incubation time of two to three weeks.
   2. It is life-threatening, irreversible, and debilitating.
   3. It is an RNA virus, spread often by food handlers infected with the virus, and has an incubation time of 15 to 50 days.
   4. It usually is not associated with jaundice, is a DNA virus, is transmitted through blood and body fluids, and often caused by sharing needles in illicit drug use.

4. Mr. Abernathy has a hereditary disease of the liver which is an autosomal recessive disorder related to copper metabolism. Which of the following disorders is this?
   1. Wilson's disease
   2. Crigler-Najjar disease
   3. Alpha-antitrypsin deficiency
   4. Hemochromatosis

Continued

5. Mr. Parker has ascites as a result of his cirrhosis condition. Which of the following is true of this condition?
   1. Refractory ascites is that which can only be treated with a splenectomy.
   2. Ascites is the accumulation of fluid in the pelvis area.
   3. A surgical shunt to divert excessive peritoneal fluid into the venous system may be attempted.
   4. Esophageal varices often result in the abdominal area specific to the ascites condition.

6. Mr. Barnes has a hepatic abscess. Which of the following is true concerning this condition?
   1. It is caused by a decrease in lecithin-cholesterol acyltransferase.
   2. It is categorized into either a macrovesicular and microvesicular disorder.
   3. It is usually caused by bacterial infection and is referred to as pyogenic hepatic abscess.
   4. It is also labeled hepatic steatosis.

7. Mrs. Williams has cancer of the liver. There are two basic types of liver cancer and they are labeled:
   1. Primary and secondary
   2. Type I and type II
   3. Stage A and stage B
   4. Organic and inorganic

8. What is the most common reason for children to have a liver transplant?
   1. Congenital hepatitis B virus
   2. Biliary atresia
   3. Cholangitis
   4. Congenital human immunodeficiency virus

9. Mrs. Adams has acute pancreatitis. Which of the following is true regarding its diagnosis?
   1. The serum laboratory tests of serum amylase and lipase are the best method of confirming acute pancreatitis.
   2. An increased alanine aminotransferase (ALT) is the best indicator for acute pancreatitis.
   3. Computed tomography (CT) scanning is the most useful test for determining the presence of pancreatitis as differentiated from other abdominal issues.
   4. Ultrasound is the most definitive manner in which to diagnose the severity of pancreatitis.

10. Mr. Hines is going to have a liver transplantation. Which of the following is true concerning this management strategy?
    1. Living donor liver transplants seldom come from parents or siblings.
    2. Cadaveric livers come from people who have been declared brain dead and have few other vital organs that are healthy.
    3. When an appropriate match has been identified, the institution has 24 hours to accept the organ.
    4. Criteria for receiving a donated liver is rigorously defined by the United Network for Organ Sharing.

REVIEW ACTIVITIES

1. Compare and contrast conjugated and unconjugated bilirubin.

2. Describe methods of assessing liver functioning.

3. Compare and contrast hepatitis A and hepatitis B.

4. Compare and contrast biliary and cardiac cirrhosis.

5. Describe your emotional feeling regarding providing care for patients who are alcoholics.

6. Describe how you would feel if you were asked to donate your liver to a relative.

7. Compare and contrast an open cholecystectomy and a laparoscopic cholecystectomy.

Visit the Contemporary Medical-Surgical Nursing online companion resource at www.delmarhealthcare.com for additional content and study aids. Click on Online Companions then select the Nursing discipline.

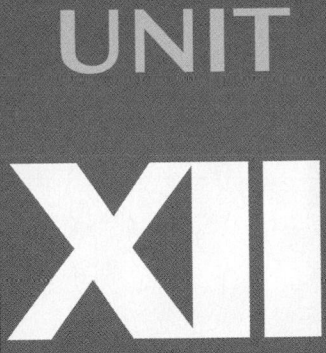

Alterations in Renal Function

Assessment of Renal Function

Irene Eaton-Bancroft, RN, MSN, CS

CHAPTER TOPICS

- Anatomy and Physiology of the Renal System

- Assessment Strategies Implemented in the Renal System

- Diagnostic Tests of the Renal System

The urinary system is critically important to the **homeostasis** (maintenance of an optimal and constant state of all body substances) of all body systems. Prevention and early recognition of system dysfunction are critical to the goal of maintaining optimal health status. The objective of this chapter is to equip the learner to assess normal renal system attributes and identify deviations from normal urinary system function.

The **renal** (pertaining to the kidney) component of the urinary system is often considered complex to understand, and its signals of dysfunction are difficult to recognize in a routine patient assessment. The learner is referred to a text on human physiology for a complete understanding of renal function. An anatomy and physiology text will supplement this chapter on renal assessment. The goal of this assessment chapter is to present anatomy and physiology from a system assessment perspective.

ANATOMY AND PHYSIOLOGY

The renal system is vital to the functioning of the human body. It is responsible for a wide variety of activities within the body and is integrated with the function of the other body systems. The renal system controls the fluid balance of the body, controls many of the metabolic processes within the body, and provides stabilization for the human body circulation. At the macrovascular level, the renal system consists of two kidneys, ureters, bladder, and urethra. In addition, the microvascular components of the renal system, such as the nephron, are presented in this chapter. The female and male urinary systems are illustrated Figure 52-1.

Kidneys

The kidneys are amazing organs with a computer-like capability to simultaneously perform multiple and complex functions. Normally, a person is born with two kidneys, though on occasion, a person is found to have a single or even a third kidney. The adult kidney is about the size of one's fist. It measures approximately 12 cm (4.5 inches) long, 6 cm (2.4 inches) wide and weighs 120–170 grams.

The kidneys are positioned in the **retroperitoneal space** (the space between the peritoneum [the membranous sac that surrounds the organs of the abdominal cavity] and the posterior abdominal wall that contains the kidneys and associated structures, the pancreas, and part of the aorta and inferior vena cava) at the level of the 12th thoracic vertebra to the 3rd lumbar vertebra with one on each side of the vertebral column. Positioned advantageously within an intact rib cage, the kidneys are offered protection from blunt trauma. The costovertebral angle (CVA), the point at which the base of the rib cage and the

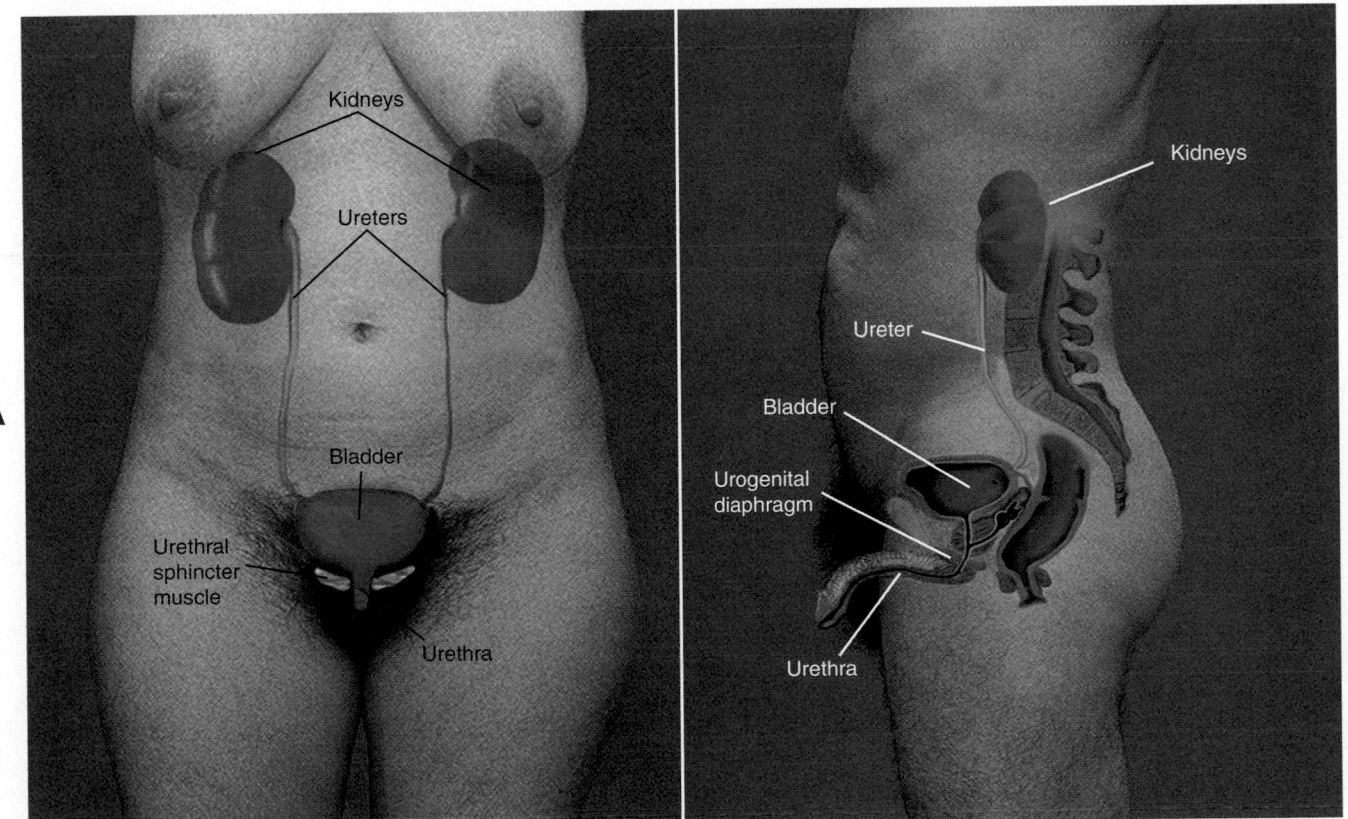

Figure 52-1 Urinary Tract: A. Female, B. Male.

spine meet, provides a landmark to locate kidney position during the physical exam. Be aware that the right kidney is positioned slightly lower than the left as it lies just under the larger right lobe of the liver. Under normal circumstance, one may not be able to palpate either kidney (Perkins & Kisiel, 2005).

A tough fibrous capsule covers and contains the kidney. Together with surrounding muscle, fascia, and fatty tissue, it offers protection to these mobile organs during times of vigorous and bouncing-type of activity. Though it is protective of the **renal parenchyma** (the cortex and medulla of the kidney, which contain the functioning units and collecting ducts of the kidney) under normal circumstances, renal capsule rigidity offers little accommodation to events such as **hydronephrosis** (dilation of the renal pelvis due to obstruction of urine flow or from ureteral reflux) secondary to postrenal obstruction. In such cases, the capsule's inability to expand increases potential for injury to the renal parenchyma due to increased intracapsular pressure and circulatory compromise to the nephrons. Acute pain in this area should prompt an expedient and thorough urological exam. The internal anatomy of the kidney is illustrated in Figure 52-2.

Blood supply to the kidney is critical from the perspective of producing hydrostatic pressure adequate for maintaining homeostasis and for the purpose of supplying oxygen and nutrients crucial to organ survival. The renal arteries branch directly from the aorta and deliver approximately 20 percent of the cardiac output to the kidneys.

The kidneys have one to two million nephrons. Microscopic in size, these functioning units produce and excrete urine to maintain homeostasis, as well as regulate or influence many physiological processes. The primary functions of the renal system are shown in Box 52-1.

Renal efficiency is amazing in that one can lose nearly 65 percent of their total kidney function before presenting symptoms of dysfunction. A person can survive easily with a single kidney. Relying on the sufficiency of one healthy

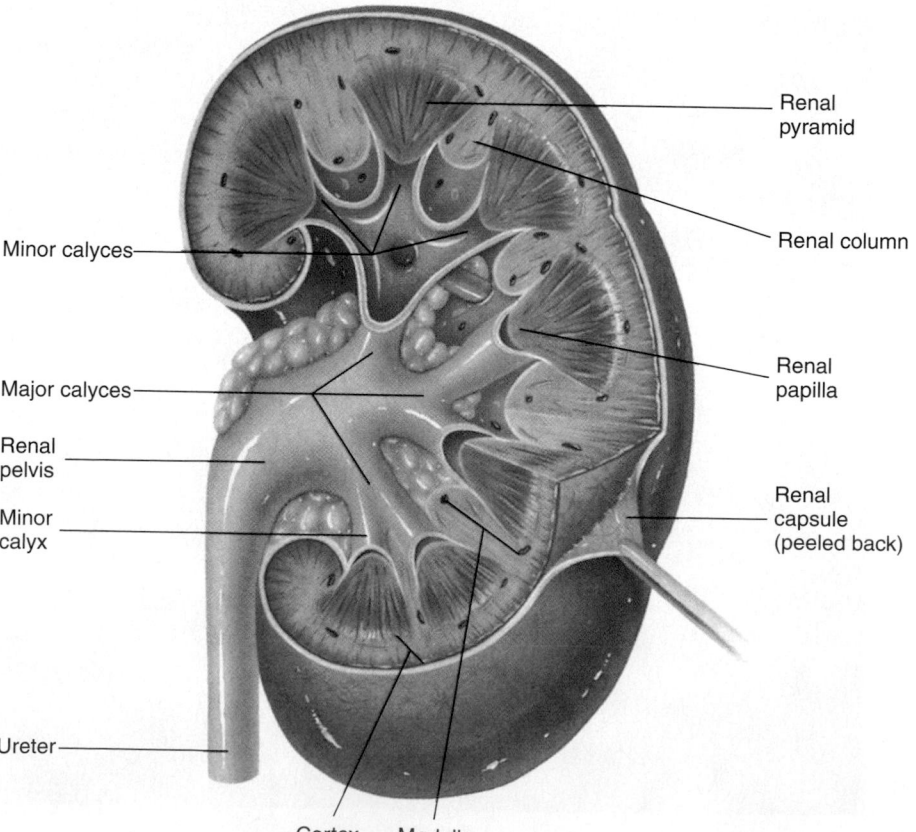

Figure 52-2 The internal anatomy of the kidney.

BOX 52-1

FUNCTIONS OF THE KIDNEY

The primary functions of the kidney are:

- Maintain fluid and electrolyte balance through excretion and reabsorption.
- Assist in blood pressure regulation through the renin-angiotensin system. A lifesaver in situations of fluid loss, this function can accelerate harm to the kidneys as they begin to fail. The mechanism of harm is release of renin by the juxtaglomerular apparatus. Timely nursing intervention in hypertensive episodes of acute renal failure are critical to recovery potential.
- Maintain chemical balance. This function is critical to maintain predictable blood levels of medication calculated on normal urinary excretion levels. The health care provider must stay alert to the potential for toxic blood levels in the event of renal function compromise.
- Maintain mineral balance. Consideration of this function is especially critical to bone health in chronic renal failure.
- Produce erythropoietin in response to low oxygen states.
- Convert vitamin D to its active enzyme form and thus influence calcium metabolism.
- Excrete waste products of protein metabolism.
- Contribute to acid-base balance. Secretion of hydrogen ions, reabsorption of bicarbonate, or generation of new bicarbonate by the kidney serve to counter acidosis and to maintain acid-base equilibrium. Adjusted renal excretion of bicarbonate ions corrects for alkalosis.

---

kidney, many have chosen to donate their second kidney. Kidney donation from living donors has expanded to include nonrelated recipients. Further information concerning kidney donation is shown in chapter 54.

Ureters

The ureter is a narrow fibromuscular tube that extends from the distal end of the renal pelvis and to the bladder. Composed of smooth muscle, the ureter propels urine toward the bladder by **peristalsis** (smooth muscle involuntary contractions that propel substances along a pathway, such as when the ureters propel urine from the kidneys to the bladder by peristaltic action). Peristaltic strength is sufficient to overcome the resistance offered by the detrusor muscle of the bladder allowing urine to pass into the bladder. Conversely, the 1 to 2 cm the ureters traverse through the detrusor muscle before emptying into the bladder prevents retrograde reflux of urine back toward the kidneys as the bladder fills.

The small diameter of the ureters contributes to easy obstruction during the passage of renal **calculi** (a substance of abnormal concretion composed of mineral salts commonly produced within the renal system) or from the external pressure of masses. Pressure receptors in the ureters and renal pelvis generate the extreme pain experienced during the passage of calculi. In addition, these receptors slow glomerular filtration when sensing high intrauretal pressures (Schafer, 2003). Slowing filtration offers a protective effect toward limiting hydronephrosis.

Urinary Bladder

The urinary bladder is a muscular sac that narrows at the base to form the bladder neck. The bladder is made up of cross-hatched smooth muscle with exceptional stretch capacity. This specific smooth muscle is referred to as detrusor muscle. Distinctively, it has tremendous capacity to stretch and then to contract in response to nervous stimuli. Normal detrusor stretch will allow as much as 500 mL bladder fill volume. Flaccid during the filling phase, the bladder contracts in response to stretch receptors and seeks to expel urine though the internal sphincter. It is at this point that both voluntary and involuntary action is needed to complete the voiding process in the continent adult (Newman, 2005).

The muscle tone of the detrusor muscle surrounding the ureter serves to occlude the ureteral orifice preventing reflux of urine toward the kidney as the bladder fills. Peristaltic pressure overcomes detrusor strength and propels urine through the detrusor area and on into the bladder. The section of the detrusor muscle involved in preventing reflux of urine into the ureter is called the ureterovesicular valve and is normally 1 to 2 cm long. Those with a shorter valve section are susceptible to reflux with subsequent enlarged ureters and intrarenal problems as a result of increased fluid pressures.

The trigone of the bladder is the triangular-shaped section of the posterior wall of the bladder just above and adjacent to the bladder neck. The trigone accommodates the orifices of the ureters at its uppermost borders while the base of this triangular area forms the bladder neck and transitions to the urethra (O'Hara, 2005). The anatomy of the urinary bladder is illustrated in Figure 52-3.

Bladder Neck (Posterior Urethra)

The bladder neck, also considered the posterior portion of the urethra, plays a critical role in continence and in dysfunctions of bladder emptying. Elastic tissue is interwoven into the detrusor muscle of this bladder/urethral section to form the internal sphincter. Smooth muscle places the internal sphincter under involuntary control via a nerve plexus originating at the second and third segment of the sacral spine. Striated muscles of the pelvic floor innervated by the pudendal nerve keep the external sphincter under voluntary control. The act of voiding in the healthy adult requires the active participation of the individual. Good muscle tone and intact innervation to the sphincters can resist the

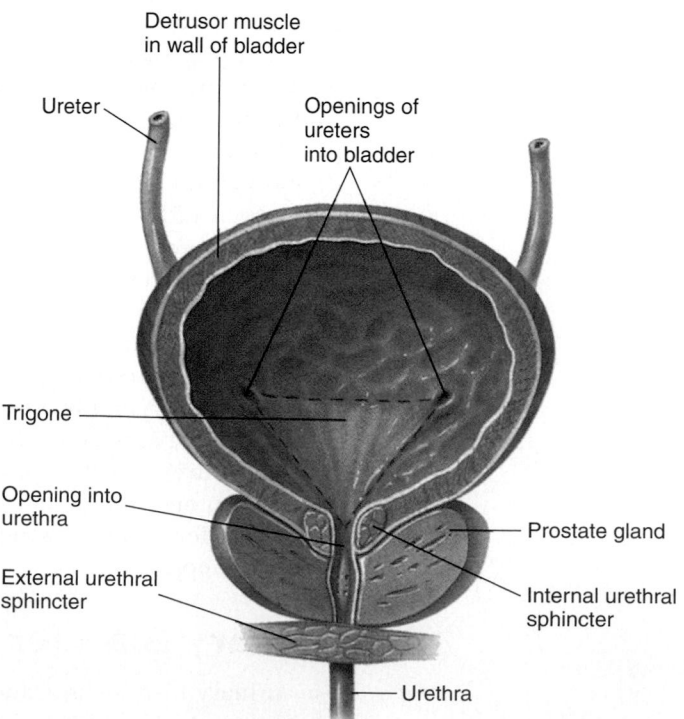

Figure 52-3 The anatomy of the urinary bladder.

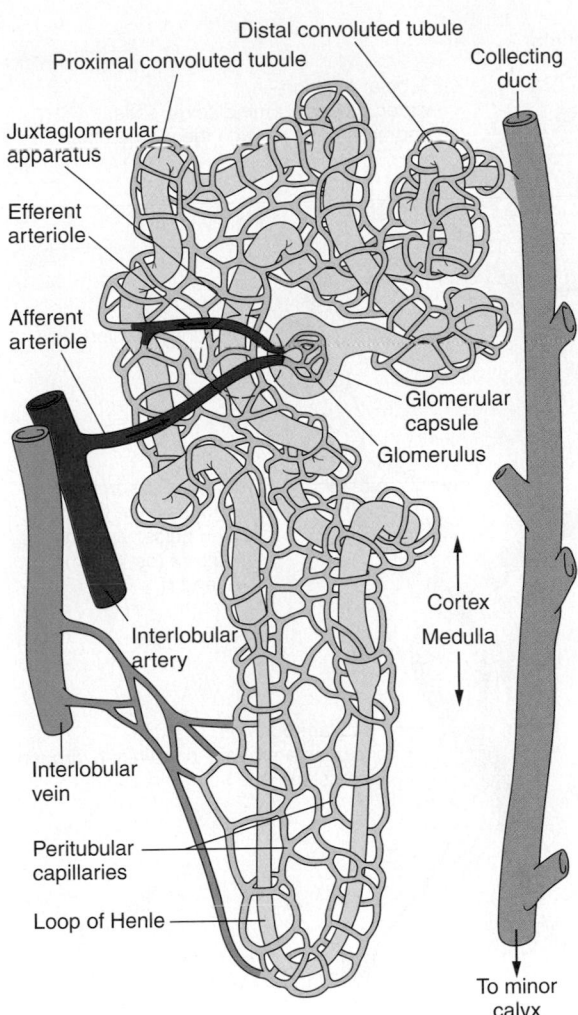

Figure 52-4 The anatomy of a nephron.

contracting detrusor and inhibit bladder emptying for a period of time, though not without discomfort as a reminder of a full bladder (O'Hara, 2005).

Commonly, problems can develop causing interference with bladder functions of urine storage or expulsion. A weak pelvic floor, particularly in cases involving the short urethra of females, can lead to incontinence. In the male, an enlarged prostate gland is the most common cause of urethral obstruction with resulting retention. Benign prostatic hypertrophy, or prostate cancer, is the most common causes of urinary retention in the male. In the female, close proximity of the urethral orifice to the vagina contributes to bacterial invasion of the urinary tract through the urethra with potential for ascending infection traveling by way of the ureter and ultimately into the kidney. These infections are labeled according to anatomic region of infection (e.g., urethritis, cystitis, **pyelonephritis,** or **nephritis**). (Note: Pyelonephritis is an infection of the ureters, and nephritis is an infection contained to the kidney.) These will be discussed in depth in chapter 54.

Nephron

The nephron is the functioning unit of the kidney. The anatomy of a nephron is illustrated in Figure 52-4. They number more than a million with cellular structure differing from section to section to accomplish the multiple and complex tasks. Each unit would seem to have two primary systems with both separate and interrelated functions. Simply stated, the tubular system collects the filtrate of water and solutes then secretes, excretes, or reabsorbs substances as necessary to maintain an internal environment in equilibrium and rid of waste products.

The vascular system of the nephron includes two capillary beds: (a) the glomerular capillary bed is shaped in the form of a tuft and sits in the first segment of the tubule, and (b) the peritubular capillary bed surrounds all portions of the tubule. Both capillary networks are vested in critical and cooperative function with the tubule. Critical to the function of both of these systems is the interstitium with functional solute concentration gradients that support the processes of both the tubule and the peritubular capillary network. The processes and structures of the nephron are presented in Figure 52-5.

Renal Tubule

The renal tubule is a complex component of the kidney. Anatomic sections of the tubule include Bowman's capsule, the proximal tubule, loop of Henle, distal tubule, and the collecting duct. Bowman's capsule, the first segment, is configured somewhat as a funnel. Bowman's capsule cradles the glomerular capillary tuft and receives the approximate 180 L/day of filtered fluids and solutes. Impermeable to protein by both size and negative charge, healthy glomerular capillaries inhibit passage of protein or blood cells into the filtrate. Interestingly, the negative charge present on each of the three glomerular capillary membranes repels the negatively charged and molecularly larger cells. Due to their negative charge or large molecular size, the presence of protein or blood cells in the urine signals problems with filtration.

The proximal and distal tubules are similarly convoluted in shape though structurally quite different. Cell structure of the proximal tubule accommodates greater reabsorption sodium, chloride, glucose, amino acids, bile salts, oxalate, urate, and catecholamines. This begins the process of creating a

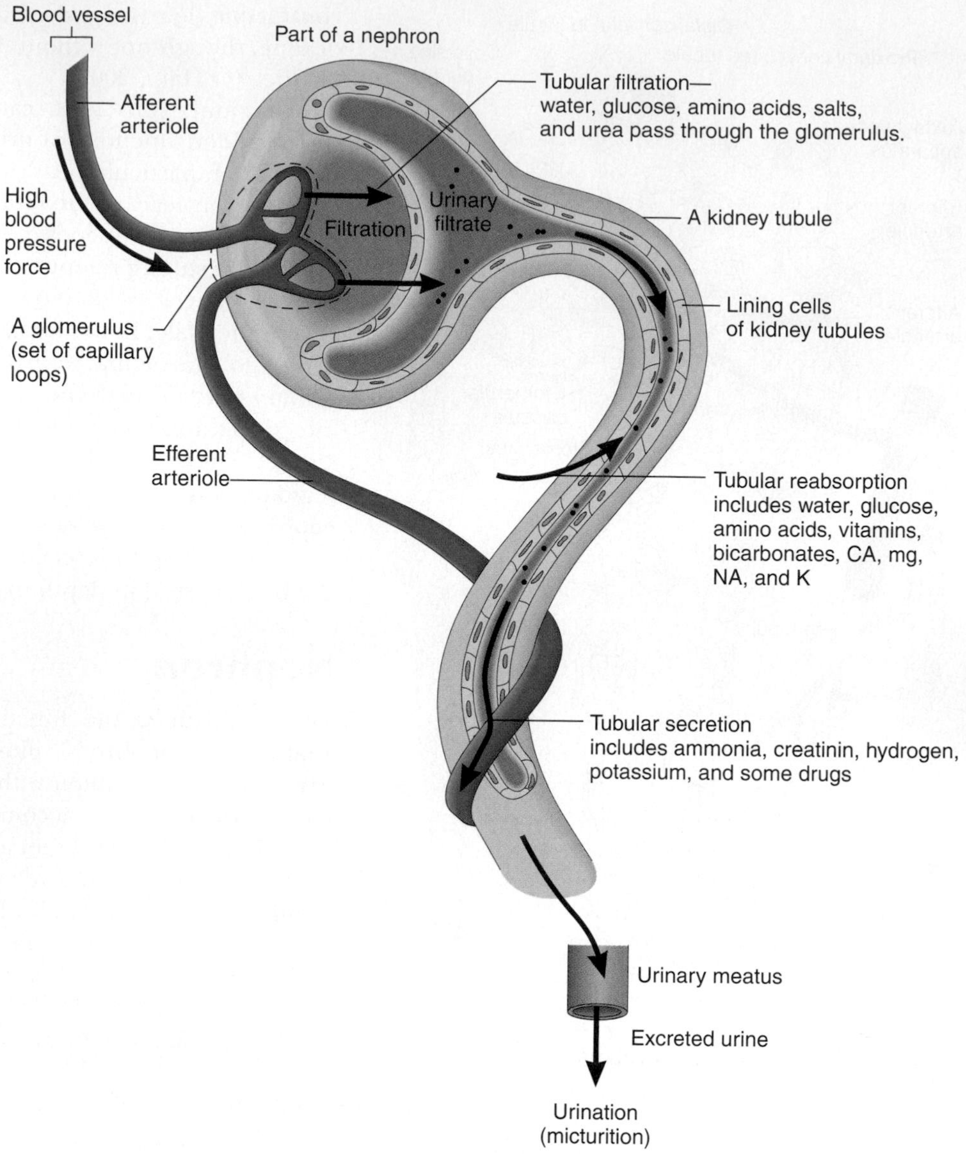

Figure 52-5 Processes and structures of the nephron.

highly concentrated renal **interstitial space,** that area surrounding the nephron loops and the peritubular capillaries, which has a high osmotic pressure due to extremely high levels of sodium. The renal interstitial space facilitates the massive volume water reabsorption required to maintain fluid balance. The interstitial space fluid environment is equipped with osmotic pressures capable of reabsorbing the approximate 165 L/day of the water filtered by the glomerular capillaries.

The loop of Henle changes cellular structure along its descending and ascending paths to create three functionally different sections. The thinner descending section facilitates large quantities of water absorption by osmosis and moderate reabsorption of solutes. Important to urine concentration, the ascending limb is highly impermeable to water. As the ascending limb of the loop of Henle thickens due to cellular structure change, the sodium pump actively moves sodium, chloride, and potassium out of the tubular fluid into the interstitial space. Large amounts of calcium, magnesium, and bicarbonate are also reabsorbed from the thick ascending limb. This solute loss creates a dilute solution in the tubule as the filtrate approaches the distal tubule. The achieved dilution is significant in setting the stage for the significant adjustments needed to accommodate the high variability of individual fluid and solute intake.

Juxtaglomerular Apparatus

The first segment of the distal tubule forms a portion of the juxtaglomerular apparatus. This is a complex of cells made up of those in the distal tubule (macula densa cells) and related cellular structure within the arterioles on either end of the glomerular capillary tuft (juxtaglomerular cells). Though often depicted as distant from one another to demonstrate the configuration of the nephron, in reality these two groups of cells are in intimate contact with one another. Macula densa cells are capable of detecting pressure or sodium solute changes and signaling the juxtaglomerular cells of the afferent arterioles to decrease resistance toward the goal of a greater filtration rate. In addition, macula densa cells stimulate renin release from the juxtaglomerular cells of the arterioles entering and exiting the glomerular tuft. Released renin initiates the angiotensin system thereby increasing the arterial blood pressure. The net result of both actions is increased glomerular filtration rate.

Blood supply to the kidney is critical from the perspective of producing hydrostatic pressure adequate for maintaining glomerular filtration and for the purpose of supplying oxygen and nutrients crucial to nephron function and survival. A renal artery branches directly from the aorta to each kidney. The artery then subdivides courses through the lobules of the kidney and ultimately forms the glomerular and peritubular capillary networks of the nephrons. The efferent arteriole separates these two capillary beds and facilitates the higher hydrostatic pressure gradients necessary for filtration in the glomerulus and the lower hydrostatic pressures in the peritubular capillaries that promote reabsorption to maintain homeostasis.

The afferent arteriole is the short vascular segment between the interlobular arteries and the glomerular capillary network in Bowman's capsule. The afferent arteriole plays a critical role in conjunction with the efferent arteriole in regulating filtering pressures and ultimately influencing systemic blood pressure through constriction, dilation or renin release. These functions are most often referred to as the autoregulatory function of the kidney.

Homeostatic balancing mechanisms are easily disturbed by events producing changes in renal perfusion, such as hypertension or vasoactive drugs, and from renin generated from within the kidney in pathological states. **Nephrotoxic** (having the ability to harm the kidney) agents, such as nonsteroidal anti-inflammatory medications and cyclosporine, are capable of compromising afferent arteriole function with the potential to impose acute renal failure by diminishing glomerular filtration and reducing the blood supply to the nephron.

Renin-Angiotensin System

It is important to understand the renin-angiotensin system and the importance of intervention in pathological states. Basic to the renin-angiotensin cycle is an understanding that renin has the capability of activating critical events. For example, when sensing low volumes of distal tubular filtrate, regardless of the cause, renin release by the juxtaglomerular cells will initiate the formation of angiotensin I, which converts to angiotensin II. Angiotensin-converting enzyme (ACE) is the catalyst in the conversion of angiotensin I to angiotensin II. The cumulative action of these three potent chemicals causes vasoconstriction and yields an increase in blood pressure. Often times, renin release is a direct result of pathology that would be further complicated by its release. One example of a pathology that activates the renin angiotensin cycle is congestive heart failure with associated decrease in renal perfusion or glomerular filtration. Another example of a condition that activates the release of renin is hypertension associated decreased glomerular filtrate. In either case, renin release is detrimental and obliges timely intervention with agents such as diuretics, ACE inhibitors, or other antihypertensive medications. The nurse is given a significant role in reversing acute renal failure when implementing protocol orders in such instances. Prudent and ethical nursing practice

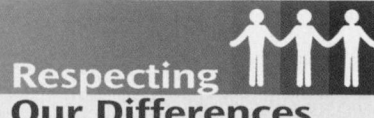

attends the clinical observations of urine output patterns, blood pressure parameters, and medication protocols (Hobbs, Irwin, & Rubner, 2005).

ASSESSMENT

The renal system is complex and vital to the human body. There are many disorders that affect the function of the renal system. The nurse must be familiar with the variety of pathologies that affect the renal system and be able to accurately assess the changes in the renal system as they occur. Initially, the health history and physical exam are the primary components of the assessment of the renal system.

Health History

Urinary tract and renal assessment must begin with a thorough health history. The nurse must gather complete information on past illnesses and family history. Hypertension, extensive cardiovascular disease, diabetes, gout, and autoimmune disease are among the more common causes of renal problems. The nurse must query for such disorders as urinary calculi, frequent urinary tract infections, congenital disorders, and stroke. In addition, the nurse must search for a history of cancer with radiation or chemotherapy. The nurse must also include the history of any hospitalizations and surgical history. General health questions should include current health status, nutrition, and work history. Be alert to symptoms suggestive of decreased kidney function. These include significantly reduced energy level, metallic taste in the mouth, anorexia, nausea, pruritus, decreased ability to concentrate, decreased urine output, and related weight gain from fluid retention (Lipman, 2005).

The nurse should ask the patient if he or she smokes and thus be more susceptible to bladder cancer. Also, the patient should be asked if he or she has an extended history of high-nitrogen and low-carbohydrate diets. This could impose abnormally high blood urea nitrogen (BUN). Also, the patient should be asked if his or her diet is excessively high in dairy products and if he or she is taking mineral supplements that may predispose him or her to calculi. And, lastly, the nurse should determine if the patient is generally well hydrated.

Assessment of Urination Patterns

Potential questions for the nurse to ask the patient when assessing renal urination are exemplified in Box 52-2.

BOX 52-2

ASSESSMENT OF URINATION PATTERNS: QUESTIONS TO ASK

Questions to ask the patient when assessing the urination patterns of the renal system

The nurse can ask the following questions when assessing the renal system:
- Is there a change in voiding patterns?
- Is there a history of incontinence, urgency, or frequency of urination?
- Does the patient have difficulty with starting the voiding process?
- Is there burning when urinating?
- What is the color of the urine?
- Has there ever been any indication of **hematuria** (blood in the urine)?
- Is there a feeling of fullness after the patient has voided?
- Is the urinary stream full or are they only able to void in dribbles?

Medication History

One important aspect of the health history for a patient with renal system dysfunction is his or her medication history. The renal system has a direct relationship in the metabolism of many medications, and the health of the renal system is vital to the use of medications for patients. The nurse should assess the medication history by asking questions regarding over-the-counter medications and any alternative therapies. It is especially important to quantify the amount and duration of nonsteroidal anti-inflammatory medication usage. This group of drugs can be especially harmful to the kidneys. Potential for damage increases in the presence of hypertension or exposure to other nephrotoxic drugs as shown in Box 52-3 (Campoy & Elwell, 2005).

Physical Examination

The physical examination of the renal examination is presented as it relates to each of the anatomic areas (e.g., skin, mouth, or abdomen). In general, weighing the patient establishes changes in weight as well as a baseline weight for further evaluation. Daily weights are critical assessment components for a patient with renal failure.

Skin

Note skin turgor for an indication of hydration state. The patient's skin could be dry and lack turgor or grossly edematous depending on the etiology within the urinary system. Observe for signs of persistent scratching as often occurs with the phosphorus or calcium imbalances of renal failure. Look for pallor or the yellow-gray cast sometimes seen in renal failure. Check the female vulva and perineum for signs of irritation from urinary incontinence or vaginal discharge. Similarly check the penis, scrotum, and perineum of the male for signs of infection or drainage.

Mouth

Check mucous membranes for signs of irritation or dryness and note breath smell. The smell of ammonia is common with **uremia** (accumulation of end-products of protein metabolism in the blood stream due to renal failure).

Abdomen

Inspect and palpate for bladder distension, masses, or enlarged kidneys as is found with renal cell cancer or **polycystic cysts** (cysts with closed sacs that develop abnormally within an organ and have a distinct enclosing membrane).

Kidneys

Palpate the kidneys at the CVA. Normally, the left kidney is not palpable. A normal right kidney may be palpable during deep inhalation. To palpate for the kidneys, place one hand under the posterior flank at the CVA and the other hand in the corresponding anterior position. Palpate deeply during

---

Red Flag

Fluid Volume Excess

The nurse must remember that a sudden increase of daily weight can indicate a sudden increase of body fluids. A weight gain of 1 kilogram would indicate retention of 1 liter of fluid. This sudden increase in body fluids could present severe cardiovascular and respiratory problems.

Skills 360°

Urinary Incontinence

Can you remember that last time that you sneezed or coughed and experienced come loss of bladder control? How did that make you feel? Did you soil your clothes? Now imagine what it must be like for a patient who has urinary incontinence on a regular basis. Interview a patient with urinary incontinence and ask him or her how it affects his or her life. Does the patient perform bathroom mapping when out in public?

BOX 52-3

POTENTIALLY NEPHROTOXIC DRUGS AND OTHER AGENTS

Potentially Nephrotoxic Drugs and Other Agents Include:

Amikacin	Chemotherapeutic agents
Gentamicin	Contrast medium
Amphotericin B	Ethylene glycol
Gentamicin	Gold and other heavy metals
Sulfonamides	Nonsteroidal anti-inflammatory drugs

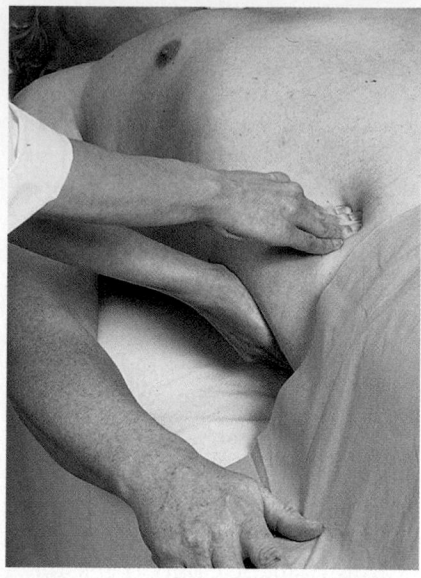

Figure 52-6 Palpation of the right kidney.

patient inspiration noting any tenderness or enlargement. To further check for tenderness in the kidney area, place one hand over the flank and strike it firmly with the fist of the other hand. Tenderness is a common finding in kidney infection as with pyelonephritis or polycystic kidneys. Palpation and percussion are illustrated in Figures 52-6 and 52-7A and B (Estes, 2006).

Lungs

Auscultate all lung fields and check for shortness of breath with rest or activity. A fluid-overloaded pulmonary capillary bed easily infiltrates the lungs with fluid as evidenced by crackles on auscultation and wet lung fields on chest X-ray. Weight, blood pressure, and lung auscultation are readily accessible nursing tools to identify and monitor fluid overload.

Bladder

Using deep palpation, the nurse can assess the bladder. First, palpate the abdomen at the midline, starting at the symphysis pubis and progressing upward to the umbilicus. If the bladder is located, palpate the shape, size, and consistency. It must be noted that an empty bladder is not usually palpable. A moderately full bladder is smooth and round, and it is palpable above the symphysis pubis. A full bladder is palpated above the symphysis pubis, and it may be close to the umbilicus. There are a variety of dysfunctions seen in bladder palpation, which are depicted in Box 52-5.

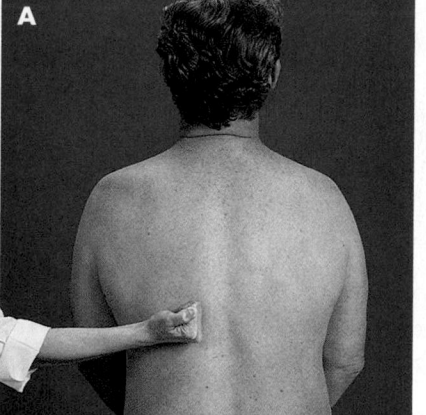

Figure 52-7 A. Direct fist percussion of the left kidney, B. Indirect fist percussion of the left kidney.

BOX 52-4

DIFFERENTIATING KIDNEY PALPATION

The distinguishing features between an enlarged liver and an enlarged kidney include:

1. The edge of the liver tends to be sharper and to extend medially and laterally, whereas the pole of the kidney is more rounded.
2. In addition, the edge of the liver cannot be captured, whereas an enlarged kidney can be.

Distinguishing features between an enlarged kidney and an enlarged spleen include:

1. A palpable notch on the medial edge of the organ favors the spleen.
2. Percussion of the spleen produces dullness, because the bowel is displaced downward; however, resonance is heard over the left kidney because of the intervening bowel.

BOX 52-5

BLADDER ABNORMALITIES

The following are the more common bladder abnormalities:

- A bladder that is nodular or asymmetrical to palpation is abnormal. A nodular bladder may indicate a malignancy. An asymmetrical bladder may result from a tumor in the bladder or an abdominal tumor that is compressing the bladder.
- Men with benign prostatic hyperplasia may be unable to completely empty their bladder because of the pressure that the enlarged prostate places on the bladder.
- Various types of urinary incontinence, due to altered mental status, muscle function, medications, and other causes can lead to incomplete bladder emptying.

DIAGNOSTIC TESTS

Adherence to specimen collection and test preparation protocols are critically important to accurately diagnose and treat urinary system disorders. In addition, patient cooperation during many of the studies is crucial. Patients must be thoroughly informed in advance of the test or assisted through the steps when they are mentally or physically dependent.

Urine Studies

Urine studies are valuable diagnostic tests to evaluate renal system function, as shown in Table 52-1.

Blood Studies

Blood studies are valuable diagnostic tests to evaluate renal system function, as shown in Tables 52-2 and 52-3.

Urinary Retention Studies

Postvoid residual of urine is obtained by either of two methods. Catheterization immediately after voiding will give an exact accounting for the volume of urine left in the bladder following voiding. As with any catheterization, there is a potential for infection. Bladder scan is a noninvasive method using ultrasound and achieves comparable results without imposing risk of infection. It is convenient and can be performed at the bedside by the nurse.

Catheterization postvoid must be done immediately after the patient voids to assess for urinary retention (Table 52-4). Sterile technique is imperative. Bladder scanning reliability requires attention to three main points: (a) Follow the operator's manual instructions. This usually requires the selection of an icon representing a male or female patient. Select the male icon for the posthysterectomy female patient. Rationale: ultrasonic adjustment accomplishes sound wave penetration through the uterus. (b) Supine position is critical to accurate results. (c) Center the urine pool image over the cross-hatch on the ultrasonic grid.

Radiographic Studies

There are a variety of radiographic studies that are used in diagnostic testing of the renal system. Each test has specific nursing implications that the nurse should know to meet the educational needs of the patient. The descriptions of the tests and the nursing care involved is provided in Table 52-5.

Renal Ultrasound (Kidney Scan)

A renal ultrasound visualizes the parenchyma and associated structures including the renal blood vessels. Doppler ultrasonography is a noninvasive test that uses ultrasound waves over the flank areas to identify occlusions of the veins or arteries. Ultrasound waves are transmitted and received from the transducer while it is placed over the circulatory system locations. The returning echoes are amplified and images are recorded on a video and strip recorder. The kidney is visualized by using the liver or the spleen as comparative structures. The renal ultrasound may be performed with an intravenous pyelogram (IVP) to define or characterize masses or lesions and can be used in people with iodine allergy (Noble & Brown, 2004).

Red Flag

Using Contrast Agents in Renal Diagnostics

Protection of renal function for patients receiving a nephrotoxic contrast agent is provided through hydration preprocedure and postprocedure. Patients with fluid restrictions or needing added protection may be given one of the following agents. (Note: expedient administration is imperative.)

1. Acetylcysteine given in doses of 600 mg by mouth twice daily starting the day before the procedure. A total of four doses are given.
2. Sodium bicarbonate is given intravenously. An alkaline environment diminishes contrast media potential for nephrotoxicity.

Red Flag

Potential Problems Associated with Renal Ultrasounds

Renal ultrasounds cannot be done over open wounds or dressings. A kidney scan must be performed before radiographic studies involving barium; if not possible, at least 24 hours must elapse between barium procedure and the kidney scan. (Note: renal biopsy may be done with ultrasound guidance.)

TABLE 52-1 Urine Studies

STUDY	PURPOSE	NURSING MANAGEMENT
Urine Dipstick	Screening urine study used primarily to identify gross abnormalities and determine need for further study	Follow instructions on the package. Store according to manufacturers guidelines to ensure test strip reliability.
		Collection is appropriate at any time of day; the first void of the day provides the optimal specimen. It is usually important to collect expediently. Send to the laboratory within one hour of the void. Avoid contamination by menses or feces.
Urine culture	Determine bacterial count and identify infecting bacteria for best choice of antibiotic. A bacterial count greater than 100,000 indicates treatable infection.	Males: Cleanse the glans penis with the appropriate cleansing solution following institutional procedure and attending any patient allergies. Retract foreskin, if present. Have the patient start to void; then collect a midstream urine sample. Keep inside of cover and container free of contamination from the hands or surroundings.
		Females: Separate the labia and cleanse the vulva as above. A catheter specimen is warranted during menses or conditions that will not allow a reliable midstream collection into a sterile container.
Timed urine collection	The most common is the 24-hour creatinine clearance to determine renal filtering efficiency. Normal clearance range is 70–140 mL/minute.	Have the patient void and discard the specimen or drain the collecting system and discard urine to start the collection. Place the collection receptacle on ice and carefully add each void to the collection. If the patient has an indwelling catheter, place the catheter bag on ice and empty regularly into the collection bottle. End the collection by having the patient void or by emptying the drainage system and adding the specimen to the collection receptacle. Label and keep on ice for delivery to the laboratory.

Voiding cystometrogram	A graphic recording of bladder filling pressure and abdominal pressure during the filling and voiding cycle. A urinary catheter is inserted into the urinary bladder for filling and emptying during the procedure. In addition, a catheter may be inserted into the vagina or rectum to measure abdominal pressures. Each has an attached manometer for measurement purposes.
	The patient will be asked about sensations while the catheter fills the bladder. A Valsalva maneuver is required at some point during the test. Alert the health care provider or technician of any patient prone to vasovagal reactions.
	Postprocedure, the patient may experience an increase in urinary symptoms from the use of the urethral catheter. Inform him or her to alert the health care provider of fever, chills, low back pain, or hematuria.
Cystography	Bladder injury and suspicion of **vesicoureteral reflux** (backward propulsion of urine through the valve the normally closes the bladder and ureteral junction to backward flow of urine) are indications for this study. Radiopaque dye is instilled via a catheter directly into the bladder. As with the voiding cystometrogram, pressure recordings can be obtained. Check for allergies to contrast media. Postprocedural hydration, unless contraindicated, is important for nephrotoxic dye excretion.

TABLE 52-2 Blood Studies

STUDY (NORMAL VALUE)	NURSING MANAGEMENT (EVALUATION AND PATIENT EDUCATION)
Blood urea nitrogen (BUN) (10–20 mg/dL)	Nonrenal causes of variance include high-protein diet, gastrointestinal (GI) bleed, rapid cell destruction as in chemotherapy or severe burns, and hydration status.
Serum creatinine normal (0.6–1.4 mg/dL)	Endogenous in source, creatinine is a by-product of muscle metabolism. It is a much more reliable indicator of renal dysfunction than is the BUN. The normal BUN/creatinine ratio is 10:1.
Sodium (135–145 mEq/L)	Abnormal levels of blood sodium are reliable indicators of intravascular hydration. Dilute or concentrated sodium indicates intravascular fluid overload (dilute) or dehydration (concentrated).
Potassium (3.5–5 mEq/L)	Serious cardiac arrhythmias or asystole are potential consequences of the high fluctuations in potassium levels associated with renal dysfunction.
Carbon dioxide content (CO_2) (22–30 mEq/L)	Indicator of metabolic acid-base balance. Variance is most commonly due to renal dysfunction. Most patients in chronic renal failure demonstrate significant metabolic acidosis.
Calcium (8.5–10.5 mg/dL)	Decreased renal secretion of phosphorus is the primary cause of hypocalcemia in renal failure. Correction is accomplished by correcting high phosphorus levels.
Phosphorus (2.5–4.5 mg/dL)	Phosphorus control is critical to prevention of renal osteodystrophy. Increased phosphorus levels result in low calcium levels and secondary hyperparathyroidism when inadequately treated.
Hematocrit (Males: 42–52 percent; Females: 35–47 percent)	Renal secretion of **erythropoietin** (**[EPO]** a hormone produced by the kidney in response to low oxygen states or a low hematocrit, which stimulates red blood cell production in the bone marrow) is compromised in renal failure and is reflected in chronically low red blood cell counts. The hematocrit is followed to adjust the dose of recombinantly produced EPO or determine need for red blood cell transfusion. Most chronic renal failure patients have hematocrit maintained in the high 20th to mid-30th percentile.

TABLE 52-3 BUN and Creatinine Levels

BUN (blood urea nitrogen)	Normal in adult 5–20 mg/dL; older adult 8–21 mg/dL; child 5–18 mg/dL	BUN measures the nitrogen fraction of urea, which is the chief end-product of protein metabolism. It is formed by the liver from ammonia and excreted by the kidney. BUN reflects protein intake, the liver's ability to metabolize, and the renal excretory ability. BUN exists in a normal ratio with serum creatinine, and they often arise together in pathological conditions of the renal system.
Creatinine	Normal in adult 0.4–1.5 mg/dL (blood) Range depends on age and gender: from as low as 52 in older females to as high as 146 in young men.	Creatinine clearance (mL/min/1.73 m²) Creatinine is a catabolic by-product of muscle energy metabolism and is excreted by the kidneys. It is dependent on muscle mass. Kidney disorders hinder creatinine excretion; creatinine clearance is the rate at which the kidneys are able to clear creatinine from the blood.

Adapted from Daniels, R. (2004). Nursing fundamentals: Caring and clinical decision making. New York: Thomson Delmar Learning.

BOX 52-6

PATIENT EDUCATION FOR A RENAL ULTRASOUND

The nurse can assist and educate the patient with a renal ultrasound by providing the following information:

- You will be positioned in a supine position. Your flank will be exposed and appropriately draped.
- Your abdomen will be lubricated with an acoustic gel.
- You will be asked to take a deep breath and hold it. This is done so that various parts of the kidney can be visualized.
- The technician will use a transducer to visualize various regions of the kidney and surrounding areas.

Source: Daniels, R. (2003). Delmar's manual of laboratory and diagnostic tests. New York: Thomson Delmar Learning.

TABLE 52-4 **Common Causes of Urinary Retention**

Bladder outlet obstruction	Prostatic enlargement
	Benign prostatic hyperplasia (BPH)
	Prostate cancer
	Prostatitis
	Bladder neck dyssynergia (dyssynergia of the smooth muscle of the sphincter mechanism)
	Detrusor sphincter dyssynergia (dyssynergia between detrusor and striated muscle of sphincter)
	Urethral stricture
	Urethral tumor (rare)
	Constipation
	Pelvic organ prolapse
	Cystocele
	Uterine prolapse
Deficient detrusor contraction strength	Transient conditions
	Fecal impaction
	Acute immobility
	Side effect of drugs, including anticholinergics and tricyclic antidepressants
	Side effect of recreational drugs, including hallucinogens
	Herpes zoster of sacral dermatomes
	Vitamin B_{12} deficiency
	Established conditions
	Lesions of the sacral spine
	Cauda equina syndrome
	Diabetes mellitus (late stages)
	Tabes dorsalis
	Poliomyelitis
	Chronic alcoholism

Adapted from Daniels, R. (2004). Nursing fundamentals: Caring and clinical decision making. New York: Thomson Delmar Learning.

Nursing Management

The correct procedures for the nurse to follow for administration of a renal ultrasound are described in Box 52-6.

Renal Biopsy

A needle biopsy via ultrasonic guided imagery offers the least intrusive method to obtain samples of the renal cortex for microscopic examination. Surgical biopsy (open biopsy) may be required. Indications for renal biopsy include unexplained renal failure, glomerular dysfunction, and transplant rejection (Mittal, Rennke, & Singh, 2005).

Nursing Management

Preprocedure, the patient will be instructed not to eat or drink for four to six hours. Forewarn of the approximate two-hour period of bedrest required for transplant graft biopsy and the four to six hours of bedrest for **native kidney**

TABLE 52-5	Radiographic Diagnostic Tests for the Renal System
STUDY	**NURSING MANAGEMENT**
KUB—abdominal X-ray study of the kidneys, ureters, and bladder	Constipation can interfere with the viewing field. The KUB show kidney size, shape, and position and presence of calculi. Hydronephrosis, cysts, and tumors may be visualized.
Computed-assisted tomography (CAT or CT) scan	Contrast media must be ingested in a brief period of time prior to going to the radiology department. Inform the patient that he or she must lie still while strapped onto a gently moving table for a considerable period of time. The table will move through a large cylindrical opening. Though alone in the room, the patient will be in voice contact with the technician. Sedation should be considered for patients with anxiety issues.
Magnetic resonance imaging (MRI)	Similar to the CAT scan, though MRI does not require contrast media. A metal screening is mandatory prior to the MRI. If the patient has had significant exposure to metal, facial X-rays will be ordered to deem the patient safe to proceed with the MRI. The patient will need an IV access and all jewelry and metal removed. Metal implants will likely exclude the patient as an MRI candidate. Claustrophobia is a real concern because of the confined space and continual loud noises while images are taken. Sedation is often needed. Noninvasive, the MRI and CT scans offer detailed images of soft tissue.
Nuclear scans	**Radioisotopes** (a compound that contains radioactive materials, which are used in nuclear scans; the activity of these tagged materials allows the study of substances as they course through the body), such as technetium or iodine, are injected prior to the study. A scintillation camera follows passage through the renal vascular system. Nuclear scans evaluate renal blood flow and renal masses. Allergies to technetium are rare; iodine allergies must be considered. Alert the patient that he or she will go to radiology for the injection and return to radiology about two hours later for the actual study. He or she will be required to lie still for about 30–45 minutes in a quiet environment. Postprocedure care: Unless the patient is fluid restricted, encourage the patient to drink liberal amounts of fluid to promote isotope excretion.
Intravenous pyelogram (IVP)	A radiopaque contrast agent is injected intravenously. This renders the urine radiopaque as the contract agent is excreted in the urine. Abnormalities of the lumen, calculi, and masses can be detected. It is imperative to check for dye allergies and to hydrate the patient for posttest dye excretion to avoid nephrotoxic damage.
Renal angiography	An invasive procedure, renal angiography evaluates renal artery stenosis, tumors, and trauma. A catheter is threaded through the femoral artery allowing direct injection of a radiopaque substance. Preprocedure, shave the groin and mark the pedal pulses. Inform the patient that he or she may feel a temporary surge of warmth when the dye is injected. Iodine allergy must be considered. Postprocedure care includes approximately four hours of bedrest, frequent vital signs, groin check for hematoma, peripheral circulation status check distal to the injection site (color, warmth, and pulses), and hydration to clear the potentially nephrotoxic contrast agent.

Source: Daniels, R. (2003). Delmar's manual of laboratory and diagnostic tests. *New York: Thomson Delmar Learning.*

(one's own kidney as opposed to a transplant graft) biopsy. Less bed rest is required for transplant biopsy due to less strain on the renal capsule with the graft located in a lower abdominal quadrant.

Postprocedure care focuses on the potential for bleeding. Nursing interventions are shown in Box 52-7.

Cystoscopy

The surgical procedure of a cystoscopy allows direct visualization via a self-contained visual lens system. An illustration of a cystoscopy is presented in Figure 52-8, while an illustration of a flexible cystoscope is presented in Figure 52-9. Although the procedure could be done under local anesthesia, gen-

---

BOX 52-7

NURSING CARE OF PATIENTS HAVING A RENAL BIOPSY

- Frequent vital signs and inspection of the biopsy site for hematoma. Typical frequency is every 15 minutes during the first hour then gradually increasing the interval if no bleeding occurs. Follow provider protocol.
- Monitor for any evidence of bleeding. Signs and symptoms include significant change in blood pressure, tachycardia, nausea or vomiting (often associated with hypotension), or a reduction in the hematocrit.
- Anything more than minimal pain. Ureteral colic could signal a clot occluding the ureter. Back pain may indicate a retroperitoneal or intrarenal bleed.
- Monitoring the urine for hematuria or clots. Serial samples of urine are saved in urinalysis tubes, dated, timed, and placed in a rack for color comparison.
- Educate the patient to avoid heavy lifting for an average of two weeks and notify the health care provider of flank pain, light-headedness or dizziness, rapid pulse, dysuria, or hematuria.

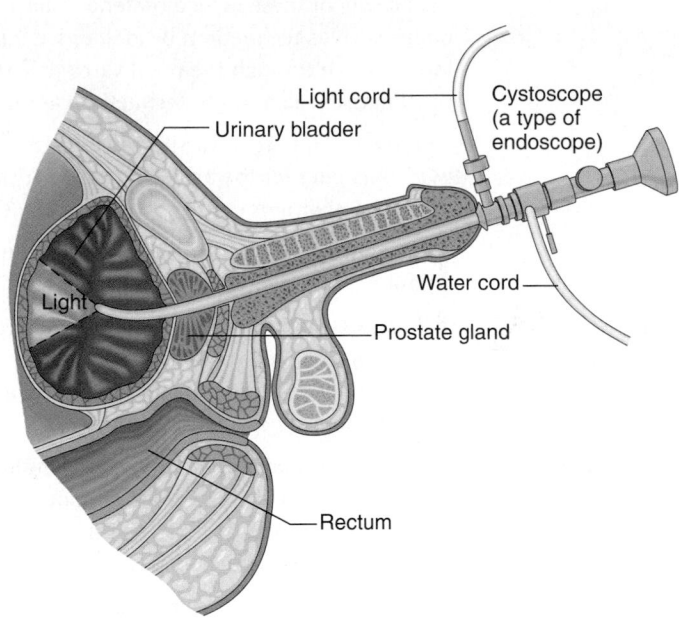

Figure 52-8 Cystoscopy.

eral anesthesia is most often chosen to prevent ureteral spasm when probing with the ureteral catheter. Complete visualization of the entire macroscopic urinary system as catheters ascend into the renal pelvis. Calculi removal, biopsy, and urine sampling from each kidney are possible with this procedure.

Nursing Management

The patient must avoid food and fluids for four to eight hours prior to the procedure if receiving general anesthesia. Postprocedural care includes monitoring the patient for urinary obstruction secondary to swelling and hematuria related to biopsy or inadvertent injury to urinary structures. Light hematuria and pain during first void(s) may not be abnormal depending on the extensiveness of the procedure (Forsyth, Shaikh, & Gunn, 2005).

The patient should be educated to notify the health care provider for problems voiding, gross hematuria, excessive pain, fever or chills, and continued **dysuria** (painful urination).

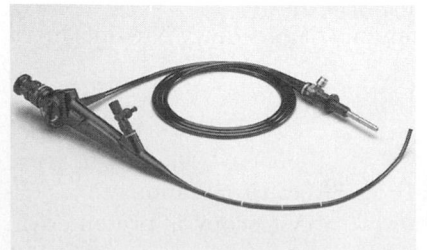

Figure 52-9 Flexible cystoscope.

KEY CONCEPTS

- The renal system controls the fluid balance of the body, controls many of the metabolic processes within the body and provides stabilization for the human body circulation.
- Composed of smooth muscle, the ureter propels urine toward the bladder by peristalsis.
- The bladder neck plays a critical role in continence and in dysfunctions of bladder emptying.
- The cumulative action seen in the renin-angiotensin cycle causes vasoconstriction and yields an increase in blood pressure.
- Hypertension, extensive cardiovascular disease, diabetes, gout, and autoimmune disease are among the more common causes of renal problems.

- Daily weight is a critical assessment components for a patient with renal failure.
- Adherence to specimen collection and test prep protocols is critically important to accurately diagnose and treat urinary system disorders.
- Serum creatinine is a by-product of muscle metabolism and is a much more reliable indicator of renal dysfunction than BUN.
- An abdominal X-ray study of the kidneys, ureters, and bladder is a KUB.
- A needle biopsy via ultrasonic guided imagery offers the least intrusive method to obtain samples of the renal cortex for microscopic examination.
- The surgical procedure of a cystoscopy allows direct visualization vial a self-contained visual lens system.

REVIEW QUESTIONS

1. Which of the following is a definitive method to monitor for bleeding into the urinary system post renal biopsy?
   1. Ask the patient if he or she has noticed blood in his or her urine
   2. Check the urine with a dipstick before discarding it
   3. Collect a small sample of each voiding and place in a rack for comparison over time
   4. Use a Foley catheter to collect a urine specimen

2. You must collect a 24-hour creatinine clearance on Mr. Jones. What will you do to begin the urine collection?
   1. Have the patient void and place the sample in the collection container
   2. Have the patient void and discard urine, noting this as the beginning of the 24-hour urine collection
   3. Wait until the patient voids to start the 24-hour urine collection
   4. All of the above are appropriate options

3. Which of the following is most appropriate intervention to protect the kidney in the presence of nephrotoxic contrast media?
   1. Hydration, administration of acetylcysteine, or administration of IV sodium bicarbonate
   2. Radiologist adjustment of nephrotoxic contrast media dosage
   3. Withhold contrast media in all cases of renal concern
   4. None of the above

4. You must send a patient for a magnetic resonance imaging (MRI) study of his kidneys. Identify two primary nursing considerations in preparation for the MRI.
   1. Coordinating the MRI with other patient care activities and informing the patient about the test
   2. Giving all scheduled medications and completing the bath before the test
   3. Report metal screening findings to the MRI department and sedate for claustrophobia before sending him or her to the MRI department
   4. Make sure the patient is NPO and hold all medications until the test is completed

5. Your patient reports, "I'm just clumsy. I dropped the cap of specimen cup on the bathroom floor, but I don't think it got dirty." What do you do now?
   1. Hope that he or she is right and send the specimen to the laboratory
   2. Discard the specimen and collect another specimen with review of instructions
   3. Clean the cover, cap the specimen, and send it to the laboratory
   4. Find a new cover to put on the specimen container and then send it to the laboratory

Continued

REVIEW QUESTIONS—cont'd

6. What position must your patient assume to obtain an accurate postvoid residual with the bladder scan?
   1. Semi-Fowler
   2. Supine
   3. Head slightly elevated
   4. Prone

7. What is the primary significance of constipation to an X-ray of the kidneys, ureters, and bladder (KUB) or other abdominal study?
   1. Resolving constipation may prevent the patient from needing the KUB.
   2. Constipation can interfere with the viewing field.
   3. The patient may have the urge to defecate during the study.
   4. There is no relationship between constipation and KUB results.

8. Identify the evidence that the kidney is an organ with high oxygen demand and the primary homeostatic organ of the body.
   1. The kidney has 2 million functioning units.
   2. The kidney filters nearly approximately 180 L water a day.

3. The kidney receives 20 percent of the cardiac output.
4. None of these are evidence of a high oxygen demand.

9. Nursing care of the patient who has had a cystoscopy include all of the following *except:*
   1. Warm sitz baths
   2. Monitor intake and output
   3. Mild analgesics for pain
   4. Restrict fluids

10. A patient is suspected to have a urinary tract infection. Which of the following laboratory tests would be appropriate to determine if an infection is present?
    1. Creatinine clearance
    2. Blood culture
    3. Residual urine
    4. Urine culture and sensitivity

REVIEW ACTIVITIES

1. State and describe the organs of the renal system.

2. Perform a concise health history related to the renal system on an adult patient.

3. Describe age-related changes seen in the renal system.

4. Describe any two of the diagnostic tests used for the renal system.

5. In the clinical setting, identify the location of (a) test strips for urinalysis; (b) specimen cups for collecting urine samples; and (c) Foley catheter kits.

Urinary Dysfunction: Nursing Management

Paul Chamberland, MSN, APRN, BC, CMSRN

Leslie H. Nicoll, PhD, MBA, RN, BC

CHAPTER TOPICS

- Urinary Tract Infections
- Interstitial Cystitis
- Pyelonephritis
- Glomerulonephritis
- Nephrotic Syndrome
- Renal Tuberculosis
- Urinary Tract Calculi (Urolithiasis)

- Renal Trauma
- Renal Vascular Disorders
- Renal Cancer
- Bladder Cancer
- Urinary Diversion
- Urinary Retention
- Urinary Incontinence

KEY TERMS

Anasarca
Cystectomy
Dysuria
Hematuria
Hydronephrosis
Hypercholesterolemia
Hypoalbuminemia
Malaise
Nephrectomy
Nephrolithiasis
Nocturia
Nosocomial
Oliguria
Proteinuria
Pyelonephritis
Ureteral strictures
Urethral strictures
Urinary tract infection (UTI)
Urolithiasis (calculi)

Urinary tract dysfunctions cover a wide spectrum. Dysfunction in any segment of the system easily creates disorder in other areas. For example, a simple bladder infection may ascend upward along the urinary tract and evolve into nephritis with significant threat to renal function. Similarly, obstruction distal to the kidney can create pressure damage to the renal parenchyma from unrelieved or repetitive episodes of **hydronephrosis** (stretching of the renal pelvis as a result of obstruction to urinary outflow). This chapter explores nursing management of infectious, noninfectious, obstructive, calculus, and vascular disorders of the entire urinary system. Surgical diversion of urinary flow into continent or incontinent systems will also be discussed. Acute and chronic renal failure will be discussed at length in chapter 54. Although these are urinary tract disorders, discussion is lengthy because of homeostatic disturbance and the extensive treatments that are involved.

URINARY TRACT INFECTION

Urinary tract infection (UTI) is an infection involving the kidneys, ureters, bladder, or urethra. Synonyms for UTI include bacteriuritis, asymptomatic bacteriuritis, bacterial cystitis, urethritis, pyelonephritis, and prostatitis. A UTI can cover a wide variety of conditions, ranging from asymptomatic infections with low bacterial counts not requiring intervention to severe infection of the kidney and sepsis with threat to survival. Early intervention has the potential to save costs, prevent significant incapacity, and save lives.

A UTI is labeled according to the region of infection. In general terms, reference is made to lower urinary tract (e.g., urethra, bladder, or prostate) and upper urinary tract infections (e.g., ureters or kidney). In addition, a UTI may be classified by events such as initial or recurrent, acute or chronic. A UTI may be identified as drug-resistant. Combinations of these labels offer critical information to the provider for assessment, care planning, and patient education purposes. For example, an initial, lower tract UTI most likely prompts a lower level of concern than does a diagnosis of a chronic, recurrent, upper tract UTI.

Further, a UTI may be classified as uncomplicated in patients without structural abnormalities or altered urodynamics or complicated in patients with a structural abnormality or altered urodynamics, or any urinary infection in males.

Epidemiology

UTIs prompt over five million office visits annually in the United States. Uncomplicated infections incur annual health care costs in excess of $350 million. UTIs are more common in females because of a shorter urethra and the proximity of the urethra to the vagina and anus (Table 53-1). Sexual intercourse and forward cleansing following defecation offer primary sources of contamination. Incidence increases in the aging female because of bladder prolapse. Recurrent infection is common.

In the male, the incidence of bladder infection is higher in the uncircumcised than in the circumcised. Incidence in all males increases with age because of problems of prostatic hypertrophy.

TABLE 53-1	**Epidemiological Factors Associated with UTI**
Incidence	Females: 12 cases per 1,000 women per year in the United States.
	Males: 0.3 cases per 1,000 men per year.
Prevalence	Females: 10–40 per 1,000 women per year.
	Males: Less than 1 per 1,000 males per year.
	Note: Asymptomatic bacteriuria occurs in up to 40 percent of elderly men and women.
Gender	Most prevalent in sexually active adult females.
	After 65 years of age, equal numbers of men and women are affected.
Age	In infants up to six months of age; UTI is more common in boys, who have a higher incidence of abnormalities of the urinary tract than girls.
	Between 1 and 65 years of age, UTI is predominantly a disease of females, presumably because of the anatomy of the female urethra, which allows bacteria to access the urinary tract relatively easily.
	Over 65 years of age, bacteriuria affects men and women roughly equally (approximately 40 percent), with the majority of infections being asymptomatic. Routine screening and treatment has not been found to decrease morbidity or mortality in this population.

Etiology

Bacteria causing a UTI usually originates from the bowel as normal flora of the host. *Escherichia coli (E. coli)* are the most common infective bacterial organism in acute cystitis and represent 80 present of all cases requiring treatment. *E. coli* bacteria are present in feces, adhere easily to the epithelium of the urinary tract, and have the capability to resist destruction by the white blood cells.

Hospital-acquired (nosocomial) infection adds a significant health care dollar burden to the public and to the institution. UTIs are of particular significance. Physical and psychological stress response to hospitalization predisposes patients to acquired infection. Hospitalized patients frequently require procedure-associated bladder catheterization. Catheter intrusion into the urinary system predisposes the patient to inoculation with bacteria-contaminated equipment or bacterial entry along the in-place catheter. In addition to *E. coli* exposure from episodes of fecal incontinence or compromised hygiene, the environment offers exposure to more virulent organisms such as *Pseudomonas* and *Staphylococcus*. More recently, interdisciplinary health faces the challenge of limiting the spread of drug-resistant organisms, such as vancomycin-resistant enterococcus (VRE). See Table 53-2 for a summary of the common causes of UTI sorted according to their frequency of occurrence.

Pathophysiology

The epithelium of the kidneys, ureter, and bladder is sterile in the healthy individual. An infection occurs when bacteria enter the urine and begin to grow. The infection usually starts at the opening of the urethra where the urine leaves the body and moves upward into the urinary tract.

Usually, the act of emptying the bladder (urinating) flushes the bacteria out of the urethra. If there are too many bacteria, this will not stop them. The bacteria can travel up the urethra to the bladder, where they can grow and cause an infection. The infection can spread further as the bacteria move up from the bladder via the ureters. If they reach the kidney, they can cause a kidney infection (pyelonephritis), which can become a serious condition if not treated promptly.

Complications of a simple lower tract infection are rare and typically involve resistant microorganisms or indicate undiagnosed structural abnormalities or abnormal urodynamics. Primary complications of complicated and resistant UTI are ascending infection and spread to the blood stream. Nephritis and sepsis place the patient at high risk have potential for chronic illness or death.

Assessment with Clinical Manifestations

In lower urinary tract infection (e.g., cystitis), the lining of the urethra and bladder becomes inflamed and irritated. The symptoms that can be seen with lower urinary tract infection include:
- **Dysuria**—Pain or burning during urination
- Frequency—More frequent urination (or waking up at night to urinate)
- Urgency—The sensation of not being able to hold urine
- Hesitancy—The sensation of not being able to urinate easily or completely (or feeling a need to urinate but only a few drops of urine come out)
- Cloudy, bad smelling, or bloody urine
- Lower abdominal pain
- Mild fever (less than 101° F [38.3° C]), chills, and not feeling well (malaise)

In upper UTI (e.g., pyelonephritis), symptoms develop rapidly and may or may not include the symptoms for a lower urinary tract infection (see Red Flag).

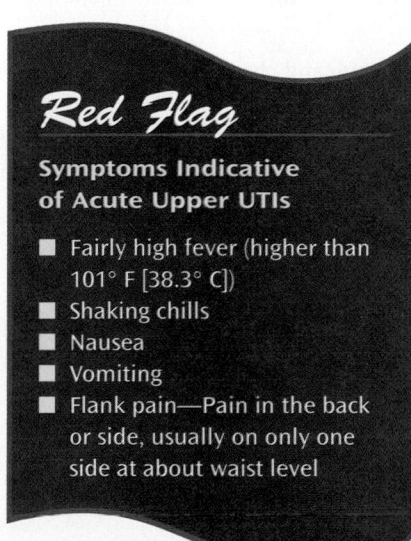

Red Flag

Symptoms Indicative of Acute Upper UTIs

- Fairly high fever (higher than 101° F [38.3° C])
- Shaking chills
- Nausea
- Vomiting
- Flank pain—Pain in the back or side, usually on only one side at about waist level

TABLE 53-2 **Causes of UTIs and Their Frequency**

Common	Gram-positive organisms:
	    Staphylococcus saprophyticus (5–15 percent)
	    Enterococcus faecalis
	Gram-negative organisms:
	    Escherichia coli (80–85 percent)
	    Klebsiella pneumoniae
	    Proteus species
	    Pseudomonas aeruginosa
	    Enterobacter species

Rare	*Salmonella* species *Mycobacterium tuberculosis* *Chlamydia trachomatis* *Candida* species Multiple microbial organisms causing infection may be found in patients with renal calculi, chronic renal abscesses, or indwelling urinary catheters
Serious	*S. aureus*—commonly a result of bacteremia producing renal or perinephric abscesses *Candida* species—found in critically ill, immunosuppressed, and chronically catheterized patients
Contributory or predisposing factors	Female gender is an independent frisk factor for UTI Recent sexual intercourse Use of spermicides or diaphragm Pregnancy Antecedent antibiotic use—antimicrobials used 15–28 days before a UTI may alter urogenital normal flora in favor of pathogen-dominated flora Obstruction of urinary tract (e.g., benign prostatic hyperplasia, tumors, or cholinergic drugs) Residual urine in bladder caused by prostatic hypertrophy, urethral strictures, cystocele, hypotonic bladder, renal calculi, urolithiasis, tumors, bladder diverticula, or anticholinergic drugs Incomplete bladder emptying caused by neurological pathology (e.g., stroke or spinal cord injuries) Retrograde urinary reflux gives an increased risk of acute and chronic pyelonephritis Urinary catheterization Mechanical instrumentation

In newborns, infants, children, and the elderly, the classic symptoms of a UTI may not be present. Other symptoms may indicate a UTI:

- Newborns—Fever or hypothermia (low temperature), poor feeding, or jaundice
- Infants—Vomiting, diarrhea, fever, poor feeding, or not thriving
- Children—Irritability, eating poorly, unexplained fever that does not go away, loss of bowel control, loose bowels, or change in urination pattern
- Elderly people—Fever or hypothermia, poor appetite, lethargy, or change in mental status

Typically pregnant women do not have unusual or unique symptoms. A urine sample should be checked during prenatal visits, because an unrecognized infection can cause pregnancy complications.

Although most people have symptoms with a UTI, some do not. The symptoms of UTI can resemble those of sexually transmitted diseases. The complete assessment of a UTI is based on information given relating to one's symptoms, medical and surgical history, medications, habits, and lifestyle (Table 53-3). A physical examination and lab tests complete the evaluation.

Diagnostic Tests

Performing a dipstick of the urine offers a quick, easy, and readily available prediction of UTI. A result that is positive for nitrates and leukocyte esterase indicate treatable infection, but it does not identify the exact location within the urinary system. To perform a dipstick test, follow instructions on the package. Verify that the dipsticks have been stored according to manufacturer's guidelines to ensure test strip reliability.

Urinalysis screens that are positive for heme, protein, leukocytes, or nitrites need further study. Collection is appropriate at any time of day; the first void of the day provides the optimal specimen. It is usually important to collect expediently. Send it to the laboratory within one hour of the void. Avoid contamination by menses or feces.

Urine culture determines bacterial count and identifies infecting bacteria for best choice of antibiotic. A bacterial count of more than 100,000 indicates treatable infection. Sensitivity may be added to the culture to determine antibacterial sensitivity or resistance. This is especially important in recurrent or complicated infections.

Collection technique for males include cleansing the glans penis with the appropriate cleansing solution following institutional procedure and attending any patient allergies. Retract foreskin, if present. Have the patient start to

---

TABLE 53-3	Clinical Assessment for UTIs: Subjective and Objective Data
Subjective Data	
Focused past health history	Previous UTIs and how treated, urinary calculi, ureteral or urethral strictures, bladder cancer or prostate problems, recent hospitalization or surgery, sexually transmitted disease, vaginal infection, diabetes, or pregnancy.
Current history	Burning on urination, urine color and odor, fever, chills, nausea or vomiting, voiding pattern and any changes. Pain character and location. Query especially for flank or low back pain, suprapubic discomfort or feeling unrelieved with voiding, bladder spasm or burning on urination, vaginal or penile discharge, and menses.
Medications	History of taking anticholinergic or antispasmodic medications. Complete listing of current medications including over-the-counter (OTC) and herbal preparations.
Personal data	Fluid and nutritional intake, hygiene habits, adherence to prescribed medications, smoking, and caffeine and alcohol intake.
Objective Data	
Systemic	Fever, chills, nausea, diarrhea, and skin turgor.
Urinary	Cloudy urine, hematuria, foul smelling urine, distension, or suprapubic or costovertebral tenderness.
Laboratory findings	Elevated white blood cell count. Urine positive for nitrites, leukocytes, red blood cells, or bacteria.

Adapted from Estes, M. (2006). Health assessment and physical examination *(3rd ed.). New York: Thomson Delmar Learning.*

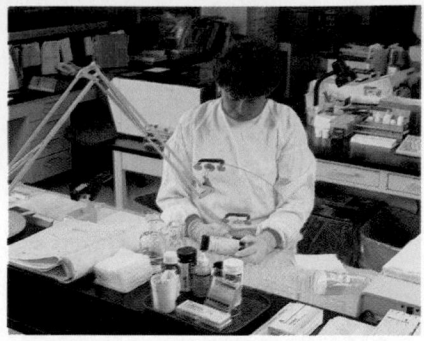

Figure 53-1 Laboratory technician examining urinalysis sample for physical, chemical, or microbiological properties from a patient with glomerulonephritis.

void then collect a midstream urine sample. Keep inside of cover and container free of contamination from the hands or surroundings. Collection technique for females include: separating the labia and cleansing the vulva. A catheter specimen is warranted during menses or conditions that will not allow a reliable midstream collection into a sterile container (Estes, 2006).

The culture is usually sent for special populations, including men, because they are less likely to get UTIs. It is not necessary to send a culture for everyone because the majority of UTIs are caused by the same bacteria. For example, a urine culture may not be required for uncomplicated cystitis in women (Figure 53-1).

Some species (e.g., *Chlamydia* and *Mycoplasma*) require special cultures to be detected. Special tests should be ordered if a patient has signs and symptoms of a UTI, but a laboratory culture fails to grow bacteria.

Imaging studies are not needed in the vast majority of patients with UTI. However, appropriate imaging studies should be done if structural abnormality or altered urodynamics are suspected. Pelvic ultrasound may be indicated in young women with pelvic tenderness, cervical discharge, and unilateral adnexal tenderness or elderly patients with abdominal pain and pyuria with no classic symptoms for UTI.

When a patient has a persistent infection that does not resolve after appropriate antibiotic therapy or suffers from recurrent infections, referral may be necessary for further tests to identify structural or functional abnormalities (Box 53-1).

BOX 53-1

SUMMARY OF DIAGNOSTIC TESTS FOR UTI

Initial Tests

- Macroscopic urinalysis: A simple, noninvasive test that should be performed on all patients suspected of having a UTI
- Dipstick nitrite tests: Detection of nitrite in urine indicates presence of nitrate-reducing bacteria. Sensitivity 0.35; specificity 0.95
- Leukocyte esterase dipstick tests: Sensitive and highly specific test for detecting greater than 10 white blood cells/mm^3 of urine (pyuria). Sensitivity 0.75-0.90; specificity 0.70
- Microscopic urinalysis: Can reveal bacteruria and pyuria
- Quantitative urine culture: Differentiates between contamination of urine and infection by quantification of bacteria; allows identification and susceptibility testing of microorganisms

Additional tests to consider if structural or functional abnormalities of the urinary tract are suspected, or with history of recurrent infections; may be performed by a specialist if warranted:

- Renal and bladder ultrasound: May demonstrate structural abnormalities
- Voiding cystourethrogram (VCUG): May demonstrate abnormalities of the collecting system, particularly vesicoureteral reflux
- Intravenous pyelogram (IVP): May demonstrate abnormal renal function, abnormalities of the collecting system, or obstruction
- Postvoid residual volume: May demonstrate significant urinary retention (greater than 100 mL is abnormal)
- Radionuclide scan: May demonstrate abnormal renal function and structure
- Cystoscopy: Allows direct visualization of bladder and distal collecting system and the collection of urine from various areas of the renal system

Adapted from Daniels, R. (2003). Delmar's manual of laboratory and diagnostic tests. *New York: Thomson Delmar Learning.*

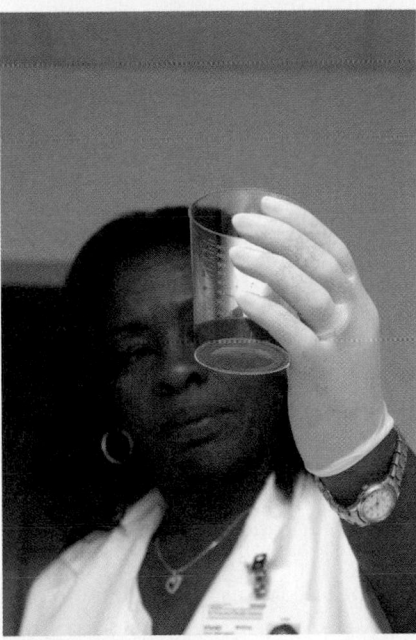

Figure 53-2 Nurse examining and measuring hematuria sample from a patient with a UTI.

Nursing Diagnoses

Based on the information gathered, examples of nursing diagnoses in the person with a UTI may include the following:

- Infection related to frequency or burning on urination, fever, elevated white blood cell count, foul-smelling urine, and suprapubic tenderness
- Impaired urinary elimination related to excessive urgency and pain with bladder filling
- Acute pain related to inflammation of urinary mucosa as evidenced by suprapubic discomfort and dysuria

Planning and Implementation

There are focused interventions to use for patients who have UTIs. The primary considerations are prevention of the UTI in the first place. Then, if a person contracts the UTI, prompt identification of the presence of the UTI is essential, followed with quick responsive antibiotic therapy (Figure 53-2). The American Urological Association (2006) is one source of referral for patients with UTIs (www.auanet.org).

Goals

The overall goals for treating a person with a UTI include: to prevent (or treat) the systemic consequences of the infection; to eradicate pathogenic organisms in the person's urine; and to prevent the recurrence of infection.

Pharmacology

It is not uncommon to have a clinically insignificant bacterial infection of this system. In such case, the patient is asymptomatic with a urinary bacterial count significantly less than 100,000 colony forming units (CFU) per milliliter. UTI are considered clinically significant and warrant treatment when presenting symptoms of UTI (irrespective of a low bacterial count) or with a bacterial count is greater than 100,000 CFU/mL. However, a health care provider should not wait to obtain the culture report before treating. Empiric antibiotic therapy should be initiated on the basis of the patient's symptoms and urinalysis results before urine culture results are obtained (Box 53-2).

Evaluation of Outcomes

Potential patient outcomes for each of the example nursing diagnoses for the patient with the UTI are shown in Table 53-4.

INTERSTITIAL CYSTITIS

The common clinical picture of interstitial cystitis (IC) presents with urgency, frequency, **nocturia** (urination at night), and dysuria in the presence of noninfected urine. **Hematuria** (blood in the urine) may be present. Pain associated with the bladder is a major complaint. IC is often confused with recurrent UTI as presenting symptoms are markedly similar. Because of its uncertain etiology, IC is regarded by many as more of a clinical syndrome than a disease entity.

Epidemiology

In general, IC affects both men and women. Although 90 percent of these people are middle-aged women, it can occur in children or older adults (Table 53-5).

PATIENT PLAYBOOK

Considerations for Patient Teaching

Health care providers should instruct all patients to completely empty the bladder when voiding; and to not put off the urge to urinate, particularly after intercourse.

It is also important to validate (or instruct, as needed) that women cleanse and dry from front-to-back when completing perineal care.

Diet

- Drinking six to eight glasses of water daily helps to prevent UTI.
- Cranberry juice may help to prevent UTI.

Sexual behavior

- Urinating before and after sexual intercourse may help to prevent UTI.
- Limiting the number of sexual partners may help to prevent UTI.

Medication history

- Always instruct the patient to finish taking the medications as the health care provider prescribed.
- Use of anticholinergic medications cautiously, as they may leave residual urine in bladder, predisposing to UTI.

Other

- If there is a family history of UTI, a genetic predisposition for bacterial adherence to bladder may be present. Awareness of and adherence to lifestyle and wellness issues, sexual behavioral practices, and dietary considerations may offer protection from UTI.
- Self-catheterization or mechanical instrumentation may introduce bacteria into urinary tract. Assist or instruct the patient on the proper and appropriate self-catheterization technique.

BOX 53-2

COMMON MEDICATIONS USED WITH PATIENTS WITH UTI

Antifolates

- Effective against common UTI pathogens except *Pseudomonas aeruginosa*. Inexpensive. Appropriate as a short course, first choice in uncomplicated UTI. Inexpensive.
- Trimethoprim-sulfamethoxazole D.S. (TMP/SMZ, Bactrim). Drink large amounts of fluids to prevent sediment in urine and calculus formation.
- Trimethoprim (Primsol, Proloprim, and Trimpex) may be prescribed alone in an attempt to limit TMP/SMZ side effects.

Fluoroquinolones

- Indicated for *Pseudomonas aeruginosa* and multidrug-resistant gram-negative infections. Expensive. Also indicated for patients with sulfa allergies.
- Ciprofloxacin (Cipro or Ciloxan) should not be administered within two hours of taking antacids.

Cephalosporins: First Generation

- Cephalexin (Biocef, Keflex, and Keftab). Typical pathogens are frequently resistant to cephalexin (20 to 30 percent nationally). Probably less effective than other alternatives for short-course (three-day) treatment, owing to its rapid clearance from urine. Is not effective in elimination of *Escherichia coli* from vaginal flora.

Penicillins

- Amoxicillin and clavulanic acid (Augmentin) is effective against beta-lactam-resistant organisms. Probably less effective than other alternatives for short-course (three-day) treatment, owing to its rapid clearance from urine. Typical pathogens are frequently resistant to amoxicillin or clavulanic acid (20 to 30 percent nationally).

Nitrofurantoin (Macrobid, Furalan, Macrodantin) attains a high concentration in the bladder because it is excreted unchanged into urine. Documented lower cure rate in short-course (three-day) treatment than other alternatives. Fifteen to 20 percent of typical organisms are resistant to nitrofurantoin. Take with food or milk to increase absorption; urine may appear dark yellow or brown.

Adapted from Broyles, B. E., Reiss, B. S., & Evans, M. E. (2007). Pharmacological aspects of nursing care (7th ed.). New York: Thomson Delmar Learning.

Etiology

The cause of this debilitating condition is not clearly known. Theories include obstruction to lymphatic flow, thrombophlebitis secondary to acute infections, prolonged arteriolar spasm, and neuropathic or endocrine dysfunction. Clearly this is a confusing anomaly. More recently, researchers are focusing on the activity of mucosal mast cells capable of releasing histamine and other irritants to the bladder mucosa.

Pathophysiology

The pathophysiology of IC is poorly understood. Various causes have been proposed, none of which sufficiently explain the differing clinical presentations, clinical courses, or responses to therapies. The most frequently cited cause of the presenting symptoms is that the bladder mucosa becomes thinned or

TABLE 53-4 UTIs: Nursing Diagnosis, Patient Outcomes, and Interventions

Patient with a UTI

Nursing Diagnosis: Acute pain related to inflammation of urinary mucosa as evidenced by suprapubic discomfort and dysuria

OUTCOMES (NOC)	INTERVENTIONS (NIC) AND RATIONALE
Pain Control (1605)	Pain Management (1400)
Uses resources appropriately.	Teach principles of pain management.
Reports changes in pain symptoms or sites to the health care professional.	Ensure that patient receives attentive analgesic care.
	Explore with patient factors that relieve or worsen pain.
Outcome Scale	Teach use of nonpharmacological techniques (heat to lower back or pubis)
1 = Never demonstrated	Perform a comprehensive assessment of pain to include location, characteristics, onset and duration, frequency, quality, intensity or severity of pain, and precipitating factors
2 = Rarely demonstrated	
3 = Sometimes demonstrated	
4 = Often demonstrated	
5 = Consistently demonstrated	

Nursing Diagnosis: Impaired urinary elimination related to UTI.

OUTCOMES (NOC)	INTERVENTIONS (NIC) AND RATIONALE
Urinary Elimination (0503)	Urinary Elimination Management (0590)
Achieves established fluid intake.	Teach patient to drink an additional eight ounces of liquid with meals, between meals, and in early evening.
Urine regains clarity and dysuria is relieved.	
1 = Never demonstrated	Consult with dietary to include additional liquids, such as soups and juices with meals.
2 = Rarely demonstrated	
3 = Sometimes demonstrated	Instruct patient to respond immediately to urge to void.
4 = Often demonstrated	Teach patient the signs and symptoms of UTI and inform of potential for recurrence.
5 = Consistently demonstrated	
	Monitor urinary elimination including frequency, consistency, odor, volume, and color.

Adapted from NANDA International. (2005a). Nursing diagnoses: Definitions & classifications 2005–2006. Philadelphia: NANDA International.

TABLE 53-5 Epidemiological Factors Associated with IC

Incidence	The incidence rate of IC is 2.6 cases per 100,000 women per year in the United States.
Prevalence	Estimated at up to 60–70 per 100,000
Frequency	1 in 4.5 women are affected; rare in men.
Race	Of patients with IC, 94 percent are white. IC appears to be slightly more common in Jewish women.
Gender	Approximately 90 percent of patients with IC are female.
Age	Median age at presentation is 40 years. IC may occur in children.
Associated medical conditions	Patients with IC are more likely to have prior gynecological surgery or a history of UTIs and are 10–12 times more likely to report childhood bladder problems. Associations exist with chronic illnesses, including inflammatory bowel disease, systemic lupus erythematosus, irritable bowel syndrome, fibromyalgia, and atopic allergy

Adapted from Rosenberg, M. T., & Hazzard, M. (2005). Prevalence of interstitial cystitis symptoms in women: A population based study in the primary care office. Journal of Urology, 174(6), 2231–2234.

denuded. The exposed detrusor muscle is progressively damaged and develops fibrosis. Losing its stretch capacity, bladder pain is elicited as the bladder fills. The irritating effect of urine constituents further elicits pain in the presence of an intact mucosa. The disease has rapid progression at onset and tends to plateau though in a debilitated state. Bladder capacity is reduced, voiding dysfunction or vesico-ureteral valvular incompetence develops. For clinical purposes, IC is often divided into two groups, ulcerative (i.e., classic) and nonulcerative (i.e., Messing-Stamey) types.

During a cystoscopic examination, a diffusely reddened appearance to the bladder surface epithelium can be seen in association with one or more ulcerative patches. These patches can also be surrounded by local areas of inflammation and mucosal ulceration (Hunner's ulcer), this being a hallmark of classic IC, and increased capillary formation resembling glomeruli (hence the term glomerulations), submucosal petechiae, and hemorrhage. These bladders demonstrate more fibrosis and scarring with progressive reduction in bladder capacity. The ulcers may become apparent only after the bladder is overdistended because areas of mucosal scarring rupture during the procedure (Ottem & Teichman, 2005). In the United States, this type of interstitial cystitis is rarely seen (less than 10 percent of cases), and some authors consider this type to be more resistant to therapy (Moldwin & Sant, 2002). The nonulcerative type of IC is characterized by similar clinical symptoms (i.e., frequency, urgency, or pelvic pain) but without the cystoscopic findings noted previously.

Genetics

Although traditionally IC has not been considered a hereditable condition, a recent study from the University of Maryland reports a higher occurrence of IC in monozygotic versus dizygotic twins, suggesting the disease has at least a partial genetic predisposition.

Assessment with Clinical Manifestations

A complete history as described for lower UTI is essential. Most importantly, it is critical to believe the patient about persistent reports of pain. People with IC have pain that ranges from mild to severe. Pain is most prominent as the bladder fills between voiding. Suprapubic pain is a common finding, but a person may also feel pain in the bladder, the urethra, the area below the umbilicus, the lower back, or the area around the vagina. Men may also feel pain in the scrotum, testes, or penis. Pain can come and go or it can be constant. It can increase during sex, and some women find that it is worse when they are having their period.

Absence of negative laboratory findings may tempt the health care provider to view the patient as a complainer and to minimize reports of pain. On the contrary, pain characteristics, frequency, duration, precipitating factors, and relieving factors are among the more important findings prompting cystoscopic examination and diagnosis. Empathetic listening and questioning are the nurse's greatest tools in treating a patient with IC. People with IC also feel the need to urinate often. Some people urinate up to 16 times a day and need to get up during the night to urinate. Whereas an urgent and frequent need to urinate combined with pain are common symptoms, not everyone has both symptoms. A person may have one but not the other. Symptoms can become worse or better over time.

Diagnostic Tests

IC is difficult to diagnose, and health care providers do not agree on the best way to identify it. No other laboratory test is definitive of or specific for IC: No urine cytology findings specifically suggest a diagnosis of IC; no serological or hematological abnormalities are known to be specific for IC; no known radiographic, ultrasonographic, or other imaging findings are specific for IC; and urodynamic studies are not helpful as part of the routine IC evaluation.

Most health care providers will begin by examining the person and asking about his or her symptoms. The first step in diagnosing IC is to rule out other diseases that cause similar symptoms. The differential diagnosis of urinary frequency, urgency, or pain is summarized in Box 53-3.

If the health care provider cannot find any other disease that is causing the person's symptoms, the provider may order or perform one of two tests commonly used to help diagnose IC. The first test often used to check for IC is cystoscopy. For this test, the procedural provider will insert a hollow tube that contains lenses and a light into the urethra and bladder. This tube, or cystoscope, allows the health care provider to directly examine the patient's bladder. In addition, most procedural providers will fill the patient's bladder with gas or liquid to test how well it can stretch.

Another common test for IC is the potassium sensitivity test. For this test, liquid that contains potassium is put into the bladder. After a few minutes, the patient will be asked to urinate. Plain water is then put into the patient's bladder. If the potassium causes more pain or a greater need to urinate than the water does, the person may have IC.

A number of other tests may be performed, depending on the patient's symptoms and medical history.

Nursing Diagnoses

Based on the information gathered, examples of nursing diagnoses in the person with IC may include the following:
- Impaired urinary elimination related to excessive urgency and pain with bladder filling
- Impaired comfort related to pain with bladder filling
- Potential for alteration in coping related to person's perception of possible chronic nature of this disease

---

BOX 53-3

DIFFERENTIAL DIAGNOSIS OF URINARY FREQUENCY, URGENCY, OR PAIN

Infectious or Inflammatory Conditions

Recurrent UTI, urethral diverticulum, infected Bartholin gland or Skene gland, vulvovestibulitis, tuberculous or eosinophilic cystitis, vaginitis (e.g., bacterial, viral [e.g., herpes]), or schistosomiasis

Gynecological Causes

Pelvic malignancy or mass (e.g., fibroid or endometrioma), endometriosis, mittelschmerz, pelvic inflammatory disease, or genital atrophy

Urological Causes

Bladder cancer or carcinoma in situ (CIS), radiation cystitis, overflow incontinence, acontractile detrusor, prostatodynia, chronic pelvic pain syndrome, bladder outlet obstruction (e.g., urinary retention with overflow incontinence), or open bladder neck (e.g., intrinsic sphincteric deficiency, urolithiasis, or urethritis)

Neurological Causes

Detrusor hyperreflexia, Parkinson disease, lumbosacral disk disease, spinal stenosis, spinal tumor, multiple sclerosis, or cerebrovascular accident

Other Possible Diagnoses

Dysfunctional voiding, vulvodynia, pelvic floor myalgia, degenerative joint disease, hernia, inflammatory bowel disease, GI neoplasm, diverticulitis, or adhesions from prior surgery

Planning and Implementation

Because no discrete pathological criteria exist for assessing and monitoring disease severity, indications and goals for treatment are based on the degree of patient symptoms. Despite considerable research, universally effective treatments do not exist, and therapy usually consists of various supportive, behavioral, and pharmacological measures. Surgical intervention is rarely indicated.

Nutrition

Some people find that changing their diet helps. Possible items to avoid include alcohol, tomatoes, spices, chocolate, caffeinated drinks, acidic foods, and artificial sweeteners.

Pharmacology

There is no general agreement about the best treatment for IC because no one knows with certainty what causes it. Many believe that each person must find a treatment that works best for him or her. There are two treatments for IC that are used by many health care providers. One is an oral agent called pentosan polysulfate sodium (Elmiron) that is taken three times a day to help the bladder heal. The other medicine for IC is a liquid solvent called dimethyl sulfoxide (abbreviated as DMSO) that is put into the bladder via a urinary catheter. It is given once or twice a week for six to eight weeks. Other drugs are sometimes given to patients with IC (Van Ophoven, Polupic, Heinecke, & Hertle, 2004). A summary of these medications is provided in Box 53-4.

BOX 53-4

COMMON MEDICATIONS USED WITH PATIENTS WITH IC

Specific for IC

Pentosan polysulfate sodium (Elmiron) is the specific for IC. Oral tablet dosage is 100 mg three times daily. The mode of action is not precisely known. It appears that Elmiron structurally and chemically resembles the lining of the bladder and offers similar protection against irritating substances. Pain reduction has been noted as soon as four weeks after the onset of treatment.

Anti-Inflammatory Agents

Cortisone acetate (Cortone, Cortone or Acetate): 100 mg daily for anti-inflammatory effect

Predinisone: 10–20 mg in divided doses daily for 21 days then in decreasing doses for another 21 days for anti-inflammatory effect

Antihistamine

Tripelennamine (Pyribenzamine): 50 mg four times a day for antihistamine effect. [Note that the side effect of this medication is bladder discomfort.]

Catheter Installation

Instillation of 50 mL of 50 percent dimethyl sulfoxide (DMSO) and letting it dwell for 15 minutes. This is repeated every two weeks and offers only symptomatic relief.

Catheter Bladder Lavage

Bladder lavage with increasing strengths of silver nitrate (1:500–1:100) for symptom relief

---

Adapted from Broyles, B. E., Reiss, B. S., & Evans, M. E. (2007). Pharmacological aspects of nursing care (7th ed.). New York: Thomson Delmar Learning.

Patient and Family Teaching for Patients with IC

The nurse should perform the following patient teaching interventions:

- Instruct the patient and family regarding signs and symptoms of upper and lower UTI.
- Instruct the patient diagnosed with IC and his or her family to distinguish between the defining characteristics of this disease and those for a UTI.
- Instruct the patient and family regarding the factors that could possibly relieve and worsen the painful episodes. Explore with the patient what was experienced with each new episode.
- Instruct the patient and family regarding the needed comfort measures.
- Review with the patient and family and explain all potentially threatening and unfamiliar procedures.
- Encourage the patient and family to identify the needed support and assist them, as appropriate, to seek and obtain it.

Health Care Resources

The International Interstitial Cystitis Patient Network Foundations offers support to patients, patient support groups, and health professionals. The latest literature, research and news are available on the World Wide Web at http://www.iicpn-foundation.org.

The Interstitial Cystitis Association (ICA) plays a vital role in research funding, disability, promoting development of new treatments, advocacy, information sharing, public awareness, and education for patients and health professionals. The association is available on the World Wide Web at http://www.ichelp.org/.

Surgery

Electrocoagulation of any splits in the bladder mucosa to relieve the painful irritation of submucosal structures may be indicated. To do this procedure, cystoscopy is required. Cystectomy with urinary diversion may be considered but only in the most severe cases. Urinary diversion is discussed later in this chapter.

Alternative Therapy

Overdistension of the bladder with water to gradually improve the capacity has been found to be successful in some cases. To do this, the person may require anesthesia. Other treatments, such as electrical stimulation or exercises to train the bladder muscles, may be prescribed. People with severe pain or major problems with urination may need surgery.

People with IC need to work with their clinical providers to find the therapy that helps them the most. Therapy can stop working over time, and most people with IC need to continue trying new therapies.

Evaluation of Outcomes

Potential patient outcomes for each of the example nursing diagnoses for the person with IC are:

- Impaired urinary elimination related to excessive urgency and pain with bladder filling. The patient is continent of urine or verbalizes satisfactory management.
- Impaired comfort related to pain with bladder filling. The patient should verbalize an adequate relief of pain along with the ability to realistically cope with the pain if it is not completely relieved.
- Potential for alteration in coping related to person's perception of possible chronic nature of this disease. The patient identifies own maladaptive coping behaviors, available resources, and support systems, describes and initiates alternative coping strategies, and describes positive results from new behaviors.

PYELONEPHRITIS

Pyelonephritis is an infection of the upper urinary tract. It may involve the ureters, renal pelvis, and the papillary tips of the collecting ducts. Unchecked, it can extend into the tubules of the nephron creating a potential for renal failure.

Etiology

Commonly, pyelonephritis is caused by urinary retention or an ascending and unresponsive lower UTI. Retained urine provides a breeding ground for bacteria. Repetitive antibacterial treatment may lead to drug resistance and extension of infection. In addition, drugs may cause necrosis of the renal papillae and sloughed papillae tissue may then cause ureteral blockage thus extension the pyelonephritis.

Renal Assessment

Subjective

The nurse can ask the following questions when obtaining a renal assessment from the patient:

- What is the general state of health?
- Is there a history of neurological deficit, diabetes, or other debilitating disease that could lead to urinary stasis, damage to the nephron, or impaired healing?
- Have there been recent hospitalizations and drug therapy?
- Is there a history of urinary calculi or prostate gland hypertrophy?
- Is there a recent history of catheterization?
- Has he or she experienced burning on urination, cloudy urine, suprapubic pain, colicky abdominal pain, or flank or back pain?
- How long have the symptoms persisted and how were they treated in the past?

Objective

The physical examination must include:

- Palpation of the abdomen for masses and tenderness.
- Palpation of CVA with a gentle tap of the fist over the kidney to elicit diagnostic discomfort in the presence of an inflammatory process.
- Urine inspection for clarity with sample collection for laboratory analysis. Key point: Catheter specimen will be necessary for females during menses or for those patients who lack the capacity to produce a reliable, noncontaminated specimen.

Pathophysiology

Prostate gland hypertrophy, masses, urinary calculi, or ureteral obstruction from sloughed papillae are common causes of urinary retention. Pooled urine promotes bacterial growth and the continuous urine pathways offer easy access for bacterial ascension to the renal pelvis. In addition, the presence of catheters or fecal incontinence increases the potential for UTI by providing an entry point for *E. coli*, one of the more common infecting organisms. Unchecked, bacteria in the urethra or bladder have easy access to the kidney via the ureters and renal pelvis.

Assessment with Clinical Manifestations

Acute pyelonephritis is described as a clinical syndrome presenting with bacteriuria accompanied by flank pain at the costovertebral angle (CVA), fever, and chills. In addition, the patient may experience painful urination, frequency, nocturia, nausea, vomiting, and colicky abdominal pain (Tolkoff-Rubin, Cotran, & Rubin, 2004). Conversely, chronic pyelonephritis may have a deceptively quiet presentation of frequency, dysuria, and nocturia. Mild, intermittent fever or intermittent back or flank pain may accompany the urinary symptoms (Kelly & Nielson, 2004).

Diagnostic Tests

There are a variety of diagnostic tests for detection of pyelonephritis. Urinalysis and urine culture may be sufficient in mild, initial cases of pyelonephritis in an uncomplicated presentation. Correct urine sample collection technique is critical to proper treatment. Catheterization may be necessary to collect a reliable specimen for the patient who is unable to stand, cleanse, and collect a midstream specimen.

Computed tomography (CT) is the standard diagnostic tool for pyelonephritis unresponsive to 72 hours of antibiotic therapy. CT is valuable in diagnosing obstructive etiology as well as identifying complications, such as perinephric abscess (Daniels, 2003).

Ultrasound is used when CT scanning is contraindicated, such as in pregnancy or in preexisting renal compromise. Renal ultrasound is used to place nephrostomy tubes for direct drainage of the renal pelvis in cases of complicated urinary obstruction.

Nursing Diagnoses

Based on the information gathered, examples of nursing diagnoses in the patient with pyelonephritis may include the following:
- Risk for imbalanced body temperature
- Pain related to ureteral colic
- Fear in response to the diagnosis of pyelonephritis
- Deficient knowledge related to completion of drug therapy, optimal fluid intake, or need to empty bladder every four hours to reduce bacterial count
- Ineffective coping related to anxiety, **malaise** (body discomfort and fatigue), and lowered activity level

Planning and Implementation

There are several strategies to providing care for patients with pyelonephritis. The implementation of these strategies may provide quick recovery and positive outcomes for the patient with this disorder.

Goals

The primary goal for providing care for pyelonephritis is to eradicate the UTI and to prevent damage to the renal parenchyma. Additionally and of equal importance, the secondary goal of preventing further infection must be promoted through patient education.

Evidence-Based Care

The nurse is positioned to play a significant role in preventing UTI. Evidence points to avoiding catheterization and early removal of catheters as critical to preventing UTI. The nurse must resist viewing catheters as nursing convenience or an easy answer to incontinence.

The nurse must always employ effective hand washing between patients to prevent patient-to-patient contamination and **nosocomial** (hospital acquired) infection. In addition, the practice of strict aseptic technique in catheter insertions and thorough, regular perineal and catheter site cleansing in the presence of a urinary catheter should be used. The nurse must practice preventive measures with prevention of an ascending UTI in mind.

Collaborative Management Including NIC

The collaborative management for pyelonephritis includes:
- Monitor vital signs and fluid balance.
- Ensure adequate hydration via an accurate intake and output record, encourage and provide at least 2 liters per day fluid intake or maintain a patent intravenous (IV) access.
- Monitor electrolytes, white blood count (WBC), blood urea nitrogen (BUN), and creatinine.
- Provide adequate pain management via usual analgesics and urinary antiseptics, such as phenazopyridine (Pyridium) or a combination urinary antiseptic or antispasmodic agent such as Urised (Urisedon or Urisedamine) or Urisept (Uriseptic).
- NIC: Assist with hygiene.

Population-Based Care

The elderly may have must be carefully assessed as they may have reduced sensation and therefore are not aware of a UTI prior to an advanced stage. The elderly may present with only minor complaints and may not have an elevation in temperature even with advanced infection.

The nurse must determine if the elderly patient uses fasting as a health practice and educate about the need for adequate fluid intake to prevent infection hypovolemia of the kidneys and bladder (Eliopoulos, 2005).

Patient and Family Teaching

The primary aspects of patient and family teaching are to educate about the importance of completing the full course of antibiotic therapy and maintaining the prescribed schedule to ensure continuous therapeutic blood levels. In addition, there needs to be information regarding the value of these above activities in preventing drug resistance. The NIC for the patient with pyelonephritis is to appraise the patient's current level of knowledge related to the disease process.

Evaluation of Outcomes

Potential patient outcomes for each of the example nursing diagnoses for the patient with pyelonephritis are:
- **Risk for imbalanced body temperature.** The patient maintains body temperature within a normal range.

- Fear in response to the diagnosis of pyelonephritis. The patient will manifest positive coping behaviors and verbalize how to effectively treat the disease and prevent its recurrence.
- Ineffective coping related to anxiety, malaise, and lowered activity level. The patient identifies own maladaptive coping behaviors, available resources, and support systems, describes or initiates alternative coping strategies, and describes positive results from new behaviors. The patient regains energy and participates in self-care.
- Acute pain related to ureteral colic or bladder spasm. Patient will verbalize maintenance of identified comfort level.
- Deficient knowledge related to completion of drug therapy, optimal fluid intake, or need to empty bladder every two hours to reduce bacterial count. The patient will verbalize the drug therapy regimen, the need to complete full dose on schedule to prevent drug resistance or continued infection. The patient will verbalize need to flush urinary system via adequate fluid intake and fully empty bladder every two hours to reduce the amount of bacteria available for growth.

GLOMERULONEPHRITIS

Glomerulonephritis is an inflammation of the glomerular capillaries. In patients with glomerulonephritis, the glomeruli become inflamed and impair the kidney's ability to filter urine. Eventually, the glomeruli become inflamed and scarred, and slowly lose their ability to remove waste and excess water from the blood to make urine. Glomerulonephritis can be acute, occurring as a sudden attack of inflammation, or chronic, which develops gradually. Glomerulonephritis can be part of a systemic disease, such as lupus or diabetes, or it can be a disease by itself, which is known as primary glomerulonephritis. Treatment varies depending on the type of glomerulonephritis that has been diagnosed.

Epidemiology

Glomerulonephritis represents 10 to 15 percent of glomerular diseases. Variable incidence has been reported in part because of the subclinical nature of the disease in more than half the affected population (Kazzi & Tehranazdeh, 2005). Incidence of poststreptococcal glomerulonephritis has fallen over the last few decades in western countries. This is believed to be a result of more rapid and effective treatment of a streptococcal infection with antibiotics, better health care delivery, and improved socioeconomic conditions. The disease remains much more common in regions such as Africa, the Caribbean, India, Pakistan, Malaysia, Papua New Guinea, and South America.

Etiology

There are many causes of glomerulonephritis. They include those related to infections, immune diseases, inflammation of the blood vessels (vasculitis), and conditions that scar the glomeruli. Often, however, the exact cause is initially unknown. Glomerulonephritis after infection includes poststreptococcal glomerulonephritis, bacterial endocarditis, and viral infections.

Poststreptococcal glomerulonephritis may develop after an infection of group A beta hemolytic streptococcus, usually in the pharynx (strep throat) or skin (impetigo). Postinfectious glomerulonephritis is becoming more uncommon because of rapid and complete antibiotic treatment of most streptococcal infections. Bacterial endocarditis is known as a cause of glomerulonephritis. Those at greatest risk are patients with a heart defect, such as a damaged or artificial heart valve. Among the viral infections that may trigger glomerulonephritis are the human immunodeficiency virus (HIV), which causes acquired immune deficiency syndrome (AIDS), and the hepatitis B and hepatitis C viruses, which affect the liver and can become chronic infections.

Systemic lupus erythematosus (SLE) is a chronic inflammatory disease and has been shown to cause glomerulonephritis. Goodpasture's syndrome is a rare immune lung disorder that may mimic pneumonia. It causes hemorrhage in the lungs as well as glomerulonephritis. Immunoglobulin A (IgA) nephropathy is characterized by recurrent episodes of blood in the urine. This condition results from deposits of the protein IgA in the glomeruli. IgA nephropathy can progress for years with no noticeable symptoms. Men seem more likely to develop this disorder than women.

Polyarteritis is a form of vasculitis that affects small and medium blood vessels in many parts of the body, including heart, kidneys, and intestines. Wegener's granulomatosis is a form of vasculitis that affects small and medium blood vessels in the lungs, upper airways, and kidneys. In both cases, the damage to the kidneys results in glomerulonephritis.

Pathophysiology

Immune complexes form in situ and deposit on the glomeruli, forming lesions. Except for poststreptococcal glomerulonephritis, the exact triggers for the formation of the immune complexes are unclear. Histopathologically, the glomerular tufts will appear swollen and infiltrated with polymorphonucleocytes. On gross examination, the kidneys may be enlarged by 50 percent.

There are a number of conditions that cause scarring of the glomeruli, including hypertension, diabetic nephropathy, and glomerulosclerosis. Hypertension damages the kidneys and impairs their ability to perform their normal functions. Glomerulonephritis can also cause high blood pressure because of its impact on kidney function. Diabetic nephropathy, also known as diabetic kidney disease, is one of the leading causes of end-stage kidney disease in the United States. It usually takes years to develop diabetic nephropathy. Damage may be slowed or prevented by in patients who maintain good control of their blood sugar. Glomerulosclerosis is characterized by scattered scarring of some of the glomeruli. This condition may result from another disease or occur for no known reason.

Chronic glomerulonephritis sometimes develops after a bout of acute glomerulonephritis, but in many patients there is no history of kidney disease. Often, the first indication of chronic glomerulonephritis is chronic kidney failure. Infrequently, chronic glomerulonephritis runs in families. In many cases, the cause is unknown.

In poststreptococcal glomerulonephritis, long-term prognosis is generally good. More than 98 percent of individuals are asymptomatic after five years. Chronic renal failure is a possibility, however, and has been reported 1 to 3 percent of the time.

For patients with other forms of glomerulonephritis, long-term outcomes generally depends on the underlying agent, which must be identified and treated and can range from complete recovery to total renal failure. In the latter case, treatment with dialysis and possibly a kidney transplant may be required. The prognosis for patients with cardiopulmonary or neurological complications is generally poorer.

Some patients become critically ill during the acute phase. Patients with anuria, nephrotic syndrome, massive proteinuria, significant hypertension, encephalopathy, or pulmonary symptoms will require hospitalization. Complications can lead to end-organ damage in the central nervous and cardiopulmonary systems. Other complications include hypertensive retinopathy, hypertensive encephalopathy, nephrotic syndrome, and chronic renal failure.

Assessment with Clinical Manifestation

In patients with poststreptococcal glomerulonephritis, there is a latent period between the streptococcal infection and the onset of signs and symptoms of acute glomerulonephritis. In general, the latent period is one to two weeks after a strep throat infection and three to six weeks after an impetigo infection (Geetha, 2004). If glomerulonephritis occurs within one to four days of a streptococcal infection, that is suggestive of preexisting renal disease.

The first clinical symptom is often dark urine, which is described as brown or tea- or cola-colored. It is caused by the hemolysis of red blood cells that have penetrated the glomerular basement membrane and have passed into the tubular system. Periorbital edema occurs suddenly. It is usually most noticeable on waking. Edema is a result of the defect in renal excretion of salt and water. The severity of the edema is not necessarily related to the degree of renal impairment. Hypertension is present in approximately 80 percent of patients. This cluster of symptoms: hematuria, edema, and hypertension, is known as nephritic syndrome. Approximately 95 percent of patients have at least two of these symptoms; 40 percent have all three.

Patients may complain of flank pain, due to stretching of the renal capsule. Approximately 10 to 50 percent of patients often have a low urine output **(oliguria)**. In this group, 15 percent have a urine output of less than 200 mL/day. Other symptoms include general malaise, weakness, and anorexia, which are present in about 50 percent of patients. Approximately 15 percent of patients complain of nausea and vomiting.

Patients with underlying systemic diseases that have caused the glomerulonephritis may present with symptoms of those diseases. For example, patients with SLE often have arthralgias or skin rashes. Patients with Wegener's granulomatosis often present with a triad of sinusitis, pulmonary infiltrates, and nephritis.

Diagnostic Tests

Laboratory tests include a complete blood count (CBC), electrolytes, including BUN and creatinine, urinalysis, and cultures of throat and skin to rule out *Streptococcus*. The BUN and creatinine will be elevated, reflecting the decrease in glomerular filtration rate. This elevation is usually transient. The urinalysis is always abnormal. Hematuria and proteinuria are present in 100 percent of cases. The specific gravity is greater than 1020 osm. Red blood cells and red blood cell casts are present in the urine. Blood cultures should be obtained in patients with fever, immunosuppression, a history of IV drug use, or those with indwelling shunts or catheters. Chest X-ray (CXR) may be necessary in patients with a cough, with or without hemoptysis.

Nursing Diagnoses

Based on the information gathered during the assessment, the following nursing diagnoses may be appropriate for the patient with glomerulonephritis:
- Excess fluid volume
- Risk for infection
- Deficient knowledge

Planning and Implementation

The management for glomerulonephritis is ideally implemented early in the disorder to prevent complications. Renal system involvement and more serious systemic problems can occur as the disorder exacerbates.

Goals

The major goals of care are to control edema and blood pressure. Therapy is symptomatic and depends on the clinical severity of the illness.

Nutrition

To control edema, the patient should be prescribed a low sodium diet (2 g per day) and placed on a fluid restriction (1 L per day). In the hospitalized patient, it is important to maintain a careful record of intake and output.

Pharmacology

In patients with positive cultures for *Streptococcus,* the infection must be treated. Penicillin is indicated in nonallergic patients. Oral penicillin G is usually prescribed as 250 mg four times a day for 7 to 10 days. Patients who are allergic to penicillin can be prescribed erythromycin, 250 mg four times a day for 7 to 10 days. Obtain throat cultures from family members and close personal contacts, and treat those who are infected.

In patients with severe edema, loop diuretics, such as furosemide (Lasix), may be prescribed. This is to increase urinary output, which will consequently improve cardiovascular congestion and hypertension. In adults, the usual dose is 20 to 40 mg orally or intravenously, given every six to eight hours. Potassium-sparing diuretics are contraindicated because of an increased risk of hyperkalemia.

Hypertension may be severe and may not be controlled by the diuretic. In this case, calcium channel blockers or angiotensin-converting enzyme (ACE) inhibitors may be prescribed. Amlodipine (Norvasc) is an example of the former and usually prescribed in a dose of 5 to 20 mg orally, twice a day. Captopril (Capoten) is an ACE inhibitor and is prescribed as 25 mg orally, two or three times per day. Total daily dose should not exceed 150 mg.

Steroids, immunosuppressive agents, and plasmapheresis are generally not indicated.

Population-Based Care

As noted above, family members and close personal contacts should have throat cultures and be treated if a streptococcal infection is present. In some areas of the world, streptococcal infection, leading to epidemics, may occur. In this case, it is recommended that close contacts and family members receive prophylactic antibiotic therapy.

Surgery

Renal biopsy may be required, especially in the following cases: (a) absence of a latent period between the streptococcal infection and acute disease; (b) anuria; (c) rapidly deteriorating renal function; (d) no improvement or continued decrease in the glomerular filtration rate at two weeks; and (e) persistent hypertension beyond two weeks. During the recovery phase, renal biopsy may be warranted if the glomerular filtration rate is not normal by four weeks or proteinuria lasts beyond six months.

Patient and Family Teaching

The patient must be taught the basics of a low-sodium diet and fluid restriction. Advise the patient to continue the diet until edema, hypertension, and urine abnormalities have resolved. If the patient is taking a diuretic, high-potassium foods, such as bananas and avocados, should be avoided.

The patient should be taught to have moderate activity until the symptoms subside; strenuous exercise can exacerbate proteinuria and hematuria. Bed rest may be required during the acute phase of the illness.

Stress to the patient the importance of follow-up care. Blood pressure should be monitored at every visit, or every month for six months, and then every six months after that. Blood work to monitor BUN and creatinine needs to be done at 2, 6, and 12 weeks, then every three months for one year. Urinalysis for hematuria and proteinuria needs to be done every two, four, and six weeks and then again at 4, 6, and 12 months. Lab values should be normal within six weeks, although it can take much longer for microhematuria in the urine to resolve.

Teach patients about their medications and side effects. Most patients will not require any medications after the acute phase of their illness, although antihypertensive medications may be required if the blood pressure remains high.

If the patient has a skin infection, stress the importance of meticulous personal hygiene.

Evaluation of Outcomes

Potential patient outcomes for each of the example nursing diagnoses for the patient with glomerulonephritis:

- Excess fluid volume. The patient with glomerulonephritis will:
  - Remain free of edema and effusion; weight will be appropriate for the patient.
  - Maintain urine output within 500 mL of intake with normal urine osmolality and specific gravity.
  - Explain measures that can be taken to treat or prevent excess fluid volume, especially diet, fluid restriction, and medications.
- Risk for infection. The patient with glomerulonephritis will:
  - Remain free from signs and symptoms of infection.
  - State symptoms of infection of which to be aware.
  - Maintain good personal hygiene.
  - State the importance of having family members tested and treated for streptococcal infection.
- Deficient knowledge. The patient with glomerulonephritis will:
  - Explain dietary and drug therapy.
  - Explain the schedule for follow-up visits and the need for long-term follow-up.
  - Discuss the need to balance activities with rest if fatigue is present.

NEPHROTIC SYNDROME

Nephrotic syndrome (nephrosis) is not a single disease but a group of symptoms. Symptoms include heavy **proteinuria** (increase in protein in the urine), **hypoalbuminemia** (decrease in albumin in the blood), edema, **hypercholesterolemia** (high serum cholesterol), and normal renal function. Nephrotic syndrome can be primary or secondary. Primary nephrotic syndrome occurs as part of a recognized systemic disease.

Epidemiology

Nephrotic syndrome is often described a disease of children and is relatively rare. It is 15 times more common in children than in adults. The reported annual incidence rate is 2 to 5 per 100,000 children younger than 16 years. The cumulative prevalence rate is approximately 15.5 per 100,000 individuals (Travis, 2005). Nephrotic syndrome prevalence is difficult to establish in adults, because the condition is usually a result of an underlying disease. In adults, diabetes mellitus is emerging as a major cause of nephrotic syndrome, thus American Indians, Hispanic (Americans), and African Americans have a higher incidence of nephrotic syndrome compared to Caucasians (Agraharkar, 2004).

BOX 53-5

PRIMARY CAUSES OF NEPHROSIS

- Collagen vascular disease, such as systemic lupus erythematosus or rheumatoid arthritis
- Sickle cell disease
- Diabetes mellitus
- Amyloidosis
- Malignancy, such as leukemia, lymphoma, Wilms tumor, or pheochromocytoma
- Toxins, such as bee sting, poison ivy or oak, or snake venom
- Medications, including probenecid, fenoprofen, captopril, lithium, or warfarin
- Heroin use

Etiology

There are both primary and secondary causes of nephrotic syndrome. Examples of primary causes are listed in Box 53-5. Secondary nephrotic syndrome occurs after an infectious disease, such as infection with group A beta-hemolytic streptococci, syphilis, malaria, tuberculosis, or viral infections, including varicella, hepatitis B, HIV, and infectious mononucleosis.

Pathophysiology

Nephrotic syndrome results from damage to the kidneys' glomeruli, the tiny blood vessels that filter waste and excess water from the blood and send them to the bladder as urine. They consist of capillaries that are fenestrated, that is, have small openings, which allow fluid, salts, and other small solutes to flow through but normally not proteins. Damage to the glomeruli from diabetes, glomerulonephritis, or even prolonged hypertension, causes the membrane to become more porous, so that small proteins, such as albumin, pass through the kidneys into urine. As protein continues to be excreted, serum albumin is decreased, which in turn decreases the serum osmotic pressure. Capillary hydrostatic fluid pressure becomes greater than capillary osmotic pressure, which results in generalized edema. As fluid is lost into the tissues, the plasma volume decreases, stimulating secretion of aldosterone to retain sodium and water, which decreases the glomerular filtration rate to retain water. This additional water also passes out of the capillaries into the tissue, leading to even greater edema.

Assessment with Clinical Manifestations

The major clinical manifestation is edema, which is the presenting symptom in about 95 percent of cases. In adults, the edema is usually present in dependent parts, such as ankles or legs, and is pitting in nature. In children, periorbital edema is common. Patients may have fluid in the pleural cavity, causing pleural effusion, or in the abdominal area, causing ascites. The edema may progress rapidly or quite slowly. Eventually, the edema is present throughout the body, which is known as **anasarca.** Some patients may notice foamy urine, due to a lowering of the specific gravity by the high amount of proteinuria. Actual urinary complaints, such as hematuria or oliguria, are uncommon. Other symptoms may include anorexia, irritability, fatigue, abdominal discomfort, and diarrhea (Travis, 2005).

When taking a history, many patients report a viral upper respiratory tract infection immediately preceding the first clinical signs of the disease but its relevance to the nephrotic syndrome is unknown. A history of prior allergic events is common. Children should be questioned about insect stings, immunizations, or poison ivy. In adults, it is important to ask about underlying diseases that may be the cause of nephrotic syndrome.

Diagnostic Tests

Laboratory tests include a urinalysis for protein and cellular elements and serum tests for protein and lipid analysis. Protein in the urine usually exceeds 100 mg/dL and values as high as 1000 mg/L are common. Protein can also be tested with a dipstick and may be as high as +3 to +4. The protein-to-creatinine ratio may vary from 1 to 20 (normal is less than 0.2). Hematuria may or may not be present. Hypoalbuminemia is common, with serum albumin levels following below 2 g/dL. Values as low as 0.5 g/dL are not uncommon. Hyperlipidemia is common and typically correlates inversely with the concentration of serum albumin. Values for lipids may remain moderately elevated for one to three months after remission of proteinuria (Daniels, 2003).

No routine imaging studies are indicated. CXR may reveal pleural effusion. The presence of pleural effusion correlates directly with the degree of edema and indirectly with the serum albumin concentration.

Nursing Diagnoses

Based on the information gathered during the assessment, the following nursing diagnoses may be appropriate for the patient with nephrotic syndrome:
- Imbalanced nutrition, less than body requirements
- Risk for infection
- Deficient knowledge

Planning and Implementation

The nurse plans a variety of strategies for caring for patients with nephritic syndrome. Nutrition and pharmacology are part of the areas of focus for the management of these patients.

Goals

The major goal of care is to preserve renal function. Secondary goals include the prevention of infection and receiving an adequate diet. In many patients, nephrotic syndrome is chronic and relapsing; they need to be taught to monitor their urine for protein and to be awareness of signs and symptoms of a recurrence of the disease.

Nutrition

In patients with nephrotic syndrome, the tubular function of the kidney to conserve sodium is not affected, thus, total body sodium is uniformly increased. Patients are often treated with glucocorticoids, which further curtails renal sodium excretion. Patients with nephrotic syndrome will usually be prescribed a sodium-restricted diet. Alterations in protein are not indicated, and fluid restriction is unnecessary unless the patient's thirst is so excessive that fluid intake is extreme.

Pharmacology

Glucocorticoid therapy has become the primary agent of choice in the treatment of patients with nephrotic syndrome. In most cases, oral prednisone or prednisolone is started in a dosage of 2 mg/kg/day. The total daily dose is usually split into two doses and given daily for four to eight weeks. Maintenance therapy should be tailored to the individual patient, with gradual weaning from the glucocorticoid.

Patients with nephrotic syndrome are at high risk for infection and immunosuppression as a result of steroid therapy, which increases this risk. If the patient becomes febrile, blood and urine cultures should be obtained. If an infection is present, it should be promptly treated with an appropriate antibiotic.

Diuretic therapy may be beneficial, especially in patients with symptomatic edema. A loop diuretic, such as furosemide, may be given orally (1–2 mg/kg/day). Patients should be carefully observed for hypovolemic shock. If the edema is severe enough to warrant IV diuretic therapy, then salt-poor albumin should be infused concurrently. The usual dose is 1 g/kg given intravenously over two to four hours.

Pneumococcal vaccine is indicated in all patients after remission is obtained.

Population-Based Care

It has been found that viral respiratory illness can initiate an exacerbation of nephrotic syndrome, therefore, the patient should avoid exposure to others with obvious respiratory tract infections.

Patient and Family Teaching

Because nephrotic syndrome can be a chronic and relapsing problem, patient education about awareness of symptoms and self-management is essential. Patients should be taught to keep a log of treatment and progress. Clinical notes, including presence, absence, or degree of edema; blood pressure; other illnesses; urine protein results; and administration of medications should all be recorded in the log on a daily basis.

Home monitoring of urine protein and albumin is an important aspect of patient education. Patients should be taught how to monitor urine protein by means of a dipstick; this should be recorded in the log. It is recommended that urine be tested daily, usually the first urine of the day. Monitoring should continue after the urine has become free of protein, during the maintenance period, and beyond. If a patient should experience a relapse, the log can give clues to the progression of the disease before edema recurs.

Evaluation of Outcomes

Potential patient outcomes for each of the example nursing diagnoses for the person with nephrotic syndrome:
- Imbalanced nutrition, less than body requirements. The patient with nephrotic syndrome will:
  - Eat a diet high low in sodium with adequate calories to meet nutritional requirements.
  - Will maintain a stable weight.
- Risk for infection. The patient with nephrotic syndrome will:
  - Remain free from signs and symptoms of infection.
  - State symptoms of infection of which to be aware.
  - State the importance of avoiding people with upper respiratory infection.
- Deficient knowledge. The patient with nephrotic syndrome will:
  - Explain dietary and drug therapy.
  - Demonstrate how to test urine for protein and maintain a clinical log.
  - Discuss the importance of monitoring ongoing health status and the need to obtain health care promptly if there is any change in status.

RENAL TUBERCULOSIS

Renal tuberculosis is the most common site of extrapulmonary tuberculosis. This infection can result in cessation and destruction of renal mass and healing can lead to strictures, obstruction, and infection, causing renal functional loss and failure. If identified early it is a completely curable condition (Casaccia, et al., 2003).

Etiology

Usually, renal tuberculosis results from silent bacillemia accompanying pulmonary tuberculosis. However, active lesions in the kidney may not manifest clinically for many years. Also, many cases remain clinically silent for years while irreversible renal destruction takes place.

Pathophysiology

The pathophysiology is that of tuberculosis and renal tuberculosis is usually secondary to tuberculosis (TB) of the lung. In a small percentage, the tubercle bacilli reaches the kidney via the bloodstream. The healing process can lead to stricture, obstruction, secondary calculi, and infection causing renal functional loss and failure.

Assessment with Clinical Manifestations

The most frequent clinical features reported have been frequency, dysuria, urgency, hematuria, and flank pain. In addition, unexplained sterile pyuria or hematuria can exist and should prompt the health care provider to undertake an evaluation for renal tuberculosis. Sometimes, patients can have a late presentation with advanced disease including renal insufficiency. Most renal tuberculosis patients are asymptomatic, and slow but continuous infection causes destruction of renal mass and the healing process leads to renal functional loss (Matsumura, Yamamoto, Hirohashi, & Kitano, 2005).

Diagnostic Tests

A detailed history including past and family history of pulmonary tuberculosis and thorough clinical examination is important. Laboratory investigations will include a urine examination with pH, acid-fast bacillus (AFB) smear, routine and AFB cultures, hemogram, serum chemistry specific to renal function (e.g., BUN and creatinine), CXR, plain abdominal X-ray, intravenous pyelogram (IVP), and tuberculin test. A CT scan is usually performed on selected patients to confirm findings on IVP and cystoscopy may be performed to get histological diagnosis (Daniels, 2003). The definitive diagnosis of tuberculosis is by culturing tubercle bacilli from urine.

Nursing Diagnoses

Based on the information gathered, examples of nursing diagnoses in the patient with renal tuberculosis may include the following:
* Acute pain as related to burning on urination
* Risk for imbalanced body temperature related to infectious process of tuberculosis

Planning and Implementation

The earlier the detection and treatment is initiated, the less the damage to the renal system. If prolonged disease, there may be renal scarring, the development of ureteral strictures, and even renal failure. The patient may require specific follow-up on the renal system to prevent complications. Specific drug therapy and nursing management are discussed in chapter 32.

Evaluation of Outcomes

Potential patient outcomes for each of the example nursing diagnoses for the patient with renal tuberculosis are:
* Acute pain as related to burning on urination. The patient should verbalize an adequate relief of pain along with the ability to realistically cope with the pain if it is not completely relieved.
* Risk for imbalanced body temperature related to infectious process of tuberculosis. The patient maintains body temperature within a normal range.

URINARY TRACT CALCULI (UROLITHIASIS)

Urolithiasis (calculi) refers to stones in the urinary tract. The formation of urinary calculi formation remains somewhat of a perplexity. The often unilateral formation of urinary stones challenges questions of environment and diet. One would assume both kidneys to be creating the same environment for stone formation. Their ability to resist the velocity urinary stream long enough to grow in size is further perplexing. Many of the people that develop renal calculi require hospitalization, and the pain associated with renal stones is often unmistakably acute.

Epidemiology

Urinary calculi afflict males more often than females at approximately a 3:1 ratio. Incidence in the United States averages 20 cases per 10,000 persons. Incidence is higher in warmer regions and is most likely related to dehydration. The incidence is primarily between 20 and 55 years of age. Whites have a greater occurrence than African Americans. Untreated, stones recur 10 percent in 1 year and up to 50 percent in 10 years. The lifetime prevalence of symptomatic **nephrolithiasis** (kidney stone disease) is approximately 10 percent in men and 5 percent in women, and more than $2 billion is spent on treatment each year.

Etiology

The etiology of renal calculi is unclear. Factors directly contributing to stone formation include an acid urine and concentration of precipitating elements in the urine. Increased rate of calcium absorption from the gut may be a more important contributory factor than is dietary intake. The likelihood of stone formation is influenced by urinary, dietary, and genetic factors as well as the presence of other medical conditions. A number of dietary factors have been associated with a reduced risk of stone formation, including higher intakes of dietary calcium, potassium, and phytate and lower intakes of animal protein, sodium, and sucrose. Systemic factors also influence risk independent of dietary intake, including higher body mass index (particularly in women), gout, and primary hyperparathyroidism (Curhan, 2005).

Pathophysiology

There are a variety of stones, each with potential to form in a different environment. Calcium composes the majority of renal stones. Struvite stones are composed of magnesium, phosphate, and ammonium and frequently present as staghorn calculi lodged in the pelvis of the kidney. Uric acid stones claim less than 5 percent of all urinary calculi. Cystine and xanthine stones are associated with hereditary factors. Indinavir, triamterene, and silicate stones are associated with medications.

Approximately 85 percent of stones in men and 70 percent in women contain calcium, most commonly as calcium oxalate. Overall, UTI or systemic disorders, such as primary hyperparathyroidism, are responsible for less than 10 percent of stones in men and 25 percent in women. The other stone types, such as cystine, uric acid, and struvite, are much less common. However, these types of stone also deserve careful attention, because recurrences are common.

A kidney stone may form when the concentrations of urinary constituents exceed their solubility. The causes of stone formation differ for different stone types. Cystine stones form only in individuals with the autosomal recessive disorder of cystinuria. Uric acid stones form only in individuals with persistently acid urine, with or without hyperuricosuria. Struvite stones form only in the setting of an upper UTI with a urease-producing bacterium. Stones may occasionally result from precipitation in the urinary tract of medications, such as acyclovir and indinavir (Curhan, 2005).

Assessment with Clinical Manifestations

The typical presentation of renal stones is sudden-onset unilateral flank pain of sufficient severity that the individual usually seeks medical attention, often at an emergency department. Although the term colic is used, this is a mis-

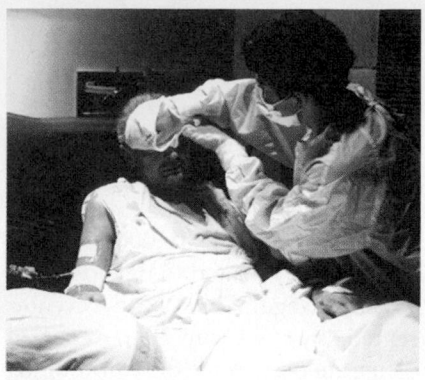

Figure 53-3 Nurse is applying cool wash cloth to man experiencing severe acute pain from renal calculi.

nomer, because the pain does not completely remit but rather waxes and wanes. The pain is often accompanied by nausea and occasionally vomiting. The pain can radiate to a variety of locations depending on the location of the stone: when the stone is in the upper ureter, pain may radiate anteriorly to the abdomen; when the stone is in the lower ureter, pain can radiate to the ipsilateral testicle in men or ipsilateral labium in women; or if the stone is lodged at the ureterovesical junction, the major symptoms may be urinary frequency and urgency. A less common acute presentation is gross hematuria without pain (Curhan, 2005). The patient may also experience the first stage of shock with cool, diaphoretic skin. In addition, the patient may develop a UTI and have the symptoms of fever, nausea, and vomiting (Figure 53-3).

Diagnostic Tests

Although the physical examination alone will not completely make the diagnosis, there are clues to help guide the evaluation. The patient will typically be in obvious pain and cannot find a comfortable position. There may be ipsilateral CVA tenderness, or in cases of obstruction with infection, signs and symptoms of sepsis may be present. In addition, the familial history may lend information to confirm renal calculi.

The serum chemistries are typically normal, but leukocytosis may be present because of stress or infection. The urinalysis classically reveals red and white blood cells and occasionally may have crystals. If the ureter is completely obstructed due to the stone, there may be no red blood cells, as no urine will be flowing from that ureter into the bladder. Clinically, patients with an asymptomatic renal stone often have microscopic hematuria.

Helical CT scan is the imaging modality of choice because of its sensitivity, ability to visualize uric acid stones (traditionally considered radiolucent), and lack of need for radiocontrast. Helical CT can detect small stones that may be missed by IV urography, which requires IV radiocontrast. Typically, CT will show a ureteral stone or evidence of recent passage whereas plain abdominal X-ray (kidney-ureters-bladder [KUB]) can miss a stone in the ureter or kidney, even if radiopaque, and provides no information on obstruction (Curhan, 2005).

Ultrasound has the advantage of avoiding radiation but can only image the kidney and possibly the proximal ureter; thus, ureteral stones are typically not seen by ultrasound.

The differential diagnosis of someone with suspected renal colic includes muscular or skeletal pain, herpes zoster, acute cholecystitis, duodenal ulcer, appendicitis, diverticulitis, pyelonephritis, abdominal aortic aneurysm, gynecological causes, ureteral obstruction due to other intraluminal factors, such as a blood clot or sloughed papilla, and ureteral stricture.

Nursing Diagnoses

Based on the information gathered, examples of nursing diagnoses in the patient with renal calculi may include the following:
- Acute pain as related to renal calculi
- Ineffective coping related to anxiety, lower activity level and the inability to perform normal activities of daily living
- Impaired urinary elimination related to renal calculi
- Risk for infection

Planning and Implementation

Renal colic is one of the most excruciating types of pain that a patient will experience; therefore, the first and foremost treatment is pain control. IV fluids are routinely given for volume repletion, and some experts believe this will increase the likelihood of stone passage, but no prospective data are available (Curhan, 2005). Overall, the management for urinary calculi focuses on relieving the pain, destroying or removing the renal stones, and preventing continued formation of calculi.

Nutrition

In general, dietary management for prevention of renal calculi focuses on changing the urine composition. Increasing fluid intake to 2.5 to 3 liters per day is advised with an intake that is spread throughout the day, as well as even drinking fluids at night.

Calcium intake is limited in regard to dietary calcium and vitamin D enriched foods. Decreasing vitamin D limits the absorption of calcium from the gastrointestinal (GI) tract. In addition, both phosphate and oxalate can also be limited from the diet.

Animal proteins are limited to prevent uric acid stones, as indicated in the Patient Playbook. Also, maintaining urine pH at higher levels (alkaline) decreases the potential development of uric acid and cystine stones. Examples of foods that alkalinize are: fruits, green vegetables, legumes, milk, and milk products.

Pharmacology

Acute pain from renal calculi is typically treated with analgesia and hydration. Evidence from many randomized controlled trials suggests that parenteral nonsteroidal anti-inflammatory drugs (NSAIDs) are as effective as narcotics in relieving the pain of renal colic. There are no clinically important differences in terms of rapidity of action or magnitude of relief. A variety of types of medications, dosages, and routes of administration have been compared, but there is no one clearly superior approach. Local active warming may also be an adjunctive treatment. Newer medications that may be effective include antispasmodics, alpha-blockers, trigger point injection with lidocaine, desmopressin, and NSAIDs combined with nitrates (Curhan, 2005).

Thiazide diuretics are often administered for calcium calculi to reduce urinary calcium excretion, which prevents further stones. Potassium citrate causes the pH of urine to move in an alkaline direction, which prevents stones from form in acidic urine (e.g., uric acid and cystine).

Surgery

Surgical options for stone removal are driven by stone size, location, and composition; urinary tract anatomy; and availability of technology. Extracorporeal shock wave lithotripsy (ESWL) is the least invasive; it is most effective for stones that are smaller than 2 cm, located in the renal pelvis, and composed of calcium oxalate dihydrate, apatite, uric acid, or struvite. If available, ESWL for acute ureteral colic may be successful and reduce the morbidity associated with stone passage (Figure 53-4).

Cystoscopic stone removal, by either basket extraction or fragmentation, is invasive but effective and can now be used to remove stones even in the kidney. Percutaneous nephrostolithotomy is more invasive but is necessary for large stone burdens or stones that cannot be removed cystoscopically and is the standard for making a patient stone free (Curhan, 2005).

The treatment of existing stones in morbidly obese individuals is challenging. The ability to image the urinary tract may be limited if the patient's size prohibits access to scanning by CT. ESWL may not be an option, as morbid obesity may impede stone localization and the ability of the shock waves to reach the calculus. Percutaneous approaches can be used but may be more difficult in the morbidly obese patient; thus, the preferred approach is ureteroscopy (Casaccia, et al., 2003).

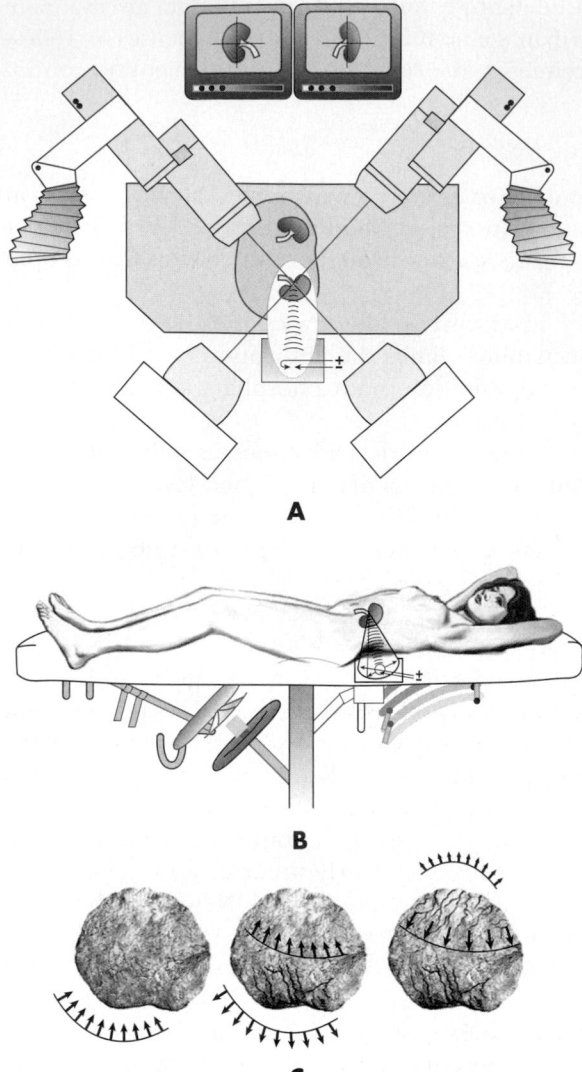

A

B

C

Figure 53-4 ESWL: A. Two X-ray beams crossing at focal point for proper positioning on stone, B. Focal point, C. Reflection of shock waves at first and second acoustical interfaces of the stone and surrounding fluid with fracture of the stone.

Evaluation of Outcomes

Potential patient outcomes for each of the example nursing diagnoses for the patient with renal calculi are:

- Acute pain as related to renal calculi. The patient should verbalize an adequate relief of pain along with the ability to realistically cope with the pain if it is not completely relieved.
- Ineffective coping related to anxiety, lower activity level, and the inability to perform normal activities of daily living. The patient identifies own maladaptive coping behaviors, available resources, and support systems, describes and initiates alternative coping strategies, and describes positive results from new behaviors.
- Impaired urinary elimination related to renal calculi. The patient is continent of urine or verbalizes satisfactory management.
- Risk for infection. The patient remains free of infection, as evidenced by normal vital signs and absence of purulent drainage from wounds, incisions, and tubes. Infection is recognized early to allow for prompt treatment.

RENAL SYSTEM TRAUMA

The kidney is the most common organ in the urinary tract to be injured by severe trauma. Trauma is injury caused by an external force that may be either blunt; such as a car accident, or penetrating, such as a gunshot wound. Blunt trauma injuries to the kidney may show no evidence of external injury, or bruises may appear over the back or abdomen where the kidney is located. Penetrating kidney injury may also be difficult to detect. For example, the external point of entry of the bullet may be small and at a distance far enough away from the location of the kidney for it not to be a consideration.

Etiology

Renal contusions, superficial cortical lacerations, and small perirenal hematomas account for 90 percent of all renal injuries. Renal injuries occur in 15 to 40 percent of patients with abdominal trauma. Blunt renal trauma can be classified according to the severity of injury and the most common is the renal contusion. The kidney can be damaged from a blow in the abdomen anteriorly, just below the rib cage, particularly in road traffic accidents, such as when the victim is thrown onto the steering column or some other projecting object. Abdominal injuries due to seat belts include 11 percent that involve the urinary tract, and half of those are renal.

Penetrating injuries (usually from gunshot or stab wounds) account for 20 percent of renal traumas in an urban setting. The damage from a bullet will depend not only on direction but also on the velocity of the missile. Also, a knife or stiletto stab can readily cut the cortex of the kidney if the weapon is driven more than three inches into the victim. Although a perirenal hematoma usually develops, the patient may not show hematuria unless the weapon has reached the calyces or renal pelvis.

There is also the possibility of iatrogenic injuries, which can occur in the passage of a catheter up the ureter (damage of renal pelvis), when a renal biopsy is done or when there is an infection carried indirectly into the renal pelvis.

Pathophysiology

The classification of renal injuries is based on the extent and depth of parenchymal lacerations, the integrity of the renal collecting system, and the status of the renal pedicle. Major renal injuries include deep cortical lacerations with or without disruption of the collecting system, comminuted renal fractures, and vascular pedicle injuries with either avulsion, intimal dissection, or traumatic occlusion. These injuries often require surgical intervention.

The most common complications in renal trauma are urinary leakage or delayed bleeding from the damage (Box 53-6). Other complications, such as the development of an abscess surrounding the kidney, can also occur. Finally, some patients develop hypertension after significant kidney trauma. This may be treated by medications, angiographically, or surgically (including removal of the kidney), if conservative treatment fails.

Assessment with Clinical Manifestations

The cardinal sign of a renal trauma is hematuria, which can be massive or microscopic, but the extent of the injury cannot be measured by the volume of hematuria or appearance of the wound. Other signs that can be present in renal trauma are lumbar and abdominal pain, sometimes with rigidity of the anterior abdominal wall and local tenderness. The health care provider should assess for such injuries as rib fractures, pelvic fractures, or vertebral injury, which can elicit renal trauma. In addition, nausea and vomiting can be present. Extensive blood loss and shock may result from retroperitoneal bleeding (Figure 53-5).

If the patient presents with a small flattening of the normal contour of the loin, a perinephric hematoma should be suspected. In the case of retroperitoneal hematoma or effusion, the renal injury may be associated with paralytic ileus, which produces a danger confusing diagnosis of intra peritoneal trauma.

Diagnostic Tests

Once injury is suspected, it is important to perform imaging studies of both kidneys to confirm clinical suspicion and determine injury severity. In past years, an X-ray in the form of an IVP was used. Currently, a CT scan with contrast is the investigation of choice to obtain a reliable and quick way of assessing kidney injury. Ultrasonography is another effective tool that may be utilized in the diag-

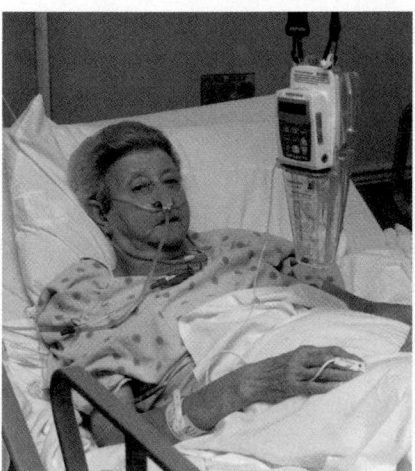

Figure 53-5 Patient with nausea while experiencing recent renal trauma.

BOX 53-6

POSSIBLE COMPLICATIONS OF RENAL TRAUMA

The most common and possible complications of renal injuries are:

- Secondary hemorrhage, usually due to infection (10 to 14 days after trauma)
- Paralytic ileus (4 to 5 days) as a result of retroperitoneal hematoma
- Hypertension as a result of the constricting effect of reorganizing perirenal hematoma
- Arterio-venous fistula
- Renal failure
- Renal atrophy
- Hydronephrosis
- Chronic pyelonephritis
- Renal calculi
- Renal artery stenosis

nosis of kidney trauma. However, it may not provide the best details of the degree of injury and may need to be supplemented by either an IVP or a CT scan.

In patients with multivisceral trauma requiring emergent laparotomy, imaging evaluation is usually limited to emergency excretory urography prior to surgery. In more stable patients, CT allows accurate diagnosis and staging of major renal injuries. CT can determine the depth of cortical laceration, the amount of infarcted renal parenchyma, the extent of perirenal hemorrhage, the status of the renal collecting system, and the vascular pedicle. Although excretory urography (ultrasonography) is the most cost-effective screening modality in the evaluation of stable patients with isolated flank trauma, its accuracy falls significantly with more severe renal injuries. The majority of patients with extensive renal injuries are not adequately staged by excretory urography alone. Therefore, contrast-enhanced CT should be performed in patients with suspected major renal trauma, multivisceral injuries, or inadequate staging with excretory urography.

Nursing Diagnoses

Based on the information gathered, examples of nursing diagnoses in the patient with renal trauma may include the following:
- Deficient fluid volume related to hematuria
- Acute pain in the lumbar and abdominal areas related to renal trauma
- Nutrition imbalance, less than body requirements, related to nausea from renal trauma

Planning and Implementation

Treatment of kidney trauma depends on the condition of the patient, the severity of kidney injury, and the presence of other injuries. If the patient's condition is stable and injury to other organ systems has been ruled out, conservative, non-surgical treatment is an option. In the cases of parenchymal lacerations, that are restricted to the cortex, the patient should be hospitalized, kept on bed rest, and given broad-spectrum antibiotics until the blood in the urine clears. When there is deep parenchymal laceration, the patient should be treated conservatively and assessed for clinical manifestations of abscess, infection, hypertension, and secondary hemorrhage. Even after discharge from the hospital, the patient needs to be monitored for the possibility of late bleeding from the injured kidney or development of high blood pressure as the result of the kidney injury.

Surgery

Patients with the more significant parenchymal lacerations (major injuries), extensive extravasation, vascular injuries, or pulsatile hematoma, will likely undergo exploratory surgery. Penetrating injuries from gunshot or stab wounds could require surgical exploration, but it is not necessary if the CT scan or arteriography show a minor injury, without extravasation of contrast medium, which confirms preservation of vascular vessels. When surgery is necessary, the aim is to try to repair and preserve the injured kidney. However, if it is not possible to save the kidney, because it is too severely injured, surgical removal of the kidney (**nephrectomy**) may be required.

Evaluation of Outcomes

Potential patient outcomes for each of the example nursing diagnoses for the patient with renal trauma are:
- Deficient fluid volume related to hematuria. The patient experiences adequate fluid volume and electrolyte balance as evidenced by urine output greater than 30 mL/hour, normotensive blood pressure, heart rate 100 beats/minute, consistency of weight, and normal skin turgor.

- Acute pain in the lumbar and abdominal areas related to renal trauma. The patient should verbalize an adequate relief of pain along with the ability to realistically cope with the pain if it is not completely relieved.
- Nutrition imbalance, less than body requirements, related to nausea from renal trauma. The patient verbalizes and demonstrates selection of foods or meals that will achieve a cessation of weight loss and weighs within 10 percent of ideal body weight.

RENAL VASCULAR DISORDERS

There are primarily three conditions of renal vascular disorders: (a) renal artery stenosis, (b) renal vein thrombosis, and (c) nephrosclerosis. Table 53-6 depicts the primary differences for each of these conditions:

RENAL CANCER

Several different types of cancer can affect the kidneys. Although it is not a common cancer overall, renal cell carcinoma is the most common kidney cancer, affecting approximately 40,000 people in the United States each year.

Epidemiology

Renal cell carcinoma accounts for approximately 3 percent of adult malignancies and 90–95 percent of neoplasms arising from the kidney. The age-adjusted incidence of renal cell carcinoma has been rising by 3 percent per year. Approximately 31,200 new cases of renal cell carcinoma were diagnosed in the year 2000, and more than 11,900 affected individuals died.

Renal cell carcinoma is more common in people of Northern European ancestry (Scandinavians) and North Americans than in those of Asian or African descent. In the United States, its incidence has been equivalent among Caucasian

---

TABLE 53-6 Renal Vascular Disorders

RENAL VASCULAR DISORDER	DESCRIPTION AND PATHOPHYSIOLOGY	CLINICAL MANIFESTATIONS	MGMT CONSIDERATIONS
Renal artery stenosis	Partial blockage of renal arteries caused by such disorders as atherosclerosis and fibromuscular hyperplasia	Hypertension (1 to 2 percent of all hypertension cases is caused by renal artery stenosis)	Renal angioplasty Surgical revascularization Nephrectomy as most critical care technique
Renal vein thrombosis	Caused by such disorders as: renal cancer, trauma, nephritic syndrome, pregnancy	Hematuria Flank pain Fever Pulmonary emboli	Corticosteroids Anticoagulants Surgical therapy (removal of thrombi)
Nephrosclerosis	Sclerosis of small vessels of kidney	Intermittent areas of ischemia from lack of blood flow Hypertension Loss of renal function, even to the extent of renal failure	Antihypertensive medication treatment Supportive mgmt if patient develops renal failure

and African Americans, but incidence among African Americans is increasing rapidly. Renal cell carcinoma is twice as common in men as in women. This condition occurs most commonly in the fourth to sixth decades of life, but the disease has been reported in younger people who belong to family clusters.

Etiology

A number of cellular, environmental, genetic, and hormonal factors have been studied as possible causal factors for renal cell carcinoma. These are shown in Box 53-7.

Pathophysiology

Renal cell carcinoma (e.g., renal adenocarcinoma and hypernephroma) is the development of cancerous changes in the cells of the renal tubules. The tissue of origin for renal cell carcinoma is the proximal renal tubular epithelium. Renal cancer occurs in both a sporadic (nonhereditary) and a hereditary form. In the past these tumors were believed to derive from the adrenal gland; therefore, the term hypernephroma often was used.

Renal cancer is staged with two different systems. The first, the Robson modification of the Flocks and Kadesky system, is uncomplicated and is used commonly in clinical practice. The Robson staging system has stages I to IV. The second system is the tumor, nodes, and metastases (TNM) classification which is endorsed by the American Joint Committee on Cancer (AJCC). The major advantage of the TNM system is that it clearly differentiates individuals with tumor thrombi from those with local nodal disease.

Genetics

Genetic studies of the families at high risk for developing renal cancer led to the cloning of genes whose alteration results in tumor formation. These genes are either tumor suppressors or oncogenes. At least four hereditary syndromes associated with renal cell carcinoma are recognized: (a) von Hippel-Lindau (VHL) syndrome, (b) hereditary papillary renal carcinoma (HPRC), (c) familial renal oncocytoma (FRO) associated with Birt-Hogg-Dube syndrome (BHDS), and (d) hereditary renal carcinoma (HRC). VHL disease is transmitted in an autosomal dominant familial multiple-cancer syndrome, which confers predisposition to a variety of neoplasms,

Assessment with Clinical Manifestations

Renal cell carcinoma symptoms include blood in the urine, abnormal urine color, flank or back pain, a lump or mass in the kidney area, abdominal pain or swelling, weight loss, testicle enlargement, fatigue, fever, and anemia. However, several less serious conditions can cause similar symptoms, including UTIs (from simple cystitis to more complex infections, such as pyelonephritis), kidney stones, or a cyst. These alternatives must be considered before establishing a diagnosis.

As renal cell carcinoma grows, it may invade organs near the kidney such as the liver, colon, or pancreas. Kidney cancer cells may also spread (metastasize) to other areas, such as the lymph nodes, brain, lungs, or bone. These advances in renal cancer lead to a wide variety of other clinical manifestations.

Diagnostic Tests

Laboratory studies in the evaluation of renal cell carcinoma should include a workup such as: urine analysis, CBC count with differential, electrolytes, renal profile, liver function tests, calcium, erythrocyte sedimentation rate (ESR), prothrombin time (PT), and activated partial thromboplastin time (APTT).

A large proportion of patients diagnosed with renal cancer have small tumors discovered incidentally on imaging studies. A number of diagnostic modalities are used to evaluate and stage renal tumors, such as, excretory urography, CT scan, ultrasonography, arteriography, venography, and magnetic resonance imaging (MRI). In addition, radiologic studies can be tailored to enable further characterization of renal masses, so that nonmalignant tumors can be differentiated from malignant ones. A bone scan is recommended for bony symptoms with elevated alkaline phosphatase level. Percutaneous cyst puncture and fluid analysis is used in the evaluation of potentially malignant cystic renal lesions detected by ultrasonography or CT imaging (Lake & Hafez, 2005).

Nursing Diagnoses

Based on the information gathered, examples of nursing diagnoses in the patient with renal cancer may include the following:
- Fear in response to the diagnosis of renal cancer
- Knowledge deficit related to the diagnosis of renal cancer
- Ineffective coping related to anxiety, lower activity level and the inability to perform normal activities of daily living

Planning and Implementation

Usually the management of renal cancer uses a combination of treatments, although surgery, including full or partial kidney removal, is the mainstay of renal cell carcinoma treatment. Other treatments, depending on individual cases, include biological therapy to trigger the body's immune system, hormone therapy, radiotherapy, chemotherapy, or arterial embolization, which blocks the blood supply to the tumor. Other treatments are under study including molecular markers and additional chemotherapy agents (Fromer, 2005). The nursing care of patients with renal cancer is illustrated in detail in chapter 15.

Pharmacology

A variety of chemotherapy agents are used in the treatment of renal cancer. Floxuridine (FUDR), 5-fluorouracil (5-FU), vinblastine, paclitaxel (Taxol), carboplatin, ifosfamide, gemcitabine, and anthracycline (doxorubicin) all have been used (Anderson, Woltman, Kovach, & Konety, 2004).

Immunotherapy stimulates the immune system to attack cancer. The most commonly used immunotherapy agents are Proleukin and interferon. The interferons (biological therapy) are natural glycoproteins with antiviral, antiproliferative, and immunomodulatory properties. The interferons have a direct antiproliferative effect on renal tumor cells (Coppin, et al., 2005).

Surgery

Surgery is always utilized for the treatment of patients with renal cell cancer unless the patient is too ill to tolerate the procedure. Currently, most health care providers think that the primary cancer should be removed even when there is widespread cancer present at diagnosis. In many patients with renal cancer, surgery alone can be curative and when the cancer is more extensive the surgery can be palliative. There also is the general concept that immunotherapy will work better if as much cancer as possible is removed before treatment. There are several surgical approaches that are utilized, depending on the extent of disease and the condition of the patient.

The most commonly performed surgery to treat renal cell cancer is radical nephrectomy. During a radical nephrectomy, the entire cancerous kidney, the attached adrenal gland, and the fatty tissue immediately around the kidney are removed. The lymph nodes around the kidney are often removed and examined under the microscope to determine if they contain cancer. Radical nephrectomy is associated with a greater than 90 percent five-year survival in patients with stage I and II cancer (Galli, Munver, Sawczuk, & Kochis, 2005).

Partial nephrectomy is performed to preserve as much normal kidney tissue as possible; however its complication rate may be slightly higher than radical nephrectomy. Open partial nephrectomy is usually the treatment of choice when radical nephrectomy may result in either immediate dialysis or a high risk for subsequent dialysis.

Laparoscopic radical nephrectomy is a surgical technique that is less extensive and invasive than a typical radical nephrectomy. Compared to open radical nephrectomy, laparoscopic radical nephrectomy involves longer operative time, less postoperative pain, shorter hospital stay, and shorter recovery time.

Tumor ablation is a process that destroys the tumor without excising it. Examples of ablative technologies include cryotherapy, interstitial radiofrequency, high-intensity focused ultrasound, microwave therapy, and laser coagulation.

Patient and Family Teaching

A vital need for nursing management of patients with renal cancer is patient teaching. Patients in the high-risk group should be made aware of the early signs and symptoms, and the need for early intervention for possible cure should be stressed. Patients in early stages who have undergone treatment should be educated about possible relapse. In addition, the consequences of the treatment strategies (e.g., chemotherapy, surgery, or radiation) are described in a thorough manner in chapter 15.

Evaluation of Outcomes

Potential patient outcomes for each of the example nursing diagnoses for the patient with renal cancer are:

- Fear in response to the diagnosis of renal cancer. The patient should manifest positive coping behaviors and verbalize a reduction in the amount of fear of having this disease.
- Knowledge deficit related to the diagnosis of renal cancer. The patient should demonstrate motivation to learn, identify perceived learning needs, and verbalize an understanding of desired content.
- Ineffective coping related to anxiety, lower activity level, and the inability to perform normal activities of daily living. The patient identifies own maladaptive coping behaviors, available resources, and support systems, describes or initiates alternative coping strategies, and describes positive results from new behaviors.

BLADDER CANCER

Bladder cancer is a common urological cancer. The most common type of bladder cancer in the United States is urothelial carcinoma, formerly known as transitional cell carcinoma (TCC). The urothelium in the entire urinary tract may be involved, including the renal pelvis, ureter, bladder, and urethra. The clinical course of bladder cancer carries a broad spectrum of aggressiveness and risk. Low-grade, superficial bladder cancers have minimal risk of progression to death; however, high-grade muscle-invasive cancers are often lethal. Smoking is the greatest single risk factor for bladder cancer and exposure to certain toxic chemicals and drugs also predispose the patient to bladder cancer.

Epidemiology

Bladder cancer is the 4th most frequently diagnosed cancer in men and the 10th most frequently diagnosed cancer in women. Most people who develop the disease are older adults with less than 1 percent of cases occurring in people younger than 40. People over the age of 70 develop the disease two to three times more often than those aged 55 and 15 to 20 times more often than those aged 30. According to the National Cancer Institute, the highest incidence of bladder cancer occurs in industrialized countries, such as the United States, Canada, and France. Incidence is lowest in Asia and South America, where it is about 70 percent lower than in the United States. An annual cohort of 300,000 to 400,000 patients with bladder cancer is reported in the United States. Bladder cancer is more prevalent in Caucasians than in African Americans and Hispanic (Americans); however, African Americans have a poorer prognosis than Caucasians (Schrag, et al., 2005).

Etiology

Cancer-causing agents (carcinogens) in the urine may lead to the development of bladder cancer. Cigarette smoking contributes to more than 50 percent of cases, and smoking cigars or pipes also increases the risk. Other risk factors include the following: age, chronic bladder inflammation, diet high in saturated fat, external beam radiation, family history of bladder cancer, infection with *Schistosoma haematobium* (parasite found in many developing countries), and treatment with certain drugs (e.g., cyclophosphamide). Exposure to carcinogens in the workplace also increases the risk for bladder cancer (Bosetti, Pira, & La Vecchia, 2005).

Pathophysiology

A review of chapter 15 addresses the pathophysiology of cancer. Almost all bladder cancers are epithelial in origin (Steinberg & Kim, 2005). The urothelium consists of a three- to seven-cell mucosal layer within the muscular bladder. Of these urothelial tumors, more than 90 percent are transitional cell carcinomas. However, up to 5 percent of bladder cancers are squamous cell in origin, and 2 percent are adenocarcinomas. The World Health Organization classifies bladder cancers as low grade (grade 1 and 2) or high grade (grade 3). Carcinoma in situ (CIS) is a flat, noninvasive, high-grade urothelial carcinoma. The most significant prognostic factors for bladder cancer are grade, depth of invasion, and the presence of CIS.

Assessment with Clinical Manifestations

Approximately 80 to 90 percent of patients with bladder cancer present with painless gross hematuria, which is the classic presentation. Consider the likelihood that patients with gross hematuria to have bladder cancer until proven otherwise. More common conditions (e.g., UTI, kidney disease, or renal calculi) also cause hematuria. Twenty to 30 percent of patients with bladder cancer experience irritative bladder symptoms (e.g., dysuria, urgency, or frequency of urination). Patients with advanced disease can present with pelvic or bony pain, lower-extremity edema from iliac vessel compression, or flank pain from ureteral obstruction.

Diagnostic Tests

Diagnosis of bladder cancer includes urological tests and imaging tests. A complete medical history is used to identify potential risk factors (e.g., smoking or exposure to dyes). Laboratory tests may include the following: BladderChek (a urine test used to detect elevated levels of a nuclear matrix protein called NMP22 to detect elevated levels of tumor markers in the urine), urinalysis with microscopy, urine cytology, and urine culture.

Various imaging tests may also be performed; IVP is the standard imaging test for bladder cancer. Other imaging tests include CT scan, MRI, bone scan, and ultrasound. If bladder cancer is suspected, cystoscopy and biopsy are performed. If the sample is positive, the cancer is staged using the TNM system. In addition, the primary procedure used for diagnosis is a cystoscopy with biopsy. Staging for bladder cancer uses the International Union Against Cancer and the American Joint Committee on Cancer Staging developed the TNM staging system, which is used to stage bladder cancer (Bassi, et al., 2005).

Nursing Diagnoses

Based on the information gathered, examples of nursing diagnoses in the patient with bladder cancer may include the following:
- Fear in response to the diagnosis of bladder cancer
- Knowledge deficit related to the diagnosis of bladder cancer
- Ineffective coping related to anxiety, lower activity level and the inability to perform normal activities of daily living
  In addition, refer to the section on renal cancer.

Planning and Implementation

Management for bladder cancer depends on the stage of the disease, the type of cancer, and the patient's age and overall health. Options include surgery, chemotherapy, radiation, and immunotherapy. In some cases, treatments are combined (e.g., surgery or radiation and chemotherapy, preoperative radiation). Further descriptions of these broad forms of management are available in chapter 15, along with specific information regarding the nursing care for patients with cancer.

Pharmacology

Chemotherapeutic drugs commonly used to treat bladder cancer include valrubicin, thiotepa, mitomycin, and doxorubicin. Side effects can be severe and include such things as: abdominal pain, anemia, bladder irritation, excessive bleeding or bruising, malaise, infection and anorexia (Manoharan, et al., 2005).

Radiation therapy is also used to relieve symptoms (called palliative treatment) of advanced bladder cancer. The typical side effects include inflammation of the rectum (proctitis), incontinence, skin irritation, hematuria, fibrosis, and impotence (Logue & McBain, 2005).

Immunotherapy (biological therapy) may be used in some cases of superficial bladder cancer. This treatment is used to enhance the immune system's ability to fight disease. A vaccine derived from the bacteria (BCG) that causes tuberculosis is infused through the urethra into the bladder, once a week for six weeks to stimulate the immune system to destroy cancer cells. Sometimes BCG is used with interferon. The side effects include inflammation of the bladder (cystitis), inflammation of the prostate (prostatitis), and flu-like symptoms.

Photodynamic therapy is a new treatment for early bladder cancer. It involves administering drugs to make cancer cells more sensitive to light and then shining a special light onto the bladder. This treatment is being studied in clinical trials.

Surgery

The type of surgery depends on the stage of the disease. In early bladder cancer, the tumor may be removed through the urethra (transurethral resection; see section on urinary diversion for more specifics of surgical intervention). Bladder cancer that has spread to surrounding tissue usually requires partial or radical removal of the bladder (cystectomy). Radical cystectomy also involves the removal of nearby lymph nodes and may require a urostomy (opening in the abdomen created for the discharge of urine). Complications include infection, urinary stones, and urine blockages. Bladder cancer has a high rate of recurrence. Urine cytology and cystoscopy are performed every three months for two years, every six months for the next two years, and then yearly (Martis, D'Elia, Diana, Ombres, & Mastrangeli, 2005).

In men, the standard surgical procedure is a cystoprostatectomy (removal of the bladder and prostate) with pelvic lymphadenectomy (removal of the lymph nodes within the hip cavity). In women, the standard surgical procedure is radical cystectomy (removal of the bladder and surrounding organs) with pelvic lymphadenectomy. Radical cystectomy in women also involves removal of the uterus (womb), ovaries, fallopian tubes, anterior vaginal wall, and urethra.

Evaluation of Outcomes

Potential patient outcomes for each of the example nursing diagnoses for the patient with bladder cancer are:

- Fear in response to the diagnosis of bladder cancer. The patient should manifest positive coping behaviors and verbalize a reduction in the amount of fear of having this disease.
- Knowledge deficit related to the diagnosis of bladder cancer. The patient should demonstrate motivation to learn, identify perceived learning needs, and verbalize an understanding of desired content.
- Ineffective coping related to anxiety, lower activity level, and the inability to perform normal activities of daily living. The patient identifies own maladaptive coping behaviors, available resources, and support systems, describes or initiates alternative coping strategies, and describes positive results from new behaviors.

In addition, refer to the section on renal cancer.

URINARY DIVERSION

Urinary diversion is a term used when the bladder is removed or diseased, or the normal structures are being bypassed and an opening is made in the urinary system to divert urine. The flow of urine is diverted through an opening in the abdominal wall. Individuals who might require urinary diversion would be those whose bladders were nonfunctional or needed to be removed either because of cancer or injury. For almost 150 years, surgeons have been performing urinary tract diversions. In 1852, Simon performed the first ureteroproctostomy on a patient with exstrophy. The procedures have since become more refined and patient outcomes have improved. Today, patients may be divided into two standard categories, those with continent diversions and those with noncontinent diversions, who require external ostomy collecting devices.

Etiology

The most common indications for urinary system diversion are as follows: bladder cancer requiring cystectomy, neurogenic bladder conditions that threaten renal function, intractable incontinence in females, chronic pelvic pain syndromes, and severe radiation injury to the bladder. The condition of the bladder, the age of the patient, the status of renal function, the pathology of ureteral dilation, and the general health of the patient are all risk factors for urinary diversion.

Assessment with Clinical Manifestations

Most often, patients who are candidates for urinary diversions present with an appearance indicating obvious illness. The typical presentation of these patients consists of easy fatigability, weakness, anorexia, weight loss, polydipsia, nausea, vomiting, and diarrhea.

The major contraindications to urinary diversion are anomalies of the bowel. For example, bowel injured by radiation should not be used for diversion. Patients with poor renal function, severe metabolic abnormalities, and significant proteinuria should not undergo diversion with continent reservoirs. Additionally, patients who lack motivation or are unable to catheterize a continent reservoir should not undergo diversion in this manner.

Diagnostic Tests

The laboratory studies assessed prior to urinary diversion are focused on assessing the patient's renal function. A minimum creatinine clearance of 60 mL/min is necessary prior to performing continent diversion. In addition, the laboratory studies for patients with urinary diversion should be primarily directed toward excluding infection and assessing metabolic status. Therefore, arterial blood gases (ABGs), complete blood count, urinalysis and urine culture, electrolytes, BUN, and creatinine are assessed.

A variety of imaging studies may be performed prior to a urinary diversion. An ultrasound is a desirable method for imaging the upper urinary tracts, because it requires no nephrotoxic agents. A nuclear scan can be used, with the main drawback being the lack of information obtained regarding the precise location of obstruction or integrity of the urinary tract. A CT scan is valuable for demonstrating the presence of urinary calculi and for assessing a ruptured continent urinary reservoir or for determining the presence of fistulous communication of the urinary tract with the GI or genital tracts. An MRI may be performed to rule out recurrent cancer in a patient who has equivocal findings on CT scan images and for imaging the drainage of a tract in a patient who is azotemic or allergic to intravenous contrast.

Planning and Implementation

Patients requiring urinary diversion often are monitored for a time by their urologist, and the decision for surgical intervention is made after conservative management fails. The topic of urinary diversion is essentially a surgical set of interventions and is discussed in the following section.

Surgery

Urinary diversions may be divided into two categories: (a) noncontinent diversions, and (b) continent diversions. Noncontinent urinary diversion into a noncontinent conduit is considered less technically demanding and is associated with the fewest postoperative complications; therefore, this technique is the criterion standard. Noncontinent urinary diversion is performed by either directly anastomosing the ureters to the anterior body wall (i.e., cutaneous ureterostomy) or using a segment of bowel to anastomose in a similar manner to the anterior wall for ostomy bag drainage. The bowels most commonly used for noncontinent conduit diversion are 15 to 25 cm of ileum, colon, and, least often, jejunum bowel segments (Deliveliotis, et al., 2005).

The second form of urinary diversion, continent urinary diversion, is subdivided into two basic types: (a) those with a surgical opening brought out of the abdomen, and (b) those in which a replacement bladder is made out of part of the intestine. Those with a new bladder are able to urinate spontaneously, whereas those patients with a surgical opening need to place a tube into the opening periodically to drain the accumulated urine. The advantage of the two types of continent urinary diversion is that no permanent ostomy bag needs to be worn. Continent urinary diversion describes all forms of urinary diversion that enable the patient to urinate at his or her own discretion without the use of any form of appliance or collecting device. All patients undergoing anticipated continent urinary diversion should be prepared for the possibility that a traditional ileal conduit might be performed (Figure 53-6). Therefore, prior to

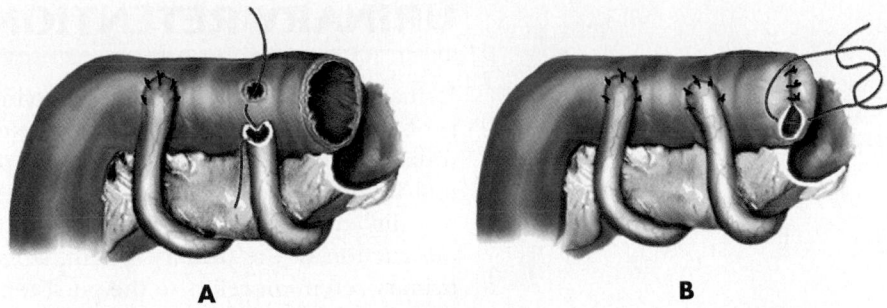

Figure 53-6 Ileal conduit: A. Ureters implanted into ileal segment, B. Closure of proximal end of ileal conduit.

the operation, the site for an external stoma should be selected in conjunction with an enterostomal therapist (Gronau & Pannek, 2005).

The removal of the bladder **(cystectomy)** will always be preceded by complete bowel preparation. A Go-Lytely one-gallon bowel preparation is administered, following a liquid dinner on the night prior to surgery. Oral antibiotics are also given to help sterilize the intestinal tract and reduce the chance of infection. All forms of urinary diversion require the placement of drainage tubes in the new bladder and the kidneys, and these will be present when the patient wakes from surgery. Certain drainage tubes will remain in place for two to three weeks postoperatively. Before removal of the drainage tubes, X-ray studies may be performed to ensure that the new bladder has healed and has no leakage. Postoperatively, patients are taught to wash out the urethral catheter at home every four to six hours. In the early postoperative period, the new bladder may hold only a small volume of urine and patients are required to empty frequently (Ludwig, et al., 2005).

Some metabolic complications that can result from use of the intestinal tract in urinary diversion are UTI, urinary stone formation, vitamin B_{12} deficiency, changes in bowel habits, and changes in pH balance. Early complications of urinary diversions include postoperative ileus or bowel obstruction, which, as a group, is more common in continent diversions. Other early complications may include ureter-bowel anastomotic leak and acute pyelonephritis. Late complications are metabolic disturbances that may result from the interaction of urine with the absorptive surface of the bowel used for the procedure. In addition, a vitamin B_{12} deficiency may develop as the terminal ileum is the exclusive site of vitamin B_{12} absorption. Patients with urinary retention usually present with abdominal pain and distension; and this condition is an emergency, and drainage of the reservoir is indicated. In addition, patients with continent reservoirs are at risk for secretory and osmotic diarrhea, depending on the length of ileum used and whether or not the ileocecal valve was resected for construction of the urinary pouch (Tolhurst, et al., 2005).

Patient and Family Teaching

The lifelong care of a stoma created with noncontinent urinary diversions may be psychologically stressful, and the nurse must provide referral services for the patient (see chapter 50 for stoma care and implications seen in lower GI managements). The patient wears an ostomy bag into which the urine continuously drains and is educated that it is still possible to participate in strenuous physical activity in addition to daily routines. Also, patients undergoing continent diversion should also be aware of the functional complications and results of this form of urinary tract reconstruction (e.g., nocturnal enuresis). Nocturnal incontinence can be expected following neobladder diversion particularly in the first six to nine months following surgery. This problem can usually be managed by external collecting devices in the male (condom catheter) or fluid restriction before bed.

Fast Forward ▶▶▶

Robotic Forms of Surgery for Urinary Diversions

The use of robotics is currently purported for a variety of surgical interventions (e.g., prostatectomy). Robotic surgery is the latest minimally invasive treatment option available for patients with localized muscle-invasive bladder cancer. The robotic laparoscopic procedure offers advantages over open radical cystectomy (removal of the bladder using a relatively large abdominal incision) in that there is a quicker recovery time and only a few small adhesive strip-sized incisions.

URINARY RETENTION

Urinary retention, or bladder-emptying problems, is a common urological problem with many possible causes. Normally, urination can be initiated voluntarily and the bladder empties completely. Urinary retention is the abnormal holding of urine in the bladder. Acute urinary retention is the sudden inability to urinate, causing pain and discomfort. Causes can include an obstruction in the urinary system, stress, or neurological problems. Chronic urinary retention refers to the persistent presence of urine left in the bladder after incomplete emptying. Urinary retention always requires medical attention, sometimes hospitalization, for treatment, symptom relief, and detection of the underlying cause. Failure to treat the condition can lead to infections or damage to the urinary tract and kidneys.

Epidemiology

Urinary retention is not an unusual condition and is more common in men than in women. The average age of patients is over 60, and hospitalization may be required for treatment.

Etiology

Urinary retention develops when the duct that drains the bladder (the urethra) becomes blocked (e.g., an enlarged prostate gland). Acute urinary retention may be caused by stones lodged in the urethra or urethral strictures (often from gonorrhea); fecal impaction, prostatitis, prostatic carcinoma, or benign prostatic hypertrophy; retroverted gravid uterus, after an operation, urethral rupture, and tumor or clots in the bladder (Lau & Lam, 2004). Any drug with anticholinergic effects or alpha adrenergic effects; such as, antihistamines, ephedrine sulfate, and phenylpropanolamine, can precipitate urinary retention. Neurological etiologies include cord lesions, spinal anesthesia, and multiple sclerosis. Patients with genital herpes may develop urinary retention from nerve involvement. Acute urinary retention has also been reported following vigorous anal intercourse.

Chronic urinary retention has a much more protracted course. It is usually relatively painless and may be reflective of renal impairment, late-onset enuresis, hypertension, and present with symptoms of bladder outflow obstruction.

Pathophysiology

As the bladder enlarges, the tension in the walls required to empty it rises in keeping with LaPlace's law so that if the bladder becomes overdistended, it is difficult or impossible to empty it naturally. The risk is greatest when production of urine is high at a time when sensation is impaired. Even if the patient is passing urine, if there is a large, palpable bladder, there is retention of urine. If the bladder is large, palpable, and tender whilst the patient complains of pain with an urge to void that cannot be fulfilled, the diagnosis is clear. If there is a mass that is not painful, it may be a bladder in chronic retention, but other considerations include a large uterus from fibroids, pregnancy, ovarian cysts, or ovarian carcinoma. It is also imperative to ascertain that failure to pass urine is not because of failure to produce urine as in acute renal failure.

Assessment with Clinical Manifestations

Acute urinary retention always presents with acute onset pain of intolerable severity, while chronic retention of urine is associated with almost no pain, and a history of gradually developing symptoms, which have suffered neglect by the

BOX 53-8

DIAGNOSTIC TESTS FOR URINARY RETENTION

- Urinalysis may give a clue to underlying UTI
- BUN and serum creatinine may reflect acute renal failure
- WBC: raised in prostatitis and UTI
- Urinalysis and electrolytes are essential as renal failure often follows chronic retention. If urinary calculus, check urate, calcium, and phosphate
- Check PSA in prostatic enlargement for carcinoma
- Renal ultrasound, IVP, urethrography

Red Flag

Catheterizing a Patient with Urinary Retention

- ▪ If the catheterization fails to drain a significant volume of urine, the diagnosis will be reconsidered.
- ▪ If there is difficulty in passing the catheter, do not use force, do not inflate catheter balloon until urine has been seen in the catheter, and do not use a catheter introducer unless adequately trained in its use.
- ▪ Note: If unable to pass a urethral catheter, the use a suprapubic puncture may be indicated.

patient. In acute urinary retention, the patient may complain of increasing dull low abdominal discomfort and the urge to urinate, without having been able to urinate for many hours. A firm, distended bladder can be palpated between the symphysis pubis and umbilicus (note: palpation can be difficult in the obese or in pregnancy). Rectal examination may reveal an enlarged or tender prostate or suspected tumor. Sometimes hematuria develops midway through bladder decompression, probably representing loss of tamponade of vessels injured as the bladder distended. This should be watched until the bleeding stops (usually spontaneously) to be sure there is no great blood loss, no other urological pathology responsible, and no clot obstruction (Elkhodair, Parmar, & Vanwaeyenbergh, 2005).

In chronic retention, the patient with chronic retention may be passing some urine. There is often retention with overflow so that the complaint is one of urinary frequency rather than inability to void. Small volumes are passed often. Painful bladder is not a complaint.

Diagnostic Tests

Typical diagnostic tests for urinary retention are shown in Box 53-8.

Nursing Diagnoses

Based on the information gathered, examples of nursing diagnoses in the patient with urinary retention may include the following:
- Urinary retention
- Acute pain as related to acute urinary retention

Planning and Implementation

Acute urinary retention may be an indication of surgical intervention. Initial management should be urethral catheterization followed by at least one voiding trial, because acute urinary retention is reversible in some patients. In the elderly, especially the male population, routine enquiry into problems of micturition that may be regarded as a normal feature of aging can permit treatment of the underlying cause before retention of urine occurs. At high risk times (e.g., postoperative or trauma), encouragement of the patient to pass urine may prevent overdistension and retention. Urine charts and awareness of failure to pass urine are essential. In addition, avoid drugs, like tricyclic antidepressants, in elderly men. The patient can be instructed to drink small volumes of water or tea or to sit in a warm bath or take a warm shower. In addition, the patient can be asked to void every three to four hours, regardless of his or her urgency (Griffiths, Fernandez, & Murie, 2004).

Evaluation of Outcomes

Potential patient outcomes for each of the example nursing diagnoses for the patient with urinary retention are:
- Urinary retention. The patient empties the bladder completely and has a residual of less than 30 mL.
- Acute pain as related to acute urinary retention. The patient should verbalize an adequate relief of pain along with the ability to realistically cope with the pain if it is not completely relieved.

URINARY INCONTINENCE

Urinary incontinence (UI), loss of bladder control, is the involuntary passage of urine. This can range from an occasional leakage of urine to a complete inability to hold any urine. There are many causes and types of incontinence and many treatment options. Treatments range from simple exercises to surgery. Women are affected by urinary incontinence more often than men. Approximately $12 to $15 billion is spent annually on UI.

Epidemiology

UI has a prevalence of 15 to 30 percent in community-residing elderly patients, 50 to 84 percent among older adults in long-term care institutions, and 33 percent in older people in acute care settings. UI affects more than 10 million Americans, 85 percent of whom are women. UI affects at least 13 million American women, with an estimated cost to society of $16 to $26 billion. UI affects up to 7 percent of children older than 5 years. Incidence is 1.4 percent of adults aged 15 to 24 years and 2.9 percent of those aged 55 to 64 years. There is no clear evidence of racial differences in prevalence of UI. Age itself is not a cause of UI; however, age-related changes may predispose or contribute to UI (e.g., diabetes, medications, sleep disturbances, restricted mobility, hormonal changes, and mentation) (American College of Obstetricians and Gynecologists, 2005).

Etiology

Incontinence may be sudden and temporary or ongoing and long term. Causes of sudden or temporary incontinence include such things as UTI, prostate infection, stool impaction from severe constipation, side effects of medications (e.g., diuretics, tranquilizers, antihistamines, and antidepressants), poorly controlled diabetes, pregnancy, or weight gain). Causes for long-term UI includes spinal injuries, urinary tract anatomical abnormalities, CVA, benign prostatic hypertrophy, pelvic prolapse in women, and bladder cancer (Madersbacher & Madersbacher, 2005).

Pathophysiology

Usually development of incontinence involves the bladder, the outlet (sphincter), or both. In bladder hyperactivity, the bladder's compliance is decreased, as seen in the decrease in the volume-pressure curve during filling or bladder contractions. Patients may have a painful bladder sensation on filling. Incontinence also can be because intermittent decreases in urethral pressure below that of bladder pressure, which occurs during abdominal straining and is unrelated to bladder hyperactivity. Episodic decrease in sphincter pressure (urethral instability) and loss of closure potential at the bladder outlet (intrinsic sphincter deficiency) are other causes of incontinence. Incontinence may be chronic and progressive, a manifestation of an underlying disease, or transient, such as that seen with a bladder infection or after childbirth. There are several different types of UI, which are shown in Box 53-9.

Assessment with Clinical Manifestations

The nurse must carry out a thorough examination, including a brief psychiatric and neurological evaluation. A goal is to eliminate any serious disease that may be the underlying cause of incontinence and any transient cause or functional impairment. The nurse can assess the abdomen, looking at the flanks and checking for masses, distended bladder after voiding, and signs of fluid overload. In addition, neurologic concerns can be fecal impaction and changes in sphincter tone. A pelvic examination is necessary for women, and the examination should be made with the patient's bladder empty to check organs and with the bladder full to check for prolapse, cystocele, rectocele, or incontinence. A stress test can assess for stress-induced leakage when the bladder is full. A stress test is performed by having the patient relax and asking the

BOX 53-9

TYPES OF INCONTINENCE

1. Stress incontinence is loss of urine with increased intra-abdominal pressure without detrusor contraction. Anatomy of the sphincter is normal, but it has lost some of its efficacy due to excessive mobility and loss of support. Stress incontinence happens when urine leaks during exercise, coughing, sneezing, laughing, lifting heavy objects, or other body movements that put pressure on the bladder. It is the most common type of bladder control problem in younger and middle-age women (Kielb, 2005).

2. Urge incontinence (true, detrusor overactivity, or reflex) is precipitous loss of urine, preceded by a strong urge to void, with increased intravesical pressure and detrusor contraction. Urge incontinence can occur in healthy persons, but it is often found in people who have chronic disorders (e.g., diabetes, stroke, or Alzheimer's disease). It is also sometimes an early sign of bladder cancer.

3. Overflow incontinence is loss of urine because of chronic urinary retention or secondary to a flaccid bladder. It usually is due to an obstructive or neuropathic lesion and occurs when small amounts of urine leak from a bladder that is always full (BPH or spinal cord injury).

4. Functional incontinence happens in many older people who have normal bladder control. They just have a hard time getting to the toilet in time because of arthritis or other disorders that make moving quickly difficult.

PATIENT PLAYBOOK

Bladder Training Techniques

The nurse instructs the patient to:

- Start by trying to not urinate for 10 minutes every time you feel an urge to urinate.
- Then try upping the waiting period to 20 minutes, with the goal to lengthen the time between trips to the toilet until you are urinating every two to four hours.
- Bladder training may also involve double voiding (urinating, then waiting a few minutes and trying to urinate again).
- When you feel the urge to urinate, relax, breathe slowly and deeply, or distract yourself with an activity.
- Nighttime bladder training may be reinforced with devices, such as moisture alarms, which wake you up when you begin to urinate. They are particularly helpful for children who wet the bed at night.
- Schedule toilet trips (timed urination) by going to the toilet according to the clock rather than waiting for the need to go (usually every two to four hours).

---

patient to cough or strain once vigorously; instantaneous leakage is typical of stress UI, delayed leakage is typical of stress-induced detrusor overactivity.

Diagnostic Tests

The history of the patient is the first assessment tool used for diagnosing UI. Then, the diagnostic tests that may be performed for UI include urinalysis, urine culture, cystoscopy, urodynamic studies (tests to measure pressure and urine flow), uroflow, and post void residual (PVR) to measure amount of urine left after urination. Other tests may be performed to rule out pelvic weakness as the cause of the incontinence. One such test is called the Q-tip test. This test involves measurement of the change in the angle of the urethra when it is at rest and when it is straining. An angle change of greater than 30 degrees often indicates significant weakness of the muscles and tendons that support the bladder.

Nursing Diagnoses

Based on the information gathered, examples of nursing diagnoses in the patient with UI may include the following:
- Impaired urinary elimination
- Deficient knowledge related to self-care and risk prevention

Planning and Implementation

The management of UI falls into four broad categories: behavioral techniques, devices, medications, and surgery. The behavioral techniques include strengthening the muscles of the pelvic floor with: bladder retraining (urinating on a schedule); Kegel exercises (voluntary contraction of the pelvic floor muscles); regulating bowels to avoid constipation; quit smoking to reduce coughing and bladder irritation; avoid alcohol and caffeinated beverages, particularly coffee, which can overstimulate the bladder; avoid foods and drinks that may irritate the bladder, like spicy foods, carbonated beverages, and citrus fruits and juices; and keep blood sugars under good control if a diabetic.

There are devices in the forms of catheters, if the behavioral methods fail or are found unacceptable. Catheters must be managed with great care to avoid infection and stone formation. The patient can use clean intermittent catheterization for problems with emptying the bladder. The catheterization techniques may be taught to the patient or family members. In addition, a condom catheter may be used when men prefer a drainage system that fits over the penis like a condom. The patient must be taught to take the same care to avoid infection as with other catheters. Condom catheters can also carry a risk of skin breakdown.

Pharmacology

Drugs commonly used to treat incontinence include anticholinergics, antidepressants, hormone replacements, and antibiotics. The anticholinergic drugs calm an overactive bladder, so they may be helpful for urge incontinence. Examples include tolterodine (Detrol), oxybutynin (Ditropan), and hyoscyamine (Levsin). These drugs can be effective at controlling incontinence, but a side effect is dry mouth. To combat dry mouth, the patient may be tempted to drink more water, which is contraindicated with the incontinence.

Antidepressants may be used to treat incontinence (e.g., imipramine). It causes the bladder muscle to relax, while causing the smooth muscles at the bladder neck to contract.

Hormone replacements are effective after menopause; a drop in estrogen can contribute to changes in the skin lining the urethra and vagina, which can contribute to the development of incontinence. Applying estrogen in the form of a vaginal cream, ring, or patch may help relieve some of the symptoms of incontinence in these women. Also, in children, nighttime incontinence may be because of a shortage of the nighttime production of a hormone called antidiuretic hormone (ADH). This hormone slows the making of urine. Therefore, a synthetic version of ADH (desmopressin [DDAVP]) is available as a nasal spray or pill for children to use before bedtime.

Antibiotics can be used if the incontinence is because of a UTI or an inflamed prostate gland (prostatitis).

Surgery

Surgery may be required to relieve an obstruction or deformity of the bladder neck and urethra. Uterine or pelvic suspension operations are sometimes needed in women. Men may require prostatectomy (removal of the prostate gland). Incontinence can sometimes be managed by artificial sphincters. These are synthetic cuffs that are surgically placed around the urethra to help retain urine. Urethral injections are another method to help keep the urethra closed. A fat-like substance (e.g., collagen) is injected into the area that surrounds the opening of the bladder into the urethra. A variety of bulking agents are available for injection.

Evaluation of Outcomes

Potential patient outcomes for each of the example nursing diagnoses for the patient with urinary incontinence are:

- Impaired urinary elimination. The patient is continent of urine or verbalizes satisfactory management.
- Knowledge deficit related to self-care and risk prevention. The patient should demonstrate motivation to learn, identify perceived learning needs, and verbalize an understanding of desired content.

Case Study

Nursing Care Plan

Mrs. Lockwell, 51 years of age and an active and energetic female, arrived at her gynecologist's office for her scheduled annual appointment. Mrs. Lockwell has had an annual gynecological evaluation for the past 7 years. She is married and has two adult children. She does not drink alcohol or smoke. She exercises three times per week at the local health club. She works as an elementary educator and has been teaching third grade for 26 years. She is active in her local church group and has an active social life. Mrs. Lockwell reports that for the past two weeks she has had to "go to the bathroom a lot and it burns when I urinate" and that her urine "smells strong and is a dark orange." When asked how much fluid she consumes daily, Mrs. Lockwell responded, "I drink one big cup of coffee in the morning, one can of diet soda at lunch, one glass of skim milk at dinner, and maybe one glass of water at bedtime." She also stated that, "My skin feels very dry and my lower back hurts."

Vital signs revealed a temperature of 37.8° C (100° F), pulse 96 beats per minute, lying blood pressure of 136/74, and a standing blood pressure of 128/70. Height is 5 feet 5 inches, and weight is 125 pounds. A urine specimen for urinalysis and for culture and sensitivity were ordered by the health care provider. The nurse observed that Mrs. Lockwell's urine was foul smelling, dark amber, cloudy, and thick. Her skin turgor revealed tenting with the shape remaining for 15 seconds. Her fluid intake for the past 24 hours was 930 mL. The urinalysis revealed a specific gravity greater than 1.030, and the culture and sensitivity report disclosed the presence of *Escherichia coli* with a sensitivity to all penicillins. Her hemoglobin was 14, hematocrit was 45 percent; and WBC count was 12,000. In addition, Mrs. Lockwell guards her lower back on movement.

Assessment

Patient is a 51-year-old female with a UTI that has existed for the past two weeks. She is febrile and has subjective complaints of pain from the infection, and her urine is concentrated, dark colored, and foul smelling.

Nursing Diagnosis 1: Impaired urinary elimination related to irritation of bladder secondary to infection as evidenced by foul smelling, dark amber, cloudy, thick urine; oral temperature 37.8° C (100° F); urine culture reveals *Escherichia coli*.

NOC: Urinary elimination; Urinary continence

NIC: Urinary elimination management

Expected Outcomes

The patient will:

1. Experience no urinary urgency as evidenced by voiding every 240 to 400 mL every 6 to 8 hours within three days of initiating treatment.
2. Report no pain or burning on urination within 24 hours of initiating treatment.
3. Be free of infection as evidenced by clear, urine that is not foul smelling, pain-free urination, WBCs between 5,000 and 10,000 within three days of initiating treatment.

Planning, Interventions, Rationales

1. Evaluate previous patterns of voiding. *Voiding patterns are unique to each patient and can vary. UTIs can cause retention, but it is more likely to cause frequency.*

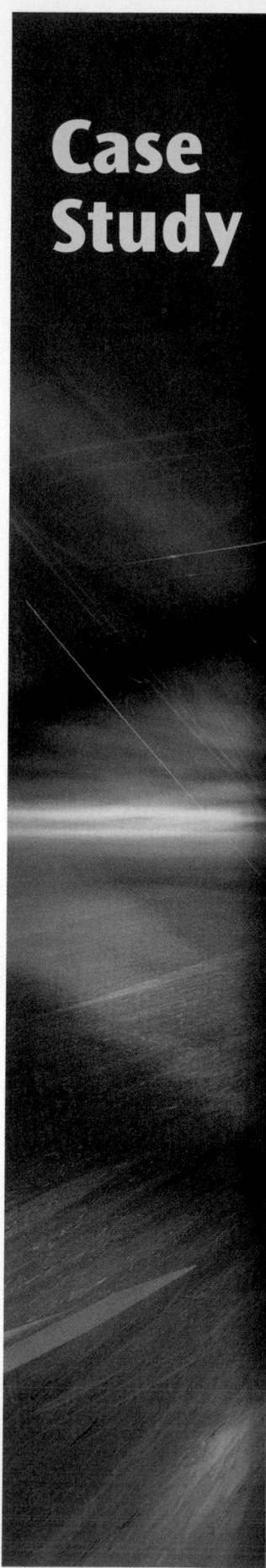

Case Study

2. Assess the balance between intake and output. *Intake greater than output may indicate retention.*

3. Monitor results of urinalysis, urine culture, and sensitivity. *Retention of urine can predispose the patient to UTIs.*

4. Every 4 hours assess patient description of pain: quality, nature, and severity using a pain rating scale. *UTIs are described as burning on urination; if renal involvement, may experience back or flank pain.*

5. Encourage fluids by offering fluids of choice every 2 hours. *Fluid intake should be 1,500 mL per 24 hours to promote renal blood flow and flush bacteria from urinary tract.*

Evaluation

Patient's urine is clear and does not smell foul, and WBC count is between 5,000 and 10,000 within three days of initiating treatment. The patient is free of urinary urgency, voids 240 to 400 mL every 6 to 8 hours within three days of initiating treatment. In addition, within 24 hours of initiating treatment, the patient rates the severity of burning on urination as a 0 on a severity rating scale of 0 to 5, with 0 being no burning and 5 severe burning on urination.

Nursing Diagnosis 2: Deficient knowledge related to lack of information about causes for UTIs and not seeking health care treatment.

NOC: Knowledge of disease process, health behaviors, health resources, infection control, treatment procedures, and treatment regimen.

NIC: Teaching: Disease process; Teaching: Individual

Expected Outcomes

The patient will:

1. Accurately verbalize measures to prevent or reduce risk of reinfection by eliminating beverages with caffeine, by consuming liquids or products that acidify urine, and by drinking at least 1,500 mL of fluids every 24 hours within 7 days of initiation of treatment and at the follow-up appointment visit.

2. Implement measures that will reduce the risk for introduction of pathogens into the urethra.

Planning, Interventions, Rationales

1. Assess knowledge of nature of UTIs. *To identify patient's knowledge and understanding of the risk factors for UTIs.*

2. Teach patient the importance of adequate fluid intake. *Keeps tissues hydrated and decrease bladder irritation.*

3. Teach patient to consume products or liquids that acidify urine (e.g., cranberry juice). *Bacteria grow poorly in acidic environment.*

4. Teach patient to avoid or reduce caffeine intake. *Caffeine is a diuretic, which may lead to dehydration.*

Evaluation

1. Patient verbalizes measures to prevent or reduce risk of reinfection by eliminating beverages with caffeine, by drinking fluids that acidify urine, and by drinking at least 1,500 mL of fluids every 24 hours within 7 days of initiation of treatment and at the follow-up appointment visit. In addition, the patient verbalizes that showering, wiping from front to back after voiding, and voiding immediately after sexual intercourse decrease the concentration of pathogens that may enter the urethra.

KEY CONCEPTS

- UTIs can cover a wide variety of conditions ranging from asymptomatic infections with low bacterial counts to severe infection of the kidney and sepsis.
- IC presents with urgency, frequency, nocturia, and dysuria in the presence of noninfected urine.
- Pyelonephritis is an infection of the upper urinary tract and may involve the ureters, renal pelvis, and the papillary tips of the collecting ducts.
- Glomerulonephritis is categorized into acute and chronic conditions.
- Nephrotic syndrome (nephrosis) is not a single disease but a group of symptoms.
- Renal tuberculosis is the most common site of extrapulmonary tuberculosis
- Many of the people that develop renal calculi require hospitalization, and the pain associated with renal stones is acute.
- The kidney is the most common organ in the urinary tract to be injured by severe trauma

- There are three conditions of renal vascular disorders: (a) renal artery stenosis, (b) renal vein thrombosis, and (c) nephrosclerosis.
- Renal cell carcinoma accounts for approximately 3 percent of adult malignancies and 90 to 95 percent of neoplasms arising from the kidney.
- Bladder cancer is the 4th most frequently diagnosed cancer in men and the 10th most frequently diagnosed cancer in women.
- Urinary diversion is a term used when the bladder is removed or diseased, and an opening is made in the urinary system to divert urine.
- Urinary retention is the abnormal holding of urine in the bladder.
- UI is the involuntary passage of urine and can range from an occasional leakage of urine, to a complete inability to hold any urine.

REVIEW QUESTIONS

1. Which of the following is true concerning the patient teaching for UTIs?
   1. Drinking 10 to 12 glasses of water daily helps to prevent UTI.
   2. Completely empty the bladder when voiding and do not put off the urge to urinate.
   3. Advise patients to use anticholinergics for their UTIs without restriction.
   4. Self-catheterization should be discouraged because of contamination problems.

2. IC is often confused with which of the following disorders, as their presenting symptoms are markedly similar?
   1. Recurrent UTI
   2. Renal cancer
   3. Renal tuberculosis
   4. Urinary retention

3. What is the most common cause of pyelonephritis?
   1. Urinary retention and ascending infection of the urinary tract
   2. Renal calculi
   3. Delayed voiding
   4. Previous UTI

4. Which of the following disorders is more common in children than in adults?
   1. Bladder cancer
   2. Pyelonephritis
   3. Nephrotic syndrome
   4. UTI

5. The nurse is performing discharge teaching for a patient who was admitted with pyelonephritis. The patient asks the nurse, "What is pyelonephritis?" Based on the nurse's knowledge, the best response would be:
   1. Pyelonephritis is an inflammation of the bladder.
   2. Pyelonephritis is a rupture of the bladder.
   3. Pyelonephritis is an infection of the kidney.
   4. Pyelonephritis is an infection of the lower urinary tract.

6. Which of the following tests are most appropriate after experiencing renal trauma?
   1. A CT scan with contrast and ultrasonography
   2. An IVP and a paracentesis
   3. A cystoscopy and histological examination
   4. Staging using the TNM system

Continued

REVIEW QUESTIONS—cont'd

7. Which of the following statements is true concerning renal cancer?
   1. BladderChek is the best lab study to confirm the presence of cancer in the bladder.
   2. The most commonly performed surgery to treat renal cell cancer is radical nephrectomy.
   3. Partial blockage of renal arteries and hypertension are the most common clinical manifestations.
   4. Renal cancer is usually secondary to tuberculosis of the lung.

8. Which of the following disorders presents with painless gross hematuria as the classic presentation?
   1. Pyelonephritis
   2. Nephrotic syndrome
   3. Bladder cancer
   4. Urinary retention

9. Which of the following uses a traditional ileal conduit for management?
   1. Continent urinary diversion
   2. Noncontinent urinary diversion
   3. Urinary retention
   4. Renal calculi

10. A patient with multiple sclerosis is unable to move about easily. Which of the following types of incontinence is the patient most likely to experience?
   1. Urge incontinence
   2. Stress incontinence
   3. Overflow incontinence
   4. Functional incontinence

REVIEW ACTIVITIES

1. Evaluate the urinalysis results of a patient in the clinical setting.

2. Describe the clinical manifestations seen in acute pyelonephritis.

3. Describe the clinical manifestations seen in patients with renal calculi.

4. Identify possible complications of renal injuries.

5. Describe the most common surgical interventions for patients with renal cancer.

Renal Dysfunction: Nursing Management

Irene Eaton-Bancroft, RN, MSN, CS

CHAPTER TOPICS

- Pyelonephritis
- Polycystic Kidney Disease
- Goodpasture Syndrome
- Rhabdomyolysis
- Acute Renal Failure
- Chronic Renal Failure

The kidneys are one of the most efficient organs in the human body. Complex in function, the kidneys maintain homeostasis of elements important to critical body functions. Sensing altered states, the kidneys are able to adjust fluid and electrolyte retention or excretion and increase excretion of protein waste products. The kidney's endocrine function allows secretion of hormones for blood pressure control in low volume output states or increased production of red blood cells in low oxygen states. In addition, the kidneys facilitate calcium absorption and metabolism through conversion of vitamin D to its enzyme form. Changes in kidney function can go relatively undetected until one has lost nearly 65 percent of total function. Signs and symptoms of renal failure are common regardless of the cause. This chapter explores the many causes of renal failure and the stages of failure. Thorough assessment and prompt, focused nursing response are critical to promote optimal recovery.

KEY TERMS

Allogeneic
Allograft
Amyloid
Anuria
Azotemia
Casts
Disequilibrium
Effluent
Fasciotomy
Hematuria
Hypervolemia
Hypovolemia
Intrarenal
Malaise
Myoclonus
Nephropathy
Normovolemia
Nosocomial
Oliguria
Parenchyma
Perinephric
Phenotypes
Postrenal
Prerenal
Proteinuria
Pyelonephritis
Xenogeneic

PYELONEPHRITIS

Pyelonephritis is an infection of the upper urinary tract. It may involve the ureters, renal pelvis, and the papillary tips of the collecting ducts. Unchecked, it can extend into the tubules of the nephron creating a potential for renal failure.

Etiology

Commonly, pyelonephritis is caused by urinary retention or an ascending and unresponsive lower urinary tract infection (UTI). Retained urine provides a breeding ground for bacteria. Repetitive antibacterial treatment may lead to drug resistance and extension of infection. In addition, drugs may cause necrosis of the renal papillae, and sloughed papillae tissue may then cause ureteral blockage and thus extension of the pyelonephritis.

Pathophysiology

Prostate gland hypertrophy, masses, urinary calculi, or ureteral obstruction from sloughed papillae are common causes of urinary retention. Pooled urine promotes bacterial growth, and the continuous urine pathways offer easy access for bacterial ascension to the renal pelvis. In addition, the presence of catheters or fecal incontinence increases the potential for UTI by providing an entry point for *Escherichia coli,* one of the more common infecting organisms. Unchecked, bacteria in the urethra or bladder have easy access to the kidney via the ureters and renal pelvis.

Assessment with Clinical Manifestations

Acute pyelonephritis is described as a clinical syndrome presenting with bacteriuria accompanied by flank pain at the costovertebral angle, fever, and chills. In addition, the patient may experience painful urination, frequency, nocturia, nausea, vomiting, and colicky abdominal pain (Tolkoff-Rubin, Cotran, & Rubin, 2004). Conversely, chronic pyelonephritis may have a deceptively quiet presentation of frequency, dysuria, and nocturia. Mild, intermittent fever, or intermittent back or flank pain may accompany the urinary symptoms (Kelly & Nielson, 2004).

Diagnostic Tests

There are a variety of diagnostic tests for detection of pyelonephritis. Urinalysis and urine culture may be sufficient in mild, initial cases of pyelonephritis in an uncomplicated presentation. Correct urine sample collection technique is critical to proper treatment. Catheterization may be necessary to collect a reliable specimen for the patient who is unable to stand, cleanse, and collect a midstream specimen.

Computed tomography (CT) is the standard diagnostic tool for pyelonephritis unresponsive to 72 hours of antibiotic therapy. CT is valuable in diagnosing obstructive etiology, as well as identifying complications, such as perinephric abscess (Daniels, 2003).

Ultrasound is used when CT scanning is contraindicated, such as in pregnancy or in preexisting renal compromise. Renal ultrasound is used to place nephrostomy tubes for direct drainage of the renal pelvis in cases of complicated urinary obstruction.

Nursing Diagnoses

Based on the information gathered, examples of nursing diagnoses in the patient with pyelonephritis may include the following:

- Risk for imbalanced body temperature

- Pain related to ureteral colic or bladder spasm
- Fear in response to the diagnosis of pyelonephritis
- Deficient knowledge related to completion of drug therapy, optimal fluid intake, or need to empty bladder every two hours to reduce bacterial count
- Ineffective coping related to anxiety, **malaise** (body discomfort and fatigue), and lowered activity level

Planning and Implementation

There are several strategies to providing care for patients with pyelonephritis. The implementation of these strategies may provide quick recovery and positive outcomes for the patient with this disorder.

Goals

The primary goal for providing care for pyelonephritis is to eradicate the UTI and to prevent damage to the renal parenchyma. Additionally and of equal importance, the secondary goal of preventing further infection must be promoted through patient education.

Evidence-Based Care

The nurse is positioned to play a significant role in preventing UTI. Evidence points to avoiding catheterization and early removal of catheters as critical to preventing UTI. The nurse must resist viewing catheters as nursing convenience or an easy answer to incontinence.

The nurse must always employ effective hand washing between patients to prevent patient-to-patient contamination and **nosocomial** (hospital acquired) infection. In addition, the nurse should practice strict aseptic technique in catheter insertions and thorough, regular perineal and catheter site cleansing in the presence of a urinary catheter. The nurse must practice preventive measures with prevention of an ascending UTI in mind.

Collaborative Management including Nursing Intervention Classifications (NIC)

The collaborative management for pyelonephritis includes:
- Monitor vital signs and fluid balance.
- Ensure adequate hydration via an accurate intake and output record, encourage and provide at least 2 liter a day fluid intake or maintain a patent intravenous (IV) access.
- Monitor electrolytes, white blood count (WBC), blood urea nitrogen (BUN) and creatinine.
- Provide adequate pain management via usual analgesics and urinary antiseptics, such as phenazopyridine (Pyridium) or a combination urinary antiseptic or antispasmodic agent, such as Urised (Urisedon or Urisedamine) or Urisept (Uriseptic).
- NIC: Assist with hygiene.

Population-Based Care

The elderly must be carefully assessed as they may have reduced sensation and therefore are not aware of a UTI prior to an advanced stage. The elderly may present with only minor complaints and may not have an elevation in temperature even with advanced infection.

The nurse must determine if the elderly patient uses fasting as a health practice and educate about the need for adequate fluid intake to prevent infection hypovolemia of the kidneys and bladder (Eliopoulos, 2005).

Patient and Family Teaching

The primary aspects of patient and family teaching are to educate about the importance of completing the full course of antibiotic therapy and maintaining the prescribed schedule to ensure continuous therapeutic blood levels. In addition, there needs to be information regarding the value of these above activities in preventing drug resistance. The NIC for the patient with pyelonephritis is to appraise the patient's current level of knowledge related to the disease process.

Evaluation of Outcomes

Potential patient outcomes for each of the example nursing diagnoses for the patient with pyelonephritis are:

- Risk for imbalanced body temperature. The patient maintains body temperature within a normal range.
- Acute pain related to ureteral colic or bladder spasm. Patient will verbalize maintenance of identified comfort level.
- Fear in response to the diagnosis of pyelonephritis. The patient should will manifest positive coping behaviors and verbalize how to effectively treat the disease and prevent its recurrence.
- Deficient knowledge related to completion of drug therapy, optimal fluid intake, or need to empty bladder every two hours to reduce bacterial count. Patient will verbalize the drug therapy regimen, the need to complete full dose on schedule to prevent drug resistance or continued infection. Patient will verbalize need to flush urinary system via adequate fluid intake and fully empty bladder every two hours to reduce the amount of bacteria available for growth.
- Ineffective coping related to anxiety, malaise, and lowered activity level. The patient identifies own maladaptive coping behaviors, available resources, and support systems, describes or initiates alternative coping strategies, and describes positive results from new behaviors. The patient regains energy and participates in self-care.

POLYCYSTIC KIDNEY DISEASE

Polycystic kidney disease is a genetically inherited kidney disease and may be autosomal dominant (ADPKD) or autosomal recessive (ARPKD). Genetic mutation causes cysts to form in the renal tubules. As the cysts enlarge, the kidney's functioning units are destroyed.

Epidemiology

Prevalence in the United States is approximately 400,000 with about 1,800 developing dialysis dependent end-stage renal disease (ESRD) each year. Polycystic kidney disease is found throughout the world and shows no preference for race or ethnicity (O'Sullivan & Torres, 2003). As polycystic kidney disease is explored regarding the nature, assessment, and treatment of this disorder, the focus will be on the autosomal dominant form as this is the form most seen in the adult population. ADPKD is commonly referred to as polycystic kidney disease.

Genetics

ADPKD is caused by genetic mutations on chromosomes 4 and 16; it is a multisystem disorder (O'Sullivan & Torres, 2003). ADPKD occurs in 1 of every 500 to 1,000 individuals. Eighty-five percent of the gene carriers will evidence the disease by their seventh decade, and 50 to 75 percent will advance to ESRD (Grantham & Winklhofer, 2004).

ARPKD, on the other hand, occurs in only 1 in every 6,000 to 55,000 individuals, is more aggressive, and usually causes patient death by age 15 (Grantham & Winklhofer, 2004).

There are two genetic types of ADPKD. ADPKD-2 is the milder of the two **phenotypes** (the expression of the genes present in an individual) of ADPKD. Patients with PKD-2 will have an onset of hypertension and develop renal failure at an older age then does the patient with PKD-1.

Pathophysiology

Cysts form in the renal tubules. As the cysts advance in number and size, the kidney becomes grossly enlarged. Enlarged cysts create pressure against the normal renal parenchyma interfering with both renal filtration and renal circulation. Stretching and occlusion of the renal tubular vasculature causes decreased filtration and renin release that leads to hypertension (Grantham & Winklhofer, 2004). The developing hypertension causes renal parenchyma fibrosis and accelerates the trajectory toward renal failure. Aggressive hypertensive control is needed to slow progression toward failure.

Polycystic kidneys have been found to be many times normal size and can weigh as much as 7 to 8 kg. Many cysts are able to actively secrete chloride and water, thus the normal fluid output seen in most cases of polycystic kidney disease. Solute clearance is compromised and will require medical management as renal function declines.

Pain, the most common presenting symptom in ADPKD, may be unilateral or bilateral and range from dull and achy to knife-like, stabbing pain. Pain is caused by blood vessel rupture with bleeding into the cyst or perinephric tissues. As the hemorrhagic cyst empties, the patient may present a sudden onset of **hematuria** (blood in the urine) ranging from mild to severe and obstructive (Grantham & Winklhofer, 2004). Gross hematuria is another source of pain.

Polycystic liver disease is the most common expression of the disease outside the kidney. Nearly 75 percent of those with ADPKD will develop cystic livers by their seventh decade. Nearly 8 percent will develop cranial aneurysms. Cysts may develop in other organs systems, such as the pancreas, arachnoid membrane, spleen, ovaries, testicles, or seminal vessels (O'Sullivan, & Torres, 2003). One can appreciate that pain and related symptoms may not follow a regular pattern.

The patient with ADPKD is susceptible to urinary obstruction from hemorrhage into large cysts, particularly those located near the renal pelvis. Advanced disease may impose renal failure and need for dialysis or transplantation.

Assessment with Clinical Manifestations

There is tremendous value to the assessment of patients with polycystic kidney disease. First, the nurse must assess the subjective components of the patient by beginning with obtaining a complete medical and family history focusing on renal disease, family history of polycystic kidney disease, pain, hematuria, increase in abdominal girth, and symptoms of UTI. Next, the nurse assesses the objective aspects of the patient with a complete physical examination, which must include careful palpation of the abdomen and costovertebral angle. Possible findings include enlarged, irregular shaped kidneys and enlarged liver with palpable cysts. The urine may be positive for blood. Proteinuria indicates an advanced stage of the disease (Grantham & Winklhofer, 2004). Any of these findings should raise one's suspicions, yet not lead to a conclusive diagnosis. Imaging studies are the most common positive identifier of PKD.

Diagnostic Tests

Ultrasound is the most useful diagnostic tool in combination with a family history or gene linkage to ADPKD. Renal ultrasound is the most reliable and least expensive test for identifying ADPKD. Advantages include avoidance of contrast media in the patient with renal disease or pregnancy.

Nursing Diagnoses

Based on the information gathered, examples of nursing diagnoses in the patient with polycystic kidney disease may include the following:

- Anxiety related to potential for renal failure and to the possibility for genetic transfer of disease to offspring
- Acute pain related to blood vessel rupture with bleeding into the cyst or perinephric tissue
- Injury, potential for related to fluid, electrolyte, and metabolic acid-base balance
- Knowledge deficit related to related genetics, disease process, and treatment regimen

Planning and Implementation

There are several strategies to providing care for patients with polycystic kidney disease. The implementation of these strategies may provide quick recovery and positive outcomes for the patient with this disorder.

Goals

Primary goals of treatment for patients with polycystic kidney disease include:

- Maintaining homeostasis in each state of renal function decline and prevent or minimize cardiovascular complications.
- The patient will feel free to express the dynamic of guilt associated with genetic disease transmission and be given appropriate resources to meet any family planning goals.
- The patient will receive support with the coping mechanism of denial in dealing with the disease.
- The patient will receive adequate pain control with consideration to need for increased doses related to drug tolerance.
- The patient will acquire full knowledge of the disease process and measures to minimize complications.

Evidence-Based Based Care

Cardiovascular complications are the primary cause of death in patients with ADPKD. Blood pressure control has proven clinically important in preventing death from left ventricular hypertrophy in the patient with ADPKD (Schrier, et al., 2002). The nurse is assigned a major therapeutic role in dispensing antihypertensive medications according to as needed within parameters medication orders (Figure 54-1).

Collaborative Management with NIC

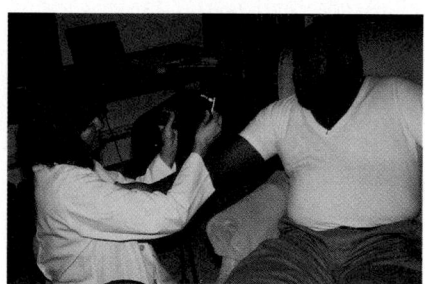

Figure 54-1 Nurse taking blood pressure of a hypertensive patient with ADPKD.

The collaborative management for polycystic kidney disease includes:

- Pain management to prevent disability from chronic pain or analgesics.
  - NIC: Notify health care provider if measures are unsuccessful or if current complaint is a significant change from patient's past experience of pain.
  - Teach patients that nonsteroidal anti-inflammatory drugs (NSAIDs) pose a hazard to remaining kidney function via further compromise to intrarenal blood flow.
  - Prepare the patient for guided ultrasound drainage of troublesome cysts or for surgical intervention, as appropriate.
- Blood pressure control to prevent complications.
  - NIC: Monitor blood pressure after patient has taken medication, if possible.
  - Early diagnosis and management of infected cysts or parenchymal infection as evidenced by fever, deep tenderness over kidney, diaphoresis, bacteremia, leukocytosis, and bacteriuria (Grantham & Winklhofer, 2004).
  - NIC: Notify health care provider if measures are unsuccessful or if current complaint is a significant change from patient's past experience of pain.
  - NIC: Monitor WBC, hemoglobin, and hematocrit levels.

- Antibiotic therapy for infected cysts. See Box 54-1 for pharmacological agents.
  - NIC: Promote adequate fluid and nutritional intake; administer antipyretic medications, as appropriate.
- Provide counseling to consider both the benefits and consequences of genetic testing in asymptomatic adult patients.
- Facilitate social work referral, as appropriate.

Health Care Resources

Emotional support and education for patients and their families are available through the Polycystic Kidney Foundation (www.PKDcure.org).

Surgery

Hemorrhagic cyst and cyst dome removal may be necessary for those individuals with frequent or obstructive episodes of bleeding. Nephrectomy may be necessary following repeated resistant infections, cysts creating uncontrollable pain, or uncontrollable hypertension with significant loss of renal function (Figure 54-2).

Patient and Family Teaching

The nurse can promote showers rather than tub baths for female patients, frequent voiding, good perineal hygiene, and voiding immediately after intercourse. The rationale is to minimize opportunity for an ascending UTI. In addition, the nurse can promote and teach to adhere to a low-sodium diet, weight control, and exercise for those patients presenting with hypertension. And, the nurse can make dietary referral, as appropriate. The nurse must be aware that a positive finding of ADPKD genes may compromise employment opportunities and prohibit health and life insurance.

Evaluation of Outcomes

Potential patient outcomes for each of the example nursing diagnoses for the patient with polycystic kidney disease are:
- Anxiety related to potential for renal failure and to the possibility for genetic transfer of disease to offspring. The patient maintains activity level within capabilities, as evidenced by normal heart rate and blood pressure during activity, as well as absence of shortness of breath, weakness, and fatigue.

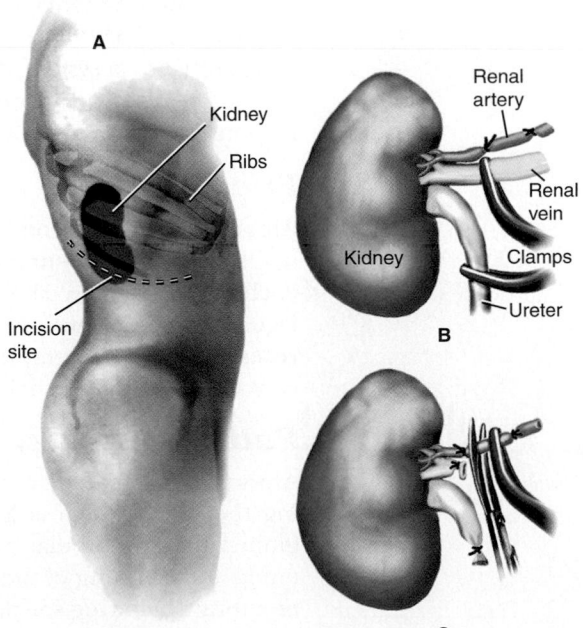

Figure 54-2 Simple nephrectomy: A. Subcostal incision, B. Renal artery ligated first, C. Renal artery transected.

- Acute pain related to blood vessel rupture with bleeding into the cyst or perinephric tissue. The patient should verbalize an adequate relief of pain along with the ability to realistically cope with the pain if it is not completely relieved.
- Injury, potential for related to fluid, electrolyte, and metabolic acid-base balance. The patient maintains adequate fluid volume, electrolyte balance, and acid-base balance as evidenced by vital signs within normal limits, clear lung sounds, pulmonary congestion absent on X-ray, resolution of edema, and arterial blood gases (ABGs) within normal limits.
- Knowledge deficit related to related genetics, disease process, and treatment regimen. The patient should demonstrate motivation to learn, identify perceived learning needs, and verbalize an understanding of desired content.

IMMUNOLOGICAL AND VASCULAR DISEASES OF THE KIDNEY

There is a group of somewhat mysterious disease phenomena that affect the renal vasculature via immune complex deposit or necrosis. Each has a potential to destroy kidney function through the common mechanism of vascular damage. Renal failure may present acutely during periods of exacerbation. With adequate treatment and response, the acute renal failure may resolve or progress with varying intensity to ESRD and chronic renal failure. The more common disorders in the group will be presented with a focus on the renal component of the disease. Note: systemic lupus erythematosus (SLE) is also a dysfunction that affects renal function and is considered in this group of disorders, but SLE is covered in detail in chapter 42. Assessment will be discussed in the sections covering acute renal failure and chronic renal failure.

Alport Syndrome

Alport syndrome is a complex genetic disorder. The genetic anomaly varies; thus patients have differing presenting syndromes. Renal dysfunction, deafness, or visual disturbance may occur dependent on genetic mutation.

Epidemiology

The genetic frequency for Alport syndrome is estimated to be one case in a population of 5,000. According to the 2005 annual data report of the United States renal data system, Alport syndrome accounts for approximately 2.5 percent of pediatric patients with ESRD In Europe, Alport syndrome may be responsible for as many as 2.3 percent of cases of ESRD.

Etiology

Alport syndrome encompasses a group of heterogeneous inherited disorders involving the basement membranes of the kidney and frequently involving the cochlea and the eye. These disorders are the result of mutations in type IV collagen genes. The mode of inheritance is X-linked in 80 percent, autosomal recessive in 15 percent, and autosomal dominant is reported in about 5 percent of individuals with Alport syndrome.

Pathophysiology

Alport syndrome may vary even within a family group. The form most affecting the renal system is X-linked Alport syndrome. Collagen anomaly in the glomerular and tubular basement membranes results in a characteristic thickening and thinning of the membrane. Focal ruptures develop in the basement membrane allowing spillage of red blood cells and protein leakage. Hematuria is a common finding. Males presenting with hematuria before age 10 commonly develop the greatest degree of renal failure (Kashtan, 2003).

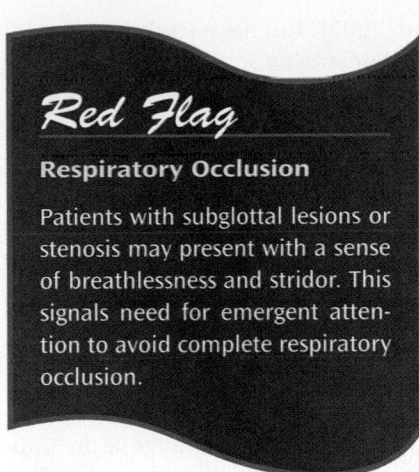

Genetics

There are three genetic forms of Alport syndrome. X-linked dominant form, autosomal recessive form, and autosomal dominant form each have differing molecular genetics. X-linked Alport syndrome accounts for approximately 80 percent of the cases (Kashtan, 2003).

Diagnostic Tests

The primary methods for diagnosing Alport syndrome are by renal biopsy and a complete family history.

Small Vessel Vasculitis: Wegener Granulomatosis

Wegener granulomatosis, Churg-Strauss' syndrome, microscopic polyangiitis, and Schönlein-Henoch purpura are a group of diseases that characteristically cause small vessel pathology. Small vessel vasculitis with inflammatory or necrotizing lesions in the vasculature is common to all of these diseases, but there may be variance in presentation. All manifest multisystem involvement in varying degrees. Renal involvement is significant in 45 to 90 percent of all cases. Wegener granulomatosis is the only one of these disorders that will discussed in this section.

Wegener granulomatosis is a multisystem disease. It presents with respiratory disease in 75 percent of the cases with classic necrotizing and cavitating lesions of the pulmonary **parenchyma** (functional elements of an organ), trachea, and subglottal region (Appel, Radhakrishnan, & D'Agati, 2004). Shortness of breath and hemoptysis may be the presenting symptoms.

Wegener granulomatosis may cause nasal crusting or septal defect, hearing loss, chronic sinusitis, or ophthalmological disorders. Fever, weakness, malaise, and cough with hemoptysis are common presenting symptoms. Renal involvement develops in up to 95 percent of all cases and is varied in the clinical presentation (Appel, et al., 2004). Evidence of renal involvement includes microscopic hematuria, **proteinuria** (protein in the urine), decreased glomerular filtration, and hypertension.

Epidemiology

The literature evidences discrepancy in incidence and demographics of this vasculitis disease set. Advances in diagnostics and knowledge of disease characteristics prompt dynamic change in available data. The collective incidence of small vessel vasculitis is 19.8 cases per million. There appears to be seasonal variance with more cases presenting in the late fall and early spring.

Incidence of Wegener granulomatosis is only slightly higher in males than in females. Peak incidence is in the fourth and fifth decades. Though more than one family member has been found to have Wegener granulomatosis, there is no conclusive evidence of genetic transmission (Appel, et al., 2004).

Etiology

There is no clear etiology of this disease group. Autoimmune humoral and cell-mediated immune responses are implicated.

Pathophysiology

Wegener granulomatosis produces granulomatous necrotizing lesions in small- and medium-sized blood vessels. A multisystem disease, Wegener granulomatosis is associated with necrosis and granulomatous inflammation of the small vessels of the respiratory tract and glomeruli (Appel, et al., 2004). Associated renal pathology includes obstruction from associated ureteral lesions with sclerotic narrowing and immunosuppression treatment-associated malignancies.

Relapse has become the major challenge in treating Wegener granulomatosis. It is postulated that the resulting granulomatous areas in the connective tissue may be the source of remission (Bacon, 2005). Intensive study is ongoing. Nurses must stay alert to changes in early diagnostics and treatment.

Assessment with Clinical Manifestations

The clinical presentation of Wegener granulomatosis varies, which affects the assessment processes. Wegener granulomatosis may be mild and obscure or present with fulminant respiratory and renal involvement. The nurse must first obtain a complete health history and perform a complete physical examination. In addition, the nurse must keep the focus broad to include those physical responses shown in the Soft Skills feature.

Diagnostic Tests

The diagnostic tests for Wegener granulomatosis are CT of the lungs, bronchoscopy with lung biopsy, and renal biopsy. In addition, the laboratory tests are antineutrophil cytoplasmic antibodies (ANCA), electrolytes, CBC, and urine studies.

Planning and Implementation

Wegener granulomatosis was formerly a lethal disease. Advances in diagnosis and treatment have decreased mortality rates but have not yet affected a cure. The primary treatment for Wegener granulomatosis is the pharmacological treatment, which uses glucocorticoids and cyclophosphamide (Appel, et al., 2004). Repeated exacerbations and related chronic health changes have resulted in considerable work disability and diminished quality of life (Reinhold-Keller, et al., 2005). Social work referral to address insurance and disability challenges is critical. Referral to or consult with the mental health nurse specialist, when available, may be of real value to this patient population.

GOODPASTURE'S SYNDROME

Goodpasture's syndrome is a glomerular basement membrane disease (GBM). Primary sites of vascular membrane destruction occur in the capillary beds of the lungs and the kidneys. Goodpasture's syndrome, by definition, must include the three characteristics of proliferative glomerulonephritis, pulmonary hemorrhage, and the presence of anti-GBM antibodies.

Epidemiology

Goodpasture's syndrome has an incidence of one in one million, occurs slightly more in males than in females, and is more prominent in Caucasians. Most diagnoses are made in the third and fifth decades (Bergs, 2005). ESRD develops in 40 to 70 percent of those with renal involvement.

Etiology

The exact cause of Goodpasture's syndrome is unknown. It is believed that the disease process may be triggered when genetically predisposed individuals are exposed to upper respiratory infection, irritants, or toxins (Bergs, 2005). Inhalation of hydrocarbon fumes, cigarette smoke, or cocaine and exposure to hair dye, metallic dust, and D-penicillamine have all been associated with syndrome exacerbations (Appel, et al., 2004).

Pathophysiology

Circulating antibodies react with antigens against type IV collagen specific to the basement membranes of glomerular and pulmonary capillaries (Appel, et al., 2004). Immune globulins deposited in the basement membranes, causing an inflammatory response, glomerulonephritis, and breakdown in the basement membrane with crescent formation. The complications of Goodpasture's syndrome include pulmonary hemorrhage, respiratory failure and dialysis dependent ESRD. Goodpasture's Syndrome carries a 50 percent mortality rate without early recognition and intervention.

Genetics

Autoimmune response has been linked to genes in q35 to q37 region of chromosome 2 (Appel, et al., 2004). It is suggested that one may have a genetic predisposition to Goodpasture's syndrome (Bergs, 2005).

Assessment with Clinical Manifestations

The primary clinical focus must be pulmonary function. The patient may first present with mild shortness of breath or severe, exsanguinating pulmonary hemorrhage (Appel, et al., 2004; Bergs, 2005). Presenting flulike symptoms of weakness, malaise, and pallor may be related to anemia secondary to chronic blood loss. Renal involvement may be evidenced by hematuria, decreased urine output, edema, and hypertension.

Diagnostic Tests

The principal indicator of Goodpasture's syndrome is laboratory finding of circulating anti-GBM antibodies, proteinuria, and iron deficiency anemia. Chest X-ray (CXR) may show hemorrhagic infiltrates, atelectasis, and pulmonary edema (Appel, et al., 2004).

Planning and Implementation

Early diagnosis and intervention have drastically decreased mortality related to Goodpasture's syndrome. Current treatment includes high dose oral or IV corticosteroid therapy to control the inflammatory process in conjunction with plasmapheresis to reduce the circulating immune complexes.

RHABDOMYOLYSIS

Rhabdomyolysis is a condition of muscle tissue destruction with release of myoglobin in the urine. It is a major cause of acute renal failure.

Etiology

A myriad of conditions contribute to rhabdomyolysis. Direct muscle injuries, drugs and toxins, infection, excessive muscular activity, ischemia, electrolyte imbalances, endocrine or metabolic disturbances, and immunological disorders are major categories of etiology. Among these categories are severe burns, crush injuries, tetanus, gas gangrene, excessive exercise, diabetic ketoacidosis, hypothermia, and polymyositis.

Pathophysiology

Lethal levels of intracellular ionized calcium occur with disruption in normal muscle structure or metabolism. Degrading enzymes are activated, causing cell death. Lysis of the cell membrane releases cell content, inclusive of myoglobin, into the system. The exact pathophysiology is unclear and believed to be a combination effect of hypovolemia, tubular toxicity, and tubular obstruction.

Safety First

Safety Considerations for Rhabdomyolysis

Health care and medical advances enable the elderly to live independently longer. Potential for falls with a period of prolonged immobility before assistance arrives expose them to the risk of rhabdomyolysis. Education and persuasion to the advantages of a personal medical alert system has the potential to minimize complications of fractures, electrolyte imbalances, or dehydration in this population. A myriad of service providers are available. Many community emergency services and or community hospitals offer these services.

Assessment of Rhabdomyolysis

The nurse must examine carefully for:

- Redness, swelling, and induration over tender or painful muscles
- Muscle stiffness or weakness varying from mild at onset to severe with the development of muscular necrosis
- Muscle paralysis that may develop with severe muscular necrosis
- Hypotension or hypertension
- Signs of hypovolemia and reduced urine output
- Dark urine from the characteristic brown debris and sediment

Safety First  **1**

Safety Considerations with Rhabdomyolysis

It has been demonstrated that many patients presenting with rhabdomyolysis do not admit to muscle pain or tenderness and do not present with swelling. This emphasizes the need for repeated patient questioning and thorough examination for early intervention and optimal recovery.

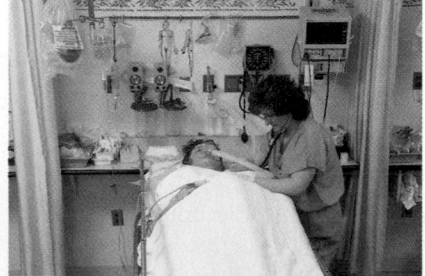

Figure 54-3 Patient in critical condition with ARF.

Genetics

Hereditary enzyme deficiencies predispose to rhabdomyolysis. They include deficiency of myophosphorylase (McArdle's syndrome), phosphofructokinase, or carnitine palmityl transferase with resultant decreased intracellular energy production.

Assessment with Clinical Manifestations

The initial data collection must include learning what the patient was doing and what the environmental conditions were prior to the onset of symptoms (Russell, 2005). An example is running an unusually long distance in hot, humid conditions with adequate hydration before, during, or after the exercise.

Diagnostic Tests

The diagnostic tests for rhabdomyolysis are primarily blood and urine. Blood studies that are used for diagnostics are elevated creatinine kinase (CK-MM) which confirm muscle injury; CK-MM which is the specific diagnostic serum marker for rhabdomyolysis; hyperkalemia is the most life-threatening consequence of muscle necrosis; hyperphosphatemia and hypocalcemia; elevated BUN and the creatinine ratio; and elevated uric acid levels. In addition, urine studies will show myoglobin, and have an acid pH and be positive for red blood cells.

Planning and Implementation

Rhabdomyolysis can cause acute renal failure, which is covered extensively later in this chapter. In addition, the primary goal for the management of rhabdomyolysis is to minimize complications and to intervene effectively as complications of muscle necrosis occur. For example, in the development of compartment syndrome requiring fasciotomy occur, the wounds must be kept infection free and the muscle tissue moist for successful closure.

ACUTE RENAL FAILURE

Acute renal failure (ARF) presents as a rapid decline in renal function. This decline may occur within a few hours or over a period of several weeks. Relatively asymptomatic, ARF is most often detected by laboratory studies. ARF is evidenced by oliguria elevated blood levels of BUN and creatinine (Brady, Clarkson, & Lieberthal, 2004).

Epidemiology

ARF occurs in approximately 5 percent of all hospital admissions and 30 percent of all intensive care unit admissions (Brady, et al., 2004). ARF contributes to an increase in morbidity and mortality in the hospitalized patient. Most patients recover from ARF. Optimal recovery is dependent on early recognition, identifying the cause, and instituting appropriate clinical management (Figure 54-3) (Toto, 2004).

Etiology

There are many causes for ARF, which are presented in the following pathophysiology section and in Table 54-1.

TABLE 54-1 Etiology of ARF

INTRARENAL CAUSES OF ACUTE OR PROGRESSIVE RENAL FAILURE	PATHOPHYSIOLOGY AND ETIOLOGY
Ischemic acute tubular necrosis (ATN)	ATN infers damage to the renal parenchyma. Multiple sources of tubular injury resulting in ATN include major and prolonged surgery, burns, overwhelming sepsis, myoglobin release, and nephrotoxic drugs. Though often associated with **hypovolemia** (insufficient intravascular fluid), ATN has occurred in states of **normovolemia** (state of normal blood volume). It is not to be confused with perfusion-deficit related ATN. Recovery potential is directly correlated to the extent of intrarenal damage (Brady, et al., 2004).
Drug toxicity	NSAIDs inhibit renal prostaglandin production thereby contribute to intrarenal vascular constriction and potential acute tubular necrosis. The potential for renal function impairment secondary to NSAIDs increases in the presence of hypovolemia, decreased arterial blood volume, or chronic renal insufficiency.
Renal artery stenosis or thrombosis	Loin pain and hematuria are the classic signs of acute renal artery occlusion. Chronic renal artery occlusion is generally asymptomatic until a precipitous event occurs. Collateral circulation from the adrenal glands will often allow chronic stenosis go undetected for some time. Causes include emboli, thrombi, hypercoagulable states, and aortic dissection or occlusion. The transplant patient may be predisposed secondary to immunosuppression or vascular rejection or constriction at the site of vascular anastomosis.
Hemolytic uremic syndrome (HUS)	Occlusion of glomerular capillaries by capillary wall thickening and thrombus formation. HUS may be associated with pregnancy as a complication of preeclampsia and may occur in the first three months postpartum. It is also seen after receiving the chemotherapeutic agent mitomycin or the antirejection medication cyclosporine.
Multiple myeloma	Protein-like **casts** (materials in a space that fills the contours of the space) in distal nephron segments, interstitial calcification, and **amyloid** (extracellular protein-like substance) deposits in nephron glomeruli and blood vessels.
Radiation nephritis	Endothelial cell swelling causes decreased intrarenal blood flow and results in tubular atrophy within the nephron.
Contrast-induced nephropathy	Ischemia resulting from dye-induced vasoconstriction is the probable cause of decreased kidney function following IV contrast media. Acute decline in renal function is seen within 24 to 48 hours of dye administration with a peak creatinine in three to five days and resolution in uncomplicated cases in about one week. At-risk populations are associated with existing renal impairment, diabetes mellitus, repeated use of contrast media, and concurrent use of nephrotoxic drugs including NSAIDs and the elderly. Preventive measures include: Infusion of 0.45% normal saline 1 mL/kg for 12 hours prior to and following contrast media Administration of oral acetylcysteine in combination with hydration (600 mg twice daily 24 hours before and after contrast media) Infusion of 154 mEq/L sodium bicarbonate as a bolus of 3 mL/kg/hour for 1 hour before the procedure and 1 mL/kg/hour for 6 hours following the procedure.

Adapted from Brady, H., Clarkson, M., & Lieberthal, W. (2004). Acute renal failure. In B. Brenner (Ed.), Brenner and Rector's the kidney (7th ed., vol. 1, pp. 1215–1292). Philadelphia: W. B. Saunders Co.; Karnib, H., & Badr, K. (2004). Microvascular diseases of the kidney. In B. Brenner (Ed.), Brenner and Rector's the kidney (7th ed., vol. 2, pp. 1601–1623). Philadelphia: W. B. Saunders Co.; Kelly, C., & Nielson, E. (2004). Tubulointerstitial diseases. In B. Brenner (Ed.), Brenner and Rector's the kidney (7th ed., vol. 2, pp. 1483–1511). Philadelphia: W. B. Saunders Co.

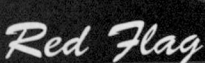

Pathophysiology

ARF is a sudden and near complete cessation of kidney function and may occur suddenly and last for days in certain situations. ARF is seen in acute care patients and may occur in other arenas of health care as well (e.g., convalescent care, home care, or out-patient care). ARF begins with oliguria, anuria, or even normal urine output. **Oliguria** (less than 400 mL per 24 hours of urine) is the most common clinical manifestation, with **anuria** (less than 50 mL per 24 hours of urine), and normal urine output being less common in occurrence. ARF can be a critical condition, and there is an associated mortality percentage even with management in the acute care settings.

The etiology of ARF is varied. Classification follows the source of failure in relation to the kidney. **Prerenal** causes of ARF are those that result in decreased blood flow to the kidney. This may be something as simple as dehydration from fluid loss or as complex as the vascular expansion of sepsis or the deficient pumping of cardiac failure. Prerenal ARF is the most common cause of ARF (Kieran & Brady, 2003). **Intrarenal** causes of ARF are intrinsic to the kidney. These include inflammation of the renal parenchyma, intrarenal vascular thrombosis, or tubular necrosis from nephrotoxic agents. **Postrenal** failure is caused by obstruction to urine flow. More commonly the obstruction is caused by an enlarged prostate gland or a calculus. There simply is no route for the urine to exit the system.

There are myriad causes of ARF. Many are presented in Table 54-1. It is important to note that any ARF event is a potential precursor to chronic renal insufficiency (CRI)) or chronic renal failure (CRF). Factors influencing resolution or progression of failure episode are early diagnosis, adequacy of treatment, and the presence of preexisting kidney disease. Major complications of ARF include hyperkalemia, hyponatremia, hypocalcemia, hyperphosphatemia, and hyperuricemia (Kieran & Brady, 2003) (Figure 54-4).

Assessment with Clinical Manifestations

The assessment for the patient with ARF needs to be comprehensive and includes the entire body system. Specific assessment components are shown in the Patient Playbook.

Diagnostic Tests

In addition to the cessation or change of urine output, there are many diagnostic tests to determine the presence of acute renal failure. The following are the diagnostic tests for ARF: plain abdominal X-ray of the kidneys, ureters and bladder (KUB) to determine calculi or renal vascular calcification; a renal ultrasound to identify renal vascular blood flow and to rule out obstruction, and a bladder scan to detect urinary retention. In addition, laboratory studies are several blood chemistry tests (e.g., BUN, serum creatinine), a basic metabolic panel (BMP), and a CBC.

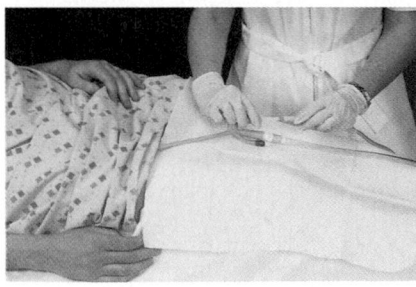

Figure 54-4 Nurse connecting irrigation tubing to irrigation port of a catheter for a postrenal cause of ARF.

Nursing Diagnoses

Based on the information gathered, examples of nursing diagnoses in the patient with ARF may include the following:
- Risk for imbalance in fluid volume
- Impaired tissue integrity related to alterations in internal regulatory function
- Risk for infection related to invasive lines and altered immune response secondary to ARF and uremic toxins
- Anxiety related to sudden change in health status
- Knowledge deficit related to disease process and related diagnostic studies

Assessment of Patients with ARF

Subjective

The nurse will gather a history with focus on hydration and medications. Questions for the nurse to ask may include:

- Have you had any nausea, vomiting, diarrhea, fever, or profuse sweating recently? Quantify the amount and duration.
- Have you felt light-headed or dizzy?
- Have you been able to drink fluids in good amounts?
- Have you experienced any change in the amount of urine or the number of times you have urinated?
- Have you noticed shortness of breath, weakness, or fatigue?
- Have you had any recent injuries?
- Have you taken any antibiotics recently?
- How much do you use NSAIDs? Name the NSAIDs: Advil, Aleve, Excedrin, ibuprofen, Indocin, Motrin, Naprosyn, Pamprin, and Voltaren.

Objective

The nurse will complete a physical examination with diagnostic studies. System alterations in acute renal failure reflect the kidneys inability to maintain homeostasis. Table 54-2 lists homeostatic losses and evidence of alteration. Table 54-3 identifies questions to ask when suspecting urinary dysfunction.

Planning and Implementation

There are many interventions and strategies for the nurse to be aware of in the management of ARF. Often patients are transferred to the critical care settings as they experience ARF, and the mortality percentages are relatively high for patients with the diagnosis of ARF.

Goals

The primary goal is to reverse the causative process with full recovery of renal function. When this is impossible, the goal is always to minimize renal compromise.

Collaborative Management including NIC

ARF presents a dynamic management challenge. The clinical presentation can rapidly change and requires intricate teamwork among health care providers. The patient can go from a state of intravascular hypovolemia to fluid overload and pulmonary edema in just a few hours and require skilled, dynamic assessment and alertness to management change. Among the considerations are:

- Treat the underlying cause of acute renal failure.
- Keep the patient informed of the disease process and the treatment plan.
- NIC: Determine patient's understanding of common medical terminology, such as *azotemia, creatinine,* and *acute renal failure.*
- Fluid replacement in primary hypovolemia and high output failure in the recovery phase.
- NIC: Offer fluids regularly throughout the day, as appropriate.
- Fluid restriction in low output failure and hypervolemia.
- Intermittent hemodialysis or continuous renal replacement therapy (Box 54-2).
- Diuretics, as appropriate and with evidence of tubular response.
- Maintain accurate intake and output records and obtain a daily weight. Day-to-day weight gain in the hospital reflects fluid gain. One liter of fluid is equivalent to 1 kilogram of weight.

BOX 54-2

CONTINUOUS RENAL REPLACEMENT THERAPY (CRRT)

Continuous renal replacement therapy (CRRT) offers lower fluid removal and solute clearance rates than intermittent HD. Hemodynamic stability is more easily attained in the hypotensive critically ill patient.

The procedure is performed in the critical care setting utilizing an inline hemofilter. Arteriovenous hemofiltration relies on the driving force of the systemic blood pressure for blood flow through the extracorporeal circuit. Venovenous hemofiltration requires a blood pump for blood flow through the extracorporeal circuit.

Vascular access is achieved by percutaneous insertion of a single-lumen catheter into a central artery and vein for arteriovenous hemofiltration. A dual-lumen catheter inserted into a central vein is sufficient for venovenous hemofiltration.

Complications include hemofilter clogging and clotting, emboli distal to arterial puncture, vascular damage, and hemorrhage.

Source: Marshall, M., & Golper, T. (2003). Other dialysis modalities. In R. Johnson & J. Feehally (Eds.), Comprehensive clinical nephrology (2nd ed., pp. 1025–1034). St. Louis, MO: Mosby.

TABLE 54-2 Alterations in ARF and the Mechanisms of the Alterations

ALTERATIONS IN ACUTE RENAL FAILURE	MECHANISM OF ALTERATION
Alterations in fluid volume	Intravascular fluid overload in oliguric states: edema, hypertension, shortness of breath, abnormal lung sounds, and acute weight gain
	Intravascular dehydration in high output failure: thirst, reduction in skin turgor, dry mucous membranes, hypotension, tachycardia, decreased urine output, and acute weight loss
Alterations in intravascular sodium (Na^+) Normal range: 135 to 145 mEq/L	Hyponatremia due to dilution in **hypervolemia** (excess intravascular fluid): disorientation, apathy, depression, depressed deep tendon reflexes, and agitation. The elderly are especially susceptible.
	Hypernatremia due to concentration in hypovolemia: thirst. Note: be alert to the development of muscle weakness, restlessness or lethargy, and coma.
Alterations in intravascular potassium (K^+) Normal range: 3.5 to 5 mmol/L	Hypokalemia in hypervolemic state because of dilution or diuretic phase of recovery because of loss. Anticipate need for potassium replacement. Watch for broad flat T waves, ST depression, or prolonged QT. The elderly and patients on digoxin or antiarrhythmic drugs are most prone to arrhythmia secondary to low potassium levels.
	Hyperkalemia in hypovolemic state because of concentration and retention. Respiratory acidosis promotes potassium movement out of the intracellular space into the extracellular space compounding hyperkalemia in any form of renal insufficiency. Hyperkalemia signals a medical emergency. Peaked T-waves characteristic of hyperkalemia. Severe and prolonged hyperkalemia will increasingly prolong the PR and QRS intervals with a potential for cardiac arrest.
Alterations in intravascular magnesium (Mg^{2+}) Normal range: 1.8 to 2.3 mg/dL	Mg^{2+} blood levels may be low because of high output kidney failure, through GI loss or dietary deficiency. All three conditions often exist in the patient with ARF. There may be no clinical signs of low magnesium levels.
	Retention of Mg^{2+} in the oliguric state can cause high blood levels of magnesium. Anticipate muscle weakness or twitching and cardiac arrhythmias when accompanied by low levels of K^+ and Ca^{2+}.
Alterations in bicarbonate	Metabolic acidosis occurs with retention of sulfuric acid and phosphoric acid from protein metabolism. As failure progresses, acidosis is compounded by retention of hydrogen ions and decreased production of bicarbonate.
Elevations in BUN and creatinine levels (azotemia)	Urea nitrogen is excreted exclusively by the kidney. Elevations may be caused by renal dysfunction, higher levels of protein catabolism, GI bleed, or severe burn or even excessive protein intake. Creatinine, on the other hand, is exogenous in source. A muscle enzyme, it is excreted exclusively by the kidney. Creatinine provides an easy, first look at kidney function.
Alteration in urine studies	Decreased sodium output as indicated by a fractional excretion of sodium of less than 1 is indicative of prerenal failure and useful in determining need for fluid challenge. Cells, casts and crystals are indicative of intrarenal damage.

Adapted from Kieran, N., & Brady, H. (2003). Clinical evaluation, management, and outcome of acute renal failure. In R. Johnson & J. Feehally (Eds.), Comprehensive clinical nephrology *(2nd ed., pp. 183–206). St. Louis, MO: Mosby; Mount, D., & Zandi-Nejad, K. (2004). Disorders of potassium balance. In B. Brenner (Ed.),* Brenner and Rector's the kidney *(7th ed., vol. 1, pp. 997–1040). Philadelphia: W. B. Saunders Co.; Pollak, M., & Yu, A. (2004). Clinical disturbances of calcium, magnesium, and phosphate metabolism. In B. Brenner (Ed.),* Brenner and Rector's the kidney *(7th ed., vol. 1, pp. 1040–1076). Philadelphia: W. B. Saunders Co.*

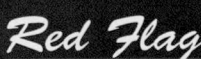

Red Flag

Hypokalemia in Renal Failure

Hypokalemia can occur in renal failure patients. The nurse must remember that hypokalemia can cause a cardiac arrest when: (a) the potassium level is less than 2.5 mEq/L, and (b) the patient is taking digitalis (an inotropic medication that strengthens the contraction of the myocardium and slows down the rate of the heart). Hypokalemia enhances the action of digitalis and therefore causes toxicity.

Red Flag

Geriatric Differences regarding Urinary Output

Older patients may have a larger amount of debris in their urine. Their urine or irrigant output must be monitoring closely for potential blockages or retention.

TABLE 54-3	Questions the Nurse Can Ask Patients Who Have Altered Patterns of Urinary Elimination Caused by Renal Dysfunction

Diurnal Voiding Habits

How long can you postpone urination?

Can you postpone urination for two hours?

Nocturia (awakening from sleep to urinate)

How many times do you wake up at night and urinate?

Does the urge to urinate interrupt your sleep?

Urinary Incontinence

Do you leak urine or lose bladder control?

Does this leakage cause any problems for you?

Urinary Retention

Do you feel you completely empty your bladder?

Have you ever been unable to urinate at all?

Do you strain to start your stream?

Does your stream start and stop?

- Monitor respiratory status; anticipate acute changes, particularly with fluid challenges or with acutely diminished urine output.
- Monitor blood chemistries and respond appropriately.
- Manage serum potassium: replacement in high output failure and restriction in low output failure. Hyperkalemia is considered a medical emergency when greater than 6.5 mmol/L (Kieran & Brady, 2003). Treatment of hyperkalemia is outlined in Box 54-3.
- Maintain blood pressure control. Hypertension: During periods of reduced tubular filtration, renin is likely secreted and the angiotensin system activated with resulting increase in blood pressure. Nursing plays an important role in maximizing recovery from ARF. Timely administration of as needed antihypertensive medications has the potential to prevent tubular necrosis or its advance.
- Maintain blood pressure control. Hypotension. In the acute setting, it is important to maintain renal perfusion. Low dose (1 to 3 mcg/kg/min) dopamine has been utilized in oliguric ARF.

Evidence-Based Care

Dopamine is the immediate precursor of norepinephrine. Low-dose dopamine has been used to increase renal perfusion by stimulating dopamine receptors by infusing a dose intended to prevent stimulation of related alpha and beta receptors (Pierce, Morris, & Clancy, 2002). Commonly referred to as renal dose dopamine, research has challenged its use in the critically patient. Tachycardia, increase in cardiac index, respiratory drive suppression, and pulmonary arteriovenous shunting have been observed in the critically ill patient (Kieran & Brady, 2003). In addition, renal dose dopamine has not been shown effective in preventing ischemic acute tubular necrosis.

The challenge to nursing is significant. Dopamine at renal doses continues in use. Many institutions have approved its use outside of the critical care units. Nurse-patient ratios in noncritical care settings range four to six or more

---

BOX 54-3

MANAGEMENT OF HYPERKALEMIA

Emergent: Regular insulin 10 units and 50 mL of 50% Dextrose intravenously; Insulin provides active transport to shift potassium from the bloodstream into the intracellular compartment. Glucose is required to prevent hypoglycemia. Frequent monitoring of blood sugar is required. Insulin and glucose are given consecutively and in the same time frame. This is a stabilizing measure only. It will usually be followed by dialysis or an exchange resin, removal of potassium from IV fluids and dietary restriction.

Sodium bicarbonate 50 mmol is given over five minutes in cases of acidosis. The addition of bicarbonate to the insulin-glucose regimen prevents continued potassium efflux from the cell in acidosis. This is a temporary measure. The acidosis must be corrected and is often accomplished by diuretic or dialysis correction of hypervolemia.

Cardiac protective: Calcium gluconate or calcium chloride (10 mL of 10% solution intravenously over five minutes) to antagonize the cardiac effect of hyperkalemia.

Intermediate: Exchange resin such as sodium polystyrene sulfonate (Kayexalate). 15 to 30 grams in 50 to 100 mL of 20% sorbitol. The exchange resin exchanges sodium ions for potassium ions in the gut. Sorbitol provides catharsis to remove the potassium complex from the gut. This is appropriate in non–life-threatening hyperkalemia. Loose bowel movements following administration and lowered serum potassium levels are indicative of successful treatment.

Maintenance: Potassium dietary restriction of 2 g/day.

Adapted from Kieran, N., & Brady, H. (2003). Clinical evaluation, management, and outcome of acute renal failure. In R. Johnson & J. Feehally (Eds.), Comprehensive clinical nephrology (2nd ed., pp. 183–206). St. Louis, MO: Mosby.

---

patients per nurse. Close observation of the respiratory, cardiovascular, and urinary systems of these ill patients need be taken seriously. Patient advocacy is critical at the sign of toxicity.

Nutrition

Dietary management in ARF requires the nurse, dietitian, and health care provider to put forth a concerted effort. Nutritional goals include preventing exacerbation of azotemia and maintaining mineral and electrolyte balance. The nutritional care for ARF involve caloric intake adequate to prevent protein catabolism and starvation ketoacidosis; protein intake restriction, except in highly catabolic patients of 0.8 to 1 g/kg/day, and phosphate restriction, as appropriate. This may require limiting dairy foods though a reduced protein diet provides phosphate restriction. In addition, there should be potassium restriction in patients at risk for hyperkalemia at 2 g/day.

Patients should be taught to avoid the following foods that are high in potassium: fresh fruits and vegetables, particularly citrus, tomatoes, and potatoes; reduce the potassium content of potatoes by boiling and replacing water during the cooking process; dried fruits and vegetables, legumes and nuts; chocolate; and protein-rich foods.

Uncovering the Evidence

ARF in Varying Regions of the World

Discussion: Although ARF is believed to be common in the setting of critical illness and is associated with a high risk of death, little is known about its epidemiology and outcome or how these vary in different regions of the world. This study's objective was to determine the prevalence, differences in etiology, illness severity, and clinical practices associated with ARF in intensive care unit (ICU) patients in multiple countries.

A prospective observational study of ICU patients who either were treated with renal replacement therapy (RRT) or fulfilled at least one of the predefined criteria for ARF from September 2000 to December 2001 at 54 hospitals in 23 countries. The main outcome measures were the occurrence of ARF, factors contributing to etiology, illness severity, treatment, need for renal support after hospital discharge, and hospital mortality.

Implications for Practice: Of 29,269 critically ill patients admitted during the study period, 1,738 had ARF during their ICU stay, including 1,260 who were treated with RRT. The most common contributing factor to ARF was septic shock (47.5 percent). Approximately 30 percent of patients had preadmission renal dysfunction. The overall hospital mortality was 60.3 percent, and dialysis dependence at hospital discharge was 13.8 percent for survivors. In conclusion, in this multinational study, the period prevalence of ARF requiring RRT in the ICU was between 5 and 6 percent and was associated with a high hospital mortality rate.

Source: Shigehiko, U., Kellum, J., Bellomo, R., Doig, G., Morimatsu, H., Morgera, S., et al. (2005). Acute renal failure in critically ill patients. JAMA, 294(7), 813–818.

Population-Based Care

The elderly are a particularly vulnerable population. Reduced glomerular capacity along with preexisting cardiac and respiratory illness makes them an easy target for ARF. Incontinence and altered mental states make early detection a challenge.

Surgery

Surgery or other invasive procedure may be implicated for the patient in ARF. Procedures include:

- Angioplasty or renal artery bypass surgery for renal artery stenosis or renal vein thrombosis.
- Ureteral stents placed by cystoscopy for obstructive conditions involving the ureters.
- Percutaneous nephrostomy tubes for obstructive conditions that will not allow ureteral stent passage. Nephrostomy tube is the treatment of choice in the obstructed patient who has hyperkalemia or sepsis (Mellon, 2003).

Patient and Family Teaching

The patient and family will have a totally new and frightening illness experience when they develop any level of renal failure. Language and tests compounded by the effects of the illness will present a confusing situation. They may need ongoing education relative to the disease process, medications inclusive of over-the-counter medication use, and nutrition.

Evaluation of Outcomes

Potential patient outcomes for each of the example nursing diagnoses for the patient with ARF are:

- Risk for imbalance in fluid volume. The patient's fluid balance is evidenced by 24-hour intake and output are balanced, orthostatic hypotension not present, normal skin turgor with moist mucous membranes, and urine-specific gravity is normal.
- Impaired tissue integrity related to alterations in internal regulatory function. The patient will improve the condition of their impaired tissue integrity as evidenced by decreased redness, swelling, and pain.
- Risk for infection related to invasive lines and altered immune response secondary to ARF and uremic toxins. The patient remains free of infection, as evidenced by normal vital signs and absence of purulent drainage from wounds, incisions, and tubes. Infection is recognized early to allow for prompt treatment.
- Anxiety related to sudden change in health status. The patient should be able to recognize the signs of anxiety, demonstrate positive coping mechanisms, and describe a reduction in the level of anxiety experienced.
- Knowledge deficit related to disease process and related diagnostic studies. The patient explains disease state, recognized need for medications, and understands treatments.

CHRONIC RENAL FAILURE

Chronic renal failure (CRF) is a progressive and irreversible decline in renal function ranging from mild with nearly normal function to ESRD requiring renal replacement therapy. The kidney disease quality initiative have classified chronic kidney disease into five stages based on glomerular filtration rate (GFR) (Table 54-4) (Nahas, 2003).

Epidemiology

CRF is a worldwide health problem. The incidence in the United States in 2000 was 252 new patients per million with a prevalence of 1,624 patients per million (Nahas, 2003). The incidence of CRF is higher in African Caribbeans, Native Americans, and Asian (Americans) and increases with aging in all populations (Winearls, 2003).

TABLE 54-4	**Stages of Chronic Kidney Disease**	
STAGE	**DESCRIPTION**	**GFR (ML/MIN/1.73M^2)**
1	Kidney damage with normal or increased GFR	Greater than or equal to 90
2	Kidney damage with mildly decreased GFR	60–89
3	Moderately decreased GFR	30–59
4	Severely decreased GFR	15–29
5	Kidney failure	Less than 15 (or dialysis)

Etiology

Diabetes mellitus and hypertension are the two most common causes of CRF in the United States. All conditions causing ARF discussed in this chapter may cause progression to CRF.

Modifiable risk factors deserve discussion. Proteinuria has been shown to exacerbate progression to CRF. Dietary modification and angiotensin-converting enzyme (ACE) inhibitors have been shown to reduce the level of proteinuria. Hypertension is less damaging to patients with proteinuria when kept at or below 125/75. Hyperglycemia is a major cause of CRF, and hyperlipidemia has been shown to hasten the progression to ESRD (Nahas, 2003). All modifiable risk factors can be better controlled by the patient and health care providers alike (Box 54-4).

Pathophysiology

The common underlying cause of progression to CRF is glomerulosclerosis (Nahas, 2003). Regardless of the initial insult, glomerulosclerosis is the end result. As the level of glomerular function declines, need for intervention increases. Failure of the kidney to maintain homeostasis has significant health implications. Cardiovascular disease is the major cause of death in the patient with ESRD.

Assessment with Clinical Manifestations

Clinical manifestations are many and varied as shown in Table 54-5.

Diagnostic Tests

There are many diagnostic tests used to determine the presence and severity of chronic kidney failure. The blood chemistries performed are: a complete blood count for general CRF, a urinalysis for cellular debris, sediment, casts, and elevated white blood cell count; and a twenty-four-hour urine collection for creatinine clearance to determine GFR. A CXR can be performed to view pulmonary status relative to fluid overload or to confirm dialysis catheter placement; and an electrocardiograph can determine the presence of severe hyperkalemia. In addition, studies relative to underlying pathologies or complications of CRF can be done.

Nursing Diagnoses

Based on the information gathered, examples of nursing diagnoses in the patient with CRF may include the following:
- Anxiety related to major health, lifestyle, role, and financial income changes
- Injury, potential for, related to alteration in homeostatic mechanism
- Imbalanced nutrition, less than body requirements, related to anorexia, nausea, vomiting, altered taste sensation, and dietary intake
- Excess fluid volume related to inability of the kidneys to excrete excess fluid, excessive daily intake, or inadequate dialysis
- Potential for injury related to phosphate clearance by pharmacological binding in the gut and highly dependent on dispensing promptly at mealtime
- Disturbed body image related to visible dialysis access, edema, and skin changes
- Readiness for enhanced family coping related to managing chronic illness and potential role changes

TABLE 54-5 Clinical Manifestations of Chronic Kidney Failure

SYSTEM	MANIFESTATION
Cardiovascular	Volume overload, hypertension, anemia-related increased cardiac output with left ventricular dysfunction, and dyslipidemia
Endocrine	Anemia secondary to decreased secretion of erythropoietin in low oxygen states. Decreased production of 1,25-dihydroxyvitamin D (calcitriol).
Skeletal	Renal bone disease related to high levels of phosphorus competing with calcium and to the kidney's decreased production of 1,25-dihydroxyvitamin D (calcitriol) and increased levels of parathyroid hormone (PTH).
Dermatological	Dry scaly skin with brown pigmentation with brownish discoloration of the nails. Pruritus is a consequence of hyperphosphatemia and thought also to be caused by histamine release.
GI	Occult blood loss, anorexia, nausea, and vomiting. Constipation is common and secondary to dietary restrictions, fluid restrictions, decreased mobility, and phosphate binders.
Hematological disturbances	Metabolic acidosis, hyperkalemia, hyponatremia secondary to dilution, hypermagnesemia, hypocalcemia, and hyperphosphatemia
Genitourinary	Hormonal changes lead to sexual dysfunction in males and infertility in females
	Menses range from severe and erratic to amenorrhea
Neurological	Uremic encephalopathy manifested as cognitive impairment in its mildest form and ranging to uremic coma
	Myoclonus (restless legs) ranging to uncontrollable twitching
	Mixed sensorimotor polyneuropathy in ESRD manifested primarily as a prickly, burning sensation
	Autonomic neuropathy causing diminished cardiovascular reflexes causing dialysis fluid removal-related hypotension
Immunological	Immunosuppression with increased risk of infection, the second cause of death in ESRD
Psychological	Anxiety and depression related to disease process, lack of knowledge, changes in lifestyle, sexual dysfunction, rising health care costs, or loss of income

Adapted from Gonzales, E., & Martin, K. (2003). Bone and mineral metabolism in chronic renal failure. In R. Johnson & J. Feehally (Eds.), Comprehensive clinical nephrology (2nd ed., pp. 873–885). St. Louis, MO: Mosby; Winearls, C. (2003). Clinical evaluation and manifestations of chronic renal failure. In R. Johnson & J. Feehally (Eds.), Comprehensive clinical nephrology (2nd ed., pp. 857–871). St. Louis, MO: Mosby.

Planning and Implementation

There are many varieties of nursing strategies for the care of patients with CRF. Providing care often involves a tremendous level of complexity for these patients. In addition, many of the problems associated with CRF are similar to ARF and have been previously discussed.

In general, the patient with CRF has three options: (a) dialysis, (b) renal transplantation, and (c) do nothing. If the patient chooses either dialysis or renal transplant, they will have implications associated with chronic care for the rest of their life. If the patient chooses to do nothing, then he or she will die from renal failure (see Ethics in Practice). The nurse must be aware that death from uremia is peaceful and should be painless. Priority is to ensure that the patient and family or significant others are comfortable with the decision (Winearls, 2003). Remember that the whole family is involved in this process. Offer consideration of their needs. Encourage breaks from the bedside vigilance while respecting the needs to be present.

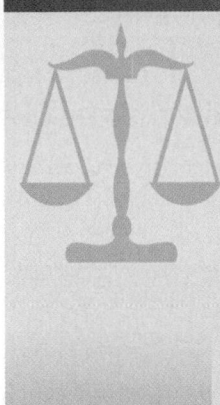

ETHICS IN PRACTICE

Patient Refuses Treatment for CRF

Probably one of the most challenging times will be allowing the patient to refuse life-dependent dialysis treatments or to cease dialysis treatments with the certain outcome of death. Refusing treatment may leave the care provider with the uncertain feeling that the patient had not really tried the therapy or that it had not been well enough explained.

The patient is told that he or she can try therapy, and it will be stopped if not acceptable. This is stressful for the patient and the care provider. If the decision is made in a depressed state, the health care provider will most likely ask for a mental health consult to establish decision reliability.

As the patient progresses into uremic coma, any stressful symptoms can be controlled. Management issues and treatment of choice include:

- Nausea and decreased appetite. Antiemetic and allow the patient to eat small, frequent meals in preference to large, regular meals. Offer snacks as visiting family members change shifts.
- Dry, crusty mouth with uremic fetor. Cleanse frequently with refreshing, mild mouth rinse.
- Twitching or clonic jerks. Benzodiazepines, such as clonazepam (Winearls, 2003).
- Breathing difficulties from pulmonary edema and acidosis. Morphine sulfate infusion.
- Supportive care to the family.

Goals

The overall goals of therapy for CRF are to halt progression to a higher level of dysfunction and to prevent or minimize complications.

Evidence-Based Care

Evidence-based care demonstrates that early intervention is critical to arresting progression in renal failure and in minimizing complications. Cardiovascular and skeletal diseases are particularly vulnerable to pathology with late intervention (Winearls, 2003). Late referral to the nephrology team places the patient at greater health risk.

Collaborative Management

CRF demands the highest level of collaborative management (Box 54-5). Competent patient self-management is pivotal in optimizing health at all stages of CRF. This is best accomplished by promoting self-efficacy (Thomas-Hawkins & Zazworsky, 2005). A concerted team effort to promote skill building and peer group modeling and support while practicing positive attitude interpreting symptoms and demonstrating a can-do attitude is essential to building patient self-efficacy.

Pharmacology

There are many medications used in the management of CRF. Examples of these medications are provided in Box 54-6.

Fast Forward ▶▶▶

ABG Monitoring

There are monitoring system for ABGs that can give a continuous ABG recording. As these machines become less expensive and more available, the many acid-base imbalances associated with kidney failure (e.g., metabolic acidosis) may be more specifically monitored. The continuous digital readout of ABGs allows the nurse in the patient with CRF to more accurately note the current status of the patient with these conditions.

BOX 54-5

NIC CARE AND CRF

NIC: Facilitate communication of concerns or feelings between patient and family or between family members.

NIC: Maintain fluid balance utilizing fluid restriction, diuretics, or dialysis.

NIC: Weight will remain within 2 to 3 kg of dry weight. Dry weight is evidenced by:

- No evidence of elevated venous jugular pressure, edema, or other signs of fluid overload.
- A predialysis blood pressure of less than 140/90.
- Low susceptibility to hypotension and cramping during the dialysis treatment.

NIC: Maintain electrolyte and mineral balance utilizing dietary restriction, phosphate binders, pharmacological therapy or dialysis.

NIC: Provide adequate nutrition. Consult with dietitian, and together provide dietary education.

NIC: Manage anemia with recombinant erythropoietin and blood transfusions, as appropriate.

NIC: Manage hyperglycemia, as necessary to maintain optimal glycemic control.

NIC: Maintain patent and infection-free dialysis access and prevent infection; maintain integrity of dialysis access.

Adapted from Farrington, K., Greenwood, R., & Ahmad, S. (2003). Hemodialysis: Mechanisms, outcome, and adequacy. In R. Johnson & J. Feehally (Eds.), Comprehensive clinical nephrology *(2nd ed., pp. 975–990). St. Louis, MO: Mosby.*

BOX 54-6

PHARMACOLOGICAL THERAPY IN CRF

- Phosphate binders (to be taken with each meal) (e.g., calcium carbonate (TUMS), calcium acetate (PhosLo), sevelamer HCl (Renagel)
- Recombinant erythropoietin (Epogen or Procrit) for CRF-related anemia. Dose adjusted for target hematocrit
- 1,25 Dihydroxyvitamin D_3 (e.g., Calcitriol, Rocaltrol)
- Water-soluble replacement because of dialysis loss: includes folate, vitamins C and B (e.g., Berocca and Nephrocap)
- Avoid magnesium-containing antacids and cathartics
- Opioids: Monitor closely for respiratory depression and adjust dose and interval, as appropriate
- Drug dose or interval adjustment is necessary for most drugs dependent on renal clearance
- Schedule daily drugs for after dialysis to prevent dialysis loss. Alternatively, check with a pharmacist for information on drugs used during dialysis.

Hemodialysis

Hemodialysis (HD) is the mainstay of RRT. The patient's blood is pumped through semipermeable capillaries in a hemodialyzer. Dialysate fluid containing a premixed concentrate of electrolytes flows countercurrent to blood flow through the intercapillary spaces of the dialyzer. Solute clearance is directly related to concentration gradient and flow rate. Prescribed fluid removal is facilitated by transmembrane pressure and the ultrafiltration capacity of the hemodialyzer. Typical HD treatment duration is three to four hours on a three times weekly schedule. Outpatients are assigned a regular time for their HD procedure at an outpatient facility (usually three times a week) or taught to do HD in their home with a dedicated partner (Figures 54-5 and 54-6).

Disequilibrium syndrome is a preventable complication of initial dialysis on a uremic patient. **Disequilibrium** refers to an imbalance in solute concentration across the blood-brain barrier. Rapid reduction in intravascular solutes can precipitate rapid fluid osmosis across the blood-brain barrier with net flow of water into the cerebrospinal space in a homeostatic attempt to equalize solute concentration. The resulting increased intracranial pressure may be evidenced by headache, nausea, vomiting, muscle twitching, and seizure. Daily initial treatments for the disequilibrium syndrome utilizing reduced dialysis blood flow rates and shorter treatment time with gradual increase of flow rate and treatment time over a few days maintains equilibrium safety.

Dialysis Vascular Access

To perform HD, there is a need to access both the arterial and venous circulation of the patient. Therefore, a temporary dialysis vascular access is achieved by insertion of a dual lumen dialysis catheter. Dialysis catheters are placed in a femoral, subclavian, or jugular vein. Insertion of a noncuffed catheter is the first choice for acute dialysis as it is easily accomplished at the bedside. Complications include subclavian stenosis, pneumothorax, venous rupture with hemorrhage, and infection. Imposed bedrest and higher infection rates are the primary disadvantage of femoral catheters (Conlon & Giblin, 2003).

Dual lumen, cuffed dialysis catheters are placed surgically for longer term use. Primary use is providing vascular access for short-term dialysis in recovering ARF or in CRF when vascular access for arteriovenous fistula (AVF) has been exhausted by complications. The dialysis catheter should be reserved for

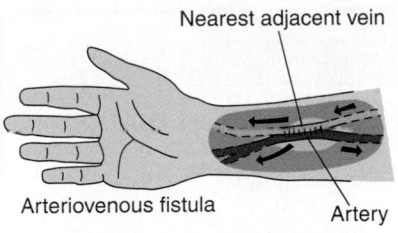

Nearest adjacent vein

Arteriovenous fistula   Artery

Edges of incision in artery and vein are
sutured together to form a common opening.

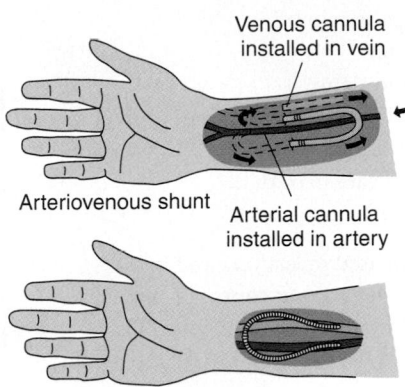

Venous cannula
installed in vein

Arteriovenous shunt   Arterial cannula
installed in artery

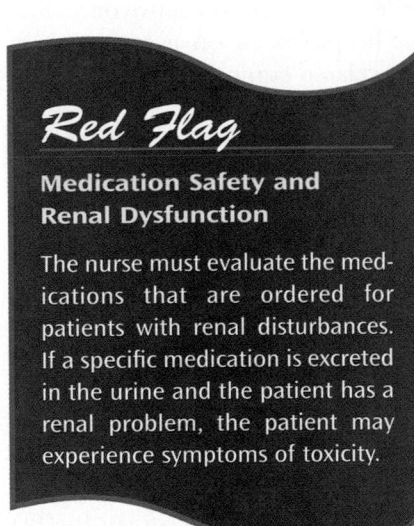

Arteriovenous vein graft

Ends of natural or synthetic graft sutured
into an artery and a vein.

Figure 54-5 HD access sites.

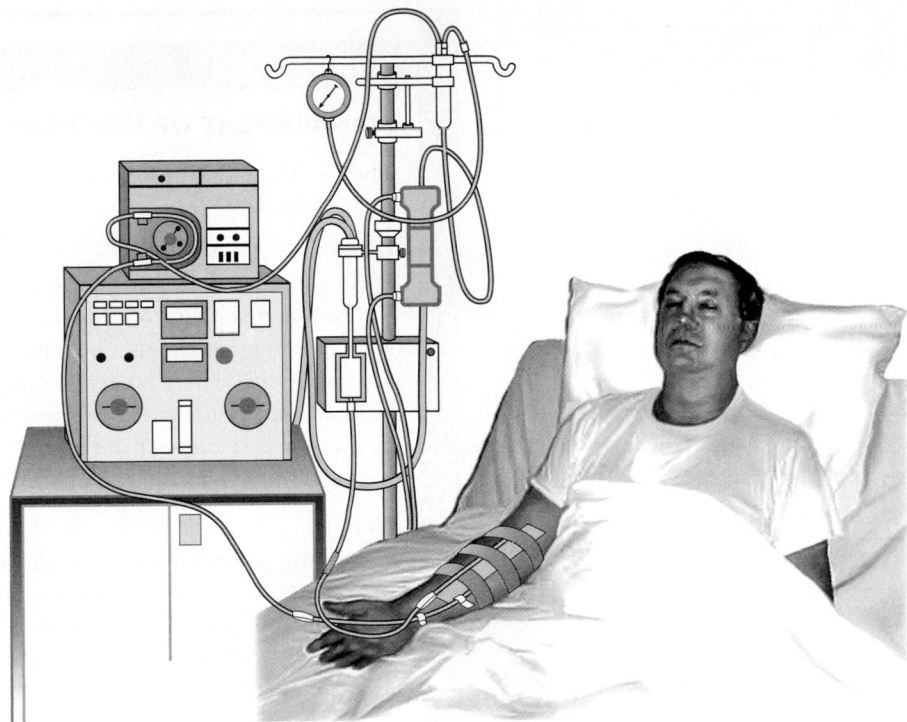

Figure 54-6 HD.

dialysis use only as it is the patient's lifeline. Meticulous care aimed at preventing dislodgement or infection is imperative (Box 54-7).

AVF is preferable for permanent dialysis vascular access. The AVF may be
created by direct anastomosis of an artery to a vein (natural or native fistula).
More commonly, a polytetrafluoroethylene (PTFE) graft is employed to create a fistula between an artery and a vein. Comprising 80 percent of the AVF
in use in the United States, PTFE grafts are advantageous in patients with
poor-quality blood vessels (Conlon & Giblin, 2003). An AVF is preferably
placed in the nondominant lower arm. Other sites include the dominant
lower arm, upper arms, and upper anterior thighs.

Complications from AVF include graft thrombosis, failure to mature
enough to allow adequate blood flow (native), infection, and arterial steal syndrome. Steal syndrome occurs with disruption of adequate blood flow to the
distal region of the extremity. Early intervention is imperative to prevent loss
of hand function. Steal syndrome is evidenced by pain, coolness, and paresthesias. Symptoms may exacerbate during the dialysis treatment. Banding to
diminish volume of blood flow diverted from the hand or ligation may be
required to preserve hand function (Conlon & Giblin, 2003).

Peritoneal Dialysis and Chronic Ambulatory Peritoneal Dialysis

Peritoneal dialysis (PD) is being used by more than 120,000 patients worldwide
(Davies & Williams, 2003). The capillaries of the peritoneal membrane allow
solute clearance down a concentration gradient between the instilled dialysate
and the plasma. Fluid removal is by osmotic gradient with dialysate dextrose
concentration providing the higher osmotic pressure. Capillary pore size will
allow some protein loss but is not large enough to allow phosphate clearance.
Phosphate binding is required.

Insertion of a Dacron cuffed, tunneled Silastic PD catheter affords easy
access. The catheter is allowed to rest for tunnel healing for approximately
one month prior to use. Meticulous exit site care according to local practice
protocols is imperative. Tunnel integrity is maintained by taping the catheter

---

BOX 54-7

MANAGEMENT OF VASCULAR ACCESS DEVICES IN DIALYSIS

The nurse should do the following when caring for patients with vascular assessment care:

Dialysis Catheter

- Maintain sterile dressing according to institution protocol.
- Confirm that caps are secure and clamps are closed.
- Prevent tugging or pulling on the catheter.
- Provide or promote meticulous patient hygiene.
- Teach patient to handle unexpected catheter dislodgement. Apply direct pressure over catheter site to control bleeding. When bleeding has ceased, cover with dry dressing and notify health care provider.

AVF

- Confirm patency; presence of thrill (palpated pulsation) and bruit (whooshing sound heard with a stethoscope) along course of the AVF.
- Nephrology precautions to prevent thrombosis and infection. This includes no blood pressure measurement, IV accesses, or laboratory blood draws on affected extremity.
- Teach patient to avoid constrictive clothing and to check fistula patency daily. Report absence of thrill or bruit promptly.
- Teach patient to handle posttreatment bleeding at cannula site: apply direct pressure for several minutes to control bleeding, apply dry dressing, and call health care provider as appropriate.

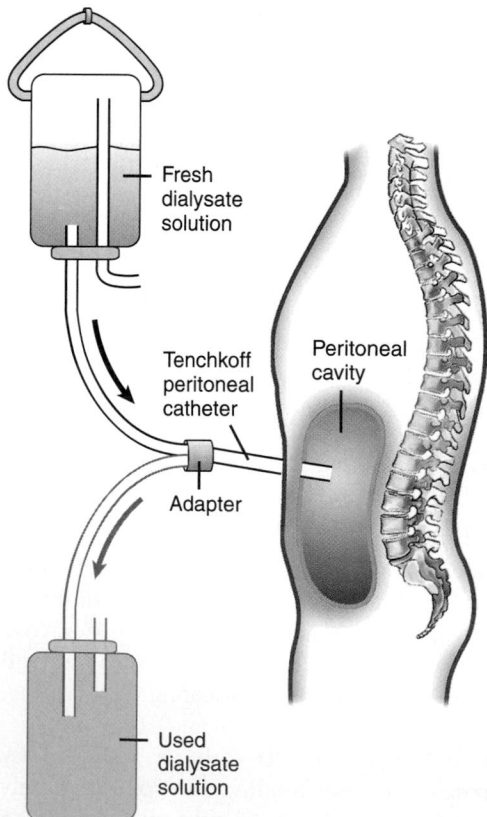

Figure 54-7 PD.

securely to the abdomen to prevent pull at the exit site. Tunnel integrity is vital to prevention of tunnel site infection and PD catheter loss. It is imperative that strict sterile technique and environmental control of circulating contaminants be practiced on every occasion when the catheter is uncapped or any related equipment is exposed to the air.

PD requires filling the peritoneal cavity with a prescribed volume of peritoneal dialysate, allowing it to dwell for a prescribed period of time then draining and discarding the **effluent** (waste materials). Continuous ambulatory peritoneal dialysis (CAPD) requires manual dialysate instillation and removal on a predetermined schedule. Continuous cyclic peritoneal dialysis is delivered by a computerized cycler. The dialysis cycler is programmed for length of therapy and desired fill volumes. The computer tracks volumes filled and drained for accurate ultrafiltration information. CAPD is usually a nighttime procedure allowing the patient to sleep through the process. CAPD requires manual fills and drains. Determining ultrafiltration volume requires weighing effluent bags.

Advantages to PD include portability (patient can perform the PD relatively easily at home or when traveling), higher level of self-efficacy and independence, daily maintenance dialysis with constant lower levels of azotemia, and moderation in dietary and fluid restrictions (Figure 54-7). Disadvantages include protein loss and potential for life-threatening peritoneal infection

Complications include changes in peritoneal vascular and interstitial structure and function, peritonitis, tunnel and exit site infection, fluid leaks, catheter malfunction, and ultrafiltration failure. While any has

---

BOX 54-8

ANTIBIOTIC THERAPY FOR PD

Antibiotic treatment of peritonitis for the patient on PD according to the Advisory Committee on Peritonitis Management of the International Society of Peritoneal Dialysis:

- Initial empirical therapy with first generation cephalosporin (cefazolin, or cephalothin). Loading dose in first bag and maintenance dose in each following bag of PD dialysate.
- Negative culture: continue cephalosporin for two weeks.

Once an organism is identified, the regimen is altered accordingly.

Adapted from Davies, S., & Williams, J. (2003). Peritoneal dialysis: Principles, techniques, and adequacy. In R. Johnson & J. Feehally (Eds.), Comprehensive clinical nephrology (2nd ed., pp. 1003–1011). St. Louis, MO: Mosby.

---

the potential for major disruption in health practices, peritonitis is probably the most important complication and cause of treatment failure (Davies & Williams, 2003). Cloudy effluent and abdominal pain are the sentinel signs of developing peritonitis and require immediate intervention. Immediate effluent sample collection for WBC count and microbiology is imperative. Empirical, intraperitoneal antibiotic treatment is usually initiated prior to culture return (Box 54-8).

Nutrition

Dietary management is crucial to minimizing disease progression and azotemia, preventing malnutrition, and preventing complications of hyperkalemia and hyperphosphatemia. The National Kidney Foundation's Kidney Disease Outcomes Quality Initiative (K/DOQI) guidelines herald nutrition as a primary determinant in ESRD patient outcomes.

Nurses have a major role in preventing malnutrition in this patient population (Wells, 2003). Assessment must include appetite, weight change, decreased muscle mass, and decreased strength and endurance are all markers of malnutrition. Positive findings coupled with a serum albumin less than 4 should prompt intervention from the health care team.

PD patients require greater amounts of protein related to protein and amino acid loss in the dialysis exchange process. In addition, daily dialysis with PD results in less electrolyte and mineral restrictions. HD patients experience some amino acid loss and may have increased catabolism. Daily dietary management includes:

- Protein intake: HD, 1.2 g/kg/day with 50 percent of high biological value; PD, 1.2 to 1.3 g/kg/day with 50 percent biological value and increases to 1.5 g/kg/day with malnutrition or peritonitis (Wells, 2003).
- Sodium is restricted in ESRD to minimize thirst. Daily recommendations are: HD, 1,000 to 3,000 mg/day; PD 2,000 to 4,000 mg/day.
- Potassium: HD, 40 to 70 mEq/day; PD 75 to 100 mEq/day.
- Phosphate: HD and PD, less than 17 mg/kg/day.
- Fluid intake: HD, 1,000 mL/day plus volume to replace any urinary output. The goal is to limit weight gain between dialysis treatments to 2 to 5 percent of the established dry weight (Wells, 2003).

Renal Transplantation

Transplantation can be both a blessing and a challenge. The health care professional experiences the excitement of successful graft function and is subjected to the trauma of graft loss or immunosuppressive complications. The recipient hopes for release from the constraints of chronic illness and resumption of a fuller life. They hope for the best and brace themselves to accept all the adverse potentials for which they have been informed.

Transplantation is not an automatic choice. Though 70 has been considered maximal age for eligibility, a good state of health will make the patient a reasonable candidate to consider (Hostima & Hilbrands, 2003). Recurrent and persistent noncompliance, acute or chronic infection, malignancy, substance abuse, unstable psychosis that would impair consent and compliance, ABO incompatibility, and a positive cross-match will render the patient ineligible for transplantation (Hostima & Hilbrands, 2003).

Patients with diabetic nephropathy and in reasonable health are prime candidates for a kidney transplant and may be considered for a pancreas or kidney transplant. It has been shown that patients with diabetic **nephropathy** (disease of the kidneys) have a better quality of life and longer term survival following transplantation (Hostima & Hilbrands, 2003).

Pretransplantation counseling and testing are completed before the patient is placed on the transplant list as eligible for a cadaver kidney (graft) or a living donor graft. The recipient undergoes extensive testing to deem them a safe immunosuppression candidate.

Transplant immunology has made successful allogeneic transplantation possible. A basic understanding of terminology and immune response facilitates appreciation and more active participation in the care of the transplant patient. **Allogeneic** signifies a genetic relationship between two individuals of the same species. An allogeneic organ is referred to as an **allograft. Xenogeneic** signifies a genetic relationship between individuals of differing species. Of interest, organ shortage is prompting research in xenogeneic transplantation.

Cell surface molecules vary in structure from individual to individual. It is this polymorphic (antigenic) phenomenon that lies at the root of the immune response to the allograft. Major histocompatibility complex (MHC), so named for the chromosomal region where encoded, evokes the most powerful rejection response. MHC in combination with the antigen presenting cell (APC) of the graft attracts cytotoxic T cells. Without intervention, this would result in graft cell death. Interestingly, graft MHC together with the presenting antigen mimics the intended receptor for the T cell and sets up a cascade of events resulting in full-scale T cell activation.

T cells are lymphocytes that mature in the thymus, thus the name T cell. T cells are divided into two classes according to their activity. CD4 T cells are classified as cytolytic. Their primary action is to kill the target cell. CD4 T cells are classified as helper cells with two primary helper activities. They stimulate B cell growth and differentiation for antibody production (humoral immunity) and secrete cytokines for phagocyte activation (Abbas & Lichtman, 2004). Cytokine release is inclusive of interleukins and tissue necrosis factor (TNF). Normally, CD4 T cells account for 50 to 60 percent, and CD8 T cells account for 20 to 25 percent of the total lymphocyte count. Significantly, each has CD3, CD4, and CD8 coreceptors on the cell surface. The CD3 coreceptor activates multiple enzymes, including calcineurin, when stimulated by the cytoplasmic tail of the other two receptors. Calcineurin is a significant target of immunosuppression.

Adhesion molecules provide another mechanism of rejection. Cells from lymphoid organs infiltrate the graft. These cells adhere to vascular endothelium and cause cytokine release (Abbas & Lichtman, 2004). Interference with this activity is another target of transplant immunosuppression.

Agents of immunosuppression and their targets are:

- Glucocorticoids: Block cytokines and migration of phagocytes indirectly block T cell activation.
- Azathioprine: Blocks DNA to prevent lymphocyte proliferation following antigenic stimulation.

- Mycophenolate: Selective inhibition of T and B lymphocyte proliferation.
- Cyclosporine: Inhibits calcineurin, blocks interleukins and TNF.
- Tacrolimus (FK506): Inhibits calcineurin and T cell activation.
- Rapamycin (Sirolimus): Inhibits T cell activation.

Cross-match and tissue typing by blood sample are utilized to align recipient with a histocompatible organ. Two primary considerations are ABO blood group antigens and human leukocyte antigens (HLA) molecules. Of the blood group type, antigen findings infer the following compatibility profile. Group A and B develop antigens to each other and to Group O; incompatible. Group O does not develop antigens against A or B, compatible donor. The rhesus Rh factor is not a concern in cross-match for organ transplantation. There is hesitation in using Group O organs for Group A or B recipients as this would diminish the organ pool for Group O recipients in this time of organ shortage.

HLA, also called MCH antigens, are found on the short arm of chromosome 6. Each set of alleles on the chromosome is called a haplotype and given a numerical designation (Abbas & Lichtman, 2004). HLA-A, HLA-B, and HLA-DR are primary concerns in organ transplantation.

Living donors include living related (biological and nonbiological), living nonrelated, paired kidney exchange, and nondirected live donation (McKay & King, 2004). The paired kidney exchange program allows willing and incompatible living donors assist the intended recipient to obtain a kidney. When two recipients have willing unmatched donors matching the opposite recipient, they may swap donors (Fisher, Kropp, & Fleming, 2005). Because of advances in immunology and continued organ shortage, live donation has increased significantly (Box 54-9).

Most often, donor nephrectomy can be accomplished by laparoscopic surgery. An approximate 2 to 3 inch incision in the lower quadrant suffices for delivering the kidney. Postoperative care follows routine postoperative guidelines. Hospital stay is minimal.

Cadaver acquired kidneys must evidence no damage by clinical testing and by history. Complete donor screening includes viral screening for all groups of hepatitis virus herpes viruses, human T cell lymphotropic virus type 1, and human immunodeficiency virus (HIV). In addition, Centers for Disease Control and Prevention (CDC) guidelines are followed to screen the donor for history of high-risk HIV behavior. Blood, urine, and sputum cultures are obtained as well as a screen for malignancy (McKay & King, 2004).

The transplanted kidney is placed in either the left or right lower abdominal quadrant anterior to the peritoneal space. The transplanted ureter is secured to the bladder wall by a technique designed to prevent urinary reflux. A urinary catheter is left in place for up to five days to allow ureteral implant healing without bladder filling. A ureteral stent may be in place if there is concern for swelling or stricture at the site of ureteral implant.

The graft may have immediate and excellent urinary output beginning in the operating room at the time of vascular anastomosis or function may be delayed for an extensive period (Figure 54-8). Ischemic acute tubular necrosis is the most common cause of delayed graft function (Magee & Milford, 2004). Managing fluid and electrolyte balance is a priority. The nurse must anticipate renal ultrasound for graft blood flow studies, graft biopsy for rejection studies, and supportive dialysis as a form of treatment (Box 54-10).

Complications include rejection, vascular thrombosis, and ureteral anastomosis failure. Renal artery thrombosis presents as an acute cessation of urine output and rapid increase in creatinine. Renal vein thrombosis may have the additional sign of sudden acute abdominal pain. The usual consequence is graft loss (Magee & Milford, 2004). Rejection presents with continuous rise in creatinine and biopsy finding of cellular or vascular changes consistent with rejection. Ureteral anastomosis failure will present

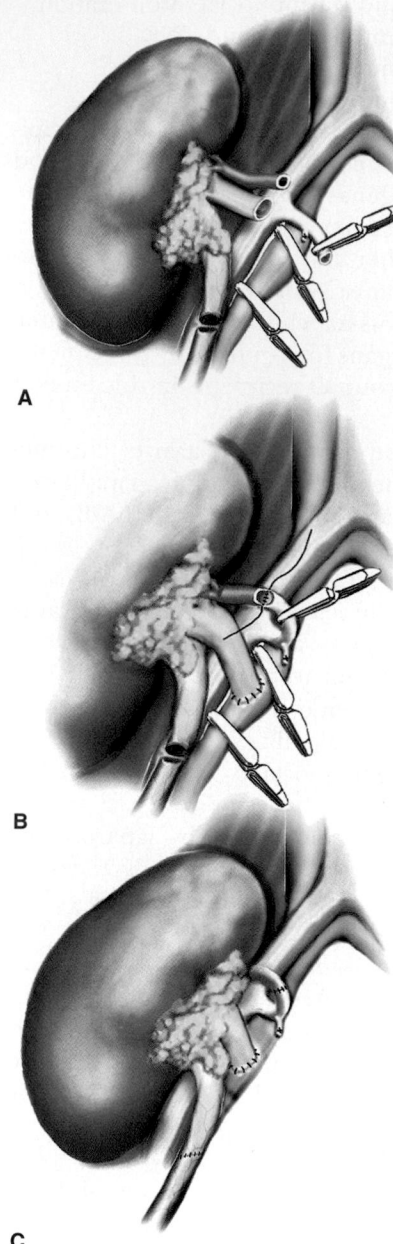

A

B

C

Figure 54-8 Renal transplantation (adult recipient): A. Iliac vessels exposed, B. Renal artery and vein anastomosis, C. Donor kidney in place.

> ## BOX 54-10
>
> ### NURSING MANAGEMENT FOR A RENAL TRANSPLANT
>
> The nurse must perform the following as part of the nursing management of a patient experiencing a renal transplant:
> - Maintain fluid balance by closely monitoring urinary output and providing expedient replacement.
> - Monitor laboratory studies for graft function and electrolyte balance.
> - Monitor for abrupt decrease in urine output or abruptly increased pain or swelling at graft site as this may be indicative of renal vascular thrombosis or acute rejection.
> - Monitor wound drainage for any signs of ureteral anastomosis failure.
> - Adhere to immunosuppression schedule and facilitate accurate timing of phlebotomy blood drawing of samples for related drug levels.
> - Monitor blood glucose and anticipate changes related to high-dose glucocorticoids.
> - Arrange for supply of medications prior to discharge to prevent any disruption in immunosuppression.
> - Teach patient medication management, follow-up protocols, signs of transplant rejection or infection and appropriate response, importance of adequate hydration, and infection prevention.
> - Offer patient support during periods of delayed graft function or graft failure.
> - Arrange postdischarge follow-up appointments.

with **perinephric** (surrounding the kidney) graft fluid collection, increased wound drainage, or rise in creatinine. Wound sample creatinine level compared to serum creatinine is the primary diagnostic tool for ureteral anastomosis failure.

There are many medications necessary for the patient following a renal transplant. In addition, there are important considerations for the patient as he or she receives his or her medications. And, there are a wide variety of side effects to consider when the patient is given these medications. Table 54-6 enumerates a number of the typical medications given to patients as they live after having a renal transplant.

Health Care Resources

There are three valuable resources for patients, families, and health care professionals. They provide up-to-date and reliable information on the latest research, understanding diseases process, and progression and state-of-the-art patient self-management.

The National Kidney Disease Education Program (NKDEP) is an initiative of the National Institute of Diabetes and Digestive and Kidney Diseases (NIDDK), National Institutes of Health (NIH), U.S. Department of Health and Human Services (DHHS). Life options is designed to help people live long and live well with kidney disease. A multidisciplinary national health care team reviews all materials presented through Life options.

Evaluation of Outcomes

Potential patient outcomes for each of the example nursing diagnoses for the patient with CRF are:
- Anxiety related to major health, lifestyle, role, and financial income changes. The patient should be able to recognize the signs of anxiety,

TABLE 54-6 Drug Therapy for Patients after a Renal Transplant

IMMUNOSUPPRESSIVE AGENTS	IMPORTANT CONSIDERATIONS	SIDE EFFECTS
Corticosteroids: IV: Methylprednisolone Oral: Prednisolone or prednisone	Be alert to tapering doses	Cataracts, infection, osteoporosis, and avascular necrosis of the head of the femur
Calcineurin inhibitors Cyclosporin (Neoral) Tacrolimus (FK506, Prograf)	Schedule phlebotomy to facilitate accurate serum level samples	Diabetes mellitus, hypertension, hyperlipidemia, nephrotoxicity, seizures and thrombocytopenia, hemolytic uremic syndrome, and gingival hyperplasia
Sirolimus (Rapamune)	Adhere strictly to 12-hour dosing	Lymphoma, malignancy, lymphocele, thrombocytopenia, and leukopenia
Azathioprine (Imuran and AZA San)	Adhere strictly to 12-hour dosing Encourage use of sun block	Bone marrow suppression, leukopenia, thrombocytopenia, and anemia; increased risk of malignancy, hepatotoxicity, and hair loss
Mycophenolate mofetil (CellCept)	Adhere strictly to 12-hour dosing	Diarrhea, increased cytomegalovirus (CMV) infection, leukopenia, and mild anemia
Thymoglobulin	Premedicate with acetaminophen, Benadryl, and corticosteroids to minimize or prevent flulike response	Thrombocytopenia, neutropenia, secondary infection, secondary malignancy, lymphoproliferative disorders, and sepsis
OKT3	Premedicate as per thymoglobulin	Pulmonary edema and acute renal failure

demonstrate positive coping mechanisms, and describe a reduction in the level of anxiety experienced.

- Injury, potential for, related to alteration in homeostatic mechanism. The patient does not experience any skin breakdown from uremia or falls from fatigue.
- Imbalanced nutrition, less than body requirements, related to anorexia, nausea, vomiting, altered taste sensation, and dietary intake. The patient verbalizes and demonstrates selection of foods or meals that will achieve a cessation of weight loss and weighs within 10 percent of ideal body weight.
- Excess fluid volume related to inability of the kidneys to excrete excess fluid, excessive daily intake, or inadequate dialysis. The patient maintains fluid balance as evidenced by skin turgor, blood pressure and weight within designated limits.
- Disturbed body image related to visible dialysis access, edema, and skin changes. The patient demonstrates enhanced body image and self-esteem as evidenced by ability to look at, touch, talk about, and care for actual or perceived altered body part or function.
- Readiness for enhanced family coping related to managing chronic illness and potential role changes. The patient and family identify own maladaptive coping behaviors, available resources, and support systems, describes or initiates alternative coping strategies, and describes positive results from new behaviors.

Financial Outcomes

CRF can be financially devastating. Many people are unable to continue employment because of work time lost to dialysis, reduced energy levels, and depression. Social work involvement is crucial. Assistance with travel arrangements to dialysis facilities, disability assistance applications, and interpretation of insurance coverage are critical at this time. Counseling is primary to facilitate adjustment to the overwhelming demands and limitations of chronic illness and family adjustment to role change.

KEY CONCEPTS

- Pyelonephritis is an infection of the upper urinary tract and may involve the ureters, renal pelvis, and the papillary tips of the collecting ducts.
- Polycystic kidney disease is a genetically inherited kidney disease and may be autosomal dominant (ADPKD) or autosomal recessive (ARPKD).
- ARF presents as a rapid decline in renal function, and this decline may occur within a few hours or over a period of several weeks.

- CRF is a progressive and irreversible decline in renal function ranging from mild with nearly normal function to ESRD requiring RRT.
- Diabetes mellitus and hypertension are the two most common causes of CRF. in the United States.
- It has been shown that patients with diabetic nephropathy (disease of the kidneys) have a better quality of life and longer term survival following transplantation.

REVIEW QUESTIONS

1. A 21-year-old woman is admitted to the hospital with a diagnosis of acute renal failure. She is oliguric and has proteinuria. She asks the nurse, "How long will it be before I start to make urine again?" Which of the following would be the correct response?
   1. This phase of renal failure will last for one to two days.
   2. This phase of renal failure will last for three to seven days.
   3. This phase of renal failure will last for one to two weeks.
   4. This phase of renal failure will last for three to four weeks.

2. You are caring for a patient who is admitted to the hospital in acute renal failure. The appearance of a U wave on the electrocardiogram (ECG) should alert you to check for which of the following laboratory values?

   1. Hyperkalemia
   2. Hypokalemia
   3. Hypernatremia
   4. Hyponatremia

3. You are caring for a man who is on hemodialysis. He has an AVF. Which of the following is expected when assessing the fistula?
   1. Ecchymotic area
   2. Enlarged veins
   3. Pulselessness
   4. Redness

4. A male patient with end-stage renal disease receives HD three times a week. You conclude that dialysis is effective when:
   1. The patient does not have a large weight gain.
   2. The patient has no signs and symptoms of infection.
   3. The patient says that he can catch up on his rest while on dialysis.
   4. The patient is able to return to work.

Continued

5. You are performing discharge teaching for a patient who was admitted with pyelonephritis. The patient asks the nurse, "What is pyelonephritis?" Based on your knowledge of pyelonephritis, your best response would be:
   1. Pyelonephritis is an inflammation of the bladder.
   2. Pyelonephritis is a rupture of the bladder.
   3. Pyelonephritis is an infection of the kidney.
   4. Pyelonephritis is an infection of the lower urinary tract.

6. A patient is admitted to your care with ARF. Which of the following must you continually assess for?
   1. Hyponatremia and hyperkalemia
   2. Decreased BUN and creatinine
   3. Alkalosis
   4. Hypercalcemia

7. A patient with CRF complains of irritating white crystals on his skin. You recognize this finding as uremic frost. Which of the following nursing actions do you take?
   1. Administer an antihistamine, because the physician would prescribe one to relieve itching
   2. Increase fluids to prevent crystal formation and decrease itching
   3. Provide skin care with tepid water and apply lotion to the skin to relieve itching
   4. Permit the patient to soak in a bathtub to remove crystals

8. Immediately following a kidney transplant, you should assess your patient for which of the following?
   1. Fluid and electrolyte imbalance
   2. Infection
   3. Hepatotoxicity
   4. Respiratory complications

9. You are caring for a patient receiving PD. You are completing the exchange by draining the dialysate. You notice it is cloudy. How do you interpret this finding?
   1. It is the normal appearance of draining dialysate.
   2. It is a sign of infection.
   3. It is an indication of an impending lower back problem.
   4. It is a sign of a vascular access occlusion.

10. You are providing patient education to a patient on CAPD. You determine that he understands is treatment when he states:
   1. I must increase my carbohydrate intake daily.
   2. I must maintain a positive nitrogen balance by decreasing protein.
   3. I must take prophylactic antibiotics to prevent infection.
   4. I must be aware of the signs and symptoms of peritonitis.

1. Describe the clinical manifestations seen in acute pyelonephritis?

2. Compare and contrast autosomal dominant (ADPKD) and autosomal recessive polycystic kidney disease (ARPKD)?

Continued

REVIEW ACTIVITIES—cont'd

3. Describe the assessment findings that may be present in Wegener granulomatosis.

5. Compare and contrast HD and CAPD.

4. What are reasons that patients with rhabdomyolysis have safety issues?

6. What would you teach a donor regarding his or her giving up a kidney in a renal transplantation?

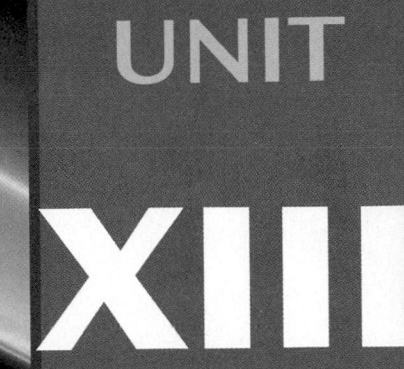

Alterations in Endocrine Function

Assessment of Endocrine Function

Martha K. Carlson, MSN

CHAPTER TOPICS

- Anatomy and Physiology of the Endocrine system

- Hormones

- Assessment of the Endocrine System

- Diagnostic Tests for the Endocrine System

The endocrine system, in conjunction with the nervous system, is responsible for the control of multiple body systems. It can be thought of as a communication system that uses hormones to help maintain homeostasis. **Hormones** are chemical messengers produced and secreted by specialized endocrine cells and released into the bloodstream to act on target cells at another location in the body. Hormones help to maintain homeostasis by regulation of metabolism and energy, cardiac output and blood pressure, reproduction, and growth and development. The hormones of the endocrine system are affected by the central nervous system (CNS); more specifically, the hypothalamus, and in turn, these hormones affect the nervous system. The hypothalamus coordinates the activity of the endocrine system through the pituitary gland using releasing hormones. Simply stated, the hypothalamus translates messages from the nervous system into chemical messengers, hormones. Hormones affect the nervous system in a variety of complex mechanisms. For example, a deficiency of thyroid hormone may result in emotional depression, and adrenaline causes increased mental activity. Hormones affect the nervous system by enhancing the rapid transmission of signals between neurons from localized synapses. The hormones cause fast outcomes and occur quickly. In contrast the endocrine system uses more generalized signals that require less energy than the synapses of the nervous system. The signals from the hormones travel by the blood stream to the specific target organs. These effects of the hormones are slower and of a longer duration than the nervous system's transmission of signals. Another system that interacts closely with the endocrine system is the immune system. Hormones secreted from the adrenal cortex regulate the immune system responses. Hormones are vital in regulating the body's internal environment.

Hormones exert their effects on target organs or tissues. A feedback system is commonly found in the endocrine system. The feedback can be direct or indirect. The most common type of feedback is negative or inhibitory, preventing excessive hormone secretion. A thermostat on a furnace controls the heat in the house by negative feedback. When the internal temperature of the house drops below a set point, the thermostat signals the furnace to turn on and produce heat. As the temperature of the house rises to a preset level, the thermostat signals the furnace to shut off. An example of negative feedback in the body is the secretion of insulin in response to rising blood glucose levels. When blood glucose levels in the body rise, **insulin,** the hormone produced by the beta cells of the pancreas to lower blood glucose, is secreted. Insulin acts on the cells, causing them to take up the excess glucose in the bloodstream. The blood glucose level then falls and insulin secretion stops. Some of the negative feedback occurring in the endocrine system is much more complex than this example, involving stimulation of more than one gland (Griffin & Ojeda, 2004).

ANATOMY AND PHYSIOLOGY

The endocrine system is comprised of the pituitary, hypothalamus, thyroid, parathyroids, pancreas, adrenals, thymus, ovaries, and testes. The endocrine system is not easily assessed as compared with other body systems. When discussing endocrine system imbalances, there are often increased or decreased variations (e.g., hyperthyroidism versus hypothyroidism).

Glands

Glands in the body are classified as endocrine or exocrine. **Exocrine glands** are those glands that secrete substances into ducts that empty into a body cavity or onto a body surface. Sweat glands and lacrimal glands (tear ducts) are examples of exocrine glands. **Endocrine glands** are those glands that produce hormones, which are secreted into the blood stream and travel to their target organs or tissues (Figure 55-1). **Target tissues** are tissues or organs in the body that are affected by specific hormones. The thyroid, parathyroid, pituitary, and adrenals are examples of endocrine glands. The pancreas is both an endocrine and an exocrine gland. Insulin and glucagon production is an endocrine function while digestive enzymes from the pancreas make up its exocrine function (Tierney, Mc Phee, & Papakakais, 2004).

Hormones

Hormones are chemicals that are produced and secreted by specific tissues or organs in the body. They travel via the bloodstream to the target organ, where they bind to specific receptors on the cell membrane or in the cell. Hormones change the metabolism of the target cells by either altering the cell membrane permeability to nutrients or by alteration of the synthesis or activation of hormones. Hormones may be either water or lipid soluble based on their chemical structure. They may stimulate an organ to release a hormone, to act, or both. Additionally, hormones can inhibit the release of other hormones and do so in a variety of locations throughout the body (Table 55-1). The pituitary produces the stimulating hormones called follicle-stimulating hormone (FSH). The hypothalamus stimulates the releasing hormones. These hormones then can change the behavior of other organs or tissues. Lipid soluble hormones (steroid and thyroid) are able to pass through cell membranes of the target organs. Hormones that are protein based are not able to pass through the cell membranes. They bind to receptors on specific cells and trigger actions with in the cell (Tierney, et al., 2004).

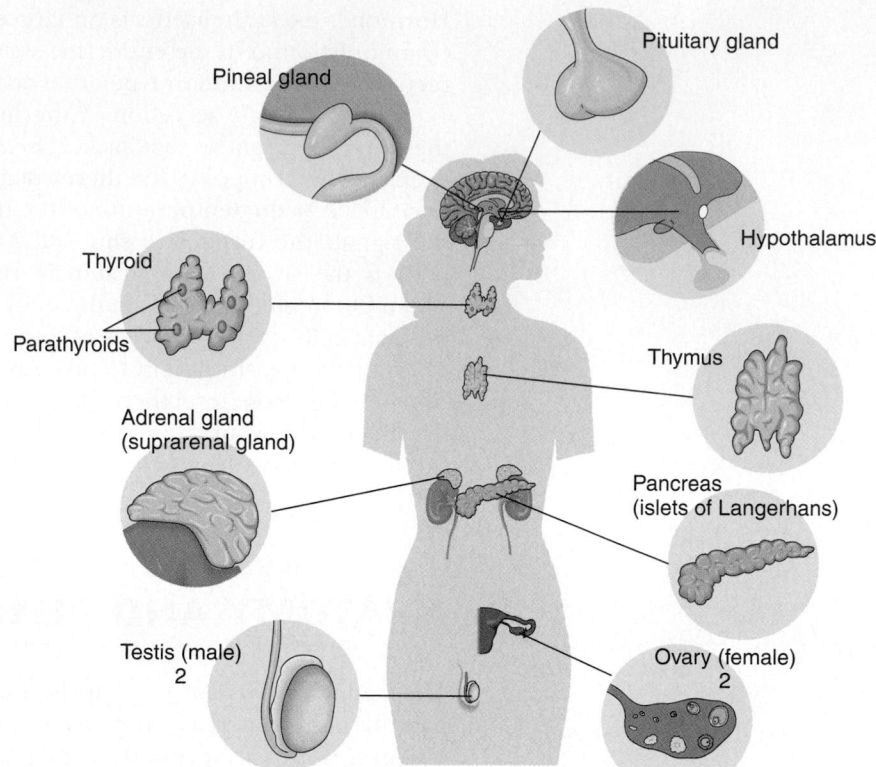

Figure 55-1 Structures of the endocrine system.

Regulation of Hormones

There are several complex mechanisms for controlling hormone levels. These body system controls are interrelated and actually are occurring simultaneously as homeostatic balances to the body system.

Negative Feedback Mechanisms

The pituitary gland and feedback mechanisms are responsible for controlling hormone levels. The majority of the feedback mechanisms are **negative feedback** (the response of a gland by increasing or decreasing the secretion of a hormone) or inhibitory, similar to a thermostat in the house. The endocrine system contains sensors that detect and alter hormone secretion to maintain balance in the body's internal environment. When the sensors detect low hormone levels, they stimulate actions that will result in an increase in hormones. Conversely, when the sensors detect elevated hormone levels, they cause a decrease in the production and release of hormones. Insulin secretion by the pancreas related to the blood glucose level is an example of negative feedback. The pancreas produces insulin when the blood glucose level rises. As the blood glucose level decreases from the insulin, the pancreas decreases the production of insulin (Greenspan & Gardner, 2004).

Positive Feedback Mechanisms

Positive feedback mechanisms occur when increasing the level of one hormone produces an increase in the level of another hormone. For example, during the follicular stage in the female menstrual cycle there is an increase in the production of estradiol. This increase in estradiol causes an increase in the production of FSH by the anterior pituitary.

Nervous System Controls

The nervous system also controls endocrine function through the CNS and the sympathetic nervous system (SNS). When stress is experienced by the body, it is detected by the CNS. The SNS then releases catecholamines that cause the

TABLE 55-1 Endocrine Gland Hormones

HORMONE	FUNCTION
Pancreas	
Glucagon	Raises blood glucose
Insulin	Lowers blood glucose
Somatostatin	Inhibits secretion of insulin, glucagon, and growth hormone from the anterior pituitary and gastrin from the stomach
Anterior Pituitary	
Thyroid-stimulating hormone (TSH)	Stimulates thyroid growth and secretion of the thyroid hormone
Adrenocorticotropic hormone (ACTH)	Stimulates adrenal cortex growth and secretion of glucocorticoids
Follicle-stimulating hormone (FSH)	Stimulates ovarian follicle to mature and produce estrogen; in the male, stimulates sperm production
Luteinizing hormone (LH)	Acts with FSH to stimulate estrogen production; causes ovulation; stimulates progesterone production by corpus luteum; in male, stimulates testes to produce testosterone
Melanocyte-stimulating hormone (MSH)	Causes increase in synthesis and spread of melanin (pigment) in skin
Growth hormone (GH)	Stimulates growth
Prolacting or lactogenic hormone	Stimulates breast development during pregnancy and milk secretion after delivery of baby
Posterior Pituitary	
Antidiuretic hormone (ADH)	Stimulates water retention by kidneys to decrease urine secretion
Oxytocin	Stimulates uterine contractions; causes breast to release milk into ducts
Thyroid Gland	
Thyroid hormone (thyroxine T_4 and triiodothyronine T_3)	Increases metabolic rate
Calcitonin	Decreases blood calcium concentration
Parathyroid Gland	
Parathyroid hormone	Increases blood calcium concentration
Adrenal Cortex	
Glucocorticoids (cortisol, hydrocortisone)	Stimulates gluconeogenesis and increases blood glucose; antiinflammatory; antiimmunity; antiallergy
Mineralocorticoids	Regulates electrolyte and fluid homeostasis
Sex hormones (androgen)	Stimulate sexual drive in females; in males, negligible effect
Adrenal Medulla	
Epinephrine (adrenalin)	Prolongs and intensifies sympathetic nervous response to stress
Norepinephrine	Prolongs and intensifies sympathetic nervous response to stress

blood pressure and heart rate to increase in an attempt to assist the body to deal with the stress more effectively. In addition, various rhythms from the brain affect the release of hormones. The circadian rhythm is an example of a 24-hour rhythm while the menstrual cycle is an example of the ultradiam rhythm, which is of longer duration.

Hypothalamus Gland

The hypothalamus can be considered the major regulating organ of the body, as it is the connection between the nervous system and the endocrine system. Input from the circulatory system and the nervous system give information to the hypothalamus about the homeostasis of the body. The hypothalamus, located centrally in the brain, secretes hormones that release or inhibit secretion of hormones from the anterior pituitary gland. The hormones from the hypothalamus are secreted in a circadian rhythmic pattern, and do not directly affect the peripheral endocrine tissues. The amount of hormones secreted by the hypothalamus is small. The hypothalamus contains neurons that produce hormones called antidiuretic hormone and oxytocin that are stored in the posterior pituitary. These neurons in the hypothalamus also interact with the brainstem, spinal cord, and limbic system.

Pituitary Gland

The pituitary gland, or hypophysis, is a small gland located under the hypothalamus in the sella turcica at the base of the brain (Figure 55-2). The pituitary gland is often labeled the master gland, because it directly or indirectly stimulates the release of a variety of hormones. It is connected to the hypothalamus by the hypophyseal stalk and is made up of two parts, the anterior stalk, the adenohypophysis, and the posterior stalk, the neurohypophysis. Hormones from the pituitary do act on the peripheral endocrine tissues. Patients with tumors of the pituitary often present with visual disturbances because of the location of the gland within the cranial vault. The pituitary response to the stimulus of the hypothalamus remains relatively constant throughout the life span with the exceptions of puberty, ovulation, and aging.

Anterior Pituitary Gland

The anterior pituitary gland is controlled by the hypothalamus and is the largest lobe of the gland (Figure 55-3). It produces more hormones than the posterior pituitary, several of which are called tropic hormones. Tropic hormones regulate the secretion of hormones by other glands. **Adrenocorticotropic hormone (ACTH)** from the anterior pituitary stimulates the secretion of corticosteroids by the adrenal cortex. Other tropic hormones secreted by the anterior pituitary include **thyroid-stimulating hormone (TSH),** FSH, and luteinizing hormone (LH). **Growth hormone (GH)** is a hormone that affects all tissues of the body, is secreted from the anterior pituitary, and is one of the counter regulatory hormones. GH is also secreted by the anterior pituitary and affects the growth of the long bones and skeletal muscles. It also plays a role in the metabolism of fat, protein, and carbohydrates. **Prolactin** is a hormone from the anterior pituitary that stimulates the breast to cause lactation.

Posterior Pituitary Gland

The posterior pituitary gland can be thought of as an extension of the hypothalamus. It is made up of nerve tissue and communicates with the hypothalamus through the median eminence. **Antidiuretic hormone (ADH)** and oxytocin are produced in the posterior pituitary. ADH regulates the reabsorption of water in the kidneys thereby regulates fluid volume. ADH secretion is controlled by the osmolality of the circulating plasma. When the osmolality of the plasma increases, sensors located in the hypothalamus are activated and ADH is released. A drop in blood pressure, orthostatic hypotension, decreased circulating blood volume, nausea, vomiting, and pain, can also trigger ADH release. When fluid volume is increased, secretion of ADH decreases, the kidneys do not reabsorb water and more dilute urine is excreted.

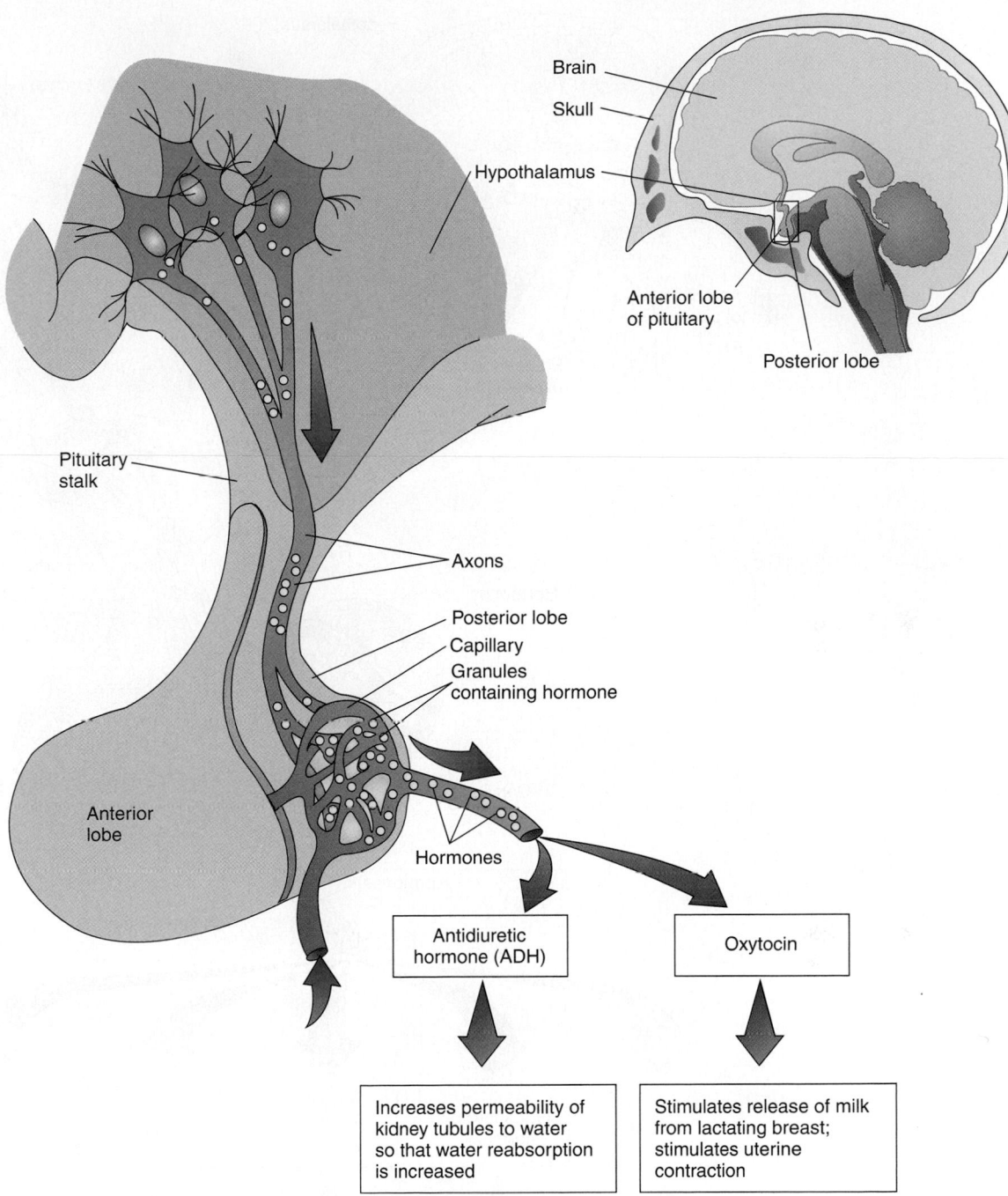

Figure 55-2 Pituitary gland.

Thyroid Gland

The thyroid gland is a vascular organ, consisting of two lobes connected by an isthmus (Figure 55-4). It is located in the anterior portion of the neck, anterior to the trachea. TSH from the anterior pituitary regulates the function of the thyroid. Hormones produced and secreted by the thyroid gland include thyroxine, triiodothyronine, and calcitonin. **Thyroxine (T_4)** is the most abundant thyroid hormone, and makes up approximately 90 percent of the thyroid hormone secretion. **Triiodothyronine (T_3)** is the most powerful thyroid hormone with 10 percent secreted by the thyroid and the remainder converted from T_4 by peripheral tissues. T_4 and T_3 are produced, stored, and released in the thyroid. A lesser amount of T_3 is produced, but it is a more potent hor-

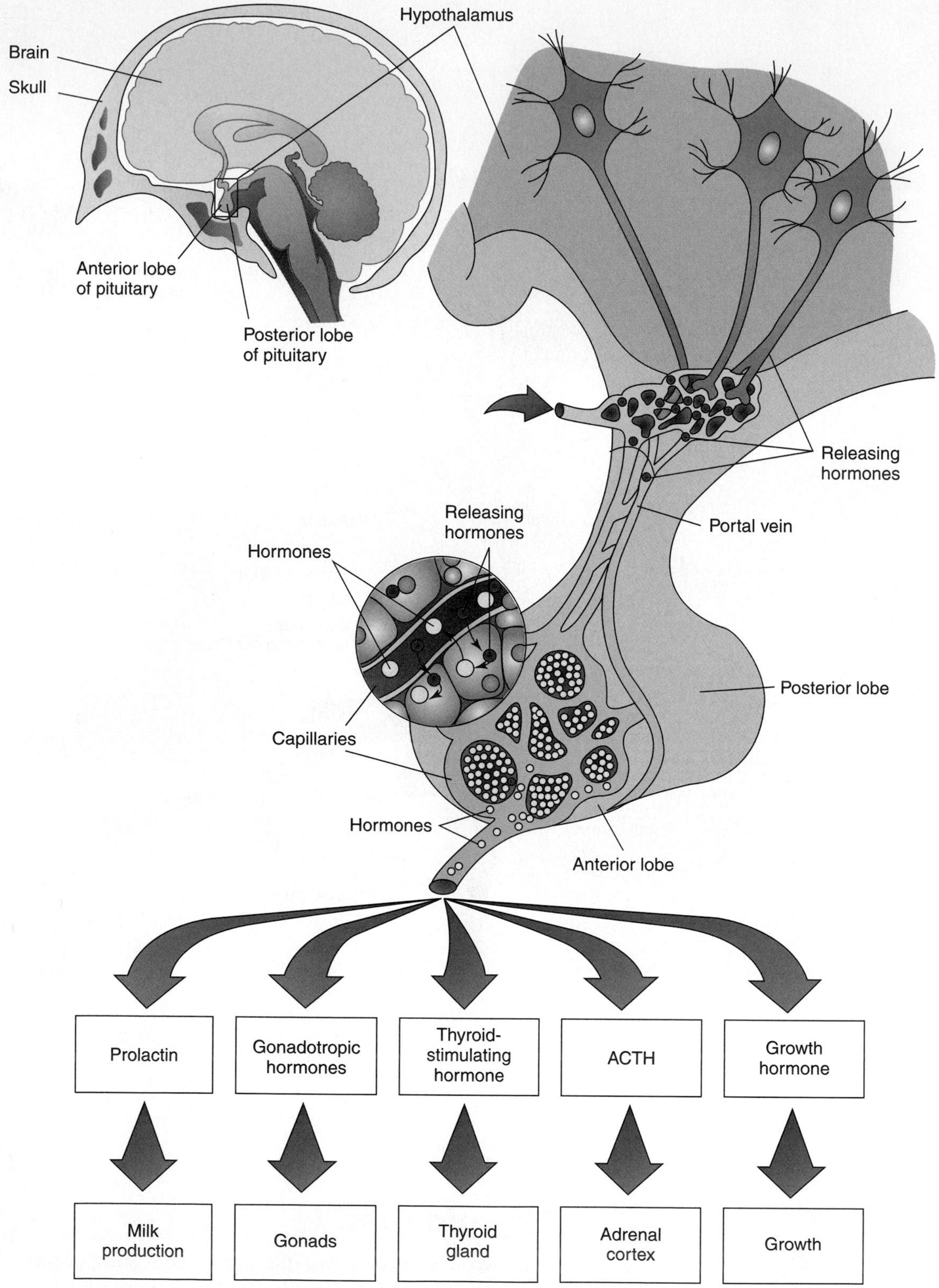

Brain

Skull

Hypothalamus

Anterior lobe
of pituitary

Posterior lobe
of pituitary

Releasing
hormones

Portal vein

Releasing
hormones

Hormones

Posterior lobe

Capillaries

Hormones

Anterior lobe

| Prolactin | Gonadotropic hormones | Thyroid-stimulating hormone | ACTH | Growth hormone |

| Milk production | Gonads | Thyroid gland | Adrenal cortex | Growth |

Figure 55-3 Anterior and posterior pituitary glands.

mone than T_4, having a greater effect on metabolism. Only about 10 percent of circulating T_3 is secreted by the thyroid gland. The remainder is converted from T_4. Synthesis of thyroid hormones requires the presence of iodine. T_3 and T_4 are lipid soluble and directly enter the cell. They affect the metabolism of lipids, metabolic rate, oxygen consumption, caloric requirements, nervous system activity, growth and development, and functions of the brain. Approximately 99 percent of the thyroid hormones are bound to plasma pro-

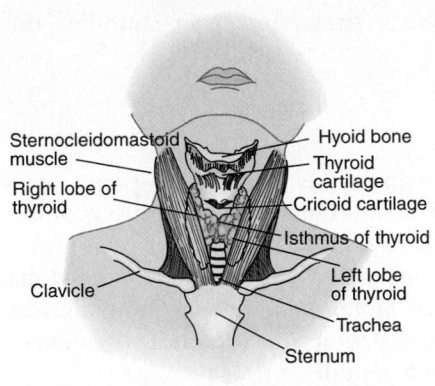

Figure 55-4 Structures of the thyroid gland.

teins. It is only the unbound or free hormones that are active and circulate within the body system (Liebert, 2003a).

Production and secretion of thyroid hormones is controlled by TSH from the anterior pituitary. The hypothalamus releases **thyroid-releasing hormone (TRH)** when circulating levels of thyroid hormones are low. TRH is the hormone that stimulates the anterior pituitary to release TSH. If the levels of circulating thyroid hormone are high, the secretion of TRH and TSH will be inhibited (Liebert, 2003b). The rate of thyroxin exchange, or turnover, changes with age, being highest in infants and children. The turnover rate of T_4 will decline to adult levels at puberty and stabilize until age 60. After age 60 the rate declines again (Greenspan & Gardner, 2004).

Calcitonin is a hormone produced by the thyroid gland when the circulating levels of calcium are elevated. Calcitonin has an inhibitory affect on the reabsorption of calcium from the bone and increases the storage of calcium in the bone. Calcitonin lowers circulating levels of calcium by promoting the excretion of calcium and phosphate by the kidneys.

Parathyroid Glands

The parathyroid glands are small glands located behind the thyroid gland and usual occur in pairs. Commonly there are four parathyroid glands. Like the thyroid, the parathyroid glands are vascular. **Parathyroid hormone (PTH)** is secreted by the parathyroids, and its main function is the regulation of the blood level of calcium in the body. The secretion of PTH is controlled by a negative feedback mechanism. PTH is secreted when serum calcium levels are low, and it is inhibited when serum calcium levels increase. PTH acts on the bone to inhibit bone formation and stimulate bone resorption, releasing phosphate and calcium in the blood. PTH stimulates the excretion of phosphate and reabsorption of calcium by the kidneys (Griffin & Ojeda, 2004).

Adrenal Glands

The two adrenal glands are located on the upper portion of each kidney. They are small vascular glands made up of a medulla and cortex. The medulla and cortex of each adrenal gland have separate and distinct functions and play a major role in the body's ability to adapt to internal and external stress.

Adrenal Medulla

The catecholamines, epinephrine, norepinephrine, and dopamine are secreted by the adrenal medulla, with epinephrine being secreted in the largest amount. Epinephrine and norepinephrine are considered hormones when they are secreted by the adrenal medulla, but they are often classified as neurotransmitters. As hormones, they are secreted and released into the circulation and act on a target organ. They play a primary role in the body's response to stress.

Adrenal Cortex

The adrenal cortex is the largest part of the gland and makes up the outer portion. It secretes steroid hormones that are classified as glucocorticoid, mineralocorticoid, and androgens. In addition, **corticosteroids** are any of the hormones, except androgen, synthesized by the adrenal cortex. Glucocorticoids (cortisol) affect the metabolism of glucose, mineralocorticoids (e.g., **aldosterone,** which is a mineralocorticoid synthesized in the adrenal cortex that functions to maintain extracellular fluid volume) maintain fluid and electrolyte balance.

Cortisol is a major glucocorticoid that functions in the regulation of blood glucose levels. By facilitating hepatic gluconeogenesis, cortisol increases blood glucose levels.

Glucocorticoids are also anti-inflammatory and play a role in the body's response to stress. Cortisol secretion is controlled by a negative feedback mechanism and the secretion of cortisol-releasing hormone (CRH) from the hypothalamus. Hypoglycemia, surgery, burns, stress, and fever stimulate the secretion of cortisol.

Pancreas Gland

The pancreas is both an endocrine and exocrine gland. The pancreas is located behind the stomach. The islets of Langerhans are the portions of the pancreas that secrete hormones. These islets are made up of four types of cells: alpha, beta, delta, and F cells. Glucagon is produced and secreted by the alpha cells, and insulin is produced and secreted by the beta cells of the pancreas. The delta cells are responsible for the production and secretion of somatostatin and the F cells secrete pancreatic polypeptide.

Glucagon

Glucagon is a hormone released from the pancreas in response to low levels of blood glucose and is a counter-regulatory hormone. Glucagon stimulates glycogenolysis, gluconeogenesis, and ketogenesis to raise the blood sugar levels.

Insulin

Insulin is a hormone produced by the beta cells of the pancreas to lower blood glucose levels. Insulin regulates the metabolism and storage of carbohydrates, fats, and proteins. Without insulin, glucose is unable to enter the cells in most tissues. The exceptions are the brain, lens of the eye, nerves, kidney tubules, and intestinal mucosa. Insulin is secreted in response to elevated blood glucose and is inhibited by hypoglycemia, glucagon, hypokalemia, and catecholamines.

At the peripheral level, insulin acts to transport glucose into the cells and triglycerides into the adipose tissue. For this reason, insulin is often referred to as a storage hormone. Insulin acts on the liver to inhibit gluconeogenesis.

Effects of Aging on the Endocrine System

Aging affects several functions of the endocrine system. The thyroid gland becomes smaller with age, decreasing the basal metabolic rate. There is an increased production of ADH resulting in more dilute urine and polyuria. The pancreas secretes less insulin, and the cells become more resistant to insulin, leading to the development of diabetes and decreased glucose tolerance. Estrogen function decreases in women leading to osteoporosis (Greenspan & Gardner, 2004).

It can be a challenge for the nurse to assess for abnormal endocrine functioning because of the presence of chronic illnesses, changes in sleep patterns that occur with normal aging, or the use of multiple medications that may affect hormone functions. Regular screenings for glucose tolerance, thyroid functioning, and calcium levels should be encouraged in the aging population.

ASSESSMENT

Effects of the endocrine system can be found in nearly every body system. The nurse uses his or her understanding of pathophysiology as a guide for assessment of this system. Following are suggestions for areas to be covered in an assessment of the endocrine system.

Subjective Data

Inquire about the energy level of the patient as the endocrine system regulates metabolism and energy production. Questions about lethargy, fatigue, increased need for sleep, and performance of activities of daily living should be assessed. The nurse should assess sleep patterns and should inquire about sleep disturbances, such as frequent awakenings. Heat and cold intolerance should also be assessed. Childhood exposure to ionizing radiation is associated with an increased risk of thyroid diseases and thyroid cancer. Use of iodine in cough medications or contrast media may increase the occurrence of hypothyroidism, hyperthyroidism, or goiter (Tierney, et al., 2004). Family history should include information about presence of thyroid disease and goiter, thyroid cancer, and diabetes. In addition, exploring whether or not the patient has ever had a crisis condition associated with their endocrine disorder is important information to obtain. An example is seen in a patient with hyperthyroidism and the condition labeled thyroid crisis (see Red Flag feature). The nurse should gather specific information regarding when the thyroid crisis occurred, what the clinical manifestations were, and what types of treatment measures were employed.

Integumentary

Questions should include assessment of hair loss (alopecia), dry skin, coarse hair, brittle nails, or changes in pigmentation. The nurse should ask patients for their history of the conditions of each of these integumentary components.

Head and Face

Inquire about puffiness of the face or eyelids, changes in the appearance of the eyes, or increased redness of the eyes. The nurse should assess for changes in the voice or enlargement of the neck. In addition, the patient needs to be assessed for alterations in self-esteem from the abnormalities often associated with endocrine disorders.

Cardiovascular

Palpitations are common with alterations in endocrine functioning. The patient should be asked if they ever "feel" his or her heart beat and if there seems to be an increase in the strength of the heartbeat. Ask if the patient feels if he or she has enough energy to complete their tasks of daily living. Inquire about exercise habits, including frequency, duration, and types of exercise.

Gastrointestinal

Common alterations include changes in weight, either loss or gain. Polydipsia, polyphagia, and polyuria occur with diabetes. Patients may also experience dysphagia with alterations in the endocrine system so assess for changes in swallowing or chewing. Assess the patient's typical daily food intake, including meals, snack, and use of supplements or vitamins. Ask about daily fluid intake including types and amounts ingested. Inquire about changes in appetite or weight.

Changes in bowel habits, constipation, and diarrhea should be assessed. Determine the patient's usual bowel habits, character of stool, use of laxatives or aids, and discomfort.

Neurological

The nervous system is closely associated with the functioning of the endocrine system, and alterations in neurological functioning are common. Common findings include tremors, memory loss, jitteriness or nervousness, and decreased sensation in the hands and feet. Depression is a common finding in the elderly patient.

Assess the patient's sleep patterns. Ask about difficulty falling asleep, number of hours per night spent sleeping, and use of sleep aids. Inquire about number of times the patient awakens at night and difficulty getting back to sleep. Is the patient bothered by nightmares? Do they feel rested when they awaken in the morning?

Genitourinary

Changes in the menstrual pattern are common in alterations of the endocrine system. Amenorrhea (absence of menses), menorrhagia (prolonged or excessive menses), and oligomenorrhea (decrease in the frequency of menses) may occur. There may also be an increase in urination (polyuria). Inquire about urinary frequency, amount, color, clarity, and odor of urine.

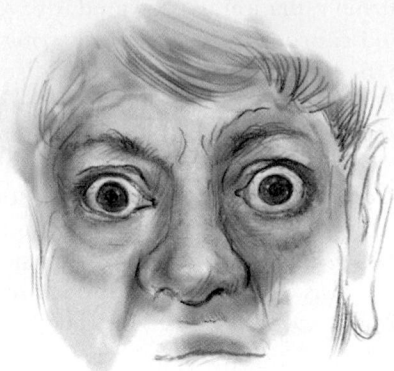

Figure 55-5 Exophthalmos of Graves' disease.

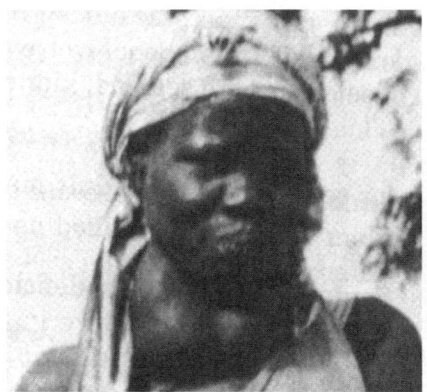

Figure 55-6 Goiter from iodine deficiency Courtesy of the Food and Agriculture Organization of the United Nations.

TABLE 55-2 Assessing the Endocrine System

SYSTEM	ASSESSMENTS
Integumentary	Skin is assessed for integrity, lesions, warmth, hair growth, pigmentation, color, and turgor.
	Hair is assessed for distribution, texture, quantity, and quality.
	Nails are assessed for color, thickness, growth, curvature, and clubbing.
Head and face	Assess the head and face for symmetry, exophthalmus, presence or absence of lid lag, periorbital, or facial edema.
Neck	Observe the neck for symmetry and position of the trachea (midline or deviated). Palpate the thyroid gland for size, symmetry, shape, consistency, and tenderness.
Heart	Inspect the anterior chest for heaves. Palpate the anterior chest for thrills and the apical impulse. Auscultate the heart sounds, noting rate, rhythm and presence of extra heart sounds.
Neurological	Assess for changes in mental status, especially in the elderly patient. Deep tendon reflexes should be assessed at the biceps, triceps, brachioradialis, patella, and Achilles tendons. Assess for presence or absence of ankle clonus. Vibratory sensation should be evaluated with a percussion hammer.

Adapted from Estes, M. (2006). Health assessment and physical examination (3rd ed.). New York: Thomson Delmar Learning.

Assess female patient's menstrual history, including age of menarche, menstrual pattern, pregnancy history, and use of contraceptives. Males and females should be assessed for interest in sexual activity or any noted changes.

Musculoskeletal

Muscle weakness and aching frequently occur and can have an impact on the patient's activities of daily living. Inquire about the patient's ability to perform the tasks of feeding, bathing, dressing, toileting, general mobility, shopping, cooking, and home maintenance tasks.

Objective Data

Vital signs, weight, nutritional status, apparent age as compared to chronological age, facial expression, and general appearance are important in the assessment of the endocrine system (Table 55-2). There are a wide variety of endocrine disturbances that exhibit themselves in identifiable appearances. For example, in hyperthyroidism, exophthalmos associated with Graves' disease causes the eyes to protrude in an obviously pathological manner (Figure 55-5). Another example is a goiter caused by hyperthyroidism as illustrated in Figure 55-6. In addition, inspection and palpation of the thyroid gland and the gonads are the two objective methods for assessing specific endocrine glands.

DIAGNOSTIC TESTS

Alterations in endocrine function are diagnosed by the use of blood and urine tests as well as radiological tests that may include computed tomography (CT) (Figure 55-7) and magnetic resonance imaging (MRI) (Table 55-3). Nursing interventions with diagnostic testing includes explanation of the procedure to the patient and significant others.

Respecting Our Differences

Assessment of Integument with Regard to Ethnic Differences

When assessing the integument of non-Caucasian patients who have endocrine disturbances, the nurse must remember the obvious differences. For example, the patient with Addison's disease (hypofunction of the Adrenal gland) in a Caucasian patient will have a bronze-colored skin. However, in an African American patient, the skin coloration related to pigmentation hormonal influences will not be as pronounced.

TABLE 55-3 Common Diagnostic Tests for Endocrine System Disorders

Pancreas Diagnostic Tests

Blood glucose, fasting blood sugar (FBS)

2-Hour postprandial glucose (2hPPG) or 2-hour post-prandial blood sugar (2hPPBS)

Glucose tolerance test (GTT)

Pituitary Gland Diagnostic Tests

Adrenocorticotropic hormone (ACTH), corticotropin

Antidiuretic hormone (ADH), vasopressin

Follicle-stimulating hormone (FSH)

Growth hormone (GH), human GH (HGH), somatotropin hormone (SH)

Growth hormone (GH) stimulation test, GH provocation test, insulin tolerance test (ITT), Arginine test

Luteinizing hormone (LH) assay

Prolactin levels (PRL)

Thyrotropin-releasing hormone (TRH) test, thyrotropin-releasing factor (TRF) test

Urine specific gravity

Long bone x-rays

Sella turcica x-ray

Computed tomography of head (CT scan of head), Computerized axial transverse tomography (CATT)

Thyroid Gland Diagnostic Tests

Antithyroid microsomal antibody, Antimicrosomal antibody, Microsomal antibody, Thyroid autoantibody, Thyroid antimicrosomal antibody

Calcitonin, HCT, Thyrocalcitonin

Serum free triiodothyronine (T_3)

Thyroid-stimulating hormone (TSH), Thyrotropin

Thyroid-stimulating hormone (TSH) stimulation test

Thyroxine index free, FTI, FT_4 Index

Thyroid Gland Diagnostic Tests—cont'd

Thyroxine, T_4, Thyroxine screen

Triiodothyronine, T_3 radioimmunoassay, T_3 by RIA

Radioactive iodine uptake, (RAIU), iodine uptake test uptake

Thyroid scan, thyroid scintiscan

Thyroid ultrasound, thyroid echogram, thyroid sonogram

Thyroid biopsy

Parathyroid Gland Diagnostic Tests

Parathyroid hormone (PTH), Parathormone

Calcium, total/ionized Ca^{++}

Phosphorus

Adrenal Glands Diagnostic Tests

Adrenocorticotropic hormone (ACTH) stimulation test, Cortisol stimulation test, Cosyntropin test

Corisol, Hydrocortisone

Dexamethasone suppression test (DST), Cortisol suppression test, ACTH suppression test

Plasma renin assay, Plasma renin activity (PRA)

Progesterone assay

Aldosterone assay

17-Hydroxycorticosteroids (17-OHCS)

17-Ketosteroids (17-KS)

Urine cortisol, Hydrocortisone

Vanillylmandelic acid (VMA) & catecholamines, VMA & epinephrine, Norepinephrine, Metanephrine, Normetanephrine, Dopamine

Adrenal angiography, Adrenal arteriogram

Adrenal venography

Computed tomography of adrenals (CAT scan of adrenal CT scan of adrenals)

Thyroid Scan

A thyroid scan utilizes a scintillation camera or scintiscanner to evaluate the thyroid gland following administration of a radioactive isotope or technetium. Hyperactive areas in the thyroid will appear as black or gray regions (hot spots) while areas of hypoactivity will appear as white (cold spots). Hot spots are generally indicative of benign nodules while malignancies will appear as cold spots (Daniels, 2003).

Nursing Management

Instruct the patient that this test evaluates the structure and function of the thyroid gland. The patient is ensured that the amount of radioactive material used is not harmful to the patient or others. Ask if the patient has received any ra-

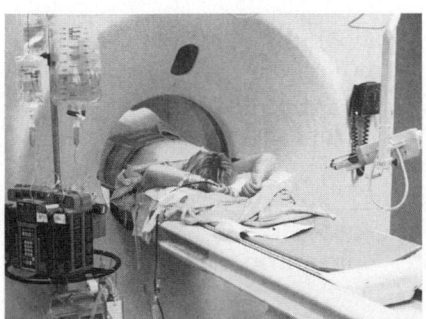

Figure 55-7 CT testing.

diographic contrasts from other diagnostic tests in the past three months as these may interfere with the scan. Patients who are taking medications with iodine (e.g., Lugol's solution, cough syrups, or multivitamins) may be instructed by the practitioner to discontinue their use for two weeks prior to the scan. Thyroid medications may be discontinued for four to six weeks prior to the scan. If I 123 or I 131 is used, the patient will be required not to eat anything (NPO) after midnight. The patient will remain NPO for 45 minutes after ingesting the isotope, and the scan is performed 24 hours later. If technetium is used, it is administered 30 minutes before the scan. IV administration eliminates the need for fasting.

Thyroid Ultrasound

Thyroid ultrasound is useful in differentiation of fluid filled cysts or tumors. It involves the use of ultrasonic pulses that are directed at the thyroid gland. The sound waves bounce back and are displayed on an oscilloscope. Fine needle aspiration or biopsy may be performed if a tumor is suspected.

Nursing Management

The procedure takes about 30 minutes and requires no special preparation. The patient just needs to be educated as to the expectations of the results of the ultrasound. In addition, young children will likely need to be restrained or potentially mildly sedated during this procedure.

Thyroid Biopsy

A biopsy may be performed as a surgical procedure, requiring general anesthesia or with the use of fine needle aspiration and local anesthesia (Liebert, 2003c). A 21-gauge needle is inserted into the thyroid nodule; tissue from the thyroid is withdrawn and placed on a slide for examination. The possibility of hematoma formation and edema postprocedure are the major complications, which may present as respiratory difficulty. If the test is to be completed using general anesthesia, the patient will be required to fast. It is common for the patient to experience a sore throat after a thyroid biopsy.

Nursing Management

Explain the test procedure and the purpose of the test. Assess for the patient's knowledge of the test. Provide preprocedure sedation and analgesia as prescribed. The older patient may find it difficult to maintain positions when required to do so for lengthy periods of time during the biopsy. Obtain a signed consent form.

KEY CONCEPTS

- The endocrine system is made up of a variety of organs that secrete hormones.
- Hormones are the chemicals produced and stored by the endocrine system that help regulate metabolism and energy.
- The hypothalamus can be considered the major regulating organ of the body.
- The pituitary gland is often labeled the master gland, because it directly or indirectly stimulates the release of a variety hormones.

- PTH is secreted by the parathyroids, and its main function is the regulation of the blood level of calcium in the body.
- The medulla and cortex of each adrenal gland have separate and distinct functions and play a major role in the body's ability to adapt to internal and external stress.
- The catecholamines, epinephrine, norepinephrine, and dopamine are secreted by the adrenal medulla.

Continued

KEY CONCEPTS—cont'd

- The adrenal cortex secretes steroid hormones that are classified as glucocorticoid, mineralocorticoid, and androgens.
- The pancreas is both an endocrine and exocrine gland.
- Glucagon is a hormone released from the pancreas in response to low levels of blood glucose and is a counter-regulatory hormone.
- Insulin is a hormone produced by the beta cells of the pancreas to lower blood glucose levels.

- Common alterations of the endocrine system include changes in weight, either loss or gain.
- Vital signs, weight, nutritional status, apparent age as compared to chronological age, facial expression, and general appearance are important in the assessment of the endocrine system.
- Alterations in endocrine function are diagnosed by the use of blood and urine tests as well as radiological tests (e.g., CT, MRI).

REVIEW QUESTIONS

1. Which of the following is *not* produced by the thyroid gland?
   1. Calcitonin
   2. T_4
   3. T_3
   4. TSH

2. What is the correct label for the body parts that secrete substances into the ducts that empty into a body cavity or onto a body surface?
   1. Endocrine glands
   2. Target tissues
   3. Exocrine glands
   4. Hormones

3. Which of the following is true of the hypothalamus gland?
   1. It is often called the master gland.
   2. It stimulates the secretion of corticosteroids.
   3. It is located in the anterior portion of the neck.
   4. It secretes hormones that release or inhibit hormones from the anterior pituitary gland.

4. Which of the following are the two major hormones secreted by the adrenal medulla?
   1. Epinephrine and norepinephrine
   2. Insulin and glucagon
   3. Cortisol and aldosterone
   4. Calcitonin and PTH

5. When blood glucose levels are elevated, the pancreas secretes insulin. When the blood glucose declines, the stimulus for the secretion of insulin decreases. This is an example of:
   1. Circadian rhythm
   2. Negative feedback
   3. Complex feedback
   4. Neural or hormonal interaction

6. All of the following statements about parathyroid hormone are correct *except:*
   1. PTH is regulated by the pituitary and hypothalamus.
   2. PTH regulates the blood level of calcium.
   3. PTH stimulates bone reabsorption.
   4. PTH stimulates the kidneys to convert vitamin D to its most active form.

7. Which organ in the endocrine system consists of two lobes, connected by an isthmus, and secretes T_4, calcitonin, and T_3?
   1. Thyroid gland
   2. Hypothalamus gland
   3. Parathyroid gland
   4. Adrenal cortex

8. Which of the following are clinical manifestations of a patient having a thyroid crisis?
   1. Chilling, coma, and dyspnea
   2. Nausea, seizures, and apprehension
   3. Fever, tachycardia, and restlessness
   4. Double vision, mental deterioration, and diarrhea

9. Which organ controls serum calcium?
   1. Adrenal gland
   2. Thyroid gland
   3. Hypothalamus gland
   4. Parathyroid gland

10. A negative feedback mechanism refers to:
    1. The response of the cardiovascular system to hormone regulation
    2. The response of a gland by increasing or decreasing the secretion of a hormone
    3. The response seen when increasing one hormone causes another hormone to increase
    4. The response of the autonomic nervous system when stimulated by the adrenal cortex

REVIEW ACTIVITIES

1. Compare and contrast the endocrine and the exocrine glands.

2. Describe a negative feedback system related to hormone control.

3. Select two of the glands in the endocrine system and describe their location and function.

4. Develop three to five questions to ask a patient regarding his or her endocrine system.

5. Perform an assessment of the thyroid gland and document your results.

Endocrine Dysfunction: Nursing Management

Joyce Campbell, RN, MSN, CCRN, FNP-C

CHAPTER TOPICS

- Hypersecretion and Hyposecretion of the Anterior Pituitary Gland

- Diabetes Insipidus

- Syndrome of Inappropriate Antidiuretic Hormone

- Hyposecretion and Hypersecretion of the Adrenal Gland

- Thyroid Disorders

- Parathyroid Disorders

KEY TERMS

Adenoma
Amenorrhea
Anovulation
Euthyroid
Galactorrhea
Gynecomastia
Hirsutism
Oligomenorrhea
Osteopenia
Panhypopituitarism
Proptosis

The endocrine system along with the nervous system influences all body functions including metabolism, maturation, growth, reproduction, and adaptation to changes within the internal environment. The endocrine system regulates body function through the secretion of chemical substances called hormones, which exert action on specific target tissue by binding to a receptor site. Disease occurs when there is hyposecretion or hypersecretion of these hormones, or when target cells become nonresponsive to the hormone (Asp, 2005).

Beginning with general pituitary dysfunction, this chapter will address each target organ and the disease entities that occur when there is hyper or hypo functioning related to hormone secretion or tissue nonresponsiveness.

HYPERSECRETION OF THE ANTERIOR PITUITARY GLAND

Pituitary dysfunction may present with a variety of clinical signs and symptoms including those related to hyposecretion or hypersecretion of the pituitary hormones and sellar turcica enlargement. The importance of the pituitary gland to system function contributes to the variety of illnesses when the gland is diseased. Ten to 15 percent of all intracranial neoplasms are pituitary adenomas (Ferri, 2005).

Hyperfunction of the pituitary gland occurs when there is excess hormonal activity. Most commonly, secretory tumors cause hypersecretion of one or more of the pituitary hormones. Autoimmune stimulation is another reason for hyperfunction of the pituitary gland.

Etiology

The most common cause of pituitary hyperfunction is a pituitary **adenoma** (a benign tumor made of epithelial cells, usually arranged like a gland), which can cause hypersecretion of prolactin, growth hormone (GH) or adrenocorticotrophin (ACTH) hormone (Jameson, 2005).

Pathophysiology

Patients who have hyperfunction of the pituitary gland may present with hormonal or neurological symptoms. Located in the sella turcica, the pituitary gland is positioned in close proximity to the cavernous sinuses, cranial nerves, and optic chiasm. Therefore, in addition to the hormonal symptoms, enlargement of the gland may cause localized symptoms, such as visual changes, cranial nerve impingement, and headache.

Hyperprolactinemia

Hyperprolactinemia is a prolactin secreting pituitary tumor. This condition is the most common pituitary tumor, accounting for 60 percent of primary pituitary tumors.

Epidemiology

Prolactin secreting tumors are more common in women. In women the tumors are usually microadenomas, which do not grow even with oral contraceptives or with pregnancy. Men more commonly have macroadenomas (Ferri, 2005).

Etiology

Etiology of hyperprolactinemia includes pituitary adenoma, primary hypothyroidism, traumatic injury, or surgery to the pituitary stalk, breast disease, estrogen therapy, pregnancy, and drugs. Renal and liver disease and hypothyroidism should also be considered a potential cause. Hyperprolactinemia is also seen in multiple sclerosis, spinal cord lesions, systemic lupus erythematosus, and other diseases. The most common cause of hyperprolactinemia is ingestion of drugs, including dopamine antagonist, haloperidol, risperidone, metoclopramide, opioids, cimetidine, verapamil (Aron, et al., 2004a).

Pathophysiology

Most commonly, prolactinomas arise from the lateral wings of the anterior pituitary. As growth of the tumor continues, the sella turcica is filled, and the normal anterior and posterior lobes are compressed. The size of the tumor varies from the more common microadenomas to large tumors, which invade the extracellular area.

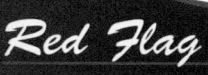

Red Flag

Visual Changes

Patients presenting with an unexplained visual field defect or bitemporal hemianopsia, or visual loss should be considered to have a pituitary or hypothalamic disorder until proven otherwise (Aron, Finding, & Tyrrell, 2004a).

Assessment with Clinical Manifestations

Clinical manifestations of hyperprolactinemia in women include **galactorrhea** (excessive secretion of milk), **amenorrhea** (absence of menstruation), **oligomenorrhea** (scanty or infrequent menstrual flow) with **anovulation** (failure to ovulate), and infertility. In men, hyperprolactinemia causes a decrease in testosterone secondary to an inhibition of gonadotropin secretion leading to decreased facial and body hair, erectile dysfunction, decrease in libido, small testicles and infertility; **gynecomastia** (enlargement of breast tissue) in the male occurs less frequency in men. Since hyperprolactinemia is associated with a decrease in estrogen, women with prolactinomas often have an estrogen deficiency with resulting symptoms of vaginal dryness, hot flashes, and more seriously **osteopenia** (a significant amount of decrease in bone mineral density), and osteoporosis. The patient may also experience weight gain, irritability, **hirsutism** (condition characterized by the excessive growth of hair or the presence of hair in abnormal places), anxiety, and depression. In some incidences, pituitary prolactinomas secrete GH simultaneously and cause acromegaly (Jameson, 2005).

Diagnostic Tests

Patients who present with symptoms of hyperprolactinemia should have a basal prolactin level, thyroid panel, and gonadal function test done. Tests to rule out renal and liver disease are advised. In addition, women with amenorrhea should have a pregnancy test. In most incidences, a PRL level of greater than 200 ng/mL is diagnostic of a prolactinoma. A prolactin level of less than 200 ng/mL does not rule out a pituitary tumor (Aron, et al., 2004a). Other causes for hyperprolactinemia should be excluded.

Computed tomography (CT) scan or magnetic resonance imaging (MRI) is recommended when prolactin levels are elevated for the purpose of identifying a microadenoma or macroadenoma. Macroadenomas are greater than 1 cm in size. Microadenomas are less than 1 cm. Tumor size usually correlates with the prolactin level (Jameson, 2005) (Box 56-1).

Nursing Diagnoses

Based on the information gathered, examples of nursing diagnoses in the patient with hyperprolactinemia may include the following:
- Disturbed body image related to gynecomastia and galactorrhea.
- Sexual dysfunction or ineffective sexuality patterns related to altered gonadal function.

Planning and Implementation

The patient will require psychosocial support to deal with altered body image and issues related to sexual function. Reversal of signs and symptoms is promising with medical or surgical treatment. Special attention must be given to instruction and preparation regarding treatment plan, (e.g., medications, surgery).

Goals

Goals of treatment include normalization of prolactin level, alleviation of the suppressive effect of gonadal function, halting of galactorrhea, and preservation of bone density (Jameson, 2005). Long-term remission is possible when the adenoma is small in size, and the prolactin levels are less than 200 ng/mL. If asymptomatic, microadenomas are usually not treated; however, close monitoring is required. For tumors larger than 2 cm, surgical treatment (see transsphenoidal resection) will usually provide an initial remission. Because there is often remaining tumor, medical interventions may be required at some time postoperatively.

Pharmacology

There are specific medications that are used to treat hyperprolactinemia. Dopaminergic medications, which stimulate dopamine receptors, are used to medically manage prolactinomas. They are capable of controlling hyperpro-

---

BOX 56-1

PROLACTIN LEVELS

Normal prolactin levels in nonpregnant women: 0–23 ng/mL or 0–23 mcg/L. Normal prolactin levels in men: 0–20 ng/mL or 0–10 mcg/L.

After fasting for 12 hours, blood for the prolactin test should be drawn between 8:00 and 10:00 a.m. It is also recommended that all prescribed medications be discontinued if possible two weeks prior to prolactin test (Daniels, 2003).

lactinemia, shrinking tumor, and restoring menses and fertility. These drugs include bromocriptine (Parlodel) and cabergoline (Dostinex). Bromocriptine, the first available dopamine agonist, has effects at both the hypothalamic and pituitary levels. Dosage is 2.5 to 10 mg a day orally in divided dosages. Side effects include postural hypotension and gastrointestinal (GI) problems. Cabergoline, (Dostinex), a newer dopaminergic agonist, is administered once or twice weekly and has fewer side effects. Ninety percent of patients have success in treatment with cabergoline (Aron, et al., 2004a).

Surgery

Conventional radiation therapy is reserved for patients who do not respond to medications or who have persistent hyperprolactinemia after surgery or medical treatment. Fifty to 60 percent of the patients experience impairment of anterior pituitary function with the radiation therapy. A newer modality for treating pituitary tumors is stereotactic radiosurgery (gamma knife). Multiple ports allow high dose ionizing radiation to be delivered with minimal irradiation to surrounding tissues (Ferri, 2005). See the National Institutes of Health Web site (www.cancer.gov) for elaboration of the gamma knife treatment procedure used for brain tumors.

Evaluation of Outcomes

Potential patient outcomes for each of the example nursing diagnoses for the patient with hyperprolactinemia are:
- Disturbed body image related to gynecomastia and galactorrhea. Patient will have resolution of gynecomastia and amenorrhea.
- Sexual dysfunction or ineffective sexuality patterns related to altered gonadal function. The patient will verbalize satisfaction with the way he or she expresses physical intimacy.

Acromegaly (Gigantism)

Acromegaly, a Greek word, *akro* (extremity) and *megas* (large) is a condition occurring in adults, that is caused by hypersecretion of the pituitary GH over a long period of time. Hypersecretion of GH in childhood causes gigantism.

Etiology

In most incidences gigantism and acromegaly are secondary to a benign tumor of the pituitary gland. Other rare causes include hypothalamus tumors producing excess GH releasing hormone (GHRH), bronchial tumors (carcinoid), and pancreatic islet cell tumors.

Epidemiology

Acromegaly occurs equally between men and women and is a rare disease with only three cases occurring per 1 million people per year. The average age for diagnosis of acromegaly is 42 years, though the duration of symptoms is usually 5 to 10 years prior to diagnosis. Diagnosis is often missed or delayed. When undiagnosed, untreated, or undertreated, there is increase morbidity and mortality due to the chronic effect of GH on body organs resulting in increase incidence of cardiovascular, cerebrovascular, respiratory disease, malignancies, and diabetes (Asp, 2005).

Pathophysiology

Most pituitary tumors, which secrete GH and cause acromegaly, are usually over 1 cm in diameter when the diagnosis is made. The tumors evolve from the outer wings of the anterior pituitary gland. In about 15 percent of the tumors, lactotrophs are present, and therefore both GH and prolactin are secreted.

Clinical manifestations of acromegaly occur due to an excess of GH, which once released into circulation stimulates production of insulin growth factor

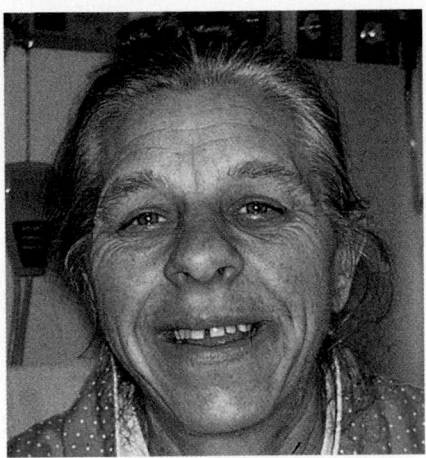

Figure 56-1 Acromegaly (note wide nose, spaced teeth, and large lips).

(IGF-1) or somatomedin C. IGF-1 is produced mainly by the liver and is the primary mediator of the growth-promoting effects of GH. In children and adolescence, gigantism occurs because GH stimulates growth in all body tissues prior to fusion of the growth plate. A child may grow to seven feet or taller. In adults, acromegaly occurs because GH causes continued growth of soft tissues and small bones of the hands and feet and the membranous bones of the skull and face (Figure 56-1). Excess GH also causes an alteration in fat and carbohydrate metabolism. The multiple effects of GH on carbohydrate metabolism include hyperglycemia, which occurs due to a decreased glucose uptake by peripheral tissues and an increased production of glucose by the liver. Rather than normal use of carbohydrates for energy, GH boosts the creation of ketones and the utilization of free fatty acids for energy. These events lead to glucose intolerance, hyperinsulinemia, and the probability of developing diabetes. Thirty percent of the patients will have some form of cardiac disease, including coronary artery disease, cardiac dysrhythmias, left ventricular hypertrophy (LVH), or cardiomyopathy (Jameson, 2005). Acromegaly has also been associated with colon polyps.

Assessment with Clinical Manifestations

There are several identifying characteristics seen in patients with acromegaly. Table 56-1 clearly represents both the history and physical findings of this disorder.

Diagnostic Tests

Diagnostic tests to determine the presence of excess GH include serum growth hormone (hGH), IGF-1, and GH suppression test. Normally growth hormone (hGH) is less than 5 ng/mL or is less than 226 pmol/L in men and is less than 10 ng/mL or is less than 452 pmol/L in women. Increased values of hGH may be associated with certain medications (e.g., glucagon, levodopa, insulin, estrogens, or oral contraceptives). In acromegaly, the hGH level is greater than 10 ng/mL (Aron, et al., 2004b). Prior to the hGH test the patient should be fasting and the test should be drawn at eight in the morning because of the circadian cycle.

TABLE 56-1 Assessment of the Patient with Acromegaly

HISTORY	PHYSICAL FINDINGS
Skin: Changes in facial features; excessive sweating	Oily skin, thickening of heal pads, acanthosis nigricans, macroglossia, hirsutism.
Neuro/HEENT: Headaches, lethargy, photophobia, headache	Prognathism (Underbite)
	Visual changes, paresthesia, carpal tunnel syndrome. Enlargement of tongue
Respiratory: Sleep apnea, hypersomnolence	Obesity
CV: History of: hypertension, atherosclerotic disease Hypercholesterolemia	LVH, cardiomyopathy
Reproductive: Decreased libido, impotence, infertility	Galactorrhea, gynecomastia
Oligomenorrhea	
GU: renal colic	
MS: arthralgias, muscle weakness	Proximal myopathy, soft tissue overgrowth
	Glucose intolerance
General: Fatigue, weight gain, and heat intolerance	

Adapted from Asp, A. (2005) Mechanisms of endocrine control. In K. Copstead & J. L. Banasik, Pathophysiology (pp. 639–645). St. Louis, MO: Elsevier Saunders.

Glucose suppression test involves measuring GH following the administration of 100 g of glucose. Normally, GH secretion is lowered to less than 2 ng/mL. A result greater than 2 ng/mL is considered conclusive of a diagnosis of acromegaly (Ferri, 2005).

Somatomedin C (SM-C): Insulin-like growth factor (IGF-1) results are interpreted according to patient's age and sex. Elevated GH levels increase IGF-1 levels and are usually diagnostic of acromegaly (Daniels, 2003). IGF-1 levels are two to three times higher in pregnancy. Additional tests include postprandial plasma glucose, serum phosphorous, and urine calcium levels, which are often elevated in the patient who has hypersecretion of GH.

Plain films will often show sellar turcica enlargement due to a pituitary tumor. Thickening of the calvarium, enlargement of the sinuses and jaw can also be seen on X-ray. An MRI will usually show tumor location and size.

Nursing Diagnoses

Based on the information gathered, examples of nursing diagnoses in the patient with acromegaly may include the following:
* Disturbed body image related to changes in skin, facial features, hair, and musculoskeletal system.
* Chronic pain related to arthralgia and myalgia from cartilage overgrowth.
* Deficient knowledge related to the disease, complications, and management.
* Sleep deprivation related to sleep apnea.

Planning and Implementation

The nurse should work with the endocrinologist or health care provider experienced in managing acromegaly. Treatment of choice is surgical removal of tumor. For patients who are not candidates for surgery treatment, elect not to have surgery, or have residual tumor following surgery, treatment may be radiotherapy or medical therapy. Conventional supervoltage irradiation successfully treats patients in 60 to 80 percent of the cases. Often there is a prolonged delay in achieving reduction of GH levels with radiotherapy. Hypopituitarism with resulting hypoadrenalism, hypogonadism, and hypothyroidism may occur with irradiation. Other complications of radiotherapy include cranial nerve dysfunction, radionecrosis, and cognitive abnormalities (Ferri, 2005). Another approach that has been used to treat tumors of the sella turcica is stereotactic technique with gamma knife.

A comprehensive plan for instruction and follow-up of the patient regarding proposed surgery or radiotherapy and prescribed medications should be implemented. Patients who are hyperglycemic due to hypersecretion of GH will need to have diabetic management involving glucose monitoring, diet, exercise, and medications to normalize glucose. Measures to prevent complications of diabetes must be implemented. Cardiovascular problems, such as hypercholesterolemia and hypertension, must be monitored closely and treated expeditiously. The nurse plays a major role in the management of the patient with acromegaly. Teaching involved in prevention and treatment of complications of the disease is of paramount importance.

Pharmacology

Octreotide is a drug that can be used to treat patients who have residual GH hypersecretion following surgery. Octreotide (Sandostatin) may be administered subcutaneously three times daily by the patient or administered intramuscularly in a long-acting form that lasts up to four weeks. Side effects may occur due to the inhibition of gastric and pancreatic function and include alteration in gastric motility, nausea, flatus, fat malabsorption, and gallstones. An alternative medication is bromocriptine (Parlodel). Though less effective than octreotide, it is less expensive and can be taken in oral form. (Ferri, 2005).

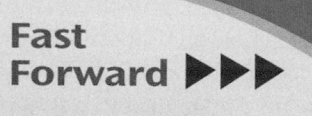

Fast Forward ▶▶▶

A Gamma Knife

A gamma knife is a new treatment modality used in the treatment of pituitary tumors. It is referred to as a stereotaxic approach for treating pituitary tumors. The stereotaxic approach is a viable alternative to radiation therapy and may continue in use in the near future. An interesting source is the National Institute of Health Web site (www.cancer.gov) for current treatment of brain tumors including gamma knife stereotaxic approach.

Surgery

Patients who undergo successful treatment for GH hypersecretion may expect a marked improvement and reversal of most signs and symptoms with successful therapy. Bone overgrowth will cease, and soft tissue bulk in extremities and facial puffiness will decrease (Aron, et al., 2004a).

Evaluation of Outcomes

Potential patient outcomes for each of the example nursing diagnoses for the patient with acromegaly are:

* Disturbed body image related to changes in skin, facial features, hair, and musculoskeletal system. Patient will relate an understanding of the cause for change in physical appearance.
* Chronic pain related to arthralgia and myalgia from cartilage overgrowth. Patient will report a decrease in skeletal muscular pain.
* Deficient knowledge related to the disease, complications, and management. Patient will verbalize understanding of disease, complications, and management.
* Sleep deprivation related to sleep apnea. Patient will report relief from symptoms of sleep deprivation.

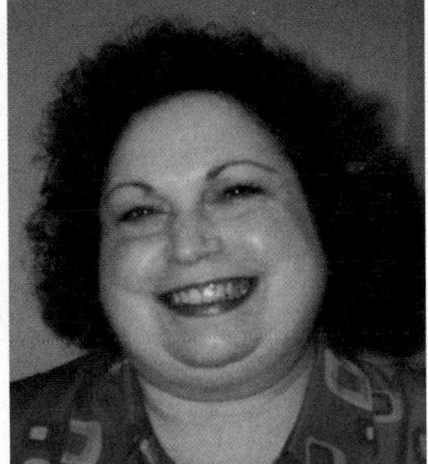

Figure 56-2 Cushing's syndrome.

Cushing's Disease (Hypercortisolism)

Hypercortisolism is most often caused by excessive production and release of ACTH by a pituitary secreting adenoma. This form of hypercortisolism is called Cushing's disease (Figure 56-2).

Epidemiology

Most commonly Cushing's disease occurs in women between 20 and 40 years of age. ACTH secreting adenomas (Cushing's disease) make up approximately 20 percent of pituitary tumors. The most common cause of Cushing's syndrome is the use of corticosteroids, which are prescribed for multiple inflammatory, immune, and numerous other conditions. Consequently, the condition of increased ACTH, which causes Cushing's disease or Cushing's syndrome (discussed later), could be included under: (a) the pituitary section from the etiology of a tumor of the pituitary gland or (b) excessive stimulation from the adrenal cortex. The clinical manifestations and management strategies are similar for either causation.

Etiology

When Cushing's disease is primary in its etiology the condition is due to a pituitary adenoma. Less often Cushing's disease may occur because of excessive corticotropic releasing hormone (CRH), which stimulates an increase in ACTH secretion. Because excess production of ACTH results in bilateral hyperplasia of the adrenal glands and hypercortisolism, the disease is often referred to as ACTH dependent. Mass effect or localized symptoms occur less frequently than other types of pituitary tumors because the adenoma is generally small, 5 to 10 mm in diameter (Aron, et al, 2004b).

Another cause for hypercortisolism is an ACTH secreting neoplasm (ectopic ACTH). The most common ACTH ectopic secreting tumor is small cell carcinoma of the lung. A nonpituitary or non-ACTH dependent hypercortisolism called Cushing's syndrome (non-ACTH dependent) is often due to the iatrogenic effects of chronic glucocorticoid therapy. Less frequent causes for Cushing's syndrome are adrenal disease, neoplasm, or hyperplasia (Aron, et al., 2004a).

Pathophysiology

Ninety percent of the patients with Cushing's disease have a pituitary adenoma. Up to 90 percent of these tumors are microadenoma (less than 10 mm). The tumors are usually basophilic or chromophobe adenomas and can appear anywhere within the anterior pituitary gland. The tumor is rarely greater than 10 mm and invasive, causing a mass effect. Malignant ACTH secreting tumors are seldom reported. Under the influence of ACTH secretion, the adrenal glands are enlarged, with thickened cortex due to hyperplasia (Aron, et al., 2004a).

Assessment with Clinical Manifestations

Clinical manifestations of hypercortisolism occurring from pituitary disease, ectopic tumor, primary disease of the adrenal gland, or iatrogenic effects of glucocorticoid are similar. Symptoms from excess cortisol and androgen are usually present. If an iatrogenic cause or other disease that causes hypercortisolism is not identified, a thorough diagnostic workup must be implemented to determine the etiology to develop a treatment plan. Many of the clinical manifestations of hypercortisolism can be interpreted as exaggeration action of cortisol, which affects glucose, protein, and fat metabolism. Some of the symptoms are easy bruising, poor wound healing, excess hair growth in females, hypertension, edema of extremities, accumulation of fat in the face (moon face), voice changes, hyperlipidemia, dysrhythmias, emotional liability, irritability, depression, poor memory, euphoria, psychosis, suicidal tendencies, protein breakdown and muscle wasting, osteopenia, osteoporosis, renal calculi, polyuria, amenorrhea in females, decrease in libido, impotence, decrease in body hair (males), protruding abdomen, subclavicular fat pads (buffalo hump), hyperinsulinemia, and abnormal glucose tolerance test. Additional clinical manifestations that may be present due to fluid and electrolyte imbalance are hypokalemia and sodium imbalances.

Diagnostic Tests

There are a number of diagnostic tests for hypersecretion of the adrenal glands: serum ACTH (elevated in hyperfunction of the pituitary; decreased in hypofunction of the pituitary), plasma cortisol, dexamethasone, ACTH suppression test, urine free cortisol (UFC) (requires 24 hour urine collection), salivary cortisol, CT and MRI of pituitary and adrenal glands, and inferior petrosal sinus sampling (IPSS). More information is provided in Box 56-2.

Nursing Diagnoses

Based on the information gathered, examples of nursing diagnoses in the patient with hypersecretion of the adrenal glands may include the following:
- Activity intolerance related to congestive heart failure, and weakness due to hypercortisolism, which causes proximal muscle weakness, decreased muscle mass, and hypokalemia.
- Disturbed body image related to appearance changes.
- Risk for infection related to altered resistance to infection due to compromised immune system, altered production of cytokines, hyperglycemia, and negative nitrogen balance.
- Risk for injury related to fractures from osteoporosis.
- Impaired skin integrity related to loss of tissue strength with increase capillary fragility.
- Ineffective sexuality patterns related to loss of libido in females secondary to elevated androgens; impotence and decreased libido in males secondary excess cortisol.

Planning and Implementation

The patient with hypercortisolism due to Cushing's disease or Cushing's syndrome presents with a complex number of problems. Priorities of care include fluid and electrolyte imbalances, which require careful monitoring for fluid excess and symptoms of electrolyte imbalance. The nurse must be prepared to monitor the patient for symptoms of heart failure and implement the medical plan of care, which may include diuretic, antihypertensive, and cardiotonic drug therapy. Providing assistance with activities of daily living is paramount,

---

BOX 56-2

ADVANCES IN DIAGNOSING PITUITARY SECRETING TUMOR

Inferior petrosal sinus sampling (IPSS), a diagnostic test that is yielding close to 100 percent accuracy is currently being done in some hospitals. The test requires the skills of an interventional radiologist (Aron, et al., 2004a). Blood leaves the pituitary gland and drains into the cavernous sinus and then on to the inferior petrosal sinuses and then into the jugular bulb and vein. Simultaneous ACTH measurement of samples of blood taken from the posterior petrosal sinus and peripheral circulation before and after CRH stimulation has high sensitivity for identifying a pituitary secreting adenoma.

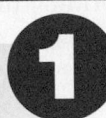

Safety First

Preventing Falls in Patients with Cushing's Disease

Safety measures to prevent falls must be implemented, because the patient is prone to fractures related to osteoporosis. Assistance with ambulation and getting in and out of bed should be included in the plan of care. Discharge planning needs to include measures to maintain a safe environment at home, including adequate lighting, clutter-free environment, and use of nonskid slippers. It is important to ensure that the patient's vision is normal or corrective lenses are available. The patient should have ongoing monitoring for fatigue, weakness, and other factors that may predispose to a fall.

because the patient may be short of breath and have activity intolerance. Weakness may also be due to hypokalemia, which requires cardiac monitoring and potassium replacement.

Special attention must be given to prevent the patient from acquiring an infection. The compromised immune system makes the patient with hypercortisolism susceptible to opportunistic or bacterial infections. Even minor wounds and infections heal slowly. The patient may not respond normally to an infection with increased body temperature and pulse rate. Even a low-grade temperature may be a red flag for the patient with hypercortisolism. The patient and significant others should be instructed to assess and report any symptoms of infection. Principles of medical and surgical asepsis must be implemented as indicated when caring for the patient.

An altered body image is of great concern for these patients. It is not uncommon for the patient's physical appearance to change to the point at which they are not recognizable. Weight gain between 25 and 100 pounds, acne, excess body hair redistribution of fat, and striae on abdomen and breast completely changes the physical appearance. Encourage the patient to explore his or her feelings. Thorough explanations about the disease and its prognosis can help the patient deal with his or her feelings.

Helping the patient to understand the cause for weight gain is important. The appetite is described as excessive by most patients. Instruction in healthy eating and measures to decrease portion size and replacement of excess eating with lower calorie snacks is important. Exercise to tolerance should be encouraged. The patient should be told that it is likely that body changes will be reversible with treatment. In addition, the patient may have to deal with cortisol induced diabetes (see chapter 57).

Pharmacology

No drugs are available to successfully suppress pituitary ACTH secretion. Ketoconazole, metyrapone, and aminoglutethimide are expensive drugs, which have been shown to have limited success in treating Cushing's disease (Aron et. al., 2004a). The initial treatment of choice is selective transsphenoidal resection with tumor removal to correct the hypercortisolism. Radiotherapy may be prescribed. In extreme cases, bilateral adrenalectomy has been done when all other therapies have failed. Lifelong hormone replacement therapy is required following the surgery.

Surgery

Transsphenoidal hypophysectomy is the treatment of choice for most pituitary adenomas (Figure 56-3). It entails a horizontal incision at the intersection of the inner part of the upper lip and the gingival extending bilaterally from the center of the upper lip and gum. From this incision, instrumentation is made underneath the nasal cartilage and splenoid sinus up to the floor of the sella turcica, where excision of the adenoma can be made (Ghoraych, 2005). Following removal of the tumor, the incision is closed and fascia or muscle obtained from the abdomen or a muscle is implanted at the surgical site to prevent leakage of cerebrospinal fluid (CSF) and assist in healing of the wound. The nasal passage is usually packed for 24 to 48 hours, and a gauze dressing is secured under the nose to absorb drainage.

A newer approach for removal of a pituitary tumor is the endonasal approach, which is considered to be less invasive, requiring no incision. A small endoscope is inserted through the nostril and into the skull base, through the splenoid sinus and into the sella turcica, where visualization of the tumor takes place. Overall recovery time is reported to be reduced.

The initial preoperative workup will usually be done on an outpatient basis. The patient should have a well-documented head-to-toe assessment to use as a

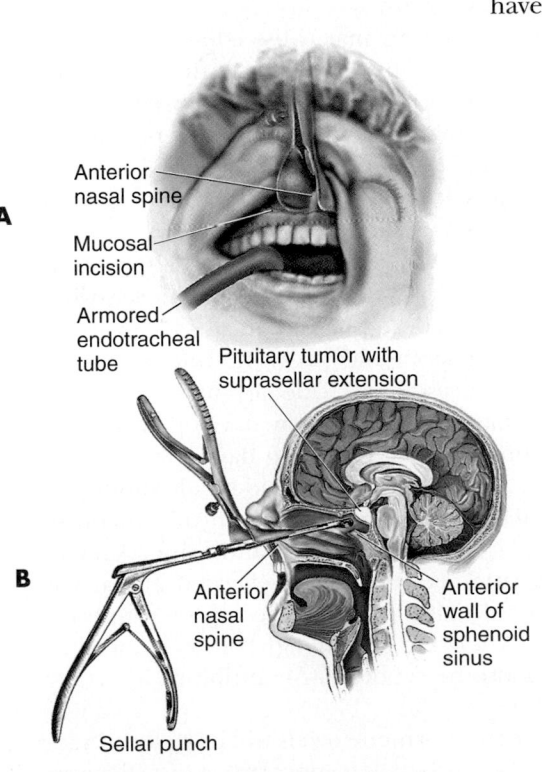

A

Anterior nasal spine

Mucosal incision

Armored endotracheal tube

Pituitary tumor with suprasellar extension

B

Anterior nasal spine

Anterior wall of sphenoid sinus

Sellar punch

Figure 56-3 Transsphenoidal approach to hypophysectomy: A. A bivalved speculum is inserted, B. The floor of the sphenoid is removed with a sellar punch.

baseline. Preoperative teaching includes informing the patient about incision sites, including both the oral incision and the donor site for removing the fascia or muscle. Discomfort regarding the packing should be explained. The necessity of receiving a liquid diet initially and use of toothettes for cleaning the teeth should be included in the teaching plan. Instructions related to deep-breathing exercises should be emphasized, along with information regarding the need for breathing through the mouth because the nostrils will be temporarily blocked. Leg exercise to prevent clot formation should be demonstrated. Diagrams and information regarding the actual procedure should be provided by the surgeon.

Following surgery the patient is positioned supine with the head of the bed elevated 30°. In addition to monitoring and ensuring that the patient has respiratory and circulatory stability postoperatively, the following potential problems should be addressed. Symptoms of meningitis or encephalitis should be addressed immediately. The patient should be monitored for signs and symptoms of infection. Clear drainage from the nasal passages or frequent swallowing (postnasally) is suggestive of a CSF leak. The patient is supplied a drip pad under the nose, which is changed as needed. Drainage amounts will vary among patients. Usually the drainage decreases within 24 hours. A CSF leak is suspected if there is an appearance of a halo ring on the dressing or if the clear drainage is positive for glucose. Lab analysis to verify that the drainage is CSF should be carried out. If it is determined that the patient has a CSF leak, bed rest with head of bed elevated should be implemented. Although, normally the leak will cease spontaneously, the patient will be at a higher risk for infection, therefore antibiotics are usually ordered. Ongoing assessment for clinical manifestations of infection is warranted. In rare situations, the patient will need additional surgery to repair the leakage site in the sella turcica. If fascia has been removed for packing, the donor site should be assessed for signs and symptoms of infection. Because the nasal passage is packed, the patient will breathe though the mouth. Frequent mouth and lip care is necessary. Liquids help to decrease the discomfort from dry mouth.

An anterior transsphenoidal hypophysectomy may cause edema or trauma to the posterior pituitary. Clinical manifestations of diabetes insipidus should be assessed. The patient's fluid status should be carefully monitored. Intake and output and daily weight are important. Neurological assessment, including cranial nerves, should be assessed initially and every hour as indicated by unit policy. Changes in neurological status may indicate an increase in intracranial pressure or other complications related to surgery.

The patient is usually discharged 48 to 72 hours after surgery. The patient should be instructed to avoid lifting, straining, stooping, blowing nose, swimming, aerobic exercise, all of which could cause pressure in the sella turcica and disrupt the healing process The nurse should stress the importance of follow-up with the endocrinologist as prescribed. Due to surgical trauma (Aron, et al., 2004b), a small percentage of patients may develop syndrome of inappropriate antidiuretic hormone (SIADH) 5 to 10 days after surgery (Prather, Forsyth, Russell, & Wagner, 2003). The patient and family should be instructed to report symptoms of SIADH including confusion, headache unrelieved by typical analgesics, and lethargy. A serum sodium and urine osmolality are used to diagnose SIADH. Serum sodium will be elevated and urine osmolality decreased. The patient should also be alerted to report symptoms of diabetes insipidus, including increased urine output, light yellow urine, and thirst. Symptoms of infection should also be reported. An antibiotic is usually prescribed for several days postsurgery.

At the follow-up appointment, pituitary hormone levels will be determined. Often patients will have transient secondary adrenocortical insufficiency requiring glucocorticoid support until the hypothalamic-pituitary-adrenal (HPA) axis recovers. If there has been total removal of the anterior pituitary, the patient will require lifelong replacement of thyroid hormone and glucocorticoids. Males will also need testosterone replacement (Aron, et al., 2004a). Follow-up MRIs will be used to monitor patient's progress.

When hypercortisolism is caused by an adrenal secreting tumor, a partial or complete removal of the adrenal gland (adrenalectomy) is usually the treatment of choice. An adrenalectomy may be done by laparoscope procedure or general surgery. General postoperative nursing care is required in addition to careful monitoring for and treatment for hypoadrenalism. If bilateral adrenalectomy is performed, the patient will require immediate and lifetime replacement of glucocorticoids and mineralocorticoids. When unilateral adrenalectomy is performed, glucocorticoid and mineralocorticoid replacement will be needed until the remaining adrenal gland regains full function.

Evaluation of Outcomes

Potential patient outcomes for each of the example nursing diagnoses for the patient with Cushing's disease (or Cushing's syndrome) are:

- Activity intolerance related to congestive heart failure, and weakness due to hypercortisolism, which causes proximal muscle weakness, decreased muscle mass, and hypokalemia. Patient will report increase in strength and will demonstrate increased participation in activities of daily living.
- Disturbed body image related to appearance changes. Patient will discuss the cause for change in body image.
- Risk for infection related to altered resistance to infection due to compromised immune system, altered production of cytokines, hyperglycemia, and negative nitrogen balance. Patient will identify ways to avoid contacting an infection.
- Risk for injury related to fractures from osteoporosis. Patient will demonstrate safety measures to help prevent a fracture.
- Impaired skin integrity related to loss of tissue strength with increased capillary fragility. Patient will maintain intact skin and not experience skin breakdown.
- Ineffective sexuality patterns related to loss of libido in females secondary to elevated androgens; impotence and decreased libido in males secondary to excess cortisol. Patient will share feelings related to altered sexuality.

HYPOSECRETION OF THE ANTERIOR PITUITARY GLAND

Hypofunction of the pituitary gland occurs with decreased hormonal activity of one or more of the pituitary hormones. When all cell types in the pituitary gland fail to synthesize and secrete hormones it is called **panhypopituitarism.**

Etiology

There are a broad number of causes for hypopituitarism, including idiopathic conditions. In the event of tumors, there are space-occupying lesions that can cause the hypopituitarism. In addition, there can be ischemic damage to the pituitary from infarctions, traumatic head injuries, and infections. There are also infiltrative diseases (e.g., sarcoidosis, hemochromatosis, and histiocytosis X) and immunological causes for the hypofunction of the pituitary gland. There can be iatrogenic causes, as well, such as surgical and radiation therapy (Aron, et al., 2004b).

Pathophysiology

Dysfunction may be caused by destruction of the anterior pituitary gland or a secondary event resulting in a shortage of hypothalamic stimulatory factors. The deficiency of stimulation to the anterior pituitary gland causes clinical manifestations congruent with an alteration in the normal function of the pituitary gland.

Assessment with Clinical Manifestations

Clinical manifestations of hypopituitarism occur in relation to the hyposecretion of the pituitary hormones, which in addition to secreting GH, controls the secretion of hormones by the ovaries, gonads, adrenal, thyroid, and parathyroid glands. Hyposecretion of GH causes decreased growth in children. In children and adults, it is associated with a diminished sense of well-being and altered level of health-related life. Hypogonadism causes amenorrhea in women and impotence in men Thyroid-stimulating hormone (TSH) deficiency causes hypothyroid symptoms similar to those of primary hypothyroidism. ACTH deficiency causes symptoms similar to those in primary adrenal failure. Often the signs of hypopituitarism are subtle and require careful attention. The patient may be mildly overweight. The face may have fine wrinkles, and the skin is fine, smooth, and pale. Pubic and body hair may be sparse, and atrophy of the genitalia may be noted. In more severe cases, the patient may have orthostatic hypotension, bradycardia, and a decreased in muscle strength (Aron, et al., 2004a).

Planning and Implementation

The nursing care plan should be focused on assessment of the patient for signs and symptoms of pituitary dysfunction. Initially the plan of care involves preparation of the patient for the test to determine the cause of the hypofunction of the pituitary gland. After the cause is identified, the patient is prepared for treatment. This may involve pituitary surgery or treatment of underlying disease. In most all incidences, hormone replacement therapy will be a priority of care. A plan of care should evolve that assists the patient to know about the importance of compliance with hormone replacement therapy.

POSTERIOR PITUITARY DISORDERS

The posterior pituitary gland secretes antidiuretic hormone (ADH). Problems can arise either because of hyposecretion of the antidiuretic hormone, which causes diabetes insipidus, or hypersecretion of ADH, which is known as SIADH. Both disorders have a pronounced effect on fluid balance.

Diabetes Insipidus

Diabetes insipidus is a disorder that occurs due either to an insufficiency of ADH, which is referred to as central diabetes insipidus, or loss of sensitivity of the nephrons of the kidney to the circulating ADH.

Etiology

Central diabetes insipidus is common following surgery for tumors of the hypothalamus or pituitary gland. Other causes are hypopituitarism, tumors, aneurysms, thrombosis, infections, and immunological disorders of the hypothalamus and pituitary gland.

Pathophysiology

When ADH is insufficient, the kidney is not adequately able to concentrate urine and there is immediate excretion of large amount of urine. When the person is conscious, thirst will be experienced because the osmoreceptors in the hypothalamus are stimulated. In turn, the patient will have induced polydipsia. Output can be more than 20 liters per day.

Assessment with Clinical Manifestations

Polyuria with daily urine ranging from 2.5 to 20, and thirst with strong preference for ice water are the two primary symptoms of diabetes insipidus. The conscious patient will experience extreme thirst, thereby drinking and helping to prevent dehydration. In an unconscious patient or patient who cannot drink, severe dehydration and hypovolemia may occur.

Diagnostic Tests

Urine osmolarity decreases to 50 to 100 mOsm/kg; serum osmolality is elevated greater than 300 mOsm/kg. Urine specific gravity will range between 1.001 and 1.005. Hypernatremia, hypercalcemia, and hypokalemia may be present (Daniels, 2003).

Nursing Diagnoses

Based on the information gathered, examples of nursing diagnoses in the patient with diabetes insipidus may include the following:
- Deficient fluid volume related to excess diuresis due to decreased ADH.
- Fatigue related to weakness secondary to hypokalemia.

Planning and Implementation

Because patients may have up to 20 liters of urinary output daily, volume replacement is a priority. Dehydration is treated by administering a hypotonic solution, such as NaCl O.45%. The flow rate is usually ordered to match the urinary output. Additional fluids may be needed to treat dehydration and hypovolemia. ADH replacement is a necessity to help resolve the fluid imbalance and to maintain fluid balance (Ferri, 2005).

Pharmacology

Aqueous pitressin (Vasopressin) may be administered subcutaneously in relation to the amount of urinary output in hospitalized patients. Desmopressin acetate a synthetic analogue of vasopressin is administered intranasally as a metered dose nasal spray or be taken orally. These agents usually control the polydipsia and polyuria in patients with central diabetes insipidus (Broyles, Reiss, & Evans, 2007). Desmopressin may be ordered for discharge maintenance if diabetes insipidus does not resolve.

Evaluation of Outcomes

Potential patient outcomes for each of the example nursing diagnoses for the patient with diabetes insipidus are:
- Deficient fluid volume related to excess diuresis due to decreased ADH. Patient will have restoration of fluid volume and electrolyte balance.
- Fatigue related to hypokalemia. Patient will demonstrate improved energy and will maintain a normal serum potassium.

Syndrome of Inappropriate Antidiuretic Hormone

Another abnormality of the posterior pituitary gland is hypersecretion of ADH, known as SIADH.

Etiology

Conditions that cause SIADH include malignant lung disease and tumors such as lymphoma and sarcoma in different organs of the body. Many central nervous system (CNS) disorders, such as infections, and trauma cause the disease. Other causes are medications that stimulate ADH release, such as thiazides, phenothiazines, vincristine, opioids, severe pain, and emotional stress. Certain endocrine diseases, such as adrenal insufficiency and hypopituitarism, are associated with SIADH.

Pathophysiology

In SIADH, the posterior pituitary gland continues to release ADH even though the normal stimulants (an increase in osmolality and hypovolemia) are not present. When plasma levels of ADH are high, hyponatremia and hypoosmolality occur. The hyponatremia, which occurs with SIADH, can lead to cerebral edema, which is the primary cause for the clinical manifestations of the illness. The urine is usually inappropriately concentrated.

Assessment with Clinical Manifestations

The patient with SIADH must be assessed for neurological symptoms that occur as a result of cerebral edema, which is related to the hypoosmolality of hyponatremia. Symptoms occurring early include headache, weakness, muscle changes, and some weight gain. Later the patient will be observed to have personality changes, hostility, and sluggish reflexes. Nausea, vomiting, and diarrhea may also be present. An impending crisis may be predicted if the patient develops confusion, lethargy, and change in respirations. When serum sodium reaches 110 mmol/L, the nurse should anticipate that seizures may occur. Additional symptoms that may occur include headache, confusion, irritability, somnolence, seizures, and coma.

Diagnostic Tests

The primary forms of diagnostic tests for SIADH are serum and urine studies. Hyponatremia and low serum osmolality (less than 280 mosm/kg) confirm the condition. And, the urine is inappropriately concentrated (greater than 100 mOsm/kg; urinary sodium is greater than 20 mmoL/d) (Daniels, 2003).

Nursing Diagnoses

Based on the information gathered, examples of nursing diagnoses in the patient with SIADH may include the following:
• Excess fluid volume related to SIADH.
• Disturbed sensory perception related to cerebral edema.

Planning and Implementation

Identifying and eliminating the underlying cause are the initial steps of treatment. Fluid restriction of 600 to 1,200 mL per day is the simplest form of treatment. Special attention must be given to nonliquid fluid intake. In the event that the patient is unable to adhere to fluid restriction, demeclocycline, an antibiotic that decreases the availability of ADH, may be prescribed. When demeclocycline is administered, water restriction is not advocated. In other situations, sodium supplements are administered along with a loop diuretic to increase urinary solute excretion (Gardner & Greenspan, 2004). Intravenous NaCl 0.9% may also be prescribed.

When the patient has acute symptomatic hyponatremia, intravenous NaCl 3% may be the treatment of choice. NaCl 3% must be administered cautiously. Rate of administration should not exceed 50 mL/hour. Rapid administration may cause fluid over load and congestive heart failure. Too rapid correction of hyponatremia may lead to central pontine myelinolysis. (Gardner & Greenspan, 2004).

Evaluation of Outcomes

Potential patient outcomes for each of the example nursing diagnoses for the patient with SIADH are:
• Excess fluid volume related to SIADH. Patient's serum sodium level will be within normal levels.
• Disturbed sensory perception related to cerebral edema. Patient will have a normal neurological assessment.

HYPOSECRETION OF THE ADRENAL GLAND

Adrenal insufficiency occurs because of one of two major reasons. Primary adrenal insufficiency results from destruction or dysfunction of the cortex of the adrenal gland. Secondary adrenal insufficiency results from deficient

ACTH secretion due to dysfunction of the pituitary-hypothalamic axis or a disorder of pituitary gland.

Epidemiology

There are five cases of Addison's disease per 100,000 population. In addition, there is a 2:1 ratio of women to men (Ferri, 2005).

Etiology

Primary adrenal insufficiency, also known as Addison's disease, is rare. The leading cause is autoimmune disease. Other causes include adrenal hemorrhage, infections, metastatic cancer or lymphoma, amyloidosis, hemochromatosis, congenital adrenal hyperplasia, familial glucocorticoid deficiency, and hypoplasia. Certain drugs, such as ketoconazole, metyrapone, aminoglutethimide, and ctomidate, have been associated with the disease. Though *Mycobacterium tuberculosis* was the leading infection in the past to cause adrenal insufficiency, in the United States today histoplasmosis is the leading infectious cause (Aron, et al., 2004a). Tuberculosis continues to be the leading cause of adrenal insufficiency worldwide. Thirty percent of patients with AIDS develop adrenal insufficiency (Ferri, 2005).

Pathophysiology

Addison's disease occurs insidiously over weeks and even months. By the time of diagnosis there is often a loss of 90 percent of the cortices of both adrenal glands. The gradual loss of adrenal function may go unnoticed because both mineralcorticoids and glucocorticoids continue to be secreted from a reserve. When the basal reserve is depleted chronic manifestations of adrenal insufficiency will manifest. An acute crisis can occur if the patient is predisposed to stressful situations, such as trauma, surgery, and the like. When the adrenals are affected by hemorrhage, both glucocorticoid and mineralocorticoid secretion is loss causing an acute adrenal crisis (Aron, et al., 2004a).

Assessment with Clinical Manifestations

Clinical manifestations of chronic adrenal insufficiency include weakness, fatigue, anorexia, GI symptoms, orthostatic hypotension, hypotension, salt craving, and hyperpigmentation. Hyperpigmentation and hyperkalemia occur only in primary hypoadrenalism. Weight loss and malnutrition can occur due to diminished appetite and nausea. The patient with secondary adrenal insufficiency may also have deficiencies in testosterone, GH, thyroxine, and ADH.

Secondary adrenal insufficiency can occur due to tumors of the hypothalamus or pituitary gland resulting in deficiency of ACTH (Table 56-2). Removal of a tumor from the pituitary gland may result in permanent deficiency in ACTH, causing cortisol and adrenal androgen deficiency. Usually in secondary adrenal insufficiency, aldosterone function is not affected. Another common cause of secondary adrenal insufficiency is the rapid withdrawal of glucocorticoid therapy. Twenty milligrams of hydrocortisone, or its equivalent, taken for longer than 7 to 10 days, has the potential for suppressing the HPA axis. If the glucocorticoid is stopped abruptly, the patient may experience an adrenal crisis (Hudak, Morton, Galle, & Fontaine, 2005).

Diagnostic Tests

In addition to the tests in Table 56-2, suppression and stimulation tests may be done to differentiate between primary and secondary insufficiency. The management of both of these types of insufficiency is linked closely to the outcomes of the diagnostic tests.

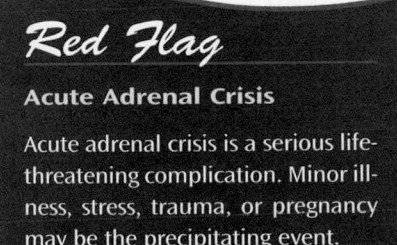

Red Flag

Acute Adrenal Crisis

Acute adrenal crisis is a serious life-threatening complication. Minor illness, stress, trauma, or pregnancy may be the precipitating event.

TABLE 56-2 **Comparison of Clinical Manifestations of Primary and Secondary Adrenal Insufficiency**

CLINICAL MANIFESTATION	PRIMARY	SECONDARY
Skin	Skin	Absent because there is a deficiency in ACTH
Hyperpigmentation due to an increase in ACTH secretion and melanocyte stimulation	Present	
Loss of axillary and pubic hair due to decrease in androgens	May occur	
Cardiovascular Hypotension with orthostatic symptoms (lower peripheral resistance)	Present	Usually not present because aldosterone secretion is usually not deficiency
Occasionally syncope due to loss of mineralocorticoid activity		Hypotension may occur in acute situations
Neurological: Anxiety and mental irritability		
GI	Present	Present
Anorexia, nausea, vomiting		
Musculoskeletal myalgias, arthralgias	Present	May occur
Reproductive amenorrhea	Often present	
Hyponatremia	Present	May occur due to water retention
Hyperkalemia	Present	Not present
Hypoglycemia	May be provoked by fasting, infection, fever, and so on	Usually not present
Deficiencies in thyroxin, testosterone, and GH	Not present because pituitary deficiency is not the problem	Possible if pituitary or hypothalamus dysfunction is present
Plasma cortisol less than 5 mg/dL at 8 a.m.	Yes	Yes
ACTH Level	Greater than 200 pg/mL	Low or normal
Antibodies	Antiadrenal antibodies present in autoimmune Addison's disease	

Adapted from Aron., D., Finding, J. Tyrell, B. (2004). Hypothalamus and pituitary. In F.S. Greenspan & D. G. Gardner (Eds.), Basic and clinical endocrinology (pp. 537–542). St. Louis, MO: Lange Medical Books.

Nursing Diagnoses

Based on the information gathered, examples of nursing diagnoses in the patient with adrenal insufficiency may include the following:
- Activity intolerance related to weakness and fatigue.
- Deficient knowledge related to disease and treatment.
- Risk for injury related to syncope from hypotension.
- Deficient fluid volume related to sodium depletion.

Planning and Implementation

The patient who presents in an adrenal crisis must be provided with aggressive care. Major goals include restoration of extracellular fluid volume, reversal of shock, and replacement of corticosteroids and mineralcorticoids. Monitor cardiovascular and respiratory status, urinary output, and neurological status every hour. Provide fluids and electrolytes to restore fluid balance and correct hypoglycemia. Electrocardiogram (ECG) monitoring should be instituted to assess the cardiac effects of hyperkalemia and hypercalcemia. Hyperkalemia and acidosis are usually corrected with replacement of fluid volume and cortisol levels. The electrolytes and creatinine should be monitor daily and as needed. Environmental stress should be minimized. Dietary assessment should be completed and caloric nutrients provided as tolerated. Nausea and anorexia should resolve with the normalizing of cortisol levels.

Goals

The following are goals for the patient with adrenal insufficiency:
- The patient will state the rationale for lifelong therapy.
- The patient will state the rationale for increasing corticosteroid dosage in the event of illness or stress.
- The patient will give the rationale for seeking medical assistance in the event that oral medication cannot be taken during time of illness.
- The patient will be normotensive.
- The patient will have a normal electrolyte profile.
- The patient will have access to a medical alert identification.

Pharmacology

Patients who have adrenal insufficiency need to be taught to adhere carefully to medication plan for hydrocortisone and fludrocortisone replacement. They will need an increase in dosage during stress or illness. With minor illness, the cortisol dose should be increased to 60 to 80 mg/day. The patient should avoid fasting and may need to increase his or her salt intake. It is recommended that the patient with adrenal insufficiency keep a kit with hydrocortisone for self-injection in an emergency and in the event that oral intake is not possible. The patient should wear a medical alert bracelet at all times. Family members need to be taught emergency care (Broyles, et al., 2007).

The patient who has adrenal insufficiency due to an ACTH insufficiency will require only glucocorticoid replacement. Mineralocorticoid replacement is not necessary. Patients who are receiving exogenous corticosteroids should be instructed to taper the dosage gradually, decreasing the dosage daily to allow the adrenal gland to return to normal function. This will help to prevent a secondary adrenal insufficiency. Patients treated with corticosteroids should be monitored for osteoporosis. A minimum maintenance dose is recommended because research shows there is a correlation between high corticosteroid dose and bone loss.

Evaluation of Outcomes

Potential patient outcomes for each of the example nursing diagnoses for the patient with adrenal insufficiency are:
- Activity intolerance related to weakness and fatigue. Patient will identify measures to conserve energy.
- Deficient knowledge related to disease and treatment. Patient will discuss pertinent information concerning the disease and treatment.
- Risk for injury related to syncope from hypotension. Patient will identify and implement measures to prevent syncope episodes.
- Deficient fluid volume related to sodium depletion. Patient will have normal fluid and electrolyte balance.

HYPERSECRETION OF THE ADRENAL GLAND (HYPERALDOSTERONISM)

An increased stimulation of the adrenal glands may lead to hyperaldosteronism. There are a variety of causes for this disorder and there are serious implications for patients with hyperaldosteronism.

Epidemiology

One to two percent of the patients who have hypertension have primary aldosteronism. It occurs more often in females (Ferri, 2005).

Etiology

Primary aldosteronism may be due to a unilateral adrenal adenoma or bilateral hyperplasia of the adrenal glands. Sixty percent of the cases are caused by an aldosterone producing adenoma. Other causes are aldosterone-producing carcinoma, glucocorticoid-suppressible hyperaldosteronism, and idiopathic hyperaldosteronism, which cause more than 30 percent of the cases (Ferri, 2005).

Pathophysiology

Involvement of the zona glomerulosa causes an increase production of aldosterone, which initiates a cascade of events that includes retention of sodium and fluid and potassium depletion. With the expansion of extracellular fluid, there is an increase in cardiac output and subsequent hypertension. As mineralocorticoid excess continues, there is an increase in total peripheral vascular resistance that contributes to the problem of hypertension (Huether, 2004).

Assessment with Clinical Manifestations

There are no characteristic physical manifestations that occur with excessive mineralocorticoids. Patients usually are diagnosed with mild to severe hypertension. Some patients may have only an elevation in diastolic pressure. Their primary complaint may be that of nonspecific loss of energy, weakness, and lassitude. In situations in which potassium depletion is more severe, dysrhythmias, decrease in gastric motility, polyuria, polydipsia, and paresthesia may be reported. Because the most common cause of hypokalemia in patients with hypertension is diuretic therapy, diuretic therapy would need to be discontinued for up to three weeks to accurately evaluate the serum potassium. Other causes of hypertension and hypokalemia must be eliminated when diagnosing hyperaldosteronism. Excessive ingestion of real licorice, oral contraceptives, Cushing's syndrome, and renal vascular disease can cause hypertension and hypokalemia (Burl, Schambelan, & Lo, 2004).

Diagnostic Tests

Urinary aldosterone excretion over a 24-hour period best measures aldosterone production. Plasma aldosterone levels should be drawn around 8:00 a.m. while the patient is supine after overnight recumbency. A plasma renin test must be done at the same time. For both urinary and serum testing for aldosterone, it is important that the patient receive normal salt intake with NaCl supplementation, because with any decrease in salt intake aldosterone production will increase causing a high serum aldosterone level and increase urinary excretion. A low plasma renin (less than 5 mcg/dL) with a 24-hour urinary test for aldosterone greater than 20 mcg/dL indicates hyperaldosteronism A plasma aldosterone greater than 20 mcg/dL supports a diagnosis of adrenal adenoma (Burl, et al., 2004).

Following a positive serum and urine test for hyperaldosteronism, a CT scan of the adrenals can identify the presence of an adenoma with 80 percent success. In the event that the CT scan is negative, adrenal vein catheterization for aldosterone or radioisotope test can be utilized for confirming diagnosis.

Nursing Diagnoses

Based on the information gathered, examples of nursing diagnoses in the patient with hyperaldosteronism may include the following:
- Fatigue related to weakness secondary to hypokalemia.
- Activity intolerance related to weakness secondary to hypokalemia.
- Decreased cardiac output related to alteration in cardiac contraction and dysrhythmias secondary to hypokalemia.
- Excess fluid volume related to sodium retention due to excess aldosterone.

Planning and Implementation

Because hypokalemia can cause cardiac conduction abnormalities, the patient with hyperaldosteronism needs to have continuous cardiac monitoring. Serum potassium levels are monitored sometimes as often as every four to six hours. Because the body cannot conserve potassium, it has to be replaced daily. Cardiac and respiratory assessment should be completed every four hours or more often as needed. Monitor vital signs in relation to activity. Daily weights and intake and output are important interventions for assessing fluid balance. Provide assistance with activities of daily living since the patient may have increasing muscle weakness related to the hypokalemia. Assess for signs and symptoms of hypertension as indicated. Lying, sitting, and standing blood pressure monitoring may be necessary if the patient has symptoms of orthostatic hypotension, which may occur with some antihypertensive medications. Discharge instructions for the patient are shown in the Patient Playbook feature.

Pharmacology

Patients with aldosterone-producing adenomas are treated with spironolactone until the blood pressure and serum K^+ are normal. Spironolactone blocks the mineralocorticoid receptor, reducing extracellular fluid volume, and promotes potassium retention. Patients diagnosed with aldosterone-producing adenoma are recommended to have a unilateral adrenalectomy if there are no contraindications. Following a unilateral adrenalectomy, blood pressure and electrolytes must be monitored frequently. Several months may elapse before blood pressure and electrolytes, particularly potassium becomes normal.

Evaluation of Outcomes

Potential patient outcomes for each of the example nursing diagnoses for the patient with hyperaldosteronism are:
- Fatigue related to weakness secondary to hypokalemia. Patient will demonstrate improved energy; potassium level will be normal.
- Activity intolerance related to weakness secondary to hypokalemia. Patient will daily increase participation in activities of daily.
- Decreased cardiac output, related to alteration in cardiac contraction and dysrhythmias secondary to hypokalemia. Patient will have normal cardiac output as indicated with normal vital signs and sinus rhythm.
- Excess fluid volume related to sodium retention due to excess aldosterone. Patient will have absence of signs and symptoms of fluid volume excess.

Pheochromocytoma

A pheochromocytoma is a tumor of the adrenal gland that secretes catecholamines. It is affecting and causes severe hypertension with those patients that are afflicted with this disorder.

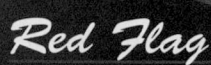

Red Flag

Diagnosing Pheochromocytomas

Consider the possibility of pheochromocytomas when the patient has severe hypertension and suspicious symptoms, such as, palpitations, diaphoresis, headache lasting minutes to hours, and chest or abdominal pain that is not explainable. More than one third of patients who have pheochromocytomas die from a stroke or cardiac arrhythmia prior to diagnosis.

Epidemiology

Though considered a rare disorder, pheochromocytomas are found in less than 0.1 percent of hypertensive individuals; autopsy suggests a higher incidence. A rare endocrine disorder, pheochromocytomas occur in two patients per million people annually. Pheochromocytomas occur most often in the fourth or fifth decade; males are more frequently affected.

Patients who should be screened for pheochromocytoma include young hypertensives, patients with symptoms of catecholamine excess, marked liability of blood pressure, family history, shock or severe hypotensive episodes with surgery, anesthesia, or antihypertensive drugs. The signs and symptoms result from persistent hypersecretion of catecholamines (epinephrine or norepinephrine) by the tumor.

Assessment with Clinical Manifestations

Most adult patients have paroxysmal symptoms that may last minutes or hours. Symptoms begin abruptly and slowly subside. Severe headache, palpitations, and profuse sweating are the most common symptoms. In addition, patients can have palpitations, chest discomfort, anxiety, visual disturbances, constipation, weight loss, and cold hands or feet. Greater than 30 percent of pheochromocytomas cause a fatal cardiac arrhythmia or stroke prior to diagnosis.

Diagnostic Tests

A single 24-hour urine specimen to measure catecholamines, specifically metanephrines, is the most common and sensitive test for diagnosing pheochromocytoma. Typically, patients with pheochromocytomas have elevations of catecholamines or metanephrines that are more than twice normal, particularly after a paroxysmal episode.

CT scan is used to detect adrenal pheochromocytomas. If not found on the adrenal gland, CT scanning is used to scan the whole pelvis, abdomen, and chest. MRI is not as sensitive but is considered a safer test because it can be done without contrast.

Nursing Diagnoses

Based on the information gathered, examples of nursing diagnoses in the patient with pheochromocytoma may include the following:
- Risk for injury related to hypertension leading to stroke and cardiovascular events.
- Anxiety related to excess catecholamines.

Planning and Implementation

Monitoring the patient's vital signs along with neurovascular, cardiac, and respiratory assessment is a priority in caring for the patient with a pheochromocytoma. Because patients may experience orthostatic hypotension, they must be instructed to rise slowly and recognize symptoms to avoid falls.

Preparing the patient psychologically and physically for upcoming surgery should be included in the plan of care. Patients need to be instructed in the rationale and side effects of medications used to control symptoms prior to surgery. The patient should have blood pressure readings in lying, sitting, and standing positions as the blood pressure medications are increased.

Postoperative complications include shock and cardiovascular collapse. Large volumes of saline or colloids may be needed to regain extracellular volume. In some incidences intravenous norepinephrine may be required. Blood glucose should be monitored. Hypoglycemia may be prevented by administering dextrose solutions.

Goals

Goals for patients with pheochromocytoma are:
- The patient will demonstrate blood pressure monitoring.
- The patient will state plan to monitor blood pressure daily and report abnormal findings.
- The patient will convey an understanding for follow-up within designated times following surgery for a 24-hour urine collection to determine fractionated catecholamines, metaphrines, and creatinine.
- Abnormal levels of catecholamines and elevation of blood pressure may indicate that the tumor has recurred and indicates a need for more thorough work-up.

Pharmacology

The risks involved with pheochromocytoma surgery are decreased by the administration of alpha-adrenergic blocking drugs. Calcium channel blockers and alpha-adrenergic blockers, such as phenoxybenzamine and angiotensin-converting enzyme (ACE) inhibitors, each may play a role in treating the hypertension occurring with a pheochromocytoma. A beta-adrenergic blocker, such as propranolol, is used for treating the symptoms, such as tachycardia, palpitations, and flushing.

Surgery

The treatment of choice is laparoscopic removal of the tumor(s) under 6 cm in diameter. With laparoscopic surgery, the patient generally has a shorter time for eating to resume, reduced postoperative pain, and fewer hospitalization days. A laparotomy may be necessary if the tumor is large and invasive.

The major postoperative complication from pheochromocytoma surgery is shock and hypoglycemia. To treat shock, large volumes of intravenous normal saline or colloids may be used. Some incidences require intravenous norepinephrine. Hypoglycemia is prevented by postoperative infusion of dextrose 5% in water at 100 mL/hour.

Evaluation of Outcomes

Potential patient outcomes for each of the example nursing diagnoses for the patient with pheochromocytoma are:
- Risk for injury related to hypertension leading to stroke and cardiovascular events. Patient's blood pressure will be within safe parameters.
- Anxiety related to excess catecholamines. Patient will report a decrease in symptoms of anxiety.

THYROID DISORDERS

Thyroid hormones influence all major body systems, thus alteration in function can have a widespread effect on the body. Patients may present with symptoms of thyroid deficiency or excess, which affect cardiac and neurological function as well as overall energy. Other patients may have thyroid enlargement. Complications of thyroid disease may be the first symptom to be identified, such as exophthalmos that occurs with Graves' disease or cardiac problems, which occur with hypothyroidism. It is not uncommon for the patient to have cardiac or mental changes because of an excess or deficit in thyroid hormone. The diagnosis may be difficult because symptoms are often insipidus and ill-defined (Greenspan, 2004).

Hypersecretion of the Thyroid Gland

Frequently seen in primary care, 0.5 percent of Americans have hyperthyroidism. Though not the same, hyperthyroidism and thyrotoxicosis are often used interchangeably. Hyperthyroidism refers to the continuous secretion of thyroid hormones by the thyroid gland with resultant abnormal elevation of triiodothyronine (T_3) and thyroxine (T_4) hormones and an abnormally low TSH level. Thyrotoxicosis is a term used for the acceleration of metabolism with toxic manifestations that occur when thyroid hormones are extremely elevated. Subclinical hyperthyroidism is a term used to define a situation in which the patient has a low TSH, normal free T_4, and free T_3 levels with few or no clinical manifestations (White, 2004).

Epidemiology

Graves' disease (diffuse toxic goiter) is the most common cause of thyrotoxicosis. This disorder occurs most often in women between and during the second through fourth decade.

Etiology

Diseases that cause overproduction of thyroid hormones include Graves' disease (diffuse toxic goiter), toxic multinodular goiter, follicular adenoma, and pituitary adenoma. Destruction of the thyroid gland with subsequent release of stored hormones occurs in lymphocytic thyroiditis and Hashimoto's thyroiditis. Administration of exogenous thyroid medications or excessive exposure of iodine in drugs, such as amiodarone or radiopaque dyes, are other causes for hyperthyroidism.

Pathophysiology

Hyperthyroid disease may occur due to overproduction of thyroid hormone or because of destruction of the thyroid gland. In Graves' disease, a TSH receptor autoantibody stimulates the thyroid gland to produce high concentrations of T_3 and T_4. The thyroid gland is enlarged and there is a marked increase in vascularity. Considered a familial disease, 50 percent of patients have close relatives who have circulating thyroid autoantibodies and 15 percent of patients have a close relative with the same diseases (Greenspan, 2004). Other autoimmune diseases that may be associated with Graves' disease are diabetes mellitus, pernicious anemia, vitiligo, and myasthenia gravis (Lingappa, 2003).

Assessment with Clinical Manifestations

The clinical manifestations of Graves' disease occur because of the excessive activity of T_3 and T_4 hormones, which cause a hypermetabolic state with an increase in oxygen consumption. There is also an increase in sympathetic nervous system activity, which suggests that the body is hyperreactive to catecholamines. All body tissues are affected, as demonstrated by the clinical manifestations described in Table 56-3. Common clinical manifestations include enlarged thyroid gland, cardiac palpitations, fatigue, excessive perspiration, heat intolerance, and weight loss without a loss of appetite, and eye changes. Eye disease (ophthalmopathy) may range from lid lag and soft tissue and extraocular muscle problems to involvement of the cornea and some vision loss.

Diagnostic Tests

There are several tests (refer to Table 56-4) used to detect thyroid disease. The most sensitive and cost-effective test is serum TSH. Combined use of the third-generation assay TSH test and T_4 provide the highest sensitivity and specificity for diagnosing thyroid disorders. An elevation of FT_4 and a suppressed TSH supports a diagnosis of hyperthyroidism. Eye signs plus an elevation of FT_4 and a suppressed TSH support a diagnosis of Graves' disease. Additional tests for Graves' disease include thyroid autoantibodies. Both Graves' disease and Hashimoto's thyroiditis will be positive for TgAb and TPO Ab, but TSH-R Ab is specific for Grave's disease (Greenspan, 2004).

TABLE 56-3 Assessment of the Patient with Thyrotoxicosis or Graves' Disease

HISTORY	PHYSICAL FINDINGS
History of other autoimmune diseases	
Medications:	Nails—ridges; discolored, splitting.
Skin: Heat intolerance. Change in temperature preference. Change in nails and hair. Pruritus	Moist warm skin. Hair loss, fine consistency. Hyperpigmentation of lower extremities. Oily skin
HEENT: Prior neck radiation, thyroid surgery, family history of thyroid disease. Presence of neck lumps, fullness, tenderness, or swelling: onset, location, size texture. Increased prominence of the eyes, difficulty swallowing. Puffiness in periorbital area. Blurred or double vision. Increase in lacrimation	Enlarged thyroid gland or goiter. Eyes: Ophthalmopathy: **Proptosis** (forward placement of the eye) (unilaterally or bilaterally), lid retraction. Diplopia, redness, congestion, conjunctival and periorbital edema.
Gritty sensation in eyes	Hyperactive reflex response
Neuromuscular: insomnia, irritability, nervousness, lethargy, or muscular weakness	Fine motor tremor
	Low bone mineral density
Skeletal:	Supraventricular dysrhythmias, atrial fibrillation, increase systolic blood, tachycardia at rest, "high output" congestive heart failure, murmur; decrease in vital capacity
CV: palpitations, tachycardia,	
Resp: shortness of breathe, exertional dyspnea	Documented high caloric intake with weight loss.
GI: Increased frequency of bowel movements. Excessive appetite with high caloric intake	
Reproductive: Diminished or scant menses	
Psychosocial: Emotional lability, mania and psychosis	
General: Fatigue, weight loss	

Adapted from Estes, M. (2006). Health assessment and physical examination (3rd ed.). New York: Thomson Delmar Learning.

Nursing Diagnoses

Based on the information gathered, examples of nursing diagnoses in the patient with hyperthyroidism may include the following:
- Anxiety related to fear of the unknown.
- Deficient knowledge related to disease and treatment (radioactive iodine therapy or surgery).

Planning and Implementation

Following assessment and diagnosis of the patient with Graves' disease, nursing management includes planning and implementation of a plan of care, which will decrease the patient's body metabolism, prevent tissue and organ damage, and restore normal body function. A collaborative approach between

TABLE 56-4 **Diagnostic Tests for Thyroid Function**

TESTS	RATIONALE
Serum T_4 Normal value: 5–12 mcg/dL	Measures by direct assay the biologically active thyroxine capable of binding with a T_3 or T_4 receptor Increased in hyperthyroidism
Serum Total T_3 Normal value: 80–200 ng/dL	Measures total amount of circulating T_3
TSH Normal 0.31–5 mLU/L	Third-generation assay is best indicator of endogenous thyroid function Undetectable or less than 10 in hyperthyroid patients is high; greater than 7 in hypothyroid patients is high. Exogenous corticosteroids and dopamine may suppress TSH
Thyroid scan	Tests the capacity of thyroid cells to trap and store iodine. Differentiates between the thyroid glands ability to trap iodine throughout the gland or whether a hypofunctioning cold nodule or hyperfunctioning hot nodule is present. Can differentiate between functioning metastasis and thyroid carcinoma
Thyroid antibodies	Antibodies against thyroid peroxidase enzyme or against thyroglobulin are frequently found in patients with Graves' disease and Hashimoto's thyroiditis
Radioactive iodine uptake (RIU)	Measures quantitatively the ability of the thyroid gland to confine radioactive iodine. The patient is administered a dosage of iodine; 24 hours later, the absorption is measured. RIU is elevated in patients with Graves' disease, multinodular goiter, or autonomous nodule
Thyroid sonogram	Distinguishes cystic from solid lesions Identify and define the size or number of thyroid nodule(s). Use for follow-up evaluation of nodules
Fine needle biopsy	Rule out cancer when nodule is present
CT scan or MRI	Diagnose substernal extension of nodule or identify deep thyroid nodules

Adapted from Daniels, R. (2003). Delmar's manual of laboratory and diagnostic tests. New York: Thomson Delmar Learning.

the nurse, health care providers, and dietitian is of paramount importance. The patient with thyrotoxicosis has several major nursing problems.

A nutrition imbalance that is often less than body requirements related to high metabolic needs is a major concern. Weight loss is often pronounced. The outcome for the patient is that the patient will have cessation of weight loss and will continue to gain until normal weight has been acquired. The patient with hyperthyroidism needs to have a thorough nutritional assessment. In collaboration with a dietitian, calorie count should be carried out and a plan be formulated for caloric intake that will meet nutritional demands.

Consultation with the dietitian to determine ways of increasing intake of high-energy foods will be beneficial. A prealbumin test helps to determine the body's protein reserve or deficit. The patient may need 4,000 to 6,000 calories a day or more to meet metabolic needs. Provision for six meals daily should be implemented. Daily weights are an essential part of the care. Interventions for nutritional needs include nutrition management.

Because of the increased energy requirements, the patient is fatigued and may be to the point of exhaustion. The patient's physical limitations should be assessed, and a plan should be developed to ensure adequate time for rest. Inform the patient that as the hypermetabolic state decreases, rest and relaxation will be easier. Interventions recommended for fatigue include energy management and sleep enhancement.

Anxiety is a common problem with the patient who has Graves' disease because to CNS irritability. Promotion of optimum rest and relaxation will assist in decreasing the patient's anxiety. Knowledge of the disease process and proposed treatment outcomes will help to decrease fears related to the symptoms that the patient is experiencing. Treatment with beta-adrenergic blockers will decrease the sympathetic response and reduce some of the symptoms of anxiety. Other interventions for anxiety include simple massage, relaxation therapy, and guided imagery.

Two major complications associated with Graves' disease are ophthalmopathy and toxic storm. Ocular manifestations including proptosis may occur as the extraocular muscles and tissue within the orbit enlarge due to infiltrative changes and edema. Paralysis of the extraocular muscles, damage to the retina and optic nerve may also occur. (Huether, 2004). The patient may experience a gritty sensation in the eye, diplopia, photophobia, lacrimation, inflammation, and edema. Catecholamine excess is thought to contribute to lid lag and stare that is associated with Graves' disease. With some patients, the eye symptoms regress as the hyperthyroidism is brought under control. Time and reassurance may be all that are needed. More severe ophthalmopathy will require aggressive therapy. Removal or destruction of the thyroid gland is recommended to prevent recurrence of thyrotoxicosis, which can reactivate residual ophthalmopathy (Greenspan, 2004). Other treatments include glucocorticoids to modify the immune response and treat the inflammation, orbital radiation therapy, plasmapheresis to remove circulating pathogenic antibodies, and decompression surgery to allow orbital tissue to expand into adjacent areas. Extraocular and or cosmetic surgery may be required to correct eyelid malposition. Minor degrees of diplopia may require special lenses.

A nursing priority in caring for the patient with ophthalmopathy is to protect the eye from injury. Nursing interventions include instructing the patient to protect the cornea against wind-borne particles, suggesting tinted or dark glasses to relieve light sensitivity, and providing artificial tears or ointment to decrease the sensation of having a foreign body in the eye. A protective shield and light taping of the lid at night with nonallergic tape may help to protect the cornea. Elevation of the head at night may help to alleviate periorbital edema.

Thyroid Crisis (Thyroid Storm)

Thyroid crisis or thyroid storm is a serious form of thyrotoxicosis, which is life-threatening. It is most likely to occur in people who have been inadequately treated or undiagnosed. Infection, stress or emotional trauma, pregnancy, comorbidity, or medications may precipitate this event. Clinical manifestations include: extremely high fever, severe neurological signs and symptoms (e.g., restlessness, delirium, agitation, psychosis, and coma) and cardiovascular problems (e.g., atrial fibrillation, heart failure, and angina). Most patients will have a high systolic blood pressure with a wide pulse pressure. One of the earliest clues to the onset of a thyroid storm is high fever and diaphoresis, which is out of proportion to an infection.

Patients with thyroid storm should be treated in the intensive care unit. It is important that expedient treatment be provided. Respiratory support should be provided immediately. Hemodynamic instability is a major priority. Intravenous access is a priority to correct volume and electrolyte depletion and administer nutrition as indicated. Vasopressors may be ordered to restore or maintain blood pressure. The nurse must be prepared to implement measures to treat congestive heart failure. Measures to reduce fever must be immediately implemented. A cooling blanket and the administration of acetaminophen as ordered is standard care.

Treatment includes adrenergic blocking drugs to interrupt the sympathetic nervous system effects. Drugs to inhibit synthesis of thyroid hormones and block production and secretion are utilized for treating thyroid storm. Because the patient may experience adrenal insufficiency with the stress related to the thyroid storm, glucocorticoids, such as hydrocortisone may be prescribed. Effort is made to identify any underlying disease that may have precipitated the storm, and antiallergy, antibiotics, and special postoperative care may be indicated. Aspirin should be avoided, because it displaces free thyroxin from protein carriers and releases more thyroxin into circulation. Heart failure may be treated with digoxin and diuretics. Plasmapheresis, or peritoneal dialysis, is emergency measures that may be implemented to remove circulating antibodies (Greenspan, 2004)

In elders the most frequent complications that present with hyperthyroidism are cardiovascular, including atrial fibrillation, congestive heart failure, angina, and acute myocardial infarction or CNS symptoms, such as apathy, depression, and confusion. A hypermetabolic state may be present with muscle wasting. Bone loss and fractures are other problems. Readjustments of medications may be necessary because an increase in metabolism may alter dose requirements (Greenspan & Resnick, 2004).

Pharmacology

Treatment of Graves' disease includes radioiodine therapy, surgery, and antithyroid medications. Newly diagnosed patients are placed on thiamazole (antithyroid drugs) medications to correct their hypermetabolic state. Examples of the thiamazole are propylthiouracil (PTU) and methimazole. These drugs are used to assist the patient to reach a euthyroid state. Young patients with small glands and mild symptoms respond most readily to medication. Outcome of therapy with the antithyroid drugs is variable. Though in many incidences the treatment is effective, there can be serious side effects to the antithyroid medications. The thioamides can cause agranulocytosis; therefore, the patients have to be monitored carefully for leukopenia. PTU can cause liver injury. Prior to the treatment, the patient should have a baseline complete blood count, comprehensive metabolic profile, including liver function test and a thyroid panel (TSH; free T_4; total T_3). PTU is the drug of choice for treating hyperthyroidism in a pregnant or breastfeeding patient, because it has limited transfer across the placenta or into breast milk. Methimazole promotes compliance because of once a day dosing. Nursing interventions for the patient receiving thioamides involve the following assessing for thrombocytopenia and hepatotoxicity; teaching the patient to report symptoms of adverse reactions: skin rash, yellowing of eyes, sore throat, chills, fever, or painful joints; reporting bruising or unexplained bleeding; and instructing patient about the importance of frequent laboratory tests to detect adverse effects and response to treatment.

In addition to the thioamides, patients can receive beta blockers (e.g., propranolol, atenolol) to decrease the beta-adrenergic activity of a stimulated thyroid gland. The beta blockers may be contraindicated for patients with congestive heart failure, asthma, or diabetes. The nurse must monitor the heart rate and blood pressure. In addition, the nurse must assist the patient alleviate symptoms of anxiety, palpitations, tremor, and heat intolerance. Side effects of

Nursing Strategies for Radioiodine Tests

The nurse should instruct the patient:

Before the test: verify that the patient is not pregnant and advise the patient to avoid pregnancy for six months and be aware that allergies to iodine do not contraindicate use.

After the test: instruct the patient to avoid sharing food and eating utensils, avoid having close contact with children and kissing for several days, flush toilet twice after use, and avoid breastfeeding.

Adapted from Grigsby, P. W. (2004). Thyroid. In C. Perez, E. Halperm, L. Brady, R. Schmidt-Ullrich (Eds.), Principles and practices of radiation oncology (pp. 211–215). New York: Lippincott, Williams & Williams.

beta blockers include nausea, headache, fatigue, insomnia, hypotension, bradycardia, and dysrhythmias.

A last type of medication to treat thyroid conditions is potassium iodide (SSKI). This medication blocks thyroid hormone release by decreasing vascularity preoperatively before thyroid surgery. The nursing implication for this medication is to assess for allergies to iodine and shellfish. In addition, the nurse can disguise the iodine taste by diluting in water or juice. Lithium carbonate may be given if prescribed as an alternative to iodine (Broyles, et. al., 2007).

Radioiodine Therapy

Radioiodine therapy is the treatment of choice in the United States for hyperthyroidism in patients over 21 years and for patients who have not responded to antithyroid therapy. Pregnant patients are absolutely contraindicated from having radioiodine therapy. Prior to 131I therapy, patients may require antithyroid agents for the purpose of obtaining a **euthyroid** state (having a normal functioning thyroid gland). To reach a euthyroid state, methimazole rather than propylthiouracil is the preferred drug, because the inhibitory effect of methimazole on radioiodine uptake dissipates in 24 hours. The antithyroid drug is stopped for five to seven days prior to the treatment with radioactive iodine. Iodine therapy may also be prescribed prior to the radioiodine therapy (see prethyroidectomy care). Prior to the therapy, a radioactive iodine uptake measurement is performed to determine the appropriate dose of 131I. Following the therapy, 80 percent of patients who are adequately treated with radioiodine therapy will develop hypothyroidism This complication of therapy actually may be considered beneficial because the patient will no longer be susceptible to Grave's disease. The patient will need to be monitored for hypothyroidism and when diagnosed be treated promptly with replacement thyroid medication (Greenspan, 2004). A variety of nursing strategies are shown in the Patient Playbook feature.

Surgery

Though surgery is rarely required for patients with thyroid disorders, a subtotal thyroidectomy may be the treatment of choice for patients with large glands or multinodular goiters or for patients who fail other treatments (Figure 56-4). Prior to surgery, the patient will be prescribed antithyroid medications to promote a euthyroid state; this usually takes around six weeks. Saturated solution of potassium iodide may be administered to reduce the vascularity of the gland (Greenspan, 2004).

Prior to thyroid surgery, the patient needs thorough preoperative teaching. An explanation regarding the medications prescribed, their action, side effects, and such should be provided. The importance of compliance to the treatment should be stressed. Ample time should be provided to answer questions. The patient will have concerns and fears about the site of the incision and the scar that may be present afterward. The patient can be reassured that minimal scarring should be present; a scarf or necklace will most likely cover the site. Complications of thyroid surgery include hypoparathyroidism, bleeding, and injury to the recurrent laryngeal nerve.

Priority in care postoperatively is prevention and detection of complications. Assess for respiratory distress, which may occur due to hemorrhage and edema, or laryngeal spasms, which may occur if there is injury to the parathyroid glands during surgery resulting in hypocalcemia and tetany. The unit code cart should be available in the event that intubation or tracheostomy is warranted.

The patient should be assessed for early symptoms of hypocalcemia. Symptoms and signs include paresthesia of the mouth, toes, fingers; generalized muscle twitching; and positive Chvostek's and Trousseau's signs. Intravenous calcium gluconate or calcium chloride should be on hand for treatment of hypocalcemia. Ionized calcium levels should be drawn to moni-

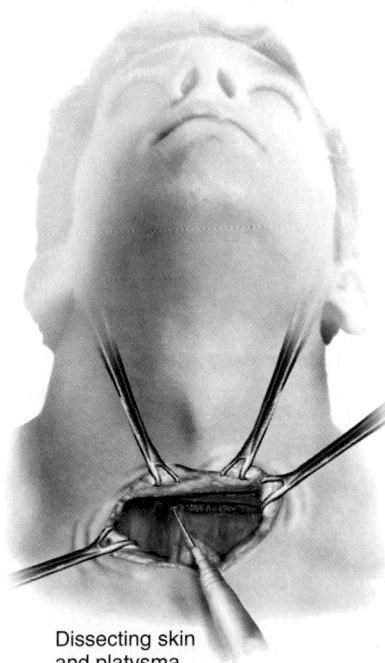

Dissecting skin and platysma

Figure 56-4 Thyroidectomy.

tor calcium. Though hoarseness may be the result of irritation due to intubation during surgery, there is potential for injury to the laryngeal nerve, which can cause permanent hoarseness.

Evaluation of Outcomes

Potential patient outcomes for each of the example nursing diagnoses for the patient with hyperthyroidism are:

- Anxiety related to fear of the unknown. Patient will report signs of anxiety and relate a decrease in symptoms of anxiety.
- Deficient knowledge related to disease and treatment (radioactive iodine therapy or surgery). Patient will verbalize an understanding of disease and treatment.

Nontoxic Goiter

Nontoxic goiter is the enlargement of the thyroid gland from TSH stimulation, which occurs due to inadequate thyroid hormone synthesis. At one time it was prevalent in the United States because of iodine deficiency. Though the problem is no longer common in the United States, because of the wide availability of iodine in food sources, there are still large areas of the world where iodine intake is deficient. Daily iodine requirements for adults range from 150 to 300 mcg a day. Other causes for nontoxic goiter include Goitrogen diet, Hashimoto's thyroiditis, neoplasm (benign and malignant), and inherited defect in thyroid hormone synthesis (Greenspan, 2004).

Thyroiditis

Thyroiditis may be classified as chronic lymphocytic (Hashimoto's) thyroiditis due to autoimmunity, subacute thyroiditis, suppurative thyroiditis, and Riedel's thyroiditis. The most common form of thyroiditis in the United States is Hashimoto's thyroiditis. A familial disease, it is six times more common in women.

Clinical manifestations of Hashimoto's thyroiditis include a diffuse, enlarged firm and nodular thyroid gland. The patient often complains of painless neck tightness. Thyroid function tests are variable. Antithyroid antibody tests are usually positive. Rarely, the patient may present with thyrotoxicosis due to destruction of thyroid tissue and sudden release of thyroid hormones. Most often the patient progresses to hypothyroidism, which is 95 percent of the time permanent.

Thyroid Nodules and Neoplasms

Other disorders of the thyroid gland are nodules and neoplasms. Either of these anomalies requires treatment and have varying levels of affects on the patients with these conditions.

Epidemiology

It is estimated that 4 percent of the adult population has a thyroid nodule, and there is a gender relationship for incidence of thyroid cancer (Greenspan, 2004). Women are more prone to thyroid nodules than men.

Etiology

Causes of thyroid nodules include: adenomas, cysts, carcinomas, multinodular goiters, Hashimoto's thyroiditis, and subacute thyroiditis (Braimon, Naaznin, Lokhandwala, & Walczak, 2003). Follicular adenoma, a solitary firm nodule, up to 5 cm, is the most common nodule occurring in the thyroid gland. It accounts for 30 percent of all nodules. In less than 10 percent of follicular adenomas, malignant change will occur. Cancer of the thyroid occurs more often in women and is rare (0.0004 percent). Cancers are classified as either papillary or follicular; these types are often mixed. Other types are Hürthle cell, anaplastic, and medulla (Table 56-5).

Predisposing factors to thyroid cancer include childhood exposure to radiation in the head or neck and genetic predisposition. Children exposed to high degrees of radiation during the Chernobyl accident have had a high incidence of thyroid cancer. Papillary and follicular cancers usually pursue a long clinical course of 15 to 20 years. Papillary cancer tends to metastasize to regional lymph nodes in the neck, and follicular thyroid cancer follows a pattern of distant metastasizes to the lung or bone (Greenspan, 2004; Lingappa, 2003).

Planning and Implementation

Patients with papillary and follicular carcinoma can be classified into high- and low-risk groups. For patients under 45 who have primary lesions that are 1 cm or less in size and no evidence of metastasis, a lobectomy is standard of care. All other patients should be considered at high risk, and a total thyroidectomy is the recommended treatment. A modified neck resection may be recommended if there is any evidence of lymphatic spread. Following surgery it is usually recommended that the patient receive radioiodine ablation therapy for any remaining thyroid tissue. See Box 56-3 for management strategies for the patient receiving high dose radioactive therapy.

Thyroid suppression therapy has been shown to reduce growth of papillary or follicular thyroid cancer. Suppression therapy involves the prescribing of levothyroxine daily. With an increase in circulating thyroid hormone, the feedback to the pituitary gland will decrease the release of TSH, thereby depressing the function of the thyroid gland and hopefully the growth of the tumor, if it is TSH dependent. Radiation therapy may also be useful in situations in which the patient does not respond to other treatments (Greenspan, 2004). The National Cancer Institute outlines the staging and treatment of thyroid cancers.

Hypothyroidism

Hypothyroidism is a clinical state in which there is a deficient production of thyroid hormone by the thyroid gland. This disorder may be primary or secondary. All body functions are affected by a thyroid deficiency, which causes an

---

TABLE 56-5 Comparison of Benign and Malignant Thyroid Lesions

	BENIGN	MALIGNANT
History	Lives in area where goiter is endemic Family history of benign goiter	Family history of thyroid medullary cancer History of irradiation of neck or head Recently diagnosed with thyroid nodule Symptoms: hoarseness or dysphagia
Sex/Age	Female sex, older women	Male; child, young adults
Clinical manifestations	Soft nodule; multinodular goiter	Firm, usually single nodule different from other thyroid tissue; vocal cord paralysis, suspected metastases, and enlarged firm nodes
Thyroid scan	Hot nodule	Cold nodule
Echo	Cyst (pure)	Solid or semicystic
Fine needle biopsy	Cytologic exam—benign	Cytologic exam malignant
Levothyroxine therapy (TSH suppression therapy)	Decrease in size	No change

Adapted from Greenspan, F. S. (2004). The thyroid gland. In F.S. Greenspan & D. G. Gardner (Eds.), Basic and clinical endocrinology (pp. 215–294). St. Louis, MO: Lange Medical Books.

BOX 56-3

CARING FOR THE PATIENT RECEIVING HIGH-DOSE RADIOACTIVE IODINE THERAPY

1. Isolation principles are employed.
2. Patient wears foot coverings when ambulating.
3. The outer door is kept closed, and the bathroom door is kept open. (Flush twice after each use.)
4. Shower and wash hands frequently.
5. Personnel and visitors must wear gloves, gown, and mask, and the patient must wear hospital gown with a "chuck" wrapped around neck (visitors are discouraged, and no children or pregnant women are allowed entry).
6. If specimen is needed, urine should be collected in a lead container.
7. At 24 hours and 48 hours the patient's radiation level is measured. The radiation level must be less than 30 mC131 prior to discharge.
8. Patients should drink copious amounts of water to promote release of radioactive iodine.
9. Male patients are instructed to sit to void.
10. Because traces of radioactive iodine remains in the urine and blood up to a week, the patient is instructed to not have close contact with children; sleep alone; avoid prolonged intimate contact; practice good personal hygiene; launder linens, towel, and clothes daily; and avoid preparing food with bare hands.

Adapted from Grigsby, P. W. (2004). Thyroid. In C. Perez, E. Halperm, L. Brady, R. Schmidt-Ullrich (Eds.), Principles and practices of radiation oncology *(pp. 211–215). New York: Lippincott, Williams & Williams.*

---

overall decline in metabolic processes. The disease may present in a range from a mild form with vague symptoms to severe symptoms, which occur with myxedema. Early in the disease the most common symptoms are fatigue, weakness, lethargy, cold intolerance, constipation, and dry skin. As the disease progresses more physical manifestations occur, including puffy face and hands, hoarseness, slow mentation, and slow reflexes.

Epidemiology

Hypothyroidism is a common disease. One and one-half percent to 2 percent of women have the disease. It occurs in 0.2 percent of the male population. More commonly it is found in the elderly patients (over 60 years); 6 percent of women and 2.5 percent of men have laboratory evidence of hypothyroidism (Ferri, 2005).

Etiology

The most common cause of hypothyroidism is Hashimoto's thyroiditis. Other primary causes are due to thyroid failure and include thyroidectomy (surgical removal of thyroid gland), radioiodine therapy resulting in destruction of the gland, or congenital defects resulting in a deficiency of thyroid hormone during infancy. Certain medications, such as lithium (a drug used to treat mania) and antithyroid drugs used in treating hyperthyroid disease, can block synthesis of thyroid hormones. Ingestion of large amounts of iodine will also result in blockage of thyroid hormone production. Products that contain iodine in abnormal amounts include kelp tablets, iodide containing cough medicines, radiographic contrast media, and the antiarrhythmic drug amiodarone, which has 75 mg of iodine per 200 mg. Rarely, hypothyroidism occurs in the United States because of iodide. Secondary causes include diseases of the pituitary gland, such as a pituitary tumor, which results in deficiency or absence of TSH. Tertiary causes include an alteration in hypothalamus function resulting in a deficiency of thyrotropin and consequential decrease in TSH (Greenspan, 2004; Huether, 2004).

Assessment with Clinical Manifestations

A careful history should be taken from the patient and family. Information is obtained regarding the patient and their history of thyroid surgery, radioiodine therapy, or previous thyroid disease. Other common symptoms, which should be checked out for thyroid disease, are fatigue and unexplained weight gain (Table 56-6).

Diagnostic Tests

A diagnosis of primary hypothyroidism is supported by a low serum FT_4 and an elevated TSH (greater than 1). T_3 results may be in the normal range. If the hypothyroidism is due to a pituitary problem, the TSH will not be elevated and the FT_4 will be low.

TABLE 56-6 **System Assessment of Patient with Hypothyroidism**

CLINICAL MANIFESTATIONS OF HYPOTHYROIDISM	RATIONALE
General	Thyroid deficiency results in general metabolic depression and alters the function of almost all body system.
Skin	An increase in the deposition of protein polysaccharide complexes lead to retention of sodium and water causing puffiness.
Dry skin, puffy skin, and thin hair. Skin may have yellow tint. Cold intolerance and sometimes decrease in body temperature.	Loss of sweat and sebaceous gland secretion causes dryness. Reduction of carotene to vitamin A may give skin a yellowish tint. Decrease in metabolic rate, oxygen consumption, and heat production with a decrease circulation to the skin contributes to cold intolerance.
HEENT: Hoarseness, large tongue	Hoarseness may occur because of accumulation of mucopolysaccharides in the larynx.
Cardiac: Bradycardia or decreased cardiac output, cardiac enlargement	Interstitial edema, nonspecific myofibrillar swelling may lead to cardiac enlargement. Insufficient thyroid hormones results in interruption of normal cardiac contraction.
Respiratory: Shallow slow respirations	Decrease in thyroid hormone alters normal ventilatory responses to carbon dioxide and hypoxia. Respiratory muscle changes occur as thyroid deficiency continues. Pleural effusions may occur with the myxedematous changes.
GI: Chronic constipation	Altered GI motility and tone with decrease in secretion of digestive juices occurs with insufficient thyroid hormones.
Renal: Impaired ability to excrete fluid	Blood flow to the kidney is reduced with resultant decrease in filtration rate.
Neuromuscular: Paresthesia, muscle weakness, diminished DTR CNS: Confusion, fatigue, slow cognition	Decrease in muscular contraction and relaxation results in slow movement. Reduction in cerebral blood flow leads to cerebral hypoxia.
Genitourinary: Severe menorrhagia anovulatory cycles, impotence, and infertility in men	Alteration in the metabolism of estrogens and androgens.
Hematological: Normocytic, normochromic, and macrocytic anemia.	Decrease in RBC production; vitamin B_{12} deficiency; inadequate iron and folate absorption related to the deficiency in thyroid hormone with resultant decrease metabolic rate and decrease in oxygen requirements.

Adapted from Greenspan, F. S. (2004). The thyroid gland. In F.S. Greenspan & D. G. Gardner (Eds.), Basic and clinical endocrinology (pp. 215–294). St. Louis, MO: Lange Medical Books; Huether, S. E. (2004). Alterations of hormonal regulation. In S. E. Huether & K. L. McCance (Eds.), Understanding pathophysiology (pp. 356–362). St. Louis, MO: Mosby.

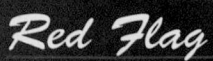

Red Flag

Subclinical Hypothyroidism

Subclinical hypothyroidism is defined as normal serum free T_3 and T_4 levels with TSH suppressed below the normal range. A detailed clinical history should be completed because patients do not generally present with overt symptoms of hypothyroidism. Patients, particularly the elderly, who have subclinical hypothyroidism are at risk for developing cardiac abnormalities, such as atrial fibrillation and osteoporosis.

Nursing Diagnoses

Based on the information gathered, examples of nursing diagnoses in the patient with hypothyroidism may include the following:

- Activity intolerance related to decrease in metabolism.
- Constipation related to decreased activity and decreased metabolic rate.
- Risk for injury related to hypersensitivity to sedatives, narcotics, and anesthetics.
- Disturbed sensory perception (numbness of the hands or feet) related to mucin deposits and nerve compression.

Planning and Implementation

When first diagnosed the patient may need assistance with activities of daily living. Fatigue and activity intolerance may be major problems. Cardiorespiratory response to activities should be monitored. Nutritional intake and sleep patterns should be also monitored and appropriate interventions taken to ensure sufficient calories and rest. Patient and family should be informed that as the medication takes effect tiredness should resolve. Constipation may have been a chronic problem if the patient has had undiagnosed hypothyroidism. Dietary assessment will help to identify nutritional needs. Discuss methods to increase dietary fiber. Encourage intake of a minimum of eight glasses of fluid daily unless contraindicated.

Cardiovascular disease is more common in patients who have hypothyroidism. Signs include bradycardia, impaired muscular contraction, and diminished cardiac output. Some patients have heart enlargement; this may be due to left ventricular dilation or pericardial effusion.

Pharmacology

The treatment of choice for hypothyroidism is levothyroxine (T_4), which is available in pure form and is inexpensive and stable. Even though only T_4 is administered, levothyroxine is converted to T_3 so that both hormones available in the tissues. Because of variable hormone content, desiccated thyroid is not satisfactory for use. Instruct patient to take oral medication one hour before a meal or two hours afterward to ensure proper absorption. Dosage will vary according to age and weight. Thyroid medications potentiate medications, such as digoxin and Coumadin. The patient should be monitored for digoxin toxicity and bleeding problems. In addition, the patient should be monitored for cardiovascular insufficiency (e.g., chest pain, shortness of breath, palpitations, tachycardia, or peripheral edema).

Evaluation of Outcomes

Potential patient outcomes for each of the example nursing diagnoses for the patient with hypothyroidism are:

- Activity intolerance related to decrease in metabolism. Patient will perform activities of daily living independently or with assistive devices as needed; patient will be free of complications of immobility, as evidenced by intact skin, absence of thrombophlebitis, and normal bowel patterns.
- Constipation related to decreased activity and decreased metabolic rate. Patient will report normal bowel elimination pattern.
- Imbalanced nutrition, more than body requirements, related to intake greater than metabolic needs. Patient will verbalize and demonstrate selection of foods or meals that will achieve and maintain weight within 10 percent of recommended body mass index.
- Impaired skin integrity related to dryness and edema secondary to movement of fluid into the interstitial tissues. Patient skin condition will show improvement as demonstrated by decreased redness, swelling, and pain.

Myxedema Coma

Myxedema is a medical emergency. The patient will present with a diminished level of consciousness due to severe hypothyroidism. Symptoms include hypothermia, hypoventilation, hypotension, and bradycardia. Preceding the coma, the patient may be depressed, confused, paranoid, and sometimes even manic.

Nursing Diagnoses

Based on the information gathered, examples of nursing diagnoses in the patient with myxedema coma may include the following:
- Impaired gas exchange related to hypercapnia or hypoxia due to hypoventilation.
- Hypothermia related to hypometabolism.
- Decreased cardiac output related to heart failure, or fluid volume deficit.

Planning and Implementation

Priorities of care for the patient with myxedema coma include respiratory and hemodynamic support. The patient will be admitted to an intensive care unit, and ventilator support is usually necessary. Respiratory and cardiovascular assessment must be provided continuously. The patient will require continuous cardiac and respiratory monitoring. Arterial blood gases should be done at intervals. Associated illnesses that may have precipitated the coma should be looked for and treated. Intravenous fluids should be given slowly because the patient may easily become overloaded with fluids. Gastric absorption of medication is poor in the myxedema patient; therefore, thyroid replacement should be administered intravenously. For patients who have had hypothyroidism for long periods and for diagnosed cardiac patients, thyroid replacement is started slowly. In the event that angina or dysrhythmias occur, the dosage is usually reduced. Therapeutic response to treatment will be indicated by increase in temperature and an improved respiratory and cerebral functioning. Patients with myxedema often have adrenal insufficiency also; therefore, glucocorticoids may be prescribed (Greenspan, 2004).

Evaluation of Outcomes

Potential patient outcomes for each of the example nursing diagnoses for the patient with myxedema coma are:
- Impaired gas exchange related to factors of hypercapnia or hypoxia due to hypoventilation. Patient's arterial blood gases will be within normal limits.
- Hypothermia related to factors of hypometabolism. Patient will have normal body temperature.
- Decreased cardiac output related to factors of heart failure and fluid volume deficit. Patient will have normal cardiac rhythm and vital signs.

HYPERPARATHYROIDISM

The parathyroid glands (normally four) are located in the neck in the posterior aspect of the thyroid gland. These small glands are easily overlooked and can be removed accidentally during thyroid surgery (Lal & Clark, 2004). When the parathyroid glands are stimulated to excess, the condition of hyperparathyroidism exists.

Epidemiology

Primary hyperparathyroidism is found in approximately 0.1 percent of adult patients examined. It occurs three times more frequently in women. Primary hyperparathyroidism accounts for about 90 percent of the cases of hypercal-

---

Red Flag

Hypothyroidism in the Elderly

Hypothyroidism may be overlooked in the elderly because euthyroid patients have similar symptoms. Elderly are more likely to present with complications of the disease, (e.g., congestive heart failure, angina, neurological problems, confusion, or depression) (Greenspan & Resnick, 2004). In addition, subclinical hypothyroidism occurs in 5 to 10 percent of elderly people. The patient should be carefully assessed for symptoms of hypothyroidism. Each person must be carefully evaluated for risk before the decision to treat is made (Huether, 2004).

cemia. Over half of cases of hyperparathyroidism occur in patients over 60 years of age.

Etiology

Hyperparathyroidism is usually sporadic and most often due to a single enlarged gland or adenoma. Other causes of hyperparathyroidism include parathyroid carcinoma and hyperplasia. Studies show that there has been a decline in cases of hyperthyroidism since 1970. Earlier detection of primary hyperparathyroidism occurs today because of incidental hypercalcemia, which is found when patients have comprehensive metabolic blood profiles. Those patients who have early detection of the disease are less likely to be symptomatic.

Pathophysiology

Hyperparathyroidism leads to excessive excretion of calcium and phosphate by the kidney. Even though parathyroid hormone stimulates the renal tubules to reabsorb calcium causing hypercalcemia, the excessive calcium in the glomerular filtrate overwhelms tubular reabsorption and results in hypercalciuria. Polyuria and polydipsia may occur as a result of the nephrogenic diabetes insipidus, which hypercalcemia can induce. Kidney stones occur in 18 percent of patients with newly diagnosed primary hyperparathyroidism. Excessive PTH can cause excessive bone reabsorption, which leads to diffuse demineralization, cystic bone lesions, and pathological fractures.

Assessment with Clinical Manifestations

Patients with hyperparathyroidism have clinical manifestations that affect many of the body's systems. Neurological symptoms can occur from mild (e.g., lethargy, fatigue, personality change, paresthesia, or depression) to severe stupor and coma. GI symptoms, such as, dyspepsia, nausea, and constipation, are also common.

Diagnostic Tests

In hyperparathyroidism, serum calcium and ionized calcium levels are elevated. A serum calcium greater than 10.9 mg/dL is the hallmark of primary hyperparathyroidism when corrected for serum albumin. When serum albumin is low, the serum calcium results may also be low, therefore ionized calcium is more accurate, because it is not bound to protein and provides a more accurate measurement of calcium. Urine calcium is also high to normal, and urine phosphorus is high. To distinguish the parathyroid from nonparathyroid causes of hypercalcemia, a parathyroid hormone assay test is warranted. A diagnosis of primary hyperparathyroidism is confirmed by a parathyroid assay test, which is high normal to elevated (Daniels, 2003).

Imaging techniques for localizing parathyroid adenomas include ultrasonography, CT, MRI, and Tc-99m MIBI studies. The expertise of the technical personnel and available equipment influence the sensitivity and specificity of the procedure. A bone survey by shoe evidence of bone resorption indicates excess of PTH. Osteitis fibrosa cystica is the classic bone disease of primary parathyroidism (Ferri, 2005).

Nursing Diagnoses

Based on the information gathered, examples of nursing diagnoses in the patient with hyperparathyroidism may include the following:
- Acute or chronic pain related to renal stone or bone discomfort.
- Risk for injury related to pathological fracture.

Planning and Implementation

Management of fluid and electrolytes is the priority problem when a patient presents with hypercalcemia. Severe hypercalcemia requires hospitalization. Intensive hydration with intravenous normal saline (fluid resuscitation with normal saline: 500 to 1,000 mL over the first hour followed by 250 to 500 mL hourly) is the treatment of choice unless contraindicated. The patient may need three to five liters of fluid each a day. Ensuring that the patient receives sodium chloride greater than 400 mEq every day is important to facilitate calcium excretion.

Patients who have mild, asymptomatic hyperparathyroidism should be followed closely by their health care provider. The patient should be encouraged to exercise and drink adequate fluids. Vitamin D and A supplements, calcium containing medications, such as antacids and laxatives, and thiazide diuretics should be avoided. Recommendations for follow-up includes serum calcium and albumin twice yearly, renal function and urine calcium once each year, and bone density every two years. There is caution in use of digitalis preparations because patients with hypercalcemia are more sensitive to toxic effects. A calcium channel blocker may be prescribed to help in preventing adverse cardiac effects from the hypercalcemia.

Surgery

Parathyroidectomy is the definitive treatment of choice leading to 95 percent cure rate of parathyroid adenoma. With parathyroid hyperplasia the cure rate is somewhat lower, because there is a 20 percent incidence of recurrent hypercalcemia. Preoperative and postoperative care is similar to the care of the patient having a thyroidectomy.

Because the parathyroid glands lie within 1 cm of the point of intersection of the recurrent laryngeal nerve, there is danger of injury with resultant hoarseness. Hypocalcemia with resulting tetany will occur if there is inadvertent removal of all parathyroid tissue. The patient needs to be observed closely the evening after surgery or on the following day. Frequent monitoring of ionized calcium is advisable. Calcium carbonate is provided orally to prevent hypocalcemia after the hypercalcemia has resolved. Intravenous calcium gluconate and calcium chloride should be available if hypocalcemia occurs. Because adequate magnesium is required for functional recovery of the remaining suppressed parathyroid glands, magnesium may be required. The patient should be monitored for hyperthyroidism immediately after parathyroid surgery because stored thyroid hormone may be released during surgery.

Evaluation of Outcomes

Potential patient outcomes for each of the example nursing diagnoses for the patient with hyperparathyroidism are:
- Acute or chronic pain related to renal stone or bone discomfort. Patient should relate that pain has been decreased and discuss measures to cope with the pain if it is not completely relieved.
- Risk for injury related to pathological fracture. Patient will not experience of fractures.

HYPOPARATHYROIDISM

By secreting PTH, the parathyroid gland and vitamin D function to maintain a normal serum calcium. Either the failure to secrete PTH or respond to PTH or vitamin D results in hypocalcemia, which is the major problem occurring with hypoparathyroidism.

Epidemiology

Hypoparathyroidism is a rare disorder, occurring equally between males and females. It is speculated that the United States has similar rates of hypoparathyroidism as does Japan, which reports 7.2 cases of idiopathic hypoparathyroid cases per one million and 3.4 cases per one million of pseudohypoparathyroidism.

Etiology

Hypoparathyroid may be familial, idiopathic, caused by infection, autoimmune disease, or surgical removal of the parathyroid glands. Hypoparathyroidism most commonly occurs following a thyroidectomy; it is usually transient, rarely, it may be permanent. Other causes of hypoparathyroidism include autoimmune syndrome, functional due to poor absorption of magnesium sulfate, and pseudohypoparathyroidism, which occurs as a result of renal resistance to parathyroid hormone.

Pathophysiology

When there is inadequate parathyroid hormone, calcium levels decrease and phosphorus levels increase. Calcium reabsorption from the bone ceases and regulation of calcium reabsorption from the renal tubules are impaired. A decrease in calcium reduces the threshold for nerve and muscle excitation so that a nerve impulse may occur by a slight stimulus along the nerve fiber. This leads to alteration in nerve transmission and in more severe incidences tetany. Serum calcium levels may be further reduced by high phosphorus levels, which impede conversion of vitamin D to its active form by inhibiting the renal enzyme that is necessary for the vitamin D to become active.

Assessment with Clinical Manifestations

Symptoms of hypoparathyroidism mirror those of hypocalcemia, and therefore are mainly due to increased neuromuscular excitability and deposition of calcium in soft tissues. Acute symptoms of hypocalcemia include numbness and tingling of lips and hands, tetany, carpopedal spasms (Trousseau's sign), Chvostek's sign, muscle and abdominal cramps, and psychological changes. Chronic clinical manifestations include lethargy, personality changes, anxiety, and blurring of vision due to cataracts. ECG may show prolonged QT intervals and T wave abnormalities.

Diagnostic Tests

Refer to the diagnostic tests section for parathyroid dysfunction.

Nursing Diagnoses

Based on the information gathered, examples of nursing diagnosis in the patient with hypoparathyroidism may include the following:
• Risk for injury related to hypocalcemia with resultant tetany

Planning and Implementation

The goal of treatment for hypoparathyroidism is to normalize calcium levels. The nurse must be prepared to recognize early symptoms of hypocalcemia. If tetany occurs, laryngospasm can result in inadequate airway calling for emergency tracheostomy. To prevent and or treat symptoms (e.g., tetany) intravenous calcium gluconate is administered. The patient will be prescribed oral calcium supplements and vitamin D for maintenance therapy. Dietary instruction for foods high in calcium should be provided. The nurse should provide a thorough explanation for the importance of compliance to the therapeutic plan.

Evaluation of Outcomes

Potential patient outcomes for each of the example nursing diagnoses for the patient with hypoparathyroidism are:
- Risk for injury related to hypocalcemia with resultant tetany. Patient will be not experience tetany and ionized calcium level will return to normal.

KEY CONCEPTS

- Hyperfunction of the pituitary gland occurs when there is excess hormonal activity.
- Hyperprolactinemia causes mainly problems with the fertility and sexual function.
- Acromegaly, though causing changes in body appearance with increase growth of body tissues, has effect on all body systems, leading to many comorbidities.
- Hypercortisolism (Cushing's disease and Cushing's syndrome) alters the function of practically all tissues and organs of the body.
- Transsphenoidal hypophysectomy is the recommended treatment for most pituitary tumors.
- Hypofunction of the pituitary gland occurs with decrease hormonal activity of one or more of the pituitary hormones.
- Both diabetes insipidus and SIADH alter fluid and electrolytes.

- Adrenal insufficiency can be life-threatening.
- An increased stimulation of the adrenal glands may lead to hyperaldosteronism.
- Pheochromocytomas are rare but have a high mortality rate because of predisposing the patient to stroke and myocardial infarction.
- An excess or decrease in available thyroid hormone alters function of all body organs.
- Hyperthyroidism refers to the continuous secretion of thyroid hormones by the thyroid gland.
- Primary hypothyroidism is usually treatable with replacement thyroid therapy.
- The treatment of choice for hyperthyroidism is radioiodine therapy.
- The major problems related to hyperparathyroidism are kidney stones and fractures.
- Hypoparathyroidism can cause hypocalcemia, which may cause tetany, a life-threatening event.

REVIEW QUESTIONS

1. When assessing a patient who is diagnosed as having acromegaly, what signs and symptoms will the nurse most likely assess? Select all that apply.
    1. Decrease in peripheral vision
    2. Hypotension
    3. Muscle weakness
    4. Large tongue

2. Which statement by a 28-year-old female patient would support a diagnosis of hyperprolactinemia?
    1. "I have progressively become hoarse over the past six months."
    2. "I am experiencing deep bone pain."
    3. "I have not had a menstrual period in 12 months."
    4. "I have had a problem with weight loss."

3. When instructing a patient who is to have a transsphenoidal hypophysectomy. What information should the nurse include?
    1. Nasal passage will be packed with gauze for 24 to 48 hours.
    2. A soft bulky head dressing will be present.
    3. A pureed diet will be provided immediately after surgery.
    4. Teeth will need brushing four to six times daily after surgery.

4. Which nursing intervention should the nurse anticipate providing for a patient with hypercortisolism?
    1. Monitoring for hypotension
    2. Fall prevention measures
    3. Assessing for symptoms of hyperkalemia
    4. Dietary instruction to promote weight gain

Continued

5. What statement by a patient with Addison's disease indicates that discharge teaching has been effective?
   1. "I will taper off of my glucocorticoid medications after I start feeling better."
   2. "The dietary supplements will help decrease my need for medications."
   3. "My glucocorticoid medications will need to be increased when I am ill or experiencing stress."
   4. "I will recognize that my symptoms are worsening when I experience extreme thirst."

6. When presenting an inservice on endocrine diseases, which statement by the nurse would be correct?
   1. Patients who have acromegaly have primary involvement of the soft tissues and joint. Major organs are spared.
   2. Patients who have diabetes insipidus should be monitored for fluid overload.
   3. Patients with hyperprolactinemia may experience breast engorgement.
   4. Patients with Cushing's syndrome often have episodes of hypotension.

7. Which outcome would be most appropriate to include in the plan of care for a patient who has been diagnosed with a pheochromocytoma?
   1. Fasting glucose will be less than 100 mg/dL
   2. Blood pressure will be within normal limits
   3. Serum sodium will be greater than 135 mg/dL
   4. ECG will demonstrate no ectopy

8. Which clinical manifestation should the nurse assess for when caring for a patient with a diagnosis of hyperthyroidism?
   1. Fine hand tremor
   2. Slow, irregular pulse
   3. Cool, pale extremities
   4. Diminished bowel sound

9. What discharge teaching would be most important for the nurse to include for the patient who is prescribed methimazole (Tapazole)?
   1. Report sore throat and fever to health care provider
   2. Take medication with full glass of water before breakfast
   3. Weight daily and record
   4. Mild headaches should be expected

10. Which statement by a patient who has received instruction about radioiodine therapy for hyperthyroidism would require further explanation by the nurse?
    1. "My infant son breastfeeds every 4 hours."
    2. "I am allergic to iodine."
    3. "I will need to flush the toilet 3 times after each use."
    4. "I will use disposable eating utensils for several days after the treatment."

11. Following a parathyroidectomy, a patient complains of numbness and tingling in the tips of the fingers and around the mouth. The nurse should anticipate the physician writing which order?
    1. Serum albumin
    2. Serum thyroxin
    3. Ionized calcium
    4. Parathyroid hormone level

12. Which therapeutic response should the nurse anticipate when vasopressin is administered?
    1. The patient relates that thirst has resolved.
    2. The patient reports that he is urinating more often.
    3. The patient states his headache has subsided.
    4. The patient demonstrates improvement in appetite.

REVIEW ACTIVITIES

1. A 21-year-old female is admitted to the floor complaining of severe abdominal pain. Routine lab work including an electrolyte panel is ordered. The lab results are as follows: Na = 115 mmol/L; K = 3.6 mmol/L; BUN = 10 mg/dL; Glucose = 126 mg/dL; Hgb = 10 g/dL; and Hct = 30%.
   a. Which lab result should require the nurse's most immediate attention?
   b. Which system assessment is a priority when the sodium is at this level?
   c. What are the priority nursing interventions when caring for a patient with SIADH?

2. A 28-year-old male patient comes to the emergency department complaining of his heart racing. After the history and physical is done, the physician plans to workup the patient for having hyperthyroidism.
   a. State one clinical manifestation that relates to the following body systems, which the nurse should assess the patient.
   Skin:
   Eyes:
   Neuromuscular:
   Respiratory:
   GI:
   Cardiovascular:
   b. Which lab test is most cost-effective and sensitive for diagnosing hyperthyroidism?
   c. What medication should the nurse anticipate the patient being prescribed to control his tachycardia.

3. A 21-year-old female patient is diagnosed as having a prolactinoma.
   a. What clinical manifestations should the nurse anticipate finding during the interview?
   b. The nurse should be aware that a patient who has an untreated prolactinoma is likely to develop what bone disease?

4. a. When caring for a patient with Cushing's syndrome, which electrolyte problem should the nurse monitor most carefully? Why?
   b. What clinical manifestations of hypokalemia should the nurse assess for?

5. Compare an alert patient who has diabetes insipidus with an unconscious patient who has diabetes insipidus. What is more likely to occur in the unconscious patient? Why? What is the priority nursing diagnosis? How is this problem corrected?

Diabetes Mellitus: Nursing Management

Martha K. Carlson, MSN

CHAPTER TOPICS

- Type 1 Diabetes
- Type 2 Diabetes
- Management of Diabetes
- Acute Complications of Diabetes
- Chronic Complications of Diabetes

Nurses will potentially encounter patients with diabetes in a wide variety of settings. Therefore it is necessary to have a fundamental knowledge of diabetes and the nursing care involved. The patient's ability to manage diabetes is an important focus for the nurse. This chapter includes information on the pathophysiology of diabetes, diagnosis and management of the disease, and acute and chronic complications. Nursing diagnoses and interventions are included along with expected outcomes.

KEY TERMS

Diabetes mellitus
Endogenous
Euglycemia
Exogenous
Glucagon
Gluconeogenesis
Glycogenolysis
Hyperesthesia
Hyperglycemia
Insulin
Lipodystrophy
Self-monitoring of blood glucose (SMBG)
Syndrome X (insulin resistance syndrome)

DIABETES MELLITUS

Diabetes mellitus refers to a group of chronic disorders of metabolism characterized by elevated blood glucose levels and disturbances in metabolism of carbohydrate, fats, and protein. Diabetes affects approximately 16 million people in the United States, and this number is expected to rise in the future. The majority of patients, approximately 1.4 million have type 1 diabetes, and the remaining 14.5 million have type 2 diabetes.

Annually nearly 18 percent of deaths in people age 25 and older is attributed to diabetes. The American Diabetes Association (ADA) places the remainder of the 16 million patients in a category of diabetes referred to as other specific types (e.g., gestational diabetes). Additionally, numerous people have impaired glucose tolerance, prediabetes, or insulin resistance. The incidence of diabetes increases with age, and there is no variation in gender. African Americans, Hispanic (Americans), Native Americans, Asian (Americans), and Pacific Islanders are at increased risk for development of diabetes. Obesity and advancing age are major contributors to the increased incidence of diabetes regardless of ethnicity or race (Cleator & Wilding, 2003).

Patients with diabetes are twice as likely to experience heart disease as the general population. The mortality rate of heart disease in patients with diabetes is six times greater in males and four times greater in females then in the general population. Type 1 diabetes results from insufficient insulin, and type 2 is a disease of insulin resistance. There has been a dramatic increase in the incidence of diabetes in the past 20 years, particularly type 2 diabetes. In the past, type 2 diabetes was thought to be a disease of adult onset. It is now common to find type 2 diabetes in children and adolescents as well. As a chronic disease, diabetes requires long-term management and is associated with subsequent development of heart disease, hypertension, stroke, kidney disease, and lower limb amputation. Patients with either type 1 or type 2 diabetes can and frequently do develop complications. Patients with diabetes are major consumers of health care, and the nurse can expect to care for them in hospitals, homes, nursing homes, schools, and communities.

It is not uncommon for patients and families to believe that diabetes treated with oral medications is less severe than diabetes treated with insulin. The nurse can play a major role in helping them understand that they do have diabetes and are not just borderline with their blood sugars.

Pathophysiology

ADA has categorized diabetes into four categories as shown in Box 57-1. Of these four types of diabetes, type 1 and type 2 are the most common. Gestational diabetes occurs with pregnancy, with the blood glucose levels typically returning to normal after delivery. These women do, however, have an increased risk of developing diabetes later in life. Impaired glucose tolerance or prediabetes exists when patients have a blood sugar that is higher than normal but not high enough to meet the criteria for diabetes. Studies indicate that many people with prediabetes can delay or even prevent the occurrence of diabetes with regular exercise and weight reduction (Fong, Aiello, Ferris, & Klein, 2004).

Type 1 Diabetes

Type 1 diabetes results from a defect or failure of the beta cells of the pancreas' islet cells. The islet cells are destroyed by an interaction of genetics and environmental factors or autoimmunity. This loss of beta cells causes an absolute lack of insulin. Historically, type 1 diabetes was called juvenile onset and thought to have an acute onset. Recent studies now suggest a genetic predis-

---

BOX 57-1

FOUR TYPES OF DIABETES MELLITUS

Type 1 diabetes mellitus

Type 2 diabetes mellitus

Gestational diabetes

Impaired glucose tolerance (prediabetes)

position with a preclinical period followed by destruction of the beta cells from autoimmune mechanisms, which results in a deficiency of insulin and hyperglycemia. Some authors suggest specific environmental factors are linked to diabetes (Mundy, 2004; Robinson, 2004). Diabetes can also result from pancreatitis or other diseases of the pancreas.

Insulin is one of the hormones produced by the pancreas (beta cells) with a function of lowering blood sugar. **Glucagon** is another hormone released by the alpha cells of the pancreas and it functions to raise blood sugar levels. Beta cell destruction is present long before the patient develops **hyperglycemia** (an elevated blood sugar level). Approximately 90 percent of the beta cells must be destroyed before hyperglycemia occurs, causing a lack of insulin. There is also an increase in glucagon production by the alpha cells of the pancreas. The hyperglycemia from lack of insulin fails to inhibit the production of glucagons. Virtually every form of diabetes is associated with elevated glucagon levels (Griffin & Ojeda., 2004).

Insulin is a storage hormone that moves glucose from the bloodstream into the cells of the liver, muscles, and fat cells. Insulin facilitates the storage of glucose as glycogen in the liver and muscle. It also helps to store fat from the diet in adipose tissue. Insulin stops the body from breaking down stores of protein, glucose, and fat.

The pancreas secretes a basal amount of insulin during times when a food is not being ingested, as during sleep or fasting. Glucagon is also secreted from the pancreas when the blood glucose levels decrease, and the liver is then stimulated to release glucose. The counter-regulatory hormones, insulin and glucagon, keep a homeostatic condition of glucose in the bloodstream.

In type 1 diabetes, there is a destruction of the beta cells of the pancreas and therefore a lack of insulin. As previously stated, the cause of type 1 diabetes is thought to be a combination of genetic, environmental, and immunological factors. Type 1 diabetes is not hereditary; however, there is a genetic predisposition for type 1 to develop in patients with certain human leukocyte antigens (HLA) types. Type 1 diabetes is consequently more common in children and adolescents but can develop at any time. Regardless of the cause, in type 1 diabetes, fasting hyperglycemia occurs as the liver continues to produce glucose. Glucose ingested in the diet is also not able to be utilized and remains in the bloodstream. As the blood glucose elevates, the kidneys are no longer able to filter it effectively, and glucose is spilled into the urine. Fluid and electrolytes are lost in the urine as well. This is referred to as an osmotic diuresis.

Insulin is required by the body for the synthesis of glucose from amino acids **(gluconeogenesis)**. It also stops the physiological process of the breakdown of stored glucose **(glycogenolysis).** With an insulin deficiency, there is no regulatory effect, and the blood sugar elevates as the cells starve. As the body breaks down fats, ketones are produced, which disrupt the acid-base balance in the body.

Type 2 Diabetes

Type 2 diabetes was previously classified as adult onset. A comparison between type 1 and type 2 diabetes is shown in Table 57-1. While patients with type 2 diabetes are generally older, there is a dramatic increase in type 2 diabetes in children and adolescents. Commonly, patients with type 2 diabetes will have insulin resistance syndrome with hypertension, central obesity, and hyperlipidemia for years before diagnosis. The major abnormalities of pathophysiology that occur in patients with type 2 diabetes are: (a) defective beta cell secretion with early loss of first phase insulin production; (b) insulin resistance in the peripheral tissues, especially muscle and liver; and (c) increased production of glucose from the liver as the disease progresses.

First phase insulin secretion inhibits the production and output of glucose by the liver. When there are defects in the beta cells, this inhibitory effect is lost, resulting in fasting hyperglycemia. The body compensates by increasing second phase insulin secretion, which results in hyperinsulinemia. The beta cells may

TABLE 57-1	Comparison of Type 1 and Type 2 Diabetes		
TYPE	**CHARACTERISTICS**	**CLINICAL MANIFESTATIONS**	**MANAGEMENT**
Type 1	Destruction of beta cells with absolute lack of insulin. Genetic predispositions and markers determine immune response. Strong hereditary link. Peak onset age 11–13. Onset may be acute, often following long preclinical period Prone to ketoacidosis	Hyperglycemia, polydipsia, polyuria, polyphagia, weight loss, and fatigue	Medications—insulin, diet, exercise, and SMBG
Type 2	Insulin resistance with insulin deficiency. Decrease in number and size of beta cells. Insidious onset. Strong genetic predisposition. Usually occurs over 40 years of age but increasing in frequency in children	Hyperglycemia, obesity, polydipsia, polyuria, skin infections, blurred vision, or fatigue. Not prone to ketosis but can develop with stress	Medications—oral agents or insulin, diet, exercise or SMBG

Adapted from DeLaune, S., & Ladner, P. (2006). Fundamentals of nursing (3rd ed.). New York: Thomson Delmar Learning.

continue to secrete high levels of insulin for years to regulate the blood glucose levels. Eventually the beta cells fail, and insulin secretion diminishes. The production of glucose from the liver increases, and then hyperglycemia results. The beta cells are not able to produce sufficient insulin for the demand but are able to produce enough to prevent the breakdown of fat and protein (ketosis).

The tissues develop a decreased sensitivity to insulin and as a result, the body produces more insulin. Hyperinsulinemia does not prevent gluconeogenesis so hyperglycemia occurs. The cells' sensitivity to insulin can decrease as much as 70 percent before fasting plasma glucose levels elevate to an abnormal level. This type 2 diabetes has a slower, more insidious onset, as long as 20 years in some cases. Although there is some uncertainty about the mechanisms of insulin resistance in the tissues, the role of obesity, especially central obesity is clear. Patients will exhibit an impaired glucose tolerance, as the beta cells are able to continue to produce enough insulin to keep the blood sugar elevated but below the level required for a diagnosis of diabetes. This slow progression of glucose tolerance manifests itself with vague symptoms of fatigue, weight gain, irritability, frequent urinary tract infections, and poor skin healing. Often, the diagnosis of type 2 diabetes is made when the patient presents for health care with a complication of the disease. Obesity is associated with type 2 diabetes because of the insulin resistance. Type 2 diabetes has a familial tendency and probably a genetic link.

Syndrome X, also known as **insulin resistance syndrome,** is a group of abnormalities of metabolism that act together to increase the risk of cardiovascular disease. Patients with syndrome X will exhibit high levels of triglycerides, insulin, hypertension, and low-density lipoproteins (LDLs), and decreased levels of high-density lipoproteins (HDLs). The risk factors for syndrome X include abdominal obesity, family history, sedentary lifestyle, gestational diabetes, polycystic ovary disease, and increased age. Programs of weight loss and exercise can prevent or delay the onset of type 2 diabetes in patients at risk for the disease.

Assessment with Clinical Manifestations

Patients with both type 1 and type 2 diabetes will present with the three Ps of diabetes (i.e., polydipsia, polyphagia, and polyuria). Type 1 diabetes is a disorder of metabolism of fat, protein, and carbohydrates. Without the presence of insulin, glucose is unable to enter the cells and remains in the bloodstream. As a result, the cells are starving, and the patient experiences hunger (polyphagia) with weight loss. The increased concentration of glucose in the circulation causes an osmotic diuresis, causing large amounts of urine to be produced (polyuria). Increased blood sugar levels will cause water to be drawn from the cells by osmosis, resulting in cellular dehydration. This triggers the thirst center in the hypothalamus, and the patient drinks large volumes of water (polydipsia). The patient will experience weight loss as the body uses proteins and fats for energy and loses fluids from the osmotic diuresis.

Type 1 diabetes typically has a rapid onset, and the patient presents with the three Ps, fatigue, and weight loss. There may be ketoacidosis present as well. Type 2 diabetes has a more insidious onset, and the patient may already have complications when presenting for health care. Symptoms that induce the patient with type 2 diabetes to seek treatment include frequent infections, delayed wound healing, or fatigue. Patients with type 2 diabetes may also experience polydipsia, polyphagia, and polyuria. Diabetics who are obese will commonly display thin muscular extremities with increased deposits of fat in the abdomen, chest, neck, and face. A waist hip/ratio of greater than 0.9 in men and greater than 0.8 in women is associated with diabetes (Tierney, McPhee, & Papakakais, 2004).

Past health history should include childhood illnesses (rubella, mumps, or other viral illnesses) recent surgery, trauma, stress or infection, pregnancy history, birth weight of infants, and history of pancreatitis. The nurse should inquire about medications used, especially diuretics, corticosteroids, and use of insulin and oral agents. A continued assessment is shown in Box 57-2.

BOX 57-2

ASSESSMENT OF PATIENTS WITH DIABETES

Nutritional—Metabolic

Assess for obesity, changes in weight, increased thirst and hunger, nausea, vomiting, delayed wound healing especially involving the feet, and daily food intake pattern.

Elimination

Inquire about constipation, diarrhea, frequency of urination, nocturia, urinary tract infections, and incontinence.

Activity—Exercise

Assess for the presence of fatigue and muscle weakness.

Cognitive—Perceptual

Assess for the presence of headache, abdominal pain, pruritus, numbness, and tingling in extremities or blurred vision.

Eyes

Inspect for vitreal hemorrhages and cataracts.

Skin

Inspect for pigmentation on legs, ulcers on feet, and loss of hair on legs and feet.

Respiratory

Assess for Kussmaul breathing (rapid, deep respirations).

Cardiovascular

Assess for weak rapid pulse and hypotension.

GI

Assess for fruity breath, vomiting, and dry oral mucous membranes.

Neurological

Assess for restlessness, confusion, stupor, coma, and altered deep tendon reflexes.

BOX 57-3

DIAGNOSTIC CRITERIA FOR DIABETES

Fasting plasma glucose level greater than 126 mg/dL

Random plasma glucose level greater than 200 mg/dL with clinical signs of diabetes

Two-hour oral glucose tolerance test greater than 200 mg/dL with a 75 g glucose load

Fast Forward ▶▶▶

Complications for People with Diabetes while Traveling

Patients with diabetes will need extra planning when they travel. Their supplies for their disease management should be readily available in carry-on luggage, including blood glucose monitoring meters, insulin, and syringes. With the increase in homeland security, the patient should bring a letter from his or her health care provider explaining the medical necessity of the syringes. The patient should bring along fast-acting carbohydrate sources to reverse hypoglycemia. Extra medications and food should be included in the event of long delays, canceled flights, and closed restaurants. Patients with diabetes should wear identification stating that they are diabetic. It is also recommended that the patient carry identification with the names of their medications and health care providers.

Diagnostic Tests

There are three standard tests used to determine the presence of diabetes, no matter what type. Diagnosis is not made on a single lab finding but is confirmed with a subsequent test (Box 57-3). If the fasting plasma glucose is elevated on one occasion, it will be confirmed by repeating the test a second day. Fasting plasma glucose is the preferred method of diagnosis. Generally a true elevation of plasma glucose is indicative of diabetes mellitus. There are factors that can elevate the blood glucose level, such as stress (surgery, trauma, general anesthesia, infections, or age), caffeine, and medications (tricyclic antidepressants, corticosteroids, or diuretics).

A patient with a random plasma glucose greater than 200 mg/dL should have a fasting plasma glucose the next day. If the fasting plasma glucose is greater than 126 mg/dL, the diagnosis of diabetes can be made, because it meets the criteria of two occasions of hyperglycemia. If the fasting plasma glucose is less than 126 mg/dL, the patient will likely be given a 75 g glucose challenge for the oral glucose tolerance test (OGTT) and a two-hour plasma glucose level drawn. If this two-hour plasma glucose is greater than 200 mg/dL, the diagnosis of diabetes can be made.

A fasting plasma glucose level is a snap shot in time, giving information about the current state of blood glucose. Another useful test is the glycosylated hemoglobin (hemoglobin A_{1C}). This test measures the amount of glucose attached to hemoglobin molecules and red blood cells over their life span of approximately 120 days. Information from this test provides assessment information about the patient's metabolic control.

The diagnosis of prediabetes is made if the fasting plasma glucose is between 110 to 125 mg/dL. Impaired fasting glucose is currently defined by the ADA as a fasting plasma glucose of 100 to 125 mg/dL. This criterion will effectively increase the number of people with prediabetes. This group may benefit from lifestyle changes of weight reduction and exercise to prevent the onset of diabetes. Screening recommendations for diabetes and prediabetes includes patients with risk factors for the disease (e.g., obesity, family history, older than age 45, or a history of gestational diabetes). Retesting is recommended in three years if the test is normal. Patients diagnosed with prediabetes or impaired glucose tolerance have a greater risk of developing diabetes in 10 years. Lifestyle modifications are recommended for this group (Burden, 2003).

Nursing Diagnoses

Patients with diabetes may have a large variety of nursing diagnoses. These diagnoses will likely change as the patient learns to manage his or her chronic illness or as other associated problems or complications arise. Based on the information gathered, examples of nursing diagnoses in the patient with diabetes may include the following:
- Deficient knowledge regarding disease process or treatment and individual care needs.
- Imbalanced nutrition less than body requirements.
- Risk for impaired adjustment.
- Risk for infection.
- Risk for disturbed sensory perception.
- Interrupted family processes.

Planning and Implementation

Nursing care for diabetes involves a combination of diet, glucose monitoring, medications, and exercise. As with any chronic disease, the patient is responsible for day-to-day management of his or her disease. Nurses play a major role in education, screening, and follow-up of patients with diabetes. The goals of

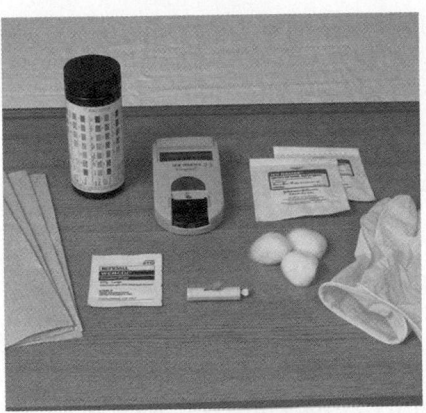

Figure 57-1 Self-monitoring blood glucose equipment.

PATIENT PLAYBOOK

Management of Diabetic People in the Home Environment

Much of the management and care of the patient with diabetes is done by the patient and family at home. The goal is to allow the patient to reach or maintain the optimal level of self-care. The diabetic patient often has difficulty reaching this goal, because patients with diabetes have an increased risk for the development of other chronic illnesses. Often the patient's visual acuity is impaired or his or her functional mobility is limited. Nursing care for diabetic patients in the home involves assessing the patient and caregiver's knowledge and technique with SMBG, insulin preparation and administration, adjustment of insulin dosage, side effects of insulin, exercise pattern, and nutritional therapy. As with any patient teaching, the nurse must first assess the patient's readiness to learn, identify barriers, and determine the meaning of the illness to the patient. It is important to identify the patient's support system and involve the family in the patient's plan of care. The family must understand the plan of care while allowing the patient to manage the disease as long as he or she are able.

nursing management are to reduce hyperglycemia and prevent or delay the onset of acute and long-term complications. Glycemic control is the most likely way to meet these goals, and it is imperative that the patient understand the management of the disease. Patients with type 1 diabetes will require insulin therapy in addition to diet and exercise. Some patients with type 2 diabetes will be successful with weight control, diet modifications, and exercise; however, the majority of patients with type 2 diabetes will require medication to control their blood sugar.

Patients just beginning to use insulin are assessed by the nurse to determine their ability to understand the relationship between insulin, food intake, and exercise. The patient must know the signs and symptoms of hypoglycemia, hyperglycemia, and the actions needed to correct them. If the patient is unable to understand or manage the care, the nurse works with the caregiver to ensure compliance. Regular evaluations of the patient's techniques with insulin therapy, including management of hypoglycemia and self-monitoring of blood glucose, are conducted. The nurse will review the patient's blood glucose log to assess patterns and glycemic control. If the patient is managing the disease with oral agents, the nursing care is similar. The nurse assesses the administration and response to the medications. The nurse must remember to advise the patient with diabetes as they live out their lives and go about their daily routines (see Fast Forward).

Blood glucose monitoring by patients has dramatically increased care in diabetes. Frequent monitoring of blood glucose levels allows the patient to adjust and manage their regimen for optimal glycemic control. Normalization of blood glucose levels helps to prevent the long-term complications of diabetes. **Self-monitoring of blood glucose (SMBG)** is a method whereby a patient tests his or her own blood glucose levels (Figure 57-1). SMBG also allows patients who take insulin the ability to detect and treat asymptomatic hypoglycemia. The Diabetes Control and Complications Trial (DCCT) determined that there are significant health benefits for patients treated with insulin that achieve normal or near normal blood glucose levels (Gordon, 2004). Based on the results of the DCCT, the recommendation from the ADA encourages the use of SMBG for daily routine monitoring, especially patients treated with insulin to maintain and prevent asymptomatic hypoglycemia. For most patients SMBG is required three times a day but the frequency may vary by individual. There are no data to suggest the optimal number of times type 2 diabetics should monitor their blood sugar, but the frequency should be enough to facilitate reaching the glycemic goals. The frequency of hyperglycemic and hypoglycemic events will be decreased with frequent SMBG. Whenever diet, exercise, or medications are modified, both type 1 and type 2 patients should increase the frequency of monitoring. Home management for diabetics is complicated and requires a great deal of instruction by nurses. This is illustrated in the patient playbook feature.

The accuracy of SMBG is dependent on the instrument and the operator. Health care providers should periodically and regularly evaluate the patient's monitoring technique. The patient should regularly use calibration and control solutions with their testing equipment to ensure accuracy of readings. The patient also needs to be taught to interpret and use the data from SMBG to achieve and maintain optimal glycemic control.

There are a variety of SMBG methods on the market. Most require application of a drop of blood from the fingertip to a reagent strip (Figure 57-2). The blood remains on the strip for a specified period of time, and the meter gives a reading of the blood glucose level. The nurse has a major role in the initial patient teaching about SMBG. Patients are instructed to keep a logbook of their blood glucose readings so patterns can be assessed. Patients should be given guidelines when to contact their health care provider. Those on intensive insulin regimens may be given algorithms to follow for changing their insulin dose based on blood glucose levels. Electronic diaries or PDAs can also

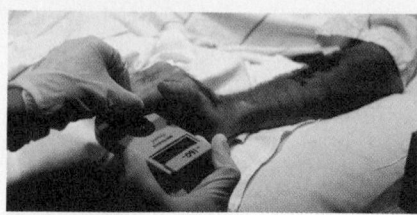

Figure 57-2 A nurse obtaining a sample of blood for glucose testing.

be used to track blood glucose results and activity levels. Data collected in this manner can be shared among patient and primary and other health care providers (Kerkenbusch, 2003).

Nutrition

Nutritional therapy is based on a well-balanced diet and is one of the mainstays in the treatment of diabetes. Because of the social and psychological issues associated with eating, this aspect of therapy can likely be one that the patient has the most difficulty controlling. A multidisciplinary health care team approach may be the most effective. There are many misconceptions about diet and diabetes, and in fact the plan of eating for diabetics is based on healthy eating, which would benefit anyone. Patients with diabetes can eat the same types of foods as people who do not have diabetes. The goals of nutritional therapy are shown Box 57-4.

Patients with type 1 diabetes will have a food plan based on activity, food intake, and insulin requirements. Patients with type 2 diabetes will have a food plan with an emphasis on maintaining blood glucose levels, lowering blood pressure, and weight reduction, as there is a high incidence of obesity. The meal plan will be formulated by the dietitian, reinforced by the nurse, and will include decreased fat intake, particularly saturated fats, and a decrease in simple sugars. Even a small weight loss of 5 to 7 percent can improve glycemic control. Weight loss can be accomplished with a program of exercise.

General dietary guidelines for patients with diabetes include the identification of the percentage of calories to come from carbohydrates, protein, and fats. Carbohydrates have the greatest effect on blood sugar, because of their rapid absorption and conversion to glucose. The ADA (2006) now recommends 60 to 70 percent of the caloric intake came from carbohydrates and monosaturated fats. This amount may vary for obese type 2 diabetics as their goals include weight loss, glucose, and lipid controls. This group of patients is taught to limit carbohydrate intake and substitute monosaturated lower cholesterol oils, such as olive oil, canola oil, or the oils in avocados and nuts. Patients with type 1 diabetes using intensive insulin therapy with near normal blood glucose levels can also use this approach. Patients are taught carbohydrate counting to administer one unit of regular or lispro insulin for 10 to 15 g of carbohydrate at a meal. Carbohydrates play a major role in the regulation of blood glucose levels. Managing carbohydrate intake can be accomplished by use of an exchange list or counting grams of carbohydrates consumed. Low-carbohydrate diets are not recommended as they are a major source for energy, water-soluble vitamins and minerals, and fiber. The current recommendation for carbohydrate intake is 45 to 65 percent of the total caloric intake.

Current recommendations for both type 1 and type 2 diabetes includes a protein intake of 15 to 20 percent of total calories and limitation of cholesterol to 300 mcg daily (Bartels, 2004). There are still no conclusions about the long-term effects of diets high in protein and low in carbohydrates (e.g., Atkins diet). While these diets produce a short-term weight loss and improve glycemia, there is no proof of long-term weight loss, and there is a concern about the effects of the diet on LDL cholesterol.

The goal for dietary fat intake for patients with diabetes is to limit saturated fats and cholesterol. Use of lower fat or fat-free foods and beverages will reduce the amount of high fat intake in the diet, and these substances are approved by the Food and Drug Administration. Regular use of these products may not reduce weight however. Polyunsaturated fats should make up approximately 10 percent of the caloric intake.

Dietary fiber has been shown to improve blood glucose levels and decrease endogenous insulin requirements. Fiber is classified as soluble or insoluble. Soluble fiber is found in legumes, some fruits, and oats. This type of fiber seems to play a larger role in reduction of blood glucose and lipid levels than insoluble fibers, but the clinical significance is probably small. Soluble fiber

Fast Forward ▶▶▶

The Use of Personal Digital Assistants (PDAs) in Blood Glucose Monitoring

Traditionally, patients recorded their blood glucose measurements using paper and pencil. The technology of PDAs offers some advantages over this traditional method of recordkeeping. Findings in a study demonstrated a significant lowering of hemoglobin A_{1C} when electronic diaries were used. The blood glucose level was tracked over a three-month period. The PDAs were able to give feedback on the amount of carbohydrate, fat, and protein in the patient's meals. This was accomplished by downloading the data via the phone lines. PDAs have also been used also in patients with migraine headaches. The technology offers promise for improving outcomes for patients with diabetes (Kerkenbush, 2003).

Respecting Our Differences

Age and the Relationship to Complications of Diabetes

Approximately 20 percent of patient's age 65 and older will have diabetes, and this number is expected to increase. Currently there are no available long-term studies of people 65 and older that examines the effects of glycemic, lipid, and blood pressure control (Fong, et al., 2004). Patients in this age-group often present with other chronic illnesses and different levels of cognitive ability that must be factored into their plan of care. Evidence suggests that greater benefits in reduction of morbidity and mortality may be possible by reduction and control of all cardiovascular risk functions instead of aiming for tight glycemic control alone. Less stringent glycemic target goals may be reasonable for older patients with advanced complications of diabetes, cognitive impairment, or other comorbidities affecting life span.

slows emptying of the stomach by forming a gel in the gastrointestinal (GI) tract. The slower rate of absorption caused by the fiber gel may contribute to lowering of the blood glucose levels. Insoluble fiber, found in whole grains, cereals, and some vegetables, increases bulk in the stools and prevents constipation in diabetes. Both types of fiber are beneficial in weight loss and produce a feeling of satiety.

Alcohol is permitted for patients with diabetes, but the patient should be aware of the affects of alcohol on diabetes. Alcohol decreases gluconeogenesis and will contribute to hypoglycemia. Additionally, alcohol has no nutritional benefits, is high in calories, and is damaging to the liver. Abuse of alcohol can make control of blood sugar more difficult, and the patient should carefully and honestly discuss this with their health care provider. Moderate use of alcohol can be incorporated into the dietary plan, if the patient has good blood sugar control. To reduce the risk of hypoglycemia from alcohol, the patient can eat carbohydrates while drinking. Alcoholic drinks provide empty calories, approximately 135 calories per drink. In addition to eating food while drinking alcohol, the patient with diabetes should drink dry, light wines, and use sugar-free mixes.

The ADA (2006) states that the clinical dietician is the team member to provide medical nutritional therapy. Often it is the nurse who is responsible for teaching dietary management to the patient and family. A useful tool is the Food Pyramid Guide, which provides visual cues to the patient about recommended amounts of foods to be eaten from each food group daily. The Food Pyramid Guide was reshaped with a new emphasis on the type of calories eaten with an emphasis on fruits, vegetables, whole grains, lower fat milk products, and exercise. Patients may also be given exchange lists, which divide foods into three main groups: carbohydrate, meat and meat substitutes, and fats. The carbohydrate group includes starches, fruit, milk, other carbohydrates, such as grains, and vegetables. The meat group is further divided into very lean, lean, medium-fat, and high-fat groups. The fat group has small serving sizes and is divided into monounsaturated, polyunsaturated, and saturated fats.

It is important for the diabetic patient and family members to learn to read food labels. Caution is advised about portion size as the serving sizes on food labels may not be the same size as those recommended in the patient's nutritional plan. The patient can compare the serving size on the food label to the serving sizes in the exchange list. They will need to check the number of grams of carbohydrate, protein, and fat in the serving size as well as the number of calories. If the food contains less than 20 calories per serving it is considered a free food.

Another way for the nurse to teach the basics of nutrition is to use the plate method. This allows the patient to visualize the portions of vegetables, meat, and carbohydrates that should fill up a 9-inch plate. At lunch and dinner, nonstarchy vegetables and meat will fill up half the plate, one fourth is 2 to 3 ounces of lean meat, and the remaining one fourth is filled with a carbohydrate. The patient should have a fruit and glass of low-fat milk to complete the meal. Breakfast is made up of one half of the plate filled with carbohydrates, one fourth filled with an optional protein, and the remaining fourth is made up of a fresh fruit and low fat milk.

It is essential to include the patient's family and significant others in the dietary teaching and planning. Identify the person who will be cooking and make sure they understand the diet. The responsibility for maintaining the diet is the patient.

Pharmacology

The storage and metabolism of carbohydrates, proteins, and fats are controlled by insulin, particularly in the liver, muscle, and adipose tissue. It is the key that unlocks the door to the cell allowing transport of nutrients inside. Because of the insulin deficiency of beta cells, patients with type 1 diabetes will require administration of **exogenous** (originating outside an organ) insulin to maintain blood glucose control. Patients with type 2 diabetes produce insulin and have functioning beta cells. Patients with type 2 diabetes may require insulin if diet, exercise, weight reduction, and oral hypoglycemics do not maintain adequate blood sugar control.

Insulin

Insulin preparations in the past were from pork or beef pancreas. Currently the majority of insulin used is human insulin. Human insulin is produced using strands of *Escherichia coli* and DNA technology. Human insulin has fewer incidences of allergic reactions than animal insulins. There are a wide variety of insulin preparations available to facilitate control of blood glucose levels and to adjust to the lifestyles of patients with diabetes. Each patient's dose of insulin is individualized to maintain **euglycemia** (a normal concentration of glucose in the blood) and avoid hyperglycemia and hypoglycemia. The measurement of insulin is units and injections are standardized with each milliliter containing 100 USP units of insulin (U100) (Broyles, Reiss, & Evans, 2007). Insulins are classified according to onset, peak action, and duration. Human insulins have a shorter duration of action than insulin from animal sources. Regular insulin is the base for all insulin preparations. Additives of protamine, zinc, and acetate buffers alter the onset, peak, and duration of insulin action. Lente insulin contains zinc; NPH insulin contains zinc and protamine. The additives in the insulin may cause allergic reactions at the injection site. The additives alter the appearance of the insulin, making it cloudy, rather than the clear appearance of regular insulin.

Lispro insulin (Humalog) is classified as an ultra short-acing insulin that peaks in one hour after subcutaneous injection, and it has a duration of action of four hours regardless of the dose. Food intake must be with in 15 minutes of injection to avoid hypoglycemia. Regular insulin is short-acting insulin with an onset of action in 30 minutes and duration of five to seven hours. Regular insulin is also administered intravenously in hyperglycemic emergencies.

Lente insulin is an intermediate-acting insulin with an onset of action in 2 hours, peak in 8 to 12 hours, and a duration of action of 18 to 24 hours. It is commonly given in two daily injections. NPH insulin is also an intermediate-acting insulin with onset and duration comparable to those of Lente. It is usually given twice daily and mixed with regular insulin to mimic the body's own insulin pattern. Premixed insulins (70% NPH, 30% Regular) are also available for patients who may have difficulty mixing insulins.

Insulin glargine (Lantus, Aventis) has a long duration of action, up to 24 hours after one subcutaneous injection. Insulin gargline is indicated for adults and children (age 6 and up) with type 1 diabetes and adults with type 2 diabetes requiring a basal (long-acting) insulin. Insulin gargline provides a constant insulin concentration similar to an insulin infusion. It requires a once daily injection at bedtime. If a patient becomes hypoglycemic with insulin gargline, the prolonged effects may delay the recovery.

Insulin is administered to mimic the body's normal insulin release and control blood glucose levels. With normal pancreatic functioning there is a continuous secretion of insulin throughout the day and night with increased secretion of insulin after eating. There are several insulin regimens used, ranging from a single dose of insulin to multiple doses requiring frequent monitoring of blood glucose. Commonly patients use a combination of short-acting and longer-acting insulin to achieve glycemic control (Table 57-2).

Insulin is administered with plastic disposable syringes that are available in 1 mL, 0.3 mL, and 0.5 mL sizes. The 0.3 mL syringe is referred to as the low-dose syringe and is popular among diabetics. Except in cases of severe insulin resistance, patients should not take more than 30 units of insulin in one injection. The syringes are available in short (8 mm) and long (12.7 mm) needle lengths, with the longer length preferable for obese patients. Patients at home may reuse the disposable syringes three to five times until the needle begins to blunt. Recapping the syringes at home after use provides sufficient sterility. It is not necessary to clean the needle with alcohol, and this practice may in fact alter the silicone coating on the needle and increase the pain with subsequent injections. Before recommending the recapping of syringes, consideration must be given to the patient's vision and manual dexterity. The patient should be taught to hold the syringe firmly in one hand and recap the needle using a straight motion of the forefinger and thumb (Figure 57-3). It is important that the syringe be stabilized to avoid needle-stick injury. Several pen-like devices are available for insulin delivery as well. These pens contain insulin cartridges and are useful for patients who are neurologically impaired.

Insulin may be given using a single type of insulin (Regular) or in a mixed dose (Regular and NPH). Longer acting insulins will have a cloudy appearance and should be rotated gently in the palms to resuspend the insulin. Insulin requires special storage considerations. As a protein, insulin is affected by heat and freezing. Extremes of temperature will alter the molecule of insulin. An insulin vial that is currently in use can be stored at room temperature as long as four weeks if the temperature of the room remains between 37 and 86 degrees.

TABLE 57-2	Types of Insulins		
TYPE	**ONSET**	**PEAK**	**DURATION**
Humalog (Lispro)	Less than 15 minutes	30–90 minutes	4 hours
Regular	30–60 minutes	2–4 hours	5–7 hours
NPH	3–4 hours	6–12 hours	18–28 hours
Lente	1–3 hours	8–12 hours	18–28 hours
Ultra Lente	4–6 hours	18–24 hours	36 hours
70/30	15–30 minutes	2–3 hours and 8–12 hours	18–24 hours
Insulin glargine	1.1 hour	5 hours	24 hours

Adapted from Broyles, B. E., Reiss, B. S., & Evans, M. E. (2007). Pharmacological aspects of nursing care (7th ed.). New York: Thomson Delmar Learning.

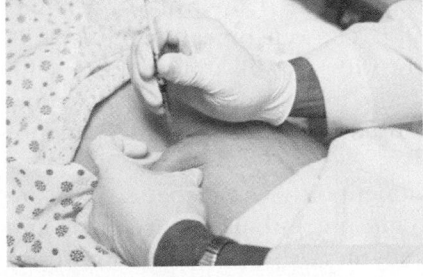

Figure 57-3 Performing a subcutaneous injection of insulin.

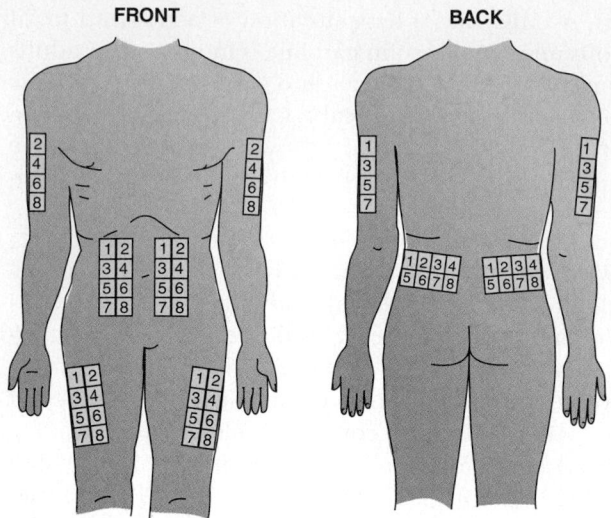

FRONT   **BACK**

Figure 57-4 Possible sites and rotation for insulin administration.

The vials should be protected from direct sunlight. Insulin not in use should be stored in the refrigerator. Insulin that is kept at room temperature is less likely to irritate the injection site than insulin that is cold.

Newly diagnosed patients requiring insulin therapy will need education on preparing and administering an insulin injection. The nurse should review insulin injection procedures with patients to ensure a correct technique as diabetes is a lifelong disease. The rate of absorption of insulin varies with the anatomic location of the injection site. Insulin is absorbed fastest from the abdomen, followed by the arm, thighs, and buttocks. Exercise of the thigh or arm will increase the absorption time and rate of onset of action. The abdomen remains the preferred site of injection because of the convenience and its good absorption rates.

Prior to the use of purified human insulins, rotation of insulin sites was a part of patient education. The rotation of sites was used to prevent **lipodystrophy,** a localized complication of insulin administration characterized by changes in the subcutaneous fat at the site of the injection. This is not a problem with human insulin, and it is no longer necessary to recommend rotation of insulin sites. Patients are instructed to inject into the abdomen and rotate the injection sites in that area (Figure 57-4).

Insulin is injected subcutaneously at a 90° angle. It is not necessary to aspirate with the injection. The needle should remain in the skin for five seconds after the injection to ensure that a complete dose of insulin has been administered. This is particularly true if an insulin pen is used. If blood or clear fluid is visible at the injection site after withdrawing the needle, pressure should be applied to the injection site for 5 to 10 seconds without rubbing. If this occurs, the patient should monitor their blood glucose more often that day. Suggestions for minimizing pain with insulin injections are shown in the Skills 360° feature.

Insulin pumps provide a continuous administration of short-acting insulin subcutaneously. These pumps are small battery operated devices that can be worn on a belt. The pump is connected to a catheter inserted in the subcutaneous tissue in the patient's abdomen. The patient will change the insertion site every 48 to 72 hours and refill the pump with insulin. The pump delivers a basal rate of insulin 24 hours a day. The user programs the pump to deliver boluses at mealtime based on the amount of carbohydrates ingested. Because the insulin pump closely mimics normal insulin secretion and uses only rapid-acting insulin, which has the least variable absorption rate, tighter glycemic control is possible. Because the insulin is absorbed more efficiently, patients often require 25 percent less insulin with a pump than with multiple daily injections. Patients who use the pump must be knowledgeable about carbohydrate counting, because the pump delivers boluses based on carbohydrates eaten at a meal. Use of a pump offers the advantage of more flexibility with mealtimes and a more normal lifestyle (Figure 57-5).

Intensive insulin therapy is another option with a goal of near normal blood glucose levels between 80 and 120 mg/dL. Multiple daily insulin injections and frequent SMBG make up this regimen. The outcomes of this type of insulin administration compares favorably with administration by insulin pump. It has the disadvantage of three or more insulin injections daily. Long-acting or intermediate-acting insulins are used for to stabilize the patient's blood glucose levels.

Oral agents are commonly used for treatment of type 2 diabetes. They are not insulin but affect the manner in which glucose and insulin are made and used by the body. It is necessary for the patient to have some **endogenous** (produced or originating from within a cell or organism) insulin for the oral hypoglycemics to take effect.

Skills 360°

Injection of Insulin

Pain with the insulin injection can be minimized by:
- Injecting insulin at room temperature.
- Ensuring no air bubbles are in the syringe prior to injection.
- Allowing topical alcohol to evaporate prior to injection.
- Using a quick wrist motion to puncture the skin quickly.
- Avoiding reuse of needles.

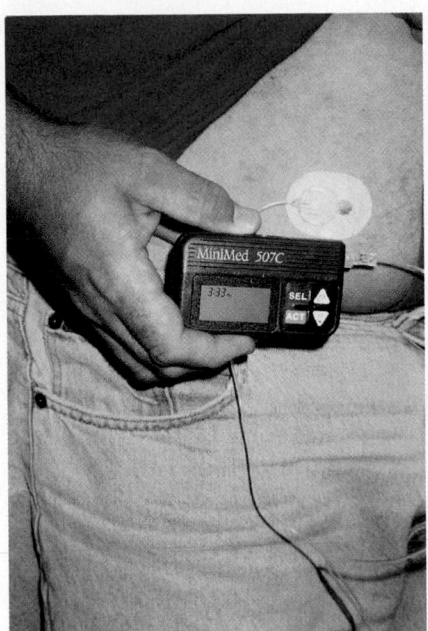

Figure 57-5 The Insulin Pump.

Sulfonylureas were introduced in the 1950s for treatment of diabetes. This classification includes Tolinase (tolazamide), Dymelor (acetohexamide), and Orinase (Tolbutamide). These drugs are referred to as first generation, because they have been used the longest. There are several second-generation sulfonylureas available today including Glucotrol and Glucotrol XL (glipizide), Micronase, DiaBeta, and Glynase (glyburide), and Amaryl (glimepiride). The second-generation drugs have a longer duration of action and fewer side effects.

Sulfonylureas act to increase the production of insulin by the pancreas, and therefore a functioning pancreas is necessary. They also improve the action of insulin at the cellular level and are thought to decrease glucose production in the liver. They tend to have better effectiveness early in the course of the disease.

Alpha glucosidase inhibitors (e.g., Precose) delay the absorption and digestion of carbohydrates in the small intestine, resulting in a smaller increase in blood glucose after eating. This classification of drugs does not alter insulin production and does not produce hypoglycemia. Because they are not absorbed systemically, they are safe to use. They can be used as monotherapy or in combination with sulfonylureas, thiazolidinediones, or meglitinide. The patient may experience hypoglycemia when used in combination with sulfonylureas and thiazolidinediones.

Biguanides (e.g., Glucophage) are another type of oral hypoglycemic agent that acts by decreasing absorption from the intestines and glucose production in the liver. Additionally, peripheral insulin sensitivity is increased. Because it does not act on the beta cells in the pancreas, there is no change in the secretion of insulin and no hypoglycemia. Lactic acidosis is a potentially serious side effect with this medication.

Meglitinide (e.g., Prandin) is another agent to lower blood glucose by stimulation of the beta cells of the pancreas. It is shorter acting than the sulfonylureas. There must be some functioning of the pancreas for this drug to be effective. It is to be taken before meals to stimulate the body to secrete insulin in response to the meal. Hypoglycemia is a side effect of meglitinide.

Thiazolidinediones (e.g., Actos, Avandia) lower insulin resistance by resensitization of the body to its own insulin and are most effective in patients with insulin resistance. They will not cause hypoglycemia when used as monotherapy, because they do not increase the production of insulin.

Patients who are using these oral hypoglycemic agents need to understand that the drugs are in addition to other types of therapy, namely diet and exercise. The patients may not always respond to the oral agents and may need to be started on insulin if the oral agents are no longer effective. Combination therapy with the oral agents is commonly used, and patients need to know the signs and symptoms of hypoglycemia (Table 57-3).

Exercise

Regular exercise is an essential part of the treatment of diabetes because of its ability to lower blood sugar and decrease cardiovascular risk factors (Blair & Church, 2003). Exercise increases the body's uptake of glucose by the muscles and therefore lowers blood sugar levels. Strength or resistance training will increase lean muscle mass and increase the metabolic rate. This is helpful in weight reduction. Exercise will aid in the reduction of cardiovascular risks by increasing HDLs and lowering cholesterol and triglyceride levels. There are additional exercise benefits resulting in decreased stress, decreased depression, and increased self-esteem.

Patients should work toward a goal of 30 minutes of exercise daily. The intensity of exercise should allow both breathing and talking with ease during the exercise. Patients can be taught to gauge the intensity of exercise by determining their desired heart range and checking the pulse to see if their heart rate falls in the target range. Target range is estimated by subtracting the patient's age from 220. This value is multiplied by 60 percent to determine the lower

TABLE 57-3 **Oral Hypoglycemics**

GENERIC (BRAND)	USUAL DOSE	ONSET TIME (HOURS)	DURATION (HOURS)
First-Generation Sulfonylureas			
tobutamide (Orinase)	500–2,000 mg divided dose	1	6–12
acetohexamide (Dymelor)	250–1,500 mg single or divided dose	1	12–24
tolazamide (Tolinase)	100–1,000 mg single or divided dose	4–6	12–24
chlorpropamide (Diabanese)	100–750 mg single dose	1	60
Second-Generation Sulfonylureas			
glipizide (Glucatrol)	2.5–40 mg single or divided dose	1–1½	10–16
glimepride (Amaryl)	1–4 mg single dose	1	24
glyburide (Diabeta, Micronase)	1.25–20 mg single or divided dose	2–4	24
Biguanides			
metformin hydrochloride (Glucophage)	500–2,500 mg two or three divided doses	24–48	6–12
Alpha-Glucosidase Inhibitors			
acarbose (Precose)	25–100 mg with meals (tid)	1	No data
miglitol (Glyset)	25–100 mg with meals (tid)	2–3	4–6
Thiazolidenediones			
troglitazone (Rezulin)	200–600 mg with a meal (qd)	2–3	No data

Adapted from Broyles, B. E., Reiss, B. S., & Evans, M. E. (2007). Pharmacological aspects of nursing care (7th ed.). New York: Thomson Delmar Learning.

limit and by 80 percent to obtain the upper limit. Patients just beginning an exercise program should use the lower limit as their target heart rate initially.

Those patients who have pacemakers, or take beta blockers, have arrhythmias, or autonomic neuropathies should use this heart rate formula with caution. The lower limit of 60 percent may overtax the heart. Patients should be taught to stop exercising and get immediate help if they experience shortness of breath, chest tightness or pain, dizziness, palpitations, or weakness.

Exercise can cause fluctuations in blood sugar levels, and the patient should be taught how to prevent these. Patients using insulin or oral medications that promote insulin secretion should be familiar with the symptoms of hypoglycemia because physical exercise lowers insulin resistance and can cause hypoglycemia for up to 48 hours after. Commonly blood glucose levels will drop between 6 and 15 hours after exercise as insulin resistance is decreased, and the muscles and liver replace the glycogen stores. The patient can reduce the risk of hypoglycemia during exercise by checking the blood sugar level before exercise and eating a carbohydrate snack for a blood sugar reading less than 100 mg/dL. It is safe to start exercise if the blood sugar level is between 100 and 200mg/dL. The patient should be taught to monitor blood glucose levels before, during, and after exercise and to eat a carbohydrate snack if the exercise session lasts longer than 60 minutes.

If the patient becomes hypoglycemic during exercise, they should immediately stop and monitor their blood sugar every 15 minutes until the level is higher than 89 mg/dL. The patient should always have a ready supply of glucose sugars and carbohydrates on hand. Exercise-induced hypoglycemia should be treated with such substances as 15 grams of carbohydrate, one half cup of fruit juice, 8 ounces of low fat milk, 6 ounces of sweetened carbonated beverage, or 4 glucose tablets.

Exercise can also cause hyperglycemia in diabetics. This typically happens when the circulating level of insulin is low and occurs more commonly in type 1 diabetes. The patient should check the blood sugar level prior to exercise. If the blood sugar level is greater than 250 mg/dL, the urine should be checked for ketones. If the ketone level in the urine is moderate to high, the patient should not exercise until the blood sugar and ketone levels are lower. Patients with type 1 diabetes can exercise with an elevated blood glucose level (250 to 300 mg/dL) as long as there are no ketones present. The blood sugar level should decrease within 15 minutes of exercise. Type 2 diabetics should not exercise if the blood sugar level is greater than 400 mg/dL. It is important to remember that type 1 diabetes is associated with ketoacidosis. Patients who participate in high-intensity physical activity may experience a transient blood glucose elevation that should fall within several hours. This elevation is a result of hormonal factors and should not be treated with insulin but should be carefully monitored.

Evaluation of Outcomes

Nutritional therapy is a mainstay in the patient's management of diabetes. The patient with diabetes should be able to maintain glycemic control utilizing their prescribed therapeutic nutritional plan. If the patient is overweight, it is expected that a slow steady weight loss will be attained using the prescribed nutritional therapy. A reduction in blood pressure may be expected with weight reduction. The patient should be able to demonstrate the selection of healthy food choices in the amounts outlined in their therapeutic nutritional plan.

There may be a localized allergic reaction at the site of the insulin injection. This is manifested as redness, tenderness, swelling, and induration or appearance of a 2- to 4-mm wheal within one to two hours after the injection. These rare reactions will occur early in the course of insulin therapy and will decrease as insulin therapy continues. Local allergic reactions are rare now with the increased use of human insulins.

Systemic allergic reactions to insulin rarely occur but may be associated with anaphylaxis. Immediately the patient will experience a localized skin reaction that increases to generalized urticaria (hives). Lipodystrophy, as previously described, can occur at the site of the injection. This reaction occurs less commonly with the use of human insulin. Fibrous, fatty changes occur at the site of repeated injections, leaving a lumpy area on the skin. Insulin injected into these scarred areas will be absorbed more slowly. In the past, lipoatrophy also occurred with repeated injections at the same site. With lipoatrophy, there is a loss of the subcutaneous fat resulting in a dimpling or pitting of the skin. Again, the occurrence of this is now rare because of the increased use of human insulins.

Respecting Our Differences

Aging and Diabetes

Geriatric patients with diabetes should be given a comprehensive geriatric history and physical in addition to a preexercise screening. Issues to be considered include an assessment of balance and gait, nutritional status, visual changes, cognitive level, and functional capacity. Elderly patients should avoid high-intensity exercise that can increase the risk of myocardial ischemia, which may be asymptomatic in diabetes. Strength training with low resistance for the legs, trunk, arms, and stomach will help to prevent functional decline and loss of muscle mass.

ACUTE COMPLICATIONS OF DIABETES

Acute complications of diabetes include hyperglycemia from too little insulin and hypoglycemia from too much insulin. In both diabetic ketoacidosis (DKA) and hyperosmolar hyperglycemic nonketotic syndrome (HHNS), there is an imbalance among circulating insulin levels and the counter regulatory hormones. The hormones stimulate increase glucose production in the liver and cause decreased utilization of glucose in the peripheral tissues. Infection is one of the most common causes for the development of DKA or HHNS. Medications affecting the metabolism of carbohydrates, such as corticosteroids or thiazides, may also contribute to the development of DKA and HHNS.

The management of both DKA and HHNS is aimed at monitoring and correcting the frequent dehydration, hyperglycemia, and electrolyte imbalances of the patient. Nurses must be able to clinically differentiate the two events. Hypoglycemia can rapidly develop causing serious threat to the patient's well-being.

Diabetic Ketoacidosis

DKA results from a marked insulin deficiency and is manifested by hyperglycemia, ketosis, acidosis, and dehydration. DKA is associated with type 1 diabetes but may also occur in type 2. It is a life-threatening medical emergency associated with a mortality rate of approximately 5 percent (Figure 57-6). Factors contributing to the development of DKA include illness, infection, inadequate management of the disease, insufficient insulin, and undiagnosed type 1 diabetes. Noncompliance with the therapeutic regimen is the most common causes of recurrent ketoacidosis (Tierney, et al., 2004).

In DKA, there is insufficient insulin to metabolize glucose, and the body begins to break down protein stores for energy. Ketones are by-products of protein breakdown and are acidic in nature. As the ketone level in the blood increases, the pH is altered, and metabolic acidosis develops.

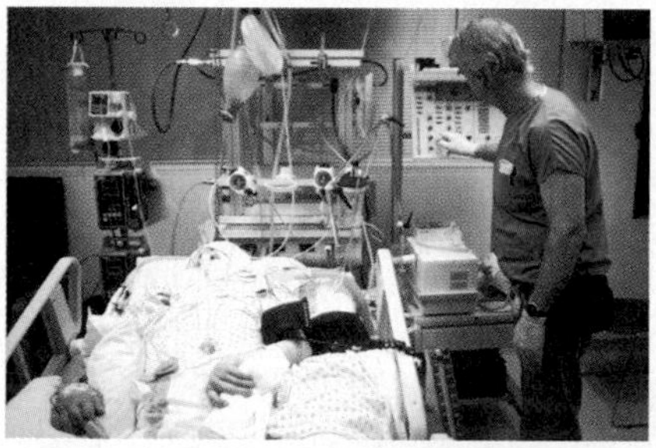

Figure 57-6 Patient on a ventilator in a critical care unit for the complication of DKA.

Assessment with Clinical Manifestations

The patient often will experience fatigue, polydipsia, and polyuria prior to the development of ketoacidosis. Nausea, vomiting, and change in the level of consciousness (LOC) can occur as well. Physical examination reveals dehydration from the hyperglycemia and the characteristic acetone or fruity odor of the breath. There is fluid and electrolyte depletion with the dehydration, and the patient will have hypotension and tachycardia. Abdominal pain is accompanied by nausea and vomiting. Kussmaul breathing is associated with DKA. The respiratory rate increases in rate and depth in an attempt to blow off the carbon dioxide accumulating with the acidosis state. Laboratory findings include hyperglycemia greater than 250 mg/dL, acidic pH in the arterial blood (less than 7.35), and low serum bicarbonate levels (less than 15 mEq/L). Ketones and glucose are present in the urine in large amounts. Serum potassium may be elevated as potassium shifts with the acidosis. Potassium levels may also be near normal or low. This represents a severe total body depletion of potassium and requires careful monitoring as the treatment of DKA will further lower the potassium levels. The patient is typically slightly hypothermic, and an infection should be suspected if an elevation in temperature is present. Hypothermia occurs because of peripheral vasodilatation and is considered a poor prognostic sign (Hurlock-Chorostecki, 2004).

Nursing Diagnoses

Based on the information gathered, examples of nursing diagnoses in the patient with diabetes may include the following:
- Deficient fluid volume related to active losses.
- Disturbed thought processes related to physiological causes.
- Risk for imbalanced body temperature related to decreased sensitivity of thermoreceptors.

Planning and Implementation

Patients with DKA can now be managed at home if the dehydration is not severe. The decision to manage the patient at home takes into consideration other accompanying symptoms, such as change in LOC, presence of fever, increased fluid losses through nausea, vomiting and diarrhea, and the ability for frequent communication with the health care practitioner.

The patient's fluid volume deficit is life-threatening and must be treated immediately. Fluid replacement of the intravascular and extravascular space is the goal of treatment. Intravenous (IV) fluids of 0.9% normal saline (NS) or 0.45% NS are used to reestablish an adequate urine output of 30 to 60 mL/hour and reverse the hypotension. When the blood glucose level is down to 250 mg/dL, 5% dextrose is added to the IV fluids to prevent hypoglycemia. Particular attention is given to correction of potassium imbalances. At the onset, the potassium levels may be high or normal, but these levels will fall with the administration of IV insulin. Insulin will move the potassium from the circulation into the cells and hypokalemia develops. This is a lethal complication of DKA. Potassium replacement will be administered to prevent hypokalemia. The potassium replacement will be started when the serum potassium level falls below 5.5 mEq/L.

Regular insulin is administered intravenously after fluid therapy has begun. Insulin will move water, potassium, and glucose into the cells. The movement of fluids into the cells acts to deplete the vascular volume. IV insulin therapy begins with a bolus of insulin, after determining that there is no hypokalemia present, followed by a continuous infusion.

Evaluation of Outcomes

Overall, DKA is resolved when the plasma glucose is less than 200 mg/dL. In addition, blood glucose levels are monitored, as are vital signs, LOC, cardiac monitoring, urine output, and O_2 saturation. The patient must be assessed for fluid volume overload with the fluid resuscitation. Potassium will be given to correct hypokalemia, and potassium levels will be closely monitored.

Hyperosmolar Hyperglycemic Nonketotic Syndrome

Patients with diabetes who produce sufficient insulin to prevent protein breakdown and ketoacidosis may not produce sufficient insulin to prevent or reverse severe hyperglycemia. HHNS is a life-threatening emergency associated with severe hyperglycemia, an osmotic diuresis, and a profound fluid volume deficit. The absence of ketosis is the distinguishing feature between DKA and HHNS.

Assessment with Clinical Manifestations

HHNS has a slower onset, days to weeks, with polydipsia, polyuria, and weakness. Blood glucose levels can rise extremely high (e.g., above 400 mg/dL), which increases the osmolality of the blood. This leads to neurological changes that include seizures, aphasia, somnolence, and coma. HHNS occurs more often in the older adult. Often these patients will have congestive heart failure and renal insufficiency. The presence of either of these will make the prognosis for the patient worse. Common precipitating factors include infection or recent surgery. The onset is frequently attributed to a decreased fluid intake. The patient will present with blood glucose levels greater than 400 mg/dL and the absence of ketones. The serum osmolality will be greater than 310 mOsm/kg, and no evidence of acidosis. The serum sodium level may be greater than 140 mEq/L.

Nursing Diagnoses

Nursing diagnoses for the patient experiencing HHNS include but are not limited to the following:
- Deficient fluid volume related to active losses.

- Risk for ineffective therapeutic regimen management.
- Disturbed sensory perception related to biochemical imbalance.

Planning and Implementation

As with DKA, fluid resuscitation is of utmost importance in treating a patient with HHNS. IV therapy is initiated with 0.9% NS if oliguria and hypotension are present. If hypotension and oliguria are not present, fluid therapy is initiated with 0.45% NS, because the patient is hyperosmolar. It is common to deliver large volumes of fluid, as much as 6 to 8 liters in the first 8 to 10 hours of therapy. When the blood glucose level reaches 250 mg/dL 5% dextrose will be added to the IV solution. A goal of therapy is maintenance of the blood glucose levels between 250 and 300 mg/dL to decrease the risk of cerebral edema. Urine output of 50 mL/hour is a goal of fluid therapy. The patient will be given IV regular insulin, but HHNS may require less insulin than DKA. If the fluid volume deficit is corrected the hyperglycemia lessens. Correction of the hypovolemia will increase the functioning of the kidneys and the excretion of glucose in the urine (Tierney, et al., 2004). Potassium imbalances occur with HHNS as insulin drives the glucose and potassium in to the cells. The patient with HHNS will have fewer problems with potassium than the patient with DKA because of the absence of acidosis. As with any administration of potassium, adequate renal function must be established.

Evaluation of Outcomes

HHNS has a higher rate of mortality than DKA because of the increased incidence in elderly patients. The elderly are at increased risk because of decreased cardiovascular functioning and the slower recognition of the onset of dehydration. The nurse will monitor the vital signs, lung sounds, cardiac rhythm, LOC, urine output, and potassium levels while caring for the patient with HHNS. Patients should be taught to care for themselves, because infection is a leading cause of DKA and HHNS.

Hypoglycemia

Another acute complication of diabetes is hypoglycemia (blood glucose levels less than 70 mg/dL). Hypoglycemia must be recognized and treated quickly, because the brain requires constant sufficient supplies of glucose to function. Hypoglycemia results from too much insulin.

Assessment with Clinical Manifestations

The patient with hypoglycemia presents with irritability, increasing confusion, tremors, hunger, sweating, weakness, and visual disturbances. The patient presentation is similar to alcohol intoxication and if not treated rapidly, coma and death may occur. Causes of hypoglycemia are too little food, too much insulin, increased exercise, or delay in eating. It is more common with insulin therapy but can occur in patients treated with oral agents as well.

Patients may not be able to recognize the symptoms of hypoglycemia (hypoglycemia unawareness). This can occur because of neuropathy in the autonomic nervous system of the diabetic. This neuropathy interferes with the release of counter-regulatory hormones by the body to compensate for the low blood sugar levels. Hypoglycemia can occur in both type 1 and type 2 diabetes (Table 57-4). Hypoglycemia unawareness is common in the elderly patients and also in patients who take beta blockers (see Red Flag feature). Patients with hypoglycemic unawareness will usually be allowed to have higher blood glucose levels to prevent undetected episodes of hypoglycemia.

A patient may exhibit symptoms of hypoglycemia in the presence of blood glucose levels that are above normal. This can occur when the blood glucose level has been extremely high and decreases rapidly. Patients may experience the symptoms of hypoglycemia when the hyperglycemia was treated aggressively.

TABLE 57-4	**Hypoglycemia in Type 1 and Type 2 Diabetes**
ONSET/CAUSE	Occurs with both type 1 and type 2 diabetes
	Rapid onset
	Too much insulin or dose error
	Insufficient food intake
RISK FACTORS	Trauma
	Illness
	Exercise
	Renal failure
	Alcohol intake
	Surgery
CLINICAL MANIFESTATIONS	Cool, moist skin
	Pallor
	Headache
	Nausea
	Sweating
	Tremors
	Hunger
	Lethargy
	Confusion
	Slurred speech
	Anxiety
TREATMENT	15 grams of fast acting carbohydrate, i.e., 3–4 glucose tablets, 4–6 ounces of fruit juice or regular soda
	Glucagon 1 mg subcutaneously or intramuscularly followed by concentrated source of carbohydrate when patient fully alert

Adapted from DeLaune, S., & Ladner, P. (2006). Fundamentals of nursing (3rd ed.). New York: Thomson Delmar Learning; Greenspan, F. S., & Gardner, D. G. (2004). Basic and clinical endocrinology (7th ed.). New York: Lange Medical Books.

Nursing Diagnoses

Nursing diagnoses for patients experiencing hypoglycemia may include but are not limited to the following:
- Imbalanced nutrition related to imbalance of food, insulin, and activity.
- Knowledge deficit regarding diabetes self-care.
- Disturbed sensory perception related to biochemical imbalance.

Planning and Implementation

Recognition of hypoglycemia is important. The blood glucose level should be assessed quickly with the onset of the first symptom. In the absence of blood glucose monitoring equipment, the patient should be treated for the hypoglycemia. If the blood glucose level is assessed at less than 70 mg/dL, treatment is begun. The patient should be given 10 to 15 g of a simple carbohydrate (fast acting), i.e., 8 ounces of low-fat milk or 4 ounces of fruit juice or a carbonated soft drink. The treatment should be moderate but quick, with the blood glucose levels monitored every 15 minutes. If the blood glucose is low (less than 70 mg/dL) after the initial treatment, the treatment is repeated. The nurse can teach the patient that 15 g of carbohydrate are given every 15 minutes until the blood glucose level is above 70 mg/dL. Once that level is reached the patient should eat a regular meal or snack and recheck the blood glucose in 45 minutes. If the hypoglycemia does not reverse after two or three doses of carbohydrates or if the swallowing is impaired, an injection of 1 mg of glucagon may be given intramuscularly or subcutaneously. Glucagon will make glucose more available by stimulating the liver to convert some glycogen stores to glucose. Foods that are sweet and contain fat should not be given, such as candy bars or cookies. The presence of fat in the food slows the absorption of the sugar. The patient may use glucose tablets or gel to treat hypoglycemia.

The patient should be assessed for reasons for the occurrence of the hypoglycemic episodes. Patient and family education may be indicated. The patient and family must recognize the danger of hypoglycemia and the potential for cognitive impairment if not treated.

Dawn Phenomenon and Somogyi Effect

The dawn phenomenon manifests itself as morning hyperglycemia present on awakening. This hyperglycemia results from predawn release of counter-regulatory hormones. It is likely that cortisol and growth hormones are factors in the occurrence of the dawn phenomenon. It is most common in adolescence and young adults.

The Somogyi effect presents as wide variations in early morning or fasting blood glucose levels. The Somogyi effect is a result of too much insulin and occurs during sleep. Too much insulin activates the counter-regulatory hormones, and gluconeogenesis and glycogenolysis occurs, resulting in hyperglycemia and ketosis. When the blood sugar is measured in the morning and hyperglycemia is present, the patient or the health care worker may increase the dose of insulin. This action is incorrect because the Somogyi effect is a result of too much insulin. The Somogyi effect causes headaches on awakening, nightmares, and night sweats. When the Somogyi effect is suspected the patient's blood sugar should be monitored between 2 and 4 a.m. to check for the presence of hypoglycemia at that time. If the patient is hypoglycemic then, the insulin dose affecting the morning blood sugar level should be reduced.

Treatment for the dawn phenomenon is an increase in insulin or an adjustment in the administration. Treatment for the Somogyi effect is less insulin. The patient and the nurse should be aware that careful assessment is necessary to determine the cause of the early morning rise in blood sugars as the treatment for Somogyi effect is different than the treatment for the dawn phenomenon.

CHRONIC COMPLICATIONS OF DIABETES

Chronic complications include macrovascular and microvascular problems. These complications include angiopathy or vessel disease, retinopathy, neuropathy, and nephropathy. These conditions are caused by damage to the large and small vessels from chronically elevated blood glucose. The risk of development of microvascular complications (e.g., integumentary problems or infections) can be dramatically decreased with optimal control of blood sugar levels. These results were achieved with an intensive insulin therapy regimen. Additionally the study indicated that intensive insulin therapy reduces the risk of retinopathy and nephropathy. Patients with diabetes require regularly scheduled follow-up treatment to prevent and monitor the occurrence of long-term complications.

Angiopathy or Vessel Disease

Macrovascular complications cause changes in the large vessels. These changes may occur in patients who do not have diabetes but are more frequent and earlier in patients who do have diabetes. As a disease of metabolism, diabetes affects the metabolism of lipids. Plaque formation from atherosclerosis is associated with diabetes. The incidence of vessel disease can be decreased with optimal glycemic control. The diseases of the larger vessels include cardiovascular, cerebral, and peripheral vascular diseases. Patients should understand the risk factors associated with macrovascular disease, because many of the risk factors are modifiable with lifestyle changes. These risk factors include obesity, smoking, sedentary lifestyle, high blood pressure, and increased fat intake. Patient education efforts should be aimed at reduction of these modifiable risk factors (refer to chapter 23 for assessment considerations).

Microvascular Complications

Microvascular complications are specific to diabetes and result from the chronic presence of hyperglycemia. The elevated blood glucose levels lead to a thickening in the capillaries and arterioles. Most common sites of occurrence include the eyes with diabetic retinopathy, the kidneys with nephropathy, and skin. These do not usually appear until the first or second decade after the onset of diabetes.

Diabetic Retinopathy

Chronic hyperglycemia causes damage to the small vessels of the retina in patients with diabetes. It is a common complication, present in approximately 60 percent of patients with type 2 diabetes and nearly every patient with type 1 diabetes for longer than 20 years. Diabetic retinopathy is the most frequent cause of new blindness among adults ages 20 to 74. During the first two decades of the disease, nearly all patients with type 1 diabetes and more than 60 percent of patients with type 2 diabetes have retinopathy.

Assessment with Clinical Manifestations

The most common form of retinopathy is nonproliferative. This manifests itself as microaneurysms in the retinal capillaries. Capillary fluid leaks from the weakened aneurysms and retinal edema occurs. If the macular area of the eye is involved, the vision will be affected.

Proliferative retinopathy is more severe, involving the vitreous humor and the retina. New blood vessels are formed in the retina as the smaller capillaries become occluded. This is called neovascularization. The new blood vessels are extremely friable (broken) and subject to hemorrhage. As the vessels tear and bleed in the vitreous, the patient's vision is changed. The patient will report the appearance of red or black lines or spots. There may be retinal detachment or involvement of the macula.

Diagnostic Tests

Examination with an ophthalmoscope allows direct visualization of the retina. A fluorescein angiograph may be performed as well to provide information about the presence and type of retinopathy. This procedure involves a venous injection of a dye that is carried throughout the body but accumulates in the vessels of the retina. The ophthalmologist is then able to visualize the retinal vessels in greater detail than with an ophthalmoscope alone. This procedure is associated with minor side effects of nausea with the injection of the dye, a yellow fluorescent color of the urine and skin for 12 to 24 hours and occasionally an allergic reaction with hives and itching. Patient instructions are shown in the patient playbook feature.

Planning and Implementation

Prevention of retinopathy is first and foremost. The importance of near normal glycemic control is stressed. The main medical treatment of diabetic retinopathy is laser photocoagulation to destroy the areas of revascularization and leaking vessels. This procedure may have a profound impact on slowing the progression of vision loss. These treatments are done on an outpatient basis, with most patients returning to usual activities of daily living the next day.

PATIENT PLAYBOOK

Instructions for a Fluorescein Angiogram

The nurse should inform the patient that is going to have a fluorescein angiogram of the following information:

- This is a painless procedure.
- The steps involved in the diagnostic test.
- The potential side effects of the procedure.
- There could be brief discomfort associated with the camera flash.

Evaluation of Outcomes

The procedure may cause some discomfort, but intense pain is rare. The patient will be pretreated with an analgesic eye drop. Occasionally patients may develop permanent visual changes from the treatment, including loss of peripheral vision or decreased ability to adapt to the dark. These changes are much less than those that result from progressive retinopathy.

If a large hemorrhage occurs in the vitreous, the blood combines with the vitreous fluid and hampers the ability of light to pass through the eye, resulting in blindness. This fluid can be removed with a drill-like instrument in a procedure called a vitrectomy. The space is then filled with saline. Patients are candidates for this surgery if the hemorrhage has persisted for six months, and they are experiencing visual loss. Vision should improve after the procedure, but a return to near normal vision is not to be expected.

Nursing care is focused on patient education regarding the importance of regular eye exams and glycemic control. The nurse emphasizes to the patient the importance of early diagnosis and treatment. If vision loss occurs, the nurse will need to incorporate the use of assistive devices to aid the patient in self-care. The patient should be reminded that retinopathy occurs after having diabetes for several years and does not indicate that the diabetes is getting worse. If the patient maintains optimal blood sugar control and optimal blood pressure, the chances for loss of vision are lessened. The patient must understand and comply with regular eye examinations.

Nephropathy

Renal disease, secondary to microvascular changes associated with diabetes, is common, accounting for approximately one half of the cases of newly diagnosed end-stage renal disease (ESRD) annually. About one quarter to one third of patients with type 1 and type 2 diabetes will exhibit nephropathy. A lesser number of type 2 diabetics progress to ESRD. Symptoms of renal disease will manifest within 10 to 15 years for type 1 diabetics and within 10 years for type 2 diabetics. Because of the slow development of type 2 diabetes, frequently patients will also develop evidence of renal disease at the time of diagnosis of type 2 diabetes. The DCCT study concluded that intensive treatment of diabetes with maintenance of hemoglobin A_{1C} levels as close to normal as possible decreased the occurrence of early signs of renal disease. Microalbuminuria was reduced by 39 percent, and albuminuria was reduced by 54 percent in that study. A similar study in the United Kingdom showed a decreased incidence of nephropathy in type 2 diabetics with good glycemic control.

When glycemic control is not adequate allowing elevated levels of blood glucose, the kidneys filtration will decrease, and protein from the blood is excreted in the urine. Protein has fluid attracting properties, and the pressure in the blood vessels of the kidneys increases. This increased blood pressure is thought to be the mechanism for nephropathy.

Assessment with Clinical Manifestations

Signs and symptoms of kidney disease are not specific to the diabetic. The diabetic patient may have an increase in the occurrence of hypoglycemia as the breakdown of insulin (exogenous and endogenous) decreases. Insulin requirements will change as a result of the kidney disease and the treatments. It is not uncommon for multiple body systems to fail as the kidney disease progresses, including visual impairment, foot ulcerations, nocturnal diarrhea, and heart failure. Patients in the early stages of renal disease will frequently develop hypertension.

Diagnostic Tests

Albumin in the urine is a hallmark of renal disease. Clinical nephropathy will develop in approximately 85 percent of patients with microalbuminuria. Albumin in the urine may be detected with a urine dipstick or 24-hour urine collection. If significant amounts of albumin are present, a blood urea nitrogen (BUN) and creatinine are obtained.

Nursing Diagnoses

Please refer to chapter 55 for specific nursing diagnoses on nephropathy conditions.

Planning and Implementation

Nursing management includes maintenance of glycemic control. Additionally, the nurse must stress prevention of urinary tract infections and management of hypertension. The nurse should adjust the patient's medications in an attempt to meet the challenging demands of decreased renal functioning. In addition, nursing care must involve nutritional changes, which will include a low-protein, low-sodium diet. Patients with microalbuminuria in excess of 30 mg in 24 hours on two consecutive tests will be started on an angiotensin-converting enzyme (ACE) inhibitor to lower the blood pressure and reduce the microalbuminuria. Another option is the use of angiotensin-receptor blocking agents and a low-protein diet.

Patients in ESRD are often placed on hemodialysis. There is a trend toward use of continuous ambulatory peritoneal dialysis for patients with diabetes. This type of dialysis allows the patient more freedom in their lifestyle. Insulin can be added to the dialysate to achieve better glycemic control. Some patients may need to increase their insulin requirements because of the glucose in the dialysate. Infection is a complication of peritoneal dialysis.

Evaluation of Outcomes

Please refer to chapter 55 for explanation of specific evaluation of outcomes for patients with nephropathy conditions.

Peripheral Neuropathy (Sensory Neuropathy)

Diabetic neuropathies involve the peripheral, autonomic, and spinal nerves. The diabetic neuropathies are a group of disorders that increase in occurrence as the diabetic patient ages and with the increasing duration of diabetes. The cause of the neuropathies is chronic elevation of blood glucose levels. The two most commonly occurring types are autonomic and sensorimotor (peripheral) neuropathy. Peripheral neuropathy most often involves the nerves of the lower extremities, affecting the body symmetrically, and proceeding proximally (Mchugh, 2004).

The peripheral neuropathies are sensory disorders that are associated with diabetes. The most common type seen in diabetes is the polyneuropathies, or bilateral sensory disorders, that begin in the toes and feet and progress upward. These conditions can become serious and lead to complete tissue destruction, gangrene, and may even require limb amputations or the development of septic shock (Figure 57-7). The presentation of symptoms will be based on the nerve fibers that are involved. In addition, infections are increased with diabetes, which also prolongs wound healing (Aragon, 2003).

Assessment with Clinical Manifestations

Assessment will reveal symptoms of generalized tingling or a prickly sensation (paresthesia) and burning sensations, particularly at night. The patient may experience **hyperesthesia** (increased sensitivity of the skin) and may report that even light pressure from bedcovers is intolerable. As the neuropathy advances, sensation in the feet decreases markedly, leaving the feet numb. This decreased sensation makes the patient susceptible to injury, as he or she is unaware of pain or pressure sensations. Peripheral neuropathy is also associated with deformities of the feet, such as Charcot's joints. Peripheral neuropathy causes atrophy of the muscles in the foot. With peripheral neuropathy, the foot assumes a rocker bottom with an abnormal weight distribution on the joints. The patient may have decreased deep tendon reflexes on exam.

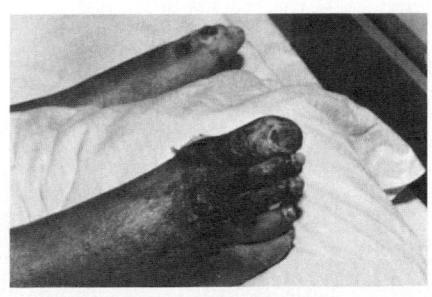

Figure 57-7 Gangrene of the toes and foot as a result of peripheral neuropathy.

Nursing Diagnoses

Nursing diagnoses for patients with diabetic neuropathies may include but are not limited to the following:

- Disturbed sensory perception, tactile, related to biochemical imbalance.
- Impaired skin integrity related to altered metabolic state.

Planning and Implementation

The best management for diabetic neuropathy is optimal glycemic control. It will be effective in some but not all cases. Symptoms are managed with medications that include topical anesthetics (e.g., capsaicin), tricyclic antidepressants (e.g., amitriptyline), and antiseizure drugs (e.g., gabapentin).

Capsaicin is produced from chili peppers. As a topical medication, it acts locally to decrease the chemicals that mediate pain. It is used with a fair amount of success when applied three to four times daily. The patient may initially experience an increase in symptoms. Within two weeks of therapy, the patients will begin to have pain relief. Tricyclic antidepressants decrease the pain sensation by inhibiting the reuptake of serotonin and norepinephrine and decrease the transmission of pain sensation at the spinal level. The exact mechanism of action of gabapentin is not understood, but it has been shown to relieve the pain of peripheral neuropathy.

Evaluation of Outcomes

Potential patient outcomes for each of the example nursing diagnoses for the patient with peripheral neuropathies are:

- Disturbed sensory perception, tactile, related to biochemical imbalance: The patient will experience not problems with peripheral neurovascular function by a specified date.
- Impaired skin integrity related to altered metabolic state: The patient will not experience any alteration in skin integrity by a specified date.

Autonomic Neuropathies

Autonomic neuropathies are widespread, and they affect nearly every body system. Essentially, the pathology of this diabetic complication is the breakdown of the autonomic nervous system.

Assessment with Clinical Manifestations

Autonomic neuropathy leads to bowel and bladder incontinence, hypoglycemic unawareness, and delayed gastric emptying (gastroparesis). Gastroparesis presents as anorexia, nausea and vomiting, feelings of fullness, and gastroesophageal reflux. The delay of absorption of food that occurs with gastroparesis can lead to the development of hypoglycemia. The effects of autonomic neuropathy on the cardiovascular system lead to postural hypotension, asymptomatic myocardial infarction, and a resting tachycardia.

Sexual functioning can be affected in males or females. Males may experience erectile dysfunction, and females may experience decreased libido. The patient may develop a neurogenic bladder with urinary retention.

Nursing Diagnoses

Potential complications or collaborative problems for the patient with autonomic neuropathies may include:

- Diarrhea.
- Constipation.
- Urinary retention.
- Decreased sexual functioning.

Planning and Implementation

Nursing management is aimed at the symptoms. No treatment is available for the painless myocardial ischemia within the cardiovascular system. Patient education should include the avoidance of strenuous exercise. Patients are cautioned about changing positions slowly in the presence of postural hypotension. Antiembolic stockings may alleviate some of the postural hypotension by decreasing the pooling of blood in the lower extremities. Gastroparesis is treated with glycemic control, a low-fat diet in small frequent feedings, and medications to increase gastric emptying (metoclopramide). If the patient experiences diarrhea from diabetes, bulk-forming agents can be used. Constipation is treated with increased fluids and fiber. Neurogenic bladder is treated by emptying the bladder every three hours and use of the Credé's method (downward pressure on the abdomen over the bladder area) Patients may need to learn self-catheterization.

Evaluation of Outcomes

Nursing care is aimed at alleviation of the symptoms. The patient may be expected to exhibit no diarrhea or constipation and increased bladder emptying.

Peripheral Vascular Complications of the Lower Extremities

The most common cause of hospitalization for the diabetic patient is the complication of the lower extremities and specifically, the foot. These complications are a result of the peripheral vascular changes that occur with diabetes, both microvascular and macrovascular (Figure 57-8). An alteration in the shape and mechanics of the foot from neuropathy contributes as well. Other risk factors include the presence of peripheral vascular disease and smoking. Patients who are male, have had diabetes for more than 10 years, have poor glycemic control, or microvascular or macrovascular complications are at increased risk of ulcerations or amputations. Peripheral vascular disease decreases the blood flow, and therefore the supply of nutrients and oxygen to the tissues. This increases the risk for infection and delays wound healing.

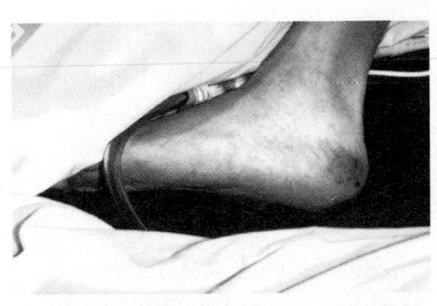

Figure 57-8 The beginnings of a pressure ulcer on the foot for the patient with diabetes can become a serious problem.

Assessment with Clinical Manifestations

Assessment for peripheral vascular dysfunction (PVD) include diminished or absent pedal pulses, cool feet, pain at rest, intermittent claudication, hair loss on the extremity, rubor of the skin (e.g., redness) when the extremity is dependent, and slower capillary filling. Doppler studies or angiography will confirm the diagnosis. The loss of sensation from peripheral neuropathy is another major risk factor for the development of foot ulcers in patients with diabetes. Loss of sensation removes the protective function of pain, and the patient is unable to sense pressure or discomfort or even injury. Pain sensation is assessed by use of a monofilament on the plantar aspect (sole) of the patient's foot.

Nursing Diagnoses

Nursing diagnoses for patients with PVD may include but are not limited to the following:

- Disturbed sensory perception, tactile, related to biochemical imbalance.
- Impaired skin integrity related to altered metabolic state.

Planning and Implementation

Early identification and prevention of risk factors is the optimal patient management. The feet of the diabetic should be assessed at every visit to a health care practitioner and inspected daily at home by the patient or family member. Sensation should be checked annually using the Semmes-Weinstein monofilament. The exam should also include an assessment of the foot structure and mechanics, the vascular status, and integrity of the skin.

Patients with neuropathy will require well-fitted shoes. If the patient has signs of increased pressure on the plantar aspect of the foot, such as calluses, redness, or warmth, cushioning with shoe inserts can be used to redistribute the pressure on the foot. Foot deformities are common in the diabetic and may require extra wide or deep shoes.

Management of PVD includes reduction or control of risk factors, especially smoking, hypertension, and elevated cholesterol levels. Patients may require surgery, including a bypass graft or amputation.

Patient and family member's knowledge and practice of foot care should be assessed regularly. Patients should be instructed to wash their feet daily with warm water and mild soap. Decreased sensation increases the risk of burn injuries; therefore the patient should first test the water temperature with his or her hands. The feet should be patted dry, particularly between the toes. Feet should be examined daily for cuts, blisters, and reddened areas. Patients are advised not to use over-the-counter (OTC) preparations to treat calluses and corns. Toe nails should be cut with the corners rounded; they are easier to trim following a bath or shower. The nails should be cut straight across to avoid ingrown toe nails. Shoes should fit properly and not be open-toed styles or high heels. Socks are to be clean cotton and colorfast. Cotton socks are more absorbent and are therefore preferable. Cuts are to be cleansed with warm water and mild soap. The use of alcohol or iodine is to be avoided. Injuries to the skin or infections are to be reported immediately to the health care provider.

Evaluation of Outcomes

Potential patient outcomes for each of the example nursing diagnoses for the patient with PVD are:

- Disturbed sensory perception, tactile, related to biochemical imbalance: The patient will not experience problems with peripheral neurovascular function by a specified date.
- Impaired skin integrity related to altered metabolic state: The patient will not experience any alteration in skin integrity by a specified date.

Skin Complications

The microangiopathy associated with diabetes increases the chances of skin changes and infections. It is common for patients with diabetes to have infections of the skin, especially *Candida albicans*. Localized skin infections, such as boils and furuncles, are common and recurrent in patients with diabetes. Often it is the history of recurrent skin infections that leads the health care provider to suspect diabetes.

Assessment with Clinical Manifestations

Assessing the skin in the diabetic patient is extremely important to his or her well-being. The appearance of the skin may change on the lower extremities. Red-yellow lesions, called necrobiosis lipoidica diabeticorum, present along the anterior aspect of the lower extremities, commonly along the shin. These spots are caused by the breakdown of collagen. Skin around the area atrophies and thins, making it susceptible to injury and ulceration. These are not common but often are present before other clinical signs of diabetes and occur more often in young women. It is common to find small brown spots along the shin. These brown spots are usually less than 1 cm in diameter and are harmless.

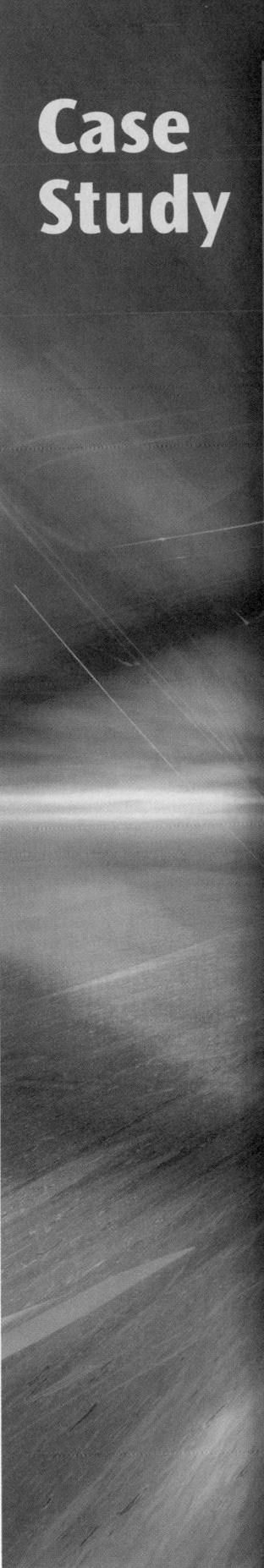

Case Study

Nursing Care Plan

Mrs. Ballenger, age 78, is hospitalized in the intensive care unit (ICU) with complications of type 1 diabetes mellitus. Most recently, she is experiencing diabetic ketoacidosis with a blood glucose of 320 mg/dL. In addition, she has coronary heart disease (CHD) from the microvascular complications of her diabetes; she has a pulmonary artery catheter to monitor his hemodynamic status. Her primary clinical manifestations from the CHD are hypertension, tachycardia, and occasional arrhythmias. At present her level of consciousness (LOC) is impaired, she is breathing with Kussmaul respirations, her breath is acetone in nature, and she is extremely fatigued.

Assessment

A 78-year-old female with complications associated with type 1 diabetes mellitus. Specifically, she has a primary diagnosis of diabetic ketoacidosis ([DKA] blood glucose = 320 mg/dL. In addition she has hypertension, atrial cardiac arrhythmias, and a decreased LOC. She is being monitored in an intensive care unit.

Nursing Diagnosis #1: Deficient fluid volume related to osmotic diuresis associated with hyperglycemia.

NOC: Electrolyte and Acid-Base Imbalance; Fluid balance; Hydration; Nutritional status; Food and fluid intake.

NIC: Fluid management; Hypovolemia management; Shock management: Volume

Expected Outcomes
The patient will:
1. Maintain a blood glucose level in the 150–180 mg/dL range within 72 hours.
2. Demonstrate no signs or symptoms of dehydration during her admission in the ICU.
3. Maintain a cardiac output in the normal range of 4–6 L/min during her admission to the ICU.

Planning/Interventions/Rationale

1. Measure blood glucose levels every hour and administer insulin per sliding scale orders. *Blood glucose levels are at a crisis level, and close monitoring prevents further complications of DKA.*
2. Evaluate cardiac output by assessing cardiac system with vital signs, hemodynamic monitor (pulmonary artery catheter), and electrophysiology. *Allows for close cardiac monitoring, which is necessary for the patient's critical condition.*
3. Assess hydration status every hour by monitoring: urine specific gravity, intake and output (hourly urine output), skin turgor, and vital signs. *Frequent assessment detects subtle changes in hydration status during the critical complication of DKA.*

Evaluation

The patient has a blood glucose within a controlled range, stable hemodynamic readings of the pulmonary artery catheter, and no clinical manifestations of dehydration during her admission to the ICU.

Nursing Diagnosis #2: Ineffective breathing pattern of Kussmaul respirations related to metabolic acidosis associated with DKA.

NOC: Respiratory status: Ventilation; Vital signs status; Respiratory status; Airway patency

NIC: Airway management; Respiratory monitoring

Case Study

Expected Outcomes

The patient will:

1. Demonstrate an effective respiratory rate of 12–16 breaths per minute with an oxygen saturation level of at least 94 percent within 24 hours.
2. Progressively regain level of consciousness within 24–48 hours.
3. Decrease sense of energy and experience less generalized fatigue within 24–48 hours.

Planning/Interventions/Rationale

1. Monitor oxygen saturation levels and assess depth or rhythm of respirations every hour. *Detects respiratory compensation during a time of the respiratory crisis of Kussmaul breathing (caused by the DKA).*
2. Assess LOC by evaluating neurological responses and patient's ability to effectively answer questions every hour. *Provides constant monitoring of neurological status.*
3. Ask patient questions regarding her level of energy and ask patient to quantify from 1–10 the level of her fatigue every hour. *Evaluates fatigue levels on constant basis.*

Evaluation

The patient has a progressive decrease in the Kussmaul breathing pattern, an increasing LOC, and an increasing level of energy.

KEY CONCEPTS

- Diabetes mellitus refers to a group of chronic disorders of metabolism characterized by elevated blood glucose levels as well as disturbances in metabolism of carbohydrate, fat, and protein.
- There are four types of diabetes mellitus: type 1 diabetes mellitus, type 2 diabetes mellitus, gestational diabetes, and impaired glucose tolerance (prediabetes).
- Insulin is one of the hormones produced by the pancreas (beta cells) with a function of lowering blood sugar.
- Glucagon is a hormone released by the alpha cells of the pancreas, and it functions to raise blood sugar levels.
- Patients with both type 1 and type 2 diabetes will present with the three Ps of diabetes (i.e., polydipsia, polyphagia, and polyuria).
- Nutritional therapy is based on a well-balanced diet and is one of the mainstays in the treatment of diabetes.
- Regular exercise is an essential part of the treatment of diabetes because of its ability to lower blood sugar and decrease cardiovascular risk factors.

- Diabetic ketoacidosis results from a marked insulin deficiency and is manifested by hyperglycemia, ketosis, acidosis, and dehydration.
- HHNS is a life-threatening emergency associated with severe hyperglycemia, an osmotic diuresis, and a profound fluid volume deficit.
- Hypoglycemia is an acute complication of diabetes where the blood glucose levels are less than 70 mg/dL.
- Chronic complications include macrovascular and microvascular problems. These complications include angiopathy or vessel disease, retinopathy, neuropathy, and nephropathy.
- Macrovascular complications in diabetes cause changes in the large vessels.
- Diabetic neuropathies involve the peripheral, autonomic, and spinal nerves.
- The most common cause of hospitalization for the diabetic patient is the complication of the lower extremities; specifically, the foot.

REVIEW QUESTIONS

1. A patient has just been admitted to the emergency department after being found disoriented at the grocery store. His medical alert bracelet indicates that he has type 1 diabetes. Which of the following clinical signs do you anticipate finding upon assessment? Check all that apply.
   1. Hyperglycemia
   2. Fruity odor of breath
   3. Tachycardia
   4. Hypertension

2. A patient with diabetes has just finished the teaching session on mixing insulins. The nurse knows that more teaching is needed when the patient:
   1. Injects air into the NPH insulin first followed by injecting air into the regular insulin vial
   2. Withdraws too much NPH insulin and injects the extra back into the Lente vial
   3. Withdraws too much regular insulin and injects the extra back into the regular insulin vial
   4. Uses separate syringes to draw up 5 units of regular insulin and 4 units of NPH

3. Which of the following lab tests offers the best information about glycemic control?
   1. HgbA$_{1C}$
   2. Fasting plasma glucose
   3. Glucose tolerance test
   4. Capillary glucose measurement

4. A patient is admitted to the hospital with DKA. The nurse can anticipate which of the following solutions will be administered initially intravenously?
   1. 5% dextrose in water
   2. Ringer's lactate
   3. 0.9% NS
   4. 5% dextrose in 0.45% NS

5. Which of the following types of insulin can be administered intravenously?
   1. Regular
   2. Lente
   3. Semi-Lente
   4. NPH

6. Diabetes is a chronic condition that requires effective long-term management. This management includes:
   1. Initial treatment of all types of diabetes with dietary modifications for a three-month time period
   2. Initial treatment of all diabetics with insulin administration to prevent complications
   3. Initial treatment of all diabetics with an oral glucose lowering agent and an exercise program
   4. Use of a glucose lowering agent, diet, and activity

7. What is the primary difference between DKA and HHNS?
   1. The absence of ketosis is the distinguishing feature.
   2. HHNS has much higher blood glucose levels.
   3. DKA has associated hyperkalemic levels.
   4. HHNS is usually caused as a reaction to previous conditions of hypoglycemia.

8. What are clinical manifestations of hypoglycemia?
   1. Severe abdominal pain, accompanied with nausea
   2. Cardiac arrhythmias
   3. Neurological responses of the parasympathetic nervous system
   4. Irritability, increasing confusion, tremors, hunger, sweating, weakness and visual disturbances

9. Which of the following is true of the dawn phenomena?
   1. It manifests itself as morning hypoglycemia.
   2. The corresponding hyperglycemia results from predawn release of counter-regulatory hormones.
   3. It is best managed by decreasing the administration amounts of insulin.
   4. The patient is not allowed to take insulin in any form when diagnosed with the dawn phenomena.

10. Which of the following is true regarding the autonomic neuropathy conditions associated with diabetic complications?
    1. They result in bradycardia and profuse diaphoresis.
    2. They are seldom seen in adult-onset diabetic conditions.
    3. They lead to bowel and bladder incontinence and delayed gastric emptying.
    4. They result in foot ulcers due to a lack of adequate circulation.

REVIEW ACTIVITIES

1. Describe what information is to be included in teaching a patient with newly diagnosed diabetes about sick day management.

2. List information to be included in teaching a patient newly diagnosed with diabetes about foot care.

3. A patient with diabetes is admitted to the emergency department with a blood sugar level of 52. The patient is still conscious. Describe the treatment that you will administer.

4. A patient with type 2 diabetes is admitted to the hospital with a diagnosis of pneumonia and is started on insulin injections. The patient questions the use of insulin, stating that he has been able to control his diabetes with pills and diet. What information should the nurse give to the patient?

5. Explain the following symptoms and their cause: polydipsia, polyphagia, and polyuria.

6. Locate a diabetes educator in your area. What are the educational requirements for the position of diabetes educator? Observe some teaching sessions with the diabetic educator and patients. What are some of the teaching strategies utilized, and how do they vary based on the age and education level of the patient? How frequently are patients seen by the diabetic educator, and how is this determined? Is a referral from a health care provider required or can the patients self refer for services? Is there an interdisciplinary team for patients with diabetes? Who makes up that team?

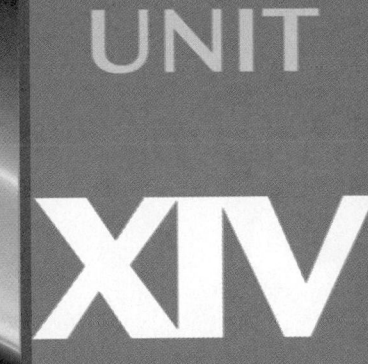

UNIT XIV

Alterations in Musculoskeletal Function

Assessment of Musculoskeletal Function

Anita M. Zehala, RN, MS, ONC, CNS

KEY TERMS

Acetylcholine
Actin filaments
Arthroscopy
Articulation
Bone scan
Bone marrow aspiration
   and biopsy
Bursae
Cancellous
Clonus
Cortical or compact (bone)
Deep vein thrombosis (DVT)
Displaced fracture
Dual energy X-ray
   absorptiometry (DEXA)
   scans
Epiphyses
Homans' sign
Hyaline
Isokinetic
Joint aspiration
Lacunae
Lamellar bone
Ligaments
Myelogram
Myosin
Osteogenesis
Osteopenia
Periosteum
Remodeling
Resorption
Sarcomere
Synovium
Tendons
Trabecular

CHAPTER TOPICS

- Anatomy and Physiology of the Bony Skeleton

- Anatomy and Physiology of Skeletal Muscles

- Musculoskeletal Assessment

- Diagnostic Studies Related to the Musculoskeletal System

The years 2000 to 2010 have been declared the Bone and Joint Decade with a goal of improving the health-related quality of life for people with musculoskeletal disorders throughout the world (Bone and Joint Decade Organization, 2004). Sanctioned by the United Nations and the president of the United States, as well as others, participants include the National Association of Orthopaedic Nurses (NAON) and the American Academy of Orthopaedic Surgeons (AAOS). Because musculoskeletal diseases affect so many lives throughout the world, one of the major efforts of the participating organizations is to increase awareness of musculoskeletal diseases. By becoming familiar with the basic anatomy and physiology and assessment of the musculoskeletal system (as well as learning about musculoskeletal dysfunction and trauma in the following two chapters) providers will be able to assist in keeping musculoskeletal diseases in the forefront. Nurses will also be able to speak with confidence regarding issues that may arise during discussions with patients and family members.

ANATOMY AND PHYSIOLOGY OF THE BONY SKELETON

The anatomy and physiology of the bone are complex and consist of multiple layers of collagen, noncollagen, protein, and mineral components. These components continually renew themselves, giving bones the strength, integrity, and structure necessary to support the human form. Bone formation is triggered by multiple sources including physical force, hormones, and genetics.

During the 19th century, surgeon Julius Wolff made an impressive discovery, known as Wolff's law, involving the formation of bone. This dynamic remodeling process called **osteogenesis** (the process of bone formation and remodeling) is thought to be a direct response to physical stresses caused by the amount and direction of physical forces placed on bones (Childs, 2002).

Macroscopic Structure of Bone

Embryonic development influences the distribution of bone cells (Schneider, Miclau, & Helms, 2002). Bones are woven in structure from infancy until 4 years of age. Woven bone is considered immature bone with collagen arranged randomly rather than in the uniform structure of lamellar bone. **Lamellar bone** (thin layer of mature bone tissue) is considered mature bone.

Four types of bones can be distinguished in the body. These types are flat, short (cuboidal), long, and irregular bones. Table 58-1 categorizes some of the bones of the body into type. Lamellar bone can be separated into two types: **cortical or compact** (dense, hard, and forms the protective exterior portion of all bones) and **cancellous, trabecular,** or spongy (inside the compact bone and porous). Cortical bone forms the hard outer layer of bone surfaces. Cancellous bone is found in the ends of the long bones (e.g., tibia) and in smaller amounts in some of the flat bones (e.g., iliac crest) (Scott & Fong, 2004).

Long bones are differentiated into three sections (Figure 58-1). The diaphysis is the shaft of a long bone, between the two ends (epiphysis), and consists of compact bone enclosing the medullary cavity or canal (the hollow tube located within the diaphysis). Within the medullary cavity is the bone marrow, in which hematopoietic activity takes place. The **epiphyses,** the widened ends of the long bone, contain mostly cancellous bone and are covered by a thin layer of cortical bone. The bone marrow system continues into the epiphyseal cavity. The metaphysis is the area of transition between the diaphysis and the epiphysis. The amount of cortical bone becomes gradually thinner as the metaphysis moves from diaphysis to epiphysis but the amount of cancellous bone increases from diaphysis to epiphysis. In the maturing child, the epiphyseal plate, or growth plate, is where active longitudinal growth occurs. The epiphyseal plate is located between the epiphysis and the metaphysis. If a fracture occurs in or through the epiphyseal plate, growth in that extremity may be delayed or stopped. When maturity is reached, the epiphyseal plate disappears when the epiphysis and the metaphysis merge (Childs, 2002).

Surrounding most bone surfaces is a layer of connective tissue containing blood vessels and osteoblasts known as the **periosteum** (Childs, 2002). The periosteum supplies nutrients to the outer portion of the cortical bone and provides a blood supply to the bone. This outer layer is essential for the repair and remodeling of bone after fractures. Within the medullary canal and cancellous bone is a layer of tissue involved in **resorption** (the removal of bone tissue by normal physiological process or as part of a pathological process such as an infection) of bone cells. This layer of tissue is known as the endosteum (the thin layer of cells lining the medullary cavity of a bone).

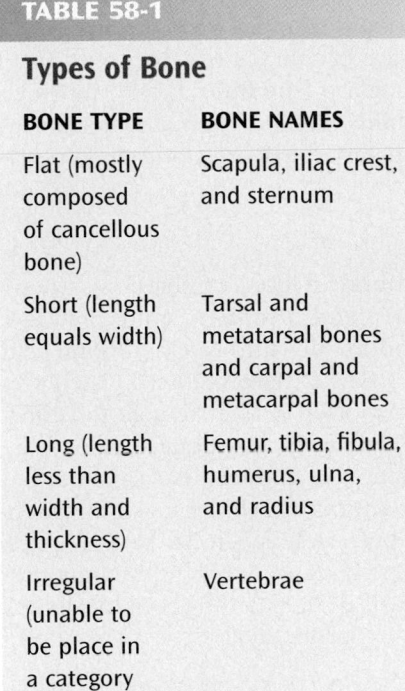

TABLE 58-1	
Types of Bone	
BONE TYPE	**BONE NAMES**
Flat (mostly composed of cancellous bone)	Scapula, iliac crest, and sternum
Short (length equals width)	Tarsal and metatarsal bones and carpal and metacarpal bones
Long (length less than width and thickness)	Femur, tibia, fibula, humerus, ulna, and radius
Irregular (unable to be place in a category listed above)	Vertebrae

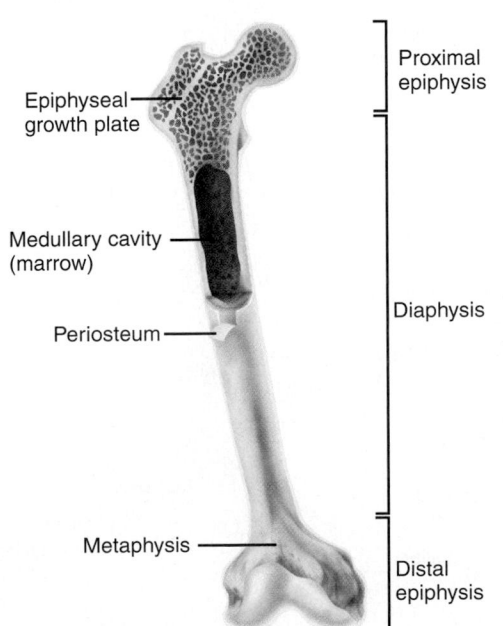

Figure 58-1 Structure of a long bone.

Microscopic Structure of Bone

Full understanding of the minute structure and physiology of the bone would take a great deal of time and effort for the nurse. Therefore, only the basic anatomy and physiology necessary for nurses to understand how a bone matures and repairs will be discussed. For a more in depth review of the anatomic makeup and physiologic processes of the bone and bone repair, refer to the references to this chapter.

Osteon (Haversian System)

Cortical bone is made up of Haversian canals or osteons (channels running through a bone in which blood vessels and nerves are located), which allow the flow of fluid throughout the bone. This fluid supplies water and nutrients to the bone. Also within the cortical bone are canaliculi, which extend from the Haversian canals to the **lacunae.** Lacunae are "the little 'lakes'" in which the mature bone cells are embedded" (Childs, 2002). The osteons are surrounded by rings of lamellae, which characterize mature bone or lamellar bone (Figure 58-2).

Cell Types

There are three characteristic cell types found in bone. Osteoblasts (bone building cells) originate from stem cells and produce bone marrow. Osteoblasts reside within the periosteum and mature into calcified bone cells (osteocytes) or remain as bone lining cells (Sims & Baron, 2002). Osteocytes are calcified mature bone cells that are transported to the lacunae to reside. Osteocytes give bone its hard structure. These cells are thought to activate bone turnover and have a part in the regulation of extracellular calcium, but the exact function is unknown. Osteoclasts demineralize bone and are responsible for resorption of osteocytes and other bony debris. Similar to osteocytes, they originate from stem cells. These cells line bones and behave in a manner similar to phagocytes. The activity of osteoclasts is regulated by both locally acting cytokines and systemic hormones (Sims & Baron, 2002).

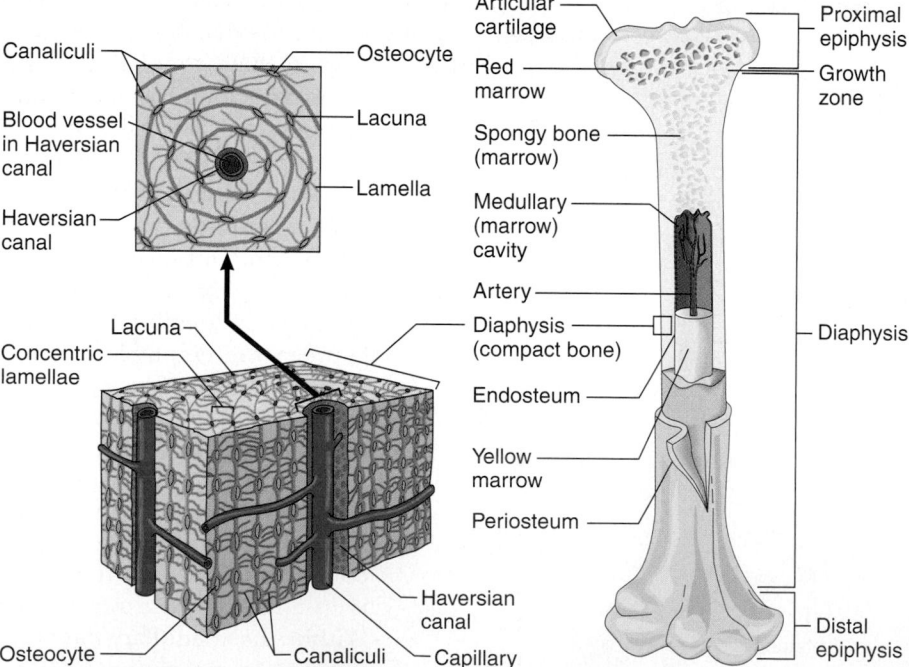

Figure 58-2 The Haversian system.

Physiological Processes

There are five physiological processes of the bone: (a) growth; (b) modeling; (c) remodeling; (d) repair; and (e) blood-bone exchange. Growth starts approximately two months after conception and continues to maturity. Lengthening and thickening of the bones occur during the growth process. The periosteum, as it becomes vascularized in utero, becomes the center of osteogenesis and continues this function throughout the life span. Modeling can be altered when genetic or nutritional circumstances affect the supply of nutrients to the bone (e.g., osteogenesis imperfecta, Paget's disease, or vitamin-deficiency rickets). Modeling also occurs in cartilage and fibrous tissue as well (Childs, 2002).

Turnover of the bone at the microscopic level is known as **remodeling.** Remodeling is a series of events continuously occurring in the bone. To maintain the structure and integrity of the bone, the bony tissue must be continually replaced. Bone cells fully replace themselves on average every 87 days. Roughly 30 percent of the total skeletal mass is renewed every year in a normal adult. There appears to be a balance of osteoclastic and osteoblastic activity that maintains and equalizes the overall skeletal mass. The exact trigger for remodeling is not known, but it is thought to occur after osteoclastic activity has occurred on the endosteal surface of the bone (Sims & Baron, 2002).

Blood-bone exchange is the physiological process in which electrolytes and acid-base substances move between the blood and bone tissue via the interstitial fluids. Bone tissue contributes to the modulation of hypercalcemia or hypocalcemia. Hydrogen ions (in acid-base balance), as well as other electrolytes, may also be influenced by tissue response within the bone. The osteocytes probably play a role in this influence (Childs, 2002).

Bone Repair/Fracture Healing

Bone repair or fracture healing occurs in much the same way as remodeling, however the trigger, such as trauma or surgery, is usually well defined. With any injury in the body, inflammation is the first stage, which occurs with an injury. Inflammation results from the ruptured blood vessels within the bone, the torn periosteum, and any damage to the surrounding soft tissue. A hematoma forms around the fracture within 24 hours. The hematoma releases hormones and inflammatory agents that stimulate the healing process. Within the hematoma, a fibrin network forms that serves as a framework for the formation of new blood vessels and cartilage. The inflammatory stage lasts several days.

In the first 24 to 48 hours after the injury, red blood cells continue to disintegrate and provide a stimulus for repair. Vascular congestion occurs and leukocytes, mainly neutrophils, invade the area causing significant edema. Approximately 48 hours after the injury, the area is flooded with macrophages to clean up remaining debris. At this time fibroblasts and chondroblasts invade the area to assist in forming a cartilage callus (new blood vessels and cartilage over the fracture site). This is stage is called the cellular proliferation stage. Chondrocytes (cartilage cells that make the structural components of cartilage), which are present in the cartilage callus, regulate the calcification of the cartilage. This usually occurs by the end of the first week. The calcified cartilage is then invaded by blood vessels and becomes resorbed by chondroblasts (a cell that arises from the mesenchyma and forms cartilage) and osteoclasts. The cartilage callus is then replaced by woven bone similar in structure to the growth plate. The callus is the beginning of bony formation but is weak.

With simple fractures the callus will reach its maximal size in two to three weeks after the injury. The callus continues to increase in strength from the precipitation of bone salts. During this time, osteoblastic and osteoclastic activity at the fracture site or injury, in response to external stresses, such as weight bearing activity, reform the bone. The ossification stage can take three to four months to complete. Remodeling also includes the growth of fine bone and the maturation of osteoblasts into osteocytes. Complete remodeling of a fracture can take months to years depending on the extent of the injury. Should the fracture be comminuted (a fracture in which the bone is splintered or crushed) or other complications be present, such as a patient with diabetes, the healing time may be increased.

Functions of Bone

The main functions of bones are to support the structure of the body, provide form, and enable movement. The skeleton is the ridged framework for the body and serves to protect the vital organs. It serves as the lever to which muscles attach. Bones store mineral, calcium and phosphate ions, lipids, and much of the hematopoietic system (the bodily system of organs and tissues, primarily the bone marrow, spleen, tonsils, and lymph nodes, involved in the production of blood), which forms new red blood cells and other blood components.

Aging and the Skeletal System

As a person ages, the physiology of the bone normally becomes thinner and weaker. This process is called **osteopenia** (the presence of less than normal amount of bone). If osteopenia is not treated it may result in osteoporosis. Osteoblastic activity slows between the ages of 30 and 40. After age 40, women lose approximately 8 percent of their bone mass every decade. In men the loss is 3 percent per decade.

ANATOMY AND PHYSIOLOGY OF SKELETAL MUSCLES

Skeletal muscle makes up the largest mass of tissue in the body and is responsible for approximately 50 percent of a person's body weight. The main functions of skeletal muscle are to produce movement, maintain posture and position, support soft tissues, guard entrances and exits to the digestive and urinary tracts, and to assist in maintaining body temperature (Scott & Fong, 2004).

Unlike cardiac and smooth muscle, skeletal muscle is voluntary. The voluntary nature of the skeletal muscle makes it unique in composition and action. Muscles are encapsulated epimysium (the external sheath of connective tissue surrounding a muscle). The long and cylindrical muscle cells contain subcellular units called myofibrils, which are surrounded by sarcoplasm (the cytoplasm of a striated muscle fiber). The myofibrils run lengthwise in the muscle and are made up of two types of subunits: myosin and actin filaments. The **myosin** (the protein that makes up the thick filaments of a myofibril) and **actin filaments** (the contractile part of a myofilament) slide together and compose the **sarcomere** (the contractile unit of the muscle). Tropomyosin and troponin are also contained within the myofibril. These components act as inhibitors to muscle contraction by preventing the interaction of myosin with actin (Childs, 2002).

The sarcoplasm reticulum releases large amounts of calcium into the vicinity of the myofibrils during contraction of the muscle. Through removal of the

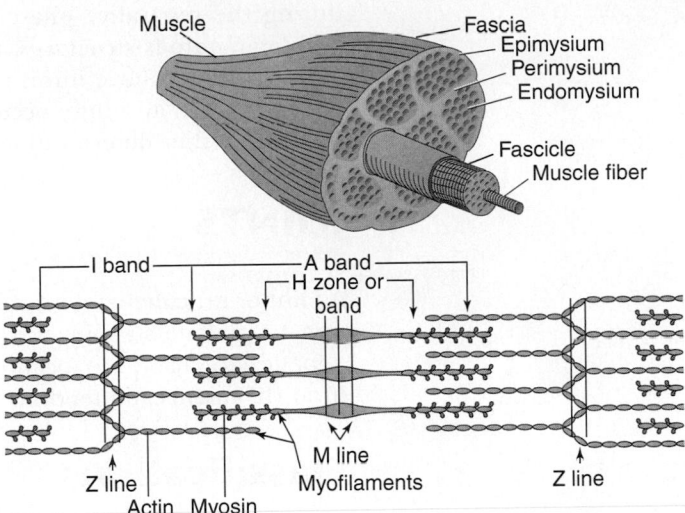

Figure 58-3 Illustration of muscle fibers.

tropomyosin-troponin block, the rise in calcium concentration initiates muscle contraction. As a result, the myosin and actin filaments slide past each other and enable myofibrillar contraction or the shortening of the sarcomere (Figure 58-3) (Childs, 2002).

Nerve and Blood Supply

There are generally one or two nerves that innervate each muscle. The nerve is necessary for the muscle to contract. When a nerve root ends within a muscle it is referred to as the neuromuscular junction. When the nerve root receives the signal from the brain to contract, **acetylcholine** (a neurotransmitter in both the central and peripheral nervous system) is released. The release of acetylcholine stimulates the sarcoplasm reticulum to release calcium and the muscle contraction begins (Childs, 2002).

Tendons, Ligaments, and Bursae

Tendons connect muscle to bone. This attachment allows the bone to move once the muscle has contracted. Tendons offer strength, extensibility, and flexibility to the muscle insertion sites.

Ligaments are strong bands of connective tissue that attach bone to bone or bone to cartilage. Ligaments help to give joints stability, guide the joint movement, and prevent excess motion within the joint (Childs, 2002).

Bursae are synovial fluid-filled sacs near joints. They are seen where tendons rub against bone, ligaments, or other tendons, as well as skin over bony prominences. Bursa provide cushion and minimize friction.

Aging and the Muscular System

In general, lean muscle mass decreases with age. Atrophy from disuse can lead to muscle wasting. Muscle contraction time is decreased in response to a reduction in acetylcholine and increased resorption of calcium. After disuse as a result of calcium resorption, fatigue is often increased and endurance decreased. Ligaments and tendons lose elasticity and resiliency. With trauma or repetitive stress, ligaments and tendons shorten, resulting in stiffness and loss of flexibility and range of motion (ROM). Furthermore, during the reparative phase, calcium can be deposited in muscle, tendon, and ligamentous structures, creating pain and further decreasing function. In light of the above information, it is essential that early rehabilitation be initiated when an injury occurs to return the patient to preinjury status and prevent further deterioration (Childs, 2002).

JOINTS

A joint or **articulation** is formed when a bone meets another bone. Joints function to provide stability and mobility. The amount of stability and mobility depend largely on the location of the joint as well as the muscular and structural (ligaments and tendons) support surrounding the joint.

Classifications

Three classes of joints can be identified according to the amount of movement allowed: synarthrosis (immovable), amphiarthrosis (slightly movable), and diarthrosis (freely movable) (Crowther, 2004). Another method of classification is based on the connective structure of the joints. Fibrin, cartilage, and **synovium** (a fibrous envelope that produces a fluid to help to reduce friction and wear in a joint) are the connective structures seen in joints. Fibrous tissue is generally found in synarthrosis joints. In amphiarthrosis joints, cartilage is the predominant connective tissue. Within the joint capsule of the diarthrosis joints is the synovium. The diarthrosis joints are the most movable and most commonly injured joints in the body.

Structural Aspects of the Diarthrosis Joint

Hyaline (articular) cartilage covers the end of each bone to reduce friction and distribute weight-bearing forces. This cartilage is either thick or thin depending on the size of the joint, the fit of the bones, and the amount of weight bearing and shearing forces to which the joint is subjected (Crowther, 2004). For example, the knee joint cartilage is thicker than the shoulder joint cartilage due to the amount of weight bearing the knee withstands.

The synovial cavity is the space between the two bones that allows movement. This cavity is surrounded by the synovial membrane and filled with synovial fluid. The synovial membrane is the smooth fragile lining of the joint capsule, which is found in the nonarticulating portions of the joint. The synovial membrane is vascular and contains phagocytic cells as well as cells that secrete hyaluronate. Hyaluronate gives the synovial fluid its viscous quality. Synovial fluid also contains an ultrafiltrated solution that lubricates the joint surfaces, provides nourishment for the articular cartilage, and covers the ends of bones. The synovial fluid contains synovial cells and leukocytes that phagocytose joint debris and microorganisms (Crowther, 2004).

Motions

Diarthrosis joints, in conjunction with muscles, tendons, ligaments, and nerves allow body movement, which enables people to perform activities of daily living.

MUSCULOSKELETAL ASSESSMENT

Limitation in movement or pain is the chief reason patients seek musculoskeletal treatment. A thorough examination of the complaint is necessary to assist the patient in the relief or abatement of the symptoms. A complete health history is important to collect when interviewing a patient. Tools needed for a musculoskeletal assessment include a goniometer, tape measure, and flashlight.

Guidelines for Assessment

The NAON publishes the *Core Curriculum for Orthopaedic Nursing*. The core curriculum lists some general guidelines to use when performing a focused orthopedic assessment (Box 58-1).

Focused Health History

When completing an adult orthopedic musculoskeletal health history, the nurse should focus on four key areas: (a) pain, (b) onset of symptoms, (c) deformity, and (d) paralysis. It is also important to consider the special circumstances of trauma and chronic conditions that may affect the musculoskeletal system.

Pain

Pain is the most common symptom associated with a musculoskeletal complaint. When assessing the patient's level of pain the nurse should ask questions that clarify the type, location, severity, duration, and precipitating or alleviating factors related to the patient's pain.

Onset of Symptoms

Knowledge of when and how the symptoms of the chief complaint first occurred helps the nurse assess the mechanism of injury. Questions to ask include: (a) What are the symptoms? (b) What occurred to cause the symptoms? (c) When did they occur? (d) Did the symptoms come on gradually or was it a sudden onset? (e) Have the symptoms gotten worse or better? (f) What have you done to treat the symptoms? (g) Where these treatments effective? (h) Has anything increased the intensity of the symptoms?

Deformity

Physical deformities can be associated with edema, pain, and stiffness. While examining the deformity the nurse may discover when the changes first appeared. The nurse may also ask questions related to heredity. Deformities occur with dislocations, fractures, sprains, and strains. The nature of inflammatory diseases can lead to multiple deformities in the joints. For example, rheumatoid arthritis may cause lateral deviations in the joints of the fingers

---

BOX 58-1

ORTHOPAEDIC ASSESSMENT GUIDELINES

1. The examination should be performed after providing privacy to the patient.
2. The patient should be dressed in a way that allows full visualization of the body and facilitates examination without needless exposure.
3. Wash your hands before beginning the examination.
4. The examination should proceed in an orderly fashion from head to toe, proximal to distal.
5. Compare one side of the body to the other, frequently alternating the assessment of one part of the body to the other side.
6. Examination should reflect the influence on activities of daily living, including impact on school and work.
7. Questions should be worded in a way that helps ascertain information. For example:
   a. Are you able to get into and out of the bathtub?
   b. Can you stand at work?
   c. Can you comb your hair?
   d. Can you lift your backpack?

Safety First

A Case Study

The victim involved in a motor vehicle accident explains to you that he was a restrained passenger in the front seat of a minivan when the accident occurred. He twisted around to the left to check on his son in the back seat at the time the van slammed into the back of the car in front of them. The air bag went off. He suffered a fractured left distal femur. On further investigation you find that the distal portion of his knee (the proximal portion of the tibia) hit a portion of the console between the front two seats. This caused the distal portion of the left femur to be pushed back while the patient's body was moving forward (even with the airbag). As a result, a tremendous amount of force was applied to the distal end of the femur going in the opposite direction of his body and resulted in a distal femur fracture. Under these circumstances, it is also important to look for complaints of hip pain as the femoral head may have been forced into the acetabulum, causing major or minor fractures in the hip joint.

and hands. Congenital anomalies can also cause deformities. The nurse should ask questions about the usual shape and position of the affected area and compare these against expected findings.

Paralysis

When examining any paralysis, the nurse needs to explore the time of onset, what limbs or areas are affected, the extent of the paralysis, and the progression or regression of the paralysis. It is also important to note the presence or absence of sensory disturbances, such as numbness or tingling.

Trauma

Trauma can be highly emotional for patients and their families. Focusing on the exact cause of the injury will help make assessment and treatment of the entire patient more effective. Some causes of trauma may include motor vehicle accidents, sports-related injuries, and physical abuse. If the trauma was emotionally disturbing, the nurse should be sensitive to the patient's physical and psychological needs. Care also needs to be taken so that the more obvious injuries do not overshadow less apparent but potentially life-threatening injuries.

When investigating a motor vehicle accident it is important to note the force and direction of the impact. These details may reveal the cause and severity of the injury. The nurse should ascertain the object(s) involved in the trauma. This information is necessary to determine the mechanism of injury.

Chronic Conditions

When completing a health history, it is important to remember that patients with chronic conditions have a unique set of needs. Health care professionals should focus questions on those directed specifically at the chronic condition (Box 58-2).

Physical Examination of the Musculoskeletal System

There are three basic maneuvers used in assessing the musculoskeletal system: (a) inspection; (b) palpation; and (c) evaluation of passive and active ROM.

BOX 58-2

HEALTH HISTORY: CHRONIC CONDITIONS

The following questions be asked when assessing a chronic problem:
- When did the symptoms begin?
- How long have the symptoms been present?
- Are the symptoms continuous or intermittent?
- How did the symptoms begin?
- What caused the symptoms?
- What helps or irritates the condition?
- What interventions have been used (both traditional and nontraditional)? What was their effect?
- What is your response to heat and cold?
- What position causes pain?
- What medications, herbs, or over-the-counter products have been used?
- What was their effect?
- What complementary or alternative therapy have been used, such as therapeutic massage, acupuncture, or aromatherapy? What was their effect?

Inspection

When performing a focused assessment involving the musculoskeletal system, the nurse needs to consider the entire body. If the patient is able to ambulate, the nurse should observe the patient's gait and ROM while entering the examination room and sitting in a chair. The nurse's assessment should focus on the patient's ROM and observed ease or discomfort associated with position changes.

Palpation

When palpating an affected area the nurse should note the firmness of the skin and muscle, any report of tenderness, warmth, texture, presence of masses under the skin (measure for accuracy, if appropriate), and crepitus (a sign of fracture). It is important to note the presence of any deformity in shape of the bone or marked changes in muscle shapes, tone, or resistance to pressure.

Neurovascular Assessment

Considered a hallmark of musculoskeletal assessment, the neurovascular assessment is a simple, yet telling method of investigating musculoskeletal complaints or assessing for complications resulting from treatment of musculoskeletal injuries. The neurovascular assessment combines a focused neurological assessment with the assessment of the vascular system.

Skills 360°

Inspection

Performing the focused assessment starts with inspecting the area where the chief complaint occurs. When inspecting look for obvious deviations, observe the contour of the musculature, the color of the skin, the presence of any scars, bruises or open areas, edema, or atrophy. You may need to use a flashlight to illuminate subtleties in contour, which can indicate edema. Always compare the area in question to the opposite side of the body. Should there be an amputation (surgical removal of a limb of the body) on the side to which you are trying to compare, ask the patient if what you observe is normal. The patient should be able to tell you if what you are observing is normal or not. For example, a male patient with a right above-the-knee amputation is complaining of left knee pain. You observe edema in the knee area. The patient should be able to tell you if this is the normal size of his knee. Remember that it is normal for the dominant upper extremity, or a limb that is used frequently in a repetitive manner, to be slightly larger than the opposite extremity.

Skills 360°

Neurovascular Assessment

Focused on the extremities, the neurovascular assessment uses the techniques of inspection and palpation. You can begin by observing the color of the skin on the toes or fingers as well as the rest of the extremity, comparing the color to that of the opposite extremity. Observe for normality of color for the patient. Palpate the most distal pulse in the affected extremity. You then need to compare that pulse to the opposite extremity, looking for a similar pulse quality in both extremities. If you are unable to compare the most distal pulses, assess the next most distal comparable pulses. For example, if the patient has a below-the-knee amputation on one extremity, use the popliteal pulses for comparison. While palpating the pulses, make note of the temperature of the skin in the foot or hand and compare this to another portion of the extremity or body to assess for consistency. If you find it difficult to feel the pulses, it is often useful to use the middle finger of your nondominant hand to attempt the palpation. This finger tends to be more sensitive then the others. Pulses which you will assess in the upper extremity include the radial, ulnar, and brachial. In the lower extremity you will assess the dorsalis pedis, posterior tibialis, popliteal, and femoral. The dorsalis pedis (often documented as the pedal pulse) is on the dorsum or top of the foot. The posterior tibialis is located behind the medial malleolus on the inside of the ankle. These two pulse points are often confusing to the beginning practitioner; therefore special care should be taken in assessment and documentation to obtain the correct assessment.

The neurological component of the neurovascular assessment evaluates both sensory and motor function. To test the sensory nerves simply ask if the patient can feel you touch his or her toes or fingers without the patient looking. In assessing motor function, ask the patient to dorsiflex and plantar flex in the lower extremity and then to make a fist, open the hand, and spread their fingers. Compare these assessments with the opposite extremity (Figure 58-4). During the assessment be sure to note differences between the extremities. In a postoperative patient, report these differences to the health care provider if it is the first time the difference has been noted, as this may be a sign of an impending complication.

Range of Motion

A unique aspect of the musculoskeletal assessment is the assessment of ROM at each joint. Joint function is essential to perform activities of daily living. There are essentially seven types of motions made by the joints: (a) flexion and extension; (b) circumduction; (c) abduction and adduction; (d) internal rotation and external rotation; (e) pronation and supination; (f) plantar flexion and dorsiflexion; and (g) inversion and eversion (Figures 58-5 through 58-9).

Measuring ROM requires the use of a goniometer to measure joint angles (Figure 58-10). For example, the knee joint when straight is at 0° of flexion. Angles can range from minus 15° in extension to as far as 130° of flexion. Table 58-2 describes the normal range of motion for joints.

Muscle Tone and Muscle Strength Grading

Muscle tone and muscle strength grading can be integrated with the assessment of ROM To assess the muscle's tone, while putting the muscle through passive ROM, the nurse should be aware of any spasticity or fasciculations (quivering) (Maher, 2002). To assess muscle strength, the nurse should ask the patient to flex the muscle and then flex the muscle again while applying resistance. It is important to also test the opposing muscle (e.g., tricep to bicep) (Figure 58-11). To assess the appropriateness of muscle strength a graded numerical scale is commonly used. See Table 58-3 for this graded scale.

Analysis of Gait

The way in which a person walks can reveal much about the musculoskeletal system. A person's gait provides evidence of pain, muscle atrophy, leg length discrepancy, as well as hip, knee, and ankle complications.

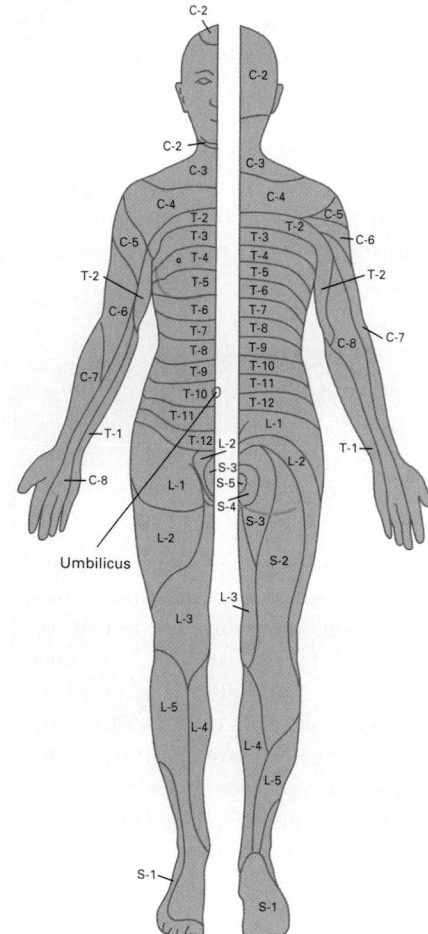

Figure 58-4 Illustration of sensory innervation of the body.

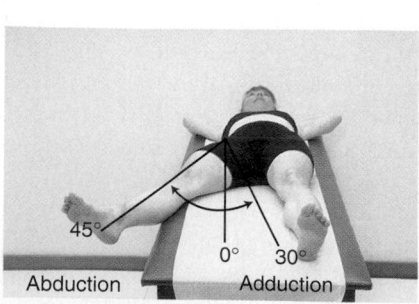

Figure 58-5 Abduction and adduction.

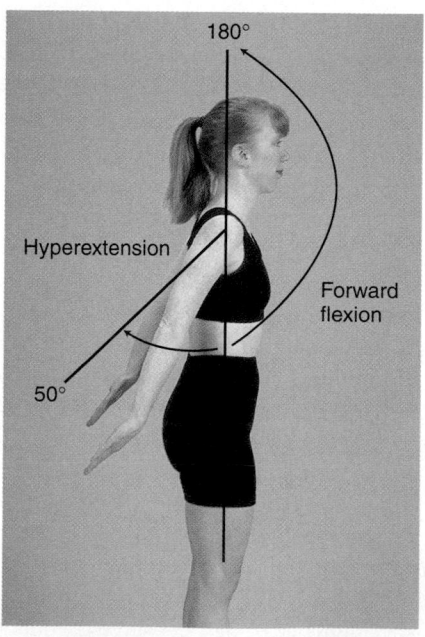

Figure 58-6 Forward flexion, hyperextension/circumduction.

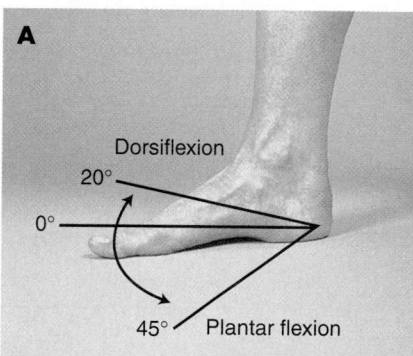

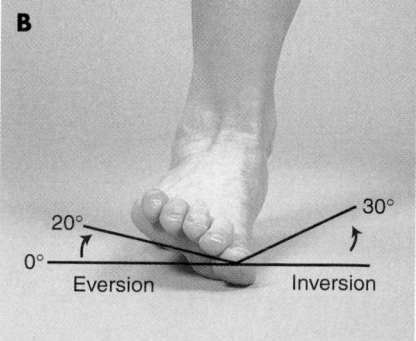

Figure 58-7 A. Plantar flexion and dorsiflexion, B. Eversion and inversion.

The gait has two phases: the stance or weight-bearing phase and the swing or non–bearing-weight phase. While the patient is walking a straight line, the nurse should note the stance phase. Particular attention should be paid to the patient's heel, how flat the foot is at midstance, and how the patient pushes off the ball of the foot. During the swing phase the nurse should assess the rate and rhythm of acceleration, midswing, and deceleration. It is important to compare the left and the right sides, looking for similarities and discrepancies during both phases of the gait.

The nurse needs to observe the alignment of the head, shoulders, spine, pelvis, knees, and feet; the rhythm of the pelvis (normal rotation during arm swing is 40° forward); the width of gap between legs (ankle to ankle should be 2 to 4 inches); the length of the step (approximately 15 inches); and the center of gravity should be midline. Any lack of coordination, use of assistive devices, such as cane or crutch, or use of equipment, such as splints or special shoes, should be noted. To observe the areas of greatest wear, the clinician should ask to see the soles of the patient's shoes. Listening to the patient walk, paying particular attention to the noises made while walking, such as the foot slapping or scraping the floor, can also reveal areas of concern in the musculoskeletal system.

Assessment of Injuries to the Musculoskeletal System

When assessing for muscle injuries or strains (occurs when a muscle or the tendon that attaches it to the bone is overstretched or torn), it is best to palpate gently from the origin (the more proximal and fixed end) to the insertion site (the end close to the center of the body). Injuries can occur throughout the muscle, but 40 percent of the injuries occur in the muscle body.

Sprains or ligamentous injuries occur because the ligament is stretched beyond its capability. The ligament is pliable but not elastic, and consequently, it is easy to sustain a ligament injury when the joint is unduly stretched.

Both muscle and ligament injuries can be classified into three different grade levels. Table 58-4 lists the grading for muscles and ligaments.

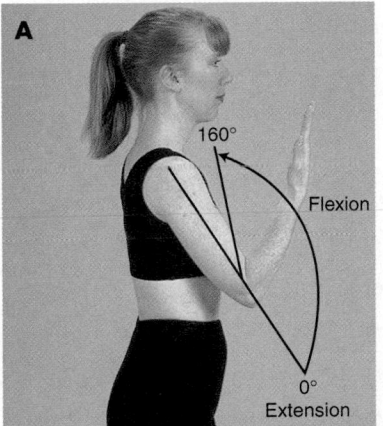

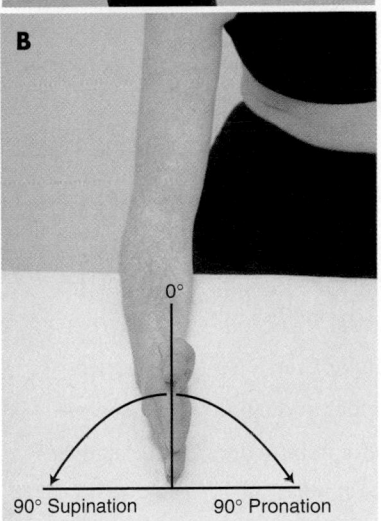

Figure 58-8 A. Elbow joint flexion and extension, B. Supination and pronation.

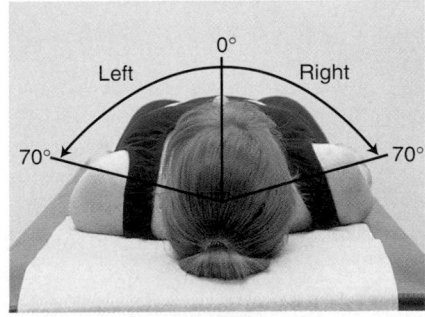

Figure 58-9 Cervical spine rotation.

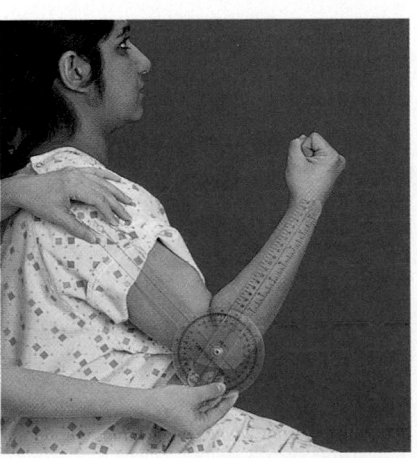

Figure 58-10 A Goniometer in use.

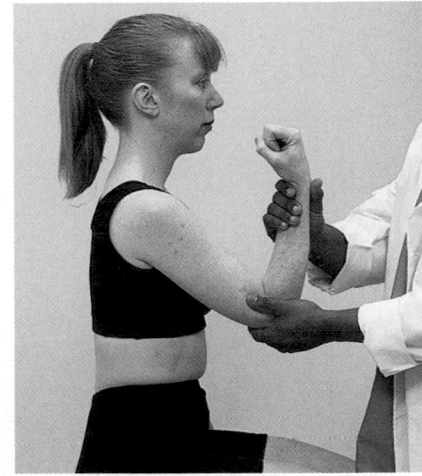

Figure 58-11 Assessment of strength in upper extremity.

Red Flag

Homans' Sign

A test that can be easily integrated into the neurovascular assessment is the **Homans' sign.** This test is used to assess for the presence of a **deep vein thrombosis** ([DVT] a blood clot in a deep vein that accompanies an artery). DVT affects mainly the veins in the lower leg. To perform this test, passively dorsiflex the patient's foot feeling for **clonus** (a slight involuntary pushing against your foot) and ask if the patient has any pain in his or her calf. A positive Homans' sign is the presence of extreme pain with or without clonus. Homans' sign is not a reliable predictor of the presence of DVT, but it is frequently used as a cursory assessment when a problem is suspected.

TABLE 58-2 Range of Motion

JOINT	RANGE OF MOTION	JOINT	RANGE OF MOTION
Cervical Spine		Radial deviation	15 degrees
Flexion	80–90 degrees	Radial deviation	15 degrees
Extension	70 degrees	Pronation	85–90 degrees
Lateral flexion	20–45 degrees	Supination	85–90 degrees
Rotation	70–90 degrees	**Hip**	
Lumbar Spine		Flexion	110–120 degrees
Flexion	40–60 degrees	Extension	10–15 degrees
Extension	20–35 degrees	Abduction	30–50 degrees
Lateral flexion	15–20 degrees	Adduction	30 degrees
Rotation	3–18 degrees	External rotation	40–60 degrees
Shoulder		Internal rotation	30–40 degrees
Flexion	160–180 degrees	**Knee**	
Extension	50–60 degrees	Flexion	0–130 degrees
Abduction	170–180 degrees	Extension	0–15 degrees
Adduction	50–75 degrees	Medial rotation	20–30 degrees
External rotation	80–90 degrees	Lateral rotation	30–40 degrees
Internal rotation	60–100 degrees	**Ankle**	
Circumduction	200 degrees	Plantar flexion	50 degrees
Elbow		Dorsiflexion	20 degrees
Flexion	140–160 degrees	Inversion	30 degrees
Extension	0–10 degrees	Eversion	20 degrees
Supination	90 degrees	Subtalar inversion	5 degrees
Pronation	80–90 degrees	Subtalar eversion	5 degrees
Wrist		Forefoot adduction	20 degrees
Flexion	80–90 degrees	Forefoot abduction	10 degrees
Extension	70–90 degrees	Great toe flexion	45 degrees
Ulnar deviation	35–45 degrees	Great toe extension	70 degrees

TABLE 58-3 Graded Muscle Strength

GRADING	DESCRIPTION	LOVETT SCALE
0	No palpable contraction of muscle	Zero (0)
1	Palpable contraction of muscle; no joint motion	Trace (T)
2	Complete range of motion (ROM) with gravity eliminated	Poor (P)
3	Complete ROM against gravity; no added resistance	Fair (F)
4	Complete ROM against gravity: some added resistance	Good (G)
5	Complete ROM against gravity with full resistance	Normal (N)

Adapted from Maher, A. B. (2002). Assessment of the musculoskeletal system. In A. B. Maher, S. W. Salmond, & T. A. Pellino (Eds.), Orthopaedic nursing (3rd ed., pp. 189–210). Philadelphia, PA: W. B. Saunders Company.

TABLE 58-4	Muscle and Ligament Injury Classification	
GRADE	**MUSCLE**	**LIGAMENT**
One	Strain–stretch on muscle fibers. Less than 10 percent muscle fibers involved.	Stretched. No tear to up to 20 percent torn.
Two	Partial tear in muscle. Palpation reveals defect. Ten to 50 percent of muscle fiber involved.	Twenty to 75 percent torn.
Three	Extensive tear or complete rupture. Fifty to 100 percent muscle fibers torn to complete rupture of the muscle.	Seventy-five percent to complete rupture of the ligament.

Adapted from Crowther, C. L. (2004). Structure and function of the musculoskeletal system. In S. E. Huether & K. L. McCance (Eds.), Understanding pathophysiology (3rd ed., pp. 1047–1070). St. Louis, MO: Mosby.

Assessment of Fractures

Although most accurately diagnosed with X-ray, if a fracture is suspected, assessment can be performed on the area by keeping the following principles in mind. A stress fracture (fracture caused by nontraumatic, cumulative overload on bone) is the most difficult to diagnose on X-ray despite the patient's ability to point to the area that hurts. There may be soft tissue swelling with painless active ROM as well as painless resisted active movement of the joint. A callous may form over the stress fracture site and may confirm the presence of a fracture. The gait may also be affected if the fracture is in the lower extremity due to pain at the fracture site with weight-bearing.

A **displaced fracture** is a fracture in which the bones have gone out of natural alignment. Immediate edema will occur with a displaced fracture. Pain may occur with movement and deformity may be seen. A fracture is considered a stable fracture if the edges of the fracture do not move. An unstable fracture is when motion is present at the fracture site causing a potential for trauma to the surrounding tissue, such as an unstable rib fracture that may puncture the lung.

Sports Injury Considerations

Whether a person is a weekend warrior or a professional athlete, sports injuries can occur at any time. Fortunately, many sports-related injuries heal without professional intervention. Guidelines to follow when deciding to see medical assistance include:

- Prolonged or nonsubsiding pain continuing two weeks after the episode.
- Any injury that occurs in or near a joint.
- Any loss of function.
- Any injury that does not heal in three weeks or in which the structure is apparently abnormal *or* any sign of infection on or under the skin, presence of pus, red streaks, swollen lymph nodes or fever.
- Any alteration in sensation, such as numbness or tingling.

The key to assessing sports injuries is to determine the severity and extent of the injury before permanent damage takes place. The following points will assist the nurse while assessing a sports-related injury: (a) because different areas of the body are developed depending on the sport, other areas may not be as developed; (b) unbalanced opposing muscle groups leave the athlete at risk to injury; and (c) it may be necessary to refer the athlete to a physician that specializes in sports-related injuries.

One of the best methods to evaluate muscle balance is to test the strength of opposing muscle groups with isometric measuring devices (muscle contraction without movement at the joint). These devices may be used for **isokinetic** exercise as well (exercise involving resistance through full range of movement).

DIAGNOSTIC STUDIES RELATED TO THE MUSCULOSKELETAL SYSTEM

Musculoskeletal assessment can be completed by physical examination. However, modern tools are available to pinpoint exact causes of musculoskeletal dysfunction and allow the diagnostician to develop thorough and complete plans of care.

Laboratory Studies

From a musculoskeletal assessment perspective, blood and urine study results show indications of disease and extent of disease progression. These studies also can be assistive in monitoring a patient's recovery from a surgical procedure or trauma. Although there are many studies that can be performed on the blood and urine, only those studies that can be used specifically in the assessment of the musculoskeletal system will be addressed here.

To monitor a patient's recovery from a surgical procedure or trauma, it is helpful to know the baseline hematology, chemistry, and coagulation studies. Blood loss is often a factor that deters a patient's ability to participate in recovery efforts postsurgery or posttrauma. Being able to compare the patient's current hemoglobin and hematocrit to preoperative levels allows the nurse to anticipate the health care provider's orders for iron supplements or administration of blood products. Basic chemistry levels allow comparisons to be made to monitor fluid balance, kidney function, and if the patient is diabetic, the reaction to the physiological stressors that the patient has endured. Elevated blood glucose levels in response to stress may necessitate a change in the patient's normal insulin or oral medication routine.

Warfarin (Coumadin) and heparin are often used as prophylactic therapy in the prevention of DVT and pulmonary embolism. Partial thromboplastin time (PTT), prothrombin time (PT), and the international normalized ratio (INR) are the laboratory values that monitor the effectiveness of aforementioned medications.

Radiographic Studies

Radiology technology has developed rapidly in recent years and has been instrumental in the diagnosis and treatment of musculoskeletal conditions. The radiographic studies described in this section are a combination of gold standard studies and new technologies to assist in making accurate diagnoses. As with the laboratory studies discussed previously, only musculoskeletal implications will be discussed for the radiologic tests presented.

Angiogram

For patients with musculoskeletal disorders, angiogram is most often used after trauma or surgery to confirm a diagnosis of a DVT or a pulmonary embolism. An angiogram is an invasive procedure that can have serious complications. A catheter is inserted in the femoral, brachial, subclavian, or carotid artery and a contrast dye is injected to visualize the vessels. The most serious complication is an embolus forming due to catheter clot formation. Another precaution to take is to assess for a potential allergy to the contrast dye. Questions about allergies to seafood, iodine, or contrast dye may prevent any allergic reactions (Kee, 2002).

Arthrography

Arthrography is a radiological examination used to diagnose complaints in the joints. Knees and shoulders are the most commonly assessed using this method. Air, contrast dye, or both are injected into the joint space to visualize the structures of the joints. Arthrography is an outpatient procedure usually done with a local anesthetic (Kee, 2002).

Preprocedure nursing interventions include reviewing the patient's medical history to obtain allergy information, obtaining signed consent, and patient teaching related to the procedure. Postprocedure interventions may include instructing the patient about the importance of limiting movement of the affected joint and maintaining compression dressings for 12 hours. Analgesia and ice may be used to reduce pain.

Bone Scan

A **bone scan** is a nuclear scan used to detect early bone disease, bone metastasis, and bone response to therapeutic regimens (Kee, 2002). Bone scans assist in detecting fractures, abnormal healing of fractures, and degenerative bone diseases (Kee, 2002). The patient is injected with the isotope because radioisotopes are used in the bone scan. Depending on the type of isotope used, the scan may take two to four hours to complete. Once the isotope is injected and has been distributed in the body, the body is scanned for hot spots. Dark spots on the scan indicate an area where the radioisotope uptake is greater, usually indicating an abnormality in that region.

Preprocedure nursing interventions include obtaining a health history, a signed consent form, and patient teaching related to the procedure. Patients are required to drink four to six glasses of water during the waiting period, remove all jewelry or metal objects, and void before the procedure. Postprocedure nursing interventions include encouraging the patient to continue increased fluid intake, observation for allergic reactions to the radioisotopes, and avoiding any other radionuclide tests for 24 to 48 hours.

Computed Tomography Scan

Also known as computed axial tomography (CAT or CT), the CT scan is a radiographic study that is 100 times more sensitive than normal X-rays (Kee, 2002). The CT scan can be done with or without contrast dye. For long bones and joints, CT scans can give a detailed examination of cross-sections of the areas examined. Defects that can be seen include tumors and fractures. Contrast may be used in joint examination. CT scans are generally tolerated well. Timing for the scan ranges from 30 to 90 minutes.

Preprocedure nursing interventions include obtaining a health history regarding possible pregnancy or allergies, a signed consent form, and patient teaching related to the procedure. The procedure requires the patient to remain still and may cause some patients to feel claustrophobic. Antianxiety medications are often helpful to alleviate these reactions. Patients are required to remove all jewelry or metal objects and void before the procedure. Postprocedure there are no physical restrictions.

Dual Energy X-ray Absorptiometry Scan

Dual energy X-ray absorptiometry (DEXA) scans measure bone density. These scans assist in the early diagnosis of osteoporosis. Using a computer analysis, the scans can determine size, thickness, and mineral content of the bone (Kee, 2002).

Preprocedure nursing interventions include obtaining a health history, a signed consent form, and patient teaching related to the procedure. Patients are required to remove all jewelry or metal objects. Postprocedure there are no physical restrictions.

Indium (White Blood Cell) Scan

The indium (white blood cell [WBC]) scan is used to detect osteomyelitis. A blood sample is obtained from the patient. An indium-111 radioisotope is then mixed with the blood to tag the WBCs. Once the blood has been mixed, it is reinfused in the patient. At 6 and 24 hours the patient's body is scanned. The scan takes 1 to 2 hours. The tagged WBCs will migrate to areas where tissue destruction from inflammation or infections is occurring (*WBC nuclear scan*, 2003)

Magnetic Resonance Imaging

Although costing approximately 30 percent more than a CT, magnetic resonance imaging (MRI) is being extensively used to confirm the diagnosis of musculoskeletal dysfunction by orthopaedic surgeons. This technique uses a magnet field and radio frequency waves that create images to be analyzed by computer technology. The computer can produce cross-sectional images, similar in detail to CT images. Kee (2002) states that MRIs are "now the most sensitive technique for defining the structure of internal organs and for detecting edema, infarction, hemorrhage, blood flow, tumors, infections, and plaques on the myelin sheath that cause Multiple Sclerosis" (p. 560). Kee also states that bone, joint, and soft tissue injuries can be seen without bone artifact and can distinguish whether a tumor is within or adjacent to a bone.

Most areas of the body can be visualized with a MRI. Because the magnets of the MRI are housed in a tubular machine that allows the magnetic field to be formed, claustrophobia can be an issue. Open MRIs are available but may not give as clear of an image as the closed system.

Preprocedure nursing interventions include obtaining a health history to determine possible pregnancy and the presence of metal implants, a signed consent form, and patient teaching related to the procedure. The procedure requires the patient to remain still and may cause some patients to feel claustrophobic. Antianxiety medications are often helpful to alleviate these reactions. Patients are required to remove all jewelry or metal objects, and void before the procedure. Postprocedure there are no physical restrictions.

Myelogram

A **myelogram** is used to diagnose defects in and around the spinal column. Using fluoroscopy and radiography, a contrast dye is injected into the subarachnoid space of the spinal canal. Defects are revealed when a smooth flow of contrast is not seen. Herniated discs, tumors, and spinal nerve root injury are examples of defects that may be seen (Kee, 2002).

Preprocedure nursing implications include obtaining a health history to determine allergies to contrast dye. Metrizamide is sometimes used as the contrast dye (water based). If it is used it is necessary to find out if the patient is taking any medications that lower the seizure threshold (phenothiazines, tricyclic antidepressants, central nervous system stimulants, or amphetamines) as metrizamide can cause seizures. Patients are often required to force fluids the night before the procedure and then have nothing by mouth (NPO) four to eight hours prior to the procedure. Other nursing interventions include obtaining a signed consent form and patient teaching related to the procedure. Patients are required to void before the procedure.

Postprocedure nursing interventions include prevention of lumbar puncture headaches and other complications. For the water-based test, the patient's head should be elevated 15 to 40° for 8 hours and then progress to supine bed rest with bathroom privileges for 16 hours. It is important to avoid phenothiazines or drugs that lower the seizure threshold. For the oil-based test the patient will be required to lie supine in bed for 12 to 24 hours. The patient may turn from side-to-side. For all patients, the nurse should encourage them to increase their fluid intake, monitor for bladder distension, perform neurological vital signs and assessments, and administer pain medications for headaches or discomfort. Possible complications include bleeding or leakage at the injection site, nausea and vomiting, headache, fever, seizure (most likely to occur 4 to 8 hours after the procedure), paralysis, arachnoiditis (inflammation of coverings of spinal cord, neck stiffness, sterile meningitis reaction, severe headache, and slow electroencephalogram [EEG] patterns), brainstem compression, and brainstem herniation.

X-rays

X-rays are the gold standard of diagnosis in the assessment of skeletal complaints. X-rays assist in the diagnosis of fractures, abnormal fracture healing, tumors, arthritic conditions, and osteomyelitis (Kee, 2002). Although brief exposure to radiation is necessary, X-rays are well tolerated by most patients.

Preprocedure nursing interventions include obtaining a health history to determine the possibility of pregnancy, a signed consent form, and patient teaching related to the procedure. Postprocedure there are no physical restrictions, but the patient may require analgesia if the procedure was prolonged.

Special Tests

Arthrometry

Arthrometry is a method used to measure and document cruciate ligament laxity of the knee both passively and actively. The arthrometer measures the distraction forces on the knee. These measurements are taken passively, actively, and manually. Measurements are taken on both the noninjured and injured knee. Surgeons use this method to diagnose anterior cruciate ligament (ACL) or posterior cruciate ligament (PCL) tears. The surgeon will evaluate and confirm ACL or PCL stability intraoperatively and postoperatively with this method of assessment.

Preprocedure nursing interventions include obtaining a health history, a signed consent form, and patient teaching related to the procedure. Postprocedure there are no physical restrictions.

Arthroscopy

Most often performed in the knee joint, an **arthroscopy** is an endoscopic procedure used to diagnose and repair meniscal, patellar, extrasynovial, and synovial diseases. Biopsies can also be performed. As with arthrography, this procedure is done on an outpatient basis. Local, spinal, or general anesthesia can be used (Kee, 2002).

Preprocedure nursing interventions include obtaining a health history to determine the possibility of pregnancy, a signed consent form, and patient teaching related to the procedure. Preprocedure medications should be administered and vital signs recorded. Patients should be instructed to remove all jewelry, contact lenses, glasses, dentures, or plates. Postprocedure, the patient will return to the recovery room for routine postoperative monitoring and assessment. Depending on type of anesthesia, activity, rehabilitation, diet, and medications may be resumed as soon as tolerated.

Bone Marrow Aspiration and Biopsy

Bone marrow aspiration and biopsy is used to examine the bone marrow for abnormal tissue growth or to monitor the progress of bone marrow disease. This procedure is performed under local anesthesia. The aspiration can be performed at the iliac crest or the sternum. Bone marrow is aspirated using a needle that is inserted into the cancellous bone (Kee, 2002).

Preprocedure nursing interventions include obtaining a health history to determine the possibility of pregnancy, a signed consent form, and patient teaching related to the procedure. Postprocedure the biopsy site should be assessed frequently for bleeding or hemorrhage and vital signs should be monitored closely. Diet, medications, and activity may be resumed as tolerated. The patient and family should be instructed to assess the site for signs of infection.

Joint Aspiration

Joint aspiration is performed to examine the synovial fluid in the joint cavity. It is also used to relieve pain in the joint resulting from edema and effusion. The procedure involves inserting a needle into the joint space and withdrawing fluid using a syringe. The fluid is then sent to the laboratory to be analyzed for infection or abnormal cells. The procedure is generally done under local anesthetic in the health care provider's office.

Preprocedure nursing interventions include patient teaching related to the procedure. Postprocedure the site will need pressure applied for 5 to 10 minutes. There are no physical restrictions.

Nerve Conduction Studies

Electromyography (EMG) measures electrical activity of skeletal muscle at rest and during voluntary muscle contraction (Kee, 2002). EMG is used to diagnose neuromuscular diseases and nerve damage. Kee states that the EMG can be used to differentiate between muscle and nerve damage. Needles are inserted into the muscle to detect electrical activity and printed as a graph. This procedure may be uncomfortable for the patient.

Preprocedure nursing interventions include obtaining a signed consent form and patient teaching related to the procedure. Patients are required to refrain from nicotine and caffeine two to three hours before the procedure. Postprocedure there are no physical restrictions.

Somatosensory Evoked Potentials (Evoked Potentials)

Somatosensory evoked potentials (SEP) are used to measure time in meters per second from the stimulation of a peripheral nerve through the response. It is used when EMG is not appropriate. This measurement documents axonal continuity when sensory potential cannot be measured due to nerve trauma. It is useful in the evaluation of radiculopathies and peripheral nerve function and the diagnosis of Charcot-Marie-Tooth disease. Electrodes are placed on the skin, stimulus is applied, and time intervals are calculated based on the time it takes from the stimulus to be given at one electrode and reach the next electrode along the peripheral nerve pathway. This procedure can be uncomfortable because of the electric nature of the stimulus.

Preprocedure nursing interventions may include patient teaching related to the procedure.

KEY CONCEPTS

- Anatomy and physiology of the bone consist of collagen, noncollagen, protein, and mineral components, which continually renew themselves.
- Bone formation is triggered by physical force, hormones, and genetics.
- There are four types of bones in the body: flat, short, long, and irregular.
- Long bones have three sections: the diaphysis, the medullary cavity, and the epiphyses.
- In the maturing child, the epiphyseal plate is the growth plate.
- Haversian canals, or osteons, allow the flow of fluid and nutrients to the bones.

Continued

KEY CONCEPTS—cont'd

- The five physiological processes of the bone are: (a) growth; (b) modeling; (c) remodeling; (d) repair; and (e) blood-bone exchange.
- Growth begins at two months after conception and continues until maturity.
- Remodeling of the bone occurs at the microscopic level through a balance of osteoclastic and osteoblastic activity.
- The main functions of the bones are to support the structure of the body, provide form, and enable movement.
- As a person ages, bones often become thinner and weaker and lean muscle mass decreases.
- A joint is formed when a bone meets another bone. It provides stability and mobility.
- The three classes of joints are synarthrosis (immobile), amphiarthrosis (slightly moveable), and diarthrosis (freely moveable).
- To reduce friction and distribute weight-bearing faces, hyaline cartilage covers the end of each bone.
- Synovial fluid lubricates joint surfaces.

- The nurse should focus on pain, onset of symptoms, deformity, and paralysis when completing an adult orthopedic musculoskeletal health history.
- The three maneuvers used in assessing the musculoskeletal system are: (a) inspection; (b) palpation; and (c) evaluation of passive and active ROM.
- Analysis of muscle tone, muscle strength, and gait are important aspects of identifying problems in the musculoskeletal system.
- Fractures can be classified as stress, displaced, stable, or unstable.
- The key to assessing sports-related injuries is to determine the severity and extent of the injury before permanent damage takes place.
- Radiographic studies are instrumental in the diagnosis and treatment of musculoskeletal conditions.
- Preprocedure nursing interventions for any testing include obtaining a health history, a signed consent form, and patient teaching related to the procedure.

REVIEW QUESTIONS

1. Wolff's law states what?
   1. The direction of growth is in opposite proportion to the amount of physical force placed on the bone.
   2. Bone forms and remodels itself in direct proportion to the amount and the direction of physical forces placed on it.
   3. Muscle tone and muscle strength increase with use.
   4. Myofibrils will contract with the release of actin and myosin.

2. A 7-year-old boy has fallen while roller-skating and fractured his radius along the epiphyseal plate. What is a likely consequence of the fracture?
   1. Fracture healing will proceed as normal and be fully remodeled in four weeks.
   2. The arm will always have a noticeable deformity, even after the fracture is healed.
   3. The fracture site has a 95 percent chance of developing an infection.
   4. Growth in the arm may be delayed or stopped.

3. All of the following statements are true regarding bone growth and remodeling *except*:
   1. Osteoblastic activity increases after the age of 30.
   2. Remodeling of a fracture can take several months to several years.
   3. Bones in children resemble cartilage more so than mature bone.
   4. The inflammation stage of fracture healing is the initial phase.

4. A few of the main functions of skeletal muscle are to (circle all that apply):
   1. Store minerals
   2. Maintain posture and body position
   3. Produce enzymes responsible for movement
   4. Guard entrances and exits to the digestive and urinary tracts

5. The mineral necessary to trigger a muscular contraction is:
   1. Potassium
   2. Calcium
   3. Magnesium
   4. None of the above

Continued

REVIEW QUESTIONS—cont'd

6. Ligaments have all the following characteristics *except*:
   1. Strong bands of connective tissue
   2. Give joints stability
   3. Elasticity
   4. Guide the joint movement

7. The three classes of joints are:
   1. Synarthrosis, amphiarthrosis, and diarthrosis
   2. Synarthrosis, biarthrosis, and amphiarthrosis
   3. Amphiarthrosis, biarthrosis, and lunarthrosis
   4. Synarthrosis, acetylarthrosis, and diarthrosis

8. Most patients come to a health care provider seeking assistance with musculoskeletal complaints because of:
   1. Obvious defects
   2. Limitation of movement
   3. Increase in the flexibility
   4. Decrease in pain

9. Physical assessment techniques used during the musculoskeletal system assessment include:
   1. Palpation and auscultation
   2. Inspection and range of motion
   3. Observation and auscultation
   4. Interview and palpation

10. Mrs. Dibble fell when getting off the bus and fractured her right ankle. The nurse is performing a neurovascular assessment (NVA). Important aspects to remember when performing a NVA are:
    1. Palpating the most distal pulse on the right lower extremity only using the nondominant hand
    2. Assessing for the patient's ability to feel the nurse touching her feet
    3. Asking the patient to dorsiflex and plantar flex her left foot only
    4. Compare the temperature of the left foot and toes to the left thigh

REVIEW ACTIVITIES

1. The patient has been diagnosed with a fractured radius and is placed in a cast. Explain to the patient why the health care provider stated the fracture would take about six weeks to heal. What would you tell the patient to look for when teaching about signs of circulatory and neurological impairment?

2. Search for a nursing article about osteoporosis, care of a patient with a joint replacement, or care of a patient with a congenital musculoskeletal problem, such as hip dysplasia, clubfoot, or muscular dystrophy. What does the article say about nursing assessment of the patient? What nursing interventions are done to minimize mobility problems? Does the article describe the collaborative nature of the relationship between the nurse and the health care provider or advanced practice nurse?

3. A neighbor tells you he has been diagnosed with bursitis in his elbow. He asks why he experiences pain when he flexes or extends his elbow. What explanation will you give?

4. Identify the orthopaedic nursing unit in your facility. Observe a nurse assessing his postoperative patient. What assessments does he perform? When performing the neurovascular assessment does he assess both extremities?

5. After being examined by the health care provider for complaints of hip and leg pain, your patient tells you that he is being scheduled for an MRI. He asks why an MRI and not a simple X-ray or CT scan. What explanation will you give him? What preparatory information can you tell him about the MRI testing procedure?

Musculoskeletal Dysfunction: Nursing Management

Anita M. Zehala, RN, MS, ONC, CNS

Debra Davis, BSN, RN

Rebecca Sears, RN

CHAPTER TOPICS

- Osteoarthritis
- Gout
- Lyme Disease
- Spondyloarthropathies Polymyositis/Dermatomyositis
- Fibromyalgia

- Metabolic Bone Disease
- Osteomyelitis
- Tumors of the Musculoskeletal System
- Spinal Disorders

KEY TERMS

Adams Bending Forward Test
Bouchard's nodes
Chondrosarcoma
Crepitus
Dactylitis
Enthesitis
Ewing's sarcoma
Fibromyalgia
Heberden's nodes
Hyperuricemia
Hypokyphosis
Keratitis
Kyphosis
Onycholysis
Osteoarthritis (OA)
Osteomalacia
Osteomyelitis
Osteoporosis
Osteosarcoma
Papilledema
Sacroilitis
Sarcoma
Scoliometer
Tendosynovial
Tophus

Musculoskeletal disorders (MSDs) affect nearly everyone. Whether a problem occurs because of overuse, sports, or an accident, there is some alteration, temporary or permanent, in a person's activities of daily living. MSDs occur in one in seven people in the United States. In a review of gender differences in upper extremity musculoskeletal disorders (UEMDs), the current literature supported the hypothesis that UEMDs did indeed occur more commonly in women than in men. Many nonfatal occupational injuries involving days away from work were MSDs. However, work-related musculoskeletal injuries occurred more often in men than women.

Because so many people are affected by MSDs, this chapter will cover the most common nontraumatic disorders in adults and children. Chapter 60 covers MSDs that are related to trauma.

OSTEOARTHRITIS

Osteoarthritis (OA) is noninflammatory degenerative joint disease characterized by degeneration of the articular cartilage, hypertrophy of bone at the margins, and changes in the synovial membrane. It is also accompanied by pain and stiffness, particularly after prolonged activity. More common than rheumatoid arthritis (RA), OA also affects the joint cavity. Unlike RA, OA is a noninflammatory arthritis. OA slowly progresses from deterioration of the articular cartilage to new bone formation in the joint margins and synovial hyperplasia and capsular thickening in diarthrodial (movable) joints. OA does not have systemic involvement.

Epidemiology

OA is the most common form of joint disease. OA, also known as degenerative joint disease (DJD), shows no favoritism with regard to race, age, or geographical area. At least 20 million adults in the United States suffer from the effects of OA. The incidence of OA increases with age, weight, and incidence of injury within a joint. The incidence of OA is twice as great in women over age 55.

Patients with OA find that physical limitations pose the greatest challenge. Seventy-eight percent of the elderly and one third of all patients report a limitation that affects performance of activities of daily living. Gait disturbance is also a common. Falls are, therefore, risks. Coping with a chronic illness, pain, and physical limitations can be challenging. Assessment of emotional and social coping is imperative.

Etiology

There are two types of OA, idiopathic (primary) and secondary. Idiopathic refers to the development of OA without any known or obvious trigger. A decrease in the quality and quantity of proteoglycans with aging is seen as an important factor that may influence the development of OA. There is evidence that idiopathic OA may be inherited as an autosomal recessive trait with gene defects causing premature cartilage destruction.

Secondary OA is the result of a known cause. Generally, the development is related to a known trauma in the area (e.g., fracture or sprain), prolonged mechanical stressors (e.g., obesity or athletics), inflammation in joint structures (not associated with RA), joint instability (e.g., damage to ligaments or tendons), neurological disorders (e.g., lost of proprioceptive reflexes leading to a tendency for abnormal movement, positioning, or weight-bearing), congenital or acquired skeletal deformities (e.g., dislocated hip or Legg-Calvé-Perthes disease), hematological or endocrine disorders (e.g., hemophilia with chronic bleeding into the joints or hyperparathyroidism with calcium loss from the bone) or selected drug use (collagen-digesting enzymes are stimulated in the synovial membrane by the drugs, such as colchicines, indomethacin, and steroids).

Sex hormones and other hormones seem to play a role in disease development and progression. For example, excessive growth hormone produces progressive overgrowth of bone and excessive parathyroid hormone results in hypercalcemia, which can produce skeletal changes. Unlike RA, OA is usually presents in only one joint (asymmetrical development).

Pathophysiology

OA occurs because of damage to articular cartilage and the metabolic response that results at the chondrocyte level. As a result of articular cartilage damage occurs, enzymes are released that breakdown the cartilage. This leads to a softening of the cartilage matrix (made up of type II collagen and pro-

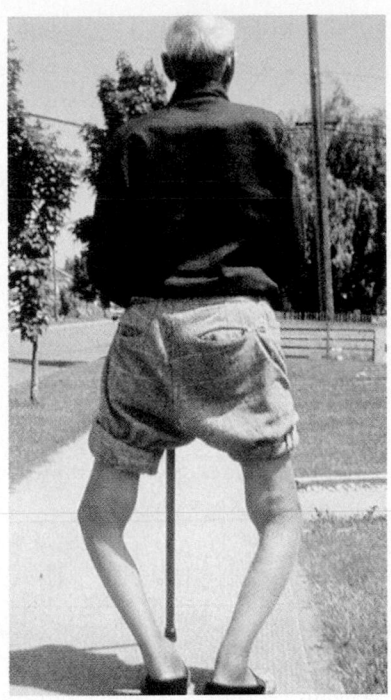

Figure 59-1 A patient with osteoarthritis of both knee joints.

teoglycans) as well as a loss of elasticity, and the cartilage becomes more fibrous. The resulting compensatory response is not enough to keep up with the destruction of the cartilage. This makes the articular surface more susceptible to joint friction.

With decreased cushioning, increased friction and tendency to become more fibrous, cartilage loses its ability to resist wear and utilize nutrients from the synovial fluid. The normally white, glistening, and smooth surface of the articular cartilage becomes yellowish, dull, and granular. The cartilage is gradually worn down to subchondral bone in the center of the joint surface. This bony friction triggers fibroblast production in the periphery of the joints, leading to the development of bone spurs in these areas.

With spurs present, the articular cartilage left in the periphery of the joint may shear off. The debris formed attracts phagocytes in to the areas, initiating an inflammatory response. This results in synovitis and an enlarged joint capsule. The inflammatory response also leads to an increase in synovial fluid production that further increases the edema in the joint. The early pain and stiffness of OA are results of the inflammatory response (Figure 59-1).

Assessment with Clinical Manifestations

Joint pain is the first and most common symptom reported by patients with OA. The joint pain is often described as aching. This symptom is what distinguishes it from other disease processes.

Physical examination will be focused on the joint(s) in which the main complaint is noted. The nurse should always compare the affected joint to the same joint in the opposite extremity. It is helpful to assess the joints most distal and proximal to the affected joint to assess if the chief complaint is actually a referred pain. For example, knee and thigh pain may be related to OA of the hip.

Patients with OA will complain of tenderness in the affected joint. Joint warmth and soft tissue swelling will indicate local inflammation—usually seen in early disease. While assessing for range-of-motion (ROM) the health care worker will note a limitation in the movement as well as **crepitus** (a crinkly, crackling, or grating feeling or sound in the joints, skin, or lungs), which is present in more than 90 percent of patients. **Heberden's nodes** (hard nodules or enlargements of the tubercles of the last phalanges of the fingers) and **Bouchard's nodes** (bony enlargements of the proximal interphalangeal joints) may develop as a result of osteophyte formation and loss of joint space (Figure 59-2). OA in the knee may lead to a varus deformity because of medial cartilage damage. Effusion around the knee can be because of synovitis. The effusion is usually only slight to moderate. Large effusions are uncommon in OA. Advanced OA in the hip can result in leg length discrepancy. This can be seen easily on a person wearing a belt—one hip is obviously higher than the other. Muscle atrophy may develop secondary to guarding of the hip.

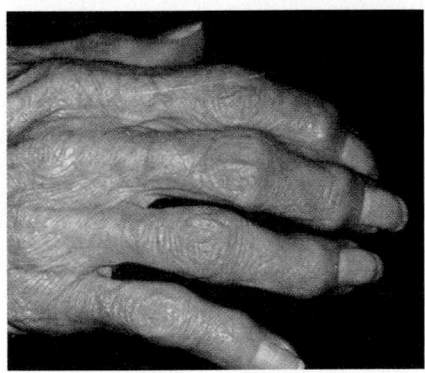

Figure 59-2 Bouchard's nodes and Heberden's nodes.

Diagnostic Testing

There is no specific laboratory test for the diagnosis of OA. Synovial aspiration may be used to rule out an infectious process if the joint is tender and swollen.

Radiographic images can confirm diagnosis. X-rays can reveal joint space narrowing, however, magnetic resonance imaging (MRI) is much more sensitive in identifying the progression of joint destruction.

Nursing Diagnoses

Based on the information gathered, examples of nursing diagnoses in the patient with OA may include:
- Acute pain.
- Chronic pain.
- Impaired physical mobility.

- Activity intolerance.
- Bathing/hygiene self-care deficit.
- Dressing/grooming self-care deficit.

Planning and Implementation

The management goals for patients with OA are to maintain joint mobility and minimize pain and inflammation. These can be accomplished by many methods, from rest to surgical joint replacement. The various options for treatment will be discussed below.

Collaborative Management

A variety of management therapies are a mainstay of recommendations by the ACR. These therapies include general aerobic type exercise as well as formal physical and occupational therapy assistance. Aerobic exercise will maintain joint mobility and muscle strength as well as assist with weight reduction, should the patient be overweight. These exercises can be done at home with a walking program at virtually no cost or in a structured environment in a gym or spa at varying costs.

Formal physical therapy does require a physician's prescription for insurance to cover some or all of the costs. Physical therapists will assess the patient's muscle strength, joint stability, and mobility; recommend heat or cold therapy; provide instruction for strength training, maintenance of joint mobility; and suggest the use of devices, such as canes or walkers (Estes, 2006). Occupational therapists can assist with joint protection and energy conservation as well as provide assistive devices and techniques for activities for daily living.

A review of literature found that home-based exercise programs were more likely to be adhered to than center-based exercise programs (gyms or with physical therapists) in the long-term (Ashworth, Chad, Harrison, Reeder, & Marshall, 2005). The literature also states that exercise of most types and intensities will assist in reducing pain and improving function in patients with osteoarthritis of the knee.

Nutrition

Many nutritional supplements have been studied examining their effect on OA. The *Alternative Medicine Review* published a review of multiple studies that looked at the effectiveness and safety of different nutritional supplements (Wang, Prentice, Vitetta, Wluka, & Cicuttini, 2004). With regard to prevention of OA, the review found that vitamin deficiencies, such as vitamin D, when treated with a vitamin supplement might play a role in preventing or treating OA (Wang, et al., 2004). The article also found that some supplements, such as avocado-soybean unsaponifiables, glucosamine, and chondroitin, may assist in providing symptom relief (pain and stiffness) and may have "structural effects" (p. 291). The theory is that these supplements may increase the lubrication in the joint.

Pharmacology

Because of the nature and cause of OA pharmacological therapy is aimed at pain control versus repair of joint damage. Traditionally, first line medication is acetaminophen for pain control. The belief is that there are fewer side effects associated with this medication (Broyles, Reiss, & Evans, 2007). Acetaminophen is available over the counter (OTC) and is inexpensive.

The next line of medication for pain management is the class of nonsteroidal anti-inflammatory drugs (NSAIDs). Nonsteroidal anti-inflammatory drugs include ibuprofen (Motrin or Advil) and naproxen sodium (Naprosyn or Aleve), diclofenac (Voltaren), and COX-2 inhibitors, such as rofecoxib (Vioxx), celecoxib (Celebrex), and valdecoxib (Bextra). Like acetaminophen, ibuprofen, and naproxen are readily available OTC and are relatively inexpensive.

Uncovering the Evidence

Treatment of OA

Discussion: The authors performed a meta-analysis comparing efficacy and safety of recommended dosages of nonsteroidal anti-inflammatory drugs with acetaminophen in the treatment of symptomatic hip and knee OA. Using a standardized form to abstract all data, Medline and EMBASE searches were performed on original clinical trials directly comparing NSAIDs with acetaminophen. Seven articles met the inclusion criteria.

NSAIDs were found to be statistically superior in reducing rest and walking pain compared with acetaminophen. They also found that safety was not statistically different between NSAID and acetaminophen groups.

Implications for Nursing Practice: There is an emphasis that includes the ability to safely recommend the use of OTC NSAIDs to patients with osteoarthritis who may find acetaminophen in ineffective for pain control.

Citation: Lee, C., Straus, W., Balshaw, R., Barla, S., Vogel, S., & Schnitzer, T. J. (2004). A comparison of the efficacy and safety of nonsteroidal antiinflammatory agents versus acetaminophen in the treatment of osteoarthritis: A meta-analysis. Arthritis and Rheumatism, 51(5), 746–754.

Diclofenac and higher doses of ibuprofen and naproxen sodium are available with a physician prescription.

Ibuprofen, naproxen and diclofenac all have been known to produce the side effect of gastrointestinal (GI) bleeding. The ACR recommends that NSAIDs be given with medications to treat or prevent GI symptoms should the patients be in a high-risk category for GI side effects.

Because of the potential side effects, a different type of NSAID was developed. Cyclooxygenase-2 (COX-2) inhibitors have fewer GI complications yet still produce the desired effects of pain relief and decreased inflammation that the NSAIDs deliver.

In cases where pain cannot be controlled with other medications, opioid analgesics (tramadol, oxycontin, hydrocodone, morphine, or diluadid) can be used to decrease pain. However, opioids do nothing to combat inflammation in the joint or surrounding musculature.

Intra-articular injections (viscosupplementation) with hyaluronic acid and glucocorticoids have been used to replace the lost synovial fluid and decrease local inflammation, respectively. ACR recommendations suggest intra-articular therapy for those patients who have been unresponsive to a program of non-pharmacological therapy and simple analgesics—especially for those who are at risk when taking NSAIDs or COX-2 inhibitors (Broyles, Reiss, & Evans, 2007). Payment from insurance companies varies for intra-articular injections.

In addition, steroid injections can be used to manage musculoskeletal disorders. They provide 2 to 6 weeks of pain relief and begin to have affects within the first 24 hours. Also, topical medication (e.g., capsacin, methylsalicylate, lidocaine patches) are recommended by the ACR.

Health Care Resources

In addition to home health nurses, physical therapists, and occupational therapists, a vocational guidance counselor can be consulted to assist with adaptations that may need to be used for those employed and have arthritis. Indeed, the changes needed for someone who is employed and has OA (or RA) can have an impact on productivity or days lost from work. A vocational guidance counselor would be able to assist the employee and the employer with the types of changes that need to be made. Most human resource departments should be able to assist in making contact with a vocational guidance counselor.

Surgery

Because the numbers of joints that can be affected by OA are numerous, only a few will be addressed below. Today, most joints can be replaced or modified in structure to return joint mobility and reduce pain.

When pain and limitations in mobility become too great for the patient, the assistance of an orthopedic surgeon is often sought. The patient's primary professional caregiver, a medical specialist (such as an internist, a pain specialist, or rheumatologist), or a concerned family member or friend often recommends the surgeon. The surgeon will need X-rays of the affected joint and sometimes an MRI to view thoroughly the source of the problem. The surgeon will interview the patient to determine if the patient has the necessary qualifications to be a candidate for surgery.

The types of surgeries that can be performed are arthroscopy, tibial osteotomy, and arthroplasty (joint replacement). Arthroscopy is used for the removal of loose bodies and resection of torn tissue when the joint space is sufficiently wide yet causing pain and mobility issues. Tibial osteotomy is employed when the patient has knee OA with a relatively small varus (inward) angle and stable ligament support (Figure 59-3). Arthroplasty is used with the patient has severe varus or valgus deformity (knock knees or bow legged), advanced OA of the hip and knee or other joint, and ineffective pain relief with other modalities. Boxes 59-1 through 59-3 provide guidance on patient care throughout the perioperative experience.

Evaluation of Outcomes

Generally OA has a good prognosis, if recommended treatment is followed. Potential outcomes for each of the example nursing diagnoses for the patient with OA are:

- Acute pain: The patient's pain should be adequately controlled, as assessed by the patient on scale of 1 to 10.

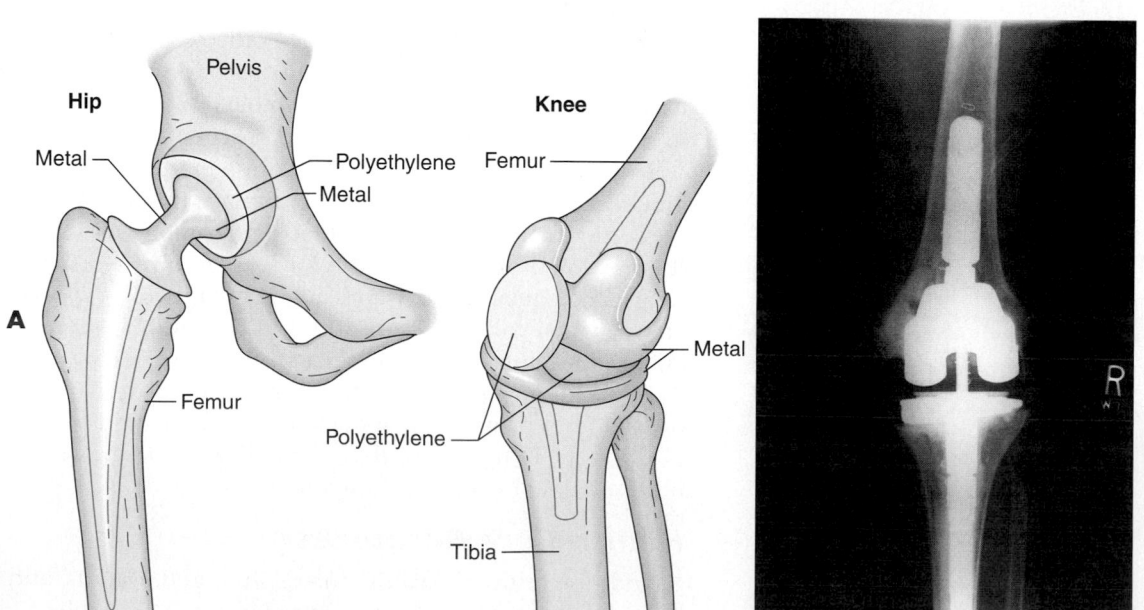

Figure 59-3 A. Total hip and knee replacement, B. Radiograph of a total knee replacement (anterior-posterior view).

BOX 59-1

CARE OF THE PATIENT WITH A TOTAL JOINT ARTHROPLASTY (PREOPERATIVE)

Assessment

- History and Physical: Gather information on past medical and surgical history. Is there any medical condition(s) that may cause postoperative concerns (e.g. hypertension, chronic obstructive pulmonary disease, or bleeding disorders)? What are the current medications taken (prescribed, OTC, and herbal or natural medications)? If the patient has had surgery in the past, was there any reaction to anesthesia? Assess patient's gait and use of any mobility devices used. What is the patient's preoperative range of motion in the affected extremity?

- Social History: Gather information regarding who the patient lives with. If the patient is alone will the person have a support individual to assist him or her in the home after surgery, will he or she go to a family member's residence after surgery, or does the patient anticipate needing to go to an extended care facility (ECF) for a short while to recover? Does the home have a first floor restroom? How many steps will the patient need to negotiate to get into the home? Does the patient have access to the necessary equipment for assistance with activities of daily living (e.g., walker, elevated toilet seat, reachers)?

- Financial Information: Are there any referrals that are needed by the insurance company? Is a social work consult necessary to assist with payment for the surgery?

Planning and Implementation

- History and Physical: Ensure patients that any medical conditions that they currently have will be addressed by the surgeon, anesthetist, and nursing staff that their other conditions will not adversely affect his recovery from surgery. Patient teaching should include what medications that patient should stop taking before surgery and when they should stop taking them. Explain the operative procedure (preoperative room, what happens during surgery and postanesthesia care unit). If available, provide written or video material that explains the surgical experience and postoperative recovery requirements that the patient can take home with him and will reinforce teaching you have already done.

- Social History: Help the patient to explore options about posthospital recovery regarding where he or she will be staying and equipment needed. Usually the hospital can provide resources for equipment for the patient. However, the patient may have relatives or friends who have had to use this type of equipment and might be able to loan or give it to the patient. Also, some churches keep such equipment that can be borrowed. If the patient anticipates going to an extended care facility after being discharged from the hospital, does he know which facility he or she would like to use? Also, consider involving social workers now or early on during the hospital stay.

- Financial Information: Make the appropriate referrals and contact the insurance company if preauthorization is necessary.

Evaluation

- History and Physical: Patient verbalizes an understanding of the basics of what will happen on the day of surgery and the general course during the hospital stay. He or she will verbalize what medications to stop taking before surgery.

- Social History: Patient verbalizes where he or she will be staying after discharge from the hospital and who will be available to assist him or her. The patient will verbalize where equipment can be obtained.

- Financial Information: Patient verbalizes any financial concerns.

BOX 59-2

IN HOSPITAL POSTOPERATIVE RECOVERY

Assessment

- Routine physical assessment consists of neurological, pulmonary, cardiac, GI, psychological, and neurovascular assessments as well as assessing the operative site. (See chapter 58 for method to perform neurovascular assessment.) Pain will also be an assessment you need to make. Arthroplasties tend to be painful (a different pain than experienced preoperatively). Adequate pain assessment and control will enhance the patient's recovery.
- Potential complications (most common): Deep vein thrombosis (DVT), wound infection, hematoma at the surgical site, neurovascular compromise, dislocation (hip).
- Also assess any patient or family concerns regarding the patient's progress.
- Assess the patient's learning of correct mobility techniques and precautions related to the specific surgery (e.g., patient verbalizes that he should not cross his legs after a total hip arthroplasty).

Planning and Implementation

- Administering pain medications, antibiotics, and anticoagulants as ordered. Emphasize to the patient that keeping pain under control will assist in the recovery process by making it easier to ambulate and rest more comfortably.
- Report any questionable assessments to the health care provider immediately to minimize adverse effects from complications.
- Generally physical therapy (PT) is the first to instruct a patient in how to get out of bed and to ambulate. Nursing is capable of doing the initial teaching but most generally reinforces the teaching of PT. Encourage the patient to gradually increase mobility, without pushing himself too far.
- Encourage patient and family to verbalize concerns and questions to you and any member of the nursing or medical staff.

Evaluation of Outcomes: Potential outcomes for the patient following surgery include:

- Patient verbalizes adequate pain control and willingly participates in therapy.
- Patient does not suffer from any postoperative complications.
- Patient's mobility steadily increases.
- Patient and family are freely able to express concerns and have concerns and questions addressed promptly.

- Chronic pain: The patient's pain should be adequately controlled, so that the patient is able to minimize disruptive effects for day-to-day living.
- Impaired physical mobility: The patient should demonstrate coordinated movement with active joint mobility. The patient should be able to perform self-care and manage activities of daily living. The patient should be able to demonstrate the proper way to transfer from bed to chair, chair to standing. The patient should be able to verbalize knowledge of prescribed activity level.
- Activity intolerance: The patient should be able to tolerate activity within normal limits and verbalize knowledge of endurance.
- Bathing/hygiene self-care deficit: The patient should demonstrate the ability to perform activities of daily living, bathing, toileting, and personal hygiene, using mobility aids if needed.
- Dressing/grooming self-care deficit: The patient should demonstrate the ability to dress.

BOX 59-3

AFTER DISCHARGE FROM THE HOSPITAL

Assessment

- Medications: Assess patient's understanding of prescribed postoperative medications and what preoperative medications the patient should continue taking after discharge.
- Mobility and exercise: Assess patient's need to obtain or maintain prescribed postoperative mobility and therapy. Does the person have a walker, crutches, or cane to for home use.
- Wound care: Assess patient's knowledge of appropriate wound care postoperatively.
- Home environment: If being discharged to a private residence, assess physical layout of the unit by asking questions. How many steps? Are there throw rugs? Are there chairs high enough to sit on (for hip patients)?
- Follow-up Care: Does the patient or caregiver understand when to see the surgeon for a follow-up appointment?

Planning and Implementation

- Medications: Teach patient which medications should be taken at home and continued. Often, antibiotics and anticoagulants are sent home with the patient. If the patient is sent home on warfarin (Coumadin), arrangements will need to be made to draw weekly or biweekly INR levels with a home health agency or a local clinic or health care provider's office. Encourage the patient to take all the prescribed antibiotics and to take the warfarin as prescribed. Caution the patient that the health care provider may change the warfarin prescription after blood tests are drawn to prevent excess bleeding. Pain medication prescriptions are most always sent home with the patient. Encourage the patient to take the pain medication about 30 minutes before exercising to keep pain to a minimum. Teach the patient about not driving when on this medication as it can cause drowsiness. Also caution the patient not to share his medications with others. Tell the patient to flush any unused pain medication down the toilet.
- Mobility and exercise: If formal therapy is prescribed, contact a home health agency to arrange this. Reinforce the necessity to increase amount of mobility each day to strengthen the muscles in the affected extremity.
- Wound care: Teach the patient appropriate wound care at home.
- Home environment: Encourage the caregiver to remove any throw rugs in the home. The health care provider will recommend how many times a patient can go up and down stairs. The rule of thumb is up and down stairs once a day for the first two weeks, then increase as the patient tolerates after that.
- Follow-up Care: Tell the patient when the surgeon wants schedule a follow-up appointment. You may make the appointment or allow the patient to do so.

Evaluation

- The patient recovers and returns to normal activities of daily living without complications.

GOUT

Gout is a metabolic disorder that primarily affects men and stems from elevated urate levels in the body. Gout has a hereditary tendency.

Epidemiology

Primary gout is more commonly found in Pacific Islanders (e.g., Filipinos or Samoans). Ninety percent of patients with secondary gout are men, generally over 30 years old. Women who develop gout are usually postmenopausal.

Etiology

As with osteoarthritis, there are two types of gout: (a) primary and (b) secondary. Primary gout is a result of excessive purine synthesis, accelerated nucleotide breakdown, or increase nucleic acid turnover. Secondary gout is a result of a known cause. The cause can be from acquired diseases (e.g., **hyperuricemia,** which is an abnormal amount of uric acid in the urine, hemolytic anemia, psoriasis, and renal insufficiency); obesity or starvation; lead toxicity; use of certain drugs (e.g., salicylates, diuretics, nicotinic acid, alcohol); or organ transplant recipients (especially renal or cardiac allografts) who take cyclosporine and diuretics. Primary gout is seen in about 90 percent of all diagnosed cases. Secondary gout only accounts for 10 percent of occurrences.

Pathophysiology

Hyperuricemia is the primary cause of the pathology of gout. Hyperuricemia is caused by an overproduction or underexcretion of uric acid. Unlike RA and OA, gout usually develops in only one joint, frequently the great toe, which accounts for 50 percent of all acute attacks. The characteristic nodule that develops is known as the **tophus.** The tophus consists of uric acid crystals. The presence of the crystals, which are not normally found in joints, causes a foreign body reaction. This leads to an acute arthritis attack.

Because of the chronic hyperuricemia, systemic problems can occur. In addition to joints, tophi can be found in cartilage, subcutaneous and periarticular tissues, tendon, bone, kidneys, as well as other areas. Kidney stones develop as a result of the elevated uric acid levels. These stones develop in 5 to 10 percent of patients with gouty arthritis. Patients with chronically elevated uric acids, especially those who are already predisposed to renal failure, can progress into chronic renal failure.

Complications

The major complications from chronic gout are soft tissue damage and deformity; joint destruction resulting in a crippling deformity; nerve compression syndrome; and nephrolithiasis and gouty nephropathy.

Assessment with Clinical Manifestations

The patient will report a rapid development (within hours) of pain and edema in the one affected joint. Pain that develops over weeks or months is more likely to be some other condition. When gathering history, the nurse should keep in mind the factors that may contribute to the development of gout (e.g., trauma, alcohol use, medications, acute illness, or family history). Physical examination will reveal swelling, pain, and decreased range of motion in the affected joint. Fever, complaints of headache, and hypertension may also be present. Tophi may be seen on external ears, hands, feet, the olecranon process and prepatellar bursas.

Diagnostic Tests

Laboratory findings will reveal the following: Uric acid levels will be elevated (7 to 10 mg/dL); urine albumin will be greater than100 mg/24 hours; urinary uric acid will be elevated; leukocytosis will be present, and there will be an elevated sedimentation rate. Radiographic studies can be useful in identifying tophi that are not visible in early disease. In chronic disease, bony abnormalities will be shown, such as the punched out erosion of bone with sclerotic borders. An overhanging rim of cortical bone may also be seen (Daniels, 2003). An MRI may be needed to differentiate tophi from infection or tumor.

Performing synovial fluid aspiration is controversial in diagnosing gout, as 80 percent of patients can be diagnosed using physical examination only. However, aspiration may have a therapeutic effect from the decompression that accompanies fluid withdraw. If differential diagnosis between septic arthritis, pseudogout, and gout is needed, the only way to confirm a diagnosis is with a synovial fluid aspiration. The fluid aspirated from a joint with gout will reveal distinctive needle-like intracellular crystals of sodium urate.

Renal and cardiovascular system evaluation is necessary because of the systemic complications from chronic hyperuricemia. This workup would include a complete blood count (CBC), serum creatinine, serum uric acid, blood urea nitrogen (BUN), and urinalysis.

Nursing Diagnoses

Based on the information gathered, examples of nursing diagnoses in the patient with gout may include:
- Acute pain.
- Chronic pain.
- Impaired physical mobility.
- Activity intolerance.
- Bathing/hygiene self-care deficit.
- Dressing/grooming self-care deficit.

Planning and Implementation

Although medication is a vital in the management and prevention of gouty arthritis, the role the nurse plays in teaching about lifestyle and nutritional changes is integral in overall management. The management goals in treating gout are to treat the arthritis symptoms first (pain and edema) and secondarily treat the hyperuricemia (Hellman & Stone, 2004).

During an acute attack, bed rest is the exercise of choice. This assists in allowing the inflammation to recede and promotes pain relief. Bed rest should be continued for approximately 24 hours. Heat, ice, and elevation will assist in relief of pain and edema during an acute attack.

Nutrition

A diet low in purines is helpful to reduce serum uric acid. Low-purine foods are refined cereals, white bread, pasta, and flour, milk and milk products, sugar, sweets, and gelatin, all fats, fruits, nuts and peanut butter, vegetables (except those listed), and cream soups. Moderate-purine foods are beef, chicken, duck, pork, and ham, shellfish (except mussels) and oysters, asparagus, mushrooms, and spinach, and kidney beans, lentils, and lima beans. High-purine foods are alcoholic beverages, anchovies, sardines, herring, mussels, codfish, scallops, trout, haddock, bacon, turkey, veal, venison, and organ meats.

Pharmacology

The medications used to treat gouty arthritis and hyperuricemia fall into four categories: (a) nonsteroidal anti-inflammatory drugs (NSAIDs); (b) gout medications; (c) corticosteroids; and (d) analgesics. Nonsteroidal anti-inflammatory medications are the drugs of choice in treating acute gout. They assist with inflammation and pain reduction. Indomethacin (Indocin) has been the traditional drug of choice. However, Hellman and Stone (2004) point out that any of the newer NSAIDs are equally effective. COX-2 inhibitors (e.g., celecoxib) work well when there is a risk of ulcer or renal problems exist.

Medications used to specifically treat the hyperuricemia have two purposes: to treat the acute attack and to assist in the prevention of further attacks. Colchicine is used for the acute attack phase. Effective within the first few hours of the attack, it is thought to work by interfering with the inflammatory response to the uric acid crystals in the joint. Unfortunately, patients poorly tolerate colchicine. Up to 80 percent of patients treated develop abdominal cramping, diarrhea, nausea, or vomiting (Hellman & Stone, 2004). Colchicine is generally used in the first 24 hours. Allopurinol, probenecid, or sulfinpyrazone (Anturane) is used to lower serum uric acid levels. Because acute attacks can happen when uric acid levels are lowered quickly, colchicine may be added to the treatment to prevent an acute attack.

Corticosteroids are used to provide symptomatic relief during acute attacks. Corticosteroids are best used when a patient is unable to take NSAIDs (Hellman & Stone, 2004). Analgesics, such as acetaminophen, may be needed to control the acute pain of gout (Broyles, Reiss, & Evans, 2007).

Patient and Family Teaching

Teaching should include proper use of medications and instruction on side effects. Dietary teaching and reinforcement are necessary. It is important to remind the patient to maintain a urinary output of 2,000 mL or more per day to minimize the precipitation of uric acid in the urinary tract (Hellman & Stone, 2004).

Evaluation of Outcomes

Generally gout has a good prognosis, if recommended treatment is followed. Potential outcomes for each of the example nursing diagnoses for the patient with gout are:

- Acute pain: The patient's pain should be adequately controlled, as assessed by the patient on scale of 1 to 10.
- Chronic pain: The patient's pain should be adequately controlled, so that the patient is able to minimize disruptive effects for day-to-day living.
- Impaired physical mobility: The patient should demonstrate coordinated movement with active joint mobility. The patient should be able to perform self-care and manage activities of daily living. The patient should be able to demonstrate the proper way to transfer from bed to chair, chair to standing. The patient should be able to verbalize knowledge of prescribed activity level.
- Activity intolerance: The patient should be able to tolerate activity within normal limits and verbalize knowledge of endurance.
- Bathing/hygiene self-care deficit: The patient should demonstrate the ability to perform activities of daily living, bathing, toileting, and personal hygiene, using mobility aids if needed.
- Dressing/grooming self-care deficit: The patient should demonstrate the ability to dress.

LYME DISEASE

Lyme disease (LD) is a multisystem inflammatory process with devastating long-term effects if not treated early or effectively (American College of Physicians, 2004). Lyme disease is a bacterial infection that occurs after the bite of an infected tick.

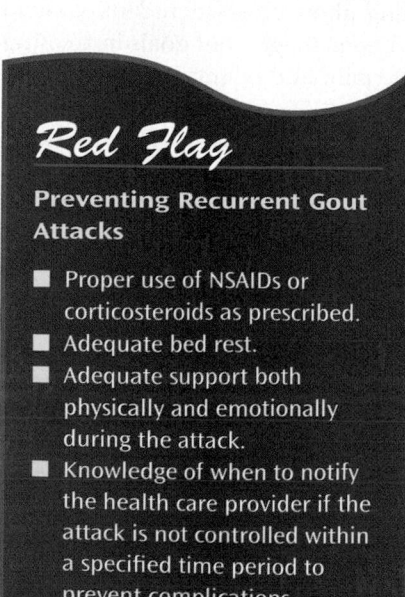

Red Flag

Preventing Recurrent Gout Attacks

- Proper use of NSAIDs or corticosteroids as prescribed.
- Adequate bed rest.
- Adequate support both physically and emotionally during the attack.
- Knowledge of when to notify the health care provider if the attack is not controlled within a specified time period to prevent complications.

Epidemiology

LD symptoms have been described since the early twentieth century (Knisley & Johnson, 2004). Until a group of children in Lyme, Connecticut developed juvenile rheumatoid arthritis, the disease was not recognized in the United States. This occurred in 1977.

The CDC reports that 23,763 cases of LD were reported in 2002, which is a 40 percent increase from 2001. It is speculated that the increase occurred because of increased deer population, increased residential development in wooded areas, tick dispersal to new areas, improved disease recognition, and enhanced reporting (Edlow, 2002). In reviewing the 2002 data, the majority of cases fell into two age-group ranges: (a) 5 to 14 years old and (b) 50 to 59 years old. The northeastern and north central states in the United States are where 95 percent of all cases were reported (CDC, 2004d).

Etiology

Lyme disease is caused by the spirochete *Borrelia burgdorferi*. It is transmitted to humans by the bite of the deer tick (Figure 59-4). The deer tick in the nymphal stage is the size of a pinhead (3.5 mm to 5.5 mm in length) (CDC, 2004d). Therefore the bite often goes unnoticed. Once the tick is attached it must remain in place 36 to 48 hours for the spirochete to be transmitted. The symptoms can develop in 7 to 14 days, but Knisley and Johnson (2004) report symptoms can begin as soon as three days or as late as 30 days after the bite.

Assessment with Clinical Manifestations

Patients will generally present with flu-like symptoms. Knisley and Johnson (2004) point out that the symptoms include but are not limited to low-grade fevers, fatigue, muscle, bone aches, chills, and malaise. Patients may or may not report a history of tick bite. They may report being physically active out of doors in the previous two to four weeks before symptoms occurred when questioned. Fifty percent to 75 percent of patients present with the classic symptom erythema migrans (EM), which is definitive of the disease (Edlow, 2002). EM presents as a circular rash that continues to grow and often resembles a bullseye.

The American College of Physicians (ACP, 2005) reports that symptoms of LD occur in three indistinct stages. Flu-like symptoms, as described above, represent the early LD stage. The second stage's symptoms reflect the spread of the bacterium throughout the body. If a patient does not get EM, then he or she may first appear to the health care provider with second-stage symptoms (early disseminated LD). These symptoms include numbness and pain in the arms and legs, paralysis of facial muscles (usually unilaterally, as in Bell's palsy), meningitis, and rarely, an abnormal heart rhythm. The third stage can occur weeks, months, or even years after infection in patients who either never received antibiotic treatment for early LD or where treatment did not kill all of the bacteria. Late LD symptoms include chronic Lyme arthritis, central nervous system (CNS) symptoms, and chronic pain in muscles or restless sleep. The arthritis symptoms revolve around bouts of pain and edema in one or more of the larger joints, but these symptoms tend to present more frequently in the knees (Edlow, 2002). Memory loss and difficulty concentrating are CNS symptoms. Arthritic symptoms may be the only clinical symptoms seen in children (Knisley & Johnson, 2004).

More serious, but rare, is ocular involvement. Symptoms range from conjunctival erythema and retinal hemorrhages to **keratitis** (inflammation of the cornea) and **papilledema** (edema of the optic disk) (Edlow, 2002).

The physical examination should include a head to toe skin assessment looking for EM. The nurse should be especially diligent when examining areas

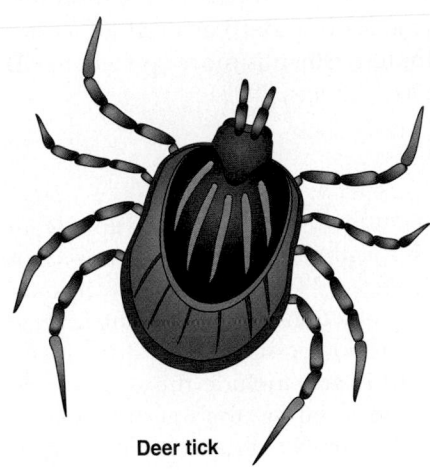

Deer tick

Figure 59-4 Lyme disease is transmitted with the help of a vector, such as the deer tick.

of the body with creases (e.g., groin and axilla). Erythema migrans is sometimes best seen when the skin is warm, such as in a bath (Knisley & Johnson, 2004). Therefore, the patient should be questioned about such occurrences when performing the examination.

Other assessments include neurological examination, assessment of range of motion, complaints of muscular pain, and a thorough cardiac examination including an electrocardiogram (ECG). Although rare, LD can cause atrioventricular block and lead to complete heart block (Knisley & Johnson, 2004).

Diagnostic Tests

Although blood tests cannot diagnose LD alone, they can be used to confirm diagnosis. LD antibody can be assessed for, but it can be positive in patients with a high rheumatoid factor. An enzyme-linked immunosorbent assay (ELISA), which tests for antibody rise, is more often used to confirm an LD diagnosis. Because the anti–*Borrelia burgdorferi* antibodies do not appear for two to six weeks after transmission, the ELISA is not performed until this time. The ELISA can show antibodies in the presence of other bacterial infections and other disease processes. A Western blot test, which is more specific to LD is performed to confirm positive ELISA tests (Daniels, 2003).

Nursing Diagnoses

Nursing diagnoses with LD will revolve around the stage of the disease in which the patient presents. Based on the information gathered, examples of nursing diagnoses for the patient with all stages of LD include activity intolerance related to fatigue or weakness; risk for infection related to longer term antibiotic use; and anxiety related to unknown progression of the disease.

Nursing diagnoses for early disseminated LD may include those similar to OA as well as disturbed body image related to facial paralysis and decreased cardiac output related to atrioventricular (AV) block. Impaired role performance and self-care deficit related to memory and concentration difficulties or chronic pain may be encountered in the late LD stage.

Planning and Implementation

LD is a curable disease, therefore the ultimate management goal is to recognize the symptoms early and start antibiotic therapy as soon as possible. If treated early, LD can be prevented from progressing to a more serious and chronic condition.

Pharmacology

Much research has been done exploring the subject of LD. In a query on the subject over 110,000 global articles were found. The articles researched and discussed identification of the responsible organism, transmission of the disease, clinical manifestations, and treatment of LD. Eppes (2003) reviewed and summarized relevant literature and found that the most effective treatment of LD was with oral antibiotics. The drug of choice is doxycycline. When doxycycline cannot be tolerated or for children less than 8 years old, amoxicillin or cefuroxime can be used orally in both the early LD stage as well as the early disseminated stage. If neurological symptoms are present, intravenous (IV) ceftriaxone is the treatment of choice in both the early disseminated stage and the late LD stage. When arthritis is present in the late LD stage, oral doxycycline is utilized. The duration of treatment is generally two to four weeks, depending on symptoms and stage.

A vaccination against LD was introduced in 1998 but was pulled from market in 2001. Controversy exists over the reason for discontinuation. Other adjuvant therapies may be helpful in controlling symptoms. Eppes (2003) suggests nonsteroidal anti-inflammatory medications can be used to assist with complaints from myalgias and arthralgias.

Surgery

When synovitis accompanies arthritic symptoms, a synovectomy may be used to reduce edema and pain in the joint.

Patient and Family Teaching

As oral antibiotic is the treatment of choice for LD, it is essential that all antibiotics be taken as prescribed, because the bacterium can live in the body for years if not completely eradicated early on (ACP, 2005).

As with any infectious disease, a prevention focus is important when providing information about LD. The CDC (2004d) recommends using personal protection measures, such as tucking pants into socks and wearing long sleeves when in areas where tick exposure is likely. The use of insect repellents on exposed skin and clothing that contains diethyl toluamide (DEET) can reduce the risk of tick attachment (CDC, 2004d). Tick checks should be done when returning from outdoor activities.

Evaluation of Outcomes

Generally LD has a good prognosis, if recommended treatment is followed. Potential outcomes for each of the example nursing diagnoses for the patient with LD are:

- Acute pain: The patient's pain should be adequately controlled, as assessed by the patient on scale of 1 to 10.
- Chronic pain: The patient's pain should be adequately controlled, so that the patient is able to minimize disruptive effects for day-to-day living.
- Impaired physical mobility: The patient should demonstrate coordinated movement with active joint mobility. The patient should be able to perform self-care and manage activities of daily living. The patient should be able to demonstrate the proper way to transfer from bed to chair, chair to standing. The patient should be able to verbalize knowledge of prescribed activity level.
- Activity intolerance: The patient should be able to tolerate activity within normal limits and verbalize knowledge of endurance.
- Bathing/hygiene self-care deficit: The patient should demonstrate the ability to perform activities of daily living, bathing, toileting, and personal hygiene, using mobility aids if needed.
- Dressing/grooming self-care deficit: The patient should demonstrate the ability to dress.

In addition, response to antibiotic and adjuvant therapy is seen in abatement of the symptoms. For those who present in the later stages of disease progression, antibiotic therapy may need to be extended to allow time to kill the bacterium and for symptoms to disappear.

SPONDYLOARTHROPATHIES

Spondyloarthropathies are a group of systemic, inflammatory, rheumatic-type syndromes. These syndromes all have common symptoms. The symptoms can make initial diagnosis challenging. The nurse's responsibility is to assess accurately the patient's complaints or lack thereof to assist in making a specific diagnosis and to provide education and support to the patient and family.

These syndromes include ankylosing spondylitis (AS), reactive arthritis (Reiter's syndrome), arthritides associated with psoriasis, Crohn's disease, and ulcerative colitis, and a form of juvenile chronic arthritis. There are also several forms of undifferentiated spondyloarthropathies that are often underdiagnosed

---

DOLLARS AND SENSE

Keeping the Cost of Treatment for LD Reasonable

Eppes' (2002) review of the LD literature found that traditional treatment with doxycycline and the minimal use of diagnostic tests for confirmation of diagnosis appeared to be the most cost-effective course when dealing with LD. Prolonged IV antibiotic therapy will add to the cost of treatment. IV therapy is utilized in the early and late disseminated stages when CNS symptoms are present and as alternatives to oral therapy.

or undiagnosed (Khan, 2002). Khan (2002) described the common features of the spondyloarthropathies: **sacroilitis** with or without spondylitis; variable inflammatory peripheral arthritis (single or multiple joints); **enthesitis** (inflammation at the bony insertion sites of ligaments and tendons); **dactylitis;** tendency for ocular inflammation; familial tendency; no rheumatoid factor; strong association with the HLA-B27 gene.

Etiology

The etiology for these syndromes is generally unknown. The majority of patients with spondyloarthropathies can identify a hereditary link or have the HLA-B27 antigen.

Pathophysiology

The mechanisms that cause inflammation in the joints and elsewhere in spondyloarthropathies are not fully understood. Similar to RA, elevated levels of T cells, macrophages and an increase in cytokine release is seen in the inflamed joints. With continued inflammation, bony erosions and new bone formation can occur. Unlike RA, there is no synovial membrane involvement. Explanation for the extra-articular symptoms may occur by the transport of triggers (T cells and others) via the lymphatic system or macrophages (Khan, 2002).

AS, reactive arthritis, and psoriatic arthritis will be described later in the chapter. General considerations for the spondyloarthropathies as a group will then be discussed.

Assessment with Clinical Manifestations

Resembling RA, arthritic symptoms will be seen worse in the morning, with complaints of pain and stiffness in the affected joint(s). The symptoms and pain will lessen within an hour and become less intense during the day. Timing of the onset of symptoms helps to identify the correct diagnosis. Symptoms of AS tends to be a gradual onset. Reactive arthritis tends to occur within four weeks after the onset of an aforementioned infection. Psoriatic arthritis is always associated with psoriasis and usually appears months to years after initial diagnosis of psoriasis. However, psoriatic arthritis can precede or occur simultaneously with the onset of skin lesions (Hellman & Stone, 2004).

Physical examination will focus on the areas of complaint. AS often shows limited motion in the back; lateral flexion and extension and forward flexion will be limited.

Reactive arthritis shows symptoms of asymmetric polyarticular complaints, with or without effusions. Again, with Reiter's syndrome the provider will see the "sausage" toes and complaints of arthritis symptoms in the knees and ankles (Khan, 2002). There will also be symptoms associated with the infectious process that precedes the arthritic symptoms. Urethritis symptoms, such as edema, redness at, and purulent drainage from, the urethral meatus may be present. Conjunctivitis or uveitis may also be seen. Psoriasis-like lesions on the soles of the feet and other body surfaces may be visible. With psoriatic arthritis sausage digits and erythema may be present in small peripheral joints. Other symptoms are psoriasis lesions and pitted and discolored nails.

When enthesitis is present in any of these syndromes, palpation along the spine will elicit tenderness. The enthesitis can also be seen with complaints of heel pain because of inflammation of the Achilles tendon and plantar fascia (Kataria & Brent, 2004). There may also be tenderness when the sacroiliac joints are palpated while the patient is flexed at the hips.

Diagnostic Testing

Diagnosis is made mainly by physical examination. X-rays in AS will show bilateral symmetrical sacroilitis and squaring of the vertebrae. As the disease progresses, total fusion of the sacroiliac joint and the involved vertebrae will occur. Eventually, spine X-rays will show a classic "bamboo spine," which is indicative of the vertebral fusion. For psoriatic arthritis, erosions may be seen in the distal interphalangeal (DIP) joints of the hands and feet.

Blood drawn to detect the presence of HLA-B27 gene is not necessary to diagnose, but it is often done to confirm the diagnosis. Rheumatoid factor may be drawn to make a differential diagnosis. Evidence of infection is frequently seen in the blood work of a patient with reactive arthritis.

Nursing Diagnoses

Based on the information gathered, examples of nursing diagnoses in the patient with spondyloarthropathies may include:

- Acute pain.
- Chronic pain.
- Impaired physical mobility.
- Activity intolerance.
- Bathing/hygiene self-care deficit.
- Dressing/grooming self-care deficit.

Planning and Implementation

The goals of care for the spondyloarthropathies involve minimizing the inflammation, maintaining functional ability, controlling pain, and minimizing the effects of systemic complications. Research on the spondyloarthropathies focuses on a wide range of subjects from causative factors to successful treatments to patients' reactions to the syndromes. Evidence will be discussed that supports multidisciplinary therapeutic interventions used with patients who have spondyloarthropathy.

As noted earlier, arthritic symptoms associated with the spondyloarthropathies are generally worse in the early morning and get better with use. Therefore, activity is a mainstay of treatment. Many studies have been done looking at the effect of exercise on the progression of symptoms, maintenance of functional ability, and patient coping.

Falkenbach (2003) found that the greater the disability in patients with AS, the greater the motivation to exercise. Ward (2002) found that functional disabilities increased as the patient's age increased and if the patient smoked. He found that the disability decreases if the patient exercised and had better social support. Intense physical therapy also increases mobility in patients for the short term.

Analay, Ozcan, Karan, Diracoglu, and Aydin (2003) studied patients to determine whether an at home exercise program would be more effective in promoting exercise than a structured program. They found that the participants in the structured program faired better and were more likely to participate.

A review of organizations with information on spondyloarthropathies (National Institute of Health, Spondylitis Association of America, The Arthritis Foundation, American College of Rheumatologists and American College of Physicians-American Society of Internal Medicine) showed unanimous agreement on the use of exercise in promoting musculoskeletal function and decreasing pain.

The use of splints, braces, and other joint support devices are not encouraged. These devices immobilize the joint, leading to further stiffness and decreased mobility as well as the potential for the development of permanent contractures. With spondyloarthropathies, rest does not decrease the symptoms.

Pharmacology

A mainstay to any treatment plan is the administration of medication. Because spondyloarthropathies share symptoms similar to RA, it is logical to believe that the medications used with RA would be effective in the treatment of the spondyloarthropathies. To some extent this is true. First-line treatment tends to be with NSAIDs. This is followed up by the use of sulfasalazine (Alzulfidine) when the NSAIDs are no longer effective in relief of the inflammatory symptoms. Kataria & Brent, (2004) reviewed five separate studies noting the positive effects of tumor necrosis factor-alpha (TNF-alpha) inhibitors (etanercept [Enbrel] and infliximab [Remicade or Centocor]) in treating the inflammation.

Disease-modifying antirheumatic drugs (methotrexate and cyclosporine) have shown some effectiveness against inflammation. Corticosteroid injections can decrease local inflammation.

Surgery

Joint replacement and stabilization may be appropriate for patients with severe arthritic symptoms. Spinal fusion can be performed when AS gets to the point of causing major functional disability.

Patient and Family Teaching

Teaching involves the proper use of medications; encouragement, and instruction in appropriate exercise therapy (with or without a therapist) and pain relief measures. Heat and cold as well as mild analgesics can be used to assist with pain relief.

Evaluation of Outcomes

Generally spondyloarthropathies have a good prognosis, if recommended treatment is followed. Potential outcomes for each of the example nursing diagnoses for the patient with spondyloarthropathies are:

- Acute pain: The patient's pain should be adequately controlled, as assessed by the patient on scale of 1 to 10.
- Chronic pain: The patient's pain should be adequately controlled, so that the patient is able to minimize disruptive effects for day-to-day living.
- Impaired physical mobility: The patient should demonstrate coordinated movement with active joint mobility. The patient should be able to perform self-care and manage activities of daily living. The patient should be able to demonstrate the proper way to transfer from bed to chair, chair to standing. The patient should be able to verbalize knowledge of prescribed activity level.
- Activity intolerance: The patient should be able to tolerate activity within normal limits and verbalize knowledge of endurance.
- Bathing/hygiene self-care deficit: The patient should demonstrate the ability to perform activities of daily living, bathing, toileting, and personal hygiene, using mobility aids if needed.
- Dressing/grooming self-care deficit: The patient should demonstrate the ability to dress.

Ankylosing Spondylitis

Ankylosing spondylitis (AS) is a chronic, progressive, inflammatory arthritis that primarily affects the synovial joints of the spine and soft tissue surrounding the spine (Chou, Lo, Kao, Jim & Cho, 2002). AS refers to fusion (ankylosis) of inflamed vertebrae (spondylitis).

Epidemiology

Ankylosing spondylitis appears more frequently in men, ages of 16 and 35. AS is seen in less than 1 percent of the U.S. population. It is three times more likely to occur in men than in women. African Americans are 25 percent more likely to develop AS than Caucasians. Five percent of AS begins in childhood. Boys develop it at a greater rate than girls. In children symptoms usually begin in the hips, knees, bottoms of heels, or big toes and may later progress to involve the spine.

Assessment with Clinical Manifestations

The typical patient has a gradual onset of symptoms of low back pain. There is often no incident that can be linked to the onset of the back pain. The pain is worse in the morning and lessens with activity. The pain may radiate to the gluteal region. A decrease in spine mobility (range of motion) will be seen as the syndrome progresses. Typically the decrease in mobility affects the lumbar spine, then moves to the sacroiliac joints, and then gradually up the spine to include the cervical spine. As the disease progresses, thoracic kyphosis is exaggerated, and the cervical spine becomes hyperextended (Kataria & Brent, 2004).

Other problems that occur with AS include: (a) uveitis (edema of the upper eyelid, excessive lacrimation, small irregular pupil, and swollen iris); (b) aortic and mitral valve dilation leading to regurgitation; and (c) fibrosis of the upper lobes of the lungs (Kataria & Brent, 2004).

Reactive Arthritis

Also known as Reiter's syndrome, reactive arthritis is associated with an infectious process, often chlamydia or enteritis secondary to gram-negative enterobacteria (Khan, 2002). Of those affected greater than two thirds have the HLA-B27 antigen. The symptoms usually appear in a series of three: nongonococcal urethritis, conjunctivitis, and arthritis. The arthritis symptoms seen usually involve the lower extremities and are asymmetrical. A classic symptom for patients with reactive arthritis is the sausage toe. The toe becomes uniformly edematous and reddened and resembles a sausage. In addition, the condition of enthesitis leads to inflammation with a tendency toward fibrosis and calcification can develop. This condition causes heel pain as a distinguishing characteristic of reactive arthritis. Low back pain is a common symptom secondary to sacroilitis. Conjunctivitis occurs in approximately 50 percent of patients (Kataria & Brent, 2004). Onset of symptoms occurs within one to four weeks after the initial infection.

Reactive arthritis is usually an acute episode. The symptoms are generally present for five days to five months. A small percentage of patients will have mild symptoms for up to a year. Fifteen to 30 percent of patients will develop chronic musculoskeletal symptoms (Khan, 2002).

Etiology

Because of wide variation in recognition and clinical severity the true incidence of reactive arthritis is difficult to assess. In Sweden the incidence was 28 reported cases in 100,000 adults (Söderlin, Börjesson, Kautiainen, Skogh, & Leirisalo-Repo, 2002). The incidences occurred equally in men and women.

Psoriatic Arthritis

Psoriatic arthritis (PsA) develops in association with the diagnosis of psoriasis. PsA is a progressive, chronic, inflammatory form of arthritis accompanied by fatigue, severe joint pain, and swelling. Psoriatic arthritis exhibits in five different patterns: arthritis in the DIP; arthritis mutans; symmetrical polyarthritis similar to RA; asymmetrical oligoarthritis; and spondyloarthropathy (Tam & Geier, 2004). Up to 60 percent of patients will often present with one typical pattern of arthritis and then transition into another pattern.

With PsA, nail lesions occur in about 80 percent of patients. These nail lesions are pitting and include **onycholysis** (the loosening of the nails starting at the border). Uveitis also tends to be present and chronic (Kataria & Brent, 2004).

Etiology

It is estimated that one million people have PsA. This is roughly 0.5 percent of the U.S. adult population. An estimated 4.5 million people have psoriasis. Psoriatic arthritis generally appears between the ages of 30 and 55 equally in men and women.

POLYMYOSITIS AND DERMATOMYOSITIS

Polymyositis (PM) and dermatomyositis (DM) are another set of autoimmune disorders that affect the musculoskeletal system. These syndromes produce muscle weakness secondary to muscle inflammation which, if left unchecked, can lead to respiratory failure and death.

Epidemiology

PM is mostly seen in adults. DM can be seen in both adults and children. The incidence of occurrence for both is 8.4 per million people in the general U.S. population. African Americans tend to develop the disorder more often than Caucasians. Women are twice as likely to develop the syndromes (Hellman & Stone, 2004).

Pathophysiology

The causes of PM and DM are not known. It is known that the autoimmune disorder causes extensive necrosis and destruction of muscle fibers. As with most autoimmune disorders, autoantibodies develop and start destroying target areas. In the case of PM, the autoantibodies (CD-8 positive cells) invade the target muscle fibers. With DM, complement C3 forms a membranolytic attack complex that is deposited in the capillaries of the muscle tissue. This complex leads to the development of edematous endothelial cells, capillary necrosis, perivascular inflammation, ischemia, and destruction of muscle fibers.

Another inflammatory myopathy can be seen that does not fit all of the diagnostic criteria of PM. Inclusion-body myositis can be sporadic, but it is less responsive to treatment (Hellman & Stone, 2004).

DM is also associated with an increased risk of cancer, especially in older adults (Hellman & Stone, 2004). The cancers seen are ovarian, in the GI tract, lung, breast, and non-Hodgkin's lymphomas.

PM and DM are sometimes seen in association with other autoimmune and connective tissue disorders (e.g., lupus). Often the symptoms overlap, making the diagnosis of new onset PM or DM challenging.

Assessment with Clinical Manifestations

The patient will present with a gradual and insidious onset of bilateral, generalized muscle weakness. Rarely is the onset acute with PM. Patients with DM often present with the characteristic rash that precedes the muscle weakness. The rash can be seen on the upper eyelids with a blue-purple discoloration (heliotrope rash), often with edema. There can also be a reddish rash on the face and anterior chest in a V shape or over the back and shoulders (which is labeled the shawl sign), knees, elbows, or malleoli. Another characteristic rash is known as Gottron rash or sign. This red rash appears on the knuckles of the hands and fingers.

Muscle weakness usually develops in a pattern. The muscle weakness starts in the proximal muscles of the arms and legs and then moves distally. Eventually, without treatment, the muscles of the fingers are affected, making fine motor movements difficult. Holding a pencil or feeding oneself is a challenging task.

Because cancer is associated with DM, cancer screening may be indicated. This is especially true if the patient is greater than 60 years of age or is in a high-risk category for cancer development.

Diagnostic Tests

There are three hallmark tests which confirm the diagnosis of PM or DM: elevated muscle enzymes, an abnormal electromyogram, and positive results in a muscle biopsy.

The muscle enzymes which specifically indicate either PM or DM are creatinine kinase (CK) and aldolase. The CK can be increased as much as 50 times the normal value for CK. These enzymes can also be monitored to indicate response to treatment.

The muscle biopsy is the definitive diagnostic test for PM and DM. In PM, the biopsy will show muscle fiber inflammation and necrosis. With DM, the inflammation is seen primarily in the perivascular areas of the muscle.

Other cancer screening diagnostic tests may need to be completed at the same time, especially for high-risk patients with DM.

Nursing Diagnoses

Based on the information gathered, examples of nursing diagnosis in the patient with PM and DM may include the following:
- Bathing/hygiene self-care deficit.
- Impaired physical mobility.
- Fear.
- Anxiety.
- Deficient knowledge.
- Risk for injury.

Planning and Implementation

The goals of therapy are to improve the ability to carry out activities of daily living by increasing muscle strength and to ameliorate extramuscular manifestations.

Pharmacology

The first-line of treatment is pharmacological care. Prednisone, in doses of 40 to 100 mg per day are prescribed for several weeks to decrease the inflammation that is causing the muscle weakness (Hellman & Stone, 2004). Prednisone is eventually tapered to a dose that effectively treats the symptoms and lowers the serum enzyme levels and is often administered on an every-other-day regimen.

Should the patient be intolerant to prednisone or the disease does not respond to the prednisone, immunosuppressive drugs are the next line of therapy. Azathioprine (Imuran or Azasan) is the most commonly used immunosuppressive agent. Other immunosuppressive therapies include methotrexate (Rheumatrex), cyclosporine (Neoral or Sandimmune), and mycophenolate mofetil (CellCept).

Collaborative Management

Therapies can be initiated to assist in regaining strength, once pharmacological therapy has been initiated. Occupational therapist may be especially helpful in the early stages to assist in providing activities of daily living equipment.

Health Care Resources

Health care providers and nurses can lend a good deal of support and information to the patient about the disease processes. There are many organizations that can lend support and encouragement for patients and their families who suffer with PM or DM. A Google search on the Internet found over 100,000 hits on PM alone. Just three organizations that were listed that had support information and access to support groups were the National Institute of Neurological Disorders and Stroke (NINDS), the Muscular Dystrophy Foundation, and the Arthritis Foundation.

Patient and Family Teaching

The focus of teaching will be disease information, medication and symptom management, safety, and for patients with DM, cancer screening. Including all applicable health care providers during the teaching phase of care ensures that all necessary aspects are covered. As the nurse, you can be a consistent contact person for questions, which is also assistive. A special contact person for the patient can coordinate care and information and clarify any questions the patient may have.

Evaluation of Outcomes

Positive patient outcomes focus on improvement of the rash and muscle weakness. Trends of decrease muscle enzymes will also show that the medication is effective. Assessing for patient reaction to the medication in the form of side effects is an important nursing responsibility.

FIBROMYALGIA

Fibromyalgia is most frequently defined as a clinical syndrome or condition involving chronic widespread diffuse musculoskeletal pain, stiffness, and tenderness. A lack of restorative or deep sleep is a prominent feature of fibromyalgia and has been described as both a contributing factor to and a symptom of the disorder (Henriksson, 2003). Fatigue and insomnia are frequently cited as accompanying features of fibromyalgia.

Fibromyalgia is a common disorder and represents the second most common disorder seen by rheumatologists in North America. The majority of sufferers are women. Although it is seen in all age-groups, prevalence appears to increase with age, reaching a peak among individuals 60 to 80 years of age (Inanici & Yunus, 2002).

Epidemiology

The incidence of fibromyalgia varies with the specifics of patient samples studied as well as the geographical location. Incidence has been described from 7 percent within the general population to 2.1 to 5.7 percent in general medical clinics or primary care practices to 10 to 20 percent in rheumatology clinics. Prevalence in Europe has been reported as between 1 to 2 percent, whereas North America reports a prevalence of 2 percent. The prevalence of fibromyalgia among women is 3.4 percent as compared to men at 0.5 percent (Inanici & Yunus, 2002).

Etiology

The etiology of fibromyalgia is unclear, although it has been suggested that the condition is not the result of a single etiological factor. The role of infectious agents as causative factors has been the subject of investigation, with Epstein-Barr virus, cytomegalovirus, human herpes virus 6, human immunodeficiency virus (HIV), and *Borrelia Burgdorferi* representing the most frequently cited organisms. The basis for an infectious origin is supported by the presence of a viral syndrome at the time of diagnosis by a reported 55 percent of patients. A genetic predisposition has been suspected but not confirmed (Inanici & Yunus, 2002).

Pathophysiology

Although some muscle abnormalities have been reported, fibromyalgia differs from other musculoskeletal disorders in its absence of clear inflammatory or structural musculoskeletal pathology. Instead, current research suggests pathology related to dysfunction within the neuroendocrine system. It is this dysfunction within the neuroendocrine system that is thought to provoke the abnormalities in pain sensitivity characteristic of fibromyalgia. Central sensitization of neurons, deficits in the functioning of the descending inhibitory system, and ongoing activity within the afferent nerves result in functional changes within the nociceptive system. A number of associated pathophysiological mechanisms responsible for the regulation of mood, sleep, and pain perception have been considered as contributory including a low serotonin level and increased substance P in the cerebrospinal fluid (Henriksson, 2003).

Abnormalities in the hypothalamic pituitary-adrenal axis are also seen. A decreased level of insulin-like growth factor 1 is common and may be a pathogenic marker in fibromyalgia. The characteristics of growth hormone deficiency, such as, diminished energy, dysphoria, impaired cognition, poor general health, reduced exercise capacity, muscle weakness, and cold intolerance parallel symptoms seen in fibromyalgia.

Fibromyalgia shares clinical features with a number of other conditions, including irritable bowel syndrome (IBS), chronic fatigue syndrome (CFS), and temporomandibular pain syndrome. Common attributes among these disorders include the increased prevalence among women, pain without tissue damage, fatigue, poor sleep, and responsiveness to similar groups of medications. Similarities are particularly striking with CFS. An estimated 70 percent of fibromyalgia patients meet the criteria for CFS. The difference appears to be largely related to the degree of pain versus the degree of fatigue experienced by the patient. Similarities between the two entities suggest the possibility of commonalities in the pathology of fibromyalgia and CFS. The evidence of central sensitization seen in fibromyalgia, CFS, IBS, and temporomandibular pain syndrome suggests central sensitization as the common physiological feature that binds these entities together and may provide clues to an underlying pathology (Inanici & Yunnus, 2002).

Assessment with Clinical Manifestations

As a clinical entity, fibromyalgia has been the subject of much debate. Historically, the subjective parameters used in the diagnosis of fibromyalgia have resulted in challenges to the existence of fibromyalgia as a distinct clinical entity. Concerns have included the subjective nature of the tender point examination, the subjective nature of chronic pain, the lack of a standardized definitive laboratory test, and the absence of clear objective pathology. Although both rheumatologists and the World Health Organization (WHO) now recognize fibromyalgia, the subjective nature of fibromyalgia continues to plague effective diagnosis and management. It is not unusual for patients to have fibromyalgia for five to seven years before a diagnosis is confirmed (Inanici & Yunus, 2002).

Diagnosis of fibromyalgia is based entirely on signs and symptoms characteristic of the syndrome. The American College of Rheumatology (ACR) established criteria in 1990 for the diagnosis of fibromyalgia based on the occurrence of both subjective and objective findings (Table 59-1). Musculoskeletal pain is typically characterized as widespread aching, in addition to tenderness on palpation with multiple tender points. Eighteen locations have been identified as common tender points in the diagnosis of fibromyalgia. The presence of at least 11 out of the 18 tender points is considered diagnostic according to ACR criteria.

A number of other clinical features and syndromes have been associated with fibromyalgia. These include restless leg syndrome, IBS, irritable bladder

---

TABLE 59-1 **Criteria for the Classification of Fibromyalgia**

History of Widespread Pain

Definition: Pain is considered widespread when all of following are present: pain in the left side of the body, pain in the right side of the body, pain above the waist, and pain below the waist. In addition, axial skeletal pain (cervical spine or anterior chest or thoracic spine or low back) must be present. In this definition, shoulder and buttock pain is considered as pain for each involved side. Low back pain is considered lower segment pain.

Pain in 11 of 18 tender point sites on digital palpation.

Definition: Pain, on digital palpitation, must be present in at least 11 of the following 18 sites:

Occiput: Bilateral at the suboccipital muscle insertions.

Low cervical: Bilateral at the anterior aspects of the intertransverse spaces at C5 to C7.

Trapezius: Bilateral at the midpoint of the upper border.

Supraspinatus: Bilateral at origins above the scapula spine near the medial border.

Second rib: Bilateral at the second costochondral junctions, just lateral to the junctions on upper surfaces.

Lateral epicondyle: Bilateral 2 cm distal to the epicondyles.

Gluteal: Bilateral in upper outer quadrants of buttocks in anterior fold of muscle.

Greater trochanter: Bilateral posterior to the trochanteric prominence.

Knee: Bilateral at the medial fat pad proximal to the joint line.

Digital palpation should be performed with an approximate force of 4 kg.

For tender point to be considered positive the subject must state that the palpation was painful.

"Tender" is not considered "painful."

For classification purposes, patients will be said to have fibromyalgia if both criteria are satisfied. Widespread pain must have been present for at least three months. The presence of a second clinical disorder does not exclude the diagnosis of fibromyalgia.

---

syndrome, interstitial colitis, headaches (particularly migraine), ocular and vestibular complaints, cognitive dysfunction, cold intolerance, multiple sensitivities, and dizziness. The coexistence of associated features supports the diagnosis of fibromyalgia in situations where only 8 to 10 tender points are noted on physical examination.

Diagnostic Tests

Although there are no definitive standardized diagnostic tests specific to the diagnosis of fibromyalgia, various laboratory tests and radiography should be performed to evaluate for any possible coexisting conditions noted by history and physical examination and to eliminate other conditions that may be responsible for the patient's symptomatology. These might include a CBC, measurement of ESR, C-reactive protein, serum electrolyte level, blood glucose level, liver enzyme tests, renal function tests, thyroid function tests, urinalysis, and various radiological exams. In some cases, a moth-eaten appearance in type 1 fibers and atrophy in type 2 fibers may be seen on muscle biopsy. An ANA, serum complement, and rheumatoid factor tests are generally not performed unless the patient shows indication of rheumatic disease (Inanici & Yunnus, 2002).

Nursing Diagnoses

Based on the information gathered, examples of nursing diagnoses in the patient with fibromyalgia may include:

- Acute pain.
- Chronic pain.
- Impaired physical mobility.
- Activity intolerance.
- Bathing/hygiene self-care deficit.
- Dressing/grooming self-care deficit.

Planning and Implementation

Central to the goal of therapy in the treatment of fibromyalgia is the alleviation of pain and the management of any associated symptoms, conditions, and contributing factors. Common approaches include both pharmaceutical and non-pharmaceutical therapy. Pharmaceutical therapy is inclusive of pain management and the medical management of coexisting conditions and symptoms. Primary to effective nonpharmaceutical management is the restoration of sleep hygiene, increasing physical fitness, and elimination of psychological distress.

Pharmacology

Analgesia, antidepressants, and muscle relaxants represent pharmaceutical therapies common in the treatment of fibromyalgia. Antidepressant therapy has been shown to improve sleep, fatigue, and pain severity in patients regardless of the presence of clinical depression. The effectiveness of NSAIDs in the treatment of pain has been debatable, although some patients have reported benefit. The most effective pharmaceutical approaches appear to employ combination therapies, such as combinations of analgesics and antidepressants or antidepressants and muscle relaxants. Amitriptyline, cyclobenzaprine, a fluoxetine and amitriptyline combination, citalopram, and tramadol have been shown to be efficacious in the treatment of fibromyalgia as reported in various research studies. Lidocaine injections into tender points can be administered to ease pain at particularly bothersome sites. A graduated and individualized approach to pharmacological therapy may be employed with doses or medications chosen to manage varying degrees of pain and other symptomatology (Inanici & Yunnus, 2002).

Nutrition

Although a specific dietary regimen has not been established in the literature, a number of concerns exist that may warrant assistance from a dietitian. Some evidence exists that implicates the role of certain foods in the exacerbation of fibromyalgia symptoms similar to what has been found with migraine and IBS. In particular the limitation of caffeine and alcohol is recommended because of their ability to act as muscle irritants. Vitamin and mineral supplements may be warranted to assist with stress, immune support, and the correction of any deficiencies. While other specific recommendations were inconclusive, agreement in the need for a healthy meal plan, avoidance of foods that patients have identified as contributory to flares, and nutritional management of coexisting conditions, such as migraine and IBS were consistently seen.

Collaborative Management

Physical deconditioning is a common feature of fibromyalgia and likely the result of physical inactivity related to patient attempts to minimize pain. The impact of physical fitness on pain has been inconsistent in studies examining the outcomes of aerobic exercise in patients with fibromyalgia. However, studies suggest that aerobic activity does contribute to improvements in physical functioning, psychological well-being, and improvements in overall quality of life. The type, duration, and intensity of the exercise program should be individualized to the needs and abilities of each patient focusing on the goal of preventing physical inactivity and improving the level of physical fitness. The added benefit of combating the muscle weakness and fatigue associated with fibromyalgia is seen with the involvement of physical therapy and cardiovascular fitness training.

The benefits of gentle low-impact aerobic exercise must be balanced with individual patient abilities to prevent the exacerbations of fibromyalgia symptoms. One suggested approach involves 3 to 5 minutes of aerobic activity per day gradually increasing to 20 to 30 minutes per day for patients who are deconditioned. A variety of methods has been suggested, including walking, bicycling, and the use of various types of home equipment. Aerobic water exercise may be best tolerated in patients who are unable to tolerate other forms of exercise. Care should be taken to avoid extremes in water temperature that may prevent patients from doing well.

Health Care Resources

The complexity of fibromyalgia demands the expertise of a comprehensive health care team including the physician, nurse, dietitian, and social worker or counselor working in collaboration with the patient and his or her family. In addition, a number of resources are available to assist patients with fibromyalgia. The Arthritis Foundation and The National Fibromyalgia Association both offer information and connecting resources.

Alternative Therapy

In addition to traditional therapy, roughly two thirds of patients with fibromyalgia seek assistance from alternative therapy. However, mind-body techniques, acupuncture, and manipulative therapies represent the only therapies supported by research as potentially beneficial in the treatment of fibromyalgia.

Patient and Family Teaching

The role of patient self-management in fibromyalgia underlines the critical importance of patient and family education. A thorough understanding related to the nature of the disease, its symptoms, variability, and the likelihood of periods of exacerbation versus remission is essential to the ongoing participation and well-being of the patient. Education should be ongoing and address the main areas of pain management, physical fitness, sleep, and psychological well-being. Pain management includes adherence to medication regimens, monitoring of pain characteristics, participation in physical activity, and prompt follow-up with health care team members regarding changes in and exacerbations of pain. Physical activity should be stressed but balanced with rest needs during periods of exacerbation. Patients should be cautioned to avoid overuse of physical activity during flares and use of the most painful muscles. Patients should be instructed to start exercise at a low level and to increase gradually on a regular basis. The keeping of an exercise diary or graph that includes exercise time, intensity, and pulse rate achievements are useful in evaluating exercise programs. Sleep can be enhanced through the avoidance of caffeine; alcohol; or heavy meals before bedtime; the elimination of disturbing factors, such as noise and light; and the establishment of a regular sleep schedule. Interventions to maintain psychological well-being may include relaxation training, coping skills training, reduction of negative pain behaviors, and the fostering of a positive attitude. A referral to counseling would be appropriate for patients struggling with anxiety and depression (Inanici & Yunus, 2002).

Evaluation of Outcomes

Fibromyalgia is a condition characterized by remissions and exacerbations. Therefore, the importance of ongoing care and follow-up can not be underestimated. Acute flares can frequently be managed with support, physical therapy, rest, and medication management. Systemic disease and other conditions may develop over time warranting a thorough evaluation of new or changes in present symptoms. Cognitive dysfunction may present as impairments in recall, concentration, and memory (Inanici & Yunus, 2002).

The impact of fibromyalgia on quality of life can be tremendous. Fibromyalgia represents a major cause of disability in the United States. As many as 25 percent of patients with fibromyalgia receive some form of disability payment or injury compensation suggesting the existence of issues with the ability to obtain and maintain suitable work environments. Self-assessments of disability parallel that of RA and OA. Pain, fatigue, and weakness are the most frequently cited causes. While most patients are able to continue working, modifications in the work environment inclusive of changes in the ergonomic structure and reductions in work hours may be required (Inanici & Yunus, 2002).

OSTEOPOROSIS

Osteoporosis is defined as being characterized by low bone mass, microarchitectural deterioration, compromised bone strength, and an increase in the risk of fracture.

Epidemiology

Based on the 2000 census data, NOF estimates that 20 percent (7.8 million) of postmenopausal Caucasian women in the United States will have osteoporosis, and 52 percent of (21.8 million) other women will have low density at the hip in 2002. Given these numbers, it is not surprising that osteoporosis is the most frequently diagnosed bone disease in humans.

Etiology

Although the exact cause of primary osteoporosis is not known, it is known that the rate of bone loss is strongly correlated with genetics, estrogen, and other risk factors, which will be discussed in further detail (Sedlak & Doheny, 2002). Secondary osteoporosis can be linked to nutritional deficiencies, endocrine function abnormalities, and disuse. Table 59-2 summarizes the known links leading to secondary osteoporosis.

Pathophysiology

As discussed in chapter 58, bone remodeling is never static. Bone formation and remodeling take place because of the balance of osteoblastic and osteoclastic activity. With osteoporosis, this activity slowly becomes less balanced, with osteopenia developing first. At about the age of 30 osteoclastic activity starts to over take osteoblastic activity. This process is more rapid during the first years after menopause and then slows down but continues throughout the rest of a female's life. Men do suffer from the effects from the imbalance, but because men generally start with a larger bone mass, the process takes longer (Crowther & McCance, 2004).

> "In normal bone, the frequency of [multicellular] unit activation, the rate of resorption and the rate of new bone formation are relatively constant, so that replacement follows resorption immediately and the amount of bone replaced equals the amount of bone resorbed. In bone affected by osteoporosis, this equilibrium can be disrupted by (1) an increase in the number of basic [multicellular] unit activated, (2) an increase in the frequency of basic [multicellular] unit activation, (3) an increase in the rate of resorption, (4) a delay in the rate of bone formation, or (5) a deficiency of cells in the [multicellular] unit. Any one of these changes will cause a net decrease in total bone mass" (Crowther & McCance, 2004, p. 1083).

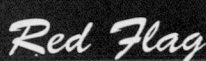

Red Flag

Risk Factors for Developing Osteoporosis and Related Fractures

The major risk factors include:
- Personal history of fracture as an adult
- History of fragility fracture in a first-degree relative
- Low body weight (less than about 127 pounds)
- Current smoking
- Use of oral corticosteroid therapy for more than three months

The minor risk factors are:
- Impaired vision
- Estrogen deficiency at an early age (younger than 45)
- Dementia
- Poor health or frailty
- Recent falls
- Low calcium intake (lifelong)
- Low physical activity
- Alcohol in amounts greater than two drinks per day

Risk Assessment Tool for Osteoporosis

1. Have either of your parents broken a hip after a minor bump or fall?
Yes   No

2. Have you broken a bone after a minor bump or fall?
Yes   No

3. Have you taken corticosteroid tablets (cortisone, prednisone, etc.) for more than three months?
Yes   No

4. Have you lost more than 3 cm (just over 1 inch) in height?   Yes   No

5. Do you regularly drink heavily (in excess of safe drinking habits)?   Yes   No

6. Do you smoke more than 20 cigarettes a day?
Yes   No

7. Do you suffer frequently from diarrhea (caused by problems such as celiac disease or Crohn's disease)?
Yes   No

For women:

1. Did you undergo menopause before the age of 45?
Yes   No

2. Have your periods stopped for 12 months or more (other than because of pregnancy)?
Yes   No

For men:

1. Have you ever suffered from impotence, lack of libido, or other symptoms related to low testosterone level?
Yes   No

Answering yes to any of these questions does not mean that you have osteoporosis. You should show this test to a health care provider or nurse practitioner and discuss the questions you have with him or her.

TABLE 59-2 Contributing Factors to Secondary Osteoporosis

Nutritional deficiencies

Vitamin C deficiency (scurvy)

Mild malabsorption syndrome (lactose intolerance)

GI and hepatic diseases (those that impair absorption of calcium, phosphate, and vitamin D)

Acid diets

Calcium-deficient diets

Chronic alcohol abuse (alcohol is a direct inhibitor of osteoblasts and may directly inhibit calcium absorption)

Endocrine function abnormalities

Hyperthyroidism

Hyperparathyroidism

Cushing's syndrome

Acromegaly

Hypogonadism

Corticosteroids

Disuse—reduces stressors on bones (Wolff's law)

Bed rest

Inactivity common in elderly

The presence of the above factors leads to an increased risk of fractures (Figure 59-5).

Assessment with Clinical Manifestations

Osteoporosis is often considered a silent disease with the first indication of a problem often being when the patient suffers a fracture. Unfortunately, this can be indicative of advanced disease. Another presenting condition most often because of osteoporosis is a decrease in height, sometimes accompanied by **kyphosis** (hunchback). Kyphosis is the result of the vertebral column becoming brittle, weak, and misshapen as the bone loses volume (Crowther & McCance, 2004).

A risk assessment is in order when osteoporosis is suspected or a familial history of osteoporosis in known. This can be done during a routine physical examination, accompanying a more focused examination or after a fracture has occurred. Knowing the amount and types of risk factors the patient has will assist the nurse in planning your teaching and anticipating health care provider orders.

Sedlak and Doheny (2002) note that an annual loss of height (approximately 0.09 percent of total height) is normal after the age of 45 They state that a loss greater than this will need investigation as height loss is often a first sign of osteoporosis. Kyphosis will be obvious on physical examination. Back pain is a common complaint.

The most common fracture sites seen with osteoporosis are the forearm, femur (hip), ribs, and spine (Crowther & McCance, 2004). Care should be taken to assess these areas assessing for pain, edema, deformity, and crepitus. Should a fracture be suspected, referral to the physician will be necessary for follow-up diagnostic studies.

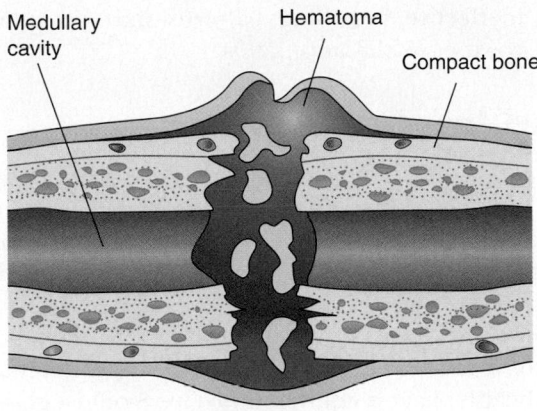

Medullary cavity Hematoma Compact bone

A. A hematoma forms from blood from ruptured vessels.

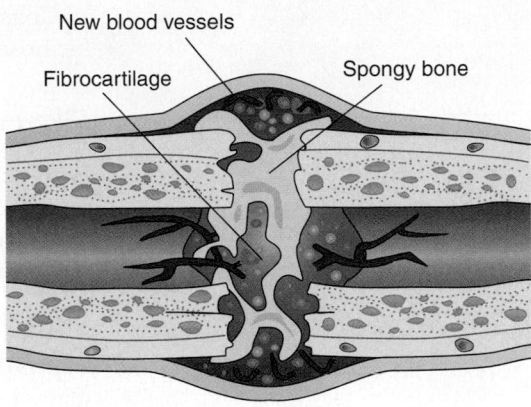

New blood vessels Fibrocartilage Spongy bone

B. Spongy bone forms close to developing blood vessels; fibrocartilage forms away from new blood vessels.

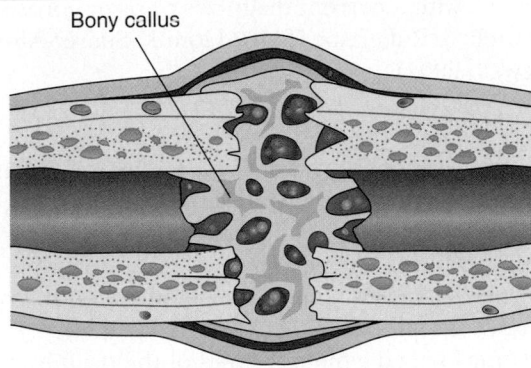

Bony callus

C. Bony callus replaces fibrocartilage.

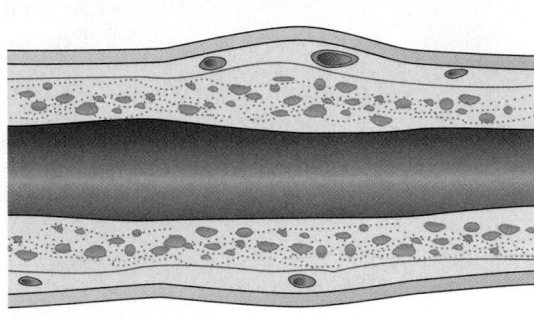

D. Excess bony tissue is removed by osteoclasts.

Figure 59-5 Steps of bone repair.

Diagnostic Tests

When a fracture is suspected, the most common test is a simple X-ray. When osteoporosis is suspected or the patient has several risk factors, measurement of bone mincral density is in order. The gold standard in determining bone mineral density and diagnosing osteoporosis is with a dual X-ray absorptiometry (DEXA) scan. Refer to chapter 58 for information on this scan.

Laboratory studies that may be conducted to assess the patient are calcium, magnesium, phosphate, vitamin D, alkaline phosphatase, and protein electrophoresis. In looking for secondary causes parathyroid hormone levels may be drawn. Further testing for thyrotoxicosis and hypogonadism may be required once a definitive diagnosis is made (Fitzgerald, 2004).

Nursing Diagnoses

A multitude of nursing diagnoses are appropriate the diagnosis of osteoporosis. For those who have just been diagnosed, deficient knowledge related to the new diagnosis of osteoporosis should be the major focus of nursing care. Anxiety related to fear of fracture may be another that may apply early on. Potential nursing diagnoses for patients with osteoporosis are:

- Impaired physical mobility (actual or high risk for) related to effects of osteoporosis
- Potential for injury related to impaired physical mobility
- Pain related to injury or effects of osteoporosis
- Alteration in nutrition: less than body requirements related to poor appetite, change in taste or smell, nutritional intake imbalance or lack of funds

Constipation and ineffective breathing patterns may be an issue when kyphosis is present (Crowther & McCance, 2004).

Planning and Implementation

With diagnosis and treatment of osteoporosis management outcomes will focus on preventing further bone loss and injuries. A multipronged approach to osteoporosis care is essential to treat the disorder and manage the sequelae of the disease process. Pharmacological, physical, and nutritional therapy will be reviewed.

Nutrition

The NIH recommends a total of 1,000 mg to 1,500 mg of calcium a day to maintain good bone health. That is equivalent to five 8-ounce glasses of milk. Most American diets do not allow for this level of calcium consumption. Therefore, calcium supplementation is necessary. It has been shown that the addition of a vitamin D supplement to the calcium can reduce the incidence of hip fractures in patients with a current diagnosis of osteoporosis (Gillespie, Avenell, Henry, O'Connell, & Robertson, 2004; Homik, Suarez-Almazor, Shea, Cranney, Wells, & Tugwell, 2004).

Pharmacology

There are several different classes of drugs used in the treatment of osteoporosis: bisphosphonates; selective estrogen receptor modulators; hormones; prescribed supplements; and skeletal anabolics. Bisphosphonates have been utilized since 1995 as inhibitors of osteoclast bone resorption (Sedlak & Doheny, 2002). The drugs in this category include alendronate sodium (Fosamax), risedronate (Actonel), and etidronate (Didronel).

Homik, et al. (2004) performed a meta-analysis of the usefulness of bisphosphonates for steroid induced osteoporosis. The findings from this review showed that bisphosphonates were effective in preventing and treating the steroid-induced bone loss at the lumbar spine and femoral neck. Other such reviews that risedronate was effective in the reduction of both vertebral and nonvertebral fractures and etidronate increased bone density in the lumbar spine and femoral neck.

Selective estrogen receptor modulators (SERM) are used for both the prevention and treatment of osteoporosis. Raloxifene (Evista) is a SERM used to "maximize the effect of estrogen on bone and minimize the negative effects on the breast and endometrium" (Sedlak & Doheny, 2002, p. 436).

Hormone replacement therapy (HRT) has become controversial because of the increased risk of breast and uterine cancer. More research is needed to look at the long-term effects and efficacy of HRT with regard to reducing bone loss versus cancer risk.

Calcitonin (Miacalcin) is a hormone that has been used in the treatment of postmenopausal and corticosteroid-induced osteoporosis. It is available both orally and as a nasal spray. Calcitonin shows a preservation of bone mass in the lumbar spine after the first year of steroid therapy when compared to placebo, but no effect was made at the femoral neck. It is suggested that more research is needed to conclude that calcitonin is effective in preventing fractures in steroid-induced osteoporosis.

A prescribed supplement that has been utilized in osteoporosis treatment is fluoride. Fluoride is known to stimulate bone formation. Fluoride should be taken with calcium. A review of the literature revealed no evidence to support that the use of fluoride prevented vertebral fractures but did show an ability to increase bone mass density at the lumbar spine.

A relatively new class of drugs used to combat osteoporosis and bone loss are skeletal anabolics. Skeletal anabolics stimulate bone formulation, produce large increases in bone mineral density, improve bone quality, and reduce bone fractures (Broyles, Reiss, & Evans, 2007).

Exercise, Physical, and Occupational Therapy

Long established as a preventive and therapeutic measure, weight-bearing exercise is a simple and low-cost treatment in the fight against osteoporosis.

Walking is the easiest therapy. Prescribed, formal exercise with the supervision of a physical therapist can be beneficial and prove to be a motivator for some. Should assistive devices be needed, an occupational therapist can be consulted. Exercises of all types (aerobics, weight-bearing, and resistance training) are effective in increasing bone mineral density (BMD) of the spine in postmenopausal women. Walking is also shown to be effective in increasing BMD in the hip.

Health Care Resources

Many local resources are available to assist patients and their families in learning about osteoporosis and its treatment. Most primary care providers (physicians and nurse practitioners) can provide good basic information. A useful source of information is a registered dietitian. As calcium supplementation is often the key in prevention of bone loss, dietitians can offer a myriad of alternatives to assist in providing the supplementation. In addition, there are also many resources available on the World Wide Web.

Surgery

See osteoarthritis for applicable surgical procedures related to fractures associated with osteoporosis.

Patient and Family Teaching

Prevention is the focus of much of the teaching associated with osteoporosis. Teaching prevention needs to start early in life to promote good nutrition habits. Family members will benefit from education and can assist the patient in applying their new found knowledge. Focuses of teaching will be on dietary needs and changes and physical activity. Handouts that a patient and family member can take home with them are useful to reinforce the messages the nurse is delivering.

When the diagnosis is confirmed, teaching should be given about the disease process, dietary needs and changes, physical activity, and any medication information that is necessary. Sedlak and Donheny (2002) add that instructions on fracture and falls prevention and pain management are needed. It is often helpful to give this abundance of information a little at a time. Information overload is always a concern. The health care worker should schedule time with the patient more than once to provide all information needed. Collaborative instruction from the physician, nurse, physical therapist, and a dietitian often assists in helping the patient get a well-rounded perspective of the disease process.

Evaluation of Outcomes

Management of osteoporosis is a lifelong process. Prevention of further bone loss is vital to prevent the sequela of fractures. Disease progression or regression can be monitored through BMD scans and biochemical markers of bone turnover found in the urine.

Fractures are the most frequent and serious complication of osteoporosis. Other problems can include weakness and fatigue from pain, kyphosis, and a risk for falls.

OSTEOMALACIA

Osteomalacia is a metabolic disease that causes poor and delayed mineralization of the bone cells in mature bones (Crowther & McCance, 2004).

Epidemiology

Fortunately, osteomalacia is rare in the United States and Western Europe. Osteomalacia is a significant problem in Great Britain, Ethiopia, Pakistan, Iran, and India. In the United States, osteomalacia secondary to vitamin D deficiency can be seen in the elderly, in premature infants with low birth weights, and in vegetarians on a strict macrobiotic diet (Crowther & McCance, 2004).

Etiology

The main cause of osteomalacia is a vitamin D deficiency. Risk factors for this deficiency include a diet deficient in vitamin D; low endogenous production of vitamin D (lack of sunlight exposure); malabsorption; renal tubule disease; and anticonvulsant therapy. Liver disease interferes with metabolism of vitamin D to its more active form, and diseases of the pancreas and biliary system cause a deficiency of bile salts needed for normal absorption of vitamin D (Crowther & McCance, 2004).

Pathophysiology

Bone cell mineralization requires adequate levels of calcium and phosphate. Vitamin D regulates the absorption of calcium ions from the intestine. Lack of vitamin D interrupts the absorption of calcium. The low calcium levels lead to the stimulation of parathyroid secretion. Although calcium levels increase, it also stimulates an increase in renal clearance of phosphate. With the ever-decreasing phosphate levels, bone cell mineralization cannot occur (Crowther & McCance, 2004).

Assessment with Clinical Manifestations

The patient generally presents with a history of generalized skeletal pain and tenderness without a history of injury. The site in which the most frequent complaint of pain is experienced is in the hips. The patient may report a reluctance to ambulate. Other complaints include low back pain, pain in the ribs, feet, and other areas. The patient will present with a waddling gait. When obtaining all history information, the provider should be sure to obtain a diet history, a medical history, and obtain a list of medications.

Diagnostic Tests

Blood tests that are obtained to assist in diagnosis are as follows: Serum calcium, phosphate, alkaline phosphatase, parathyroid hormone, 25-hydroxy vitamin D, as well as BUN and creatinine (Daniels, 2003).

Bone densitometry and X-rays will be performed to examine the extent of the disease. In adults with sporadic onset hypophosphatemia, hyperphosphatemia, or low serum 1, 25 hydroxy D levels, a tumor may be suspected, and an MRI of the whole body is recommended (Daniels, 2003).

Nursing Diagnoses

Based on the information gathered, examples of nursing diagnoses for the patient with osteomalacia may include the following:
- Impaired physical mobility related to osteomalacia.
- Risk for impaired skin integrity related to compromised tissue perfusion.
- Acute pain as related to osteomalacia.

Planning and Implementation

The goals of therapy are to prevent osteomalacia and to prevent further bone loss in already established disease.

Nutrition

Milk fortified with vitamin D is readily available in the United States. An 8-ounce glass of milk provides 25 percent of the recommended daily allowance (RDA) of vitamin D and 50 percent of the RDA for calcium.

Pharmacology

To prevent a vitamin D deficiency, sunlight exposure and vitamin D supplementation are recommended. The RDA of vitamin D is 10 g (400 international units) per day. Patients with low sunlight exposure, the RDA is 1,000 international units per day. Patients taking phenytoin (Dilantin), the RDA for prophylactic treatment is 50,000 international units orally every two to four weeks (Fitzgerald, 2004). Vitamin D is available OTC or by prescription.

For established osteomalacia, the deficiency is treated with ergocalciferol (D$_2$) 50,000 international units orally one or two times per week for 6 to 12 months, then 1,000 international units per day. For malabsorption problems the dose is 25,000 to 100,000 international units per day. In addition, the patients will receive calcium citrate (0.4 to 0.6 g of elemental calcium) or calcium carbonate (1 to 1.5 g of elemental calcium) per day (Fitzgerald, 2004).

For osteomalacia secondary to hypophosphatemia, aluminum-containing antacids are discontinued. Patients with renal tubule acidosis are given bicarbonate therapy. For idiopathic hypophosphatemia or hyperphosphatemia, oral phosphate supplements are used on an ongoing basis with calcitriol (Rocaltrol) given to combat decreased calcium absorption caused by the oral phosphate (Fitzgerald, 2004).

Patient and Family Teaching

Teaching about the disease itself will need to be initiated. Medication and nutrition education will focus on prevention with vitamin D and sunlight exposure or correction of deficiencies or other causes of the osteomalacia. Proper dosage and schedule will be the focal points for the medication teaching. For sunlight exposure, encourage the use of sunblock, explaining that the sunblock will not stop the necessary exposure to stimulate vitamin D production.

Evaluation of Outcomes

Fortunately, osteomalacia is treatable, and therefore the prognosis for patients who suffer from osteomalacia is good. Complications can include fractures and bone growth deformities.

Financial Outcomes

Fortunately the prevention and treatment of osteomalacia is relatively inexpensive, especially if caused by a dietary deficiency. Expenses can be high if the deficiency is secondary to other disease processes (e.g., renal tubule disease with dialysis required).

PAGET'S DISEASE

Paget's disease is the second most common bone disease after osteoporosis in the United States. It often goes undiagnosed until the disease is in the advanced stages. It is difficult to diagnosis, because the pain associated with Paget's disease is similar to arthritis. Paget's disease is a chronic bone disorder with no definitive cure. However, an early diagnosis along with effective treatment can lessen the impact of the disease and decrease the complications associated with Paget's disease (The Paget Foundation, 2005).

Epidemiology

Paget's disease is rare before the age of 40 and increases with age with an incidence of 1.5 to 8 percent of the population over the age of 50. It affects men slightly more than women. It is more commonly seen in people of Anglo-Saxon ancestry, and it is rarely seen in people of Asian, Indian, and Scandinavian descent (The Paget Foundation, 2005). Overall, the incidence of Paget's disease has been declining. The reason for this is unknown.

Etiology

The cause of Paget's disease remains unknown. However, Paget's disease tends to run in families and several genes have been linked to the disorder, but no specific abnormality can explain Paget's disease. Paramyxovirus has also been linked to the etiology of Paget's disease, but once again there is a lack of conclusive evidence (Binder, 2003).

Pathophysiology

Paget's disease begins with an increase in bone absorption. To compensate for this, bone formation increases along with bone remodeling. This newly formed bone is highly vascular and weak, which leads to deformity and fractures. The areas most often affected are the long bones, pelvis, lumbar vertebrae, and skull (Maher, Salmond, & Pellino, 2002).

Assessment with Clinical Manifestations

Assessment should begin with a thorough history including family incidence of Paget's disease and previous fractures. Patients with Paget's disease are often asymptomatic. For patients who experience symptoms, the most common symptom is pain in the hip and pelvis. The pain is often described as a deep aching that worsens with weight bearing. The patient may also have deficits in hearing, vision, swallowing, speech, movement of eye and facial muscles, and balance (Maher, Salmond, & Pellino, 2002).

Physical examination begins with inspection of the skeleton for deformities. Bowing of the long bones of the arms and legs is a common finding. Bowing of the tibia can cause increased pain to the knee and ankle and an increased risk of fracture. The skull is often enlarged with the bone becoming soft and thick. In more advanced cases, the spine may also show kyphosis or scoliosis. Palpation of the skin over areas of Pagetic bone may reveal areas that are warm to touch because of the increased blood flow to the newly formed bone (Maher, Salmond, & Pellino, 2002).

Diagnostic Tests

An increase in serum alkaline phosphatase (ALP) is often the first indicator that the patient's symptoms are associated with Paget's disease and not arthritis. Normal serum ALP is 30 to 115 international units/L. A slightly higher level is often found in a patient with a healing fracture. However, values two to three times the normal amount indicates Paget's disease. ALP is an enzyme produced by bone, liver, and the intestines. It can further be broken down into isoenzymes to pinpoint the origin of the enzyme. An increase in the bone-specific ALP (bAP) indicates an increase in bone formation. There are also several markers for bone formation, turnover, and reabsorption that can be detected in the urine. These include calcium, hydroxyproline, N-telopeptide, and deoxypyridinolines (The Paget Foundation, 2005). However, these are less sensitive than serum bAP.

X-rays and a bone scan are the two diagnostic studies used in the diagnosis on Paget's disease. Bones affected by Paget's disease have characteristic features that show well on X-ray. Early in the disease osteolytic lesions are observed in the long bones and the skull. As the disease progresses, the bones become enlarged with coarse and irregular borders (Maher, Salmond, & Pellino, 2002). A radioactive bone scan is a more sensitive diagnostic tool. A radioactive bisphosphonate is injected intravenously. This substance collects in areas of bone where there is an increase in blood flow and bone formation. This test is used to determine the full extent of the disease.

Nursing Diagnoses

Based on the information gathered, examples of nursing diagnoses in the patient with Paget's disease may include:
- Acute pain.
- Chronic pain.
- Impaired physical mobility.
- Activity intolerance.
- Bathing/hygiene self-care deficit.
- Dressing/grooming self-care deficit.

In addition, based on information gathered, examples of nursing diagnoses for the patient with Paget's disease may include the following shown in Table 59-3. This table shows additional nursing diagnoses, NIC, and NOC classifications that may be applicable for patients with Paget's disease.

Planning and Implementation

The three major areas of focus for a patient diagnosed with Paget's disease are symptom management, limiting disability, and complication prevention. In the past only patients with symptoms were treated. Now, the standard is to treat all patients with active disease including asymptomatic patients. Active disease is defined as ALP level twice the upper limit of normal (Rakel & Bope, 2003). Treatment of Paget's disease may not correct existing damage to hearing, deformities to bone, or osteoarthritis caused by the disease. The goal is to prevent any further complications by restoring the normal pattern of new bone formation. Treatment of Paget's disease is comprised of four main options that are used in conjunction with each other. These options are physical therapy, pharmacological therapy, analgesics, and surgery.

Also, although Paget's disease is an incurable disease, there are few life-threatening complications. The prescribed treatment is usually effective in decreasing pain and slowing the progression of the disease. Fractures usually develop in the weight-bearing portion of long bones and may start out as stress fractures. Neurological complications are also seen because of the pagetic bone pressing on nerves and include hearing loss, changes in vision, impairment of the eye and facial muscles, and problems with swallowing, speech, and

TABLE 59-3	Nursing Diagnoses, NIC, and NOC Classifications for Paget's Disease	
NURSING DIAGNOSIS	**NURSING INTERVENTION CLASSIFICATIONS (NIC)**	**NURSING OUTCOMES CLASSIFICATIONS (NOC)**
Potential injury	Fall prevention	Fall prevention behavior
	Environment management	
Fear related to potential injury	Anxiety reduction	Fear self-control
	Coping enhancement	
	Security enhancement	

balance (Maher, et al., 2002). Other neurological complications may include hydrocephalus, radicular neuropathies, and spinal stenosis.

The pagetic bone is highly vascularized and prone to bleeding. Because of this there is a potential complication of hemorrhage and an increase in blood loss during bone surgery. Bisphosphonates may be given prior to surgery to reduce the bleeding from the operative bone during the surgery (Rakel & Bope, 2003).

Another potential complication of Paget's disease is hypercalcemia. It is imperative that the patient continues with weight-bearing exercises to keep the bones strong. Any amount of prolonged bed rest, especially after surgery, will increase bone demineralization and hypercalcemia. Hypercalcemia can contribute to hypertension, weakness, urinary lithiasis, or mild bowel disturbances (Rakel & Bope, 2003).

Pharmacology

Pharmacological therapy is a major component of the treatment plan. Antiresorptive agents inhibit osteoclastic activity therefore suppressing bone turnover. Calcitonin was the first osteoclastic inhibitor to be used in the treatment of Paget's disease. It is a hormone that binds to the osteoclast receptor site and inhibits bone resorption and turnover. It is given as a subcutaneous injection, and it is expensive. Because of these two disadvantages, this treatment is not widely used any more unless the patient is unable to tolerate other medications. Bisphosphonates are other types of antiresorptive agents used to slow the progression of Paget's disease and to treat the bone pain associated with the disease. They can also be used prior to surgery to reduce the bleeding from the bone that is being repaired (Rakel & Bope, 2003). The disadvantage of these medications is that they must be taken orally on waking with a full glass of water on an empty stomach, and the patient must stay upright for 30 minutes after taking the medication. These instructions must be followed to reduce the risk of reflux that may cause esophagitis. Food, milk, and other dairy products prevent the absorption of this drug; therefore, the patient must take the medication on an empty stomach. Hypocalcemia is a potential side effect; therefore the patient should be taking oral calcium and vitamin D. Refer to Table 59-4 for a list of bisphosphonates.

Exercise, Physical, and Occupational Therapy

Physical therapy is another vital component in the treatment of Paget's disease. The focus of physical therapy is to improve muscle strength and to promote mobility by encouraging weight-bearing exercises, which may improve bone strength. Occupational therapy along with physical therapy may help the patient become more functional and independent by providing advice on assistive devices used for activities of daily living and for walking aids, heels lifts, and corsets (Maher, Salmond, & Pellino, 2002). Physical therapy may also help control chronic pain.

Surgery

Surgery may be a necessary treatment option for some patients. Surgery may include repair of a pathological fracture, realignment of the knee to decrease pain, total joint arthroplasty for arthritic changes from the disease process. It is important to mobilize the patient as soon as possible and to avoid bed rest. Periods of immobilization can lead to bone demineralization and hypercalcemia, which can further increase the patient's risk of pathological fractures (Rakel & Bope, 2003).

Patient and Family Teaching

Patient and family teaching begins with education regarding the disease process and support for the patient and family as they cope with the impact the disease may have on the patient's quality of life. Another important component

TABLE 59-4	Bisphosphonates used with Paget's Disease	
DRUG	**DOSE**	**SPECIAL INSTRUCTIONS**
Etidronate (Didronel)	200–400 mg once daily for six months; 400 mg dose is preferred	Available in oral form Must be taken with six to eight ounces of water on an empty stomach No food, beverages, or other medication two hours before or after dose Treatment should not exceed six months Repeat courses can be given after a three to six month rest period
Pamidronate (Aredia)	30 mg intravenously over four hours for three consecutive days	Available in IV form only May be readministered as needed
Alendronate (Fosamax)	40 mg once daily for six months	Available in oral form Must be taken on an empty stomach, with six to eight ounces of water, in the morning. No food, beverages, or other medication for 30 minutes after dose. Do not lie down for at least 30 minutes after taking dose.
Tiludronate (Skelid)	400 mg once daily for three months	Available in oral form Must be taken on an empty stomach with six to eight ounces of water. It may be taken any time during the day, as long as there is no food, beverage, or other medication taken two hours before or after the dose.
Risedronate (Actonel)	30 mg once daily for two months	Available in oral form Must be taken on an empty stomach, with six to eight ounces of water. No food, beverages, or other medication for 30 minutes after dose. Do not lie down for at least 30 minutes after taking dose.

Adapted from Broyles, B. E., Reiss, B. S., & Evans, M. E. (2007). Pharmacological aspects of nursing care (7th ed.). New York: Thomson Delmar Learning.

of teaching is medication administration. The patient needs to know the potential side effects of the prescribed medications and the correct way to take these medications to decrease the risk of these side effects. Another area of needed information is in regard to pain management. Simple strategies like anti-inflammatory drugs and nonnarcotic analgesics may be all that are needed to reduce the patient's bone pain (Rakel, & Bope, 2003). Positioning and following the treatment modalities may also decreased the patient's pain.

Evaluation of Outcomes

Generally Paget's disease has a good prognosis, if recommended treatment is followed. Potential outcomes for each of the example nursing diagnoses for the patient with Piaget's disease are:

- Acute pain: The patient's pain should be adequately controlled, as assessed by the patient on scale of 1 to 10.

- Chronic pain: The patient's pain should be adequately controlled, so that the patient is able to minimize disruptive effects for day-to-day living.
- Impaired physical mobility: The patient should demonstrate coordinated movement with active joint mobility. The patient should be able to perform self-care and manage activities of daily living. The patient should be able to demonstrate the proper way to transfer from bed to chair, chair to standing. The patient should be able to verbalize knowledge of prescribed activity level.
- Activity intolerance: The patient should be able to tolerate activity within normal limits and verbalize knowledge of endurance.
- Bathing/hygiene self-care deficit: The patient should demonstrate the ability to perform activities of daily living, bathing, toileting, and personal hygiene, using mobility aids if needed.
- Dressing/grooming self-care deficit: The patient should demonstrate the ability to dress.

OSTEOMYELITIS

Osteomyelitis is a serious infection of the bone that is often difficult to treat. Osteomyelitis can be categorized as acute or chronic, which occurs when the symptoms are present for longer than three months.

Epidemiology

Acute osteomyelitis occurs commonly in children under 13 (1 in 5,000) (Zorn, 2001). Forty percent of all cases occur in children under age 20, with 35 percent of cases occurring in adults over age 50. Chronic osteomyelitis is responsible for one to three percent of all hospital admissions and occurs after orthopaedic surgery from 0.5 to 1.5 percent of the time (Zorn, 2001). The most common site is the tibia, following an open fracture.

Etiology

Osteomyelitis can stem from an infection that has spread through the blood to the site of infection (site varies with the individual). It can also be caused by a soft tissue infection that spreads to the bone. It is also associated with patients who have diabetes or vascular problems. With these patients the site of infection is often the foot or ankle (Hellman & Stone, 2004).

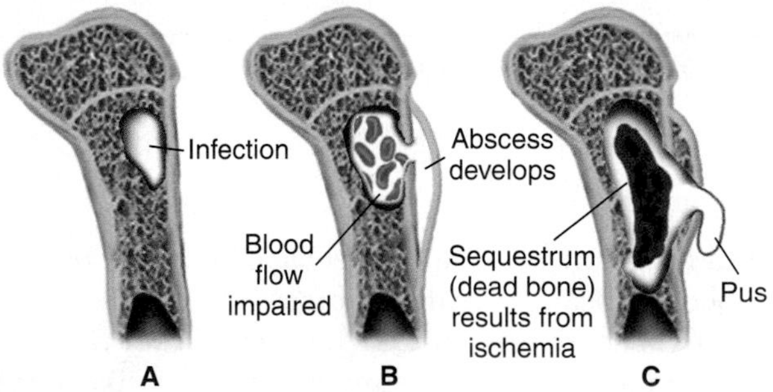

Figure 59-6 Pathology and progression of osteomyelitis: A. Osteomyelitis, B. Without early treatment, an abscess forms, C. Bone dies (sequestrum) and pus forms.

Pathophysiology

The infection is spread through the bloodstream to the medullary canal. Cellulitis develops in the bone marrow. As the infection develops, bacteria and white blood cells cause exudate to form and pressure increases within the medullary canal. The infection continues to invade the inner layers of the bone until it spreads to the periosteum leading to necrosis and devascularization of the cortex of the bone (Zorn, 2001) (Figure 59-6).

Assessment with Clinical Manifestations

In acute osteomyelitis the patient will have manifestations of acute infection. There may be a report of recent acute infection, puncture wound, mild trauma, or obvious fracture. Adults may present with history of diabetes, vascular insufficiency, or other process that leads to a compromised immune system.

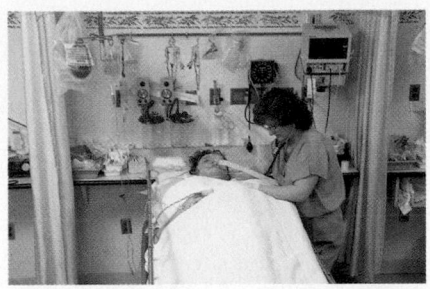

Figure 59-7 Acute osteomyelitis has caused an uncontrolled infectious process in this patient is in an ICU.

Children present with a variety of symptoms. Infants will present with symptoms that range from irritability to pseudoparalysis or signs of sepsis. Most children will complain of localized pain. Younger children may refuse to use the affected extremity.

Chronic osteomyelitis patients will present with mild systemic symptoms, have periods of remissions and exacerbations, pain (from mild to severe), and soft tissue abscesses and draining wounds may occur. There will generally be a history of surgery or trauma to the affected extremity or site. There may be a previous history of acute osteomyelitis, and the patient may have continued or intermittent symptoms. These patients may also have histories of immune system compromise. Fever is common with acute osteomyelitis but not with the chronic form of the infection.

Complications of osteomyelitis include loss of function of the joint above or below the infection, leg-length discrepancies or deformities, and renal insufficiency or hearing loss related to nephrotoxic or ototoxic antibiotics (Figure 59-7).

Diagnostic Tests

There are a variety of diagnostic tests for both acute and chronic osteomyelitis. These diagnostics are shown in Box 59-4.

Nursing Diagnoses

Based on the informative gathered, examples of nursing diagnoses for the patient with osteomyelitis may include the following:
- Acute or chronic pain due to the osteomyelitis.
- Fear due to the diagnosis of osteomyelitis.
- Impaired physical mobility due to the osteomyelitis.
- Risk for impaired skin integrity related to compromised tissue perfusion.
- Deficient knowledge related to self-care and risk prevention.

Planning and Implementation

Management goals are to eliminate the infection and prevent complications.

BOX 59-4

DIAGNOSTIC TESTING FOR OSTEOMYELITIS

Acute Osteomyelitis

- X-rays will not show changes until 10 to 14 days after the infection occurs
- Sedimentation rate and white blood cells will be elevated
- Blood cultures are positive in about half of the samples
- Bone scans will be positive in the area of the infection
- Bone wound cultures will need to be taken to identify the microorganism present

Chronic Osteomyelitis

- X-rays will show bone and soft tissue changes
- Sedimentation rate will be mildly to moderately elevated
- May see a minimal elevation of white blood count and mild anemia
- C-reactive protein will be elevated
- CT scans will show changes in the bone and can show pockets of exudates
- Wound cultures will need to be take

Pharmacology

Traditional pharmacological therapy is for four to six weeks of IV antibiotic therapy based on the results of wound cultures for acute osteomyelitis. Chronic osteomyelitis is treated with six to eight weeks of oral antibiotic therapy, based on the wound culture results (Hellman & Stone, 2004).

Surgery

Localized wound debridement will be necessary to rid the site of the necrotic bone.

Patient and Family Teaching

Teaching will be focused on the disease process and management.

Evaluation of Outcomes

Potential patient outcomes for each of the example nursing diagnoses for the patient with osteomyelitis are:

- Acute or chronic pain due to the osteomyelitis. The patient should verbalize an adequate relief of pain along with the ability to realistically cope with the pain if it is not completely relieved.
- Fear due to the diagnosis of osteomyelitis. The patient should manifest positive coping behaviors and verbalize a reduction in the amount of fear of the having this disease.
- Impaired physical mobility due to the osteomyelitis. The patient should perform physical activity independently or with assistive devices as needed. In addition, the patient should be free of complications of immobility, as evidenced by intact skin, absence of thrombophlebitis, and normal bowel patterns.
- Risk for impaired skin integrity related to compromised tissue perfusion. The condition of the skin should be improved as evidenced by decreased redness, swelling, and pain.
- Deficient knowledge related to self-care and risk prevention. The patient should demonstrate motivation to learn, identify perceived learning needs, and verbalize an understanding of desired content.

TUMORS OF THE MUSCULOSKELETAL SYSTEM

Tumors of the musculoskeletal system can arise in any of the structures that make up this system. They are classified as either benign or malignant and are found in children and adults. A malignant neoplasm of the musculoskeletal system is called a **sarcoma**. According to the American Cancer Society, in 2005 there will be an estimated 11,990 newly diagnosed cases of cancer of the bones, joints, and soft tissues. The estimated number of deaths for musculoskeletal cancers in 2005 is 4,700.

Primary Bony and Soft Tissue Tumors

Primary bone cancers are rare. There are an estimated 2,500 new case of primary bone cancer each year. Primary bone cancers are generally considered pediatric cancers. Most cases are diagnosed between the ages of 10 and 25. **Osteosarcoma** is the most common type of primary bone cancer. Other primary bony tumors include **Ewing's sarcoma** (a diffuse endothelioma or endothelial myeloma forming a fusiform swelling on a long bone) and **chondrosarcoma** (cartilaginous sarcoma). These tumors are aggressive and tend to recur if not completely excised. They also tend to metastasize to the lungs early in the disease process especially if they are high-grade tumors.

Malignant soft tissue tumors arise from or resemble connective tissues of the body. These tissues include muscle, fat, cartilage, fibrous tissue, **tendosynovial** tissue, vessels, and peripheral nerves. Most soft tissue malignancies are considered intermediate in nature, meaning that they tend to be locally aggressive but have a low-to-moderate tendency to metastasize to distant areas. These primary soft tissue tumors occur twice as often as primary bone sarcomas and are seen more often in men than in women. They are seen in the lower extremity 45 percent of the time and the upper extremity 15 percent of the time. They are seen less often in the head and neck, retroperitoneum, abdomen, chest wall, and in the connective tissue of organs. Soft tissue sarcomas are typically seen in the older adult with the exception of rhabdomyosarcoma, which is typically seen in children and young adults.

Epidemiology

Bony sarcomas are considered pediatric cancers. They are usually diagnosed in people ages 10 to 25 years. Soft tissue sarcomas usually occur in adults over the age of 55 (Maher, et al., 2001). Sarcomas appear in males slightly more often than females. There is a second peak of osteosarcoma in the seventh decade, which is most likely due with osteosarcomas association with Paget's disease. Secondary chondrosarcomas can also appear later in life from benign cartilage lesions.

Etiology

The exact cause of primary sarcomas is not known, and there are no definitive risk factors. Factors that may play a role in the development of sarcomas are previous high-dose irradiation, exposure to chemicals, prior treatment with chemotherapy drugs, immunosuppression, preexisting bone conditions (Paget's disease), and skeletal maldevelopment. Environmental factors, such as trauma or a past injury, have also been associated with the development of primary sarcomas (Maher, et al., 2002).

Pathophysiology

As the sarcoma grows, it forms a ball-like mass that penetrates the bony cortex (Wittig, et al., 2002). High-grade tumors are aggressive and quickly metastasize to the lung. Once this occurs, the prognosis worsens.

Assessment with Clinical Manifestations

Clinical symptoms of a bony sarcoma include a dull, aching pain that worsens at night. Often, the pain may be associated with a prior injury. Other symptoms may include swelling, localized enlargement of the extremity, fever, night sweats, and occasionally, pathological fracture. In early stages of soft tissue sarcomas there are often no symptoms. Symptoms start to appear once the tumor has grown enough to put pressure on surrounding structures, such as nerves and muscles causing pain.

During the physical examination a mass may be visible. It may be firm and warm to the touch. It can be painless, or the patient may have some localized tenderness around the mass. Range of motion of the adjacent joints may be compromised. The patient may also have a limp or a decrease in muscle strength if the tumor is located in the lower extremity. It is important to note the size of the mass and to compare it to the bilateral extremity or side.

Diagnostic Tests

The definitive diagnostic test for a sarcoma is a biopsy. In most cases a percutaneous needle biopsy is recommended. It is minimally invasive, associated with lower risk of infection, contamination, and postbiopsy fractures (Wittig, et al., 2002). In osteosarcoma a plain film X-ray will show a destructive lesion with a mixture of osteolytic and osteoblastic areas. Staging of the tumor is important in planning course of treatment. MRI and computed tomography (CT) scans are used to determine the local extent of the disease. Plain film X-rays, CT scans of the chest, and a bone scan are used to check for metastases to the lungs and other bone. A bone marrow aspirate is also used to check for metastasis in the bone marrow.

Blood tests may reveal an elevation in serum lactate dehydrogenase and ALP levels due to the increase in bone formation and cell turnover. This elevation is seen in about 50 percent of patients, so it is not useful in the diagnosis of sarcoma. However, it has been linked to a poorer prognosis.

Nursing Diagnoses

Based on the informative gathered, examples of nursing diagnoses for the patient with sarcomas may include the following:
- Acute or chronic pain due to the sarcoma.
- Fear due to the diagnosis of sarcoma.
- Impaired physical mobility due to the sarcoma.
- Risk for impaired skin integrity related to compromised tissue perfusion.
- Deficient knowledge related to self-care and risk prevention.

Planning and Implementation

The overall goal of treatment of sarcoma is to destroy or remove the tumor from the primary site and to treat any metastatic lesions. Prior to 1970, treatment of choice for sarcoma was amputation. For Ewing's sarcoma the treatment varied from other sarcomas because of the tumor's response to radiation therapy. However, sarcomas still had an overall mortality rate of 70 to 80 percent because of metastases to the lung. With the improvement in chemotherapy, radiotherapy, and surgical techniques, amputation is only seen in advanced stages of the disease, and the survival rate is 70 percent. Limb-sparing surgery is the standard of care with chemotherapy and radiation if tumor is radiation sensitive, before and after surgery to shrink the tumor and to decrease the risk of the tumor returning or metastasis occurring. Amputations are only necessary in about 5 percent of cases. Some of the contraindications for limb-sparing surgery include inability to achieve wide surgical margins, invasion of major neurovascular structures, patients with extensive skin involvement, pathological fractures, and sepsis (Hosalkar & Dormans, 2004).

The current treatment of osteosarcoma involves a course of chemotherapy before surgery. This shrinks the size of the tumor and kills the microscopic metastases before they have a chance to multiply. A second round of chemotherapy is administered to the patient after surgery to ensure that any cells left behind are destroyed. Surgery may not always be a viable option if the location of the tumor is axial (involving spine or pelvis) or if the surgery will result in an amputation. In these cases, radiotherapy for local control may be another option for some patients who respond to chemotherapy.

Complications of bony sarcoma include weakened bone and pathological fractures. Other complications are related to reconstructive surgery and can include prosthetic loosening, infection, and mechanical failure (Wittig, et al., 2002). Infection can be a serious complication if it delays chemotherapy or radiation treatment. Delaying adjuvant therapy could increase the patient's risk of metastasis and local recurrence. Another complication for some patients who have undergone a resection involving the lymph system is lymphedema. Lymphedema may also be a complication of radiation therapy.

Pharmacology
Table 59-5 lists common chemotherapy drugs used to treat sarcoma.

Exercise, Physical, and Occupational Therapy
Therapy following a limb-sparing surgery or an amputation is crucial in allowing the patient to obtain the highest level of function possible and independence in daily activities. The rehabilitation program is initiated by the physical and occupational therapist. However, the nurse plays an important role by reinforcing the program and ensuring the patient is adequately

TABLE 59-5 **Common Chemotherapy Drugs Used in Treatment of Sarcoma**

CLASSIFICATION AND DRUG NAME	ACTION	NURSING IMPLICATIONS
Methotrexate	A folate antimetabolite that inhibits enzyme production for DNA synthesis, leading to strand breaks or premature chain termination	Follow with leucovorin and calcium rescue
		Mucositis is common, mouth care is needed
		Photosensitivity precautions needed
		Patient to avoid multivitamins that contain folic acid
Cisplatin	Causes cross-linkage and breaks in the DNA helix strand, thereby inhibiting DNA replication	Hold drug if serum creatinine is greater than 1.5 mg/dL to prevent renal damage.
Dacarbazine	Causes cross-linkage and breaks in the DNA helix strand, thereby inhibiting DNA replication	Flu-like syndrome may occur up to seven days after drug administration
		Dacarbazine can cause severe pain and burning at injection site.
Ifosfamide	Causes cross-linkage and breaks in the DNA helix strand, thereby inhibiting DNA replication	Always administer Ifosfamide with Mesna to prevent hemorrhagic cystitis.
Dactinomycin	Binds with DNA inhibiting DNA and RNA	Dactinomycin is a vesicant.
Doxorubicin	Binds with DNA inhibiting DNA and RNA	Doxorubicin is a vesicant.
Vincristine	Prevents formation of mitotic spindles, preventing cell division	Cardiotoxicity, check baseline ejection fraction.
		May cause flare reaction.
		Vincristine is a vesicant.
		Assess for peripheral neuropathy
		Constipation is a common side effect

Adapted from Broyles, B. E., Reiss, B. S., & Evans, M. E. (2007). Pharmacological aspects of nursing care (7th ed.). New York: Thomson Delmar Learning.

medicated for pain prior to therapy to maximize the patient's participation during the therapy session.

Alternative Therapy

Alternative and complementary therapy are becoming more popular in the treatment of cancer. Some therapies have shown to increase quality of life, but others have been shown to do harm or interfere with the traditional medical regimen. Nutrition and dietary supplements are becoming more commonplace. The goal of these therapies may be to strengthen the immune system, increase energy, promote cell health, or ease the side effects associated with chemotherapy or radiation therapy. Other complementary or alternative therapy may be used to treat pain, such as massage or acupuncture. It is important for the nurse to encourage the patient to discuss openly other therapy the patient is using and to document these on the medical record.

Patient and Family Teaching

Patient and family teaching starts with the initial diagnosis of the sarcoma. The patient and family may be overwhelmed with all of the new information related to the diagnosis and treatment options. After the physician initially speaks with the family and patient regarding the diagnosis, the nurse should be available to explain things with simpler terms, answer questions, or just to offer support. This education with the patient and family is ongoing and continuous. The patient and family may need to hear the information more than once and may need to have it presented in different ways using printed material, pictures, or audiovisual modalities.

Evaluation of Outcomes

After the initial treatment phase the patient will need to continue follow-up with the orthopedic or medical oncologist. Radiographic tests will be ordered on a routine basis to monitor for local recurrence and metastatic disease.

Metastatic Tumors

Metastatic tumors of the bone are detrimental consequences of cancer. Metastatic tumors greatly affect the patient's quality of life and increase morbidity (Wilfred & Muttarak, 2002). They are more commonly seen than primary bone sarcomas.

Epidemiology

The three most common sites of metastases in order of occurrence are the lung, liver, and bone (Reich, 2003). The primary cancers that most frequently metastasize to the bone are breast, prostate, kidney, thyroid, and lung. Ninety percent of metastatic bone lesions are found on the vertebrae, pelvis, proximal parts of the femur, ribs, proximal part of the humerus, and skull.

Pathophysiology

Malignant tumor cells tend to break off from the primary site and travel through the bloodstream or through the lymphatic system to other areas. The tumor can also invade nearby tissues as the tumor grows beyond the normal limits of the primary site. Metastatic bone lesions can be categorized into three different categories: osteolytic, osteoblastic, and mixed. Osteolytic lesions occur in patients with multiple myeloma due to the osteoclastic activity caused by excessive proteins. Osteoblastic lesions are areas where new bone has grown over existing bone and are seen in patients with prostate cancer. The last type of lesion is called mixed osteoblastic and osteolytic and are seen most often in patients with breast cancer.

Assessment with Clinical Manifestations

The number one symptom of bone metastases is pain. The pain is usually described as a dull, aching pain that increases at night and with weight bearing. Other complications that can be caused by metastatic bone disease include hypercalcemia, myelosuppression, pathological fractures, and spinal cord compression (Reich, 2003).

Diagnostic Tests

Diagnostic testing begins with X-rays; however, X-rays can only detect large lesions. Therefore, skeletal scintigraphy (bone scan) is the standard in staging and monitoring bone metastases. The disadvantage of a bone scan is that while it is sensitive in detecting bone metastases, it is unable to provide information regarding the type of lesion (Wilfred & Muttarak, 2002). Plain film radiography is the standard in characterizing the type of lesion seen on bone scan and in determining the response of the bone. Positron emission tomography (PET) scan is another option in detecting and staging bone metastases.

However, it is unclear if the sensitivity of PET scan is comparable to the bone scan (Folgelman, Cook, Israel, & Van der Wall, 2005).

Nursing Diagnoses

Based on the informative gathered, examples of nursing diagnoses for the patient with bone metastases may include the following:

- Acute or chronic pain due to the bone metastases.
- Fear due to the diagnosis of bone metastases.
- Impaired physical mobility due to the bone metastases.
- Risk for impaired skin integrity related to compromised tissue perfusion.
- Deficient knowledge related to self-care and risk prevention.

Planning and Implementation

The management goals of treatment for metastatic bone disease are pain control, prevention of complications, and remission through a multimodal approach. Therapy, much like those for primary bone tumors, includes pain medication, hormone therapy, chemotherapy, surgery, radiation therapy, and the use of bisphosphonates.

Radiotherapy is the first treatment used for a bone lesion. An external beam of radiation is used to kill the tumor cells directly at the site of the lesion. In a review of 43 studies, radiotherapy has been shown to be clearly effective in providing pain relief in patients with metastatic bone disease (Licata, 2005).

Bisphosphonates, however, have not been proven as effective in reducing pain associated with bone metastases. In a review of over 50 randomized controlled studies, the results show modest pain relief at best. Therefore, bisphosphonates are not used as first-line therapy for pain relief. Bisphosphonates may be used in the treatment of bone metastases to prevent complications, such as pathological fractures, and to prevent new osteolytic lesions (Licata, 2005).

Evaluation of Outcomes

Potential patient outcomes for each of the example nursing diagnoses for the patient with bone metastases are:

- Acute or chronic pain due to the bone metastases. The patient should verbalize an adequate relief of pain along with the ability to realistically cope with the pain if it is not completely relieved.
- Fear due to the diagnosis of bone metastases. The patient should manifest positive coping behaviors and verbalize a reduction in the amount of fear of the having this disease.
- Impaired physical mobility due to the bone metastases. The patient should perform physical activity independently or with assistive devices as needed. In addition, the patient should be free of complications of immobility, as evidenced by intact skin, absence of thrombophlebitis, and normal bowel patterns.
- Risk for impaired skin integrity related to compromised tissue perfusion. The condition of the skin should be improved as evidenced by decreased redness, swelling, and pain.
- Deficient knowledge related to self-care and risk prevention. The patient should demonstrate motivation to learn, identify perceived learning needs, and verbalize an understanding of desired content.

SPINAL DISORDERS

Spinal disorders are relatively common and require assistance from the health care team. The more common ones are scoliosis, kyphosis, lordosis, and spinal stenosis (Figure 59-8).

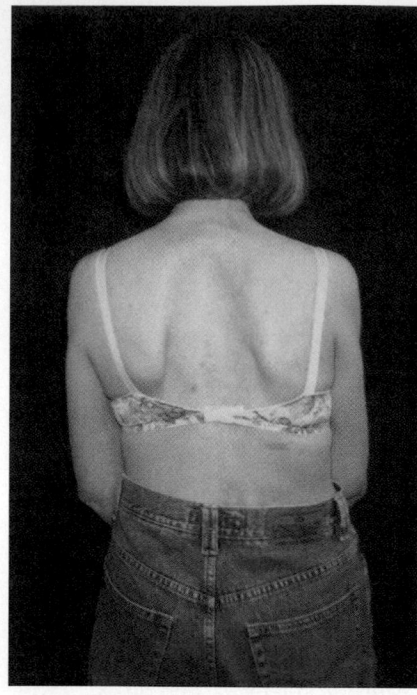

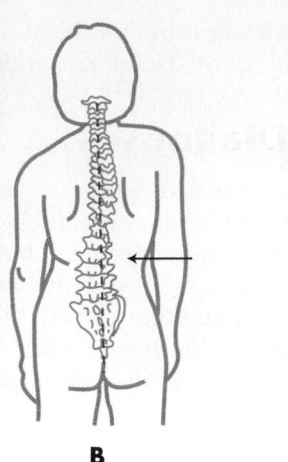
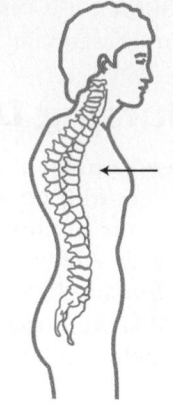
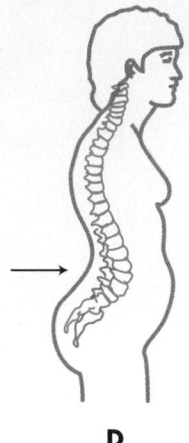
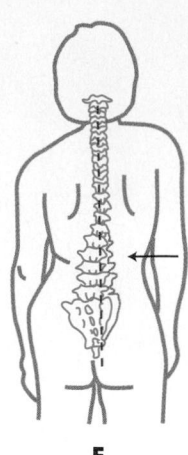

B C D E

Figure 59-8 Abnormalities of the spine: A. Scoliosis, B. Scoliosis, C. Kyphosis, D. Lordosis, and E. List.

Scoliosis

Scoliosis is defined as a spinal deformity that is characterized by a lateral curve, spinal rotation causing rib asymmetry, and thoracic **hypokyphosis** (less than normal curvature in the thoracic spine) (Hockenberry &Brown, 2003).

Epidemiology

An estimated 2 to 3 percent of 10 to 16 year-olds are affected by curvatures of 10 degrees or more.

Etiology

Scoliosis can be congenital or developmental during infancy or childhood. Most often it is detected early in adolescence. The cause of scoliosis is most often unknown but can be associated with a number of neuromuscular disorders.

Assessment with Clinical Manifestations

Scoliosis is seldom seen before the age of 10 and parents will be referred to a health care provider after a school screening; or they may notice uneven pant lengths or skirt hems (Hockenberry & Brown, 2003). Pain is usually not an issue until the deformity has progressed.

The physical assessment technique used in school screenings is known as the **Adams Bending Forward Test** (a test to assess for scoliosis). The patient, wearing only underwear, bends forward at the waist with both arms hanging toward the floor, palms together. Viewing the patient from behind, the health care worker observes the back for curvature by observing the symmetry of the shoulders, scapulae, flank shapes, hip heights, and pelvis. A **scoliometer** (an instrument for measuring curves, especially those in lateral curvature of the spine) can be used to measure the trunk rotation during the Adams Test (Figure 59-9). Authors do note that the reliability of these tests are questionable but do not make recommendations for other screening tools (Hockenberry & Brown, 2003; Slote, 2002).

Diagnostic Tests

Standing spinal X-rays are performed, and curvature is measured. The amount of curvature noted determines actual diagnosis and the degree of deformity. It will also help to determine the type of treatments recommended (Hockenberry & Brown, 2003).

Nursing Diagnoses

Based on the informative gathered, examples of nursing diagnoses for the patient with scoliosis may include the following:
- Acute or chronic pain due to the scoliosis.
- Fear due to the diagnosis of scoliosis.

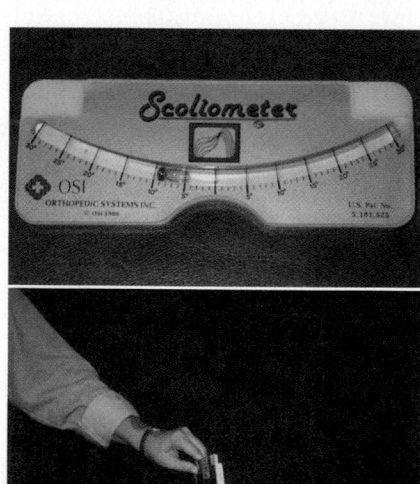

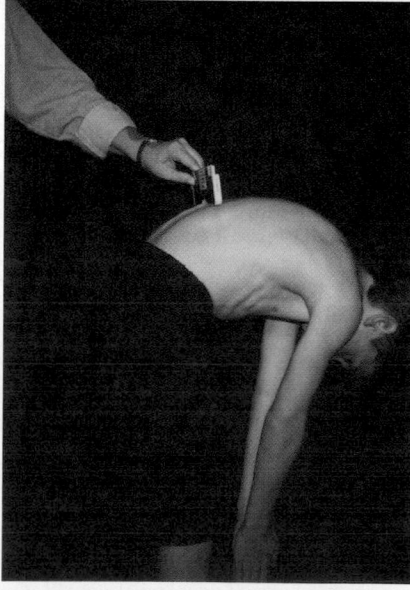

Figure 59-9 Use of scoliometer.

- Impaired physical mobility due to the scoliosis.
- Risk for impaired skin integrity related to compromised tissue perfusion.
- Deficient knowledge related to self-care and risk prevention.

Planning and Implementation

The goal of treatment, whether surgical or nonsurgical, is to correct the deformity and prevent complications. For mild curvature, exercise and bracing are the treatments of choice. Exercise is used in conjunction with bracing. Bracing allows the scoliosis progression to be stopped or slowed because of the limitation in truncal mobility. Usually utilized in growing children, braces are used until the child reaches maturity (Hockenberry & Brown, 2003). Two types of braces are used: the Boston brace and the thoracolumbar sacral orthotic (TLSO).

Left untreated, scoliosis can lead to back pain, compromised cardiopulmonary function, GI tract disturbances, and gait abnormalities. Surgical complications include postoperative paralysis, paralytic ileus, and urinary retention (Hockenberry & Brown, 2003). A long-term complication may be a failure in the hardware used in the surgery. This failure can be include broken hardware or failure of the hardware to stay in place, sometimes due to poor bone quality, although this is more frequent in older people after a spinal fusion.

Surgery

Spinal fusion is used to fuse the vertebrae to correct the curvature as well as the rotation of the spine. Surgery is recommended for curves greater than 40 degrees with continued development of the curve over time (Slote, 2002). Fusion of the vertebrae is performed two vertebrae above the curve and two vertebrae below the curve. Bracing is continued after the surgery to provide additional support while recovery takes place.

Patient and Family Teaching

Patient and family teaching include defining the disorder, discussion of treatment for the level of severity (may include bracing and exercise or surgery options), and understanding of the developmental support (both social and emotional) for the child.

Evaluation of Outcomes

Potential patient outcomes for each of the example nursing diagnoses for the patient with scoliosis are:
- Acute or chronic pain due to the scoliosis. The patient should verbalize an adequate relief of pain along with the ability to realistically cope with the pain if it is not completely relieved.
- Fear due to the diagnosis of scoliosis. The patient should manifest positive coping behaviors and verbalize a reduction in the amount of fear of the having this disease.
- Impaired physical mobility due to the scoliosis. The patient should perform physical activity independently or with assistive devices as needed. In addition, the patient should be free of complications of immobility, as evidenced by intact skin, absence of thrombophlebitis, and normal bowel patterns.
- Risk for impaired skin integrity related to compromised tissue perfusion. The condition of the skin should be improved as evidenced by decreased redness, swelling, and pain.
- Deficient knowledge related to self-care and risk prevention. The patient should demonstrate motivation to learn, identify perceived learning needs, and verbalize an understanding of desired content.

In addition, successful interventions provide the successful outcomes of halting the progress of the spinal curvature and supporting the growing body into an anatomically correct position. Other successful outcomes include adequate coping by the patient and family with the treatment of the disorder. Slote (2002) emphasizes psychological support and empowering the patient.

Family and peer support groups can take a proactive role in the patient's emotional and physical healing by providing the support and empowerment the patient needs. The involvement of these support groups can and will make the relatively long treatment and recovery period a positive experience, especially after surgery.

Kyphosis

Kyphosis (posterior curvature of the thoracic spine) is abnormal when the curvature of the thoracic spine is greater than 45 degrees. Kyphosis often results from osteoporosis (hunchback) or AS. Treatment can be accomplished with bracing or spinal fusion should the defect cause cardiopulmonary problems or pain.

Spinal Stenosis

Spinal stenosis is a degeneration of the spine that causes narrowing of the spinal canal secondary to bony overgrowth (osteophytes) at the facet joints, hypertrophy of the ligaments supporting the spine, or protrusion of intervertebral disks (Hellman & Stone, 2004). The most common site of stenosis is the lumbar region of the spine. The result of the narrowing of the canal is impingement on the nerves and subsequent low back pain and/or leg pain as well as leg fatigue and reduced physical activity tolerance.

The incidence of spinal stenosis increases with age. Spinal stenosis can be a complication of many processes traumatic back injury, arthritis, or Paget's disease.

Assessment with Clinical Manifestations

The patient will usually present with a gradual onset of difficulty walking or low back pain. Pain may also radiate down one leg. The patient may complain of the inability to stand or sit in one position for long because of the pain or fatigue (Hellman & Stone, 2004). A neurological assessment may be unremarkable. Gait assessment may reveal unsteadiness or a limp.

Diagnostic Tests

An MRI is the most useful diagnostic tool when spinal stenosis is suspected.

Nursing Diagnoses

Based on the information gathered, examples of nursing diagnoses in the patient with spinal stenosis (and other spinal disorders) may include the following:
- Chronic and acute pain related to spinal stenosis.
- Activity intolerance.
- Ineffective coping.
- Ineffective role performance.

Planning and Implementation

The goals of treatment are to reduce pain and return the patient to normal physical activity. Exercises to strengthen back muscles and flexibility are often prescribed. These exercises can be done in conjunction with a therapist's or nurse's instruction or by simple written instructions.

Nutrition
Weight loss is recommended to reduce the lumbar lordosis that causes strain on the back. A consult with a dietitian may be in order.

Surgery
To treat continuing pain, a decompression laminectomy may be performed. The laminectomy relieves the pressure within the spinal canal and reduces the pain. Some patients may need to have a spinal fusion in order to stabilize the

spine. Refer to the section on scoliosis for more on spinal fusions. Risks of surgical complications increase with age and comorbid conditions. The potential postoperative complications are: hematoma, dural tears, spinal cord injury, nonunion of the fusion, infection, and delayed wound healing.

Patient and Family Teaching

Teaching will revolve around the disease process, the prescribed exercises and pain medications as well as the importance of weight control. Teaching may also need to be done regarding potential surgical options.

Evaluation of Outcomes

A review of the literature found that patients with mild symptoms of spinal stenosis did better with conservative treatment whereas patients with moderate to severe symptoms did better with surgical treatment (Snyder, Doggett, & Turkelson, 2004). However, a study performed on long-term effects of spinal fusions in lumbar spinal stenosis showed that although the surgical group had initially better results than the nonsurgical group, the benefit of surgery decreased with time (Chang, Singer, Wu, Keller, & Atlas, 2005).

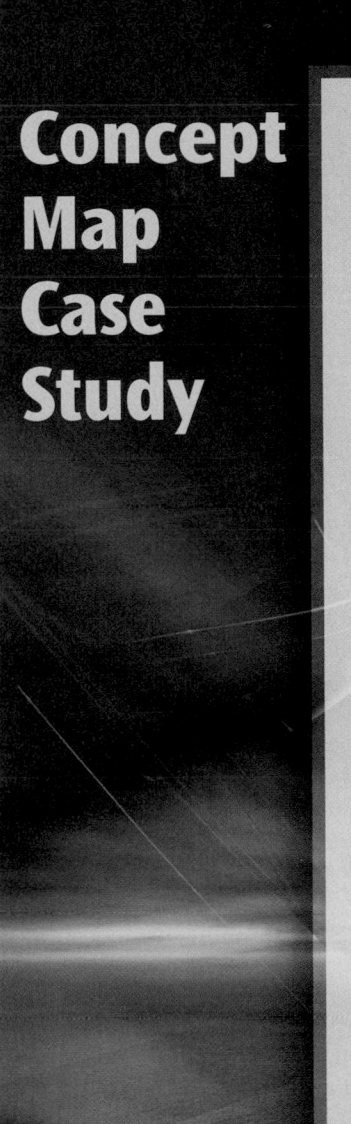

Concept Map Case Study

Mr. Juan Rodriguez

Juan Rodriguez, age 76, is a retired schoolteacher. He is widowed and lives alone in the home that he and his wife shared for 37 years. His two adult sons and their wives live in the city, and they visit him at least once each week. His two grandchildren attend college in another state. A cleaning woman comes to his home every two weeks. Mr. Rodriguez enjoys his independence, still drives his car, attends his church regularly, and likes to garden. He manages the routine cooking and household tasks rather well. He also belongs to a group of retired teachers that has breakfast meetings once a month.

Mr. Rodriguez has hypertension and is taking daily doses of lisinopril, an angiotensin-converting enzyme (ACE) inhibitor medication, of 40 mg and pravastatin, an antilipemic medication, of 10 mg, and low-dose aspirin of 81 mg. He takes Tylenol (over-the-counter) for arthritis pain. He is scheduled for cataract surgery next month.

Yesterday, he tripped and fell when he was retrieving his mail from the post box by his driveway. He felt a sharp pain in his right hip and leg and was unable to get up. His next door neighbor heard his shouts for help and ran out to assist him. She notified Mr. Rodriguez's son and called 911. After being examined in the emergency department, he was diagnosed with a femoral neck fracture. He was transferred to the orthopedic unit and was scheduled for a total hip replacement (arthroplasty).

Postoperative orders include: thigh high support hose, an indwelling catheter (for two to three days), legs must remain abducted, and Mr. Rodriguez cannot be turned. The wound dressing and Hemovac drainage must be assessed. He has an intravenous (IV) fluid running. Intake and output are to be measured. Narcotic analgesics will be administered via a patient controlled analgesia device (PCA) for the first two days with transition to oral analgesics the third day, if needed. Heparin is to be administered via IV as a prophylactic measure against thrombophlebitis. Vital signs and neurovascular status of the lower extremities are to be evaluated on a routine basis.

Concept Map Case Study

Note: There is a current trend for using clinical pathways for managing the interdisciplinary care for total hip replacement. Patients can usually return to their regular presurgical diet on the second postoperative day. Hospitalization for this type of surgery is four to five days. The patient is usually discharged to a rehabilitation facility for a period of time. Physical and occupational therapies and education related to transferring techniques, weight bearing, exercises, modifications in the home, and so on begins early in the postoperative treatment time. The nurse is also involved in education and monitoring the patient's progress. The recovery period is approximately four to six weeks. As you respond to the discussion questions for this case study, consider the special needs of the geriatric patient as they relate to the holistic mental, physical, spiritual, environmental, and safety needs. Refer to the sample concept map for assistance in designing a map for Mr. Rodriguez. Add concepts where you believe they belong. (Note: some concepts may belong in more than one area.)

Suggested References

Current Nurses Drug Guide or Pharmacology Text
Current Medical/Surgical Nursing Text
Nanda International. (2005). *NANDA nursing diagnoses: Definitions and classification 2005–2006.* Philadelphia: Author.

1. Describe the potential complications due to immobility. What are the nursing actions to prevent these complications?
2. What precautions should be taken when transferring Mr. Rodriguez from the bed to a chair?
3. What clinical manifestations (respiratory, gastrointestinal, mental, and so on) would alert you to the adverse side effects of the narcotic medications?
4. Describe discharge instructions that you would provide for Mr. Rodriguez.
5. If you were assigned to evaluate Mr. Rodriguez's home what safety precautions or adaptations would you suggest to minimize falls and to promote his progress toward independent living?

KEY CONCEPTS

- OA occurs because of damage to articular cartilage and the metabolic response that results at the chondrocyte level.
- Patients with gout will report a rapid development (within hours) of pain and edema in the one affected joint.
- LD is preventable by taking simple precautions.
- The common features of the spondyloarthropathies are sacroilitis variable inflammatory peripheral arthritis, enthesitis, dactylitis, tendency for ocular inflammation, familial tendency, no rheumatoid factor, and strong association with the HLA-B27 gene.

- There are three hallmark tests which confirm the diagnosis of polymyositis or dermatomyositis: elevated muscle enzymes; an abnormal electromyogram; and positive results in a muscle biopsy.
- Fibromyalgia is most frequently defined as a clinical syndrome or condition involving chronic widespread diffuse musculoskeletal pain, stiffness, and tenderness.
- Osteoporosis is the most frequently diagnosed bone disease in humans.
- The main cause of osteomalacia is a vitamin D deficiency and is rare in the United States.

Continued

KEY CONCEPTS—cont'd

■ Paget's disease is a chronic bone disorder character-ized by weakened bone structure with no definitive cause or cure.

■ Musculoskeletal infections can have devastating results if not treated promptly or completely.

■ Primary bone cancers are rare. Metastatic tumors of the bone are detrimental consequences of cancer and are more common than primary bone cancers.

■ For mild scoliosis curvature, exercise and bracing are the treatments of choice. For greater curves, spinal fusion is used.

■ Spinal stenosis causes impingement on the nerves and subsequent low back pain or leg pain, as well as leg fatigue and reduced physical activity tolerance.

REVIEW QUESTIONS

1. Mrs. Jones is newly diagnosed with osteoarthritis of her knees. She told you the health care provider prescribed acetaminophen or ibuprofen for pain. She asks you how she can afford this medication. Your best response would be:
   1. "Dr. Cho thinks your pain is only minimal, and the cheap drugs are a good way to keep you out of the office."
   2. "Dr. Cho knows that these medications will help your pain and are relatively inexpensive and available over-the-counter at your local grocery or pharmacy."
   3. "I'll call the social worker."
   4. "Dr. Cho knows that these medications are covered by insurance and you shouldn't worry."

2. Mr. Cooper, a 65 year-old white male, has just been diagnosed with gout. Your teaching would include instructions to:
   1. Check his feet everyday for ulcers
   2. Avoid alcohol and turkey
   3. Avoid fats and milk products
   4. Take his antigout medications only when his toe hurts

3. Your patient is admitted for an appendectomy and states he has been suffering with Reiter's syndrome. You remember that patient's with Reiter's syndrome can present with all of the following symptoms *except:*
   1. The patient's eyes may be red and irritated.
   2. One of your patient's toes may be swollen and red.
   3. Your patient will complain of headaches.
   4. Your patient will complain of low back pain.

4. Your 55-year-old female patient with ankylosing spondylitis has been taking NSAIDs for years and finds these are no longer effective. A disease-modifying antirheumatic drug (DMARD) is now being prescribed. You tell you patient the following about DMARDs:

   1. They will help to increase the lubrication in the joint.
   2. They are analgesics.
   3. They assist with reducing inflammation.
   4. They should be taken with milk.

5. A 10-year-old boy is brought into your clinic. The parents state he has been complaining of pain in his knees and elbows for the past couple of days. On physical examination you find a bullseye-shaped rash on his upper back. Which of the following do you suspect?
   1. LD
   2. Reactive arthritis
   3. Fibromyalgia
   4. Extra pulmonary tuberculosis

6. A 59-year-old female is presenting to the clinic for a workup for suspected fibromyalgia. You know the following about fibromyalgia:
   1. The patient will have pulmonary function tests performed.
   2. The patient will be tested for rheumatoid factor and serum complement.
   3. The patient will be tested for electrolyte panel and ESR.
   4. The patient will have a liver biopsy.

7. A 67-year-old female presents with progressively worsening pain in the lower back with numbness and pain down the right leg. She reports she has lost about an inch in height over the last 10 years. You suspect spinal stenosis because:
   1. Spinal stenosis causes impingement of the nerve roots and can lead to back and leg pain.
   2. Disc space in the spinal column shrinks with spinal stenosis causing height loss.
   3. She was a long distance runner in her earlier years and the constant jarring from running causes spinal stenosis.
   4. Her X-rays show hypokyphosis.

Continued

8. A woman who has had rheumatoid arthritis for several years is admitted to the hospital. On physical examination of this patient, you should expect to find:
   1. Asymmetrical joint involvement
   2. Heberden's nodes
   3. Obesity
   4. Small joint involvement

9. A 50-year-old man has suffered from low back pain and sciatica for over two years. He is admitted to the hospital for evaluation and treatment of this problem. A thorough assessment of his level of discomfort from low back pain is important primarily because:
   1. This will provide a baseline for later comparison.
   2. This is a method for identifying patients with low back neurosis.
   3. Patients who have pain localized to the back and radiating to one extremity are probably not candidates for surgery.
   4. Surgery is contraindicated for patients who have had pain for less than two years.

10. A 52-year-old woman has RA and is taking prednisone. In creating a teaching plan, you will be certain to tell the patient which of the following?
    1. The patient should expect to be on corticosteroids for the rest of her life.
    2. It may take three to six months for the patient to notice any effect from the medication.
    3. The patient should notify the health care provider of any stomach upset.
    4. The patient should avoid bananas and spinach while she is taking this drug.

REVIEW ACTIVITIES

1. During a rotation in the operating room, ask to see an orthopedic surgery (preferably a joint replacement). What were there surgical instruments like? Did they look familiar? If you were present for a joint replacement how was the surgical team dressed? How was the patient placed during surgery? Was there any type of traction put on the patient during this surgery?

2. Visit the orthopedic nursing unit in your hospital. Does your hospital have a designated orthopedic nursing unit? What types of patient's do you see admitted? Why are these types of patient's admitted and others not? How long is the typical stay for an orthopedic patient after joint replacement?

Continued

3. Your patient with osteoarthritis is concerned about the long-term effects of the disease. What can you tell the patient about the prognosis to allay any fears? What support programs are available to the patient or her family? How can you assess the patient's acceptance of this information?

4. Perform a search on the World Wide Web for information about Lyme disease. Look at both sites directed toward laypersons and medical personnel. What sort of information do you see? Is the information factual on the layperson sites? Who sponsors these sites? How can you tell if they are reliable sources? What information can you give to your patients about searching for medical information on the web?

Visit the Contemporary Medical-Surgical Nursing online companion resource at www.delmarhealthcare.com for additional content and study aids. Click on Online Companions then select the Nursing discipline.

Musculoskeletal Trauma: Nursing Management

Rebecca Sears, RN

Anita M. Zehala, RN, MS, ONC, CNS

CHAPTER TOPICS

- Sports Injuries
- Overuse Syndrome/Repetitive Motion Injuries
- Shoulder Dislocations
- Rotator Cuff Tears
- Lateral Epicondylitis
- Carpal Tunnel Syndrome
- Patellar Tendonitis
- Knee Ligament Injuries
- Meniscal Injuries
- Ankle Sprain
- Achilles Tendon Injuries
- Plantar Fasciitis
- Stress Fractures
- Fractures
- Hip Fractures
- Complications
- Amputation

KEY TERMS

Ankle sprain
Arthroscopy
Closed reduction
Compartment syndrome
Cryotherapy
Drawer test
Fascia
Fasciotomy
Fracture
Inversion stress test
Lateral epicondylitis
Mechanism of injury
Microtrauma
Occult fracture
Overuse syndrome
Phalen's maneuver
Phantom limb sensation
Prosthesis
Radiculopathy
RICE
Rotator cuff tears
Sports medicine
Thenar
Tinel's sign
Valgus
Varus

U nintentional trauma is the leading cause of death for Americans between the ages of 1 and 44. Overall, unintentional injuries are the fifth leading cause of death for all age-groups. Males are injured two to three times more often than females, however, after the age of 65 this trend reverses, and females sustain more injuries than males (National Center for Health Statistics, 2004). Motor vehicle accidents are the leading cause of unintentional injuries for all age groups, followed by poisonings and falls. Sports injuries and occupational injuries are also a musculoskeletal concern. In 2002, 2.5 million workplace injuries and illnesses resulted in either days away from work, job transfer, or job restrictions (National Center for Health Statistics, 2004). Injuries place a heavy burden on our health care system and it resources. According to a 2000 report from the Center for Disease Control and Prevention (CDC), the United States spent $117 billion on medical expenditures related to injuries. This is equal to 10 percent of the total amount of medical expenditures for 2000. On an annual basis, injuries accounted for 9 million inpatient hospital days, 36 percent of total visits to the emergency department, and 1.8 million discharges, with fractures being the most common type of injury (National Center for Health Statistics, 2004).

SPORTS INJURIES

Sports medicine can be defined as the application of professional knowledge to the understanding, prevention, treatment, and rehabilitation of sports-related and exercise-related problems. It entails a multidisciplinary team approach, including the health care providers, nurses, physical therapists, athletic trainer, coaches, and exercise physiologists. The initial treatment of sports-related injuries consists of protection, rest, ice, compression, and elevation **(RICE),** and pain control. The rehabilitation phase begins when the pain is gone, and the injury is healed. The overall goal of rehabilitation is to return the patient back to preinjury status, and in the case of the competitive athlete, back to full participation in the sport activity. Rehabilitation consists of four areas of focus: full range of motion of the joint, optimal flexibility, strength, and endurance.

OVERUSE SYNDROME/REPETITIVE MOTION INJURIES

Overuse syndrome (also called repetitive motion injuries or cumulative trauma disorders) is caused by a repetitive motion or sustained exertion, causing **microtrauma** to the involved tissue (usually a muscle or tendon). The injured tissue is not given sufficient time to rest and heal before being subjected to more stress, which leads to pain, swelling, fatigue, and numbness. Overuse syndrome is an umbrella term and is used to describe many work-related injuries and injuries seen in athletes. The injury can take weeks or years to develop, and the symptoms may start to appear gradually. Many factors play a role in development of these injuries (Box 60-1).

Many occupations and sports have also been associated with a high level of overuse syndromes. These are listed in Box 60-2.

DISLOCATION OF THE SHOULDER

The shoulder is an important joint and is used in most activities of daily living. Therefore when it is injured it can cause disability and great inconvenience to the patient and family.

Epidemiology

In 2002, 12.3 million people in the United States visited a health care provider for a shoulder-related problem. Shoulder dislocations account for almost 50 percent of all joint dislocations. About 90 percent are anterior dislocations and 2 to 10 percent are posterior dislocations. In younger patients the dislocation is caused by direct trauma and sports injuries. In the elderly the number one cause is a fall and a fracture is also commonly sustained (Quillen, Wuchner, & Hatch, 2004).

BOX 60-1

FACTORS ASSOCIATED WITH OVERUSE SYNDROME

Repetitive tasks

Forceful exertions

Exposure to vibration

Exposure to cold temperatures

Awkward positioning

Poor ergonomics and work place design

Lack of job satisfaction

Physiological makeup

Boredom at work

BOX 60-2

OCCUPATIONS AND SPORTS WITH HIGH INCIDENCE OF OVERUSE SYNDROME

Grocery store clerks

Computer keyboard operators

Dental hygienists

Frozen food workers

Assembly line workers

Health care workers

Meat packers and butchers

Professional dancers

Musicians

Etiology

The **mechanism of injury** for an anterior dislocation is a fall on an outstretched hand and arm that is abducted and externally rotated. It can also be caused by a direct blow to the posterior humerus. In a posterior dislocation, the force is applied while the arm is adducted and internally rotated.

Pathophysiology

The shoulder joint is a ball-and-socket joint, which allows a great amount of range and movement, but because of this, it is more vulnerable to dislocation. The shoulder is supported by the joint capsule, cartilage, and the muscles of the rotator cuff. In most adults the cause of a shoulder injury is a traumatic force. In the older adult, collagen fibers have fewer cross-links, which makes the shoulder joint weaker and more likely to dislocate (Price & Wilson, 2005).

Complications

After conservative treatment, recurrent dislocation can occur in 67 to 97 percent of cases with a higher incidence occurring in patients younger than 30 years. Athletes also have a higher incidence of recurring dislocation (82 percent) when compared to nonathletes (30 percent) (Welsh & Veenstra, 2004). Many studies have shown that early surgical treatment may prevent recurring dislocation (Davy & Drew, 2002).

Assessment with Clinical Manifestations

Assessment begins with a history of the traumatic event, including the position of the arm before and after the event. History of a prior dislocation is a risk factor for future dislocations. During the physical assessment any movement of the affected arm will cause severe pain because of muscle spasms. The affected arm is often guarded and cradled with the contralateral arm. The affected shoulder will appear lower, and the humeral head can be palpated in the front of the shoulder (Welsh & Veenstra, 2004). A neurovascular assessment is extremely important. Any changes in pulses, color, temperature, or sensation to the limb may be because of the impingement of the axillary nerves and radial artery. See chapter 58 for instructions on how to perform a neurovascular assessment.

Diagnostic Tests

Radiographic films are often used to confirm diagnosis and to assess for any accompanying fractures. However, relocation of the shoulder should not be delayed because of diagnostic testing. The longer the time between injury and relocation, the more difficult the relocation can become.

Nursing Diagnoses

Based on the information gathered, examples of nursing diagnoses, interventions, and outcomes in the patient with upper extremity trauma include:
- Acute pain.
- Risk for peripheral neurovascular dysfunction.
- Impaired physical mobility.
- Anxiety.
- Bathing/hygiene self-care deficit.
- Dressing/grooming self-care deficit.

Planning and Implementation

Closed reduction should be accomplished as soon as possible after the injury. As time passes, the muscles in the shoulder will become more spastic, and the joint itself will become more inflamed and swollen making reduction more difficult. Sedation and analgesics are often used in addition to a muscle relaxant to make reduction easier. Traditionally, treatment after reduction follows a conservative approach. The affected shoulder is immobilized in a sling for four to six weeks. External rotation and abduction is avoided (Welsh & Veenstra, 2004). After the initial rest period, rehabilitation is started, which includes strengthening of the shoulder girdle, flexibility, and regaining full range of motion.

ROTATOR CUFF TEARS

Rotator cuff tears are a common cause of shoulder pain in the adult population. They are most commonly seen in adults over the age of 40 years. In younger patients they are seen following a traumatic event or a sports-related injury (Fischer, 2005). The rotator cuff is made up of four muscles: the supraspinatus, infraspinatus, teres minor, and subscapularis (Figure 60-1).

The primary function of the rotator cuff is providing stability to the shoulder joint. It also provides some movement to the shoulder.

Epidemiology

The incidence of full thickness tears range from 5 to 40 percent and increases with age (Malanga, Andrus, & Bowen, 2004).

Etiology

Injury to the rotator cuff can occur by direct trauma, such as a fall, motor vehicle accident, or shoulder dislocation, or it can be caused by an overuse syndrome as seen in sports and activities that require extensive overhead movements

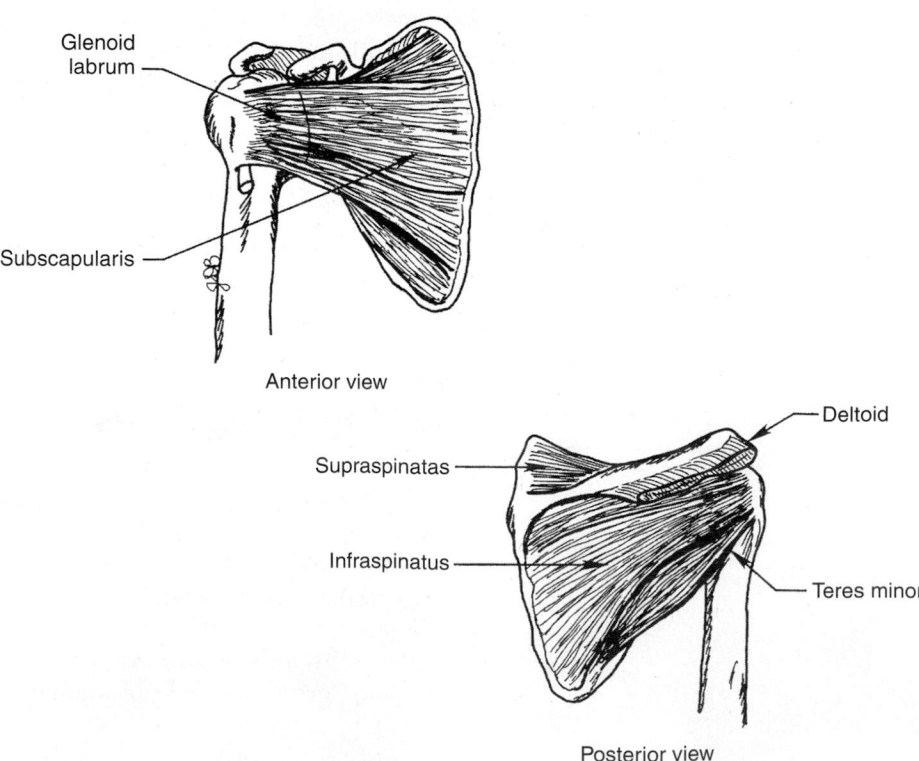

Anterior view

Posterior view

Figure 60-1 Rotator cuff tear.

(Quillen, et al., 2004). In overuse syndromes, poor posture, improper technique, and direct injury cause swelling and microtears to the muscles. If the microtrauma continues, eventual rupture of the rotator cuff can result. Rotator cuff tears are most commonly seen in sports that requires extensive use of the upper extremities, such as baseball, softball, tennis, swimming, and volleyball.

Assessment with Clinical Manifestations

A detailed history of the injury is needed to help rule out other causes of the symptoms, such as **radiculopathy** of the cervical nerves and pain that is of cardiac origin (Malanga, et al., 2004). History should include onset of pain, description of symptoms, and aggravating factors.

The physical assessment begins with inspection and comparison of the shoulder with the contralateral shoulder, noting any swelling, muscle atrophy, or asymmetry. Palpation will reveal localized tenderness. Assessment of the strength and range of motion (both passive and active) is important in determining the existence of a rotator cuff injury. With a rotator cuff tear, pain and reduced range of motion are experienced when the arm is abducted and externally rotated.

Diagnostic Tests

Diagnostic testing includes plain radiographs to view the bony structures of the shoulder and magnetic resonance imaging (MRI) to detect the size, location, and severity of the tear (Malanga, et al., 2004).

Nursing Diagnoses

Based on the information gathered, examples of nursing diagnoses, interventions, and outcomes in the patient with a rotator cuff tear include:
- Acute pain.
- Potential for impaired neurovascular status.
- Impaired physical mobility.

Planning and Implementation

The goals of treatment during the initial phase of the injury are rest and immobilization. Overhead activity is restricted, and a sling is usually worn. Pendulum exercises are started to reduce loss of range of motion (Quillen, et al., 2004). Ice, nonsteroidal anti-inflammatory drugs (NSAIDs), and acetaminophen are also used during this time to relieve inflammation and pain. During the recovery phase, physical therapy focuses on restoration of the range of motion, strengthening, proprioception, and joint stability (Malanga, et al., 2004).

Surgical Procedures

Surgical treatment is usually indicated for partial-thickness and full-thickness tears in active patients when three to six months of conservative treatment have failed to improve pain and function (Malanga, et al., 2004). Competitive athletes usually have better outcomes with surgical treatment (Quillen, et al, 2004). For smaller tears, the surgical procedure is usually performed by **arthroscopy.** The rotator cuff is derided, and measures may be taken to increase the subacromial space to prevent recurrence. For larger tears the procedure is performed using an open surgical technique.

Patient and Family Teaching

Patient teaching should focus on the rehabilitation plan of care. It is extremely important to stress to the patient the reasoning behind the program and why certain exercises may not be preformed until healing has occurred to protect the surgical site and to prevent fibrosis and reinjury to the rotator cuff.

Evaluation of Outcomes

Potential patient outcomes for each of the example nursing diagnoses for the patient with a rotator cuff tear are:

- Acute pain. The patient should verbalize an adequate relief of pain along with the ability to realistically cope with the pain if it is not completely relieved.
- Potential for impaired neurovascular status. The patient will have intact nervous system as evidenced by normal movement and sensation.
- Impaired physical mobility. The patient should perform physical activity independently or with assistive devices as needed. In addition, the patient should be free of complications of immobility, as evidenced by intact skin, absence of thrombophlebitis, and normal bowel patterns.

LATERAL EPICONDYLITIS

Lateral epicondylitis, or tennis elbow, is a common injury seen in athletes and in the general population. It is an overuse injury that involves the extensor/supinator muscles that attach to the distal humerus.

Epidemiology

Lateral epicondylitis has been seen in up to 50 percent of tennis players. The risk of injury increases with the hours of play and with the age of the athlete. Prevalence in relation to occupation varies widely from 1.6 to 23.1 percent (Hong, et al., 2003). There are no differences between men and women (Owens, et al., 2004).

Etiology

Although tennis is most commonly associated with lateral epicondylitis, any activity involving an extensive amount wrist extension or supination can cause lateral epicondylitis, such as many different manufacturing workplace activities. In younger patients, lateral epicondylitis tends to be associated with tennis and other sport activities, and in older patients, it is associated with occupational causes. In regard to tennis players, risk factors include improper technique, size of racquet handle, and racquet weight (Owens, Murphy, & Kuklo, 2004).

Pathophysiology

Although named lateral epicondylitis, many studies have failed to find evidence of an inflammatory process (Hong, Durand, & Loisel, 2003). The cause has been attributed to microinjuries with an inadequate repair response leading to macroscopic tearing and structural failure of the tendon (Owens, et al., 2004).

Assessment with Clinical Manifestations

The most common presenting symptom is pain at the lateral aspect of the elbow and in the forearm that is exacerbated with use (Owens, et al., 2004). The ability to grip is also impaired, thus everyday activities become difficult (Hong, et al., 2003).

Tenderness slightly distal to epicondyle is found with palpation of the elbow. Wrist extension and supination against resistance will cause an increase in pain; however, wrist flexion and pronation will not. The chair raise test examines the patient's ability to grip and lift. The patient stands behind a chair and places their hands on the chair back. The patient then attempts to raise the chair. If pain is experienced over the lateral elbow, lateral epicondylitis may be present (Owens, et al., 2004).

Diagnostic Tests

As with many overuse and sport injuries, the diagnosis is based on clinical findings during the examination of the patient. X-rays may be useful in ruling out other causes of elbow pain, such as osteochondral loose bodies and osteophytes (bone spurs). If the condition is chronic, calcification of the tendon may also be seen on X-ray. MRI can also be useful in the diagnosis, but usually it is not needed.

Nursing Diagnoses

Based on the information gathered, examples of nursing diagnoses, interventions, and outcomes in the patient with lateral epicondylitis include:
- Acute pain.
- Potential for impaired neurovascular status.
- Impaired physical mobility.

Planning and Implementation

The goal of treatment is to return the patient to preinjury status. Most patients respond to conservative treatment, which includes avoiding the activity that causes the pain, bracing and splinting of the elbow and wrist, and use of NSAIDs for short-term pain relief.

Once the patient is no longer experiencing pain, rehabilitation therapy can begin with strengthening exercises (Owens, et al., 2004). The first phase is stretching of the wrist with the elbow extended. This includes flexion, extension, and rotation of the wrist. The next phase is strengthening of the wrist using light weights in both extension and flexion. Forearm pronation and supination is then added along with having the patient squeeze a tennis ball.

If the patient is still experiencing symptoms after six months of conservative treatment, surgery is needed. The procedure is usually performed on an outpatient basis. Debridement of the muscle, removal of the portion of diseased epicondyle, and release of the tendon is performed.

Once the patient's strength is back to baseline, the focus of therapy turns to prevention of further injury to the elbow. Education on correct technique, equipment in relation to sports, and modification of occupational activities is important in preventing further irritation to the lateral elbow.

Evaluation of Outcomes

Potential patient outcomes for each of the example nursing diagnoses for the patient with a lateral epicondylitis are:
- Acute pain. The patient should verbalize an adequate relief of pain along with the ability to realistically cope with the pain if it is not completely relieved.
- Potential for impaired neurovascular status. The patient will have intact nervous system as evidenced by normal movement and sensation.
- Impaired physical mobility. The patient should perform physical activity independently or with assistive devices as needed. In addition, the patient should be free of complications of immobility, as evidenced by intact skin, absence of thrombophlebitis, and normal bowel patterns.

CARPAL TUNNEL SYNDROME

Carpal tunnel syndrome (CTS) is a median nerve entrapment neuropathy. It is the most common compression neuropathy of the upper extremity.

Epidemiology

CTS is most often seen between the ages of 30 and 60. Women are five times as likely to experience CTS as men (Wright, 2003).

Etiology

CTS is seen in conjunction with many other conditions. It is often seen during pregnancy, premenstrual period, and menopause; suggesting a hormonal link. It is also seen in patients with a history of arthritis, lipomas, ganglion, and after a fracture or trauma to the hand or wrist (Figure 60-2). Diabetes mellitus impairs peripheral nerve conduction and repair, therefore CTS is commonly seen in these patients as well (Kennedy & Zochodne, 2005). Anything that may cause the tendons of the wrist to become inflamed or swollen can also place pressure on the median nerve. Besides these above conditions, CTS is also associated with repetitive motion of the hand and wrist. Any activity where hand use is vigorous and routine can lead to CTS. The activities that have been associated with CTS are computer keyboarding or typing, playing a musical instrument, driving a motor vehicle or motorcycle, and flying a plane. There is also an increase in incidence in occupations that subject workers to a cold environment, such as meat packers, butchers, and frozen food workers (Falkiner & Myers, 2002).

Pathophysiology

The carpal tunnel is a canal in the wrist made up of the carpal bones and the transverse carpal ligament through which the flexor tendons and median nerve pass through to the hand. It is located at the base of the palm. CTS is the result of increased pressure inside the canal, which causes ischemia to the medial nerve. The damaged nerve is unable to function properly resulting in impaired nerve conduction, paresthesia, muscle weakness, and pain to the wrist and hand.

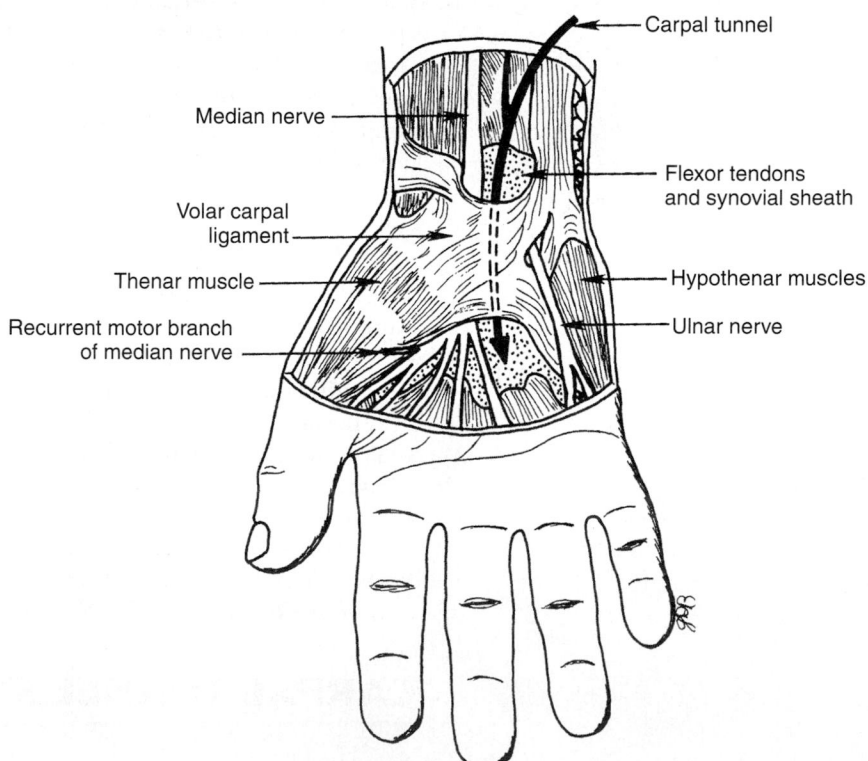

Figure 60-2 Carpal tunnel syndrome.

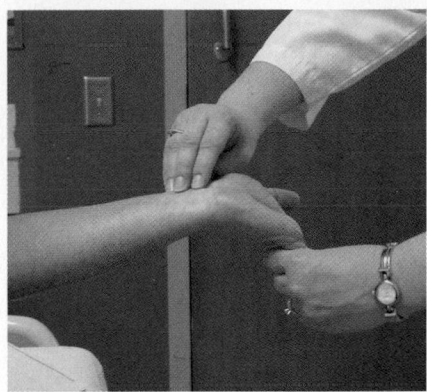

Figure 60-3 Tinel's sign.

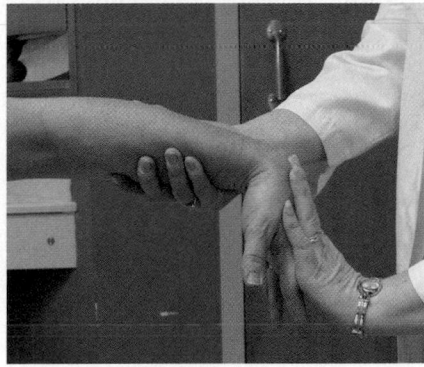

Figure 60-4 Phalen's maneuver.

Assessment with Clinical Manifestations

The diagnosis of CTS begins with a thorough history of symptoms. The patient may present with a combination of paraesthesia, numbness, and pain. The pain is usually described as a deep aching, or throbbing that is diffuse in nature and radiates up the forearm (Wright, 2003). The pain typically worsens at night. To attribute these symptoms to CTS, they must occur in the areas of the hand supplied by the median nerve, which includes the palmar aspect of the thumb, index finger, middle finger, and radial half of the ring finger. The patient may also report that the symptoms improve when the affected hand is placed in a dependent position and is shaken. This is known as the "flick test" (Katz & Simmons, 2002).

The physical examination consists of two classic tests to determine if the medial nerve has been compromised. The **Tinel's sign** (Figure 60-3) is a way to determine if the nerve is irritated. The area over the median nerve is lightly tapped. If the patient experiences a sensation of tingling or "pins and needles" the test is positive. The **Phalen's maneuver** (Figure 60-4) is more sensitive in the diagnosis of CTS. In this test the patient's wrist is put into flexion for 30 seconds. If the patient experiences a burning, tingling, or numbness the test it considered positive. Loss of two point discrimination along the area of the hand supplied by the median nerve and **thenar** (the palm of the hand or the sole of the foot) atrophy are late signs of CTS (Katz & Simmons, 2002).

Diagnostic Tests

Diagnostic testing is only used to confirm the diagnosis of CTS. Electromyography is used to test the function of the nerve. A mild electric current is used to stimulate the median nerve to see if there is a delay in motor response, which could indicate CTS.

Planning and Implementation

Conservative treatment starts with splinting of the affected wrist. The splint is used to maintain the wrist in the neutral position. This is important especially during sleep. Activity modifications along with exercises of the wrist may help to alleviate symptoms as well. If after four to six weeks of conservative treatment, symptoms remain or worsen, or the patient has thenar muscle atrophy or weakness, corticosteroid injection is recommended (Wright, 2003).

Pharmacology

If the symptoms are mild, NSAIDs are used to decrease the inflammation of the tendon and to help with pain control.

Health Care Resources

Annually, estimated 3 of every 10,000 workers lost time from work and half of these workers missed more than 10 days of work because of CTS. The average lifetime cost of carpal tunnel syndrome, including medical bills and lost time from work, is estimated to be about $30,000 for each injured worker (National Institute of Neurological Disorders and Stroke, 2002).

Surgery

If conservative treatment, including corticosteroid injection, does not improve symptoms after three months, surgery is considered. Surgical options include an open release of the ligament either by a mini or standard incision or by endoscopic surgery. It is performed on an outpatient basis using a regional block. After surgery, the patient is placed in a splint with instructions on range of motion exercises of the fingers. After, a few days, the splint is removed and more active physical therapy may begin. Most patients return to work within

2 to 14 days depending on the type of occupation and surgery. There is some debate over the use of surgery versus corticosteroid injection. In a study comparing the two treatments local steroid injections showed a slightly better outcome in the short term, but at 12 months, the outcomes for both groups were comparable (Ly-Pen, Andreu, de Blas, Sanchex-Olaso, & Millan, 2005).

Alternative Therapy

In a study by O'Connor, Marshall, & Massey-Westropp (2005), 21 trials comparing nonsurgical treatments for CTS other than steroid injection were reviewed. The results showed that there is significant short-term benefit from oral steroids, splinting, ultrasound, yoga, and carpal tunnel mobilization. However, magnet therapy, laser acupuncture, exercise, or chiropractic care did not show a significant benefit in symptom relief when compared to placebo or control.

Patient and Family Teaching

Patient teaching focuses on changes in ergonomics when completing daily activities. Teaching the patient proper hand and wrist alignment and stretching exercises can improve the symptoms and prevent further problems. Relaxing the force of grip on pens and other objects and taking frequent short breaks can also dramatically reduce the symptoms.

PATELLAR TENDINOPATHY

Patellar tendinopathy, also known as jumper's knee, is seen in athletes who participate in activities that require a lot of jumping, such as basketball and volleyball. It can be a challenge to treat the athlete, whether professional or recreational, and in some cases, he or she will no long be able to participate in those activities that cause the pain.

Epidemiology

Patellar tendinopathy occurs in 20 percent of jumping athletes and affects men twice as often as females (Hyman, et al., 2005).

Etiology

Patellar tendinopathy is caused by functional stress overload that is applied to the patellar tendon with jumping (Hyman, Malanga, & Alladin, 2005). Risk factors include overtraining, jumping on hard surfaces, poor quadriceps and hamstring flexibility, and poor jumping or landing technique (Hyman, et al., 2005).

Pathophysiology

In the past, patellar tendinopathy was thought to be an inflammatory process, but now it is thought to be a degenerative process from overuse (Peers & Lysens, 2005). When strain is applied to the tendon, microinjuries occur. If the amount of injuries outnumbers the ability of the tendon to repair itself, the tendon will start to degenerate (Hyman, et al., 2005).

Assessment with Clinical Manifestations

Patients usually describe anterior knee pain with an aching quality to it. It usually has an insidious onset, and most athletes will not be able to remember a specific precipitating event but may remember noticing the pain during an increase in activity or training. The extent of functional impairment is also important to assess. If the athlete is unable to participate in activities that require jumping, or if the pain continues long after the activity has ended, the tendinopathy may be more severe (Peers & Lysens, 2005).

During palpation of the knee joint, point tenderness may occur at the inferior patella pole and hamstring and quadriceps tightness may also be present (Hyman, et al., 2005). Range of motion should still be within normal limits.

Diagnostic Tests

Radiographic imaging is rarely needed to make a diagnosis, but it may be used to exclude other bony abnormalities (Hyman, et al., 2005). Ultrasound and MRI can also be used to visualize a degenerative process in the patella tendon (Peers & Lysens, 2005).

Nursing Diagnoses

Based on the information gathered, examples of nursing diagnoses, interventions and outcomes in the patient with inflammatory and connective tissue disorders include:

- Acute pain
- Impaired physical mobility
- Anxiety

Planning and Implementation

The goal of treatment is getting the patient back to preinjury state. Most patients respond to conservative management, which includes avoiding jumping and squatting. The patient should be encouraged to do other exercises that do not cause pain to the knee. Total immobilization of the knee joint is contraindicated because of risk of muscle or joint contracture (Hyman, et al., 2005). Physical therapy consists of strengthening and stretching programs for the quadriceps and hamstring muscles to help prevent the injury from returning. Surgical repair is only recommended if pain and functional disability remains after six months of conservative treatment (Hyman, et al., 2005).

Pharmacology

NSAIDs are used more for acute pain relief than for their anti-inflammatory properties, because inflammation is not part of the disease process. Corticosteroids are used only when conservative treatment has failed, and the pain is disrupting performance in a sport activity because of the risk of further damaging the tendon (Hyman, et al., 2005).

Evaluation of Outcomes

Potential patient outcomes for each of the example nursing diagnoses for the patient with patellar tendinopathy are:

- Acute pain: The patient should verbalize an adequate relief of pain along with the ability to realistically cope with the pain if it is not completely relieved.
- Impaired physical mobility: The patient should perform physical activity independently or with assistive devices as needed. In addition, the patient should be free of complications of immobility, as evidenced by intact skin, absence of thrombophlebitis, and normal bowel patterns.
- Anxiety: The patient should be able to recognize the signs of anxiety, demonstrate positive coping mechanisms, and describe a reduction in the level of anxiety experienced.

LIGAMENT INJURIES

Two set of ligaments in the knee provide a four-plane stability force to the knee. The collateral ligaments and are located on each side of the knee. The medial collateral ligament (MCL) connects the femur to the tibia and protects the knee from **valgus** (lateral) stress and external rotation. The lateral collateral ligament (LCL) connects the femur to the fibula and provides protection from **varus** (medial) forces. The other set of ligaments are called the cruciate ligaments and are located inside the knee joint and crisscross as they connect the femur to the tibia. The anterior cruciate ligament (ACL) is located in the front of the knee and prevents the tibia from excessive anterior movement. The posterior cruciate ligament (PCL) is located in the back of the knee (Figure 60-5).

Etiology and Pathophysiology

The MCL is the most commonly injured ligament (Gundel, 2004). The injury occurs when the foot is firmly planted and a direct valgus force is applied to the knee or the leg sustains an external rotational force. This injury is commonly seen in athletes who participate in football or basketball. The LCL is rarely injured, but if exposed to a contact varus force while the foot is planted, an injury can occur.

An ACL tear can result from several different mechanisms of injury. A sudden change in direction with the foot planted, sudden deceleration with some or no knee flexion, landing from a jump or by a direct valgus stress applied to an externally rotated leg. Any sport or activity that requires pivoting, twisting, rapid deceleration, or contact are associated with ACL injury, including basketball, football, skiing, soccer, and volleyball. ACL and meniscal injuries often coexist. The PCL is rarely injured, and the usual mechanism of injury involves an anterior force to the tibia with the knee flexed. This type of injury is commonly referred to as a dashboard injury.

Epidemiology

According to the American Academy of Orthopaedic Surgeons, more than eight million people visit an orthopaedic surgeon each year because of pain and other problems associated with the knee. Souryal and Adams (2005) reviewed several epidemiological studies and estimated that about 1 in 3,000 people sustain an ACL injury every year in the United States. Female athletes sustain injury to the ACL 3 to 10 times more frequently than male counterparts.

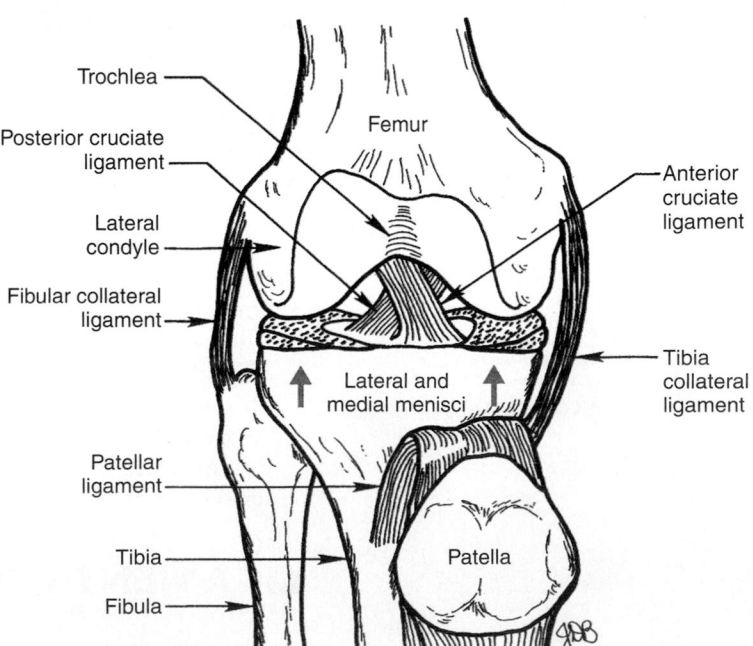

Figure 60-5 Normal anatomy of the knee with ligaments.

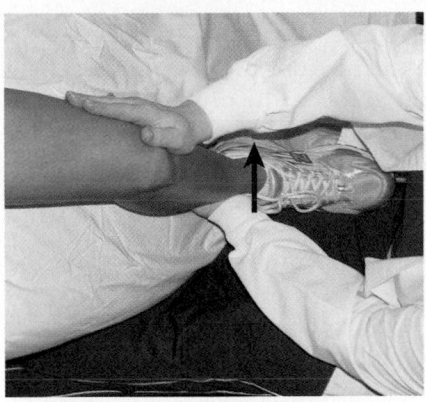

Figure 60-6 Varus stress test.

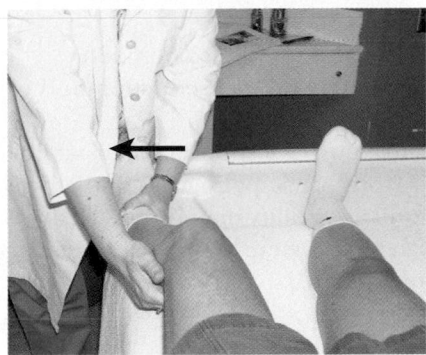

Figure 60-7 Valgus stress test.

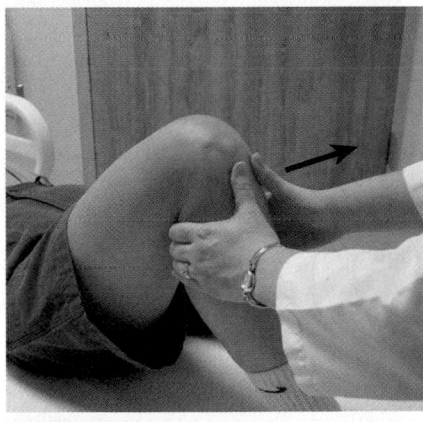

Figure 60-8 Drawer test.

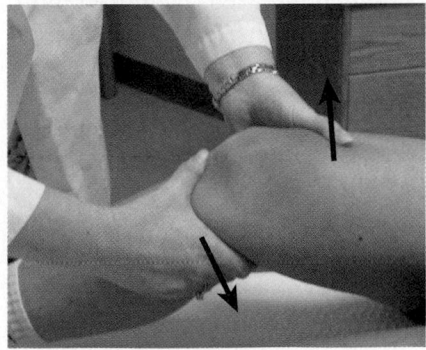

Figure 60-9 Lachman's test.

The reasons for the gender difference are not known, but many studies have linked possible factors, such as size and strength of the athlete and anatomical and hormonal differences.

Assessment

A history of the traumatic event is helpful in the diagnosis of a ligament injury. Details of how the injury occurred, position of the knee and foot, and any sounds of popping or tearing should be explored. Physical assessment begins with inspecting and comparing both knees while the patient sits, walks, stands, and is supine. Assess for the presence of pain, swelling, and any difficulty walking. Localized tenderness at the site of injury and joint effusion are often present during palpation of the knee joint. Stability of the knee is also an important area of assessment. The valgus stress test and varus stress tests are used to assess the stability of the LCL and MCL and the Drawer and Lachman stress tests are used to assess the stability of the ACL and PCL (Figures 60-6 through 60-9).

Diagnostic Tests

Plain radiographs are used when a clinically significant fracture is suspected. MRI is used to view both the soft tissue and the bone to further confirm the diagnosis of a ligament injury.

Nursing Diagnoses

Based on the information gathered, examples of nursing diagnoses, interventions, and outcomes in the patient with ligament injury include:
- Acute pain
- Impaired physical mobility
- Anxiety

Planning and Implementation

The goal of treatment is obtaining the best functional level possible. Return to preinjury status and ability to participate in high level sport activity is an indicator of successful treatment (Kvist, 2004). Immediately following the injury, ice and elevation are recommended until the patient can be seen by a health care professional. The decision to treat the ligament tear by conservative measures versus surgical repair involves consideration of many factors, such as severity of the tear, patient's age, level of athletic activity, occupation, and lifestyle expectations. Conservative treatment includes RICE and rehabilitation. Severe ACL tears are usually treated with surgical repair.

Early rehabilitation is the key to success whether or not the treatment plan includes surgical repair or conservative treatment with the rehab program being similar to both groups (Souryal & Adams, 2005). Early range-of-motion, strengthening, and flexibility exercises are the cornerstone of the rehab program. The patient must be committed to the program to achieve a successful outcome and return to preinjury status.

Surgery

Surgical repair of the ACL can be performed either by arthroscopy or by open incision. Repair may include reconstruction of the ACL by using a piece of the patellar tendon or a portion of the hamstring muscle. In some cases a synthetic material is used. Recommending that the patient wear a brace when involved in strenuous sport activity remains controversial. The theory behind this practice is that the brace will protect the knee from recurrence of a ligament injury, However, McDevitt, et al. (2004) showed that there was no difference in the rate of recurrence of injury with or without functional bracing.

Patient and Family Teaching

Successful rehabilitation requires a commitment from the patient. Teaching the patient and family on why it is important to follow the program and not to participate in activities until cleared by the health care provider is needed to gain the full benefit of the therapy program.

Evaluation of Outcomes

Potential patient outcomes for each of the example nursing diagnoses for the patient with knee ligament injury are:

- Acute pain: The patient should verbalize an adequate relief of pain along with the ability to realistically cope with the pain if it is not completely relieved.
- Impaired physical mobility: The patient should perform physical activity independently or with assistive devices as needed. In addition, the patient should be free of complications of immobility, as evidenced by intact skin, absence of thrombophlebitis, and normal bowel patterns.
- Anxiety: The patient should be able to recognize the signs of anxiety, demonstrate positive coping mechanisms, and describe a reduction in the level of anxiety experienced.

The main complication of a knee ligament injury is symptomatic instability of the knee, which may inhibit the patient from participating in competitive sports at the same level prior to injury. Chronic instability may also cause damage to the other structures of the knee, such as the menisci and the articular surfaces of the joint, which may lead to osteoarthritis.

MENISCAL INJURIES

The menisci are crescent-shaped pieces of fibrocartilage found inside of the knee joint. The function of the menisci are to absorb the loading forces the knee joint experiences during movement and weight bearing and aid in maintaining the stability of the joint.

Epidemiology

The incidence of acute meniscal tears is 60 per 100,000, with a 60 percent incidence of degenerative meniscal tears after age 60 years.

Etiology

Meniscal injuries are caused by a rotational force as the flexed knee is moving toward extension. When the foot is planted, the femur is internally rotated and a valgus force is applied to the flexed knee, the medial meniscus is at risk for injury. If the femur is externally rotated and a varus force is applied, the lateral meniscus is at risk. The medial meniscus is injured more often than the lateral. The reason for this has to do with the way the menisci are attached inside the joint capsule. The medial meniscus is more tightly tethered to the tibial plateau and therefore is less able to move when a force is applied. Because of this, it is torn more easily than the lateral meniscus. The peripheral third of the meniscus has minimal blood supply, which limits its ability to heal when torn or injured. The most common location of injury is in the posterior section, with longitudinal tears being the most common type. A history of a previous meniscal injury predisposes the menisci to additional injury from a lesser force than in a healthy knee. Also with aging the menisci start to degenerate, placing them at higher risk for tears and injury (Miller, 2003).

Assessment with Clinical Manifestations

If a specific traumatic event caused the symptoms, a detailed history of the trauma, with positioning of the leg, foot, and knee is helpful in determining a diagnosis. The patient may remember hearing a popping or tearing sound at the time of the injury. If the tear is degenerative, the onset of pain may be more gradual, or it may have been caused by minimal movement such as rising from a squatting position (Miller, 2003). Symptoms can include pain over the area of the injury, swelling, stiffness, locking, catching or popping of the knee, and buckling of the knee.

During the physical assessment, the most common finding is tenderness along the joint line. Inspect the knee for joint effusion, comparing it with the contralateral knee. Meniscal injuries usually accompany ligament injuries, so stability of the knee should also be assessed (refer to section on ligament injuries).

Diagnostic Tests

Plain radiographs are used to rule out fractures and other possible causes of symptoms, but they are of little value in diagnosing torn menisci. MRI is highly specific and sensitive in the diagnosing of a tear.

Nursing Diagnoses

Based on the information gathered, examples of nursing diagnoses, interventions and outcomes in the patient with meniscal injuries include:
- Acute pain
- Impaired physical mobility
- Anxiety

Planning and Implementation

The goals of treatment are to return the patient back to preinjury status and restoring full strength and range of motion to the knee. Traumatic meniscal tears are usually treated with surgical repair. If the tear is small and of degenerative origin, conservative treatment is tried first. Conservative treatment includes the use of RICE, with strict activity restriction. A knee immobilizer is used for four to six weeks or until the pain and swelling has subsided. Once this occurs rehabilitation can begin. If the pain and swelling continue and locking of the knee is present surgery is considered.

During conservative treatment isometric exercises are used to maintain strength of the leg and to help in the rehabilitation process once the brace is removed (Miller, 2003). During the rehabilitation phase, the focus is on quadriceps strengthening and range of motion. Full return to participation in sports is usually three to six months (Miller, 2003).

For small tears, surgery usually entails suturing of the tear or partial removable when suturing is not an option. It is performed by arthroscopy and on an outpatient basis. Removal of the entire meniscus is avoided when possible due to the risk of developing osteoarthritis later in life (Englund, Roos, & Lohmander, 2003; Miller, 2003).

The patient teaching focuses on the rehabilitation program and ways to protect the knee from future injury. Following the therapy and exercise regimen is stressed to get the patient back to preinjury state. Explaining to the patient theory behind the rehabilitation will help in compliance. Strategies for future injury prevention includes having strong thigh and hamstring muscles, stretching before and after exercise, wearing shoes that fit properly and that are appropriate for the activity the patient is doing, and when skiing, ensuring that ski bindings are set correctly by a trained professional so that skis release with a fall.

Evaluation of Outcomes

Potential patient outcomes for each of the example nursing diagnoses for the patient with meniscal injuries are:

- Acute pain: The patient should verbalize an adequate relief of pain along with the ability to realistically cope with the pain if it is not completely relieved.
- Impaired physical mobility: The patient should perform physical activity independently or with assistive devices as needed. In addition, the patient should be free of complications of immobility, as evidenced by intact skin, absence of thrombophlebitis, and normal bowel patterns.
- Anxiety: The patient should be able to recognize the signs of anxiety, demonstrate positive coping mechanisms, and describe a reduction in the level of anxiety experienced.

ANKLE SPRAIN

Ankle sprain is extremely common, occurring at a rate of one injury per 10,000 people per day (Struijs & Kerkhoffs, 2005). They occur in both athletes and nonathletes and in people of all ages.

Etiology

The ligaments of the ankle act as stabilizers by preventing the ankle from movements, such as twisting, turning, or rolling of the foot. When the ankle is displaced or a sudden force is applied the ligaments are stretched beyond their normal stretching capacity and a sprain of the ligament occurs. The most common type of ankle sprain is a lateral sprain. The mechanism of injury is a combination of plantar flexion and inversion. Medial ankle sprains are less common but can occur with excessive eversion and dorsiflexion of the foot.

Ankle sprains are categorized according to severity (Table 60-1.)

TABLE 60-1 Ankle Sprain		
GRADE OF SPRAIN	**TYPE OF TEAR**	**SYMPTOMS**
Grade I (mild)	Partial tear	No instability
		Mild tenderness, minimal swelling
		Able to bear weight and walk
Grade II (moderate)	Partial disruption of one or more ligaments	Mild instability
		Tenderness and swelling more diffuse
		May or may not be able to bear weight
Grade III (severe)	Complete disruption of at least one ligament	Moderate to severe instability
		Severe swelling inability to bear weight

Source: Gehrig, L. (2005). Sprained ankle. Retrieved on September 26, 2005, from http://orthoinfo.aaos.org/.

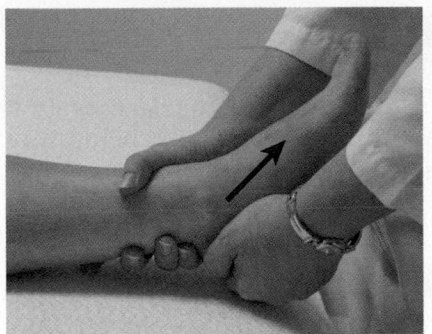

Figure 60-10 Anterior drawer test.

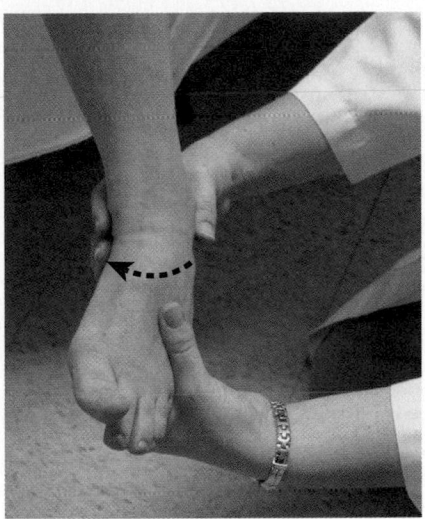

Figure 60-11 Inversion stress test.

Assessment with Clinical Manifestations

Assessment begins with a history of how the injury occurred. The patient may remember hearing a pop or a snap at the time of injury. Have the patient describe the exact motion of the foot and ankle and the position of the foot before and after the traumatic event. It is also important to ask about previous injuries to the ankle. In chronic ankle problems little force is needed to reinjure the ligaments.

The physical examination begins with observation of the joint for any gross deformities that may indicate a fracture. The amount of swelling is best determined 24 hours after the initial injury. Minimal swelling immediately after the injury may not be a reliable indication of the severity of the injury. Physical assessment should also include neurovascular status, range of motion, and presence of crepitus. Palpation of the ankle will reveal tenderness. The anterior **drawer test** and the **inversion stress test** are used in determining the stability of the ankle joint (Figures 60-10 and 60-11).

Diagnostic Tests

Plain radiographic films are useful in ruling out fractures in the ankle and foot, but are only indicated when a fracture is suspected by the presence of tenderness in the posterior half of the lower fibula and tibia or in the fifth metatarsal and if the patient is unable to bear weight. For symptoms that persist for more than six weeks, a computed tomography (CT) or a MRI is indicated to further rule out other complications.

Nursing Diagnoses

Representative nursing diagnoses for the patient with an ankle sprain include:
* Acute pain
* Impaired mobility

Planning and Implementation

The immediate goals of treatment are to prevent swelling and to maintain range of motion to the ankle joint. Immediate interventions include RICE. The amount of weight bearing to the ankle will be determined by the amount of pain. Crutches may be needed for two to three days to allow for rest of the ankle joint and to relieve pain. For more sever sprains cast boots or air splints may be used. Ice should be immediately applied. Apply for 20 to 30 minutes three to four times a day. An elastic bandage should be used to further reduce the amount of swelling and to provide support to the joint. Finally, the ankle is elevated above the level of the heart for the first 48 hours after injury to facilitate venous and lymph drainage.

Rehabilitation starts at one or two weeks after the injury. The focus is on restoring the range of motion and strengthening the ankle joint to prevent complications of chronic instability. Proprioception and flexibility training is also important improve balance and to prevent recurring injury to the joint.

Complications usually result from returning to activities too soon and not allowing the ankle to fully heal. Complications may include abnormal proprioception, imbalance, weakness, and instability of the ankle joint. A chronic ankle sprain is defined as frequently respraining of the ligaments and having symptoms for more than four to six weeks. Surgery may be indicated if the joint remains unstable after several months of conservative treatment.

Pharmacology

Anti-inflammatory drugs, such as NSAIDS, may be used to control pain and inflammation.

ACHILLES TENDON INJURIES

The Achilles tendon is the strongest tendon in the body (McGuigan & Aierstok, 2005). It absorbs large stresses during running and jumping. The tendon itself moves in two directions, lengthening and concentric contracting. This puts it at a higher risk for injury and degenerative changes.

Epidemiology

Tendon ruptures occur in men three times as often as in women. The peak incidence of rupture is in middle age.

Etiology

Injury to the Achilles tendon is seen in athletes that participate in activities that require a lot of running, jumping, and stop and go movements, such as tennis and basketball. Tendonitis is seen more commonly seen in runners from overuse and repetitive loading of the tendon. Rupture of the tendon is more commonly seen in tennis and basketball players. Many ruptures are also seen in middle age adults who lead sedentary lives who participate in physical activity (Koike, et al., 2004). There has also been a link between the use of fluoroquinolone antibiotics and Achilles tendonitis.

Pathophysiology

The Achilles tendon is located in the posterior distal third of the lower extremity. It attaches the calf muscles to the calcaneus. The blood supply to the distal portion of the tendon is poor, which predisposes this area to a higher incidence of injury. Tendonitis is seen more often in the proximal portion of the tendon and is two to three times more common than rupture (McGuigan & Aierstok, 2005). Tendonitis can result from a sudden and persistent change in the tightness of the tendon. This change causes pain and inflammation. An example of this is a woman who routinely wears high-heeled shoes and begins to wear athletic shoes while doing physical activity

Rupture of the tendon is thought to be caused by a combination of earlier injury and degenerative and regenerative changes (Koike, et al., 2004).

Assessment with Clinical Manifestations

A detailed history of the pain is necessary to make a accurate diagnosis. Tendonitis initially causes pain after physical activity. If the patient continues with activity the tendonitis will progress and cause pain during physical activity (Koike, et al., 2004). Patient with a rupture may describe a sharp severe pain and hearing a popping sound at the time of injury followed by difficulty walking.

The ankle, foot, and tendon should be inspected for deformity and swelling. On palpation, tenderness, local heat, crepitation, and a possible nodule may be present. With a rupture a gap between the tendon and the heel may also be palpated. The Thompson test is used to help in diagnosis of a rupture. The foot will normally plantar flex when the calf is squeezed just distal to the maximum girth. In a patient with a ruptured tendon the foot does not plantar flex (Koike, et al., 2004).

Diagnostic Tests

A plain radiographic film will not pick up a tendon injury. If the tendonitis is chronic, calcium deposits may be seen (McGuigan & Aierstok, 2005). MRI is often used and will show inflammation, tearing, and degenerative changes.

However, ultrasound may be the best method of visualizing the tendon because of the availability and low cost (Koike, et al., 2004).

Nursing Diagnoses

Nursing diagnoses for a patient with an injury to the Achilles tendon include:
- Acute pain
- Impaired mobility

Planning and Implementation

Treatment of tendonitis begins with resting the tendon. A heel lift or fracture boot is often used to decrease the stress on the tendon (McGuigan & Aierstok, 2005). **Cryotherapy** (cold therapy) is also used to decrease inflammation and swelling. Early treatment is crucial in preventing chronic tendonitis, which may predispose the patient to a rupture.

Tendon rupture is also treated nonoperatively. The patient is placed in a cast or brace with the foot in plantar flexion for up to six weeks. Surgical repair is indicated when the tendon ends have receded and in athletes who want to retain strength and power with plantar flexion (Koike, et al., 2004). Surgical treatment also requires cast immobilization. Physical therapy is a crucial part of the treatment plan if the patient is to return to preinjury state. The exercise regimen focuses on strengthening of the lower leg and ankle (McGuigan & Aierstok, 2005). Rehabilitation usually takes five to six months.

It is important to teach the patient the importance of following the treatment course. It may be difficult for athletes to abstain from activity to rest the tendon. However, it is important for the athlete to understand the consequences of too much activity, which may include chronic tendonitis and rupture. Once the rehabilitation phase is over, it is important to teach the patient the importance of proper warm up and conditioning before participation in high-impact sports and running to prevent another injury.

There is no hard evidence in the literature to support a consensus in the treatment of acute and chronic tendonitis (McLauchlan & Handoll, 2005). However, the goal of treatment is to return the patient back to preinjury status. This goal may be more important for an athlete than for the average individual.

Pharmacology

NSAIDs are usually helpful in the treatment of tendonitis. Steroid injections are not recommended (McGuigan & Aierstok, 2005).

Evaluation of Outcomes

Potential patient outcomes for each of the example nursing diagnoses for the patient with tendonitis are:
- Acute pain: The patient should verbalize an adequate relief of pain along with the ability to realistically cope with the pain if it is not completely relieved.
- Impaired mobility: The patient should perform physical activity independently or with assistive devices as needed. In addition, the patient should be free of complications of immobility, as evidenced by intact skin, absence of thrombophlebitis, and normal bowel patterns.

PLANTAR FASCIITIS

Plantar fasciitis is a common cause of heel pain and mobility problems from young athletes to the elderly.

Etiology

The exact cause of plantar fasciitis is unknown, but many factors may be involved. Risk factors include obesity, low arches (pes planus), reduced dorsiflexion of the ankle, and occupations that require prolonged standing (Roxas, 2005). In athletes, risk factors can include running on hard surfaces, changing the intensity or duration of an exercise or training program, and improper footwear. In the elderly, poor muscle strength of the foot and ankle and a decrease in the body's ability to heal may also play a role.

Pathophysiology

The plantar fascia extends from the heel to the toes. When the arch of the foot is flattened during walking or running the fascia is stretched. Plantar fasciitis is thought to be a degenerative process from repeated trauma that has caused microinjuries or microtears to the fascia. Inflammation of the fascia may or may not be present.

Assessment with Clinical Manifestations

The diagnosis of plantar fasciitis relies on a detailed history of symptoms. Most patients will report heel pain that is usually worse in the morning or after a prolonged period of inactivity. The pain tends to improve through out the day but may increase again at night, especially if the patient is on his or her feet all day. Recent changes in a training or exercise program, foot wear, and weight should also be explored.

The patient may experience pain and tenderness with palpation of the heel and foot. The pain may be exacerbated by passive dorsiflexion of the toes or by having the patient stand on their tip toes. Signs of inflammation, such as swelling, redness, and warmth in the area, may or may not be present.

Diagnostic Tests

Plain radiographs and bone scan may be useful in ruling out other causes of heel pain, such as a stress fracture of the heel. However, the diagnosis of plantar fasciitis is usually based on clinical assessment alone.

Nursing Diagnoses

Representative nursing diagnoses for the patient with plantar fasciitis include:
* Acute pain
* Impaired mobility

Planning and Implementation

Plantar fasciitis is considered a self-limiting condition, which means that even without treatment the symptoms will subside. However, it can take 6 to 18 months before plantar fasciitis is resolved. Because of this, treatment is focused on relieving the symptoms and returning the patient back to original baseline. Treatment begins with rest, avoidance of intense weight-bearing activity, avoidance of walking barefoot on hard surfaces, and replacing old footwear with better fitting footwear. Ice may also be use to reduce pain and inflammation after activity.

Physical and occupational therapy play a major role in the treatment of plantar fasciitis. Stretching and strengthening programs can help to correct functional risk factors, such as muscle weakness and inflexibility of the foot and ankle. Night splinting and orthotics may also be useful in more severe cases.

Vitamin C and zinc are essential components in connective tissue repair; therefore, a deficiency may contribute to changes seen in plantar fasciitis.

More research is needed to discover the full impact of vitamin C and zinc in plantar fasciitis (Roxas, 2005).

The surgical intervention of a plantar fascia release is performed only when all other therapies have failed. Complications that can occur with surgical intervention include nerve damage, which may cause a small amount of numbness to the heel area, wound infection, and osteomyelitis. An acquired flatfoot deformity may also develop requiring the patient to wear supportive footwear with good heel support.

Pharmacology

Oral NSAIDs may be useful in temporarily relieving the pain and inflammation, however, they are not curative (Roxas, 2005). Corticosteroid injections are usually given for chronic heel pain that has not responded to conservative treatment. There are many risk factors and potential complications with the use of locally injected corticosteroids, such as weakening and rupture of the fascia and atrophy of the fat pad that cushions the heel (Tallia & Cardone, 2003).

Teaching begins with the treatment course. It is important for the patient to truly rest the foot and avoid intense weight-bearing activity, to be successful in resolving plantar fasciitis. Teaching proper stretching before and after intense weight-bearing activity may be useful in preventing plantar fasciitis from recurring. Also, selecting proper footwear, which offers good arch support and cushioning may also prevent a recurrence of plantar fasciitis.

Evaluation of Outcomes

Potential patient outcomes for each of the example nursing diagnoses for the patient with plantar fasciitis are:

- Acute pain: The patient should verbalize an adequate relief of pain along with the ability to realistically cope with the pain if it is not completely relieved.
- Impaired mobility: The patient should perform physical activity independently or with assistive devices as needed. In addition, the patient should be free of complications of immobility, as evidenced by intact skin, absence of thrombophlebitis, and normal bowel patterns.

STRESS FRACTURES

Stress fractures are a common sports-related injury. They are most commonly seen in the metatarsals and tibia, and less commonly in the fibula, calcaneus, femur, and pelvis. Stress fractures in the upper extremities and in the ribs are not as common as in the lower extremity. Stress fractures of the tibia occur in the distal third of the bone and are more common in activities that involve running and jumping. Stress fractures in the metatarsals occur most frequently in the distal second or third metatarsals. These fractures are commonly seen in military recruits and in runners. Stress fractures of the calcaneus are often misdiagnosed as plantar fasciitis. They can occur at any age and are a common cause of chronic heel pain. Stress fractures of the femur are often seen in endurance athletes and are difficult to diagnosis. They also have a high incidence of complications, such as nonunion, complete fracture, and avascular necrosis (Sanderlin & Raspa, 2003). Stress fractures that occur with normal activity are called insufficiency fractures and are caused by an underlying bone disease, such as osteoporosis.

Epidemiology

Stress fractures are more commonly seen in track and field sports. In one study, 20 percent of track and field athletes developed a stress fracture, and these stress fractures made up 20 percent of the total injuries experienced by these athletes. Many studies have also shown that stress fractures occur more often in women, especially in those who diet or exercise to the point of amenorrhea. Stress fractures tend to recur. In one study 60 percent of those with a stress fracture had a history of a previous stress fracture.

Etiology

Stress fractures frequently occur in preseason training or when there is a rapid increase in the amount or speed of activity or training or a significant increase in distance with running. They are seen in athletes who participate in tennis, track and field, gymnastics, and basketball. For risk factors, see Box 60-3.

Pathophysiology

Stress fractures occur as a result of repetitive use injury. There are two theories that may explain the development of stress fractures. The first theory is when there is an increase in activity there is a delay in the remodeling of the bone cells. The osteoclasts eats away the old bone, but the osteoblasts take a few weeks to lay down new bone cells. During this period the bone may be more at risk for microfractures, which can go on to form stress fractures. The second theory focuses on the repetitive stress on the bone at the insertion point of the muscles which can stress the bone to the point of fracture (Sanderlin & Raspa, 2003).

Assessment with Clinical Manifestations

The assessment begins with a detailed history of the pain. The patient may report an insidious onset of pain that is dull with activity. The pain usually subsides with rest and returns with the causative activity. The patient usually cannot remember a specific incidence of trauma to the injured area. Exploring recent changes in exercise and training programs can also offer clues that the injury is a stress fracture.

Palpation will reveal local tenderness at the fracture site. Redness and swelling may also be observed. The pain may be reproducible with weight bearing or with stress to the injured bone.

Diagnostic Tests

Plain radiographs may not reveal a fracture until two to four weeks after injury (Martinez & Tsai, 2004). Bone scans and MRI are more sensitive in detecting stress fractures (Martinez & Tsai, 2004; Sanderlin & Raspa, 2001).

Nursing Diagnoses

Nursing diagnoses for the patient with a stress fracture include:
- Acute pain
- Impaired mobility

Planning and Implementation

The goals of treatment focus on conservative therapies to returning the patient back to preinjury state or in the case of an athlete, back to participating in sport activity. The first step is resting the involved bone for six to six weeks. This includes complete avoidance of the activity that causes pain or a significant reduction of that activity followed by a gradual return (Martinez & Tsai, 2004). Substitution of a non–weight-bearing exercise or activity may be used to allow the athlete from becoming deconditioned, such as swimming. Patients who experience pain with walking may be placed in a walking cast or a short leg brace to achieve rest.

Rehabilitation consists of a stretching and flexibility program, cross training, and a gradual return to the offending activity. The use of air casting may be beneficial in returning the athlete to preinjury state sooner (Rome, Handoll, & Ashford, 2005).

Surgery is indicated for stress fractures that are displaced or that fail conservative treatment as indicated by nonunion or delayed union. The best cure for stress fractures is prevention (Box 60-4).

Pharmacology

There is some controversy on whether anti-inflammatory drugs should be used in the treatment of stress fractures. There is thought that to heal properly the bone needs to go through an inflammatory process. The use of NSAIDs may in fact lead to a higher incidence of nonunion. More research is needed in this area before a definitive decision can be made (Wheeler & Batt, 2005).

Evaluation of Outcomes

Potential patient outcomes for each of the example nursing diagnoses for the patient with stress fractures are:

- Acute pain: The patient should verbalize an adequate relief of pain along with the ability to realistically cope with the pain if it is not completely relieved.
- Impaired mobility: The patient should perform physical activity independently or with assistive devices as needed. In addition, the patient should be free of complications of immobility, as evidenced by intact skin, absence of thrombophlebitis, and normal bowel patterns.

FRACTURES

A **fracture** is defined as any disruption in the continuity of a bone. The fracture can result from a direct blow or from an indirect force. A fracture occurs when the bone is exposed to more stress than it can absorb. The amount of force or stress needed to cause a fracture depends on several factors including size and density of bone, the type and mount of force, and individual biological factors, such as age and underlying disease. As an individual gets older, bone becomes more brittle, and less force is needed to cause a fracture. A pathological fracture occurs when bone is weakened by an underlying disease process, and the force needed to cause a fracture is less than what is needed for normal, healthy bone. Refer to Box 60-5 for causes of pathological fractures.

Epidemiology

According to the National Center for Health Statistics, 17,789 deaths in 2002 were attributed to fractures (2004). Between the years 2000 and 2002 the average annual number of emergency department visits for nonfatal fractures was 3,894,000 with 992,000 of these patients requiring hospitalization.

Pathophysiology

Fractures are classified by how they look on a plain radiograph and by clinical assessment. Anatomy is used to describe the bones involved, the location within the bone and if any articular surface was involved. Description also includes any displacement, angulations, or rotations that may have occurred as seen on the radiograph. Shortening, fragmentation, and soft tissue involvement are also included in the description of a fracture (see Figure 60-12 for types of fractures).

Fractures can be classified as complete or incomplete. A complete fracture is a break across the entire section of bone producing two bone fragments. An incomplete fracture occurs through only one cortex of the bone. Fractures are also described as closed or open. A closed fracture has intact skin over the site of injury while an open fracture has a break in the skin over the injury, which may have been caused by the mechanism of injury or the bone fragments themselves. An open fracture places the patient at a higher risk for infection because of contamination of the wound. See Table 60-2 for classification of types of open fractures.

Complications of fractures can be divided into immediate and delayed complications. Immediate complications include shock, fat, embolism, compartment syndrome, deep vein thrombosis, pulmonary embolism, and infection.

Delayed complications include joint stiffness, malunion, delayed union, nonunion, and refracture. Joint stiffness can result from edema, joint contractures, and immobilization. It is most common in fractures that involve the upper extremities. Malunion occurs when the fracture has healed in an abnormal position or alignment. It is caused by improper reduction or inadequate immobilization. A malunion can impair how the bone functions in several ways. It can cause irregular weight bearing in a joint, which can lead to arthritis. If the malunion occurs in the lower extremities it can interfere with the patient's gait, balance, and coordination (Whittle, 2003). Many malunions do not impede function and therefore are not surgically repaired even if a visual deformity is present. Surgical repair is considered when a deficit in function is present.

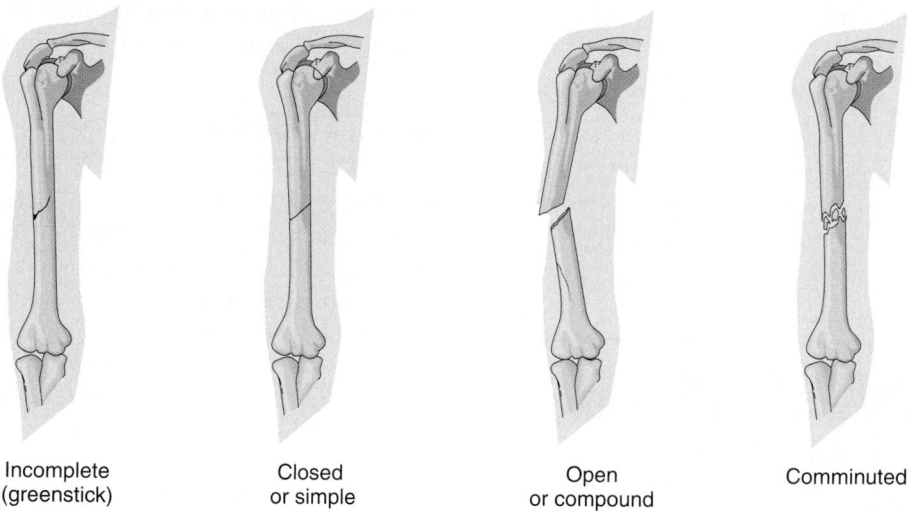

| Incomplete (greenstick) | Closed or simple | Open or compound | Comminuted |

Figure 60-12 Types of fractures.

TABLE 60-2	Classification of Open Fractures
Type I	Length of wound less than 1 cm, low-energy injury, clean
Type II	Length of wound longer than 1 cm, low-energy injury, clean
Type III	Length of wound longer than 1 cm with significant soft tissue damage, fracture is comminuted, high-energy trauma
Type III A	Sufficient soft tissue to cover bone, no reconstruction surgery is needed for closure
Type III B	Damage to soft tissue is extensive requires reconstruction surgery for wound closure
Type III C	Any open fracture associated with arterial damage. Requires involvement of vascular surgeon.

Delayed union is diagnosed when healing has not advanced for three months to one year after the fracture has occurred. It is usually treated with a cast that allows as much function of the limb as possible. In the lower extremities a snug walking cast is often used that will promote healing (Lavelle, 2003). Delayed union can be a sign of infection or in the case of internal fixation a fracture at the site of the fixation. Once the cause is identified and solved, conservative treatment is usually successful (Lavelle, 2003). If conservative treatment fails, then the delayed union is treated as a nonunion.

A nonunion is when healing at the site of the fracture has ceased and union is highly unlikely. Factors that may lead to nonunion are a poor metabolic or nutritional state, overall poor health, low activity level, tobacco or alcohol intake, and having an open fracture. Surgery is required for healing to take place. The fragments are realigned and a bone graft is inserted. Another option for treatment of certain types of nonunion and malunion is the use of external fixation to achieve solid union and to correct any deformities and limb-length discrepancies caused by the nonunion or malunion (Katsenis, Bhave, Paley, & Herzenberg, 2005).

Assessment with Clinical Manifestations

Assessment begins with emergency management and the basic principles of trauma care. The initial primary assessment focuses on the general condition of the patient, which includes airway maintenance, bleeding or shock management, and stabilization of any life-threatening injuries. In multiple traumas, most fractures are not life-threatening so their management is a second priority. Once the patient is stabilized, assessment of the fracture can begin with focus on neurovascular status and pain (Keany, 2005). The mechanism of injury and a detailed description of the accident can help determine the nature and extent of the fracture and can also lead to injuries that otherwise might be missed.

Physical assessment starts with observing for any ecchymosis, edema, deformity, or other soft tissue injury, which may point to a possible fracture site. Other abnormal findings may include muscle spasms, tenderness, pain, numbness, loss of function, abnormal movement, or crepitus. If a femur or hip fracture is suspected the lower extremity may appear shortened and externally rotated (Keany, 2005). Assessment for hypovolemic shock should be completed when a femoral, tibial, or pelvic fracture is suspected because of the possibility of high-volume blood loss and the risk for exsanguinations. Signs and symptoms of hypovolemic shock include hypotension, tachycardia, tachypnea, and dyspnea.

A peripheral neurovascular assessment should be performed and documented on a frequent basis. This comprehensive examination should include a vascular assessment, comparing color, temperature, capillary refill, peripheral pulses, and edema of the involved extremity to the contralateral extremity whenever possible. The peripheral neurological examination includes assessing sensation and function. Assessment of pain is also important in determining the location of injury and the severity. Pain will increase in severity until the fracture is mobilized.

Diagnostic Tests

Radiographs should include the joint above and below the suspected fracture in order to see the extent of the injury. The patient who has sustained multiple trauma should also have a CT scan of the chest and pelvis to rule out the possibility of further injury.

Nursing Diagnoses

Nursing diagnoses for the patient with a stress fracture include:
- Acute pain
- Impaired mobility

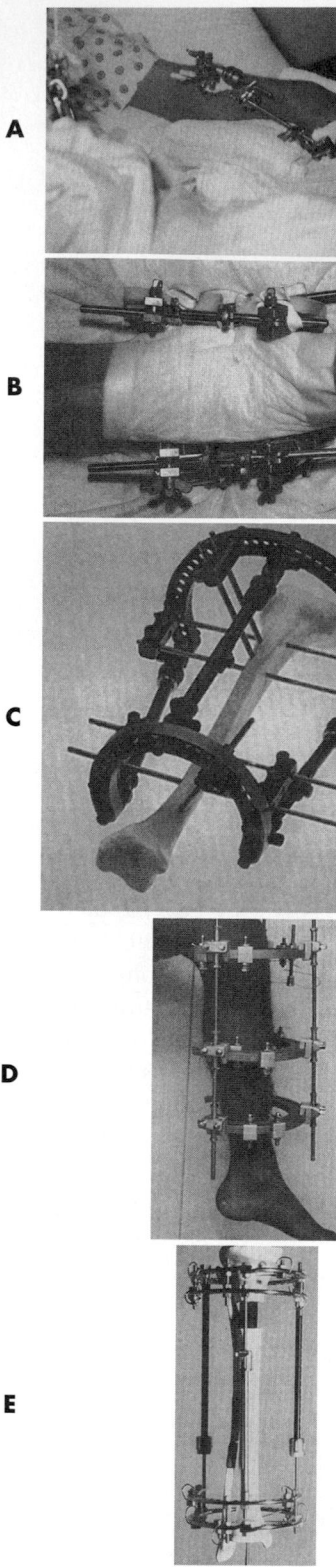

Figure 60-13 Examples of external fixation devices: A. Hoffman external fixation to the forearm, B. To the tibia and fibula, C. Ace-Fischer external fixator, D. Monticelli-Spinelli external fixator, E. Ilizarov external fixator.

Planning and Implementation

The primary goals for fracture management are the prevention of complications and the return to preinjury state. In emergency treatment, the first step is covering any open wounds or fractures with a sterile normal saline dressing to control bleeding and prevent further contamination. The next step for a closed or open fracture is splinting. Whenever possible, this should be accomplished before moving the patient. The purpose of splinting is to minimize bleeding, edema, and pain. Splinting can also prevent further injury to the tissues and structures surrounding the fracture, such as nerves, vessels, muscles, and tendons. Complications from improper handling or splinting can include increase bleeding, a significant increase in pain, and a decrease in sensation and function, which may be temporary or permanent. The incidence of fat embolism and shock are also increased.

Depending on the type of fracture, location, and other associated injuries, treatment may include closed or open reduction, internal or external fixation, amputation, or a combination of the above. If the fracture is stable and the bone fragments are properly aligned, the patient is placed in a splint or cast to maintain alignment as healing occurs.

Management of a displaced fracture starts with reduction. Reduction is the manipulation of bone segments to obtain proper natural alignment of the bone involved. It can be a painful procedure; therefore, local anesthesia or sedation may be required. Reduction can be accomplished by several different methods. Closed reduction is when manual traction is applied to move the bone segments back into alignment. Realignment is confirmed with a radiograph and then a splint or cast is applied to keep the bone segments in place. When a cast or splint is applied it usually immobilizes the joint below and above the fracture site to maintain immobilization of the fracture segments.

Open reduction is the realignment of bone segments under direct visualization through an incision. Open reduction is indicated for fractures with multiple bone segments, for widely separated bone segments, or when there is soft tissue in between the bone segments. For unstable fractures casts may not be adequate in maintaining bone alignment. Complications of not maintaining proper alignment include nonunion, delayed union, or displacement of the fracture segments. Casts also immobilize the muscles and joints next to the fracture site causing weakness, wasting, stiffness, and contractures (Gugenheim, 2004). Because of these disadvantages, internal fixation is often used for unstable fractures. Internal fixation is a surgical procedure where the surgeon implants metal wires, plates, rods, pins, screws, or nails to support the bone directly. Open reduction and internal fixation is contraindicated when there is an active infection, fractures that have multiple bone fragments, or severe osteoporosis. There are several disadvantages to internal fixation as well. It is an invasive procedure and introduces a foreign body into the patient. It is also difficult to eliminate contamination in open fractures and places the patient at higher risk for infection. It also can cause osteoporosis of the bone directly surrounding the hardware because of stress shielding (Gugenheim, 2004).

Another option in the treatment of fractures is external fixation (Figure 60-13). External fixation is the use of percutaneous pins or wires that is connected to a rigid external frame. The advantages of external fixation are listed in Box 60-6.

Patient and Family Teaching

Patient and family education begins with the type of injury and treatment options. Once a treatment option is chosen, education focuses on the treatment plan, normal bone healing, care of immobilization devices (e.g., splints, casts, external fixators), use of assistive devices, and signs and symptoms of complications.

It is important to assess the patient's and family's readiness to learn. Look for teachable moments, when the patient and family are most ready to learn. This is

BOX 60-6

ADVANTAGES OF EXTERNAL FIXATION

Minimally invasive procedure

Allows for acute and gradual fracture reduction

Immediate motion of the joints above and below the fracture

Direct visualization of soft tissue

Allows for treatment of soft tissue injuries surrounding fracture

Can be used to treat chronic infections, contractures, limb length discrepancy, acute nonunion fractures, or fractures with extensive soft tissue injury

Once healing has been accomplished, the pins or wires and external frame are removed leaving no foreign material in the extremity

Adapted from Gugenheim, J. J. (2004). External fixation in orthopedics. Journal of the American Medical Association, 291, *2122–2124.*

Uncovering the Evidence

Discussion: The National Association of Orthopaedic Nurses (NAON) has developed this guideline to present evidence-based recommendations for the care of the skin around the skeletal pin site using current knowledge gleamed from critical reviews of research literature and from expert opinion. CINAHL and MEDLINE databases were searched from 1995 through mid-2004. Only seven studies were found that linked a method of pin site care to infection rates. These studies were diverse in populations studied and definitions of infection. Therefore, the authors concluded through a meta-analysis of these studies that there is insufficient evidence on which to recommend a particular pin site care method. The evidence did provide a basis for recommendations on several actions over others until more specific answers are offered through additional research. The use of the expert panel also provided a basis for these recommendations as well. These recommendations are:

- Pins located in areas with considerable soft tissue should be considered at greater risk for infection.
- After the first 48 to 72 hours (when drainage may be heavy), pin sites care should be done daily or weekly for sites with mechanically stable bone-pin interfaces.
- Chlorhexidine 2 mg/mL solution may be the most effective cleansing solution for pin site care.
- Patients or their families should be taught pin site care before discharge from the hospital. They should be required to demonstrate whatever care needs to be done and should be provided with written instructions that include signs and symptoms of infection.

Implications for Practice: Nursing implications from this study is to be more diligent in pin site care in areas where there is more soft tissue, perform pin site care on a routine basis either daily or weekly, use of chlorhexidine 2 mg/mL as the preferred solution and to make sure the patient and family is knowledgeable in pin site care and in knowing what signs and symptoms to report to the orthopedic surgeon.

Source: Holmes, S. B., & Brown, S. J. (2005). Skeletal pin site care: National Association of Orthopaedic Nurses guideline for orthopaedic nursing. Orthopaedic Nursing, 24(2), *99–107.*

usually when the patient's pain is best controlled and the level of distraction is low (Hohler, 2004). Start with assessing what the patient already knows and build on it, giving information in small amounts so the patient and family have time to absorb the information and think of questions. Teaching is a team effort, passing on to the next nurse where the patient and family is in their educational needs will help to provide continuity. It is also important to evaluate what the patient and family has learned. This is best achieved by asking open-ended questions.

Physical therapy and occupational therapy play pivotal roles in the rehabilitation and in the prevention of complications. The physical therapist will teach the patient the proper technique for using assistive devices, such as walkers or crutches. Exercises are also important to build and maintain muscle strength and endurance. The occupational therapist's role is important in making sure the patient is as independent as possible with activities of daily living. There are many aids that may help the patient maintain his or her independence with dressing, such as dressing sticks, shoe horns, sock aids, and reachers.

PATIENT PLAYBOOK

Casts

The nurse can instruct the patient to care for their cast by the following:

Plaster casts

The type of cast hardens within 5 to 10 minutes, but may take two to three days to completely dry.

To move or reposition the cast, use the palms of your hands to prevent denting the cast.

Place the cast on a soft, flexible surface to prevent the cast from flattening until fully dry.

Reposition the cast every 2 hours to help the cast dry.

If weight bearing is allowed, do not do so until the cast is completely dry, usually about 48 hours.

Keep the cast dry.

Synthetic casts (Fiberglass)

The type of cast will harden rapidly, so you can bear weight (if allowed) within 30 minutes after application.

If the surface of the cast is rough, a sock or stockinette can be applied to protect the skin on the opposite limb, and to prevent it from snagging on clothes or blankets.

It can be immersed in water but check with your health care provider first. To dry the cast, use a hair dryer on a low heat setting.

Helpful hints for both types of casts

If you are not allowed to get the cast wet, protect it well with a waterproof covering, such as plastic bag. Place a cloth at the top of the cast and tape the plastic bag into place.

If the cast does become wet or damp, dry it using a towel and a hair dryer on a low heat setting.

Elevate the limb above the level of the heart whenever possible to decrease swelling.

Do not scratch under your cast or poke anything down into the cast to scratch. The skin under the cast can become irritated and an infection can develop. Instead, if itching occurs, try knocking on the cast or use a hair dryer on a low heat setting.

Inspect the cast daily, looking for cracks, soft spots, excessive flaking, or flattening.

When to call the physician

Numbness or tingling to the fingers or toes or any part of the limb.

Extreme pain not relieved by prescribed medication.

Extreme tightness of the cast.

Swollen or discolored fingers or toes.

Cracks, soft spots, or any other problems with the integrity of the cast.

Foul odor from the cast.

Hot spots which may point to an infection.

Source: Altizer, L. (2004). Casting for immobilization. Orthopedic Nursing, 23(2), 136–141.

Evaluation of Outcomes

Potential patient outcomes for each of the example nursing diagnoses for the patient with fractures are:

- Acute pain: The patient should verbalize an adequate relief of pain along with the ability to realistically cope with the pain if it is not completely relieved.
- Impaired mobility: The patient should perform physical activity independently or with assistive devices as needed. In addition, the patient should be free of complications of immobility, as evidenced by intact skin, absence of thrombophlebitis, and normal bowel patterns.

HIP FRACTURES

Hip fractures are one of the most serious health consequences of falls and are the most frequently seen injury requiring hospitalization. The problem is on the rise and is only expected to become a larger health concern for several reasons. First of all the general life expectancy of the general population is increasing along with the escalation of the total number of people over the age of 65. Secondly, the number of people age 65 or older living in nursing homes is also rising. In 1997, 1.5 million people lived in nursing homes, and by 2030 that number is expected to increase to 3 million. In 2002, nearly 13,000 people over the age of 65 and older died of fall-related injuries. Many, if not most, of these falls, and the injuries caused by the fall, are preventable. When a hip fracture occurs in people younger than 50 years of age it is usually the result of contact sports, industrial accidents, or motor vehicle accidents. This type of trauma is classified as high energy as compared to a fall, which is a low-energy trauma. Osteoporosis is a major contributing factor to the cause of hip fractures from falls. Low bone mineral density is one of the most consistent risk factors in predicting hip fractures in older women. In one study women with a low bone mineral density were three times more likely to sustain a hip fracture than women who had a higher bone mineral density. See chapter 59 for more information on osteoporosis. However, the normal aging process may also have a component in the cause of hip fractures as well. As a person ages and is less active, there is not as much mechanical load to the femur. This causes the bone to thin and weaken making a hip fracture more likely (Mayhew, et al., 2005). Other factors that increases fracture risk include lack of physical activity or exercise in the last year, reduced vision, and a fall within the last year.

Epidemiology

Based on the 2000 census, there are 360,000 to 480,000 fractures a year that are fall-related. This equals to about one in three people over the age of 64 falling each year. Women are more likely to sustain a hip fracture from a fall at a rate of 4:1. Caucasian men have the highest death rate because of a fall, followed by Caucasian women, African American men, and African American women.

Pathophysiology

The hip is classified as a ball-and-socket joint. The classification of hip fractures is based on the anatomical location of the fracture within the hip. The fracture may occur in the femoral head, neck, intertrochanter, subtrochanter, or acetabular area. Treatment depends on the location of the fracture. With a femoral neck fracture, blood supply to the femoral head may be disrupted placing the patient at risk for avascular necrosis (AVN) and degenerative changes to the femoral head especially if the fracture is displaced. Therefore this type of fracture is treated with a hemiarthroplasty. With a hemiarthroplasty, the entire head and neck of the femur is replaced with an implant. If the fracture is not displaced internal fixation with a cannulated screw is the treatment of choice (Altizer, 2005). Intertrochanteric fractures are usually repaired with a nail fixation. Subtrochanteric fractures are usually treated with an intramedullary nailing.

Complications

Infection can severely disrupt the patient's rehabilitation. Function and range of motion to the affected joint or bone can be compromised. The fracture healing process slows or stops completely, because the cells normally involved in fracture repair are now focused on fighting the infection. Patient characteristics that may increase the risk of infection include diabetes mellitus, nicotine use, steroid use, malnutrition, prolonged preoperative hospital stay, and a perioperative blood transfusion.

Inspection and observation of the incision area includes looking for erythema, edema, drainage, and tenderness. Another clue that an infection may be present is the presence of persistent pain in the joint area especially with movement (Altizer, 2005). Other signs and symptoms may include elevated sedimentation rate (ESR), progressive narrowing of the joint space on X-ray, loss of bone density, or loosening of the internal fixation devices (Altizer, 2005).

Assessment with Clinical Manifestations

Assessment begins with a history of the fall and a general medical history, including past fractures and presence of osteoporosis.

The physical assessment starts with the basics of trauma care. Refer to the section on fractures for detailed information. The fractured extremity is usually shortened and externally rotated. There may also be bruising and swelling in the groin area and inner thigh. A neurovascular assessment is critical in making sure that there is no compromise of the nerves or blood vessels in that extremity.

Diagnostic Tests

Radiographs should include a two-dimensional view of the hip including a right-angle view of the site to diagnosis the anatomical location of the fracture. An oblique view may also be helpful in determining any rotation and the extent of displacement (Altizer, 2005). The views should also include the joint above and below the site of injury to rule out any further fractures. Not all hip fractures are easily diagnosed with an X-ray. An **occult fracture** is defined as a fracture that does not show up on plain radiographic films until the healing process begins and calcification is seen. If the patient is experiencing hip pain, difficulty bearing weight, and difficulty ambulating, a nuclear bone scan or a MRI may be useful in determining the presence of a fracture (Lubovsky, Liebergall, Mattan, Weil, & Mosheiff, 2005). CT has not been proven to be effective in the diagnosis of occult hip fractures (Lubovsky, et al., 2005). Failure to diagnose the fracture can lead to serious consequences, including displacing of a stable fracture and a longer, more complicated surgery and rehabilitation.

Nursing Diagnoses

Nursing diagnoses for the patient with a hip fracture include:
- Acute pain
- Impaired mobility

Planning and Implementation

The goal of treatment is to return the patient back to his or her preinjury level of functioning. This is completed by surgical intervention and an intensive rehabilitation program.

Physical therapy and occupational therapy play important roles in helping the patient achieve preinjury state. The patient will need an exercise program to strengthen the muscles of the injured extremity as well and to increase endurance. Teaching the patient the correct use of assistive devices and providing dressing tools will help the patient regain independence.

Patient and family teaching should focus on fall and fracture prevention. If the patient is returning to the community, either to his or her own home or to a family member's home, interventions can include gait training and a long-term exercise program, review of current medications focusing on the use of psychotropic medications, and use of proper assistive devices. For patients going to a long-term or assisted living, interventions also include staff education programs. To further reduce the risk of falls, the environment should be assessed and hazards removed. Things that can be done to decrease the risk of falling include removing throw rugs and clutter in the hallway, placing nonslip mats on the shower floor, installing grab bars next to the toilet and shower, installing handrails on both sides of stairs, and improving the lighting throughout the house and outside in the garage and porch. The patient should also see his or her health care provider yearly for a routine assessment of risk factors and should have his or her vision tested yearly as well. A bone mineral density test should be completed and measures taken to raise levels if they are low.

Evaluation of Outcomes

Unfortunately the prognosis for recovery from a hip fracture is not always positive. Patients who are age 75 and older are four to fives times more likely to be admitted into a nursing home for a year or longer. Many patients never get back to their preinjury level and sustain complications because of immobility, such as pneumonia, pulmonary embolism, and future fall-related injuries. Half of older adults who suffer a hip fracture never regain their previous level of functioning and an estimated 13,000 people die each year from complication of a hip fracture.

Potential patient outcomes for each of the example nursing diagnoses for the patient with a hip fracture are:

- Acute pain: The patient should verbalize an adequate relief of pain along with the ability to realistically cope with the pain if it is not completely relieved.
- Impaired mobility: The patient should perform physical activity independently or with assistive devices as needed. In addition, the patient should be free of complications of immobility, as evidenced by intact skin, absence of thrombophlebitis, and normal bowel patterns.

COMPARTMENT SYNDROME

A compartment is an area in the body where muscles, nerves, and blood vessels are enclosed within tissue, such as bone or fascia. **Fascia** is a nonelastic connective tissue that covers and separates muscles, tendons, and ligaments.

A total of 46 compartments are found throughout the body with a total of 36 found in the limbs. The most common compartments affected are the anterior compartment of the leg and the volar compartment of the forearm. Acute **compartment syndrome** can be caused by either an increase in the amount of contents inside the compartment or a decrease in the size of the compartment itself. Pressure inside the compartment can be caused by trauma especially fractures of the tibia and other long bones, severe crush syndrome, and hypotension. Peripheral vascular disease also increases the risk of compartment syndrome. See Box 60-7 for a list of causes of acute compartment syndrome.

Chronic or exertional compartment syndrome is seen with exercise and overuse that cause inflammation and edema. It is seen in long distance runners, new military recruits, or patients who have made a major change in activity. The result is an increase in pressure, which causes an aching pain and tightness. It is usually relieved by rest and rarely causes permanent damage.

The rest of this section discusses acute compartment syndrome only.

Pathophysiology

When there is an increase in pressure inside the compartment no matter the cause, the result is ischemia, which causes damage to the nerves, muscles, and blood vessels. This causes a secondary elevation in the venous pressure, which obstructs blood outflow. This viscous cycle will evidentially increase pressure inside the compartment to the point that it supersedes arterial pressure, and the compartment is left without a blood supply. If the blood flow is not returned within a period of time usually four to eight hours, the structures inside the compartment will die. The result is a Volkman's contracture (Figure 60-14).

BOX 60-7

CAUSES OF ACUTE COMPARTMENT SYNDROME

Trauma

Fractures

Crush injuries

Hypothermia

Snake or spider bites

Burns

External pressure

Positioning

Tourniquets

Tight dressings

Casts

Splints

Excessive traction

Bleeding

Vascular injury

Coagulopathies

Venous obstruction

IV infiltration

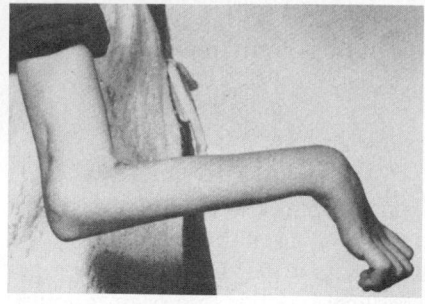

Figure 60-14 Volkman's contracture.

Assessment with Clinical Manifestations

Signs and symptoms may occur as soon as 30 minutes after the ischemia begins. Early recognition of the signs and symptoms are critical in preserving the limb. The classical symptoms include the 6 P's: pain, paresthesia, paresis, pressure, pallor, and pulselessness. The two earliest symptoms are pain disproportionate to the injury especially on passive stretching on the long muscle inside the affected compartment and a change in sensation distal to the ischemic compartment. Late symptoms include pallor, paralysis, tight or rigid compartment, and pulselessness. Neurovascular and pain assessments should be performed at least every four to eight hours for all orthopedic patients and more often, such as every one to two hours in the immediate postoperative phase. The health care provider should be notified right away if the patient develops any of the signs or symptoms of compartment syndrome.

Diagnostic Tests

Direct measurement of the pressure inside the compartment can confirm diagnosis. The measurement can be preformed by a wick, continuous infusion, or by an injection method.

A normal compartment pressure is 0 to 10 mm Hg. Compartment syndrome is diagnosed when the diastolic pressure minus the intracompartment pressure is less than or equal to 30 mm Hg.

Goals

The primary goal is prevention. This includes making sure that edema and bleeding within the compartment is minimized by preventing motion at the fracture site and minimizing soft tissue damage. This can be accomplished by splinting, traction, early closed reduction with casting, and when needed, early internal fixation. Elevating the limb to the level of the heart will also help to decrease edema in the affected limb. Elevation above the level of the heart is contraindicated, because this makes it more difficult for arterial blood flow to enter into the compartment.

Once compartment syndrome is suspected the goals of treatment include relieving the pressure in the compartment, restoring blood flow back to the structures inside the compartment and preserving the function of the limb. If the patient has a constrictive cast, splint, or dressing, the first step in relieving pressure and restoring blood flow is to bivalve the cast and loosen the underlying dressings or splints. Ice should be avoided once compartment syndrome is suspected, because it will further decrease blood flow and mask symptoms of pain. Fluid balance should also be monitored carefully, and fluids replaced as needed to ensure an adequate blood volume and arterial pressure. If the above interventions do not relieve the pressure in the compartment, a **fasciotomy** is the next step. A fasciotomy is the surgical opening of the fascia that surrounds the affected compartment. The incision is usually done length wise and the wound is left open to allow the contents of the compartment to decompress. Wet dressings are applied, and once the swelling subsides closure is accomplished. Complications of a fasciotomy include loss of fracture stabilization, necrosis of the bone, delayed union or nonunion, and infection.

FAT EMBOLISM SYNDROME

Fat embolism syndrome (FES) is seen following trauma in the presence of long bone fractures, pelvic fractures, multiple fractures, and intramedullary manipulation during internal fixation procedure. The most common causes are fractures of the pelvis, femur, tibia, or ribs (Fort, 2003). FES occurs when fat globules are released into the bloodstream and travel to the lungs and brain where they produce ischemia and inflammation. It is a serious complication of trauma and can lead to acute respiratory insufficiency, thrombocytopenia, deteriorating mental status, and death. The incidence of FES is 1 to 2 percent with tibia or femoral shaft fractures. The incidence rises to 5 to 10 percent when there are fractures of both the tibia and femoral shaft or multiple fractures as seen in pelvic fractures. The mortality rate ranges from 10 to 20 percent (Kirkland, 2005).

Pathophysiology

There are two different theories on the cause of FES. The first theory is that fat globules are released from the marrow of injured bone or injured soft tissues and enter the venous circulation through torn veins at the site of injury. The fat droplets deposit in other parts of the body including the lungs, brain, kidney, retina, or skin and cause damage to these areas. The second theory is a biochemical theory, and it proposes that hormonal changes due to trauma trigger the release of free fatty acids into the circulation, such as chylomicrons, a type of lipoprotein. The chylomicrons join together to form fat globules that deposit through out the body. This theory helps to describe how nontraumatic FES can occur (Goer & Lacey, 2005; Kirkland, 2005).

The severity of FES depends on the amount of fat released into the circulation and the overall health of the patient. The patient is at high risk for hypovolemia, shock, hypoxia, and right-sided heart failure.

Assessment with Clinical Manifestations

The most critical period for the occurrence of FES is 24 to 72 hours after the injury. The classical symptoms are hypoxemia, changes in mental status, and petechiae on the upper body. Seizures may also occur. Rales or rhonchi may be auscultated throughout the lung fields. Other signs and symptoms may include use of accessory muscles, tachypnea, dyspnea, restlessness, apprehension, anxiety, agitation, or confusion (Fort, 2003). Gurd's criteria are used to diagnosis the presence of FES. It is named after a health care provider who established the system for diagnosing FES (Box 60-8).

Diagnostic Tests

Arterial blood gases will show an initial drop of the $PaCO_2$ due to hyperventilation, but as the compensatory mechanisms fail, $PaCO_2$ will rise and metabolic acidosis will occur.

Chest x-ray (CXR) films will show diffuse bilateral infiltrates. CT scan of the brain may show diffuse fatty infiltrates as well.

Planning and Implementation

The first priority is to prevent FES from occurring. This includes proper splinting of the fractured long bone, avoiding unnecessary handling of the fracture, and early reduction. Other ways to protect the lungs is to have the patient cough and breathe deeply and regularly to minimize atelectasis and improve pulmonary function, provide adequate oxygenation, maintain adequate hydration to prevent shock, protect kidneys, and prevent mobilization of fat, and record baseline assessments and frequently assess patient for changes in condition (Goer & Lacey, 2005).

Once FES develops, treatment is supportive and focused on preserving oxygenation. Supplemental oxygen is provided and intubation and mechanical ventilation may be necessary. Prevention of shock is another focus. Maintaining adequate circulatory volume is a must. Adequate blood pressure is also critical to ensure that the body is receiving the necessary oxygen. Hypotension is treated immediately and aggressively.

BOX 60-8

GURD'S CRITERIA FOR DIAGNOSIS OF FES

The diagnosis is made in the presence of one major and three minor criteria or in the presence of two major and two minor criteria.

Major Criteria

Nonpalpable reddish brown petechial rash over upper body in a vest distribution

Respiratory symptoms: hypoxia with a PaO_2 less than 60 mm Hg, pulmonary edema, bilateral CXR changes, tachypnea, and dyspnea

Cerebral changes: agitation, seizures, or coma

Minor Criteria

Tachycardia

Temperature greater than 101.3° F (38.5° C)

Retinal hemorrhages

Fat globules in the urine or sputum

Sudden decrease in hemoglobin and hematocrit levels and platelet count

Increase in sedimentation rate

VENOUS THROMBOEMBOLISM

Deep vein thrombosis (DVT) and pulmonary embolism (PE) together are known as venous thromboembolism (VTE). They are major causes of morbidity and mortality in the orthopedic patient. A thrombosis is a blood clot in a vessel, when this clot breaks off and travels through the circulatory system to the lungs it is called a PE. The rate of fatal PE in orthopedic patients who do not receive any antiembolism prevention is 40 percent in total joint replacements or multiple trauma patients. Risk factors are based on Virchow's triad: trauma to the vessel, venous stasis, and hypercoagulability (Box 60-9).

Pathophysiology

Virchow's triad, which is damage to vessels, venous stasis, and hypercoagulability, contributes to the formation of the thrombosis. Injury to the vessel initiates the clotting cascade and platelet aggregation. Venous stasis develops from immobility caused by the injury itself or by the treatment. This causes the clotting factors to accumulate. Finally, the injury itself or the surgical treatment can cause hemorrhage, shock, or hypothermia, which modifies the coagulability of the blood (Fort, 2003).

Assessment with Clinical Manifestations

The diagnosis of a DVT can be difficult. The signs and symptoms are often nonspecific, and some patients have no signs or symptoms at all. The most common symptoms are pain and tenderness at or below the site of the thrombosis. The patient may describe the pain as aching, cramping, sharp, dull, severe, or mild. During the physical assessment, swelling at or below the site of the thrombosis may be present. If tenderness or pain is associated with the presence of swelling, a DVT may be present. The site may also be red and warm to touch. Homans' sign is not a reliable predictor of the presence of a thrombosis.

The signs and symptoms of a PE include unexplained dyspnea and chest pain. Other signs and symptoms may include hypoxia, apprehension, confusion, and anxiety. Breath sounds are often diminished, but rales and wheezes may also be heard. Cough, fever, diaphoresis, and hemoptysis are other less common symptoms.

Diagnostic Tests

Venous ultrasound is a sensitive and accurate diagnostic test in diagnosing the presence of a DVT. It is noninvasive and can be preformed at the bedside. Venous Doppler is also done at the bedside and is noninvasive, but it is not as sensitive and may provide false readings. Other available diagnostic tests include venography and impedance plethysmography. Both have disadvantages and are not used as often as the ultrasound and Doppler methods.

A ventilation/perfusion (V/Q) scan is often the first test ordered when a PE is suspected. The gold standard is a pulmonary angiogram, but the V/Q scan is less invasive and readily available. The V/Q test measures two areas. The first is ventilation. During this part, the patient inhales a radiolabeled gas and then X-rays are taken looking at the distribution of the gas throughout the lung fields. The second part looks at the perfusion to the lung fields. This involves injection of radiolabeled albumin into the circulatory system and X-rays are taken to show the distribution of blood flow to the lungs. A normal V/Q scan can effectively rule out a PE. Large perfusion defects that do not show up on the ventilation scan are associated with a high probability for a PE.

Planning and Implementation

The primary goal is the prevention of the DVT. This is achieved by using a mechanical form and an anticoagulant method of prophylaxis (Geerts, et al., 2004). The mechanical methods include early ambulation, elevation of the foot of the bed with the knees in extension, ankle exercises, graded compression elastic stockings, and intermittent external pneumatic compression devices. Anticoagulation choices include warfarin, unfractionated heparin, low molecular weight heparin, and aspirin. Aspirin alone is not recommended without a mechanical method (Geerts, et al., 2004).

One a DVT is suspected, the treatment goals turn to preventing additional clots, and to prevent the movement of the clot to the lungs (PE). The traditional therapy for a DVT is intravenous (IV) unfractionated heparin (Fort, 2005). This requires frequent monitoring and blood tests to monitor the level of the activated partial thromboplastin time (APTT). Platelet counts are also monitored for the presence of thrombocytopenia. Low molecular weight heparins are now being used as well in the treatment of a DVT. They do not require the IV access or the high level of monitoring as unfractionated heparin does, so often the patient does not need to be in an acute hospital setting. Oral warfarin is started within 24 hours after heparin therapy is initiated. The therapeutic international normalized ratio (INR) is 2 to 3, with a goal of 2.5. Patients receiving anticoagulants need to be monitored carefully for signs and symptoms of bleeding. This includes changes in mental status and monitoring stool, urine, and emesis for the presence of blood. The patient is usually on bedrest until a therapeutic APTT is achieved. Elevation of the leg is recommended, but the use of other mechanical devices, such as compression stockings and pneumatic devices, should be stopped to prevent a PE.

Treatment of a PE includes anticoagulation with unfractionated heparin. Even though it does not have the ability to dissolve clots, it prevents new clots and emboli. Oral warfarin is started within three days of initiation of heparin therapy. Thrombolytic therapy may also be indicated in the presence of a large PE. Thrombolytic therapy hastens clot lysis, promotes pulmonary tissue reperfusion, and can reverse right-sided heart failure. Other treatments include insertion of a vena cava filter and a pulmonary embolectomy.

AMPUTATION

Amputation is the oldest of surgical procedures. Advancements in surgical technique and prosthetic design have been motivated by the consequences of war. There have also been major advances in microvascular surgery, antibiotic therapy, treatment for musculoskeletal tumors, and orthopedic reconstructive surgery that have allowed for limb salvage in many cases where amputation would have been performed in the past. The only absolute indication for amputation is irreversible ischemia either caused by disease or trauma.

Epidemiology

According to the latest information from the National Limb Loss Information Center ([NLLIC]2002), there are approximately 1.2 million people living in the United States without at least one limb and about 185,000 hospital discharges related to an amputation every year. The number of new cases of amputation is highest in the diabetic patient population with 1 in every 185 diabetic patients undergoing an amputation of a digit or limb (NLLIC, 2002). Congenital limb deficiency rate is 2.6 per 10,000 live births (NLLIC, 2002).

Etiology

The most frequent indication for elective lower extremity amputation is peripheral vascular disease, with over half of the amputations attributed to diabetes mellitus (National Limb Loss Information Center, 2002). Trauma is the leading cause of amputation in the younger population and is more common in men because of higher exposure to vocational and recreational hazards. Amputation may also be indicated in thermal or electrical burns, severe frostbite, and gangrene. Malignant tumors may also warrant amputation, but this is less common because advances in limb salvage. Refer to chapter 60.

Pathophysiology

In peripheral vascular disease the muscle group involved (usually the calf muscle) does not receive adequate arterial blood supply either caused by obstruction or occlusion. In diabetes mellitus, this is caused by arteriosclerosis. This will evidentially lead to irreversible ischemia. In trauma, every effort is made to salvage the limb, with the only absolute indication for amputation being irreparable vascular injury.

A hematoma may form at the incision site and can delay wound healing and can also predispose the patient to infection. A hematoma can be prevented by using a drain for the first 24 to 48 hours after surgery and by using a dressing with good compression to the stump. If a hematoma does develop, it is treated conservatively with a compression dressing. If this fails the patient may be taken back to surgery to evacuate the hematoma.

Infection is also another risk associated with amputation. It is more commonly seen in patients with peripheral vascular disease, especially those with diabetes mellitus. Antibiotics can be used, but a debridement may be necessary to manage the infection.

Assessment with Clinical Manifestations

If the amputation is from chronic disease, the patient's history should include past medical history to find the cause of the amputation or impending amputation. If the cause is because of peripheral vascular disease, assess the patient for a history of intermittent claudication which includes pain (usually in the calf muscles) with activity that is relieved by rest. Also ask the patient about the presence of pain in the toes and feet at rest that improves with placing the extremity in a dependent position. If the cause is from trauma or burns, the mechanism of injury is obtained.

Physical examination starts with a thorough neurovascular assessment of the affected extremity and also of the opposite extremity. Refer to chapter 59 for instructions on how to perform a neurovascular assessment. Further assessment should include observing for discoloration of the ankles, edema, skin integrity, presence of ulcerations, presence or absence of hair on the legs, and presence of any necrosis or gangrene. Another assessment technique is the elevation-dependency test, which assesses collateral arterial blood supply. If there is a sudden blanching with elevation and significant redness when the leg is placed in a dependent position, poor collateral circulation is present (Chojnowski, 2005).

After the amputation, the postoperative assessment should include pain level, limb color, temperature, and presence of drainage and edema. Inspect the stump, making sure the stitches or staples are intact and the incision is well approximated. Mild serosanguineous drainage, edema, and inflammation may be expected, but if there is excessive edema or drainage, heat, or odor, an infection may be suspected and the health care provider should be contacted.

Diagnostic Tests

A noninvasive diagnostic test commonly used is the ankle-brachial index. This test compares the blood pressure of the arm with the leg using a Doppler ultrasound device (Rice, 2005). The most common invasive test is the angiogram. During an angiogram, radiopaque dye is injected into a blood vessel and then radiographs are taken in rapid succession to determine the size and shape of the vessel.

Nursing Diagnoses

Based on the information gathered, examples of nursing diagnoses in the patient with an amputation may include the following:

- Acute pain
- Impaired physical mobility

Planning and Implementation

With vascular disease the goals of treatment is to restore the circulation to the limb (femoropopliteal bypass) if this fails and additional bypass surgery is not possible, or the patient's pain cannot be controlled then amputation is the next step. The goal of treatment then becomes providing the patient with the highest level of functioning. To achieve this, the amputation is preformed at the most distal level that has sufficient blood supply to allow for healing.

In the traumatic amputation, the primary goal is to salvage and reattach the limb. Many guidelines and scoring systems have been established to aid in determining, which limbs are salvageable. One of the most widely used scoring system is the mangled extremity severity score (MESS) (Table 60-3).

When the amputation is performed due to trauma, the contaminated tissue must be derided and irrigated to reduce the risk of infection. Often this type of amputation will be left open to allow further debridement, and skin flaps are closed at a later time. If there is not enough tissue to create flaps to close the wound, bone revision and skin grafting may be necessary.

No matter if the amputation was caused by chronic disease, trauma, or other causes, the patient will need to adapt and accept the changes in physical appearance and functionality. Common reactions that patients may experience include postamputation depression, anxiety, feelings of vulnerability, and changes in body image, social support changes, and grief (Rybarczyk, Edwards, & Behel, 2004). Nurses are in a vital position to offer emotional support to the patient and family and to assess for depression and inadequate coping (Norris & Spelic, 2002). The patient should be encouraged to express his or her emotions and be allowed to convey grief. This will promote a full recovery by helping the patient reach his or her maximum functional level. Several factors may influence the progress and quality of coping. These include individual values and interpretations, access to health care technologies, social support, life experiences, and self-esteem (Norris & Spelic, 2002). Referrals for further treatment should be offered if the patient is struggling or exhibiting inadequate coping mechanisms. Information on local support groups and other resources should also be made available to the patient with the help of the social services department.

Patient and family teaching is crucial in the achievement of the treatment goals. The first decision the patient may need to make in a traumatic amputation is whether to attempt limb salvage (if this is an option) or to have an immediate amputation with a prosthetic fitting. With limb salvage the patient may need multiple surgical procedures to obtain soft tissue coverage. External fixation may also be necessary. Other possible complications with limb salvage are infection, nonunion, or loss of a muscle flap. The patient may also be at

TABLE 60-3 Mangled Extremity Severity Score

TYPE	CHARACTERISTICS	INJURIES	POINTS
A. Skeletal and Soft Tissue Injury			
1	Low energy	Stab wounds	1
		Simple closed fractures	
		Small caliber gunshot wounds	
2	Medium energy	Open or multiple fractures	2
		Dislocations	
		Moderate crush injuries	
3	High injury	Close range shotgun	3
		High-velocity gunshot wounds	
4	Massive crush	Logging, railroad, or oil rig accidents	4
		Gross contamination	
		Tissue avulsion	
B. Shock			
1	Normotensive	Blood pressure stable in field and in operating room	0
2	Transient hypotensive	Blood pressure unstable in field but responsive to intravenous fluids	1
3	Prolonged hypotensive	Systolic blood pressure less than 90 mm Hg in field and responsive to IV fluids only in operating room	2
C. Limb Ischemia			
1	None	Pulse present, perfusion normal	0[a]
2	Mild	Diminished pulses without signs of ischemia	1[a]
3	Moderate	No pulse by Doppler, sluggish capillary refill, paresthesia, diminished motor activity	2[a]
4	Advanced	Pulseless, paralyzed, and numb without capillary refill	3[a]
D. Age			
1	0–30 years		0
2	30–50 years		1
3	50+ years		2

[a]Points are doubled for ischemia greater than 6 hours.
Score less than 7 means that the patient has a salvageable extremity.
Score 7 or greater means that the patient has a nonsalvageable extremity.

higher risk for chronic pain, drug addiction, and greater financial difficulties. Even with all the advances in limb salvage, the patient also needs to realize that the procedure may fail and may require an amputation or the patient may end up with a limb that is not functional.

Care of the stump is important in preventing skin breakdown and to provide a good fit for the **prosthesis.** A daily skin care routine of cleansing and inspecting for redness, abrasions, and any skin breakdown is essential. Until the incision has healed the patient will need an analgesic about 30 minutes prior to stump care and dressing change. Instruct the patient to wash the stump with a mild soap and warm water. The stump must be dried thoroughly before applying a dressing, compressive bandage, or shrinking device. Often the patient can leave the stump open to air for about 10 minutes to allow the stump to dry completely. This time also allows the patient the opportunity to look at the stump and aid in acceptance. The next step in stump care is massage. This is performed on a routine basis as well to desensitize the residual limb. It also prevents adherence of the underlying tissue to the skin, which can cause complications once the prosthesis is worn. The patient should be encouraged to perform stump care and massage to increase the patient's independence and to help the patient accept the amputation. Immediately after surgery a sterile dressing is kept in place along with a compressive bandage. The compressive bandage should be applied using a figure eight method (Figure 60-15) with the greatest compression applied to the distal end of the stump to prevent edema. Instruct the patient to be cautious in using clips or pins in securing the compression dressing because of the risk of causing cuts or abrasions on the residual limb.

Before the patient is fitted for the prosthesis, a stump shrinker is used to decrease edema and to shape the residual limb for the prosthesis. To prevent other complications, such as hemorrhage, neurovascular damage, infection, abduction, external rotation, and flexion contractures, guidelines for positioning the stump must be followed. In the first 24 hours after surgery the limb

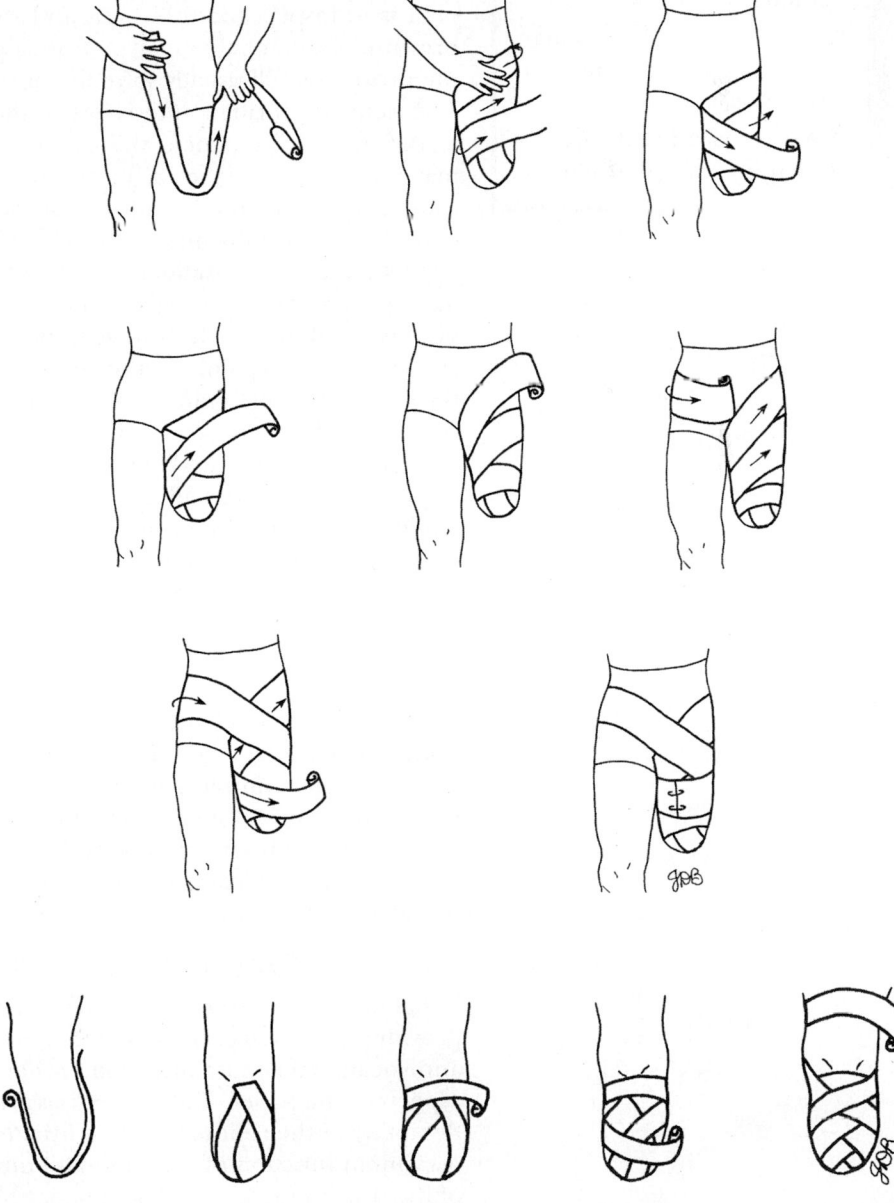

Figure 60-15 Illustration of a figure eight method of wrapping a stump.

BOX 60-10

GUIDELINES FOR POSITIONING A STUMP.

Keep residual limb elevated on a padded surface at the level of chair or toilet

Do not place pillows under the stump or bend the knee of the bed

Position legs close together

Change position every hour in a chair and every two hours in bed

Encourage use of trapeze

Lie flat on back several times a day for 10 to 20 minutes

Avoid use of pillow under stump, do not elevate past level of chair cushion

Avoid excessive hip abduction, flexion, or external rotation

can be elevated to reduce edema. After this initial period of time the stump should not be elevated or propped up with pillows because of the risk of causing contractures. A dependent position should be also avoided to help with circulation and prevention of increasing edema. While the patient is sitting in the chair or on the toilet the stump should be maintained on a padded surface at the same level as the chair or toilet. Instruct the patient to keep legs positioned together to prevent hip abduction. The patient should be encouraged to change position every hour while in the chair and every two hours while in bed. The patient can achieve this through using a trapeze. The patient should also be instructed to lie prone several times a day for 10 to 20 minutes to promote hip extension and prevent hip flexion contractures. A summary of guidelines is listed in Box 60-10.

Contractures can be prevented by good positioning. Refer to Box 60-10 for instructions on properly positioning the stump. If a contracture does occur, the prosthesis can be modified to adapt. In severe cases surgical release may be necessary.

There are several types of pain that the patient may experience after the postoperative pain has subsided. Residual limb pain or chronic stump pain may be because of several factors. The first step in assessing the cause of the pain is to inspect the prosthesis and stump. Look for any areas of abnormal pressure or edema that may indicate a poor-fitting prosthesis. Modification of the prosthesis will usually solve the problem.

A neuroma formation too close to the end of the stump can cause irritation to the nerve. The patient will experience a neuropathic type of pain, which may include burning, or a sharp shooting pain. Treatment starts with modification of the prosthesis and the use of pain medication, but if this is unsuccessful, the neuroma may need to be removed.

Phantom limb sensations are when the patient has the perception that the limb is there. They are not painful and should be expected. Over time the sensations will diminish. If these sensations are painful, then they are referred to as phantom limb pain. Most patients describe these pains as tingling, burning, throbbing, itching, cramping, stabbing, or shocking, and the pains are localized to the distal area of the limb (Talu & Erdine, 2005). The pain can be continuous or intermittent. Phantom limb pain is experienced by 50 to 80 percent of patients who have had an amputation. In many patients the pain will eventually dissipate, but for some it is ongoing. Various medications have been used in the treatment of phantom limb pain. Most narcotics are not useful because this type of pain is neuropathic in nature. The most commonly used drugs are antidepressants and anticonvulsants. Other medications that have been found effective are beta blockers, calcitonin, and ketamine. Other therapies that have been used in the treatment of phantom limb pain include nerve blocks, transcutaneous electrical nerve stimulation (TENS), acupuncture, neurostimulation, and neuroablation (Talu & Erdine, 2005). Other techniques include guided imagery, music therapy, biofeedback, and distraction. Although there is no psychological component in the cause of phantom pain, anxiety may increase the pain sensation because of the release of noradrenalin and adrenalin. Therefore, anxiolytic medications may be useful along with other stress reducing techniques to decrease this reaction.

Exercise, Physical, and Occupational Therapy

Rehabilitation is a true team effort and includes the patient, nurse, health care provider, prosthetist, physical therapist, occupational therapist, psychologist, and vocational counselor. A comprehensive approach is needed to address all aspects of the patient's life. Exercises are used to increase muscle strength and flexibility in the residual limb and the other extremities. The goal is to obtain maximum function of the residual limb as well as allowing for maximum use of the prosthesis. A pool program may help the patient achieve these goals and increase endurance, strength, balance, coordination, and mobility. The type of prosthesis chosen depends on the level of amputation, the patient's lifestyle and occupation, and patient preference. Age, agility, weight, endurance, general medical condition, and mobility are also considered. Gait training is initiated with the use of parallel bars and is progressed to crutches and then to a cane. Other important aspects of therapy are walking on uneven surfaces, mastering stairs, and learning how to fall and how to get up.

Evaluation of Outcomes

Potential patient outcomes for each of the example nursing diagnoses for the patient with an amputation are:

- Acute pain: The patient should verbalize an adequate relief of pain along with the ability to realistically cope with the pain if it is not completely relieved.
- Impaired physical mobility: The patient should perform physical activity independently or with assistive devices as needed. In addition, the patient should be free of complications of immobility, as evidenced by intact skin, absence of thrombophlebitis, and normal bowel patterns.

KEY CONCEPTS

- Unintentional trauma is the leading cause of death for Americans between the ages of 1 and 44.
- The initial treatment of sports related injuries consists of protection, RICE, and pain control.
- Patient teaching should focus on the importance of adherence to the rehabilitation schedule to achieve the best functional outcome.
- Treatment for a shoulder dislocation includes immediate closed reduction and immobilization for four to six weeks followed by rehabilitation.
- Surgical repair for a rotator cuff repair is indicated for partial-thickness and full-thickness tears in active patients once a six-month trial of conservative treatment as failed.
- The common signs and symptoms of carpal tunnel syndrome are paraesthesia, numbness, and a deep aching or throbbing pain that worsens at night to the area innervated by the median nerve (palmar aspect of the thumb, index finger, middle finger, and radial half of the ring finger).
- The most common complication after a knee ligament injury is instability of the knee.
- Meniscal injuries of the knee are caused by rotational forces as the flexed knee is moving toward extension.
- Achilles tendon injuries are most often seen in athletes whose sport or activity involves a great deal of running, jumping, and stop-and-go movements. The prognosis for an Achilles tendon rupture is good.
- Plantar fasciitis is a self-limiting condition; however, it may take 6 to 18 months before the symptoms resolve.

- Stress fractures can result from repetitive use or may be a result of an underlying pathological condition, such as osteoporosis.
- The primary goals in the management of a fracture are the prevention of complications and a return to preinjury states of function.
- The advantages of external fixation over internal fixation and immobilization with a cast include acute and gradual reduction, immediate mobility of adjacent joints, and direct visualization of soft tissues.
- Injuries from falls are a major health concern for the elderly population.
- In the elderly population the prognosis for a full recovery from a hip fracture is poor with many never returning to preinjury status.
- The first signs and symptoms of compartment syndrome are extreme pain with passive stretching and change in sensation distal to the affected compartment.
- The signs and symptoms of a PE are unexplained dyspnea, chest pain, and a feeling of apprehension or anxiety.
- Common reactions that a patient may experience after an amputation include depression, anxiety, feelings of vulnerability, changes in body image, and grief.
- It is important for the nurse to encourage the amputee to express his or her feelings and to provide the patient with additional resources, such as support groups.
- The majority of patients who have had an amputation will experience phantom limb pain; however, chronic phantom limb pain is rare.

REVIEW QUESTIONS

1. The home health nurse is teaching a patient with osteoporosis about reducing the risk for falls. Which of the following recommendations is not necessary to include in the teaching plan?
   1. Installing grab bars in the bathroom
   2. Use of nightlights
   3. Installing railings to both sides of stairs
   4. Removing wall-to-wall carpeting

2. A patient enters the emergency department for a lower leg injury. There is a visible deformity to the lower aspect of the leg, and it appears shorter than the other leg. The area is painful, swollen, and beginning to show signs of bruising. The nurse understands that the patient has experienced a:
   1. Contusion
   2. Sprain
   3. Fracture
   4. Strain

3. The nurse witnesses a patient fall in the bathroom, and the patient is now lying on the floor. The nurse suspects that the hip may be fractured. Which of the following interventions is of the highest priority of the nurse?
   1. Immobilize the leg before moving the patient
   2. Notify the patient's family of the fall
   3. Call the radiology department for an X-ray
   4. Reassure the patient that everything will be alright

4. Which of the following is *not* true concerning a plaster cast?
   1. The patient will need to keep the cast dry
   2. The patient will be able to bear weight on the cast in 30 minutes
   3. The cast can be elevated to the level of the heart
   4. The cast will give off heat as it dries

5. The patient has a fiberglass cast and asks the nurse when the patient will be able to walk on the cast. The nurse tells the patient:
   1. In 30 minutes
   2. In 8 hours
   3. In 24 hours
   4. In 48 hours

6. The nurse is assessing a patient with a fiberglass cast to the lower leg. Which of the following signs and symptoms is indicative of an infection?
   1. Coolness and pallor of the extremity
   2. Diminished pedal pulse
   3. Pain with passive stretching of toes
   4. Presence of a hot spot on the cast

7. Which of the following patients is at most risk for FES?
   1. A patient with a hip fracture
   2. A patient with a sprained ankle
   3. A patient with a mid shaft femur fracture
   4. A patient with a shoulder dislocation

8. Which of the following symptoms is not indicative of FES?
   1. Restlessness
   2. Decrease in pedal pulses
   3. Dyspnea
   4. Petechial rash over chest

9. Which of the following symptoms are early indicators of compartment syndrome?
   1. Pulselessness and pallor
   2. Swelling at the site and inability to move joints
   3. Fever and erythema
   4. Pain with passive motion and loss of sensation

10. Which of the following diagnostic tests is used for the diagnosis of a pulmonary embolism?
    1. Ventilation/perfusion scan (V/Q scan)
    2. CXR
    3. Nuclear bone scan
    4. MRI

11. Which of the following interventions is not appropriate for caring for a stump postoperatively?
    1. Allow patient to lay prone every day for 20 to 30 minutes
    2. Elevate the stump on two to three pillows
    3. Encourage patient to look at stump
    4. Remove and rewrap ACE bandage or elastic stump shrinker three to four times a day

REVIEW ACTIVITIES

1. Complete a rotation visit an outpatient rehabilitation facility. What type of injuries do the patients have? What treatments have they had? What type of exercises are they doing with the therapist? What activity restrictions do they have?

2. Complete a rotation visit to an emergency department that receives a high number of trauma patients. What kinds of trauma patients are seen? What treatments did the paramedics give the patients in the field? How did they immobilize any fractures that are seen?

3. Visit an inpatient orthopaedic unit. How many hip fracture patients are admitted? What is the ratio of hip fracture patients to other types of orthopaedic patients? Describe the type of hip fractures seen and the surgical treatment used to fixate the fractures. Does the surgeon give a rationale for the surgical treatment chosen? If not, list why you think that particular surgical treatment was chosen? Which surgical procedures require that the patient follow hip precautions?

4. Develop a teaching plan for an elderly patient who is at risk for falls. How do you personalize the plan for the individual patient? List some of the important questions you would ask the patient. What are the main elements of the teaching plan?

5. Perform a search of the local resources available for a patient who has recently undergone an amputation. How would you find these resources? What vital people would you ask? What Web sources are available? Who sponsors these sites? How can you tell if these sites are reliable sources?

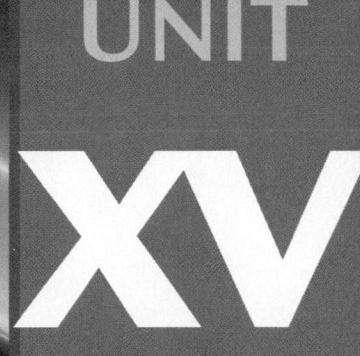

Alterations in Reproductive Function

Assessment of Reproductive Function

Mary Fry, PhD, RN

CHAPTER TOPICS

- Anatomy and Physiology of the Male and Female Reproductive Systems

- Sexual Response Cycle

- Assessment of Reproductive and Sexual Function

- Diagnostic Studies of Reproductive Function

Reproductive health assessment should be a part of every complete physical assessment. Reproductive health issues are relevant to lifestyle, healthy intimate relationships, and reproductive choices to bear children or prevent unintended pregnancies. Reproductive system dysfunction and disease take a high and costly toll in loss of life, infertility, and epidemic numbers of sexually transmitted infections, as well as the emotional stresses of **sexual dysfunction** and intimate relationship problems. Because of the sensitive nature of sexual concerns, health care providers must first become comfortable with their own sexuality and develop a professional manner in addressing sexual concerns with patients so that patients are able to initiate discussion of any reproductive health concerns they are experiencing.

ANATOMY AND PHYSIOLOGY

When comparing males and females, many of the structures and functions of the reproductive systems are more similar than different, with the exception of women's unique role of pregnancy and birth and the associated menstrual cycling. Healthy sexuality, sexual function, and reproductive function are integral with, and dependent on, overall health and emotional well-being.

Male Reproductive System

The primary functions of the male reproductive system are (a) production of sperm, (b) transport and deposit of sperm in the female reproductive tract, and (c) secretion of testosterone. The testes are the primary reproductive organs. Testosterone is necessary for the development of reproductive functions of **spermatogenesis** (formation of mature functional spermatozoa from the testes, usually beginning during puberty and continuing throughout the life of the adult male), sexual libido, and secondary sex characteristics of the male. The secondary reproductive organs are the ducts (epididymis, vas deferens, ejaculatory ducts, and the urethra), sex glands (prostate gland, bulbourethral gland, and seminal vesicles), and the external genitalia (scrotum and penis) (Figure 61-1).

Testes

The testes are two oval, firm, smooth organs that produce spermatozoa and testosterone. They are 4 to 5 cm long and 2 to 3 cm wide. The testes are suspended from the body by the spermatic cord, which contains the vas deferens and testicular blood and lymph vessels and nerves. Each testicle is covered by a sac derived from the peritoneum acquired during its descent from the abdomen during fetal development. Under the sac each testis is surrounded by a thick capsule of collagenous connective tissue. The posterior surface of

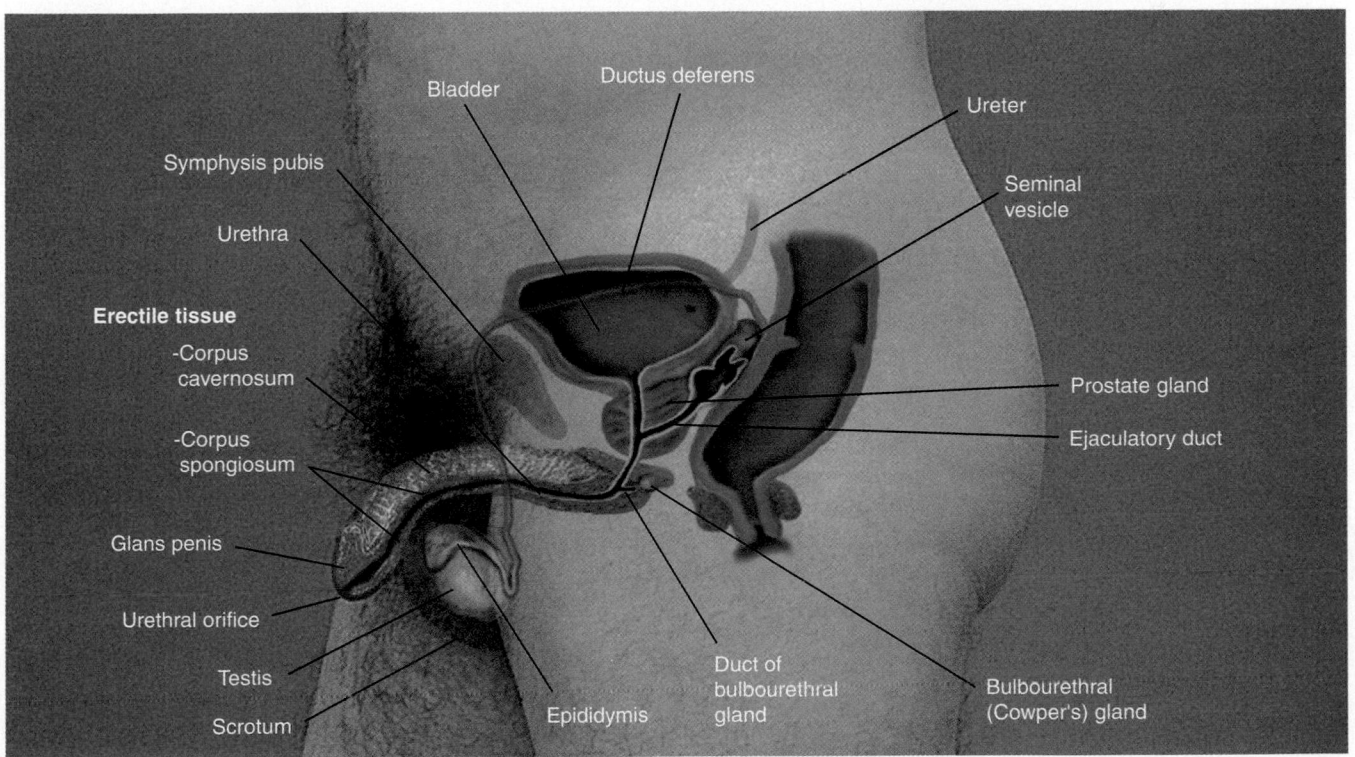

Figure 61-1 Male genitalia.

the sac is thickened to form the mediastinum from which septa extend into the gland to separate it into about 250 lobules. Each lobule is filled with 1 to 4 seminiferous tubules, connective tissue, vascular supply, lymphatic vessels nerves, and interstitial cells.

Spermatozoa are produced within the seminiferous tubules. The interstitial cells produce testosterone. Within each testis there are about 200 meters of seminiferous tubules accounting for 80 to 90 percent of the testicular mass. Seminiferous tubules contain a lining of germ cells and specialized Sertoli cells that partially envelop and nurture the developing **gametes** (a mature male or female reproductive cell). The Sertoli cells are joined to one another by tight junctions so that substances cannot freely flow from the blood to the tubular lumen. This testis-blood barrier is important in protecting the sperm from antibodies in the blood. Follicle-stimulating hormone (FSH) from the pituitary gland stimulates Sertoli cells to produce androgen-binding protein, which is excreted into the lumen of the tubule. This provides for a high concentration of testosterone within the lumen necessary for spermatogenesis. The rete testes, a meshwork of ducts, collect sperm from the seminiferous tubules. The sperm are transported to the epididymis by testicular fluid pressure, ciliary action, and contraction of the efferent ductules.

Epididymis and Vas Deferens

The epididymis is a hood-like structure lying on the top and back side of each testis. It consists of about 6 meters of tightly coiled tubule. As they travel through the epididymis over 12 days, spermatozoa are functionally and morphologically readied for fertilization. The sperm leave the epididymis during sexual arousal and travel through the vas deferens that propels sperm forward by muscular peristaltic contractions into the ejaculatory duct. Supported within the spermatic cords, the vas deferens is continuous with the tail of the epididymis, passing through the superficial inguinal ring, inguinal canal, and deep inguinal ring to reach the posterior surface of the bladder, where it joins with the duct of the seminal vesicle to form the ejaculatory duct.

Seminal Vesicles

The seminal vesicles are glandular sacs that reside behind the bladder. The thick alkaline fluid secreted by the glandular epithelium of the seminal vesicle contributes about 60 percent of the seminal fluid volume. This fluid is rich in fructose, citric acid, amino acids, proteins, and prostaglandins for the health and nutrition of the sperm.

Prostate Gland

The prostate gland is located in front of the rectum just under the bladder and surrounds a portion of the urethra. The prostate is comprised of 30 to 50 branched glands, weighing about 20 g and measuring 4 by 2 by 3 cm. It is surrounded by a fibroelastic capsule that penetrates the gland to divide it into lobes. The capsule and the stroma within the gland contain smooth muscle cells capable of contracting to expel the prostatic fluid. The ejaculatory ducts join the urethra within the prostate gland. The prostate gland produces a milky alkaline fluid rich in citric acid, spermine, cholesterol, phospholipids, fibrinogenase, fibrinolysin, zinc, and acid phosphatase, and other proteins. The alkalinity helps to neutralize the acidity of the male urethra and female vagina. It contributes about 30 to 35 percent of the total seminal fluid volume.

The central portion of the prostate contains pseudostratified epithelium. The peripheral zone is composed of stratified epithelium, occupies some 70 percent of the gland's volume, and is the most prevalent site of prostatic cancer. The prostate cells, as well as prostate cancer cells, produce a protein called prostate specific antigen (PSA), which is used as a biomarker for metastatic cancer of the prostate. The transitional zone between these types of tissue is the most common site of benign prostatic hyperplasia. Benign prostatic hypertrophy (BPH) occurs in about 50 percent of men over the age of 50 years. The prostate remains normal size until the age of 40 or 50 when, in some men, in association with decreasing testosterone, it degenerates without any symptoms.

Bulbourethral Glands

The bulbourethral glands (Cowper's) are two pea-sized glands located just below the prostate gland. They are connected to the urethra by small ducts. During sexual arousal the glands secrete alkaline mucus into the penile urethra. The alkalinity of the mucus protects sperm by neutralizing any residual acidic urine in the urethra.

Penis

The penis functions as the external male sex organ and also a passageway for urine. Its structure consists of two dorsally paired corpus cavernosa, and one ventrally located corpus spongiosum that surrounds the urethra. These three cylindrical masses are wrapped in thick membranous sheaths and are surrounded by a loose layer of skin. The corpus spongiosum expands at the terminal end to form the glans penis. The erectile tissues are composed of venous spaces lined with epithelial cells separated by connective tissue and smooth muscle cells. The arterial supply to the penis originates at the internal pudendal arteries. Nutritive arteries supply oxygen and nutrients to the vascular tissues. Other arteries empty directly into the erectile tissues, and when activated by sexual arousal greatly increase the flow into the penis. The glans is highly innervated with sensory neurons that are sensitive to contact and friction during sexual stimulation, which may result in pleasure sensations, erection, orgasm, and ejaculation of semen. The glans is naturally covered by a retractable foreskin. As newborns many men had the foreskin removed in a procedure called circumcision for religious or sociocultural reasons.

Spermatogenesis

Male contribution to reproduction is through spermatogenesis, a process that requires endocrine regulation from the hypothalamus and pituitary interacting with interstitial cells within the testes to produce, mature, and eject sperm in sufficient numbers to effectively fertilize the ovum in the female. The process of mating requires that the penis becomes erect through sexual stimulation and that erection is maintained for penetration and ejaculation into the female vagina. These complex functions require functional endocrine, neurological, and vascular interactions within the male genitalia. Psychological, relational, and sociocultural factors can also play important roles in creating healthy sexual responses for many men.

Spermatogenesis is the process of sperm generation in the seminiferous tubules in the testes. When the male enters puberty, the gonadotropin-releasing hormone (GnRH) produced by the hypothalamus is received by the anterior pituitary gland, which in turn releases FSH and luteinizing hormone (LH). FSH establishes the function of the Sertoli cells in the interstitial tissue of the testes and stimulates mitotic division of spermatogonia. Sertoli cells also regulate sperm production by producing inhibin, which provides negative feedback to reduce pituitary FSH. LH increases testosterone production by the interstitial cells in the interstitial tissue of the testes. Testosterone in turn promotes Sertoli cell function and maintains spermatogenesis.

The process of spermatogenesis takes 70 days for cells to mature in an orderly process along the length of the seminiferous tubules. It occurs in three phases: (a) proliferation of the stem cell spermatogonia by mitotic division, (b) production of the haploid gamete by meiotic division, and (c) morphological maturation of spermatids into spermatozoa. Mature males continue to produce spermatozoa throughout their lives, with several hundred million sperm produced each day.

Spermatogonia are labile and can be affected by seasonal hormonal and temperature cycles, disease, trauma, or heat. As external structures, the testes are able to maintain a lower than core body temperature necessary for healthy sperm production. Spermatozoa that are not ejaculated die and are reabsorbed within the body.

Semen Production

Semen is composed of secretions produced by the testes, seminal vesicles, prostate gland, and bulbourethral glands. Normal ejaculate volume is between 2 and 6 mL, 60 percent of the volume from the seminal vesicles, 30 to 35 percent from the prostate gland, and a small amount of the volume from sperm and bulbourethral secretions. Normal semen pH is 7.2 to 8.0. Prostatic secretion is more acidic, and seminal vesicle fluid is alkaline due to the presence of fructose. Infections can increase the alkalinity of semen.

Androgen Hormone Production

The male sex hormones are called **androgens.** Most androgens are produced by the testes, although the adrenal cortex also produces a small amount. Testosterone, the primary androgen, is responsible for the growth and development of the masculine characteristics. It directly influences the maturation of the male sex organs. After puberty, sperm development and sexual drive, as well as erectile function are maintained by testosterone. The secondary male sex characteristics (facial hair patterns, thickened vocal chords, and increased muscle mass) are also under the influence of testosterone. Testosterone secretion appears to decline slowly and continuously throughout adult life in men, with plasma levels decreasing about 35 percent between 20 and 85 years of age.

Because testosterone is the main hormonal mediator of libido, when testosterone levels decline, sexual desire decreases. Testosterone also has a critical role in stabilizing the levels of intracavernosal nitric oxide synthase, the enzyme responsible for triggering the nitric oxide cascade required to have an erection.

Erection and Ejaculation

Healthy erectile response requires functional neurological and vascular systems. The neural pathways involved in erection are located in the sacral segments of the spinal cord between the S3 and T12 vertebrae. Input from sensory endings in the genitalia and descending tracts carrying impulses generated from erotic stimuli are integrated in the spinal cord. Sensory signals from physical stimulation of the penis are sent via the pudendal nerve to the erection center. Incoming signals activate connector nerve cells, which in turn stimulate nearby parasympathetic neurons. These neurons then transmit erection-inducing signals from the sacral spine to the endothelial linings of penile arterioles. Endothelial linings of the arterioles in the corpus cavernosa release nitric oxide, which activates the enzyme guanylate cyclase, which in turn increases cyclic guanosine monophosphate (American Association of Clinical Endocrinologists Male Sexual Dysfunction Task Force, 2003). The smooth muscles in the arterioles relax and allow increased inflow of blood. This reflex arc needs to remain intact for an erection to be possible. When these systems are functioning, the male has the ability to achieve and maintain an erection of sufficient duration and firmness to complete satisfactory intercourse through vaginal penetration as desired.

Pharmacological treatments of erectile dysfunction, such as sildenafil (Viagra), target the enzymatic processes in the epithelium of the erectile tissues. Erectile functions may be affected by injury and disease factors, such as lumbar neurological injuries; vascular disease affecting large or small vessels, neurological conditions, such as multiple sclerosis, Parkinson's disease, peripheral neuropathies, and endocrine disorders.

Ejaculation is the reflexive phenomenon that ejects the seminal fluid through the penis. Ejaculation is usually preceded by erection of the penis and can occur during copulation, masturbation, or as a nocturnal emission. Effective sexual stimulation of the penis results in buildup of neural excitation to a critical level. When the threshold is reached, several internal events are triggered. Ejaculation occurs in two stages. In the emission phase, the prostate, seminal vesicles, and upper portions of the vas deferens undergo contractions bringing the seminal fluids into the ejaculatory ducts and prostatic urethra. The urethral sphincters (to the bladder and below the prostate) trap the seminal fluid in the urethral bulb. The male experiences this as a sense that orgasm is imminent.

The second stage of ejaculation, called the expulsion phase, occurs when strong, rhythmic contractions of pelvic muscles that surround the urethral bulb and root of the penis expel the collected semen through the urethra. The external sphincter below the prostate relaxes while the internal sphincter remains contracted to prevent the escape of urine.

Although male orgasm is associated with ejaculation, these processes are not one and the same, nor do they necessarily occur together. Prior to puberty, orgasms may not involve ejaculation. If several orgasms occur within a sexual encounter, some orgasms may be nonejaculatory. Some men may experience retrograde ejaculation into the bladder with little or no ejaculation from the penis, particularly after prostate surgery if internal sphincter damage has occurred.

Female Reproductive System

The primary functions of the female reproductive system are (a) production of ova, (b) secretion of hormones, (c) pregnancy and birth of a fetus, and (d) breastfeeding the infant. The main reproductive organs of the female are the ovaries, oviducts, uterus, vagina, external genitalia, and breasts.

The female reproductive functions of **ovulation,** pregnancy, birth, and lactation are regulated by a complex neuroendocrine process referred to as the reproductive axis. The hypothalamus, pituitary gland, and ovaries function to produce hormones that interact to regulate the **menstrual cycle;** facilitate the maturation and release of ova; maintain an enriched endometrial lining in the uterus, which is shed and replenished monthly; maintain the endometrium in response to embryonic hormones in pregnancy; and interact with placental-fetal hormones that sustain the pregnancy, prepare for lactation, and produce milk to meet infant nutritional needs after birth. Because of the complex and multiple levels of function, when menstrual disorders and or fertility issues arise it is sometimes difficult to determine the cause because dysfunctions in the system may occur at any of the functional levels.

Ovaries

The ovaries are solid, paired, oval bodies about 3 cm long by 1.5 cm wide. Each ovary is divided into a medulla and a cortex. The medulla is composed of loose connective tissue, blood vessels, lymphatics, and nerves. The cortex is composed of Graafian vesicles, which contain the ovum. At birth the ovaries contain between 2 to 4 million ova. Most of these ova will degenerate across time until there are only 300,000 to 400,000 ova present at puberty. These begin maturing one or more at a time during monthly menstrual cycling after the age of puberty through to menopause. The woman may release fewer than 500 mature ova during monthly ovulation across her reproductive years.

Fallopian Tubes

The fallopian tubes are 8 to 14 cm long, extending from a fimbriated end over the ovary to a narrowed insertion point in the upper uterine wall. The lumina are internally continuous with the uterine cavity. The fimbriae create a small current that pulls ova released from the ovaries into the tube. The tubes are lined with longitudinal ciliated and secretory columnar epithelial cells. Along with the cilia, the fallopian tubes produce contractions that can move the ovum toward the uterus, a 2- to 3-day journey. Secretory cells provide nutrients for the ovum during transport. Fertilization of the ovum usually occurs within the fallopian tube.

Uterus

The uterus is a hollow, pear-shaped, muscular organ, approximately 7.5 cm long by 5 cm wide by 2.5 cm thick. The walls of the uterus are composed of three layers: the external peritoneum, the middle muscular myometrium, and the internal endometrium. Its size varies slightly according to **parity** (the number of viable births) a woman has experienced.

The fundus or body of the uterus is covered by the peritoneal layer, which separates the uterus from the abdominal cavity. The lining flows from the uterus on the anterior side to form a pouch with the bladder wall called the vesicouterine pouch. On the posterior side, the peritoneal lining forms the rectouterine pouch (Douglas' cul-de-sac) between the uterus and the vaginal-rectal wall. The uterus is held into position by several ligaments. The round ligaments extend laterally from the uterine wall and down to the internal inguinal ring, through the inguinal canal where they blend with the labia majora. The broad ligaments are folds of peritoneum that envelope the fallopian tubes and extend to the lateral pelvic wall. The uterosacral ligaments extend posteriorly from the uterus to the sacrum. The body of the uterus is usually flexed anteriorly but may also be retroflexed.

The myometrium of the uterus is formed by three overlapping layers of smooth muscles that are interlaced with blood vessels. These muscles stretch and grow in size to accommodate a growing fetus, contract at intervals during labor to expel the fetus, and then contract tightly to minimize bleeding after childbirth. The smooth muscle cells shrink in size after childbirth, allowing the uterus to return to normal size within a few weeks.

The inner endometrial layer of the uterus is composed of tubular glands and arteries that can be divided into two functional segments. The outer layer is built up each month under the influence of estrogen and progesterone to form a rich nutrient bed prepared to receive a fertilized ovum. This portion is shed during the menstrual period when fertilization of an ovum did not occur. The base of epithelial and glandular cells remains in tact, supplying the replicative cells to regenerate the lining after menstruation.

Cervix

The cervix is the portion of the uterus that extends into the vagina. The cervix is composed of fibrous, muscular, and elastic tissue and is lined by simple columnar and stratified squamous epithelium. The fibrous connective tissue is the predominant component. Smooth muscle, making up about 15 percent of the cervix, is mainly located in the upper portion. The vaginal portion has rare smooth muscle fibers.

The cervical canal is approximately 2.5 cm long and provides the passageway for sperm to enter the uterus and menstrual flow to exit the uterus. The internal os of the cervical canal is located at the junction with the uterine corpus. The endocervical surface and the infolding that create glands are lined by a simple columnar mucin-producing epithelium. The cervical mucus is subject to profound cyclic changes. Under estrogen stimulation, the endocervical secretions are profuse, watery, and alkaline, facilitating sperm penetration. During the postovulatory phase, secretions are scant, thick, and acid, contain numerous leukocytes, and act as a barrier for sperm penetration. The external os is located centrally on the vaginal portion of the cervix. The os is circular in women who have not borne children and is slit-like in women who have borne children.

The outer cervix is covered with squamous epithelium. Where the endocervical glandular epithelium joins the squamous epithelium is the transformational zone known as the squamocolumnar junction. The clinical identification of the transformation zone is important, because almost all cervical squamous neoplasia and their precursors begin in this area. During the reproductive period, the transformation zone is located on the exposed portion of the cervix and can be visualized.

Vagina

The vagina is a 7.5- to 10-cm canal that extends upward and backward from the vulva to the uterus. It is situated behind the bladder and in front of the rectum and its axis forms an angle of over 90 degrees with that of the uterus. Its walls are ordinarily in contact, and the usual shape of its lower part on transverse section is that of a collapsed H. It is constricted at its commencement, dilated in the middle, and narrowed near its uterine extremity. It surrounds the vaginal portion of the cervix, its attachment extending higher up on the posterior than on the anterior wall of the uterus. The recess behind the cervix is called the posterior fornix, while the smaller recesses in front and at the sides are called the anterior fornix and lateral fornix.

The vagina consists of an internal mucous lining and a muscular coat separated by a layer of erectile tissue. The mucosal lining is stratified squamous epithelium. The epithelium contains elastic fibers and a rich venous and lymphatic network. Although the vaginal mucosa contains no glands, its surface is lubricated by cervical mucus and by direct transudate through the mucosa during sexual stimulation. Secretions from the vaginal epithelial cells contain glycogen and liquid. The amounts of glycogen and transudates secreted by the vaginal mucosa are influenced by ovarian hormones. Normal vaginal flora, particularly *Lactobacillus acidophilus,* interact with the glycogen to produce lactic acid, maintaining an acidic pH of 4 to 5 in the vagina. This acidity reduces susceptibility to vaginal infections.

The vaginal mucous membrane is continuous above with that lining the uterus. The presence of longitudinal ridges along with numerous transverse ridges, or rugae, on the vaginal wall allows the vagina to be highly distensible during intercourse and the birth process. The submucosa is loose erectile tissue, containing numerous large veins, which by their anastomoses form a plexus, together with smooth muscular fibers derived from the muscular coat. The muscular coat consists of two layers: an external longitudinal layer and an internal circular layer. The longitudinal fibers are continuous with the superficial muscular fibers of the uterus.

Vaginal tissues receive their blood supply from uterine arteries and sometimes branches of the internal iliac artery. Blood returns to the venous system through veins that empty into the internal iliac veins. Lymphatic drainage is via the external and internal iliac lymph nodes and superficial inguinal lymph nodes. The muscles of the pelvic floor provide important support to the vagina and uterus.

External Genitalia

The external genitalia, also known as the vulva, extend from the mons pubis anteriorly to the anus posteriorly and laterally to the inguinal-gluteal folds. The vulva include the mons pubis, the clitoris, the labia majora and minora, the hymen, Bartholin's and Skene's glands and ducts, and the vaginal introitus (Figure 61-2).

Mons Pubis

The mons pubis is a fatty layer covered with coarse pubic hair, lying over the pubic bone. It provides some protective padding during intercourse. Touch and pressure on the mons can be sexually pleasurable because of the presence of numerous nerve endings.

Labia Majora and Labia Minora

The labia majora are tissue folds covered by hair-bearing skin and contain both smooth muscle and fat. The labia majora fuse anteriorly with the mons pubis and posteriorly with the perineum. The skin of the labia majora is usually darker that the skin of the thighs. The nerve endings and underlying fatty

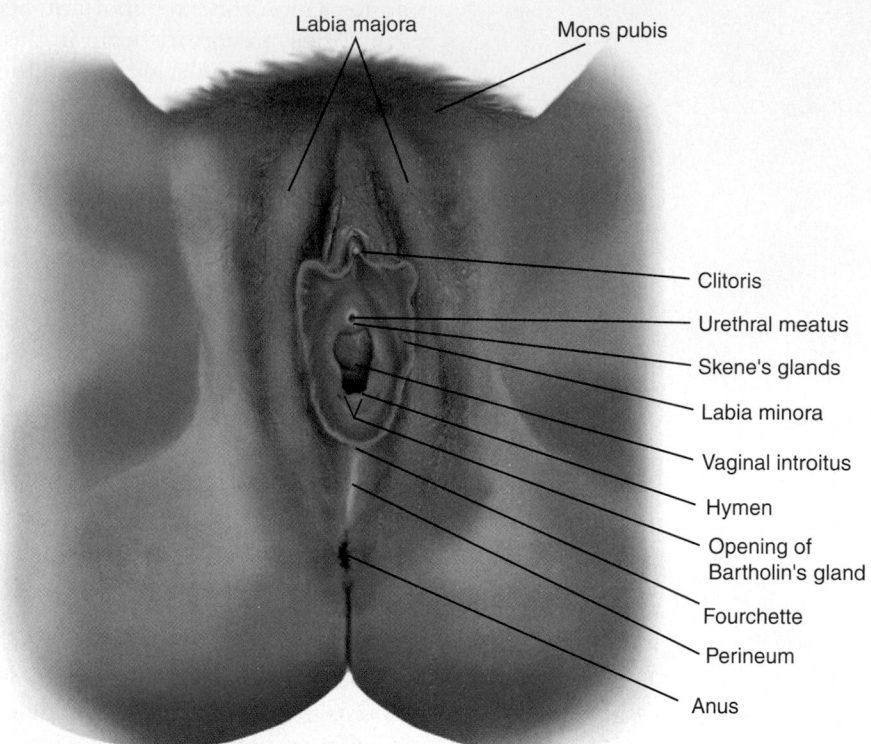

Figure 61-2 External female genitalia.

tissue are similar to those in the mons. Vestibular bulbs analogous to the corpus spongiosum in the male lie behind the folds of the labia majora.

The labia minora are smaller thin folds covered by skin that bears no hair laterally and by vaginal mucosa medially. The folds fuse anteriorly to form the hood or prepuce of the glans of the clitoris. Posteriorly along the lower edge of the vaginal opening, the labia minora form a thin, flat tissue called the fourchette. The labia minora are devoid of fat but are rich in elastic fibers and blood vessels forming erectile tissue. Sebaceous glands are present on both surfaces of minora and produce thick cheesy secretions called smegma.

Clitoris

The clitoris is analogous to the male phallus. It is comprised of a glans, a shaft, and crura. The glans is the portion externally visible just under the hood formed by the labia minora. The glans is highly sensitive to touch, resulting in sexual arousal and pleasure. The clitoral shaft is composed of vascular erectile tissue that engorges with blood during sexual arousal. The crura divide in two conjoined cavernous bodies, which branch near the base of the clitoris and lie along the pubic bone behind the labia majora. The corpora cavernosa are composed of endothelial lined lacunar spaces, cavernosal arteries, smooth muscle, and connective tissue similar to these structures in the male penis. Although other sexual organs, both male and female, have combined functions of reproduction and waste elimination, the only known function of the clitoris is arousal and sexual pleasure. This exclusive purpose of the clitoris for sexual pleasure confounds notions in some cultures that women are less sexual than men.

Hymen

The hymen is a fold of mucous membrane that partially marks the introitus or entrance to the vagina. It may appear smooth in nonparous women. In parous women, it may have irregular tags because of stretching and small lacerations during birth. Occasionally the hymen may completely or partially occlude the vaginal opening. If the occlusion interferes with menstrual flow or sexual activity, a surgical incision may be necessary to open it. Contrary to assumptions in some cultures, the degree of intactness of the hymen cannot be used to prove or disprove virginity or history of sexual intercourse.

Perineum

The perineum is the area of smooth skin between the vaginal introitus and the anus, composed of vascular tissue and nerve tissue. A transverse fold of mucous membrane called the posterior fourchette is formed by connecting the ends of the labia minora. It may disappear after initiation of sexual intercourse and childbearing, leaving the vulva more open.

Paraurethral (Skene's) Glands

The paraurethral glands (Skene's), equivalent to the prostate in the male, are composed of mucus-secreting columnar epithelium. The openings are located just inside of, and on the posterior area of, the urethra. The glands can become infected by bacteria present in the vulvar area.

Bulbourethral (Bartholin's) Glands

The vestibular glands (Bartholin's), equivalent to the bulbourethral (Cowper's) glands in the male, are located on each side of the vestibule of the vagina inside the labia minora. These glands are composed of alveoli lined with columnar cells that produce mucus that is excreted through small ducts near the vaginal opening. Mucus produced by these glands may contribute somewhat to vaginal lubrication during sexual activity. The glands are usually not palpable unless infection occludes the ducts creating an abscess or cyst.

Breasts

The breasts are mammary glands that produce milk to nourish an infant after birth. As such, they function as accessories to the reproductive process and are considered part of the secondary female sex characteristics. Their growth, development, and functions are regulated by hormonal influences from the hypothalamus, pituitary gland, and the ovaries. Breasts also function as organs for sexual arousal in some cultures and can be responsive to sexual stimuli.

Extending from the second to the sixth ribs, the breasts are dome-shaped and are composed of alveolar glands clustered in 15 to 20 lobes separated from each other by interlobular septa. Each lobe is drained by a lactiferous duct that opens at the tip of the nipple. The nipple, located centrally on the dome of the breast, contains nerve endings and erectile tissue. The nipple is surrounded by the areola, a pigmented area that contains sebaceous glands (Montgomery's). Usually the nipple protrudes from the areola, though in some women one or both nipples may be flat or inverted. Inverted nipples may cause some problems with initiation of breastfeeding.

Fibrous and fatty tissue surrounding the glandular tissue provides support and accounts for the varying sizes and shapes in the breasts of different women. Part of the mammary gland may extend along the inferolateral edge of the pectoralis major toward the axilla (armpit), forming an axillary tail (of Spence). Approximately 50 percent of breast cancer tumors are located in this portion of breast tissue.

Under the influence of increasing estrogen production during puberty, the glandular and ductal tissues undergo growth and development. With menstrual cycling, some women experience tenderness and fullness in the breast tissue related to increased production of ovarian hormones. Over half of women 30 to 50 years of age may experience benign fibrocystic changes in their breasts. These usually recede after menopause.

Changes in the breast occur during pregnancy. Increasing amounts of estrogen and progesterone are secreted first by the corpus luteum of the ovary and later by the placenta. Progesterone works along with the estrogen to complete the development of the alveoli. After birth, prolactin hormone from the pituitary gland initiates milk production. In response to nerve stimulation of the nipple, oxytocin is released from the posterior pituitary gland and induces smooth muscles surrounding the alveoli and within the ductal system to contract and bring the milk down from the glands during suckling by the infant.

Menarche

Menarche refers most specifically to the initiation of the first menstrual period. Menarche results from a rapid maturation of the reproductive axis. The average age of menarche is around 12 years of age, though it can range from 9 to 16 years of age. Age of onset is mediated by genetics, race, and possibly nutritional and socioeconomic status.

The functions of the menstrual cycle are mediated by the hypothalamus, which begins to secrete GnRH directly to the pituitary gland. The pituitary is stimulated to produce FSH, which is picked up by the ovaries where a number of primary **oocytes** (the early or primitive ovum before it has developed completely) begin the maturational process. Granulosa and thecal cells surrounding these oocytes increase in number and form the follicles. Usually one follicle exceeds the others in size and activity. The follicles that have lagged behind in their development atrophy, and those oocytes die and are absorbed. The maturing follicle continues to expand, pushing through to the exterior wall of the ovary. The granulosa cells surrounding the ovum produce estrogen in increasing amounts along with lower levels of progesterone.

Under the influence of a second pituitary hormone, LH, and along with peak levels of FSH, the follicle ruptures releasing the ovum coated with follicular fluid into the peritoneal cavity. The fimbriated ends of the fallopian tube create currents that pull the ovum into the tube. The follicular cells at the site of ovulation, now called the corpus luteum, continue to produce estrogen and even higher levels of progesterone. These hormones are picked up by endometrial tissue that continues to grow in vascularity and glandular activity. The follicular cells also produce inhibin, a glycoprotein, which provides negative feedback to the pituitary gland to decrease the production of FSH.

If fertilization of the ovum has not occurred, approximately 10 to 12 days after ovulation the corpus luteum decreases its production of estrogen and progesterone. The dropping levels of these ovarian hormones cause the vessels of the endometrial lining to constrict resulting in cellular death and the sloughing of the endometrial lining in menses. The drop in estrogen now creates a negative feedback to the hypothalamus to increase production of GnRH, which again stimulates release of FSH from the pituitary gland and the menstrual cycle begins again.

If the ovum has been fertilized, the developing zygote produces human chorionic gonadotropin (hCG). The hCG is picked up by the ovary, causing the corpus luteum to continue production of estrogen and progesterone for several more weeks until the placenta can produce levels of estrogen and progesterone sufficient to maintain the pregnancy.

Estrogen and progesterone produced by the ovaries are also responsible for the development of female secondary sex characteristics, such as the development of the mammary glands, feminine patterns of fat distribution, and pubic and body hair patterns. During pregnancy these hormones also contribute to the growth of the uterus and increased vascularization of the breasts, pelvic, and perineal tissues.

Menopause

Menopause specifically refers to the last menses, which marks the end of the menstrual cycling. This event occurs between the ages of 40 and 58 and occurs within the perimenopausal period, or **climacteric,** which occurs two to eight years prior to menopause and up to one year after the final menses. The quality and quantity of follicular development undergoes decline about 20 to

25 years after menarche. Variation in the menstrual cycle length may be related to anovulation or irregular maturation of follicles. A shorter menstrual cycle is the most common change that occurs during the perimenopausal period.

Because there is a decrease in the number of functional follicles that respond to FSH, the follicular phase of the menstrual cycle shortens and may become anovulatory. The luteal phase remains fairly constant at 14 days. Although fertility declines, women may still conceive during the perimenopausal period. As the follicular tissue becomes more resistant to gonadotropin stimulation along with a decreased production of inhibin, which regulates, particularly, LH, there are increases in production of FHS and LH.

Hypothalamic-pituitary insensitivity to estrogen feedback may also play a significant role in perimenstrual symptoms (Weiss, Skurnick, Goldsmith, Santoro, & Park, 2004). Symptoms such as hot flashes and sleep disturbances occur more commonly in perimenopausal women and are related to decreasing levels of estrogen and increasing levels of LH. However, early in the perimenopausal phase, levels of LH are higher in perimenopausal women even in the presence of estrogen levels similar to younger women. Elevated FSH and LH levels lead to stromal stimulation of the ovary, which increases the production of estrone levels and decreases estradiol levels. With fewer functioning follicles, inhibin levels also drop during this time causing further rises in FSH levels.

Systems affected by the perimenopausal phase include neuroendocrine, cardiovascular, genitourinary, skeletal, and skin and hair. Hot flashes are defined as transient periods of intense heat in the upper body, arms, and face, which are followed by flushing of the skin and sweating. Core body temperature may drop a degree or two after the hot flash because of heat lost through increased blood flow to the skin and evaporation. From 40 to 70 percent of women experience hot flashes and of these 10 to 20 percent may seek attention from their health care professional. Hot flashes may be experienced for months or years but average around three years for most women. Hot flashes may disturb sleep patterns and result in fatigue, irritability, and negative impact on life activities. It remains unclear whether hot flashes are caused by the high levels of FSH and LH or low levels of estrogen and inhibin. It is possible that both of these factors may be required to increase the incidence of hot flashes (Whiteman, Staropoli, Benedict, Borgeest, & Flaws, 2003).

The risk of atherosclerotic disease, including coronary heart disease increases with age. Women demonstrate lower incidences of cardiovascular diseases than men before age 50. However, after the age of 50 the incidence of disease increases until women's rates are similar to the rate in men. Total cholesterol, low-density lipoprotein (LDL) cholesterol, and triglyceride levels increase after menopause, whereas high-density lipoprotein (HDL) cholesterol levels decline, promoting atherosclerosis.

Vaginal mucosal thinness and dryness progresses later in the perimenopausal period and is related to estrogen withdrawal. Skin and hair changes may also be noted. The incidence of osteoporosis increases substantially after menopause. The cause is not fully understood but may be related to loss of estrogen influence on parathyroid activity and production of the active form of vitamin D, resulting in bone reabsorption.

SEXUAL RESPONSE CYCLE

The sexual response is a complex interplay between psychological and physiological factors. Humans usually move from sexual neutrality to interactive sexual behavior for reasons related to enhancement of emotional closeness, desire to increase a sense of attractiveness and attraction to a partner, and a desire to share sexual pleasure. Masturbation or self-stimulation is more commonly related to sexual tension or hunger. Sexual desires, or at least willingness to be receptive to sexual stimuli, are important cognitive components to sexual arousal, which may also require adequate levels of gonadal hormones to maintain libido.

Physiologically, sexual function is dependent on functional endocrine, neurological, and vascular systems. During puberty, male testosterone levels increase approximately 10 to 20 times, triggering the maturation of male genitalia, secondary sex characteristics, and behavioral changes, particularly a fourfold increase in sexual activity. Clinical literature shows that testosterone levels directly and indirectly influence the fundamental components of male sexual function including sex drive, erectile function, and ejaculation. Although testosterone levels are much lower in women, the presence of testosterone in women seems important in maintaining libido. Changes in testosterone levels through puberty in the female have not been documented. A woman's testosterone level begins to decline in the perimenopause (5 to 10 years before menopause) and tends to stabilize at lower levels several years after menopause.

The two fundamental physiological responses to effective sexual stimulation that occur in both males and females are vasocongestion and **myotonia** (tonic spasm of a muscle or temporary rigidity). Vasocongestion is the engorgement of blood in the genital and breast tissue in response to sexual stimuli. Myotonia refers to building muscle tension in the muscles of the pelvic floor and throughout the body. Myotonia is evident in the facial grimaces, spasmodic contractions of the hands and feet, and the muscular spasms that occur during orgasm. These responses follow the same general pattern regardless of the method of sexual stimulation. Masters and Johnson (1966) first distinguished four phases in the physiological sexual response pattern in both males and females: excitement, plateau, orgasm, and resolution. These phases, as well as some variations in male and female expression of the phases are described in Table 61-1. Kaplan (1985) adds the psychological phase of desire to the response cycle.

Healthy and safe sexuality involves intentional decisions to live a lifestyle that maintains maximum health for reproduction if and when one might desire to become a parent. This includes establishing a healthy intimate relationship, preventing unintentional impregnation, and planning pregnancy when the decision is mutual and the couple is prepared for the role of parenting, as well as avoidance of contracting or spreading sexually transmitted infections.

Male Sexual Response Cycle

The physiological components of male sexual response include erection, orgasm, and ejaculation. These components are discussed here as a basis for understanding both sexual function and dysfunction as these are related to selected treatment protocols. An erection is a process coordinated by neural input generated from sensory erotic and fantasy experiences and stimulation of sensory endings in the genitalia. The penis is maintained in a flaccid state by sympathetic nervous system stimulation of the penile blood vessels and smooth muscle contractions within the vessel walls of the lacunar spaces of the cavernosa of the penile shaft. When the penis is flaccid the intralacunar smooth muscle is in a contracted state, and the tone is maintained by norepinephrine. When a male becomes sexually aroused vasodilator impulses are delivered by the parasympathetic nervous system. Dilation of the arterioles of the penis and relaxation of the smooth muscles of the lacunar spaces cause the erectile tissue of the penis to fill with blood. The veins are compressed by this engorgement so that outflow is blocked. The effect of these vascular changes is to increase penile distension. The testes also experience increased blood flow and increase 50 percent in size during sexual arousal.

When fully distended, the penis is rigid and capable of penetrating the vagina, facilitating sperm deposits into the vaginal vault with ejaculation. The

TABLE 61-1 Physiological Phases of the Sexual Response Cycle

MALE RESPONSES	FEMALE RESPONSES	SHARED RESPONSES
Excitement		
Penis becomes erect. Erection may be partially lost and regained during a prolonged phase. Testes enlarge and elevate. Scrotum tightens, flattens, and skin thickens. When fully distended, the penis is rigid and capable of penetration.	Clitoris swells, glans becomes tumescent, and shaft increases in diameter and length. Vagina lubricates and expands. Uterus elevates and breasts enlarge.	Myotonia spreads; some evidence of involuntary muscle activity. Heart rate increases in direct proportion to rising sexual tension. Sex flush may be visible in some women. Nipples become erect.
Plateau		
Erection is stabilized. Increase in penile circumference at coronal ridge. Full testicular elevation; enlargement of testes reaches 50 percent over unstimulated size. Secretions from Cowper's appear at urethral opening.	Continued vaginal expansion; uterine and cervical elevation. Development of orgasmic platform. Retraction of clitoris under labial hood. Secretions of Bartholin's gland. Further enlargement of breasts.	Increased muscle tension; superficial and deep vasocongestion. Rapid respiration and increase in heart rate and blood pressure; hyperventilation may be present. Sex flush appears in some men, becomes more pronounced in women.
Orgasm		
Contractions of vas deferens, seminal vesicles, prostate gland moves sperm and semen to penile bulb; emission phase of orgasm. Contractions of pelvic floor muscles around urethral bulb causes ejaculation of semen and creates sensations of orgasm	Contractions of muscles of pelvic floor and uterus create sensations of orgasm	Same pelvic floor muscles are contracting in men and women. Length and strength of orgasmic responses are similar in men and women. Hyperventilation and increased heart rate and blood pressure and sex flush continue.
Resolution		
Loss of most of penile erection within 30 seconds. Testes descend into relaxed scrotum. Refractory period limits the return of an erection and orgasm.	Loss of vaginal and clitoral vasocongestion. Clitoris returns to prestimulated position. With continued stimulation vasocongestion and myotonia may recur for multiple orgasms.	Loss of muscle tension and nipple erection. Sex flush disappears. Heart rate, breathing, and blood pressure return to normal.

Adapted from Kaplan, H. S. (1985). Comprehensive evaluation of disorders of sexual desire. *Washington, DC: American Psychiatric Press.*

firmness in the erection may come and go within a sexual encounter as the male's focus on his own sensations vary, such as when his attention is given to his partner. As he nears orgasm the erection stabilizes. Following orgasm arterial blood flow into the penis decreases to nonaroused levels, vasocongestion is relieved, and the penis becomes flaccid.

Although an erection is basically a physiological response, it also involves psychological components. In healthy sexual relationships, sexual interactions with a desired partner can involve intense emotional feelings of intimacy and attachment along with the personal pleasure from the experience. When other psychological issues are involved within the relationship or within the individual, altered sexual responsiveness can inhibit erectile functions.

Ejaculation is a neurophysiological reflexive process by which semen is expelled through the penis to the outside of the body. When effective sexual stimulation of the penis results in a buildup of neural excitation to a critical level, several internal physiological events are triggered in the ejaculatory process. During the emission phase of the process, the ampulla of the vas deferens, the seminal vesicles, and the prostate gland undergo contractions. The contractions eject the glandular secretions into the urethral bulb. Two sphincters, one located where the urethra exits the bladder and the other below the prostate, enclose the semen in the urethral bulb. Next, in the expulsion phase, the collected semen is expelled out of the urethra by strong, rhythmic contractions of the pelvic floor muscles that surround the urethral bulb and the root of the penis. The external sphincter relaxes, allowing the semen to pass through, while the internal sphincter remains contracted to prevent the loss of urine.

Orgasm is the series of contractions of the levator ani and pubococcygeus muscles of the pelvic floor and is associated with pleasure and the release of the sexual tension. The first few muscular contractions are quite strong and occur at close intervals. Most of the seminal fluid is expelled in spurts with each contraction. Several more muscular contractions occur in decreasing intensity and frequency. The entire expulsion stage may last from 3 to 10 seconds.

Following orgasm the blood flow decreases and the vasocongestion is relieved, a process known as **detumescence.** Detumescence begins within seconds of the orgasm, but may take 10 to 30 minutes to return the penis to a flaccid nonaroused state. If orgasm is not experienced, the release of vasocongestion may take longer. The male may also experience aching in the testes until the testicular vasocongestion is relieved.

Female Sexual Response Cycle

Although the anatomical appearance of female genitalia differs from male genitalia, the physiological sexual response is the same within analogous tissues and includes sexual arousal, lubrication, and orgasm. In the nonaroused state, the clitoral body and vaginal smooth muscles are under contractile tone. Following sexual stimulation, the neurogenic and endothelial release of nitric oxide relaxes the smooth muscles in the clitoral cavernosum and coiled arteriolar smooth muscles. Increased arterial inflow creates increased intracavernosal pressure and clitoral engorgement resulting in the extrusion of the glans clitoris and enhanced sensitivity.

Within the vaginal wall, neurotransmitters including nitric oxide and vasoactive intestinal peptide (VIP) are released modulating vaginal vascular and nonvascular smooth muscle relaxation. Dramatic increase in capillary flow in the submucosa leads to production of 3 to 5 mL of vaginal transudate that provides vaginal lubrication. Vaginal smooth muscle relaxation results in increased vaginal length and diameter, especially in the distal two thirds of the vagina.

Because the cavernous bodies in the female lie out along the pelvic floor, rather than being contained within a shaft of skin as in males, engorgement of these spongy tissues is less visible. Vasocongestion can be visualized through magnetic resonance imaging (MRI) during sexual arousal in the female, demonstrating that clitoral and cavernous tissues doubles in size (Maravilla, et al., 2005). The female can experience a more diffuse vasocongestion than males.

During orgasm, the female experiences a series of rhythmic, rapidly occurring contractions of the orgasmic platform, the outer third of the vagina and the engorged tissues surrounding it. Females experience a variety of orgasmic responses from intense contractions of the pelvic floor muscles to mild contractions that are perceived as pleasurable and relieve sexual tension, though release of vasocongestion may take longer. A mild orgasm may be accompanied by 3 to 5 contractions; intense orgasms may continue for 12 or more contractions. The intervals between contractions lengthen in duration after the first few and intensity diminishes progressively.

Following orgasm, the vasocongestion is relieved and both the outer third and inner two thirds of the vagina return to their unstimulated state. The vagina loses its deep coloration and regains its normal appearance about 10 to 15 minutes after an orgasm. If the female does not experience orgasm, relief of vasocongestion may take longer and may result in dull aching heaviness similar to premenstrual abdominal heaviness.

Interactive Sexual Intimacy

Adequate functioning of the neurological and vascular systems is important in physiological sexual responsiveness. Establishing and maintaining a positive interpersonal relationship with one's sexual partner also contributes to sexual interest, desire, and willingness to participate in sexual intimacy. Cognitive components, such as negative past experiences, anxiety, emotional distress, and depression, may influence the ability to respond to sexual situations with sexual arousal and to experience sexual satisfaction as desired or expected. When a patient or a couple expresses concerns about sexual functioning, contributing factors within the individual or within the couple relationship should be explored. If serious personal or relationship issues are present the patient or couple should be referred to counseling.

Sexual Dysfunction

Sexual dysfunction is a disturbance or disorder in desire, excitement, or orgasm of the sexual response cycle. Sensory arousal combines with emotional arousal and conscious thoughts to trigger and interdependently direct the hormonal, neurological, and circulatory systems that develop and maintain the sexual response cycle. Thus, levels of performance and satisfaction may vary situationally, relationally, and across the life span related to aging or disease. Sexual dysfunction may be caused by factors such as the patient's perception and beliefs about gender role or aging. Sexual functioning must always be examined in the context of the whole person and the intimate partner relationship not just physical or psychological status.

Physical, Medical, or Surgical Causes of Sexual Dysfunction

Patients who have chronic illness, physical disability, or episodic acute illness often have difficulties with sexual functioning. Although physical demands of sexual activity are high, there are rarely significant restrictions on sexual activities. However, couples may need to alter their usual sexual patterns and activities to accommodate any limitations they may experience. Psychological effects on sexual functioning may result from disinterest, anxiety, fatigue, pain, or misconceptions about their ability to experience sexual activities (Nusbaum, Hamilton, & Lenahan, 2003).

Chronic medical illnesses tend to disrupt the desire and arousal phases of sexual response. Negative body image and perception of self as a sexual being may result from medical diagnoses and required lifestyle changes. Neurological disorders can potentially affect desire, arousal, and orgasm. Treatments of chronic illnesses can also interfere with sexual functioning. Many drugs contribute to changes in sexual response. Antihypertensive and psychotropic drugs particularly affect arousal and possibly disrupt orgasm. Sometimes alternative drugs can be prescribed that have less effect on sexual functioning. But when selected drugs are essential, the patient may require information on alternative ways to experience intimacy. Surgery may disrupt sympathetic and parasympathetic neural pathway.

Substance-Induced Sexual Dysfunction

Substance-induced sexual dysfunction can affect any stage of the sexual response cycle. For diagnosis, a link needs to be established between a clinically diagnosed sexual dysfunction and a specific substance, legal or illegal. Diagnostic criteria include the following: (a) the sexual dysfunction must cause

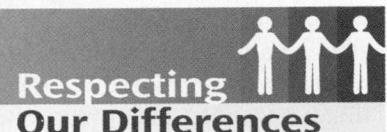

Respecting Our Differences

Reproductive Issues Accompanying Aging

Fecundity and fertility are reduced as both males and females grow older. A woman's fertility starts to decline in her late 20s, and for men, fertility begins to drop after age 35. A woman is born with her lifetime supply of ova, which diminishes to about 300,000 by the time she reaches puberty. By the time she reaches her late 30s, the risks of abnormal haploid cell division and other chromosomal abnormalities increase. As men and women approach middle age, chronic disorders, such as diabetes mellitus and hypertension, may reduce fertility in both men and women and increase the risks associated with childbearing in women. In association with chronic conditions, the incidence of miscarriage increases with age as does preterm birth and low-birth-weight babies. Medications used to treat some health conditions may also interfere with sexual function and fertility, and some pose risks of congenital anomalies.

marked distress or interpersonal difficulty; (b) the condition may involve impaired desire, arousal, or orgasm, or sexual pain and is fully explained by the direct effects of the substance; and (c) the recurring or persistent dysfunction is not better accounted for by a dysfunction that is not substance induced. Both psychotropic drugs and somatotropic drugs may have side effects that can produce sexual dysfunction.

A significant number of prescribed drugs, combinations of prescribed drugs, or over-the-counter (OTC) drugs are known to affect sexual functioning (e.g., antiandrogens, antiarrhythmics, anticholinergics, antihistamines, corticosteroids, decongestants, and diuretics). Sexual side effects of some drugs may be present in some patients and not in others. Health care practitioners must review the known side effects of drugs taken by patients, providing information as indicated. If patients are unaware of potential side effects, the cause of the sexual dysfunction may be assumed to be unrelated to medication and not be reported to the practitioner. Patients with chronic diseases who must take more that one medication regularly are particularly susceptible. The effects can range from a simple additive effect (the effect on one medication added to the effect of the other) to a synergistic effect (the effects of two or more drugs creating a third, enhanced, and often unpredictable effect). Patients should be informed to not mix some medically prescribed drugs or OTC medications with alcohol or illegal substances.

As with all psychoactive drugs, the patient's psychological well-being and environment can affect the outcome of the drug activity. Antidepressants, tranquilizers, barbiturates, and alcohol are all central nervous system depressants, reducing or slowing down neurological functioning. Mild tranquilizers and alcohol are sometimes used to reduce anxiety and improve mood in an attempt to enhance sexual desire and induce a relaxed, less inhibited state of mind. In higher doses, these drugs may impair the patient's judgment, impacting sexual decisions, or the drugs may decrease the ability to function sexually. Narcotic medications usually create a loss of sexual desire, arousal, and orgasm.

Psychological Issues

Childhood learning shapes many fundamental attitudes, values, and beliefs about sexuality. The need for close bonding with other humans and the need for sensual touch are present from birth to death. When life experiences fail to meet these needs in healthy ways, psychological issues can result that impact psychosexual development and negatively influence intimate relationships. Psychological issues affecting sexual functioning may be related to sexual ignorance, fear of failure, or communication or relationship issues with a partner. Life issues such as restrictive upbringing, rigid gender roles, traumatic sexual experiences, or conflict with sexual orientation also can contribute to sexual dysfunction. Sometimes psychological factors can be resolved with information and education; other times professional psychiatric counseling may be required.

ASSESSMENT

Sexuality is an integral component of physical and emotional health for all people, incorporating gender identity, self-worth, the ability to establish healthy intimate relationships, and expressions of sexual behaviors. Thus, all patients should be provided opportunity to discuss sexual concerns that are related to health issues. All women of reproductive age should be assessed for the need for contraception, assistance with pregnancy planning, and sexual practices that may place them at risk for sexually transmitted diseases (STDs). Adolescent males and females are particularly vulnerable to STDs because of greater likelihood of inadequate education and self comfort, and the social skills necessary to practice safer sexual behaviors. Because STDs can have serious impacts on reproductive function, as well as be life-threatening, sexual practices must be assessed for all patients. Patients deemed at risk must be screened for STDs and be provided education regarding safer sex behaviors.

Populations known to be at higher risk for STDs are adolescent women age 15 to 19 years and young adults (male and female) aged 20 to 24 years. Rates of human immunodeficiency virus (HIV) infection remain high, especially among minority populations. Of newly diagnosed HIV infections in the United States during 2005, the Centers for Disease Control and Prevention (CDC) estimated that approximately 62 percent were men who were infected through sexual contact with other men, 51 percent were African Americans, 31 percent were Caucasians, and 17 percent were Hispanic (Americans). Studies of HIV infection among young men who have sex with men (MSM) in the mid- to late-1990s revealed high rates of HIV prevalence, incidence, and unrecognized infection, particularly among young African American MSM. Although some populations, such as lesbian women and older adults, are sometimes assumed to be at lower risks for STDs and unsafe sexual practices, there is sufficient incidence to mandate that all patients need to be assessed.

General Health and Medical History

Sexual health concerns should be included in a matter-of-fact manner in the general review of body systems. If health care professionals do not inquire about sexual concerns, patients may believe them to be unimportant, insignificant, or not amenable to treatment. These concerns are often not addressed because of discomfort or anxiety on the part of the health care provider, which can leave the patient unable to bring up issues of a sexual nature. Health care providers must learn to be comfortable and nonjudgmental in asking questions about sexuality and responding to issues that arise from questioning the patient or from the patient's efforts to address concerns. The health care provider should initiate the discussion to let the patient know that sexuality is an important aspect of health.

When basic questions about sexuality are included in preconsultation questionnaires that are given to patients, the patients may feel more comfortable about discussing concerns. Questions should be sensitive but direct enough to clarify issues. Emphasizing the commonality of concerns about sexual functioning may ease patient discomfort. In a patient who has arthritis, for example, the health care practitioner may begin by saying "It is common for people who have arthritis to notice changes in their sexual lives. Has your pain affected your sexual activity?" Often patients become more comfortable when the practitioner begins with open questions, such as "How can I help you?" and "What do you think is the cause of the difficulty?"

Sexual Health History

Depending on the complexity and severity of a sexual concern, a brief sexual history may be adequate (Box 61-1). With more severe concerns, a comprehensive history may be indicated. The patient may need to be referred to a psychiatrist, psychologist, or sexual counselor.

Intimate Partner Violence

The rate of family violence is approximately 2 victims per 1,000 U.S. residents age 12 or older. Family violence accounts for about 1 in 10 violent victimizations. intimate partner violence (IPV) occurs in some degree across all social, economic, religious, and cultural groups (Heise & Garcia-Moreno, 2002). Women and those in families living below the poverty line are more likely to be affected. In the study 30 percent of the women who had married or had lived with a man as part of a couple reported violence by a husband or male

PATIENT PLAYBOOK

Promoting Optimal Health of the Reproductive System

The nurse can suggest the following to instruct the female patient how to promote optimum reproductive health:

- Become comfortable with your own body. Examine your genitals to become familiar with normal appearance and to note any changes, such as inflammation, lesions, or masses.
- Become familiar with the amount, color, consistency, and odor of your normal daily discharge. If the discharge changes, consult a health care provider
- Maintain a record of your menstrual cycle.
- Be actively involved in your own health care. Wash the vulva daily with warm soapy water and avoid douching, scented hygiene sprays, and perfumed soaps.
- Never force vaginal penetration. Make sure your vagina is well-lubricated before inserting anything into it and be careful about what you insert into your vagina.
- Be sure that a condom is used during sexual intimacy when there may be any risk of exposure to STDs or unintended pregnancy if permitted by religious beliefs.

The nurse can suggest the following to instruct the male patient how to promote optimum health:

- Become comfortable with your own body. Examine your genitals to become familiar with normal appearance and to note any changes.
- Be actively involved in your own health care. Seek out information. Ask questions. If you are at risk, seek regular checkups.
- Retracting the foreskin when intact, wash your genitals daily with warm soapy water.
- Urination before and after intercourse can help to reduce urinary tract infections (UTIs).
- Be sure that a condom is used during sexual intimacy when there may be any risk of exposure to STDs or unintended pregnancy. You are fully responsible to protect yourself and to protect your partner.
- Do not progress from anal intercourse to vaginal intercourse without first washing your penis. If a condom is used, the condom should be changed.
- Strive to be in a mutually satisfying, infection-free relationship with one person.
- If you desire or intend to become a parent, select behaviors and a lifestyle that maintains fertility.

Adapted from Stewart, E. G., & Spencer, P. (2002). The V book: A doctor's guide to complete vulvovaginal health. *New York: Bantam.*

BOX 61-1

SHORT FORM OF SEXUAL HISTORY

- Are you currently sexually active: with one, or more than one, partner? Male, female, or both?
- Is sex satisfying to you? For your partner?
- How has your present illness (concern) affected your sexual functioning?
- Do you experience any pain during vaginal penetration? Under what circumstances? Is vaginal dryness a problem?
- Do you have difficulty achieving an orgasm when you want to? If so, in what situations?

Pertinent Questions for Postmenopausal Women

- Has your interest in sexual activity changed?
- Do you have discomfort with intercourse?
- Do you lubricate adequately with sexual stimulation?
- Is your partner able to have an erection? Maintain an erection?
- Are you taking hormone replacement therapy? Other medications?

Adapted from Estes, M. (2006). Health assessment and physical examination *(3rd ed.). New York: Thomson Delmar Learning.*

cohabitant. All adult and teenage women should be routinely screened for IPV. The possibility of abuse should also be considered in elder adults, same sex relationships, and men. Of note is that 11 percent of women living with another woman reported IPV. Approximately 15 percent of males living with a male intimate partner report IPV compared with 7.7 percent of males who were married or living with a woman as a couple. American Indian/Alaska Native women and men report more violence than do other cultural groups. Hispanic (American) women are more likely to report instances of intimate partner rape. Barriers to screening for domestic violence include the assumption of time constraints, care provider discomfort with the topic, discomfort about offending the patient, and perceptions of powerlessness to change the situation. Prevention and early intervention can occur by routinely asking simple and direct nonjudgmental questions regarding abuse and sexual assault (Box 61-2).

Screening for violence must be based on more than observed injuries. Psychological abuse or unseen injuries may also be occurring. Previous health care visits should be monitored for a pattern of injuries, history of abuse or assault, chronic pelvic pain, headaches, irritable bowel syndrome, depression, substance use, suicide attempts, and anxiety. Such symptoms may be warning signs of IPV. However, violence can exist in the absence of warning signs in the patient's medical history or behavior. Patients may not present with symptoms, especially those who experience psychological or emotional abuse. They may conceal what they are experiencing out of shame or fear. Thus, it is essential to screen every patient routinely. Partner control is often an important factor in violence and abuse. Thus, it is essential to ask questions in private, apart from the partner and apart from children, family, or friends. Behaviors of the partner during a health care visit that may be indicative of abuse include never leaving the patient's side, being over solicitous, being hostile and demanding, or answering questions for the patient. The patient must be assessed for safety and ensured that they are not in immediate danger.

When IPV is occurring, the patient may present with a flat affect or as frightened, depressed, or anxious. Symptoms of posttraumatic stress disorder (PTSD), such as dissociation, psychic numbing, or negative responses to touch, may be present in severe cases. Abused women may appear overly compliant and may have learned not to question authority. Conversely, because of the fear and shame associated with the abuse and the possibility of its detection, an abused woman may exhibit distrust of health care providers.

In cases where violence is identified, findings must be documented in the patient's chart. Explanations about issues of confidentiality must be given, but awareness of any state mandatory reporting laws is important. Most states have mandatory reporting laws that require health care providers to contact local domestic violence and child protection agencies. Patients must be informed of any such requirement when abuse is documented. The patient's options should be reviewed with him or her and referrals provided.

Sexual Abuse and Assault

According to the National Violence Against Women Survey, 1 in 6 women and 1 in 33 men in the United States have experienced an attempted or completed rape at some time in their lives. Immediate physical and psychological trauma must be addressed. Pregnancy and sexually transmitted diseases can result from sexual assault. Long-lasting physical symptoms and illnesses have been associated with sexual abuse and assault. Symptoms may include chronic pelvic pain, gastrointestinal (GI) disorders, and a variety of chronic pain disorders, including headaches and back pain.

Sexual violence victims exhibit immediate reactions that can include shock, disbelief, fear, confusion, and anxiety; symptoms associated with PTSD. Longer term effects of PTSD, which may continue for months or become chronic, include anxiety, nervousness, phobias, sleep disturbances, substance abuse, depression, alienation, flashbacks, emotional detachment, and sexual dysfunction. Recognition of the uniqueness of each individual's expression of outcomes is important in understanding their trauma and facilitating their healing.

People who have experienced sexual assault are more likely than those who are not victims to express risky behavior patterns that make them vulnerable to further victimization. Such behaviors include having unprotected sex, having sex at a younger age, and having multiple sexual partners. Other victims may use alcohol, drugs, or overeating to cope with their stress. Women, particularly those under age 18 or minority women are significantly more likely to experience sexual assault.

Physical Examination of Male Genitalia

Unless the male patient seeks health care for a reproductive or genital tract problem, physical examination of the genitalia may not be performed, depending on the health care setting and age of the patient. Some male patients may be embarrassed or anxious about assessment of their genitalia. Before beginning the examination the health care practitioner should consider the patient's cultural background and what beliefs or attitudes he may have about the examination. His culture may prohibit female practitioners from examining him. The patient's level of apprehension should be addressed, ensuring him as necessary that this is normal. The assessment techniques should be explained. If an erection occurs in response to touch during the examination, this should be explained in a professional and matter-of-fact manner as a common response. The examination should take place in a comfortable room that ensures privacy and freedom from interruptions. After undressing, the patient may be asked to lie supine on an examination table or stand in front of the seated examiner. Clean gloves should be worn to prevent spread of infection.

The examiner notes the secondary sex characteristics and assesses appropriateness for developmental stage, including distribution of pubic hair, size of penis, size of scrotum, and size and descent of testes. Presence of pubic lice, scabies, or lesions is noted. The foreskin, glans, and shaft of the penis are inspected for lesions, swelling, and inflammation. If the patient is uncircumcised, he is asked to retract the foreskin. The foreskin should retract easily and completely over the glans. The glans should appear smooth, with the urinary meatus located centrally at the distal tip. The glans is compressed between the thumb and forefinger to determine whether any discharge is present. Any discharge should be considered abnormal and a specimen for culture should be obtained. The shaft of the penis is palpated noting tenderness, hard areas under the skin, or signs of inflammation.

The examiner can ask the patient to hold the penis to one side for inspection of the size and shape of the scrotum. Using the thumb and two fingers, the examiner should gently palpate the scrotum, testes, epididymis, and spermatic cord for size, shape, consistency, tenderness, and presence of masses. The testes should have smooth borders, with the epididymis extending from the posterior surface. This portion of the examination can be used to teach the patient about monthly testicular self-examination (TSE), encouraging him to palpate his own testes while the shape and contours are explained to him. The spermatic cord is palpated on each side along its length from the epididymis to the inguinal ring noting nodules or swelling.

The final assessment of the male reproductive system is inspection of the rectum and prostate. The patient may be positioned in a knee-chest position, lying in a lateral position with knees flexed, or standing and leaning over the examining table. The anal area is visually examined for lesions, ulcerations, or fissures. Then the examiner gently inserts a lubricated index finger through the anus in direction of the umbilicus. The prostate gland is palpated through the anterior rectal wall, noting the size, shape, and consistency of the lateral posterior lobes. The contour is symmetrical and bilobed, with a palpable vertical groove in the center. The prostate should feel firm, smooth, slightly mobile and tender.

Commonly, some patients may experience the urge to urinate when the gland is being palpated. All male patients over 50 years of age should have the prostate gland examined annually by digital rectal examination (DRE). Because only the posterior lobes are palpable, when prostatic tumors or hypertrophy is suspected, additional diagnostic tests may be necessary.

Abnormal findings of the male reproductive system are most often related to benign or malignant growths or inflammations and lesions associated with infections. Penile growths or masses related to malignancy may be nodular or ulcerated. Chancre lesions are indurated, smooth, and disk-like in appearance. Chancroids are more papular to irregular-shaped ulcerations that drain pus. Condyloma may be flat, wart-like nodules or elevated, fleshy, elongated projections. Painful vesicles, erosions, or ulcers may be indicative of herpes, chancroid, or other inflammatory infections. Painless, singular, small erosions with eventual lymphadenopathy may be related to lymphogranuloma venereum or cancer.

Scrotal masses with localized swelling and tenderness unilaterally or bilaterally can be indicative of epididymitis, orchiditis, or testicular torsion. Incarcerated intestinal hernia is evidenced by a tender or painful swelling up through the groin. Hydroceles present as unilateral or bilateral translucent scrotal swelling without much pain. Spermatoceles are firm and within the epididymal tissue, varicoceles, dilations of the veins that drain the testes, palpate as cordlike or wormlike in texture. Testicular cancer tends to be a firm and nodular unilateral mass.

Penile discharge indicative of infections, such as chlamydia or gonorrhea, can be clear to purulent and minimal to copious. Urination may or may not be painful. The presence of macules or papules on the penis or scrotum may indicate scabies or pubic lice. Cultures must be taken whenever infections are suspected.

Gynecological Examination of the Female

Assessment of the female reproductive system consists of breast examination, inspection and palpation of the external genitalia, speculum assessment of the internal genitalia, collection of specimens for laboratory analysis, bimanual examination, and rectovaginal assessment. The patient may be apprehensive about the examination. If the patient is anxious, explanations of each step of the process, along with relaxation and breathing techniques, can be provided as the examination proceeds. Women experiencing their first pelvic examination and women who have a history of sexual abuse or assault may benefit from the presence of a support person during the examination. The examination should take place in a comfortable room that ensures privacy and freedom from interruptions.

Breasts are first examined by visual inspection for size, shape, contour, and symmetry (see chapter 63). The skin of the breasts, areolae, and nipples are inspected for color, pigmentation, vascularity, surface characteristics, discharge, and lesions. The breasts are inspected in various postures for bilateral pull, symmetry, and contour. The breast tissue and axillary nodes are palpated for lesions or masses. Instruction in breast self-examination (BSE) should be provided to women who have not yet been instructed. The examination provides the opportunity to have the patient feel her own breast tissue and recognize the usual textures of her own breast tissue. Review of the procedure and the regularity of practice should be included in all subsequent health visits.

During the gynecological examination, with the patient in recumbent position, the abdomen is palpated for symptomatic or asymptomatic abdominal or pelvic masses. The masses may originate from reproductive, GI, or renal organs. Gynecological masses, such as ovarian, adnexal, or uterine masses, may be differentiated through the bimanual pelvic portion of the examination.

The mons pubis and vulva are observed for hair distribution, age-appropriate development, skin coloration, and condition. The labia majora and minora are inspected and palpated for pigmentation and surface characteristics. The skin pigmentation of the labia majora is slightly darker than the patient's general skin. The labia minora should be dark pink and moist, with no evidence of nodules, tenderness, drainage, or lesions. The clitoris is noted and should be smooth, pink, and moist, about the size of a pea.

The urethral meatus should be centrally located and close to, or slightly within, the vaginal introitus. The vaginal introitus may be a thin vertical slit or a larger orifice with irregular edges from hymenal remnants related to vaginal birth. The skin surface of the perineum between the vaginal introitus and the anus should appear smooth and free from lesions. An episiotomy scar may be present in some women who have given birth vaginally. The anus is inspected for color and lesions, including hemorrhoids.

The Skene's glands are located in the periurethral area and are not visible. The glands are palpated by placing the index finger into the vagina, exerting pressure on the anterior vaginal wall and milking the glands toward the vaginal opening. The glands should be tender and without discharge. If discharge is present, a specimen should be obtained for culture.

Next the Bartholin's glands are palpated. These glands are not visible but are located in the posterolateral portion of the labia majora. Using the thumb and index finger, the examiner can palpate the perineal tissue between the vaginal wall and the lower portion of the labia majora. The surface should appear smooth and pink, and it should be tender, without discharge.

If there is a history of incontinence or discomfort in a woman who has had children, then the examiner can assess vaginal wall tone. While holding the labia apart, the patient is asked to bear down and to cough. The vaginal wall is observed for bulging indicative of a cystocele, rectocele, or uterine prolapse, which may be the result of injury, childbirth, or age.

Speculum Examination

Every woman should have a Papanicolaou (Pap) smear as part of a complete pelvic examination beginning when she becomes sexually active or reaches 18 years of age but no later than 21 years. These examinations should continue throughout her reproductive years. Current guidelines from the National Cancer Institute recommend that Pap tests need not be repeated within two years of a prior negative test (Sawaya, et al., 2003). Women ages 65 to 70 who have had at least three normal Pap tests and no abnormal Pap tests in the last 10 years may decide, after talking with their health care practitioner, to stop having Pap tests (National Cancer Institute, 2003).

The internal organs of the pelvis are examined bimanually. The patient is placed in a lithotomy position with Trendelenburg and draped (Figure 61-3). With clean gloves, the middle and index fingers are gently placed in the vagina. The vaginal wall is palpated for surface characteristics and discomfort. The wall should be smooth and nontender. The cervix is located with the fingers of the internal hand. The hand on the abdominal should gently hold the uterus downward against the internal hand so that the cervix and vaginal fornices can be palpated. The cervix should feel smooth, slightly round, and firm. It is located in the midline position and slightly mobile in either direction without causing discomfort. The examiner moves the fingers in the vagina into the anterior fornix while positioning the other hand on the abdomen "trapping" the uterus between the two hands to assess its position, size, shape, and mobility. The ovaries may not always be palpable, but if felt, they should feel smooth, firm and ovoid. Oviducts are soft and normally not palpable. The rectovaginal portion of the examination involves palpating the rectal wall for surface characteristics, such as masses, fistulas, fissures, or tenderness. The posterior wall

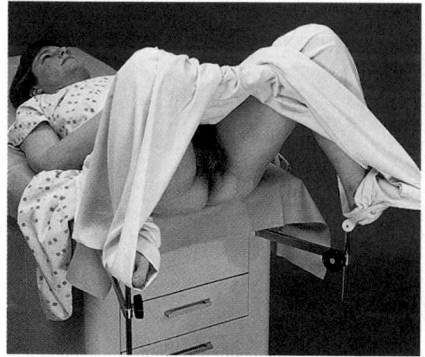

Figure 61-3 Patient positioning and draping for gynecological examination.

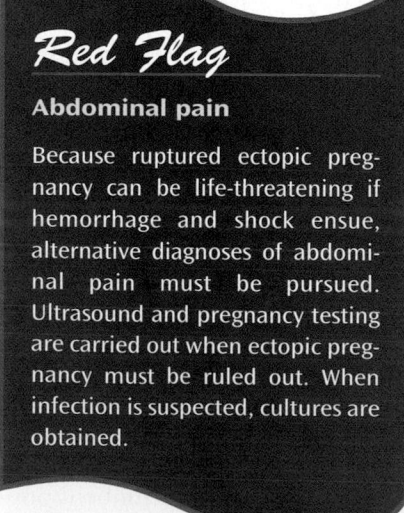

Red Flag

Abdominal pain

Because ruptured ectopic pregnancy can be life-threatening if hemorrhage and shock ensue, alternative diagnoses of abdominal pain must be pursued. Ultrasound and pregnancy testing are carried out when ectopic pregnancy must be ruled out. When infection is suspected, cultures are obtained.

PATIENT PLAYBOOK

Pap Test

The nurse can instruct the patient in the following prior to her Pap test:

- Schedule your examination when you are not menstruating (ideally 10 to 20 days after the first day of the last menstrual period).
- For 2 days before the test, avoid douching, vaginal creams, or jellies.
- You will be asked to empty your bladder before the examination, and you will put on a patient gown.
- The examiner will wear gloves during the examination.
- The speculum should be warmed and lubricated using warm water, and you will be asked to bear down, while breathing slowly.
- The cervix is examined for color, shape, modules, masses, erosions, discharge, or bleeding.
- Specimens are obtained cytological studies, if indicated, and a specimen for culture obtained from any suspicious discharge.

Adapted from Estes, M. (2006). Health assessment and physical examination (3rd ed.). New York: Thomson Delmar Learning.

of the uterus is palpated by stabilizing the cervix with the internal hand and palpating with the abdominal hand. As the internal fingers are withdrawn, the anal sphincter is evaluated for tone.

Abnormal Findings

Common abnormalities of the female reproductive system notable on assessment include vulvar or vaginal discharges, erythema, masses or lesions, and abdominal masses, pain, or tenderness. Candidiasis may present as vulvovaginal discharge that is odorless and plaque-like in consistency, accompanied by itching and inflammation. Bacterial vaginosis also creates vulvar irritation but with a grayish, copious, "fishy," malodorous discharge. Bloody discharge not directly associated with menstruation may be caused by trauma or vaginal, cervical, or uterine infections. With the use of some lower dosage oral contraceptives, or during the first few cycles of oral contraceptive use until the hormonal cycle adapts, breakthrough bleeding may occur. Vulvar erythema may often be related to vulvovaginal sexually transmitted infections. Vulvovaginal lesions associated with genital herpes may present with a reddened base, painful vesicles, or ulcerations. Herpes lesions may be on the labial folds, surrounding or inside the vestibule, on the vaginal walls, or on the cervix. Genital warts are nontender, soft, flat or fleshy growths that may be warty in appearance. Chancres are indurated, firm ulcers that tend to be nonpainful. Abdominal pain or tenderness may result from ectopic pregnancy, salpingitis, endometritis, pelvic inflammatory disease (PID), cystitis, ovarian cysts, or abscesses that may or may not have ruptured.

DIAGNOSTIC TESTS

The reproductive system has many disorders that require extensive diagnostic tests to determine the nature of the dysfunction. In general, there are specific tests for the male and specific tests for the female. Males have unique serum tests of such areas as the prostate gland and semen. Females have diagnostic tests of specific areas that are unique to their gender; such as the cervix and breast. This section of the chapter will examine the diagnostic tests for each gender separately.

Male Diagnostic Tests

Studies for assessment of health and disease in the male reproductive system include diagnosing infection, fertility issues, sexual dysfunction, structural abnormalities, and tissue masses. When indications of genitourinary infection are present, discharge or lesions may be swabbed or aspirated to obtain potential microorganisms for microscopic examination. To obtain a urethral smear, the male patient should not urinate prior to specimen collection. A small swab is inserted into the urethra. An anoscope is used to collect a rectal smear specimen and sample areas containing pus.

The smear of a specimen to which a gram stain is applied can distinguish gram-positive from gram-negative bacteria. A gram stain can provide important diagnostic information concerning the type of organisms present and the appropriate therapy to initiate while waiting for other test results. The gram stain is used to aid in the diagnosis of gonorrhea and candidal infections and in the assessment of urethritis, proctitis, and other infections characterized by a discharge.

Infections within the urethra, prostate, and bladder can contribute to urogenital dysfunction. Urinalysis detects bacteria, white blood cells, and red blood cells. Patient complaints, such as pain related to tissue inflammation, pain or irritation during voiding, bladder spasms, or alterations in urinary elimination, should be assessed by urinalysis. A clean-catch specimen may also be collected for examination.

Analysis of the semen for quality and presence of sperm is a primary diagnostic tool in infertility assessment. Semen specimens are obtained by masturbation into a sterile wide-mouthed container after two to five days of abstinence. The specimen must be analyzed within two hours of collection. Usually, two to three specimens, each separated by at least a month, are analyzed to ensure a meaningful evaluation. An obstruction of the ejaculatory duct is usually implied when **azoospermia** (absence of spermatozoa in the semen) is coupled with low ejaculate volume of nonclotting watery fluids that are fructose-negative. If the vasa are palpable, a transrectal ultrasonography (TRUS) can be diagnostic. Patients who are not azoospermic but are **oligospermic,** or have low sperm motility with a low semen volume, may have partial ejaculatory duct obstruction or retrograde ejaculation. Retrograde ejaculation is commonly seen in diabetics, as well as in men who have had transurethral surgery at, or near, the bladder neck. To assess for retrograde ejaculation a postejaculatory urine specimen is obtained. The specimen is obtained by first having the patient empty his bladder, then ejaculate. Following ejaculation the patient voids again into a separate container. Computer-assisted semen analysis (CASA) is available but is primarily used as a research tool and does not provide information that alters therapy at this time.

Prostate fluid is assessed when bacterial infection is suspected to be localized in the prostate gland. To obtain a specimen from the lower urinary tract for culture, the patient is asked to urinate a few drops into a sterile container. Then a midstream urine sample is collected in a second container. A prostate examination and massage are performed, and the prostate fluid is collected for culture and microscopic examination. The patient is then asked to urinate into a third container. A diagnosis of chronic bacterial prostatitis is made if the bacterial count of the postmassage urine sample is ten-fold higher than in the first urine samples.

DRE is performed by the practitioner to detect abnormalities of the prostate gland. Abnormalities such as induration, marked asymmetry, and frank nodularity are associated with clinically significant intracapsular prostate tumors. The examination can be performed in any of three positions: the patient can stand with flexed hips and lean over an examination table, lie on his side and curl inward, or kneel, face-down on top of the examination table. The examiner inserts the index finger into the rectum and palpates the prostate, which is situated between the examining finger and the symphysis pubis. While the DRE may detect abnormalities present in the posterior and lateral aspects of the glands, masses located on the anterior surface cannot be directly palpated. Used alone, DRE has been shown to miss approximately 40 percent of cancers detected during an initial screening (Daniels, 2003).

Basic endocrine evaluation includes measurement of serum testosterone and FSH, LH, and prolactin. LH abnormalities are rare and thus, LH levels need be obtained only in men with abnormal testosterone levels. Elevated serum FSH can result from impaired secretion of inhibin, which is produced by the Sertoli cell and provides feedback at the pituitary and hypothalamus to turn off FSH secretion. Elevated serum FSH can imply abnormalities in the seminiferous epithelium and subsequently spermatogenesis. Prolactin, another pituitary hormone, may affect fertility by decreasing LH production, resulting in a decrease in testosterone and subsequently, decreased libido. Low levels of FSH, LH, and testosterone are also diagnostic of hypogonadotropic hypogonadism resulting in a delay or failure in the onset of puberty and therefore poorly developed secondary sexual characteristics and small, firm testes. Serum estrogens, prolactin, and adrenal steroids are only measured if clinically indicated due to low serum testosterone, decreased libido, gynecomastia, or a history of precocious puberty.

PSA testing is used to evaluate men at risk for prostate cancer, to assist in pretreatment staging of prostate cancer, to monitor the posttreatment, and manage treatment of this disease. Produced exclusively by the epithelial cells of the prostate, periurethral, and perirectal glands, PSA is excreted by normal, hyperplastic, and malignant cells of the prostate. PSA increases yearly after age 40, but especially after age 50, by approximately 3 percent per year in healthy 60-year-olds without cancer. In conjunction with the DRE, PSA is used to investigate or evaluate an enlarged prostate gland or masses palpable on the prostate gland when cancer is suspected. PSA levels are determined in a 5-mL blood specimen, and a PSA reading of 4 nanograms and below is considered normal. A reading of up to 10 nanograms may be an indication of cancer. Men with PSA levels of 4.1 to 9.9 nanograms should undergo prostate biopsy. PSA levels may be repeated three or more times over a period of one to three years to determine PSA velocity. This can indicate the potential presence of prostate cancer and the need for a prostate biopsy before the total PSA becomes abnormally elevated. If the PSA increase is greater than 0.75 ng/mL over the last year, prostate cancer is likely present.

Prostate biopsy is the primary screening test for prostate cancer, though less than 25 percent of all biopsies contain cancer. Prostatic biopsy is performed by inserting a needle through the perineum (external) or via the rectum through the rectal wall to penetrate areas of nodularity or induration of the prostate. Multiple random needle biopsies may be performed to determine if a tumor is multifocal.

Ultrasonography measures and records high-frequency sound waves as they pass through tissues of variable density. Ultrasonography helps to identify masses greater than 3 cm, such as tumors within the prostate or nodal enlargement associated with metastasis or infections. Ultrasonography can also determine the adequacy of arterial circulation in the genital organs. TRUS is performed to view prostate tissue and is usually carried out in conjunction with prostatic biopsy.

After pathological confirmation of prostate cancer, MRI is used to determine the staging of the cancer. MRI can determine the extent of malignant involvement by exhibiting capsular penetration, seminal vesicle and neurovascular invasion, regional lymph node metastasis, or diffuse body metastasis.

In patients with PSA levels of 20 nanograms and higher, a radionuclide bone scan is done to rule out metastasis. Radionuclide can also localize in soft tissue areas, demonstrating calcification as well as infarction, inflammation, trauma, and tumor. Computed tomography (CT) scan detects grossly enlarged lymph nodes but does not provide clear pictures of intraprostatic features.

Testicular biopsy is used to determine if men with either azoospermia or severe oligospermia have an absence or deficiency of sperm production or whether obstruction is present at some point along the pathway from seminiferous tubule to ejaculatory duct. The procedure may also be performed to confirm presence of neoplastic tissue. Under local anesthesia, a 3- to 4-mm incision is made through the scrotum into the testis exposing about a pea-sized sample of seminiferous tubule. The procedure is often carried out in an operative setting where the patient may undergo immediate exploration and microsurgical reconstruction or sperm retrieval for immediate use in an in vitro fertilization (IVF) or intracytoplasmic sperm injection (ICSI) cycle or cryopreservation.

Cavernosometry and cavernosography are procedures that evaluate the flow of blood and pressure functions of the penis. These tests assess the integrity of the arterial and venous circulatory systems of the penis during an erection. Local anesthesia and an intracavernosal injection of a vasoactive drug are given prior to initiation.

Duplex ultrasonography is used to diagnose marked arterial insufficiency as the major cause of erectile dysfunction. Duplex ultrasonography entails high-resolution sonography with pulsed Doppler blood flow analysis to evaluate the penile arterial status. An injected vasodilator drug (e.g., papaverine hydrochloride, phentolamine mesylate, and prostaglandin E_1) is given prior to the test to enhance assessment of arterial or venous insufficiency.

The penile brachial index (PBI) is calculated by comparing the penile systolic blood pressure, determined by a Doppler, with the brachial systolic blood pressure at rest and after exercise. An intracavernosal injection of a vasoactive drug may be administered prior to the test. The normal range for PBI is equal to or more than 0.75, while abnormal range for PBI is equal to or less than 0.6. A PBI that is not within the normal range may indicate a vascular cause of erectile dysfunction.

Female Diagnostic Tests

This section will examine the diagnostic tests that are specific to disorders of the reproductive system of the female. Studies for assessment of health and disease in the female reproductive system include diagnosing infection, fertility issues, sexual dysfunction, structural abnormalities, and tissue masses. To begin, mammography is a radiographic image of the breast to screen for cancerous lesions in the breast tissue. The U.S. Preventive Services Task Force (USPSTF) recommends screening mammography, with or without clinical breast examination (CBE), every one to two years for women age 40 and older (U. S. Department of Health and Human Services, Agency for Health Care Research and Quality, 2002). Mammography, in combination with breast self-examination (BSE) and breast examinations during routine physical assessment, detects about 85 to 90 percent of existing breast cancers. The health history of women at increased risk for breast cancer (family history, genetic tendency, and past breast cancer) should be evaluated to determine the benefits and limitations of starting mammography screening earlier, having additional tests (breast ultrasound or MRI), or having more frequent examinations. Abnormalities of the breast determined by mammography or palpation should be further evaluated by fine needle biopsy or core needle biopsy that provides a larger sample, to determine the histology of the tissue mass or lesion. These procedures may be performed under local anesthesia in a clinic setting. Ultrasound may be used to guide the placement of the needle to targeted areas. If cancer is diagnosed, further treatment, such as surgery, chemotherapy, hormone therapy, or radiation, is also initiated.

Screening, particularly for STDs, can be performed by culture of blood samples, lesions, or any discharge from the reproductive tract. Chlamydia and gonorrhea are the two most common STD infections of the female reproductive tract. Both produce similar symptoms and may occur simultaneously. Because symptoms may be asymptomatic or mild, periodic screening is recommended among sexually active women.

Cervical cytological screening (Pap smear) is used to detect cancer and precursors of cancer in the uterine cervix. A sampling of exfoliated cells from the cervix is examined microscopically using a technique developed by Papanicolaou in 1942, thus, the current abbreviated name of Pap smear. Widespread use of Pap smears in routine gynecological screening in the United States has reduced deaths from cervical cancer by 75 percent. A description of the Pap test (e.g., speculum exam) and instructions to patients were described previously in the chapter. Women with atypical Pap smear results and evidence of high-risk type HPV should receive further evaluation with colposcopy.

Colposcopy involves examination of the cervix, the vagina, and at times, the vulva with magnification using a colposcope, a special binocular microscope and light system that magnifies the mucosal surfaces. A 3 percent solution of acetic acid is applied to improve the contrast between tissue types. Photographs for future reference and biopsy samples may be taken of any lesions that appear to be abnormal or suggestive of dysplasia or invasive cancer.

A culdoscopy is the examination of the viscera of the female pelvic cavity after introducing a flexible endoscope via the posterior vaginal fornix. It is use as a diagnostic procedure for infertility and for pelvic pain. Surgical procedures, such as tubal ligation, excision of an ovarian cyst, lysis of adhesions, and biopsy of endometriosis, may also be performed using culdoscopy. These procedures can be done using local, regional, or general anesthesia.

When cervical cytological studies reveal atypical squamous cells, a diagnostic excisional procedure should be carried out by the health care practitioner to obtain a specimen from the cervical transformation zone and endocervical canal for histological evaluation and to remove the area of cervical dysplasia. The specimen may be collected by several methods, including laser conization, cold-knife conization (CKC), loop electrosurgical excision (LEEP), and loop electrosurgical excision of transformational zone (LEETZ). All these procedures create a raw wound on the cervix and bleeding may require cauterization. Laser conization is performed with a carbon dioxide laser. The procedure may be performed with the use of colposcopy, which allows precise determination of the margins of the cervical lesion. Cold knife cone biopsy is the surgical excision of a wedge-shaped portion of the ectocervix and endocervix, including the removal of the entire squamocolumnar junction of the cervix. LEEP uses high-frequency electromagnetic currents to obtain a specimen by passing a thin wire loop through the transformation zone of the cervix approximately 1 cm in depth (Figure 61-4).

When abnormal uterine bleeding occurs an endometrial biopsy is performed to differentially diagnose hormonal imbalances or an anatomical cause for bleeding (e.g., polyps, hyperplasia, or cancer). The procedure involves taking a small sample of endometrial tissue from the inside of the uterus by inserting an endometrial suction catheter through the cervix and into the fundus of the uterus, where suction is applied to the catheter as it is gently rotated within the uterus. Endometrial tissue is collected by this process and sent for microscopic examination. In infertility treatment, endometrial biopsy is performed to evaluate the endometrial changes indicative of normal

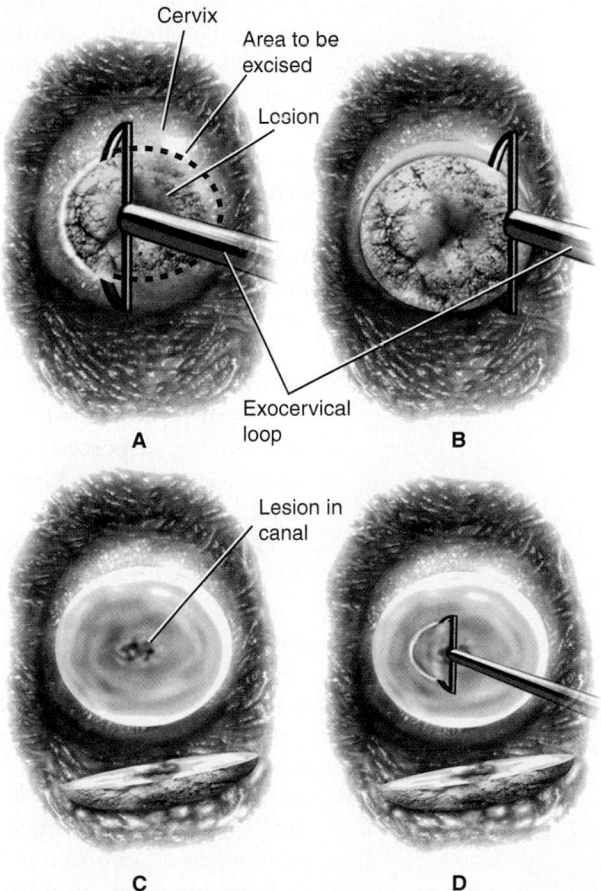

Figure 61-4 Cervical conization—LEEP technique: A. Path of electrosurgical loop through distal cervix, B. Loop near completion of excision, C. Lesion identified in cervix, D. Loop excision of lesion.

endometrial growth and cycling to determine endometrial readiness to accept embryo transplants.

Dilation and curettage (D & C) is a surgical procedure in which the cervical canal is dilated using dilators of graduated size and the endometrial tissue of the uterus is scraped out using a sharp curette. This procedure may be performed to evaluate infertility, to treat endometrial hyperplasia and other abnormal uterine bleeding, and as an abortion procedure.

Menstrual cycling, sexual responses, fertility, pregnancy, and menopause are all regulated by complex interactive endocrine activities involving the pituitary, ovaries, uterus, and other endocrine systems. When there are indications of abnormal functioning in any of these processes, there are a range of diagnostic endocrine studies that may be performed. FSH and LH studies are performed using a serum specimen and immunoassay. These studies are indicated in a range of reproductive disorders and assessments of abnormal functional patterns (gonadal failure, menstrual disturbances, and infertility). Estrogen and progesterone levels may be measured to determine the presence of dysfunction (e.g., gonadal dysfunction, menstrual abnormalities, or responses to hormone replacement therapy). Testosterone levels in women are normally 10 percent of the levels found in men. Levels in perimenopausal women may fall slightly more in relationship to age than to menopausal status.

Pregnancy tests are designed to detect hCG, a hormone produced by the placenta, using immunochromatographic assay. In normal pregnancy, hCG can be detected in serum as early as seven days following conception, doubling every 1.3 to 2 days and reading 100 mIU/mL at the first missed menstrual period. Serum levels less that 5 mIU/mL indicate that the woman is not pregnant. When using hCG-based urine tests, including those available OTC, the highest possible screening sensitivity conducted on the first day of a missed period is 90 percent. Pregnancy tests also assist in the diagnoses of suspected ectopic pregnancy, threatened abortion, incomplete abortion, and hCG-producing tumors.

Pelvic organs and tissues can be visualized by a range of endoscopic examinations. These procedures are usually performed on an outpatient basis even when performed under general anesthesia. Instructions for endoscopy may include bowel preparation and clear liquids or fasting on the day of the procedure. Postoperative instructions include the expectation of abdominal or referred pain and vaginal bleeding or discharge. Normal activities often are resumed within two to three days. Because these procedures are invasive, abdominal pain, fever, significant bleeding, or nausea and vomiting may indicate complications and need to be reported to the care provider immediately.

For reproductive assessments, laparoscopy using a fiberoptic scope may be performed to inspect the uterus, oviducts, ovaries, and lower pelvic region. Common indications for laparoscopy are unexplained pelvic pain, infertility procedures, suspected endometriosis, or ovarian masses. Procedures that can be performed under laparoscopic visualization include tubal sterilization, lysis of adhesions caused by endometriosis, and uterine fibroidectomy.

Hysteroscopy is a procedure in which direct visual examination of the uterus is used to investigate reproductive system problems, such as dysfunctional uterine bleeding, uterine fibroids, or suspected uterine cancer. The patient is given a local anesthetic and placed in the lithotomy position. Either carbon dioxide or fluid is inserted into the uterine cavity, and the hysteroscope is inserted through the vagina into the uterus. The uterine cavity is inspected for abnormalities and biopsies may be taken. Problems diagnosed with hysteroscopy include the cause of abnormal bleeding; fibroid tumors that arise within the uterine cavity; intrauterine polyps; location of a lost intrauterine device, uterine abnormalities, such as a uterine septum, bicornate uterus and, in some cases, endometrial cancer.

Basal body temperature (BBT) is a noninvasive method of determining the probable time of ovulation as well as determining ovulatory versus anovulatory cycles. The patient should use a digital basal thermometer and chart her oral temperatures taken after at least five hours of sleep and before arising from bed. A slight drop in temperature often occurs just before ovulation. After ovulation the temperature raises 0.2° to 0.4° C (0.4° to 0.8° F) and remains up through the remainder of the menstrual cycle. Records should be kept for at least three months to ascertain ovulation patterns.

The patient is taught to collect vaginal mucus using toilet tissue or her fingers and to document changes throughout her menstrual cycle. Before ovulation and after ovulation the cervical mucus is normally scant, thick, sticky, and opaque. When this ovulatory phase mucus is present, it indicates that ovulation has likely occurred. Postcoital examination of cervical mucus is used to evaluate the characteristics of cervical mucus and sperm function. Assessments include characteristics of the cervical mucus, correlated with the phase of the woman's menstrual cycle and with the number, morphology, motility, and ability of the sperm to cross the cervical mucus. The test should be scheduled one to two days before ovulation is anticipated and within two to three hours after intercourse.

When the female patient is experiencing infertility or recurrent pregnancy loss, the uterine cavity is evaluated through hysteroscopy, hysterosalpingogram, or sonohysterography. Hysterosalpingography involves instillation of contrast media through the cervix into the uterine cavity and out into the oviducts to determine abnormalities. The recent development of the falloposcope has increased the use of falloposcopy in evaluation of the oviducts in the infertile patient (American Infertility Association, 2005). Saline infusion sonohysterography (SHG) creates an image of the uterus and uterine cavity using ultrasonography after sterile saline is instilled into the uterine cavity. The purpose of SHG is to detect abnormalities of the uterus and endometrial cavity (e.g., abnormal uterine bleeding, infertility, or recurrent spontaneous miscarriage). The procedure begins with a transvaginal ultrasound examination. The uterine cavity is filled with sterile saline to improve the detail of the images of the uterine cavity. Pelvic ultrasound may be performed transabdominally, transvaginally, or endovaginally in women and transrectally in men. In reproductive system assessment in women pelvic ultrasound is most often used to examine the uterus and ovaries and, during pregnancy, to monitor the health and development of the embryo or fetus. Sonography can assist in determining the causes of pelvic pain, abnormal bleeding, or other menstrual problems and identifying palpable masses, such as ovarian cysts, uterine fibroids, and ovarian or uterine cancers.

A CT scan is an X-ray procedure that combines many X-ray images with the aid of a computer to generate cross-sectional views and three-dimensional images of the internal organs and structures of the body. A CT scan is used to define normal and abnormal structures in the body, as well as to accurately guide the placement of instruments or treatments during procedures. For reproductive assessment, CT scans are used to verify the presence or absence of tumors, infection, or abnormal anatomy, as well as to assist in certain procedures, such as biopsies of suspicious masses, draining of abscesses, or removal of fluids for diagnostic tests.

MRI uses radiofrequency waves and a strong magnetic field to provide clear and detailed images without exposing pelvic organs and tissues to radiation. MRIs can contrast uterine myometrium and endometrium; identify evidence of endometriosis; differentiate cervical, epithelial, and mucous tissue; and differentiate ovarian cysts and masses.

Prevention and control of STDs is based on education and counseling of persons at risk, identification of infected people, effective diagnosis and treatment of infected persons, evaluation and treatment of sex partners, and preexposure vaccinations of people at risk for vaccine-preventable STDs. As part of the clinical interview, health care providers can obtain a sexual history from their patients. If risk factors are identified, providers should encourage patients to adopt safer sexual behaviors. Patients seeking treatment or screening for STDs

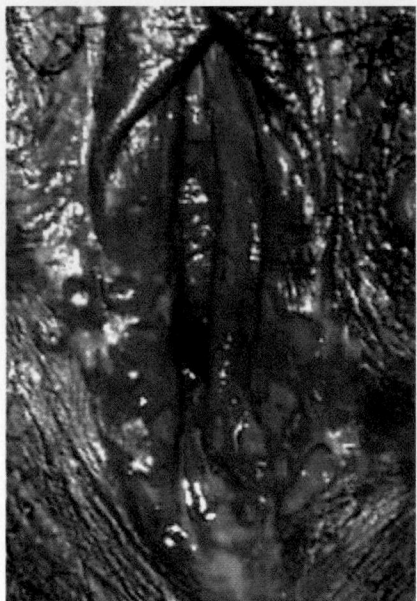

Figure 61-5 Primary HSV, first episode. Serology tests are negative for HSV. Copyright GlaxoSmithKline. Used with permission.

may expect evaluation for all common STDs (e.g., *Chlamydia trachomatis, Neisseria gonorrhoeae,* syphilis, herpes simplex virus [HSV], human papillomavirus, HIV).

A number of STDs can be diagnosed by point of care testing (POCT), which is defined as testing performed outside of clinical laboratories. This may be particularly relevant in clinical settings that provide care to transient populations, patients who may not be motivated to return for care after confirmation of an STD, or with patients who do not have access to regular health care. However, most STD POCT should be verified by additional standard testing within a clinical laboratory. In addition, physical examination can detect STD abnormalities (Figure 61-5). Most patients whose STDs are treatable with antibiotics should return for a test of cure, ensuring that the treatment regimen was effective.

Laboratory-based tests are available for many of the STD disorders. POCT has long included the gram-stained smear for *N. gonorrhoeae* and *C. trachomatis.* In addition, cultures are also performed on endocervical swab specimens in the female, or for male patients, on an intraurethral swab specimen. Specimens may also be obtained from rectal or pharyngeal swab specimens. The screening tests for syphilis are the Venereal Disease Research Laboratory (VDRL) and rapid plasma reagin (RPR) tests that detect a rise in antibody titers following infection (U.S. Department of Health and Human Services, Centers for Disease Control and Prevention, 2003).

KEY CONCEPTS

- The primary functions of the male reproductive system are production, transport, and deposit of sperm and secretion of testosterone.
- The primary functions of the female reproductive system are production of ova, secretion of hormones, pregnancy and birth of a fetus, and breastfeeding an infant.
- The physiological components of male sexual response include erection, orgasm, and ejaculation.
- Adequate functioning of the neurological and vascular systems is important in physiological sexual responsiveness.
- Sexual dysfunction is a disturbance or disorder in desire, excitement, or orgasm of the sexual response cycle.
- Sexuality is an integral component of physical and emotional health for all people, incorporating gender identity, self-worth, the ability to establish healthy intimate relationships, and expressions of sexual behaviors.

- Sexual violence victims exhibit immediate reactions that can include shock, disbelief, fear, confusion, and anxiety, symptoms associated with PTSD.
- Assessment of the female reproductive system consists of breast examination, palpation of the external genitalia, speculum assessment, laboratory analysis, bimanual examination, and rectovaginal assessment.
- Women with specific concerns about premenstrual symptoms, irregular menstrual cycles, or dysmenorrhea should be assessed for further diagnostic work.
- Assessment of the male reproductive system includes self testicular examination, laboratory analysis, prostate examination, and palpation of external genitalia.

REVIEW QUESTIONS

1. Sperm generation in the male is dependent on testosterone production, which is mediated by which pituitary gland hormones?
   1. Gonadotropin-releasing hormone and FSH
   2. FSH and LH
   3. Gonadotropin-releasing hormone and Sertoli hormone
   4. LH and Sertoli hormone

2. Menstruation is the result of:
   1. Withdrawal of human chorionic gonadotropin
   2. Decreasing production of LH and progesterone
   3. Decreasing production of estrogen and progesterone by the corpus luteum
   4. Withdrawal of FSH and LH

3. In both the male and female body, the fundamental physiological responses to effective sexual stimulation are:
   1. Vasocongestion and muscle tension (myotonia)
   2. Erections and increased blood pressure and heart rate
   3. Lubrication from the Cowper's gland and the Bartholin's glands
   4. Excitement and plateau

4. Why is it essential for the health care practitioner to address sexual health concerns in routine health assessment?
   1. To ensure the patient that sexual health concerns are an important aspect of health
   2. To ensure the patient that sexual concerns can be discussed in the health care setting
   3. To provide opportunity to discuss preventive sexual health lifestyles with the patient
   4. All of the above

5. Which of the following questions is not part of a sexual history?
   1. Are you currently sexually active?
   2. Is sex satisfying to you?
   3. How has your present illness (concern) affected your sexual functioning?
   4. Which sexual positions do you prefer?

6. Which of the following symptoms is commonly associated with sexually transmitted infections in the male?
   1. Penile discharge with pain on urination
   2. Difficulty initiating a steady urine stream
   3. Heavy tenderness in the scrotum

7. A 22-year-old woman returns to the health clinic with her concerns about pelvic pain. Although her pelvic examination revealed no apparent abnormalities beyond the general tenderness, the nurse notes bruises on her upper arms and chest. An important question to ask would be:
   1. Are your injuries work-related?
   2. Do you bruise easily? Does your family have a history of a clotting disorder?
   3. Violence is a problem for many women. Has someone been hurting you?
   4. Have you been raped?

8. Which of the following descriptions of vaginal discharge is indicative of possible bacterial vaginosis?
   1. Odorless, white, opaque mucus that is sticky
   2. Copious, green, frothy, somewhat malodorous discharge
   3. Odorless, plaque-like patches accompanied by vulvar redness
   4. Copious, gray, malodorous, or "fishy" odor discharge

9. A 3-cm nodule was palpated during the digital rectal examination of the prostate gland? What diagnostic tests would be recommended to evaluate the nodule?
   1. Prostate ultrasonography, biopsy of nodule, and PSA
   2. PSA, serum testosterone level, and MRI
   3. MRI, serum testosterone level, and PSA
   4. Prostate ultrasonography and serum testosterone level

10. The Pap smear as part of routine pelvic assessment of the female patient examines what specific tissue for potential precancerous or cancerous changes?
    1. The transformation zone between columnar epithelial cells of the cervical canal and the squamous cells covering the outer cervix
    2. The squamous cells of the cervix on the posterior surface and along the posterior fornix of the vagina
    3. The cervical mucus, which contains sloughed cells from the uterine lining as well as the cervical canal
    4. Any cervical lesions showing evidence of HPV

Continued

REVIEW QUESTIONS—cont'd

11. What is the rationale for teaching an 18-year-old male how to perform self-examination of his genitals?
    1. Self-examination can prevent him from acquiring an STD.
    2. Testicular torsion is a surgical emergency that requires prompt identification and treatment.
    3. Self-examination can help determine when he has achieved fully developed genitalia.
    4. Testicular cancer is the most common type of cancer in young men.

12. A female patient indicated that she has sex with multiple partners and she does not use condoms because she is on oral contraceptives. Which of the following responses is most appropriate?
    1. How long have you been on oral contraceptives?
    2. You should avoid sex until you are married.
    3. Even though you are on oral contraceptives, you should use condoms to protect yourself from sexually transmitted disease.
    4. How well do you know your partners?

REVIEW ACTIVITIES

1. Role-play taking a sexual health history with a peer to increase your comfort in asking appropriate questions.

2. Provide nursing care for a person of the opposite gender who is close to your age. Describe the potential difficulties of patient education regarding self-examinations that are characteristic of reproductive function (e.g., TSE, BSE).

3. Describe the sexual response cycle to a peer and afterward discuss together the areas that you believe will be somewhat uncomfortable for you to verbalize with a patient.

4. Compare four diagnostic tests in the reproductive system, which are performed with a male.

5. Compare four diagnostic tests in the reproductive system, which are performed with a female.

Female Reproductive Dysfunction: Nursing Management

Mary Franklin, MSN, CNM

CHAPTER TOPICS

- Menstrual Disorders
- Reproductive Tract Infections
- Benign Reproductive Tract Conditions
- Female Genital Mutilation
- Reproductive Tract Malignancies
- Infertility
- Sexual Dysfunction

The female reproductive system is complicated both in terms of anatomical structures and of hormonal regulation. A result of that complexity, reproductive dysfunctions are common. Nurses play a crucial role in the care of women with reproductive dysfunctions, and there is strong nursing collaboration with other disciplines that also provide care for women. Nurses with basic clinical preparation, advanced practice nurses, and certified nurse midwives work in the area of women's reproductive health care. The social and psychological consequences of female reproductive dysfunctions require skilled and sensitive nursing care. The topics discussed in this chapter are menstrual disorders, reproductive tract infections, benign reproductive tract conditions, female genital mutilation, reproductive tract malignancies, infertility, and sexual dysfunction.

KEY TERMS

Anovulation
Condyloma
Didelphic
Dysfunctional uterine bleeding (DUB)
Dysmenorrhea
Dyspareunia
Endometriosis
Imperforate hymen
Leiomyomata
Menopause
Menorrhagia
Metrorrhagia
Müllerian dysgenesis
Myomectomy
Oligomenorrhea
Perimenopause
Primary amenorrhea
Primary anorgasmia
Secondary amenorrhea
Secondary anorgasmia
Vaginitis

MENSTRUAL DISORDERS

Menstrual disorders are varied and have many different consequences in females. The menstrual disorders included in this section are: dysmenorrhea, amenorrhea, menopause, and premenstrual disorders.

Dysmenorrhea

Dysmenorrhea or pain during the menstrual cycle, affects 75 percent of menstruating women, and 90 percent of adolescents experience it with the onset of ovulatory cycles. Menstrual pain is commonly described by women as a cramping pain but may also include backache and leg pain. The release of prostaglandin hormone with the onset of menses is a main factor in dysmenorrhea. Increased prostaglandin release also accounts for the nausea, sweating, and bowel emptying experienced by some women at the start of their cycles.

Dysmenorrhea is not as common in the first 12 to 24 months after menarche, before cycles become ovulatory. Dysmenorrhea occurring with the first few menstrual cycles can be caused by an outflow obstruction and should be evaluated. **Leiomyomata** (benign smooth muscle tumors of the uterus commonly called fibroids), infection, ovarian cysts (globular sacs on the ovaries that are filled with fluid or semisolid material), or **endometriosis** (growth of the functioning endometrial tissue that lines the uterus somewhere outside of the uterus) may cause a significant worsening or new onset of dysmenorrheal (Figure 62-1). Therefore, dysmenorrhea not responsive to nonsteroidal anti-inflammatory drugs (NSAIDs) or combined oral contraceptives must be evaluated.

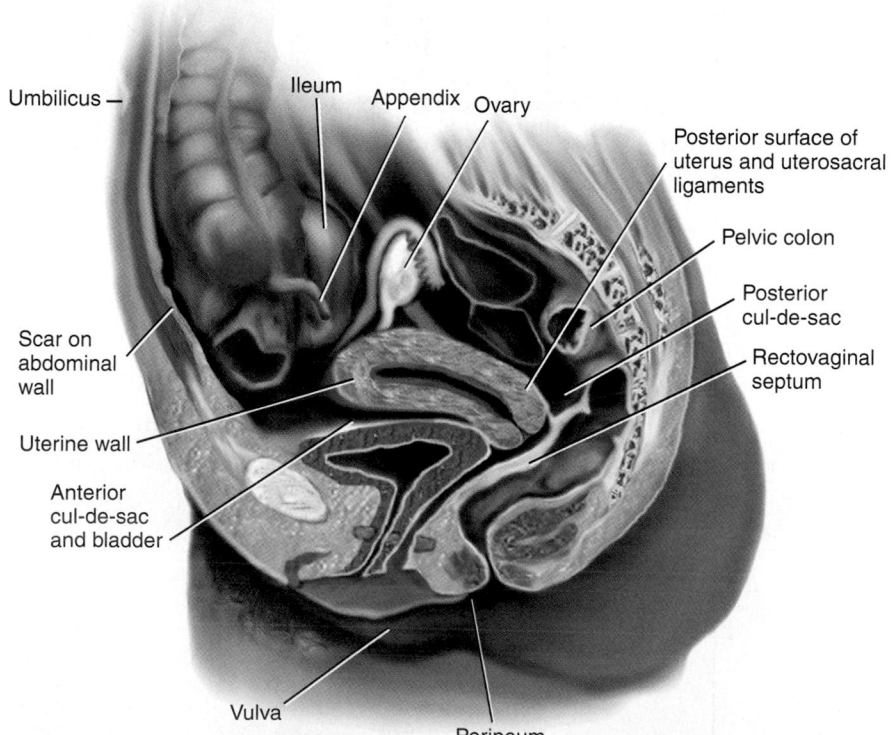

Figure 62-1 Common areas of endometriosis.

Amenorrhea

The average age of menarche in the United States is 12.8 years. In **primary amenorrhea** menstrual cycles have not started by age 16. In **secondary amenorrhea** menstrual cycles start normally but then stop. Of prime importance in evaluating any woman with amenorrhea is ruling out pregnancy.

Distinguishing primary from secondary amenorrhea is done to rule out the structural abnormalities that only need to be considered in primary amenorrhea. Primary amenorrhea can be caused by a congenital absence of a part of the reproductive tract, such as the ovaries, uterus, or vagina. Another cause is when the hymenal opening at the exit of the vagina does not form **(imperforate hymen),** and there is no exit from the vagina. Imperforate hymen occurs in 1 in 1,000 women. When imperforate hymen is the only abnormality menstrual cycles occur normally, but menstrual flow cannot be released to the outside and considerable pain and pelvic distension occurs. Treatment of imperforate hymen is excision of the hymen. This is usually a simple office procedure, performed under local anesthesia, which provides immediate resolution of the problem without sequelae.

Amenorrhea, either primary or secondary, can also occur because of disruptions in the hypothalamic system, elevated prolactin levels, thyroid disorders, premature ovarian failure, lack of sufficient body fat, or as a side effect of medication, stress, surgery, or local trauma. Unexplained secondary amenorrhea that lasts three months or longer or **oligomenorrhea** (menstrual cycles that occur farther apart than usual) of nine cycles or less per year needs evaluation (Practice Committee of the American Society for Reproductive Medicine, 2004). Amenorrhea is sometimes an expected event not requiring evaluation. Breastfeeding women will commonly be amenorrheic for up to 10 months postpartum. Amenorrhea is an expected and sometimes desired side effect of medications such as long-acting progesterone contraceptives and gonadotropin-releasing hormone (GnRH) agonists.

Athletes and women with anorexia nervosa can be amenorrheic if fat comprises less than 10 percent of their body. The female athlete triad includes the following three components: a menstrual disorder (amenorrhea or oligomenorrhea), an eating disorder, and decreased bone mineral density (Sherman & Thompson, 2004). Obese women also have a higher incidence of amenorrhea. Excessive scraping of the uterine lining with curettage, usually after childbirth or abortion, can cause permanent damage to the uterine lining and an absence of further menstruation. This is called Asherman's syndrome.

Women with amenorrhea always have **anovulation** (failure of the ovaries to grow or failure to release ova) except when amenorrhea is caused by a structural problem (American College of Obstetricians and Gynecologists [ACOG], 2002). Treatment of amenorrhea depends on its cause. Correcting pituitary disorders, thyroid disorders, or gaining sufficient body fat usually results in a resumption of menses.

For women with a hypothalamic disorder, progesterone therapy can be used to initiate a cycle. For example, a course of 10 mg of Provera for 10 days may be prescribed. Most amenorrheic women without other disorders will have a cycle within two weeks of taking Provera. If Provera alone does not initiate a cycle, particularly if amenorrhea is long-standing, estrogen therapy to prime the endometrium prior to taking Provera may prove effective. If there is no menses with estrogen followed by progesterone therapy, then expert consultation is required. Continued therapy for amenorrhea includes repeated courses of Provera, or hormonal contraceptives, to induce a cycle at least once every three months. Provera therapy will not protect against a pregnancy. If conception is desired, ovulation induction may be required.

Menopause

The average age of natural **menopause** (cessation of menses) in the United States is 51.4 years, with an age range of 42 to 58 years. By the time women are in their early 50s, 90 percent will have experienced menopause. Smoking accelerates the age of menopause by 1.5 to 2 years. That means that about 50 million women are currently in the menopausal transition or in menopause. Women are considered to be menopausal if they have not had a menstrual cycle for 12 months. Cessation of menstrual cycles is caused by cessation of ovarian function and estrogen depletion. When life expectancy was age 50, few women experienced menopause. With an average life expectancy of 70 to 80 years, women now spend up to one third of their life in menopause.

The **perimenopause** transition includes the 5 to 10 years before menses cease. As the ovaries begin to decline in function, hormonal fluctuations are common. Women may have irregular cycles and some inconsistent menopausal symptoms. Anovulatory menses is common.

The depletion of estrogen with onset of menopause can lead to vasomotor symptoms including hot flashes and night sweats, difficulty with memory and concentration, sleep disturbances, skin changes, vaginal dryness, and an increased risk of osteoporosis and cardiovascular disease. The incidence and severity of hot flashes is variable, although most hot flashes are mild to moderate and decrease in intensity and frequency over time. Women typically report that hot flashes last six months to 2 years, although some women report hot flashes for as long as 10 years. Increased environmental temperatures, higher body mass index (BMI), cigarette smoking, sedentary lifestyle, and lower socioeconomic status (SES) have all been related to an increased incidence of hot flashes (North American Menopause Society [NAMS], 2004).

In the past, replacement of estrogen was considered beneficial for women's health, not only in terms of symptom relief, but also for prevention of cardiovascular disease and osteoporosis. It was routine to offer and encourage women to take estrogen therapy as they became postmenopausal. In July, 2002, a large study of postmenopausal estrogen and progesterone therapy was ended early when investigators found an increased risk of coronary heart events, stroke, breast cancer, and pulmonary embolism (Writing Group for the Women's Health Initiative Investigators, 2002). In 2004 the Food and Drug Administration (FDA) evaluated the research evidence and decided to require a boxed warning of harm for estrogen/progesterone formulations. They strongly recommend that estrogen preparations not be used to prevent

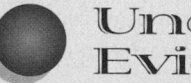

Uncovering the Evidence

Perimenopausal Symptoms and Age

Discussion: In this study of 418 women ages 30 to 50, the authors found that the following perimenopausal symptoms increased with age: sleeplessness, moodiness, depression, and poor concentration. Headache ranked first among symptoms for severity. The study subjects did not often recognize the symptoms of perimenopause.

Implications for Practice: Education and anticipatory guidance for women entering perimenopause should be included in women's health care.

Source: Lyndaker, C., & Hulton, L. (2004). The influence of age on symptoms of perimenopause. Journal of Obstetric, Gynecologic, and Neonatal Nursing, 33(3), 340–347.

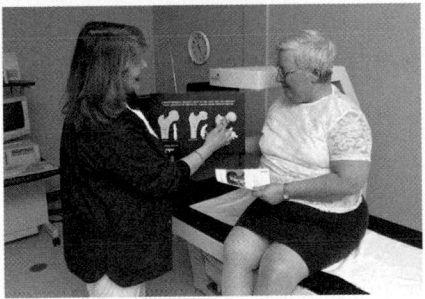

Figure 62-2 As women approach menopause, osteoporosis prevention education is critical in promoting optimal health.

coronary disease or osteoporosis. In addition, the following recommendations are made for using estrogen therapy:

- Estrogen and progesterone should not be used to prevent coronary events, strokes, or osteoporosis.
- There are risks with the use of postmenopausal estrogen, and each woman must have an individual assessment of whether the benefits outweigh the risks.
- Estrogen therapy is the most effective relief for vasomotor symptoms and vaginal dryness, but estrogen should be used for the shortest amount of time and in the lowest doses and with full knowledge of risks and benefits.

Estrogen therapy should be done on an individual basis, taking into consideration a woman's complete health and family history, particularly her risk for cardiovascular disease and breast cancer. When estrogen therapy is prescribed for a woman who still has her uterus, progesterone therapy must also be prescribed to reduce the risk of endometrial cancer.

Topical vaginal therapy is an effective treatment for vaginal atrophy and dryness. Vaginal rings, cream, and tablets are available. Vaginal lubricants, moisturizers, and maintaining regular sexual activity can help relieve and prevent vaginal dryness. Progesterone therapy to protect the endometrium is not necessary when only vaginal therapy is used. Ultra-low-dose estradiol therapy in a transdermal patch (Meno star) has been developed to prevent osteoporosis. This therapy is not indicated to relieve the vasomotor symptoms.

Risk reduction for heart disease and osteoporosis must be part of the health care of menopausal women (Figure 62-2). This includes education on diet, exercise, calcium and vitamin D intake, and screening for cholesterol and bone density. Other therapies for osteoporosis prevention and treatment should be considered for women not taking hormone therapy.

In addition to natural menopause, women of all ages can experience surgical menopause induced by oophorectomy, the surgical removal of one or both ovaries. Women with removal of the uterus without removal of the ovaries will experience amenorrhea without other accompanying menopausal symptoms until the ovaries stop functioning at the usual age of menopause, because the ovaries continue to produce estrogen. When the ovaries are removed, either with or without the uterus, amenorrhea and menopausal symptoms begin immediately. The therapies for treating vasomotor symptoms in women experiencing surgical menopause are the same as for women experiencing natural menopause except that progesterone therapy is not required if estrogen is prescribed. The decision to use estrogen therapy for women experiencing surgical menopause must be made on an individual basis, taking into account the woman's age, significance of symptoms, and health status.

Premenstrual Syndrome and Premenstrual Dysphoric Disorder

Premenstrual syndrome (PMS) is a collection of symptoms associated with the last half of the menstrual cycle and usually relieved shortly after the onset of menstruation. Symptoms can be physical, such as bloating, headache, and breast tenderness or mental and emotional, such as irritability, depression, anxiety, food cravings, and mood swings. Social withdrawal and difficulty concentrating may also be present. The symptoms are severe enough to prompt 30 to 40 percent of women with PMS to seek treatment (Reid & Bruce, 2003). To diagnose PMS, charting of symptoms is helpful to establish a pattern of symptoms clustered in the last half of the cycle and relieved shortly after the onset of menses.

Premenstrual dysphoric disorder (PMDD) is a form of PMS with more severe emotional symptoms. Only 3 to 8 percent of women have PMDD. PMDD has not been officially adopted as a diagnosis by the American Psychiatric Association but has been identified as a proposed diagnosis requiring further study. The main symptoms of PMDD are markedly depressed mood, marked anxiety, marked affective lability, and decreased interest in activities. To establish a diagnosis these symptoms should have occurred during the last week of the luteal phase of the menstrual cycle during most cycles in the previous 12 months. The symptoms begin to resolve during the week of menses and are always absent in the week after the menses. PMS and PMDD resolve once menopause occurs.

To diagnose PMDD, five or more of the following symptoms must have been present most of the time during the last week of the luteal phase:
- Feeling sad, hopeless, or self-deprecating
- Feeling anxious
- Mood swings or tearfulness
- Persistent irritability
- Anger and increased conflicts in relationships
- Feeling fatigued, lethargic, or lacking in energy
- Marked changes in appetite with binges or food cravings
- Increased sleep or insomnia
- Feeling overwhelmed
- Physical symptoms
- Suicidal thoughts

When these symptoms are severe enough to impair the ability to function in everyday life, evaluation by a health care provider is needed. It is important to distinguish PMDD from clinical depression, anxiety, or panic disorders or the premenstrual exacerbation of an underlying psychiatric disorder. The hallmark of PMDD is that there is always a symptom-free period every month. Diagnosis of PMS and PMDD is done with charting of symptoms each month for at least three months and exclusion of other diseases.

Polycystic Ovary Syndrome

Polycystic ovary syndrome (PCOS) is an endocrine disorder usually characterized by multiple ovarian cysts, oligomenorrhea or amenorrhea, hirsutism, acne, obesity, and infertility. Alopecia and hypertension may also be present. The incidence of PCOS is approximately 5 to 10 percent, making it the most common endocrine disorder in women of childbearing age. A recent study conducted in Alabama of 400 premenopausal women found an incidence of 6.6 percent (Azziz, et al., 2004). PCOS is considered to be an endocrine disorder involving insulin resistance and higher than usual testosterone levels.

The exact cause of PCOS is not known, but genetic mutations are being studied, because there is a strong genetic tendency for PCOS. Women with PCOS may have male or female relatives with adult-onset diabetes, elevated triglyceride levels, and hypertension and female relatives with infertility, hirsutism, and menstrual disorders (McKittrick, 2002). Women with PCOS should also have testing for diabetes and hyperlipidemia, because they are at risk for diabetes and coronary artery disease due to insulin resistance.

Lifestyle recommendations for PCOS include weight loss as a first priority, exercise including aerobic and weight resistance training, identifying and correcting behavioral impediments to healthy eating and exercising, adding 1,000 to 1,500 mg of calcium and a multivitamin supplement to their diet, and avoiding smoking. Correcting insulin resistance with metformin can result in resumption of regular menstrual cycles and fertility. Metformin plus clomiphene citrate to induce ovulation is also used to induce ovulation to achieve pregnancy. Combined oral contraceptives regulate menstruation, reduce androgen levels, and help clear acne.

Hair removal products help with hirsutism. Topical eflornithine HCL (Vaniqa) reduces unwanted facial hair in women (Cowan & Graham, 2003). Studies have shown that a significant problem with PCOS is body image and self-esteem. Depression or emotional lability are common and may be related to insulin resistance, physical symptoms of androgen excess, such as hirsutism and acne, or infertility. A small qualitative study in the United Kingdom found that women with PCOS felt abnormal as women because of hirsutism, disordered menstruation, and infertility (Varcoe, 2002).

Dysfunctional Uterine Bleeding

Dysfunctional uterine bleeding (DUB) is defined as abnormal uterine bleeding in the absence of pathology and includes **menorrhagia** (prolonged or excessive, but regular, menses), **metrorrhagia** (bleeding between menstrual cycles), and postmenopausal bleeding. DUB is often related to anovulation and is therefore common at both ends of the age spectrum. Adolescents often have irregular cycles in the first year or two of initiating cycles, and women in the perimenopause often have irregular or disordered bleeding. Anovulation results in continued endometrial growth without progesterone-induced bleeding and results in unpredictable bleeding in terms of both timing and volume. Assessment of DUB includes a careful history. Menstrual cycles that are shorter than 21 days in length or longer than 7 days in duration are usually considered abnormal. Menorrhagia affects 15 to 20 percent of women who have DUB.

One defining characteristic of DUB is the absence of reproductive pathology. DUB may be caused by thyroid disorders, hormonal imbalances, clotting disorders, or as a side effect of medications, among other etiologies. Abnormal uterine bleeding that can be associated with pathology is distinct from DUB and can be caused by polyps (small tumor like growths that project from mucous membrane), leiomyomata, infection, carcinomas, local trauma, ovarian cysts (globular sacs on the ovaries filled with fluid or semisolid material), and pregnancy complications.

When DUB occurs in adolescents, inherited clotting disorders, such as platelet disorders, prothrombin deficiencies, idiopathic thrombocytopenia, and von Willebrand's disease should be considered. The incidence of von Willebrand's disease is approximately 1 percent of the population. There is a clear genetic component for von Willebrand's disease, so a family history should be obtained. Leukemia should be ruled out in adolescents with menstrual hemorrhages. Perimenopausal and postmenopausal bleeding should be a cause to suspect reproductive tract carcinomas until these are excluded.

The incidence of endometrial cancer increases with age, therefore all women over age 40 need evaluation of anovulatory bleeding with endometrial biopsy. Endometrial biopsy, typically done in the outpatient setting, involves removing a sample of the uterine lining. Usually, no anesthesia is required for the procedure. A thin catheter is placed through the cervical canal into the endometrium, and a small amount of endometrial lining is removed and sent to the pathology lab for examination. If dilation of the cervix is necessary to allow for passage of the catheter, then a local anesthetic, either a topical spray or injectable anesthesia is used. The patient commonly experiences menstrual-like cramping during and for a short time following the procedure. Endometrial biopsy may be performed by a physician, an advanced practice nurse, or a physician's assistant.

Therapy for DUB depends on the cause of the disordered bleeding. Initial treatment is often antiprostaglandin therapy with NSAIDs or cyclooxygenase inhibitors. An antiprostaglandin is started with the first day of the cycle and continued throughout the menses. Treatment may include hormonal therapies, such as combined or progesterone-only oral contraceptives, injectable progesterone or GnRH agonists, the levonorgestrel-containing intrauterine system, destruction of the uterine lining using heat or laser, or treatment of fibroids. Tranexamic acid, a fibrinolytic agent, has been studied in the United Kingdom, Pakistan, and Australia and has shown to be an effective treatment for DUB.

Endometrial ablation, or destruction of the uterine lining with heat, results in amenorrhea for 50 percent of women. Endometrial ablation is done under general anesthesia, and patient satisfaction with the procedure is 90 to 95 percent. Hysterectomy, surgical removal of the uterus, also has high patient satisfaction ratings for relief of dysfunctional bleeding (Kuppermann, et al., 2004).

Acute uterine hemorrhage commonly occurs during a spontaneous abortion or in prolonged perimenopausal bleeding but may also occur secondary to uterine fibroids or other uterine conditions. Hemorrhage that occurs in the postpartum or postoperative period is classified as a complication rather than as a reproductive dysfunction. Most commonly, a woman presents at the emergency department with a complaint of uncontrolled vaginal bleeding. The treatment for acute vaginal hemorrhage involves stabilizing the patient and making a rapid decision whether to implement medical therapy or operative therapy. The unstable patient usually requires an immediate dilatation of the cervix and removal of the uterine lining by scraping (dilatation and curettage [D & C]), to stop the hemorrhage. Hysterectomy is always a consideration, especially if childbearing is not an issue and there is a failure of medical therapy.

If the patient is stable, fluids, blood, and high-dose intravenous (IV) conjugated estrogens, 25 mg, are administered every four hours until the hemorrhage stops. High-dose estrogens have three actions that stop uterine hemorrhage: initiation of endometrial proliferation, increase in clotting factors, and promotion of platelet clumping and clotting at the capillary level.

Nursing management of the woman experiencing acute uterine hemorrhage includes a rapid assessment of status including vital signs, amount of visible hemorrhage, skin turgor, presence and location of pain, level of consciousness and orientation, and the possibility of pregnancy. The physician is immediately notified and IV fluid therapy is initiated. Lab work for complete blood count, clotting indices, pregnancy hormone level, and type and cross-match is obtained. Administration of blood products and medications is done according to the physician's orders. Urinary catheterization may be required to most accurately monitor intake and output. Continuous monitoring of vital signs, intake and output, and level of consciousness is done until the patient has either stopped hemorrhaging and is stable, or is transferred to surgery. Support of the patient and family includes explanation of procedures and treatment, relieving anxiety, and helping the patient and family be prepared for surgery, if necessary.

Endometriosis

Endometriosis is a condition involving implantation of segments of endometrium outside of the uterus in the pelvis or abdomen. These implants behave as though they were located within the uterus. They bleed during the menstrual cycle and cause internal bleeding, pain, inflammation, and scarring. There are theories about how the endometrium becomes implanted outside the uterus, but there is no one explanation of how this happens. Implants can be on the ovaries, on the pelvic wall, on the fallopian tubes, on the colon, or elsewhere in the peritoneal cavity. Occasionally the implants occur in remote areas of the body.

Typically endometriosis is diagnosed between the ages of 25 and 35 and affects between 5 and 15 percent of women of reproductive age (Denny, 2004). Endometriosis among family members is common, and patients with an affected first-degree relative have 10 times the risk of developing endometriosis. Infertility affects 30 to 40 percent of women with endometriosis and is more common as the disease progresses. Symptoms are quite varied, depend on the location of the endometrial implants, and can include pelvic pain, severe dysmenorrhea, **dyspareunia** (painful intercourse), abnormal uterine bleeding, and infertility. Intestinal symptoms of abdominal cramping and diarrhea or constipation can also occur.

Diagnosis of endometriosis can be quite difficult, because there are no specific tests short of surgery to confirm the diagnosis. This means that there is often a delay in diagnosis, and a delay of several years between onset of symptoms and diagnosis is common. Once other causes for pain have been excluded, laparoscopic surgery is considered for diagnosis and removal of the implants.

If pregnancy is desired, conception is advised as soon as possible after surgery, because endometrial implants tend to recur and the best chance for successful conception is immediately after surgery. Hormonal therapy, such as Provera, norethindrone, depo-medroxyprogesterone acetate (DMPA), danazol, or leuprolide, can also be used. A limiting factor in leuprolide therapy is the cost—each three-month injection can cost $1,400 or more. Surgical treatments include excising implants or ablating them with laser. Hysterectomy is also a treatment option.

Assessment with Clinical Manifestations

When assessing patients with actual or potential menstrual disorders, a careful history is most important. Women should be asked about their age at menarche, the date of the first day of last menstrual period (LMP), length of cycles and any recent changes, number of days of bleeding, amount of bleeding during cycles (light, moderate, or heavy), presence of clots, and any intermenstrual bleeding. Every woman should be encouraged to write down the days she has bleeding each month. Reviewing a history of bleeding days may reveal that a bleeding pattern that a woman thought was abnormal is just a variation of normal. Women can be assisted to determine cycle length by calculating the number of days between the first day of bleeding and the day before menses starts again.

Asking direct and concrete questions about the number of tampons or sanitary pads used, the amount of bleeding on each tampon or pad, and the presence or absence of clots gives a good indication of the amount of blood loss. Pain should be evaluated as to location, type, severity, relieving and aggravating factors, any changes in pain over time, and other symptoms associated with the pain. Women with painful cycles need to be asked questions about the impact of pain on their functioning and activities of daily living, as well as about the therapies that they use to treat the pain.

A history should be obtained about the type of contraception being used, recent surgeries or traumas, medications, chronic illness, family history—particularly of bleeding disorders, endometriosis and PCOS—usual type of physical activity, and eating disorders. Women should be asked about any constitutional symptoms, such as weight loss or gain, hot flashes, night sweats, heat or cold intolerance, fatigue, or insomnia. Queries regarding medications should include over-the-counter (OTC) medicines and herbal therapies, as well as prescription medications.

The treatment of menstrual disorders often changes depending on a woman's age and desires for childbearing, so women should be asked if they are currently planning a pregnancy, have a need for contraception, or have completed their families. It is important not to assume that all younger women want to become pregnant and that women over 35 with multiple children have completed their families. Women should be asked about the effect of their menstrual disorder on work and activities, relationships, sleep patterns, eating patterns, elimination patterns, and sexual interest and function. Pregnancy must be ruled out in cases of amenorrhea or irregular bleeding, and all women should be asked about the possibility of pregnancy. The history is not usually relied on to determine pregnancy status, however, and a routine pregnancy test is often ordered even if women deny sexual activity.

Diagnostic Tests

Diagnostic testing for dysmenorrhea includes a pelvic exam, cultures for gonorrhea (a sexually transmitted infection of the cervix caused by *Neisseria gonorrhoeae*), and chlamydia (a sexually transmitted infection of the cervix caused

Skills 360°

Reproductive Health History

Nurses, as well as patients, may feel uncomfortable about discussing reproductive health history. Here are some suggestions for helping to desensitize the history process. Nurses often use open-ended history questions, but in assessing menstrual cycles more directed questioning may be helpful. Helping women remember when their last menstrual cycle started may include use of a calendar, or questions such as "Your birthday was last month; was your period before or after your birthday?" When obtaining a reproductive history it is important to use language that is inclusive and non-judgmental. Use phrases such as "your sexual partner" rather than "your husband." Avoid assumptions. If you ask "How many children do you have?" you may get an answer that is not the same as the answer to the question "How many pregnancies have you had?" Using a brief preface to the section of reproductive history questions paves the way for the history section and can make the patient more receptive to the questions. Here is an example of an introduction: "I'm going to ask you a series of questions about female health issues. The answers to these questions help give us an idea of your complete health status. If you don't understand the question I am asking or feel uncomfortable giving me an answer, please let me know."

by *Chlamydia trachomatis*), and ultrasound, if structural abnormalities are a concern. Diagnostic tests for amenorrhea include the physical and pelvic examination and lab studies, such as a pregnancy test, prolactin level (to rule out prolactin-stimulating tumor), thyroid-stimulating hormone (TSH) level (to rule out thyroid disease), and follicle-stimulating hormone (FSH) level (to rule out premature ovarian failure). Ultrasound may be indicated if absence of reproductive organs is suspected as a cause of primary amenorrhea.

Menopause is diagnosed by a physical with a pelvic examination. FSH and estradiol levels can be drawn if the diagnosis of menopause is uncertain. Screening for osteoporosis risk (bone density scan), hyperlipidemia risk (cholesterol level), and breast cancer (mammogram) may be indicated.

No specific diagnostic tests exist for endometriosis short of laparoscopy. The diagnosis of endometriosis is made by eliminating other causes of pelvic pain, so cultures for infection, ultrasound, physical, and pelvic examination are often performed. A physical examination and pelvic exam are performed to diagnose PCOS. Lab testing may include testosterone level, insulin level, glucose testing, and serum dehydroepiandrosterone sulfate (DHEAS). Ultrasound can be done to verify polycystic ovaries but is not required for diagnosis.

PMS and PMDD are diagnosed by reviewing symptom diaries and excluding other causes of physical or emotional symptoms. Evaluation of DUB includes physical and pelvic examinations. Lab studies include a complete blood count and TSH. Diagnostic tests may include pregnancy testing, pelvic exam and Pap smear, ultrasound examination, saline-infusion sonogram, hysteroscopy, endometrial biopsy, D & C, and laparoscopy. Saline-infusion sonogram is an ultrasound study performed in the outpatient ultrasound area. A thin catheter is inserted through the cervix into the uterus, and saline is injected into the uterine cavity. The saline expands the endometrial cavity and helps with visualization of any anomalies. No anesthesia is typically needed unless dilation of the cervix is required.

Hysteroscopy is a procedure done in the operating room. It may be performed under local, regional, or general anesthesia and may be done in conjunction with D & C or laparoscopy. The cervix is dilated and the hysteroscope is inserted through the cervix into the uterus. Liquid or gas is used to improve visualization. Using light through the hysteroscope, the health care provider can directly view the uterine cavity and the opening of the fallopian tubes into the uterus.

D & C is done under regional or general anesthesia in the operating room. The cervix is dilated and the health care provider uses one or more instruments to scrape out the lining of the uterus. Samples of the uterine lining are often sent to the pathology lab for examination. D & C may provide both diagnosis and treatment of DUB. Lab work for DUB may include prolactin level, TSH, FSH, complete blood count, and screening for von Willebrand's disease.

Nursing Diagnoses

Based on the information gathered, examples of nursing diagnoses in the patient with menstrual disorders may include the following:

- Anxiety related to the impact of menstrual dysfunction on relationships, daily functioning, plans for childbearing, or implications of the disease.
- Deficient knowledge related to relief measures available for dysmenorrhea, range of normal menstrual patterns, or changes in health status associated with menopause.
- Acute or chronic pain related to dysmenorrhea or pain of endometriosis.
- Disturbed body image related to negatively viewing physical changes associated with PCOS.

Planning and Implementation

Care of the patient with menstrual disorders includes education, support, therapeutic interventions, and prevention measures. Collaborative management of the patient with dysmenorrhea requires evaluation by a physician, advanced practice nurse, or physician's assistant. Once other disorders are eliminated, relief of dysmenorrhea with prescription and nonprescription pain relief can be ordered by the evaluating provider. The nurse provides patient education about relief measures for dysmenorrhea, side effects and instructions for medications ordered, and symptoms that should prompt contact with the health care provider.

The patient with amenorrhea also needs a full evaluation. If the athletic triad is present, physical therapists can be an important part of the health care team in terms of making the assessment and its treatment and prevention (Papanek, 2003). Psychological counseling can be helpful for women with eating disorders. Nutritionists can assist with diet counseling for women with anorexia-related amenorrhea. Women with primary amenorrhea caused by imperforate hymen will need a hymenectomy performed in the physician's office by a gynecologist. Women with primary amenorrhea caused by congenital absence of reproductive organs will need consultation with a gynecologist and reproductive endocrinologist. A management plan for amenorrhea is outlined by the evaluating provider. The nurse provides the patient with education about the plan, when menses may be expected, the contraceptive effect (if any) of the medication provided, and what symptoms should prompt contact with the health care provider.

The patient in menopause needs an evaluation by a health care provider. A management plan for menopause is outlined by the evaluating provider. A nutritionist may assist the woman in modifying her diet to reduce vasomotor symptoms. The nurse plays an important role in education for women in menopause, because many of the health care interventions for women in menopause include strategies to maintain health and prevent symptoms and disease.

The patient with PMS/PMDD symptoms requires evaluation by a physician, advanced practice nurse, or physician's assistant. Psychological counseling may help with relationship issues and communication difficulties. A management plan for PMS/PMDD is outlined by the evaluating provider. The nurse provides the woman with PMS/PMDD education about monitoring her cycles, adjunctive therapies to relieve symptoms, and symptoms that should prompt contact with their health care provider.

The patient with PCOS needs an evaluation by a physician, advanced practice nurse, or physician's assistant. Consultation with an endocrinologist may be required. A nutritionist can assist the woman with PCOS in planning meals and snacks to reduce cravings and promote weight loss, and provide education and support. Psychological counseling may be helpful for women experiencing anxiety or self-esteem issues as well as those women with eating disorders. Spiritual counseling may be helpful for those with PCOS that has an effect on fertility. The nurse provides education, especially about the long-term implications of PCOS for the woman's overall health. The nurse also helps the patient problem-solve to maximize compliance to the treatment regimen and achieve the patient's goals such as fertility.

The patient with DUB requires an evaluation by a physician, advanced practice nurse, or physician's assistant. Gynecologists will perform hysteroscopy, laparoscopy, or other indicated surgery, such as hysterectomy. Hematologists may be consulted for women with von Willebrand's disease or other hematological disorders. If surgery is indicated, the nurse provides preoperative and postoperative care and education. The nurse also gives prescribed medications and monitors the patient for resolution of DUB. Nursing care includes educating women about monitoring cycles, adjunctive therapies to relieve symptoms, and symptoms that should prompt contact with the health care provider.

Women on antipsychotic medications may have prolactin abnormalities causing amenorrhea and may need hormonal therapy to have regular cycles (Miller, 2004). Women with cystic fibrosis can have amenorrhea related to poor weight gain and delayed puberty. Women with cystic fibrosis also may have congenital absence of pelvic organs (Jarzabek, et al., 2004). Chronic debilitating diseases, such as uncontrolled diabetes, end-stage renal disease, cancers, acquired immune deficiency syndrome (AIDS), or malabsorption, can result in amenorrhea from anovulation, probably caused by stress-induced hormonal changes (Practice Committee of the American Society for Reproductive Medicine, 2004).

Women with endocrine disease, cancer, systemic lupus erythematosus (SLE), anemia, or infection may have cyclical aggravation of their symptoms. Women with trauma or who have surgery can have short-term menstrual disturbances in their recovery phase. Inherited clotting disorders, such as idiopathic thrombocytopenia and von Willebrand's disease, can be the cause of DUB in adolescents. Migraines, asthma, allergies, and seizure disorders may be exacerbated during the premenstrual phase of the cycle, and it is important to distinguish between one of these aggravated conditions and PMDD.

Nutrition

Calcium-intake and a healthy diet should be addressed for postmenopausal women. Adequate intake of vitamin B_6, vitamin B_{12}, folic acid, and magnesium during the menopause are necessary to prevent cardiovascular disease and prevent osteoporosis. It is prudent for postmenopausal women to take a multivitamin supplement. For women with PMS/PMDD and physical symptoms, nutritional counseling on a diet low in salt, refined carbohydrates, caffeine, and alcohol, and increased calcium intake as well as small frequent meals may be beneficial. Supplementation with calcium, magnesium, vitamin B_6, and vitamin E may be helpful.

It is important to assess the learning needs of postmenopausal patients before giving advice or teaching about lifestyle recommendations. Although calcium intake is typically low in women older than 50, some women have a diet high in dairy products and do not need calcium supplementation. Women with adequate dietary calcium instead need messages of positive reinforcement about their calcium intake. In addition, some women have medical conditions in which calcium supplementation is not advised or a particular calcium supplement is not advised. Women with hypercalcemia or a history of calcium kidney stones may be advised not to take a calcium supplement. Women with diabetes need to consider their calcium supplement carefully, because some calcium supplements contain sugars. Tailoring the basic message of adequate calcium intake to the particular patient improves the effectiveness of teaching and enhances patient compliance (Roth, 2007).

Weight loss and regular exercise are recommended as part of the treatment regimen for PCOS. If obesity is present, weight loss is the first priority in treating PCOS. Nutrition counseling should include correcting behavioral impediments to healthy eating and advise adding 1,000 to 1,500 mg of calcium and a multivitamin supplement.

Pharmacology

There are five classes of medications used in the pharmacological management of menstrual disorders. The first class of medications used in treatment of menstrual disorders is the hormones. The second class of medications includes the pain relievers used to treat dysmenorrhea and menorrhagia. The third class of medications includes the selective serotonin reuptake inhibitors (SSRIs) used to treat PMS/PMDD and the mood disorders of menopause. The fourth class of medications includes the antihyperglycemic drug used to treat insulin resistance in PCOS. The final class of drugs includes the topical cream used to prevent unwanted facial hair in PCOS. Table 62-1 summarizes the medications used to treat menstrual disorders.

Surgery

DUB may be treated with endometrial ablation or hysterectomy. Endometriosis may be diagnosed and treated laparoscopically or with hysterectomy. Hysterectomy may include removal of only the body of the uterus without the cervix (partial hysterectomy) or the total uterus (complete hysterectomy).

TABLE 62-1	**Medications Used to Treat Menstrual Disorders**	
DRUG	**INDICATION**	**SIDE EFFECTS**
Hormones		
Estrogen (Alora, Climara, FemPatch; Ogen; Premarin; Estrace; Estratab, etc.)	Suppression of vasomotor symptoms Prevention of urogenital atrophy	Breast tenderness; nausea; depression; headache; bleeding or spotting
Progestin (Provera; Hylutin; Aygestin; Megace; Depo Provera; Mirena; etc.)	DUB Amenorrhea Endometriosis	Breast tenderness; irregular bleeding
Combo oral contraceptives (Ortho Novum; Norinyl; Ovcon; Levlen; Modicon; Necon; Nelova; Estrostep; etc.)	Suppression of vasomotor symptoms Prevention of urogenital atrophy DUB Amenorrhea	Breast tenderness; nausea; depression; headache; bleeding or spotting
GnRH agonists (Lupron)	DUB Endometriosis	Amenorrhea; hot flashes; headache; vaginal dryness; reversible bone loss
Danazol (Danocrine)	Endometriosis	Weight gain; acne; hirsutism; deepening of voice
Nonsteroidal Anti-inflammatory Agents		
Motrin; Advil; Orudis; Mylan; Anaprox; Aleve; Ponstel; etc.	Relief of dysmenorrhea and menorrhagia	Gastric upset; heartburn; nausea; bleeding; renal impairment
Selective Serotonin Reuptake Inhibitors		
Celexa; Prozac; Luvox; Zoloft; Lexapro; Paxil	Relief of PMS/PMDD Relief of menopausal mood disorders	Irregular heartbeat; blood pressure changes
Hypoglycemic Drugs		
Glucophage	Reduce insulin resistance in PCOS	Nausea; vomiting; diarrhea; abdominal pain; decreased appetite
Topical Cream		
Vaniqa	Prevention/treatment of hirsutism in PCOS	Skin irritation; folliculitis

Adapted from Broyles, B., Reiss, B., & Evans, M. (2007). Pharmacological aspects of nursing care (7th ed.). New York: Thomson Delmar Learning.

Removal of the ovaries and fallopian tubes is called a salpingo-oophorectomy. The hysterectomy may be performed abdominally. Removal of the uterus, ovaries, and fallopian tubes through the abdominal incision is called total abdominal hysterectomy and bilateral salpingo-oophorectomy (TAH and BSO). Hysterectomy may also be performed vaginally. During a vaginal hysterectomy, the laparoscope can be used to help with visualization and removal of organs. This is called laparoscopically assisted vaginal hysterectomy (LAVH).

Nursing care for patients undergoing hysterectomy includes preoperative and postoperative care. Preoperative care includes patient education about the surgical procedure, anticipatory guidance about expected recovery and monitoring for complications, and assessing the patient's feelings about the loss of the uterus and childbearing ability. Nursing interventions to reduce anxiety and improve knowledge are most important. Postoperative nursing care is discussed in detail in chapter 22.

Alternative Therapy

Dysmenorrhea can often be relieved by drugs that have antiprostaglandin activity, such as NSAIDs. Other relief measures include heat and exercise. Studies have found fish oil to be of some benefit in dysmenorrhea relief, and preliminary studies from Germany found that magnesium supplementation reduced prostaglandin levels and relieved pain (Health Gate Data Corp, 2003). Supplementation with thiamine (vitamin B_1) or calcium has shown some effect on dysmenorrhea and herbal therapies, such as black cohosh, have been proposed as relief measures. Acupuncture and biofeedback have been shown to be of some benefit (Sidani & Campbell, 2002).

The dramatic shift away from traditional hormone therapy has led to a proliferation of alternative therapy to treat the vasomotor symptoms of menopause including black cohosh, evening primrose oil, soy supplements, vitamin E, antidepressants, such as venlafaxine, paroxetine, or fluoxetine, the anticonvulsant gabapentin, antihypertensives clonidine, methyldopa, or Bellergal (Fitzpatrick, 2003; NAMS, 2004). Acupuncture and yoga have been used to treat the vasomotor symptoms of menopause. Lifestyle modifications recommended to relieve hot flashes include reducing the environmental temperature and dressing in layers, increasing physical activity, weight reduction, smoking cessation, and relaxation techniques.

Botanical therapy with chasteberry, black cohosh, gingko biloba, or St. John's wort has been used to relieve PMS and PMDD symptoms (Girman, Lee, & Kligler, 2003; Sidani & Campbell, 2002). Evening primrose oil has been used to treat PMS. For emotional symptoms, psychological therapy, education and counseling about communication strategies may help with relationship issues. Relaxation therapy, biofeedback, guided imagery, cognitive behavior therapy, light therapy, massage, and yoga have all been used to treat PMS. Lifestyle changes, such as increased exercise, quitting smoking and stress management, may also help relieve symptoms. Acupuncture may be of some benefit for women with PCOS and anovulation. Complementary treatment options for endometriosis may include traditional Chinese medicine, nutritional approaches, homeopathy, allergy management, and immune therapy.

Patient and Family Teaching

Patients and their family need to be taught to recognize normal and abnormal menstrual patterns. When dysmenorrhea occurs, teaching of the most effective pain management strategies is needed. Information on procedures to evaluate and treat menstrual disorders may become necessary. Once diagnosed, the implications for altered health status with PCOS or menopause should be taught to both patients and their family.

All women need to know that any postmenopausal bleeding is an abnormal finding that must be reported to their health care provider. When surgery is required, the nurse should teach postoperative care. Patients and their family need to anticipate the possibility of disrupted menstrual cycles following trauma, surgery, or selected treatment regimens.

Evaluation of Outcomes

Potential patient outcomes for each of the example nursing diagnoses for the patient with menstrual disorders are:

- Anxiety related to the impact of menstrual dysfunction on relationships, daily functioning, plans for childbearing, or implications of the disease. The patient should be able to recognize the signs of anxiety, demonstrate positive coping mechanisms, and describe a reduction in the level of anxiety experienced.
- Deficient knowledge related to relief measures available for dysmenorrhea, range of normal menstrual patterns, or changes in health status associated with menopause. The patient should demonstrate motivation to learn, identify perceived learning needs, and verbalize an understanding of desired content.
- Acute or chronic pain related to dysmenorrhea or pain of endometriosis. The patient should verbalize an adequate relief of pain along with the ability to realistically cope with the pain if it is not completely relieved.

- Disturbed body image related to negatively viewing physical changes associated with PCOS. The patient demonstrates enhanced body image and self-esteem as evidenced by ability to look at, touch, talk about, and care for actual or perceived altered body part or function.

INFECTIONS

Vaginitis and Bartholin's (Skene's) gland infections are the most common vaginal infections. These infections are sometimes considered sexually transmitted diseases ([STDs] contagious diseases usually contracted through sexual contact), because the causative organisms may be passed to sexual partners. Many infections develop without sexual contact and sexual partners do not always become infected.

Vaginitis

Strictly defined, **vaginitis** is inflammation of the vagina, and the term is commonly used for any vaginal inflammation, regardless of the underlying etiology. Vaginal infections are one of the most common reasons that women seek gynecological care. The three most common types of vaginitis are candida, bacterial vaginosis (BV), and trichomoniasis. Candidal vaginal infections are commonly known as yeast infections. Ninety percent of vaginal yeast is caused by *Candida albicans*. Candida infections can be caused by a shift in vaginal flora (such as with antibiotic administration) or a change in vaginal pH, or an environment conducive to yeast growth (a high blood sugar or suppressed immune system). Glucose tolerance testing for diabetes and human immunodeficiency virus (HIV) screening are recommended for women with chronic candida infections. Routine douching for hygiene purposes has been shown to double the risk of contracting vaginitis and to increase the risk of pelvic inflammatory disease (PID) and endometritis and should be discouraged. Itching is a hallmark presenting symptom. Typically there is thick, white discharge that is adherent to the vaginal walls. Treatment is with either oral or vaginal antifungal preparations. Exogenous lactobacillus either orally or vaginally can be used to prevent and treat chronic candida infections (Jeavons 2003; Reid & Bruce, 2003).

BV is a condition of an overgrowth of the bacteria normally present in the vagina. BV is the most common vaginal infection in women of reproductive age. The cause of BV is not clearly understood, although it rarely occurs in women who are not sexually active. It is often associated with douching, having a new sex partner, or having multiple partners. BV can be spread through contact with a female sex partner. Presenting symptoms are discharge that is white or gray, thin, watery and with an odor. Treatment is with oral or vaginal metronidazole (Flagyl) or clindamycin (Cleocin). Male sex partners generally do not need treatment, because men do not seem to get BV; so treating partners is not generally helpful in preventing recurrences. Female partners may need treatment. BV has been associated with premature rupture of membranes and preterm labor, and pregnant women with BV should be treated. Women with a history of preterm labor, particularly with preterm rupture of membranes, should have a wet mount to check for BV.

Trichomoniasis is infection with a small parasite, *Trichomonas vaginalis*. Trichomonas can be transmitted through sex with either men or women, although men rarely have symptoms. An estimated 7.4 million cases occur each year in men and women (CDC, 2004g). Trichomonads reside in the female vagina, urethra, bladder, and Skene's glands. Presenting symptoms is discharge that is frothy and may be green or white. Irritation or itching is common. Treatment is with metronidazole (Flagyl). Male and female partners must be treated to prevent reinfection.

Although trichomoniasis can be transmitted through sexual contact, candida and BV are not usually classified as infections that can be transmitted by sexual contact. However, this depends on women's sexual practices. Women can transfer candida and BV to female sexual partners. Histories should be taken in a nonjudgmental way that allows women the opportunity to share all their pertinent sexual information and get their questions answered.

Vaginal infections and cystitis share many of the same symptoms, and the organisms that cause vaginitis may also infect the urethra and Skene's glands. Infections with the herpes virus, a virus that produces small, transient fluid-filled blisters on skin and mucous membrane, can have dysuria as the presenting symptom. A careful history can help reveal those women with dysuria who need more than an evaluation for cystitis. Women with dysuria must have an evaluation for vaginitis if their urinalysis or culture is negative or inconclusive for cystitis or if their history and symptoms suggest an underlying or coexisting vaginitis or vulvitis.

Bartholin's or Skene's Gland Infection

The Bartholin's and Skene's glands may become obstructed, inflamed, or infected. In women without a cervix, the urethra and Skene's glands may be the primary site of infection for gonorrhea, caused by the bacterium *N. gonorrhoeae* or chlamydia, caused by the bacterium *C. trachomatis*. A Bartholin's cyst is an obstruction of the duct causing an enlargement of the Bartholin's gland. The enlargement may be significant, but it is typically soft and painless or mildly uncomfortable. Treatment of Bartholin's cysts primarily involves hot soaks with water and observation. Some women have minor enlargements of the Bartholin's glands that persist but are without symptoms and do not in any way obstruct the vaginal entrance, and these do not need treatment.

When the Bartholin's glands become infected the symptoms include pain, progressive enlargement of the gland, redness of the skin around the gland, exquisite tenderness to the touch and, often, induration. If there is an opening in the gland to the skin, there may be purulent or bloody discharge around the gland. The pain and gland enlargement are usually progressive until the contents are released through the skin, either naturally or through surgical draining. Gonorrhea and chlamydia are common causes of Bartholin's gland abscesses, so culture of the gland contents and antibiotic treatment are indicated. If the infection is more than superficial long-term or multiple antibiotic treatments may be indicated.

The Skene's glands can be a site for STDs, particularly gonorrhea, chlamydia, and trichomoniasis. The Skene's glands are assessed during a pelvic examination. With one finger in the vagina, the Skene's gland is milked between the examining finger and the vagina. If there is an infection, purulent discharge will be noted coming out of the glands. Culture of this discharge may be helpful and antibiotics are indicated. If trichomoniasis is suspected because there is a concomitant vaginal infection, then metronidazole should resolve the Skene's infection as well as the vaginal infection.

Sexually Transmitted Disease

Sexually transmitted diseases (STD) are infections that include gonorrhea, chlamydia, syphilis (caused by the spirochete *Treponema pallidum*), human papillomavirus ([HPV] the cause of genital warts), herpes virus infections, hepatitis B (a form of viral hepatitis), and human immunodeficiency virus (HIV). Gonorrhea and chlamydia typically infect the cervix in women. These infections are most common in young women under the age of 24. Having multiple partners increases the risk of contracting an STD. The location of the transformation zone of the cervix in adolescents and young women makes their cervices more susceptible to STD infections. The CDC estimates that 700,000 people in the United States have gonorrhea each year.

Gonorrhea is a bacterial infection that infects the cervix, anus, or throat. Many women are asymptomatic, but if women have symptoms they can include a purulent vaginal or cervical discharge, dysuria, and abdominal pain. Gonorrhea is treated with antibiotics. Antibiotic-resistant strains of gonorrhea are a recurrent problem. Treatment for gonorrhea shifted away from penicillin when penicillin-resistant strains of gonorrhea became prevalent. Gonococcal strains may also be resistant to spectinomycin (Trobicin) and fluoroquinolones. Changes in antibiotic treatments have so far kept pace with the resistant strains.

Chlamydia is caused by the bacteria *C. trachomatis*. It infects the cervix, urethra, anus, or pharynx. Chlamydia is the most frequently reported bacterial STD in the United States. An estimated 2.8 million Americans are infected each year. For both gonorrhea and chlamydia, partner notification and treatment are important. The CDC recommends that all sexually active women under age 25 have annual screening cultures for chlamydia.

Blood-borne infections include hepatitis B, syphilis, and HIV. HIV is discussed in chapter 42. Hepatitis B can be spread by sexual contact and contact with infected blood. Symptoms of hepatitis B include jaundice, fatigue, nausea, anorexia, and weight loss. Hepatitis B can resolve or can become a chronic infection, and treatment with antiviral drugs is sometimes needed.

Syphilis is caused by the bacteria *Treponema pallidum*. Syphilis is contracted by direct contact with a syphilis sore or by contact with syphilis-infected blood. Primary syphilis is characterized by a painless genital ulcer. This will resolve without treatment. If syphilis progresses to the secondary stage, symptoms usually include a rash on the palms of the hands and soles of the feet. Tertiary syphilis is characterized by brain and nervous system involvement.

Herpes Simplex Virus

The CDC estimates that one out of every five people over age 12 in the United States has had a genital herpes infection caused by the *Herpes simplex* virus (HSV). The number of Americans diagnosed with a genital herpes infection increased by 30 percent between the late 1970s and the early 1990s. Herpes virus type 1 and type 2 both cause identical genital herpes viral infections. Of all the HSV genital infections, 75 to 85 percent are caused by type 2 herpes virus and 15 to 25 percent are caused by type 1. One-third of women ages 20 to 45 have been exposed to the type 2 herpes virus. Of all women with antibodies to the type 2 herpes virus, 60 to 85 percent never have a recognized genital infection.

Symptoms of HSV can be significant or mild and subtle and usually include blisters that break open and form a sore or an ulcer. This ulcer is painful and often causes dysuria. It usually occurs three to seven days after exposure. Initial outbreaks often include flu-like symptoms of malaise, fever, swollen inguinal lymph nodes, and muscle aches. Subsequent outbreaks are usually not as painful, they do not last as long, the symptoms are usually more localized, and women do not have as many accompanying symptoms. Transmission of type 2 herpes virus usually occurs from sexual contact with someone who has type 2 genital herpes. More women than men are likely to have infection with type 2 herpes virus, possibly because transmission of the type 2 virus is more common from men to women than it is from women to men (CDC, 2004c).

Transmission of type 1 herpes virus can occur from sexual contact with someone who has type 1 genital herpes but can also happen from genital-to-oral contact, because type 1 herpes virus also causes oral lesions or cold sores. Type 1 lesions tend to recur less frequently, but the diagnosis and treatment is the same. Diagnosis is obtained by culturing the lesion. The herpes virus resides in the nerve ganglia between outbreaks, and it is not possible to eradicate the virus. Transmission of the virus is possible even if lesions are not present, and condoms are not as effective at preventing the transmission of the herpes virus as they are at preventing the transmission of infections that affect mucous membranes.

Human Papillomavirus

The human papillomavirus (HPV) is associated with genital warts and cervical cancer (a neoplasm of the uterine cervix). The CDC (2004) estimates that 20 million people currently have HPV. HPV is present in 30 to 45 percent of women. The link between HPV and cervical cancer is clear. Regular Papanicolaou test, or Pap smears, help detect precancerous lesions and allow for treatment. The increase in the performance of routine screening Pap smears accounts for the 74 percent decline in the incidence of cervical cancer between 1955 and 1992 (American Cancer Society [ACS], 2004b).

There are more than 100 different strains of HPV virus, and types 16, 18, 31, 33, and 35 are considered high risk and are associated with high-grade cervical dysplasia (atypical or abnormal cervical cells) and cervical cancer. The prevalence of HPV decreases with increasing age. HPV viral infection is usually asymptomatic. Women may have genital warts (**condyloma**) present. All types of HPV virus can cause abnormalities in Pap smears, but the presence of a high-risk type of HPV indicates that those Pap smear abnormalities need close follow-up. Along with traditional Pap smear testing, HPV genetic typing (HPV digene) is done for mildly abnormal Pap smears, using either the original sample or by obtaining a sample just for HPV typing.

Each year approximately 3.5 million women in the U.S. (7 percent of all women obtaining Pap smears) have an abnormal result requiring follow-up or evaluation. Postmenopausal women are less likely to have significant cervical abnormalities with Pap smears that only show atypical cells. Pap smear test results are reported as one of the following: negative for intraepithelial lesions (normal), atypical squamous cells of undetermined significance (ASCUS), low-grade squamous intraepithelial lesion (LGSIL), high-grade squamous intraepithelial lesion (HGSIL), carcinoma-in-situ, and invasive cervical cancer.

A more unusual finding is atypical glandular cells of undetermined significance (AGUS). Premenopausal women with AGUS are more at risk for cervical

Safety First

Pap Smear Follow-up

Having a plan to manage Pap smears is not sufficient to ensure that patients get appropriate treatment and follow-up. If a system is not in place to ensure that Pap smear results are received from the pathology lab, women can have progression of cervical lesions and more extensive disease at time of treatment. An example of a problem with Pap smear follow-up is as follows. A patient went to her gynecologist's office for a yearly Pap smear. All her Pap smears up to this point had been normal. In this gynecology office, nurses were responsible for keeping a log book, recording all Pap smears that went to the lab, and logging in all results as they returned. The log book was not checked in a timely fashion, and it was not noticed that this patient's Pap smear results were never logged in. The patient returned the following year for her annual examination, and the results of that Pap smear showed HGSIL. When the previous year's Pap smear result was obtained from the lab, it showed LGSIL that could have been treated before progression to a high-grade lesion. The nurses in

the office instituted the following procedures to fix this problem:

- The pathology lab was contacted and asked to send out a follow-up letter to the office asking for confirmation that patients with results of LGSIL or worse had been notified.
- The nurses established a schedule to check the Pap log book on a daily basis.
- Patient postcards indicating normal test results were sent out as the normal Pap smear results came into the office. Patients were instructed to call the office in four weeks to find out their results if they had not received a postcard.
- Charts of patients with abnormal Pap smears were covered with a green folder to remind the health care providers that the patients with green charts had an abnormal Pap smear.

Red Flag

Emergency Treatment of TSS

Immediate treatment for TSS includes hospital admission, removal of tampon or diaphragm, IV fluids to maintain blood pressure, and antibiotics. Intubation, vasopressors, and dialysis may all be indicated. There is a 3 percent incidence of fatality with supportive therapy. Antibiotics reduce the recurrence rate from 30 to 50 percent. Nursing management of the patient with TSS includes removal of the tampon or diaphragm, rapid assessment of vital signs and level of consciousness and orientation, and immediate notification of the physician. Lab work is drawn for complete blood count, clotting functions, sedimentation rate, and chemistries as indicated. IV fluids, blood products, and antibiotics are administered as ordered by the health care provider. Insertion of a urinary catheter may be required to monitor intake and output. Close monitoring of vital signs and level of consciousness continues until the patient is stable or transferred.

abnormalities, and postmenopausal women with AGUS are more at risk for endometrial hyperplasia and cervical cancer. Treatment is often required for cervical lesions associated with high risk HPV. However, in adolescent or postmenopausal women with LGSIL on Pap smear testing, it is possible to avoid aggressive treatment and expectantly follow Pap smears.

Pelvic Inflammatory Disease

The CDC estimates that one million women each year have pelvic inflammatory disease (PID), an inflammatory condition of the female pelvic organs. PID can lead to abscess formation, scarring and occlusion of the fallopian tubes, reinfection, and chronic pelvic pain. Scarring of the fallopian tubes can lead to infertility and risk of ectopic pregnancy. Fallopian tube occlusion associated with untreated chlamydia infections is a major cause of infertility.

PID is a common cause of hospitalization for young women. It is an expensive illness in terms of costs for hospitalization, medications, follow-up, and risks for infertility. The symptoms of PID include abdominal pain, fever, elevated white count, purulent cervical discharge, acute cervical pain on palpation, and adnexal tenderness or enlargement.

Treatment of PID includes antibiotic therapy. Outpatient antibiotic therapy can be considered for a compliant patient with the ability to return for close follow-up, but hospitalization is considered if these conditions cannot be met because the risk for tubo-ovarian abscess and significant morbidity associated with untreated or inadequately treated PID is great. The criteria for inpatient treatment of PID can be seen in Box 62-1.

Management of PID includes treatment of the infection, close follow-up, partner evaluation and treatment, and education to maximize compliance with therapy and followup to prevent reinfection. Possible intravenous treatment regimens for PID are cefotetan, cefoxitin plus doxycycline, clindamycin plus gentamicin, ofloxacin, levofloxacin with or without metronidazole, ampicillin/sulbactam plus doxycycline.

Toxic Shock Syndrome

Toxic shock syndrome (TSS) is an acute illness caused by toxin-producing *Staphylococcus aureus* bacteria. Six percent of women carry *S. aureus* in their vagina, but only 2 percent of women have the type capable of producing the toxin. TSS is highly associated with menstruation and tampon use but has also occurred in the postpartum and postoperative periods. It has also been described with contraceptive diaphragm use. All women should avoid prolonged and overnight use of tampons, although this is of uncertain effectiveness.

Symptoms include a high fever greater than 102° F (38.9° C), a diffuse rash, falling blood pressure, systemic symptoms of nausea, vomiting, diarrhea, myalgia, hyperemia of mucous membranes, possibly disorientation, and coma. Blood urea nitrogen (BUN), creatinine, and liver enzymes are elevated and thrombocytopenia is present.

Complications

PID is the most common serious complication of chlamydia. Up to 40 percent of untreated women with chlamydia will develop PID. Chlamydia-associated PID is a common cause of infertility. Reiter's syndrome, which is a combination of arthritis, skin lesions, inflammation of the eye, and urethra, is a rare complication. Women with chlamydia are up to five times more likely to be infected with HIV, if exposed (CDC, 2004a). If left untreated, complications of gonorrhea can include PID, perihepatic inflammation, or gonococcal arthritis. Neonatal eye infections with gonorrhea and chlamydia are also possible if the mother has an untreated infection at the time of delivery. Untreated chlamydia can also cause neonatal pneumonia.

Chronic hepatitis is a complication of hepatitis B infections. Irreversible brain and nervous system impairment is a consequence of untreated syphilis that progresses to tertiary syphilis. Infants can also contract hepatitis B and congenital syphilis during birth if the mother is infected and untreated. An infant that comes in contact with an active herpes outbreak during delivery may contract systemic neonatal herpes infection. A woman with an active genital herpes virus infection at the time of labor is recommended to deliver by cesarean section to reduce this risk. Cervical cancer is a complication of HPV infection.

Assessment with Clinical Manifestations

In evaluating women for infections a nonjudgmental history needs to be taken. Information is obtained about the specific symptoms and their timing, any symptoms the sexual partner may have, an assessment of the possibility of pregnancy, and any history of infections. Pain must be evaluated as to location, type, severity, and relieving and aggravating factors, any changes in pain over time, and other symptoms associated with pain. The history for patients with infections should include the number of sexual partners and whether those partners are male, female, or both, and the types of sexual contact. Information on contraceptive method, LMP, any chronic illness, and routine medications should be obtained. Information on the timing and results of the last Pap smear is important to obtain.

Diagnostic Tests

The diagnosis of vaginitis involves taking a small sample of the vaginal discharge during a speculum examination, checking the pH, and examining the discharge under the microscope. The discharge is mixed with normal saline to prevent drying of the sample and placed on a microscope slide. This is called a wet mount and is examined under the microscope for the presence of trichomonads, bacteria-studded epithelial cells indicative of bacterial vaginosis called clue cells, and budding forms of yeast called hyphae. After this examination, a drop of potassium hydroxide is added to the discharge and the "whiff test" is performed to check for the presence of a fishy odor indicative of BV. The sample with potassium hydroxide can then be examined under the microscope for hyphae, as these are easier to identify in the potassium hydroxide sample.

Diagnosis of gonorrhea or chlamydia is made by taking a swab from the area of sexual contact and sending the specimen to be cultured. Visual inspection is necessary to diagnose external infections and genital warts. Other diagnostic tests include Pap smears, colposcopy with biopsies, and the pelvic exam. Cultures for HSV are obtained as indicated. The HPV digene test is done as indicated. Blood testing is done to detect syphilis, hepatitis B, and HIV infections. When one STD is diagnosed, it is important to test for the other sexually transmitted infections as the presence of one makes a woman more susceptible to others. TSS is diagnosed by site-specific cultures for *S. aureus* and exclusion of other illnesses such as Rocky Mountain spotted fever, leptospirosis, and measles (Daniels, 2003).

Women with AGUS Pap smears are usually evaluated with colposcopy and endometrial biopsy. Diagnosis of cervical pathology with HPV infection usually includes colposcopy, cervical biopsy, and endocervical curettage. Colposcopy is the use of a microscope to evaluate the cervix. The cervix is usually washed with an acetic acid solution, because this aids in the detection of lesions. Cervical biopsies are usually taken through the colposcope from the site of abnormalities. Colposcopy and Pap smears are ideally done at least 24 hours after any douching, use of tampons, intercourse, or use of vaginal medications. An endocervical scraping or curettage is generally also done during colposcopy, except if the patient is pregnant. A small amount of bleeding or discharge is normal after colposcopy, but continued bleeding, fever, chills, severe lower abdominal pain, or malodorous discharge should be reported.

Nursing Diagnoses

Based on the information gathered, examples of nursing diagnoses in the patient with infections of the reproductive system may include the following:
- Acute pain related to HSV, PID, or other painful infection.
- Risk for infection, reinfection, or infecting others related to sexually transmitted infections.
- Deficient knowledge related to knowledge of disease transmission and prevention.

Planning and Implementation

Care of the patient with gynecological infections include education, support, therapeutic interventions, and prevention measures. An advanced practice nurse, physician's assistant, or physician performs a pelvic examination, obtains cultures, wet mount, or other diagnostic tests, and orders antibiotics or antifungal therapy. For women who are hospitalized with acute infections, infectious disease specialists may be consulted. Advanced practice nurses or physician's assistants may perform colposcopy, but physicians are usually responsible for treatment of abnormal cervical pathology. An oncologist may be consulted for significant cervical pathology. The nurse administers therapies as ordered and assists with diagnostic tests. The nurse is responsible for monitoring women who are hospitalized with infections, including response to therapy and readiness for discharge. A crucial role for nurses is patient education.

Women with diabetes and altered immune systems from diseases, such as HIV, are more prone to yeast vaginitis. Women with chlamydia infections are more susceptible to HIV. Immunosuppressed women are more likely to have significant cervical abnormalities with Pap smears that only show atypical cells, and immunosuppressed women are more likely to be infected with high risk types of HPV.

Nutrition

Lactobacillus has been proposed as a preventive for candidal yeast infections. Lactobacillus can be obtained by eating yogurt, as a supplement, or in applications directly to the vagina. Lysine supplementation has been shown to reduce the frequency and intensity of herpes virus infections.

Pharmacology

The medications used to treat gynecological infections can be found in Table 62-2.

Population-Based Care

Control of sexually transmitted infections depends on partner identification, notification, and treatment. Measures to make notification and treatment of partners easier include preprinted cards that can be given to sexual contacts with information from health care providers on the specific infection and treatment needed. Screening programs for STDs and other infections, such as HIV, should be concentrated in the populations where these infections are most prevalent. Screening all women under age 25 for gonorrhea and chlamydia may help reduce the incidence of PID and infertility. With a few exceptions, all adolescents in the United States can consent to STD screening and treatment without parental notification or consent (Workowski & Levine, 2002).

TABLE 62-2 **Medications for Gynecological Infections**

DRUG	INDICATION	SIDE EFFECTS
Antifungal		
Monistat; Terazol; Mycelex; Femstat; Nystatin; Diflucan	Treatment of candida vaginitis and candida vulvitis	Nausea; abdominal pain; headache; local irritation
Antibacterial		
Flagyl; Cleocin	Treatment of trichomoniasis and bacterial vaginosis	Nausea; vomiting; GI upset; metallic taste
Penicillin G; Doxycycline; Tetracycline	Treatment of syphilis	Nausea; vomiting; GI upset; discoloration of teeth
Azithromycin, Erythromycin, Doxycycline	Treatment of chlamydia	Nausea; vomiting; GI upset; hepatic injury
Cefixime; Ciprofloxacin; Spectinomycin	Treatment of gonorrhea	Nausea; vomiting; skin rash; dizziness; headache
Antiviral		
Zovirax; Famvir; Valtrex	Treatment of HSV lesions	Nausea; vomiting; GI upset
Wart Removal Agents		
Podocon; Tri-chlor; Condylox; Aldara	Treatment of condyloma caused by HPV	Skin irritation

Adapted from Broyles, B., Reiss, B., & Evans, M. (2007). Pharmacological aspects of nursing care (7th ed.). New York: Thomson Delmar Learning.

Health Care Resources

Syphilis, gonorrhea, chlamydia, and HIV are infections reportable to local health departments in every state. Health departments have the responsibility to prioritize the infections to track and to carry out personal notification and treatment of partners. Since the early 1980s, most health departments have concentrated their resources on partner notification and treatment for HIV and AIDS.

Surgery

Surgery is not commonly needed to treat infections. When surgical draining is performed on Bartholin's gland infections, the skin is cleansed with Betadine, local anesthetic is usually injected, and an incision is made with a scalpel to allow for draining. A syringe may be used to release as much of the gland's contents as possible and to collect a sample for culture. It is important that the skin not close before all the contents of the gland have released or the infection may not resolve, so packing is sometimes done. Whether or not packing is done, close follow-up must be done to ensure that the Bartholin's gland infection resolves. Surgery may be required to remove a tubo-ovarian abscess associated with PID. Treatment for cervical abnormalities caused by HPV includes cryotherapy, loop electrosurgical excision procedure (LEEP), cone biopsy, electrocautery, laser and, rarely, hysterectomy.

Cryotherapy involves freezing the cervical lesion using the colposcope for visualization. Typically, no anesthesia is needed for cryotherapy, and it is done as an outpatient procedure. The LEEP procedure involves the use of a thin wire loop with an electric current that removes a thin layer of surface cells. LEEP is done as an outpatient procedure. A speculum is inserted, the colposcope is used, and the cervix is cleaned with an acetic acid solution. The cervix is anesthetized. The LEEP is used to remove a thin layer of surface cells, and Monsel's solution is used to ensure hemostasis, if necessary. Vaginal bleeding, mild cramping, and a brownish-black discharge from the Monsel's solution are expected side effects. Patients should consult their health care provider if heavy bleeding, severe abdominal pain, fever, chills, or malodorous discharge is experienced. If pregnancy occurs after a LEEP procedure is done, cervical competency may need to be assessed by ultrasound during the pregnancy.

A cone biopsy is done under general anesthesia. A cone-shaped piece of tissue is removed from the cervix with a small knife or a laser. Cervical tissue regenerates in four to six weeks. One concern after conization is the ability of the cervix to be competent with a subsequent pregnancy. If more than one cone biopsy has been done, the risk of incompetent cervix increases.

Alternative Therapy

Lactobacilli recolonization to treat and prevent yeast vaginitis and BV with yogurt and lactobacillus capsules is done by oral and intravaginal administration. Betadine vaginal suppositories or douches have been used to treat BV. Vaginal boric acid capsules, 600 mg/day at bedtime for two weeks, have been successfully used as treatment for recurrent or chronic yeast infections. Boric acid is not recommended for use during pregnancy.

Tea tree oil has been used as an antifungal and antibacterial. Garlic, one clove wrapped in unbleached gauze, and crushed before vaginal insertion nightly for six nights has been used to treat yeast vaginitis. Supplementation with L-lysine, vitamin C, and zinc has been used to prevent recurrent HSV infections. Herbal therapy with an herb from the rain forest of Peru, cat's claw, has been used to prevent recurrent HSV infections.

Patient and Family Teaching

Along with treatment of the woman, partner identification, notification, treatment, and ways to prevent reinfection must be discussed. Prevention of reinfection includes avoiding contact with untreated partners, use of condoms, and avoiding sexual contact if symptoms (e.g., HSV) are present. Patient education to avoid reinfection is an integral part of therapy. Male condoms are an effective prevention for the spread of HIV, if they are used consistently and correctly, and they can reduce the risk of spreading other infections, such as gonorrhea, chlamydia, and trichomoniasis. Condoms are most effective in preventing infections transmitted by contact with mucosal surfaces, such as HIV, gonorrhea, chlamydia, and trichomoniasis. They are less effective in preventing those infections transmitted by skin contact, such as HSV, HPV, and syphilis. Incorrect use, not breakage, is usually the cause of condom failure (CDC, 2002a).

Patient teaching includes education on disease transmission and prevention, avoidance of douching, use of condoms for STD prevention, completing the course of antibiotic therapy even if symptoms have resolved, symptoms that indicate medical evaluation is necessary, and importance of regular Pap screening. Patients may need explicit instructions on the use of vaginal medications. The use of a demonstration applicator for vaginal medications may be helpful. Patients should be made aware of the limitations on the use of condoms and the correct application of condoms. If one sexually transmitted infection is diagnosed, patients must be advised to obtain testing for the other infections.

Evaluation of Outcomes

Evaluation of outcomes allows the nurse to determine the effectiveness of interventions and change or refocus care as needed.

- Acute pain related to HSV, PID, or other painful infection. The patient should verbalize an adequate relief of pain along with the ability to realistically cope with the pain if it is not completely relieved.
- Risk for infection, reinfection, or infecting others related to sexually transmitted infections. The patient remains free of infection, as evidenced by normal vital signs and absence of purulent drainage from wounds, incisions, and tubes. Infection is recognized early to allow for prompt treatment.
- Deficient knowledge related to knowledge of disease transmission and prevention. The patient should demonstrate motivation to learn, identify perceived learning needs, and verbalize an understanding of desired content.

STRUCTURAL ABNORMALITIES AND BENIGN CONDITIONS

There are many structural abnormalities and benign conditions of the female reproductive system. Women have a variety of clinical manifestations and complications related to these disorders. The conditions included in this section are: polyps, pelvic relaxation, anatomic deviation, leiomyomata, and ovarian cysts.

Polyps

Polyps are fleshy growths on the cervix or in the endometrial cavity. Cervical polyps can be found in approximately 4 percent of all gynecology patients. Polyps may be located on the exterior or exocervix, in the cervical canal, or in the endometrial cavity. Polyps are usually asymptomatic. If symptoms do occur, they include bleeding and unusual vaginal discharge. Carcinoma with polyps is rare. Polyps are treated by removal. This is accomplished by grasping the polyp with a ring forceps and twisting it off, usually a painless procedure. In pregnancy, stable and benign polyps are followed conservatively by observation only, so that minimal disruption of the cervix occurs prior to delivery. In postmenopausal women, cervical polyps can be associated with endometrial polyps that can cause postmenopausal bleeding, so a diagnosis of cervical polyps may warrant further evaluation, such as uterine ultrasound or endometrial biopsy.

Pelvic Relaxation

Urethrocele is defined as relaxation of the anterior vaginal wall causing prolapse of the urethra into the vagina. Cystocele is relaxation of the anterior vaginal wall causing prolapse of the bladder neck or bladder into the vagina. Urethrocele and cystocele are associated with parity or childbearing. The greater number of pregnancies with a high percentage resulting in vaginal births increases the likelihood that some degree of pelvic relaxation will have occurred. The symptoms of urethrocele and cystocele are a sensation of suprapubic fullness or pressure, stress incontinence, urgency to void, and a feeling of incomplete emptying after voiding.

Management of urethrocele and cystocele includes teaching of Kegel's exercises (a regimen of isometric exercises to increase contractility of the vaginal introitus), pessary insertion, estrogen cream to correct vaginal atrophy if there are no contraindications, and operative repair. Pessaries are devices of different shapes that are inserted into the vagina to provide support to relaxed pelvic structures. Pessaries are typically left in and removed on a regular basis for cleaning and reinsertion. This is done either by the patient or by a health care provider. The use of vaginal therapy to minimize irritation is helpful when a pessary is used. Either estrogen vaginal cream or Trimo-San cream can be used. Trimo-San cream modulates the pH of the vagina and helps prevent bacterial infection and irritation.

Rectocele is defined as relaxation of the posterior vaginal wall causing prolapse of the rectum into the vagina. Symptoms of rectocele include a feeling of pressure in the vagina, constipation, and a sensation of incomplete rectal emptying. Rectoceles are also associated with parity. Therapy for rectocele includes instruction in Kegel's exercises, estrogen vaginal cream to correct vaginal atrophy if there are no contraindications, and operative management.

Enterocele is defined as the herniation of the intestines into the space between the vagina and the rectum. Enteroceles are difficult to diagnosis and are usually found during operative repairs for other conditions of pelvic relaxation. The treatment for an enterocele is operative repair.

Uterine prolapse is caused by relaxation of the support structures holding up the uterus. The result is the descent of the uterus into the vagina. The symptoms of uterine prolapse are a feeling of something falling out of the vagina, and the cervix may eventually be seen protruding from the vagina. Temporary descent of the cervix may occur immediately following a vaginal delivery, but it usually corrects itself within a few weeks after delivery. Urination and defecation changes are also common.

Uterine prolapse often occurs in conjunction with cystocele or rectocele. If the cervix appears low in the vagina but is not visible from the outside, no therapy is needed unless symptoms are present. Therapy is often indicated for the cervix that is visible external to the vagina, because irritation and ulcerations of the cervix can occur. Therapy includes insertion of pessaries to hold the uterus up and surgical repair, usually including hysterectomy. These conditions of pelvic relaxation can be present singly or in any combination. Risk factors for pelvic relaxation include obesity, family history of pelvic relaxation, and parity.

Leiomyomata

Commonly called uterine fibroids, leiomyomata are benign growths originating from the smooth muscle cells of the uterus. Fibroids may be single or multiple, small or large, and are located within the uterine cavity, in the muscle wall of the uterus itself, or external to the uterus. Leiomyomata are the most common solid pelvic tumors in women, and 20 to 40 percent of women have fibroids during their childbearing years. Fibroids are the most common reason for hysterectomy in the United States. Leiomyomata are estrogen-dependent tumors, and they predictably shrink during menopause (Wallach & Vlahos, 2004).

Most women with fibroids do not have symptoms. If women do have symptoms, the most common ones are excessive menstrual bleeding and pelvic pressure. Increased dysmenorrhea may be associated with fibroids. Depending on the location of the fibroid, gastrointestinal (GI) or urinary symptoms may be present. Constipation, increased abdominal girth, urinary retention, and dyspareunia may all be present. Uterine leiomyomata located in the uterine cavity may be associated with infertility and pregnancy loss. Asymptomatic fibroids need no therapy.

Symptomatic fibroids can be evaluated with ultrasound or hysterosalpingography. The choice of therapy depends on factors, such as age, desires for childbearing, severity of symptoms, size, number, and location of fibroids, and associated medical conditions. Fibroids can be followed expectantly, managed with medical therapy, removed with preservation of the uterus (**myomectomy**), reduced or destroyed by eliminating the blood supply to the fibroid through interventional radiology (uterine artery embolization), or treated by hysterectomy. Medical therapy with hormones can include progestins (either oral or injectable), combined estrogen-progesterone oral contraceptives, or GnRH analogues, such as leuprolide. Medical management should be adjusted individually for each woman. Costs and side effects of medical management may limit their use long-term.

Unless infertility or recurrent losses are an issue, women do not need to have fibroids removed to prevent possible pregnancy complications. Additional surveillance of pregnancy may be indicated if the placenta is implanted over the fibroid (Lefebvre, et al., 2003). When acute hemorrhage happens in women with fibroids, medical management, D & C, or hysteroscopy may be considered, but hysterectomy may be needed to control the hemorrhage.

Ovarian Cysts

Ovarian cysts are a common finding. There are follicular cysts, corpus luteum cysts, dermoid cysts, and endometriomas. Follicular cysts form in the first half of the menstrual cycle. The dominant follicle fails to ovulate, becomes fluid-filled, and does not regress right away. Follicular cysts are typically fluid-filled cysts within the ovaries that last up to two months and spontaneously resolve. Most follicular ovarian cysts are asymptomatic, have no known specific cause, and do not require treatment.

Follicular ovarian cysts usually occur during the childbearing years. If symptoms occur, they include pelvic pain, dyspareunia, abnormal menstruation or amenorrhea, and abdominal bloating, and distension. Follicular ovarian cysts can present with signs of rupture and intraperitoneal bleeding. Treatment includes combined oral contraceptives, which help resolve and prevent the reoccurrence of ovarian cysts. However, use of estrogen and progesterone oral contraceptives may not be an acceptable alternative for women with chronic illnesses, such as migraines, diabetes, and cardiovascular disease. If cysts do not resolve spontaneously, surgical removal may be indicated.

Corpus luteum cysts form in the last half of the menstrual cycle. They are less common but are often filled with blood and fluid. Rupture is possible, but most regress spontaneously. Persistent corpus luteum cysts are associated with menstrual irregularities and often amenorrhea. There may be cramping abdominal pain on the same side of the abdomen as the cyst, or if rupture has occurred, sharp, generalized abdominal pain is present. The pain may radiate to the back, shoulders, or legs, and bladder or rectal discomfort is possible.

Dermoid cysts are benign complex cystic growths that commonly contain different kinds of tissue such as fat, hair, and teeth. They are ovarian germ cell tumors and are the most frequent ovarian tumor in women under age 20. The peak incidence is ages 20 to 40. Dermoids are often asymptomatic, but pressure, achiness, or abdominal pain may be present.

Endometriomas (or chocolate cysts) are formed when endometrial tissue attaches to the outside of the ovary. They are usually associated with endometrial implants elsewhere in the pelvis. Endometriomas contain old blood. They are typically painful and cause dysmenorrhea and dyspareunia. Endometriomas may need to be removed through a laparoscopic procedure or during laparotomy.

Genetics

Any defect in the development of the müllerian system, typically before the eighth week of embryonic development, can result in structural or functional defects in the reproductive system. There may be congenital absence of the ovaries, fallopian tubes, uterus, or vagina. **Müllerian dysgenesis** is defined as abnormally developed or absent uterus, cervix, or upper part of the vagina. Ovaries, however, are present and develop normally.

Congenital absence of the ovaries is called ovarian agenesis or Turner's syndrome. Women with Turner's syndrome have an absence of one of the X chromosomes in all body cells caused by a lack of disjunction of the sex chromosomes. The typical woman with Turner's syndrome is short in stature and has neck webbing, lateral placement of the nipples on the chest, and an absence of breast development. Axillary and pubic hair is also lacking. Turner's syndrome is associated with coarctation of the aorta and absence of one kidney, but these typical features may not be present.

There are other chromosomal abnormalities that cause abnormal reproductive function. People with 46XY karyotypes have feminine or ambiguous genitalia with intra-abdominal testes. Breast development takes place, but the vagina is a blind pouch and there is no uterus or ovaries and no axillary or pubic hair. When an XY karyotype is detected the reproductive tissue is usually removed, because of the high risk of malignant changes, and hormone therapy is started. Sex-hormone insensitivity is associated with the 46XY karyotype.

Absent or anomalous fallopian tube formation results from failure of müllerian duct fusion. Tubal absence usually occurs with absence of the uterus. Any complete absence of ovaries, tubes, or uterus results in infertility. The absence of the uterus is usually diagnosed when primary amenorrhea exists and is identifiable during a pelvic examination. Absence of a vagina is rare, with an incidence of 1 in 4,000 to 1 in 10,000. The absence of a vagina is usually accompanied by absence of a uterus, caused by failure of müllerian duct fusion during embryonic development (ACOG, 2002).

Patients with absence of the vagina and uterus have a normal 46XX karyotype, normal ovarian formation and function, and normal secondary sex characteristics. Agenesis of the vagina is usually diagnosed as a consequence of primary amenorrhea and must be distinguished from sex-hormone insensitivity, a low-lying transverse vaginal septum, and imperforate hymen. Patients with vaginal agenesis may also have other congenital anomalies of the urinary tract and skeleton. Psychological support is necessary, and the adolescent with vaginal agenesis needs to be aware of the implications of the disorder. A normal sex life is possible with construction of a neovagina, but infertility is a consequence of the disorder. Harvesting of the woman's eggs and pregnancy achieved through surrogacy is a possibility for these patients.

Imperforate hymen is the most common müllerian duct defect and is a disorder of descent of the müllerian ducts. The hymenal membrane does not regress and obstructs the lower vagina, causing accumulation of menstrual blood behind the hymen.

Duplication of the müllerian system also exists. Deviations in the normal fusion of the müllerian duct buds result in duplication of all or part of the uterus, cervix, or upper vagina. Estimates are that müllerian duct defects occur in 1 in 700 women. Most of these defects are asymptomatic.

If a **didelphic,** or duplicated, uterus and cervix are present, fertility and childbirth are usually not affected, as long as both uteri and cervices communicate with a vagina and have a normal intrauterine cavity. The unicornuate uterus usually also has no affect on pregnancy, except that it may take longer to conceive if there is only one tubal connection with the uterus. Bicornuate uterus or uterus with septum may complicate fertility and pregnancy outcome if there is not sufficient space in the endometrial cavity to allow the pregnancy to implant, grow, and develop. Uterine septi are disorders of müllerian duct descent and are frequently associated with recurrent spontaneous pregnancy losses. Therefore, septi may need to be removed to allow for sufficient uterine function.

Assessment with Clinical Manifestations

Assessment includes a complete history and physical assessment with questions about menstrual cycles, pain symptoms, pregnancy history, and family history. Information about plans for future childbearing is crucial in developing plans for treatment of fibroids, pelvic relaxation, and other disorders where hysterectomy may be indicated for definitive treatment. Physical assessment includes observation of external genital features and in the case of suspected genital developmental abnormalities, assessment of secondary sex characteristics.

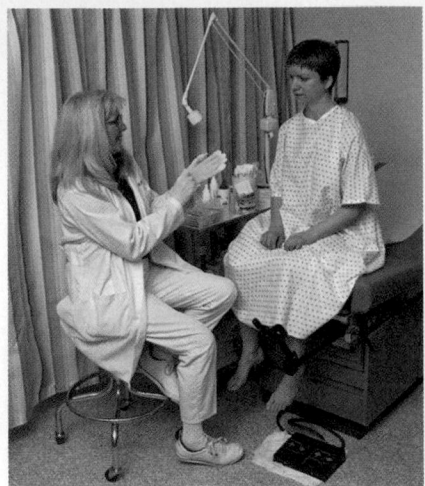

Figure 62-3 The nurse and patient prepare for a pelvic examination.

A comprehensive pelvic examination is the most helpful assessment for structural abnormalities and benign conditions.

Diagnostic Tests

The diagnosis of urethrocele and cystocele is made by observing a soft bulging mass of the anterior vaginal wall during a speculum or pelvic examination (Figure 62-3). Straining or coughing makes the bulging mass more apparent. If a urethrocele or cystocele is suspected, it is helpful to use only the posterior half of the speculum, insert it into the vagina and place downward pressure. This allows for unobstructed observation of the anterior vaginal wall.

Diagnosis of rectocele is made by observing a soft, bulging mass of the posterior vaginal wall during a speculum examination. To evaluate the rectocele, the posterior half of the speculum is inserted along the anterior vaginal wall and upward traction is applied, allowing for unobstructed observation of the posterior vaginal wall. Having the patient cough or strain will make the bulge in the posterior vaginal wall more apparent. Uterine prolapse may be diagnosed by observing the cervix protruding from the vaginal opening, but it is usually diagnosed by observing descent of the cervix into the vagina during a speculum examination.

Diagnostic tests for fibroids and structural abnormalities may include ultrasound, saline infusion sonogram, and hysterosalpingogram (HSG). An HSG is an X-ray study of the interior of the fallopian tubes and uterus. It is typically done to evaluate tubal patency and the structure of the uterine cavity. With the patient lying on an X-ray table, a speculum is inserted into the vagina, the cervix is numbed with an anesthetic, a thin tube is inserted through the cervix into the uterus, and then dye is inserted through the uterus into the fallopian tubes. X-rays are then taken, and the progress of the dye through the tubes is monitored. An HSG typically takes 10 to 20 minutes to perform. Rare complications of an HSG include infection or a recurrence of a chronic infection, allergic reaction to the dye, bleeding, and damage to the uterine wall or fallopian tubes. If fibroids are symptomatic, a complete blood count may be needed to assess the severity of anemia and the urgency for treatment. Chromosomal studies may be indicated if congenital structural abnormalities are suspected (Daniels, 2003).

Diagnostic tests for ovarian cysts include a pelvic exam, ultrasound examination, and serum hCG levels to rule out pregnancy. Lab tests may also include tumor markers, such as cancer antigen 125 (CA125) and alpha fetoprotein (AFP) to rule out ovarian cancer, a malignant neoplasm of the ovaries. Endometriomas are usually evaluated with ultrasound and possibly other imaging such as magnetic resonance imaging (MRI) or computerized tomography (CT) scan, or direct visualization with laparoscopy. Hysteroscopy can be used for diagnosis or treatment of disorders, such as abnormal uterine bleeding, infertility due to a structural uterine defect, repeated miscarriages due to structural defect, adhesions, polyps, fibroids, or displaced intrauterine devices.

Nursing Diagnoses

Based on the information gathered, examples of nursing diagnoses in the female patients with structural abnormalities may include the following:
- Situational low self-esteem or risk for situational low self-esteem related to physical changes and infertility associated with structural abnormalities.
- Disturbed body image related to negatively viewing physical changes associated with structural abnormalities.
- Acute or chronic pain associated with ovarian cysts.
- Impaired urinary elimination related to relaxed pelvic support.

Planning and Implementation

Care of the patient with structural abnormalities includes education, support, therapeutic interventions, and prevention measures. The initial physical and pelvic examination may be performed by an advanced practice nurse, physician's assistant, or physician. Any of these providers can order initial ultrasound or imaging studies and can remove cervical polyps. Gynecologists generally perform surgery to correct structural abnormalities, ovarian cysts, fibroids, and pelvic relaxation, although a urogynecological specialist may be consulted for reconstruction involving the urinary system. Physical therapists may be involved in bladder training and pelvic therapy to treat pelvic relaxation. Psychological or spiritual counseling may be helpful for women with congenital anatomical deviations, particularly those affecting fertility and body image. Patient education and patient preparation for any testing may be ordered. The nurse provides preoperative and postoperative care and discharge instructions, and plays a crucial role in teaching Kegel's exercises.

Uterine prolapse is associated with intra-abdominal pressure. This can come from ascites, pelvic, or intra-abdominal tumors, sacral nerve disorders (particularly injuries to S1 through S4), or diabetic neuropathy. Increased abdominal pressure and uterine prolapse can also be associated with coughing, such as occurs in chronic bronchitis, asthma, or bronchiectasis.

In a New York study of elderly women with chronic medical conditions undergoing pelvic reconstructive surgery, the women had no mortality and no significant morbidity. The women did find that the corrective surgery provided an immediate, substantial, and long-lasting improvement to the quality of life. The conclusion of the investigators was that pelvic reconstructive surgery should be an option even for women with chronic medical conditions (Vetere, Putterman & Kesselman, 2003). Conditions of pelvic relaxation are associated with parity and multiple vaginal births.

Nutrition

Women with fibroids may need nutritional counseling regarding foods that are a high source of iron to correct iron-deficiency anemia. Women with symptomatic pelvic relaxation who are obese may benefit from nutritional counseling for weight loss.

Pharmacology

Estrogen vaginal cream is indicated to relieve vaginal atrophy and improve symptoms associated with cystocele, rectocele, and uterine prolapse. The GnRH agonist leuprolide is used in treating fibroids to correct anemia and shrink fibroids, particularly prior to surgical intervention. Combined estrogen and progesterone oral contraceptive are used in the treatment of fibroids and the prevention and treatment of follicular ovarian cysts. Progesterone therapy, both oral progesterone and long-acting intramuscular progesterone are used in the treatment of fibroids. The hormonal therapies that may be used are listed previously in Table 62-1.

Surgery

Cervical polyps that cannot be removed in the outpatient setting and endometrial polyps may require surgical removal (Box 62-2). Anatomical structural defects may need to be corrected or removed surgically. The absence of a vagina can be corrected with surgical reconstruction or dilation of the blind pouch with dilators. Creating the vagina with dilators takes several months of progressive dilation (ACOG, 2002). Surgery to create a vagina is an option if dilation is unsuccessful or not a preferred option. Symptomatic pelvic relaxation is often treated with anterior or posterior repair, usually with hysterectomy. Fibroids may be treated with

---

BOX 62-2

INDICATIONS FOR SURGICAL MANAGEMENT OF FIBROIDS

- Abnormal bleeding not responsive to medical therapy
- High level of suspicion of malignancy
- Growth of fibroids after menopause
- Infertility from distortion of the uterine cavity, particularly if there are recurrent pregnancy losses
- Symptoms that interfere with quality of life
- Urinary tract symptoms from obstruction
- Iron deficiency anemia from chronic blood loss

removal of only the fibroids in the uterus-sparing myomectomy or with removal of fibroids along with the entire uterus in hysterectomy. Uterine artery embolization is not a surgical procedure but is an intervention performed by a radiologist.

If surgery is contemplated, a course of leuprolide may be prescribed to shrink the fibroids and correct anemia before surgery is performed. Hysterectomy is a definitive treatment, for a woman who has completed their childbearing and is associated with a high level of patient satisfaction (Lefebvre, et al., 2003). Women choosing uterine artery embolization must be carefully counseled that they preserve their uterus, but long-term data on effectiveness, potential fertility, pregnancy outcomes, and patient satisfaction are not complete. Ovarian cysts may be removed with minimal disruption to the ovary or may be accomplished by complete removal of the ovary or associated hysterectomy.

Alternative Therapy

Pessaries are a nonsurgical alternative used to treat all the pelvic relaxation disorders. Each pessary has a specific function and specific directions for fitting and removal. The choice of the appropriate type of pessary is made by the care provider who fits the pessary. The pessary can be inserted and then removed and cleaned at intervals by the patient or by a health care provider. Vaginal therapeutic creams can be used to prevent vaginal irritation from the pessary. Trimo-San cream can be used to adjust the vaginal pH and prevent bacterial infection, and estrogen cream can be used to prevent atrophy. If pessary removal and cleaning is done in the gynecology office, the vagina and cervix should be inspected for unusual discharge, bleeding, or areas of irritation.

Patient and Family Teaching

Teaching includes information about the patient's specific diagnosis, particularly if there are implications for fertility. Teaching should also include information on treatment options, instruction in the use of pessaries, and medication instruction. If surgery is indicated, preoperative and postoperative teaching is indicated. Ways to cope with pain and pain relief measures should be reviewed. Teaching Kegel exercises is an important part of the treatment plan for problems of pelvic relaxation. Recognition of symptoms indicating the need for medical attention should be reviewed with women who have asymptomatic cervical polyps, fibroids, and ovarian cysts.

Evaluation of Outcomes

Potential patient outcomes for each of the example nursing diagnoses for the patient with structural abnormalities and benign conditions are:
- Situational low self-esteem or risk for situational low self-esteem related to physical changes and infertility associated with structural abnormalities. The patient demonstrates acceptance of self and condition of infertility.
- Disturbed body image related to negatively viewing physical changes associated with structural abnormalities. The patient demonstrates enhanced body image and self-esteem as evidenced by ability to look at, touch, talk about, and care for actual or perceived altered body part or function.
- Acute or chronic pain associated with ovarian cysts. The patient should verbalize an adequate relief of pain along with the ability to realistically cope with the pain if it is not completely relieved.
- Impaired urinary elimination related to relaxed pelvic support. The patient is continent of urine or verbalizes satisfactory management.

FEMALE GENITAL MUTILATION

Female circumcision (FC) or female genital mutilation (FGM) involves removal of part or all of the external genital structures. Removal of the clitoris and labia minora is the most common type of procedure. FC and FGM comprise all

Kegel Exercises

The nurse should instruct the patient in the following to perform Kegel exercises:

- Locate the pubococcygeus muscle by placing your finger inside your vagina and tightening the muscle around your finger.
- If you are unwilling, or unable, to place your finger in your vagina, an alternative approach is to contract the muscles around your anus, without contracting the buttocks or abdominal muscles, as if you were attempting to stop the passage of gas.
- Hold the contraction to a count of 10 and then release.
- Contract the muscle using both slow muscle squeezes and fast muscle squeezes.
- Repeat the muscle contraction-relaxation cycle 10 to 20 times in a row.
- The exercise should be repeated three times a day.
- After six weeks, symptom improvement should be noted.
- These exercises can be done while performing everyday tasks, such as standing in line, doing dishes, and driving.

procedures involving partial or total removal of the external female genitalia or other injury to the female genital organs whether for cultural, religious, or other nontherapeutic reasons. The World Health Organization (WHO) estimates that between 100 and 140 million women, particularly in African countries, are affected. FGM also occurs in Asia and the Middle East. Female emigrants from these countries who have undergone the procedure can also be found in Europe, Australia, Canada, and the United States.

Immediate health consequences associated with FGM include pain, difficulty with urination, infection, and hemorrhage. Hemorrhage and infection can cause subsequent shock and death. Later health consequences include pain, infection, sexual dysfunction, urinary incontinence, scarring, and childbirth complications (Nour, 2004). Dyspareunia and psychosexual dysfunctions are common. The United Nations Children's Fund, the United Nations Population Fund, and the WHO have jointly issued a statement that FC and FGM cause unacceptable harm and issued a call for the elimination of this practice worldwide.

Nursing care for women who have had FGM must include an understanding of the physical and psychological effects of the procedure. Vaginal exams and gynecological procedures may be painful and produce anxiety, and women require sensitive, empathetic care. Women may suffer anxiety, depression, and impairment to psychosexual and psychological health. The FGM procedure itself may cause a direct or indirect barrier to childbirth because of scarring or infectious complications, resulting in a long or obstructed labor. Episiotomy often relieves soft tissue obstruction, and episiotomy and lacerations are the most common complication of labor and birth with FGM. Increased postpartum pain and postpartum hemorrhage may be present. Fear of labor and birth may be evident. Urinary retention may happen during labor.

Assessment with Clinical Manifestations

Culturally competent providers should care for women with FGM to the extent possible. Assessment must be tactful and respectful of the cultural and religious roots of FGM practices. Assumptions about the effect of FGM on a woman's self-esteem or body image must not be made. The nurse needs to explore the woman's view of FGM and any implications for her emotional, psychological, and sexual health. The type of mutilation must be ascertained to understand what physical effects can be expected as a result of it. Any symptoms relating to FGM, such as urinary problems, pain, or infection, should be elicited. The nurse must assess for the immediate complications of FMG including pain, difficulty with urination, infection, as well as hemorrhage, shock, and death. Later complications include pain, infection, sexual dysfunction, urinary incontinence, scarring, and childbirth complications (Nour, 2004).

Diagnostic Tests

Diagnosis of female mutilation involves inspection of the external genitalia. The care provider confirms which parts have been excised and determines any scarring or restriction of function that is evident. In addition, related laboratory tests, radiologic tests, or CT scans can also confirm the presence of injury.

Nursing Diagnoses

Based on the information gathered, examples of nursing diagnoses in the patient with female mutilation may include the following:

- Chronic pain related to the FGM procedure or its sequelae.
- Impaired urinary elimination related to FGM.
- Disturbed body image related to changes in external genitalia.
- Sexual dysfunction related to alterations in external genitalia.

Planning and Implementation

Care of the patient with female genital mutilation includes education, support, therapeutic interventions, and prevention of complications. Psychological counseling, particularly with a counselor who is culturally competent, can be invaluable in helping patients who have experienced FGM (Box 62-3). Mutilating procedures can be associated with religious practices, and a spiritual advisor may be helpful to the woman experiencing complications. A physician or nurse-midwife may need to surgically revise the FGM outcome to assist in childbirth and relieve symptoms. FGM is closely associated to the woman's culture of origin and may have religious significance. Childbirth may be associated with complications of FGM, if there is perineal trauma and repair. Patient teaching should include hygiene measures that will minimize urinary tract infections (UTIs) and knowledge of symptoms requiring medical evaluation. There is no special nutritional therapy for FGM, although a diet that is generally well-balanced will help make tissues as strong as possible for any healing that must occur as a result of childbirth and make urinary infection less likely. Surgery may be necessary to revise FGM to relieve symptoms, particularly during and after childbirth.

Pharmacology

There is typically no medical therapy indicated for FGM. If recurrent urinary infections are a concern, prophylactic antibiotics can be used to prevent UTIs. If disruption and repair of FGM was performed during childbirth, a short-term course of topical estrogen cream may assist with healing and prevent atrophy and scarring.

Population-Based Care

The prevalence of FGM will vary in areas of the country. Areas with large numbers of emigrants from Africa will likely have more women with FGM. Women with FGM are reluctant to seek care, particularly from care providers unfamiliar with FGM, as they are afraid they will be subject to embarrassing questions and painful examinations.

Evaluation of Outcomes

Potential patient outcomes for each of the example nursing diagnoses for the patient with FGM are:
- Chronic pain related to the FGM procedure or its sequelae. The patient should verbalize an adequate relief of pain along with the ability to realistically cope with the pain if it is not completely relieved.
- Impaired urinary elimination. The patient is continent of urine or verbalizes satisfactory management.
- Disturbed body image related to changes in external genitalia. The patient demonstrates enhanced body image and self-esteem as evidenced by ability to look at, touch, talk about, and care for actual or perceived altered body part or function.
- Sexual dysfunction related to alterations in external genitalia. The patient will verbalize satisfaction with the way they express physical intimacy.

MALIGNANCIES

There are several gynecological malignancies with different prognoses, clinical manifestations, and consequences for the patient. This section will examine the following malignancies: vulvar, vaginal, cervical, endometrial, and ovarian cancers. In general, refer to chapter 15 for more information regarding the various types of management strategies for patients that have cancer.

Vulvar Cancer

Vulvar cancer is a malignant neoplasm of the vulvar tissue that accounts for 4 percent of all cancers of the female reproductive tract. Over 90 percent of vulvar cancers are squamous cell cancers. These cancers begin with precancerous changes confined to the epithelial layer called vulvar intraepithelial neoplasia (VIN). VIN can be further divided into VIN1, VIN2, and VIN3. VIN1 is the earliest stage of precancerous changes, and VIN3 is the latest stage toward cancerous changes. Not all women with VIN will progress to vulvar cancer, but it is difficult to determine which lesions will progress and which will not, so all women with VIN are treated.

Melanomas account for 2 to 4 percent of vulvar cancers. A small percentage of vulvar cancers develop from the glands, particularly the Bartholin's glands, and these are called adenocarcinomas. When vulvar cancer is detected early the prognosis is good. If lymph nodes are not affected the five-year survival rate is 90 percent. When lymph node involvement is present, the five-year survival rate drops to 50 to 70 percent. Risk factors for vulvar cancer include HPV infection, smoking, HIV infection, VIN, lichen sclerosis, other genital cancers, and a personal or family history of melanoma. Lichen sclerosis is a skin condition which makes the skin thin and atrophic, and therefore susceptible to cancerous changes. Women with vulvar cancer usually are symptomatic. When symptoms are present they include persistent vulvar itching, vulvar skin color changes, a white warty bump or sore that does not heal, new darkly pigmented mole, or an atypical mole.

Vaginal Cancer

Primary vaginal cancers are much rarer than other cancers of the genital tract. Only about 3 percent of genital tract cancers are vaginal. Squamous cell carcinomas account for 85 to 90 percent of vaginal cancers, most occurring in the upper area of the vagina near the cervix. Adenocarcinomas account for 5 to 10 percent of vaginal cancers.

Adenocarcinomas are usually found in women over 50 years of age. Clear cell carcinoma is a specific type of adenocarcinoma typically found in younger women with diethylstilbestrol (DES) exposure. The risk for vaginal cancer increases with age. More than half the women diagnosed with vaginal cancer are over age 60. Other risk factors include vaginal adenosis (replacement of the usual squamous lining of the vagina with glandular cells) caused by DES exposure, HPV infection, cervical cancer, and smoking.

Vaginal intraepithelial neoplasia (VAIN) is an indicator of precancerous changes. VAIN is diagnosed with colposcopy and treated with laser surgery or topical chemotherapy. VAIN is usually asymptomatic, but lesions may be noted during a routine examination or on colposcopy. Vaginal cancers are usually symptomatic, and if symptoms are present, they include abnormal vaginal discharge, abnormal vaginal bleeding, a vaginal mass, or dyspareunia. Dysuria, constipation, or pelvic pain may occur with advanced disease.

Cervical Cancer

Most cervical cancer originates in the transformation zone between the endocervical canal and the ectocervix. Squamous cell carcinomas account for 80 to 90 percent of cervical cancers, with the rest being adenocarcinomas. Most cervical cancer is diagnosed in women in their postreproductive years, and half of all cancers are diagnosed in women between 35 and 55 years of age. The five-year survival rate for the earliest stage of cancer is 92 percent, and the overall five-year survival rate is 71 percent.

The most important risk factor for cervical cancer is infection with high-risk type HPV. The likelihood of contracting an HPV infection increases with the

Fast Forward ▶▶▶

HPV Vaccination

In the future, vaccines may be available to immunize young women against HPV. A clinical trial for a vaccine against HPV type 16 showed 100 percent effectiveness over an 18-month study. One cost-benefit analysis estimated that vaccinating 12-year-old girls and doing Pap screening every three years would result in a 92 percent reduction of cervical cancer (Goldie, et al., 2004).

first sexual contact occurring at an early age, having multiple partners, and having sexual contact with uncircumcised men. Although HPV infection must be present, other risk factors for cervical cancer include smoking, HIV infection, past or current chlamydia infection, obesity, low SES, multiple pregnancies, DES exposure, and family history of cervical cancer (ACS, 2004c). Most cervical cancer is asymptomatic. If symptoms are present, they can include abnormal vaginal discharge or vaginal bleeding, particularly after intercourse, and dyspareunia.

The ACS (2004b) has identified four factors that influence the quality of life that people with cancer have: physical, social, psychological, and spiritual. Women with cervical cancer are often concerned about: the opportunity for pregnancy, fear of recurrence, the presence of pain, sexual problems, fatigue, guilt for behaviors that caused the cancer or delayed screening or treatment, changes in physical appearance, depression, sleep disorders, changes in activities of daily living, the impact on finances, and the effect on their relationships with loved ones.

Endometrial Cancer

Most endometrial cancers are adenocarcinomas. Cancer of the endometrium is the most common cancer of the female reproductive system. Women over age 40 account for 95 percent of all women with endometrial cancer. The five-year survival rate for all types of endometrial cancer is 84 percent. The lifetime probability for a woman to develop endometrial cancer is 1 in 38 (ACS, 2004d).

Risk factors for endometrial cancer include early age at menarche, late menopause, infertility or nulliparity, obesity, use of tamoxifen, estrogen therapy unopposed by progesterone, ovarian tumors, a diet high in animal fat, diabetes, age greater than 40, family history of hereditary nonpolyposis colon cancer, breast or ovarian cancer, and prior pelvic radiation therapy. Tamoxifen is a selective estrogen receptor modulator (SERM) used as adjunctive therapy for breast cancer and to prevent breast cancer in women at high risk. Tamoxifen therapy is associated with endometrial proliferation, hyperplasia, polyp formation, and endometrial cancer. The risk is two to three times that of women the same age not taking tamoxifen. Women taking tamoxifen should be closely monitored for endometrial hyperplasia and should have a gynecological examination once a year. In addition, women taking tamoxifen should be educated about the risks of endometrial proliferation and cancer and be educated about warning signs, such as unusual vaginal discharge and unusual spotting or bleeding.

Oral contraceptives protect against the risk of developing endometrial cancer, as does taking progesterone therapy along with estrogen replacement therapy. If hyperplasia develops, treatment with progesterone and D & C can prevent development of endometrial cancer. The main symptom of endometrial cancer is irregular vaginal bleeding, primarily postmenopausal bleeding. Weight loss, the presence of pelvic pain, and a pelvic or an abdominal mass may also be present in the late stages.

Ovarian Cancer

Excluding nonmelanoma skin cancers, ovarian cancer is the fifth most common cancer in women and the second most common female reproductive cancer. Epithelial ovarian carcinomas account for 85 percent of ovarian cancers (ACS, 2004c). The lifetime probability for women to develop ovarian cancer is 1 in 59.

Most ovarian cancers occur in women after menopause. Half of all ovarian cancers are in women over the age of 63. More women die from ovarian cancer than from cervical and uterine cancer combined. Risk factors for ovarian cancer include increased age; early menstruation; late menopause; no children or first child after age 30; prolonged use of clomiphene citrate to induce ovulation; family history of breast, ovarian, or colorectal cancer; personal history of breast cancer; possibly postmenopausal estrogen therapy; and possibly the use of talcum powder.

Ovarian cancers are often asymptomatic. If symptoms occur, they include abdominal pain and swelling, bloating, nausea, vomiting, indigestion, change in bowel or bladder habits, unexplained weight loss, leg and back pain, and pelvic pain (ACOG, 2002, ACS, 2004c). The breast cancer genes BRCA1 and BRCA2 are associated with a high risk of breast and ovarian cancer. These two genes are responsible for about 9 percent of all cases of ovarian cancer. If there is a family history of breast and ovarian cancer, consideration should be given to offering genetic counseling and testing for the BRCA1 and BRCA2 genes, because prophylactic treatments can be offered for women carrying these genes. Hereditary ovarian cancer accounts for 5 to 10 percent of all ovarian cancers. The lifetime risk of developing ovarian cancer for a woman with the BRCA1 or BRCA2 gene is 15 to 45 percent. If prophylactic treatments are not done, regular screening with pelvic examinations, ultrasound, and CA125 is indicated. Oral contraceptives, hysterectomy, tubal ligation, having a child before age 30, and prolonged breastfeeding all offer a protective effect against ovarian cancer (ACS, 2004c).

Assessment with Clinical Manifestations

The nursing assessment of a patient with a genital cancer should include a complete health history, including the presence of any chronic illness, the possibility of pregnancy, any lifestyle issues that may need to be addressed, such as smoking, the woman's age and plans for childbearing, and relationship support. Family history should also be obtained, particularly the history of breast or ovarian cancer. Refer to chapter 15 for further development of the assessment of patients with cancer.

Diagnostic Tests

Diagnostic tests include colposcopy with cervical biopsy, endocervical curettage, and possibly cone biopsy for evaluation of cervical cancer. Diagnosis of endometrial cancer is usually done by endometrial biopsy or D & C. Ultrasound evaluation may also be helpful. Ultrasonography, other imaging such as MRI or CT scan, and tumor markers such as hCG, CA125, and AFP are used to evaluate ovarian cancer.

Ultrasound and CA125 tests are not recommended as routine screening for women without risk factors because CA125 may be falsely positive, and as many as half of all women with ovarian cancer have a falsely reassuring CA125 result. CA125 is not recommended for premenopausal women, because an elevated level of CA125 may be associated with benign conditions, such as leiomyomata, PID, endometriosis, adenomyosis, pregnancy, and even menstruation (ACOG, 2002). Vulvar and vaginal cancer are evaluated with direct inspection, colposcopy, and tissue biopsy. Other imaging or lymph node biopsy may be necessary. Staging of cancers may include imaging studies such as CT or MRI, chest X-ray, and intravenous pyelogram (IVP).

Nursing Diagnoses

Based on the information gathered, examples of nursing diagnoses in the patient with malignancies may include the following:
- Anxiety related to loss of reproductive function and fear of cancer.
- Altered body image related to surgical changes in genital organs.
- Acute pain related to treatment for genital cancer.
- Deficient knowledge for self-care related to diagnosis or treatment of cancer.
- Sexual dysfunction related to anxiety, altered body image, or treatments for cancer.

Planning and Implementation

Care of the patient with a gynecological malignancy includes education, support, therapeutic interventions, and prevention measures. Treatment of reproductive cancers requires a team approach including nurses, gynecological surgeons, oncologists, physical therapists, nutritionists, sex therapists, and psychological counselors. A diet low in animal fat has been proposed to reduce the risk of certain types of cancer. Women with reproductive tract cancers should be encouraged to regularly eat green, leafy vegetables. Cervical cancer is more prevalent in women who are obese, who smoke, who have HIV or chlamydia, have low SES, and in women with DES exposure, or a family history of cervical cancer. When a diagnosis of cervical cancer is made in a woman who is pregnant, the woman may choose early termination or may choose to continue the pregnancy and obtain treatment after delivery. Endometrial cancer is more common in women with infertility, diabetes, a family history of hereditary nonpolyposis colon cancer, or prior pelvic irradiation. Women with breast cancer are at risk and are at an additional risk if they have used tamoxifen to treat the breast cancer. Ovarian cancer also contributes to the risk of endometrial cancer. Ovarian cancer is more common in women with a family history of ovarian or breast cancer and in women with infertility, particularly with prolonged use of clomiphene citrate to stimulate ovulation. Most reproductive cancers are treated surgically or with radiation. Chemotherapeutic agents also may be used, which are discussed in chapter 15.

Population-Based Care

Minority women are more likely to develop cervical and endometrial cancer, and Caucasian women are more likely to develop ovarian cancer. Vietnamese women have the highest rates of incidence of cervical cancer. The cervical cancer death rate for African Americans is twice that of the national average. Hispanic (American) women and American Indian women also have higher death rates than Caucasian women. Caucasian women have a higher risk of developing and dying from ovarian cancer than do African American women. African American women are twice as likely to die from endometrial cancer as are white women (ACS, 2004c).

Health Care Resources

In August 1990, Congress enacted the Breast and Cervical Cancer Mortality Prevention Act. This act authorized the CDC to establish programs to increase breast and cervical cancer screening among low-income women who are uninsured. The current priority of the cervical cancer screening project is to target women who have never had a Pap smear or have not had a Pap smear for five years or longer.

Surgery

Treatment for reproductive cancers may include surgery, chemotherapy, and radiation therapy. Treatment for cervical cancer often involves surgery, which may include local laser excision, cryosurgery, or cone biopsy if the cancer is in the earliest stages and the woman wants to preserve her fertility. Typically, early cervical cancer is treated with hysterectomy, although pelvic exenteration (removal of the uterus and pelvic structures, lymph nodes, bladder, vagina, rectum, and part of the colon) may be necessary for recurrent cervical cancer. Radiation or chemotherapy may be used for more extensive cervical cancer.

Surgery for endometrial cancer involves hysterectomy and potentially, removal of the ovaries. Surgery for ovarian cancer usually involves removal of the ovaries and uterus. Treatment for vulvar cancer may include laser or surgical excision, vulvectomy, pelvic exenteration, radiation, or chemotherapy. Treatment of vaginal cancer may involve radiation, chemotherapy, or surgery. Local excision may be done for small lesions. If the vagina needs to be removed, a replacement vagina is reconstructed from a graft.

Patient and Family Teaching

Patient and family teaching is extremely important for patients with malignancies of the female reproductive system. For example, an important part of the teaching for women with ovarian cancer is the information that a strong family history of breast and ovarian cancer may indicate the presence of the BRCA1 or BRCA2 gene, and the possibility for other family members to be offered genetic counseling, testing, and prophylactic treatment. Teaching includes information on the specific diagnosis. Lifestyle modifications that can reduce the risk of recurrence, such as smoking cessation, should be discussed. Patients may need information on treatment options. Preoperative and postoperative teaching will also need to be done.

Women undergoing vulvectomy have specific educational needs. Such women may experience discomfort from tight clothing after a vulvectomy. The vaginal opening looks different and scarring may be present; this may cause sexual difficulties for women if they fear their partner's reaction. This may be particularly true for women who enjoy oral stimulation as part of sex. Women who have a vulvectomy have difficulty reaching orgasm and may have numbness in their genital area. Light touching and lubrication may help irritation.

Scar tissue may narrow the entrance to the vagina, causing painful penetration. Vaginal dilators can assist with stretching the vaginal opening. If lymph nodes have been removed, women may have swelling of their genital areas or legs. This can result in pain, fatigue, and difficulty with intercourse. Nurses need to assist women to anticipate problems and help them with communication skills and solving difficulties. Partner education and support is, of course, essential. Sexual issues need to be explored with women who have had vaginal reconstruction. The replacement vagina has no natural lubrication, and sensation during intercourse is varied and different.

Evaluation of Outcomes

Evaluation of outcomes allows the nurse to determine the effectiveness of interventions and change or refocus care as needed.

- Anxiety related to loss of reproductive function and fear of cancer. The patient should be able to recognize the signs of anxiety, demonstrate positive coping mechanisms, and describe a reduction in the level of anxiety experienced.
- Altered body image related to surgical changes in genital organs. The patient demonstrates enhanced body image and self-esteem as evidenced by ability to look at, touch, talk about, and care for actual or perceived altered body part or function.
- Acute pain related to treatment for genital cancer. The patient should verbalize an adequate relief of pain along with the ability to realistically cope with the pain if it is not completely relieved.
- Deficient knowledge for self-care related to diagnosis or treatment of cancer. The patient should demonstrate motivation to learn, identify perceived learning needs, and verbalize an understanding of desired content.
- Sexual dysfunction related to anxiety, altered body image, or treatments for cancer. The patient will verbalize satisfaction with the way they express physical intimacy.

INFERTILITY

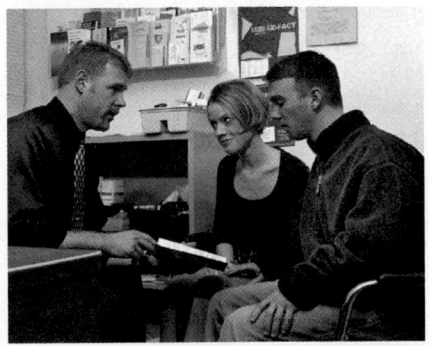

Figure 62-4 An important element in fertility counseling is sharing information with both members of the concerned couple.

Infertility must be considered as the problem of the couple, not an individual, and must be evaluated as such (Figure 62-4). Approximately 14 percent of couples will have difficulty conceiving. Infertility is a concern for 2.7 million U.S. women. The definition of infertility is one year of unprotected intercourse without conception.

The male factor in infertility accounts for 30 percent of infertility, anovulation for 25 percent, tubal damage for 20 percent, and unexplained factors for 25 percent. Among women with anovulation, 70 percent have PCOS. Regular menstrual cycles of 22 to 35 days with premenstrual symptoms and dysmenorrhea suggest that ovulation is occurring. Infertility is associated with a higher (above 27) BMI.

Anovulation may be caused by PCOS, disorders of the hypothalamic system, hyperprolactinemia, and premature ovarian failure. If hypothalamic disruption is caused by a low BMI of less than 20, weight gain may result in the resumption of normal menses and ovulation (ACOG, 2002). Much of infertility treatment includes support and counseling.

Assessment with Clinical Manifestations

The nursing assessment includes questions about pregnancy history, menstrual cycle characteristics, timing of intercourse, and length of time patient and partner have been attempting pregnancy. A complete medical history should be obtained including medication use (prescription, OTC, and herbal), chronic illness, and any surgeries. A social history should be obtained including the use of cigarettes, marijuana, other recreational drugs, and alcohol. A history should be obtained to screen for tubal patency. If there is a history of STDs, PID, ruptured appendix, exposure to DES, or previous pelvic surgery, hysterosalpingography should be considered (ACOG, 2002). DES is a form of estrogen that was given to women from 1940 to 1971 to prevent spontaneous abortion. The daughters of mothers who took DES are at increased risk to develop clear cell adenocarcinoma of the vagina and other reproductive problems.

The partner's history should be obtained including any pregnancies with a prior partner, chronic illness and medication use, surgical history, history of any trauma to the testes or radiation therapy, any use of recreational substances, alcohol, smoking, and type of underwear worn. A family history including questions about endometriosis, PCOS, and infertility should be obtained. Occasionally, the process of obtaining the nursing assessment will uncover an underlying explanation for failure of conception. Sometimes this explanation will be as simple as couples not having an opportunity to have sex at midcycle because of work schedules and not understanding that conception only occurs when ovulation happens.

Diagnostic Tests

A semen analysis for the male partner should be conducted at the beginning of the evaluation of the woman for infertility. The first goal in assessing a woman for infertility is diagnosis of ovulation or anovulation. Laboratory methods to determine ovulation include basal body temperature (BBT) charting; measurement of urine luteinizing hormone (LH), the test used in OTC ovulation predictor kits; measurement of luteal phase serum progesterone; and endometrial biopsy. Serial ultrasounds can be used to identify the growth and rupture of ovarian follicles. The BBT record is reviewed after three months and used in conjunction with ovulation prediction kits to determine the ovarian cycle. If ovulation is occurring, and the semen analysis is normal, the next step is usually to ensure tubal patency with HSG. HSG is discussed in the section on structural abnormalities.

Nursing Diagnoses

Based on the information gathered, examples of nursing diagnoses in the patient with infertility may include the following:
- Anxiety related to inability to conceive.
- Altered body image related to inability to fulfill role as woman.
- Deficient knowledge related to infertility.

Planning and Implementation

Care of the patient with infertility includes education, support, therapeutic interventions, and prevention measures. The nurse caring for a woman experiencing infertility generally collaborates with a primary care practitioner who evaluates and manages the overall care plan and process. This might be a physician, advanced practice nurse, or physician's assistant. If surgery is necessary, this is performed by the general gynecologist or reproductive specialist. Referral to reproductive endocrinologists or fertility specialists may be necessary. Psychological and spiritual counseling is often helpful to support the couple through the process. It is important to verify with the couple at each step that continuing with the plan is what they wish to do. Each couple will have their own financial and emotional threshold for continuing with the infertility process and it is important not to assume what each couple will decide.

Women with PCOS or endometriosis have a higher risk of infertility. For these women, it is not generally advisable to wait an entire year before seeking consultation about infertility. Patients with a diagnosis of PCOS or endometriosis will benefit from anticipatory guidance about trying for pregnancy and the interventions that can maximize their success. Women with other chronic illnesses may find conceiving difficult because of anovulation, fatigue, lack of sexual desire, or use of medications that are contraindicated in pregnancy.

Women with chronic illnesses who are contemplating pregnancy should consult the health care provider managing their chronic illness about taking medication that is effective yet the safest for pregnancy. Women sometimes seek evaluation of infertility because their partners have a chronic illness with a related decrease in sexual functioning. If the patient has a BMI over 30, or diabetes is suspected, testing for diabetes is indicated before attempting to

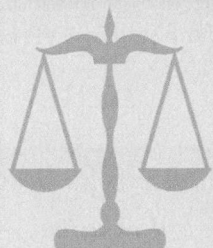

ETHICS IN PRACTICE

Multifetal Pregnancy Reduction

If the result of infertility treatment is a multiple gestation of more than two fetuses, the couple may need to make difficult choices about carrying a multiple pregnancy or selectively terminating one or more fetuses. Selectively terminating one or more fetuses from a multiple pregnancy is called multifetal pregnancy reduction. The ethical decisions to be made regarding selective reduction of fetuses are difficult for the parents and for their health care providers.

Patients who have gone through extensive time, testing, and procedures to become pregnant may be faced with the following choices: terminate the entire pregnancy, continue the pregnancy and take the risk of delivering severely preterm infants with a high likelihood of neonatal mortality and morbidity, or have selective reduction performed in an effort to decrease the risks of delivering extremely preterm babies. The decision is especially difficult if the parents do not agree on a plan. The plan that parents make in the hypothetical case of what if there is a multiple pregnancy may not be a plan they can live with once a multiple gestation pregnancy is a reality. Spiritual advice from religious advisers may help some couples, as well as talking with couples who have had to make similar choices.

induce ovulation. Diabetes mellitus should be controlled prior to trying for pregnancy to reduce the risks of congenital defects (ACOG, 2002).

Pharmacology

Clomiphene citrate is used to induce ovulation. When clomiphene citrate is used, most successful pregnancies occur within the first three cycles of using the clomiphene, and almost all occur within six months of initiating its use. Gonadotropins (LH and FSH or only FSH) can be used to treat anovulation in women with PCOS, and combined LH and FSH treatment can be used to treat anovulation in women with hypothalamic disorders. Metformin can be used in PCOS, along with clomiphene citrate to induce ovulation if indicated. Dopamine-agonist drugs, such as bromocriptine, pergolide, and cabergoline, are used to induce ovulation in women with hyperprolactinemia. The drugs in Table 62-3 are used in the treatment of infertility.

Health Care Resources

Some health insurance plans cover infertility services, usually to a set end point or to a dollar amount. The most expensive types of infertility evaluation and treatment are not usually covered by health care insurance. This limits infertility treatment to those who can pay for the procedures.

Surgery

Surgery may be used to correct blocked fallopian tubes, for artificial insemination, for egg retrieval, and for in vitro fertilization (IVF). If ovulation is not occurring, then treatment is ovulation induction. If ovulation induction does not work, then options include artificial insemination, or directly introducing sperm into the cervix, uterus, or fallopian tubes. The sperm used may be the woman's partner's sperm, referred to as artificial insemination husband (AIH) or donor sperm, referred to as artificial insemination donor (AID).

IVF involves inducing ovulation, removing the eggs, fertilizing them and then implanting the fertilized eggs inside the uterus. Zygote intrafallopian transfer (ZIFT) involves the same steps as IVF, but the fertilized eggs are transferred into

---

TABLE 62-3 **Medications Used in the Treatment of Infertility**

DRUG	INDICATION	SIDE EFFECTS
Ovulation Inducer		
Clomid; Milophene; Serophene	Induction of ovulation in conditions of anovulation	Vasomotor symptoms; lower abdominal tenderness; nausea; headache; ovarian cysts
Gonadotropins		
Gonal-F; Bravelle Follistim; Profasi; Pergonal; Choron; Ovidrel; etc.	Induction of ovulation in PCOS or hypothalamic dysfunction	Ovarian hyperstimulation; increased risk of multiple gestation
Dopamine Agonists		
Parlodel; Permax; Dostinex	Ovulation induction in women with hyperprolactinemia	Hypotension; nausea

Note: Metformin is also used in infertility treatment associated with PCOS.
Adapted from Broyles, B., Reiss, B., & Evans, M. (2007). Pharmacological aspects of nursing care (7th ed.). New York: Thomson Delmar Learning.

the fallopian tube instead of into the uterus. Gamete intrafallopian transfer (GIFT) involves induction of ovulation, harvesting the eggs, mixing the eggs with sperm, and implanting the egg-sperm combination in the fallopian tube for fertilization to occur within the tube.

Women may have complications from surgical procedures, such as infection or hemorrhage. The process of evaluation and treatment for infertility can be a significant stressor for the couple and can lead to relationship difficulties and psychological trauma.

Alternative Therapy

Yoga has been described as an adjunctive therapy to help with relaxation, making decisions, and feeling positive about treatment choices. Multivitamin supplements and acupuncture have been suggested to increase fertility.

Patient and Family Teaching

There is much helpful teaching that can maximize couples' chances of conceiving. Women should be taught how to predict their ovulation and time intercourse for maximum success. Women and their partners should be counseled to stop smoking cigarettes and marijuana, drinking alcohol, and using other illicit substances. The partner should be encouraged to wear boxer shorts because tighter, restrictive underwear reduces sperm counts. Women should be given clear guidance on when to present for an evaluation, based on their age, history, and likelihood of conceiving.

Evaluation of Outcome

Potential patient outcomes for each of the example nursing diagnoses for the patient with infertility are:

* Anxiety related to inability to conceive. The patient should be able to recognize the signs of anxiety, demonstrate positive coping mechanisms, and describe a reduction in the level of anxiety experienced.
* Altered body image related to inability to fulfill role as woman. The patient demonstrates enhanced body image and self-esteem as evidenced by ability to look at, touch, talk about, and care for actual or perceived altered body part or function.
* Deficient knowledge related to infertility. The patient should demonstrate motivation to learn, identify perceived learning needs, and verbalize an understanding of desired content.

SEXUAL DYSFUNCTION

Sexual dysfunction is any disorder of the female sexual system, including dysfunctions of desire, arousal, orgasm, or pain. By definition, sexual dysfunction results in personal distress and has an effect on interpersonal relationships. Risk factors associated with sexual dysfunction are emotional problems or difficulties coping with stress, deterioration in economic standing, history of sexual trauma, and lower educational levels. Fatigue and emotional exhaustion can contribute to sexual dysfunction.

Sexual dysfunction may occur in up to 35 percent of U.S. women (Walton & Thorton, 2003). Lack of libido is the most common reported symptom. In postmenopausal women, decreased lubrication, decreased arousal, difficulty achieving orgasm, and pain with intercourse are commonly reported. Frequency of sexual activity and desire for sexual activity both decrease in the menopausal years and may relate to the increase in dyspareunia.

A lack of sexual desire (sexual arousal disorder) is the persistent or recurrent deficiency of sexual desire sufficient to maintain sexual excitement that causes personal distress. Depression is often associated with lack of libido. The lack of sexual desire should first be treated by correcting psychological, relationship, and situational issues, such as mental or physical exhaustion. A healthy lifestyle with exercise and rest may help correct a lack of desire, but the woman may need to be referred for professional counseling.

Disorders of sexual arousal can result from a lack of vaginal lubrication, poor genital vascularity, or neurological conditions. Sexual arousal disorders may be caused by physical factors, such as insufficient foreplay, lack of vaginal lubrication, lack of vaginal muscle relaxation, decreased sensitivity of external genitalia, pelvic trauma, medication use, or postsurgical changes. Sexual arousal disorders may also be caused by psychological factors, such as emotional distraction or inability to relax.

An orgasmic disorder is the persistent or recurrent difficulty in obtaining orgasm. Orgasmic disorders are associated with communication difficulties with the partner, negative attitudes toward masturbation, and greater sexual guilt. Women who have never achieved orgasm (**primary anorgasmia**) may need referral to a sex therapist. **Secondary anorgasmia** (loss of the ability to achieve orgasm in a woman who was previously orgasmic) may result from depression or medications used to treat depression. Changing from SSRIs to bupropion may provide relief. Pelvic floor rehabilitation can be used to correct secondary anorgasmia caused by surgery or menopause.

Pain disorders include dyspareunia, vaginismus, vulvar vestibulitis syndrome, and nonsexual pain. Dyspareunia is recurrent or persistent genital pain associated with sex. Dyspareunia can be caused by endometriosis, vulvar vestibulitis syndrome, interstitial cystitis, atrophy of genital tissues, infection, or adhesions. Smoking may decrease blood flow to the vagina and make atherosclerotic changes in the pelvic blood vessels worse and should be discouraged. Women with pain disorders may have suffered sexual trauma in the past.

Vaginismus is the recurrent or persistent involuntary spasm of the muscles at the entrance of the vagina, interfering with penetration and causing pain and personal distress. Vulvar vestibulitis syndrome (VVS) is characterized by pain on insertion of the penis into the vagina, redness at the vaginal entrance, and tenderness when pressure is exerted within the vaginal vestibule. VVS is one of the most common causes of dyspareunia for women of childbearing age. There is no specific etiology for VVS. A careful history and physical must be done if VVS is suspected. Any vaginal infection must be diagnosed and treated, particularly if chronic candida infection is present (Graxiottin & Brotto, 2004).

Assessment with Clinical Manifestations

History taking from a woman with sexual dysfunction should use gender inclusive terminology so that heterosexuality is not assumed. The interview should be private—this may be an issue in the hospital setting—and confidentiality must be ensured (Figure 62-5). Assessment includes a complete history to include the timing of the symptoms and their history; the presence of any chronic illness; injuries; surgical and psychiatric history; the relationship dynamics and the level of partner support; as well as any medications, alcohol use, recreational drug use or therapies that may interfere with sexual activity. A complete history and a physical need to be done for women with pain disorders. Pain may be associated with endometriosis, pelvic adhesions, interstitial cystitis, or postmenopausal atrophic vaginitis. A medication history is important. The partner's sexual functioning must also be assessed.

Diagnostic Tests

Inspection of external genitalia is performed, and areas of tenderness are assessed. Vaginal atrophy is assessed with a speculum exam. The presence of vaginismus is evaluated by examination with a finger. The presence of pain should be evaluated. If possible, the pain should be reproduced. Muscle tone

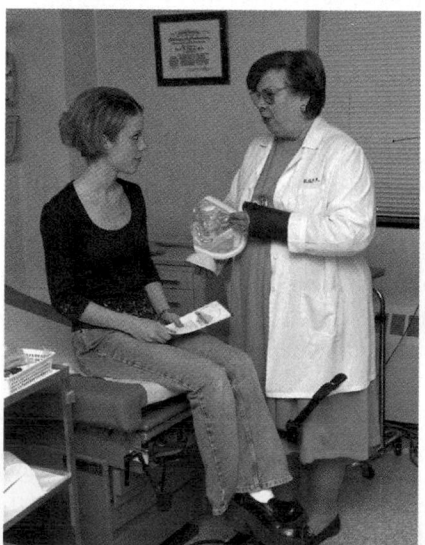

Figure 62-5 Nurses play an important role in helping patients understand their sexual health and development.

and strength are evaluated during the pelvic examination. If vaginal atrophy or thyroid disorders are suspected, lab work for estrogen levels and thyroid hormone profiles need to be drawn. Testosterone levels are often drawn before testosterone supplementation is considered.

Nursing Diagnoses

Based on the information gathered, examples of nursing diagnoses in the patient with sexual dysfunction may include the following:

- Sexual dysfunction related to a specific etiology.
- Risk for situational low self-esteem related to sexual difficulties.
- Chronic pain related to vulvar vestibulitis.

Planning and Implementation

Care of the patient with sexual dysfunction includes education, support, therapeutic interventions, and prevention measures. The woman with sexual dysfunction should have a gynecological examination by a health care provider with experience in sexual dysfunction. Psychological counselors and sex therapists are often involved in developing the management plan. Physical therapists may be involved in pelvic physical therapy including biofeedback and strength, relaxation, and exercise training. Gynecologists may evaluate and treat some aspects of sexual dysfunction, and urologists may need to be consulted to correct interstitial cystitis or urethral disorders. The nursing role in sexual dysfunction includes patient support, education, and referral, as indicated.

Women with chronic illnesses or surgery may have sexual dysfunction. Postoperative pain from surgery to correct incontinence or prolapse may be associated with dyspareunia. Women with endometriosis commonly have dyspareunia. Lack of sexual desire can be a consequence of medical conditions or psychological or emotional disorders. Neurological conditions can cause a disorder of sexual arousal or the inability to achieve orgasm. Lack of sexual arousal can be the result of medical or surgical treatment, pelvic floor disorders, or a lack of ability to relax the pelvic floor muscles.

The inability to achieve orgasm may be caused by nerve injury from pelvic surgery or spinal cord injury. The use of beta-adrenergic blockers, central nervous system (CNS) depressants, anticholinergics, or antidepressants can have sexual side effects. Depression is often associated with decreased libido. Vascular effects related to sexual arousal are noted in women with hypertension, smoking, high cholesterol levels, and cardiac disease. Women with arthrosclerosis may have decreased pelvic blood flow and decreased lubrication and clitoral engorgement. Cardiovascular disease may indirectly interfere with sexual activity due to dyspnea. Impaired pelvic floor muscles from episiotomy or significant lacerations with poor healing may contribute to muscular dysfunction leading to vaginismus and sexual pain disorder.

If sexual dysfunctions are not treated, disorders may become progressive, multifaceted, and difficult to treat. Relationships and self-esteem may suffer. Sexual pain syndromes can become chronic pain syndromes that are difficult to treat.

Pharmacology

Postmenopausal women may have relief of atrophic changes with estrogen therapy. Estrogen can be administered with creams, tablets, or a vaginal ring. Women with bilateral oophorectomy and postmenopausal women may benefit from testosterone therapy. Tricyclic antidepressants, such as amitriptyline, and the anticonvulsant gabapentin have also been used to treat VVS (Graxiottin & Brotto, 2004). A common dosage schedule for amitriptyline is 10 to 25 mg orally, with the dose increased, up to three times a day if necessary. Table 62-4 displays the drugs used to treat sexual dysfunction.

TABLE 62-4	**Medications Used to Treat Sexual Dysfunction**	
DRUG	**INDICATION**	**SIDE EFFECTS**
Androgens		
Delatestryl; Depo-Testosterone; Testopel; Testim; AndroGel; Danazol	Increase sexual desire, arousal, activity, and orgasm frequency	Acne; hirsutism; voice deepening; clitoromegaly; lipoprotein alterations
Impotence Agents		
Viagra	Treatment of orgasmic disorders or sexual dysfunction	Potentiates nitrates; headache

Note: Oral and topical estrogen therapy is used to treat atrophy of vaginal tissues. Adapted from Broyles, B., Reiss, B., & Evans, M. (2007). Pharmacological aspects of nursing care (7th ed.). New York: Thomson Delmar Learning.

Population-Based Care

Hispanic (American) women have less incidence of sexual dysfunction. Caucasian women have a slightly higher incidence of pain disorders, and almost twice as many African American women have a lack of sexual desire when compared to Caucasian women.

Alternative Therapy

The clitoral therapy device is an FDA approved therapy to treat sexual arousal disorder. It is a battery-powered vacuum device that enhances clitoral blood flow and clitoral enlargement, improving sexual arousal. Several herbal formulations are marketed to promote libido and sexual arousal. Sentia contains epimedium, damiana leaf, dodder seed, black cohosh, isoflavones, valeriana root, ginger root, gingko biloba, bayberry fruit, licorice root, capsicum pepper, and red raspberry leaf. Avlimil contains sage leaf, red raspberry leaf, kudzu root extract, red clover, capsicum pepper, licorice root, bayberry fruit, damiana leaf, valeriana root, ginger root, and black cohosh.

Treatment of sexual disorders may include behavior modification. Exercise improves body image, decreases depression, increases libido, and increases testosterone levels. Strength training exercise may benefit postmenopausal women who have decreased desire. Pelvic floor rehabilitation includes Kegel's exercises, vaginal weights, biofeedback, or pelvic floor physical therapy. Cognitive behavioral therapy, Kegel's exercises, relaxation, and biofeedback have been used for VVS.

Women with vaginismus may benefit from pelvic-floor physical therapy and psychological counseling. Muscle relaxation and progressive vaginal dilation may be used to treat vaginismus. Muscle relaxation, is taught by having the patient isolate and concentrate on the musculature during an examination, and practice contracting and relaxing the vaginal muscles. Dilators are available commercially or tampons of increasing diameter can be used. The dilators or tampons are placed in the vagina for 15 minutes twice a day by the patient to facilitate muscle relaxation and dilation. Reactive muscle tension of the pelvic floor may be treated by teaching relaxation, use of lubricants, self-stretching with dilators, Kegel's exercises, and massage. Physical therapy with relaxation and biofeedback may also be effective. Pain may be treated with surface electroanalgesia, local injection of interferon, topical anesthetics, SSRIs, or oral analgesia. Couples' sex therapy and cognitive behavioral therapy has also been used to treat VVS.

Patient and Family Teaching

Patients should be taught to recognize signs of sexual dysfunction and be made aware that treatment is available. It is important to assist patients to recognize the goals of therapy. Explanations of how treatments such as physical therapy may help correct sexual dysfunction are also important.

Evaluation of Outcomes

Potential patient outcomes for each of the example nursing diagnoses for the patient with sexual dysfunction are:

- Sexual dysfunction related to a specific etiology. The patient will verbalize satisfaction with the way they express physical intimacy.
- Risk for situational low self-esteem related to sexual difficulties. The patient demonstrates enhanced body image and self-esteem as evidenced by ability to look at, touch, talk about, and care for actual or perceived altered body part or function.
- Chronic pain related to vulvar vestibulitis. The patient should verbalize an adequate relief of pain along with the ability to realistically cope with the pain if it is not completely relieved.

Case Study

Nursing Care Plan

Tim and Karen, both 61 years old, have been married for 32 years. For the past several years Karen has suffered from increasingly painful osteoarthritis. She is in the hospital after receiving a right knee replacement. As you are reviewing her discharge plans, Tim comments that now he hopes they can be intimate again. When you ask for clarification, Karen blushes and states that she avoids sex, because it is so painful for her.

Assessment

A married couple who are having difficulty in their sexual activities for a variety of reasons. They do not communicate well and are not open in their expressions regarding their sexual activities. In addition, the wife has osteoarthritis that causes her to have pain and consequently this interrupts her outlook on sexual behaviors.

Nursing Diagnosis 1: Ineffective sexual patterns related to painful and swollen joints

NOC: Risk of Ineffective role performance; Situational low self-esteem; Sexual dysfunction

NIC: Sexual counseling

Expected Outcomes

The patient will:
1. Verbalize a sexually satisfying relationship with spouse by second counseling appointment.
2. Acknowledge strategies to decrease pain by end of first counseling appointment.

Case Study

Planning, Interventions, Rationales

1. Explore with patient current methods used to enhance sexual function, including open communication. *Increases knowledge level.*
2. Encourage patient to take a hot bath or shower prior to sexual activity. *Potentially increases libido.*
3. Apply anti-inflammatory creams over joints prior to sexual activity. *Decreases pain during sexual activities and increases satisfaction during sexual intercourse.*
4. Explores alternative positions for sexual activity. *Decreases the amount of strain on arthritic joints.*
5. Explore the best time of day for sexual activity. *Pain may be lowest in the morning or after gentle physical activity.*

Evaluation

After two months, Tim and Karen both verbalize satisfaction with sexual function. Morning is the best time for Karen to participate in sexual intercourse, after taking ibuprofen followed by a hot shower and gentle range of motion exercises. The couple is most satisfied with a side-lying position for sex. They have also incorporated more massage and touch in sexual activity, lengthening the amount of foreplay and leading to more satisfactory sexual activity for both Tim and Karen. Both also acknowledge that improved communication has lead to less misunderstandings and frustrations.

KEY CONCEPTS

- The female reproductive system is complicated both in terms of anatomical structures and hormonal regulation.
- Pregnancy must always be the first consideration in women with the complaint of amenorrhea or dysfunctional bleeding.
- Women with endometriosis commonly experience a delay in diagnosis and this increases the emotional distress associated with the disease.
- The hallmark of PMS/PMDD is a symptom-free period with every cycle shortly after the menstrual cycle begins.
- Routine douching for hygiene purposes increases the risk for vaginal infection and should be discouraged.
- Antiviral therapy can be used to both treat HSV outbreaks and to help prevent outbreaks.
- Uterine fibroids are the most common solid pelvic tumor in women and the most common reason for hysterectomy.
- Some structural abnormalities of the reproductive tract have implications for childbearing.
- Pessaries are a nonsurgical option used in treating pelvic relaxation disorders.

- FGM is commonly associated with urinary complications.
- Cervical cancer rates have dramatically decreased because of routine Pap smear screening.
- The breast cancer genes (BRCA1 and BRCA2) are associated with the development of ovarian cancer.
- Most reproductive cancers in the early stages are treated surgically.
- Surgeries for reproductive tract cancers are associated with significant psychological, sexual, and body image issues.
- The top three reasons for infertility are male factors, anovulation, and tubal damage or obstruction.
- Anovulation caused by PCOS can often be corrected with the use of metformin and clomiphene citrate.
- Loss of libido is the most common sexual dysfunction.
- Diagnosis and treatment of sexual dysfunction is important to prevent complications and progression of the disorders.
- Amitriptyline is a useful treatment for VVS.
- Physical therapy can be a useful treatment for some sexual dysfunctions.

REVIEW QUESTIONS

1. A patient complains of dysmenorrhea. Which of the following are nonprescription relief measures you can suggest that she try?
   1. Heat, exercise, NSAIDs, and oral contraceptives
   2. Oral contraceptives, vitamin E, and COX-2 inhibitor
   3. Aspirin, soy supplements, and NSAIDs
   4. Heat, exercise, and NSAIDs

2. A 30-year-old patient has severe dysmenorrhea that suddenly started two cycles ago. Which of the following might be an explanation for this?
   1. Ovarian cancer
   2. Imperforate hymen
   3. Fibroids
   4. Late-onset menarche

3. What of the following is not a long-term health implication for a woman diagnosed with PCOS?
   1. Cervical cancer
   2. Hyperlipidemia
   3. Insulin resistance and diabetes
   4. Infertility

4. What is the first priority for managing PCOS?
   1. Inducing ovulation with clomiphene citrate
   2. Weight loss
   3. Checking cholesterol level
   4. Tracking menstrual cycles with a calendar

5. If a woman is experiencing menopausal symptoms and does not want to take hormone therapy, which intervention can you recommend that she try to reduce hot flashes?
   1. Dress in layers
   2. Reduce the environmental temperature
   3. Exercise
   4. Black cohosh supplements
   5. All of the above

6. What is the most common serious consequence of untreated chlamydia?
   1. Neonatal eye infection
   2. Arthritis
   3. Infertility related to tubal damage of PID
   4. Cervical cancer

7. Which of the following messages should be included in the patient teaching session for women who have been diagnosed with an STD?
   1. Condoms are not a perfect protection against STDs.
   2. Take all medication until it is gone.
   3. Sexual partners should be contacted and treated.
   4. Keep all follow-up appointments.
   5. All of the above

8. Most hysterectomies in the United States are performed for what indication?
   1. Cervical cancer
   2. Vaginal infections
   3. PCOS
   4. Fibroids

9. You are providing nursing care for a teenager who has just been diagnosed with a didelphic reproductive system. She asks you about the implications for pregnancy. Which of the following is the correct answer?
   1. Pregnancy is not possible, but adoption or surrogate pregnancy is an option.
   2. Pregnancy is possible, but there is a high risk of complications and the pregnancy will have to be closely monitored.
   3. Pregnancy is possible, but conception may take longer than usual.
   4. Pregnancy is not usually affected as long as there are two separate uteri, cervices, and vaginas that open to the outside.

10. A woman comes into the family practice office where you work. She has been trying to conceive for eleven months without success. What diagnostic testing might be included in the initial evaluation for this patient?
    1. BBT and semen analysis
    2. HSG and BBT
    3. Semen analysis and D & C
    4. Ultrasound and HSG

11. Cervical cancer is associated with what virus?
    1. HSV
    2. Coxsackie virus
    3. Rubella
    4. HPV

12. What accounts for the large decrease in cervical cancer seen in the last half of the 20th century?
    1. Increased hysterectomy rate
    2. Improved antibiotics
    3. Increased incidence of regular Pap smear screening
    4. Improved nutrition

13. Women with strong family histories of ovarian and breast cancer may need to be referred for genetics counseling. What role does genetics play in the development of ovarian cancer?
    1. The ovarian cancer gene has been isolated and is responsible for developing ovarian cancer.
    2. The breast cancer genes are associated with the development of ovarian cancer.

Continued

REVIEW QUESTIONS—cont'd

3. The gene that makes women susceptible to HPV infection increases the risk for developing ovarian cancer.
4. Ovarian cancer is inherited through the paternal cell line.

14. What is the most common reproductive cancer in women?
    1. Vaginal
    2. Vulvar
    3. Endometrial
    4. Ovarian

15. Which of the following is the most common complication of FGM?
    1. Urinary complications
    2. Infertility
    3. Delayed menopause
    4. Vulvar cancer

16. Which of the following is the most common sexual dysfunction?
    1. Vaginismus
    2. Anorgasmia
    3. Dyspareunia
    4. Decreased libido

REVIEW ACTIVITIES

1. Write a sample patient education sheet on PCOS.

2. Interview a patient who is going to have or has had a hysterectomy. About what issues is she most concerned?

3. Write sample nursing diagnoses and expected outcomes for a patient who has been diagnosed with PCOS.

4. Find out the incidence of cervical cancer for your local community or state. Can you suggest any improvements that could be made in local cervical cancer screening programs?

5. Interview five postmenopausal women. What are their attitudes about hormone therapy for menopausal symptoms?

Visit the Contemporary Medical-Surgical Nursing online companion resource at www.delmarhealthcare.com for additional content and study aids. Click on Online Companions then select the Nursing discipline.

Breast Alterations: Nursing Management

Ruth Grendell, MSN, RN

Marilyn Moorhouse, RN, MSN

CHAPTER TOPICS

- Anatomy and Physiology of the Breast
- Assessment and Diagnosis of Breast Problems of the Breast
- Breast Disorders
- Mammoplasty
- Breast Cancer

KEY TERMS

Atypia
Breast augmentation
Fibroadenomas
Galactorrhea
Gynecomastia
Intraductal papilloma
Lumpectomy
Mammary duct ectasia
Mammoplasty
Mastalgia
Mastitis
Mastodynia
Paget's mammary disease
Periductal mastitis
Supernumerary nipples

Although breast disease can occur in the male, such disease is primarily viewed as a female issue. Both the male and the female breast is commonly associated with physical beauty and perceived as a symbol of sexuality and sexual desire. The female breast is also viewed as a symbol of motherhood and nurturing. Most societies place considerable significance on the cosmetic appearance of the breast, making it difficult to separate the social aspects from the physical aspects of breast disorders. Alterations of the breast can generate negative perceptions of body image, which in turn, can negatively impact the individual's feelings about self-worth. Therefore, addressing the social and psychological implications of breast alterations is essential. This chapter addresses the pathology, collaborative treatment, and nursing care of diseases and conditions that affect the breast.

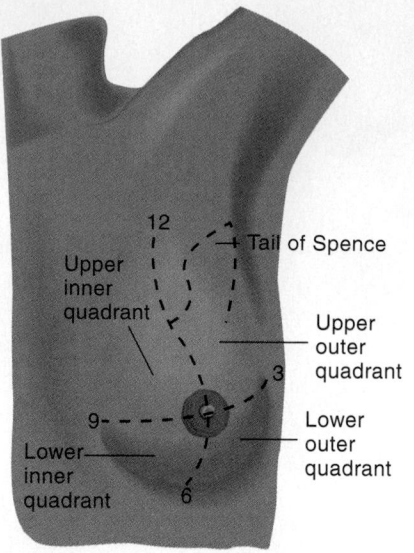

Figure 63-1 Quadrants of the left breast.

ANATOMY AND PHYSIOLOGY OF THE BREAST

The sole physiological function of the female breast, or mammary gland, is to secrete milk for nourishment of an infant. This function is directed and mediated by the same hormones that regulate the reproductive system, and the breast is considered an accessory organ of that system. Each breast is composed of a mound of glandular, adipose, and fibrous tissue located between the third and seventh ribs of the anterior chest wall. For ease in locating structures or areas of the breast, it is conceptually divided into four quadrants. Figure 63-1 shows the quadrants of the left breast. The quadrants of the right breast are a mirror image of those of the left breast.

The breasts are supported by the pectoralis major muscles shown in Figure 63-2 and by fibrous bands called Cooper's ligaments. The ligaments are suspensory ligaments that extend in a radial fashion from the outer boundaries of the breast to the nipple area, similar in configuration to the spokes of a wheel. The ligaments divide the breast into 15 to 20 breast lobes of lactiferous (milk-carrying) ducts and help to shape the breast. The ligaments are attached to the deep layer of the subcutaneous fascia of the dermis. The skin of the breast is attached to the superficial connective and glandular tissues. This is an important contributing factor to visualizing the movement of the skin over the breast during self-examination.

Each woman's breasts are shaped differently. Individual breast appearance is influenced by the volume of a woman's breast tissue and fat, her age, her history of pregnancies and lactation, her heredity, the quality and elasticity of her breast skin, and the influence of hormones. Normal anatomy on a mammogram will image differently depending on a woman's weight, age, and the presence of surgical scars or implants, as well as the amount of fatty tissue in her breasts. The Cooper's ligaments also affect the image of the glandular tissue seen on the mammogram (Daniels, 2003). Because the breast is made up

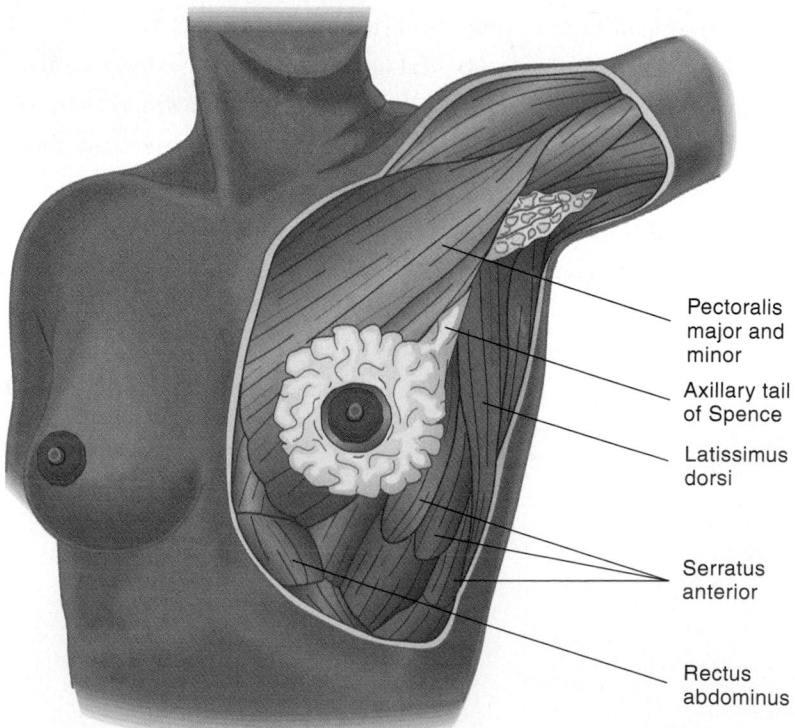

Figure 63-2 Muscles supporting the breast.

of tissues with different textures, it may not have a smooth surface and often feels lumpy. This irregularity is especially noticeable when a woman is thin and has little breast fat to soften the contours; it becomes less obvious after menopause when the cyclic changes and endocrine stimulation of the breast have ceased and the glandular tissue.

Breast Alterations during Maturational Phases

Breasts undergo significant changes during specific maturational phases of a person's life. Initially, there are changes in the breast that correlate with the onset of hormonal influences. Later, various changes in the way breast tissue develops may occur related to pregnancy, lactation, and during menopause. The growth and development stages of the human body and the changes in breast tissue are detailed in the following section.

Effects of Hormones on Breast Tissue

The breast is responsive to a complex interplay of hormones that cause the breast tissue to develop, enlarge, and produce milk. The three major hormones affecting the breast are estrogen, progesterone, and prolactin. These hormones cause glandular tissue in both the breast and the uterus to change during a woman's menstrual cycle. Because of reduced hormonal levels, the breasts are less full for one to two weeks after menstrual flow. Therefore, it may be easier to detect breast lumps during this time. Reduction of hormonal levels is also responsible for the breast's return to its prepregnant state after breastfeeding is concluded.

Changes at Birth

Both female and male infants are born with rudimentary breast tissue that has ducts lined with epithelium. An inspection should reveal a symmetrical location of the nipples in the mid-clavicular line at the fourth to sixth ribs of the anterior chest. Infrequently, small dark spots on the chest may indicate undeveloped nipples and areola called **supernumerary nipples** that can be mistaken for moles. The presence of the extra nipples may be associated with congenital renal or cardiac anomalies (Littleton & Engebretson, 2002).

Changes at Puberty and Adolescence

The release of follicle-stimulating hormone (FSH), luteinizing hormone (LH), and prolactin from the pituitary gland in females at puberty stimulates the release of estrogen from the ovaries. The estrogen stimulates the growth of the ductile system in the breasts. At the onset of the ovulation cycles progesterone is released stimulating the growth of the ductile system and the secretory epithelium of the alveoli. Breast development is the first pubertal change for females. The female breast assumes the characteristic contour by the time of adolescence. Feelings of fullness and discomfort in the breasts are common during the menstrual cycle.

Changes during Pregnancy

Changes in the breast during pregnancy are significant because of the increased levels of estrogen and progesterone. The alveolar epithelium and the ductile system are being prepared for the lactation process. The cellular changes that occur are considered to be beneficial in altering the susceptibility to estrogen-influenced changes in later life.

Prolactin, a hormone secreted by the anterior pituitary gland stimulates the secretion of milk by the alveolar cells. The release of oxytocin from the posterior pituitary gland influences the ejection of the milk from the alveolar cells to the ductile system. Suckling by the infant further stimulates ejection of the milk by providing feedback to the hypothalamus and on to the posterior pituitary.

Leakage of milk often occurs during the later stages of pregnancy. Following the termination of breastfeeding, a woman may have milk leakage for a period of three months to a year until the hormones return to the nonlactating level. Leakage can also occur from overzealous stimulation of the breast even when the woman is not pregnant.

Changes with Menopause

The levels of estrogen and progesterone are gradually reduced at the onset of menopause. The breasts lose glandular tissue; the lobular-alveolar structures atrophy; adipose tissue, connective tissue, and the ducts remain. The breasts decrease in mass and become pendulous. Estrogen supplements after menopause can cause continued lumpiness. As discussed previously, the breast glands drain into a collecting system of ducts that go to the base of the nipple. The ducts then extend through the nipple and open on its outer surface. In addition to serving as a channel for milk, these ducts are often the source of breast problems. Experts now believe that most breast cancer begins in the lining of the ducts and sometimes the milk glands. Benign fibrocystic changes also originate from these ducts.

Gynecomastia in Males

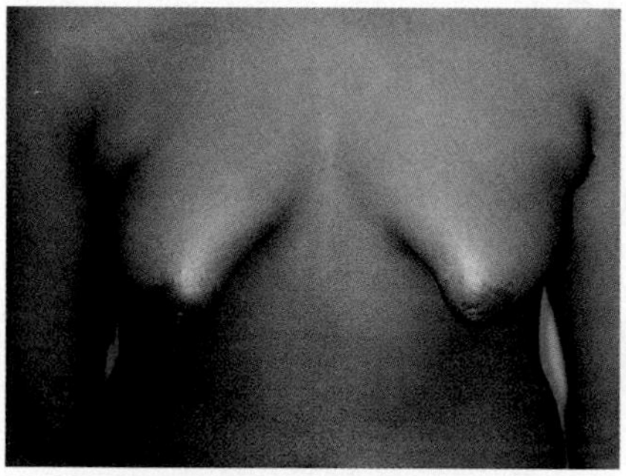

Figure 63-3 Gynecomastia. *Courtesy of Steven M. Lynch, M.D.*

Gynecomastia, a Greek word meaning woman-like breasts, is used to describe the enlargement of male breast tissue shown in Figure 63-3. Although gynecomastia in men is not often talked about, it can occur in 40 to 60 percent of all males. Gynecomastia may be transitory at birth, arise at puberty, and then gradually subside, or it may occur later in life. There may be multiple causes. For instance, digoxin is weakly estrogenic and can cause gynecomastia in some men. Spironolactone, a diuretic, can also cause gynecomastia. Breast development in the male is frequently caused by a shift in the estrogen/androgen ratio because of increased circulating estrogens or decreased circulating androgens. Pseudo-gynecomastia is the enlargement of the male breast because of an increase in fatty tissue. Gynecomastia can result in feelings of embarrassment or feelings of increased self-consciousness in individuals who are affected. Plastic surgery to reduce the glandular tissue or breast fat is an option.

ASSESSMENT AND DIAGNOSIS OF BREAST PROBLEMS

Nurses are instrumental in the education and assessment of women and men with breast disorders. Nurses are also pivotal sources of education and assessment of all individuals for prevention of cancer. Understanding the normal physiology of the breast and the steps in the examination process is essential to providing care for this population.

Examination of the Breast

Examination of the breast is performed in both the upright and supine positions. The examination involves bilateral inspection and palpation of the breasts, areola, axillary, and supraclavicular areas. Adequate lighting is needed for optimal examination, with the woman standing or sitting with hands on hips and disrobed to the waist. Visual inspection focuses on the contour and symmetry of the breasts; skin changes, such as scaling, puckering, dimpling, or scars; the position of nipples; nipple discharge or retraction; and presence or absence of masses.

Variations between breasts are not uncommon, but the breasts should be fairly symmetrical. Findings should include the surface contours of both breasts being round and the skin being smooth, with uniform and matching skin tone. The areola can range from pink to dark brown depending on

BSE

The nurse needs to teach BSE using clear and understandable methods and terminology. The following is one example:

1. First the patient must be advised that BSE should be performed once a month, eight days following menses or on any given fixed date. Advise the patient to avoid the time when her breasts might be tender because menstruation or ovulation. Encourage her to put the BSE on her calendar and include her significant other in the process.

2. Think "B" (bed): Show the patient how to palpate her breast while supine in bed using the palmar surfaces of her fingers. She should start by placing her right arm over her head and palpating the right breast with the left hand, moving in concentric circles from the periphery inward and including the periphery, tail of Spence, and areola. Finally, instruct the patient to squeeze the nipple to examine for discharge. Using the reverse procedure, the woman should examine the other breast.

3. Think "S" (standing): Instruct the patient to repeat the above palpation method while standing.

4. Think "E" (examination before a mirror): The patient should stand in front of a mirror and examine her breasts for symmetry, retractions, dimpling, inverted nipples, or nipple deviation with her arms at her sides, then with her arms raised over head, and finally, with her hands pressed into her hips.

hormonal factors and normal skin tone. Vascular patterns should be diffuse and symmetrical. Pregnant, obese, or fair-skinned individuals may have hypervascular patterns on examination. Unilateral or focal patterns are considered abnormal and are generally produced by dilated superficial veins that may occur in malignant conditions because of increased blood flow to the area (Estes, 2006).

The areola and nipples are inspected for shape and size. Both areolae and nipples are generally equal in size. Montgomery tubercles may be irregularly spaced around the areola. Nipples should be soft and smooth and usually point in the same direction. If the nipples have been inverted since puberty, it is considered normal. If, however, nipple inversion is a new change, investigation must take place.

Dimpling, a sign of possible underlying tumor, can be detected by asking the woman to slowly raise both arms over her head. The tension created in the breast by contracting the pectoral muscle makes any dimpling evident. Retraction can be assessed with the woman sitting with both hands at waist level with her palms pressed together. For large breasts, have the woman lean forward while standing. This allows the nurse to watch the movement of the breasts to assess that there is no fixation of the breasts to the chest wall.

Palpation of the breasts begins with the lymph nodes. The axillary, subclavicular, and supraclavicular lymph nodes are palpated for firmness and for lumps. While the patient is encouraged to relax the muscles in the arm, the provider palpates the axilla for enlarged nodes. The palpation then progresses down along the chest wall, the anterior border of the axilla, along the posterior border of the axilla, and along the inner aspect of the upper arm.

The supraclavicular nodes are palpated with the woman sitting with the neck flexed slightly forward and turned slightly to the side. The primary purpose of palpation is to discover masses. The examination needs to be completed in a systematic manner. Developing a specific system used for each patient is necessary to ensure all areas of the breast are palpated. The upper outer quadrant of the breast to the axilla (tail of Spence) is an area that needs to be evaluated well. The greatest proportion of malignancies is found in this area of the breast. The breast examination should be completed with the woman in the sitting and supine positions with the provider using the pads of the fingers to palpate. This is done first with the patient sitting with arms down at the sides and then with the patient in the supine position with the arm of the side being examined raised over the head. If a mass is felt, the mass should be identified by the location, size, shape, consistency, distance from the nipple, and quadrant. Nipple discharge is best assessed in the upright position. Collection of the liquid can be done by bringing a slide in contact with the fluid.

The last portion of the breast examination is the patient demonstrating breast self-examination (BSE) as shown in Figure 63-4. This provides an opportunity for teaching, answering questions, and enforcing the importance of monthly self-examinations.

BREAST DISORDERS

The majority of breast disorders are benign. However, it is imperative that breast disorders are diagnosed accurately and treated early to have the most optimal outcome. The emotional distress that a potential breast disorder creates in the patient with breast alteration symptoms is significant. Even when the final diagnosis is of a benign nature, the period of waiting for confirmation can be a time of intense fear and anxiety. Unfortunately, some women delay seeking health care attention because of their fear of a dreaded diagnosis. The following discussion is related to several of the benign breast problems.

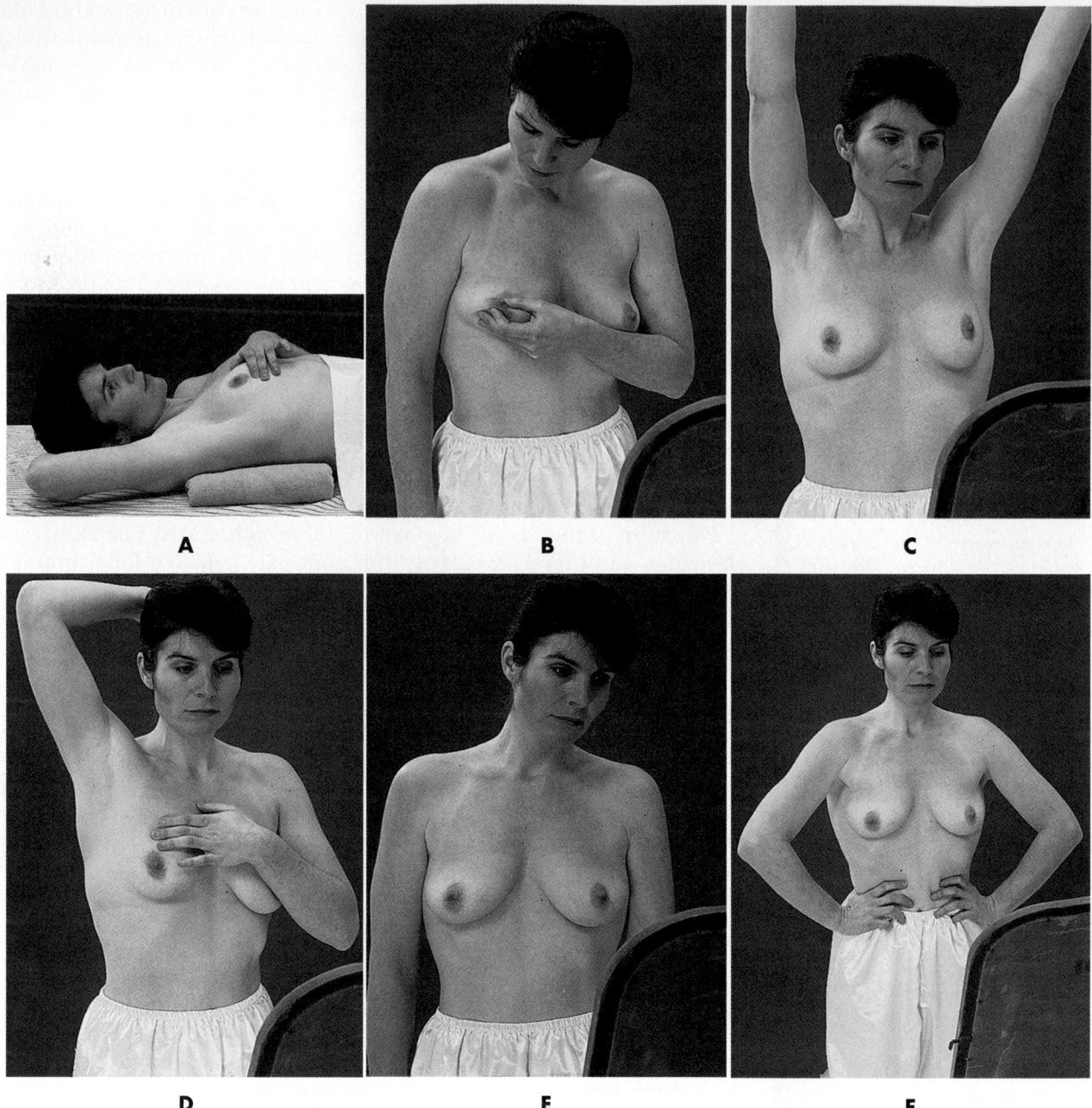

Figure 63-4 Breast Self-Examination (BSE).

Mastodynia and Mastalgia

Mastodynia and **mastalgia** are used synonymously to refer to breast pain, the most common breast complaint. However, pain is not generally associated with breast cancer. Women with cyclic premenstrual mastodynia also may have lumpy breasts about one week prior to the menses. Examination is performed to rule out any problems. A well-fitting supportive brassiere worn particularly during jogging and other vigorous exercise may be helpful. Decreasing the intake of coffee may also be beneficial.

Nipple Disorders

There are three primary pathological conditions of the nipple: (a) bleeding, (b) discharge, and (c) fissures. A bloody discharge is generally produced when there is an increase of pressure in the areola. Usually, bleeding in this manner

Skills 360°

Cultural Influences on Breast Examination

The women's health nurse practitioner is to conduct a well-woman examination on a 31-year-old new patient. The woman made this appointment at the insistence of her husband, who wants to begin a family. The woman has been in the United States four years and has never had a well-woman checkup. She comes from a culture that highly respects women's privacy and modesty. The female nurse practitioner spends 12 minutes explaining the examination and what the woman will experience. In addition, the equipment that will be used is shown to the patient. The patient has no questions, so the nurse leaves the room to let the patient undress in privacy. The nurse returns a few minutes later to find the woman wearing the paper gown. The nurse tells the patient that the breast examination will be performed first. The nurse inspects the woman's breasts. As soon as the nurse begins to palpate the breasts, the patient grabs the gown around herself, stands up, and states that she has had enough for the day.

The nurse practitioner suspects that the woman may be feeling offended, because the nurse practitioner touched her breasts. The nurse practitioner asks the woman whether she is feeling upset about having her breasts manually examined. In addition, the nurse practitioner expresses respect for the woman's cultural beliefs and empathy for the woman's feelings. The nurse practitioner encourages the woman to talk about her beliefs to better understand how the examination might be modified to be acceptable, drawing the woman out about whether doing the examination through a fabric or with another person from her own culture present might be an option. Through using a soft, caring tone of voice the nurse practitioner attempts to elicit suggestions for alternative approaches from the woman herself, without frightening her with admonitions about what she is risking if she refuses the breast examination.

Red Flag

Examining Nipple Discharge

If a woman is found to have abnormal nipple discharge:

1. Don gloves before proceeding with the assessment.
2. Note the following: color, odor, consistency, amount, whether it is unilateral or bilateral, whether it is spontaneous or provoked.
3. With a sterile, cotton-tipped swab, obtain a sample of the discharge so that a culture and sensitivity, as well as a gram stain can be obtained.
4. Consider checking the sample for occult blood.
5. Follow your institution's guidelines for sample preparation.

---

is because of a benign condition, but it may accompany malignancy. Bleeding can also occur from trauma to the breast that causes blood to be released through the nipple. Generally, if bleeding is noticed, women should be encouraged to seek their health care professional's consultation immediately to pursue diagnostics.

Discharge from the nipples, other than lactation, can be related to several possible causes. For example, cancer, pituitary adenoma, cystitis, and a variety of medications can cause fluid discharge from the nipples. Some discharge may be normal in many women, but following up on any discharge is the responsibility of the health care provider. The discharge will be examined to see if it is lactation products, sanguine discharge, or infectious products.

Fissures of the nipple are ulcers that most commonly develop in lactating women. In the presence of fissures, the patient should wash the breast and nipple area carefully with water, massage with lanolin, and expose to air to dry. If the fissure is too painful or bleeding occurs, the lactating woman may be advised to stop breastfeeding. Referral to a lactation specialist should be suggested.

Fibrocystic Changes

Fibrocystic change is the most frequently occurring pathological breast problem. The etiology of fibrocystic conditions is unknown, but there is some evidence that it is related to hormonal regulation. Typical changes include fluid-filled cysts that are round, soft or hard, and movable. The cysts may increase in size premenstrually. These changes are most common during the childbearing years but can also occur after menopause. Breast tenderness and pain may be present, but there should not be any nipple discharge. If nipple discharge is noted a health care provider should be contacted. For women with fibrocystic changes it is critically important to do monthly BSEs to be familiar with the breast tissue so that any change is noticed as soon as possible. Although this is often called a disease, it is classified as a condition. There is no specific treatment for fibrocystic breast changes. Aspiration of a cyst may be necessary depending on the symptoms it causes. A biopsy is performed if the cyst recurs after an aspiration procedure. Fibrocystic disease is considered to be a risk factor for breast cancer when there it is accompanied by cellular proliferation and **atypia** (deviation from the standard cell form). Regular examinations by a health care professional and regular mammograms are recommended in addition to BSEs (Estes, 2006).

Fibroadenoma

Fibroadenomas are benign, fibrous growths, or tumors, of the glandular epithelium in breast tissue. They usually occur in women between the ages of 15 and 30 years. These growths are generally solid, painless, rubbery masses that do not attach to any structures in the breast. The movability of the tumor is its most distinctive characteristic, and it can be diagnosed by cytology. The tumor may form a dense stroma (a collection of serosanguineous fluid). A fibroadenoma is usually removed surgically using a local anesthetic.

Galactorrhea

Galactorrhea is the secretion of a white, milk-like fluid in a nonlactating breast. This may be because of vigorous nipple stimulation; medications, such as exogenous hormones, blood pressure medications, or antidepressants; herbal preparations, including nettle, fennel, anise, fenugreek seed, and blessed thistle; street drugs, such as opiates and marijuana; internal hormonal imbalance; or local chest infection or trauma. Large amounts of prolactin hormone from a pituitary tumor may also be the cause. Galactorrhea is usually benign. A health care provider should be contacted for further assessment if the breast liquid is reddish or blood-tinged (serosanguineous).

Cyst

Cysts are fluid-filled sacs. The cause of a cyst is unknown, and the majority of cysts are not harmful. Cysts may cause pain and may disappear spontaneously. Surgical removal may be necessary if the cysts continue to be problematic and painful.

Abscess

An abscess of the breast is a collection of pus resulting from infection. Antibiotics are given and local comfort measures are used to relieve pain. In some cases, draining the cyst may be necessary.

Intraductal Papilloma

Intraductal papilloma is a small, benign tumor that grows within the terminal portion of a solitary milk duct of the breast. Papillomas occur in women mainly between the ages of 25 and 55, and the cause is unknown. Solitary intraductal papillomas are usually not precancerous. They are usually too small to palpate but often cause serosanguineous nipple discharge. In the presence of serosanguineous discharge, it is required that malignancy be ruled out. Surgical excision is the primary treatment.

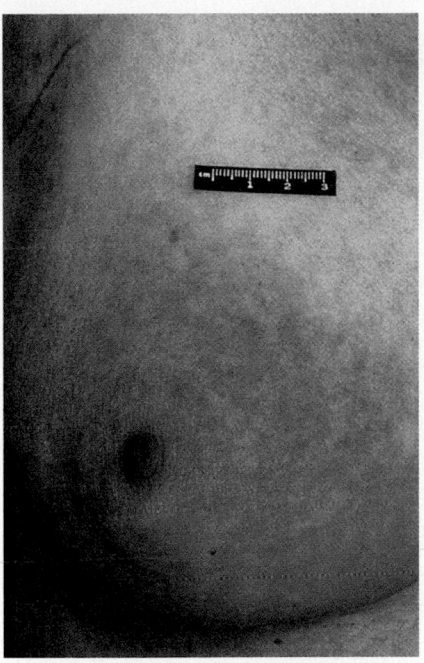

Figure 63-5 Inflamed breast with erythema.

Mastitis

Mastitis is inflammation of the breast. It can be caused from irritation, injury, or infection, and while it most commonly occurs within the first three months after childbirth, it can occur at any age. Mastitis can develop at any time so long as a woman is breastfeeding. Causes of mastitis during breastfeeding include bacterial or, occasionally, fungal infections, poorly fitting bras, and breastfeeding in only one position. The sentinel symptoms of mastitis include erythema (usually wedge-shaped redness with swelling), pain, and breast tissue that feels warm to touch accompanied by general malaise and fever. An inflamed breast with erythema is shown in Figure 63-5. Cracked nipples also commonly accompany mastitis. The treatment includes warm compresses, continued breastfeeding to completely empty the affected breast, antibiotics, pain medications, bed rest, increased fluid intake, and improved support. If an abscess forms, it may be necessary to drain the breast. Nursing care and education of the woman with mastitis is essential. Reassurance that the baby will not be affected by continued breastfeeding from the inflamed breast or from the medications being given can ease the concerns of the mother.

Periductal Mastitis

Periductal mastitis is an inflammation of the breast that can occur in nonlactating older women. Milk ducts near the nipple become inflamed and breast pain results. There may be other changes noted including a mass, dimpling, and nipple retraction. There is a great need to be followed by a health care provider. Treatment includes antibiotics and, in some cases, surgery. Thorough examination is recommended as breast cancers can present in this manner.

Inflammatory breast cancer can be confused with mastitis. This is a rapidly growing, aggressive, deadly cancer, and treatment needs to be initiated quickly. One differentiating symptom between mastitis and inflammatory breast cancer is fever. The woman with mastitis generally complains of a fever.

Mammary Duct Ectasia

Mammary duct ectasia is a noncancerous condition of the breast in which the milk ducts beneath the nipple become dilated and sometimes inflamed. It occurs most often in women during or after menopause. Causes may include smoking, hormonal changes, vitamin A deficiency, or inverted nipples. Symptoms include breast and nipple tenderness, dirty white or greenish nipple discharge, breast redness, and a lump. This condition may improve without treatment, but more often, antibiotics, warm compresses and excision of the affected ducts are needed.

Breast Tumor

A breast tumor that is precancerous or cancerous usually is evident as a white area on a mammogram even before it can be palpated. In cases where the tumor is cancerous, it may appear as a white area with radiating arms. A cancerous tumor may have no symptoms, or it may cause swelling, tenderness, and discharge from the nipple or indentation of the nipple called retraction. Nipple retraction is shown in Figure 63-6. There may be a dimpled appearance to the skin over the tumor. A breast biopsy is the choice to determine whether a lesion is cancerous.

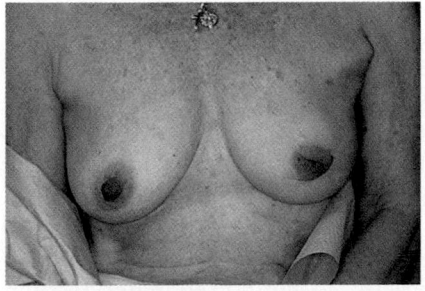

Figure 63-6 Nipple retraction of left breast.
Courtesy of Steven M. Lynch, M.D.

Paget's Mammary Disease

Paget's mammary disease is an uncommon skin cancer characterized by a chronic eczema-like rash of the nipple and adjacent areolar skin. It most commonly occurs between 50 and 60 years of age and is much more common in women than in men. Paget's mammary disease is associated with an underlying cancer, either in situ carcinoma of the breast or a more widespread infiltrating cancer, although this is sometimes difficult to detect on clinical examination or by mammogram.

Most patients go to their health care provider with the chief complaint of an itchy rash in the breast area. Additional symptoms may include nipple discharge that is often bloody, redness, scaling, inversion or ulceration, and swelling around the nipple. The diagnostic workup includes a skin biopsy to determine the presence or absence of Paget's cells. Mammography may also be helpful in assessing the patient for underlying breast cancer. Because Paget's disease is associated with underlying cancer the diagnostic workup must be extensive.

MAMMOPLASTY

Mammoplasty is a surgical procedure to increase or decrease the size or shape of the breast. It is usually considered an elective procedure. Generally speaking, there are two categories of mammoplasty: (a) breast augmentation and (b) breast reduction. Both of these interventions are discussed in the following section.

Breast Augmentation

Many women who seek **breast augmentation** (surgical enlargement of the breasts) are young individuals who are dissatisfied with the appearance of their breasts. However, mature women also choose to have breast revisions for various reasons. Health care providers need to be nonjudgmental toward the woman's desire to alter the appearance of her breasts as she strives to alter her body image. It is also important to be aware of the cultural values placed on the woman's breasts. The number of women seeking breast augmentation has increased steadily over the past 10 years. Breast augmentation is the most popular cosmetic procedure performed by plastic surgeons in the United States (American Cancer Society, 2004a). From a historical perspective, the American Society of Plastic Surgeons (2002) reported that 206,354 breast augmentation surgeries had been performed in 2001. This represents a 56 percent increase from 1998 and a 533 percent increase since 1992.

Many factors influence a woman's decision to seek breast augmentation. Included in the decision-making process is consideration of at least five factors: (a) intrapsychic or internal motivation that is affected by body image, feelings about physical appearance, female identity, focused dissatisfaction with breast appearance, and quality of life; (b) interpersonal reasons related to the importance of breasts in social or romantic situations; (c) available information about breast augmentation; (d) medical risks, including pain and complications; and (e) the out-of-pocket cost of cosmetic surgery.

Over the centuries women have attempted to create the look of a full bosom. This look was initially attempted through the modification of clothing as early as 3,000 B.C. Minoan women used primitive corsets and bras to enhance breast contour. With the exception of brief periods of time in the 15th and 20th centuries when the fashion was to attempt to deemphasize the size of the female breast, large breasts have been one of the standards that define beauty in society.

In the 18th century women underwent disfiguring and painful surgeries to enhance the breasts. These procedures were invasive and used materials such as rubber, glass, ivory, and metal as implants. Not only were these procedures unsuccessful in enhancing breast size, the procedures caused many medical problems for the women who underwent these surgeries. Interest in breast enlargement continued and other materials were used for injection in to the breasts. These included olive oil, paraffin, and petroleum jelly. Again, the outcomes were extremely negative, resulting in complications and terrible cosmetic results.

In 1992 silicone breast implants were banned because of concerns with potential leaking, physical symptoms, and nonspecific illnesses in women with such implants. Saline implants soon replaced the banned silicone implants. There has been an increasing number of women who have undergone breast augmentation surgery with saline implants. In 1999 the Institute of Medicine released the investigational results of silicone breast implants and concluded that there is no association between autoimmune disease or other health problems and silicone breast implants.

Investigators have become increasingly concerned regarding the ability to accurately screen and diagnosis women for breast cancer after they have undergone breast augmentation surgery. It has been suggested that women who have undergone breast augmentation are at higher risk for presenting with advanced disease. The studies have been limited by small sample sizes and have reported conflicting findings. A multicentered study found that the sensitivity level for screening women with breast augmentation was significantly lower than for those without augmentation. Another study found that sensitivity was significantly higher in women with augmentation than without and that there was no significant difference for asymptomatic women diagnosed with breast cancer with or without breast augmentation on the basis of tumor characteristics, i.e., stage, invasiveness of the disease, nodal status tumor size, or estrogen receptor status (Miglioretti, et. al., 2004). This study identified that breast augmentation does present difficulties with accurately diagnosing women with breast cancer on mammography. However, the study also suggests that women with breast augmentation are no more likely to be diagnosed with advanced disease than women without augmentation.

Breast augmentation techniques have improved over the past decade. The size of the incision has decreased and the materials used are less toxic to the patient. The use of saline-filled implants has decreased the potential for connective tissue or autoimmune diseases. However, saline implants still carry a risk for potential complications including infection, hematoma, and hypertrophic scarring. Such complications are estimated to occur in 1 to 3 percent of all surgeries. More frequent complications include mammographic interference; breastfeeding problems; decrease in, or loss of, nipple sensation; and capsular contracture. The occurrence rate for these issues is 10 to 35 percent of surgical cases. The latter complications may occur immediately after surgery or may take years to surface.

The current prostheses are safe, durable, and seamless silicone rubber casings filled with saline, dextran, or silicone. Soybean oil implants are sometimes used. This implant has an outer shell of silicone filled with highly refined soybean oil. (X-rays can easily penetrate the implant to allow for better visualization of the underlying breast tissues.) The prosthesis is placed beneath existing breast tissue or beneath the pectoralis muscle. The incision may be made under the breast or around the nipple. Mammography is performed prior to the surgery to rule out breast cancer in women older than 35 years of age or in younger women with a family history of cancer or with a suspicious lump. The surgery is usually performed under general anesthesia as an outpatient procedure, but the patient may stay overnight in the hospital. Drains are usually placed in the surgical wound to prevent hematoma formation. The drains are removed two to three days postoperatively if the drainage is normal.

Postoperative complications can occur including changes in sensation or the development of a hematoma, infection, or leakage from the prosthesis, but the complication that occurs in as many as 70 percent of cases is formation of fibrous sacs of collagen, or scar tissue, around the implant that contract and compress the breast into the shape of a hard, round ball. The breast becomes hard, immobile, painful, and distorted. This generally happens within the first six months after surgery and is beginning to be considered a natural outcome by researchers, rather than a complication. Breast massage may be prescribed to deter such scar tissue formation. The woman's temperature should be monitored, and sterile dressings changed as needed. The health care provider may instruct the woman to wear a supportive brassiere continuously for a few days.

Breast Reduction

Surgical breast reduction is performed to relieve the neck and shoulder pain that can lead to degenerative nerve changes because of overly large breasts. Large breasts can also interfere with daily activities, such as writing, typing, or driving a car, and it may be difficult to find appropriate clothing. Overly large breasts may be a source of embarrassment and affect the woman's self-esteem and self-image. Breast reduction can have psychological as well as physiological benefits. The reduction consists of removing wedges of tissue from the upper and lower quadrants of the breast. Excess skin is removed, and the nipple and areola are repositioned on the breast. The woman may be able to breastfeed if a large amount of tissue is not removed and the nipples remain connected during the surgery.

Nursing Diagnoses

Nursing diagnoses that may be appropriate for a woman with mammoplasty may include the following:
- Disturbed body image related to mammoplasty.
- Fear in response to diagnosis of breast cancer.
- Ineffective coping related to uncertainty and anxiety regarding surgical outcome and compromised ability to perform normal activities of daily living postoperatively.

Planning and Implementation

During the nursing assessment of the patient undergoing a breast-related diagnostic workup, problems that require management by other health care disciplines, such as medicine, physical therapy, nutrition, or pharmacy, may be discovered. The nurse is responsible for recognizing the need for collaboration across the health care team and for initiating team action. Nurses are able to bridge the issues and coordinate care, as well as monitor the response of the patient and inform the specific disciplines involved. The opportunity to case manage a patient, minimize complications, and promote the patient's safe passage along the health care continuum are important aspects of the collaborative process. The nursing care required for patients with breast diagnoses includes significant emphasis on social and psychological support. In addition to the need for emotional support, the opportunity for teaching and enhancing health management in relationship to breast health is paramount.

Evaluation of Outcomes

Potential patient outcomes for each of the example nursing diagnoses for the patient with mammoplasty are:
- Disturbed body image related to mammoplasty. The patient demonstrates enhanced body image and self-esteem as evidenced by ability to look at, touch, talk about, and care for actual or perceived altered body part or function.
- Fear in response to diagnosis of breast cancer. The patient should manifest positive coping behaviors and verbalize a reduction in the amount of fear of the having this disease.
- Ineffective coping related to uncertainty and anxiety regarding surgical outcome and compromised ability to perform normal activities of daily living postoperatively. The patient identifies her own maladaptive coping behaviors, available resources and support systems, describes and initiates alternative coping strategies, and describes positive results from new behaviors.

BREAST CANCER

It has only been within the last 20 years that breast cancer and treatment have been openly discussed. Well-known women have been sharing their personal experiences with breast cancer, treatment and the importance of early detection by discussing their stories with the media. This disease is no longer kept a secret as it was previously.

Epidemiology

Breast cancer is the most common type of cancer in women and is a major public health problem in the United States, with one in eight women expected to be diagnosed sometime during their lives. In 2004 the number of reported cases of invasive breast cancer in the United States was 217,440. This number includes only 1,450 men. In women, breast cancer is the most frequently diagnosed nonskin cancer. In addition to invasive breast cancer 59,390 cases of cancer in situ were documented in 2004. The increase in reporting and detection is directly related to the use of screening mammography and the ability to detect breast lesions before they can be palpated.

Breast cancer rates have continued to increase since the 1980s with some slowing in the 1990s. The increased incidence of breast cancer in women 50 years of age and older has persisted. Most breast abnormalities are benign, do not grow uncontrollably, and are not life-threatening. Careful evaluation must take place to ensure an accurate diagnosis.

Etiology

Although men are diagnosed with breast cancer, it remains a predominately female disease. Besides being female, age is the most important risk factor for breast cancer. Currently, a woman in the United States has a 13.2 percent, or one in eight, chance of developing breast cancer in her lifetime. The rate of breast cancer has gradually increased over the past 30 years, in part because of longer life expectancies and also that more women are diagnosed with breast cancer because of improved screening techniques.

A personal history of cancer has been shown to increase the risk of breast cancer. Women with a family history of breast cancer of a first-degree relative have an increased risk. The risk increases if more than one relative has a positive family history, and the risk also increases inversely to the age of that relative at the time of diagnosis. It is estimated that 5 to 10 percent of breast cancer cases result from inherited mutations or alterations in the breast cancer susceptibility genes, BRAC1 and BRAC2. These mutations are found in less than 1 percent of the population. Some women who know they carry one of the genes use the information to decide whether to use medication (e.g., tamoxifen) prophylactically. It is impossible to predict if or when these women may be diagnosed with breast cancer, and it is uncertain as to whether genetic predisposition and other factors combine to increase an individual's risk.

Risk factors related to diet, exercise, alcohol consumption, or immune system issues are thought to make a difference in the risk of contracting breast cancer. Environment is also being studied as a source of risk for the development of breast cancer. Some pesticides have chemical similarities to estrogen and may actually attach to receptor sites in the same manner as estrogen.

Caucasian women continue to have the highest breast cancer rates. However, African American women have later diagnostic testing and poorer responses to treatment. This population often enters treatment at later stages of the disease, thus negatively influencing the outcomes and life expectancy of those diagnosed and treated.

Hormones are thought to increase breast cancer risk by affecting cell proliferation, damaging deoxyribonucleic acid (DNA) and promoting cancer cell growth. Early menarche (younger than 12 years of age) and later menopause (older than 50 years of age), older age at first full-term pregnancy (older than 30 years of age), and fewer number of pregnancies are thought to impact a woman's risk by affecting the endogenous reproductive hormones (Kumle, et al., 2003). Recent use of oral contraceptives may increase the risk of breast cancer, but women who have not used oral contraceptives for 10 years have the same risk as those who have never used hormones. Use of hormone replacement therapy (HRT) has been shown to increase breast cancer risk with a higher risk associated with the duration of use (Li, Malone, & Porter, 2003). When given to women without a uterus, estrogen alone does not increase the risk of developing breast cancer as much as HRT does (Beral, 2003). Breastfeeding has consistently been shown to decrease a woman's risk of breast cancer slightly, with greater benefit for those who breastfeed for a longer duration.

Increased weight or obesity increases the risk of postmenopausal women for breast cancer. Some studies suggest that weight gain during adulthood increases the risk. The rationale for this association is that in postmenopausal women fat produces circulating estrogen, and an increase in fatty tissue can therefore increase estrogen levels and the potential for developing breast cancer. A study by the American Cancer Society showed that overweight women are 1.3 to 2.1 times more likely to die from breast cancer compared to women of normal weight (Calle, Rodriguez, Walker-Thurmond, & Thun, 2003).

Alcohol intake is consistently associated with an increased risk of breast cancer. Studies have suggested that the equivalent of two drinks, or 24 ounces, of alcohol per day may increase breast cancer risk by 21 percent. This risk is dose dependent, and it does not matter what type of alcohol beverage is consumed. It is thought that the increase is attributed to an increase in androgen and estrogen levels.

Smoking has continued to be controversial. In a recent report from Reuters regarding a study from Canada, the investigator calculates that women who smoke have a 46 percent increased risk of breast cancer and that women exposed to passive smoke have an overall increased risk of 27 percent. Physical activity has been suggested to provide a small amount of protection against breast cancer. A recent study suggests that regular exercise, regardless of intensity, may reduce the risk of breast cancer in postmenopausal women (McTiernan, Kooperberg, & White, 2003).

Pathophysiology

Some cancers are classified as in situ, which means they have not spread beyond the area where they began. In situ breast cancer is confined within the ducts (ductal carcinoma in situ or DCIS) or lobules (lobular carcinoma in situ or LCIS). Nearly all cancers at this stage can be cured. Many oncologists believe that lobular carcinoma is not a true cancer, but that it is an indicator of increased risk for developing invasive cancer at a later date.

The remaining breast cancers are invasive or infiltrating. This type of cancer begins in the lobules or ducts of the breast and then spreads through the duct or gland wall to invade the surrounding fatty breast tissue. The degree of seriousness of invasive carcinoma depends on the stage of the disease and the extent to which it has spread when it is diagnosed. Two different staging or classifications of tumors are used. The American Joint Committee on Cancer (AJCC) uses stages I, II, III, or IV with stage I being an early stage, and stage IV being an advanced stage based on information about the tumor size, lymph node involvement, and the presence or absence of distant metastases (American Cancer Society, 2004a). A broader system used for staging of most cancers is known as the SEER summary stage system. The SEER classifications are local stage (confined to the breasts, regional stage (tumors that have spread to surrounding tissue or nearby nodes), and distant stage (cancers that have metastasized to distant organs.

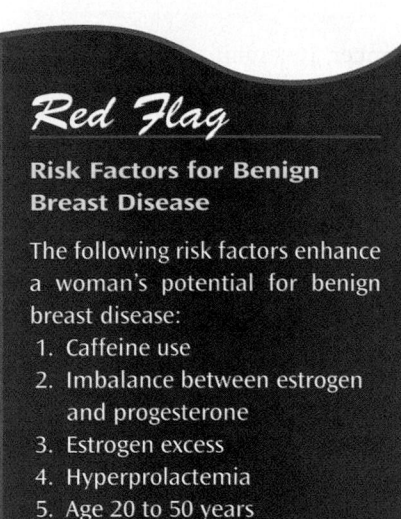

Red Flag

Risk Factors for Benign Breast Disease

The following risk factors enhance a woman's potential for benign breast disease:
1. Caffeine use
2. Imbalance between estrogen and progesterone
3. Estrogen excess
4. Hyperprolactemia
5. Age 20 to 50 years

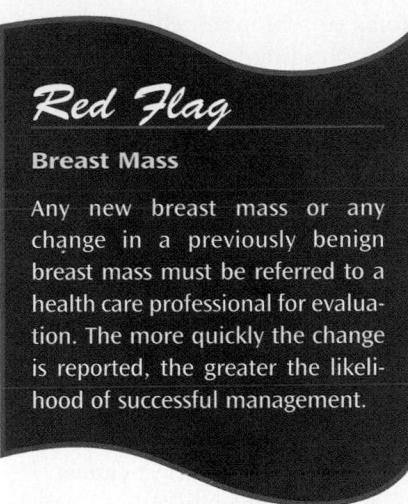

Red Flag

Breast Mass

Any new breast mass or any change in a previously benign breast mass must be referred to a health care professional for evaluation. The more quickly the change is reported, the greater the likelihood of successful management.

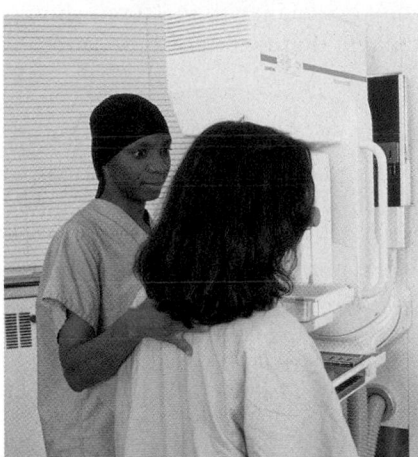

Figure 63-7 The patient is being positioned for a mammogram by a radiology technologist.

Diagnostic Tests

There are several primary tests used to diagnose alterations of the breast in addition to physical examination. The most common are mammography, ultrasonography, and biopsy. This section will discuss the specifics of these tests.

Mammography

Mammography is low dose X-ray visualization of the internal structures of the breast. It is highly accurate. Mammography has been shown to significantly increase the early detection of breast cancers and thus the ability to initiate treatment at an earlier stage of the disease. Mammography is the single most effective method for early detection of breast cancer. On average, mammography will detect about 80 to 85 percent of breast cancers in asymptomatic women. Testing is a little more accurate in postmenopausal than in premenopausal women. There is a 5 to 10 percent false-positive reporting requiring further testing. Figure 63-7 shows a woman being positioned for a mammography examination.

Recommended screening intervals are based on the duration of time a breast cancer is detectable by mammography before symptoms develop. Many breast cancers are not diagnosed until they become large, more advanced cancers because too much time lapses between mammography examinations. In an effort to detect breast cancer while it is optimally treatable, women are having mammograms at earlier ages. There are some studies that question the use of mammography and that suggest that mammograms have the potential to increase a woman's risk of developing breast cancer. Some researchers are questioning whether radiation exposure at earlier ages might be related to earlier development of the disease.

Recent reports from the behavioral risk factor surveillance system found that 61.5 percent of U.S. women age 40 and older have had a mammogram within the past year. A woman with less than a high school education, who has no health insurance, or who is a recent emigrant to this country is much less likely to have had a recent mammogram. While utilization of mammograms in general has been increasing, women below the poverty level are less likely to have had a mammogram within the last two years (Miglioretti, et al., 2004).

Breast Ultrasound

The increased use of breast ultrasonography has paralleled the augmented use of screening mammography. Unlike mammography, however, ultrasonography is not an effective screening tool; it is mainly used in the office setting for further characterization and biopsy of breast masses and suspicious axillary nodes. However, ultrasonography is particularly useful for differentiating cystic from solid breast lesions. Sonographically, simple cysts tend to be oval or lobulated and anechoic (echo free) with well-defined borders. Solid masses are characterized sonographically with respect to shape, compressibility, height-width ratio, margins, internal echo pattern, and presence of shadowing versus posterior enhancement. Carcinomas are typically hypoechoic (echoes are weaker than normal) with masses that are taller than they are wide, irregular borders, and broad acoustic shadowing. As with mammography, some malignancies cannot be visualized with ultrasonography. Therefore all clinically suspicious breast masses should undergo biopsy. In the operating room, ultrasonography can help the surgeon locate and excise nonpalpable breast lesions and achieve clean lumpectomy margins. It is also being used to guide various investigational tumor-ablating procedures.

Biopsy

Cytological, or tissue, diagnosis of a palpable breast mass may be obtained by means of fine needle aspiration (FNA) biopsy, core needle biopsy, and open incisional or excisional biopsy. Needle biopsy techniques are less invasive, less costly, and more expeditious than open biopsy, but they are significantly more likely to yield false-negative results. The choice of a biopsy technique should be individualized on the basis of the clinical and radiographic features of the lesion, the experience of the health care provider, and the patient's condition and preference.

Fine Needle Aspiration Biopsy

FNA biopsy permits the sampling of cells from breast lesions for cytological analysis. It is an appropriate first step in the evaluation of dominant breast masses, but it requires substantial experience on the part of both the operator and the cytopathologist. FNA biopsy is usually the diagnostic procedure of choice for T3 and T4 primary lesions, as well as chest wall and axillary recurrences for which systemic chemotherapy or irradiation is indicated as the first treatment modality. Because of sampling error, the procedure is less useful in evaluating small masses and areas of vague thickening or nodularity. In addition, it often cannot reliably distinguish invasive from noninvasive cancer.

Discrete masses discovered on physical examination may be either cystic or solid. Unless previous ultrasonographic examination has shown the mass to be solid, the needle used should be large enough (20 or 21 gauge) to permit aspiration of potentially viscous fluid if the lesion proves to be cystic. If the mass is known to be solid, a smaller needle (22 to 25 gauge) is sufficient for obtaining diagnostic tissue and will cause the patient less discomfort. For sufficient suction to be generated, a syringe with a capacity no smaller than 10 mL should be used. A variety of syringe holders are available that facilitate application of suction with a single hand.

Image-Guided Core Needle Biopsy

Needle biopsy techniques are increasingly being used to diagnose nonpalpable breast lesions. In general, FNA biopsy of nonpalpable lesions is inadvisable because of its high false negative rate. Little is lost by attempting an FNA biopsy of a palpable lesion in the office setting, but performing a stereotactic or ultrasound-guided FNA biopsy of a nonpalpable mass carries a significant cost in terms of time, patient discomfort, and expense. The diagnostic accuracy currently achievable with FNA biopsy in this setting does not justify this cost. Consequently, image guided core needle biopsy is the preferred approach for needle biopsy of nonpalpable lesions.

In choosing core needle biopsy, both patient and health care provider must be comfortable with the fact that the lesion will only be sampled rather than excised, recognize that the possibility of a sampling error that will cause the examiner to miss the lesion is higher with core needle biopsy than with open biopsy, and realize that equivocal findings will necessitate follow-up with open biopsy. The trade-off for these limitations is that core needle biopsy generally costs less than open biopsy, takes less time, and leaves only a tiny scar. After a core needle diagnosis of malignancy, the surgeon may proceed directly to wide local excision and will often be able to obtain clean margins with a single open procedure.

Open Biopsy

The vast majority of open breast biopsies are now performed with either local anesthesia alone or local anesthesia with intravenous sedation (monitored anesthesia care). General anesthesia is reserved for situations in which multiple lesions must be excised and the amount of local anesthetic required would exceed the maximum safe dose.

Open biopsy incisions should generally be curvilinear and should be placed directly over the lesion to minimize tunneling through breast tissue. Resection of a portion of overlying skin is not necessary unless the lesion is extremely superficial. In case the lesion proves to be malignant, all open biopsy incisions should also be oriented so that they can be excised with any subsequent lumpectomy or mastectomy incision. Accordingly, if an open biopsy is to be done at an extremely lateral or medial site, it may be best approached via a radial incision placed over the lesion rather than via a more vertical curvilinear incision.

Stereotactic Versus Ultrasound Guided Core Needle Biopsy

Whenever feasible, core needle biopsy is performed with ultrasonographic guidance that permits real-time documentation of needle position within the lesion. Stereotactic mammography guided core needle biopsy is performed if the lesion is not visualized ultrasonographically. Stereotactic biopsy is appropriate for lesions that are favorably located within the breast for achieving stable positioning in the biopsy window of the machine. Lesions close to the chest wall or the areola may not be accessible to stereotactic biopsy and are best approached via open biopsy with needle localization.

Clustered microcalcifications may also be approached by stereotactic core needle biopsy. If the cluster is not large enough for calcifications to remain to guide subsequent wide excision if a malignancy is found, a clip should be placed to mark the biopsy site. Alternatively, if the surgeon has experience with breast ultrasonography, this imaging modality may be used intraoperatively to identify the hematoma that results from stereotactic core needle biopsy.

As is the case for open biopsy of palpable lesions, the vast majority of needle-localized breast biopsies are now performed with local anesthesia or local anesthesia with intravenous sedation. General anesthesia is reserved for excision of multiple lesions or other special circumstances. The lesion to be excised is localized by inserting a thin needle and a fine wire under mammographic or ultrasonographic guidance immediately before surgery. To facilitate incision placement, images should be sent to the operating room with the wire entry site indicated on them. With superficial lesions, the wire entry site is usually close to the lesion and thus may be included in the incision. With some deeper lesions, the wire entry site is on the shortest path to the lesion and so may still be included in the incision. The incision is placed as directly as possible over the mass to minimize tunneling through breast tissue. Once the incision is made, a core of tissue is excised around and along the wire in such a way as to include the lesion. This process is easier and involves less excision of tissue if the localizing wire has a thickened segment several centimeters in length that is placed adjacent to, or within, the lesion. The surgeon then follows the wire itself into the breast tissue until the thick segment is reached. Only then is the excision extended away from the wire to include the lesion in a fairly small tissue fragment.

Nursing Diagnoses

Based on the information gathered, examples of nursing diagnoses in the patient with breast cancer may include the following:
- Acute pain as related to breast surgery.
- Fear in response to the diagnosis of breast cancer.
- Ineffective coping related to anxiety, lower activity level and the inability to perform normal activities of daily living.
- Activity intolerance related to fatigue after breast surgery.

Planning and Implementation

There are a variety of treatment modalities for cancer of the breast. These treatment choices are divided into those that do not require surgery and those requiring surgical intervention.

Nonsurgical Treatment

Systemic therapy includes hormonal and biological therapy and chemotherapy. This is called neoadjuvant treatment, and it has been found to be as effective as adjuvant therapy given after surgery to kill any undetected cancer cells that may

Fast Forward ▶▶▶

Diagnostic Tests That Are Definitive for Breast Cancers

There are several forms of diagnostic tests that are currently being used for the refinement of diagnoses related to breast cancers. These tests are continuing to be studied for their effectiveness and likely will progress to more specific value in the near future.

Ductal Lavage

The majority of breast cancers originate from the epithelium of the mammary ducts. Ductal lavage is a method of recovering breast duct epithelial cells for cytological analysis via a microcatheter that is inserted into the duct. It has several promising potential applications, such as identifying high-risk women, predicting risk with the help of molecular markers, monitoring the effectiveness of chemopreventive agents as evidenced by regression of cellular atypia, and delivering drugs directly into the ducts. At present, however, ductal lavage remains investigational and its predictive value and clinical utility await further definition.

Ductoscopy

Advances in endoscopic technology have made visualization and biopsy of the mammary ducts possible. Mammary ductoscopy is a procedure in which a microendoscope is employed to directly visualize the ductal lining of the breast and to provide access for retrieval of epithelial cells by means of lavage. At present, this technology is only available at a few centers, and as with all new technological developments, there is a learning curve associated with its application.

Ductoscopy is currently being evaluated for use in three main areas: (a) evaluation of patients with pathological nipple discharge; (b) evaluation of high-risk patients; and (c) evaluation of breast cancer patients to determine the extent of intraductal disease and, perhaps, define the extent of resection more precisely. Further study will be required to determine the precise role of this investigational technique in the evaluation and management of breast disease (Lind, Smith, & Souba, 2005).

---

have migrated to other parts of the body. This therapy often shrinks the tumor enough to make surgical removal possible. In some cases this neoadjuvant therapy has decreased tumor size enough to allow women whose larger tumors would require mastectomy to have breast conserving surgery instead.

Herceptin biological therapy is a monoclonal antibody that directly targets the HER2 protein of breast tumors and offers significant survival benefit for some women with metastatic disease. It is currently being used to treat women with late stage, recurring cancer. It has been suggested that women with early cancers may also benefit from this therapy.

Radiation therapy may be used to destroy cancer cells remaining in the breast, chest wall, or axilla after surgery. The ability to more accurately target radiation therapy has increased dramatically over the past decade, thus decreasing radiation therapy side effects. When used in conjunction with surgery and chemotherapy, long-term survival has been improved in women with lymph node positive disease.

Surgery

There are several surgical options for primary treatment of breast cancer. It should be emphasized that for most patients, wide local excision (lumpectomy) to microscopically clean margins coupled with axillary dissection and radiation therapy yields long-term survival equivalent to that associated with modified radical mastectomy. Currently, indications for mastectomy include patient preference, inability on the part of the surgeon to achieve clean margins without unacceptable deformation of the remaining breast tissue, the presence of multiple primary tumors, previous chest wall irradiation, pregnancy, and the presence of severe collagen vascular disease (e.g., scleroderma). Nonmedical indications for mastectomy include the lack of access to a radiation therapy facility and any other patient factors that would prevent completion of a full course of radiation therapy.

Lumpectomy

Lumpectomy, also referred to more precisely as wide local excision or partial mastectomy, involves excision of all cancerous tissue to microscopically clean margins. Reexcision or lumpectomy without axillary dissection may be performed with the patient under local anesthesia, but sedation or general anesthesia is usually advisable if a significant amount of tissue is to be excised or if there is tenderness from a previous biopsy. Lumpectomy with axillary dissection usually calls for general anesthesia, but it may be performed with thoracic epidural anesthesia supplemented by local anesthesia as needed.

Like open breast biopsy incisions, lumpectomy incisions should generally be curvilinear, should be placed directly over the lesion, and should also be oriented so as to be included within a subsequent mastectomy incision if margins prove positive. Extremely lateral or medial incisions may be better approached via a radial incision placed over the lesion. Because accurate assessment of margins is of central importance in a lumpectomy, it is critical that the incision be long enough to allow removal of the specimen in a single piece rather than in several pieces (Lind, et al., 2005).

Along with the mass itself, it is generally necessary to remove a 1- to 1.5-cm margin of tissue that appears normal beyond the edge of the palpable tumor or, if excisional biopsy has already been performed, around the biopsy cavity. In the case of nonpalpable lesions diagnosed via needle biopsy, the position of the lesion must be determined by means of wire localization, and 2 to 3 cm of tissue should be excised around the wire to obtain an adequate margin. The specimen should be oriented by the surgeon and the margins inked by the pathologist; this orientation is useful if reexcision is required to achieve clean margins. Reexcision of any close margins may be performed during the same surgical procedure if the specimen margins are assessed immediately by the pathologist. Surgical clips may be left in the lumpectomy site before closure to assist the radiation oncologist in planning the radiation boost to the tumor bed.

Minimally Invasive Ablative Techniques

The next step in the evolving application of less invasive techniques to breast cancer is to determine whether ablative local therapies can be effective substitutes for extirpative local therapies. Cryotherapy, laser ablation, radiofrequency ablation (RFA), and focused ultrasound ablation have all been studied as means of eradicating small breast cancers (Simmons, 2003). In most of these techniques a probe is placed percutaneously into the breast lesion under the guidance of an imaging modality, and tumor cell destruction is achieved by means of either heat or cold.

Cryotherapy has been successfully used for some time in the treatment of nonresectable liver tumors. It kills tumor cells by disrupting the cellular membrane during the freeze/thaw cycle. Unfortunately, early results of studies evaluating cryotherapy in breast cancer patients indicate that it does not always achieve complete tumor destruction. In addition, ultrasonographic monitoring of cell death may not be precise enough to allow accurate determination of the adequacy of treatment.

Laser ablation causes hyperthermic cell death by delivering energy through a fiberoptic probe inserted into the tumor. Because of the precise targeting required, ensuring complete tumor destruction has proved difficult with this technique.

RFA is a minimally invasive thermal ablation technique in which frictional heat is generated by intracellular ions moving in response to alternating current. Currently, RFA appears to be the most promising ablative method for small breast cancers. Like cryotherapy, RFA has also been extensively used to treat liver tumors. The RFA probe is percutaneously placed in the tumor under imaging guidance, and a star-shaped set of electrodes is extruded from the tip of the probe. Postprocedural MRI may help confirm complete tumor destruction, not only after RFA, but also after other ablative techniques as well.

Experience with ablative breast therapies is still relatively scant, and these techniques remain investigational. To date, most of the studies examining ablative breast cancer techniques have been single institution pilot studies involving highly selected patients with small, well-defined lesions who do not have extensive intraductal cancer or multifocal disease. In addition, these techniques have been restricted to lesions that are neither superficial nor deep, so as to avoid injury to the skin or the chest wall. Most of the initial ablative series involved subsequent surgical excision to obtain histological evidence of cell death. Unfortunately, when ablative therapies are used alone, the benefits of pathological assessment of the specimen, including evaluation of margin status, are lost; and positive surgical margins are associated with increased local recurrence rates. Preliminary data from the initial studies demonstrate acceptable short-term results, but the long-term results must be evaluated against those of standard breast conservation techniques (Simmons, 2003). The minimally invasive ablative techniques clearly are technically feasible, and they appear to offer some potential advantages, but it remains to be determined to what extent they are oncologically appropriate.

Lymphatic Mapping and SLN Biopsy

The histological status of the axillary nodes is the single most important predictor of outcome for breast cancer patients. Traditionally, axillary dissection has been a routine part of the management of breast cancer, but it has become clear that axillary dissection can be associated with sensory morbidities and lymphedema. The growing recognition of the morbidity of axillary dissection, together with the increasing ability of mammography to detect smaller and smaller node-negative tumors, gave rise to the need for a less morbid axillary procedure. Lymphatic mapping and SLN biopsy is a minimally invasive method of determining occult lymph node metastasis that is less morbid and more accurate than axillary dissection. SLN biopsy is based on the principle that the SLN is the first node to which tumor spreads; thus, if the SLN is tumor free, patients can be spared the morbidity associated with axillary dissection (Lind, et al., 2005).

The technique of SLN biopsy continues to evolve, but at present, the most common method of identifying the SLN employs both a vital dye and a radionuclide. Lymphatic mapping is a critical part of the procedure. A radionuclide is injected before surgery and dynamic gamma camera imaging is subsequently employed to delineate sites of drainage. Several imaging series examining various sites of injection (peritumoral, intradermal, and subareolar) concluded that the breast and its overlying skin may drain to the same few SLNs. In the operating room, a vital blue dye is injected (usually peritumorally), and the breast is massaged to stimulate lymphatic flow. The surgeon then makes a small incision in the axilla and uses a handheld gamma probe to remove lymph nodes that are "hot" (i.e., radioactive), blue, or both. At the time of breast surgery, the SLN can be examined by means of frozen section analysis or touch-print cytology. If metastases are present in the SLN, axillary dissection may then be performed.

Because SLN biopsy involves analysis of only one or two nodes, the pathologist can carry out a more intensive pathological examination than would be possible with a standard axillary lymphadenectomy specimen containing multiple nodes. Newer techniques (e.g., immunohistochemical and molecular assays) can also be used to identify micrometastases that light microscopy would fail to detect, but the therapeutic and prognostic significance of tumor cells identified by such means remains unclear.

Because there is a learning curve for SLN biopsy, the success rate varies with the surgeon's experience. Accordingly, it is recommended that surgeons first learning the technique use axillary dissection as a backup for the first 20 procedures to gain experience in identifying the SLN. Surgeons competent in SLN biopsy should be able to identify the SLN with better than 85 percent accuracy and a false-negative rate lower than 5 percent. (Classe, Curtet, & Campion, 2003). Currently, axillary dissection is recommended for patients who have a positive SLN; however, prospective, randomized trials are required to determine to what extent this step is necessary in SLN-positive patients. A number of studies have confirmed that the absence of metastases in the SLN reliably predicts the absence of metastases in the remaining axillary nodes.

SLN biopsy has also been employed in DCIS patients. Women with DCIS have high survival rates without undergoing any axillary procedure, and there is concern that indiscriminate application of SLN biopsy to these patients may result in unnecessary axillary dissection and subsequent systemic chemotherapy. Therefore, SLN biopsy should be limited to (a) patients with extensive DCIS in whom percutaneous biopsy may have missed areas of invasion and (b) patients with extensive DCIS who are undergoing mastectomy that would preclude SLN biopsy if occult invasive disease were found on pathological examination. The SLN identification rates and false-negative rates reported when SLN biopsy is performed after neoadjuvant chemotherapy are similar to those seen when the procedure is performed after diagnosis, but before systemic chemotherapy. Contraindications to SLN biopsy include the presence of palpable axillary nodes suggestive of metastatic disease, the presence of large or locally advanced breast cancers, prior axillary surgery, and pregnancy or lactation.

Axillary Dissection

Before the advent of SLN biopsy, axillary dissection was routinely performed in breast cancer patients; it provided prognostic information that guided subsequent adjuvant therapy, it afforded excellent local control, and it may have contributed a small overall survival benefit. Axillary dissection for clinically node-negative breast cancer includes resection of level I and level II lymph nodes and the fibrofatty tissue within which these nodes lie. The superior border of the dissection is formed by the axillary vein laterally and the upper extent of level II nodes medially; the lateral border of the dissection is formed by the latissimus dorsi from the tail of the breast to the crossing point of the axillary vein; the medial border is formed by the pectoral muscles and the anterior serratus muscle; and the inferior border is formed by the tail of the breast. Level II nodes are easily removed by retracting the greater and smaller pectoral muscles medially; it is not necessary to divide or remove the smaller pectoral muscle. In general, level III nodes are not removed unless palpable disease is present.

Mastectomy

The goal of a mastectomy is to remove all breast tissue, including the nipple and the areola, while leaving well-perfused, viable skin flaps for primary closure or reconstruction. This is the case whether the mastectomy is performed for treatment of breast cancer or for prophylaxis in high-risk patients. Proper skin incisions and good exposure throughout the procedure are the important components of a well-performed mastectomy. The borders of dissection extend superiorly to the clavicle, medially to the sternum, inferiorly to where breast tissue ends on the costal margin below the inframammary fold, and laterally to the border of the latissimus dorsi. The fascia of the greater pectoral muscle forms the deep margin of the dissection and should be removed with the specimen.

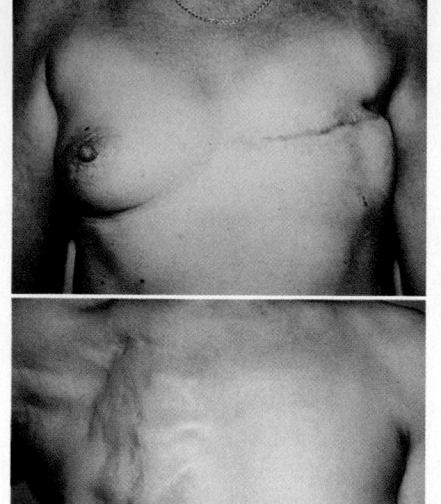

Figure 63-8 Mastectomy patients. *Courtesy of Steven M. Lynch, M.D.*

Mastectomy usually calls for general anesthesia, but it may be performed with thoracic epidural anesthesia supplemented by local anesthesia as needed. When a simple mastectomy is to be performed in a frail patient for whom general anesthesia poses unacceptable risks (particularly if the patient is elderly and has a narrow-based, pendulous breast), local anesthesia with sedation is appropriate.

Simple mastectomy is performed: (a) to treat DCIS; (b) as a prophylactic measure; (c) as a follow-up to lumpectomy and axillary dissection if lumpectomy margins are positive for malignancy; (d) to treat local recurrence of breast cancer after lumpectomy, node dissection, and irradiation; and (e) in elderly patients in whom coexisting medical conditions or other factors constitute contraindications to axillary dissection. Simple mastectomy is also indicated for treatment of sarcomas of the breast, because lymphatic spread to axillary nodes is not part of the natural history of this disease (Lind, et al., 2005).

Modified radical mastectomy is performed to treat invasive breast cancer when (a) there are contraindications to breast preservation or (b) the patient or the health care provider prefers mastectomy. Simple mastectomy in conjunction with SLN biopsy is an increasingly common alternative to modified radical mastectomy for patients with clinically negative axillary nodes. If the nodes are positive for tumor on pathological examination, the surgeon may then elect to perform a completion axillary dissection. Postoperative views of two patients who underwent mastectomy are shown in Figure 63-8.

An increasingly popular approach for women requiring mastectomy is skin-sparing mastectomy (SSM) (Hultman & Daiza, 2003). This procedure consists of resection of the nipple-areola complex, any existing biopsy scar, and the breast parenchyma, followed immediately by breast reconstruction. It is somewhat demanding technically in that the effort expended in preserving the skin makes it difficult for the oncologist to ensure removal of as much breast tissue as possible. Because the inframammary fold is preserved and a generous skin envelope remains after SSM, cosmetic results after reconstruction are optimized. SSM is oncologically safe and is not associated with an increased incidence of local recurrence. The recurrences that do occur typically develop below the skin flaps and thus are easily detectable. Deep recurrences beneath the reconstruction are comparatively uncommon. Patients with locally advanced breast cancer are not appropriate candidates for SSM with immediate reconstruction. In general, immediate reconstruction should be reserved for patients at low risk for postoperative adjuvant therapies.

Breast Reconstruction

Advances in reconstructive techniques have made breast reconstruction increasingly popular. Reconstruction may be done either at the time of the mastectomy (immediate reconstruction) or later (delayed reconstruction). It is well recognized that immediate breast reconstruction after mastectomy is safe, does not significantly delay subsequent administration of chemotherapy or radiation therapy, and does not prevent detection of recurrent disease. Either implants or autologous tissue may be used in reconstruction.

The option of breast reconstruction is presented to the mastectomy patient by her breast surgeon during preoperative discussion of mastectomy or in the case of delayed reconstruction, during follow-up after an earlier mastectomy. The patient, the plastic surgeon, and the oncologist or general surgeon will decide among the several reconstruction options available: implants with tissue expansion, the transverse rectus abdominis myocutaneous (TRAM) flap, the latissimus dorsi myocutaneous flap, and various free flaps on the basis of patient preference and lifestyle, the availability of suitable autologous tissue, and the demands imposed by any additional cancer therapies required. Familiarity with the strengths and drawbacks of these reconstruction options facilitates this decision.

Perhaps the simplest method of reconstruction is to place a saline-filled implant beneath the greater pectoral muscle and the anterior serratus muscle to recreate a breast mound as shown in Figure 63-9. Even after SSM, the greater pectoral muscle is usually so tight that unless the patient is small-breasted, expansion of this muscle and the skin is necessary before an implant that matches the opposite breast can be inserted. Serial expansions are performed on an outpatient basis: saline is injected into the expander every 10 to 14 days until an appropriate size has been attained. A second operative procedure is then required to exchange the expander for a permanent implant. A nipple and an areola are constructed at a later date (Lind, et al., 2005).

The major advantage of implant reconstruction is that there is no need to harvest autologous tissue, and the patient is spared the discomfort, scarring, and loss of muscle function that would occur at the donor site. Accordingly, implant reconstructions are commonly performed in patients who require bilateral mastectomies and reconstructions. The initial operating time is significantly shorter for implant reconstruction than for autologous tissue reconstruction, and there is no need for autologous blood donation or transfusion. Hospital stay and recuperation time are also significantly shorter. The main drawbacks are the prolonged time and the multiple office visits required to achieve a symmetrical reconstruction if tissue expansion is required and the necessity of a second surgical procedure to place the permanent implant. In addition, the final cosmetic result often is not as good as what can be achieved with autologous tissue reconstruction, and it may deteriorate over time as a consequence of capsule formation or implant migration (Lind, et al., 2005). The implant-reconstructed breast is significantly firmer than the contralateral breast. The life expectancy of currently available saline implants has not been established, but it may be less than a decade, which means that many patients who have received or are receiving implants may need replacements at some point. Patients who have previously undergone irradiation of the breast or the chest wall may have tissue that cannot be adequately expanded and thus is unsuitable for implant reconstruction.

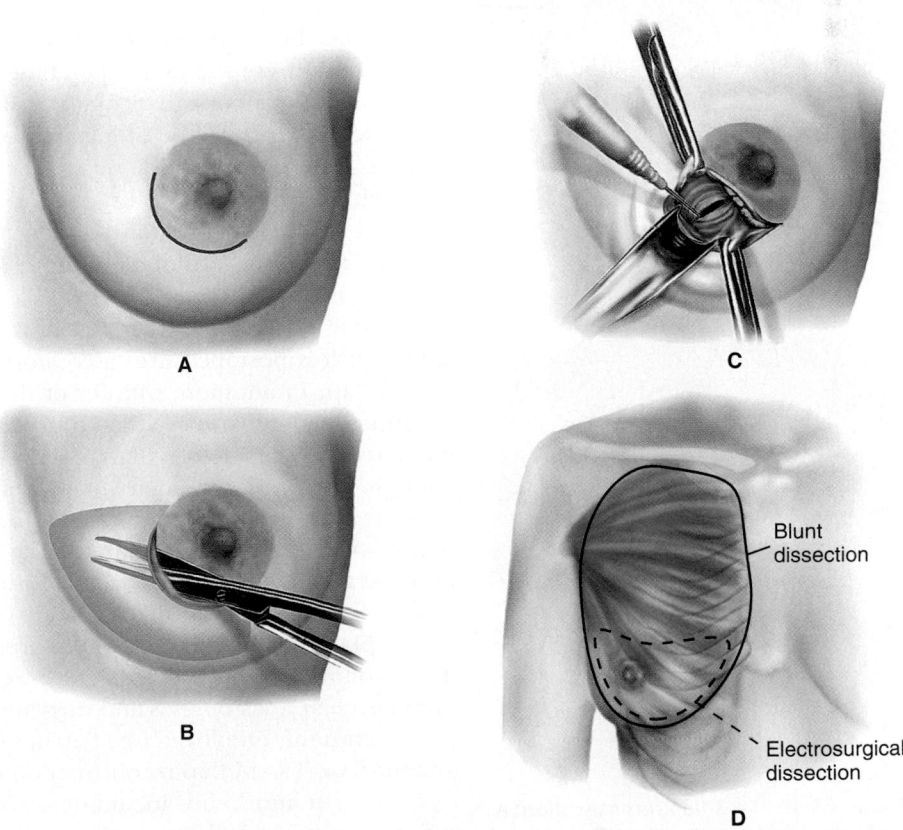

Figure 63-9 Augmentation mammoplasty: A. Areolar incision, B. Creation of pocket, C. Pectoral muscle incision, D. Implant position.

A second approach to reconstruction is to transfer vascularized muscle, skin, and fat from a donor site to the mastectomy defect. The most commonly used myocutaneous flaps are the TRAM flap and the latissimus dorsi flap. Use of the free TRAM flap is advocated by certain centers. Other free-flap options, including the free gluteus flap, are used in special circumstances, such as when other donor sites are unsuitable.

The major advantage of autologous tissue reconstruction is that it generally yields a superior cosmetic result. Often the size and shape of the opposite breast can be matched immediately with no need for subsequent office or operative procedures. The reconstructed breast has a soft texture that is similar to that of the contralateral breast. In addition, the cosmetic result is stable over time. The main drawbacks are the magnitude of the surgical procedure required for the reconstruction (involving both a prolonged operating time and longer inpatient hospitalization); the potential need for autologous blood donation or transfusion; and the pain, scarring, and loss of muscle function that arise at the donor site. Smokers and patients with significant vascular disease may not be ideal candidates for autologous tissue reconstruction. Partial necrosis of the transferred flap may create firm areas, while on rare occasions complete necrosis and consequent loss of the flap can occur (Lind, et al., 2005).

A number of factors are considered in choosing between the TRAM flap and the latissimus dorsi flap. In a TRAM flap reconstruction, the contralateral rectus abdominis is transferred along with overlying skin and fat to create a breast mound. This procedure yields a flatter abdominal contour, but it calls for a long transverse abdominal incision and necessitates repositioning of the umbilicus (Lind, et al., 2005). A major advantage of the TRAM flap is that it can provide enough tissue to match all but the largest contralateral breasts. Some patients, however, such as those who have undergone an abdominal procedure that compromises the TRAM flap's vascular supply, are not ideal candidates for TRAM flap reconstruction. Postoperative discomfort is greater with TRAM flap reconstruction than with other flap reconstructions because of the extent of the abdominal portion of the procedure. In young, healthy, and motivated patients who require bilateral reconstructions it is often possible to perform two TRAM flap procedures in the same operation (Hultman & Daiza, 2003).

In a latissimus dorsi myocutaneous flap reconstruction, the ipsilateral latissimus dorsi is transferred along with overlying skin and fat to create a breast mound. Either a horizontal or a vertical donor site incision may be made on the back. The operative technique for the latissimus dorsi flap reconstruction is complex. Patients who have undergone irradiation of the breast, chest wall, or axilla (including irradiation of the thoracodorsal vessels) may not be eligible for this procedure.

A major advantage of the latissimus dorsi flap is that its donor site is associated with less postoperative discomfort than the abdominal donor site of the TRAM flap. In addition, transfer of the latissimus dorsi results in substantially less functional impairment than transfer of the rectus abdominis. A drawback of the latissimus dorsi flap is that in many women, the latissimus dorsi is not bulky enough to provide symmetry with the contralateral breast. In such cases, an implant must be added to the flap to match the size and shape of the opposite breast, which means that the drawback of the implant's limited life span is added to the drawbacks already associated with autologous tissue reconstruction.

Free flap reconstruction options are utilized primarily when other autologous and implant reconstruction options are not available, do not provide sufficient tissue volume, or have failed. They are more complex procedures, requiring microvascular anastomoses and carrying a higher risk of total flap loss. The two most commonly employed free flap options are the free TRAM flap and the free gluteus flap. TRAM flap reconstruction is shown in Figure 63-10.

Donor site morbidity, including postoperative pain, wound healing complications, decreased abdominal muscle strength, and hernia formation, is a prime disadvantage of pedicled or free TRAM flap reconstruction. As a result,

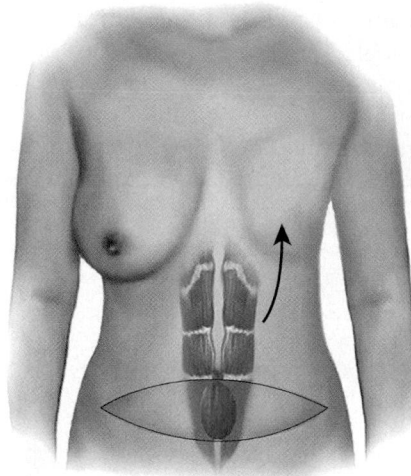

A

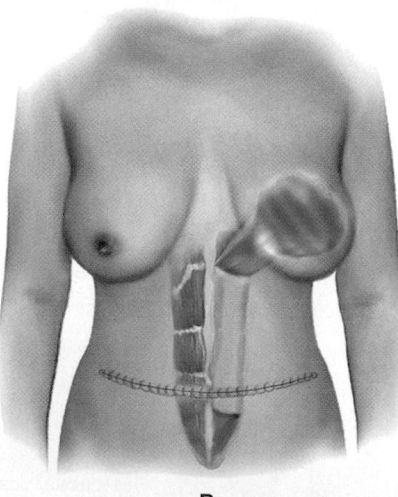

B

Figure 63-10 TRAM flap reconstruction: A. Abdominal incision, B. TRAM flap rotated into position.

muscle-sparing alternatives to autogenous breast reconstruction have been developed, such as the deep inferior epigastric perforator (DIEP) flap (Craigie, Allen, DellaCroce, & Sullivan, 2003). In this approach, free flaps are used that comprise skin and fat alone, without the rectus abdominis. Avoidance of muscle sacrifice in the abdomen ultimately translates into greater patient satisfaction, but careful patient selection is essential to optimize outcomes. The disadvantages of the DIEP flap include the considerable technical expertise and long operating time required, as well as the greater potential for flap loss, because this flap has a more tenuous blood supply than the standard TRAM (Lind, et al., 2005).

Evaluation of Outcomes

Potential patient outcomes for each of the example nursing diagnoses for the patient with breast cancer are:

- Acute pain as related to breast surgery. The patient should verbalize an adequate relief of pain along with the ability to realistically cope with the pain if it is not completely relieved.
- Fear in response to the diagnosis of breast cancer. The patient should manifest positive coping behaviors and verbalize a reduction in the amount of fear of the having this disease.
- Ineffective coping related to anxiety, lower activity level, and the inability to perform normal activities of daily living. The patient identifies own maladaptive coping behaviors, identifies available resources and support systems, describes or initiates alternative coping strategies, and describes positive results from new behaviors.
- Activity intolerance related to fatigue after breast surgery. The patient maintains activity level within capabilities, as evidenced by normal heart rate and blood pressure during activity, as well as absence of shortness of breath, weakness, and fatigue.

KEY CONCEPTS

- The sole physiological function of the breast, or mammary gland, is to secrete milk for nourishment of the infant.
- There are varying ways that the breast tissue develops during pregnancy, lactation, and during menopause.
- Gynecomastia is frequently caused by a shift in the estrogen/androgen ratio because of increased circulating estrogens or to decreased circulating androgens.
- The breast exam involves bilateral inspection and palpation of the breasts, areola, axillary, and supraclavicular areas.
- The majority of breast disorders are benign, but it is imperative that breast disorders are diagnosed accurately and treated early to have the most optimal outcome.
- There are three primary pathological conditions of the nipple: (a) bleeding, (b) discharge, and (c) fissures.
- Fibrocystic breast changes are the most frequently occurring pathological breast problem.

- Mastitis (inflammation or infection) of the breast may be caused from irritation, injury, or infection and most commonly occurs within the first three months after childbirth; however it can occur at any age.
- Mammoplasty is a surgical procedure to increase or decrease the size or shape of the breast and is usually considered an elective procedure.
- Surgical breast reduction is performed to relieve the neck and shoulder pain that can lead to degenerative nerve changes due to overly large breasts.
- Breast cancer is the most common type of cancer in women and is a major public health problem in the United States, with one in eight women expected to be diagnosed sometime during their lifetime.
- In situ breast cancer is confined within the ducts (ductal carcinoma in situ, DCIS) or lobules (lobular carcinoma in situ).
- Cytological (tissue) diagnosis of a palpable breast mass may be obtained by means of FNA biopsy, core needle biopsy, or open incisional or excisional biopsy.

Continued

KEY CONCEPTS—cont'd

- Lumpectomy is a wide local excision or partial mastectomy that involves excision of all cancerous tissue to microscopically clean margins.
- The goal of a mastectomy is to remove all breast tissue, including the nipple and the areola, while leaving well-perfused, viable skin flaps for primary closure or reconstruction.

- Breast reconstruction may be done either at the time of the mastectomy (immediate reconstruction) or later (delayed reconstruction).

REVIEW QUESTIONS

1. The three major hormones that cause the breast tissue to develop, enlarge, and produce milk are:
   1. Estrogen, progesterone, and LDH
   2. Progesterone, FSH, and estrogen
   3. Estrogen, progesterone, and prolactin
   4. LDH, FSH, and MSH

2. Which of the following is true concerning an examination of the breast?
   1. Only examine the patient in the supine position
   2. Variations between breast size is not uncommon, but breasts should be fairly symmetrical.
   3. Dimpling of the nipples on large-breasted women is best detected by having the woman lean backward.
   4. Palpation of the breasts begins with the nipples.

3. Which of the following is true concerning pathological conditions of the nipples?
   1. Bleeding in the discharge generally suggests malignancy.
   2. A variety of medications can cause fluid discharge from the nipples.
   3. Fissures in the nipples are most often caused by puberty.
   4. It is not necessary for health care providers to follow-up on discharge from the nipples.

4. Which of the following is correct regarding changes and disorders of the breast?
   1. Fibrocystic breast changes involve the secretion of a white, milk-like fluid in a nonlactating breast.
   2. Fibroadenomas are benign, fibrous growths of the glandular epithelium in breast tissue.
   3. Intraductal papillomas usually occur in women over the age of 60.
   4. Mastitis occurs in all ages of women, but primarily at puberty in adolescence.

5. Which of the following is true concerning the risk factors for breast cancer?
   1. Other types of cancer history have no correlation with breast cancer.
   2. Environment is not a risk factor for breast cancer.
   3. Ethnicity is a risk factor for breast cancer.
   4. Hormones are not a risk factor for breast cancer.

6. Which of the following is true of a breast biopsy?
   1. A fine needle aspiration biopsy permits the sampling of cells from breast lesions.
   2. FNA biopsy of nonpalpable lesions has the highest level of accuracy for diagnostics.
   3. Open biopsies usually are performed under a general anesthetic.
   4. Stereotactic mammography-guided biopsy is performed only if the lesion is easily visualized.

7. Ms. Jones has a ductoscopy. Which of the following is true of this test?
   1. It involves recovering breast duct epithelial cells for cytological analysis.
   2. It is particularly useful in evaluating patients with nipple discharge.
   3. It is not diagnostic in patients who are in the high-risk category for cancer.
   4. It is predictive of whether or not the patient may not be a good risk for breast augmentation.

8. Which of the following is the least invasive form of surgery?
   1. Modified radical mastectomy
   2. Simple mastectomy
   3. Lumpectomy
   4. Skin-sparing mastectomy

Continued

REVIEW QUESTIONS—cont'd

9. Which of the following is the single most important predictor of outcome for breast cancer patients?
   1. The age of the patient
   2. The presence of nipple discharge at the time of diagnosis
   3. The histological status of the axillary nodes
   4. The presence of mastitis and an infection process upon diagnosis

10. What is the major advantage of implant reconstruction of the breast using a prosthetic saline-filled implant?
    1. It is less expensive.
    2. It does not require harvesting of autologous tissue and a loss of muscle function.
    3. It allows for fewer office visits and additional surgical interventions.
    4. It lasts virtually forever and therefore does not require surgical revision.

REVIEW ACTIVITIES

1. Describe the changes in the breast tissue during the maturational phases of a woman.

2. Teach a patient how to perform a BSE.

3. Evaluate the differences in cultures as related to breast examinations.

4. Describe the history of breast augmentation surgery.

5. Describe one of the common diagnostic methods for determining alterations of the breast.

6. Compare and contrast minimally ablative techniques to breast cancer.

Male Reproductive Dysfunction: Nursing Management

Pam Hamre, RN, MS, CNM

CHAPTER TOPICS

- Prostatitis
- Benign Prostatic Hyperplasia
- Prostate Cancer
- Testicular Disorders
- Disorders of the Penis and Urethra

Disorders of the male reproductive system can impact the urinary system, as well as the emotional stability and social lifestyle of the patient and his family across the life span. Regardless of whether such disorders involve minor inconveniences or major lifestyle and self-concept issues, assessing problems of the reproductive system requires gentle and thoughtful therapeutic communication that is open, frank, and educational with close attention to detail. The nurse must constantly be alert to verbal and nonverbal indicators of patients' sensitivity or embarrassment about their genitals, their sexual behaviors, and conditions that could be interpreted as assaults on their masculinity.

KEY TERMS

Balanitis
Balanoposthitis
Embolization
Epididymitis
Epispadias
Hypospadias
Infertility
Orchitis
Paraphimosis
Phimosis
Posthitis
Priapism
Prostatitis
Spermatocelectomy
Testicular self-examination (TSE)
Urethritis
Urethroplasty
Urethrotomy
Varicocele
Varicocelectomy
Vasectomy

PROSTATITIS

Prostatitis is inflammation of the prostate gland. The inflammation is classified as either acute or chronic, by the causative agent (bacterial or nonbacterial), and by whether the patient is aware or unaware of symptoms. If there is an acute infectious process present, the condition is termed acute bacterial prostatitis. If the infection is recurrent, it is termed chronic bacterial prostatitis. In the absence of demonstrable infection, prostatitis is classified as chronic nonbacterial prostatitis or chronic pelvic pain syndrome (CPPS). In the absence of symptoms, prostatitis is classified as asymptomatic inflammatory prostatitis (AIP) (Theodorescu & Krupski, 2005).

Epidemiology

Approximately 50 percent of men experience symptoms of prostatitis at some time in their life, with the highest incidence occurring between ages 35 and 65. However, only about 10 percent of prostatitis is bacterial in origin. When the prostate gland becomes inflamed and enlarges, creating pressure on the bladder, urinary symptoms result.

Etiology

The most common causes for prostatitis are bacteria, mycoplasma, and fungi. In addition, other causes are urethral strictures and prostatic hyperplasia. The most common bacterial cause is *Escherichia coli* and is usually carried from the urethra to the prostate. In cases of bacterial prostatitis, common bowel bacteria (*E. coli*, *Enterobacter*, or *Enterococcus*) or sexually transmitted organisms (*Chlamydia trachomatis* or *Gonococcus*) invade the prostate by ascending the urethra.

Pathophysiology

Chronic prostatitis can create hard nodules of scarring on the prostate gland, that can be mistaken for prostate cancer on digital rectal examination (DRE) and that can cause chronic pelvic pain. Nonbacterial prostatitis is thought to be either an autoimmune disorder or the result of neurological damage to tissues surrounding the prostate during bacterial prostatitis.

Assessment with Clinical Manifestations

Prostatitis is usually characterized by acute onset of urinary burning, frequency, urgency, and dysuria. Patients with bacterial prostatitis often experience fever and malaise. Pain experienced in the testes, rectum, low back, or perineum may also be present. The assessment for prostatitis includes questions that are shown in the Patient Playbook.

Diagnostic Tests

A variety of diagnostic tests can be used to verify prostatitis. Urethral and prostatic secretions may be tested for the presence of white blood cells and cultured for organisms. Diagnosis of bacterial prostatitis is made by culturing spontaneous or expressed urethral discharge, or prostate fluid (Daniels, 2003). Urine can also be cultured to detect which bacteria is the causative organism. Prostate fluid is obtained by collecting a clean, divided specimen. The patient voids about 20 mL, the amount of urine lying in the urethra, and then prostatic massage is performed until the prostate secretions are collected. The patient then voids again to provide a specimen containing a combination of bladder urine and prostate secretions. The presence of cytotoxic T-cells in the expressed prostate fluid may indicate an autoimmune inflammatory response, indicative of nonbacterial prostatitis.

PATIENT PLAYBOOK

Assessment of Prostatitis

The nurse can ask the patient the following questions in assessing for the presence of prostatitis:

- When did the dysuria begin?
- Were there precipitating factors for the urinary frequency and urgency?
- Is urethral discharge present, and if so, what color is it?
- When were malaise and fever noticed?
- What is your sexual history, including episodes of unprotected intercourse or sexual contact with partners with sexually transmitted infections?

Nursing Diagnoses

Based on the information gathered, examples of nursing diagnoses in the patient with prostatitis may include the following:

- Pain related to prostatic enlargement and inflammation.
- Risk for imbalanced body temperature secondary to acute bacterial prostatitis.
- Risk for infection related to prostatitis.

Planning and Implementation

If the prostatitis is bacterial in nature, elimination of the bacteria causing the infection is the primary goal. The secondary goal is to eliminate the pain and urinary symptoms. Prevention of chronic pain is a third goal. In addition to the primary health care provider and nurse, the team of health care providers may need to include several other professionals. A pharmacist and an infection control provider may help manage the infection. Mental health professionals may be needed to assist the patient to cope with emotional distress. A public health nurse or social worker may need to carry out case finding if the infection was sexually transmitted.

Pharmacology

Medications prescribed for prostatitis are dependent on the cause of the inflammation. In the case of bacterial prostatitis, ciprofloxacin (Cipro) and doxycycline are commonly utilized. A severe infection may require intravenous (IV) antibiotics and hospitalization. Acetaminophen or ibuprofen may be used to control fever and pain. Nonsteroidal anti-inflammatory drugs (NSAIDs) are optimally effective because of their anti-inflammatory properties and thus are more commonly recommended for those patients who can tolerate them (Broyles, Reiss, & Evans, 2007).

Patient and Family Teaching

Teaching focuses on eradication of the infection and helping the patient feel more comfortable. The nurse needs to ensure that the patient understands and accepts the importance of careful adherence to the treatment plan and the importance of completing the antibiotic regimen, because prostatitis is prone to recur. Patients should be given written and verbal information on the cause of their prostatitis. If a sexually transmitted infectious organism is found to be the bacteria involved, state mandates regarding notification of sexual partners must be implemented.

Comfort may be enhanced by sitz baths and avoiding long periods in a sitting position. Foods and beverages that have diuretic action or that increase prostatic secretions, such as alcohol, coffee, tea, chocolate, cola, and spices, should be avoided. The patient also needs to be cautioned to avoid sexual arousal and intercourse while the acute infection persists.

Evaluation of Outcomes

Potential patient outcomes for each of the example nursing diagnoses for the patient with prostatitis are:

- Pain related to prostatic enlargement and inflammation. The patient should verbalize an adequate relief of pain along with the ability to realistically cope with the pain if it is not completely relieved.
- Risk for imbalanced body temperature secondary to acute bacterial prostatitis. The patient maintains body temperature within a normal range.
- Risk for infection related to prostatitis. The patient remains free of infection, as evidenced by normal vital signs and absence of purulent drainage from wounds, incisions, and tubes. Infection is recognized early to allow for prompt treatment.

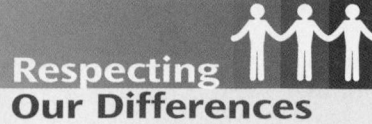

Respecting Our Differences

Prostate Enlargement and Elderly Males

BPH is obviously common among elderly males. Nurses must make certain that they do not assume that the patient with BPH is accepting his disorder without reservations. The nurse must remember to communicate well with the patient and ask open-ended questions regarding how the patient feels about the new diagnosis. In addition, the nurse must remember that issues of sexuality and incontinence may be of great importance to the patient, even though the patient is elderly.

BENIGN PROSTATIC HYPERPLASIA

Benign prostatic hyperplasia (BPH) is enlargement of the prostate gland because of an overgrowth in the number of cells. The enlargement of the prostate creates pressure on the neck of the bladder, requiring intrabladder pressures to be higher than normal to overcome the prostate pressure so that urine can be released. The increased pressure exerted on the neck of the bladder is responsible for the symptoms of BPH that together are referred to as prostatism: weak and dribbling urine stream, difficulty in starting the stream of urine, nocturia, and voiding small amounts frequently.

Epidemiology

BPH is a common condition affecting middle-aged and elderly men and the greatest risk factor for BPH is age. According to the National Cancer Institute virtually all men over age 50 have some degree of prostatic hyperplasia resulting in enlargement of the prostate gland. In addition, 50 percent of men over age 60 and 90 percent of men over age 70 have symptomatic BPH (National Cancer Institute, 2005d). Family history may also have a contributory effect. Men of southern European descent have the highest risk, while men of Asian and Scandinavian descent have a slightly lower risk. When men do not recognize that prostatic hyperplasia is a normal aging process for which effective treatment is available they may not seek treatment.

Pathophysiology

The prostate gland normally undergoes two periods of active growth. At puberty the prostate doubles in size, and at about age 25 additional growth of the prostate begins to occur. This latter growth is ongoing and over time, develops into BPH. As the cells continue to replicate they crowd against the urethra, causing the urinary stream difficulties. The additional prostatic tissue results in an abnormally high total amount of dihydrotestosterone (DHT), causing the smooth muscle cells of the urethra and prostate tissue to spasm slightly. The spasms further increase the difficulty in voiding.

The hyperplastic prostate cells are not precancerous. Hyperplasia creates an enlargement of the prostate that is soft in consistency in an inward expansion of the transitional portion of the prostate tissue that wraps around the urethra. In contrast, prostate cancer is usually firm and nodular to palpation and is located in the periphery of the prostate gland.

Assessment with Clinical Manifestations

Assessment for BPH involves taking a careful history about urinary function. The ease with which the stream of urine is started, the strength of the stream, the perceived amount of urine eliminated each voiding, along with the patient's sense about whether his bladder is completely emptying and the presence of nocturia or dribbling are important indicators of urethral compression. A DRE is performed to assess the size and consistency of the prostate.

Diagnostic Tests

The primary concern when evaluating BPH is the potential for having a malignancy of the prostate. To assist in differentiating BPH from prostate cancer a prostate specific antigen (PSA) blood test is also obtained to rule out prostate cancer. Rectal ultrasonography of the prostate may be undertaken if prostate cancer is suspected. A postvoiding bladder scan may be done to assess how effectively the bladder is emptying, and a cystoscopy may be performed to assess the degree of urethral compression and bladder wall integrity. Renal function tests, such as creatinine, may be done to ascertain any renal impairment secondary to elevated retrograde pressure.

Nursing Diagnoses

Based on the information gathered, examples of nursing diagnoses in the patient with BPH may include the following:

- Risk for infection from frequent urinary tract infections.
- Impaired urinary elimination related to BPH.
- Risk for disturbed sleep pattern secondary to nocturia.

Planning and Implementation

The goal of treatment for BPH is a reduction in prostate size that improves bladder outflow and decreases urinary system issues. The primary methods of correcting this disorder are surgery and management with medications. In general, the health care provider is also concerned that the condition does not become malignant, and the patient will be evaluated based on preventing cancer from developing.

Surgery

BPH is often treated through surgical removal of the hypertrophied prostate tissue. Transurethral resection of the prostate (TURP) is the most common procedure used. The surgery is usually performed under regional anesthesia and involves laser ablation of prostatic tissue during cystoscopy. Resection of the prostate can also be accomplished using a laser to vaporize or necrotize prostate tissue with less bleeding than occurs with the traditional TURP.

Following the surgery a double lumen indwelling catheter is placed into the urinary bladder. Normal saline is instilled through one lumen of the catheter

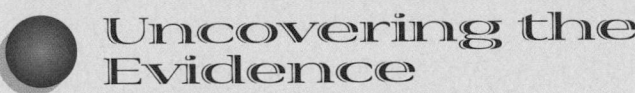

Uncovering the Evidence

Quality of Life While Living with Prostate Cancer

Discussion: The aim of the study was to investigate men with prostate cancer and BPH in comparison with men from the general population. In addition, the study investigated the impact of micturition problems on quality of life.

The samples consisted of 155 men with prostate cancer, 131 with BPH, and 129 from the general population. Micturition problems were assessed with four different instruments. Parametric and nonparametric statistics were applied. The findings revealed that the most troublesome urinary problems were leakage, feelings of discomfort, and disrupted urinary function, and frequency. Men with urological diagnosis had more micturition problems, fatigue, and sleeping difficulties than men from the general population, but the cancer diagnosis did not add to the problems. Role and social functioning (prostate cancer), emotional functioning (BPH), and grade of fatigue (general population) showed itself vital for overall quality of life.

Implications for Practice: The results of this study show that assistance in solving issues of micturition problems, fatigue, and sleeping disturbances may contribute to maintenance of role, social, and emotional aspects of life.

Source: Jakobsson, L., Loven, L., Hallberg, I. R. (2004). Micturition problems in relation to quality of life in men with prostate cancer or benign prostatic hyperplasia: Comparison with men from the general population. Cancer Nursing, 27(3), 218–229.

and flows into the bladder, where it flushes or washes out the blood that oozes from the operative site. The second lumen of the catheter drains the saline, blood, and urine out of the bladder. Immediately postoperatively, the urine is bright red, and the saline must be run in fast enough to prevent clotting of the blood within the bladder that could plug the outflow holes of the catheter. Large 5 liter bags of 0.9% saline are used for this continuous bladder irrigation. The presence of the catheter often creates bladder spasms that are treated with antispasmodic medications.

An alternative to a TURP is transurethral microwave procedure (TUMP). In this hour-long outpatient procedure the enlarged prostatic tissue that impinges into the urethra is heated to 111° F (43.8° C) through a transurethral catheter, while a water cooling system protects the urethra from damage. This microwave therapy does not achieve a cure of the BPH and does not correct incomplete emptying of the bladder. TUMP merely reduces the urinary flow symptoms. A third surgical procedure is the transurethral needle ablation (TUNA). In this procedure low-level radiofrequency energy is emitted through twin needles to burn away the enlarged prostate tissue impinging the urethra. TUNA improves urine flow and relieves urinary symptoms with fewer side effects than TURP.

Pharmacology

Medications can be used instead of surgery in the treatment of mild to moderate BPH. Commonly used medications include nonselective alpha blockers, such as terazosin (Hytrin), alfuzosin (Uroxatral), and doxazosin (Cardura). These medications do not decrease the size of the hypertrophic cells but instead create smooth muscle relaxation of the bladder neck and prostate (Broyles, et al., 2007). Such muscle relaxation leads to an almost immediate improvement in urinary flow. The nonselective alpha blockers can cause orthostatic hypotension. Tamsulosin (Flomax) is a highly selective alpha blocker that maximizes urinary flow with fewer side effects. Finasteride is an antiandrogen agent that prevents conversion of testosterone to DHT helping to shrink the hyperplastic cells. However, finasteride may cause erectile dysfunction and gynecomastia (breast enlargement).

Alternative Therapy

The herb saw palmetto (*Serenoa repens*) has been shown to improve urinary tract symptoms. Saw palmetto has fewer side effects (e.g., orthostatic hypotension, and erectile dysfunction) than the traditional medications. In addition, using the herbal therapy is much less expensive and may have reliable results.

Patient and Family Teaching

Patient teaching for BPH initially focuses on conservative measures to control the primary symptoms associated with impaired urinary flow. Establishment of a consistent medication routine, avoidance of large quantities of late evening fluid intake, and emptying the bladder immediately before going to bed can help to control nocturia that interrupts restful sleep. In social situations, emptying the bladder regularly can help avoid sudden onset of urgency. If surgery becomes the treatment plan, teaching the patient and family what will happen on the day of surgery, how he will feel postoperatively, what treatments will be used postoperatively, and how long he can expect to be hospitalized become paramount.

Evaluation of Outcomes

Potential patient outcomes for each of the example nursing diagnoses for the patient with BPH are:
- Risk for infection from frequent urinary tract infections. The patient remains free of infection, as evidenced by normal vital signs and absence of purulent drainage from wounds, incisions, and tubes. Infection is recognized early to allow for prompt treatment.

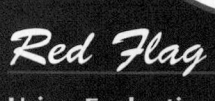

Red Flag

Urine Evaluation

It is especially important to alert the patient and family that the urine will normally appear bloody for several hours postoperatively. The patient and family should be taught to assess for clinical manifestations of low blood volume (e.g., fatigue, skin pallor, or tachycardia), in which case the health care provider should be notified.

- Impaired urinary elimination related to BPH. The patient is continent of urine or verbalizes satisfactory management.
- Risk for disturbed sleep pattern secondary to nocturia. The patient is able to sleep without wakefulness and awakens rested in the morning.

PROSTATE CANCER

Prostate cancer is a condition in which the cells of the prostate gland become abnormal in their morphology. Prostate cancer is the second most commonly diagnosed cancer in men. Only skin cancer is more common. About 70 percent of men diagnosed with this disease are over the age of 65. It has been estimated that 80 percent of the men over age 80 have prostate cancer. A total of 232,090 new cases of prostate cancer and 30,350 deaths from the disease occurred in 2005 (National Cancer Institute, 2005d).

Epidemiology

African American men die from prostate cancer twice as often as Caucasian men. Asian (American) men generally have low rates of prostate cancer. Men of northern European descent have the highest incidence of this disease. There is a 2 to 11 percent increase in risk of developing the disease if a first-degree relative has also had it. However, this risk factor only accounts for 5 to 10 percent of prostate cancer cases. As for other correlates for causation of cancer itself, refer to chapter 15.

Pathophysiology

As in most cancers, prostate cancer develops when the rate of cell division is greater than the rate of cell death. Prostate cancer begins most commonly in the outer portion of the prostate gland. It is accepted that most prostatic cancers are preceded by the development of prostatic intraepithelial neoplasia, characterized by rapid proliferation of both glandular and ductal tissues. These epithelial abnormalities are thought to progress in terms of degree of abnormality and tissues involved until cellular changes are extensive and widespread. Most of the prostate cancer cases are multifocal with multiple areas of simultaneous cancer development. Therefore multiple biopsies (6 to 12) are required for optimal diagnostic detection. Bone is the most common site of metastases (The Prostate Cancer Foundation, 2004).

Assessment with Clinical Manifestations

Incontinence is a common first symptom in men, but it is not unusual for younger men to experience no symptoms. Men over the age of 50 are recommended to have an annual screening digital rectal examination (DRE) (Figure 64-1). Prostate cancer is suspected when the DRE reveals an enlarged, nodular, and hard prostate gland.

Another screening tool used for men over age 50 is the serum PSA. The normal PSA level gradually increases with age so the level at which the PSA is considered abnormal is dependent on the patient's age (Table 64-1).

It must be remembered that conditions, such as BPH, and even recent sexual activity will cause an elevated PSA. Most health care provider will progress to biopsy when the PSA is greater than 4.0 (Dreicer, 2004).

Diagnostic Tests

Transrectal ultrasonography is useful for differentiating between BPH and prostate cancer. A definitive diagnosis is accomplished through biopsy, which is usually a needle biopsy of multiple sites obtained transrectally under ultrasound guidance. Based on the analysis of the biopsy results, the

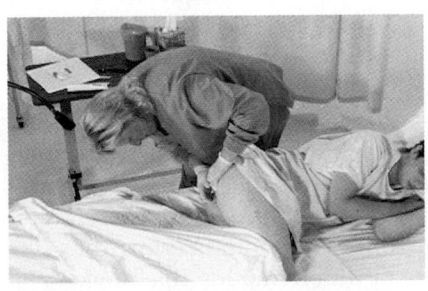

Figure 64-1 Nurse performing a DRE.

TABLE 64-1 PSA Levels

Normal PSA Levels Across Age Ranges

Age younger than 40	40–50	51–60	61–70	Older than 70
Less than 2 ng/mL	Less than 2.5 ng/mL	Less than 3.5 ng/mL	Less than 4.5 ng/mL	Less than 6.5 ng/mL

Elevated PSA Levels

0.25 ng/mL	2.6–10 ng/mL	10.1–19.9 ng/mL	More than 20 ng/mL
Low	Mildly elevated	Moderately elevated	Significantly elevated

Adapted from Daniels, R. (2003). Delmar's manual of laboratory and diagnostic tests. New York: Thomson Delmar Learning; Dreicer, R. (2005). Prostate cancer. Retrieved July 19, 2006, from http://www.clevelandclinicmeded.com.

TABLE 64-2 Gleason Grading System

GLEASON GRADE	1	2	3	4	5
Prostate tissue	Closely packed, well-defined glands	Less uniformly shaped glands	Irregular glands of varying shape	Mass of fused glands	Few if any glands, little difference

Adapted from National Cancer Institute. (2004d). National Cancer Institute cancer facts radiation therapy for cancer: Questions and answers. Retrieved June 16, 2006, from http://cis.nci.nih.gov.

TABLE 64-3 Cancer Staging System

STAGE A OR T1	STAGE B OR T2	STAGE C OR T3	STAGE D OR T4
Not palpable during DRE, confined to prostate	Palpable during DRE, confined to prostate	Palpable, spread beyond prostate but not to other organs	Palpable, spread to organs and often distant sites such as bones or lymph nodes

Adapted from American Joint Committee on Cancer. (2002). Staging systems. Retrieved June 16, 2005, from http://training.seer.cancer.gov.

cancer is then graded and staged. Grading refers to the aggressiveness of the cancer, while staging refers to the localization or spread of the disease. The Gleason Grading System is a commonly used scale for grading prostate cancer (Table 64-2).

At least two separate biopsy specimens are graded based on their differentiation from normal prostate cells. The scores of the two specimens are then added to obtain a score of 2 to 10. A tumor score less then 4 is considered a low-grade cancer that is well differentiated. A score of 5 to 7 is considered an intermediate-grade cancer with moderate differentiation. A score of 8 or greater indicates a high-grade cancer with poor differentiation that tends to be growing rapidly (Theodorescu & Krupski, 2005).

Staging of prostate cancer designates how far beyond the prostate the cancer has spread (Table 64-3). The stage of a cancer often dictates what type of treatment is recommended. Staging is usually reported with either an A to D system or a numeric system. Ultimately, the size of the tumor, how rapidly it is growing, the age of the patient, and the treatment combine to determine life expectancy.

Nursing Diagnoses

Based on the information gathered, examples of nursing diagnoses in the patient with cancer of the prostate may include the following:
- Risk for impaired urinary elimination.
- Fear secondary to the diagnosis of cancer.
- Deficient knowledge related to self-care and risk prevention.

Planning and Implementation

The management strategies for cancer of the prostate are varied with the staging of the cancer and its virility. Treatment options for prostate cancer usually take an interdisciplinary approach and are based on the grade and stage of the disease, as well as the age of the patient. The typical therapies are surgery, medications, and radiation. In general, surgery has good success with treating prostate cancer when surgery is indicated. And, often the growth of the cancer of the prostate is slow enough, that when the cancer is less advanced, and diagnosed early, the patient has a good survival rate with treatment. The primary goal in the treatment of prostate cancer is to prevent the spread of the disease. Nursing care must also focus on assisting the patient to manage the physical and emotional implications of incontinence and impotence.

Radiation Therapy

Radiation therapy is commonly used to treat prostate cancer. Traditional external beam radiation is used, as is intensity modulated radiation therapy (IMRT). IMRT applies computer technology to plan and administer three-dimensional radiation treatment that is both powerful and more specific to the tumor tissue, sparing surrounding tissue. Brachytherapy is the implantation of radioactive seeds directly into the tumor. Brachytherapy is indicated when the tumor is confined to the prostate. About 25 percent of patients experience impotence following definitive radiation therapy (National Cancer Institute, 2005d).

Surgery

The standard surgical procedure for treating early stage, potentially curable prostate cancer in a patient with greater than 10 years' life expectancy is the radical prostatectomy. In this procedure the entire prostate gland and seminal vesicles are removed along with several lymph nodes. Radical prostatectomy can be done via a transabdominal, laparoscopic, transperitoneal or extraperitoneal route (Figure 64-2). Postoperative urinary incontinence occurs in 5 to 10 percent of patients, and sexual impotence can be anticipated because of the risk for nerve damage during manipulation of tissues while accessing the posterior prostate. Currently, there is a newer form of robotic surgery for a prostatectomy. This method is more expensive and has qualifying criteria for those that could have this form of surgery. The robotic method has fewer postoperative complications, and the patient returns to normal activities of daily living more quickly than the suprapubic or other surgical approaches.

Pharmacology

In cases of metastatic or recurrent prostate cancer, androgen deprivation therapy through the use of orchiectomy or medications that suppress the release of luteinizing hormone, such as leuprolide, goserelin, and triptorelin, is sought to decrease or eliminate the availability of testosterone. Approximately 90 percent of cases are tumors dependent on testosterone. Chemotherapy, most often with taxane-based medications, is also commonly used in treating prostate cancer. For general information on chemotherapy, refer to chapter 15.

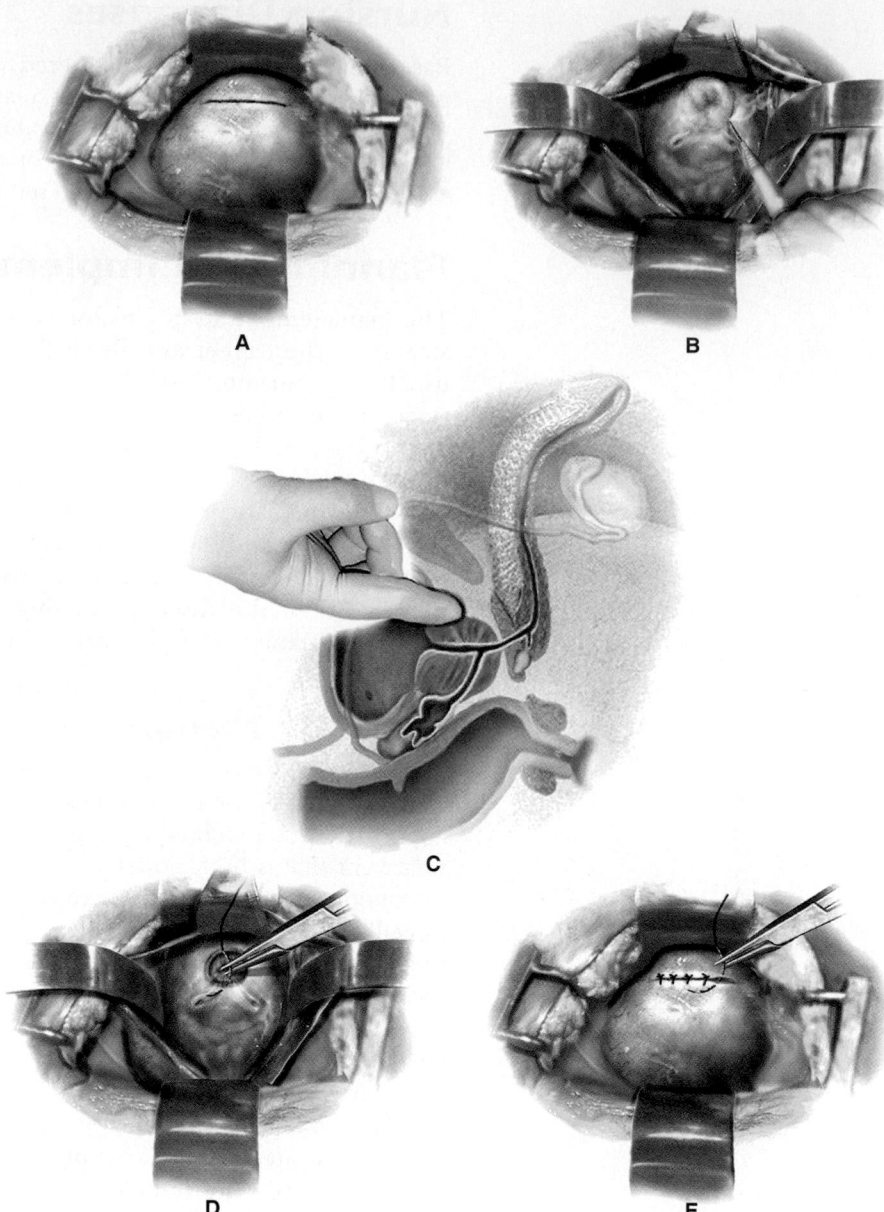

Figure 64-2 Suprapubic prostatectomy: A. Bladder exposed through low transverse incision, B. Bladder entered, C. Blunt dissection of prostate, D. Prostate fossa sutured to bladder mucosa.

Alternative Therapy

Alternative therapy for treatment of prostate cancer includes the herb saw palmetto and oral ingestion of shark or bovine cartilage. The use of these substances results in a decrease in the size of the prostate. Human studies using cartilage administration trials reveal improved outcomes with use of cartilage, but none of the studies was done exclusively on patients with prostate cancer. The study can be reviewed at http://www.cancer.gov.

Patient and Family Teaching

As with any patient with a diagnosis of malignancy teaching must be sensitive, as well as thorough and accurate. Information may need to be provided repeatedly over several sessions when the patient's (or family's) anxiety, fear, and pain are barriers to his being able to focus on the teaching. Facilitating open discussion about an uncertain future, as well as about the important private functions and behaviors associated with urination and sexuality can be challenging. The nurse may need to open such discussions by suggesting some ways the patient must be feeling or some issues that must be concerning to the patient (Mayo Clinic, 2003). Pain management, fluid intake, nourishment, catheter care, perineal muscle exercises to help manage incontinence, wound care, symptoms to report to the health care provider (e.g., infection, bleeding, urinary bladder pain, or leg pain), recommended activity level, fatigue management, and feelings of hopelessness or embarrassment could all be fertile areas for teaching both the patient and those who support him.

Evaluation of Outcomes

Potential patient outcomes for each of the example nursing diagnoses for the patient with cancer of the prostate are:

- Risk for impaired urinary elimination. The patient is continent of urine or verbalizes satisfactory management.
- Fear and anxiety secondary to the diagnosis of cancer. The patient should be able to recognize the signs of anxiety, demonstrate positive coping mechanisms, and describe a reduction in the level of anxiety experienced.
- Deficient knowledge related to self care and risk prevention. The patient should demonstrate motivation to learn, identify perceived learning needs, and verbalize an understanding of desired content.

TESTICULAR CANCER

Cancer of the testes is the most common form of cancer in men ages 15 to 35. It is estimated that 8,010 new cases will be diagnosed in the United States in 2005, resulting in 390 deaths (National Cancer Institute, 2005d). Rates of testicular cancer have more than doubled in the past 40 years, but mortality rates have decreased 60 percent. Testicular cancer is highly treatable and usually a form of curable cancer.

Epidemiology

Scandinavian and Swiss men have the highest incidence, while African and Asian men have the lowest; the United States is in the midrange. Men with untreated congenital cryptorchidism (undescended testis) have a 10 to 40 times increased risk of testicular cancer. Males who have an XXY genotype also have an increased risk of developing testicular cancer and men who were exposed to diethylstilbestrol (DES) in utero may also face a higher risk. At the time of diagnosis, 60 percent of testicular cancers are localized, 24 percent regionalized, and 14 percent have spread to lymph nodes or other organs.

Pathophysiology

The two types of testicular cancer are germinal and nongerminal. Germinal tumors grow from the germinal cells of the testes and may be seminomas or nonseminomas. Seminomas are the most common, are susceptible to treatment by radiation, and have upward of a 90 percent treatment success rate, because they tend to remain localized. The nonseminomas are also referred to as germ cell tumors, are cancers of remaining embryonic tissue, and include choriocarcinoma, yolk sac carcinoma, and teratoma. These are rapid-growing tumors. Nongerminal tumors originate in epithelium. Approximately 95 percent of testicular cancers are germinal and of those, approximately 40 percent are seminomas.

Assessment with Clinical Manifestations

The most common presentation is an otherwise healthy male with a painless lump in the testicle. Testicular self-examination (TSE) is one of the best methods of detecting testicular cancer in its beginning stages (reviewed more specifically later in this section). The appropriate diagnosis and treatment can be delayed if the practitioner merely suspects testicular trauma and prescribes watchful waiting to allow a suspected trauma to resolve spontaneously.

Diagnostic Tests

Painless enlargement of a testis is generally diagnostic of testicular cancer. Transillumination of the scrotum can detect thickened areas or lumps that are potential areas of cancer. However, this is a nonspecific approach and generally regarded as a screening tool. Scrotal ultrasonography more definitively evaluates testicular lumps. An initial needle biopsy of the lump is usually undertaken, although some surgeons will proceed directly to lumpectomy in young patients with negative computerized tomography (CT) scans. The CT scan is performed to detect metastases to other organs, especially to the pelvis and lungs (Daniels, 2003). Lymphangiography can identify lymph node involvement.

Nonseminoma tumors produce alpha fetoprotein (AFP), beta human chorionic gonadotropin (hCG), and lactate dehydrogenase (LDH.) Immunocytochemical analyses are used to identify the malignant cells that produce them. These serum markers are measured at the time of diagnosis and after treatment; if the levels rise after treatment, cancer remains or has recurred and additional treatment is required. Staging of the cancer is based on a variety of factors, including location and spread of the primary tumor, involvement in regional lymph nodes, presence or absence of distant metastases, and the levels of serum tumor markers.

Nursing Diagnoses

Based on the information gathered, examples of nursing diagnoses in the patient with testicular cancer may include the following:

- Fear in response to the diagnosis of testicular cancer.
- Ineffective coping related to anxiety, lower activity level, and the inability to perform normal activities of daily living.
- Disturbed body image related to testicular cancer.

Planning and Implementation

The first nursing goal related to testicular cancer is early detection, which is best accomplished through regular **testicular self-examination (TSE)** (a method of a male assessing their testicles for any changes as a preventive measure against testicular cancer) (Estes, 2006). This technique should be taught to young men, and should be performed on a monthly basis (Figure 64-3). The goal of medical treatment is to eradicate the existing disease and prevent metastases. It is important to note that testicular cancer with multiple metastases is still curable. The well publicized case of bicyclist Lance Armstrong illustrates the value of early management.

Most commonly treatment involves surgery, either lumpectomy or orchiectomy (surgical removal of at least the affected testicle) (Figure 64-4). Nonseminoma tumors are more difficult to stage via CT scanning, and surgical lymph node dissection is frequently required. Patients who have been treated for cancer in one testicle have a 2 to 5 percent rate of recurrent disease in the remaining testicle within 25 years of treatment (National Cancer Institute, 2005d). External beam radiation is also commonly utilized, especially for less invasive cases. Chemotherapy is utilized prior to surgery in patients with symptomatic metastases and after surgery in many cases. All treatment options will at least temporarily decrease sperm production, which may lead to subfertility or infertility after treatment. Prior to the onset of treatment many men will

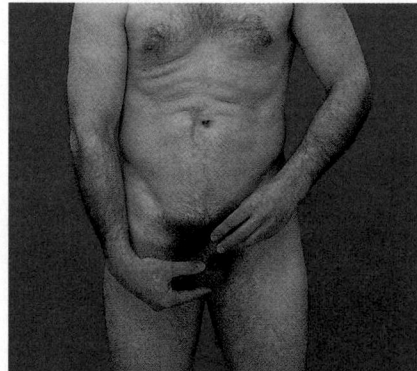
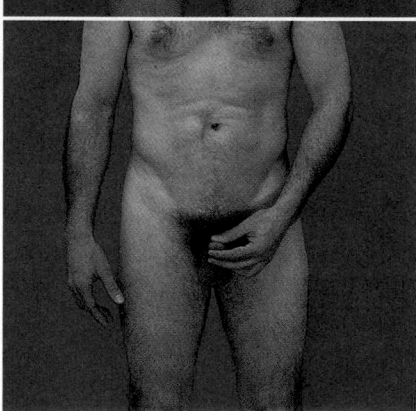

Figure 64-3 Performing a TSE.

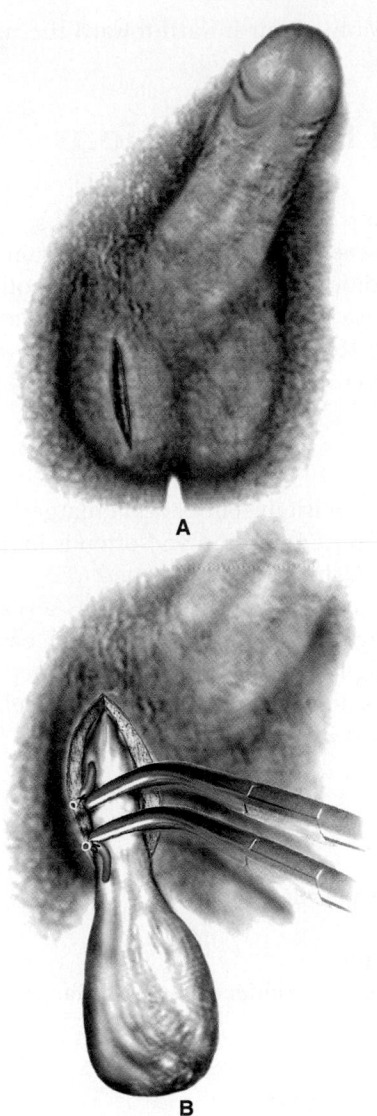

Figure 64-4 Simple orchiectomy: A. Scrotal incision, B. Removal of testicle.

choose to donate and store sperm in a commercial sperm banking facility for use when fertility is desired.

Pharmacology

Testicular cancers are quite successfully treated with chemotherapy. Cisplatin (Platinol) is the most successful chemotherapeutic agent for testicular cancer (National Cancer Institute, 2005d). Bleomycin (Blenoxane) vinblastine (Velban), and ifosfamide (Ifex) are other chemotherapy medications that usually achieve remission. Combined chemotherapy, radiation therapy, and surgery are notable for success even after metastasis is evident.

Patient and Family Teaching

In addition to teaching the patient and family about the positive prognosis for eradication of testicular cancer, the nurse needs to teach them about comfort measures. After the surgical intervention, ice and a scrotal support may help relieve discomfort during recovery.

Evaluation of Outcomes

Potential patient outcomes for each of the example nursing diagnoses for the patient with testicular cancer are:

* Fear in response to the diagnosis of testicular cancer. The patient should manifest positive coping behaviors and verbalize a reduction in the amount of fear of the having this disease.
* Ineffective coping related to anxiety, lower activity level and the inability to perform normal activities of daily living. The patient identifies own maladaptive coping behaviors, available resources and support systems, describes or initiates alternative coping strategies, and describes positive results from new behaviors.
* Disturbed body image related to testicular cancer. The patient demonstrates enhanced body image and self-esteem as evidenced by ability to look at, touch, talk about, and care for actual or perceived altered body part or function.

TESTICULAR TORSION

Testicular torsion is a condition where the testis twists on the spermatic cord within the scrotum, creating venous, lymphatic, and arterial obstruction leading to occlusion with resultant hypoxia of the testicle. The development of testicular torsion may be related to sexual activity or exercise but can also occur during sleep. Testicular torsion is a urological emergency. Incidence in the United States is approximately 1 in 4,000, with the left testicle more commonly involved.

Epidemiology

Testicular torsion occurs most commonly in adolescents and almost always prior to the age of 30. Patients describe a rapid onset of acute pain with scrotal edema developing rapidly after the onset of pain.

Pathophysiology

Testicular torsion is more common in men who have bell clapper deformity, a condition where the tunica vaginalis does not anchor normally to the posterior scrotum. This deformity, which occurs in approximately 12 percent of males, allows the testicle to swing like a bell clapper inside the scrotum. The freedom of movement can lead to torsion. Most torsions occur inward toward the midline of the body.

Assessment with Clinical Manifestations

The primary symptomatology with testicular torsion is the acute pain experienced in the testicular region. The nurse must assess the patient for his subjective response to the pain and have the patient verbalize the level of their pain on the 1 to 10 pain scale (see chapter 16). In addition, the nurse can assess for other clinical manifestations of pain (e.g., hypertension, facial grimacing, or diaphoresis). And, the nurse can assess the patient for their restriction of movement and whether their activities of daily living are affected by the testicular torsion.

Diagnostic Tests

Men with testicular torsion present with an exquisitely tender and enlarged testicle. The affected testicle is usually in a horizontal position and often is higher in the scrotum than the nonaffected testicle. Urinalysis is performed to rule out urinary tract involvement. C-reactive protein levels may be elevated as a result of the inflammatory response to hypoxia. The diagnosis is largely clinical, based on the symptoms. Although diagnostic imaging studies can be performed to assess testicular blood flow, many believe ordering such examinations delays treatment and subsequently decreases the possibility for testicular salvage.

Nursing Diagnoses

Based on the information gathered, examples of nursing diagnoses in the patient with testicular torsion may include the following:
- Acute pain related to testicular torsion.
- Impaired physical mobility secondary to pain.
- Potential for disturbed body image related to orchiectomy secondary to testicular torsion.

Planning and Implementation

The goal of testicular torsion treatment is to untwist the spermatic cord and thus reestablish normal blood flow to the testicle quickly so that the testicle can be salvaged. In the emergency department, the testicle may be manually untwisted to promote blood flow to the testicle; two or three twists may be required to replace the testicle to anatomic position. This procedure is successful in 30 to 70 percent of cases. Orchiopexy is a surgical procedure where the testicle is untwisted on the spermatic cord, and the testicle is then sutured to the scrotum on two sides to prevent recurrence. If surgical treatment occurs within 6 hours of the onset of pain, the testicle is salvaged at least 80 percent of the time; if treatment is delayed 12 hours or more, the hypoxia of the testicle progresses to necrosis and thus the testicle must be removed. Analgesics are the medications used to treat the pain of testicular torsion and to treat postoperative pain. No medications will cure the torsion. Patient teaching is focused on providing comfort. Application of ice and use of a scrotal support can be recommended.

Evaluation of Outcomes

Potential patient outcomes for each of the example nursing diagnoses for the patient with testicular torsion are:
- Acute pain related to testicular torsion. The patient should verbalize an adequate relief of pain along with the ability to realistically cope with the pain if it is not completely relieved.

- Impaired physical mobility secondary to pain. The patient should perform physical activity independently or with assistive devices as needed. In addition, the patient should be free of complications of immobility, as evidenced by intact skin, absence of thrombophlebitis, and normal bowel patterns.
- Potential for disturbed body image related to orchiectomy secondary to testicular torsion. The patient demonstrates enhanced body image and self-esteem as evidenced by ability to look at, touch, talk about, and care for actual or perceived altered body part or function.

ORCHITIS

Orchitis is acute inflammation of the testes, usually as a result of infection and most commonly during concurrent **epididymitis,** infection of the epididymis. Orchitis can be caused by viral, spirochetal, parasitic, or bacterial infections. In the United States, orchitis is most often a result of having contracted a sexually transmitted infection, such as chlamydia (responsible for about 30 percent of orchitis cases) or gonorrhea. Mumps is the most common viral cause of orchitis, with the orchitis occurring four to seven days after the onset of mumps in about 30 percent of males who experience puberty and then contract mumps. Mumps is particularly devastating to men because approximately 30 percent of men who suffer orchitis will develop testicular atrophy and subsequent sterility (Gilbert, 2004). Orchitis can also develop secondary to urinary tract instrumentation, such as an indwelling urinary catheter or cystoscopy.

Pathophysiology

Infection of the genitourinary tract can progress to infection of the testis. The infection causes inflammation, which in turn creates edema. The causative organism in men under age 35 is most often gonorrhea or chlamydia. In men over age 35 and in sexually active gay men the causative organism is more likely to be gram-negative bacteria (Mycyk & Moyer, 2004).

Assessment with Clinical Manifestations

Symptoms of orchitis include fever with painful erythema and edema of the groin, testicles, and scrotum. Pain is often exacerbated by movement or straining for a bowel movement. Dysuria, urethral discharge, and blood in the semen may also be present. Although dysuria can be severe with chlamydia or gonorrhea, there usually is no mechanical blockage of the bladder from orchitis, thus urinary retention is rarely a problem (American Urologic Association, 2004).

Diagnostic Tests

There are several diagnostic tests used to confirm orchitis. There is not a single laboratory study or test that is positive for orchitis. Rather, a compilation of the following tests confirms the presence of orchitis. A complete blood count (CBC) is performed to assess for an elevated white count indicative of infection. When a bacterial cause is suspected, urine and urethral discharge cultures are done to identify the bacteria. Doppler ultrasonography is used to verify increased blood flow to the testis, a sign of inflammation, and rule out testicular torsion.

Nursing Diagnoses

Based on the information gathered, examples of nursing diagnoses in the patient with orchitis may include the following:
- Pain secondary to orchitis.
- Risk for imbalanced body temperature secondary to orchitis.

Planning and Implementation

The goal of management for orchitis is first to identify the organism involved and then treat the underlying cause of the infection. The secondary goal is alleviation of symptoms. While awaiting the lab results to verify the organism involved, broad-spectrum antibiotics may be initiated based on the suspected causative organism as determined from the patient's history. Viral causes have no direct treatment. Common antibiotics for treatment of chlamydia are oral doxycycline or azithromycin (Zithromax). Common antibiotics for gonorrhea treatment include intramuscular (IM) ceftriaxone (Rocephin) or oral (PO) ciprofloxacin (Cipro) or ofloxacin (Floxin). Trimethoprim (Bactrim DS) and sulfamethoxazole (Septra DS) are commonly used for urinary tract infections (Broyles, et al., 2007). NSAIDs may be used to decrease inflammation and pain. Patient teaching is directed toward rapid and effective relief of the symptoms. Bed rest is advised and elevation of the scrotum may decrease pain. Cold packs applied to the area may also decrease pain.

Evaluation of Outcomes

Potential patient outcomes for each of the example nursing diagnoses for the patient with orchitis are:

- Pain secondary to orchitis. The patient should verbalize an adequate relief of pain along with the ability to realistically cope with the pain if it is not completely relieved.
- Risk for imbalanced body temperature secondary to orchitis. The patient maintains body temperature within a normal range.

EPIDIDYMITIS

Epididymitis is inflammation of the epididymis and vas deferens. Inflammation of the epididymis and vas deferens usually develops secondary to bacterial infection in the urinary tract or prostatitis, most commonly chlamydia or gonorrhea. Rarely, noninfectious chemical epididymitis can occur from backflow of urine into the vas deferens during heavy lifting or straining. The epididymis is located like a hood on the top of the testis, extending down the posteriolateral side to the juncture of the vas deferens. That location causes epididymitis to present much like orchitis.

Most cases occur in adults and can be either unilateral or bilateral, but most cases are unilateral. Acute epididymitis presents with a rapid onset of severe symptoms. Chronic epididymitis tends to have a longer, more gradual onset and may never be completely eradicated. As in orchitis, inflammation creates fever along with pain and edema in the scrotum and groin. Chronic epididymitis usually presents only with pain in the scrotum; edema is not usually present (American Urologic Association, 2004).

As in orchitis, bacteria from sexually transmitted infections or urinary tract infections ascend into the epididymis and into the vas deferens. Because of their proximal location, infections of the epididymis and testis often occur simultaneously. For that reason the assessment, diagnostic tests, nursing diagnoses, planning and implementation, and patient and family teaching for epididymitis are identical to those for orchitis (see preceding section).

HYDROCELE, HEMATOCELE, AND SPERMATOCELE

Hydrocele is a fluid-filled sac located along the spermatic cord and within the scrotum. It is a fairly common finding in newborns. This condition may accompany an inguinal hernia, develop from an adjacent infection, or develop secondary to a systemic infection, such as mumps. Trauma to the scrotum may cause hydrocele, especially in older men. Hematocele is similar to hydrocele, but is a blood-filled sac. Spermatocele is a cyst-like structure within the scrotum that contains fluid and dead sperm cells.

Pathophysiology

During fetal development the testes form in the low abdomen and descend along the inguinal canals. If a canal fails to close properly, peritoneal fluid can flow into the scrotum, creating a hydrocele. If hydrocele occurs later in life, the cause is thought to be either overproduction of fluid associated with inflammation, or from reabsorption problems because of lymphatic or venous obstruction (Gilbert, 2003). Hematocele usually results from direct scrotal trauma and is painful. The etiology of spermatocele development is unknown. It has been hypothesized that the condition develops as a result of epididymal duct obstruction that results in a bulging cyst of fluid and sperm.

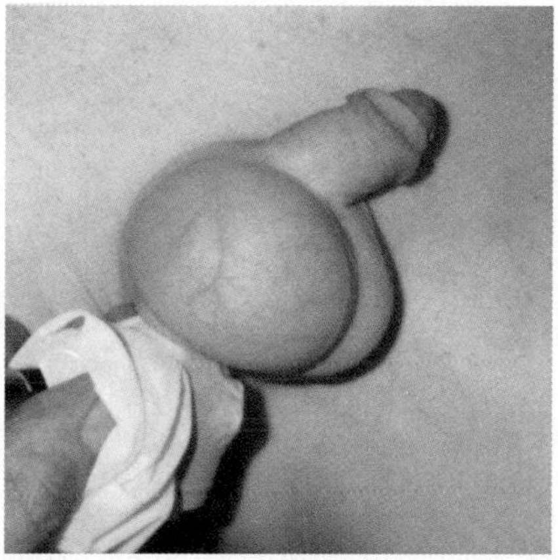

Assessment with Clinical Manifestations

Hydrocele, hematocele, and spermatocele all present with painless swelling or bulging in the scrotum. Hydroceles transilluminate clearly (Figure 64-5), whereas an inguinal hernia, hematocele, and spermatocele do not. The condition is usually unilateral, and the affected side feels much like a water-filled balloon to palpation. If a large amount of fluid is present, the testis can be difficult to palpate. Spermatocele often palpates as a discrete firm mass in the scrotum, located at the epididymis.

Figure 64-5 Transillumination of a hydrocele.

Diagnostic Tests

Scrotal ultrasonography accurately detects these conditions and is used to differentiate among the three conditions. A history of scrotal trauma, systemic illness, or orchitis and epididymitis can help identify the underlying etiology.

Nursing Diagnoses

Based on the information gathered, examples of nursing diagnoses in the patient with any of these cysts may include the following:
- Risk for pain secondary to treatment of hydrocele or hematocele.
- Risk for body image disturbance related to diagnosis.

Planning and Implementation

Most often no treatment is undertaken for these cysts. In the newborn most cases of hydrocele resolve spontaneously within a few months after birth. When treatment is undertaken, it is usually surgery with the goal is to improve comfort or to promote spermatogenesis.

Surgery

In older men, if a hydrocele or hematocele becomes uncomfortably large or disrupts blood flow, surgical repair may be undertaken. Spermatocele may also become significantly uncomfortable and require treatment. Surgical correction may be undertaken if infertility is associated with the spermatocele. Surgical removal of the spermatocele (**spermatocelectomy**) is performed under local anesthesia.

Sclerotherapy is an alternative to surgical treatment. Sclerotherapy is done by inserting a large-bore needle into the spermatocele, aspirating the contents thoroughly, and then injecting a substance that causes inflammation. The inflammatory response causes scarring of the spermatocele to prevent reformation. Approximately 32 percent of patients undergoing sclerotherapy for treatment of spermatocele require a second treatment for complete resolution of the condition (Alsakafi & Kuznetsov, 2004). Analgesics are usually the medications used to manage any of these conditions.

Evaluation of Outcomes

Potential patient outcomes for each of the example nursing diagnoses for the patient with any of these cysts are:
- Risk for pain secondary to treatment of hydrocele or hematocele. The patient should verbalize an adequate relief of pain along with the ability to realistically cope with the pain if it is not completely relieved.
- Risk for body image disturbance related to diagnosis. The patient demonstrates enhanced body image and self-esteem as evidenced by ability to look at, touch, talk about, and care for actual or perceived altered body part or function.

VARICOCELE

Varicocele is a group of varicose veins within the scrotum. A varicocele can enlarge during increased intra-abdominal pressure during a Valsalva maneuver, such as a sneeze or bowel movement.

Pathophysiology

It has been hypothesized that the varicocele has a torturous system of enlarged blood vessels within the scrotum that develops along the spermatic cord as a result of incompetent valves in the left internal spermatic vein. This group of vessels often increases in size with age. **Infertility** or subfertility often occurs in conjunction with varicocele because the increased blood flow in the varicocele raises the scrotal temperature beyond 93.2° F (34° C), the ideal temperature for spermatogenesis.

Assessment with Clinical Manifestations

Pain and tenderness in the scrotum and inguinal discomfort may be evident. About 10 percent of the male population, however, has an asymptomatic varicocele of which they are unaware. When palpated, a varicocele often feels like a bag of worms that is apparent when the patient is upright and greatly diminishes or disappears when the patient is supine.

Diagnostic Tests

The patient with a varicocele disorder is identified primarily by confirmation with the patient history. In addition, scrotal ultrasonography can assist in diagnosis, as can Doppler ultrasonography.

Nursing Diagnoses

Based on the information gathered, examples of nursing diagnoses in the patient with varicocele dysfunction may include the following:
- Acute pain related to the varicocele.
- Deficient knowledge related to self-care and risk prevention.
- Disturbed body image related to infertility.

Planning and Implementation

The goal of therapy is primarily to improve comfort. A secondary goal may be to improve or preserve fertility. The treatment undertaken varies with the age of the patient, the size of the varicocele, the amount of discomfort present, and whether infertility is an issue. If the patient is experiencing discomfort, surgical removal of the varicocele (**varicocelectomy**) may be undertaken. Varicocelectomy is done under local anesthesia and involves ligating the internal spermatic vein. **Embolization** can also be undertaken. Embolization involves introduction of an angiocatheter into the internal spermatic vein, fluoroscopic visualization of the vein, and insertion of steel or platinum springs or detachable silicone balloons into the beginning of the venous defect to correct the dysfunction. Medications used in the treatment of varicocele are primarily analgesics.

Patient and Family Teaching

Teaching for varicocele is focused on postoperative comfort measures. Cold packs to control edema and bleeding from the operative site and elevating the scrotum usually contribute to improved comfort. The nurse needs to ensure that the patient recognizes signs of bleeding or infection that must be reported to the care provider.

Evaluation of Outcomes

Potential patient outcomes for each of the example nursing diagnoses for the patient with varicocele dysfunction are:

- Acute pain related to the varicocele. The patient should verbalize an adequate relief of pain along with the ability to realistically cope with the pain if it is not completely relieved.
- Deficient knowledge related to self-care and risk prevention. The patient should demonstrate motivation to learn, identify perceived learning needs, and verbalize an understanding of desired content.
- Disturbed body image related to infertility. The patient demonstrates enhanced body image and self-esteem as evidenced by ability to talk about and care for actual or perceived altered body part or function and express feelings regarding potential infertility.

VASECTOMY

Vasectomy is surgical sterilization of men through removal, ligation, or destruction of a small portion of the vas deferens to prevent passage of sperm to the urethra. Approximately 500,000 men in the United States choose vasectomy as permanent birth control each year (Johnsen & Davis, 2005.) There is mixed and indefinite evidence linking vasectomy to prostate and testicular cancer.

Assessment with Clinical Manifestations

The most important aspect of assessing a patient prior to vasectomy is to be certain that he understands the permanent nature of the procedure and under no circumstances wants additional children. Men who are uncertain about their decision, considering having children in the future, making the decision during times of great life change, or are undergoing the procedure because of coercion by their partners should be counseled to reconsider their decision. Sperm banking prior to undergoing the procedure may be a consideration.

Nursing Diagnoses

Based on the information gathered, examples of nursing diagnoses in the patient having a vasectomy may include the following:
- Acute pain related to the vasectomy.
- Fear and anxiety related to actual or potential lifestyle changes from the vasectomy.

Planning and Implementation

The goal of a vasectomy is permanent sterilization with minimum side effects. The surgery is performed on an outpatient basis under local anesthesia. A small one-fourth inch incision is made on each side of the scrotum, a portion of the vas deferens is lifted up through the incision and a small section of the vas deferens is removed. The ends of the vas deferens are then cauterized, ligated, or crushed. The vas deferens is then replaced into the scrotum. One small suture is placed to close the incision. In the no-incision method, a puncture is made in the scrotum, the vas deferens is pulled through the puncture wound, and the rest of the surgery proceeds as in the incisional method, except that no suture is needed. Recanalization of the vas deferens can occur if there is leakage into the scrotum from the severed end of the proximal vas deferens. The medications used for vasectomy are primarily analgesics. If necessary, antibiotics are used to treat infection.

Patient and Family Teaching

The nurse's teaching for a vasectomy focuses on comfort measures that promote both physical and psychological health. Initial use of ice packs to control postoperative bleeding and edema and cotton jockey type briefs to provide scrotal support followed by warm sitz baths has been demonstrated to be useful. The patient needs to feel confident that any postoperative edema and discoloration are normal and temporary. The nurse needs to provide the signs and symptoms of infection and of bleeding in writing for the patient's reference, along with instructions about how to notify the health care provider if such symptoms become evident. It is important that the nurse validates that the patient and the partner understand the difference between sterility and impotence and that there will be no effect on sexual capability (erection or ejaculation); that there will be no noticeable change in the amount or consistency of ejaculate, but that it will contain no sperm; that the patient's body will simply reabsorb the sperm; and that vasectomy does not protect against sexually transmitted diseases. The patient will need to be instructed to use contraceptives until all sperm are cleared from the distal vas deferens. The health care provider may order an examination of ejaculate for the presence of sperm approximately one month postoperatively.

Evaluation of Outcomes

Potential patient outcomes for each of the example nursing diagnoses for the patient having a vasectomy are:
- Acute pain related to the vasectomy. The patient should verbalize an adequate relief of pain along with the ability to realistically cope with the pain if it is not completely relieved.
- Fear and anxiety related to actual or potential lifestyle changes from the vasectomy. The patient should be able to recognize the signs of anxiety, demonstrate positive coping mechanisms, and describe a reduction in the level of anxiety experienced.

CRYPTORCHIDISM

Cryptorchidism is also referred to as undescended testes when it is present at birth. In about 70 percent of cases, one testicle has not descended fully and either remains in the inguinal canal or the abdomen. Cryptorchidism occurs in about 3 percent of males and is the most common pediatric genital abnormality. The condition affects about 30 percent of preterm males, because the testis normally descends into the scrotum toward the end of 28 to 40 weeks gestation (Kolon, 2005).

Pathophysiology

Mechanical or hormonal obstruction to the descent of the testes occurs in utero. During the first trimester the testes are formed and migrate into the inguinal canal under the influence of testosterone. If there is inadequate production of testosterone the testes may not descend. If the epididymis does not develop normally the testes will not descend. Occasionally the testes are located ectopically or not within the inguinal canal. Cryptorchidism may occur concurrently with other conditions including Wilms' tumor, cerebral palsy, hypospadias, abnormal epididymis, and abdominal wall defects, such as gastroschisis or omphalocele (hernia of the navel).

Assessment with Clinical Manifestations

The testes may be palpable or nonpalpable. If they are palpable, they are located in the inguinal canal and will usually descend by one year of age. Nonpalpable testes are associated with higher degrees of epididymal abnormalities. Approximately 9 percent of male infants with nonpalpable testes actually have absent testes. Such absence is thought to be caused by a late prenatal vascular occlusion that resulted in hypoxia and necrosis of the testes.

Diagnostic Tests

Cryptorchidism is identified with a thorough assessment of the testes of the patient. In addition, ultrasonography of the groin, pelvis, and lower abdomen usually reveal the location of the testes.

Nursing Diagnoses

Based on the information gathered, examples of nursing diagnoses in the patient with cryptorchidism may include the following:
- Acute pain related to the vasectomy.
- Fear and anxiety related to actual or potential lifestyle changes from the vasectomy.

Planning and Implementation

The goal of care is permanent appropriate location of the testes with surgical intervention. Orchiopexy is the surgical procedure to relocate the testis down through the inguinal canal into the scrotum, where it is anchored. If spontaneous resolution of cryptorchidism does not occur by around one year of age, orchiopexy is usually performed. This procedure is undertaken to prevent progressive failure of spermatogenesis that occurs in undescended testes because of the increased core temperature in the abdomen as compared to the scrotum and to allow earlier detection of testicular cancer if it occurs.

In addition, human chorionic gonadotropin may be given IM to promote bilateral testicular descent. From 250 to 1,000 international units is administered IM (dosage varies by age of the patient) two to three times per week for up to six weeks (Broyles, et al., 2007).

Patient and Family Teaching

The nurse is responsible for providing the parents of a child with an orchiopexy with a written list of the signs and symptoms of bleeding and of infection, as well as information about how to contact a care provider in the event that those symptoms become evident. Comfort measures such as the appropriate application of ice to the scrotal area and use of a soft support are important. It is also critical that the nurse provide information and reassurance to the parents adequate to ensure that parent/child attachment is completed.

Evaluation of Outcomes

Potential patient outcomes for each of the example nursing diagnoses for the patient with cryptorchidism are:
- Acute pain related to the vasectomy. The patient should verbalize an adequate relief of pain along with the ability to realistically cope with the pain if it is not completely relieved.
- Fear and anxiety related to actual or potential lifestyle changes from the vasectomy. The patient should be able to recognize the signs of anxiety, demonstrate positive coping mechanisms, and describe a reduction in the level of anxiety experienced.

PHIMOSIS AND PARAPHIMOSIS

Phimosis is the inability of the foreskin to be stretched and retracted over the glans of the penis. Phimosis can occur congenitally or be acquired as a result of infection or edema. It is important to note that the foreskin is not retractable at birth but becomes retractable usually between two and four years of age. Nearly all infant males have enough movement in the foreskin prepuce that the urethral meatus is visible and urine can flow out. By age 16 less than 1 percent of uncircumcised males continue to experience phimosis (Cantus, 2004).

Congenital phimosis is present at birth and can cause urinary retention when the urethral opening is covered by unretractable foreskin. Acquired phimosis usually develops in situations where penile hygiene to cleanse normal secretions is inadequate and balanitis (inflammation) and adhesions develop. Thickened secretions become encrusted with urinary salts and calcify, forming calculi in the prepuce. Eventually, uncorrected phimosis may predispose the patient to the development of cancer of the penis. Acquired phimosis can result if the foreskin is forcibly retracted and inflammation results. Foreskin piercing can lead to acquired phimosis if infection accompanies the piercing. Phimosis only becomes a surgical emergency when the urethral opening is covered and urine is unable to escape. Surgical correction of phimosis is circumcision.

Paraphimosis is the entrapment of the retracted foreskin behind the glans penis of an uncircumcised male. Paraphimosis is characterized by edema of the foreskin, pain, and erythema. Foreskin piercing can lead to development of paraphimosis if pain from the piercing prevents replacement of a retracted foreskin.

Pathophysiology

The foreskin of an infant is not retractable until the progression of keratinization of the epithelial tissues located between the foreskin and the glans is complete. In acquired phimosis, long-term poor hygiene resulting in chronic balanitis causes fibrotic tissue to form near the prepuce, which adheres the foreskin to the glans. Paraphimosis develops when the foreskin has been retracted for an extended period of time. As edema of the foreskin develops, edema and venous engorgement of the glans quickly follow.

Assessment with Clinical Manifestations

Phimosis, whether congenital or acquired, is diagnosed when the foreskin is not able to be retracted behind the glans penis. Paraphimosis is diagnosed when the foreskin is not able to be replaced over the glans after being retracted.

Diagnostic Tests

Phimosis and paraphimosis are identified by clinical history and assessment. In addition, there are no specific diagnostic tests available to determine the presence of phimosis or paraphimosis.

Nursing Diagnoses

Based on the information gathered, examples of nursing diagnoses in the patient with phimosis and paraphimosis may include the following:
- Impaired urinary elimination.
- Pain related to paraphimosis.

Planning and Implementation

In the case of congenital phimosis the primary goal is to explain to parents and caretakers of the male infant that an unretractable foreskin is a normal finding. This is especially important if the father of the child is circumcised and has no personal experience with care of an uncircumcised penis. In the case of acquired phimosis and paraphimosis, the main goal is that the patient will learn and consistently practice good hygiene.

Surgery

If urinary obstruction exists, either circumcision or dorsal slit surgery is performed to free the urethral opening and allow for urine to flow. If paraphimosis is not resolvable through lubrication of the glans and manual replacement of the foreskin because of inflammation or extensive edema, dorsal slit surgery may be required to restore foreskin mobility.

Patient and Family Teaching

In the case of congenital phimosis without urinary obstruction, adequate education of parents of newborn males must include information on foreskin care including: the foreskin will not be retractable yet; complete retractability of the foreskin can take several years to develop; no parental manipulation of the foreskin is required; forcible retraction of the foreskin can cause paraphimosis; hygiene of the retractable foreskin and glans involves retraction, cleaning, and replacement of the foreskin. In acquired phimosis the patient must be instructed in appropriate hygiene and antibiotic treatment, if balanitis is present. With paraphimosis, appropriate penile and foreskin hygiene must be taught, including the need to both retract and replace the foreskin.

Evaluation of Outcomes

Potential patient outcomes for each of the example nursing diagnoses for the patient with phimosis and paraphimosis are:
- Impaired urinary elimination. The patient is continent of urine or verbalizes satisfactory management.
- Pain related to paraphimosis. The patient should verbalize an adequate relief of pain along with the ability to realistically cope with the pain if it is not completely relieved.

BALANITIS AND POSTHITIS

Balanitis is inflammation of the glans penis. Balanitis usually occurs in uncircumcised or partially circumcised males. **Posthitis** is inflammation of the foreskin and thus only occurs in uncircumcised or partially circumcised males. If posthitis occurs concurrently with balanitis, the condition is termed **balanoposthitis.**

Etiology

Usually a bacterial infection is the causative agent for balanitis and posthitis. In extreme cases urinary obstruction can occur as a result of balanitis. Phimosis can also occur. Balanitis accounts for 11 percent of adult visits to urology clinics (Leber, 2005). Diabetes is the most common cause of balanitis, but chemical irritation from soaps or other products applied to the penis can also be to blame. Right-sided congestive heart failure (CHF) can also contribute to balanitis because of the edema that develops as a result of the CHF. In cases of morbid obesity, hygiene may be extremely difficult or impossible to perform, resulting in balanitis. In addition, if the foreskin is not retracted, the glans then cleaned, and the foreskin replaced, balanitis can occur. Bacterial, viral, or fungal infections can create balanitis.

Pathophysiology

The pathology of these infection-induced conditions is primarily the result of the inflammatory processes. Thus, the initiation of the typical infection increases in swelling of fluids to the areas of infection, warmth and redness in the areas of the infection, and other cellular responses to the inflammation of these conditions.

Assessment with Clinical Manifestations

The typical clinical manifestations for balanitis and posthitis include penile discharge, pain, erythema, and edema. In addition, it is important that the history includes hygienic practices along with the onset and severity of symptoms.

Diagnostic Tests

Diagnostic tests include culture of any discharge present to identify the causative organism involved. A wet mount to detect fungi is performed and serology for syphilis may also be obtained. If the patient is known, or suspected, to be diabetic, serum glucose or hemoglobin A_{1C} may be ordered as part of a comprehensive diabetes workup.

Nursing Diagnoses

Based on the information gathered, examples of nursing diagnoses in the patient with balanitis and posthitis may include the following:
- Impaired urinary elimination related to phimosis secondary to balanitis.
- Pain related to balanitis.

Planning and Implementation

In order that appropriate treatment can be quickly undertaken, identification of the causative organisms is the first goal. Prevention of recurrence is another goal and must be directed at the appropriate cause. Medications that treat the causative organism are utilized. If bacterial infection is suspected, topical antibiotic ointments, such as Neosporin, are used. If fungal infection is detected, topical clotrimazole (Lotrimin) is applied twice daily. Patients are instructed to retract the foreskin and soak in warm water daily to thoroughly clean the glans. Appropriate treatment of causative organisms should be undertaken. If phimosis leading to urinary obstruction is present, dorsal slit surgery may be required.

Evaluation of Outcomes

Potential patient outcomes for each of the example nursing diagnoses for the patient with balanitis and posthitis are:
- Impaired urinary elimination related to phimosis secondary to balanitis. The patient is continent of urine or verbalizes satisfactory management.
- Pain related to balanitis. The patient should verbalize an adequate relief of pain along with the ability to realistically cope with the pain if it is not completely relieved.

URETHRITIS

Urethritis is inflammation of the urethra, which most commonly occurs with a genitourinary tract infection but can also be due to trauma. Posttraumatic urethritis occurs in up to 20 percent of men who must self-catheterize for urinary elimination and is 10 times more common with latex catheters than with silicone catheters. Urethritis can accompany other infectious processes, such as orchitis or prostatitis or even otitis media. Symptoms include dysuria, penile discharge, and erythema.

Pathophysiology

Urethritis inflammation secondary to cystitis is frequently caused by gram-negative bacteria, but sexually transmitted infections, such as gonorrhea and chlamydia, comprise at least 80 percent of urethritis cases. Both gonorrhea and chlamydia will often present initially as urethritis, because the urethra is the portal of entry for the infectious organisms. Sudden onset of dysuria with penile discharge is suggestive of either gonococcal or chlamydial infection. Traumatic urethritis can lead to urethral stricture.

Assessment with Clinical Manifestations

Urethritis is assessed by evaluating the onset of symptoms, sexual history, and medical history including self-catheterization. Temperature and white blood cell count should be assessed for elevations that suggest the presence of urethritis. Urinary frequency or urgency are rarely present in males with urethritis, and suggest, instead, prostatitis. The penis must be palpated for painful localized fluctuant areas that may indicate abscess formation.

Diagnostic Tests

Diagnostic tests for urethritis include urine culture if cystitis or prostatitis is also suspected, and urethral discharge culture or polymerase chain reaction testing for suspected gonorrhea and chlamydia infections. A retrograde urethrogram may be ordered if a foreign body is suspected.

Nursing Diagnoses

Based on the information gathered, examples of nursing diagnoses in the patient with urethritis may include the following:
- Impaired urinary elimination related to urethritis.
- Pain related to urethritis.

Planning and Implementation

The goals of care for urethritis are to prevent recurrence and complications and to encourage compliance with the treatment regimen to ensure a complete cure of the infection. In addition, appropriate antibiotic therapy is administered. Common antibiotics for treatment of chlamydia are oral doxycycline or azithromycin (Zithromax). Common antibiotics for gonorrhea treatment include IM ceftriaxone (Rocephin) or PO ciprofloxacin (Cipro) or ofloxacin (Floxin). Trimethoprim and sulfamethoxazole (Bactrim DS or Septra DS) are commonly used for urinary tract infections. NSAIDs may be used to decrease inflammation and pain (Broyles, et al., 2007).

Traumatic urethritis cases should be managed by an urologist to help prevent complications such as urethral stricture. Patient education on safer sex practices, including monogamy and consistent use of condoms, should be provided for patients with suspected or documented cases of sexually transmitted infections. Patients should also be educated about the need to complete the entire course of antibiotics to achieve complete eradication of the infection.

Evaluation of Outcomes

Potential patient outcomes for each of the example nursing diagnoses for the patient with urethritis are:
- Impaired urinary elimination related to urethritis. The patient is continent of urine or verbalizes satisfactory management.
- Pain related to urethritis. The patient should verbalize an adequate relief of pain along with the ability to realistically cope with the pain if it is not completely relieved.

URETHRAL STRICTURE

Urethral stricture is a narrowing or stenosis of the urethra. The main symptom is difficulty voiding and a noticeably decreased urine stream that can develop either gradually or suddenly. Dysuria, pelvic pain, and increased urinary frequency or urgency are also often present. The risk factors for development of urethral stricture are men who have experienced multiple episodes of urethritis, prostatitis, sexually transmitted infections, BPH, or trauma to the urethra (including instrumentation). Rarely, complete urinary obstruction develops.

Pathophysiology

Urethral stricture is caused by inflammation. Severe or repeated episodes of inflammation can lead to the development of fibrotic scar tissue, which in turn, narrows the urethral diameter as the scarring builds up. Recurrence is high after treatment (Gilbert, 2004).

Assessment with Clinical Manifestations

The description of the onset of symptoms and presence of risk factors (e.g., self-catheterization or recent instrumentation) must be assessed. In addition, the patient history is important to evaluate the clinical manifestations for suspected urethral stricture.

Diagnostic Tests

Diagnostic tests for suspected urethral stricture include urinary flow rate, ultrasound postvoiding residue measurement, urinalysis with culture, tests for gonorrhea and chlamydia. Also if indicated either a retrograde urethrogram or cystoscopy is performed for confirmation of urethral stricture.

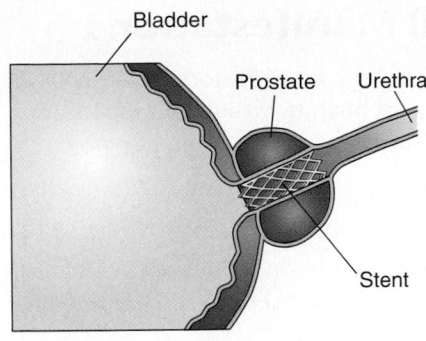

Figure 64-6 Urethral stent.

Nursing Diagnoses

Based on the information gathered, examples of nursing diagnoses in the patient with urethral stricture may include the following:

- Impaired urinary elimination secondary to urethral stricture.
- Deficient fluid volume related to lack of oral fluid intake secondary to lengthy, painful urination.

Planning and Implementation

The primary goal for the management of urethral stricture is to facilitate urinary drainage to prevent urinary stasis, which can lead to a urinary tract infection or to hydronephrosis. Treatment is usually successful, but there is a high rate of recurrence of stricture. With small strictures, urethral dilation can be accomplished by inserting gradually increasing diameter instruments into the stricture until normal diameter is achieved. A urethral stent may be placed using a cystoscopic approach (Figure 64-6). If urinary retention has developed as a result of the severity of the stricture, a suprapubic urinary catheter may be placed. **Urethrotomy** (an opening in the urethra) can decrease the stricture size, at least on a temporary basis. This procedure involves direct visualization of the urethra through an endoscope to create small longitudinal incisions through the fibrotic scar tissue.

Open **urethroplasty** may need to be performed. This procedure involves removing the diseased portion of the urethra and inserting a new urethra that is constructed using other tissue. In some cases, a urinary diversion is created so that self-catheterization can be performed through the abdominal wall. Medications are usually not helpful in treatment of urethral stricture.

Evaluation of Outcomes

Potential patient outcomes for each of the example nursing diagnoses for the patient with an urethral stricture are:

- Impaired urinary elimination secondary to urethral stricture. The patient is continent of urine or verbalizes satisfactory management.
- Deficient fluid volume related to lack of oral fluid intake secondary to lengthy, painful urination. The patient experiences adequate fluid volume and electrolyte balance as evidenced by urine output greater than 30 mL/hour, normotensive blood pressure, heart rate 100 beats/minute, consistency of weight, and normal skin turgor.

EPISPADIAS AND HYPOSPADIAS

Both epispadias and hypospadias are congenital malformations involving the location of the urethral meatus. Misplacement or malformation occurs in approximately 1 in 300 male births. When the urinary meatus is located along the superior (upper) aspect of the penis, the condition is referred to as **epispadias.** When the urinary meatus is located along the inferior (lower) aspect of the penis, the condition is referred to as **hypospadias.** Either variant can occur anywhere along the length of the penis but occur most commonly on the glans of the penis. Aside from controlling urinary flow direction, the greatest problem with epispadias and hypospadias is infertility, because sperm will be deposited in the vagina rather than near the cervix. Most cases of epispadias and hypospadias are considered a nuisance and not a threat to health.

Pathophysiology

The pathophysiology of both epispadias and hypospadias is an incomplete closure of the urethra during fetal development. The urethral opening then forms prior to the tip of the glans. The farther from the glans the urethral opening occurs, the more complex the surgical repair will be.

Assessment with Clinical Manifestations

Assessment is based on clinical findings and the patient history. The defect of both epispadias and hypospadias is apparent at birth by visualizing the location of the foreskin prepuce in relationship to the glans penis.

Diagnostic Tests

The diagnosis of epispadias and hypospadias is made on visualization and clinical assessment. Other diagnostic tests are usually not required, because diagnosis is based on clinical findings alone.

Nursing Diagnoses

Based on the information gathered, examples of nursing diagnoses in the patient with epispadias and hypospadias may include the following:
- Deficient knowledge related to the diagnosis of epispadias and hypospadias.
- Disturbed body image related to abnormal genital formation.

Planning and Implementation

The goals of care for epispadias or hypospadias are to promote acceptance of this anomaly by the parents and to facilitate normal penile function during voiding and sexual intercourse. If the defect is midshaft or lower, or if there are multiple urethral openings, surgery for urethral reconstruction is done before the child is 2 years of age. Circumcision will not be performed on infants with these defects, because the foreskin needs to be preserved so that it can be used as a tissue graft during reconstructive surgery.

Evaluation of Outcomes

Potential patient outcomes for each of the example nursing diagnoses for the patient with epispadias and hypospadias are:
- Deficient knowledge related to the diagnosis of epispadias and hypospadias. The patient should demonstrate motivation to learn, identify perceived learning needs, and verbalize an understanding of desired content.
- Disturbed body image related to abnormal genital formation. The patient demonstrates enhanced body image and self-esteem as evidenced by ability to look at, touch, talk about, and care for actual or perceived altered body part or function.

PEYRONIE'S DISEASE

Peyronie's disease is the formation of dense fibrotic scar tissue plaques in the corpora cavernosa, the tissue that engorges with blood during penile erection. These plaques lack flexibility and cause the penis to curve during erection, sometimes to the point of making intercourse impossible. This condition affects about 1 to 3 percent of men, most commonly between the ages of 40 and 65. Acute onset cases often follow trauma, but gradual onset cases often have no known history of trauma. The condition is most common in men of northern European descent, uncommon in men of African descent, and rare in men of Asian descent (Cornell University Department of Urology, 2005).

Pathophysiology

The pathophysiology of Peyronie's disease is not fully understood. It is hypothesized that trauma to the penis creates localized bleeding that, in turn, leads to inflammation. The inflammatory process becomes fibrotic plaques as the red cells are reabsorbed and the inflammation resolves. These plaques are inflexible and occur between the tunica and the corpus cavernosa. About 30 percent of men with Peyronie's disease will also develop fibrotic areas in other parts of their bodies, such as Dupuytren's contracture of the hand. There is a familial tendency toward Peyronie's (National Kidney and Urologic Diseases Information, 2003).

Assessment with Clinical Manifestations

A history of the onset of symptoms including progression must be obtained. Cases can range from a mild nuisance to those causing severe pain during erection and difficulty with penile penetration for intercourse. Symptoms can be slow in progression or develop overnight.

Diagnostic Tests

Diagnostic tests are usually not indicated, because the diagnosis is made on clinical findings. An important physical finding is inability to stretch the penis. The presence of plaques significantly decreases the ability of the penis to stretch.

Nursing Diagnoses

Based on the information gathered, examples of nursing diagnoses in the patient with Peyronie's disease may include the following:
- Deficient knowledge related to Peyronie's disease.
- Sexual dysfunction secondary to Peyronie's disease.

Planning and Implementation

The primary goal of treatment for Peyronie's disease is to maintain sexual function and activity in patients. Urologists believe that the majority of cases will resolve spontaneously within one to two years and do not require treatment (Peyronie's Disease, 2003). In severe cases, surgical removal of the plaque may be performed. Medications are generally not effective in treating Peyronie's disease.

Evaluation of Outcomes

Potential patient outcomes for each of the example nursing diagnoses for the patient with Peyronie's disease are:
- Deficient knowledge related to Peyronie's disease. The patient should demonstrate motivation to learn, identify perceived learning needs, and verbalize an understanding of desired content.

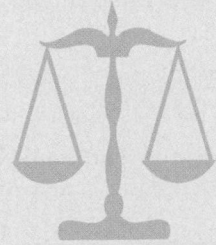

ETHICS IN PRACTICE

Aberrant Sexual Practices

The nurse must be careful and nonjudgmental in providing care for the patient with Peyronie's disease. An objective recording of the patient's description of symptoms is essential, because trauma to the penis may have been caused by aberrant sexual practices. In addition, the patient may be sensitive or embarrassed by the dysfunction and without sensitivity to communication and emotions, the patient may not feel open enough to share information with the nurse. Ethically, the nurse is bound to not have a condemning voice tone or visual responses that allow the patient to feel they are not being supported.

• Sexual dysfunction secondary to Peyronie's disease. The patient will verbalize satisfaction with the way he expresses physical intimacy.

CANCER OF THE PENIS (BOWEN'S DISEASE)

Penile cancer is usually squamous cell carcinoma. It is a rare condition, affecting about 1,000 men per year in the United States and Europe combined. Cancer of the penis accounts for 0.4 to 0.6 percent of all malignancies. However, penile cancer represents 20 to 30 percent of malignancies in Asia, Africa, and South America. About 48 percent of penile cancers occur on the glans, 21 percent occur on the prepuce, 9 percent affect the glans and the prepuce, and about 2 percent occur on the penile shaft. Up to 75 percent of patients diagnosed with this cancer also have phimosis (Brosman, 2004.) Penile cancer rarely occurs in men who were circumcised as newborns.

Pathophysiology

Genital herpes and human papillomavirus (HPV) infections are associated with increased rates of penile cancer. Penile intraepithelial neoplasia progresses to penile cancer in about 15 percent of cases. The cancer initially is a small lesion that can be flat, slightly raised, or crater-like in appearance and that enlarges over time. Lesions that are 5 cm in diameter or broader or that cover 75 percent or more of the penile shaft tend to have more metastases to lymph nodes and a lower survival rate (Brosman, 2004). The lesions tend to be painless. Because of the rich blood and lymphatic supplies to the penis, metastases occur readily. Death occurs within two years in untreated patients. Cure rates of 82 to 85 percent have been reported in patients undergoing treatment who have one to three nodes involved (Brosman, 2004).

Assessment with Clinical Manifestations

Patients reporting lesions or sores on their penis that do not heal should be examined. The patient needs to be evaluated regarding their pain level and subjective acceptance and understanding of their disorder.

Diagnostic Tests

Biopsy is used to definitively diagnose cancer. MRI or CT may be obtained in men with positive biopsies to determine lymph node involvement. The Jackson Classification system is commonly used to determine the grade of the cancer (Table 64-4).

Nursing Diagnoses

Based on the information gathered, examples of nursing diagnoses in the patient with cancer of the penis may include the following:

TABLE 64-4 **Jackson Classification System That Grades Cancer of the Penis**

STAGE I (A)	STAGE II (B)	STAGE III (C)	STAGE IV (D)
Confined to glans or prepuce	Extends onto shaft	Operable inguinal metastasis	Involves adjacent structures, associated with inoperable inguinal metastasis or distant metastasis

Adapted from Brosman, S. (2004). Penile cancer. Retrieved June 23, 2006, from http://www.emedicine.com.

- Deficient knowledge related to cancer of the penis.
- Sexual dysfunction secondary to cancer of the penis.

Planning and Implementation

The goal of penile cancer treatment is to remove the cancer while it is still in a small and localized stage retaining normal or nearly normal, residual penile function. Up to 50 percent of patients will delay seeking care when lesions develop because of embarrassment or fear. Care may not be sought until odor from necrosis and infection is evident. Treatment is determined by the size of the lesion and ranges from laser ablation to excisional biopsy to partial or total penectomy. Circumcision is recommended as a part of therapy to improve access to and visualization of lesions. Radiation therapy is often performed instead of penectomy because of the psychological aspects of such surgery. External beam radiation tends to require high doses and can result in fistula or stricture formation. Brachytherapy has fewer side effects. Cisplatin, bleomycin, methotrexate, and fluorouracil are chemotherapeutic medications that are often used either alone or in conjunction with radiation therapy.

Evaluation of Outcomes

Potential patient outcomes for each of the example nursing diagnoses for the patient with cancer of the penis are:
- Deficient knowledge related to cancer of the penis. The patient should demonstrate motivation to learn, identify perceived learning needs, and verbalize an understanding of desired content.
- Sexual dysfunction secondary to cancer of the penis. The patient will verbalize satisfaction with the way they express physical intimacy.

ERECTILE DYSFUNCTION

Erectile dysfunction (ED) is the inability to create or to maintain an erection of the penis for the purpose of intercourse. The term most commonly used for this condition is impotence, but ED is being used more often by the lay public as a result of ED medication advertising.

Etiology

Diabetes is the most common endocrine disease that leads to ED, but pituitary tumors and thyroid disease can also be culprits. Stroke, aging, and chronic renal failure also affect blood flow to the penis. Multiple sclerosis and other neuropathies damage the nerves that serve the penis and can also be associated with ED, as can Parkinson's. Medications, such as psychoactive agents and anticholinergics, and chemicals can also affect penile erection. Cigarette smoking markedly decreases penile blood flow, as do alcohol and marijuana. Beta blockers and calcium channel blockers used in the treatment of hypertension can cause ED, as can most medications used for prostate gland enlargement. About 1 percent of men with abdominal aneurysms also have ED.

Pathophysiology

The exact physiology of penile erection is only partially understood. The cause of ED can be psychogenic or physiological. Psychogenic erectile dysfunction is complex, may be related to anxiety or fatigue, and can be temporary or long term. Physiologically, parasympathetic nerve impulses and hormones, such as epinephrine, norepinephrine, acetyl choline, prostaglandins, and nitric oxide, work together to dilate small arteries in the penis sending blood to engorge the corpora cavernosa, causing the penis to become firm and stand upright. Physiological ED is often related to impaired arterial circulation. Arteries within the penis or the arteries in the pelvis leading to the penis may be partially occluded, resulting in insufficient blood flow to the corpora cavernosa to achieve or to sustain firm erection. Thus, erectile dysfunction can be an indicator of systemic atherosclerotic disease.

Assessment with Clinical Manifestations

The complex interdependent psychophysiologic nature of ED requires a detailed physical, psychological, and sexual history and examination. A history of the symptoms and the progression of symptoms is important, clarifying details as appropriate.

Diagnostic Tests

The majority of men presenting with ED do not require a detailed workup. However, a number of investigations exist to determine the cause of a patient's ED. Such investigations include: vascular testing, such as duplex ultrasound and dynamic infusion cavernosometry or cavernosography; neurological testing, such as a biothesiometry, somatosensory evoked potentials and pudendal electromyography; and nocturnal penile tumescence and rigidity analysis. Much debate has been conducted on the indications for such investigations. Adjunctive investigations are reserved for the following groups of patients: (a) patients who are potentially curable: this group includes patients with a high risk for primarily psychogenic ED, patients with endocrinopathy, young males with traumatically induced pure arteriogenic ED, and young males with isolated crural venous leak; (b) patients with penile curvature prior to undergoing penile reconstructive surgery; and (c) medicolegal cases (Cornell University Department of Urology, 2005).

Nursing Diagnoses

Based on the information gathered, examples of nursing diagnoses in the patient with ED may include the following:
- Deficient knowledge related to ED.
- Sexual dysfunction secondary to ED.

Planning and Implementation

The management for ED is complicated and requires sensitive communication and care by the nurse. In general, the overall goal of ED treatment is to achieve a functional erection. Nonpharmacological treatment options include vacuum devices that fit over the penis and when negative pressure is created, blood is drawn into the penile shaft. Once the penis is erect a constriction band is placed around the base of the shaft to maintain the firmness. Surgically placed penile implants are also available. The inflatable prosthesis has a reservoir and pump that are located in the scrotum and used to inflate or deflate the penis. The semirigid rod (Small-Carrion) prosthesis creates a permanent partial erection.

Pharmacology

Medications used to treat ED include oral selective enzyme inhibitors, such as sildenafil (Viagra), vardenafil (Levitra), and tadalafil (Cialis) taken 30 minutes to eight hours prior to sexual activity. However, 30 to 50 percent of men with low serum testosterone levels do not respond to Viagra alone and require concomitant testosterone replacement therapy. Side effects of Viagra may include headache, flushing, and blue-tinged vision. Viagra is

Skills 360°

Therapeutic Communication with Patients Who Have ED

The nurse must remember to be professional when communicating with patients who have ED. The nurse should think through his or her own feelings of either embarrassment or being uncomfortable when discussing the sexuality issues with patients who have ED. In addition, the nurse can also make referrals to sexuality counselors or social workers whose specialty is working with patients who have sexual disorders. In general, the nurse needs to appear objective, yet empathetic to the patient in open discussions regarding the ED issue.

contraindicated for patients on nitrate therapy and patients who have retinopathy. Yohimbine (Yohimbine or Yocon) must be taken for six to eight weeks to see results.

The selective enzyme inhibitors are contraindicated in patients with angina, a history of myocardial infarction or cerebrovascular accident in the last six months, unstable hypertension, and those taking nitrites or alpha blockers. Injections into the corpus cavernosa of prostaglandin (Caverject) or phentolamine (Regitine) successfully creates erection in 80 percent of patients in 5 to 15 minutes and should only be used every four to seven days. Urethral suppositories (alprostadil) containing prostaglandin (Muse) will produce erection in about 60 percent of men. Vasoactive agents, such as alprostadil or papaverine may be injected directly into the penis (Broyles, et al., 2007).

Patient and Family Teaching

Patient education regarding ED requires sensitivity from the nurse. An open and communicating relationship is essential between the patient and the health care provider. One aspect of the teaching is about potential side effects of medications used to treat ED. Information about how to contact a health care provider in case of an untoward reaction to a medication must also be provided. The patient and his partner must be supported as they learn to adapt their sexual practices to use of a prosthesis. The signs and symptoms of migration of a prosthesis must be clearly understood by the patient and his partner, and the nurse may find it useful to collaborate with a sex therapist. Referral to Impotence Anonymous (I-anon), a 10-step program, may also be indicated.

Evaluation of Outcomes

Potential patient outcomes for each of the example nursing diagnoses for the patient with ED are:
- Deficient knowledge related to ED. The patient should demonstrate motivation to learn, identify perceived learning needs, and verbalize an understanding of desired content.
- Sexual dysfunction secondary to ED The patient will verbalize satisfaction with the way they express physical intimacy.

PRIAPISM

Priapism is the presence of a prolonged, often painful, penile erection. Two types exist: arterial high-flow and veno-occlusive. Veno-occlusive priapism is seen most often in men with sickle cell disease. About 40 percent of men with sickle cell disease report having had at least one episode of priapism, with peak incidence between the ages of 19 and 21. Priapism can also occur as a side effect to the use of intracavernosal injections of medication used to treat ED.

Etiology

Conditions that are associated with the development of priapism include sickle cell, leukemia, amyloidosis, malaria, carbon monoxide poisoning, black widow spider bites, and spinal anesthesia. Many medications can also cause priapism. These include the psychotropic medications, especially chlorpromazine (Thorazine), trazodone (Desyrel), thioridazine (Mellaril), and citalopram (Celexa). Hydralazine (Apresoline), metoclopramide (Reglan), omeprazole (Prilosec), hydroxyzine (Vistaril), prazosin (Minipress), and other calcium channel blockers, have also been implicated in causing priapism. Androstenedione

(Andro), often used to enhance athletic ability, can also create priapism. Cocaine, marijuana, ecstasy, and methamphetamines are illicit drugs that can cause priapism.

Pathophysiology

In priapism, the corpora cavernosa remains engorged with blood because of malfunctioning of the valve system that controls the onset and release of erections. There are two main types of priapism: arterial high-flow priapism and veno-occlusive priapism. Arterial high-flow priapism is rare, is usually painless and occurs when a cavernosa artery has ruptured, usually secondary to penetrating or blunt trauma to the penis. Due to arterial spasm or clot formation, the priapism may not develop immediately after trauma. Veno-occlusive priapism is painful and occurs when a vein is occluded which prevents cavernosa drainage. If not treated promptly, the venous occlusion can create the formation of fibrotic tissue within a few hours, which in turn can lead to the loss of ability to achieve an erection (Carey, 2004).

Assessment with Clinical Manifestations

A thorough review of medical history, onset of symptoms, history of trauma, and current legal and illicit medication use is crucial to understanding the underlying causes of priapism. The nurse will need to use therapeutic communication carefully and support the patient while asking questions in obtaining a history of the condition.

Diagnostic Tests

Obviously, the priapism is recognized upon observational assessment. However, laboratory studies including CBC and coagulation studies are indicated to rule out leukemia and detect coagulopathy. Doppler flow studies can help differentiate between high-flow and veno-occlusive priapism. In cases suspected to be caused by arterial high-flow, penile artery angiography may be obtained (Daniels, 2003).

Nursing Diagnoses

Based on the information gathered, examples of nursing diagnoses in the patient with priapism may include the following:
- Deficient knowledge related to priapism.
- Sexual dysfunction secondary to priapism.

Planning and Implementation

The goal of treating priapism is to resolve the condition before the fibrotic changes take place and cause permanent damage that leaves the patient unable to achieve erection in the future. Ice packs to the perineum will resolve some cases. Most cases require pharmacological intervention or other procedures. Selective embolization of problematic arteries is sometimes utilized. The treatment most commonly used is to aspirate 20 to 30 mL of blood by inserting a large-bore needle on a large syringe into the corpus cavernosa; multiple puncture sites and aspirations are usually required. This procedure is performed after penile nerve block has been achieved.

Pharmacology

There are a variety of medications used to manage priapism (Table 64-5). These medications have different results and are managed by the symptomatic response of the patient.

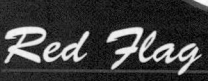

Red Flag

Priapism in the Emergency Department

The patient with priapism may seek the emergency department and when he is first admitted, the patient may be embarrassed about his condition. The nurse must solicit information from the patient, while working with the patient using good therapeutic communication skills. It is necessary to find out what medications the patient has been taking and if there are other potential causative agents that need to be identified quickly.

TABLE 64-5 Medications in Management of Priapism

MEDICATION	MECHANISM OF ACTION	DOSE
Metaraminol bitartrate	Strong arterial vasoconstrictor	100–500 mcg per dose, up to 10 doses administered in a dilute solution (1 mL of phenylephrine to 499 mL of saline 0.9%) 10–20 mL per dose via intracavernosal injection every 5–10 minutes.
Ethylene blue	Smooth muscle relaxant	1–2 mg/kg IV slowly over 5 minutes
Phenylephrine (Neo-Synephrine)	Arteriole vasoconstrictor	100–500 mcg per dose, up to 10 doses; use 10–20 mL of 20 mcg/mL solution via intracavernosal injection every 10 minutes
Metaraminol (Aramine)	Arterial vasoconstriction	0.5–1 mg intravenously; repeat after 5 minutes
Terbutaline (Brethaire, Bricanyl)	Smooth muscle relaxant	5 mg by mouth every 15 minutes for three doses 0.25–0.50 mg subcut every 15 minutes for three doses

Adapted from Broyles, B. E., Reiss, B. S., & Evans, M. E. (2007). Pharmacological aspects of nursing care (7th ed.). New York: Thomson Delmar Learning.

Evaluation of Outcomes

Potential patient outcomes for each of the example nursing diagnoses for the patient with priapism are:

- Deficient knowledge related to priapism. The patient should demonstrate motivation to learn, identify perceived learning needs, and verbalize an understanding of desired content.
- Sexual dysfunction secondary to priapism. The patient will verbalize satisfaction with the way he expresses physical intimacy.

KEY CONCEPTS

- Prostatitis is classified as either acute or chronic.
- BPH is a common condition affecting middle-aged and elderly men, and the greatest risk factor for BPH is age.
- Prostate cancer is the second most commonly diagnosed cancer in men.
- Painless enlargement of a testis is generally diagnostic of testicular cancer.
- Testicular torsion is a condition where the testis twists on the spermatic cord with resultant hypoxia of the testicle.
- Orchitis can be caused by viral, spirochetal, parasitic, or bacterial infections.
- Epididymitis usually develops secondary to bacterial infection in the urinary tract or prostatitis.
- Hydrocele, hematocele, and spermatocele all present with painless swelling or bulging in the scrotum.
- Varicocele is a group of varicose veins within the scrotum.
- Vasectomy is surgical sterilization of men to prevent passage of sperm to the urethra.
- Cryptorchidism is also referred to as undescended testes when it is present at birth.
- Phimosis, paraphimosis, balanitis, and posthitis are disorders of the glans penis and foreskin of the penis.
- Urethritis most commonly occurs with a genitourinary tract infection but can also be due to trauma.
- Urethral stricture causes difficulty voiding and a noticeably decreased urine stream.
- Epispadias and hypospadias are congenital malformations involving the location of the urethral meatus.
- Peyronie's disease is the formation of dense fibrotic scar tissue, which is the tissue that engorges with blood during penile erection.
- Penile cancer is a rare condition and seldom occurs in men who were circumcised as newborns.
- The cause of erectile dysfunction can be psychogenic or physiological.
- Priapism is the presence of a prolonged, often painful, penile erection.

REVIEW QUESTIONS

1. Which of the following is true concerning the diagnosis of prostatitis?
   1. It is identified primarily by a 24-hour urine specimen.
   2. It is diagnosed by culturing spontaneous or expressed urethral discharge or prostate fluid.
   3. It is falsely diagnosed in the presence of prostatic massage.
   4. It is a condition that is clearly identified with serum changes in a CBC.

2. Which of the following is true concerning the surgical treatment of benign prostatic hyperplasia?
   1. TUMP is an alternative treatment that heats the prostate tissue.
   2. TURP is seldom performed on the aged, due to complications.
   3. TUNA involves freezing the prostate to decrease the nature of its inflammation.
   4. Resection of the prostate is not normally performed if other procedures can be employed.

3. Which of the following is true concerning the staging and classification of prostate cancer?
   1. The normal PSA range for under 40 years of age is less than 4 to 6 ng/mL.
   2. The Gleason grading system is usually used for hematological cancers but not prostate cancer.
   3. At least two separate biopsy specimens are graded based on their differentiation from normal prostate cells.
   4. A score of D is less invasive than a score of B in the cancer staging system.

4. Which of the following is true concerning orchitis?
   1. There is a single blood test that will test positive in the presence of orchitis.
   2. Orchitis is usually asymptomatic.
   3. Orchitis involves an active inflammation of the epididymis and vas deferens.
   4. Antibiotics are normally given in the management of orchitis.

5. Which of the following is true concerning the condition of a varicocele?
   1. It is normally present in one testicle and causes infertility.
   2. It is the presence of varicose veins seen in the extremities of persons who have inguinal hernias.
   3. It often causes infertility or subfertility as a clinical manifestation.
   4. It can be removed with surgery and is managed this way if the patient is experiencing discomfort.

6. Which of the following is true of balanitis?
   1. It is usually caused by a bacterial infection.
   2. It is the entrapment of the retracted foreskin behind the glans penis of an uncircumcised male.
   3. It is an inflammation of the foreskin.
   4. It is the inability of the foreskin to be stretched and retracted over the glans of the penis.

7. Which of the following is true concerning a urethral stricture?
   1. It is an incomplete closure of the urethra during fetal development.
   2. It causes changes in the tissue that engorges with blood during penile erection.
   3. It has a main symptom of difficulty voiding and a noticeably decreased urine stream.
   4. It is not managed well with a urethral stent.

8. Which of the following is not true of penile cancer?
   1. The Jackson classification system grades cancer of the penis.
   2. Genital herpes and HPV infections are associated with increased rates of penile cancer.
   3. The goal of penile cancer treatment is to leave the tumor in place, as it is slow growing and seldom causes problems.
   4. Radiation therapy is often performed instead of penectomy because of the psychological aspects of such surgery.

9. Which of the following is true of ED?
   1. The medications used to treat ED usually have to be administered 24 hours prior to sexual intercourse.
   2. Parasympathetic nerve impulses and hormones work together to cause the penis to become firm in an erection.
   3. There are no nonpharmacological measures that can be used to treat ED.
   4. Prosthetic devices do not work well for most patients.

10. Which of the following is true concerning priapism?
    1. It is best treated with a surgical penile implant.
    2. It is often accompanied with a fever, chills, and nausea.
    3. It is differentiated with the use of Doppler flow studies.
    4. It is often caused as a complication of urethral surgery.

REVIEW ACTIVITIES

1. Select a patient with benign prostatic hyperplasia and discuss his knowledge of the disorder and the typical surgical interventions that are used in its management.

2. Teach a male patient to perform a TSE.

3. Write the subjective reflections that would accompany your thoughts and feelings about suddenly being diagnosed with cancer. Then, discuss with a peer how you would both approach a patient who was newly diagnosed with prostate cancer.

4. Develop a teaching plan to share with your peers for a patient with ED.

5. Describe the assessment and management for a patient with priapism.

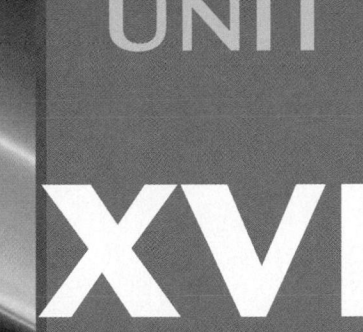

Special Considerations in Medical and Surgical Nursing

Multisystem Failure

Ruth Grendell, MSN, RN

CHAPTER TOPICS

- Immune Inflammatory
  Responses

- Shock Syndrome

- Systemic Inflammatory
  Response Syndrome (SIRS)

- Disseminated Intravascular
  Coagulation (DIC)

- Acute Respiratory Distress
  Syndrome (ARDS)

- Multiple Organ Dysfunction
  Syndrome (MODS)

The human body is composed of thousands of interacting and interdependent systems that regulate body functions. Many of the cellular functions are under genetic control, including cell structure and replication. Other systems integrate the functions of different organ systems. The body fluids that surround the cells and the various organ systems provide the pathways for exchange between the internal and external environments. The physiological processes are carefully coordinated to promote homeostasis and to oppose any disruptive change. Many of these autonomic functions occur without our knowledge until something within the process is altered. On the other hand, when the body receives an insult from either the internal or external environment, certain body systems interact to counteract any detrimental effect the insult might have. If successful, the threat is minimized or eliminated and the homeostatic state returns. However, if there is widespread inflammatory response to a severe insult, several organs can be involved. An insult can be anything that triggers the body's protective inflammatory response, such as trauma, surgery, anesthesia, burns, cardiovascular disorders, renal or liver disease, pancreatitis, gastrointestinal (GI) disorders, drugs, allergic reactions, shock, infection, and various pulmonary problems. When the body systems become overwhelmed the cascade of events can be described as a domino effect, which is when one system malfunctions, the other systems are adversely affected as well.

The person is also exposed to emotional stressors, which include the possibility of hospitalization and time in the intensive care unit or surgery, receiving blood transfusions, and being without the normal intake of food and fluids. These are all events that can have consequences on recovery. Anxiety over the outcome of the illness and spiritual distress associated with the fear of suffering and possible death can also influence the patient's psychological and physiological responses. The family processes are often interrupted, causing distress and potential alterations in coping with the events surrounding the ill person's condition. Cultural influences must also be taken into consideration in the plan of care. The nurse, as an important member of a multidisciplinary team, must understand the various changes in these life-threatening situations and be able to respond promptly and appropriately to help avoid complications, secondary multiple organ dysfunction or multiple organ failure (MOF), and death. The nurse must also support the patient and family during the crisis, thus ensuring that a holistic plan of care is provided. This chapter provides an overview of the natural protective responses that are constantly defending the body from foreign substances and abnormal cells that may develop within the body, the pathophysiological responses of the body to an insult, and the current evidence-based standards for therapeutic interventions for the patient and family members.

INFLAMMATORY IMMUNE RESPONSE

The immune system is made up of several types of immune cells and the central and peripheral lymphoid bodies. The **inflammatory immune response (IIR),** is a response that is composed of several body systems, which are constantly on alert to detect nonself and harmful intruders from the normal cells and proteins in the body. The immune system also has the ability to remember a foreign agent and to develop a heightened response during a subsequent exposure. When regulation of the immune response is controlled, the response is protective; however, when the immune response is exaggerated, the consequences can be undesirable and dangerous.

The acute phase of the IIR occurs almost immediately following an insult to the body (Box 65-1). The purposes of this innate protective response are to control bleeding, remove waste products, limit infection, and promote healing. IIR responses cause local vasodilation to aid in delivering an increased blood flow and to bring neutrophils, macrophages (the major phagocytic cells of the immune system), and clotting factors to the damaged area. The body is usually economical in the use of only the required responses that will minimize tissue damage. Minor injuries or insults elicit a transient response; more serious injuries involve a sustained response that may occur for several days and can damage the vessels in the area of injury.

A prolonged response causes an increase in permeability of the capillaries. The **endothelium,** which is the cellular tissue that lines the blood and lymphatic vessels, the heart, and various other body cavities, is a prominent contributor to the activation of the IIR (Box 65-2). The endothelial cells are metabolically active and produce several compounds that affect vascular lumen and anticoagulation of platelets. Damage to the endothelium results in a loss of anticoagulation factors and can result in the development of thrombi or major hemorrhage.

Capillary permeability results in the release of several inflammatory mediators from the damaged area that attracts the elements, which will fight invading microorganisms or minimize blood loss and further injury and promote healing. Mediators are bioactive substances that stimulate physiological change in cells. The most prominent mediators are histamine, kinins, prostaglandins, and cytokines, such as interleukin-1 (IL-1). IL-1 is released by almost all nucleated cells and activates the growth and function of neutrophils, lymphocytes (including killer cells), and macrophages. Killer cells are part of the immune system

---

BOX 65-1

CARDINAL SIGNS OF THE INFLAMMATORY RESPONSE

The local reaction to an injury was first described by Celsus, an early Roman physician.

Cardinal signs were termed as:

Rubor (redness)

Tumor (swelling)

Calor (heat)

Dolor (pain)

The Greek physician, Galen, added a fifth cardinal sign:

Function laesa (loss of function)

BOX 65-2

CHARACTERIZATIONS OF CHRONIC INFLAMMATION

Chronic inflammation is characterized by:

- A prolonged state of inflammation that may last for weeks, months, or years usually caused by persistent irritants that are resistant to phagocytosis (digestion and destruction) and other inflammatory mechanisms.
- The release of macrophages and lymphocytes instead of neutrophils to the damaged area.
- Chronic elevation of white blood cells, low-grade fever, and pain.
- Proliferation of fibroblasts (cells involved in development of connective tissue) rather than exudates (fluids containing pus or serum).
- Great risk for scar formation and deformity (Scar tissue often replaces normal connective tissue).
- Potential formation of granuloma: a tumor or growth composed of macrophages that are unable to destroy foreign bodies and some mycobacteria, which results in the formation of a mass surrounding the foreign body that is eventually encapsulated by a dense membrane of connective tissue that isolates it.
- Causative agents include: foreign bodies, e.g., asbestos, viruses, some bacteria, fungi, and larger parasites, e.g., tubercle bacillus, mycobacterium of leprosy, treponema of syphilis, and actinomyces, and tissues surrounding healing fractures.

Adapted from Rizzo, D. (2006). Fundamentals of anatomy and physiology *(2nd ed.). New York: Thomson Delmar Learning.*

---

surveillance network and are automatically programmed to kill foreign cells, such as cancer and virus-infected cells. It also promotes the release of other mediators, such as the complement system (a complex cascade of more than 20 serum proteins) that influence the antigen-antibody response. The mediators increase the permeability of capillary membranes, thus leading to the classic signs of swelling, edema, redness, and heat and pain. Loss of function is because of localized swelling and the release of the chemical mediators.

When the IIR is localized as in wound healing, or systemically capable of restoring metabolic function, healing will take place without complications. However, if the IRR response is not regulated, the system goes into overdrive and is considered to be pathogenic. This heightened response can result in uncontrolled intravascular inflammation and an increase in vascular permeability. The mediators can become toxic to other cells, thus damaging tissues, vessels, and organs, and result in hypoxia. An insufficient oxygen level to meet the body's demands will result in a switch from aerobic to anaerobic metabolism by the body cells.

Anaerobic metabolism results in the formation of lactic acid as a by-product of glucose metabolism. Anaerobic metabolism is not as efficient as aerobic metabolism; waste products accumulate, and the presence of lactic acid contributes to muscle fatigue. Failure of the sodium/potassium pump due to metabolic acidosis allows sodium, which is normally in the intravascular area, to enter cells as potassium leaves cells. Fluid follows sodium into the cells causing swelling and release of intracellular enzymes, thus preventing the cells from their normal functions. Calcium also enters the cells and blocks the use of phosphorus, a component of adenosine triphosphate (ATP) that is present in all cells and needed for producing energy. The cells eventually burst and die. Hyperkalemia, or excess potassium in the blood, can cause cardiac arrhythmias

---

BOX 65-3

SEQUENCE OF EVENTS INVOLVING ANAEROBIC METABOLISM AND METABOLIC ACIDOSIS

Anaerobic metabolism and metabolic acidosis

Inefficient cellular metabolism, accumulation of waste products, production of lactic acid, and muscle fatigue

Failure of sodium/potassium pump

Influx of sodium and water into cell	Outflow of potassium into blood stream
Swelling and release of cellular enzymes	Hyperkalemia
Calcium enters the cells	Potential cardiac arrhythmias and muscle weakness

Phosphorus not available to form ATP to produce energy for cell functions.

Cells eventually burst and die

Multiple organ failure process begins when a large number of cells die

Adapted from Edwards, S. (2002). Physiological insult/injury: Pathophysiology and consequences. British Journal of Nursing, 11(4), 263–277.

---

and possible muscle weakness. If the metabolic acidosis process continues and cannot be reversed, organ dysfunction and failure will occur (Box 65-3).

NEUROENDOCRINE SYSTEM RESPONSE

The neuroendocrine protective response to an insult is also closely linked to the immune response and tissue function. This response occurs as the cytokines (lymphokines and monokines) are released from the injury site. In fact IL-1 may be the linking factor between the immune response and stimulation of the neuroendocrine system. The principal elements include the sympathetic nervous system, the hypothalamus, pituitary and the adrenal glands that are involved in the typical "fight or flight" response to a threat. The sympathetic nervous system secretes the catecholamines adrenaline and noradrenaline. Adrenaline stimulates the heart and metabolic activities resulting in increased heart rate, cardiac output, metabolic rate, dilated bronchioles, and elevated blood glucose levels (Figure 65-1). Noradrenaline aids peripheral vascular constriction that helps to shunt circulating blood temporarily from nonessential organs to essential organs, such as the brain and heart, and to skeletal muscles. The major effect of the catecholamines is to increase glucose production and activation of platelets. However, if the catecholamine levels continue to rise, they could contribute to hyperglycemia, resistance to insulin, cardiac arrhythmias, and possible cardiac arrest.

The release of hormones into the blood stream is regulated by a negative feedback system. The activated sympathetic system and release of IL-1 interrupt the normal feedback process and trigger the hypothalamus to release

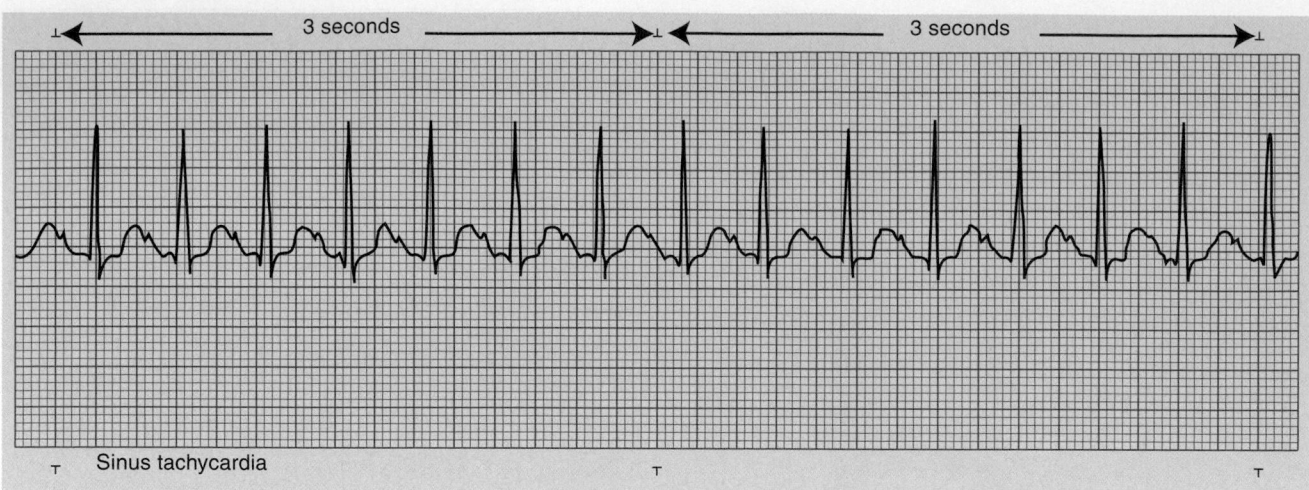

Sinus tachycardia

Heart rate 140 (Tachycardia)

Figure 65-1 Adrenaline causes the heart rate to develop tachycardia in the neuroendocrine response.

corticotrophin-releasing hormone (CRH). This signals the pituitary gland to secrete the adrenocorticotrophic hormone (ACTH) that stimulates the release of cortisol from the cortex of the adrenal gland. Cortisol (a) assists in the breakdown, or catabolism, of fats and proteins into simple substances; (b) assists in the synthesis of glucose from noncarbohydrate elements, such as fats and amino acids from proteins; and (c) converts glycogen that is stored in the liver into glucose. These processes take place primarily in the liver and help maintain blood glucose levels that are needed for the energy to conduct physiological processes. Cortisol also enhances adrenaline's influence on vascular constriction to aid in distribution of nutrients and energy sources where they are needed.

The purposes for the release of stress hormones following an insult to the body are to aid in restoring balance to the systems and to prevent secondary complications including loss of fluids, hypotension, and infection. The close link between the stress response and the sympathetic nervous system results in the release of a large amount of adrenaline into the blood stream in the attempt to defend the body from the stressor or insult. Stress hormones are also involved in the release of mineralocorticoids, such as aldosterone, when fluids are lost due to fluid shifts to interstitial spaces or hemorrhage. The primary function of mineralocorticoids is the regulation of the electrolyte balance, particularly potassium and sodium in the extracellular fluids.

THE RENAL RESPONSE

Loss of fluid or blood will lead to a decrease in kidney perfusion. The kidneys respond by releasing the enzyme renin. Renin splits angiotensinogen (a serum globulin formed in the liver) to angiotensin I, a vasopressor substance that is later converted in the lungs to angiotensin II. Angiotensin II stimulates the release of noradrenaline resulting in vasoconstriction, an increase in blood pressure, and thus a potential delivery of blood, nutrients, and oxygen to the deprived kidneys and other organs. Angiotensin II also stimulates the release of the mineralocorticoid aldosterone that aids the reabsorption of sodium and water by the kidneys and an increase in excretion of potassium. This process helps with an increase in intravascular volume, an increase in venous return, cardiac output, and blood pressure and clearance of potassium leaked from damaged cells. Angiotensin II also stimulates the posterior pituitary gland to release the antidiuretic hormone (ADH), which aids in water reabsorption and a decrease in urinary output (Box 65-4).

BOX 65-4

CASCADE OF PHYSIOLOGICAL EVENTS FOLLOWING AN INSULT TO THE BODY

Primary Injury

Trauma, surgery, anesthesia, burns, circulatory disorders, myocardial infarction, renal or liver disease, pancreatitis, gastrointestinal [GI] disorders, drugs, allergic reactions, shock, infection, deep vein thrombosis [DVT], and pulmonary embolism.

Systemic Inflammatory Immune Response (IIR)

Protective Measures
Release of inflammatory mediators from damaged tissue to area of need (histamine, kinins, prostaglandins, complement, and cytokines—interleukin-1).

Overdrive Response
Uncontrolled intravascular inflammation.
Increase in vascular permeability
Mediators can become toxic to other cells and contribute to hypoxic damage to organs.
Coagulation/microvascular thrombosis & altered tissue perfusion.

Secondary Response
Suppressed immune system infection—potential sepsis
Shock

Endothelial Response

The endothelium consists of flat cells that line the blood and lymphatic vessels, the heart, and various other body cavities. The cells are metabolically active and produce several compounds that affect the vascular lumen, anticoagulation and are closely linked to the IIR.

Protective Measures
Prevents excessive blood loss and isolates the injured site

Overdrive Responses
When damaged, anticoagulant properties are lost

Neuroendocrine Response

Response is to the release of cytokine (lymphokines and monokines) and other IIR mediators. Stimulation of hypothalamus, pituitary, and adrenal gland creates a highly complex series of events that affect cardiovascular system.

Protective Measures
Stimulation of sympathetic system and release of catecholamines (adrenaline and noradrenaline)

Increase in heart beat and cardiac output; metabolic rate and blood glucose dilation of bronchioles
Peripheral vasoconstriction; blood shifted temporarily from nonessential organs to brain, heart, and skeletal muscles.

Release of cortisol (as anti-inflammatory agent).
Enhances adrenaline's vasoconstrictive effects to ensure nutrients are supplied to tissues.
Release of adrenocorticotrophic hormone (ACTH) from adrenal cortex.
Release of mineralocorticoids to help regulate electrolytes.

Overdrive Responses
Excess circulating catecholamines
Increase in oxygen consumption
Rise in blood glucose
Arrhythmias, possible cardiac arrest.

Cardiovascular Response

Protective Measures
Increase in rate and strength of cardiac contractions to increase cardiac output

Overdrive Responses
Inflammatory mediators circulate and can alter endothelial integrity

Increased myocardial oxygen demand and possible arrhythmias
Cardiac depression

Systemic thrombosis or gross hemorrhage—DIC

Continued

BOX 65-4

CASCADE OF PHYSIOLOGICAL EVENTS FOLLOWING AN INSULT TO THE BODY—cont'd

Neuroendocrine Response—cont'd

Respiratory Response

Protective Measures

Increase in rate and depth of breathing to enhance gas exchange and to counteract metabolic acidosis

Overdrive Responses

Tachypnea

$PaCO_2$ less than 32 mm Hg

Alveolar damage

Pulmonary edema

Respiratory distress

Secondary Responses—Stress

Stress is related to increased sympathetic nervous system arousal and involves a wide physiological response. Many

Protective Measures

Presence of adrenaline in attempt to protect body from stressors (flight or fight response).

Presence of cortisol

stressors act synergistically rather than cumulatively.

Overdrive Responses

Prolonged emotional demands

Can produce stress ulcers, reduced wound healing, reduced cardiac function, and reduced immune response

Loss of balance between neurological, endocrine, and immune systems

Shock

The shock syndrome is a systemic condition when the peripheral blood flow is inadequate to provide sufficient

blood to the heart for normal function and transport of oxygen to all organs and tissues.

Adapted from Hardaway, R. (2006). Traumatic shock. Military Medicine, 171(4), 278–279; Ren, J., & Wu., S. (2006). A burning issue: Do sepsis and systemic inflammatory response syndrome (SIRS) directly contribute to cardiac dysfunction? Frontiers in Bioscience, 11, 15–22.

SHOCK SYNDROME

The **shock syndrome** is a systemic condition in which the peripheral blood flow is inadequate to provide sufficient blood to the heart for normal function and transport of oxygen to all organs and tissues. The mean arterial blood pressure (MABP) is inadequate to meet the needs of the tissues (Bench, 2004). Any factor that affects blood volume, blood pressure, or cardiac function can quickly exhaust energy resources and can initiate the complex shock syndrome. Common causes include hemorrhage, drug reaction (or allergic reaction to an antigen), trauma, pulmonary embolism, myocardial infarction, dehydration, heat stroke, and infection. There is some degree of shock with every insult or injury to the body. For example, an emotional response to an injury can induce syncope, or fainting, due to a transient inadequate blood supply to the brain.

The shock syndrome, or acute circulatory failure, has traditionally been classified according to etiology into five categories: anaphylactic, cardiogenic, hypovolemic, neurogenic, and septic (Table 65-1). A functional classification defines the types of shock as: hypovolemic, transport, obstructive, and cardiogenic. Anaphylactic, neurogenic, and sepsis shock are integrated into the transport classification. Regardless of the initiating event, there are four phases involved: initial, compensatory, progressive, and refractory. Progression from one stage to the other is dependent on the patient's health status, duration of the insult, response to therapy, and the correction of the underlying cause. The end result is always the same; tissues fail to receive oxygen and nutrients and are unable to eliminate waste products (Walsh, 2005).

TABLE 65-1 Traditional and Functional Classifications of Shock States	
Impaired oxygen delivery and altered oxygen consumption is common to all shock states.	
TRADITIONAL CLASSIFICATION	**FUNCTIONAL CLASSIFICATION**
Neurogenic—loss of sympathetic tone	*Transport*—loss of sympathetic tone, anemia, and histamine release
Low hemoglobin (a form of distributive or transport shock)	Endotoxin release
Anaphylactic—hypersensitivity reaction (a form of distributive or transport shock)	
Septic—caused by microorganisms (a form of distributive or transport shock)	
Cardiogenic—diminished forward pumping capability, ischemia, and irregularity in heart beat	*Cardiogenic*—diminished forward pumping capability, ischemia, and irregularity in heart beat
Hypovolemic—loss of intravascular volume and low cardiac output	*Hypovolemic*—loss of intravascular volume and low cardiac output
	Obstructive—barriers to blood flow
	Pulmonary embolus (artery blocked), tension pneumothorax, cardiac tamponade, or great vessels kinked

Adapted from Walsh, C. (2005). Multiple organ dysfunction syndrome after multiple trauma. Orthopaedic Nursing, 24(5), 324–335.

The Four Stages of the Shock Syndrome

The initial stage of the shock syndrome is marked by a decrease in cardiac output and impaired tissue perfusion. In the absence of oxygen, the cells switch to the anaerobic metabolism as a source of energy. However the formation of lactic acid contributes to muscle weakness and cell damage. The body attempts to remedy the problem by initiating the homeostatic mechanisms during the compensatory stage (e.g., the person may hyperventilate to eliminate the effects of acidosis), activation of the sympathetic nervous system causes the heart to beat faster, and blood is shifted to critical organs. As the shock process progresses, cellular damage prevents cells from functioning (Figure 65-2), and every system in the body is affected and is referred to as **multiple organ dysfunction syndrome (MODS)** or MOF. Finally, during the refractory stage, the body can no longer respond to therapy. The shock condition is considered irreversible. Because of the seriousness of the shock syndrome, most hospitalized patients receive care in the specialized intensive care units. The principle collaborative treatment goals are to identify and treat the underlying cause of the shock syndrome, deliver oxygen to the tissues, promote utilization of oxygen by the tissues, maintain surveillance for complications, and provide comfort and emotional support (Box 65-5) (Bench, 2004).

Planning and Implementation

In 2003, scientists representing 11 international organizations developed research-based guidelines for treatment of severe sepsis and septic shock to improve outcomes. The guidelines are clinically tested, updated annually, and updated as often as new information becomes available (Box 65-6). In general, hospitals continue to improve their abilities to manage critical incidents with patients (see Fast Forward feature). In addition, there are general assessments and interventions for patients with the shock syndrome (Box 65-7).

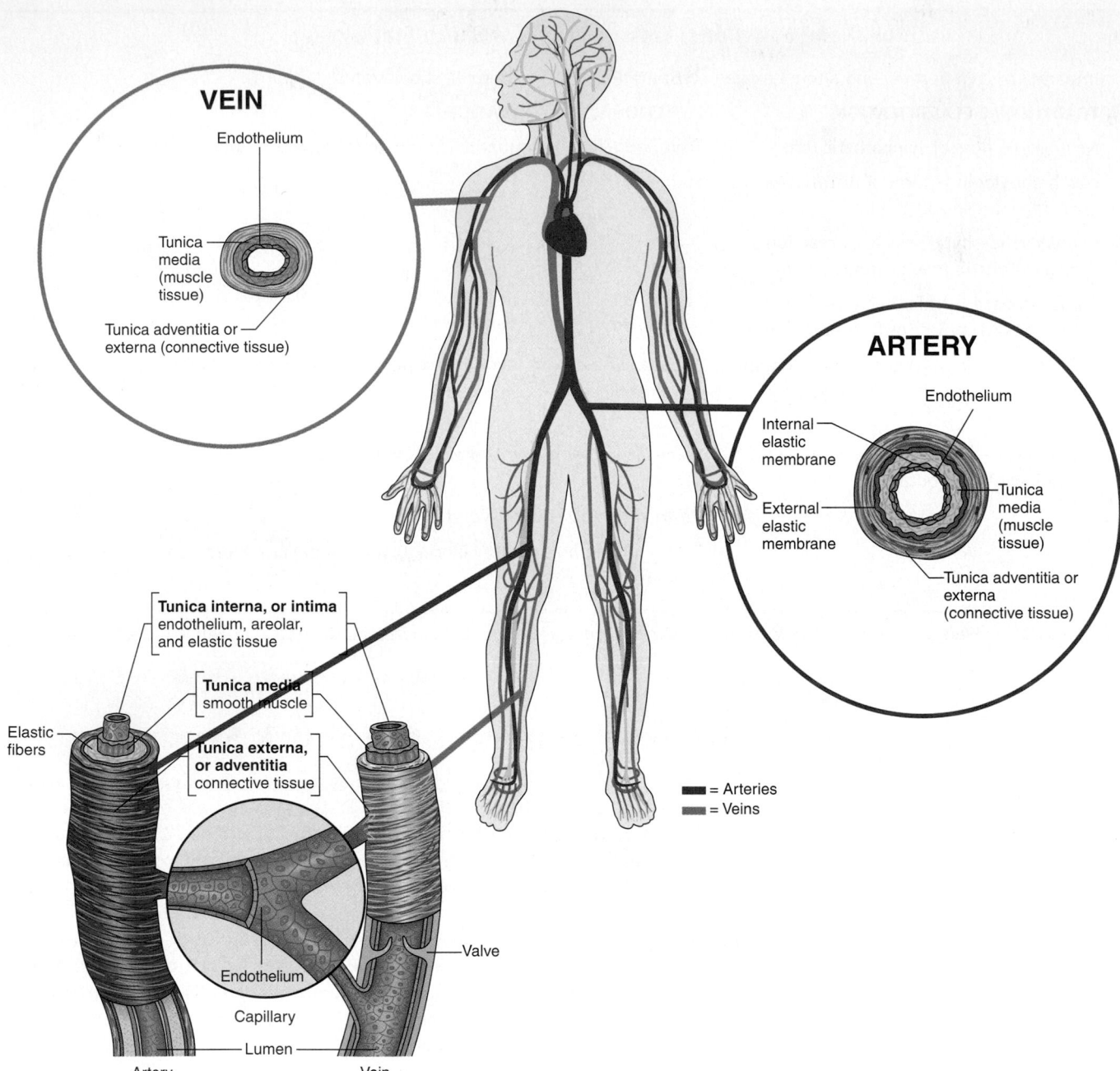

Figure 65-2 Generalized dilation of the blood vessels will cause a decrease in blood pressure as the affected fluid compartments become too enlarged.

Pediatric patients are more likely to need intubation because of low functional residual capacity and because intravenous (IV) access is difficult. Fluid resuscitation is based on weight with recommendation of 40–60 mL/kg or higher.

HYPOVOLEMIC SHOCK

The shock process is initiated by many types of injuries. These methods of initiating the shock syndrome are divided into five primary categories (hypovolemic cardiogenic, neurogenic, septic, and anaphylactic) as described in the following section. First, hypovolemic shock occurs when there is a lack of circulating fluid volume in the intravascular space. This type of shock can occur

Fast Forward ▶▶▶

100,000 Lives Campaign

The Institute for Healthcare Improvement ([IHI] 2005) reported that more than 2,600 hospitals across the United States have made a commitment to implement changes to improve patient care and to prevent avoidable deaths. The guidelines cover interventions to prevent adverse drug responses, to prevent surgical site and central venous line infections, and ventilation-associated pneumonias. Other interventions will be added and an evaluation of the outcomes of the campaign efforts is being assessed.

From IHI. (2005). 100,000 Lives Campaign. Retrieved June 14, 2006, from http://www.ihi.org.

BOX 65-5

ASSESSMENT AND DIAGNOSIS OF SHOCK

Common clinical manifestations of the shock syndrome will vary according to the underlying cause, the stage of shock, and the individual person's response to shock. The exact course of events can be variable. Each person must be assessed individually prior to any intervention.

- Regardless of the type of shock, it leads to a systolic blood pressure (SBP) less than 90 mm Hg and narrowing of pulse pressure that is inadequate to meet the tissue needs. (SBP may be elevated initially.)
- Early shock symptoms are subtle requiring close surveillance to avoid overlooking their presence.
- All persons in shock are at risk of deterioration in status. Prompt intervention is required.
- Nurses must have a clear understanding of the pathophysiology of the different etiologies of shock.
- In all instances of shock following a trauma incident, consider hypovolemia or hemorrhage unless proven otherwise.
- Shock is a frightening experience for the patient and family. Effective psychological support is essential.

Symptoms include:

- Hypothermia
- Tachycardia or bradycardia
- Rapid thready pulse, slow capillary refill, or collapse of superficial veins in extremities
- Altered mental status—dissociation from normal thought processes, detached, a feeling of numbness, and impaired sensory-emotional response. Loss of consciousness, restlessness, anxiety, irritability, and weakness may be present.
- Clinical findings correlated with organs compromised by inadequate oxygen supply and the phases of the shock syndrome.

Examples:

 a. Skin: cold, clammy, cyanotic, poor capillary refill, or warm dry skin due to pooling of blood in extremities. Cyanosis (circumoral, earlobes, finger tips, or toes).
 b. Kidneys: decreased urine output; anuria, or oliguria.
 c. Lungs: dyspnea, crackles, or wheezes
 d. GI system: thirst, dry mucous membranes; nausea and vomiting; or decreased bowel sounds

Adapted from Bench, S. (2004). Clinical skills: Assessing and treating shock: A nursing perspective. British Journal of Nursing, 13(12), 715–721.

---

with any loss of fluids in a manner that decreases the circulating plasma to effectually decrease blood pressure. A patient in hypovolemic shock can either lose fluids from the body or into different body fluid compartments and result in hypovolemic shock. Hypovolemia from whatever cause is the most common type of shock.

Etiology

Conditions that contribute to hypovolemic shock include dehydration, severe burn injuries, loss of intravascular volume, vasodilation due to neurogenic shock (loss of sympathetic tone), anaphylactic shock (release of histamine), and septic shock (release of endotoxin). Other contributing factors include

> **BOX 65-6**
>
> ## MANAGEMENT OF SEPTIC SHOCK
>
> ### Research recommendations for treatment include:
>
> The early goal-directed resuscitation procedures for the septic patient should be started during the first six hours after recognition of the problem.
>
> - Use of diagnostic studies to identify the causative organism before administering antibiotics.
> - Early administration of broad-spectrum antibiotics (usually a 7 to 10 day course).
> - Ongoing physical assessment and reassessment of response to therapy.
> - Administration of appropriate fluids.
> - Administration of vasopressor medications.
> - Administration of stress dose steroid therapy for septic shock. There is some concern about administering high-dose steroids.
> - Use of recombinant activated protein C for patients with severe sepsis and at high risk for death. May be contraindicated if patient has coronary artery disease or acute hemorrhage.
> - Establish hemoglobin target of 7 to 9 g/dL; appropriate use of blood products.
> - Use of protective oxygen ventilation (low tidal volume) level to avoid lung damage. Follow protocols for weaning from mechanical ventilation and sedation or analgesia.
> - Place patient in semirecumbent position unless contraindicated.
> - Maintain blood glucose level less than 150 mg/dL after the patient is stable. Patients are at greater risk of hypoglycemia with aggressive glucose control methods.
> - Monitor diagnostic studies for fluid and electrolyte balance, bicarbonate levels.
> - Apply deep vein thrombosis (DVT) and stress ulcer prevention measures.
>
> *Adapted from Dellinger, R., Carlet, J., Masur, H., Gerlach, H. (2004). Surviving sepsis campaign guidelines for management of severe sepsis and septic shock.* Critical Care Medicine, *32(3), 858. Retrieved June 23, 2006, from www.survivingsepsis.com.*

vomiting, diarrhea, nasogastric suction, diuretic therapy, diabetes insipidus, trauma, surgery, and hyperglycemic osmotic diuresis.

Pathophysiology

An actual loss of fluid from the body, such as whole blood, is referred to as **absolute hypovolemia.** Normally, fluids in the intracellular and extracellular spaces remain the same and allow movement of water, electrolytes, and other substances to move back and forth. **Relative hypovolemia** refers to the shifting of fluid from the intravascular space to the extravascular, or interstitial, space that can result from a loss of intravascular integrity or increased capillary permeability or a decreased colloidal osmotic pressure.

Third spacing is the accumulation of fluid in the extracellular and intracellular spaces and in a third body, such as the intestine, that does not support circulation (Diehl-Oplinger & Kaminski, 2004). These events lead to a decrease in venous return to the heart and an eventual decrease in cardiac output and inadequate oxygen supply to body tissues.

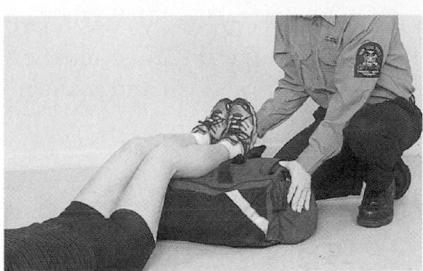

Figure 65-3 Elevation of the lower half of the body serves to allow increased blood flow to the brain and vital organs.

BOX 65-7

ASSESSMENT AND CARE OF SHOCK SYNDROME

The nurse should monitor signs and symptoms associated with alterations in body response to shock complications. Initially, the first responder should manage the patient with the immediate care interventions for patients suspected of the shock syndrome (e.g., position patient to maximize oxygen return to the brain, monitor pulse and breathing rates, keep normothermic, and administer oxygen) (Figure 65-3).

Initial Compensatory Stage

Body mechanisms are triggered to maintain adequate blood pressure and tissue perfusion. Subtle changes in baseline may be observed. Monitor heart rate and pulse, blood pressure, central venous pressure (CVP), respiratory rate core, peripheral temperature, and urinary output. Pulse oximetry may also be performed. Arterial gases are monitored for accurate assessment. Blood sampling for urea and electrolyte levels, full blood count, and glucose levels may also be performed. Elevated glucose levels are present with release of stress hormones such as cortisol.

Progressive Stage

Compensating mechanisms begin to fail. Symptoms are evident of inadequate organ perfusion. A full assessment should be done to identify any signs of blood or fluid loss, fluid shift as in ascites, infection, vomiting, or inadequate fluid intake.

Decompensated Stage

Failure of compensating mechanisms. No response to treatment. There is a great risk of cardiac arrest. A rising serum lactate is an indicator of inadequate tissue perfusion due to metabolic acidosis. Low arterial oxygen content, chest pain, cardiac dysrhythmias, altered level of consciousness (LOC), or low urinary output. MAPB cannot be maintained without assistance.

Adapted from Bench, S. (2004). Clinical skills: Assessing and treating shock: A nursing perspective. British Journal of Nursing, 13(12), 715–721.

Assessment with Clinical Manifestations

In hypovolemic shock, the compensatory systems attempt to maintain cardiac output. Initially, heart and respiratory rate increase and the depth of respirations increase to improve oxygenation; vasoconstriction is initiated to increase blood pressure. Later, urine output declines, and the skin becomes pale and cool with delayed capillary refill. Mental status changes due to poor oxygenation include disorientation, restlessness, anxiousness, and decreased levels of consciousness. As these compensatory mechanisms become overwhelmed (usually with the loss of 30–40 percent or 1,500–2,000 mL of fluid) tissue perfusion is impaired. Clinical manifestations include hypotension and possible orthostatic changes in blood pressure. Cardiac output will be diminished and pressures will be low in the right atrium, the pulmonary artery, and the left ventricle because of the diminished blood volume return. In shock caused by anemia or hemorrhage, hematocrit and hemoglobin levels will be low. Respiratory distress will be evident; metabolic acidosis and **hypoxemia** are present. Hypoxemia, a decreased concentration of oxygen in the blood, is measured by arterial oxygen partial pressure (PaO_2). With the loss of 40 percent or more of fluid volume, the compensatory systems fail completely (Box 65-8). Symptoms of MODS develop (Walsh, 2005). Nursing diagnoses and evaluation of outcomes are shown in Table 65-2. A listing of manifestations and management can be found in Box 65-8 and Box 65-9, respectively.

Planning and Implementation

Hypovolemic shock is treated aggressively to correct the cause and to rapidly restore perfusion to the body tissues, especially the brain and heart. Administration of fluids is usually dependent on the type of fluid that is lost.

TABLE 65-2 Examples of Nursing Diagnoses, NIC, and NOC Related to All Shock Syndromes

NANDA NURSING DIAGNOSES	NURSING INTERVENTIONS (NIC)	EXPECTED PATIENT OUTCOMES (NOC)
Airway		
Impaired gas exchange (related to specific cause)	Shock management	Respiratory status:
	Airway management	Airway patency, gas exchange, ventilation stabilization
Impaired spontaneous ventilation	Airway insertion and stabilization	
	Resuscitation	
	Ventilation assistance	
Cardiac		
Decreased cardiac output (related to specific cause)	Cardiac care, acute	Cardiac pump effectiveness
	Cardiac precautions	Circulation status effective
	Vital signs monitoring	
Fluids		
Deficient fluid volume	Fluid and electrolyte management	Electrolyte and acid-base balance
Risk for deficient fluid volume	Acid-base management (metabolic/respiratory)	Energy conservation
Risk for fluid imbalance	Blood products administration	
	Hypovolemia management	
	Intravenous therapy	
Tissue Perfusion		
Imbalanced nutrition, less than body requirements	Nutrition management	Tissue perfusion (cardiac, cerebral, peripheral, or pulmonary)
Ineffective tissue	Implement fluid management strategies	
Perfusion (related to: renal, cerebral, cardiopulmonary, gastrointestinal, or peripheral)		Nutritional status: biochemical measures controlled
Mental		
Acute confusion	Cerebral perfusion promotion	Anxiety control
Spiritual distress	Anxiety reduction	Hope
Anxiety	Coping enhancement (patient and family)	Coping appropriate (patient and family)
Ineffective coping		Knowledge: disease process
Output		
Impaired urinary elimination	Urinary elimination management	Urinary elimination adequate

Adapted from DeLaune, S., & Ladner, P. (2006). Fundamentals of nursing (3rd ed.). New York: Thomson Delmar Learning; Walsh, C. (2005). Multiple organ dysfunction syndrome after multiple trauma. Orthopaedic Nursing, 24(5), 324–335.

BOX 65-8

SELECTED MANIFESTATIONS OF HYPOVOLEMIC SHOCK

Tachycardia

Pulse pressure narrows as the diastolic increases

Tachypnea and increase in depth of respirations (may gasp for breath)

Decline in urine output

Skin pale, cool, delayed capillary refill

Jugular veins appear flat

Decreased cerebral perfusion and a change in level of consciousness (LOC)

Disoriented, confused, restless, anxious, or irritable

BOX 65-9

MANAGEMENT OF HYPOVOLEMIC SHOCK

The nurse should:

- Implement measures to minimize fluid loss.
- Monitor fluid replacement process. This includes insertion and management of large diameter intravenous (IV) catheters, IV lines and connections; administration of prescribed fluids and medications. Also, the nurse must understand the advantages, limitations, and the implications associated with the different types of fluid. Blood products can initiate a secondary shock due to infection and anaphylaxis. Observe for local or generalized rash and urticaria. Document and report findings.
- Monitor vital signs (including bradycardia or tachycardia); temperature changes, pulmonary artery pressure (PAP); pulmonary artery wedge pressure (PAWP), which measures pulmonary artery and left ventricle pressures; right atrial pressure (RAP). Positioning the patient with legs elevated, trunk flat, and head and shoulders above the chest (modified Trendelenburg position).
- Monitor for manifestations of fluid overload, such as changes in respirations or respiratory distress; assess lung sounds for crackles and rhonchi; assess changes in heart sounds and heart rate; and monitor urinary output (usually via retention catheter).
- Monitor laboratory results (Check for alterations in the coagulation process, white blood cell [WBC] level for infection and hemoglobin and hematocrit levels).
- Observe patient for signs of infection (IV insertion site and lungs).
- Monitor mental status, changes in skin condition or appearance.
- Administer analgesics.
- Provide positions for comfort; provide a calm environment.
- Limit activities to promote conservation of oxygen supply.
- Educate patient and family regarding measures to reduce anxiety.

The choices include crystalloid or colloid solutions or a combination of both. The military antishock trousers (MAST) are used in severe crisis to assist in controlling hemorrhage and to provide blood pressure support. Another garment, the pneumatic antishock garment (PASG) fits like a pair of trousers and covers the lower extremities and the trunk. This intervention is often used in the prehospital management of trauma victims.

The primary goals of are to minimize fluid loss, to enhance fluid replacement (Table 65-3), and to monitor the patient responses to interventions. Identification of patients at risk for hypovolemic shock and careful monitoring of fluid balance are important prevention strategies.

CARDIOGENIC SHOCK

Cardiogenic shock results in the failure of either the right or left ventricle or both to provide an adequate delivery of oxygen to the body tissues due to a weakened forward pumping function of the heart. Precipitating factors can be a myocardial infarction, irregular rate or rhythm, or cardiomyopathy. This type of shock commonly occurs when more than 40 percent of the myocardium is irreversibly damaged.

TABLE 65-3 Types of Parenteral Fluid Replacement

SOLUTION CLASSIFICATION	SOLUTION EXAMPLES	UTILIZATION	PRECAUTIONS
Crystalloids—solutions that mimic the body's extracellular fluid	*Isotonic* (same tonicity as plasma) 0.9% Saline Ringer's solution Ringer's lactate solution *Hypotonic* 0.45% saline *Hypertonic* 3–5% saline Concentrated dextrose in water added to amino acid solutions.	Use for fluid losses due to vomiting, diarrhea, surgery, and prior to blood transfusion To move fluid into intracellular compartment Use when sodium restriction is required Use to relieve cellular edema and correct hypoglycemia and provide calories	Monitor for fluid excess or overload. Monitor patient closely. Overload can cause intravascular fluid depletion, hypotension, cellular edema, and tissue damage. Raise risk for volume overload. Monitor closely, especially persons with heart failure.
Colloids: contain undissolved protein, sugar, and starch molecules that are too large to pass through capillary walls	Albumen (5% isotonic with no clotting components) Albumen 25%	Use to expand intravascular volume. Have same effects as hypertonic crystalloid solutions. Given in smaller volumes	Monitor closely because solutions have longer duration of action.
Blood and blood products	Whole blood Packed RBCs Plasma	Whole blood used to replace red blood cells (RBCs), white blood cells (WBCs), platelets, and plasma Replace RBCs and delivery of oxygen to tissues Replace albumin, globulins, antibodies, proteins, and clotting factors	Rarely used if more than 24 hours old. Monitor for allergic reactions. *Can trigger anaphylactic shock* Administer over one to two hours or within four hours.
Pharmaceutical plasma expanders	Dextran Mannitol (sugar/alcohol substance dissolved in 0.9% saline)	Draws water into the intravascular space Decrease intracranial pressure due to cerebral edema, reverse cerebrospinal fluid buildup; lower intraocular pressure. Produces osmotic diuresis	Monitor closely for fluid volume deficit.

Adapted from Diehl-Oplinger, L., & Kaminski, M. (2004). Choosing the right fluid to counter hypovolemic shock. Nursing, 34(3), 52–54.

Pathophysiology

In cardiogenic shock there is an impaired forward pumping function with a decreased stroke volume and decreased cardiac output of the left ventricle. This dysfunction results in a backup of blood into the pulmonary system causing edema and impaired gas exchange. Therefore, a reduction in oxygenated arterial blood further decreases tissue perfusion throughout the body and is followed by metabolic acidosis.

Assessment with Clinical Manifestations

Clinical manifestations of right ventricle failure are associated with systemic venous congestion (e.g., fatigue, dependent edema, jugular vein distension, liver engorgement, ascites, or cyanosis). The patient in cardiogenic shock may exhibit a heart rate greater than 100 beats per minute, a weak, thready pulse, diminished heart sounds and dysrhythmias, tachypnea and adventitious lung sounds, cool, pale, moist skin, and chest pains. Renal failure is evident by a decreased urine output, and there is a decreased level of consciousness due to hypoperfusion of brain tissue. Cardiopulmonary collapse may be the cause of death (Johnson, 2005). Review Table 65-2 for nursing diagnoses and evaluation of outcomes.

Edema and weight gain are also prominent clinical manifestations of cardiogenic shock (Box 65-10). Edema is most often developed in dependent areas of the body. Accumulation of 1 liter of fluid is evidenced by a weight gain of 1 kg or 2.2 pounds. A weight gain of 2 pounds in 24 hours or 5 pounds in a week is considered as a sign of additional heart or kidney failure. Daily monitoring of the patient's weight, intake, and output is an important assessment tool. Recall that an intake that exceeds output indicates a positive fluid balance that can result in fluid volume overload. The reverse condition occurs when output (due to fever, increased perspiration, vomiting, diarrhea, gastric suction, or diuretic therapy) exceeds fluid intake. Urine output and insensible fluid losses, such as perspiration, stool, and water vapor from lungs can vary from 750–2,400 mL/day. Elimination of 30 mL per hour or 400 mL/day is considered to be an approximate estimate of renal function. Central venous pressure (CVP) and arterial pressure measures can accurately reflect alterations in vascular volume returning to and being ejected from the heart. The nurse can also assess fluid status by assessing the skin turgor, moisture of mucous membranes, presence of edema or ascites, diaphoresis, low-grade fever, neck and hand vein engorgement, "crackles" in lungs, dyspnea, tachycardia, blood pressure changes, S_3 and S_4 sounds, headache, blurred vision, vertigo on rising, papilledema, and mental changes (Estes, 2006).

Planning and Implementation

Treatment includes an aggressive approach to treat the underlying cause, to enhance the pumping mechanism of the heart, and to improve tissue perfusion. Procedures are dependent on whether cardiogenic shock is caused by right-sided or left-sided heart failure. The goals of treatment for right-sided heart failure are directed toward improving right ventricular stroke volumes and to restore filling of the left ventricle. Examples include vasodilators, such as nitroglycerin, fluids, vasopressors (e.g., dopamine to support an appropriate blood pressure), and the use of IV medications, such as dobutamine, to stimulate more forceful contractions of the heart. The goals of treatment for left-sided heart failure are to increase the left ventricle contractions and to prevent the progression of right-sided heart failure. Examples of treatments include supplemental oxygen, mechanical intubation, and administration of diuretics and inotropic drugs to increase ventricle contractility and cardiac output. Cardiac monitoring and close observation are essential. Analgesics are given to relieve pain and to decrease myocardial oxygen demand. Morphine is frequently used to improve coronary perfusion by dilating the coronary vessels and to alleviate pain and anxiety. The intra-aortic balloon pump (IABP) is used to improve the oxygen supply to the myocardium. The ventricular assist device (VAD) is used as a temporary measure to replace the function of the left ventricle, allowing it to rest and heal. In some instances, coronary angioplasty and coronary artery bypass grafting is performed.

BOX 65-10

SELECTED MANIFESTATIONS OF CARDIOGENIC SHOCK

Hypotension—Systolic blood pressure less than 90 mm Hg

Heart rate greater than 100 beats per minute

Weak thready pulse

Diminished heart sounds

Change in level of consciousness (LOC)

Cool, pale, moist skin

Urine output less than 30 mL/hour

Chest pain

Dysrhythmias

Tachypnea

Crackle breath sounds

Decreased cardiac output

BOX 65-11

NURSING INTERVENTIONS FOR A PATIENT IN CARDIOGENIC SHOCK

The nurse should:
- Administer the prescribed fluids and medications.
- Administer supplemental oxygen and monitoring patient response.
- Monitor vital signs; observe for thready pulse, change in heart sounds, chest pain; changes in respirations or respiratory distress; assess lung sounds for crackles and rhonchi.
- Monitor patients on intra-aortic balloon pump (IABP) for complications, e.g., formation of emboli, infection, aortic rupture, improper balloon placement, function, or rupture, bleeding, and complications related to the cannulated extremity.
- Monitor laboratory results and intake and output.
- Monitor mental status, changes in skin condition or appearance.
- Administer analgesics to diminish the myocardial oxygen consumption.
- Provide positions for comfort; provide a calm environment.
- Educate patient and family regarding measures to reduce anxiety.
- Limit activities to promote conservation of oxygen supply.
- Additional interventions are similar to management of patients in hypovolemic shock.

Nursing interventions for a patient in cardiogenic shock include (a) promoting adequate supply of oxygen to the myocardium, (b) limiting myocardial consumption of oxygen, and (c) monitoring the patient's responses to interventions. For specific nursing interventions refer to Box 65-11.

ANAPHYLACTIC SHOCK

Almost any substance can cause a hypersensitivity response involving the interaction of an antibody and antigen. The antigen substances can consist of several foods including eggs and milk, shellfish, peanuts, chocolate, strawberries and tomatoes; food additives; diagnostic agents, such as iodine; blood, gamma globulin; vaccines and antitoxins; latex allergies; molds or fungus, animal dander and hair; drugs, insect stings, and venoms.

Pathophysiology

When the body is exposed to a foreign substance, or antigen, the immune system creates antibodies against it. The antibodies will recognize the specific antigen when the body is exposed to it a second time, and they attempt to destroy the antigen via **phagocytosis** (surrounding and destruction of particulate matter by phagocyte cells). This process serves as an important bodily defense mechanism against infection by microorganisms and against occlusion of mucous surfaces or tissues by foreign particles and tissue debris. Anaphylactic shock is caused by an exaggerated widespread antibody response following a previous exposure to the antigen. It can be life-threatening due to constricted bronchioles, acute respiratory distress, severe hypotension, tachycardia, hypovolemia, and inadequate blood supply to body tissues. Edema of the airways, particularly the larynx impedes airflow to the lungs.

The antibody-antigen response triggers the mast cells to release the mediators histamine, eosinophilic chemotactic factor of anaphylaxis (ECF-A), neutrophilic chemotactic factor of anaphylaxis (NCF-A), proteinases, heparin, serotonin, leukotrienes prostaglandins, and platelet-activating factor (PAF).

Assessment with Clinical Manifestations

Responses in anaphylactic shock include vasodilation, increased capillary permeability, broncho-constriction and inflammation, and stimulation of nerve endings in cutaneous tissues that produce sensations of warmth, itching, and pain. Some patients complain of abdominal cramping. Constriction of coronary vessels causes severe myocardial depression. Venous return from peripheral tissues is impaired. Decreased oxygen supply to the cellular tissues leads to impaired cellular metabolism. Death often results from airway obstruction or cardiovascular collapse or both. This is a form of transport shock in the functional classification (Walsh, 2005).

Reports of latex (natural rubber product) allergy, especially in health care, have increased in recent years. The frequent use of latex gloves to prevent the transmission of infections places individuals with hypersensitivities at risk for developing minor to serious problems. An alert was published by the National Institute for Occupational Safety and Health (NIOSH) in 1997, which provided information on the problem, and they made available a pamphlet describing prevention measures, The hypersensitivity reactions are to the proteins in the latex itself or to chemicals added to the rubber during harvesting. It is also believed that the proteins could be trapped in the powder. The most common reaction is contact dermatitis resulting in skin rashes, hives, flushing, itching, nasal, eye, or sinus problems. When the gloves are changed, the powder can become airborne and inhaled; for susceptible individuals, asthma may be the result. Some individuals with latex-induced asthma have had life-threatening anaphylactic reactions.

A comprehensive history is a valuable tool in the prevention of anaphylactic shock. A detailed description of the patient's allergies should be clearly documented and communicated to other health care personnel. Anyone can experience anaphylaxis to a foreign substance; however, it is more common in people who have a history of allergies and previous anaphylactic reactions. Patients with asthma also have a heightened immune response. The nurse must be able to anticipate the typical allergic reactions (Box 65-12) to an antigen substance and be able to intervene in this life-threatening event. Refer to Table 65-2 for nursing diagnoses and evaluation of outcomes.

Planning and Implementation

The care for anaphylactic shock begins with prevention. Preventive measures include avoiding the use of latex gloves, using gloves with no powder, avoiding the use of oil-based hand creams, and washing the hands with soap and water and drying thoroughly after wearing gloves. Frequent cleaning of areas where dust containing powder should be done. Individuals with hypersensitivity to latex should wear an alert bracelet and have an Epi-Pen which is an injectable vial of epinephrine.

Nurses should be aware that other latex products are balloons, condoms, catheters, clothing elastic, carpet backing, some upholstery materials, and dishwashing gloves. Some medication vials have latex stoppers; administration of the medication can produce a severe reaction in people with hypersensitivities. Assessment of the patient's allergy history is important. Reactions are more prevalent for individuals with dermatitis, eczema, rhinitis, and asthma. Susceptible individuals may also react to avocados, bananas, chestnuts, kiwi fruit, and poinsettia plants (Hamilton, Brown, Veltri, Feroli, Primeau, Schauble, et al., 2005; Hathaway, 2005; McNulty, 2005; Smith, Wallace, & Smith-Campbell, 2004).

Nursing interventions for a patient in anaphylactic shock include a wide variety of management strategies. A priority is facilitating ventilation by ensuring a patent airway, positioning the patient, and instructing the patient to breathe slowly and deeply. Then the nurse must observe for dyspnea, hoarseness, and stridor, which are early signs of laryngeal edema. In addition, the

BOX 65-12

CLINICAL MANIFESTATIONS OF ANAPHYLACTIC SHOCK

Hypotension

Tachycardia

Decreased cardiac output

Stridor

Wheezing

Rales and rhonchi

Dysphagia

Pruritus—Urticaria

Erythema

Angioedema

Restlessness, uneasiness, apprehension, and anxiety

Decreased level of consciousness (LOC)

Nausea, vomiting, and diarrhea

Incontinence or vaginal bleeding

Complaints of feeling warm, dyspneic, itching, abdominal cramping, and pain

nurse must monitor the vital signs and assess for common manifestations of decreased cardiac output (e.g., hypotension, rapid pulse, cyanosis, or dysrhythmias). The nurse also must monitor the effectiveness of prescribed oxygen therapy (Note: immediate oxygenation may be by a nonrebreather mask, and endotracheal intubation or tracheostomy may be necessary). To correct the fluid compartment issues, the nurse will likely insert a large diameter IV catheter, administering the prescribed fluids and medications, and monitor the flow of fluids. The patient must be positioned with his or her legs elevated and head and shoulders above the chest. Administration of medications may be given to relieve itching. The patient may be provided warm soaks to skin and gloves (if needed) to discourage scratching. Due to the likelihood of renal failure and renal dysfunction, the patient is monitored for a cessation of urinary output. In general the patient's and family's teaching needs are important (e.g., spiritual, psychological, and emotional needs). Last discharge planning must be implemented throughout the patient's hospitalization. The patient must be educated on how to avoid future anaphylactic reactions, instructed to wear a medical alert bracelet, and carry information that lists allergies (Smith, et al, 2004).

Goals

The primary goals of treatment include removal of the antigen if possible, reversing the effects of the biochemical mediators, and promoting adequate tissue perfusion. Support to the patient's airways is provided by administering supplemental oxygen, intubation, and mechanical ventilation if needed. In some instances, the patient may experience respiratory or cardiac arrest and cardiopulmonary resuscitation is initiated.

Pharmacology

Medications, such as IV epinephrine or via an endotracheal tube, are given to promote bronchodilation and vasoconstriction and to prevent further secretion of the mediators. Benadryl (diphenhydramine hydrochloride) is given to block the release of histamine, and corticosteroids are administered to prevent or reduce inflammation and to help stabilize the capillary membranes. Crystalloid (balanced salt solutions, such as normal saline, lactated Ringer's, and 5% glucose in water) or colloid solutions, such as hetastarch, mannitol, and dextran, which contain oncotic substances to expand intravascular volume, are given as fluid replacement. Lactated Ringer's solution contains sodium, potassium calcium chloride, and lactate. It is contraindicated for people with renal or liver disease or in lactic acidosis. Inotropic and vasoconstrictor drugs are often given to increase myocardial contraction and to reverse vasodilation. Box 65-13 includes information on pharmacological shock.

NEUROGENIC SHOCK

Neurogenic shock is usually a transient condition that occurs in the absence or suppression of sympathetic nervous system tone and is considered in the functional hypovolemic shock classification. This type of shock can be caused by anything that disrupts the transmission of an impulse to the hypothalamus, the sympathetic vasomotor center in the brain, or anything that blocks the outflow of the sympathetic response.

Pathophysiology

Loss of sympathetic tone results in massive peripheral vasodilation, loss of temperature regulation, loss of sympathetic tone to the heart, and diminished baroreceptor response to changes in blood pressure. The skin temperature becomes the same as the room temperature (poikilothermia), and because of the inability to sweat, the skin feels dry to the touch. There is an increased risk of developing deep vein thrombosis (DVT) in the lower extremities. Neurogenic shock often occurs with a spinal cord injury above the midthoracic region when blood vessels lose the ability to constrict, and continuing parasympathetic impulses allow vasodilation (Figure 65-4). Blood pools in the peripheral veins, venous return to the right side of the heart is inadequate, and cardiac output is decreased. Other causes include central nervous system (CNS) dysfunction, spinal anesthesia, and drugs. The end result is a decrease in delivery of oxygenated blood to body tissues.

Assessment with Clinical Manifestations

Neurogenic shock has similar clinical manifestations as those listed in the opening section of the discussion of shock syndrome. In addition, the following are typical manifestations of neurogenic shock: hypotension, bradycardia, hypothermia, warm dry skin, decreased cardiac rate and output, decreased venous return, and flaccid paralysis below spinal injury. These signifying manifestations are those that are specific to neurogenic shock and somewhat different by comparison. The paralysis and warm, dry skin are not seen commonly with the other types of shock conditions. In addition, neurogenic shock is not the same as autonomic dysreflexia, which is described in detail in chapter 36. Refer to Table 65-2 for nursing diagnoses and evaluation of outcomes.

Planning and Implementation

Fluid distribution is disrupted throughout the body; therefore the goal is to establish circulatory blood volume, administer appropriate fluids, and monitor fluid overload. Inotropic and vasoconstrictor drugs are often given to increase sympathetic tone and myocardial contraction and to reverse vasodilation if

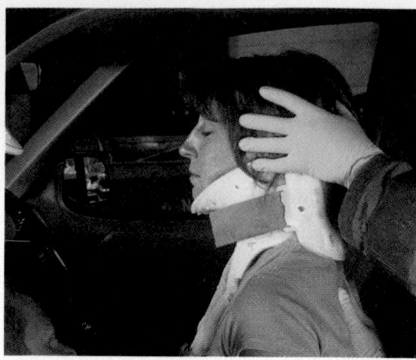

Figure 65-4 Spinal cord injuries often precede neurogenic shock.

sufficient tissue perfusion is still present. A low dose of a corticosteroid is often given to minimize inflammation (Ahrens & Vollman, 2004). Atropine is given to counteract bradycardia due to parasympathetic overstimulation of the heart. Temporary cardiac pacing may be necessary to assist in cardiac output. Assessment using the Glasgow Coma Scale is important if there is cerebral damage, and the patient must be closely monitored for further deterioration in multiple systems (Bench, 2004).

Priority nursing interventions are focused on treating the hypovolemia, promoting normal body temperature, preventing hypoxemia, and monitoring for dysrhythmias. Identification of patients at risk for neurogenic shock and careful monitoring of fluid balance are important prevention strategies. Patients are at risk of DVT because of venous pooling in the lower extremities. The nurse must administer prescribed fluids and monitor patient's response to compensate for the fluid imbalances in the neurogenic shock. The nurse must monitor for manifestations of fluid overload, such as changes in respirations or respiratory distress; assess lung sounds for crackles and rhonchi; assess changes in heart sounds and heart rate; and monitor urinary output usually via retention catheter. In addition, the nurse should monitor specific laboratory results (e.g., coagulation factors, white blood cell [WBC] levels for infection, and hemoglobin or hematocrit levels). Due to the nature of the neurogenic shock, the patient must be observed for signs of infection (e.g., IV insertion site and lungs). The nurse must monitor for evidence of DVT, including leg and foot edema and measurement of calf and thigh circumference. The application is to use prescribed antiembolic stockings or sequential pneumatic stockings, provide passive range of motion exercises, and administer prescribed anticoagulation therapy. To avoid severe complications, the nurse should also assess for signs of pulmonary embolism (e.g., shortness of breath, respiratory distress, and chest pain). Limit activities to promote conservation of oxygen supply. The patient is monitored in regard to his or her mental status, changes in skin condition and appearance. Comfort measures are employed to minimize anxiety and spiritual distress. Last, the patient and family are educated regarding measures to reduce anxiety.

SEPTIC SHOCK

Sepsis is a systemic response to infection that involves the systemic inflammatory process resulting in endothelial dysfunction and altered circulation and coagulation. Severe sepsis is associated with one or more organ dysfunctions because of hypotension or hypoperfusion of tissues. Symptoms may include lactic acidosis, oliguria, and acute changes in mental status.

Pathophysiology

Septic shock is a complex systemic response that involves action of cellular and humoral (body fluids and components of the immune system) against any type of microorganism that invades the body, including gram-negative and gram-positive bacteria, fungi, and viruses. Gram-negative bacteria are considered to be a major cause of septic shock. The microorganisms secrete endotoxins that stimulate capillary permeability and release of mediators which results in increased complement activity, leukopenia, and leukocytosis. Diagnostic studies can confirm the presence of infection; however, in some cases, the source of infection is not identified. Dilation of the vascular bed affects cardiac function and the coagulation cascade, resulting in disseminated intravascular coagulation (DIC) can be triggered by septic shock.

Assessment with Clinical Manifestations

Early symptoms may include a rising core temperature, increase in WBC count, or a rise in C-reactive protein. Manifestations often mimic the criteria established for systemic inflammatory response syndrome (SIRS). A patient

DOLLARS AND SENSE

Financial Impact of Sepsis

Severe sepsis causing multiple organ malfunctions has affected 3,234,000 people worldwide since 2001, with an estimated death rate of 927,000 people. It currently affects 750,000 Americans each year and is the cause of more than 200,000 deaths. Sepsis is the leading cause of death in intensive care units. It is estimated that annual costs in the United States are more than $15 billion. Sepsis is expected to affect one million people by the end of the decade as the population ages. It has increased for children and adults in the last 20 years. Proposed causes are overuse of antibiotics and development of drug-resistant microbes. Health care providers are also able to diagnose signs and symptoms much earlier than they were previously.

Adapted from Bridges, E., & Dukes, S. (2005). Cardiovascular aspects of septic shock: Pathophysiology, monitoring, and treatment. Critical Care Nurse, 25(2), 14–16, 18–20.

history is important for identifying the possible etiology. Potential etiologies of septic shock include: bowel surgery, severe malnutrition, multiple antibiotic therapy or immunosuppressant therapy, prolonged hospitalization, and exposure to nosocomial infection (Kleinpell, 2005).

The patient exhibits at least two signs of SIRS and at least one organ is dysfunctional or has failed. Additional manifestations include chills, hypotension, widened pulse pressure, decreased skin perfusion, and decreased urine output. In addition, the patient with sepsis will often experience significant edema or positive fluid balance (greater than 20 mL/kg over 24 hours), a decreased capillary refill or mottling, hyperglycemia (plasma glucose greater than 120 mg/dL in the absence of diabetes, and a decreased bicarbonate (HCO_3), and an unexplained change in mental status (Kleinpell, 2005). Refer to Table 65-2 for the nursing diagnoses and evaluation of outcomes.

Planning and Implementation

Identification and elimination of the cause as soon as possible are paramount in the treatment of septic shock. Blood cultures are taken, and antibiotic therapy is initiated as soon as possible to prevent the progression to severe sepsis and shock. Supplemental oxygen and respiratory or ventilation support is provided, and the patient is transferred to a critical care unit if necessary. IV access is established, and fluid is administered to improve blood pressure. Inotropic medications, such as dobutamine, are often prescribed to assist with the force of cardiac contractions. Cardiac monitoring (electrocardiogram [ECG]) for possible dysrhythmias is initiated. Antipyretic therapy is administered to relieve fever after consideration is given to the stage of fever and the patient status. Strict universal precautions and prevention of secondary infection are important aspects of care. Prophylactic measures are taken to avoid DVT and stress ulcers. Steroids are administered for patients who have relative adrenal insufficiency.

Sepsis can develop quickly. The nurse must be skilled in recognizing dysfunction of any organ to prevent the progression of severe sepsis. The pulmonary and cardiovascular systems are the most common to show early signs of dysfunction. However, by the time that severe sepsis is recognized, it has already affected many areas of the body. Arterial blood pressure is the best indicator of blood flow. Appropriate tissue oxygenation is indicated by a normal blood pressure and a normal central venous pressure (about 60–75 percent). This means

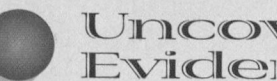

Uncovering the Evidence

New Drug Reduces Mortality in Severe Sepsis

Discussion: International clinical trials were conducted to evaluate the effectiveness of drotrecogin alfa, activated (Xigris) to improve survival in severe sepsis based on the theory that the drug could minimize the affects of the inflammatory response to infection. The drug, which is a recombinant form of human activated protein C, mimics the human protein that (a) inhibits the production of thrombin and prevents clot formation, (b) inhibits the release of plasminogen activator inhibitor-1, and (c) blocks thrombin formation. Therefore, the microvascular thrombi that form can be broken down, and perfusion of tissues would be improved as well potential restoration of organ function. The study consisted of a large double-blind, placebo controlled international study. Xigris is the first drug found to improve survival in severe sepsis. There is a risk of bleeding, although only slightly higher than in patients receiving a placebo. Approximately 80 percent of the drug's effects will be cleared from the system within 30 minutes.

Implications for Practice: Although, Xigris has proven to be beneficial, the costs are prohibitive, at $6,800 for a 96-hour infusion. Strict guidelines have been established for the use of the treatment.

Adapted from Ahrens, T., & Vollman, K. (2003). Severe sepsis management: Are we doing enough? Critical Care Nurse, 24(Suppl 2), 2–16.

that approximately 25–40 percent of oxygen is available in the blood to be extracted by the tissues to support metabolism.

The primary goals are to provide the prescribed antibiotics, fluids, and vasopressor drugs, preventing secondary infections, monitoring the fluid and electrolyte balance, and assessing the patient's response to care. The nurse must be constantly alert to subtle changes that can indicate a progression of the septic process.

Therapeutic nursing interventions for patients with septic shock include implementing standard precautions and monitoring diagnostic reports, including blood glucose levels, clotting dysfunction (e.g., activated partial thromboplastin time [APTT], and international normalized ratio [INR], or prothrombin time [PT], and platelets abnormalities). The nurse must also manage the airway, administer oxygen, supervise ventilatory support, and monitor the patient's response to airway management. The nurse must administer prescribed medications and assess the patient's response, followed by documenting the findings and providing information to appropriate team members. The administration of fluid and nutritional therapy (including blood product administration), along with monitoring and recording intake and output, is essential to the patient's positive progression. In addition, the nurse must provide comfort measures, such as warm blankets or cooling methods, and provide emotional support. Last, the patient and his or her family need education regarding the management strategies that are employed and measures to reduce anxiety.

SYSTEMIC INFLAMMATORY RESPONSE SYNDROME

Recall that infection need not be present for the IIR to be initiated. However, an uncontrolled acute inflammatory response that causes inflammation in multiple organs that are remote from the original insult is defined as the systemic inflammatory response syndrome (SIRS). Conditions commonly associated with SIRS include infection, pancreatitis, ischemia, multiple trauma, hemorrhagic shock, aspiration of gastric contents, massive transfusions, and host defense deficiencies. Regardless of the cause of the insult, the body responses are similar. If the process cannot be contained, there is an increased activation of the inflammatory cells, including the neutrophils, macrophages, and lymphocytes; additional damage to the vascular endothelium, deterioration in transport of nutrients to the organs, and subsequent complication of MODS (Walsh, 2005). The symptoms defining SIRS are shown in Box 65-14.

The WBC values will vary depending on the presence of an active infection, how many of the metabolic processes occur simultaneously, and whether protein supplies are depleted. Transition from SIRS to dysfunction of multiple organs greatly increases the risk of mortality. Four factors are associated with this transition. These factors include: (a) failure to control the source of the inflammation or infection, (b) persistent hypoperfusion due to prolonged shock status, (c) the presence of necrotic tissue (e.g., an abscess), and (d) altered cellular oxygen consumption (hypermetabolism).

DISSEMINATED INTRAVASCULAR COAGULATION

Disseminated intravascular coagulation (DIC) is a pathological form of the normal localized coagulation response to injury. DIC occurs as a result of disease or injury and spreads throughout the body actually damaging organs and tissues. It alters the clotting process so that both excessive clotting and hemorrhage can occur. For example, severe crush injuries, burns, and sepsis cause cell and blood vessel injury, platelet aggregation, and release of thromboplastin into the blood stream. Circulation is impaired due to the microvascular clots. Without oxygen and nutrients, cells will die and release mediators that will activate the inflammatory process. Hypoxia and acidosis and shock occur. Systems commonly affected by DIC are the skin, lungs, kidneys, the CNS, and GI system. DIC is often associated with septic shock, some viral, bacterial, and protozoal infections, respiratory and cardiogenic shock states, hemorrhaging during pregnancy (Figure 65-5), placenta abruption, retained dead fetal tissue, heat stroke, liver disease, and some snake bites.

There may be a delay in determining internal hemorrhaging. All drainage and GI output, mucous membranes, eyes, nose, and mouth should be observed for the presence of blood. Petechiae and purpura of the skin may be early symptoms of hemorrhage. Blood pressure changes, rapid and thready pulse, decreased level of consciousness are additional indicators.

Careful handling of the patient when changing positions and performing procedures is important as these activities can produce bleeding. Avoiding sharp objects, such as razors and intramuscular injections, will be necessary. Constipation and straining should be prevented to minimize potential bleeding. Fluid replacement with crystalloid and colloid solutions and blood products are also indicated (Walsh, 2005; Edwards, 2002).

ACUTE RESPIRATORY DISTRESS SYNDROME

Acute respiratory distress syndrome (ARDS), formerly called adult respiratory distress syndrome, is classified as noncardiac pulmonary edema with increased permeability of the alveolar-capillary membrane due to injury to the pulmonary vasculature or the airways (see chapter 32). The alveoli fill with fluid, thus minimizing or prohibiting gas exchange. It is a sudden progressive pulmonary disorder that is manifested by severe dyspnea, hypoxemia, and diffuse bilateral infiltrates.

BOX 65-14

CLINICAL MANIFESTATIONS OF SIRS

At least two or more of the following symptoms will be present in SIRS:

- Fever greater than 38° C (98.6°F) or less than 36° C (96°F) or inability to maintain a normal temperature
- Tachycardia greater than 90 beats per minute
- Tachypnea—Respiratory rate greater than 20 per minute or a PaCO$_2$ less than 32 mm Hg
- Elevated white blood cell (WBC) count (greater than 12,000 cells/μL) **or**
- Inability to create WBCs (count is less than 4,000/μL) or too many immature WBCs

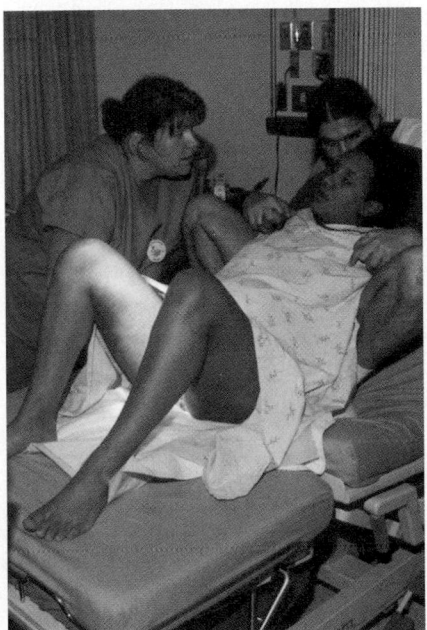

Figure 65-5 DIC can result after delivery with excess bleeding or placenta abruption.

Etiology

ARDS is caused by a variety of clinical events and often occurs in previously healthy people. (Synonyms are shock lung, wet lung, posttraumatic lung, congestive atelectasis, capillary leak syndrome, and adult hyaline membrane disease). Risk factors include direct injury from aspiration, near-drowning, inhalation of smoke and other toxic gases, pneumonia, radiation, drug toxicity, and severe chest trauma. Indirect injuries include sepsis, pneumonia, cardiopulmonary bypass (CPB), embolism, severe pancreatitis, SIRS, DIC, and shock states. ARDS is a major cause of morbidity and death in intensive care units. The risk is dependent on the condition of the host and the etiological factors. The acute phase can resolve or progress to fibrosis. Survivors are usually young, and gradual return of adequate pulmonary function may occur over a year's time. People are usually at greater risk for diminished pulmonary function, fatigue, and repeated respiratory problems (Allen & Parsons, 2005).

Diagnostic Tests

The following diagnostic criteria are recommended by the American-European Consensus Committee on ARDS based solely on pulmonary gas exchange:
- ARDS is defined by ratio of PaO_2 to fraction of inspired oxygen (FiO_2) of 200 or less regardless of positive end-expiratory pressure (PEEP) needed to support oxygenation. (a ratio less than or equal to 300 mm Hg defines acute lung injury)
- Acute (abrupt) onset.
- Development of new bilateral infiltrates on chest X-ray (CXR).
- Pulmonary artery occlusion pressure (PAOP) of 18 mm Hg or less or no clinical evidence of left atrial hypertension.

Nursing Diagnoses

Based on the information gathered, examples of nursing diagnoses in the patient with ARDS may include the following:
- Impaired gas exchange related to decreased passage of gases between the alveoli of the lungs and the vascular system.
- Decreased cardiac output related to alterations in preload.
- Imbalanced nutrition: less than body requirements related to lack of exogenous nutrients or increased metabolic demand.

Planning and Implementation

Collaborative management for ARDS consists of treating the underlying cause, promoting gas exchange, providing oxygen therapy, and preventing complications. The patient is intubated and placed on mechanical ventilation that limits and controls the amount of pressure in the lungs and helps prevent further trauma to the lungs. PEEP is used to facilitate oxygenation because the hypoxemia associated with ARDS if frequently unresponsive to oxygen therapy. Nursing management includes facilitating oxygenation and ventilation, providing comfort and emotional support, and monitoring the patient for complications.

Evaluation of Outcomes

Potential patient outcomes for each of the example nursing diagnoses for the patient with ARDS are:
- Impaired gas exchange related to decreased passage of gases between the alveoli of the lungs and the vascular system: The patient maintains optimal gas exchange as evidenced by normal arterial blood gases (ABGs) and alert responsive mentation or no further reduction in mental status.

- Decreased cardiac output related to alterations in preload: The patient maintains blood pressure within normal limits; warm dry skin; regular cardiac rhythm; clear lung sounds; and strong bilateral, equal peripheral pulses.
- Imbalanced nutrition: less than body requirements related to lack of exogenous nutrients or increased metabolic demand: The patient verbalizes and demonstrates selection of foods or meals that will achieve a cessation of weight loss and weighs within 10 percent of ideal body weight.

MULTIPLE ORGAN DYSFUNCTION SYNDROME

Multisystem failure has been called multiple system organ failure (MSOF), MOF, and MODS. Whatever the term, the meaning is the same; it is the evidence of a progressive inflammatory response in an acutely ill patient, which has caused more than one of the body's organs to fail, and homeostasis cannot be maintained without intervention (Walsh, 2005). There is usually a precipitating event, such as aspiration or septic shock, which is associated with hypotension.

Assessment with Clinical Manifestations

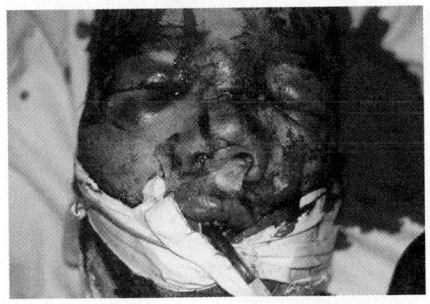

Figure 65-6 Critical head injuries often place a patient at risk for MODS. (Courtesy of Dr. Kevin Reilly, Albany Medical Center, Albany, NY.)

In MODS the patient often is in a crisis, and his or her management has included fluid administration. Following resuscitation with appropriate fluids and vasopressors, the patient appears to be doing well for a short period of time; then a sequence of systemic inflammatory events begins with manifestations of low grade fever, tachycardia, dyspnea, an increase in neutrophils and WBCs, elevated glucose levels, and then signs of infiltrates on the CXR may be seen. Renal and hepatic lab results are relatively normal in the initial stages. Dyspnea progresses and often requires mechanical intubation. Some deterioration in mental status is evident. An example of renal dysfunction includes a creatinine level more than 2 mg/dL and an output of less than 480 mL in a 24-hour period. Renal failure would require dialysis. The outcome may be irreversible, and the end is death over a period of hours to days unless the patient receives complex medical and nursing interventions, and even then, mortality is high. MODS may be responsible for approximately 80 percent of all mortality in the critical care unit and is a leading cause of late mortality after trauma (Figure 65-6).

The findings from classic studies conducted by Knaus, Draper, Wagner and Zimmerman (1986, 1993) to predict the severity of a disease and risk of death are frequently used to diagnose multiple organ dysfunctions. The acute physiology and chronic health evaluation (APACHE II) criteria includes the number of alterations in cardiac, respiratory, renal, hematological, neurological, and hepatic organ failure, age, and preexisting illnesses or diseases as predictive measures.

PRIMARY MULTIPLE ORGAN DYSFUNCTION

Primary multiple organ dysfunction is directly related to an insult, such as a major trauma to the chest or following aspiration or as the result of inhaled fumes or smoke. Primary MODS usually develops quickly. The inflammatory process can trigger the widespread SIRS that places the patient at risk for secondary organ dysfunctions.

Assessment with Clinical Manifestations

Primary MODS begins with disorders such as toxic shock. Toxic shock is a toxin-mediated multisystem disease and is a form of septic shock caused by *Staphylococcus aureus* or group A streptococcus (GAS), an aerobic gram-positive

Uncovering the Evidence

Validation of a Severity of Illness Measure

Discussion: The study purpose is to validate the effectiveness of the APACHE classification system to predict outcomes for severely ill patients admitted to the intensive care unit. The methods included collecting clinical and recorded data, which was conducted in a major U.S. hospital. The subjects were 833 severely ill patients who had been consecutively admitted on an emergency basis to a medical intensive care unit. Nonoperative patients were chosen. Data was collected 24 hours after admission by two former intensive care unit nurses. Data consisted of alterations in seven major organs. Criteria were weighted on a scale of 0 to 4. The weighted sum of 33 potential physiological measures was used as the predictive criteria. Most of the admitted patients had scores on 8–25 of the 33 potential measures, having one or more indications of individual organ failures. The study occurred over a 27-month period. Detailed information was also collected on preadmission data, including age and illnesses. Analysis of physiological data was through regression analysis, and comparison was made with the preadmission data. The findings revealed there was a significant stable association between age, severity of illness, and rate of survival. Similar findings were found with comparison of data from other hospitals. The decline in cardiopulmonary reserve capacity due to age and the incidence of chronic illnesses were closely associated with the mortality outcome predictive scores of the APACHE scale.

Implications for Practice: The APACHE scale can be a useful tool for diagnosis purposes and for suggesting appropriate interventions. The tool will also be useful in further research. Note: the APACHE scale continues to be used as a diagnostic tool and predictor of outcome for severely ill patients with organ dysfunctions.

Wagner, D., Knaus, W., & Draper, E. (1983). Statistical validation of a severity of illness measure. American Journal of Public Health, 73(8), 878–885.

organism. The initial site of infection is the skin or soft tissue, and the infection is easily transferable. It has also occurred in children who have been exposed to the varicella virus and has occurred in young menstruating women who used vaginal tampons. Approximately half of the reported cases have occurred in men and nonmenstruating women. Initial flu-like symptoms, such as high fever, headache, vomiting and diarrhea, hyperactive bowel sounds and abdominal pain, muscle and joint pain, and general malaise, are present. The patient may have a strawberry tongue, an erythematous macular rash, which progresses to desquamation (peeling) of the skin in 7 to 10 days. The disease can cause necrotizing fasciitis (severe infection of the superficial or deep fascia that surrounds muscles of an extremity or the trunk), and spontaneous gangrene of muscle tissue that may require surgical intervention and amputation of limbs. There is a high mortality rate (Walsh, 2005).

SECONDARY MULTIPLE ORGAN DYSFUNCTION

Secondary multiple organ dysfunction is the result of failure of organs that were not affected by the initial insult. Each of the organ systems are affected by and contribute to the exaggerated inflammatory process.

Assessment with Clinical Manifestations

Typical manifestations for secondary multiple organ dysfunction are described in Box 65-15. Refer to Table 65-2 for nursing diagnoses and evaluation of outcomes.

Planning and Implementation

The goals of collaborative management of MODS are to protect the affected organs from further damage, to use aggressive management of sources of infection, to control the mediators of inflammation, and to provide nutritional support that will facilitate metabolic processes and promote homeostasis. Discussing life-sustaining therapies and end-of-life issues with family of critically ill patients is often a necessary component in the plan of care. Nurses are important in meeting these goals.

BOX 65-15

CLINICAL MANIFESTATIONS IN SECONDARY MULTIPLE ORGAN DYSFUNCTION

- Pulmonary edema due to destruction of the alveolar-capillary membrane; hypoxemia due to maldistribution of oxygenated blood; deterioration in breath sounds; and development of crackles and wheezes. Restlessness and dyspnea are evident.
- Tachycardia is initiated in attempt to increase cardiac output; hypotension is due to vasodilation; skin will be flushed, warm to touch due to vasodilation; altered level of consciousness (LOC) is result of decreased cerebral perfusion; urine output is decreased.
- Neurological dysfunction is indicated by restlessness, insomnia, or confusion that can progress to coma as result of cerebral edema. Muscles become rigid; tremors may be present.
- Gastrointestinal dysfunction results from damage to the endothelium lining; normal intestinal flora may escape into the circulation causing systemic infection, particularly of the lung; manifestations include diarrhea, bloody stools, abdominal distension, increase in stomach acidity, and development of stress ulcers.
- Manifestations of hepatic dysfunction include jaundice and impaired mental status (encephalopathy). Diagnostic tests reveal elevated bilirubin and serum glutamic-pyruvic transaminase (SGPT) or L-lactate dehydrogenase (LDH) levels, decreased albumin, and plasma proteins.
- Pancreatic dysfunction indicators include decreased insulin production and hyperglycemia; the release of proteolytic enzymes from dying cells contributes to the inflammatory process in other organs. Nausea, vomiting, and pain are present along with abdominal distension. Lipase and amylase levels are elevated.
- Renal dysfunction caused by ischemia is indicated by oliguria, elevated creatinine and BUN levels, and inability to concentrate urine, electrolyte abnormalities, hypertension, and buildup of toxins.
- Hematological dysfunction (DIC) is manifested by simultaneous bleeding and coagulation. The skin, lungs, and kidneys are the most commonly involved organs. Prothrombin time is prolonged. Signs of hypoxia are evident.

From Kidd, P. (2005). Multiple organ dysfunction syndrome. In K. Wagner & P. Kidd (Eds.), High acuity nursing *(pp. 312–324). New Jersey: Prentice Hall.*

Guidelines include ongoing careful assessment to detect manifestations of early changes in organ function, progressive inflammation and infection, and patient responses to interventions. Nursing priorities include preventing development of secondary infections, adherence to universal safety precaution standards, facilitating delivery of oxygen to the tissues, and limiting tissue oxygen demand, providing fluid and nutritional support, and providing comfort measures and emotional support (Walsh, 2005).

Severely ill patients are exposed to a variety of stressors in the critical care setting and often are unable to cope. They have a loss of autonomy and control over the environment and the loss of privacy and dignity. The feeling of powerlessness can be overwhelming. Spiritual distress is often related to the threat of death and questioning the meaning of suffering in relation to a personal belief system. The person may express anger to God or another supreme being or have self-blame feelings or express regret for being unable to practice belief rituals. Holistic care involves meeting the spiritual needs and alleviating the person's responses to stress.

Patients in intensive care are exposed to light, noise, and the general activity of the unit, which can be disturbing or even threatening. Sleep deprivation occurs due to pain, discomfort, and the environment. The patient is separated from his or her family and friends. Intubated patients cannot verbally express their needs. The sequence and accumulation of stressors, impact of medications and diminished cerebral perfusion, and fluid and electrolyte imbalances can result in acute confusion and delirium, often referred to as intensive care unit psychosis, often referred to as ICU-itis. Confused individuals may be aware of these changes in mental status and believe that they are losing their minds. Manifestations of confusion can resemble symptoms of dementia; therefore differentiation between the two conditions is more difficult (Grendell, 2004). Refer to the nursing interventions described for management of patients with septic shock.

POPULATIONS AT RISK

Several factors place individuals at risk for systemic infections, potential sepsis, and organ failure, including environmental situations, acute and chronic illnesses, hypersensitivities to antigens, genetic predisposition for altered immune function, autoimmune diseases, and acquired immune deficiency. A minor infection, such as the flu or a urinary tract infection, can be the initial source of sepsis for anyone.

Wounds, burns, vehicle accident injuries, and bullet wounds are also potential sources (Figure 65-7). Many trauma events involve injuries to the chest head, spinal cord, and bone fractures as well as breaks in skin integrity and hemorrhage. Burns and near-drowning incidents can cause damage to multiple organs. A trauma incident that requires surgery, blood transfusions, and other invasive measures also place the patient at risk for infection, sepsis, and secondary MODS. The hospital environment adds additional risk factors. Nosocomial (hospital acquired) infections, which are more difficult to treat than community acquired infections, are due to the presence of drug-resistant microorganisms and the compromised condition of the ill hospitalized patient (International Sepsis Forum, 2003).

Secondary, or opportunistic, infections can rapidly progress to sepsis in the extremely young (especially premature infants) and in elderly individuals who have limited immune resources to counteract infections. The immune system is also impaired by an underlying infection, addictive use of alcohol and drugs, smoking or exposure to smoke, hypersensitivities to environmental allergens, malnutrition, and chronic illnesses, such as anemia, hepatic disease, chronic fatigue, and one or more organ dysfunction. Other examples include individuals with a colostomy or ileostomy who become dehydrated due to diarrhea caused by a GI infection, individuals with a

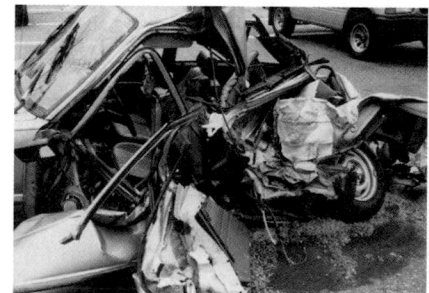

Figure 65-7 Severe motor vehicle crashes often result in multiple injuries, which creates at risk populations for shock syndromes and MODS. (Courtesy of Craig Smith)

tracheostomy, and individuals with cancer who receive chemotherapy or radiation therapy.

Autoimmune diseases, such as diabetes mellitus, rheumatoid arthritis, multiple sclerosis, hemolytic anemia, glomerulonephritis, myasthenia gravis, and systemic lupus erythematosus, are conditions where the body does not recognize the tissue as a part of the self. These problems initiate their own inflammatory process in the attempt to invade and destroy the nonself tissues. Some autoimmune diseases, such as Hashimoto's thyroiditis, attack only the thyroid tissue, and non-Hodgkin's lymphoma arises directly from the thymus gland thus adversely influencing the immune system. These conditions place the individual at high risk for succumbing to infections. Other examples include acquired immune deficiency infections, such as human immunodeficiency virus [HIV] and acquired immune deficiency syndrome [AIDS], which greatly increase the individual's susceptibility to opportunistic infections. Kaposi's sarcoma, a vascular malignancy that is usually seen initially on the skin or mucous membranes, has become closely associated with AIDS. In later stages, the lungs can be affected.

Graft rejection involves the activation of the immune response against a transplanted organ that the body recognizes as nonself. Side effects of immunosuppressant therapy can be life-threatening. Infection can be a major problem following a transplant, and repeated courses in antibiotic therapy can place the patient at risk for a super infection such as *Clostridium difficile* or *Candida*, or drug-resistant bacteria. The patient is also at risk for cytomegalovirus (CMV) infection within a few months of the transplant.

KEY CONCEPTS

- An insult can be anything that triggers the body's IIR.
- The purposes of the IIR are to control bleeding, remove waste products, to limit infection, and to promote healing.
- The shock syndrome is a systemic condition when the peripheral blood flow is inadequate to provide sufficient blood to the heart for normal function and transport of oxygen to all organs and tissues.
- Manifestations of shock will vary according to the underlying cause, the stage of shock, and the individual person's response to shock. Each person must be assessed individually prior to any intervention.
- The four phases of the shock syndrome are the initial phase, the compensatory phase, multiple organ dysfunction phase, and the refractory phase.
- The principle collaborative treatment goals are to identify and treat the underlying cause of the shock syndrome, deliver oxygen to the tissues, promote utilization of oxygen by the tissues, maintain surveillance for complications, and provide comfort and emotional support.
- Hypovolemic shock occurs when there is a lack of circulating fluid volume in the intravascular space.
- Cardiogenic shock results in the failure of either the right or left ventricle or both to provide an adequate delivery of oxygen to the body tissues due to a weakened forward pumping function of the heart.

- Anaphylactic shock is caused by an exaggerated widespread antibody response following a previous exposure to an antigen.
- Neurogenic shock is usually a transient condition that occurs in the absence or suppression of sympathetic nervous system tone.
- Septic shock is a complex systemic response that involves action of cellular and humoral against any type of microorganism that invades the body including gram-negative and gram-positive bacteria, fungi, and viruses.
- An uncontrolled acute inflammatory response that causes inflammation in multiple organs, which are remote from the original insult, is defined as SIRS.
- DIC is a pathological form of the normal localized coagulation response to injury. DIC occurs as a result of disease or injury and spreads throughout the body actually damaging organs and tissues.
- ARDS is a noncardiac pulmonary edema with increased permeability of the alveolar-capillary membrane due to injury to the pulmonary vasculature or the airways. ARDS is a major cause of morbidity and death in intensive care units.
- MODS is the evidence of a progressive inflammatory response in an acutely ill patient that has caused more than one of the body's organs to fail and homeostasis cannot be maintained without intervention.

REVIEW QUESTIONS

1. Biological mediators produce:
   1. Increased capillary permeability
   2. Aspiration
   3. Hyperthermia
   4. Hypoglycemia

2. Hypovolemic shock state is produced by:
   1. Pulmonary emboli
   2. Anemia
   3. Carbon monoxide poisoning
   4. Third spacing of body fluids

3. Manifestations of anaphylactic shock include:
   1. Systolic blood pressure greater than100 mm Hg
   2. Warm, moist skin
   3. Bradycardia and hypotension
   4. Stridor and wheezing

4. Which of the following organ systems is among the most common to fail in severe sepsis?
   1. Gastrointestinal system
   2. Cardiovascular system
   3. Renal system
   4. Neurological system

5. The primary purpose for providing crystalloid solutions is to:
   1. Supplement hemoglobin concentrations
   2. Prevent right ventricular failure
   3. Restore fluid volumes and increase preload
   4. Minimize organ oxygen demand

6. DIC plays a role in the inflammatory process by:
   1. Promoting movement of bacteria into the general system
   2. Decreasing oxygen supplies to cells

   3. Limiting biological mediator release
   4. Increasing vascular resistance

7. What manifestations would indicate a reversal of the shock process?
   1. A heart rate of 90 beats per minute
   2. A blood pressure of 130/70
   3. A respiratory rate of 24 per minute
   4. A urine output of 225 cc per hour

8. All of the individuals below are at risk for developing MODS as the result of a severe insult to the body. Which one would have the greatest risk?
   1. A person who smokes
   2. A 75-year-old individual
   3. A person with congestive heart failure
   4. A person with renal dysfunction

9. Which of the following is the most important factor for increasing oxygen supply?
   1. Decreasing cardiac preload
   2. Administration of appropriate fluids
   3. Administration of vasoconstrictor medications
   4. Maximizing optimal cardiac output

10. Noncardiogenic-pulmonary edema may result from:
    1. Decrease in surfactant
    2. Shunting of blood to nonventilated areas
    3. Alterations in the alveolar-capillary membrane
    4. Increased cardiac output

REVIEW ACTIVITIES

1. What are the gastrointestinal (including hepatic, gallbladder, and pancreas) responses during the sustained IIR response and shock conditions? Use http://www.medicalfacts.org as a resource.

2. Discuss why there has been an increase in the number of sepsis cases within the last two decades.

Continued

REVIEW ACTIVITIES—cont'd

3. Get a copy of Ahrens, T., & Vollman, K. (2003). Severe sepsis management: Are we doing enough? *Critical Care Nurse* Oct. (Suppl),24(2–16).
   a. What are the ethical issues related to the use of Xigris?
   b. Read the case studies at the end of the article. Use the nursing process to develop a plan of care for these patients.

4. Access the Web site for the United States. Center for Disease Control (CDC) at: http://www.cdc. Review the links to the FEMA fact sheet and the American Red Cross Health and safety tips related to the consequences of exposure to extreme heat. Develop a plan to share this information with someone.

5. Access the Web site for the Institute for Healthcare Improvement at: http://www.ihi.org. View the PowerPoint presentation on the six-month update of the 100,000 lives campaign. Note the six changes that have been proposed to save lives. Read the press release. Listen to the informational call recording that gives an overview of the campaign.

6. Access the International Sepsis Forum Web site at: www.sepsisforum.org. You can download the free educational booklet for families. It is available in Dutch, English, French, German, Italian, Portuguese, and Spanish.

7. Access the non-Hodgkin's lymphoma Web site at: http://www.lymphomafocus.org. View videos and transcripts for information about this disease. A case study is also presented.

8. To learn more about Vytex TM, the safe latex material, access http://www.vytex.com. Read the information there that is in a pdf format.

Mass Casualty Care

Heather Freiheit, RN, BSN, EMT-P

CHAPTER TOPICS

- Emergency Nursing
- Triage
- Mass Casualty Incidents
- Incident Command
- Hospital Operation Plans

- Personal Protective Equipment
- Hazardous Materials
- Biological Warfare
- Blast Injuries
- Stress Reactions

E mergency nursing is a unique aspect of the nursing profession. No matter the emergency department (ED) size, trauma level, or geographical location, the ED nurse must be ready to care for anything that comes through the doors at a moment's notice. ED nurses must be capable of providing care across the developmental continuum. This group of specialized nurses must be prepared to care for a women giving birth, care for a 70-year-old patient suffering a myocardial infarction (MI), resuscitate a 30-day-old infant, assist with a lumbar puncture, provide emotional support to the families, and everything in between. Frequently EDs are referred to as an environment of controlled chaos because of their ever-changing environment. No one can predict when the next patient will arrive, or the severity of their injury or illness; this is why EDs utilize a **triage system,** which is a method to rank or classify patient's illnesses or severity of injury.

KEY TERMS

Acute respiratory distress
  syndrome (ARDS)
Anaphylaxis
Antiphagocytic
Centrifugal
Coagulopathies
Compartment syndrome
Coronavirus
Crash cart
Critical incident
Epidemiological
  investigation
Exanthema
High efficiency particulate
  air (HEPA) filter
Intradermal route
Macrophages
Macular rash
Malaise
Mass casualty incident
  (MCI)
Mitigation
Myalgia
Nuchal
Preparedness
Prodrome phase
Rhabdomyolysis
Rigors
Rye ergot
Stridor
Triage system
Vesicular rash

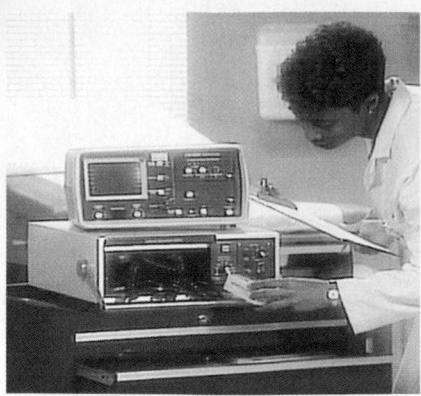

Figure 66-1 Crash cart.

EMERGENCY NURSING

EDs in the early 20th century always had dedicated nurses and were not joined by dedicated ED physicians until the 1970s. Prior to that time, many EDs were staffed by unsupervised residents, who in turn, were oriented and guided through their ED rotations by experienced ED nurses (Schriver, Talmadge, Chuong, & Hedges, 2003).

Over the last 40 years, ED nurses have been instrumental in establishing ED-specific policies and procedures. For example, registered nurse (RN) Anita Dorr developed the **crash cart** (mobile cart with defibrillator, resuscitation equipment, and medications used when patients go into cardiac arrest) (Figure 66-1), originally called the crisis cart in 1967. In 1970 the Emergency Nurses Association (ENA) was created. The ENA established the nationally recognized Certificate of Emergency Nursing and the *Journal of Emergency Nursing*, helping to establish emergency nurses as a recognized profession.

With health care in crisis, more uninsured patients than ever, a decreasing availability of medical doctors (MDs), and poor insurance reimbursement, patients are not able to establish care with a primary care physician, leaving the EDs as the safety net. Additionally, the population is growing while hospitals are closing, placing an even greater burden on emergency departments. Because of the federal regulation, Emergency Medical Treatment and Labor Act (EMTALA), hospitals cannot turn anyone away until it has been established the patient does not have a serious medical condition. These increasing patient volumes overwhelm EDs, forcing patients to be cared for on gurneys in the hallways. As hospitals build larger EDs to help care for this increasing patient population, they must be designed to allow for influxes of large numbers of patients, patients who may be contaminated with hazardous chemicals, requiring decontamination, as well as multiple trauma victims. These patients may arrive via ambulance, helicopter, taxi, or even their own private vehicles, and departments must have acceptable routes and entrances for all (Figure 66-2).

EDs have become the major diagnostic and resuscitation site for Americans. Emergency nursing has had to keep up with the expanded role and diverse patient populations. The knowledge base, complexity, and technical skill set have grown tremendously, and emergency nurses are required to have many additional specialty certifications. These courses usually are advanced cardiac life support (ACLS), pediatric advanced life support (PALS), trauma nursing core curriculum (TNCC), or their equivalents.

The philosophy of emergency medicine is to stabilize patients, alleviate pain or symptoms, and frequently to refer the patient to a specialist for follow-up, or to admit the patient for further care. There are some minor illnesses or injuries that may not require any further follow-up, such as rashes, ear infections, strains, and sprains. Although EDs refer patients for follow-up care with a primary care physician, frequently the patient returns to the ED, because he or she has no insurance and cannot afford to pay up front to be evaluated by the referral doctor.

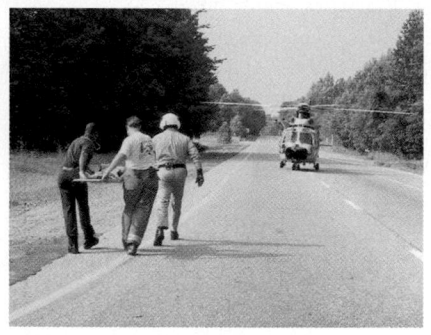

Figure 66-2 Transportation of a patient via a helicopter. Courtesy of Craig Smith.

The nurse, patient, and the family or caregiver, must take a collaborative approach to provide the best patient management during the ED visit. The average length of stay for an ED patient is less than three hours, which creates a challenge when developing a nursing plan of care. A nurse in triage will perform a brief assessment, but the primary nurse is responsible for completing a full assessment when the patient is taken back to a room. Based on the patient's chief complaint, vital signs, and the findings from the assessment the nurse can formulate nursing diagnoses. The RN works collaboratively with the physician to decide the patient's plan of care, but the RN is responsible for implementing the plan. Throughout the implementation of the plan the RN evaluates the effectiveness of the interventions. Based on evaluations of her findings, the RN will advise the physician, and the plan will be revised. ED nurses work closely with ED physicians side by side day after day. This close work environment has helped foster comradeship between these two profes-

Uncovering the Evidence

Discussion: This one-year study looked at ambulatory visits to EDs in the United States during 2002. The data was collected from the 2002 National Hospital Ambulatory Medical Care Survey (NHAMCS), a national probability sample survey conducted by the Centers for Disease Control and Prevention (CDC) and the Health Care Statistics Division. In this study, 396 hospitals were asked to participate, and 376 completed the survey (an overall response rate of 94.9 percent). The following highlights were discovered.

ED visits increased 23 percent between 1993 through 2002, but the number of available EDs decreased by almost 15 percent.

Overall ED utilization rate per population increased by 9 percent; from 35.7 visits per 100 in 1992 to 38.9 visits per 100 in 2002.

The mean age of ED patients rose from 33 in 1992 to 35.6 in 2002; but patients over 75 years of age had the highest rate of ED visits at 61.1 visits per 100.

In 2002, abdominal pain, chest pain, fever, and headache were leading patient complaints. Two thirds of ED patients spend between 1 and 6 hours in an ED with an average of 3.2 hours.

Implications for Practice: This data shows that EDs throughout the United States are being used more frequently and are becoming busier and busier. Because 15 percent of the nation's EDs have closed over the last nine years, this has left fewer remaining open EDs to care for all of these patients, leading to longer patient wait times and stays in the ED. As a result of all of these changes, EDs are becoming more overwhelmed, including the need to divert ambulances to other EDs. More elderly patients are being seen in the EDs, and they tend to require more extensive workups and are more acutely ill than younger patients. It is becoming increasingly difficult to transfer patients out of the ED and get them admitted to an inpatient bed because of full inpatient units and limited available nurses. This leads to ED holding these patients for 24 hours or even longer. Due to EMTALA, EDs cannot turn away or refuse evaluation to any walk-in patients, which leads to overcrowded departments, long waits, patients in the hallways, ambulance diversions, and a stressful work environment for ED nurses. ED managers and educators are discovering their nurses must also have training in inpatient documentation, procedures, and care standards because they are holding these patients and care must be continued.

As these trends continue, administrators must be proactive, changing hospital-wide systems to assist EDs in obtaining beds for admissions and create system efficiencies to help reduce patient through-put times for EDs to be able to care for this continued increase in patient volume.

Source: McCaig, L., & Burt, C. (2004). National hospital ambulatory medical care survey: 2002 emergency department summary. *USDHHS Publication No. (PHS) 2004-125004-0226-0302. Hyattsville, MD: U. S. Department of Health & Human Services.*

---

sions and has strengthened patient care through open two-way communication channels (Figure 66-3)

TRIAGE

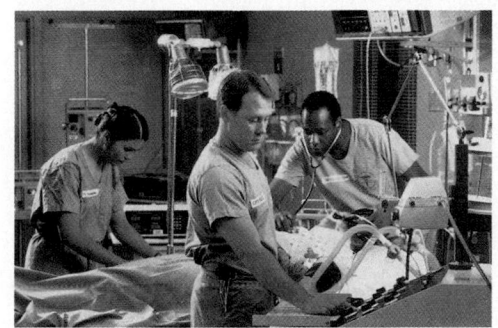

Figure 66-3 ED nurses working with a physician. Courtesy of U. S. Government, as represented by the Secretary of the Army.

Triage stems from a French word meaning "to sort." Triage is the process of rapidly assessing patients and assigning them a classification or priority for care. Triage was first used to prioritize care for injured soldiers in France in the 1800s. It was not until the 1900s, when inner city hospital EDs started to become crowded, that hospital triage was adopted in the United States (Ihlenfeld, 2003). Triage was then perfected by the American military during the Korean and Vietnam wars with Mobile Army Surgical Hospitals (MASH) units.

The objectives of a triage system are to (a) identify patients who require immediate care, (b) use space and resources efficiently, (c) facilitate patient flow into the ED, (d) provide assessment and reassessment of patients, (e) alleviate fear and anxiety of patients or visitors, (f) improve guest relations, and (g) initiate legal accountability. Triage is usually performed by a RN who completes a rapid assessment of the patient's chief complaint, vital signs, overall appearance and mentation, pain level, and psychosocial needs to

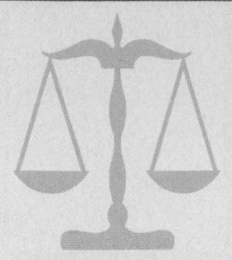

ETHICS IN PRACTICE

Family members and EDs will have different philosophies as to whether family members should be allowed to wait in the examination room during resuscitation of a cardiac arrest. Some hospitals still do not allow family to be present at all in the room during a cardiac arrest, although this practice is being challenged.

EDs are being encouraged to allow family to be present during resuscitations or at least brought in after the initial first few minutes. This practice is encouraged for a variety of reasons:

- This allows family members to see that everything is being done for their loved ones.
- This also may help loved ones choose to have the resuscitation stopped after they are educated on what has been done, the lack of patient response, and see the futility of the efforts.
- When families are present during resuscitation, they also are less apt to pursue legal actions, because they have seen what was done and had a chance to have their questions answered.

DOLLARS AND SENSE

The Financial Implications of On-Call Specialists in the ED

In November of 2003, the Centers for Medicare and Medicaid Services (CMS) revised the EMTALA regulations. In these revised regulations CMS acknowledged that the demands on health care providers are becoming overwhelming, and there is a need to balance available health care providers with ED call coverage. EDs must maintain a list of on-call health care specialists, but MDs are being allowed to take calls at more than one ED at a time. Additionally, on-call specialists are being allowed to limit the amount of call time they are available. This leniency for on-call specialist coverage combined with reduced health care provider payment from insurance companies, higher malpractice insurance, and a growing number of uninsured patients, is affecting ED patient access to specialized care in a timely fashion. Frequently, this results in patients being transferred to another ED to receive care from the needed specialist. Delays in care may lead to greater injury or disability for patients, which may have been prevented or mini-mized if treatment had been administered in a timely fashion. For example, a previously healthy 55-year-old male patient arrives with chest pain and ST elevation indicative of a MI. If the ED does not have a cardiologist on call, the patient cannot be immediately taken for a heart catheterization and possible intervention. If it takes two hours for the patient to be transferred to an ED with a cardiologist, the patient has two hours of cardiac muscle damage that could have been prevented. If this was extensive muscular damage and the man is disabled and can no longer be work, he begins drawing from Social Security for an injury that may have been prevented. Health care professionals, health care providers, policy makers, and the government must work together to find ways and ensure specialized physicians are on-call and available to all. This may be accomplished through capping malpractice insurance, lobbying for affordable health care, and establishing fair compensation for health care providers.

adequately determine the patient's acuity and assign him or her a priority level of care. Triage scales are based on the severity of the patient's injury or illness. There are a variety of triage scales used in EDs, but they all rate the patient's severity and classify the order in which the patient is to be seen as: Level I, II, or III; critically ill, intermediate, or low risk; and urgent, emergent, or stable (Ihenfeld, 2003).

Currently, most EDs use a three-tiered system, although this is changing to a five-tiered system because of a more reliable and consistent triage level. The five-tiered system looks not only at the patient's acuity, but it also helps to predict the number of resources the patient will require. The highest priority or the most emergent conditions involve the potential for loss of life or limb without immediate intervention. These conditions may include unresponsive patients, **anaphylaxis** (a widespread severe allergic reaction that may be life-threatening), or stroke-like symptoms. Urgent patients are defined as those having an acute condition that requires prompt evaluation and may include fractures without neurovascular compromise, abdominal pain, or nosebleeds. Nonurgent patient conditions are those in which there is not a risk of deterioration and care can be delayed. Examples include dermatitis (inflammation of the skin either from allergic reaction or direct contact with an irritant; redness, itching, and blisters may occur), medication refills, toothaches, or sprains, and strains. Triage RNs are challenged with assessing the order in which patients need to be evaluated by an ED doctor. It is the RN's responsibility to assess each patient and assign his or her triage level. These RNs are frequently challenged with an overwhelming number of patients requesting emergency care. It is recommended that the most experienced ED RNs perform triage. For some patients with life-threatening illnesses, it is an expert RN who will be able to recognize the subtle symptoms underlying the patient's complaint.

In assessing their patients, the triage nurse needs to be aware of the some risks. First, a nurse runs the risk of failing to recognize and care for patients in extreme pain, and the RN must also not judge whether the patient is or is not exaggerating his or her pain. Second, a nurse runs the risk of failing to recognize and appropriately triage high-risk chief complaints, such as chest pain, neurological changes, or headaches. Third, a nurse runs the risk of not getting complete vital signs. Fourth, a nurse runs the risk of not reevaluating patients placed in the waiting room. Last, a nurse runs the risk of incomplete or lack of documentation regarding triage assessment and reassessment.

Triage is not to be mistaken for a medical screening exam (MSE). EMTALA requires a MSE for all patients presenting to an ED requesting treatment or evaluation. EMTALA mandates that a MSE be completed to protect patients with life-threatening illnesses or injury from being refused medical treatment by ED as a result of the patient's lack of insurance coverage or inability to pay. A MSE determines whether the patient has an emergency medical condition or not. If an emergency condition exists, the patient must be treated and cannot be transferred or referred to another hospital until they are stabilized. A physician, nurse practitioner, or physician's assistant completes these exams. A MSE includes the patient's initial triage information and includes a focused examination of the appropriate system related to the chief complaint. For example, a patient with a fever and sore throat would have their throat examined to assess if there is an emergent condition, such as epiglottitis (a bacterial infection causing rapid inflammation of the epiglottis; this inflammation may completely occlude the airway and lead to death) or a peritonsillar abscess (pus collects behind the tonsils from an infection causing compression of the uvula, and this may lead to airway obstruction), before the decision can be made to refer them to a primary health care provider or clinic.

START Method of Triage

In the early 1980s, the simple triage and rapid treatment (START) was developed as a method to quickly triage multiple patients. The START method is a nationally recognized triage system that can be initiated in the prehospital setting and

Fast Forward ▶▶▶

Nurses Future Role in the ED of Small Hospitals

Because of a decreasing availability of ED physicians in rural hospitals and an increasing patient volume, the CMS adapted their regulations and now a RN may perform a MSE, which is a new philosophy for hospitals. Currently, EDs around the nation are exploring if and how they will implement this. If ED nurses are to begin performing the MSEs, they must have a system in place that dictates which health care provider they consult if the nurse feels the patient has a life-threatening issue or if the nurse has a question.

carried into the hospital environment. Three patient criteria are evaluated: ventilation, pulses and perfusion, and neurological status. In the event of multiple casualties, using the START method, each patient assessment is completed in less than 60 seconds. This enables the nurse to determine the number of causalities, the severity of their injuries, and to rapidly mobilize the necessary resources.

The traditional way of triaging patients is based on caring for the most critical patients first. In dealing with a mass casualty incident (MCI), the triage philosophy is to first provide care to those patients most likely to survive (Ihlenfeld, 2003). In other words, do the greatest good for the most; patients most severely injured will be cared for last. Similarly, this MCI philosophy is similar to what is used in military triage situations. This change in philosophy may be uncomfortable to nursing personnel who want to care for all patients or to first care for those most severely injured. It is to be remembered that resources and systems will be overwhelmed during a MCI or disaster. Following the MCI philosophy, the ED will provide care to the greatest number of injured. Four colors are used to identify four categories of patients that require triaging: (a) green is used to identify patients who need minimal health care, (b) yellow is used to identify patients who need health care, but not immediately and not at a high acuity of injury, (c) red is used to identify patients who need health care immediately and are life threatened, and (d) black is used to identify patients who are going to die. As a further explanation, it is vital to identify patients who will do well with minimal care (green and some yellows), those who most likely will die even with care (black), and focus immediate resources and rapid intervention for those who will benefit the most (reds and some yellows). In disaster settings, health care providers have an obligation to treat as many people as possible that have the best chance of survive. During a MCI, in these resource-constrained situations clinicians must prioritize victims (Burkle, 2002). On the average day, ED nurses are familiar with triaging patients but during a MCI or disaster, even the most experienced triage RN will become overwhelmed.

Patients who are initially triaged at the scene of a MCI must receive the same rapid triage by a RN or MD on arrival at the ED. This assessment determines if the patient's triage criteria have changed, for example, from yellow to red.

Military Triage

Depending on the event, the military uses two different types of triage methods: tactical and nontactical. These methods are similar to other triage systems as they are intended to balance the human lives at stake, the level of resources available, and the realistic capabilities of medical personnel on the scene (Table 66-1).

MASS CASUALTY INCIDENT

Most experts agree it is not a matter of if, but rather of when the next MCI will occur. A **mass casualty incident (MCI)** is defined as an influx of victims that overwhelms the hospital and affects the institutions capability to care for this influx of victims. Unfortunately, in recent years, hospitals have had resources challenged with a rapid influx of patients: the World Trade Center bombing of 1993, the events of September 11, 2001, the anthrax events in fall of 2001, the Florida hurricanes of 2004, and the disaster associated with hurricane Katrina in 2005 (Box 66-1). Hospitals must be prepared for a MCI 24 hours a day, seven days a week. No one knows when, where, or what will be the cause of the next event. What is known is it has happened before, it will happen again, and there will be injured survivors.

The American College of Emergency Physicians defines a disaster as "when the destructive effects of natural or man-made forces overwhelm the ability of a given area or community to meet the demand of health care" (Mothershead, 2003). A MCI has large numbers of injured and dead, but the community infrastructure remains intact (Mothershead, 2003). A MCI will tax the hospital and

KATRINA DISASTER

The Katrina hurricane disaster in August 2005 was the deadliest and costliest hurricane in the history of the United States. There were 1,836 fatalities and an estimated expense of $75 billion. President George W. Bush declared a state of emergency in three states two days prior to landfall of the Class V hurricane. The mayor of New Orleans, Ray Nagin, ordered a mandatory evacuation on August 28, and the Superdome was used as a shelter for 26,000 people. Overall, Katrina revealed the difficulty in implementing a large-scale disaster plan. The Federal Emergency Management Agency (FEMA) drew tremendous criticism over the ensuing months, and people demanded a better federal plan for disasters. The Katrina disaster signaled the importance of continued progression and development of better planning for the future of mass casualty incidents.

Source: Knabb, R., Rhome, J., & Brown, D. (2005, August 23–30). Tropical cyclone report: Hurricane Katrina. National Hurricane Center. Retrieved on May 30, 2006, from www.nhc.noaa.gov.

TABLE 66-1 Tactical vs. Non-Tactical Triage

Tactical Triage Utilized in Combat-type Settings

Class I:	Patients with minor injuries that can be treated in an ambulatory outpatient basis.
Class II:	Patients whose injuries require immediate intervention to sustain life but require minimum amount of time, personnel, and supplies initially.
Class III:	Definitive treatment can be delayed without threat to life or limb.
Class IV:	Patients with extensive injuries that would require extensive treatment beyond the immediate medical capabilities. Caring for these victims would jeopardize other victims.

Nontactical Triage (Similar to Tactical Triage, but the Four Priority Classes Are Different)

Priority I:	Patients with correctable life-threatening illnesses or injury.
Priority II:	Patients with serious but not life-threatening injuries or illnesses.
Priority III:	Patients with minor injuries.
Priority IV:	Patients who are dead or fatally injured.

Triage during a disaster is an ongoing process that is based on trying to save the most patients possible. There will be instances when a patient may have the potential to survive but dedicating the personnel and resources to that individual most likely will compromise others.

Source: Integrated Publishing. (2004). Triage. Retrieved June 21, 2006, from http://infodotinc.com.

prehospital systems, whereas a mass casualty event or disaster usually destroys the community support systems and leads to the influx of an overwhelming number of patients. During a MCI or a disaster, the goal is to quickly identify those patients who have stable, minor injuries and can wait for care (green patients), those patients who will most likely die even with immediate interventions (black patients), and to focus care and resources on those patients who will benefit from rapid care and interventions (red and yellow patients).

What constitutes an MCI for one institution is not necessarily true for another. During a MCI, a hospital is challenged with a large volume of sick or injured patients, creating a discrepancy between available hospital resources and the number of patients arriving. The characteristics of the facility, such as the hospital's size, advanced preparation and training, combined with available resources, number of ED beds, radiology resources, operating room (OR) suites, and number of critical care beds, will help determine if a hospital will be overwhelmed. The facility characteristics combined with the specific event will help individual hospitals decide if they need to activate their disaster plan to manage the incident. Fortunately, the United States has never experienced an event where thousands of patients are sick or injured in one community and needing care. Unfortunately, with the current terrorist cells, it is possible this type of MCI to occur at any time and health care facilities and their communities must be prepared for this to occur (Ihlendfeld, 2003).

INCIDENT COMMAND

When a disaster or MCI occurs, it results in the hospital's normal day-to-day operations being interrupted for long periods of time and involves extensive man hours. To operate effectively and efficiently, a hospital must have preestablished response plans in place and be familiar with how to initiate and use them. The Incident Command System (ICS) is a system utilized to help manage large-scale events where areas of responsibility are assigned to personnel for coordination. Originally, the ICS was created to help manage the large numbers of firefighters utilized on wilderness fire scenes. This system was so successful it has since been restructured for hospital use, known as the hospital emergency incident command system (HEICS). The HEICS is extremely practical and creates a valid instrument for assisting hospitals during times of disasters and complex problem situations. The HEICS includes five functional branches of command, finance and planning, operations, logistics, and subunits may be established off of each branch depending on the disaster. The ICS can be implemented in varying levels, depending on the type of incident, the number of potential victims, and the estimated length of an event.

Hospital Emergency Incident Command System

The HEICS was initially tested in the early 1990s by six hospitals in Orange County, California. In 1992, HEICS was refined and distributed to hospitals around the world (Greater New York Hospital Association, 2002). Following the 1993 Northridge earthquake in California, HEICS was utilized successfully by hospitals damaged in the earthquake. Implementation of the HEICS provides the following advantages: a consistent algorithm for organizing information, controlling and coordinating the influx and movement of patients, and the distribution of required staff, supplies, and resources. HEICS also allows for a manageable span of control for the assigned group leaders and a consistent way of communication using common terminology. HEICS is a flexible program, which can be expanded on or scaled down, depending on the magnitude of the event. During large-scale events, preset roles fulfilled staffed by a variety of personnel to allow for periods of rest. HEICS also provides an organized means of successfully transferring the command process to relieve the incident command staff.

Following HEICS guidelines, the role of incident commander (IC) is preassigned, and this position is implemented immediately after notification of an event. Without an IC, staff takes independent actions that are not in coordination with one another. These uncoordinated actions lead to rapid chaos and potential patient compromise or staff injury. Depending on the type and time of the event, the IC may initially be a department manager or the house supervisor, although the IC role is transferred on to an administrator as early as possible.

Like the prehospital incident command system (ICS), the HEICS system has four components: finance, logistic, operations, and planning (FLOP). The IC appoints chiefs to these components, and the chiefs then designate directors and unit leader for each subunit. This structure and distribution of assignments limits individuals' span of control and helps obtain adequate documentation and tracking of the event. HEICS provides both a framework for standardized roles internally and allows a universal network between hospitals, police, fire, emergency medical services (EMS) agencies, and the city or county emergency operations center. This system supports effective communication between these agencies using common terminology and standardized roles (Figure 66-4). For example, during a county-wide MCI, the material and supply unit officer from one hospital can call the material and supply unit officer from another hospital to check on mask availability of N-95 masks, thus coordinating resources.

HEICS Activator

Both internal and external events can lead to the initiation of the ICS. Internal events occur within the hospital and can prevent the hospital from functioning normally, compromising patient care. Examples of internal events include

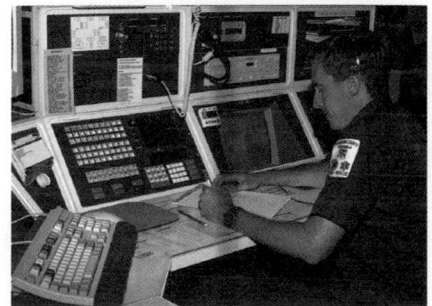

Figure 66-4 Communication among agencies is facilitated by complex technological centers.

a main water pipe rupturing or fire. External events take place outside of the hospital and lead to a large influx of patients arriving at the ED. Disasters may be both internal and external, such as an earthquake or tornado. As soon as the hospital's ED receives notification of a MCI or disaster, the hospital's disaster plan is activated; this pulls additional staff from other areas of the hospital to assist ED staff in caring for the influx of sick or injured patients. In the case of possible infectious disease outbreak, as soon as the hospital's ED starts to see patients experiencing similar signs and symptoms, the disaster plan is initiated. When the hospital disaster plan is activated, outside agencies may need to be contacted so to as alert them to the hospital's limited capabilities.

Incident Command Education

It is imperative that hospitals have a preestablished incident command structure that is integrated with the hospital disaster plan. Personnel must be familiar with the hospital's ICS and understand their role during a disaster or MCI. Unless hospitals provide training and drills for staff, having a disaster plan will not be beneficial as staff will be unfamiliar with the plan. In these drills, a variety of potential scenarios must be practiced including: nuclear, biological, natural disasters, and loss of power or water. The Joint Commission on Accreditation of Healthcare Organizations ([JCAHO] 2006a) Environment of Care Standard EC.1.4 requires hospitals have an emergency management plan that addresses four phases of emergency management: **preparedness** (activities which build the hospital's capacity to manage the effects of an emergency or disaster), **mitigation** (activities a hospital undertakes to help lessen the severity and impact of potential emergencies that may affect operations or services provided by a hospital), response, and recovery. Standard EC.2.9.1 states the hospital response plan must be practiced twice a year, and at least once a year there must be an influx of victims through the ED. Following the terrorist attacks of September, 2001, JCAHO added the requirement that hospitals practice communication and coordination with other agencies and hospitals in the community in preparation for a large-scale event.

For all personnel to be included and familiar with the procedures, drills take place on day/evening/night shifts and weekends. Additionally, specific staff is trained and able to perform decontamination of patients exposed to hazardous chemicals or biological toxins and this drill is practiced at least once a year. In these drills, leadership personnel are usually placed into the IC roles, whereas patient care providers will most likely be continuing to care for patients. For the HEICS to work effectively, staff needs to understand the IC structure and needs to accept a reporting structure and different lines of authority with which they are accustomed to (Greater New York Hospital Association, 2002). Additional staff is generally sent to the ED to assist with the initial influx of patients. If hospitals have had frequent disaster drills to practice their different roles in a disaster, employees will be comfortable working in the ED to care for patients.

HOSPITAL OPERATIONS PLAN

Hospital operation plans (ps plans) are made up of many components that allow hospitals to be prepared for a variety of unusual incidents. These plans include sections on HEICS, disasters, bioterrorism, chemical, and radiation emergencies and are used by staff and IC as guides during events.

Hospital emergency operation plans need to include elements of preparedness, response, mitigation, and recovery. The plan must incorporate strategies to care for a large influx of patients for up to 72 hours, as it may be this long before assistance from the government can arrive. Additional supplies will be made available to hospitals from national stockpiles as early as 24 hours but may take as long as 72 hours. The time it takes for these resources to be mobilized and arrival depends on the extent of the event and national priority of the community requesting resources. Operation plans must also include the hospitals available supply of on site antibiotics, antidotes, ventilators, respirators, and other supplies needed to care for victims of a MCI. The plans must also have contingencies to acquire additional supplies to survive 24 to 72 hours until the arrival of federal assistance, also known as disaster medical assistance teams (DMATs). DMAT teams are made up of physicians, nurses, and EMTs who are transported to large-scale events to help in triaging, stabilization, transport, and patient treatment (Mothershead, 2003). Hospital operation plans must have established working relationships between other area hospitals, police and EMS and fire agencies, and the city or county emergency operations center. Communication plans need to have interoperability or the ability of different hospitals and public safety agencies to communicate with one another in real time. This helps to coordinate patient transport and communication with community members about the location of their loved ones. One way to help interoperability is for all entities involved to use the ICS.

A terrorist event or even a food-borne illness outbreak may be covert or overt. Hospital ops plans need to have established systems to expedite disease reporting of suspected outbreaks to both internal infection control practitioners and the county health department. Having established communication plans with the community and media prior to an event allows for quicker dissemination of important information to the general public.

In addition to hospital employees' phone numbers, these ops plans should include important external resource phone numbers, such as local health department, Federal Bureau of Investigation (FBI) field office, CDC infection control and bioterrorism branch, local hazardous materials (HazMats) team, and contracted supply and pharmaceutical suppliers. The hospital ops plan must also include the process for hospital evacuation and meeting places along with alternate care sites for the patients, supplies, and medical records (Box 66-2).

PERSONAL PROTECTIVE EQUIPMENT

Personal protective equipment (PPE) refers to the clothing and respiratory equipment required to protect staff from chemical, biological, or infectious threats. EDs must have PPE available to personnel who will be caring for these individuals. Patient care providers need access to the correct and adequate amounts of PPE. If a large-scale biological event were to occur, PPE would be needed by all ED staff with the means to rapidly replenish stock. Prior to any event, ED personnel must know how and when to correctly use the PPE and the location of where it is stored. The type of PPE required depends on the event or suspected disease. Some diseases require standard precautions, whereas others require expanded precautions. In addition to PPE, the nurse will need to follow the guidelines for standard precautions and expanded precautions (i.e., contact precautions, droplet precautions, airborne infection, and isolation precautions). Refer to chapter 11 for a review of these guidelines.

HAZARDOUS MATERIALS

Hazardous materials (HazMats) are materials that have the potential to harm a person or the environment (Figure 66-5). Caring for patients who have been contaminated with HazMats is extremely challenging for staff. ED staff are required to care for contaminated patients knowing they may potentially be exposing themselves to the chemical. Even without the threat of a terrorist attack, the potential for a HazMat patient arriving at an ED is great. More than four billion tons of chemicals are transported across the United States, stemming from over 100,000 different locations, and involving over one million

---

BOX 66-2

HOSPITAL OPERATION PLAN CRITERIA

Hospital disaster plans should include information on the following topics:

- Recognition and notification
- Assessment of hospital capabilities
- Personnel recall back to work
- Establishment of incident command
- Maintenance of accurate records
- Public relations
- Equipment supply and resupply

Adapted from Mothershead, J. (2003). Disaster planning. Retrieved June 27, 2006, from http://emedicine.com; Ihlenfeld, J. (2003). A primer on triage and mass casualty events. Dimensions of Critical Care, Nursing, 22(5), 204–209.

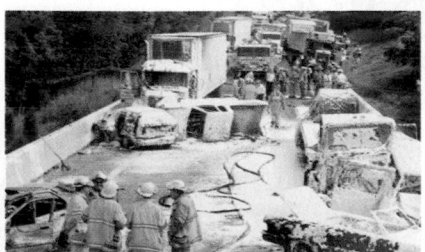

Figure 66-5 HazMats cause a type of crisis that has specific implications for health care providers and persons dispatched to the accident scene.

> **BOX 66-3**
>
> **COMPONENTS OF HOSPITAL HAZMAT EMERGENCY RESPONSE PLAN**
>
> - Identify local facilities producing, using or storing hazardous materials
> - Have designated hospital, community, and industrial coordinators
> - Have established mechanism of early notification
> - Establish training programs including EMS and fire departments
> - Have established decontamination area and equipment
>
> *Adapted from Cox, Robert. (2003). Hazmat. Retrieved June 14, 2006, from http://www.emedicine.com.*

workers yearly (Cox, 2003). Review of past HazMat events show that most exposures occurred at facilities where the chemicals were stored or produced. In 13 percent of these HazMat incidences, the patients also had traumatic injuries and were taken to the trauma center. Not only do hospitals need to have decontamination plans in place and practice them, they also need to be familiar with the chemicals produced and stored in their area (Box 66-3).

ED personnel must be aware they may not have any previous warning of a contaminated patient's arrival, and these patients may come to the ED in a private vehicle. It is the triage nurse's responsibility to know how to recognize a contaminated patient and immediately direct him or her to the decontamination area. Many of these HazMat chemicals have the potential to close EDs down because of contamination from the chemical. ED nurses learn early that the top priority in dealing with a HazMat situation is to protect themselves, other patients, and the department. An ED nurse cannot help a contaminated patient if the nurse is suffering injuries from being exposed himself or herself to the contaminated substance. To assist with patient decontamination, ED staff needs to wear specific PPE to prevent their own exposure. Hospitals select which level of protection will be best for their staff based on their HazMat risk assessments, regulatory requirements, and recommendations from local experts. Level B protection will usually suffice for most hospital staff that may be involved in initial decontamination and care of contaminated patients. There are three different levels of PPE for HazMat per Occupational Safety and Health Administration (OSHA) as shown in Box 66-4.

Decontamination

Hospitals are required to have dedicated areas in which to decontaminate patients who have been exposed to chemicals. Three different decontamination tiers are required: a small designated area for a few patients, an area that can be quickly set up for medium-sized events, and an area or plan for large-scale events. Internal decontamination rooms are usually used for one to four patients and need a dedicated external entrance, negative pressure air with dedicated **High efficiency particulate air (HEPA) filters** (a filter used to remove submicron particulate matter from the air), HazMat compatible wastewater containment, tables or gurneys for washing patients, and accessible storage for staff PPE. Commonly, outdoor areas are utilized for medium to large-scale events, because these areas do not require dedicated air handling and ventilation systems. These areas will require heated water and special water containment tanks to protect the environment and the community. If the event is small, the ED will receive help from the local fire department HazMat team. During large-scale events, the local HazMat teams will be unavailable, and the EDs will need to perform patient decontamination independently.

BOX 66-4

OSHA PPE LEVELS

Level A—Provides the highest level of respiratory and skin protection. It is resistant to chemicals and impermeable to gases and vapors. This suit is used with a self-contained breathing apparatus (SCBA) or an air supplied respirator. This is the level recommended to be worn with unknown agents but is the most cumbersome for staff and is usually only worn by HazMat teams.

Level B—This suit provides respiratory protection but does not provide a fully enclosed environment. It may allow chemical vapors to permeate the suit. Although this suit is not as cumbersome as a Level A suit, it is still challenging for care providers to wear.

Level C—This suit provides splash protection and is chemical resistant, but a respirator must still be worn. With this level PPE, the chemical or agent must be known, because an agent-specific cartridge needs to be placed in the respirator to filter out that particular agent.

Adapted from Occupational Safety and Health Administration. (2005). Safety and health topics: Personal and protective equipment. *Retrieved June 24, 2006, from www.osha.gov.*

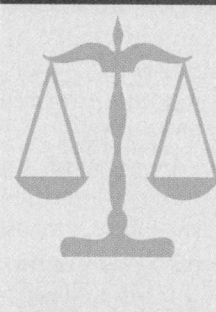

ETHICS IN PRACTICE

Preparation for an Outbreak of an Infectious Agent

Health care providers may be faced with being asked to work during an infectious agent outbreak. This may pose an ethical dilemma where they nurse is torn between staying at home, caring and protecting for her family versus going to work and potentially exposing himself or herself to a contagious disease. ED nurses must ask themselves this question in advance so they will not be in a dilemma if this situation arises. Hospitals should consider providing prophylactic medication to health care workers' families if there was an outbreak.

BIOLOGICAL WARFARE AND BIOLOGICAL AGENTS

The global biological warfare threat must be taken seriously. There are at least 10 countries worldwide known to have offensive biological weapons programs. Biological warfare was used as early as the 6th century B.C. with the Assyrians poisoning enemy wells with **rye ergot** (a fungus from the rye plant causing hallucinations, gastrointestinal [GI] upset, and a form of gangrene if ingested). Since the breakup of the former Soviet Union, it is known that vials of the smallpox virus are unaccounted for and are presumed to be in the hands of possible terrorists. To protect the welfare of the health care workers, other patients, and the community, management of patients with a known or possible infectious disease must be well organized and rehearsed. The hospital operations plan needs to specify designated, preestablished areas in the hospital or an off-site location to cohort contagious patients whose illness creates a hazard to the community.

Biological weapons include bacteria, viruses, and toxins and are placed into groupings based on how dangerous they are, the ease of dissemination or transmission, and the degree of, public panic and social disruption they could cause. The A-list consists of the agents considered to be of the highest risk. The A-list bacterial agents include: anthrax, brucellosis, bubonic plague, and tularemia. Viral agents of concern are: smallpox, Venezuelan equine encephalitis, and the viral agents known to cause hemorrhagic fevers. Botulism and ricin are two biological toxins of concern.

Health care workers, especially ED personnel, may be the first people to see an increase in patients with similar signs or symptoms and become suspicious of an epidemiological outbreak. ED nurses need to be alert for these patterns and diagnostic clues that may be indicative of an outbreak, whether accidental or intentional (Box 66-5).

It is imperative that any suspicion is reported immediately to both the hospital infection control staff and the local health department so rapid diagnosing may occur. As soon as a pattern is suspected, an **epidemiological investigation** (study looking at a specific disease, its distribution, and initial source) is initiated. This investigation helps in identifying the agent, and it will also help to institute the correct medical treatment modalities as rapidly as possible and alert others of the outbreak. Treatment must begin as early as possible to provide the best chance of survival and prevent continued spread or contamination. Nurses need to be familiar with the early signs or symptoms of these infectious diseases and must know the mode of transmission to protect themselves and other patients (Table 66-2) (Stilp, 2004).

Identification of the causative agent will take longer and be more difficult if the specimen must be sent to remote laboratories for identification. Not all laboratories are able to handle suspected contagious disease specimens, especially the A-list diseases, and these specimens may need to be sent to specialized labs for diagnosis (Refer to Table 66-3). Specimen packaging and transport must be coordinated with the sending lab, CDC, and FBI to ensure safe transport. Therefore, as a result of delayed laboratory diagnosis, initial identification and treatment may rely on the presenting signs or symptoms and public health information through syndrome surveillance (Burkle, 2002).

BOX 66-5

POTENTIAL BIOLOGICAL WARFARE CLINICAL PRESENTATIONS

- Gastroenteritis of apparent infections etiology
- Pneumonia with the sudden death of a healthy adult
- Widened mediastinum in a febrile patient with no other explanation
- Rash of synchronous vesicular or pustular lesions
- Acute neurological illness with fever
- Advancing cranial nerve impairment with progressive generalized weakness
- Higher than usual number of patients with fever, urinary, and GI complaints
- Multiple patients with similar complaints from a common location
- An endemic disease appearing during an unusual time of year

Adapted from Burkle, F. (2002). Mass casualty management of a large scale bioterrorism event: An epidemiological approach that shapes triage decisions. Emergency Medicine Clinics of North America, 20(2), 409–436.

TABLE 66-2 Isolation Guidelines

	Bacterial Agents	Anthrax	Brucellosis	Cholera	Glanders	Bubonic plague	Pneumonic plague	Tularemia	Q fever	Viruses	Smallpox	Venez. equine encephalitis	Viral hemorrhagic fever	Biological Toxins	Botulism	Ricin
Isolation Precautions																
Standard precautions for all aspects of patient care		X	X	X	X	X	X	X	X		X	X	X		X	X
Contact precautions (gown and gloves; wash hands after each patient encounter)			X^c	X^a	X^a						X		X			
Airborne precautions (negative pressure room and N-95 masks for all individuals entering the room)											X		X^b			
Droplet precautions (surgical mask)							X									
Patient Placement																
No restrictions		X	X	X	X			X	X			X			X	X
Cohort like patients when private room unavailable				X^c	X^a	X	X				X		X			
Private room				X^c	X^a	X^a	X				X		X			
Negative pressure											X		X^b			
Door closed at all times											X		X^b			
Patient Transport																
No restrictions		X	X	X	X	X		X	X		X				X	X
Limit movement to essential medical purposes only				X^c	X^a	X^a	X^a					X^a	X			
Place mask on patient to minimize dispersal of droplets							X^a					X^a	X^b			
Discontinuation of Isolation																
48 hours of appropriate antibiotic and clinical improvement							X									
Until all scabs separate											X					
Until skin decontamination completed (1 hour contact time)																
Duration of illness				X^c	X^a	X^a							X			

^{a}Contact precautions needed only if the patient has skin involvement (bubonic plague: draining bubo) or until decontamination of skin is complete.

^{b}A surgical mask and eye protection should be worn if you come within three feet of patient. Airborne precautions are needed if patient has cough, vomiting, diarrhea, or hemorrhage.

^{c}Contact precautions needed only if the patient is diapered or incontinent.

Adapted from Stilp, R. (2004). Biological weapons and emergency preparedness, Part I. *Retrieved June 27, 2006, from nsweb.nursingspectrum.com.*

TABLE 66-3	Laboratory Biosafety Levels
Biosafety Level I	These labs work with microorganisms not known to cause disease in healthy humans.
Biosafety Level II	These labs work with microorganisms that are of moderate risk to humans and the environment. Frequently the agents cause childhood diseases, to which the laboratory personnel have built up immunity or can be vaccinated against. Most hospital labs are biosafety level II.
Biosafety Level III	These labs work with infectious agents, which can cause serious or lethal disease, via the inhalation route. Personnel frequently wear respirators when performing these tests.
Biosafety Level IV	These labs work with infectious agents with a high potential of aerosol-transmitted diseases. Personnel wear a one-piece positive pressure suit that is ventilated by a life support system protected by HEPA filtration.

Adapted from Richmond, J. (2006). The 1, 2, 3s of biosafety levels. Retrieved June 24, 2006, from www.cdc.gov.

Triage stemming from a bioterrorism event (BT) will be less like standard triage and more like disaster triage. Patient care will be directed to rapidly treat those patients who have the greatest likelihood of survival as it will be difficult to successfully treat multiple patients with advanced signs or symptoms. ED staff will need to think beyond the current case, look into the future and consider the available resources and potential number of victims. Care will first be given to those with the greatest chance of survival, not necessarily the sickest. If the disease is contagious, the triage nurse's first goal will be to prevent the spread of secondary infection. To prevent secondary infection, the basic reproduction rate of the disease needs to be reduced.

Decreasing the contact rate between people will help prevent secondary infection although staff behaviors and hospital policies may need to be changed. First, adequate PPE must be worn at all times and hand washing must occur between every patient contact. Prophylactic antibiotics and vaccinations may have some benefit depending on the causative agent, and staff may be advised to receive these medications for their protection. Patients, staff, and even hospitals may need to be quarantined to help limit the epidemic (Burkle, 2002). Unlike victims of trauma, it may not always be obvious which patients were truly exposed to biological agents versus those who are worried well. Hospital ops plans must have preestablished disease-specific criteria to help assess which patients need treatment versus those who need monitoring or just emotional support. Victims who need surveillance will need to be grouped together and monitored for developing symptomatology and to initiate treatment if they become ill.

Smallpox

Smallpox is caused by the virus ortho pox and has two forms, variola major and variola minor, with major being the most common and deadly. In 1980, the World Health Organization (WHO) declared smallpox eradicated worldwide, and routine vaccination was stopped, and the supply of smallpox vaccine was destroyed. Much of the current population has not been vaccinated, or if vaccinated, they have not received routine booster shots.

Epidemiology

As a result most of the world is without smallpox immunity. Unfortunately, smallpox is thought to have the potential to become a biological weapon, and the extent of worldwide clandestine smallpox virus is unknown.

Etiology

Smallpox is usually spread through prolonged face-to-face contact and may also be spread via direct contact with contaminated items. The average incubation period for smallpox is 12 days but ranges anywhere between 7 and 19 days. Patients are contagious from rash onset until all the scabs have sepa-

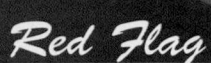

Red Flag

Recognizing Smallpox

You must be prepared to recognize a **vesicular rash** (a raised blistering rash), **exanthema** (breaking out in a rash), and immediately take the appropriate isolation and droplet precautions. The hospital's infection control practitioners must be involved as early as possible, because one confirmed smallpox case could be a worldwide emergency.

rated. In some cases patients may be contagious after exposure but prior to the onset of the rash during the **prodrome phase** (the beginning clinical manifestations that a person has for an upcoming illness). It is for this reason that patients who exhibit the rash or who have been exposed are quarantined and respiratory precautions taken.

Assessment with Clinical Manifestations

Patients will initially present with an acute onset of **malaise** (a vague feeling of not being quite right or ill at ease), **rigors** (a muscular tremor caused by a chill), vomiting, headache, backache, and a high fever. This is the prodrome phase and lasts two to four days. The prodrome phase is followed by the **macular rash** (a rash with flat red spots) rash stage, which begins as small red spots on the tongue and in the mouth. These spots then break open in the patient's mouth and throat, and it is during this time that the patients are most contagious. Within 24 hours, the rash spreads to the patient's face, arms, legs, and then hands and feet. Although chickenpox and smallpox have many similarities, the distinguishing characteristic between the two is that the smallpox rash is **centrifugal** (extends outward away from the center) with a greater abundance on the extremities and face. Patients with smallpox will also have the rash on the palms of their hands and soles of their feet. Around day four the rash is raised, the lesions fill with a thick opaque fluid, develop a depression that resembles a belly button, and become round and firm to the touch. Around 10 days from the rash onset, scabs will begin to form. Approximately two-and-a-half weeks after onset, the scabs will start to fall off. After all of the scabs have fallen off, the patient is no longer contagious (CDC, 2006e).

Diagnostic Tests

Smallpox may be diagnosed by culturing the pustules, although there are only a few labs in the United States that are equipped to diagnose the ortho pox virus. The CDC will advise how the samples need to be sent (CDC, 2006e).

Nursing Diagnoses

Based on the information gathered, examples of nursing diagnoses in the patient with smallpox may include the following:
- Disturbed body image related to the smallpox rash.
- Impaired tissue integrity related to damage from the smallpox rash.
- Risk for infection related to tissue destruction from the smallpox virus.

Planning and Implementation

Smallpox is a disease that is spread from person-to-person contact. In addition, it is a highly contagious disorder with grave consequences in the event of its spread. Therefore, the plan of care is highly focused on prevention of the disease and careful assessment of potential persons who could contract the smallpox virus. Smallpox is spread via direct contact with infected body fluids or other contaminated objects, such as linen. It is also spread via the respiratory route with face-to-face contact. Individuals caring for suspected or known smallpox patients must use standard, droplet, and airborne precautions, and PPE (Box 66-6).

Pharmacology

Although at this time a smallpox vaccination does exist, there is not a large enough supply to immunize the world's population. Currently pharmaceutical companies are working to create a supply large enough for worldwide immunization. The vaccination is administered via the **intradermal route** (an injection into the skin).with a bifurcated needle, which leaves a circular scar (scarification). Refer to Figure 66-6 that shows a vaccination, which may be administered prophylactically or within seven days of a known exposure. There is no specific pharmacological treatment for smallpox, and management is supportive. In large outbreak smallpox, patients may be cared for at home with family providing the supportive care.

> **BOX 66-6**
>
> **IMPORTANT FACTS REGARDING SMALLPOX VACCINATION**
>
> Administered by bifurcated needle.
>
> A vesicle appears at the vaccination site five to seven days after inoculation with surrounding erythema and induration.
>
> This lesion will scab over and heal one to two weeks later.
>
> Common side effects include a low-grade fever and axillary lymphadenopathy.
>
> Rare side effects include secondary inoculation of the virus to other areas, such as the face, eyelid, other people, or systemic spread of the virus (generalized vaccinia).
>
> *Adapted from Centers for Disease Control and Prevention. (2006e). Small pox disease overview. Retrieved June 24, 2006, from www.cdc.gov.*

Patient Family Teaching

Education will need to be provided to family who will be caring for smallpox patients at home. Hospitals should have home care instructions available prior to any event in multiple languages.

Evaluation of Outcomes

Potential patient outcomes for each of the example nursing diagnoses for the patient with the smallpox virus are:

- Disturbed body image. The patient will demonstrate enhanced body image and self-esteem as evidenced by the ability to look at, touch, talk about, and care for the area of the smallpox sites.
- Impaired tissue integrity. The condition of the impaired tissue caused by the smallpox virus improves as evidenced by a decreased redness, swelling, and pain.
- Risk for infection. The patient remains free of infection, as evidenced by normal vital signs and the absence of purulent drainage from the smallpox areas. In addition, the potential area of infection is recognized early to allow for prompt treatment.

Plague

Yersinia pestis bacterium causes three forms of the plague: bubonic, septicemic, and pneumonic. The bubonic form is passed from infected fleas and then migrates into the patient's lymph nodes, known as a bubo, a swollen, painful node. Left untreated, the patient develops septicemic plague, which is often fatal. Less than 20 cases of bubonic plague are seen each year and are usually found in the southwestern United States (CDC, 2004e). During the 1950s and 1960s, the Soviet and U.S. governments worked with *Y. pestis* to create a biological weapon and were able to create an aerosolized organism. This, combined with the contagious nature of the pneumonic form, makes it particularly dangerous if it is released.

Assessment with Clinical Manifestations

Pneumonic plague is a pulmonary infection, which arises from either inhalation of the organism, primary plague, or spreads to the lungs from septicemic plague. Symptoms develop acutely between one to six

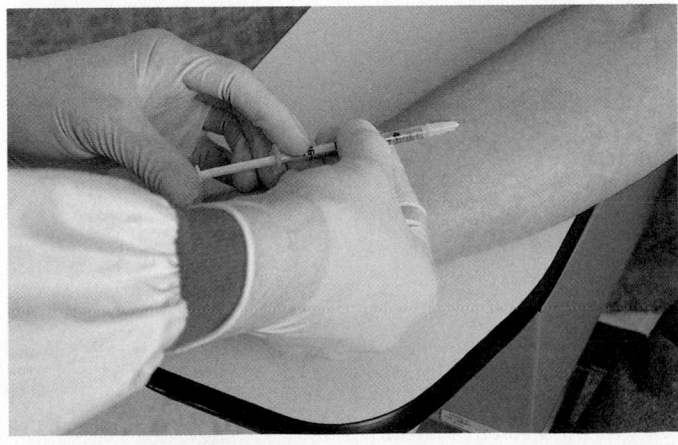

Figure 66-6 Administering vaccination.

days after exposure to pneumonic plague. Symptoms include fever, chills, malaise, myalgias, headache, nausea, vomiting, diarrhea, and abdominal pain. Within 24 hours of the initial symptoms, the patient develops a cough with bloody sputum. Without treatment, the disease progresses rapidly to respiratory and circulatory collapse. The mortality of pneumonic plague is almost 100 percent, unless treatment is initiated within 24 hours of infection (Stilp, 2004).

Diagnostic Tests

Plague must be suspected with a large influx of previously healthy patients who have fulminant gram-negative pneumonia. Definitive diagnosis is made via culture of the organism from sputum and blood samples (CDC, 2004e).

Nursing Diagnoses

Based on the information gathered, examples of nursing diagnoses in the patient with the plague may include the following:
- Impaired gas exchange related to altered oxygen supply and CO_2 exchange from the plague.
- Risk for imbalanced body temperature related to the febrile condition evidenced during plague.
- Ineffective breathing pattern related to the pulmonary complications caused by plague.

Planning and Implementation

The plague is a relatively rare disorder, but when it does manifest itself, it generally presents with respiratory complications. Therefore, the care needs to initially focus on the assessment and detection of the presence of the disease. If the disease does exist in the patient, the respiratory assessment and potential oxygenation status of the patient needs managing. Because pneumonic plague is spread via droplets, these patients will need to be isolated or grouped together, and ED nurses must utilize standard and droplet precautions when caring for these patients.

Pharmacology

Antibiotic therapy must be started as soon as culture samples are taken. Streptomycin is the drug of choice, but gentamicin, tetracycline, and chloramphenicol are also effective when streptomycin is not available. Individuals who have been exposed to pneumonic plague need to be started on doxycycline as a prophylaxis (Broyles, Reiss, & Evans, 2007). Currently there is no vaccine available for plague.

Evaluation of Outcomes

Potential patient outcomes for each of the example nursing diagnoses for the patient with the plague are:
- Impaired gas exchange due to altered oxygen supply and CO_2 exchange. The patient maintains optimal gas exchange as evidenced by normal arterial blood gases (ABGs) and has alert mentation or no further reduction in mental status.
- Risk for imbalanced body temperature. The patient maintains body temperature within a normal range.
- Ineffective breathing pattern. The patient's breathing pattern is maintained as evidenced by eupnea, normal skin color, and regular respiratory rate and patterns.

Ebola

The Ebola virus is a Filovirus that has had at least 20 known outbreaks since the 1960s. This virus has been prepared as a biological weapon and is of great concern because of its extreme destructive nature and the high mortality rates associated with its occurrence.

Epidemiology

It is hypothesized that this virus is initially passed to humans via infected animals native to Africa. Initially, diagnosing Ebola may be difficult because of the non-specific symptoms, and therefore, the nurse must be astute to the patient's travel history, especially to Africa. If a large number of patients with Ebola-like symptoms are seen outside of Africa, biological warfare must be considered.

Etiology

Viral hemorrhagic fevers (VHFs) make up a group of illnesses caused by viruses from several similar families: arena viruses, Filoviruses, bunyaviruses, and flaviviruses. These four viruses are similar in that they are all RNA viruses and depend on an animal or insect host, as the natural reservoir for their survival. Humans are infected when they come into contact with one of these infected hosts (CDC, 2004b).

Assessment with Clinical Manifestation

Filoviridae virus causes Ebola hemorrhagic fever. The incubation period of Ebola ranges from 2 to 21 days. The initial symptoms begin abruptly with fever, headache, myalgias, sore throat, and weakness. Patients then develop abdominal pain, diarrhea, and vomiting (CDC, 2004b). Patients may also develop **coagulopathies** (disorders that lead to abnormal clotting of the blood), generalized internal and external hemorrhage, hypotension, and shock, because this virus targets the vascular beds.

Diagnostic Tests

A diagnosis of Ebola may be confirmed through antigen-capture enzyme linked immunosorbent assay (ELISA), IgM ELISA, and virus isolation blood tests. Because of the contagiousness of this virus, specimens must be sent to a Biolevel-4 (BL-4) lab for analysis. The CDC will advise how to package and transport the specimen.

Nursing Diagnoses

Based on the information gathered, examples of nursing diagnoses in the patient with Ebola may include the following:
- Risk for deficient fluid volume related to diarrhea and bleeding associated with Ebola.
- Diarrhea related to the Ebola virus.
- Acute pain related to the Ebola virus.

Planning and Implementation

Supportive management for a disease with no treatment or cure is the obvious recommendation from the CDC. The patient, his family, the community of focus, and health care workers need substantial teaching to illicit appropriate and timely responses to this rare but deadly disease. Ebola is spread from affected humans through direct contact with body fluids. Nurses must be cautious, because contaminated objects, such as needles, can also spread this virus. In Africa the virus has been spread from patient to caregivers who were not wearing PPE and passed via the aerosol route. Patients who are suspected of having VHF must be placed in a private isolation room with a separate anteroom for changing into PPE and patient equipment and supply storage. Standard precautions along with airborne precautions must be used for all of these patients. Additionally, if the patient has a prominent cough or loss of body fluids, the nurse must wear a respirator.

Pharmacology

There is no known specific treatment for Ebola, treatment is aimed at supportive care and treating specific symptomatology. Volume replacement may be needed for blood loss; pressor agents are frequently used to help maintain blood pressure; and ventilators may be required to help maintain oxygenation.

Evaluation of Outcomes

Potential patient outcomes for each of the example nursing diagnoses for the patient with Ebola are:

- Risk for deficient fluid volume related to diarrhea and bleeding associated with Ebola. The patient should experience fluid volume and electrolyte balance as evidenced by a urine output of greater than 30 mL/hour, normal blood pressure and heart rate, a consistency of general body weight, and normal skin turgor.
- Diarrhea related to the Ebola virus. The patient should defecate a soft, formed stool with no more than a frequency of three times a day.
- Acute pain related to the Ebola virus. The patient should verbalize an adequate relief of pain along with the ability to realistically cope with the pain if it is not completely relieved.

Anthrax

Anthrax is considered the greatest bioterrorism threat. In recent attacks, anthrax has been used as a scare tactic as well as a true threat. The organism of concern is *Bacillus anthracis,* anthrax, which is a genetic gram-positive bacterium (CDC, 2006a). The ease of obtaining the organism and relative ease of dispensing anthrax are the primary reasons for fearing this pathological threat of terrorist activity.

Epidemiology

There are three forms of anthrax: cutaneous, inhaled, and GI. Cutaneous anthrax develops from direct contact with spores usually from infected animals or animal products, such as wool. Inhalation of aerosolized anthrax spores leads to respiratory anthrax. Consumption of undercooked meat contaminated with the spores lead to the GI form. WHO estimates that if 50 kg of anthrax spores were dispersed over a 2-kilometer line upwind from a city with a population of 500,000, within three days 125,000 people would be infected and 95,000 people could die (CDC, 2006a).

Etiology

The pulmonary **macrophages** (a type of white blood cell that ingests and helps destroy foreign material) carry the spores to the tracheobronchial or mediastinal lymph nodes. This organism then produces an **antiphagocytic** (something that destroys the neutrophils and macrophages function) capsule, which produces lethal toxins leading to the release of *B. anthracis* into the blood stream, causing overwhelming septicemia. Anthrax spores resist environmental destruction, tolerate aerosolization well, and are 2 to 6 microns in diameter, the perfect setup for attachment to the respiratory mucosa.

Assessment with Clinical Manifestations

The average incubation period of inhalation of anthrax is 1 to 6 days, but it has been dormant for up to 43 days. After the incubation period, the patient complains of nonspecific flu-like symptoms, such as headache and a nonproductive cough. After 1 to 3 days, many patients have a brief period when they feel better but then rapidly deteriorate with high fever, dyspnea, **stridor** (a high-pitched harsh sound heard on inhalation due to narrowing of the airway), cyanosis, and shock. Chest x-rays (CXRs) may show a widened mediastinum. One hundred percent of inhalation anthrax patients will die if there is no treatment, and there is 95 percent mortality rate if treatment is not begun within 48 hours.

Diagnostic Tests

Anthrax should be suspected when patients present with the signs and symptoms outlined, and gram-positive bacilli are seen on peripheral blood smear. Aerobic blood culture growth of large number of gram-positive bacilli is a preliminary diagnosis of *Bacillus* species.

Nursing Diagnoses

Based on the information gathered, examples of nursing diagnoses in the patient with anthrax may include the following:

- Ineffective breathing pattern related to the respiratory problems caused by the anthrax.
- Ineffective tissue perfusion related to decreased systemic vascular resistance in anthrax condition.
- Risk for imbalanced body temperature related to the febrile condition evidenced during anthrax disorder.

Planning and Implementation

It is critical to diagnose the presence of the anthrax virus in people suspected of having the virus. The more immediate the identification of the disease, the higher the correlation of successful antibiotic therapy. In addition, the patient, family, the community of focus, and health care workers need substantial teaching to calm their fears related to a widespread contaminant and potential terrorist threat. Because anthrax has a low potential for person-to-person transmission, standard precautions are adequate.

Pharmacology

If anthrax is suspect after obtaining blood cultures, it is recommended to immediately start ciprofloxacin (Cipro) IV. Oral Cipro is recommended for postexposure treatment. This should be started as early as possible to all people exposed, including health care workers. In confirmed anthrax cases, exposed personnel should also be immunized (CDC, 2006a).

Evaluation of Outcomes

Potential patient outcomes for each of the example nursing diagnoses for the patient with the anthrax organism are:

- Ineffective breathing pattern related to the respiratory problems caused by the anthrax. The patient's breathing rhythm is maintained as shown by normal unlabored breathing, normal skin color, and verbalizing comfort in the breathing.
- Ineffective tissue perfusion related to decreased systemic vascular resistance in anthrax condition. The patient should maintain good tissue perfusion to the essential organs, as demonstrated by strong peripheral pulses, normal arterial blood gases, and an alert level of consciousness (LOC).
- Risk for imbalanced body temperature. The patient maintains body temperature within a normal range.

Severe Acute Respiratory Syndrome

Severe acute respiratory syndrome (SARS) is a newly recognized infectious disease. SARS was first recognized in the Guangdong Province in southeastern China in 2002 and is the first new infectious disease of the 21st century. WHO issued a global warning about the appearance of SARS in March of 2003 (File, 2004).

Epidemiology

This disease spread worldwide in early 2003. SARS gained global notoriety, because it is a highly contagious infectious disease with a high mortality rate and is easily transmitted to health care workers. SARS led to the disruption of health care delivery systems worldwide and has even caused hospital closures because of outbreaks (CDC, 2004f). This disease is particularly challenging because so little is known about it.

Etiology

SARS is caused by a new **coronavirus,** a virus that normally only leads to upper respiratory infection. No one understands why this virus now has turned deadly. This virus has been found in humans, in civet cats, and a raccoon dog (considered human delicacies in Guangdong Province). This suggests the virus can be passed from animal to human (File, 2004). Researchers are trying to learn why some individuals exposed to the SARS virus live, and others will die. Deaths from SARS are more prevalent in the elderly population but young, healthy individuals have also died from SARS.

Assessment with Clinical Manifestations

SARS patients initially complain of a prodrome phase with onset of fever (38° C [100.4° F] or greater), chills, rigors, **myalgia** (pain in the muscles), and headache, symptoms similar to influenza, although patients deny having sneezing or runny nose. Three to seven days later patients develop lower respiratory tract symptomatology and pneumonia with a nonproductive cough. Twenty percent of SARS patients will then develop **acute respiratory distress syndrome (ARDS)** (an acute syndrome that leads to pulmonary insufficiency from accumulation of fluid in the alveolar sacs and requires ventilatory support). After exposure, the average incubation period for developing SARS is 6 to 10 days. Because SARS is a new illness, many facts are still unknown about the disease. With each outbreak, more epidemiological, prevention, and treatments will be found.

Diagnostic Tests

The coronavirus causing SARS can be identified through a reverse transcription polymerase chain test. Blood or nasal samples are taken to look at the virus' DNA strand. Patients with SARS will also have identifiable coronavirus antibodies in their blood. The virus can also be identified via fluid or tissue culture.

Nursing Diagnoses

Based on the information gathered, examples of nursing diagnoses in the patient with SARS may include the following:
- Impaired gas exchange due to damage to alveolar-capillary membrane, change in lung compliance.
- Acute pain related to the headache condition associated with SARS.
- Fear in response to the diagnosis of SARS.

Planning and Implementation

The SARS disorder requires a worldwide preventive goal as the disease presents itself in a given region. Emphasis on patient education related to traveling and immigration should be emphasized. Once the disease is suspected, then the focus for identifying the disease and subsequent support of the patient, family, and community is necessary. ED personnel may be the first care providers to be suspicious of SARS when triaging or caring for a patient. To protect themselves, transmission of the infection must be prevented at the first point of contact. The following recommendations can be practiced for all patients visiting an ED: post signs, in appropriate language for the EDs clientele, at all entrances, asking patients to inform personnel if they have signs of a respiratory infection, to cover their mouth when coughing, to dispose of tissues, and to wash their hands frequently (Box 66-7) (CDC, 2004f). During periods of increased respiratory illnesses, triage nurses should provide masks to patients with a cough and provide a separate waiting room for these patients. Additionally, health care workers should practice droplet precautions using N-95 masks, along with standard precautions when in close contact with patients with respiratory illness. It is also theorized that the virus may be spread via contaminated objects, making it imperative that nurses practice stringent hand hygiene.

Pharmacology

There is no specific treatment for SARS, but current recommendations include supportive care (such as ventilatory support) and broad-spectrum antimicrobials.

Red Flag

SARS

During periods of known SARS outbreak, triage nurses must also screen all patients with respiratory illness for the following risk factors:

Within the last 10 days has the patient traveled to mainland China, Hong Kong, Taiwan, or areas where outbreak is occurring or close contact with an ill person who has traveled to these areas?

Is the patient a health care worker who has been caring for patients with respiratory illness? Is the patient a laboratory staff person where live SARS virus exists? If any of these are true, the patient needs to be immediately placed in isolation with droplet precautions.

BOX 66-7

INFECTION CONTROL PRECAUTIONS FOR POTENTIAL SARS PATIENTS

Place patient in a negative-pressure isolation room.

Maintain a log of all persons who enter room.

Restrict visitors.

Restrict number of personnel caring for the patient.

All health care workers must practice hand hygiene, standard, and airborne precautions.

Limit cough inducing treatments, such as sputum induction or suction.

Avoid using noninvasive positive-pressure ventilation.

Educate all individuals caring for these patients to immediately seek treatment if they develop SARS symptoms.

Quarantine personnel who were exposed to patient without respiratory protection.

Adapted from Koller, D., Nicholas, D., Goldie, R., Gearing, R., & Selkirk, E. (2006). When family-centered care is challenged by infectious disease: Pediatric health care delivery during the SARS outbreaks. Qualitative Health Research, 16(1), 47–60.

Fast Forward ▶▶▶

Pharmacological Management of SARS

As with any other infectious disease it is important to educate health care workers on required infection control measures to protect themselves and others. Staff must not only understand the importance of basic infection control measures, they must practice it. During the 2003 SARS outbreak, health care workers were not following hand hygiene and isolation recommendations, and they were not using PPE correctly (CDC, 2004f). Despite worldwide research efforts, an effective treatment regimen has not been found. Recently preliminary studies found that the antiviral drug combination of lopinavir and ritonavir and ribavirin have prevented serious complications and even death. Research continues with the hope of Food and Drug Administration (FDA) approval for this use.

Evaluation of Outcomes

Potential patient outcomes for each of the example nursing diagnoses for the patient with SARS are:

- Impaired gas exchange due to damage to alveolar-capillary membrane, change in lung compliance. The patient maintains optimal gas exchange as evidenced by normal arterial blood gases (ABGs) and has alert mentation or no further reduction in mental status.
- Acute pain related to the headache condition associated with SARS. The patient should verbalize an adequate relief of pain along with the ability to realistically cope with the pain if it is not completely relieved.
- Fear in response to the diagnosis of SARS. The patient should manifest positive coping behaviors and verbalize a reduction in the amount of fear of the having this disease.

West Nile Virus

The West Nile virus (WNV) was first identified in Africa in the 1930s and was first documented in the United States in 1999. There was an epidemic in New York City in 1999, and patients were seen with what was first diagnosed as meningitis. Since that time, there have been increasing numbers of WNV reported on a worldwide basis.

Epidemiology

By 2004 all 50 states had confirmed human WNV cases totaling over 9,800 and over 250 deaths (Mayo Foundation for Medical Education and Research, 2004). Frequently individuals have been infected with the virus and have no signs or symptoms or may have complained of mild, virus-like illness. But WNV may lead to serious complications, including encephalitis, meningitis, or meningoencephalitis, and even death in the elderly and patients with other chronic medical diseases.

Etiology

WNV is a single-stranded RNA virus, a member of the Flaviviridae family. This virus survives in nature via biological transmission between blood feeding hosts (CDC, 2006f). Birds are the main reservoir for WNV. When a mosquito bites an infected bird, the mosquito then becomes the vector and passes the virus to humans via mosquito bites. Less than 1 percent of individuals bitten by an infected mosquito will become seriously ill. West Nile virus has been documented being passed from contaminated blood and organs, but it is not passed via the airborne route (Mayo Foundation for Medical Education and Research, 2004).

Assessment with Clinical Manifestations

Most people who have been bitten by an infected mosquito will have no signs or symptoms. Approximately 20 percent of bite victims will manifest a mild infection and complain of fever, headache, myalgias, backache, anorexia, GI disturbance, swollen lymph nodes, and a mild rash. One percent of patients bitten will develop a life-threatening illness manifested by high fever, stiff neck, severe headache, change in mentation, seizures, Parkinsonism, decreased coordination, partial paralysis, and coma (Mayo Foundation for Medical Education and Research, 2004).

Diagnostic Tests

The most common test for WNV is to measure for antibodies that are produced in blood. If the patient is presenting with encephalitis or meningitis symptomatology, a lumbar puncture will be performed to look for the virus presence in the patient's cerebrospinal fluid (CSF).

Nursing Diagnoses

Based on the information gathered, examples of nursing diagnoses in the patient with WNV may include the following:
- Acute pain as related to **nuchal** (a stiff painful neck due to irritated meninges) rigidity, inflammation of meninges, and headache.
- Fear in response to the diagnosis of WNV.
- Risk for imbalanced body temperature.
- Risk for infection related to the WNV.

Planning and Implementation

The WNV requires a worldwide preventive goal as the disease presents itself in a given region. Emphasis on patient education related to traveling and immigration should be emphasized. Once the disease is suspected, then the focus for identifying the disease and subsequent support of the patient, family, and community is necessary. WNV cannot be spread by direct person-to-person contact, and therefore standard precautions are all that are required when caring for a patient with WNV.

Patient and Family Teaching

ED nurses can help provide education to patients about decreasing their risk of exposure to infected mosquitoes. Patients must be taught to use mosquito repellant with diethyltoluamide (DEET), wear long pants and long sleeve shirts during evening hours, and spend evening hours indoors in late summer and early fall. Removal of stagnate water around the house will also help decrease the number of mosquitoes.

Evaluation of Outcomes

Potential patient outcomes for each of the example nursing diagnoses for the patient with the WNV are:
- Acute pain as related to nuchal rigidity, inflammation of meninges, and headache. The patient should verbalize an adequate relief of pain along with the ability to realistically cope with the pain if it is not completely relieved.

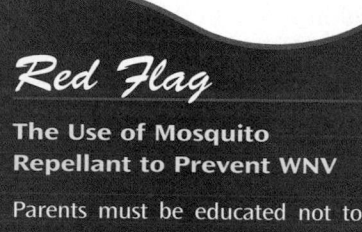

Red Flag

The Use of Mosquito Repellant to Prevent WNV

Parents must be educated not to use mosquito repellent containing DEET on children less than 2 months of age. Instead, the infant's stroller should be covered with mosquito netting (CDC, 2006f).

- Fear in response to the diagnosis of WNV. The patient should manifest positive coping behaviors and verbalize a reduction in the amount of fear of the having this disease.
- Risk for imbalanced body temperature. The patient maintains body temperature within a normal range.
- Risk for infection related to the WNV. The patient remains free of infection as evidenced by normal vital signs and an absence of inflammatory manifestations. In addition, an infection is recognized early for prompt management.

BLAST INJURIES

The majority of terrorist attacks in the United States, Atlanta Olympics and Oklahoma City, involve conventional weapons including bombs and missiles (CDC, 2003b). Victims of blast injuries have semipredictable injury patterns and injury severity predictors. Bombs are known to have a one third to two thirds injury split. One third of the victims will be critically injured and two thirds will be mildly injured, treated, and released.

The ED nurse must understand that injuries from explosions create a unique pattern of injury. There are four mechanisms of injury: primary, secondary, tertiary, and quaternary (Table 66-4). When a device explodes, it creates a blast wave (primary); the intense overpressurization force, which is created from the explosion of a device. This primary explosion affects the body's hollow organs.

Blast lung is the most common primary fatal injury among initial blast survivors. ED nurses will usually see this injury with the initial evaluation, but cases have been reported up to 48 hours after the event. Blast lung is characterized by a triad of apnea, bradycardia, and hypotension and produces a characteristic butterfly pattern on CXR. Abdominal injuries may be initially overlooked or hidden until the patient develops an acute abdomen or sepsis. If there is a traumatic amputation, the patient may have associated multisystem injuries. The ED nurse should not become focused on the gory injury but must perform a thorough systems assessment to rule out other injuries. Because the primary blast affects air-filled organs, air embolism is seen frequently and may present as MI, stroke, blindness, deafness, spinal cord injury (SCI), or vascular clotting. If the patient was trapped under debris, acute renal failure or **rhabdomyolysis**

TABLE 66-4	**Blast Injury Patterns**		
CATEGORY	**CHARACTERISTICS**	**BODY PART AFFECTED**	**INJURY TYPE**
Primary	From blast wave	Gas-filled structures most likely the lung, GI tract, and middle ear	Blast lung (pulmonary barotraumas) tympanic rupture
			Abdominal hemorrhage and rupture
			Globe (eye) rupture
			Concussion
Secondary	Results from flying debris and bomb fragments	Any body part may be affected	Penetrating or blunt injuries
Tertiary	Results from patient being thrown from blast wave	Any body part may be affected	Fracture and traumatic amputation
			Closed and open brain injury
Quaternary	All injuries, illness not related to first, second, or third mechanism; includes exacerbation or complication of existing conditions	Any body part may be affected.	Burns
			Crush injury
			Respiratory problems due to smoke or dust
			Angina
			Hypertension

Adapted from Centers for Disease Control and Prevention (2003b). Explosion and blast injuries: A primer for clinicians. Retrieved June 13, 2006, from www.cdc.gov/.

(destruction of skeletal muscle cells which causes the release of myoglobin), or **compartment syndrome** (develops when muscle is damage from a traumatic event and swells cutting off circulation; if this pressure is not released, permanent muscle and nerve damage may occur) may be present. The patient may also have burn injuries from the explosive device (CDC, 2003b).

STRESS REACTIONS

Caring for victims of a MCI, whether it stems from a traumatic event, terrorism, natural disaster, or civil unrest will not only affect the victims, their families, the patient care providers, witnesses, and many others from the community. In addition to the physical injuries and depending on the event, victims may also suffer the loss of their loved ones, friends, pets, home, place of employment, and personal possessions. ED nurses will have to manage both injured disaster victim along with the worried well suffering from emotional distress, even if they were not directly affected by the event.

Traumatic events are marked by a sense of horror, helplessness, serious injury or threat of injury, or death. Following any traumatic event, it is a normal response for individuals to experience stress reactions, and the body's response to stress may affect a person's emotional, psychological, physical, or spiritual states. Individuals will have varying degrees of emotional or physical responses when exposed to a traumatic episode; these may include feelings of fear, grief, depression, nausea, vertigo, loss of appetite, change in sleep patterns, or social withdrawal (Table 66-5). These responses will be most prevalent the first days after the event and normally subside and resolve within 10 to 30 days (CDC, 2003a).

It is imperative for hospital ops plans to include established preincident crisis intervention plans that can be activated at the onset of an event to help care for their staff members. In events where there is the potential for transmission of the disease or chemical to the caregiver, staff will have the added fear of transmission or contraction of the disease. Hospital plans need to incorporate available resources and mobilization of counselors or pastors. In addition, hospitals should have coordinated preevent training with these individuals including defusing and debriefing techniques. During the event, staff who are triaging and caring for victims need to be evaluated throughout their shift to assess their emotional and physical stability. Individuals in the hospital's incident command should also be assessed for emotional stability due to the extreme pressure they can experience. Hospital plans should also include follow up for staff and victims. Postevent crisis intervention cannot be a one-time event but must be over a continuum.

The nurse plays an important role when interacting with the victims of a traumatic event and should encourage the patient to talk about their reactions

TABLE 66-5	Common Responses to a Traumatic Event		
COGNITIVE	**EMOTIONAL**	**PHYSICAL**	**BEHAVIORAL**
Poor concentration	Shock	Nausea	Suspicion
Confusion	Numbness	Lightheaded	Irritability
Disoriented	Overwhelmed	Dizzy	Withdrawn
Memory loss	Insecure	Headaches	Silent
Indecisive	Volatile emotions	Sleeplessness	Substance abuse

Adapted from Centers for Disease Control and Prevention (2003a). Coping with a traumatic event. *Retrieved June 16, 2006, from www.cdc.gov/.*

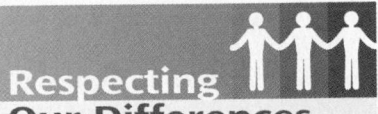

Respecting Our Differences

Cultural Backgrounds and Disasters

ED nurses must understand that patients with different cultural backgrounds may act and respond differently to disasters or traumatic events. It is imperative for the ED nurse to be familiar with the cultural groups in their communities and understand their norms, traditions, spiritual practices, and grieving process to provide the best care for these patients. Being familiar with these cultural practices will allow you to provide the best support, education, and counseling to your patients.

BOX 66-8

SIGNS AND SYMPTOMS OF PTSD

Nightmares or flashbacks of the event

Feelings of guilt

Numbing of emotions

Detachment or estrangement from friends and family

Decreased interest in previous activities or hobbies

Feelings of hopelessness or helplessness

Difficulty concentrating

Difficulty sleeping

Substance abuse

Severe depression

Hyperarousal: panic, rage, extreme irritability

Adapted from National Center for PTSD. (2003). What is post-traumatics stress disorder? Retrieved June 23, 2006, from www.ncptsd.org/facts.

---

when they are ready. Survivors respond best when the ED nurse offers eye contact, calm presence, and utilizes therapeutic listening skills. The patient needs validation that his or her reactions are normal and to be encouraged to follow normal routines, find ways to relax, eat healthy, sleep or rest quietly, and identify and utilize support systems. Frequently victims will need to have ongoing counseling to help the recovery process.

Each age-group is vulnerable to stress and may respond in different ways. Children think and process information differently than adults and will have different responses than adult patients. The age of the child will determine their understanding of the event. The nurse must understand the child's developmental stage to effectively deal with the child's psychological response. Reassurance will help children cope with traumatic events, and younger children will need a lot of cuddling. When a child asks questions, they need to be answered honestly, but do not dwell on the frightening details. Children must be encouraged to express their feelings not only through conversation, but also through drawing, painting, and play. Parents need to be encouraged to maintain normal household routines but limit children's viewing of television news coverage. Like adults, children need to be given the opportunity to discuss their feelings. The nurse should use age appropriate terms letting the child know it is okay to feel scared, sad or worried. Children respond to the emotional state of their caretaker, and the nurse needs to maintain a calm demeanor while caring for these children. It is important for the nurse to educate the child's parents that the psychological trauma does not go away immediately after the event and may continue to resurface for two years post event.

Posttraumatic Stress Disorder

Although it is normal for many people to experience stress reactions following a traumatic event, these responses should begin to subside within 10 days and resolve within 30 days. When these symptoms do not subside and begin interfering with a person's daily life, this is defined as posttraumatic stress disorder (PTSD). PTSD is an intense physical and psychological response to a traumatic event that lasts for weeks, months, or even years after the event. This disorder can occur in any age, socioeconomic class, gender, or any cultural group.

Pathophysiology

Both biological and physiological changes are seen with the patients suffering from PTSD. Changes are found with both the central and autonomic nervous systems; the hippocampus does not function as it should and the amygdala has abnormal activation possibly leading to flashbacks. The sympathetic nervous system becomes hyperaroused leading to sleep abnormalities and an overactive startle reflex (National Center for PTSD, 2003). Patients suffering from PTSD also have been found to have abnormal cortisol, epinephrine, and norepinephrine levels. In addition to PTSD, these patients frequently experience depression, anxiety disorder, or substance abuse which compounds their symptomatology.

Assessment with Clinical Manifestations

There are a wide variety of clinical manifestations associated with PTSD, which are illustrated in Box 66-8.

Planning and Implementation

PTSD is treated by a variety of psychotherapy support groups and medications. The patient should be referred to someone who is knowledgeable about trauma and disasters. The ED nurse must be aware of the signs and symptoms of PTSD and plan patient treatment with these in mind. Frequently, patients with PTSD are evaluated for depression and will need to be assessed and monitored for suicidal behaviors while in the ED. Some individuals will respond to cognitive therapy, group therapy, and exposure therapy. Selective serotonin reuptake inhibitors (SSRIs), like Prozac or Zoloft, are commonly found to be beneficial for treatment modalities for these individuals.

ED nurses have selected a highly rewarding field in which to work, but they have also selected a specialty that takes place in a demanding and stressful environment. These nurses place themselves in stressful situations daily, ranging from potential exposure to contagious disease, interacting with violent and verbally abusive patients, gruesome injuries, and traumatic deaths. ED nurses cannot choose which types of patients arrive in their department. Many of these patients die unexpectedly, and frequently these deaths involve a traumatic event. ED nurses quickly realize many of these deaths could have been prevented and were unnecessary.

Crises are a normal part of the ED nurse's day. This ongoing state of crisis places ED nurses at risk for developing PTSD. This may develop from one particular horrific event, such as caring for victims of the September 11th terrorist attack or the Columbine school shooting. Frequently though, PTSD arises from the accumulation of stress, which evolves from caring for single isolated events over time.

All people react to and respond differently to stress. These responses may be altered by a variety of things, such as the individual's psychological and emotional fatigue, coping style, and previous experiences combined with their closeness to the event. If the nurse caring for a 4-year-old critically injured child also has a child that age, it is likely that the nurse will experience increased stress compared with a nurse with no children.

Advance warning of the incoming patients and their injury or acuity level will help the ED nurse to prepare for what is arriving and begin to utilize coping strategies. When the brain receives input, it tries to file it in the appropri-

Skills 360°

Prevention of Pediatric Trauma Deaths

Up to 50 percent of the pediatric traumatic deaths are considered preventable. ED nurses commonly choose to become involved in community education to help stop these needless deaths. This may include education regarding bicycle, skateboard, and motorcycle helmet use, car seat safety, water safety, and bike rodeos. Frequently EDs give out free helmets and car seats to low-income families who visit their department. As an ED nurse it is essential you are educated on the required safety guidelines to provide injury prevention education to your patients or direct them to appropriate resources during every visit. ED nurses must take advantage of this captive audience to help promote safe and healthy children.

Respecting Our Differences

The Effects of Trauma on Children

Children are more vulnerable to the effects of an infectious disease or traumatic injury because of their physiological status. Children have a faster respiratory rate than adults, and therefore will receive more inhaled agent than adults. A child's skin is thinner, which offers less protection from absorption, and they have a larger surface to mass ratio than adults. They also have a smaller circulating blood volume with less tolerance to volume loss from bleeding, vomiting, or diarrhea (American Academy of Pediatrics, 2002). Children cannot be considered little adults, and medication and antidote doses will be different from the standard adult doses. Hospitals must have the correct pediatric and neonatal medication concentrations available. If a child requires decontamination he or she presents an even greater challenge because of his or her rapid heat loss and increased risk for hypothermia. EDs should create special treatment areas for pediatric victims. Disaster drills must include pediatric victims so staff will be familiar caring for them. Hospital operation plans need to include provisions for psychological support to these young victims.

Children depend on daily routines and when these routines are interrupted, especially because of a disaster, the child may become anxious. Following a disaster, children are fearful that the event will occur again, that they will be separated from their family, that someone will be killed, or that they will be left alone. Additionally, children may have lost a special comfort measure, such as a blanket or stuffed animal, which adults may consider insignificant, but for the child it has an emotional attachment. This loss combined with a traumatic event may lead to the child having nightmares, becoming easily upset, or even reverting to younger behaviors, such as bedwetting. The child may be afraid to leave his or her family, and some children may even believe he or she was the cause of the event.

Uncovering the Evidence

Traumatic Brain Injury

Discussion: The purpose of this study was to explore the relationship of child abuse following a natural disaster, specifically looking at traumatic brain injury (TBI). The study concluded that TBI increased in those counties most affected by Hurricane Floyd six months post disaster compared to those counties predisaster. Cases of inflicted TBI, intra-cranial injury, in children ≤ 2 years, with admission to an ICU or death from September 1998 to December 2001 in North Carolina were reviewed. A Poisson regression modeling calculated the rate ratios of injury for each geographical area by time period. It was found there was a five-fold increase for injury inflicted to children ≤ 2 years in counties more severely affected versus those less affected.

Implications for Practice: Disasters lead to increased stress related to the event. They also lead to stress from disruption of the community's social structure, loss of home, jobs, and financial hardship. Nurses need to realize the opportunities for providing parents with resources for support and need to be given immediately after the event and in the ensuing months. Parents must be educated on coping techniques and when and who to call when they are feeling overwhelmed. The ED nurse must remember to maintain a high index of suspicion when caring for children with closed head injuries or with decreased LOCs, especially in areas recently experiencing a disaster.

Citation: Keenan, H., Marshall, S., Nocera, M., & Runyan, D. (2004). Increased incidence of inflicted traumatic brain injury in children after a natural disaster. American Journal of Preventive Medicine, 26(3), 189–193.

ate place. When the nurse knows in advance the type of patient that is coming in, the brain is better able to help the nurse prepare for the horrific case. Thus, a grotesquely disfiguring injury does not seem as bad as when the nurse has time to prepare for it emotionally.

ED nurses tend to utilize two separate sides of their brain when caring for a **critical incident** (a patient or event that causes a stress reaction in the health care worker) patient. If ED nurses were to react emotionally every time they were exposed to critical incidents, it would be extremely difficult for them to perform their job. The ED nurse utilizes their professional side to help remain calm and care for the patient at hand. All the while the nurse's emotional side is absorbing the sights, sounds, and smells of the event and is creating an imprint or memory. The professional side helps the nurse to function on autopilot at times, even relying on rote memory to achieve the desired outcomes. The professional side, all the while, is helping to keep the emotional side pushed aside or "stuffed" until it can surface after the event.

During resuscitation much of the nurse's brain is busy multitasking. The brain is taking in all that is occurring, evaluating actions, and anticipating what tasks need to be performed next. If an unanticipated sight, smell, or sound occurs, such as a parent screaming as he or she is brought into the resuscitation room, the brain cannot buffer or file this normally. This unanticipated impulse is randomly placed in the memory core of the brain, the hippocampus.

ED nurses must be proactive in trying to protect themselves from the development of PTSD. Nurses must learn how to deal with routine stress to care for themselves and coworkers. They must eat well-balanced meals, drink plenty of water, and limit caffeine and sugar intake. Regular exercise (at least 30 minutes four times a week) will help rid the body of toxic chemicals that are released dur-

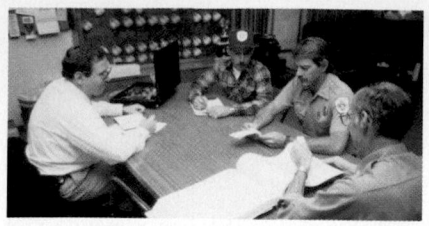

Figure 66-7 A critical incident stress management debriefing is an invaluable setting to assist health care workers, such as the phlebotomist, deal with the impact of a stressful event.

ing stressful situations. Staying rested and having consistent sleep patterns will help prevent psychological and emotional fatigue and better prepare the nurse to respond to stressful events. After being involved with the care of a patient from a critical incident, it is imperative the nurse be allowed a few minutes to decompress before moving on to care for the next patient. This will allow the nurse to cry, pray, meditate, or just have a few minutes of self-reflection and processing of the recent events. At the completion of the shift the nurse needs to take time to talk with coworkers, friends, or family to also help process the events.

Critical Incident Stress Management

Many health care professionals utilize critical incident stress management (CISM) to help decrease the stress reactions and prevent PTSD. CISM teams are made up of emergency professionals and mental health workers who have been trained in leading defusing and debriefings.

Defusing allow the staff to talk about their feelings and process their emotions and also provides an opportunity for the nurse to be educated on normal stress responses versus prolonged responses. Defusing occur as a one-on-one between a team member and the health care provider immediately or shortly after the event. This technique is employed when only one or two individuals are having difficulties with the case. Debriefings are more formalized and all health care providers are invited to attend from the EMS dispatchers to the phlebotomists (Figure 66-7). Debriefings usually occur within 24 to 96 hours after the event and take place over a two- to three-hour period. Debriefings are not critiques of the case but a chance for every team member to tell his or her story and discuss how he or she are feeling (Box 66-9). It is important for ED managers to provide support and shift coverage for any staff members to attend if they are working the day of the debriefing.

ED staff may not want to attend the debriefings, because they believe they will be considered as weak if they cannot cope. In addition, these nurses may feel that they should be able to stuff all of their emotions, because death is part of their job. If nurses do not care for themselves and take advantage of theses debriefings, they will eventually suffer from burnout and may even develop PTSD.

BOX 66-9

THE EIGHT PHASES OF A DEBRIEFING

- Introduction phase: ground rules are established, the process is explained, introductions are made, and the individuals role in the event is explained.
- Fact phase: individuals provide facts of the case. Introduction of these facts frequently fills in missing answer for other care providers.
- Thought phase: touching on the individual's emotional aspects begins in the phase.
- Reaction phase: usually felt to be the most intense phase, participants are asked to answer, "how did you react to the incident?" Individuals may just choose to listen instead of answer.
- Symptom phase: various symptoms that people are experiencing are discussed and validated.
- Teaching phase: members are educated on stress reactions and techniques to decrease these reactions are explored.
- Reentry phase: this is the closure phase.
- Follow-up phase: the CISM team may follow-up with individuals postdebriefing to ensure they are feeling better.

Adapted from Pulley, S. (2004). Critical incident stress management. Retrieved July 6, 2006, from http://www.emedicine.com.

BOX 66-10

MANAGING YOUR STRESS DURING A DISASTER

- Develop a buddy system with another coworker.
- Eat small, frequent, healthy snacks.
- Drink lots of water.
- Take breaks.
- Stay in touch with family or friends.
- Support your coworkers.
- Take a few minutes to defuse each shift.

Adapted from National Center for PTSD. (2003). What is post-traumatic stress disorder? Retrieved June 23, 2006, from http://www.ncptsd.org.

Skills 360°

Nurses Attending a Debriefing

ED nurses may not want to attend the debriefing, because they feel they are not affected by the critical event or case. All caregivers involved in the case should attend the debriefing, because they have a piece of the puzzle that may help another health care worker. For instance, the ED nurse has cared for a child involved in a house fire, the child and her sister were asleep in bunk beds. The child on the top bunk died, but the child on the bottom bunk survived. The ED nurse cannot understand why one child died and the other child lived. During the debriefing the firefighters on the scene told their part of the story and described the burned bedroom; thereby answering the nurse's questions. Ultimately this helped the nurse to cope, process, and recover form the horrific event (Box 66-10).

KEY CONCEPTS

- EDs are becoming America's safety net for patient care.
- Because of a short length of stay it is challenging for ED nurses to develop a collaborative plan of care.
- A triage system is one in which priorities for care are developed.
- The START method allows for rapid triage, less than 60 seconds, of multiple patients.
- During an MCI, the triage philosophy changes to providing care first to those most likely to survive versus providing care first to the most critical.
- A disaster is defined as the destructive effects of natural or manmade forces overwhelm the ability of a given area or community to meet the demands of health care.
- The ICS is a system utilized to help manage large-scale events.
- HEICS helps provide a consistent algorithm for organizing information, controlling and coordinating the influx of patients, distribution of required staff, supplies, resources, and communication.
- JCAHO requires hospitals to have an emergency management plan that addresses four phases: preparedness, mitigation, response, and recovery.
- Hospital ops plans need to address internal and external disasters, bioterrorism, and chemical and radiation emergencies.

- DMAT teams will be deployed to large-scale disasters and comprise MDs, nurses, EMTs, and social workers.
- HazMats have the potential to harm a person or the environment.
- There are three OSHA-approved levels of protection. Level A offers the highest level of protection.
- Biological agents include bacteria, viruses, and toxins. The A-list is those agents considered the largest threat.
- Smallpox patient are contagious until all of the scabs have fallen off.
- The mortality of *Yersinia* plague is almost 100 percent if treatment is not started within 24 hours of infection.
- If a large number of patients with Ebola-like symptoms are seen in the United States, biological warfare should be suspected.
- All of the patients suffering from inhalation anthrax will die without treatment.
- WNV is passed to humans via contaminated mosquitoes. Individuals will experience a variety of emotional and physical responses when exposed to a traumatic event.
- PTSD is an intense physical and psychological response to a traumatic event that lasts weeks, months, or years after exposure to a traumatic event.
- Defusing occurs one-on-one briefly after an event, whereas debriefings occur with larger groups after the event.

REVIEW QUESTIONS

1. Biological weapons are considered the ultimate weapon, because they:
   1. Can cause mass casualties
   2. Are inexpensive and relatively easy to produce
   3. Can be quite difficult to detect
   4. Can be disseminated at great distances
   5. All of the above

2. Which statement about smallpox is *false*?
   1. Vaccines exist for smallpox and chicken pox.
   2. Skin lesions are synchronous in development for both smallpox and chicken pox.
   3. Both diseases are contagious via the aerosol route spread between people.
   4. With smallpox, patients can develop a rash on their palms and soles of feet.

3. Patients with illnesses caused by biological warfare agents can be cared for by using standard precautions.
   1. True
   2. False

4. A patient with severe life-threatening injuries who most likely will not survive would be triaged as:
   1. Blue
   2. Yellow
   3. Black
   4. Red

5. Symptoms of PTSD usually begin to develop by:
   1. 1 week
   2. 1 year
   3. 3 months
   4. 13 months

6. All individuals who experience a traumatic event will suffer from PTSD.
   1. True
   2. False

7. Airborne precautions should be used:
   1. When the patient is coughing.
   2. At all times
   3. Never, not an infection control definition
   4. When the patient is vomiting.

8. The HEICS provides the following, except:
   1. Way organize information
   2. Controlling and coordinating patient influx and movement
   3. A new way to treat smallpox
   4. Manageable span of control

9. Pneumonic plague occurs because of:
   1. Chemical
   2. Virus
   3. Bacteria
   4. Fungi

10. Triage is the act of:
    1. Discharging a patient for follow-up
    2. Prioritizing the patient's priority for care
    3. Providing a medical screening exam
    4. Admitting a patient to the intensive care unit

11. If a patient arrives to the ED with insecticide on him or her, the ER nurse does not need to be worried.
    1. True
    2. False

12. All of the following are true about SARS except:
    1. It is caused by a virus.
    2. It is not contagious.
    3. It originated in China.
    4. Patient's complain of a prodrome phase.

REVIEW ACTIVITIES

1. Visit the ED at your next clinical rotation and ask to review their triage guidelines. See if they use a three-tiered or five-tiered system.

2. Ask your instructor to find out when the hospital is performing their next disaster drill. Ask if you can observe the ED staff during a drill.

3. Review the hospital's disaster policy or packet and review your role as a student or a new RN. Familiarize yourself with their ICS.

4. Locate the PPE on every unit you are practicing on—make sure you know what size N-95 mask you are and that you have been fit tested.

5. Research your communities CISM team members and go and talk with one of them regarding critical incident stress debriefings.

6. Ask your clinical instructor to let you have time in the ED during your rotation.

Appendix A
Concept Mapping

Concept mapping is the process of analyzing the meaning of interrelationships among several concepts. Concept mapping has many synonyms including cognitive mapping, mind mapping, concept trees, and semantic networking (Beitz, 1998). A **concept map** is a graphic design that provides a visual picture of the analytical thinking process and interpretation of the information (Kathol, Geiger, & Hartig, 1998). The major concept is usually placed in the center of the map. Concepts or words related to the major concept are situated around it in categories or clusters. The concept clusters are linked to the major concept by lines, arrows, or significant words similar to the connecting roads and topographical areas between cities on a geographical map. Concept maps have three characteristics: hierarchical structure, chains or links, and clustering (Bietz, 1998).

The mapping process is associated with problem-solving learning. Educators have found concept mapping to be an innovative teaching method that promotes critical thinking, communication, categorization of information, and self-directed learning. The tool is relatively new to nursing; however, it has been used for several years in a variety of disciplines, including education and education psychology, business, medicine, the social sciences, and research (Beitz, 1998; Kathol, et al., 1998).

In nursing education, the concept map is primarily used as an alternative to the traditional linear care plan. Visual learners particularly value the map design, because it provides a visuo-spatial illustration of patient information. Creating the map assists students in gaining a holistic perspective of the patient, the health problem, and all the contributing factors, as well as realizing the implications for each phase of the nursing process (Alexander, McDaniel, Baldwin, & Money, 2002; Beitz, 1998; Kathol, et al., 1998; Mueller, Johnston, & Bligh, 2001; Schuster, 2000).

CREATING A CONCEPT MAP

Concept maps can be simple or elaborate and creatively designed, and either handwritten or computer generated. An entire page is used, usually in landscape form. The patient's name and the reason for entering the

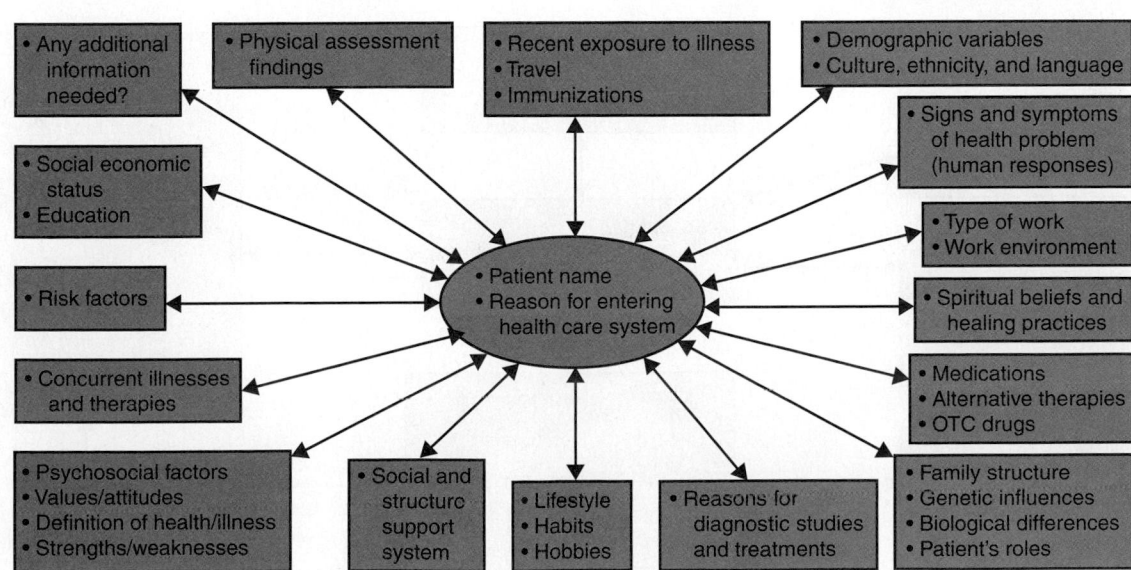

Figure A-1 Concept mapping patient information.

health care system are placed in the center of the diagram. Patient information is gathered through assessment, interviews with the patient or others, and review of the patient's record. The information can be clarified by reviewing texts, professional journal articles, and other literature. All concepts are analyzed for a possible connection to each other. Clusters of similar or related patient information are linked to the patient according to the best fit envisioned by the mapmaker. As concepts are added, the relationships and links may change (Figure A-1). Color coding is often used to sort and categorize the information and to signify priority needs and nursing actions. Arrows identify the direction of the connecting links among the various concepts and the relationship of the patient's responses to the health problem (Heinrich, Karner, Gagline, & Lambert, 2002; Kathol, et al., 1998; King & Shell, 2002).

Concept mapping also includes the organization of patient information within the phases of the nursing process to demonstrate the connections to the plan of care (Figure A-2 is an example). The end product is a unique representation "of an individual's health status as well as those concepts that affect the individual, such as social, cultural, ethnicity, and psychosocial state" (King & Shell, 2002, p. 36). Each map is considered a unique representation of the learner's ability to link theory to clinical practice.

PREPARATION FOR CONCEPT MAPPING

Students must have an understanding of the concepts and principles of the life sciences and a working knowledge of the nursing process prior to creating concept maps. Concept mapping can be introduced by mapping one's plan to visit a specific area or by creating a map of one's personal experiences and their effects on learning. These activities facilitate the transition to using nursing concepts in planning care. Case studies aid students in designing a map that illustrates the connections between clusters of information and selecting appropriate nursing diagnoses, patient outcomes, and nursing activities. Other helpful activities are mapping the effects of nursing concepts, such as immobility, oxygenation, pain, or anxiety on a patient's systems, and correlating the effects of a medication or therapy to a nursing diagnosis (King & Shell, 2002; Mueller, et al., 2001).

CLINICAL APPLICATION

Students learn the practice of clinical nursing by relating concepts, drawing on past learning and experience, and organizing conceptual meanings that make sense to them (Kathol, et al., 1998). A simple, or micromap is often used as a worksheet for a clinical day. Throughout the day, the instructor and student can evaluate where new information should be added and where changes need to be made. An updated version of the map is completed following the clinical experience.

ADVANTAGES OF CONCEPT MAPPING

Concept mapping enhances motivation and facilitates the learning process (Beitz, 1998). Critical thinking skills can be used for developing creative pictorial designs, such as placing concepts related to a respiratory problem in a lung-shaped map, inserting patient information related to a urinary problem within a kidney shape, or

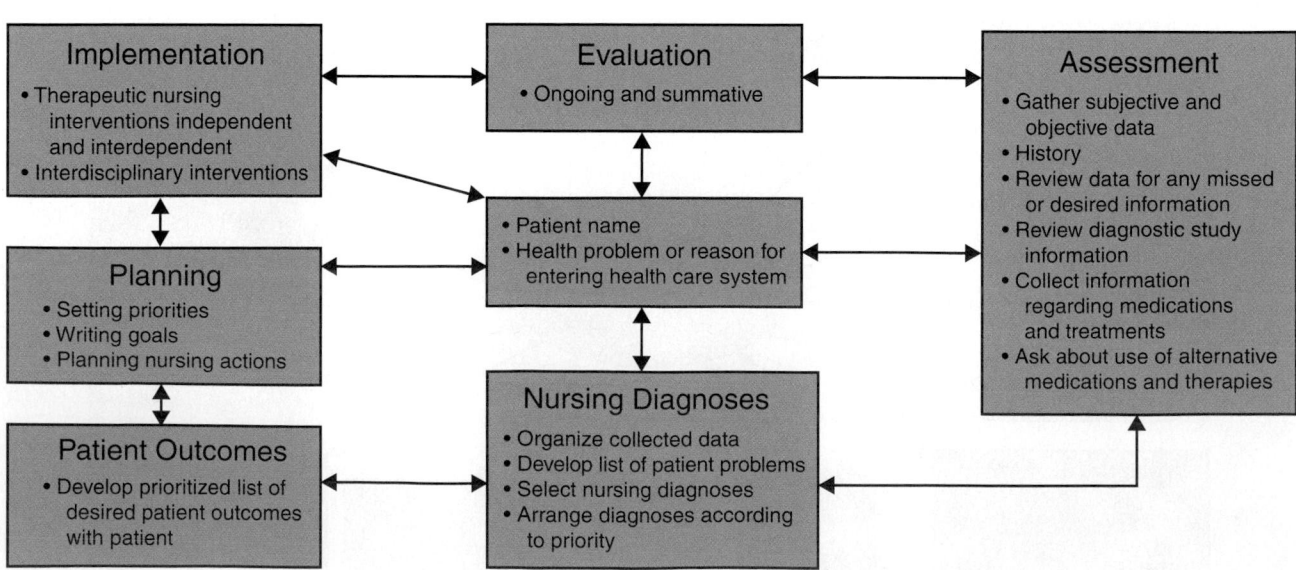

Figure A-2 Concept mapping.

drawing a map of the country of origin for content related to a patient from a different culture. Concept mapping can be an individual or group activity in the classroom or clinical settings for short-term or long-term assignments. Simple maps can be expanded throughout the curriculum to include more complex ideas, such as ethical/legal and leadership/management issues. They can also be used as study guides and for evaluation purposes. Concept mapping can be used as a curriculum matrix to track major concepts and themes, thus illustrating to faculty and students how the concepts and subject matter of the various courses are related to each other (Beitz, 1998; Heinrich et al., 2002). It also correlates well with the current emphasis on research and evidence-based practice (Burns & Grove, 2001; King & Shell, 2002).

DISADVANTAGES OF CONCEPT MAPPING

Because there are many ways to demonstrate connections between concepts, concept mapping may be difficult for individuals who believe there is only one way.

The mapping process may also be challenging for people who think in a linear manner. Mapping may not be appropriate for all areas of learning. Concept mapping is a time-consuming activity; however, computer graphics facilitate the development process. Educators must value its importance and take time to prepare students to use the mapping process.

APPLICATION

Concept map case studies are included in this text to assist in learning the process of concept mapping. Statements and questions are listed as prompts for developing a concept map. However, the mapmaker is encouraged to be creative.

Appendix B
English/Spanish Words and Phrases

Being able to say a few words or phrases in the patient's language is one way to show that you care. It lets the patient know that you as a nurse are interested in the individual. There are three rules to keep in mind regarding the pronunciation of Spanish words.

- If a word ends in a vowel, or in *n* or *s*, the accent is on the next to the last syllable.
- If the word ends in a consonant other than *n* or *s*, the accent is on the last syllable.
- If the word does not follow these rules, it has a written accent over the vowel of the accented syllable.

Courtesy phrases, names of body parts, and expressions of time and numbers are included in this section for quick reference. The English version will appear first, followed by the Spanish translation and Spanish pronunciation.

COURTESY PHRASES

Please	Por favor	Por-fah-**vor**
Thank you	Gracias	**Grah**-the-as
Good morning	Buenos días	Boo-**ay**-nos **dee**-as
Good afternoon	Buenas tardes	Boo-**ay**-nas **tar**-days
Good evening	Buenas noches	Boo-**ay**-nas **no**-chays
Yes/No	Sí/No	See/No
Good	Bien	Be-en
Bad	Mal	Mahl
How many?	Cuántos?	Coo-ahn-tos?
Where?	Dónde?	**Don**-day?
When?	Cuándo?	Coo-**ahn**-do?

BODY PARTS

abdomen	el abdomen	el ab-doh-men
ankle	el tobillo	el to-**beel**-lyo
anus	el ano	el **ah**-no
anvil (incus)	el yunque	el **yoon**-kay
appendix	el apéndice	el ah-**pen**-de-thay
aqueous humor	el humor acuoso	el oo-**mor** ah-coo-o-so
bladder	la vejiga	lah vah-**nee**-gah
brain	el cerebro	el thay-**ray**-bro
breast	el pecho	el **pay**-cho

buttock	la nalga	lah **nahl**-gah
calf	la pantorrilla	lah pan-tor-**reel**-lyah
cervix	la cerviz	lah ther-**veth**
cheek	la mejilla	lah mah-**heel**-lyah
chin	la barbilla	lah bar-**beel**-lyah
choroid	la coroidea	lah co-ro-e-**day**-ah
ciliary body	el cuerpo ciliar	el coo-**err**-po the-le-**ar**
clitoris	el clitoris	el **clee**-to-ris
coccyx	el coxis	el **coc**-sees
conjunctiva	la conjuntiva	lah con-hoon-**tee**-vah
cornea	la córnea	lah **cor**-nay-ah
penis	el pene	el **pay**-nay
prostate gland	la próstata	lah **pros**-ta-tah
pupil	la pupila	lah poo-**pee**-lah
rectum	el recto	el **rec**-to
retina	la retina	lah ray-**tee**-nah
sclera	la esclerótica	lah es-clay-**ro**-te-cah
scrotum	el escroto	el es-**cro**-to
seminal vesicle	la vesícula seminal	lah vay-**see**-coo-lah say-me-**nahl**
shoulder	el hombro	el **om**-bro
small intestine	el intestino delgado	el in-tes-**tee**-no del-**gah**-do
spinal cord	la médula espinal	lah **may**-doo-lah es-pe-**nahl**
spleen	el bazo	el **bah**-tho
stirrup (stapes)	el estribo	el es-**tree**-bo
stomach	el estómago	el es-**toh**-mah-go
temple	la sien	lah se-**ayn**
testis	el testículo	el tes-**tee**-coo-lo
thigh	el muslo	el **moos**-lo
thorax	el tórax	el **to**-rax
tongue	la lengua	lah **len**-goo-ah
trachea	la tráquea	lah **trah**-kay-ah
upper extremities	las extremidades superiores	las ex-tray-me-**dahd**-es soo-pay-re-**or**-es
ureter	el uréter	el oo-**ray**-ter
uterus	el útero	el **oo**-tay-ro
vagina	el vagina	lah vah-**hee**-nah
vitreous humor	el humor vítreo	el oo-**mor vee**-tray-o
wrist	la muñeca	lah moo-**nyay**-cah

EXPRESSIONS OF TIME, CALENDAR, AND NUMBERS

after meals	después de comer	des-poo-**es** day co-**merr**
at bedtime	al acostarse	al ah-cos-**tar**-say
before meals	antes de comer	**ahn**-tes day co-**merr**
daily	el diario	el de-**ah**-re-o

date	la fecha	lah **fay**-chah
day	el día	el **dee**-ah
every hour	a cada hora	ah **cah**-dah o-rah
hour (time)	la hora	lah o-rah
how often	cada cuánto tiempo	**cah**-dah coo-**ahn**-to te-**em**-po
noon	el mediodía	el may-de-o-**dee**-ah
now	ahora	ah-**o**-rah
once	una vez	**oo**-nah veth
today	hoy	**oh**-e
tomorrow	mañana	mah-**nyah**-nah
tonight	esta noche	**es**-tah **no**-chay
week	la semana	lah say-**mah**-nah
year	año	**a**-nyo
Sunday	el domingo	el do-**meen**-go
Monday	el lunes	el **loo**-nes
Tuesday	el martes	el **mar**-tes
Wednesday	el miércoles	el me-**err**-co-les
Thursday	el jueves	el hoo-**ay**-ves
Friday	el viernes	el ve-**err**-nes
Saturday	el sábado	el **sah**-bah-do
zero	cero	**thay**-ro
one	uno	**oo**-no
two	dos	dose
three	tres	trays
four	cuatro	coo-**ah**-tro
five	cinco	**theen**-co
six	seis	**say**-ees
seven	siete	se-**ay**-tay
eight	ocho	**o**-cho
nine	nueve	noo-**ay**-vay
ten	diez	de-**eth**

NURSING CARE SENTENCES AND QUESTIONS

What is your name?
¿Cómo se llama usted?
¿**Co**-mo say **lyah**-mah oos-**ted?**

I am a student nurse.
Soy estudiante enfermero(a).
Soy es-too-de-**ahn**-tay en-fer-**may**-ro(a).

My name is . . .
Mi nombre es . . .
Mee **nom**-bray es . . .

Do you need a wheelchair?
¿Necesita usted una silla de rueda?
¿Nay-thay-**se**-ta oos-**ted oo**-nah **seel**-lyah day roo-**ay**-dah?

How do you feel?
¿Cómo se siente?
¿**Co**-mo say se-**ayn**-tah?

When is your family coming?
¿Cuándo viene su familia?
¿Coo-**ahn**-do vee-**en**-nah soo fah-**mee**-le-ah?

This is the call light.
Esta es la luz para llamar a la enfermera.
Es-tah es lah looth **pah**-ra lyah-**mar** a lah en-fer-**may**-ra.

If you need anything, press the button.
Si usted necesita algo, oprima el botón.
See oos-**ted** nay-thay-**se**-ta **ahl**go o-pre-**ma** el bo-**tone.**

Do not turn without calling the nurse.
No se voltee sin llamar a la enfermera.
No say **vol**-tay seen lyah-**mar** a lah en-fer-**may**-ra.

The side rails on your bed are for your protection.
Los rieles del costado están para su protección.
Los re-**el**-es del cos-**tah**-do es-**tahn pah**-ra soo pro-tec-the-**on.**

Please do not try to lower or climb over the side rail.
Por favor no pretenda bajarlos (barjarlas) o treparse sobre ellos.
Por fah-**vor** no pray-**ten**-dah ba-**har**-los o tray-**par**-say **so**-bray **ayl**-lyos.

The head nurse is . . .
La jefa de enfermeras es . . .
La **hay**-fay day en-fer-**may**-ras es . . .

Do you need more blankets or another pillow?
¿Necesita usted más frazadas u otra almohada?
¿Nay-thay-**si**-ta oos-**ted** mahs frah-**thad**-dahs oo **o**-trah al-mo-**ah**-dah?

You may not smoke in the room.
No se puede fumar en el cuarto.
No say poo-**ay**-day foo-**mar** en el coo-**ar**-to.

Do you want me to turn on (turn off) the lights?
¿Quiere usted que encienda (apague) la luz?
¿Ke-**ay**-ray oos-**ted** day en-the-**en**-dah (a-**pah**-gay) lah looth?

Are you thirsty?
¿Tiene usted sed?
¿Tee-**en**-nah oos-**ted** sayd?

Are you allergic to any medication?
¿Es usted alérgico(a) a alguna medicina?
¿Es oos-**ted** ah-**lehr**-hee-co(a) ah ah-**goo**-nah nay-de-**thee**-nah?

You may take a bath.
Usted puede bañarse.
Oos-**ted** poo-**ay**-day bah-**nyar**-say.

Do not lock the door, please.
No cierre usted la puerta con llave, por favor.
No the-**err**-ray oos-**ted** lah poo-**err**-tah con **lyah**-vay por-fah-**vor.**

Call if you feel faint or in need of help.
Llame si usted se siente débil o si necesita ayuda.
Lyah-mah see oos-**ted** say se-**ayn**-tah **day**-bil o see nay-thay-**se**-ta ah-**yoo**-dah.

Call when you have to go to the toilet.
Llame cuando tenga que ir al inodoro.
Lyah-mah coo-**ahn**-do **ten**-gah kay eer al in-o-**do**-ro.

I will give you an enema.
Le pondré una enema.
Lay pon-**dray oo**-nah ay-**nay**-mah.

Turn on your left (right) side.
Voltese a su lado izquierdo (derecho).
Vol-**tay**-say ah soo **lah**-do ith-ke-**er**-do(dah) (day-**ray**-cho[cha]).

Here is an appointment card.
Aqui tiene usted una tarjeta con la información escrito.
Ah-**kee** tee-**en**-nah oos-**ted oo**-nah tar-**hay**-tah con lah in-for-mah-the-**on** es-**cree**-to.

You are going to be discharged (released) today.
A usted le van a dar de alta hoy.
Ah oos-**ted** lay vahn ah dar day **ahl**-tah **oh**-e.

How did this illness begin?
¿Cómo empezó esta enfermedad?
¿**Co**-mo em-pa-**tho es**-tah en-fer-may-**dahd?**

Is the pain better after the medicine?
Siente usted alivio depués de tomar la medicina?
¿Se-**ayn**-tah oos-**ted** al-**lee**-ve-o des-poo-**es** day to-**mar** lah may-de-**thee**-nah?

Where is the pain?
¿Qué la duele? (or) ¿Dónde le duele?
¿Kay lah doo-**ay**-le? (or) ¿**Don**-day lay doo-**ay**-le?

Do you have pains in your chest?
¿Tiene usted dolores in el pecho?
¿Tee-**en**-nah oos-**ted** do-**lor**-es en el **pay**-cho?

Are you in pain now?
¿Tiene usted dolores ahora?
¿Tee-**en**-nah oos-**ted** do-**lor**-es ah-**o**-rah?

Is it constant pain or does it come and go?
¿Es un dolor constante or va y vuelve?
¿Es oon do-**lor** cons-**tahn**-tay o vah ee voo-**el**-vah?

Is there anything that makes the pain better?
¿Hay algo que lo alivie?
¿**Ah**-ee **ahl**-go kay lo al-**le**-ve?

Is there anything that makes the pain worse?
¿Hay algo que lo aumente?
¿**Ah**-ee **ahl**-go kay lo ah-oo-**men**-tay?

Where do you feel the pain?
¿Dónde siente usted el dolor?
¿**Don**-day se-**ayn**-tah oos-**ted** el do-**lor?**

Point to where it hurts.
Apunte usted por favor, adonde le duele.
Ah-**poon**-tay oos-**ted** por fah-**vor** ah-**don**-day lay doo-**ay**-le.

Show me where it hurts.
Enséñeme usted donde le duele.
En-**say**-nah-may oos-**ted don**-day lay doo-**ay**-le.

Is the pain sharp or dull?
¿Es agudo o sordo el dolor?
¿Es ah-**goo**-do o **sor**-do el do-**lor?**

Do you know where you are?
¿Sabe usted donde esta?
¿Sah-**bay** oos-**ted don**-day es-**tah?**

You are in a hospital.
Usted está en el hospital.
Oos-**ted** es-**tah** en el os-pee-**tahl.**

You will be okay.
Usted va a estar bien.
Oos-**ted** vah a es-**tar be**-en.

Do you have any drug reactions?
¿Tiene usted alguna sensibilidad a productos químicos?
¿Te-**en** nah oos-**ted** al-**goo**-nah sen-se-be-le-**dahd** a pro-**dooc**-tos **kee**-me-cos?

Have you seen another doctor or native healer for this problem?
¿Ha visto usted a otro médico o curandero tocante a este problema?
¿Ah **vees**-to oos-**ted** a **o**-tro **may**-de-co o coo-ran-**day**-ro to-**cahn**-tay a **es**-ah pro-**blay**-mah?

Have you vomited?
¿Ha vomitado usted?
¿Ah vo-me-**tah**-do oos-**ted?**

Do you have any difficulty in breathing?
¿Tiene usted alguna dificultad para respirar?
Te-**en**-nah oos-**ted** ah-**goo**-nah de-fe-cool-**tahd pah**-ra res-pe-**rar?**

Do you smoke?
¿Fuma usted?
¿Foo-**mar** oos-**ted?**

How many per day?
¿Cuántos al día?
¿Coo-**ahn**-tos al **dee**-ah?

For how many years?
¿Por cuántos años?
¿Por coo-**ahn**-tos **a**-nos?

Do you awaken in the night because of shortness of breath?
¿Se despierta usted por la noche por falta de respiración?
¿Say des-pee-**err**-tah oos-**ted** por lah **no**-chay por **fahl**-tah day res-pe-rah-the-**on?**

Is any part of your body swollen?
¿Tiene usted alguna parte del cuerpo hinchada?
¿Te-**en**-nah oos-**ted** ah-**goo**-nah **par**-tay del coo-**err**-po in-**chah**-da?

How much water do you drink daily?
Cuántos vasos de agua bebe usted diariamente?
¿Coo-**ahn**-tos **vah**-sos day **ah**-goo-ah **bay**-be oos-**ted** de-ah-re-ah-**men**-tay?

Are you nauseated?
¿Tiene náusea?
¿Te-**en**-nah **nah**-oo-say-ah?

Are you going to vomit?
¿Va a vomitar?
¿Vah a vo-me-**tar?**

When was your last bowel movement?
¿Cuánto tiempo hace que evacúa usted?
¿Coo-**ahn**-to te-**em**-po **ah**-the kay ay-vah-**coo**-ah oos-**ted?**

Do you have diarrhea?
¿Tiene usted diarrea?
¿Te-**en**-nah oos-**ted** der-ar-**ray**-ah?

How much do you urinate?
¿Cuánto orina usted?
¿Coo-**ahn**-to o-**re**-nah oos-**ted?**

Did you urinate?
¿Orino usted?
¿O-re-**no** oos-**ted?**

What color is your urine?
¿De qué color es la orina?
¿Day kay co-**lor** es lah o-**re**-nah?

Call when you have to go to the toilet.
Llame usted cuando tenga que ir al inodoro.
Lyah-mah oos-**ted** coo-**ahn**-do **ten**-gah kay eer al in-o-**do**-ro.

I need a urine specimen from you.
Necesito una muestra de orina de usted.
Nay-thay-**se**-to **oo**-nah moo-**ays**-trah day o-**re**-nah day oos-**ted.**

We will put a tube in your bladder so that you can urinate.
Le pondremos un tubo en la vejiga para que puede orinar.
Lay pon-**dray**-mos un **too**-be en lah vay-**hee**-gah **pah**-rah kay poo-**ay**-day o-re **nar.**

When was your last menstrual period?
¿Cuándo fue se última menstruación?
¿Coo-**ahn**-do foo-**ay** soo **ool**-te-mah mens-troo-ah-the-**on?**

Are you bleeding heavily?
¿Está sangrando mucho?
¿Es-tah san-**grahn**-do **moo**-cho?

Take off your clothes, please.
Desvístase usted, por favor.
Des-**ves**-tah-say oos-**ted** por-fah-**vor.**

Just relax.
Relaje usted el cuerpo.
Ray-**lah**-he oos-**ted** el coo-**err**-po.

I am going to listen to your chest.
Voy a escucharle el pecho.
Voye a es-coo-**char**-lay el **pay**-cho.

Let me feel your pulse.
Déjeme tomarle el pulso.
Day-ha-me to-**mar**-lay el **pool**-so.

I am going to take your temperature.
Voy a tomarle la temperatura.
Voye a to-**mar**-lay lah tem-pay-rah-**too**-rah.

Lie down, please.
Acuéstese, por favor.
Ah-coo-**es**-tah-say por fah-**vor**.

Do you understand?
¿Me comprende usted?
¿May com-**pren**-day oos-**ted**?

That's right.
Así. Bien.
Ah-**see**. **Be**-en.

You are doing very well.
Usted va muy bien.
Oos-**ted** vah **moo**-e **be**-en.

Do not take any medicine from home.
No tome usted ninguna medicina traída de su casa.
No **to**-may oos-**ted** nin-**goon**-ay may-de-**thee**-nah trah-**ee** dah day soo **cah**-sah.

I am going to give you an injection.
Voy a ponerle una inyección.
Voye a po-**nerr**-lay **oo**-nah in-yec-the-**on**.

Take a sip of water.
Tome usted un traguito de agua.
To-may oos-**ted** un trah-**gee**-to day **ah**-goo-ah.

Very good. That was fine.
Muy bien. Excelente.
Moo-e **be**-en. Ex-thay-**len**-tay.

Don't be nervous.
No se ponga nervioso(a).
No say **pon**-gah ner-ve-**o**-so(ah).

Do you feel dizzy?
¿Se siente vertigo?
¿Say see-**ayn**-tah **verr**-to-go?

Please lie still.
Quédese inmóvil, por favor.
Kay-day-say in-**mo**-veel por fah-**vor**.

You must drink lots of liquids.
Usted debe tomar muchos liquidos.
Oos-**ted** **day**-bay to-**mar** **moo**-chos **lee**-ke-dos.

Appendix C
Symbols and Abbreviations

Symbols

~	similar		>	greater than
≅	approximately		<	less than
@	at		%	percent
√	check		+	positive
Δ	change		–	negative
↑	increased		♀	female
↓	decreased		♂	male
=	equals		△₁△₂△₃	trimester of pregnancy (one triangle
#	pounds			for each trimester)

Abbreviations

2,3-DPG	2,3-diphosphoglycerate		AONE	Association of Nurse Executives
AACN	American Association of Colleges of Nursing		AORN	Association for Operating Room Nurses
			APN	advanced practice nurse
AAOHN	American Association of Occupational Health Nurses		APRN	advanced practice registered nurse
			APTT	activated partial thromboplastin time
AARP	American Association of Retired Persons		AST	aspartate aminotransferase
ABG	arterial blood gas		AT	axillary temperature
A/C	alternative/complementary		ATP	adenosine triphosphate
Acetyl-CoA	acetyl coenzyme A		ATSDR	Agency for Toxic Substances and Disease
ADA	Americans with Disabilities Act			Registry
ADAMHA	Alcohol, Drug Abuse, and Mental Health Administration		BCR	bulbocavernosus reflex
			BMI	body mass index
ADH	antidiuretic hormone		BMR	basal metabolic rate
ADL	activities of daily living		BN	bachelor's degree in nursing
ADP	adenosine diphosphate		BP	blood pressure
ADR	adverse drug reactions		BScN	bachelor of science in nursing (in Canada)
AEB	as evidenced by		BSE	breast self-examination
AGF	angiogenesis factor		BSN	bachelor of science in nursing
AHA	American Hospital Association		BUN	blood urea nitrogen
AHNA	American Holistic Nurses Association		C	Celsius; also called centigrade
AHRQ	Agency for Health Care Research and Policy		CAT	computerized adaptive testing
			CAUSN	Canadian Association of University Schools of Nursing
AIDS	acquired immunodeficiency syndrome			
AJN	*American Journal of Nursing*		CBC	complete blood count
AMB	as manifested by		CBE	charting by exception
ANA	American Nurses Association		CDC	Centers for Disease Control and
ANS	autonomic nervous system			Prevention

CEUs	continuing education units	HCFA	Health Care Financing Administration
CHD	coronary heart disease	Hct	hematocrit
CLIA	Clinical Laboratory Improvement Act	HDL	high-density lipoprotein
cm	centimeter	HEPA	high efficiency particulate air
CMS	Centers for Medicare & Medicaid Services	Hgb	hemoglobin
CNA	Canadian Nurses Association	HIS	hospital information system
CNATS	Canadian Nurses Association Testing Service	HIV	human immunodeficiency virus
		HMO	health maintenance organization
CNM	certified nurse midwife	HPN	home parenteral nutrition
CNO	community nursing organization	HQIA	Healthcare Quality Improvement Act
CNS	central nervous system	HRSA	Health Resources and Services Administration
CNS	clinical nurse specialist		
CO$_2$	carbon dioxide	HSV-2	herpes simplex virus 2
COBRA	Consolidated Omnibus Budget Reconciliation Act	HT	healing touch
		IHS	Indian Health Service
COPD	chronic obstructive pulmonary disease	IM	intramuscular
CPK	creatine phosphokinase	in	inch
CPM	continuous passive motion	I&O	intake and output
CPN	central parenteral nutrition	IOM	Institute on Medicine
CPR	cardiopulmonary resuscitation	IPPB	intermittent positive-pressure breathing
CPT	chest physiotherapy	IRA	individual retirement account
CQI	continuous quality improvement	IV	intravenous
CRNA	certified registered nurse anesthetist	IVP	intravenous pyelogram
CSF	cerebrospinal fluid	JCAHO	Joint Commission on Accreditation of Healthcare Organizations
CST	computerized clinical simulation testing		
CT	computed tomography	kcal	kilocalorie
CVA	cerebrovascular accident	kg	kilogram
DDS	doctor of dental science	LAS	localized adaptation syndrome
DHHS	Department of Health and Human Services	lb	pound
		LDH	lactic dehydrogenase
dL	deciliter; also abbreviated dl	LDL	low-density lipoprotein
DNR	do not resuscitate	LLQ	left lower quadrant
DNSc	doctorate of nursing in science	LOC	level of consciousness
DRGs	diagnosis-related groups	LPN	licensed practical nurse
DSN	doctorate of science in nursing	LUQ	left upper quadrant
DUS	Doppler ultrasound stethoscope	LVN	licensed vocational nurse
DVT	deep vein thrombosis	m	meter
ECG	electrocardiogram (also known as an EKG)	MA	master of arts degree
EEG	electroencephalogram	MAC	mid-upper-arm circumference
EN	enteral nutrition	MAR	medication administration record
EPA	Environmental Protection Agency	MD	doctor of medicine
EPO	exclusive provider organization	MDR	multidrug-resistant
ESR	erythrocyte sedimentation rate	mEq	milliequivalent
ET	ear canal temperature	mEq/L	milliequivalent per liter
F	Fahrenheit	mg	milligram
FAF	fibroblast-activating factor	MH	malignant hyperthermia
FAS	fetal alcohol syndrome	MI	myocardial infarction
FDA	Food and Drug Administration	mL	milliliter; also abbreviated ml
FiO$_2$	fraction of inspired oxygen	mm	millimeter
ft	feet	mm Hg	millimeters of mercury
g	gram	MN	master's degree in nursing
GAS	general adaptation syndrome	mOsm	milliosmole; also spelled milliosmol
GCS	Glasgow Coma Scale	mOsm/L	milliosmole per liter
gH	drop	MRI	magnetic resonance imaging
GI	gastrointestinal	MRSA	methicillin-resistant *Staphylococcus aureus*
GNP	gross national product	MSN	master of science in nursing
HBD	alpha-hydroxybutyrate dehydrogenase	NACGN	National Association of Colored Graduate Nurses
HBV	hepatitis B virus		

NANDA	North American Nursing Diagnosis Association		PO	*per os* (by mouth)
NCEP	National Cholesterol Education Program		POMR	problem-oriented medical record
NCLEX	National Council Licensing Examination		POR	problem-oriented record
NCLEX-PN	National Council Licensure Examination for Practical Nurses		PPN	peripheral parenteral nutrition
			PPO	preferred provider organization
NCLEX-RN	National Council Licensure Examination for Registered Nurses		PPS	prospective payment system
			prn	*pro re nata* (as needed)
NCNR	National Center for Nursing Research		PRO	peer review organization
NCSBN	National Council of State Boards of Nursing		PSRO	professional standards review organization
NIC	Nursing Interventions Classification		PT	physical therapist
NIH	National Institutes of Health		PT	prothrombin
NINR	National Institute of Nursing Research		PT	prothrombin time
NLN	National League for Nursing		PTSD	posttraumatic stress disorder
NMDS	Nursing Minimum Data Set		PTT	partial thromboplastin
NP	nurse practitioner		PURT	prompted urge response toileting
NPO	*non per os* (nothing by mouth—to eat or drink)		q	every
			QA	quality assurance
			R	respiration
NS	nutrition support		RAS	reticular activating system
NST	nutritional support team		RBC	red blood cell
OAM	Office of Alternative Medicine		RD	registered dietitian
OBRA	Omnibus Budget Reconciliation Act		RDA	recommended dietary allowance
OR	operating room		RDDA	recommended daily dietary allowances
OSHA	Occupational Safety and Health Administration		RHC	Rural Health Clinic
			RLQ	right lower quadrant
OT	occupational therapist		RN	registered nurse
OT	oral temperature		RNA	registered nurse's assistant
OTC	over-the-counter		ROM	range-of-motion
oz	ounce		RPCH	rural primary care hospital
P	pulse		RPh	registered pharmacist
PO$_2$	partial pressure of oxygen in a mixture of gasses, or in solution		RT	rectal temperature
			RT	related to
PO$_2$	partial pressures of oxygen		RT	respiratory therapist
PA	physician's assistant		RUQ	right upper quadrant
PaO$_2$ (PAO$_2$)	partial pressure of oxygen dissolved in arterial blood plasma		S-CDTN	Self-Care Deficit Theory of Nursing
			SA	sinoatrial node
PAP	Papanicolaou test		SAECG	signal-averaged electrocardiography
PAT	pulmonary artery temperature		SaO$_2$	percent saturation of arterial blood (hemoglobin) with oxygen
PC	potential complication			
PCA	patient-controlled analgesia		SBC	school-based clinic
PCO$_2$	partial pressure of carbon dioxide dissolved in arterial blood plasma		SI	*le Système International d'Unités* (the international system of units)
PCP	primary care provider			
PEG	percutaneous endoscopic gastrostomy		SL	sublingual
PERRLA	pupils equal, round, reactive to light, and accommodation		SLT	social learning theory
			SMDA	Safe Medical Devices Act
			SMI	sustained maximum inspiration
pH	hydrogen ion concentration of a solution		SO	source-oriented charting
PID	pelvic inflammatory disease		SOAP	Subjective data, Objective data, Assessment, Plan
PIE	problem, intervention, evaluation			
PIEE	pulsed irrigation enhanced evacuation		SOAPIE	Subjective data, Objective data, Assessment, Plan, Implementation, Evaluation
PKU	phenylketonuria			
PMR	progressive muscle relaxation		STD	sexually transmitted disease
PMS	premenstrual syndrome		SUI	stress urinary incontinence
PN	parenteral nutrition		SW	social worker
PNI	psychoneuroimmunology		T	temperature
PNS	peripheral nervous system		TEFRA	Tax Equity Fiscal Responsibility Act

TENS	transcutaneous electrical nerve stimulation	UHDDS	uniform hospital discharge data set
TMJ	temporomandibular joint	USPHS	United States Public Health Service
TNA	total nutrient admixture	VA	Veterans Affairs
TPN	total parenteral nutrition	VLDL	very low-density lipoprotein
TQM	total quality management	V/Q	ventilation/perfusion mismatch
TSE	testicular self-examination	VRE	vancomycin-resistant enterococci
TT	therapeutic touch	WBC	white blood cell
UAP	unlicensed assistive personnel	WIC	Women, Infants, and Children

Appendix D
NANDA Nursing Diagnoses 2005–2006

Activity Intolerance
Risk for Activity Intolerance
Impaired Adjustment
Ineffective Airway Clearance
Latex Allergy Response
Risk for Latex Allergy Response
Anxiety
Death Anxiety
Risk for Aspiration
Risk for Impaired Parent/Infant/Child Attachment
Autonomic Dysreflexia
Risk for Autonomic Dysreflexia
Disturbed Body Image
Risk for Imbalanced Body Temperature
Bowel Incontinence
Effective Breastfeeding
Ineffective Breastfeeding
Interrupted Breastfeeding
Ineffective Breathing Pattern
Decreased Cardiac Output
Caregiver Role Strain
Risk for Caregiver Role Strain
Impaired Verbal Communication
Readiness for Enhanced Communication
Decisional Conflict (Specify)
Parental Role Conflict
Acute Confusion
Chronic Confusion
Constipation
Perceived Constipation
Risk for Constipation
Defensive Coping
Ineffective Coping
Readiness for Enhanced Coping
Ineffective Community Coping
Readiness for Enhanced Community Coping
Compromised Family Coping
Disabled Family Coping
Readiness for Enhanced Family Coping
Risk for Sudden Infant Death Syndrome
Ineffective Denial
Impaired Dentition

Risk for Delayed Development
Diarrhea
Risk for Disuse Syndrome
Deficient Diversional Activity
Energy Field Disturbance
Impaired Environmental Interpretation Syndrome
Adult Failure to Thrive
Risk for Falls
Dysfunctional Family Processes: Alcoholism
Interrupted Family Processes
Readiness for Enhanced Family Processes
Fatigue
Fear
Readiness for Enhanced Fluid Balance
Deficient Fluid Volume
Excess Fluid Volume
Risk for Deficient Fluid Volume
Risk for Imbalanced Fluid Volume
Impaired Gas Exchange
Anticipatory Grieving
Dysfunctional Grieving
Risk for Dysfunctional Grieving
Delayed Growth and Development
Risk for Disproportionate Growth
Ineffective Health Maintenance
Health-Seeking Behaviors (Specify)
Impaired Home Maintenance
Hopelessness
Hyperthermia
Hypothermia
Disturbed Personal Identity
Functional Urinary Incontinence
Reflex Urinary Incontinence
Stress Urinary Incontinence
Total Urinary Incontinence
Urge Urinary Incontinence
Risk for Urge Urinary Incontinence
Disorganized Infant Behavior
Risk for Disorganized Infant Behavior
Readiness for Enhanced Organized Infant Behavior
Ineffective Infant Feeding Pattern
Risk for Infection

Risk for **I**njury
Risk for Perioperative-Positioning **I**njury
Decreased **I**ntracranial Adaptive Capacity
Deficient **K**nowledge
Readiness for Enhanced **K**nowledge (Specify)
Risk for **L**oneliness
Impaired **M**emory
Impaired Bed **M**obility
Impaired Physical **M**obility
Impaired Wheelchair **M**obility
Nausea
Unilateral **N**eglect
Noncompliance
Imbalanced **N**utrition: Less than Body Requirements
Imbalanced **N**utrition: More than Body Requirements
Readiness for Enhanced **N**utrition
Risk for Imbalanced **N**utrition: More than Body
  Requirements
Impaired **O**ral Mucous Membrane
Acute **P**ain
Chronic **P**ain
Readiness for Enhanced **P**arenting
Impaired **P**arenting
Risk for Impaired **P**arenting
Risk for **P**eripheral Neurovascular Dysfunction
Risk for **P**oisoning
Post-Trauma Syndrome
Risk for **P**ost-Trauma Syndrome
Powerlessness
Risk for **P**owerlessness
Ineffective **P**rotection
Rape-Trauma Syndrome
Rape-Trauma Syndrome: Compound Reaction
Rape-Trauma Syndrome: Silent Reaction
Impaired **R**eligiosity
Readiness for Enhanced **R**eligiosity
Risk for Impaired **R**eligiosity
Relocation Stress Syndrome
Risk for **R**elocation Stress Syndrome
Ineffective **R**ole Performance
Sedentary Life Style
Bathing/Hygiene **S**elf-Care Deficit
Dressing/Grooming **S**elf-Care Deficit
Feeding **S**elf-Care Deficit
Toileting **S**elf-Care Deficit
Readiness for Enhanced **S**elf-Concept
Chronic Low **S**elf-Esteem

Situational Low **S**elf-Esteem
Risk for Situational Low **S**elf-Esteem
Self-Mutilation
Risk for **S**elf-Mutilation
Disturbed **S**ensory Perception (Specify: Visual,
  Auditory, Kinesthetic, Gustatory, Tactile, Olfactory)
Sexual Dysfunction
Ineffective **S**exuality Patterns
Impaired **S**kin Integrity
Risk for Impaired **S**kin Integrity
Sleep Deprivation
Disturbed **S**leep Pattern
Readiness for Enhanced **S**leep
Impaired **S**ocial Interaction
Social Isolation
Chronic **S**orrow
Spiritual Distress
Risk for **S**piritual Distress
Readiness for Enhanced **S**piritual Well-Being
Risk for **S**uffocation
Risk for **S**uicide
Delayed **S**urgical Recovery
Impaired **S**wallowing
Effective **T**herapeutic Regimen Management
Ineffective **T**herapeutic Regimen Management
Readiness for Enhanced Management of **T**herapeutic
  Regimen
Ineffective Community **T**herapeutic Regimen
  Management
Ineffective Family **T**herapeutic Regimen Management
Ineffective **T**hermoregulation
Disturbed **T**hought Processes
Impaired **T**issue Integrity
Ineffective **T**issue Perfusion (Specify Type: Renal,
  Cerebral, Cardiopulmonary, Gastrointestinal,
  Peripheral)
Impaired **T**ransfer Ability
Risk for **T**rauma
Impaired **U**rinary Elimination
Readiness for Enhanced **U**rinary Elimination
Urinary Retention
Impaired Spontaneous **V**entilation
Dysfunctional **V**entilatory Weaning Response
Risk for Other-Directed **V**iolence
Risk for Self-Directed **V**iolence
Impaired **W**alking
Wandering

Appendix E
Standard Precautions

STANDARD PRECAUTIONS
FOR INFECTION CONTROL

Wash Hands (Plain Soap)
Wash after touching **blood, body fluids, secretions, excretions**, and **contaminated items**. Wash immediately **after gloves are removed** and **between patient contacts**. Avoid transfer of microorganisms to other patients or environments.

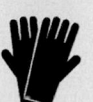

Wear Gloves
Wear when touching **blood, body fluids, secretions, excretions**, and **contaminated items**. Put on **clean** gloves just **before touching mucous membranes** and **nonintact skin**. Change gloves between tasks and procedures on the same patient after contact with material that may contain high concentrations of microorganisms. Remove gloves promptly after use, before touching noncontaminated items and environmental surfaces, and before going to another patient, and wash hands immediately to avoid transfer of microorganisms to other patients or environments.

Wear Mask and Eye Protection or Face Shield
Protect mucous membranes of the eyes, nose, and mouth during procedures and patient–care activities which are likely to generate **splashes** or **sprays** of **blood, body fluids, secretions**, or **excretions**.

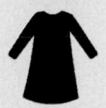

Wear Gown
Protect skin and prevent soiling of clothing during procedures that are likely to generate **splashes** or **sprays** of **blood, body fluids, secretions**, or **excretions**. Remove a soiled gown as promptly as possible and wash hands to avoid transfer of microorganisms to other patients or environments.

Patient-Care Equipment
Handle used patient–care equipment soiled with **blood, body fluids, secretions**, or **excretions** in a manner that prevents skin and mucous membrane exposures, contamination of clothing, and transfer of microorganisms to other patients and environments. Ensure that reusable equipment is not used for the care of another patient until it has been appropriately cleaned and reprocessed and single use items are properly discarded.

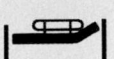

Environmental Control
Follow hospital procedures for routine care, cleaning, and disinfection of environmental surfaces, beds, bedrails, bedside equipment, and other frequently touched surfaces.

Linen
Handle, transport, and process used linen soiled with **blood, body fluids, secretions**, or **excretions** in a manner that prevents exposures and contamination of clothing and avoids transfer of microorganisms to other patients and environments.

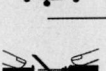

Occupational Health and Blood-Borne Pathogens
Prevent injuries when using needles, scalpels, and other sharp instruments or devices; when handling sharp instruments after procedures; when cleaning used instruments; and when disposing of used needles.

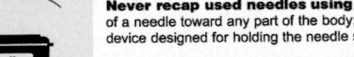

Never recap used needles using both hands or any other technique that involves directing the point of a needle toward any part of the body; rather, use either a one-handed "scoop" technique or a mechanical device designed for holding the needle sheath.

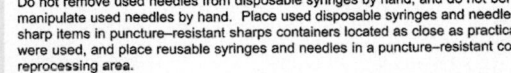
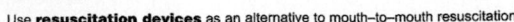

Do not remove used needles from disposable syringes by hand, and do not bend, break, or otherwise manipulate used needles by hand. Place used disposable syringes and needles, scalpel blades, and other sharp items in puncture–resistant sharps containers located as close as practical to the area in which the items were used, and place reusable syringes and needles in a puncture–resistant container for transport to the reprocessing area.

Use **resuscitation devices** as an alternative to mouth–to–mouth resuscitation.

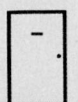

Patient Placement
Use a **private room** for a patient who contaminates the environment or who does not (or cannot be expected to) assist in maintaining appropriate hygiene or environmental control. Consult Infection Control if a private room is not available.

The information on this sign is abbreviated from the HICPAC Recommendations for Isolation Precautions in Hospitals.

Form No. **SPR**   BREVIS CORP., 3310 S 2700 E, SLC, UT 84109   © 1996 Brevis Corp.

Courtesy of the Brevis Corporation

Glossary

12-lead electrocardiogram (ECG) A standardized recording of the electrical activity of the heart and may be used to detect heart irregularities, lack of oxygen to parts of the heart, and enlargement of the chambers.

A

A waves Plateau waves seen and related to severe intracranial hypertension. A waves have a range of 50 to 100 mm Hg.

abscess Collection or cavity of fluid, such as pus or cellular debris, which developed as result of an inflammatory response.

absolute hypovolemia Shock condition that occurs with the actual loss of fluid from the body including whole blood.

absorption A pharmacokinetic process that accounts for the movement of the drug from the site of administration into the bloodstream.

access Ability to obtain affordable health care when needed.

acculturation Process of learning the norms, beliefs, and behavioral expectations of a group.

acetylcholine A neurotransmitter in both the central and peripheral nervous system.

achalasia A motility disorder from failure of smooth muscle to relax or the absence of muscular contraction of the lower esophagus.

acidemia A decreased arterial pH, less than 7.35.

acne Results from thickening of the follicular opening, increased sebum production, the presence of bacteria, and the host's inflammatory response.

acquired immunity Refers to immunity that is not present at birth and develops as a result of exposure to pathogens; also called adaptive or specific immunity.

actin filaments The contractile part of a myofilament.

actinic keratoses Changes because of exposure to ultraviolet light (sun) Considered as premalignant lesion.

active euthanasia Someone other than the patient performs an action that ends the patient's life.

acute abdomen Refers to a constellation of clinical signs and symptoms usually best treated by surgery. Abrupt onset of abdominal pain; a potential medical emergency involving one of the abdominal organs, i.e., appendicitis.

acute respiratory distress syndrome (ARDS) Classified as noncardiac pulmonary edema with disruption of the alveolar-capillary membrane due to injury to the pulmonary vasculature or the airways (formerly called adult respiratory distress syndrome).

Adams Bending Forward Test A test used to assess for scoliosis.

adaptation (adjustment) The ongoing process of modifying one's behavior in changed circumstances or in an altered environment to fulfill psychological, physiological, and social needs.

addiction A compulsive disorder in which an individual becomes preoccupied with obtaining and using a substance, the continued use of which results in a decreased quality of life.

adducts Free radicals that can bind closely with the patient's healthy tissues and create hybrid molecules.

adenoma A benign (not malignant) tumor made of epithelial cells, usually arranged like a gland.

adjuvant A remedy that enhances the effect of another therapy.

adjuvant therapy Treatment given after the primary treatment to increase the chances of a cure. Adjuvant therapy may include chemotherapy, radiation therapy, hormone therapy, or biological therapy.

adrenergic stress response The physical and psychological responses to threatening environmental stimuli and the rapid release of epinephrine (adrenalin) from the sympathetic nervous system.

adrenocorticotropic hormone (ACTH) Hormone released from the anterior pituitary that stimulates the secretion of corticosteroids by the adrenal cortex.

adult daycare Provides health, social, and recreational services to adults who require supervision during family absence.

advance directives Written documents that allow a person to state, in advance, specific decisions about how he or she wants his or her own health care managed if he or she becomes incapacitated and is unable to communicate.

adverse effects Negative response to a drug, can range from mild to life-threatening.

aerophagia Excessive amounts of air are swallowed.

affective domain Area of learning that involves attitudes, beliefs, and emotions.

afterload The load that the ventricular muscle exerts when it is pushing its contents into the aorta.

agency Capacity for intentional action.

Agency for Healthcare Research and Quality (AHRQ) A federally funded U.S. government agency established by Congress in 1989 to support research designed to improve the quality of health care, reduce its cost, improve patient safety, decrease medical errors, and broaden access to essential health care service.

ageusia Loss or impairment of taste.

agglutination Occurs when an antibody links to the same epitope on two different antigens; appears in the blood as clumping.

agranulocytosis Severe neutropenia, with less than 200 cells/μm.

airborne transmission Infectious material trapped in dust and carried on air currents.

airway pressure release ventilation (APRV) Two levels of pressures to ventilate the patient.

akinesia The loss of movement.

alaryngeal voice Alternative methods of speaking that do not include the larynx; method used by patients who have their larynx removed.

aldosterone A mineral corticoid synthesized in the adrenal cortex; functions to maintain extracellular fluid volume.

alkalemia An increased arterial pH, more than 7.45.

allele One of two or more different genes containing specific inheritable characteristics that occupy corresponding positions on paired chromosomes.

allergen A substance that induces an allergic reaction.

allogeneic A remedy that replaces a patient's blood or bone marrow with blood or bone marrow from a donor.

allogeneic transplantation Stem cells from a sibling or unrelated donor with matching human leukocyte antigens (HLA).

allograft Skin graft.

allograft or homograft transplant *See* allogenic transplantation.

allopathic Mainstream, orthodox, conventional medical practice in the United States.

alopecia The loss of hair.

alpha-fetoprotein (AFP) A fetal protein produced in the yolk sac of the embryo for the first six weeks of gestation and then by the fetal liver.

altruism Unselfish concern for the welfare of others.

amblyopia A reduction in visual acuity caused by cerebral blockage of visual stimuli, which can develop in the eye affected by strabismus.

amenorrhea Absence of menstruation most commonly caused by an underlying hypothalamic-pituitary-endocrine dysfunction or a congenital abnormality or acquired abnormalities of the reproductive tract.

amplification The end result of the process in the formation of the erythrocyte whereby one rubriblast can form 14 to 16 erythrocytes.

amyloid Extracellular protein-like substance.

anabolism The constructive part of metabolism concerned especially with macromolecular synthesis.

analgesia Insensitivity to pain.

anaphylaxis Immediate, life-threatening hypersensitive allergic reaction.

anasarca Generalized edema is associated with malnutrition, terminal illness, and metabolic fluid overload problems.

anastomosis Surgical union of parts and especially hollow tubular parts.

androgens The male sex hormones.

anesthesia Absence of touch sensation.

anesthesia care provider Anesthesiologist or nurse anesthetist who delivers anesthesia to patients in surgical settings.

aneuploid A chromosome number that is not an exact multiple of the haploid number resulting in an extra or a missing chromosome.

aneurysm A permanent bulging and stretching of an artery, in which the dilation is two times or greater the size of the artery.

angina pectoris Pain in the chest.

angiogenesis The establishment of blood supply through formation of new blood vessels.

angioneurotic edema A condition associated with allergies and histamine release in which large welts develop below the surface of the skin, especially around the eyes and lips. The welts may also affect the hands, feet, and throat.

anion gap The portion of negatively charged ions not measured with routine laboratory studies.

anions Negatively charged particles.

ankle sprain When the ankle is displaced or a sudden force is applied, the ligaments are stretched beyond their normal stretching capacity and a sprain of the ligament occurs.

annular Ring-shaped (superficial fungal infections, such as ringworm, pityriasis rosea, seborrheic dermatitis, psoriasis, and others).

anosmia Loss or impairment of smell.

anovulation Failure to ovulate.

anthropophilic Human source.

antibodies Proteins produced by plasma cells that recognize and bind to a specific antigen.

anticipatory grieving Intellectual and emotional responses and behaviors by which individuals work through the process of modifying self-concept based on the perception of potential loss.

anticipatory stress A concern or worry about a potential problem or the uncertain outcome of a future event and the inability to control one's future.

anticoagulants Pharmaceuticals that prevent further clot formation in the body.

antidiuretic hormone (ADH) Hormone produced in the posterior pituitary and regulates the reabsorption of water in the kidneys, thereby regulating fluid volume.

antigen A substance that stimulates an immune response.

antigen presenting cells (APCs) Cells that ingest antigens, digest them, and display the epitope to stimulate immune response.

antineoplastic A drug that prevents, kills, or blocks the growth and spread of cancer cells.

antiphagocytic Something that destroys the function of the neutrophils and macrophages.

anuria Less than 50 mL per 24 hours of urine.

aphakic vision Absence of the crystalline lens of the eye.

aphasia Impairment in the ability to speak or comprehend.

apheresis Procedure that consists of withdrawal of blood from a donor, removal of one or more components (as plasma, blood platelets, or white blood cells) from the blood, and transfusion into patients with low platelet or white blood cell counts; the remaining blood is transfused back into the donor.

aphonia Loss of voice.

aphthous stomatitis Ulcerative conditions of the gums and mucous membranes; are labeled mouth ulcers.

apneustic breathing A pattern of respirations characterized by a prolonged inspiratory phase, followed by expiration apnea (the rate of apneustic breathing is usually 1:5 cycles per minute).

apoptosis An intact regulation of physiological cell death, which protects the organism from the development of a cancerous tumor.

approximated Wound edges also called borders, or margins, that are well connected without gaps.

arcus senilis Lipid deposition on the periphery of the cornea.

aromatherapy The therapeutic use of concentrated essences or essential oils that have been extracted from plants and flowers to stimulate, uplift, relax, or soothe by promoting balance between the sympathetic and parasympathetic nervous systems.

arrhythmias Deviations from normal cardiac rhythm.

arteriosclerosis Hardening of the arteries and defined as a thickening and solidifying of the endothelial lining of the walls in small arteries and arterioles.

arthroscopy A diagnostic test performed in the knee joint; an arthroscopy is an endoscopic procedure used to diagnose and repair meniscal, patellar, extrasynovial, and synovial diseases.

articulation Where a bone meets another bone to form a joint.

ASA scale Evaluation method used by anesthesiologists to determine risk of patients undergoing surgical procedures.

ascending cholangitis An infection in the gallbladder that moves in the direction of the liver.

ascites The accumulation of fluid in the peritoneal cavity.

asepsis Practice of ensuring that bacteria are excluded from open sites during surgery, wound dressing, blood sampling, and other medical procedures.

assessment The first step in the nursing process that involves the systematic collection, verification, organization, interpretation, and documentation of data for use by health care professionals.

assisted living Provides personal, social and health care, plus 24-hour supervision.

assisted suicide Similar to active euthanasia; often associated with a health care provider assisting another to end his or her own life.

astereognosis Lack of ability to identify objects by touch.

astigmatism Occurs when there is an unequal curve of the cornea and the light rays are bent unevenly.

ataxia A lack of muscle coordination.

atherogenesis Developmental process of the atherosclerotic lesion.

atherosclerosis Atherosclerosis begins as fatty streaks of the arterial wall in adolescence, progressing to hard fatty plaques that narrow and "harden" the arteries lumen in adulthood.

atopic dermatitis (AD) A hereditary and chronic skin disorder; also called eczema.

atopy A personal or familial tendency to become sensitized and produce immunoglobulin E (IgE) antibodies in response to ordinary exposure to allergens.

atresia Absence or closure of a natural passage of the body.

atypia Deviation from the standard cell form.

auditory Pertaining to the sense of hearing.

auditory learners Style of learning in which an individual learns by hearing.

aura Sensation that occurs immediately before a disorder, such as a migraine headache or a seizure.

auricle (pinna) The external ear.

auscultation Listening to sounds produced by the body, which are created by movement of air or fluid.

autoantibody An antibody that reacts against a person's own tissue.

autograft A permanent graft where a piece of skin from a remote unburned area of the body and transplants it to cover the burn wound.

autoimmunity The loss of tolerance (self-tolerance) of the body's antigenic markers on cells.

autologous The collection and storage of blood or blood components from a patient for subsequent transfusion to that same person.

autologous donation Occurs when a patient's own blood or blood products are donated 72 hours or more prior to surgery in anticipation of the need for blood or blood product replacement during surgery.

autologous transplantation Transplant of the patient's own stem cells.

autolytic debridement Uses moist wound dressings maintain a natural level of moisture, facilitating a normal inflammatory response.

automaticity When a group of cardiac cells have the ability to generate an electrical impulse spontaneously.

autonomic dysreflexia Disordered discharge of autonomic responses, which results in massive discharge of sympathetic responses.

autonomously Independent provision of primary health care.

autonomy Self-rule that is free from controlling influence by others and from limitation, such as inadequate understanding.

autosomes Any chromosome other than the sex chromosomes.

axis The imaginary line drawn between two electrodes.

ayurveda A healing system based on Hindu philosophy, which embraces the concept of an energy force in the body that seeks to maintain balance or harmony.

azoospermia Absence of spermatozoa in the semen.

azotemia A build up of nitrogenous waste products.

B

B waves Waves seen with intracranial pressures of 20 to 50 mm Hg.

balanitis Inflammation of the glans penis.

balanoposthitis A condition in which posthitis occurs concurrently with balanitis.

bariatric therapy Specialization dealing with patients who are overweight or obese.

barium An oral preparation that allows roentgenographic visualization of the internal structures of the digestive tract.

barium enema A rectal infusion of barium sulfate.

baroreceptors Pressure sensitive receptors located primarily in the arch of the aorta, which sense the pressure generated in the arteries by the pumping action of the heart.

barotrauma An injury to the lungs as a result of increased air pressure in the lungs.

basic human needs Need that must be met for survival.

basophils Granulocytes that attack fungi.

beneficence Requires that actions are of benefit to others.

bereaved People mourning a loss.

bioavailability Percentage of the drug that is available to achieve its intended effect in the body.

biofeedback A mechanism of providing feedback of physiological process to help patients learn how to manipulate those responses through mental activity.

biotechnology Use of data and techniques of engineering to solve problems related to natural organisms.

Biot's (ataxic) breathing The presence of an abnormal pattern of breathing, which is characterized by totally irregular rate and depth of respirations with periods of apnea.

blepharitis Inflammation of the hair follicles (cilia) and glands along the edges of the eyelids.

blood pressure Force exerted by the blood against the walls of the blood vessel to maintain tissue perfusion during rest and activity.

body mass index (BMI) Formula using weight and height to determine the percentage of total body fat.

bone marrow aspiration and biopsy A diagnostic test used to examine the bone marrow for abnormal tissue growth or to monitor the progress of bone marrow disease.

bone scan A diagnostic nuclear scan used to detect early bone disease, bone metastasis, and bone response to therapeutic regimens.

borborygmi sounds Loud, hyperactive bowel tones.

borborygmus Hyperactive bowel sounds.

Bouchard's nodes In rheumatoid arthritis, bony enlargements of the proximal interphalangeal joints.

brachytherapy The treatment with radioactive sources placed into or near the tumor or affected area.

bradykinesia Slowness in performing spontaneous movements.

bradypnea An abnormally slow rate of breathing.

brain dead Loss of consciousness, brainstem reflexes, and respiration with essentially flat electroencephalograms.

brash water Occurs when the mouth suddenly fills with saliva; secondary to reflex salivary secretion stimulated by acid back flow into the esophagus.

breakthrough pain Acute flares of pain when medication or therapy does not relieve all of the pain.

breast augmentation Surgical enlargement of the breasts.

bronchophony The presence of distinct, clear, and relatively loud sounds heard over areas of the lung in which the normal alveoli are filled with fluid or replaced by solid tissue.

bruit An adventitious sound of venous or arterial origin heard during auscultation.

Buerger's disease An occlusive disease mostly located in small to medium-sized arteries and occasionally in veins. Though commonly found in the upper and lower distal extremities, it is associated with clot formation and fibrosis of the vessel wall. In prolonged cases, large extremities vessels may be affected.

buffy coat An area that is light-colored and contains the mostly white blood cells seen in a test tube that is centrifuged or allowed to stand.

bullae Enlarged airspaces that do not contribute to ventilation but occupy space in the chest.

bullous myringitis The presence of an infectious vesicle and inflammation of the tympanic membrane caused by the organism *Mycoplasma pneumoniae*.

burn shock Massive fluid shifts of plasma, electrolytes, and proteins into the burn wound causing the inability of the circulatory system to meet the needs of cells, tissues, and vital organs.

burrows Linear lesions produced by tunneling of animal parasite, such as in scabies.

bursae Synovial fluid-filled sacs near a joint.

C

C waves Small waves seen with pressures less than 20 mm Hg.

cachexia A breakdown of muscle mass resulting from rapid weight loss or a general wasting due to illness or stress.

calcitonin A hormone produced by the thyroid gland when circulating calcium levels are elevated.

calculi A substance of abnormal concretion composed of mineral salts commonly produced within the renal system.

cancellous Found in the ends of the long bones and in smaller amounts in some of the flat bones.

carbuncles Aggregates of infected follicles originating deep in the dermis and subcutaneous tissue.

cardiac index The patient's cardiac output divided by the patient's body surface area.

cardiac output (CO) Total blood flow through the systemic or pulmonary circulation per minute.

cardiogenic shock Shock that occurs when inadequate oxygen and nutrients are supplied to the tissues because of severe left ventricular failure.

carditis Inflammation of the heart.

caregiver role strain Caregiver's felt difficulty in performing the family caregiver role.

carrier An individual who is heterozygous for a normal gene and an abnormal gene.

casts Accumulation of materials in a space that fills the contours of the space.

catabolism Destructive metabolism involving the release of energy and resulting in the breakdown of complex materials within the organism.

cations Positively charged particles.

cell-mediated immunity Refers to immunity that is mediated by T lymphocytes.

cellular components The parts of the blood that are derived from the stem cell. These include erythrocytes, granulocytes, platelets, B lymphocytes, and T lymphocytes.

cellulitis Generalized inflammation of the deeper connective tissue.

centering Bringing body, mind, and emotions to a quiet, focused state of consciousness; being still and nonjudgmental.

centrifugal Extends outward away from the center.

cephalalgia Headache.

cerebral perfusion pressure The pressure at which cerebral tissue is perfused. It is calculated by subtracting the intracranial pressure from the mean arterial pressure.

cerebrovascular accident ([CVA] stroke) Damage to the brain due to lack of blood flow.

cerumen A thick, wax-like substance secreted by the sweat glands within the ear canal.

chakra A concentrated area of energy of which there are seven primary centers in the physical body according to Hindu belief.

cheilosis Small fissures at the corners of the mouth.

chemoembolization An embolizing drug impregnated with chemotherapy drugs to deliver a concentrated dose directly to the area close to the tumor.

chemokines Chemicals that attract other cells, particularly leukocytes.

chemotaxis Response to a chemical stimulant to attract white blood cells to a specific site.

Cheyne-Stokes breathing The presence of an abnormal pattern of breathing, characterized by alternating periods of crescendo-decrescendo depth of breathing with periods of apnea.

cholangitis Inflammation of the bile duct.

cholecystitis Inflammation of the gallbladder.

cholelithiasis Gallstones.

cholestasis Any condition that impedes bile flowing freely through the bile ducts.

cholesteatoma A cyst that contains an accumulation of squamous epithelium, keratin, and other debris.

chondrosarcoma A cartilaginous sarcoma.

chorea Abnormal and excessive involuntary movements.

chromosomes Thread-like structures within the nucleus of a cell that carry the genes.

chyme The contents of the stomach, which are semiliquid.

climacteric The perimenopausal period.

clinical decisions Decisions that promote the optimal clinical response in a patient.

clinical ethics Ethical issues that impact patient care.

clinical practice guidelines (CPGs) Systematically developed statements to assist clinicians and patients in making decisions about appropriate health care for specific clinical circumstances.

clonus A slight involuntary pushing against the foot.

closed reduction External manipulation of a fracture, which forces it into alignment.

clubbing An abnormal enlargement of the distal phalanges.

coagulopathies Disorders that lead to abnormal clotting of the blood.

Cochrane Collaboration Global nonprofit and independent collaborative founded in 1993 in the United Kingdom that disseminates evidence summaries for use by clinicians, health policy makers, and consumers of health care.

Cochrane library Subscription service repository of full text reports and abstracts of evidence summaries.

code of ethics Principles that guide professional practice.

cognitive domain Learning by understanding the material that is presented with the mind.

colectomy Surgical operation to remove all or part of the colon.

collective bargaining Process where employer and worker representatives negotiate conditions of employment.

coma depasse Irreversible coma.

comedones Plugged secretions of horny material retain within a pilosebaceous follicle.

compartment syndrome Swelling in the soft tissues and muscles that in turn cause compromised circulation to that area.

competence Individual's demonstrated command of a body of knowledge or skills and the ability to consistently perform to a standard and achieve a desired outcome.

complement A cascade of proteins in serum that, when activated, attract more leukocytes to the site of activation, encourage phagocytosis, and lyse pathogen cell membranes.

complementary and alternative medicine (CAM) Therapy that has a focus beyond specific symptom management.

complementary therapy Otherwise known as alternative therapy; methods of medicine that are not Western based but that offer alternative ways to accomplish health care goals. Examples include massage therapy and hypnosis.

compliance The distensibility or elasticity of the lung that decreases as lung tissue becomes stiffer.

concept map A special form or diagram used for exploring knowledge and gathering and sharing information.

concussion Mild form of brain injury.

conductivity The ability of the cardiac cells to transmit an impulse.

condyloma Genital warts caused by the human papillomavirus (HPV).

conscious sedation A drug-induced depression of consciousness during which patients respond purposefully to verbal commands, either alone or accompanied by light tactile stimulation.

consensual response Pupillary constriction on the opposite pupil.

constipation Straining at stool with the production of hard stools, decreased frequency, and a feeling of not completely evacuating the colon.

contact dermatitis An acute or chronic skin inflammation triggered in the epidermis by contact with a specific antigen or irritant.

contextual features Social, economic, and cultural factors that make each person a unique individual.

continuing care Provides ongoing care for disabilities, chronic diseases, or permanent changes in functional capacity.

continuous mandatory ventilation (CMV) Breaths are delivered at preset intervals, regardless of patient effort. This mode is used most often in the paralyzed or apneic patient because it can increase the work of breathing if respiratory effort is present.

continuous positive airway pressure (CPAP) Pressure that adds to the functional residual capacity in patients who are spontaneously breathing.

continuous quality improvement (CQI) Application of scientific process analysis methods to improve quality and productivity.

contractility The capability of muscle fibers to shrink.

contracture Shortening of a muscle.

conventional medicine The common medical practice in the United States by medical doctors, doctors of osteopathy, and their adjunct practitioners: nurses, physical therapists, and social workers.

convulsion The abnormal motor response or jerking movements that occur during a seizure.

coping Conscious or unconscious methods used to deal with, and attempt to overcome, problems and difficulties such as stressful events, violence, and illness.

coping efficacy Perceived effectiveness of the coping effort to manage a stressful event.

cor pulmonale Hypertrophy or failure of the right ventricle resulting from disorders of the lungs, pulmonary vessels, or chest wall.

corneal reflex Stimulation of the trigeminal nerve (cranial nerve V) causes this protective blink.

coronary artery bypass grafting (CABG) A surgery where veins and arteries are used as conduit to bypass the coronary artery stenosis.

coronavirus A virus that normally only leads to upper respiratory infection.

cortical or compact (bone) The hard outer layer of bone surfaces.

corticosteroids Any of the hormones, except androgen, synthesized by the adrenal cortex.

cortisol A major glucocorticoid that functions in the regulation of blood glucose levels.

cough To expel air from the lungs suddenly and noisily to keep the respiratory passages free from irritating material.

counterpulsation The synchronization of the intra-aortic balloon pump to assist the heart according to the cardiac cycle.

crash cart Mobile cart with defibrillator, resuscitation equipment, and medications used when patients go into cardiac arrest.

crepitus A crinkly, crackling, or grating feeling or sound in the joints, skin, or lungs.

critical access hospital (CAH) Provides outpatient, emergency, and inpatient services in a rural area.

critical incident A patient or event that causes a stress reaction in the health care worker.

cryopexy Freezing of the retinal tear area.

cryotherapy The use of ice or cold water over an injury site to decrease inflammation.

cultural assimilation Individuals from a minority group are absorbed by the dominant culture and take on the characteristics of the dominant culture.

cultural awareness A conscious learning process in which people become appreciative of and sensitive to the cultures of others.

cultural competence The complex integration of knowledge, attitudes, and skills that enable the nurse to provide culturally appropriate health care.

cultural context Environment or situation that is relevant to the care, beliefs, values, and practices of the culture under study.

cultural diversity The difference among people that results from ethnic, racial, and cultural variables.

cultural encounter The process that encourages individuals to engage directly in cross-cultural interactions with people from culturally diverse backgrounds.

cultural knowledge The process of understanding the vital aspects of a groups' culture as it relates to health and health care practices.

cultural skill The ability to collect relevant cultural data regarding health histories and performing culturally specific assessments.

culture The knowledge, values, beliefs, art, morals, law, customs, and habits of the members of a society.

culture for caring Ideas, customs, skills, and arts of a work group that are transferred, communicated, or passed along to succeeding generations of health care workers.

Cushing response A late sign of increasing intracranial pressure with signs of slowing respirations, slowing heart rate, and increasing blood pressure.

cystectomy Removal of the bladder.

cytokines Chemicals that affect the way other cells behave.

cytotoxic (killer) T cells Lymphocytes that lyse host cells infected with a virus; also called CD8 T cells.

D

dactylitis An inflammatory affection of the fingers.

dead space That portion of ventilation that does not participate in gas exchange.

debridement A mechanical method of eliminating necrotic tissue.

deep partial-thickness burn Also called second-degree burn; a burn that involves the entire epidermis and the lower two thirds of the dermis.

deep sedation/analgesia A drug-induced depression of consciousness during which patients cannot be easily aroused but respond purposefully following repeated or painful stimulation.

deep vein thrombosis (DVT) A blood clot in a deep vein that accompanies an artery.

defibrillation Delivering an electrical shock to the heart so that it completely depolarizes the cardiac cells in an effort to terminate ventricular fibrillation.

dehiscence The separation of a wound or scar. A rupture or splitting open, as of a surgical wound or of an organ or structure to discharge its contents as splitting open.

deletion The loss of varying amounts of genetic material that is detectable at the DNA or chromosomal level.

demargination A process whereby the granulocytes can suddenly leave the peripheral tissues.

dendritic cells Large phagocytic antigen presenting cells that activate T cells.

deontology Philosophy concerned with the moral duty and obligation of an action rather than the action's outcome.

deoxyribonucleic acid (DNA) The molecular basis of heredity, consisting of purine and pyrimidine nucleotides arranged in two long strands, twisted about each other to form a double helix.

depolarization Electrical changing in the interior of an excitable cell from negative to positive, which results in an action potential.

dermatomal Localized into a dermatome supplied by one or more dorsal ganglia (herpes zoster and segmental vitiligo).

dermatome The body region supplied by a pair of a dorsal root ganglia.

detumescence The process that occurs following orgasm where the blood flow decreases and the vasocongestion is relieved.

diabetes mellitus A chronic metabolic disorder characterized by hyperglycemia (elevated blood sugar levels) related to a lack of insulin, lack of effects of insulin, or a combination.

diapedesis Cells squeeze through pores in capillary wall.

diaphoresis Profuse sweating.

diarrhea An increase in the liquid state of the stool.

diastolic blood pressure Phase in the cardiac cycle when the heart is at rest.

didelphic Duplication; usually refers to two uteri, two cervices, and two vaginas.

differentiation A process involving constant turnover of new cells of the epidermis.

diffusion The movement of solutes from an area of high concentration to an area of low concentration.

dimorphic Existing in two shapes or forms.

diploid Two complete sets of chromosomes, double the number present in gametes (ova or sperm cells). In humans, the diploid number is 46.

diplopia Double vision.

direct calorimetry A measurement of energy expended by measuring temperature changes in a closed structure.

direct contact transmission Body surface to body surface contact.

direct response Pupillary constriction on the pupil being tested.

directed or controlled coughing Cough technique to expectorate sputum and avoid fatigue associated with undirected, forceful coughing that consists of slow, maximal inspiration followed by breath holding for several seconds and then two or three coughs.

disaccharides A class of sugars, which yields two monosaccharide molecules through hydrolysis.

disease prevention or health protection Behavior motivated by a desire to actively avoid illness, detect it early, or maintain functioning within the constraints of an illness.

disequilibrium An imbalance in solute concentration across the blood brain barrier.

displaced fracture A fracture in which the bones have gone out of natural alignment.

disseminated Spread over a large area of the body, tissue, or organ.

disseminated intravascular coagulation (DIC) Clotting and bleeding disorder that results from the generation of tissue factor activity within the blood. This trigger of the coagulation cascade quickly leads to significant thrombin production, which perpetuates its own formation and results in bleeding.

distress Stressor that is perceived as negative or stress that produces a negative response; a certain level of negative stress is needed for growth and development.

distribution The movement of the drug, after absorption into the bloodstream, to the site of intended action.

diverticula Sac-like outpouches of mucosa through the muscular layer of the bowel.

diverticulosis When there are multiple infected diverticula that result in pathology.

do not resuscitate (DNR) A health care provider's order that there be no attempt to restart a failed heartbeat or apply cardiopulmonary resuscitation.

domains of nursing The four main areas of nurses' practice, which includes clinical practice, education, administrative practice, and research.

dominant culture Group whose values prevail within a society.

double effect Palliative therapy, itself, hastens death.

drawer test An assessment technique used to diagnose rupture of cruciate ligaments.

Dressler's syndrome Inflammation of the pericardium that can occur 2 to 10 weeks after a myocardial infarction.

droplet transmission Particles propelled through the air.

dual energy X-ray absorptiometry (DEXA) scans Diagnostic tests that assist with the early diagnosis of osteoporosis.

Durable Power of Attorney for Health Care (DPAHC) Advance directive that appoints an agent or proxy decision maker to make health care decisions for a person who has lost decisional capacity.

dysarthria Difficulty in oral movement to form words.

dyscrasia Nonspecific term for blood disease.

dysdiadochokinesia The inability to perform rapidly alternating movements.

dysesthesia Burning or tingling.

dysfunctional uterine bleeding (DUB) Abnormal uterine bleeding not caused by malignancy, inflammation, or pregnancy.

dysgeusia Disturbed sense of taste.

dysmenorrhea Pain associated with menstruation.

dysmetria Impaired judgment of distance, range, speed, and force of movement.

dyspareunia Painful intercourse.

dyspepsia An uncomfortable feeling in the upper abdominal region.

dysphagia Difficulty swallowing.

dyspnea Difficulty breathing.

dysrhythmia A disturbance in rhythm.

dyssynergy A lack of coordinated muscle movement.

dysthymia A low-level depression that can last at least two years, and if left untreated, can lead to more severe depression.

dysuria Painful urination.

E

echocardiogram A noninvasive test in which ultrasound is used to reflect cardiac structures. It can be performed at rest or in conjunction with a stress test.

ectopy Heartbeat arising from a location other than the sinoatrial node on a monitor screen.

ectropion When the lower eyelid is turned away from the globe of the eye.

eczematoid Lesion suggesting inflammation with tendency to thickening, oozing, vesiculation, or crusting (related to eczema).

edema An abnormal collection of fluid in the interstitial spaces between cells resulting in a lifting and separating of the layers of the skin.

effluent Waste materials.

egophony The presence of loud, nasal, and "bleating" sounds when auscultating the lungs.

ejection fraction (EF) An index that estimates contractile function of the left ventricle. The expected ejection fraction is 60 to 70 percent.

electrolytes Charged particles found in body fluids.

emboli A blood clot or other particle (plaque) that break loose and block blood vessels.

embolization Introduction of an angio catheter to visualize the internal spermatic vein, to correct dysfunction of the spermatic vein.

emmetropia In normal vision the light falls onto the retina without any distortion or abnormal bending of the light.

empowerment To assist or encourage a person to be involved in decision making and development of the plan of care; the ability to assume self-care management.

endemic Restricted to a particular region, community, or group of people.

endocarditis Inflammation of the endocardium.

endocardium The membrane that lines the cavities of the heart and forms part of the heart valves.

endocrine glands Those glands that produce hormones that are secreted into the bloodstream and travel to their target organs or tissues.

endogenous Produced or originating from within a cell or organism.

endometriosis Ectopic growth of functioning endometrial tissue.

endorphins Peptides secreted in the brain that boost mood and help fight depression and pain.

endothelium The layer that lines the blood and lymphatic vessels, the heart, and various other body cavities is a prominent contributor to the activation of the inflammatory immune response. Cells produce several compounds that affect the vascular lumen and platelets.

endotracheal intubation The passage of tube into the trachea through either the mouth or nares to maintain an open airway or facilitate mechanical ventilation.

enterokinase An enzyme that hastens effective digestion.

enterprises Organized systems of any size in any location that provide any type of health care for compensation.

enthesitis Traumatic disease occurring at the insertion of muscles where recurring concentration of muscle stress provokes inflammation with a tendency toward fibrosis and calcification.

entropia An eye that deviates inward.

entropion When the lower eyelid is turned in toward the globe of the eye.

enucleation Surgical removal of an eye.

environmental control Relationships between people and nature and a person's perceived ability to control activities of nature.

enzymatic debridement Accomplished using a chemical debriding agent.

eosinophil A granulocyte that helps to control the inflammatory process.

epidemiological investigation Study looking at a specific disease, its distribution, and initial source.

epididymitis Infection of the epididymis.

epilepsy Chronic recurrent pattern of seizures.

epiphyses The widened ends of the long bone.

epispadias The urinary meatus is located along the superior (upper) aspect of the penis.

equianalgesia The provision of equal analgesic effects in changing from one drug and/or delivery method to another or choosing a different delivery method.

ergonomics Science that seeks to adapt work or working conditions to suit the worker.

erythromelalgia A burning sensation in the digits of the extremities.

erythropoietic Relating to the formation of red blood cells.

erythropoietin (EPO) A hormone produced by the kidney in response to low oxygen states or a low hematocrit, which stimulates red blood cell production in the bone marrow.

eschar Burned skin that is dead and must be removed before healing can occur.

escharotomy Incision through full-thickness circumferential burn tissue to restore and maintain circulation or chest expansion.

esotropia Convergent strabismus.

ethics The study of philosophical ideals of right and wrong behavior.

ethics of care Belief that health care professionals have a moral obligation and duty to provide care to those in need.

ethnicity A cultural group's perception of themselves (group identity). This self-perception influences how the group's members are perceived by others.

ethnocentrism Belief that one's own culture is superior to all others.

eugenics The selection and recombination of genes already existing in the gene pool.

euglycemia A normal concentration of glucose in the blood.

euploidy A term referring to the correct number of chromosomes in a cell.

eupnea The presence of normal respirations, or normal rate and depth of breathing.

eustachian tube A tube that connects the middle ear to the nasopharynx.

eustress A certain level of positive stress that is needed for growth and survival.

euthanasia Practice in which a person other than the patient directly administers medication that causes the death of a patient.

euthenics (euphenics) The techniques for correcting defects in individuals after they have been born.

euthyroid Having a normal functioning thyroid gland.

evidence-based practice (EBP) Process through which scientific evidence is identified, appraised, and applied in health care interventions.

evidence summary Report of the state of scientifically produced knowledge that is developed using rigorous methods to synthesize knowledge across a number of research studies so that study variations and contradictory study results can be understood in a single conclusion statement.

Ewing's sarcoma A diffuse endothelioma or endothelial myeloma forming a fusiform swelling on a long bone.

exacerbation A sudden increase in the seriousness of the disease with greater intensity in signs and symptoms, which lasts from minutes to hours or days.

exanthema Breaking out in a rash.

excitability The capacity for that cell to depolarize in response to an electrical impulse.

exocrine glands Those glands that secrete substances into ducts that empty into a body cavity or onto a body surface.

exogenous Originating outside an organ.

exotropia (wall eyes) An eye that deviates outward.

expiratory reserve volume (ERV) The maximal amount of gas that can be expired at the end of a normal exhalation.

expressive aphasia (Broca's aphasia) A condition in which a patient cannot express what he or she wants to say.

extracellular fluid (ECF) The fluid located between cells and includes interstitial and intravascular fluid.

extravasation The inadvertent administration of vesicant into the surrounding tissues.

extrinsic distortion Occurs when the interpreter is improperly prepared.

exudate Accumulated fluid in a cavity.

F

fascia An inelastic connective tissue that covers and separates muscles, tendons, and ligaments.

fasciotomy Incision through a fibrous layer that separates muscles.

fast pain (rapid pain) Pain that originates in the free endings of the large myelinated nerve fibers of the skin; such pain respond to strong pressure and high temperature, thus eliciting the withdrawal reflex.

fecalith Hard mass of fecal material.

fibroadenomas Benign fibrous growths or tumors of the glandular epithelium in breast tissue.

fibromyalgia A disorder characterized by muscle pain, stiffness, and easy fatigability.

first pass effect After absorption, oral drugs are transported via hepatic portal circulation to the liver, where they are metabolized (broken down) before they can pass into the general circulation.

flatulence Gas formed within the gastrointestinal tract and expelled via the rectum.

foam cell Engorged lipid-laden macrophages that are the major component of the fatty streak.

focused assessment An assessment that is limited in scope to focus on a particular need or health care problem or potential health care risk.

folliculitis Acute inflammation of the hair follicle caused by physical irritation, infection, or chemical irritation.

fracture A break in a bone.

fremitus The feeling of vibration, which will be increased or decreased in certain conditions.

fulguration Destruction of tissue using high-frequency electric sparks.

full-thickness burn Also called third-degree burn; involves the entire epidermis and dermis that extends to subcutaneous tissue and possibly muscle and bone.

furuncles (boils) Localized bacterial infections that can manifest as painful, indurated, or fluctuant, fluid-filled masses.

G

galactorrhea Excessive secretion of milk.

gametes A mature male or female reproductive cell.

gender identity The biological sex of male, female, or intersexed.

gender role The masculine or feminine role adopted by a person, which is often culturally and socially determined.

gene A segment of a DNA molecule that is the heredity unit that occupies a fixed chromosomal locus.

gene therapy The process of treating or curing a genetic disorder by providing the affected individual with an intact, functional copy of the gene in question.

general inhibition syndrome (GIS) "Possum" response to stress because of overstimulation of the parasympathetic nervous system (PNS) as a means of survival or a paralyzing or numbing effect when facing a life-threatening event; a state of panic or freezing.

genetic counseling The interaction between health care provider and patient to manage the human problems associated with the occurrence, or risk of occurrence, of a genetic disorder in a family.

genetic engineering Changing a particular molecule in the structure of the gene, either to eliminate a certain bad trait or to improve the genotype.

genetic screening Population screening for a genetic variation or mutation, for example, PKU screening at birth.

genetic testing Testing of an individual at significant risk because of family history or because of presentation of symptoms, for example chromosome abnormalities.

genogram A family tree related to health history.

genomics The study of genome composition, structure, and function in combination with environmental factors that has led to the discovery of numerous health care products.

genotype The genetic constitution or blueprint of an individual, the gene pairs that are inherited from the parents.

global aphasia A condition in which a patient has both expressive and receptive aphasia.

globalization Organized or established worldwide.

glossitis An inflammation of the tongue.

glucagon A hormone released from the pancreas in response to low levels of blood glucose and is a counterregulatory hormone.

gluconeogenesis The process of the liver converting predominant amino acids to glucose in the fasting state.

glycogen hydrolysis Conversion of stored glycogen into usable glucose to meet the immediate energy needs of the body.

glycogen synthesis Conversion of glucose to glycogen that can be stored in preparation of times of fasting.

glycogenolysis The physiological process of the breakdown of stored glucose to raise blood sugar levels.

grading The degree of malignancy or cell differentiation of the tumor cells.

granulocytes Class of leukocytes with prominent granules.

granuloma A mass of inflamed granulation tissue.

graphesthesia Identify letters, numbers, or shapes drawn on hand.

grief resolution An adjustment to actual or impending loss.

gross domestic product (GDP) Total value of final goods and services produced in a year within the United States.

growth hormone (GH) Hormone that affects all tissues of the body, is secreted from anterior pituitary, and is one of the counterregulatory hormones.

gynecomastia Breast enlargement in men.

H

half-life The time required for the body, tissue, or organ to metabolize or make inactive half the amount of a substance taken in.

haploid One complete set of chromosomes. The haploid number in humans is 23.

haptens An antigen that does not cause an immune response unless bound to a carrier molecule.

harvesting A procedure to collect tissue such as the spongy bone marrow from inside bones containing stem cells.

healing touch (HT) An energy-based therapeutic therapy that alters the energy field through the use of touch.

health A state and a process of being and becoming an integrated and whole person.

health care Care related to all states of health from severe illness and injury to supreme good health; diagnosis and treatment of disease and strategies that maintain and improve health.

health care system Network of individuals, technologies, and processes that provide and support health care.

health insurance Insurance policy that provides payment for benefits of a covered sickness or injury. Included under this definition are various types of insurances, such as accident insurance, disability insurance, medical expense insurance, and accidental death insurance.

health maintenance Behavior directed toward maintaining a current level of health.

health maintenance activities The activities or behaviors an individual performs to maintain or improve a current level of health.

health maintenance organizations (HMOs) Type of managed care plan where access to care is controlled by a primary care provider and coverage is limited to the approved medical services, administered by a network of health care providers, hospitals, skilled nursing facilities, and other providers included in the plan. Emphasis is on prevention.

health promotion Process undertaken to increase levels of wellness in individuals, families, and communities.

heartburn (pyrosis) A substernal burning sensation often radiating to the neck that is experienced within one hour of eating or one to two hours after reclining.

Heberden's nodes Hard nodules or enlargements of the tubercles of the last phalanges of the fingers.

Heinz bodies Degraded hemoglobin.

helper T cells Lymphocytes that orchestrate the immune response; also called CD4 T cells. There are two subclasses TH1 and TH2.

hemarthrosis Untreated bleeding into the joint.

hematochezia Stools containing red blood rather than tarry stools.

hematoma Excessive bleeding that occurs around a wound site as a result of broken blood vessels from trauma or surgery.

hematomas A swelling noted in tissue, caused by extravasated blood.

hematopoiesis The ability to maintain the body's blood supply and its components.

hematopoietic Pertaining to the formation of blood or blood.

hematuria Blood in the urine.

hemiparesis Weakness on one side of the body.

hemiplegia Inability to move of one side of the body.

hemoglobinuria Hemoglobin in the urine.

hemolysis Destruction of red blood cells.

hemoptysis Indicates either the presence of frank blood or blood-streaked sputum.

hemorrhagic stroke When a blood vessel bursts leaking blood into brain tissue or surrounding spaces.

hemosiderosis A condition in which iron is toxic to the cells.

hemovac A type of surgical drain with a piece that connects to a mechanical suction device.

hepatomegaly Enlarged liver, palpated below the level of the ribs.

hereditary angioedema (HAE) An inherited abnormality of the immune system that causes swelling, particularly of the face, and abdominal cramping.

heterograft (xenograft) A graft of skin obtained from another species.

high-density lipoprotein (HDL) The substance that transports plasma cholesterol away from atherosclerotic plaques and to the liver for metabolism and excretion and is considered "good" cholesterol because increased levels decrease the tendency to CAD.

high efficiency particulate air (HEPA) filter Filter used to remove submicron particulate matter from the air.

hirsutism Condition characterized by the excessive growth of hair or the presence of hair in abnormal places.

histamine A chemical released by the immune system during allergic reactions.

histocompatibility leukocyte antigens (HLA) A complex set of proteins on the surface membrane of human nucleated cells, tissues, and blood cells (except red blood cells).

holism The concept that the whole is greater than the sum of its parts. Holism encompasses consideration of the physiological, psychological, sociocultural, intellectual, and spiritual aspects of each individual.

Homans' sign Dorsiflexing the foot, causing pain in the calf.

homeopathy Treatment of disease with minute drug doses to activate an illness that then stimulates the body's normal defense system to eliminate illness.

homeostasis Physiological and psychological equilibrium or balance.

homograft A graft of skin obtained from a cadaver 6 to 24 hours after death that is used as a temporary graft.

homonymous hemianopsia Inability to see out of one half of both eyes, and the visual field cut.

hope A feeling expressed as future-oriented, which allows the person to set goals, devise strategies for achieving the desired goals, and a sense of being in control.

hormones The chemicals produced and stored by the endocrine system that help regulate metabolism and energy, cardiac output and blood pressure, reproduction, and growth and development.

hospice Provides end-of-life care for patients and their families.

hospice care Coordinated program of palliative care services with a goal of attaining the highest possible quality of life for patients and their families at the end of life and continuing through the bereavement period.

human leukocyte antigen (HLA) MHC class I.

humectants Substances that promote moisture in skin.

humoral-mediated immunity Refers to immunity that is mediated by B lymphocytes, plasma cells, and antibodies.

hyaline Cartilage that covers the end of each bone to reduce friction and distribute weight-bearing forces.

hydronephrosis Dilation of the renal pelvis because of an obstruction of urine flow or from ureteral reflux.

hypalgesia Diminished sensitivity to pain.

hyperalgesia (allodynia) A state of neural supersensitivity where a slight painful stimulus can be interpreted as very painful.

hypercapnia An accumulation of $PaCO_2$ in the blood, indicating hypoventilation.

hypercholesterolemia High serum cholesterol.

hyperesthesia Increased sensitivity of the skin.

hypergesia Increased sensitivity to pain.

hyperglycemia An elevated blood sugar level.

hyperlipidemia Elevated blood cholesterol levels.

hyperopia (farsightedness) Occurs when the light passing through the eye is focused behind the retina when looking a close objects.

hyperplasia Increase in number.

hypersensitive response An extreme physical response to an allergen, in which large amounts of IgE are produced.

hypertension Sustained elevation of blood pressure.

hypertonic A solution with a concentration higher than that of blood.

hypertrophic Increase in size of an organ or structure secondary to inflammation or overgrowth of cells not related to tumor formation.

hypertrophy Abnormal enlargement, increase in size and mass, of a body part or organ.

hyperuricemia An abnormal amount of uric acid in the urine.

hypervolemia Excess intravascular fluid.

hypesthesia Diminished sense of touch.

hypoalbuminemia Decrease in albumin in the blood.

hypocapnia Less than normal $PaCO_2$ in the blood, indicating hyperventilation.

hypogeusia Diminished taste sensitivity.

hypokyphosis Less than normal curvature in the thoracic spine.

hypospadias The urinary meatus is located along the inferior (lower) aspect of the penis.

hypotany Low intraocular pressure.

hypotension Blood pressure lower than needed for adequate tissue perfusion and oxygenation.

hypothermia Condition where the body temperature falls to less than 36° C (96.8° F). It is classified as mild, if not less than 32° C (89.6° F).

hypotonic A solution with a concentration less than that of blood.

hypovolemia Insufficient intravascular fluid.

hypoxemia A decrease in PaO_2 below 80 mm Hg.

hypoxia A general term for decrease in tissue oxygenation.

I

icterus Yellow coloration in the sclera of the eye.

idiopathic A disease state that arises from an unknown cause.

idiopathic pain Spontaneous or unpredictable breakthrough pain.

ileus Refers to intestinal obstruction because of a partial or complete arrest of intestinal peristalsis; also known as paralytic or adynamic ileus.

illness care Care aimed at relieving the discomfort of disease.

imagery The use of one's sense to create an image in one's mind.

immune response A body response to an antigen that occurs when lymphocytes identify the antigenic molecule as foreign and induce the formation of antibodies and lymphocytes capable of reacting with it and rendering it harmless.

immunity The quality or state of being immune; a condition of being able to resist a particular disease through preventing development of a pathogenic microorganism or by counteracting the effects of its products.

immunodeficiency Inability to produce a normal complement of antibodies or immunologically sensitized T cells especially in response to specific antigens.

immunogen A particle that can cause an immune response.

immunoglobulins (IG) The class of proteins that antibodies belong to. Body manufactures five isotopes: IgM, IgD, IgG, IgA, and IgE.

immunotherapy The process of introducing allergens to the body by injection for the purpose of increasing immunity.

imperforate hymen Congenital malformation of the hymenal ring resulting in lack of a vaginal opening.

inborn error of metabolism A condition in which the metabolism of an organism is abnormal because of the presence of one, or a pair of, abnormal alleles.

incentive spirometer A machine used to allow patients a quantifiable aid in deep breathing postoperatively.

incidence The number of new cases of a condition, symptom, death, or injury that arise during a specific period of time such as a month or a year.

indirect calorimetry A method for estimating energy expenditure by measuring oxygen consumption and carbon dioxide production.

indirect contact transmission Inanimate object involved in transfer.

infertility The inability to conceive within one year when a couple is engaging in unprotected sexual intercourse at the appropriate times in the female's menstrual cycle.

infiltration Inadvertent administration of a solution into the surrounding tissues.

inflammation A nonspecific response to any foreign invader involving the immune system.

inflammatory immune response (IIR) A response that is composed of several body systems that are constantly on alert to detect nonself and harmful intruders from the normal cells and proteins in the body.

informed consent A patient's authorization for care based on full disclosure of risks, benefits, alternatives, and consequences of refusal.

innate immunity Immunity that is inherent within a species and develops regardless of exposure.

inspection Careful, systematic visual observation.

inspiratory reserve volume (IRV) The maximal amount of gas that can be inspired at the end of a normal inspiration.

insulin Hormone produced by the beta cells of the pancreas to lower blood glucose levels.

integrated care delivery system Network of organizations that provides a coordinated continuum of services to a defined population and that is willing to be held clinically and fiscally accountable for the outcomes and health status of the population served.

integrative review Alternative term for an evidence summary.

integrative therapy Therapy that combines conventional medical therapies with complementary alternative medicine (CAM) therapies for which there is some high-quality scientific evidence of safety and effectiveness.

interdisciplinary team Clearly defined group of members of specific disciplines who work collaboratively to develop a coordinated plan of care.

interferons (IFNs) Proteins formed when cells are exposed to invaders such as viruses that are able to activate other components of the immune system.

interleukins (IL) Generic name for cytokines released by leukocytes.

interstitial fluid The fluid located between cells.

interstitial space The area surrounding the nephron loops and the peritubular capillaries, which has a high osmotic pressure due to extremely high levels of sodium. The renal interstitial space facilitates the massive volume water reabsorption required to maintain fluid balance.

intra-aortic balloon pump A catheter with an oblong balloon on the end that eases the workload on the patient's heart by decreasing afterload and coronary perfusion.

intracellular fluid (ICF) The fluid located inside each cell.

intracranial pressure (ICP) The amount of pressure placed on the structures within the brain.

intractable pain Pain that is refractory or resistant to some or all forms of treatment.

intradermal route An injection into the skin.

intraductal papilloma Small benign tumor that grows within the terminal portion of a solitary milk duct of the breast.

intraoperative The operative period from entry into the operating suite through departure from the post-anesthesia care unit (PACU).

intrarenal Occurring within the kidney.

intrathecal Within the spinal canal, the space between the double-layered covering or lining of the brain and spinal cord.

intravascular fluid The fluid located inside the blood vessels, excluding the fluid inside the cells in the blood vessels.

intrinsic distortion Occurs when information is passed on from one person to another through an interpreter.

intussusception Invagination, or telescoping, of one part of the intestine into itself.

inverse ratio ventilation Ventilating the patient with a longer inspiratory time as compared to the expiratory time.

inversion stress test A physical examination test used to assess for ankle joint laxity. It is performed by bracing the heel with left hand, inverting the foot with right hand, and comparing to the opposite side.

ischemic stroke Damage to the brain due to a clogged artery.

isokinetic Exercise involving resistance through full range of movement.

isotonic Solution that has the same osmotic pressure as the referent solution (e.g., plasma).

J

jaundice Yellow pigmentation of the skin and sclera.

joint aspiration A procedure performed to examine the synovial fluid in the joint cavity and to relieve pain in the joint resulting from edema and effusion.

Joint Commission on Accreditation of Hospitals (JCAHO) An independent, not-for-profit organization that sets standards for measuring health care quality. Accredited hospitals receive an on-site review every three years.

justice Requires that like cases are treated in like fashion.

K

karyotype A photomicrograph of the chromosomes of an individual that have been arranged in the standard classifications system by group and size.

keratinization A process that is used by epidermal tissue to replenish itself.

keratitis Inflammation of the cornea.

keratometry Measurement of the cornea.

kernicterus Yellow discoloration and degenerative lesions in the central nervous system causing brain damage.

kinesthesia The ability to perceive the movement of one's body.

kinesthetic learners Learning style in which a person processes information by experiencing the information or by touching and feeling.

knowledge transformation Five sequential steps that convert primary research knowledge to evidence that a specific health care intervention achieves positive clinical outcomes.

Kupffer cells Specialized reticuloendothelial cells of the liver, which belong to the monocyte-macrophage system.

Kussmaul breathing The presence of abnormally deep and rapid respirations, with the presence of a fruity odor to the breath.

kyphoscoliosis A combination of kyphosis and scoliosis.

kyphosis An exaggeration of thoracic spine convexity.

L

labyrinth A complex, closed, fluid-filled system of interconnecting tubes in the inner ear.

lacunae Reservoirs in which the mature bone cells are embedded.

lamellar bone The thin layer of mature bone tissue.

laminar airflow Filtered air circulating in parallel-flowing planes.

lancinating Stabbing or piercing.

laparoscopic cholecystectomy A surgical procedure using a laparoscope to remove the gallbladder.

laparoscopy A diagnostic procedure where the peritoneal cavity (pelvis and abdomen) are examined.

laparotomy Surgical incision made in the wall of the abdomen.

lateral epicondylitis Pain over the lateral epicondyle of the humerus or head of the radius. Also called tennis elbow.

latex allergy An immediate type of hypersensitive reaction to latex exposure.

lavage The irrigation (wash out) of the stomach contents.

learning Process of assimilating information with a resultant change in behavior.

learning plateaus Peaks in effectiveness of teaching and depth of learning.

learning style Way in which an individual incorporates new information.

leiomyomata Benign smooth muscle tumors of the uterus commonly called fibroids.

length of stay (LOS) Length of time a patient remains hospitalized, an outcome variable that refers to the efficiency of a health care delivery system.

lentigines Flat brown spots seen on aged exposed skin.

lesions Circumscribed altered area of tissue that should be treated as abnormal finding.

leukapheresis The removal of blood to collect specific blood cells; the remaining blood is returned to the body.

leukocytes General name for all white blood cells.

leukopenia A decrease in the total circulating white blood cells.

Levine's sign Clenched fist over the chest is the universal sign for angina.

liberty Independent from coercion.

lichenification Thickening of the epidermis.

ligaments Strong bands of connective tissue that attach bone to bone or bone to cartilage.

lipodystrophy A localized complication of insulin administration characterized by changes in the subcutaneous fat at the site of the injection.

liver lobule The functional unit of the liver.

liver sweats The movement of plasma from the lymphatic system into this potential space in the abdomen.

living will (LW) Advance directive that allows a person to document specifically what medical treatment they wish, or do not wish, to have.

locus The position of a gene on a chromosome.

long-term care Extended assistance for the chronically ill, mentally ill, or disabled.

low-density lipoprotein (LDL) The main lipid component of the atherosclerotic plaque and is considered "bad" cholesterol because increased levels reflect increased tendency to CAD.

lower motor neuron Motor pathway that originates in the spinal cord and continues on as spinal nerves sending impulses to the peripheral areas of the body.

lumpectomy Wide local excision or partial mastectomy that involves excision of all cancerous tissue to microscopically clean margins.

lymphadenopathy Painless lymph node enlargements from obstruction and pressure.

lymphocytes Primary cells in the immune response.

M

macronutrients Carbohydrate, protein, and lipids.

macrophages Phagocytic cells found in tissues.

macules Flat circumscribed changes of the skin (flat nevi, café au lait spots, vitiligo, telangiectases or capillary hemangiomas).

macular rash A rash with flat red spots.

major surgery Operations that involve risk to life in some way, such as those involving multiple systems, or that require long periods of time in the operating suite.

malaise Body discomfort and fatigue.

malignant Cells that invade and destroy nearby tissues and spread to other parts of the body.

malignant hyperthermia (MH) Life-threatening, acute pharmacogenic disorder, developing during or after a general anesthesia.

malrotation Failure during embryonic development of normal rotation of all or part of an organ or system.

mammary duct ectasia Noncancerous condition of the breast in which the milk ducts beneath the nipple become dilated and sometimes inflamed.

mammoplasty Surgical procedure to increase or decrease the size or shape of the breast.

managed care organizations (MCOs) Groups implementing health care using managed care concepts including pre-authorization of treatment, utilization review, and a fixed network of care providers.

mandatory minute ventilation (MMV) A mode of ventilation that allows the ventilator to adjust its breaths based on the patient's minute ventilation.

mass casualty incident (MCI) An influx of patients that overwhelms a hospital and affects its capability to care for patients.

mastalgia Breast pain.

mastitis Inflammation or infection of the breast.

mastodynia Breast pain.

mastoidectomy An incision of the mastoid sinuses.

mastoiditis Infectious process of the mastoid sinuses.

mechanical debridement Uses gauze dressings to remove necrotic or devitalized tissue from wounds.

mechanical ventilation A means of providing ventilatory assistance by a mechanical device.

mechanism of injury The manner in which an injury occurs.

Medicaid Program that pays for medical assistance for certain individuals with low income and resources. It is jointly funded by federal and state governments.

medical futility When a particular therapy offers no medical benefit.

Medicare National health insurance program for people age 65 years and older, people under aged 65 with disabilities, and people with end-stage renal disease. Medicare provides coverage to approximately 40 million Americans.

Medicare Hospice Benefit Reimbursement benefit provided by the federal government for hospice services.

meditation A mind-body technique by which an individual can consciously quiet the mind by focusing one's attention in order to control some functions of the sympathetic nervous system.

meiosis A series of two specialized divisions of diploid germ cells to produce four gametes containing the haploid number of chromosomes.

menarche Initial menstrual period, normally occurring between 9 and 17 years of age.

menopause Permanent cessation of menstrual activity, usually occurring between 35 and 55 years of age.

menorrhagia Cyclic menstrual bleeding that is abnormally long or heavy.

menstrual cycle Periodically recurring series of changes associated with uterine endometrial growth in preparation for fertilization and shedding of endometrium when fertilization has not occurred.

meta analysis Statistical procedure used to summarize the results of research across multiple research reports.

metabolic syndrome Diagnosed when three or more factors such as high blood pressure, abdominal obesity, high triglyceride levels, low high-density lipoprotein (HDL) cholesterol and high fasting blood glucose levels are present.

metabolism or biotransformation Biotransformation process in which the drug is broken down by enzymes to a form that can be excreted from the body. The primary organ of metabolism is the liver. The chemical changes in living cells by which energy is provided for vital processes and activities, and new material is assimilated.

metastasis Spread of cancerous tumor to other distant locations.

metrorrhagia Bleeding at times other than normal menstrual cycle.

microtrauma Trauma to muscles, tendons, ligaments, and bones on a microscopic level.

minimal sedation (anxiolysis) Drug-induced state during which patients respond normally to verbal commands. Although cognitive function and coordination may be impaired, ventilatory and cardiovascular functions are unaffected.

minor surgery Operations that do not involve risk to life in some way, such as those that involve one system that can be done in a short period of time or can be performed in a health care provider's office.

minority group Ethnic, racial, or religious group that constitutes less than a numerical majority of the total population.

mitigation Activities a hospital undertakes to help lessen the severity and impact of potential emergencies that may affect operations or services provided by a hospital.

mitosis Somatic cell division resulting in the formation of two cells, each with the same chromosome complement as the parent cell.

mitral facies A florid appearance with cyanosed cheeks.

mixed venous oxygen saturation (SvO$_2$) A measurement of the amount of hemoglobin saturated with oxygen compared to the total amount of hemoglobin in the pulmonary artery.

modulation Alteration in the level of pain intensity (by either increasing or inhibiting it), including the processing of incoming impulses from the sensory nerve to the dorsal horn of the spinal cord; modulation also occurs via descending messages originating in the midbrain and sent to the dorsal horn.

monoclonal antibodies Genetically engineered immunosuppressive agents that are used in combination with other drugs to prevent graft rejection.

monocytes Phagocytic cells found in the blood.

monosaccharides Simple sugar molecules not decomposable by hydrolysis.

moral distress Occurs in response to awareness of the right and moral action, coupled with inability to carry out that action.

morals Customs or habits that are ethically correct.

morbidity The number of ill persons in relationship to a specific population.

mortality The ratio of the number of deaths in a given population.

mosaicism Tissue composed of cells of two different genotypes or karyotypes.

motivation The internal drive or externally arising stimulus to action or thought.

mucositis An inflammation and ulceration of the lining of the mouth, throat, or gastrointestinal (GI) tract most commonly associated with chemotherapy or radiotherapy for cancer.

Müllerian dysgenesis Malformation of the embryonic duct that becomes the fallopian tubes, uterus, and vagina.

multiple organ dysfunction syndrome (MODS) Evidence of a progressive inflammatory response has caused more than one of the body's organs to fail. The presence of altered organ function in an acutely ill patient such that homeostasis cannot be maintained without intervention.

Murphy's sign Pain on deep inspiration when an inflamed gallbladder is palpated by pressing the fingers under the rib cage.

music-thanatology A holistic and palliative method for using music to help dissipate obstacles to patients' peaceful transition to death.

mutation A permanent change in genetic material.

myalgia Pain in the muscles.

myectomy Excision of a portion of the muscle.

myelogram A diagnostic test used to determine defects in and around the spinal column.

myelosuppression A decrease in the production of red blood cells, platelets, and some white blood cells by the bone marrow. Also, inhibition of the production of blood cells, a bone marrow function.

myocardial infarction (MI) Prolonged ischemia, 20 minutes or more, that results in myocardial cellular death.

myocarditis An inflammation of the myocardium.

myoclonus Twitching or clonic spasms of a muscle or group of muscles.

myomectomy Surgical removal of fibroid tumors in the wall of the uterus.

myopia (nearsightedness) Occurs when the light passing through the eye is overbent or overrefracted.

myosin The protein that compose the thick filaments of a myofibril.

myotonia Tonic spasm of a muscle or temporary rigidity.

myringoplasty Plastic surgery of the tympanic membrane.

myringotomy Incision into the tympanic membrane.

N

nadir The period of time following chemotherapy, usually 7 to 10 days after chemotherapy, when blood counts drop, thereby increasing susceptibility to infection or bleeding.

narrative review Less rigorous form of summary process used in nursing.

nasal airway A soft, flexible tube that is inserted into the nasal passage to maintain an open airway.

National Guideline Clearinghouse Searchable database of nearly 1,500 clinical practice guidelines.

native kidney One's own kidney as opposed to a transplant graft.

negative feedback Response of a gland by increasing or decreasing the secretion of a hormone.

neoadjuvant Adjunctive or adjuvant therapy given prior to the primary (main) therapy.

neoangiogenesis Development of new blood vessels.

neoplasm An abnormal mass of cells, can be benign or malignant.

nephrectomy Surgical removal of the kidney.

nephritis Infection contained to the kidney.

nephrolithiasis Kidney stone disease.

nephropathy Disease of the kidneys.

nephrotoxic Having the ability to harm the kidney.

neuralgia Pain associated with peripheral nerves, which follows the course of nerves.

neuropathies Dysfunctions of the peripheral nervous system.

neuropeptides Amino acids produced in the brain and other sites in the body that act as chemical communicators.

neurotransmitters Chemical substances produced by the body that facilitate nerve impulse transmission.

neutropenia A decreased number of circulating neutrophils, usually less than 1,500 cells/μm.

neutrophils Chief phagocytic cell of early inflammatory response.

nociceptive pain Pain that occurs when there is normal processing of the pain impulse.

nociceptor A free nerve endings that is a receptor for painful (noxious) stimuli. Nociceptors are found in almost all types of tissue.

nocturia Urination at night.

nodules Circumscribed elevated, usually solid lesions (fibromas, neurofibromas, xanthomas, erythema nodosum, and various benign or malignant growths).

nonmaleficence Use of ability, judgment, or skill to help someone else without intent to cause injury or harm.

normovolemia State of normal blood volume.

nosocomial Infection acquired in a health care facility.

nuchal A stiff painful neck due to irritated meninges.

nutraceuticals Any natural substance found in plant or animal foods that acts as a protective or healing agent.

nystagmus An involuntary rhythmic movement of the eyes in a back and forth or cyclical movement.

O

objective data Data that are observable and measurable.

occult fracture A fracture that does not show up on plain radiographic films until the healing process begins and calcification is seen.

odynophagia Pain that is experienced when a person swallows.

oligomenorrhea Menstrual cycles occurring farther apart than usual.

oligospermic Having low sperm motility with a low semen volume.

oliguria Low urine output.

oncogenes Cancer susceptibility genes. When altered or mutated proto-oncogenes promote tumor formation or growth.

oncotic pressure Osmotic pressure because of proteins.

onycholysis The loosening of the nails starting at the border.

oocytes The early or primitive ovum before it has developed completely.

opportunistic Organism causing disease in a host whose resistance to fight infection is diminished.

oppression Rules, modes, and ideals of one group are imposed on another group.

opsonization A process that coats a foreign substance and makes it more susceptible to phagocytosis.

oral airway A stiff plastic tube that prevents the tongue from sliding back into the pharynx and blocking the airway.

orchitis Acute inflammation of the testes.

orthostatic hypotension Hypotension occurring when changing position from supine to upright.

osmolality The number of solutes per kilogram of fluid.

osmolarity The number of solutes per liter of fluid.

osmosis The movement of water from an area of low concentration of solutes (low osmolality) to an area of high concentration of solutes (high osmolality).

osmotic pressure The ability of a solution to draw fluid across a semipermeable membrane.

ossicles Three tiny bones (in the middle ear) that play a crucial role in the transmission of sound.

osteoarthritis (OA) Noninflammatory degenerative joint disease characterized by degeneration of the articular cartilage, hypertrophy of bone at the margins, and changes in the synovial membrane.

osteogenesis The process of bone formation and remodeling.

osteomalacia A condition marked by softening of the bones with pain, tenderness, muscular weakness, anorexia, and loss of weight, resulting from deficiency of vitamin D and calcium.

osteomyelitis Inflammation of the bone caused by a pyogenic organism.

osteopenia A significant amount of decrease in bone mineral density.

osteoporosis A reduction in the amount of bone mass, leading to fractures after minimal trauma.

osteosarcoma Malignant tumor of bone.

ostomy A surgically created opening made between the intestine and the abdominal wall.

otalgia Ear pain.

otitis media An inflammation of the middle ear.

otorrhea Liquid discharge or drainage from the ear.

otosclerosis A progressive hearing loss of predominately low tones.

ototoxic A substance that damages the acoustic nerve or hearing mechanism.

outcome variables Consequences of care delivery categorized as humanistic, financial, and clinical.

overuse syndrome An injury to musculoskeletal tissues affecting the upper extremity or cervical spine, resulting from repeated movement, temperature extremes, overuse, incorrect posture, or sustained force or vibration. Also called repetitive motion injuries or cumulative trauma disorders.

ovulation Periodic maturation and release of an ovum from a follicle on the ovary.

oxyhemoglobin dissociation curve
A relationship between the partial pressure of oxygen in the blood and the saturation of hemoglobin with oxygen.

P

P wave Graphic representation of atrial depolarization.

Paget's mammary disease
Uncommon skin cancer characterized by a chronic eczema-like rash of the nipple and adjacent areolar skin.

pain An unpleasant sensory and emotional experience arising from actual or potential tissue damage or described in terms of such damage.

pain scales scales used to quantify patient's pain so that consistent relief measures can be taken.

pain threshold The lowest intensity of a painful stimulus perceived by the individual as pain.

pain tolerance The degree of pain that an individual is willing to endure.

palliation The process of easing symptoms and maximizing quality of life when cure or control is not possible.

palliative care Active total care of patients whose disease is not responsive to curative treatment.

palpation The use of the sense of touch to assess texture, temperature, moisture, organ location and size, vibrations and pulsations, swelling, masses, and tenderness.

palpebrae Eyelids that cover and protect the eyes by covering the anterior aspect of the eyes.

panhypopituitarism Defective or absence of function of the entire pituitary gland.

papillary reflex Stimulation of cranial nerve II that causes direct and consensual reactions to light.

papilledema A swelling of the optic disc.

papules Elevated circumscribed lesions (elevated nevi, verrucae, molluscum contagiosum, and individual lesions of lichen planus).

paracentesis The aspiration of fluid from the abdominal cavity.

paraphimosis The entrapment of the retracted foreskin behind the glans penis of an uncircumcised male.

paraplegia Paralysis involving the lower extremities.

parathyroid hormone (PTH)
Hormone that is secreted by the parathyroids and is not controlled by the pituitary and hypothalamus but by negative feedback.

parenchyma Functional elements of an organ.

paresthesia Numbness, tingling, or prickling sensation.

parity The number of viable births.

passive euthanasia Omission of an action, thereby allowing death to occur.

patient controlled analgesia (PCA)
Devices that can be used by the patient to deliver pain medications (usually via intravenous [IV] route) as needed.

peak drug level Time it takes for the drug to reach its highest concentration in the blood.

pediculosis Infection by human lice.

pediculosis pubis Infection in pubic area by lice.

pedigrees Diagrammatic representations of a family history indicating the affected individuals and their relationship to proband or index case.

percent solution A measure of parts per hundred.

perception A person's sense and understanding of the world.

percussion Short tapping strokes on the surface of the skin to create vibrations of underlying organs.

percutaneous coronary interventions (PCI) Category of procedures performed during the cardiac angiography using catheters, balloons, and devices to treat atherosclerotic lesions (e.g., percutaneous transluminal coronary angioplasty [PTCA]).

perfusion The exchange of oxygen and carbon dioxide at the alveolar-capillary level.

pericarditis An inflammation of the pericardium.

pericardium A double-layered serous membrane that surrounds the heart.

periductal mastitis Inflammation of the breast that can occur in nonlactating older women.

perimenopause Five- to 10-year period before menopause.

perinephric Surrounding the kidney.

perioperative Inclusive term to denote preoperative, intraoperative, and postoperative periods.

periosteum The outer portion of the cortical bone that supplies nutrients and a blood supply to the bone.

peripheral vascular resistance (PVR) The pressure against the flow of blood to or from the arteries or veins outside the chest.

peristalsis Successive waves of involuntary contraction passing along the walls of a hollow muscular structure (as the esophagus or intestine) and forcing the contents onward.

petechiae Small, pinpoint hemorrhages.

phagocytosis Process by which foreign substances are ingested and destroyed.

Phalen's maneuver A physical test involving flexion of the fully extended hand at the wrist to aid in the diagnosis of carpal tunnel syndrome.

phantom limb sensation When the patient has the perception of a limb that is no longer there. If the patient feels pain it is known as phantom limb pain.

pharmaceutic Phase that an oral drug disintegrates and dissolves into a form that can be used by the body.

pharmacodynamics Phase that describes the biochemical and physiological effects the drug has on the body.

pharmacogenomics The study of how an individual's genetic inheritance affects the body's response to drugs.

pharmacokinetics Phase that describes how drugs are acted on in the body from ingestion to elimination, includes the processes of absorption, distribution, metabolism (biotransformation), and excretion.

pharmacology The scientific study of drugs and their origins, actions on, and interactions with, living things through chemical processes.

phenotype The physical, biochemical, and physiological nature of an individual as determined by the genotype and the environment. It is the outward expression of the individual's genes.

philosophy Statement of beliefs that is the foundation for one's thoughts and actions.

phimosis The inability of the foreskin to be stretched and retracted over the glans of the penis.

phlebitis Inflammation of a vein.

phlebostatic axis Location at the midpoint of the anterior and posterior chest at the fourth intercostal space. This is the point at which transducers should be leveled for hemodynamic parameters.

photoaging Degenerative changes in connective tissue caused by chronic exposure to ultraviolet A (UVA).

photoallergic Sensitivity to light that causes allergic reactions.

photochemotherapy UVA therapy combined with oral or topical 8-methoxypsoralen.

phototherapy The treatment of certain dermatological conditions with artificially produced, nonionizing UV light.

phototoxic Rapidly developing non-immunologic skin reaction when exposed to light.

physical dependence Body is dependent on a substance and abrupt cessation or reduction in the dose may result in withdrawal symptoms.

physician-assisted suicide Medical hastening of death by a physician in consultation with a terminally ill patient.

phytonutrients Chemicals found in plants that act as protective or healing agents.

pica Craving for substances other than food, such as dirt, clay, starch, or ice cubes.

pigmentation Color of the skin (produced by melanocytes in the epidermis).

plaques Elevated disc-shaped lesions (psoriasis, lichen simplex or chronicus neurodermatitis).

plasma The liquid portion of the circulation system.

plasma half-life (t $_{1/2}$) The time required to eliminate one half of the ingested medication after administration.

plasmapheresis (plasma exchange) Plasma is removed from the patient and replaced with the fresh frozen plasma.

pleuritic chest pain Discomfort detected on expiration or inspiration caused by an inflammation of the lining of the lungs.

pneumothorax A collection of air in the pleural cavity may occur as a result of trauma, tuberculosis, or chronic respiratory diseases. This collection of air leads to a collapse of all or part of a lung.

polycystic cysts Cysts with closed sacs that develop abnormally within an organ and have a distinct enclosing membrane.

polycythemia An abnormal increase in the number of red blood cells.

polypharmacy Situation in which multiple drugs are prescribed to treat a variety of conditions.

positive end expiratory pressure (PEEP) A ventilator setting that adds pressure at the end of expiration to keep alveoli open and enable gas exchange.

posthitis Inflammation of the foreskin.

postoperative Takes the patient from the time of departing from the surgical suite through the length of their hospital stay and beyond.

postrenal Occurring after the kidney.

posttraumatic stress disorder (PTSD) A psychological reaction that occurs after experiencing a highly stressing event, such as wartime combat, physical violence, or a natural disaster.

Power of Attorney for Health Care Legal document that allows the patient to choose a person called a health care proxy or agent to make decisions about the patient's medical care when the patient is unable to do so for himself or herself.

PR interval An estimate of the amount of time it takes the impulse to travel from the SA node through the AV node, the bundle of His, and the main part of the left bundle branch.

prana The life force of the Indian culture that is believed to fill the body with a vital energy.

preferred provider organization (PPO) Type of managed care plan in which members receive more coverage if they choose health care providers approved by or affiliated with the plan.

preload The amount the myocardial fibers are stretched at the end of diastole. This stretch reflects the amount of pressure and volume in the ventricle immediately preceding systole.

preoperative Prior to the intraoperative period or events leading up to entry into the surgical suite.

preparedness Activities that build the hospital's capacity to manage the effects of an emergency or disaster.

prerenal Occurring prior to the kidney.

presbyopia A loss of near acuity (near vision) as the lens loses its elasticity and accommodation of the lens fails.

presbyphagia Dysphagia in the elderly.

prevalence The number of current cases of a disease in a specific population at a given time period.

preventive care Focuses on health promotion, including educational and preventive programs designed to promote healthy lifestyles.

priapism The presence of a prolonged, often painful, penile erection.

primary amenorrhea Failure of the menstrual cycles to begin.

primary anorgasmia Never having achieved orgasm.

primary brain tumor The growth originated in the brain or central nervous system.

primary care Basic, routine health care.

primary immune response Occurs when an antigen is initially introduced into the system. It involves both mast cell degranulation and activation of plasma proteins, i.e., complement, clotting factors, and kinin (polypeptides that increase blood flow and permeability of small blood capillaries).

primary intention Utilizes normal repair processes.

primary multiple organ dysfunction Directly related to an insult, such as a major trauma.

prions Protein-containing infectious agents.

process variables Refers to how care is provided, under what circumstances, and how patients are moved into, through, and out of the health care system.

proctocolectomy Surgical removal of the rectum together with part or all of the colon.

prodrome phase The beginning clinical manifestations that a person has for an upcoming illness.

prolactin A hormone from the anterior pituitary that stimulates the breast to cause lactation.

prophylactic Preventing or contributing to the prevention of disease.

proprioception Awareness and coordination of movement and position of the body, head, and limbs.

proptosis Forward placement of the eye.

prostatitis Inflammation of the prostate gland.

prosthesis A replacement of a missing body part, such as an extremity.

protein binding Process in which the drug, once absorbed into the bloodstream, attaches itself to a protein molecule (usually albumin) to be transported to it site of action.

proteinuria Increase in protein in the urine.

pruritus Dermatological symptom described as itching and a desire to scratch.

psoriasis T cell–mediated inflammatory disease characterized by epidermal hyperplasia (overproduction of epidermal tissue) usually localized in certain regions of the body.

psychomotor domain Area of learning that involves performance of motor skills.

psychoneuroimmunoendocrinology (PNIE) A multidisciplinary paradigm involving mind-body medicine that emerged in 1955, and is sometimes referred to as psychoneuroimmunology.

psychoneuroimmunology (PNI) An emerging field of science that studies the complex relationship between the mind and body, specifically the cognitive/affective system in the brain, the neurological system, and the immune system.

ptosis Drooping of the eyelid.

pulmonary artery (PA) catheter A long balloon-tipped catheter that is positioned in the pulmonary artery and monitors different pressures in the heart.

pulse pressure Difference between systolic and diastolic blood pressure.

pulsus alternans Alternating weak and strong heart beats.

pulsus paradoxus Pathological decrease in systolic blood pressure by 10 mm Hg or more on inspiration.

Purkinje fibers Conductive fibers that help to spread the electrical impulses of throughout the ventricular muscle. They have an inherent rate of 15 to 40 beats per minute.

purulent Containing the detritus of white blood cell activity within an infectious process usually.

purulent sputum A light green to yellowish white fluid formed in infected tissue and consists of white blood cells, cellular debris, and necrotic or dead tissue.

pustules Circumscribed elevations containing purulent exudates (pustular psoriasis, bromoderma or small pox).

pyelonephritis Infection of the ureters and kidney.

pyrosis A substernal burning sensation often radiating to the neck; commonly called heartburn.

Q

QRS complex Graphic representation of ventricular depolarization.

QT interval Graphic representation of the amount of time it takes for ventricular depolarization and repolarization.

quadriplegia (tetraplegia) Paralysis involving upper and lower extremities.

R

race A grouping of people based on biological similarities.

racism Form of oppression defined as discrimination directed toward individuals who are misperceived to be inferior because of biological differences.

radiculopathy A term used to specifically describe pain and other symptoms, like numbness, tingling, and weakness, in arms or legs that are caused by a problem with nerve roots.

radioisotope A compound that contains radioactive materials that are used in nuclear scans; the activity of these tagged materials allows the study of substances as they course through the body.

radiotherapy The use of X-rays and other forms of radiation in treatment.

Raynaud's disease Venous disease caused by unilateral vasospasm of the upper and lower extremities. Bilateral vasospasm is identified as Raynaud's disease, usually occurs in the age group over 30 and is equally distributed between genders.

rebound hypertension Rapid increase in blood pressure after abrupt stopping of medication.

receptive aphasia (Wernicke's aphasia) A condition in which a patient is unable to understand what is being said or what is written.

receptor Site on the cell membrane that can be occupied by a drug to cause an effect within the body.

recessive trait A trait that is expressed only when an individual is homozygous for that specific gene.

referred pain The transfer of visceral pain sensations and deep somatic pain via the autonomic nervous system to a body surface at a distance from the actual origin.

refractory ascites Ascites that cannot be effectively managed with normal therapies.

regeneration Replacement of damaged or lost tissue with more of the same tissue. Only the epidermis and superficial dermis are capable of regeneration.

relative hypovolemia A shifting of fluid from the intravascular space to the extravascular space that can result from a loss of intravascular integrity, increased capillary permeability, or a decreased colloidal osmotic pressure.

relaxation response A state of increased arousal of the parasympathetic nervous system, which leads to a relaxed physiological state.

remodeling A continuously occurring process in the bone that maintains the structure and integrity of the bone.

remote assessment Use of technology such as video links or teleconferencing to allow for health care personnel and patients to transmit assessment information over long distances.

renal Pertaining to the kidney.

renal parenchyma The cortex and medulla of the kidney that contain the functioning units and collecting ducts of the kidney.

repolarization Electrical change in the interior of an excitable cell following depolarization in which the inside of the cell becomes more negatively charged.

residual volume (RV) The amount remaining in the lungs and airways after a maximal expiration.

resilience Dynamic process that involves protective factors such as effective problem-solving strategies and adaptability to situations that the person cannot control or change.

resorption The removal of bone tissue by normal physiological process or as part of a pathological process, such as an infection.

resting energy expenditure A measurement of resting metabolic rate expressed as kilocalories per 24 hours.

restorative care Follow-up postoperative care, home care, and rehabilitation.

reticuloendothethial (RE) system Phagocytic system composed of monocytes and macrophages.

retroperitoneal space The space between the peritoneum (the membranous sac that surrounds the organs of the abdominal cavity) and the posterior abdominal wall that contains the kidneys and associated structures, the pancreas, part of the aorta, and inferior vena cava.

review of literature Less rigorous form of summary process used in nursing.

review of systems (ROS) A brief account from a patient of any recent signs of symptoms associated with any of the body systems.

rhabdomyolysis Destruction of skeletal muscle cells that causes the release of myoglobin.

rhinitis A seasonal or year-round immunoglobulin E (IgE)-mediated inflammation of the nasal mucosa; may be infectious, inflammatory, or allergic in nature.

rhinitis medicamentosa Rebound congestion of the nasal mucous membranes caused by overuse of decongestant nasal sprays.

rhinorrhea Thin, watery discharge from the nose.

rhonchi Bubbling or gurgling sounds heard primarily on expiration and indicate fluid in the larger airways.

RICE The acronym used for Rest, Ice, Compression, and Elevation when treating a sprain.

right to die Belief that humans have a basic right to die.

rights-based ethics Proscribes that there are specific human rights to specific human goods.

rigors A muscular tremor caused by a chill.

rotator cuff tears Refers to tears in one or more of the four muscles that form a single tendon in the shoulder. The rotator cuff is responsible for circumduction and internal and external rotation of the shoulder.

rye ergot A fungus from the rye plant causing hallucinations, gastrointestinal upset, and a form of gangrene if ingested.

S

SA node Primary pacemaker of the heart with an inherent rate of 60 to 100 beats per minute.

sacroilitis Inflammation of the sacroiliac joint.

sarcoma A form of cancer that arises in the supportive tissues such as bone, cartilage, fat, or muscle.

sarcomere The contractile unit of the muscle.

sarcopenia Age-related decreases in muscle mass.

schistocytes Fragmented red blood cells.

Schwartze's sign Rosy or reddish-blue color of the tympanic membrane related to vascular changes.

science The most reliable source of knowledge on which to base clinical decisions.

science of research synthesis Field of science that generates evidence summaries to provide state-of-the-science conclusions about knowledge thus far developed.

scoliometer An instrument for measuring curves, especially those in lateral curvature of the spine.

scoliosis An abnormal lateral curvature of the spine.

secondary amenorrhea Cessation of the menstrual cycles after they are established in the absence of pregnancy.

secondary anorgasmia Loss of the ability to achieve orgasm in a woman who was previously orgasmic.

secondary intention Heals by spread of granulation.

secondary multiple organ dysfunction The result of failure of organs that were not affected by the initial insult.

secondary or specific antibody response Includes the activation of B cells and the memory cells (IgG, IgM, IgA, and IgE); and activation of T cells, cytotoxic (killer) cells, lymphokine-producing cells, helper cells, and suppressor cells.

sedation Reduction of anxiety, stress, irritability, or excitement by the administration of a sedative agent or drug.

seizure Brief episode of abnormal electrical activity in the brain.

self-efficacy Perceived capability of mastering difficult situations and the ability to actively control one's own destiny; closely linked to a positive self-esteem and internal locus of control.

self-monitoring of blood glucose (SMBG) A method whereby a patient tests his or her own blood glucose levels.

semipermeable membranes Separation between two areas that allows movement of some fluids or solutes.

sepsis A systemic inflammatory response to an infection.

sequela Any abnormality following or resulting from a disease or injury or treatment.

serum The liquid part of blood after coagulation.

serum sickness A type III hypersensitivity reaction that results from the injection of heterologous or foreign protein or serum.

sex roles Culturally determined patterns associated with being male or female.

sexual dysfunction Unsatisfactory enjoyment of sex or inability to participate in sexual intimacy as desired because of multiple causes, including lack of sexual interest, impaired sexual arousal (erectile dysfunction in the male, lack of lubrication in the female), or inability to achieve orgasm.

sexuality Human characteristic that refers not just to gender but to all the aspects of being male or female, including feelings, attitudes, beliefs, and behavior.

shaman A folk healer priest who uses natural and supernatural forces to heal others, has an extensive knowledge of herbs, is skilled in many forms of healing, and serves as guardian of the spirits.

shamanism A form of spiritual healing that refers to the practice of entering altered states of consciousness with the intent of helping others to enhance healing and well-being. The shaman connects with spiritual guides and seeks healing on behalf of others.

shock syndrome A systemic condition when the peripheral blood flow is inadequate to provide sufficient blood to the heart for normal function and transport of oxygen to all organs and tissues.

short stay surgery Usually preplanned, nonemergency procedures with an expected hospital or surgical center stay of less than 23 hours.

shunting That portion of the cardiac output that does not exchange with alveolar air.

side effects Expected physiological effects of a drug that are not related to the desired drug effect.

sinusoids Specialized capillaries found only in the liver and are identified by specific types of cells.

slow pain Pain originating in the endings of the smaller unmyelinated nerves that has a throbbing or aching quality.

social support The person's perception of, and the degree of satisfaction with, support systems.

solutes Particles contained within the fluid that contribute to the concentration or osmolality of the fluid.

somatic (parietal) pain Pain that originates from the bone, joints, muscles, skin, or connective tissue. Sharp or knife-like in character, usually precisely located to the affected areas.

somesthesia Awareness of body; derived from the Greek words meaning body and sensation.

somnolence Prolonged drowsiness or sleepiness.

spermatocelectomy Surgical removal of the spermatocele.

spermatogenesis Formation of mature functional spermatozoa from the testes, usually beginning during puberty and continuing throughout the life of the adult male.

spinal shock A loss of all motor and sensory function, generally occurring after spinal cord injury.

spirituality Relationship with one's self, a sense of connection with others, and a relationship with a higher power or divine source.

sports medicine The application of professional knowledge to the understanding, prevention, treatment, and rehabilitation of sports- and exercise-related problems.

staging The extent or spread of the tumor within the body from the site of origin.

standard precautions Actions to be used with all patients to reduce risk of transmission of disease.

stapedectomy Removal of the stapes and replacing the stapes with a prosthetic device.

state-of-the-science review Less rigorous form of summary process used in nursing.

status asthmaticus Severe and persistent asthma that does not respond to conventional therapy and that may lead to respiratory failure.

steatorrhea Pale-yellow, greasy, fatty stool, or chronic watery diarrhea.

stereognosis Identify objects by touch.

stereotactic radiotherapy (SRS) Noninvasive use of computers and radiation to target tumor cells within the brain.

stereotyping Expectation that all people within the same racial, ethnic, or cultural group act alike and share the same beliefs and attitudes.

stomatitis The inflammation of the soft tissues in the mouth resulting in mouth sores. It is a common side effect of chemotherapy, radiation therapy, and some biological therapy.

strabismus (tropia) When one muscle is weak resulting in one eye deviating from the other when the eyes are focused on an object.

stress The body's reaction to any stimulus.

stridor Inspiratory wheezing.

structural variables Organizational features or participant characteristics that have an impact on organizational performance.

stye (hordeolum) A localized inflammatory swelling of one or more of the glands of the eyelid.

subarachnoid hemorrhage Blood that leaks into the subarachnoid space.

subclavian steal syndrome Occurs when the subclavian artery is occluded, and blood flow is diminished or obstructed to the upper extremities.

subculture Group of people within the dominant group who are functionally unified by factors, such as status, ethnic background, residence, religion, or education and whose experiences differ from those of the dominant group.

subjective data Data from the patient's point of view that may include feelings, perceptions, and concerns.

superficial burn Also called a first-degree burn; it only involves the epidural layer of the skin.

superficial partial-thickness burn Also called a second-degree burn; it involves the entire epidermis and the upper third of the dermis.

supernumerary nipples Small dark spots on the chest that may indicate undeveloped nipples and areola.

suppurative cholangitis A condition when pus is produced in the biliary tract.

surrogate decision maker Agent or proxy who is legally able to make health care decisions for another who has lost the capacity to do so for himself or herself.

sycosis Inflammation of the entire hair follicle.

sycosis barbae Inflammation of the entire hair follicle that is traumatized by shaving.

synchronized cardioversion Delivering an electrical shock to the heart that is synchronized to the patient's R wave.

synchronized intermittent mandatory ventilation (SIMV) The ventilator delivers preset breaths in coordination with the respiratory effort of the patient. Spontaneous breathing is allowed between breaths.

syndrome X Classic angina symptoms without angiographic evidence of CAD.

syndrome X (insulin resistance syndrome) A group of abnormalities of metabolism that act together to increase the risk of cardiovascular disease.

synergy model Combination of factors that each multiplies the effects of the other(s), rather than merely adding to them.

syngeneic transplant Blood or tissue donated by an identical twin.

synovium A fibrous envelope that produces a fluid to help to reduce friction and wear in a joint.

system Set of parts linked in orderly and logical interdependence that function together as a synergistic unit.

systematic review Newer term for an evidence summary.

systemic inflammatory response syndrome (SIRS) Widespread uncontrolled acute inflammatory response to a severe insult.

systolic blood pressure Blood pressure measured at the moment of contraction.

T

T wave Graphic representation of ventricular repolarization.

tachypnea An abnormally rapid rate of breathing.

Tao Traditional spiritual belief system of the Chinese. The belief that everything is the Tao, and the Tao is everything leads to the understanding of oneness in all things in nature.

target tissues Tissues or organs in the body that are affected by specific hormones.

teaching Active process in which one individual shares information with another as a means to facilitate behavioral changes.

teaching-learning process Planned interaction that promotes a behavioral change that is not a result of maturation or coincidence.

teaching strategies Techniques employed by the teacher to promote learning.

telangiectasia Dilatation of small blood vessels on the cheeks, nose, and ears, as well as pigmental changes, such as freckles from exposure to sun light.

teleology Evaluation of final causes.

tendons Connect muscle to bone and allow bone to move once the muscle has contracted.

tendosynovial Pertaining to the tendon insertion in the joint near the synovial membrane.

tenesmus Distressing but ineffectual urge to evacuate the rectum.

teratogens Agents that produces or increases the incidence of congenital malformations.

terminal illness One in which there is no possibility for a cure, resulting in the decline of the patient's physical condition and then death.

tertiary care Includes acute and complex interventions.

tertiary intention Wound requires suturing of granulation layers.

testicular self-examination (TSE) A method of a male assessing his testicles for any changes as a preventive measure against testicular cancer.

thenar Refers to the palm of the hand or the sole of the foot.

therapeutic range Serum drug level that lies between the minimum effective concentration and the toxic concentration. Level to be maintained to achieve desired affects and avoid symptoms of toxicity.

therapeutic touch (TT) Assessing alterations in a person's energy field and using a hand to direct energy to achieve a balanced energy state.

thermoregulation A patient's status in relation to internal temperature control.

third spacing The accumulation of fluid in the extracellular and intracellular spaces and in a third body, such as the intestine, that does not support circulation.

thrombophlebitis The inflammation of a vein accompanied by the formation of thrombus (blood clot), which can be dislodged and lead to pulmonary emboli. Deep vein thrombosis (DVT) is a term often used for this venous complication, which most commonly occurs in the deep veins of the lower extremities.

thrombus Blood clot that blocks a blood vessel.

thyroid-releasing hormone (TRH) The hormone that stimulates the anterior pituitary to release TSH.

thyroid-stimulating hormone (TSH) A hormone produced from the anterior pituitary that regulates the function of the thyroid.

thyroxine (T$_4$) The most abundant thyroid hormone; makes up approximately 90 percent of the thyroid hormone secretion.

tic douloureux Trigeminal neuralgia; dysfunction causing pain along the pathway of the fifth cranial nerve.

tidal volume (Vt) The amount of air in and out of the lungs with a normal breath.

tineas Fungal infections.

Tinel's sign A tingling sensation produced by pressing on or tapping the nerve that has been damaged or is regenerating following trauma.

tinnitus A ringing, buzzing, or jingling sound in the ear.

tolerance Occurs when a higher dose of a drug (e.g., an opioid) is required to achieve the desired effect.

tophus A chalky deposit of sodium urate occurring in gout, tophi forms most often around joints in cartilage, bone, bursae, and subcutaneous tissue and in the external ear, producing a chronic foreign body inflammatory response.

total parenteral nutrition (TPN) The intravenous (IV) administration of nutrients to patients through a central venous catheter.

total quality management (TQM) Structured systematic process for organizational planning and implementation of CQI.

toxoid A toxin that has had the active portion removed but can still be recognized by the immune system.

trabecular The porous cavity found inside the compact bone.

tracheostomy Operation of cutting into the trachea usually for insertion of a tube to overcome tracheal obstruction.

tracheostomy tube A tube placed by surgical incision into the trachea and secured by sutures to maintain an open airway or facilitate long-term mechanical ventilation.

transcellular fluid Fluid that is in neither the intracellular nor extracellular space, and includes cerebrospinal fluid, joint fluid, and the fluid within the gastrointestinal tract.

transduction The initiation of the pain stimulus.

transient ischemic attack (TIA) Temporary loss of blood flow to the brain that results in temporary loss of function.

translocation The transfer of a segment of one chromosome to a nonhomologous chromosome. When no material is lost or gained, the translocation is said to be balanced.

transmission The process of carrying the pain information along the axon of a sensory nerve to the CNS.

transmission routes Ways by which microorganisms reach the body.

tremor Rhythmic, purposeless, quivering muscle movement.

trends The general direction or prevailing tendency in following a general course.

triage system A method to rank or classify patient's illnesses or severity of injury.

triggers Cause the release of inflammatory mediators from the bronchial mast cells, macrophages, and epithelial cells and lead to recurrent episodes of wheezing, breathlessness, chest tightness, and coughing.

triiodothyronine (T$_3$) The most powerful thyroid hormone; 10 percent secreted by thyroid and the remainder converted from T$_4$ by peripheral tissues.

trisomies Three of a given chromosome instead of the usual pair.

trocar A large-bore abdominal paracentesis needle.

trough drug level Minimum blood serum level of a drug reached immediately before the next scheduled dose.

tubercles Nodules or swelling of lymphocytes and epithelioid cells that forms the lesions seen in tuberculosis.

tumor markers Substances that are expressed by the tumor or by normal tissue in response to a tumor.

tumor necrosis factor Inflammatory biochemical that is produced in response to various stressors.

tumor suppressor gene A gene that can block or suppress the development of cancer.

tumors Larger and deeper circumscribed solid lesions; they can be benign or malignant.

turgor The skin's elasticity, resilience, and hydration.

tympanometry A test performed to detect abnormalities in the middle ear, such as fluid, eustachian tube dysfunction, or problems with the ossicles.

tympanosclerosis Formation of fibrous tissue around the ossicles preventing vibratory movement.

U

upper motor neuron The descending motor pathway, which originates in the brain and synapse with lower motor neurons in the spinal cord.

uremia Accumulation of end-products of protein metabolism in the bloodstream due to renal failure.

ureteral strictures A narrowing of the lumen of the ureter.

urethral strictures A narrowing of the lumen of the urethra.

urethritis Inflammation of the urethra.

urethroplasty A procedure that removes the diseased portion of the urethra and inserts a new urethra constructed from other tissue.

urethrotomy An opening in the urethra.

urinary tract infection (UTI) An infection involving the kidneys, ureters, bladder, or urethra.

urolithiasis (calculi) Refers to stones in the urinary tract.

urticaria A hypersensitive dermatological manifestation in response to the release of histamine in an antigen-antibody reaction.

utilitarian Belief that an action should be of benefit to the greatest number of people affected by the action.

V

vaginitis Inflammation of the vagina.

valgus Bending or twisting outward from the midline of the body.

valvular regurgitation Backward flow of blood through a heart valve.

valvular stenosis A narrowing or constriction of the diameter of a bodily passage or orifice.

valvuloplasty Plastic surgery performed to repair a valve in the body.

varicocele A group of varicose veins within the scrotum.

varicocelectomy Surgical removal of the varicocele.

varicose veins Tortuous varicosities, in which the veins are dilated and lack surrounding muscle support.

varus Bending or twisting inward toward the midline of the body.

vasectomy Surgical sterilization of men through removal, ligation, or destruction of a small portion of the vas deferens to prevent passage of sperm to the urethra.

vector-borne transmission Infectious material carried by living organism tissue from base of wound.

venous stasis ulcers Erosions of the skin because of lack of blood flow to the extremity, which leads to skin necrosis, open wounds, and black, hardened skin known as eschar.

ventilation The movement of air in and out of the lungs.

ventilator weaning The gradual withdrawal of ventilatory support.

ventricular assist device (VAD) A mechanical device designed to eliminate the workload on the left ventricle, right ventricle, or both and is designed for long-term therapy unlike the intra-aortic balloon pump.

vertigo A sensation or feeling of a loss of equilibrium, sometimes referred to as spinning or whirling.

vesicant An intravenous (IV) medication that causes blisters and tissue injury when it escapes into surrounding tissue. Vesicatory refers to causing blisters.

vesicles Sharply circumscribed, elevated fluid-containing vesicle lesions (herpes, dyshidrosis, pompholyx, varicella, or contact dermatitis).

vesicoureteral reflux Backward propulsion of urine through the valve that normally closes the bladder and ureteral junction to backward flow of urine.

vesicular rash A raised, blistering rash.

visceral pain Pain that originates from any of the large interior organs that occupy a body cavity (cranial, thoracic, abdominal, or pelvic).

visual learners Style of learning in which people learn by processing information by seeing.

vital capacity (VC) The volume of air in and out of the lungs with maximal inspiratory effort and maximal expiratory effort.

volume control ventilation Delivers breaths at a preset target volume.

volvulus A twisting of the intestine on itself that causes obstruction.

W

wellness care Care focused on prevention of illness and promotion of health.

wheals Solid superficial elevations usually in response to pruritus conditions (insect bites, urticaria, or allergic reactions).

wheezes Musical sounds heard primarily on expiration and indicate narrowing of the larger airways, with either spasm or secretions.

wheezing A whistling sound when breathing out related to airway constriction.

workforce diversity Differences in attributes or belief system among members of the workforce.

X

xanthelasma A yellow, lipid-rich plaque present on the eyelids.

xenogeneic A genetic relationship between individuals of differing species.

xerosis Abnormal dryness of skin, mucous membranes, or conjunctiva.

xerostomia Dry mouth.

Z

zone of coagulation Area of the burn that has the most contact with the causative agent, causing coagulated cellular necrosis.

zone of hyperemia Area peripheral to the zone of stasis characterized by viable cells with minimal injury.

zone of stasis Area peripheral to the zone of coagulation characterized by injured viable cells with compromised blood flow.

zoophilic Animal source.

Review Questions Answers

Chapter 1

1. 3. Rationale: Historically, nurses provided comfort care. As knowledge expanded nurses took on aspects of illness care directed by physicians. Nurses then focused on wellness care as their own practice. Care directed at either illness or wellness is known as health care. Nurses now seek to provide evidence-based care.
2. 4. Rationale: As the body of scientific knowledge grew, no single physician could know all there was to know about all illnesses. Specialty practices emerged, fractionating care and the traditional close physician-patient relationship.
3. 1. Rationale: An increasing amount of legislation is regulating health care.
4. 3. Rationale: The Medicare and Medicaid amendments to the Social Security Act initiated the era of health care reform.
5. 2. Rationale: Scholarly publication is an expectation, but is not an *essential* feature of professional nursing as defined by American Nurses Associations.
6. 1. Rationale: Poultices are no longer commonly used, and the other options are bogus.
7. 4. Rationale: Food preparation, biomedical engineering, faith healing, and meditation are not required areas of knowledge or skill for nurses.
8. 2. Rationale: 1, 3, and 4 are bogus answers.
9. 3. Rationale: Although there is some evidence that fresh flowers may harbor undesirable organisms, there is currently no ban on them.
10. 3. Rationale: Blackouts related to chemical dependence are varying lengths of time when an intoxicated individual interacts with others without later memory of the interactions.

Chapter 2

1. 4. Rationale: The most reliable source of knowledge on which to base clinical decisions is state-of-the-science knowledge from integrated rigorous research.
2. 2. Rationale: The Knowledge Hurdles and Solutions matrix articulated by Stevens rates the volume and complexity of science and technology as a primary hurdle to overcome to move research into practice.
3. 4. Rationale: The primary premise underlying knowledge transformation is that such transformation is necessary before research results are useable in clinical decision making.
4. 3. Rationale: A major feature of EBP is that it is heavily interdisciplinary.
5. 3. Rationale: All of the other Web sites are bogus.
6. 4. Rationale: The ACE Star Model developed by Stevens depicts knowledge transformation through five sequential steps.
7. 2. Rationale: In 2001 Glasziou, Irwig, Bain, & Colditz articulated the six essential steps in conducting a systematic review: (a) formulate the question, (b) locate relevant studies, (c) select and appraise the studies, (d) summarize and synthesize the results across studies, (e) interpret the findings, and (f) update the review regularly.
8. 1. Rationale: Using evidence in our care increases certainty and predictability in the effect of the practice on the outcome of that practice. There are a growing number of evidence summaries available to effect transformation of evidence into use for clinical decision making by practitioners across multiple disciplines and multiple levels of practice. It is predicted that the public will soon demand that care not only be more error aversive, but that it be evidence-based.
9. 3. Rationale: While all of the answers are desirable changes in health care delivery, in 2001 the Institute of Medicine identified 20 priority areas for quality improvement according to three criteria. The number two criterion was improvability by using evidence to close gaps between best practice and usual care.

10. 1. Rationale: While the other concepts reflect the essence of the applied science of nursing, those concepts lack the essential aspects needed to make the transformation of research into practice a widespread reality.

Chapter 3

1. 2. Rationale: A learning plateau is a peak in the effectiveness of the teaching process.
2. 3. Rationale: The cognitive domain describes learning by understanding the material that is presented with the mind.
3. 4. Rationale: When the nurse allows the patient with diabetes to give an injection to a synthetic material that is similar to a real arm it is labeled a demonstration.
4. 3. Rationale: Kinesthetic learning takes place a person can physically do something.
5. 1. Rationale: Self-efficacy is when a person believes that his or her actions ("puts her mind to it") will have the desired effect.
6. 3. Rationale: Repetition is the best strategy in teaching new information for the memory impaired.
7. 2. Rationale: A lack of perception is experienced when a person does not accept the factual information regarding his or her health practices (in this instance).
8. 3. Rationale: Two basic components of health maintenance are health promotion and disease prevention.
9. 3. Rationale: Imposing a health policy that an individual must follow is not a health promotion strategy.
10. 3. Rationale: Basic human needs are the psychological dimension made up of those characteristics of self-esteem, feelings of security, and those feelings that create a sense of belonging.

Chapter 4

1. 4. Rationale: All of the elements of cultural competency result in incorporating cultural preferences into nursing practice.
2. 4. Rationale: Ethnocentrism is the belief that one's own culture is superior to all others.
3. 2. Rationale: Cultural assessment tools include assessing the family structure, traditional preferences, and medical context, all parts of the cultural assessment tool.
4. 3. Rationale: Poverty status is highly correlated with health risk factors.
5. 2. Rationale: Culture refers to the knowledge, beliefs, behaviors, ideas, attitudes, values, habits, customs, languages, symbols, rituals, ceremonies, and practices that are unique to a particular group of people.

6. 1. Rationale: All ethnic groups have shown an increase in numbers for several decades and will continue to do so.
7. 2. Rationale: Biological differences, (differences in enzymes and genetics) increase the potential for certain diseases, interactions with medications, foods (e.g., lactose intolerance).
8. 4. Rationale: Extrinsic distortion occurs when the interpreter is improperly prepared.
9. 4. Rationale: Racism is defined as a form of oppression or discrimination of people perceived as inferior.
10. 1. Rationale: A magicoreligious belief system is based on the concept that health and illness are determined by supernatural forces.

Chapter 5

1. 4. Rationale: The principle of beneficence requires that a clinical intervention benefits a patient, (e.g., in some way adds value to that patient's health).
2. 2. Rationale: Utilitarian is identified as the ethical theory that supports the "greatest good for the greatest number." This is the philosophy of giving levodopa to this patient with Parkinson's disease.
3. 2. Rationale: Professional codes of ethics focus on behavior between care providers and patients, as well as between care providers themselves. The codes seek behavior that is respectful and protects others from both external and internal harm secondary to one's behavior.
4. 1. Rationale: Moral distress in nursing occurs when the nurse is aware of the right and moral action to take in a given patient situation but is unable to carry out that action because of external restrictions.
5. 4. Rationale: This law protects patients' basic rights to privacy and their control over the disclosure of their personal health information.
6. 4. Rationale: The mother is focused on the quality of life of her child and has weighed that against medical treatments or interventions for her child.
7. 3. Rationale: The principle of double effect occurs when the intended use of palliative pain therapy has the unintended effect of hastening a person's death.
8. 5. Rationale: Advance directives for health care may be either written documents, such as a living will and durable power of attorney, or a verbal statement of preference for what a person wants done and when it is to be done.

9. 1. Rationale: The Nuremberg Code grew out of the revelations of research atrocities carried out by Nazi physicians on prisoners of war during World War II. The war ended in 1945, and the trials of war criminals followed soon after.

10. 2. Rationale: If a person has the mental capacity to make specific decisions about his or her health care, he or she is autonomous to do so, and health care providers must honor such decisions even though they may not personally or professionally agree with those decisions.

Chapter 6

1. 3. Rationale: Older adults usually underreport their symptoms. Everyone over 65 does not necessarily have two chronic health problems; not all older adults have diabetes.

2. 2 and 3. Rationale: Obesity is not primarily due to overeating; current trends indicate that obesity rates are climbing for all age-groups.

3. 1. Rationale: Smoking has been linked to persons of lower levels of education and social economic status. Smoking has actually decreased for pregnant women.

4. 1. Rationale: Most persons who attempt or commit suicide have been seen by a nonmental health care professional; symptoms are not easy to recognize, because the symptoms vary a great deal; the primary reason for suicide ideation is loss of something meaningful in the person's life, such as loss of relationship, a job, death of a loved one, and posttraumatic stress disorders.

5. 2. Rationale: The population of older women will continue to surpass the number of older men, although longevity has increased for both genders; a majority of the frail elderly will be cared for at home by family caregivers; older Hispanic (Americans) will be the largest racial/ethnic group by 2030.

6. 4. Rationale: The syndrome is related to abdominal obesity, hypertension, high triglyceride and low high-density lipoprotein (HDL) cholesterol levels, and high fasting blood glucose levels; the risk can be present at all age levels; The syndrome can contribute to coronary artery disease (CAD).

7. 2. Rationale: The other racial/ethnic groups may be at risk for hypertension, but the incidences are higher for African Americans, especially males.

8. 3. Rationale: None of the other statements ensure that safe measures will be taken. Selecting someone to perform cosmetic procedures on the basis of cost can be disastrous. Cosmetic procedures should be performed by qualified professionals (health care providers) certified by a national organization.

9. 2 and 3. Rationale: The goal is for a 50 to 75 percent of excess weight over a period of time; bariatric surgery is performed for a select group of people who meet the criteria that includes a comprehensive medical, psychological, nutritional, and surgical evaluation by a multidisciplinary team.

10. 1. Rationale: Life expectancy has increased for both genders and will continue to do so as the baby boomer generation ages. These individuals are more active and have the benefit of health promotion programs through their young and middle adult years. Women still live longer than men; the median income of older adults falls between $11,400 for females and $19,400 for males. Over 3.6 million older adults live below the poverty level, and Medicare benefits may decrease in the future.

Chapter 7

1. 4. Rationale: A tenet of hospice and palliative care is that the values and morals of the patients and families determine the best courses of action.

2. 2. Rationale: A component of therapeutic communication is an acknowledgement of difficulties faced by patients and caregivers. It is inappropriate to assume full knowledge of another person's feelings. Many individuals do not have a belief in heaven. There is no specific timeline for grief to be resolved.

3. 3. Rationale: Dyspnea is a subjective symptom best evaluated by the patient's description of the difficulty breathing.

4. 2. Rationale: A change in the breathing pattern is the universal sign of imminent death.

5. 4. Rationale: Fixed, dilated pupils are the most reliable sign of death.

6. 3. Rationale: Hospice care is indicated when the patient has a disease that is not responsive to curative treatments.

7. 1, 2, and 3. Rationale: The patient can receive hospice and palliative care services if he or she is in the hospice or home setting.

8. 1, 2, and 4. Rationale: Values and behaviors may vary among members of a given group.

9. 1, 2, 3, 4, and 5. Rationale: All listed are integral members of the team.

10. Power of Attorney for Health Care. Rationale: Advanced Directives include two documents: the Living Will and the Power of Attorney for Health Care. The Living Will provides written evidence of the patient's wishes regarding life-sustaining procedures. The Power of Attorney for Health Care allows the patient to choose an agent to make decisions about medical care when the patient is unable to do so.

Chapter 8

1. 4. Rationale: Because it is the critical nature of potential suicide.
2. 1. Rationale: There is no reason to have the patient in a patient gown to evaluate mental status.
3. 3. Rationale: Relieving the headache is an alleviating factor.
4. 2. Rationale: The patient's statement evidences this symptom as the primary reason for seeking health care.
5. 2. Rationale: The question defines an ecomap.
6. 3. Rationale: This is the best response given and is a valid nursing intervention for a spiritual problem.
7. 2. Rationale: This is the label for the definition provided in the question.
8. 4. Rationale: The elevator is not legally appropriate.
9. 1. Rationale: This test is designed for evaluating comatose patients.
10. 2. Rationale: This is the correct order for assessment.
11. 4. Rationale: This variable is the only one that can be altered.

Chapter 9

1. 1, 4; Rationale: Cri-du-chat syndrome and Down syndrome are conditions that are caused by the involvement of an entire chromosome. Neural tube defects are considered to be multifactorial, because they occur as a result of genetic and environmental factors. Sickle cell disease and achondroplasia are caused by because a defect of a single gene so they are considered to be unifactorial.
2. 3. Rationale: Answer 1 is the definition for mutation; answer 2 is the definition for phenotype; and answer 4 is the definition for karyotype.
3. 2. Rationale: Haploid refers to having one complete set of unpaired chromosomes. The haploid number in humans is 23.
4. 3. Rationale: In autosomal recessive inheritance, each parent carries a gene alteration for the condition, such as CF. Each child of those parents has a 25 percent chance to inherit the altered gene from both parents and will have manifestations of the condition.
5. 2. Rationale: An isolated neural tube defect usually occurs as a result of genetic and environmental factors and so is multifactorial in origin.
6. 3. Rationale: Genetic testing of children is indicated to make a diagnosis for conditions in which early intervention and treatment can be

initiated. This is the case for Down syndrome. Being a carrier of a gene for CF does not pose a health risk to a child so is not indicated. HD is an adult-onset disorder for which there is currently no available treatment. Testing for HD is not indicated in children, until they have reached the age of 18 when such testing can be offered if risk exists.
7. 4. Rationale: Amniocentesis and CVS are prenatal diagnostic procedures. The prenatal AFP multiple marker testing is a genetic screening test to identify pregnancies at increased risk for neural tube defects and chromosomal abnormalities. Ultrasound evaluation is used to screen a pregnancy for major congenital malformations.
8. 4. Rationale: Nurses have a role in all of these activities: identifying individuals for whom genetic testing is available; referring individuals for genetic testing; and assessing the impact of genetic test results on the individual and the family.
9. 1. Rationale: BRCA1 and 2 are markers for hereditary breast and ovarian cancer not an indication of hypersensitivity to allergens. Phagocytes, eosinophils, and basophils are terms associated with white blood cells but they are not indicators of the immune system.
10. 2. Rationale: Both heredity and environmental triggers play a role in the development and expression of allergies and asthma making it a complex multifactorial disorder not a single gene disorder.

Chapter 10

1. 1. Rationale: Her behavioral response to her altered body image will be influenced by the reactions of others. There is not sufficient information in the case scenario to assume that 2, 3, or 4 is true.
2. 4. Rationale: She may be accepting the outcome as a result of fate or because external circumstances. 1, 2, and 3 are incorrect; (1) there is no indication that she is repressing her anxiety, (2) she has misinterpreted information, or (3) that she is depressed.
3. 3. Rationale: 1, 2, and 4 are incorrect. (1) Fear and depression are common reactions following discovery of a breast lump. (2) Many husbands do have problems adjusting to their wife's altered body image. (4) Married women do not have less difficulty adjusting than single women.
4. 4. Rationale: This is a major principle of self-care management. 1, 2, and 3 are incorrect. (1) Physical activity prior to bedtime does not help

to induce sleep. (2) Mild antianxiety medications can be a temporary solution that do not help to alleviate the underlying response to stress. (3) Informing the patient about hospital routines may facilitate the patient's feeling of losing control.

5. 2. Rationale: Gaining additional information will help to clarify how Jane feels and what coping mechanisms she has used to adapt to the loss of her mother and to adapt to a new manner of life. The nurse can assist Jane to make healthy decisions. 1, 3, and 4 are incorrect. (1) There is nothing to indicate that Jane is angry. (3) Asking Jane how the nurse can help her does not help Jane to search for her own inner strengths and support systems that can lead to self-care management of her life. (4) Stating that you understand how the other person feels is not totally truthful. Each person's perception of reality is unique. This is a response that can limit further expression or discussion of the person's grieving process.

6. 3. Rationale: Denial is a temporary ego defense mechanism used to protect the person from the full impact of the stressful situation/diagnosis. 1, 2, and 4 are incorrect. (1) Fantasy is an internal visualization of memories and their interpretation. (2) Undoing is an action taken to un do or to neutralize an original action. (4) Rationalization is selecting a substitute reason for the real reasons for personal behavior.

7. 4. Rationale: (1) Mr. Aiken does not have a realistic perception of his problem. (2) His perception and manner of coping are not pathological. His behavior is one of free choice. (3) He is not making a conscious secondary appraisal of the situation.

8. 2. Rationale: Rivalry with siblings is a typical behavior that occurs in normal family dynamics. Bobbie may even compete with his siblings for additional attention from his mother. (1) A drop in scholastic grades, (3) disturbance in relations with peers, and (4) a feeling of loss of personal internal control over the family situation are common responses to a stressful disintegration of the family structure.

9. 4. Rationale: (1) People often use the excuse that smoking makes them feel better for not quitting, because the initial response to nicotine is bronchodilation. (2) Refusal to quit is another frequent excuse because of the fear associated with the grieving process over loss of a pleasurable habit. (3) Denial of the severity of his condition is, also, an attempt to retain control over his life situation.

10. 3. Rationale: (1) There have been three health care revolutions over the past 30 years. (2) The current health care system is focused on illness, rather than wellness. (3) Web-based information continues to face scrutiny as to its accuracy and validity.

Chapter 11

1. 2. Rationale: Neutrophils are the first leukocytes attracted to an injured tissue.

2. 2. Rationale: This is the correct order for these events in an inflammatory response.

3. 1. Rationale: The classic sign of swelling seen in the inflammatory process results from leakage of plasma into the injured area.

4. 2. Rationale: This is the most likely cause of fever that is seen in a patient with an infectious disease.

5. 2. Rationale: Chronic inflammation is not caused by a response to a normal body substance such as low density lipoprotein lodged in excess in an arteriole wall.

6. 3. Rationale: This is a nursing teaching strategy to reduce the development of an antibiotic resistant organism.

7. 2. Rationale: A patient with a known infection must be managed by using standard precautions.

8. 4. Rationale: This is not a risk factor for delayed wound healing.

9. 3. Rationale: This fills the wound in healing by primary intention.

10. 1. Rationale: The steroid drug impedes macrophage migration, which delays wound healing if a person has been taking a steroid drug.

11. 3. Rationale: Rest and immobilization are important to wound healing because they prevent further injury to area.

Chapter 12

1. 3. Rationale: Swelling and weight gain are signs of fluid volume excess. Although the child may need increased diaper changes because of diarrhea, those are not a sign of fluid volume deficit. Depressed fontanelles occur in young children with fluid volume deficit.

2. 2. Rationale: Although all of these patients might experience fluid volume deficit, the most at risk are patients at the extreme of age, either young or old; in this case the 82-year-old patient.

3. 2. Rationale: Mental status is rarely affected in a fluid excess without a change in osmolality. Postural vital signs are most important in patients with fluid volume deficit. Urine output may be increased or decreased, depending on the cause of the fluid excess. Weight is an important indicator of fluid balance.

4. 1. Rationale: Patients with hyponatremia are at high risk for seizures. Vital sign assessment is important, but patient safety takes priority. Frequent oral care would be important in a patient with hypernatremia or fluid volume deficit. Cardiac monitoring is important in hyperkalemia or hypokalemia.

5. 2. Rationale: D_5W is a hypotonic intravenous (IV) solution. While administration of large volumes of any IV solution may result in fluid volume excess, a hypotonic IV solution also places the patient specifically at risk for hyponatremia. Fluid volume deficit is not a risk of IV fluid administration.

6. 4. Rationale: Weighing the patient and measuring edema are important interventions in patients with fluid volume excess. However, the priority intervention is to reduce the cause of the excess, in this case, the IV fluid. Capillary refill is an important assessment but is not specific for assessing fluid balance.

7. 4. Rationale: The major risk associated with a low potassium level is cardiac dysrhythmia. Chvostek's sign is associated with hypocalcemia. Although blood pressure may be affected by cardiac dysrhythmia, it is not specific to potassium balance. Edema is associated with fluid balance.

8. 1. Rationale: Kayexalate is indicated for the removal of excess potassium. K-Lor is a potassium supplement indicated for patients with hypokalemia. Kaopectate is an antidiarrheal medicine, and Keflex is an antibiotic.

9. 3. Rationale: While hypocalcemia may affect cardiac rhythm, Trousseau's sign is most specific to calcium balance. Urine output and weight are important assessment parameters for fluid balance.

10. 1. Rationale: Cardiac arrest is associated with tissue hypoxia and development of lactic acidosis. This causes a metabolic acidosis.

11. 1. Rationale: The ABGs reveal respiratory acidosis. A primary intervention is to increase ventilation through deep breathing and removal of secretions. Although vital sign and cardiac assessment are important, increasing ventilation will help resolve the problem. Leg exercises may be encouraged to prevent deep vein thrombosis, but are not related to the ABGs presented in this scenario.

12. 1. Rationale: Removal of gastric acids may result in metabolic alkalosis. The patient unable to access water is at risk for fluid volume deficit and hypernatremia. The infant is at risk for fluid volume excess. The patient experiencing a stroke is not at risk for a specific fluid, electrolyte, or acid-base imbalance.

13. 1. Rationale: The PCO_2 is low, indicating alkalosis. To compensate, the body has excreted excess bicarbonate, and the HCO_3 is low. This compensation has returned the pH within normal range.

Chapter 13

1. 1. Rationale: The cephalic vein can be a found along the thumb side of the wrist. Basilic vein can be found running along the little finger side of the arm. The vein that runs along the inner aspect of the forearm is the median vein. The dorsal metacarpal veins can be found on the back of the hand.

2. 3. Rationale: Tonicity is the ability to cause fluid movement across membranes. Osmosis is the movement of fluid through a semipermeable membrane. Hypertonicity refers to solutions that cause fluid to move out of the cell resulting in shrinking of the cells.

3. 2. Rationale: Hypotonic solution causes fluid to move into the cells leading to swelling and in some cases bursting. An isotonic solution causes no fluid shift between compartments as it has the same tonicity as plasma. Hypertonic solutions cause fluid to move out of the cell resulting in shrinking of the cells. Tonic refers to the ability to cause fluid movement across membranes.

4. 2. Rationale: Magnesium is important in the transmission of neuromuscular impulses. Too much magnesium may cause respiratory muscle depression leading to respiratory depression and arrest. Calcium is found mostly in teeth and bones and is involved in blood coagulation. It is also involved in muscle contraction and nerve impulse transmission. Potassium is necessary for the transmission of nerve impulses, cardiac rhythms, and muscle contraction. Chloride is found in the blood and in the stomach combined with other substances.

5. 4. Rationale: It is the correct steps of venipuncture.

6. 1. Rationale: Chemical phlebitis occurs when the medication itself causes irritation of the vein wall. Mechanical phlebitis occurs when the cannula causes the vein to become inflamed. Phlebitis can be present without infection and typically presents as a hard cord. Extravasation

refers to the leakage of a vesicant into the surrounding tissue. A vesicant is a medication that can cause tissue damage if infused outside of the vein into the surrounding tissue. Infiltration refers to the infusion of a fluid or medication into the surrounding tissue. An occluded or blocked cannula will not cause phlebitis.

7. 3. Rationale: CDC as well as, the Infusion Nurses Society recognize the distal one third of the superior vena cava as the preferred location for a central venous catheter. All other locations are considered peripheral locations.

8. 1, 3, 4. Rationale: The other response is IV solution and not blood components.

9. 3. Rationale: The five rights are: right medication, right patient, right dose, right time, and right route.

10. 3. Rationale: The skin of an older adult is thinner, has less subcutaneous fat, and is more fragile. Consider the mental status of an older adult when obtaining consent or providing patient education. The location of an intravenous site may limit a patient's mobility, but this will not affect the nurse's assessment of the site.

11. 2. Rationale:

Ratio Proportion	Formula method	
10 mg:1 mL = 6 mg: X	X (G) = $\underline{6\ mg}$ (D)	1 = $\underline{6}$ = 6 ÷
10 mgX = 6 mL		10 = 0.6 mL
X = 0.6 mL		

12. 1. Rationale:

Ratio Proportion	Formula method
1,000 mL:24 mL = X:1 hr	$\underline{1,000\ mL}$ X × mL/hour =
24 mLX = 1,000 mL	41.6 mL/hour or 42
X = 41.6 mL/hr or 42 mL/hr	

Chapter 14

1. 4. Rationale: European herbalism is not as widely known or accepted, lacking the long tradition of Ayurvedic, TCM, and Native American shamanism.

2. 2, 4, and 5. Rationale: Integrative medicine involves the use of CAM therapies with conventional medicine. Naturopathic medicine is a form of CAM therapies that involves homeopathy, herbs, etc. Allopathic, Western, and Orthodox are all synonyms with conventional medicine, which is geared toward the use of medications or surgery to treat disease.

3. 3. Rationale: Neurobiology is a current field of study that focuses on physiology of the biology of the nervous system. Psychoimmunology and neuroimmunology omit an important component of CAM therapies—the mind-body connection. Psychoneuroimmunology studies how the mind, nervous system, and immune system all interact to promote wellness.

4. 3. Rationale: Traditional Chinese medicine and shiatsu come from Chinese origins. Shamanism comes from Native American and other indigenous peoples. Ayurvedic comes from Hindu and Indian tradition.

5. 3. Rationale: Research from the NCCAM has demonstrated acupuncture to be most cost-effective in management of osteoarthritis. It additionally improves range of motion of the knee.

6. 2, 3. Rationale: While friends may be useful in finding practitioners, they may recommend someone based on whether they liked them rather than their effectiveness or competence. Patients may be able to take herbs and prescription medications at the same time, but they should check with their pharmacists first. If they are told they cannot take both, some patients may only take herbs, denying themselves necessary medications. Patients should tell their primary care provider all CAM therapies in which they engage. They should also make sure their CAM provider is properly trained, educated, certified, or licensed.

7. American Holistic Nurses Association. Rationale: The American Holistic Nurses Association is an organization dedicated to helping nurses get education, training, and resources for integration of CAM therapies into their practice. They also provide certification for holistic nursing practice and publish a journal dedicated to holistic nursing practice.

8. 2. Rationale: Nightingale first wrote about nature acting on the patient and nursing's role in her *Notes on Nursing*. The other leaders have made major contributions to holistic nursing practice, but based on principles espoused by Nightingale.

9. 3, 4, and 5. Rationale: In most states, hypnosis requires certification, licensure, or licensure as a specified practitioner, e.g., psychologist or nurse practitioner (NP). Reiki requires attunements by a Reiki master and practitioners receive a certificate, although the states do not regulate Reiki practitioners. All states that allow

acupuncture require licensure as acupuncturists, with the exception that allows health care providers or chiropractors to practice acupuncture by virtue of their medical license. Relaxation and imagery are common interventions that can be performed by any nurse and to not require any special certification or licensure.

10. 2. Rationale: Tomatoes and tomato sauce contain lycopene. Red chili peppers contain capsaicin. Apples, pears, and prunes are most beneficial for their fiber pectin. Citrus fruits, broccoli, and most other vegetables are the most common sources of ascorbic acid.

11. 5. Rationale: Aloe vera is a common ingredient in lotions and topical applications for treatment of sunburn or light skin abrasions. Evening primrose is effective for eczema, eucalyptus for respiratory decongestion, chamomile for anxiety, and celery seed for edema.

12. 4. Rationale: Milk thistle works well for persons with hepatitis or cirrhosis, both diseases of the liver.

13. 1, 4. Rationale: Gingko and brewer's yeast are known to increase bleeding risks. Aloe vera may enhance potassium loss. Licorice root may increase blood pressure and alter antihypertensive effects of some medications.

14. 2. Rationale: National Center for Complementary and Alternative Medicine was specifically developed to provide research resources for the study of the effectiveness of CAM therapies. American Holistic Nurses Association and American Association for Oriental Medicine are designed to provide a professional organization for its practitioners. National Institute of Arthritis and Musculoskeletal and Skin Diseases may provide research support for CAM therapies, but it would be incidental support. Most of its research support is for conventional medical treatment of arthritis, musculoskeletal, and skin disorders.

Chapter 15

1. 2. Rationale: T stands for size on a range from 0 to 4, 2.5 is T2 range. N represents the amount of regional lymph node involvement with a range from 0 to 4; N1 identifies involvement in one region. M represents presence of metastasis, either M0 or M1. The designation (x) for T, N, or M signifies undetermined.

2. 3. Rationale: Common sites for metastasis related to primary breast cancer are the lungs and the bone.

3. 3. Rationale: The focus of primary prevention is to prevent the disease. The focus of secondary prevention is early detection and screening to detect disease early. The focus of tertiary prevention is to prevent reoccurrence of disease or to limit disability associated with the disease. Thus, 3 is the correct answer, a focus on screening or self-exam for testicular cancer.

4. 3. Rationale: Nadir is defined as the period of time when blood counts reach their lowest point. The absolute neutrophil count is a value that represents the absolute amount of neutrophils (a type of white blood cell) in the blood.

5. 3. Rationale: Markings should not be removed until all therapy is completed. Application of cold may damage the irradiated area. This is external beam radiation therapy, not brachytherapy, therefore precautions as noted in 4 are not indicated. 3 is the best answer. Damage to the skin must be avoided and many over-the-counter creams have alcohol, or other drying agents contained. The best approach is to consult the oncology provider about which creams or lotions may be used.

6. 3. Rationale: Doxorubicin (Adriamycin) is a chemotherapeutic agent that is administered intravenously. To provide optimum safety, all intravenous (IV) chemotherapeutic agents should be managed as if all are vesicants. Therefore, special precautions should be taken, which would include use of the chemotherapy spill kit that should be present on the nursing unit.

7. 4. Rationale: In caring for a patient undergoing brachytherapy or a patient with an implanted radiotherapeutic device, the nurse must observe the three cardinal rules for radiation therapy: Time, distance, and shielding. Mrs. Brown will be on bedrest to prevent dislodgement of the radioactive implant, and all three rules must be addressed.

8. 4. Rationale: Neupogen is a colony-stimulating factor administered prior to the nadir to stimulate the production of neutrophils. Thus the focus for response would be on neutrophils, rather than red blood cells. A normal neutrophil count ranges from 2,200–7,000 mm^3. Effectiveness would be reflected in the higher neutrophil count.

9. 1. Rationale: Skin cells are naturally rapidly dividing cells, as such the normal skin cells are at risk of damage in the area which received external beam radiation therapy. When skin cells are damaged or weakened, dehiscence and evisceration are possible complications. The correct response to this item is specific to the external beam radiation and the abdominal surgery.

10. 1. Rationale: Is the only option in which all are correct according to the American Cancer Society guidelines.

Chapter 16

1. 4. Rationale: The correct response is 4, because the purpose of myelinated nerve fibers is to provide an electrical insulator to increase the speed of an impulse.

2. 3. Rationale: The correct response is 3, because the latest version of the gate control theory suggests that the control mechanism is influenced by internal analgesic substances.

3. 2. Rationale: The correct response is 2, because transduction of pain refers to the initiation of an electrical activity due to the impact of noxious stimuli.

4. 4. Rationale: The correct response is 4, because allodynia is a term that refers to hypersensitivity to a noxious stimulus.

5. 3. Rationale: The correct response is 3, because the autonomic nervous system is a major part of the CNS that regulates homeostasis or equilibrium of the body's internal environment.

6. 1. Rationale: The correct response is 1, because endogenous opioid peptides are chemicals that are released as needed to assist in modulating pain sensations.

7. 3. Rationale: The correct response is 3, because the best description for the cause of nociceptive pain is when there is no injury or malfunction of the nerve transmission process.

8. 4. Rationale: The correct response is 4, because an example of neuropathic pain is phantom limb pain.

9. 3. Rationale: The correct response is 3, because NSAIDs provide analgesia by blocking the production of prostaglandins.

10. 3. Rationale: The correct response is 3, because the cornerstone of effective pain management is patient and family education.

Chapter 17

1. 3. Rationale: The most important action the nurse can take is to check the patient's blood sugar. This data will determine the next action.

2. 4. Rationale: Glyburide is a sulfonylurea antidiabetic agent. There is a cross-sensitivity with sulfa drugs. The nurse must assess for any allergy to sulfa drugs prior to administration.

3. 2. Rationale: Anticoagulants are contraindicated for patients with potential for active bleeding. A recent history of gastric ulcers would make the patient at high risk for hemorrhage.

4. 3. Rationale: The major adverse effects of antilipemics drugs are related to altered liver function. The nurse monitors laboratory results that include elevated transaminase.

5. 1. Rationale: Theophylline is a methylxanthine bronchodilator used to treat obstructive lung diseases, such as asthma and chronic obstructive pulmonary disorder (COPD).

6. 3. Rationale: H_2 blockers are effective in blocking both volume and acidity of stomach acid. This group of drugs is used to treat duodenal ulcers, gastric ulcers, hypersecretory conditions, and gastric reflux disease (GERD).

7. 1. Rationale: The ability of digoxin to slow the heart rate is called a negative chronotropic effect. The release of calcium ions causes more forceful myocardial contraction that is termed a positive inotropic effect.

8. 4. Rationale: Unrelieved anginal pain may indicate an impending myocardial infarction (MI) and warrants emergency intervention.

9. 2. Rationale: A common side effect and potential adverse effect of diuretic therapy is hypokalemia. Potassium is frequently prescribed to prevent this adverse effect. The nurse should monitor potassium levels carefully.

10. 3. Rationale: Only drug taken by the oral route are subject to first pass metabolism in the liver.

11. 4. Rationale: Drug half-life is defined as the time it takes for half the absorbed dose to be eliminated from the body. It takes three to five half-lives to reach steady state.

12. 4. Rationale: Though age is a factor to consider, it is the function of the liver and kidneys that affect pharmacokinetic processing of medication. The nurse should obtain baseline laboratory studies of renal and liver function prior to initiating medications.

13. 2. Rationale: Ototoxicity that can include permanent hearing loss is a serious adverse effect of aminoglycoside therapy. The nurse should monitor for early signs of hearing loss.

14. 4. Rationale: Mouth sores, diarrhea, and vaginal itching are clinical manifestations of a fungal superinfection, a common adverse effect of anti-infective therapy. The nurse should notify the physician and obtain orders for treatment of this infection.

Chapter 18

1. 4. Rationale: Donabedian's classic model for evaluating quality identifies three vectors of quality: structure, process, and outcome.

2. 2. Rationale: Primary care is delivered through ambulatory outpatient agencies.

3. 1. Rationale: The three components of the synergy model are patient characteristics, nurse competencies, and safe passage.

4. 1. Rationale: Medicaid is the national health insurance program that pays for medical assistance for certain people with low income. Medicaid is administered by the state government.

5. 3. Rationale: The proportion of the gross national product dedicated to health care has been climbing for many years and currently consumes the highest percentage of all products tracked.

6. 1. Rationale: Congress passed a prescription drug payment system in the summer of 2006, but there is insufficient funding for a complete reimbursement program.

7. 3. Rationale: The hospital report card deals with measurement of acute care hospital quality and thus, tertiary care.

8. 2. Rationale: The board of trustees oversees administrative and operational processes. JCAHO evaluates clinical care processes for compliance with established standards of care for the purpose of accreditation. Positive clinical outcomes are, in part, the result of nurses accepting responsibility for providing the nursing care needed by a patient.

9. 2. Rationale: Nursing homes and hospice provide continuing care; childhood immunizations constitute preventive care.

10. 2. Rationale: Medicare is the national health insurance program for those age 65 years and over, so neither 1 nor 4 are correct.

Chapter 19

1. 2. Rationale: Sedation will help to slow the patient's respiratory rate and help the respiratory alkalosis.

2. 1. Rationale: PEEP causes increased intrathoracic pressure, which in turn decreases venous return, and can cause a pneumothorax.

3. 2. Rationale: The other situations cause the high-pressure alarm to sound.

4. 1, 3, 4, 5, 6; Rationale: 2 causes the low exhaled tidal volume alarm to sound.

5. 1. Rationale: The patient should not be requiring high amounts of oxygen prior to extubation.

6. 1. Rationale: Nitroprusside can cause rapid changes in blood pressure. Blood pressure should be monitored every five minutes.

7. 1. Rationale: The intra-aortic balloon pump deflates during systole.

8. 4. Rationale: The pulmonary artery catheter passes through the tricuspid valve and then the pulmonic valve.

9. 4. Rationale: SVR is an indirect measurement of afterload.

10. 4. Rationale: Patients who are hypovolemic will have low right atrial pressures.

11. 1. Rationale: Pulmonary artery wedge pressure is an indirect measurement of left ventricular performance.

Chapter 20

1. 2. Rationale: As an initial response, it always wise to seek clarification of complex questions, especially when the preoperative nurse is dealing with information that is likely not to have clear-cut answers. Patients may draw unusual conclusions during times that are stressful, such as the preoperative period.

2. 1. Rationale: Spirituality is the attempt to provide meaning within life's events. Religious faith has a slightly more specific definition.

3. 2. Rationale: In some cases, it might be unwise to have the preoperative patient closely examining and interpreting each vital sign reading as well as heart rhythm tracings. Nurses might want to ask for clarification of circumstances in which this would be done.

4. 4. Rationale: Electronic record keeping will always hold the potential for patients' private information to be captured by those without a need to know and without patient consent.

5. 4. Rationale: On a two-day stay and noncomplex surgery, it might be unwise for the patient to focus energy on work-related matters.

6. 2, 4, 5. Rationale: Lung removal and CABG are major surgeries because the chest cage is usually opened. Disruption to the underlying tissues, extended length of time for completion of surgery, and the likelihood of intensive care stays indicate that these are not minor. Total hip replacement also involves major tissue disruption and mobility interruption.

7. 2. Rationale: This is a recall test item. Refer to definitions within the chapter.

8. 4. Rationale: All are reasons to delay the patient's arrival in the surgery holding area. Some may lead to cancellation of surgery because the patient may not have been capable of informed consent, may not be stable physically, or may not want to go through with surgery at this time.

9. 1. Rationale: To be absolutely sure that the surgical team is positive about the correct site or correct side of the body, the patient's placing a mark is best. Lessons of the past indicate that reliance on documents or the surgeon's memory may lead to unfortunate patient consequences.

10. 3. Rationale: Only the registered nurse is permitted to perform and document physical assessment of patients.

11. 1, 2, 4. Rationale: Age, immunosuppression (even if mild at the time of surgery), and long-term respiratory compromise will increase the general risks for anesthesia and surgery.

12. 3. Rationale: This is a recall test item. Refer to discussion in the chapter.

13. 2. Rationale: There are exceptions to highest ER prioritization always centering on preservation of life. There will be instances in which the terminally ill patient will report in to the ER for ease of access to other hospital services.

Chapter 21

1. 1. Rationale: Items above the level of the draped patient are within the sterile field.

2. 1. Rationale: Shoe covers are needed for infection prevention purposes.

3. 5. Rationale: All are true for standard infection-control precautions.

4. 4. Rationale: All are methods of hand hygiene.

5. 5. Rationale: Hand washing indications include: when gloves are removed and before leaving the operating room, when hands are visibly soiled, and before patient care.

6. 1. Rationale: A jacket with long sleeves does not provide protection from blood splatter or body fluids.

7. 2. Rationale: Wearing gloves does not replace the need for hand washing.

8. 3. Rationale: All instruments need cleaning even if they do not have visible contamination.

9. 5. Rationale: All answers are true regarding monitoring the correct functioning of a sterilizer.

10. 3. Rationale: Light amplification by the stimulated emission of radiation (LASER).

11. 5. Rationale: All are early signs of MH.

12. 1. Rationale: Activation of the emergency medical code team is a main step in the emergency treatment of MH.

13. 1. Rationale: The differential diagnosis of MH includes: external heating, septicemia, thyrotoxicosis, pheochromocytoma, anaphylaxis, respiratory problems, pulmonary emboli, and myopathy

14. 4. Rationale: Monitoring of the patient suspected to have MH includes ECG, blood pressure, CO_2 monitoring, pulse oximeter, temperature, creatininase, electrolytes, and blood gas analysis.

Chapter 22

1. 2. Rationale: Not knowing a caller's identity means that the RN may be discussing confidential information with an unauthorized individual.

2. 1. Rationale: ABC's (airway, breathing, and circulation) are always the top priority to ensure preservation of life.

3. 4. Rationale: Indicates the patient is having mental status changes. Not only could this indicate fluid and electrolyte imbalance or low blood counts, it is a safety hazard.

4. 1. Rationale: Because somnolent patients often respond to simple stimulation, this should be the RN's first action, especially if family members are at the bedside

5. 2. Rationale: Indicates hematoma.

6. 2. Rationale: The nurse should medicate the patient, because the morphine given in PACU wears off in about one hour.

7. 2. Rationale: Should the patient's cardiorespiratory system be in distress from heavy blood loss, this will be indicated by signs of shock such as altered level of consciousness, rapid heart rate, and falling blood pressure.

8. 1, 2, 3. Rationale: Answers 4 and 5 are expected findings in the postoperative abdominal surgery patient.

9. 3. Rationale: This patient has early onset insulin dependent diabetes and is more likely to experience difficulty with wound healing.

10. 3. Rationale: Indicates the patient does not understand the purpose of the compression stockings.

11. 1. Rationale: The standard of care for the postoperative patients is that they will have at least 200 mL of output within six hours of surgery.

12. 1. Rationale: With the abdominal surgical patient, full (regular) diet is indicated when the patient is able to pass flatus. Flatus will be passed long before the patient is ready to have a bowel movement and indicates a functioning gastrointestinal tract.

13. 3. Rationale: The RN should try to avoid teaching when patients are distracted and involved with other activities.

14. 1. Rationale: Failure to assess the patient's readiness to learn is one of the most common mistakes made by the novice teacher.

Chapter 23

1. 1, 2. Rationale: Platelets and fibrinogen are used in hemostasis.

2. 1. Rationale: Pallor is best assessed in the mucous membranes and conjunctivae. The skin is normally a pinkish color in various skin colors.

3. 3. Rationale: The valve closing makes the loudest sound until normal physiological conditions; therefore the sound is transmitted to the chest wall.

4. 3. Rationale: Diastole is correlated with ventricular filling.

5. 4. Rationale: In children and young adults, the sound of the blood entering the ventricles may be transmitted to the chest wall, but after the early 20s the sound is associated with heart failure.

6. 2. Rationale: S_2 is the sound associated with closure of the aortic valve.

7. 1. Rationale: S_1 is the sound associated with closure of the mitral valve.

8. 4. Rationale: A physiological split of S_2 is from closure of the pulmonic valve, which is best auscultated in the second ICS on the left side of the sternum.

9. 3. Rationale: The mitral area and the apical pulse are the fifth ICS midclavicular line.

10. 2. Rationale: A scale of I to VI is the standard scale for assessing heart murmurs.

Chapter 24

1. 4. Rationale: These are all risk factors for coronary artery disease.

2. 3. Rationale: Chest pressure lasting greater than 20 minutes not relieved by rest is not a typical stable angina symptom.

3. 4. Rationale: Unstable angina, STEMI, and NSTEMI are included in the clinical spectrum of ACS.

4. 2. Rationale: The atherogenesis of coronary artery disease does not begin with unstable plaque.

5. 2. Rationale: Initial diagnostic studies in the setting of an acute MI include an ECG and exercise stress test.

6. 4. Rationale: Aspirin, beta blockers, and nitroglycerin are common medications used for CAD and ACS.

7. 5 nursing diagnoses for patients with angina and MI are:
   - Acute pain (angina) related to the imbalance between myocardial oxygen supply and demand.
   - Ineffective tissue perfusion related to myocardial ischemia and decreased cardiac output.
   - Anxiety related to pain, perceived threat of death, possible lifestyle changes, and diagnosis of CAD.
   - Activity intolerance related to angina, pulmonary congestion, fatigue, and inadequate tissue perfusion.

   - Ineffective therapeutic regimen management related to lack of knowledge related to disease process, prognosis, and treatment strategies.

8. Components of patient education for patients with stable angina are:
   - Understanding of cardiac condition
   - Chest pain management
   - Activity
   - Medications
   - Risk factor modification
   - Diet
   - Signs and symptoms to report to the physician

9. The goals of therapy for stable angina are to improve the quality of life by decreasing episodes of angina and ischemia and increase the quantity of life by preventing progression to myocardial infarction and death.

10. The goals of therapy for acute MI are to limit myocardial damage and prevent complications and recurrent events.

Chapter 25

1. 3. Rationale: Cardiac catheterization is a procedure used to help identify causes and degree of heart failure. The procedure is performed by placing a catheter through a vein that leads to the heart. An angiogram, also called a left heart catheterization, is a procedure in which the arterial system is accessed. An x-ray is taken during a cardiac catheterization procedure to allow visualization of the internal anatomy of the heart and blood vessels after the intravascular introduction of radiopaque contrast medium (dye) and can assist in measurement of pulmonary artery pressure (Murthy, 2004). A biopsy is the retrieval of a part of the heart muscle that is sent for laboratory testing.

2. 1. Rationale: Signs of left-sided heart failure may reveal dysrhythmic heart rate, tachycardia, heart murmurs, extra heart sounds, lung crackles, and decreased basilar lung sounds (Kang, 2004). An increase in the work of breathing, an increase in the rate of respirations, and an increase in the depth of respiration all indicate strain on the system in situations like heart failure. The pulse increases in an effort to pump oxygen into the body, but it will be weak and ineffective. Left-sided heart failure may present as the following symptoms: shortness of breath, paroxysmal nocturnal dyspnea, palpitations, tachycardia, cough with frothy blood-tinged mucus, fatigue, weakness, syncope, weight gain, fluid retention, and oliguria.

3. 2. Rationale: In left-sided heart failure, the left ventricle loses its ability to effectively pump oxygenated blood into the systemic circulation leaving the body starving for oxygen and nutrients (Kang, 2004).

In right-sided heart failure, the right ventricle loses its ability to pump efficiently and causes blood that would normally be pumped through the heart into the lungs, and errantly backs up into the systemic circulation. This back up of blood causes congestion that can affect the liver, the gastrointestinal tract, and the periphery (arms and legs) (Hart, 2004). The decrease in peripheral oxygenation, (not pulmonary venous congestion that the question asked about), will reveal ashen skin, cyanotic nail beds, and circumoral pallor. Eventually, the heart will not receive enough oxygen to function properly. The jugular neck veins will distend.

In heart failure in general, an increase in the work of breathing, an increase in the rate of respirations, and an increase in the depth of respiration all indicate strain on the system.

4. 4. Rationale: The more pumping and harder the heart works, the more oxygen that is required for the body to continue working hard. Respiratory support consists of nonrebreathing oxygen by mask to relieve hypoxemia and dyspnea.

5. 4. Rationale: ACE inhibitors work by decreasing the pressure the heart must overcome to eject blood from the heart by interfering with the renin-angiotensin-aldosterone system. This interference results blocking the conversion of angiotensin I to angiotensin II in the kidney, causing a decreased aldosterone, increased sodium excretion, and in peripheral vasodilatation that allows for decreased pressure-causing volume in the heart and a decrease in blood pressure (Jessup & Brozena, 2003).

6. 1. Rationale: Characteristic of acute heart failure is an abnormal accumulation of fluid in the lungs. This fluid disperses into all available lung spaces, even those that are used for oxygen exchange. This alteration in the ability of the lungs to perform their oxygenation function results in a rapid onset of symptoms such as panic, anxiety, shortness of breath, cough, and restlessness. Shortly, the pulse increases in an effort to pump oxygen into the body, but it will be weak and ineffective. A back up of blood will ensue and the jugular neck veins will distend.

7. 4. Rationale: Weight reduction is suggested for those obese HCM patients, moderation in alcohol intake is suggested, and flu vaccination is considered. HCM patients are encouraged to avoid overexertion, acute loss of body fluid volume, situations that may predispose one to fainting, hot showers or water immersion, and medication that quickly drops blood pressure.

8. 1. Rationale: Heart muscle disease is called cardiomyopathy and is a problem with the physical shape of the muscle. Heart muscle inflammatory dysfunction is called carditis; an inflammation of the heart muscle.

9. 1. Rationale: Heart transplantation is necessary for some who have severe alteration in the heart's ability to pump effectively. Still other possible treatments include electrical cardioversion, pacemaker insertion, and implantable defibrillator.

10. 2. Rationale: The lung sounds and breath sounds will become moist and noisy with frothy (sometimes pink) sputum. The patient may manifest signs of confusion. These symptoms are ominous and require immediate intervention.

Chapter 26

1. 3. Rationale: This is the appropriate method of calculating a heart rate from a strip when it is irregular. 1 and 4 are only appropriate methods to calculate heart rate when the rhythm is regular.

2. 1. Rationale: Sodium ions move into the cell to initiate depolarization.

3. 4. Rationale: The nurse should establish unresponsiveness prior to initiating CPR.

4. 4. Rationale: Asking the patient to cough may cause a vagal response, which would slow the heart rate down.

5. 1. Rationale: The electrical rhythm is normal sinus rhythm, but the patient has no pulse. The interpretation should be PEA, in which case CPR should be started.

6. 4. Rationale: The patient is not suffering from hemodynamic instability at this time. It is important to continue to monitor the patient in a sinus bradycardia.

7. 2, 4, 5. Rationale: Each of these are possible treatments for ventricular tachycardia with a pulse.

8. 2. Rationale: Epinephrine will be given after three unsuccessful defibrillation attempts in ventricular fibrillation.

9. 4. Rationale: Ventricular arrhythmias are primarily interpreted by analyzing the QRS complex as it represents ventricular depolarization.

10. 4. Rationale: The health care provider assesses and manages breathing by using positive-pressure ventilations.

Chapter 27

1. 1. Rationale: Patients with bleeding disorders need to be assessed for risks and contraindications associated with the disease prior to the start of anticoagulant therapy.
2. 3. Rationale: These are classic symptoms of thoracic-aortic aneurysm, related to the pressure of the aneurysm on the esophagus and laryngeal nerve.
3. 2. Rationale: Uncontrolled bleeding after 10 minutes must be reported to the physician, as excessive bleeding can indicate hypercoagulation.
4. 1. Rationale: INRs must be taken on a consistent basis to monitor the effectiveness of the Coumadin, and the blood level is in therapeutic and safe range.
5. 2. Rationale: The patient is demonstrating symptoms of prolonged bleeding time. Coumadin should be held and an INR drawn for evaluation.
6. 1. Rationale: Frank bleeding is a side effect of t-PA, and has a three times greater incidence of bleeding than heparin.
7. 1. Rationale: Heparin does not dissolve clots, but prevents further clot formation and is reversed quickly with protamine sulfate.
8. 2. Rationale: Venous ulcers have edema at the site, irregular margins, and pink ulcer beds.
9. 1. Rationale: Fever, abdominal pain, and dyspnea are the three major symptoms of pulmonary embolism.
10. 4. Rationale: Decreased blood flow leads to tissue necrosis and infection.

Chapter 28

1. 4. Rationale: Target organ damage that can occur from uncontrolled hypertension includes kidney dysfunction and left ventricular hypertrophy.
2. 3. Rationale: When teaching a patient how to control hypertension, the nurse must recognize that lifestyle modifications are indicated for all patients with hypertension.
3. 2. Rationale: Renin is secreted into the blood by the kidney structure known as the juxtaglomerular apparatus.
4. 1. Rationale: The secretion of antidiuretic hormone (ADH) is stimulated by decreased venous return.
5. 3. Rationale: A patient with a blood pressure of 200/141 mm Hg would have a hypertensive emergency
6. 1. Rationale: Patient teaching for modifiable risk factor reduction should include dietary factors.
7. 2. Rationale: ACE inhibitors such as captopril (Capoten) and enalapril (Vasotec) decrease both blood pressure and peripheral vascular resistance by blocking the conversion of angiotensin I to angiotensin II.
8. 2. Rationale: The interval between the first and second heart sounds is ventricular systole.
9. 3. Rationale: Afterload is the force that the left ventricle must generate to eject its blood volume.
10. 1. Rationale: Pulsus paradoxus is a sign of cardiac tamponade
11. 2. Rationale: Bupropion is a non–nicotine-containing therapy used to support smoking cessation.
12. 1. Rationale: 118/78 is considered a normal B/P according to the JNC VII guidelines.
13. 2. Rationale: A cause of secondary hypertension is hypothyroidism.

Chapter 29

1. 1. Rationale: The three components of the hematology system are: bone marrow, blood cells, and plasma.
2. 2. Rationale: As the three primary classes for anemias are: 1) bleeding, which results in RBC loss; 2) hemolytic anemia, which is caused by RBC destruction; and 3) hypoproliferative, which results from defective RBC production.
3. 2. Rationale: As thalassemia is prevalent in populations from specific areas of descent (China, Philippines, Thailand, Mediterranean ancestry, African Americans), and the other three responses are incorrect.
4. 3. Rationale: Because a cobalamin deficiency is labeled a vitamin B_{12} deficiency.
5. 1. Rationale: Because plasmapheresis is the primary treatment for thrombocytopenia.
6. 3. Rationale: Because DIC is the correct label and is described as the clotting disorder that consumes the clotting factors and causes patients to have clotting difficulties.
7. 4. Rationale: Because primary polycythemia is the type of polycythemia that is more common in European Jewish persons than the other forms of polycythemia.
8. 2. Rationale: Because acute myelogenous leukemia affects persons of all ages, and the other responses are false.
9. 3. Rationale: Because CML is characterized by the presence of the Philadelphia chromosome.
10. 2. Rationale: As bone pain is the distinguishing clinical manifestation for multiple myeloma.

Chapter 30

1. 2. Rationale: Crackles is the best description of adventitious breath sounds as described.
2. 3. Rationale: It is a false statement.
3. 4. Rationale: All four answers are correct.
4. 3. Rationale: This is the best response, because response b is false.
5. 3. Rationale: PaO_2 is the best method of assessing oxygenation status.
6. 2. Rationale: This is the correct definition for shunting.
7. 1. Rationale: The correct interpretation of the blood gases is respiratory acidosis.
8. 1. Rationale: Barrel chest can be seen in chronic obstructive lung disease and normal aging.
9. 1. Rationale: Low flow oxygen delivery systems include the use of entrainment of room air and the use of the mouth and nose as a reservoir.
10. 2. Rationale: Employment history and occupational exposure are vital data in determining prior existing conditions despite current employment status.
11. 3. Rationale: Vesicular breathing is most frequently seen in usual and normal breathing.
12. 3. Rationale: Pulsus paradoxus is described as a drop in blood pressure on inspiration.

Chapter 31

1. 3. Rationale: The most important information to give a patient about prevention with allergic rhinitis is to avoid the triggers that bring about the allergic episode. Triggers include things, such as dust, pollen, cigarette smoke, pet dander, or foods.
2. 4. Rationale: Signs and symptoms of rhinitis are the same regardless of the triggering event. Common clinical manifestations of rhinitis are rhinorrhea, nasal congestion, nasal itchiness, and sneezing are classical features. Headache and cough may be seen. If the patient presents with pyrexia (fever), further assessment should be performed to look for an infectious component.
3. 2. Rationale: The most common side effect in the second-generation antihistamines is urinary retention. The nurse should hold the medication until the health care provider can be notified.
4. 1. Rationale: Proper instructions for instilling nasal spray include tilting the head slightly forward, inhaling gently and evenly, spray once in each side of the nose and wait about 15 to 20 seconds before instilling another spray, and avoid blowing the nose after administration to enhance its effects on the mucous membranes.

5. 3. Rationale: Decongestant nasal sprays will help relieve nasal congestion by reducing the inflammation in the nasal passages. However, they should not be used for more than three consecutive days because of the risk of rhinitis medicamentosa, a rebound congestion that can be worse than the original congestion the patient was experiencing.
6. 4. Rationale: Research demonstrates the limited use of antibiotics in eradicating sinus infections. They have been overused and have lead to resistance of many bacterial organisms. Decongestants help reduce nasal swelling, loosen congestion, and promote drainage within the sinus cavities. Antihistamines have not been shown to be of benefit in treating sinusitis. There is insufficient evidence to support the use of wetting agents, mucolytics, or expectorants.
7. 3. Rationale: Fever and yellow secretions indicate the generalized response of inflammation.
8. 1. Rationale: Thick secretions are best cleared from the airways by drinking plenty of fluids to facilitate expectoration. Measures to help drain the sinuses include warm packs, irrigating the sinuses, and taking decongestants as needed.
9. 4. Rationale: It is often difficult to distinguish viral and bacterial pharyngitis. Fever and cervical adenopathy are generally more pronounced in streptococcal pharyngitis. Other characteristics that are most reliable predictors of streptococcal pharyngitis are tonsillar exudate and the absence of cough. The presence of three of these criteria has a specificity and reliability of 75 percent.
10. 3. Rationale: Patients must understand the importance of reporting frank bleeding from the surgical site. Secondary bleeding is more common than immediate postoperative bleeding and can occur 5 to 8 days after the surgery. The patient is instructed to start with liquids and progress to soft foods for the first few days. The patient should avoid gargling, coughing, straining, and smoking for 10 days.
11. 3. Rationale: Physical examination in a patient with a peritonsillar abscess reveals a displaced tonsil toward the center of the throat by the abscess, the soft palate is erythematous and swollen, and the uvula is edematous and displaced to the opposite side.
12. 3. Rationale: Complaints from a bed partner about snoring and daytime sleepiness often indicate the presence of obstructive sleep apnea. The nurse needs to ask about the onset of other symptoms, such as memory loss, personality changes, morning headaches, fatigue, nocturia, or gastric reflux.

13. 4. Rationale: The priority interventions for patients who have sustained a fracture of the nose are to control bleeding and swelling. Other important measures include pain relief, assessing for symmetry, and reducing anxiety and fear.

14. 2. Rationale: Cancer in the glottic area is usually found early because the patient complains of a change in the voice. The voice becomes raspy, harsh, or lower in pitch because of tumor impingement on the vocal cords.

15. 1. Rationale: Radiation therapy causes changes in the head and neck. Xerostomia, or dry mouth, occurs because radiation interferes with the ability of the parotid gland to produce mucus.

Chapter 32

1. 4. Rationale: *Pneumocystis carinii* pneumonia is a type of fungal infection that often affects immunocompromised patients.

2. 2. Rationale: Latent TB is diagnosed when a person presents with a positive PPD, has no clinical picture of active disease, and CXR is normal. 1 is incorrect because active disease is different than latent disease. 3 is incorrect as extrapulmonary TB disease can present within the bones but usually exist only with advanced disease circumstances. 4 is incorrect because TB disease is no longer latent if it becomes active.

3. 4. Rationale: Exposure of TB requires close frequent contact and exposure will not be present on a PPD until six weeks after inhalation of pathogen. To ensure employee safety a nurse should always report on the job injury or potential harm. Monitoring any signs or symptoms of active disease will minimize exposure to others and provide quick treatment interventions.

4. 1. Rationale: The two leading risk factors for aspiration include alcohol and mental status changes.

5. 3. Rationale: The primary reason for aspiration of pneumonia pathogens is aspiration of oropharyngeal secretions. Mechanical ventilation and enteral feedings place the patient at risk for pneumonia through aspiration or inhalation of pathogens. 1 is incorrect as the acquiring of TB disease is due to prolonged contact with a person with active disease. 2 is incorrect because there is no indication or clinical presentation that the patient has a pneumothorax. 4 is incorrect as Cor pulmonale occurs when the pulmonary blood pressure due to chronic effects of disease or pulmonary embolism.

6. 3. Rationale: A nurse should complete a patient assessment for any changes in condition, such as a soiled dressing, chest tube dislodgment, and symptoms of respiratory distress or pain. Drainage system is evaluated next and includes adequate tube connections, unclamped tubing, adequate water in the water seal chamber, and drainage amount. Next the nurse will check the water seal for air leaks and finally the suction control chamber if wall suction is being used. A gently constant bubbling should be present. Answers 2, 3, and 4 are missing aspects of the above components.

7. 4. Rationale: Chest tubes allow air or fluid to leak out on expiration but on inspiration the chest tube closes preventing fluid or air from moving into the pleural cavity. 1 is incorrect as chest tubes do not allow air and fluid to move in and out of the pleural space during both expiration and inspiration, doing so would make the chest tube dysfunctional. 2 is incorrect s chest tubes should never be clamped for longer than a few minutes and only during a chest drainage device change. 3 is incorrect, as the nurse should never reinsert chest tube devices, as this is a defined health care provider tack. Clamping of chest tubes is unacceptable practice.

8. 1. Rationale: Spontaneous pneumothorax occurs in men between the ages of 20 to 40, with thin men at high risk. Patients presenting with any trauma will have tachycardia and an elevated blood pressure as the body attempts to compensate for the injury. Swallowing breathing occurs due to the collapse lungs effects and pain with breathing. Lack of any impact injury rules out other causes for the pneumothorax. Answers 2 and 4 are incorrect, because pneumonia or tuberculosis could be a possibility but the fact that there is not a fever and the absence of cough present makes the nurse look at other options. Answer 3 is incorrect as fractured ribs could have occurred, but there is not report of trauma.

9. 2. Rationale: As a result of direct blunt force trauma to the chest and broken ribs the patient is at risk for a pneumothorax. 1 is incorrect as flail chest occurs with rib fractures of three or more ribs and an unstable or nonworking thoracic cage. 3 is incorrect as cor pulmonale is a result of a chronic disease process not an acute injury. 4 is incorrect because trauma is the reason for the ER visits not infection. However, pneumonia may occur as a complication to the pulmonary injury.

10. 4. Rationale: Includes all of the above interventions. Patients who use a medication pump are at risk and must be able to troubleshoot problems, have adequate supplies, complete routine medical workup, and know when and how to call for assistance.

Chapter 33

1. 1,950 mg; convert the patient's weight from pounds to kilograms by dividing 143 pounds by 2.2 kg. This equals 65 kg. Next multiply the 65 kg by 25 mcg. This equals 1,950 mg.

   143 lb/2.2 kg = 65 kg.

   65 kg × 25 mcg = 1,950 mg

2. 1, 2. Rationale: Signs and symptoms of right-sided heart failure include jugular venous distension and hepatomegaly. Dyspnea, crackles, and tachycardia are signs of left-sided heart failure.

3. 4. Rationale: In a patient with COPD, the stimulus to breathe is low oxygen levels. Frequent nursing observations are necessary to see how the patient tolerates low-flow oxygen administration. 1 is incorrect. Humidification is necessary, but this is not the most important nursing intervention. 2 is incorrect, because patients with COPD and hypoxemia need oxygen. 3 is incorrect, because the patient with COPD will probably need to be placed in high-Fowler's position, but this is not the most important nursing intervention.

4. 1. Rationale: The medication should be administered with food, such as milk and crackers to prevent gastrointestinal (GI) irritation. Options 2, 3, 4 are appropriate instructions regarding the use of this medication.

5. 4. Rationale: Pursed-lip breathing facilitates maximal expiration for patients with obstructive lung disease. This type of breathing allows better expiration by increasing airway pressure that keeps air passages open during exhalation. Options 1, 2, and 3 are not the purpose of this breathing.

6. 3. Rationale: The patient should be instructed to hold his or her breath at least 5 to 10 seconds before exhaling the mist. Options 1, 2, and 4 are accurate instructions regarding the use of the inhaler.

7. 3. Rationale: The development of an IgE is a strong predisposing factor for developing asthma. The other responses are false.

8. 2. Rationale: Decreased wheezing in a patient with asthma may be incorrectly interpreted as a positive sign when, in fact, it may signal an inability to move air. A "silent chest" is an ominous sign during an asthma episode. With treatment, increased wheezing may actually signal that the child's condition is improving. The normal pulse rate is 60 to 80 beats per minute. Warm, dry skin indicates improvement in condition, as the patient is normally diaphoretic during exacerbations.

9. 4. Rationale: In a sweat test, sweating is stimulated on the child's forearm with pilocarpine, the sample is collected on absorbent material, and the amounts of sodium and chloride are measured. A chloride level greater than 60 mEq/L is considered to be a positive test result. A chloride level of 40 mEq/L is suggestive of cystic fibrosis (CF) and requires a repeat test.

10. 1. Rationale: Tobramycin (TOBI) is an aerosolized medication and the best antibiotic used to treat lower respiratory tract infections in patients with CF. The other three responses are false.

Chapter 34

1. 2. Rationale: When grading muscle strength, a score of 1 indicates a trace of contraction.

2. 1. Rationale: When the nurse is performing the Romberg test he or she should instruct the patient to close his or her eyes and remain still.

3. 3. Rationale: The patient who has difficulty choosing the right words and responds hesitantly is displaying symptoms of expressive aphasia.

4. 2. Rationale: When an adult has a Babinski's it indicates upper motor neuron disease.

5. 3. Rationale: The ability to recognize an object's shape is known as stereognosis.

6. 4. Rationale: Paralysis of lateral gaze indicates a lesion of cranial nerve VI.

7. 4. Rationale: Stimulation of the parasympathetic nervous system results in relaxation of the urinary sphincters.

8. 4. Rationale: When preparing a patient for an EEG, the nurse should tell the patient that bright lights will be used during the procedure.

9. 2. Rationale: The consensual pupillary response is tested by directing a light toward one eye and observing the pupil on the opposite side.

10. 4. Rationale: One way to test the vestibular function of the acoustic nerve (CN VIII) is to rub your fingers together near the patient's ears.

11. 2. Rationale: The trapezius muscle squeeze is the technique recommended for eliciting a response to peripheral pain.

12. 1. Rationale: Cerebrospinal fluid (CSF) is reabsorbed into the venous system via the arachnoid villi.

13. 3. Rationale: The significance of the blood-brain barrier is that it limits the transmission of substances from the blood to the brain.

Chapter 35

1. 1. Rationale: The type of CVA (stroke) that occurs when a blood vessel in the brain becomes clogged, usually by plaque build up is an ischemic stroke.
2. 3. Rationale: The modifiable risk factor in the prevention of a stroke is obesity. A patient can take steps to lose weight by diet modification and exercise. Age, sex, and family history cannot be changed to prevent a stroke.
3. 4. Rationale: An important nursing intervention when caring for a patient receiving tPA is to watch for decreased level of consciousness and increase in blood pressure.
4. 2. Rationale: A CT scan is usually the radiological test first administered to a patient suspected of having a stroke.
5. 2. Rationale: A primary brain injury is caused by an external force. Often a primary brain injury is a result of direct trauma to the brain. ICPs, an abnormal growth of brain tissue, and internal force are all things that occur within the brain to cause brain damage. These are considered secondary brain injuries.
6. 1. Rationale: A moderate brain injury is characterized by a loss of consciousness ranging from a few minutes to hours to days.
7. 1. Rationale: One of the most important things to tell person teaching 7-year-olds on preventing brain injury is to always wear a helmet when riding your bike or skateboard or rollerblading.
8. 4. Rationale: When a patient is evaluated using the Glasgow Coma Scale and the patient responds only to pain by withdrawing his or her hand and cursing frequently, this patient would score a 9 (the patient responds to pain only (2), withdraws from pain (4), and curses frequently (3). 2 + 4 + 3 = 9).
9. 3. Rationale: This patient may be developing a intracerebral bleed or cerebral edema, which is an emergency. The family should seek medical attention immediately.
10. 4. Rationale: Mannitol is an osmotic diuretic and is often used to decrease ICP.
11. 1. Rationale: Risk for infection is the most important nursing diagnosis for an open skull fracture because of the potential for bacteria to enter the brain directly through the opening.

12. 2. Rationale: Benign brain tumors are slow-growing and noncancerous tumors. Malignant brain tumors are cancerous and fast-growing.
13. 3. Rationale: A secondary brain tumor means that the cancer originated somewhere else in the body and spread to the brain.
14. 2. Rationale: The most common form of brain tumor is a glioma.
15. 3. Rationale: Stereotactic radiotherapy uses radiation with or without invasive surgery to deliver a precise dose of radiation to a specific location within the brain. It can only be used for small, benign tumors.

Chapter 36

1. 2. Rationale: A patient who has a C6 SCI will respond with "I will be able to feed myself" if the patient understands the teaching about the long-term effects of the injury.
2. 1, 3, 4. Rationale: Loss of pain and temperature sensation on the opposite side, loss of motor function (paralysis) on the same side as the injury, and loss of position sense and vibration on same side as the injury are what the patient experiences with an incomplete spinal cord injury resulting in Brown Séquard syndrome.
3. 2. Rationale: If the new SCI patient responds that there is often a period of spinal shock, and it is difficult to determine if the paralysis will be permanent. When it resolves there can be some regaining of abilities.
4. 4. Rationale: Carbamazepine (Tegretol) is the first choice of treatment for trigeminal neuralgia.
5. 4. Rationale: High-frequency hearing loss is not generally present in a patient with Ménière's disease.
6. 1. Rationale: The nurse seeing a patient with Ménière's disease in the clinic for the first time should first assess for a history of taking thyroid supplements.
7. 2. Rationale: Burning and tingling pain are worse during the nighttime in pain associated with carpal tunnel syndrome.
8. 4. Rationale: A positive Phalen's sign for carpal tunnel syndrome is indicated by pain and tingling experienced on flexion of the wrist at a right angle for one minute.
9. 1. Rationale: Emergency treatment with methylprednisolone for a patient with an SCI must be instituted within the first 8 hours after injury.
10. 1. Rationale: A patient with a cervical SCI that has an upper motor neuron lesion will need the administration of baclofen for spasticity.

11. 2. Rationale: The priority nursing action for a patient with an SCI experiencing a pounding headache and blood pressure of 220/120 indicating autonomic dysreflexia is to check for distended bladder or kinked catheter tubing.

Chapter 37

1. 4. Rationale: A patient who has a migraine headache would be sensitive to sound.
2. 2. Rationale: Nursing documentation of seizure activity should be highly descriptive and detailed.
3. 2. Rationale: The teaching plan for a patient with epilepsy should include wearing a medical alert bracelet.
4. 1. Rationale: Dairy products are food products potentially associated with migraine attacks.
5. 2. Rationale: Two distinguishing features of migraine are family history of headaches and headache-related disability.
6. 3. Rationale: The most common clinical manifestation reported by a patient with myasthenia gravis is weakness on exertion.
7. 4. Rationale: Dopamine is the neurotransmitter that is decreased in patients with Parkinson's disease.
8. 3. Rationale: The priority safety intervention when protecting the patient having a seizure is positioning the patient to prevent aspiration of secretions.
9. 1. Rationale: Atropine is the drug that must be kept at the bedside of patient's with myasthenia gravis.
10. 4. Rationale: An abnormal plantar reflex is commonly seen with upper motor neuron lesions.
11. 1. Rationale: The brief sensory experience that occurs prior to the onset of seizure is called the prodromal phase.

Chapter 38

1. 2. Rationale: A disorder of his palpebrae is a problem with the eyelids.
2. 3. Rationale: The extraocular muscles are innervated by cranial nerves III, IV, and VI.
3. 1. Rationale: The parasympathetic nervous system causes the pupils to constrict.
4. 4. Rationale: A congenital defect that causes color vision problems is due to a dysfunction in the cones.
5. 3. Rationale: The Snellen chart is responsible for testing visual acuity.
6. 2. Rationale: Yellow, lipid rich plaque lesion on the eyelid is labeled xanthelasma.

7. 3. Rationale: A left eye that does not constrict when light is shined in the right eye is labeled a problem associated with a consensual response.
8. 2. Rationale: When using the ophthalmoscope, the red numbers indicate posterior eye problems.
9. 4. Rationale: Purulent drainage coming from the ear is described as otorrhea.
10. 1. Rationale: A conduction problem of both ears is tested with a Weber test, which evaluates whether sounds are heard centrally or on one side.

Chapter 39

1. 3. Rationale: Color blindness is not one of the three main ocular movement dysfunctions.
2. 1. Rationale: Cataract describes the condition asked for in the question.
3. 3. Rationale: Tonometry is the diagnostic test used to reveal the presence of eye pressure.
4. 3. Rationale: The condition described in the question is age-related macular degeneration.
5. 2. Rationale: Assessment of the patient with an impaled object is the priority.
6. 1. Rationale: Melanoma is the most common cause of ocular cancer.
7. 2. Rationale: Keratoconus is caused by rubbing the eyes profusely.
8. 1. Rationale: Hyperopia is the condition corrected with convex corrective lens.
9. 3. Rationale: Hordeolum is the label for the condition described in the question.
10. 4. Rationale: Decreasing daily intake of water is not an appropriate nursing intervention for keratoconjunctivitis sicca.

Chapter 40

1. 2. Rationale: Patients with sensorineural hearing loss have difficulty hearing in noisy environments. The patient with conductive loss is able to hear in these environments. Mixed would also have difficulty hearing in noisy environments.
2. 4. Rationale: Patients with conductive hearing loss have difficulty hearing all pitches and therefore are able to hear in noisy environments, talk softer because they hear their voices as louder, and their speech is clear not distorted.
3. 4. Rationale: Commonly patients experience some vertigo after surgery and therefore need assistance with ambulation. The patient should lie on the unoperated ear; coughing can cause postoperative complications and should be discouraged. The patient cannot be ensured that his hearing will be normal after the operation.

4. 3. Rationale: High doses of aspirin can cause tinnitus, and the patient should report this finding to the health care provider. Tinnitus does not occur with normal aging process, increasing the sound to drown out the ringing will not solve the problem, because it is most likely caused by the aspirin. Performing a Rinne or Weber test will not detect cause of tinnitus.

5. 3. Rationale: Patients with Meniére's disease have sensorineural hearing loss and experience vertigo and tinnitus.

6. 1. Rationale: External ear canals that are blocked by cerumen should be gently irrigated. An individual should not place anything into the canal, such as cotton-tipped swabs. Curettes can cause damage to the canal or tympanic membrane and therefore should not be used. It is not necessary to refer a patient with cerumen to a specialist.

7. 1, 5. Rationale: When communicating with a person who has a hearing deficit speaking loudly or yelling will not help the patient and may cause anxiety. The light source should be placed behind the patient, not the nurse. When it is placed behind the nurse the light tends to glare into the patient's face, making it difficult to read lips or watch facial expressions. When having to repeat a word or phase, another phase should be used. Communicate in clear simple words.

8. 2. Rationale: Most hearing aids will increase the volume of sound but will not make it clearer. The hearing aid is an assistive device and will not return the patient's hearing to normal.

9. 1. Rationale: Normal hearing is measured at 0–15 dB; anything above that range indicates some loss.

10. 1. Rationale: Patient who experiences a loud blast for greater than 20 seconds can have permanent hearing loss.

11. 1, 2. Rationale: OSHA recommends that workers are tested on hiring and yearly and monitoring sound levels on a regular basis. Training and education is mandated yearly. It is not necessary for all employees to wear noise protection only the ones who are exposed to high levels.

12. 2. Rationale: Frequent attacks of vertigo, tinnitus, nausea, vomiting, and intermittent hearing loss are classic signs in Meniére's disease. Presbycusis is a degenerative hearing loss associated with the aging process and has constant loss. Otosclerosis is also a steady decrease in hearing related to the formation of spongy bones around the oval window. Mastoiditis is inflammation of the mastoid process located behind the ear, and the patient does not experience hearing loss.

Chapter 41

1. 2. Rationale: Bone marrow suppression will most likely be reflected in the immune system, but neither detecting nor signaling bone marrow is one of the immune system's roles.

2. 2, 3. Rationale: Both macrophages and dendritic cells process ingested antigen and present it to lymphocytes. Neutrophils and natural killer cells do not.

3. 1, 2, 3, 4. Rationale: Antigens are defined as a substance that can bind to a specific antibody. Haptens are a kind of antigen. Immunogens are any substance that cause an immune reaction, and therefore will eventually cause antibody production. Complement is part of the immune system and may be activated by binding to an antibody.

4. 1. Rationale: Neutrophils are phagocytes, ingesting bacteria to destroy them. Basophils and natural killer cells are exocytotic. Plasma cells produce lymphocytes.

5. 4. Rationale: Dendritic cells and macrophages both activate lymphocytes, but dendritic cells are more potent activators than macrophages.

6. 1, 4. Rationale: Bone marrow and the thymus gland are considered primary lymphoid organs, because they are the site of lymphocyte maturation.

7. 4. Rationale: The innate immune system initiates inflammation. The other answers are characteristics of the acquired immune system.

8. 2. Rationale: Family history of measles is not relevant to giving injections, although a personal history may be.

9. 4. Rationale: Angioedema is the only adverse reaction listed that is a hypersensitivity reaction.

10. 4. Rationale: Heart transplant usually results in destruction of the thymus gland either by mutilation or excision. The spleen and tonsils are both secondary lymphoid tissues.

11. 1, 2. Rationale: Both bacterial infection and MI are associated with elevated neutrophil count.

12. 1. Rationale: Health history provides the framework with which to interpret the physical examination and laboratory values.

Chapter 42

1. 3. Rationale: Patients tend to focus on lifestyle changes in the early stages of a chronic disease.

2. 4. Rationale: The goal of HAART is to avoid viral resistance for each drug.

3. 2. Rationale: The early clinical manifestations of GVHD are skin rash and pruritus.

4. 3. Rationale: Monoclonal antibodies are genetically engineered immunosuppressant drugs.

5. 3. Rationale: Hypersensitivity disorders are because of a heightened immune response to an antigen.

6. 2. Rationale: The reversible form of SLE is because of a reaction to drugs, such as oral contraceptives (e.g., Levora).

7. 1. Rationale: Cell-mediated immunity is initiated by specific antigen recognition by T cells.

8. 2. Rationale: Passive immunity involves inoculation with vaccine containing live or killed infectious organisms.

9. 2. Rationale: Sero-conversion antibodies to HIV are detected by diagnostic studies with in one to three months or more after exposure to HIV.

10. 4. Rationale: Criteria used to diagnose AIDS in an individual with HIV includes development of an opportunistic cancer.

Chapter 43

1. 1. Rationale: The elimination and challenge diet is the cornerstone for treatment of food allergy.

2. 2. Rationale: Intramuscular epinephrine (adrenaline) is the most effective drug in treating anaphylaxis. Epinephrine by inhalation is less effective.

3. 3. Rationale: Swelling around the eyes and or mouth (angioedema) is an initial response to latex allergy. The cascade of symptoms can progress rapidly to anaphylaxis.

4. 1. Rationale: Production of IgE levels to specific allergens tends to be an inherited trait.

5. 3. Rationale: Bee and wasp stings are the most common causes of anaphylaxis. The risk of hyposensitization is balanced against the much larger risk of being stung again.

6. 4. Rationale: The "wheal and flare" skin reaction is visible within 5 to 10 minutes in a positive response to an allergen.

7. 3. Rationale: Drug reactions are a common source of allergic response. The risk of a drug reaction is greater when the drug is given parenterally, rather than orally.

8. 3. Rationale: Dermatitis often appears in this distribution first.

9. 4. Rationale: The parental route gives a larger dose in a shorter period of time.

10. 3. Rationale: Bronchial hyperreactivity is a classic symptom of asthma.

Chapter 44

1. 3. Rationale: The epidermis replenishes itself by a process labeled as keratinization.

2. 4. Rationale: Cells that are responsible for skin pigmentation are melanocytes.

3. 2. Rationale: Neoangiogenesis, a process during the wound healing process is the responsibility of endothelial cells.

4. 2. Rationale: The major function of the subcutaneous tissue is to provide padding over body joints and other internal structures.

5. 3. Rationale: Regeneration of skin is accomplished by replacing damaged tissue with the same cell type.

6. 4. Rationale: Repeated or prolonged insults to tissues can result in development of pressure sores.

7. 1. Rationale: The substances that control the proliferation and differentiation of cells are known as: growth factors.

8. 2. Rationale: In assessment of an edematous area, the nurse should palpate for temperature changes, tenderness, and mobility.

9. 3. Rationale: A teenager with severe acne decides that he does not want to participate in the swimming exercises that are part of the physical education course at his school. This is an example of social isolation related to anticipatory fear of rejection.

10. 1. Rationale: Patient teaching for older adults should include information about avoiding the use of potent topical steroids because decreased vascularity in the skin decreases capacity to clear medications from the system.

Chapter 45

1. 4. Rationale: The appropriate cleansing agent is dependent on the underlying etiology of the problem. Necrotic or devitalized tissue left in the wound will impede healing. A moist wound environment must be provided and maintained for healing to take place.

2. 3. Rationale: Dermatological dysfunctions are complicated and require a multifocused care plan that may include topical and systemic medications, dietary and lifestyle adjustments, and specialized procedures of multidisciplinary team members.

3. 1. Rationale: A lesion's being visually evident does not necessarily make the etiology readily identifiable.

4. 4. Rationale: There are multiple etiologies for dermatological dysfunctions and all of the possible answers are among them.

5. 2. Rationale: Photoaging is the multiple damaging effects the ultraviolet B radiation of the sun has on skin.

6. 4. Rationale: Contact dermatitis is treated upon identification of the sensitizing substance and controlling the symptoms.

7. 1. Rationale: Fungal infections, also known as tineas, are the most common dermatological problems encountered by health care professionals.

8. 2. Rationale: Rosacea has an insidious onset, develops between 30 and 50 years of age, affects more women than men, and is more common in fair-skinned persons.

9. 3. Rationale: All other answers are fabrications.

10. 4. Rationale: Pruritus is a symptom, not a disease and can accompany both healing and infection.

Chapter 46

1. 4. Rationale: Increased capillary permeability may cause hypovolemic shock in large total body surface area burns.

2. 1. Rationale: The rule of nines refers to a method used to estimate the total body surface burned.

3. 2. Rationale: A superficial partial-thickness burn includes color pink, area moist, blisters large, and pain sensation intact.

4. 4. Rationale: Absence of skin leads to loss of protective barrier against fluid loss, hypermetabolic state increases insensible fluid loss, and increased respirations raise insensible fluid loss through moisture evaporation from the lungs.

5. 1. Rationale: Wounds that appear moist and pale with sluggish capillary refill and white in color can be classified as deep partial.

6. 1. Rationale: The fluid shift in burn shock is primarily water, electrolytes, and albumin.

7. 2. Rationale: Face = 4.5; anterior chest = 18; bilateral forearms = (4.5 + 4.5) = 9; total = 31.5 or 32 percent.

8. Formula = 4 mL × % TBSA × weight in kg. 4 mL × 32% TBSA × 70 kg = 8,960 mL.

9. Half of the total volume is to be infused over the first eight hours: 8,960/2 = 4,480.
4,480/8 = 560 mL/hour

10. Half of the total volume is to be infused over the next 16 hours.
8,960/2 = 4,480
4,480/16 = 280 mL/hour

Chapter 47

1. 2. Rationale: Saliva is a product of exocrine glands in the oral cavity that lubricates the mouth and begins the digestive process.

2. 4. Rationale: The spleen is the organ that is located in the left upper quadrant.

3. 3. Rationale: Acute pain in the abdomen is labeled as an acute abdomen.

4. 4. Rationale: Auscultation is performed first when performing an abdominal assessment so that the sounds produced from percussion and palpation do not alter what is auscultated.

5. 3. Rationale: Normally the liver does not descend beyond 1 to 2 cm of the costal margin and is not palpable during an assessment.

6. 3. Rationale: Conscious sedation allows patients to respond to verbal commands throughout the procedure.

7. 2. Rationale: Murphy's sign is the assessment technique that is not used to asses for ascites.

8. 3. Rationale: A positive Murphy's sign indicates an inflammatory process associated with cholecystitis.

9. 2. Rationale: The assessment technique for flexing the patient's right leg at the hip and the knee is at a right angle and then internally and externally rotating the patient's leg and observing the patient's reaction is called an obturator muscle test.

10. 4. Rationale: The low-pitched sound that is auscultated in the abdomen and caused by turbulent blood flow is called a bruit.

11. 4. Rationale: Secretin testing is used to determine if a patient has incipient chronic pancreatitis.

Chapter 48

1. 2. Rationale: The Institute of Medicine recommended 45–65 percent of calories from carbohydrate, 20–35 percent of calories from fat, and 10–35 percent of calories from protein. The ranges allow for healthy eating with a flexible approach and allow for a higher intake from fat, provided that fat intake is mostly polyunsaturated.

2. 3. Rationale: Indirect calorimetry estimates energy expenditure by measuring oxygen consumed and carbon dioxide produced. (1) A calorie count estimates food intake over a period of one to three days; (2) there is no known blood test which determines the amount of calories burned; and (4) intake and output records are normally recorded in an acute care setting and are not related to indirect calorimetry.

3. 4. Rationale: BMI Categories: Underweight = less than 18.5, Normal weight = 18.5–24.9, Overweight = 25–29.9, Obesity = BMI of 30 or greater.

4. 3. Rationale: Maintaining a consistent intake of foods high in vitamin K will help to maintain a stable INR. Increasing or decreasing intake of foods high in vitamin K can affect the blood's

clotting ability and may result in an unnecessary change in warfarin dose.

5. 2. Rationale: A "ng" feeding is a nasogastric enteral feeding in which the tube is placed from the nose to the stomach.

6. 2. Rationale: The head of the bed should be elevated 30 degrees when a patient is being fed enterally. (1) Utilizing parenteral nutrition instead of enteral nutrition does not offer fewer complications and is not indicated when the patient can be fed enterally; and (3) blenderizing foods and putting them through a tube feeding in the hospital is contraindicated because of the potential for infection, difficulty getting the correct consistency, and decreased ability to deliver adequate nutrition to the patient.

7. 1, 2, 3, and 4. Rationale: These are indications that the patient's nutritional status is improving and are not indicators of nutrition risk.

8. 1. Rationale: Prealbumin is one of the laboratory measures of visceral protein stores. 2, 3, and 4 are abnormal lab values but are not indicators of visceral protein stores.

9. 1. Rationale: Elderly people have decreased total body water, often have impaired thirst mechanisms and may have difficulty accessing adequate food and fluid.

10. 2. Rationale: Nutrition plays a vital role in the prevention of chronic disease. (1) The incidence of obesity and diabetes are both increasing; (3) poor nutrition and overweight are risk factors for developing type 2 diabetes. Type 1 diabetes is thought to be an autoimmune disease and is not correlated with body weight; and (4) lifestyle is more a factor in the development of chronic diseases such as type 2 diabetes than genetics.

Chapter 49

1. 3. Rationale: Odynophagia is the correct label for symptoms related to erosion of the esophagus.

2. 2. Rationale: Somatic pain is the correct label for GI pain that is specific to a region of the body.

3. 3. Rationale: Burning mouth syndrome is a constant burning sensation of the tongue.

4. 4. Rationale: A PEG tube is sutured in place and has complications such as bleeding, infection, or peritonitis.

5. 2. Rationale: Pain in the esophagus from esophagitis can be confused as cardiac pain.

6. 1. Rationale: GERD is characterized by heartburn after meals, some regurgitation of fluids that are foul tasting when the patient is full, and the patient often is not able to lie down comfortably just after eating.

7. 3. Rationale: A hiatal hernia is the most likely condition when the patient is pregnant and experiencing pyrosis and regurgitation after eating her meals.

8. 1. Rationale: Fresh fruits and vegetables are appropriate foods to eat when there is a family history of stomach cancer.

9. 3. Rationale: Acute episodes of diarrhea that are sudden in occurrence; after a gastric surgery is most likely dumping syndrome.

Chapter 50

1. 3. Rationale: Intussusception is due to telescoping of a loop of bowel into a lower loop of bowel.

2. 2. Rationale: Assessment of Crohn's disease would include evidence of weight loss and anemia.

3. 3. Rationale: Teaching strategies for patients who have IBS would focus on dietary modifications.

4. 3. Rationale: IBS is best described as a functional bowel disorder with no signs of pathology present.

5. 1. Rationale: Modifications in the daily diet to alleviate IBS symptoms include a high soluble fiber diet.

6. 4. Rationale: An important change in lifestyle to aid in minimizing IBS symptoms is eating slowly.

7. 3. Rationale: Acidic chime from the stomach that flows into the duodenum is neutralized by the alkaline liquid secreted from the jejunum cells.

8. 3. Rationale: Serotonin is a neurochemical mediator that has been implicated in the transmission of pain in the GI tract.

9. 2. Rationale: IBS in the United States and other developed countries is more prevalent in women.

10. 4. Rationale: IBS symptoms can exacerbate following dietary intolerances.

Chapter 51

1. 3. Rationale: The definition of gluconeogenesis is the synthesis of glucose from amino acids during times of fasting.

2. 2. Rationale: The thymus is the organ that an endoscopic retrograde cholangiopancreatography (ERCP) does not inspect.

3. 3. Rationale: Hepatitis A is an RNA virus, spread often by food handlers infected with the virus, and has an incubation time of 15 to 50 days.

4. 1. Rationale: Wilson's disease is a hereditary disease of the liver, which is an autosomal recessive disorder related to copper metabolism.

5. 3. Rationale: A management strategy for ascites associated with cirrhosis is a surgical shunt, which diverts excessive peritoneal fluid into the venous system.

6. 3. Rationale: A hepatic abscess is usually caused by bacterial infection and is referred to as pyogenic hepatic abscess.

7. 1. Rationale: The two basic types of liver cancer are labeled primary and secondary.

8. 2. Rationale: The most common reason for children to have a liver transplant is biliary atresia.

9. 3. Rationale: The diagnosis for acute pancreatitis best made with computed tomography (CT) scanning in differentiating the pancreatitis from other abdominal issues.

10. 4. Rationale: Criteria for receiving a donated liver is rigorously defined by the United Network for Organ Sharing.

Chapter 52

1. 3. Rationale: Collect a small sample of each voiding and place in a rack for comparison over time. This allows the nurse to assess changes in color and determine the presence of blood in the urine.

2. 2. Rationale: Have the patient void and discard urine, noting this as the beginning of the 24-hour urine collection. A 24-hour urine specimen is a collection of all urine produced in 24-hour period. The collection should begin with an empty bladder.

3. 1. Rationale: Hydration, administration of acetylcysteine, or administration of IV sodium bicarbonate. Hydration is vital to protection of renal function. Patients with fluid restriction may require the additional agents.

4. 3. Rationale: Report metal screening findings to the MRI department and sedate for claustrophobia before sending him or her to the MRI department. Patients with significant exposure to metal may not be able to have an MRI.

5. 2. Rationale: Discard the specimen and collect another specimen with review of instructions. This is the only way to ensure that the specimen is not contaminated.

6. 2. Rationale: Supine position, which is critical to ensure accurate results.

7. 2. Rationale: Constipation can interfere with the viewing field, which can lead to inaccurate results.

8. 3. Rationale: The kidney receives 20 percent of the cardiac output through the renal arteries that comes directly from the aorta.

9. 4. Rationale: The patient should be encouraged to force fluids not restrict fluid intake.

10. 4. Rationale: Urine culture and sensitivity, which is used to diagnose bacterial infections of the urinary tract.

Chapter 53

1. 2. Rationale: Completely empty the bladder and do not put off the urge to urinate. Fully emptying the bladder promptly discourages the incubation of bacteria in the urinary tract.

2. 1. Rationale: Common presenting symptoms for both IC and recurrent UTI include urgency, frequency, nocturia, and dysuria.

3. 1. Rationale: Urinary retention and ascending infection of the urinary tract, both of which predispose the patient to develop a bacterial infection.

4. 3. Rationale: Nephrotic syndrome, which is 15 times more common in children than in adults.

5. 3. Rationale: Pyelonephritis is an inflammation or infection of the kidney or kidney pelvis.

6. 1. Rationale: A CT scan and ultrasound are the most appropriate methods to identify the source and extent of renal trauma.

7. 2. Rationale: Removal of the diseased organ is the best approach to treat renal cancer.

8. 3. Rationale: Bladder cancer most commonly presents without pain but with gross hematuria.

9. 1. Rationale: Continent urinary diversion uses a traditional ileal conduit.

10. 4. Rationale: Functional incontinence is likely in patients with multiple sclerosis who may experience impaired mobility.

Chapter 54

1. 3. Rationale: The oliguric period in acute renal failure usually lasts one to two weeks.

2. 2. Rationale: U waves on the electrocardiogram are associated with hypokalemia.

3. 2. Rationale: Leaking of arterial blood into an AV fistula causes the veins to enlarge, so they are easier to access for hemodialysis.

4. 4. Rationale: It is imperative for the patient to maintain an adequate fluid status as evidenced by normal weight and to remain infection free. The primary nursing goal is to help the patient maintain a positive self-image and continue to be a productive member of society.

5. 3. Rationale: Pyelonephritis is an inflammation or infection of the kidney or kidney pelvis.

6. 1. Rationale: The most common findings in acute renal failure include elevations in BUN and creatinine, metabolic acidosis, hyponatremia, hyperkalemia, hypocalcemia, and hypophosphatemia.

7. 3. Rationale: Appropriate skin care for patients with uremic frost is bathing with tepid water and applying oils to reduce dryness and itching.

8. 1. Rationale: Immediate assessments to be performed for a kidney recipient are fluid and electrolyte status, intake and output, and hypotension.

9. 2. Rationale: Peritonitis is usually caused by *Staphylococcus*. The first indication of peritonitis is cloudy dialysate.

10. 4. Rationale: Peritonitis is a life-threatening complication of continuous ambulatory peritoneal dialysis, which is manifested by abdominal pain and distension, diarrhea, vomiting, and fever. Antibiotics are given as treatment not prophylactically.

Chapter 55

1. 4. Rationale: TSH is not produced by the thyroid gland.

2. 3. Rationale: The exocrine glands are responsible for secreting substances into the ducts that empty into a body cavity or onto a body surface.

3. 4. Rationale: The hypothalamus gland secretes hormones that release or inhibit hormones from the anterior pituitary gland.

4. 1. Rationale: Epinephrine and norepinephrine are the two major hormones secreted by the adrenal medulla.

5. 1. Rationale: Circadian rhythm is an example of negative feedback is seen in the relationship between insulin and blood glucose levels.

6. 1. Rationale: The PTH is regulated by negative feedback.

7. 1. Rationale: The thyroid gland is the organ in the endocrine system that consists of two lobes, connected by an isthmus, and secretes thyroxine, calcitonin, and triiodothyronine.

8. 3. Rationale: Fever, tachycardia, and restlessness are clinical manifestations of a patient having a thyroid crisis.

9. 4. Rationale: The parathyroid gland controls serum calcium.

10. 2. Rationale: A negative feedback mechanism refers to the response of a gland by increasing or decreasing the secretion of a hormone.

Chapter 56

1. 1, 3, 4. Rationale: These are the symptoms seen in a patient with acromegaly.

2. 3. Rationale: Not having a menstrual period for a year would support a diagnosis of hyperprolactinemia.

3. 1. Rationale: Patient education for a transsphenoidal hypophysectomy would include information regarding the nasal passage being packed with gauze for 24 to 48 hours.

4. 2. Rationale: Fall prevention measures are important for the nurse to anticipate when caring for a patient with hypercortisolism.

5. 3. Rationale: Patient with Addison's disease needs to know that their glucocorticoid medications need to be increased during times of illness or stress.

6. 3. Rationale: Patients with hyperprolactinemia may experience breast engorgement.

7. 2. Rationale: Patient with pheochromocytoma needs to have their blood pressure within normal limits, as this condition causes hypertension.

8. 1. Rationale: Fine hand tremor is indicative of hyperthyroidism.

9. 1. Rationale: Patient taking methimazole (Tapazole) needs to report a sore throat and fever to their health care provider.

10. 1. Rationale: Breastfeeding is contraindicated with a patient involved in radioiodine therapy for hyperthyroidism.

11. 3. Rationale: Ionized calcium is the correct therapy for changes following a parathyroidectomy that cause numbness and tingling in the tips of the fingers and around the mouth.

12. 1. Rationale: Vasopressin causes thirst to be resolved.

Chapter 57

1. 1, 2, and 3. Rationale: Clinical manifestations of type 1 diabetes are hyperglycemia, fruity odor of breath, and tachycardia.

2. 2. Rationale: The nurse knows that more teaching is needed when the patient who is mixing insulin withdraws too much NPH insulin and injects the extra back into the Lente vial.

3. 1. Rationale: HgbA$_{1C}$ is the lab test that offers the best information about glycemic control.

4. 3. Rationale: When a patient is admitted to the hospital with DKA the nurse can anticipate that 0.9% NS will be administered.

5. 1. Rationale: Regular insulin can be administered intravenously.

6. 4. Rationale: The long term management of diabetes includes the use of a glucose lowering agent, diet, and activity.

7. 1. Rationale: The primary difference between DKA and HHNS is the absence of ketosis.

8. 4. Rationale: Clinical manifestations of hypoglycemia are irritability, increasing confusion, tremors, hunger, sweating, weakness, and visual disturbances.

9. 2. Rationale: The corresponding hyperglycemia seen in the dawn phenomena results from predawn release of counter-regulatory hormones.

10. 3. Rationale: The autonomic neuropathy conditions associated with diabetic complications lead to bowel and bladder incontinence and delayed gastric emptying.

Chapter 58

1. 2. Rationale: Wolff's law states that bone forms and remodels itself in direct proportion to the amount and the direction of physical forces placed on it.
2. 4. Rationale: In a maturing child, the epiphyseal plate, or growth plate, is where active longitudinal growth occurs (until the age of maturity). If a fracture occurs in or through the epiphyseal plate, growth in that extremity can be delayed or stopped. When maturity is reached the epiphyseal plate merges the epiphysis and the metaphysis and the epiphyseal plate completely disappears.
3. 1. Rationale: Osteoblastic activity slows down between the ages of 30 and 40. After age 40, women lose approximately 8 percent of their bone mass every decade. In men the loss is 3 percent per decade.
4. 2, 4. Rationale: The main functions of skeletal muscle are to produce movement, maintain posture and body position, support soft tissues, guard entrances and exits to the digestive and urinary tracts, and to assist in maintaining body temperature.
5. 2. Rationale: During muscle contraction, the sarcoplasm reticulum releases large amounts of calcium into the vicinity of the myofibrils. This sudden rise in calcium concentration within the sarcoplasm initiates muscle contraction by removing the tropomyosin-troponin block.
6. 3. Rationale: Ligaments help to give joints stability, guide the joint movement, and prevent excess motion within the joint.
7. 1. Rationale: Classified according to the amount of movement, three classes of joints can be identified: synarthrosis (immovable), amphiarthrosis (slightly movable), and diarthrosis (freely movable).
8. 2. Rationale: When an individual seeks assistance with a musculoskeletal complaint, it is generally because the complaint has caused a limitation in movement or pain.
9. 2. Rationale: There are three basic maneuvers used in assessing the musculoskeletal system: inspection, palpation, and assessment of range of motion (passive and active).
10. 2. Rationale: When performing a NVA you should always compare one extremity to another to observe for abnormalities.

Chapter 59

1. 2. Rationale: Acetaminophen (Tylenol) and ibuprofen (Advil) are both available over-the-counter and are relatively inexpensive. The nurse corrected Mrs. Jones perception that these were prescription medications and provided additional information.
2. 2. Rationale: Alcohol and turkey contain purine, which can aggravate gout.
3. 3. Rationale: Headaches are not a symptom of Reiter's syndrome.
4. 3. Rationale: DMARDs also reduce inflammation, as do NSAIDs, and may provide relief when NSAIDs are no longer effective.
5. 1. Rationale: A bullseye rash is the classic symptom of LD.
6. 3. Rationale: Baseline screening for fibromyalgia includes an electrolyte panel and ESR as markers of the inflammatory process that is occurring.
7. 1. Rationale: Spinal stenosis causes a narrowing of the spinal column where the nerves exit. Pressure on the nerves results in pain.
8. 4. Rationale: Small joint involvement is common in rheumatoid arthritis. All the other symptoms are seen in osteoarthritis but not rheumatoid arthritis.
9. 1. Rationale: A baseline assessment of neurological signs is made so that deviation from the database can be noted. Once a pain assessment is complete, a plan for pain management can be developed.
10. 3. Rationale: High dosage or long-term use of corticosteroids is associated with the development of gastric ulcers.

Chapter 60

1. 4. Rationale: Installing grab bars and hand rails on both sides of stairs along with improving the lighting in and around the house can decrease the risk of falling.
2. 3. Rationale: The signs and symptoms of a fracture include ecchymosis, edema, deformity, other soft tissue injury, muscle spasms, tenderness, pain, numbness, loss of function, abnormal movement, or crepitus.
3. 1. Rationale: The purpose of immobilizing or splinting the fractured limb is to minimize bleeding, edema, pain, and prevent further injury to the tissues and structures surrounding the fracture. Complications from improper handling or splinting can include increase bleeding, a significant increase in pain, and a

decrease in sensation and function, which may be temporary or permanent. The incidence of fat embolism and shock are also increased.

4. 4. Rationale: The patient may not bear weight on the cast until it is fully dry. For a plaster cast this is about 48 hours after application.

5. 1. Rationale: Fiberglass casts dry within 30 minutes of application.

6. 4. Rationale: Signs and symptoms of an infection under a cast include odor, purulent drainage, and areas of the cast that are warmer than other areas (hot spots).

7. 3. Rationale: FES is more prevalent in patients who have sustained long bone fractures, fractures of the ribs and pelvis, or multiple fractures.

8. 2. Rationale: The signs and symptoms of FES are hypoxemia, changes in mental status, petechiae on the upper body, seizures, use of accessory muscles, tachypnea, dyspnea, restlessness, apprehension, anxiety, agitation, or confusion.

9. 4. Rationale: These symptoms occur early in the disease process. The others listed (pulselessness, pallor, inability to move joints, and swelling) are late signs, and fever and erythema are indicative of an infection.

10. 1. Rationale: This test is less invasive than a pulmonary angiogram and is readily available.

11. 2. Rationale: This should be avoided, because it might cause a flexion contracture of the extremity.

Chapter 61

1. 2. Rationale: Sperm generation in the male is dependent on testosterone production, which is mediated by FSH and LH.

2. 3. Rationale: Menstruation is the result of decreasing production of estrogen and progesterone by the corpus luteum.

3. 1. Rationale: In both the male and female body, the fundamental physiological responses to effective sexual stimulation are vasocongestion and muscle tension (myotonia).

4. 4. Rationale: All of the answers are correct.

5. 4. Rationale: That question does not pertain to any prospective that might help a health care provider assess a medical situation.

6. 1. Rationale: The symptom commonly associated with sexually transmitted infections in the male is penile discharge with pain on urination.

7. 3. Rationale: The question "Violence is a problem for many women. Has someone been hurting you"? is a very important question to ask.

8. 4. Rationale: The description of vaginal discharge that is indicative of possible bacterial vaginosis is that it is copious, gray, malodorous, or "fishy" odor discharge.

9. 1. Rationale: The diagnostic tests recommended to evaluate the nodule are prostate ultrasonography, biopsy of nodule, and PSA.

10. 1. Rationale: The Pap smear examines the transformation zone between columnar epithelial cells of the cervical canal and the squamous cells covering the outer cervix.

11. 4. Rationale: The rationale for teaching an 18-year-old male how to perform self-examination of his genitals is that testicular cancer is the most common type of cancer in young men.

12. 3. Rationale: It is the best response for a female patient that has indicated she has sex with multiple partners and she does not use condoms, because she is on oral contraceptives.

Chapter 62

1. 4. Rationale: Nonprescription relief measures for dysmenorrhea include heat, exercise, and NSAIDs.

2. 3. Rationale: Dysmenorrhea that is suddenly worse may indicate the presence of endometriosis, fibroids, ovarian cysts, or infection.

3. 1. Rationale: The health implications for PCOS are insulin resistance leading to glucose intolerance and diabetes, infertility, and hyperlipidemia.

4. 2. Rationale: Weight reduction is the first priority in the management of PCOS.

5. 5. Rationale: Women experiencing vasomotor symptoms of menopause may be helped by the following interventions: wearing layered clothing, reducing the environmental temperature, increased exercise, weight reduction, smoking cessation if applicable, and relaxation techniques.

6. 3. Rationale: The most common serious complication of untreated chlamydia is infertility associated with tubal infection.

7. 5. Rationale: Educational messages for women with a diagnosis of an STD should include the following concepts:
   • The only way to completely prevent transmission of STD is to abstain from sex.
   • Condoms provide some protection against STDs but must be used consistently and correctly.
   • Condoms are most effective in preventing infections such as human immunodeficiency virus (HIV), gonorrhea, chlamydia, and trichomoniasis transmitted by contact with mucous membranes. They are less effective in preventing those infections transmitted by skin contact, such as herpes simplex virus (HSV), human papillomavirus (HPV), and syphilis.
   • If one STD is diagnosed, infection with another STD is likely and testing for all STDs is advised.

- It is important to take all the prescribed antibiotics, even after symptoms resolve.
- It is important not to have any sexual contact with an untreated infected partner.
- It is important to keep follow-up appointments.

8. 4. Rationale: Fibroids are the most common reason for hysterectomy.

9. 4. Rationale: Didelphic reproductive anomalies are generally associated with normal pregnancy outcomes, as long as there are two functional uteri, cervices, and vaginas that communicate to the outside.

10. 1. Rationale: The initial workup for infertility should include a semen analysis and charting of BBT to diagnose ovulation.

11. 4. Rationale: HPV is the virus associated with cervical cancer.

12. 3. Rationale: The decline in cervical cancer incidence is directly related to the increased use of Pap smear screening.

13. 2. Rationale: The BRCA1 and BRCA2 genes are associated with an increased risk of ovarian cancer.

14. 3. Rationale: Endometrial cancer is the most common reproductive cancer in women.

15. 1. Rationale: Urinary complications are the most common complications of FGM.

16. 4. Rationale: Lack of libido is the most common sexual dysfunction.

Chapter 63

1. 3. Rationale: The other acronyms are not hormones that act on the breast.

2. 2. Rationale: Women should be examined in the upright and supine positions; dimpling is best detected with the woman raising both arms over her head; and palpation of the breasts begins with the lymph nodes.

3. 2. Rationale: Bleeding from the nipples can be caused by trauma including fissures, as well as malignancy; fissures are associated with nipple trauma during suckling and increase the risk of mastitis; and discharge from the nipples is only normal during lactation and rarely, as a result of strong massage. Therefore, discharge under other circumstances needs to be evaluated by a health care professional.

4. 2. Rationale: Fibrocystic breast changes are typically fluid-filled cysts within the breasts; intraductal papillomas occur mainly in women between the ages of 25 and 55; and mastitis occurs primarily within the first three months after childbirth.

5. 3. Rationale: Personal or first-degree family history of any cancer is correlated with increased risk for breast cancer; exposure to various environmental pollutants such as pesticides that have chemical similarities to estrogen may behave like estrogen, increasing risk of breast cancer; and hormones are thought to increase breast cancer by effecting cell proliferation, causing DNA damage and promoting cell growth.

6. 1. Rationale: FNA biopsy of nonpalpable lesions is less useful because of sampling error; the vast majority of open biopsies are performed with either local anesthesia alone or local anesthesia with intravenous sedation; and stereotactic mammography-guided biopsy is performed only if the lesion is not visualized ultrasonographically.

7. 2. Rationale: Ductoscopy is employed to directly visualize the ductal lining of the breast; it is being evaluated for use with high-risk patients; and it is being evaluated for use in resection.

8. 3. Rationale: Lumpectomy is a wide local excision or partial mastectomy. All other procedures listed involve removal of the entire breast.

9. 3. Rationale: The histological status of the axillary nodes is the single most important predictor of outcome for breast cancer patients.

10. 2. Rationale: Cost comparisons were not provided in the chapter; fewer office visits and additional surgical interventions refers to breast reconstruction not breast augmentation; and saline implants have not been in use long enough to know how long they will last, but they may need to be replaced after 10 years.

Chapter 64

1. 2. Rationale: Prostatitis is diagnosed by culturing spontaneous or expressed urethral discharge or prostate fluid.

2. 1. Rationale: TUMP is an alternative treatment that heats the prostate tissue.

3. 3. Rationale: At least two separate biopsy specimens are graded based on their differentiation from normal prostate cells.

4. 4. Rationale: Antibiotics are normally given in the management of orchitis.

5. 4. Rationale: A varicocele can be removed with surgery and is managed this way if the patient is experiencing discomfort.

6. 1. Rationale: Balanitis is usually caused by a bacterial infection.

7. 3. Rationale: A urethral stricture has a main symptom of difficulty voiding and a noticeably decreased urine stream.

8. 3. Rationale: The goal of penile cancer treatment is to remove the tumor as soon as it is detected.
9. 2. Rationale: Parasympathetic nerve impulses and hormones work together to cause the penis to become firm in an erection.
10. 3. Rationale: Priapism is differentiated with the use of Doppler flow studies.

Chapter 65

1. 1. Rationale: Biological mediators produce increased capillary permeability.
2. 4. Rationale: Hypovolemic shock state is produced by the third spacing of fluids.
3. 4. Rationale: Manifestations of anaphylactic shock include stridor and wheezing.
4. 2. Rationale: The cardiovascular system is the most common organ system to fail in severe sepsis.
5. 3. Rationale: The primary purpose for providing crystalloid solutions is to restore fluid volumes and increase preload.
6. 2. Rationale: DIC plays a role in the inflammatory process by decreasing oxygen supplies to cells.
7. 4. Rationale: A urine output of 225 cc per hour is the manifestation that would indicate a reversal of the shock process.
8. 3. Rationale: Congestive heart failure places an individual at the greatest risk for developing MODS.
9. 4. Rationale: Maximizing optimal cardiac output is the most important factor for increasing oxygen supply.
10. 3. Rationale: Noncardiogenic-pulmonary edema may result from alterations in the alveolar-capillary membrane.

Chapter 66

1. 5. Rationale: Biological weapons may cause mass casualties. They are easy to produce and inexpensive. Currently, biological weapons cannot be easily detected and may disseminated over large areas.
2. 2. Rationale: Smallpox develops as a centrifugal rash.
3. 2. Rationale: Many agents are contagious and require contact or respiratory precautions.
4. 3. Rationale: A patient with severe life-threatening injuries who most likely will not survive would be triaged as black.
5. 3. Rationale: People still experiencing stress reactions after 3 months should seek medical or psychological follow-up.
6. 2. Rationale: Not all individuals who experience a traumatic event will suffer from PTSD.
7. 1. Rationale: Airborne precautions are used when the patient is coughing, and the suspected organism is small in diameter.
8. 3. Rationale: All other answers are true.
9. 3. Rationale: Pneumonic plague occurs because of bacteria.
10. 2. Rationale: Triage is the act of prioritizing the patient's priority of care.
11. 2. Rationale: Patients with insecticide on them are considered to be contaminated with a hazardous chemical and require decontamination. Patients with hazardous materials on them who enter an emergency department may expose everyone to a potential harmful chemical.
12. 2. Rationale: SARS is contagious.

Review Activities Answers

Chapter 1

1. This activity provides insight into the kinds of legislation that may directly or indirectly impact health care or nursing practice.

2. This activity assists the reader to gain understanding about how legislators inform the positions they take on health care bills.

3. Nurses observe shortcomings of the health care system 24/7 and are in an excellent position to identify "what if" situations. An innovation in health care delivery could be born out of this brainstorming activity.

4. It is not unusual for someone to "dump" feelings of anger, frustration, fear, or fatigue from an object of high risk for retribution to an object of lower risk for retribution. Those objects may be quite independent of each other. We all need to step back from negative situations and examine what might be influencing the negative behavior.

5. Some state boards of nursing and attorneys general take punitive action against nurses who are chemically dependent, and other states consider chemical dependence to be an illness and provide supportive assistance toward recovery. Such support may include a recovery program and long-term random testing.

Chapter 2

1. There is no specific solution to this activity, because the reader is free to pursue a questionable practice from the reader's clinical experience. The reader might choose to look for research evidence that raising the upper half of side rails is just as effective at preventing patient falls as raising the entire side rail. The activity is meant to provoke skepticism in the reader about the effectiveness of a nursing intervention and engender a spirit of curiosity about whether the activity is supported by evidence that can be found in a rigorous database.

2. Similarly, there is no specific solution to this activity, because the reader is directed to choose the topic. The activity is meant to demonstrate whether there is congruence between the databases on any identical topic.

3. A conclusion that the reader might draw is that one database is more useful to the nurse than the other. Such usefulness might be based on the breadth of subjects included, the clarity of the content, or the transferability of the content to practice.

4. If the reader finds the site useful a decision about whether a change in personal practice or a change in the practice guidelines of a health care enterprise is indicated. If a change is indicated based on solid scientific evidence, the reader will need to consider how best to implement the change.

5. It is anticipated that the reader will become aware of the value of evidence for improving nursing practice and of the potential impact that an individual nurse might make in the application of knowledge for nursing practice.

Chapter 3

1. Cognitive domain: patient understanding how the kidneys work

   Affective domain: patient having a caring attitude toward his or her spouse who is ill

   Psychomotor domain: patient is able to change his or her ostomy appliance without assistance

2. Anxiety, anger, pain, and fatigue are four barriers to learning. The following are the interventions for each:

   Anxiety: inform the patient that the surgery will cure his or her inflammation of the appendix

   Anger: allow the patient to vent his or her emotions regarding his or her new diagnosis of cancer

   Pain: ask the patient to rate his or her pain from 0 to 10

   Fatigue: schedule rest periods every hour so the patient can recover from his or her malaise

3. A combination of teaching methods increases the potential for learning.

4. Student will self-reflect on his or her own learning needs.

5. Student will develop a flow sheet that diagrams a simple teaching plan for a patient in the clinical setting

6. The student should choose two learning needs of a patient in his or her clinical setting and describe interventions for each learning need.

7. The nursing implications for Maslow are based on identifying the priority of the patient needs. This allows the nurse to set priorities and to seek interventions that will most benefit the patient.

8. The student will interview another student and ask if there is a relationship between any physical manifestations and his or her attitudes. In addition, the student will ask the peer if he or she feels better physically when he or she is mentally relaxed or vice versa.

9. The student will interview five people and ask them how they know when they are healthy. The student will also list the determinants of their health.

10. The student will list those things that motivate him or her regarding choosing healthy behaviors. In addition, the student will reflect on how these factors can assist him or her working with patients in health promotive interventions.

Chapter 4

1. Culture refers to knowledge, beliefs, behaviors, ideas, attitudes, values, habits, customs, languages, symbols, rituals, ceremonies, and practices that are unique to a particular group of people. Ethnicity, on the other hand, is a cultural group's perception of themselves or group identity. This self-perception influences how others perceive the group's members.

2. The factors that contribute to the multiculturalism environment in the United States revolve primarily around the fact that the U.S. population has shown an increase in ethnic and racial diversity during the last half of the 20th century, especially in the last three decades. Immigration from Latin America, Asia, and the Pacific Islands has contributed to the growing U.S. diversity. The population of races that are different from the Caucasian or African American populations has demonstrated significant growth, but Caucasians continue to be the most numerous race. In addition, Hispanic (Americans) are the fastest growing ethnic minority, having more than doubled from 1980 to 2000. Factors that contribute to the tremendous growth include high

levels of immigration and high fertility levels. Also, the percentage of Asian (American) and Pacific Islander populations more than doubled to 3.8 percent in 2000. The Caucasian population has shown a noticeable proportional decrease in the total U.S. population. Last, the 2000 census was the first time that individuals were allowed to identify themselves as being of more than one race.

3. Discuss how a nurse can provide culturally and linguistically competent nursing care. Even when both patient and nurse speak the same language, communication problems may occur because of varying cultural contexts in which words have different meanings to different people. Therefore, the nurse needs to be aware of all aspects of communication among cultures. Also, utilizing a qualified interpreter is imperative to achieving communication when the nurse and patient do not speak the same language, regardless of the practice domain or site. In addition, the nurse must remember that nonverbal communication can be culturally misunderstood through the presence, or absence, of eye contact.

4. This is best applied in the practicum and laboratory settings. You can refer to an assessment text and develop questions to ask patients. In addition, you can discuss the topic with peers and work on the questions together.

5. This is best applied in the practicum and laboratory settings. You can refer to an assessment text and develop questions to ask patients. In addition, you can discuss the topic with peers and work on the questions together.

6. This is best applied by exploring the Web site provided (i.e., http://erc.msh.org) to learn more about Kleinman's explanatory health model. After visiting the Web site develop questions that could have been asked of the Hmong family described in *The spirit catches you and you fall down* by Ann Fadiman (1997).

Chapter 5

1. Implemented by contacting the chairperson of an IRB and discussing your impressions in class.

2. Implemented by contacting the chairperson of an ethics committee and discussing your impressions in class.

3. Performed in the practicum setting with the identification of an ethical dilemma and an appropriate ethical theory.

4. Evaluated by obtaining a copy of advanced directives, completing the form, and sharing your emotional thoughts related to filling out the form with your classmates.

5. Active euthanasia would support a person other than the patient to make the decision of do-not-resuscitate the patient. This is in contrast with passive euthanasia, which would withhold resuscitative measures from a patient who is in the terminal stages of physical life. The passive euthanasia would honor the patient's request to withhold lifesaving measures, but health care providers would not intentionally withhold treatment against the patient's desires.

Chapter 6

1. Best accomplished by accessing the Robert Havinghurst information at: http://personalwebs.oakland.edu and then interviewing a middle-aged or older adult who has or had siblings and summarizing the findings. The student will examine the interview related to the birth order of the siblings of the interviewee, the four stages of life, and the aspects of sibling relationships into the adult years.

2. Best accomplished by accessing the body mass index (BMI) measuring instrument at: http://www.consumer.gov/weightloss.bmi.htm. The BMI is calculated and then identify the risk factors you may have. In addition, determine the BMI of a family member and compare those risk factors with your own.

3. Best applied by accessing the Activity Pyramid at: http://www.mypyramid.gov/pyramid. Then design an exercise program for the inactive individual and include how to overcome potential barriers to an exercise program, such as lack of time, no convenient access to exercise center, etc.

4. Accomplished at the Activity Pyramid site, and reviewing all the topics inside the pyramid. Review the information for kids, for professionals, and my pyramid tracker and review the new dietary pyramid guidelines. Plan a menu for one day for you that meets the guidelines.

5. Best accomplished by locating the tool kit to prevent senior falls provided by the National Center for Injury and Prevention and Control at: http://www.cdc.gov/ncipc. In addition, an interview with a friend or family member who is living independently in the community is performed. And the tool kit to assess vision and balance capability is performed. Identify whether there is any assistance needed, if any, for accomplishing activities of daily living or impaired activities of daily living. Explore what safety features should be addressed in the home environment as addressed in the tool kit guidelines.

6. Applied by reviewing the tips for care of aging parents provided by the National Safety Council at http://www.nsc.org. A poster is prepared using these tips and presenting the information to a small community group (such as a church group or parent-teacher association [PTA]).

7. Accomplished by reviewing the techniques to improve patient safety (TIPS) provided by the Joint Commission Resources at: http://www.doody.com/TIPS and clicking on Obese Patients. Then a summary report of the strategies is written.

8. Best performed by accessing one of the resources and writing a brief report on the mission or services provided.

Chapter 7

1. If the nurse has been employed at the enterprise for several years, a variety of hospice and palliative care situations have probably been experienced, some particularly rewarding and perhaps others that have been quite challenging. There are patients or families who stand out in every nurse's memory, but those who stand out for the hospice and palliative care nurse may do so for reasons that are different from your experiences. Because students do not generally have an opportunity for clinical experience in a hospice or palliative care setting, learning about that aspect of nursing from someone who may feel passionately about the care could spark your interest in a unique area of practice.

2. If you choose to access a site providing health care policy information, you may discover that something you or your colleagues do routinely is actually regulated. Such a discovery ought to provoke a change in your practice or that of those nurse colleagues with whom you may share the information. In addition, your interest in health care policy may be sparked, and you may venture into the political advocacy arena.

3. One of the most advantageous ways to learn about ethnic and religious beliefs is through the firsthand application of those who hold them. Nuances, variations from region to region, and experiences that have shaped the actual practice of someone you know can put "life" into what otherwise might be considered irrelevant concepts. Consideration of others' beliefs and practices in comparison to your own might also suggest interesting practices that you may try out.

   Understanding the rationale for people's beliefs and behaviors directly from them may help you to better respect their diversity.

4. Patients and families who have a long track record of open or closed communication tend to continue that communication pattern during end-of-life interaction. If you observe closed communication that could be regretted after death, it would be appropriate for you to consult your care team colleagues and include interventions by an expert to try to support more open communication between the patient and the family.

5. The Jehovah's Witnesses forbade organ transplant in 1967 but reversed that decision in 1980. Organ transplant and organ donations are considered matters of individual choice. There is no biblical injunction against taking in body tissue or bone as there is against taking in blood.

Chapter 8

1. Health perception/health management pattern: 4, 10
   Nutrition metabolic pattern: 6
   Elimination pattern: 5
   Activity-exercise pattern: 2, 3, 7
   Sleep-rest pattern: 4
   Self-perception/self-concept pattern: 4
   Role-relationship pattern: 1, 8
   Sexuality/reproductive pattern: 1
   Coping/stress tolerance pattern: 4, 8
   Value/belief pattern: 9

2. O: "What brings you to the clinic today?"

   O: "I spoke with your primary care physician who made the referral for your hospital admission."

   W: "The last time we met, you told me you were on a diet. I see that your clothes fit much looser and that your face appears thinner. How much weight have you lost?"

   C: "I have completed the physical examination and our time is about up."

3. Open ended: "How many children do you have?"
   Open ended: "How what are your thoughts about having surgery?"
   Open ended: "What questions do you have about your new medication?"

4. The issue is her unwillingness to allow her family to be informed. The primary duty of the nurse is to the patient and to protecting her confidentiality. Professional code of conduct: If the potential for harm to another is serious, this confidentiality may be breached. A prudent and professional approach for the nurse is to explore the reasons for withholding this information from her siblings

Chapter 9

1. The nurse could explain to Martha the CF is an autosomal recessive inherited condition. Because Martha's sister has had a child with CF she is a carrier. This means that Martha's chance to be a carrier is increased (one in two chance). It would be appropriate to discuss with Martha that carrier testing for CF are available to help further define Martha's actual carrier status. If Martha decides to have carrier testing for CF and is found to be a carrier, then carrier testing would be offered to her husband. If both Martha and her husband are identified to be CF carriers, then prenatal diagnosis (e.g., amniocentesis) would be discussed. In this situation, the nurse's role is identifying individuals for whom genetic testing is available and referring individuals for genetic testing.

2. Because Mrs. R. is 35 years old, she has a higher risk for having a baby born with a chromosomal abnormality, such as Down syndrome. It would be appropriate to discuss prenatal diagnosis, such as amniocentesis. Before talking with Mrs. R. about her increased chance to have a baby with a chromosomal abnormality and the availability of prenatal diagnosis, the nurse would want to assess Mrs. R's health beliefs—how she views pregnancy, prenatal testing, and disability—whether prenatal testing is something she would consider. You could provide her with information about maternal age risks and prenatal testing in Spanish and refer her to Web sites with culturally appropriate descriptions of the testing.

3. Ann's personal and family history of depression suggests that this condition is inherited in an autosomal dominant manner with affected individuals in multiple generations. Ann is referring to pharmacogenomic testing—testing an individual to determine their particular genotype before prescribing a particular medication at a particular dose. You could respond to Ann by explaining that pharmacogenomic testing is increasingly available to individualize treatment and avoid adverse effects. You could refer Ann to her psychiatrist for further discussion about specific testing that would be appropriate for her.

4. You could explain to Susan that the constellation of congenital heart defects, cleft palate, and learning and speech issues in multiple generations does suggest the possibility of an inherited genetic condition or syndrome. You could offer Susan a referral to a geneticist for further genetic evaluation and counseling to determine whether there is an identifiable genetic condition in the

family and whether diagnostic and prenatal diagnostic testing is available to Susan.

5. Jane's family history of early-onset breast and ovarian cancer suggest the presence of a hereditary breast or ovarian cancer syndrome that is inherited in the family in an autosomal dominant manner. As the nurse practitioner, you could explain to Jane that genetic testing for hereditary breast ovarian cancer is now available to individuals and families at increased risk. You could offer Jane a referral for further genetic evaluation and counseling so that she can have the option to pursue genetic testing for hereditary breast or ovarian cancer.

Chapter 10

1. It is important to emphasize to the patient that there are common responses to stress, particularly as related to a crisis such as cancer. Describe that some of the potential physiological responses are increased heart rate, heart palpitations, diaphoresis, and rapid respirations. Educate the patient that some of the potential psychological responses are depression, worry, frustration, anger, and anxiety. In addition, explain that elderly patients are particularly prone to confusion.

2. Identifying the role of caregiver stress is essential for the family providing care to an elderly relative. Explain that stress causes a wide range of physiological and psychological as described in activity 1 and that the care providers should first accept these responses. Then describe to the family the need to adapt to their stress responses and identify constructive coping mechanisms to their stress.

3. From Orem's theory, explain that the recent surgery has caused stress, and encourage the patient to self-evaluate the surrounding stressors and the environment. Assist the patient in identifying the necessity for understanding what elements of the situation are under the patient's control. Encourage the patient to carefully follow the suggested nursing interventions that can effectively reduce stress. In addition, the nurse needs to consider the patient's self-care needs when providing patient education and implementing the plan of care.

4. Student evaluates stress level and develops a written plan for reducing stress.

5. Student evaluates their interview with a peer and writes an evaluation of the effectiveness of their coping strategies.

Chapter 11

1. This will be accomplished in student's clinical practice.

2. This will be accomplished in student's clinical practice.

3. This will be accomplished in student's clinical practice.

4. The following guidelines are to be followed when caring for any patient:
   - Nonsterile gloves must be worn when touching any body fluid, secretions, or contaminated items. Hands must be washed after removing the gloves.
   - Masks, eye protection, and face shields should be used when there is a possibility of splashes or sprays of body fluids reaching the face of the health care worker. The level of protection is determined by the degree of exposure expected.
   - Gowns should be worn to protect the health care person's skin and clothing when exposure to blood, body fluids, secretions, or excretions. The gown is to be removed prior to leaving the patient's room, and hands should be washed after removal of the gown.
   - Patient care equipment exposed to body fluids or excretions should be handled so that any contamination is removed prior to use with another patient.
   - Each facility must have procedures for the cleaning of all equipment and environmental surfaces.
   - Linens should be handled, transported, and then cleaned to prevent transfer of possible organisms to others. Adequate laundry facilities will be sufficient to destroy any possible pathogens.
   - All sharp instruments must be handled in a way to prevent injury to any person. Needles are not removed from syringes after use and are placed in a puncture-proof container.
   - Sharp instruments must be cleaned and disposed of with care.

5. a. The nurse should survey the skin of the wound area for: signs of inflammation, the type of drainage, the size, and depth of wound.
   b. The nurse should monitor the appropriate laboratory tests to monitor the process of wound healing (e.g., white blood cells/differential counts, hemoglobin/hematocrit levels, wound culture).
   c. Ensure appropriate nutrition that is vital to promoting wound healing. Protein is needed to supply the amino acids required to build new tissue.

d. Maintain a moist environment that encourages reepitheliazation and wound healing.

e. Mechanical debridement when the amount of nonviable tissue in the wound is minimal.

f. To maintain optimal conditions for wound healing, care must be taken to prevent further injury.

Chapter 12

1. One liter of fluid weighs one kilogram. A diuresis of 2,500 mL will be evidenced by a weight loss of approximately 2.5 kg. The weight today will be 59.5 kg.

2. Answers vary based on patient selected.

3. Patients with fluid volume deficit need isotonic fluid replacement. Appropriate intravenous (IV) solutions include normal saline and Ringer's lactate.

4. Patients with increased secretion of ADH will have retention of water and reduced urine output. The retention of water will dilute the bloodstream and will be indicated by a low serum osmolality and hyponatremia.

5. A patient with intracellular dehydration needs hypotonic IV solutions. This will make the extracellular fluid compartment hypotonic in relation to a concentrated intracellular space. As a result, fluid will shift from the extracellular space into the intracellular compartment correcting the intracellular dehydration.

Chapter 13

1. Practice demonstrating in a laboratory setting and then apply setting up intravenous (IV) infusion equipment in the practicum setting.

2. Infiltration is caused from fluid leaking into the interstitial space, and it causes swelling, pain, skin pallor, and coolness to touch. Phlebitis is caused by something that inflames the vein and has clinical manifestations of swelling, pain, skin redness, and warmth.

3. Correctly and accurately setting the IV rate is done first by practicing the skills in the laboratory setting and then applied in the practicum setting. The nurse preceptor or clinical faculty person should supervise the process.

4. Patients are indicated for TPN when they are not able to either mechanically eat enough to be well nourished or who are malnourished from a disease process. In addition, patients who are indicated for TPN are also those who have poor swallowing abilities and those who have some type of neurological deficiency.

5. This is evaluated in the clinical practicum setting and should be done under the supervision of the clinical faculty or nurse preceptor.

Chapter 14

1. The students will be able to know how the individual perceives acupuncture as a means to promote health or ease symptoms of illness.

2. The activity will provide new insight to the purpose of physical therapy, especially the use of therapeutic massage. Preparation of the report will assist the student to reflect on the experience, use communication skills during the interview, analyze the article(s), and practice writing skills in preparing the report.

3. This activity involves critical thinking and problem-solving skills as well as creative thinking skills in developing the case study and designing a holistic patient-centered care plan.

4. This activity involves the student in actively investigating the items that are available to the public. It also involves research to determine what interactions, if any, between the product ingredients and medications and food. Creating the poster and considering how it would create awareness is an appropriate teaching/learning strategy for fellow students or a public group.

5. The student will learn to develop appropriate questions to use in an informal survey and will be able to obtain information about the use of CAM. Higher level cognitive skills will be used in analyzing the findings. Preparing the report involves the use of critical thinking and communication skills.

Chapter 15

1. Many times the woman's activities focus around taking care of others and assuming roles as wife, mother, and possibly an employee. The woman now becomes a patient. Examine the impact of the cancer care waiting times, such as in clinics or doctors offices. Examine the effects of fatigue on running a household and taking kids to after school activities. For the woman, the usual patterns are gone, and role reversal occurs from caretaker to patient. It might help to tell others; even though the public's understanding of cancer is generally improving, some prejudices and wariness remain and she may be concerned about this for her spouse and children. Problems that occur within any family can be the most difficult to handle simply, because she cannot go home to escape them. Some family members may deny the reality of

cancer or refuse to discuss it. Her children may be asked also to behave exceptionally well, to play quietly, or contribute to household chores. The children may receive less attention, and some will fear the loss of their parent. It may help if a favorite relative or family friend can devote extra time and attention to the children, who need comfort and reassurance, affection, guidance, and discipline.

2. Effective communication is a critical skill for nurses. Nurses also need to assume responsibility for lifelong learning. Effective communication using multiple techniques expands options for continuing learning and for communicating with patients when they are outside of the clinical setting. Good communication facilitates groups and individuals sharing their ideas and experiences. E-mail, teleconferencing, and videoconferencing help to bridge some of the geographical barriers, but nurses need to become comfortable in using these tools. Identify a group, such as a class team or course section. Group members can lead review and response to selected topics in a threaded discussion format. Examples: prepare an environmental assessment of a local environment. The activity can include a comparative evaluation of the relative toxicity of common household products or selected chemotherapeutic agents the nurse may encounter on the unit. Discussion points: Using material safety data sheets (MSDS) available from the Internet; product inserts; poison control information service; include opportunities for interpretation and understanding of graphical and statistical information.

How can we overcome the barriers or obstacles that stand in the way of pursuing good health habits and medical screening or intervention? Post a cancer case study, pose questions; accurate answers or creative problem solving questions earn points or awards. Issues: health beliefs and practices are intertwined intimately with cultural and familial traditions, how might this effect screening and early detection of breast and cervical cancer. Much emphasis of cancer care is related to screening for early detection. Many in our society have limited health care access, does this create discrimination of service. Access is more than availability. Access includes consideration of distance, trust, and cost. How might these situations impact a woman needing annual breast cancer screening?

3. Preparation is the key to a successful work reentry. Reintegration planning includes consideration of the patient, the family, and the employer.

For the patient: have the patient keep a log so that he has some idea of how long he can tolerate activity and begin with brief time intervals at the job. Discuss how he will handle coworkers'

reactions to any changes in appearance. Discuss plans for protection of exposure to office communicable illnesses. Allow time for patient to discuss concerns about returning.

Employer: Offer to have someone from the care team contact the employer to respond to concerns. Possible work concerns: effect of medication on performance; any behavior changes from medication or treatment; anticipated physical tolerance; contact plan in case of complications; what to do if health issues occur at work; special considerations needed for return. The employee may benefit from flextime, job sharing, or telecommuting.

Family: Talk with the family early on about the importance of communicating with friends, coworkers, and the employer during the course of the illness, so they are ready to transition the patient back. Family should have a clear contact plan that they can share if they need to be contacted suddenly on the patient's return. Other planning topics for discussion: observing for signs and symptoms of fatigue of side effects; fears they may have about the patient's ability to return to activities of daily living; and planning for dietary or treatment needs during the work shift.

4. Some risk factors for cancer (like family history) are out of your control, but you can control some of the important risk factors for most types of cancer, such as your exposure to sunlight and tanning beds. Research supports that ultraviolet (UV) light damages the deoxyribonucleic acid (DNA) in cells. Usually body repairs this damage but occasionally a cell mutates during the repair process, accumulation of these mutated cells can result in cancer.

Fun in the sun: UV exposure; controllable; tanning beds versus outdoor exposure; skin and eye issues; sunscreens. Severe sunburn increases your risk of developing melanoma. In fact, five doses of sunburn while you are young can double your risk of developing this deadly disease later in life. Mild sunburn or tanning is also not acceptable. Myth: tanning bed exposure is safe, if you do not burn you do not do damage. There is no safe way to expose yourself to the sun without increasing your risk of skin cancer. It is actually worse to go to the tanning parlor and get a little bit each day than it is to get infrequent sunburn. Myth: if you use sunscreen you will not get skin cancer. Sunscreens are useful in reducing skin cancer risk, but they can not provide total protection from UV rays. Sunscreen is not a substitute for seeking shade, wearing protective clothing and avoiding the midday sun, when rays are strongest. In addition, sunscreen is not recommended for infants under six months of age. Skin cancer is not sexy.

Cigarette ads. Facts: Smoking causes lung cancer. As soon as you stop smoking, your risk of lung cancer starts to go down; smoking is a risk factor for all cancers associated with the larynx, oral cavity, and esophagus. Myth: smoking pipes and cigars is OK. Fact: other forms of tobacco, such as cigars, chewing tobacco, and snuff can also cause cancer; like cigarette smoking, the risks from cigar smoking increase with increased exposure. Myth: smoking low tar cigarettes is safe. Fact: research shows that people who cut back, or switch to low tar cigarettes, may often inhale more deeply and can be just as addicted to nicotine as people who smoke more; filtered and low tar cigarettes might reduce risk slightly, but most smokers cancel this out by taking more puffs, deeper puffs or smoking more cigarettes. If you smoke with your buddies, be prepared to die of cancer with your buddies.

5. This is best applied in the practicum setting by providing care for a patient with cancer. Journal your thoughts and discuss your reflections with peers in clinical seminar and laboratory settings.

Chapter 16

The activities have been structured around World Wide Web sites to encourage the reader to actively research the many resources that are available. Some of the Web sites have interactive programs. Some of the materials can be downloaded free of charge and can be used as patient instructional materials. The various activities also stimulate critical thinking and can easily be used as individual or group assignments as part of the course requirements or as extra-activities.

Chapter 17

1. Digoxin: Highly protein bound and has many drug-to-drug interactions. If given with warfarin (Coumadin, also highly protein bound), the amount of free drug is increased, and both drugs can produce adverse effects because of changes in their levels. Changes in nutritional status (decrease in albumin and decreases receptor sites) and electrolytes can affect drug levels.

   Tetracycline: Avoid administration with milk products, because it will form inactive compounds. Administer on an empty stomach. Use with caution in patients with renal impairment.

2. Develop a nursing care plan for a patient with emphasis on pharmacological interventions. Discuss the clinical manifestations of a specific medical disorder, such as congestive heart failure. Identify the selected medications used (digoxin and furosemide [Lasix]), baseline laboratory monitoring (electrolytes and renal function), informed consent and medication teaching, first dose monitoring (hypotension), and evaluation (improvement in lung sounds, respiratory effort, and edema).

3. Set up scenario for student that includes a patient (put an armband on the patient), a medication administration record (MAR), and a medication. Student should demonstrate getting the medication, checking the label, and then checking it against the MAR. The MAR should be taken to the patient, the MAR checked with the patient armband, and once again with the medication. Student should ask about allergies prior to administering medication. Administer medication. Document on the MAR and if needed in the nurses notes (for as needed medications).

4. Side effects are predictable effects of the prescribed medication. These effects can be either desirable or undesirable. An example of a desirable effect might be the sedation that results with antihistamines may help improve sleep if taken at bedtime. An undesirable effect of the same medication might be the sedation when the patient needed to be alert for daily activities. Adverse effects are not predictable or desirable. They pose potentially life-threatening problems and require the medication to be discontinued.

5. An example cited in the text was the death caused to the patient by administering intravenous (IV) medication too fast. Can be prevented by looking up the drug prior to administering to determine recommended time to push medication.

   Other errors that are documented include errors that result from drugs having similar names (wrong drug) and patients that have similar names (wrong patient).

6. Monitor drug levels. Observe patient for side effects and adverse effects. Carefully monitor drug efficacy.

7. Assess for allergies, drug, and food. If there is evidence of hypersensitivity response, stay with patient and notify physician immediately. Maintain airway and prepare to administer epinephrine. An antihistamine, such as Benadryl, may be ordered for a milder reaction. Monitor patients for a period of time after giving medications, such as penicillin.

Chapter 18

1. Individuals form opinions based on their own experiences. This activity encourages the reader to look outside of personal experiences to gain understanding about others' experiences with the

health care system and how those experiences may have promoted differing perceptions about the health care system from his or her own perceptions. It also encourages the reader to develop the habit of considering the perceptions of others.

2. As the American cultural demographic becomes more diverse, it becomes essential for health care providers to develop skills in culturally competent care. Exposing the reader to Web sites like this tool box not only gives them an enjoyable way to learn, it may also introduce them to a new resource.

3. Nurse theorists, such as Nightingale and Henderson, as well as other nurse leaders, acknowledge that the environment for care can make a significant impact on the quality of care outcomes. Nurses can gauge the tone of the environment for care through their senses and make a judgment about the level and quality of care being provided.

4. The synergy model is a relatively new concept. In striving for exemplary patient care and, perhaps, magnet status agencies ought to consider the impact that implementation of synergy concepts could make toward accomplishment of such goals. This activity provides an opportunity for the reader to teach.

5. A common concern is whether needed health care can be easily accessed. Nurses are often sought to answer such a question for patients and their families. Having such knowledge at hand can facilitate choices for care that ensure safe passage through the health care agency system.

Chapter 19

1. The patient is at risk for oxygen toxicity with the FiO_2 at 70 percent. The patient is also on too high of a tidal volume for his weight. This puts the patient at risk for respiratory alkalosis and barotrauma. Other complications associated with mechanical ventilation are ventilator-associated pneumonia, tracheal damage, anxiety, and problems with communication, stress ulcers, and fluid retention.

2. Respiratory alkalosis; possible ventilator changes may include reduction of the FiO_2, reduction of the tidal volume, or ventilator rate. Depending on the patient's respiratory rate, the patient may also need sedation.

3. The patient's room should be kept as dark as possible and quiet. Nursing cares should be spaced to allow for rest periods. The patient's vital signs should be monitored frequently to assess for changes associated with increasing intracranial

pressure or changes in temperature. Complete neurological assessments should be completed to monitor for increases in intracranial pressure. The patient should be monitored for seizure activity and should be on antiepileptic medication to prevent seizures. The patient may be receiving diuretic therapy to prevent increases in cerebral edema. The patient's head should be kept in a neutral position to allow for venous drainage that helps to prevent increases in intracranial pressure. The patient's oxygenation should be carefully monitored to ensure adequate oxygenation of brain cells.

4. The family will be fearful and wanting information on prognosis and current status. The intensive care unit environment can also be intimidating to the family. The nurse can explain the intravenous (IV) lines and therapies. The nurse can give some information on current status (for example, blood pressure) and the need for mechanical ventilation. The nurse should also encourage the family to talk to the patient and let him know they are at the bedside. The physician can also be contacted to talk to the family. Financial concerns are common when the family has a loved one in the intensive care unit. The cost of intensive care unit care combined with not working can be a concern for the patient and family. Contacting social services may be helpful in this area. The family is also probably wondering if the patient will be able to work any more at all. Again, social services may be helpful. They will need teaching regarding initial home care needs and medications the patient will be started on. Information on the general floor will also be helpful. It would be helpful to have a nurse from the floor come to the intensive care unit to meet the patient and explain some of the floor routine. The patient may be fearful of having another cerebrovascular accident (CVA). The nurse can reassure the patient with regard to blood pressure control and monitoring of vital signs while the patient is on the floor.

5. The critical care nurse should acknowledge the difficulty of the situation and the grief the family members are experiencing. The nurse should then offer to arrange a meeting for the family members with the health care team to help them in making this decision. Other support services available to the family are the social services, clergy, and other medical staff. The ethics committee is also available for consult if there is indecision among family members. The role of the critical care nurse in this process is to administer analgesics and sedatives prior to extubation to prevent air hunger and distress. The nurse will also provide support and comfort to the family, information on what will

occur during the process of extubation, and what to expect after the discontinuation of life support. Comfort measures for the patient should continue to be a priority after mechanical ventilation has been withdrawn. The nurse should stay with the family as needed and until the time of death if appropriate.

Chapter 20

1. Decisional conflict, impaired comfort, risk for acute pain, risk for delayed surgical recovery, fear, and many others.

2. Some preoperative care trends would be inside-the-body biofeedback and monitoring systems with implanted chips and miniaturized intervention systems, distance monitoring leading up to the time of surgery through streaming video and digital diagnostics. Other trends will be greater levels of assertion by preoperative nurses in relation to protection of patient decision making, autonomy, and protection.

3. End-of-life and beginning-of-life issues will continue to be predominant bioethical issues. Modern technology will continue to advance to a point at which decisions will center on quality of life rather than strictly prolonging life through surgical means or medical adjustment through internal biofeedback mechanisms.

4. The nurse may safely advise the patient or family to use certain steps to investigate a health care provider or health care facility match with the patient's surgical and recovery needs. The nurse may want to avoid personally endorsing one health care provider over another. To choose a health care provider, advise the patient to trace degree-granting institutions, publications, board certification, hospitals granting staff privileges, and finally word of mouth. To choose a hospital or surgical center, investigate hospital size (recall the 300 to 500 bed sizes mentioned in the chapter), whether the hospital is university-affiliated, and whether the hospital or medical center has a national reputation. In addition look for Magnet Status, presence of a trauma center and critical care unit(s). Finally, rely on personal observation through previsits or the experience of acquaintances.

5. Recall that major surgery involves greater than minimal risk to life in some way, such as happens with surgeries involving multiple systems or that require long periods of time in the operating suite. Minor surgery involves minimal risk to life, one body system, and minimal incision length and depth. Minor surgery can be done in a short period of time, often in a health care provider's office or freestanding surgical center. Such surgical procedures as laparoscopic appendectomy or laparoscopic cholecystectomy have largely replaced the full-incision procedure. Knee arthroscopy for repair purposes may yield the same result as knee surgery requiring more extensive incision and healing time. Many dental, eye-ear-nose-throat, and urological procedures are now done in outpatient or short-stay centers as compared with the norm of 20 to 30 years ago.

6. Procedures that require long, deep incisions and full anesthesia (as a way to relax musculature) commonly require transfusion. Examples are gastrointestinal surgery and orthopedic procedures, such as hip replacement. Cardiac or respiratory procedures that require opening and spreading the bones of the thorax would also require transfusion. Family and patient will want to be informed of preoperative self-donation possibilities or family donation. Inform patients and family that modern blood-screening techniques have greatly decreased the chance of acquiring any blood-borne pathogens, such as hepatitis or human immunodeficiency virus (HIV).

7. The nurse who is teaching in the immediate period leading up to surgery will want to consult the printed or online surgical schedule to give patient and family probable time of surgery. In addition, tell the family that the patient will leave for surgery at least an hour prior to the scheduled time. Sometimes the patient's time will be delayed because of an emergency. Sometimes the time will be advanced because of a cancellation. The nurse will describe the need for diet modification and sleep assist the evening before surgery. In addition, hygiene and changing to a hospital gown without jewelry or other personal items is usually a mandate with major surgery. The patient should practice postoperative leg exercises, painless repositioning techniques, and incentive spirometry use or deep breathing. The nurse will describe IV lines, catheters, dressings or casts, pumps, monitors, and other paraphernalia that might be present in the immediate postoperative period. The nurse should be aware of whether the agency's PACU has a ward-like appearance or seems more patient-friendly.

8. Opioids, amnesiacs, anticholinergics, antacids or proton pump inhibitors, muscle relaxants, and antibiotics are some of the more commonly encountered preoperative drugs.

9. Those with pulmonary compromise; immune system suppression or compromise; neuroendocrine disorders, such as myasthenia gravis or multiple sclerosis; hepatic disease, such as

cirrhosis or hepatitis; or chronic renal problems are at increased perioperative risk. Those with diabetes mellitus and those with chronic pancreatitis are also at risk. Those with cardiovascular disorders and patients at extreme ends of the age spectrum may be at increased risk. The disabled and those who are obese, addicted, or alcoholic present challenges, as do those with unstable psychiatric situations

Chapter 21

1.

Risk for infection	Limit and control traffic
	Use standard precautions
Risk for impaired skin integrity	Keep skin clean and dry
	Pad bony prominences
Risk of injury related to surgical environment	Shield from radiation sources
	Limit exposure to laser beam
Risk of hypothermia	Monitor room temperature and humidity
	Monitor patient vital signs, labs, intake and output

2. Appropriate nursing interventions for the care of patients with MH:
   - Hyperventilation with 100 percent O_2
   - Deepen anesthesia with opioids and sedatives, muscle relaxation with a nondepolarizing relaxant
   - Stop trigger, remove vaporizer
   - Prepare dantrolene perfusion
   - Antiarrhythmic therapy with beta blocker (esmolol 0.25 mg/kg intravenously.) or lidocaine (1 mg/kg intravenously.)
   - Cooling: for example, ice water through a nasogastric tube
   - Additional monitoring: arterial catheter, central venous catheter, swan-Ganz-catheter, urinary catheter

3. Errors: Surgery performed on the wrong patient, or the wrong surgical site, or the wrong side (if a bilateral option is present), or the wrong surgery is performed. Medication errors also exist as potential surgical problems.

   Prevention methods: Avoid performing multiple procedures on multiple parts of a patient during a single surgical encounter; failure to include the patient or family members and significant others when identifying the correct site; use of abbreviations related to the surgical procedure, site, or laterality; problems related to illegible handwriting; and incomplete or inaccurate communication among members of the surgical team.

4. Factors associated with electrical safety in the OR:
   - The ESU settings should always be confirmed verbally with the operator. Good practice is to always use the lowest possible power settings.
   - Manufacturer's instructions should be followed and approved instruments or electrodes should be used.
   - The ESU generator must be mounted securely on a cart or boom to prevent falling.
   - Items should not be placed on top of the generator—especially potentially dangerous items, such as fluids.
   - The ESU foot pedal should be kept in an impervious bag. Fluid from blood and irrigation solutions can cause a shock.

5. A sterile object remains sterile only when touched by another sterile object.

   Check for sterility by checking expiration dates, intactness and integrity of outer wraps, and sterilization indicators inside the package.

   Only sterile objects may be placed on a sterile field. If there is a question of sterility, it is considered contaminated or nonsterile.

   A sterile object or field out of the range of vision or an object held below a person's waist is contaminated.

   Reduce air currents around a sterile object by not reaching across a sterile field, keep doors and curtains closed, and move sterile objects as little as possible on a sterile field.

   When a sterile surface comes in contact with a wet, contaminated surface, the sterile object or field becomes contaminated by capillary action.

   Keep caps of open sterile bottles right side up; avoid splashing or spillage when pouring liquids.

   Keep tips of sterile instruments pointed down; keep hands up after performing a surgical hand scrub.

6. Factors that contribute to perioperative hypothermia:
   - Decreased metabolic heat production
   - Increased environmental heat loss
   - Redistribution of heat within the body
   - Induced inhibition of thermoregulation during surgical procedures
   - Patient's physical status
   - Type of anesthesia used
   - Body fat and length and type of surgical device

Chapter 22

1. The top priorities immediately after surgery center on airway, breathing pattern, tissue oxygenation (sensed through the pulse oximeter or with nursing observation), cardiac function, peripheral vascular

perfusion, renal perfusion, level of consciousness, body temperature regulation, and pain. Others might be electrolyte balance, correcting severe blood loss, and safety.

2. Pain and diminished sleep may be continuing problems. Nursing interventions derived from the Nursing Intervention Classification (NIC) system as described in other chapters are numerous. Medication, together with measures to decrease anxiety may be helpful with pain control. Arranging an environment free from disturbing stimuli might also be helpful. There is always the potential for wound or respiratory infection. Care with pulmonary measures, such as incentive spirometry and respiratory therapy, are helpful measures for the postoperative patient. Careful wound care and patient education are useful, and control of nutrition and fluid-electrolyte balance will help to avert infection. Delivery of ordered antibiotics is needed for those with active infection. Alterations in activity or gait problems may make it difficult for some patients to resume previous levels of independence. Consistent patient exercise by nursing or physical therapy will allow the patient to experience reassuring levels of progress in most cases. Knowledge deficit or home difficulties may make it more difficult for the recovering patient to make the transition to home care. Again, the nurse will deal with some matters directly, using consultation with social services or, in many cases, the entire discharge planning team.

3. Some possibilities include slowing your speech and activity patterns. Match your pace to that desired by the senior patient. Another style change involves carefully assessing readiness of the older patient to engage in physical activity or in learning activities. Biorhythms of the older patient may be different from those of younger people. Assess sensory changes and be sure to note vision or hearing difficulties. The older patient will often have difficulty clearing certain medications from the body. This is important in the case of antibiotics or perhaps with analgesics or soporifics. The nurse may want to allow the older patient to sleep in before the breakfast hour and to turn in for sleep earlier in the evening than what would work with a younger person.

4. List four possible complications for the patient recovering from surgery. Using the priorities list and the NANDA taxonomy, one can extrapolate likely life-threatening complications, such as ineffective breathing, airway disruption, air exchange problems, cardiovascular inefficiency, or excessive blood loss. Altered mental status may be a disturbing possibility for family and patient alike.

There are many other possibilities in the immediate postoperative period. Beyond the first 24 hours, hemorrhage or hematoma may be complications. Infection of wound or respiratory system is another complication that may ensue beyond the day of surgery.

5. Typical dilemmas involve management of extended recuperation needs with senior citizens. These can be traumatic for patient and spouse. Sometimes there is a dilemma when one is unable to live free without the other. Other dilemmas might involve the delivery of negative findings and the need for later nursing support. These are difficult situations and call for thorough assessment of patient and family responses, a delicate touch, and, often, calling clergy or some of the psychologists who are familiar with assisting with adaptation under difficult circumstances. There is sometimes, although rarely, a reluctance of family to support the delivery of negative prognoses. There may be conflict when the health care provider wants to fully brief the patient on probable outcome.

6. Acute pain, hypothermia, risk for aspiration, ineffective breathing pattern, impaired gas exchange, imbalanced fluid volume (risk for), decreased cardiac output (risk for), impaired tissue integrity, and many more.

7. The best measures will be demonstration of methods for keeping the dressing dry during hygiene activities. In the hospital, plastics can be temporarily placed over the old dressing prior to showering, if the surgeon has given permission for a shower. The patient should be instructed in careful hand washing and told to do that at home prior to working with the dressing and wound. The nurse should talk the patient or designated family through a dressing change, or preferably two. In addition, the nurse will observe as the patient or family member empties the JP and recharges the vacuum. What to do in case of disrupting the drain should be covered as well as observations that necessitate a call to the health care provider.

Chapter 23

1. The formations of the cells of blood come from a stem cell that differentiates into erythrocytes, granulocytes, platelets, B lymphocytes, and T lymphocytes

2. The oxygen in the erythrocyte is carried on hemoglobin; iron is a component of the hemoglobin molecule.

3. The white blood cells include granulocytes, which include the neutrophil, eosinophils, basophils, and the lymphocytes.

4. Granulocytes are formed to respond to infections and inflammation. Phagocytosis is a method used to control foreign substance by ingesting the particle. Neutrophils respond to bacterial infections. Eosinophils are more likely to be associated with infections from parasites and are more likely to be involved in allergies. Basophils are produced in the bone marrow and go to the peripheral blood and can and migrate to the tissues; in the tissues they are called mast cells. The mast cells release prostaglandins, leukotrienes, heparin, and histamine.

5. Platelets come from megakaryocytes that form thousands of platelets, which do not have nuclei but have many receptors that respond to stimuli that make the platelet sticky for forming a platelet plug.

6. The flow of blood through the heart is as follows: The blood returns to the heart from the inferior and superior vena cave and enters into the right atrium; it then flows over the tricuspid valve into the right ventricle. It then flows through the pulmonic valve into the pulmonary arteries into the pulmonary veins and enters the left atrium. When it leaves the left atrium it travels through the mitral valve into the left ventricle. As it leaves the left ventricle it is ejected through the aortic valve into the aorta and out to systemic circulation.

7. Evaluate heart sounds on a patient in the clinical practicum setting.

8. Complete a cardiovascular assessment in the clinical practicum setting.

Chapter 24

1. Mr. Anthony has stable angina (the chest pain is relieved with rest), which is likely caused by atherosclerosis because of his genetic influences, his hypertension, and his smoking. The anginal pain is caused by the irritation of lactic acid on nerve fibers from anaerobic metabolism.

2. Evaluation of this activity will take place as the student presents his or her materials to a group of student peers.

3. This experience will enhance your ability to have knowledge about diagnostic tests and the ability to share education with patients.

4. Locating local support programs will prepare you for referring patients to appropriate programs. Attending a class will give you a better understanding of the content and location while developing valuable contacts for the future.

5. Working with an advanced practice nurse in the care of the cardiac patient will provide you with a wealth of information and practice approaches to the care of the cardiac patient. This experience will also give you a better understanding of these nursing roles.

Chapter 25

1. Heart valves function much like full-length, one-directional swinging western-style bar room doors work. They allow free flow of blood in one direction. Regurgitation occurs when the valves are unable to close appropriately because of continued pressure in the ventricles, improper fitting of the valve's leaflets because of inflammation, weakness of the valves from illness, improperly shaped leaflets because of infection, and degeneration of the surface of the leaflets. Regurgitation allows some of the blood to flow back through the valve, in the opposite direction of the way the blood is meant to flow. The term stenosis is used to describe the valve's inability to properly open. This dilemma causes a reduction in the amount of blood that is allowed through the valves and a resultant increase in blood volume that remains in the heart chamber.

2. While most cases of mitral valve prolapse remain asymptomatic, some patients have symptoms such as fatigue, shortness of breath, light-headedness, dizziness, syncope, palpitations, chest pain, and anxiety. In extreme cases, the stretching of the leaflet can expand too far, and the result is sudden death.

   Assessment of mitral regurgitation often results in the patient remaining asymptomatic. When symptoms do occur, they are often vague and nonspecific and can present as fatigue, generalized weakness, dyspnea with or without exertion, palpitations, and cough. Auscultation of the heart may (or may not) reveal a systolic murmur. Palpation of the pulse may (or may not) reveal an irregular rhythm.

   Assessment of a mitral stenosis patient may reveal no symptoms or may reveal dyspnea on exertion, fatigue, and cough with hemoptysis. History often reveals chest pain, rheumatic fever, and dysphasia (Horenstein, Petersen, & Walters, 2002). Inspection may reveal a prominent wave in the jugular venous pulse, and in late stages, signs of peripheral edema, enlarged liver, ascites, and mitral facies—a florid appearance with cyanosed cheeks (if pulmonary hypertension has developed). Palpation may reveal a displace apex beat because of the enlarged right ventricle with a right ventricular heave. Auscultation of the heart may reveal a diastolic murmur and a displace apex beat. Palpation of the pulse may reveal an irregular rhythm (Saver, Hodgson, Van Norman, & Bahler, 2004).

Assessment of aortic regurgitation often reveals an asymptomatic patient. A patient history may reveal increased dyspnea on exertion, fatigue, and paroxysmal nocturnal dyspnea. Some patients may state an awareness of forceful pulsations in the upper thorax and head regions because of an increased force with which the left ventricle is required to perform. Cardiac auscultation may reveal a diastolic murmur. Upon palpation, the nurse may be able to palpate increase in intensity of carotid and temporal pulses. A hallmark sign of aortic regurgitation is a palpable pulse that is intense and then quickly weakens. The pulse pressure, the difference between the systolic blood pressure and diastolic blood pressure, described above, widens (Singh, Sharma, Nanda, Reddy, & Strom, 2004).

Assessment of aortic stenosis often reveals an absence of symptoms, whereas advanced aortic stenosis, characterized by a decrease in blood flow to the brain, results in multiple assessment findings. Dyspnea on exertion is common. Dizziness, syncope, and angina are frequently found when oxygen supplies have decreased in aortic stenosis patients. Auscultation reveals a systolic murmur, and palpation reveals a thrill.

3. Commissurotomy, a common form of valvuloplasty, is the procedure used to separate fused valve leaflets by cutting or manually pulling apart the leaflets.

Balloon valvuloplasty, a type of commissurotomy, is a cardiac catheterization laboratory procedure in which a balloon is inflated, which stretches the valve open, and separates the fused leaflets. Then the balloon is deflated and removed.

Annuloplasty is a procedure used to strengthen the junction of the leaflets to the heart muscle.

Leaflet repair is considered when the leaflets are elongated or ballooning. In the leaflet repair, the extra tissue of the leaflet is removed.

Chordoplasty is the repair of the chordae tendineae of the mitral valve. This involves repairing the defect in the shape of the chordae tendineae that causes regurgitation.

Valve replacement consists of removing the diseased valve and replacing it with a donor valve (prosthesis).

4. Nursing management of the heart valve repair or replacement surgical patient occurs in a critical care unit. Management consists of hemodynamic monitoring, anesthesia recovery, wound care, and patient teaching.

Hemodynamic monitoring involves maintaining blood pressure through administration of IV fluids and hemodynamic medications. Also important to hemodynamic monitoring is the monitoring and treatment of cardiac dysrhythmias. Anesthesia recovery involves assessment of the neurological, respiratory, and cardiovascular systems. Wound assessment and management is also important.

Patient teaching requires a simple explanation of the anatomy of heart, the functioning of coronary arteries, and explanation of surgery. Purpose of medications and side effects are also important for educating the patient. Clear explanations of the purpose for long-term anticoagulant therapy and antibiotic prophylaxis are necessary.

5. Treatment for mild symptoms includes controlling volume overload through monitoring sodium and fluid intake. Dietary restrictions of salt are recommended. Fluid intake may also be restricted. These restrictions, whether recommended in isolation or with other treatments, make up the most basic concept of volume control in the treatment of heart failure.

6. Monitoring of oxygenation via pulse oximetry and arterial blood gases is one of the more important of nursing management activities. Positioning the patient for maximum cardiovascular functioning is also important. If possible, patients should dangle legs to decrease the venous return to the heart. The head of the bed should remain elevated so that there is a decrease in the amount of lung surface area affected by the increased fluid volume. Also important in nursing management of patients with congestive heart failure is reassurance and anxiety reduction. At a time when the heart is working its hardest, anxiety can cause more work for the heart.

7. Nursing management includes assessment of symptoms: Assessment of heart failure is best accomplished through a holistic approach of gathering data from a health history, a thorough physical exam with attention paid to the cardiovascular and pulmonary systems, and objective measurement of various body parts and function.

Oxygenation measures, respiratory effort, rate, and depth of respiration on exertion and at rest provide significant information about patients with heart failure.

Nursing management includes administration and monitoring of therapeutic regimen; monitoring of oxygenation via pulse oximetry and arterial blood gases is one of the more important of nursing management activities.

Nursing management includes measuring treatment effectiveness: Evaluation of therapeutic regimens is optimal when outcomes are measurable. Generally, the objective evaluation of heart failure interventions should include an increase in oxygenation, an increase in cardiac and peripheral perfusion, a cardiovascular and peripheral vascular volume balance, an increase in activity levels, a decrease in cardiac workload, a decrease in work of breathing, a decreased anxiety level, maintenance of optimal vital signs, and an increase in quality sleep and rest.

Nursing management includes providing physiological and psychological support: reassurance and anxiety reduction. At a time when the heart is working its hardest, anxiety can cause more work for the heart.

8. Dilated cardiomyopathy (DCM), a disease of the heart muscle, results in a dilated heart chamber, which expands much the way a balloon expands. DCM results in a decreased ability for the heart to pump strongly and forcefully.

Hypertrophic cardiomyopathy (HCM) is an increase in the size and thickness of the heart muscle. The sheer size of the hypertrophic heart muscle decreases the volume of blood that can be accommodated in the heart's chambers. Likewise, the size and thickness of the hypertrophic heart muscle disallows timely cardiac relaxation that is necessary for quick blood filling of the heart chambers.

Arrhythmogenic right ventricular cardiomyopathy (ARVC) is a disease of the cardiac muscle in which the heart muscle is replaced by fibrous scar and fatty tissue. The right ventricle is more likely to be affected. The progressive loss of heart muscle affects the hearts electrical functioning, which leads to alteration in the hearts ability to effectively pump.

Restrictive cardiomyopathy (RCM) is a disease of the ventricular heart muscle in which the muscle walls become stiff but not necessarily thickened. The cause is not known, but metabolic disorders, sequela of radiation therapy, and family history of cardiomyopathy have been identified as causes in some people.

9. Maslow's Hierarchy of Needs for the following nursing diagnoses:
   a. Physiological: risk for ineffective respiratory function related to excessive secretions secondary to cardiopulmonary dysfunction.
   b. Safety: activity intolerance related to insufficient knowledge of adaptive techniques needed secondary to impaired cardiac function.
   c. Esteem: anxiety related to powerlessness and vulnerability.

10. Maslow's Hierarchy of Needs for the following nursing diagnoses:
   a. Physiological necessity: risk for ineffective respiratory function related to decreased respiratory depth.

   b. Physiological comfort: pain related to friction rub and inflammatory process.
   c. Safety: activity intolerance related to insufficient knowledge of adaptive techniques needed secondary to impaired cardiac function.

Chapter 26

1. Steps necessary in this activity include: (a) Take the defibrillator to the patient's bedside; (b) Attach the monitor or defibrillator pads to the patient's chest; (c) Turn the monitor power on and view rhythm; (d) Confirm ventricular fibrillation; (e) Charge the defibrillator to 200 joules; (f) Make sure everyone is clear of the patient and equipment and then deliver the shock; (g) Confirm continued presence of ventricular fibrillation then reshock. The intravenous (IV) supplies are typically kept in a drawer of the crash cart with IV solutions kept on the bottom of the crash cart. Frequently, emergency medications are kept in the top drawer of the crash cart.

2. Causes of sinus tachycardia in this patient could include pain, fever, hypoxia, and hypovolemia. The treatment of sinus tachycardia would be to identify why the patient is experiencing the rhythm, then to treat the underlying cause.

3. The steps of analyzing a rhythm strip are: (a) Determine the rate; (b) Determine the rhythm; (c) Determine the presence of P waves; (d) Measure the PR interval; (e) Measure the QRS interval; (f) Measure the QT interval.

4. This is answered by spending time in an acute care agency and observing in a telemetry or critical care setting.

5. The ventricular arrhythmias are generally more pathological for the patient, as these arrhythmias are more affecting to the cardiac output. The ventricle is the more significant muscle as associated with delivery of blood throughout the circulatory system.

Chapter 27

1. The concept map for a patient with abdominal aortic aneurysm is located on the following page.

2. Characteristics of decreased oxygen, related to peripheral vascular disease are:
   1. Altered sensation of the skin
   2. Brittle nail beds
   3. Thin/sparse hair
   4. Delayed healing
   5. Decreased or diminished pulses
   6. Skin discoloration, including pale
   7. Coolness of the skin

CONCEPT MAP

Patient: 54-Year-Old Male with Aortic Abdominal Aneurysm

2: Pain, back and abdominal

- R/T: statement of pain 8 of 10 scale
- AEB: need for quite environment
- AEB: need for antihypertensive medications
- AEB: need for pain medications
- AEB: no pressure or physical exam of the abdomen

1. Ineffective tissue perfusion: tissues distal to the aneurysm:

- R/T: interruption of blood flow to lower extremities
- AEB: pulsation and bruit noted in abdominal region
- AEB: neuro exam q4
- AEB: diminished pulses bilateral legs
- BP: 174/98
- AEB: need for antihypertensive medication
- AEB: lab results: list all labs R/T AAA
- AEB: abdominal X-ray demonstrating mass

4: Fear and anxiety:

- R/T: actual and potential serious complications
- AEB: lack of knowledge of the risk factors leading to AAA
- AEB: education of diagnostic test results
- AEB: need for education of surgical risks
- AEB: need for post-op instructions
- AEB: need for lifestyle changes

Reason for seeking health care:
Nausea, vomiting, back pain, abdominal pressure, legs bluish color

3. Risk for impaired skin integrity

- R/T: compromised tissue perfusion distal to the aneurysm
- AEB: bedrest
- AEB: diminished bilateral popliteal, dorsalis pedis, and pedal pulses
- AEB: parenthesis of lower extremities
- AEB: need to place on fall precautions

5. Imbalanced nutrition: more than body requirement:

- R/T: ht: 5'10" weight 215 lb
- AEB: high cholesterol diet history
- AEB: lack of exercise history
- AEB: list all labs R/T unbalanced diet
- AEB: need for replacement fluids and nutrients while experiencing N/V

Possible complications:

Hemorrhage
Aortic dissection
Hypovolemic shock
Decreased oxygen supply to tissues distal to the aneurysm

Preexisting conditions:

Hx of smoking
Hypertension
Diet high in cholesterol
Overweight

3. The following should be included in the nurse's assessment of the patient when being discharged:
   1. Knowledge of the plan of care
   2. Accurate return demonstration of skills needed to care for self
   3. Knowledge of self-care activities to prevent long-term complications
   4. Express the importance of health promotion activities and health screening
   5. Plan for physical support, either during recovery or continuous
   6. Financial assessment, patient has the finances to care for self
   7. Home safety assessment, prevention of falls and other hazards

4. The following are the primary teaching points for Coumadin administration:
   a. Coumadin is an anticoagulant, or blood thinner, which slows the normal blood clotting process. It can prevent clots form forming, but cannot dissolve blood clots which have already formed.
   b. Do not stop or increase your medication in any way or add other medications, including over the counter medications, without consulting your health care provider (physician or nurse practitioner). Many medications can alter the way Coumadin works, including increased bleeding, and interfere with the desired effects of your anticoagulant.
   c. Coumadin is taken once a day and your blood is tested routinely for the effectiveness of Coumadin. This monitoring is important as your health care provider will adjust the strength of your medication according to the results of the blood test.
   d. You should wear a Medic Alert bracelet stating you are taking this drug and are at an increased risk for bleeding.
   e. Common side effects include: stomach bloating and cramps; loss of hair and skin rashes; orange-yellow discoloration of the urine. If these side effects are persistent or irritating, notify your health care provider.
   f. Report the following side effects to your health care professional: unusual bleeding when brushing your teeth; excessive bleeding form an injury; excessive bruising; black, tarry stools; cloudy, dark urine; sore throat, fever, or chills; and headaches or dizziness
   g. Avoid: contact sports; using a straight razor; and foods high in vitamin K (dark green, leafy vegetables such as spinach).

5. Three NOC goals related to the following nursing diagnoses are: tissue perfusion, peripheral, ineffective.

Chapter 28

1. a. 1. Weight loss using DASH diet
      2. Aerobic exercise
      3. Smoking cessation
      4. Moderation of alcohol intake
      5. Salt restriction
   b. 1. The DASH diet is rich in grains, fruits, vegetables, and low-fat dairy products. The plan limits fat, saturated fat, and cholesterol while providing plentiful amounts of fiber, potassium, calcium, and magnesium. Multiple research studies have shown a reduction in blood pressure of 8 to 14 mm Hg in patients with hypertension who follow the DASH diet.
      2. The JNC VII advises all patients who are physically able to participate in regular aerobic physical activity for at least 30 minutes per day, most days of the week. Exercise strengthens muscles and at the same time opens up arteries to allow for more nutrients and oxygen to flow into the tissues. The combination of a stronger, more efficient heart and blood vessels that are more open leads to lower blood pressure.
      3. Tobacco is the single greatest cause of disease and premature death in the United States and is responsible for more than 400,000 deaths per year. Patients with high blood pressure who also use tobacco products are two to three times more likely to develop cardiovascular disease. Exposure to secondhand smoke, also called environmental tobacco smoke, is also a serious health hazard.
      4. Moderation is the best method for controlling alcohol intake. Excessive alcohol intake increases blood pressure and the calories have no nutritional value.
      5. It has been estimated that the average daily intake of sodium for individuals in the United States is between 4,000 and 6,000 mg. The majority of sodium intake is from food, and many foods naturally contain some sodium. Most sodium ingestion comes from commercially processed foods and meal preparation at home.
   c. Altered health maintenance R/T lack of knowledge of pathology, complications, and management of hypertension
      Ineffective coping R/T effects of chronic illness and major changes in lifestyle
      Ineffective sexuality patterns related to side effects of medications
      Risk for ineffective therapeutic regimen management R/T noncompliance with treatment
      Risk for ineffective coping R/T inability to cope with chronic disease

2. Subjective Data

   a. age, height, weight, allergies

   b. chronic diseases (DM, HTN, COPD)

   c. alcohol, tobacco, caffeine, drug use

Objective Data

   a. body build, general appearance

   b. blood pressure, heart rate, respirations

   c. level of consciousness

3. Causes of secondary hypertension

   Chronic kidney disease

   Renal artery stenosis

   Congenital narrowing of the aorta

Diagnostic test(s)

   Estimated GFR, MRA

   Doppler flow study

   CT angiography

4. Address the risk factors that apply to the patient, and identify realistic goals for the patient to decrease their hypertension. Refer to question 1b for further educational information.

5. Pharmacological therapy usually begins with a diuretic. Diuretics are divided into several classes: loop, potassium sparing, thiazide, and thiazide-like. The first diuretics usually used are thiazide diuretics. In addition, diuretics are the preferred treatment for isolated systolic hypertension in older adults. Aldosterone receptor blockers (such as spironolactone) prevent the effects of aldosterone on the kidneys and this allows the kidneys to remove the extra sodium and water.

Chapter 29

1. Iron deficiency anemia develops when there is a loss of iron that becomes inadequate for red blood cell production. It is the most common type of anemia and is particularly common in the elderly.

   Folic acid deficiency anemia results from a lack of folic acid. Folic acid deficiency anemia is found in the chronically undernourished, such as alcoholics, drug abusers, and the elderly. Consumption of alcohol increases folic acid requirements. In addition, pregnancy increases the need for folic acid.

2. The types of diagnostic tests to confirm DIC are CBC, platelet count, schistocytes (fragmented RBCs), prolonged coagulation studies (PT, PTT, thrombin time), and increased fibrin degradation products.

3. Hemophilia A, a factor VIII deficiency known as classic hemophilia, affects 1 in 10,000 males. It is transmitted to the offspring as a cross-linked recessive disorder from mothers to sons. The defect of hemophilia A on the X chromosome could cause the deficiency of factor VIII or its production.

Hemophilia C, also known as factor XI deficiency, is also an autosomal recessive disorder. It primarily affects the population of Ashkenazi Jews and is somewhat rare based on the narrow population that is affected. The clinical manifestations are related to the prolonged partial thromboplastin time and are basically the same as for the previously other forms of hemophilia. Often these patients are identified in the perioperative arena with prolonged bleeding during or after surgery.

4. Acute leukemia is characterized by abrupt onset and rapid progression. The two types of acute leukemia are: (1) Acute myeloid leukemia (AML), which affects people of all ages, and (2) Acute lymphocytic leukemia (ALL), which most commonly affects children under 15.

   Chronic leukemia has a gradual onset, a prolonged clinical course, and relatively long survival. There are two types of chronic leukemia: (1) Chronic myeloid leukemia (CML), which affects people at all ages, and (2) Chronic lymphocytic leukemia (CLL), which rarely strikes before age 45 and most victims are over 65.

5. Autologous stem cell transplantation is a common management therapy in the cancer of the blood disorders. This procedure consists of patients undergoing peripheral stem cell collections after stimulation with granulocyte colony-stimulating factor (G-CSF), with or without a dose of mobilization chemotherapy. Once adequate stems cells are collected, high-dose melphalan is administered, followed by the infusion of the previously harvested stem cells. In general, high-dose therapy with autologous transplant may improve the survival rates of those patients who have the treatment.

6. This activity would be performed in the student nurse clinical practicum experience.

Chapter 30

1. Mrs. Hastings will require about two months to completely recover from her bout with pneumonia. Because she is weakened, her mobility and endurance may be decreased, and she is at increased risk for falls. Because her family members are unavailable during the day to assist her with activities of daily living, she may benefit from an adult daycare program or visits from a home health team. Because she may experience a relapse, she should be closely monitored for any signs of respiratory infection or increasing fatigue, alterations in mental status, or changes in overall health. By supporting her efforts to remain in her

home, her independence will be preserved while she is receiving the care she requires. She should be instructed to rest frequently, take her entire course of antibiotics, use effective hand hygiene, keep her follow-up appointment with her health care provider, and avoid crowds, those with illnesses, contact with infants and small children, hypothermia, and secondhand smoke. Referral to a case manager, social services provider, and home health nurse will be helpful in her recovery.

2. Mr. and Mrs. Myers are both experiencing health problems because of cigarette smoking. Mr. Myers is at substantially increased risk for additional lung problems because he is exposed daily to additional cigarette smoke that caused his respiratory disease. He is at risk of experiencing a respiratory emergency, because his ability to exchange oxygen at the alveolar capillary level is severely compromised. Because of his increasing dyspnea at rest, he will probably require maintenance oxygen in his home. Both Mr. and Mrs. Myers should be instructed about the importance of keeping all flames away from oxygen. Also, Mrs. Myers should be instructed to avoid any cigarette smoking inside her house and in the area adjacent to her windows in her yard. Smoking cessation should also be reexplored. Mr. Myers may develop mobility and self-care limitations because of chronic dyspnea. Further, he may become depressed because of his activity limitations. As cold weather develops, the windows in their house will probably be opened less frequently, so the accumulation of tobacco smoke in drapes, furniture, and carpets will cause additional problems. Also, heat from the furnace will dry the indoor air, making it more difficult for Mr. Myers to mobilize his respiratory secretions. He should be instructed to use a humidifier in the house all winter if the furnace is on. He should also be instructed to avoid long intervals of bed rest; avoid exposure to cold, dry air; and drink plenty of fluids to assist in mobilization of his secretions. In teaching this couple, use of visual materials and repeating instructions will be helpful. Instructions should be provided over several visits, and you should plan to follow-up with written instructions in large print that can be left in their house.

3. Because Mrs. Myers seems to have some cognitive and memory problems, she may be experiencing symptoms of confusion, delirium, hearing loss, or dementia. New learning will be difficult for her to grasp with any of these conditions. Those with problems related to thinking, memory, or hearing loss are not suitable to prepare medications for themselves or others. Mrs. Myers should be evaluated for the above problems. In the interval, Mr. Myers should receive medication assistance from a reliable family member or a home health nurse. Because of his endurance and visual problems, he should not set up his medications at this time. Whenever teaching is ongoing, all sources of distraction, such as the television or outside noise should be eliminated. Teaching in the morning may work better because fatigue set in less soon after arising.

4. Nearly every place Irma visits has known triggers for asthma. In the country or in many rural areas, pollen, dust, and molds are common. In the local grocery store, she may come in contact with those experiencing colds or flu or have secondary exposure to cleaning agents used in the store. Her weekly trip to the city library may produce breathing difficulties in the presence of smog. Further, the resale shop may cause breathing problems if mold, mildew, dust, or dry cleaning products are in the air. Exertion is a known trigger for many with asthma, so exercising at the health club may also produce wheezing and bronchospasms associated with asthma. The pet groomer is also a known trigger for asthma, because debris from fleas, dander from dog skin, and fur or hair from grooming will likely be floating in the air. Irma should be advised to medicate prior to contact with these sources of irritation, minimize contact, and consider eliminating sources of irritation from her weekly routines.

5. Ask Mr. Jeffers to hold his breath while you auscultate him.

Chapter 31

1. Nursing Diagnoses as set forth by the North American Nursing Diagnosis Association (NANDA), for a patient with upper airway infection may include the following, as well as others:

- Activity intolerance
- Ineffective airway clearance
- Acute pain
- Deficient knowledge

2. Suggested NIC for the nursing diagnoses are:
   Activity intolerance is related to fever, fatigue, or a compromised immune system. The patient experiences insufficient physiological energy to complete or endure required or desired daily activities.

- Self-care assistance
- Energy management
- Environmental management
- Sleep enhancement

Ineffective airway clearance is related to inflammation of the mucous membranes and rhinorrhea.

- Airway management
- Cough enhancement
- Fluid management

Acute pain is related to congestion, cough, and fever.

- Analgesic administration
- Environmental management
- Medication administration
- Heat/cold application

Deficient knowledge

- Health education
- Teaching—Disease process
- Teaching—Medication
- Behavior modification

3. Evidence-based medical research has shown the limited efficacy of antibiotic use in eradicating infection. This is due in part because of the overuse of antibiotics with subsequent bacterial organism resistance. Newer drugs are more costly, and studies have not demonstrated superiority of one antibiotic over another in eradicating infection. However, the amount of organism resistance in an area must be considered when selecting an antibiotic. The benefits of antibiotic therapy must be weighed against the potential for adverse effects. There is limited evidence that antibiotics (including amoxicillin, cephalosporins, and macrolides) for 7 to 10 days are effective in the treatment of radiologically or bacteriologically confirmed acute maxillary sinusitis.

If infection with a bacterial agent is confirmed, antibiotics are indicated for 7 to 10 days. First-line drugs of choice are amoxicillin (Amoxil), and trimethoprim/sulfamethoxazole (Bactrim).

4. Standard throat cultures have fallen out of favor because of their inability to distinguish active infection from the carrier state, unpredictability between lab and user, and the fact that results are rarely available in time to decrease symptoms. On the other hand, rapid antigen testing takes about 5 to 7 minutes to obtain results and treatment can begin immediately.

5. Epistaxis is classified on the basis of the primary bleeding site as anterior or posterior. Hemorrhage is most commonly anterior, originating from the nasal septum. A common source of anterior epistaxis is Kiesselbach plexus, a network of vessels on the anterior portion of the septum just superior to the posterior end of the nasal vestibule. Posterior hemorrhage originates in the posterior nasal cavity or nasopharynx, usually below the posterior half of the inferior turbinate or roof of the nasal cavity.

Management of nosebleeds depends on the location of the bleeding site. A nasal speculum is used to access the location of the bleeding. For nosebleeds originating from the anterior portion of the nose, direct pressure may be the only treatment that is needed. The patient is shown how to lean forward slightly while pinching the soft outer portion of the nose against the nasal septum for about five to ten minutes continuously. If this proves unsuccessful, additional treatment is indicted. If the source of bleeding can be visualized, an application of silver nitrate may help to stop the bleeding. Cotton pledgets soaked in 4% topical cocaine solution or a solution of 4% lidocaine and topical epinephrine (1:10,000) can be placed into the nasal cavity. They should remain in place for 10 to 15 minutes.

If bleeding is occurring from the posterior portion of the nasal cavity, packing must be used to stop the bleeding. Commonly used treatments include traditional nasal packing, nasal tampons or balloons, or prefabricated nasal sponges.

Nasal packing may be left in place for two to five days. Oral antibiotics and analgesics may be prescribed.

6. A clear association has been made between smoking, excess alcohol ingestion, and the development of laryngeal cancer. A direct correlation exists between the amount of smoking and the chance of developing laryngeal cancer. Alcohol has been found to be a synergistic agent, increasing the risk up to 100-fold in individuals who smoke and ingest alcohol over nonsmokers and nondrinkers. Other carcinogens associated with the risk of laryngeal cancer include exposure to wood dust, paint fumes, asbestos, mustard gas, tar products, leather, and metals. Other contributing factors in the development of laryngeal cancer include constant straining of the voice, a weak immune system (such as in acquired immune deficiency syndrome [AIDS]), human papillomavirus (HPV), nutritional deficiencies (such as vitamin B, A, retinoids), and gastroesophageal reflux disease (GERD).

7. Esophageal speech involves the patient being able to take air into the mouth and swallow or force the air into the esophagus by locking the tongue to the roof of the mouth. Forcing the air into the esophagus causes the walls of the esophagus and pharynx, as well as the returning air, to vibrate, producing a low-pitched sound. The tongue, lips, and mouth then form this sound into words. The process is similar to a burp or belch. The advantage

to this method is that the sound is more normal than speech produced by mechanical devices. It is less costly than other methods, because there is no equipment to buy. A disadvantage to this method it that it is more difficult to learn than speech produced with special devices and it may be harder to understand. It is important to remind the patient that it can take months to perfect this form of artificial speech.

Tracheoesophageal speech is similar to esophageal speech, but a valve is placed in the tracheal stoma to divert the air into the esophagus. The procedure is called a tracheoesophageal puncture (TEP) and may be performed at the same time as the laryngectomy. The procedure creates an opening between the trachea and the esophagus. A one-way valve is inserted into the stoma and allows air to pass from the trachea into the esophagus, while preventing food from entering the trachea. To produce speech, the patient covers the opening and forces the air into the esophagus and out of the mouth. This allows the patient to produce sound in the same way as esophageal speech, but the sound produced is much more like natural speech. Tracheoesophageal speech is successful in 80 to 90 percent of patients and is a widely accepted form of alaryngeal communication because it is fairly easy to learn. The valve can be removed and cleaned to prevent mucus from occluding the opening.

Mechanical speech may be used while the patient is learning esophageal speech or tracheoesophageal speech or if they have been unsuccessful at either of these methods. Speech production occurs by means of an electrical device that is powered by batteries (electrolarynx) or by air (pneumatic larynx). The electrolarynx is a handheld device, that when placed against the neck, causes sound to travel through the neck into the mouth. A pneumatic larynx is held over the stoma and uses air instead of batteries to make it vibrate. The sound travels to the mouth through a plastic tube. Both methods produce a mechanical sounding voice that may be difficult to understand. The advantage to mechanical speech is that communication is relatively

Chapter 32

1. This is best applied in the practicum setting with the selection of a patient that has a diagnosis of pneumonia.

2. When there is a 5-mm induration, it suggests that the patient could have one of the following: recent contact, an immunocompromised person, and an abnormal chest X-ray. When there is a 10-mm induration, it suggests that the person has diabetes mellitus, renal insufficiency, a recent gastrectomy, corticosteroid therapy, people who traveled within the past 5 years to a country with TB, and substance abusers in treatment programs. The latter is a greater severity within these potential problems.

3. The patient is assessed and diagnostic tests reveal that they have a lung abscess. Then, the treatment goals focus on minimizing further tissue damage, promoting effective airway breathing, removal of secretions, and treatment of infection. The patient will be then be prescribed antibiotic therapy to reduce the infection quickly. Bronchodilators could be used to expand the bronchi allowing removal of secretions through the use of an inhaled mist. There will also be a focus on improving his respiratory condition (e.g., oxygen therapy, rest periods when ambulating, and effective pain control) and assessing the results of the interventions. Chest physiotherapy and postural drainage will also be used to improve his condition.

4. This is be implemented in the clinical setting. Be honest with yourself and share your feelings with your classmates. Ask them and your clinical preceptor to assist you in creating strategies for your professional role with this disorder in a patient.

5. The fractured ribs can be singular in nature or multiple. The patient would have acute pain on inspiration and would naturally splint his or her rib cage area during his or her breathing. Unless the fractured ribs cause bleeding or internal organ damage, they are usually not a high priority in relationship to the viability of the patient. On the other hand, a flail chest involves the fracture of several ribs that are usually in a segment together. The patient typically has chest pain, dyspnea, tachypnea, and tachycardia. This patient will be more compromised than just fractured ribs and have more of a respiratory distressed condition.

Chapter 33

1. Tell the patient with COPD that the pulmonary rehabilitation program has educational, psychosocial, behavioral, and physical components. Identify what some of these components are. Let your patient know that he or she will set the pace. He or she will not be asked to do anything that he or she is unable to do. Let him or her verbalize his or her concerns and get his or her feelings out. Give him or her accurate information to reduce his or her fear. The patient can expect classes in anatomy and physiology of the lung, changes with COPD, medications, home oxygen therapy, nutrition, importance of regular exercise,

respiratory therapy, smoking cessation, symptom alleviation, infection prevention, sexuality, coping with COPD, communicating with the health care team, advance directives, living wills, and health care alternatives for the future.

2. This will best be answered by observation in a practicum setting. The pulmonary rehabilitation program also teaches the patient to pace activities through the day and use assistive devices to decrease energy expenditure. Measure this patient's outcomes with a tool, such as the Medical Outcomes Study Short Form.

3. This will best be applied in a practicum setting by developing a relationship with a patient and family that has cystic fibrosis (CF). In addition, accessing the Web site for the CF Foundation will complete this question.

4. This will be applied in a practicum setting by assessing and evaluating a patient with asthma.

5. This will be applied by observing a respiratory therapist in clinical setting as he or she cares for the three types of COPD patients.

6. This will be answered by evaluating CF on the identified Web site for the CF Foundation.

Chapter 34

1. The three neurotransmitters in the basal ganglia and their impact on motor function are:
   - acetylcholine—excitatory; stimulates the release of γ-aminobutyric acid (GABA);
   - GABA—excitatory and inhibitory; chorea develops with low levels;
   - dopamine—inhibits release of GABA; tremor and gait disturbances develop with low levels.

2.

SYSTEM	SYMPATHETIC RESPONSE	PARASYMPATHETIC RESPONSE
Neurological	Pupils dilated	Pupils normal size
	Heightened awareness	
Cardiovascular	Increased heart rate	Decreased heart rate
	Increased myocardial contractility	Decreased myocardial contractility
	Increased blood pressure	

SYSTEM	SYMPATHETIC RESPONSE	PARASYMPATHETIC RESPONSE
Respiratory	Increased respiratory rate	Bronchial constriction
	Increased respiratory depth	
	Bronchial dilation	
Gastrointestinal	Decreased gastric motility	Increased gastric motility
	Decreased gastric secretions	Increased gastric secretions
	Increased glycogenolysis	Sphincter dilation
	Decreased insulin production	
	Sphincter contraction	
Genitourinary	Decreased urine output	Normal urine output
	Decreased renal blood flow	

3. The six major portions of the physical assessment of the neurological system are mental status, cranial nerve exam, sensory exam, motor exam, cerebellar exam, and reflex exam.

4. The follow-up nursing interventions after a computed tomography (CT) scan are:
   a. Teaching by the nurse should begin with a description of the CT scanner. When contrast media is planned, identification of any allergies to the media, shellfish, or iodine, may require premedication. Instruct the patient on the importance of lying still during the procedure. Identify any need for sedation due to anxiety. The patient is not usually ordered to have nothing by mouth (NPO). A peripheral intravenous (IV) site may need to be implemented.
   b. The patient is placed flat on a movable table. His or her head is secured in a holding device. The table moves in and out of the cylindrical scanner. A noncontrast series of pictures are taken first. If contrast is ordered, it is administered intravenously, and the series is repeated. The entire procedure usually takes approximately 10–40 minutes.

Continued

c. If given, the nurse should monitor for any delayed reaction to contrast media When contrast media is used, the diuresis that results may require replacement fluids.

5. The student would observe several neurological diagnostic studies in the practicum setting.

Chapter 35

1. a. What type, size, and grade is the tumor? This helps to identify if the tumor is benign or malignant, the types (gliomas, meningioma, etc.), and if malignant, how much it will spread.
   b. What types of treatment options are available for this type of tumor? This question will help determine whether treatment will be surgical, radiation, chemotherapy, or a combination of all three.
   c. What is my prognosis? This helps the patient determine the next step and assist with planning.
   d. Should I see any special physicians? A patient may need to consult with a neurosurgeon, neuro-oncologist, and neuro-radiation specialist for treatments.
   e. Where can I receive this treatment? This is important for the patient to know if they will need to travel outside of the area or can remain close to family and friends for treatment.

2. Topics to include in the presentation are: (a) Helmets are an important part of recreational sports and (b) Motor vehicle crashes cause the most head injuries and is the leading cause of brain injury in teenagers. This is usually due to alcohol, drugs, inexperienced drivers, and speeding.

3. Some important nursing interventions to include are:
   a. Importance of seeking help from family, friends, and community resources.
   b. Importance of taking care of himself of herself—getting out of the house to do whatever helps the patient to relax (e.g., exercise, crafts, etc.).
   c. Promoting independence for the patients, as much is as possible.
   d. Joining support groups.

4. Some appropriate nursing interventions for this patient are: (a) Keep environment structured, (b) Orient frequently, (c) Maintain a safe environment, (d) Monitor self-care but should be able to perform with moderate assistance, (e) Keep active by attending structure programs, (f) Keep consistent with behavior modification techniques, and (g) adopt a reward system.

5. Interventions to assist a patient in modifying various risk factors for a stroke are outlined as follows:

a. Hypertension: exercise, decrease salt intake, stress management, and administer antihypertensives.
b. Hypercholesterolemia: decrease saturated fats in diet, increase vegetables and fruits, and administer lipid reducing medications.
c. Atrial fibrillation: administer anticoagulants.
d. Obesity: significant diet modification, exercise, and counseling.
e. Smoking: participate in a smoking cessation program.
f. Drugs and alcohol: eliminate illicit drugs and alcohol.
g. Diabetes: control blood sugars and education regarding the complications of diabetes.

Chapter 36

1. Interviewing a patient and family members will provide an understanding of the physical limitations and psychosocial adjustments that both patients and their families must make. The physical adjustments of the living environment are significant and will help the nurse understand how to anticipate the care that patients will need when they go home. The nursing care worksheet focuses on self-care limitations and will help the nurse understand what type of self-care assistance will be needed by the patient and what the family can anticipate.

2. The improvement of neurological function after administration of methylprednisolone occurs because of the reduction of edema to the area of injury. It is also thought to occur because of the effect of the methylprednisolone on the reduction of leukocytes to the area along with a decrease in free fatty acid production. Steroid treatment also inhibits breakdown of phospholipids, improving blood flow to the spinal cord and stopping the inflammatory response, thereby avoiding further injury to the spinal cord. Methylprednisolone has been shown to counter many of the injury cascades that cause injury to the spinal cord. These injury cascades include the emergent phase of spinal shock, which includes spinal edema and inflammation processes.

3. A teaching plan should include assessment of risk factors, especially work history related to word processing and keyboarding activities. Teaching should include proper positioning of hands and wrists, proper height of keyboard, wrists off the surface of the desk and support through the use of gel devices. Teaching to athletes should emphasize rest and immobilization of the wrist if experiencing

symptoms. Nonsteroidal anti-inflammatory medications will be helpful in these situations.

4. Neurological assessment of motor and sensory function is a priority after the surgery, as well as careful assessment for the development of a headache, which may indicate a subdural hematoma. Administration of dexamethasone for the prevention and treatment of edema associated with the spinal cord tumor and surgery will be an aspect of postoperative care, along with administration of antacids to protect the gastrointestinal (GI) tract from the adverse effects of corticosteroids. Careful assessment of urinary and bowel elimination and progression to self-care activities will also be included in the postoperative care of this patient.

5. This Web site provides a wealth of information for health care providers and for patients and family members. It is important for nurses to know the research to be able to talk with patients who are knowledgeable about care.

Chapter 37

1. Tension-type headache is caused by irritation of the pain-sensitive structures of the brain. The intracranial structures include portions of the trigeminal (CN V), facial (CN VII), glossopharyngeal (CN IX), vagus (CN X), upper cervical nerves, the large arteries, and the venous sinuses. When the sensory receptors of the muscles, tendons, joints, and skin are stimulated, they transmit pain messages to the pain-sensitive areas of the brain. Tension-type headaches may be episodic or chronic.

   Migraine is characterized by vasodilation of the dural blood vessels, resulting in stimulation of the trigeminal nerve pain pathways. Then neuropeptides, involved in pain transmission, are released. The neuropeptides make the vasodilation worse and sensitize the brainstem, causing the associated symptoms of light, sound, movement, and odor sensitivity.

Medications to Treat Headaches

TENSION-TYPE HEADACHE	MIGRAINE HEADACHE	CLUSTER HEADACHE
Nonnarcotic analgesics	*Nonnarcotic analgesics*	*100 percent O$_2$/ facemask*
Caffeine		Ergot alkaloids
Narcotic combinations	Narcotic analgesics	Triptans
		Intranasal lidocaine

Medications to Treat Headaches—*cont'd*

TENSION-TYPE HEADACHE	MIGRAINE HEADACHE	CLUSTER HEADACHE
Nonnarcotic analgesics	*Nonnarcotic analgesics*	*100 percent O$_2$/ facemask*
Antidepressants	Triptans	Capsaicin
	Ergot alkaloids	Nonnarcotic analgesics
		Narcotic analgesics
		Calcium channel blockers
Beta blockers	Beta blockers	Corticosteroids
	Calcium channel blockers	Anticonvulsants
	Antidepressants	

Cluster headache is similar to a migraine headache; however, the triggers are different. The triggers include vasodilating agents (nitroglycerine), histamine, alcohol, and nicotine. Acetylcholine is believed to play a role in the parasympathetic symptoms.

2. Withholding treatment refers to never starting a treatment. Withdrawing treatment refers to stopping a treatment once it has been started. The deciding factor is whether the decision is consistent with the patient's or surrogate's interests and preferences. If the surrogate decides to withhold the tube feedings, the health care provider must respect the decision. Administering the tube feeding against the surrogate's wishes would violate their autonomy.

3. Parkinson's disease is a slowly progressive degenerative neurological disorder caused by the loss of nerve cell function in the basal ganglia. The basal ganglia includes the substantia nigra, striatum, globus pallidus, subthalamic nucleus, and the red nucleus. Loss of nerve cells in the substantia nigra causes a reduction of dopamine production. Dopamine is the neurotransmitter essential for control of posture, supporting the body in an upright position, and voluntary motions.

4. Meal planning to promote medication effectiveness; provide verbal cues to chew food thoroughly; teach caregivers the Heimlich maneuver; match food consistency to ability to swallow; and schedule meals when patient is well rested.

5. The student would compare any three of the neurological degenerative disorders described in the chapter, as related to pathophysiology.

Chapter 38

The solutions to the review activities are demonstrated in the assessment of patients in practicum settings.

Chapter 39

1. Student will accomplish this in an applied clinical setting.

2. Student will accomplish this in an applied clinical setting.

3. Student will accomplish this in an applied clinical setting.

4. Student will accomplish this in an applied clinical setting.

5. (a) Remember to assess the patient for priority injuries first, (b) leave the object in place and stabilize the patient's head, (c) place a cup over the impaled object and tape in place, and (d) transport the patient in a safe and efficient manner remembering to not allow the impaled object to move.

6. a. Myopia is nearsightedness, which occurs when the light passing through the eye is overbent or overrefracted. Objects that are viewed up close are clear and distant objects are unclear. Myopia is treated with corrective lens that redirects the light to the retina by changing the angle of the light. These corrective lens' are cut biconcave.

   b. Hyperopia, or farsightedness, occurs when the light passing through the eye is focused behind the retina when looking a close objects. As a result, images up close are unclear, but images over 20 feet distant are clear. Hyperopia is treated with convex corrective lens that redirects the light to the retina.

   c. Astigmatism occurs where the light is spread over a diffuse area. Astigmatism occurs when there is an unequal curve of the cornea, and the light rays are bent unevenly. The exact cause of astigmatism is unknown, although there is some familial pattern. Astigmatism is treated with corrective lens in a cylindrical shape.

7. Hordeolum is an inflamed sweat gland, which is reddened, swollen, and tender to touch and is also called a stye.

   Chalazion is a small benign tumor similar to a sebaceous cyst, hordeolum, or even a sebaceous carcinoma.

   Blepharitis is an inflammation of the hair follicles (cilia) and glands along the edges of the eyelids.

Conjunctivitis, also called pink eye, can be the result of exposure to allergens or irritants and as such is not contagious.

Keratitis is an inflammation and ulceration of the cornea.

8. Reading devices with increased bifocal power; monocular microscopes ("near telescopes"); handheld magnifiers; stand magnifiers; illuminated magnifiers; closed circuit televisions; large print newspapers, magazines, and other reading materials; dial markers on the gauges of appliances; self-threading needles; books on tape; talking clocks and watches.

Chapter 40

1. Preparing the patient for surgery is an important part of nursing care. Communicating clear expectations before surgery will help alleviate fears. Stressing that manipulation of the auditory system may interfere with hearing and take some time before hearing is restored. Other teaching should include avoiding anything that will interfere with the function of the eustachian tube (blowing nose, cough, sneeze), not lying on the surgical side, and ways in which the nurse and patient will communicate after surgery.

2. Learning as much as possible is important to be able to counsel the patient of potential resources in their own community. The nurse is a valuable contact person for patients with a hearing deficit to obtain information on what services are accessible and also make a useful tool when encountering a patient or family member who has auditory dysfunction.

3. The more information that the nurse has, the more he or she will be able to provide to the patient. The Internet has a wealth of information, and the nurse should be able to decipher fact from fiction. Many elderly patients are not computer savvy and need assistance in finding the best resource to meet their needs.

4. There are so many types of hearing aids that the nurse should become familiar with as many types as possible to assist the patient in the office or hospital. Visiting the audiologist will also give the nurse a valuable resource person when needed.

5. Putting yourself in another's shoes is an ideal way to get a picture of what the patient may be experiencing. Using both an ear muff and plugs will block out the most sound, and the nurse will be able to identify with a person having auditory dysfunction. This experience will also give the students a chance to experiment with different ways to communicate without hearing sounds.

Chapter 41

1. You should empathize with the patient, assessing her knowledge of SLE and its diagnosis. Educating the patient about both the disease and the testing is essential, as fear of the unknown is the worst kind of fear. She should be informed that the tests will show if she has inflammation not associated with an infection and whether she has antinuclear antibodies. She should also be informed that her symptoms are nonspecific, and the tests will help to determine what is wrong with her. She should be advised that although ANA is associated with SLE, it can be caused by other things.

2. Increased UTI in an elderly male patient is most likely associated with decreased urine output and decreased bladder sensitivity and possibly prostate hypertrophy. Other things that should be assessed include the urine for proteinuria, hematuria, and glycosuria (diabetes).

3. The allergy should be posted prominently in the patient's room. Nonlatex gloves should be placed in the patient's room, as well as nonlatex versions of any other bandages or instruments that may be needed in their care. Stethoscopes should be covered in a protective sleeve. The patient should be educated in the differences in appearance between common latex and nonlatex supplies. The patient should be instructed to be assertive if latex products are being used.

4. The exact requirements may vary, but your patient will most likely require proof of all the childhood immunizations, including MMR, HIB, hepatitis B, polio, tetanus, and varicella. In addition, she will also need a PPD. Booster shots will likely be needed for MMR and tetanus/diphtheria, if she did not have them when she started college as a freshman.

5. Sexual behaviors and risk should be addressed, as well as any past STDs or possible exposures. The nature of the tests to be performed should be explained as well as the procedures for picking up the results of the test. Any concerns or fears should be dealt with as empathetically as possible.

Chapter 42

1. A case study about HIV/AIDS would need to be available. Students will gain additional knowledge about the various drugs used in treatment of HIV/AIDS and also learn more about the disease process.

2. Allows students to study several diagnostic tests that are used for patients with immune disorders. In addition, the focus of patient education is beneficial to the student in addressing the practical needs of the patient.

3. Provides current update and exploration of internet resources and national guidelines for HIV/AIDS.

4. Allows student to consider the psychosocial or physical or spiritual aspects of a chronic immune disease and how to interact with patients.

5. Promotes critical thinking about safety measures for patients with immune disorders and procedures to follow for employees who have accidental exposure to HIV-contaminated fluids.

6. Provides the opportunity for students to research information on immune disorders, which are presented in this immune chapter.

Chapter 43

1. Examples of hypersensitivity type 1 allergic response are:
   a. Anaphylaxis
   b. Atopic asthma
   c. Atopic eczema
   d. Drug allergy
   e. Acute rhinitis

2. The patient and family communication should include a discussion of learning to anticipate triggers and practicing avoidance. Asthma triggers irritate the lungs and produce mucus, inflammation, and tightening of the bronchial tubes. Common triggers for asthma include:

   • Pollen: keep windows and doors closed, and use air conditioning to keep pollen out.

   • Dust mites: use special coverings for mattresses and pillows. Remove carpets, rugs and drapery in bedrooms. Wash bedding in hot water.

   • Toys should not include stuffed animals.

   • Keep humidity between 30–40 percent.

   • Use a vacuum cleaner with a filter. Change filter and bag often.

   • Animal hair and dander: Pet removal is best. If around pets, keep them out of bedrooms, and off furniture.

   • Mold: Try to eliminate mold in the environment. Dehumidifiers can help. Avoid freshly cut grass.

   • Environment: Avoid cigarette smoke and all other types of smoke. When outdoor air quality is poor, stay indoors. Cover the nose and mouth during cold weather.

   • Exercise: Perform slow warm-ups and cool-downs and be sure to use asthma medication approximately 10 minutes before beginning an exercise routine.

3. Four categories for potential allergens that may cause anaphylaxis in hypersensitive patients are:
   - Drugs
   - Insect venoms
   - Foods
   - Animal serums
   - Blood products
   - Contrast media

4. Food allergy is treated by avoiding the foods that trigger the reaction. By excluding certain foods, (milk, soy, or wheat) from the diet, the patient with a food allergy can gradually reintroduce the eliminated foods back into the diet and evaluate potential for allergic response to the reintroduced food.

5. Exposure to an allergen initiates a humoral response. Immunoglobulin E (IgE) molecules specific to an antigen attach to cell surface receptors on mast cells. The mast cell's response includes the release of histamine, a hormone that causes vasodilation and an increase in permeability of blood vessel walls. The release of histamine creates the clinical manifestations of an allergic reaction.

6. Avoiding the allergen is the best treatment. Other treatments include treating the symptoms with antihistamines, decongestants, and corticosteroids applied by nasal spray. Secondary infections indicated by facial pain or a greenish-yellow discharge may require antibiotic therapy.

7. Atopy refers to an individual being prone to develop allergies because of a genetic state of hyper-responsiveness to sensitizing agents. If a person inherits this tendency from parents who are allergic, they have a hyper-responsive immune system that will produce large quantities of IgE on the second or subsequent exposure to an allergen. These individuals may develop a number of allergies. The spectrum of their allergic conditions may include asthma, food allergies, drug allergies, eczema, and so on.

Chapter 44

1. Best applied in the practicum setting by interviewing three persons of different cultural backgrounds. This activity permits the student to apply a holistic perspective of skin conditions and to use critical thinking skills in comparing information from different cultures.

2. Best applied with a small group of peers, either in a laboratory or practicum setting. This activity involves the use of several skills—critical thinking, problem solving, creativity—and if it is a group activity, it can be an exercise for working as a team. It also permits the student to use a holistic approach to understanding the physiological and psychosocial-spiritual aspects of an individual.

3. This activity can be done in a learning laboratory setting with peers or alone. The activity involves the student in considering the various environmental factors that contribute to skin disorders, the risks involved, and the development of patient teaching strategies.

4. This activity is best performed using an assessment text, along with interviewing or assessing an older person (e.g., friend of family or relative). It involves developing an organized approach for assessment, use of interview skills, review of information about etiology of older adult skin damage, and interaction with an older adult, and use of communication skills.

5. This activity is best performed while accessing the Web site at: http://www.aad.org. Click on Public Resource Center, then click on Skincarephysicians. com. The student can then review the information and develop an instruction pamphlet based on the answers to questions posed on the specific skin disorder.

6. This activity is best performed while accessing the Web site at: http://www.aad.org. Click on Public Resource Center, click on Kids Connection. This is an especially good activity for students who enjoy computer resources. There is a wealth of information at the American Academy of Dermatology Web site. The specific activities will increase knowledge about the various skin disorders and allow the students to be creative in completing the projects. Accessing the Web site will also provide additional resources for learning.

Chapter 45

1. Because dermatological dysfunctions are most often managed in private practices the observational experience is meant to expose the student to typical dermatological dysfunctions and to the typical management of those dysfunctions, both by physicians and by nurses. There are no right or wrong observations.

2. Examples of nursing diagnoses are:
   - Acute pain R/T contact dermatitis: Assess pain on regular basis. Teach principles of pain management. Administer pharmacological methods of pain relief.
   - Impaired skin integrity R/T radiation: Assess skin on regular basis. Remove adhesive tape and debris.

Keep bed linens clean, dry, and wrinkle free. Apply topical medications, as appropriate. Document skin condition.

- Imbalanced nutrition: Less than body weight R/T body weight 20 percent or more under ideal. Complete a nutritional assessment. Weigh patient at regular intervals. Monitor caloric and nutrient intake. Offer nutritional supplements, as needed.

- Disturbed body image R/T skin lesions: Determine patient's body image expectations. Assist patient to discuss changes. Facilitate contact with individuals with similar changes.

- Risk for infection R/T tissue destruction and increased environmental exposure: Monitor for signs and symptoms of infection. Maintain asepsis. Inspect skin and mucous membranes for redness, erythema, or drainage. Provide appropriate skin.

3. The two main herpetic infections are: (a) Herpes simplex virus-1 (HSV-1) and (b) herpes simplex virus-2 (HSV-2). HSV-1 is generally associated with oral cold sores and fever blisters, and HSV-2 is associated with genital infections. Both types of infections are becoming more common and may be related to oral-genital sexual contact. Treatment of HSV consists of cool, moist compresses of Burrow's solution, controlling secondary infections, and systemic or topical antivirals that may include Acyclovir, Famvir, or Valtrex. Treatment of herpes zoster centers on pain control and antiviral therapy. Antiviral medications must be started within 72 hours of the onset of the rash or pain. Pain can be severe enough to require nerve blocks. Selection and dosage of medications is determined according to the needs of the individual patient. The same antiviral drugs used to treat HSV are used to treat herpes zoster.

4. This is best evaluated in class and seminar settings. The strategies for treatment are the preventive strategies of covering up the areas easily burned, using protective lotions or creams to block the sun rays, and close observation of the skin for symptoms of sunburn.

5. This is applied in the seminar and laboratory settings by assessing one another and interviewing peers for their reactions and comments to their wart conditions. In addition, reviewing the pathophysiology and management strategies together can increase the knowledge level of all involved.

Chapter 46

1. Complaints of pain would be the ideal assessment indicator for distinguishing a partial-thickness from a full-thickness burn. Partial-thickness burns have intact pain receptors and nerve endings therefore pain is sensed. Pain receptors and nerve endings are destroyed in full-thickness burns and pain is not sensed (this is why escharotomy, a surgical incision, does not require an anesthestic).

2. *Withdrawal* nursing approaches include: avoid forcing patient to deal with situation, provide supportive environment, and provide ongoing information on status and care. *Denial* nursing approaches include: support patient, avoid forcing patient to deal with fears, answer questions honestly, and provide information in small doses over time. *Regression* nursing approaches include: avoid attacking and responding negatively to behavior exhibited, acknowledge patient's difficulty in coping, and encourage and reward positive behaviors and independence. *Anger and hostility* nursing approaches include: encourage verbalization of frustration, avoid responding directly to anger, provide choices and control, and assist patient to search for meaning to injury. *Depression* nursing approaches include: acknowledge the loss and focus the patient on realistic expectations.

3. Develop a fire escape plan. Keep exit routes free of clutter and have two escape routes. Do not include windows with bars in the escape routes. All windows with bars should have a quick release feature for easy removal. Keep whistle by bed to alert rescuers where you are or to warn others of fire. The fire department will place a sticker in your bedroom window to assist firefighters in locating you should a fire occur. Keep eyeglasses, keys, flashlight, and telephone near your bedside in case of an emergency. People using oxygen should not smoke or be near fire with oxygen in use. Smokers should use large deep ashtrays and never smoke in bed. Set hot water heater thermostat at 120° F or less with installation of valves in the bathrooms that regulate water temperature. Turn handles of pans to back of stove when cooking. Do not wear clothing with loose sleeves when cooking. Double-check that the stove is off after cooking.

4. Emergent phase: The goals of management include psychosocial adjustment of the patient, the prevention of scars and contractures, and the resumption of preburn activity, including work, family, and social roles. This phase may take years or even last a lifetime.

5. Appearance

Superficial Partial Injury
   Blisters that will increase in size
   Blanches with fingertip pressure and color returns when pressure returns
   Moist

Deep Partial Injury
   Blisters present slower to increase in size
   Blanching decreased, prolonged
   Less moisture
   Color

Superficial Partial Injury
   Pink

Deep Partial Injury
   Pale, mottled with dull, white, tan, cherry red areas

Healing Time

Superficial Partial Injury
   5 to 21 days, no grafting

Deep Partial Injury
   21 to 35 days without complications
   May convert to full-thickness and require grafting

Chapter 47

1. The major organs of the gastrointestinal (GI) tract include the hollow organs from the mouth to the anus; the pancreas that through its exocrine function produces digestive enzymes, and the liver and biliary systems, which achieve important metabolic, digestive, and absorption functions.

2. Perform a concise GI health history by examining the following areas:

   (a) family history, (b) past abdominal history and current problems, (c) eating habits, (d) nutritional assessment, (e) evaluating dysphagia or heartburn (pyrosis), (f) assessing nausea or vomiting, (g) assessing any abdominal pain, and (h) describing any medications taken in any form, particularly those that might influence the GI tract.

3. The physiological processes that are involved during the act of vomiting are: (a) stimulation of afferent input to the vagal fibers, which stimulates serotonin 5 via the splanchnic autonomic fibers, (b) stimulation of the vestibular system (CN VII), which increases histamine H_1 and muscarinic cholinergic receptors, (c) stimulation of the central nervous system (CNS) centers, which are located in the center dorsal part of the medulla oblongata, and (d) stimulation of the chemoreceptor trigger zone (CTZ) located in the floor of the fourth ventricle (outside of the blood-brain barrier).

4. Perform the three primary tests for appendicitis, which are:
   a. Rebound tenderness (Blumberg's sign): A positive response may mean peritoneal irritation. The tips of the fingers are pressed gently into the abdominal wall then suddenly withdrawn. A painful response is positive. Cutaneous hyperesthesia is elicited in the area of the skin over an appendix that is inflamed.
   b. Iliopsoas muscle test: The patient is asked to flex the right thigh (raises the right leg) against resistance (pushing down over the lower part of the thigh)—the patient will experience pain in the pelvis because of irritation of the iliopsoas muscle.
   c. Obturator muscle test: The patient flexes the right thigh (raises the right leg) to 90 degrees. Holding the ankle, the leg is rotated internally and externally. Pelvic pain is produced is the muscle is inflamed.

5. Choose any two of the diagnostic tests from this chapter and describe their use.

Chapter 48

1. A great resource for this patient is the American Diabetes Association at www.diabetes.org. Although this patient has not been diagnosed as being diabetic, the Web site lists community events and resources, has an online bookstore, and has a section on diabetes prevention. The patient should check with his or her health care provider to see if he or she can start a moderate exercise program. Keeping food records, decreasing portion sizes, and reading labels are actions the patient can take to improve his or her diet.

2. Utilize the BMI chart. The National Heart, Lung, and Blood Institute, www.nhlbi.nih.gov, has information on their Web site called "Aim for a Healthy Weight." Under this section, there is information on exercise, shopping, menu planning, and other helpful tips. Information can also be obtained by mail:

   NHLBI Information Center

   P.O. Box 30105

   Bethesda, MD 20824-0105

   Phone: 301-592-8573

   Fax: 301-592-8563

3. Patients with increased protein needs who might need a higher protein enteral feeding include patients with protein losses from wounds, fistulas, and hypercatabolic patients, such as burn patients.

4. If you are doing a clinical rotation or are employed by a hospital, ask for a copy of the policy on nutrition screening and assessment. JCAHO accredited hospitals are required to screen for nutrition risk and have a process in place to further assess at-risk patients.

5. Causes of the rise in childhood obesity include inadequate physical activity, along with a more sedentary lifestyle, including more hours spent

watching television. In addition, children often over-consume high calorie foods.

6. To help your elderly patients in the hospital maintain their nutritional status be on the alert for any problems with chewing, swallowing, or mouth pain and contact the health care provider when these problems are noted. Patients, who are underweight or who have had weight loss and are not diabetic, may benefit from between meal supplements. A dietitian consult can be helpful if these interventions are not successful.

Chapter 49

1. Have the patient look in a mirror and check for symmetry, the presence of lumps, swelling, or bumps. Then have him or her assess the skin on his or her face and look for moles, sores, or growths that have changed in size or color. Continue to teach the patient to check his or her neck and chin for any lumps, tenderness, or swelling. Tell the patient to assess the lips for sores or color changes and to inspect his or her mouth area with a flashlight and note areas of discoloration and to look for lumps, swelling, or bumps. Finally, instruct the patient to contact his or her dentist if he or she sees anything unusual in his or her self-exam.

2. The student would contact the speech pathology department and follow them in an observational capacity as they work with their patients.

3. The student would gain permission to watch an endoscopy and then describe the procedure.

4. The nurse should instruct the patient to (a) eat small meals at any given setting and avoid eating two to three hours before sleeping, (b) wash the throat with water after each meal, (c) sit in a semi-Fowler's position if lying down after eating, (d) avoid irritating food substances, and (e) quit smoking.

5. The patient often experiences upper epigastric pain, particularly if his or her stomach is empty. In addition, he or she may describe certain foods as causing him or her to have more pain, or he or she could describe the manifestations to be worse during stressful situations. In addition, the patient may be able to point to a specific area of the abdomen as the origin of his or her pain.

6. Initially, a genuine concerned attitude is portrayed by the nurse. Then, the nurse should express to the patient that it is important for the patient to ask whatever questions he or she has of his or her health care providers. The nurse can ask who the patient has for support systems and whether he or she would like the nurse to be there when telling these people about the new diagnosis. The nurse can move toward describing the types of supportive care that are typically presented for patients with cancer of the stomach (e.g., pharmacology, surgery). The nurse must remember to not answer with generalizations or statements, which ignore the severity of the new diagnosis.

Chapter 50

1. This will be accomplished in student classroom or lab setting.

2. This will be accomplished in the practicum setting.

3. This will be accomplished in the practicum setting.

4. The etiology of peritonitis can be a postoperative inflammatory infection, ruptured appendix, abdominal fistulas that have resulted in infection, and any other condition that allows contamination of the peritoneal area. The potential effects of peritonitis are septic shock, MODS, and SIRS. The typical clinical manifestations are hypotension, tachycardia, severe febrile condition, renal failure, and decreasing level of consciousness and mentation.

5. The etiology and risk factors for the development of herniations of the bowel are any conditions which increase intraabdominal pressure (e.g., ascites, portal hypertension), inflammatory bowel disorders, and cancer of the bowel. The management strategies for inguinal hernia repair are those that are typical for recovering abdominal surgeries (e.g., monitor vital signs for potential respiratory problems, monitor the healing of the wound area, deep breathing exercises, and active or passive range of motion. In addition, many of these surgeries are short-term surgeries and may allow the patient to be discharged within 24 hours of the surgery, which makes patient teaching important.

6. The etiology and risk factors for the development of hemorrhoids are employment that has a lack of mobility and sitting in one position for long periods of time (e.g., truck driving, grocery clerks, officer personnel); peripheral vascular disorders; and genetic predisposition to circulatory dysfunction. The clinical manifestations are internal or external bleeding of the rectal tissue, painful bowel movements with bleeding, uncomfortable when in a sitting position, chronic anemia, decreased hematocrit or hemoglobin, swelling and protrusion of the hemorrhoids in the anorectal region.

Chapter 51

1. Conjugated bilirubin (direct bilirubin) is bound to molecules while unconjugated bilirubin (indirect bilirubin) is not bound to another molecule. Total bilirubin lab tests reflect the amount of conjugated plus unconjugated bilirubin in the blood.

2. The nurse can physically palpate and percuss the liver as one method of assessing the size and location of the liver boundaries. In addition, serum tests are performed to screen patients with no symptoms. In addition, bile fluid examinations, endoscopy, liver biopsies, ultrasound, computed tomography (CT), magnetic resonance imaging (MRI), nuclear medicine, angiogram, and radiological tests can be performed.

3. Hepatitis A is spread via fecal-oral routes, is shorter in duration, and can be prevented with medical asepsis methods of care. Hepatitis B is transmitted with blood and body fluids, causes lifelong destruction to the patient and has relatively high mortality and morbidity rates.

4. Biliary cirrhosis results from blocked bile ducts, which cause congestion, inflammation, and damage to the tissue in the liver. Infants are affected when they are born with biliary atresia, which deprives the bile of avenues of exit from the liver and ultimately causing tissue damage. In adults, inflamed or blocked bile ducts can occur with scarring results.

   Cardiac cirrhosis occurs when blood flow out of the liver is restricted by severe right-sided heart failure. When that blood is not able to exit at a predictable rate, liver engorgement occurs and the pressure in the liver vasculature increases, causing venous congestion, anoxia or hypoxia, and hepatic cell necrosis.

5. The student would describe his or her feelings regarding caring for patients with alcoholism.

6. The student would describe his or her feelings if he or she were asked to donate his or her liver to a relative.

7. The laparoscopic cholecystectomy has a faster recovery time, fewer complications, and fewer bile duct injuries than the open cholecystectomy. In this operation, a small incision is made at the umbilicus plus three other puncture sites. A laparoscope with video camera and laser technology is introduced, and the gallbladder is dissected from the surrounding organs, drained of fluid and stones, and removed through the incision at the umbilicus.

   The open cholecystectomy can be performed when the laparoscopic technique fails, there are stones that are inaccessible to the laparoscope, or other surgeries are required at the same time (as in treating trauma). The gallbladder is dissected and removed, the cystic duct is ligated, and a T-tube is inserted into the common bile duct to keep it patent.

Chapter 52

1. The structures are the kidney, ureter, bladder, urethra, nephron, and tubule structure of the kidney.

   The kidney is responsible for ultrafiltration; the ureter is the structure that allows for flow of kidney fluids from the kidney to the bladder; the bladder is a small sac-like organ that collects urine; the nephron is the functional unit of the kidney; the tubule structure is responsible for the transport within the kidney.

2. Student-directed activity in a clinical setting.

3. Decreased muscle tone and elasticity in the ureters, bladder, urinary sphincter, and surrounding structures resulting in problems of incontinence; prostatic hyperplasia in the male resulting in urinary retention; decreased functioning nephrons and glomerular filtration rate. This may be reflected in slightly higher blood levels of urea nitrogen and creatinine; nocturia may become a result from problems of retention or from decreases in renal concentration.

4. Examples of diagnostic tests are renal biopsy, renal ultrasound, and intravenous pyelogram. The renal biopsy obtains a physical cellular example from the kidney for further examination. The renal ultrasound is a noninvasive test that provides images of the kidney and surrounding structures. The intravenous pyelogram is a radioactive dye study that allows for visualization of the function.

5. It is important to know the location of supplies and equipment so you can be efficient in your work in the clinical setting.

Chapter 53

1. The student will perform this activity in the clinical course arena.

2. Acute pyelonephritis presents with bacteriuria accompanied by flank pain at the costovertebral angle, fever, and chills. In addition, the patient may experience painful urination, frequency, nocturia, nausea, vomiting, and colicky abdominal pain.

3. The typical presentation of renal stones is sudden-onset unilateral flank pain, which usually causes the individual to seek medical attention. The pain does not completely remit but rather waxes and wanes. The pain is often accompanied by nausea and

occasionally vomiting. The pain can radiate to a variety of locations depending on the location of the stone. When the stone is in the upper ureter, pain may radiate anteriorly to the abdomen. When the stone is in the lower ureter, pain can radiate to the ipsilateral testicle in men or ipsilateral labium in women. If the stone is lodged at the ureterovesical junction, the major symptoms may be urinary frequency and urgency. A less common acute presentation is gross hematuria without pain. The patient may also experience the first stage of shock with cool, diaphoretic skin. In addition, the patient may develop a urinary tract infection and have the symptoms of fever, nausea, and vomiting.

4. Possible complications associated with renal injuries are secondary hemorrhage, usually due to infection (10 to 14 days after trauma), paralytic ileus (4 to 5 days) as a result of retroperitoneal hematoma, hypertension as a result of the constricting effect of reorganizing perirenal hematoma, arterio-venous fistula, renal failure, renal atrophy, hydronephrosis, chronic pyelonephritis, renal calculi, and renal artery stenosis.

5. The most commonly performed surgery to treat renal cell cancer is radical nephrectomy. During a radical nephrectomy, the whole kidney along with the cancer, the attached adrenal gland, and the fatty tissue immediately around the kidney are removed. The lymph nodes around the kidney are often removed and examined under the microscope to determine if they contain cancer. Partial nephrectomy is performed to preserve as much normal kidney tissue as possible; however its complication rate may be slightly higher than radical nephrectomy. Open partial nephrectomy is usually the treatment of choice when radical nephrectomy may result in either immediate dialysis or a high risk for subsequent dialysis. Laparoscopic radical nephrectomy is a surgical technique that is less extensive and invasive than a typical radical nephrectomy. Compared to open radical nephrectomy, laparoscopic radical nephrectomy involves longer operative time, less postoperative pain, shorter hospital stays and shorter recovery time.

Chapter 54

1. Acute pyelonephritis presents with bacteriuria accompanied by flank pain at the costovertebral angle, fever, and chills. In addition, the patient may experience painful urination, frequency, nocturia, nausea, vomiting, and colicky abdominal pain.

2. Autosomal dominant polycystic kidney disease (ADPKD) is caused by genetic mutations on chromosomes 4 and 16. A multisystem disorder, ADPKD occurs in 1 of every 500 to 1,000 individuals. Eighty-five percent of the gene carriers will evidence the disease by their seventh decade and 50 to 75 percent will advance to end-stage renal disease.

    ARPKD, on the other hand, occurs in only 1 in every 6,000 to 55,000 individuals, is more aggressive and usually causes patient death by age 15.

3. • Upper and lower respiratory symptoms including hoarseness, shortness of breath, cough, hemoptysis or nasal drainage; and inspect for nasal crusting or septal defect
   • Recent hearing deficit, tinnitus, pain; inspect ear for drainage, or perforation of the tympanic membrane
   • Sinus infection; pain or tenderness over the sinuses
   • Visual disturbances or conjunctivitis
   • Joint and muscle aches
   • Changes in urine quantity and quality

4. It has been demonstrated that many patients presenting with rhabdomyolysis do not admit to muscle pain or tenderness and do not present with swelling. This emphasizes the need for repeated patient questioning and thorough examination for early intervention and optimal recovery.

5. HD is more definitive in its abilities to filter the blood than CAPD. In addition, HD is monitored thoroughly by a trained clinician and is performed in a dialysis center.

    CAPD, on the other hand, is cheaper, can be performed by a family member or care provider at home, and allows the patient to be more flexible in where they perform the CAPD (e.g., the patient could travel and carry the equipment to perform the CAPD "on the road"). Potential disadvantages for CAPD include protein loss and potential for life-threatening peritoneal infection.

6. The donor should know that it is fundamental that they have disclosed everything that is pertinent and that they have been completely truthful to those asking questions prior to kidney donation (e.g., presence of HIV and illicit drugs). In addition, the donor needs to be told that they will have to undergo major surgery to have the kidney removed. However, donor nephrectomy can be accomplished by laparoscopic surgery, which involves an approximate 2 to 3 inch incision in the lower quadrant suffices for delivering the kidney.

Chapter 55

1. Endocrine glands are ductless glands that secrete specific hormones into the blood stream for circulation to their target cells. Examples of endocrine glands include the hypothalamus, pituitary, thyroid, parathyroid, thymus, adrenal glands, pancreas, ovaries in the females, and testes in the male.

   Exocrine glands empty their secretions into ducts that transport the secretions to specific locations. Examples of exocrine glands include the salivary and sweat glands. The pancreas is both an endocrine and an exocrine gland. The islets of Langerhans make up the endocrine portion of the pancreas, regulating the control of blood glucose.

   As an exocrine gland the pancreas secretes digestive enzymes through ducts that empty into the duodenum.

2. An example of negative feedback in the body is the secretion of insulin in response to rising blood glucose levels. When blood glucose levels in the body rise, insulin is secreted by the islet cells of the pancreas. Insulin acts on the cells, causing them to take up the excess glucose in the bloodstream. The blood glucose level then falls, and insulin secretion stops.

3. Hypothalamus is located at the base of the forebrain near the thalamus and regulates the anterior pituitary hormones.

   Thyroid is located in the neck, inferior to the larynx and cricoid cartilage and regulates the rate of metabolism.

   Parathyroids are located in the lobes of the thyroid and regulate levels of calcium and phosphate.

   Adrenal glands are located above each kidney and regulate metabolism, blood pressure, sodium, and potassium levels.

   Pancreas is located between the duodenum and the spleen and regulates blood glucose levels.

4. Do you have enough energy to perform your normal daily tasks?

   Have you experienced any changes in your appetite or weight?

   Have you noticed any changes in your ability to tolerate heat or cold?

   Have you noticed any changes in your sleep?

   Do you have any difficulty with concentration?

   Have you noticed any changes in the beating of your heart?

   Have you had any changes in your usual bowel patterns?

   Have you noted any changes in your skin or hair?

   Are your belts or rings tighter than normal?

5. Thyroid is not enlarged, symmetrical, smooth, and nontender.

Chapter 56

1. a. Solution: Na = 115 mmol/L
   b. Solution: Neurological. The sodium level indicates dilutional hyponatremia, which can cause cerebral edema resulting in alteration in cognitive and sensory/motor function. As the sodium level drops, the patient may even seizure.
   c. Solution: 1. Ongoing neurological and fluid volume status; 2. Implementing fluid restriction as indicated; 3. Careful monitoring of intake and output; and 4. Cautious administration of NaCl 3%.

2. a. Solution:

   Skin: Oily skin, hyperpigmentation of lower extremities, hair loss, and moist warm skin.

   Eyes: Proptosis (forward placement of the eyes), lid retraction, or puffiness in periorbital area. Blurred or double vision.

   Neuromuscular: Fine hand tremor, hyperactive reflex response, nervousness, muscular weakness.

   Respiratory: Shortness of breath, exertional dyspnea.

   GI: Weight loss even with high caloric intake; Diarrhea.

   Cardiovascular: Palpitations, tachycardia, dysrhythmias, or hypertension.
   b. Solution: TSH (Thyroid-stimulating hormone) and a T_4 (Thyroxin) are recommended for initial diagnosing of hyperthyroidism.
   c. Solution: Beta blocker, i.e., propranolol or atenolol

3. a. Solution: Change in menstrual cycle: amenorrhea or oligomenorrhea; galactorrhea; or infertility.
   b. Solution: Because of the estrogen deficiency that accompanies hyperprolactinemia, women often develop osteopenia and osteoporosis.

4. a. Solution: Potassium. In Cushing's disease, an excess of mineral corticoids leads to retention of sodium and potassium loss.
   b. Solution: 1. Cardiac dysrhythmias; 2. Muscle weakness; 3. Decrease in gastrointestinal motility; and 4. Polyuria.

5. Solution: A patient who is alert will be thirsty and request water or other drinks, thereby maintaining fluid balance. An unconscious patient will readily

become dehydrated with fluid and electrolyte replacement. Another problem is that elderly people sometimes lose their thirst sensation and are not sensitive to their need for fluids.

Chapter 57

1. Acute illnesses, even a viral infection or upper respiratory infection, can affect the blood sugar level. This occurs as the counter regulatory hormones respond to the stress of the illness. The patient should be taught to continue eating his or her regular meal plan and increase the amount of fluids that do not have calories, i.e., water and decaffeinated fluids. They should monitor their blood glucose every four hours and take their insulin or oral agents as prescribed. If the blood sugar level rises above 240 mg/dL, the urine should be checked for ketones every three to four hours. If moderate to large amounts of ketones are present in the urine, the health care provider should be contacted. If nausea and vomiting prevents the normal food intake, the glucose lowering agents should be continued as pre-scribed. If possible, fluids with carbohydrates should be ingested, such as regular soft drinks without caffeine, fruit juices, and soups. If the patient is not able to keep anything down, the health care provider should be notified. It is important that the patient understand to continue the glucose lowering agents during illness, either insulin or oral hypoglycemics, as the counter regulatory hormones will produce an elevation in blood glucose.

2. Feet should be inspected daily for signs of redness and pressure. If the patient is unable to do this, it should be done by a significant other. Cuts can be cleansed with warm water and mild soap. Do not use any over-the-counter antiseptics on cuts. Cover the cut with a clean dressing that does not apply pressure. Continue to observe the area for signs of infection. Socks should be white absorbent cotton or colorfast. It is important to check the temperature of the water to avoid burn injuries. Wash the feet daily in warm water using a mild soap. Dry thoroughly between the toes. Pat the feet dry, do not rub. Toenails should be cut straight across. No commercial preparations are to be used for removal of corns or calluses. Shoes should fit properly without any pressure areas and should not have open toes or heels. The patient should not go barefoot.

3. The blood sugar level is below 70 mg/dL indicating that the patient is hypoglycemic and requires immediate intervention. Because the patient is still responsive and able to swallow, 15 grams of a fast-acting carbohydrate such as 8 ounces of low-fat milk or 4–6 ounces of regular soft drink or fruit juice are given orally. Glucose tablets or gels may also be used in this situation as the patient is able to swallow. The blood sugar is reassessed 15 minutes after the carbohydrates are ingested. This is repeated until the blood sugar level rises above 70 mg/dL. The patient is then given a regularly scheduled meal or snack, and the blood glucose is reassessed in 45 minutes.

4. When patients with diabetes experience an acute illness, the body reacts to this stress by activating the counter-regulatory hormones. The counter-regulatory hormones increase blood sugar levels. It is common to see hospitalized patients on insulin therapy even though they do not require it at home. When the patient heals and returns home, he or she can expect to return to his or her usual management.

5. Polydipsia, polyphagia, and polyuria are symptoms that occur with hyperglycemia. Polyphagia (increased eating) is a result of the cells starving as there is not sufficient insulin present to move the food into the cells. Polyuria (frequent urination) and polydipsia (increased thirst) result from the osmotic effect of hyperglycemia. The thirst center is stimulated to reduce the concentration by increasing fluid intake, and the kidneys increase urination in an attempt to reduce the concentration on glucose.

6. The student will need to communicate with the diabetic educator to answer the specific questions for this question.

Chapter 58

1. Explain to the patient that a fracture goes through various stages of healing. The first stage takes several days to complete. The next stage, when new bone cells start to grow, can take up to a week to get started. The third stage occurs when the callus starts to form. The callus grows and becomes stronger for the next several weeks. By the end of the six weeks, the callus has strengthened enough to allow return to normal activity. The fracture area is still healing and may take three to four months to return to its previous strength. During this time the patient may feel tinges or aches at the healing fracture site, but this is completely normal.

When teaching your patient about signs of circulatory and neurological impairment, review the neurovascular assessment. Show the patient how to check for proper movement in the hands and fingers or feet and toes. Teach the patient and his or her care providers how to check pulses and capillary refill. Inform the patient to report any numbness, tingling, or edema that is not relieved with 30 minutes of elevation of the extremity. Also teach the patient to feel the foot or hand for warmth. He or she should report these findings to a health care provider. Provide a handout to reinforce teaching and for discharge.

2. The quality of a nursing article depends on how applicable the information is to daily patient care. In the nursing article found, did the article address nursing assessment of the patient? Nursing articles should address nursing assessment and compare normal and abnormal findings for the particular topic investigated. The article should address what nursing interventions are done to minimize complications. Additionally, the article should address the collaboration necessary between the nurse and the health care provider or advanced practice nurse to determine the best plan of care. Also, patient or family involvement should be included during the discussion of plan of care.

3. Inform the neighbor with bursitis that a bursa is a fluid-filled sac under a tendon near the joint that provides cushioning and minimizes friction between the tendon and other structures in the joint. With bursitis the fluid-filled sac is swollen, and the cushioning over the joint is interrupted. This causes the tendon to rub on the bone, a ligament, or another tendon leading to pain.

4. During the assessment of a postoperative orthopedic patient, observe the nurse performing head-to-toe assessments. The nurse should be assessing for the following: level of consciousness; alertness and orientation; lung and heart sounds; bowel sounds; and a neurovascular assessment on the affected extremity or full neurological assessment that includes bilateral hand grasps, bilateral dorsiflexion, and plantar flexion for spine surgery. While performing the neurovascular assessment the nurse should assess both extremities to compare and contrast sides, looking for differences that may indicate neurovascular impairment related to the operative procedure.

5. Tell the patient that a magnetic resonance imaging (MRI) is the most sensitive technique for outlining structures in the body. The MRI can determine whether a tumor is within or adjacent to a bone. Computed tomography (CT) scans are not as sensitive and X-rays only show the surface structure of the bone, not what is happening inside the bone itself. In preparing the patient for the procedure, the nurse is responsible asking about metal implants and ensuring the consent form has been signed. A female patient should be asked about her pregnancy status. All patients need to remove jewelry. Explain the procedure and the length of the procedure. This depends on how many images the health care provider needs, but it generally takes 30 minutes. Determine if the patient gets claustrophobic. Some patients need to be lightly sedated because of anxiety. Unless the patient has had sedation, there are no special precautions needed after the procedure.

Chapter 59

1. Watching orthopedic surgery is like being in your father's workshop. You will see saws, hammers, screws, bolts, and other equipment. This is the equipment used to repair fractures and remove damaged bone tissue and make room for prostheses that will replace a joint surface. During join replacement you will notice that the team is dressed in what might be referred to as space suits, complete with helmets and air hoses for cooling the team member off. Because of the vascularity of the joint and susceptibility to infection, the surgeons wear these suits to protect the patient from infection. When working on an extremity, it is often suspended with tape and gauze to keep the extremity in the correct position to facilitate the surgery. Often the extremity is exsanguinated using ace wraps to minimize blood loss. The type of traction used in surgery is skin traction to keep the bone ends apart before or during the procedure.

2. Today, true orthopedic nursing units are vanishing. Quite often the service is coupled with another surgical service. Specialty hospitals are becoming more popular. There are several purely orthopaedic institutions across the United States. The types of patients seen on an inpatient unit are typically hospitalized after joint replacements or traumas. These patients are generally hospitalized, because they need special nursing care to assist in their recovery. This special care includes administration of antibiotics, establishing anticoagulant therapy, monitoring the patient's response, and ensuring the patient can perform mobility tasks safely (getting in and out of a bed or chair and ambulating with assistive devices). Other types of orthopedic surgery are generally done on an outpatient basis, because they do not require the special skills of a nurse to recover successfully. The typical length of stay for a joint replacement of the lower extremity is three to four days. These patients do not generally need to go to an extended care facility after discharge.

3. Tell your patient with osteoarthritis that although there is no cure for the disease, control can be obtained and they can live normal and active lives

with a few lifestyle changes. You can refer your patient to a local chapter of the Arthritis Foundation or other local arthritis support groups to assist in the physical and emotional coping that is required. When assessing acceptance of the information you provide, ask your patients what plans they may have to contact the organization. You can also make a follow-up phone call. You can offer support at that time and ask if she contacted the agency. Sometimes, patients just need encouragement to seek the assistance that will make their lives easier.

4. When obtaining information from the World Wide Web, you need to take many things into consideration, such as whether or not the information is from a reliable source and is accurate. Two sources that can assist in knowing about the reliability and accuracy of the information is the Health on the Net Foundation (http://www.hon.ch or http://www.hon.ch/HONcode/Conduct.html). This international foundation reviews Web sites for accuracy and reliability. They have a distinctive logo that they apply to a Web site homepage if they feel the information meets the standards of the foundation. Please visit one of the two sites to see the logo. Bobby Watchfire is a web accessibility desktop testing tool designed to help expose barriers to accessibility and encourage compliance with existing accessibility guidelines, including Section 508 of the U.S. Rehabilitation Act and the W3C's Web Content Accessibility Guidelines (WCAG). You can find this at http://www.watchfire.com. They rate Web sites according to the amount of compliance met to the Section 508 standards.

Chapter 60

1. Visiting an outpatient rehabilitation facility will give the student exposure to a wide variety of sports-related injuries not normally seen on an inpatient basis. They will be able to see firsthand what treatments are used for specific injuries and will be able to see the work involved with rehabilitation. It is also important to realize what limitations these patients must live with until their rehabilitation is complete.

2. Visiting an emergency department will expose the student to a wide variety of trauma. The student should focus on the initial treatments given in the field especially how any fractures are splinted and immobilized.

3. Visiting an inpatient orthopaedic unit will expose the student to patients who have sustained hip fractures. Describing the type of fracture along with the surgical treatment will help the student link the

two together with the rationale on why that particular treatment was chosen. This activity will also help the student link which patients need to follow hip precautions.

4. Developing a teaching plan on fall prevention will help the student to focus on fall prevention strategies and to focus on how an elderly patient learns best. The student should include adult learning principles into the plan. It should also help the student to bring to fruition the risk factors that places a patient at risk for falls. Having the student list important questions will help to clarify and organize the main elements of the teaching plan.

5. It is important for the student to realize the value of being a patient advocate. To be an advocate the student must be able to find information that the patient may need and to be able to use available resources available to the nurse to bring the resources, such as a support group, and the patient together. The student must also be able to recognize quality Web sources and to be able to tell a patient how to find a quality Web source as well.

Chapter 61

1. Best applied in a laboratory setting with a peer. Use a nursing assessment text and develop a list of questions to ask in a sexual health history.

2. Best performed in a practicum setting by providing nursing care for a person of the opposite gender who is close to your age. Afterward, discuss with your peers the potential difficulties of patient education regarding self-examinations that are characteristic of reproductive function. Ideally, find a peer of the opposite gender and get his or her perspective on how he or she would feel having these types of questions asked of him or her. Remember, your goal is to increase your knowledge level to enhance your abilities to be comfortable with the topic.

3. Best applied in laboratory or seminar settings. Review the sexual response cycle before the discussion with a peer to increase your knowledge level in the content area.

4. Compare four of the varied diagnostic tests in the reproductive system that are performed with a male (e.g., urethral smear, urinalysis, semen analysis, digital rectal examination (DRE), endocrine evaluation of various hormones, and prostate-specific antigen [PSA] levels).

5. Compare four diagnostic tests in the reproductive system, which are performed with a female (e.g., mammography, blood cultures, Pap smear, colposcopy, culdoscopy, and endometrial biopsy).

Chapter 62

1. The patient education sheet should include most of the following elements:

   - Description of PCOS as an endocrine disorder with insulin resistance as its main pathology.
   - List of symptoms women may experience including hirsutism, high body mass index (BMI), acne, and infertility.
   - Descriptions of the lifestyle changes that may help relieve symptoms, including weight loss, exercise, calcium supplementation, and avoiding smoking.
   - List of medications that might be used to treat PCOS including oral contraceptives, metformin, clomiphene citrate, and topical eflornithine HCL.
   - Web sites and other patient resources.

2. Concerns for a hysterectomy patient may include:

   - Pain and pain relief issues
   - Returning to regular daily activities
   - Effects on sexual response
   - Response to loss of childbearing including grief, loss, or relief
   - Need for education about physical changes associated with hysterectomy

3. Sample nursing diagnoses for patient with PCOS:

   - Anxiety related to infertility
   - Disturbed body image related to physical changes associated with PCOS
   - Risk for situational low self-esteem related to changes in body image

   Expected outcomes for patient with PCOS:

   - Relief of anxiety
   - Improved body image
   - Improved self-esteem

4. Cervical cancer incidence by state can be found at the Centers for Disease Control and Prevention (CDC) Web site: http://www.cdc.gov/. Local cervical cancer incidence may be obtained from the American Cancer Society (ACS) or local health departments. Recommendations for improvement in cervical cancer screening programs may include screening women most at risk, e.g., those in sexually transmitted disease (STD) clinics; offering screening along with other services, e.g., mammograms or emergency department visits; and using a variety of providers to do screenings (nurse practitioners and physicians' assistants, along with physicians).

5. Postmenopausal women have a variety of attitudes about hormone therapy. Many women who were happily taking therapy in 2002 were distressed to learn about potential side effects and recommendations to reduce or stop therapy. Many other women have always been reluctant to take hormones and avoided any postmenopausal therapy. Other women are conflicted. They do not want to increase their risks for serious health conditions, but need effective relief of menopausal symptoms that interfere with activities of daily living and relationships. Interviewing postmenopausal women should give nursing students an idea of the range of opinions about hormone therapy and an insight into the controversy surrounding this topic.

Chapter 63

1. At birth there is rudimentary breast tissue that has ducts lined with epithelium. During puberty, or adolescence, there is a release of follicle-stimulating hormone (FSH), luteinizing hormone (LH), and prolactin that stimulates the release of estrogen from the ovaries. The estrogen stimulates the growth of the ductile system in the breasts, and the breast assumes the characteristic contour. During pregnancy, estrogen, progesterone and prolactin prepare the breast for lactation. At menopause, the breasts lose their glandular tissue because of decreased levels of estrogen and progesterone.

2. Patients need to first be advised that BSE should be performed once a month, eight days following menses or on any given fixed date. Advise the patient to avoid the time when her breasts might be tender because of menstruation or ovulation. Encourage her to put the BSE on her calendar and include her significant other in the process.

   Second, think B (bed): Show the patient how to palpate her breast while supine in bed using the palmar surfaces of her fingers. She should start by placing her right arm over her head and palpating the right breast with the left hand, moving in concentric circles from the periphery inward and including the periphery, tail of Spence, and areola. Finally, instruct the patient to squeeze the nipple to examine for discharge. Using the reverse procedure, she should examine the other breast.

   Third, think S (standing): Instruct the patient to repeat the above palpation method while standing.

   Fourth, think E (examination before a mirror): The patient should stand in front of a mirror with her arms at her sides, then with her arms raised over head, and finally with her hands pressed into her hips and in each position examine her breasts for symmetry, retractions, dimpling, inverted nipples, or nipple deviation.

3. This is performed in the clinical setting and should identify such topics as privacy issues, importance of

the gender of the health care provider, and clear communication encouraged by the health care provider.

4. The first surgeries for breast augmentation occurred in the 18th century with poor results. Throughout the 1990s the use of silicone implants for augmentation had varying results, but techniques have greatly improved since that time. Saline-filled implants have decreased some risks, but still have some complications. Breast augmentation surgeries continue to be evaluated and are being taken more seriously as improved techniques are employed.

5. A description needs to be given of one of the following: physical examination, mammography, ultrasonography, or biopsy.

6. A description is given for each of the following: cryotherapy, laser ablation, radiofrequency ablation (RFA), and focused ultrasound ablation. In most of these a probe is placed under the skin into the breast lesion under the guidance of an imaging modality, and tumor cell destruction is achieved by means of either heat or cold.

Chapter 64

1. This is performed in the clinical practicum setting with the selection of a patient with benign prostate hypertrophy. Discuss your findings with your peers in clinical seminar and laboratory settings.

2. Teach a TSE to a male patient. Introduce yourself in the clinical setting and describe the rationale for performing this procedure. Provide the patient time to ask questions and use information from an assessment text to support your techniques of examination.

3. Take notes in a reflective journal and perhaps selecting a patient with cancer would assist you in this activity. Then meet with a peer who shares your clinical course with you and ask open-ended questions regarding his or her feelings if he or she were to be diagnosed with cancer. Encourage open communication and be honest in stating how you would really feel if you were suddenly diagnosed with cancer.

4. This is best applied in a laboratory setting, and you can use a peer to simulate being the patient. Then share how you would bring up the initial topic of ED with the patient. Ask your peer to evaluate how you ask your questions and specifically to critique whether or not you appear to be comfortable and at ease in sharing your information.

5. This is best applied in a laboratory setting, and you can use a peer to simulate being the patient. Focus on techniques of therapeutic communication for discussing the priapism with the patient. Ask the peer to simulate asking you difficult questions and have the peer be hesitant to bring up the subject. Then, practice discussing the disorder using verbal techniques to make the patient be comfortable with this topic.

Chapter 65

The activities have been structured around World Wide Web sites to encourage the reader to actively research the many resources that are available. Some of the Web sites have interactive programs. Some of the materials can be downloaded free of charge and can be used as patient instructional materials. The various activities also stimulate critical thinking and can easily be used as individual or group assignments as part of the course requirements or as extra activities. Some of the articles include case studies related to the shock syndrome and multiple organ dysfunction.

Chapter 66

1. Reviewing an emergency department (ED) triage criteria will help one to become familiar with guidelines. This will also help to give some ideas as to what type of injuries or illnesses as triaged at what level.

2. Observing or even participating in a disaster drill is a wonderful way to see how hospitals implement their disaster policies and incident command. Disaster drill observation also will show how triage differs in a disaster versus every day triage.

3. This will allow the student to know what will be expected if he or she was in clinical if the hospital disaster plan was initiated and how the event would be run.

4. As a student, one must develop practices to protect oneself from contagious diseases. This includes knowing where to locate and how to use the appropriate personal protective equipment (PPE) for the disease.

5. Talking with CISM team members will give you a better understanding of the team members' roles. Familiarization with this process will make one more comfortable attending a debriefing if the situation arose.

6. There is no better way to experience ED nursing than have clinical time in the department.

References

Abbas, A., & Lichtman, A. (2004). *Basic immunology: Functions and disorders of the immune system* (2nd ed.). Philadelphia: W. B. Saunders Co.

Abu AlRub, R. (2004). Job stress, job performance, and social support among hospital nurses. *Journal of Nursing Scholarship, 36*(1), 73–78.

Ackley, B. J., & Ladwig, G. B. (2004). *Nursing diagnosis handbook: A guide to planning care* (6th ed.). St. Louis, MO: Mosby.

Adams, H. P., Adams, R. J., Brott, T., del Zoppo, G. J., Furlan, A., Goldstein, L. B., et al. (2003). Guidelines for the early management of patients with ischemic stroke: A scientific statement from The Stroke Council of the American Stroke Association. *Stroke, 34*(4), 1056–1083.

AdminaStar Federal. (2003). *Explanation of reimbursement rates under Critical Access Hospitals (CAH)*. Washington, DC: Critical Access Hospital Certified Manual.

Aggarwal, S., (2003). Portal vein thrombosis complicating neonatal hepatic abscess. *Indian Pediatrics, 40*(10), 997–1001.

Agraharkar, M. (2004, September). *Nephrotic syndrome*. Retrieved January 25, 2006, from http://www.emedicine.com.

Ahrens, T., & Sona, C. (2003). Capnography application in acute and critical care. *AACN Clinical Issues, 14*, 123–132.

Ahrens, T., & Vollman, K. (2003). Severe sepsis management: Are we doing enough? *Critical Care Nurse, 24*(Suppl 2), 2–16.

Ahrens, T., & Vollman, K. (2004). Low dose steroid replacement in severe sepsis. *Critical Care Nurse, 24*(2), 16.

Aiken, L. H., Clarke, S. P., Sloane, D. M., Sochalski, J., & Silber, J. H. (2002). Hospital nurse staffing and patient mortality, nurse burnout, and job dissatisfaction. *The Journal of the American Medical Association, 288*(16), 1987–1993.

Ait-Khaled, N., & Enarson D. (2006). Management of asthma: The essentials of good clinical practice. *International Journal of Tuberculosis and Lung Disease, 10*(2), 133–137.

Alarcon Segovia, D., Alarcon-Riquelme, M., Cardiel, M., Caeiro, F., Massardo, L., Villa, A., et al. (2005). Familial aggregation of systemic lupus erythematosus, rheumatoid arthritis, and other autoimmune diseases in 1,177 lupus patients form the GLADEL cohort. *Arthritis and Rheumatism, 52*(4), 1138–1147.

Alden, N., Rabbits, A., & Yurt, R. (2005). Burn injury in patients with dementia: An impetus for prevention. *Journal of Burn Care and Rehabilitation, 26*(3), 267–271.

Alderson, P., Green, S., & Higgins, J. P. T. (Eds.). (2003). Cochrane reviewers' handbook 4.2.2. In *The Cochrane Database of Systematic Reviews* (1), 2004. Chichester, UK: John Wiley & Sons.

Aldridge, M. (2005). Decreasing parental stress in the pediatric intensive care unit: One unit's experience. *Critical Care Nurse, 25*(6), 40–50.

Alexander, J., McDaniel, G., Baldwin, M., & Money, B. (2002). Promoting, applying, and evaluating problem-based learning in the undergraduate nursing curriculum. *NLN Perspectives, 23*(5), 248–254.

Allen, D. (2004). Reading the signs. *Nursing Older People, 16*(4), 6.

Allen, G. (2005). Evidence for practice. Conversion from laparoscopic to open cholecystectomy. *AORN Journal, 81*(3), 690, 693.

Allen, G., & Parsons, P. (2005). Acute lung injury: Significant treatment and outcome. *Current Opinion in Anesthesiology, 18*(2), 209–215.

The ALLHAT Officers and Coordinators for the ALLHAT Collaborative Research Group. (2002). Major outcomes in high-risk hypertensive patients randomized to angiotensin-converting enzymes inhibitor or calcium channel blocker vs diuretic: The antihypertensive and lipid-lowering treatment to prevent heart attack trial (ALLHAT). *Journal of the American Medical Association, 288*, 2981–2997.

Almefty, R., Webber, B., & Arnautovic, K. (2006). Intraneural perineurioma of the third cranial nerve: Occurrence and identification. Case report. *Journal of Neurosurgery, 104*(5), 824–827.

Alsakafi, N., & Kuznetsov, D. (2004). *Spermatocele*. Retrieved July 1, 2006, from http://www.emedicine.com.

Altizer, L. (2004). Casting for immobilization. *Orthopedic Nursing, 23*(2), 136–141.

Altizer, L. (2005). Hip fractures. *Orthopaedic Nursing, 24*(4), 283–292.

Altman, G. (2004). *Delmar's fundamental and advanced nursing skills* (2nd ed.). New York: Thomson Delmar Learning.

Altman, G. B., & Taylor, S. C. (2004). Assessing immediate postoperative care. In G. B. Altman (Ed.), *Delmar's fundamental and advanced nursing skills* (2nd ed., pp. 510–519). Albany, NY: Thomson Delmar Learning.

Amado, M., & Portnoy, J. (2006). Recent advances in asthma management. *Missouri Medicine, 103*(1), 60–64.

Ambuel, B., Hamlett, K., Marx, C., & Blumer, J. (1992). Assessing distress in pediatric intensive care environments: The comfort scale. *Journal of Pediatric Psychology, 17*(1), 95–109.

American Academy of Allergy, Asthma, and Immunology. (2002). *Practice parameters for the diagnosis and management of sinusitis.* Retrieved December 17, 2004, from http://www.aaaai.org.

American Academy of Allergy, Asthma, and Immunology. (2006). *Fact sheets.* Retrieved July 8, 2006, from www.aaaai.org.

American Academy of Dermatology. (2002). Actinic keratoses and skin cancer. *Dermatology Nursing, 16*(6), 397–399.

American Academy of Dermatology. (2006). *Aging skin.* Retrieved July 22, 2006. from http://www.aad.org.

American Academy of Orthopaedic Surgeons. (2003). *Orthopaedic fast facts.* Retrieved September 5, 2006, from http//orthoinfo.aaos.org.

American Academy of Otolaryngology-Head and Neck Surgery (AAO-HNS). (2002a). *Fact sheet: Antibiotics and sinusitis.* Retrieved December 17, 2004, from http://www.entnet.org/healthinfo/sinus/antibiotics_sinusitis.cfm.

American Academy of Otolaryngology-Head and Neck Surgery (AAO-HNS). (2002b). *Fact sheet: Sinusitis: Special considerations for aging patients.* Retrieved December 17, 2004, from http://www.entnet.org/healthinfo/sinus/aging_patients.cfm.

American Academy of Otolaryngology-Head and Neck Surgery (AAO-HNS). (2002c). *Fact sheet: Sinus surgery.* Retrieved December 17, 2004, from http://www.entnet.org/healthinfo/sinus/sinus_surgery.cfm.

American Academy of Otolaryngology-Head and Neck Surgery (AAO-HNS). (2002d). *Doctor, explain tonsils and adenoid.* Retrieved August 25, 2004 from, http://www.entnet.org/healthinfo/throat/tonsils.cfm.

American Academy of Pediatrics. (2002). *The youngest victims: Disaster preparedness to meet childrens' needs.* Retrieved June 23, 2006, from aap.org/terrorism.htm.

American Association of Clinical Endocrinologists Male Sexual Dysfunction Task Force. (2003). Medical guidelines for clinical practice for the evaluation and treatment of male sexual dysfunction: A couple's problem—2003 update. *Endocrine Practice, 9*(1), 77–95.

American Association of Colleges of Nursing. (1997). *Peaceful death document.* Retrieved June 15, 2006, from www.aacn.nche.edu/publications/deathfin.htm.

American Association of Colleges of Nursing. (October, 2004). *Position statement on the practice doctorate in nursing.* Retrieved October 3, 2005, from www.aacn.nche.edu/DNP/DNPpositionstatement.htm.

American Association of Critical Care Nurses. (2002) *Critical care nursing fact sheet.* Retrieved May 21, 2004, from www.aacn.org.

American Association of Critical Care Nurses. (2003). *General information regarding certification.* Retrieved May 7, 2004, from www.aacn.org.

American Association of Critical Care Nurses and AACN Certification Corporation. (2003). Safeguarding the patient and the profession: The value of critical care nurse certification. *American Journal of Critical Care, 12*(5), 154–164.

American Brain Tumor Association. (2004a). *A primer of brain tumors: A patient's reference* (8th ed.). Retrieved June 13, 2006, from www.abta.org.

American Brain Tumor Association. (2004b). *Focusing on treatment: Chemotherapy.* Retrieved June 14, 2006, from www.abta.org.

American Brain Tumor Association. (2004c). *Focusing on treatment: Surgery.* Retrieved June 13, 2006, from www.abta.org.

American Burn Association. (2005). *Advanced burn life support course: Provider's manual.* Chicago: Author.

American Cancer Society. (2003). Cancer reference information: Overview: Laryngeal and hypopharyngeal cancer. Retrieved June 10, 2004, from http://www.cancer.org/docroot/CRI/CRI_2_1x.asp?rnav=criov&dt=23.

American Cancer Society. (2004a). *Cancer facts and figures.* Atlanta, GA: Author.

American Cancer Society. (2004b). *Detailed guide to cervical cancer.* Retrieved August 30, 2004, from http://www.cancer.org/docroot/CRI/CRI_2_3x.asp?dt=8.

American Cancer Society. (2004c). *Detailed guide to endometrial cancer.* Retrieved October 14, 2004 from http://www.cancer.org/docroot/CRI/CRI_2_3x.asp?dt=11.

American Cancer Society. (2004d). *Ovarian cancer.* Retrieved August 30, 2004, from http://www.cancer.org/docroot/CRI/CRI_0.asp.

American Cancer Society. (2004e). *Overview: Lung cancer.* Retrieved August 16, 2006, from http://www.cancer.org.

American Cancer Society. (2004f). *Understanding radiation therapy: A guide for patients and families.* Retrieved March 22, 2005, from http://www.cancer.org.

American Cancer Society. (2004g). *What are the key statistics for brain and spinal cord tumors? Cancer Reference Information.* Retrieved June 13, 2006, www.cancer.org.

American Cancer Society. (2006a). *Stomach (gastric) cancer* (p. 1). Retrieved June 25, 2006, from www.cancer.gov.

American Cancer Society. (2006b). *Surveillance research.* Retrieved October 4, 2006, from http://www.cancer.org.

American Cancer Society. (2006c). Retrieved June 24, 2006, from www.cancersociety.com.

American Chronic Pain Association. (2004). *Nurses' pain awareness kit.* Retrieved from www.theacpa.org.

American College for Emergency Physicians. (2004). Code of ethics. Policy statement. *Annals of Emergency Medicine, 43*(5), 686–694.

American College of Obstetricians and Gynecologists. (2002). *Nonsurgical diagnosis and management of vaginal agenesis.* ACOG Committee Opinion: No. 274, 82–85.

American College of Obstetricians and Gynecologists. (2005). Urinary incontinence in women. *Obstetrics and Gynecology, 105*(6), 1533–1545.

American College of Physicians. (2005). *Lyme disease: A patient guide.* Retrieved September 5, 2006, from www.acponline.org.

American College of Rheumatology. (2004). *New pulmonary hypertension guideline challenges use of common medications.* Retrieved September 16, 2004, from http://www.rheumatology.org.

American Diabetes Association. (2006). Retrieved June 23, 2006, from www.diabetes.org.

American Heart Association. (2001). Heart association science advisory: Lyon diet heart study. Benefits of a Mediterranean-style, National Cholesterol Education Program/American Heart Association step I dietary pattern on cardiovascular disease. *#71-0202 Circulation, 1*(103), 1823–1825.

American Heart Association. (2003). *Heart disease and stroke statistics—2004 update.* Dallas, TX: American Heart Association.

American Heart Association. (2004a). *Heart disease and stroke statistics—2004 update.* Retrieved June 24, 2006, from www.aha.com.

American Heart Association (2004b). *Primary or unexplained pulmonary hypertension.* Retrieved September 16, 2004, from http://www.americanheart.org.

American Heart Association. (2004c). *Pulmonary hypertension.* Retrieved July 17, 2006, from http://www.americanheart.org.

American Heart Association. (2005). *Heart disease and stroke statistics.* Dallas: Author.

American Heart Association. (2006a). *American heart association 2005 guidelines for CPR and ECC.* Retrieved July 3, 2006, from www.americanheart.org.

American Heart Association. (2006b). *Heart failure: Understanding heart failure.* Retrieved June 26, 2006, from www.americanheart.org.

American Heart Association. (2006c). *Inflammation heart disease and stroke: The role of C-reactive protein.* Retrieved June 23, 2006, from www.americanheart.org.

American Holistic Nursing Association. (2006). (p. 14). Retrieved June 23, 2006, from www.ahna.org.

American Hospital Association. (1980). *A patient's bill of rights.* Chicago: Author.

American Hospital Association. (1992). Catalog no. 157759. Retrieved July1, 2005, from www.aha.org.

American Hospital Association. (2005, December 8). *AHA News Now.*

American Infertility Association. (2005). *Focus on fertility.* Retrieved June 23, 2006, from http://www.focusonfertility.org.

American Joint Committee on Cancer. (2002). *Staging systems.* Retrieved June 16, 2005, from http://training.seer.cancer.gov.

American Lung Association. (2003a). *Bronchietasis fact sheet.* Retrieved August 15, 2006, from http://www.americanheart.org.

American Lung Association. (2003b). *Facts about lung cancer.* Retrieved June 30, 2004, from http://www.lungusa.org.

American Lung Association. (n.d.a). *Freedom from smoking online.* Retrieved August 30, 2005, from http://www.lungusa.org.

American Lung Association. (n.d.b). *Open airways for schools.* Retrieved August 30, 2005, from http://www.lungusa.org.

American Lung Association. (n.d.c). *Special reports.* Retrieved August 30, 2005, from http://www.lungusa.org.

American Lung Association. (n.d.d). *Tobacco control and teens.* Retrieved August 30, 2005, from http://www.lungusa.org.

American Lung Association Epidemiology and Statistic Unit Research and Scientific Affairs. (2004). *Trends in lung cancer and morbidity and mortality.* Retrieved June 30, 2004, from http://www.lungusa.org.

American Medical Association. (1999). Medical futility in end-of-life care. *Journal of the American Medical Association, 281,* 937–941.

American Medical Association. (2003). Pain management: The online series. Retrieved from www.ama-cmeonline.com.

American Medical Association. (2004). News from the AMA: *Giving antibiotics within four hours of arrival at a hospital improved outcomes for older patients with pneumonia.* Retrieved September 16, 2004, from http://www.medem.com.

American Nurses Association. (1992a). *Position statement on active euthanasia.* Washington, DC: Author.

American Nurses Association. (1992b). *Position statement on nursing and the patient self determination act.* Washington, DC: Author.

American Nurses Association. (1992c). *Position statement on nursing care and do-not-resuscitate decisions.* Washington, DC: Author.

American Nurses Association. (1992d). *Position statement on foregoing nutrition and hydration.* Washington, DC: Author.

American Nurses Association. (1995). *Nursing: A social policy statement.* Washington, DC: Author.

American Nurses Association. (2001). *Code of ethics for nurses with interpretive statements.* Silver Spring, MD: American Nurses Publishing. Retrieved August 5, 2006, from www.nursingworld.org.

American Nurses Association. (2003a). *Nursing's social policy statement* (2nd ed.). Washington, DC: Author.

American Nurses Association. (2003b). *Position statement on pain management and control of distressing symptoms in dying patients.* Retrieved July 12, 2005, from Nursebooks.org.

American Nurses Association. (2003c). *Social policy statement on pain symptom management of the dying patient.* Retrieved from www.nursingworld.org.

American Nurses Association. (2006). *Code of ethics for nurses with interpretive statements.* Washington DC: American Nurses Publishing.

American Nurse Credentialing Center. (2005). Retrieved June 15, 2005, from http://www.nursingworld.org/ancc.

American Organization of Nurse Executives. (2004, April 9). *AONE eNews Update.*

American Pain Foundation. (2004). Retrieved from www.painfoundation.org.

American Sleep Apnea Association. (2004). *What is sleep apnea?* Retrieved June 10, 2004, from http://www.sleepapnea.org.

American Society for Aesthetic Plastic Surgery. (2006). *What's new in plastic surgery?* Retrieved July 26, 2006, from http://www.surgery.org.

American Society of Anesthesiologists. (2004). *Continuum of depth of sedation definitions of general anesthesia and levels of sedation/analgesia.* Oklahoma: ASA House of Delegates.

American Society of Plastic Surgeons. (2002). *National clearinghouse of plastic surgery statistics 2002 report.* Arlington Heights, IL: Author.

American Spinal Injury Association. (2004). Retrieved July 13, 2006, from http://www.asia-spinalinjury.org.

American Stroke Association. (2004, June 24). Long-term outlook good for carotid stenting to prevent stroke. Fifth World Stroke Congress meeting report. *Stroke News.* Retrieved June 13, 2006, from http://www.strokeassociation.org.

American Thoracic Society, Center for Disease Control, & Infectious Disease Society of America. (2003). *Treatment of tuberculosis.* MMWR. Retrieved September 16, 2004, from http://www.cdc.gov.

American Urologic Association. (2004, February). *Orchitis and epididymitis.* Retrieved June 1, 2006, from http://www.urologyhealth.org.

American Urological Association. (2006). *Urologic diseases in America.* Retrieved July 16, 2006, from www.auanet.org.

Analay, Y., Ozcan, E., Karan, A., Diracoglu, D., & Aydin, R. (2003). The effectiveness of intensive group exercise on patients with ankylosing spondylitis. *Clinical Rehabiliation, 17*(6), 631–636.

Andersen, B., Kallehave, F., & Andersen, H. (2004). *Antibiotics versus placebo for prevention of postoperative infection after appendectomy* [Electronic version: Cochrane Review]. Retrieved December 15, 2004, from http://www.cochrane.org.

Anderson, B. (2005). Nutrition and wound healing: The necessity of assessment. *British Journal of Nursing, 14*(19); *Tissue Viability Supplement:* S30, S32, S34.

Anderson, D., Woltman, M., Kovach, G., & Konety, B. (2004) Long-term treatment of metastatic renal-cell carcinoma with fluorouracil. *Lancet Oncology, 5*(11), 690–692.

Anderson, R. (2005). *Psychoneuroimmunoendocrinology review and commentary. Townsend Letter for doctors and patients.* Retrieved August 2, 2006, from www.learnnet.co.nz.

Anderson-Shaw, L. (2003). The unilateral DNR order—one hospital's experience. *Journal of Nursing Administration's Healthcare, Law, Ethics, and Regulation, 5*(2), 42–46.

Andres, E., Affenberger, S., Zimmer, J., Vinzio, S., Grosu, D., Pistol, G., et al. (2006). Current hematological findings in cobalamin deficiency. A study of 201 consecutive patients with documented cobalamin deficiency. *Clinical and Laboratory Haematology, 28*(1), 50–56.

Andres, E., Loukili, N. H., Noel, E., Kaltenbach, G., Abdelgheni, M. B., Perrin A. E., et al. (2004). Vitamin B_{12} (cobalamin) deficiency in elderly patients. *Canadian Medical Association Journal, 171*(3), 251–259.

Andrews, E., & Fleischer, A. (2005). Sonography for deep venous thrombosis: Current and future applications. *Ultrasound Quarterly, 21*(4), 213–225.

Andrews, M. M., & Boyle, J. S. (2002). *Transcultural concepts in nursing care* (4th ed.). Philadelphia: Lippincott, Williams & Wilkins.

Andrews, M., & Boyle, J. (2003). *Transcultural concepts in nursing care* (5th ed.). Philadelphia: Lippincott, Wilkins, & Williams.

Angus, F., & Burakoff, R., (2003). The percutaneous endoscopic gastrostomy tube: Medical and ethical issues in placement. *The American Journal of Gastroenterology, 98*(200), 272–277.

Antai-Otong, D. (2003). *Psychiatric nursing: Biological and behavioral concepts.* Clifton Park, NY: Thomson Delmar Learning.

Antman, E. M., Anbe, D. T., Armstrong, P. W., Bates, E. R., Green, L. A., Hand, M., et al. (2004). ACC/AHA guidelines for the management of patients with ST-elevation myocardial infarction-executive summary. *Circulation, 110*(5), 588–641.

Anzueto, A., & Niederman, M. S. Diagnosis and treatment of rhinovirus respiratory Infections. (2003). *Chest, 123*(5), 1664–1672.

Appel, G., Radhakrishnan, J., & D'Agati, V. (2004). Secondary glomerular disease. In B. Brenner (Ed.), *Brenner and Rector's the kidney* (7th ed., vol. 1, p. 1381). Philadelphia: W. B. Saunders Co.

Aragon, D., Ring, C., & Covelli, M. (2003). The influence of diabetes mellitus on postoperative infections. *Critical Care Nursing Clinics of North America, 15*(1), 125–136.

Arnstein, P. (2005). Accurate assessment is key to effective pain management: taking the fifth (vital sign). *RN, 68*(1), 12.

Aron, D., Finding. J., & Tyrell, B. (2004a). Glucocorticoids and adrenal androgens. In F.S. Greenspan & D. G. Gardner (Eds.), *Basic and clinical endocrinology* (pp. 534–543). St. Louis, MO: Lange Medical Books.

Aron, D., Finding, J., & Tyrell, B. (2004b).Hypothalamus and pituitary. In F. S. Greenspan & D. G. Gardner (Eds.), *Basic and clinical endocrinology* (pp. 537–542). St. Louis, MO: Lange Medical Books.

Aronson, B. S., & Marquis, M. (2004). Care of the adult patient with cystic fibrosis. *Medsurg Nursing, 13*(3), 143–154; quiz 155.

Arthritis Food Guide. (2006). *Arthritis today on call: Safe foods for gout.* Retrieved September 5, 2006, from http://arthritis-guide.com.

Artinian, N. (2003). The psychosocial aspects of heart failure. *American Journal of Nursing, 103*(12), 32–41.

Artinian, N. (2004). Innovations in blood pressure monitoring. *American Journal of Nursing, 104*(8), 52–59.

Asbury, E., & Collins, P. (2005). Cardiac syndrome X. *International Journal of Clinical Practice, 59*(9), 1063–1069.

Ashworth, N. L., Chad, K. E., Harrison, E. L., Reeder, B. A., & Marshall, S. C. (2005). Home versus center based physical activity programs in older adults. *The Cochrane Database of Systematic Reviews 2005.* Art. CD004017. Pub 2. DOI:0.1002/14651858.CD004017.pub2.

Asp, A. (2005) Mechanisms of endocrine control. In K. Copstead & J. L Banasik, *Pathophysiology* (pp. 639–645). St. Louis, MO: Elsevier Saunders.

Association for the Advancement of Medical Instrumentation. (2005). *Standards. Sterilization in health care facilities (part 1) and sterilization equipment (part 2).* Arlington, VA: AAMI Publications.

Association of Operating Room Nurses. (2005a). Recommended practices for electrosurgery. In *Standards, recommended practices and guidelines* (pp. 248–250). Denver: AORN.

Association of Operating Room Nurses. (2005b). Recommended practices for surgical attire. In *Standards, recommended practices and guidelines.* Denver: AORN.

Association of Operating Room Nurses. (2006). *Standards, recommended practices, and guidelines with official AORN statements. 2006 Edition.* Denver: AORN.

Assouline-Dayan, Y., Chang, C., Greenspan, A., Shoenfeld, Y., & Gershwin, M. E. (2002). Pathogenesis and natural history of osteonecrosis. *Seminars in Arthritis Rheumatism, 32*(2), 94–124.

Astin, J. (2004). Mind-body therapies for the management of pain. *Clinical Journal of Pain, 20*(1), 27–32.

Astin, J. A., & Forys, K. (2004). Psychosocial determinants of health and illness: Integrating mind, body and spirit. *Advances in Mind-Body Medicine, 20*(4), 14–21.

Attarian, S., Vedel, J., Pouget, J., & Schmied, A. (2006). Cortical versus spinal dysfunction in amyotrophic lateral sclerosis. *Muscle and Nerve, 33*(5), 677–690.

Aufort, S., Charra, L., Lesnik, A., Bruel, J., & Taourel, P. Multidetector CT of bowel obstruction: Value of postprocessing. *European Radiology, 15*(11), 2323–2329.

Ayers, D. (2004). Melanoma. *Nursing, 34*(4), 52–53.

Azziz, R., Woods, K., Reyna, R., Key, T., Knochenhauer, E., & Yildiz, B. (2004). The prevalence and features of the polycystic ovary syndrome in an unselected population. *Journal of Clinical Endocrinology and Metabolism, 89,* 2745–2749.

Bacon, P. (2005). The spectrum of Wegener's granulomatosis and disease relapse. *The New England Journal of Medicine, 352*(4), 330-332.

Bader, M., Littlejohns, L., & March, K. (2003). Brain tissue oxygen monitoring in severe brain injury II: Implications for critical care teams and case study. *Critical Care Nurse, 23*(4), 29–43.

Badesch D. B., Abman S. H., Ahearn G. S., Barst R. J., McCrory D. C., Simonneau G., et al. (2004). Medical therapy for pulmonary arterial hypertension: ACCP evidenced based clinical practice guidelines. *Chest*(1 Suppl), *126,* 35S–62S.

Badke, M. B., Shea, T. Z., Miedaner, J. A., & Grove C. R. (2004). Outcomes after rehabilitation for adults with balance dysfunction. *Archive Physical Medicine Rehabilitation, 85,* 227–233.

Baier, F. (2006). The Medicare prescription drug benefit: Understanding the benefits and the gaps in this new coverage. *American Journal of Nursing, 106*(6), 66–72.

Bailey, D., & Dresser, G. (2004). Natural products and adverse drug interactions. *Canadian Medical Association Journal, 170*(10), 1531–1532.

Bakas, T., Austin, J. K., Jessup, S. L., Williams, L. S., & Obsert, M. T. (2004). Time and difficulty of tasks provided by family caregivers of stroke survivors. *Journal of Neuroscience Nursing, 36*(2), 95–106.

Baker, D. (2005, October 5). Teens having casual sex earlier, study says. *San Diego Union Tribune,* p. A5.

Baker, J. J. (2002). Medicare payment system for hospital inpatients: Diagnosis-related groups. *The Journal of Health Care Finance, 28*(3), 1–13.

Bandman, E., & Bandman, B. (2002). *Nursing ethics through the life span* (4th ed.). Princeton, NJ: Prentice Hall.

Bandura, A. (1977). *Social learning theory.* Englewood Cliffs, NJ: Prentice Hall.

Baron, R., & Schwartzstein, R. (2004). *Diseases of the chest wall.* Retrieved June 25, 2006, from http://www.uptodate.com.

Barone, C., Pablo, C., & Barone, G. (2004). Postanesthetic care in the critical care unit. *Critical Care Nurse, 24*(1), 38–45.

Bartels, D., (2004). Adherence to oral therapy for type 2 diabetes: Opportunities for enhancing glycemic control. *Journal of the American Academy of Nurse Practitioners, 16*(1), 8–16.

Bartholomay, M., Finn, S., Rounds, A., Bigelow, R., Barrett E., & Coakley A., et al. (2006). Uncovering practice differences related to the care of indwelling and external tunneled catheters across practice settings in a large academic medical center. *Oncology Nursing Forum, 33*(2), 419–420.

Bassi, P., De Marco, V., De Lisa, A., Mancini, M., Pinto, F., Bertoloni, R., et al. (2005). Non-invasive diagnostic tests for bladder cancer: A review of the literature. *Urologia Internationalis, 75*(3), 193–200.

Battais, F., Mothes, T., Moneret-Vautrin, D., Pineau, F., Kanny, G., Popineau, Y., et al. (2005). Identification of IgE-binding epitopes on gliadins for patients with food allergy to wheat. *Allergy, 60*(6), 815–821.

Battleman, D. S., Callahan M., & Thaler, H. T. (2002). Rapid antibiotic delivery and appropriate antibiotic selection reduced length of hospital stay of patients with community acquired pneumonia. *Archives of Internal Medicine, 167*(6), 682–688.

Bee, H., & Boyd, D. R. (2003). *The developing child* (10th ed.). New York: Allyn & Bacon.

Beebe, R., & Funk, D. (2001). *Fundamentals of emergency care.* New York: Thomson Delmar Learning.

Beers, M. H., & Berkow, R. (2004). *The Merck manual of diagnosis and therapy* (17th ed.). West Point, PA: Merck & Co.

Beese-Bjurstrom, S. (2004). Hidden danger: Aortic aneurysm and dissections. *Nursing, 34*(2), 36–42.

Behin, A., Hoang-Xuan, K., Carpentier, A. F., & Delattre, J. (2003). Primary brain tumors in adults. *Lancet, 361*(9354), 323–331.

Beitz, J. (1998). Concept mapping: Navigating the learning process. *Nurse Educator, 23*(5), 35–41.

Bell, G., & Sander, J. (2002, April 11). The epidemiology of epilepsy: the size of the problem. *Seizure, 10*(Suppl A), 306–316.

Bench, S. (2004). Clinical skills: Assessing and treating shock. A nursing perspective. *British Journal of Nursing, 13*(12), 715–721.

Benisty J. I. (2002). *Pulmonary hypertension.* Retrieved September 16, 2004, from http://circ.ahajournals.org.

Benner, E., Mosley, R., Destache, C., Lewis, T., Jackson-Lewis, V., Gorantla, S., et al. (2004). Therapeutic immunization protects dopaminergic neurons in a mouse model of Parkinson's disease. *Proceedings of the National Academy of Sciences of the USA, 101*(25), 9435–9440.

Benson, A. B., III, Ajani, J. A., Catalano, R. B., Engelking, C., Kornblau, S. M., Martenson, J. A., Jr., et al. (2004). Recommended guidelines for the treatment of cancer treatment-induced diarrhea. *Journal of Clinical Oncology, 22*(14), 2918–2926.

Beral, V. (2003). Breast cancer and hormone-replacement therapy in the Million Women Study. *Lancet, 362*(9382), 419–427.

Berardino, M., Morrone, O., Sciacca, P.F., Rosato, R., Ciccone, G. & Massaro, F. (2004). Discharge criteria from intensive care unit in brain injured patients. *Acta Neurochir (Wein), 146*(5), 453–456.

Beresford, I. J. M., Parsons, A. A., & Hunter, A. J. (2003). Treatments for stroke. *Expert Opinions on Emerging Drugs, 8*(1), 103–122.

Berg, F. M., Tymoczko, J. L., & Stryer, L. (2002.) *Biochemistry* (5th ed.). New York: W. H. Freeman and Company.

Bergren, M. (2004). Information technology: HIPAA-FERPA revisited. *Public Health Nursing, 20*(2), 107–112.

Bergs, L. (2005). Immunology: Goodpasture syndrome. *Critical Care Nurse, 25*(5), 50–58.

Bergstrom, N., & Braden, B. (2002). Predictive validity of the Braden Scale among black and white subjects. *Nursing Research, 51*(6), 398–403.

Berman, B. M., Lao, L., Langenberg, P., Lee, W. L., Gilpin, A. M. K., & Hochberg, M. C. (2004). Effectiveness of acupuncture as adjunctive therapy in osteoarthritis of the knee: A randomized, controlled trial. *Annals of Internal Medicine, 141*(12), 901–910.

Berry, T., & Shooner, K. (2004). Family history: The first genetic screen. *The Nurse Practitioner, 29*(11), 14–23.

Beth Israel Deaconess Medical Center. (2004). *WebMD clinical trial services.* Retrieved June 10, 2005, from http://my.webmd.com.

Beyea, S. C. (Ed.). (2002). *The perioperative nursing data set* (2nd ed.). Denver: AORN, Inc.

Bialous, S., & Sarna, L. (2004). Sparing a few minutes for tobacco cessation. *American Journal of Nursing, 104*(12), 54–60.

Binder, I. B. (2003). Paget's disease. *Journal of Endodontics, 29*(11), 720–723.

Birgen, M., Harris, S., Lindbaek, M., & Oslo, N. (2004). Cochlear implants and health status: A comparison with other hearing-impaired patients. *Annals Otology Rhinology and Laryngology, 113,* 914–921.

Bishop, A. H., & Scudder, J. R., (Eds.). (1985). *Caring, curing, coping: Nurse, physician, patient relationships.* Birmingham, AL: University of Alabama Press.

Bisno, A. L., Gerber, M. A., Gwaltney, Jr, J. M., Kaplan, E. L., & Schwartz, R. H. (2002). Practice guidelines for the diagnosis and management of group A streptococcal pharyngitis. *Clinical Infectious Diseases; Infectious Diseases of America, 35*(2), 113–125.

Bisson, J., & Andrew, M. (2005). Psychological treatment of post-traumatic stress disorder (PTSD). *The Cochrane Database of Systematic Reviews* (2), CD003388.

Biton, V., & Tabak, N. (2003). The relationship between the application of the nursing ethical code and nurses' satisfaction. *International Journal of Nursing Practice, 55*(3), 140–157.

Black, J., & Hawks, J. (2004). *Medical-surgical nursing: Clinical management for positive outcomes* (7th ed.). Philadelphia: W. B. Saunders.

Blair, S., & Church, T. (2003). The importance of physical activity and cardiorespiratory fitness for patients with type 2 diabetes. *Diabetes Spectrum, 16*(4), 236–240.

Blais, K., Hayes, J., Kozier, B., & Erb, G. (2002). *Professional nursing practice: Concepts and perspectives* (4th ed.). New Jersey: Prentice Hall.

Blood type facts. (2006). Retrieved July 11, 2006, from http://www.bloodbook.com.

Bloom, B. S. (1977). *Taxonomy of educational objectives: The classification of educational goals, Handbook I: Cognitive domain.* New York: Longman.

Blumenthal, D., Prais, D., Bron-Harlev, E., & Amir, J. (2004). Possible association of Guillain-Barre syndrome and hepatitis A vaccination. *Pediatric Infectious Disease Journal, 23*(6), 586–588.

Blumenthal, M., Brinkman, J., Dinda, K., Goldberg, A. & Wolkschlaegear, B. (2004). *The ABC clinical guide to herbs.* New York: Hawthorne Press, Inc.

Bluvol, A. (2003). The Codman Award Paper: Quality of life in stroke survivors and their spouses: Predictors and clinical implications for rehabilitation teams. *AXON, 25*(2), 10–19.

Bodnar, L., Cogswell, M., & McDonald, T. (2005). Have we forgotten the significance of postpartum iron deficiency? *American Journal of Obstetrics and Gynecology, 193,* 36–44.

Boehm, M., Olive, M., True, A. L., Crook, M. F., San, H., Qu, X., et al. (2004). Bone marrow-derived immune cells regulate vascular disease through a p27Kip1-dependent mechanism. *Journal of Clinical Investigation, 114*(3), 419–426.

Bogardus, S. T., Yueh, B., & Shekelle, P. (2003). Screening and management of adult hearing loss in primary care: Clinical applications. *JAMA, 289*(15), 1986–1990.

Bonadonna, R. (2003). Meditation's impact on chronic illness. *Journal of Holistic Nursing Practice, 17*(6), 309–319.

Bonaiuti, D., Shea, B., Iovine, R., Negrini, S., Robinson, V., Kemper, H. H., et al. (2004). Exercise for preventing and treating osteoporosis in postmenopausal women (Cochrane review). In *The Cochrane Database of Systematic Reviews.* Chichester, UK: John Wiley & Sons, Ltd.

Bone and Joint Decade Organization. (2004, April). *Osteoporosis in Men.* Retrieved September 20, 2004, from http://www.boneandjointdecade.org.

Borneman, T., Stahl, C., Ferrell, B., & Smith, D. (2002). The concept of hope in family caregivers of cancer patients at home. *Journal of Hospice and Palliative Nursing, 4*(1), 21–33.

Boruchoff, S., & Weinstein, M. (2004). *Sputum cultures.* Retrieved June 25, 2006, from http://www.uptodate.com.

Bosen, D. M., & Flemming, M. A. (2003). Beyond ECGs: Understanding electrophysiology testing, part 1. *Nursing, 32*(11), 1–5.

Bosetti, C., Pira, E., & La Vecchia, C. (2005). Bladder cancer risk in painters: A review of the epidemiological evidence, 1989–2004. *Cancer Causes and Control, 16*(9), 997–1008.

Botstein D., & Risch N. (2003). Discovering genotypes underlying human phenotypes: past successes for Mendelian disease, future approaches for complex disease. *Nature Genetics, 33*(Suppl), 228–237.

Boudreaus, E., Edmond, S., & Race, S. (2003) Ethnicity and asthma among children presenting to the emergency department. *Pediatrics III,* (5), e615–e621.

Boyington, A. R., Wildemuth, B. M., Dougherty, M. C., Hall, E. P. (2005). Development of a computer-based system for continence health promotion. *Nursing Outlook, 52*(5), 241–247.

Boyle, E. (2006). Visual impairment reduces functional status of elderly patients. *Ocular Surgery News, 24*(1), 73–74.

Bracken, M. B. (2004). Steroids for acute spinal cord injury. *The Cochrane Database of Systematic Reviews* (2), CD001046. DOI: 10.1002/14651858.

Bradley, J., & Davis, K. (2003). Orthostatic hypotension. *American Family Physician, 68*(12), 2393–2398.

Brady, H., Clarkson, M., & Lieberthal, W. (2004). Acute renal failure. In B. Brenner (Ed.), *Brenner and Rector's the kidney* (7th ed., vol. 1, pp. 1215–1292). Philadelphia: W. B. Saunders Co.

Braimon, J. C., Naaznin, L., & Walczak, M. (2003). In T. M. Buttaro, J. Trybulski, P. P. Bailey, & J. Sandberg-Cook (Eds.), *Primary care: A collaborative practice* (pp. 112–116). St. Louis, MO: Mosby.

Brain Injury Association of America. (2004). *Support adequate finding of the traumatic brain injury act in FY 2005.* McLean, VA: Author.

Brain Injury Association of America. (2006). Retrieved June 13, 2006, from www.biausa.org.

Brain Tumor Society. (2004). *Patient resources.* Retrieved June 15, 2006, from www.tbts.org.

Braun, A., Roth, R., & McGinniss, M. (2003). Technology challenges in screening single gene disorders. *European Journal of Pediatrics, 162*(Suppl 1), S13–S16.

Brenner, M., Hoistad, D., & Hain, T. (2004). Prevalence of thyroid dysfunction in patients with Meniere's Disease. *Archives of Otolaryngology—Head and Neck Surgery, 130*(2), 226–228.

Bretler, S. J. (2004). Traumatic brain injury. *RN, 67*(4), 32–37.

Bridges, E., & Dukes, S. (2005). Cardiovascular aspects of septic shock: Pathophysiology, monitoring, and treatment. *Critical Care Nurse, 25*(2), 14–16, 18–20, 24, 26–28, 30–32, 34–36, 38–40.

Brill, J., (2004). Trends in pain syndrome diagnostic technology. *Practical Pain Management, 4*(4), 12–19.

Brookes, M. J., & Green, J. R. B. (2004). Maintenance of remission in Crohn's disease: Current and emerging therapeutic options. *Drugs, 64*(10), 1069–1089.

Brooks, G. A., Butte, N. F., Rand, W. M., Flatt, J. P., & Caballero, B. (2004). Chronicle of the Institute of Medicine physical activity recommendation. *American Journal of Clinical Nutrition, 79*(5), 921S–930S.

Brors, D., & Bodmer D. (2004). New aspects of inner ear research. *Hospital Medicine, 65*(7), 392–395.

Brosman, S. (2004). *Penile cancer.* Retrieved June 23, 2006, from http://www.emedicine.com.

Brouwer-DudokdeWit, A., Savenue, A., Zoeteweij, M., Maat-Kievit, A., & Tibben, A. (2002). A hereditary disorder in the family and the family life cycle: Huntington Disease as a paradigm. *Family Process, 41*(4), 677–692.

Brown, A. E., Elting, L., Freifeld, A. G., Greene, J. N., Ito, J. I., King, E. K., et al. (2002, May). *Fever and neutropenia treatment guidelines for patients with cancer (Version 1).* Retrieved June 10, 2005, from http://www.nccn.org.

Brown, B. B., Grigsby, J., Walsh, A. C., & Kaye, K. (2002). *Mental capacity: Legal and medical aspects of assessment and treatment* (2nd ed.). New York: Clark.

Brown, B. J. (2004). Reconstructing healthcare in a global marketplace. *Nursing Administration Quarterly, 28*(2), 81–82.

Brown, C. (2003). Surgical treatment of trigeminal neuralgia. *Association of periOperative Registered Nurses, 78*(5), 743–762.

Brown, D., & McCormack, B. (2005). Developing postoperative pain management: Utilising the Promoting Action on Research Implementation in Health Services (PARIHS) framework. *Worldviews on Evidence-Based Nursing, 2*(3), 131–141.

Brown, D. R., Ludwig, R., Buck, G. A., Durham, D., Shumard, T., & Graham, S. S. (2004). Health literacy: Universal precautions needed. *Journal of Allied Health, 33*(2), 150–155.

Brown, K. (2003). *Emergency dysrhythmias: EKG injury patterns.* New York: Thomson Delmar Learning.

Brown University School of Medicine Center for Gerontology and Health Services Research. (2000). *Facts in dying: Policy-relevant data on care at the end of life.* Retrieved July 12, 2005, from www.chsr.brown.edu/dying/usa.

Browning, A. (2006). Exploring advanced directives. *Journal of Christian Nursing, 23*(1): 34–39.

Broyles, B. E., Reiss, B. S., & Evans, M. E. (2007). *Pharmacological aspects of nursing care* (7th ed.). New York: Thomson Delmar Learning.

Brunner, E., Thorogood, M., Rees, K., & Hewitt, G. (2006). Dietary advice for reducing cardiovascular risk. *The Cochrane Database of Systematic Reviews* (1), CD002128.

Buckley, J., & Herth, K. (2004). Fostering hope in terminally ill patients. *Nursing Standard, 19*(10), 33–41.

Bukstein, D., Elder, M. A., Larsen, J., & Mellon, M. (2003). *Clearing the air: Effective management of asthma and allergic rhinitis. A special edition of patient care for the nurse practitioner.* Montvale, NJ: Thomas Medical Economics Company.

Bullard, K. M., & Rothenberger, D. A. (2005). Colon, rectum and anus. In F. C. Brunicardi (Ed.), *Schwartz's principles of surgery* (8th ed., pp. 1055–1117). New York: McGraw Hill.

Bullock, S., & Manias, E. (2002). The educational preparation of undergraduate nursing students in pharmacology: a survey of lectures' perceptions and experiences. *Journal of Advanced Nursing, 40*(1), 7–16.

Bunge, M., & Pearse, D. (2003). Transplantation strategies to promote repair of the injured spinal cord.

Journal of Rehabilitation Research and Development, 40(4) (Suppl), 1–8.

Bunn, K., & Roberts, I. for the WHO Pre-Hospital Trauma Care Steering Committee. (2004). Spinal immobilization for trauma patients. *The Cochrane Database of Systematic Reviews* (2, 4), CD002803. DOI: 10.1002/14651858.

Bunnell, R. E., Nassozi, J., Marum, E., Mubangizi, J., Malamba, S., Dillon, B., et al (2005). Living with discordance: Knowledge, challenges, and prevention strategies of HIV discordant couples in Uganda. *AIDS Care, 17*(8), 999–1012.

Burden, M., (2003). Diabetes: Signs, symptoms and making a diagnosis. *Nursing Times, 99*(1), 30–32.

Burckhardt, C. S. (2005). Educating patients: Self-management approaches. *Disability and Rehabilitation, 27*(12), 703–709.

Burkhardt, M. A., & Nathaniel, A. K. (2002). *Ethics and issues in contemporary nursing* (2nd ed.). New York: Thomson Delmar Learning.

Burkle, F. (2002). Mass casualty management of a large scale bioterrorism event: An epidemiological approach that shapes triage decisions. *Emergency Medicine Clinics of North America, 20*(2), 409–436.

Burl, D., Schambelan, M., & Lo, J. (2004). Endocrine hypertension. In F. S. Greenspan & D. G. Gardner (Eds.), *Basic and clinical endocrinology* (pp. 414–438). St. Louis, MO: Lange Medical Books.

Burns, N., & Grove, S. (2001). *Cognitive mapping in the practice of nursing research conduct, critique & utilization* (4th ed.). Philadelphia: W. B. Saunders.

Burns, V. E., Carroll, D., Drayson, M., Whitham, M., & Ring, C. (2003). Life events, perceived stress and antibody response to influenza vaccination in young, healthy adults. *Journal of Psychosomatic Research, 55*(6), 569–572.

Buscemi, N., Vandermeer, B., Friesen, C., Bialy, L., Tubman, M., Ospina, M., et al. (2005). *Manifestations and management of chronic insomnia in adults. Summary, evidence report technology assessment: Number 125.* AHRQ Publication Number 05-E021-1. Retrieved June 15, 2005, from http://www.ahrq.gov/clinic/epcsums/insomnsum.htm.

Bush, N., & Griffin-Sobel, J. (2003). Acute postoperative pain management and malfunctioning epidural catheter. *Oncology Nursing Forum, 30*(2), 227–228.

Butcher, G. (2003). *An illustrated colour text: Gastroenterology.* London: Churchill Livingstone.

Butterworth, C. E. (1974). The skeleton in the hospital closet, *Nutrition Today, 9*(2), March/April, 4.

Byars, L. (2002). Neutropenia risk assessment and management in the ambulatory care setting. *Oncology Support Care, 1*, 27–39.

Byock, I. (1997). *Dying well: The prospect for growth at the end of life.* New York: Riverhead Books.

Calder, L., Balasubramanian, S., & Stiell, I. (2004). Lack of consensus on corneal abrasion management results of a national survey. *Canadian Journal of Emergency Medicine, 6*(6), 402–407.

Calgary Health Region. (2004). *Decision-making for enteral feeding tube placement in adult patients: The development of a guideline for decision making, final report.* Retrieved July 11, 2006, from http://www.crha-health.ab.ca.

Calianno, C., & Jakubek, P. (2006). Wound and skin care. Wound bed preparation: Laying the foundation for treating chronic wounds, part I. *Nursing, 36*(2), 70–71.

Calle, E., Rodriguez, C., Walker-Thurmond, K., & Thun, M. (2003). Overweight, obesity, and mortality form cancer in a prospectively studied cohort of U.W. adults. *New England Journal of Medicine, 348*(17), 1625–1638.

Calne, S., & Kumar, A. (2003). Nursing care of patient's with late-stage Parkinson's disease. *Journal of Neuroscience Nursing, 35*(5), 242–251.

Campbell, M., & Torrance, C. (2005). Coronary angioplasty: Impact on risk factors and patients' understanding of the severity of their condition. *Australian Journal of Advanced Nursing, 22*(4), 26–31.

Campbell, T. (2004). Nurses are vital to those living with a chronic disease. *Nursing Spectrum, 43*(12), 34.

Campos, L., Meng, Z., Hu, G., Chiu, D., Ambron, R., & Martin, J. (2004). Engineering novel spinal circuits to promote recovery after spinal injury. *The Journal of Neuroscience, 24*(9), 2090–2101.

Campoy, S., & Elwell, R. (2005). Pharmacology and CKD: How chronic kidney disease and its complications alter drug response. *American Journal of Nursing, 105*(9), 60–72.

Cancer Research UK. (2004). *General side effects of chemotherapy drugs.* Retrieved June 9, 2005, from http://www.cancerhelp.org.uk.

Cancer Source. (2003). *Grading toxicities from chemotherapeutic agents.* Retrieved June 10, 2005, from http://www.cancersourcern.com.

Candela, L., & Yucha, C. (2004). Renal regulation of extracellular fluid volume and osmolality. *Nephrology Nursing Journal, 31*(4), 397–404, 444.

Cannon, C. P., Braunwald, E., McCabe, C. H., Rader, D. J., Rouleau, J. L., Belder, R., et al. (2004). Intensive versus moderate lipid lowering with statins after acute coronary syndromes. *New England Journal of Medicine, 350*(15), 1495–1504.

Cantus, S. (2004). *Phimosis and paraphimosis.* Retrieved July 2, 2006, from http://www.emedicine.com.

Capriotti, T. (2004). The "alphabet" of rheumatoid arthritis therapy. *Nursing, 13*(6), 920–928.

Carding, P., Welch, A., Owen, S., & Stafford, F. (2001) Surgical voice restoration. *The Lancet, 357*, 1463–1465.

Cardiomyopathy Association. (2006). *Which cardiomyopathy?* Retrieved June 26, 2006, from www.cardiomyopathy.org.

Carey, M. (2004). *Priapism.* Retrieved August 4, 2005, from http://www.emedicine.com.

Carpenito, L. J. (2004). *Nursing diagnosis: Application in clinical practice* (10th ed.). Philadelphia: Lippincott, Williams & Wilkins.

Carpenito-Moyet, L. J. (2005). *Nursing diagnosis: Application to clinical practice* (10th ed.). Philadelphia: Lippincott, Wilkins and Williams.

Carson, J. S., Burke, F. M., & Hark, L. A. (2004). *Cardiovascular nutrition: Disease management and prevention.* Chicago: American Diabetic Association.

Carter, K., Dufour, L., & Ballard, C. (2004). Identifying secondary skin lesions. *Nursing, 34*(1), 68.

Carter-Templeton, H. (2005). Malignant hyperthermia. *Nursing, 35*(6), 88.

Carver, C. (2005). Enhancing adaptation during treatment and the role of individual differences. *Cancer, 104*(11 Suppl), 2602–2607.

Casaccia, M., Torelli, P., Fontana, I., Panaro, F., & Valente, U. (2003). Laparoscopic bilateral hand-assisted nephrectomy: End-stage renal disease from tuberculosis, an unusual indication for nephrectomy before transplantation. *Surgical Laparoscopy Endoscopy and Percutaneous Techniques, 13*(1), 59–62.

Casebeer, L., Strasser, S., Spettell, C., Wall, T., Weisman, N., Ray, M., et al. (2003). *Designing tailored web-based instruction to improve physician's preventative practices.* Retrieved September 8, 2006, from www.jmir.org.

Casseb, J., Da Silva, D., & Alberto, J. (2005). Structured intermittent therapy with 7 day cycles of HAART for chronic HIF infections: A pilot study. *AIDS Patient Care and STDs, 19*(7), 425–429.

Castro, M. G., Cowen, R., Williamson, I. K., David, A., Jimenez-Dalmaroni, M. J., Yuan, X., et al. (2003). Current and future strategies for the treatment of malignant brain tumors. *Pharmacology and Therapeutics, 98*(1), 71–108.

Catalano, J. (2003). *Nursing now! Today's issues, tomorrow's trends* (3rd ed.). Philadelphia: F. A. Davis.

Cavanaugh, B. (2003). *Nurse's manual of laboratory and diagnostic tests.* Philadelphia: F. A. Davis Company.

Celik, S., Aksoy, G., & Akyolcu, N. (2004). Nursing role on preventing secondary brain injury. *Accident and Emergency Nursing, 12*(2), 94–98.

Center for Disease Control, National Center for Infectious Diseases. (2006). *All about Hantaviruses.* Retrieved June 23, 2006, from www.cdc.gov.

Centers for Disease Control and Prevention. (2002a). Hysterectomy surveillance—United States, 1994–1999. *Morbidity Mortality Weekly Report, 51*(SS05), 1–8.

Centers for Disease Control and Prevention. (2002b). Trends in tuberculosis morbidity–United States 1992–2002. Retrieved July 31, 2004, from http://www.cdc.gov.

Centers for Disease Control and Prevention. (2003a). *Coping with a traumatic event.* Retrieved June 16, 2006, from www.cdc.gov.

Centers for Disease Control and Prevention. (2003b). *Explosion and blast injuries: A primer for clinicians.* Retrieved June 13, 2006, from www.cdc.gov.

Centers for Disease Control and Prevention. (2003c). *New pediatric growth charts.* Retrieved June 16, 2005, from http://www.cdc.gov.

Centers for Disease Control and Prevention. (2004a). *Chlamydia fact sheet.* Retrieved July 30, 2006, from http://www.cdc.gov.

Centers for Disease Control and Prevention. (2004b). *Ebola hemorrhagic fever and viral hemorrhagic fever.* Retrieved July 3, 2006, from www.cdc.gov.

Centers for Disease Control and Prevention. (2004c). *Genital herpes fact sheet.* Retrieved July 30, 2006, from http://www.cdc.gov.

Centers for Disease Control and Prevention. (2004d). Lyme disease—United States, 2001–2002. *MMWR, 53*(17), 365–369.

Centers for Disease Control and Prevention. (2004e). *Questions and answers about plague.* Retrieved June 27, 2006, from www.cdc.gov.

Centers for Disease Control and Prevention. (2004f). *Severe acute respiratory syndrome. Supplement I: Infection control in healthcare, home and community settings.* Retrieved June 11, 2006, from http://www.cdc.gov.

Centers for Disease Control and Prevention. (2004g). *Trichomonas fact sheet.* Retrieved July 30, 2006, from http://www.cdc.gov.

Centers for Disease Control and Prevention. (2005a). *Healthy people 2010: Focus areas at a glance.* Retrieved on June 29, 2006, from www.cdc.gov.

Centers for Disease Control and Prevention. (2005b). *HIV/AIDS.* Retrieved June 25, 2006, from www.cdc.gov.

Centers for Disease Control and Prevention. (2006a). *Anthrax.* Retrieved June 22, 2006, from www.bt.cdc.gov.

Centers for Disease Control and Prevention. (2006b). Asthma prevalence and control characteristics by race/ethnicity—United States 2006. *Morbidity and Mortality Weekly Report, 53*(7), 1.

Centers for Disease Control and Prevention (2006c). *CDC fast stats. Stroke and cerebrovascular disease.* Retrieved June 17, 2006, from http://www.cdc.gov.

Centers for Disease Control and Prevention. (2006d). *Skin cancer guidelines.* Retrieved July 5, 2006, from http://www.cdc.gov.

Centers for Disease Control and Prevention. (2006e). *Small pox disease overview.* Retrieved June 24, 2006, from www.cdc.gov.

Centers for Disease Control and Prevention. (2006f). *West Nile virus.* Retrieved July 11, 2006, from http://www.cdc.gov.

Centers for Medicare and Medicaid Services. (2004). *The specifications manual for national hospital quality measures.* Retrieved May 18, 2005, from http://cms.hhs.gov/quality/hospital.

Centers for Medicare and Medicaid Services. (2005). *Health United States 2005.* Retrieved March 30, 2006, from http://www.cms.hhs.gov.

Centers for Medicare and Medicaid Services. (2006). *HIPPA insurance reform.* Retrieved from http://www.cms.hhs.gov.

Centers for Medicare and Medicaid Services. (n.d.). *Statistics and data.* Retrieved August 30, 2005, from http://www.cms.hhs.gov.

Certification for adult, pediatric and neonatal critical care nurses. (2003). Retrieved May 7, 2004, from www.aacn.org.

Cesari, M., Penninx, B. W., Newman, A. B., Kritchevsky, S. B., Nicklas, B. J., Sutton-Tyrrel, K., et al. (2003). Inflammatory markers and cardiovascular disease (The Health, Aging and Body Composition [Health ABC] Study). *The American Journal of Cardiology, 92*(5), 522–528.

Chaiyakunapruk, N., Veenstra, D., Lipsky, B., & Saint, S. (2002). Chlorhexidine compared with povidone-iodine solution for vascular catheter-site care: A meta-analysis. *Annals of Internal Medicine, 136*(11), 792–801.

Chalela, J., & Kasner, S. (2004). *Cardiac and respiratory complications of stroke*. Retrieved June 25, 2006, from http://www.uptodate.com.

Chally, P. S., & Hough, M. C. (2005). Nursing ethics. In K. Chitty, *Professional nursing: Concepts and challenges* (4th ed., pp. 212–227). St. Louis, MO: Elsevier.

Chambers, S., & Isenberg, D. (2005). Anti-B cell therapy (rituximab) in the treatment of autoimmune disease. *Lupus, 14*(3), 210–214.

Champagne, C. (2006). Dietary interventions on blood pressure: The dietary approaches to stop hypertension (DASH) trials. Prevention of nutrition-related chronic diseases: Scientific foundations and community interventions. Fifth Nestle Nutrition Conference, Mexico City, Mexico, October 7–8, 2004. *Nutrition Reviews, 64* (2 Part 2): S53–56.

Chang, B. S., & Lowenstein, D. H. (2003). Practice parameter: Antiepileptic drug prophylaxis in severe traumatic brain injury. Report of the Quality Standards Committee of the American Academy of Neurology. *Neurology, 60,* 10–16. Retrieved June 13, 2006, from www.guideline.gov.

Chang, Y., Singer, D. E., Wu, Y. A., Keller, R. B., & Atlas, S.J. (2005). The effect of surgical and nonsurgical treatment on longitudinal outcomes of lumbar spinal stenosis over 10 years. *Journal of American Geriatrics Society, 53*(5), 785–792.

Chapman, E. (2002). The social and ethical implications of changing medical technologies: The views of people living with genetic conditions. *Journal of Health Psychology, 7*(2), 195–206.

Chaudhry B., Capicatto M., & O'Brien A., (2002). Mystery of the dark green sputum: Lung abcess. *Post Graduate Medicine, 112*(3), 75–76, 82.

Chavis, S., & Duncan, L. (2003). Home study program: Pain management: Continuum of care for surgical patients. *Association of Operating Room Nurses Journal, 78*(3), 382–383, 385–386, 389–394, 396–399.

Cherkin, D. C., Sherman, K. J., Deyo, R. A., & Shekelle, P. G. (2003). A review of the evidence for the effectiveness, safety, and cost of acupuncture, massage therapy, and spinal manipulation for back pain. *Annals of Internal Medicine, 138*(11), 898–906.

Childs, S. G. (2002). Anatomy and physiology of the musculoskeletal system. In A. B. Mahler, S. W. Salmond, & T. A. Pellino (Eds.), *Orthopaedic nursing* (3rd ed., pp. 152–174). Philadelphia, PA: W. B. Saunders Company.

Chiller T. M., Galgiani J. N. & Stevens D. A. (2003). Coccidioidomycosis. *Infectious Disease Clinics of North America, 17*(1), 41–57.

Chinnock, P., & Roberts, I. (2004). Gangliosides for acute spinal cord injury. *The Cochrane Database of Systematic Reviews* (3), CD004444. DOI: 10.1002/14651858.

Chobanian, A. V., Bakris, G. L., Black, H. R., & Cushman, W. C. (2003). The seventh report of the joint national committee on the prevention, detection, evaluation, and treatment of high blood pressure: The JNC 7 report. *Journal of the American Medical Association, 289*(19), 2560–2571.

Chojnowski, D. (2003). "GOLD" standards for acute exacerbation in COPD. *Nurse Practitioner, 28*(5), 26–35; quiz 36–37.

Chojnowski, D. (2005). Peripheral arterial disease: Danger! Slow blood flow ahead. *Nursing Made Incredibly Easy, 3*(4), 4–17.

Chopra, D., & Simon, D. (2002). *Grow younger, live longer. 10 ways to reverse aging*. New York: Three Rivers Press.

Chou, L., Lo, S. Kao, M., Jim, Y., & Cho, D. (2002). Ankylosing spondylitis manifested by spontaneous anterior atlantoaxial subluxation. *American Journal of Physical Medicine & Rehabilitation, 81*(12), 952–955.

Christopher, K. (2003). Transtracheal oxygen catheters. *Clinics in Chest Medicine, 24*(3), 485–510.

Chrvala, C. A., & Bulger, R. J. (1999). *Leading health indicators for Healthy People 2010: Final report*. Division of Health Promotion and Disease Prevention, Institute of Medicine. Washington, DC: National Academy Press.

Ciarleglio, L., Bennett, R., Williamson, J., Mandell, J., & Marks, J. (2003). Genetic counseling throughout the life cycle. *The Journal of Clinical Investigation, 112*(9), 1280–1286.

Cicatiello, J. (2004). Reconstructing healthcare in a global marketplace. *Nursing Administration Quarterly, 28*(2), 83–85.

Cioffi, J. (2005). Nurses' experiences of caring for culturally diverse patients in an acute care setting. *Contemporary Nurse, 20*(1), 78–86.

Civetta, J. (1996). Futile care or caregiver frustration? A practical approach. *Critical Care Medicine, 24*(2), 346–351.

Clark, P., Drain, M., & Malone, M. (2004). *Addressing patients' emotional and spiritual needs*. Oakbrook Terrace, IL: Joint Commission Resources.

Clark, P. C., & King, K. B. (2003) Comparison of family caregivers: Stroke survivors vs. persons with Alzheimer's disease. *Journal of Gerontological Nursing, 32*(5), 45–55.

Classe, J., Curtet, C., & Campion, L. (2003). Learning curve for the detection of axillary sentinel lymph node in breast cancer. *European Journal of Surgical Oncology, 29,* 426.

Cleator, J., & Wilding, J. (2003). Obesity and diabetes. *Nursing Times, 99*(15), 54–55.

Cleveland Clinic. (2004). *What you need to know about living with pulmonary hypertension*. Retrieved September 16, 2004, from http://www.clevelandclinic.org.

Cochrane Database of Systematic Reviews. (2004). *Postoperative radiotherapy for non-small cell lung cancer*. Retrieved September 16, 2004, from http://www.cochrane.org.

Cohen, J., & De LaMare, J. (2002). *Health care costs: Fact sheet*. Retrieved June 17, 2006, from www.ahcpr.gov.

Cohen, M. R. (2005). Labetalol crisis: Speed kills. *Nursing, 35*(2), 18.

Cohen, S. M., Labadie, R. F., Dietrich, M.S., & Haynes, D. S. (2004). Quality of life in hearing-impaired adults: The role of cochlear implants and hearing aids. *Otolaryngology-Head and Neck Surgery, 131,* 413–422.

Collemer, S. (2004). *Too hot to handle*. Retrieved March 18, 2006, from http://www.aanet.org.

Collins, F. S., Green, E. D., Guttmacher, A., & Guyer, M. S. (2003). A vision for the future of genomics research: A blueprint for the genomic era. *Nature, 422*(24), 835–847.

Cole, E. (2005). *The Last Word.* U.S. Food, and Drug Administration. Retrieved March 10, 2005, from www.fda.gov.

Cole, S., & Dunne, K. (2004). Continuing professional development. *Hodgkin's lymphoma. Nursing Standard, 18*(9), 46–52, 54–55.

Colombo, A., Solberg, B., Vanderhoeft, E., Ramsay, G., & Schouten, H. (2005). Measurement of nursing care time of specific interventions on a hematology-oncology unit related to diagnostic categories. *Cancer Nursing, 28*(6), 476–480.

Comer, S. (2005). *Delmar's critical care nursing care plans* (2nd ed.). Clifton Park, NY: Thomson Delmar Learning.

Commission on Classification and Terminology of the International League against Epilepsy. (1981). Proposal for revised clinical and electroencephalographic classification of epileptic seizures. *Epilepsia, 22,* 489–501.

Conboy, L., Patel, S., Koptchuk, T., Gottlieb, B., Eisenberg, D., & Acevedo-Garcia, D. (2005). Types of complementary and alternative medicines: An analysis based on nationally representative sample. *Alternative and Complementary Medicine, 11*(6), 977–994.

Conlon, P., & Giblin, L. (2003). Vascular access for dialysis. In R. Johnson & J. Feehally (Eds.), *Comprehensive clinical nephrology* (2nd ed., pp. 957–965). St. Louis, MO: Mosby.

Cook, L. (2003). Staying current on defibrillator therapy. *Nursing, 33*(11), 44–46.

Coppin, C., Porzsolt, F., Awa, A., Kumpf, J., Coldman, A., & Wilt, T. (2005). Immunotherapy for advanced renal cell cancer. *The Cochrane Database of Systematic Reviews* (4), ID #CD001425.

Corey, H. (2003). Stewart and beyond: New models of acid-base balance. *Kidney International, 64,* 777–787.

Corley, M. C., (2002). Nurse moral distress: A proposed theory and research agenda. *Nursing Ethics, 9*(6), 635–650.

Cornell University Department of Urology. (2005). *Peyronie's disease.* Retrieved June 3, 2006, from http://www.cornellurology.com.

Cowan, J., & Graham, M. (2003, November). Polycystic ovary syndrome: More than a reproductive disorder. *Patient Care Nurse Practitioner,* 6–15.

Coward, L. J., Featherstone, R. L., & Brown, M. M. (2004). Percutaneous transluminal angioplasty and stenting for carotid artery stenosis. *The Cochrane Database of Systematic Reviews (Oxford).* ID # CD000515.

Cox, Robert. (2003). *Hazmat.* Retrieved June 14, 2006, from http://www.emedicine.com.

Craigie, J., Allen, R., DellaCroce, F., & Sullivan, S. (2003). Autogenous breast reconstruction with the deep inferior epigastric perforator flap. *Clinical Plastic Surgery, 30,* 359.

Crimlisk, J., & Grande, M. (2004). Neurologic assessment skills for the acute medical surgical nurse. *Orthopaedic Nursing, 23*(1), 3–9.

Criste, A. (2002). Gender and pain. *American Association of Nurse Anesthetists, 70*(6), 475–481.

Cross, C. (2004). Seizures: Regaining control. *RN, 67*(12), 44–51.

Crowther, C. L. (2004). Structure and function of the musculoskeletal system. In S. E. Huether & K. L. McCance (Eds.), *Understanding pathophysiology* (3rd ed., pp. 1047–1070). St. Louis, MO: Mosby.

Crowther, C. L., & McCance, K. L. (2004). Alterations of musculoskeletal function. In S. E. Huether & K. L. McCance (Eds.), *Understanding pathophysiology* (3rd ed., pp. 1071–1116). St. Louis, MO: Mosby.

Cua, I. H. Y., & George, J. (2005). Non-alcoholic fatty liver disease. *Hospital Medicine, 66*(2), 106–111.

Cuddy, M. (2005). Treatment of hypertension: Guidelines from JNC 7 (The Seventh Report of the Joint National Committee on Prevention, Detection, Evaluation, and Treatment of High Blood Pressure). *Journal of Practical Nursing, 55*(4), 17–23.

Cullen, L., Titler, M., & Drahozal, R. (2003). Family and pet visitation in the critical care unit. *Critical Care Nurse, 23*(5), 62–65.

Cullen, R. D., Higgins, C., Buss, E., Clark, M., Pillsbury, H. C., & Buchman, C. A. (2004). Cochlear implantations in patients with substantial residual hearing. *Laryngoscope, 114,* 2218–2223.

Cumbie, S., Conley, V., & Berman, M. (2004). Advanced practice nursing model for comprehensive care with chronic illness: Model for promoting process engagement. *Advances in Nursing Science, 27*(1), 70–80.

Cummins, R. (2003) *Advanced cardiac life support provider manual.* Dallas: American Heart Association.

Curhan, G. (2005). Clinical crossroads: conferences with patients and doctors. A 44-year-old woman with kidney stones. *Journal of the American Medical Association, 293*(9), 1107–1114.

Curley, M. (1998). Patient-nurse synergy: Optimizing patient outcomes. *American Journal of Critical Care, 7*(1), 64–72.

Curtis, S., Kolytolo, C., & Broome, M. (2004). Somatosensory function and pain. In C. Porth (Ed.), *Pathophysiology: Concepts of altered health states,* 6th ed. (pp. 245–251). Philadelphia: Lippincott.

Czernin, J., Gambhir, S., Brunken, R., & Schelbert, H. (2004). *Tutorial: Clinical PET-Cardiology.* Retrieved September 25, 2004, from http://laxmi.nuc.ucla.edu:8000/lpp/clinpetcardio/evaluation.html#Evaluation.

D'Antonio, J. (2004). You can lessen leukemia's toll. *Nursing, 34*(7), *Hospital Nursing,* 1–4.

D'Antonio, J. (2005). Chronic myelogenous leukemia. *Clinical Journal of Oncology Nursing, 9*(5), 535–538, 561–563.

D'Arcy, Y. (2004). Using technology to help alleviate pain. *Nursing Management, 35*(11), 45–47.

D'Arcy, Y. (2005). Pain management standards, the law, and you. *Nursing, 35*(4), 17.

Daller, J. A. (2004). *Heart valve surgery.* Retrieved August 29, 2004, from http://www.nlm.nih.gov/medlineplus/ency/article/002954.htm.

Dang, D., Johantgen, M., Pronovost, P., Jenckes, M., & Bass, E. (2002). Postoperative complications: Does intensive care unit staff nursing make a difference? *Heart and Lung, 31*(3), 219–228.

Daniels, R. (2003). *Delmar's manual of laboratory and diagnostic tests.* New York: Thomson Delmar Learning.

Daniels, R. (2004). *Nursing fundamentals: Caring and clinical decision making.* New York: Thomson Delmar Learning.

Darovic, G. (2004). *Handbook of hemodynamic monitoring* (2nd ed.). St. Louis, MO: Saunders.

Davidoff, T. Q., & Cunningham, M. (2004, May). *Sinusitis, acute.* Retrieved August 5, 2004, from http://www.emedicine.com/med/topic2555.htm.

Davies, P., & Galer, B. (2004). Review of lidocaine patch 5% studies in the treatment of postherpetic neuralgia. *Drugs, 64*(9), 937–947.

Davies, S., & Gilmore, A. (2003). The role of hydroxyurea in the management of sickle cell disease. *Blood Reviews, 17,* 99–109.

Davies, S., & Williams, J. (2003). Peritoneal dialysis: Principles, techniques, and adequacy. In R. Johnson & J. Feehally (Eds.), *Comprehensive clinical nephrology* (2nd ed., pp. 1003–1011). St. Louis, MO: Mosby.

Davila, R. E., Rajan, E., Adler, D., Hirota, W. K., Jacobson, B. C., Leighton, J. A., et al. (2005). ASGE Guideline: The role of endoscopy in the diagnosis, staging, and management of colorectal cancer. *Gastrointestinal Endoscopy, 61*(1), 1–7.

Davy, A. R., & Drew, S. J. (2002). Management of shoulder dislocations—Are we doing enough to reduce the risk or recurrence? *Injury, 33,* 775–779.

de la Chica, R., Ribas, I., Giraldo, J., Egozcue, J., & Fuster, C. (2005). Chromosomal instability in amniocytes from fetuses of mothers who smoke. *Journal of the American Medical Association, 293,* 1212–1222.

Deaton, C., Bennett, J. A., & Riegel, B. (2004). State of the science for care of older adults with heart disease. *Nursing Clinics of North America, 39*(3), 495–528.

Deb, S., & Crownshaw, T. (2004). The role of pharmacotherapy in the management of behavioral disorders in traumatic brain injury patients. *Brain Injury, 18*(1), 1–31.

DeFrances, C. J., & Hall, M. J. (2004, May 21). 2002 national hospital discharge survey. *CDC Advance Data from Vital and Health Statistics, 342*(3), 1–27.

DeLaune, S., & Ladner, P. (2006). *Fundamentals of nursing* (3rd ed.). New York: Thomson Delmar Learning.

Delta Society. (2005). *Animal assisted therapy.* Retrieved August 2, 2006, from http://www.deltasociety.org.

Dellinger, R., Carlet, J., Masur, H., Gerlach, H. (2004). Surviving sepsis campaign guidelines for management of severe sepsis and septic shock. *Critical Care Medicine, 32*(3), 858. Retrieved June 23, 2006, from www.survivingsepsis.com.

Deliveliotis, C., Papatsoris, A., Chrisofos, M., Dellis, A., Liakouras, C., & Skolarikos, A. (2005). Urinary diversion in high-risk elderly patients: Modified cutaneous ureterostomy or ileal conduit? *Urology, 66* (2), 299–304.

DeMarini, D., & Preston, R. (2005). Smoking while pregnant: Transplacental mutagenesis of the fetus by tobacco smoke. *Journal of the American Medical Association, 293,*1264–1265.

Demling, R. (2005). The role of anabolic hormones of wound healing in catabolic states. *Journal of Burns and Wounds.* Retrieved May 31, 2006, from www.journalofburnsandwounds.com.

Dempski, K. M., & Killion, S. W. (2001). *Legal & ethical issues in nursing.* Thorofare, NJ: SLACK, Inc.

Denis, L., Namey, M., Costello, K., Frenette, J., Gagnon, N., Harris, C., et al. (2004). Long term treatment optimization in individuals with multiple sclerosis using disease-modifying therapies: A nursing approach. *Journal of Neuroscience Nursing, 36*(1), 10–22.

Denkins, B. A. (2005). My side. Are we really helping? The problem of dual diagnoses, homelessness, & hospital-hopping. *Journal of Psychosocial Nursing and Mental Health Services, 43*(11), 48–50.

Dennis, M. V. (2003). Digital photographs in the ED: Images of an accident can offer ED staff a clearer picture of the cause and extent of victims' injuries. *The American Journal of Nursing, 103*(12), 44–46.

Dennis, V. (2004). *Electrosurgical safety and your staff.* Retrieved July 31, 2005, from http://www.encision.com.

Denny, E. (2004). Women's experience of endometriosis. *Journal of Advanced Nursing, 46*(6), 641–648.

Deodato, F., Boenzi, S., Rizzo, C., Abeni, D., Caviglia, S., Bartuli, A., et al. (2004). Inborn errors of metabolism: An update on epidemiology and on neonatal-onset hyperammonemia. *Acta Paediatrica, S445*(93), 18–21.

DeVault, K., & Castell, D. (2005). Updated guidelines for the diagnosis and treatment of gastrointestinal reflux disease. *American Journal of Gastroenterology, 100*(1), 190–200.

Diehl-Oplinger, L., & Kaminski, M. (2004). Choosing the right fluid to counter hypovolemic shock. *Nursing, 34*(3), 52–54.

Diepgen, T., & Mahler, V. (2002). The epidemiology of skin cancer. *British Journal of Dermatology, 146*(Suppl 61), 1–6.

Dieterich, M. (2004). Dizziness. *Neurology, 10*(3), 154–164.

Dixon, L. (2002). Postoperative complications and the older adult. *Geriatric Nursing, 23*(11), 203.

DNAdirect. (2006). *Genetic testing.* Retrieved July 10, 2006, from www.dnadirect.org.

Dochterman, J. M., & Bulechek, G. M. (2004). *Nursing interventions classification (NIC)* (4th ed.). St. Louis, MO. Mosby.

Doe Report. (2005). *Burn injuries. The Doe report medical reference library.* Retrieved March 1, 2006, from http://www.doeroport.com.

Doganci, L., Odabasi, Z., & Turan, M. (2003). Dangerous to link a hepatatrophic etiology to a neurologic illness. *American Journal of Physical Medicine and Rehabilitation, 82*(7), 563.

Donabedian, A. (1966). Evaluating the quality of medical care. *Milbank Memorial Fund Quarterly, 44*(3 Suppl), 166–206.

Donabedian, A. (1998). The quality of care: How can it be assessed? *Journal of the American Medical Association, 260*(12), 1743–1748.

Doughty, D. (2004). Skin integrity and wound healing. In R. Daniels (Ed.), *Nursing fundamentals: Caring and clinical decision making* (pp. 165–170). New York: Thomson Delmar Learning.

Douglas, R. M., Chalker, E. B., & Treacy, B. (2004, February). *Vitamin C for preventing and treating the common cold.* Retrieved June 17, 2004, from http://www.cochrane.org/cochrane/revabstr/ab000980.htm.

Drake, A. D., & Carr, M. M. (2003, February). *Tonsillectomy.* Retrieved August 25, 2004, from http://www.emedicine.com/ent/topic315.htm.

Dreger, V., & Tremback, T. (2002). Optimize patient health by treating literacy and language barriers. *Association of Operating Room Nurses Journal, 75*(2), 280–293.

Dreicer, R. (2005). *Prostate cancer.* Retrieved July 19, 2006, from http://www.clevelandclinicmeded.com.

Drug prices. (2006). Retrieved July 3, 2006, from www.drugstore.com.

Drumm, C., Bruner, J., & Minutillo, A. (2004). Plague comes to New York. *American Journal of Nursing, 104*(8), 61–64.

Druz, D. (2005). Recognizing signs, symptoms could lead to a more accurate diagnosis in diplopia. *Ocular Surgery News, 23*(8), 124–125.

Duke, J. (2002). *The green pharmacy.* Emmaus, PA: Rodale Press.

Dunn, L. (2005). New blood. *Nursing Standard, 20*(4), 69.

Dweyer M. K., & Uhl T. L. (2003). A traumatic pneumothorax as a result of a rib fracture in a college baseball player. *Orthopedics, 26*(7), 726–729.

Ebersole, P., Hess, P., & Luggen, A. (2004). *Toward healthy aging* (6th ed.). St. Louis, MO: Mosby.

Eckert, M., & Jones, T. (2002). How does an implantable cardioverter defibrillator (ICD) affect the lives of patients and their families. *International Journal of Nursing Practice, 8,* 152–157.

Edelman, C. L., & Mandle, C. L. (2002). *Health promotion throughout the life span* (5th ed.). St. Louis, MO: Mosby.

Edgar, D. (2004). Advances in genetics: Implications for children, families, and nurses. *Pediatric Nursing, 16*(6), 26–29.

Edlow, J. A. (2002). Tick-borne diseases, lyme. *eMedicine Journal, 3*(4). Retrieved September 5, 2006, from http://www.emedicine.com.

Edwards, D., & Burnard, P. (2003). A systematic review of stress and stress management interventions for mental health nurses. *Journal of Advanced Nursing, 42*(2), 169–200.

Edwards, S. (2002). Physiological insult/injury: Pathophysiology and consequences. *British Journal of Nursing, 11*(4), 263–277.

Eggenberger, S., & Nelms, T. (2004). Artificial hydration and nutrition in advanced Alzheimer's disease: Facilitating family decision-making. *Journal of Clinical Nursing, 13,* 661–667.

Eggenberger, S., Grassley, J., Restrepo, E. (2006). Culturally competent nursing care for families: Listening to the voices of Mexican-American women. *The Online Journal of Issues in Nursing, 11*(3). Retrieved from www.nursingworld.org.

Ehlers, V. (2002). Republic of South Africa: Policies and politics guide nurses' application of genetic technology in public health settings. *Policy, Politics, & Nursing Practice, 3*(2), 149–159.

Eichner, J., Dunn, S., Perveen, G., Thomson, D., Stewart, K., & Stoehla, B. (2002). Apolipoprotein E polymorphism and cardiovascular disease: A huge review. *American Journal of Epidemiology, 155,* 487–495.

El-Alfy, M., & El-Sayed, M. (2004). Overwhelming postsplenectomy infection: Is quality of patient knowledge enough for prevention? *Hematology Journal, 5*(1), 77–80.

Eliopoulos, C. (2005). *Gerontological nursing* (6th ed.). Philadelphia: Lippincott Williams & Wilkins.

Elkhodair, S., Parmar, H., & Vanwaeyenbergh, J. (2005). The role of the IPSS (International Prostate Symptoms Score) in predicting acute retention of urine in patients undergoing major joint arthroplasty. *Surgeon, 3*(2), 63–65.

Emanuel, E., Crouch, R., Arras, J., Moreno, J., & Grady, C. (2003). *Ethical and regulatory aspects of clinical research.* Baltimore, MD: Johns Hopkins University Press.

Eng, J., Krishnan, J., Segal, J., Bolger, D., Tamariz, L., Streiff, M., Jenckes, M., & Bass, E. (2004). Accuracy of CT in the diagnosis of pulmonary embolism: A systematic literature review. *American Journal of Roentgenology, 183,* 1819–1827.

Englund, M., Roos, E. M., & Lohmander, L. S. (2003). Impact of type of meniscal tear on radiographic and symptomatic knee osteoarthritis: A sixteen-year followup of meniscectomy with matched controls. *Arthritis and Rheumatism, 48,* 2178–2187.

Enns, G., & Packman, W. (2002). The adolescent with an inborn error metabolism: Medical issues and transition to adulthood. *Adolescent Medicine, 13*(2), 315–329.

Enright, P. (2004). *Overview of pulmonary function testing.* Retrieved June 25, 2006, from http://www.uptodate.com.

Epel, E. S., Blackburn, E. H., Lin, J., Dhabhar, F. S., Adler, N. E., Morrow, J. D., et al. (2004). Accelerated telomere shortening in response to life stress. *Proceedings of the National Academy of Science USA, 101*(49), 17312–17315.

Eppes, S. C. (2003). Diagnosis, treatment, and prevention of Lyme disease in children. *Pediatric Drugs, 5*(6), 363–372.

Erikson, E. (1963). The eight stages of man. In *Childhood and society* (2nd ed.) (pp. 247–274). New York: WW. Norton.

Erlen, J. (2004). HIPAA—clinical and ethical considerations for nurses. *Orthopaedic Nursing, 23*(6), 410–413.

Estes, M. (2006). *Health assessment and physical examination* (3rd ed.). New York: Thomson Delmar Learning.

Estiarte R., Colome, J. J., Artes, E., & Jimenez, F. J. (2003). Drug utilization study in patients with Crohn's disease in Spain. *European Journal of Gastroenterology and Hepatology, 15*(4), 355–362.

Estores, I. (2003). The consumer's perspective and the professional literature: What do persons with spinal cord injury want? *Journal of Rehabilitation Research and Development, 40*(4), 1–6.

Etchegary, H. (2006). Genetic testing for Huntington's disease: How is the decision taken? *Genetic Testing, 10*(1), 60–67.

Evans, L. S., & Hancock, B. W. (2003). Non-Hodgkin lymphoma. *Lancet, 362*(9378), 139–146.

Evered, A. (2003). Hypothermia: Risk factors and guidelines for nursing care. *Nursing Times, 99*(49), 40–43.

Everett, B., & Salamonson, Y. (2005). Differences in postoperative opioid consumption in patients prescribed patient-controlled analgesia versus intramuscular injection. *Pain Management Nursing, 6*(4), 137–144.

Eysteinsdottir, J. H., Freysdottir, J., Haraldsson, A., Stefansdottir, J., Skaftadottir, I., Helgason, H., et al. (2004). The influence of partial or total thymectomy during open heart surgery in infants on the immune function later in life. *Clinical and Experimental Immunology, 136*(2), 349–355.

Fadiman, A. (1997). *The spirit catches you and you fall down.* New York: Noonday Press.

Falkenbach, A. (2003). Disability motivates patients with ankylosing spondylitis for more frequent physical exercise. *Archives of Physical Medicine and Rehabilitation, 84*(3), 382–383.

Falkiner, S., & Myers, S. (2002). When exactly can carpal tunnel syndrome be considered work related? *ANZ Journal of Surgery, 72*(3), 204–209.

Faris, R., Flather, M., Purcell, H., Henein, M., Poole-Wilson, P., & Coats, A. (2002). Current evidence supporting the role of diuretics in heart failure: A meta analysis of randomised controlled trials. *International Journal of Cardiology, 82*(2), 149–158.

Farooq, S., & Fear, C. (2003). Working through interpreters. *Advances in Psychiatric Treatment, 9,* 104–109.

Farrington, K., Greenwood, R., & Ahmad, S. (2003). Hemodialysis: Mechanisms, outcome, and adequacy. In R. Johnson & J. Feehally (Eds.), *Comprehensive clinical nephrology* (2nd ed., pp. 975–990). St. Louis, MO: Mosby.

Fecci, P. E., Mitchell, D. A., Archer, G. E., Morse, M. A., Lyerly, H. K., Bigner, D. D., et al. (2003). The history, evolution, and clinical use of dendritic cell-based immunization strategies in the therapy of brain tumors. *Journal of Neurooncology, 64*(1–2), 161–176.

Feder, B. J., & Zeller, T. (2004). *Identity badge worn under skin approved for use in health care.* Retrieved July 4, 2006, from http://www.nytimes.com.

Felberg, R. A., & Naidech, A. (2003). The five Ps of acute ischemic stroke treatment: Parenchyma, pipes, perfusion, penumbra, and prevention of complications. *The Ochsner Journal, 5*(1), 5–10.

Ferlito, A., Silver, C. E., Howard, D. J., Laccourreye, O., Rinaldo, A., & Owen, R. (2000). The role of partial laryngeal resection in current management of laryngeal cancer: A collective review. *Acta Oto-Laryngolica, 120,* 456–466.

Ferri, F. (2005). *Ferri's clinical advisor.* Philadelphia: Lippincott, Williams & Wilkins.

Ferri, F. F., Saver, D. F., Mugge, R. E., Leickly, F. E., Millman, B., & Fox, R. (2004, August). *Allergic rhinitis.* Retrieved December 17, 2004, from http://www.firstconsult.com.

Fields, L., Burt, V., Cutler, J., Hughes, J., Roccella, E., & Sorlie, P. (2004). The burden of adult hypertension in the United States 1999–2000: A rising tide. *Hypertension, 44,* 398–404.

File, T. (2004). The challenge of SARS: A clinical review. *The Journal of Respiratory Disease, 25*(4), 147–155.

Fine, P. (2005). The evolving and important role of anesthesiology in palliative care. *Anesthesia and Analgesia, 100*(1), 183–188.

Fine, R., & Mayo, T. (2003). Resolution of futility by due process: Early experience with the Texas Advance Directives Act. *Annals of Internal Medicine, 138*(9), 743–746.

Fischer, S. J. (2005). *Rotator cuff tears.* Retrieved on September 28, 2005, from http://orthoinfo.aaos.org.

Fitzgerald, P. A. (2004). Endocrinology. In L. M. Tierney, S. J. McPhee, & M. A. Papidakis (Eds.), *Current medical diagnosis and treatment* (43rd ed., pp. 1062–1145). New York: McGraw-Hill.

Fitzpatrick, L. (2003). Alternatives to estrogen. *Medical Clinics of North America, 87*(5), 1091–1113.

Flegal, K., Carroll, M., Ogden, C., & Johnson, C. (2002). Prevalence and trends in obesity among U.S. adults, 1999–2000. *Journal of the American Medical Association, 288,* 1723–1727.

Fleischmann, D., & Rubin, G. (2005). Quantification of intravenously administered contrast medium transit through the peripheral arteries: Implications for CT angiography. *Radiology, 236*(3), 1076–1082.

Flynn, B. (1997). Partnerships in health cities and communities: A social commitment for advanced practice nurses. *Advanced Practice Nursing Quarterly, 2*(4), 1–6.

Foley, E. (2005). HIV/AIDS and African immigrant women in Philadelphia: Structural and cultural barriers to care. *AIDS Care, 17*(8), 1030–1043.

Foley, M. (2004). Update on needlestick and sharps injuries. *American Journal of Nursing, 104*(8), 96.

Folgelman, I., Cook, G., Israel, O., Van der Wall, H. (2005). Positron emission tomography and bone metastases. *Seminar Nuclear Medicine, 35*(2), 135–142.

Folmer, R. L., Martin, W. H., & Shi, Y. (2004). Tinnitus: Questions to reveal the cause, answers to provide relief. *The Journal of Family Practice, 53,* 532–540.

Folstein, M., Folstein, S., & McHugh, P. (1975). Mini-mental state: A practical method for grading the cognitive state of patients for the clinician. *Journal of Psychiatric Research, 12*(3), 189–198.

Fong, D., Aiello, L., Ferris, F., & Klein, R. (2004). Retinopathy in diabetes. *Diabetes Care, 7*(1), 84–87.

Food and Nutrition Board, National Academy of Sciences. (2004). *Dietary reference intakes table.* Retrieved June 24, 2006, from http://www.iom.edu.

Forsyth, I., Shaikh, S., & Gunn, I (2005). The nurse cystoscopist: Extending the role. *British Journal of Perioperative Nursing, 15*(8), 342–345.

Fort, C. W. (2003). Can you solve the mystery? The patient might have DVT . . . or is it FES? *Nursing Made Incredibly Easy, 1*(2), 10–16.

Fortinash, K., & Holoday-Worret, P. (2004). *Psychiatric mental health nursing* (3rd ed.). St. Louis, MO: Mosby.

Frantz, R. (2004). *Chronic wound healing.* Retrieved August 13, 2004, from www.nursing.uiowa.edu/sites/chronicwound/.

Frasco, P., Sprung, J., & Trentman, T. (2005). The impact of the joint commission for accreditation of healthcare organization's pain initiative on perioperative opiate consumption and recovery room length of stay. *Anesthesia-Analgesia, 100*(1), 162–168.

Frawley, P. M., & Habashi, N. (2001). Airway pressure release ventilation: Theory and practice. *AACN Clinical Issues, 12*(2), 234–246.

Frazel, J. (2004). Optimize migraine management in primary care. *Nurse Practitioner, 29*(4), 22–33.

Frazier, S., Moser, D., Daley, L., McKinley, S., Riegel, B., Garvin, B., et al. (2003). Critical care nurses' beliefs about and reported management of anxiety. *American Journal of Critical Care, 12*(1), 19–27.

Friedman, S. L., McQuaid, K. R., & Grendell, J. H. (2003). *Current diagnosis and treatment in gastroenterology* (2nd ed.). New York: Lange Medical Books.

Friedrich, M. (2002). Preserving privacy, preventing discrimination becomes the province of genetics experts. *Journal of the American Medical Association, 288,* 815–816.

Frith, M. (2006). Acne scarring: Current treatment options. *Dermatology Nursing, 18*(2), 130–134.

Fromer, M. (2005). Metastatic kidney cancer: Prognosis still poor, but new treatment options on horizon. *Oncology Times, 27*(3), 16, 19–20.

Fry, S., & Johnstone, M. (Eds.). (2002). *International Council of Nurses Ethics in nursing practice A guide to ethical decision-making.* Malden, MA: Blackwell Publishing.

Frye, R., Tamer, M. A., & Kunha, B. A. (2005). *Bacterial overgrowth syndrome.* Retrieved June 25, 2006, from http://www.emedicine.com.

Fryer, D., & McIntosh S. (2005). A simplified history of anesthesia. *Dissector, 32*(4), 14–16.

Funk, S. G., Tournquist, E. M., & Champagne, M. T. (1989). A model for improving the dissemination of nursing research. *Western Journal of Nursing Research, 11*(3), 361–367.

Furlanetto, D., Crighton, A., & Topping, G. (2006). Differences in methodologies of measuring the prevalence of oral mucosal lesions in children and adolescents. *Journal of Pediatric Dentistry, 16*(1), 31–39.

Furness, S. (2005). Shifting sands: Developing cultural competence. *Practice, 17*(4), 247–256.

Fuster, V., Alexander, R. W., O'Rourke, R. A. (2004). *Hurst's the heart* (11th ed.). New York: McGraw-Hill Medical Publishing Division.

Gaberson, K. B., Schroeter, K., Killen, A. R., & Valentine, W. A. (2003).The perceived value of certification by certified perioperative nurses. *Nursing Outlook, 51*(6), 273–277.

Gahart, B., & Nazareno, A. (2002). *Intravenous medications* (18th ed.). St. Louis, MO: Mosby.

Gaitatzis, A., & Patsalos, P. (2002). Preconception counseling of women with epilepsy. *Pulse, 62*(30), 29–32.

Gajic, O., Dzik, W., & Toy, P. (2006). Fresh frozen plasma and platelet transfusion for nonbleeding patients in the intensive care unit: benefit or harm? *Critical Care Medicine, 34*(5 Suppl), S170–S173.

Galli, B., Munver, R., Sawczuk, I., & Kochis, E. (2005). Laparoscopic radical nephrectomy in renal cell carcinoma. *Urologic Nursing, 25*(2), 83–87, 133.

Gallup Organization. (2006). Nurses top list in honesty and ethics again in Gallup poll. Retrieved June 26, 2006, from www.gallup.com.

Gambrell, M., & Flynn, N. (2004). Seizures 101. *Nursing, 34*(8), 36–41.

Gammon, R. (2004) *Measurement of arterial blood gases.* Retrieved June 25, 2006, from http://www.uptodate.com.

Ganong, W. F. (2003). *Review of medical physiology* (21st ed.). San Francisco: Lange Medical Books/McGraw Hill.

Ganong, W. (2005). *Review of medical physiology* (22nd ed.). New York: McGraw-Hill.

Ganz, P. A., Greendale, G. A., Petersen, L, Kahn, B., & Bower, J. E. (2003). Breast cancer in your women: Reproductive and late health effects of treatment. *Journal of Clinical Oncology, 21,* 4184–4193.

Garber, S. L., & Rintala, D. H. (2003). Pressure ulcers in veterans with spinal cord injury: A retrospective study. *Journal of Rehabilitation Research and Development, 40*(5), 433–442.

Gardner, D., & Greenspan, F. (2004). Endocrine emergencies. In F.S. Greenspan & D. G. Gardner (Eds.), *Basic and clinical endocrinology* (pp. 829–842). St. Louis, MO: Lange Medical Books.

Gates, G. A., Feeney, M. P., & Higdon, R. J. (2003). Word recognition and the articulation index in older listeners with probable age-related auditory neuropathy. *Journal of American Academy of Audiology, 14*(4), 574–581.

Gawande, A. A., Studdert, D. M., Orav, E. J., Brennan, T. A., & Zinner, M. J. (2003). Risk factors for retained instruments and sponges after surgery. *New England Journal of Medicine, 348,* 229–235.

Geerts, W. H., Pineo, G. F., Heit, J. A., Bergqvist, D., Lassen, M. R., Colwell, C. W., et al. (2004). Prevention of venous thromboembolism: The seventh ACCP conference on antithrombotic and thrombolytic therapy. *Chest, 126*(3 Suppl), 338S–400S.

Geetha, D. (2004, November). *Poststreptococcal glomerulonephritis.* Retrieved January 27, 2006, from http://www.emedicine.com/med/topic889.htm.

Gehrig, L. (2005). *Sprained ankle.* Retrieved on September 26, 2005 from http://orthoinfo.aaos.org.

Geisbert, T. W., Hensley, L. E., Larsen, T., Young, H. A., Reed, D. S., Geisbert, J. B., et al. (2003). Pathogenesis of Ebola hemorrhagic fever in cynomolgus macaques: Evidence that dendritic cells are early and sustained targets of infection. *American Journal of Pathology, 163*(6), 2347–2370.

Gentlesk, P. J., & McCabe, J. (2004). *Acute pericarditis.* Retrieved June 24, 2006, from www.emedicine.com.

Gentry, C. (2005). *New program lifts safety at hospital.* Retrieved October 21, 2005, from http://www.tampatrib.com/Business/MGBAJFSCOFE.html.

Germond, C., Figueredo, A., Taylor, B. M., Micucci, S., & Zwaal, C. (2004). *Postoperative adjuvant radiotherapy and/or chemotherapy for resected stage II or II rectal cancer.* Practice guideline Report #2-3. (Program in evidence-based care). Toronto, Ontario: Cancer Care.

Geslak, J. (2005). When resources are scarce, consider growing your own. *AORN Journal, 82*(2), 244, 246–249.

Ghoraych, B. (2005). *Trans-sphenoid approach to the sella turcica.* Retrieved June 23, 2006, from www.ghorayeb.com.

Giammattei, J., Blix, G., Marshak, H. H., Willitzer, A. O., & Pettitt, D. J. (2003). Television watching and soft drink consumption: Associations with obesity in 11 to 13 year old schoolchildren. *Archives of Pediatric and Adolescent Medicine, 157*(9), 882–886.

Gibson, R. L., Burns, J. L., & Ramsey, B. W. (2003). Pathophysiology and management of pulmonary infections in cystic fibrosis. *American Journal of Respiratory and Critical Care Medicine, 168*(8), 918–951.

Giger, J. N., & Davidhizar, R. E. (2004). *Transcultural nursing: Assessment and intervention* (4th ed.). St. Louis, MO: Mosby.

Gilbert, S. (2003). *Hydrocele.* Retrieved July 10, 2006, from http://www.nlm.nih.gov.

Gilbert, S. (2004). *Orchitis.* Retrieved July 19, 2006, from http://www.nlm.nih.gov.

Gilchrist, D., & Hall, J. (2002). Medical genetics: An approach to the adult with a genetic disorder. *Canadian Medical Association Journal, 167*(9), 1021–1029.

Giles, W., Thompson, M., Champion, S., Grégoire, S., Meban, D., Patel, L., et al. (2005). *MacIntosh common symptoms and signs in gastroenterology.* Retrieved July 11, 2006, from http://gastroresource.com.

Gill, D., Davies, L., Pringle, I., & Hyde, S. (2004). The development of gene therapy for diseases of the lung. *Cellular and Molecular Life Sciences, 61*(3), 355–368.

Gill, J. M., Quisel, A. M., Rocca, P. V., & Walters, D. T. (2003). Diagnosis of systemic lupus erythematosus. *American Family Physician, 68*(11), 2179–2186.

Gillespie, L. D., Gillespie, W. J., Robertson, M. C., Lamb, S. E., Cumming, R. G., & Rowe, B. H. (2005). *Interventions for preventing falls in elderly people.* Oxford, UK: The Cochrane Database of Systematic Reviews.

Gillespie, W. J., Avenell, A., Henry, D. A., O'Connell, D. L., & Robertson, J. (2004). Vitamin D and vitamin D analogues for preventing fractures associated with involutional and post-menopausal osteoporosis (Cochrane review). In *The Cochrane Database of Systematic Reviews.* Chichester, UK: John Wiley & Sons, Ltd.

Gines, P., Guevara, M., Arroyo, V., & Rodes, J. (2003). Hepatorenal syndrome. *Lancet, 362*(9398), 1819–1827.

Girman, A., Lee, R., & Kligler, B. (2003). An integrative medicine approach to premenstrual syndrome. *American Journal of Obstetrics and Gynecology, 188*(5 Suppl), S56–65.

Glass, J. M., Lyden, A. K., Petzke, F., Stein, P., Whalen, G., Ambrose, K., et al. (2004). The effect of brief exercise cessation on pain, fatigue, and mood symptom development in healthy, fit individuals. *Journal of Psychosomatic Research, 57*(4), 391–398.

Glassroth, C. (2004). Successful migraine management: Patient-customized care. *Clinician Reviews, 14*(5), 56–61.

Glasziou, P., Irwig, L., Bain, C., & Colditz, G (2001). *Systematic reviews in health care: A practical guide.* Cambridge, UK: Cambridge University Press.

Goer, T., & Lacey, S. (2005). Bone up on fat embolism syndrome. *Nursing, 23*(4), 1–4.

Golash, V., & Willson P. (2005). Early laparoscopy as a routine procedure in the management of acute abdominal pain: A review of 1,320 patients. *Surgical Endoscopy, 19*(7):882–885.

Goldberg, B. (2002). *Alternative medicine: The definitive guide.* Tiburon, CA: Future Medicine Publishing.

Goldberg, B., & Goldberg, M. (2002). *Alternative medicine: The definitive guide.* Berkeley, CA: Celestial Arts.

Goldberg, D. (2004). *Photodamaged skin.* New York: Marcel Dekker.

Goldberg, J. P., Belury, M. A., Elam, P., Finn, S. C., Hayes, D., Lyle, R., et al. (2004). The obesity crisis: Don't blame it on the pyramid. *Journal of the American Dietetic Association, 104*(7), 1141–1147.

Goldberg, S. (2004). Tuberculosis. *Clinics in Family Practice, 6*(1), 175.

Goldhaber, S. Z., Dunn, K., Gerhard-Herman, M., Park, J. K., & Black, P. (2002). Low rate of venous thromboembolism after craniotomy for brain tumor using multimodality prophylaxis. *Chest, 122*(6), 1933–1937.

Goldie, S., Kohli, M., Grima, D., Weinstein, M., Wright, T., Bosch, F., et al. (2004). Projected clinical benefits and cost-effectiveness of a human papillomavirus 16/18 vaccine. *Journal of the National Cancer Institute, 96*(8), 604–614.

Goldrick, B. (2004). Emerging infections: MRSA, VRE, and VRSA. *American Journal of Nursing, 104*(8), 50.

Gonzales, E., & Martin, K. (2003). Bone and mineral metabolism in chronic renal failure. In R. Johnson & J. Feehally (Eds.), *Comprehensive clinical nephrology* (2nd ed., pp. 873–885). St. Louis, MO: Mosby.

Goodal, D., & Etters, L. (2005). The therapeutic use of music on agitated behavior in those with dementia. *Journal of Holistic Nursing Practice, 19*(6), 97–104.

Gordon, M. (1994). *Nursing diagnosis: Process and application* (3rd ed.). St. Louis, MO: Mosby.

Gordon, M. (1997). *Manual of nursing diagnoses.* St. Louis, MO: Mosby.

Gordon, M. (2002). *Manual of nursing diagnosis* (10th ed.). St. Louis, MO: Mosby.

Gordon, P. A. (2004). Effects of diabetes on the vascular system: Current research evidence and best practice recommendations. *Journal of Vascular Nursing, 22*(1), 2–13.

Gosselin, B. J. (2004, July). *Peritonsillar abscess.* Retrieved August 25, 2004, from http://www.emedicine.com/med/topic2803.htm.

Gottlieb, M., & Furman, J. (2004). *Successful management and surgical closure of chronic and pathological wounds using Integra®.* Retrieved May 1, 2006, from http://www.journalofburnsandwounds.com.

Gowen, G. (2003). Long tube decompression is successful in 90% of patients with adhesive small bowel obstruction. *The American Journal of Surgery, 185,* 512–515.

Greco, K., & Mahon, S. (2003). Genetics nursing practice enters a new era with credentialing. *The Internet Journal of Advanced Nursing Practice, 5*(2), 1523–6064.

Grady, D. (2006). *Studies suggest two major diseases have close links: Alzheimer's, diabetes tolls seen rising.* Retrieved July 17, 2006, from http://www.alz.org.

Graham, T. A. D. (2002). Diagnosis and treatment of pharyngitis in adults. *CJEM Journal Club, 4*(6), 429–430.

Grantham, J., & Winklhofer, F. (2004). Cystic diseases of the kidney. In B. Brenner (Ed.), *Brenner and Rector's the kidney* (7th ed., vol. 2, pp. 1743–1775). Philadelphia: W. B. Saunders Co.

Grauer, K., & Ruskin, J. (2004, February). Palpitations and arrhythmias: Benign or threatening? *Patient Care,* 30–36.

Graxiottin, A., & Brotto, L. (2004). Vulvar vestibulitis syndrome: A clinical approach. *Journal of Sex and Marital Therapy, 30,* 125–139.

Gray, E. (2005). Understanding the role of the glaucoma specialist nurse. *Nursing Times, 101*(38), 32–34.

Grayson, M. (2004). The open organization. *Hospitals and Health Networks, 78*(10), 36–44.

Greater New York Hospital Association. (2002). *Do you know your incident command system?* Retrieved July 5, 2006, from http://www.gnyha.org.

Green, D., Hartwig, D., Chen, D., Soltysik, R., Yarnold, P. (2003). Spinal cord injury risk assessment for thromboembolism. *American Journal of Physical Medicine and Rehabilitation, 82*(12), 950–956.

Green, H. J., Pakenham, K. I., & Gardiner, R. A. (2005). Objective and cognitive deficits associated with cancer: Implications for health professionals. *Psychology, Health, and Medicine, 10*(2), 145–160.

Green, R. (2005). Toward a full theory of moral status. *American Journal of Bioethics, 5*(6), 44–46.

Greenland, P., Knoll, M. D., & Stamler, J., Neaton, J., Dyer, A., Garside, D., et al. (2003). Major risk factors for cardiovascular disease as antecedents of fatal and nonfatal coronary heart disease events. *Journal of the American Medical Association, 290*(7), 891–897.

Greenspan, F. S. (2004). The thyroid gland. In F. S. Greenspan & D. G. Gardner (Eds.), *Basic and clinical endocrinology* (pp. 215–294). St. Louis, MO: Lange Medical Books.

Greenspan, F. S., & Gardner, D. G. (2004). *Basic and clinical endocrinology* (7th ed.). New York: Lange Medical Books.

Greenspan, F. S., & Resnick, N. M. (2004). Geriatric endocrinology. In F. S. Greenspan & D. G. Gardner (Eds.), *Basic and clinical endocrinology* (pp. 543–548). St. Louis, MO: Lange Medical Books.

Grendell, R. (2004). Psychosocial alterations. In L. Urden, K. Stacy, & M. Lough (Eds.), *Priorities in critical care nursing* (pp. 172–181). St. Louis, MO: Mosby.

Griffin, J. E., & Ojeda, S. R. (2004). *Textbook of endocrine physiology* (5th ed.). New York: Oxford Press.

Griffiths, R., Fernandez, R., & Murie, P. (2004). Removal of short-term indwelling urethral catheters: The evidence. *Journal of Wound Ostomy Continence Nurses Society, 31*(5), 299–308.

Grigsby, P. W. (2004). Thyroid. In C. Perez, E. Halperm, L. Brady, R. Schmidt-Ullrich (Eds.), *Principles and practices of radiation oncology* (pp. 211–215). New York: Lippincott, Williams & Williams.

Gronau, E., & Pannek, J. (2005). Acute urinary retention in ileum conduit urinary diversion. *Urology, 65*(3), 593.

Gruenwald, J. (2004). *PDR for herbal medicines* (3rd ed.). Montvale, NJ: Medical Economics Co., Inc.

Gruffydd, E., & Randle, J. (2006). Alzheimer's disease and the psychosocial burden for caregivers. *Community Practitioner, 79*(1), 15–18.

Grundy, S. M., Cleeman, J. I., Merz, C. B., Brewer, B., Clark, J. T., Hunninghake, D. B., et al. (2004). Implications of recent trials for national cholesterol education program adult treatment panel III guidelines. *Circulation, 110*(2), 227–239.

Gugenheim, J. J. (2004). External fixation in orthopedics. *Journal of the American Medical Association, 291,* 2122–2124.

Guillet, G., Guillet, M., & Dagregorio, G. (2005). Allergic contact dermatitis from natural rubber latex in atopic dermatitis and the risk of later Type I allergy. *Contact Dermatitis, 53*(1), 46–51.

Gundel, J.C. (2004). *Medial collateral knee ligament injury.* Retrieved on September 28, 2005, from http://www.emedicine.com/sports/topic73.htm.

Guttmacher, A. E., & Collins, F. S. (2002). Genomic medicine: A primer. *New England Journal of Medicine, 347*(19), 1512–1520.

Guyton, A., & Hall, J. (2001). *Pocket companion to textbook of medical physiology* (10th ed). Philadelphia: W. B. Saunders Company.

Guyton, A., & Hall, J. (2006). *Textbook of medical physiology* (11th ed.). Philadelphia: W. B. Saunders.

Haas, F. (2005). Clinical. Understanding the legal implications of living wills. *Nursing Times, 101*(3), 18–24, 34–37.

Haas, K. (2004). Who will make room for the intersexed? *American Journal of Law and Medicine, 30*(1), 41–68.

Habel, M. (2004, January 6). The hospitalized older adult: Entering a danger zone. *Nurseweek,* pp. 22–23.

Hadaway, L. C. (2002, August). IV infiltration, not just a peripheral problem. *Nursing, 32*(1), 36–42.

Hader, C., & Guy, J. (2004). Your hand in pain management. *Nursing Management, 35*(11), 21–27.

Hagerty, B., & Patusky, K. (2004). Mood disorders: Depression and mania. In K. Fortinash & P. Holoday-Worret (Eds.), *Psychiatric mental health nursing* (3rd ed., pp. 324–341). St. Louis, MO: Mosby.

Hall, D. (2004). Work-related stress of registered nurses in a hospital setting. *Journal for Nurses in Staff Development, 20*(1), 6–14.

Hamilton, R. G., Brown, R. H., Veltri, M. A., Feroli, E. R., Primeau, M. N., Schauble, J. F., et al. (2005). Administering pharmaceuticals to latex allergic patients from vials containing natural rubber latex closures. *American Journal of Health System Pharmacy, 62*(17), 1822–1828.

Hamilton, R. J., Bowers, B. J., & Williams, J. K. (2005). Disclosing genetic test results to family members. *Journal of Nursing Scholarship, 37*(1), 18–24.

Hanks-Bell, M., Halvey, K., & Paice, J. (2004). Pain assessment and management in aging. *Online Journals in Nursing, 9*(3), 1–18.

Hardaway, R. M. (2006) Traumatic shock. *Military Medicine, 171*(4), 278–279.

Hark, L., & Morrison, G. (2003). *Medical nutrition and disease: A case-based approach.* Malden, MA: Blackwell Publishing.

Harkness, K., Smith, K., Taraba, L., MacKenzie, C., Gunn, E., & Arthur, H. (2005). Effect of a postoperative telephone intervention on attendance at intake for cardiac rehabilitation after coronary artery bypass graft surgery. *Heart and Lung, 34*(3), 179–186.

Harman, L. (2003). Attitudes toward genetic testing: Gender, role, and discipline. *Topics in Health Information Management, 24*(1), 50–58.

Harper, D. G., Arsura, E. L., Bobba, R. K., Reddy, C. M., Sawh, A. K. (2005). Acquired color blindness in an elderly male patient from recurrent metastatic prostate cancer. *Journal of the American Geriatrics Society, 53*(7), 1265–1267.

Hart, J. A. (2004). Right-sided heart failure. Retrieved June 24, 2006, from http://www.nlm.nih.gov.

Hathaway, L. (2005). Anaphylaxis. *Nursing, 35*(1), 46–47.

Havener, G., Roth, M., Arakere, R., & Barenfanger, K. (2005). *Effective investigation and control of an aspergillosis outbreak in a regional burn unit.* Retrieved May 1, 2006, from http://www.journalofburnsandwounds.com.

Hawkley, L. C., & Cacioppo, J. T. (2003) Loneliness and pathways to disease. *Brain, Behavior, and Immunity, 17*(Suppl 1), S98–S105.

Hayes, D. (2004). Phosphorus: Here, there, everywhere. *Nursing Made Incredibly Easy! 2*(6), 36–41.

He, L., Zhou, D., Wu, B., Li, N., & Zhou, M. (2004). Acupuncture for Bell's palsy. *The Cochrane Database of Systematic Reviews* (1), CD002914.

Headley, A. A., Ogden, C. L., Johnson, C. L., Carroll, M. D., Curtain, L. R., & Flegal, K. M. (2004). Prevalence of overweight and obesity among U.S. children, adolescents, and adults, 1999–2002. *Journal of the American Medical Association, 291*(23), 2847–2850.

Health Gate Data Corp. (2003). *Dysmenorrhea.* Retrieved September 6, 2004, from http://iHerb.com.

HealthGrades. (2005). *Medical errors gap widens between best and worst hospitals: Healthgrades study.* Retrieved June 26, 2005, from www.healthgrades.com.

Healthy People 2010. (2004). *About healthy people 2010.* Retrieved May 14, 2005, from http://www.healthypeople.gov.

Heck, R. K., & Carnesale, P. G. (2003). General principles of amputations. In S. T. Canale (Ed.), *Campbell's operative orthopaedics* (vol. 1, 10th ed., pp. 537–554). Philadelphia: Mosby.

Heffner, J. E. (2003). Chronic obstructive pulmonary disease: Translating new understanding into improved patient care. *Respiratory Care, 48*(12), 1184.

Heidary, N., & Cohen, D. (2005). Hypersensitivity reactions to vaccine components. *Dermatitis, 16*(3), 115–120.

Heinrich, C., Karner, K., Gaglione, B., & Lambert, L. (2002). Order out of chaos: The use of a matrix to validate curriculum integrity. *Nurse Educator, 27*(3), 136–140.

Heinz, D. (2004). Hospital nurse staffing and patient outcomes. *Dimensions of Critical Care Nursing, 23*(1), 44–50.

Heise, L., & Garcia-Moreno, C. (2002). *Violence by intimate partners. World report on violence and health.* Geneva: World Health Organization.

Hellman, D. B., & Stone, J. H. (2004). Arthritis & musculoskeletal disorders. In L.M. Tierney, S. J. McPhee, & M. A. Papidakis (Eds.), *Current medical diagnosis and treatment* (43rd ed., pp. 1062–1145). New York: McGraw-Hill.

Henderson, V. (1939). *Principles and practices of nursing.* New York: Macmillan.

Henderson, V. (1966). *The nature of nursing.* New York: Macmillan.

Henderson, V. (1991). *The nature of nursing: Reflections after 25 years.* New York: National League for Nursing.

Henderson, V., & Nite, G. (1978). *Principles and practice of nursing* (6th ed.). New York: Macmillan.

Henneman, E., Dracup, K., Ganz, T., Molayeme, O., & Cooper, C. (2002). Using a collaborative weaning plan to decrease duration of mechanical ventilation and length of stay in the ICU for patients receiving long-term ventilation. *American Journal of Critical Care, 11*(2), 132–140.

Hennessy, B. T., Hanrahan, E. O., & Daly, P. A. (2004). Non-Hodgkin lymphoma: An update. *Lancet Oncology, 5*(6): 341–353.

Henriksson, K. G. (2003). Fibromyalgia—From syndrome to disease. Overview of pathogenic mechanisms. *Journal of Rehabilitative Medicine, 43*, 89–94.

Hess, D., & Kacmarek, R. (2002). *Essentials of mechanical ventilation* (2nd ed.). New York: McGraw-Hill.

Hicken, B., & Tucker, D. (2002). Impact of genetic risk feedback: Perceived risk and motivation for health protective behaviors. *Psychology, Health, and Medicine, 7*(1), 25–36.

Hietanen, A., Era, P. Sorri, M., & Heikkiness, N. (2004). Changes in hearing in 80 year old people: A 10 year followup study. *International Journal of Audiology, 43*, 126–135.

Highfield, M. (2000). Providing spiritual care to patients with cancer. *Clinical Journal of Oncology Nursing, 4*(30), 115–120.

Higo, R., Tayama, N., Nitou, T., Watanabe, T., & Ugawa, Y. (2003). Videofluoroscopic and manometric evaluation of swallowing function in patients with multiple system atrophy. *Annals of Otology, Rhinology & Laryngology, 112*(7), 630–636.

Hildebrandt, L., Fracchia, J., Driscoll, J., & Giroux, P. (2002). Comparison of post-pyloric versus gastric enteral formula administration. *Topics in Clinical Nutrition, 17*(3), 44–51.

Hill, M., Hughes T., & Milford C. (2005). Treatment for swallowing difficulties (dysphagia) in chronic muscle disease. *The Cochrane Database of Systematic Reviews (Oxford)* (2), CD004303.

Hillman, T., Arriaga, M., & Chen, D. (2003). Intratympanic steroids: Do they acutely improve hearing in cases of cochlear hydrops? *Laryngoscope, 113*(11), 1903–1907.

Hillman, T., Chen, D., & Arriaga, M. (2004). Vestibular nerve section versus intratympanic gentamicin for Meniere's disease. *Laryngoscope, 114*(2), 216–222.

Hinkle, J. (2004). Potential new drug for spinal cord injury. *Journal of Neuroscience Nursing, 36*(1), 49.

Hinson, G. (2005). *Shock management.* Retrieved July 12, 2006, from http://www.cdi.pub.ro.

Hitchcock, J., Schubert, P., & Thomas, S. (2003). *Community health nursing: Caring in action* (2nd ed.). New York: Thomson Delmar Learning.

Hohler, S. E. (2004). Tips for better patient teaching. *Nursing, 34*(7), 7–8.

Hobbs, F., & Stoops, N. (2002). Demographic trends in the 20th century, *U.S. Census Bureau, Census 2000*

Special Reports, Series CENSR-4. Washington, DC: U.S. Government Printing Office.

Hobbs, F., Irwin, P., & Rubner, J. (2005). Evidence-based treatment of hypertension: What's the role of angiotensin II receptor blockers? *British Journal of Cardiology, 12*(1), 65–70.

Hockenberry, M. J., & Brown, J. (2003). Conditions caused by defects in physical development. In D. Wilson, M. L. Winkelstein, & N. E. Kline. *Wong's nursing care of infants and children* (7th ed., pp. 1757–1831). St. Louis, MO: Mosby.

Hoffman, M., & Monroe, D. (2005). Rethinking the coagulation cascade. *Current Hematology Reports, 4*(5), 391–396.

Hollinworth, H. (2005). The management of patients' pain in wound care. *Nursing Standard, 20*(7), 65–66, 68, 70.

Holmes, S. B., & Brown, S. J. (2005). Skeletal pin site care: National Association of Orthopaedic Nurses guideline for orthopaedic nursing. *Orthopaedic Nursing, 24*(2), 99–107.

Holmes, T. H., & Rahe, R. H. (1967). The social readjustment rating scale. *Journal of Psychosomatic Medicine, 11*(14), 213–218.

Holoday-Worret, P. (2004). Foundations of psychiatric mental health nursing. In K. Fortinash & P. Holoday-Worret (Eds.), *Psychiatric mental health nursing* (3rd ed., pp. 225–234). St. Louis, MO: Mosby.

Homik, J., Suarez-Almazor, M. E., Shea, B., Cranney, A., Wells, G., & Tugwell, P. (2004). Calcium and vitamin D for corticosteroid-induced osteoporosis (Cochrane Review). In *The Cochrane Database of Systematic Reviews.* Chichester, UK: John Wiley & Sons, Ltd.

Homs, M., Steyerberg, E., Eijkenboom, W., & Siersema, P. (2006). Predictors of outcome of single-dose brachytherapy for the palliation of dysphagia from esophageal cancer. *Brachytherapy, 5*(1), 41–48.

Hong, Q. N, Durand, M. J., & Loisel, P. (2003). Treatment of lateral epicondylitis: Where is the evidence? *Joint Bone Spine, 71,* 369–373.

Honkus, V. (2003). Sleep deprivation in critical care units. *Critical Care Nurse Quarterly, 26*(3), 179–189.

Horenstein, M. S., Pettersen, M., & Walters, H. L. (2002). *Mitral stenosis.* Retrieved June 24, 2006, from www.emedicine.com.

Horowitz, A., Brennan, M., Reinhardt, J. P. (2005). Prevalence and risk factors for self-reported visual impairment among middle-aged and older adults. *Research on Aging, 27*(3), 307–326.

Horstman, J. (2006). *Tai Chi. Arthritis foundation news.* Retrieved August 14, 2006, from http://www.arthritis.org.

Hosalkar, H., & Dormans, J.P. (2004). Limb sparing surgery for pediatric musculoskeletal tumors. *Pediatric Blood Cancer, 42*(4), 295–310.

Hospice Foundation of America. (2003). Retrieved June 24, 2006, from http://www.hospicefoundation.org.

Hospice and Palliative Nurses Association Board of Directors. (2004). *Artificial nutrition and hydration in end-of-life care.*

Hospital Compare. (2005). *Hospital compare.* Retrieved May 18, 2005, from http://www.hospitalcompare.hhs.gov.

Hostima, A., & Hilbrands, L. (2003). Evaluation of renal transplant donor and recipient. In R. Johnson & J. Feehally (Eds.), *Comprehensive clinical nephrology* (2nd ed., pp. 1071–1091). St. Louis, MO: Mosby.

Hoyt, K. S., & Haley, R. J. (2005). Innovations in advanced practice: Assessment and management of eye emergencies. *Topics in Emergency Medicine, 27*(2), 101–117.

Huckleberry, Y. (2004). Nutritional support and the surgical patient. *American Journal of Health-System Pharmacy, 61*(7), 671–684.

Hudak, C. M., Morton, P., Galle, B., & Fontaine, D. (2005). *Critical care nursing: A holistic approach.* Philadelphia: Lippincott, Williams & Wilkins.

Hudson, M. M., Mertens, A. C., Yasui, Y., Hobbie W., Chen, H., Gurney, J. G., et al. (2003). Health status of adult long-term survivors of childhood cancer: A report from the childhood cancer survivor study. *Journal of American Medical Association, 290*(12), 1583–1592.

Huether, S. E. (2004). Alterations of hormonal regulation. In S. E. Huether & K. L. McCance (Eds.), *Understanding pathophysiology* (pp. 356–362). St. Louis, MO: Mosby.

Hultman, C., & Daiza, S. (2003). Skin-sparing mastectomy flap complications after breast reconstruction: Review of incidence, management, and outcome. *Annals of Plastic Surgery, 50*(3), 249.

Hughes, F., Bryan, K., & Robbins, I. (2005). Relatives' experiences of critical care. *Nursing in Critical Care, 10*(1), 23–30.

Hughes, S. C., & Martin, D. E. (2005). Traditional IV catheters: To be or not to be, that is the question! *American Society of Anesthesiologists, 69*(3), 14–15.

Hurlock-Chorostecki, C. (2004). Managing diabetic ketoacidosis: The role of the ICU nurse in an endocrine emergency. *Canadian Association of Critical Care Nurses, 15*(1), 18–22.

Hurskainen, R., Teperi, J., Rissanen, P., Aalto, A., Grenman, S., Kivela, A., et al. (2004). Clinical outcomes and costs with the levonorgestrel-releasing intrauterine system or hysterectomy for treatment of menorrhagia: Randomized trial 5-year follow-up. *Journal of the American Medical Association, 291,* 1456–1463.

Hurwitz, S. R. (2004). *Plantar fasciitis.* Retrieved on December 7, 2005, from http://www.emedicine.com/orthoped/topic542.htm.

Huston, J., & Brox, G. (2004). Professional ethics at the bottom line. *The Health Care Manager, 23*(3), 267–272.

Hyman, G., Malanga, G. A., & Alladin, I. (2005). *Jumper's knee.* Retrieved on September 6, 2005, from http://www.emedicine.com/sports/topic56.htm.

Ibrahim, M., Wurpel, J., & Gladson, B. (2003). Intrathecal baclofen: A new treatment approach for severe spasticity in patients with stroke. *Journal of Neurologic Physical Therapy, 27*(3), 142–148.

Ignatavicius, D., & Workman, M. (2006). *Medical-surgical nursing: Critical thinking for collaborative care* (5th ed.). St. Louis, MO: Elsevier Saunders.

Ihlenfeld, J. (2003). A primer on triage and mass casualty events. *Dimensions of Critical Care, Nursing, 22*(5), 204–209.

Imke, S. (2003). Parkinson's disease: More than meets the eye. *Advance for Nurse Practitioners, 11*(9), 42–54.

Inadomi, J., Sampliner, R., Lagergren, J., Lieberman, D. Fendrick, & Vakil, N. (2003). Screening and surveillance for Barrett esophagus in high-risk groups: A cost-utility analysis. *Annals of Internal Medicine, 138*(3), 176–186.

Inanici, F., & Yunus, B. M. (2002, August). Fibromyalgia syndrome: Diagnosis and management. *Hospital Physician*, 53–66.

Indian Health Service. (n.d.a). *About IHS*. Retrieved August 30, 2005, from p://www.ihs.gov.

Indian Health Service. (n.d.b). *Appropriations*. Retrieved August 3, 2005, from http://www.ihs.gov.

Institute for Clinical Systems Improvement. (2003). *Diagnosis and initial treatment of ischemic stroke.* Retrieved June 17, 2006, from www.guideline.gov.

Institute for Healthcare Improvement. (2005). 100,000 lives campaign. Retrieved June 25, 2006, from http://www.ihi.org.

Institute of Medicine. (2000). *To err is human: Building a safer health system.* Washington, DC: National Academy Press.

Institute of Medicine. (2001). *Crossing the quality chasm: A new health system for the 21st century.* Washington, DC: National Academy Press.

Institute of Medicine. (2002). Dietary reference intakes for energy, carbohydrate, fiber, fat, fatty acids, cholesterol, protein, and amino acids. Washington, DC: National Academy Press.

Institute of Medicine. (2003). *Priority areas for national action: Transforming health care quality.* Washington, DC: National Academy Press.

Integrated Publishing. (2004). *Triage.* Retrieved June 21, 2006, from http://infodotinc.com.

International Headache Society. (2004). The international classification of headache disorders (2nd ed.). *Cephalalgia, 24* (Suppl 1), 1–160.

International Sepsis Forum. (2003). *The critical care forum.* Retrieved June 28, 2006, from www.sepsisforum.org.

Isowa, T., Ohira, H., & Murashima, S. (2004). Reactivity of immune, endocrine and cardiovascular parameters to active and passive acute stress. *Biological Psychology, 65*(2), 101–120.

Ives, J. R. (2005). New chronic EEG electrode for critical/ intensive care unit monitoring. *Journal of Clinical Neurophysiology, 22*(2), 119–123.

Izzo, J., & Black, H. (2003). *Hypertension primer* (3rd ed.). Dallas: American Heart Association.

Jablonski, A., & Wyatt, G. (2005). A model for identifying barriers to effective symptom management at the end of life. *Journal of Hospice and Palliative Nursing, 7*(1), 23–26.

Jacobs, B., Neil, N., & Aboulafia, D. (2005). Retrospective analysis of suspending HAART in selected patients with controlled HIV replication. *AIDS Patient Care and STDs, 19*(7), 429–438.

Jacox, A., Carr, D., & Payne, R. (1994). *Management of pain. Clinical practice guidelines.* No. 9, AHCPR Publication No. 94-0592. Rockville, MD: Agency for Health Care Policy and Research, U.S. Department of Health and Human Services, Public Health Service.

Jakobsson, L., Loven, L., & Hallberg, I. R. (2004). Micturition problems in relation to quality of life in men with prostate cancer or benign prostatic hyperplasia: Comparison with men from the general population. *Cancer Nursing, 27*(3), 218–229.

Janeway, C. A., Jr., Travers, P., Walport, M., & Shlomchik, M. J. (2004). *Immunobiology, the immune system in health and disease* (6th ed.). New York: Garland Science Publishing.

Janssen, I., Katzmarzyk, P., & Ross, R. (2004). Waist circumference and not body mass index explains obesity-related health risk. *American Journal of Clinical Nutrition, 79*, 379–384.

Jarzabek, J., Zbucka, M., Pepinski, W., Szamatowicz, J., Domitrz, J., Janica, J., et al. (2004). Cystic fibrosis as a cause of infertility. *Reproductive Biology, 4*(2), 119–129.

Jarzyna, D. (2005). Opioid tolerance: A perioperative nursing challenge. *MEDSURG Nursing, 14*(6), 371–377.

Jeavons, H. (2003). Prevention and treatment of vulvovaginal candidiasis using exogenous *Lactobacillus. Journal of Obstetric, Gynecologic, and Neonatal Nursing, 32*, 287–296.

Jemal, A. (2003). Cancer statistics. *CA: A Cancer Journal for Clinicians, 53*(1), 5–26.

Jenkins, J. F., & Lea, D. H. (2004). *Nursing care in the genomic era: A case-based approach.* Sudbury, MA: Jones & Bartlett Publishers.

Jenner, P., & Olanow, C. W. (2006). The pathogenesis of cell death in Parkinson's disease. *Neurology, 66*(10 Suppl 4), S24–S36.

Jeremitsky, E., Omert, L., Dunham, M., Protetch, J., & Rodriguez, A. (2003). Harbingers of poor outcome the day after severe brain injury: Hypothermia, hypoxia, and hypoperfusion. *The Journal of Trauma, Injury, Infection, and Critical Care, 54*(2), 312–319.

Jessup, M., & Brozena, S. (2003). Medical progress: Heart failure. *New England Journal of Medicine, 348*(20), 2007–2018.

Jirillo, E., Mastronardi, M. L., Altamura, M., Munno, I., Miniello, S., Urgesi, G., et al. (2003). The immunocompromised host: Immune alterations in splenectomized patients and clinical implications. *Current Pharmaceutical Design, 9*(24), 1918–1923.

Johns Hopkins Institutes. (2003). *Economic impact of the Johns Hopkins Institutes in Maryland.* Silver Springs, MD: Johns Hopkins University and Johns Hopkins Medicine.

Johnsen, J., & Davis, J. (2005). *All about vasectomy.* Retrieved July 16, 2006, from http://www.plannedparenthood. org.

Johnson, K. (2005). Shock states. In K. Wagner, P. Kidd, & K. Johnson (Eds.), *High acuity nursing.* New Jersey: Prentice Hall.

Johnson, K., Nicol, T., & Kraus, N. (2005). Brain stem response to speech: A biological marker of auditory processing. *Ear and Hearing, 26*(5), 424–434.

Johnstone, C., Farley, A. & Hendry, C. (2005). The physiological basis of wound healing. *Nursing Standard, 19*(43), 59–65.

Joint Commission on Accreditation of Healthcare Organizations (JCAHO) and National Pharmaceutical Council (NPC). (2003). Monograph: Improving the Quality of Pain Management through Measurement and Action.

Joint Commission on Accreditation of Healthcare Organizations. (2004). *2004 national patient safety goals.* Retrieved February 7, 2005, from http://jcaho.org.

Joint Commission for Accreditation of Healthcare Organizations. (2005). *Accreditation manual.* Chicago: Author.

Joint Commission on Accreditation of Healthcare Organizations (2006a). *Emergency management standards EC.1.4 and EC.2.9.1.* Retrieved June 18, 2006, from http://www.jcrinc.com.

Joint Commission on Accreditation of Healthcare Organizations. (2006b). *Focus areas.* Retrieved May 22, 2006, from http://www.soros.org/initiatives/pdia/focusareas/grants/grantees/royal1994.

Joint Commission on Accreditation of Healthcare Organizations. (n.d.). *Critical access hospitals.* Retrieved August 4, 2005, from http://www.jcaho.org.

Joint Commission on Accreditation of Hospitals and Healthcare Organizations. (2004). *Provision of care, treatment, and services. Comprehensive accreditation manual for hospitals.* Oakbrook Terrace, IL: Author.

Jones, A. (2005). The role of hope in serious illness and dying. *European Journal of Palliative Care, 12*(1), 28–31.

Jones, D. (2005). Savings sharing. *Journal of Nursing Administration, 35*(4), 199–204.

Jones, J. (1993). *Bad blood: The Tuskegee syphilis experiment.* New York: The Free Press.

Jones, L., & Bagnall, A. (2004). Spinal injuries centres (SICs) for acute traumatic spinal cord injury. *The Cochrane Database of Systematic Reviews* (4), CD: 004442.

Jones, R. (2004). Relationships of sexual imposition, dyadic trust, and sensation seeking with sexual risk behavior in young urban women. *Research and Nursing Health, 27*(3), 185–197.

Jones, R. C., Hodgson, J. M., Bahler, R. C., & Orford, J. (2004). *Mitral valve prolapse.* Retrieved June 24, 2006, from www.firstconsult.com.

Jong, P., Demers, C., McKelvie, R. S., & Liu, P. P. (2002). Angiotensin receptor blockers in heart failure: Meta-analysis of randomized controlled trials. *Journal of the American College of Cardiology, 39*(3), 463–470.

Joo, Y., Park, C., Lee, W., Kim, H., Choi, S., Cho, C., et al. (2004). Primary non-Hodgkin's lymphoma of the common bile duct presenting as obstructive jaundice. *Journal of Gastroenterology, 39*(7), 692–696.

Jubran, A. (2004). Pulse oximetry. *Intensive Care Medicine, 30*(11), 2017–2020.

Julian, D. (2001). The evolution of the coronary care unit. *Cardiovascular Research, 51*(4), 621–624.

Jungles, S. L. (2004). Video wireless capsule endoscopy: A diagnostic tool for early Crohn's disease. *Gastroenterology Nursing, 27*(4), 170–175.

Jurgens, G., & Graudal, N. (2006). Effects of low sodium diet versus high sodium diet on blood pressure, renin, aldosterone, catecholamines, cholesterols, and triglyceride. *The Cochrane Database of Systematic Reviews* (1), CD004022.

Kaiser Permanente (n.d.). *Press room.* Retrieved September 5, 2005, from https://newsmedia.kaiserpermanente.org/kpweb/homepage.do.

Kanellos, M. (2004). *Human chips more than skin deep.* Retrieved August 23, 2006, from http://zdnet.com.com.

Kang, S. (2004). *Left-sided heart failure.* Retrieved June 24, 2006, from http://www.nlm.nih.gov.

Kang, S., Bergfeld, W. Gottlieb, A., Hickman, J., Humeniuk, J., Kempers, S., et al. (2005). Long-term efficacy and safety of Tretinoin emollient cream 0.05% in treatment of photo damaged skin. *American Journal of Clinical Dermatology, 6*(4), 245–253.

Kaplan, H. S. (1985). *Comprehensive evaluation of disorders of sexual desire.* Washington, DC: American Psychiatric Press.

Kaptanoglu, E., Beskonakli, E., Okutan, O., Surucu, H., & Taskin, Y. (2003). Effect of magnesium sulphate in experimental spinal cord injury: Evaluation with ultrastructural findings and early clinical results. *Journal of Clinical Neuroscience, 10*(3), 329–334.

Karcioglu, O., Oskara, E., Civancr, M., & Ozucclik, N. (2003). Resuscitation of a Jehovah's Witness with multiple injuries without blood: Right to die? *The Internet Journal of Emergency and Intensive Care Medicine, 7*(1).

Karnath, B. (2002). Smoking cessation. *American Journal of Medicine, 112*(5), 399–405.

Karnib, H., & Badr, K. (2004). Microvascular diseases of the kidney. In B. Brenner (Ed.), *Brenner and Rector's the kidney* (7th ed., vol. 2, pp. 1601–1623). Philadelphia: W. B. Saunders Co.

Kashtan, C. (2003). Alport and other familial glomerular syndromes. In R. Johnson & J. Feehally (Eds.), *Comprehensive clinical nephrology* (2nd ed., pp. 627–637). St. Louis, MO: Mosby.

Kasper, D. L., Braunwald, E., Fauci, A. S., Hauser, S. L., Longo, D. L., & Jameson, J. L. (2005). *Harrison's principles of internal medicine* (16th ed.). New York: McGraw-Hill.

Kataria, R. K., & Brent, L. H. (2004). Spondyloarthropathies. *American Family Physician, 69*(12), 2853–2860.

Kathol, D., Geiger, M., & Hartig, J. (1998). Clinical correlation map: A tool for linking theory and practice. *Nurse Educator, 23*(4), 31–34.

Katkin, J. P. (2002). Clinical manifestations and diagnosis of cystic fibrosis. *Up to Date, 10*(1).

Katsenis, D., Bhave, A., Paley, D., & Herzenberg, J. (2005). Treatment of malunion and nonunion at the site of an ankle fusion with the Ilizarov apparatus. *The Journal of Bone and Joint Surgery, 87*-A, 302–309.

Katz, A., Davis, P., & Findlay, S. S. (2002). Ask and ye shall plan: A health needs assessment of a university population. *Canadian Journal of Public Health [Revue Canadienne de Sante Publicque], 93*(1), 63–66.

Katz, J. N., & Simmons, B. P. (2002). Carpal tunnel syndrome. *New England Journal of Medicine, 346*(23), 1807–1812.

Katz, M. J. (2004). Medical problems: Brief reviews. Glaucoma. *Journal of Pharmacy Technology, 20*(5), 318–320.

Kazzi, A. A., & Sheeks, P. (2004, August). *Peritonsillar abscess.* Retrieved August 25, 2004, from http://www.emedicine.com/emerg/topic417.htm.

Kazzi, A. A., & Tehranazdeh, A. D. (2005, October). *Acute glomerulonephritis.* Retrieved January 27, 2006, from http://www.emedicine.com/EMERG/topic219.htm.

Keany, J. E., (2005). *Femur fractures.* Retrieved on September 28, 2005, from http://www.emedicine.com/orthoped/topic193.htm.

Kee, J. L. (2002). *Laboratory and diagnostic tests with nursing implications* (6th ed.). Upper Saddle River, NJ: Prentice Hall.

Kee, J. L, Paulanka, B., & Purnel, L. (2004). *Fluid and electrolytes with clinical applications: A programmed approach* (7th ed.). New York: Thomson Delmar Learning.

Keenan, H., Marshall, S., Nocera, M., & Runyan, D. (2004). Increased incidence of inflicted traumatic brain injury in children after a natural disaster. *American Journal of Preventive Medicine, 26*(3), 189–193.

Keithley, J. K., & Swanson, B. (2004). Enteral nutrition: An update on practice recommendations. *Medsurg Nursing, 13*(2), 131–134.

Kelly, C., & Nielson, E. (2004). Tubulointerstitial diseases. In B. Brenner (Ed.), *Brenner and Rector's the kidney* (7th ed., vol. 2, pp. 1483–1511). Philadelphia: W. B. Saunders Co.

Kelly, J. P., Kaufman, D. W., Kelley, K., Rosenberg, L., Anderson, T. E., & Mitchell, A. A. (2005). Recent trends in use of herbal and other natural products. *Archives of Internal Medicine, 165,* 281–286.

Kennedy, J. M., & Zochodne, D. W. (2005). Impaired peripheral nerve regeneration in diabetes mellitus. *Journal of the Peripheral Nervous System, 10*(2), 144–158.

Kennedy, W. (2004). Beneficence and autonomy in nursing: a moral dilemma. *British Journal of Perioperative Nursing, 14*(11), 500–506.

Kerfoot, K. M. (2004). Synergy from the vantage point of the development and transformation. *Excellence in nursing knowledge.* Indianapolis, IN: Sigma Theta Tau Press.

Kerkenbush, N. (2003). The emerging role of electronic diaries in the management of diabetes mellitus. *AACN Clinical Issues, 14*(3), 371–378.

Kern, L. (2004). Postoperative atrial fibrillation: New directions in prevention and treatment. *Journal of Cardiovascular Nursing, 19*(2), 103–115.

Keshav, S. (2004). *The gastrointestinal system at a glance.* Malden, MA: Blackwell Science.

Khan, M. A. (2002). Update on Spondyloarthropathies. *Annals of Internal Medicine, 136*(12), 896–907.

Khoury, M., McCabe, L., & McCabe, E. (2003). Population screening in the age of genomic medicine. *New England Journal of Medicine, 348*(1), 50–58.

Kidd, P. (2005). Multiple organ dysfunction syndrome. In K. Wagner & P. Kidd (Eds.), *High acuity nursing* (pp. 312-324[0]). New Jersey: Prentice Hall.

Kielb, S. (2005). Stress incontinence: Alternatives to surgery. *International Journal of Fertility of Women's Medicine, 50*(1), 24–29.

Kieran, N., & Brady, H. (2003). Clinical evaluation, management, and outcome of acute renal failure. In R. Johnson & J. Feehally (Eds.), *Comprehensive clinical nephrology* (2nd ed., pp. 183–206). St. Louis, MO: Mosby.

Kim, B. W., Wang, H. J., Jeong, I. H., Ahn, S. I., & Kim, M. W. (2005). Metastatic liver cancer: A rare case. *World Journal of Gastroenterology, 11*(27), 4281–4284.

Kim, H., Schwartz-Barcott, D., Tracy, S., Fortin, J., & Sjostrom, B. (2005). Strategies of pain assessment used by nurses on surgical units. *Pain Management Nursing, 6*(1), 3–9.

King, A. B., & LeMaire, G. J. (2002). Managing anticoagulation in patients with atrial fibrillation. *Nurse Practitioner, 27*(9), 17–23.

King, I. (1971). *Toward a theory for nursing: General concepts of human behavior.* New York: John Wiley and Sons.

King, M., & Shell, R. (2002). Teaching and evaluating critical thinking with concept maps. *Nurse Educator, 27*(5), 214–216.

King, R. (2004). Nurses perceptions of their pharmacology educational needs. *Journal of Advanced Nursing, 45*(4), 392–400.

King, T. (2004). *Basic principles and techniques of bronchoalveolar lavage.* Retrieved June 25, 2006, from http://www.uptodate.com.

Kinsel, B. (2005). Resilience as adaptation in older women. *Journal of Women and Aging, 17*(3), 23–39.

Kinton, L., Johnson, M., Smith, S., Farrell, F., Stevens, J., Rance, J., et al. (2002). Partial epilepsy with pericentral spikes: A new familial epilepsy syndrome with evidence for linkage to chromosome 4p15. *Annals of Neurology, 51*(6), 740–749.

Kirkland, L. (2005). *Fat embolism.* Retrieved on October 5, 2005, from http://www.emedicine.com/med/topic652.htm.

Kleinbeck, S. V. M. (2002) Revising the perioperative nursing data set. *AORN Journal, 75*(3), 602–610.

Kleinpell, R. (2005). Working out the complexities of severe sepsis. *The Nurse Practitioner, 30*(4), 43–48.

Klijn, C. J. M., & Hankey, G. J. (2003). Management of acute ischemic stroke: New guidelines from the American Stroke Association and European Stroke Initiative. *Lancet, 2,* 698–701.

Knabb, R., Rhome, J., & Brown, D. (*2005, August 23–30*). *Tropical cyclone report: Hurricane Katrina.* National Hurricane Center. Retrieved May 30, 2006, from www.nhc.noaa.gov.

Knaus, W., Draper, E., Wagner, D., & Zimmerman, J. (1986). An evaluation of outcome from intensive care in major medical centers. *Annals of Internal Medicine, 104*(3), 410–419.

Knaus, W., Draper, E., Wagner, D. & Zimmerman, J. (1993). Variation in mortality in length of stay in ICUs. *Annals of Internal Medicine, 118*(10), 753–762.

Knisley, J., & Johnson, M. (2004). Lyme disease: Knowledge is the best prevention. *The Nurse Practitioner, 29*(8), 34–37, 39–40, 43–45.

Knoops, K. T. B., de Groot, L. C. P. G. M., Kromhout, D., Perrin, A., Moreiras-Varela, O., Menotti, A., et al. (2004). Mediterranean diet, lifestyle factors and 10 year mortality in elderly European men and women: The HALE project. *Journal of the American Medical Association, 292*(12), 1433–1439.

Knowles, J. (1977). *Doing better and feeling worse: Health in the United States.* New York: McGraw-Hill.

Knowles, M. S. (1984). *The adult learner: A neglected species* (3rd ed.). Houston: Gulf Publishing.

Koch, T., & Hudson, S. (2000). Older people and laxative use: Literature review and pilot study report. *Journal of Clinical Nursing, 9*(4), 516–525.

Koike, Y., Uhthoff, H. K., Ramachandran, N., Doherty, G.P., Lecompte, M., Backman, D.S., et al. (2004). Achilles tendinopathy. *Critical Reviews in Physical and Rehabilitation Medicine, 16*(2), 109–132.

Koller, D., Nicholas, D., Goldie, R., Gearing, R., & Selkirk, E. (2006). When family-centered care is challenged by infectious disease: Pediatric health care delivery during the SARS outbreaks. *Qualitative Health Research, 16*(1), 47–60.

Kolon, T. (2005). *Crytporchidism.* Retrieved June 2, 2006, from http://www.emedicine.com.

Koppel, R., Metlay, J., Cohen, A., Abaluck, B., Localio, A., Kimmel, S., et al. (2005). Physician order entry systems in facilitating medication errors. *Journal of the American Medical Association, 293*(10), 1197–1203.

Korsten, M., Fajardo, N., Rosman, A., Creasey, G., Spungen, A., & Bauman, W. (2004). Difficulty with evacuation after spinal cord injury: Colonic motility during sleep and effects of abdominal wall stimulation. *Journal of Rehabilitation Research & Development, 41*(1), 95–100.

Kostis, J., Wilson, A., Freudenberger, R., Cosgrove, N., Pressel, S., & Davis, B. (2005). Long-term effect of diuretic-based therapy on fatal outcomes in subjects with isolated systolic hypertension with and without diabetes. *American Journal of Cardiology, 95*, 29–35.

Kraft, M., Btaiche, I., Sacks, G., & Kudsk, K. (2005). Treatment of electrolyte disorders in adult patients in the intensive care unit. *American Journal of Health-System Pharmacy (AJHP), 62*(16), 1663–1682.

Kreiger, D. (1993). *Accepting your power to heal: The personal practice of therapeutic touch.* Santa Fe, NM: Bear & Company Publishing.

Kreiger, D. (2002). *Therapeutic touch as transpersonal healing.* New York: Lanterns Books.

Kübler-Ross, E. (1969). *On death and dying.* New York: Macmillan.

Kuehn, B. M. (2005). Inflammation suspected in eye disorders. *JAMA: Journal of the American Medical Association, 294*(1), 31–32.

Kullmann, D. (2003). Epilepsy genetics. *Drugs Today, 39*(9), 725–732.

Kumle, M., Weiderpass, E., Braatan, T., Persson, I., Adami, H., & Lund, E. (2003). Use of oral contraceptives and breast cancer risk: The Norwegian-Swedish Women's Lifestyle and Health Cohort Study. *Cancer Epidemiologic Biomarkers Preview, 11*(11), 1375–1381.

Kuppermann, M., Varner, R., Summitt, R., Learman, L., Ireland C, Vittinghoff, E., et al. (2004). Effect of hysterectomy vs medical treatment on health-related quality of life and sexual functioning: The medicine or surgery (Ms) randomized trial. *Journal of the American Medical Association, 291*, 1447–1455.

Kuwabara, S. (2004). Guillain-Barre syndrome: Epidemiology, pathophysiology and management. *Drugs, 64*(6), 597–610.

Kuziemsky, C., Laul, F., & Leung, R. (2005). A review on diffusion of personal digital assistants in healthcare. *Journal of Medical Systems, 29*(4), 335–342.

Kvist, J. (2004). Rehabilitation following anterior cruciate ligament injury: Current recommendations for sport participation. *Injury Clinic, 34*(4), 269–280.

Lafleur, K. J. (2004). Tackling med errors with technology. *RN, 67*(5), 29–35.

Laheij, R. J., Sturkenboom, M. C., Hassing, R., Dieleman, J. Stricker, H. C., Jansen, J. (2004). Risk of community-acquired pneumonia and use of gastric acid-suppressive drugs. *Journal of the American Medical Association, 292*, 1955–1960.

Lake, A., & Hafez, K. (2005). Renal cell carcinoma: Controversies in prognosticators. *Contemporary Urology, 17*(8), 13, 15–16, 19–22.

Lal, G., & Clark, O. H.(2004). Endocrine surgery. In F. S. Greenspan & D. G. Gardner (Eds.), *Basic and clinical endocrinology* (pp. 364–367). St. Louis, MO: Lange Medical Books.

Lam, G. M., & Mobarhan, S. (2004). Central obesity and elevated liver enzymes. *Nutrition Reviews, 62*(10), 394–399.

Lampert, R., McPherson, C., Clancy, J., Caulin-Glaser, T., Rosenfeld, L., & Batsford, W. (2004). Gender differences in ventricular arrhythmia recurrence in patients with coronary artery disease and implantable cardioverter-defibrillators. *Journal of the American College of Cardiology, 43*(12), 2293–2299.

Landro, L. (2006, July 26). The new force in walk-in clinics. *The Wall Street Journal,* D1, D2.

Lane, D., Lip, G., & Beevers, D. (2005). Ethnic differences in cardiovascular and all-cause mortality in Birmingham, England: The Birmingham factory screening project. *Journal of Hypertension, 23*(7): 1347–1353.

Lang, L. (2004) Environmental impact on hearing: is anyone listening? *Environmental Health Perspectives, 102*, 102–111.

Lapin, C., & Lapin, A. (2003, March). *Airway clearance techniques for the CF team.* Paper presented at the Seventeenth North American Cystic Fibrosis Conference, Anaheim, CA.

LaPointe, M., & Haines, S. (2004). Fibrinolytic therapy for intraventricular hemorrhage in adults. *The Cochrane Database of Systematic Reviews (Oxford)* (2), CD003692.

LaPointe, M., & Haines, S. (2006). Fibrinolytic therapy for intraventricular hemorrhage in adults. *The Cochrane Database of Systematic Reviews* (1), CD003692.

Larson, E., Shadlen, M., Wang, L., McCormick, W., Bowen, J., Teri, L., et al. (2004). Survival after initial diagnosis of Alzheimer's disease. *Annals of Internal Medicine, 140*(7), 501–509.

Lashley, F. (2005). *Genetics in clinical nursing practice* (3rd ed.). New York: Springer Publishing Company.

Lau, H., & Lam, B. (2004). Management of postoperative urinary retention: a randomized trial of in-out versus overnight catheterization. *ANZ Journal of Surgery, 74*(8), 658–661.

Lavelle, D. G. (2003). Delayed union and nonunion of fractures. In S. T. Canale (Ed.), *Campbell's operative orthopaedics* (vol. 3, 10th ed., pp. 3125–3165). Philadelphia: Mosby.

Lawn, C., Weir, F., & McGuire, W. (2006). Base administration or fluid bolus for preventing morbidity and mortality in preterm infants with metabolic acidosis. *The Cochrane Database of Systematic Reviews* (1), CD003215.

Lazarus, R. (1990). Theory-based stress management. *Psychological Inquiry, 1*(1), 3–13.

Lazarus, R., & Folkman, S. (1987). *Stress, appraisal and coping.* New York: Springer.

Lea, D. H., & Smith, R. S. (2003). *The genetics resource guide.* Scarborough, ME: Foundation for Blood Research.

Leber, S. (2005). *Balanitis.* Retrieved June 2, 2006, from http://www.emedicine.com.

Lebovidge, J., Stone, K., Twarog, F., Raiselis, S., Kalish, L., Bailey, E., et al. (2006). Development of a preliminary questionnaire to assess parental response to children's food allergies. *Annals of Allergy, Asthma, & Immunology, 96*(3), 472–477.

Lee, L. (2004). Improving the quality of patient discharge from emergency settings. *The British Journal of Nursing, 13*(7), 412–421.

Lee, C., Straus, W., Balshaw, R., Barla, S., Vogel, S., & Schnitzer, T. J. (2004). A comparison of the efficacy and safety of nonsteroidal antiinflammatory agents versus acetaminophen in the treatment of osteoarthritis: A meta-analysis. *Arthritis and Rheumatism, 51*(5), 746–754.

Lee, S. B. (2005). *When will we cure cancer? Sooner rather than later, for a surprising number of malignancies. Others, we may just have to live with.* Retrieved April 20, 2005, from http://www.time.com.

Lefebvre, G., Vilos, G., Allaire, C., Jeffrey, J., Arneja, J., Birch, C., et al. (2003). The management of uterine leiomyomas. *Journal of Obstetrics and Gynaecology Canada, 25*, 396–418.

Lehne, R. (2004). *Pharmacology for nursing care.* St. Louis, MO: W.B. Saunders.

Leininger, M. (1978). *Transcultural nursing: Concepts, theories, and practice.* New York: John Wiley and Sons.

Leininger, M., & McFarland, M. (2006). *Culture care diversity and universality: A worldwide nursing theory.* Sudbury, MA: Jones and Bartlett.

Lemke, D. M. (2004). Riding out the storm: Sympathetic storming after traumatic brain injury. *Journal of Neuroscience Nursing, 36*(1), 4–9.

Leon, T. G., & Pase, M. (2004, June). Essential oncology facts for the float nurse. *Medsurg Nursing, 13*(3), 165–171, 189.

Leonard, G. D., Brenner, B., & Kemeny, N. E. (2005). Neoadjuvant chemotherapy before liver resection for patients with unresectable liver metastases from colorectal carcinoma. *Journal of Clinical Oncology, 23*(9), 2038–2048.

Leonard, T. (2005, October 18). New tuberculosis drug therapy could cut treatment time. Associated Press news release *San Diego Union Tribune*, p. A8.

Leske, J. (2002). Interventions to decrease family anxiety. *Critical Care Nurse, 22*(6), 61–65.

Letizia, M., Creech, S., Norton, E., Shanahan, M., & Hedges, L. (2004). Barriers to caregiver administration of pain medication in hospice care. *Journal of Pain and Symptom Management, 27*(2), 114–124.

Levinson, D. J., Darrow, C. N., Klein, E. B., Levinson, M. H., & McKee, B. (1978). *The seasons of a man's life.* New York: Knopf.

Lewis, J. (2002). Genetics in perinatal nursing: Clinical applications and policy considerations. *Journal of Obstetric, Gynecologic, and Neonatal Nursing, 31*(2), 188–192.

LexiComp, Inc. (2005). New drugs: Ziconotide. Retrieved from www.lexi.com/web/content/newdrugs.

Leydig, E. J. (2005) Are you endangering your patients? *RN, 68*(2), 29–31.

Li, C., Malone, K., & Porter, P. (2003). Relationship between long durations and different regimens of hormone therapy and risk of breast cancer. *Journal of the American Medical Association, 289*(24), 3254–3263.

Li, W., Keegan, T., Sternfeld, B., Sidney, S., Quesenberry, Jr., & Kelsey, J. (2006). Outdoor falls among middle aged and older adults: A neglected public health problem. *American Journal of Public Health, 96*(7), 1192–1200.

Liao, D. (2003). Management of acne. *The Journal of Family Practice, 52*(1), 43–51.

Liberati, A., D'Amico, R., Pifferi, S., Torri, V., & Brazzi, L. (2004). Antibiotic prophylaxis to reduce respiratory tract infections and mortality in adults receiving intensive care (Cochrane Review). *The Cochrane Database of Systematic Reviews* (3), 2004; (1), CD000022.

Licata, A. A. (2005). Discovery, clinical development, and therapeutic uses of bisphosphonates. *The Annals of Pharmacotherapy, 39*(4), 668–677.

Lieberman, B. (2006, August 1). Vaccine may offer immunity to obesity. *San Diego Union Tribune*, p. B3, 8.

Liebert, M. (2003a). Free thyroxine (FT4) and free triiodothyronine (FT3) estimate tests. *Thyroid, 13*(1), 21–32.

Liebert, M.(2003b). Thyroid autoantibodies (TPOAb, TgAB and TRAb). *Thyroid, 13*(1), 45–56.

Liebert, M. (2003c). Thyroid fine needle aspiration (FNA) and cytology. *Thyroid, 13*(1), 80–86.

Lim, K., & Morgenthaler, T. (2005). Defining obstruction or restriction remains the goal: Pulmonary function tests. Part 1: Applying the basics. *Journal of Respiratory Diseases, 26*(1), 26–28, 29–30, 32.

Lind, D., Smith, B., & Souba, W. (2005). Breast procedures. *ACS Surgery; Principles and Practice.* Retrieved July 5, 2005, from www.WebMD.com.

Lingappa, V. R. (2003). Disorders of the hypothalamus and pituitary gland. In S. J. McPhee, V. R. Lingappa, &

W. F. Ganong (Eds.), *Pathophysiology of disease* (pp. 367–374). New York: McGraw–Hill.

Linton, M. F., Major, A. S., & Fazio, S. (2004). Proatherogenic role for NK cells revealed. *Arteriosclerosis, Thrombosis, and Vascular Biology, 24*(6), 992–994.

Lipman, M. (2005). Earlier detection of kidney problems. *Consumer Reports on Health, 17*(4), 11.

Litman, R. S., & Rosenberg, H. (2005). Malignant hyperthermia: Update on susceptibility testing. *Journal of the American Medical Association, 293*(23), 2918–2924.

Littleton, L., & Engebretson, J. (2002). *Maternal, neonatal, and women's health nursing.* Clifton Park, NY: Thomson Delmar Learning.

Livingston, E. (2004). Procedure incidence and in-hospital complication rates of bariatric surgery in the United States. *The American Journal of Surgery, 188*(2), 105–110.

Livneh, H., & Martz, E. (2003). Psychosocial adaptation to spinal cord injury as a function of time since injury. *International Journal of Rehabilitation Research, 26*(3), 191–200.

Lledo, J. B., Roig. M. P., Bertomeu, C. A., Santafe, A. S., Lafargue, M. G., & Espinosa, R. G. (2005). Preoperative predictive factors of ambulatory laparoscopic cholecystectomy. *Ambulatory Surgery, 12*(1), 45–49.

Lloyd-Jones, D. M., Nam, B. H., D'Agostino, R. M., Levy, D., Murabito, J. M., Wang, T. J., et al. (2004). Parental cardiovascular disease is a risk factor for cardiovascular disease in middle-aged adults: A prospective study of parents and offspring. *Journal of the American Medical Association, 291*(18), 2204–2220.

Loftus, B. (2005). Neuropathic pain. Retrieved from www.lofutsmd.com/articles/pain.

Logan, R., & Delaney, B. (2001). ABC of the upper gastrointestinal tract: Implications of dyspepsia for the NHS. *British Medical Journal, 323*, 675–677.

Logue, J., & McBain, C. (2005). Radiation therapy for muscle-invasive bladder cancer: Treatment planning and delivery. *Clinical Oncology (Royal College of Radiologists), 17*(7), 508–513.

Lord, S. R., Castell, S., Corcoran, J., Dayhew, J., Matters, B., Shan, A., et al. (2003). The effect of group exercise on physical functioning and falls in frail older people living in retirement villages: A randomized, controlled trial. *Journal of the American Geriatrics Society, 51*(12), 1685–1692.

Louw, G., & Pinkerton, C. R. (2005). Interventions for early stage Hodgkin's disease in children. *The Cochrane Database of Systematic Reviews (Oxford)*, (3), 34–41.

Lozano, A. (2003). Surgery for Parkinson's disease the five W's: Why, who, what, where, and when. *Advances in Neurology, 91*, 303–307.

Lubovsky, O., Liebergall, M., Mattan, Y., Weil, Y., & Mosheiff, R. (2005). Early diagnosis of occult hip fractures MRI versus CT scan. *International Journal of the Care of the Injured, 36*(6), 788–792.

Ludwig, A., Inampudi, L., O'Donnell, M., Kreder, K., Williams, R., & Konety, B. (2005). Two-surgeon versus single-surgeon radical cystectomy and urinary diversion: Impact on patient outcomes and costs. *Urology, 65*(3), 488–492.

Lumley, J., Oliver, S. S., Chamberlain, C., & Oakley, L. (2005). Interventions for promoting smoking cessation during pregnancy. *Cochrane Pregnancy and Childbirth Group, The Cochrane Database of Systematic Reviews.* Cochrane Library (3). Chichester, UK: Wiley & Sons, Ltd.

Lundin, S. C., Paul, H., & Christensen, J. (2000). *Fish! A remarkable way to boost morale and improve results.* New York: Hyperion.

Luo, C. C. (2005). Spinal cord compression secondary to metastatic non-Hodgkin's lymphoma: A case report. *Archives of Physical Medicine and Rehabilitation, 86*(2), 332–334.

Ly-Pen, D., Andreu, J. L., de Blas, G., Sanchez-Olaso, A., & Millan, I. (2005). Surgical decompression versus local steroid injection on carpal tunnel syndrome: A one year, prospective, randomized, open, controlled clinical trial. *Arthritis and Rheumatism, 52*, 612–619.

Lyndaker, C., & Hulton, L. (2004). The influence of age on symptoms of perimenopause. *Journal of Obstetric, Gynecologic, and Neonatal Nursing, 33*(3), 340–347.

Madersbacher, H., & Madersbacher, S. (2005). Men's bladder health: Urinary incontinence in the elderly (Part I). *Journal of Men's Health and Gender, 2*(1), 31–37.

Magnusson, M., Sundelin, C., & Westerlund, M. (2006). Identification of health problems at 18 months of age—a task for physicians or child health nurses? *Child: Care, Health and Development, 32*(1): 47–54.

Maher, A. B. (2002). Assessment of the musculoskeletal system. In A. B. Maher, S. W. Salmond, & T. A. Pellino (Eds.), *Orthopaedic nursing* (3rd ed., pp. 189–210). Philadelphia, PA: W. B. Saunders Company.

Maher, A. B., Salmond, S. W. & Pellino, T. A. (2002). *Orthopedic nursing.* Philadelphia: W.B. Saunders Company.

Majewski, W. (2005). Long-term outcome, adhesions, and quality of life after laparoscopic and open surgical therapies for acute abdomen: Follow-up of a prospective trial. *Surgical Endoscopy, 19*(1), 81–90.

Makoul, G., & Clayman, M. L. (2006). An integrative model of shared decision making in medical encounters. *Patient Education and Counseling, 60*(3), 301–312.

Malanga, G. A., Andrus, S. G., & Bowen, J. (2004). *Rotator cuff injury.* Retrieved on September 28, 2005, from http://www.emedicine.com/sports/topic115.htm.

Mangan, P. (2005). Recognizing multiple myeloma. *Nurse Practitioner: American Journal of Primary Health Care, 30*(3), 14–18, 23–24, 26–29.

Mangram, A. J., et al. (2005). *Guideline for prevention of surgical site infection.* Retrieved on June 21, 2006, from www.cdc.gov.

Manias, E., Bucknall, T., Botti, M. (2005). Nurses' strategies for managing pain in the postoperative setting. *Pain Management Nursing, 6*(1), 18–29.

Manoharan, M., Reyes, M., Kava, B., Singal, R., Kim, S., & Soloway, M. (2005). Is adjuvant chemotherapy for bladder cancer safer in patients with an ileal conduit than a neobladder? *BJU International, 96*(9), 1286–1289.

Mantone, J. (2005). Critical time at rural hospitals. *Modern Healthcare, 35*(10), 22.

Mapes, T., & Zembaty, J. (1986). *Biomedical ethics* (2nd ed.). St. Louis, MO: McGraw-Hill.

Maravilla, K., Cao, Y., Heiman, J., Yang, C., Garland, P., Peterson, B., et al. (2005). *Journal of Urology, 173*(1), 162–166.

Marcus, P. (2004). Anxiety and related disorders. In K. Fortinash & P. Holoday-Worret (Eds.), *Psychiatric mental health nursing* (3rd ed., pp. 112–123) St. Louis, MO: Mosby.

Marik, P., & Zaloga, G. (2003). Gastric versus post-pyloric feeding: A systematic review. *Critical Care, 7*(3), 46–51.

Marshall, M., & Golper, T. (2003). Other dialysis modalities. In R. Johnson & J. Feehally (Eds.), *Comprehensive clinical nephrology* (2nd ed., pp. 1025–1034). St. Louis, MO: Mosby.

Martin, A. (2001). Should continuous lateral rotation therapy replace manual turning? *Dimensions of Critical Care Nursing, 20*(1), 42–49.

Martinez, J. M., & Tsai, A. M. (2004). *Stress fractures.* Retrieved on September 26, 2005, from http://www.emedicine.com/orthoped/topic446.htm.

Martins, P., Pratschke, J., Pascher, A., Fritsche, L., Frei, U., Neuhaus, P., et al. (2005). Age and immune response in organ transplantation. *Transplantation, 79*(2), 127–132.

Martis, G., D'Elia, G., Diana, M., Ombres, M., & Mastrangeli, B. (2005). Prostatic capsule- and nerve-sparing cystectomy in organ-confined bladder cancer: Preliminary results. *World Journal of Surgery, 29*(10), 1277–1281.

Martynowicz M. A., & Prakash U. B. S. (2002). Pulmonary blastomycosis: An appraisal of diagnostic techniques. *Chest, 121*(3), 768–773.

Maslow, A. (1970). *Motivation and personality* (2nd ed.). New York: Harper & Row.

Mason, J. (2003). Being around for a long time: How one woman with heart failure learned to live again. *American Journal of Nursing, 103*(12), 35.

Masoudi, F. A., & Krumholz, H. M. (2003). Polypharmacy and comorbidity in heart failure. *British Journal of Medicine, 327*(7414), 513–514.

Masters, W., & Johnson, V. (1966). *Human sexual response.* Boston: Little, Brown.

Mastin, T. (2003, September). Recognizing and treating non-infectious rhinitis. *Journal of the American Academy of Nurse Practitioners, 15,* 398–409.

Mathur, P. (2004). *An overview of medial thorascopy.* Retrieved June 25, 2006, from http://www.uptodate.com.

Matsumura, N., Yamamoto, K., Hirohashi, R., & Kitano, S. (2005). Renal tuberculosis mimicking hydronephrosis. *Journal of Internal Medicine, 44*(7), 768.

Mayer, S., & Chong, J. (2002). Critical care management of increased intracranial pressure. *Journal of Intensive Care Medicine, 17*(2), 55–67.

Mayer, V. (2004). The challenges of managing dysphagia in brain-injured patients. *British Journal of Community Nursing, 9*(2), 67–73.

Mayhall, G. C. (2004). Ventilator-associated pneumonia or not? Contemporary Diagnosis. *Emerging Infectious Disease Journal, 7*(2), 11.

Mayhew, P. M., Thomas, C. D., Clement, J. G., Loveridge, N., Beck, T. J., Bonfield, W., et al. (2005). Relation between age, femoral neck cortical stability, and hip fracture risk. *Lancet, 366*(9480), 129–135.

Mayo Clinic. (2003). *Tips for coping with a cancer diagnosis.* Retrieved June 10, 2006, from http://www.cnn.com.

Mayo Clinic. (2004, October). *Chronic sinusitis.* Retrieved December 17, 2004, from http://www.mayoclinic.com.

Mayo Clinic. (2005). *Tips for coping with a cancer diagnosis.* Retrieved June 10, 2006, http://www.mayoclinic.com/health/cancer-diagnosis/HQ01306.

Mayo Foundation for Medical Education and Research. (2004). *Severe acute respiratory syndrome.* Retrieved June 17, 2006, from http://www.cnn.com.

Max, A., Gattuso, J., Hinds, P., Norman, G., Price, R., Whitmore-Sisco, L., et al. (2003). Developing nursing care guidelines for children with Hodgkin's disease. *European Journal of Oncology Nursing, 7*(4), 253–258.

McCafferty, M., Sorbellini, D., & Cianci, P. (2002). Telemetry to home: Successful discharge of patients with ventricular assist devices. *Critical Care Nurse, 22*(3), 43–51.

McCaffery, M., and Pasero, C. (2004). *Pain: Clinical Manual,* 2nd ed. St. Louis, MO: Mosby.

McCaffrey, R., Frock, T. & Garguilo, H. (2003). Understanding chronic pain and the mind-body connection. *Holistic Nursing Practice, 17*(6), 281–287.

McCaig, L., & Burt, C. (2004). *National hospital ambulatory medical care survey: 2002 emergency department summary.* USDHHS Publication No. (PHS) 2004-125004-0226-0302. Hyattsville, MD: U. S. Department of Health & Human Services.

McCain, N., Gray, D., Walter, J., & Robins, J. (2005). Implementing a comprehensive approach to the study of health dynamics using the psychoneuroimmunology paradigm. *Advances in Nursing Science, 28*(4), 320–332.

McCance, K., & Huether, S. (2005). *Pathophysiology: The biological basis for disease in adults and children* (5th ed.). St. Louis, MO: Mosby.

McCloskey, J., & Bulechek, G. (2000). *Nursing interventions classification (NIC)* (3rd ed.). St. Louis, MO: Mosby.

McCullough, F. (2005). Book review: Nutrition and the eye. *Journal of Human Nutrition and Dietetics, 18*(4), 321.

McDaniel, J. (2005). Alternative approach. CO_2 may not be the enemy. *Virginia Nurses Today, 13*(3), 9.

McDermott, F. T., Rosenfeld, J. V., Laidlaw, J. D., Cordner, S. M., & Tremayne, A. B. (2004). Evaluation of management of road trauma survivors with brain injury and neurologic disability in Victoria. *Journal of Trauma: Injury, Infection, and Critical Care, 56*(1), 137–149.

McDevitt, E. R., Taylor, D. C., Miller, M. D., Gerber, J. P. Ziemke, G., Hinkin, D. et al. (2004). Functional bracing after anterior cruciate ligament reconstruction: A prospective, randomized, multicenter study. *The American Journal of Sports Medicine, 32*(8), 1887–1892.

McDonald, J. (2005, June 7). Supreme Court decision trumps California law. *San Diego Union Tribune,* pp. A-1, 8.

McDonald, S., Hetrick, S., & Green, S. (2004). Pre-operative education for hip or knee replacement (Cochrane Review). In: *The Cochrane Database of Systematic Reviews* (4). Chichester, UK: John Wiley & Sons, Ltd.

McElligott, J. M., Greenwald, B. D., & Watanabe, T. K. (2003). Congenital and acquired brain injury. New frontiers: Neuroimaging, neuroprotective agents, and complimentary medicine. *Archives of Physical Medicine and Rehabilitation, 84*(Suppl 1), S18–S22.

McGhee, B., & Bridges, M. (2002). Monitoring arterial blood pressure: What you may not know. *Critical Care Nurse, 22*(2), 60–79.

McGlinchey, D. (2004). *Lockheed developing military health tracking system.* Retrieved June 28, 2006, from http://www.govexec.com.

McGuigan, F. X., & Aierstok, M. D. (2005). Disorders of the Achilles tendon and its insertion. *Current Opinion in Orthopaedics, 16*(2), 65–71.

McGwin, G., Hall, T. A., Searcey, K., Modjarrad, K., Owsley, C. (2005). Cataract and cognitive function in older adults. *Journal of the American Geriatrics Society, 53*(7), 1260–1261.

McHugh, J. (2004). Diabetes and peripheral sensory neurons: What we don't know can hurt us. *AACN Clinical Issues, 15*(1), 136–149.

McKelvie, R. (2003). Heart failure. In F. Godlee (Ed.), *Clinical evidence concise,* (vol. 10, pp. 19–22). London: BMJ Publishing Group.

McKenzie, S. B. (2005). Advances in understanding the biology and genetics of acute myelocytic leukemia. *Clinical Laboratory Science,18*(1), 28–37, 57–59.

McKittrick, M. (2002). Diet and polycystic ovary syndrome. *Nutrition Today, 37*(2), 63–69.

McLauchlan, G. J., & Handoll, H. G. (2005). Interventions for treating acute and chronic Achilles tendinitis. *The Cochrane Database of Systematic Reviews* (4).

McNulty, M. (2005). Vyster unveils new natural rubber latex. *Rubber and Plastic News, 35*(1), 5.

McTiernan, A., Kooperberg, C., & White, E. (2003). Recreational physical activity and the risk of breast cancer in postmenopausal women: The Women's Health Initiative Cohort Study. *Journal of the American Medical Association, 290*(10), 1331–1336.

Mechem, C. (2004). *Pulse oximetry.* Retrieved June 25, 2006, from http://www.uptodate.com.

Medline Plus. (2005a). *Energy preservation.* Retrieved July 20, 2005, from www.nlm.nih.gov/medlineplus.gov.

Medline Plus. (2005b). *National Library of Medicine: National Institutes of Health.* Retrieved from www.medlineplus.gov.

Medline Plus. (2006). *Definitions of prevalence and incidence.* Retrieved July 20, 2006, from http://www.nih.gov/medlineplus.

Mellon, J. K. (2003). Urological issues for the nephrologist. In R. Johnson & J. Feehally (Eds.), *Comprehensive clinical nephrology* (2nd ed., pp. 759–767). St. Louis, MO: Mosby.

Menzin, J., Lang, K., Earle, C., & Glendenning, A. (2004). Treatment patterns, outcomes and costs among elderly patients with chronic myeloid leukemia: A population-based analysis. *Drugs and Aging, 21*(11), 737–746.

Meric-Berstam, F., & Pollock, R. E. (2005). Oncology. In F. C. Brunicardi (Ed.), *Schwartz's principles of surgery* (8th ed., pp. 249–294). New York: McGraw Hill.

Merikangans, K., & Risch, N. (2003). Will the genomics revolution revolutionize psychiatry? *American Journal of Psychiatry, 160,* 625–635.

Merten, G., Burgess, P., Gray, L., Holleman, J., Roush, T., Kowalchuk, G., et al. (2004). Prevention of contrast-induced nephropathy with sodium bicarbonate. *Journal of the American Medical Association, 291*(19), 2328–2334.

Metules, T., & Bauer, J. (2005). Unstable angina: Is your care up to snuff? *RN, 68*(2), 22–28.

Michelson, P. E. (2005). Common visual problems: Symptoms and treatment, part I two-part article. *Annals of Long-Term Care, 13*(8), 17–22.

Middleton, L., Dimond, E., Calzone, K., Davis, J., & Jenkins, J. (2002). The role of the nurse in cancer genetics. *Cancer Nursing, 25*(3), 196–208.

Miglioretti, D., Rutter, C., Geller, C., Cutter, G., Barlow, W., Rosenberg, R., et al. (2004). Effect of breast augmentation on the accuracy of mammography and cancer characteristics. *Journal of the American Medical Association, 291*(4), 442–450.

Miller, F. G., & Moreno, J. D. (2005). The state of research ethics: A tribute to John C. Fletcher. *Journal of Clinical Ethics, 16*(4), 355–364.

Miller, K. (2004). Management of hyperprolactinemia in patients receiving antipsychotics. *CNS Spectrums, 8*(Suppl 7), 28–32.

Miller, N. R., & Newman, N. J. (2004). The eye in neurological disease. *Lancet, 364*(9450), 2045–2054.

Miller, R. H. (2003). Knee injuries. In S. T. Canale (Ed.), *Campbell's operative orthopaedics* (vol. 3, 10th ed., pp 2165–2337). Philadelphia: Mosby.

Milligan, L. (2006). Epidemiology and cancer. *Advance for Nurses, 3*(15), 15–17.

Millman, R., & Kramer, N. (2004) *Polysomnography in the diagnostic evaluation of sleep apnea.* Retrieved June 25, 2006, from http://www.uptodate.com.

Milstead, J. A., & Furlong, E. (2006). *Handbook of nursing leadership: Creative skills for a culture of safety.* Sudbury, MA: Jones and Bartlett.

Minden, P. (2002). Humor as focal point of therapy for psychiatric patients. *Holistic Nursing Practice, 16*(4), 775–786.

Mion, L. (2003). Care provided for older adults: Who will provide? *Online Journal of Issues in Nursing 1*(2), 99–109.

Mitchell, A., & Parish, T. (2005). Using combination therapy for smoking cessation. *Clinician Reviews, 15*(5), 40–45.

Mitchell, R. A., Hasbrouch, L., Ingram, M. E., Dunaway, C. & Annest, J. L. (2003). Public health and aging: Nonfatal physical assault-related injuries among persons aged > 60 years treated in hospital emergency departments United States, 2001. *Morbidity and Mortality Weekly Report, 52*(5), 812–816.

Mittal, B., Rennke, H., & Singh, A. (2005). The role of kidney biopsy in the management of lupus nephritis. *Current Opinion in Nephrology and Hypertension, 14*(1), 1–8.

Miyamoto, R., Houston, D., & Bergeson, T. (2005). Cochlear implantation in deaf infants. *Laryngoscope, 115*(8), 1376–1380.

MMWR. (2004, September 10). *Recommendations and reports: Indicators for chronic disease surveillance.* Centers for Disease Control, 53 (RR11), 1-6, Atlanta: Author.

Mohapatra, S., Lockey, R., & Shirley S. (2005). Immunobiology of grass pollen allergens. *Current Allergy and Asthma Reports, 5*(5), 381–387.

Mohr, D., & Pelletier, D. (2006). A temporal framework for understanding the effects of stressful life events on inflammation in patients with multiple sclerosis. *Brain, Behavior, & Immunity, 20*(1), 27–36.

Mokdad, A., Ford, E., Bowman, B., Dietz, W., Vinevor, F., Bales, V., et al. (2003). Prevalence of obesity, diabetes and obesity: Related health risk factors. *Journal of American Medical Association, 289*, 76–79.

Moldwin R. M., & Sant G. R. (2002). Interstitial cystitis: A pathophysiology and treatment update. *Clinical Obstetrics and Gynecology, 45*(1), 259–272.

Mollaret, P., & Goulon, M. (1959). Le coma depasse (memoire preliminaire). *Revue Neurologique (Paris), 101*, 3–5.

Monarch, K. (2002, November/December). Legal aspects of infusion practice. *Journal of Infusion Nursing, 25*(6), S21–S30.

Montague, A. (1986). *Touching: The human significance of the skin* (3rd ed.). New York: Perennial Library.

Montbriand, M. J. (2005). Herbs or natural products that may cause cancer and harm part four of a four-part series [Online exclusive]. *Oncology Nursing Forum, 32*(1). Retrieved June 10, 2005, from http://www.ons.org.

Moore, Z. & Cowman, S. (2006). Wound cleansing for pressure ulcers. *The Cochrane Database of Systematic Reviews*, CD004983.

Moran, T. A., & Viele, C. S. (2005). Normal clotting. *Seminars in Oncology Nursing, 21*(4 Suppl 1), 1–11.

Mothershead, J. (2003). *Disaster planning.* Retrieved June 27, 2006, from http://emedicine.com.

Mount, D., & Zandi-Nejad, K. (2004). Disorders of potassium balance. In B. Brenner (Ed.), *Brenner and Rector's the kidney* (7th ed., vol. 1, pp. 997–1040). Philadelphia: W. B. Saunders Co.

Mueller, A., Johnston, M., & Bligh, D. (2001). Mind-mapped care plans: A remarkable alternative to traditional nursing care plans. *Nurse Educator, 26*(2), 75–80.

Mueller, H., & Hawkins, D. (2006). Trouble-shooting hearing aid fitting issues: the case of the missing "ping." *Hearing Journal, 59*(1), 10, 12, 14–15.

Mueller, P., Hook, C., & Hayes, D. (2003). Ethical analysis of withdrawal of pacemaker or implantable cardioverter-defibrillator support at the end of life. *Mayo Clinic Procedures, 78*, 959–963.

Mukand, J. A., Guilmette, T. J., & Tran, M. (2003). Rehabilitation for patients with brain tumors. *Critical Reviews in Physical and Rehabilitation Medicine, 15*(2), 99–111.

Muller, U., & Golden D., (2004). Immunotherapy for hymenoptera venom and biting insect hypersensitivity. *Clinical Allergy Immunology, 18*, 441–559.

Mulrow, C. (1994). Rationale for systematic reviews. *British Medical Journal, 309*, 597–599.

Mulrow, C. D., & Oxman, A. D. (Eds.). (1994; updated 2004). Cochrane Collaboration Handbook. In *The Cochrane Database of Systematic Reviews. The Cochrane Collaboration.* Oxford, UK: Update Software.

Mundy, A. (2004). Clinical updates. New updates in diabetes. *The Journal of Continuing Education in Nursing, 35*(2), 54–55.

Munro, C. L., & Grap, M. J. (2004). Oral health and care in the intensive care unit: State of the science. *American Journal of Critical Care, 13*(1), 25-33.

Murphy, F. (2005). Myths and realities in acute wound-care. *Practice Nurse, 30*(4), 52–53.

Murphy, J. (2003). Pharmacological treatment of acute ischemic stroke. *Critical Care Nurse, 26*(4), 276–282.

Murphy, K., Hopp, R., Kittelson, E., Hansen, G., Windle, M., & Walburn, J. (2006). Life-threatening asthma and anaphylaxis in schools: A treatment model for school-based programs. *Annals of Allergy, Asthma, & Immunology, 96*(3), 398–405.

Murthy, T. H. (2004). *Cardiac catheterization.* Retrieved June 24, 2006, from http://www.nlm.nih.gov.

Mustalish, S. H. (2002). Avoiding allergic reactions in children from botanical medicines. *Integrative Medicine Consult, 1*, 6.

Mutsch, M., Zhou, W., Rhodes, P., Bopp, M., Chen, R., Linder, T., et al. (2004). Use of the inactivated intranasal influenza vaccine and the risk of Bell's palsy in Switzerland. *New England Journal of Medicine, 350*(4), 896–903.

Mycyk, M., & Moyer, P. (2004). *Orchitis.* Retrieved August 1, 2005, from http://www.emedicine.com.

Myer, G., Brunner, H., Melson, P., Paterno, M., & Ford, T. (2005). Specialized neuromuscular training to improve neuromuscular function and biomechanics in a patient with quiescent juvenile rheumatoid arthritis. *Physical Therapy, 85*(8), 791–802.

Mythen, M. (2004). Postoperative gastrointestinal tract dysfunction. *Anesthesia-Analgesia, 100*(1), 196–204.

Nahas, M. (2003). Progression of chronic renal failure. In R. Johnson & J. Feehally (Eds.), *Comprehensive clinical nephrology* (2nd ed., pp. 843–856). St. Louis, MO: Mosby.

NANDA International. (2005a). *Nursing diagnoses: Definitions and classification 2005–2006.* Philadelphia: NANDA International.

NANDA International. (2005b). Nursing diagnosis: Disturbed energy field. In *Nursing diagnoses: Definitions and classification 2005–2006.* Philadelphia: Author.

National acute care nurse practitioner certification exam. (2003). Retrieved May 7, 2004, from www.aacn.org.

National Association of Orthopaedic Nurses. (2006). *Osteoporosis: Bone anabolic agents revolutionize bone loss and bone disease therapies.* Retrieved September 6, 2006, from www.orthonurse.com.

National Asthma Education and Prevention Program. (2002). *Executive summary expert panel report: Guidelines for the diagnosis and treatment of asthma–update on select topics* (No. 02-5075). Bethesda, MD: National Institutes of Health.

National Cancer Institute. (2003a). *Hormone replacement.* Retrieved July 20, 2006, from http://www.cancer.gov.

National Cancer Institute. (2003b). *Laryngeal cancer.* Retrieved December 17, 2004, from http://www.nci. nih.gov/cancertopics/pdq/treatment/laryngeal/ healthprofessional.

National Cancer Institute. (2003c). *What you need to know about cancer of the larynx.* Retrieved December 17, 2004 from, http://www.nci.nih.gov/cancertopics/wyntk/ larynx.

National Cancer Institute. (2004a). *Antioxidants and cancer prevention: Questions and answers.* Retrieved June 10, 2005, from http://www.cancer.gov.

National Cancer Institute. (2004b). *Biological therapy.* Retrieved June 10, 2005, from http://www.nci.nih.gov.

National Cancer Institute. (2004c). *Bone marrow transplantation and peripheral blood stem cell transplantation: Questions and answers.* Retrieved June 10, 2005, from http://cis.nci.nih.gov.

National Cancer Institute. (2004d). *National Cancer Institute cancer facts radiation therapy for cancer: Questions and answers.* Retrieved March 25, 2005, from http://cis.nci.nih.gov.

National Cancer Institute. (2004e). *Radiation enteritis.* Retrieved June 10, 2005, from http://www.cancer.gov.

National Cancer Institute. (2005a). *Gastrointestinal complications (PDQ).* Retrieved June 10, 2005, from http://www.nci.nih.gov.

National Cancer Institute. (2005b). *Gastrointestinal complications: National Cancer Institute's common toxicity criteria for grading severity of diarrhea.* Retrieved June 10, 2005, from http://www.nci.nih.gov.

National Cancer Institute. (2005c). *NCI/PDQ patients: Nutrition in cancer care.* Retrieved June 10, 2005, from http://www.oncolink.com.

National Cancer Institute. (2005d). *Prostate cancer.* Retrieved July 31, 2006, from http://www.nci.nih.gov.

National Cancer Institute. (2006). *Stomach cancer: NCI Drug Dictionary.* Retrieved June 25, 2006, from www.nic.gov.

National Cancer Institute's Cancer Information Service. (2005). *HIV/AIDS prevention home: Basic statistics overview.* Retrieved June 11, 2006, from http://cis. nci.nih.gov.

National Center for Complementary and Alternative Medicine (NCCAM). (2002). *What is complementary and alternative medicine?* Publication No. D156. Bethesda, MD: Author.

National Center for Complementary and Alternative Medicine. (2005). *Get the Facts. What is complementary and alternative medicine (CAM)?* Retrieved August 26, 2006, from http://www.nccam.nih.gov.

National Center for Complementary and Alternative Medicine. (2006). (p. 11). Retrieved June 23, 2006, from http://nccam.nih.gov.

National Center for Health Statistics. (2002, October 25). *Data tables for vaccine.* Retrieved June 30, 2004, from http://www.cdc.gov.

National Center for Health Statistics. (2004). *Health, United States, 2004 with chartbook on trends in the health of Americans.* Retrieved on July 5, 2005, from http://www.cdc.gov/nchs/data/hus/hus04.pdf.

National Center for Health Statistics. (2005). *Fact sheet on mortality: Adolescent and young adults.* Retrieved July 17, 2006, from http://www.cdc.gov.

National Center for Health Statistics. (2006a). *About healthy people 2010.* Retrieved August 25, 2006, from www.cdc.gov.

National Center for Health Statistics. (2006b). *Health, United States, 2005: 29th report on the health status of the nation.* Retrieved July 12, 2006, from http://www. cdc.gov/nchs.

National Center for PTSD. (2003). *What is post-traumatic stress disorder.* Retrieved June 23, 2006, from http:// www.ncptsd.org.

National Cholesterol Education Program. (2004). Implications of recent clinical trials for the national cholesterol education program adult treatment panel III guidelines. Retrieved June 24. 2006, from http://www.nhibi.nih.bov/guidelines/cholesterol.

National Collaborating Centre for Nursing and Supportive Care. (2004). *Clinical practice guideline for the assessment and prevention of falls in older people.* Retrieved June 15, 2005, from http://www.guideline.gov.

National Committee for Quality Healthcare (n.d.). *The environment right now.* Retrieved June 15, 2005, from www.ncqhc.org/execinstitute/rightnow.cfm.

National Comprehensive Cancer Network. (2005). *Clinical practice guidelines in oncology.* Retrieved June 10, 2005, from http://www.nccn.org.

National Guideline Clearinghouse. (2002, October 21). *Evidence-based guidelines for weaning and discontinuation of ventilatory support.* Retrieved September 18, 2004, from www.guideline.gov.

National Guideline Clearinghouse. (2003). *Screening for lung cancer.* Retrieved June 30, 2004, from http:// www.guideline.gov.

National Health System. (2005a). *Center for evidence-based medicine. Glossary.* Retrieved July 11, 2005, from http://www.minervation.com/cebm2.

National Health System. (2005b). *Levels of evidence.* Retrieved July 11, 2005, from http://cebm.jr2. ox.ac.uk.

National Heart, Lung, and Blood Institute. (2004a). *Health information center.* Retrieved June 24, 2006, from www.nhlbi.nih.gov.

National Heart, Lung, and Blood Institute. (2004b). *What is pulmonary arterial hypertension.* Retrieved September 16, 2004, from http://www.nhlbi.nih.gov.

National Heart, Lung, and Blood Institute. (2006a). *High blood cholesterol: What you need to know.* Retrieved July 31, 2006, from http://www.nhbi.nih.gov.

National Heart, Lung, and Blood Institute. (2006b). *What is heart failure?* (pp. 1–11). Retrieved June 25, 2006, www.nhlbi.nih.gov.

National Institute of Allergy and Infectious Diseases. (2002, April). *Sinusitis.* Retrieved December 17, 2004, from http://www.niaid.nih.gov.

National Institute of Arthritis and Musculoskeletal and Skin Diseases (NIAMS). Handout on health: Systemic lupus erythematosus (pp. 1–40). Retrieved June 26, 2006, from http://www.niams.nih.gov.

National Institute of Neurological Disorders and Stroke. (2002). *Carpal tunnel syndrome fact sheet.* Retrieved on September 28, 2005, from http://www.ninds.nih.gov/disorders/carpal_tunnel/detail_carpal_tunnel.htm.

National Institute of Neurological Disorders and Stroke. (2006). Retrieved June 16, 2006, from www.ninds.nih.gov.

National Institute of Nursing Research. (n.d.). *About NINR.* Retrieved June 1, 2005, from www.ninr.nih.gov.

National Institutes of Health. (2004a). *Frequently asked questions about acupuncture.* Bethesda, MD: National Institutes of Health.

National Institutes of Health. (2004). *My Pyramid.* U.S.D.A. NIH Publication No. 04-4006, Bethesda, MD: Author.

National Institutes of Health, National Heart, Lung, and Blood Institute. (1998). *Clinical guidelines on the identification, evaluation, and treatment of overweight and obesity in adults. The evidence report.* NIH Publication No. 98-4083, Bethesda, MD: Author.

National Kidney and Urologic Diseases Information Clearinghouse. (2003). *Peyronie's disease.* Retrieved July 13, 2006, from http://kidney.niddk.nih.gov.

National Limb Loss Information Center. (2002). *Limb amputations.* Retrieved on October 15, 2005. from http://www.amputee-coalition.org.

National Marrow Donor Program. *How the NMDP helps patients* (pp. 1–4). Retrieved June 26, 2006, from http://www.marrow.org.

National Sleep Foundation. (2004). *Sleep apnea.* December 17, 2004, from http://www.sleepfoundation.org/publications/sleepap.cfm.

National Stroke Association. (2006). *People with atrial fibrillation increase stroke risk by 500%.* Retrieved June 21, 2006, from http://www.stroke.org.

Needleman, J., Buerhaus, P., Mattke, S., Stewart, M., & Zelevinsky, K. (2002). Nurse-staffing levels and the quality of care in hospitals. *New England Journal of Medicine, 346*(22), 1715–1722.

Nelson, J. (2005). Families and bioethics: Old problems, new themes. *Journal of Clinical Ethics, 16*(4), 299–302.

Nelson, R., Edwards, S., & Tse, B. (2004). Prophylactic nasogastric decompression after abdominal surgery. *The Cochrane Database of Systematic Reviews* (3), CD004929.

Nelson, S. (2004). The search for the good in nursing? The burden of ethical expertise. *Nursing Philosophy, 5*(1), 12–22.

Net income increased by 2.5% on international sales growth. (2006, July 18). *The Wall Street Journal,* A9.

Neuhauser, D. (2003). The coming third healthcare revolution: Personal empowerment. *Quality Management in Healthcare, 12*(3), 171–184.

Neuman, B. (1982). *The Neuman systems model. Application to nursing education and practice.* Norwalk, CT: Appleton-Century-Crofts.

Neurnberger, P. (1981). *Freedom from stress: A holistic approach.* Honesdale, PA: The Himalayan International Institute of Yoga Science and Philosophy.

Neville, K. (2003). Uncertainty in illness: An integrative review. *Orthopaedic Nursing, 22*(3), 206–214.

New Haven Hospice. (2006). Retrieved August 31, 2006, from www.hospice.com.

New Zealand Guidelines Group. (2003). *Prevention of hip fracture amongst people aged 65 years and over.* Retrieved June 15, 2005 from http://www.nzgg.org.nz/.

Newman, D. (2005). Assessment of the patient with an overactive bladder. *Journal of WOCN, 32*(3 Suppl 1), S5–10, S24–26.

Nguyen, L., Mohr, W., Ahrenholz, D., & Solem, L. (2004). Treatment of hydrofluoric acid burn to the face by carotid artery infusion of calcium gluconate. *Journal of Burn Care and Rehabilitation, 25*(5), 421–424.

Nicholas, J., & Geers, A. (2006). The process and early outcomes of cochlear implantation by three years of age. In P. E. Spencer & M. Marschark (Eds.), *Advances in the Development of Spoken Language by Deaf Children* (pp. 124–129). New York: Oxford University Press.

Nicholson, B. (2003). Diagnosis and management of neuropathic pain: A balanced approach to treatment. *Journal of the American Academy of Nurse Practitioners* (Suppl 150), 3–9.

Nienhuis, A., Hanawa, H., Sawai, N., Sorrentino, B., & Persons, D. (2003). Development of gene therapy for hemoglobin disorders. *Annals of the New York Academy of Science, 996*(1), 101–111.

Nietsch, H. H., & Kowdley, K. V. (2004). Review: Magnetic resonance cholangiopancreatography is accurate for diagnosing biliary disease. *ACP Journal Club, 141*(1), 25.

Nightingale, F. (1859). *Notes on nursing: What it is and what it is not.* London: Harrison Pall Mall.

Nightingale, F. (1860). *Notes on nursing: What it is and what it is not.* London: Harrison and Sons.

Nightingale, F. (1969 [1859]). *Notes on nursing what it is and what it is not.* New York: Dover Publications.

Noble, K. (2003). Name that tube. *Nursing, 33*(3), 56–62.

Noble, V., & Brown, D. (2004). Renal ultrasound. *Emergency Medicine Clinics of North America, 22*(3), 641–659.

Noga, S. J. (2004). 93-year-old man with non-Hodgkin's lymphoma. *Advanced Studies in Medicine, 4*(3B), S202–204, S207–209.

Nogueira, S., & Appling, S. (2000). Breast cancer: Genetics, risks, and strategies. *Nursing Clinics of North America, 35*(3), 663–670.

Nolan, P. (2006). What to do until the music therapist arrives: Developing therapeutic activities using music. *Journal of Holistic Nursing Practice, 20*(1), 37–40.

Norris, J., & Spelic, S. S. (2002). Supporting adaptation to body image disruption. *Rehabilitation Nursing, 27*(1), 8–11.

North American Nursing Diagnosis Association. (2005). *Nursing diagnoses: Definitions and classifications 2005–2006.* Philadelphia: Author.

North American Menopause Society (NAMS). (2004). Treatment of menopause-associated vasomotor symptoms: Position statement of the North American Menopause Society. *Menopause: The Journal of the North American Menopause Society, 11*(1), 11–33.

Norton, L. B., Peipert, J. F., Zierler, S., Lima, B., & Hume, L. (1995). Battering in pregnancy: An assessment of two screening methods. *Obstetrics and Gynecology, 85*(3), 321–325.

Nosek, L. J. (1986). Explanation of hospital stay by nursing diagnoses, medical diagnoses, and social position. *Dissertation Abstracts International, 47*(07B), 00215. (University Microfilms No. AAG8622844).

Nosek, L. J. (2004). Globalization's costs to healthcare: How can we pay the bill? *Nursing Administration Quarterly, 28*(2), 116–121.

Nosek, L. J., & Androwich, I. M. (2003). Basic clinical health care economics. In P. Kelly-Heidenthal (Ed.), *Nursing leadership and management* (pp. 32–58). Albany, NY: Thomson Delmar Learning.

Nosek, M., Hughes, R., Howland, C., Young, M. Mullen, P, & Shelton, M. (2004). The meaning of health for women with physical disabilities. A qualitative analysis [Electronic version]. *Family and Community Health, 27*(1), 6–21.

Nour, N. (2004). Female genital cutting: Clinical and cultural guidelines. *Obstetrical and Gynecological Survey, 59*(4), 272–279.

Nowlin, A. (2005). The promise of stem cells. *RN, 68*(4), 48–53.

Nurse Healers-Professional Associates, Inc. (2005). *Therapeutic touch process.* Retrieved August 2, 2006, from http://therapeutictouch.org.

Nurseweek. (2004). *A nurse's guide to pain management.* Retrieved June 14, 2006, from www.nurseweek.com.

Nursing law case on point. Nurse terminated for botching sponge count denied U.I. benefits. (2005). *Nursing Law's Regan Report, 45*(11), 4.

Nusbaum, M., Hamilton, C., & Lenahan, P. (2003). Chronic illness and sexual functioning. *American Family Physician, 67*(2), 347–354.

O'Brien, J. G., Chennubhotla, S. A., & Chennubhotla, R. V. (2005). Treatment of edema. *American Family Physician, 71*(11), 2111–2118.

O'Connell, B., Baker, L., & Prosser, A. (2003). The educational needs of caregivers of stroke survivors in acute and community settings. *Journal of Neuroscience Nursing, 35*(1), 21–28.

O'Conner, A., & Besner, G. (2004). *Burns a surgical perspective.* Retrieved April 8, 2006, from www.emedicine.com.

O'Connor, D., Marshall, S., & Massey-Westropp, N. (2005). *Non-surgical treatment (other than steroid injection) for carpal tunnel syndrome.* Retrieved on September 28, 2005, from http://www.cochrane.org/reviews/en/ab003219.html.

O'Hara, M. (2005). A case-based review of overactive bladder. *Clinical Advisor, 8*(7), 38, 40–41, 45.

O'Sullivan, D., & Torres, V. (2003). Autosomal dominant polycystic kidney disease. In R. Johnson & J. Feehally (Eds.), *Comprehensive clinical nephrology* (2nd ed., pp. 598–609). St. Louis, MO: Mosby.

Occupational Safety and Health Administration. (2005). *Safety and health topics: Personal and protective equipment.* Retrieved June 24, 2006, from www.osha.gov.

Office of the Robert Wood Johnson Foundation. (2001). *Advanced practice nurses' role in palliative care; a position statement from American nursing leaders. Promoting excellence in end-of-life care: A national program.* Bozeman, MT: University of Montana.

Olson, T. (2004). The geriatric client. In R. Daniels (Ed.), *Nursing fundamentals: Caring and clinical decision making* (pp. 83–88). New York: Thomson Delmar Learning.

Oregon Death with Dignity Act. (1997). *Oregon Revised Statute 127800-127,* 897.

Orem, D. E. (1995). *Nursing: Concepts of practice* (5th cd.). St. Louis, MO: Mosby-Yearbook.

Orens, J. B. (2004) Listing the patient: Deciding when transplantation is the only viable life-sustaining option. *Advances in Pulmonary Hypertension.* Retrieved June 30, 2004, from http://www.phassociation.org/.

Otchy, D., Hyman, N. H., Simmang, C., Anthony, T., Buie, W.D., Cataldo, P., et al. (2004). Practice parameters for colon cancer. *Diseases of the Colon and Rectum, 47*(8), 1269–1284.

Otlowski, M., & Williamson, R. (2003). Ethical and legal issues and the "new genetics." *Medical Journal of Australia, 178*(11), 582–585.

Ottem, D. P., & Teichman, J. M. (2005). What is the value of cystoscopy with hydrodistention for interstitial cystitis? *Urology, 66*(3), 494–499.

Ouellet, L., Hodgins, M., Pond, S., Knorr, S., & Geldart, G. (2003). Post-discharge telephone follow-up for orthopaedic surgical patients: a pilot study. *Journal of Orthopaedic Nursing, 7*(2), 87–93.

Owens, B. D., Murphy, K. P., & Kuklo, T. R. (2004). *Lateral epicondylitis.* Retrieved on September 7, 2005, from http://www.emedicine.com/orthoped/topic510.htm.

Oxman, M., Levin, M., Johnson, G., Schmader, K. Straus, S., Gclb, L., et al. (2005). A vaccine to prevent herpes zoster and post-herpetic neuralgia in older adults. *New England Journal of Medicine, 352,* 2271–2284.

Ozer, H., & Diasio, R. B. (2004). Perspectives in the treatment of colorectal cancer. *Seminars in Oncology, 31*(6 Suppl 15), 14–18.

Pacini, C. M. (2004). Synergy: A framework for professional development and transformation. *Excellence in nursing knowledge.* Indianapolis, IN: Sigma Theta Tau Press.

Palmer, D., Mulhall, K., Thompson, C., Severson, E., Santos, E., & Saleh, K. (2005). Total knee arthroplasty in juvenile rheumatoid arthritis. *Journal of Bone and Joint Surgery (Am), 87*(7), 1510–1514.

Papakakais, M. A. (2006). *Current medical diagnosis and treatment* (45th ed.). New York: Lange Medical Books/McGraw-Hill.

Papanek, P. (2003). The female athlete triad: An emerging role for physical therapy. *The Journal of Orthopaedic and Sports Physical Therapy, 33*(10), 594–614.

Parker, E., Donato, L., & Dalgleish, D. (2005). Effects of added sodium caseinate on the formation of particles in heated milk. *Journal of Agricultural and Food Chemistry, 53*(21), 8265–8272.

Pavlovsky, S., & Lastiri, F. (2004). Progress in the prognosis of adult Hodgkin's lymphoma in the past 35 years through clinical trials in Argentina: A GATLA experience. *Clinical Lymphoma, 5*(2), 102–109.

Payton, C. (2005). Referral diagnosis and management of dysphagia. *Pulse, 65*(8), 64–65.

Pearson, R. L., Kabongo, M. L., Ejnes, Y. D., & Bahler, R. C. (2004). *Aortic valvular stenosis.* Retrieved June 24, 2006, from www.firstconsult.com.

Peck, S. (2005). Is it really Hodgkin's disease? *CURE: Cancer Updates, Research and Education, 4*(1), 45.

Pediatric Alert. (2004). Thalidomide for severe juvenile rheumatoid arthritis. *Pediatric Alert, 29*(24), 143–144.

Peers, K. H. E., & Lysens, R. J. J. (2005). Patellar tendinopathy in athletes: Current diagnosis and therapeutic recommendations. *Sports Medicine, 35*(1), 71–87.

Pelletier, K. (2004). *The best alternative medicine.* New York: Simon & Shuster.

Pelletier, K. (2004). Mind-body medicine in ambulatory care: An evidence-based assessment. *Journal of Ambulatory Care Management, 27*(1), 25–42.

Pender, N., Murdaugh, C., & Parsons, M. (2002). *Health promotion in nursing practice* (4th ed.). Upper Saddle River, NJ: Prentice Hall.

Perez, R., Chen, J. M., & Nedzelski, J. M. (2004). The status of the contralateral ear in established unilateral Meniere's disease. *Laryngoscope, 114*(8), 1373–1376.

Perkins, C., & Kisiel, M. (2005). Renal nursing. Utilizing physiological knowledge to care for acute renal failure. *British Journal of Nursing, 14*(14), 768–773.

Perron, A. D. (2003). Chest pain in athletes. *Clinics in Sports Medicine, 22*(1), 37–50.

Persiani, R., Biondi, A., Buccelletti, F., Rausei, S., Silveri, N. (2006). Unusual acute abdomen: To operate or not to operate? *Lancet, 367*(9521), 1548.

Philipp, C. S., Faiz, A., Dowling, N., Dilley, A., Michaels, L. A., Ayers, C., et al. (2005). Age and the prevalence of bleeding disorders in women with menorrhagia. *Obstetrics and Gynecology, 105*(1), 61–66.

Phillips, M. (2003). Genetics of hearing loss. *MEDSURG Nursing, 12*, 386–390, 411.

Phillips, N. (2004). *Berry and Kohn's operating room technique* (12th ed.). New York: Mosby.

Pierce, J., Morris, D., & Clancy, R. (2002). Understanding renal dose dopamine. *Journal of Infusion Nursing, 25*(6), 365–371.

Pierie, J. P., Muzikansky, A., Tanabe, K. K., & Ott, M. J. (2005). The outcome of surgical resection versus assignment to the liver transplant waiting list for hepatocellular carcinoma. *Annals of Surgical Oncology, 12*(7), 552–560.

Pilnick, A., & Coleman, T. (2003). "I'll give up smoking when you make me better": Patient's resistance to attempts to problematise smoking in general practice (GP) consultants. *Social Science Medicine, 57*, 135–145.

Pitchford, P. (2002). *Healing with whole foods: Asian traditions and modern nutrition.* Berkeley, CA: North Atlantic Books.

Plantinga, L., Natowicz, M., Kass, N., Hull, S., Gostin, L., & Faden, R. (2003). Disclosure, confidentiality, and families: Experiences and attitudes of those with genetic versus nongenetic medical conditions. *American Journal of Medical Genetics, 199C*(1), 51–59.

Platt, T., Parrish, K., & Hostler, D. (2004). A prospective and qualitative prehospital comparison of head immobilization devices, Prehospital Care Research Forum EMS Today, JEMS supplement. Retrieved September 8, 2006, from www.jems.com.

Plewa, M., & Worthington, R. (2004). *Mitral valve prolapse.* Retrieved June 24, 2006, from www.emedicine.com.

Plomin, R., & Spinath, F. (2004). Intelligence: Genetics, genes, and genomics. *Journal of Personality and Social Psychology, 86*(1), 112–129.

Plonk, W. M. (2005). To PEG or not to PEG. *Practical Gastroenterology, 29*(7), 16–31.

Poirier, P. (2006). The relationship of sick leave benefits, employment patterns and individual characteristics to radiation therapy related fatigue. *Oncology Nursing Forum, 33*(3), 593–601.

Pollak, M., & Yu, A. (2004). Clinical disturbances of calcium, magnesium, and phosphate metabolism. In B. Brenner (Ed.), *Brenner and Rector's the kidney* (7th ed., vol. 1, pp. 1040–1076). Philadelphia: W. B. Saunders Co.

Polovich, M. (2004). Safe handling of hazardous drugs. *Online Journal of Issues in Nursing 19*(3), Manuscript 5. Retrieved June 10, 2005, from http://www.nursingworld.org.

Pontali, E. (2005). Facilitating adherence in highly active antiretroviral therapy in children with HIV infections: What are the issues and what can be done. *Pediatric Drugs, 7*(3), 137–149.

Porth, C. (2003). *Pathophysiology: Concepts of altered health states* (5th ed.). Philadelphia: Lippincott, Williams & Wilkins.

Porth, C. (2004). *Pathophysiology: Concepts of altered health states* (6th ed.). Philadelphia: Lippincott.

Porth, C. (2005). *Pathophysiology: Concepts of altered health states* (7th ed.). Philadelphia: Lippincott, Williams & Wilkins.

Potts, H. W. (2005). Online support groups: An overlooked resource for patients. *Health Information on the Internet,* (44), 6–8.

Potts, N., & Mandleco, B. (2002). *Pediatric nursing: Caring for children and their families.* New York: Thomson Delmar Learning.

Powell, H., & Gibson, P. G. (2004). Options for self-management education for adults with asthma (Cochrane Review). In *The Cochrane Database of Systematic Reviews* (1). Chichester, UK: John Wiley & Sons, Ltd.

Powers, P. (2003). Empowerment as treatment and the role of health professionals. *Advances in Nursing Science, 26*(3), 227–237.

Practice Committee of the American Society for Reproductive Medicine. (2004). Current evaluation of amenorrhea. *Fertility and Sterility, 82*(1), 266–272.

Prather, S. H., Forsyth, L. W., Russell, K. D., & Wagner, V. L. (2003). Caring for the patient undergoing transsphenoidal surgery in the acute care setting: an alternative to critical care. *Journal of Neuroscience Nursing, 35*(5), 270–275.

Prevost, S. (2004). Improve pain management. In S. Hegyvary (Ed.), *Working Paper on Grand Challenges in*

Improving Global Health. Journal of Nursing Scholarship, 36(2), 96–101.

Price compare: Antibiotics. (2006). Retrieved August 13, 2006, from destinationrx.com.

Price, D. D., & Wilson, S. R. (2005) *Dislocations, shoulders.* Retrieved on September 27, 2005, from http://www.emedicine.com/emerg/topic148.htm.

Price, P. (2004). *Surgical technology for the surgical technologist* (2nd ed.). New York: Thomson Delmar Learning.

Price, S. A., & Wilson, L. M. (2003). *Pathophysiology: Clinical concepts of disease process.* (6th ed.). St. Louis, MO: Mosby.

Prince, M., Christensen, E., & Gluud, C. (2005). Glucocorticosteroids for primary biliary cirrhosis. *The Cochrane Database of Systematic Reviews* (3), ID #CD003778.

Prochazka, A., Kick, S., Steinbrunn, C., Miyoshi, T., & Fryer, G. (2004). A randomized trial of nortriptyline combined with transdermal nicotine for smoking cessation. *Archives of Internal Medicine, 164,* 2229–2233.

The Prostate Cancer Foundation. (2004). *Report to the nation on prostate cancer.* Retrieved July 17, 2006, from http://www.prostatecancerfoundation.org.

Proust, M. (2002 [1920]). The guermantes way. Translated by M. Treharne. New York: The Penguin Group.

Pruitt, B., & Jacobs, M. (2005). Caring for a patient with asthma. *Nursing, 33*(2), 48–51.

Pruitt, W., & Jacobs, M. (2004). Take a deep breath and conquer your fear of mechanical ventilation. *Nursing Made Incredibly Easy, June/July,* 10–21.

Public broadcasting system (PBS) interview, 89.7 FM, January 4, 2006.

Puddu, P., Cravero, E., & Puddu, G., Muscari A. (2005). Genes and atherosclerosis: At the origin of the predisposition. *International Journal of Clinical Practice, 59*(4), 462–472.

Pui, C.H., Cheng, C., Leung, W., Rai, S. N., Rivera, G. K., Sandlund, J. T., et al. (2003). Extended follow-up of long-term survivors of childhood acute lymphoblastic leukemia. *New England Journal of Medicine, 349*(7), 640–649.

Pulley, S. (2004). *Critical incident stress management.* Retrieved July 6, 2006, from http://www.emedicine.com.

Pumphrey, R. S. (2003). Fatal posture in anaphylactic shock. *Journal of Allergy Clinical Immunology, 112,* 451–452.

Punch, J., Joseph, A., & Rakerd, B. (2004). Most comfortable and uncomfortable loudness level: Six decades of research. *American Journal of Audiology, 13,* 144–157.

Puntillo, K., Wild, L., Morris, A., Stanik-Hutt, J., Thompson, C., & White, C. (2002). Practices and predictors of analgesic interventions for adults undergoing painful procedures. *American Journal of Critical Care, 11*(5), 415–429.

Purnell, L. D., & Paulanka, B. J. (2005). *Guide to culturally competent health care.* Philadelphia: F. A. Davis.

Quillen, D. M., Wuchner, M., & Hatch, R. (2004). Acute shoulder injuries. *American Family Physician, 70*(10), 1947–1954.

Raak, R., & Raak, A. (2003). Work attendance despite headache and its economic impact: A comparison between two workplaces. *Headache, 43,* 1097–1101.

Radimer, K., Bindewald, B., Hughes, J., Ervin, B., Swanson, C., & Picciano, M. F. (2004). Dietary supplement use by US adults: Data from the national health and nutrition examination survey, 1999–2000. *American Journal of Epidemiology, 160*(4), 339–349.

Rakel, R. E. & Bope, E. T. (2003). *Conn's current therapy 2003.* Philadelphia: Elsevier Science.

Ramachandran, V., & Shorvon, S. (2003). Clues to the genetic influences of drug responsiveness in epilepsy. *Epilepsia, 44*(Suppl 1), 33–37.

Ramadan, H. H. (2004). Surgical management of chronic sinusitis in children. *Laryngoscope, 114*(12), 2103–2109.

Raman, S., Somasekar, K., Winter, R. K., & Lewis, M. H. (2004). Are we overusing ultrasound in non-traumatic abdominal pain? *Postgraduate Medical Journal, 80* 177–179.

Rambaldi, A., & Gluud, C. (2005). Propylthiouracil for alcoholic liver disease. *The Cochrane Database of Systematic Reviews* (3), ID #CD002800.

Ramee, S. R., Subramanian, R., Felberg, R. A., McKinley, K. L., Jenkins, J. S., Collins, T. J., et al. (2004). Catheter-based treatment for patients with acute ischemic stroke ineligible for intravenous thrombolysis. *Stroke, 35*(5), 1–3.

Randolph, T. R. (2004). Advances in acute lymphoblastic leukemia. *Clinical Laboratory Science, 17*(4), 235–245, 247–249.

Ray, R. (2004, February 9). A distressing link between chronic stress, Alzheimer's. *Nurseweek,* p. 6.

Ray, W. A., Murray, K. T., Meredith, S., Narasimhulu, S. S., Hall, K., & Stein, C. M. (2004). Oral erythromycin and the risk of sudden death from cardiac causes. *New England Journal of Medicine, 351*(11), 1089.

Razek, O. A., & Poe, D. (2004, June). *Sinusitis, chronic, medical treatment.* Retrieved December 17, 2004, from http://www.emedicine.com/ent/topic338.htm.

Redaelli A., Laskin, B. L., Stephens, J. M., Botteman, M. F., & Pashos, C. L. (2004). The clinical and epidemiological burden of chronic lymphocytic leukaemia. *European Journal of Cancer Care, 13*(3), 279–287.

Redaelli A., Laskin B. L., Stephens, J. M., Botteman, M. F., & Pashos C. L. (2005). A systematic literature review of the clinical and epidemiological burden of acute lymphoblastic leukaemia (ALL). *European Journal of Cancer Care, 14*(1), 53–62.

Reddy, L. S. (2004). Heads up on cerebral bleeds. *Nursing Made Incredibly Easy! 2*(3), 8–17.

Reeves, S., Havidich, J., & Tobin, P. (2004). Conscious sedation of children with propofol is anything but conscious. *Pediatrics, 114*(1 Suppl), e74–e76.

Registered Nurses Association of Ontario. (2005, March). *Prevention of falls and fall injuries in the older adult.* Toronto, ON: Author.

Rehabilitation Institute of Chicago. (n.d.). *Research.* Retrieved August 30, 2005, from http://www.ric.org.

Reich, C. D. (2003) Advances in the treatment of bone metastases. *Clinical Journal of Oncology Nursing, 7*(6), 641–646.

Reiche, E. M., Nunes, S. O., & Morimoto, H. K. (2004). Stress, depression, the immune system, and cancer. *Lancet Oncology, 5*(10), 617–625.

Reid, G., & Bruce, A. (2003). Urogenital infections in women: Can probiotics help? *Postgraduate Medical Journal, 79*(934), 428–432.

Reinhold-Keller, E., Herlyn, K., Wagner-Bastmeyer, R., Gutfleisch, J., Peter, H., Raspe, H., et al. (2005). Effect of Wegener's granulomatosis on work disability, need for medical care, and quality of life in patients younger than 40 years at diagnosis. *Arthritis and Rheumatism, 47*(3), 320–325.

Reis, J., Breslin, M., Lezzoni, L., & Kirschner, K. (2004). *It takes more than ramps to solve the crisis of health care for people with disabilities.* Chicago: Rehabilitation Institute of Chicago.

Ren, J., & Wu, S. (2006). A burning issue: Do sepsis and systemic inflammatory response syndrome (SIRS) directly contribute to cardiac dysfunction? *Frontiers in Bioscience, 11,* 15–22.

Rhiner, M., Palos, G., & Termini, M. (2004). Managing breakthrough pain: A clinical review with three case studies using oral transmucosal fentanyl citrate. *Clinical Journal of Oncology Nursing, 8*(5), 507–512.

Rice, J. (2002). *Medications and mathematics for the nurse* (9th ed.). New York: Thomson Delmar Learning.

Rice, K. (2005). How to measure ankle/brachial index. *Nursing, 35*(1), 56–57.

Richmond, J. (2006). *The 1, 2, 3s of biosafety levels.* Retrieved June 24, 2006, from www.cdc.gov.

Richmond, T., & Thompson, H. (2002).Quality care in challenging circumstances: A patient with a spinal cord injury. *Journal of Neuroscience Nursing, 34*(11), 44-48.

Riddington, C., & Wang, W. (2002). Blood transfusion for preventing stroke in people with sickle cell disease. *The Cochrane Database for Systematic Reviews* (1), CD003146.

Ridker, P., Cook, N., Lee, I., Gordon, D., Gaziano, J., Manson, J., et al. (2005). A randomized trial of low-dose aspirin in the primary prevention of cardiovascular disease in women. *New England Journal of Medicine, 352*(13), 1293–1304.

Riggs, J. M. (2004). New therapies for heart failure. *RN, 67*(3), 28–33.

Rintala, D., Robinson-Whelen, S., & Matamoros, R. (2005). Subjective stress in male veterans with spinal cord injury. *Journal of Rehabilitation Research and Development, 42*(3), 291–304.

Ripamonti, C., & Mercadante, S. (2004). How to use octreotide for malignant bowel obstruction. *Journal of Supportive Oncology, 2*(4), 357–364.

Ristig, M., Drechsler, H., & Powderly, W.G. (2005). Hepatic steatosis and HIV infection. *AIDS Patient Care and STDs, 19*(6), 356–365.

Ritchey, C. (2005). Advice of counsel. Documentation puts nurse on solid legal ground. *RN, 68*(2), 21, 46, 58–59.

Rizzo, D. (2006). *Fundamentals of anatomy and physiology* (2nd ed.). New York: Thomson Delmar Learning.

Robbins, J., Gangnon, R., Theis, S., Kays, S., Hewitt, A., & Hind, J. (2005). The effects of lingual exercise on swallowing in older adults. *Journal of American Geriatric Society, 53*(9), 1483–1489.

Robert Woods Johnson Hospital. (2006). *RWJUH is one of only four hospitals in the nation to be awarded Magnet Status in nursing excellence three times.* Retrieved July 9, 2006, from www.rwjuh.edu.

Roberts, J., LaRusse, S., Katzen, H., Whitehouse, P., Barber, M., Post, S., et al. (2003). Reasons for seeking genetic susceptibility testing among first-degree relatives of people with Alzheimer disease. *Alzheimer Disease and Associated Disorders, 17*(2), 86–93.

Roberts, K. (2003). Treating asthma in the zone. *American Journal of Nursing, 103*(11), 118–119.

Robinson, P. (2004). Nurse-led diabetes care. *Community Practitioner, 77*(3), 82–84.

Robinson, P. (2005). Is surgery safe for a patient with hemophilia? *Nursing, 35*(5), *Hospital Nursing,* 1–3.

Robinson-Smith, G. (2002). Self-efficacy and quality of life after stroke. *Journal of Neuroscience Nursing, 34*(2), 91–98.

Rodgers, R. W. (2004). Hearing loss and wax occlusion in older people. *Practice Nursing, 15,* 290–294.

Rodrigue, N., Cote, R., Kirsh, C., Germain, C., Couturier, C., & Fraser, R. (2002). Meeting the nutritional needs of patients with severe dysphagia following a stroke: An interdisciplinary approach. *AXON, 23*(3), 31–37.

Rodriguez, D. A. (2002). *Conceptualizations of health and illness in Mexican American children, ages 8–12: An ecological perspective.* Phd. Diss., University of California, San Francisco.

Rogers, B. (2005). Looking at lymphoma and leukemia. *Nursing, 35*(7), 56–64.

Rome, K., Handoll, H. G., & Ashford, R. (2005). *Interventions for preventing and treating stress fractures and stress reactions of bone of the lower limbs in young adults.* Retrieved on August 5, 2005, from www.tees.ac.uk.

Rosenberg, M. T., & Hazzard, M. (2005). Prevalence of interstitial cystitis symptoms in women: A population based study in the primary care office. *Journal of Urology, 174*(6), 2231–2234.

Rosenberg, S., Prusiner, S., DiMauro, R., Barchi, E., & Nestler, J. (2003). *The molecular and genetic basis of neurologic and psychiatric disease* (3rd ed.). Philadelphia: Butterworth-Heinemann.

Roth, R. (2007). *Nutrition and diet therapy* (9th ed.). New York: Thomson Delmar Learning.

Rothenhaus, T. (2003, May). *Epistaxis.* Retrieved September 7, 2004, from http://www.emedicine.com/emerg/topic806.htm.

Rothrock, J., McEwen, D., & Smith, D. (Eds.). (2003) *Alexander's care of the patient in surgery* (12th ed.). St. Louis, MO: Elsevier.

Rovig, G. W. (2004). Hearing health risk in a population of aircraft carrier flight deck personnel. *Military Medicine, 169*(6), 429–432.

Rowley, J., & Lorenzo, N. (2004, February). *Obstructive sleep apnea.* Retrieved June 10, 2004, from http://www.emedicine.com/neuro/topics419.htm.

Roxas, M. (2005). Plantar fasciitis: Diagnostic and therapeutic considerations. *Alternative Medicine Review, 10*(2), 83–93.

Roy, C., & Andrews, H. (1991). *The Roy adaptation model: The definitive statement.* Norwalk, CT: Appleton & Lange.

Roy, C., & Andrews, H. (1999). *The Roy adaptation model* (2nd ed.). Stamford, CT: Appleton & Lange.

Royal Victoria Hospital/Montreal. (2006). Retrieved August 31, 2006, from www.royalvictoriahospital/Montreal.

Rubber ducks at sea. (2003, August 1). *USA Today,* 14A.

Rudnicke, Cheryl. (2003, January/February). Transfusion alternatives. *Journal of Infusion Nursing, 26*(1), 29–33.

Rudy, S., & Parham-Vetter, P. (2003). Percutaneous absorption of topically applied medication. *Dermatology Nursing, 15*(2), 145–152.

Russell, T. (2005). Acute renal failure related to rhabdomyolysis: Pathophysiology, diagnosis, and collaborative management. *Nephrology Nursing Journal, 32*(4), 409–417.

Rybarczyk, B., Edwards, R., & Behel, J. (2004). Diversity in adjustment to a leg amputation: Case illustrations of common themes. *Disability and Rehabilitation, 26*(14), 944–953.

Sackett, D. L., Straus, S. E., Richardson, W. S., Rosenberg, W., & Haynes, R. B. (2000). *Evidence-based medicine: How to practice and teach EBM* (2nd ed.). Edinburgh, UK: Churchill Livingstone.

Sadovich, J. (2005). Work excitement in nursing: An examination of the relationship between work excitement and burnout. *Nursing Economics, 23*(2), 55, 91–96.

Sahn, S. (2004). *Diagnostic thoracentesis.* Retrieved June 25, 2006, from http://www.uptodate.com.

Saiman, L., & Siegel, J. (2003). Infection control recommendations for patients with cystic fibrosis: Microbiology, important pathogens, and infection control practices to prevent patient-to-patient transmission. *American Journal of Infection Control, 31*(3 Suppl), S1–S62.

Saldanha, J., Heath, A., Lelie, N., Pisani, G., & Yu, M.Y. (2005). Collaborative Study Group. A World Health Organization International Standard for hepatitis A virus RNA nucleic acid amplification technology assays. *Vox Sanguinis, 89*(1), 52–58.

Sample, S. (2003). A modern-day Florence Nightingale: Hollie's story. In C. Smeltzer & F. Vlasses (Eds.), *Ordinary people, extraordinary lives: The stories of nurses* (pp. 8–9). Indianapolis, IN: Sigma Theta Tau International.

Sanderlin, B. W., & Raspa, R. F. (2003). Common stress fractures. *American Family Physician, 68*(8), 1527–1532.

Satake, K., Lou, J., & Lenke, L. (2004). Migration of mesenchymal stem cells through cerebrospinal fluid into injured spinal cord tissue. *Spine, 29*(18), 1971–1979.

Satou, G. M., & Herzbert, G. (2004). *Heart failure, congestive.* Retrieved June 24, 2006, from www.emedicine.com.

Saunders, S., & Edwards, B. (2004). How dermatology units can improve psychological wellbeing. *Nursing Standard, 18*(21), 33–37.

Saver, D. F., Demetroulakos, J. L., Groves, M. J., Millman, B., & Mugge, R. E. (2004, September). *Cancer of the larynx.* Retrieved December 20, 2004, from http://www.firstconsult.com.

Saver, D. F., Ferri, F. F., Murray, J. L., & Demetroulakos, J. L. (2004, December). *Sinusitis.* Retrieved December 17, 2004, from http://www.firstconsult.com.

Saver, D. F., Hodgson, J. M., Van Norman, G. A., & Bahler, R. C. (2004). *Mitral stenosis.* Retrieved June 24, 2006, from www.firstconsult.com.

Savoy, N. (2005). Triage decisions. Differentiating stridor in children at triage: It's not always croup. *Journal of Emergency Nursing, 31*(5), 503–510.

Sawaya, G. F., McConnell, K. J., Kulasingam, S. L., Lawson, H. W., Kerlikowske, K., Melnikow, J., et al. (2003). Risk of cervical cancer associated with extending the interval between cervical cancer screenings. *New England Journal of Medicine, 349*(16), 1501–1509.

SBAR technique for communication: A situational briefing model. (2005). Retrieved September 2, 2006[0] from www.ihi.org.

Scarlet, C. (2006). Anaphylaxis. *Journal of Infusion Nursing, 29*(1), 39–44.

Schafer, J. (2003). *Essential medical physiology.* San Diego, CA: Elsevier Academic Press.

Schaffer, S., & Yucha, C. (2004). The relaxation response can play a role in managing chronic and acute pain. *American Journal of Nursing, 104*(8), 75–82.

Scheinman, M., Calkins, H., Gillette, P., Klein, R., Lerman, B., Morady, F., et al. (2003). NASPE policy statement on catheter ablation: Personnel, policy, procedures, and therapeutic recommendations. *Pacing and Clinical Electrophysiology, 26*(3), 789–799.

Scherger, J. E., O'Hanlon, K. M., Jones, R. C., Hodgson, J. M., Bahler, R. C., & Frances, R. J. (2004). *Aortic regurgitation.* Retrieved June 24, 2006, from www.firstconsult.com.

Schieken, L. S. (2002). Asthma pathophysiology and the scientific rationale for combination therapy. *Allergy and Asthma Proceedings, 23*(4), 247–251.

Schleder, B.J. (2003). Taking charge of ventilator-assisted pneumonia. *Nursing Management, 34*(8), 27–32

Schneider, R. A., Miclau, T., & Helms, J. A. (2002). Embryology of bone. In R. H. Fitzgerald, H. Kaufer, & A. L. Malkani (Eds.), *Orthopaedics* (pp. 143–146). St. Louis, MO: Mosby.

Schrag, D., Mitra, N., Xu, F., Rabbani, F., Bach, P. Herr, H., et al. (2005). Cystectomy for muscle-invasive bladder cancer: Patterns and outcomes of care in the Medicare population. *Urology, 65*(6), 1118–1125.

Schrier, R., McFann, K., Johnson, A., Chapman, A., Edelstein, C., Brosnahan, G., et al. (2002). Cardiac and renal effects of standard versus rigorous blood pressure control in autosomal-dominant polycystic kidney disease: Results of a seven-year prospective randomized study. *Journal of the American Society of Nephrology, 13*(7), 1733–1739.

Schriver, J., Talmadge, R., Chuong, R., & Hedges, J. (2003). Emergency nursing historical, current and futures roles, *Journal of Emergency Nursing, 29,* (5).

Schroeder, K., Fahey, T., & Ebrahim, S. (2004). *Interventions for improving adherence to treatment in patients with high blood pressure in ambulatory settings.* The Cochrane Database of Systematic Reviews (2), CD004804.

Schroeter, K. (2003). Ethics in perioperative practice: Patient advocacy. *AORN Journal, 75*(6), 941–949.

Schulder, M., Sernas, T., & Karimi, R. (2003). Thalamic stimulation in patients with multiple sclerosis: Long-term follow-up. *Stereotactic and Functional Neurosurgery, 80*(1–4), 48–55.

Schulz, A., Caldwell, C., & Foster, S. (2003). "What are they going to do with the information?" Latino/Latina and African American perspectives on the Human Genome Project. *Health Education and Behavior, 30*(2), 151–169.

Schuster, P. (2000). Concept mapping: Reducing clinical care plan paperwork and increasing learning. *Nurse Educator, 25*(2), 78–91.

Schutte, D. (2002). Evidence-based protocol: Identification, referral, and support of older adults with genetic conditions. *Journal of Gerontological Nursing, 28*(2), 6–14.

Scileppi, P. A. (2005). *Values for interpersonal communication: How then shall we live?* Belmont, CA: Star Publishing Company, Inc.

Scott, A. N. & Fong, E. (2004). *Body structures and functions* (10th ed.). Clifton Park, NY: Thomson Delmar Learning.

Scully, J. A. (2000). Life event checklists: Revisiting the social readjustment rating scale after 30 years. *Educational and Psychological Measurement, 60*(6), 864–876.

Sedlak, C. A., & Doheny, M. O. (2002). Metabolic conditions. In A. B. Maher, S. W. Salmond, & T. A. Pellino (Eds.), *Orthopaedic nursing* (3rd ed., pp. 423–467). Pitman, NJ: W.B. Saunders Company.

Sellman, S. (2005). Disease of disguise: Learning about lyme. *Canadian Journal of Health and Nutrition, 275*(15), 76–78.

Selye, H. (1956). *The stress of life.* New York: McGraw-Hill.

Selye, H. (1991). History and present status of the stress concept. In A. Monat & R. Lazarus (Ed.), *Stress and coping: An anthology* (pp. 154–168). New York: Columbia University Press.

Seventh Report of Joint National Commission on Prevention, Detection and Treatment of Hypertension (JNC7). (2006). *Hypertension.* Retrieved July 29, 2006, from http://www.cdc/dhhs.

Sever, P. S., Dahlof, B., Poulter, N. R., Wedel, H., Beevers, G., Caulfield, M., et al. (2003). Prevention of coronary and stroke events with atorvastatin in hypertensive patients who have average or lower-than-average cholesterol concentrations, in the Anglo-Scandinavian cardiac outcomes trial-lipid lowering arm (ASCOT-LLA). *Lancet, 361*(9363), 1149–1158.

Shabbir, J., Ridgway, P. F., Lynch, K., Law, C. E., Evoy, D., O'Mahoney, J. B., et al. (2004). Administration of analgesia for acute abdominal pain sufferers in the accident and emergency setting. *European Journal of Emergency Medicine, 11*(6), 309–312.

Shah, R. K., & Shapshay, S. (2003, July). *Acute laryngitis.* Retrieved August 25, 2004, http://www.emedicine.com/ent/topic353.htm.

Shapiro, J., & Bowles, K. (2002). Nurses' and consumers' understanding of and comfort with the patient self-determination act. *Journal of Nursing Administration, 3210*, 503–508.

Sharp Health Care. (2004). (p. 7). Retrieved June 23, 2006, from http://www.sharp.com.

Shatnawi, N., & Bani-Hani, K. (2005). Unusual causes of mechanical small bowel obstruction. *Saudi Medical Journal, 26*(10), 1546–1550.

Shaw, S. (2006). Nursing and supporting patients with chronic pain. *Nursing Standard, 20*(19), 60–66, 68.

Sheehan, C. (2004). *Ambulances may get virtual doctors.* Retrieved July 5, 2006, from http://www.eweek.com.

Sheffield, P., Smith, A., & Fife, C. (2004). *Wound care practices.* Flagstaff, AZ: Best Publishing Company.

Sheikh, A., & Panesar, S.S. (2003). Effective prescribing for rhinitis. *Practice Nurse, 25*(9), 46–50

Sheldon, L. K. (2004). *Communication for nurses: Talking with patients.* Thorofare, NJ: Slack.

Sherman, R. T., & Thompson, R. A (2004). The female athlete triad. *The Journal of School Nursing, 20*(4), 197–202.

Shigehiko, U., Kellum, J., Bellomo, R., Doig, G., Morimatsu, H., Morgera, S., et al. (2005). Acute renal failure in critically ill patients. *Journal of the American Medical Association, 294*(7), 813–818.

Ship, A. N. (2005). Clinical crossroads: Update. A 50-year-old man with hepatitis C and cirrhosis needing liver transplantation, 18 months later. *Journal of the American Medical Association, 293*(16), 128–134.

Shortell, S., & Kaluzny, A. (2000). *Health care management: Organization design and behavior.* New York: Thomson Delmar Learning.

Shriners' Hospitals for Children. (n.d.). *Shrine facts and statistics.* Retrieved August 30, 2005, from http://www.shrinershq.org.

Shuey, K., & Brant, J. (2004). Test your knowledge. Hypercalcemia of malignancy: part II. *Clinical Journal of Oncology Nursing, 8*(3), 321–323.

Sibell, D., Colantonio, A., & Stacey B. (2005). Successful use of spinal cord stimulation in the treatment of severe Raynaud's disease of the hands. *Anesthesiology, 102*(1), 225–227.

Sidani, M., & Campbell, J. (2002). Gynecology: Select topics. *Primary Care, 29*, 297–321.

Sieger, C., Arnold, J., & Ahronheim, J. (2002). Refusing artificial nutrition and hydration: Does statutory law send the wrong message? *Journal of the American Geriatrics Society, 50*(3), 544–550.

Sigma Theta Tau International. *Arista 3 Executive Summary Report.* Retrieved June 23, 2006, from http://www.nursingsociety.org.

Simmons, P. (2003, June). A primer for nurses who administer blood products. *MedSurg Nursing, 12*(6), 184–190.

Simmons, R. (2003). Ablative techniques in the treatment of benign and malignant breast disease. *Journal of the American College of Surgery, 197*(2), 334.

Simms, L. M., Price, S. A., & Ervin, N. E. (2000). *Professional practice of nursing administration* (3rd ed.). Albany, NY: Thomson Delmar Learning.

Sims, J. M. (2003). Guidelines for treating asthma. *Dimensions of Critical Care Nursing, 22*(6), 247–250.

Sims, N., & Baron, R. (2002). Bone: Structure, function, growth and remodeling. In R. H. Fitzgerald, H. Kaufer,

& A. L. Malkani (Eds.), *Orthopaedics* (pp. 147–159). St. Louis, MO: Mosby.

Singh, G. K. & Miller, B. A. (2004). Health, life expectancy, and mortality patterns among immigrant populations in the United States. *Canadian Journal of Public Health, 95*(3), 114–121.

Singh, V. N., Sharma, R. K., Nanda, N. C., Reddy, H., & Strom, J. (2004). *Aortic regurgitation*. Retrieved June 24, 2006, from www.emedicine.com/radio/topic45.htm.

Sisk J. E., Whang, W., Butler, J. C., Sneller V. P., & Whitney, C. G. (2003). Cost effectiveness of vaccination against invasive pneumococcal disease among people 50 through 64 years of age: Role of comorbid conditions and race. *Annals of Internal Medicine, 138*(12), 960–968.

Sismanis, A. (2005). Diagnostic and management dilemma of sudden hearing loss. *Archives of Otolaryngology-Head & Neck Surgery, 131*(8), 733–734.

Skirton, H., & Patch, C. (2002). *Genetics for healthcare professionals: A lifestage approach*. Oxford, UK: BIOS Scientific Publishers Limited.

Sloman, R., Rosen, G., Rom, M., & Shir, Y. (2005). Nurses' assessment of pain in surgical patients. *Journal of Advanced Nursing, 52*(2), 125–132.

Slota, M., Shearn, D., Potersnak, K., & Haas, L. (2003). Perspectives on family-centered, flexible visitation in the ICU setting. *Critical Care Medicine, 31*(5), S362–S366.

Slote, R. J. (2002). Psychological aspects of caring for the adolescent undergoing spinal fusion for scoliosis. *Orthopaedic Nursing, 21*(6), 19–31.

Smith, B., Ivnik, M., Owens, B., McDougall, J., & Dierkhising R. (2005). Use of an interactive health communication application in a patient education center. *Journal of Hospital Librarianship, 5*(1), 41–49.

Smith, D. H., Meaney, D. F., & Shull, W. H. (2003). Diffuse axonal injury in head trauma. *Journal of Head Trauma Rehabilitation, 18*, 307–316.

Smith, H., & Connolly, M. (2003). Evaluation and treatment of dysphagia following stroke. *Topics in Geriatric Rehabilitation, 19*(1), 43–59.

Smith, J. (2006). Debridement of diabetic foot ulcers. *The Cochrane Database of Systematic Reviews* (1), CD003556.

Smith, J. E., & Perez, C. L. (2004, July). *Nasal fractures*. Retrieved August 20, 2004, from http://www.emedicine.com/radio/topic468.htm.

Smith, K., Wallace, A., & Smith-Campbell, B. (2004). What you should know about latex allergy. *Nurse Practitioner, 29*(12), 24.

Snider, G. L. (2003). Nosology for our day: Its application to chronic obstructive pulmonary disease. *American Journal of Respiratory and Critical Care Medicine, 167*(5), 678–683.

Snyder, D. L., Doggett, D., & Turkelson, C. (2004). Treatment of degenerative lumbar spinal stenosis. *American Family Physician, 70*(3), 517–520.

Snyder, M. C., & Lydiatt, W. M. (2003, October). *Glottic cancer*. Retrieved December 20, 2004, from http://www.emedicine.com/ent/topic688.htm.

Sobajima, S., Kim, J., Gilbertson, L., & Kang, J. (2004) Gene therapy for degenerative disc disease. *Gene Therapy, 11*(4), 390–401.

Söderlin, M. K., Börjesson, O., Kautiainen, H., Skogh,T., & Leirisalo-Repo, M. (2002). *Annals of the Rheumatic Diseases, 61*(1010), 911–915.

Soderman, M., Andersson, T., Karlsson, B., Wallace, M. C., & Edner, G. (2003). Management of patients with brain arteriovenous malformations. *European Journal of Radiology, 46*(3), 105–205.

Sole, M., Lamborn, M., & Hartshorn, J. (2001). *Introduction to Critical Care Nursing*. Philadelphia: W. B. Saunders Company.

Soriano-Sarabia, N., Leal, M., Delgado, C., Molina-Pinelo, S., De Felipe, B. Ruiz-Mateos, E., et al. (2005). Effect of hepatitis C virus coinfection on humoral immune alterations in naive HIV-infected adults on HAART: A three year follow-up study. *Journal of Clinical Immunology, 25*(3), 296–302.

Souryal, T., & Adams, K. (2005). *Anterior cruciate ligament injury*. Retrieved on September 29, 2005, from http://www.emedicine.com/pmr/topic3.htm.

Spandorfer, P., Alesandrini, E., Joffe, M., Localio, R., & Shaw, K. (2005). Oral versus intravenous rehydration of moderately dehydrated children: A randomized, controlled trial. *Pediatrics, 115*(2), 295–301.

Spector, R. E. (2004). *Cultural diversity in health and illness* (6th ed.). Upper Saddle River, NJ: Prentice Hall.

Spee, R., & Floyd, N. (2005). The person behind the pain. *Perspectives, 29*(3), 17–20.

Speroff, L., & Clarkson, T. (2003). Is tibolone a viable alternative to HT? *Contemporary OB/GYN, 48*, 54–68.

Spratto, G., & Woods, A. (2003). *PDR nurses' drug handbook*. Clifton Park, NY: Thomson Delmar Learning.

Spratto, G. R., & Woods, A. L. (2007). *2007 PDR Nurse's Drug Handbook*. New York: Thomson Delmar Learning.

Stabile, G., Bertaglia, E., Senatore, G., De Simone, A., Zerbo, F., Carreras, G., et al. (2003). Feasibility of pulmonary vein ostia radiofrequency ablation in patients with atrial fibrillation: A multicenter study. *Pacing and Clinical Electrophysiology, 26*, 284–287.

Stain, S. (2005). Gastrointestinal conditions. *Journal of the American College of Surgeons, 201*(6), 940–947.

Stanford Stroke Awareness. (2002). Stroke Awareness Part II: Diagnosis and treatment options. Retrieved June 24, 2006, from www.stanford.edu.

Stanik-Hutt, J. (2003). Pain management in the critically ill. *Critical Care Nurse, 23*(2), 99–103.

Stanley, M., Blair, K., & Beare, P. (1999). *Gerontological nursing. Promoting successful aging with older adults*. Philadelphia: F. A. Davis.

Stark, P. (2004). *Computed tomographic and positron emission tomographic scanning of pulmonary nodules*. Retrieved June 25, 2006, from http://www.uptodate.com.

Staylor, A. (2005). *Heart failure therapy: Past, present, and future*. Retrieved June 24, 2006, from www.medscape.com.

Steefel, L. (2004). Race against time. *Nursing Spectrum Midwest Edition, 5*(1), 8–9.

Steinberg, G. D., & Kim, H. L. (2005). *Bladder cancer.* Retrieved June 27, 2006, from http://www.emedicine.com/med/topic2344.htm.

Steiner, M., DeWalt, D., & Byerley, J. (2004). Is this child dehydrated? *Journal of the American Medical Association, 291,* 2746–2754.

Stenson, A., Charalambous, T., Divadwa, L., Pemba, L., Du Toit J. D., Baggaley, R., et al. (2005). Evaluation of antiretroviral therapy (ART) related counseling in a workplace base on ART implementation program, South Africa. *AIDS Care, 17*(8), 949–957.

Stetler, C. B., & Marram, G. (1976). Evaluating research findings for applicability in practice. *Nursing Outlook, 24*(9), 559–563.

Stone, P. (2005). ST-segment analysis in ambulatory ECG (AECG or Holter) monitoring in patients with coronary artery disease: Clinical significance and analytic techniques. *Annals of Noninvasive Electrocardiology, 10*(2), 263–278.

Stroud, M., Duncan, H., & Nightingale, J. (2003). Guidelines for enteral feeding in adult hospital patients. *Gut, 52*(Suppl VII), vii1–vii12.

Stuart, G. (2004). *Principles and practice of psychiatric nursing* (7th ed.). St. Louis, MO: Mosby.

Stuart, M., & Nagel, R. (2004). Sickle-cell disease. *Lancet, 364,* 1343–1360.

Stevens, K. R. (2004). *ACE star model of knowledge transformation.* Retrieved May 1, 2005, from www.acestar.uthscsa.edu.

Stewart, E. G., & Spencer, P. (2002). *The V book: A doctor's guide to complete vulvovaginal health.* New York: Bantam.

Stilp, R. (2004). *Biological weapons and emergency preparedness, Part I.* Retrieved June 27, 2006, from http://nsweb.nursingspectrum.com.

Stocking, J. (2005). *Initial assessment and resuscitation.* Retrieved March 5, 2006, from http://www.astna.org.

Struijs, P., & Kerkhoffs, G. (2005, November 1). *Ankle sprain. BMJ Clinical Evidence.* Retrieved November 1, 2006, from http://www.clinicalevidence.com/ceweb/conditions/msd/1115/1115_background.jsp#REF7.

Sunderamoorthy, D., & Chaudhury, M. (2003). An uncommon peripheral nerve injury after penetrating injury of the forearm: The importance of clinical examination. *Emergency Medicine Journal, 20,* 565–566.

Supportive Care Guidelines Group. (2004) Neuro-oncology Disease Site Group. Taos, N.M., Laetsch, N. S., Wong, R. K. S., & Laperriere N. Management of brain metastases: Role of radiotherapy alone or in combination with other treatment modalities [full report]. *Cancer Care Ontario (CCO)* Mar. (35), Practice guideline report; no.13–4.

Svehla, C. J., & Anderson-Shaw, L. (2006). Hospital ethics committees: Is it time to expand our access to managed care organizations? *JONA's Healthcare Law, Ethics, and Regulation, 8*(1), 15–19.

Swartz, C. (2004). *Prevention plan and model for posttraumatic stress disorder (PTSD) from burns.* Retrieved May 1, 2006, from www.journalofburnsandwounds.com.

Swearingen, P., & Keen, J. (2001). *Manual of critical care nursing.* St. Louis, MO: Mosby.

Tablan, O. C., Anderson, L. J., Besser, R., Bridges, C., & Hajjeh, R. (2004). Guidelines for preventing health care-associated pneumonia 2003: Recommendations of CDC and the Healthcare Infection Control Practices Advisory Committee. Retrieved September 16, 2004, from http://www.cdc.gov/.

Talhari, C., Angerstein, W., Becker, J., Ruzicka, T., & Megahed M. (2005). Long-standing oral ulcers. *Lancet, 365*(9463), 1002.

Talley, N. (2005). *Dyspepsia and functional dyspepsia: Unraveling an enigma. Digestive disease week; Functional gastrointestinal disorders.* Retrieved June 25, 2006, from http://www.medscape.com.

Tallia, A. F., & Cardone, D. A. (2003). Diagnostic and therapeutic injection of the ankle and foot. *American Family Physician, 68,* 1356–1362.

Talu, G. K., & Erdine, S. (2005). Intrathecal morphine and bupivacaine for phantom limb pain: A case report. *Pain Practice, 5*(4), 55–57.

Tam, A., & Geier, K. A. Psoriatic arthritis. *Orthopaedic Nursing, 23*(5), 311–314.

Tambor, E., Bernhardt, B., Rodgers, J., Holtzman, N., & Geller, G. (2002). Mapping the human genome: An assessment of media coverage and public reaction. *Genetics in Medicine, 4*(1), 31–36.

Tantravahi, U., & Wheeler, P. (2003). Molecular genetic testing for prenatal diagnosis. *Clinics in Laboratory Medicine, 23*(2), 481–502.

Taricco, M., Adone, R., Pagliacci, C., & Telaro, E. (2004). Pharmacological interventions for spasticity following spinal cord injury. *The Cochrane Database of Systematic Reviews* (2), CD:001131.

Tate, D. M. (2003). Cultural awareness: Bridging the gap between caregivers and Hispanic patients. *Journal of Continuing Education in Nursing, 34*(5), 213–217.

Taylor, S. C., & Altman, G. B. (2004). Administering preoperative care. In G. B. Altman (Ed.), *Delmar's fundamental and advanced nursing skills* (2nd ed., pp. 491–499). Albany, NY: Thomson Delmar Learning.

Terzioglu, F., & Dinc, L. (2004). Nurses' views on their role in genetics. *Journal of Obstetric, Gynecologic, and Neonatal Nursing, 33*(6), 756–764.

Theodorescu, D., & Krupski, T. (2005). *Prostate cancer: Biology, diagnosis, pathology, staging, and natural history.* Retrieved July 31, 2006, from http://www.emedicine.com.

Thomas, B. J., & Powers, R. D. (2002, July). *Pharyngitis, bacterial.* Retrieved September 25, 2004, from http://www.emedicine.com/med/topic1811.htm.

Thomas-Hawkins, C., & Zazworsky, D. (2005). Self-management of chronic kidney disease. Patients shoulder the responsibility for day-to-day management of chronic illness. How can nurses support their autonomy? *American Journal of Nursing, 105*(10), 40–48.

Thompson, B., & Hales, C. (2004). *Clinical manifestations of and diagnostic strategies for acute pulmonary embolism.* Retrieved June 25, 2006, from http://www.uptodate.com.

Thomson Micromedex Healthcare Series. Retrieved July 24, 2005, from www.thomson.com/hcs.

Thurkettle, M. (2003). Shifting the healthcare paradigm: The case manager's opportunity and responsibility. *Case Management, 8*(4), 160–165.

Tierney, L. M., McPhee, S. J., & Papadakis, M. A. (2003). *Current medical diagnosis and treatment* (42nd ed.). Stamford, CT: Lange Medical Books/McGraw-Hill.

Tierney, L. M., McPhee, S. J., & Papakakais, M. A. (2004). *Current medical diagnosis and treatment* (43rd ed.). New York: Lange Medical Books.

Tilton, D. (2006). Central venous access device infections in the critical care unit. *Critical Care Nursing Quarterly, 29*(2), 117–122.

Tolhurst, S., Rapp, D., O'Connor, R., Lyon, M., Orvieto, M., & Steinberg, G. (2005). Complications after cystectomy and urinary diversion in patients previously treated for localized prostate cancer. *Urology, 66*(4), 824–829.

Tolkoff-Rubin, N., Cotran, R., & Rubin, R. (2004). Urinary tract infection, pyelonephritis, and reflux nephropathy. In B. Brenner (Ed.), *Brenner and Rector's the kidney* (7th ed., vol. 2, pp. 423–454). Philadelphia: Saunders.

Tolkoff-Rubin, N., Cotran, R., & Rubin, R. (2004). Urinary tract infection, pyelonephritis, and reflux nephropathy. In B. Brenner (Ed.), *Brenner and Rector's the kidney* (7th ed., vol. 2, pp. 626–631). Philadelphia: W. B. Saunders Co.

Tomey, A. M., & Alligood, M. R. (1998). *Nursing theorists and their work* (4th ed.). St. Louis, MO: C. V. Mosby.

Topf, M., & Thompson, S. (2001). Interactive relationships between hospital patients' noise-induced stress and other stress with sleep. *Heart and Lung, 30*(4), 237–243.

Topol, E. J. (2005). *Acute coronary syndrome.* New York: Marcel Dekker.

Torpy, J. M. (2005). JAMA patient page: Malignant hyperthermia. *Journal of the American Medical Association, 293*(23), 2958.

Toto, R. (2004). Approach to the patient with kidney disease. In B. Brenner (Ed.), *Brenner and Rector's the kidney* (7th ed., vol. 1, pp. 1079–1106). Philadelphia: W. B. Saunders Co.

Townes, D. A. (2004). Biliary tract disease. *Emergency Medicine, 36*(2), 17–19.

Toyoda, H., Kumada, T., Kiriyama, S., Sone, Y., Tanikawa, M., Hisanaga, Y., et al. (2005). Comparison of the usefulness of three staging systems for hepatocellular carcinoma. *American Journal of Gastroenterology, 100*(8), 1764–1771.

Transitions. (2006). *Bernice Neugarten's life times theory.* Retrieved July 25, 2006. from http://www.transitionalonestop.org.

Travis, L. (2005). *Nephrotic syndrome.* Retrieved January 25, 2006, from http://www.emedicine.com.

Trethewey, P. (2004). Systemic lupus erythematosus. *Dimensions of Critical Care Nursing, 23*(3), 111–115.

Tsai, S., Lin, Y., & Wu, S. (2005). The effect of cardiac rehabilitation on recovery of heart rate over one minute after exercise in patients with coronary artery bypass graft surgery. *Clinical Rehabilitation, 19*(8), 843–849.

Tuckett, A. G. (2004). Truth-telling in clinical practice and the arguments for and against: A review of the literature. *Nursing Ethics, 11*(5), 500–513.

Tullman, D. F., & Dracup, K. (2005). Knowledge of heart attack symptoms in older men and women at risk for acute myocardial infarction. *Nursing Research, 25*(1), 33–39.

Tusaie, K., & Dyer, J. (2004). Resilience: A historical review of the construct. *Holistic Nursing Practice, 18*(1), 3–10.

Udeh, E. (2005). Alvimopan: A peripherally selective opioid mu receptor antagonist. *Formulary, 40,* 176–183.

Ullman E. A., Donley L. P., & Brady W. J. (2003). Pulmonary trauma: Emergency department evaluation and management. *Emergency Medicine Clinics of North America, 21*(2), 291–313.

United States Public Health Service. (1990). *Healthy people 2000: National health promotion and disease prevention objective.* [Conference edition summary]. Washington, DC: U.S. Government Printing Office.

The University of Alabama National SCI Statistical Center. (2006). Retrieved July 16, 2006, from http://www.spinalcord.uab.edu.

University of California Los Angeles Library (UCLA). (2004). *Gate Control Theory.* Retrieved from http://www.library.ucla.

University of California San Diego Healthcare (UCSD). (2003). Chronic pain. Retrieved from http://community.healthgate.com.

Uphold C. R., & Graham, M. V. (2003). *Clinical guidelines in adult health* (3rd ed.). Gainesville, FL: Barmarrae Books.

Uren, N., Odbert, R., & Davey, P. (2002). *Heart failure.* Retrieved June 24, 2006, from www.netdoctor.co.uk.

U.S. Bureau of the Census. (2003). *United States—Selected social characteristics.* Retrieved June 17, 2005, from http://servlet/MYPTable.

U.S. Department of Agriculture. (2005). *Dietary guidelines for Americans.* Washington, DC: Author.

U.S. Department of Health and Human Services. (2000). *Healthy People 2010: Understanding and improving health.* Retrieved May 5, 2006, from http://www.healthpeople.gov.

U.S. Department of Health and Human Services. (2000, November). Objectives for improving heart disease and stroke. In *Healthy People 2010 Part A* (2nd ed.). Retrieved June 13, 2006, from http://www.healthypeople.gov.

U.S. Department of Health and Human Services. (2003). *Cancer and the environment* (National Institute of Health Publication No. 03-2039). Retrieved June 10, 2005, from http://www.cancer.gov.

U.S. Department of Health and Human Services. (2004). *HHS Fact Sheet.* Retrieved June 17, 2005, from http://raceandhealth.hhs.gov.

U.S. Department of Health and Human Services. (2005). *Dietary guidelines for Americans.* Washington, DC: Author.

U.S. Department of Health and Human Services, Agency for Health Care Research and Quality. (2002).

Screening for breast cancer, AHRQ Pub. No. 03-507A. Retrieved June 12, 2006, from http://www.ahrq.gov.

U.S. Department of Health & Human Services, Centers for Disease Control and Prevention. (2003). *Recommendations for public health surveillance of syphilis in the United States division of STD prevention March 2003.* Retrieved July 22, 2006, from http://www.cdc.gov.

U.S. Department of Health and Human Services Office of Minority Health. (2000). *National standards for culturally and linguistically appropriate services in health care.* Retrieved June 17, 2005, from http://www.omhrc.gov.

U.S. Food and Drug Administration. (1997). Summaries of "Dear health professional" letters and other safety notifications. Retrieved March 31, 2005, from http://www.fda.gov.

U.S. Food and Drug Administration. (2006). Retrieved from www.fda.gov.

U.S. National Library of Medicine, & National Institute of Health. (2004). *Lung cancer-non small cell.* Retrieved June 30, 2004, from http://www.nlm.nih.gov.

VA Health Care. (n.d.). *Research and development.* Retrieved August 30, 2005, from http://www.1.va.gov/health.

VA Health System. (n.d.). *A history of supporting veterans.* Retrieved August 30, 2005, from http://www.va.gov/history.

VA National Center for Patient Safety. (n.d.). *NCPS.* Retrieved August 3, 2005, from http://www.patientsafety.gov.

Vakil, N., Talley, N., Moayyedi, P., & Fennerty, M. (2005). The diagnostic value of alarm features in predicting upper gastrointestinal malignancy in dyspeptic patients: Systematic review and meta-analysis. *Gastroenterology, 128*(Suppl 2), A80.

Vallerand, A., Reily-Doucet, C. Hasenau, S., & Templin, T. (2004). Improving cancer pain management by homecare nurses. *Oncology Nursing Forum, 31*(4), 809–816.

Vadhan-Raj, S., Schreiber, F., Thomas, L. C., Gandhi, J., Hong, J. J., Gregory, S. A., et al. (2003). Every-2-week darbepoetin alfa improves fatigue and energy rating scores in cancer patients undergoing chemotherapy. *Journal of Supportive Oncology, 1*(Suppl 1), 1–8.

Valk, P., Verhaak, R., Beijen, M., Erpelinck, C., van Doorn-Khosrovani, S., Boer, J., et al. (2004). Prognostically useful gene-expression profiles in acute myeloid leukemia. *New England Journal of Medicine, 350,* 1617–1628.

Values, Ethics and Rationing in Critical Care (VERICC) Task Force. (2005). *ICU cost burdens.* Retrieved from http://www.vericc.org.

Van Campen, L., Morata, T., Kardous, C., Gwin, K., Wallingford, K., Dallaire, J., et al. (2005). Ototoxic occupational exposures for a stock car racing team: I. Noise surveys. *Journal of Occupational & Environmental Hygiene, 2*(8), 383–390.

Van Dijk, M., Peters, W., & van Deventer, P. (2005). The COMFORT behavior scale. *American Journal of Nursing, 105*(1), 33–35.

Van Ophoven, A., Pokupic, S., Heinecke, A., & Hertle, L. (2004). A prospective, randomized, placebo controlled, double-blind study of amitriptyline for the treatment of interstitial cystitis. *Journal of Urology, 172*(2), 533–536.

Varcoe, C. (2002). 'The thief of womanhood': Women's experience of polycystic ovarian syndrome. *Social Science and Medicine, 54,* 349–361.

Varricchio, C. (2004). *ACS: A cancer source book for nurses* (8th ed.). Sudbury, MA: Jones and Bartlett Publishers.

Vavilala, M. S., Bowen, A., Lam, A. M., Uffman, J. C., Powell, J., Winn, H. R., et al. (2003). Blood pressure and outcome after severe pediatric traumatic brain injury. *Journal of Trauma: Injury, Infection and Critical Care, 55*(6), 1030–1044.

Verive, M. (2004). Hypokalemia. What are the causes of hypomagnesemia? [Electronic version]. *Journal of Family Practice, 54,* 174–176.

Vermeulen, H., Ubbink, D., Goossens, A., de Vos, R., & Legemate, D. (2006). Dressings and topical agents for surgical wounds healing by secondary intention. *The Cochrane Database of Systematic Reviews* (1), CD003554.

Verschuur, E., Homs, M., Steyerberg, E., Haringsma, J., Wahab, P., Kuipers, E., et al. (2006). A new esophageal stent design (Niti-S stent) for the prevention of migration: A prospective study in 42 patients. *Gastrointestinal Endoscopy, 63*(1), 134–140.

Veterans Affairs. (n.d.). *Veteran data and information.* Retrieved August 30, 2005, from http://www.va.gov/data.

Vetere, P., Putterman, S., & Kesselman, E. (2003). Major reconstructive surgery for pelvic organ prolapse in elderly women, including the medically compromised. *Journal of Reproductive Medicine, 48*(6), 417–421.

Vrabec, J. (2003). Herpes simplex virus and Meniere's disease. *Laryngoscope, 113*(9), 1431–1438.

Vuckovic, S., Gardiner, D., Field, K., Chapman, G. V., Khalil, D., Gill, D., et al. (2004). Monitoring dendritic cells in clinical practice using a new whole blood single-platform TruCOUNT assay. *Journal of Immunological Methods, 284*(1–2), 73–87.

Vorenberg, S. (2005, April 11). Chemicals released by brain signal pain. *San Diego Union-Tribune,* pp. 1–6 (from Scripps Howard News Service.).

Wagner, L. I., & Cella, D. (2004). Fatigue and cancer: Causes, prevalence, and treatment approaches. *British Journal of Cancer, 91*(5), 822–828.

Wahlgren, N. G., & Ahmed, N. (2004). Neuroprotection in cerebral ischemia: Facts and fancies-the need for new approaches. *Cerebrovascular Disease, 17*(Suppl 1), 153–166.

Waites, K. B., Canupp, K. C., Armstrong, S., & DeVivo, M. J. (2004). Effect of cranberry juice on bacteriuria and pyuria in persons with neurogenic bladder secondary to spinal cord injury. *Journal of Spinal Cord Medicine, 27*(1), 35-40.

Wakata, N., Nemoto, H., Sugimoto, H., Nomoto, N., Konno, S., Hayashi, N., et al. (2004). Bone density in myasthenia gravis patients receiving long-term prednisolone therapy. *Clinical Neurology and Neurosurgery, 106,* 139–141.

Wallach, E., & Vlahos, N. (2004). Uterine myomas: An overview of development, clinical features, and management. *Obstetrics and Gynecology, 104*, 393–406.

Walsh, C. (2005). Multiple organ dysfunction syndrome after multiple trauma. *Orthopaedic Nursing, 24*(5), 324–335.

Walsh, D., Nelson, K. A., & Mahmoud, F. A. (2003). Established and potential therapeutic applications of cannabinoids in oncology. *Support Care Cancer, 11*, 137–143.

Walters, R. (2005). What's a nurse to do? How the Health Insurance Portability and Accountability Act of 1996 impacts a nurse's (or any other healthcare provider's) ex parte discussion of protected health information in medical malpractice cases. *JONA's Healthcare Law, Ethics, and Regulation, 7*(1): 21–34.

Walton, B., & Thorton, T. (2003). Female sexual dysfunction. *Current Women's Health Reports, 3*, 319–326.

Wang, K., Wongkeesong, M., & Buttar, N. (2005). American gastroenterological association medical position statement: Role of the gastroenterologist in the management of esophageal carcinoma. *Gastroenterology, 128*(2), 1468–1470.

Wang, Y., Prentice, L. F., Vitetta, L., Wluka, A. E., & Cicuttini, F. M. (2004). The effect of nutritional supplements on osteoarthritis. *Alternative Medicine Review, 9*(3), 275–296.

Waninger, K. (2004). Management of the helmeted athlete with suspected cervical spine injury. *The American Journal of Sports Medicine, 32*(20), 1331–1350.

Ward, M. M. (2002). Predictors of the progression of functional disability in patients with ankylosing spondylitis. *Journal of Rheumatology, 29*(7), 1420–1425.

Warm, E., & Weissman, D. (2002, March). *The legal liability of undertreatment of pain. Fast facts and concepts #63. End-of-life physician resource center.* Retrieved May 17, 2005, from www.eperc.mcw.edu.

Watkins, L. O. (2004). Epidemiology and burden of cardiovascular disease. *Clinical Cardiology, 27*(6 Suppl 3), 2–6.

Watkinson, S. (2005). Visual impairment in older people: The nurse's role. *Nursing Standard, 19*(17), 45–52, 54.

Watret, L. (2005). Teaching wound management: A collaborative model for future education. *World Wide Wounds, 8*(15), 13–16.

Watson, D., & Rivkin, A. (2004, July). *Rhinoplasty, septoplasty.* Retrieved September 7, 2004, from http://www.emedicine.com/ent/topic128.htm.

WBC (nuclear) scan. (2003, October 17). *Medical Tests and Procedures.* Retrieved September 2, 2004, from http://www.mercksource.com.

Weiger, W., & Eisenberg, D. (2002). *Easing the treatment.* Retrieved May 25, 2006, from www.keepmedia.com.

Weijer, C., & Miller, P. (2004). Protecting communities in pharmacogenetic and pharmacogenomic research. *Journal of Pharmacogenomics, 4*(1), 9–16.

Weil, A. (2005). *Healthy aging: A lifelong guide to your physical and spiritual well-being.* New York: Alfred Knopf.

Weiss, G., Skurnick, J. H., Goldsmith, L. T., Santoro, N. F., & Park, S. J. (2004). Menopause and hypothalamic-pituitary sensitivity to estrogen. *Journal of the American Medical Association, 292*, 2991–2996.

Weiss, J. (2005). A journey in holistic growth. *Journal of Holistic Nursing, 23*(4), 434–440.

Wells, C. (2003). Optimizing nutrition in patients with chronic kidney disease. *Nephrology Nursing Journal, 30*(6), 637–648.

Welsh, S., & Veenstra, M. (2004). *Shoulder dislocations.* Retrieved on September 26, 2005, from http://www.emedicine.com/orthoped/topic440.htm.

Wener, K. (2004). *Endocarditis.* Retrieved June 24, 2006, from www.nlm.nih.gov.

Westerbrook, G.J. (2005, May 23). Methadone for pain management. *Nurseweek*, pp. 8–9.

Wheaton, J., & Pinkstaff, S. (2006). Atherosclerotic vascular disease and diabetes in the older adult part I: Understanding pathogenic mechanisms and identifying risk factors. *Clinical Geriatrics, 14*(1), 17–24, 25.

Wheeler, P., & Batt, M. E. (2005). Do non-inflammatory drugs adversely affect stress fracture healing? A short review. *British Journal of Sports Medicine, 39*(2), 65–69.

White, G. (2005). *Equipment theory for respiratory care* (4th ed.). Clifton Park, NY: Thomson Delmar Learning.

White, L., & Duncan, G. (2002). *Medical-surgical nursing: An integrated approach* (2nd ed.). New York: Thomson Delmar Learning.

White, R. D. (2004). Hyperthyroidism: Current standards of care. *Consultant, 44*(8), 24–27.

Whiteman, M. K., Staropoli, C. A., Benedict, J. C., Borgeest, C., & Flaws, J. A. (2003). Risk factors for hot flashes in midlife women. *Journal of Women's Studies, 12*(5), 459–472.

Whitman, S. C., Rateri, D. L., Szilvassy, S. J., Yokoyama, W., & Daugherty, A. (2004). Depletion of natural killer cell function decreases atherosclerosis in low-density lipoprotein receptor null mice. *Arteriosclerosis, Thrombosis, and Vascular Biology, 24*(6), 1049–1054.

Whitney, J., & Parkman, S. (2004). The effect of postoperative physical activity on tissue oxygen and wound healing. *Biological Research in Nursing, 6*(2), 79–89.

Whittle, A. P. (2003). Malunion of fractures. In S. T. Canale (Ed.), *Campbell's operative orthopaedics* (vol. 3, 10th ed., pp. 3071–3124). Philadelphia: Mosby.

Whyte, J., Hart. T., Vaccaro, M., Grieb-Neff, P., Risser, A., Polansky, M., et al. (2004). Effects of methylphenidate on attention deficits after traumatic brain injury. *American Journal of Physical Medicine and Rehabilitation, 83*(6), 401–420.

Wilbanks, B., Wakim, J., Daicoff, B., & Monterde, S. (2005). Hyperkalemia-induced residual neuromuscular blockade: A case report. *AANA Journal, 73*(6): 437–441.

Wilkes, G. (2004). Anemia in cancer care. *CancerSourceRN.* Retrieved June 10, 2005, from http://www.cancersourcern.com.

Wilkinson, C. (2005). Interventions for asymptomatic retinal breaks and lattice degeneration for preventing retinal detachment. *The Cochrane Database of Systematic Reviews (Oxford)* (4), ID #CD003170.

Wilkinson, J. M. (2005). *Nursing diagnosis handbook.* Upper Saddle River, NJ: Prentice Hall.

Williams, R. (2006). Have your say. *Nursing Management, 13*(4), 38.

Wills Eye. (n.d.a). *Pioneering technology.* Retrieved August 2, 2005, from http://www.willseye.org.

Wills Eye. (n.d.b). *Charitable giving.* Retrieved August 2, 2005, from http://www.willseye.org.

Wilson, B.A., Shannon, M.T., & Stang, C.L. (2005). *Nurses drug guide.* Upper Saddle River, NJ: Pearson–Prentice Hall.

Wilson, C., Anderson, D., Toms, S., Fleetwood, J. & Phelps, J. (2006). Family-witnessed resuscitation in a family-centered critical care unit. *American Journal of Critical Care, 15*(3), 343–344.

Wilson, J. (1973). *Environment and birth defects.* New York: Academic Press.

Wilson, L. M. (1999). Healthy people—a new millennium: Progress and comparison on the Healthy People 2000 and Healthy People 2010 objectives. *JONAs Healthcare Law, Ethics, and Regulation, 1*(2), 29–32.

Winearls, C. (2003). Clinical evaluation and manifestations of chronic renal failure. In R. Johnson & J. Feehally (Eds.), *Comprehensive clinical nephrology* (2nd ed., pp. 857–871). St. Louis, MO: Mosby.

Winegarden, C. (2005). From "prehypertension" to hypertension? Additional evidence. *Annals of Epidemiology, 15*(9), 720–725.

Winer, N., & Sowers, J. R. (2004). Epidemiology of diabetes. *Journal of Clinical Pharmacology: Incidence of Diabetes, 44,* 397–405.

Winslow, C., & Rozovsky, J. (2003). Effect of spinal cord injury on the respiratory system. *American Journal of Physical Medicine and Rehabilitation, 82,* 803–814.

Winters, B. D., & Dorman, T. (2006). Rapid response teams. *Contemporary Critical Care, 4*(3):1–10.

Wisniewski, A. (2003). Chronic bronchitis and emphysema: Clearing the air. *Nursing, 33*(5), 46–49.

Withrow, S. (2004). *Healthcare IT: Adopt guidelines for electronic consultations.* Retrieved June 25, 2006, from CNET_Networks_Member_Services@newsletter.online.com.

Witt, M. E., Haas, M., Marrinan, M. A., & Brown, C. N. (2003). Understanding stereotactic radiosurgery for intracranial tumors, seed implants for prostate cancer, and intravascular brachytherapy for cardiac restenosis. *Cancer Nursing, 26*(6), 494–502.

Wittig, J. C., Bickels, J., Priebat, D., Jelinek, J., Kellar-Garney, K., Shmookler, B., et al. (2002). Osteosarcoma: A multidisciplinary approach to diagnosis and treatment. *American Family Physician, 65*(6), 1123–1132.

Wlnlk, L.W. (2006, January 8). Who works hardest. Intelligence Report, *Parade,* 20.

Wojnicki-Johansson, G. (2001). Communication between nurse and patient during ventilator treatment: Patient reports and RN evaluations. *Intensive and Critical Care Nursing, 17*(1), 29–39.

Wong, P. F., Gilliam, A. D., Kuman, S., Shenfine, J., O'Dair, G. N. & Leaper, D. J. (2005). Antibiotic regimens for secondary peritonitis of gastrointestinal origin in adults. *The Cochrane Database of Systematic Reviews* (2), CD004539.

Woodruff, D. (2006). Deciphering diagnostics. Take these 6 easy steps to ABG analysis. *Nursing Made Incredibly Easy! 4*(1), 4–7.

Woods, A. (2004). Loosening the grip of hypertension. *RN, 34*(12), 36–43.

Workowski, K., & Levine, W. (2002). *Sexually transmitted disease guidelines 2002.* Retrieved August 30, 2004, from http://www.cdc.gov.

World Health Organization. (2002). *World health report 2002: Reducing risks, promoting health lifestyles.* Geneva Switzerland. Retrieved September 18, 2006, from www.who.org.

World Health Organization. (2004a). Breakthrough (episodic) vs. baseline (persistent) pain in cancer. (Interview with Dr. S. Mercadante). *Cancer Pain Release, 17*(4).

World Health Organization. (2004b). *Stroke now and in the future.* Retrieved June 12, 2006, from http://www.who.int.2.

World Health Organization. (2005a). *Palliative care.* Retrieved May 18, 2005, from www.who.int/about/en/.

World Health Organization. (2005b). *The world health report 2000—Health systems: Improving performance.* Retrieved March 21, 2005, from www.who.int/whr/2000.

World Health Organization. (2006). (p. 13). Retrieved June 23, 2006, from http://www.who.int.

Worley, C. (2004). Assessment and terminology: Critical issues in wound care. *Dermatology Nursing, 16*(5), 451–452, 457.

Worley, C. (2005). "So, what do I put on this wound?" Making sense of the wound dressing puzzle: Part I. *Dermatology Nursing, 17*(2), 143–144.

Wormald, R., Evans, J., Smeeth, L., & Henshaw K. (2005). Photodynamic therapy for neovascular age-related macular degeneration. *The Cochrane Database Systematic Reviews (Oxford)* (4), ID #CD002030.

Wozniak, R. H. (1992). *Mind and body: René Descartes to William James.* Bethesda, MD and Washington DC: National Library of Medicine and American Psychological Association.

Wright, C., Kerzin-Storrar, L., Williamson, P., Fryer, A., Njindou, A., Quarrell, O., et al. (2002). Comparison of genetic services with and without genetic registers: Knowledge, adjustment, and attitudes about genetic counseling among probands referred t three genetic clinics. *Journal of Medical Genetics, 39*(12), 84.

Wright, L. (2005). *Spirituality, suffering, and illness: Ideas for healing.* Philadelphia: F. A. Davis.

Wright, P. E. (2003). Carpal tunnel, ulnar tunnel, and stenosing tenosynovitis. In S. T. Canale (Ed.), *Campbell's operative orthopaedics* (vol. 3, 10th ed., pp. 3761–3778). Philadelphia: Mosby.

Writing Group for the Women's Health Initiative Investigators. (2002). Risks and benefits of estrogen plus progestin in healthy postmenopausal women: Principal results from the Women's Health Initiative randomized controlled trial. *Journal of the American Medical Association, 288,* 321–333.

Yamada, Y. (2005). *Handbook of gastroenterology* (2nd ed.). Philadelphia: Lippincott, Williams & Wilkins.

Yang, C., Wang, H., Wang, Z., Du, H., Tao, D., Mu, X., et al. (2005). Risk factors for esophageal cancer: A case-control study in South-western China. *Asian Pacific Journal of Cancer Prevention, 6*(1), 48–53.

Yeates, E., Singer, M., & Morton, A. (2004). Salt and water: A simple approach to hyponatremia. *Journal of the Canadian Medical Association, 170*(3), 365–369.

Yellen, E. A., & Ricard, R. (2005). The effect of a preadmission videotape on patient satisfaction. *AORN Journal, 81*(4), 831–840, 842, 845.

Yezierksi, R., Radson, E., & Vanderah, T. (2004). Understanding chronic pain. *Nursing, 34*(4), 22–23.

Yoshitatsu, S., Sambuughin, N., & Muldoon, S. (2004). Malignant hyperthermia genetic testing in North America working group meeting. *Anesthesiology, 100*(2), 464–465.

Young, M. (2003). Preparing dermatology nurses: Biologic therapies for psoriasis. *Dermatology Nursing, 15*(2), 413–423.

Yueh, B., Shapiro, N, MacLean, C. H., & Shekelle, P. (2003). Screening and management of adult hearing loss in primary care: Scientific review. *JAMA, 289*(15), 1976–1985.

Zavarella, M., Leblebicioglu, B., Claman, L., & Tatakis, D. (2006). Unilateral severe chronic periodontitis associated with ipsilateral surgical resection of cranial nerves V, VI, and VII. *Journal of Periodontology, 77*(1), 142–148.

Zepf, B. (2003). Exercise prescription for patients with claudication. *American Family Physician, 67*(5), 1072.

Zevitz, M. E. (2004). *Heart failure.* Retrieved June 24, 2006, from www.emedicine.com.

Zorn, K. F. (2001). Infections. In D. C. Schoen (Ed.), *NAON: Core curriculum for orthopaedic nursing* (4th ed., pp. 189–204). Pitman, NJ: Anthony J. Jannetti, Inc.

Index

Page numbers followed by "f" denote figures and "t" denote tables. Page numbers followed by "b" indicate boxed text.

IMPORTANT! READ CAREFULLY: This End User License Agreement ("Agreement") sets forth the conditions by which Thomson Delmar Learning, a division of Thomson Learning Inc. ("Thomson") will make electronic access to the Thomson Delmar Learning-owned licensed content and associated media, software, documentation, printed materials, and electronic documentation contained in this package and/or made available to you via this product (the "Licensed Content"), available to you (the "End User"). BY CLICKING THE "I ACCEPT" BUTTON AND/OR OPENING THIS PACKAGE, YOU ACKNOWLEDGE THAT YOU HAVE READ ALL OF THE TERMS AND CONDITIONS, AND THAT YOU AGREE TO BE BOUND BY ITS TERMS, CONDITIONS, AND ALL APPLICABLE LAWS AND REGULATIONS GOVERNING THE USE OF THE LICENSED CONTENT.

1.0   SCOPE OF LICENSE

1.1   Licensed Content. The Licensed Content may contain portions of modifiable content ("Modifiable Content") and content which may not be modified or otherwise altered by the End User ("Non-Modifiable Content"). For purposes of this Agreement, Modifiable Content and Non-Modifiable Content may be collectively referred to herein as the "Licensed Content." All Licensed Content shall be considered Non-Modifiable Content, unless such Licensed Content is presented to the End User in a modifiable format and it is clearly indicated that modification of the Licensed Content is permitted.

1.2   Subject to the End User's compliance with the terms and conditions of this Agreement, Thomson Delmar Learning hereby grants the End User, a nontransferable, nonexclusive, limited right to access and view a single copy of the Licensed Content on a single personal computer system for noncommercial, internal, personal use only. The End User shall not (i) reproduce, copy, modify (except in the case of Modifiable Content), distribute, display, transfer, sublicense, prepare derivative work(s) based on, sell, exchange, barter or transfer, rent, lease, loan, resell, or in any other manner exploit the Licensed Content; (ii) remove, obscure, or alter any notice of Thomson Delmar Learning's intellectual property rights present on or in the Licensed Content, including, but not limited to, copyright, trademark, and/or patent notices; or (iii) disassemble, decompile, translate, reverse engineer, or otherwise reduce the Licensed Content.

2.0   TERMINATION

2.1   Thomson Delmar Learning may at any time (without prejudice to its other rights or remedies) immediately terminate this Agreement and/or suspend access to some or all of the Licensed Content, in the event that the End User does not comply with any of the terms and conditions of this Agreement. In the event of such termination by Thomson Delmar Learning, the End User shall immediately return any and all copies of the Licensed Content to Thomson Delmar Learning.

3.0   PROPRIETARY RIGHTS

3.1   The End User acknowledges that Thomson Delmar Learning owns all rights, title and interest, including, but not limited to all copyright rights therein, in and to the Licensed Content, and that the End User shall not take any action inconsistent with such ownership. The Licensed Content is protected by U.S., Canadian and other applicable copyright laws and by international treaties, including the Berne Convention and the Universal Copyright Convention. Nothing contained in this Agreement shall be construed as granting the End User any ownership rights in or to the Licensed Content.

3.2   Thomson Delmar Learning reserves the right at any time to withdraw from the Licensed Content any item or part of an item for which it no longer retains the right to publish, or which it has reasonable grounds to believe infringes copyright or is defamatory, unlawful, or otherwise objectionable.

4.0   PROTECTION AND SECURITY

4.1   The End User shall use its best efforts and take all reasonable steps to safeguard its copy of the Licensed Content to ensure that no unauthorized reproduction, publication, disclosure, modification, or distribution of the Licensed Content, in whole or in part, is made. To the extent that the End User becomes aware of any such unauthorized use of the Licensed Content, the End User shall immediately notify Thomson Delmar Learning. Notification of such violations may be made by sending an e-mail to delmarhelp@thomson.com.

5.0   MISUSE OF THE LICENSED PRODUCT

5.1   In the event that the End User uses the Licensed Content in violation of this Agreement, Thomson Delmar Learning shall have the option of electing liquidated damages, which shall include all profits generated by the End User's use of the Licensed Content plus interest computed at the maximum rate permitted by law and all legal fees and other expenses incurred by Thomson Delmar Learning in enforcing its rights, plus penalties.

6.0   FEDERAL GOVERNMENT CLIENTS

6.1   Except as expressly authorized by Thomson Delmar Learning, Federal Government clients obtain only the rights specified in this Agreement and no other rights. The Government acknowledges that (i) all software and related documentation incorporated in the Licensed Content is existing commercial computer software within the meaning of FAR 27.405(b)(2); and (2) all other data delivered in whatever form, is limited rights data within the meaning of FAR 27.401. The restrictions in this section are acceptable as consistent with the Government's need for software and other data under this Agreement.

7.0   DISCLAIMER OF WARRANTIES AND LIABILITIES

7.1   Although Thomson Delmar Learning believes the Licensed Content to be reliable, Thomson Delmar Learning does not guarantee or warrant (i) any information or materials contained in or produced by the Licensed Content, (ii) the accuracy, completeness or reliability of the Licensed Content, or (iii) that the Licensed Content is free from errors or other material defects. THE LICENSED PRODUCT IS PROVIDED "AS IS," WITHOUT ANY WARRANTY OF ANY KIND AND THOMSON DELMAR LEARNING DISCLAIMS ANY AND ALL WARRANTIES, EXPRESSED OR IMPLIED, INCLUDING, WITHOUT LIMITATION, WARRANTIES OF MERCHANTABILITY OR FITNESS OR A PARTICULAR PURPOSE. IN NO EVENT SHALL THOMSON DELMAR LEARNING BE LIABLE FOR: INDIRECT, SPECIAL, PUNITIVE OR CONSEQUENTIAL DAMAGES INCLUDING FOR LOST PROFITS, LOST DATA, OR OTHERWISE. IN NO EVENT SHALL THOMSON DELMAR LEARNING'S AGGREGATE LIABILITY HEREUNDER, WHETHER ARISING IN CONTRACT, TORT, STRICT LIABILITY OR OTHERWISE, EXCEED THE AMOUNT OF FEES PAID BY THE END USER HEREUNDER FOR THE LICENSE OF THE LICENSED CONTENT.

8.0   GENERAL

8.1   Entire Agreement. This Agreement shall constitute the entire Agreement between the Parties and supercedes all prior Agreements and understandings oral or written relating to the subject matter hereof.

8.2   <u>Enhancements/Modifications of Licensed Content</u>. From time to time, and in Thomson Delmar Learning's sole discretion, Thomson Delmar Learning may advise the End User of updates, upgrades, enhancements and/or improvements to the Licensed Content, and may permit the End User to access and use, subject to the terms and conditions of this Agreement, such modifications, upon payment of prices as may be established by Thomson Delmar Learning.

8.3   <u>No Export</u>. The End User shall use the Licensed Content solely in the United States and shall not transfer or export, directly or indirectly, the Licensed Content outside the United States.

8.4   <u>Severability</u>. If any provision of this Agreement is invalid, illegal, or unenforceable under any applicable statute or rule of law, the provision shall be deemed omitted to the extent that it is invalid, illegal, or unenforceable. In such a case, the remainder of the Agreement shall be construed in a manner as to give greatest effect to the original intention of the parties hereto.

8.5   <u>Waiver</u>. The waiver of any right or failure of either party to exercise in any respect any right provided in this Agreement in any instance shall not be deemed to be a waiver of such right in the future or a waiver of any other right under this Agreement.

8.6   <u>Choice of Law/Venue</u>. This Agreement shall be interpreted, construed, and governed by and in accordance with the laws of the State of New York, applicable to contracts executed and to be wholly preformed therein, without regard to its principles governing conflicts of law. Each party agrees that any proceeding arising out of or relating to this Agreement or the breach or threatened breach of this Agreement may be commenced and prosecuted in a court in the State and County of New York. Each party consents and submits to the nonexclusive personal jurisdiction of any court in the State and County of New York in respect of any such proceeding.

8.7   <u>Acknowledgment</u>. By opening this package and/or by accessing the Licensed Content on this Web site, THE END USER ACKNOWLEDGES THAT IT HAS READ THIS AGREE-MENT, UNDERSTANDS IT, AND AGREES TO BE BOUND BY ITS TERMS AND CONDI-TIONS. IF YOU DO NOT ACCEPT THESE TERMS AND CONDITIONS, YOU MUST NOT ACCESS THE LICENSED CONTENT AND RETURN THE LICENSED PRODUCT TO DELMAR LEARNING (WITHIN 30 CALENDAR DAYS OF THE END USER'S PURCHASE) WITH PROOF OF PAYMENT ACCEPTABLE TO THOMSON DELMAR LEARNING, FOR A CREDIT OR A REFUND. Should the End User have any questions/comments regarding this Agreement, please contact Thomson Delmar Learning at delmarhelp@thomson.com.

StudyWare™ to Accompany Contemporary Medical-Surgical Nursing

Minimum System Requirements

- Operating System: Microsoft Windows 98 SE, Windows 2000, or Windows XP
- Processor: Pentium PC 500 MHz or higher (750 Mhz recommended)
- Memory: 64 MB of RAM (128 MB recommended)
- Screen Resolution: 800 × 600 pixels
- Color Depth: 16-bit color (thousands of colors)
- Disk Space: Minimum of 10 MB free
- Macromedia Flash Player 9. The Macromedia Flash Player is free, and can be downloaded from http://www.adobe.com/products/flashplayer/

Installation Instructions

1. Insert disc into CD-ROM drive. The StudyWare™ installation program should start automatically. If it does not, go to step 2.
2. From My Computer, double-click the icon for the CD drive.
3. Double click the *setup.exe* file to start the program.

Technical Support

Telephone: 1-800-477-3692, 8:30 A.M.-5:30 P.M. Eastern Time
Fax: 1-518-881-1247
E-mail: delmarhelp@thomson.com

StudyWare™ is a trademark used herein under license.

Microsoft® and Windows® are registered trademarks of the Microsoft Corporation.

Pentium® is a registered trademark of the Intel® Corporation.